LIPPINCOTT
MANUAL OF
NURSING PRACTICE

LIPPINCOTT
MANUAL OF NURSING PRACTICE

Eleventh Edition

SANDRA M. NETTINA, MSN, ANP-BC
Nurse Practitioner and Founder
Prime Care House Calls
West Friendship, Maryland

 Wolters Kluwer

Philadelphia • Baltimore • New York • London
Buenos Aires • Hong Kong • Sydney • Tokyo

Acquisitions Editor: Nicole Dernoski
Editorial Coordinator: Lindsay Ries
Development Editor: Lisa Marshall
Production Project Manager: Linda Van Pelt
Manufacturing Coordinator: Kathleen Brown
Prepress Vendor: SPi Global

Eleventh Edition

Library of Congress Cataloging-in-Publication Data
Names: Nettina, Sandra M., editor.
Title: Lippincott manual of nursing practice / [edited by] Sandra M. Nettina.
Other titles: Manual of nursing practice
Description: Eleventh edition. | Philadelphia : Wolters Kluwer, [2019] | Includes bibliographical
    references and index.
Identifiers: LCCN 2018030662 | ISBN 9781496379948 (hardback)
Subjects: | MESH: Nursing Care | Handbooks
Classification: LCC RT51 | NLM WY 49 | DDC 610.73—dc23 LC record available at
https://lccn.loc.gov/2018030662

CCS0818

Dedicated to the nurses who teach, educate, mentor, precept, and support new and future

nurses. Whether you are a paid educator or a natural role model who assists with clinical

training in addition to all your other duties, you are needed and appreciated.

The art of nursing must be experienced and nurtured within students and recent graduates.

Quality care is not gleaned from science alone. Our profession depends on all those

who have followed in the footsteps of the Lady with the Lamp...

to improve the health of individuals and the quality of health care.

CONTENTS

PART FIVE
PSYCHIATRIC NURSING

APPENDICES

PART FIVE
PSYCHIATRIC NURSING

APPENDICES

CONTRIBUTORS AND REVIEWERS

CONTRIBUTORS

CHAPTER 1　Nursing Practice and the Nursing Process
Christine Nelson-Tuttle, DNS, APRN, PNP-BC
Associate Professor of Nursing
D'Youville College
Buffalo, New York

CHAPTER 2　Standards of Care and Ethical and Legal Issues
Marianne Chiafery, DNP, MS Clinical Bioethics, PNP-C
Assistant Professor
University of Rochester School of Nursing
SOM Division of Bioethics and Humanities Ethics Consult Service
Rochester, New York

CHAPTER 3　Health Promotion and Preventive Care
Sandra M. Nettina, MSN, ANP-BC
Nurse Practitioner and Founder
Prime Care House Calls
West Friendship, Maryland

CHAPTER 4　Genetics and Health Applications
Yvette P. Conley, PhD
Associate Professor of Nursing and Human Genetics
University of Pittsburgh
Pittsburgh, Pennsylvania

CHAPTER 5　Adult Physical Assessment
Sandra M. Nettina, MSN, ANP-BC
Nurse Practitioner and Founder
Prime Care House Calls
West Friendship, Maryland

CHAPTER 6　Intravenous Therapy
Courtney Edwards, MSN, MPH, RN, CCRN, CEN, TCRN
Trauma Outreach Education, Injury Prevention and Research Manager
Rees-Jones Trauma Center Parkland Health & Hospital System
Dallas, Texas

CHAPTER 7　Perioperative Nursing
Claudia G. King, BSN, CNOR, RNFA
Clinical Mentor/Educator, Surgical Services
Carroll Hospital Center
Westminster, Maryland

CHAPTER 8　Cancer Nursing
DeClue Riley, MSN, CRNP
Nurse Practitioner
Johns Hopkins Kimmel Cancer Center
Baltimore, Maryland

CHAPTER 9　Care of the Older Adult or Adult with Disabilities
Elizabeth Galik, PhD, CRNP, FAAN, FAANP
Associate Professor
School of Nursing
University of Maryland
Baltimore, Maryland

Ann A. Scheve, MS, RN
Clinical Faculty
College of Nursing
Villanova University
Villanova, Pennsylvania

CHAPTER 10　Respiratory Function and Therapy
Lorie Dambaugh, DNP, CNS, RN, ACCN-AG
Assistant Professor of Nursing
St. John Fisher College
Rochester, New York

CHAPTER 11　Respiratory Disorders
Chris Garvey, MSN, MPA, FNP, FAACVPR
Manager, Pulmonary and Cardiac Rehabilitation
Seton Medical Center
Daly City, California
Nurse Practitioner
Sleep Disorders Center
University of California at San Francisco
San Francisco, California

CHAPTER 12   Cardiovascular Function and Therapy

CHAPTER 13   Cardiac Disorders
Joy Malanyaon, RN, BSN, CCRN
Johns Hopkins Hospital
Baltimore, Maryland

Ann Marie Cullen, RN, MSN, CCNS, CCRN
Clinical Nurse Specialist
Cardiac Care Unit
Johns Hopkins Hospital
Baltimore, Maryland

Dzifa Dordunoo, PhD, RN, MSN, CCRN
Assistant Professor
University of Victoria
Victoria, British Columbia, Canada

Mary Grace Nayden, RN, BSN
Nurse Clinician III, Discharge Planner
Johns Hopkins Hospital
Baltimore, Maryland

CHAPTER 14   Vascular Disorders
Theresa E. DeVeaux, RN, MS, ACNP
Nurse Practitioner
University of Maryland Community
Medical Group
Vasular Center at UM
Baltimore Washington Medical Center
Baltimore, Maryland

Christine Owen, RN, MS, ACNP
Nurse Practitioner
University of Maryland Community
Medical Group
Vasular Center at UM
Baltimore Washington Medical Center
Baltimore, Maryland

CHAPTER 15   Neurologic Disorders
Denise Miller Niklasch, DNP, ANP, CNRN
Neurocritical Care Nurse Practitioner
Medical College of Wisconsin
Milwaukee, Wisconsin

Donna Avanecean, DNP, FNP-BC, CNRN
APRN Neuro Oncology
Cancer Center
Hartford Hospital
Hartford, Connecticut

CHAPTER 16   Eye Disorders
Agueda Lara-Smalling, BSN, MPH
Nurse Reviewer-Research
Michael E. DeBakey VA Medical Center
Houston, Texas

CHAPTER 17   Ear, Nose, and Throat Disorders
Doreen Frances Gagné, MS, CRNP, CORLN
Otolaryngology Nurse Practitioner
Summit ENT and Hearing Services
Chambersburg, Pennsylvania

Carol Sailese Maragos, MSN, CRNP, CORLN
Otolaryngology Nurse Practitioner
Johns Hopkins Hospital
Baltimore, Maryland

CHAPTER 18   Gastrointestinal Disorders
Dawn L. Piercy, MS, NP, CCRC
Senior Nurse Practitioner and Clinical Trials Manager
Duke University Medical Center
Durham, North Carolina

CHAPTER 19   Hepatic, Biliary, and Pancreatic Disorders
Natalie Masco Dixon, DNP, RN, FNP-C
Assistant Professor
Wegmans School of Nursing
St. John Fisher College
Rochester, New York

CHAPTER 20   Nutritional Problems
Karen Flanders, MSN, NP-C, APRN, BC, CBN
Metabolic and Bariatric Surgery Nurse Practitioner
Massachusetts General Hospital Weight Center
Boston, Massachusetts

CHAPTER 21   Renal and Urinary Disorders
Dorene Holcombe, CRNP
Department of Nephrology
Johns Hopkins University
Baltimore, Maryland

Caprice Warren, CM-DRN, BSN, RN
Financial Pre-certification Nurse Specialist
Johns Hopkins Hospital
Baltimore, Maryland

Rosmond Lynch, BSN, RN
NC 3
Johns Hopkins Hospital
Baltimore, Maryland

CHAPTER 22   Gynecologic Disorders
Kylene Abraham, DNP, APRN, RNC-OB
Assistant Professor of Nursing
Wegmans School of Nursing
St. John Fisher College
Rochester, New York

Nancy Wilk, DNS, WHNP-C
Assistant Professor of Nursing
Wegmans School of Nursing
St. John Fisher College
Rochester, New York

CHAPTER 23   Breast Conditions
Susan Fischera, MSN, FNP-BC
Nurse Practitioner
Southeastern Surgical Group
Tallahassee, Florida

CHAPTER 24   Endocrine Disorders
Jessica Horst, FNP-c
Transition of Care Coordinator
Portneuf Medical Center
Pocatello, Idaho

CHAPTER 25   Diabetes Mellitus and Related Disorders
Lucia M. Novak, MSN, ANP-BC, BC-ADM
Adjunct Assistant Professor
Uniformed Services
University of the Health Sciences
Bethesda, Maryland
Director
Riverside Diabetes Center
Riverside Medical Associates, P.A.
Riverdale, Maryland

CHAPTER 26   Hematologic Disorders
Rebekah Zonozy, RN, MSN, CPNP
Pediatric Nurse Practitioner
Hematology Oncology Department
Cook Children's Hospital
Fort Worth, Texas

CHAPTER 27   Transfusion Therapy and Blood and Marrow Stem
Cell Transplantation
Rebekah Zonozy, RN, MSN, CPNP
Pediatric Nurse Practitioner
Hematology Oncology Department
Cook Children's Hospital
Fort Worth, Texas

CHAPTER 28   Asthma and Allergy
Sayda Major, RN, MSN, ACNP-BC
Nurse Practitioner, Hospitalist Medicine
Parkland Health and Hospital System
Dallas, Texas

CHAPTER 29   HIV Infection and AIDS
Lisa M. Wolf, RN, ACRN, JD
Clinical Nurse
AIDS Unit
Johns Hopkins University Hospital
Baltimore, Maryland

CHAPTER 30   Connective Tissue Disorders
Victoria Ruffing, RN-BC
Director of Patient Education
Johns Hopkins Arthritis Center
Johns Hopkins University
Baltimore, Maryland

CHAPTER 31   Infectious Diseases
Anne M. Caston-Gaa, RN, MSN, MPH
Nurse Clinician
Johns Hopkins Hospital
Baltimore, Maryland

Melanie Gavin, M(ASCP), CIC
Infection Control Epidemiologist
Johns Hopkins University
Baltimore, Maryland
Medical University of South Carolina
Charleston, South Carolina

CHAPTER 32   Musculoskeletal Disorders
Peggy Barksdale, MSN, RN, CNS-BC, OCNS-C
Clinical Nurse Specialist
National Association of Clinical Nurse Specialists
National Association of Orthopaedic Nurses
Indianapolis, Indiana

CHAPTER 33   Dermatologic Disorders
Lisa S. Ball, PhD, APRN, FNP-BC
Associate Professor
Nursing Department
Daemen College
Amherst, New York

CHAPTER 34   Burns
Stephanie A. Campbell, MS, RN, CCRN-K
Burn Program Manager
Parkland Regional Burn Center
Parkland Health & Hospital System
Dallas, Texas

CHAPTER 35   Emergent Conditions
Rebecca Roloff, MS, FNP-BC, APRN
Clinical Assistant Professor
D'Youville College, FNP program
Nurse Practitioner in Emergency Medicine
Oishei Children's Hospital
Buffalo, New York

CHAPTER 36   Maternal and Fetal Health

CHAPTER 37   Nursing Management During Labor and Delivery

CHAPTER 38   Care of Mother and Neonate During the
Postpartum Period

CHAPTER 39   Complications of the Childbearing Experience
Kylene Abraham, DNP, APRN, RNC-OB
Assistant Professor of Nursing
Wegmans School of Nursing
St. John Fisher College
Rochester, New York

Susan M. McCarthy, DNP, APRN, EFM-C
Professor of Nursing
Finger Lakes Community College
Canandaigua, New York

CHAPTER 40   Pediatric Growth and Development

CHAPTER 41 Pediatric Physical Assessment
Christine Nelson-Tuttle, DNS, APRN, PNP-BC
Associate Professor of Nursing
D'Youville College
Buffalo, New York

CHAPTER 42   Pediatric Primary Care
Elyse Borsuk, APRN, MSN, CPNP-PC
Lecturer/Clinical Liaison
School of Nursing
Yale University
West Haven, Connecticut

CHAPTER 43   Care of the Sick or Hospitalized Child
Jocelyn Gmerek, MSN, PNP-C
Pediatric Nurse Practitioner
General Surgery
Children's Hospital of Philadelphia
Philadelphia, Pennsylvania

Mary Kate Klarich, MSN, PNP-C
Pediatric Nurse Practitioner
General Surgery
Children's Hospital of Philadelphia
Philadelphia, Pennsylvania

CHAPTER 44   Pediatric Respiratory Disorders
Mary Beth Lyons
Clinical Nurse Specialist
PICU and Pediatrics
Maria Fareri Children's Hospital
Valhalla, New York

CHAPTER 45   Pediatric Cardiovascular Disorders
Wendy Hou, MSN, RN
Golisano Children's Hospital at Strong
University of Rochester Medical Center
Rochester, New York

CHAPTER 46   Pediatric Neurologic Disorders
Maria Zak, MN, NP-Pediatrics
Nurse Practitioner
Division of Neurology
The Hospital for Sick Children
Adjunct Professor
Lawrence S. Bloomberg Faculty of Nursing
University of Toronto
Toronto, Ontario, Canada

Valerie W. Chan, BScN, RN, CNN
Neurology Clinic Nurse
The Hospital for Sick Children
Toronto, Ontario, Canada

CHAPTER 47   Pediatric Eye and Ear Problems
Zoe Strough O'Brien, MS, PNP-C
Pediatric Nurse Practitioner
Children's Pediatricians and Associates
Gaithersburg, Maryland

CHAPTER 48   Pediatric Gastrointestinal and Nutritional Disorders
Ellen Thomen Clore, MSN, CPNP-AC
Pediatric Nurse Practitioner
Children's National Medical Center
Washington, District of Columbia

Erin Garth, MSN, PNP-BC
Pediatric Nurse Practitioner
Children's National Medical Center (formerly)
Washington, District of Columbia

CHAPTER 49   Pediatric Renal and Genitourinary Disorders
Abby Varghese, RN(EC), NP-PHC
Nurse Practitioner
Division of Urology
The Hospital for Sick Children
Toronto, Ontario, Canada

April Cherian, NP (Pediatric)
CKD Program
Division of Nephrology
Hospital for Sick Children
Toronto, Ontario, Canada

CHAPTER 50   Pediatric Metabolic and Endocrine Disorders
Christine Nelson-Tuttle, DNS, APRN, PNP-BC
Associate Professor of Nursing
D'Youville College
Buffalo, New York

CHAPTER 51   Pediatric Oncology
Tamara Gray
PhD Student
School of Nursing
Johns Hopkins University
Baltimore, Maryland

CHAPTER 52   Pediatric Hematologic Disorders
Barbara Ehrenreich, RN, MSN, CPNP
Pediatric Nurse Practitioner
Pediatric Bone Marrow Transplant Coordinator
Division of Pediatric Hematology, Oncology, and Stem Cell
    Transplantation
Maria Fareri Children's Hospital at Westchester Medical Center
Valhalla, New York

CHAPTER 53   Pediatric Immunologic Disorders
Georgina MacDougall, RN
HIV Clinic Nurse Coordinator
The Hospital for Sick Children
Toronto, Ontario, Canada

Audrey Bell-Peter, RN, MN
Rheumatology Nurse Coordinator
The Hospital for Sick Children
Toronto, Ontario, Canada

Holly Convery, BScN, NP-Primary Care
Clinic Nurse
Division of Rheumatology
The Hospital for Sick Children
Toronto, Ontario, Canada

Brenda Reid, RN, MN
Clinical Nurse Specialist
Immunology/Allergy
The Hospital for Sick Children
Toronto, Ontario, Canada

CHAPTER 54   Pediatric Orthopedic Problems

Catherine M. Haut, DNP, CPNP-AC, CPNP-PC, CCRN
Pediatric Nurse Practitioner
Pediatrix Medical Group
The Herman and Walter Samuelson Children's Hospital at Sinai Hospital
Baltimore, Maryland

CHAPTER 55   Pediatric Integumentary Disorders

Stephanie A. Campbell, MS, RN, CCRN-K
Burn Program Manager
Parkland Regional Burn Center
Parkland Health & Hospital System
Dallas, Texas

Lisa S. Ball, PhD, APRN, FNP-BC
Associate Professor
Nursing Department
Daemen College
Amherst, New York

CHAPTER 56   Developmental Disabilities

Christine Nelson-Tuttle, DNS, APRN, PNP-BC
Associate Professor of Nursing
D'Youville College
Buffalo, New York

CHAPTER 57   Problems of Mental Health

Matthew R. Sorenson, PhD, RN
Interim Director
School of Nursing
DePaul University
Chicago, Illinois

REVIEWERS

Jorie Klein, BSN, RN
Director, Trauma Program
Rees-Jones Trauma Center at Parkland
Dallas, Texas

Barbara J. Pitto, RN, DNC
Registered Nurse 4
Vanderbilt University Medical Center
Nashville, Tennessee

Elizabeth Turcotte, RN-BC, ONC
Nurse Manager
Orthopedic Institute of Central Maine at Maine Medical Center
Lewiston, Maine

PREFACE

The world's ever-changing technology and health care systems have challenged nurses more than ever over the past 10 years. I firmly believe, however, that to improve health we cannot forget the past. Fundamental tasks such as nursing assessment and documentation are more important than ever. Care of the patient from hospital to home and across all settings is essential to reduce cost and improve outcomes. Health care today must mirror the past, with the patient at center, in the home, or transitioning to home, in one's own family and community system, rather than as a mere cog in the wheel of a large health care system.

Following the publication of the *Lippincott Manual of Nursing Practice*, 10th edition, I moved my clinical practice into the home health arena, with the firm belief that this is where I could use my 40 years of nursing experience to make the greatest difference in people's health and quality of life. While I exclusively provide medical care in the home and assisted living facilities, I am active in coordination of care for the patient across settings. While a major focus is prevention of hospital admission, I am alert for care needs that become greater than even a highly skilled home health team can meet. When a patient is admitted, I stay involved to help with the transition to rehabilitation settings and back to home. When a patient at home needs more supervision or assistance with activities of daily living than can be provided, I assist with the transition to a long-term care setting. This is what nurses do, whatever the patient needs, and our skills can be used in all settings.

Now I present the 11th edition of the *Lippincott Manual of Nursing Practice* with that focus. This manual is meant to guide students and nurses across all care settings, to provide whatever the patient needs, according to established standards of practice, but not forgetting the caring interactions that nurses do so well.

ORGANIZATION

This new edition continues to follow a basic outline format for easy readability and access of information. The subheadings continue to follow a medical model—Pathophysiology and Etiology, Clinical Manifestations, Diagnostic Evaluation, Management, and Complications—and a nursing process model—Nursing Assessment, Nursing Diagnoses, Nursing Interventions, Community and Home Care Considerations, Patient Education and Health Maintenance, and Evaluation: Expected Outcomes. Medical model information is presented because nurses need to understand the medical disorder, diagnostic workup, and treatment that are the basis for nursing care. The nursing process section provides a practical overview of step-by-step nursing care for almost any patient scenario.

This edition is divided into five parts to present a comprehensive reference for all types of nursing care. Part One discusses the role of the nurse in the health care delivery system. It comprises chapters on Nursing Practice and the Nursing Process, Standards of Care and Ethical and Legal Issues, Health Promotion and Preventative Care, and Genetics and Health Applications.

Part Two encompasses medical–surgical nursing. General topics are presented in Unit I, including Adult Physical Assessment, Intravenous Therapy, Perioperative Nursing, Cancer Nursing, and Care of the Older Adult or Adult with Disability. Units II through XII deal with body system function and dysfunction and the various disorders seen in adult medical and surgical nursing.

Part Three covers Maternity and Neonatal Nursing. Chapters include Maternal and Fetal Health, Nursing Management during Labor and Delivery, Care of the Mother and Newborn during the Postpartum Period, and Complications of the Childbearing Experience. Chapters reflect the routine childbearing experience as well as frequently encountered high-risk situations and problems that may arise for the mother as well as the infant.

Part Four focuses on Pediatric Nursing. Chapters are divided into two units. One unit covers General Practice Considerations, comprising Pediatric Growth and Development, Pediatric Physical Assessment, Pediatric Primary Care, and Care of the Sick or Hospitalized Child. The other unit contains chapters based on body systems to describe the various disorders and corresponding nursing care seen in pediatric nursing.

Part Five discusses Psychiatric Nursing. Entries follow the *Diagnostic and Statistical Manual of Mental Disorders*, Fifth Edition, classification of mental illness. Treatments and nursing management for each are discussed.

Sandra M. Nettina, MSN, ANP-BC

NEW TO THIS EDITION

New and Expanded Material

Information has been added to or extensively updated throughout chapters in these areas:

Chapter 1—new section on transitional care, the concept of ensuring coordination and continuity of care when a patient moves from one care setting to another.

Chapter 3—updated U.S. Preventive Services Task Force screening guidelines

Chapter 4—introduction of precision health care

Chapter 5—streamlined to highlight the most frequently used nursing assessment techniques

Chapter 6—IV therapy extensively updated

Chapter 8—survivorship care added

Chapter 10—extensive updating

Chapter 11—extensive updating

Chapter 12—extensive updating

Chapter 13—extensive updating

Chapter 15—extensive updating

Chapter 19—extensive updating

Chapter 20—eating disorders section expanded

Chapter 23—magnetic resonance imaging screening, hormonal treatment

Chapter 25—American Diabetic Association updates

Chapter 29—extensive updating

Chapter 34—extensive updating

Chapter 36-38—extensive updating with emphasis on improving outcomes

Chapter 42—expanded information

Chapter 45—new medications and treatment information

Chapter 46—new medications and treatment information

Chapter 47—risk factors for eustachian tube dysfunction

Chapter 53—extensive updating on pediatric immunodeficiency and other disorders

Chapter 57—reclassification of disorders according to DSM 5

You will find updated information on diagnostic tests and medical care for almost every entry. Nursing care has also been updated to reflect new treatments and best practice information.

Transitional Care

Added to this edition is the concept of transitional care, or ensuring coordination and continuity of care when a patient moves from one care setting to another, as in moving from an inpatient setting to home, or across health states such as from curative to palliative care or from pediatric care to adult care. The purpose is to provide support during the transition and improve health outcomes. At every episode of transition, there are critical nursing assessment, intervention, and education opportunities to help facilitate the transition. In each chapter, we have included a new logo item, Transitional Care Alert, which highlights important nursing care in specific transitions.

Graphics

To streamline the book, we have removed Procedure Guidelines from the print edition. Important points from the procedures have been added to text, and Procedure Guidelines can be found in online editions. Many new figures, boxes, and tables have been added or updated.

It has been my pleasure preparing the 11th edition of the *Lippincott Manual of Nursing Practice* for you. I hope that it will serve you well in providing patient care across all settings.

Sandra M. Nettina, MSN, ANP-BC

ACKNOWLEDGMENTS

I would like to thank past and present reviewers and contributors and the entire Lippincott Williams & Wilkins team for their contribution to the *Lippincott Manual of Nursing Practice*, 11th edition. Lisa Marshall, developmental editor, has been instrumental in guiding and supporting me in this project. Lindsay Ries, editorial assistant, has been invaluable in directing the day-to-day logistics and activities behind the scenes. Bruce Hobart kept the chapters, and all of us involved, moving through production. Christine Nelson-Tuttle as my associate clinical editor provided complete oversight of the pediatric chapters and many other aspects of the project. Everyone involved has come to respect the enormity of the task and how each step affects the next. I am proud of our accomplishment.

LIPPINCOTT
MANUAL OF
NURSING PRACTICE

PART ONE

NURSING PROCESS AND PRACTICE

1
Nursing Practice and the Nursing Process

NURSING PRACTICE
Basic Concepts in Nursing Practice

Since Florence Nightingale developed the first model for nursing education in 1873, the role of the professional nurse and nursing scope of practice has evolved. Emphasis now is focused on evidence-based nursing care and preventive health practices. Understanding basic concepts in nursing practice, such as roles of nursing, theories of nursing, licensing, and legal issues, helps enhance performance.

Definition of Nursing

1. Nursing is an art and a science.
2. Earlier emphasis focused on care of the sick patient; now, the promotion of health is stressed.
3. American Nurses Association (ANA) definition (1980): Nursing is the diagnosis and treatment of the human response to actual and potential health problems.

Roles of Nursing

Whether in a hospital-based or community health care setting, nurses assume three basic roles:
1. Practitioner—involves actions that directly meet the health care and nursing needs of patients, families, and significant others; includes staff nurses at all rungs of the clinical ladder, advanced practice nurses, and community-based nurses.
2. Leader—involves actions, such as deciding, relating, influencing, and facilitating, that affect the actions of others and are directed toward goal determination and achievement; may be a formal nursing leadership role or an informal role periodically assumed by the nurse. Leadership roles may occur outside the typical nurse–patient relationship, in areas of advocacy in health policy where the focus is on improving the health of large populations of people.
3. Researcher—involves actions taken to implement studies to determine the actual effects of nursing care to further the scientific base of nursing; may include all nurses, not just academicians, nurse scientists, and graduate nursing students.

Theories of Nursing

1. Nursing theories help define nursing as a scientific discipline of its own.
2. The elements of nursing theories are uniform: nursing, patient, environment, and health—also known as the *paradigm* or *model* of nursing.
3. Nightingale was the first nursing theorist; she believed the purpose of nursing was to put the patient in the best condition for nature to restore or preserve health.
4. Theories range from broad to limited in scope.
   a. Grand nursing theories are the broadest and most abstract; they pertain to all nursing situations but are limited in directing or explaining nursing care.
   b. Middle-range nursing theories bridge grand theory with nursing practice; they can generate theoretical research and nursing practice strategies.
   c. Nursing practice theories (microrange) are limited in scope; they provide framework for nursing interventions and predicted outcomes in specific nursing situations.
5. More recent nursing theorists include the following:
   a. Levine—nursing supports a patient's adaptation to change because of internal and external environmental stimuli.
   b. Orem—nurses assist the patient to meet universal, developmental, and health deviation self-care requisites.
   c. Roy—nurses manipulate stimuli to promote adaptation in four modes: physiologic, self-concept, role function, and interdependence relations.
   d. Leninger—model of transcultural nursing; nurses should provide culturally specific care.
   e. Pender—nurses promote healthy behavior through a preventive model of health care.
   f. Rogers—nurses promote harmonious interaction between the patient and environment to maximize health; both are four-dimensional energy fields.
6. In recent years, the priority of interprofessional care has resulted in many nursing research initiatives to utilize other health care theories not specifically designated as nursing theorists.

Nursing in the Health Care Delivery System

1. Technology, education, society values, demographics, and health care financing all have an impact on where and how nursing is practiced.
   a. As the population ages, chronic disease rates rise and health care utilization increases.
   b. Chronic diseases are responsible for 7 of 10 deaths each year, and treating people with chronic diseases accounts for 86% of health care costs in the United States.
   c. The World Economic Forum estimates that chronic diseases account for almost two thirds of all deaths worldwide—and 80% of these now occur in low- and middle-income countries. By 2030, more people in these countries will die from heart attacks and strokes than from infectious diseases.
2. Health promotion and prevention strategies such as immunizations, health education, and screening tests aimed at reducing the incidence of infectious disease, injuries, and chronic illness save health care dollars and improve well-being. Nurses are well prepared for implementing health promotion strategies.
3. A nursing faculty shortage may challenge the ability of nursing to meet the needs of the expanded patient population.
   a. US nursing schools turned away almost 70,000 qualified applicants from baccalaureate and graduate nursing programs in 2014 because of an insufficient number of faculty, clinical sites, classroom space, clinical preceptors, and budget constraints.
   b. Almost two thirds of the nursing schools report faculty shortages as a reason for not accepting all qualified applicants into baccalaureate programs.
4. Advanced practice nurses are utilized as primary care and acute care providers because of a shortage of physicians. The Institute of Medicine 2010 report "The Future of Nursing" called for removal of regulatory barriers so nurses could practice to the full extent of their education and scope of practice.

Advanced Practice Nursing

1. Registered professional nurses with advanced training, education, and certification are allowed to practice in expanded scope.
2. This includes nurse practitioners, nurse-midwives, nurse-anesthetists, and clinical nurse specialists.
3. Scope of practice and legislation vary by state.
   a. Clinical nurse specialists are included in advanced practice nurse (APN) legislation in at least 27 states (some of these include only psychiatric/mental health clinical nurse specialists).
   b. Nurse practitioners have some type of prescriptive authority in all 50 states and the District of Columbia.
   c. In most cases, nurse practitioners are now eligible for Medicare reimbursement across the United States at 85% of the physician fee schedule and are eligible for Medicaid reimbursement in most states.
   d. Many states give full practice authority to APNs through the board of nursing with no requirement for physician oversight or collaboration required.
4. Master's degree preparation is the current requirement for most APN roles; however, many certificate programs have trained APNs in the past 40 years. In addition, doctoral programs are becoming increasingly desired, with emphasis on the practice role of APNs.
5. In Canada and other countries, the growth of the number of APNs in practice has been slower than in the United States, except for midwives in many cases.

Licensing, Certification, and Continuing Education

1. Every professional registered nurse must be licensed through the state board of nursing in the United States to practice in that state or the College of Nursing to practice in a Canadian province.
2. Although the state primarily regulates and restricts practice, the framework for scope of practice actually depends on a four-tier hierarchy: (1) the ANA Scope and Standards for Nursing Practice, (2) the particular state Nurse Practice Act, (3) the facility policies and procedures where the nurse is practicing, and (4) the nurse with her or his individual self-determination and competencies. Indeed, it is the nurse's responsibility to maintain competency and practice within the appropriate scope.
3. Continuing education requirements vary depending on state laws, facility policies, and area of specialty practice and certification. Continuing education units can be obtained through a variety of professional nursing organizations and commercial educational services.
4. Many professional nursing organizations exist to provide education, certification, support, and communication among nurses; for more information, contact your state nurses' association, state board of nursing, or the ANA, 8515 Georgia Avenue, Suite 400, Silver Spring, MD 20910, 800-274-4ANA, *www.nursingworld.org*.
5. Nursing curriculum and the nursing role have expanded to meet the demands of an aging, chronically ill population, advanced technology in the acute care setting, and expanding preventive strategies and community-based care to promote a healthier population. A wide variety of certifications offered through the American Nurses Credentialing Center (*www.nursecredentialing.org*) acknowledge advanced preparation of nurse practitioners, clinical nurse specialists, home health nurses, case management nurses, and many other specialties.

Management/Leadership in Nursing

1. There is a need to transform the health care workplace to better provide optimal health care to all patients. The transformation of health care will require nurses educated and actively using interprofessional collaborative processes, translation of knowledge, and motivation into the highest level of nursing care performance.
2. The Doctor of Nursing Practice (DNP) was introduced in 2005 to ensure that nursing can meet the demands of the changing health care system with the highest level of scientific knowledge and practice expertise.
   a. The American Association of Colleges of Nursing has proposed that the DNP replace the master's degree as preparation for advanced practice nursing; however, this is still up for debate.
   b. There are almost 300 DNP programs in the United States and more than 100 developments.

3. A recent addition to the certification arena is that of the clinical nurse leader, which has a master's degree requirement. It is defined as a nursing generalist whose role is to improve the quality of nursing care. The clinical nurse leader provides direction at the point of care, collaborates with the health care team, provides risk assessment, and implements quality improvement strategies based on evidence-based practice.

4. Challenges will exist in translating educational concepts in management and leadership into effective and relevant practices used by individuals in health care teams.

Safe Nursing Care

Patient Safety

1. Adequate nursing staffing is essential to reduce nurses' dissatisfaction, burnout, and high turnover rates, as well as reduce patient mortality. Studies have linked inadequate staffing to increased patient mortality.
   a. A recent retrospective observation study at a Magnet hospital identified an average patient exposed to three nursing shifts with below staffing resulted in 6% higher risk of mortality than patients with no below-target mortality.
   b. The American Nursing Association campaign, "Safe Nursing Saves Lives," advocates that hospitals set staffing levels on each unit based on patient acuity, number of patient, nursing skills, support staff, and technology (*http://www.nursingworld.org/MainMenuCategories/ThePracticeofProfessionalNursing/NurseStaffing*).

 EVIDENCE BASE Lee, S., & Scott, L. (2018). Hospital nurses' work environment characteristics and patient safety outcomes: A literature review. *Western Journal of Nursing Research, 40*(1), 121–145.

2. The Institute of Medicine (IOM) of the National Academies has focused on deficient health care systems as the cause of medical errors that are preventable and result in more than 50% of adverse events and patient deaths. The IOM offers recommendations for improving systems and processes in health care organizations to ultimately improve patient safety. For more information, refer to the website *www.iom.edu*.

3. The Agency for Healthcare Research and Quality has compiled a wide array of patient safety literature as a resource for all types of health care providers and settings, available at *http://psnet.ahrq.gov/default.aspx*.

4. The Joint Commission is also committed to improving safety for patients in health care organizations. The National Patient Safety Goals were implemented in 2003 to help address specific concerns for patient safety by health care setting, including ambulatory care, long-term care, behavioral health care, home care, hospital, laboratory services, and office-based surgery. New goals are introduced yearly with suggested performance measures to meet the goals. These are available at *www.jointcommission.org/standards_information/npsgs.aspx*. See Box 1-1 for selected National Patient Safety Goals.

Personal Safety

1. Nurses may be at risk for personal harm in the workplace. The ANA has sponsored initiatives to improve nurses' personal

---

BOX 1-1	National Patient Safety Goals: Hospital Program*

Use at least two patient identifiers when providing care, treatment, and services.

Ensure the correct patient gets the correct blood when they get a blood transfusion.

Report critical results of tests and diagnostic procedures on a timely basis.

Label all medications, medication containers, and other solutions on and off the sterile field in perioperative and other procedural settings.

Reduce the likelihood of patient harm associated with the use of anticoagulant therapy.

Make improvements to ensure that alarms on medical equipment are heard and responded to in a timely manner.

Maintain and communicate accurate patient medication information.

Comply with either the current Centers for Disease Control and Prevention (CDC) hand hygiene guidelines or the current World Health Organization (WHO) hand hygiene guidelines.

Implement evidence-based practices to prevent health care–associated infections because of multidrug-resistant organisms in acute care hospitals.

Implement evidence-based practices to prevent central line–associated bloodstream infections.

Implement evidence-based practices for preventing surgical site infections.

Implement evidence-based practices to prevent indwelling catheter-associated urinary tract infections (CAUTI).

Identify patients at risk for suicide.

Conduct a preprocedure verification process.

Mark the procedure site.

A time-out is performed before the procedure.

See www.jointcommission.org/assets/1/6/NPSG_EPs_Scoring_HAP_20110706.pdf for elements of performance. https://www.jointcommission.org/standards_information/npsgs.aspx.

safety. The Position Statement: Risk and Responsibility in Providing Nursing Care acknowledges that there may be limits to the personal risk a nurse can assume in providing care in any clinical setting.

2. The Centers for Disease Control and Prevention estimates that 380,000 health care workers are injured by needles and other sharps each year, increasing the risk of hepatitis B, hepatitis C, and human immunodeficiency virus. Nurses sustain the largest percentage of these injuries. The ANA's "Safe Needles, Save Lives" (*www.needlestick.org*) campaign was key in promoting the use of safety devices. Nurses and other health care workers are protected by the Needlestick Safety and Prevention Act (P.L. 106-430), which requires health care organizations to use needleless or shielded-needle devices, obtain input from clinical staff in the evaluation and selection of devices, educate staff on the use of safety devices, and have an exposure control plan.

3. The physical work environment, which includes patient-handling tasks such as manual lifting, transferring, and repositioning patients, can also place nurses at risk for musculoskeletal disorders such as back injuries and shoulder strains.

The ANA's "Handle with Care" campaign (*www.nursing-world.org/handlewithcare*) aims to prevent such injuries and to promote safe patient handling through the use of technology and assistive patient-handling equipment and devices.

Culturally Competent Care

 EVIDENCE BASE Darnell, L., & Hickson, S. (2015j. Cultural competent patient-centered nursing care. *Nursing Clinics of North America, 50*(1), 99–108.

The changing demographics of the United States, Canada, the United Kingdom, and other countries bring a diverse array of individuals with varying cultures and beliefs into nursing practice. Nurses must provide culturally competent care by expanding their knowledge about different cultures. Cultural competence involves learning a new set of attitudes, behaviors, and skills to help the nurse provide care effectively in cross-cultural situations. See Box 1-2, Standards of Practice for Culturally Competent Nursing Care. The Transcultural Nursing Society (TCNS) was founded in 1975 by Madeleine Leininger with a focus on human caring.

Culturally congruent and competent care results in improved health and well-being for people worldwide. TCNS offers a peer-reviewed evidence-based journal, educational courses, and many other resources to provide information about the values, beliefs, and traditions of various cultures (*www.tcns.org*). However, the nurse must always use caution and avoid generalizing and stereo-typing patients. Culturally competent care begins with an individualized patient assessment, including the patient's own definition of health and expectations for care. Based on this assessment and application of a set of standards, the nurse can develop an individualized care plan.

THE NURSING PROCESS

The nursing process is a deliberate, problem-solving approach to meeting the health care and nursing needs of patients. It involves assessment (data collection), nursing diagnosis, planning, implementation, and evaluation, with subsequent modifications used as feedback mechanisms to promote the resolution of the nursing diagnoses. The process as a whole is cyclical, with the steps being interrelated, interdependent, and recurrent.

BOX 1-2   Transcultural Nursing Standards of Practice

1. **Social Justice:** Professional nurses shall promote social justice for all. The applied principles of social justice guide decisions of nurses related to the patient, family, community, and other health care professionals. Nurses will develop leadership skills to advocate for socially just policies.

2. **Critical Reflection:** Nurses shall engage in critical reflection of their own values, beliefs, and cultural heritage to have an awareness of how these qualities and issues can impact culturally congruent nursing care.

3. **Transcultural Nursing Knowledge:** Nurses shall gain an understanding of the perspectives, traditions, values, practices, and family systems of culturally diverse individuals, families, communities, and populations for whom they care, as well as knowledge of the complex variables that affect the achievement of health and well-being.

4. **Cross-Cultural Practice:** Nurses shall use cross-cultural knowledge and culturally sensitive skills in implementing culturally congruent nursing care.

5. **Health Care Systems and Organizations:** Health care organizations should provide the structure and resources necessary to evaluate and meet the cultural and language needs of their diverse clients.

6. **Patient Advocacy and Empowerment:** Nurses shall recognize the effect of health care policies, delivery systems, and resources on their patient populations and shall empower and advocate for their patients as indicated. Nurses shall advocate for the inclusion of their patient's cultural beliefs and practices in all dimensions of their health care when possible.

7. **Multicultural Workforce:** Nurses shall actively engage in the effort to ensure a multicultural workforce in health care settings. One measure to achieve a multicultural workforce is through strengthening of recruitment and retention effort in the hospital and academic setting.

8. **Education and Training:** Nurses shall be educationally prepared to promote and provide culturally congruent health care. Knowledge and skills necessary for ensuring that nursing care is culturally congruent shall be included in global health care agendas that mandate formal education and clinical training, as well as required ongoing, continuing education for all practicing nurses.

9. **Cross-Cultural Communication:** Nurses shall use culturally competent verbal and nonverbal communication skills to identify client's values, beliefs, practices, perceptions, and unique health care needs.

10. **Cross-Cultural Leadership:** Nurses shall have the ability to influence individuals, groups, and systems to achieve positive outcomes of culturally competent care for diverse populations.

11. **Policy Development:** Nurses shall have the knowledge and skills to work with public and private organizations, professional associations, and communities to establish policies and standards for comprehensive implementation and evaluation of culturally competent care.

12. **Evidence-Based Practice and Research:** Nurses shall base their practice on interventions that have been systematically tested and shown to be the most effective for the culturally diverse populations that they serve. In areas where there is a lack of evidence of efficacy, nurse researchers shall investigate and test interventions that may be the most effective in reducing the disparities in health outcomes.

Adapted with permission from Douglas, MK (2011). Standards of Practice for Culturally Competent Nursing Care: 2011 Update. The Journal of Transcultural Nursing, 22(4), 317–333. © 2011 Sage Publishing.

Steps in the Nursing Process

Assessment—systematic collection of data to determine the patient's health status and to identify any actual or potential health problems. (Analysis of data is included as part of the assessment. For those who wish to emphasize its importance, analysis may be identified as a separate step of the nursing process.)

Nursing diagnosis—identification of actual or potential health problems that are amenable to resolution by nursing actions.

Planning—development of goals and a care plan designed to assist the patient in resolving the nursing diagnoses.

Implementation—actualization of the care plan through nursing interventions or supervision of others to do the same.

Evaluation—determination of the patient's responses to the nursing interventions and of the extent to which the goals have been achieved.

Assessment

1. The nursing history.
   a. Subjective data obtained by interviewing the patient, family members, or significant other and reviewing past medical records.
   b. Provides the opportunity to convey interest, support, and understanding to the patient and to establish a rapport based on trust.
2. The physical examination.
   a. Objective data obtained to determine the patient's physical status, limitations, and assets.
   b. Should be done in a private, comfortable environment with efficiency and respect.

Nursing Diagnosis

 EVIDENCE BASE Herdman, H., & Kamitsuru, S. (2018). *NANDA Nursing Diagnoses: Definitions and classifications, 2018–2020, 11th ed.* New York: Thieme.

1. The process of making a clinical judgment about experiences or responses to health problems or life processes, based on an individual, family, or community and done through patient assessment rather than picked from a list of medical diagnoses.
2. Used to determine the appropriate plan of care (ie, to select nursing interventions that will achieve desired outcomes).
3. Nursing diagnoses are based on the NANDA International taxonomy, which is a standardized nursing language that includes evidence-based definitions, defining characteristics, and etiologic factors.
   a. Nursing diagnoses continue to be developed and refined by NANDA International and the University of Iowa Center for Nursing Classification and Clinical Effectiveness.
   b. There are currently 235 nursing diagnoses grouped in 13 domains (see Box 1-3). Nursing diagnoses are listed throughout this book associated with medical diagnoses and other health conditions, but in reality, nursing diagnoses are formulated through individualized patient assessment.

Planning

See Nursing Care Plan 1-1 (page 7).

See Nursing Care Plan 1-1 (page 7).

BOX 1-3	NANDA International Domains of Nursing

Health Promotion
Nutrition
Elimination and Exchange
Activity/Rest
Perception/Cognition
Self-Perception
Role Relationships
Sexuality
Coping/Stress Tolerance
Life Principles
Safety/Protection
Comfort
Growth/Development

 EVIDENCE BASE De Carvalho, E., Eduardo, A., Romanzini, A., Simao, T., Zamarioli, C., Garguio, D., & Herdman, T. (2018). Correspondence between NANDA international nursing diagnoses and outcomes as proposed by the nursing outcomes classification. *International Journal of Nursing Knowledge, 29*(1), 66–78.

1. Assign priorities to the nursing diagnoses. Highest priority is given to problems that are the most urgent and critical.
2. Establish goals or expected outcomes derived from the nursing diagnoses.
   a. Specify short-term, intermediate, and long-term goals as established by nurse and patient together.
   b. Goals should be specific, measurable, and patient-focused and should include a time frame.
   c. The Nursing Outcomes Classification developed by the University of Iowa College of Nursing Center is a comprehensive, standardized nursing language of outcomes used to evaluate the effects of nursing interventions. Each of the approximately 490 outcomes includes a list of indicators and is linked to NANDA I nursing diagnoses.
3. Identify nursing interventions as appropriate for goal attainment.
   a. An intervention is defined as any treatment, based on clinical judgment and knowledge, that a nurse performs to enhance patient/client outcomes.
   b. Include independent nursing actions as well as collaborative interventions based on medical orders.
   c. Should be detailed to provide continuity of care.
   d. Nursing Interventions Classification (NIC) is a standardized language describing treatments performed by nurses in all settings and specialties. More than 550 NIC interventions have been developed through the University of Iowa College of Nursing. NIC is organized into 30 classifications and 7 domains and includes physiologic and psychosocial interventions as well as interventions for illness prevention and treatment. NIC interventions serve a role in documentation, possibly coding, and reimbursement for nursing care in the future.
4. Formulate the nursing care plan. The nursing care plan may be a component of the interdisciplinary/collaborative care plan for the patient.
   a. Include nursing diagnoses, expected outcomes, interventions, and a space for evaluation.

NURSING CARE PLAN 1-1

Example of a Nursing Care Plan

Mr. John Preston, a 52-year-old businessperson, was admitted with chest pain; rule out myocardial infarction. He had experienced substernal chest pain and weakness in his arms after having lunch with a business associate. The pain had lessened by the time he arrived at the hospital. The nursing history revealed that he had been hospitalized 5 months previously with the same complaints and had been told by his physician to go to the emergency department if the pain ever recurred. He had been placed on a low-fat diet and had stopped smoking. Physical examination revealed that Mr. Preston's vital signs were within normal limits. He stated that he had feared he was having a "heart attack" until his pain subsided and until he was told that his electrocardiogram was normal. He verbalized that he wanted to find out how he could prevent the attacks of pain in the future. The physician's orders on admission included activity as tolerated, low-cholesterol diet, and nitroglycerin 0.4 mg (1/500 g) sublingually as needed.

NURSING DIAGNOSIS

Acute Pain related to angina pectoris/rule out myocardial ischemia

GOAL

Short-term: Relief of pain.
Intermediate: Inclusion of healthy lifestyle measures that decrease myocardial ischemia.
Long-term: Compliance with therapeutic regimen.

Expected Outcomes	Nursing Intervention	Critical Time*	Actual Outcomes (Evaluation)
• Blood pressure (BP), pulse (P), and respiration (R) will remain within normal limits.	Monitor BP, P, R q4h.	24 h	• BP: stable at 116 to 122/72 to 84 • P: stable at 68 to 82 • R: stable at 16 to 20
• Patient will remain free from chest pain.	Assess frequency of chest pain and precipitating events.	24 h	• Denies chest pain; able to walk length of hall, eat meals, and visit with family and friends without chest discomfort.
• Will tolerate dietary regimen. • Will not experience chest pain after meals. • Will maintain normal bowel elimination. • Will have intake of 1,500 to 2,000 mL fluid/day.	Encourage food and fluid intake that promotes healthy nutrition, digestion, and elimination and that does not precipitate chest pain: light, regular meals; foods low in cholesterol; 1,500 to 2,000 mL fluid/day.	24 h	• Denies chest pain after meals; no constipation or diarrhea; fluid intake 1,700 to 2,100 mL/day.
• Will identify foods low in cholesterol and those foods that are to be avoided. • Will select well-balanced diet within prescribed restrictions.	Request consultation with dietitian. Reinforce diet teaching.	48 h	• Dietitian reviewed diet restrictions with patient and wife; wife counseled in meal planning. Patient selects and eats a balanced diet consisting of foods low in cholesterol.
• Will identify activities and exercises that could precipitate chest pain: those that require sudden bursts of activity and heavy effort. • Will identify emotionally stressful situations; will explain the necessity for alternating periods of activity with periods of rest.	Encourage alterations in activities and exercise that are necessary to prevent episodes of anginal pain.	48 h	• Patient and wife have identified activities and situations that should be avoided; patient and wife have studied their usual daily routine and have made plans to alter the routine to allow for rest periods; teenage son has volunteered to assist with strenuous home maintenance chores.
• Will describe action, use, and correct administration of nitroglycerin.	Teach about nitroglycerin regimen.	24 h	• Patient has accurately stated action, use, and dosage of nitroglycerin; demonstrated correct administration.

*These times have not been standardized but are individualized according to the patient's needs.

b. May use a standardized care plan—check off appropriate data and fill in target dates for expected outcomes and frequency and other specifics of interventions.

c. May use a protocol that gives specific sequential instructions for treating patients with a particular problem, including who is responsible and what specific actions should be taken in terms of assessment, planning, interventions, teaching, recognition of complications, evaluation, and documentation.

d. May use a care path or clinical pathway (also called *care map* or *critical pathway*) in which the nurse as case manager is responsible for outcomes, length of stay, and use of equipment during the patient's illness; includes the patient's medical diagnosis, length of stay allowed by diagnostic-related group (DRG), expected outcomes, and key events that must occur for the patient to be discharged by that date. Key events are not as specific as nursing interventions but are categorized by day of stay and who is responsible (nurse, physician, other health team member, patient, family).

e. May also use a computerized care plan that is based on assessment data and allows for the selection of nursing interventions and establishment of expected outcomes.

f. Nursing concept maps are similar and may be used to plan and prioritize care.

Implementation

1. Coordinate activities of patient, family, significant others, nursing team members, and other health team members.
2. Delegate specific nursing interventions to other members of the nursing team as appropriate.
   a. Consider the capabilities and limitations of the members of the nursing team.
   b. Supervise the performance of nursing interventions.
3. Record the patient's responses to nursing interventions precisely and concisely.

Evaluation

Determines the success of nursing care and the need to alter the care plan.
1. Collect assessment data.
2. Compare patient's actual outcomes to expected outcomes to determine to what extent goals have been achieved.
3. Include the patient, family, or significant other; nursing team members; and other health team members in the evaluation.
4. Identify alterations that need to be made in the goals and the nursing care plan.

Continuation of the Nursing Process

1. Continue all steps of the nursing process: assessment, nursing diagnosis, planning, implementation, and evaluation.
2. Continuous evaluation provides the means for maintaining the viability of the entire nursing process and for demonstrating accountability for the quality of nursing care rendered.

CARE ACROSS SETTINGS
Community and Home Health Concepts

The home care nurse functions in the home and community, outside the walls of health care facilities. The role is more independent, and the basic concepts of home health are different from hospital

or outpatient nursing. With the emphasis on promoting patients quickly from the acute care settings to care in the home, descriptions and requirements for community health nurses have evolved. Theses nurses may work with one specific population based on care needs or developmental stages (wound care, pediatric patients) or care through all stages and nursing needs. Although some nurses focus on individual patients (and their families or support persons), some nurses focus on improving the overall health of an entire population of persons.

Roles and Duties of the Home Care Nurse

1. The home care nurse maintains a comprehensive knowledge base of the health of the patient.
2. The home care nurse performs an extensive evaluation of the patient's medical history, physical condition, psychosocial well-being, living environment, and support systems.
3. The home care nurse functions independently, recommending to the primary or specialty health care provider what services are needed in the home.
4. The home care nurse coordinates the services of other disciplines, such as physical therapy, occupational therapy, nutrition, and social work.
5. The home care nurse oversees the entire treatment plan and keeps the health care provider apprised of the patient's progress or lack of progress toward goals.
6. The home care nurse acts as a liaison between patient, family, caregivers, and the primary health care provider and other members of the health care team.
7. The home care nurse may function as supervisor of home health aides who provide direct daily care for the patient.
8. The home care nurse must honor the same patient rights as a health care facility.

Skills for Home Care Nursing

1. Good rapport building—to engage the patient, family, and caregivers in goal attainment.
2. Clear communication—to provide effective teaching to family and caregivers, to relate assessment information about the patient to the health care provider, and to share information with the home care team.
3. Flexibility—ability to care for a variety of patients in diverse home care settings with multiple health care conditions requiring nursing care.
4. Cultural competence—knowledge and appreciation of the cultural norms being practiced in the home. Cultural practices may affect family structure, communication, and decision-making in the home; health beliefs, nutrition, and alternative health practices; and spirituality and religious beliefs.
5. Accurate documentation—record keeping in home care is used for reimbursement of nursing services, accreditation and regulatory review, and communication among the home care team.

Reimbursement Issues

1. Skilled home health services are reimbursed by Medicare, Medicaid, and a variety of commercial insurances and managed care plans.
2. In recent years, many health care services have changed from reimbursement from volume-based reimbursement to more focus on outcomes.
3. Some patients are willing to pay out of pocket for additional services not covered by insurance because of the well-established

value of home care services compared with more expensive hospital and nursing home services.

4. Services are reimbursed by Medicare Part A if they meet the following criteria:
    a. Need is documented in a face to face visit by a health care provider; plan of care must be signed by a physician.
    b. Services are intermittent or needed on a part-time basis.
    c. The patient is homebound.
    d. The services required are skilled (need to be provided by a licensed nurse, physical therapist, or speech therapist or by an occupational therapist, social worker, or home health aide along with the service of a nurse).
    e. The services requested are reasonable and medically necessary.
5. The home health nurse must evaluate the case and ensure that these criteria apply. This information must be documented so reimbursement will not be denied.

Transitional Care

Transitional care is the concept of ensuring coordination and continuity of care when a patient moves from one care setting to another. This may include between settings such as acute care hospital to skilled nursing facility or from an inpatient setting to home. It may also occur across levels of care within a setting such as from an intensive care unit to general medical unit or across health states such as from curative to palliative care or from pediatric care to adult care. The purpose is to provide support during the transition and improve health outcomes.

1. Patients experiencing a care transition experience a period of vulnerability that may contribute to high rate of health care services with potential adverse outcomes.
2. Transitional care services are a set of actions, essentially time-limited, which are added to usual care or primary care services that are designed to ensure health care continuity and best possible outcomes for at-risk populations.
3. At-risk individuals, particularly the elderly and those with chronic disease, may experience physical, emotional, and behavioral barriers to receiving optimal quality and safe care.
4. Transitional care services include logistical arrangements, education of the patient and family, and coordination among the health professionals.
5. Current transitional care programs are designed to reduce 30-day hospital readmission rates to save health care system dollars.

Home Health Practice

The nursing process is carried out in home care as it is in other nursing settings. Patient interactions are structured differently than in the hospital because the nurse will interact with the patient intermittently and in the intimate home environment. Many procedures and nursing interventions are implemented in a similar manner as other nursing settings, as outlined in the rest of this book. Major concerns of the home care nurse are patient teaching, infection control, and safety maintenance.

The Home Care Visit

1. The initial home care visit should be preceded by information gathering and an introductory phone call to the patient.
2. Extensive assessment is carried out at the first visit, including complete medical and psychosocial history, physical examination, home environment assessment, nutritional assessment, medication review, and current treatment plan review.

3. Once assessment (gathered from multiple sources) is complete, nursing diagnoses are formed. The plan of care must be adaptable to the specific home dynamics.
4. Outcome planning (goal setting) is done with the patient, family, and caregivers involved.
5. The plan is implemented over a prescribed time period (the certified period of service). Interventions may be:
    a. Cognitive—involves patient teaching.
    b. Psychosocial—reinforces coping mechanisms, supports caregivers, and reduces stress.
    c. Technical—entails procedures, such as wound care and catheter insertion.
6. Evaluation is ongoing at every visit and by follow-up phone calls to adjust and refine the care plan and frequency of service.
7. Recertification for continued service, discharge, or transfer (to a hospital or nursing home) ultimately occurs.

Patient Teaching

1. Patient teaching is directed toward the patient, family, caregivers, and involved significant others.
2. Patient teaching is usually considered skilled and is therefore reimbursable. Topics may include the following:
    a. Disease process, pathophysiology, and signs and symptoms to monitor treatment.
    b. Administration of injectable medication or complex regimen of oral medications.
    c. Diabetic management for a patient newly diagnosed with diabetes.
    d. Wound or ostomy care.
    e. Catheterization.
    f. Gastrostomy and enteral feedings.
    g. Management of peripheral or central intravenous catheters.
    h. Use of adaptive devices for carrying out activities of daily living and ambulation.
    i. Transfer techniques and body alignment.
    j. Preparation and maintenance of therapeutic diet.
3. Barriers to learning should be evaluated and removed or compensated for.
    a. Environmental barriers, such as noise, poor lighting, and distractions.
    b. Personal barriers, such as sensory deficits, poor reading skills, and drowsiness.
4. The teaching plan should include the three domains of learning:
    a. Cognitive—sharing of facts and information.
    b. Affective—addressing the patient's feelings about the disease and treatment.
    c. Psychomotor—discussing performance of desired behavior or steps in a procedure.
5. Documentation of patient teaching should be specific and include the degree of patient competence of the procedure.
6. Patient teaching plans may include review of teaching started in the hospital and may take several sessions to implement successfully.
7. Patient teaching plans should include significant support persons (family or other persons important to the patient) who will assist the patient in obtaining or maintaining optimal health outcomes.

Infection Control

1. Nosocomial infection rates are much lower in home care, but patients are still at risk for infection because of weakened immune systems and the variability of a clean or sterile environment at home.

2. The nurse should assess and maintain a clean environment.
   a. Make sure that clean or sterile supplies are readily available when needed.
   b. Make sure that contaminated supplies are disposed of promptly and properly.
      i. Needles should be disposed of in a safe and secure container (usually kept in the home [until full]), which can be disposed of through the home health agency or the patient's pharmacy.
      ii. Supplies, such as dressings, gloves, and catheters, should be securely bagged and disposed of in small amounts through the regular trash collection at the patient's home. However, biohazardous waste disposal may be necessary in some cases.
3. The nurse should be aware of all methods of transmission of infection and implement and teach preventive practices.
4. The nurse must perform ongoing assessment for signs and symptoms of infection and teach the patient, family, and caregivers what to look for.
5. The nurse should be aware of community-acquired infections that may be prevalent in certain populations, such as tuberculosis, human immunodeficiency virus infection, hepatitis, and sexually transmitted diseases.
   a. Teach preventive practices.
   b. Encourage and institute screening programs.
   c. Report infections according to the local public health department policy.
6. Encourage and provide vaccination for the patient and household contacts for influenza, pneumococcal pneumonia, hepatitis B, and others as appropriate.

 NURSING ALERT Above all else, model and teach good hand-washing practice to everyone in the home.

Ensuring Safety

1. Continually assess safety in the home, particularly if the patient is very ill and the care plan is complex.
2. Assess for environmental safety issues—cluttered spaces, stairs, throw rugs, slippery floors, poor lighting.
3. Assess for the patient's personal safety issues—sensory deficits, weakness, problems with eating or swallowing.
4. Assess safety in the bathroom—handrails, bath mat, raised toilet seat, water temperature.
5. Assess safety in the kitchen—proper refrigeration of food, ability to shop for and cook meals, oven safety.
6. Be alert for abuse and neglect, especially of children, dependent elders, and women.
7. Check equipment for electrical and fire safety and that it is being used properly.
8. Be continually cognizant of your own safety—get directions, travel during daylight hours, wear seat belts, do not enter suspicious areas without an escort, be alert to your surroundings.

SELECTED REFERENCES

American Association of Colleges of Nursing. (2016, April). The doctor of nursing practice fact sheet. Available: *www.aacn.nche.edu/media-relations/fact-sheets/dnp*

American Association of Colleges of Nursing. (2016). Annual state of the schools. Available: *www.aacn.nche.edu/publications/AnnualReport15.pdf*

American Nurses Association. (2014). ANA's handle with care. Available: *www.nursingworld.org/MainMenuCategories/WorkplaceSafety/Healthy-Work-Environment/SafePatient/SPHM-Self-Assessment-Resource*

American Nurses Association. (2015). *Position statement: Risk and responsibility in providing nursing care.* Silver Spring, MD: Author.

American Nurses Credentialing Center. (2017). Certification and renewals. Available: *www.nursecredentialing.org/Certification*

Andrew, M. A., & Boyle, J. S. (2015). *Transcultural concepts in nursing care* (7th ed.). Philadelphia, PA: Lippincott Williams & Wilkins.

Bender, M. (2016). Conceptualizing clinical nurse leader practice: An interpretive synthesis. *Journal of Nursing Management, 24,* E23–E31.

Bumpus, S., Brush, B., Wheeler, J., Pressler, S., Eagle, K., & Rubenfire, M. (2016). Cost analysis of an advanced practice registered nurse transitional care model for cardiac patients. *Nursing Economics, 34*(5), 236–241.

Buurman, B., Parlevliet, J., Allore, H., Blok, W., van Deelen, B. A.,... de Rooij, S. E. (2016). Comprehensive geriatric assessment and transitional care in acutely hospitalized patients: The transitional care bridge randomized clinical trial. *JAMA Internal Medicine, 176*(3), 302–309.

Carpenito, L. J. (2016). *Nursing diagnosis: Applications to clinical practice* (15th ed.). Philadelphia, PA: Lippincott Williams & Wilkins.

Cato, D. (2018). Expanding the Global footprint of safe quality care. *Arizona Nurse, 71*(1), 11.

Centers for Medicare and Medicaid Services (2016). *National health expenditure projections 2016–2025.* Baltimore, MD: Office of the Actuary, National Health Statistics Group. Available: *www.cms.gov/Research-Statistics-Data-and-Systems/Statistics-Trends-and-Reports/NationalHealthExpendData/Downloads/proj2016.pdf*

Chavez, E., & Yoder, L. (2015). Staff nurse clinical leadership: A concept analysis. *Nursing Forum, 50*(2), 90–100.

Darnell, L., & Hickson, S. (2015). Cultural competent patient-centered nursing care. *Nursing Clinics of North America, 50*(1), 99–108.

De Carvalho, E., Eduardo, A., Romanzini, A., Simao, T., Zamarioli, C., Garguio, D., & Herdman, T. (2018). Correspondence between NANDA international nursing diagnoses and outcomes as proposed by the nursing outcomes classification. *International Journal of Nursing Knowledge, 29*(1), 66–78.

Herdman, H. & Kamitsuru, S. (2018). *NANDA nursing diagnoses: Definitions and classifications, 2018–2020,* 11th ed. New York: Thieme.

Joint Commission (2016). Hospital 2017 national patient safety goals. Available: *www.jointcommission.org/hap_2017_npsgs/*

Kaiser Family foundation. (2017). Data note: Americans' challenges with healthcare costs. Available: http://kff.org/health-costs/poll-finding/data-note-americans-challenges-with-health-care-costs/

Marion, L., Douglas, M., Lavin, M., Barr, N., Gazaway, S. H., Thomas, E., & Bickford, C. (2017). Implementing the new ANA standard 8: Culturally congruent practice. *Online Journal of Issues in Nursing, 22*(1), 1.

Markey, K., Tilki, M., & Taylor, G. (2018). Understanding nurses' concerns when caring for patients from diverse cultural and ethnic backgrounds. *Journal of Clinical Nursing, 27*(1/2), 259–268.

McFarland, M. R., & Wehbe-Alamah, H. (2017). *Transcultural nursing: Concepts, theories, research, and practice* (7th ed.). New York: McGraw-Hill.

Murray, M., Sundin, D., & Cope, V. (2018). New graduate registered nurses' knowledge of patient safety and practice: A literature review. *Journal of Clinical Nursing, 27*(1/2), 31–47.

Lee, S., & Scott, L. (2018). Hospital nurses' work environment characteristics and patient safety outcomes: A literature review. *Western Journal of Nursing Research, 40*(1), 121–145.

National Quality Forum. (2015). *Safe practices for better healthcare: 2015 update.* Washington, DC: Author.

O'Connor, M., Arcamone, A., Amorin, F., Hoban, M. B., Boyd, R. M., Fowler, L.,... Fitzpatrick, M. L. (2016). Exposing baccalaureate nursing students to transitional care. *Home Healthcare Now, 34*(9), 491–499.

Parry, A., Barriball, K., & While, R. (2015). Factors contributing to registered nurse medication administration error: A narrative review. *International Journal of Nursing Studies, 52*(1), 403–420.

Peters, J. (2017). Role of transitional care measures in the prevention of readmission after critical illness. *Critical Care Nurse, 37*(1), e10–e17.

Ray, M. (2016). *Transcultural caring dynamics in nursing and health care.* Philadelphia, PA: Davis.

U.S. Department of Health and Human Services. (2017). Center for Linguistic and Cultural Competency in Health. Available: *https://minorityhealth.hhs.gov/omh/browse.aspx?lvl=1&lvlid=6*

2

Standards of Care and Ethical and Legal Issues

INTRODUCTION

Professional nurses occupy the front lines of the health care arena. So it is no surprise that nurses are members of the health care team patients trust most with their health and welfare. Along with this privilege, nurses carry equal duties of responsibility and accountability to follow ethical principles and standards of care integral to the profession. Continued efforts must be made from within the profession to systematically and deliberately apply evidence-based research data to daily practice, thereby increasing patient safety, improving outcomes, and reducing harm and adverse events. Transformation of the professional culture within the health care system gives nurses at the bedside the incentive to join in these efforts as full partners with colleagues in health care. Additional measures might include protocol implementation, preceptor performance review, peer review, continuing education, patient satisfaction surveys, and the implementation of risk management techniques. However, in certain instances, either despite or in the absence of such internal mechanisms, claims are made for an alleged injury or alleged malpractice liability. Although the vast majority of claims may be without merit, many professional nurses may have to cope with the unfamiliar legal system. Application of ethical principles and standards of care will be beneficial to prevent such situations. Therefore, it is preferable for the nursing profession to incorporate ethical and legal principles and protocols in daily practice to assure patient safety and excellent standards of patient care.

ETHICAL CORE CONCEPTS

Clinical ethics literature identifies four principles and values that are integral to the professional nurse's practice: the nurse's ethical duty to respect the patient's autonomy and to act with beneficence, nonmaleficence, and justice.

Respect for the Individual and Autonomy

1. Respect for the individual's autonomy incorporates principles of freedom of choice, self-determination, and privacy.
2. The professional nurse's duty is to view and treat each individual as an autonomous, self-determining person with the freedom to act in accordance with self-chosen, informed goals, as long as the action does not interfere or infringe on the autonomous action of another.
3. Numerous institutions and health care organizations have developed patient rights statements and policies that impact nursing care.
   a. The National League of Nursing (NLN) has developed an Education Competencies Model for all educational levels of nursing, which names the core values as caring, diversity, ethics, excellence, holism, integrity, and patient centeredness.
   b. The American Nurses Association (ANA) has developed and updated a Code of Ethics for Nurses, which states, "The nurse in all professional relationships practices with compassion with respect for the inherent dignity, worth, and uniqueness of every individual, unrestricted by considerations of social or economic status, personal attributes, or the nature of health problems."

 EVIDENCE BASE National League of Nursing. (2015). *The NLN education competencies model.* New York, NY: Author.
American Nurses Association. (2015). *Code of ethics for nurses with interpretive statements (code for nurses).* Silver Spring, MD: Author.

Beneficence

The principle of beneficence affirms the inherent professional aspiration and duty to help promote the well-being of others and, often, is the primary motivating factor for those who choose a career in the health care profession. Health care professionals aspire to help people achieve a better life through an improved state of health.

Nonmaleficence

1. The principle of nonmaleficence complements beneficence and obligates the professional nurse not to harm the patient directly or with intent.
2. In the health care profession, this principle is often actualized with the complementary principle of beneficence because it is common for the nurse to cause pain or expose the patient to risk of harm when such actions are justified by the benefits of the procedures or treatments.
3. It is best to seek to promote a balance of potential risk-induced harms with benefits, with the basic guideline being to strive to maximize expected benefits and minimize possible harms. Therefore, nonmaleficence should be balanced with beneficence.

Justice

1. Justice, or fairness, relates to the distribution of services and resources.
2. As the health care dollar becomes increasingly scarce, justice seeks to allocate resources fairly and treat patients equally.
3. Dilemmas arise when resources are scarce and insufficient to meet the needs of everyone. How do we decide fairly who gets what in such situations?
4. One might consider whether it is just or fair for many people not to have funding or access to the most basic preventive care, whereas others have insurance coverage for expensive and long-term hospitalizations.
5. Along with respect for people and their autonomy, the complex principle of justice is a culturally accepted principle in countries such as the United States. Nonetheless, the application of justice is complex and often challenging.

ETHICAL DILEMMAS

Conflicting Ethical Principles

1. Ethical dilemmas arise when two or more ethical principles are in conflict.
2. Such dilemmas can best be addressed by applying principles on a case-by-case basis once all available data are gathered and analyzed.
3. Clinicians should network with their colleagues and consider establishing multidisciplinary ethics committees to provide guidance.

Ethics Committees

1. Ethics committees identify, examine, and promote resolution of ethical issues and dilemmas and strive to:
   a. Protect the patient's rights.
   b. Protect the staff and the organization.
   c. Review decisions regarding clinical standards of practice and policy development.

   d. Improve the quality of care and services.
   e. Serve as educational resources to staff.
   f. Build a consensus on ethical issues with other professional organizations.
2. Addressing and resolving ethical dilemmas is usually a challenging decision shared with the clinical staff.

Examples of Ethical Dilemmas and Possible Responses

Unsafe Nurse-to-Patient Ratio

1. A pattern of unsafe nurse-to-patient ratio can be caused by temporary or long-term staffing problems.
2. A series of actions to best resolve the problem may include the following:
   a. Address the unsafe situation verbally and in writing to the unit charge nurse with copies to the nursing supervisor.
   b. Work up the administrative chain of command as indicated.
   c. This will likely prompt action by the facility, such as creating an as-needed pool of nurses to call for such situations, hiring more staff, or, in the interim, securing contracts with outside nursing agencies and utilizing agency nursing personnel.
3. Tolerance by staff nurses employed under such circumstances will preclude appropriate resolution and will leave the nurse open to unsafe practice and unmet patient needs, potentially increasing the risk of liability.
4. Although the employer is liable for the acts of the employee performed within the scope of employment, the nurse will not be exonerated should a patient's care be compromised in a setting of an unsafe nurse-to-patient ratio.

Nonresponse by Physician

1. A patient arrives to the rehabilitation unit at 9 P.M. with numerous positive criteria for falling, including poor short-term memory, daily use of a diuretic, daily use of a sleep aid, a history of a fall within the preceding 2 months, and known vision impairment.
   a. Patient is oriented to time, place, and person, his new room, facility bed, and call light use.
   b. The nurse instructs patient to summon her if he needs to void or otherwise get out of bed, at least until he becomes familiar with his new environment.
   c. Upon returning to patient's room 10 minutes later, the nurse finds patient out of bed, arranging his clothes in his closet, standing in a pool of urine on the floor.
   d. The nurse weighs the risks and benefits of restraint use and determines whether alternatives are available. She calls the physician for a restraint order if patient continues to jeopardize his safety. The nurse intends to ask the physician for an order with clear specification of the least restrictive method of restraint, the duration, circumstances, frequency of monitoring, and reevaluation if it differs from facility policy. However, the physician does not return her calls.
   e. The nurse documents her initial assessment of the patient, her nursing diagnoses, the orientation to room and equipment provided to the patient, the circumstances wherein she found the patient out of bed, and her repeated messages for the physician and the lack of a return telephone call.

2. Again, a series of actions may resolve the problem or at least prevent injury to the patient. Address this situation with intermediate measures while waiting for the physician's return call:
   a. Raise side rails on the patient's bed.
   b. Move patient to a room close to the nurse's station.
   c. Place a sign on patient's room door and above the bed identifying him as being at risk for falling.
   d. Place a sign above the bed instructing personnel to raise the bed's side rails fully before leaving patient's room.
   e. Check on the patient frequently during the first 24 hours, reminding him of the call light, its use, and the need to call the nurse before getting out of bed.
   f. If available, assign a patient care technician to stay with the patient.
3. Call the patient's family, advising them of your concern about the patient's safety, and discuss the issue of restraints with them. Discuss the risk for falling and prevention of fall-induced injury versus the restriction of the patient's freedom of movement about the room.
4. Document ongoing assessments of potential problems, calls to the physician, and discussions with family members.
5. Apply restraints according to the policy of the rehabilitation unit until an order is secured from the physician.
   a. Consult facility policy on restraint use.
   b. Secure an order from the physician for restraints to be used as needed, including specific criteria outlined in step 1d.
6. Reassess the patient's need for diuretic and sleep aid or sedative use. Discuss discontinuation of any unnecessary medications that increase the patient's degree of confusion or risk for falling, if possible.

Inappropriate Orders

1. A 74-year-old patient with a diagnosis of pneumonia is presently on a general medical ward for treatment and close monitoring. She is becoming increasingly anxious and dyspneic during your shift. Her heart rate is mildly increased. A house officer is summoned to evaluate this change in clinical status.
   a. The house officer, unfamiliar with the patient, spends 2 minutes reviewing the chart, quickly examines the patient, and orders a sedative to be administered stat and, as needed, every 4 hours.
   b. You tell the house officer that you heard decreased breath sounds in the left, lower lung and ask him to order some diagnostic tests, such as a chest x-ray and arterial blood gas analysis, and share your concern that administering a sedative to the patient may mask the underlying cause of the anxiety, lead to further respiratory compromise, and delay diagnosis and treatment of the underlying clinical problem. Nevertheless, he leaves the unit.
   c. Based on your evaluation of the situation, concerns about patient safety, and your role as patient advocate, you decide not to give the sedative ordered by the house officer.
2. Although you cannot automatically follow an order you think is unsafe, you cannot just ignore a medical order either.
   a. Document the scenario described above in the patient's chart, contact the resident on call, and notify your supervising nurse.
   b. If the resident on call agrees with the house officer's assessment, call the attending physician to discuss your concerns, obtain appropriate stat orders, and notify the house officer and resident of the attending physician's orders and the actions taken.

c. Notify all involved medical and nursing personnel of the patient's status.
d. Document accurately, clearly, succinctly, and in a timely fashion.
3. Your actions reflect concern about the best interest of the patient, and although they may yield negative behaviors by the house officer or resident, it is more important to prevent potential harm to the patient.

LEGAL ASPECTS OF PROFESSIONAL NURSING PRACTICE
Accountability

1. Integral to the practice of any profession is the inherent need to be responsible for actions taken and for omissions.
2. The professional nurse must be proactive and take all appropriate measures to ensure that professional practice is not lacking, remiss, or deficient in any area or way.
3. Useful proactive measures include the following:
   a. Maintain familiarity of relevant, current facility policies, procedures, and regulations as they apply to the nurse's practice and specialty area.
   b. Provide for self-audit.
   c. Provide for peer review to assess reasonableness of care in a particular setting for a particular problem.
   d. Work with local nursing organizations to assure that local standards of practice are met.
   e. Examine the quality (accuracy and completeness) of documentation.
   f. Establish collegial working relationships with colleagues wherein honest constructive criticism and discussion are welcomed for the greater goal of quality patient care.
4. Local standards of practice normally align with those of nationally accepted standards.

Advocacy

The professional nurse has the duty to:
1. Promote what is best for the patient, as perceived by the patient and/or his surrogate.
2. Ensure that the patient's needs are met and a therapeutic environment is maintained.
3. Protect the patient's rights, including confidentiality and informed consent, among others.

Confidentiality

1. The patient's privacy is consistent with the Hippocratic Oath and with the law as part of the constitutional right to privacy.
2. Although the professional nurse should assure the patient of confidentiality, limits on this standard must be clarified and discussed with the patient at the earliest opportunity.
3. It is imperative to clearly understand the process of informed consent and the legal standard for disclosure of confidential patient information to others.
4. The Medical Record Confidentiality Act of 1995, a federal statute, is the primary federal law governing the use of health treatment and payment records. Several practical guidelines include the following:
   a. Respect the individual's right to privacy when requesting or responding to a request for a patient's medical records.

b. Always require a signed medical authorization and consent form to release medical records and information to protect and respect patient–provider privilege statutes.

c. Discuss confidentiality issues with the patient and establish consent. Address concerns or special requests for information not to be disclosed.

5. Based on the Health Insurance Portability and Accountability Act (HIPAA), the Department of Health and Human Services issued guidelines in 1996 to protect the confidentiality of individually identifiable health information. The rule:

a. Limits the use and disclosure of certain individually identifiable health information.

b. Gives patients the right to access their medical records.

c. Restricts most disclosure of health information to the minimum needed for the intended purpose.

d. Establishes safeguards and restrictions regarding the use and disclosure of records for certain public responsibilities, such as public health, law enforcement, and research.

e. Provides for criminal or civil sanctions for improper uses or disclosures.

6. The exceptions or limits to confidentiality include situations in which society has judged that the need for information outweighs the principle of confidentiality. However, legal counsel should be consulted because these decisions are made on a case-by-case basis and broad generalizations cannot be assumed.

7. It may be appropriate to breach confidentiality on a limited basis in situations such as the following:

a. If a patient reveals intent to harm him- or herself or another individual, it is imperative to protect the patient and third parties from such harm.

b. A clinician employed by a company, school, military unit, or court has split allegiances, and the patient should be so advised at the appropriate time.

c. Court orders, subpoenas, and summonses in some states may require the clinician to release records for review or testify in court. However, legal counsel should be consulted first to ensure that complying with these orders does not violate HIPAA.

d. Most insurance companies, health maintenance organizations, and governmental payers require participants to sign a release of their records to the payers.

e. When a patient places his or her medical condition at issue, such as in personal injury cases, worker's compensation, or in various other cases of patients claiming injuries for which they are seeking compensation from any entity or organization.

f. Many states have laws requiring clinicians to report the incidence of certain diseases, deaths, and other vital statistics.

g. Criminal codes in many states require reporting gunshot wounds, incidents of rape, and incidents of child, spousal, or elder abuse if they have reasonable cause to suspect abuse.

Informed Consent

1. The doctrine of informed consent has become a fundamentally accepted principle governing the relationship between professional nurses and all other health care providers and patients.

2. Informed consent relates to the patient's right to accept or reject treatment by a nurse or any other health care provider and is a right of all legally competent adults or emancipated minors.

3. In the majority of circumstances, informed consent is obtained for medical or surgical procedures to be performed by physicians. Therefore, it is the duty of the physician to inform the patient of alternative treatments, the nature of the procedure, and benefits and potential risks. Oftentimes, especially when the patient is hospitalized, the nurse is required to witness the patient's signature before the procedure. It is prudent for the nurse to note witness to signature directly next to the patient's signature.

4. Emancipated minors are individuals who are under age 18 and married, are parents of their own children, or are self-sufficiently living away from the family domicile with parental consent.

5. In the case of a minor, informed consent would be obtained from the legal guardian.

6. In the case of individuals incapable of understanding medical treatment issues, informed consent must be obtained through a responsible person such as a guardian or surrogate.

7. The nurse has the duty to verify that the physician or other health care provider has explained each treatment or procedure in a language the patient (or the responsible person) can comprehend; has warned the patient of any material risks, dangers, or harms inherent in or collateral to the treatment; and has advised the patient of available alternatives. This enables the patient to make an intelligent and informed decision and choice about whether to undergo treatment.

8. The informed consent should be obtained before rendering the treatment or performance of the procedure. For more information on informed consent for patient's surgery, see Chapter 7, page 86.

9. The nurse must document that the informed consent was obtained and that the patient demonstrated understanding of the information.

10. A witness signature is desirable and may be required by some health care institutions.

 NURSING ALERT With the increasing cultural diversity of our patient population, it is prudent and ethically obligatory to obtain an interpreter for the patient if there is a reasonable chance that the patient will not understand explanations in the English language.

Scope of Practice, Licensure, and Certification

1. The professional nurse's scope of practice is defined and outlined by the State Board of Nursing that governs practice. The National Council of State Boards of Nursing and the NLN have developed standards that guide each State Board in the development of their licensure requirements and scope of practice rules.

2. Licensure is granted by an agency of state government and permits individuals accountable for the practice of professional nursing to engage in the practice of that profession while prohibiting all others from doing so legally.

3. Certification is provided by a nongovernmental association or agency and certifies that a person licensed to practice as a professional nurse has met certain predetermined standards described by that profession for specialty practice, thereby assuring the patient that a person has mastered a body of knowledge and acquired the skills in a particular specialty.

4. The mechanisms for achieving certification and maintaining a specialty certification vary by association and certifying body, such as a specified number of hours of clinical practice, continuing education, peer review, periodic self-assessment examination, or reexamination.

5. The American Nurses Credentialing Center is one certifying body that provides specialty certification (*www.nursecredentialing.org* or 800-284-2378). Credentialing protects the public by recognizing professional nurses who have successfully completed an approved course of study and achieved a level of specialized knowledge and skill to hold specialized positions.

Standards of Practice

General Principles

1. The practice of professional nursing has standards of practice setting minimum levels of acceptable performance for which its practitioners are accountable.
   a. The authority for the practice of nursing is based on a social contract that acknowledges rights and responsibilities, along with mechanisms for public accountability.
   b. These standards provide patients with a means of measuring the quality of care they receive.

2. Standards of practice were developed by the ANA and have been updated regularly to include general standards as well as standards for each nursing specialty. A copy can be purchased from the ANA publications office (*www.nursesbooks.org* or 800-637-0323).
   a. These standards describe what nursing is, what nurses do, and the responsibilities for which nurses are accountable.
   b. Professional nurses are to be guided by the generic standards applicable to all nurses in all areas of practice as well as by specialty area standards.

3. Various specialty groups have developed their own additional standards, but addressing these exceeds the scope of this chapter. The professional nurse needs to be familiar with all standards applicable to her or his own practice areas.

4. Standards and parameters also provide a source of legal protection for the practicing nurse.
   a. Standards and parameters typically consist of a simple, realistic series of steps that would be applicable given the same or similar clinical scenario.
   b. Standards and parameters should outline the minimum requirements for safe care and need to be updated as scientific knowledge changes.

5. A deviation from the protocol should be documented in the patient's chart with clear, concise statements of the nurse's decisions, actions, and reasons for the care provided, including any apparent deviation. This should be done at the time the care is rendered because passage of time may lead to a less than accurate recollection of the specific events.

6. Informal or volunteer practice must be consistent with the applicable standard of care. Documentation that the care rendered was the standard of practice within a community or state may afford the practitioner a degree of protection. Informal or volunteer care still needs to comply with the applicable standard of care.

Common Departures from the Standards of Nursing Care

Legal claims most commonly made against professional nurses include the following departures from appropriate care: failure to assess the patient properly or in a timely fashion, follow physician orders, follow appropriate nursing measures, communicate information about the patient, adhere to facility policy or procedure, document appropriate information in the medical record, administer medications as ordered, and follow physician's orders that should have been questioned or not followed, such as orders containing medication dosage errors (see Box 2-1).

BOX 2-1   Common Legal Claims for Departure from Standards of Care

- Failure to monitor or observe a patient's clinical status adequately
- Failure to monitor or observe a change in a patient's clinical status
- Failure to communicate or document a significant change in a patient's condition to appropriate professional
- Failure to obtain a complete nursing history
- Failure to formulate or follow the nursing care plan
- Failure to perform a nursing treatment or procedure properly
- Failure to provide a safe environment and to protect the patient from avoidable injury
- Failure to implement a physician's, advanced practice nurse's, or physician assistant's order properly or in a timely fashion
- Failure to administer medications properly and in a timely fashion or to report and administer omitted doses appropriately
- Failure to observe a medication's action or adverse effect
- Failure to prevent infection

- Failure to obtain help for a patient not receiving proper care from a physician or other health care provider
- Failure to report that a patient is not receiving proper care from a physician or other health care provider
- Failure to use equipment properly
- Failure to evaluate or identify a patient at high risk for falling or to plan and implement a fall prevention program appropriate to the individual patient
- Failure to apply restraints when indicated and ordered
- Failure to apply restraints in a proper manner
- Using equipment that is known to be defective
- Failure to make prompt, accurate entries in a patient's medical record
- Altering a medical record without noting it as a correction with signature, date, and time of change
- Failure to adhere to facility policy or procedural guidelines
- Following medical orders that should not have been followed such as medication dosage errors
- Failure to act as a patient advocate, such as not questioning illegible or incomplete medical orders or not questioning discharge when a patient's clinical status warrants

Quality Assurance and Adverse Event Reduction

1. A quality assurance program creates and implements a systematic, deliberate, and ongoing mechanism for the evaluation and monitoring of professional nursing practice aimed at performance improvement and adverse event reduction. Many facilities follow the National Database of Nursing Quality Indicators program, implemented by the ANA. It is a database that is updated regularly to track progress in providing quality care in certain areas, including pressure ulcers, falls, hospital-acquired infections, and restraint prevalence.
2. In 2007, the U.S. Centers for Medicare and Medicaid Services announced that Medicare would be ending payments to facilities for the increased costs attributable to preventable, facility-acquired conditions, including pressure ulcers, catheter-associated urinary tract infections, vascular catheter–associated infections, coronary artery bypass graft–related mediastinitis, and injuries such as dislocations and fractures. More recently, payment will be withheld for patients readmitted within 30 days after hospital discharge for conditions such as heart failure and acute myocardial infarction. More than ever before, nurses delivering care at the front lines are critical partners in promoting quality care, preventing adverse events, and saving avoidable expenditure of health care dollars.
3. Integral to the creation of such a proactive program are the following key factors:
   a. Create an atmosphere of interprofessional collegiality.
   b. Develop and implement the consistent application of new policies and procedures for quick, easy, and, if possible, anonymous error reporting, with protection from disciplinary action.
   c. Support employees involved in serious errors, adopting a nonpunitive attitude.
   d. Acknowledge the need for system-wide improvement and for centralization of information. Doing so ensures maximal benefit to the patients of health care and to all disciplines involved in the delivery of care.
   e. Introduce scientifically valid quality and safety solutions universally throughout the health care system, allowing for sharing of successful strategies and measures and reward systems.
   f. These actions would promote the delivery of high-quality care, a sense of responsibility and accountability, as well as ongoing self- and peer-auditing, thus yielding greater trending, analysis, problem-solving, and system-wide refinements.
4. Consequently, the use of a quality assurance program effectively reduces the professional nurse's exposure to liability, identifies educational needs, and improves the documentation of the care provided.
5. The components of quality assurance include the following:
   a. Structure—focuses on the organization of patient care.
   b. Process—focuses on tests ordered and procedures performed.
   c. Outcome—focuses on the outcome, such as absence of complications, timely discharge, patient satisfaction, or mortality data.
6. Mechanisms to incorporate in quality assurance programs may include the following:
   a. Patient satisfaction surveys to assess nurse interactions and maintain open lines of communication between the provider and the patient.
   b. Peer review to recognize and reward care delivered, raise the expectations for higher standards of practice within a community, and discourage practice beyond the scope of legal authority.
   c. Audit of clinical records to determine how well-established criteria were met by the care rendered.
   d. Utilization review to evaluate the extent to which services or resources were used as measured against a standard.

Management of Liability

1. The sources of legal risk in a professional nurse's practice include patient care, procedures performed, quality of documentation, violation of confidentiality, among others.
2. Liability can be minimized by the application of risk management systems and activities, which are designed to recognize and intervene to reduce the risk of injury to patients and subsequent claims against professional nurses.
3. Risk management systems and activities are based on the premise that many injuries to patients are preventable.

Malpractice

1. Nursing malpractice refers to a negligent act of a professional nurse engaged in the practice of that profession.
2. Although negligence embraces all negligent acts, malpractice is a specific term referring to negligent conduct in the rendering of professional services.
3. There is no guaranteed way to avoid a medical malpractice suit short of avoiding practicing as a professional nurse. Even the best nurses have been named as defendants.
4. A diligent and reflective nurse can reduce the risks of malpractice by consistently incorporating the following four elements into her or his practice:
   a. Excellent communication skills, with consistent efforts to elicit and address the expectations and requests of the patient.
   b. Sincere compassion for each patient.
   c. Competent practice.
   d. Accurate and complete charting with notations of any deviations from the applicable standard of care with the specific reasons (eg, the patient refused chest radiograph because of personal time constraint) and, if applicable, the patient's noncompliance.
5. Generally, the professional nurse has the duty to:
   a. Exercise a degree of diligence and skill that is ordinarily exercised by other professional nurses in the same state and specialty of practice.
   b. Apply such knowledge with reasonable care.
   c. Keep up to date and informed of approved standards of care in general use.
   d. Exercise best judgment in rendering care to the patient.
6. Some states apply a geographic standard, referred to as a locality rule, which asserts that providers in remote rural areas may have less access to continuing education and various technology and equipment than their colleagues in urban areas. However, because communication and transportation continue to improve rapidly, the locality rule is becoming obsolete.

Burden of Proof for Malpractice

The plaintiff has the burden of proving four elements of malpractice, usually by means of expert testimony.

Duty

1. The plaintiff has a burden to prove that a nurse–patient relationship did, in fact, exist and, by virtue of that relationship, the nurse had the duty to exercise reasonable care when undertaking and providing treatment to the patient.
2. Limits and obligations of duty include the following:
   a. This duty exists only when there is a nurse–patient relationship.
   b. The professional nurse is not obligated to enter into a nurse–patient relationship with any individual.
   c. Professional nurses generally have the right to decide to whom they will provide professional services and may request to be reassigned to another patient if the nurse–patient relationship is strained, the nurse feels unsafe, or the treatment plan is a gross violation of the nurse's ethical or religious values.
   d. Nurses have limits on their rights to decide; however, they cannot refuse to treat a patient who has relied reasonably on the nurse's apparent willingness to treat all in need (eg, the emergency department in a general facility that advertises its emergency services) and may not abandon an established patient.
   e. If a professional nurse wishes to terminate an established relationship with a patient, an alternative with an equivalent level of nursing services must be made available to the patient in a timely fashion.

 NURSING ALERT The professional nurse must use caution when offering telephone advice for which there is no charge; there have been reported cases of patients successfully suing providers because they reasonably relied on the telephone advice of a nurse that caused them to delay seeking care and sustain permanent injuries as a result.

Breach of Duty

1. The plaintiff has the burden to establish that the professional nurse violated the applicable standard of care in treating the patient's condition.
2. The plaintiff must establish by way of expert professional nurse testimony that the "negligent" nurse failed to conform to the applicable standard of care or provided nursing care that fell below the level of care that would have been provided by a prudent and diligent nurse under the same circumstances.

Proximate Cause

1. The plaintiff has the burden of establishing a causal relationship between the breach in the standard of care and the patient's injuries.
2. If a breach in standard of care did not cause the alleged injuries, there is no proximate cause.

Damages

The plaintiff has the burden of establishing the existence of damages to the patient as a result of malpractice.

Malpractice Insurance

1. Malpractice insurance will not protect the professional nurse from charges of practicing outside the scope of practice if he or she is practicing outside the legal scope of practice permitted within the state.
2. It is critical that the nurse know the exact scope of practice permitted in his or her jurisdiction.

3. It is universally recommended that all professional nurses carry their own liability insurance coverage. This affords one's own legal representation and an attorney who will be looking out solely for the nurse's best interests. Such coverage is recommended over and above the legal coverage and representation afforded by the employer's coverage.
4. Coverage should be by occurrence, rather than claims-made terms. Occurrence policies cover the nurse whenever the occurrence of the care took place, even if the nurse is no longer employed at that location or the policy is not active at the time the claim is made.

Telephone Triage, Advice, and Counseling

1. The use of telephone triage, advice, and counseling has become increasingly prevalent as health care providers have attempted to meet and satisfy the health care needs of their patients, increase access to care, and improve continuity of care while limiting scheduled appointments to those truly requiring a patient–physician or other health care provider interaction.
2. Health care professionals who provide telephone services must keep in mind that they are legally accountable for gathering an accurate and complete history, application of appropriate protocols for diagnostic impressions, appropriate consultation with other health care providers, advice and counseling given, and facilitation of timely and appropriate access to treatment facilities or referral to specialists to those in need.
3. Internet and other means of electronic communication are becoming acceptable but present concerns for privacy.
4. A number of legal concepts of relevance to telephone triage are outlined in the next section.

Confidentiality

Just as in face-to-face interactions, all information exchanged during a telephone interaction is privileged and is to be used only in the context of the advice being sought, with the sole purpose of providing the most appropriate and timely care needed by the patient.

Implied Relationships

Even if the professional nurse providing telephone advice has never had face-to-face interaction with the patient, the telephone interaction itself will establish a formal and legally binding nurse–patient relationship, for which the practitioner will be accountable legally.

Information Retrieval

1. The professional nurse has the duty to provide advice and counsel in the context of all medical data available to the practice from within the patient's medical record.
2. Therefore, a rapid method for the retrieval of medical record data should be established and integrated into the telephone component of all practices.
3. Telephone advice must not be provided in a vacuum of knowledge about the patient's past history.
4. Because limited time will usually preclude the gathering of all data available in the medical record, advice rendered without the benefit of all known medical history is more subject to error.

Respondeat Superior

1. Employers are held accountable, legally responsible, and liable for all inappropriate advice provided by their employees and all damages that may result.
2. Therefore, employers must be responsible for educating and training employees and updating protocols.

Vicarious Liability

1. Although similar to the concept of respondeat superior, vicarious liability is a broader concept in that a professional nurse providing telephone advice or counseling may be viewed as a representative of the facility physician, practice group, or facility, thereby binding them legally for all acts of omission or commission and damages that result.
2. Thus, if telephone advice and counsel are rendered by an LPN, RN, or unlicensed personnel, the nurse, health care facility, or physicians in the practice may be viewed by a court as vicariously liable for inappropriate advice provided and all resulting damages to the patient.
3. This underscores the reasons for limiting this practice to well-trained nurses, physicians, and other health care providers and following carefully devised office protocols and standards.
4. The professional nurse must be encouraged to consult briefly with the in-office physician or other health care providers to reduce the possibility of advice that is not appropriate or is in error.

Negligent Supervisor

1. This concept relates to the failure of a supervising physician or other health care provider to provide the needed guidance and direction to the telephone advice nurse, despite a prevailing understanding, practice, or policy obligating this supervision.
2. This scenario usually overlaps with respondeat superior or vicarious liability.

Negligence

1. Any telephone assessment and advice rendered must be in accordance with the generally accepted standards and protocols.
2. Violation of the applicable standards of practice or care is considered to be negligent.
3. Evidence of standards of care is established by:
   a. Publications on the topic.
   b. Community practices.
   c. Generally accepted professional and evidence-based guidelines or treatises on the topic.

Abandonment

1. This concept becomes operational when a patient calls or comes in to report symptoms, seek advice, or request an on-site evaluation or treatment, and this communication is documented or otherwise established as fact, but the telephone advice nurse fails to follow through with the professional component of the interaction (advice).
2. However, unless an undesirable outcome with serious and permanent damages occurs due to the absence of follow-through by the telephone practitioner, it is doubtful that a legal claim could be brought successfully against the practitioner.

Successful Telephone Practice

1. Policies aimed at minimizing the risk of an untoward outcome resulting from telephone advice, triage, and counseling should be established in every practice.
2. Policies should include protocol use, telephone practitioner training and education, use of an established patient database, communication with a physician or other health care provider, and appropriate documentation of interaction.
3. See Box 2-2 for components of a successful telephone advice practice.

BOX 2-2 Components of Successful Telephone Practice

- Apply standardized protocols and guidelines for the most frequently reported chief complaints.
- Train nurses in proper history taking, protocol or guideline utilization, and documentation.
- Apply a computer-based approach to manage the telephone encounters to complement existing protocols and guidelines to improve the process and documentation of the encounter.
- Implement a quality assurance system to ensure a regular review of telephone logs.
- Discuss problem cases with telephone advice nurses and perform outcome surveys.
- Maintain a constant availability of physicians and other health care providers to provide consultative assistance to the telephone advice nurse as needed.
- Ensure an ongoing review and revision of protocols and policies to eliminate or improve on problematic policies and protocols.
- Schedule patients with serious problems as soon as possible.
- Ask and confirm that the patient understands and feels comfortable with the plan at the end of the telephone interaction.
- Invite the patient for an after-hours visit if he or she is uncomfortable with receiving home care instructions or with waiting until the next day to see the physician or other health care provider.
- Encourage patients to call back if their condition worsens or if they have additional questions.
- Advise patients to contact their health care provider the next day if the problem has not improved.
- Document succinctly the components of the telephone interaction, including the chief complaint, history of present illness, past medical history, allergies, home care or other instructions given, confirmation of the patient's understanding and comfort with the advice given, emergency precautions provided, and follow-up plans.

4. The telephone advice nurse must gather and document certain fundamental information from the patient seeking health care advice or treatment. Although the following list is presented, it is not intended to limit inquiry or imply that the list is exhaustive. The inquiry and documentation must minimally include the following:

    a. Date and time of the call.
    b. Caller information including the name of the patient, relationship to the patient, telephone number with area code, when and where the caller may be reached for return calls, and alternative telephone numbers with area code for backup.
    c. Chief complaint.
    d. History of present illness, with brief description of onset, symptoms, treatment used to date, effectiveness or lack thereof of measures attempted, and aggravating or alleviating factors.
    e. Whether the patient has had this problem before and, if so, when, diagnosis, and method of resolution.
    f. If female, last menstrual period, method of birth control, and follow-up to rule out pregnancy.
    g. Past medical history and other medical problems.
    h. Allergies.
    i. Likely differential diagnosis based on the established protocols and guidelines being utilized by the organization or facility.
    j. Impact of the problem on the caller or patient.
    k. Accessibility of alternative sources of health care.
    l. Nurse's perception of the patient's vulnerability.
    m. Nurse's perception of the patient's understanding and comfort with the plan of care and follow-up plans.

SELECTED REFERENCES

American Nurses Association. (2015). *Code of ethics for nurses with interpretive statements (code for nurses)*. Silver Spring, MD: Author.

American Nurses Association. (2016). *Nursing scope and standards of practice*. Available: *http://nursingworld.org/sop*

Baker, J. (2017). Nursing research, quality improvement and evidence based practice. *AORN Journal, 105*(1), 3–5.

Balestra, M. (2017). Electronic health records: Patient care and ethical and legal implications for nurse practitioners. *The Journal for Nurse Practitioners, 13*(2), 105–111.

Centers for Medicare and Medicaid Services. (2016). *Outcome measures*. Available: *www.cms.gov/Medicare/Quality-Initiatives-Patient-Assessment-Instruments/HospitalQualityInits/OutcomeMeasures.html*

Cohen, L. T., Millock, P. J., Asheld, B., & Lane, B. (2015). Are employers responsible for an employee's unauthorized review of a patient's confidential health information? *Journal of the American College of Radiology, 12*(4), 412–414.

Farmer, L., & Lundy, A. (2017). Informed consent: Ethical and legal considerations for advanced practice nurses. *The Journal for Nurse Practitioners, 13*(2), 124–130.

Gallup (2017). Honesty/Ethics in Professions. Retrieved *http://news.gallup.com/poll/1654/honesty-ethics-professions.aspx*

Gerard, L., Boyle, D., Simon, M., Dunton, N., & Gajewski, B. (2016). Reliability and validity of the NDNQI injury falls measure. *Western Journal of Nursing Research, 38*(1), 111–128.

Institute of Medicine. (2011). *Health IT and patient safety: Building safer systems for better care*. Washington, DC: Author.

Landry, J. (2017). Delivering culturally sensitive care to LGBTQI patients. *The Journal for Nurse Practitioners, 13*(5), 342–347.

Lo, Bernard (2013). *Resolving ethical dilemmas: A guide for clinicians* (5th ed.). New York, NY: Lippincott Williams & Wilkins.

Moffat-Bruce, S., Ferdinand, F., & Finn, J. (2016). Patient safety: Disclosure of medical errors and risk mitigation. *Annals of Thoracic Surgery, 102*, 358–362.

National Council of State Boards of Nursing. (2016). *Nurse practice act, rules and regulation*. Author. Available: *www.ncsbn.org/nurse-practice-act.htm*

National League of Nursing. (2018). *http://www.nln.org/professional-development-programs/competencies-for-nursing-education*

National League of Nursing. (2012). *Outcomes and competencies for graduates of practical/vocational, diploma, baccalaureate, master's, practice doctorate and research*. New York, NY: Wolters Kluwer.

Press Ganey. (2016). Nursing quality (NNDQI). Available: *www.pressganey.com/solutions/clinical-quality/nursing-quality*

Teitelbaum, J., & Wilensky, S. (2017). *Essentials of health policy and law* (3rd ed.). Burlington, MA: Jones & Bartlett Learning, LLC.

Westrick, S. J., & Jacob, N. (2016). Disclosure of errors and apology: Law an ethics. *Journal for Nurse Practitioners, 12*(2), 120–126.

3

Health Promotion and Preventive Care

CONCEPTS IN PROMOTION AND PREVENTION

 See additional online content: Patient Education Guidelines 3-1–3-4.

Principles of Health Promotion

Health promotion is defined as the actions taken to develop a high level of wellness and is accomplished by influencing individual behavior and the environment in which people live.

Levels of Prevention

1. Disease prevention is aimed at avoiding problems or minimizing problems once they occur.
   a. Primary prevention is the total prevention of a condition.
   b. Secondary prevention is the early recognition of a condition and the measures taken to speed recovery.
   c. Tertiary prevention is the care given to minimize the effects of the condition and prevent long-term complications.
2. Preventive care should involve assessment for people at risk for specific disorders.

Healthy People 2020

 EVIDENCE BASE Office of Disease Prevention and Health Promotion, USDHHS. (2018). Healthy People 2020. Available: *www.healthypeople.gov*. Updated February 5, 2018.

1. Health promotion goes beyond prevention to help people manage their health and live longer and feel better.
2. Health promotion has become a priority since the U.S. Department of Health and Human Services (DHHS) initiated its Healthy People 2000 campaign in 1990.
3. For the Healthy People 2010 campaign, launched in 2000, 23% of the campaign's stated objectives were reached or exceeded, whereas 48% of the stated objectives were approached. The two major goals of Healthy People 2010 were to enhance life expectancy while improving quality of life and to reduce health disparities due to gender, race and ethnicity, income and education, disabilities, and other factors.

4. Healthy People 2020 consists of 42 topic areas with 1,200 objectives. Leading health indicators (LHIs) were chosen as a subset of objectives indicating priority health issues (see Box 3-1, page 21). At midcourse review, 4 (15.4%) LHIs had met or exceeded their target and 10 (38.5%) showed improvement.
5. The framework for Healthy People 2030 has been developed with the vision: A society in which all people achieve their full potential for health and well-being across the lifespan.

Nursing Role in Health Promotion

1. Nurses have played key roles in prevention in such areas as prenatal care, immunization programs, occupational health and safety, cardiac rehabilitation and education, and public health care and early intervention.
2. Nurses in all settings can meet health promotion needs of patients, whether their practice is in a hospital, a clinic, a patient's home, a health maintenance organization, a private office, or a community setting. Health promotion is primarily accomplished through patient education, an independent function of nursing.
3. Health promotion should occur through the life cycle, with topics focused on infancy, childhood, adolescence, adulthood, and older adults. Specific preventive services are evidence based and recommended by the United States Preventive Services Task Force (USPSTF) (*www.ahrq.gov/clinic/prevenix. htm*), the Canadian Task Force on Preventive Health Care (*www.canadiantaskforce.ca/index.html*), the National Institute for Health and Clinical Excellence (*www.nice.org.uk*) in the United Kingdom, as well as other agencies (see Table 3-1).
   a. For infancy, teach parents about the importance of prenatal care, basic care of infants, breast-feeding, nutrition, and infant safety (see Chapter 42).
   b. For childhood, stress the importance of immunizations, proper nutrition to enhance growth and development, and safety practices, such as use of car seats and seat belts, fire prevention, and poison-proofing the home (see Chapter 42).
   c. For adolescence, focus on motor vehicle safety; avoidance of drug, alcohol, and tobacco use; sexual decision making and contraception; and prevention of suicide.
   d. For adulthood, teach patients about nutrition, exercise, and stress management to help them feel better; also teach

BOX 3-1	Healthy People 2020 Leading Health Indicators

- Persons with medical insurance
- Persons with a usual primary care provider
- Adults receiving colorectal cancer screening
- Adults with hypertension whose blood pressure (BP) is under control
- Persons with diagnosed diabetes with A1c > 9%
- Children receiving the recommended doses of vaccines
- Air Quality Index > 100
- Children exposed to secondhand smoke
- Injury deaths
- Homicides
- All infant deaths
- Total preterm live births
- Suicide
- Adolescents with a major depressive episode
- Adults meeting aerobic physical activity and muscle-strengthening requirements
- Obesity among adults
- Obesity among children and adolescents
- Mean daily intake of total vegetables
- Children, adolescents, and adults who visited the dentist
- Sexually active females receiving reproductive health services
- Knowledge of serostatus among human immunodeficiency virus (HIV)-positive persons
- Students graduating from high school 4 years after starting
- Adolescents using alcohol or illicit drugs
- Adult binge drinking
- Adult cigarette smoking
- Adolescent cigarette smoking

cancer-screening techniques, such as breast and testicular self-examination, and risk factor reduction for the leading causes of death—heart disease, stroke, cancer, and chronic lung disease.

e. For older adults, stress the topics of nutrition and exercise to help people live longer and stay fit, safety measures to help them compensate for decreasing mobility and sensory function, and ways to stay active and independent (see Chapter 9).

Theories of Behavior Change

Lifestyle changes that promote wellness and reduce or prevent illness are often difficult to accomplish. Although education and support by nurses are key, lifestyle changes are ultimately up to the patient. Nurses should understand the concepts and processes related to behavior change to help direct interventions for successful outcomes in individual patients or groups.

Health Belief Model

The health belief model identifies perceptions that influence an individual's behavior. Nurses can inquire about a patient's perceptions in three areas to individualize education and interventions.

1. The first perception is susceptibility to and seriousness of disease or threat of illness. This most directly influences whether a person will take action.
2. The perceived benefit of taking action also affects behavior change.
3. Any perceived barriers to change may prevent or impede action.

Transtheoretical Model

The transtheoretical model of behavior change developed by Prochaska and DiClemente identifies six predictable stages of change. The stages may cycle back and forth several times before

Table 3-1	Preventive Services Recommended by the USPSTF

The USPSTF recommends that clinicians discuss these preventive services with eligible patients and offer them as a priority. All these services have received an "A" (strongly recommended) or "B" (recommended) grade from the Task Force.

RECOMMENDATION	MEN	WOMEN	PREGNANT WOMEN	CHILDREN
Abdominal aortic aneurysm, screening (1)	✓			
Alcohol misuse screening and behavioral counseling interventions	✓	✓	✓	
Aspirin for the primary prevention of cardiovascular events (2)	✓	✓		
Asymptomatic bacteriuria in adults, screening (3)			✓	
BRCA-related cancer in women, screening (4)		✓		
Breast cancer, preventive medications (5)		✓		
Breast cancer, screening (6)		✓		
Breast-feeding, counseling (7)		✓	✓	
Cervical cancer, screening (8)		✓		
Chlamydial infection, screening (9)		✓	✓	
Colorectal cancer, screening (10)	✓	✓		
Congenital hypothyroidism, screening (11)				✓
Depression (adults), screening (12)	✓	✓		
Falls in older adults (13)	✓	✓		
Folic acid supplementation (14)		✓		
Gestational diabetes mellitus, screening (15)			✓	
Gonococcal ophthalmia, prophylactic medication (16)				✓
Gonorrhea, screening (17)		✓		
Hearing loss in newborns, screening (18)				✓
Hepatitis B virus in pregnant women, screening (19)			✓	
Hepatitis C virus in adults, screening (20)	✓	✓	✓	✓
High blood pressure in adults, screening	✓	✓		

(continued)

Table 3-1 Preventive Services Recommended by the USPSTF (*Continued*)

RECOMMENDATION	MEN	WOMEN	PREGNANT WOMEN	CHILDREN
Human immunodeficiency virus (HIV), screening (21,22)	✓	✓	✓	✓
Iron deficiency anemia, prevention (23)				✓
Iron deficiency anemia, screening (24)			✓	
Lipid disorders in adults, screening (25)	✓	✓		
Lung cancer, screening (26)	✓	✓		
Major depressive disorder in children and adolescents, screening (27)				✓
Obesity in adults, screening (28)	✓	✓		
Obesity in children and adolescents, screening (29)				✓
Osteoporosis, screening (30)		✓		
Phenylketonuria, screening (31)				✓
Sexually transmitted infections, counseling (32)	✓	✓		
Sickle cell disease in newborns, screening (33)				✓
Skin cancer, counseling (34)	✓	✓	✓	✓
Syphilis infection in pregnant women, screening			✓	
Tobacco use in adults (35)	✓	✓	✓	
Tobacco use in children and adolescents (36)				✓
Visual impairment in children, screening (37)				✓

1. *One-time screening by ultrasonography in men aged 65 to 75 who have ever smoked.*
2. *When the potential harm of an increase in gastrointestinal hemorrhage is outweighed by a potential benefit of a reduction in myocardial infarctions (men aged 45 to 79 years) or in ischemic strokes (women aged 55 to 79 years).*
3. *Pregnant women at 12 to 16 weeks' gestation or at first prenatal visit, if later.*
4. *Refer women whose family history is associated with an increased risk for deleterious mutations in BRCA1 or BRCA2 genes for genetic counseling and evaluation for BRCA testing.*
5. *Engage in shared, informed decision making and offer to prescribe risk-reducing medications, if appropriate, to women aged ≥35 years without prior breast cancer diagnosis who are at increased risk.*
6. *Biennial screening mammography for women aged 50 to 74 years. Note: The Department of Health and Human Services, in implementing the Affordable Care Act, follows the 2002 USPSTF recommendation for screening mammography, with or without clinical breast examination, every 1 to 2 years for women aged 40 and older.*
7. *Interventions during pregnancy and after birth to promote and support breast-feeding.*
8. *Screen with cytology every 3 years (women aged 21 to 65) or co-test (cytology/HPV testing) every 5 years (women aged 30 to 65).*
9. *Sexually active women aged 24 or younger and other asymptomatic women at increased risk for infection. Asymptomatic pregnant women aged 24 and or younger and others at increased risk.*
10. *Adults aged 50 to 75 using fecal occult blood testing, sigmoidoscopy, or colonoscopy.*
11. *Newborns.*
12. *When staff-assisted depression care supports are in place to assure accurate diagnosis, effective treatment, and follow-up.*
13. *Provide intervention (exercise or physical therapy and/or vitamin D supplementation) to community-dwelling adults ≥65 years at increased risk for falls.*
14. *All women planning or capable of pregnancy take a daily supplement containing 0.4 to 0.8 mg (400 to 800 mcg) of folic acid.*
15. *Asymptomatic pregnant women after 24 weeks of gestation.*
16. *Newborns.*
17. *Sexually active women, including pregnant women aged 25 and younger, or at increased risk for infection.*
18. *Newborns.*
19. *Screen at first prenatal visit.*
20. *Persons at high risk for infection and adults born between 1945 and 1965.*
21. *All adolescents and adults aged 15 to 65 years and others who are at increased risk for HIV infection and all pregnant women.*
22. *Asymptomatic women of childbearing age; provide or refer women who screen positive to intervention services.*
23. *Routine iron supplementation for asymptomatic children aged 6 to 12 months who are at increased risk for iron deficiency anemia.*
24. *Routine screening in asymptomatic pregnant women.*
25. *Men aged 20 to 35 and women over age 20 who are at increased risk for coronary heart disease; all men aged 35 and older.*
26. *Asymptomatic adults aged 55 to 80 years who have a 30-pack-year smoking history and currently smoke or have quit smoking within the past 15 years.*
27. *Adolescents (aged 12 to 18) when systems are in place to ensure accurate diagnosis, psychotherapy, and follow-up.*
28. *Patients with a body mass index of 30 kg/m² or higher should be offered or referred to intensive, multicomponent behavioral interventions.*
29. *Screen children aged 6 years and older; offer or refer for intensive counseling and behavioral interventions.*
30. *Women aged 65 years and older and women under age 65 whose 10-year fracture risk is equal to or greater than that of a 65-year-old white woman without additional risk factors.*
31. *Newborns.*
32. *All sexually active adolescents and adults at increased risk for STIs.*
33. *Newborns.*
34. *Children, adolescents, and young adults aged 10 to 24 years.*
35. *Ask all adults about tobacco use and provide tobacco cessation interventions for those who use tobacco; provide augmented, pregnancy-tailored counseling for those pregnant women who smoke.*
36. *Provide interventions to prevent initiation of tobacco use in school-aged children and adolescents.*
37. *Screen children aged 3 to 5 years.*

Agency for Healthcare Research and Quality. (2014). The guide to clinical preventive services, 2014: Recommendations of the US Preventive Services Task Force. Author. Available: www.uspreventiveservicestaskforce.org/Page/Name/tools-and-resources-for-better-preventive-care.

change is complete. Education and interventions can be aimed at moving the patient onto the next stage or back into the cycle if a lapse occurs.

1. Precontemplation—no intention to change; may deny that there is a problem; may blame others for any problems.
2. Contemplation—acknowledgment that there is a problem; willing to change but may be ambivalent or anxious about change.
3. Preparation—explores options; actively plans to change; may go public with intent.
4. Action—overtly making a change; substituting desired behavior for old behavior.
5. Maintenance—continuing the change; may devalue old behavior; lapse may occur.
6. Termination—takes on a new self-image; old behavior is no longer a threat.

Patient Teaching and Health Education

Health education is included in the American Nurses Association Standards of Care and is defined as an essential component of nursing care. It is directed toward promotion, maintenance, and restoration of health and toward adaptation to the residual effects of illness.

Learning Readiness

1. Assist the patient in physical readiness to learn by trying to alleviate physical distress that may distract the patient's attention and prevent effective learning.
2. Assess and promote the patient's emotional readiness to learn.
   a. Motivation to learn depends on acceptance of the illness or that illness is a threat, recognition of the need to learn, values related to social and cultural background, and a therapeutic regimen compatible with the patient's lifestyle.
   b. Promote motivation to learn by creating a warm, accepting, positive atmosphere; encouraging the patient to participate in the establishment of acceptable, realistic, and attainable learning goals; and providing constructive feedback about progress.
3. Assess and promote the patient's experiential readiness to learn.
   a. Determine what experiences the patient has had with health and illness, what success or failure the patient has had with learning, and what basic knowledge the patient has on related topics.
   b. Provide the patient with prerequisite knowledge necessary to begin the learning process.

Teaching Strategies

1. Patient education can occur at any time and in any setting; however, you must consider how conducive the environment is to learning, how much time you are able to schedule, and what other family members can attend the teaching session.
2. Use a variety of techniques that are appropriate to meet the needs of each individual.
   a. Lecture or explanation should include discussion or a question-and-answer session.
   b. Group discussion is effective for individuals with similar needs; participants commonly gain support, assistance, and encouragement from other members.
   c. Demonstration and practice should be used when skills need to be learned; ample time should be allowed for practice and return demonstration.
   d. Teaching aids include books, pamphlets, pictures, slides, videos, tapes, and models and should serve as supplements to verbal teaching. These can be obtained from government agencies, such as the Department of Health and Human Services, the Centers for Disease Control and Prevention, and the National Institutes of Health; nonprofit groups, such as the American Heart Association or the March of Dimes; various Internet health Web sites; or pharmaceutical and insurance companies.
   e. Reinforcement and follow-up sessions offer time for evaluation and additional teaching, if necessary, and can greatly increase the effectiveness of teaching.
3. Document patient teaching, including what was taught and how the patient responded; use standardized patient teaching checklists if available.

Health Literacy

1. Health literacy is the ability to read, understand, and act on health information.
2. Health literacy goes beyond ability to read; it encompasses the following processes:
   a. Being able to follow instructions on prescription bottles.
   b. Understanding follow-up and referral appointment information.
   c. Understanding consent forms.
   d. Reading and understanding informational brochures and other instructions.
   e. Being able to negotiate the complex health care system.
3. According to the Institute of Medicine's report "A Prescription to End Confusion," poor health literacy is a stronger predictor of a person's health than age, income, employment status, education level, or race.
4. Vulnerable groups include people over 65 years of age, minorities and immigrants, low-income populations, and people with chronic mental and physical conditions.
5. The majority of Americans read at an eighth-grade level, and 20% read at a fifth-grade level or below. Most health-related materials are written at a 10th-grade reading level.
6. Clear communication between patients and health care professionals is critical. Nurses can assess patient literacy skills, use level-appropriate language and written materials, and help patients ask the right questions. The Ask Me 3 program, designed by the Partnership for Clear Health Communication, encourages patients to ask and understand the answers to the following questions:
   a. What is my main problem?
   b. What do I need to do?
   c. Why is it important for me to do this?

Selected Areas of Health Promotion

Counsel patients about proper nutrition, smoking cessation, physical activity, relaxation, and sexual health to promote well-being.

Nutrition and Diet

 EVIDENCE BASE U.S. Department of Health and Human Services and U.S. Department of Agriculture. (December 2015). 2015–2020 Dietary Guidelines for Americans (8th ed.). Available: *http://health.gov/ dietaryguidelines/2015/guidelines.*

1. Poor diet and sedentary lifestyle are linked to cardiovascular disease, type 2 diabetes, hypertension, osteoporosis, and some cancers.
2. The U.S. DHHS and the U.S. Department of Agriculture recommend and update dietary guidelines every 5 years. These guidelines, combined with physical activity, should enhance the health of most individuals. For more information on these guidelines, see *www.dietaryguidelines.gov.*
3. The 2015–2020 guidelines recommend a healthy eating pattern that accounts for all foods and beverages within an appropriate calorie level.
4. A healthy eating pattern includes the following:
   a. A variety of vegetables from all subgroups—dark green, red and orange, legumes (beans and peas), starchy, and other.
   b. Fruits, especially whole fruits.
   c. Grains, at least half of which are whole grains.
   d. Fat-free or low-fat dairy, including milk, yogurt, cheese, and/or fortified soy beverages.
   e. A variety of protein foods, including seafood, lean meats and poultry, eggs, legumes (beans and peas), and nuts, seeds, and soy products.
   f. Oils.
5. A healthy eating pattern limits the following:
   a. Consume less than 10% of calories per day from added sugars.
   b. Consume less than 10% of calories per day from saturated fats.
   c. Consume less than 2,300 milligrams (mg) per day of sodium.
   d. If alcohol is consumed, it should be consumed in moderation—up to one drink per day for women and up to two drinks per day for men—and only by adults of legal drinking age.
6. Children and adults of all ages should also meet physical activity guidelines to maintain healthy body weight and reduce the risk of chronic disease.
7. Educate patients about the five basic food groups, optimum weight, calorie requirements, and ways to increase fiber and decrease fat in the diet.
8. Teach patients to add fiber to the diet by choosing whole-grain breads and cereals; raw or minimally cooked fruits and vegetables (especially citrus fruits, squash, cabbage, lettuce and other greens, beans); and any nuts, skins, and seeds. Fiber can also be increased by adding several teaspoons of whole bran to meals each day or taking an over-the-counter fiber supplement, such as psyllium, as directed.
9. Encourage patients to keep food diaries and review them periodically to determine if other adjustments should be made.
10. If weight loss is desired, have the patient weigh in monthly, and review the diet and give praise or corrective advice at this visit. Many people, especially women, respond to group therapy that focuses on education, support, and expression of feelings related to overeating.

NURSING ALERT Encourage all patients to follow up closely with their health care providers if they are following any type of diet. Any diet that is unbalanced may require vitamin supplementation and alter biochemical processes such as cholesterol metabolism and fluid balance.

Smoking Prevention and Cessation

 EVIDENCE BASE PDQ® Screening and Prevention Editorial Board. (2017). *PDQ Cigarette Smoking.* Bethesda, MD: National Cancer Institute. Available: *www.cancer.gov/about-cancer/causes-prevention/risk/ tobacco/quit-smoking-hp-pdq. Updated April 27, 2017.*

1. Smoking is the leading cause of preventable deaths in the United States, with 480,000 deaths per year and many more living with a smoking-related illness such as cancer, heart disease, peripheral vascular disease, or chronic obstructive pulmonary disease (COPD).
2. Not smoking promotes health by increasing exercise tolerance, enhancing taste bud function, and avoiding facial wrinkles and bad breath. A 15% reduction all-cause mortality is seen in heavy smokers subjected to intensive clinical cessation interventions.
3. Smoking prevention education should begin during childhood and be stressed during adolescence, a time when peer modeling and confusion over self-image may lead to smoking.
4. Smoking cessation can be accomplished through an individualized, multidimensional program that includes the following:
   a. Information on the short- and long-term smoking effects.
   b. Behavioral therapy including practical behavior-modification techniques to help break the habit—gum chewing, snacking on carrot and celery sticks, or sucking on mints and hard candy to provide oral stimulation; working modeling clay, knitting, or other ways to provide tactile stimulation; avoiding coffee shops, bars, or other situations that smokers frequent; delaying each cigarette and recording each cigarette in a log before it is smoked; and incentive plans such as saving money for each cigarette not smoked and rewarding oneself when a goal is reached.
   c. Use of medications designed to reduce physical dependence and minimize withdrawal symptoms, including a long- (patch) or short-acting (gum, lozenge, inhaler or nasal spray) nicotine replacement product, varenicline, bupropion, or a combination of products. Nortriptyline and clonidine may also be prescribed.
   d. Use of support groups, frequent reinforcement, and follow-up. Encourage additional attempts if relapse occurs.
   e. There is not sufficient evidence to recommend the e-cigarette, hypnosis, acupuncture, or other alternative techniques.
5. Although the benefits of quitting are greater the earlier one quits, it is never too late to quit. Even quitting after the diagnosis of cancer improves prognosis and reduces the risk of a second cancer.
6. Many resources are available. For more information, call 1-800-QUIT-NOW or see *www.CDC.gov/tobacco.*

Exercise and Fitness

1. Regular exercise as part of a fitness program helps achieve optimal weight, control BP, increase high-density lipoprotein, lower risk of coronary artery disease, increase endurance, and improve the sense of well-being.
2. Long-term goals of regular exercise include decreased absenteeism from work, improved balance and reduced disability among older adults, decreased osteoporosis and fracture risk, and reduced health care costs.
3. Most health benefits occur with at least 150 minutes of physical activity a week, or 30 minutes of moderate-intensity

physical activity (in addition to usual activity) most days of the week. Greater benefits can be obtained by increasing intensity and duration of activity.

   a. Children and adolescents should do 60 minutes of physical activity daily that is age appropriate and includes aerobic, muscle-strengthening, and bone-strengthening activities.

   b. For additional health benefits such as managing or losing weight, adults should increase their aerobic activity to 300 minutes (5 hours) of moderate-intensity or 150 minutes (2.5 hours) of vigorous-intensity aerobic activity weekly.

   c. Muscle-strengthening activities that involve all major muscle groups two or more days a week provide additional benefits.

   d. Older adults and those with disabilities should engage in physical activities as their conditions allow. Generally the benefits of physical activity outweigh potential risks.

4. Suggest walking, jogging, bicycling, swimming, water aerobics, and low-impact aerobic dancing as good low- to moderate-intensity exercise, performed three to five times per week for 45 minutes. Walking can be done safely and comfortably by most patients if the pace is adjusted to the individual's physical condition. Use of weights is important for muscle strengthening throughout the life span.

   a. Exercise programs should include 5- to 10-minute warm-up and cool-down periods with stretching activities to prevent injuries.

   b. Full intensity and duration of exercise should be increased gradually over a period of several weeks to months.

5. Advise patients to stop if pain, shortness of breath, dizziness, palpitations, or excessive sweating is experienced.

6. Advise patients with cardiovascular, respiratory, and musculoskeletal disorders to check with their health care provider about specific guidelines or limitations for exercise.

 GERONTOLOGIC ALERT Older adults who are at risk for falling should do exercise that maintains or improves balance.

 NURSING ALERT Severe cases of COPD, osteoarthritis, or coronary disease are contraindications for unsupervised exercise; check with the patient's health care provider to see if a physical therapy or occupational therapy referral would be helpful.

Relaxation and Stress Management

1. *Stress* is a change in the environment that is perceived as a threat, challenge, or harm to the person's dynamic equilibrium. In times of stress, the sympathetic nervous system is activated to produce immediate changes of increased heart rate, peripheral vasoconstriction, and increased BP. This response is prolonged by adrenal stimulation and secretion of epinephrine and norepinephrine and is known as the "fight-or-flight" reaction.

2. A limited amount of stress can be a positive motivator to take action; however, excessive or prolonged stress can cause emotional discomfort, anxiety, possible panic, and illness.

3. Prolonged sympathetic–adrenal stimulation may lead to high BP, arteriosclerotic changes, and cardiovascular disease; stress has also been implicated in acute asthma attack, peptic ulcer disease, irritable bowel syndrome, migraine headaches, and other illnesses.

4. Stress management can help patients control illnesses, improve self-esteem, gain control, and enjoy life more fully.

5. Stress management involves the identification of physiologic and psychosocial stressors through assessment of the patient's education, finances, job, family, habits, activities, personal and family health history, and responsibilities. Positive and negative coping methods should also be identified.

6. Relaxation therapy is one of the first steps in stress management; it can be used to reduce anxiety brought on by stress. Relaxation techniques include the following:

   a. Relaxation breathing—the simplest technique that can be performed at any time. The patient breathes slowly and deeply until relaxation is achieved; however, this can lead to hyperventilation if done incorrectly.

   b. Progressive muscle relaxation—relieves muscle tension related to stress. The patient alternately tenses and then relaxes muscle groups until the entire body feels relaxed.

   c. Autogenic training—can help relieve pain and induce sleep. The patient replaces painful or unpleasant sensations with pleasant ones through self-suggestions; may require extensive coaching at first.

   d. Imagery—uses imagination and concentration to take a "mental vacation." The patient imagines a peaceful, pleasant scene involving multiple senses. It can last as long as the patient chooses.

   e. Distraction—uses the patient's own interests and activities to divert attention from pain or anxiety and includes listening to music, watching television, reading, singing, knitting, coloring, doing crafts or projects, or physical activities.

7. To assist patients with relaxation therapy, follow these steps:

   a. Review the techniques and encourage a trial with several techniques of the patient's choice.

   b. Teach the chosen technique and coach the patient until effective use of the technique is demonstrated.

   c. Suggest that the patient practice relaxation techniques for 20 minutes per day to feel more relaxed and to be prepared to use them confidently when stress increases.

   d. Encourage the patient to combine techniques such as relaxation breathing before and after imagery or progressive muscle relaxation along with autogenic training to achieve better results.

8. Additional steps in stress management include dealing with the stressors or problem areas and increasing coping behaviors.

   a. Help the patient to recognize specific stressors and determine if they can be altered. Then develop a plan for managing that stressor, such as changing jobs, postponing an extra class, hiring a babysitter once per week, talking to the neighbor about a problem, or getting up 1 hour earlier to exercise.

   b. Teach the patient to avoid negative coping behaviors, such as smoking, drinking, using drugs, overeating, cursing, and using abusive behavior toward others. Teach positive coping mechanisms, such as continued use of relaxation techniques and fostering of support systems—family, friends, church groups, social groups, or professional support groups.

Sexual Health

1. Because sexuality is inherent to every person and sexual functioning is a basic physiologic need of human beings, nurses can help patients gain knowledge, validate normalcy, prepare

for changes in sexuality throughout the life cycle, and prevent harm gained through sexual activity.

2. Education about sexuality should begin with school-age children, increase during adolescence, and continue through adulthood.

3. Topics to cover include the following:
   a. Relationships, responsibilities, communication.
   b. Normal reproduction—the menstrual cycle, ovulation, fertilization, sperm production.
   c. Prevention of unwanted pregnancy (approximately 1 million teen pregnancies occur in the United States each year) and sexually transmitted diseases (STDs).

4. The Centers for Disease Control and Prevention estimates that there are approximately 19 million new STD infections each year, which cost the U.S. health care system $16.4 billion annually and cost individuals even more in terms of acute and long-term health consequences.
   a. The number of cases of gonorrhea is declining and the number of cases of chlamydia is increasing (probably due to increased screening), but still only about half of people at risk for STDs are screened.
   b. Chlamydia, gonorrhea, and syphilis are reportable to state and local health departments; however, other STDs such as human papillomavirus (HPV) and herpes simplex virus are prevalent and cause chronic effects. Complications of STDs include pelvic inflammatory disease, infertility, serious vital organ damage in the case of tertiary syphilis, cervical cancer in the case of HPV, and increased risk of contracting HIV.
   c. Nurses are in a key position to teach prevention through abstinence and barrier protection, identify cases through screening for earlier treatment, and reduce the burden of these serious and often chronic diseases.

5. Use and refer patients to such resources as the American Sexual Health Association (*www.ashastd.org*) and Centers for Disease Control and Prevention Health Topics A to Z: (*www.cdc.gov/health/default.htm*).

SELECTED REFERENCES

Agency for Healthcare Research and Quality. (2014). *The guide to clinical preventive services, 2014: Recommendations of the US Preventive Services Task Force.* Author. Available: *www.uspreventiveservicestaskforce.org/Page/Name/tools-and-resources-for-better-preventive-care*

Committee on Health Literacy. (2004). *Health literacy: A prescription to end confusion.* Washington, DC: National Academies Press.

National Comprehensive Cancer Network. (2017). NCCN Clinical Practice Guidelines in Oncology. Smoking Cessation. Version 2.2017.

National Patient Safety Foundation. (2016). Ask Me 3. Available: *www.npsf.org/for-healthcare-professionals/programs/ask-me-3*

Office of Disease Prevention and Health Promotion. (2018). *Physical activity.* Washington (DC): U.S. Department of Health and Human Services; Updated 2/6/2018. Available at: *http://www.health.gov/paguidelines*

Office of Disease Prevention and Health Promotion, USDHHS. (2018). Healthy People 2020. Available: *www.healthypeople.gov.* Updated February 5, 2018.

PDQ® Screening and Prevention Editorial Board. (2017). *PDQ cigarette smoking.* Bethesda, MD: National Cancer Institute. Available: *www.cancer.gov/about-cancer/causes-prevention/risk/tobacco/quit-smoking-hp-pdq.* Updated April 27, 2017.

Raphaelidis, L. (2016). Maintaining weight loss: Lessons from the national weight control registry. *Journal for Nurse Practitioners, 12*(4), 286–287.

Rizer, C.A., & Lusk, M.D. (2017). Screening and initial management of alcohol misuse in primary care. *The Journal for Nurse Practitioners, 13*(10), 660–666.

Smith, S.L., Smith, C., Cheatham, M., & Smith, H.G. (2017). Electronic cigarettes: A burn case series. *The Journal for Nurse Practitioners, 13*(10), 693–699.

U.S. Department of Health and Human Services. (2008). *Physical Activity Guidelines for Americans.* Washington, DC: U.S. Department of Health and Human Services; 2008. Available: *www.health.gov/paguidelines*

U.S. Department of Health and Human Services and U.S. Department of Agriculture. (December 2015). 2015–2020 Dietary Guidelines for Americans (8th ed.). Available: *http://health.gov/dietaryguidelines/2015/guidelines*

U.S. Department of Health and Human Services, Centers for Disease Control and Prevention. (2017). STD surveillance 2016. Atlanta, GA: author.

U.S. Preventive Services Task Force. (2017). Seventh annual report to congress on high-priority evidence gaps for clinical preventive services. December 2017. Available: *https://www.uspreventiveservicestaskforce.org/Page/Name/seventh-annual-report-to-congress-on-high-priority-evidence-gaps-for-clinical-preventive-services*

U.S. Preventive Services Task Force. (2018). Final recommendation statement: screening for ovarian cancer. February 2018. Available: *https://www.uspreventiveservicestaskforce.org/Announcements/News/Item/final-recommendation-statement-screening-for-ovarian-cancer*

4
Genetics and Health Applications

HUMAN GENETICS

Human genetics, as it pertains to health care, is the study of the etiology, pathogenesis, and natural history of human conditions that are influenced by genetic factors. Genetic factors extend beyond the limited view of solely distinct genetic syndromes to encompass influences on health, the occurrence of complex disorders, individual biologic responses to illness, potential treatment and medical management approaches, and strategies for prevention or cure.

This tremendous realization is apparent through the accomplishments of initiatives such as the Human Genome Project. This 15-year international collaborative effort was completed in 2003. One significant goal of the Human Genome Project was to identify the approximately 25,000 human genes. These advances and the associated knowledge will continue to affect the delivery of health care and nursing practice significantly. Genetic evaluations, screening, testing, guided treatment, family counseling, and related legal, ethical, and psychosocial issues are increasingly becoming daily practice for many nurses.

The impact of genetics on nursing is significant. In 1997, the American Nurses Association (ANA) officially recognized genetics as a nursing specialty. This effort was spearheaded by the International Society of Nurses in Genetics (ISONG), which also initiated credentialing for the Advanced Practice Nurse in Genetics and the Genetics Clinical Nurse. ANA and ISONG have collaborated in the establishment of a scope and standards of practice for nurses in genetics practice. Essential Nursing Competencies and Curricula Guidelines for Genetics and Genomics were finalized in 2006 with Outcome Indicators established in 2008. The 2nd edition was published in 2009, "Essentials of Genetic and Genomic Nursing: Competencies, Curricula Guidelines, and Outcome Indicators." They reflect the minimal genetic and genomic competencies for every nurse regardless of academic preparation, practice setting, role, or specialty. In 2012, the ANA and ISONG published "Essential Genetic and Genomic Competencies for Nurses with Graduate Degrees." A copy of both of these documents is available through the ANA Web site (*www.nursingworld.org /genetics*).

The purpose of this chapter is to provide the nurse with practical information, resources, representative examples, and professional considerations critical to integration of genetics knowledge into nursing practice.

Underlying Principles

Readers are encouraged to use the Talking Glossary of Genetic Terms available through the National Human Genome Research Institute to supplement the terms provided here. This glossary can be found at *www.genome.gov/glossary*.

Cell: The Basic Unit of Biology

1. Cytoplasm—contains functional structures important to cellular functioning, including mitochondria, which contain extranuclear deoxyribonucleic acid (DNA) important to mitochondrial functioning.
2. Nucleus—contains 46 chromosomes in each somatic (body) cell or 23 chromosomes in each germ cell (egg or sperm) (see Figure 4-1, page 28).

Chromosomes

1. Each somatic cell with a nucleus has 22 pairs of autosomes (the same in both sexes) and 1 pair of sex chromosomes.
2. Females have two X sex chromosomes; males have one Y sex chromosome and one X sex chromosome.
3. Normally, at conception, each individual receives one copy of each chromosome from the maternal egg cell (1 genome, also called haploid) and one copy of each chromosome from the paternal sperm cell (1 genome), for a total of 46 chromosomes (2 genomes, also called diploid).
4. *Karyotype* is the term used to define the chromosomal complement of an individual (eg, 46, XY), as is determined by laboratory chromosome analysis.
5. Each chromosome contains a different number of genes, with a range of approximately 300 to 3,000 genes.

Genes

1. The basic unit of inherited information.
2. Each copy of the human genome in the nucleus has about 20,000 genes. Cells also have some nonnuclear genes located within the mitochondria within the cytoplasm.
3. Alternate forms of a gene are termed *alleles*.
4. For each gene, an individual receives one allele from each parent and thus has two alleles for each gene on the autosomes and also on the X chromosomes in females.

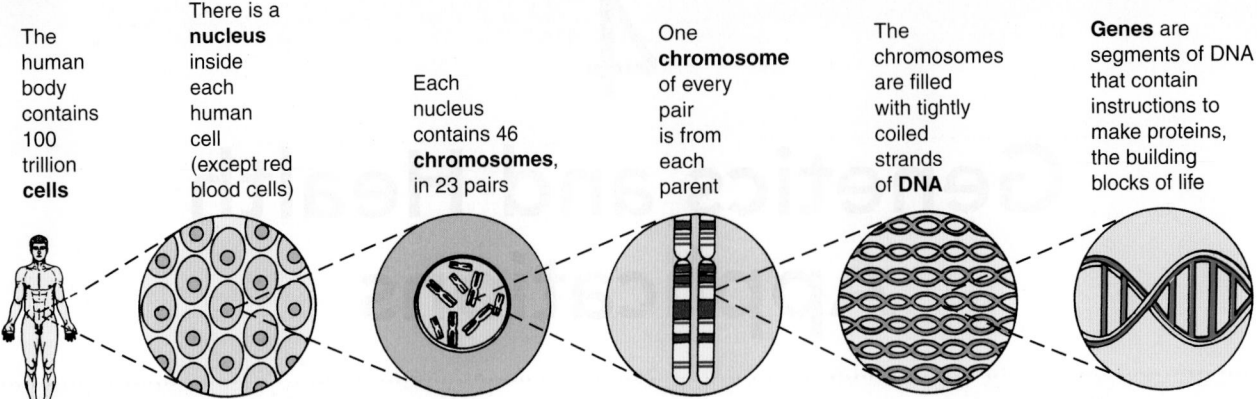

The
human
body
contains
100
trillion
cells

There is a
nucleus
inside
each
human
cell
(except red
blood cells)

Each
nucleus
contains 46
chromosomes,
in 23 pairs

One
chromosome
of every
pair
is from
each
parent

The
chromosomes
are filled
with tightly
coiled
strands
of **DNA**

Genes are
segments of DNA
that contain
instructions to
make proteins,
the building
blocks of life

Figure 4-1. Cells, chromosomes, DNA, and genes.

5. Males have only one X chromosome and, therefore, have only one allele for all genes on the X chromosome; they are hemizygous for all X-linked genes.
6. At any autosomal locus, or gene site, an individual can have two identical alleles (homozygous) for that locus or can have two different alleles (heterozygous) at a particular locus.
7. *Genotype* refers to the constitution of the genetic material of an individual; for practical purposes, it is commonly used to refer to a particular base or bases in the DNA, for example, the gene for sickle cell disease, the gene for cystic fibrosis, or the gene for familial polyposis.
8. *Phenotype* refers to the physical or biochemical characteristics an individual manifests regarding expression of the presence of a particular feature, or set of features, associated with a particular gene.
9. Each gene is composed of a unique sequence of DNA bases.

DNA: Nuclear and Mitochondrial

1. Human DNA is a double-stranded helical structure comprised of four different bases, the sequence of which codes for the assembly of amino acids to make a protein—for example, an enzyme. These proteins are important for the following reasons:
   a. For body characteristics such as eye color.
   b. For biochemical processes such as the gene for the enzyme that digests phenylalanine.
   c. For body structure such as a collagen gene important to connective tissue and bone formation.
   d. For cellular functioning such as genes associated with the cell cycle.
2. The four DNA bases are adenine, guanine, cytosine, and thymine (A, G, C, and T).
3. A change, or mutation, in the coding sequence, such as a duplicated or deleted region, or even a change in only one base, can alter the production or functioning of the gene or gene product, thus affecting cellular processes, growth, and development.
4. DNA analysis can be done on almost any body tissue (blood, muscle, skin) using molecular techniques (not visible under a microscope) for mutation analysis of a specific gene with a known sequence or for DNA linkage of genetic markers associated with a particular gene.

Normal Cell Division

1. Mitosis occurs in all somatic cells, which, under normal circumstances, results in the formation of cells identical to the original cell with the same 46 chromosomes.

2. Meiosis, or reduction division, occurs in the germ cell line, resulting in gametes (egg and sperm cells) with only 23 chromosomes, one representative of each chromosome pair.
3. During the process of meiosis, parental homologous chromosomes (from the same pair) pair and undergo exchanges of genetic material, resulting in recombinations of alleles on a chromosome and thus variation in individuals from generation to generation.

CLINICAL APPLICATION
Genetic Disorders

Presentations warranting genetic consideration include intellectual disability, birth defects, biochemical or metabolic disorders, structural abnormalities, multiple miscarriages, and family history of the same or related disorder.

Examples of disorders that result from abnormalities of chromosomes or genes or that are, at least in part, influenced by genetic factors are described in Table 4-1.

Classification of Genetic Alterations
Chromosomal
1. The entire chromosome or only part can be affected. This is usually associated with birth defects and intellectual disability because there are extra or missing copies of all genes associated with the involved chromosome.
   a. Numerical—abnormal number of chromosomes because of nondisjunction (error in chromosomal separation during cell division). Examples are Down and Klinefelter syndromes.
   b. Structural—abnormality involving deletions, additions, or translocations (rearrangements) of parts of chromosomes. Examples are Prader-Willi and Angelman syndromes.
2. May involve autosomes or sex chromosomes.

Single Gene or Pair of Genes
1. Manifestations are specific to cells, organs, or body systems affected by that gene.
2. Autosomal dominant—presence of a single copy of an abnormal gene results in phenotypic expression.
   a. These genes may involve proteins of a structural nature such as collagen. Affected individuals are usually of normal intelligence.

Table 4-1 Selected Genetic Disorders

DISORDER AND INCIDENCE	CHARACTERISTICS	ETIOLOGY AND RECURRENCE RISKS	CONSIDERATIONS AND COMMENTS
Chromosomal Disorders			
Autosomal			
Down syndrome (Trisomy 21) 1 in 700 neonates; incidence increases with advanced maternal age (eg, risk at maternal age 25 is 1 in 1,350; at age 35, 1 in 384; at age 45, 1 in 28)	Brachycephaly: oblique palpebral fissures; epicanthal folds; Brushfield spots; flat nasal bridge; protruding tongue; small, low-set ears; clinodactyly; simian crease; congenital heart defects; hypotonia; intellectual disability; growth retardation; dry, scaly skin; increased risk for childhood leukemia and early-onset Alzheimer disease	• Extra copy of number 21 chromosome (total of three copies). • 94% of cases are trisomy (karyotype 47, +21) for three distinct number 21 chromosomes because of nondisjunction (failure of chromosomal separation during meiosis); recurrence risk 1%, plus maternal age–related risk if older than age 35. • 4% of cases have a translocation—the extra number 21 is attached to another chromosome, usually a number 13 or number 14; half of these translocations are new occurrences, and the other half are inherited from a parent. • 2% of cases are mosaic—affected individual has two different cell lines, one with the normal number of chromosomes and the other cell line trisomic for the number 21 chromosome; because of a postconception error in chromosomal division during mitosis.	• Recurrence risk for parents of affected are dependent on one or more of the following: chromosomal type of disorder, maternal age, parental karyotype, family history, and sex of transmitting parent and other chromosome involved (if translocation). • May demonstrate nuchal thickening prenatally on ultrasound examination. • Associated with moderate intellectual disability. • No phenotypic differences between trisomy Down syndrome and translocation Down syndrome. • Chromosome analysis should be performed on all persons with Down syndrome. • Prenatal maternal serum screening can adjust risk for the pregnancy. See page 1458 for nursing care.
Trisomy 13 (Patau syndrome) 1 in 5,000 live births	Holoprosencephaly; cleft lip or palate, or both; abnormal helices; cardiac defects; rocker-bottom feet; overlapping positioning of fingers; seizures; severe intellectual disability	• Extra number 13 chromosome (total of three copies): Either trisomy form, because of nondisjunction, with less than a 1% recurrence risk, or translocation form, with recurrence risk less than that of translocation Down syndrome and dependent on other factors, including chromosomes involved.	• 44% die within the first month; 18% survive first year of life.
Trisomy 18 (Edwards syndrome) 1 in 6,000 live births	Small for gestational age (may be detected prenatally); feeble fetal activity; weak cry; prominent occiput; low-set, malformed ears; short palpebral fissures; small oral opening; overlapping positioning of fingers (fifth digit over fourth, index over third); nail hypoplasia, short hallux; cardiac defects; inguinal or umbilical hernia; cryptorchidism in males; severe intellectual disability	• Extra number 18 chromosome (total of three copies): Majority due to nondisjunction resulting in three distinct chromosome 18s with less than 1% recurrence risk.	• Most trisomy 18 conceptions miscarry; 90% die within first year of life.

(continued)

Table 4-1   Selected Genetic Disorders (*Continued*)

DISORDER AND INCIDENCE	CHARACTERISTICS	ETIOLOGY AND RECURRENCE RISKS	CONSIDERATIONS AND COMMENTS
Sex Chromosome			
Klinefelter syndrome 1 in 700 males; 47, XXY abnormality in 90%; other 10% have more than two X chromosomes in addition to the Y chromosome or have mosaicism (about 20%)	Body habitus may be tall, slim, and underweight; long limbs; gynecomastia; small testes; inadequate virilization; azoospermia or low sperm count; cognitive defects; behavioral problems	• Because of nondisjunction during meiosis, except for cases of mosaicism, which are due to mitotic nondisjunction.	• No distinguishing features prenatally. • Diagnosis may not be suspected or pursued before puberty. • Diagnosis in childhood is beneficial in planning for testosterone replacement therapy, in addition to accurate understanding of learning or behavioral problems. • Tend to be delayed in onset of speech, have difficulty in expressive language, may be relatively immature, may have history of recurrent respiratory infections.
Turner syndrome (45, X) 1 in 2,500 female births	Webbing of neck and short stature; lymphedema of hands and feet as neonate; congenital cardiac defects (especially coarctation of the aorta); low posterior hairline; cubitus valgus; widely spaced nipples; underdeveloped breasts; immature internal genitalia (eg, streak ovaries); primary amenorrhea; learning disabilities	• About 50% because of a nondisjunctional error during meiosis (karyotype 45, X); 20% are mosaic because of nondisjunction during mitosis; 30% have two X chromosomes, but one is functionally inadequate (eg, because of presence of abnormal gene); generally a sporadic occurrence.	• Webbing of neck and short stature may be detected prenatally by ultrasound. • Early diagnosis enhances optimal health care management (eg, planning for administration of growth hormone therapy, estrogen replacement). • Psychosocial implications associated with short stature, delayed onset of puberty. • Infertility associated with ovarian dysgenesis; oocyte donation and adoption are generally the only options for having children. See page 1461.
Microdeletion/Microduplication			
Fragile X syndrome 1 in 3,600 males; 1 in 4,000 females	Motor delays; hypotonia; speech delay and language difficulty; hyperactivity; classic features including long face, prominent ears, and macroorchidism manifest around puberty; autism (about 7% of males); intellectual disability in most males; learning disabilities in most affected females	• Mutation in the FMR-1 gene, represented as a large DNA expansion of a normally present trinucleotide. • Carrier mother of an affected male has a 50% risk for future affected males and 50% chance of transmitting the FMR-1 X chromosome to a daughter who would be a carrier, may be unaffected, or manifest features associated with the fragile X syndrome and has a 50% chance of transmitting that gene to future offspring.	• Expansion of DNA in the region of the gene that houses a CpG island results in methylation of the DNA resulting in the gene being "shut down," and the protein normally made by the gene is not made resulting in the phenotype. Testing involves DNA analysis to characterize the size of the DNA expansion. Testing for methylation status of the DNA increases sensitivity. • Phenotypic expression of this gene in males and females is variable; genetic mechanisms determining expression of this gene are very complicated. • Fragile X should be considered in the differential diagnosis of any male with intellectual disability who is undiagnosed; it is the most common intellectual disability in males.

Table 4-1   Selected Genetic Disorders (Continued)

DISORDER AND INCIDENCE	CHARACTERISTICS	ETIOLOGY AND RECURRENCE RISKS	CONSIDERATIONS AND COMMENTS
Microdeletion/Microduplication			
Prader-Willi syndrome Estimated incidence 1 in 15,000	Hypotonia and poor sucking ability in infancy; almond-shaped palpebral fissures; small stature; small, slow growth of hands or feet; small penis, cryptorchidism; insatiable appetite, behavioral problems developing in childhood; below-normal intelligence or intellectual disability	• Cytogenetic microdeletion in chromosome 15q11 to 13 identified in 50% to 70% of cases; deletion associated with paternally inherited number 15 chromosome. • Generally sporadic occurrence; empiric recurrence risk 1.6%.	• Consider diagnosis in infants presenting with hypotonia and sucking problems where etiology is unknown. • Associated with lack of a functioning paternal gene at this locus; presents clinical evidence for the necessity of two functioning genes, both a maternal and paternal contribution. • Another distinct entity, termed *Angelman syndrome*, is associated with a deletion of the maternal contribution in this same cytogenetic region; it is also associated with mental deficiency but with a different phenotypic presentation.
Mendelian Disorders—Single Gene			
Autosomal Dominant			
Achondroplasia 1 in 10,000 live births Increased incidence associated with advanced paternal age (>40)	Megalocephaly; small foramen magnum and short cranial base with early sphenooccipital closure; prominent forehead; low nasal bridge; midfacial hypoplasia; small stature; short extremities; lumbar lordosis; short tubular bones; incomplete extension at the elbow; normal intelligence	• Autosomal dominant inheritance; 80% to 90% are due to a new mutation and neither parent is affected. • An affected parent has a 50% risk to transmit the gene to each child.	• Hydrocephalus can be a complication of achondroplasia and may be masked by megalocephaly. • Risk for apnea secondary to cervical spinal cord and lower brain stem compression because of alterations in shape of cervical vertebral bodies; respiratory problems are also a risk because of the small chest and upper airway obstruction. • Can be diagnosed prenatally by ultrasound.
Osteogenesis imperfecta (Type 1) 1 in 15,000 live births	Blue sclerae; fractures (variable number); deafness may occur	• Defect in the procollagen gene associated with decreased synthesis of a constituent chain important to collagen structure. • Can occur as a new mutation in that gene or can be inherited from a parent who has a 50% recurrence risk to transmit the gene; most severe cases represent a sporadic occurrence within a family.	• There are at least four general classifications of osteogenesis imperfecta, each with varying clinical severity, presentation, and pattern of genetic transmission. • Treatment with calcitonin and fluoride may be beneficial in reducing the number of fractures.
Breast and breast/ovarian cancer syndrome Accounts for 5% to 10% of breast cancer	Breast cancer (usually, but not exclusively, early-age onset, premenopausal); ovarian cancer	• Mutation in the BRCA1 or BRCA2 gene; poses increased susceptibility (not certainty) for breast (31% to 78%) and/or ovarian (3% to 54%) cancer.	• Studies have also noted increased risk for prostate cancer and colon cancer in some families; also an association between male breast cancer and BRCA2 mutations. • Individuals from Ashkenazi Jewish ancestry are at increased risk for mutations in BRCA1 and BRCA2.

(continued)

Table 4-1   Selected Genetic Disorders (*Continued*)

DISORDER AND INCIDENCE	CHARACTERISTICS	ETIOLOGY AND RECURRENCE RISKS	CONSIDERATIONS AND COMMENTS
Autosomal Dominant			
Familial adenomatous polyposis (FAP) Accounts for about 1% of colon cancer	Associated with multiple adenomatous colorectal polyps (classic: >100; atypical: <100), desmoid tumors, other GI polyps, jaw cysts; family history of polyps or colorectal cancer; polyps progress to cancer; polyps can be present in childhood	• Mutations in the APC gene (a tumor suppressor gene). The majority of APC mutations result in a truncated protein. • Mutations in the MUTYH gene (a DNA repair gene). The majority of mutations in MUTYH result in an amino acid change.	• Genetic testing (protein truncation testing is available). If mutation is identified in affected person, relatives can be tested for the same finding. Relatives at risk, whether by family history or by genetic testing, should start cancer screening by age 18, if not earlier, if there are symptoms or as a baseline. Screening includes colonoscopy and ophthalmologic examination.
Autosomal Recessive			
Sickle cell disease 1 in 400 live births of African Americans	Physically normal in appearance at birth; hemolytic anemia and the occurrence of acute exacerbations (crises), resulting in increased susceptibility to infection and vascular occlusive episodes	• Point mutation in the beta globin gene resulting in an altered gene product; red blood cells susceptible to sickling at times of low-oxygen tension. • Parents of an affected individual are both unaffected carriers of one abnormal copy of the beta globin gene (sickle cell trait); together have a 25% risk for recurrence in any offspring.	• 1 in 10 African Americans is a carrier of the beta globin gene mutation; population screening is indicated for these individuals. • Unaffected siblings of an affected individual have two-thirds, or 67%, risk to have the sickle cell trait and should be screened. • See page 1376 for nursing care. • Prenatal testing is available through DNA analysis from specimen obtained during chorionic villus sampling or amniocentesis.
Cystic fibrosis (CF) 1 in 2,500 live births (predominantly white)	Phenotypically normal at birth; may present with meconium ileus (10%) as neonate or later with persistent cough, recurrent respiratory problems, gastrointestinal complaints, malnutrition, abdominal pain, or infertility	• Mutation in the CF transmembrane conduction regulator gene on chromosome 7 results in an abnormality of a protein integral to the cell membrane. • Healthy parents of an affected individual are both considered obligate carriers of one copy of the abnormal CF gene; thus, together, they have a 25% recurrence risk with each conception.	• 1 in 25 White from Northern European ancestry; 1 in 58 Hispanic White; and 1 in 61 African Americans is a carrier of a CF gene mutation. • Many different mutations have been identified within the CF gene, the most common of which is Delta-F508, which accounts for about 70% of CF mutations. CF screening can identify about 85% of all CF mutations, but the rate of detection varies by ancestry (94% in Ashkenazi Jewish population; 88% in non-Hispanic Whites; 72% in Hispanic Whites; 64% in African Americans; and 49% in Asian Americans). • "General population" screening is recommended by the American College of Obstetrics and Gynecology. • DNA analysis of the CF gene is advised for affected individuals and relatives of persons with CF. • See page 1191 for nursing care.

Table 4-1 Selected Genetic Disorders (*Continued*)

DISORDER AND INCIDENCE	CHARACTERISTICS	ETIOLOGY AND RECURRENCE RISKS	CONSIDERATIONS AND COMMENTS
Autosomal Recessive			
Tay-Sachs disease 1 in 3,600 Ashkenazi Jews	Normal at birth; progressive neurodegenerative manifestations, including loss of developmental milestones and lack of central nervous system maturation; cherry-red spot on macula	• Mutation in the gene for hexosaminidase A, an enzyme important to cellular metabolic processes, results in accumulation of metabolic by-products within the cell (especially brain), impairing functioning and causing the neurodegenerative effects. • Parents of an affected individual are both considered unaffected obligate carriers of one copy of the Tay-Sachs disease gene; together, they have a 25% risk of recurrence in their offspring.	• About 1 in 25 Ashkenazi Jews is a carrier of the Tay-Sachs gene; about 1 in 17 French Canadians is a carrier of an abnormal Tay-Sachs gene (different mutation from that of the Jewish ancestry); persons of these ancestries should be screened. • No treatment available; results in death in childhood. • Prenatal and preimplantation testing are available.
X-Linked Recessive			
Duchenne muscular dystrophy (DMD) 1 in 3,500 males	Phenotypically normal at birth; dramatically elevated creatinine kinase level (detectable as early as age 2 days); hypertrophy of the calves; history of tendency to trip and fall (at about age 3); Gowers sign (tendency to push off oneself when getting up from a sitting position)	• DNA mutation, generally a deletion, detectable in 70% of affected males. • Carrier females have a 25% risk, with each pregnancy, to have an affected male, a 25% risk to have a carrier female, a 25% chance to have a healthy male, and a 25% chance to have a healthy noncarrier female.	• 1 in 1,750 females is a carrier of the DMD gene. • In the case of an isolated affected male, the mother has a two-thirds statistical risk that she is a carrier of the DMD gene and a one-third chance that her affected son developed as the result of a new mutation in that gene (she is not a carrier). • DNA testing is recommended for affected males; once type of gene mutation is known in that family, prenatal diagnosis and evaluation of potential female carriers can be carried out. • DNA analysis may provide clues as to expected clinical severity.
Hemophilia A 1 in 5,000 males	Phenotypically normal at birth; bleeding tendency (ranging from frequent spontaneous bleeds associated with the severe form to bleeding only after trauma associated with the mild form)	• Deficiency of Factor VIII (antihemophilic factor) because of abnormality in this gene located on the X chromosome. • Carrier females have a 25% risk, with each pregnancy, to have an affected son, a 25% risk to have a carrier daughter, and a 25% chance each to have a healthy unaffected daughter or son. • Mates of affected males should be tested for carrier status. If the female is not a carrier, the affected male will not have any affected children.	• Frequency of carrier females is about 1 in 3,500. • The severe form occurs in about 48% of cases. • Moderate cases account for 31%. • The mild form accounts for 21% of cases. • See page 1384 for nursing care.

(continued)

Table 4-1 Selected Genetic Disorders (*Continued*)

DISORDER AND INCIDENCE	CHARACTERISTICS	ETIOLOGY AND RECURRENCE RISKS	CONSIDERATIONS AND COMMENTS
X-Linked Recessive			
Glucose-6-phosphate dehydrogenase (G6PD) Frequency varies by ancestry (ie, 11% to 12% of male live births of African American origin and 60% to 70% of Kurdish Jewish origin)	Phenotypically normal at birth; many remain asymptomatic throughout life; may manifest acute hemolysis associated with exposure to outside factors (eg, certain medications)	• Abnormality of the G6PD gene on the X chromosome. • Carrier females have a 25% risk, with each pregnancy, to have an affected male and 25% risk to have a carrier female.	• Be aware of drugs, such as antimalarial drugs or sulfonamides, or chemicals, such as phenylhydrazine (used in silvering mirrors, photography, soldering), associated with hemolysis in G6PD-deficient individuals.
Multifactorial Disorders			
Neural tube defects 1 in 1,000 live births	Abnormalities of neural tube closure, ranging from anencephaly to myelomeningocele to spina bifida occulta	• Probably several genetic factors may predispose certain individuals or families to susceptibility, but certain environmental (eg, prolonged hyperthermia or folate deficiency) and other unknown factors play an additive rule in surpassing an arbitrary threshold, placing the developing fetus at risk. • Recurrence risk for isolated neural tube defects range between 1% and 5%.	• Recurrence risk for isolated neural tube defects is dependent on the severity of the defect (ie, a defect in the neurulation [the cranial end of the neural tube] vs. cannulation [the development of the caudal end]) and if there is a positive family history. • Maternal screening can be performed prenatally (after 14 weeks' gestation) through alpha-fetoprotein levels in maternal serum. • Can be associated with chromosomal or genetic disorders.
Cleft lip and/or cleft palate 1 in 1,000 live births	Unilateral or bilateral; cleft lip and cleft palate may occur together or in isolation	• Failure of migration and fusion of the maxillary processes during embryogenesis. • Recurrence risk for first-degree relatives of a person with an isolated cleft lip or cleft palate ranges between 2% and 6%.	• Clefting can occur as an isolated congenital abnormality or be one component of a syndrome, genetic defect, or chromosome abnormality, the latter three of which are associated with a recurrence risk specific to that disorder. • Recurrence for isolated cleft lip or palate is dependent on the type of cleft, the sex of the affected individual, and the family history. See page 1271.

b. Can be inherited from one parent, whose physical manifestations can vary, depending on the specific disorder and the gene's penetrance and expressivity (eg, neurofibromatosis).

c. Can arise as a result of a new mutation in that gene in the affected individual.

d. An individual with an autosomal dominant gene has a 50% chance of transmitting that gene to all offspring.

3. Autosomal recessive—requires that both alleles at a gene locus be abnormal for an individual to be affected.

a. These genes are frequently important to biochemical functions, such as the breakdown of phenylalanine. Depending on the gene and the nature of the mutation, affected individuals may be of normal intelligence or have intellectual disability.

b. Generally, two healthy parents of an affected child are considered obligate carriers (unaffected) of one copy of the abnormal gene.

c. Such a carrier couple has a 25% chance, with each pregnancy, to have an affected child, a 50% chance for the child to be an unaffected carrier, and a 25% chance for the child to be an unaffected noncarrier.

4. X-linked recessive—because of one or more abnormal genes on the X chromosome.

a. These genes may be important to structure or biochemical function. Depending on the gene and the nature of the mutation, affected individuals may be of normal intelligence or have intellectual disability.

b. Recessively inherited, in most cases, meaning that two abnormal genes are required to be affected. However, only one abnormal gene needs to be present for a male to be affected because males are hemizygous for all X-linked genes, as in Duchenne muscular dystrophy.

   c. Females are typically only carriers of X-linked recessive disorders because the presence of a corresponding normal gene on the other X chromosome in a female produces enough gene products for normal functioning. Carrier females can be affected to varying degrees in certain circumstances. Incidence of females affected with X-linked recessive conditions is possible and usually have an affected father and a carrier mother.

   d. A carrier female has a 25% chance, with each pregnancy, to have an affected son, a 25% chance to have a carrier daughter, a 25% chance to have an unaffected son, and a 25% chance to have an unaffected noncarrier daughter.

   e. A male with an abnormal X-linked gene who has children with a noncarrier female will transmit that gene to all of his daughters, who will be carriers of that gene (usually unaffected); none of his sons will inherit his abnormal X-linked gene because they receive his Y chromosome.

5. X-linked dominant—relatively rare.

   a. Mutations in these genes are usually lethal to male conceptions, as in Rett syndrome.

   b. Depending on the gene and the nature of the mutation, affected females may be of normal intelligence or have intellectual disability. An example is incontinentia pigmenti.

6. Mitochondrial—genes whose DNA is within the mitochondria, which are located in the cytoplasm, not in the nucleus and therefore do not follow Mendelian laws of inheritance.

   a. Many of these genes are associated with respiratory functions within mitochondria and thus affect energy capacity of cells. Disorders may be manifested by diminished strength in the involved tissue or myopathy.

   b. Essentially are maternally inherited because the egg cell contains the cytoplasmic material that is involved in the zygote; the sperm cell contributes mainly only nuclear DNA.

   c. Varying phenotypes, depending on the number and distribution of abnormal mitochondrial genes.

   d. Males and females can have mitochondrial conditions, but males transmit few, if any, mitochondrial genes to their offspring.

Multifactorial

1. Caused by multiple genetic factors in addition to other nongenetic influences (eg, environmental).

2. Because of the genetic components, affected individuals or close relatives are at an increased risk, compared with the general population, to have an affected child or develop the condition themselves.

3. Elimination of known nongenetic risk factors or proactive treatment regimen in some conditions can reduce risk for occurrence (eg, diet modification to manage hypercholesterolemia, cessation of smoking to reduce risk of cancer, or weight control and exercise to prevent type 2 diabetes in susceptible individuals).

Precision Health Care

Precision health care is the tailoring of health care to the individual patient. Data informing the health care provider to enable precision health care to a patient include information about their lifestyle, environment, and genetic makeup (ie, genetic variations drive a lot of the variability in how patients respond to medications) or the genetic makeup of their diseased cells (ie, using information on gene expression in cancer cells to prognosticate and select targeted therapies). This is a rapidly evolving area of health care on which genomics is having a huge impact. The National Institutes of Health website provides a timely resource for information about the Precision Medicine Initiative at *www.nih.gov/research-training/allofus-research-program*.

Genetic Counseling

Genetic counseling is a communication process that deals with human problems associated with the occurrence or recurrence of a genetic disorder in a family or individual at increased risk for a condition that has a genetic component because of factors such as ancestral background or the results of screening tests. For these individuals or families, specific concern exists about risk associated with a certain problem or because of the relationship to someone who is affected (the proband). Several steps occur in the genetic evaluation, including obtaining and reviewing the medical history and records of the affected, eliciting the family history with special attention to factors pertinent to the diagnosis in the proband, evaluating and examining the affected (if available and indicated), ordering appropriate tests and interpreting results, and then meeting with the person seeking the consultation and/or the proband.

Goals of Genetic Counseling

Assist the patient and proband to:

1. Comprehend the medical facts, including the diagnosis, the possible course of the disorder, and the available management.

2. Understand the inheritance of the disorder, susceptibility to a condition, and the risk of recurrence in specified relatives.

3. Understand the options for dealing with the risk of recurrence.

4. Choose a course of action that seems appropriate to the individuals involved; consider their risk, family goals, and religious beliefs and act in accordance with that decision.

5. Make the best possible adjustment to the disorder.

6. Understand the individual risks and the types of testing available and assist with interpretation and follow-up of test results.

Identify People in Need of Genetic Assessment and Counseling

1. Parents of a child with a birth defect, intellectual disability, or known or possible genetic disorder.

2. Any individual with a genetic or potentially genetic disorder.

3. People with a family history of intellectual disability, birth defects, genetic disorder, or condition that tends to run in the family.

4. Pregnant women who will be age 35 or older at the time of delivery.

5. Couples of ancestral/ethnic origin known to be at an increased risk for a specific genetic disorder.

6. Couples who have experienced two or more miscarriages.

7. Pregnant women who have an elevated or low maternal serum screening test result such as alpha-fetoprotein (AFP).

8. Women who have been exposed to drugs or infections during pregnancy.

9. Couples who are related to each other.

10. Couples who are identified as carriers of autosomal recessive conditions through screening.

11. People who are concerned about the risk for a genetic disorder.

Genetic Screening, Testing, and Research

Screening

1. Screening is the level of testing offered to large populations (eg, neonate) or to high-risk segments of the population at increased risk of being carriers (such as individuals from African ancestry, Ashkenazi Jewish ancestry, and Mediterranean ancestry) to identify individuals with a genetic disorder, increased risk for abnormality, or carriers of a genetic disorder.
2. Criteria include that the test itself must be reliable, appropriate to the designated population, and cost-effective and that the condition being tested must be treatable or that early identification will enhance quality of life.
3. Neonate screening varies among facilities and states; however, all states and facilities test for a minimum of 30 conditions including phenylketonuria, hypothyroidism, sickle cell disease, and galactosemia, with most states testing for up to 50 or more conditions.
4. Prenatal screening includes multiple-marker screening that uses maternal serum to test AFP level alone or the triple screen (includes measurement of maternal serum AFP, beta-human chorionic gonadotropin, and estriol). A fourth protein, inhibin-A, measured by some laboratories, is called the quadruple screen. These tests are typically conducted after 14 weeks' gestation and can identify pregnancies at increased risk for neural tube defects (NTD), Down syndrome, trisomy 13 (Patau syndrome), and trisomy 18 (Edwards syndrome).

 EVIDENCE BASE National Newborn Screening and Genetic Resource Center. (2018). Resources on newborn screening including the national newborn screening status reports. Available: *http://genes-r-us.uthscsa.edu.*

Testing

1. Biochemical testing is done on body tissue or fluid to measure enzyme levels and activity.
2. DNA testing is done on blood or tissue samples to look for a gene mutation or to study DNA linkage.
3. Chromosomal testing is done on nucleated cells (usually white blood cells) or other tissue for detection of various conditions, such as extra, missing, deleted, duplicated, or rearranged chromosomes.

Prenatal Testing

1. Chorionic villus sampling—for chromosomal and DNA testing; done at 9 to 12 weeks' gestation.
2. Amniocentesis—for chromosomal, biochemical, and DNA testing as early as 11 to 13 weeks' gestation (early amniocentesis); AFP measures can be done starting at 14 weeks' gestation.
3. Ultrasound—for dating pregnancy and assessing fetal structures, placenta, amniotic fluid, and nuchal translucency.
4. Acetylcholinesterase—for testing amniotic fluid for suspected NTD.
5. Fetoscopy—for obtaining fetal blood samples or visualizing details of fetal structures; done during the second trimester.
6. Percutaneous umbilical blood sampling—for obtaining fetal blood; done during second trimester.

Preimplantation Diagnosis

1. Requires *in vitro* fertilization so that embryos can form in the laboratory. One or two cells are removed from the embryo and sent for genetic testing. Only embryos lacking the genetic composition for disease are placed into the womb for further development.
2. Useful if the embryo is at an increased risk for a specific genetic condition, for example, an autosomal/X-linked recessive, autosomal/X-linked dominant, or chromosomal condition.

Research

1. Testing is performed to further understand the genetics of a disorder, biochemical process, or individual response to therapies.
2. Genetic research is *not* clinical testing and may have no clinical value to the patient's case.
3. There is ongoing and extensive research on cancer susceptibility genes, genetic abnormalities present in different cancer types, and genes related to therapeutic response to medications.

Additional Genetic Testing Consideration

DNA banking—extraction and storage of one's DNA from blood through a qualified genetics laboratory; requires informed consent, proper collection, and prompt handling.

Nursing Roles and Responsibilities

1. Recognize or suspect genetic disorders by their physical characteristics and clinical manifestations.
2. Demonstrate an understanding of the relationship of genetics and genomics to health, prevention, screening, diagnostics, prognostics, selection of treatment, and monitoring of treatment effectiveness.
3. Create a genetic pedigree (diagram of the family history), including cause of death and any genetically linked ailments (see Figure 4-2).
4. Explain those aspects of diagnosis, prognosis, and treatment that affect the patient and family. Relate information that parents, affected or at-risk individuals, and caregivers need to know to plan for the care of the patient.
5. Clear up misconceptions and allay feelings of guilt.
6. Assist with the diagnostic process by exploring medical and family history information, using physical assessment skills, procuring samples for testing, and developing a plan of care that incorporates genetic and genomic assessment information.
7. Enhance and reinforce self-image and self-worth of parents, child, or the individual at risk for or presenting with a genetic condition.
8. Advocate for clients' access to genetic/genomic services and resources, including support groups.
9. Refer and prepare family for genetic counseling.
   a. Inform that prenatal testing does not mean termination of pregnancy (eg, it may confirm that the fetus is not affected, thus eliminating worry throughout pregnancy, although the determination of an abnormality is also a possibility).
   b. Encourage parents and patient to allow adequate time to deliberate on a course of action (eg, they should not rush into a test without full knowledge of what the results can and can't tell, nor should they rush to make future reproductive decisions such as tubal ligation because in a few years, they may want more children).
   c. Remain nonjudgmental.

Figure 4-2. Genetic pedigree of a patient with breast cancer. Maternal side only is shown; however, both maternal and paternal sides are assessed. Genetic risk may run through either side.

10. Check with the state (eg, state health department) or with the Centers for Disease Control and Prevention (*www.cdc.gov*) for information and resources regarding neonatal testing required and state regulations on genetic testing and research.

11. Recognize that there are many ethical, legal, psychosocial, and professional issues associated with obtaining, using, and storing genetic information.
    a. Be aware of associated professional responsibilities, including informed consent, documentation in medical records, medical releases, and individual privacy of information.
    b. Refer to federal legislation (Genetic Information Nondiscrimination Act of 2008 and Health Insurance Portability and Accountability Act, 1997) that deals with protection from genetic discrimination in medical insurance; individual state legislation; genetics professional societies (see below); and the World Health Organization document on ethical considerations in genetic testing and services.

12. Refer for further information and support to:
    • March of Dimes: *www.modimes.org*
    • International Society of Nurses in Genetics: *www.isong.org*
    • Genetic Alliance: *www.geneticalliance.org*
    • Oncology Nursing Society: *www.ons.org*
    • National Society of Genetic Counselors: *www.nsgc.org*
    • CDC Public Health Genomics: *www.cdc.gov/genomics*
    • American Nurses Association, Genetics: *www.nursingworld.org/genetics*

SELECTED REFERENCES

American Nurses Association. (2018). Educational genetics resources. Available: *http://www.nursingworld.org/MainMenuCategories/EthicsStandards/Resources/Genetics-1*

Consensus Panel on Genetic/Genomic Nursing Competencies. (2009). Essentials of genetic and genomic nursing competencies, curricula guidelines, and outcomes indicators (2nd ed.). Silver Spring, MD: American Nurses Association. Available: *www.nursingworld.org/genetics*

Greco, K. E., Tinley, S., & Seibert, D. (2012). Essential genetic and genomic competencies for nurses with graduate degrees. Silver Spring, MD: American Nurses Association and International Society of Nurses in Genetics. Available: *www.nursingworld.org/genetics*

International Society of Nurses in Genetics and American Nurses Association. (2007). *Statement on the scope and standards of genetics clinical nursing practice.* Washington, DC: American Nurses Publishing.

Komen, S. G. (2018). Inherited gene mutations. Available: *http://ww5.komen.org/BreastCancer/InheritedGeneticMutations.html*

McKusick-Nathans Institute for Genetic Medicine, Johns Hopkins University and National Center for Biotechnology Information, National Library of Medicine. (2018). Online Mendelian Inheritance in Man, OMIM (TM). Available: *www.ncbi.nlm.nih.gov/omim*

Metcalfe, K., Lubinski, J., Lynch, H. T., Ghadirian, P., Foulkes, W. D., Kim-Sing, C., … Narod, S. A. (2010). Family history of cancer and cancer risks in women with BRCA1 or BRCA2 mutations. *Journal of the National Cancer Institute, 102*(24), 1874–1878.

National Human Genome Research Institute. (2018). All about the Human Genome Project. Available: *www.genome.gov/10001772/all-about-the--human-genome-project-hgp/*

National Newborn Screening and Genetic Resource Center. (2018). Resources on newborn screening including the national newborn screening status reports. Available: *http://genes-r-us.uthscsa.edu/*

Nussbaum, R. L., McInnes, R. R., & Willard, H. F. (2015). *Genetics in medicine* (8th ed.). Philadelphia, PA: Elsevier.

Silbert-Flagg, J., & Pillitteri, A. (2017). *Maternal and child health nursing* (8th ed.). Philadelphia, PA: Wolters Kluwer.

GENERAL HEALTH
CONSIDERATIONS

5

Adult Physical Assessment

PART TWO

MEDICAL-SURGICAL NURSING

5

Adult Physical Assessment

THE PATIENT HISTORY
General Principles

1. The first steps in caring for a patient are to establish a relationship and gather information.
2. In all patient encounters, the assessment process begins with thorough and accurate history taking, thorough review of the patient record, interviewing the patient, and obtaining information from other individuals.
3. Use good communication skills, to elicit comprehensive health history and establish rapport with the patient simultaneously.

Interviewing Techniques

1. Provide privacy in as quiet a place as possible and see that the patient is comfortable.
2. Begin the interview with a courteous greeting and an introduction. Address the patient as *Mr.*, *Mrs.*, or *Ms.* and shake hands if appropriate. Explain who you are and the reason for your presence.
3. Make sure that facial expressions, body movements, and tone of voice are pleasant, unhurried, and nonjudgmental and that they convey the attitude of a sensitive listener so the patient will feel free to express thoughts and feelings.
4. Use open-ended questions and avoid narrowing the discussion or reassuring the patient prematurely (before you have adequate information about the problem). This only cuts off discussion; the patient may then be unwilling to expand on a problem causing concern.
5. Be alert for cues or suggestions by the patient that may require you to explore more by asking more pointed questions.
6. Guide the interview so the necessary information is obtained in a timely manner. Controlling a rambling patient is often difficult, but, with practice, it can be done without jeopardizing the quality of the nurse–patient relationship.

Components
Identifying Information

1. Supply date and time of the interview. Review data about the patient if already in the record or obtain patient's name, address, telephone number, race, ethnicity, religion, birth date, and age.
2. Obtain name of referring practitioner, insurance data, and name and contact information of informant(s) other than the patient. Note reliability of an informant if necessary.
3. Explain the reasons why the information is needed to help put the patient at ease.

Chief Complaint

1. Obtain a brief statement of the patient's primary problem or concern in the patient's own words, including the duration of the complaint, for example, "hacking cough × 3 weeks."
2. Purpose is to allow the patient to describe his or her own problems and expectations with little or no direction from the interviewer and to identify the overriding problem for which the patient is seeking help (there may be numerous complaints).
3. To obtain information, ask the patient a direct question, such as "For what reason have you come to the facility?" or "What is your primary health concern at this time?"
   a. Avoid confusing questions, such as "What brings you here?" ("The bus.") or "Why are you here?" ("That's what I came to find out.")
   b. Ask how long the concern or problem has been present, for example, whether it has been hours, days, or weeks. If necessary, establish the time of onset precisely by offering such clues as "Did you feel this way a month (6 months or 2 years) ago?"

4. Write down what the patient says using quotation marks to identify patient's words.

History of Present Illness

1. Obtain a detailed chronological picture, beginning with the time the patient was last well (or, in the case of a problem with an acute onset, the patient's condition just before the onset of the problem) and ending with a description of the patient's current condition.
2. If there is more than one important problem, describe each in a separate, chronologically organized paragraph in the written history of present illness.
3. Investigate the chief complaint by eliciting more information through the use of the mnemonic "OLD CARTS":
   a. **O**nset (setting, circumstances, rapidity, or manner in which it began).
   b. **L**ocation (exact place where the symptom is felt, radiation pattern).
   c. **D**uration (how long; if intermittent, the frequency and duration of each episode).
   d. **C**haracter/course (nature or quality of the symptom, such as sharp pain, interference with activity, how it has changed or evolved over time; ask to describe a typical episode).
   e. **A**ggravating/associated factors (medications, rest, activity, diet; associated nausea, fever, and other symptoms).
   f. **R**elieving factors (lying down, having bowel movement).
   g. **T**reatments tried (pharmacologic and nonpharmacologic methods attempted and their outcomes).
   h. **S**everity (the quantity of the symptom; eg, how severe on scale of 1 to 10).
4. Alternately, use the mnemonic PQRST: **p**rovocative/palliative factors, **q**uality/quantity, **r**egion/radiation, **s**everity, **t**iming.
5. Obtain OLD CARTS data for all the major problems associated with the present illness, as applicable.
6. Clarify the chronology of the illness by asking questions and summarizing the history of present illness for the patient to comment on.

Past Medical History

1. Determine the background health status of the patient, including present status, recent health conditions, and past health conditions, that will serve as a basis for nursing care planning for holistic patient care.
2. General health and lifestyle patterns—sleeping pattern; diet; stability of weight; usual exercise and activities; use of tobacco, alcohol, illicit drugs.
3. Childhood illnesses, such as infectious diseases (if applicable).
4. Immunizations—childhood vaccines; adult vaccines including hepatitis, human papillomavirus, influenza, tetanus, herpes zoster, and pneumococcal vaccines.
5. Operations—surgical procedure, indication, approximate date, any complications.
6. Previous hospitalizations—facility, approximate date, diagnosis, treatment.
7. Injuries—approximate date, treatment, outcome.
8. Major acute and chronic illnesses (any serious or prolonged illnesses not requiring hospitalization)—dates, symptoms, course, treatment.
9. Medications—prescription drugs from all providers (including ophthalmologist and dentist); nonprescription drugs including vitamins, supplements, and herbal products; include dosage, length of use, and adherence.
10. Allergies—environmental allergies, food allergies, drug reactions; give type of reaction (hives, rhinitis, local reaction, angioedema, anaphylaxis).
11. Obstetric history (may appear in review of systems).
    a. Pregnancies, miscarriages, abortions.
    b. Describe course of pregnancy, labor, and delivery; date, place of delivery.
12. Psychiatric history (may appear in review of systems)—treatment by a mental health provider, diagnosis, date, medications.

Family History

1. Purpose is to present a picture of the patient's family health, including that of grandparents, parents, brothers, sisters, aunts, and uncles because some diseases show a familial tendency or are hereditary.
2. Include age and health status (or age at and cause of death) of maternal and paternal grandparents, parents, and siblings.
3. History, in immediate and close relatives, of heart disease, hypertension, stroke, diabetes, gout, kidney disease or stones, thyroid disease, pulmonary disease, blood problems, cancer (types), epilepsy, mental illness, arthritis, alcoholism, obesity.
4. Genetic disorders, such as hemophilia or sickle cell disease.
5. Age and health status of spouse and children.

Review of Systems

1. Purpose is to obtain detailed information about the current state of the patient and significant past symptoms, or lack of symptoms, patient may have experienced related to a particular body system.
2. May give clues to diagnosis of multisystem disorders or progression of a disorder to other areas.
3. Include subjective information about what the patient feels or sees with regard to the major systems of the body.
   a. General constitutional symptoms—fever, chills, night sweats, malaise, fatigability, recent weight loss or gain.
   b. Skin—rash, itching, change in pigmentation or texture, sweating, hair growth and distribution, condition of nails, skin care habits, protection from sun.
   c. Skeletal—problems of joints, muscles, or bones including pain, stiffness, deformity, restriction of motion, swelling, redness, heat, cramping.
   d. Head—headaches, dizziness, syncope, head injuries.
   e. Eyes—vision, pain, diplopia, photophobia, blind spots, itching, burning, discharge, glaucoma, cataracts, glasses or contact lenses worn, date of last eye appointment.
   f. Ears—hearing acuity, earache, discharge, tinnitus, vertigo, history of tubes or infection.
   g. Nose—sense of smell, frequency of colds, obstruction, epistaxis, postnasal discharge, sinus pain or therapy, use of nose drops or sprays (type and frequency).
   h. Teeth—pain; bleeding, swollen or receding gums; recent abscesses, extractions; dentures; dental hygiene practices, last dental examination.
   i. Mouth and tongue—soreness of tongue or buccal mucosa, ulcers, swelling.
   j. Throat—sore throat, tonsillitis, hoarseness, dysphagia.
   k. Neck—pain, stiffness, swelling, enlarged glands or lymph nodes.
   l. Endocrine—goiter, thyroid tenderness, tolerance to heat and cold, changes in skin pigmentation, libido, polyuria,

polydipsia, polyphagia, hormone therapy, unexplained weight change.

m. Respiratory—pain in the chest with breathing, dyspnea, wheezing, cough, sputum, hemoptysis, risk factors, and testing for tuberculosis.

n. Cardiovascular—chest pain, palpitations, dyspnea, orthopnea (note number of pillows required for sleeping), history of heart murmur, edema, cyanosis, claudication, varicose veins, exercise tolerance, blood pressure (if known), history of blood clots.

o. Hematologic—anemia, tendency to bruise or bleed, any known abnormalities of blood cells.

p. Lymph nodes—enlargement, tenderness, drainage.

q. Gastrointestinal—appetite, food intolerance, belching, heartburn, nausea, vomiting, hematemesis, bowel habits, diarrhea, constipation, flatulence, stool characteristics, hemorrhoids, jaundice, use of laxatives or antacids, history of ulcers or other conditions, previous diagnostic tests such as colonoscopy.

r. Urinary—dysuria, pain, urgency, frequency, hematuria, nocturia, oliguria, hesitancy, dribbling, decrease in size or force of stream, passage of stones, incontinence.

s. Male reproductive—puberty onset, sexual activity, use of condoms, libido, sexual dysfunction, history of sexually transmitted diseases (STDs).

t. Female reproductive—pattern and characteristics of menses, libido, sexual activity, pregnancies, methods of contraception, STD protection.

u. Breasts—pain, tenderness, discharge, lumps, mammograms, breast self-examination.

v. Neurologic—loss of consciousness, seizures, confusion, memory, cognitive function, incoordination, weakness, numbness, paresthesia, tremors.

w. Psychiatric—how patient views self, mood, sadness, depression, anxiety, irritability, obsessive thoughts, compulsions, suicidal or homicidal thoughts, hallucinations.

Personal and Social History

1. Explore the patient's family structure and habits to identify resources an individual has to aid in coping with the situation and determine what health promotion activities may improve health.
2. Determine personal status—birthplace, education, position in the family, education level, job status, satisfaction with life situations, personal concerns.
3. Identify habits and lifestyle patterns.
   a. Sleeping pattern, number of hours of sleep, difficulty sleeping.
   b. Exercise, activities, recreation, hobbies.
   c. Nutrition and eating habits (diet recall for a typical day).
   d. Alcohol—frequency, amount, type; CAGE questionnaire—positive response may indicate problem drinking:
      i. Have you ever thought you should **C**ut down on your drinking?
      ii. Have you ever been **A**nnoyed by criticism of your drinking?
      iii. Have you ever felt **G**uilty about your drinking?
      iv. Do you drink in the morning (ie, an **E**ye-opener)?
   e. Caffeine—type and amount per day.
   f. Illicit drugs (illegal or improperly used prescription or over-the-counter medications).

g. Tobacco—past and present use, type (cigarettes, cigars, chewing, snuff), pack, years.
h. Sexual habits (can be part of genitourinary history)—relationships, frequency, satisfaction, number of partners in past year and lifetime, STD and pregnancy prevention.
4. Home conditions.
   a. Marital status, nature of family relationships.
   b. Financial—source of income, health insurance.
   c. Living arrangements, type of housing.
   d. Involvement with agencies (name, caseworker).
   e. History of abuse—physical, intimate partner, sexual.
5. Environmental exposure—through work or other activities, including exposure to stress, noise, chemicals, pollution.
6. Culture—important in coping and health practices.
7. Religion/faith—may affect some treatment decisions.

Ending the History

When you have completed the history, it is often helpful to say, "Is there anything else you would like to tell me?" or "What additional concerns do you have?" This allows the patient to end the history by saying what is on his or her mind and what concerns the patient most.

PHYSICAL EXAMINATION
General Principles

1. Conduct a complete or partial physical examination following a careful comprehensive or problem-related history.
2. Make sure the exam takes place in a quiet, well-lit room with consideration for patient privacy and comfort.

Approaching the Patient

1. When possible, begin with the patient in a sitting position so both the front and back can be examined.
2. Completely expose the part to be examined, but drape the rest of the body appropriately.
3. Conduct the examination systematically from head to foot so as not to miss observing any system or body part.
4. While examining each region, consider the underlying anatomic structures, their function, and possible abnormalities.
5. Because the body is bilaterally symmetric for the most part, compare findings on one side with those on the other.
6. Explain all procedures to the patient while the examination is being conducted to avoid alarming or worrying the patient and to encourage cooperation.

Techniques of Examination and Assessment

Use the following techniques of examination, as appropriate, for eliciting findings.

Inspection

1. Begin on your first encounter with the patient to observe behavior and physical appearance in a systematic manner.
2. Use your eyes to inspect each part of the body with the appropriate light and exposure for characteristics such as symmetry, color, enlargement or swelling, and deformity.

Table 5-1 Five Basic Notes Produced by Percussion

	RELATIVE INTENSITY	RELATIVE PITCH	RELATIVE DURATION	EXAMPLE LOCATION
Flatness	Soft	High	Short	Thigh
Dullness	Medium	Medium	Medium	Liver
Resonance	Loud	Low	Long	Normal lung
Hyperresonance	Very loud	Lower	Longer	Emphysematous lung
Tymphany	Loud	High*	*	Gastric air bubble

*Distinguished mainly by its musical timbre.
Adapted from Bickley, L. S. (2016). Bates' guide to physical examination and history taking (12th ed.). Philadelphia, PA: Lippincott Williams & Wilkins.

Palpation

1. Use your fingertips or palms to touch the region or body part just observed for temperature, texture, tenderness, and moisture in a systematic manner.
2. With experience, you will be able to determine abnormal consistency and pinpoint tender areas.

Percussion

1. By setting underlying tissues in motion, percussion helps in determining the density of the underlying tissue and whether it is air-filled, fluid-filled, or solid.
2. Audible sounds and palpable vibrations are produced, which you can distinguish as five basic notes of percussion, differing in sound, pitch, duration, and intensity (see Table 5-1).
3. To perform percussion, follow these steps:
   a. Hyperextend the middle finger of your left hand, pressing the distal portion and joint firmly against the surface to be percussed.
      i. Other fingers touching the surface will damp the sound.
      ii. Be consistent in the degree of firmness exerted by the hyperextended finger as you move it from area to area or the sound will vary.
   b. Cock the right hand at the wrist, flex the middle finger upward, and place the forearm close to the surface to

be percussed. The right hand and forearm should be as relaxed as possible.
   c. With a quick, sharp, relaxed wrist motion, strike the extended left middle finger with the flexed right middle finger, using the tip of the finger, not the pad. Aim at the end of the extended left middle finger (just behind the nail bed) where the greatest pressure is exerted on the surface to be percussed.
   d. Lift the right middle finger rapidly to avoid damping the vibrations.
   e. The movement is at the wrist, not at the finger, elbow, or shoulder; use the lightest touch capable of producing a clear sound.

Auscultation

1. You will use a stethoscope to augment your sense of hearing. Earpieces should be comfortable, the length of the tubing should be 10 to 15 inches (25 to 38 cm), and the head should have a diaphragm and a bell.
2. Use the bell to detect low-pitched sounds such as certain heart murmurs.
3. Use the diaphragm for high-frequency sounds such as breath sounds.
4. Try to minimize extraneous sounds produced by clothing, hair, and movement of the head of the stethoscope.

text continues on page 69

Adult Physical Assessment

EQUIPMENT
- Cotton applicator stick
- Flashlight
- Oto-ophthalmoscope
- Reflex hammer
- Safety pin
- Sphygmomanometer
- Stethoscope
- Thermometer
- Tongue blade
- Tuning fork
- Additional items may include disposable loves and lubricant for rectal examination and a speculum for examination of female pelvis.

Technique	Findings

VITAL SIGNS

Important: Many major therapeutic decisions are based on the vital signs; therefore, accuracy is essential.

Temperature

Oral, axillary, and temporal artery (forehead) temperature are measured routinely as a substitute for core body temperature. Tympanic membrane (ear) readings are considered inaccurate.

A rectal temperature is the most accurate but may be contraindicated with some rectal problems and cardiac arrhythmias.

Temperature—may vary with the time of day and method used (axillary slightly lower). 98.6°F (37°C) is considered normal oral temperature, but range is 96.4 (35.8) to 99.1 (37.3).

Rectal temperature is higher than oral by 0.7°F to 0.9°F (0.4°C to 0.5°C).

Pulse

Palpate the radial pulse and count for at least 30 seconds.

If the pulse is irregular, count for a full minute and note the number of irregular beats per minute.

Note whether the beat of the pulse against your finger is strong or weak, bounding or thready.

Pulse—Normal adult pulse is 60 to 80 beats/minute; regular in rhythm. Elasticity of the arterial walls, blood volume, and mechanical action of the heart muscle are some of the factors that affect the strength of the pulse wave, which normally is full and strong.

Respiration

Count the number of respirations for 15 seconds and multiply by 4. Count longer for better accuracy if abnormality detected.

Note rhythm and depth of breathing.

Respiration—Normally 16 to 20 respirations per minute.

Blood pressure

Measure the blood pressure (BP) in both arms. Document the patient's position.

Palpate the systolic pressure before using the stethoscope to detect an auscultatory gap.*

Apply the cuff firmly; if it is too loose, it will give a falsely high reading.

Use an appropriate-sized cuff: a pediatric cuff for children; a large cuff or a leg cuff for obese people.

The cuff should be approximately 1 inch (2.5 cm) above the antecubital fossa.

Normal BP is less than 120/80 mm Hg.

A difference of 5 to 10 mm Hg between arms is common.

Systolic pressure in lower extremities is usually 10 mm Hg higher than reading in upper extremities.

Going from a recumbent to a standing position can cause the systolic pressure to fall 10 to 15 mm Hg and the diastolic pressure to rise slightly (by 5 mm Hg).

HEIGHT, WEIGHT, AND WAIST CIRCUMFERENCE

Determine the patient's height and weight. Use a measuring device rather than asking the patient for recent measurements.

Determine waist circumference by using tape measure just above the umbilicus at the narrowest point.

Height and weight can be used to determine body mass index.

Waist circumference is an independent risk factor for cardiovascular disease. Normal is ≤40 inches (102 cm) for men and ≤35 inches (88 cm) for women.

*Auscultatory gap:
1. The first sound of blood in the artery is usually followed by continuous sound until nothing is audible with the stethoscope.
2. Occasionally, the sound is not continuous and there is a gap after the first sound, after which the sound of blood in the vessel is heard again.
3. If one uses only the auscultatory method and pumps the cuff up until the sound is no longer heard, it is possible, when there is a gap in the sound or when the sound is not continuous, to get a falsely low systolic reading.

Adult Physical Assessment (*Continued*)

Technique	Findings
GENERAL APPEARANCE Begin observation on first contact with the patient; continue throughout the interview systematically. ***Inspection*** Observe for: race, gender, general physical development, nutritional state, mental alertness, affect, evidence of pain, restlessness, body position, clothes, apparent age, hygiene, grooming. Use smell and hearing as well as sight.	 Careful observation of the general state of the individual provides many clues about a person's body image, how he or she behaves, and also some idea of how well or ill he or she is.
SKIN Examine the skin as you proceed through each body system. ***Inspection*** Observe for: skin color, pigmentation, lesions (distribution, type, configuration, size), jaundice, cyanosis, scars, superficial vascularity, hydration, edema, color of mucous membranes, hair distribution, nails. ***Palpation*** Examine skin for temperature, texture, elasticity, turgor, and superficial tenderness.	 "Normal" varies considerably depending on racial or ethnic background, exposure to sun, complexion, and pigmentation tendencies (such as freckles). Nails are present and smooth and cared for in some way. The skin is normally warm, slightly moist, and smooth and returns quickly to its original shape when picked up between two fingers and released. There is a characteristic hair distribution over the body associated with gender and normal physiologic function.
HEAD ***Inspection*** Observe for: symmetry of face, configuration of skull, hair color and distribution, scalp. ***Palpation*** Examine: hair texture, masses, swelling or tenderness of scalp, configuration of skull.	 Normally, the skull and face are symmetric, with distribution of hair varying from person to person. (However, determine by history if there has been any change.) The scalp should be free of flaking, with no signs of nits (small, white louse eggs), lesions, deformities, or tenderness.

EYES AND VISION

Equipment

- Snellen chart for visual acuity (see page 433)
- Ophthalmoscope for advanced examination

Bickley, L. (2016). *Bates' guide to physical examination and history taking* (12th ed.) Philadelphia: Lippincott Williams & Wilkins. Photograph by Barbara Proud.

continued on following page

Adult Physical Assessment (Continued)

Technique	Findings
EYES AND VISION (Continued)	

Inspection

1. Globes (eyeballs)—for protrusion.
2. Palpebral fissures (oval opening between the upper and lower eyelids)—for width and symmetry.

3. Lid margins—for scaling, secretions, erythema, position of lashes.

4. Bulbar and palpebral conjunctivae—for congestion and color. Bulbar conjunctiva—membranous covering of the sclera (contains blood vessels). Palpebral conjunctiva—membranous covering of the inside of the upper and lower lids (contains blood vessels).

5. Sclerae and iris—for color.
6. Pupils—for size, shape, symmetry, reaction to light and accommodation (ability of the lens to adjust to objects at varying distances).

7. Eye movement—extraocular movements, nystagmus, convergence. (Nystagmus: rapid, lateral, horizontal, or rotary movement of the eye; convergence: ability of the eye to turn in and focus on a very close object.) (See neurologic system, page 65.)

8. Gross visual fields—by confrontation. (See neurologic system, page 65.)
9. Visual acuity—check with a Snellen chart (with and without glasses).

2. Palpebral fissures—appear equal when eyes open. Normally, upper lid covers small portion of iris and lower lid margin is just below the junction of cornea and sclera (limbus). Ptosis—drooping of the upper eyelid.

3. Lid margins—are clear; the lacrimal duct openings (puncta) are evident at the nasal ends of the upper and lower lids.

   Eyelashes—normally are evenly distributed and turn outward.

4. Bulbar conjunctiva—normally, transparent blood vessels may become dilated and produce the characteristic "bloodshot" eye.

   Palpebral conjunctivae—are pink and clear.

   Conjunctivitis—inflammation of the conjunctival surfaces.

5. Sclerae—should be white and clear.
6. Pupils—normally constrict with increasing light and accommodation. Pupils are normally round and can range in size from very small ("pinpoint") to large (occupying the entire space of the iris).

7. Extraocular movement—movement of the eyes in conjugate fashion. (Six muscles control the movement of the eye.) Eyes normally move in conjugate fashion, except when converging on an object that is moving closer.

   Nystagmus—may be seen briefly on lateral movement as a result of eye fatigue; however, vertical nystagmus or prolonged nystagmus should be evaluated.

   Convergence—fails when double vision occurs, usually 4 to 6 inches (10 to 15 cm) from the nose.

8. Peripheral vision—is full (medially and laterally, superiorly and inferiorly) in both eyes.
9. Normal vision—20/20.

   Myopia—nearsightedness.

   Hyperopia—farsightedness.

Palpation

1. Determine the strength of the upper lids by attempting to open closed lids against resistance.
2. Palpate globes through closed lids for tenderness and tension.

1. The examiner should not be able to open the lids when the patient is squeezing them shut.
2. Globes normally are not tender when palpated.

Fundoscopic examination

Advanced assessment technique, which visualizes the cornea, lens, and retina for abnormalities.

EARS AND HEARING

Equipment

- Tuning fork
- Otoscope

Adult Physical Assessment (*Continued*)

Technique	Findings

EARS AND HEARING (*Continued*)

To examine with otoscope

1. Hold the helix of the ear and gently pull the pinna upward and back toward the occiput to straighten the external canal.
2. Gently insert the lighted otoscope, using an earpiece that is a comfortable size for the patient.
3. Once the otoscope is in place, put your eye up to the eyepiece and examine the external canal.

Inspection

1. Pinna—examine for size, shape, color, symmetry, placement on the head, lesions, and masses.
2. External canal—examine with the otoscope for discharge, impacted cerumen, inflammation, masses, or foreign bodies.
3. Tympanic membrane—examine for color, luster, shape, position, transparency, integrity, and scarring.
4. Landmarks—note cone of light, umbo, handle and short process of the malleus, pars flaccida, and pars tensa. Gently move the otoscope to observe the entire drum. (Cerumen may obscure visualization of the drum.)

Palpation

Pinna—examine for tenderness, consistency of cartilage, swelling.

2. External canal—is normally clear with perhaps minimal cerumen.

3. Tympanic membrane and landmarks.

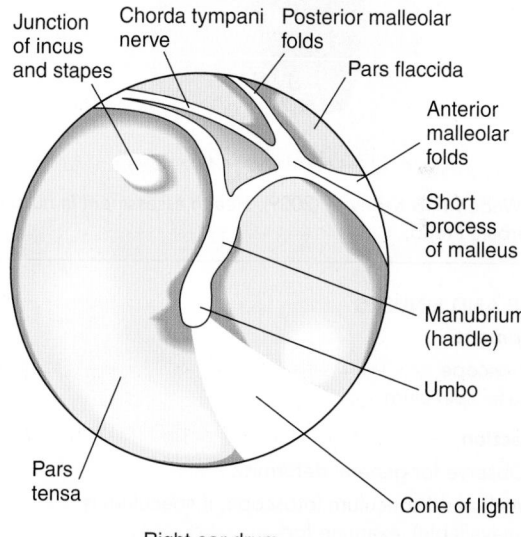

Right ear drum

Smeltzer, S., & Bare, B. (2006). *Brunner and Suddarth's textbook of medical-surgical nursing* (11th ed.). Philadelphia, PA: Lippincott Williams & Wilkins.

continued on following page

Adult Physical Assessment (*Continued*)

Technique	Findings

EARS AND HEARING (*Continued*)

Mechanical tests

1. Test each ear for gross hearing acuity using a whispered word or a watch. Cover the ear not being tested.

2. Weber test—test for lateralization of vibration. Tap the tuning fork against a hard surface to make it vibrate. Then, place the tuning fork in the center of the scalp near the forehead (**A**). (Also see Chapter 17.)

3. Rinne test—compares air and bone conduction.
   a. Place the vibrating tuning fork on the mastoid process behind the ear and have the patient tell you when the vibration stops (**B**).
   b. Then, quickly hold the buzzing end of the tuning fork near the ear canal and ask if patient can hear it (**C**).

1. A person with normal hearing can hear a whispered word from approximately 15 feet (4.5 m) and a watch from 1 foot (30 cm). The patient should hear the sound equally well in both ears; that is, there is no lateralization.

2. Sound should be heard equally in both ears.

3. Sound should be heard after vibration can no longer be felt; that is, air conduction is greater than bone conduction. Lateralization and conduction findings are altered by damage to the cranial nerve VIII and damage to the ossicles in the middle ear.

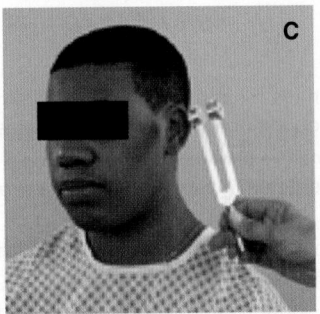

A-C. Weber, J., & Kelley, J. (2009). *Health assessment in nursing* (4th ed.). Philadelphia, PA: Lippincott Williams & Wilkins. Photographs by Barbara Proud.

NOSE AND SINUSES

Equipment

- Otoscope
- Nasal speculum

Inspection

1. Observe for general deformity.
2. With nasal speculum (otoscope, if speculum is unavailable), examine for:
   a. Nasal septum (position and perforation)
   b. Discharge (anteriorly and posteriorly)
   c. Nasal obstruction and airway patency
   d. Mucous membranes for color

1. External features vary but are generally symmetrical.

Nasal septum—is normally straight and not perforated.
Discharge—none should be present.
Airways—are patent.
Mucous membranes—are normally pink.

Adult Physical Assessment (*Continued*)

Technique	Findings

NOSE AND SINUSES (*Continued*)

e. Turbinates for color and swelling

Weber, J., & Kelley, J. (2003). *Health assessment in nursing* (2nd ed.). Philadelphia, PA: Lippincott Williams & Wilkins. Photograph by Barbara Proud.

Turbinates—three bony projections on each lateral wall of the nasal cavity covered with well-vascularized, mucous-secreting membranes. They warm the air going into the lungs and may become swollen and pale with colds and allergies.

Tenderness of sinuses may indicate sinusitis. (Weber, J., & Kelley, J. [2006]. *Health assessment in nursing* [3rd ed.]. Philadelphia, PA: Lippincott Williams & Wilkins. Photographs by Barbara Proud.)

Palpation

Sinuses (frontal and maxillary)—for tenderness.

Frontal—direct manual pressure upward toward the wall of the sinus. Avoid pressure on eyes.

Maxillary—with thumbs, direct pressure upward over lower edge of maxillary bones.

MOUTH

Equipment

- Flashlight
- Tongue blade
- Gloves
- Gauze sponges

Inspection

1. Observe lips for color, moisture, pigment, masses, ulcerations, fissures.

Smeltzer, S., & Bare, B. (2000). *Brunner and Suddarth's textbook of medical-surgical nursing* (9th ed.). Philadelphia, PA: Lippincott Williams & Wilkins.

2. Use tongue blade and penlight to examine:
   a. Teeth—number, arrangement, general condition.
   b. Gums—for color, texture, discharge, swelling, retraction.

   c. Buccal mucosa—for discoloration, vesicles, ulcers, masses.
   d. Pharynx—for inflammation, exudate, masses.

Teeth—an adult normally has 32 teeth.

Gums—commonly recede in adults. Bleeding is fairly common and may result from trauma, gingival disease, or systemic problems (less common).

Buccal mucosa and pharynx are pink to reddish brown with some color variation.

continued on following page

Adult Physical Assessment (Continued)

Technique	Findings

MOUTH (Continued)

    e. Tongue (protruded)—for size, color, thickness, lesions, moisture, symmetry, deviations from midline, fasciculations.

    f. Salivary glands—for patency.

      i. Parotid glands

      ii. Sublingual and submaxillary glands

    g. Uvula—for symmetry when patient says "ah."

    h. Tonsils—for size, ulceration, exudates, inflammation.

    i. Breath—for odor.

    j. Voice—for hoarseness.

Findings (Mouth):

Tongue—is normally midline and covered with papillae, which vary in size from the tip of the tongue to the back. (The circumvallate papillae are large and posterior.)

Parotid glands—open in the buccal pouch at the level of the upper teeth halfway back.

Sublingual and submaxillary glands—open underneath the tongue.

Uvula—should be midline.

Lingual tonsils—can often be seen on the posterior portion of the tongue.

Odor of breath—may indicate dental caries.

Palpation

1. Examine the oral cavity with a gloved hand for masses and ulceration. Palpate beneath the tongue and laterally explore the floor of the mouth.

2. Grasp the tongue with a gauze sponge to retract it; inspect the sides and undersurface of the tongue and the floor of the mouth.

Findings (Palpation):

1. Entire oral cavity should be pink and without ulcers, deep-red color, lesions, palpable masses, or swelling. An indurated mass raises the suspicion of malignancy.

Weber, J., & Kelley, J. (2006). *Health assessment in nursing* (3rd ed.). Philadelphia, PA: Lippincott Williams & Wilkins. Photograph by Barbara Proud.

NECK

Equipment

- Stethoscope

Inspection

1. Inspect all areas of the neck anteriorly and posteriorly for muscular symmetry, masses, unusual swelling or pulsations, and range of motion.

2. Thyroid—ask the patient to swallow and observe for movement of an enlarged thyroid gland at the suprasternal notch.

3. Muscular strength.

    a. Cervical muscles—have the patient turn his chin forcefully against your hand.

    b. Trapezius muscles—exert pressure on the patient's shoulders while he or she shrugs the shoulders.

Findings (Neck):

1. Range of motion—normally, the chin can touch the anterior chest, and the head can be extended at least 45 degrees from the vertical position and can be rotated 90 degrees from midline to side.

2. Thyroid—is not usually visible, except in extremely thin people.

3. Strength—see "Findings, cranial nerve XI," page 67.

Adult Physical Assessment (*Continued*)

Technique	Findings

NECK (*Continued*)

Palpation

1. Palpate the 10 areas for cervical lymph nodes as shown here.

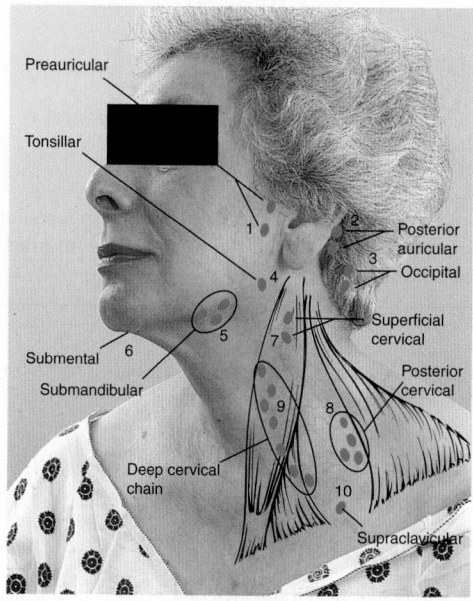

Timby, B. K., & Smith, N. E. (2017). *Introductory medical-surgical nursing* (12th ed.). Philadelphia, PA: Lippincott Williams & Wilkins. Photograph by Barbara Proud.

2. Trachea—palpate at the sternal notch. Place one finger along the side of the trachea and note the space between it and the sternomastoid. Compare to the other side.
3. Thyroid—palpate for size, symmetry, and consistency.
   a. Stand behind the patient and have him flex the neck slightly to relax the muscles.
   b. Place the fingertips of both hands on either side of the trachea just below the cricoid cartilage. Have the patient swallow and feel for any glandular tissue rising under your fingertips.
   c. Palpate the area over the trachea for the isthmus and laterally for the right and left lobes.
   d. Note any enlargement, nodules, masses, or consistency.

1. Cervical nodes—in the adult, the cervical lymph nodes are not normally palpable unless the patient is very thin, in which case the nodes are felt as small, freely movable masses. Tender nodes suggest inflammation; hard, fixed nodes suggest malignancy.

2. Trachea—should be midline. Spaces measured by fingers should be symmetrical. Tracheal deviation may be caused by neck mass or problems within the chest.
3. If the thyroid is palpable, it is normally smooth, without nodules, masses, or irregularities. Enlargement, asymmetry, or nodules require further evaluation.

Weber, J., & Kelley, J. (2006). *Health assessment in nursing* (3rd ed.). Philadelphia, PA: Lippincott Williams & Wilkins. Photograph by Barbara Proud.

continued on following page

Adult Physical Assessment (Continued)

Technique	Findings

NECK (Continued)

Palpation (continued)

4. Carotid arteries
   a. Palpate the carotids one side at a time.
   b. The carotids lie anterolaterally in the neck—avoid palpating the carotid sinuses at the level of the thyroid cartilage just below the angle of the jaw because this may cause slowing of heart rate.
   c. Note the symmetry of pulsations, strength, and amplitude, as well as any abnormal thrill.

4. A thrill (humming-like vibration) usually indicates arterial narrowing.

Auscultation

1. Use the diaphragm of the stethoscope to listen for bruits (murmur-like sound) over the carotid arteries.

1. A bruit may indicate arterial narrowing with turbulent blood flow. A cardiac murmur may also be referred to the carotid arteries.

LYMPH NODES

1. Lymph nodes are normally nonpalpable or felt as small, nontender, freely moveable masses.

Inspection

Additional lymph nodes are examined when the region of the body is examined; for example, the inguinal nodes are inspected when the abdomen is examined. Observe size and shape.

Lymph nodes are usually not visible unless enlarged or inflamed.

Palpation

1. Supraclavicular and infraclavicular nodes (usually palpated during neck or chest exam). Palpate for size, shape, mobility, consistency, tenderness, and warmth.
2. Axillary nodes (usually done during breast exam).
   a. Examine the patient while patient is sitting.
   b. Place the patient's arm at his side and examine the apex of the patient's axilla. (Use the fingers of your right hand to examine the left axilla and vice versa.)
   c. Rotate the examining hand so the fingers can palpate the anterior and posterior axillary fossae pressing against the chest wall. Press against the humerus bone in the axilla to examine the lateral fossa for nodes. Conclude the axillary examination by moving the fingers from the apex of the axilla downward in the midline along the chest wall.

1. Supraclavicular and infraclavicular nodes—not normally palpable. Enlargement may indicate a thoracic problem.

2. Axillary nodes—normally nonpalpable. Enlargement may occur with a breast or arm problem.

location of epitrochlear node

3. Inguinal nodes—are located in the groin and are usually examined when the abdomen is examined.

4. Epitrochlear nodes—are palpated just above the medial epicondyle, between the biceps and triceps muscles.

3. Inguinal nodes—a few may be felt. Enlargement and acute tenderness may indicate a genital or lower extremity problem.

4. Epitrochlear nodes—not normally palpable. Enlargement may indicate an arm or systemic problem.

Adult Physical Assessment (*Continued*)

Technique	Findings

BREASTS (MALE AND FEMALE)

Female breast

Inspection

(With the patient sitting, arms relaxed at sides.)

1. Inspect the areolae and nipples for position, pigmentation, inversion, discharge, crusting, and masses. Extra, or supernumerary, nipples may occur normally, most commonly in the anterior axillary region or just below the normal breasts.

2. Examine the breast tissue for size, shape, color, symmetry, surface, contour, skin characteristics, and level of breasts. Note any retraction or dimpling of the skin.

3. Ask the patient to elevate her hands over her head; repeat the observation.

4. Have the patient press her hands to her hips; repeat the observation.

Palpation

(This is best done with the patient in a recumbent position.)

1. The patient with pendulous breasts should be given a pillow to place under the ipsilateral scapula of the breast being palpated, so the tissue is distributed more evenly over the chest wall.

2. The arm on the side of the breast being palpated should be raised above the patient's head.

3. Palpate one breast at a time, beginning with the "asymptomatic" breast if the patient complains of symptoms.

4. To palpate, use the palmar aspects of the fingers in a rotating motion, compressing the breast tissue against the chest wall. Don't forget to include the "tail" of the breast tissue, which extends into the axillary region in the upper outer quadrant of the breast.

5. Note skin texture, moisture, temperature, or masses.

6. Gently squeeze the nipple and note any expressible discharge.

7. Repeat the examination on the opposite breast and compare findings.

Male breast

Examination of the male breast can be brief but may be important.

1. Observe the nipple and areola for ulceration, nodules, swelling, or discharge.

2. Palpate the areola for nodules and tenderness.

3. Palpate axillary lymph nodes (see page 52).

Findings

1. The *nipples* should be at the same level and protrude slightly. An *inverted nipple* (one that turns inward), if present since puberty, may be normal.

   A *supernumerary nipple* usually consists of a nipple and a small areola and may be mistaken for a mole.

2. Breast size—in the female, it is not uncommon to find a difference in the size of the two breasts. Normal asymmetry has usually been present since puberty and is not a recent phenomenon.

3. If there is a mass attached to the pectoral muscles, contracting the muscles will cause retraction of the breast tissue.

3. This allows the examiner to palpate the "normal" breast first and then compare the "symptomatic" breast to it.

4. Breast texture—varies according to the amount of subcutaneous tissue present.
   a. In young females, tissue is fairly soft and homogeneous; in postmenopausal women, tissue may feel nodular or stringy.
   b. Consistency also varies with menstrual cycle, being more nodular and edematous just prior to menstruation.

5. Masses—If a mass is palpated, its location, size, shape, consistency, mobility, and associated tenderness are reported.

6. Discharge—In the normal nonpregnant or nonlactating female, there is usually no nipple discharge.

1. There should be no discharge.

2. Enlargement of glandular tissue is gynecomastia, related to hormone imbalance.

continued on following page

Adult Physical Assessment (*Continued*)

Technique   Findings

THORAX AND LUNGS

Use anatomic landmarks to perform and document assessment of the thorax, keeping in mind the underlying structures of the lungs and heart.

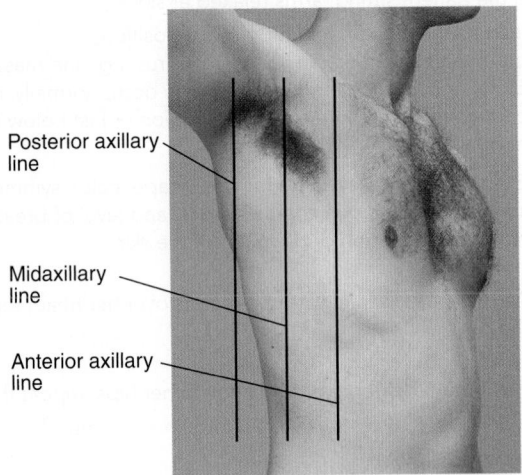

Bickley, L. (2008). *Bates' guide to physical examination and history taking* (10th ed.). Philadelphia, PA: Lippincott Williams & Wilkins.

Posterior thorax and lungs

Begin the examination with the patient seated; examine posterior chest and lungs.

Inspection

1. Inspect the spine for mobility and any structural deformity.
2. Observe the symmetry of the posterior chest and the posture and mobility of the thorax on respiration. Note any bulges or retractions of the costal interspaces on respiration or any impairment of respiratory movement.
3. Note the anteroposterior diameter in relation to the lateral diameter of the chest.

2. The thorax is normally symmetric; it moves easily and without impairment on respiration. There are no bulges or retractions of the intercostal spaces, which may indicate respiratory distress.
3. The anteroposterior diameter of the thorax in relation to the lateral diameter is approximately 1:2.

Palpation

1. Palpate the posterior chest with the patient sitting; identify areas of tenderness, masses, and inflammation.
2. Palpate the ribs and costal margins for symmetry, mobility, and tenderness and the spine for tenderness and vertebral position.

2. On palpation, there should be no tenderness; chest movement should be symmetric and without lag or impairment. Tenderness may indicate musculoskeletal strain, fracture, or other problems.

3. To assess respiratory expansion, place thumbs at the level of the 10th vertebra. With hands held parallel to the 10th ribs as they grasp the lateral rib cage, ask the patient to inhale deeply. Observe the movement of the thumbs while feeling the range and observe the symmetry of the hands.

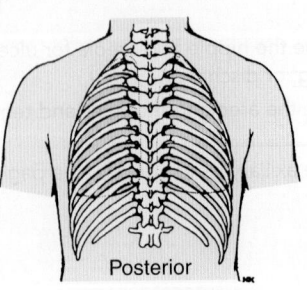

Adult Physical Assessment (Continued)

Technique	Findings

THORAX AND LUNGS (Continued)

4. To elicit tactile *fremitus* (palpable vibrations transmitted through the bronchopulmonary system on speaking).
   a. Ask the patient to say "99"; palpate and compare symmetric areas of the lungs with the ball of one hand. Begin at the upper lobes and move downward.
   b. Note any areas of increased or decreased fremitus.
   c. If fremitus is faint, ask the patient to speak louder and in a deeper voice.

4. Posteriorly, fremitus is generally equal throughout the lung fields. It may be increased near the large bronchi because of consolidation of tissue resulting from pneumonia. It may be decreased or absent anteriorly and posteriorly when vocal loudness is decreased, when posture is not erect, or when excessive tissue or underlying structures are present or in cases of pneumothorax and other pathology.

Percussion

As with palpation, the posterior chest is optimally percussed with the patient sitting.

1. Percuss symmetric areas, comparing sides.

1. Percussion normally reveals resonance over symmetric areas of the lung. Percussion sound may be altered by poor posture or the presence of excessive tissue.

2. Begin across the top of each shoulder and proceed down between the scapulae and then under the scapulae, both medially and laterally in the axillary lines.

3. Note and localize any abnormal percussion sound.

3. Dullness may indicate mass or consolidation because of pneumonia.

4. For diaphragmatic excursion, percuss by placing the pleximeter (stationary) finger parallel to the approximate level of the diaphragm below the right scapula. (See diagram on the right.)
   a. Ask the patient to inhale deeply and hold his breath; percuss downward to the point of dullness. Mark this point.
   b. Let the patient breathe normally, and then, ask patient to exhale deeply; percuss upward from the mark to the point of resonance.
   c. Mark this point and measure between the two marks—normally 2 to 2½ inches (5 to 6 cm).
   d. Repeat this procedure on the opposite side of the chest.

4. The lower border of the lungs is approximately at the level of the 10th thoracic spinous process on normal respiration. Unilateral abnormality of decreased excursion may indicate pleural effusion, atelectasis, or paralysis of one side of the diaphragm.

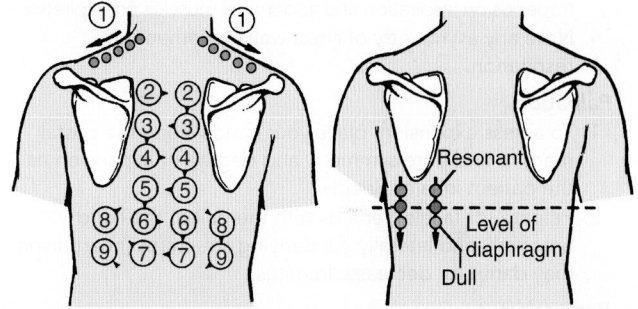

Auscultation

Aids in assessing airflow through the lungs, the presence of fluid or mucus, and the condition of the surrounding pleural space.

1. Have the patient sit erect.*
2. With a stethoscope, listen to the lungs as the patient breathes more deeply than normally with the mouth open. (Let the patient pause, as needed, to avoid hyperventilation.)
3. Place the stethoscope in the same areas on the chest wall as those percussed, and listen to a complete inspiration and expiration in each area.
4. Compare symmetric areas methodically from the apex to the lung bases.

On auscultation, breath sounds vary according to proximity of the large bronchi.
  – They are louder and coarser near the large bronchi and over the anterior.
  – They are softer and much finer (vesicular) at the periphery over the alveolae.
Breath sounds also vary in duration with inspiration and expiration. Sounds may normally decrease in obese individuals.

Note: If the patient is unable to sit without assistance for examination of the posterior chest and lungs, position him or her first on one side and then on the other as you examine the lung fields.

continued on following page

Adult Physical Assessment (Continued)

Technique	Findings

THORAX AND LUNGS (Continued)

5. It should be possible to distinguish three types of normal breath sounds as indicated in the following table.

5. Pathology will alter the normal bronchial, bronchovesicular, and vesicular breath sounds. Adventitious sounds include crackles, wheezes, and rhonchi.

Breath Sounds	Duration of Inspiration and Expiration	Pitch of Expiration	Intensity of Expiration	Normal Location
Vesicular	Inspiration > Expiration	Low	Soft	Most of lungs
Bronchovesicular	Inspiration = Expiration	Medium	Medium	Near the main stem bronchi (below the clavicles and between the scapulae, especially on the right)
Bronchial or tubular	Expiration > Inspiration	High	Usually loud	Over the trachea

Adapted from Bickley, L. S. (2008). Bates' guide to physical examination and history taking (10th ed.). Philadelphia: Lippincott Williams & Wilkins.

Anterior Thorax and Lungs

The patient should be recumbent with his or her arms at sides and slightly abducted.

Inspection

1. Inspect the chest for any structural deformity.
2. Note the width of the costal angle.

3. Observe the rate and rhythm of breathing, any bulging or retraction of intercostal spaces on respiration, and use of accessory muscles of respiration (sternocleidomastoid and trapezius on inspiration and abdominal muscles on expiration).
4. Note any asymmetry of chest wall movement on respiration.

Palpation

1. To assess expansion, place your hands along the costal margins and note symmetry and degree of expansion as the patient inhales deeply.
2. Palpate for tactile fremitus with the ball of the hand anteriorly and laterally. (Underlying structures [heart, liver] may damp, or decrease, fremitus.)

Percussion

1. With patient's arms resting comfortably at sides, percuss the anterior and lateral chest. Begin just below the clavicles and percuss downward from one interspace to the next, comparing the sound from the interspace on one side with that of the contralateral interspace.
2. Displace the female breast so breast tissue does not damp the vibration. Continue downward, noting the intercostal space where hepatic dullness is percussed on the right and cardiac dullness on the left.
3. Note the effect of underlying structures.

2. The angle at the tip of the sternum is determined by the right and left rib margins at the xiphoid process. Normally, the angle is less than 90 degrees.
3. There are no bulges or retractions of the intercostal spaces.

4. The thorax is normally symmetric and moves easily without impairment on respiration.

1. Hands should separate slightly on inspiration.

2. Vibration should be felt somewhat symmetrical. It may be necessary to displace the female breast gently.

1. Resonance is heard over most of the lungs.

2. A tympanic sound is produced over the gastric air bubble on the left somewhat lower than the point of liver dullness on the right.

3. Percussion over heart will produce a dull sound. The upper border of the liver will be percussed on the right side, producing a dull note.

Percussion of anterior thorax

① Flat ③ Resonant
② Dull ④ Tympanic

Auscultation

Listen to the chest anteriorly and laterally for the distribution of resonance and any abnormal or adventitious sounds.

Adult Physical Assessment (*Continued*)

Technique	Findings

HEART

1. Landmarks in relation to the sternum and the ribs are used during examination to yield the most information about function of the heart and its valves.
   a. In locating the intercostal spaces, begin by identifying the angle of Louis, which is felt as a slight ridge approximately 1 inch (2.5 cm) below the sternal notch, where the manubrium and the body of the sternum are joined.
   b. The 2nd ribs extend to the right and left of this angle.
   c. Once the 2nd rib is located, palpate downward and obliquely away from the sternum to identify the remaining ribs and intercostal spaces.

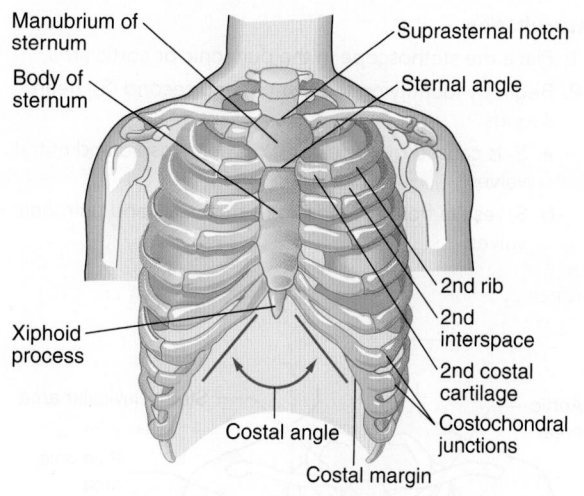

Inspection

1. Inspect the precordium for any bulging, heaving, or thrusting.
2. Look for the apical impulse in the 5th or 6th intercostal space at or just medial to the midclavicular line.
3. Note any other pulsations. Tangential lighting is most helpful in detecting pulsations.

1. Normally, there are no bulges or heaves; these indicate pathology.
2. An apical impulse may or may not be observable.
3. There should be no other pulsations.

Palpation

1. Use the ball of the hand to detect vibrations, or "thrills," which may be caused by murmurs. (Use the fingertips or palmar surface to detect pulsations.)

1. There should be no thrills or other pulsations. (Thrills are vibrations caused by turbulence of blood moving through valves that are transmitted through the skin, which feels similar to a purring cat.)

2. Proceed methodically through the examination so no area is omitted. Palpate for thrills and pulsations in each area (aortic, pulmonic, tricuspid, mitral).
   a. Begin in the aortic area (2nd right intercostal space, close to the sternum) and proceed to the pulmonic area (2nd left intercostal space) and then downward to the apex of the heart. (The mitral area is considered the apex of the heart.)
   b. In the tricuspid area, use the palm of the hand to detect any heaving or thrusting of the precordium (tricuspid area—5th intercostal space next to the sternum).
   c. In the mitral area (5th intercostal space, at or just medial to the midclavicular line), palpate for the apical beat; identify the point of maximal impulse (PMI) and note its size and force.

Ordinarily, no heaving of the ventricle is felt except, possibly, in the pregnant female.

The apical pulse should be felt approximately in the 5th intercostal space, at or just medial to the midclavicular line. In a young, thin person, it is a sharp, quick impulse no larger than the intercostal space. In an older person, the impulse may be less sharp and quick. An apical impulse displaced laterally may indicate left ventricular hypertrophy.

Percussion

1. Outline the heart border or area of cardiac dullness.
   a. The left border generally does not extend beyond 4, 7, and 10 cm left of the midsternal line in the 4th, 5th, and 6th intercostal spaces, respectively.
   b. The right border usually lies under the sternum.
2. Percuss outward from the sternum with the stationary finger parallel to the intercostal space until dullness is no longer heard. Measure the distance from the midsternal line in centimeters.

continued on following page

Adult Physical Assessment (Continued)

Technique	Findings

HEART (Continued)

Auscultation

1. Place the stethoscope in the pulmonic or aortic area.
2. Begin by identifying the first (S_1) and second (S_2) heart sounds.
   a. S_1 is caused by the closing of the tricuspid and mitral valves.
   b. S_2 results from the closing of the aortic and pulmonic valves.

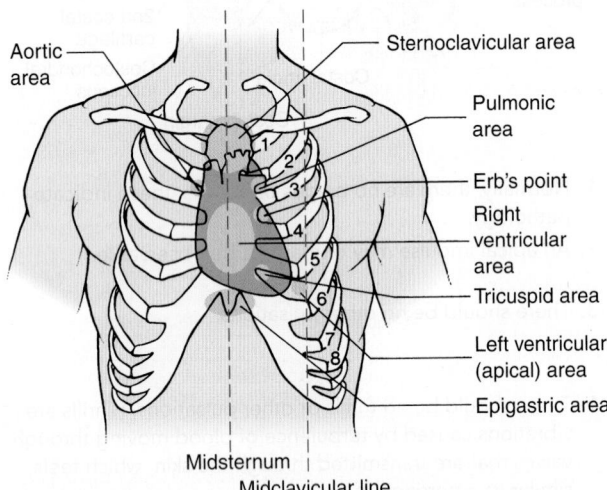

Smeltzer, S., & Bare, B. (2000). *Brunner and Suddarth's textbook of medical-surgical nursing* (9th ed.). Philadelphia, PA: Lippincott Williams & Wilkins.

3. Once the heart sounds are identified, count the rate and note the rhythm as discussed under vital signs. If there is an irregularity, try to determine if there is any pattern to the irregularity in relation to the intervals, heart sounds, or respirations.
4. Once rate and rhythm are determined, listen in each of the four areas and at Erb's point (3rd left interspace, close to the sternum) systematically, first with the diaphragm (detects higher-pitched sounds) and then with the bell (detects lower-pitched sounds). In each area, listen to S_1 and then to S_2 for intensity and splitting.

2. The two sounds are separated by a short systolic interval; each pair of sounds is separated from the next pair by a longer, diastolic interval. Normally, two sounds are heard—"lub, dub."
   – In the aortic and pulmonic areas, S_2 is usually louder than S_1. In this way, each of the paired sounds can be distinguished from the other.
   – In the tricuspid area, S_1 and S_2 are of almost equal intensity and, in the mitral area, S_1 is often slightly louder than S_2.

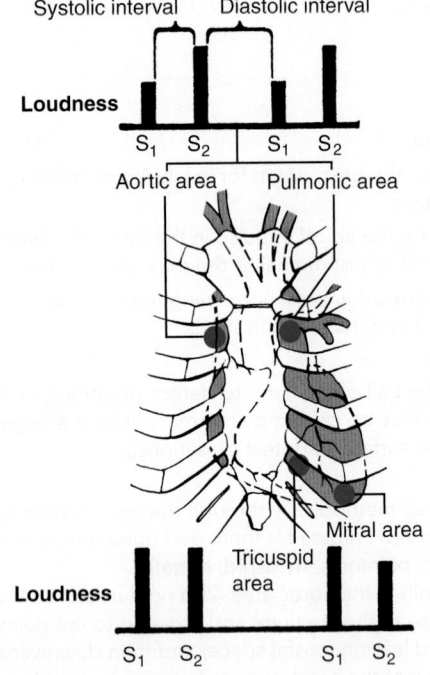

3. Normally, the heart sounds are regular, with a rate of 60 to 80 beats/minute (in the adult). In the athlete or jogger, the resting pulse may be between 40 and 60 beats/minute.
4. An extra "woosh" sound between S_1 and S_2 indicates systolic murmur; between S_2 and S_1 indicates a diastolic murmur. Note the area of its greatest intensity (aortic, pulmonic, mitral, tricuspid). An extra sound of short duration usually indicates an S_3 or S_4 gallop. Occasionally, there may be a splitting of S_2 in the pulmonic area. This is normal. Splitting of S_2 (two contiguous sounds are heard instead of one) is best heard at the end of inspiration, when right ventricular stroke volume is sufficiently increased to delay closure of the pulmonic valve *slightly* behind closure of the aortic valve.

Adult Physical Assessment (*Continued*)

Technique	Findings

PERIPHERAL CIRCULATION

Jugular veins

Evaluation of jugular venous distention is most useful in patients with suspected compromise of cardiac function.

Inspection	
1. Inspect neck for internal jugular venous pulsations.	1. Jugular venous pulsations can be distinguished from carotid pulsations by the following chart:

Internal Jugular Pulsations	Carotid Pulsations
Rarely palpable	Palpable
Soft, undulating quality, usually with two or three outward components (a, c, and v waves)	A more vigorous thrust with a single outward component
Pulsation eliminated by light pressure on the vein just above the sternal end of the clavicle	Pulsation not eliminated
Level of pulsation barely descends with inspiration	Pulsation not affected by inspiration
Pulsations vary with position	Pulsations are unchanged by position

From Bickley, L. S. (2008). Bates' guide to physical examination and history taking (10th ed.). Philadelphia: Lippincott Williams & Wilkins.

2. Note the highest point at which pulsations are seen and measure the vertical line between the point and the sternal angle. With the head raised 30 degrees, the internal jugular venous pulsations should not be visible more than 1 inch (2.5 cm) above the sternal angle. Increased level of internal jugular pulsations indicates right heart failure.

Morton, P. G., & Fontaine, D. K. (2017). *Critical care nursing* (11th ed.). Philadelphia, PA: Lippincott Williams & Wilkins.

Extremities

Inspection	
1. Observe skin over extremities for color, hair distribution, pallor, rubor, and swelling.	1. Extremities should be symmetrically even in color, warmth, and moisture, without swelling. Swelling of feet may occur after prolonged standing or sitting but will disappear when extremity is elevated (dependent edema).
2. Inspect for any visible vessels.	2. Faint veins may be visible, but tortuous and bulging veins may be abnormal.

Palpation	
1. Note the temperature of the skin over extremities, comparing one side to the other.	1. Temperature varies but should not be very warm or very cool.
2. Palpate pulses (radial, femoral, posterior tibial, dorsalis pedis), comparing symmetry from side to side.	2. Absence of peripheral pulses indicates peripheral vascular disease.

Left: Bickley, L. (2016). Bates' *guide to physical examination and history taking* (12th ed.). Philadelphia, PA: Lippincott Williams & Wilkins.
Right: Rosdahl, C. B., & Kowalski, M. T. (2016). *Textbook of basic nursing* (11th ed.). Philadelphia, PA: Lippincott Williams & Wilkins.

continued on following page

Adult Physical Assessment (Continued)

Technique	Findings

PERIPHERAL CIRCULATION (Continued)

Weber, J., & Kelley, J. (2006). *Health assessment in nursing* (3rd ed.). Philadelphia, PA: Lippincott Williams & Wilkins. Photograph by Barbara Proud.

3. Palpate the skin over the tibia for edema by squeezing the skin for 30 to 60 seconds. Run the pads of your fingers over the area pressed and note indentation. If indentation is noted, repeat the procedure, moving up the extremity, and note the point at which no more swelling is present.

Weber, J., & Kelley, J. (2006). *Health assessment in nursing* (3rd ed.). Philadelphia, PA: Lippincott Williams & Wilkins. Photograph by Barbara Proud.

3. Edema is usually graded from trace to 3+ or 4+ pitting. Trace is a slight indentation that disappears in a short time. Grade 3+ or 4+ is deep pitting that does not disappear readily. At best, these are subjective measurements, which are tried and confirmed through practice and comparison of findings with associates.

ABDOMEN

1. Make sure the patient has an empty bladder and is lying comfortably with arms at sides. Bend the knees to help relax the abdominal muscles if necessary.
2. Expose the abdomen fully. Make sure your hands and the stethoscope diaphragm are warm.
3. Be methodical in visualizing the underlying organs as you inspect, auscultate, percuss, and palpate each quadrant or region of the abdomen.

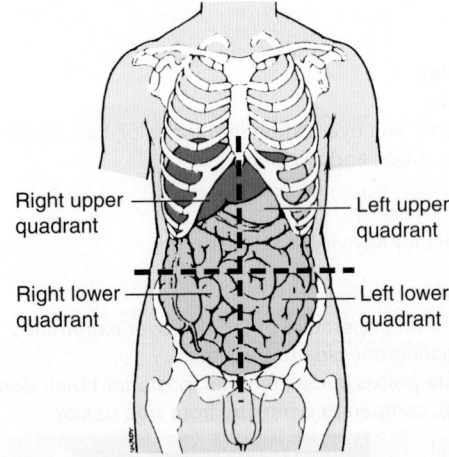

Right upper quadrant — Left upper quadrant

Right lower quadrant — Left lower quadrant

Inspection

1. Observe the general contour of the abdomen (flat, protuberant, scaphoid, or concave; local bulges). Also, note symmetry, visible peristalsis, and aortic pulsations.
2. Check the umbilicus for contour or hernia and the skin for rashes, striae, and scars.

1. The abdomen may or may not have any scars and should be flat or slightly rounded in the nonobese person. Slight pulsation may be noted.

Adult Physical Assessment (Continued)

Technique	Findings

ABDOMEN (Continued)

Auscultation

1. This is done before percussion and palpation because palpation may alter the character of bowel sounds.
2. Note the frequency and character of bowel sounds (pitch, duration).
3. Listen over the aorta, renal arteries (upper quadrants), and iliac arteries (lower quadrants) for bruits.

2. Anywhere from 5 to 35 bowel sounds per minute. May have familiar sound of "growling."
3. Bruits indicate arterial narrowing.

Percussion

1. Percussion provides a general orientation to the abdomen.
2. Proceed methodically from quadrant to quadrant, noting tympany and dullness.
3. In the right upper quadrant (RUQ) in the midclavicular line, percuss the borders of the liver.
   a. Begin at a point of tympany in the midclavicular line of the right lower quadrant (RLQ) and percuss upward to the point of dullness (the lower liver border); mark the point.
   b. Percuss downward from the point of lung resonance above the RUQ to the point of dullness (the upper border of the liver); mark the point.
   c. Measure in centimeters the distance between the two marks in the midclavicular line (the liver span).
   d. Tympany of the gastric air bubble can be percussed in the left upper quadrant over the anterior lower border of the rib cage.

2. Tympany usually predominates, possibly with scattered areas of dullness because of fluid and feces.
3. Percussion of the liver should help guide subsequent palpation. The liver border in the midclavicular line should normally range from 2½ to 4½ inches (6 to 11 cm).

Gastric gas bubble
Midclavicular line

4. Assess for an enlarged spleen by percussing the lowest interspace of the right anterior axillary line (should be tympanic). Ask the patient to take a deep breath and repeat (should still be tympanic).

4. Change in percussion note to dullness on inspiration indicates an enlarged spleen.

Palpation

1. Perform light palpation in an organized manner to detect any muscular resistance (guarding), tenderness, or superficial organs or masses.
2. Perform deep palpation to determine location, size, shape, consistency, tenderness, pulsations, and mobility of underlying organs and masses.
3. Move slowly and gently from one quadrant to the next to relax and reassure the patient.
4. Use two hands if the abdomen is obese or muscular, with one hand on top of the other. The upper hand exerts pressure downward, whereas the lower hand feels the abdomen.

1. Tenderness and involuntary guarding indicate peritoneal inflammation.
2. Rebound tenderness (pain on quick withdrawal of the fingers following palpation) suggests peritoneal irritation, as in acute appendicitis.
3. Palpate painful areas last.

continued on following page

Adult Physical Assessment (*Continued*)

Technique	Findings

ABDOMEN (*Continued*)

Liver

1. Palpate the liver by placing the left hand under the patient's lower right rib cage and the right hand on the abdomen below the level of liver dullness. Press gently inward and upward with your fingertips while the patient takes a deep breath.

1. A normal liver edge may be palpable as a smooth, sharp, regular surface. An enlarged liver will be palpable and may be tender, hard, or irregular.

Spleen

1. Place your left hand around and under the patient's left lower rib cage and press your right hand below the left costal margin inward toward the spleen while the patient takes a deep breath.

1. A normal spleen is usually not palpable. Be sure to start low enough so as not to miss the border of an enlarged spleen.

Kidney

1. Next, palpate for the left and right kidneys.

1. The kidney is usually felt only in people with very relaxed abdominal muscles (the very young, the aged, and multiparous women). The right kidney is slightly lower than the left.

2. Place the left hand under the patient's back between the rib cage and the iliac crest.

3. Support the patient while you palpate the abdomen with the right palmar surface of the fingers facing the left side of the body.

4. Palpate by bringing the left and right hands together as much as possible slightly below the level of the umbilicus on the right and left.

5. If the kidney is felt, describe its size and shape and note any tenderness.

5. The kidney is felt as a solid, firm, smooth elastic mass.

6. Costal vertebral angle tenderness is palpated with the patient sitting, usually during the examination of the posterior chest. Locate the costal vertebral angle in the flank region and strike firmly with the ulnar surface of your hand. Note any tenderness over the area.

6. There should be no costal vertebral angle tenderness. If found may indicate kidney infection.

Aorta

1. Palpate for the aorta with the thumb and index finger.

1. The aorta is soft and pulsatile.

2. Press deeply in the epigastric region (roughly in the midline) and feel with the fingers for pulsations, as well as for the contour of the aorta.

Other Findings

1. Palpation of the RLQ may reveal the part of the bowel called the *cecum*.

1. The cecum will be soft.

2. The sigmoid colon may be palpated in the lower left quadrant.

2. The sigmoid colon is ropelike and vertical and, if filled with feces, may be quite firm.

3. The inguinal and femoral areas should be palpated bilaterally for lymph nodes.

3. Often, small inguinal nodes are present; they are nontender, freely movable, and firm.

MALE GENITALIA AND HERNIAS

This part of the examination requires wearing gloves and is best done with the patient standing. (A hernia is the protrusion of a portion of the intestine through an abnormal opening.)

Inspection

1. With the groin and genitalia exposed, inspect the pubic hair distribution and the skin of the penis.

2. Retract the foreskin, if present.

2. The foreskin of the penis, if present, should be easily retractable.

Adult Physical Assessment (*Continued*)

Technique	Findings

MALE GENITALIA AND HERNIAS (*Continued*)

3. Observe the glans penis and the urethral meatus. Note any ulcers, masses, or scars.

4. Note the location of the urethral meatus and any discharge.

5. Observe the skin of the scrotum for ulcers, masses, redness, or swelling. Note size, contour, and symmetry. Lift the scrotum to inspect the posterior surface.

6. Inspect the inguinal areas and groin for bulges (with and without the patient bearing down, as though having a bowel movement).

Palpation

1. Palpate any lesions, nodules, or masses, noting tenderness, contour, size, and induration. Palpate the shaft of the penis for any induration (firmness in relation to surrounding tissues).

2. Palpate each testis and epididymis separately between the thumb and first two fingers, noting size, shape, consistency, and undue tenderness (pressure on the testis normally produces pain).

3. Palpate the spermatic cord, including the vas deferens within the cord, from the testis to the inguinal ring.

4. Palpate for inguinal hernias, using the left hand to examine the patient's left side and the right hand to examine the patient's right side.
   a. Insert the right index finger laterally, invaginating the scrotal sac to the external inguinal ring.
   b. If the external ring is large enough, insert the finger along the inguinal canal toward the internal ring and ask the patient to strain down, noting any mass that touches the finger.

5. Palpate the anterior thigh for a herniating mass in the femoral canal. Ask the patient to strain down. (The femoral canal is not palpable; it is a potential opening in the anterior thigh, medial to the femoral artery below the inguinal ligament.)

---

3. The skin of the glans penis is smooth, without ulceration.

4. The urethral meatus normally is located ventrally on the end of the penis. Normally, there is no discharge from the urethra.

5. The scrotum descends approximately 1½ inches (4 cm) in the adult; the left side is often larger than the right side.

1. There should be no nodules or tenderness.

2. The testes are usually rubbery and of approximately equal size. The epididymis is located posterolaterally on each testis and is most easily palpable on the superior portion of the testis.

3. There should be no nodules or tenderness.

4. Normally, there is no palpable herniating mass in the inguinal area.

Anterior superior spine

Inguinal ligament

External inguinal ring

Bickley, L. (2003). *Bates' guide to physical examination and history taking* (8th ed.). Philadelphia, PA: Lippincott Williams & Wilkins.

5. Ordinarily, there is no palpable mass in the femoral area.

FEMALE GENITALIA

Wearing gloves, observe the external genitalia for abnormalities such as lesions, discharge, or bulging of the vagina. Gently separate the labia to continue visual inspection, noting any tenderness.

RECTUM

Equipment

- Glove
- Lubricant

continued on following page

Adult Physical Assessment (Continued)

Technique	Findings

RECTUM (Continued)

Position patient on left side with knees drawn up toward chest and drape so that buttocks are exposed. Men may also stand and bend over the edge of the exam table with toes pointed inward. Women may be examined in lithotomy position at the end of a pelvic examination. (Change gloves to prevent cross-contamination.)

Inspection

Spread the buttocks and inspect the anus, perianal region, and sacral region for inflammation, nodules, scars, lesions, ulcerations, or rashes. Ask the patient to bear down; note any bulges.

In males and females, the perianal and sacrococcygeal areas are dry, with varying amounts of hair covering them. Anal and perianal lesions include hemorrhoids, abscesses, skin tags, and sexually transmitted genital lesions.

Palpation

1. Palpate any abnormal area noted on inspection.
2. Lubricate the index finger of the gloved hand. Rest the finger over the anus as the patient bears down, and as the sphincter relaxes, insert your finger slowly into the rectum.

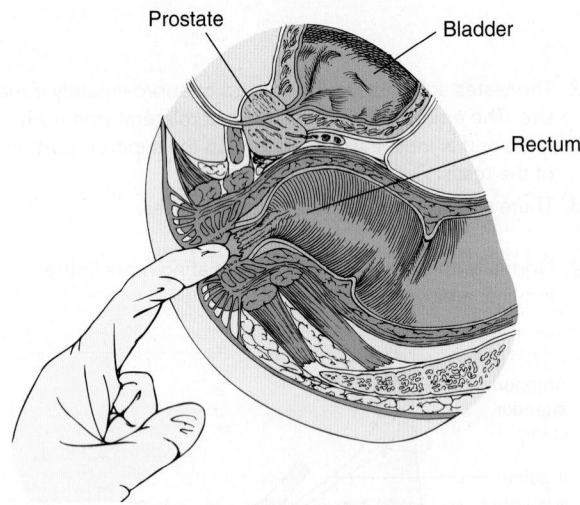

Weber, J., & Kelley, J. (2006). *Health assessment in nursing* (3rd ed.). Philadelphia, PA: Lippincott Williams & Wilkins.

3. Note sphincter tone, any nodules or masses, or tenderness.

4. Insert the finger further and palpate the walls of the rectum laterally and posteriorly while rotating your index finger. Note irregularities, masses, nodules, tenderness.
5. Anteriorly, palpate the two lateral lobes of the prostate gland in males and its median sulcus for irregularities, nodules, swelling, or tenderness.
6. If possible, palpate the superior portion of the lateral lobe, where the seminal vesicles are located. Note induration, swelling, or tenderness.
7. Just above the prostate anteriorly, the rectum lies adjacent to the peritoneal cavity. If possible, palpate this region for peritoneal masses and tenderness.
8. In the female, anteriorly, the cervix, and perhaps a retroverted uterus, may be felt.
9. Continue to insert the finger as far as possible and have the patient bear down so more of the bowel can be palpated.
10. Gently withdraw your finger. Any fecal material on the glove should be tested for occult blood.

3. The anal canal is approximately 1 inch (2.5 cm) long; it is bordered by the external and internal anal sphincters, which are normally firm and smooth.
4. The wall of the rectum in males and females is smooth and moist.

5. The male prostate gland is approximately 1 inch (2.5 cm) long, smooth, regular, nonmovable, nontender, and rubbery.
6. The seminal vesicles are generally not palpable unless swollen.

7. No masses or tenderness should be palpable.

8. Anteriorly, the cervix is round and smooth.

10. There is normally no occult blood in the stools.

Adult Physical Assessment (*Continued*)

Technique	Findings

MUSCULOSKELETAL SYSTEM

General approach

1. Examine the muscles and joints, keeping in mind the structure and functions of each.
2. Observe and palpate joints and muscles for symmetry and examine each joint individually as indicated.
3. The examination is performed with the joints both at rest and in motion, moving through a full range of motion; joints and supporting muscles and tissues are noted.

3. Joints should move freely without resistance or pain.

Inspection

1. Inspect the upper and lower extremities for size, symmetry, deformity, and muscle mass.
2. Inspect the joints for range of motion (in degrees), enlargement, redness.
3. Note gait and posture; observe the spine for range of motion, lateral curvature, or any abnormal curvature.
4. Observe the patient for signs of pain during the examination.

Palpation

1. Palpate the joints of the upper and lower extremities and the neck and back for tenderness, swelling, warmth, any bony overgrowth or deformity, and range of motion.
2. Hold the palm of your hand over the joint as it moves, or move the joint through the fullest range of motion and note any crepitation (crackling feeling within the joint).
3. Palpate the muscles for size, tone, strength, any contractures, and tenderness.
4. Palpate the spine for bony deformities and crepitation. Gently tap the spine with the ulnar surface of your fist from the cervical to the lumbar region and note any pain or tenderness.

NEUROLOGIC SYSTEM

Equipment

- Safety pin
- Cotton
- Tuning fork
- Reflex hammer
- Flashlight
- Tongue blade
- Vision screener
- Cloves, coffee, or other scented items

The screening neurologic exam or any of its components can be performed with the patient in either the sitting or supine position and may be incorporated into examination of other regions of the body. Rather than using palpation, percussion, and auscultation, the examiner uses inspection and special testing to assess the components of mental status, cranial nerves, cerebellar function, motor function, sensation, and deep tendon reflexes.

continued on following page

Adult Physical Assessment (*Continued*)

Technique	Findings

NEUROLOGIC SYSTEM (*Continued*)

Mental status

1. Determine level of consciousness by speaking the patient's name loudly and gently shaking the patient, if necessary.

2. The patient's ability to remember is also evaluated as the history is taken; ask for his or her past medical history (long-term memory) and dietary habits: "What did you eat for breakfast?" (intermediate memory).

3. Cognition and ideational content are evaluated throughout the history by what the patient says and by his or her articulateness, consistency, and reliability in reporting events.

4. Affect or mood is evaluated by observing the patient's verbal and nonverbal behavior in response to questions asked, sudden noises, and interruptions. For example, does the patient laugh or smile when talking about normally sad events, or is he or she easily startled by unexpected noises?

1. Normally, the individual is alert, knows who he or she is and where he or she lives, and can tell you the date.

2. The patient remembers recent and past events consistently and willingly admits forgetting something. Older adults often have much better long-term memory than recent memory.

3. There is no evidence of delusions or hallucinations.

4. Mood should be appropriate to the content of the conversation.

Cranial nerves (CN)

1. Test the olfactory nerve (first CN) by occluding one nostril and having the patient (with eyes closed) identify a common substance by smell; repeat on the opposite side.

2. Evaluate the optic nerve (second CN) by testing visual acuity via a Snellen chart and testing visual fields.
   a. Have the patient cover right eye with the right hand. (You cover your left eye with your left hand.)
   b. Stand approximately 2 feet (60 cm) from the patient and have him or her fix gaze on your nose.
   c. Bring two wagging fingers in from the periphery (in a plane equidistant from the patient and you) in all quadrants of the visual field and ask the patient to tell you when he or she sees your wagging fingers.

3. Test the oculomotor (3rd CN), trochlear (4th CN), and abducens (6th CN) together. They control the movements of the extraocular muscles of the eye—the superior and inferior oblique and the medial and lateral rectus muscles. The oculomotor nerve also controls pupillary constriction.
   a. Hold your index finger approximately 1 foot (30 cm) from the patient's nose. Ask the patient to hold head steady.
   b. Ask the patient to follow your finger with his or her eyes.
   c. Move your finger to the right as far as the patient's eye moves. Before bringing your finger back to the center, move it up and then down so that the patient glances up and peripherally and then down and peripherally.
   d. Repeat the test, moving your finger to the left.

4. Test the trigeminal nerve (5th CN). which controls muscles of mastication and has a sensory component that controls sensations of the face.
   a. Test the motor component by having the patient clench teeth while palpating the temporal and masseter muscles of the jaws with both hands.
   b. Test the sensory component by having the patient close eyes and touch one side of the face then the other (forehead, cheek, chin). (Always demonstrate to the patient how you are testing sensation—to avoid startling the patient and to encourage cooperation.)

5. Test the facial nerve (7th CN) by observing facial expression and symmetry of facial movement. Ask the patient to frown, close eyes, and smile.

1. The patient should be able to identify common smells such as cinnamon and coffee.

2. Normal vision (with glasses or contact lenses) is at or near 20/20. Assuming your visual fields are grossly normal, the patient and you should see the wagging fingers approximately simultaneously. (The patient's peripheral vision should approximate the examiner's.)

a. Muscle strength in the face should be present and should be symmetric.

b. Sensation should be present and symmetrical.

5. The facial muscles should look symmetric when the patient frowns, closes eyes, and smiles. Notice particularly the symmetry of the nasolabial folds.

Adult Physical Assessment (Continued)

Technique	Findings

NEUROLOGIC SYSTEM (Continued)

6. Evaluate the acoustic nerve (8th CN) cochlear branch by testing hearing (see page 48) and vestibular branch by performing the Romberg test for equilibrium. Have the patient stand erect with eyes closed and feet close together.

7. Test the glossopharyngeal (9th CN) and vagus nerve (10th CN) together (they both have a motor portion innervating the pharynx).
   a. Ask the patient to say "ah" and observe the movement of the uvula and palate (10th CN).
   b. Gently use a tongue blade to check the presence of the gag reflex (9th CN).

8. Evaluate the spinal accessory nerve (11th CN), which mediates the sternocleidomastoid and upper portion of the trapezius muscles.
   a. Ask the patient to turn head to the side against resistance while you apply pressure to the jaw.
   b. Palpate the sternocleidomastoid muscle on the opposite side.
   c. Have the patient shrug shoulders while you place your hands on his or her shoulders and apply slight pressure.

9. Evaluate the hypoglossal nerve (12th CN), which innervates muscles of the tongue by noting articulation and by having the patient stick out the tongue, noting any deviation or asymmetry.

Cerebellar function

1. Observe posture and gait.
2. Ask the patient to walk forward (and then backward) in a straight line.
3. To test for muscle coordination in the lower extremities, have the patient run the right heel down the left shin and vice versa.
4. To test coordination in upper extremities, have the patient close eyes and touch the nose with the index finger (starting position: arms outstretched) first left, then right, in rapid succession.

Motor function

1. Evaluate muscle mass, tone, strength, and any abnormal movements (tics, fasciculations, twitching). May be done with musculoskeletal exam.
   a. Test muscle tone by noting the resistance the muscle offers to movement on passive motion.

   b. Test muscle strength by asking the patient to actively resist your movement to flex or extend their various muscle groups. Grade muscle strength as follows: 0 = no muscle contraction, 1 = faint muscle contraction, 2 = active movement of body part with gravity eliminated, 3 = active movement against gravity, 4 = active movement against gravity and some resistance, 5 = active movement against full resistance without fatigue.

Findings

6. Slight swaying may occur, but the patient should not fall. (Stand close to the patient so you can assist if he or she begins to fall.)

   a. The palate and uvula should move symmetrically without deviation.
   b. The gag reflex should be present, and there should be no difficulty in swallowing.

8. Neck and shoulder muscle strength should be symmetric.

9. The patient should speak clearly and tongue should be symmetric and should not deviate.

2. The patient should be able to perform all the tests described with smooth, even movement and without losing balance.

4. The normal person can do this with rapid, smooth movements without undershooting or overshooting the target.

Normally, abnormal movements are not present either at rest or with movement.

   a. Generally, there is slight resistance to passive movement of muscles as opposed to flaccidity (no resistance) or rigidity (increased muscle tone).
   b. Strength will vary from person to person, but 5 on a scale of 0 to 5 is considered normal. It should be equal bilaterally.

continued on following page

Adult Physical Assessment (*Continued*)

Technique	Findings

NEUROLOGIC SYSTEM (*Continued*)

Sensory function

1. Test sensitivity to light touch (cotton), pain (pinprick), vibration (tuning fork), and discrimination. Compare both sides of the body.

   a. Ask the patient to close eyes. Brush the skin with a piece of cotton (on the back of hands, forearms, upper arms, dorsal portion of foot laterally and medially, and along the tibia and thigh laterally and medially). Ask the patient to indicate when he or she feels the cotton and to compare the sensation bilaterally.

    a. Patient should feel light touch bilaterally.

   b. Use a safety pin; touch the skin as lightly as possible to elicit a sharp sensation. (Alternately, temperature discrimination can be tested.)

    b. Pain should be felt bilaterally, or warm and cold can be differentiated.

   c. Test vibration sense by placing a vibrating tuning fork on a distal interphalangeal joint of the finger, then of the great toe, and ask if they feel vibration. If they are unable to feel vibration, move proximally to the next bony prominence. (Alternately, position sense can be tested by moving a toe up or down.)

    c. The patient should be able to detect vibration or position if there is no peripheral neuropathy. (If the patient is unsure if they can feel vibration, touch the fork to stop vibration and ask the patient to tell you when it stops).

   d. Test discrimination (which also depends on an intact cortex) by placing a small object such as a paper clip in the hand (stereognosis), using the blunt end of a pen to draw a number in the palm (graphesthesia), or using an open paper clip to touch the skin with 1 or 2 points alternately (two-point discrimination).

    d. The patient should be able to identify object, number, or one- or two-point stimulation.

Deep tendon reflexes

1. Make sure the patient is relaxed and extremity is supported for all reflex testing. If the patient is not relaxed and you cannot elicit reflexes, have the patient grasp hands and contract arm muscles to relax the lower extremities or tap feet on the floor to relax the upper extremities.

    1. Amplitude of the reflex may vary for different tendons but is equal bilaterally.

2. Test biceps reflex by striking indirectly.

   a. Place your right thumb on the patient's right biceps tendon (located in the antecubital fossa) with the patient's arm slightly flexed.

   b. Strike your thumb with the pointed end of the hammer head. Hold the hammer loosely so it pivots in your hand when it is moved with a wrist action.

   c. Strike your thumb with the least amount of pressure needed to elicit the reflex.

    c. The forearm may move, and your thumb should feel the tendon jerk.

3. Test the triceps tendon by using the pointed end of the hammer.

Adult Physical Assessment (*Continued*)

Technique	Findings

NEUROLOGIC SYSTEM (*Continued*)

    a. Have the patient hang arm freely while you support it with your nondominant hand or rest the slightly flexed arm in the patient's lap.

    b. With the elbow flexed, strike the tendon directly, using the pointed end of the hammer.

4. Test the brachioradialis tendon by striking the forearm with the flat end of the hammer about 1 inch (2.5 cm) above the wrist over the radius.

5. Test the quadriceps reflex by having the patient sit with legs hanging over the edge of the table or lay down while you support the legs at the knee (slightly bent), and strike the tendon with the pointed end of the hammer just above the patella.

b. The forearm should move slightly.

4. There should be slight flexion and supination of the forearm.

Bickley, L. (2016). *Bates' guide to physical examination and history taking* (12th ed.). Philadelphia, PA: Lippincott Williams & Wilkins. Photograph by Barbara Proud.

6. The foot should move downward into your hand.

6. Test the Achilles reflex by supporting the foot in dorsiflexed position and tapping the Achilles tendon with the flat end of the hammer.

Lynn, P. (2010). *Taylor's Clinical Nursing Skills* (3rd ed.). Philadelphia, PA: Lippincott Williams & Wilkins. Photograph by Barbara Proud.

7. Stroke the sole of the patient's foot with a flat object such as a tongue blade to test the plantar reflex.

7. Toes normally flex. Dorsiflexion of the great toe and fanning of the other toes is known as a positive Babinski response and indicates a central nervous system problem.

SELECTED REFERENCES

Bickley, L. S. (2016). *Bates' guide to physical examination and history taking* (12th ed.). Philadelphia, PA: Wolters Kluwer.

Bijur, P. E., Shah, P. D., & Esses, D. (2016). Temperature measurement in the adult emergency department. *Emergency Medicine Journal, 33*(12), 843–847.

Ewing, J. A. (1984). Detecting alcoholism: The CAGE questionnaire. *Journal of the American Medical Association, 252*(14), 1905–1907.

Jarvis, C. (2015). *Physical examination and health assessment* (7th ed.). Philadelphia, PA: Elsevier.

Jensen, S. (2014). *Nursing health assessment: A best practice approach* (2nd ed.). Philadelphia, PA: Lippincott Williams & Wilkins.

Johnstone, C., (2018). How to undertake a nutritional assessment in adults. *Nursing Standard, 32*(22), 41–45.

Lippincott Williams & Wilkins. (2010). *Professional guide to signs and symptoms* (6th ed.). Philadelphia, PA: Author.

Lippincott Williams & Wilkins. (2012). *Assessment made incredibly easy* (5th ed.). Philadelphia, PA: Author.

Niven, D. J., Gaudet, J. E., Laupland, K. B., Mrklas, K. J., Roberts, D. J., & Stelfox, H. T. (2015). Accuracy of peripheral thermometers for estimating temperature: A systematic review and meta-analysis. *Annals of Internal Medicine, 163*(10), 768–777.

Osborne, S., Douglas, C., Reid, C., et al. (2015). The primacy of vital signs–Acute care nurses' and midwives' use of physical assessment skills: A cross sectional study. *International Journal of Nursing Studies, 52*(5), 951–962.

Sliwinski, M., Mogle, J., Hyun, J., Munoz, E., Smyth, J., & Lipton, R., (2018). Reliability and Validity of Ambulatory Cognitive Assessments. *Assessment, 25*(1), 14–30.

Wald, A., & Garber, C., (2018). A Review of Current Literature on Vital Sign Assessment of Physical Activity in Primary Care. *Journal of Nursing Scholarship, 50*(1), 65–73.

6

Intravenous Therapy

GENERAL CONSIDERATIONS

Goals

The goals of intravenous (IV) therapy are to:
1. Provide hydration and/or correction of electrolyte imbalances in the patient who cannot maintain an adequate oral intake.
2. Administer safe and effective infusions of medications by using the appropriate vascular access.
3. Administer blood components and/or blood products.
4. Provide for invasive patient hemodynamic monitoring.
5. Provide nutrition while resting the GI tract.

Physiologic Assimilation of Infusion Solutions

Principles

1. Tissue cells (such as epithelial cells) are surrounded by a semipermeable membrane.
2. Cell membrane permeability refers to the ability of the cellular membrane to allow substances such as water to pass freely, whereas charged ions, such as sodium, cannot cross the membrane and are trapped on one side.
3. Osmotic pressure is the "pulling" pressure demonstrated when water moves through the semipermeable membrane of tissue cells from an area of weaker concentration to stronger concentration of solute (eg, sodium ions and blood glucose). The end result is dilution and equilibration between the intracellular and extracellular compartments.
4. Total body water (TBW), depending slightly on age, gender, and race, comprise 45% to 60% of a person's weight. Total body water is the sum of intracellular fluid (about 2/3 TBW) and extracellular fluid volume (about 1/3 TBW). Extracellular fluid volume (EFV) is a composition of interstitial fluid (about 2/3 of EFV) and intravascular volume (about 1/3 of EFV).
5. Extracellular compartment fluids primarily include plasma and interstitial fluid.

Types of Intravenous Fluids

Intravenous fluids include colloids and crystalloids. See Table 6-1.
1. Colloid solutions contain large proteins or molecules that cannot pass through the cellular semipermeable membrane. Colloids increase intravascular volume by drawing fluid into the intravascular space via oncotic pressure. Common natural colloids include red blood cells, plasma, and albumin. Common synthetic colloids include dextran and hetastarch.
2. Crystalloid fluid contains electrolytes but lack large proteins and molecules. Crystalloid fluid is capable of passing through a semipermeable membrane. Classified according to their "tonicity," crystalloids are isotonic, hypotonic, or hypertonic solutions.

Isotonic

A solution that exerts the same osmotic pressure as that found in plasma. This fluid will distribute evenly between the intravascular and intracellular space. This type of fluid is typically administered to replace extracellular fluid losses to expand intravascular volume.
1. 0.9% sodium chloride solution (normal saline, NS).
2. Lactated Ringer solution (LR).
3. Dextrose 5% in water (D_5W).

Hypotonic

A solution that exerts less osmotic pressure than that of blood plasma. Administration of this fluid generally causes dilution of plasma solute concentration and forces water to move into cells to reestablish intracellular and extracellular equilibrium; cells will then rehydrate.
1. 0.45% sodium chloride solution (half NS).
2. 0.33% sodium chloride solution (one-third NS).

Hypertonic

A solution that exerts a higher osmotic pressure than that of blood plasma. Administration of this fluid increases the solute concentration of plasma, drawing water out of the cells and into the extracellular compartment to restore osmotic equilibrium; cells will then shrink.
1. D_5W in lactated Ringer solution (D_5LR).
2. D_5W in normal saline solution.
3. D_5W in 0.45% (half normal) saline solution (only slightly hypertonic because dextrose is rapidly metabolized and renders only temporary osmotic pressure).

Table 6-1	Composition of Selected Intravenous Solutions						
SOLUTION	**TONICITY**	**NA⁺ (MEQ/L)**	**K⁺ (MEQ/L)**	**CL⁻ (MEQ/L)**	**CA⁺⁺ (MEQ/L)**	**BUFFER**	**PH**
Lactated Ringer (LR)*	Isotonic	130	4	109	3	28 lactate	6.5
0.9% normal saline (NS)	Isotonic	154	0	154	0	0	—
D5W	Isotonic	0	0	0	0	0	4.5
D5LR	Slightly hypertonic	130	4	109	3	28 lactate	5
D5NS	Hypertonic	154	0	154	0	0	4
3% NS	Hypertonic	513	0	513	0	0	—
0.45% NS	Hypotonic	77	—	7	—	0	5.3
5% D and 0.45% NS†	Slightly hypertonic	77	—	77	—	0	4

*Lactate converts to bicarbonate in the liver.
†5% dextrose metabolizes rapidly in the blood and, in reality, produces minimal osmotic effects.
DW, dextrose in water; NS, normal saline.

4. Dextrose 10% in water ($D_{10}W$).
5. Dextrose 20% in water ($D_{20}W$).
6. 3% or 5% sodium chloride solution.
7. Hyperalimentation solutions.

Uses and Precautions with Common Types of Infusions

See Table 6-2, for signs and symptoms of water excess or deficit.
1. D_5W.
   a. Used to replace water (hypotonic fluid) losses, supply some caloric intake, or administer as carrying solution for numerous medications.
   b. Should be used cautiously in patients with water intoxication (hyponatremia, syndrome of inappropriate antidiuretic hormone release).
   c. Should not be used as concurrent solution infusion with blood or blood components.
2. Normal saline solution (0.9% NS or NaCl).
   a. Commonly used resuscitative crystalloid used to replace isotonic fluid losses, administer with blood components, or treat patients in hemodynamic shock.
   b. Should be used cautiously in patients with isotonic volume excess such as heart or renal failure patients; monitor for hyperchloremic acidosis with resuscitation uses.
   c. Inexpensive.
3. Lactated Ringer solution (LR).
   a. Commonly used resuscitative crystalloid used to replace fluid losses, replenish specific electrolyte losses, and moderate metabolic acidosis.
   b. Use cautiously in patients with liver failure.
4. Hypertonic saline solution (3% NS or NaCl).
   a. Acts as a plasma volume expander by increasing the movement of intracellular and interstitial water into the intravascular space.
   b. Risk of hypernatremia and requires careful monitoring, particularly of patient's neurologic status.

TYPES OF INTRAVENOUS MEDICATION ADMINISTRATION

There are three intravenous routes of administration: bolus or "IV push," intermittent infusion, and continuous infusion.

IV "Push" (Bolus)

IV "push" (or *IV bolus*) refers to the administration of a medication from a syringe directly into an ongoing IV infusion or may be given directly into a vein by way of an intermittent access device (saline or heparin lock).

Table 6-2	Signs and Symptoms of Water Excess or Deficit	
SITE	**WATER EXCESS**	**WATER DEFICIT**
Central nervous system	• Muscle twitching • Hyperactive tendon reflexes • Convulsions • Increased intracranial pressure, coma	• Sleepiness • Apathy • Restlessness • Weakness • Delirium • Coma
Cardiovascular	• Elevated venous pressure • Increased cardiac output • High pulse pressure • Heart gallop • Rales, pulmonary edema	• Tachycardia • Orthostatic hypotension, hypotension • Flat neck veins • Cool, clammy skin
Gastrointestinal	• Anorexia, nausea, and vomiting • Edema of stomach, colon, and mesentery	• Anorexia • Thirst • Silent ileus
Tissues	• Increased salivation, tears • Watery diarrhea • Subcutaneous pitting edema	• Decreased saliva and tears • Dry, sticky mucous membranes • Red, swollen tongue • Flushed skin • Decreased skin turgor • Sunken eyes
Other	• None	• Decreased temperature

Indications

1. When a rapid concentration of a medication in the patient's bloodstream is needed (eg, cardiopulmonary resuscitative procedures).
2. When quicker response from a medication is required (eg, furosemide or digoxin).
3. To administer "loading" doses of a drug that will be continued by way of infusion (eg, heparin, pain medications).
4. To reduce patient discomfort by limiting the need for intramuscular injections.
5. To avoid incompatibility problems that may occur when several medications are mixed in one bottle/bag.
6. To deliver medications or solutions to patients unable to take them orally (eg, unresponsive patients) or intramuscularly (eg, coagulation disorder).
7. Cost-effective method—no need for extra tubing or syringe pump.

Precautions and Recommendations

1. Before medication administration, review order and confirm patient identification and allergies. Be familiar with facility policies and guidelines regarding how, where, and by whom IV push medications or solutions can be given.
2. Use aseptic technique when preparing and administering IV push medications and accessing the vascular device.
3. Determine the correct (safest) rate of administration. Consult the pharmacy or pharmaceutical text. Most medications are given slowly (rarely in less than 1 minute); sometimes as long as 30 minutes is required. Too rapid administration may result in serious adverse effects.
4. Dilute the drug as indicated by manufacturer or pharmacy references with the appropriate dilutant. Many medications are irritating to veins and require sufficient dilution. Caution during this process because of the associated increased risk for medication errors and contamination of sterile IV medications or solutions.
5. If withdrawing IV push medications from a glass ampule, use a filter needle or straw unless the specific drug precludes their use. Unless the medication or solution is prepared at the patient's bedside for immediate administration without any break in the process, appropriately label all nurse-prepared syringes of IV push medications or solutions.
6. Perform an appropriate assessment of the patient. This includes an evaluation of the prescribed therapy for the patient's age and clinical condition, rights of medication administration (right patient, medication name, dose, route, time), and reason for medication or solution treatment. Assess the vascular site and ensure patency of the IV line by aspirating for positive blood return and encountering no resistance when manually flushing the vascular access device. Ascertain the dwell time of the catheter. For infusion of vesicants, a catheter placement of 24 hours or less is advisable.
7. If your facility uses barcode technology, scan your identification (ID) badge, the patient's ID bracelet, and the medication's barcode.
8. If IV push is to be given with an ongoing IV infusion or to follow another IV push medication, check pharmacy for possible incompatibility. It is always wise to flush the IV tubing or cannula with saline before and after administration of a drug.
9. Use a needleless connector that is closest to the patient to allow the medication or solution to reach the central circulation as soon as possible with a minimal amount of flushing.

Needleless connectors protect health care providers by eliminating the need for needles and subsequent needlestick injuries when attaching syringes and/or administration sets to the vascular access device.

10. Monitor the patient's reaction to the medication during and after administration.
    a. Be alert for major adverse effects, such as anaphylaxis, respiratory distress, tachycardia, bradycardia, or seizures. If this occurs, stop the medication and notify the health care provider. Institute emergency procedures as necessary.
    b. Assess for minor adverse effects, such as nausea, flushing, skin rash, or confusion. If this occurs, stop medication and notify the health care provider.

 NURSING ALERT Unless its use would result in a clinically significant delay and potential patient harm (eg, medication administration during cardiopulmonary resuscitation), barcode scanning or similar technology is recommended immediately prior to medication or solution administration as an effective error reduction strategy.

11. Monitor the vascular access site for any signs of infiltration or extravasation.

Intermittent Infusions

Intermittent intravenous infusions are a medication or solution administered over a set period of time at prescribed intervals. An intermittent infusion may be given through an intermittent access device (saline lock) or "piggybacked" to a continuous IV infusion as a secondary medication.

Intermittent Access Device (Saline Lock)

1. This intermittent infusion device permits the administration of periodic IV medications and solution without continuous fluid administration.
2. Needleless connectors protect health care providers by eliminating the need for needles and subsequent needlestick injuries when attaching syringes and/or administrations sets to the vascular access device.
3. Prepare for medication or solution administration by confirming patient and order as required by facility procedure and perform appropriate hand hygiene.
4. Provide patient education regarding medication or solution. Encourage patient to report any discomfort at the IV site including pain, burning sensation, or swelling noted.
5. Maintain aseptic technique throughout the procedure.
6. Ensure patency of saline lock with normal saline flush prior to administration of medication or solution. Do not force if resistance is felt.
7. When administering the medication or solution, use a timer with a second hand to inject according to facility policy and manufacturer recommendations. Use a push–pause method to inject the medication.
8. After administration of the medication or solution, flush the saline lock with normal saline at the same rate as the medication administration to ensure that all medication remaining in the saline lock or extension tubing is administered at the appropriate rate and to prevent future contact incompatibilities.
9. Observe for expected therapeutic effect and potential adverse effects.

NURSING ALERT Medication errors are often a result of calculation errors, drug preparation errors, human errors, and transcription inaccuracy. Unusual dosages or unfamiliar medication or solutions should always be confirmed with the health care provider and pharmacist before administration. Ultimately, the nurse is accountable for the medication or solutions administered.

Secondary Medication Administration ("Piggyback")

1. Means of administering a medication or solution by way of an established primary infusion line.
2. Needleless connectors protect health care providers by eliminating the need for needles and subsequent needlestick injuries when attaching syringes and/or administration sets to the vascular access device.
3. Prepare for medication or solution administration by confirming patient and order as required by facility procedure and perform appropriate hand hygiene.
4. Provide patient education regarding medication or solution. Encourage patient to report any discomfort at the IV site including pain, burning sensation, or swelling noted.
5. Maintain aseptic technique throughout the procedure.
6. Prime the secondary tubing and use the extension hook.
   a. If using gravity infusion, hang the secondary medication higher than the primary IV solution bag. Use the roller clamp or flow regulators to calculate infusion rate.
   b. If using an electronic infusion device, set an appropriate rate.
7. When a backcheck valve is present on the primary tubing, it:
   a. Permits the primary infusion to flow after the medication has been administered.
   b. Prevents air from entering the system.
   c. Prevents secondary fluid from "running dry."
   d. Permits less mixing of primary fluid with secondary solution.
8. Always select the assess port closest to the insertion site of the vascular access device.
9. Use of an electronic infusion device or flow regulator will permit rate changes between primary and secondary infusions.
10. Never administer a solution or medication through a continuous IV line that is infusing blood, blood products, heparin IV, insulin IV, cytotoxic medications, or parenteral nutrition solutions.
11. A volume-controlled intermittent set is a device attached below the primary infusion to regulate the secondary medication or solution. These devices are used most often for children, older adults, or critically ill patients where fluid volume is a concern.

Continuous Infusion

Continuous infusion is the IV infusion of a medication or solution over several hours to days. Use of an electronic infusion device with dose-error technology is recommended.

1. Prepare for medication or solution administration by confirming patient and order as required by facility procedure and perform appropriate hand hygiene.
2. Provide patient education regarding medication or solution. Encourage patient to report any discomfort at the IV site including pain, burning sensation, or swelling noted.
3. Maintain aseptic technique throughout the procedure.

Use of Infusion Control Devices

Infusion control devices allow for the infusion of large and small volumes of IV solution or medication with accuracy over a determined time period at prescribed intervals, reducing the risk of rapid infusion. Use of infusion control devices should be based on the needs and factors of the patient, type of vascular access device, and health care setting. Electronic infusion devices with dose-error reduction systems are preferred. The nurse must be competent in the use of all available equipment.

Types

Manual Control Flow Regulator
1. Delivers a prescribed fluid volume per hour.
2. To be used for lower-risk infusions.
3. Nonautomated and requires manual adjustment of a regulator clamp to administer correct flow rate.

Electronic Infusion Devices
1. Deliver a prescribed fluid volume per hour.
2. Often, incorporate dose-error reduction technologies to minimize adverse patient situations.
3. Divided into large-volume and small-volume devices.
4. Indicated for continuous infusions of chemotherapy, hyperalimentation, fluid and electrolytes in patients at risk for fluid overload, infant and pediatric therapies, and most medications.
5. Some electronic infusion devices are designed to be used at a patient's bedside, whereas other, called ambulatory infusion pumps, are designed to be portable or wearable.

Blood and Fluid Warmers
Used when attempting to avoid or treat hypothermia, during cardiopulmonary bypass, when the patient is known to have cold agglutinins, or during replacement of large blood volumes.

Power Injectors
1. Used to deliver specific amounts of contrast media at a specified rate/time during radiological diagnostic procedures. Radiological contrast media are to be considered vesicant solutions with the potential to cause severe tissue injury in the setting of infiltration/extravasation.
2. Vascular access device must be able to withstand pressure of 300 psi or greater to be compatible with power injectors.

Nursing Responsibilities

1. Continuous or intermittent infusions must be monitored by the nurse to ensure accurate delivery.
2. Follow the manufacturer's instructions carefully when using administration tubing sets or inserting tubing into an electronic infusion device.
3. Eliminate all air from the administration tubing set before connecting it to the patient's vascular access device.
4. Continue to check the patient regularly for complications, such as infiltration or infection, and not rely solely on the electronic infusion device pressure alarms.
5. Ensure that infusion therapy is initiated, changed, or discontinued based upon the order of the prescribing health care provider.
6. Explain the purpose of the device and the alarm system to the patient and/or caregivers. Added machines in the room can evoke greater anxiety in the patient and family.
7. For rapid administration of solutions and blood or blood products, avoid using needleless connectors. Instead connect directly to the hub of the vascular access device because needleless connectors can greatly reduce flow rates.
8. Adhere to all manufacturers' guidelines regarding product use.

Vascular Access Device Selection

Selecting the appropriate vascular access device is based on the needs of the patient, particularly the prescribed therapy and duration of therapy, as well as characteristics of the patient including age, comorbidities, and vascular characteristics.

Short Peripheral Catheters

1. These catheters are inserted into the dorsal and ventral surfaces of the upper extremities, including the metacarpal, cephalic, basilic, and median veins.
2. These catheters are intended for short-term therapy—typically less than 6 days.
3. The smallest gauge short peripheral catheter that can accommodate the prescribed therapies and patient's needs should be selected.
4. Therapies not appropriate for short peripheral catheters include continuous vesicant therapy, parenteral nutrition, and infusions with a pH less than 5 or greater than 9 or with an osmolality greater than 600 mOsm/L.

Midline Catheters

1. These catheters are inserted into the basilic, cephalic, or median cubital veins and extend 3 to 8 inches (7.5 to 20 cm) up the arm with the proximal tip resting in the upper arm just distal to the axillary arch.
2. Per manufacturing guidelines, may need to be routinely replaced every 28 to 30 days.
3. They are considered deep peripheral and not appropriate for continuous vesicant therapy such as hyperosmolar solutions, parenteral nutrition, and some antibiotics, such as erythromycin and nafcillin, as well as infusions with a pH less than 5 or greater than 9 or with an osmolality greater than 600 mOsm/L.
4. Avoid use in patients with a history of thrombosis, hypercoagulability, and decreased venous flow or in the setting of vein preservation such as with end-stage renal disease.
5. Ultrasound guidance is recommended to decrease the risks of cannulation failure, arterial puncture, hematoma, and pulmonary complications.

 NURSING ALERT Avoid placing vascular access devices in the veins of an upper extremity on the same side as a previous breast surgery with axillary lymph node dissection, after radiation therapy to that side, in the setting of lymphedema, or in an extremity affected by cerebrovascular accident, because risk is greater for infectious and thrombotic complication.

Central Venous Access Devices

Indications

1. Physiologic instability of the patient and/or complexity of infusion therapies.
2. Continuous vesicant or irritant therapy, chemotherapy, or parenteral nutrition medication.
3. Invasive hemodynamic monitoring.
4. History of difficult peripheral venous access because of extensive previous IV therapy, surgery, or previous tissue damage where vascular site selection is limited or the use of ultrasound guidance has failed.
5. Long-term IV therapy—weeks, months, or years.

Types

See Figure 6-1.

1. Central catheter—nontunneled; commonly called *percutaneous*.
   a. Has one to four lumens.
   b. Dwell time usually less than 1 month.
   c. May be inserted in femoral, jugular, or subclavian veins. To minimize the risk of catheter-related infections and thrombotic complications in adult patients, the subclavian vein is preferred. However, in patients with advanced kidney disease, the subclavian site to prevent subclavian stenosis and preserve the site for hemodialysis.
   d. Ultrasound guidance is recommended to decrease the risks of cannulation failure, arterial puncture, hematoma, and pulmonary complications.

 NURSING ALERT Prior to the initiation of medication or solution therapy, ensure the appropriate placement of all central vascular catheters radiographically or by other imaging technology.

2. Central catheter—tunneled.
   a. A tunneled catheter is inserted into a central vein (usually the subclavian, then the superior vena cava) and subcutaneously tunneled to an exit site approximately 4 inches (10 cm) from the insertion site.
   b. A Dacron cuff is located approximately ¾ to 1 inch (2 to 3 cm) from the exit site, providing a barrier against microorganisms.
   c. Examples of the tunneled catheters in current use are Hickman™, Broviac™, and Groshong™.
3. Peripheral inserted central catheter (PICC).
   a. Inserted in basilic, median cubital, brachial, or cephalic veins in adult patients; additional sites are available in neonate and pediatric patients.
   b. PICCs placed in the median cubital vein tend to follow the cephalic vein to central placement. Observe carefully for pain and tenderness because the cephalic vein is smaller than the basilic.
   c. Used in patients in acute, long-term, and home care settings.
   d. May be inserted by nurses with special training or interventional radiologists.
   e. PICC tip placement must be located in superior vena cava (verified by x-ray). Tip placement in subclavian or innominate vein contraindicated for hyperosmolar solutions (hyperalimentation).
   f. Ultrasound guidance is recommended for placement to improve first-attempt success and decrease adverse events.
   g. PICC insertion site and hub should be covered by a transparent dressing.
   h. Extension tubing must be clamped when no solution is being infused. Tape it securely to the patient's arm.
   i. Measure upper arm circumference before and after insertion and as clinically indicated to assess for edema and possible infiltration/extravasation or deep vein thrombosis. Take this measurement 10 cm above the antecubital fossa. Positive pressure flushing will keep PICC from clotting.
4. Central implanted vascular device.
   a. A subcutaneous pocket is formed and a reservoir is placed; a catheter is attached to the reservoir and tunneled subcutaneously and inserted into a central vein (usually, the

Figure 6-1. Types of central venous catheters for long-term venous access. **(A)** Implantable venous access port. **(B)** Peripherally inserted central catheter (PICC). **(C)** Tunneled central venous catheter.

catheter tip is in the superior vena cava). This device cannot be seen exteriorly.

b. Central implanted vascular devices are typically used in patients who require intermittent long-term infusion therapy such as with chemotherapy.

c. Examples of implanted devices in current use include the Port-A-Cath™, Mediport™, Infuse-A-Port™, Bard Port systems, and Groshong Port™.

 NURSING ALERT If central catheters are placed too deeply and extend into the right atrium, an irregular heartbeat may result. Monitor heart rhythm and notify the health care provider immediately.

 EVIDENCE BASE Infusion Nursing Society (INS). (2016). Infusion therapy standards of practice nursing standards of practice. *Journal of Infusion Nursing, 349*(1S).

Alternative Infusion Devices

1. Intraspinal access devices
   a. Access devices placed in the epidural, intrathecal, or ventricular spaces.
   b. Anticipate intraspinal infusion administration that requires pain management, chemotherapies, or spasticity control.
   c. Administer only preservative-free medications or solutions.
2. Intraosseous (IO) access devices
   a. Access devices placed in the marrow of the bone.

b. Anticipate intraosseous infusion for emergent and nonemergent use in patients with limited or no vascular access.

3. Subcutaneous access devices
   a. Anticipate subcutaneous access for administration of isotonic solutions for treatment of mild to moderate dehydration or continuous opioid administration.
   b. Use hyaluronidase to facilitate the dispersion and absorption of medications or solutions in adults and pediatric patients.

NURSING ROLE IN INTRAVENOUS THERAPY

Initiating an IV Line

Intravenous therapy is an invasive procedure and should be ordered only when necessary. Nurses must be familiar with the procedure as well as the equipment involved in initiating an IV to provide effective therapy and prevent complications. See Standards of Care Guidelines 6-1, page 76.

 See additional online content: Procedure Guidelines 6-1–6-4.

Selecting a Vein

1. Verify the order for IV therapy and explain the procedure to the patient.

STANDARDS OF CARE GUIDELINES 6-1
IV Therapy

To prevent adverse effects of IV therapy, perform the following assessments and procedures:

- Before starting IV therapy, consider the indication for intravenous therapy including duration of therapy, type of infusion, condition of veins, and medical condition of the patient to assist in choosing IV site and type of catheter.
- Ensure competence in initiating the type of IV therapy to be utilized and familiarity with facility policy and procedure before initiating therapy.
- After initiation of IV therapy, monitor the patient frequently for:
  - Signs of infiltration or sluggish flow.
  - Signs of phlebitis or infection.
- Correct solution, medication, volume, and rate.
- Dwell time of catheter and need to be replaced.
- Condition of catheter dressing and frequency of change.
- Fluid and electrolyte balance.
- Signs of fluid overload or dehydration.
- Patient satisfaction with mode of therapy.

This information should serve as a general guideline only. Each patient situation presents a unique set of clinical factors and requires nursing judgment to guide care, which may include additional or alternative measures and approaches.

---

2. Select a vein suitable for venipuncture.
   a. Back of hand—metacarpal veins (see Figure 6-2A). Avoid digital veins, if possible.
      i. Advantages: Veins in location are easily visualized and palpated. Selection of this site permits arm movement. Should successive venipuncture be needed, another location higher up the arm may be utilized.
      ii. Disadvantages: Caution when selecting this site in the older adult because of thin skin and inadequate tissue often occurring in this area. When possible, select the nondominant hand.
   b. Forearm—basilic (along the ulnar side of the forearm) or cephalic (along the radial side of the forearm) vein (see Figure 6-2B).
      i. Advantages: These are larger veins that allow for more rapid infusion. Hand can be used freely.
      ii. Disadvantages:

   c. Inner aspect of elbow, antecubital fossa—intermediate median basilic and intermediate median cephalic; used for relatively short-term infusion.
      i. Advantages: Well supported by subcutaneous tissue preventing vein mobility; deeper and more tolerant to caustic substances.
      ii. Disadvantages: Prevents bending of arm; median basilic and cephalic veins are not recommended for chemotherapy because of the potential for extravasation and poor healing, resulting in impaired joint movement; should be reserved for intermediate- or long-term indwelling catheters.

> **! NURSING ALERT** Avoid selecting areas of flexion for placement of intravascular access. Areas of flexion are at an increased risk for adverse events because of the superficial presentation of arteries and nerves and are more likely to result in infiltration/extravasation, thrombophlebitis, arterial puncture, and nerve injury.

Posterior (dorsal)

- Accessory cephalic vein
- Cephalic vein
- Basilic vein
- Dorsal venous arch
- Dorsal metacarpal veins
- Intercapitular veins

A

Anterior (palmar)

- Cephalic vein
- Accessory cephalic vein
- Intermediate (median) cephalic vein
- Cephalic vein
- Intermediate (median) antebrachial vein
- Basilic vein
- Intermediate (median) basilic vein
- Perforating veins

B

Figure 6-2. **(A)** Superficial veins, dorsal aspect of the hand. **(B)** Superficial veins, forearm. (Smeltzer, S., and Bare, B. [2000]. Brunner and Suddarth's textbook of medical-surgical nursing [9th ed.]. Philadelphia, PA: Lippincott Williams & Wilkins.)

d. Lower extremities—great saphenous vein at the ankle, superficial dorsal plexus, dorsal venous arch, or medial marginal vein of the foot.
   i. Advantages: The lower division of the great saphenous vein is frequently used in infants and toddlers.
   ii. Disadvantages: May require explicit orders from the health care provider because thrombosis occurs more frequently than in veins of the upper extremities; irregular absorption may occur due to the increased number of valves present in the lower extremities causing infusions to potentially pool.

> **NURSING ALERT** Selection of lower extremity sites for venipuncture in patients with diabetes or peripheral vascular disease is not recommended because of the increased risk of phlebitis, thrombosis, infection, and potential for poor healing.

3. Be prepared to use central veins in the following cases:
   a. When medications and infusions are hypertonic or highly irritating, requiring rapid, high-volume dilution to prevent systemic reactions and local venous damage (eg, chemotherapy and hyperalimentation).
   b. When peripheral blood flow is diminished (eg, shock) or when peripheral vessels are not accessible (eg, obese patients).
   c. When hemodynamic monitoring is desired.
   d. When moderate- or long-term fluid therapy is expected.

> **NURSING ALERT** Ultrasound-guided vascular access as compared to cannulation by anatomic landmarks and/or acoustic Doppler is significantly safer for the patient and improves efficiency and effectiveness of the clinician.

Methods of Distending a Vein

1. Apply a tourniquet (soft nonlatex) at least 2 to 6 inches (5 to 15 cm) above the planned insertion site, fastening it with a slipknot or hemostat, in a manner to impede venous flow but allowing for arterial circulation. Alternately apply a blood pressure cuff (keep pressure just below systolic pressure).
2. Apply manual compression above the site where the cannula is to be inserted.
3. Position the extremity lower than the level of the heart, having the patient open and close his or her fist, and lightly stoke the vein downward.
4. Lightly tap the vein site; this is to be done gently so the vein is not injured.
5. Apply warmth to site by using a warm dry towel or heat pack.

Selecting Needle or Catheter

1. Use the smallest gauge catheter suitable for the type and location of the infusion to minimize trauma to the vein.
2. Refer to Table 6-3, Types of Short Peripheral Cannulas, to assist in selecting the most appropriate catheter type. If a blood transfusion is to be given, use a larger-bore catheter, preferably 18G or larger.
3. Consider local anesthetic agents to minimize pain while obtaining vascular access.
   a. Agents include topical vapocoolant sprays, topical transdermal agents, intradermal lidocaine, and pressure-accelerated lidocaine.
   b. May cause collapse of desired veins, allergic reactions, and increase cost of the procedure.
   c. Warm compresses can mitigate the vasoconstrictive effects of local anesthetics.
4. Do not leave steel-winged devices in place; they are for single-dose administration only.
5. Use catheters manufactured with protective devices to guard against needlestick injuries (see Figure 6-3).

Table 6-3 Types of Short Peripheral Cannulas

CANNULA TYPE	PURPOSE	APPROXIMATE MAXIMUM FLOW RATE WITH GRAVITY	VOLUMES
24 gauge Yellow/lime	Infants; pediatric patients; older adults; patient with difficult venous access	23 mL/min	Small
22 gauge Blue	Infants; pediatric patients; older adults; small veins	22–50 mL/min	Small
20 gauge Pink	Adult; most infusion therapies; commonly used	55–80 mL/min	Medium
18 gauge Green	Fluid replacement; blood transfusion; for use with a contrast-based radiographic study; commonly used	100–120 mL/min	Large
16 gauge Gray	Rapid fluid replacement; blood transfusion	150–240 mL/min	Large
14 gauge Orange/brown	Rapid fluid replacement; blood transfusion	250–300 mL/min	Extra large
Medial (blue) and proximal (white) lumen of triple-lumen catheter 18 gauge	Fluid replacement; blood transfusion; medication administration	26 mL/min	Large
Distal (brown) lumen of the triple-lumen catheter 16 gauge	Fluid replacement; blood transfusion; medication administration; hemodynamic monitoring	52 mL/min	Large

Before activation

Activation button
Push off tab
Needle inside catheter
Safety barrel
Finger grip
Flash chamber

After activation

Activation button
Safety barrel
Push off tab
Flash chamber
Spring
Finger grip
Needle retracted into barrel

Figure 6-3. The activation button is pressed after the catheter is in the vein so that the needle will retract into the safety barrel while catheter remains in the vein.

Cleaning the Infusion Site

 EVIDENCE BASE Infusion Nursing Society (INS). (2016). Infusion therapy standards of practice nursing standards of practice. *Journal of Infusion Nursing*, 349(1S).

1. If skin is dirty, clean the infusion site thoroughly with soap and rinse.
2. Clean the IV site with an effective topical antiseptic according to facility protocol.
   a. The preferred skin antiseptic is chlorhexidine solution used in an outward, circular scrubbing manner following manufacturer's instructions. Allow to dry completely.
   b. Caution with chlorhexidine in premature infants and infants under 2 months of age because of increased risks of skin irritation and chemical burns.
   c. Alcohol swabs, povidone–iodine, or tincture of iodine may be used in the same outward circular scrubbing manner where chlorhexidine is contraindicated. Allow to dry completely.

 DRUG ALERT Iodine solutions may cause allergic reactions in some patients. The patient should be assessed for iodine allergies before use.

Use of Stabilization Devices

Stabilizing vascular access devices can prevent unintentional dislodgement and adverse complications. Do not rely on vascular access device dressings such as a transparent semipermeable membrane or gauze as a means for stabilization.

Infusion Tubing

1. Drip chambers.
   a. A "microdrip" system delivers 60 drops/mL and is used when small volumes are being delivered (eg, less than 50 mL/hour); this reduces the risk of clotting the IV line because of slow infusion rates.
   b. The "macrodrip" system delivers 10, 15, or 20 drops/mL and is used to deliver solution in large quantities or at fast rates.
2. Vented tubing should be used with standard glass bottles; this permits air to enter the vacuum in the bottle and displace solution as it flows out. Nonvented tubing should be used for IV bags and glass bottles that have a built-in air vent.
3. Filters help minimize the risk of contamination from certain microorganisms and particulate matter.
   a. Filters are found "in line" on conventional IV, blood, and parental nutrition tubing and are preferred because they reduce the risks of contamination. An additional filter is needed for mannitol and may be needed for other solutions based on facility protocol.
   b. "Add-on" filters should be located as close to the insertion site as possible and be changed with administration set changes.
4. Most electronic infusion pumps require specialized tubing to fit their particular pumping chamber. Need for such a device should be determined before initiating infusion therapy.
   a. If added tubing length is required (especially for children and restless patients), extension tubing is available; this should be added at the time of IV setup.
   b. Secondary administration tubing sets are used for administration of intermittent, "piggyback," medications that are connected to the port closest to the drip chamber.
   c. Special-coated tubing, designed to prevent leaching of polyvinyl chloride, is used for delivering medications, such as nitroglycerin, paclitaxel, and cyclosporine.
   d. Add-on devices such as single- and multilumen extension sets, extension loops, needleless connectors, inline filters, manual flow-control devices, and stopcocks should be used only when clinically indicated. Use systems that minimize the manipulation and reduce multiple components to limit potential contamination and change with each new administration set.
5. Administration tubing set change—label with date, time opened, and initials.
   a. Primary and secondary continuous tubing administration sets used for medications and solutions other than lipids, blood, or blood products should be changed no more frequently than every 96 hours but at least every 7 days.
   b. Intermittent tubing administration sets should be changed every 24 hours.
   c. Tubing administration sets used for parenteral nutrition solutions should be replaced every 24 hours or with each new container.
   d. Tubing administration sets used for intravenous fat emulsions should be replaced every 12 hours or with each new container.
   e. Tubing administration sets used for blood or blood products should be changed every 2–4 units of blood or every 4 hours.

Adjusting Rate of Flow

The health care provider prescribes the flow rate. The nurse is responsible for regulating and maintaining the proper rate. When initiating an infusion, consider using smart pumps with dose-error reduction software as an effective error-reducing strategy.

Patient Determining Factors

When determining flow rates, consider patient factors such as age, acuity and severity of the illness/injury, type of therapy, dosing considerations, and health care setting.

1. Age—fluids should be administered slowly in the very young and elderly.
2. Condition—a patient in hypovolemic shock requires greater amounts of fluids, whereas the patient with heart or renal failure should receive fluids judiciously.
3. Tolerance to solutions—fluids containing medications causing potential allergic reactions or intense vascular irritation (eg, potassium chloride) should be well diluted or given slowly.
4. Prescribed fluid composition—efficacy of some drugs is based on speed of infusion (eg, antibiotics); rate for other solutions is titrated to the patient's response to them (eg, dopamine, nitroprusside, heparin).

System Determining Factors

1. Gauge of IV catheter.
2. Pressure gradient—the difference between two levels in a fluid system.
3. Friction—the interaction between fluid molecules and surfaces of inner wall of tubing.
4. Diameter and length of tubing.
5. Height of column of fluid.
6. Characteristics of fluid.
   a. Viscosity.
   b. Temperature—refrigerated fluids may cause diminished flow and vessel spasm; bring fluid to room temperature before infusion.
7. Vein trauma, clots, plugging of vents, venous spasm, and vasoconstriction.
8. Flow-control clamp derangement.
   a. Some clamps may slip and loosen, resulting in a rapid, or "runaway," infusion. Many tubings now have safety clamps to prevent this rapid infusion.
   b. Plastic tubing may distort, causing "creep" or "cold flow"—the inside diameter of tubing will continue to change long after clamp is tightened or relaxed.
   c. Marked stretching of tubing may cause distortions of tubing and render clamp ineffective (may occur when patient turns over and pulls on a short tubing).
9. If there is any question about the rate of fluid administration, check with the health care provider.

 GERONTOLOGIC ALERT Be aware that veins are more likely to roll within the loose tissue beneath the skin, collapse, and become irritated in older adults. Also, fluid overload may be more pronounced, making IV therapy more difficult and potentially dangerous.

Calculation of Flow Rate

1. Most infusion rates are given at a certain volume per hour.
2. Delivery of the prescribed volume is determined by calculating necessary drops per minute to deliver the volume.
3. Drops per milliliter will vary with commercial parenteral sets (eg, 10, 15, 20, or 60 drops/mL). Check manufacturer's instructions. Most macrodrip sets delivers 10 to 20 drops/mL and microdrip sets 60 drops/mL.
4. Calculate the infusion rate using the following formula:

$$\text{Drop/minute} = \frac{\text{total volume} \times \text{infused drops/mL}}{\text{total time for infusion in minutes}}$$

Example: Infuse 150 mL of D$_5$W in 1 hour (set indicates 10 drops/mL)

$$\frac{150 \times 10}{60 \text{ minutes}} = 25 \text{ drops/minute}$$

5. The nurse hanging a new IV solution should write the date, time, and her or his initials on the container label.

 NURSING ALERT To avoid leaks, never write directly on the IV bag. Do not use magic markers because they are absorbed into the plastic bag and possibly into the solution. Write on the label or tape using a regular pen.

Vascular Access Maintenance and Removal

Maintaining Patency

Flush vascular access device with normal saline and aspirate blood prior to each infusion to assess catheter function as well as after each infusion to clear the infused medicine from the catheter lumen and to prevent potential contact of incompatible medicines. Flushing intermittent peripheral catheters with normal saline is equivalent to flushing with heparin in maintaining catheter patency and complication rates. Flush volume of 10 mL may remove fibrin deposits, drug precipitate, and other debris from the lumen to ensure patency. See Box 6-1.

Assess vascular access frequently for signs of infiltration, infection, phlebitis, and other complications.

Removal of Vascular Access Device

1. Assess vascular access daily as part of the patient's overall plan of care, with the goal of removal as soon as possible.

BOX 6-1	Flushing Intravenous Access

1. Locked vascular access devices must be flushed before and after medication or solution administration.
2. Flushing with prefilled syringes is preferred over nurse-filled syringes. Do not use intravenous solution containers (bags or bottles) as a "flush" bag.
3. Flush all vascular access devices with preservative-free 0.9% sodium chloride (NS). If bacteriostatic 0.9% sodium chloride is used, limit volume to less than 30 mL per 24-hour period to reduce potential toxic effects of benzyl alcohol, the preservative used. However, facilities should have an established standardized locking solution for each patient population that should be used.
4. Use a push–pause method to inject the medication. Do not force if resistance is met, rather evaluate for patency or complications of the vascular access.
5. Recommendation is to flush at least two times the volume of the catheter and add-on devices, usually 10 mL. An adequate flush volume removes debris, fibrin deposits, and medication/solution in the catheter and port reservoir to reduce the risk of clotting and infection.

2. Realize that vascular access devices should be removed with any signs and symptoms of complications, however working in coordination with the health care team to avoid delays in medically necessary treatments.

3. In the event of infiltration/extravasation of a short peripheral or midline catheter, stop the infusion immediately, detach all administration sets, and determine if a vesicant extravasation has taken place before removing the vascular access device.

Evaluation, Documentation, Patient Education, and Quality Improvement

Documentation and Patient Education

1. Documentation must contain accurate, factual, and complete information regarding the initial and ongoing assessment, nursing diagnosis or problems, interventions, and patient's response to those interventions.

2. Documentation specific to intravenous therapy should include, but is not limited to, the following:
   a. Date and time of cannula insertion.
   b. Site and preparation of insertion.
   c. Number of cannulation attempts.
   d. Size and type of inserted cannula.
   e. Dressing.
   f. Tolerance of the procedure.
   g. Monitoring of the site.
   h. Date and time of cannula removal.
   i. Identification and management of complications.

3. The clinician is responsible for educating the patient and/or caregiver about intravenous therapies. This education should include such topics as the plan of care, purpose and/or goals of treatment, intravascular device-related care, and potential complications. The teaching methods and any learning materials provided should be sensitive to the preferred learning style of the patient considering such factors as developmental and cognitive level, health literacy, cultural influences, or readiness to learn.

Evaluation and Quality Improvement

1. Quality improvement programs include the surveillance, aggregation, analysis, and reporting of intravenous-related patient quality indicators.

2. Adverse events must be recognized and documented to minimize health care–associated infections related to intravenous therapy.

3. Clinician practice, processes, and/or systems should be evaluated to identify areas for improvement.

Complications of IV Therapy

 GERONTOLOGIC ALERT Providing intravascular therapy for special populations including older adult patient requires competency in the clinical management of such populations and understanding of anatomic and physiologic differences, safety considerations, implications for vascular access device management, and infusion administration. Older adults have more fragile peripheral veins and surrounding tissue and may be at risk for circulatory overload.

Infiltration/Extravasation

Cause

1. Dislodgment of the IV cannula from the vein. Infiltration is the unintentional infusion of nonvesicant medications or solutions into the surrounding tissue; whereas, extravasation is the unintentional infusion of a vesicant into the surrounding tissues.

Clinical Manifestations

1. Discomfort or pain, depending on nature of solution.
2. Swelling, blanching, and coolness of surrounding skin and tissues.
3. Fluid flowing more slowly or ceasing.
4. Absence of blood backflow in IV catheter and tubing.

Preventive Measures

1. Select the most appropriate vascular access device and insertion site.
2. Make sure that the IV and distal tubing are secured sufficiently with tape to prevent movement.
3. Splint the patient's arm or hand as necessary.
4. Assess the vascular access device for functionality routinely and prior to use.

Nursing Interventions

1. Stop infusion immediately and remove the IV needle or catheter.
2. In the event of infiltration/extravasation of a short peripheral or midline catheter, stop the infusion immediately and detach all administration sets. Remove the vascular access device, however if extravasation has occurred, aspirate from the catheter hub prior to catheter removal to remove as much of the medication or solution from the catheter lumen and subcutaneous tissue as possible.
3. If a vasoconstrictor agent (eg, norepinephrine bitartrate, dopamine), vesicant (various chemotherapy agents, potassium chloride, etc.), or irritant (determined by facility) has extravasated, initiate emergency local treatment as directed to limit the potential damage to subcutaneous tissue by the medication or solution. Serious tissue injury, necrosis, and sloughing may result if actions are not taken.
4. To localize the medication or solution in the tissues and reduce inflammation, apply dry, cold compresses to the area; or to to increase blood flow and disperse the medication, apply dry compresses, per facility protocol.
5. Document assessments and interventions.

Phlebitis

Causes

1. Injury to the vein that occurs during venipuncture or caused from prolonged needle or catheter use or using too large of a catheter for the selected vein.
2. Poor aseptic technique.
3. Irritation to vein because of rapid infusions or irritating solutions (eg, hypertonic glucose solutions, cytotoxic agents, strong acids or alkalis, potassium, antibiotics, and others); smaller veins are more susceptible.
4. Clot formation at the end of the needle or catheter because of slow infusion rates or inadequate hemodilution of medications or solutions.
5. More commonly seen with synthetic polyurethane catheters than synthetic silicone catheters or steel needles.

Clinical Manifestations

1. Pain and tenderness to palpation at intravenous site that will progress to extending along the path of the cannula and vein.

2. Redness, swelling, warmth, induration, or purulence at intravenous site; the vein may appear as a red streak above the insertion site.
3. Palpable venous cord.

Preventive Measures
1. Routinely assess the vascular access site with a standardized tool for signs and symptoms of phlebitis.
2. Anchor the needle or catheter securely at the insertion site.
3. Use large veins for irritating fluid because of higher blood flow, which rapidly dilutes the irritant.
4. Sufficiently dilute irritating agents before infusion.

Nursing Interventions
1. Apply warm compresses to stimulate circulation and promote absorption, counteracting venoconstriction caused by phlebitis.
2. Elevate the extremity.
3. Consider removal of the vascular access device.
4. Consider other pharmacologic interventions such as analgesics, anti-inflammatory agents, or corticosteroids as necessary.
5. Document assessments and interventions.
6. Participate in facility quality improvement activities regarding phlebitis occurrence rates. One formula that can be used is:

$$\frac{\text{Number of phlebitis incidents}}{\text{Total number of IV peripheral catheters}} \times 100$$

$$= \% \text{ peripheral phlebitis}$$

 EVIDENCE BASE Infusion Nursing Society (INS). (2016). Infusion therapy standards of practice. *Journal of Infusion Nursing, 39*(1S).

Catheter-Associated Bloodstream Infections

Causes
1. Underlying thrombophlebitis increases risk 18-fold.
2. Contaminated equipment or infused solutions (see Figure 6-4).
3. Prolonged placement of an IV device (catheter or needle, tubing, solution container).
4. Nonsterile IV insertion or dressing change.
5. Cross-contamination by the patient with other infected areas of the body.
6. A critically ill or immunosuppressed patient is at greatest risk of bacteremia.

Clinical Manifestations
1. Possible signs of local infection at vascular access insertion site (eg, redness, pain, edema, foul drainage).
2. Elevated temperature, chills.
3. Nausea, vomiting.
4. Elevated white blood cell (WBC) count.
5. Malaise, increased pulse.
6. Backache, headache.
7. May progress to septic shock with profound hypotension.

Preventive Measures
1. Follow the same measures as outlined for thrombophlebitis.
2. Strict adherence to hand hygiene and the use of aseptic techniques with maximal barrier precautions during insertion and dressing changes remain the most important measure for the prevention of catheter-associated bloodstream infections.

Figure 6-4. Potential mechanisms for contamination of IV infusion systems.

3. Ensure appropriate cleaning products are used to cleanse the skin prior to insertion of the cannula. Chlorhexidine is preferred and has been shown to reduce the rate of infections.

 TRANSITIONAL CARE ALERT Hand hygiene, personal protective equipment, and safe injection practices using aseptic technique form the basis of standard precautions. Appropriate infection control measures are essential in preventing complications and ensuring the delivery of efficient, high-quality care across care settings, and ultimately so the patient can remain at home.

4. Choose appropriate sites for catheter insertion.
5. Replacing intravenous catheters when clinically indicated, rather than routine replacement every 72 to 96 hours, demonstrates no increased patient risk of thrombophlebitis or infection. An exception to this is when adherence to aseptic technique cannot be assured (eg, insertion during a medical emergency) at which time, the catheter should be replaced as soon as possible but no longer than 48 hours after insertion.
6. Use antimicrobial-impregnated central venous catheters where the expected dwell time is greater than 5 days or in patients with high risk of infections such as neutropenic, burn, or critically ill patients.

7. Change catheter administration sets at appropriate intervals. Continuous IV administration sets should be changed every 96 hours when the medications or solutions do not contain lipids, blood, or blood products. When the catheter administration sets contain lipids, blood, or blood products, the catheter administration set should be changed every 24 hours. Intermittent IV administration sets including secondary sets and add-on devices should be changed no more frequently than at 72- to 96-hour intervals.

8. Do not allow medications and solutions to hang longer than 24 hours. Lipid-containing solutions should be completed within 24 hours of hanging the solution. Lipid emulsions should be completed within 6 to 12 hours of hanging the solution. Blood or other blood products should be completed within 4 hours of hanging the solution. Maintain integrity of the infusion system at all times.

9. Ensure proper vascular access site assessment and care. Change the IV dressing on a routine basis and immediately if it becomes damp, loosened, or soiled.
   a. Gauze dressing that prevents visualization of the site should be changed every 48 hours.
   b. Transparent semipermeable dressing should be changed every 7 days.

10. Use passive disinfection caps containing disinfecting agents (eg, isopropyl alcohol), which result in reduced intraluminal microbial contamination and decreases the rates of catheter-associated bloodstream infection.

11. Ensure removal of catheters when no longer essential.

 NURSING ALERT When accessing the port of a vascular access device, vigorously scrub—not wipe—the hub of the catheter for 15 seconds with alcohol or clorhexidine solution.

Nursing Interventions

1. Discontinue infusion and consider removal of vascular access device. A peripheral venous device with signs and symptoms of infection and erythema extending at least 1 cm from the insertion site, induration, exudate, and fever with no other source of infectious process should be removed. Collaboration with the health care team is needed to determine whether a central venous access device can be salvaged or necessitates removal.

2. If purulent exudate is present, obtain a sample for culture and gram staining.

3. With removal of the vascular access device, cut off the tip of the catheter with sterile scissors; place in a dry, sterile container; and immediately send it to the laboratory for culture and gram staining.

4. Assess for and provide necessary measures to maintain patient's stability.

5. Start appropriate antibiotic therapy immediately after receiving orders and obtaining all additional specimens for culture and gram staining.

6. Document assessments and interventions.

Circulatory Overload

Cause

1. Delivery of excessive amounts of IV fluid (greater risk exists for older patients, infants, or patients with cardiac or renal insufficiency).

Clinical Manifestations

1. Increased BP and pulse.
2. Increased CVP, venous distention (engorged jugular veins).
3. Headache, anxiety.
4. Shortness of breath, tachypnea, coughing.
5. Pulmonary crackles.
6. Chest pain (if history of coronary artery disease).

Preventive Measures

1. Assess patient for existing heart or kidney condition. Be particularly vigilant in the high-risk patient.
2. Closely monitor the infusion flow rate, and use electronic infusion devices in patients at greater risk.
3. Keep accurate intake and output records.
4. Splint the arm or hand if the IV flow rate fluctuates too widely with movement.

Nursing Interventions

1. If circulatory overload is suspected, notify health care provider, sit patient up for easier breathing, and anticipate reduced IV infusion rate and additional medication therapy.
2. Monitor closely for worsening clinical condition.

Air Embolism

Causes

1. A greater risk exists in central venous lines, when air enters catheter during tubing changes (air sucked in during inspiration because of negative intrathoracic pressure).
2. Air in tubing delivered by IV push or infused by infusion pump.

Clinical Manifestations

1. Sudden onset of dyspnea, breathlessness, elevated respiratory rate.
2. Chest pain, hypotension, elevated heart rates.
3. Altered mental status, altered speech.
4. Changes in facial appearance, paralysis.

Preventive Measures

1. Clear all air from tubing before infusion to patient.
2. Change solution containers before they run empty.
3. Ensure that all connections are secure. Use Luer-lock connections or administration sets with air-eliminating filters unless contraindicated.
4. Use appropriate technique with removal of central venous access devices.
5. When removing a central venous access device, place the patient in supine or Trendelenburg position unless contraindicated so that the insertion site is at or below the level of the heart.
6. Instruct the patient to bear down (Valsalva maneuver) during catheter withdrawal unless contraindicated.

Nursing Interventions

1. Immediately prevent additional air from entering the bloodstream by closing, kinking, clamping, or covering the existing vascular access device or insertion site with an air-occlusive dressing.
2. Immediately turn the patient on left side and lower the head of the bed; in this position, air will become trapped in the right side of the heart.
3. Notify the health care provider immediately.
4. Administer oxygen as needed and support the medical stability of the patient.
5. Document assessments and interventions.

Mechanical Failure (Sluggish Flow or Occlusion)

Causes
1. Malposition of the catheter including the cannula lying against the side of the vein, cutting off fluid flow or infiltration of the catheter.
2. Clot at the end of the catheter or needle.
3. External mechanical causes such as inking of the tubing or catheter, clogged filter, or needless connector.

Clinical Manifestations
1. Inability to withdraw blood or sluggish blood return.
2. Sluggish IV flow or frequent occlusion alarms on electronic infusion devices.
3. Signs of infiltration/extravasation.

Preventive Measures
1. Asses the functionality of the vascular access device routinely.
2. Use appropriate flushing procedures.
3. Secure the IV well with tape and an armboard, if necessary.

Nursing Interventions
1. Assess for mechanical causes of occlusion.
2. Reposition the catheter by pulling back on the cannula slightly because it may be lying against the vein wall valve or bifurcation.
3. Reposition the patient's extremity in which the vascular access device is placed.
4. Lower the solution container to below the level of patient's heart and observe for blood backflow.
5. If using an electronic infusion device, assess its functionality.
6. Consider the need for a catheter-clearing agent or thrombolytic agent in collaboration with the health care team.
7. Consider the need to remove the vascular access device.

Hemorrhage

Causes
1. Loose connection of tubing or injection port.
2. Inadvertent removal of peripheral or central catheter.
3. Anticoagulant therapy.

Clinical Manifestations
1. Oozing or trickling of blood from IV site or catheter.
2. Hematoma.

Preventive Measures
1. Cap all central lines with Luer-lock adapters and connect Luer-lock tubing to the cap—not directly to the line.
2. Secure catheters. Use transparent dressing when possible for peripheral and central catheters. Tape the remaining catheter lumens and tubing in a loop so tension is not directly on the catheter.
3. Keep pressure on sites where catheters have been removed—a minimum of 10 minutes for a patient taking anticoagulants.

Venous Thrombosis

Causes
1. Infusion of irritating solutions.
2. Infection along catheter may preclude this syndrome.
3. Fibrin sheath formation with eventual clot formation around the catheter. (This clot will eventually occlude the vein.)
4. Patient factors including a medical history of a hypercoagulable state (eg, cancer, diabetes, or end-stage renal failure), history of deep vein thrombosis, surgical or trauma patients, critical care patients, and extremes of age.
5. Stasis of blood in the intravenous catheter.

Clinical Manifestations
1. Swelling and pain in the area of catheter or in the extremity proximal to the insertion site.
2. Slowing of IV infusion or inability to draw blood from the central line.
3. Palpable lump in the cannulated vessel.

Preventive Measures
1. Select appropriate vascular access device and site location.
2. Ensure proper dilution of irritating substances.
3. Ensure proper placement of vascular access device.
4. Institute nonpharmacological strategies for thrombosis prevention if possible such as early patient mobility and adequate hydration.
5. Prophylaxis with anticoagulant therapies as ordered by the health care team.

Nursing Interventions
1. If venous thrombosis is suspected, notify health care provider, anticipate evaluation and therapeutic anticoagulant dose, and support the patient.

SELECTED REFERENCES

Bhave, G., & Neilson, E. G. (2011). Volume depletion versus dehydration: How understanding the difference can guide therapy. *American Journal of Kidney Diseases*, 58(2), 302–309.

Centers for Disease Control and Prevention (CDC). (2017). Summary of recommendations: Guidelines for the prevention of intravascular catheter-related infections 2011. Available: *https://www.cdc.gov/infectioncontrol/guidelines/bsi/recommendations.html*

Centers for Disease Control and Prevention. (2011). *Guidelines for the prevention of intravascular catheter-related infections, 2011.* Atlanta, GA: Author.

Charron, K. (2012). Decreasing central line infections and needlestick injury rates: Combining best practice and introducing a Luer-activated intravenous therapy system and antimicrobial intravenous connector. *Journal of Infusion Nursing*, 35(6), 370–375.

Crowley, M., Brim, C., Proehl, M., et al. (2012). Emergency nursing resource: Difficult intravenous access. *Journal of Emergency Nursing*, 38(4), 335–343.

Edwards, C., & Johnson, C. (2012). Evaluation of a Luer-activated intravenous administration system. *Journal of the Association for Vascular Access*, 17(4), 200–207.

Hadaway, L. (2012). Short peripheral intravenous catheters and infections. *Journal of Infusion Nursing*, 35(4), 230–240.

Hugill, K. (2017). Preventing bloodstream infection in IV therapy. *British Journal of Nursing*, 26(14), S4–S10.

Infusion Nursing Society (INS). (2016). Infusion therapy standards of practice. *Journal of Infusion Nursing*, 39(1S).

Lamperti, M., Bodenham, A. R., Pittiruti, M., et al. (2012). International evidence-based recommendations on ultrasound-guided vascular access. *Intensive Care Medicine*, 38, 1105–1117.

O'Grady, N. P., Alexander, M., Burns, L. A., et al. (2011). Guidelines for the prevention of intravascular catheter-related infections, 2011. Available: *http://www.cdc.gov/hicpac/pdf/guidelines/bsi-guidelines-2011.pdf*

Parker, S. I. A., Benzies, K. M., Hayden, K. A. (2017). A systematic review: Effectiveness of pediatric peripheral intravenous catheterization strategies. *Journal of Advanced Nursing*, 73(7), 1570–1582.

Phillips, L. D. (2014). *Manual of IV therapeutics: Evidence-based practice for infusion therapy* (6th ed.). Philadelphia, PA: Davis.

Schnock, K. O., Dykes, P. C., Albert, J., et al. (2017). The frequency of intravenous medication administration errors related to smart infusion pumps: A multihospital observational study. *British Medical Journal Quality and Safety*, 26, 131–140.

Shastay, A. D. (2016). Evidence-based safe practice guidelines for I.V. push medications. *Nursing*, 46(10), 38–44.

Smith, J. S., Irwin, G., Viney, M., et al. (2012). Optimal disinfection times for needleless intravenous connectors. *Journal of the Association for Vascular Access*, 17(3), 137–143.

Vizcarra, C., Cassutt, C., Corbitt, N., et al. (2014). Infusion Nursing Society (INS) position paper: Recommendations for improving safety practices with short peripheral catheters. *Journal of Infusion Nursing*, 37(2), 121–124.

Webser, J., Osborne, S., Rickard, C. M., & New, K. (2013). Clinically-indicated replacement versus routine replacement of peripheral venous catheters. *Cochrane Database System Review*, (4), CD007798.

7
Perioperative Nursing

OVERVIEW AND ASSESSMENT

*See additional online content: Patient
Education Guidelines 7-1.*

Introduction

Perioperative nursing is a term used to describe the nursing care provided during the total surgical experience of the patient: preoperative, intraoperative, and postoperative.

Preoperative phase—from the time the decision is made for surgical intervention to the transfer of the patient to the operating room.
Intraoperative phase—from the time the patient is received in the operating room until admitted to the postanesthesia care unit (PACU).
Postoperative phase—from the time of admission to the PACU to the follow-up evaluation.

An *anesthesia care provider* is a professional who can administer and monitor anesthesia during a surgical procedure; he or she may be a licensed physician board certified in anesthesia (anesthesiologist) or a certified registered nurse anesthetist.

Types of surgery include the following:

Elective—The scheduled time for surgery is at the convenience of the patient; failure to have surgery is not catastrophic (eg, superficial cyst).
Required—The condition requires surgery within a few weeks (eg, cataract).
Urgent—Necessitates surgery as soon as possible but may be delayed for a short amount of time (eg, internal fixation of fracture).
Emergent—The situation requires immediate surgical attention without delay (eg, intestinal obstruction). This must be done to save life or limb or functional capacity.

Common abdominal incisions are pictured in Figure 7-1.

Perioperative Safety

The safety and welfare of patients during surgical intervention is a primary concern. Patients entering the perioperative settings are at risk for infection, impaired skin integrity, altered body temperature, fluid volume deficit, and injury related to positioning and chemical, electrical, and physical hazards.

The Surgical Care Improvement Project (SCIP), National Safety Goals for Surgery, and Enhanced Recovery After Surgery (ERAS) programs have resulted in major improvements in clinical outcomes. Care protocols are developed based on evidence of best practice. Examples include practices as apparent as proper identification and early mobilization, as well as proper antibiotic use, minimally invasive surgery, and multimodal approaches to resolving issues.

EVIDENCE BASE The Joint Commission. (2018). Hospital: 2018 National Patient Safety Goals. Available: *www.jointcommission.org/hap_2017_npsgs.*
The Joint Commission. (2018). Surgical Care Improvement Project. Available: *www.jointcommission.org/surgical_care_improvement_project.*

Surgical Care Improvement Project

1. The Surgical Care Improvement Project (SCIP), a national quality partnership interested in improving surgical care by significantly reducing surgical complications, is a coalition of health care organizations that has developed evidence-based interventions that have proven effective.
   a. The goal is to reduce surgical complications by 25%.
   b. Implementing nursing interventions at the earliest stage possible of a developing complication is also of utmost importance.
2. SCIP measures that have been shown to be effective include the following:
   a. Prophylactic antibiotic received within 1 hour prior to surgical incision.
   b. Prophylactic antibiotic discontinued within 24 hours after surgery end time.
   c. Cardiac surgery patients with controlled postoperative serum glucose.
   d. Surgery patients with appropriate hair removal.

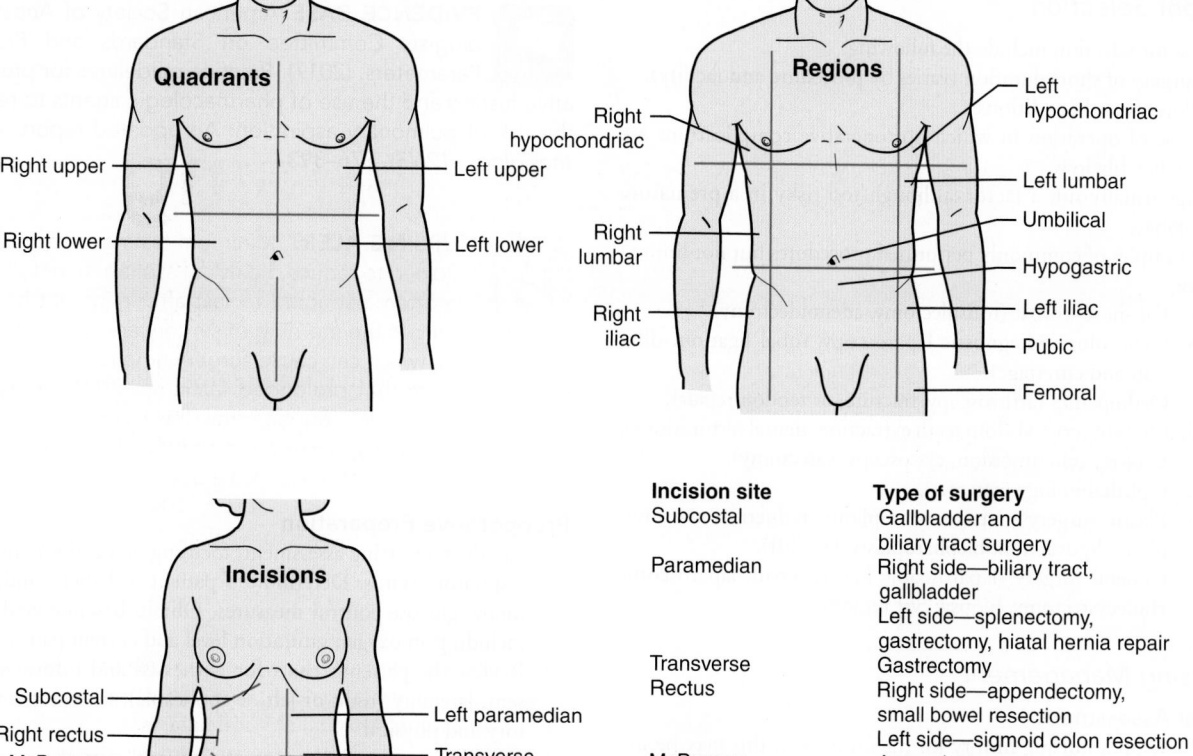

Incision site	Type of surgery
Subcostal	Gallbladder and biliary tract surgery
Paramedian	Right side—biliary tract, gallbladder
	Left side—splenectomy, gastrectomy, hiatal hernia repair
Transverse	Gastrectomy
Rectus	Right side—appendectomy, small bowel resection
	Left side—sigmoid colon resection
McBurney	Appendectomy
Midline (lower)	Female reproductive tract
Suprapubic (low-transverse, Pfannenstein)	Gynecologic surgery

Figure 7-1. Regions and incisions of the abdomen.

e. Urinary catheter removed on postoperative day 1 or postoperative day 2 with day of surgery being day 0.
f. Patients continue beta-blockers on day of surgery.
g. Appropriate venous thromboembolism prophylaxis and treatment.

National Patient Safety Goals

1. Prevent infection—use hand cleaning guidelines from the Centers for Disease Control and Prevention or the World Health Organization.
   a. Use proven guidelines to prevent infections that are difficult to treat.
   b. Use proven guidelines to prevent infection of the blood from central lines.
   c. Use proven guidelines to prevent infection after surgery.
   d. Use proven guidelines to prevent infections of the urinary tract caused by catheters.
2. Prevent mistakes in surgery—make sure the correct surgery is done on the correct patient at the correct place on the patient's body.
   a. Mark the correct place on the patient's body where the surgery is to be done.
   b. Pause before surgery to make sure a mistake is not being made.

Enhanced Recovery after Surgery

Multimodal perioperative care pathways designed to achieve early recovery after surgical procedures by maintaining preoperative organ function and reducing the profound stress response following surgery.

Ambulatory Surgery

Ambulatory surgery (same-day surgery, outpatient surgery) is a common occurrence for certain types of procedures. The office nurse is in a key position to assess patient status, plan the perioperative experience, and monitor, instruct, and evaluate the patient.

Advantages

1. Reduced cost to the facility and insuring and governmental agencies.
2. Reduced psychological stress to the patient.
3. Less incidence of hospital-acquired infection.
4. Less time lost from work by the patient and minimal disruption of the patient's activities and family life.

Disadvantages

1. Less time to assess the patient and perform preoperative teaching.
2. Less time to establish rapport between the patient and health care personnel.
3. Less opportunity to assess for late postoperative complications. (This responsibility is primarily with the patient, although telephone and home care follow-up is possible.)

Patient Selection

Criteria for selection include the following:
1. Surgery of short duration (varies by procedure and facility).
2. Noninfected conditions.
3. Type of operation in which postoperative complications are predictably low.
4. Age usually not a factor, although too risky in a premature neonate.
5. Examples of commonly performed procedures but not limited to:
   a. Ear–nose–throat (tonsillectomy, adenoidectomy)
   b. Gynecology (diagnostic laparoscopy, tubal ligation, dilation and curettage).
   c. Orthopedics (arthroscopy, fracture, or tendon repair).
   d. Oral surgery (wisdom teeth extraction, dental restorations).
   e. Urology (circumcision, cystoscopy, vasectomy).
   f. Ophthalmology (cataract).
   g. Plastic surgery (mammary implants, reduction mammoplasty, liposuction, blepharoplasty, face-lift).
   h. General surgery (laparoscopic hernia repair, laparoscopic cholecystectomy, biopsy, cyst removal).

Nursing Management

Initial Assessment

1. Develop a nursing history for the outpatient; this may be initiated in the health care provider's office. The history should include the patient's physical and psychological status. You will also inquire about allergies, tobacco, alcohol, and drug use; disabilities or limitations; current medications (including over-the-counter drugs, vitamins, supplements, and herbal products); current health conditions (focus should be on cardiovascular and respiratory problems, diabetes, and renal impairments); and any past surgeries and/or problems with anesthesia.
2. Ensure availability of a signed and witnessed informed consent that includes correct surgical procedure and site.
3. Explain any additional laboratory studies needed and state why.
4. Begin health education with the following instructions:
   a. Notify the health care provider and surgical unit immediately if you get a cold, have a fever, or have any illness before the date of surgery.
   b. Arrive at the specified time.
   c. Restrict food and fluid before surgery according to facility protocol to prevent aspiration of gastric contents. Based on scientific evidence, the American Society of Anesthesiologists has issued guidelines for elective procedures recommending the following:
       i. Clear liquids—minimum fasting of 2 hours.
       ii. Breast milk—minimum fasting of 4 hours.
       iii. Infant formula—minimum fasting of 6 hours.
       iv. Nonhuman milk—minimum fasting of 6 hours.
       v. Light meal—minimum fasting of 6 hours.
   d. Do not wear makeup or nail polish.
   e. Wear comfortable, loose clothing and low-heeled shoes.
   f. Leave valuables or jewelry at home.
   g. Brush your teeth in morning and rinse but do not swallow any liquid.
   h. Shower the night before or day of the surgery.
   i. Follow the health care provider's instructions for taking medications, including over-the-counter medications and supplements.
   j. Have a responsible adult accompany you and drive you home; have someone stay with you for 24 hours after the surgery.

EVIDENCE BASE American Society of Anesthesiologists Committee on Standards and Practice Parameters. (2017). Practice guidelines for preoperative fasting and the use of pharmacologic agents to reduce the risk of pulmonary aspiration: An updated report. *Anesthesiology, 126*(3), 376–393.

NURSING ALERT Minimum fasting times must be followed to reduce the risk of aspiration, but patients are often instructed to fast after midnight because schedule changes the morning of surgery are possible due to cancellations, which can cause surgery time to be moved forward. Be aware that prolonged fasting before surgery may result in undue thirst, hunger, irritability, headache, and possibly dehydration, hypovolemia, and hypoglycemia.

Preoperative Preparation

1. Conduct a nursing assessment, focusing on cardiovascular and respiratory status. Determine if patient is diabetic and, if so, follow glucose control measures. Obtain baseline vital signs, including an oxygen saturation level and current pain score.
2. Review the patient's chart for witnessed and informed consent, laterality (right or left, if applicable), lab work, and history and physical.
3. Verify correct patient, correct site, and correct procedure. Consider "time out" and SCIP measures, including marking of incision.
4. Make sure the patient has followed food and fluid restrictions, has removed all jewelry and dentures, and is appropriately dressed for surgery.
5. Perform medication reconciliation. Certain home meds may be taken, especially beta-blockers. Check with health care provider and have patient take with a sip of water.
6. Inform anesthesia provider if patient is taking any herbal supplements.
7. Administer preprocedural medication, if applicable.

Postoperative Care

1. Check vital signs, including oxygen saturation, temperature, and pain score.
2. Administer oxygen, if necessary.
3. Change the patient's position and progress activity—head of bed elevated, dangling, and walking. Watch for dizziness or nausea.
4. Ascertain, using the following criteria, that the patient has recovered adequately to be discharged:
   a. Vital signs stable and returned to preoperative level.
   b. Stands without excessive dizziness and able to walk short distances.
   c. Pain score within tolerable level (usually less than 3 required).
   d. Able to drink fluids.
   e. Oriented to time, place, and person.
   f. No evidence of respiratory distress.
   g. Has the services of a responsible adult who can escort the patient home and remain with patient.
   h. Understands postoperative instructions and takes an instruction sheet home.

Informed Consent (Operative Permit)

Informed consent (operative permit) is the process of informing the patient about the surgical procedure, that is, risks and possible complications of surgery and anesthesia. Consent is obtained by the surgeon. This is a legal requirement. Hospitals usually have a standard operative permit form approved by the hospital's legal department.

Purposes

1. To ensure that the patient understands the nature of the treatment, including potential complications and alternative treatment or procedures.
2. To indicate that the patient's decision was made without pressure.
3. To protect the patient against unauthorized procedures and to ensure that the procedure is performed on the correct body part.
4. To protect the surgeon and facility against legal action by a patient who claims that an unauthorized procedure was performed.

Adolescent Patient and Informed Consent

1. An emancipated minor is usually recognized as one who is not subject to parental control. Regulations vary by jurisdiction but generally include:
   a. Married minor.
   b. Those in military service.
   c. Minor who has a child.
2. Most states have statutes regarding treatment of minors.
3. Standards for informed consent are the same as for adults.

Procedures Requiring Informed Consent and Time Out

1. Any surgical procedures whether major or minor.
2. Entrance into a body cavity, such as colonoscopy, paracentesis, bronchoscopy, cystoscopy, or lumbar puncture.
3. Radiologic procedures, particularly if a contrast material is required (such as myelogram, magnetic resonance imaging with contrast, angiography).
4. All procedures requiring any type of anesthesia, which includes cardioversion.

Obtaining Informed Consent

1. Before signing an informed consent document, the patient should:
   a. Be told in clear and simple terms by the surgeon what is to be done, the risks and benefits, as well as any alternatives to the surgery or procedure. The anesthesia care provider will explain the anesthesia plan and possible risks and complications.
   b. Have a general idea of what to expect in the early and late postoperative periods.
   c. Have a general idea of the time involved from surgery to recovery.
   d. Have an opportunity to ask any questions may be necessary.
   e. Sign a separate form for each procedure or operation may be necessary.
2. Written permission is required by law and a witness may be required according to facility policy.
3. Signature is obtained with the patient's complete understanding of what is to occur; it is obtained before the patient receives sedation and is secured without pressure or duress.
4. For a minor (or a patient who is unconscious or irresponsible), permission is required from a responsible family member—parent, legal guardian, or court-appointed guardian.
5. For a married emancipated minor, permission from the spouse is acceptable when the patient is declared incapable.
6. If the patient is unable to write, an "X" is acceptable.
7. In an emergency, permission by way of telephone is acceptable with two witnesses.

Surgical Risk Factors and Preventive Strategies

Obesity

Danger

1. Increases the difficulty involved in the technical aspects of performing surgery; risk for wound dehiscence is greater.
2. Increases the likelihood of infection because of compromised tissue perfusion.
3. Increases the potential for postoperative pneumonia and other pulmonary complications because obese patients chronically hypoventilate.
4. Increases demands on the heart, leading to cardiovascular compromise.
5. Increases the risk for airway complications.
6. Alters the response to many drugs and anesthetics.
7. Decreases the likelihood of early ambulation.

Therapeutic Approach

1. Encourage weight reduction if time permits.
2. Anticipate postoperative obesity-related complications.
3. Be extremely vigilant for respiratory complications.
4. Carefully splint abdominal incisions when moving or coughing.
5. Be aware that some drugs should be dosed according to ideal body weight versus actual weight (owing to fat content) to prevent toxicity, including digoxin, lidocaine, aminoglycoside antibiotics, and theophylline.
6. Be aware that obese patients require higher doses of antibiotics to achieve effective tissue levels.
7. Avoid intramuscular (IM) injections in morbidly obese individuals (IV or subcutaneous routes preferred).
8. Never attempt to move an impaired patient without assistance or without using proper body mechanics.
9. Obtain a dietary consultation early in the patient's postoperative course.

Poor Nutrition

Danger

1. Greatly impairs wound healing (especially protein and calorie deficits and a negative nitrogen balance).
2. Increases the risk of infection.

Therapeutic Approach

1. Any recent (within 4 to 6 weeks) weight loss of 10% of the patient's normal body weight or decreased serum albumin should alert the health care staff to poor nutritional status and the need to investigate as to the cause of the weight loss.
2. Attempt to improve nutritional status before and after surgery. Unless contraindicated, provide a diet high in proteins, calories, and vitamins (especially vitamins C and A); this may require enteral and parenteral feeding.
3. Review a serum prealbumin level to determine recent nutritional status.
4. Recommend repair of dental caries and proper mouth hygiene to prevent infection.

Fluid and Electrolyte Imbalance

Danger

Can have adverse effects in terms of general anesthesia and the anticipated volume losses associated with surgery, causing shock and cardiac dysrhythmias.

NURSING ALERT Patients undergoing major abdominal operations (such as colectomies and aortic repairs) often experience a massive fluid shift into tissues around the operative site in the form of edema (as much as 1 L or more may be lost from circulation). Watch for the fluid shift to reverse (from tissue to circulation) around the 3rd postoperative day. Patients with heart disease may develop failure because of the excess fluid "load."

Therapeutic Approach

1. Assess the patient's fluid and electrolyte status.
2. Rehydrate the patient parenterally and orally as prescribed.
3. Monitor for evidence of electrolyte imbalance, especially Na^+, K^+, Mg^{++}, and Ca^{++}.
4. Be aware of expected drainage amounts and composition; report excess and abnormalities.
5. Monitor the patient's intake and output; be sure to include all body fluid losses.

Aging

Danger

1. Potential for injury is greater in older people.
2. Be aware that the cumulative effect of medications is greater in the older patient.
3. Medications in the usual dosages, such as morphine, may cause confusion, disorientation, and respiratory depression.

Therapeutic Approach

1. Consider using lesser medication doses for desired effect.
2. Anticipate problems from chronic disorders such as anemia, obesity, diabetes, and hypoproteinemia.
3. Adjust nutritional intake to conform to higher protein and vitamin needs.
4. When possible, cater to their set patterns in older patients, such as sleeping and eating.

Presence of Cardiovascular Disease

Danger

1. May compound the stress of anesthesia and the operative procedure.
2. May result in impaired oxygenation, cardiac rhythm, cardiac output, and circulation.
3. May also produce cardiac decompensation, sudden arrhythmia, thromboembolism, acute myocardial infarction (MI), or cardiac arrest.
4. Holding cardiac medications, particularly beta-blockers, may have negative impact on cardiac status.

Therapeutic Approach

1. Frequently assess heart rate and blood pressure (BP) and hemodynamic status and cardiac rhythm, if indicated.
2. Avoid fluid overload (oral, parenteral, blood products) because of possible MI, angina, heart failure, and pulmonary edema.
3. In compliance with SCIP measures, make sure the patient has not held beta-blocker prior to surgery. Administer with a sip of water.
4. Prevent prolonged immobilization, which results in venous stasis. Monitor for potential deep vein thrombosis (DVT) or pulmonary embolus.
5. Encourage position changes but avoid sudden exertion.
6. Use antiembolism stockings and/or sequential compression device intraoperatively and postoperatively.
7. Note evidence of hypoxia and initiate therapy.

 EVIDENCE BASE American Society of PeriAnesthesia Nurses. (2017). *2017–2018 perianesthesia nursing: Standards, practice recommendations, and interpretive statements.* Cherry Hill, NJ: Author.

Presence of Diabetes Mellitus

Danger

1. Hypoglycemia may result from food and fluid restrictions and anesthesia.
2. Hyperglycemia and ketoacidosis may be potentiated by increased catecholamines and glucocorticoids because of surgical stress.
3. Chronic hyperglycemia results in poor wound healing and susceptibility to infection.
4. Research has shown that surgical patients have better outcomes when glucose levels are well controlled throughout the surgical process.

Therapeutic Approach

1. Recognize the signs and symptoms of ketoacidosis and hypoglycemia, which can threaten an otherwise uneventful surgical experience. Dehydration also threatens renal function.
2. Monitor blood glucose and be prepared to administer insulin, as directed, or treat hypoglycemia.
3. Confirm what medications the patient has taken and what has been held. Facility protocol and provider preference vary, but the goal is to prevent hypoglycemia. If the patient is NPO (nothing by mouth), oral agents are usually withheld and insulin may be ordered at 75% of the usual dose.
4. Reassure the diabetic patient that when the disease is controlled, the surgical risk is no greater than it is for the nondiabetic patient.

DRUG ALERT Rare reports of lactic acidosis have raised concerns about the use of metformin in the perioperative period. Metformin is usually held 48 hours before surgery and restarted when full food and fluid intake has restarted and normal renal function has been confirmed.

Presence of Alcoholism

Danger

The additional problem of malnutrition may be present in the presurgical patient with alcoholism. The patient may also have an increased tolerance to anesthetics.

Therapeutic Approach

1. Note that the risk of surgery is greater for the patient who has chronic alcoholism.
2. Anticipate the acute withdrawal syndrome within 72 hours of the last alcoholic drink.

Presence of Pulmonary and Upper Respiratory Disease

Danger

1. Chronic pulmonary illness may contribute to hypoventilation, leading to pneumonia and atelectasis.
2. Surgery may be contraindicated in the patient who has an upper respiratory infection because of the possible advance of infection to pneumonia and sepsis.
3. Sleep apnea in the perioperative patient provides a great risk to anesthesia and must be noted and assessed prior to surgery.

Therapeutic Approach

1. Patients with chronic pulmonary problems, such as emphysema or bronchiectasis, should be evaluated and treated prior to surgery to optimize pulmonary function with bronchodilators, corticosteroids, and conscientious mouth care, along with a reduction in weight and smoking and methods to control secretions.
2. Patients with obstructive sleep apnea should be evaluated by an anesthesia provider prior to surgery. General anesthesia should be avoided if possible. Patients should bring continuous positive airway pressure (CPAP) machines to the hospital for use postanesthesia.
3. Opioids should be used cautiously to prevent hypoventilation. Patient-controlled analgesia is preferred.
4. Oxygen should be administered to prevent hypoxemia (low liter flow in chronic obstructive pulmonary disease).

Concurrent or Prior Pharmacotherapy

Danger

Hazards exist when certain medications are given concomitantly with others (eg, interaction of some drugs with anesthetics can lead to hypotension and circulatory collapse). This also includes the use of many herbal substances. Although herbs are natural products, they can interact with other medications used in surgery.

Therapeutic Approach

1. An awareness of drug therapy is essential.
2. Notify the health care provider and anesthesia provider if the patient is taking any of the following drugs:
   a. Certain antibiotics.
   b. Antidepressants, particularly monoamine oxidase inhibitors, and St. John's wort, an herbal product.
   c. Phenothiazines.
   d. Diuretics, particularly thiazides.
   e. Corticosteroids.
   f. Anticoagulants, such as warfarin or heparin, or medications or herbals that may affect coagulation, such as aspirin, feverfew, Ginkgo biloba, nonsteroidal anti-inflammatory drugs, ticlopidine, and clopidogrel.

PREOPERATIVE CARE
Patient Education

Patient education is a vital component of the surgical experience. Preoperative patient education may be offered through conversation, discussion, the use of audiovisual aids, demonstrations, and return demonstrations. It is designed to help the patient understand the surgical experience to minimize anxiety and promote full recovery from surgery and anesthesia. The educational program may be initiated before hospitalization by the physician, nurse practitioner or office nurse, or other designated personnel. This is particularly important for patients who are admitted the day of surgery or who are to undergo outpatient surgical procedures. The perioperative nurse can assess the patient's knowledge base and use this information in developing an IPOC (interdisciplinary plan of care), for an uneventful perioperative course.

Teaching Strategies

Obtain a Database

1. Determine what the patient already knows or wants to know. This can be accomplished by reading the patient's chart, interviewing the patient, and communicating with the health care provider, family, and other members of the health care team.
2. Ascertain the patient's psychosocial adjustment to impending surgery.
3. Determine cultural or religious health beliefs and practices that may have an impact on the patient's surgical experience, such as refusal of blood transfusions, burial of amputated limbs within 24 hours, or special healing rituals.

Plan and Implement Teaching Program

1. Begin at the patient's level of understanding and proceed from there.
2. Plan a presentation, or series of presentations, for an individual patient or a group of patients.
3. Include family members and significant others in the teaching process.
4. Encourage active participation of patients in their care and recovery.
5. Demonstrate essential techniques; provide the opportunity for patient practice and return demonstration.
6. Provide time for and encourage the patient to ask questions and express concerns; make every effort to answer all questions truthfully and in basic agreement with the overall therapeutic plan.
7. Provide general information and assess the patient's level of interest in or reaction to it.
   a. Explain the details of preoperative preparation and provide a tour of the area and view the equipment when possible.
   b. Offer general information on the surgery. Explain that the health care provider is the primary resource person.
   c. Notify the patient when surgery is scheduled (if known) and approximately how long it will take; explain that afterward the patient will go to the PACU. Emphasize that delays may be attributed to many factors other than a problem developing with this patient (eg, previous case in the operating room may have taken longer than expected or an emergency case has been given priority).
   d. Let the patient know that his or her family will be kept informed and that they will be told where to wait and when they can see the patient; note visiting hours.
   e. Explain how a procedure or test may feel during or afterward.
   f. Describe the PACU and what personnel and equipment the patient may expect to see and hear (specially trained personnel, monitoring equipment, tubing for various functions, and a moderate amount of activity by nurses and health care providers).
   g. Stress the importance of active participation in postoperative recovery.
8. Use other resource people: health care providers, therapists, chaplain, and interpreters.
9. Document what has been taught or discussed as well as the patient's reaction and level of understanding.
10. Discuss with the patient the anticipated postoperative course (eg, length of stay, immediate postoperative activity, follow-up visit with the surgeon).

Use Audiovisual Aids if Available

1. Videotapes or computer programs are effective in giving basic information to a single patient or group of patients. Many facilities provide a television channel dedicated to patient instruction.
2. Booklets, brochures, and models, if available, are helpful.
3. Demonstrate any equipment that will be specific for the particular patient. Examples:
   a. Drains and drainage bags.
   b. Monitoring equipment.
   c. Side rails.
   d. Incentive spirometer.
   e. Sequential compression device.

General Instructions

Preoperatively, the patient will be instructed in the following postoperative activities. This will allow a chance for practice and familiarity.

Incentive Spirometry

Preoperatively, the patient uses a spirometer to measure deep breaths (inspired air) while exerting maximum effort. The preoperative measurement becomes the goal to be achieved as soon as possible after the operation.

1. Postoperatively, the patient is encouraged to use the incentive spirometer about 10 to 12 times per hour.
2. Deep inhalations expand alveoli, which prevents atelectasis and other pulmonary complications.
3. There is less pain with inspiratory concentration than with expiratory concentration such as with coughing.

Coughing

Coughing promotes the removal of chest secretions. Instruct the patient to:

1. Interlace fingers and place hands over the proposed incision site; this will act as a splint during coughing and not harm the incision.
2. Lean forward slightly while sitting in bed.
3. Breathe, using the diaphragm.
4. Inhale fully with the mouth slightly open.
5. Let out three or four sharp "hacks."
6. With the mouth open, take in a deep breath and quickly give one or two strong coughs.
7. Secretions should be readily cleared from the chest to prevent respiratory complications (pneumonia, obstruction).

 NURSING ALERT Incentive spirometry, deep breathing, and coughing, as well as certain position changes, may be contraindicated after some surgeries (eg, craniotomy and eye or ear surgery).

Turning

Changing positions from back to side-lying (and vice versa) stimulates circulation, encourages deeper breathing, and relieves pressure areas.

1. Help the patient to move onto his or her side if assistance is needed.
2. Place the uppermost leg in a more flexed position than that of the lower leg, and place a pillow comfortably between the legs.
3. Make sure that the patient is turned from one side to the back and onto the other side every 2 hours.

Foot and Leg Exercises

Moving the legs improves circulation and muscle tone.

1. Have the patient lie supine; instruct the patient to bend a knee and raise the foot—hold it a few seconds, and lower it to the bed. Alternately, have the patient do ankle pumps by flexing and pointing feet 20 times.
2. Repeat above about five times with one leg and then with the other. Repeat the set five times every 3 to 5 hours.
3. Then, have the patient lie on one side and exercise the legs by pretending to pedal a bicycle.
4. Suggest the following foot exercise: trace a complete circle with the great toe.

Evaluation of Teaching Program

1. Observe the patient for correct demonstration of expected postoperative behaviors, such as foot and leg exercises and special breathing techniques.
2. Ask pertinent questions to determine the patient's level of understanding.
3. Reinforce information when necessary.

Preparation for Surgery

 EVIDENCE BASE Mehta, J. A., Sable, S. A., & Nagral, S. (2015). Updated recommendations for control of surgical site infection. *Annals of Surgery*, 261(3), e65.
World Health Organization. (2016). *Global guidelines on the prevention of surgical site infections*. Geneva: Author.

Skin Antisepsis

1. Human skin normally harbors transient and resident bacterial flora, some of which are pathogenic. Skin cannot be sterilized without destroying skin cells.
2. The attributes of an appropriate surgical skin antiseptic require the ability to significantly reduce microorganisms, provide broad-spectrum activity, be fast acting, and have a persistent effect.
   a. Preoperative bathing with chlorhexidine reduces pathogenic organisms on the skin. Using multiple showers or showers immediately before coming to the operating room substantially reduces skin organisms.
   b. Cleansing with a bactericidal-impregnated sponge just before operation will provide additional reduction in skin bacteria.
3. The Centers for Disease Control and Prevention recommends that hair not be removed near the operative site unless it will interfere with surgery. The skin is easily injured during shaving that often results in a higher rate of postoperative wound infection.
4. If required, hair removal should be done by clipping, not shaving, and should be performed within 2 hours of surgery. Scissors may be used to remove hair greater than 3 mm in length.
5. For head surgery, obtain specific instructions from the surgeon concerning the extent of shaving.

Gastrointestinal Tract

1. Preparation of the bowel is imperative for patients undergoing intestinal surgery because escaping bacteria can invade adjacent tissues and cause sepsis.
   a. Cathartics and enemas remove gross collections of stool (eg, GoLYTELY).
   b. Oral antimicrobial agents (eg, neomycin, erythromycin) suppress the colon's potent microflora.
   c. Enemas "until clear" are generally not necessary. If ordered, they are given the night before surgery. Notify the health care provider if the enemas never return clear.
2. Solid food is withheld from the patient for 6 hours before surgery. Patients having morning surgery are kept NPO overnight. Clear fluids (water) may be given up to 4 hours before surgery depending on facility protocols.

Genitourinary Tract

A medicated douche may be prescribed preoperatively if the patient is to have a gynecologic or urologic operation.

Preoperative Medication

1. Administration of systemic prophylactic perioperative antibiotics is among one of the most important steps in preventing surgical site infection, which are the most common and

costly type of hospital-acquired infections. It is estimated that 60% are preventable through evidence-based protocols.

2. Redosing of antibiotics during long procedures and when there is excessive blood loss, and discontinuation within 24 hours after surgery end time (48 hours for cardiac surgeries) is recommended.

 DRUG ALERT *Antibiotics should be administered just before surgery—preferably 1 hour (2 hours for vancomycin and fluoroquinolones) before an incision is made—to be effective when bacterial contamination is expected.*

3. There is a risk, however, of an increase in *Clostridium difficile* diarrheal infections because of antibiotic use.

Administering "On-Call" Medications

1. Have the medication ready and administer it as soon as the call is received from the operating room.
2. Proceed with the remaining preparation activities.
3. Indicate on the chart or preoperative checklist the time when the medication was administered and by whom.

Admitting the Patient to Surgery

Final Checklist

The Comprehensive Surgical Checklist from Association of periOperative Registered Nurses (AORN) combines the World Health Organization and the Joint Commission measures for patient preparedness. It may be customized for use in any setting or may be used in addition to a facility's specific checklist that the nurse is also responsible for (see Figure 7-2).

Identification and Verification

This includes verbal identification by the perioperative nurse while checking the identification band on the patient's wrist and written documentation (such as the chart) of the patient's identity, the procedure to be performed (laterality, if indicated), the specific surgical site marked by the surgeon with indelible ink, the surgeon, and the type of anesthesia. These are all patient safety goals as outlined by the Joint Commission.

Review of Patient Record

Check for inclusion of the fact sheet; allergies; history and physical; completed preoperative checklist; laboratory values, including most recent results, pregnancy test, if applicable; electrocardiogram (ECG) and chest x-rays, if necessary; preoperative medications; and other preoperative orders by either the surgeon or anesthesia care provider.

Consent Form

All nurses involved with patient care in the preoperative setting should be aware of the individual state laws regarding informed consent and the specific facility policy. Obtaining informed consent is the responsibility of the surgeon performing the specific procedure. Consent forms should state the procedure, various risks, and alternatives to surgery, if any. It is a nursing responsibility to make sure the consent form has been obtained with the patient or guardian's signature and that it is in the chart.

Patient Preparedness

1. NPO status.
2. Proper attire (clean gown and hair covering) and clean linen.
3. Skin preparation, if ordered.
4. IV line started with correct gauge needle.

5. Dentures or plates removed.
6. Jewelry, piercings, contact lenses, and glasses removed and secured in a locked area or given to a family member.
7. Allow the patient to void.

Transporting the Patient to the Operating Room

1. Adhere to the principle of maintaining the comfort and safety of the patient.
2. Accompany operating room attendants to the patient's bedside for introduction and proper identification.
3. Assist in transferring the patient from bed to stretcher (unless the bed goes to the operating room floor).
4. Complete the chart and preoperative checklist; include laboratory reports and x-rays as required by facility policy or the health care provider's directive.
5. Make sure that the patient arrives in the operating room at the proper time.

The Patient's Family

1. Direct the patient's family to the proper waiting room where magazines, television, and beverages may be available.
2. Tell the family that the surgeon will probably contact them there after surgery to inform them about the operation.
3. Inform the family that a long interval of waiting does not mean the patient is in the operating room the whole time; anesthesia preparation and induction take time, and after surgery, the patient is taken to the PACU.
4. Tell the family what to expect postoperatively when they see the patient—tubes, monitoring equipment, and blood transfusion, suctioning, and oxygen equipment.

INTRAOPERATIVE CARE

 NURSING ALERT Nursing competencies for intraoperative care include ACLS/PALS, moderate sedation, intralipid protocol, recognition of signs and symptoms of toxicity including cardiac arrhythmias and seizures, pharmacology of local anesthetic agents, and neurovascular/neurological checks. Nurses should be familiar with each type of block performed, its therapeutic effects, associated side effects, possible adverse reactions associated with the specific block performed, and any indicated emergency interventions. These competencies are necessary to ensure the patient's optimal safety during the perioperative patient experience.

Anesthesia and Related Complications

The goals of anesthesia are to provide analgesia, sedation, and muscle relaxation appropriate for the type of operative procedure as well as to control the autonomic nervous system.

Common Anesthetic Techniques

Moderate Sedation

EVIDENCE BASE Association of periOperative Registered Nurses. (2017). *Recommended practice for managing the patient receiving moderate sedation/analgesia.* Denver, CO: Author.

COMPREHENSIVE SURGICAL CHECKLIST

Blue = World Health Organization (WHO)   Green = The Joint Commission - Universal Protocol 2016 National Patient Safety Goals   Teal = Joint Commission and WHO

PREPROCEDURE CHECK-IN	SIGN-IN	TIME-OUT	SIGN-OUT
In Preoperative Ready Area	**Before Induction of Anesthesia**	**Before Skin Incision**	**Before the Patient Leaves the Operating Room**
Patient or patient representative actively confirms with registered nurse (RN):	**RN and anesthesia professional confirm:**	Initiated by designated team member: All other activities to be suspended (except in case of life-threatening emergency)	**RN confirms:**
Identity ☐ Yes Procedure and procedure site ☐ Yes Consent(s) ☐ Yes Site marked ☐ Yes ☐ N/A by the person performing the procedure **RN confirms presence of:** History and physical ☐ Yes Preanesthesia assessment ☐ Yes Nursing assessment ☐ Yes Diagnostic and radiologic test results ☐ Yes ☐ N/A Blood products ☐ Yes ☐ N/A Any special equipment, devices, implants ☐ Yes ☐ N/A	Confirmation of the following: identity, procedure, procedure site, and consent(s) ☐ Yes Site marked ☐ Yes ☐ N/A by person performing the procedure Patient allergies ☐ Yes ☐ N/A Pulse oximeter on patient ☐ Yes Difficult airway or aspiration risk ☐ No ☐ Yes (preparation confirmed) Risk of blood loss (> 500 mL) ☐ Yes ☐ N/A # of units available _____ Anesthesia safety check completed ☐ Yes **Briefing:** All members of the team have discussed care plan and addressed concerns ☐ Yes	Introduction of team members ☐ Yes **All:** Confirmation of the following: identity, procedure, incision site, consent(s) ☐ Yes Site is marked and visible ☐ Yes ☐ N/A **Fire Risk Assessment and Discussion** ☐ Yes (prevention methods implemented) ☐ N/A Relevant images properly labeled and displayed ☐ Yes ☐ N/A Any equipment concerns ☐ Yes ☐ N/A **Anticipated Critical Events** **Surgeon:** States the following: ☐ Critical or nonroutine steps ☐ Case duration ☐ Anticipated blood loss **Anesthesia professional:** Antibiotic prophylaxis within 1 hour before incision ☐ Yes ☐ N/A Additional concerns ☐ Yes ☐ N/A **Scrub person and RN circulator:** Sterilization indicators confirmed ☐ Yes Additional concerns ☐ Yes ☐ N/A **RN:** Documented completion of time out ☐ Yes	Name of operative procedure: _____ Completion of sponge, sharp, and instrument counts ☐ Yes ☐ N/A Specimens identified and labeled ☐ Yes ☐ N/A Equipment problems to be addressed ☐ Yes ☐ N/A **Discussion of Wound Classification** ☐ Yes **To all team members:** What are the key concerns for recovery and management of this patient? _____ _____ _____ _____ **Debriefing with all team members:** Opportunity for discussion of – team performance – key events – any permanent changes in the preference card June 2016

Include in Preprocedure check-in as per institutional custom:
Beta blocker medication given
☐ Yes ☐ N/A
Venous thromboembolism prophylaxis ordered
☐ Yes ☐ N/A
Normothermia measures
☐ Yes ☐ N/A

The Joint Commission does not stipulate which team member initiates any section of the checklist except for site marking. The Joint Commission also does not stipulate where these activities occur. See the Universal Protocol for details on the Joint Commission requirements.

Figure 7-2. Comprehensive surgical checklist. (Reprinted with permission from AORN.org. Copyright © 2016, AORN, Inc, 2170 S. Parker Road, Suite 400, Denver, CO 80231. All rights reserved. www.aorn.org/guidelines/clinical-resources/tool-kits/correct-site-surgery-tool-kit/aorn-comprehensive-surgical-checklist.)

1. A specific level of sedation that allows patients to tolerate unpleasant procedures by reducing the level of anxiety and discomfort, previously known as conscious sedation.
2. The patient achieves a depressed level of consciousness (LOC) and altered perception of pain while retaining the ability to respond appropriately to verbal and tactile stimuli.
3. Cardiopulmonary function and protective airway reflexes are maintained by the patient.
4. Knowledge of expected outcomes is essential. These outcomes include, but are not limited to:
   a. Maintenance of consciousness.
   b. Maintenance of protective reflexes.
   c. Alteration of pain perception.
   d. Enhanced cooperation.
5. Adequate preoperative preparation of the patient will facilitate achieving the desired effects.
6. Nurses caring for patients receiving moderate sedation should be specially trained in the agents used for moderate sedation, such as midazolam and fentanyl, and should be skilled in advanced life support. Many facilities have strict regulations and training requirements for staff handling such patients.
7. Nurses working in this setting should also be aware of the regulations from the board of nursing in the state they are practicing concerning the care of patients receiving anesthesia and should be compliant with state advisory opinions, declaratory

rules, and other regulations that direct the practice of the registered nurse.
8. Patients who are not candidates for conscious sedation and require more complex sedation should be managed by anesthesia care providers.

Monitored Anesthesia Care

1. Light to deep sedation that is monitored by an anesthesia care provider.
2. The patient is asleep but arousable.
3. The patient is not intubated.
4. The patient may receive local anesthesia and oxygen, is monitored, and receives sedation and analgesia. Midazolam, fentanyl, alfentanil, and propofol are frequently used in monitored anesthesia care procedures.

General Anesthesia

1. A reversible state consisting of complete loss of consciousness. Protective reflexes are lost.
2. With the loss of protective reflexes, the patient's airway needs to be maintained. This can be done by endotracheal intubation or insertion of a laryngeal mask airway (LMA).
   a. For certain, short, and uncomplicated surgeries (eg, myringotomies), the insertion of a breathing tube may not be necessary, and the airway is maintained manually with a jaw thrust/chin-lift.

b. Endotracheal (ET) intubation is facilitated by the use of a laryngoscope. The ET tube is inserted into the trachea and passed through the vocal cords. A cuff is then inflated, thus ensuring a secure airway where no secretions from the oral cavity can enter the lungs.

c. LMA does not require a laryngoscope for insertion and is inserted only to the entrance of the trachea. Although LMA does not provide a totally protected airway, it is non-invasive and more gentle on the tissue.

3. General anesthesia consists of three phases: induction, maintenance, and emergence.

4. Induction can be accomplished either by parenteral or inhalation route. Common agents for IV induction are propofol and phenobarbital. In addition to the induction agent, a potent analgesic is also often added (eg, fentanyl) to potentiate the induction agent as well as provide analgesia. Patients can also reach an unconscious state by inhaling a potent, short-acting volatile gas, such as sevoflurane. Once the patient is asleep, and if the surgical procedure so requires, a muscle relaxant is given and the ET tube is inserted.

5. Maintenance is accomplished through a continuous delivery of the inhalation agent, or an IV infusion of an agent, such as propofol, to maintain an unconscious state. Intermittent doses of an analgesic are given as needed as well as intermittent doses of a muscle relaxant for longer surgeries.

6. Emergence occurs at the end of the surgery when the continuous delivery of either the gas or the IV infusion is stopped and the patient slowly returns to a conscious state. If muscle relaxants are still in effect, they can be reversed with neostigmine to allow for adequate muscle strength and return of spontaneous ventilations. A nerve stimulator can be used to assess if adequate muscle control has returned before extubation of the trachea.

 NURSING ALERT During emergence, the patient is very sensitive to any stimuli. Keep noise levels to a minimum, and refrain from manipulating the patient during this stage.

Regional Anesthesia

1. Anesthesia block is achieved by injecting a local anesthetic, such as lidocaine or bupivacaine, in close proximity to appropriate nerves. It may be spinal, epidural, or peripheral block.

2. Nursing responsibilities include being familiar with the drug used and maximum dose that can be given, knowing signs and symptoms of toxicity, and maintaining a comfortable environment for the conscious patient.

3. *Spinal anesthesia* is the injection of a local anesthetic into the lumbar intrathecal space. The anesthetic blocks conduction in spinal nerve roots and dorsal ganglia, thereby causing paralysis and analgesia below the level of injection.

4. *Epidural anesthesia* involves injecting local anesthetic into the epidural space. Results are similar to spinal analgesia but with a slower onset.
   a. Often, a catheter is inserted for continuous infusion of the anesthetic to the epidural space.
   b. The catheter may be left in place to provide postoperative analgesia as well.

5. *Peripheral nerve block* is achieved by injecting a local anesthetic into a bundle of nerves (eg, axillary plexus) or into a single nerve to achieve anesthesia to a specific part of the body (eg, hand or single finger).

Intraoperative Complications

1. Hypoventilation and hypoxemia—because of inadequate ventilatory support.
2. Oral trauma (broken teeth, oropharyngeal or laryngeal trauma)—because of difficult ET intubation.
3. Hypotension—because of preoperative hypovolemia or untoward reactions to anesthetic agents.
4. Cardiac dysrhythmia—because of preexisting cardiovascular compromise, electrolyte imbalance, or untoward reactions to anesthetic agents.
5. Hypothermia—because of exposure to a cool ambient operating room environment and loss of normal thermoregulation capability from anesthetic agents.
6. Peripheral nerve damage—because of improper positioning of the patient (eg, full weight on an arm) or use of restraints.
7. Malignant hyperthermia.
   a. This is a rare reaction to anesthetic inhalants (notably sevoflurane, enflurane, isoflurane, and desflurane) and the muscle relaxant succinylcholine.
   b. Caused by abnormal and excessive intracellular accumulations of calcium with resulting hypermetabolism, increased muscle contraction, and elevated body temperature.
   c. Treatment consists of discontinuing the inhalant anesthetic, administering IV dantrolene, and applying cooling techniques (eg, cooling blanket, iced saline lavages).
8. Local anesthesia systemic toxicity (LAST)
   a. This is an adverse outcome that occurs when the serum level of local anesthesia increases to an unsafe level.
   b. It is important for the nurse to recognize signs and symptoms. CNS symptoms usually present first (patient has metallic taste, numbness of the tongue and lips, tinnitus, confusion, agitation, and seizures) followed by cardiac symptoms.
   c. Lipid emulsion (20%) therapy must be administered intravenously bolus 100 mL over 2 to 3 minutes for >70 kg patient and bolus 1.5 mL/kg for >70 kg patient. Learn more about LAST protocol at *www.lipidrescue.org*.

 EVIDENCE BASE Fencl, J. L. (2015). Local anesthetic systemic toxicity: Perioperative implications. *AORN Journal, 101*(6), 697–700.

 NURSING ALERT Recognize malignant hyperthermia immediately so that inhalant anesthesia can be discontinued and treatment measures started, to prevent seizures and other adverse effects.

POSTOPERATIVE CARE
Postanesthesia Care Unit

To ensure continuity of care from the intraoperative phase to the immediate postoperative phase, the circulating nurse or anesthesia care provider gives a thorough report to the PACU nurse. See Standards of Care Guidelines 7-1 (page 94). This report should include the following:

1. Type of surgery performed and any intraoperative complications.
2. Type of anesthesia (eg, general, local, sedation).
3. Drains and type of dressings.
4. Presence of ET tube or type of oxygen to be administered (eg, nasal cannula, T piece).
5. Types of lines and locations (eg, peripheral IV, central line, arterial line).

Postanesthesia care unit (PACU) care is geared toward recognizing the signs of distress and anticipating and preventing postoperative difficulties. Carefully monitor the patient coming out of general anesthesia until:

- Vital signs are stable and are within normal range.
- The patient has no signs of respiratory distress and can maintain his or her own airway.
- Reflexes have returned to normal.
- Pain is under control and at a tolerable level for the patient.
- The patient is responsive and oriented to time and place.

This information should serve as a general guideline only. Each patient situation presents a unique set of clinical factors and requires nursing judgment to guide care, which may include additional or alternative measures and approaches.

6. Catheters or tubes, such as a urinary catheter or T tube.
7. Administration of blood, colloids, and fluids and electrolytes.
8. Drug allergies and pertinent medical history.
9. Preexisting medical conditions.
10. Intraoperative course, including any complications or instability in the patient's vital signs.

Initial Nursing Assessment

Before receiving the patient, note the proper functioning of monitoring and suctioning devices, oxygen therapy equipment, and all other equipment. The following initial assessment is made by the nurse in the PACU:

1. Verify the patient's identity, the operative procedure, and the surgeon who performed the procedure.
2. Obtain vital signs, including pulse oximetry and temperature.
3. Evaluate airway status, noting any stridor or snoring respirations. Capnography may be used to assess adequate oxygenation as well.
4. Evaluate respiratory status, including rate and effort, and auscultate breath sounds.
5. Assess circulatory status, noting skin color, peripheral pulses, and ECG monitor.
6. Observe LOC and orientation to time and place.
7. Evaluate condition of surgical dressings and drains, and check IV lines and infusing fluids and/or IV medications. Initial surgical dressing is usually maintained for 48 hours.
8. Determine patient's pain level using a 1 to 10 scale.
9. Review the health care provider's orders.

NURSING ALERT It is important for the nurse to be able to communicate in the patient's language to provide an accurate assessment. An interpreter must be obtained when necessary.

Initial Nursing Diagnoses

- Ineffective Airway Clearance related to effects of anesthesia.
- Impaired Gas Exchange related to ventilation–perfusion imbalance.
- Risk for unstable glucose level related to uncontrolled diabetes and stress of surgery.
- Ineffective Tissue Perfusion (Cardiopulmonary) related to hypotension postoperatively.

- Risk for Imbalanced Body Temperature related to medications, sedation, and cool environment.
- Risk for Deficient Fluid Volume related to blood loss, food and fluid deprivation, vomiting, and indwelling tubes.
- Acute Pain related to surgical incision and tissue trauma.
- Impaired Skin Integrity related to invasive procedure, immobilization, and altered metabolic and circulatory state.
- Risk for Injury related to sensory dysfunction and physical environment.
- Disturbed Sensory Perception related to effects of medications and anesthesia.

Initial Nursing Interventions

Maintaining a Patent Airway

1. Closely monitor the patient arriving with an oral or nasal airway in place until fully awake.
2. Monitor for return of cough and gag reflex. When the patient is awake and able to protect his or her own airway, the oral or nasal airway can be discontinued.
3. Early initiation of CPAP in the PACU is beneficial for patients exhibiting hypoxemia, apnea, and frequent severe airway obstruction because of obstructive sleep apnea.

Maintaining Adequate Respiratory Function

1. Encourage the patient to take deep breaths to aerate the lungs fully and prevent atelectasis; use an incentive spirometer to aid in this function.
2. Assess lung fields frequently through auscultation.
3. Periodically evaluate the patient's LOC—response to name or command. *Note:* Alterations in cerebral function may suggest impaired oxygen delivery.
4. Administer humidified oxygen to reduce irritation of airways and facilitate secretion removal.

Maintaining Glycemic Control

1. Check serum glucose on arrival to PACU and monitor as indicated.
2. For patients who are diabetic, administer insulin and follow protocols to keep serum glucose levels between 120 and 160 mg/dL. Studies show that normalizing blood glucose for the first 2 to 3 days postoperatively reduces the incidence of deep wound infections comparable to that in nondiabetic patients.

Promoting Tissue Perfusion

1. Monitor vital signs (BP, pulse, respiratory rate, and oxygen saturation) according to protocol, normally every 15 minutes while in the PACU. Monitor ECG tracing for arrhythmias.
   a. Report variations in BP, heart rate, respiratory rate, and cardiac arrhythmias.
   b. Evaluate pulse pressure to determine status of perfusion. (A narrowing pulse pressure indicates impending shock.)
2. Monitor intake and output closely.
3. Recognize the variety of factors that may alter circulating blood volume, such as blood loss during surgery and fluid shifts after surgery.
   a. Recognize early symptoms of shock or hemorrhage: cool extremities, decreased urine output (less than 30 mL/hour), slow capillary refill (greater than 3 seconds), decreased BP, narrowing pulse pressure, and increased heart rate.
4. Intervene to improve tissue perfusion.
   a. Initiate oxygen therapy or increase fraction of inspired oxygen of existing oxygen delivery system.
   b. Increase parenteral fluid infusion, as prescribed.

c. Place the patient in the shock position with his or her feet elevated (unless contraindicated).

d. See Chapter 35 for more detailed consideration of shock.

Stabilizing Thermoregulatory Status

1. Monitor temperature every 15 minutes and be alert for development of both hypothermia and hyperthermia.
2. Report a temperature more than 101.5°F (38.6°C) or less than 95°F (35°C).
3. Monitor for postanesthesia shivering that, although common in hypothermic patients, may also occur in normothermic patients, especially those who received inhalants during anesthesia. It represents a heat-gain mechanism, which drastically increases oxygen demand.
4. Provide warm blankets for patients feeling cold.
5. Provide active warming with forced warm air for hypothermic patients.

Maintaining Adequate Fluid Volume

1. Administer IV, as ordered.
2. Monitor intake and output.
3. Monitor electrolytes and recognize evidence of imbalance, such as nausea, vomiting, and weakness.
4. Evaluate mental status and skin color and turgor.
5. Recognize signs of fluid imbalance.
   a. Hypovolemia—decreased BP, decreased urine output, decreased central venous pressure (CVP), and increased pulse.
   b. Hypervolemia—increased BP; changes in lung sounds, such as crackles in the bases; changes in heart sounds (eg, S_3 gallop); and increased CVP.
6. Evaluate IV sites to detect early infiltration. Restart lines immediately to maintain fluid volume.

Promoting Comfort

1. Assess pain by observing behavioral and physiologic manifestations (change in vital signs may be a result of pain); have the patient rate pain on a scale of 1 to 10.
2. Administer analgesics and document efficacy.
3. Position the patient to maximize comfort.

Minimizing Complications of Skin Impairment

1. Perform handwashing before and after contact with the patient.
2. Inspect dressings routinely and reinforce them, if necessary.
3. Record the amount and type of wound drainage (see "Wound management," page 103).
4. Turn the patient frequently and maintain good body alignment.

Maintaining Safety

1. Keep the side rails up until the patient is fully awake.
2. Protect the extremity into which IV fluids are running so that the needle will not become accidentally dislodged.
3. Avoid nerve damage and muscle strain by properly supporting and padding pressure areas.
4. Be aware that patients who have received regional anesthesia may not be able to complain of an injury, such as the pricking of an open safety pin or a clamp that is exerting pressure.
5. Check the dressing for constriction.
6. Determine the return of motor control following regional anesthesia—indicated by how the patient responds to a request to move a body part.

Minimizing Sensory Deficits

1. Know that the ability to hear returns more quickly than other senses as the patient emerges from anesthesia.
2. Avoid saying anything in the patient's presence that may be disturbing; the patient may appear to be sleeping but still consciously hears what is being said.
3. Explain procedures and activities at the patient's level of understanding.
4. Minimize the patient's exposure to emergency treatment of nearby patients by drawing the curtains and lowering your voice and noise levels.
5. Treat the patient as a person who needs as much attention as the equipment and monitoring devices.
6. Respect the patient's feeling of sensory deprivation and overstimulation; make adjustments to minimize this fluctuation of stimuli.
7. Demonstrate concern for and an understanding of the patient and anticipate his or her needs and feelings.
8. Tell the patient repeatedly that the surgery is over and that he or she is in the PACU.

Evaluation: Expected Outcomes

- Absence of respiratory distress.
- Lung sounds clear to auscultation.
- Glucose less than 160 mg/dL.
- Vital signs stable and within preoperative ranges.
- Body temperature more than 95°F (35°C) and less than 101.5°F (38.6°C).
- IV infusion patent; urine output 50 to 60 mL/hour.
- Adequate pain control.
- Wound/dressing intact without excessive drainage.
- Side rails up; positioned carefully; moving extremities appropriately.
- Quiet, reassuring environment maintained.

Transferring the Patient from the PACU

Each facility may have an individual checklist or scoring guide used to determine a patient's readiness for transfer. The above evaluation criteria must be met before transfer.

Transfer Responsibilities

1. Relay appropriate information to the unit nurse regarding the patient's condition. Use an approved method of communication such as SBAR (situation, background, assessment, and recommendations). Point out significant needs, vital signs (trends and most recent set), fluid therapy, incision and dressing requirements, intake needs, urine output, and color and amount of any drainage.
2. Physically assist in the transfer of the patient.
3. Orient the patient to the room, attending nurse, call light, and therapeutic devices.

Postoperative Discomforts

Most patients experience some discomforts postoperatively. These are usually related to the general anesthetic and the surgical procedure. The most common discomforts are nausea, vomiting, restlessness, sleeplessness, thirst, constipation, flatulence, and pain.

Postoperative Nausea and Vomiting (PONV)

Causes

1. Occurs in many postoperative patients.
2. Most commonly related to inhalation anesthetics (nitrous oxide) and opioid use.
3. Can result from an accumulation of fluid or food in the stomach before peristalsis returns.
4. May occur as a result of abdominal distention, which follows manipulation of abdominal organs.

Preventive Measures

EVIDENCE BASE American Society of PeriAnesthesia Nurses. (2017). *2017–2018 perianesthesia nursing standards and practice recommendations.* Cherry Hill, NJ: Author.

1. Insert a nasogastric (NG) tube intraoperatively for operations on the GI tract to prevent abdominal distention, which triggers vomiting.
2. Evaluate patient preoperatively for risk factors for PONV, such as being female, being a nonsmoker, and having a history of motion sickness.

Nursing Interventions

1. Encourage the patient to breathe deeply to facilitate elimination of anesthetic.
2. Support the wound during retching and vomiting; turn the patient's head to the side to prevent aspiration.
3. Discard vomitus and refresh the patient—provide mouthwash and clean linens.
4. Provide small sips of a carbonated beverage such as ginger ale, if tolerated or permitted.
5. Report excessive or prolonged vomiting so the cause may be investigated.
6. Maintain an accurate intake and output record and replace fluids as ordered.
7. Detect the presence of abdominal distention or hiccups, suggesting gastric retention.
8. Administer antiemetic agents such as ondansetron or promethazine as directed; be aware that some of these drugs may potentiate the hypotensive effects of opioids.

DRUG ALERT Suspect idiosyncratic response to a drug if vomiting is worse when a medication is given (but diminishes thereafter).

Thirst

Causes

1. Inhibition of secretions by medication with atropine.
2. Fluid lost by way of perspiration, blood loss, and dehydration because of NPO status.

Preventive Measures

Unfortunately, postoperative thirst is a common and troublesome symptom that is usually unavoidable due to anesthesia. The immediate implementation of nursing interventions is most helpful.

Nursing Interventions

1. Administer fluids parenterally or orally, if tolerated and permitted.
2. Offer ice chips.
3. Apply a moistened gauze square over lips occasionally to humidify inspired air.
4. Allow the patient to rinse mouth with mouthwash.

Constipation and Gas Cramps

Causes

1. Trauma and manipulation of the bowel during surgery as well as opioid use.
2. More serious causes: peritonitis or abscess.

Preventive Measures

1. Encourage early ambulation to aid in promoting peristalsis.
2. Provide adequate fluid intake to promote soft stools and hydration.
3. Advocate proper diet to promote peristalsis.
4. Encourage the early use of nonopioid analgesia because many opiates increase the risk of constipation.
5. Assess bowel sounds frequently.

Nursing Interventions

1. Ask the patient about any usual remedy for constipation and try it, if appropriate.
2. Insert a gloved, lubricated finger and break up the fecal impaction manually, if necessary.
3. Administer an oil retention enema (180 to 200 mL), if prescribed, to help soften the fecal mass and facilitate evacuation.
4. Administer a return flow enema (if prescribed) or a rectal tube to decrease painful flatulence.
5. Administer GI stimulants, laxatives, suppositories, and stool softeners, as prescribed.

Postoperative Pain

Pain is a subjective symptom, in which the patient exhibits a feeling of distress; stimulation of, or trauma to, certain nerve endings cause pain. Pain is one of the earliest symptoms that the patient expresses on return to consciousness. Maximal postoperative pain occurs directly after surgery and usually diminishes significantly by 48 hours.

Clinical Manifestations

1. Autonomic.
   a. Elevation of BP.
   b. Increase in heart and pulse rate.
   c. Rapid and irregular respiration.
   d. Increase in perspiration.
2. Skeletal muscle.
   a. Increase in muscle tension or activity.
3. Psychological.
   a. Increase in irritability.
   b. Increase in apprehension.
   c. Increase in anxiety.
   d. Attention focused on pain.
   e. Complaints of pain.
4. The patient's reaction depends on:
   a. Previous experience.
   b. Anxiety or tension.
   c. State of health.
   d. Ability to be distracted.
   e. Meaning that pain has for the patient.

Preventive Measures

1. Reduce anxiety because of anticipation of pain.
2. Teach patient about pain management.
3. Review analgesics with patient and reassure that pain relief will be available quickly.
4. Establish a trusting relationship and spend time with patient.

Nursing Interventions

Use Basic Comfort Measures

1. Provide therapeutic environment—proper temperature and humidity, ventilation, and visitors.
2. Massage patient's back and pressure points with soothing strokes—move patient gently and with prewarning.
3. Offer diversional activities, soft music, or favorite television program.

4. Provide for fluid needs by giving a cool drink; offer a bed pan.
5. Investigate possible causes of pain, such as bandage or adhesive that is too tight, full bladder, a cast that is too snug, or elevated temperature indicating inflammation or infection.
6. Instruct the patient to splint the wound when moving.
7. Keep bedding clean, dry, and free from wrinkles and debris.

Recognize the Power of Suggestion
1. Provide reassurance that the discomfort is temporary and that the medication will aid in pain reduction.
2. Clarify patient's fears regarding the perceived significance of pain.
3. Assist patient in maintaining a positive, hopeful attitude.

Assist in Relaxation Techniques
Imagery, meditation, controlled breathing, self-hypnosis or suggestion (autogenic training), and progressive relaxation.

Apply Cutaneous Counterstimulation
1. Vibration—a vigorous form of massage that is applied to a nonoperative site. It lessens the patient's perception of pain. (Avoid applying this to the calf because it may dislodge a thrombus.)
2. Heat or cold—apply to the operative or nonoperative site as prescribed. This works best for well-localized pain. Cold has more advantages than heat and fewer unwanted adverse effects (eg, burns). Heat works well with muscle spasm.

Give Analgesics as Prescribed in a Timely Manner
1. Instruct the patient to request an analgesic before the pain becomes severe.
2. If pain occurs consistently and predictably throughout a 24-hour period, analgesics should be given around the clock—avoiding the usual "demand cycle" of dosing that sets up eventual dependency and provides less adequate pain relief.
3. Administer prescribed medication to the patient before anticipated activities and painful procedures (eg, dressing changes).
4. Monitor for possible adverse effects of analgesic therapy (eg, respiratory depression, hypotension, nausea, skin rash). Administer naloxone to relieve significant opioid-induced respiratory depression.
5. Assess and document the efficacy of analgesic therapy.

Pharmacologic Management

Oral and Parenteral Analgesia
1. Surgical patients are commonly prescribed a parenteral analgesic for 2 to 4 days or until the incisional pain abates. At that time, an oral analgesic, opioid, or nonopioid will be prescribed.
2. Although the health care provider is responsible for prescribing the appropriate medication, it is the nurse's responsibility to make sure the drug is given safely and assessed for efficacy.

 NURSING ALERT The patient who remains sedated because of analgesia is at risk for complications such as aspiration, respiratory depression, atelectasis, hypotension, falls, and poor postoperative course.

 DRUG ALERT Opioid "potentiators," such as hydroxyzine, may further sedate the patient.

Patient-Controlled Analgesia (PCA)
1. Benefits.
   a. Bypasses the delays inherent in traditional analgesic administration (the "demand cycle").

b. Medication is administered by IV, producing more rapid pain relief and greater consistency in patient response.
   c. The patient retains control over pain relief (added placebo and relaxation effects).
   d. Decreased nursing time in frequent delivery of analgesics.
2. Contraindications.
   a. Generally, patients younger than age 10 or 11 (depends on the weight of the child and facility policy).
   b. Patients with cognitive impairment (delirium, dementia, mental illness, hemodynamic or respiratory impairment).
3. A portable PCA device delivers a preset dosage of opioid (usually morphine). An adjustable "lockout interval" controls the frequency of dose administration, preventing another dose from being delivered prematurely. An example of PCA settings might be a dose of 1 mg morphine with a lockout interval of 6 minutes (total possible dose is 10 mg/hour).
4. Patient pushes a button to activate the device.
5. Instruction about PCA should occur preoperatively; some patients fear being overdosed by the machine and require reassurance.

Epidural Analgesia
1. Requires injections of opioids into the epidural space by way of a catheter inserted by an anesthesiologist under aseptic conditions (see Figure 7-3).
2. Benefit: provides for longer periods of analgesia.
3. Disadvantages.
   a. The epidural catheter's proximity to the spinal nerves and spinal canal, along with its potential for catheter migration, makes correct injection technique and close patient assessment imperative.
   b. Adverse effects include generalized pruritus (common), nausea, urinary retention, respiratory depression, hypotension, motor block, and sensory or sympathetic block. These adverse effects are related to the opioid used (usually, a preservative-free morphine or fentanyl) and catheter position.
4. Strict sterile technique is necessary when inserting the epidural catheter.
5. Opioid-related adverse effects are reversed with naloxone.
6. The nurse ensures proper integrity of the catheter and dressing.

Postoperative Complications

Postoperative complications are a risk inherent in surgical procedures. They may interfere with the expected outcome of the surgery and may extend the patient's hospitalization and convalescence. The nurse plays a critical role in attempting to prevent complications and in recognizing their signs and symptoms immediately.

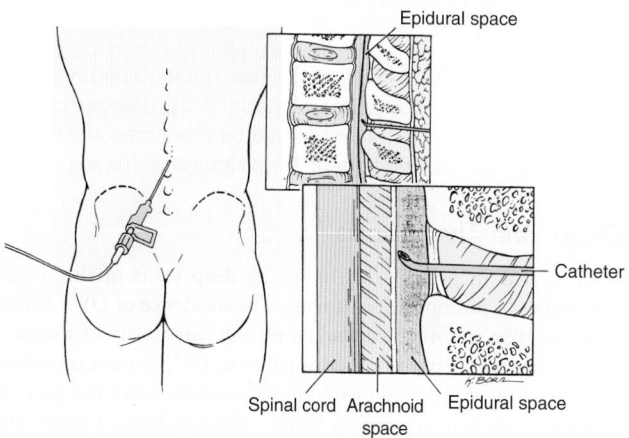

Figure 7-3. Epidural catheter placement.

NURSING ALERT Notify the surgeon if there is any deviation from the normal expected outcomes postoperatively.

Shock

Shock is a response of the body to decreased tissue perfusion, culminating, eventually, in cellular hypoxia and death. (See Chapter 35 for classification and emergency management of shock.)

Preventive Measures

1. Have blood available if there is any indication that it may be needed.
2. Accurately measure any blood loss and monitor all fluid intake and output.
3. Anticipate the progression of symptoms on earliest manifestation.
4. Monitor vital signs per facility protocol until they are stable.
5. Assess vital sign deviations; evaluate BP in relation to other physiologic parameters of shock and the patient's premorbid values. Orthostatic pulse and BP are important indicators of hypovolemic shock.
6. Prevent infection (eg, indwelling catheter care, wound care, pulmonary care) to minimize the risk of septic shock.

Hemorrhage

Hemorrhage is the escape of blood from a ruptured blood vessel. Hemorrhage from an arterial vessel may be bright red in color and come in spurts, whereas blood from a vein is dark red and comes in a steady flow. Hemorrhage may be external or internal (concealed).

Clinical Manifestations

1. Apprehension; restlessness; thirst; cold, moist, pale skin; and circumoral pallor.
2. Pulse increases, respirations become rapid and deep ("air hunger"), and temperature drops.
3. With progression of hemorrhage:
   a. Decrease in cardiac output and narrowed pulse pressure.
   b. Rapidly decreasing BP, as well as hematocrit and hemoglobin (if hypovolemic shock is due to hemorrhage).

Nursing Interventions and Management

1. Treat the patient as described for shock (see Chapter 35).
2. Inspect the wound as a possible site of bleeding. Apply pressure dressing over an external bleeding site.
3. Increase the IV fluid infusion rate and administer blood as directed and as soon as possible.
4. Administer 100% oxygen.

 NURSING ALERT Numerous, rapid blood transfusions may induce coagulopathy and prolonged bleeding time. The patient should be monitored closely for signs of increased bleeding tendencies after transfusions.

Deep Vein Thrombosis

DVT occurs in pelvic veins or in the deep veins of the lower extremities in postoperative patients. The incidence of DVT varies between 10% and 40% depending on the complexity of the surgery or the severity of the underlying illness. DVT is most common after hip surgery, followed by retropubic prostatectomy and general thoracic or abdominal surgery. Venous thrombi located above the knee are considered the major source of pulmonary emboli.

Causes

1. Injury to the intimal layer of the vein wall.
2. Venous stasis.
3. Hypercoagulopathy and polycythemia.
4. High risks include obesity, prolonged immobility, cancer, smoking, estrogen use, advancing age, varicose veins, dehydration, splenectomy, and orthopedic procedures.

Clinical Manifestations

1. Most patients with DVT are asymptomatic.
2. Pain or cramp in the calf or thigh, progressing to painful swelling of the entire leg.
3. Slight fever, chills, and perspiration.
4. Marked tenderness over the anteromedial surface of the thigh.
5. Intravascular clotting without marked inflammation may develop, leading to phlebothrombosis.
6. Circulation distal to the DVT may be compromised if sufficient swelling is present.

Preventive Measures and Management

1. Hydrate patient adequately postoperatively to prevent hemoconcentration.
2. Encourage leg exercises and ambulate patient as soon as permitted by surgeon.
3. Avoid restricting devices, such as tight straps, that can constrict and impair circulation.
4. Avoid rubbing or massaging calves and thighs.
5. Instruct the patient to avoid standing or sitting in one place for prolonged periods and crossing legs when seated.
6. Refrain from inserting IV catheters into legs or feet of adults.
7. Assess distal peripheral pulses, capillary refill, and sensation of lower extremities.
8. Check for positive Homans sign—calf pain on dorsiflexion of the foot, present in nearly 30% of DVT patients.
9. Prevent the use of bed rolls or knee gatches in patients at risk because there is danger of constricting the vessels under the knee.
10. Initiate anticoagulant therapy IV, subcutaneously, or orally as prescribed.
11. Prevent swelling and stagnation of venous blood by applying appropriately fitting compression stockings or wrapping the legs from the toes to the groin with compression bandage.
12. Apply external pneumatic compression intraoperatively to patients at highest risk of DVT. Pneumatic compression can reduce the risk of DVT by 30% to 50% (see Figure 7-4).
13. Mechanical prophylaxis by having the patient perform foot pumps also provides an alternative to chemical agents in the prevention of thromboembolic disease. The use of foot pumps is safe and patient compliance may be enhanced.

Figure 7-4. Pneumatic compression. Pressures of 35 to 20 mm Hg are sequentially applied from the ankle to the thigh, producing an increase in blood flow velocity and improved venous clearing.

Pulmonary Complications

Causes and Clinical Manifestations
1. Atelectasis.
   a. Incomplete expansion of the lung or portion of it occurring within 48 hours of surgery.
   b. Attributed to the absence of periodic deep breaths.
   c. A mucus plug closes a bronchiole, causing the alveoli distal to the plug to collapse.
   d. Symptoms are typically absent but may include mild to severe tachypnea, tachycardia, cough, fever, hypotension, and decreased breath sounds and chest expansion of the affected side.
2. Aspiration.
   a. Caused by the inhalation of food, gastric contents, water, or blood into the tracheobronchial system.
   b. Anesthetic agents and opioids depress the central nervous system, causing inhibition of gag or cough reflexes.
   c. NG tube insertion renders upper and lower esophageal sphincters partially incompetent.
   d. Gross aspiration has 50% mortality.
   e. Symptoms depend on the severity of aspiration and may be silent or become evident within minutes, including tachypnea, dyspnea, cough, bronchospasm, wheezing, rhonchi, crackles, hypoxia, and frothy sputum.
3. Pneumonia.
   a. An inflammatory response in which cellular material replaces alveolar gas.
   b. In the postoperative patient, most commonly caused by gram-negative bacilli because of impaired oropharyngeal defense mechanisms.
   c. Predisposing factors include atelectasis, upper respiratory infection, copious secretions, aspiration, dehydration, prolonged intubation or tracheostomy, history of smoking, and impaired normal host defenses (cough reflex, mucociliary system, alveolar macrophage activity).
   d. Symptoms include dyspnea, tachypnea, pleuritic chest pain, fever, chills, hemoptysis, cough (rusty or purulent sputum), and decreased breath sounds over the involved area.

Preventive Measures
1. Report evidence of upper respiratory infection to the surgeon.
2. Suction nasopharyngeal or bronchial secretions if the patient cannot clear his or her own airway.
3. Use proper patient positioning to prevent regurgitation and aspiration.
4. Recognize the predisposing causes of pulmonary complications:
   a. Infections—mouth, nose, sinuses, and throat.
   b. Aspiration of vomitus.
   c. History of heavy smoking and chronic pulmonary disease.
   d. Obesity.
5. Avoid oversedation.

Nursing Interventions and Management
1. Monitor the patient's progress carefully on a daily basis to detect early signs and symptoms of respiratory difficulties.
   a. Slight temperature, pulse, and respiration elevations.
   b. Apprehension and restlessness or a decreased LOC.
   c. Complaints of chest pain, signs of dyspnea, or cough.
2. Promote full aeration of the lungs.
   a. Turn the patient frequently.
   b. Encourage the patient to take 10 deep breaths hourly, holding each breath to a count of five and exhaling.
   c. Use a spirometer or other device that encourages the patient to ventilate more effectively.
   d. Assist the patient in coughing in an effort to bring up mucus secretions. Have patient splint chest or abdominal wound to minimize discomfort associated with deep breathing and coughing.
   e. Encourage and assist the patient to ambulate as early as the health care provider will allow.
3. Initiate specific measures for particular pulmonary problems.
   a. Provide cool mist or heated nebulizer for the patient exhibiting signs of bronchitis or thick secretions.
   b. Encourage the patient to take fluids to help "liquefy" secretions and facilitate expectoration (in pneumonia).
   c. Elevate the head of the bed and ensure proper administration of prescribed oxygen.
   d. Prevent abdominal distention—NG tube insertion may be necessary.
   e. Administer prescribed antibiotics for pulmonary infections.

Pulmonary Embolism

Causes
1. Pulmonary embolism (PE) is caused by the obstruction of one or more pulmonary arterioles by an embolus originating somewhere in the venous system or in the right side of the heart.
2. Postoperatively, the majority of emboli develop in the pelvic or iliofemoral veins before becoming dislodged and traveling to the lungs.

Clinical Manifestations
1. Sharp, stabbing pains in the chest.
2. Anxiousness and cyanosis.
3. Pupillary dilation and profuse perspiration.
4. Rapid and irregular pulse becoming imperceptible—leads rapidly to death.
5. Dyspnea, tachypnea, and hypoxemia.
6. Pleural friction rub (occasionally).

Nursing Interventions and Management
1. Administer oxygen with the patient in an upright sitting position (if possible).
2. Reassure and calm the patient.
3. Monitor vital signs, ECG, and arterial blood gases.
4. Treat for shock or heart failure, as needed.
5. Give analgesics or sedatives, as directed, to control pain or apprehension.
6. Prepare for anticoagulation or thrombolytic therapy or surgical intervention. Management depends on the severity of the PE.

 NURSING ALERT Massive PE is life-threatening and requires immediate intervention to maintain the patient's cardiorespiratory status.

Urinary Retention

Causes
1. Occurs postoperatively, especially after operations of the rectum, anus, vagina, or lower abdomen.
2. Often seen in patients having epidural or spinal anesthesia.
3. Caused by spasm of the bladder sphincter.
4. More common in male patients because of inherent increases in urethral resistance to urine flow.
5. Can lead to urinary tract infection and possibly renal failure.

Clinical Manifestations
1. Inability to void or voiding small amounts at frequent intervals.
2. Palpable bladder.
3. Lower abdominal discomfort.

Preventive Measures and Management
1. Help patient to sit or stand (if permissible) because many patients are unable to void while lying in bed.
2. Provide patient with privacy.
3. Run tap water—frequently, the sound or sight of running water relaxes spasm of bladder sphincter.
4. Use warmth to relax sphincters (eg, a sitz bath or warm compresses).
5. Notify health care provider if the patient does not urinate regularly after surgery.
6. Administer antispasmodic as directed to reduce painful bladder spasm.
7. Catheterize only when all other measures are unsuccessful. SCIP recommends removing an indwelling catheter within 24 hours. Use of bladder scanner can reduce the need for catheterization by checking for residual urine noninvasively.

 NURSING ALERT Recognize that when a patient voids small amounts (30 to 60 mL every 15 to 30 minutes), this may be a sign of an overdistended bladder with "overflow" of urine.

Intestinal Obstruction

Intestinal obstructions result in a partial or complete impairment to the forward flow of intestinal contents. Most obstructions occur in the small bowel, especially at its narrowest point—the ileum. (See page 515 for a full discussion of intestinal obstruction.)

Preventive Measures and Management
1. Monitor for adequate bowel sound return after surgery. Assess bowel sounds and the degree of abdominal distention (may need to measure abdominal girth); document these findings every shift.
2. Monitor and document characteristics of emesis and NG drainage.
3. Relieve abdominal distention by passing a nasoenteric suction tube as ordered.
4. Replace fluid and electrolytes.
5. Monitor fluid, electrolyte (especially potassium and sodium), and acid–base status.
6. Administer opioids judiciously because these medications may further suppress peristalsis.
7. Prepare the patient for surgical intervention if the obstruction continues unresolved.
8. Closely monitor the patient for signs of shock.
9. Provide frequent reassurance to the patient; use nontraditional methods to promote comfort (touch, relaxation, imagery).

Wound Infection

Wound infections are the second most common health care–related infection. The infection may be limited to the surgical site (60% to 80%) or may affect the patient systemically.

Causes
1. Exposed tissues during long operations, operations on contaminated structures, gross obesity, old age, chronic hypoxemia, and malnutrition are directly related to an increased infection rate.
2. The patient's own flora is most commonly implicated in wound infections (*Staphylococcus aureus*).
3. Other common culprits in wound infection include *Escherichia coli*, *Klebsiella*, *Enterobacter*, and *Proteus*.
4. Wound infections typically present 5 to 7 days postoperatively.

5. Factors affecting the extent of infection include:
   a. Type, virulence, and quantity of contaminating microorganisms.
   b. Presence of foreign bodies or devitalized tissue.
   c. Location and nature of the wound.
   d. Amount of dead space or presence of hematoma.
   e. Immune response of the patient.
   f. Presence of adequate blood supply to wound.
   g. Presurgical condition of the patient (eg, age, alcoholism, diabetes, malnutrition).

Clinical Manifestations
1. Redness, excessive swelling, tenderness, and warmth.
2. Red streaks in the skin near the wound.
3. Pus or other discharge from the wound.
4. Tender, enlarged lymph nodes in the axillary region or groin closest to the wound.
5. Foul smell from the wound.
6. Generalized body chills or fever.
7. Elevated temperature and pulse.
8. Increasing pain from the incision site.

 GERONTOLOGIC ALERT Older adults do not readily produce an inflammatory response to infection, so they may not present with fever, redness, and swelling. Increasing pain, fatigue, anorexia, and mental status changes are signs of infection in older patients.

 NURSING ALERT Mild, transient fevers appear postoperatively as a result of tissue necrosis, hematoma, or cauterization. Higher sustained fevers arise with the following four most common postoperative complications: atelectasis (within the first 48 hours), wound infections (in 5 to 7 days), urinary infections (in 5 to 8 days), and thrombophlebitis (in 7 to 14 days).

Preventive Measures and Management
1. Preoperative.
   a. Encourage the patient to achieve an optimal nutritional level. Enteral or parenteral alimentation may be ordered preoperatively to reduce hypoproteinemia with weight loss.
   b. Reduce preoperative hospitalization to a minimum to avoid acquiring nosocomial infections.
2. Operative.
   a. Follow strict sterile technique throughout the operative procedure.
   b. When a wound has exudate, fibrin, desiccated fat, or nonviable skin, it is not approximated by primary closure but through secondary (delayed) closure.
3. Postoperative.
   a. Keep dressings intact, reinforcing if necessary, until prescribed otherwise.
   b. Use strict sterile technique when dressings are changed.
   c. Monitor and document the amount, type, and location of drainage. Ensure that all drains are working properly. (See Table 7-1 for expected drainage amounts from common types of drains and tubes.)
4. Postoperative care of an infected wound.
   a. The surgeon removes one or more stitches, separates the wound edges, and looks for infection using a hemostat as a probe.
   b. A culture is taken and sent to the laboratory for bacterial analysis.
   c. Wound irrigation may be done; have an aseptic syringe and saline available.

Table 7-1 Expected Drainage from Tubes and Catheters and Catheters

DEVICE	SUBSTANCE	DAILY DRAINAGE
• Foley catheter • Ileal conduit • Suprapubic catheter	Urine	500–700 mL/24 hr first 48 hr; then 1,500–2,500 mL/24 hr
• Gastrostomy tube	Gastric contents	Up to 1,500 mL/24 hr
• Chest tube	Blood, pleural fluid, air	Varies: 500–1,000 mL first 24 hr
• Ileostomy	Small bowel contents	Up to 4,000 mL in first 24 hr; then <500 mL/24 hr
• Miller-Abbott tube	Intestinal contents	Up to 3,000 mL/24 hr
• NG tube	Gastric contents	Up to 1,500 mL/24 hr
• T tube	Bile	500 mL/24 hr

d. A drain may be inserted or the wound may be packed with sterile gauze.

e. Antibiotics are prescribed.

f. Wet-to-dry dressings may be applied (see page 103).

g. If deep infection is suspected, the patient may be taken back to the operating room.

Wound Dehiscence and Evisceration

Causes

1. Commonly occurs between the 5th and 8th day postoperatively when the incision has weakest tensile strength; greatest strength is found between the 1st and 3rd postoperative day.
2. Chiefly associated with abdominal surgery.
3. This catastrophe is commonly related to:
   a. Inadequate sutures or excessively tight closures (the latter compromises blood supply).
   b. Hematomas and seromas.
   c. Infections.
   d. Excessive coughing, hiccups, retching, and distention.
   e. Poor nutrition and immunosuppression.
   f. Uremia and diabetes mellitus.
   g. Steroid use.

Preventive Measures

1. Apply an abdominal binder for heavy or elderly patients or those with weak or pendulous abdominal walls.
2. Encourage the patient to splint the incision while coughing.
3. Monitor for and relieve abdominal distention.
4. Encourage proper nutrition with emphasis on adequate amounts of protein and vitamin C.

Clinical Manifestations

1. Dehiscence is indicated by a sudden discharge of serosanguineous fluid from the wound.
2. Patient complains that something suddenly "gave way" in the wound.
3. In an intestinal wound, the edges of the wound may part and the intestines may gradually push out. Observe for drainage of peritoneal fluid on dressing (clear or serosanguineous fluid).

Nursing Interventions and Management

1. Stay with patient and have someone notify the surgeon immediately.
2. If the intestines are exposed, cover with sterile, moist saline dressings.
3. Monitor vital signs and watch for shock.
4. Keep patient on absolute bed rest.

5. Instruct the patient to bend the knees, with head of the bed elevated in semi-Fowler position to relieve abdominal tension.
6. Assure patient that the wound will be properly cared for; attempt to keep patient calm and relaxed.
7. Prepare patient for surgery and repair of the wound.

Psychological Disturbances

Depression

1. Cause—perceived loss of health or stamina, pain, altered body image, various drugs, and anxiety about an uncertain future.
2. Clinical manifestations—withdrawal, restlessness, insomnia, nonadherence to therapeutic regimens, tearfulness, and expressions of hopelessness.
3. Nursing interventions and management.
   a. Clarify misconceptions about surgery and its future implications.
   b. Listen to, reassure, and support the patient.
   c. If appropriate, introduce the patient to representatives of ostomy, mastectomy, or amputee support groups.
   d. Involve the patient's family and support people in care; psychiatric consultation is obtained for severe depression.

Delirium

1. Cause—prolonged anesthesia, cardiopulmonary bypass, drug reactions, sepsis, alcoholism (delirium tremens), electrolyte imbalances, and other metabolic disorders.
2. Clinical manifestations—disorientation, hallucinations, perceptual distortions, paranoid delusions, reversed day–night pattern, agitation, and insomnia; delirium tremens often appears within 72 hours of last alcoholic drink and may include autonomic overactivity—tachycardia, dilated pupils, diaphoresis, and fever.
3. Nursing interventions and management.
   a. Assist with the assessment and treatment of the underlying cause (restore fluid and electrolyte balance, discontinue the offending drug).
   b. Reorient the patient to environment and time.
   c. Keep surroundings calm.
   d. Explain in detail every procedure done to the patient.
   e. Sedate the patient, as ordered, to reduce agitation, prevent exhaustion, and promote sleep. Assess for oversedation.
   f. Allow extended periods of uninterrupted sleep.
   g. Reassure family members with clear explanations of the patient's aberrant behavior.
   h. Have contact with the patient as much as possible; apply restraints to the patient only as a last resort if safety is in question and if ordered by the health care provider.

WOUND CARE

 See additional online content: Procedure Guidelines 7-1 and 7-2.

Wounds and Wound Healing

A *wound* is a disruption in the continuity and regulatory processes of tissue cells; *wound healing* is the restoration of that continuity. Wound healing, however, may not restore normal cellular function.

Wound Classification

Mechanism of Injury

1. Incised wounds—made by a clean cut of a sharp instrument, such as a surgical incision with a scalpel.
2. Contused wounds—made by blunt force that typically does not break the skin but causes considerable tissue damage with bruising and swelling.

3. Lacerated wounds—made by an object that tears tissues, producing jagged, irregular edges; examples include glass, jagged wire, and blunt knife.
4. Puncture wounds—made by a pointed instrument, such as an ice pick, bullet, or nail.

Degree of Contamination

1. Clean—an aseptically made wound, as in surgery, that does not enter the alimentary, respiratory, or genitourinary tracts.
2. Clean-contaminated—an aseptically made wound that enters the respiratory, alimentary, or genitourinary tracts. These wounds have slightly higher probability of wound infection than do clean wounds.
3. Contaminated—wounds exposed to excessive amounts of bacteria. These wounds may be open (avulsive) and accidentally made or may be the result of surgical operations in which there are major breaks in sterile techniques or gross spillage from the gastrointestinal tract.
4. Infected—a wound that retains devitalized tissue or involves preoperatively existing infection or perforated viscera. Such wounds are often left open to drain.

Physiology of Wound Healing

The phases of wound healing—inflammation, reconstruction (proliferation), and maturation (remodeling)—involve continuous and overlapping processes.

Inflammatory Phase (Lasts 1 to 5 Days)

1. Vascular and cellular responses are immediately initiated when tissue is cut or injured.
2. Transient vasoconstriction occurs immediately at the site of injury, lasting 5 to 10 minutes, along with the deposition of a fibrinoplatelet clot to help control bleeding.
3. Subsequent dilation of small venules occurs; antibodies, plasma proteins, plasma fluids, leukocytes, and red blood cells leave the microcirculation to permeate the general area of injury, causing edema, redness, warmth, and pain.
4. Localized vasodilation is the result of direct action by histamine, serotonin, and prostaglandins.
5. Polymorphic leukocytes (neutrophils) and monocytes enter the wound to engage in destruction and ingestion of wound debris. Monocytes predominate during this phase.
6. Basal cells at the wound edges undergo mitosis; resultant daughter cells enlarge, flatten, and creep across the wound surface to eventually approximate the wound edges.

Proliferative Phase (Lasts 2 to 20 Days)

1. Fibroblasts (connective tissue cells) multiply and migrate along fibrin strands that are thought to serve as a matrix.
2. Endothelial budding occurs on nearby blood vessels, forming new capillaries that penetrate and nourish the injured tissue.
3. The combination of budding capillaries and proliferating fibroblasts is called *granulation tissue.*
4. Active collagen synthesis by fibroblasts begins by the 5th to 7th day, and the wound gains tensile strength.
5. By 3 weeks, the skin obtains 30% of its preinjury tensile strength, intestinal tissue about 65%, and fascia 20%.

Remodeling Phase (21 Days to Months or Years)

1. Scar tissue is composed primarily of collagen and ground substance (mucopolysaccharide, glycoproteins, electrolytes, and water).
2. From the start of collagen synthesis, collagen fibers undergo a process of lysis and regeneration. The collagen fibers become more organized, aligning more closely to each other and increasing in tensile strength.

3. The overall bulk and form of the scar continue to change once maturation has started.
4. Typically, collagen production drops off; however, if collagen production greatly exceeds collagen lysis, keloid (greatly hypertrophied, deforming scar tissue) will form.
5. Normal maturation of the wound is clinically observed as an initial red, raised, hard immature scar that molds into a flat, soft, and pale mature scar.
6. The scar tissue will never achieve greater than 80% of its pre-injury tensile strength.

Types of Wound Healing

(See Figure 7-5.)

First Intention Healing (Primary Closure)

1. Wounds are made sterile by minor debridement and irrigation, with a minimum of tissue damage and tissue reaction; wound edges are properly approximated with sutures.
2. Granulation tissue is not visible and scar formation is typically minimal (keloid may still form in susceptible people).

Secondary Intention Healing (Granulation)

1. Wounds are left open to heal spontaneously or are surgically closed at a later date; they need not be infected.
2. Examples in which wounds may heal by secondary intention include burns, traumatic injuries, ulcers, and suppurative infected wounds.
3. The cavity of the wound fills with a red, soft, sensitive tissue (granulation tissue), which bleeds easily. A scar (cicatrix) eventually forms.

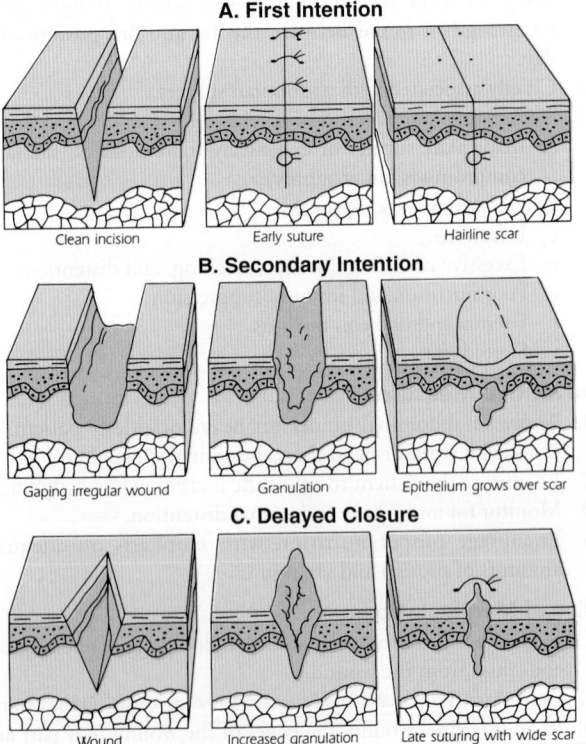

A. First Intention

Clean incision   Early suture   Hairline scar

B. Secondary Intention

Gaping irregular wound   Granulation   Epithelium grows over scar

C. Delayed Closure

Wound   Increased granulation   Late suturing with wide scar

Figure 7-5. Classification of wound healing. **(A)** First intention: A clean incision is made with primary closure; there is minimal scarring. **(B)** Second intention: The wound is left open so that granulation can occur; a large scar results. **(C)** Delayed closure: The wound is initially left open and later closed when there is no further evidence of infection. (Smeltzer, S., & Bare, B. [2000]. *Brunner and Suddarth's textbook of medical-surgical nursing* [9th ed.]. Philadelphia, PA: Lippincott Williams & Wilkins.)

4. In infected wounds, drainage may be accomplished by the use of special dressings and drains. Healing is thus improved.
5. In wounds that are later sutured, the two opposing granulation surfaces are brought together.
6. Secondary intention healing produces a deeper, wider scar.

Wound Management

Many factors promote wound healing, such as adequate nutrition, cleanliness, rest, and position, along with the patient's underlying psychological and physiologic state. Of added importance is the application of appropriate dressings and drains.

Dressings

Purpose of Dressings
1. To protect the wound from mechanical injury.
2. To splint or immobilize the wound.
3. To absorb drainage.
4. To prevent contamination from bodily discharges (feces, urine).
5. To promote hemostasis, as in pressure dressings.
6. To debride the wound by combining capillary action and the entwining of necrotic tissue within its mesh.
7. To inhibit or kill microorganisms by using dressings with antiseptic or antimicrobial properties.
8. To provide a physiologic environment conducive to healing.
9. To provide mental and physical comfort for the patient.
10. To encourage healing by applying localized subatmospheric pressure at site of wound as in negative pressure dressings.

Advantages of Not Using Dressings
When the initial dressing on a clean, dry, and intact incision is removed, it is often not replaced; this may occur within 24 hours after surgery.
1. Permits better visualization of the wound.
2. Eliminates conditions necessary for growth of organisms (warmth, moisture, and darkness).
3. Minimizes adhesive tape reaction.
4. Aids bathing.

Types of Dressings
1. Dry dressings.
   a. Used primarily for wounds closing by primary intention.
   b. Offers good wound protection, absorption of drainage, and aesthetics for the patient and provides pressure, if needed, for hemostasis.
   c. Disadvantage—they adhere to the wound surface when drainage dries. (Removal can cause pain and disruption of granulation tissue.)
2. Wet-to-dry dressings.
   a. These are useful for infected wounds that must be debrided and closed by secondary intention.
   b. Gauze saturated with sterile saline (preferred) or an antimicrobial solution is packed into the wound, eliminating dead space.
   c. The wet dressings are then covered by dry dressings (gauze sponges or absorbent pads).
   d. As drying occurs, wound debris and necrotic tissue are absorbed into the gauze dressing by capillary action.
   e. The dressing is changed when it becomes dry (or just before). If there is excessive necrotic debris on the dressing, more frequent dressing changes are required.
3. Wet-to-wet dressings.
   a. Used on clean open wounds or on granulating surfaces. Sterile saline or an antimicrobial agent may be used to saturate the dressings.

b. Provides a more physiologic environment (warmth, moisture), which can enhance the local healing processes as well as ensure greater patient comfort. Thick exudate is more easily removed.
c. Disadvantage—surrounding tissues can become macerated, there is an increased risk for infection, and bed linens become damp.

Types of Surgical Dressing Supplies
1. Hydrophobic occlusive (petroleum gauze).
   a. This is an impermeable, nonadhering dressing that protects wounds from air- and moisture-borne contamination.
   b. It is used around chest tubes and any fistula or stoma that drains digestive juices.
   c. It is relatively nonabsorptive.
2. Hydrophilic permeable (oil-based gauze, Telfa pads).
   a. Allows drainage to penetrate the dressing but remains somewhat nonadhering.
   b. For wounds with light to moderate exudate.
   c. Oil-based gauze used on abraded and open ulcerated or granulating wounds.
   d. May also be used to pack "caverns and sinuses" of large open wounds.
   e. Telfa pads are generally reserved for simple, closed, stable wounds.
3. Dressing sponges (general-use gauze sponges).
   a. Gauze sponges come in various sizes (most commonly 2" × 2", 4" × 4") and may be used for simple dry dressings, wet-to-dry dressings, or wet-to-wet dressings. Gauze allows for better absorption of drainage and necrotic wound debris.
4. All-absorbent combined dressing.
   a. Large (5" × 9", 8" × 10") cotton-filled dressing that is typically used as an "overdressing," covering gauze or hydrophilic dressings for added wound protection, stabilization of dressings, and drainage absorption.
   b. May also be used unaccompanied over intact surgical wounds.
5. High-bulk gauze bandage ("fluffs")—primarily used for packing large wounds that are undergoing healing by secondary intention.
6. Drain sponge—a gauze sponge with a premade slit, which makes the dressing highly suitable for drain sites and tracheostomy sites.
7. Transparent film dressing.
   a. Highly elastic dressing, adjusts exceptionally well to body contours. It is permeable to oxygen and water vapor but generally impermeable to liquids and bacteria.
   b. Controversies (related to incidence of infection) have reduced its use.
   c. Most common indications include covering arterial and venous catheter sites as well as protecting vulnerable skin exposed to shearing forces.
   d. Commonly used for surgical wounds over gauze dressing to replace tape.
8. Silver-impregnated dressing.
   a. Highly effective for difficult-to-heal wounds. They are available in many sizes and should be placed directly on the wound without any topical ointment.
   b. These may replace need for wet-to-dry or wet-to-wet dressings.
9. Negative pressure wound therapy—promotes healing by applying a vacuum through a special sealed dressing.
   a. Evacuates wound fluid, stimulates granulation tissue, and decreases bacterial colonization.
   b. Contraindicated on patients with active bleeding or taking anticoagulants.

c. NPWT has different interface materials, safety features, and recommended applications by manufacturers. The use is dependent on wound type, provider's preference for gauze or foam packing, and product available.

Drains

Purpose of Drains

1. Drains are placed in wounds only when abnormal fluid collections are present or expected to decrease pooling of body fluids in wound.
2. Drains are usually placed in compartments (eg, joints and pleural space) that are intolerant to fluid accumulation and have large blood supply (eg, neck and kidney), in areas of large superficial tissue dissection (eg, the breast), or in infected wounds.
3. Collection of body fluids in wounds can be harmful in the following ways:
   a. Provides culture media for bacterial growth.
   b. Causes increased pressure at surgical site, interfering with blood flow to area.
   c. Causes pressure on adjacent areas.
   d. Causes local tissue irritation and necrosis (because of fluids such as bile, pus, pancreatic juice, and urine).

Wound Drainage

1. Drains are commonly made of latex, polyvinyl chloride, or silicone and placed within either wounds or body cavities.
2. Drains placed within wounds are typically attached to portable (or, rarely, wall) suction with a collection container.
   a. Examples include the Hemovac, Jackson-Pratt, and Surgivac drainage systems.
3. Drains may also be used postoperatively to form hollow connections from internal organs to the outside to drain a body fluid, such as the T tube (bile drainage), nephrostomy, gastrostomy, jejunostomy, and cecostomy tubes.
4. Drains create a portal for entry and exit of infectious microorganisms; therefore, the risk of infection exists.
5. Drains within wounds are removed when the amount of drainage decreases over a period of days or, rarely, weeks.
6. Body fluid drains are often left in for longer periods of time.
   a. Careful handling of these drains and collection bags is essential.
   b. Accidental early removal may result in caustic drainage leaking within the tissues.
   c. The risk is reduced within 7 to 10 days when a wall of fibrous tissue has been formed.
7. The amount of drainage varies with the procedure. Drains are commonly not needed on some surgical procedures (eg, appendectomy, cholecystectomy, abdominal hysterectomy), which usually have minimal wound drainage.

 NURSING ALERT The greatest amount of drainage is expected during the first 24 hours; closely monitor dressing and drains.

Nursing Process Overview

 EVIDENCE BASE Leaper, D., & Edmiston, C. (2017). World Health Organization: global guidelines for the prevention of surgical site infection. *Journal of Hospital Infection*, 95(2), 135–136.

Nursing Assessment

The wound should be assessed every 15 minutes while the patient is in the PACU. Thereafter, the frequency of wound assessment is determined by the nature of the wound, the degree of drainage, and the facility protocol. Assessment and documentation of the wound's status should occur at least every shift until the patient is discharged.

Determine the following, which will affect wound healing:

1. What type of surgery did the patient have?
2. Was hemostasis in the operating room effective?
3. Has the patient received blood to sustain an adequate hematocrit (and promote perfusion to wound)?
4. What is the patient's age?
5. What is the nutritional status? What was it preoperatively?
   a. Is current intake of protein and vitamin C adequate?
   b. Is the patient obese or cachectic?
6. What underlying medical conditions does the patient have, and what medications is he or she taking that could affect wound healing (eg, diabetes mellitus, steroids)?
7. How long has the patient been hospitalized preoperatively? (Longer preoperative facility stays can increase complications.)
8. How is the wound held together?
   a. Staples, nylon sutures, adhesive strips, tension sutures, surgical skin glue.
   b. If the wound is left open, how is it being treated? Is granulation tissue present?
9. Are drains in place? What kind? How many?
   a. Is portable suction being used?
   b. Is the amount of drainage consistent with the nature of surgery?
10. What kinds of dressings are being used?
    a. Are they saturated?
    b. Is the amount and type of drainage consistent with nature of the surgery?
11. How does the wound appear?
    a. Is there evidence of edema, irritation, inflammation?
    b. Are the wound edges well approximated?
    c. Is the wound clean and dry?
12. How does the patient appear?
    a. Are there signs of wound pain or discomfort?
    b. Is fever or elevated white blood cell count present?
    c. Does the patient express concern about the wound and potential disfigurement?
13. Does the patient understand the purpose of wound therapies, and can he or she or his or her family effectively carry out discharge instructions about wound care?

Nursing Diagnoses

- Risk for Infection related to surgical wound.
- Impaired Tissue Integrity related to surgical wound.
- Acute Pain related to wound dressing procedures.

Nursing Interventions

Preventing Infection

1. Prior to the first dressing change (usually performed by the surgeon), reinforce the dressing when saturated.
2. Gather supplies (dressings, tape, scissors, sterile saline solution, cotton swabs, extra gauze and culture materials if indicated).
3. Explain procedure to the patient. Provide privacy and comfort by premedicating for pain.
4. Wash your hands thoroughly and don gloves. Ensure strict aseptic technique during dressing changes.

5. Remove the old dressings and assess the wound. Loosen all tapes gently. Place dressings in disposable bag. Assess the wound for future documentation noting any redness, swelling, exudate, warmth, bleeding, swelling, or discoloration.
6. Culture the wound if necessary, using sterile technique. Wear sterile gloves. Dab the wound using the culture swab attempting saturation. Place it in the tube. Prepare and label this specimen and send to the lab.
7. Using sterile gloves, clean around the wound edges with saline moist gauze. Do not go over the area with the same gauze. Repeat as necessary with a fresh gauze until all the areas are clean.
8. Dress the wound with sterile gauze and secure with tape. Use minimal amount of tape to assure adhesive.
9. Discard contaminated items, ensure the patient's comfort, and document the procedure.

Enhancing Tissue Integrity Through Healing
1. Assess the patient's nutritional intake; consult with the patient's health care provider if supplemental nutritional intake is required.
2. Minimize strain on the incision site:
   a. Use appropriate tape, bandages, and binders.
   b. Have the patient splint abdominal and chest incision when coughing.
   c. Instruct the patient in proper way to get out of bed while minimizing incision strain (eg, for abdominal incision, have the patient turn on one side and push self up with the dependent elbow and the opposite hand).
3. Assess and accurately document the condition of the incision site each shift.

Relieving Pain
1. Give the patient prescribed medication before painful dressing changes.
2. Continue to assess for pain at incision site.
3. Consider nonpharmacologic pain relief, such as use of music therapy, relaxation exercises, and acupressure, as indicated.

Patient Education
Before discharge, instruct the patient and family on techniques and rationale for wound care.
1. Report immediately to the health care provider if the following signs of infection occur:
   a. Redness, marked swelling, tenderness, and increased warmth around wound.
   b. Pus or unusual discharge and foul odor from wound.
   c. Red streaks in the skin near wound.
   d. Chills or fever (over 100°F [37.8°C]).
2. Follow the directives of the health care provider regarding activity allowances.
3. Keep the wound clean (the patient may shower unless contraindicated by the health care provider; avoid tub bathing until sutures or staples are removed); never vigorously rub near the suture line; pat dry.
   a. Sutures that have been placed need to be removed or may be absorbable. Gently cleanse one to two times daily. Dab dry.
   b. Staples if used will need to be removed after 7 to 14 days. Keep the site clean and dry.
   c. Skin glue, which may be used, allows for good approximation of tissue. Keep the wound clean, and remove glue with medical adhesive removing wipes according to your doctor's instruction.

4. Contact your health care provider for follow-up appointment.
5. Report to the health care provider if after 2 months the incision site continues to be red, thick, and painful to pressure (probable beginning of keloid formation).

Evaluation: Expected Outcomes
- No signs of infection.
- Wound edges well approximated without gaping.
- Pain at level 1 or 2.

POSTOPERATIVE DISCHARGE INSTRUCTIONS
It is of primary importance that the nurse makes sure that the patient has been given specific and individualized discharge instructions. These should be written by a provider and reinforced verbally by the nurse. A provider telephone contact should be included as well as information regarding follow-up care and appointments. The instructions should be signed by the patient, provider, and nurse, and a copy becomes part of the patient's chart. Forms and procedures for discharge instructions may vary per facility.

Patient Education
Rest and Activity
1. It is common to feel tired and frustrated about not being able to do all the things you want; this is normal.
2. Plan regular naps and quiet activities, gradually increasing your exercise over the following weeks.
3. When you begin to exercise more, start by taking a short walk two or three times per day. Consult your health care provider if more specific exercises are required.
4. Climbing stairs in your home may be surprisingly tiring at first. If you have difficulty with this activity, try going upstairs backward ("scooching") on your "bottom" until your strength has returned.
5. Consult your health care provider to determine the appropriate time to return to work.

Eating
1. Follow dietary instructions provided at the facility before your discharge.
2. Your appetite may be limited or you may feel bloated after meals; this problem should lessen as you become more active. (Some prescribed medications can cause this.) If symptoms persist, consult your health care provider.
3. Eat small, regular meals and make them as nourishing as possible to promote wound healing.

Sleeping
1. If sleeping is difficult because of wound discomfort, try taking your pain medication at bedtime.
2. Attempt to get sufficient sleep to aid in your recovery.

Wound Healing
1. Your wound will go through several stages of healing. After initial pain at the site, the wound may feel tingling, itchy, numb, or tight (a slight pulling sensation) as healing occurs.
2. Do not pull off any scabs because they protect the delicate new tissues underneath. They will fall off without any help when ready. Change the dressing according to the surgeon's instructions.

Bowels

1. Irregular bowel habits can result from changes in activity and diet or the use of some drugs.
2. Avoid straining because it can intensify discomfort in some wounds; instead, use a rocking motion while trying to pass stool.
3. Drink plenty of fluids and increase the fiber in your diet through fruits, vegetables, and grains, as tolerated.
4. It may be helpful to take a mild laxative. Consult your health care provider if you have any questions.

Bathing and Showering

1. You may get your wound wet 3 days after your operation if the initial dressing has been changed (unless otherwise advised).
2. Showering is preferable because it allows for thorough rinsing of the wound.
3. If you are feeling too weak, place a plastic or metal chair in the shower so you can be seated during showering.
4. Be sure to dry your wound thoroughly with a clean towel and dress it as instructed before discharge.

Clothing

1. Avoid tight belts and underwear and other clothes with seams that may rub against the wound.
2. Wear loose clothing for comfort and to reduce mechanical trauma to wound.

Driving

1. Ask your health care provider when you may resume driving. Safe driving may be affected by your pain medication. In addition, any violent jarring from an accident may disrupt your wound.

Bending and Lifting

1. How much bending, stretching, and lifting you are allowed depends on the location and nature of your surgery.
2. Typically, for most major surgeries, you should avoid lifting anything heavier than 5 pound for 4 to 8 weeks.
3. It is ideal to obtain home assistance for the first 2 to 3 weeks after discharge.

SELECTED REFERENCES

American Diabetes Association. (2016). Standards of medical care in diabetes. *Diabetes Care, 39*(Suppl. 1), S1–S106.

American Diabetes Association. (2017). Summary of revisions: Standards of medical care in diabetes. *Diabetes Care, 41*(Suppl. 10), S4–S6.

American Society of Anesthesiologists Committee on Standards and Practice Parameters. (2017). Practice guidelines for preoperative fasting and the use of pharmacologic agents to reduce the risk of pulmonary aspiration. An updated report. *Anesthesiology, 126*(3), 376–393.

American Society of PeriAnesthesia Nurses. (2017). Evidence based clinical practice guidelines for the promotion of normothermia. Available: www.aspan.org/Clinical-Practice/Clinical-Guidelines for the ASPAN Clinical Practice Guidelines.

American Society of PeriAnesthesia Nurses. (2017). *2017–2018 perianesthesia nursing standards, practice recommendations and interpretative statements.* Cherry Hill, NJ: Author.

Anesthesia Screening for Obstructive Sleep Apnea. (2016). *ARC Journal of Anesthesiology, 1*(2), 6–12.

Anon, (n.d.). *National Patient Safety Goals® | Joint Commission.* [online]. Available at: https://www.jointcommission.org/standards_information/npsgs.aspx. [Accessed 27 February 2018].

Anon, (n.d.). *TJC Publishes 2018 National Patient Safety Goals.* [online]. Available at: https://www.americandatanetwork.com/2018/01/tjc-publishes-2018-national-patient-safety-goals/ [Accessed 27 February 2018].

Association of periOperative Registered Nurses. (2017). *AORN recommended practices for monitoring the patient receiving intravenous sedation.* Denver, CO: Author.

Association of periOperative Registered Nurses. (2016). Guideline at a glance: Skin antisepsis. *AORN Journal, 104,* 273–276.

Association of periOperative Registered Nurses. (2017). *Recommended practice for managing the patient receiving moderate sedation/analgesia.* Denver, CO: Author.

Association of periOperative Registered Nurses. (2018). *AORN standards and recommended practices* (18th ed.). Denver, CO: Author.

Balinowski, H., & Lopez, C. (2013). Improving patient safety through pre-anesthesia screening for obstructive sleep apnea utilizing the STOP-Bang questionnaire. *Journal of PeriAnesthesia Nursing, 28*(3), e27.

Cirocchi, R., Georgi, P., Mutafchiyski, V., et al. (2017). Negative pressure wound therapy versus healing by secondary intention in pressure ulcers. *Negative Pressure Wound Therapy Journal, 4*(2), 4.

Dubos, K. E. (2017). Why now? Managing obstructive sleep apnea in the ambulatory setting. *Journal of PeriAnesthesia Nursing, 32*(1), 64–65.

El-Boghdadly, K., & Chin, K. (2017). Local anesthetic systemic toxicity. *Obstetric Anesthesia Digest, 37*(1), 12–13.

Fencl, J. L. (2016). Guideline implementation: Moderate sedation/analgesia. *Association of periOperative Registered Nurses Journal, 103*(5), 500–511.

Goode, V., & Phillips, E. (2016). A patient safety dilemma: Obesity in the surgical patient. *AANA Journal, 84*(6), 404–412.

Guideline at a glance: Moderate sedation/analgesia. (2017). *AORN Journal, 105*(6), 638–642.

Harrelson, B., & Fencl, J. (2016). Care of the surgical patient with obstructive sleep apnea. *AORN Journal, 103*(4), 443–437.

Karuppaiah, I. (2017). Role of prophylactic antibody to prevent the surgical site infections—A study in a tertiary care hospitals. *Journal of Medical Science And clinical Research, 05*(06), 23698–23706.

Kibler, V., Hayes, R., Johnson, D., et al. (2012). Cultivating quality: Early postoperative ambulation: Back to basics. *American Journal of Nursing, 112*(4), 63–69.

Leaper, D., & Edmiston, C. (2017). World Health Organization: Global guidelines for the prevention of surgical site infection. *Journal of Hospital Infection, 95*(2), 135–136.

Ljungqvist, O., Scott, M., & Fearon, K. (2017). Enhanced recovery after surgery. *JAMA Surgery, 152*(3), 292.

Manivannan, B., Gowda, D., Bulagonda, P., et al. (2018). Surveillance, auditing, and feedback can reduce surgical site infection dramatically: Toward zero surgical site infections. *Surgical Infections, 19*(3). https://doi.org/10.1089/sur.2017.272.

Martindell, D. (2012). The safe use of negative-pressure wound therapy. *American Journal of Nursing, 112*(6), 59–62.

Maurice, E. (2015). Timely discharge from the ambulatory surgical setting. *AORN Journal, 102*(2), 185–191.

Norman, G., Dumville, J., Mohapatra, D., et al. (2016). Antibiotics and antiseptics for surgical wounds healing by secondary intention. *Cochrane Database of Systematic Reviews, 3,* CD011712.

Raimond, E., Pelissier A., Etienette, M., et al. (2017). Use of negative pressure wound therapy after vulvar carcinoma case studies. *Journal of Wound Care, 26*(2), 72–74.

Rothrock, C. J. (2015). *Alexander's care of the patient in surgery* (15th ed.). St. Louis, MO: Mosby.

Scott, A., Stonemetz, J., Wasey, J., et al. (2016). Compliance with surgical care improvement project for body temperature management (SCIP Inf-10) is associated with improved clinical outcome. *Survey of Anesthesiology, 60*(2), 82–83.

Steenhagen, E. (2016). Enhanced recovery after surgery: It's time to change practice! *Nutrition in Clinical Practice, 31*(1), 18–29.

The Joint Commission. (2018). *Hospital: 2018 National patient safety goals.* Available: www.jointcommission.org/hap_2018_npsgs/

The Joint Commission. (2017). *Surgical care improvement project.* Available: www.jointcommission.org/surgical_care_improvement_project.

Talec, P., Gaujoux, S., & Samama, C. (2016). Early ambulation and prevention of post-operative thrombo-embolic risk. *Journal of Visceral Surgery, 153*(6), S11–S14.

Toon, C., Lusuku, C., Ramamoorthy, R., Davidson, B., & Gurusamy, K. (2015). Early versus delayed dressing removal after primary closure of clean and clean-contaminated surgical wounds. *Cochrane Database of Systematic Reviews, 2015*(9), Art. No.: CD010259.

Yokoe, D. S. (2018). The surgical care improvement project redux: Should CMS revive process of care measures for prevention of surgical site infections? In G. Bearman, S. Munoz-Price, D. Morgan, R. Murthy (Eds.). *Infection prevention.* New York: Springer.

8
Cancer Nursing

OVERVIEW AND ASSESSMENT

Cancer is a large group of malignant diseases characterized by a lack of controlled growth and the ability to spread to distant sites.

The malignant cell is able to invade the surrounding tissue and regional lymph nodes. Primary cancer usually has a predictable natural history and pattern of spread.

Metastasis is the secondary growth of the primary cancer in another organ. The cancer cell migrates through a series of steps to another area of the body. Metastasis begins with local invasion followed by detachment of cancer cells that disseminate via the lymphatics and blood vessels and eventually establish a secondary tumor in another area of the body. Lymph nodes are often the first site of distant spread (see Figure 8-1).

Etiology, Detection, and Prevention

Epidemiology

 EVIDENCE BASE American Cancer Society. (2018). Cancer-facts-figures-2018. Available: *www.cancer. org/Research/CancerFactsFigures/CancerFacts Figures/cancer-facts-figures*
American Cancer Society. (2015). Global facts and figures. Available: *www.cancer.org/Research/CancerFactsFigures/ GlobalCancerFactsFigures/global-facts-figures-2nd-ed*

1. According to the American Cancer Society (ACS), there will be 1,735,350 predicted new diagnoses of invasive cancer diagnosed in the United States in 2018. This does not include basal and squamous cell skin cancers as well as noninvasive cancers or DCIS (ductal carcinoma *in situ*).
2. According to the International Agency for Research on Cancer, there were 14.7 million new cancer cases in 2016 worldwide. This number is expected to rise as developing countries adopt Western lifestyles such as smoking and lack of exercise.
3. Although the death rate continues to decline, cancer is the second leading, under heart disease, cause of death in the United States, with 729, 000 predicted for 2018.
4. There are multiple factors that can lead to the development of cancer.
   a. Spontaneous transformation of the cell where no causative agent is identified.
   b. Exposure to a chemical or other carcinogen.
   c. Genetic mutations or alterations.
   d. Exposure to virus.
5. Age is the most outstanding risk factor for cancer.
   a. Cancer incidence increases progressively with age.
   b. Approximately 87% of people diagnosed with cancer are over age 50.
   c. Prostate, lung and bronchus, and colorectal cancers account for 32% of all cases in men. For women, the three most commonly diagnosed cancers are breast, lung and bronchus, and colorectal, representing one half of all cases; breast cancer alone is expected to account for 30% all new cancer diagnoses in women.
6. Forty two percent of all cancers in the United States are related to lifestyle habits (eg, smoking, alcohol consumption, diet, physical activity) and environmental carcinogens.
   a. Tobacco is the single greatest cause of cancer-related deaths and is attributed to more than 480,000 deaths annually from various cancers and 42,000 from secondhand smoke.
   b. Excessive alcohol intake is associated with cancers of the mouth, larynx, throat, esophagus, and liver, especially when combined with smoking. In addition, regular consumption of alcohol is associated with an increased risk of breast cancer. This may be due to alcohol-induced increases in circulating estrogens.
   c. Being overweight or obese is clearly linked with an increased risk of many cancers, including cancers of the breast (in postmenopausal women), colon and rectum, endometrium, esophagus, kidney, and pancreas. Overweight and obesity may also be associated with increased risk of gallbladder, liver, cervical, and ovarian cancer, non-Hodgkin lymphoma, and multiple myeloma.
   d. Exposure to carcinogens, such as asbestos, benzene, and radiation, increases the risk of developing certain types of cancer.
   e. Solar ultraviolet radiation exposure is related to an increased risk of skin cancers.
7. There is a hereditary predisposition to specific forms of cancers that have been linked to certain events within a gene (eg, BRCA1 and BRCA2 in breast cancer; MLH1, MSH2, and MSH6 in colon cancer).
8. Infections and viruses are associated with an increased risk of certain forms of cancer.
   a. Human papillomavirus (HPV)—cervical cancer, anal cancers, upper airway cancers.

Venous system
Cancer cells may travel through the veins, often to the liver and the lungs.

Superior mesenteric artery and vein

Middle colic vein

Transverse colon

Lymph nodes

Ascending colon

Lymphatic system
Cancer cells may move through this series of channels from the tissues to lymph nodes and eventually, via the circulatory system, to distant sites.

Primary cancer

Seeding
Cancer may penetrate the wall of an organ, move into a body cavity, and spread throughout that area.

Figure 8-1. How cancer spreads. Cancer cells may invade nearby tissues or metastasize (spread) to other organs. Cancer cells may move to other tissues by any or all of three routes: venous, lymphatic, or seeding. (Springhouse. [2001]. *Anatomical chart company atlas of pathophysiology* [1st ed.]. Philadelphia, PA: Lippincott Williams & Wilkins.)

b. Epstein-Barr virus—lymphoma, nasopharyngeal cancers, gastric cancer, Kaposi sarcoma.
c. Cytomegalovirus—Kaposi sarcoma, colon cancer.
d. Human immunodeficiency virus (HIV)—Kaposi sarcoma, lymphoma.
e. Human T-lymphocyte virus—T-cell lymphoma/leukemia.
f. Hepatitis B and C—hepatocellular cancer.
g. *Helicobacter pylori*—gastric lymphoma (possibly).
9. Five-year survival rates are increasing with improved therapy and earlier detection.
10. Ongoing genetic research is searching for the ability to correct and modify hereditary susceptibility.
11. Patterns of incidence and death rates vary with sex, age, race, and geographic location (see Table 8-1).

Nutrition, Physical Activity, and Cancer

 EVIDENCE BASE American Cancer Society. (2017). American Cancer Society guidelines on nutrition and physical activity for cancer prevention: Reducing the risk of cancer with healthy food choices and physical activity. Available: *www.cancer.org/healthy/eat-healthy-get-active/acs-guidelines-nutrition-physical-activiy-cancer-prevention/guidlelines.*
U.S. Department of Health and Human Services and U.S. Department of Agriculture. (2015). 2015—2020 dietary guidelines for Americans (8th ed.). Available: *http://health.gov/dietaryguidelines/2015/guidelines.*

1. Lifestyle does influence the risk of cancer. Among nonsmokers, dietary choices and physical activity are the most important modifiable risks of cancer. The ACS and the U.S. Department of Health and Human Services have established guidelines on nutrition and physical activity to promote optimal health and prevent cancer.
2. Achieve and maintain a healthy weight.
   a. Be as lean as possible throughout life without being underweight.
   b. Avoid excessive weight gain at all ages.
c. Limit the consumption of high-calorie foods and beverages.
3. Adopt a physically active lifestyle.
   a. Adults should engage in 150 minutes of moderate intensity or 75 minutes of vigorous activity each week, preferably spread throughout the week.
   b. Children and adolescents should engage in 60 minutes/day of moderate to vigorous physical activity each day, with vigorous intensity activity at least 3 days a week.
   c. Limit sedentary behavior such as sitting, lying down, and watching TV and other forms of screen-based entertainment.
   d. Doing any intentional physical activity above usual activities can have many health benefits.
4. Consume a healthy diet, with emphasis on plant sources.
   a. Choose foods and drinks in amounts that help achieve and maintain a healthy weight.
   b. Eat at least 2½ cups of vegetables and fruits daily.
   c. Choose whole grains over processed (refined) grains.
   d. Limit intake of processed and red meats.
   e. Limit alcoholic beverages to no more than 2 drinks per day for men and 1 drink per day for women.
5. ACS recommendations for community action:
   a. Increase access to healthful foods in schools, worksites, and communities.
   b. Changes in public policy and community environment that help individuals make smart food choices and portion sizes to help maintain a healthy weight.
   c. Provide safe, enjoyable spaces for physical activity in schools.
   d. Provide for safe, physically active transportation (such as biking and walking) and recreation in communities.

Detection and Prevention

Primary prevention and secondary prevention are effective measures in decreasing mortality and morbidity of many cancers. Most cancers, however, are diagnosed after reported symptoms. The ACS recommends specific primary and secondary prevention measures to reduce an individual's risk of cancer death.

Table 8-1 Leading New Cancer Cases and Deaths: 2018 Estimates

ESTIMATED NEW CASES*		ESTIMATED DEATHS	
MALE	FEMALE	MALE	FEMALE
Prostate 164,690 (19%)	Breast 266.120 (30%)	Lung and bronchus 83,550 (27%)	Lung and bronchus 70,500 (25%)
Lung and bronchus 121,680 (14%)	Lung and bronchus 112,350 (12%)	Colon and rectum 27,390 (9%)	Breast 40,920 (14%)
Colon and rectum 75,610 (8%)	Colon and rectum 64,640 (8%)	Prostate 29,430 (8%)	Colon and rectum 23,240 (8%)
Urinary bladder 62,380 (7%)	Uterine corpus 63,230 (7%)	Pancreas 23,020 (7%)	Pancreas 21,310 (7%)
Melanoma of the skin 55,150 (6%)	Thyroid 40,900 (5%)	Liver and intrahepatic bile duct 20,540 (6%)	Ovary 14,070 (5%)
Kidney and renal pelvis 42,680 (5%)	Melanoma of the skin 36,120 (4%)	Leukemia 14,270 (4%)	Uterine corpus 11,350 (4%)
Non-Hodgkin lymphoma 41,730 (5%)	Non-Hodgkin lymphoma 32,950 (4%)	Esophagus 12,850 (4%)	Leukemia 10,100 (4%)
Leukemia 35,030 (4%)	Leukemia 27,270 (3%)	Urinary bladder 12,520 (4%)	Liver and intrahepatic bile duct 9,660 (3%)
Oral cavity and pharynx 37,160 (4%)	Pancreas 26,240 (3%)	Non-Hodgkin lymphoma 11,510 (4%)	Non-Hodgkin lymphoma 8,400 (3%)
Liver and hepatic bile duct 30,610 (3%)	Kidney and renal pelvis 22,660 (3%)	Kidney and renal pelvis 10,010 (3%)	Brain and other nervous system 7,340 (3%)
All sites 856,370 (100%)	All sites 878,980 (100%)	All sites 323,630 (100%)	All sites 286,010 (100%)

*Excludes basal and squamous cell skin cancers and in situ carcinoma except urinary bladder.

Primary Prevention

The assessment or reduction of risk factors before the disease occurs:

1. Make appropriate lifestyle changes.
2. Stop smoking.
3. Limit alcohol intake.
4. Eat a healthy diet as outlined above.
5. Be physically active: maintain a healthy weight and follow exercise guidelines outlined above.
6. Avoid sun exposure, especially during the hours of 10 A.M. and 4 P.M., and cover exposed skin with sunscreen with a skin protection factor of 15 or higher.
7. Those at high risk for certain cancers should consider genetic counseling and testing.
8. Chemoprevention—the use of natural or synthetic substances to reduce the risk of developing cancer.
   a. Aspirin—can decrease the risk of colorectal cancer.
   b. Tamoxifen and raloxifene—can reduce the risk of breast cancer in women who are at high risk by nearly 50%.
   c. Finasteride—may reduce the risk of prostate cancer.
   d. COX-2 inhibitors—may reduce the risk of colorectal cancer.
   e. Metformin—may decrease the risk of breast, colon, and possibly other cancers.
   f. Statins—may reduce the risk of prostate, lung, colorectal, and breast cancers.
9. Vaccinations—HPV causes most cervical, vulvar, vaginal, anal, and oropharyngeal cancers in women and most oropharyngeal, anal, and penile cancers in men. These could be prevented by HPV vaccinations. The Advisory Committee on Immunization Practices in conjunction with the Centers for Disease Control and Prevention has established guidelines on the use of this vaccine.
   a. Routine HPV vaccination is recommended for males and females ages 11 to 13 in two doses; may begin as early as age 9.
   b. For persons initiating vaccination on or after their 15th birthday, 3 doses are recommended.
   c. HPV vaccination is not currently recommended for persons over age 27.
   d. Screening for cervical cancer should continue in both vaccinated and unvaccinated women according to current ACS early detection guidelines.

 EVIDENCE BASE The Advisory Committee on Immunization Practices. (2018). General recommendations on immunizations. Available: www.cdc.gov/vaccines/pubs/ACIP-list.htm.

Secondary Prevention

 EVIDENCE BASE Smith, R., Andrews, K. et al. (2016). Cancer screening in the United States, 2017: A review of current American Cancer Society guidelines and current issues in cancer screening. *CA_Cancer journal for Clinicians, 67,* 100–121.

1. The goal of screening is early detection to improve overall outcome and survival. Performing routine screening tests should be based on whether these tests are adequate to detect a potentially curable cancer in an otherwise asymptomatic person and are also cost-effective.
2. Screening should be based on an individual's age, sex, family history of cancer, ethnic group or race, previous iatrogenic factors (prior radiation therapy or drugs such as DES), and history of exposure to environmental carcinogens. See Table 8-2 for ACS recommendations for screening.

Diagnostic Evaluation

1. Complete medical history and physical examination, radiographic evaluation based on the affected body system, laboratory evaluation, and biopsy.
2. Biopsy of tumor site to determine pathologic diagnosis. Biopsy results are used to determine the histology and/or grade of a tumor, which is a prerequisite for planning definitive therapy. Additional cellular and genetic features are also used to form a final diagnosis and guide treatment.
   a. Fine-needle aspiration (FNA)—technique in which cells are aspirated from the tumor using a needle and syringe. FNA cannot distinguish invasive from noninvasive malignancy. Negative results do not rule out malignancy. However, it is inexpensive, causes little discomfort, and can be performed in an outpatient or office setting.
   b. Needle core—needle biopsies are performed with a large-bore needle. This technique retrieves a small piece of intact tumor tissue, which yields enough tissue to adequately diagnose most tumor types. It is highly accurate and can be performed in an office or outpatient setting.
   c. Open biopsy—may be required for some lesions to determine a definitive diagnosis. This is done in the operating room, is more expensive, and requires a longer period of recovery. The biopsy may be incisional, sampling only part of the tumor, or excisional, removing the total tumor.
3. Classification of tumor type is based on tissue and cellular staining. Differences in cytoplasmic and nuclear staining distinguish one cell type from another and identify their stage of differentiation. The grade of the tumor (rating of 1 to 4) is based on how well differentiated the tissue or cells appear or how closely tumor cell resemble normal cells. The higher the grade, the less differentiated it is, which is associated with poorer prognosis.
4. Flow cytometry testing of tumor tissue determines the deoxyribonucleic acid (DNA) content and indicates potential risk of recurrence.
5. Special stains are performed to determine specific markers or proteins that may help guide treatment (ie, estrogen and progesterone receptors for breast cancer).
6. Laboratory tests—including complete blood count (CBC) with differential; platelet count; and blood chemistries, including liver function tests, blood urea nitrogen (BUN), and creatinine—are done to determine baseline values.
   a. Further testing depends on cancer diagnosis.
7. Blood markers (carcinoembryonic antigen, PSA, CA 15-3, CA 125) may be appropriate to follow response to therapy.
8. Imaging procedures—chest x-ray, nuclear medicine scan, CT scanning, magnetic resonance imaging (MRI), and positron-emission tomography (PET) are used to determine evidence or extent of metastasis.

Table 8-2 ACS Recommendations for the Early Detection of Cancer in Average-Risk, Asymptomatic Individuals

CANCER SITE	POPULATION	TEST OR PROCEDURE	FREQUENCY
Breast	Women, ages 40–54 yr	Mammography	Women should undergo regular screening mammography starting at age 45 yr; women aged 45 to 54 yr should be screened annually; women should have the opportunity to begin annual screening between ages 40 and 44 yr
	Women, aged >55 yr	Mammography	Women aged ≥55 should transition to biennial screening or have the opportunity to continue screening annually; women should continue screening mammography as long as their overall health is good and they have a life expectancy of ≥10 yr
Cervix	Women, ages 21–29 yr	Pap test	Cervical cancer screening should begin at age 21 yr; for women ages 21–29 yr, screening should be done every 3 yr with conventional or liquid-based Pap tests; for women ages 30–65 yr, screening should be done every 5 yr with both the HPV test and the Pap test (preferred) or every 3 yr with the Pap test alone (acceptable); women aged >65 yr who have had ≥3 consecutive negative Pap tests or ≥2 consecutive negative HPV and Pap tests within the last 10 yr, with the most recent test occurring in the last 5 yr, and women who have had a total hysterectomy (for a benign condition) should stop cervical cancer screening; women at any age should not be screened annually by any screening method.
	Women, ages 30–65 yr	Pap test and HPV DNA test	
	Women, ages 66+	Pap test and HPV DNA test	
	Women who have had a total hysterectomy	Pap test and HPV DNA test	
Colorectal	Men and women, ages ≥50 yr, for all tests listed	Guaiac-based fecal occult blood test (gFOBT) with at least 50% test sensitivity for cancer, or fecal immunochemical test (FIT) with at least 50% test sensitivity for cancer, or	Annual: Testing stool sampled from regular bowel movements with adherence to manufacturer's recommendation for collection techniques and number of samples is recommended; "throw in the toilet bowl" FOBTs are also not recommended; compared with guaiac-based tests for the detection of occult blood, immunochemical tests are more patient friendly and are likely to be equal or better in sensitivity and specificity; there is no justification for repeating FOBT in response to an initial positive finding; patients should be referred to colonoscopy
		Multitarget stool DNA test, or	Every 3 yr, per manufacturer's recommendation
		Flexible sigmoidoscopy (FSIG), or	Every 5 yr. FSIG can be performed alone, or consideration can be given to combining FSIG performed every 5 yr with a highly sensitive gFOBT or FIT performed annually.

Table 8-2   ACS Recommendations for the Early Detection of Cancer in Average-Risk, Asymptomatic Individuals *(Continued)*

CANCER SITE	POPULATION	TEST OR PROCEDURE	FREQUENCY
		DCBE, or	Every 5 yr.
		Colonoscopy	Every 10 yr.
		CT colonography	Every 5 yr.
Endometrial	Women, at menopause		At the time of menopause, women at average risk should be informed about the risks and symptoms of endometrial cancer and strongly encouraged to report any unexpected bleeding or spotting to their physicians.
Lung	Current or former smokers ages 55–74 yr in good health with at least a 30-pack-year history	Low-dose helical CT (LDCT)	Clinicians with access to high-volume, high-quality lung cancer screening, and treatment centers should initiate a discussion about annual lung cancer screening with apparently healthy patients ages 55–74 yr who have at least a 30-pack-year smoking history and who currently smoke or have quit within the past 15 yr; a process of informed and shared decision-making with a clinician related to the potential benefits, limitations, and harms associated with screening for lung cancer with LDCT should occur before any decision is made to initiate annual lung cancer screening; smoking cessation counseling remains a high priority for clinical attention in discussions with current smokers, who should be informed of their continuing risk of lung cancer; screening should not be viewed as an alternative to smoking cessation.
Prostate	Men, ages ≥50 yr	DRE and PSA	Men who have at least a 10-yr life expectancy should have an opportunity to make an informed decision with their health care provider about whether to be screened for prostate cancer, after receiving information about the potential benefits, risks, and uncertainties associated with prostate cancer screening. Prostate cancer screening should not occur without an informed decision-making process.

ACS, American Cancer Society; BSE, breast self-examination; CBE, clinical breast examination; CT, computed tomography; DCBE, double-contrast barium enema; DRE, digital rectal examination; FOBT, fecal occult blood test; FIT, fecal immunochemical test; FSIG, flexible sigmoidoscopy; gFOBT, guaiac-based toilet bowl FOBT tests; HPV, human papillomavirus; Pap, Papanicolaou; PSA, prostate-specific antigen.

Staging

Staging is necessary at the time of diagnosis to determine the extent of disease (local vs. metastatic), to determine prognosis, and to guide proper management.

1. The American Joint Committee on Cancer (AJCC) has developed a simple classification system that can be applied to all tumor types. It is a numeric assessment of tumor size (T), presence or absence of regional lymph node involvement (N), and presence or absence of distant metastasis (M) (see Box 8-1).
2. No standard evaluation exists for all cancers. Workup depends on the patient, tumor type, symptoms, and medical knowledge of the natural history of that cancer.

PROCEDURES AND TREATMENT

The method of treatment depends on the type of malignancy, the specific histologic cell type, stage, presence of metastasis, and condition of the patient. It is important to have ongoing discussions with the patient regarding the goals of therapy and whether those goals are achievable. The four modalities of treatment are surgery, chemotherapy/hormonal therapy, radiation therapy, and biologic therapy or a combination of these modalities. Many clinical trials are available to evaluate the effectiveness of a new drug or other therapy. Refer patients who are interested in clinical trials to CancerTrials at *https://www.cancer.gov/about-cancer/treatment/clinical-trials.*

Surgical Management

Surgical management may be curative to remove all or a portion of the primary tumor, it may be the only treatment a patient requires or it may be used in conjunction with other modalities, or it may be used in the palliative setting to alleviate symptoms.

Types of Surgical Procedures

The role of surgery can be divided into several approaches: preventive, primary surgery, cytoreductive, salvage treatment, palliative treatment, and reconstructive.

1. Preventive/prophylactic surgery—removal of lesions that, if left in the body, are at risk of developing into cancer; for example, resection of polyps in the rectum or mastectomy in women who are at high risk.
2. Primary surgery—complete surgical removal of a malignant tumor and may include regional lymph nodes and neighboring structures. This can be performed laparoscopically in some cases.
3. Cytoreductive surgery—partial removal of bulk of disease. This is performed when the spread of tumor precludes the removal of all disease. In some cases, this approach improves survival when used in combination with chemotherapy (ie, ovarian cancer).
4. Salvage treatment—use of an extensive surgical approach to treat a local recurrence.

BOX 8-1   AJCC Classification System of Tumors

T—primary tumor
Tx—primary cannot be evaluated
T0—no evidence of primary tumor
Tis—carcinoma *in situ*
T1, T2, T3, T4—increasing size and/or local extent of primary tumor

N—presence or absence or regional lymph node involvement
Nx—regional lymph nodes are unable to be assessed
N0—no regional lymph node involvement
N1, N2, N3—increasing involvement of regional lymph nodes

M—absence or presence of distant metastasis
Mx—unable to assess
M0—absence of distant metastasis
M1—presence of distant metastasis

5. Palliative treatment—attempts to relieve the complications of cancer (eg, obstruction of the GI tract, pain produced by tumor extension into surrounding nerves).
6. Reconstructive/rehabilitative surgery—repair of defects from previous radical surgical resection; can be performed early (breast reconstruction) or delayed (head and neck surgery).

Chemotherapy

Chemotherapy is the use of antineoplastic drugs given systemically that may promote tumor cell destruction by interfering with cellular function and reproduction.

Principles of Chemotherapy Administration

1. The intent of chemotherapy is to destroy as many tumor cells as possible with minimal effect on healthy cells.
2. Cancer cells depend on the same mechanisms for cell division as normal cells. Damage to those mechanisms leads to cell death.
3. Chemotherapy is utilized in different clinical settings:
   a. Adjuvant chemotherapy is the use of systemic treatment following surgery and/or radiation therapy. Adjuvant therapy is given to patients who have no evidence of residual disease but who are at high risk for relapse. The justifications for adjuvant chemotherapy are the high recurrence rate after surgery for apparently localized tumors, the inability to identify cured patients at the time of surgery, and the failure of therapy to cure these patients after recurrence of disease.
   b. Neoadjuvant chemotherapy is the use of systemic treatment prior to primary surgery or radiation. The goal is to shrink or downstage the primary tumor to improve the effectiveness of surgery as well as control/eradicate microscopic cancer cells. For example, patients with large breast tumors can preserve the breast and undergo lumpectomy instead of mastectomy. The goal of therapy is to decrease the amount of tissue that needs to be removed as well as to attempt to maximize cure potential.
   c. High-dose/intensive therapy is the administration of high doses of chemotherapy, usually in association with growth factor support before bone marrow transplant/stem cell rescue.
   d. Palliative chemotherapy is used when a cure is not possible to control the cancer and minimize side effects from the disease.

4. Chemotherapeutic agents can be effective on any stage of the cell life cycle. This is the reproductive process ion both normal and malignant cells. The cell cycle is divided into five stages:
   a. G0 (gap 0) resting phase: Cells are not dividing in this stage and, for the most part, are refractory to chemotherapy.
   b. G1 (gap one) postmitotic phase: Ribonucleic acid (RNA) and proteins (enzymes for DNA synthesis) are manufactured.
   c. S (synthesis) phase: DNA is replicated in preparation for cell division.
   d. G2 (gap two) premitotic phase: This is a short period; protein and RNA synthesis occurs, and the mitotic spindle apparatus is formed.
   e. M (mitosis) phase: In an extremely short period, the cell divides into two identical daughter cells.
5. Routes of administration
   a. Oral
   b. Subcutaneous
   c. Intravenous (IV) push (bolus) or infusion over a specified period
   d. Intramuscular
   e. Intrathecal/intraventricular—given by injection via an Ommaya reservoir or by lumbar puncture
   f. Intra-arterial
   g. Intraperitoneal cavity
   h. Intravesical—into uterus or bladder
   i. Topical
6. Most drug dosage is based on surface area (mg/m²) in both adults and children. Some agents are based on AUC (area under the curve), which refers to the amount of drug exposure over time or the total drug concentration in plasma over a period of time.
7. Most chemotherapeutic agents have dose-limiting toxicities that require nursing interventions (see Table 8-3, pages 114 to 117). Chemotherapy predictably affects normal, rapidly growing cells (eg, bone marrow, GI tract lining, hair follicles). It is imperative that these toxicities be recognized early by the nurse. Patient education is very important to minimize hospital admission and readmissions.

Chemotherapy Administration Safety Standards

 EVIDENCE BASE Oncology Nursing Society. (2014). *Chemotherapy and biotherapy guidelines and recommendations for practice* (4th ed.). Pittsburgh, PA: Author.

1. Specialized education, preparation, and training of the oncology nurse who administers chemotherapy and biotherapy are essential and ensure a safe level of care for patients. The Oncology Nursing Society (ONS) offers the ONS/Oncology Nursing Credentialing Center (ONCC) Chemotherapy Biotherapy Certificate Course and provides up-to-date resources. See Standard of Care Guidelines 8-1 (page 113) for a checklist of the competency required by ONS.
2. The American Society of Clinical Oncology's (ASCO) quality oncology practice initiative certification program requires that hospitals, infusion centers, and physician practices comply with safety standards for chemotherapy administration.
3. Check with your hospital/institutional policy on handling and administering antineoplastic drugs.
4. Cytotoxic drugs are considered hazardous to health care workers. A safe level of occupational exposure is unknown. It is important to adhere to practices to minimize occupational exposure.

STANDARD OF CARE GUIDELINES 8-1
Administering IV Chemotherapy

ONS Chemotherapy Administration Competency Evaluation

Prior to Administration
1. Coordinates time of administration with pharmacy and others as needed.
2. Verifies signed consent for treatment.
3. Verifies laboratory values are within acceptable range and reports to the provider as needed.
4. Performs independent double check of original orders with a second RN for accuracy of
   a. Protocol or regimen
   b. Agents
   c. Calculated body surface area
   d. Patient dose
   e. Schedule
   f. Route.
5. Verifies that patient education, premedication, prehydration, and other preparations are completed.

Administration
1. Compares original order to dispensed drug label at the bedside with another RN.
2. Verifies patient identification.
3. Applies gloves and gown and uses safe handling precautions.

4. Verifies adequacy of venous access and appropriate IV site selection.
5. Checks patency of IV and flushes with 5 to 10 mL normal saline.
6. Demonstrates safe administration
   a. Pushes through side arm or at hub closest to the patient, checks patency every 2 to 5 mL.
   b. Verifies appropriate rate of administration.
7. Demonstrates appropriate monitoring/observation for specific acute drug effects.
8. Verbalizes appropriate action in the event of extravasation.
9. Verbalizes appropriate action in the event of hypersensitivity reaction.

After Administration
1. Flushes line with enough fluid to clear IV tubing of drug.
2. Removes peripheral IV device or flushes/maintains vascular access device.
3. Disposes of chemotherapy waste according to policy.
4. Documents medications, education, and patient response.
5. Communicates posttreatment considerations to the patient, caregivers, and appropriate personnel.

Guidelines for Personal Protective Equipment

1. Gloves—wear two pairs of disposable gloves that are powder-free and have been tested for use with hazardous drugs. Avoid latex drugs because of potential latex sensitivity. Remove outer glove first, turning them inside out to prevent contaminated outer surfaces from touching the inner gloves. Remove the inner gloves last after discarding all contaminated items. Do not reuse gloves.
2. Gowns—wear a disposable, lint-free gown made of low-permeability fabric. The gown should have a solid front, long sleeves, tight cuffs, and back closure. The inner glove should be worn under the gown cuff and the outer glove should extend over the gown to protect the skin. Gown and gloves are meant for single use only.
3. Respirators—wear a National Institute for Occupational Health and Safety–approved respirator mask when there is a risk of aerosol exposure such as when administering chemotherapy or cleaning a spill. Surgical masks do not provide adequate protection.
4. Eye and face protection—wear a face shield and/or mask that provides splash protection whenever there is a possibility of splashing.
5. Wear personal protective equipment whenever there is a risk of chemotherapy being released into the environment such as preparation or mixing of chemotherapy, spiking/priming IV tubing, administering the drug, and when handling body fluids or chemotherapy spills.

Personal Safety to Minimize Exposure

1. Prepare cytotoxic drugs in a vertical laminar flow hood.
2. Wash hands before donning PPE and change gloves after each use, tear, puncture, or medication spill or after every 60 minutes of wear. Wash hands after removing PPE.
3. Vent vials with filter needle to equalize the internal pressure or use negative-pressure techniques.

4. Wrap gauze or alcohol pads around the neck of ampules when opening to decrease droplet contamination.
5. Wrap gauze or alcohol pads around injection sites when removing syringes or needles from IV injection ports.
6. Use puncture- and leak-proof containers for noncapped, non-clipped needles.
7. Prime all IV tubing with normal saline or other compatible solution to reduce exposure.
8. Use syringes and IV tubing with Luer locks (which have a locking device to hold needle firmly in place).
9. Label all syringes and IV tubing containing chemotherapeutic agents as hazardous material.
10. Place an absorbent pad directly under the injection site to absorb any accidental spillage.
11. Do not eat, drink, or chew gum while preparing or handling chemotherapy agents.
12. Keep all food and drink away from preparation area.
13. Avoid hand-to-mouth or hand-to-eye contact while handling chemotherapeutic agents or body fluids of the patient receiving chemotherapy.
14. If any contact with the skin occurs, immediately wash the area thoroughly with soap and water.
15. If contact is made with the eye, immediately flush the eye with water and seek medical attention.
16. Spill kits should be available in all areas where chemotherapy is stored, prepared, and administered.

Safe Disposal of Antineoplastic Agents, Body Fluids, and Excreta

1. Discard gloves and gown into a leak-proof container, which should be marked as contaminated or hazardous waste.
2. Use puncture- and leak-proof containers for needles and other sharp or breakable objects.

text continues on page 118

Table 8-3 | Frequently Used Chemotherapeutic Agents

CLASSIFICATION	MEDICATION NAME	ROUTE OF ADMINISTRATION	COMMON THERAPEUTIC USES
Alkylating Agents	Altretamine	PO	Ovarian cancer
	Cyclophosphamide	IV or PO	Lymphomas, leukemias, and a variety of solid tumors
	Busulfan	IV or PO	Chronic myelocytic leukemia, bone marrow transplantation
	Carboplatin	IV or IP	Ovarian cancer
	Chlorambucil	PO	Chronic lymphocytic leukemia, Hodgkin disease
	Cisplatin	IV	Ovarian, testicular, bladder, cervical, non–small cell lung cancer, esophageal
	Dacarbazine	IV or IM	Malignant melanoma, Hodgkin lymphoma, sarcomas
	Ifosfamide	IV	Testicular, lymphoma, sarcomas, ovarian, bone
	Melphalan	IV or PO	Multiple myeloma, ovarian, malignant melanoma
	Oxaliplatin	IV	Colorectal cancers
	Temozolomide	PO	Glioblastoma, astrocytoma, melanoma
	Thiotepa	IV, IM, SC, IT	Breast, ovarian, bladder, lymphomas, bone marrow transplantation
Antibiotics	Bleomycin	IV, SC, IM	Head and neck cancers, cervical, lymphomas, testicular, Hodgkin's
	Dactinomycin	IV	Ewing sarcoma, Wilms tumor, testicular
	Daunorubicin	IV	Leukemias
	Doxorubicin	IV	Breast, ovarian, prostate, thyroid, lung, head and neck cancers, leukemia
	Doxorubicin liposomal	IV	Ovarian, breast, AIDS-related sarcoma
	Epirubicin	IV	Breast cancer
	Mitomycin	IV	Pancreatic, stomach, colon, lung, bladder, esophageal
	Mitoxantrone	IV	Prostate acute myelocytic leukemia
Camptothecins	Irinotecan	IV	Colorectal
	Topotecan	IV	Ovarian, cervical, small cell lung cancer

COMMON TOXICITIES	NURSING CONSIDERATIONS
Nausea, vomiting, peripheral neuropathy, myelosuppression	Do not open capsules
Nausea, vomiting, diarrhea, myelosuppression, alopecia, lethargy, hemorrhagic cystitis	Ensure adequate hydration (2–3 L /d). Have patients void frequently to avoid hemorrhagic cystitis
Pulmonary fibrosis, hypertension, tachycardia, myelosuppression, alopecia, skin pigmentation	Instruct patients to take on an empty stomach to decrease nausea/ vomiting. Monitor blood counts
Myelosuppression particularly platelets, alopecia, hypersensitivity reaction	Have emergency medications available for possible hypersensitivity reactions
Myelosuppression, nausea, vomiting, skin reactions, seizures	Contraindications in patients with a history of seizures
Nausea, vomiting, myelosuppression, nephrotoxicity, hypersensitivity reactions, low electrolytes	Monitor renal function and electrolytes. Have emergency medications available for possible hypersensitivity reactions
Nausea, vomiting, myelosuppression, alopecia, rash	Irritant—may cause tissue necrosis if extravasated
Hemorrhagic cystitis, nausea, vomiting, myelosuppression, confusion, encephalopathy	Always given in conjunction with mesna to decrease risk of hemorrhagic cystitis
Myelosuppression, nausea, vomiting	Vesicant—Avoid extravasation
Nephrotoxicity, hypersensitivity reactions, peripheral neuropathy, nausea, vomiting, myelosuppression	Monitor for peripheral neuropathy. Instruct patients to avoid consuming cold beverages for 3–4 d to avoid laryngopharyngeal dysaesthesias
Myelosuppression, nausea, vomiting, headache, photosensitivity	Contraindicated in patients with sensitivity to dacarbazine. Instruct patients to avoid sun exposure for several days
Myelosuppression, nausea, vomiting, rash, fever	
Skin reaction, pulmonary fibrosis, fever, allergic reaction, alopecia, stomatitis	Administer a test dose in patient with lymphoma as they seem to have a higher incidence of allergic reactions
Myelosuppression, nausea, vomiting, alopecia, venoocclusive disease of the liver, skin rash, and fever	Vesicant—avoid extravasation
Myelosuppression, nausea, vomiting, alopecia, cardiomyopathy, red urine, radiation recall	Vesicant—avoid extravasation. Monitor cardiac function
Cardiomyopathy, alopecia, red urine, radiation recall, nausea, vomiting, red urine	Vesicant—avoid extravasation 550 mg/m^2 lifetime dose
Myelosuppression, nausea, vomiting, mucositis, diarrhea, alopecia, radiation recall	Similar to Adriamycin, less cardiotoxic
Myelosuppression, nausea, vomiting, alopecia, heart failure, radiation recall, red urine	Vesicant—avoid extravasation
Delayed myelosuppression, nausea, vomiting, alopecia, mucositis, renal and pulmonary dysfunction	Vesicant—avoid extravasation
Myelosuppression, tachycardia, mucositis, nausea, vomiting, alopecia	May turn urine blue-green
Diarrhea, myelosuppression	Monitor for severe diarrhea that may require delays or dose reduction
Myelosuppression, alopecia, diarrhea, headache, fatigue	

(continued)

Table 8-3   Frequently Used Chemotherapeutic Agents (Continued)

CLASSIFICATION	MEDICATION NAME	ROUTE OF ADMINISTRATION	COMMON THERAPEUTIC USES
Plant alkaloids (vinca alkaloids)	Vinblastine	IV	Hodgkin lymphoma, Kaposi sarcoma, testicular, bladder, prostate, renal cell
	Vincristine	IV	Lymphoma, acute leukemia, neuroblastoma, multiple myeloma, testicular
	Vinorelbine	IV	Non–small cell lung, breast, cervical, ovarian cancer
	Etoposide	IV or PO	Small cell lung, testicular cancer
	Teniposide	IV	Childhood acute lymphocytic leukemia, adult neuroblastoma
Antimetabolites	Azacitidine	SC, IV	MDS
	Methotrexate	IV, IM, IT, or PO	Lymphoma, acute lymphoblastic leukemia, breast, bladder, sarcoma
	Cytarabine	IV, SC, IT, IM	Hodgkin and non-Hodgkin lymphoma, acute myelogenous leukemia, acute lymphoblastic leukemia
	5-Fluorouracil	IV or topical	Breast, colorectal, anal, gastroesophageal, hepatocellular, pancreatic, head and neck cancer
	6-Mercaptopurine	PO	Acute lymphoblastic leukemia
	Thioguanine	PO	Acute myelogenous leukemia, acute lymphoblastic leukemia
	Fludarabine	IV or PO	Chronic lymphocytic leukemia, non-Hodgkin lymphoma
	Pemetrexed	IV	Non–small cell lung cancer
	Gemcitabine	IV	Pancreatic, non–small cell lung, breast, bladder, ovarian, sarcoma, Hodgkin lymphoma
Taxanes	Paclitaxel	IV	Breast, ovarian, non–small cell lung, bladder, esophagus, cervical, gastric, head and neck sarcoma
	Docetaxel	IV	Breast, gastric, head and neck, prostate, non–small cell lung, ovarian cancer
	Ixabepilone	IV	Breast cancer
Miscellaneous	Asparaginase	IM	ALL
	Hydroxyurea	PO	CML, myeloma
	Eribulin	IV	Breast cancer
	Ixabepilone	IV	Breast cancer

IM, intramuscular; IP, intraperitoneal; IT, intrathecal; IV, intravenous; PO, by mouth; SQ, subcutaneous.

COMMON TOXICITIES	NURSING CONSIDERATIONS
Myelosuppression, alopecia, peripheral neuropathy, bone pain	Vesicant—avoid extravasation
Constipation, nausea, vomiting, alopecia, bone pain	Vesicant—avoid extravasation; monitor for severe constipation
Alopecia, diarrhea, nausea, neuropathy	Distal neuropathies, extravasation, and necrosis; should consider central access
Myelosuppression, nausea, alopecia, mucositis	Monitor renal function
Myelosuppression, nausea, vomiting, diarrhea, alopecia	Can cause hypersensitivity reactions
Myelosuppression, nausea, vomiting, elevated serum creatinine	Administration should occur within 1 hr of reconstitution
Mucositis, diarrhea, myelosuppression, acute renal failure, pneumonitis	High doses require concomitant use of leucovorin and IV fluids
Nausea, vomiting, myelosuppression, cerebellar ataxia, lethargy	Side effects are dose dependent; higher doses are associated with profound myelosuppression, GI toxicity, and neurotoxicity
Nausea, vomiting, diarrhea, mucositis, myelosuppression, neurotoxicity, photosensitivity	Instruct patients to avoid sun exposure, use sunscreen. Leucovorin may be used concomitantly
Myelosuppression, nausea, vomiting, diarrhea, hepatotoxicity	Instruct patients to take on an empty stomach
Myelosuppression, nausea, vomiting, mucositis, diarrhea, hepatotoxicity	Instruct patients to take on an empty stomach
Myelosuppression, mild nausea, vomiting, fever, interstitial pneumonitis	Monitor pulmonary function tests
Myelosuppression, renal, and liver toxicities	Must be given with folic acid starting 1 wk prior to infusion
Nausea, vomiting, myelosuppression, flulike syndrome, fever	Warn patients of flulike symptoms that can occur the day following treatment
Myelosuppression, peripheral neuropathy, myalgias, alopecia, fatigue	Observe closely for hypersensitivity reaction; premedication required with dexamethasone, diphenhydramine, and H2 blocker requires non-PVC IV tubing
Myelosuppression, edema, alopecia, nail changes, peripheral neuropathy	Treatment with dexamethasone prior to and for 2 d after can minimize edema
Myelosuppression, fatigue, neuropathy, nausea, vomiting, diarrhea, myalgias	Observe closely for hypersensitivity reaction; premedication required with dexamethasone, diphenhydramine, and H2 blocker requires non-PVC IV tubing
Anaphylaxis, nausea, vomiting, hypercalcemia, fever, renal toxicity	Observe closely for anaphylaxis
Myelosuppression, nausea, vomiting, fever	Do not open capsules
Neutropenia, peripheral neuropathy	Not compatible with D5W
Peripheral neuropathy, myelosuppression, fatigue	Avoid St. John's wort. Monitor for hypersensitivity reaction

Table 8-4 Management of Chemotherapy Extravasation

CHEMOTHERAPEUTIC AGENT	ANTIDOTE	NURSING INTERVENTION
Anthracyclines (doxorubicin, epirubicin, daunorubicin)	Dexrazoxane	Apply ice, but remove at least 15 min before dexrazoxane. Dose of dexrazoxane is based on body surface area and should be administered IV in an area other than the extravasation site, opposite arm: Day 1: 1,000 mg/m² Day 2: 1,000 mg/m² Day 3: 500 mg/m²
Alkylating agents (nitrogen mustard, cisplatin)	Sodium thiosulfate	Prepare ¼ molar solution and inject 2 mL for each milligram of chemotherapy suspected to have extravasated. Inject solution subcutaneously in the site using a 25G needle (change the needle with each injection). Apply ice for 6–12 hr following sodium thiosulfate injection.
Vinca alkaloids (vincristine, vinblastine, vinorelbine)	Hyaluronidase	Inject 1 mL of hyaluronidase locally as five separate injections subcutaneously into the extravasated area. Apply moderate heat for 15–20 min at least four times daily for the first 24–48 hr to disperse drug and minimize pain.
Taxanes (paclitaxel, docetaxel)	No known antidote	Apply ice for 15–20 min at least four times daily for the first 24 hr.
Antibiotics	None	Apply ice for 15–20 min at least four times daily for the first 24 hr.

3. Linens contaminated with chemotherapy or excreta from patients who have received chemotherapy within 48 hours should be contained in specially marked hazardous waste bags.
4. Wear nonsterile nitrile gloves for disposing of body excreta and handling soiled linens within 48 hours of chemotherapy administration.
5. In the home, wear gloves when handling bed linens or clothing contaminated with chemotherapy or patient excreta within 48 hours of chemotherapy administration. Place linens in a separate, washable pillow case. Wash separately in hot water and regular detergent.

 DRUG ALERT It is imperative that the nurse be alert for immediate complications that patients may experience during or shortly after cytotoxic therapy.

Extravasation
1. Occurs when the vesicant chemotherapy leaks out of the blood vessel and into the surrounding tissue resulting in:
   a. Blistering, begins within 3 to 5 days.
   b. Peeling and sloughing of skin, begins within 2 weeks.
   c. Tissue necrosis, usually in 2 to 3 weeks.
   d. Damage to tendons, nerves and joints.
   e. Functional and sensory impairment of the area.
   f. Disfigurement.
   g. Loss of limb.
2. Steps to take if extravasation is suspected:
   a. STOP infusion of the vesicant.
   b. Disconnect the IV tubing from the IV device. DO NOT remove the IV device or port needle.
   c. Attempt to aspirate residual vesicant from the IV using a small syringe.
   d. Remove the IV or port needle.
   e. Assess the site of extravasation.
   f. Assess symptoms experienced by the patient.
   g. Notify the patient's provider.

h. Initiate appropriate management measures in accordance with type of agent (see Table 8-4).

Chemotherapy Follow-Up
1. Document drug dosage, site, and any occurrence of extravasation, including estimated amount of drug.
2. Observe regularly after administration for pain, erythema, induration, and necrosis, and notify the appropriate health care provider as indicated.
3. Monitor for other adverse effects of infusion.
   a. Patient may describe sensations of pain or pressure within the vessel, originating near the venipuncture site or extending 3 to 5 inches (7.5 to 12.5 cm) along the vein.
   b. Discoloration or red streak following the line of the vein (called a flare reaction, common with doxorubicin) or darkening of the vein (with 5-fluorouracil).
   c. Itching, urticaria, muscle cramps, or pressure in the arm, caused by irritation of surrounding subcutaneous tissue.

Adverse Effects of Chemotherapy

All chemotherapy drugs have adverse effects. Adverse effects are exacerbated if the patient is elderly, has comorbid conditions, or has impaired renal or hepatic function.

Adverse effects of chemotherapy are graded on a scale of 0 to 5, with 0 being no toxicity and 5 resulting in death. Scoring of adverse effects will determine if a delay in therapy is necessary, dose modification is necessary, or cessation of therapy must occur.

Alopecia
1. Most chemotherapeutic agents cause some degree of alopecia. This is dependent on the drug dose, half-life of drug, and duration of therapy.
2. Most commonly occurs on the scalp but can occur anywhere on the body.
3. Usually begins 1 to 3 weeks after administration of chemotherapy. Regrowth takes about 3 to 5 months.

4. Emotionally difficult for patients. Encourage patients to verbalize their feelings.
5. The use of scalp hypothermia and tourniquets is highly controversial.

Anorexia

1. Chemotherapy changes the reproduction of taste buds.
2. Absent or altered taste can lead to a decreased food intake.
3. Concurrent renal or hepatic disease can increase anorexia.

Diarrhea

1. Defined as loose or watery stool. If left untreated, can lead to severe dehydration, electrolyte imbalances, hospitalizations, and treatment delays.
2. Cause is multifactorial, but up to 90% of all patients receiving chemotherapy can experience diarrhea.

Fatigue

The cause of fatigue is generally unknown but can be related to anemia, weight loss, altered sleep patterns, and emotional stress.

Nausea and Vomiting

1. Caused by the stimulation of the vagus nerve by serotonin released by cells in the upper GI tract.
2. Incidence depends on the particular chemotherapeutic agent and dosage.
3. Patterns of nausea and vomiting:
   a. Anticipatory—conditioned response from repeated association between therapy and vomiting; can be prevented with adequate antiemetic control.
   b. Acute—occurs 0 to 24 hours after chemotherapy administration.
   c. Delayed—can occur 1 to 6 days after chemotherapy administration; nausea is often worse than vomiting.

Mucositis

1. Caused by the destruction of the oral mucosa, causing an inflammatory response.
2. Initially presents as a burning sensation with no changes in the mucosa and progresses to significant breakdown, erythema, and pain of the oral mucosa.
3. Consistent oral hygiene is important to avoid infection.

Neutropenia

1. Defined as an absolute neutrophil count (ANC) of $1,500/mm^3$ or less.
2. Primary dose-limiting toxicity of chemotherapy.
3. Risk of infection is greatest with an ANC less than $500/mm^3$.
4. Caused by suppression of the stem cell.
5. Usually occurs 7 to 14 days after administration of chemotherapy but depends on the agent used.
6. Can be prolonged.
7. Patients should be taught to avoid infection through proper handwashing and hygiene and avoiding those with illness. Eliminating raw meats, seafood, eggs, or unwashed vegetables is also recommended.
8. Patients need to be monitored and treated promptly for fever or other signs of infection.
9. Can be prevented with the use of growth factors (eg, granulocyte colony-stimulating factor [CSF], pegfilgrastim).

Anemia

1. Caused by suppression of the stem cell or interference with cell proliferation pathways.
2. May require red blood cell transfusion or injection of erythropoietin or darbepoetin.

Thrombocytopenia

1. Caused by suppression of megakaryocytes.
2. Incidence depends on the agent being used.
3. Risk of bleeding is present when platelet count falls below $50,000/mm^3$.
4. Risk is high when count falls below $20,000/mm^3$.
5. Risk is critical when count falls below $10,000/mm^3$.
6. Patient should be taught to avoid injury (eg, no razors), vaginal douches, rectal suppositories, and dental floss during the period of thrombocytopenia.
7. May require platelet transfusions if count drops below $20,000/mm^3$.

Hypersensitivity Reactions

1. Nearly all of the available chemotherapeutic agents can produce hypersensitivity reactions (HSRs) in at least an occasional patient, and some cause reactions in 5% or more of patients receiving the drug. There are several agents (L-asparaginase, paclitaxel, docetaxel, teniposide, and carboplatin) for which HSRs are frequent enough to be a major form of treatment-limiting toxicity.
2. The mechanism is unknown for most of the chemotherapeutic agents.
3. Signs and symptoms include hives, pruritus, back pain, shortness of breath, hypotension, and anaphylaxis.
4. All unexpected drug reactions should be reported to the manufacturer.

Nursing Assessment

Skin and Mucous Membranes

1. Inspect for pain, swelling with inflammation or phlebitis, necrosis, or ulceration.
2. Inspect for skin rash and characteristics (eg, whether pruritus is general or local).
3. Assess areas of erythema and associated tenderness or pruritus. Instruct the patient to avoid irritation to skin, sun exposure, or irritating soaps.
4. Assess changes in skin pigmentation.
5. Note reports of photosensitivity and tearing of the eyes.
6. Assess condition of gums, teeth, buccal mucosa, and tongue.
   a. Determine whether any taste changes have occurred.
   b. Check for evidence of stomatitis, erythematous areas, ulceration, infection, or pain on swallowing.
   c. Determine whether the patient has any complaints of pain or burning of the oral mucosa or on swallowing.

GI System

1. Assess for frequency, timing of onset, duration, and severity of nausea and vomiting episodes before and after chemotherapy.
   a. Usually occurs from 0 to 24 hours after chemotherapy but may be delayed. Anticipatory vomiting may occur after first course of therapy. Can be initiated by various cues, including thoughts, smell, or even sight of the medical personnel.
2. Observe for alterations in hydration and electrolyte balance.
3. Assess for diarrhea or constipation.
   a. Ascertain any changes in bowel patterns.
   b. Discuss the consistency of stools.
   c. Consider the frequency and duration of diarrhea (the number of stools each day for the number of days).
   d. Evaluate dietary changes or use of medications such as opioids or 5-HT3 blockers that have had an impact on diarrhea or constipation.

4. Assess for anorexia.
    a. Discuss taste changes and changes in food preferences.
    b. Ask about daily food intake and normal eating patterns.
5. Assess for jaundice, right upper quadrant abdominal pain, changes in the stool or urine, and elevated liver function tests that indicate hepatotoxicity.
6. Monitor liver function tests and total bilirubin.

Hematopoietic System

 NURSING ALERT Fever greater than 101°F (38.3°C) in a patient with an ANC less than 500/mm³ is an emergency requiring immediate administration of antibiotics.

1. Assess for neutropenia—ANC less than 500/mm³.
    a. Assess for any signs of infection (pulmonary, integumentary, central nervous system, GI, and urinary).
    b. Auscultate lungs for adventitious breath sounds.
    c. Assess for productive cough or shortness of breath.
    d. Assess for urinary frequency, urgency, pain, or odor.
    e. Monitor for elevation of temperature above 101°F (38.3°C) and chills.
2. Assess for thrombocytopenia—platelet count less than 50,000/mm³ (mild risk of bleeding); less than 20,000/mm³ (high risk of bleeding).
    a. Assess skin and oral mucous membranes for petechiae and bruises on extremities.
    b. Assess for signs of bleeding (including nose, urinary, rectal, or hemoptysis).
    c. Assess for blood in stools, urine, or emesis.
    d. Assess for signs and symptoms of intracranial bleeding if platelet count is less than 20,000/mm³; monitor for changes in level of responsiveness, vital signs, and pupillary reaction.
3. Assess for anemia.
    a. Assess skin color, turgor, and capillary refill.
    b. Ascertain whether patient has experienced dyspnea on exertion, fatigue, weakness, palpitations, or vertigo. Advise rest periods as needed.

Respiratory and Cardiovascular Systems

1. Assess lung sounds.
2. Assess for pulmonary fibrosis, evidenced by a dry, nonproductive cough with increasing dyspnea. Patients at risk include those over age 60, smokers, those receiving or having had pulmonary radiation, those receiving a cumulative dose of bleomycin, or those with any pre-existing lung disease.
3. Assess for signs and symptoms of heart failure or irregular apical or radial pulses.
4. Verify baseline cardiac studies (eg, electrocardiogram, multiple-gated acquisition scan/ejection fraction) before administering cardiotoxic chemotherapy such as doxorubicin.

Neuromuscular System

1. Determine whether the patient is having difficulty with fine motor activities, such as zipping pants, tying shoes, or buttoning a shirt.
2. Determine the presence of paresthesia (tingling, numbness) of fingers or toes.
3. Evaluate deep tendon reflexes.
4. Evaluate the patient for weakness, ataxia, or slapping gait.

5. Determine impact on activities of daily living and discuss changes.
6. Discuss symptoms of urinary retention or constipation.
7. Assess for ringing in ears or decreased hearing acuity.

Genitourinary System

1. Monitor urine output.
2. Assess for urinary frequency, urgency, or hesitancy.
3. Evaluate changes in odor, color, or clarity of urine sample.
4. Assess for hematuria, oliguria, or anuria.
5. Monitor BUN and creatinine.

Nursing Diagnoses

- Risk for Infection related to neutropenia.
- Risk for Bleeding related to thrombocytopenia.
- Fatigue related to anemia.
- Imbalanced Nutrition: Less Than Body Requirements related to adverse effects of therapy.
- Impaired Oral Mucous Membranes related to stomatitis.
- Ineffective Protection and risk for hypersensitivity reaction related to chemotherapy.
- Disturbed Body Image related to alopecia and weight loss.

Nursing Interventions

Preventing Infection

1. Monitor vital signs every 4 hours; report occurrence of fever greater than 101°F (38.3°C) and chills.
2. Provide patient education.
    a. Instruct patient to report signs and symptoms of infection:
        i. Fever greater than 101°F (38.3°C) and/or chills.
        ii. Mouth lesions, swelling, or redness.
        iii. Redness, pain, or tenderness at rectum.
        iv. Change in bowel habits.
        v. Areas of redness, swelling, induration, or pain on skin surface.
        vi. Pain or burning when urinating or odor from urine.
        vii. Cough or shortness of breath.
    b. Reinforce good personal hygiene habits (routine bathing [preferably a shower], clean hair, nails, and mouth care).
    c. Avoid contact with people who have a transmittable illness.
    d. Encourage deep breathing and coughing to decrease pulmonary stasis.
3. Avoid performing invasive procedures—rectal temperatures, enemas, or insertion of indwelling urinary catheters.
4. Monitor white blood cell (WBC) count and differential.
5. Be aware that hematologic nadirs (lowest level) generally occur within 7 to 14 days after drug administration. Length of myelosuppression depends on specific drug. Institution of further therapy usually depends on an adequate WBC count and ANC.
6. Calculate ANC to determine the number of neutrophils capable of fighting an infection by:

$$\text{Total WBC count} \times (\% \text{ polys} + \% \text{ bands}) = \text{ANC}$$
$$\text{Example: } 700 \times (10\% + 5\%) = 105.$$

   Interpretation: 105 of the 700 WBCs are neutrophils and capable of fighting an infection (indicates severe neutropenia).
7. Administer prophylactic antibiotics, as prescribed (if WBC count is less than 500).
8. Administer growth factors, as prescribed: subcutaneous (SC) filgrastim 5 mcg/kg starting 24 hours after chemotherapy for 5 to 10 days for neutropenia prophylaxis or pegfilgrastim

6 mg SC for a single dose 24 hours after chemotherapy. Should also be administered with subsequent courses of chemotherapy to hasten neutrophil maturity.

Preventing Bleeding

1. Avoid invasive procedures when platelet count is less than 50,000/mm³, including IM injections, suppositories, enemas, and insertion of indwelling urinary catheters.
2. Apply pressure on injection sites for 5 minutes.
3. Monitor platelet count; administer platelets as prescribed.
4. Monitor and test all urine, stools, and emesis for blood.
5. Provide patient education.
   a. Instruct patient to avoid straight-edge razors, nail clippers, and vaginal or rectal suppositories.
   b. Avoid intercourse when platelet count is less than 50,000/mm³.
   c. Encourage patient to blow his or her nose gently.
   d. Avoid dental work or other invasive procedures while thrombocytopenic.
   e. Avoid the use of nonsteroidal anti-inflammatory drugs (NSAIDs), aspirin, and aspirin-containing products.

Minimizing Fatigue

1. Monitor blood counts (hemoglobin and hematocrit).
2. Administer blood products as prescribed.
3. Administer growth factors as prescribed, such as erythropoietin or darbepoetin.
4. Provide patient education and counseling.
   a. Information about fatigue.
   b. Reassurance that treatment-related fatigue does not mean your cancer is worse.
   c. Why fatigue and shortness of breath may occur.
   d. Suggestions for ways to cope with fatigue.
      i. Encourage aerobic and strength-training exercise. Balance activity and rest.
      ii. Plan frequent rest periods between daily activities; take naps that do not interrupt nighttime sleep.
      iii. Set priorities and delegate tasks to others.
   e. Stress management.
   f. Explain that blood transfusions, if given, are a part of therapy and not necessarily an indication of a setback.
   g. Observe skin color.
   h. Monitor nutritional status.

TRANSITIONAL CARE ALERT Oncology patients are very complex. The most common admission diagnosis includes chemotherapy-related side effects, infectious causes, anemia, and dehydration. Prevention is a key responsibility of the nurse in any setting. Prior to discharge, a coordinated effort between social work, case management, and the medical and nursing teams is critical to prevent readmissions. This includes discharge education, adherence to medications, and attention to outpatient follow-up appointments.

Promoting Nutrition

EVIDENCE BASE National Comprehensive Cancer Network. (2017). Clinical practice guidelines in oncology: Version 2.2017 Antiemesis. Available: *www.nccn.org*.

1. Prevention of nausea/vomiting is the goal. Administer antiemetics before chemotherapy and on a routine schedule (not as needed).
2. Be aware that antiemetic combinations are more effective than single agents.
3. For highly emetogenic chemotherapy regimens greater than 90% frequency of emesis:
   a. Serotonin (5-HT3) antagonist.
      i. Ondansetron, 16 to 24 mg PO or 8 to 12 mg (maximum 32 mg) IV day 1, then 8 mg PO tid for 2 to 3 days or
      ii. Granisetron, 2 mg PO or 1 mg PO bid or 0.01 mg/kg (maximum 1 mg) IV day 1, then daily for 2 to 3 days or
      iii. Dolasetron, 100 mg PO, then daily for 2 to 3 days or
      iv. Palonosetron, 0.25 mg IV day 1, and
   b. Corticosteroid—dexamethasone, 12 mg PO or IV day 1, then 8 mg PO or IV days 2 to 4.
   c. Neurokinin 1 agonist.
      i. Aprepitant, 125 mg PO day 1, then 80 mg PO daily days 2 and 3 or
      ii. Fosaprepitant, 150 mg IV day 1 only, or
      iii. Rolapitant 180 mg PO once.
   d. Include an as-needed antiemetic, such as metoclopramide, prochlorperazine, dexamethasone, or lorazepam.
4. For moderately emetogenic regimens:
   a. Premedicate with aprepitant, 125 mg PO (for selected high-risk patients); dexamethasone, 12 mg PO or IV and a 5-HT3 antagonist, such as palonosetron, 0.25 mg IV, or ondansetron, 16 to 24 mg PO or 8 to 12 mg; or ± lorazepam, 0.5 to 2 mg either PO or IV or sublingual every 4 to 6 hours prn.
   b. On days 2 to 4: aprepitant, 80 mg PO on days 2 and 3 (if used on day 1); dexamethasone, 8 mg IV or PO daily plus a 5-HT3 agonist, such as ondansetron, PO bid; granisetron, 1 to 2 mg PO or 1 mg PO bid; or dolasetron, 100 mg PO
   c. Include an as-needed antiemetic, such as prochlorperazine or lorazepam.
5. For low emetogenic regimens:
   a. Dexamethasone, 12 mg PO or IV daily, or
   b. Prochlorperazine, 10 mg PO or IV every 4 to 6 hours or 15 mg spansule PO every 8 to 12 hours, or
   c. Metoclopramide, either 20 to 40 mg PO every 4 to 6 hours or 1 to 2 mg/kg IV every 3 to 4 hours; ± diphenhydramine, 25 to 50 mg PO or IV every 4 to 6 hours; or ± lorazepam, 0.5 to 2 mg PO or IV every 4 to 6 hours.
6. Extrapyramidal reactions occur frequently in patients under age 30 and over age 65. Treat dystonic reactions with diphenhydramine; treat restlessness with lorazepam.
7. Consider alternative measures for relief of anticipatory nausea, such as relaxation therapy, imagery, acupuncture, and distraction.
8. Encourage small, frequent meals appealing to patient preferences, but including high calories and proteins. Provide a high-protein supplement as needed.
9. Discourage smoking and alcoholic beverages, which may irritate mucous membranes.
10. Encourage fluid intake to prevent constipation.
11. Monitor intake and output, including emesis.
12. Consult dietitian about patient's food preferences, intolerances, and individual dietary interventions.
13. Recognize that the patient may have alterations in taste perception, such as a keener taste of bitterness and loss of ability to detect sweet tastes.

Minimizing Stomatitis

1. Report signs of infection—erythematous areas, white patches, ulcers.
2. Encourage good oral hygiene.
   a. Soft nylon-bristled toothbrush, brush two to three times daily, rinse frequently.
   b. Floss once daily.
3. Encourage the use of oral agents to promote cleansing, debridement, and comfort. Mouthwashes with more than 25% alcohol should be avoided.
4. Assess the need for antifungal, antibacterial, or antiviral therapy (each infection has a different appearance).
5. Administer local oral therapy, such as combinations with viscous lidocaine, for symptomatic control and maintenance of calorie intake.

Preventing and Managing Hypersensitivity Reactions

1. Be alert for signs of allergic reactions such as pruritus, urticaria, and difficulty breathing as well as back pain. The situation may worsen suddenly to hypotension and anaphylaxis.
2. Stop the medication or infusion immediately, notify the health care provider, and monitor the patient closely. Treatment is supportive and dependent on type of reaction and its severity.
   a. Do not administer the agent again if there was a severe reaction resulting in significant hypotension.
   b. Premedicate the patient with antihistamine or corticosteroid, as directed, if there is a history of moderate reaction.

Strengthening Coping for Altered Body Image

1. Reassure patient that hair will grow back; however, it may grow back a different texture or different color.
2. Suggest wearing a turban, wig, or headscarf, preferably purchased before hair loss occurs. Many insurance companies will pay for a wig with a prescription.
3. Encourage patient to stay on therapeutic program.
4. Be honest with patient.

Patient Education and Health Maintenance

1. Make sure patient uses good hygiene, knows the symptoms of infection to report, and avoids crowds and people with infection while neutropenic.
2. Advise patient to avoid using a razor blade to shave, contact sports, manipulation of sharp articles, use of a hard-bristle toothbrush, and passage of hard stool to prevent bleeding while thrombocytopenic.
3. Advise women to report symptoms of vaginal infection because of opportunistic fungal or viral infection.
4. Encourage patient participation in plan for chemotherapy and to set realistic goals for work and activities.
5. Assure patient that changes in menses, libido, and sexual function are usually temporary during therapy.

Evaluation: Expected Outcomes

- Afebrile, no signs of infection.
- No bruising or bleeding noted; stool and urine heme test negative.
- Denies shortness of breath or severe fatigue.
- Tolerates small, frequent meals following antiemetic.
- No oral lesions or pain on swallowing.
- No urticaria, shortness of breath, or change in vital signs.
- Wears turban and expresses feelings about body image.

Radiation Therapy

Radiation therapy is the use of high-energy x-rays or other radiation particles to treat malignant diseases. Radiation with sufficient energy to disrupt atomic structures by ejecting orbital electrons is called ionizing radiation. The goal of radiation is to deliver a precisely measured dose of irradiation to a defined tumor volume with minimal damage to surrounding healthy tissue. This results in eradication of tumor, high quality of life, and prolongation of survival and allows for effective palliation or prevention of symptoms of cancer, with minimal morbidity. Over the past 20 years, advances have been made in imaging and treatment delivery, allowing for improved targeting and increased sparing of normal tissues.

General Considerations

1. Different irradiation doses are required for tumor control, depending on tumor type and the number of cells present. Varying radiation doses can be delivered to specific portions of the tumor (periphery vs. central portion) or to the tumor bed in cases in which all gross tumor has been surgically removed.
2. Treatment portals must adequately cover all treatment volumes plus a margin.

Goals of Therapy

1. Curative—when there is a probability of long-term survival after adequate therapy, some adverse effects of therapy, although undesirable, may be acceptable.
2. Palliative—when there is no hope of survival for extended periods, radiation can be used to palliate symptoms, primarily pain. Lower doses of irradiation (75% to 80% of curative dose) can control the tumor and palliate symptoms without excessive toxicity.

Principles of Therapy

1. Radiosensitivity is the sensitivity of cells, tissues, or tumors to radiation. Rapidly dividing cells are most sensitive.
2. Radioresistance is the lack of tumor response to radiation because of tumor characteristics (slow growing, less responsive), tumor cell proliferation, and circulation. Radiation is most effective during the mitotic stage of the cell cycle.
3. Radioresistant tumors: Many tumors are resistant to radiation, such as squamous cell, ovarian, soft tissue sarcoma, and gliomas. Many other tumors can become resistant after a period of time. Normal radioresistant tissues include mature bone, cartilage, liver, thyroid, muscle, brain, and spinal cord.
4. Role of oxygen: The presence of oxygen enhances radiation. Without oxygen, chemical damage to DNA may be repaired. Giving multiple, daily doses allows reoxygenation and enhances radiosensitivity. The dose should allow for repair of normal tissues.
5. Tissue tolerance dose is the amount of radiation that a healthy cell can receive and still function. This is what limits the dose of radiation one can receive.
6. Tumor size is a major factor in response to radiation therapy. Smaller tumors are more responsive than larger tumors.

Types of Radiation Therapy

There are generally two types of ionizing radiation: teletherapy and brachytherapy and several ways in which it is delivered.

1. Teletherapy is most commonly delivered through a linear accelerator machine. And there are a number of techniques used to administer teletherapy.
    a. Intraoperative radiation therapy—given during surgery for tumors that are not completely operable or are at high risk for recurrence. Examples include gynecological malignancies and colorectal cancers.
    b. Stereotactic radiation (radiosurgery)—used for brain tumors where the radiation beam is delivered precisely to the tumor itself sparing surrounding healthy brain tissue. This can be administered through gamma knife technology. The patient's head is placed into a frame that is secured to the cranium with screws. Scanning technology allows for precise and accurate delivery of radiation.
    c. Intensity-modulated radiation therapy (IMRT)—uses radiation beams of varying intensities to deliver different doses of radiation to small areas of tissue at the same time. This is used most commonly in brain, head, and neck tumors and lung tumors.
    d. Image-guided radiation therapy—uses repeated imaging scans (obtained via CT, MRI, or PET) during treatment to identify changes in a tumor's size and location because of treatment and to allow the position of the patient or the planned radiation dose to be adjusted, as needed. Repeated imaging can increase the accuracy of radiation treatment and may allow reductions in the planned volume of tissue to be treated, thereby decreasing the total radiation dose to normal tissue.
    e. Tomotherapy—type of image-guided IMRT. A tomotherapy machine is a hybrid between a CT imaging scanner and an external beam radiation therapy machine. Tomotherapy machines can capture CT images of the patient's tumor immediately before each treatment, to allow for precise tumor targeting and sparing of normal tissue.
2. Brachytherapy uses seeds, wires, or catheters to deliver radiation directly to or adjacent to the tumor bed. This technique delivers less radiation to adjacent normal tissue, but it requires direct tumor access. It may be temporary or permanent. The permanent type remains in place with gradual decay. The implant procedure is performed under local or general anesthesia and is typically used for breast and prostate cancers.
    a. Intracavitary therapy utilizes radioactive material that is inserted into a cavity such as the vagina, as in cancer of the uterine cervix.
    b. Other forms of brachytherapy are systemic irradiation (parenteral or IV), oral ^{131}I for thyroid cancer, or intraperitoneal radiation.

Chemical and Thermal Modifiers of Radiation
1. Radiosensitization is the use of medications to enhance the sensitivity of the tumor cells.
2. Radioprotectors increase therapeutic ratio by promoting repair of normal tissues.
3. Hyperthermia is combined with radiation. Uses a variety of sources (ultrasound, microwaves) and produces a greater effect than radiation alone. It is usually applied locally or regionally immediately after radiation.

Units for Measuring Radiation Exposure or Absorption
1. Centigray (cGy) is a unit of radiation dose absorbed by the body equal to one hundredth of a gray; formerly called a rad (eg, 1 cGy equals 1 rad). Gray (Gy) is the unit of absorbed radiation dose equal to 100 rad.

2. Hyperfractionated radiation therapy is the division of the total radiation dose into smaller daily doses. Administering fractions allows treatment of tumor cells while giving healthy cells time to repair themselves.

Nature and Indications for Use
Used alone or in combination with surgery or chemotherapy, depending on the stage of disease and goal of therapy.
1. Adjuvant radiation therapy—used in combination with other treatment modalities, such as chemotherapy or surgery, when a high risk of local recurrence or large primary tumor exists.
2. Curative radiation therapy—used in anatomically limited tumors (retina, optic nerve, certain brain tumors, skin, oral cavity). Course is usually longer and the dose higher.
3. Palliative—for treatment of symptoms.
    a. Provides excellent pain control for bone metastasis.
    b. Used to relieve obstruction.
    c. Relief of neurologic dysfunction for brain metastasis.
    d. Given in short, intensive courses.

Treatment Planning
1. Evaluation of tumor extent (staging), including diagnostic studies before treatment.
2. Define the goal of therapy (cure or palliation).
3. Select appropriate treatment modalities (irradiation alone or combined with surgery, chemotherapy, or both).
4. Treatment planning is known as simulation. This is the process of aiming and defining radiation beams to meet the goals of prescribed therapy.
    a. Simulation is used to accurately identify target volumes and sensitive structures. CT simulation allows for accurate three-dimensional treatment planning of target volume and anatomy of critical normal structures.
    b. Treatment aids (eg, shielding blocks, molds, masks, immobilization devices, compensators) are extremely important in treatment planning and delivery of optimal dose distribution. Repositioning and immobilization devices are critical for accurate treatment.
    c. Lead blocks are made to shape the beam and protect normal tissues.
    d. Skin markings are applied to define the target and portal. These are generally replaced later by permanent tattoos.
5. Usual schedule is Monday through Friday.
6. Actual therapy lasts minutes. Most time is spent on positioning.
7. Determine optimal dose of irradiation and volume to be treated, according to anatomic location, histologic type, stage, potential regional nodal involvement (and other tumor characteristics), and normal structures in the region.

Complications

Complications depend on the site of radiation therapy, type of radiation therapy (brachytherapy or teletherapy), total radiation dose, daily fractionated doses, and overall health of the patient. Adverse effects are predictable, depending on the normal organs and tissues involved in the field.

Acute Adverse Effects
1. Fatigue and malaise.
2. Skin: may develop a reaction as soon as 2 weeks into the course of treatment.
    a. Erythema—may range from mild to severe.
    b. Dry desquamation—shedding of the skin.

c. Moist desquamation—shedding of the skin to reveal moist, edematous skin underneath. Areas having folds, such as the axilla, under the breasts, groin and gluteal fold, are at an increased risk because of increased warmth and moisture.

d. Folliculitis—infection of the hair follicles, which may result in pustule formation.

3. GI effects: nausea and vomiting, diarrhea, and esophagitis.
4. Oral effects: changes in taste, mucositis, dryness, and xerostomia (dryness of mouth from lack of normal secretions).
5. Pulmonary effects: dyspnea, productive cough, and radiation pneumonitis (usually occurs 1 to 3 months after radiation to the lung).
6. Renal and bladder effects: cystitis and urethritis.
7. Cardiovascular effects: damage to vasculature of organs and thrombosis (heart is relatively radioresistant).
8. Recall reactions: acute skin and mucosal reactions when concurrent or past chemotherapy (doxorubicin, dactinomycin).
9. Bone marrow suppression: more common with pelvic or large bone radiation.

Chronic Adverse Effects

After 6 months with variability in time of expression:

1. Skin effects: fibrosis, telangiectasia, permanent darkening of the skin, and atrophy.
2. GI effects: fibrosis, adhesions, obstruction, ulceration, and strictures.
3. Oral effects: permanent xerostomia, permanent taste alterations, and dental caries.
4. Pulmonary effects: fibrosis.
5. Renal and bladder effects: radiation nephritis and fibrosis.
6. Second primary cancer: patients who have received combined radiation and chemotherapy with alkylating agents have a rare risk of developing acute leukemia.

Nursing Assessment

1. Assess skin and mucous membranes for adverse effects of radiation.
2. Assess GI, respiratory, and renal function for signs of adverse effects.
3. Assess patient's understanding of treatment and emotional status.

Nursing Diagnoses

- Risk for Impaired Skin Integrity related to radiation effects.
- Ineffective Protection related to brachytherapy.

Nursing Interventions

Maintaining Optimal Skin Care

1. Inform the patient that some skin reaction can be expected but that it varies from patient to patient. Examples include dry erythema, dry desquamation, wet desquamation, epilation, and tanning.
2. Do not apply lotions, ointments, or cosmetics to the site of radiation unless prescribed.
3. Discourage vigorous rubbing, friction, or scratching because this can destroy skin cells. Apply ointments as instructed by health professionals.
4. Avoid wearing tight-fitting clothing over the treatment field; prevent irritation by not using rough fabric such as wool and corduroy.
5. Take precautions against exposing the radiation field to sunlight and extremes in temperature.

6. Do not apply adhesive or other tape to the skin.
7. Avoid shaving the skin in the treatment field.
8. Use lukewarm water only and mild soap when bathing.

Ensuring Protection from Radiation

1. To avoid exposure to radiation while the patient is receiving therapy, consider the following:
   a. Time—exposure to radiation is directly proportional to the time spent within a specific distance to the source.
   b. Distance—amount of radiation reaching a given area decreases as resistance increases.
   c. Shield—sheet of absorbing material placed between the radiation source and the nurse decreases the amount of radiation exposure.
2. Individual monitoring devices should be worn by personnel exposed to radiation or radioactive material.
3. Take appropriate measures associated with sealed sources of radiation implanted within a patient (sealed internal radiation).
   a. Follow directives on precaution sheet that is placed on the charts of all patients receiving radiotherapy.
   b. Do not remain within 3 feet (1 m) of the patient any longer than required to give essential care.
4. Know that the casing material absorbs all alpha radiation and most beta radiation but that a hazard concerning gamma radiation may exist.
5. Do not linger longer than necessary in giving patient care, even though all precautions are followed.
6. Be alert for implants that may have become loosened (those inserted in cavities that have access to the exterior); for example, check the emesis basin following mouth care for a patient with an oral implant.
7. Notify the radiation therapist of any implant that has moved out of position.
8. Use long-handled forceps or tongs and hold at arm's length when picking up any dislodged radium needle, seeds, or tubes. Never pick up a radioactive source with your hands.
9. Do not discard dressings or linens unless you are sure that no radioactive source is present.
10. After the patient is discharged from the facility, it is a good policy for the radiologist to check the room with a radiograph or survey meter to be certain that all radioactive materials have been removed.
11. Continue radiation precautions when a patient has a permanent implant, until the radiologist declares precautions unnecessary.

Evaluation: Expected Outcomes

- Skin without breakdown or signs of infection.
- Radiation precautions maintained.

Biologic Therapy

Biologic therapy is targeted cancer treatment. It has emerged as an important modality of cancer treatment and one where intensive research is actively being conducted. The goal is to produce antitumor effects through the action of natural host defense mechanisms. It is capable of altering the immune system with either stimulatory or suppressive effects. The underlying principle is that the primary function of the immune system is to detect and eliminate substances that are recognized as "nonself." This represents the most promising new cancer treatment approach since the development of chemotherapy.

Types of Immunotherapy

Cytokines

Cytokines are soluble proteins produced by mononuclear cells of the immune system (usually the lymphocytes and monocytes) that have regulatory actions on other cells in the immune system. Cytokines produced by lymphocytes are referred to as *lymphokines*, and cytokines produced by monocytes are referred to as *monokines*.

1. Examples of cytokines include interleukins, interferons, CSFs, and tumor necrosis factor.
2. Many other biologic agents are currently under investigation.

Antibody Therapy

Monoclonal antibodies work on cancer cells in the same way natural antibodies work, by identifying and binding to the target cells. They then alert other cells in the immune system to the presence of the cancer cells.

1. Promotes targeting cells through antibody–antigen response.
2. Monoclonal antibodies may be used alone or in combination with chemotherapy.
3. Examples of monoclonal antibodies include:
   a. Rituximab—a murine/human chimeric monoclonal antibody specific for the CD20 surface marker on B cells. It is approved for the treatment of relapsed or refractory low-grade/follicular non-Hodgkin lymphoma.
   b. Ibritumomab—combines the targeting power of monoclonal antibodies with the cell-damaging ability of localized radiation. It is developed to recognize and attach to substances on the surface of certain cells and deliver cytotoxic radiation directly to the cancerous cells.
   c. Trastuzumab—a recombinant DNA–derived humanized monoclonal antibody that selectively binds with high affinity in a cell-based assay to the extracellular domain of the human epidermal growth factor receptor 2 protein (HER2). It is approved for the treatment of patients with early stage and advanced metastatic breast cancer whose tumors overexpress the HER2 protein.
   d. Cetuximab—binds to extracellular EGRF resulting in inhibition of cell growth and induction of apoptosis.
   e. Bevacizumab—binds to and inhibits the activity of human VEGF to its receptors blocking proliferation and formation of new blood vessels that supply tumor cells.
   f. Panitumumab—inhibits the binding of ligand to the EGFR receptor resulting in inhibition of cell growth.
   g. Alemtuzumab—recognizes the CD52 antigen expressed on malignant and normal B lymphocytes. It has come to be used therapeutically in B-cell malignancies.
4. Potential adverse effects of monoclonal antibodies include dyspnea and mild wheezing, fever and chills, headache, rash, nausea and vomiting, tachycardia, bleeding, and allergic reactions.

Other Types of Immunotherapy

1. Virus immunotherapy—uses viruses to deliberately infect the cancer cell, which in turn triggers an immune response against the infected cancer cell.
2. Immune checkpoint inhibitors—these drugs block tumor cells from inactivating T cells. This allows the T cell to remain active and fight the tumor cells. Examples include nivolumab and pembrolizumab.

Nursing Assessment

1. Review patient's record or obtain history from the patient to determine site of cancer, previous cancer therapies, current medications, and other medical conditions.
2. Assess current cardiovascular and respiratory status.
3. Assess patient's understanding of immunotherapy and associated toxicities.
4. Assess for common side effects of immune system stimulation, including fever, chills, body aches, nausea, vomiting, and fatigue, as well as serious and potentially life-threatening adverse reactions, including dyspnea, wheezing, tachycardia, bleeding, hypotension, and anaphylaxis.

Nursing Diagnoses

- Hyperthermia as an adverse effect of immunotherapy.
- Ineffective Tissue Perfusion related to capillary permeability leak syndrome (third spacing of fluid) caused by immunotherapy.

Nursing Interventions

Controlling Hyperthermia

1. Discuss the overall goal of immunotherapy, expected adverse effects, and the method of administration.
2. Instruct the patient to report fever, chills, diarrhea, nausea and vomiting, itching, or weight gain.
3. Administer or advise self-administration of antipyretics, such as acetaminophen for fever.
4. Emphasize that adverse effects are temporary and will usually cease within 1 week after treatment ends.

Maintaining Tissue Perfusion

1. Monitor vital signs at least every 4 hours for hypotension, tachycardia, tachypnea, and fever.
   a. Instruct the patient to remain in bed if blood pressure is low.
   b. Monitor apical heart rate.
2. Assess respirations for rate and depth, and auscultate breath sounds for evidence of pulmonary edema.
3. Assess for signs of restlessness, apprehension, discomfort, or cyanosis, which may indicate respiratory distress.
4. Administer oxygen as prescribed.
5. Maintain patent IV line and administer serum albumin as prescribed.
6. Check extremities for warmth, color, and capillary refill.

Evaluation: Expected Outcomes

- Relief of fever after medication.
- Blood pressure stable and lungs clear.

SPECIAL CONSIDERATIONS IN CANCER CARE

Pain Management

Pain related to cancer may be caused by direct tumor infiltration of bones, nerves, viscera, or soft tissue, as well as by therapeutic measures (surgery, radiation). Pain is the most common symptom associated with cancer and has a negative impact on a patient's functional status and quality of life. Cancer pain can be controlled with medication in 80% to 95% of patients, and there is increasing evidence that survival is linked to pain management. See Appendix D, page 1508 for more information on pain management.

Oncologic Emergencies

Oncologic emergencies are a group of life-threatening metabolic syndromes or abnormalities associated with cancer and/or cancer treatment.

Septic Shock

Septic shock is a systemic disease associated with the presence and persistence of pathogenic microorganisms or their toxins in the blood. It is characterized by hemodynamic instability, abnormal coagulation, and altered metabolism.

Risk Factors

1. Neutropenia, ANC less than 500.
2. Patients who are neutropenic longer than 7 days most susceptible.
3. Patients with HIV and concomitant neutropenia.
4. Prolonged hospitalization.
5. Older patients.
6. Patients with comorbid conditions, such as diabetes and pulmonary diseases.

Clinical Manifestations

1. Fever greater than 100.5°F (38.3°C).
2. Warm, flushed, dry skin.
3. Hypotension.
4. Tachycardia.
5. Tachypnea.
6. Decreased level of consciousness.
7. Patients will not have the usual symptoms of infection because of the lack of neutrophils. For example, skin infections may manifest as subtle rash or erythema. Urinary tract infections may be asymptomatic and patients with lung infections may be without pulmonary infiltrates.

Diagnostic Evaluation

1. Vital signs.
2. Culture—blood, urine, stool, sputum, central and peripheral IV lines, and any open wounds to determine source and type of infection.
3. Chest x-ray—to detect underlying pneumonia.
4. CT scans as necessary.
5. Arterial blood gas analysis—decreased pH reflects acidosis.
6. BUN and creatinine—elevated because of decreased circulating blood volume.
7. CBC with differential—elevated WBC count with shift to left.

Management

1. Antibiotics are started immediately; broad-spectrum antibiotics are given until organism is identified.
2. IV fluids and plasma expanders are used to restore circulating volume.
3. CSFs are administered to increase ANC.
4. Vasopressors are administered to support blood pressure.
5. Oxygen is administered, as needed, to prevent tissue hypoxia.
6. Vital signs, respiratory status, urine output, and any signs of bleeding are monitored carefully.
7. Complications, such as renal failure, respiratory failure, cardiac failure, metabolic acidosis, and disseminated intravascular coagulation, are treated aggressively.

Spinal Cord Compression

Spinal cord compression (SCC) is the result of tumor compression on the dural sac. This can result in neurologic impairment or permanent loss of function if not treated immediately.

Incidence

1. Affects 5% of all terminal cancer patients in the last 2 years of their lives with less than a 6-month median survival from diagnosis.
2. Lung, breast, and prostate cancer account for 15% to 20% of all cases.
3. Multiple myeloma, non-Hodgkin lymphoma, and renal carcinoma account for 5% to 10% of cases.

Clinical Manifestations

1. Cervical spine.
   a. Vertigo.
   b. Radicular pain in neck and back of head that is aggravated by neck flexion.
   c. Upper extremity weakness.
   d. Sensory loss in area of weakness (ie, paresthesia, numbness).
   e. Abnormal deep tendon reflexes.
   f. Gastric hypersecretion and paralytic ileus.
2. Thoracic spine.
   a. Local or radicular pain (or both).
   b. Lower extremity weakness.
   c. Sensory loss below the level of the lesion.
   d. Band of hyperesthesia at dermatome of tumor site.
   e. Impaired bladder or bowel control.
3. Lumbar spine.
   a. Local or radicular pain (or both).
   b. Lower extremity weakness and paralysis.
   c. Atrophy of lower extremity muscles.
   d. Sensory loss below level of the lesion.
   e. Urinary symptoms (hesitancy, retention), constipation, or bowel incontinence.
4. Weakness and unsteadiness may be noted before changes in motor function. (Progression is usually rapid with foot drop and impaired ambulation. Urgent investigation and treatment are crucial to minimize the risk of paraplegia. The degree of weakness and ability to walk at presentation are important clinical predictors of outcome.)
5. Changes in sensation—paresthesia, numbness, tingling. (Severity usually mirrors the severity of motor weakness.)

 NURSING ALERT Any abnormal neurologic symptoms in a patient with cancer should be considered an SCC until proven otherwise.

Diagnostic Evaluation

1. Neurologic examination—early diagnosis is important.
2. X-ray of the painful site—may be abnormal; can be used as an initial screen for complaints of back pain.
3. Bone scan—more sensitive to bony metastasis than x-ray to detect abnormal vertebral bodies.
4. MRI—most useful in detecting spinal cord lesions. The entire spine can be viewed. Immediately indicated if radiculopathy or myelopathy is present or x-rays are abnormal.

Management

1. Treatment is usually palliative because it is associated with metastatic disease.
2. Treatment goals are to relieve pain, minimize complications, and preserve or restore neurologic function.
3. Corticosteroids are the initial treatment until more definitive treatment can be instituted, reduce inflammation and swelling at site, increase neurologic function, and relieve pain.
   a. A loading dose of dexamethasone is usually given followed by tapering doses over a period of weeks.
   b. Steroids must be tapered and not abruptly discontinued.
   c. Monitor patient's glucose levels during dexamethasone treatment because it can cause hyperglycemia.

4. Radiation therapy to the tumor on spinal column is the most common treatment. Radiation is effective with 70% of patients having improvement in pain and function.
5. Surgery is considered when tumors are not radiosensitive or located in an area that has been previously radiated. It is also indicated for spinal instability.

Complications

1. Respiratory impairment, including pneumonia and atelectasis.
2. Mobility impairment, foot drop, skin impairment, and postural hypotension.
3. Sensory losses creating safety concerns.
4. Bladder or bowel dysfunction.

Patient Education

1. Facilitate referral to home care services for nursing assessment, nursing intervention, and rehabilitation for residual deficits.
2. Facilitate referral to appropriate outpatient services, including physical therapy, occupational therapy, and psychosocial support.
3. Provide instruction about safety issues for residual sensory deficits (eg, test bath water temperature, careful use of extreme hot or cold).

Hypercalcemia

Hypercalcemia is an elevated serum calcium level above 11 mg/dL. It results when bone resorption exceeds both bone formation and the ability of the kidneys to excrete extracellular calcium released from the bones.

Incidence

1. The most common life-threatening disorder associated with malignancy; occurs in 20% to 30% of patients at some point in their illness.
2. Occurs most commonly in patients with carcinoma of the lung, breast, and renal cells; multiple myeloma; and adult lymphomas.
3. Can occur with or without skeletal metastasis, but more than 80% of patients do have bony disease.
4. Associated with a poor prognosis.

Clinical Manifestations

1. Signs and symptoms may vary, depending on the severity, and may be nonspecific and insidious.
   a. Early symptoms include anorexia, weakness, polyuria, polydipsia, and fatigue.
   b. Late symptoms include apathy, irritability, profound muscle weakness, nausea, vomiting, constipation, pruritus, lethargy, and confusion.
2. A rapid and life-threatening increase in calcium may cause dehydration, renal failure, coma, and death.

Diagnostic Evaluation

1. Serum calcium level greater than 11 mg/dL in adults, but ionized calcium of greater than 1.29 mmol/L is the most reliable test.
2. Electrolyte levels, BUN, and creatinine are obtained to determine hydration status and renal function.
3. ECG may show shortening of the QT interval and prolongation of the PR interval.

Management

1. Management includes treating the primary malignancy with chemotherapy, surgery, or radiation.
2. Acute, symptomatic hypercalcemia should be treated as an emergency.

3. Hydration and diuresis—IV normal saline (0.9% NaCl) is the initial treatment for patients with acute hypercalcemia and clinical symptoms to dilute the calcium and promote its renal excretion. Diuresis is induced with furosemide. (Thiazide diuretics aggravate hypercalcemia and should be avoided.)
4. Pharmacotherapy includes:
   a. Bisphosphonates—primary drug therapy, administered IV; pamidronate or zoledronic acid inhibits osteoclast resorption in the bone.
   b. Calcitonin—used in combination with glucocorticoids and inhibits bone resorption. It has a rapid onset but a short duration of action. Used most commonly in patients with multiple myeloma. It should not be used for longer than 72 hours.
   c. Denosumab—a monoclonal antibody that should be used in the setting of hypercalcemia at least 7 days after bisphosphonates.

Nursing Interventions

1. Prevent and detect hypercalcemia early.
   a. Recognize patients at risk and monitor for signs and symptoms, such as nausea and vomiting, constipation, lethargy, and anorexia.
   b. Emphasize importance of mobility to minimize bone demineralization and constipation.
   c. Instruct patient on the importance of adequate hydration.
2. Administer normal saline infusions as prescribed.
3. Administer medications as prescribed.
4. Maintain accurate intake and output; observe for oliguria or anuria.
5. Take vital signs every 4 hours, especially apical pulse and blood pressure.
6. Monitor electrolyte values and renal function.
7. Assess mental status.
8. Assess cardiorespiratory status for signs of fluid overload.

Superior Vena Cava Syndrome

Superior vena cava syndrome (SVCS) is obstruction and thrombosis of the superior vena cava caused by direct compression by a tumor or an enlarged lymph node, resulting in impaired venous drainage of the head, neck, arms, and thorax.

Incidence

1. Eighty percent to 95% of patients with SVCS are cancer patients.
2. Eighty percent of cases arise from advanced lung cancer, specifically small cell lung cancers, and 15% from lymphoma.
3. Other malignancies associated with SVCS are thymoma and breast cancer.

Clinical Manifestations

1. Signs and symptoms may vary, depending on the degree of obstruction and how rapidly the obstruction occurs.
2. A rapid onset of SVCS is dramatic and potentially life threatening and requires immediate intervention.
3. Facial edema is found in 80% of cases and is the most common initial finding.
4. Early symptoms include progressive dyspnea, cough, feeling of fullness in the head, difficulty buttoning shirt collar (Stoke sign), dysphagia and hoarseness, and chest pain.
5. Cyanosis and edema of the head and upper extremities may be apparent. Collateral circulation with dilated chest wall veins may be visible.

6. Late symptoms include respiratory distress, headache, vision disturbances, dizziness and syncope, lethargy, irritability, and mental status changes.
7. Pleural effusion on chest x-ray may also be seen.

Diagnostic Evaluation

1. CT scan is the most common imaging technique used to diagnose SVC syndrome.

Management

1. Radiation therapy and corticosteroids are the gold standard of treatment for SVCS to reduce tumor size and relieve pressure. Most patients experience a relief of symptoms within the first 4 days of therapy.
2. Chemotherapy may be used in conjunction with radiation. Specific chemotherapeutic agents depend on the tumor type.
3. Surgery is rarely used because of the associated high morbidity and mortality risks.
4. Percutaneous stent placement—an expandable stent may be placed inside the superior vena cava to keep it patent. Anticoagulants are also used in conjunction.
5. Thrombolytic and anticoagulant therapy may be used if a thrombus is suspected or to prevent the formation of a thrombus; must be used within the first 7 days to be effective.
6. Oxygen is given for relief of dyspnea and maintenance of tissue oxygenation.
7. Analgesics and tranquilizers are used for discomfort and anxiety.

Nursing Interventions

1. Administer oxygen, as prescribed, to relieve hypoxia.
2. Place patient in Fowler position—facilitates gravity drainage and reduces facial edema.
3. Limit patient's activity and provide a quiet environment.
4. Reassure patient that cyanotic color and facial edema will subside with treatment.

Psychosocial Components of Care

Nursing Assessment

1. Assess lifestyle before illness. How did patient solve other problems?
2. Assess for signs of anxiety and coexistence of depression: agitation and restlessness, sleep disturbances, excessive autonomic activity, weight gain or loss, mood changes.
3. What activities of daily living can patient perform?
4. What changes in lifestyle have resulted from cancer and its treatment?
5. Determine patient's perception of the disease and treatment.
6. Evaluate available social support; who is the most significant other?
7. Ask patient if any complementary or alternative medicine (CAM) modalities are being utilized for cancer treatment. Be aware that many patients seek herbal and other remedies despite lack of scientific evidence of any benefit. Encourage patient and family to discuss CAM use with health care provider to ensure safety.
8. Try to gain a sense of emotional strengths and potential problem areas. Ask if patient and family have a plan for end-of-life care as appropriate.

Nursing Diagnoses

- Anxiety related to complex disease process, treatment options, and prognosis.
- Ineffective Coping related to life-altering disease process.
- Fear of Death and dying.

Nursing Interventions

Reducing Anxiety

1. Establish and sustain an unhurried approach to give the patient time to organize fears, thoughts, and feelings.
2. Allow patient to share feelings about having cancer.
3. Reflect and amplify insights and judgments; try to reduce anxiety through reflection and reorientation.
4. Recognize feelings of losing control.
5. Discuss methods of stress reduction (imagery, relaxation).
6. Discuss the positive aspects of treatment.
7. Encourage expression of positive emotions—emphasis on living in the here and now, greater appreciation of life.
8. Reinforce effective coping behaviors.
9. Encourage patient to join a support group. Refer to local chapter of the ACS, call 1-800-ACS-2345 or visit *www.cancer.org*.
10. Remain available as problems arise. Give patient telephone numbers of people to call when needed.
11. Initiate referrals for additional rehabilitation and psychosocial services as appropriate.

Promoting Effective Coping

1. Encourage patient and family members to enroll in cancer education program.
2. Encourage patient to learn everything about treatment plan because this promotes a sense of control.
3. Provide expert physical care and teach patient about care.
4. Assist patient in strengthening support system (family, friends, visitors, health care staff and volunteers, support groups)—strengthens self-esteem through the experience of feeling accepted and valued.
5. Help patient readjust expectations and goals to promote ongoing adjustment.
6. Support patient in coping mechanisms chosen.

Allaying Fear of Death and Dying

1. Educate patient and family about prognosis and end-of-life choices, as outlined by patient's health care provider. Be direct, stating the statistics but stressing the positive aspects of the situation.
2. Assess and respect patient's beliefs.
3. Help patient and family agree on goals.
4. Facilitate emotional support for patient.
5. Provide bereavement support to survivors.

Evaluation: Expected Outcomes

- Discusses feelings; practices stress reduction.
- Patient and family attend cancer education program.
- Asks questions about prognosis and sets goals for care.

Survivorship

With earlier diagnosis and better treatment, more and more patients are surviving and living beyond cancer. Recent estimates show that as of 2016, the number of cancer survivors has surpassed 16 million. This expected continual increase in cancer survivors has put a strain on the health care delivery system. Primary care providers and oncologists have not been able to keep up with the growing number of patients who have completed their therapy.

The oversight of a health care provider is important as patient's transition from active cancer care to survivorship. Sadly, many needs of cancer survivors are not being met. In 1986, the National Coalition for Cancer Survivors was created to address these issues. Nearly two decades later, accredited cancer centers are now required to have survivorship programs. Nurses are uniquely positioned to help transform care survivorship care and improve the quality of care and patient outcomes.

Principles of Survivorship Care

1. Survivorship care is the process of learning how to live through cancer and beyond.
2. The goals cancer survivorship programs as recommended by the ASCO include the following:
   a. Prevention of recurrent and new cancers.
   b. Surveillance for cancer spread or recurrence.
   c. Assessment of late medical and psychological effects of therapy.
   d. Adherence and interventions for consequences for cancer and its treatment.
   e. Coordination between specialist and other health care providers.
3. There are different models of survivorship programs. Most include a transition visit at the end of treatment. During this visit, current symptoms are addressed and patients are provided a survivorship care plan and education to include prevention of recurrent and new cancers, surveillance and late effects, health promotion, and a follow-up plan.
4. These visits are often conducted by physicians and/or nurse practitioners. Nurses, however, have a pivotal role in survivorship programs. As patients often receive care from each of the treatment disciplines (medical oncology, surgical oncology, radiation oncology), nurses have the skills to integrate, coordinate care, and serve as the patient advocate. Nurses possess the skills and knowledge to educate and manage treatment-related side effects.

Management and Nursing Interventions

1. Realize that patients themselves have a difficult time adjusting to life after cancer treatment. They are often challenged with long-term side effects, both physical and psychological.
2. Provide education regarding the symptoms of recurrence, identification of late side effects, and an adoption of healthy lifestyle changes.
3. Ensure the patient has a knowledgeable provider that specifically addresses survivorship needs, and coordinate referrals to specialists as needed.

Palliative Care

Palliative cancer care is the integration of therapies that address the multiple issues that cause cancer patients and their families suffering. It is the care of the whole person along the illness trajectory, not just the end of life, to promote quality of life and relieve suffering. Palliative care comprises the management of pain, as well as other physical, psychological, and spiritual problems, and may be integrated into anticancer treatment and life-prolonging therapy. The hospice model of palliative care provides intensive end-of-life care, bereavement services, and support of the family after death of a loved one. Although palliative care is appropriate for many cancer patients, it is not limited to cancer; many neurologic, cardiac, pulmonary, and other types of disorders call for palliative care in their more severe or advanced forms.

There are facility- and community-based programs as well as inpatient facilities and home care services (including hospice). Care of patients with advanced illness, such as cancer, and dealing with death and dying is an integral part of oncology nursing.

Palliative care has been added to most medical and nursing schools across the country in recent years.

Principles of Palliative Care

1. Palliative care is an interdisciplinary team approach, including experts from medicine, nursing, social work, the clergy, and nutrition. This team approach is needed to make the necessary assessments and to institute appropriate interventions.
2. The essential components of palliative care are relief of symptom distress, improved quality of life, opening of communication on a regular basis with patients to provide appropriate care on their terms, and psychosocial support for patients and families.
3. The goal is to provide comfort and maintain the highest possible quality of life for as long as possible.
4. The traditional focus of palliative care is not on death but on a compassionate, specialized care for the living. It is based on a comprehensive understanding of patient suffering and focuses on providing effective pain and symptom management to seriously ill patients while improving quality of life.

End-of-Life Care

- Hospice and palliative care provide care during progressive illness, but hospice eligibility begins only when a patient has a life expectancy of 6 months or less. In contrast, palliative care begins when the patient has been diagnosed with a life-limiting illness. It recognizes that the goals of care may change, but the focus is always on quality of life.
- Unfortunately, hospice is equated with care of the dying, causing it to be underutilized; thus, many patients only live a few days to a week after contacting hospice.
- It has been shown that early referral to palliative care and hospice not only improves patient's symptoms and quality of life but also improves survival.
- Hospice care and palliative care offer end-of-life care, which can be achieved by:
   a. Enhancing physical well-being through effective symptom management: pain, nausea, vomiting, constipation, sleeplessness.
   b. Enhancing psychological well-being through management of anxiety, depression, fear, denial, and hopelessness. Rather, happiness, enjoyment, and leisure are promoted.
   c. Enhancing social well-being by addressing financial burden, caregiver burden, roles and relationships, affection and sexual function, and concerns about appearance.
   d. Enhancing spiritual well-being through minimization of suffering and instead focusing on religious beliefs, hope, and meaning.

Management and Nursing Interventions

1. Provide pain relief, symptom control (dyspnea, nausea, constipation, anxiety, agitation), and prevention of complications.
2. Encourage patient and family to exceed their current situation.
   a. Encourage patient and family to pursue enjoyable activities.
   b. Assist patient and family to focus on present and past joys.
   c. Share positive and hope-inspiring stories.
3. Facilitate participation in religious or spiritual activities.
4. Encourage families to minimize social isolation.
5. Provide private time for relationships.
6. Discuss end-of-life issues early in patient's treatment plan.

7. Encourage patients to express their preferences about end of life in the form of a legal document.
   a. Advance directives, such as medical orders for life-sustaining treatment or health care proxy and durable power of attorney, allow for the refusal of further treatment or authorize a family member or friend to make decisions for the patient (see page 159).
   b. After discussion with the patient and family, the primary care provider in an inpatient setting can write orders based on the directives such as "do not resuscitate."
8. Make referrals for respite care, counseling, pastoral care, and bereavement services, as needed.
9. Assist patients and families with decisions for withholding or withdrawing life-sustaining therapies and transfer in and out of inpatient settings by explaining such therapies and clarifying how they fit with the goals of care.
10. Promote ethical practice by organizing interdisciplinary rounds on patients with end-of-life care issues, setting up a partnership in care with family members, collaborating with other nurses who have been through similar situations, and consulting with the ethics committee within your facility.

NURSING ALERT It is important for health care professionals to have open and frank discussions with patients about their preferences regarding end-of-life care. This discussion should not occur during a life-threatening event when patients and families are stressed and feel rushed to make a decision.

SELECTED REFERENCES

American Cancer Society. (2017). American Cancer Society guidelines on nutrition and physical activity for cancer prevention: Reducing the risk of cancer with healthy food choices and physical activity. Available: *https://www.cancer.org/healthy/eat-healthy-get-active/acs-guidelines-nutrition-physical-activity-cancer-prevention/guidelines.html*

American Cancer Society. (2016). Global facts & figures. Available: *www.cancer.org/Research/CancerFactsFigures/GlobalCancerFactsFigures/index*

American Cancer Society. (2018). Cancer facts & figures. Available: *https://www.cancer.org/content/dam/cancer-org/research/cancer-facts-and-statistics/annual-cancer-facts-and-figures/2018/cancer-facts-and-figures-2018.pdf*

American Joint Committee on Cancer. (2017). *Cancer staging manual* (8th ed.). Philadelphia, PA: Springer International Publishing.

Cancer.Net. Available: *https://www.cancer.gov/about-cancer/treatment/clinical-trials*

Centers for Disease Control and Prevention (2018). Vaccine schedules. Available: *https://www.cdc.gov/vaccines/schedules/hcp/index.html*

Chan, A. T. (2016). Metformin for cancer prevention: A reason for optimism. *The Lancet Oncology, 17*(4), 407–409.

Denmark-Wahnefried, W., Rogers, L., Alfano, C., et al. (2015). Practical clinical interventions for diet, physical activity, and weight control in cancer survivors. *CA—Cancer Journal for Clinicians, 65*, 167–189.

Devita, V. T., Lawrence, T. S., & Rosenberg, S. A. (2014). *Cancer: Principles and practice of oncology* (10th ed.). Philadelphia, PA: Wolters Kluwer.

Gonzoles-Rodrigues, E. (2016). Immune checkpoint inhibitors: Review and management of endocrine adverse events. *The Oncologist, 21*, 1–13.

Hui, D., & Bruera, E. (2014). A personalized approach to assessing and managing pain in patients with cancer. *Journal of Clinical Oncology, 32*(16), 1640–1646.

Lawrence, H. K., Doyle, M. S., McCullough, M., et al. (2012). American Cancer Society guidelines on nutrition and physical activity for cancer prevention: Reducing the risk of cancer with healthy food choices and physical activity. *CA—Cancer Journal for Clinicians, 62*, 30–67.

National Comprehensive Cancer Network. (2016). Clinical practice guidelines in oncology: Version 2.2016 Antiemesis. Available: *www.nccn.org*

National Comprehensive Cancer Network. (2018). Clinical practice guidelines in oncology. Available: *www.nccn.org*

Neuss, M. N., Polovich, M., & McNiff, K. (2013) Updated American Society of Clinical Oncology/Oncology Nursing Society Chemotherapy Administration Safety standards including standard for the safe administration and management of oral chemotherapy. *Oncology Nursing Forum, 40*(3), 225–233.

Oncology Nursing Society. (2012). *Manual for radiation oncology nursing practice and education* (4th ed.). Pittsburgh, PA: Author.

Oncology Nursing Society. (2014). *Chemotherapy and biotherapy: Guidelines and recommendations for practice* (4th ed.). Pittsburgh, PA: Author.

Patrignani, P., & Patrrona, C. (2016). Aspirin and Cancer. *Journal of the American College of Cardiology, 68*(9), 967–976.

Pi, J., Kang, Y., Smith, M., et al. (2016). A review in the treatment of oncologic emergencies. *Journal of Oncology Pharmacy Practice, 22*(4), 625–638.

Powell, L. L., & Seibert, S. M. (2017). Cancer survivorship, models and care plans: A status update. *Nursing Clinics of North America, 52*, 193–209.

Salins, N., Ramanjulu, R., Patra, L., et al. (2016). Integration of early specialist palliative care and patient related outcomes: A critical review of evidence. *Indian Journal of Palliative Care, 22*(3), 252–257.

Smith, R., Andrews, K. et al. (2017). Cancer screening in the United States, 2017: A review of current American Cancer Society guidelines and current issues in cancer screening. *CA_Cancer journal for Clinicians, 67*, 100–121.

Stricker, C. T., & O'Brien, M. (2014). Implementing the commission on cancer standards for survivorship care plans. *Clinical Journal of Oncology Nursing, 18*(1), 15–22.

Visavanathan, K., Hurley, P., Bantug, E., et al. (2013). Use of pharmacologic interventions for breast cancer risk reduction: American society of clinical oncology clinical practice guideline. *Journal of Clinical Oncology, 31*(23), 2942–2962.

Yarbro, C. H., Wujciki, D., & Gobel, B. H. (2018). *Cancer nursing: Principles and practice* (8th ed.). Boston, MA: Jones & Bartlett.

9

Care of the Older Adult or Adult with Disabilities

OVERVIEW AND ASSESSMENT

A comprehensive geriatric evaluation (CGE) is essential to understand the holistic health needs of older adults. The CGE is performed by an interdisciplinary team, which typically includes a geriatric nurse, geriatrician, and social worker. Other members of the team may include a pharmacist, physical therapist, occupational therapist, and dietitian. The Hartford Institute for Geriatric Nursing provides many tools for assessment of older adults on their website (*www.consultgerirn.org/resources*).

Normal Changes of Aging

There are a number of normal age-related changes that occur in all major systems of the body. These may present at different times for different people. It is important to be able to differentiate between normal and abnormal changes in older adults and to educate patients and families about these differences.

Vision

Characteristics
1. Decreased visual acuity.
2. Decreased visual fields, resulting in decreased peripheral vision.
3. Decreased dark adaptation.
4. Elevated minimal threshold of light perception.
5. Presbyopia (farsightedness) because of decreased visual accommodation from loss of lens elasticity.
6. Decreased color discrimination because of the yellowing of the lens; short wavelength colors, such as blues and greens, are more difficult to see.
7. Increased sensitivity to glare.
8. Decreased depth perception.
9. Decreased tear production.
10. Be aware that patients with decreased vision can experience feelings of depression or anxiety.

Assessment Findings
1. Arcus senilis—deposits of lipid around the eye, seen as a white circle around the iris; causes no vision impairments.
2. Cataracts—clouding of the normally clear lens of the eye. (This results in lens thickening and decreased permeability; noted on examination with an ophthalmoscope; fuzziness of vision, like looking through wax paper. Cataracts cause blurring, sensitivity to light, and/or double vision.)
3. Macular degeneration—because of damage to macula that results in loss of central vision. (Objects seem blurred or distorted or are not seen.)
4. Glaucoma—increased intraocular pressure with tonometer testing. (Results in blurring, colored "halos" around lights, pain or redness of eyes, loss of peripheral vision.)
5. Smaller pupil size.
6. Complaints of decreased ability to read, discomfort from light, changes in depth perception, falls, collisions, difficulty handling small objects, difficulty with activities of daily living (ADLs), and tunnel vision.
7. Dry, red eyes.
8. Vitreous floaters, which are lightning flashes in the visual field.

Nursing Considerations and Teaching Points
1. Make sure objects are in the patient's visual field, and do not move objects around.
2. Use large lettering to label medications and any distributed written information.
3. Allow the person more time to focus and adjust to the environment.
4. Avoid glare—may help to wear sunglasses.
5. Use nightlights to help with dark adaptation problems.
6. Use red and yellow to stimulate vision.
7. Mark the edges of stairs and curbs to help with depth perception problems.
8. Use microspiral telescopes or magnifying glasses and high-intensity lighting.

9. Encourage yearly eye examination and/or refer for examination if vision changes worsen (flashing lights in fields or "veil over the eye").
10. Encourage use of isotonic eyedrops as needed for dry eyes.
11. Encourage use of low vision aids, such as magnifying lens, light filtering lens, telescopic lenses, or electronic devices.
12. If patient reports depression or anxiety, refer patient for further evaluation of symptoms.
13. Refer patients to the following resources for vision impairments:
    - Prevent Blindness America
      800-331-2020
      www.preventblindness.org
    - American Foundation for the Blind
      800-232-5463
      www.afb.org
    - American Council of the Blind
      800-242-8666
      www.acb.org
    - National Institutes of Health Low Vision & Blindness Educational Resources
      http://health.nih.gov/topic/LowVisionBlindness

Hearing

Characteristics

1. Approximately 30% to 50% of people older than age 65 have significant hearing loss.
2. Two major types of hearing disorders are common in the older population.
   a. Sensorineural—progressive, irreversible bilateral loss of high-tone perception often associated with aging. This results in difficulty with discriminating sounds. Sound waves reach the inner ear but are not properly transmitted to the brain.
   b. Conduction deafness—results from blockage or impairment of the mechanical movement in the outer or middle ear (also a pathologic condition). Sound waves are not conducted to the inner ear, resulting in sounds that are muffled.
3. Hearing loss in older adults is usually a combined problem. The majority of the loss is due to auditory nerve changes or deterioration of the structures of the ear. There may also be nerve damage beyond the ear. Presbycusis and central deafness can result in permanent hearing loss; conduction deafness is reversible.
4. Usual progression from high-tone or high-frequency loss to a general loss of both high and low tones.
5. Consonants (higher-pitched sounds) are not heard well.
6. Hearing loss increases with age and is greater in men.
7. Increase in the sound threshold (ie, greater sound needed to stimulate the older adult).
8. Decreased speech discrimination, especially with background noise.
9. Cerumen impaction, the most common cause of conductive hearing loss, is reversible.

Assessment Findings

1. Increased volume of patient's own speech.
2. Turning of head toward speaker.
3. Requests of a speaker to repeat.
4. Inappropriate answers, but otherwise cognitively intact.
5. The person may withdraw, demonstrate a short attention span, and become frustrated, angry, and depressed.
6. Lack of response to a loud noise.

Nursing Considerations and Teaching Points

1. Be aware that hearing loss can impact the safety and quality of life for older adults in many ways. For example, the older adult may not hear instructions, alerting signals, telephones, or oncoming traffic. Hearing loss can contribute to social isolation and lower self-esteem.
2. Suggest hearing testing with an audiologist for further evaluation and consideration of an assistive device.
3. Face the person directly so he can lip-read.
4. Use gestures and objects to help with verbal communication.
5. Touch the person to get his or her attention before talking.
6. Speak into the patient's "good ear."
7. *Do not shout.* Shouting increases the tone of the voice, and older adults are unable to hear these high tones. Try speaking in a deeper or lower tone of voice.
8. Speak slowly and clearly.
9. Suggest amplifiers on telephones and alarms.
10. Allow the person more time to answer your questions.
11. Evaluate the person's ear canals regularly and assist with cerumen removal. Cerumen removal is facilitated by:
    a. Use of ceruminolytic agents, such as carbamide peroxide, 10 drops in the affected ear twice per day for 5 days, followed by flushing the ear with warm water via a 50-mL irrigation syringe or an electronic irrigation device.
    b. Careful use of an ear spoon to mechanically remove cerumen.
12. Refer patients to the following organizations:
    - American Speech–Language–Hearing Association: *www.asha.org*
    - HearingLoss.com: *www.hearingloss.com*
    - National Institute on Deafness and Other Communication Disorders: *www.nidcd.nih.gov/health/hearing/pages/older.aspx*

Smell

Characteristics

1. Changes in smell (olfaction) are due to nasal sinus disease preventing odors from reaching smell receptors, a decrease in nerve fibers, chronic injury from infections, or bleeding.
2. Discrimination of fruity odors seems to persist the longest.
3. Generally, olfaction decreases in men more than in women.

Assessment Findings

1. Inability to notice unpleasant odors, such as fire, body odor, or excessive perfume.
2. Decreased appetite.

Nursing Considerations and Teaching Points

1. Age-related changes can impact safety and quality of life. For example, an older individual may not be able to recognize the smell of smoke or gas.
2. The inability to smell food may cause a decrease in the consumption of nutritious food.
   a. At mealtimes, name food items and give the person time to think of the smell/taste of the food.
   b. Suggest use of stronger spices and flavorings to stimulate sense of smell.

Taste

Characteristics

1. Taste buds decrease with age, especially in men. People over age 60 have lost half of their taste buds. By age 80, only one sixth of the taste buds remain.

2. Taste buds are lost from the front to the back (ie, sweet and salty tastes are lost first, whereas bitter and sour tastes remain longer).

Assessment Findings

1. Complaints that food has no taste.
2. Excessive use of sugar and salt.
3. Inability to identify foods.
4. Decrease in appetite and weight loss.
5. Decreased pleasure from food.

Nursing Considerations and Teaching Points

1. Age-related changes can impact safety. For example, the older individual may not be able to detect spoiled food.
2. Serve food attractively, and separate different types of foods.
3. Vary the texture of foods.
4. Encourage good oral hygiene.
5. Season food.

Kinesthetic Sense

Characteristics

1. With age, the receptors in the joints and muscles that tell us where we are in space lose their ability to function. Therefore, there is a change in balance.
2. Walking with shorter step length, less leg lift, a wider base, and a tendency to lean forward.
3. With age, less ability to stop a fall from occurring.

Assessment Findings

1. Alterations in posture, ability to transfer, and gait.
2. Complaint of dizziness.

Nursing Considerations and Teaching Points

1. Position items within reach.
2. Give person more time to move.
3. Take precautions to prevent falls.
4. Suggest physical therapy with balance training after periods of prolonged immobility.

Cardiovascular

Characteristics

1. With age, the valves of the heart become thick and rigid as a result of sclerosis and fibrosis, compounding any cardiac disease already present.
2. Blood vessels also become thick and rigid, resulting in elevated blood pressure, which is present in half of the US population over age 65.
3. Maximum heart rate and aerobic capacity decrease with age.
4. Slower response to stress. Once the pulse rate is elevated, it takes longer to return to baseline.
5. Decline in maximum oxygen consumption.
6. About 50% of older adults have an abnormal resting electrocardiogram.
7. Subtle changes in artery walls result in a less flexible vasculature.
8. Decreased baroreceptor sensitivity.

Assessment Findings

1. High blood pressure (BP) over age 60 requiring treatment is greater than or equal to 150/90 mm Hg and greater than or equal to 140/90 for adults with diabetes and kidney disease.
2. Prolonged tachycardia may occur following stress.

 EVIDENCE BASE James, P. A., Oparil, S., Carter, B. L., et al. (2014). Evidence-based guideline for the management of high blood pressure in adults. Report from the panel members appointed to the Eighth Joint National Committee (JNC 8). *JAMA, 311*(5), 507–520.

Nursing Considerations and Teaching Points

1. Encourage regular BP evaluation as well as lifestyle modifications and medication adherence, if indicated, for hypertension.
2. Check for postural BP changes to detect orthostatic hypotension and prevent falls. Instruct patients to rise slowly from lying to sitting to standing.
3. Encourage longer cooldown period after exercise to return to baseline cardiac function.
4. Encourage moderate physical activity: walking, biking, or swimming for 30 minutes five times per week (150 minutes per week), in addition to muscle strengthening exercises two times a week.

Pulmonary

Characteristics

1. With age, there is a weakening of the intercostal respiratory muscles, and the elastic recoil of the chest wall diminishes.
2. There is no change in total lung capacity; however, residual volume and functional residual capacity increase.
3. Partial pressure of oxygen decreases with age because of ventilation–perfusion mismatches. However, older adults are not hypoxic without coexistent disease.
4. There is a decrease in the mucus transport/ciliary system. Therefore, there is decreased clearance of mucus and foreign bodies, including bacteria.

Assessment Findings

1. Prolonged cough, inability to raise secretions.
2. Increased frequency of respiratory infections.

Nursing Considerations and Teaching Points

1. Older adults who are undergoing surgical treatment should engage in deep breathing exercises.
2. Teach measures to prevent pulmonary infections—avoid crowds during cold and flu season, wash hands frequently, and report early signs of infection.
3. Avoid smoking and exposure to secondhand smoke.
4. Encourage annual flu vaccine and pneumonia vaccine at age 65 or as needed.

Immunologic

Characteristics

1. The function of T-cell lymphocytes, such as cell-mediated immunity, declines with age because of involution and atrophy of the thymus gland.
2. Decreased T-cell helper activity; increased T-cell suppressor activity.
3. Declining B-cell function as a result of T-cell changes.

Assessment Findings

1. More frequent infections.
2. Increased incidence of many types of cancer.

Nursing Considerations and Teaching Points

1. Teach older adults that they are at increased risk of infection, cancer, and autoimmune disease; therefore, routine follow-up and screening are essential.
2. Encourage healthy lifestyle practices to maintain optimal health.

Neurologic

Characteristics

1. There is gradual loss in the number of neurons with age, but no major change in neurotransmitter levels.
2. Some brain tissue atrophy is normal and does not relate to cognitive impairment.
3. Decrease in muscle tone, motor speed, and nerve conduction velocity.
4. Decrease in gait speed of 1.6% per year after age 63; decreased step length, stride length, and arm swing.

Assessment Findings

1. Decreased position and vibration sense.
2. Diminished reflexes, possible absent ankle jerks.
3. Complaint of falls and impaired balance.
4. Wide-based gait with decreased arm swing.

Nursing Considerations and Teaching Points

1. Because gait, strength, and sensory changes, it is essential to teach older adults fall-prevention techniques.
2. Teach environmental safety techniques, including nonslip surfaces, securely fastened handrails, sufficient light, glare-free lights, avoidance of low-lying objects, chairs of the proper height with armrests, skidproof strips or mats in the tub or shower, toilet and tub grab bars, elevated toilet seats.
3. Refer for home safety evaluations, which may be available through state and local health departments. A home safety checklist can be obtained from the National Safety Council at *www.nsc.org*.

 TRANSITIONAL CARE ALERT Using Electronic Health Care Records can help reduce hospital readmissions and improve outcomes for older adults. When nurses worked with IT departments to design input data such as evidence-based assessment tools and decision support tools, several nurse sensitive quality measures improved. An expert decision support system developed by nurses was embedded within the nursing admission assessment identified older adults who needed postacute care, which reduced hospital readmission rates.

 EVIDENCE BASE Bowles, K. H., Hanlon, A., Holland, D., Potashnik, S. L., & Topaz, M. (2014). Impact of discharge planning decision support on time to readmission among older adult medical patients. *Professional Case Management, 19*(1), 29–38.

Musculoskeletal

Characteristics

1. Declining muscle mass and endurance with age, although deconditioning may be an associated factor.
2. Decreased bone density, less so in men than in women.
3. Decreased thickness and resiliency of cartilage, with a resulting increase in the stiffness of joints.
4. Bone resorption exceeds bone formation, resulting in a decline in bone density.
5. Injuries to the cartilage accumulate with age.

Assessment Findings

1. Muscle atrophy.
2. Increased incidence of fractures.
3. Complaint of joint stiffness in absence of arthritis.
4. Decreased bone density (less than 2.5 standard deviations below normal).

Nursing Considerations and Teaching Points

1. Early intervention to encourage regular exercise (including weight-bearing exercise and resistance training) in older adults is important to prevent exacerbation of these normal changes.
2. Encourage increased intake of calcium and vitamin D and decreased alcohol and nicotine use.

Community and Home Care Considerations

1. Encourage older adults to engage in 30 minutes of moderate physical activity, including walking, biking, or swimming, at least five times per week, in addition to muscle strengthening exercises at least two times a week.
2. For older adults who will be exercising at less than 80% of the maximum heart rate (220 − age), stress testing before starting an exercise program is not needed.
3. To help with adherence to the exercise program, older adults should be encouraged to exercise at a set time, to relieve pain before exercising, and to do an activity they enjoy. Provide positive reinforcement for those who do exercise, and continually reinforce the benefits of exercise (increased bone strength, cardiovascular fitness, decreased risks of falls, overall sense of well-being).

Endocrine

Characteristics

1. Decreased secretion of trophic hormones from the pituitary gland.
2. Blunted growth hormone release during stress.
3. Elevated vasopressin (antidiuretic hormone); exaggerated response to osmotic challenge.
4. Elevated levels of follicle-stimulating hormone and luteinizing hormone because of reduced end-organ response.
5. Decreased insulin secretion after meals; this may be a function of weight or genetic factors.

Assessment Findings

Usually asymptomatic.

Nursing Considerations and Teaching Points

1. Encourage routine screening for elevated blood glucose—both fasting and postprandial.
2. Provide education about a well-balanced diet.

Reproductive

Characteristics

1. In women, menopause leads to decreases in the size of the ovaries and hormone production. This results in uterine involution, vaginal atrophy, and loss of breast mass.
2. With age, there is increased risk in females of cystocele, rectocele, and uterine prolapse.
3. In men, testosterone production and secretion decrease with age. However, serum levels may be in the low-normal range through age 80.

Assessment Findings

1. Vaginal dryness, painful intercourse.
2. Atrophic vaginitis.
3. Urinary incontinence.

Nursing Considerations and Teaching Points

1. Suggest the use of additional lubrication during sexual intercourse.

2. Advise sexually active older men that spermatogenesis may continue into advanced age.
3. Address risks and benefits of time-limited hormone replacement therapy for symptomatic relief related to menopause.
4. Refer patient for further evaluation for urinary incontinence

Renal and Body Composition

Characteristics
1. Increased body fat and decreased lean muscle mass, even when weight remains stable.
2. Decreased renal function, measured by the glomerular filtration rate, or creatinine clearance.
3. Despite reduced total body creatinine because of decreased muscle mass in the older adult, serum creatinine often remains within normal range. This is because of decreased elimination of creatinine by the kidneys.
4. About 10% decline in creatinine clearance per decade after age 40; however, relatively unchanged serum creatinine.

Assessment Findings
1. Usually asymptomatic.
2. Increased incidence of anemia.

Nursing Considerations and Teaching Points
1. Be aware that although serum creatinine may be within normal range, creatinine clearance may be decreased. To obtain an accurate creatinine clearance in an older adult, the following formula may be used: (140 – age) (weight [kg])/(72) (serum creatinine [mg/dL]).
2. Drugs that are cleared through the kidneys may be given in decreased dosage. Adverse effects and toxicity must be closely monitored.
3. Consider the advantages and disadvantages of drug management for anemia associated with renal disease.

Skin

Characteristics
1. Thinning of all three layers of the skin—epidermis, dermis, and subcutaneous tissue—leads to greater fragility of the skin and decreased ability of the skin to function as a barrier to external factors.
2. Fewer melanocytes and decreased tanning.
3. Less efficient thermoregulation of heat because of fewer sweat glands.
4. Drier skin because the decreased number of sebaceous glands results in reduced oil production.
5. Other changes in aging skin include reduced sensory input, decreased elasticity, and impaired cell-related immune response.

Assessment Finding
1. Dry, irritated skin.

Nursing Considerations and Teaching Points
1. Excessive use of soap, which can be drying to the skin, should be avoided.
2. Careful skin evaluation and lubrication are necessary to prevent fissures and breakdown.
3. Heat regulation needs to be controlled by proper clothing and avoidance of extreme temperatures.
4. Avoid direct application of extreme hot or cold to skin because damage may occur without feeling it.
5. Encourage use of sunscreen during all outdoor activities.

Community and Home Care Considerations
Xerosis (dry skin) is a common problem for older adults. Treatment should include:
1. Drinking 2,000 mL of liquid daily.
2. Total body immersion in warm water (90°F to 105°F [32.2°C to 40.6°C]) for 10 minutes.
3. Use of nonperfumed soap without hexachlorophene.
4. Application of emollient, particularly those with alpha-hydroxy acids, after bathing and at bedtime.

Hematopoietic

Characteristics
1. Unchanged number of stem cells of all three cell lines; however, bone marrow cellularity is decreased by 33% during adult life.
2. Declining marrow activity, especially in response to stress, such as with blood loss or infection.

Assessment Finding
Asymptomatic.

Nursing Considerations and Teaching Points
1. Anemia and granulocytopenia are not normal consequences of aging and should be investigated.
2. Teach patients that there is no need to take oral iron unless there is an actual documented decrease in iron levels.
3. Encourage oral B_{12} and folate replacement to manage associated anemias.

Altered Presentation of Disease

Characteristics
1. In part because of the physiologic changes that occur with aging, the manifestations of illness in the older patient are less dramatic than in younger patients.
2. Most older adults have at least one chronic condition. These coexisting conditions can complicate the evaluation of new symptoms.
3. Some risk factors make it more likely that they will present with an altered presentation of disease: over age 85, multiple comorbid conditions, taking over five medications, and having cognitive or functional impairment.

 EVIDENCE BASE Smith, C. M., Cotter, V. T. (2016). Age-related changes in health. In M. Boltz, E. Capezuti, T. Fulmer, & D. Zwicker (Eds.), *Evidence-based geriatric nursing protocols for best practice* (5th ed., pp. 23–41). New York, NY: Springer Publishing Company.

Assessment Findings
1. The classic indicators of disease are usually absent or disorders present atypically (see Table 9-1).
2. Older people are less likely to report new symptoms but, rather, attribute them to aging or existing conditions. Many older adults minimize symptoms because of fears of hospitalization or health care costs.

Nursing Considerations and Teaching Points
1. Have a high index of suspicion for underlying illness if the older adult presents with an acute change in cognition, behavior, or function.

Table 9-1 Atypical Presentation of Disorders in the Older Adult

DISORDER	ATYPICAL PRESENTATION
Acute intestinal infection	• Abdominal pain may be absent. • May present with acute confusional state, leukocytosis, and acidosis
Appendicitis	• Pain may be diffuse, not localized in the right lower quadrant.
Biliary disease	• Confusion, declining function, and other nonspecific symptom • Abnormal liver function tests may be only sign.
Heart failure	• Initially, may have change in mental status and fatigue
Hyperthyroidism	• Apathy, palpitations, weight loss, weakness
Hypothyroidism	• Presents with weight loss
Myocardial infarction	• Chest pain may be absent. • May present with syncope, dyspnea, vomiting, or confusion
Perforated ulcer	• Rigidity may be absent until late.
Pneumonia	• May present with confusion • Fever and cough may be absent
Pulmonary embolism	• May present with change in mental status • May not have fever, leukocytosis, or tachycardia
Septicemia	• May be afebrile
Systemic lupus erythematosus	• Pneumonitis, subcutaneous nodules, and discoid lesions are more common. • Malar rash, Raynaud phenomenon, and nephritis are less common.
Urinary tract infection	• Confusion

Functional Assessment

Functional assessment is the measurement of a patient's ability to complete functional tasks and fulfill social roles, specifically addressing a patient's ability to complete tasks ranging from simple self-care to higher-level activities. It provides the nurse with objective data to help determine the older adult's needs and plan interventions. Across the United States, there is an imperative to reduce hospital readmissions. Many programs have been successful. A common feature in most of the programs is the need to complete a functional assessment

Purpose

1. Functional assessment is essential in the care of the older adult because it:
   a. Offers a systematic approach to assessing older adults for deficits that commonly go undetected.
   b. Helps the nurse to identify problems and utilize appropriate resources.
   c. Provides a way to assess progress and decline over time.
   d. Helps the nurse evaluate the safety of the patient's ability to live alone.
2. Functional status includes the evaluation of sensory changes, ability to complete ADLs and instrumental ADLs, gait and balance problems, and elimination.

Instruments to Measure Functional Ability

1. Functional status may be assessed by several methods: self-report, direct observation, or family report. Direct observation is the method of choice, when possible.
2. The instrument chosen should be based on the specific goal or purpose for the evaluation. For example, if the focus is on basic self-care and mobility, the Barthel index should be used. See page 161 for reference (Mahoney & Barthel).
3. The Katz Index for Activities of Daily Living and Instrumental Activities of Daily Living is another rating scale for measuring

functional ability. Use this scale to determine level of independence of the older adult and repeat periodically to compare level of functioning over time. See page 161 for reference (Katz, et al.).
4. Performance measures, such as the Tinetti Gait and Balance measure or the Chair Rise test, can be used to evaluate higher-level functioning. Consult with a physical therapist.

Psychosocial Assessment

Altered Mental Status

1. Assessment of mental status to detect altered cognition involves examination of memory, perception, communication, orientation, calculation, comprehension, problem solving, thought processes, language, executive function, visual–spatial abilities, abstraction, attention, aphasia, and apraxia.
2. Assessment can be facilitated by use of cognitive screening tools. A commonly utilized instrument is the Mini-Mental State Examination (MMSE), a 30-point cognitive screening instrument that assesses orientation to time and place, registration and recall, calculation, language skills, and visual–spatial abilities.
3. The total possible score is 30. A score of 24 to 30 suggests intact cognitive function; 20 to 23, mild cognitive impairment; 16 to 19, moderate cognitive impairment; and 15 or less, severe cognitive impairment. The MMSE can help to follow the patient's cognition over time and assess for acute and/or chronic changes.
4. Although success on scales such as this has been associated with language abilities, education, and socioeconomic status, this scale continues to be used as an appropriate screening tool for abnormal cognitive function.
5. Another cognitive screening instrument is the Mini-Cog examination, which is composed of a three-item recall and the clock drawing test (CDT). The Mini-Cog can be administered under 3 minutes, does not appear to be affected by the patient's education or language abilities, and has been

successfully used to screen for dementia across a variety of clinical settings. The Mini-Cog can be administered as follows:

   a. Tell the patient to listen carefully and remember and repeat three unrelated words.
   b. Tell the patient to draw the face of a clock including numbers and hands to read a specific time. The CDT is considered normal if all numbers are present in the correct sequence and position and the hands display the requested time.
   c. Ask the patient to repeat the three previously stated words.
   d. Unsuccessful recall of all three items suggests dementia. Successful recall of all three items suggests intact cognition. An abnormal CDT with one to two errors on recall suggests dementia. A normal CDT with one error on recall suggests no dementia.

6. Assessment of altered mental status or behavior may elicit criteria that lead to a diagnosis of dementia. It is essential to differentiate dementia from delirium (which is treatable and reversible).

7. *Delirium* is a change in mental status that is abrupt in onset and is commonly because of an underlying medical condition, such as infection, electrolyte imbalance, medication intolerance or toxicity, cardiac decompensation, or hypoxia.

   a. Occurs early, and the behavior is variable hour to hour. May be superimposed upon dementia making identification difficult.
   b. Clouded, altered, or fluctuating level of consciousness (lethargic to hypervigilant), short attention span, and disturbed sleep–wake cycle. Hallucinations (sensory experiences without a stimulus) are common.
   c. Reversible with treatment of the underlying cause; however, individuals with an unrecognized and prolonged episode of delirium may not return to their previous cognitive baseline.
   d. Underrecognized and is associated with morbidity and mortality among older adults.

8. *Dementia* has a gradual onset. Behavior is usually consistent, and disorientation occurs late. Consciousness is not clouded, attention span is generally not reduced, and day–night reversal of sleep–wake cycles can occur rather than hour-to-hour variation. Delusions (fixed false beliefs) are more common than hallucinations.

Social Activities and Support

1. Social support for older adults is generally instrumental, informational, or emotional. The social environment is important with regard to recovery of acute medical problems and management of chronic illness.

2. Elicit information by asking such questions as:
   a. How often do you socialize with others?
   b. With whom do you socialize?
   c. What type of activities do you enjoy?
   d. Do you enjoy socializing?
   e. Who can you call for help?
   f. Do you know of any church or community groups you can call for help?

Emotional and Affective Status

Characteristics

1. Depression may occur for the first time in older age and has been related to the many changes that occur with aging:
   a. The independence of one's children.
   b. Adjusting to new routines associated with retirement.
   c. The loss of roles, income, spouse, friends, family, home, pets, functional ability, health, and ability to participate in leisure activities such as reading.
   d. Ageist messages from society supporting and encouraging the value of youth.

2. Depression may also be associated with underlying illnesses, such as Alzheimer disease, Parkinson disease, and stroke, and by medications, such as antihypertensives (beta-blockers), antiarthritics, and antianxiety agents.

3. Depression is usually difficult to identify in the older adult because the presentation is different than in younger people. Obtain the following information to assess for depression:
   a. Complaints of insomnia, weight loss, anorexia, and constipation (vegetative symptoms).
   b. Presence of anhedonia (lack of joy in usually pleasurable activities).
   c. Decrease in concentration, memory, and decision-making (pseudodementia syndrome).
   d. Other somatic complaints, such as decreased appetite, musculoskeletal aches and pains, chest pain, and fatigue.
   e. History of chronic illness or other health problems.
   f. Current medications.

4. Evaluate depression using the Geriatric Depression Scale as a screening tool for older adults without or with mild cognitive impairment. The Cornell Scale for Depression in Dementia can be used as a screening tool for older adults with dementia.

5. Suicide is sometimes associated with depression, with suicides being especially high in older white men. Assess for suicide risk.

6. Pain is underdetected and may be undertreated in older adults and can contribute to depressive symptoms. Assess pain by asking and observing the patient, and provide appropriate measures to make patient more comfortable.

Nursing and Patient Care Considerations

1. Treatment of depression should be given to older adults and includes medications, psychotherapy, and, in some cases, electroconvulsive therapy.

2. Complement other therapeutic measures by providing opportunities to increase the patient's self-esteem.
   a. Encourage participation in meaningful activities.
   b. Promote the patient's positive self-image.
   c. Help the patient develop a sense of mastery.
   d. Encourage reminiscence of meaningful past events.

3. Help patient identify and use social supports.

4. For behavioral problems (agitation, combative behavior, or irritability) consider options such as aromatherapy, music therapy, pet therapy, relaxation techniques, massage, or physical activity.

Motivation in Older Adults

Characteristics

1. Motivation is an important variable in the older adult's ability to recover from any disabling event and the ability to maintain his or her highest level of wellness.

2. Understanding individual motivational factors for engaging in health promotion activities like exercise is an approach that can improve adherence. It is possible to evaluate a patient's motivation to comply with a given treatment plan and adopt interventions to help to improve the older adult's motivation.

3. Factors that influence motivation in an older adult include:
   a. Needs such as hunger.
   b. Past experiences, specifically with health care providers.
   c. Negative attitudes toward aging.
   d. Self-efficacy expectations or the belief in one's ability to perform a specific activity.
   e. Outcome expectations or the belief that if a specific activity is performed there will be an expected outcome.
   f. The cost of performing a specific activity in terms of time, money, pain, fatigue, or fear.
   g. Internal factors, such as sensory changes, cognitive status, resilience and adverse drug effects.
   h. External factors, such as social norms (particularly if those norms conflict with treatment) and the influence of social supports.
4. Problems in motivation because of age-related differences include:
   a. A shift from achievement motivation to conservative motivation.
   b. Establishment of meaningful rewards for older people, because of losses.
   c. Greater significance placed on the meaning of a task; it must be meaningful to the older person.
   d. Evidence that older adults do not do well on tasks if they are asked to do them rapidly, under a time limit, or in a stressful situation.
   e. Increased importance placed on the cost of participating in an activity; fear of failing can be expressed either as increased anxiety or decreased willingness to take risks.
5. The Motivation Wheel (see Figure 9-1) can be used to evaluate motivation in the older adult.
   a. Motivation is influenced by beliefs about physical and emotional benefits, mastery experiences, individualized care, social support, the environment, goals, physical sensations, and new activities.
   b. Motivation can be increased by strengthening beliefs about potential benefits, providing opportunities for mastery, identifying individualized care approaches and goals, using social supports, accessing supportive environments, decreasing unpleasant sensations, and trying new activities.

Figure 9-1. The wheel that moves.

Nursing and Patient Care Considerations

1. Strategies to improve motivation include:
   a. Establish whose motives are being discussed. Involve the patient, family, and health care providers in setting patient-centered goals.
   b. Explore with patient any indication of fear or other unpleasant sensation associated with the activity, such as pain or fatigue, and implement interventions to decrease these unpleasant sensations.
   c. Evaluate the spokes of the wheel to consider the many factors that influence motivation and implement interventions as appropriate.
   d. Encourage patient to verbally express emotional factors associated with the activity.
   e. Examine the setting for the desired behavior to occur. Is the environment too stressful, too dark, or too noisy?
   f. Attempt to use role models. Older adult role models can change ageist attitudes and stimulate patients to perform the desired behavior.
   g. Set small goals to be met either daily or each shift. This provides frequent rewards.
   h. Do not be afraid to use yourself. Research has indicated that being nice, demonstrating caring, using humor, verbal encouragement, and support, can all help motivate the older adult.
2. Educate the older adult about the benefits of the activity, whether these are physical or psychological.

 EVIDENCE BASE Smaerup, M., Gronvall, E., Larsen, S. B., et al. (2017). Exercise gaming: a motivational approach for older adults with vestibular dysfunction. *Disability and Rehabilitation: Assistive Technology, 12*(2), 137–144.

HEALTH MAINTENANCE

 EVIDENCE BASE United States Preventive Services Task Force. (2017). The guide to clinical preventive services: Recommendations of the U.S Preventive Services Task Force. Available: *https://www.uspreventiveservicestaskforce.org/Page/Name/recommendations*.

Primary Prevention

The goal of health promotion and disease prevention is to add more quality years to life. There are three levels of health promotion and disease prevention.

Primary prevention is the prevention of disease before it occurs. Primary prevention can be broken down into counseling, immunizations, and chemoprophylaxis.

Counseling

1. Encourage smoking cessation.
   a. Approximately 8% of people in the United States age 65 and older are smokers.
   b. Tobacco use has been linked to heart disease; peripheral vascular disease; cerebrovascular disease; chronic obstructive pulmonary disease; cancer such as lung, bladder, and esophageal malignancies; and numerous other health problems that decrease quality of life or cause premature death.
   c. Although much damage has been done to the lungs and blood vessels by many years of smoking, older adults can still benefit from smoking cessation by increasing quality of life.

d. The US Preventive Service Task Force recommends the "5-A" behavioral counseling framework as a useful strategy for engaging patients in smoking cessation discussions: (1) Ask about tobacco use; (2) Advise to quit through clear personalized messages; (3) Assess willingness to quit; (4) Assist to quit; and (5) Arrange follow-up and support.

2. Encourage physical activity.
   a. It has been stated that 75% of older Americans are inactive.
   b. It has been recommended that older adults participate in regular physical activity for 30 minutes, 5 days a week, especially aerobic activities that promote cardiovascular fitness, such as walking, cycling, or swimming.
   c. Refer to a physical, occupational, or rehabilitation therapist. An individualized exercise prescription should be developed and cleared with the health care provider.

3. Identify alcohol abuse in older adults.
   a. The consequences of alcoholism include liver disease, gastrointestinal (GI) bleeding, and motor vehicle accidents.
   b. Question older adults about drug or alcohol abuse. Although current street drug use is less common, prescription drug abuse may be occurring or alcohol may be used for pain.
   c. Recognize the signs and symptoms of alcohol abuse in older adults (see Box 9-1).
   d. Refer for counseling.

4. Evaluate and counsel on dental health.
   a. Dental problems in older adults include missing teeth, ill-fitting dentures, periodontal disease, and tooth decay.
   b. Dental problems commonly lead to poor eating habits, apathy, and fatigue.
   c. Regular dental care should be encouraged to improve nutrition and the quality of life.

Immunizations

 EVIDENCE BASE Centers for Disease Control and Prevention. (2016). *Advisory Committee for Immunization Practices (ACIP) recommendations.* Atlanta, GA: CDC. Available: *www.cdc.gov/vaccines/pubs/ACIP-list.htm#pcv.*

1. Pneumococcal pneumonia is a significant cause of mortality and morbidity in older adults.
   a. There are two vaccines that prevent pneumococcal disease: pneumococcal conjugate vaccine (PCV13) and pneumococcal polysaccharide vaccine (PPSV23). The CDC recommends that two pneumococcal vaccines be given to all people age 65 or over. A dose of PCV13 should be given first, followed by a dose of PPSV23 at least 1 year later. Individuals who have been previously vaccinated with PPSV23 should receive a dose of PCV13 at least 1 year following their most recent dose of PPSV23.

| BOX 9-1 | Signs of Alcohol Abuse in Older Adults |

- Difficulty with gait and balance.
- Acute change in cognition.
- Frequent falls or accidents.
- Change in drinking patterns.
- Poor nutritional intake.
- Poor hygiene and self-care.
- Lack of physical exercise.

---

b. The above vaccination schedule is also recommended for individuals aged 19 to 64 who smoke or who have functional or structural asplenia or immunocompromising conditions.

2. Influenza may cause significant complications in older adults. Annual influenza vaccination is recommended for all people over age 6 months without contraindications (eg, egg allergy).
   a. The intranasal live-attenuated influenza vaccine has not been approved for individuals 50 years of age or older.
   b. Several antiviral agents are effective against influenza. These agents can be effective in ameliorating symptoms if given within 48 hours of onset of illness.

3. Tetanus–diphtheria (Td) immunization is an important but frequently forgotten component of health maintenance, especially in older adults.
   a. The mortality rate of tetanus exceeds 50% in those over age 65.
   b. Combined tetanus–diphtheria boosters should be given every 10 years; no age for discontinuation has been stated.
   c. Because of an increase in pertussis cases, a single dose of acellular pertussis is also recommended as a component (Tdap) for adults aged 65 years and older who anticipate having close contact with an infant less than 12 months of age and who previously have not received Tdap. Tdap can be administered regardless of interval since the last tetanus booster.
   d. For those with no history of immunization or unknown immunization status, a primary series should be initiated, consisting of two doses of tetanus–diphtheria vaccine at least 4 weeks apart, followed by a third dose 6 to 12 months later.

4. A single dose of the herpes zoster vaccine is recommended for older adults to prevent the dermatologic reoccurrence of varicella and the possible painful sequela known as postherpetic neuralgia.
   a. Age is the most important factor in the development of herpes zoster, with a large increase beginning between age 50 and 60, and about 50% of people experience herpes zoster by age 85.

Chemoprophylaxis

1. The risk and benefits of oral anticoagulation therapy should be considered for older adults at risk of cardiovascular disease, particularly stroke. The United States Preventive Services Task Force (USPSTF) strongly recommends that clinicians discuss aspirin therapy with patients at risk for coronary heart disease.
   a. Contraindicated if patient is at risk for GI bleeding.
   b. Should be discussed with older adults with regard to prevention of deep vein thrombosis, nonvalvular atrial fibrillation, cardiomyopathy, valvular heart disease, mechanical prosthetic heart valves, and acute myocardial infarction.

2. Calcium, vitamin D, and other agents, such as selective estrogen receptor modulators or bisphosphonates, may be considered for those at risk for osteoporosis.

Secondary Prevention

Secondary prevention is the detection of disease in an early stage for best treatment outcomes, such as cancers, cardiovascular disease, osteoporosis, and tuberculosis.

Screening Recommendations

 EVIDENCE BASE United States Preventive Services Task Force. (2016). *The guide to clinical preventive services: Recommendations of the U.S Preventive Services Task Force.* Available: *www.uspreventiveservices-taskforce.org/index.html.*

Age alone is not a criterion as to when to stop screening. Rather, the patient and health care provider should discuss values, expectations, functional status, and quality of life. A guide to shared decision-making for cancer screening is available at the USPSTF website at *www.uspreventiveservicestaskforce.org/3rduspstf/shared/sharedba.htm.*

The USPSTF has made the following recommendations for cancer screenings for older adults:

1. The precise age at which to discontinue screening mammography is uncertain. No clinical trials have been conducted on women over age 74. Furthermore, although older women face a higher probability of developing breast cancer, they also have a greater chance of dying from other causes.
2. Regarding cervical cancer, it is appropriate for older women to discontinue cervical cancer screening after age 65 only if they have had adequate recent screening with normal results and are not at high risk for cervical cancer.
3. The age to discontinue colorectal cancer screening has not been determined; however, the USPSTF recommends against routine colorectal cancer screening in adults ages 75 to 85, unless there are conditions that support screening for these individuals.
4. The USPSTF states that there is insufficient evidence to recommend for or against screening for prostate cancer. Older men and men with other significant medical conditions who have a life expectancy of fewer than 10 years are unlikely to benefit from the prostate-specific antigen test and digital rectal examination.

Tertiary Prevention

Tertiary prevention addresses the treatment of established disease to avoid complications and death. The major areas of focus for the older adult are preventing the complications of immobility and rehabilitation

Preventing Complications of Immobility

Positioning

1. The goal of frequent position changes is to prevent contractures, stimulate circulation and prevent pressure sores, prevent thrombophlebitis and pulmonary embolism, promote lung expansion and prevent pneumonia, and decrease edema of the extremities. Changing position from lying to sitting several times per day can help prevent changes in the cardiovascular system, which is known as *deconditioning.*
2. The recommendation is to change body position at least every 2 hours and, preferably, more frequently in patients who have no spontaneous movement.

 EVIDENCE BASE Lozano-Montoya, I., Velez-Diaz-Pallares, M., Abraha, I., et al. (2016). Nonpharmacologic interventions to prevent pressure ulcers in older patients: An overview of systematic reviews (Software ENgine for the Assessment and optimization of drug and non-drug Therapy in Older peRsons [SENATOR] definition of Optimal evidence-based Non-drug Therapies in Older People [ONTOP] Series). *Journal of the American Medical Directors Association*, 17(4), 370.e1–370.e10.

Proper Body Alignment

1. Dorsal or supine position
   a. The head is in line with the spine, both laterally and anteroposteriorly.
   b. The trunk is positioned, so flexion of the hips is minimized to prevent hip contracture.
   c. The arms are flexed at the elbow with the hands resting against the lateral abdomen.
   d. The legs are extended in a neutral position with the toes pointed toward the ceiling.
   e. The heels are suspended in a space between the mattress and the footboard to prevent heel pressure.
   f. Trochanter rolls are placed under the greater trochanters in the hip joint areas.
2. Sidelying or lateral position
   a. The head is in line with the spine.
   b. The body is in alignment and is not twisted.
   c. The uppermost hip joint is slightly forward and supported by a pillow in a position of slight abduction.
   d. A pillow supports the arm, which is flexed at both the elbow and shoulder joints.
3. Prone position
   a. The head is turned laterally and is in alignment with the rest of the body.
   b. The arms are abducted and externally rotated at the shoulder joint; the elbows are flexed.
   c. A small, flat support is placed under the pelvis, extending from the level of the umbilicus to the upper third of the thigh.
   d. The lower extremities remain in a neutral position.
   e. The toes are suspended over the edge of the mattress.

Therapeutic Exercise

1. It has been reported that there is a daily loss of 1% to 1.5% of initial strength in an immobilized older adult.
2. The goals of therapeutic exercise are to develop and retrain deficient muscles, to restore as much normal movement as possible to prevent deformity, to stimulate the functions of various organs and body systems, to build strength and endurance, and to promote relaxation.
3. Perform passive range-of-motion (ROM) exercise.
   a. Carried out without assistance from the patient.
   b. The purpose is to retain as much joint ROM as possible and to maintain circulation.
   c. Move the joint smoothly through its full ROM (see Box 9-2, pages 141 to 144). Do not push beyond the point of pain.
4. Perform active assistive ROM.
   a. Carried out by the patient with the encouragement and/or assistance of the nurse.
   b. The purpose is to encourage normal muscle function.
   c. Support the distal part and encourage the patient to take the joint actively through its ROM.
   d. Give only the amount of assistance necessary to accomplish the action.
5. Encourage active ROM.
   a. Accomplished by the patient without assistance.
   b. The purpose is to increase muscle strength.
   c. When possible, active exercise should be done against gravity.
   d. Encourage the patient to move the joint through the full ROM without assistance.
   e. Make sure that the patient does not substitute another joint movement for the one intended.
   f. Other active forms of exercise include turning from side to side, turning from back to abdomen, and moving up and down in bed.

BOX 9-2 Range of Motion

SHOULDER

ELBOW

(continued)

BOX 9-2   Range of Motion (*Continued*)

WRIST

THUMB

FINGERS

BOX 9-2   Range of Motion (*Continued*)

ANKLE

TOES

HIP

(continued)

BOX 9-2	Range of Motion (*Continued*)

KNEE

CERVICAL SPINE

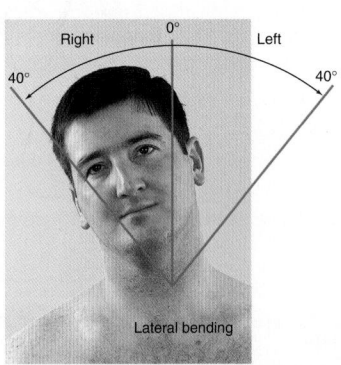

Weber, J., & Kelley, J. (2006). Health Assessment in Nursing (3rd ed.). Philadelphia, PA: Lippincott Williams & Wilkins. Photographs by Barbara Proud.

6. Assist with resistive exercise.
   a. Carried out by the patient working against resistance produced by either manual or mechanical means.
   b. The purpose is to increase muscle strength.
   c. Encourage the patient to move the joint through its ROM while you or someone else provides slight resistance at first and then progressively increases resistance.
   d. Weights may be used and are attached at the distal point of the involved joint.
   e. The movements should be done smoothly.
7. Teach isometric or muscle-setting exercise.
   a. Involve alternately contracting and relaxing a muscle while keeping the part in a fixed position; performed by the patient.
   b. The purpose is to maintain strength when a joint is immobilized.
   c. Teach the patient to contract or tighten the muscle as much as possible without moving the joint.
   d. The patient holds the position for several seconds and then relaxes.

Geriatric Rehabilitation and Restorative Care

Characteristics
1. The primary goal is restoring the older adult to maximum functional level.
2. Multidisciplinary service involving input from the primary care provider; nursing personnel; physical, occupational, speech, and recreational therapists; social worker; psychologist; and dietitian.
3. Rehabilitation and restorative nursing involves developing a rehabilitation philosophy of care.
   a. Patients are encouraged, and allowed sufficient time, to perform as much of their personal care as possible.
   b. Goals are set *with* the patient rather than *for* the patient.
   c. Prevention of further impairment is imperative.

d. Focus on skin and wound care, regaining or maintaining bowel and bladder function, independent medication use, good nutritional status, psychosocial support, an appropriate activity–rest balance, and patient and family education.

 EVIDENCE BASE Resnick, B., Galik, E., Wells, C., et al. (2015). Optimizing physical activity among older adults post trauma: Overcoming system and patient challenges. *International Journal of Orthopedic and Trauma Nursing, 19*(4), 194–206.

Nursing and Patient Care Considerations

1. Impaired cognitive function may have an impact on the quality of rehabilitation.
   a. Assess for physical problems that may exacerbate cognitive dysfunction (eg, infection, adverse drug effects, metabolic or circulatory problems, or fatigue).
   b. Provide innovative measures to encourage ambulation, active ROM, and increased function; provide frequent verbal cues and large-print reminders; focus on basic self-care abilities and activities that are consistent with the individual's past life experiences.
   c. Implement appropriate safety measures, such as bed side rails, proper lighting, appropriate staffing, and avoidance of chemical and physical restraints.
2. Disability has a tremendous impact on patient's body image and requires an adjustment by patient. Be aware of the stages of psychological reaction the patient may undergo.
   a. Period of confusion, disorganization, and denial.
   b. Period of depression or anxiety and grief.
   c. Period of adaptation and adjustment.
3. Interventions in rehabilitation nursing include:
   a. Provide an atmosphere of acceptance.
   b. Identify and encourage positive coping patterns.
   c. Encourage socialization and participation in group activities.
   d. Give positive reinforcement and feedback about progress.
   e. Involve families as much as possible.
4. Use suggested interventions to motivate older adult to engage in functional activities and exercise.

Community and Home Care Considerations

1. Family or significant other caring for the older adult at home can have a major impact on the rehabilitation process.
   a. Assist family or significant other to face the reality of the patient's disability and to set appropriate and achievable goals.
   b. Involve family or significant other in the decision-making and in the patient's care for them to develop and practice the skills necessary for the patient to reach rehabilitation goals.
   c. Help extend and enlarge family's or significant other's skills by teaching problem solving, treatment needs of the patient, ways to communicate to health care providers, and the use of community resources.
   d. Assess the level of caregiver fatigue or burnout (see Box 9-3).
2. For the older adult living independently:
   a. Encourage adherence to a regular exercise program, which includes aerobic exercise, stretching, and strength training to maintain optimal function.
   b. The Centers for Disease Control and Prevention recommends that all adults should accumulate at least 150 minutes of moderate-intensity physical activity (walking, biking, swimming, etc.) per week and strength training (heavy gardening, yoga, lifting weights, resistance exercises) at least 2 days a week.

BOX 9-3	Caregiver Strain Index

Instructions given to the caregiver: I am going to read a list of things that other people have found to be difficult in caring for patients after they come home from the hospital. Would you tell me whether any of these apply to you? (Give the examples.)

Score one point for "yes" and zero for "no"

1. Sleep is disturbed (eg, because _____ is in and out of bed or wanders around at night).
2. It is inconvenient (eg, because helping takes so much time or it is a long drive over to help).
3. It is a physical strain (eg, because of lifting in and out of a chair).
4. It is confining (eg, because helping restricts free time or cannot visit).
5. There have been family adjustments (eg, because helping has disrupted routine or there has been no privacy).
6. There have been changes in personal plans (eg, had to turn down a job or could not go on vacation).
7. There have been other demands on my time (eg, from other family members).
8. There have been emotional adjustments (eg, because of severe arguments).
9. Some behavior is upsetting (eg, incontinence; _____ has trouble remembering things; _____ accuses others of taking things).
10. It is upsetting to find that _____ has changed so much from before (eg, _____ is a different person from before).
11. There have been work adjustments (eg, because of having to take time off).
12. It is a financial strain.
13. It has been completely overwhelming (eg, because of worry about _____ or concerns about how to continue to manage).

Scoring: Total score of 7 or more suggests a greater level of stress.

Robinson, B. C. (1983). Validation of a caregiver strain index. *Journal of Gerontology, 38*(3), 344–348. ©1983 The Gerontological Society of America.

c. Older adults can meet the physical activity recommendations with the following sample schedule:
  i. Aerobic exercise: brisk walking 5 days per week for at least 30 minutes.
  ii. Flexibility: stretch every day.
  iii. Strength training: do strength-building activities 2 to 3 days per week that involve all major muscle groups.
d. For further information on exercise for older adults living independently, see *www.cdc.gov/physicalactivity/everyone/guidelines/olderadults.html*.

SPECIAL HEALTH PROBLEMS OF THE OLDER ADULT
Altered Response to Medication

Adults over age 65 consume 30% to 40% of all prescription drugs and over-the-counter drugs. Age-related changes predispose older adults to problems with adverse drug effects.

Pathophysiology and Etiology

1. Drug absorption is affected by such age-related changes as:
  a. Decreased gastric acid.
  b. Decreased GI motility.
  c. Decreased gastric blood flow.
  d. Changes in GI villi.
  e. Decreased blood flow and body temperature in rectum.
2. Drug distribution is affected by:
  a. Decreased body size.
  b. Decreased water content in the body.
  c. Increased total body fat.
  d. Drugs distributed in water have a higher concentration in older adults (eg, gentamicin).
  e. Drugs distributed in fat have a wider distribution and less intense but prolonged effect (eg, phenobarbital).
3. Drug metabolism in the older adult:
  a. Is altered by a decrease in liver size, blood flow, enzyme activity, and protein synthesis.
  b. Requires more time than in younger adults. Therefore, there is increased drug activity time in drugs that are metabolized in the liver (eg, propranolol, theophylline).
4. Excretion of drugs is altered in older adults because of the following renal changes:
  a. Decreased renal tubular function and blood flow.
  b. This causes a decrease in renal filtration and an increase in blood levels of drugs that are excreted through the kidneys (eg, cimetidine).

 DRUG ALERT Drugs that may have severe adverse effects in elderly patients include anticholinergics (antihistamines, tricyclic antidepressants, drugs for treating urinary incontinence), nonsteroidal anti-inflammatory drugs (NSAIDs), any drug with a long half-life, and drugs with action on the central nervous system (CNS).

Nursing Assessment

1. Drug toxicities in older adults are different than they are in younger people.
2. Fewer symptoms may be identified, and they may develop slower; however, the reactions may be more pronounced and further advanced once they do present.
3. Behavioral and cognitive adverse effects are more common in older adults because the blood–brain barrier becomes less effective; the first reaction to a drug is confusion.
4. Many potential adverse drug effects are not identified because they are attributed to old age; fatigue, dementia, anorexia, or indigestion as adverse drug effects may not be reported.
5. Allergic reactions to drugs increase with age because of a greater likelihood of earlier exposure.

Nursing and Patient Care Considerations

1. Maintain awareness that the older adult is at greater risk for adverse drug reactions.
  a. This risk increases from 6% when two drugs are taken to 50% when five different drugs are taken and to 100% when eight or more drugs are taken.
2. Assess patient's ability to follow medication regimen by evaluation of:
  a. Cognition.
  b. Ability to read drug labels.
  c. Hand and muscle coordination.
  d. Swallowing difficulty.
  e. Lifestyle patterns, specifically smoking and alcohol use.
  f. Cultural beliefs toward medication.
  g. Ability to afford medication.
  h. Caregiver involvement in medication administration; assess caregiver if indicated.
3. Identify problems in the use of medications, such as:
  a. Lack of knowledge about drugs.
  b. Multiple medications and difficult administration techniques.
  c. Caregiver misunderstanding of medication use.
4. Appropriate interventions for safe drug use include:
  a. Obtain a complete drug history.
  b. Reinforce verbal instructions with written instructions using large-print and simple wording. If necessary, use color-coding rather than drug names.
  c. Write what the drug is used for and what the adverse effects can be.
  d. Make sure patient or caregiver can open the medication container.
  e. Arrange medication schedules to coincide with regular activity, such as eating (if appropriate for that drug). Simplify the drug regimen as much as possible.
  f. If necessary, arrange a check-off system using a chart to ensure adherence or weekly pill box.
  g. If possible, visibly evaluate all medications in the home, or ask patient to bring all medications for evaluation.
  h. Encourage patient to check expirations dates and discard all old or unneeded medications.
  i. Encourage patient to store medications in original containers in a dry, dark place.
  j. Encourage patient to avoid over-the-counter (OTC) medication without checking with the primary care provider before use.
  k. Encourage patient to report adverse drug effects.
  l. Work with prescribing caregiver and patient to maintain a medication regimen that follows the principles for geriatric drug use; start dosages low and go slow, use only necessary medications, titrate the dose to patient response, simplify the regimen, and have frequent reevaluations of the medication regimen.

Community and Home Care Considerations

1. Ask the patient or family to bring in all the patient's medications for clinic or office visits or whenever the patient goes to a facility to obtain an accurate medication history.
2. Ask the patient what vitamins, minerals, herbal supplements, and other OTC products are being used. Many patients do not consider these medications and will not readily supply the information unless specifically asked.
3. Alert patients and family members that many "natural" products sold over the counter still may cause adverse reactions and toxicity as well as interactions with other drugs.
4. Warn patients and families that many complementary and alternative medicine (CAM) therapies do not have proven effectiveness despite advertisements. CAM should be used as an adjunct to conventional therapy, and the patient should notify all health care providers of supplements and therapies being used.

Altered Nutritional Status

 EVIDENCE BASE Bowles, K. H., Dykes, P., & Demiris, G. (2015). The use of health information technology to improve care and outcomes for older adults. *Research in Gerontological Nursing, 8*(1), 5–10.

There is growing evidence that a balanced diet along with other health promotion behavior contribute to longevity. However, normal age-related changes, behavioral changes, and pathologic conditions may lead to malnutrition in the older adult.

Pathophysiology and Etiology

1. Changes in the oral cavity, including loss of teeth, diminished saliva production, and difficulty with mastication, may cause decreased food intake.
2. A decrease in gastric secretion with reduced pepsin hinders protein digestion and iron, vitamin B_{12}, calcium, and folic acid absorption; there are no significant changes in the small or large bowel.
3. Sensory changes involving taste and smell cause anorexia.
4. Psychosocial factors including changes in living situation, widowhood, depression, loneliness, decreased choice of food for institutionalized older adults, need to adhere to special diets, socioeconomic status, and ability to obtain and prepare food all impact what is eaten.
5. Alcohol use interferes with the absorption of B-complex vitamins. Additionally, alcohol is high in calories and low in nutritional value.
6. Medications can alter nutrition by directly decreasing absorption and utilization of nutrients. Indirectly, medications can result in anorexia, xerostomia, dysgeusia, and early satiety.
7. Dysphagia, which commonly occurs after stroke, intubation, or head and neck surgery, or is related to Parkinson disease and dementia, may cause decreased food intake.
8. With age, there is a decrease in energy needs because of a decrease in muscle mass (total caloric need decreases by 30%).

Nursing Assessment

1. Be alert for patients who complain of difficulty swallowing and difficulty managing saliva. Watch for coughing after swallowing, sounding "wet" after eating, and pocketing food in the cheeks.
2. Assess for absent or diminished gag reflex.
3. Assess for a 10% weight loss over 6 months (marasmus) or weight loss along with low serum albumin levels (kwashiorkor), which are signs of protein-energy malnutrition.
4. Determine if cholesterol level is below 130 mg/dL, which also may indicate malnourishment.

Nursing and Patient Care Considerations

1. Educate older adult and family or significant other about basic nutritional requirements and on overcoming barriers that interfere with optimal nutrition.
   a. The Required Dietary Allowances for healthy older adults are the same as that for younger adults, with three exceptions: decreased caloric intake, decreased protein intake (1 g/kg), and decreased iron requirements for postmenopausal women.
2. Encourage good mouth care.
3. Encourage patients to avoid alcohol if possible; refer for counseling if necessary and compensate for the nutritional consequences of alcohol abuse with liquid supplements, B vitamins.
4. Review all prescription and OTC medications with patients, and evaluate the influence of these on nutritional status.
5. If food procurement, preparation, and enjoyment are a problem, identify community resources to offer assistance in obtaining food and community meals.
6. In large facility settings, environmental factors may influence food enjoyment. Encourage socialization when eating, and try to minimize the negative effects of disruptive people and/or settings. Try to improve aesthetics.
7. To compensate for age-related changes in taste and smell, encourage use of low-sodium food additives.
8. Encourage proper body position (eg, sitting upright during mealtimes) and staying up for 30 minutes after eating to help with digestion.
9. If possible, encourage five to six small meals per day rather than three large meals.
10. If appropriate, encourage family to bring in favorite foods for patient.
11. Position food on the plate so that if there is visual neglect, or impairment, patient is best able to see the food served.
12. Identify patients with dysphagia and obtain a referral to a speech therapist.
    a. Work with the speech therapist and primary health care provider to determine what consistency of food is safe for patient to swallow. If patient is unable to swallow, thin liquids, slushes, puddings, or applesauce should be given to ensure adequate hydration.
    b. Use good compensatory techniques if indicated. These include sitting upright, tucking and turning the head, placing the food on the unaffected side of the tongue, swallowing twice to clear the pharyngeal tract, tucking the chin to the chest, and bringing the tongue up and back and holding the breath to swallow.
    c. Write out swallowing instructions for patient and family and educate family regarding the importance of maintaining these precautions.

Community and Home Care Considerations

1. Encourage the older adult at home to eat a well-balanced diet to maintain an optimal nutritional state.
2. Suggest vitamin preparations with the fewest number of minerals and vitamins needed to prevent interactions and avoid megadoses.

3. Advise taking calcium carbonate, iron, and zinc at least 2 hours apart and taking vitamins at the same time daily.

4. Advise taking iron on an empty stomach and taking fat-soluble vitamins (A, D, E, and K) with food.

5. Educate about different types of calcium preparations:
   a. Calcium carbonate is more difficult to absorb on an empty stomach; it needs an acidic environment to enhance absorption. The percent of calcium absorbed decreases as the calcium load increases; therefore, calcium carbonate absorption is greatest in doses of 500 mg or less, with food.
   b. Because calcium citrate is highly soluble in acid, it is better absorbed on an empty stomach. The citrate form does not need gastric acid for absorption.
   c. Calcium lactate can be absorbed at various pHs and does not need to be taken with food for absorption.

Urinary Incontinence

 EVIDENCE BASE Dowling-Castronovo, A., & Broadway, C. (2016). Urinary incontinence. In M. Bolts, E. Capezuti, T. Fulmer, & D. Zwicker (Eds.), *Evidence-based geriatric nursing protocols for best practice* (5th ed., pp. 343–349). New York, NY: Springer Publishing Company.

Approximately 13 million Americans suffer from urinary incontinence. Approximately 35% of older adults admitted to an acute care hospital will develop urinary incontinence. The prevalence increases significantly for older adults living in nursing homes; it is estimated that up to 90% of residents in nursing homes are incontinent of urine.

Pathophysiology and Etiology

1. There are five basic types of urinary incontinence:
   a. Stress—an involuntary loss of urine with increases in intra-abdominal pressure. Usually caused from weakness and laxity of pelvic floor musculature or bladder outlet weakness.
   b. Urge—involves leakage of urine because of inability to delay voiding after sensation of bladder fullness is perceived. This is associated with detrusor hyperactivity, CNS disorders, or local genitourinary conditions.
   c. Overflow—because of a leakage of urine resulting from mechanical forces on an overdistended bladder. This results from mechanical obstruction or hypomobility of the detrusor muscle.
   d. Mixed—symptoms of both stress and urge incontinence secondary to both an overactive detrusor and pelvic floor/urethral incompetence.
   e. Functional—involves urinary leakage associated with inability to get to the toilet because of cognitive and/or physical functioning.

Nursing Assessment

Because of the prevalence and increased incidence of incontinence in older adults, it is imperative that nurses include urine function in their assessments.

1. Identify reversible causes of incontinence using the DRIP acronym:
   D—Delirium, especially new-onset delirium.
   R—Restricted mobility, retention.
   I—Infection (especially sudden-onset cystitis), inflammation (such as atrophic vaginitis or urethritis), impaction (fecal).

P—Polyuria (from poorly controlled diabetes or diuretic treatment), pharmaceuticals (including psychotropics, anticholinergics, alpha-agonists, beta-agonists, calcium channel blockers, opioids, alpha-antagonists, and alcohol).

2. Evaluate lower urinary tract function.
   a. Stress maneuvers are evaluated by asking the patient, with a full bladder, to cough three times while standing. Observe for urine leakage.
   b. Check for postvoid residual by inserting a 12- or 14-French straight catheter a few minutes after the patient voids or use a portable ultrasound bladder scanner to measure postvoid urine residual.
   c. Evaluate bladder filling by leaving the straight catheter in place and using a 50-mL syringe to fill the bladder with sterile water. Hold the syringe about 6 inch (15 cm) above the pubic symphysis. Continue to fill the bladder in 25-mL increments until the patient feels the urge to void. Observe for involuntary bladder contractions. These contractions are detected by continuous upward movement of the column of fluid in the absence of abdominal straining.

Nursing and Patient Care Considerations

1. For stress or urge incontinence, teach Kegel (pelvic muscle) exercises.
   a. Teach the patient to first practice stopping the stream of urine while voiding to identify proper contraction of the pubococcygeal muscle; contraction will result in stopping flow, and relaxation allows flow.
   b. Once proper contraction is verified, advise patient to practice contraction of the muscle for 3 seconds and then relaxation of the muscle for 3 seconds in sets of 15 three times per day.
   c. The exercise can be practiced anywhere at any time because it involves contraction of an internal muscle; encourage patient to try them sitting, standing, and lying down. The abdomen should be relaxed, and no movement should be visible by doing Kegel exercises.

2. Assist with biofeedback that involves the use of bladder, rectal, or vaginal pressure recordings to train patients to contract pelvic floor muscles and relax the abdomen.

3. Institute a behavioral training program, using bladder records, biofeedback, and pelvic floor exercises for patients with stress or urge incontinence.

4. Institute other interventions such as:
   a. Bladder retraining—progressive lengthening or shortening of voiding intervals to restore the normal pattern of voiding; this is useful after period of immobility or catheterization.
   b. Scheduled toileting—using a fixed toileting schedule to prevent wetting episodes for patients with urge or functional incontinence.
   c. Habit training—involves using a variable toileting schedule based on patient's pattern of voiding; also incorporates positive reinforcement.
   d. Prompted voiding—includes regular prompts to void every 1 to 2 hours with positive reinforcement.
   e. Appropriate use of incontinence aids, such as pads or diapers.
   f. Judicious use of medications to help control urge incontinence. These include oxybutynin and tolterodine, among others. Contraindicated in urinary or gastric retention, myasthenia gravis, and uncontrolled glaucoma. Monitor carefully for anticholinergic effects—dry mouth, heat intolerance, urine retention, constipation, drowsiness, dry eyes, blurred vision.

Urine Retention

EVIDENCE BASE Park, J. & Palmer, M. H. (2015). Factors associated with incomplete bladder emptying in older women with overactive bladder symptoms. *Journal of the American Geriatrics Society, 63*(7), 1426–1431.

Urine retention is a common problem in the older adult, commonly related to a neurologic or other underlying condition.

Pathophysiology and Etiology

1. Frequently encountered in the acute care setting, postcatheterization, after stroke, in diabetics because of atonic neuropathic bladder, because of fecal impaction, and in males with prostatic enlargement.
2. The patient with urine retention may void small amounts or may be incontinent continuously because of overflow of urine.
3. Patients with urine retention will usually have incontinence during the night.
4. Urine retention may also be caused or aggravated by drugs with anticholinergic properties, such as levodopa or tricyclic antidepressants, especially amitriptyline. Other commonly prescribed drugs, such as alpha-agonists, beta-agonists, and calcium channel blockers, can cause urinary retention.

GERONTOLOGIC ALERT Urine retention may cause urinary tract infection, which can lead to poor outcomes for older adult.

Nursing Assessment

1. Take a complete history and perform a physical examination to rule out causes of urine retention.
2. Understand and identify the risk factors for urinary retention.
3. Monitor for a distended bladder and perform postvoid catheterization; there is no consensus of the upper or lower limits of a postvoid residual. However, residual of greater than 100 mL of urine is often used as a sign of urine retention.

Nursing and Patient Care Considerations

1. Remove fecal impaction to help patient regain bladder function.
2. If prostatic disease is suspected, appropriate referral is necessary.
3. Encourage male to use the standing position and female to use the sitting position to facilitate urinary flow; provide privacy.
4. Teach "double voiding." Finish voiding and then reposition oneself to void again. Also teach Credé method: have the patient massage the area of the abdomen directly over the bladder to "milk" the bladder to express any residual urine.
5. Evaluate medication regimen and discuss with health care provider the necessity or substitution of offending medication.
6. If no underlying condition is suspected, attempt intermittent catheterizations every 8 hours, in combination with regular voiding attempts by patient. If there is no response in 2 weeks (ie, no decrease in postvoid residuals), referral to a urologist may be necessary for medical management of the urine retention.

Fecal Incontinence

Fecal incontinence is an inability to voluntarily control the passage of gas or feces. It occurs in an estimated 15% of women and 6% to 10% of men who live in the community and in an estimated 45% of older adults who live in nursing homes.

EVIDENCE BASE Any, U. U., Vaughan, C. P., Burgio, K. L., et al. (2016). Shared risk factors for constipation, fecal incontinence, and combined symptoms in older U.S. adults. *Journal of the American Geriatrics Society, 64*(11), e183–e188.

Pathophysiology and Etiology

1. Fecal continence depends on normal rectal and anal sensation, rectal reservoir capacity, and internal and external sphincter mechanisms.
2. In institutionalized older adults, fecal impaction is a primary cause of fecal incontinence because of stool leaking around a fecal mass.
3. In noninstitutionalized older adults, fecal incontinence is commonly associated with dysfunction of one of the anorectal continence mechanisms, such as impaired contractile strength of the sphincters and lower rectal volume capacity. Stroke and spinal cord injuries cause loss of sensation in the rectal area.
4. Sometimes, functional or cognitive impairment and depression may inhibit motivation and the ability to remain continent.
5. Commonly, no cause can be determined for the fecal loss, and it is believed that the incontinence may be due to a degenerative injury to the pudendal nerve.

Nursing Assessment

1. Assess overall function, cognition, and affect.
2. Assess baseline bowel status through health history or observation.
3. Assess severity and frequency of symptoms, including quantity of fecal incontinence.
4. Perform a rectal examination to check for impaction or decreased rectal sphincter tone.
5. If the fecal incontinence is diarrheal in nature, stool evaluation for leukocytes, culture and sensitivity, ova and parasites, and *Clostridium difficile* may be indicated.

Nursing and Patient Care Considerations

1. Increase dietary fiber in an attempt to add bulk to the stool to stimulate regular defecation, if there is no infection and no impaction present.
2. Try antidiarrheals such as loperamide, as directed, for managing diarrhea.
3. Try to set up a regular bowel evacuation pattern once an impaction is detected and removed. This includes regular toileting times, set preferably after breakfast, and increased fluid and fiber intake. Use laxatives only as a last resort.
4. In bedbound patients, increased fiber in the diet is contraindicated. These patients may require a bisacodyl suppository or an enema to help with rectal evacuation two to three times per week.

5. Treat those with neurogenic fecal incontinence, such as patients with spinal cord injuries and poststroke, to induce fecal evacuation at regularly scheduled times.

6. Administer glycerin or bisacodyl suppository two to three times per week before breakfast (to use the normal gastrocolic reflex that starts after the first meal of the day) to help induce a complete rectal evacuation and decrease stool incontinence.

Community and Home Care Considerations

1. Explain to patient and family that it is not necessary to have bowel movements every day.

2. Advise avoidance of laxatives, which may induce diarrhea.

3. Encourage fibrous foods that stimulate the bowel to be eaten daily, preferably at breakfast, such as stewed prunes, citrus fruits, and bran cereals. Make sure that help is available to toilet patient when the urge to defecate is felt.

4. Recommend a home remedy to maintain regular bowel movements: 3 tbsp applesauce, 2 tbsp bran, and 1 tbsp prune juice mixed, refrigerated, and given at least 1 tbsp each morning.

Pressure Ulcers

 EVIDENCE BASE Ayello, E. A., & Sibbald, R. G. (2016). Nursing standard of practice protocol: Pressure ulcer prevention & skin tear prevention. In M. Boltz, E. Capezuti, T. Fulmer, & D. Zwicker (Eds.), *Evidence-based geriatric nursing protocols for best practice* (5th ed.). New York, NY: Springer Publishing Company.

Haesler, E. (Ed.), National Pressure Ulcer Advisory Panel, European Pressure Ulcer Advisory Panel and Pan Pacific Pressure Injury Alliance. (2014). *Prevention and Treatment of Pressure Ulcers: Quick Reference Guide*. Osborne Park, Western Australia: Cambridge Media.

Pressure ulcers (decubitus ulcers) are localized ulcerations of the skin or deeper structures. They most commonly result from prolonged periods of bed rest in acute- or long-term care facilities; however, they can develop within hours in the compromised individual (see Figure 9-2).

Pathophysiology and Etiology

Factors in the Development of Pressure Ulcers

1. Pressure of 70 mm Hg applied for longer than 2 hours can produce tissue destruction; healing cannot occur without relieving the pressure.

2. Friction contributes to pressure ulcer development by causing abrasion of the stratum corneum.

3. Shearing force, produced by sliding of adjacent surfaces, is particularly important in the partial sitting position. This force ruptures capillaries over the sacrum.

4. Moisture on the skin results in maceration of the epithelium.

Risk Factors for Pressure Ulcers

1. Bowel or bladder incontinence.
2. Malnourishment or significant weight loss.
3. Edema, anemia, hypoxia, or hypotension.
4. Neurologic impairment or immobility.
5. Altered mental status, including delirium or dementia.

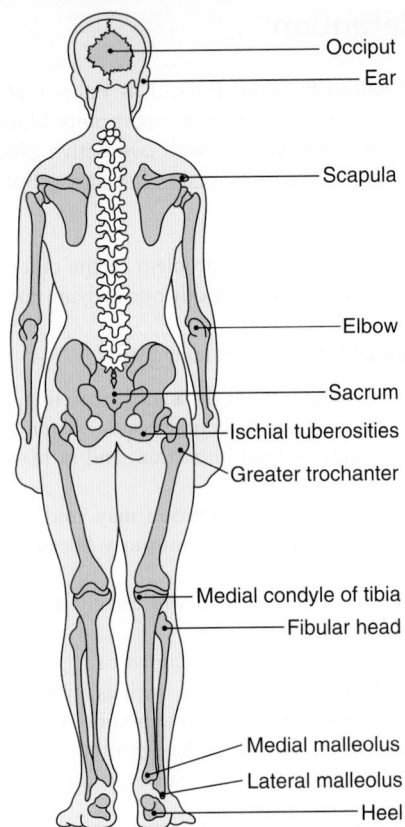

Figure 9-2. Areas susceptible to pressure ulcers. (Smeltzer, S., & Bare, B. [2000]. *Brunner and Suddarth's textbook of medical-surgical nursing* [9th ed.]. Philadelphia, PA: Lippincott Williams & Wilkins.)

Nursing Assessment

1. Assess for risk factors for pressure ulcer development and alter those factors, if possible.

2. Assess skin of the older adult frequently for the development of pressure ulcers. The Braden Scale for Predicting Pressure Sore Risk is one of the most commonly used instruments for predicting the development of pressure ulcers (*www.braden-scale.com*). The Braden Scale assesses pressure ulcer risk in six areas: sensory perception, skin moisture, activity, mobility, nutrition, and friction/shear.

3. Stage the ulcer so appropriate treatment can be started. The National Pressure Ulcer Advisory Panel advocates the following staging system (see Figure 9-3).

   a. Stage I—intact skin with nonblanchable redness of a localized area, usually over a bony prominence.

   b. Stage II—partial thickness loss of dermis presenting as a shallow open ulcer with a red–pink wound bed, without slough; may also present as an intact or open/ruptured serum-filled blister.

   c. Stage III—full-thickness tissue loss, with subcutaneous fat that may be visible but bone, tendon, or muscle is not exposed; may include undermining and tunneling. Slough may be present but does not obscure the depth of tissue loss.

   d. Stage IV—full-thickness tissue loss with exposed bone, tendon, or muscle; slough or eschar may be present on some parts of the wound bed; often includes undermining and tunneling.

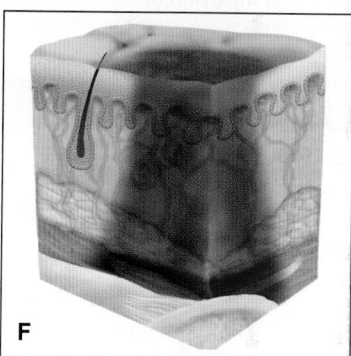

Figure 9-3. International NPUAP/EPUAP pressure injury stages. **(A)** Stage I—nonblanchable erythema. **(B)** Stage II—partial thickness skin loss with exposed dermis. **(C)** Stage III—full-thickness skin loss. **(D)** Stage IV—full-thickness skin and tissue loss. **(E)** Unstageable pressure injury—obscured full thickness skin and tissue loss. **(F)** Deep tissue pressure injury—persistent non-blanchable deep red, maroon, or purple discoloration. (2016 NPUAP Pressure Injury Staging Illustrations from http://www.npuap.org/resources/educational-and-clinical-resources/pressure-injury-staging-illustrations/. Used with permission of the National Pressure Ulcer Advisory Panel March 2018. © NPUAP.)

   e. Unstageable—full-thickness tissue loss in which the base of the ulcer is covered by slough and/or eschar in the wound bed.

   f. Suspected deep tissue injury—a localized area of intact skin or blood-filled blister, maroon or purple in color, caused by damage of the underlying soft tissue from shear or pressure.

Nursing and Patient Care Considerations

Prevent Pressure Ulcer Development

1. Provide meticulous care and positioning for immobile patients.

   a. Inspect skin several times daily.

   b. Wash skin with mild soap, rinse, and pat dry with a soft towel.

   c. Lubricate skin with a bland lotion to keep skin soft and pliable.

   d. Avoid poorly ventilated mattress that is covered with plastic or impermeable material.

   e. Employ bowel and bladder programs to prevent incontinence.

   f. Encourage ambulation and exercise.

   g. Promote nutritious diet with optimal protein, vitamins, and iron.

2. Teach older adult and family or significant other the importance of good nutrition, hydration, activity, positioning, and avoidance of pressure, shearing, friction, and moisture.

Relieve the Pressure

1. Avoid elevation of head of bed greater than 30 degrees.

2. Reposition every 2 hours.

3. Use special devices to cushion specific areas (especially bony areas), such as flotation rings, lamb's wool or fleece pads, convoluted foam mattresses, booties, or elbow pads. Lift heels off the bed in bedbound patients. Do not use donut devices.

4. Use an alternating-pressure mattress or air-fluidized bed for patients at high risk to prevent or treat pressure ulcers.

5. Provide for activity and ambulation as much as possible.

6. Advise frequent shifting of weight and occasional raising of buttocks off chair while sitting.

Clean and Debride the Wound

1. Use normal saline for cleaning and disinfecting wounds.
2. Apply wet-to-dry dressings or enzyme ointments for debridement as directed or assist with surgical debridement.

Treat Local Infection

1. Avoid obtaining wound cultures because open wounds are always colonized with bacteria, unless there is evidence of systemic infection or progressive local infection such as cellulitis.
2. Apply topical antibiotics to locally infected pressure ulcer as prescribed.

Cover the Wound

1. Cover the wound with a protective dressing as this minimizes disruption of migrating fibroblasts and epithelial cells and results in a moist, nutrient-rich environment for healing to occur.
   a. Polyurethane thin film dressings can be used for superficial low-exudate wounds. They are air and water permeable but do not absorb exudate.
   b. Hydrocolloids can provide padding to wounds but can lead to maceration; they are not oxygen permeable.
   c. Polyurethane foam/membrane dressings absorb exudate and are oxygen permeable.
   d. Hydrogel dressings are multilayered and include properties of both hydrocolloids and polyurethane (see Table 9-2 for comparison of selected occlusive dressings).

Osteoporosis

Osteoporosis is a condition in which the bone matrix is lost, thereby weakening the bones and making them more susceptible to fracture. Bone mineral density is 2.5 standard deviations below the peak bone density for young adults (T score –2.5). Decrease in bone density of 1.5 to 2.5 below young adult is termed *osteopenia* (T score –1.5 to –2.5). It is the most age-related metabolic bone disorder.

Pathophysiology and Etiology

1. The rate of bone resorption increases over the rate of bone formation, causing loss of bone mass.
2. Calcium and phosphate salts are lost, creating porous, brittle bones.
3. Occurs most commonly in postmenopausal women but may also occur in men.
4. Other factors include:
   a. Age.
   b. Inactivity.
   c. Chronic illness.
   d. Medications, such as corticosteroids, excessive thyroid replacement, cyclosporine.
   e. Calcium and vitamin D deficiency.
   f. Family history.
   g. Smoking and alcohol use.
   h. Diet—caffeine has been linked as a risk factor.

Table 9-2	Comparison of Selected Occlusive Dressing			
DRESSING TYPE	**EXAMPLES**	**APPROPRIATE USE**	**ADVANTAGES**	**DISADVANTAGES**
Absorption	Debrisan Hydrophilic Beads	• Stage II–V ulcer with drainage	• Absorbs drainage and deodorizes wound	• Need to change dressing 1–2 times daily
Hydrocolloid	DuoDerm	• Stage I–II ulcer	• Provides padding • Easy to apply • Water impermeable • No skin excoriation	• Poor absorptive capacity • Poor oxygen exchange • Messy residue • Pressure areas possible
Polyurethane	OpSite, Tegaderm	• Nondraining wounds	• Transparent • Self-adhesive • Oxygen permeable	• No absorptive capacity • May cause excoriation • Difficult to apply
Polyurethane membrane	Mitraflex	• Skin tears • Tape burns • Blisters • Stage II ulcers • Low-moderate exudate wounds	• Good absorptive ability • Good oxygen exchange • Water impermeable • May debride	• May cause excoriation
Polyurethane foam	Epi-Lock	• Skin tears • Tape burns • Blisters • Stage II ulcers • Low to moderate exudate wounds	• Good absorptive ability • Good oxygen exchange • Water impermeable • May debride • No skin excoriation	• Nonadhesive
Hydrogel	Vigilon, Biofilm	• Stage I–III	• No skin excoriation • Transparent • Some ability to absorb drainage • Easy to apply	• Difficult to apply • Nonadherent
Debriding enzyme	Elase, Travase	• Stage III–IV	• Acts against devitalized tissue • Not appropriate for hard, dry eschar	• May damage healthy tissue

i. Race—whites and Asians have higher-risk incidence.
j. Body type—small frame/short stature, low body fat.

Clinical Manifestations

1. Asymptomatic until later stages.
2. Fracture after minor trauma may be first indication. Most frequent fractures associated with osteoporosis include fractures of the distal radius, vertebral bodies, proximal humerus, pelvis, and proximal femur (hip).
3. May have vague complaints related to aging process (stiffness, pain, weakness).
4. Estrogen deficiency may be noted.

Diagnostic Evaluation

1. X-rays show changes only after 30% to 60% loss of bone.
2. Dual-energy x-ray absorptiometry (DEXA) scanning shows decreased bone mineral density (T score −2.5 or worse).
3. Serum and urine calcium levels are normal.
4. Serum bone matrix Gla protein (a marker for bone turnover) is elevated.
5. Bone biopsy shows thin, porous, otherwise normal bone.

Management

Management is primarily preventive.
1. Identify patients at risk for fractures.
2. Reduce modifiable risk factors through improved diet, smoking cessation, decreased alcohol consumption, and other healthy lifestyle choices.
3. Adequate intake of calcium—1.2 g/day—may be preventive.
4. Adequate intake of vitamin D.
   a. Vitamin D plays a major role in calcium absorption and bone health. With age, there is decreased ability to take in vitamin D through the skin; therefore, replacement is recommended.
   b. Food sources are milk products, egg yolks, fish, and liver; however, dietary intake of vitamin D is limited.
   c. Vitamin D can be manufactured in the skin through sunlight exposure; however, this may be limited by cloud cover, latitude, season and skin cancer prevention methods that limit exposure.
   d. Recommended daily allowance for adults age 70 and over is 800 international units.
5. Weight-bearing exercise (eg, walking) throughout life.
6. Hormone replacement therapy is no longer recommended for osteoporosis prevention or treatment because the risks outweigh the benefits.
7. Raloxifene, an estrogen receptor agonist, is an alternative to estrogen. Not as effective as estrogen, but does show some benefit in preserving bone density. No increase in risk of breast cancer.
8. Calcitonin administered by nasal spray may help prevent spinal fracture. Adverse effect is nasal burning and a runny nose.
9. Bisphosphonates, such as risedronate, alendronate, and ibandronate, bind to and inhibit osteoclast action, remain active on bone resorptive surfaces for 3 weeks, and do not impede normal bone formation.
   a. Associated with improved bone density and decreased hip and spinal fracture rate.
   b. They must be taken with fluid but not food, and patient must remain upright for 30 minutes after taking pill to prevent esophagitis.

c. Long-acting injectables such as zoledronic acid and teriparatide are protective for women at high risk for fractures and helpful in increasing bone mass in men who are on long-term glucocorticoid therapy.
10. Parathyroid hormone teriparatide utility is limited because it requires daily subcutaneous injections.
11. Prevention of falls in older adults helps to prevent fractures.

EVIDENCE BASE Cosman, F., de Beur, S. J., LeBoff, M. S., et al. (2014). Prevention and treatment of osteoporosis. *Osteoporosis International, 25,* 2359.

Complications

1. Fractures.
2. Progressive kyphosis, loss of height (see Figure 9-4).
3. Chronic back pain from compression fracture.

Nursing Assessment

1. Obtain history of risk factors for osteoporosis, fractures, and other musculoskeletal disease.
2. Assess risk for falls and fractures—sensory or motor problems, improper footwear, lack of knowledge of safety precautions, and so forth. See Table 9-3, for assessment factors and interventions.

Nursing Diagnosis

Chronic Pain related to vertebral compression fractures in late stages of osteoporosis

Figure 9-4. Progressive kyphosis in osteoporosis. (Anatomical Chart Company.)

Table 9-3 Assessment Factors and Interventions to Decrease Risk of Falls	
KNOWN RISK FACTORS	**SPECIFIC INTERVENTIONS TO DECREASE INDIVIDUAL RISK**
History of falls	• Identify the patient as being at risk for falls: May use sticker on chart or door, inform families and other care providers of increased risk.
Fear of falling	• Encourage patient to verbalize feeling. • Strengthen self-efficacy related to transfers and ambulation by providing verbal encouragement about capabilities and ability to perform safely.
Bowel and bladder incontinence	• Set up regular voiding schedule (every 2 hr or as appropriate based on patient need). • Monitor bowel function and encourage sufficient fluids and fiber (eight 8-oz glasses daily and 24 g of fiber). • Utilize laxatives as appropriate.
Cognitive impairment	• Evaluate patient for reversible causes of cognitive impairment or delirium and eliminate causes as relevant. Monitor patient with cognitive impairment at least hourly with relocation of the patient such that nursing staff can observe and monitor regularly. • Encourage family member to hire staff or stay with patient continuously. • Utilize monitoring devices if available (ie, bed/chair or exit alarms) rather than restraint.
Mood	• Encourage verbalization of feeling. • Evaluate patient's ability to concentrate and learn new information. • Encourage participation in daily activities. • Utilize alternative interventions, such as massage, aromatherapy, pet and plant therapy, and music or exercise.
Dizziness	• Monitor lying, sitting, and standing blood pressures and continually evaluate for factors contributing to dizziness. • Encourage adequate fluid intake (eight 8-oz glasses daily). • Set up environment to avoid movements that result in dizziness or vertigo. • Decrease or avoid alcohol use.
Functional impairment, immobility, impaired gait	• Encourage participation in personal care activities at highest level (ie, if possible encourage ambulation to bathroom rather than use of bed pan). • Refer to physical and occupational therapy as appropriate. • Facilitate adherence to exercise program when indicated. • Maintain safe and appropriate use of assistive device.
Medications	• Review medications with primary health care provider and determine need for each medication. • Make sure that medications are being used at lowest possible dosages to obtain desired result.
Medical problems	• Work with primary health care provider to augment management of primary medical problem, such as Parkinson disease, heart failure, or anemia.
Environment	• Remove furniture if patient cannot be seated with feet reaching the floor. • Remove clutter. • Make sure furniture and any assistive devices used are in good condition. • Make sure lighting is adequate. • Make sure safety bars are available in the bathroom.

Nursing Interventions

Reducing Pain

1. Administer opioid analgesics, as ordered, for acute exacerbations of pain.
2. Encourage replacement with nonopioid pain relievers as soon as possible to avoid drowsiness, possible addiction.
3. Assist with putting on back brace and ensure proper fit. Encourage use as much as possible, especially while ambulatory.
4. Encourage compliance with physical therapy appointments and practicing exercises at home to increase muscle strength surrounding bones and to relieve pain.

 GERONTOLOGIC ALERT Be alert for alcohol use combined with other CNS depressants in older adults. With advanced age, there is a reduction in

lean body mass, an increase in body fat, a decrease in water content, and a decrease in the gastric alcohol dehydrogenase enzyme. This results in an increase in the blood alcohol level in older individuals compared to younger individuals per unit of alcohol consumed, especially in women. Alcohol use, particularly when combined with opioids or sedative hypnotics, is commonly associated with falls in these individuals.

Patient Education and Health Maintenance

1. Encourage exercise for all age groups. Teach the value of walking daily throughout life to provide stress required for strong bone remodeling.
2. Provide dietary education in relation to adequate daily intake of calcium (1,200 mg). Calcium can be obtained through milk and dairy products, vegetables, and supplements. Anyone with

a history of urinary tract calculi should consult with health care provider before increasing calcium intake.

3. Encourage use of combined calcium and vitamin D replacement. Avoid massive doses of vitamin D, however, because this may be harmful.
4. Encourage young women at risk to maximize bone mass through nutrition and exercise.
5. Suggest that perimenopausal women confer with their health care provider about the need for calcium supplements and estrogen therapy.
6. Alert patients to resources such as the National Osteoporosis Foundation (*www.nof.org*).

Community and Home Care Consideration

 EVIDENCE BASE U.S. Preventive Services Task Force. (2015). Final Update Summary: Osteoporosis: Screening. Available: www.uspreventiveservices-taskforce.org/Page/Document/UpdateSummaryFinal/osteoporosis-screening?ds=1&s=osteoporosis.

1. Encourage screening according to the USPSTF guidelines for all women over age 65 and women over age 60 at increased risk through DEXA of the femoral neck, with rescreening at approximately 2-year intervals.
2. Identify women at high risk for osteoporotic fractures in the community—frail, older white or Asian women with poor dietary intake of dairy products and little exposure to sun—and provide education and safety measures to prevent falls and fracture.
3. Make sure that diet contains maximal calcium. Teach family and caregivers how to read labels, encourage dairy products, and add powdered milk to foods as possible. Use skim milk if cholesterol and fat intake is a consideration.
4. Make sure that supplements and other medications are being taken properly.
   a. Patient teaching is critical in dosing of bisphosphonates to prevent esophagitis. Patient must take this upon waking with 6 to 8 oz of water, at least 30 minutes before ingesting first food of the day, and must remain upright for 30 minutes after taking the medication. Weekly or monthly dosing increases compliance.
   b. Calcitonin nasal spray dose is one spray in one nostril once per day; alternate nostrils each day.
5. Teach strategies to prevent falls. Assess home for hazards (eg, scatter rugs, slippery floors, extension cords, inadequate lighting).
6. Obtain physical and occupational therapy consultations, as needed, to encourage use of walking aids when balance is poor and to improve muscle strength.

Evaluation: Expected Outcomes

- Pain tolerable with nonopioid analgesics; no new fractures.
- Received screening and understands prevention measures.

Alzheimer Disease

The most common form of dementia is characterized by progressive impairment in memory, cognitive function, language, judgment, perception, and learned motor skills. Ultimately, patients cannot perform self-care activities and become dependent on caregivers.

Pathophysiology and Etiology

1. Gross pathophysiologic changes in the brain include cortical atrophy most prominent in the frontal and temporal lobes, enlarged ventricles, and atrophy of the hippocampus.
2. Microscopically, changes occur in the proteins of the nerve cells of the cerebral cortex and lead to accumulation of neurofibrillary tangles composed of the tau protein and neuritic plaques composed of the amyloid protein (deposits of protein and altered cell structures on the interneuronal junctions) and granulovascular degeneration. There is loss of cholinergic nerve cells, which are important in memory, function, and cognition.
3. Biochemically, neurotransmitter systems are impaired.
4. The cause is unknown, but advanced age, female gender, family history of AD, and head trauma with a loss of consciousness are risk factors. Indeed, research has identified four specific genes involved in predisposition to Alzheimer's. Genes on chromosomes 1, 14, and 21 have been implicated in the causation of early-onset Alzheimer disease, whereas the #4 allele of the apolipoprotein gene on chromosome 19 appears to be associated with the development of Alzheimer disease after age 65.
5. Viruses, environmental toxins, cerebrovascular disease, and educational level may also play a role.

Clinical Manifestations

1. Disease onset is subtle and insidious. Initially, a gradual decline of cognitive function from a previously higher level may be noticed. Short-term memory impairment and problems with executive functioning (planning and organizing) is commonly the first characteristic in earliest stages of the disease. Patients are forgetful and have difficulty learning and retaining new information. In addition to memory impairment, at least one of the following functional deficits is present:
   a. Language disturbance (aphasia, may be receptive, expressive or both).
   b. Visual processing and recognition difficulty (agnosia).
   c. Inability to perform skilled motor activities, such as dressing and walking (apraxia).
   d. Poor abstract reasoning and concentration.
2. Patients may have difficulty planning meals, managing finances, using a telephone, or driving without getting lost. Other classic signs include personality changes, such as irritability and suspiciousness, personal neglect of appearance, and disorientation to time and place.
3. The following clinical manifestations are typical in the middle stage of Alzheimer disease:
   a. Repetitive actions (perseveration).
   b. Nocturnal restlessness.
   c. Apraxia (impaired ability to perform purposeful activity).
   d. Aphasia (impaired ability to speak).
   e. Agraphia (inability to write).
4. With disease progression, signs of frontal lobe dysfunction appear, including loss of social inhibitions and loss of spontaneity. Delusions, hallucinations, aggression, and wandering behavior often occur in the middle and late stages.
5. Patients in the advanced stage of Alzheimer disease require total care. Symptoms may include:
   a. Urinary and fecal incontinence.
   b. Emaciation.
   c. Resistance to care

    d. Inability to walk.

    e. Decreased responsiveness to verbal and physical stimulation.

    f. Difficulty swallowing (dysphagia).

Diagnostic Evaluation

1. Detailed patient history with corroboration by an informed source to determine cognitive and behavioral changes, their duration, and symptoms that may be indicative of other medical or psychiatric illnesses.
2. Noncontrast computed tomography (CT) scan to rule out other neurologic conditions, such as a stroke or tumor. Magnetic resonance imaging and single-photon emission CT may be used.
3. Neuropsychological evaluation, including some form of mental status assessment, to identify specific areas of impaired mental functioning in contrast to areas of intact functioning.
4. Laboratory tests include complete blood count, sedimentation rate, chemistry panel, thyroid-stimulating hormone, test for syphilis, urinalysis, serum B_{12}, folate level, and test for human immunodeficiency virus to rule out infectious or metabolic disorders.
5. Commercial assays for cerebrospinal fluid tau protein and beta-amyloid are available, but their use is limited. Genetic testing is available, but its use is controversial. Three disease genes and one gene indicating susceptibility have been identified.

Management

1. Primary goals of treatment for Alzheimer disease are to optimize functional abilities and improve quality of life by enhancing mood, cognition, and behavior. No curative treatment exists. Treatment includes pharmacologic and nonpharmacologic approaches.
2. Cholinesterase inhibitors were the first treatment for cognitive impairment of Alzheimer disease. These drugs improve cholinergic neurotransmission to help delay decline in cognition and function over time. There is also evidence that cholinesterase inhibitors may be helpful in decreasing agitated behaviors common in dementia.

    a. Donepezil is widely used in mild to moderate cases because it can be given once daily and is well tolerated; starting at 5 mg at bedtime and increased to 10 mg after 4 to 6 weeks. In patients with moderate to severe Alzheimer disease, the dose of Donepezil may be increased to 23 mg daily; however, there is an increased risk of adverse gastrointestinal side effects at this higher dose. Donepezil has also been shown to be beneficial in individuals with severe dementia.

    b. Galantamine is given with food in dosage of 4 to 12 mg twice per day. Should be restarted at 4 mg bid if interrupted for several days. Dose should be reduced in cases of renal or hepatic impairment. Razadyne ER is an extended-release formula that can be given in once-daily dosing with dose ranges from 8 to 24 mg/day.

    c. Rivastigmine is given 1.5 mg twice per day with meals and increased up to 6 to 12 mg/day. Rivastigmine is also available in an oral solution and a patch form. Use of the Rivastigmine patch is associated with fewer gastrointestinal side effects than oral use.

 DRUG ALERT Cholinesterase inhibitors were initially aimed at improving memory and cognition. These drugs, however, seem to have an important impact on the behavioral changes that occur in patients with cognitive impairment. Specifically, research studies have demonstrated that use of cholinesterase inhibitors improves the apathy, disinhibition, pacing, and hallucinations commonly noted in dementia. Be alert for drug interactions with NSAIDs, succinylcholine-type muscle relaxants, cholinergic and anticholinergic agents, drugs that slow the heart, and other drugs that are metabolized by the hepatic CYP2D6 or CYP3A4 pathways.

3. Memantine, an N-methyl D-aspartate-receptor antagonist, is approved for moderate to severe Alzheimer disease. The immediate release dosage is 10 mg bid, and the extended-release dosage begins at 7 mg once a day and is gradually increased to a maximum dose of Memantine XR 28 mg once a day. The drug can be used with a cholinesterase inhibitor because it works by regulating the neurotransmitter, glutamate.
4. Studies indicate that other drugs, such as estrogen and NSAIDs, have not proven helpful in treatment and prevention of Alzheimer disease.
5. Patients with depressive symptoms should be considered for antidepressant therapy.
6. Nonpharmacologic treatments used to optimize cognition and behavior include environmental manipulation that decreases stimulation, pet therapy, aromatherapy, massage, music therapy, and exercise.
7. If nonpharmacologic approaches have been applied consistently and have failed to adequately reduce the frequency and severity of behavioral symptoms that have the potential to cause harm to the patient or others, then the introduction of medications such as antipsychotics, benzodiazepines, anticonvulsants, antidepressants, and sedatives may be appropriate but will still need to be carefully and routinely monitored over time.

    a. The risk and potential benefits of any medication must be discussed with the patient (when appropriate) and/or the patient's family/decision maker.

    b. The minimum amount of a medication should be used for the shortest time possible.

 DRUG ALERT Be aware that no medications are specifically approved by the FDA to treat the neuropsychiatric and behavioral symptoms of individuals with dementia. Antipsychotics have been linked to higher risk of death among older adults with dementia. This led the FDA to issue a black box warning for antipsychotic use in dementia.

Complications

1. Increased incidence of functional decline.
2. Injury because of lack of insight, hallucinations, and confusion.
3. Malnutrition because of inattention to mealtimes and hunger or lack of ability to prepare meals or feed self.

Nursing Assessment

1. Perform cognitive assessment for orientation, insight, abstract thinking, concentration, memory, and verbal ability.
2. Assess for changes in behavior and ability to perform ADLs.

3. Evaluate nutrition and hydration; check weight, skin turgor, and meal habits.
4. Assess motor ability, strength, muscle tone, and flexibility.

Nursing Diagnoses

- Disturbed Thought Processes related to physiologic disease process.
- Risk for Injury because of loss of cognitive abilities.
- Insomnia Secondary to disease process.
- Caregiver Role Strain related to physical needs and behavioral manifestations of the disease process.

Nursing Interventions

Improving Cognitive Response

1. Simplify the environment: reduce noise and social interaction to a level tolerable for the patient.
2. Maintain a predictable, structured routine, decrease the number of choices available to the patient, use pictures to identify activities, and use structured group activities.
3. Encourage active participation in care as tolerated and provide positive feedback for tasks that are accomplished.
4. Provide opportunities for physical activity alternating with rest periods.
5. Avoid confrontations and arguments. Follow the patient's direction and individualize care as much as possible.
6. Maintain consistency in interactions and introduce new people slowly.

Preventing Injury

1. Avoid restraints, but maintain observation of the patient as necessary.
2. Provide for adequate lighting to avoid misinterpretation of the environment.
3. Remove unneeded furniture and equipment from the room.
4. Provide medical alert identification such as bracelet.
5. Make sure patient has nonslip shoes or slippers that are easy to put on.
6. Encourage use of assistive safety devices, such as handrails and shower chairs.
7. Ensure physical activity as tolerated and ROM exercises to maintain mobility.

Ensuring Adequate Rest

1. Attempt to limit the use of medications that act on the CNS, such as anxiolytics and antipsychotics; however, if used, monitor for clinical response and potential adverse effects, including increased confusion, excess sedation, parkinsonism, extrapyramidal symptoms, and cardiovascular events.
2. Provide periods of physical exercise to expend energy.
3. Support normal sleep habits and bedtime rituals.
   a. Keep regular bedtime.
   b. Have patient change into pajamas at bedtime.
   c. Allow desired bedtime activity, such as snack, warm non-caffeinated beverage, listening to music, or prayer.
4. Maintain quiet, relaxing environment to avoid confusion and agitation.

Supporting Caregiver

1. Encourage caregiver to discuss feelings.
2. Encourage caregiver to maintain own health and emotional well-being.
3. Stress the need for relaxation time or respite care.

4. Assist the caregiver in finding resources, such as community or church groups, social service programs, or facility-based support groups.
5. Assess caregiver's stress and refer for counseling.
6. Support decision to place patient in a long-term care facility.

Community and Home Care Considerations

1. Encourage regular medical checkups with attention to health maintenance every 3 to 6 months to provide ongoing medical surveillance of patient and stamina of caregivers. Include influenza vaccine and ensure that patient has had pneumococcal pneumonia vaccine.
2. Discuss advance directives for patients and discuss long-term placement options in anticipation of future needs to help family members adjust and plan arrangements.
3. Encourage patients to be involved in social and intellectual activities as long as possible, such as family events, exercise, and recreational activities and sharing the newspaper and other forms of media.
4. Assist caregivers to modify the home environment for safety, and advise families of safety hazards such as wandering and driving a car. Encourage use of door locks, electronic wander-alert guards, and registration with the "Safe Return" program through the Alzheimer's Association or local police department.
5. Remind family members of possible dangers around the house as patient becomes less responsible for behavior. Encourage caregivers to reduce the temperature of the hot water heater, remove dials from stove and other electrical appliances, remove matches and lighters, and safely store away tools and other potentially dangerous items.

Patient Education and Health Maintenance

1. Encourage activities that provide physical exercise and repetitive movement but that require little thought, such as dancing, painting, doing laundry, or vacuuming.
2. Teach patient and family to eliminate stimulants, such as caffeine, and maintain good nutrition.
3. Discuss with the family the need to organize finances and to make advanced directive decisions and guardianship arrangements before they are needed to allow the patient input into the process.
4. OTC products, such as ginkgo biloba, have gained popularity; however, their clinical benefits have not been demonstrated to be better than placebo in well-designed randomized clinical trials. Although high doses of vitamin E (2,000 international units) have shown to delay nursing home placement by a few months, there is no evidence of cognitive improvements, and doses higher than 400 international units have been associated with bleeding and cardiovascular events. Families should be encouraged to discuss their use with the health care provider and not abandon conventional treatment.
5. For additional information, refer families to:
   Alzheimer's Association: *www.alz.org*.
   Alzheimer's Disease Education and Referral Center: *www.nia.nih.gov/Alzheimers*.

Evaluation: Expected Outcomes

- Participates in ADL without agitation or resistance.
- Remains free from injury.
- Sleeps 6 to 8 hours a night with a 1-hour rest period twice per day.
- Caregiver reports using support systems and community resources.

LEGAL AND ETHICAL CONSIDERATIONS

Restraint Use

Since the Nursing Home Reform Act took effect in October 1990, long-term care facilities throughout the United States have been required to follow guidelines emphasizing individualized, less restrictive care for residents.

The goal should be to minimize restraint use. This is a challenge, yet there are many nursing strategies that can be implemented to help reduce restraint use. And, although most nurses cite the rationale for placing a restraint on a patient is for patient safety, there is little evidence that patient safety or a reduction in injuries is actually achieved.

There are many alternative approaches to care as well as how to minimize risks associated with falls, as outlined at *https://consultgeri. org/geriatric-topics/physical-restraints* and *https://consultgeri.org/try-this/dementia/issue-d1* and *https://consultgeri.org/patient-symptoms/ pulling-out-tubes*.

Guidelines

1. The following are the federal requirements for the use of restraints based on the 1987 Omnibus Budget Reconciliation Act.
2. These guidelines must be met in any long-term care facility that participates in Medicare or Medicaid. However, these guidelines are useful for health care providers working with older adults in all settings.
   a. The resident has the right to be free from any physical restraints imposed or psychoactive drug administered for purposes of discipline or convenience and not required to treat the resident's medical symptoms.
   b. Physical restraints are any manual method of physical or mechanical device, material, or equipment attached or adjacent to the resident's body that the person cannot remove easily, which restricts freedom of movement or access to one's body (includes leg and arm restraints, hand mitts, soft ties or vest, wheelchair safety bars, and geriatric chairs).
   c. There must be a trial of less restrictive measures unless the physical restraint is necessary to provide life-saving treatment.
   d. The resident or legal representative must consent to the use of restraints.
   e. Residents who are restrained should be released, exercised, toileted, and checked for skin redness every 2 hours.
   f. The need for restraints should be re-evaluated periodically.
   g. The specific facility will have to develop policies and procedures for the appropriate use of restraints and psychoactive drugs.
   h. Primary health care providers will have to write appropriate orders for restraints and psychoactive drugs.
3. The most frequently reported reason for nurses' use of restraints is to prevent patients from harming themselves or others. Specifically, they are used to prevent falls and prevent removal of catheters or IV lines.
4. Multiple studies have found that restraints actually increase incidence of falls, can result in patient strangulation, can increase patient confusion, can cause pressure ulcers and nosocomial infections, can decrease functional ability, and can result in social isolation.
5. In regard to the patient's personal and social integrity, restraints have resulted in emotional responses of anger, fear, resistance, humiliation, demoralization, discomfort, resignation, and denial.

Alternative Interventions Instead of Restraints

1. Evaluate those patients who are considered to be in need of a restraint. Evaluation should include physical function and cognitive status (see page 136), elimination history, history of falls, vision impairment, BP (specifically evaluating for orthostatic hypotension), and medication use.
2. Attempt to correct any problems identified in the evaluation, such as vision impairment or unsafe gait.
3. Use the evaluation to determine patients at high risk of falling (eg, those with confusion, orthostatic hypotension, multiple medication regimens, and altered gait).
4. Use interventions as alternatives to restraints as outlined in Box 9-4.

BOX 9-4 **Techniques to Prevent Falls as Alternative to Restraints**

FOR ALL PATIENTS

- Familiarize patient with environment (ie, identify call light or bell to ring, label the bathroom, kitchen, closet).
- Have patient demonstrate ways to obtain help if needed.
- Place bed in low position with brakes locked if possible, or mattress on the floor.
- Make sure that footwear is fitted and nonslip and is used properly.
- Determine appropriate use of side rails based on cognitive and functional status.
- Utilize nightlight.
- Keep floor surfaces clean and dry.
- Keep room uncluttered and make sure that furniture is in optimal condition.
- Make sure patient knows where personal possessions are and can safely access them.
- Ensure adequate handrails in bathroom (commode, shower, and tub), room, and hallway.
- Establish a care plan to maintain bowel and bladder function.
- Evaluate effects of medications that increase the patient's risk of falling.
- Encourage participation in functional activities and exercise at patient's highest possible level and refer to physical therapy as appropriate.
- Monitor patient regularly and encourage safe activities.

FOR PATIENTS AT HIGH RISK FOR FALLING WHEN WALKING INDEPENDENTLY

- Use specially designed chairs that make independent transfer difficult.
- Use a chair alarm and bed alarm when the patient cannot be visually supervised.
- Institute physical therapy and increased exercise activities to help strengthen muscles and improve function.
- For the patient who interferes with treatment, evaluate the need for invasive treatments. When such treatments are essential, use mittens or gloves rather than restraints.
- For the patient who wanders, provide an exercise program or establish a bounded environment in which the person can ambulate freely.
- For aggressive and agitated patients, be aware that restraints may only make the behavior worse. Provide a low-stimulus environment, consistent caregivers, and appropriate medications to help control the agitation. Music therapy has also been shown to decrease aggressive behavior.

Advance Directives

The 1990 Patient Self-Determination Act, which requires that patients be asked about the existence of advanced directives at the time of enrollment into a health care facility, has increased awareness of older adults' rights to determine their own care. Based on the ethical principle of autonomy (a person's privilege of self-rule), advance directives provide a clear and detailed expression of a person's wishes for care. Providing an older adult with the opportunity to discuss their end-of-life plans is helpful. A four-step process includes initiating a discussion, facilitating the discussion, completing the document, and updating.

Durable power of attorney is now called *health care proxy*. It involves the designation of another person to make health care decisions for an incapacitated person. Many states have official documents that can be downloaded from their websites with detailed information about advanced directives and health care proxy.

 EVIDENCE BASE Farber-Post, M., Boltz, M. (2016). Advance care planning. In M. Boltz, E. Capezuti, T. Fulmer, & D. Zwicker (Eds.), *Evidence-based geriatric nursing protocols for best practice* (5th ed., pp. 691–701). New York, NY: Springer Publishing Co.

Types of Advance Directives

Living Wills

1. Living wills were the first and most widespread type of advance directive.
2. They were proposed as a mechanism for refusing "heroic" or unwanted medical intervention for the dying person.
3. They allow a person to state in writing that certain life-sustaining treatments should be withdrawn or withheld when that person is dying and unable to directly communicate his or her wishes.
4. Living wills only allow for the refusal of further treatment. They are not precise in terms of directives and focus only on the patient who is clearly terminally ill.

Health Care Proxy

1. This document appoints a proxy to act on behalf of another person, provides guidance for the proxy, and endures even when the maker is incapacitated.
2. This is always a written document.
3. The document states the preferences and perhaps even the values of its maker. It outlines the types of decisions the person would want to have made on his behalf.
4. Because no health care proxy document can cover all situations, the document should name a person who has the task of ensuring that the patient's wishes are honored. The proxy has the responsibility to interpret the document and extrapolate its contents to situations not specifically covered.

Medical Orders for Life Sustaining Treatment (MOLST)

1. Many states are beginning to implement a standard health care provider order form that indicates patient choices for a variety of life-sustaining treatment and is used across health care facilities.
2. MOLST (also known as Physician Orders for Life Sustaining Treatment—POLST) is important for patients with serious health conditions who:
   a. Want to avoid or receive any or all life-sustaining treatment.
   b. Are residents of long-term care facilities.
   c. Might die within a year.
3. Completion of the MOLST begins with a conversation or a series of conversations between the patient, patient's health care agent or surrogate, primary care provider, and specialist care provider.
4. The health care provider should help delineate the patient's goals for care, review possible treatment options on the entire MOLST form, and facilitate informed medical decision-making.
5. The completed form can then also be used as a medical order across health care settings, from emergency personnel responding to the patient at home and to the staff of an intensive care unit.

Nursing and Patient Care Considerations

1. Under the Patient Self-Determination Act, all patients who enter a Medicare- or Medicaid-certified facility, nursing home, or home health agency must:
   a. Be provided with information about the state's laws and the facility's policies regarding advance directive.
   b. Be asked if they have advance directives.
   c. Have their advance directives placed in their medical record.
2. Education of patients and families is essential in helping them to understand the difference between living wills, MOLST, or health care proxy and determining which document best suits their needs.
3. Patients and families need to be educated about what is involved in undergoing various life-sustaining procedures so they can make a decision regarding their future treatment.
4. Patients need to be informed that they can have more than one advance directive. That is, if a patient has a living will but is not terminally ill, encourage the patient to obtain a health care proxy to ensure that health care wishes will be met in any situation.

Community and Home Care Considerations

1. Information about completing advance directives can be obtained by contacting the National Palliative Care and Hospice Organization at *www.caringinfo.org*.
2. Instruct older adults that they will be allowed to record their wishes about various types of medical treatments, and let them appoint a proxy for if and when they are unable to make those decisions on their own.

Advocacy for Persons with Disabilities

There are an estimated 54 million Americans, not all of whom are older adults, with disabilities. Disability may strike any age group, ethnic or racial origin, and socioeconomic group. Nurses must not only provide skilled physical care to reduce complications and enhance the rehabilitation potential of disabled persons, they must also act as advocates to help these individuals transcend their disabilities to be as independent, functional, and self-actualized as possible. The United States Surgeon General's Call to Action to Improve the Health and Wellness of Persons with Disability requests that all health care providers do the following:

- Give each patient the information necessary to live a long and healthy life.
- Listen and respond to the patient's health concerns.
- Communicate clearly and directly.
- Take the time needed to meet the patient's health care needs.

Definition of Disability

1. A disability can be viewed as any restriction or lack of ability to perform activities in a manner that is normal for most people.
2. The Americans with Disabilities Act (1990) defines a disability as a physical or mental impairment that substantially limits one or more major life activities. A person can also be disabled if there is a record of such an impairment or is regarded as having such an impairment.
3. Handicap is an outdated term; there should be no reason for an individual with a disability to be handicapped. A handicap is a disadvantage resulting from an impairment that limits or prevents fulfillment of a role.

Disability Laws

1. There were many laws enacted in the United States in the 20th century to provide funding for health care, education, and vocational rehabilitation.
   a. Initial laws were limited and focused on groups, such as wounded soldiers, injured workers, and veterans.
   b. The Social Security Act of 1935 broadened vocational rehabilitation to cover civilians and gave rehabilitation a permanent legislative basis.
   c. Medicare and Medicaid were created in 1965 as an amendment to the Social Security Act to provide health insurance and benefits to individuals based on age, presence of disability, and low income. Medical and nursing care are covered.
2. The Rehabilitation Act of 1973 was the first federal law in the United States to protect persons with a disability from discrimination.
   a. This law focused on access to public buildings and transportation, discrimination in the workplace, and independent living situations.
   b. However, this law only applied to facilities and programs supported by the federal government and did not affect the private sector.
3. The Americans with Disabilities Act of 1990 amended previous legislation and made it illegal to discriminate against individuals with disabilities in the private sector as well as the public sector. Areas of focus are:
   a. Employers with 15 or more employees must provide qualified individuals with disabilities an equal opportunity to benefit from employment, including the hiring, training, promotion, and other privileges of employment. Employers are required to provide reasonable accommodations for the known physical or mental limitations of otherwise qualified individuals, so long as accommodations do not cause undue hardship to the employer.
   b. All state and local government institutions are required to provide equal opportunities for individuals with disabilities to take part in all programs, services, and activities, regardless of federal funding status.
   c. Public accommodations, which calls for the removal of barriers in public places that may be owned by private entities, such as restaurants, shops, hotels, and private schools. In addition, courses and examinations related to educational programs must be provided in a manner accessible to all despite obstacles such as hearing, vision, or speech limitations.
   d. Telecommunication relay services are required in all areas to allow those with hearing and speech limitations to communicate with others through a third party.

Problems for Persons with Disabilities

1. Psychosocial adaptation to a disability is an ongoing process that progresses through stages: shock, denial, depression, ambivalence, and adaptation. It may become stalled at one or more stages and not reach adaptation.
2. Caregiver and family strain because of loss of income, hopelessness, and physical and mental exhaustion from taking over roles and responsibilities from the person with a disability may impede successful rehabilitation.
3. Despite laws, persons with disabilities are still discriminated against when applying for jobs and educational programs. To get around the laws, employers and educational systems may list multiple physical requirements of a job or program that are meant to discourage disabled persons from applying or that would prompt failure, even though these physical requirements may have nothing to do with the actual job.
4. In addition to physical barriers at workplaces and educational institutions, persons with disabilities must overcome tremendous attitude barriers. Once a disability is known, stereotyping and prejudice may overshadow a person's potential.

Nursing Interventions for Advocacy

1. Become familiar with Medicare and Medicaid regulations and coverage in the United States and assist patients with the medical forms.
   a. Medicare is available to individuals with a disability after 2 continuous years of disability with inability to work. Medicare is provided through the federal government and is not driven by income level.
   b. Medicare does cover health care provider visits, hospitalizations, and medications, but does not cover some durable medical equipment.
   c. Eligibility for Medicaid is based on income level and how many persons are in the household and is controlled by the state and local government. This may cover very-low-income people with disabilities.
2. Help individuals in the United States understand the eligibility for Social Security disability income if their medical condition lasts for 1 year or longer and they are unable to perform substantial employment. The individual must have worked within the last 5 years and have adequate employment credits.
3. Become aware of social services in your geographic area, both through government and charitable programs, such as public transportation that will transport individuals who use wheelchairs to medical appointments.
4. Assist patients in obtaining prescription drugs through discounted and free programs that may be available through pharmaceutical companies to those who do not have limited prescription coverage. Contact pharmaceutical companies directly or *www.ppaRx.com* Partnership for Pharmaceutical Assistance) for eligibility requirements and applications.
5. If your facility is not fully accessible for persons with disabilities, advocate for structural changes that allow access.
6. When providing care for a person with a disability, always ask if you can assist and allow the individual to direct your assistance. Most individuals with disabilities know what works for them and what causes the least amount of discomfort.
7. Be aware that an individual with an acquired disability goes through an adjustment phase that can be compared with bereavement. Allow the individual time and respect for where they are in the process. Denial can last a year or more and they must be supported, not pushed, to move on in the process.

8. Be aware of your own biases and attitudes toward individuals with a disability. Refrain from stereotyping. Also be aware that not all disabilities are visible (eg, mental illness or impairment from a head injury). Treat all persons with respect and understanding.

9. Encourage sensitivity training in your facility for all employees to ensure compassionate care and polite interactions with all individuals with a disability.

10. Utilize the following resources for additional information and support:
    - Americans with Disabilities Act: *www.ada.gov*
    - Centers for Disease Control and Prevention; Disability and Health: *www.cdc.gov/ncbddd/disabilityandhealth/index.html*
    - Youreable (products, services, and information for disabled persons): *www.youreable.com*
    - National Organization on Disability: *www.nod.org*
    - National Council on Disability: *www.ncd.gov*
    - Association of Rehabilitation Nurses: *www.rehabnurse.org*
    - ExceptionalNurse.com (resources for nurses with disabilities): *www.exceptionalnurse.com*

SELECTED REFERENCES

Abraha, I., Rimland, J. M., Trotta, F., et al. (2016). Non-pharmacological interventions to prevent or treat delirium in older patients: Clinical practice recommendations the SENATOR-ONTOP series. *Journal of Nutrition, Health & Aging, 20*(9), 927–936.

Aguado, T. M., Barratt, J., Beard, J. R., Blomberg, B. B., Chen, W. H., Hickling, J., … Ortiz, J. R. (2017). Report on WHO meeting on immunization in older adults. *Vaccine, 36*(7), 921–931.

Anderson, J. G., Lopez, R. P., Rose, K. M., & Specht, J. K. (2017). Nonpharmacological strategies for patients with early-stage dementia or mild cognitive impairment: A 10-year update. *Research in Gerontological Nursing, 10*(1), 5–11.

Andy, U. U., Vaughan, C. P., Burgio, K. L., et al. (2016). Shared risk factors for constipation, fecal incontinence, and combined symptoms in older U.S. adults. *Journal of the American Geriatrics Society, 64*(11), e183–e188.

Blustein, J., Weinstein, B. E., & Chodosh, J. (2018). Tackling hearing loss to improve the care of older adults. *British Medical Journal, 360*, k21.

Buys, D. R., Campbell, A. D., Godfryd, A., et al. (2017). Meals enhancing nutrition after discharge: Findings from a pilot randomized controlled trial. *Journal of the Academy of Nutrition and Dietetics, 117*(4), 599–608.

By the American Geriatrics Society 2015 Beers Criteria Update Expert Panel. (2015). American Geriatrics Society 2015 updated Beers Criteria for potentially inappropriate medication use in older adults. *Journal of the American Geriatrics Society, 63*(11), 2227–2246.

Carey, R. M., & Whelton, P. K. (2018). Prevention, detection, evaluation, and management of high blood pressure in adults: Synopsis of the 2017 American College of Cardiology/American Heart Association Hypertension Guideline. *Annals of Internal Medicine, 168*(5):351–358.

Cornelius, R., Herrn K. A., Gordon, D. B., Kretzer, K., & Butcher, H. K. (2017). Evidence-based practice guideline: Acute pain management in older adults. *Journal of Gerontological Nursing, 43*(2):18–27.

Del Signore, A. (2016). Self-management of LUTS: Behavioral changes following continence workshops for older women. *Annals of Long Term Care, 24*(8), 9.

Earner, G., Taheri, A., Chenn, S., Daviduck, Q., Chambers, T., Shi, X., & Khadarro, R. G. (2018). Comprehensive geriatric assessment for older people admitted to a surgical service. *Cochrane Database Systematic Review,1*:CD012485.

Farber-Post, L., & Boltz, M. (2016). Advanced care planning. In M. Boltz, E. Capezuti, T. Fulmer, & D. Zwicker (Eds.), *Evidence-based geriatric nursing protocols for best practice* (5th ed., pp. 691–692–701). New York: Springer Publishing Company.

Hanlon, J. T., Perera, S., Newman, A. B., et al. (2017). Potential drug-drug and drug-disease interactions in well-functioning community-dwelling older adults. *Journal of Clinical Pharmacy and Therapeutics, 42*(2), 228–233. *https://doi.org/10.1111/jcpt.12502*

Katz, S., Ford, A. B., & Moskowitz, R. W., et al. (1963). Studies of illness in the aged: The Index of ADL: A standardized measure of biologic and psychosocial function. *Journal of the American Medical Association, 185*, 914–919.

Kim, L. D., Koncilja, K., & Nielsen, C. (2018). Medication management in older adults. *Cleveland Clinic Journal of Medicine, 85*(2), 129–135.

Lach, H. W. (2016). Changing the practice of physical restraint use in acute care. *Journal of Gerontological Nursing, 42*(2), 17–26.

Lanctôt, K. L., Amatniek, J., Ancoli-Israel, S., et al. (2017). Neuropsychiatric signs and symptoms of Alzheimer's disease: New treatment paradigms. *Alzheimer's and Dementia: The Journal of the Alzheimer's Association, 3*(3):440–449.

Lozano-Montoya, I., Vélez-Díaz-Pallarés, M., Abraha, I., et al. (2016). Nonpharmacologic interventions to prevent pressure ulcers in older patients: An overview of systematic reviews (The Software ENgine for the Assessment and optimization of drug and non-drug Therapy in Older peRsons [SENATOR] Definition of Optimal Evidence-Based Non-drug Therapies in Older People [ONTOP] Series). *Journal of the American Medical Directors Association, 17*(4), 370.e1–370.e10.

Mahoney, F., & Barthel, D. (1965). Functional evaluation: The Barthel index. *Maryland State Medical Journal, 14*, 62–72.

Nylén, P., Favero, F., Glimne, S., et al. (2014). Vision, light and aging: A literature overview on older-age workers. *Work, 47*(3), 399–412.

O'Connor, M., Hanlon, A., Mauer, E., et al. (2017). Identifying distinct risk profiles to predict adverse events among community-dwelling older adults. *Geriatric Nursing, 38*(6), 510–519.

O'Connor, M., Murtaugh, C. M., Shah, S., et al. (2016). Patient characteristics predicting readmission among individuals hospitalized for heart failure. *Medical Care Research & Review, 73*(1), 3–40.

Park, J., & Palmer, M. H. (2015). Factors associated with incomplete bladder emptying in older women with overactive bladder symptoms. *Journal of the American Geriatrics Society, 63*(7), 1426–1431.

Pilotto, A., Cella, A., Pilotto, A., et al. (2017). Three decades of comprehensive geriatric assessment: Evidence coming from different healthcare settings and specific clinical conditions. *Journal of the American Medical Directors Association, 18*(2), 192.e1–192.e11.

Rausch, A., Caljouw, M. A. A., & van der Ploeg, E. S. (2017). Keeping the person with dementia and the informal caregiver together: A systematic review of psychosocial interventions. *International Psychogeriatrics, 29*(4), 583–593.

Resnick, B., Galik, E., Wells, C. L., et al. (2015). Optimizing physical activity among older adults post trauma: Overcoming system and patient challenges. *International Journal of Orthopaedic and Trauma Nursing, 19*(4), 194–206.

Smaerup, M., Grönvall, E., Larsen, S. B., et al. (2017). Exercise gaming—A motivational approach for older adults with vestibular dysfunction. *Disability and Rehabilitation Assistive Technology, 12*(2), 137–144.

Smeltzer, S. C., Mariani, B., de Mange, E. P., et al. (2016). Perceptions of persons with disability of their experience as standardized patients. *Nursing Research, 65*(2), E89–E90.

Talley, K. M. C., Wyman, J. F., Olson-Kellogg, B., et al. (2016). Reliability and validity of two measures of toileting skills in frail older women without dementia. *Journal of Gerontological Nursing, 42*(9), 16–20.

The Hartford Institute for Geriatric Nursing. (n.d.) Unable to control urine. ConsultGeri. Available: *https://consultgeri.org/patient-symptoms/unable-control-urine*. Retrieved on February 19, 2017.

Vaughan, C. P., Markland, A. D., Smith, P. P., Burgio, K. L., & Kuchel, G. A; American Geriatrics Society/National Institute on Aging Urinary Incontinence Conference Planning Committee and Faculty. (2018). Report and research agenda of the American Geriatrics Society and National Institute on Aging bedside-to-bench conference on urinary incontinence in older adults: A translational research agenda for a complex geriatric syndrome. *Journal of the American Geriatrics Society, 66*, 773–782.

10

Respiratory Function and Therapy

OVERVIEW AND ASSESSMENT

 See additional online content: Procedure Guidelines 10-1 and 10-2.

Respiratory Function

The major function of the pulmonary system (lungs and pulmonary circulation) is to deliver oxygen (O_2) to cells and remove carbon dioxide (CO_2) from the cells (gas exchange). The adequacy of oxygenation and ventilation is measured by partial pressure of arterial oxygen (PaO_2) and partial pressure of arterial carbon dioxide ($PaCO_2$). The pulmonary system also functions as a blood reservoir for the left ventricle when it is needed to boost cardiac output, as a protector for the systemic circulation by filtering debris/particles, and as a provider of metabolic functions such as surfactant production and endocrine functions.

Terminology

1. Alveolus—air sac where gas exchange takes place.
2. Apex—top portion of the upper lobes of the lungs.
3. Base—bottom portion of the lower lobes of the lungs, located just above the diaphragm.
4. Bronchoconstriction—constriction of smooth muscle surrounding bronchioles.
5. Bronchus—large airways; lung divides into right and left bronchi.
6. Carina—a ridge at the base of the trachea that separates the right and left mainstem bronchi.
7. Cilia—hairlike projections on the tracheobronchial epithelium, which aid in the movement of secretions and removal of debris.
8. Compliance—ability of the lungs to distend and change in volume relative to an applied change in pressure (eg, emphysema—lungs very compliant; fibrosis—lungs noncompliant or stiff).
9. Dead space—ventilation that does not participate in gas exchange; also known as wasted ventilation when there is adequate ventilation but no perfusion, as in pulmonary embolus or pulmonary vascular bed occlusion. Normal dead space is 150 mL.
10. Diaphragm—primary muscle used for respiration; located just below the lung bases; it separates the chest and abdominal cavities.
11. Diffusion (of gas)—movement of gas from area of higher to lower concentration.
12. Dyspnea—subjective sensation of breathlessness associated with discomfort, often caused by a dissociation between motor command and mechanical response of the respiratory system as in:
    a. Respiratory muscle abnormalities (hyperinflation and airflow limitation from chronic obstructive pulmonary disease [COPD]). Abnormal ventilatory impedance (narrowing airways and respiratory impedance from COPD or asthma).

b. Abnormal breathing patterns (severe exercise, pulmonary congestion or edema, recurrent pulmonary emboli).

c. Arterial blood gas (ABG) abnormalities (hypoxemia, hypercarbia).

13. Hemoptysis—the expectoration of blood or of blood-stained sputum from the larynx, trachea, bronchi, or lungs.

14. Hypoxemia—PaO_2 less than normal, which may or may not cause symptoms. (Normal PaO_2 is 80 to 100 mm Hg on room air.)

15. Hypoxia—insufficient oxygenation at the cellular level because of an imbalance in oxygen delivery and oxygen consumption. (Usually causes symptoms reflecting decreased oxygen reaching the brain and heart.)

16. Mediastinum—compartment between lungs containing lymph and vascular tissue that separates left from right lung.

17. Orthopnea—shortness of breath when in reclining position.

18. Paroxysmal nocturnal dyspnea—sudden shortness of breath associated with sleeping in recumbent position.

19. Perfusion—blood flow, carrying oxygen and CO_2 that passes by alveoli.

20. Pleura—serous membrane enclosing the lung; composed of visceral pleura, covering all lung surfaces, and parietal pleura, covering chest wall and mediastinal structures, between which exists a potential space.

21. Pulmonary circulation—network of vessels that supply oxygenated blood to and remove CO_2-laden blood from the lungs.

22. Pulmonary hypertension—an increase in pressure in the pulmonary arteries, pulmonary vein, or pulmonary capillaries.

23. Respiration—inhalation and exhalation; at the cellular level, a process involving uptake of oxygen and removal of CO_2 and other products of oxidation.

24. Shunt—adequate perfusion without ventilation, with deoxygenated blood conducted into the systemic circulation, as in pulmonary edema, atelectasis, pneumonia, and COPD.

25. Surfactant—lipid–protein complex secreted by alveolar cells that reduces surface tension of pulmonary fluids and aids in elasticity of pulmonary tissue. Plays a role in the barrier against the entry of pathogens.

26. Ventilation—is the process by which oxygen and CO_2 are transported to and from the lungs.

27. Ventilation–perfusion (V/Q) imbalance or mismatch—imbalance of ventilation and perfusion; a cause for hypoxemia. V/Q mismatch can be due to:

a. Blood perfusing an area of the lung where ventilation is reduced or absent.

b. Ventilation of parts of the lung that is not perfused.

Subjective Data

Explore symptoms retrieved from the patient's description of an event through characterization and history taking to help anticipate needs and plan care. Encourages the patient to give a full description of the onset, the course, and the character of the problem and any factors that aggravate or relieve it.

Dyspnea

EVIDENCE BASE Chen, Y., Coxson, H., & Reid, W. D. (2016). Reliability and validity of the brief fatigue inventory and dyspnea inventory in people with chronic obstructive pulmonary disease. *Journal of Pain and Symptom Management, 52*(2), 298–304.

1. Characteristics—Is the dyspnea acute or chronic? Has it occurred suddenly or gradually? Is more than one pillow required to sleep? Is the dyspnea progressive, recurrent, or paroxysmal? Walking how far leads to shortness of breath? How does it compare to the patient's baseline level of dyspnea? Ask patient to rate dyspnea on a scale of 1 to 10, with 1 being no dyspnea and 10 being the worst imaginable. What relieves and what aggravates the dyspnea?

2. Associated factors—Is there a cough associated with the dyspnea and is it productive? What activities precipitate the shortness of breath? Does it seem to be worse when upset? Is it influenced by the time of day, seasons, and/or certain environments? Does it occur at rest or with exertion? Any fever, chills, night sweats, ankle/leg swelling? Any change in body weight?

3. History—Is there a patient history or family history of chronic lung disease, cardiac or neuromuscular disease, cancer, problems with blood clotting, or immunocompromise? What is the smoking history?

4. Significance—Sudden dyspnea could indicate pulmonary embolus, pneumothorax, myocardial infarction (MI), acute heart failure, or acute respiratory failure. In a postsurgical or postpartum patient, dyspnea may indicate pulmonary embolus or edema. Orthopnea can be indicative of heart disease or COPD. If dyspnea is associated with a wheeze, consider asthma, COPD, heart failure, or upper airway obstruction. When dyspnea occurs in combination with fatigue, pulmonary hypertension may exist. Metabolic disorders, psychiatric conditions, and neuromuscular disorders may also contribute to dyspnea.

Chest Pain

1. Characteristics—Is the pain sharp, dull, stabbing, or aching? Is it intermittent or persistent? Is the pain localized or does it radiate? If it radiates, where? How intense is the pain? Are there factors that alleviate or aggravate the pain, such as position or activity?

2. Associated factors—What effect do inspiration and expiration have on the pain? What other symptoms accompany the chest pain? Is there diaphoresis, shortness of breath, or nausea?

3. History—Is there a smoking history or environmental exposure? Has the pain ever been experienced before? What was the cause? Is there a preexisting pulmonary or cardiac diagnosis? Has there been recent trauma?

4. Significance—Chest pain related to pulmonary causes is usually felt on the side where pathology arises, but it can be referred. Dull persistent pain may indicate carcinoma of the lung, whereas sharp, stabbing pain usually arises from the pleura. Dyspnea with pleuritic chest pain indicates clinically significant pulmonary embolism.

Cough

EVIDENCE BASE Irwin, R., French, C., Lewis, Z. S., et al. (2014). Overview of the management of cough: Chest guideline and expert panel report. *Chest, 146*(4), 885–889.

1. Characteristics—Is the cough dry, hacking, loose, barky, wheezy, or more like clearing the throat? Is it strong or weak? How frequent is it? Is it worse at night or at any time of day? Does the intensity change on days off from work? Is there

seasonal variation? Is it aggravated by food intake or exertion? Is it alleviated by any medication? How long has it been going on?

2. Associated factors—Is the cough productive? If so, what is the consistency, amount, color, and odor of the sputum? Is there hemoptysis? How does sputum compare to the patient's baseline? Is it associated with shortness of breath, pain, or nausea?

3. History—Is there a smoking history? Is the smoking current or in the past? Has there been any environmental or occupational exposure to dust, fumes, or gases that could lead to cough? Are there past pulmonary diagnoses, asthma, rhinitis, allergy, or exposure to allergens, such as pollen, house dust mites, animal dander, birds, mold or fungi, cockroach waste, and irritants (smoke, odors, perfumes, cleaning products, exhaust, pollution, cold air)? Has there been prolonged exposure to dampness, chemical sanitizers, cobalt or other hard metals, beryllium, asbestos, dusts from coal, wood, or grains? Does the patient have a history of acid reflux, postnasal drip or use an angiotensin-converting enzyme inhibitor with a common adverse effect of cough? Has there been a concurrent voice change? Has the patient recently traveled outside the country? Can the patient identify any specific triggers? Is the patient immunocompromised?

4. Significance—A dry, irritative cough may indicate viral respiratory tract infection. A cough at night should alert to potential left-sided heart failure, asthma, or postnasal drip worsening at night. A morning cough with sputum might be bronchitis. A cough that is less severe on days off from work may be related to occupational or environmental exposures. A patient with severe or changing cough should be evaluated for bronchogenic carcinoma. Consider bacterial pneumonia if sputum is rusty and lung tumor if it is pink-tinged. A profuse pink frothy sputum could be indicative of pulmonary edema. A cough associated with food intake could indicate problems with aspiration. A dry cough may be associated with pulmonary fibrosis. History of recent travel may be associated with infection from a source not commonly identified in the United States.

Hemoptysis

1. Characteristics—Is the blood from the lungs? It could be from the GI system (hematemesis) or upper airway (epistaxis). Is it bright red and frothy? How much? Is onset associated with certain circumstances or activities? Was the onset sudden, and is it intermittent or continuous?

2. Associated factors—Was there an initial sensation of tickling in the throat? Was there a salty taste or burning or bubbling sensation in the chest? Has there been shortness of breath, chest pain, or difficulty with exertion?

3. History—Was there any recent chest trauma or respiratory treatment (chest percussion)? Does the patient have an upper respiratory infection, sinusitis, or recent epistaxis? Has the patient used cocaine or other illicit drugs?

4. Significance—Hemoptysis can be linked to pulmonary infection, pulmonary edema, COPD, lung carcinoma, abnormalities of the heart or blood vessels, pulmonary artery or vein abnormalities, or pulmonary emboli and infarction. Small amounts of blood-tinged sputum may be from the upper respiratory tract, and regurgitation of blood comes from a GI bleed.

Objective Data

The process in which data relating to the patient's problem are obtained through direct physical examination, including observation, palpation, percussion, auscultation; laboratory analysis; radiologic and other studies.

 EVIDENCE BASE Heuer, A., & Scanlan, C. (2017). *Wilkins clinical assessment in respiratory care* (8th ed.). St. Louis, Mo: Mosby.

Key Observations

1. What is the respiratory rate, depth, and pattern? Are accessory muscles being used? Is the patient breathing through the mouth or pursing lips during exhalation? Is sputum being expectorated, and what is its appearance and odor?

2. Is there an increase in the anterior to posterior chest diameter, suggesting air trapping?

3. Is there obvious orthopnea or splinting?

4. Is there clubbing of the fingers, associated with bronchiectasis, lung abscess, empyema, cystic fibrosis, pulmonary neoplasms, and various other disorders?

5. Is there central cyanosis indicating possible hypoxemia or cardiac disease? Are mucous membranes and nail beds pink?

6. Are there signs of tracheal deviation, as seen with pneumothorax?

7. Are the jugular veins distended? Is there peripheral edema or other signs of cardiac dysfunction?

8. Does palpation of the chest cause pain? Is chest expansion symmetrical? Any change in tactile fremitus or egophony?

9. Is percussion of lung fields resonant bilaterally? Is diaphragmatic excursion equal bilaterally?

10. Are breath sounds present and equal bilaterally? Are the lung fields clear or are there rhonchi, wheezing, crackles, stridor, or pleural friction rub? Does auscultation reveal egophony, bronchophony, or whispered pectoriloquy?

Laboratory Studies

Arterial Blood Gas Analysis

Description

1. An ABG is a laboratory test that measures (PaO_2) oxygen tension, ($PaCO_2$) carbon dioxide tension, acidity (pH), oxyhemoglobin saturation SaO_2, and bicarbonate (HCO_3). This provides a means of assessing the adequacy of ventilation.

2. Allows assessment of body's acid–base (pH) status, indicating if acidosis or alkalosis is present, whether acidosis or alkalosis is respiratory or metabolic in origin, and whether it is compensated or uncompensated.

3. Used for diagnostic evaluation and evaluation of response to clinical interventions (oxygen therapy, mechanical ventilation, noninvasive ventilation, etc.).

Nursing and Patient Care Considerations

1. Blood can be obtained from any artery but is usually drawn from the radial, brachial, or femoral site. It can be drawn directly by percutaneous needle puncture or accessed by way of indwelling arterial catheter. Determine facility policy for qualifications for ABG sampling and site of arterial puncture.

2. If the radial artery is used, an Allen test must be performed before the puncture to determine if collateral circulation is present.

3. Arterial puncture should not be performed through a lesion, through or distal to a surgical shunt, or in area where peripheral vascular disease or infection is present.

4. Absolute contraindications include an abnormal modified Allen test, severe peripheral vascular disease of the artery being sampled, active Raynaud syndrome, and local infection at the arterial site.

5. Coagulopathy or medium- to high-dose anticoagulation therapy may be a relative contraindication for arterial puncture.

6. Results may be affected by recent changes in oxygen therapy, suctioning, or positioning.

7. Interpret ABG values by looking at trends for the patient as well as the following normal values:
   a. PaO_2—partial pressure of arterial oxygen (80 to 100 mm Hg).
   b. $PaCO_2$—partial pressure of arterial carbon dioxide (35 to 45 mm Hg).
   c. SaO_2—arterial oxygen saturation (greater than 95%).
   d. pH—hydrogen ion concentration or degree of acid–base balance (7.35 to 7.45).
   e. (HCO_3^-)—bicarbonate primarily a metabolic buffer (22 to 26 mEq/L).

Sputum Examination

Description

1. Sputum may be obtained for evaluation of gross appearance, microscopic examination, Gram stain, culture and sensitivity, acid-fast bacillus, and cytology.
   a. The direct smear shows presence of white blood cells and intracellular (pathogenic) bacteria and extracellular (mostly nonpathogenic) bacteria.
   b. Gram stain shows whether bacteria is gram-positive or gram-negative and can be used to guide therapy until culture and sensitivity results are available.
   c. The sputum culture is used to identify presence of specific pathogens; sensitivity determines drug efficacy and serves as a guide for drug treatment (ie, choice of antibiotic).
   d. Acid-fast smears detect presence of pathogens such as *Mycobacterium tuberculosis.*
   e. Cytology identifies abnormal and possibly malignant cells.

Nursing and Patient Care Considerations

1. Patients receiving antibiotics, steroids, and immunosuppressive agents for a prolonged time may have periodic sputum examinations because these agents may give rise to opportunistic pulmonary infections.

2. It is important that the sputum be collected correctly and that the specimen be sent to a laboratory immediately. Allowing it to stand in a warm room will result in overgrowth of organisms, making identification of pathogen difficult; this also alters cell morphology. A series of three early morning specimens is needed for acid-fast bacillus examination. Cytology samples should be collected in container with fixative solution.

3. Sputum can be obtained by various methods:
   a. Deep breathing and coughing.
      i. An early morning specimen obtained prior to eating or drinking yields best sample of deep pulmonary secretions from all lung fields.
      ii. Have patient clear nose and throat and rinse mouth with plain water—to decrease contamination by oral and upper respiratory flora.
      iii. Position patient upright or in high Fowler's unless contraindicated. Instruct patient to take several deep breaths, exhale, and perform a series of short coughs.
      iv. Have patient cough deeply and expectorate the sputum into a sterile container.
      v. If patient is unable to produce specimen, increasing oral fluid intake may be useful (unless on fluid restriction).
   b. Induction through use of ultrasonic or hypertonic saline nebulization.
      i. Patient inhales mist through mouth slowly and deeply for 10 to 20 minutes.
      ii. Nebulization increases the moisture content of air going to lower tract; particles will condense on tracheobronchial tree and aid in expectoration.
   c. Suctioning—aspiration of secretions via mechanical means; must be used with caution because it may cause bleeding, cardiac dysrhythmias, and increased intracranial pressure.
      i. Tracheal, through endotracheal (ET) or tracheostomy tube.
      ii. Nasotracheal (NT), through nose and into back of throat or trachea.
   d. Bronchoscopy with bronchoalveolar lavage, in which 60 to 100 mL, is instilled and aspirated from various lung segments. Sedation and/or anesthesia is required.
   e. Gastric aspiration (rarely necessary since advent of ultrasonic nebulizer).
      i. Nasogastric (NG) tube is inserted into the stomach, approximately 50 mL sterile water is instilled, and swallowed pulmonary secretions are siphoned out.
      ii. Useful only for culture of tubercle bacilli, not for direct examination.
      iii. Must be done as soon as patient wakes up in the morning
   f. Transtracheal aspiration involves passing a needle and then a catheter through a percutaneous puncture of the cricothyroid membrane. Transtracheal aspiration bypasses the oropharynx and avoids specimen contamination by mouth flora.

4. Generally, a sputum sample of 15 mL is adequate for laboratory testing.

Pleural Fluid Analysis

Description

1. Pleural fluid is continuously produced and reabsorbed, with a thin layer normally in the pleural space. Abnormal pleural fluid accumulation (effusion) occurs in diseases of the pleura, heart, or lymphatics. The pleural fluid is studied, with other tests, to determine the underlying cause.

2. Obtained by aspiration (thoracentesis) or by tube thoracotomy. See Figure 10-1.

3. The fluid is examined for cancerous cells, cellular makeup, chemical content, and microorganisms.

4. Pleural cavity contains 10 to 20 mL clear yellow (serous) fluid that lubricates the surfaces of the pleura, the thin membrane that lines the chest cavity and surrounds the lungs. A pleural effusion is an abnormal collection of this fluid.

5. The test is performed to determine the cause of a pleural effusion and to relieve associated shortness of breath.

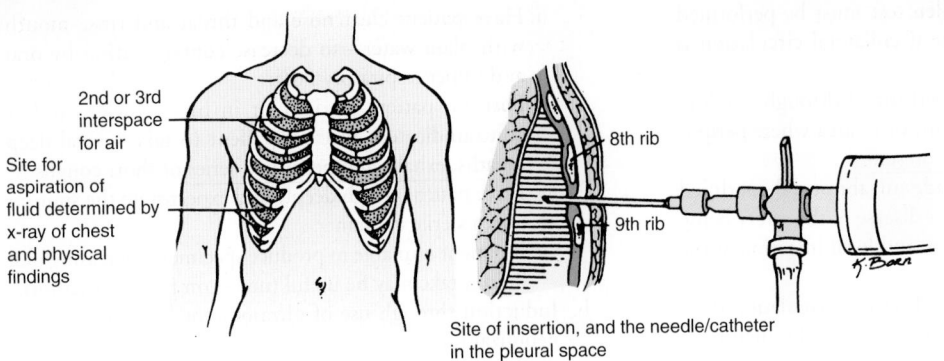

Figure 10-1. Thoracentesis for removal of pleural effusion and pleural fluid analysis.

2nd or 3rd interspace for air

Site for aspiration of fluid determined by x-ray of chest and physical findings

8th rib

9th rib

Site of insertion, and the needle/catheter in the pleural space

Nursing and Patient Care Considerations

1. If done at bedside, prepare the patient by assisting to a supported upright position with lateral and posterior thorax of particular side exposed or in side-lying position with head of bed elevated 30 to 45 degrees and arm overhead. Support the patient through the process.
2. Observe and record total amount of fluid withdrawn, nature of fluid, and its color and viscosity.
3. Prepare sample of fluid and ensure transport to the laboratory.
4. A chest x-ray may be done before or after the fluid is withdrawn.
5. Patient should not cough, breathe deeply, or move while fluid is being withdrawn.
6. Instruct patient to inform provider immediately if sharp chest pain or shortness of breath occurs.

Radiology and Imaging

Chest X-Ray

Description

1. Normal pulmonary tissue is radiolucent and appears black on film. Thus, densities produced by tumors, foreign bodies, and infiltrates can be detected as lighter or white images.
2. Commonly, two views—posterior–anterior and lateral—are obtained.
3. This test shows the position of normal structures, displacement, and presence of abnormal shadows. It may reveal pathology in the lungs in the absence of symptoms.

Nursing and Patient Care Considerations

1. Should be taken upright if patient's condition permits. Assist technician at bedside in preparing patient for portable chest x-ray.
2. Encourage patient to take deep breath, hold breath, and remain still as x-ray is taken.
3. Make sure that all jewelry, electrocardiogram (ECG) or monitor leads, and metal objects (including metal-containing transdermal patches) in x-ray field are removed so as not to interfere with film.
4. Consider the contraindication of x-rays for pregnant patients.

Computed Tomography Scan

Description

1. Cross-sectional x-rays of the lungs are taken from many different angles and processed through a computer to create three-dimensional images. This three-dimensional imaging provides more complete diagnostic information than the two-dimensional x-ray.
2. It may be used to define pulmonary nodules and pulmonary abnormalities or to demonstrate mediastinal abnormalities and hilar adenopathy.

Nursing and Patient Care Considerations

1. Describe test to patient and family, including that table will slide into doughnut-shaped scanner and patient must lie still during test. The test usually takes about 30 minutes but may take longer.
2. Be alert to allergies to iodine or other radiographic contrast media that might be used during testing.
3. For scans performed with contrast, informed consent and IV access required. Patient should take nothing by mouth (NPO) for 4 hours prior to scan. Blood urea nitrogen and creatinine should be evaluated 24 to 48 hours before test or according to facility protocol.
4. Hydrate patient well to facilitate excretion of contrast, if used.
5. Check regarding weight limit of equipment prior to scanning bariatric patients.
6. Consider the contraindication of radiologic studies for the pregnant patient, especially computed tomography (CT) scans with contrast media.

Magnetic Resonance Imaging

Description

1. Noninvasive procedure that uses a powerful magnetic field, radio waves, and a computer to produce detailed pictures of the organs, soft tissue, bone, and other internal structures.
2. Provides contrast between various soft tissues and is performed to:
   a. Assess abnormal growths, including cancer of the lungs or other tissues inadequately assessed with other imaging modalities.
   b. Determine stage of cancer, including tumor size, extent, and degree to which cancer has spread.
   c. Visualize lymph nodes and blood vessels.
   d. Assess disorders of the vertebrae, ribs, and sternum.
3. Traditional radiographic contrast media are not used but gadolinium injection or ingestion may be necessary, depending on patient's medical history and anatomy to be imaged.
4. It is helpful to synchronize the magnetic resonance imaging (MRI) picture to the ECG in thoracic studies.
5. The hazards of MRI during pregnancy are unknown, although ionizing radiation (x-ray) is not used during MRI.

Nursing and Patient Care Considerations

1. Explain procedure to patient and assess ability to remain still in a closed space; sedation may be necessary if the patient is claustrophobic. The test takes approximately 1 hour.
2. Evaluate patient for contraindications to MRI: implanted devices, such as implanted defibrillators that may malfunction; cochlear implants; or metallic surgical clips used on brain aneurysms.
3. Devices that may interfere with the exam or potentially pose a risk include artificial heart valves, implanted drug infusion ports, infusion catheters, intrauterine devices, pacemakers and neurostimulators, metallic implants such as prosthetic valves or joints, and metal pins, screws, plates, or surgical staples.
4. Make sure that all jewelry, ECG or monitor leads, hearing aids, pins/hairpins, removable dental work, and metal objects (including metal-containing transdermal patches) are removed.
5. Kidney disease and sickle cell anemia may contraindicate MRI with contrast material.
6. Check with MRI technician about the use of equipment, such as ventilator or mechanical IV pump, in MRI room.
7. Earplugs may be used to muffle loud thumping and humming noises during imaging.
8. Evaluate the patient for claustrophobia, and teach relaxation techniques to use during test or advocate for use of open MRI. Be ready to administer sedation, if necessary.
9. Check regarding size capacity of equipment prior to scanning bariatric patients.
10. It is recommended that nursing mothers not breastfeed for 36 to 48 hours after MRI with contrast.

Positron Emission Tomography Scan

Description

1. Physiologic images are obtained, based on the detection of radiation from the emission of positrons. Positrons are tiny particles emitted from a radioactive isotope–administered IV to the patient. Radioactivity localizes in the area(s) being scanned and is detected by positron emission tomography (PET). Different colors or degrees of brightness on a PET image represent different levels of tissue or organ function.
2. Radioisotope is administered 30 to 90 minutes prior to scan via IV or inhalation.
3. Distinguishes between benign and malignant lung nodules.

Nursing and Patient Care Considerations

1. Describe test to patient and family, including that table will slide into doughnut-shaped scanner and patient must lie still during test. The test usually takes 30 to 45 minutes.
2. Isotope has a short half-life and is not considered a radiologic hazard.
3. Encourage fluids to facilitate excretion of isotope.
4. Consider the contraindication of radiologic studies for the pregnant or breastfeeding patient.
5. Test results may be inaccurate for diabetic patients or for patients who have eaten within a few hours prior to the scan if blood glucose or insulin levels are not normal.

Pulmonary Angiography

Description

1. An imaging method used to study pulmonary vessels and pulmonary circulation.
2. For visualization, radiopaque medium is injected by way of a catheter in the main pulmonary artery rapidly into the vasculature of the lungs. Films are then taken in rapid succession after injection.
3. It is considered the "gold standard" for diagnosis of pulmonary embolus, but spiral CT scanning can also be effectively used.

Nursing and Patient Care Considerations

1. Determine whether patient is allergic to radiographic contrast media, describe the procedure, and obtain informed consent.
2. Patient may be kept NPO for 4 to 8 hours prior to procedure.
3. Instruct patient that injection of dye may cause flushing, cough, and a warm sensation.
4. Pulse, blood pressure (BP), and respirations are monitored during the procedure.
5. After the procedure, make sure pressure is maintained over access site and monitor pulse rate, BP, and circulation distal to the injection site.
6. Patient may be advised to keep extremity straight for up to 12 hours after the procedure.
7. Necessity of test should be carefully evaluated in patients with bleeding disorders and pregnant women.

Ventilation–Perfusion Scan

Description

1. A pair of nuclear scan tests using inhaled and injected radioisotopes to measure breathing (ventilation) and blood flow (perfusion) in all areas of the lungs. The two tests may be performed either separately or together.
2. Perfusion scan is done after injection of a radioactive isotope. It measures blood perfusion through the lungs and evaluates lung function on a regional basis.
3. Ventilation scan is done after inhalation of radioactive gas (eg, xenon with O_2), which diffuses throughout the lungs. It indicates how well air reaches all parts of the lung.
4. Usually performed to detect pulmonary embolus. Also useful in evaluating advanced pulmonary disease (COPD), detecting abnormal circulation (shunts) in the pulmonary blood vessels, evaluating lung function, and identifying fibrosis.
5. Is also referred to as *V/Q scan* because the initials are used in mathematical equations that calculate air and blood flow.

Nursing and Patient Care Considerations

1. Determine if patient is allergic to radiographic dye before V/Q scan.
2. Explain the procedure to patient and encourage cooperation with inhalation and brief episodes of breath holding.
3. Contraindicated in patients with primary pulmonary hypertension.
4. False positives may occur in patients with vasculitis, mitral stenosis, and pulmonary hypertension and when tumors obstruct a pulmonary artery with airway involvement, fatty tissues, and presence of parasites.
5. False negatives are associated with partially occluded vessels.

Other Diagnostic Tests

Bronchoscopy

EVIDENCE BASE Paradis, T., Dixon, J., & Tieu, B. (2016). The role of bronchoscopy in the diagnosis of airway disease. *Journal of Thoracic Disease, 8*(12), 3826–3837.

Description

1. The direct inspection and observation of the upper and lower respiratory tract through fiberoptic (flexible) or rigid broncho-scope as a means of diagnosing and managing inflammatory, infectious, and malignant diseases of the airway and lungs including airway injury and obstruction by a foreign body tumor or mass.
2. Flexible fiberoptic bronchoscopy allows for more patient comfort and better visualization of smaller airways, including nasal passages. It is usually performed using local anesthesia with or without moderate sedation. Fluoroscopy may be needed to facilitate specimen collection. Used for therapeutic and diagnostic procedures such as:
   a. Bronchoalveolar lavage.
   b. Endobronchial or transbronchial biopsies.
   c. Cytologic wash or brush.
   d. Transbronchial needle aspiration.
   e. Endobronchial ultrasound.
   f. Autofluorescence bronchoscopy.
   g. Balloon dilation.
   h. Endobronchial laser ablation.
   i. Electrocautery.
   j. Photodynamic therapy.
   k. Brachytherapy.
   l. Some types of stent placement.
3. Rigid bronchoscopy, often requires general anesthesia with adequate sedation and muscle relaxants, may be combined with flexible bronchoscopy for better access to distal airways. Diagnostic and therapeutic indications include:
   a. Bleeding or hemorrhage into the airway.
   b. Foreign body extraction.
   c. Deeper biopsy specimen collection than can be obtained fiberoptically.
   d. Dilation of tracheal or bronchial strictures.
   e. Relief of airway obstruction.
   f. Insertion of stents.
   g. Tracheobronchial laser therapy or other mechanical tumor ablation.

Nursing and Patient Care Considerations

1. Check that an informed consent form has been signed and that risks and benefits have been explained to the patient.
2. Make sure that IV access is present and patent.
3. Absolute contraindications include uncorrectable coagulopathy, severe refractory hypoxemia, unstable hemodynamic status, facial trauma, and unstable cervical spine. Patients with increased risk are those with MI within past 6 weeks, head injuries susceptible to increased intracranial pressures (ICP), and known or suspected pregnancy (because of possible radiation exposure).
4. Review and follow facility policy and procedure for anesthesia and sedation.
5. Administer prescribed medication to reduce secretions, block the vasovagal reflex and gag reflex, and relieve anxiety. Give encouragement and nursing support.
6. Restrict fluid and food, as ordered, before procedure to reduce risk of aspiration when reflexes are blocked. Patient may be kept NPO for 4 hours prior to flexible bronchoscopy with minimal sedation; if deeper sedation is used, patient's time on NPO is extended.
7. Remove dentures, contact lenses, and other prostheses.
8. After the procedure:
   a. Monitor cardiac rhythm and rate, BP, and level of consciousness (LOC).
   b. Monitor respiratory effort and rate.
   c. Monitor oximetry.
   d. Withhold ice chips and fluids until patient demonstrates gag reflex.
   e. Monitor patient's perceptions of pain, discomfort, and dyspnea.
9. Promptly report cyanosis, hypoventilation, hypotension, tachycardia or dysrhythmia, hemoptysis, dyspnea, and decreased breath sounds.
10. Provide outpatients with specific instructions regarding signs and symptoms of complications and what to do if they arise.

 NURSING ALERT After bronchoscopy, be alert for complications, such as pneumothorax, dysrhythmias, laryngospasm, and bronchospasm.

Lung Biopsy

Description

1. Procedures used for obtaining histologic material from the lung to aid in diagnosis include:
   a. Transbronchial biopsy—biopsy forceps inserted through bronchoscope and specimen of lung tissue obtained.
   b. Transthoracic needle aspiration biopsy—specimen obtained through needle aspiration under fluoroscopic guidance.
   c. Open lung biopsy—specimen obtained through small anterior thoracotomy; used in making a diagnosis when other biopsy methods have not been effective or are not possible.

Nursing and Patient Care Considerations

1. Obtain permission for consent, if required.
2. Observe for possible complications, including pneumothorax, hemorrhage (hemoptysis), and bacterial contamination of pleural space.
3. A chest x-ray should be done 1 hour after transbronchial biopsy to exclude pneumothorax.
4. See "Bronchoscopy" (page 167) or "Thoracic Surgeries" (page 184) for postprocedure care.

Pulmonary Function Tests

 EVIDENCE BASE Cheung, H., & Cheung, L. (2015). Coaching patients during pulmonary function testing. A practical guide. *Canadian Journal of Respiratory Therapy*, 51(3), 65–68.

Description

1. Pulmonary function tests (PFTs) are used to detect and measure abnormalities in respiratory function and quantify severity of various lung diseases. Such tests include measurements of lung volumes, ventilatory function, diffusing capacity, gas exchange, lung compliance, airway resistance, and distribution of gases in the lung.
2. Ventilatory studies (spirometry) are the most common group of tests.
   a. Requires electronic spirometer, water spirometer, or wedge spirometer that plots volume against time (timed vital capacity).

Table 10-1 Pulmonary Function Tests

TERM	SYMBOL	DESCRIPTION	REMARKS
Vital capacity	VC	Maximum volume of air exhaled after a maximum inspiration	• VC < 10–15 mL/kg suggests need for mechanical ventilation • VC > 10–15 mL/kg suggests ability to wean
Forced vital capacity	FVC	Total volume of air a patient is able to exhale for the total duration of the test during maximal effort	• Reduced in obstructive disease (COPD) because of air trapping and restrictive disease • Reflects airflow in large airways
Forced expiratory volume in 1 sec	FEV_1	Volume of air exhaled in the first second of the performance of the FVC	• Reduced in obstructive disease (COPD) because of air trapping • Reflects airflow in large airways
Ratio of FEV_1/FVC	FEV_1/FVC	FEV_1 expressed as a percentage of the FVC. The percentage of FVC expired in 1 sec	• Decreased in obstructive disease • Normal in restrictive disease
Forced midexpiratory flow	$FEF_{25\%-75\%}$	Average flow during the middle half of the FVC	• Reflects airflow in small airways • Smokers may have change in this test before other symptoms develop
Peak expiratory flow rate	PEFR	Most rapid flow during a forced expiration after a maximum inspiration	• Used to measure response to bronchodilators, airflow obstruction in patients with asthma
Maximal voluntary volume	MVV	Volume of air expired in a specified period (12 sec) during repetitive maximal effort	• An important factor in exercise tolerance • Decreases in neuromuscular diseases

b. Patient is asked to take as deep a breath as possible and then to exhale into spirometer as completely and either slowly or as forcefully as possible, depending on the type of test.

c. Results are compared with normals for patient's age, height, and sex (see Table 10-1).

d. A reduction in the vital capacity, inspiratory capacity, and total lung capacity may indicate a restrictive form of lung disease (disease because of increased lung stiffness).

e. An increase in functional reserve capacity, total lung capacity, and reduction in flow rates usually indicate an obstructive flow because of bronchial obstruction or loss of lung elastic recoil.

3. Lung volumes are determined by asking the patient to inhale a known concentration of inert gas, such as helium or 100% oxygen, and measuring concentration of inert gas or nitrogen in exhaled air (dilution method) or by plethysmography.

a. Yields thoracic volume (total lung capacity, plus any unventilated blebs or bullae).

b. An increased residual volume is found in air trapping because of obstructive lung disease.

c. A reduction in several parameters usually indicates a restrictive form of lung disease or chest wall abnormality.

4. Diffusing capacity measures lung surface effective for the transfer of gas in the lung by having patient inhale gas containing known low concentration of carbon monoxide and measuring carbon monoxide concentration in exhaled air. Difference between inhaled and exhaled concentrations is related directly to uptake of carbon monoxide across alveolar–capillary membrane. Diffusing capacity is reduced in interstitial lung disease, emphysema, pneumonectomy, pulmonary embolus, and anemia.

Nursing and Patient Care Considerations

1. Instruct the patient in correct technique for completing PFTs; coach the patient through test, if needed. Appropriate interpretation requires adequate patient cooperation and effort and accurate equipment. Instruct patient not to use oral or inhaled bronchodilator (eg, albuterol), caffeine, or tobacco at least 4 to 6 hours before the test (longer for long-acting bronchodilators).

2. Used with caution in patients with hemoptysis of unknown origin; pneumothorax; unstable cardiovascular status; recent MI or pulmonary embolus; thoracic, abdominal, or cerebral aneurysm; or recent eye, thoracic, or abdominal surgery.

3. Using a noseclip for all spirometric maneuvers is strongly recommended.

4. Although forced expiratory volume in the first second of a forced vital capacity is the "gold standard" for diagnosing airway obstruction, there is no single cutoff value separating normal from abnormal. This determination is based more on trending of individual results.

Pulse Oximetry

Description

1. Noninvasively provides an estimate of arterial oxyhemoglobin saturation by using selected wavelengths of light to determine the saturation of oxyhemoglobin. Oximeters function by passing a light beam through a vascular bed, such as the finger or earlobe, to determine the amount of light absorbed by oxygenated (red) and deoxygenated (blue) blood.

2. Calculates the amount of arterial blood that is saturated with oxygen (SaO_2) and displays this as a percentage.

3. Provides indication only of oxygenation, not ventilation.

4. Indications include:

a. Monitor adequacy of oxygen saturation; quantify response to therapy.

b. Monitor unstable patient who may experience sudden changes in blood oxygen level.

c. Evaluation of need for home oxygen therapy.

d. Determine supplemental oxygen needs at rest, with exercise, and during sleep.

e. Need to follow the trend and need to decrease number of ABG sample drawn.

5. The oxyhemoglobin dissociation curve allows for correlation between SaO_2 and PaO_2 (see Figure 10-2).

a. Increased body temperature, acidosis, and increased phosphates (2,3-DPG) cause a shift in the curve to the right, thus increasing the ability of hemoglobin to release oxygen to the tissues.

b. Decreased temperature, decreased 2,3-DPG, and alkalosis cause a shift to the left, causing hemoglobin to hold on to the oxygen, reducing the amount of oxygen being released to the tissues.

6. Increased bilirubin, increased carboxyhemoglobin, low perfusion, or SaO_2 less than 80% may alter light absorption and interfere with results.

NURSING ALERT There is a potential error in SaO_2 readings of ±2% that can increase to greater than 2% if the patient's SpO_2 drops below 80%. Oximeters rely on differences in light absorption to determine SaO_2. At lower saturations, oxygenated hemoglobin appears bluer in color and is less easily distinguished from deoxygenated hemoglobin. ABG analysis should be used in this situation.

Figure 10-2. The oxyhemoglobin dissociation curve shows the relation between the partial pressure of oxygen and the oxygen saturation. At pressures greater than 60 mm Hg, the curve is essentially flat with blood oxygen content not changing with increases in the oxygen partial pressure. As oxygen partial pressures decrease in the slope of the curve, the oxygen is unloaded to peripheral tissue as the hemoglobin's affinity decreases. The curve is shifted to the right by an increase in temperature, 2,3-DPG, or $PaCO_2$, or a decrease in pH and to the left by the opposite of these conditions.

Nursing and Patient Care Considerations

1. Assess patient's hemoglobin. SaO_2 may not correlate well with PaO_2 if hemoglobin is not within normal limits.

2. Remove patient's nail polish because it can affect the ability of the sensor to correctly determine oxygen saturation, particularly polish with blue or dark colors.

3. Correlate oximetry with ABG values and then use for single reading or trending of oxygenation (does not monitor $PaCO_2$).

4. Display heart rate should correlate with patient's heart rate.

5. To improve quality of signal, hold finger dependent and motionless (motion may alter results) and cover finger sensor to occlude ambient light.

6. Assess site of oximetry monitoring for perfusion on a regular basis because pressure ulcer may occur from prolonged application of probe. Rotate probe every 2 hours.

7. Device limitations include motion artifact, abnormal hemoglobins (carboxyhemoglobin and methemoglobin), intravenous (IV) dye, exposure of probe to ambient light, low perfusion states, skin pigmentation, nail polish or nail coverings, and nail deformities such as severe clubbing.

8. Document inspired oxygen or supplemental oxygen and type of oxygen delivery device.

9. Accuracy can be affected by decreased peripheral perfusion, ambient light, IV dyes, nail polish, deeply pigmented skin, cold extremities, hypothermia, patients in sickle cell crisis, jaundice, severe anemia, and use of antibiotics such as sulfas.

10. In patients with COPD, oxygen saturation levels may remain unchanged, even though CO_2 levels may be rising as the patient becomes acidotic. Pulse oximetry will not detect this deterioration.

11. Contraindicated for monitoring patients who have high levels of arterial carboxyhemoglobin, such as fire victims.

Capnometry/Capnography

Description

1. Used to noninvasively determine and monitor end-tidal carbon dioxide ($ETCO_2$)—the amount of CO_2 that is expired with each breath—via colorimetric indicator.

2. $ETCO_2$ is displayed as a capnogram (a waveform that may be time-based or volume-based and a numeric reading).

3. Normally, 2 to 5 mm Hg less than $PaCO_2$ in adults, with the difference being greater in the presence of lung disease, or increase in dead space, and can be used as an indirect estimate of V/Q mismatching for the lung.

4. Indicated for monitoring severity of pulmonary disease and monitoring response to therapy; evaluating efficacy of mechanical ventilatory support; monitoring adequacy of pulmonary, systemic, and coronary blood flow; and assessing metabolic rate and/or alveolar ventilation.

5. A standard in anesthesia care, it is being increasingly used in the critical care setting as well as in emergency care via pocket-sized models.

Nursing and Patient Care Considerations

1. Draw ABGs initially to correlate $ETCO_2$ with $PaCO_2$ and to establish the gradient between $PaCO_2$ and $ETCO_2$.

2. Accuracy of measurement can be affected by alterations in breathing pattern or tidal volume (V_T), breathing frequency, presence of freon from metered-dose inhalers, contamination of the system by secretions or condensate, low cardiac output, use of antacids or carbonated beverages, and leaks around tracheal tube cuffs or uncuffed tubes.

3. Does not evaluate pH or oxygenation.
4. Effective for confirming ET tube placement and for monitoring CO_2 in patients who tend to retain CO_2 (eg, COPD).
5. Not a reliable method for determining inadvertent pulmonary placement of gastric tubes.
6. Clean and disinfect sensors and monitors as per manufacturer's instructions.

Exhaled Breath Condensate

 EVIDENCE BASE Konstaninidi, E., Lappa, A., Tzortzi, A., & Panagiotis, B. (2015). Exhaled breath condensate: Technical and diagnostic aspects. *The Scientific World Journal, 2015*, 435160.

Description
1. Emerging as a source for determining biomarkers of lung disease mainly from the lower respiratory tract. Exhaled breath condensate (EBC) is a matrix of exhaled particles and droplets in which biomarkers may be identified, such as:
   a. Volatile (acetic acid, formic acid, ammonia) and nonvolatile compounds.
   b. Very-low- and low-molecular-weight compounds.
   c. Polypeptides.
   d. Proteins.
   e. Nucleic acids.
   f. Lipid mediators.
   g. Inorganic molecules.
   h. Organic molecules.
   i. Redox relevant molecules.
   j. pH relevant molecules.
   k. Cytokines and chemokines.
2. Currently, there is no gold standard—either invasively or noninvasively—for determining absolute concentrations with which EBC can be easily compared.
3. The pH of EBC depends on disease state, ranging from 3.5 to 9.0, which can affect the reactivity and stability of other biomarkers being assayed.

Nursing and Patient Care Considerations
1. Collect condensate sample. Collection methods vary, depending on specific biomarkers to be analyzed. Ten minutes of tidal breathing yields 1 to 2 mm of sample; smaller sample sizes may be adequate for analysis of only one or two biomarkers.
2. Be aware that lower airway condensate may be contaminated by particles from oral and retropharyngeal mucosa.
3. Saliva trapping systems may be used with drooling patients to reduce salivary contamination.

GENERAL PROCEDURES AND TREATMENT MODALITIES

 See additional online content: Procedure Guidelines 10-3–10-24.

Artificial Airway Management

 EVIDENCE BASE Burns, S. (2014). *AACN essentials of critical care nursing* (3rd ed.). New York, NY: McGraw Hill.

Airway management may be indicated in patients with loss of consciousness, facial or oral trauma, aspiration, tumor, infection, copious respiratory secretions, respiratory distress, and the need for mechanical ventilation. See Figure 10-3.

Types of Airways
1. Oropharyngeal airway—curved plastic device inserted through the mouth and positioned in the posterior pharynx to move tongue away from palate and open the airway.
   a. Usually for short-term use in the unconscious patient or may be used along with an oral ET tube.
   b. Not used if recent oral trauma, surgery, or if loose teeth are present.
   c. Does not protect against aspiration.
   d. Not recommended for use in alert patients because the device may trigger the gag reflex and induce vomiting
2. Nasopharyngeal airway (nasal trumpet)—soft rubber or plastic tube hollow inserted through nose into posterior pharynx.
   a. Facilitates frequent nasopharyngeal suctioning.
   b. Useful in the semiconscious patient as an adjunct to help maintain airway patency
   c. Use extreme caution with patients on anticoagulants or bleeding disorders.
   d. Select size that is slightly smaller than diameter of nostril and slightly longer than distance from tip of nose to earlobe.
   e. Check nasal mucosa for irritation or ulceration, and clean airway with hydrogen peroxide and water.
3. Laryngeal mask airway—composed of a tube with a cuffed masklike projection at the distal end; inserted through the mouth into the pharynx; seals the larynx and leaves distal opening of tube just above glottis.
   a. Easier placement than ET tube because visualization of vocal cords is not necessary.
   b. Provides ventilation and oxygenation comparable to that achieved with an ET tube.
   c. Cannot prevent aspiration because it does not separate the GI tract from the respiratory tract.
   d. May cause laryngospasm and bronchospasm.
   e. Greater likelihood of misplacement.
4. Combitube—double-lumen tube with pharyngeal lumen and tracheoesophageal lumen; pharyngeal lumen has blocked distal end and perforations at pharyngeal level; tracheoesophageal lumen has open upper and lower end; large oropharyngeal balloon serves to seal mouth and nose; distal cuff seals the esophagus or trachea.
   a. Very seldom used in the hospital setting because of complications.
5. Endotracheal tube—flexible tube inserted through the mouth or nose and into the trachea beyond the vocal cords that acts as an artificial airway. Preferred method for trauma, medical emergencies, short-term complex patient.
   a. Maintains a patent airway.
   b. Allows for deep tracheal suction and removal of secretions.
   c. Permits mechanical ventilation.
   d. Inflated balloon seals off trachea so aspiration from the GI tract cannot occur.
   e. Generally easy to insert in an emergency, but maintaining placement is more difficult so this is not for long-term use.
6. Tracheostomy tube—firm, curved artificial airway inserted directly into the trachea at the level of the second or third tracheal ring through a surgically made incision.
   a. Permits mechanical ventilation and facilitates secretion removal.

Distal lumen

Pharyngeal
balloon

Proximal
lumen

Pharyngeal
perforations

Distal cuff

Blind distal end

Open distal end

D

Figure 10-3. Types of airways: **(A)** oropharyngeal airway, **(B)** nasopharyngeal airway (nasal trumpet), **(C)** laryngeal mask airway, **(D)** combined tub.

b. Can be for long-term use.
c. Bypasses upper airway defenses, increasing susceptibility to infection.
d. Allows the patient to eat and swallow.

> **NURSING ALERT** Position patient on side and suction oral cavity frequently to prevent aspiration of oral secretions or vomitus when an oral airway is in place.

> **NURSING ALERT** Nasopharyngeal airways may obstruct sinus drainage and produce acute sinusitis. Be alert to fever and facial pain.

Endotracheal Tube Insertion

1. Orotracheal insertion is technically easier because it is done under direct visualization with a laryngoscope. Disadvantages are increased oral secretions, decreased patient comfort, difficulty with tube stabilization, and inability of patient to use lip movement as a communication means.

2. NT insertion may be more comfortable to the patient and is easier to stabilize. Disadvantages are that blind insertion is required; possible development of pressure necrosis of the nasal airway, sinusitis, and otitis media.

3. Tube types vary according to length and inner diameter, type of cuff, and number of lumens.
   a. Usual sizes for adults are 6.0, 7.0, 8.0, and 9.0 mm.
   b. Most cuffs are high volume, low pressure, with self-sealing inflation valves, or the cuff may be of foam rubber.
   c. Most tubes have a single lumen; however, dual-lumen tubes may be used to ventilate each lung independently (see Figure 10-4).

4. May be contraindicated when glottis is obscured by vomitus, bleeding, foreign body, or trauma or cervical spine injury or deformity.

Tracheostomy Tube Insertion

1. Tube types vary according to presence of inner cannula and presence and type of cuff (see Figure 10-5).
   a. Tubes with high-volume, low-pressure cuffs with self-sealing inflation valves; with or without inner cannula.
   b. Fenestrated tube.

Figure 10-4. (A) Endotracheal tubes: single-lumen and double-lumen endotracheal tube. When the double-lumen tube is used **(B)**, two cuffs are inflated. One cuff (*1*) is positioned in the trachea and the second cuff (*2*) in the left mainstem bronchus. After inflation, air flows through an opening below the tracheal cuff (*3*) to the right lung and through an opening below the bronchial cuff (*4*) to the left lung. This permits differential ventilation of both lungs, lavage of one lung, or selective inflation of either lung during thoracic surgery. (Republished with permission of John Wiley and Sons, Inc., from *Anesthesia for thoracic procedures*, Marshall, B, E., Longnecker, D. E., & Fairley, H. B. [Eds.], Blackwell Scientific, 1988.)

c. Foam-filled cuffs.
d. Speaking tracheostomy tube.
e. Tracheal button or Passy-Muir valve.
f. Silver tube (rarely used).
2. Vary according to length and inner diameter in millimeters. Usual sizes for an adult are 5.0, 6.0, 7.0, and 8.0.
3. Tracheostomy is usually planned, either as an adjunct to therapy for respiratory dysfunction or for longer-term airway management when ET intubation has been used for more than 14 days.
4. May be done at the bedside in an emergency when other means of creating an airway have failed.

Indications for Endotracheal or Tracheostomy Tube Insertion

1. Acute respiratory failure, central nervous system (CNS) depression, neuromuscular disease, pulmonary disease, chest wall injury.
2. Upper airway obstruction (tumor, inflammation, foreign body, laryngeal spasm).
3. Anticipated upper airway obstruction from edema or soft tissue swelling because of head and neck trauma, some postoperative head and neck procedures involving the airway, facial or airway burns, decreased LOC.
4. Need for airway protection (vomiting, bleeding, or altered mental status).
5. Aspiration prophylaxis.
6. Fracture of cervical vertebrae with spinal cord injury; requiring ventilatory assistance.

Complications of Endotracheal or Tracheostomy Tube Insertion

1. Laryngeal or tracheal injury.
   a. Sore throat, hoarse voice.
   b. Glottic edema.
   c. Trauma (damage to teeth or mucous membranes, perforation or laceration of pharynx, larynx, or trachea).
   d. Aspiration.
   e. Laryngospasm, bronchospasm.
   f. Ulceration or necrosis of tracheal mucosa.
   g. Vocal cord ulceration, granuloma, or polyps.
   h. Vocal cord paralysis.
   i. Postextubation tracheal stenosis.
   j. Tracheal dilation.
   k. Formation of tracheal–esophageal fistula.
   l. Formation of tracheal–arterial fistula.
   m. Innominate artery erosion.
2. Pulmonary infection and sepsis.
3. Dependence on artificial airway.

Nursing Care for Patients with Artificial Airways

General Care Measures

1. Handwashing and application of application of alcohol gel should be followed before and after all procedures.
2. Ensure adequate ventilation and oxygenation through the use of supplemental oxygen or mechanical ventilation as indicated.

Cuffless: nonfenestrated (left) and fenestrated (right). Tracheostomy plug to allow breathing through upper airway is also shown.

Cuffed: fenestrated (left) and nonfenestrated (right) with inner cannula and obturator for insertion. Percutaneous tracheostomy inducer (bottom).

Speaking valve.

Figure 10-5. Types of tracheostomy tubes. (© 2018 Medtronic. All rights reserved. Used with the permission of Medtronic.)

3. Assess breath sounds every 2 hours. Note evidence of ineffective secretion clearance (rhonchi, crackles), which suggests need for suctioning.

4. Provide adequate humidity when the natural humidifying pathway of the oropharynx is bypassed.

5. Provide adequate suctioning of oral secretions to prevent aspiration and decrease oral microbial colonization.

6. Use clean technique when inserting an oral or nasopharyngeal airway, and take it out and clean it with hydrogen peroxide and rinse with water at least every 8 hours.

7. Perform oral care every 2 to 4 hours with soft toothbrush or swabs and prepackaged oral care kits. Frequent oral care will aid in prevention of ventilator-associated pneumonia. The patient's lips should be kept moisturized to prevent them from becoming sore and cracked.

8. Ensure that aseptic technique is maintained when inserting an ET or tracheostomy tube. The artificial airway bypasses the upper airway, and the lower airways are sterile below the level of the vocal cords.

9. Elevate the patient to a semi-Fowler's or sitting position, when possible; these positions result in improved lung compliance. The patient's position, however, should be changed at least every 2 hours to ensure ventilation of all lung segments and prevent secretion stagnation and atelectasis. Position changes are also necessary to avoid skin breakdown.

10. If an oral or nasopharyngeal airway is used, turn patient's head to the side to reduce the risk of aspiration (because there is no cuff to seal off the lower airway).

Nutritional Considerations

1. Consciousness is usually impaired in patient with an oropharyngeal airway, so oral feeding is contraindicated.

2. To enhance comfort, remove a nasopharyngeal airway in the conscious patient during mealtimes.

3. Recognize that an ET tube holds the epiglottis open. Therefore, only the inflated cuff prevents the aspiration of oropharyngeal contents into the lungs. The patient must not receive oral feeding. Administer enteral tube feedings or parenteral feedings, as ordered.

4. Administer oral feedings to a conscious patient with a tracheostomy, usually with the cuff inflated. The inflated cuff prevents aspiration of food contents into the lungs but causes the tracheal wall to bulge into the esophageal lumen and may make swallowing more difficult. Patients who are not on mechanical ventilation and are awake, alert, and able to protect the airway are candidates for eating with the cuff deflated. Utilize a speech therapist to evaluate the patient's ability to eat.

5. Patients should receive thickened rather than regular liquids; this will assist in effective swallowing.

 NURSING ALERT Consider the patient's nutritional needs early in the process of intubation so nutritional status does not decline further. It is difficult to wean patients who have compromised nutritional status.

Cuff Maintenance

1. ET tube cuffs should be inflated continuously and deflated only during intubation, extubation, and tube repositioning.

2. Tracheostomy tube cuffs also should be inflated continuously in patients on mechanical ventilation or continuous positive airway pressure (CPAP).

3. Tracheostomized patients who are breathing spontaneously may have the cuff inflated continuously (in the patient with decreased LOC without ability to fully protect airway), deflated continuously, or inflated only for feeding if the patient is at risk of aspiration.

4. Monitor cuff pressure every 4 hours.

External Tube Site Care

1. Secure an ET tube so it cannot be disrupted by the weight of ventilator or oxygen tubing or by patient movement.
   a. Use strips of adhesive tape or Velcro straps wrapped around the tube and secured to tape on patient's cheeks or around the back of patient's head.
   b. Replace when soiled or insecure or when repositioning of tube is necessary.
   c. Position tubing so traction is not applied to ET tube.

2. Perform tracheostomy site care at least every 8 hours using 0.9%NS, and change tracheostomy ties when soiled and according to facility policy.
   a. Make sure ventilator or oxygen tubing is supported so traction is not applied to the tracheostomy tube.

3. Have available at all times at the patient's bedside a replacement ET tube in the same size as patient is using, resuscitation bag, oxygen source, and mask to ventilate the patient in the event of accidental tube removal. Anticipate your course of action in such an event.
   a. ET tube—know location and assembly of reintubation equipment including replacement ET tube. Know how to contact someone immediately for reintubation.
   b. Tracheostomy—have extra tracheostomy tube, obturator, and hemostats at bedside. Be aware of reinsertion technique, if facility policy permits, or know how to contact someone immediately for reinserting the tube.

 NURSING ALERT In the event of accidental ET or tracheostomy tube removal, use a bag/mask resuscitation device to ventilate the patient by mouth while covering tracheostomy stoma. However, if the patient has complete upper airway obstruction, a gaping stoma, or a laryngectomy, mouth-to-stoma ventilation must be performed.

Psychologic Considerations

1. Assist patient to deal with psychological aspects related to artificial airway.

2. Recognize that patient is usually apprehensive, particularly about choking, inability to communicate verbally, inability to remove secretions, uncomfortable suctioning, difficulty in breathing, or mechanical failure.

3. Explain the function of the equipment carefully.

4. Inform patient and family that speaking will not be possible while the tube is in place, unless using a tracheostomy tube with a deflated cuff, a fenestrated tube, a Passy-Muir speaking valve, or a speaking tracheostomy tube.
   a. A Passy-Muir valve is a speaking valve that fits over the end of the tracheostomy tube. Air that is inhaled is exhaled through the vocal cords and out through the mouth, allowing speech.

5. Develop with patient the best method of communication (eg, sign language, lip reading [alphabet, picture, writing boards]).
   a. Patients with tracheostomy tubes or nasal ET tubes may effectively use orally operated electrolarynx devices.
   b. Devise a means for patient to get the nurse's attention when someone is not immediately available at the bedside, such as call bell, soft-touch call bell hand-operated bell, or rattle.
6. Anticipate some of patient's questions by discussing "Is it permanent?" "Will it hurt to breathe?" "Will someone be with me?"
7. If appropriate, advise patient that as condition improves, a tracheostomy button may be used to plug the tracheostomy site. A tracheostomy button is a rigid, closed cannula that is placed into the tracheostomy stoma after removal of a cuffed or uncuffed tracheostomy tube. When in proper position, the button does not extend into the tracheal lumen. The outer edge of the button is at the skin surface and the inner edge is at the anterior tracheal wall.

 NURSING ALERT With the use of artificial airways, remember the patient may use a call bell, but he or she will not be able to communicate verbally (unless device is used to allow speech).

Community and Home Care Considerations

1. Teach patient and/or caregiver procedure. Patient will need to use stationary mirror to visualize tracheostomy and perform procedure.
2. Suctioning patient in the home: whenever possible, patient and/or caregiver should be taught to perform procedure. Patient should use controlled cough and other secretion-clearance techniques.
3. Preoxygenation and hyperinflation before suctioning may not be routinely indicated for all patients cared for in the home. Preoxygenation and hyperinflation are based on patient need and clinical status.
4. Normal saline should not be instilled unless clinically indicated (eg, to stimulate cough).
5. Clean technique and clean examination gloves are used. At the end of suctioning, the catheter or tonsil tip should be flushed by suctioning recently boiled and cooled, or distilled, water to rinse away mucus, followed by suctioning air through the apparatus. The outer surface may be wiped with alcohol or hydrogen peroxide. The catheter and tonsil tip should be air-dried and stored in a clean, dry place. Generally, suction catheters should be discarded after 24 hours. Tonsil tips may be boiled and reused.
6. Care of tracheostomy stoma: clean with half-strength hydrogen peroxide (diluted with sterile water) and wipe with sterile water or sterile saline.

Mobilization of Secretions

The goal of airway clearance techniques is to improve clearance of airway secretions, thereby decreasing obstruction of the airways. This serves to improve ventilation and gas exchange. Patients with respiratory disorders, neuromuscular disorders, or CNS disorders, such as loss of consciousness that may impair respiratory function, typically require help with mobilization and removal of secretions. Increased amount and viscosity of secretions and/or inability to clear secretions through the normal cough mechanism may lead to pooling of secretions in lower airways. Pooling of secretions leads to infection and inadequate gas exchange. Secretions should be removed by coughing or, when necessary, by suctioning. However, routine suctioning should be avoided. Auscultation and visual inspection of the patient should be used to determine the need for suctioning. Secretions can be mobilized through the chest physical therapy measures of postural drainage, directed cough, positive expiratory pressure (PEP), high-frequency oscillation (oral devices such as Flutter or Acapella device, or chest devices such as the Vest) mucus clearance devices, autogenic drainage, intrapulmonary vibration, percussion and vibration, and other secretion-clearance measures.

Nasotracheal Suctioning

1. Intended to remove accumulated secretions or other materials that cannot be moved by the patient's spontaneous cough or less-invasive procedures. Suctioning of the tracheobronchial tree in a patient without an artificial airway can be accomplished by inserting a sterile suction catheter lubricated with water-soluble jelly through the nares into the nasal passage, down through the oropharynx, past the glottis, and into the trachea.
2. NT suction is a blind, high-risk procedure with uncertain outcome. Complications include mechanical trauma, hypoxia, dysrhythmias, bradycardia, increased BP, vomiting, increased ICP, and misdirection of catheter.
3. Contraindications include:
   a. Bleeding disorders, such as disseminated intravascular coagulation, thrombocytopenia, leukemia.
   b. Laryngeal edema, laryngeal spasm.
   c. Esophageal varices.
   d. Tracheal surgery.
   e. Gastric surgery with high anastomosis.
   f. Myocardial infarction.
   g. Occluded nasal passages or nasal bleeding.
   h. Epiglottitis.
   i. Head, facial, or neck injury.
4. May cause trauma to the nasal passages.
   a. Do not attempt to force the catheter if resistance is met.
   b. Report if significant bleeding occurs.
5. Insert a nasal airway if repeated suctioning is necessary to protect the nasal passages from trauma.
6. Be alert for signs of laryngeal edema because of irritation and trauma.
   a. Stop if suctioning becomes difficult or if the patient develops new upper airway noise or obstruction.
   b. Duration of the suctioning should be limited to less than 15 seconds.

 NURSING ALERT NT suctioning should not be routinely performed. Only indicated when other methods to remove secretions from airway have failed.

Suctioning Through an Endotracheal or Tracheostomy Tube

1. Ineffective coughing may cause secretion collection in the artificial airway or tracheobronchial tree, resulting in narrowing of the airway, respiratory insufficiency, and stasis of secretions.
2. Assess the need for suctioning at least every 2 hours through auscultation of the chest.
3. Ventilation with a manual resuscitation bag will facilitate auscultation and may stimulate coughing, decreasing the need for suctioning.
4. Maintain sterile technique while suctioning.
5. Administer supplemental 100% oxygen through the mechanical ventilator or manual resuscitation bag before, after, and between suctioning passes to prevent hypoxemia.
6. Closed-system suctioning may be done with the suction catheter contained in the mechanical ventilator tubing. Ventilator disconnection is not necessary so positive end-expiratory pressure (PEEP) is maintained, sterility is maintained, risk of exposure to body fluids is eliminated, and time is saved. However, studies have not demonstrated that closed-system suctioning is more effective when compared to open suctioning in actually removing secretions.

Community and Home Care Considerations

1. Encourage patient to use directed cough or other airway clearance technique prior to suctioning. Auscultate the lungs to assess need for suctioning.
2. Teach caregivers to suction in the home situation using a clean technique, rather than sterile. Wash hands well before suctioning.
3. Put on fresh examination gloves for suctioning, and reuse catheter after rinsing it in warm water.
4. Be aware that appropriate and aggressive airway clearance will assist in preventing pulmonary complications, thus lessening the need for hospitalization.
5. Hazards and complications are the same for the home care patient as they are for a hospitalized patient.

Chest Physical Therapy

 EVIDENCE BASE Pathmanathan, N., Beaumont, N., & Gratrix, A. (2015). Respiratory physiotherapy in the critical care unit. *British Journal of Anesthesia*, *15*(1), 20–25.
Strickland, S. L., Rubin, B. K., Drescher, G. S., et al. (2013). AARC clinical practice guideline: Effectiveness of nonpharmacologic airway clearance therapies in hospitalized patients. *Respiratory Care, 58*(12), 2187–2193.

Breathing Exercises

1. Techniques used to compensate for respiratory deficits and conserve energy by increasing efficiency of breathing. Have patient breathe in through the nose and out through the mouth at a ratio of 1:2.
2. The overall purposes for doing breathing exercises are:
   a. To relax muscles, relieve anxiety, and improve control of breathing.
   b. To eliminate useless, uncoordinated patterns of respiratory muscle activity.
   c. To slow the respiratory rate.
   d. To decrease the work of breathing.
   e. To improve efficiency and strength of respiratory muscles.
   f. To improve ventilation and oxygen saturation during exercise.
3. Diaphragmatic abdominal breathing is used primarily to strengthen the diaphragm, which is the main muscle of respiration. It also aids in decreasing the use of accessory muscles and allows for better control over the breathing pattern, especially during stressful situations and increased physical demands.
4. Pursed-lip breathing is used primarily to slow the respiratory rate and assist in emptying the lungs of retained CO_2. This technique is always helpful to patients, but especially when they feel extreme dyspnea because of exertion.
5. Breathing exercises are most helpful to patients when practiced and used on a regular basis.

 NURSING ALERT For patients with severe COPD, evidence does not support the use of diaphragmatic breathing because this type of breathing may result in hyperinflation as a result of increased dyspnea and fatigue.

Percussion and Vibration

1. Postural drainage uses gravity and, possibly, external manipulation of the thorax to improve mobilization of bronchial secretions, to enhance matching of ventilation and perfusion, and to normalize functional residual capacity.
2. Indicated for difficulty with secretion clearance, evidence of retained secretions, and lung conditions that cause increased production of secretions such as bronchiectasis, cystic fibrosis, chronic bronchitis, and emphysema.
3. Contraindicated in undrained lung abscess, lung tumors, pneumothorax, diseases of the chest wall, lung hemorrhage, painful chest conditions, tuberculosis, severe osteoporosis, increased ICP, uncontrolled hypertension, and gross hemoptysis.
4. Percussion is movement done by "clapping" the chest wall in a rhythmic fashion with cupped hands or a mechanical device directly over the lung segments to be drained. The wrists are alternately flexed and extended so the chest is cupped or clapped in a painless manner. A mechanical percussor may be used to prevent repetitive motion injury. Research is mixed on the benefit of this technique.
5. Vibration is the technique of applying manual compression with oscillations or tremors to the chest wall during the exhalation phase of respiration. Research is mixed on the benefit of this technique.

Postural Drainage

1. Gravity-assisted positions, deep breathing, chest clapping, shaking or vibration to assist in the removal of bronchial secretions from affected lung segments to central airways (see Figure 10-6).
2. The patient is positioned so the diseased areas are in a near vertical position, and gravity is used to assist drainage of the specific segments.
3. The positions assumed are determined by the location, severity, and duration of mucus obstruction.
4. The exercises are usually performed two to four times daily, before meals and at bedtime. Each position is held for 3 to 15 minutes.
5. The procedure should be discontinued if tachycardia, palpitations, dyspnea, or chest pain occurs. These symptoms may indicate hypoxemia. Discontinue if hemoptysis occurs.

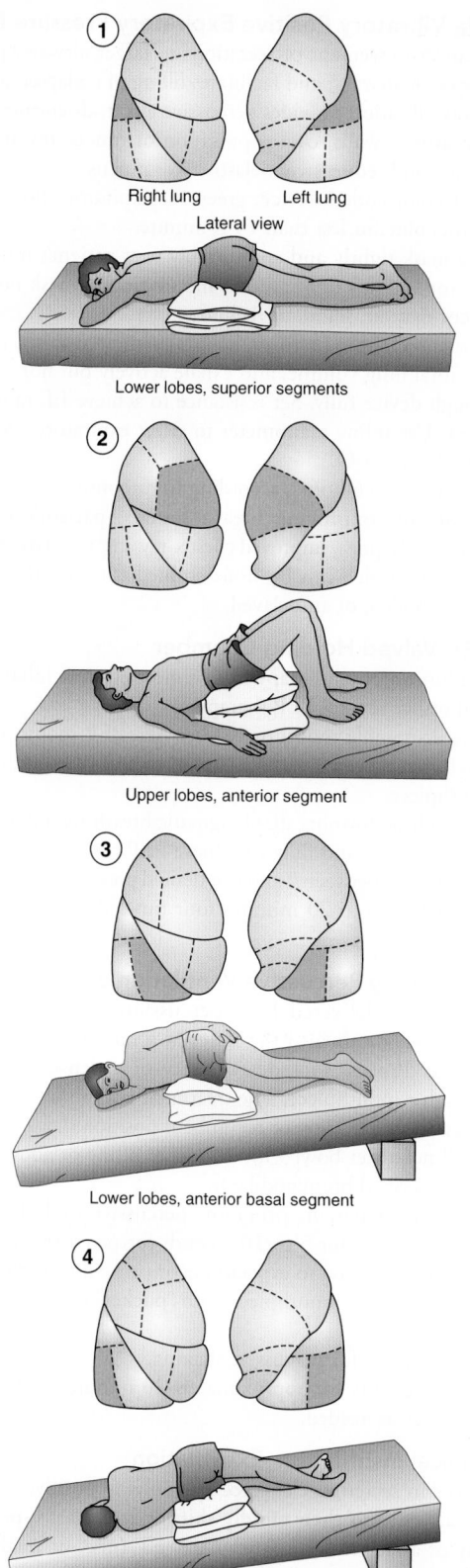

Figure 10-6. Postural drainage positions. Anatomic segments of the lung with four postural drainage positions. The numbers relate the position to the corresponding anatomic segment of the lung. (Smeltzer, S., & Bare, B. [2000]. *Brunner and Suddarth's textbook of medical-surgical nursing* [9th ed.]. Philadelphia, PA: Lippincott Williams & Wilkins.)

6. Contraindications include increased ICP, unstable head or neck injury, active hemorrhage with hemodynamic instability or gross hemoptysis, recent spinal surgery or injury, empyema, bronchopleural fistula, rib fracture, flail chest, and uncontrolled hypertension.

7. Bronchodilators, mucolytic agents, water, or saline may be nebulized and inhaled, or an inhaled bronchodilator may be used before postural drainage and chest percussion to reduce bronchospasm, decrease thickness of mucus and sputum, and combat edema of the bronchial walls, thereby enhancing secretion removal.

8. Perform secretion-clearance procedures before eating or a minimum of 1 hour after eating.

9. Make sure patient is comfortable before the procedure starts and as comfortable as possible while he or she assumes each position.

10. Auscultate the chest to determine the areas of needed drainage.

11. Encourage the patient to deep-breathe and cough after spending the allotted time in each position (normally 3 to 15 minutes).

12. Encourage diaphragmatic breathing throughout postural drainage; this helps widen airways so secretions can be drained.

 NURSING ALERT Postural drainage and chest percussion may result in hypoxia and should only be used if secretions are believed to be present.

Forced Expiratory Technique

1. Used to enhance effects of a spontaneous cough and compensate for physical limitations. Used for secretion clearance, atelectasis, prophylaxis against postoperative pulmonary complications, routine bronchial hygiene for cystic fibrosis, bronchiectasis, and chronic bronchitis and to obtain sputum specimen for diagnostic analysis.

2. Procedure includes a forced expiratory technique of two to three "huffs" (forced expirations), from mid- to low-lung volume, with glottis open, followed by a period of relaxed, controlled diaphragmatic breathing. Explain to the patient that to huff cough is the same maneuver that fogs eyeglasses. The forced expiration can be augmented by brisk adduction of the upper arms to self-compress the thorax.

3. Contraindications include increased ICP or known intracranial aneurysm, as well as acute or unstable head, neck, or spinal injury.

Manually Assisted Cough

The external application of mechanical pressure to the epigastric region coordinated with forced exhalation. This procedure may improve cough efficiency in those individuals with neuromuscular weakness or structural defects of the abdominal wall.

Positive Expiratory Pressure

1. Positive back pressure is created in the airways when the patient breathes in and out 5 to 20 times through a flow resistor or fixed orifice device.

2. During prolonged exhalation against positive pressure, peripheral airways are stabilized while air is pushed through collateral pathways (pores of Kohn and canals of Lambert) into distal lung units past retained secretions.

3. Expiratory airflow moves secretions to larger airways to be removed by coughing.
4. The pressure generated can be monitored and adjusted with a manometer (usually ranges from 10 to 20 cm H_2O).
5. Active exhalation with an inspiratory-to-expiratory (I:E) ratio of 1:3 or 1:4 is suggested.
6. The cycle is repeated until secretions are expelled, usually within 20 minutes or less if patient tires.

Autogenic Drainage

1. Controlled breathing used at three lung volumes, beginning at low-lung volume to unstick mucus, moving to midlung volume to collect mucus, and then to high-lung volume to expel mucus.
2. This method may be difficult for some patients to learn and to perform independently.
3. Can be performed in a seated position.

Flutter Mucus Clearance Device

1. Provides PEP and high-frequency oscillations at the airway opening. Provides approximately 10 cm H_2O positive airway pressure.
2. The flutter valve is a pipe-shaped device with an inner cone and bowl loosely supporting a steel ball. The bowl containing the steel ball is covered by a perforated cap.
3. Indications include atelectasis, bronchitis, bronchiectasis, cystic fibrosis, and other conditions producing retained secretions.
4. Mucus clearance is based on:
   a. Vibration of the airways, which loosens mucus from airway walls.
   b. Intermittent increase in endobronchial pressure that keeps airways open.
   c. Acceleration of expiratory airflow to facilitate upward movement of mucus.
5. Contraindications include pneumothorax and right-sided heart failure.
6. Directions:
   a. Patient should be seated upright with chin tilted slightly upward to further open airway.
   b. Instruct patient to inhale slowly to three fourths of normal breath.
   c. Place flutter in mouth with lips firmly sealed around stem or mouthpiece.
   d. Position flutter at horizontal level or raise bulb end up to 30 degrees for greater force.
   e. Instruct patient to hold breath for 2 to 3 seconds.
   f. Exhale through flutter at moderately fast rate, keeping cheeks stiff. Urge to cough should be suppressed.
   g. Repeat for 5 to 10 more breaths.
7. Have patient perform same technique with one to two forced exhalations to generate mucus elimination and huff coughs as needed.
8. Generally used for 10 to 20 breaths with device followed by several directed coughs, repeating series four to six times or for 10 to 20 minutes up to four times daily.
9. Clean flutter device every other day by disassembling and using a liquid soap and tap water. Disinfect regularly by soaking cleaned disassembled parts in one part alcohol to three parts tap water for 1 minute; rinse, wipe, reassemble, and store.

Acapella Vibratory Positive Expiratory Pressure Device

1. Enhances movement of secretions to larger airways, prevents collapse of airways, and facilitates filling of collapsed alveoli.
2. Airway vibration provides percussive effect, disengages mucus from airway walls, causes pulsation of mucus toward larger airways, and reduces viscoelasticity of mucus.
3. Select color-coded device: green for expiratory flow ≥15 L/minute, blue for less than 15 L/minute.
4. Place mask tightly and comfortably over patient's mouth and nose (or seal lips tight around mouthpiece if mask not used). Patient may sit, stand, or recline.
5. Instruct patient to perform diaphragmatic breathing, inhale to near-total lung volume, and exhale actively but not forcefully through device fully. Set resistance to achieve I:E ratio of 1:3 to 1:4. Use inline manometer to select expiratory pressure of 10 to 20 cm H_2O.
6. Use every 1 to 6 hours, according to response.
7. Assessment: improving breath sounds, patient's report of improved dyspnea, improved chest x-ray, improved oxygenation.
8. Acapella Choice can be disassembled for cleaning in dishwasher, boiled, or autoclaved.

AeroPEP Valved Holding Chamber

1. Combines aerosol therapy from a metered-dose inhaler with a fixed orifice resister PEP therapy.
2. Place disposable mouthpiece over AeroPEP mouthpiece and attach manometer. Instruct patient to seal lips tightly around mouthpiece.
3. Although performing diaphragmatic breathing, inhale fully.
4. Exhale actively and fully to achieve PEP of 10 to 20 cm H_2O. Set AeroPEP between 0 and 6 at desired pressure on manometer.
5. Repeat for up to 20 minutes four times daily or as clinically indicated.

Intrapulmonary Percussive Ventilation or Percussionaire

1. Therapy is delivered by a percussionator, which delivers minibursts of air into the lungs at a rate of 100 to 300 per minute. Process includes delivery of a dense aerosol mist through a mouthpiece. The treatment lasts about 20 minutes.
2. Patient uses in sitting or recumbent position.
3. Instill nebulizer bowl with 20 mL of saline or aqueous water and prescribed bronchodilator.
4. Clinician or patient programs percussive cycle by holding down a button for 5 to 10 seconds for percussive inspiratory cycle and releasing to expectorate or pause during therapy.
5. Seal lips around mouthpiece with "pucker" to minimize cheek flapping.
6. Observe chest for percussive shaking.
7. Use twice daily for approximately 20 minutes with increased frequency as needed.

Mechanical Insufflation–Exsufflation

1. Assists in secretion clearance by applying positive pressure to the airway and then rapidly shifting to negative pressure by way of a face mask, mouthpiece, ET tube, or tracheostomy tube to increase cough effectiveness.
2. Used in patients with impaired cough who are unable to clear secretions.

Electrical Stimulation of the Expiratory Muscles

Electrical stimulation of the abdominal muscles to increase cough effectiveness. An advantage is that presence of a caregiver is not required.

The Vest Airway Clearance System

1. Enhances secretion clearance through high-frequency chest wall oscillation. High-frequency compression pulses are applied to the chest wall by way of an air pulse delivery system and inflatable vest.
2. Variable-frequency large-volume air pulse delivery system attached to inflatable vest. Pressure pulses that fill the vest and vibrate the chest wall are controlled by a foot pedal. Pulse frequency ranges from 5 to 25 Hz and pressure in the vest ranges from 28 to 39 mm Hg.
3. A foot or hand control starts and stops pulsations.
4. Treatment length usually 10 to 30 minutes. Therapy should include a break at least every 10 minutes for directed cough. Use twice daily, with increased frequency as needed.

Community and Home Care Considerations

1. Nebulizer tubing and mouthpiece can be reused at home repeatedly. Recommend thorough rinsing with warm water after each use, shake off excess water, and let air-dry.
2. Twice-weekly cleaning should include washing with liquid soap and hot water, followed by 30-minute soak in one part white vinegar and two parts tap water, and then rinsing with tap water, air-drying, and storing in a clean, dry place.

Administering Oxygen Therapy

 EVIDENCE BASE Singh, L. T., Sharara, R., Leap, J., & Singh, A. (2016). Management of respiratory failure. *Critical Care Nursing Quarterly, 39*(2), 94–109.

Oxygen is an odorless, tasteless, colorless, transparent gas that is slightly heavier than air. It is used to treat or prevent symptoms and manifestations of hypoxia. Oxygen can be dispensed from a cylinder, piped-in system, liquid oxygen reservoir, or oxygen concentrator. It may be administered by nasal cannula, transtracheal catheter, nasal cannula with reservoir devices, or various types of face masks, including CPAP mask. It may also be applied directly to the ET or tracheal tube by way of a mechanical ventilator, T-piece, or manual resuscitation bag. The method selected depends on the required concentration of oxygen, desired variability in delivered oxygen concentration (none, minimal, moderate), and required ventilatory assistance (mechanical ventilator, spontaneous breathing).

Methods of Oxygen Administration

1. Nasal cannula—nasal prongs that deliver low or high flow of oxygen.
   a. Requires nose breathing.
   b. Cannot deliver oxygen concentrations much higher than 40%.
2. Simple face mask—mask that delivers moderate oxygen flow to nose and mouth. Delivers oxygen concentrations of 40% to 60%.
3. Venturi mask—mask with device that mixes air and oxygen to deliver constant oxygen concentration.
   a. Total gas flow at the patient's face must meet or exceed peak inspiratory flow rate. When other mask outputs do not meet inspiratory flow rate of patient, room air (drawn through mask side holes) mixes with the gas mixture provided by the face mask, lowering the inspired oxygen concentration.
   b. Venturi mask mixes a fixed flow of oxygen with a high but variable flow of air to produce a constant oxygen concentration. Oxygen enters by way of a jet (restricted opening) at a high velocity. Room air also enters and mixes with oxygen at this site. The higher the velocity (smaller the opening), the more room air is drawn into the mask.
   c. Mask output ranges from approximately 30% to 50% oxygen.
   d. Virtually eliminates rebreathing of CO_2. Excess gas leaves through openings in the mask, carrying with it the expired CO_2.
4. Partial rebreather mask—has an inflatable bag that stores 100% oxygen.
   a. On inspiration, the patient inhales from the mask and bag; on expiration, the bag refills with oxygen and expired gases exit through perforations on both sides of the mask and some enters bag (see Figure 10-7A).

Figure 10-7. **(A)** Airflow diagram with partial rebreathing mask. **(B)** Airflow diagram with non-rebreathing mask. *Arrows* indicate direction of flow.

b. High concentrations of oxygen (50% to 75%) can be delivered.

c. Often used to conserve oxygen supply during patient transport.

5. Nonrebreathing mask (see Figure 10-7B)—has an inflatable bag to store 100% oxygen and a one-way valve between the bag and mask to prevent exhaled air from entering the bag.

   a. Has one-way valves covering one or both of the exhalation ports to prevent entry of room air on inspiration.

   b. Has a flap or spring-loaded valves to permit entry of room air should the oxygen source fail or patient needs exceed the available oxygen flow.

   c. Optimally, all the patient's inspiratory volume will be provided by the mask/reservoir, allowing delivery of nearly 100% oxygen.

6. Transtracheal catheter—accomplished by way of a small (8 French) catheter inserted between the second and third tracheal cartilage.

   a. Does not interfere with talking, drinking, or eating and can be concealed under a shirt or blouse.

   b. Oxygen delivery is more efficient because all oxygen enters the lungs.

   c. Requires surgical procedure with temporary stent until tract is healed.

7. Continuous Positive Airway Pressure mask—used to provide expiratory and inspiratory positive airway pressure in a manner similar to PEEP and does not require ET intubation.

   a. Has an inflatable cushion and head strap designed to tightly seal the mask against the face. See Figure 10-8.

   b. A PEEP valve is incorporated into the exhalation port to maintain positive pressure on exhalation.

   c. High inspiratory flow rates are needed to maintain positive pressure on inspiration.

8. Bilevel positive airway pressure (BiPAP) mask—a combination of inspiratory and expiratory pulmonary artery pressure (PAP) often used to avoid intubation and mechanical ventilation.

   a. Preset pressure to be delivered during inspiration and preset pressure to be maintained during expiration.

   b. Mask with airtight seal is used, similar to CPAP.

9. T-piece (Briggs) adapter—used to administer oxygen to patient with ET or tracheostomy tube who is breathing spontaneously.

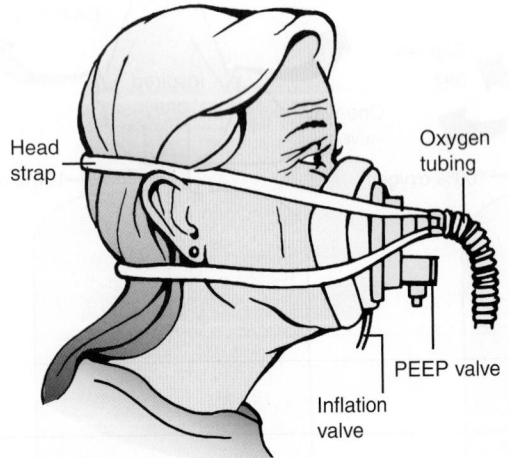

Figure 10-8. CPAP mask with airtight seal.

a. High concentration of aerosol and oxygen delivered through wide-bore tubing.

b. Expired gases exit through open reservoir tubing.

10. Manual resuscitation bag—delivers high concentration of oxygen to patient with insufficient inspiratory effort.

    a. With mask, uses upper airway by delivering oxygen to mouth and nose of patient.

    b. Without mask, adapter fits on ET or tracheostomy tube.

    c. Usually used in cardiopulmonary arrest, hyperinflation during suctioning, or transport of ventilator-dependent patients.

Nursing Assessment and Interventions

1. Assess need for oxygen by observing for symptoms of hypoxia:

   a. Tachypnea.

   b. SaO_2 less than 88%.

   c. Tachycardia or dysrhythmias (premature ventricular contractions).

   d. A change in LOC (symptoms of decreased cerebral oxygenation are irritability, confusion, lethargy, and coma, if untreated).

   e. Cyanosis occurs as a late sign ($PaO_2 \leq 45$ mm Hg).

   f. Labored respirations indicate severe respiratory distress.

   g. Myocardial stress—increase in heart rate and stroke volume (cardiac output) is the primary mechanism for compensation for hypoxemia or hypoxia; pupils dilate with hypoxia.

2. Obtain ABG values and assess the patient's current oxygenation, ventilation, and acid–base status.

3. Administer oxygen in the appropriate concentration and device.

   a. Low concentration (24% to 28%)—may be appropriate for patients prone to retain CO_2 (COPD, drug overdose), who are dependent on hypoxemia (hypoxic drive) to maintain respiration. If hypoxemia is suddenly reversed, hypoxic drive may be lost and respiratory depression and, possibly, respiratory arrest may occur. Monitor $PaCO_2$ levels.

   b. High concentration ($\geq 30\%$)—appropriate in patients not predisposed to CO_2 retention.

   c. Ensure proper use and fit of oxygen delivery device-cannula or mask, with oxygen flow rate according to manufacturer's instructions.

4. Monitor response by oximetry and/or ABG sampling.

5. Increase or decrease the inspired oxygen concentration, as appropriate.

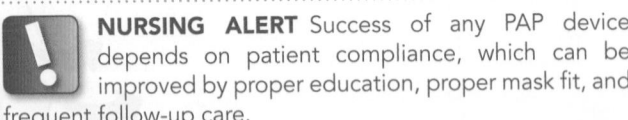 **NURSING ALERT** Success of any PAP device depends on patient compliance, which can be improved by proper education, proper mask fit, and frequent follow-up care.

NURSING ALERT All Joint Commission–accredited hospitals must be smoke free; however, other facilities and homes where oxygen is used may allow smoking. Make sure that no smoking is permitted where oxygen is used.

Community and Home Care Considerations

1. Indications for supplemental oxygen based on Medicare reimbursement guidelines:

a. Documented hypoxemia: In adults: PaO_2 = 55 torr or SaO_2 ≤ 88% when breathing room air, or PaO_2 56 to 59 torr or SaO_2 ≤ 89% in association with cor pulmonale, heart failure, or polycythemia with hematocrit greater than 56%.

b. Some patients may not qualify for oxygen therapy at rest but will qualify for oxygen during ambulation, exercise, or sleep. Oxygen therapy is indicated during these specific activities when SaO_2 is demonstrated to fall to ≤88%.

c. Determine oxygen prescription for rest, exercise, and sleep, and instruct patient and caregiver to follow these flow rates.

2. Precautions in the home:

a. In COPD with presence of CO_2 retention (generally because of chronic hypoxemia), oxygen administration at higher levels may lead to increased $PaCO_2$ level and decreased respiratory drive.

b. Fire hazard is increased in presence of higher than normal oxygen concentrations. Instruct patient and caregiver of home oxygen precautions:

i. Post no smoking signs. Instruct on avoidance of cigarettes within 6 feet of oxygen.

ii. Avoid potential electrical sparks around oxygen (shave with blade razor instead of electric razor; keep away from heat sources).

iii. Keep oxygen at least 6 feet (1.8 m) from any source of flame.

c. Power failure may lead to inadequate oxygen supply when an oxygen concentrator is used without backup tank.

d. Oxygen tanks must be secured in stand to prevent falling over.

e. Improper use of liquid oxygen (touching liquid) may result in burns.

3. Oxygen delivered by way of tracheostomy collar or T tube should be humidified.

4. Oxygen concentrators extract oxygen from ambient air and should deliver oxygen at concentrations of 85% or greater at up to 4 L/minute.

5. Liquid oxygen is provided in large reservoir canisters with smaller portable units that can be transfilled by patient or caregiver. Liquid oxygen evaporates from canister when not in use.

6. Compressed gas may be supplied in large cylinders (G or H cylinders) or smaller cylinders (D or E cylinders) with wheels for easier movement.

7. All oxygen delivery equipment should be checked at least once daily by patient or caregiver, including function of equipment, prescribed flow rates, remaining liquid or compressed gas content, and backup supply.

Mechanical Ventilation

 EVIDENCE BASE Singh, L. T., Sharara, R., Leap, J., & Singh, A. (2016). Management of respiratory failure. *Critical Care Nursing Quarterly, 39*(2), 94–109.
Burns, S. (2014). *AACN critical care nursing* (3rd ed.). New York, NY: McGraw-Hill.

The mechanical ventilator device functions as a substitute for the bellows action of the thoracic cage and diaphragm. The mechanical ventilator can maintain ventilation automatically for prolonged periods. It is indicated when the patient is unable to maintain safe levels of oxygen or CO_2 by spontaneous breathing even with the assistance of other oxygen delivery devices.

Clinical Indications

Mechanical Failure of Ventilation

1. Neuromuscular disease.
2. CNS disease.
3. CNS depression (drug intoxication, respiratory depressants, cardiac arrest).
4. Inefficiency of thoracic cage in generating pressure gradients necessary for ventilation (chest injury, thoracic malformation).
5. When ventilatory support is needed postoperatively.

Disorders of Pulmonary Gas Exchange

1. Acute respiratory failure.
2. Chronic respiratory failure.
3. Left-sided heart failure.
4. Pulmonary diseases resulting in diffusion abnormality.
5. Pulmonary diseases resulting in V/Q mismatch.
6. Acute lung injury.

Underlying Principles

1. Variables that control ventilation and oxygenation include:
   a. Ventilator rate—adjusted by rate setting.
   b. V_T—volume of gas required for one breath (mL/kg).
   c. Fraction of inspired oxygen concentration (FiO_2)—set on ventilator and measured with an oxygen analyzer.
   d. Ventilator dead space—circuitry (tubing) common to inhalation and exhalation; tubing is calibrated.
   e. PEEP—set within the ventilator or with the use of external PEEP devices; measured at the proximal airway.
2. CO_2 elimination is controlled by V_T, rate, and dead space.
3. Oxygen tension is controlled by oxygen concentration and PEEP (also by rate and V_T).
4. In most cases, the duration of inspiration should not exceed exhalation.
5. The inspired gas must be warmed and humidified to prevent thickening of secretions and decrease in body temperature. Sterile or distilled water is warmed and humidified by way of a heated humidifier.

Types of Ventilators

Negative Pressure Ventilators

1. Applies negative pressure around the chest wall. This causes intra-airway pressure to become negative, thus drawing air into the lungs through the patient's nose and mouth.
2. No artificial airway is necessary; patient must be able to control and protect own airway.
3. Indicated for selected patients with respiratory neuromuscular problems or as adjunct to weaning from positive pressure ventilation.
4. Examples are the iron lung and cuirass (shell unit) ventilator.

Positive Pressure Ventilators

During mechanical inspiration, air is actively delivered to the patient's lungs under positive pressure. Exhalation is passive. Requires use of a cuffed artificial airway.

1. Pressure cycled.
   a. Delivers selected gas pressure during inspiratory phase.
   b. Volume delivered depends on lung compliance and resistance.
   c. Use of volume-based alarms is recommended because any obstruction between the machine and lungs that allows a buildup of pressure in the ventilator circuitry will cause the ventilator to cycle, but the patient will receive no volume.
   d. Exhaled tidal volume is the variable to monitor closely.
2. Volume limited.
   a. Designated volume of air is delivered with each breath regardless of resistance and compliance. Usual starting volume is 6 to 8 mL/kg.
   b. Delivers the predetermined volume regardless of changing lung compliance (although airway pressures will increase as compliance decreases). Airway pressures vary from patient to patient and from breath to breath.
   c. Pressure-limiting valves, which prevent excessive pressure buildup within the patient-ventilator system, are used. Without this valve, pressure could increase indefinitely and pulmonary barotrauma could result. Usually equipped with a system that alarms when selected pressure limit is exceeded. Pressure-limited settings terminate inspiration when reached.

Modes of Operation

Controlled Ventilation
1. Patient receives a predetermined number and volume of breaths/minute.
2. Provides a fixed level of ventilation, but will not cycle or have gas available in circuitry to respond to patient's own inspiratory efforts. This typically increases work of breathing for patients attempting to breathe spontaneously.
3. Generally used for patients who are unable to initiate spontaneous breaths.

Assist/Control
1. Inspiratory cycle of ventilator is activated by the patient's voluntary inspiratory effort and delivers a preset full volume.
2. Ventilator also cycles at a rate predetermined by the operator. Should the patient not initiate a spontaneous breath, or breathe so weakly that the ventilator cannot function as an assistor, this mandatory baseline rate will provide a minimum respiratory rate.
3. Indicated for patients who are breathing spontaneously, but who have the potential to lose their respiratory drive or muscular control of ventilation. In this mode, the patient's work of breathing is greatly reduced.

Synchronized Intermittent Mandatory Ventilation (SIMV)
1. Allows patient to breathe at his or her own rate and volume spontaneously through the ventilator circuitry.
2. Periodically, at a preselected time, a mandatory breath is delivered. The ventilator delivers the mandatory breath in synchrony with the patient's inspiratory effort.
3. If no inspiratory effort is delivered, the ventilator will deliver a mandatory breath at a scheduled time.
4. Gas provided for spontaneous breathing flows continuously through the ventilator.
5. Ensures that a predetermined number of breaths at a selected V_T are delivered each minute.
6. Indicated for patients who are breathing spontaneously, but at a V_T and/or rate less than adequate for their needs. Allows the patient to do some of the work of breathing.

Pressure Support
1. Augments inspiration to a spontaneously breathing patient.
2. Maintains a set positive pressure during spontaneous inspiration.
3. The patient ventilates spontaneously, establishing own rate, V_T, and inspiratory time.
4. Pressure support may be used independently as a ventilatory mode or used in conjunction with CPAP or synchronized intermittent mandatory ventilation.

Positive Pressure Ventilation Techniques

Positive End-Expiratory Pressure
1. Maneuver by which pressure during mechanical ventilation is maintained above atmospheric at end of exhalation, resulting in an increased functional residual capacity. Airway pressure is therefore positive throughout the entire ventilatory cycle.
2. Purpose of PEEP is to increase functional residual capacity (or the amount of air left in the lungs at the end of expiration). This aids in:
   a. Increasing the surface area of gas exchange.
   b. Preventing collapse of alveolar units and development of atelectasis.
   c. Decreasing intrapulmonary shunt.
   d. Improving lung compliance.
   e. Improving oxygenation.
   f. Recruiting alveolar units that are totally or partially collapsed.
3. Benefits:
   a. Because a greater surface area for diffusion is available and shunting is reduced, it is often possible to use a lower FiO_2 than otherwise would be required to obtain adequate arterial oxygen levels. This reduces the risk of oxygen toxicity in conditions such as acute respiratory distress syndrome (ARDS).
   b. Positive intra-airway pressure may be helpful in reducing the transudation of fluid from the pulmonary capillaries in situations where capillary pressure is increased (ie, left-sided heart failure).
   c. Increased lung compliance resulting in decreased work of breathing.
4. Hazards:
   a. Because the intrathoracic pressure is increased by PEEP, venous return is impeded. This may result in:
      i. Decreased cardiac output and decreased oxygen delivery to the tissues (especially noted in hypovolemic patients).
      ii. Decreased renal perfusion.
      iii. Increased intracranial pressure.
      iv. Hepatic congestion.
   b. The decreased venous return may cause antidiuretic hormone formation to be stimulated, resulting in decreased urine output.
5. Precautions:
   a. Monitor frequently for signs and symptoms of respiratory distress—shortness of breath, dyspnea, tachycardia, chest pain.
   b. Monitor frequently for signs and symptoms of pneumothorax (increased PAP, increased size of hemothorax, uneven chest wall movement, hyperresonant percussion, distant or absent breath sounds).
   c. Monitor for signs of decreased venous return (decreased BP, decreased cardiac output, decreased urine output, peripheral edema).
   d. Abrupt discontinuance of PEEP is not recommended. The patient should not be without PEEP for longer

than 15 seconds. The manual resuscitation bag used for ventilation during suction procedure or patient transport should be equipped with a PEEP device. In-line suctioning may also be used so that PEEP can be maintained.

e. Intrapulmonary blood vessel pressure may increase with compression of the vessels by increased intra-airway pressure. Therefore, central venous pressure (CVP), PAP, and pulmonary capillary wedge pressure may be increased. The clinician must bear this in mind when determining the clinical significance of these pressures.

Continuous Positive Airway Pressure

1. Assists the spontaneously breathing patient to improve oxygenation by elevating the end-expiratory pressure in the lungs throughout the respiratory cycle.
2. May be delivered through ventilator circuitry when ventilator rate is at "0" or may be delivered through a separate CPAP circuitry that does not require the ventilator.
3. Indicated for patients who are capable of maintaining an adequate V_T, but who have pathology preventing maintenance of adequate levels of tissue oxygenation or for sleep apnea.
4. CPAP has the same benefits, hazards, and precautions noted with PEEP. Mean airway pressures may be lower because of lack of mechanical ventilation breaths. This results in less risk of barotrauma and impedance of venous return.

Newer Modes of Ventilation

Inverse Ratio Ventilation

1. I:E ratio is greater than 1, in which inspiration is longer than expiration.
2. Potentially used in patients who are in acute severe hypoxemic respiratory failure. Oxygenation is thought to be improved.
3. Very uncomfortable for patients; need to be heavily sedated.
4. Pressure-controlled inverse ratio ventilation—used in ARDS and acute lung injury.
5. Pressure-regulated volume control ventilator mode is a volume-targeted mode used in acute respiratory failure that combines the advantages of the decelerating inspiratory flow pattern of a pressure-control mode with the ease of use of a volume-control (VC) mode.

Airway Pressure Release Ventilation

1. Ventilator cycles between two different levels of CPAP.
2. The baseline airway pressure is the upper CPAP level and the pressure is intermittently released.
3. Uses a short expiratory time.
4. Used in severe ARDS/acute lung injury.

Noninvasive Positive Pressure Ventilation

1. Uses a nasal or face mask or nasal pillows. Delivers air through a volume- or pressure-controlled ventilator.
2. Used primarily in the past for patients with chronic respiratory failure associated with neuromuscular disease. Now is being used successfully during acute exacerbations. Some patients are able to avoid invasive intubation. Other indications include acute or chronic respiratory distress, acute pulmonary edema, pneumonia, COPD exacerbation, weaning, and postextubation respiratory decompensation.
3. Can be used in the home setting. Equipment is portable and relatively easy to use.
4. Eliminates the need for intubation; preserves normal swallowing, speech, and the cough mechanism.

5. May include BiPAP, which is essentially pressure support with CPAP. The system has a rate setting as well as inspiratory and expiratory pressure setting.

High-Frequency Ventilation

1. Uses very small V_T (dead space ventilation) and high frequency (rates greater than 100/minute).
2. Gas exchange occurs through various mechanisms, not the same as conventional ventilation (convection).
3. Types include:
   a. High-frequency oscillatory ventilation.
   b. High-frequency jet ventilation.
4. Theory is that there is decreased barotrauma by having small V_T and that oxygenation is improved by constant flow of gases.
5. Successful with infant respiratory distress syndrome, much less successful with adult pulmonary complications.

Nursing Assessment and Interventions

1. Monitor for complications:
   a. Airway aspiration, decreased clearance of secretions, ventilator-acquired pneumonia, tracheal damage, and laryngeal edema.
   b. Impaired gas exchange.
   c. Ineffective breathing pattern.
   d. ET tube kinking, cuff failure, mainstem intubation.
   e. Sinusitis.
   f. Pulmonary infection.
   g. Barotrauma (pneumothorax, tension pneumothorax, subcutaneous emphysema, pneumomediastinum).
   h. Decreased cardiac output.
   i. Atelectasis.
   j. Alteration in GI function (stress ulcers, gastric distention, paralytic ileus).
   k. Alteration in renal function.
   l. Alteration in cognitive–perceptual status.
2. Suction the patient as indicated.
   a. When secretions can be seen or sounds resulting from secretions are heard with or without the use of a stethoscope.
   b. After chest physiotherapy.
   c. After bronchodilator treatments.
   d. Increased peak airway pressure in mechanically ventilated patients that is not due to the artificial airway or ventilator tube kinking, the patient biting the tube, the patient coughing or struggling against the ventilator, or a pneumothorax.
3. Provide routine care for patient on mechanical ventilator, including good oral care and repositioning to prevent ventilator-associated pneumonia. Provide humidity to help mobilize secretions.
4. Assist with the weaning process, when indicated (patient gradually assumes responsibility for regulating and performing own ventilations).
   a. Patient must have acceptable ABG values, no evidence of acute pulmonary pathology, and must be hemodynamically stable.
   b. Obtain serial ABGs and/or oximetry readings, as indicated.
   c. Monitor very closely for change in pulse and BP, anxiety, and increased rate of respirations.
   d. The patient is awake and cooperative and displays optimal respiratory drive.
5. Once weaning is successful, extubate and provide alternate means of oxygen.

6. Extubation will be considered when the pulmonary function parameters of V_T, VC, and negative inspiratory pressure are adequate, indicating strong respiratory muscle function.

Community and Home Care Considerations

Patients may require mechanical ventilation at home to replace or assist normal breathing. Ventilator support in the home is used to keep patient clinically stable and to maintain life.

1. Candidates for home ventilation are those patients who are unable to wean from mechanical ventilation and/or have disease progression requiring ventilator support. Candidates for home mechanical ventilator support:
   a. Have a secure artificial airway (tracheostomy tube).
   b. Have FiO_2 requirement ≤40%.
   c. Are medically stable.
   d. Are able to maintain adequate ventilation on standard ventilator settings.
2. Patients may choose not to receive home ventilation. Examples of inappropriate candidates for home ventilation include patients who:
   a. Have a FiO_2 ≥ 40%.
   b. Use PEEP greater than 10 cm H_2O.
   c. Require continuous invasive monitoring.
   d. Lack a mature tracheostomy.
   e. Lack able, willing, appropriate caregivers, and/or caregiver respite.
   f. Lack adequate financial resources for care in home.
   g. Lack adequate physical facilities:
      i. Inadequate heat, electricity, sanitation.
      ii. Presence of fire, health, or safety hazards.
3. For patients on mechanical ventilation in the home, a contract and relationship with a home medical equipment company and home nursing agency must be developed to provide:
   a. Care of ventilator-dependent patient.
   b. Provision and maintenance of equipment.
   c. Timely provision of disposable supplies.
   d. Ongoing monitoring of patient and equipment.
   e. Training of patient, caregivers, and clinical staff on proper management of ventilated patient and use and troubleshooting of equipment.
4. Equipment required:
   a. Appropriate ventilator with alarms (disconnect and high pressure).
   b. Power source.
   c. Humidification system.
   d. Manual resuscitation bag with tracheostomy adapter.
   e. Suction equipment.
   f. Replacement tracheostomy tubes.
   g. Supplemental oxygen, as medically indicated.
   h. Communication method for patient.
   i. Backup charged battery to run ventilator during power failures.
5. Lay caregiver training and return demonstration must include the following:
   a. Proper setup, use, troubleshooting, maintenance, and cleaning and infection control of equipment and supplies.
   b. Appropriate patient assessment and management of abnormalities, including cardiopulmonary resuscitation, response to emergencies, and power and equipment failure.
6. Potential complications include:
   a. Patient deterioration, decannulation, and need for emergency services.
   b. Equipment failure and malfunction.
   c. Psychosocial complications, including depression, anxiety, and/or loss of resources (caregiver, financial, detrimental change in family structure or coping capacity).
7. Communication is essential with local emergency medical services (fire, police, rescue) and utility (telephone, electric) companies from whom the patient would need immediate and additional assistance in event of emergency (eg, power failure, fire).

Thoracic Surgeries

Thoracic surgeries (see Table 10-2) are operative procedures performed to aid in the diagnosis and treatment of certain pulmonary conditions and when performing surgery that compromises the integrity of the thoracic cavity. Procedures include thoracotomy, video-assisted thoracoscopy, decortication, lung volume reduction surgery, lobectomy (see Figure 10-9, page 185), pneumonectomy, segmental resection, and wedge resection. These procedures may or may not require chest drainage immediately after surgery.

 NURSING ALERT Meticulous attention must be given to the preoperative and postoperative care of patients undergoing thoracic surgery. These operations are wide in scope and represent a major stress on the cardiorespiratory system.

Preoperative Management

Goal is to maximize respiratory function to improve the outcome postoperatively and reduce risk of complications.

1. Encourage the patient to stop smoking to restore bronchial ciliary action and to reduce the amount of sputum, and likelihood of postoperative atelectasis, by decreasing secretions and increasing oxygen saturation.
2. Teach an effective coughing technique.
   a. Sit upright with knees flexed and body bending slightly forward (or lie on side with hips and knees flexed if unable to sit up).
   b. Splint the incision with hands or folded towel.
   c. Take three short breaths, followed by a deep inspiration, inhaling slowly and evenly through the nose.
   d. Contract abdominal muscles and cough twice forcefully with mouth open and tongue out.
   e. Alternate technique—huffing and coughing—is less painful. Take a deep diaphragmatic breath and exhale forcefully against hand; exhale in a quick, distinct pant, or "huff."
3. Humidify the air to loosen secretions.
4. Administer bronchodilators to reduce bronchospasm.
5. Administer antimicrobials for infection.
6. Encourage deep breathing with the use of incentive spirometer to prevent atelectasis postoperatively.
7. Teach diaphragmatic breathing.
8. Carry out chest physical therapy and postural drainage to reduce pooling of lung secretions (see page 176).
9. Evaluate cardiopulmonary status for risk and prevention of complication.
10. Encourage activity to improve exercise tolerance.
11. Diagnostic studies may include PFT, chest x-ray, ECG, ABGs, serum electrolytes, CBC, and coagulation studies.

Table 10-2 Thoracic Surgery Types

TYPE	DESCRIPTION	INDICATIONS
Exploratory thoracotomy	*Internal view of lung* • Usually posterolateral parascapular but could be anterior incision • Chest tubes after procedure	May be used to confirm carcinoma or for chest trauma (to detect source of bleeding)
Lobectomy	*One-lobe removal* • Thoracotomy incision at site of lobe removal • Chest tubes after procedure	Used when pathology is limited to one area of lung: bronchogenic carcinoma, giant emphysematous blebs or bullae, benign tumors, metastatic malignant tumors, bronchiectasis, and fungal infections
Pneumonectomy	*Removal of an entire lung* • Posterolateral or anterolateral thoracotomy incision • Sometimes there is a rib resection • Normally no chest drains or tubes because fluid accumulation in empty space is desirable	Performed chiefly for carcinoma but may be used for lung abscesses, bronchiectasis, or extensive tuberculosis. *Note: Right lung is more vascular than left; may cause more physiologic problems if removed*
Segmentectomy (segmental resection)	• *Removal of one or more lung segments. Segments function as individual units*	Used when pathology is localized (such as in bronchiectasis) and when the patient has preexisting cardiopulmonary compromise
Wedge resection	*Removal of small, localized lesion that occupies only part of a segment.* • Incision made without regard to segments • Chest tubes after procedure	Performed for random lung biopsy and small peripheral nodules Considered when less invasive tests have failed to establish a diagnosis May be used as a therapeutic procedure
Thoracoscopy	*Direct visualization of pleura with thoracoscope via an intercostal incision* • Medical under sedation or local anesthesia; allows for visualization and biopsy • Video-assisted thoracoscopic surgery (VATS) under general anesthesia; multiple puncture sites and video screen allow for visualization and manipulation of the pleura, mediastinum, and lung parenchyma	VATS may be used for lung biopsy, lobectomy, resection of nodules, repair of fistulas
Decortication	*Removal or stripping of thick fibrous membrane from visceral pleura* • Use of chest tube drainage system postoperatively	Empyema unresponsive to conservative management
Thoracotomy not involving lungs	• Incision into the thoracic cavity for surgical procedures on other structures	Used for hiatal hernia repair, open-heart surgery, esophageal surgery, tracheal resection, aortic aneurysm repair
Lung volume reduction surgery (LVRS)	• Involves reducing lung volume by multiple wedge excisions or VATS	Performed in advanced bullous emphysema, α^1-antitrypsin emphysema

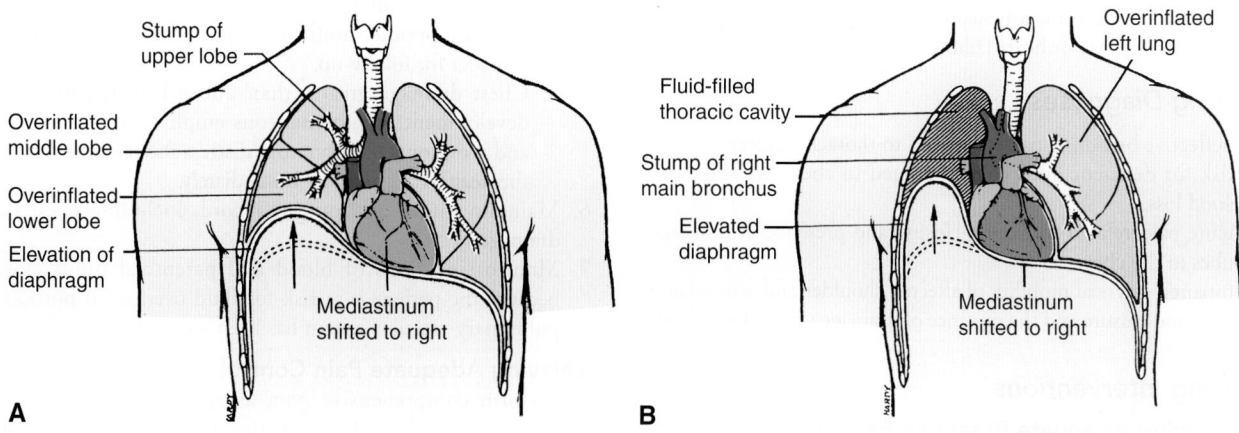

Figure 10-9. Operative procedures. **(A)** Lobectomy. **(B)** Pneumonectomy.

12. Administer medications and limit sodium and fluid to improve heart failure, if indicated.
13. Correct anemia, dehydration, and hypoproteinemia with IV infusions, tube feedings, and blood transfusions as indicated.
14. Give prophylactic anticoagulant, as prescribed, to reduce perioperative incidence of deep vein thrombosis and pulmonary embolism.
15. Provide teaching and counseling.
    a. Orient the patient to events that will occur in the postoperative period—coughing and deep breathing, suctioning, chest tube and drainage system, oxygen therapy, ventilator therapy, pain control, leg exercises, and range-of-motion (ROM) exercises for affected shoulder.
16. Make sure that patient fully understands surgery and is emotionally prepared for it; verify that informed consent has been obtained.

Postoperative Management

1. Use mechanical ventilator and/or supplemental oxygen until respiratory function and cardiovascular status stabilize. Assist with weaning and extubation.
2. Auscultate chest, monitor vital signs, monitor ECG, and assess respiratory rate and depth frequently. Arterial line, CVP, and pulmonary artery catheter are usually used.
3. Monitor ABG values and/or SaO_2 frequently.
4. Monitor and manage chest drainage system to drain fluid, blood, clots, and air from the pleura after surgery (see page 188). Chest drainage is usually not used after pneumonectomy because it is desirable that the pleural space fills with an effusion, which eventually obliterates the space.

Complications

1. Hypoxia—assess for restlessness, tachycardia, tachypnea, and elevated BP.
2. Postoperative bleeding—monitor for restlessness, anxiety, pallor, tachycardia, and hypotension.
3. Pneumonia; atelectasis—monitor for fever, chest pain, dyspnea, changes in lung sounds on auscultation.
4. Bronchopleural fistula from disruption of a bronchial suture or staple; bronchial stump leak.
    a. Observe for sudden onset of respiratory distress or cough productive of serosanguineous fluid.
    b. Position with the operative side down.
    c. Prepare for immediate chest tube insertion and/or surgical intervention.
5. Cardiac dysrhythmias (usually occurring 3rd to 4th postoperative day); MI or heart failure.

Nursing Diagnoses

- Ineffective breathing pattern related to thoracic surgery.
- Risk for deficient fluid volume related to chest drainage and blood loss.
- Acute pain related to wound closure and presence of drainage tubes in the chest.
- Impaired physical mobility of affected shoulder and arm related to wound closure and the presence of drainage tubes in the chest.

Nursing Interventions

Maintaining Adequate Breathing Pattern

1. Monitor rate, rhythm, depth, and effort of respirations.

2. Auscultate chest for adequacy of air movement to detect bronchospasm, consolidation.
3. Monitor pulse oximetry and obtain ABG analysis and pulmonary function measurements as ordered.
4. Monitor LOC and inspiratory effort closely to begin weaning from ventilator as soon as possible.
5. Suction, as needed, using meticulous aseptic technique.
6. Elevate the head of the bed 30 to 40 degrees when patient is oriented and BP is stabilized to improve movement of diaphragm and alleviate dyspnea.
7. Encourage coughing and deep-breathing exercises and use of an incentive spirometer to prevent bronchospasm, retained secretions, atelectasis, and pneumonia.
8. Provide optimal pain relief to promote deep breathing, turning, and coughing.

 NURSING ALERT Tracheobronchial secretions are present in excessive amounts in postthoracotomy patients because of trauma to the tracheobronchial tree during operation, diminished lung ventilation, and diminished cough reflex.

 NURSING ALERT Look for changes in color and consistency of suctioned sputum. Colorless, fluid sputum is not unusual; opacification or coloring of sputum may mean dehydration or infection.

Stabilizing Hemodynamic Status

1. Evaluate BP, pulse, and respiration every 15 minutes or more frequently as indicated; extend the time intervals according to the patient's clinical status.
2. Monitor heart rate and rhythm by way of auscultation and continuous ECG because dysrhythmias are frequently seen following thoracic surgery.
3. Monitor CVP for prompt recognition of hypovolemia and for effectiveness of fluid replacement.
4. Monitor cardiac output and pulmonary artery systolic, diastolic, and wedge pressures. Watch for subtle changes, especially in the patient with underlying cardiovascular disease.
5. Assess chest tube drainage for amount and character of fluid.
    a. Chest drainage should progressively decrease after first 12 hours.
    b. Prepare for blood replacement and possible reoperation to achieve hemostasis if bleeding persists.
    c. Chest tube drainage in excess of 1,000 to 1,200 mL per 24-hour period should be reported to the health care provider for follow-up.
    d. Chest drainage greater than 200 mL in the first hour, development of subcutaneous emphysema, or any signs and symptoms of respiratory distress should be reported to the health care provider immediately.
6. Maintain intake and output record, including chest tube drainage.
7. Monitor infusions of blood and parenteral fluids closely because the patient is at risk for fluid overload if portion of pulmonary vascular system has been reduced.

Achieving Adequate Pain Control

1. Perform comprehensive pain assessment including onset, location, duration, characteristics, precipitating factors, and response to interventions.

2. Provide appropriate pain relief—pain limits chest excursions, thereby decreasing ventilation. Severity of pain varies with type of incision and with the patient's reaction to and ability to cope with pain. Usually, a posterolateral incision is the most painful.
3. Give opioids (usually by continuous IV infusion or by epidural catheter by way of patient-controlled analgesia pump) for pain relief, as prescribed, to permit patient to breathe more deeply and cough more effectively. To avoid respiratory and CNS depression, do not give too much opioid; patient should be alert enough to cough.
4. Assist with intercostal nerve block or cryoanalgesia (intercostal nerve freezing) for pain control as ordered.
5. Position for comfort and optimal ventilation (head of bed elevated 15 to 30 degrees); this also helps residual air to rise in upper portion of pleural space where it can be removed by the chest tube.
   a. Patients with limited respiratory reserve may not be able to turn on unoperated side because this may limit ventilation of the operated side.
   b. Vary the position from horizontal to semi-erect to prevent retention of secretions in the dependent portion of the lungs.
6. Encourage splinting of incision with pillow, folded towel, or hands, while turning, changing position, or coughing.
7. Teach relaxation (nonpharmacologic) techniques, such as progressive muscle relaxation and imagery, to help reduce pain.

 NURSING ALERT Evaluate for signs of hypoxia thoroughly when anxiety, restlessness, and agitation of new onset are noted before administering as-needed sedatives.

Increasing Mobility of Affected Shoulder
1. Begin ROM exercise of arm and shoulder on affected side immediately to prevent ankylosis of the shoulder ("frozen" shoulder).
2. Perform exercises at time of maximal pain relief.
3. Encourage patient to actively perform exercises three to four times per day, taking care not to disrupt chest tube or invasive lines (ie, IV).

Patient Education and Health Maintenance
1. Advise that there will be some intercostal pain for several weeks, which can be relieved by local heat and oral analgesia. Many patients experience intercostal pain up to 1 year following surgery.
2. Advise that weakness and fatigability are common during the first 3 weeks after a thoracotomy, but exercise tolerance will improve with conditioning.
3. Suggest alternating walking and other activities with frequent short rest periods. Walk at a moderate pace and gradually extend walking time and distance.
4. Encourage continuing deep-breathing exercises for several weeks after surgery to attain full expansion of residual lung tissue.
5. Instruct on maintaining good body alignment to ensure full lung expansion.
6. Advise that chest muscles may be weaker than normal for 3 to 6 months after surgery. Patient must avoid lifting more than 10 pound (4.5 kg) until complete healing has taken place.
7. Any activity that causes undue fatigue, increased shortness of breath, or chest pain should be stopped immediately.

8. Because all or part of one lung has been removed, warn patient to avoid respiratory irritants (smoke, fumes, and high level of air pollution).
   a. Avoid irritants that may cause coughing spasms.
   b. Sit in nonsmoking areas in public places.
9. Encourage patient to receive an annual influenza vaccine and obtain a pneumococcal pneumonia vaccine.
10. Encourage patient to keep follow-up visits.
11. Instruct patient to prevent respiratory infections by frequent handwashing and avoiding others with respiratory infections.

Evaluation: Expected Outcomes
- Respirations with normal range, adequate depth; lungs clear; ABG values and SaO_2 within normal limits.
- BP, CVP, and pulse within normal limits for individual.
- Coughs and turns independently; reports relief of pain.
- Performs active ROM of affected arm and shoulder; reports improved exercise tolerance.

Chest Drainage

Chest drainage is the insertion of a tube into the pleural space to evacuate air or fluid and/or help regain negative pressure. Whenever the chest is opened, there is loss of negative pressure in the pleural space, which can result in collapse of the lung. The collection of air, fluid, or other substances in the thoracic cavity can compromise cardiopulmonary function and cause collapse of the lung.

It is necessary to keep the pleural space evacuated postoperatively and to maintain negative pressure within this potential space. Therefore, during or immediately after thoracic surgery, chest tubes/catheters are positioned strategically in the pleural space, sutured to the skin, and connected to a drainage apparatus to remove the residual air and fluid from the pleural or mediastinal space. This assists in the reexpansion of remaining lung tissue.

Chest drainage can also be used to treat spontaneous pneumothorax or hemothorax/pneumothorax caused by trauma (see Table 10-3). Sites for chest tube placement are:
1. For pneumothorax (air)—second or third interspace along midclavicular or anterior axillary line.
2. For hemothorax (fluid)—sixth or seventh lateral interspace in the midaxillary line.

Principles of Chest Drainage
1. Many types of commercial chest drainage systems are in use, most of which use the water-seal principle. The chest tube/catheter and collecting tubing is attached to a chest drainage system using a one-way valve principle. Water acts as a seal and permits air and fluid to drain from the chest. However, air cannot reenter the chest cavity.

Table 10-3	Indications for Chest Tube Use
INDICATION	**ACCUMULATING SUBSTANCE**
Pneumothorax	Air
Hemothorax	Blood
Pleural effusion	Fluid
Chylothorax	Lymphatic fluid
Empyema	Pus

Figure 10-10. Chest drainage systems. **(A)** Strategic placement of a chest catheter in the pleural space. **(B)** Three types of mechanical drainage systems. **(C)** A Pleur-evac operating system: (*1*) the collection chamber, (*2*) the water seal chamber, and (*3*) the suction control chamber. The Pleur-evac is a single unit with all three bottles identified as chambers.

2. Chest drainage can be categorized into three types of mechanical systems (see Figure 10-10). There are numerous types of chest drainage units available including dry suction systems.

One-Bottle Water-Seal System
1. The end of the collecting tube is covered by a layer of water, which permits drainage of air and fluid from the pleural space, but does not allow air to move back into the chest. Functionally, drainage depends on gravity, on the mechanics of respiration, and, if desired, on suction by the addition of controlled vacuum.
2. The tube from the patient extends approximately 1 inch (2.5 cm) below the level of the water in the container. There is a vent for the escape of any air that may be leaking from the lung. The water level fluctuates as the patient breathes; it goes up when the patient inhales and down when the patient exhales.
3. At the end of the drainage tube, bubbling may or may not be visible. Bubbling can mean either persistent leakage of air from the lung or other tissues or a leak in the system.

Two-Bottle Water-Seal System
1. The two-bottle system consists of the same water-seal chamber, plus a fluid-collection bottle.
2. Drainage is similar to that of a single unit, except that when pleural fluid drains, the underwater-seal system is not affected by the volume of the drainage.
3. Effective drainage depends on gravity or on the amount of suction added to the system. When vacuum (suction) is added to

the system from a vacuum source, such as wall suction, the connection is made at the vent stem of the underwater-seal bottle.
4. The amount of suction applied to the system is regulated by the wall gauge.

Three-Bottle Water-Seal System
1. The three-bottle system is similar in all respects to the two-bottle system, except for the addition of a third bottle to control the amount of suction applied. Recent research has shown that suction may actually prolong an air leak by pulling air through the opening that would otherwise heal on its own.
2. The amount of suction is determined by the depth to which the tip of the venting glass tube is submerged in the water and level of water in the suction chamber or setting of a dial—depending on the system in use.
3. In the three-bottle system (as in the other two systems), drainage depends on gravity or the amount of suction applied. The mechanical suction motor or wall suction creates and maintains a negative pressure throughout the entire closed drainage system.
4. The manometer bottle regulates the amount of negative pressure transmitted back to the patient from the suction/vacuum device. This is accomplished through the use of a water or dry system that down-regulates the suction/vacuum applied.
5. In the commercially available systems, the three bottles are contained in one unit and identified as "chambers" (see Figure 10-10C). The principles remain the same for the commercially available products as they do for the glass bottle system.

6. First chamber acts as the collection chamber and receives fluid and air from the chest cavity through the collecting tube attached to the chest tube.

7. Second chamber acts as the water-seal chamber with 2 cm of water acting as a one-way valve, allowing drainage out but preventing backflow of air or fluid into the patient.

8. Third chamber applies controlled suction. The amount of suction is regulated by the volume of water (usually 20 cm) in the chamber, not the amount of suction or bubbling with a water system. In a dry suction control system no water is used, no bubbling occurs, and a restrictive device or regulator is used to dial the desired negative pressure (up to 40 cm suction).

> **NURSING ALERT** When the motor or the wall vacuum is turned off, the drainage system should be open to the atmosphere so that intrapleural air can escape from the system. This can be done by detaching the tubing from the suction port to provide a vent.

Nursing and Patient Care Considerations

1. Assist with chest tube insertion.
2. Assess patient's pain at insertion site and give medication appropriately. If patient is in pain, chest excursion and lung inflation will be hampered. Medicate for pain as needed. Assess for effectiveness and respiratory depression.
3. Maintain chest tubes to provide drainage and enhance lung reinflation. Ensure the tubing does not loop, kink, or restrict movements of the patient.
4. Maintain integrity of insertion site, observing for drainage, redness, impaired healing, and subcutaneous emphysema.
5. Make sure there is fluctuation of the fluid level in the drainage container ("tidaling"). Fluctuation will stop if a dependent loop develops or the tubing is obstructed by blood clots or fibrin and when the lung is reexpanded.

> **NURSING ALERT** Clamping of chest tubes is not recommended because of the increased danger of tension pneumothorax from rapid accumulation of air in the pleural space. Clamp only momentarily to change the drainage system. Check for leaks to assess the patient's tolerance for removal of the chest tube (perhaps up to 24 hours).

> **NURSING ALERT** Milking and stripping of chest tubes to maintain patency are not recommended. This practice has been found to cause significant increases in intrapleural pressures and damage to the pleural tissue. New chest tubes contain a nonthrombogenic coating, thus decreasing the potential for clotting. If it is necessary to help the drainage move through the tubing, apply a gentle squeeze-and-release motion to small segments of the chest tube between your fingers.

SELECTED REFERENCES

Ambrosino, N., Makhabah, D. (2014). Physiotherapy in the ICU. *Respiratory Therapy*. Available: *http://www.rtmagazine.com/2014/07/physiotherapy-icu/*

American Association for Respiratory Care. (2007). Clinical practice guidelines. Bronchoscopy assisting—2007 revision and update. *Respiratory Care*, 52(1), 74–80.

American Association for Respiratory Care. (2007). Clinical practice guidelines. Removal of endotracheal tube. *Respiratory Care*, 52(1), 81–93.

American Association for Respiratory Care. (2007). Clinical practice guidelines. Removal of the endotracheal tube—2007 revision and update. *Respiratory Care*, 52(1), 81–93.

American Association for Respiratory Care. (2010). Clinical practice guidelines. Endotracheal suctioning of mechanically ventilated patients with artificial airways. *Respiratory Care*, 55(6), 758–764.

American Heart Association. (2015). *Highlights of the 2015 American Heart Association guidelines update for cardiopulmonary resuscitation and emergency cardiovascular care*. Dallas, TX: Author.

American Society of Anesthesiologists. (2013). Practice guidelines for management of the difficult airway: An updated report by the American society of anesthesiologists task force on management of the difficult airway. *Anesthesiology*, 118(2), 251–270.

Bailey, P. (2016). Continuous oxygen delivery systems for infants, children, and adults. *UpToDate*. Available: *https://www.uptodate.com/contents/continous-oxygen-delivery-systems-for-infants-adults-children*

Bailey, P. (2017). Continuous oxygen delivery systems for infants, children and adults. *UpToDate*. Available: *http://www.uptodate.com/contents/continuous-oxygen-delivery-systems-for-infants-children-and-adults*

Burns, S. (2014). *AACN essentials of critical care nursing* (3rd ed.). New York: McGraw-Hill.

Chen, Y., Coxson, H., & Reid, W. D. (2016). Reliability and validity of the brief fatigue inventory and dyspnea inventory in people with chronic obstructive pulmonary disease. *Journal of Pain and Symptom Management*, 52(2), 298–304.

Cheung, H., & Cheung, L. (2015). Coaching patients during pulmonary function testing. A practical guide. *Canadian Journal of Respiratory Therapy*, 51(3), 65–68.

Conaway, M., Bleck, T., Burns, S., et al. (2012). The Relationship of 26 clinical factors to weaning outcome. *American Journal of Critical Care*, 21, 52–59.

Courey, A., & Hyzy, R. (2017). Overview of mechanical ventilation. *UpToDate*. Available: *www.uptodate.com*

Dawson, D. (2014). Essential principles: Tracheostomy care in the adult patient. *British Association of Critical Care Nurses*, 19(2), 63–72.

Hanlon, P. (2017). Patient monitoring: Capnography and capnometry applications. *The Journal for Respiratory Care Practitioners*, 30(7), 18–19.

Hess, D. (2016). Delivery of inhaled medications in adults. *UpToDate*. Available: *https://www.uptodate.com/contents/delivery-of-inhaled-medications-in-adults*

Hess, D., & Kacmerek, R. (2014). *Essentials of mechanical ventilation* (3rd ed.). New York, NY: McGraw-Hill.

Heuer, A., & Scanlan, C. (2017). *Wilkins clinical assessment in respiratory care* (8th ed.). St. Louis, MO: Mosby.

Irwin, R. S., French, C. T., Lewis, S. Z., et al. (2014). Overview of the management of cough: CHEST guideline and expert panel report. *Chest*, 146(4), 885–889.

Johnson, A., & Crumlet, H. (2017). *Critical care nursing certification: Preparation, review and practice exam* (7th ed.). New York: McGraw-Hill.

Kodali, B. (2014). *Capnography.com*. Available: *www.capnography.com*

Konstaninidi, E., Lappa, A., Tzortzi, A., & Panagiotis, B. (2015). Exhaled breath condensate: Technical and diagnostic aspects. *The Scientific World Journal*, 2015, 435160. Available: *https://www.hindawi.com/journals/tswj/2015/435160/abs/*

MacIntyre, N. R., Galvin, W. F., Mishoe, S. C., Hess, D. R., et al. (2016). *Respiratory care: Principles and practice* (3rd ed.). Sudbury, MA: Jones & Bartlett.

Mejia, A., Montero, J., Vasquez-Caicido, M., et al. (2016). Radiological evaluation and endovascular treatment of hemoptysis. *Current Problems in Diagnostic Radiology*, 45(3), 215–224.

Morris, L., Whitmer, A., & McIntosh, E. (2013). Tracheostomy care and complications in the intensive care unit. *Critical Care Nurse*, 33(5), 18–30.

National Heart Lung and Blood Institute. (2015). Pulmonary Hypertension. Available: *https://www.nhlbi.nhi.gov/healthtopics/pulmonary-hypertension*

Orlewicz, M. (2016). Double lumen endotracheal tube placement. *Medscape Drugs and Diseases*. Available: *http://emedicine.medscape.com/article/1999993-overview*

Paradis, T., Dixon, J., & Tieu, B. (2016). The role of bronchoscopy in the diagnosis of airway disease. *Journal of Thoracic Disease*, 8(12), 3826–3837.

Pathmanathan, N., Beaumont, N., & Gratrix, A. (2015). Respiratory physiotherapy in the critical care unit. *British Journal of Anesthesia*, 15(1), 20–25.

Reamy, B., Willams, P., & Odom, M. R. (2017). Pleuritic chest pain: Sorting through the differential diagnosis. *American Family Physician*, 96(5), 306–312.

Singh, L. T., Sharara, R., Leap, J., & Singh, A. (2016). Management of respiratory failure. *Critical Care Nursing Quarterly*, 39(2), 94–109.

Sokol, G., Vilozni, D., Hakimi, R., et al. (2015). The short-term effect of breathing tasks via an incentive spirometer on lung function compared with autogenic drainage in subjects with cystic fibrosis. *Respiratory Care, 60*(12), 1819–1825.

Strickland, S. L., Rubin, B. K., Drescher, G. S., et al. (2013). AARC clinical practice guideline: Effectiveness of nonpharmacologic airway clearance therapies in hospitalized patients. *Respiratory Care, 58*(12), 2187–2193.

Theodore, A. (2015). Arterial blood gases. *UpToDate*. Available: *www.uptodate.com/contents/arterialbloodgases*

Wang, C. H., Tsai, J.C., Chen, S. F., et al. (2017). Normal saline instillation before suctioning: A meta analysis of randomized control trials. *Australian Critical Care, 30*(5), 260–265.

Weinberger, S., & Silverstri, R. (2016). Treatment of subacute and chronic cough in adults. *UpToDate*. Available: *www.uptodate.com/contents/treatment-of-subacute-and-chronic-cough-in-adults*

Wiegand, D. J. (2016). *AACN procedure manual for critical care* (7th ed.). Philadelphia, PA: Elsevier Saunders.

11

Respiratory Disorders

ACUTE DISORDERS

See additional online content: Procedure Guidelines 11-1.

Respiratory Failure

Respiratory failure is a failure of the one or both of the respiratory system's gas exchange systems: oxygenation (hypoxemia respiratory failure) and carbon dioxide elimination (hypercapnic respiratory failure).

Hypoxemic respiratory failure (type I) is characterized by arterial oxygen (PaO_2) level below 60 mm Hg (hypoxemia) with a normal (40 mm Hg) or low arterial carbon dioxide level ($PaCO_2$). It is the most common form of respiratory failure, usually associated with acute diseases of the lung generally involving fluid collection or collapse of alveolar units. Examples include cardiogenic or noncardiogenic pulmonary edema, pneumonia, and pulmonary hemorrhage.

Hypercapnic respiratory failure (type II) is characterized by an arterial carbon dioxide ($PaCO_2$) level of greater than 50 mm Hg. Hypoxemia is common while breathing room air. The pH depends on the bicarbonate level, which, in turn, is dependent on the duration and degree of hypercapnia.

Respiratory failure may be further classified as acute, chronic, or both. Acute respiratory failure is characterized by life-threatening abnormalities in arterial blood gases (ABGs) and acid–base levels, whereas chronic respiratory failure abnormalities may be less dramatic and more insidious.

Classification

Acute Respiratory Failure

1. Characterized by hypoxemia (PaO_2 less than 60 mm Hg) or hypercapnia ($PaCO_2$ greater than 50 mm Hg) and acidosis (pH less than 7.35).
2. Occurs rapidly, usually in minutes to hours or days.

Chronic Respiratory Failure

1. Characterized by hypoxemia and/or hypercapnia with a normal pH (7.35 to 7.45).

2. Occurs over a period of days, months, or years, allowing activation of compensatory mechanisms, including renal bicarbonate retention (normal, approximately 22 to 26 mEq/L) with normalization of pH (or only slightly decreased, approximately 7.30 to 7.34).

Combined Acute and Chronic Respiratory Failure

1. Characterized by an abrupt increase in the degree of hypoxemia and/or hypercapnia in patients with preexisting chronic respiratory failure.
2. May occur during or following acute upper respiratory infection, pneumonia, exacerbation, or without obvious cause.
3. Extent of deterioration is best assessed by comparing the patient's present ABG levels with previous ABG levels (patient baseline).

Pathophysiology and Etiology

Hypoxemic Respiratory Failure

Characterized by a decrease in PaO_2 and normal or decreased $PaCO_2$.

1. The primary problem is inability to adequately oxygenate blood, resulting in hypoxemia, because of an abnormality in one or more parts of the respiratory system, central nervous system (CNS), respiratory muscles, or chest wall.
2. Hypoxemia occurs because damage to the alveolar–capillary membrane causes leakage of fluid into the interstitial space or into the alveoli and slows or prevents movement of oxygen from the alveoli to the pulmonary capillary blood.
   a. Damage is either widespread (eg, acute respiratory distress syndrome [ARDS]) or relatively localized (eg, lobar pneumonia), resulting in decreased or absent ventilation in affected areas of the lung.
   b. Consequences are severe ventilation–perfusion mismatch and shunt (perfusion without ventilation).
3. Hypocapnia may result from hypoxemia and decreased pulmonary compliance or stiffness because of fluid within the lung.
   a. Change in compliance reflexively stimulates the increased ventilation.
   b. Ventilation is also increased as a response to hypoxemia.

4. Ultimately, if treatment is unsuccessful, $PaCO_2$ will increase and the patient will experience both an increase in $PaCO_2$ and a decrease in PaO_2.

5. Etiology includes the following:
   a. Cardiogenic or noncardiogenic pulmonary edema, pneumonia, and pulmonary hemorrhage.
   b. ARDS. The four main causes of ARDS are aspiration, pneumonia, sepsis, and trauma. However, there are numerous other causes of lung injury including pancreatitis, smoke inhalation, and near drowning.
   c. Hypercapnic respiratory failure: drug overdose, neuromuscular disease, chest wall abnormalities, asthma, and chronic obstructive pulmonary disease (COPD).

Ventilatory Failure without Underlying Lung Disease

Characterized by a decrease in PaO_2 that is proportional to the increase in $PaCO_2$ and a decrease in pH.

1. The primary problem is insufficient respiratory center stimulation or insufficient chest wall movement, resulting in alveolar hypoventilation.
2. Hypercapnia occurs because impaired neuromuscular function or chest wall expansion limits the amount of carbon dioxide removed from the lungs.
   a. The primary problem is not the lungs. The patient's minute ventilation (tidal volume [V_T] × respiratory rate) is insufficient to allow normal alveolar gas exchange.
3. Carbon dioxide (CO_2) not excreted by the lungs combines with water (H_2O) to form carbonic acid (H_2CO_3). This predisposes to acidosis and a fall in pH.
4. Hypoxemia occurs as a consequence of inadequate ventilation and hypercapnia. When $PaCO_2$ rises, PaO_2 falls unless supplemental oxygen is used.
5. Etiology includes the following:
   a. Insufficient respiratory center activity (drug intoxication, eg, opioid overdose, oversedation, general anesthesia; vascular disorders, such as cerebral vascular insufficiency, brain tumor; trauma, such as head injury, increased intracranial pressure).
   b. Insufficient chest wall function (neuromuscular disease, such as Guillain-Barré syndrome, myasthenia gravis, amyotrophic lateral sclerosis, poliomyelitis; chest wall trauma resulting in multiple fractures; spinal cord trauma; kyphoscoliosis).

Ventilatory Failure with Intrinsic Lung Disease

Characterized by a decrease in PaO_2, increase in $PaCO_2$, and decrease in pH.

1. The primary problem is acute exacerbation or chronic progression of previously existing lung disease, resulting in CO_2 retention.
2. Hypercapnia occurs because of damage to the lung parenchyma primarily caused by chronic airway obstruction (chronic bronchitis, emphysema, or severe asthma). This limits the amount of CO_2 removed by the lungs because the lungs are hyperinflated and poorly perfused.
3. The CO_2 not excreted by the lungs combines with H_2O to form H_2CO_3. This predisposes to acidosis with a fall in pH.
4. Hypoxemia occurs due to hypoventilation and hypercapnia. In addition, damage to the lung parenchyma and/or airway obstruction limits the amount of oxygen that enters the pulmonary capillary blood.
5. Etiology includes the following:
   a. COPD, chronic bronchitis, emphysema.
   b. Severe asthma.
   c. Cystic fibrosis.

Clinical Manifestations

1. Hypoxemia—restlessness, agitation, dyspnea, disorientation, confusion, delirium, loss of consciousness.
2. Hypercapnia—headache, somnolence, dizziness, confusion.
3. Tachypnea initially; when no longer able to compensate, bradypnea.
4. Accessory muscle use.
5. Asynchronous respirations.

 NURSING ALERT Obtain ABG levels whenever the history or signs and symptoms suggest that the patient is at risk for developing respiratory failure. Initial and subsequent values should be recorded, so comparisons can be made over time. The need for ABG analysis can be decreased by continuous oximetry monitoring of oxygen saturation (SpO_2). Correlate oximeter values with ABG values and then use oximeter for trending. Be aware that oximetry does not measure $PaCO_2$ and pH, important determinants of respiratory acidosis.

Diagnostic Evaluation

1. ABG analysis—shows changes in PaO_2, $PaCO_2$, pH, and possibly HCO_3 from patient's normal levels or PaO_2 less than 60 mm Hg, $PaCO_2$ greater than 50 mm Hg, and pH less than 7.35.
2. Pulse oximetry—decreasing SpO_2 (less than 90%).
3. End-tidal CO_2 monitoring—elevated (greater than 40 mm Hg or greater than 5 mm Hg above $PaCO_2$).
4. Complete blood count, serum electrolytes, chest x-ray, urinalysis, electrocardiogram (ECG), and blood and sputum cultures—to aid in determination of underlying cause and patient's condition.

Management

Hypoxemia is the major acute concern impacting organ function. Once corrected with stable ventilation and hemodynamics, identification and correction of underlying causes is essential and used to direct treatment.

1. Oxygen therapy to correct hypoxemia.
2. Turn patient regularly and mobilize when clinically stable to improve ventilation and oxygenation. When appropriate, early ambulation of the patient.
3. Bronchodilators and possibly corticosteroids to reduce bronchospasm and inflammation.
4. Diuretics for pulmonary vascular congestion or pulmonary edema.
5. Ventilatory support using mechanical ventilation or noninvasive positive pressure ventilation using a face mask.

 NURSING ALERT Unless mechanically ventilated, high-flow oxygen in COPD patients with CO_2 retention is contraindicated because it may cause depression of the respiratory center drive. In this population, the drive to breathe may be hypoxemia.

Complications

1. Oxygen toxicity if prolonged high FiO_2 required (≥ 0.80 for ≥ 3 days).
2. Barotrauma from mechanical ventilation intervention—damage to alveoli causing extra-alveolar air, primarily caused by the use of nonphysiologic tidal volumes (greater than 8 mL/kg predicted body weight).

Nursing Assessment

See Standards of Care Guidelines 11-1.

1. Note objective signs suggesting increased work of breathing that include some combination of the following: tachypnea, pronounced use of sternocleidomastoid muscles, tracheal tugging, nasal flaring, sternal retractions (or intercostal muscle retraction) recruitment of abdominal muscles during exhalation, and diaphoresis. Patient may also complain of dyspnea ("can't catch my breath," "my breathing is hard," etc.).
2. Assess breath sounds.
   a. Diminished or absent sounds may suggest inability to ventilate the lungs sufficiently to prevent atelectasis. Decreased breath sounds may be common in moderate to severe COPD.
   b. Crackles may indicate ineffective airway clearance and fluid in the lungs.
   c. Wheezing indicates narrowed airways and bronchospasm.
   d. Rhonchi and crackles suggest ineffective secretion clearance.
3. Assess level of consciousness (LOC) and ability to tolerate increased work of breathing.
   a. Confusion and lethargy.
   b. Rapid shallow breathing, abdominal paradox (inward movement of abdominal wall during inspiration), and accessory muscle retractions suggest inability to maintain adequate minute ventilation.
4. Assess for signs of hypoxemia and hypercapnia.
5. Analyze ABG and compare with previous values.
   a. If the patient cannot maintain a minute ventilation sufficient to prevent CO_2 retention, pH will fall.
   b. Mechanical ventilation or noninvasive ventilation may be needed if pH falls to 7.30 or below.
6. Determine vital capacity (VC) and respiratory rate, and compare with values indicating the need for mechanical ventilation:

   a. VC less than 15 mL/kg.
   b. Respiratory rate greater than 30 breaths/minute.
   c. Negative inspiratory force less than –30 cm H_2O.
   d. Refractory hypoxemia.
7. Determine hemodynamic status through assessment of blood pressure (BP), heart rate, pulmonary wedge pressure, cardiac output, and SvO_2, and compare with previous values. If patient is on mechanical ventilation with positive end-expiratory pressure (PEEP), venous return may be limited, resulting in decreased cardiac output.

Nursing Diagnoses

- Impaired Gas Exchange related to inadequate respiratory center activity, chest wall movement, airway obstruction, and/or fluid in the lungs.
- Ineffective Airway Clearance related to increased, tenacious, and/or retained secretions.

Nursing Interventions

Improving Gas Exchange

1. Administer oxygen to maintain PaO_2 of 60 mm Hg or SaO_2 greater than 90% using devices that provide increased oxygen concentrations (aerosol mask, partial rebreathing mask, nonrebreathing mask, noninvasive positive pressure ventilation, or mechanical ventilation).
2. Administer diuretics and, as indicated, antibiotics and/or cardiac medications as ordered for underlying disorder.
3. Monitor fluid balance by intake and output measurement, daily weight, and direct measurement of pulmonary capillary wedge pressure to detect hypovolemia or hypervolemia.
4. Provide measures to prevent hypoventilation and atelectasis, and promote chest expansion and secretion clearance, such as incentive spirometer, nebulization, head of bed elevated 30 degrees, turn frequently, out of bed when clinically stable.
5. Monitor adequacy of alveolar ventilation by frequent measurement of SpO_2, ABG levels, respiratory rate, and forced vital capacity (FVC).
6. Compare monitored values with criteria indicating the need for mechanical ventilation (see above in Nursing Assessment section). Report and prepare to assist with noninvasive ventilation or intubation and initiation of mechanical ventilation, if indicated.

Maintaining Airway Clearance

1. Where indicated, administer medications to increase alveolar ventilation—bronchodilators to reduce bronchospasm and corticosteroids to reduce airway inflammation.
2. Teach slow, pursed-lip breathing to reduce dyspnea and improve oxygen saturation. Secretion clearance techniques may be considered for retained secretions.
3. Promote effective cough with positioning, deep breathing, and bronchodilators if ordered. If cough effort is poor and/or ineffective for mucus clearance, suction patient, if needed, to assist with removal of secretions.
4. If the patient becomes increasingly lethargic, cannot cough or expectorate secretions, and cannot cooperate with therapy, or if pH falls below 7.30, despite the use of the above therapy, report and prepare to assist with intubation and initiation of mechanical ventilation.

Patient Education and Health Maintenance

1. Instruct patient with preexisting pulmonary disease to seek early intervention for infections to prevent acute respiratory failure, pneumonia, and exacerbations.

STANDARDS OF CARE GUIDELINES 11-1
Respiratory Compromise

When caring for patients at risk for respiratory compromise, consider the following assessments and interventions:

- Monitor closely and document complete assessments. Evaluate closely for any changes in clinical assessments.
- Perform thorough systematic assessment, including mental status, vital signs, respiratory status, and cardiovascular status.
- Evaluate for signs of hypoxia when anxiety, restlessness, confusion, or aggression of new onset are noted. Do not administer sedatives unless hypoxia has been ruled out by performing respiratory assessment.
- Notify appropriate health care provider of significant findings of hypoxia: SpO_2 < 92%, cyanosis, circumoral pallor, rapid and shallow respirations, abnormal breath sounds, change in behavior or level of consciousness (LOC). Request assessment and intervention by health care provider, as indicated.
- Use extreme caution in administering sedatives and opioids to patients at risk for respiratory compromise.

This information should serve as a general guideline only. Each patient situation presents a unique set of clinical factors and requires nursing judgment to guide care, which may include additional or alternative measures and approaches.

2. Teach patient about medication regimen.
   a. Return demonstrate proper technique for inhaler use.
   b. Actions, dosage, and timing of medications.
   c. Monitoring for adverse effects of oral corticosteroids to report to health care provider: weight gain because of fluid retention and/or increased appetite, hyperglycemia, mood changes, insomnia, bruising, fragile skin, and vision changes because of cataracts or glaucoma.

Community and Home Care Considerations

1. Encourage patients at risk, especially older adults and those with preexisting lung disease, to get pneumococcal pneumonia and annual influenza vaccination.
2. All adults aged 65 years and older should receive the 13-valent pneumococcal conjugate vaccine (PCV13), in addition to the 23-valent pneumococcal polysaccharide vaccine (PPSV23). PCV13 is recommended for all adults aged 65 years and older who were not previously vaccinated with it, followed by PPSV23 12 months later.
3. Encourage annual immunization for influenza in persons 6 months and older.
4. Intranasal live attenuated vaccine is an alternative for people ages 5 to 49 without chronic conditions, human immunodeficiency virus (HIV), or asthma.

 EVIDENCE BASE Center for Disease Control and Prevention. (2016). Prevention and control of seasonal influenza with vaccines: Recommendations of the Advisory Committee on Immunization Practices—United States, 2016–17 Influenza Season. *MMWR, 65*(5), 1–54.

Kobayashi, M., Bennett, N. M., Gierke, R., Almendares, O., Moore, M. R., Whitney, C. G., & Pilishvili, T. (2015). Intervals between PCV13 and PPSV23 vaccines: Recommendations of the Advisory Committee on Immunization Practices (ACIP). *MMWR, 64*(34), 944–947.

Evaluation: Expected Outcomes

- ABG values within patient's normal limits.
- Decreased secretions; lungs clear.

Acute Respiratory Distress Syndrome

ARDS or acute *lung injury* results from acute insult at the level of the alveoli leading to severe hypoxemia and decreased pulmonary compliance. Hallmarks of ARDS include a risk factor for ARDS (eg, sepsis, trauma, pancreatitis), severe hypoxemia with the need for high FiO_2, decreased lung compliance, bilateral pulmonary infiltrates, and absence of cardiogenic pulmonary edema. Mortality is 55% and improves with early intervention.

Pathophysiology and Etiology

1. Pulmonary and/or nonpulmonary insult to the alveolar–capillary membrane causing protein-rich fluid leakage into interstitial and alveolar spaces, resulting in edema.
   a. Inflammation in the interstitium and alveolar space promotes atelectasis and lung damage.
   b. This is associated with severe hypoxemia and reduced pulmonary compliance.
   c. Fibroproliferative state is often accompanied by capillary thrombosis, lung fibrosis, and neovascularization follows.

Figure 11-1. Pathogenesis of ARDS.

2. Diffuse alveolar damage with ventilation–perfusion (V/Q) mismatch caused by shunting of blood (see Figure 11-1).
3. Mechanisms are unclear. Acute lung injury includes both pulmonary capillary endothelium and alveolar epithelium. Etiologies are numerous and can be pulmonary or nonpulmonary. Predisposing factors include (but are not limited to):
   a. Infections, including sepsis, pneumonia (usually bacterial or aspiration).
   b. Shock (any cause), trauma, pulmonary contusion, near drowning, direct or indirect lung injury, burns, pancreatitis.
   c. Inhaled agents—smoke, high concentration of oxygen, corrosive substances.
   d. Major surgery including coronary artery bypass graft, fat emboli, lung or bone marrow transplantation, transfusion of blood products, reperfusion pulmonary edema.

Clinical Manifestations

1. Acute onset of severe dyspnea, tachypnea, tachycardia, use of accessory muscles, cyanosis.
2. Increasing requirements of oxygen therapy. Hypoxemia refractory to supplemental oxygen therapy.
3. Scattered crackles and rhonchi heard on auscultation.
4. Decreased pulmonary compliance, evidenced by increasing pressure required to ventilate patient on mechanical ventilator.

Diagnostic Evaluation

1. Diagnosis is based on clinical, hemodynamic, and oxygen criteria. The hallmark signs for ARDS include acute-onset, severe hypoxemia, despite increasing oxygen therapy, and chest x-ray exhibiting bilateral infiltrates.
2. Pulmonary artery catheter readings show pulmonary artery wedge pressure greater than 18 mm Hg, absence of left atrial hypertension, and no clinical signs of heart failure.

Management

1. Current ARDS treatment is primarily supportive. The underlying cause for ARDS should be determined so appropriate treatment can be initiated.
2. Mechanical ventilation is nearly always required to decrease work of breathing and improve oxygenation.
   a. Low V_T by mechanical ventilation (6 mL/kg of predicted body weight) reduces mortality compared to high-volume ventilation.
   b. Protective ventilation (ie, maximum inspiratory pressure of less than 35 cm) should be instituted.
   c. PEEP should be used to improve PaO_2 (keeps the alveoli open, thereby improving gas exchange). Therefore, a lower oxygen concentration (FiO_2) may be used to maintain satisfactory oxygenation.
3. Fluid management must be maintained. The patient may be hypovolemic because of the movement of fluid into the interstitium of the lung. Pulmonary artery catheter monitoring and inotropic medication can be helpful.
4. Medications are aimed at treating the underlying cause. Corticosteroids are used infrequently because of controversial benefits.
5. Adequate nutrition should be initiated early and maintained.

NURSING ALERT The treatment for ARDS is aimed at maximizing clinical stability and managing symptoms, but the underlying cause must be treated or ARDS will not resolve. Supportive measures assist the patient while the underlying cause is being treated.

Complications

1. Infections, such as pneumonia, sepsis.
2. Respiratory complications, such as pulmonary emboli, barotrauma, oxygen toxicity, subcutaneous emphysema, or pulmonary fibrosis.
3. GI complications, such as stress ulcer, ileus, pancreatitis.
4. Cardiac complications, such as decreased cardiac output and dysrhythmias.
5. Renal failure, disseminated intravascular coagulation.
6. Multiorgan failure and sepsis, which may result in death.
7. Cognitive impairment.

Nursing Interventions

Care is similar to patient with respiratory failure (page 191) and pulmonary edema (page 304). Also see "Mechanical Ventilation" section, page 181.

Acute Bronchitis

Acute bronchitis is an inflammation of the airways resulting from infection (viral, bacterial) or an irritant (smoke, gastric acid). The inflammation causes airway narrowing and congestion, with increase in secretions.

Pathophysiology and Etiology

1. Primarily viral etiology, such as rhinovirus, respiratory syncytial virus (RSV), and influenza.
2. Bacterial etiology more common in people with underlying pulmonary disease.
3. Exposure to irritants may be acute or chronic.
4. Airways become inflamed, narrowed, and congested with increased mucus production.

Clinical Manifestations

1. Dry cough, which may become productive with clear to purulent sputum.
2. Rhinorrhea, sore throat, and nasal congestion may precede and accompany lower respiratory tract symptoms.
3. Occasional pleuritic chest pain and fever.
4. Diffuse rhonchi and crackles and occasional wheezing heard on auscultation.

Diagnostic Evaluation

1. Chest x-ray—no evidence of infiltrates or consolidation.
2. Sputum Gram stain and culture have limited value.
3. Spirometry to determine FVC, forced expiratory volume in 1 second (FEV_1), and FEV_1/FVC ratio, which may indicate underlying airflow limitation as found in COPD (chronic bronchitis +/or emphysema).

Management

1. Antibiotic therapy is normally avoided due to predominantly viral cause of infection. If bacterial infection is present or strongly suspected, or for patients with underlying COPD, antibiotics are usually prescribed based on community resistance patterns and patient history and physical examination.
2. Hydration and humidification.
3. Secretion clearance interventions for retained or excess mucus (may include controlled cough, positive expiratory pressure [PEP] valve therapy, chest physical therapy) and mobilization.
4. Bronchodilators for bronchospasm, secretion clearance, and treatment of airflow obstruction if present.

Table 11-1	Commonly Encountered Pneumonias	
TYPE	**ORGANISM RESPONSIBLE**	**MANIFESTATIONS**
Bacterial		
Streptococcal pneumonia (pneumococcal pneumonia) (60% of community-acquired pneumonia)	• *Streptococcus pneumoniae*	• May be history of previous respiratory infection • Sudden onset, with shaking and chills • Rapidly rising fever; tachypnea • Cough, with expectoration of rusty or green (purulent) sputum • Pleuritic pain aggravated by cough • Chest dull to percussion; crackles, bronchial breath sounds **GERONTOLOGIC ALERT** Confusion and/or increase in respiratory rate may be only presenting feature in older patient.
Staphylococcal pneumonia	• *Staphylococcus aureus*	• Commonly, history of viral infection, especially influenza • Insidious development of cough, with expectoration of yellow, blood-streaked mucus • Onset may be sudden if patient is outpatient • Fever, pleuritic chest pain, progressive dyspnea • Pulse varies; may be slow in proportion to temperature
Pneumonia because of gram-negative enteric bacilli	• *Klebsiella* species, *Pseudomonas* organisms, *Escherichia coli*, *Serratia*, *Proteus* species	• Sudden onset with fever, chills, dyspnea • Pleuritic chest pain and production of purulent sputum
Legionella species	• *Legionella pneumophila*	• High fever, chills, cough, chest pain, tachypnea • Respiratory distress
Haemophilus influenza pneumonia *Moraxella catarrhalis* pneumonia	• *H. influenzae* • *M. catarrhalis*	• Abrupt onset of coughing, fever, chills, tachypnea
Atypical and Nonbacterial		
Mycoplasma or chlamydial pneumonia (*Legionella pneumoniae* may also be included in this category)	• *Mycoplasma pneumoniae, Chlamydia trachomatis*, or *L. pneumophila*	• Gradual onset; severe headache; irritating hacking cough producing scanty, mucoid sputum • Anorexia; malaise • Fever; nasal congestion; sore throat
Viral pneumonia	• Influenza viruses • Parainfluenza viruses • Respiratory syncytial viruses • Rhinoviruses • Adenovirus • Varicella, rubella, rubeola, herpes simplex, cytomegalovirus, Epstein-Barr virus	• Cough • Constitutional symptoms may be pronounced (severe headache, anorexia, fever, and myalgia)

CLINICAL FEATURES	TREATMENT*	COMPLICATIONS
• Usually involves one or more lobes • Chest x-ray shows consolidation of affected areas • Common community-acquired pneumonia as well as seen in nursing home residents, alcoholics, smokers, those with chronic obstructive pulmonary disease (COPD), IV drug use, early human immunodeficiency virus (HIV), endobronchial obstruction	• Penicillin nonresistant: MIC < 2 mg/mL • Penicillin G, amoxicillin • Penicillin resistant: MIC > 2 mg/mL • Agents chosen on the basis of susceptibility, including cefotaxime, ceftriaxone, fluoroquinolone	• Shock • Pleural effusion • Superinfections • Pericarditis • Otitis media
• Commonly seen in facility setting; during influenza epidemics; in IV drug abuse; and COPD, smokers, bronchiectasis • These infections commonly lead to necrosis and destruction of lung tissue • Treatment must be vigorous and prolonged owing to disease's tendency to destroy the lungs • Organism may develop rapid drug resistance • Prolonged convalescence usual	• Methicillin susceptible: antistaph penicillins, cefazolin, clindamycin • Methicillin resistant: vancomycin or TM-SMX for methicillin-resistant *S. aureus*	• Effusion/pneumothorax • Lung abscess • Empyema • Meningitis
• Infection usually occurs from aspiration of pharyngeal flora into bronchioles. • Seen in persons with severe illness; among the more common causes of hospital-acquired pneumonia	• Enterobacteriaceae: third-generation cephalosporin, carbapenem (drug of choice if extended-spectrum beta-lactamase producer) beta-lactam/beta-lactamase inhibitor, fluoroquinolone • *Pseudomonas aeruginosa:* antipseudomonal beta-lactam *plus* ciprofloxacin or levofloxacin or aminoglycoside, aminoglycoside *plus* ciprofloxacin or levofloxacin	• Early necrosis of lung tissue with rapid abscess formation • High mortality
• Peak incidence in people over age 50 who are cigarette smokers and have underlying diseases that increase susceptibility to infection or who have been on a cruise ship in the past 2 wk	• Fluoroquinolone, azithromycin, doxycycline	• Respiratory failure
• Common in smokers and former smokers • May affect healthy young adults • X-ray may show consolidation • Often seen in early HIV and may be first indication of endobronchial tumor	• Non–beta-lactam-producing organisms: amoxicillin, fluoroquinolones, doxycycline, azithromycin, clarithromycin • Beta-lactam–producing organisms: second- or third-generation cephalosporins, amoxicillin clavulanate, fluoroquinolones, doxycycline, azithromycin, clarithromycin	• High mortality in patients with underlying disease (cancer, COPD) • Pleural effusion common
• Occurs most commonly in children and young adults, as well as in older adults in community or hospital setting • Rise in serum complement–fixing antibodies to the organism • More common in COPD and in smokers	• For mycoplasma or *Chlamydophila pneumoniae:* macrolides, fluoroquinolones • For *Legionella:* fluoroquinolones, azithromycin, doxycycline	• Persisting cough, meningoencephalitis, polyneuritis, monoarticular arthritis, pericarditis, myocarditis • Chlamydial pneumonia has been implicated in cardiac atheromatous lesions in some patients
• In majority of patients, influenza begins as an acute coryza and myalgias; others have bronchitis and pleurisy, whereas still others develop GI symptoms • Risk of developing influenza related to crowding and close contact with groups	• Treat symptomatically • Prophylactic vaccination recommended for high-risk persons (over age 65; chronic cardiac or pulmonary disease, diabetes, and other metabolic disorders) • For influenza virus: oseltamivir, zanamivir	• Persons with underlying disease have increased risk of complications, primary influenzal pneumonia, and secondary bacterial pneumonia • Bacterial superinfection • Pericarditis • Endocarditis

(continued)

Table 11-1 Commonly Encountered Pneumonias (*Continued*)

TYPE	ORGANISM RESPONSIBLE	MANIFESTATIONS
Pneumocystis jiroveci pneumonia (PCP)	• *P. jiroveci*	• Insidious onset • Increasing dyspnea and nonproductive cough • Tachypnea; progresses rapidly to intercostal retraction, nasal flaring, and cyanosis • Lowering of arterial oxygen tension • Chest x-ray will reveal diffuse, bilateral interstitial pneumonia
Fungal pneumonia	• *Aspergillus fumigatus*	• Fever, productive cough, chest pain, hemoptysis • Chest x-ray reveals a broad range of abnormalities from infiltration to consolidation, cavitation, and empyema

* *Patients with CAP should be treated a minimum of 5 days and should be afebrile for 48 to 72 hours and clinically stable before discontinuing antibiotics.*

5. Symptom management for cough and fever.
6. Management of irritants through acid reflux therapy, smoking cessation, and use of air filter.

Nursing Assessment

1. Obtain history of respiratory infection, course, and length of symptoms.
2. Assess severity of cough and characteristics of sputum production.
3. Auscultate chest for diffuse rhonchi and crackles as opposed to localized crackles usually heard with pneumonia.
4. Obtain medical history including COPD, GERD, smoking history, and exposure to irritants.

Nursing Diagnosis

• Ineffective Airway Clearance related to sputum production.

Nursing Interventions

Establishing Effective Airway Clearance

1. Supportive care with symptom management is usually first line in otherwise healthy patients. For those with bacterial infections and/or underlying COPD, administer or teach self-administration of antibiotics, as ordered.
2. Encourage mobilization of secretions through patient mobilization and, possibly, hydration, effective cough technique, and, if needed, the use of secretion clearance devices such as PEP and, possibly, chest physical therapy. Educate patient that beverages with caffeine or alcohol do not promote hydration.
3. If ordered, administer or teach self-administration of inhaled bronchodilators to reduce bronchospasm and enhance secretion clearance.
4. Caution patients on the use of over-the-counter cough suppressants, antihistamines, and decongestants that may cause drying and retention of secretions. Cough preparations containing the mucolytic guaifenesin may be appropriate.

Patient Education and Health Maintenance

1. Instruct patient about medication regimen, including the completion of the full course of antibiotics, if prescribed, and the effects of food or alcohol on the absorption of the selected medications. If patient is not being treated with antibiotics, reassure patient that full recovery without antibiotic treatment occurs in most cases, but to advise health care provider if symptoms do not improve.
2. Encourage patient to seek medical attention for shortness of breath, severe fatigue, and worsening condition.
3. Advise patient that a dry cough may persist after bronchitis because of irritation of the airways. A bedside humidifier and avoidance of dry environments may help. Humidifiers must be cleaned frequently to avoid growth of mold.
4. Encourage patient to discuss complementary and alternative therapies with health care provider. When questioned, some people use garlic as an antimicrobial. Other herbs that many believe to be helpful for asthma and bronchitis are echinacea, eucalyptus, and thyme; however, there are no definitive studies that show benefit. Because herbal products and supplements are not standardized, and may be mixed with other ingredients, safety and effectiveness cannot be ensured.

Evaluation: Expected Outcomes

• Coughs up clear secretions effectively.

Pneumonia

Pneumonia is an inflammatory process, involving the terminal airways and alveoli of the lung, caused by infectious agents (see Table 11-1, pages 196–198). It may be classified according to its causative agent.

Pathophysiology and Etiology

1. Community-acquired pneumonia (CAP) is a common infectious disease often caused by the bacteria *Streptococcus pneumoniae*, *Haemophilus influenzae*, and *Moraxella catarrhalis*, as well as the viruses rhinovirus and influenza.
2. Development of CAP may be due to a defect in host defenses, exposure to a virulent microorganism, or an overwhelming exposure. An organism gains access to the lungs through aspiration of oropharyngeal contents, by inhalation of respiratory secretions from infected individuals, via the bloodstream, or from direct spread to the lungs as a result of surgery or trauma.
3. Risk factors include altered mental status, smoking, alcohol use, hypoxemia, toxic inhalations, pulmonary edema, uremia,

CLINICAL FEATURES	TREATMENT*	COMPLICATIONS
• Usually seen in host whose resistance is compromised; most common opportunistic infection in AIDS in the United States • Organism invades the lungs of patients who have suppressed immune system (from AIDS, cancer, leukemia) or after immunosuppressive therapy for cancer, organ transplant, or collagen disease • Frequently associated with concurrent infection by viruses (cytomegalovirus), bacteria, and fungi	• TMP-SMX; dapsone with trimethoprim, clindamycin with primaquine • Pentamidine methanesulfonate	• Patients are critically ill • Prognosis guarded because it is usually a complication of a severe underlying disorder
• Neutropenic individual most susceptible • May develop Aspergillus as a superinfection • Often seen in late HIV disease	• Amphotericin B; itraconazole	• High mortality rate • Invades blood vessels and destroys lung tissue by direct invasion and vascular infarction

malnutrition, bronchial obstruction, advanced age, immunosuppression, heart disease, underlying lung disease (cystic fibrosis, bronchiectasis, COPD, ciliary dysfunction, lung cancer), viral respiratory infection, and history of pneumonia.

   a. Immunocompromised patients include those receiving corticosteroids, immunosuppressants, chemotherapy, or radiotherapy; those with cancer, HIV infection, acquired immunodeficiency syndrome (AIDS), and alcoholism; those who are intravenous (IV) drug users; and those undergoing organ transplantation.

   b. These people have an increased risk of developing overwhelming infection. Infectious agents include aerobic and anaerobic gram-negative bacilli, *Staphylococcus*, *Nocardia*, fungi, *Candida*, viruses such as cytomegalovirus, *Pneumocystis jiroveci*, reactivation of tuberculosis (TB), and others.

4. When bacterial pneumonia occurs in a healthy person, it may be preceded by a viral illness.

5. Other predisposing factors include conditions interfering with normal secretion clearance of the lung, such as tumor, general anesthesia, postoperative immobility; depression of the CNS from drugs, neurologic disorders, alcohol; and intubation.

6. Pneumonia may be divided into three groups:

   a. Community acquired, because of several organisms.

      i. "Typical" organisms include *Streptococcus pneumoniae* (most common organism), *Haemophilus influenzae*, *Staphylococcus aureus*, *Moraxella catarrhalis*, anaerobes, and aerobic gram-negative bacteria, and rhinovirus and influenza virus.

      ii. Atypical pneumonia may be caused by *Legionella* species, *Mycobacterium pneumoniae*, and *Chlamydophila pneumoniae*.

   b. Health care–associated pneumonia, also known as hospital or nursing home acquired (nosocomial), due primarily to gram-negative bacilli and staphylococci. HCAP includes patients who have recently been hospitalized within 90 days of the infection, resided in a nursing home or long-term care facility, or received parenteral antimicrobial therapy, chemotherapy, or wound care within 30 days of pneumonia.

   c. Pneumonia in the immunocompromised person.

7. People older than age 65 have a high rate of mortality, even with appropriate antimicrobial therapy.

 NURSING ALERT Recurring pneumonia commonly indicates underlying disease, such as cancer of the lung, multiple myeloma, bronchiectasis, or COPD.

Clinical Manifestations

For most common forms of bacterial pneumonia:

1. Typical bacterial CAP typically presents with fever, dyspnea, fatigue, and productive cough and often with pleuritic chest pain.
2. Pleuritic chest pain may be aggravated by respiration/coughing.
3. Dyspnea and tachypnea use of accessory muscles of respiration and fatigue.
4. Tachycardia may be present.

Diagnostic Evaluation

1. Chest x-ray shows a discernible infiltrate and presence/extent of pulmonary disease, typically consolidation.
2. Gram stain and culture and sensitivity of sputum are reliable and diagnostic if performed on a well-collected specimen without saliva contamination (excess squamous epithelial cells are present if saliva contamination) and if a predominant organism is present.

   a. Many patients, especially elderly persons, are not able to produce an adequate suitable sputum sample.

   b. Endobronchial specimens should be obtained from intubated patients.

   c. CAP is often diagnosed presumptively, without culture, but should be investigated for specific pathogens that would significantly alter standard management decisions, based on sputum culture (Gram stain typically shows few or no predominant organisms in atypical CAP).

3. Indications for sputum culture include:

   a. All patients requiring intubation and mechanical ventilation.

   b. Nonventilator patients with risk factors for *Pseudomonas aeruginosa* or other multidrug-resistant gram-negative enteric pathogen infection, including severe COPD, use of chronic oral corticosteroids, and those with active alcohol abuse.

c. Nonventilator patients with risk factors for *Staphylococcus aureus*, including end-stage renal disease, receiving hemodialysis, history of injection drug use, cavitary pulmonary infiltrates, and acute postinfluenza pneumonia.

4. Pretreatment blood samples for culture to detect bacteremia should be obtained from patients with admission to intensive care unit, cavitary lesion on chest x-ray, leukopenia, active alcohol abuse, chronic severe liver disease, asplenia, positive pneumococcal urinary antigen test, or pleural effusion.

5. Immunologic tests may be ordered to detect microbial antigens in serum, sputum, and urine.

6. Severity-of-illness scores, such as the CURB-65 criteria (confusion, uremia, respiratory rate, low BP, age 65 or greater), or pneumonia severity index can be used to identify patients with CAP who may be candidates for outpatient treatment.

Management

1. Antimicrobial therapy—depends on empiric recommendations and/or laboratory identification of causative organism and sensitivity to specific antimicrobials.

2. Oxygen therapy, if patient has inadequate gas exchange.

3. Patients with hypoxemia or respiratory distress who are refractory to oxygen should receive a cautious trial of noninvasive ventilation unless they require immediate intubation because of severe hypoxemia or acute respiratory failure.

4. Low V_T ventilation (6 mL/kg ideal body weight) for diffuse bilateral pneumonia or ARDS.

5. Early mobilization when clinically stable reduces length of facility stay.

6. Assess influenza and pneumococcal vaccination status, and if not currently vaccinated or status uncertain, perform prior to hospital discharge.

7. Advise and assist with smoking cessation in currently smoking patients.

8. Respiratory hygiene measures, including the use of hand hygiene and masks or tissues for patients with cough, should be used in outpatient settings and EDs to reduce the spread of respiratory infections.

Complications

1. Pleural effusion.
2. Sustained hypotension and shock, especially in gram-negative bacterial disease, particularly in older patients.
3. Empyema.
4. Superinfection: pericarditis, bacteremia, and meningitis.
5. Delirium—considered a medical emergency.
6. Atelectasis—because of mucus plugs.
7. Delayed resolution.

Nursing Assessment

1. Take a careful history to help establish etiologic diagnosis. Local epidemiology and patient travel history, history of exposures, and local or national outbreaks may help in pneumonia identification.
   a. History of recent respiratory illness, complete medical history, and social history including risk factors for pneumonia.
   b. Presence of purulent sputum, increased amount of sputum, fever, chills, pleuritic pain, dyspnea, and tachypnea.
   c. Any pattern of family illness.
   d. Medications (including recent antibiotics) and allergies.
2. Observe for dyspnea, excess fatigue, change in mental status, anxiety, or respiratory distress.

3. Auscultate for crackles overlying affected region and for bronchial breath sounds when consolidation (filling of airspaces with exudate) is present.

Nursing Diagnoses

- Impaired Gas Exchange related to decreased ventilation secondary to inflammation and infection involving distal airspaces.
- Ineffective Airway Clearance related to excessive tracheobronchial secretions.
- Acute Pain related to inflammatory process, infection, and dyspnea.
- Risk for Injury secondary to complications.

Nursing Interventions

Improving Gas Exchange

1. Observe for dyspnea, hypoxia, cyanosis, and confusion, indicating worsening condition.
2. Follow ABG levels/SpO_2 to determine oxygen need and response to oxygen therapy.
3. Administer oxygen at concentration to maintain PaO_2/SpO_2 at acceptable level. Hypoxemia may be due to abnormal V/Q mismatch with shunt in affected lung segments.
4. Use caution with high concentrations of oxygen in patients with COPD, particularly with evidence of CO_2 retention; use of high oxygen concentrations may worsen alveolar ventilation in some patients by depressing the patient's only remaining ventilatory drive. If high concentrations of oxygen are given, monitor alertness and PaO_2 and $PaCO_2$ levels for signs of CO_2 retention.
5. Place patient in an upright position as tolerated to obtain greater lung expansion and improve aeration. Frequent turning and increased activity (up in chair, ambulate as tolerated) should be employed if clinically stable.

Enhancing Airway Clearance

1. If ordered, obtain freshly expectorated sputum for Gram stain and culture initially prior to antibiotic treatment. Early morning specimens are preferable for subsequent specimens. Instruct the patient as follows:
   a. Perform oral care and rinse mouth with water to minimize contamination by normal flora.
   b. Breathe deeply several times.
   c. Cough deeply and expectorate raised sputum into sterile container.
2. Auscultate the chest for crackles and rhonchi. Encourage patient to deep breath and cough to reduce retained secretions that interfere with gas exchange. Suction as necessary.
3. Encourage increased fluid intake, unless contraindicated, to replace fluid losses caused by fever, diaphoresis, dehydration, and tachypnea.
4. Humidify oxygen over 4 L/minute to reduce dryness of mucus membranes.
5. Employ PEP device use, huff cough, and possibly chest wall percussion and postural drainage, when appropriate, to loosen and mobilize secretions.
6. When clinically stable, mobilize patient to improve ventilation and secretion clearance and reduce risk of atelectasis and worsening pneumonia.

Relieving Pleuritic Pain

1. Place patient in a comfortable position (semi-Fowler's) for resting and breathing; encourage frequent change of position to prevent pooling of secretions in lungs and atelectasis.
2. Demonstrate how to splint the chest while coughing.
3. Avoid suppressing a productive cough.

4. Administer prescribed nonsedating analgesic agent to relieve pain.
5. Use comfort measures to improve symptom control.
6. Encourage modified bed rest during febrile period.
7. Watch for abdominal distention or ileus, which may be due to swallowing of air during intervals of severe dyspnea. Insert a nasogastric (NG) or rectal tube, as directed.

 GERONTOLOGIC ALERT Sedatives, opioids, and cough suppressants should be used cautiously in older patients because of their tendency to suppress cough and gag reflexes and respiratory drive. Also, provide or encourage frequent oral care for pneumonia prevention.

Monitoring for Complications

1. Be aware that fatal complications may develop during the early period of antimicrobial treatment.
2. Monitor temperature, pulse, respiration, BP, oximetry, mentation, and for evidence of dyspnea at regular intervals to assess the patient's response to therapy.
3. Auscultate lungs and heart. Heart murmurs or friction rub may indicate acute bacterial endocarditis, pericarditis, or myocarditis.
4. Employ special nursing surveillance for patients with:
   a. Alcoholism, COPD, and immunosuppression—these people as well as older patients may have little or no fever.
   b. Chronic bronchitis—it may be difficult to detect subtle changes in condition because the patient may have seriously compromised pulmonary function and regular mucus production.
   c. Epilepsy—pneumonia may result from aspiration after a seizure.
   d. Delirium—may be caused by hypoxia, meningitis, and alcohol withdrawal.
5. Assess these patients for unusual behavior, alterations in mental status, stupor, and heart failure.
6. Assess for resistant fever or return of fever, potentially suggesting bacterial resistance to antibiotics.

 NURSING ALERT Delirium causes and treatment must be identified to control symptoms and prevent exhaustion and cardiac failure. Prepare for lumbar puncture, if indicated, to rule out meningitis, which may be lethal. Mild sedation should be considered with caution.

Patient Education and Health Maintenance

1. Advise patient to complete entire course of antibiotics.
2. Advise patient that fatigue and weakness may persist after pneumonia.
3. Once clinically stable, encourage gradual increase in activities to improve ventilation and reduce hazards of immobility.
4. Encourage breathing exercises to clear lungs and promote full expansion and function.
5. Explain that a chest x-ray is usually taken 4 to 6 weeks after recovery to evaluate lungs for clearing and detect any tumor or underlying cause.
6. Advise smoking cessation. Cigarette smoke destroys tracheobronchial cilial action, which is the first line of defense of lungs, also irritates mucosa of bronchi, and inhibits function of alveolar scavenger cells (macrophages).
7. Advise the patient to keep up natural resistance with good nutrition, adequate rest, and physical activity, when tolerated.

One episode of pneumonia may make the patient susceptible to recurring respiratory infections.

8. Instruct patient to avoid fatigue, sudden extremes in temperature, and excessive alcohol intake, which lower resistance to pneumonia.
9. Assess for and facilitate vaccination with pneumococcal and influenza vaccines (see pages 193 to 194). Influenza vaccine is associated with reduced hospitalizations for pneumonia, influenza, and death in community-dwelling older adults.
10. Advise avoidance of contact with people with upper respiratory infections for several months after pneumonia resolves.
11. Respiratory and hand hygiene includes frequent handwashing, especially after contact with others.

Evaluation: Expected Outcomes

- Cyanosis and dyspnea reduced; ABG levels and SaO_2 improved.
- Coughs effectively; absence of crackles.
- Appears more comfortable; free of pain.
- Fever controlled; no signs of resistant infection.

Aspiration Pneumonia

Aspiration is the inhalation of oropharyngeal secretions and/or stomach contents into the lower airways. It may lead to acute pneumonia.

Pathophysiology and Etiology

1. Loss of protective airway reflexes (swallowing, cough) may be caused by altered state of consciousness, alcohol or drug overdose, seizures, stroke, head trauma, general anesthesia, intercranial mass or lesion, during resuscitation procedures, seriously ill or debilitated patients, and abnormalities of gag and swallowing reflexes.
2. Other conditions and risk factors associated with aspiration include the following:
   a. Esophageal strictures and diverticula, head and neck neoplasms, tracheoesophageal fistula, and gastroesophageal reflux.
   b. Multiple sclerosis, dementia, Parkinson disease, myasthenia gravis, and pseudobulbar palsy.
   c. Intubation, tracheostomy, endoscopy, and bronchoscopy.
   d. Obstetric patients—from general anesthesia, lithotomy position, delayed emptying of the stomach from enlarged uterus, and labor contractions.
   e. Gastrointestinal conditions—hiatal hernia, intestinal obstruction, abdominal distention, nasogastric or feeding tube, and gastric or postpyloric tube feedings.
   f. Prolonged vomiting or recumbent position.
3. Effects of aspiration depend on volume and character of aspirated material.
   a. Gastric acid causes a chemical pneumonitis.
   b. Bacteria from the oropharynx causes aspiration pneumonia.
   c. Oil (mineral oil or vegetable oil) causes exogenous lipoid pneumonia.
   d. Foreign body may cause an acute respiratory emergency and may predispose the patient to bacterial pneumonia.
   e. Many cases of pneumonia result from aspiration of pathogens from the oral cavity or nasopharynx caused by *Streptococcus pneumoniae*, *Haemophilus influenza*, *Staphylococcus aureus*, and gram-negative bacteria. These bacteria are relatively virulent so that only a small inoculum is required to result in a pneumonia. The aspiration episode may be subtle.

 GERONTOLOGIC ALERT Oropharyngeal dysphagia has been found in the majority of elderly patients (mean age, 84 years).

Clinical Manifestations

1. Tachycardia and fever.
2. Dyspnea, cough, and tachypnea.
3. Hypoxemia and cyanosis.
4. Decreased breath sounds, rales, pleural friction rub, and dullness to percussion overconsolidation.
5. Purulent sputum.

Diagnostic Evaluation

1. Chest x-ray may be normal initially; with time, shows consolidation and other abnormalities.

Management

1. Clearing the obstructed airway.
   a. If foreign body is visible, it may be removed manually.
   b. Suction trachea/ET tube—to remove particulate matter.
   c. Optimize secretion clearance and manage hypoxia with supplemental oxygen.
2. Antimicrobial therapy or specific therapy depending on material aspirated.
3. Laryngoscopy/bronchoscopy may be performed for aspiration of solid material.
4. Oxygen therapy and assisted ventilation if adequate oxygenation cannot be maintained.
5. Fluid volume replacement and correction of acidosis for correction of hypotension and shock.

Complications

1. Lung abscess and empyema.
2. Necrotizing pneumonia.
3. ARDS.

Nursing Assessment

1. Assess for airway obstruction and hypoxemia.
2. Assess for development of fever, foul-smelling sputum, and congestion.
3. Assess LOC, gag reflex, swallowing ability, and other risk factors for aspiration.

Nursing Diagnoses

- Impaired Gas Exchange related to decreased ventilation secondary to inflammation and infection involving distal airspaces.
- Ineffective Airway Clearance related to excessive tracheobronchial secretions.
- Acute Pain related to inflammatory process and dyspnea.
- Risk for Injury secondary to complications.

(See pages 196 to 201 for nursing interventions.)

Additional Nursing Interventions

1. Carefully monitor patients at risk for aspiration.
2. Elevate head of bed for debilitated patients, for those receiving tube feedings, and for those at risk for aspiration.
3. For patients with feeding tubes, make sure tube is positioned properly and tube is patent.
   a. Give tube feedings slowly, with head of bed elevated. Check for residual volume.
   b. Check position of tube in the stomach before feeding.
   c. Check seal of cuff of tracheostomy or ET tube before feeding.
4. Keep the patient in a fasting state before anesthesia (at least 8 hours).
5. Feed patients with impaired swallowing slowly, and make sure that no food is retained in the mouth after feeding.

 NURSING ALERT Morbidity and mortality rates of aspiration pneumonia remain high even with optimum treatment. Prevention is the key to the problem.

Pulmonary Embolism

Pulmonary embolism (PE) refers to the obstruction of one or more pulmonary arteries by a thrombus (or thrombi) usually originating in the deep veins of the legs, the right side of the heart, or, rarely, an upper extremity, which becomes dislodged and is carried to the pulmonary vasculature.

Acute PE is a common form of venous thromboembolism (VTE) leading to V/Q mismatch, increase in pulmonary vascular resistance, pulmonary artery pressure, right heart workload and heart failure, decrease in cardiac output, and shock. Pulmonary infarction refers to necrosis of lung tissue because of reduction in blood supply.

Pathophysiology and Etiology

1. Obstruction, either partial or full, of pulmonary arteries, which causes decrease or absent blood flow; therefore, there is ventilation but no perfusion (V/Q mismatch).
2. Hemodynamic consequences:
   a. Increased pulmonary vascular resistance.
   b. Increased pulmonary artery pressure (PAP).
   c. Increased right-sided heart workload to maintain pulmonary blood flow.
   d. Right-sided heart failure.
   e. Decreased cardiac output.
   f. Decreased BP.
   g. Shock.
   h. Risk of hypoxemia.
3. Pulmonary emboli can vary in size and seriousness of consequences.
4. Predisposing factors include the following:
   a. Stasis and prolonged immobilization.
   b. Concurrent phlebitis.
   c. Heart failure and stroke.
   d. Injury to vessel wall.
   e. Coagulation disorders and hypercoagulable state.
   f. Malignancy.
   g. Advancing age, estrogen therapy, and oral contraceptives.
   h. Fracture of long bones.
   i. Obesity.

 NURSING ALERT Be aware of high-risk patients for pulmonary embolism—immobilization, trauma to the pelvis (especially surgical) and lower extremities (especially hip fracture), obesity, history of thromboembolic disease, varicose veins, pregnancy, heart failure, myocardial infarction (MI), malignant disease, postoperative patients, and older patients.

Clinical Manifestations

1. Rapid onset of dyspnea at rest, pleuritic chest pain, cough, syncope, delirium, apprehension, tachypnea, diaphoresis, and hemoptysis. Onset may be prolonged and presentation more subtle if obstruction is partial.
2. Chest pain with apprehension and a sense of impending doom occur when most of the pulmonary artery is obstructed.
3. Tachycardia, rales, fever, hypotension, cyanosis, heart gallop, and loud pulmonic component of S_2 (split S_2).
4. Calf or thigh pain, edema, erythema, tenderness, or palpable cord (signs suggestive of deep vein thrombosis).

NURSING ALERT Have a high index of suspicion for pulmonary embolus if there is a subtle or significant deterioration in the patient's condition and unexplained cardiovascular and pulmonary findings.

Diagnostic Evaluation

1. Thoracic imaging: V/Q scan (possibly using single-photon emission computed tomography) or helical contrast-enhanced computed tomography (CT).
2. Pulmonary angiography if noninvasive testing is inconclusive or not candidate for noninvasive testing. Contrast studies should be avoided in persons who are pregnant or have advanced renal failure.
3. D-Dimer assay for low to intermediate probability of pulmonary embolism.
4. ABG levels—decreased PaO_2 is usually found, because of perfusion abnormality of the lung.
5. Chest x-ray—normal or possible wedge-shaped infiltrate.

Management

Emergency Management

For massive pulmonary embolism, the goal is to stabilize cardiorespiratory status.

 NURSING ALERT Massive pulmonary embolism is a medical emergency; the patient's condition tends to deteriorate rapidly. There may be a profound decrease in cardiac output, with an accompanying increase in right ventricular pressure.

1. Oxygen is administered to relieve hypoxemia, respiratory distress, and cyanosis and to dilate pulmonary vasculature.
2. An infusion is started to open an IV route for drugs and fluids.
3. Vasopressors, inotropic agents such as dopamine, and antiarrhythmic agents may be indicated to support circulation if the patient is unstable.
4. ECG is monitored continuously for findings suggestive of right-sided heart failure, which may have a rapid onset. Changes may include sinus tachycardia, Q waves, late T-wave inversion, S wave in lead I, right bundle-branch block, right axis deviation, atrial fibrillation, and T-wave changes.
5. Small doses of IV morphine may be given to relieve anxiety, alleviate chest discomfort (which improves ventilation), and ease adaptation to mechanical ventilator, if this is necessary.
6. Pulmonary angiography, thoracic imaging, hemodynamic measurements, ABG analysis, and other studies are carried out.

Subsequent Management: Anticoagulation and Thrombolysis

1. Anticoagulant therapy includes subcutaneous low molecular weight heparin (LMWH), IV or subcutaneous unfractionated heparin (UFH) with monitoring, unmonitored weight-based subcutaneous UFH, or subcutaneous fondaparinux.
2. Anticoagulants stop further thrombus formation and extend the clotting time of the blood; they do not dissolve clots.
   a. UFH is given as IV loading dose usually followed by continuous pump or drip infusion or given intermittently every 4 to 6 hours.
   b. Dosage adjusted to maintain the partial thromboplastin time (PTT) at 1½ to 2 times the pretreatment value (if the value was normal).
   c. Protamine sulfate may be given to neutralize heparin in the event of severe bleeding.

3. Oral anticoagulation with warfarin is usually used for follow-up anticoagulant therapy after heparin therapy has been established and interrupts the coagulation mechanism by interfering with the vitamin K–dependent synthesis of prothrombin and factors VII, IX, and X.
   a. Dosage is controlled by monitoring serial tests of international normalized ratio (INR), achieving 2.0 to 3.0 as the norm.
   b. Fresh frozen plasma (FFP) should be given for emergent reversal of INR greater than 9 (2 units FFP for patients with low to moderate risk of bleeding, 4 units for those with high risk).
   c. Vitamin K may be given orally when INR is greater than 5, in addition to holding doses of coumadin, or by slow IV infusion for significant bleeding.
4. Thrombolytic (fibrinolytic) agents, such as streptokinase, may be used in patients with massive pulmonary embolism.
   a. Effective in lysing recently formed thrombi.
   b. Improved circulatory and hemodynamic status.
   c. Administered IV in a loading dose followed by constant infusion.
5. Newer clot-specific thrombolytics (tissue plasminogen activator, streptokinase activator complex, single-chain urokinase) are preferred.
   a. Activate plasminogen only within thrombus itself rather than systematically.
   b. Minimize occurrence of generalized fibrinolysis and subsequent bleeding.
6. Absolute contraindications to fibrinolytics include any prior intracranial hemorrhage, known structural intracranial cerebrovascular disease such as arttriovenous malformation, known intracranial neoplasm, ischemic stroke within 3 months, suspected aortic dissection, bleeding, recent surgery of spinal canal or brain, and recent closed head or facial trauma. Caution should be the used in patients greater than 75 years, current use of anticoagulation, pregnancy, no compressible vascular punctures, traumatic or prolonged cardiopulmonary resuscitation, recent internal bleeding, history of severe hypertension, current systolic BP greater than 180 or diastolic BP greater than 110, dementia, remote ischemic stroke, and major surgery within 3 weeks.
7. Graduated compression stockings with 30 to 40 mm Hg compression, knee-high, and sized to fit help dilate deep veins and decrease swelling and venous ulcers that can develop due to postthrombosis syndrome and reduce risk of recurrent DVT and PE.

 GERONTOLOGIC ALERT Consider the patient's age and INR level in dosing of anticoagulation therapy. Older patients will usually need a decreased dosing regimen.

Surgical Intervention

1. When anticoagulation and thrombolysis are contraindicated or patient has recurrent embolization or develops serious complications from drug therapy.
2. Placement of transvenously inserted intraluminal filter in inferior vena cava to prevent migration of emboli (see Figure 11-2); inserted through femoral or jugular vein by way of catheter.
3. Embolectomy (removal of pulmonary embolic obstruction), either by open surgical embolectomy or catheter embolectomy with fragmentation.

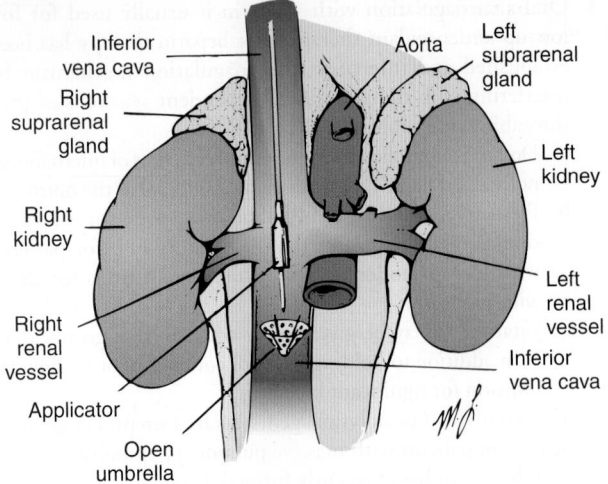

Figure 11-2. Insertion of umbrella filter in inferior vena cava to prevent pulmonary embolism. Filter (compressed within an applicator catheter) is inserted through an incision in the right internal jugular vein. The applicator is withdrawn when the filter fixes itself to the wall of the inferior vena cava after ejection from the applicator.

 EVIDENCE BASE Poterucha, T. J., Bergmark, B., Aranki, S., et al. (2015). Surgical pulmonary embolectomy. *Circulation, 132,* 1146–1151.

Complications

1. Bleeding as a result of treatment.
2. Respiratory failure.
3. Chronic thromboembolic pulmonary hypertension (CTEPH) and cor pulmonale.

Nursing Assessment

1. Take nursing history with emphasis on onset and severity of dyspnea and nature of chest pain, as well as PMH for contraindications to thrombolytic therapy.
2. Examine the patient's legs carefully. Assess for swelling of the leg, duskiness, warmth, pain on pressure over gastrocnemius muscle, and pain on dorsiflexion of the foot (positive Homans sign), which indicate thrombophlebitis as source.
3. Monitor respiratory rate—may be accelerated out of proportion to degree of fever and tachycardia.
   a. Observe rate of inspiration to expiration.
   b. Percuss for resonance or dullness.
   c. Auscultate for friction rub, crackles, rhonchi, and wheezing.
4. Auscultate heart; listen for splitting of second heart sound.
5. Evaluate results of INR for patients on anticoagulants and report results that are outside of therapeutic range promptly; anticipate a dosage change.

Nursing Diagnoses

- Ineffective Breathing Pattern related to acute increase in alveolar dead airspace and possible changes in lung mechanics from embolism.
- Ineffective Tissue Perfusion (Pulmonary) related to decreased blood circulation.
- Acute Pain (pleuritic) related to congestion, possible pleural effusion, and possible lung infarction.

- Anxiety related to dyspnea, pain, and seriousness of condition.
- Risk for Injury related to altered hemodynamic factors and anticoagulant therapy.

Nursing Interventions

Correcting Breathing Pattern

1. Assess for hypoxia, dyspnea, headache, restlessness, apprehension, pallor, cyanosis, and behavioral changes.
2. Monitor vital signs, ECG, oximetry, and ABG levels for adequacy of oxygenation.
3. Monitor patient's response to IV fluids/vasopressors.
4. Monitor oxygen therapy—used to relieve hypoxemia.
5. Prepare patient for assisted ventilation when hypoxemia does not respond to supplemental oxygen. Hypoxemia is due to ventilation/perfusion mismatch.

Improving Tissue Perfusion

1. Closely monitor for shock—decreasing BP, tachycardia, and cool, clammy skin.
2. Monitor prescribed medications given to preserve right-sided heart filling pressure and increase BP.
3. Maintain patient on bed rest during acute phase to reduce oxygen demands and risk of bleeding.
4. Monitor urinary output hourly because there may be reduced renal perfusion and decreased glomerular filtration.
5. Provide antiembolism compression stockings with 30 to 40 mm Hg of compression.

Relieving Pain

1. Watch patient for signs of discomfort and pain.
2. Ascertain if pain worsens with deep breathing and coughing; auscultate for friction rub.
3. Give morphine, as prescribed, and monitor for pain relief and signs of respiratory depression.
4. Position with head of bed slightly elevated (unless contraindicated by shock) and with chest splinted for deep breathing and coughing.
5. Evaluate patient thoroughly for signs of hypoxia when anxiety, restlessness, and agitation of new onset are noted, before administering as-needed sedatives. Consider calling health care provider when these signs are present, especially if accompanied by cyanotic nail beds, circumoral pallor or cyanosis, and increased respiratory rate.

Reducing Anxiety

1. Correct dyspnea and relieve physical discomfort.
2. Explain diagnostic procedures and the patient's role; correct misconceptions.
3. Listen to the patient's concerns; attentive listening relieves anxiety and reduces emotional distress.
4. Speak calmly and slowly.
5. Do everything possible to enhance the patient's sense of control.

Intervening for Complications

1. Be alert for bleeding—related to anticoagulant or thrombolytic therapy. Major bleeding may occur from GI tract, brain, lungs, nose, and genitourinary (GU) tract.
2. Perform stool guaiac test to detect occult blood loss.
3. Monitor platelet count to detect heparin-induced thrombocytopenia.
4. Minimize risk of bleeding by performing essential ABG analysis on upper extremities; apply digital compression at puncture site for 30 minutes; apply pressure dressing to previously involved sites; check site for oozing.

5. Maintain patient on strict bed rest during thrombolytic therapy; avoid unnecessary handling.
6. Discontinue infusion in the event of uncontrolled bleeding.
7. Notify health care provider on call immediately for change in LOC or sensation or ability to follow commands, move limbs, or respond to questions with clear articulation. Intracranial bleed may necessitate discontinuation of anticoagulation promptly to avert massive neurologic catastrophe.
8. Be alert for shock from low cardiac output secondary to resistance to right-sided heart outflow or to myocardial dysfunction because of ischemia.
   a. Assess for skin color changes, particularly nail beds, lips, earlobes, and mucous membranes.
   b. Monitor BP, pulse, and SpO_2.
   c. Measure urine output.
   d. Monitor IV infusion of vasopressor or other prescribed agents.

 TRANSITIONAL CARE ALERT Follow-up nursing care involves anticoagulant management and early identification of complications to prevent readmission. Patients presenting with unexplained dyspnea, exercise intolerance, or clinical evidence of right-sided heart failure should be evaluated for CTEPH with echocardiogram 6 weeks after an acute PE to screen for persistent pulmonary hypertension. Risk factors for CTEPH include multiple episodes of PE, larger perfusion defect, younger age, female gender, and genetic propensity.

Patient Education and Health Maintenance

1. Advise patient of the possible need to continue taking anticoagulant therapy for 6 weeks up to an indefinite period as well as safety considerations and drug and food interactions with anticoagulants.
2. Train regarding food and drug interactions if taking warfarin.
3. Teach about signs of bleeding, especially of the gums and nose, bruising, and blood in urine and stools.
4. For patients on anticoagulants, instruct to use soft toothbrush, avoid shaving with blade razor (use electric razor instead), and avoid aspirin-containing products. Notify health care provider of bleeding or increased bruising.
5. Warn against taking medications unless approved by health care provider because many drugs interact with anticoagulants.
6. Instruct patient to tell dentist about taking an anticoagulant.
7. Warn against inactivity for prolonged periods or sitting with legs crossed to prevent recurrence.
8. Warn against sports/activities that may cause trauma or injury to legs and predispose to a thrombus.
9. Encourage wearing a MedicAlert bracelet, identifying patient as anticoagulant user.
10. Instruct patient to lose weight, if applicable; obesity is a risk factor.
11. Discuss contraceptive methods with patient, if applicable; females with history of pulmonary embolus are advised against taking hormonal contraceptives.

Evaluation: Expected Outcomes

- Verbalizes less shortness of breath.
- Vital signs stable; adequate urinary output.
- Reports freedom from pain.

- Appears more relaxed; sleeping at long intervals.
- Progresses without major bleeding or other complications.

Tuberculosis

Tuberculosis (TB) is an infectious disease caused by bacteria (*Mycobacterium tuberculosis*). It is usually spread from person to person through droplet aerosolization (droplet nuclei). It usually infects the lung but can occur at virtually any site in the body.

Pathophysiology and Etiology

Transmission

1. The term *Mycobacterium* is descriptive of a bacterium that resembles a fungus. The organisms multiply at varying rates and are characterized as acid-fast aerobic organisms that can be killed by heat, sunshine, and ultraviolet light.
2. TB is an airborne disease transmitted by droplet nuclei, usually from within the respiratory tract of an infected person who exhales them during coughing, talking, sneezing, or singing.
3. When a susceptible person inhales the droplet-containing air, the organism is carried into the lung to the pulmonary alveoli.
   a. About 2½ to 12 weeks after initial TB infection, TB testing (purified protein derivative [PPD] or quantiFERON blood test) is positive; however, most people who become infected do not develop clinical illness because the body's immune system brings the infection under control.
   b. Some bacilli remain viable in the body for years, such as with LTBI. Persons with LTBI have no symptoms and are not infectious.
4. Persons at increased risk for TB include close contacts of persons with active TB; persons travelling from Africa, Asia, Eastern Europe, Latin America, and Russia; residents of high-risk congregate settings (correctional facilities, long-term care facilities, and homeless shelters); health care workers exposed to high-risk patients; and infants and children or adolescents exposed to high-risk adults.
5. Of concern in controlling TB in the United States is the prevalence of infection among foreign-born persons residing in the United States, delays in detecting and reporting pulmonary TB, and deficiencies in identifying and screening close contacts and persons with LTBI who are at risk for progression to active TB. The population at risk for progression include the following:
   a. Those who are HIV positive.
   b. Those who have acquired TB infection within last 2 years.
   c. Children younger than age 4.
   d. Those with already immunocompromised conditions such as silicosis; diabetes mellitus; chronic renal failure; leukemia, lymphoma, and carcinoma of the head, neck, or lung; 10% or more below ideal body weight; prolonged corticosteroid use; use of tumor necrosis factor–alpha (TNF-α) antagonists; organ transplant; intestinal bypass or gastrectomy; and history of untreated or inadequately treated TB.

Pathology

1. The bacilli of TB infect the lung, forming a tubercle (lesion).
2. The tubercle:
   a. May heal, leaving scar tissue.
   b. May continue as a granuloma, then heal, or be reactivated.
   c. May eventually proceed to necrosis, liquefaction, sloughing, and cavitation.

3. The initial lesion may disseminate tubercle bacilli by extension to adjacent tissues, by way of the bloodstream, the lymphatic system, or through the bronchi.
4. Extrapulmonary TB occurs more commonly in children and immunocompromised individuals and can involve lymph nodes, bones, joints, pleural space, pericardium, CNS, GI tract, GU tissue, and the peritoneum.

Clinical Manifestations

Patient may be asymptomatic or may have insidious symptoms that may be ignored.
1. Constitutional symptoms.
   a. Fatigue, anorexia, weight loss, low-grade fever, and night sweats.
   b. Some patients have acute febrile illness, chills, and flulike symptoms.
2. Pulmonary signs and symptoms.
   a. Cough (insidious onset) progressing in frequency and producing mucoid or mucopurulent sputum and hemoptysis.
   b. Chest pain and dyspnea (suggest extensive involvement).
3. Extrapulmonary TB: pain, inflammation, and dysfunction in any of the tissues infected.

Diagnostic Evaluation

1. Testing for suspected TB infection includes sputum smear evaluated by microscopy for acid-fast bacilli (AFB) following Center for Disease Control and Prevention guidelines. Three sputum specimens are collected 8 to 24 hours apart with one being an early morning specimen.
   a. Results of sputum sample are needed to drive decisions regarding the discontinuation of isolation precautions for patients with suspected TB in health care settings.
   b. For patients with a diagnosis of TB, decisions regarding discontinuation of precautions should be based on sputum smear (ie, three consecutive negative smears) and other clinical criteria.
   c. In patients unable to produce sputum, induction with hypertonic saline should be attempted.
2. Sputum culture—a positive culture for *M. tuberculosis* confirms a diagnosis of active TB infection and can detect drug-resistant strains.
3. Chest x-ray to determine the presence and extent of disease.
4. Tuberculin skin test (PPD or Mantoux test)—inoculation of tuberculin purified protein derivative into the intradermal layer of the inner aspect of the forearm. It is used to detect *M. tuberculosis* infection, past or present, active or inactive (latent).
   a. Skin reaction is observed 48 to 72 hours after injecting 0.1 mL of PPD intradermally. Inspect and palpate for induration and measure the maximum transverse diameter.
   b. An induration of 5 or more millimeters is considered positive in HIV-infected persons, recent contact of a person with TB disease, persons with chest x-ray changes consistent with prior TB, organ recipients, and persons immunosuppressed for other reasons.
   c. An induration of 10 or more millimeters is considered positive in recent immigrants (less than 5 years) from high-prevalence countries, injection drug users, those exposed to high-risk congregate settings, mycobacteriology laboratory personnel, other clinical conditions considered high risk, children less than 4 years of age, infants, children, and adolescents exposed to adults in high-risk categories.

   d. An induration of 15 or more millimeters is considered positive in any person, including persons with no known risk factors for TB. However, targeted skin testing programs should only be conducted among high-risk groups.
5. QuantiFERON TB Gold blood assay for *Mycobacterium tuberculosis* may serve as an alternative to PPD, but does not distinguish between active and latent TB.
   a. Unaffected by past exposure to BCG vaccine.
   b. Negative tests should be interpreted with caution in the immunocompromised, those at high risk for TB, and children.

 EVIDENCE BASE Centers for Disease Control and Prevention. (2016). Tuberculin skin testing. Available: *www.cdc.gov/tb/publications/factsheets/testing/skintesting.htm.*

 NURSING ALERT Cavitation on chest x-ray, positive sputum AFB smear, and ongoing cough increase the risk of infection transmission.

Management

See Table 11-2.
1. In patients with active TB, a combination of drugs to which the organisms are susceptible is given to destroy viable bacilli as rapidly as possible and to protect against the emergence of drug-resistant organisms.
2. Current recommended regimen of uncomplicated, previously untreated pulmonary TB is an initial phase of 2 months of bactericidal drugs, including isoniazid (INH), rifampin, pyrazinamide (PZA), and ethambutol (EMB). This regimen should be followed until the results of drug susceptibility studies are available, unless there is little possibility of drug resistance.
   a. If drug susceptibility results are known and organism is fully susceptible, EMB does not need to be included.
   b. For children whose visual acuity cannot be monitored, EMB is not normally recommended except with increased likelihood of INH resistance or if the child has upper lobe infiltration and/or cavity formation.
   c. Because of increasing frequency of global streptomycin resistance, streptomycin is not considered interchangeable with EMB unless organism is known to be susceptible to streptomycin.
   d. PZA may be withheld in patients with severe liver disease, gout, and, possibly, pregnancy.
   e. Adverse effects, including liver injury, have been noted with rifampin and pyrazinamide in a once-daily or twice-weekly combination; therefore, this combination is not recommended for the treatment of latent TB infection.
3. Follow with 4 months of isoniazid and rifampin. Six months of therapy is usually effective for killing the three populations of bacilli: those rapidly dividing, those slowly dividing, and those only intermittently dividing.
4. Sputum smears may be obtained every 2 weeks until they are negative; sputum cultures do not become negative for 3 to 5 months.
5. Rifabutin is used as a substitute for rifampin if the organism is susceptible to rifabutin and for patients taking medications that may interact with rifampin.
6. Second-line drugs—such as cycloserine, ethionamide, streptomycin, amikacin, kanamycin, capreomycin, para-aminosalicylic

Table 11-2 Recommended Drugs for the Initial Treatment of Tuberculosis in Adults

DRUG	DOSAGE FORMS	DAILY DOSE	TWICE-WEEKLY DOSE	THRICE-WEEKLY DOSE	MAJOR ADVERSE EFFECTS
Isoniazid	• Tablets: 50 mg, 100 mg, 300 mg • Syrup: 50 mg/5 mL • Vials: 1 g	5 mg/kg PO or IM (maximum 300 mg)	15 mg/kg (maximum 900 mg) (can also be given once per week)	15 mg/kg (maximum 900 mg)	Paresthesias, nausea, vomiting, elevated liver transaminases peripheral neuropathy, hepatitis, hypersensitivity, hepatotoxicity, seizures, irritability, lack of concentration, lupuslike syndrome
Rifampin	• Capsules: 150 mg, 300 mg • Syrup: formulated from capsules, 10 mg/mL	10 mg/kg PO (maximum 600 mg)	10 mg/kg (maximum 600 mg)	10 mg/kg (maximum 600 mg)	Red-orange discoloration of body fluids, nausea, vomiting, anorexia, hepatitis, elevated liver transaminases, febrile reaction, purpura (rare), pruritus and rash, caution regarding drug interactions
Pyrazinamide	• Tablets: 500 mg	20 to 25 mg/kg PO	40 to 50 mg/kg	30 to 40 mg/kg (maximum 3 g)	Anorexia, rash, urticaria, nausea, vomiting, hepatotoxicity, hyperuricemia, arthralgias, acute gouty arthritis
Ethambutol	• Tablets: 100 mg, 400 mg	15 to 20 mg/kg	240 to 250 mg/kg	25 to 35 mg/kg	Optic neuritis (decreased red-green color discrimination, decreased visual acuity), peripheral neuritis, joint pain, anorexia, nausea, vomiting, skin rash

acid, and some fluoroquinolones—are used in patients with resistance, for retreatment, and in those with intolerance to other agents. Patients taking these drugs should be monitored by health care providers experienced in their use.

7. Extensively drug-resistant tuberculosis (XDR TB) is a relatively rare type of multidrug-resistant tuberculosis resistant to almost all oral drugs used to treat TB, including isoniazid, rifampin, fluoroquinolones, and at least one of the three injectable drugs (ie, amikacin, kanamycin, or capreomycin). XDR TB is of special concern for persons with HIV infection and/or immunocompromised persons because of increased risk of infection and mortality.

8. For people with suspected LTBI, treatment should begin after active TB has been ruled out (see Table 11-3). The usual treatment regimen for LTBI is isoniazid 300 mg PO daily for 9 months. To prevent neurotoxicity, pyridoxine 25 to 50 mg daily is also recommended.

DRUG ALERT Adverse reactions to anti-TB drugs may be significant. Monitor liver function tests and instruct patients to seek immediate medical attention if signs or symptoms of hepatitis occur (nausea, emesis, anorexia, jaundice, dark urine, light grey or clay colored stool, and/or abdominal pain).

EVIDENCE BASE Centers for Disease Control and Prevention. (2016). Treatment Options for Latent Tuberculosis Infection (LTBI). Available: www.cdc.gov/tb/publications/factsheets/treatment/LTBItreatmentoptions.htm.

Table 11-3 Drug Therapy for Latent Tuberculosis Infection

DRUG	DURATION (MONTHS)	INTERVAL	MINIMUM DOSES
Isoniazid	9	Daily	270
		Twice weekly	76
Isoniazid	6	Daily	180
		Twice weekly	52
Rifampin	4	Daily	120
Rifampin/ pyrazinamide	Generally should not be offered for treatment of LTBI	—	—

Adapted from Centers for Disease Control and Prevention. (2016). Treatment options for latent tuberculosis infection (LTBI). Available: www.cdc.gov/tb/publications/factsheets/treatment/LTBItreatmentoptions.htm.

Complications

1. Pleural effusion.
2. TB pneumonia.
3. Other organ involvement with TB.
4. Serious reactions to drug therapy.

Nursing Assessment

1. Obtain history of exposure to TB.
2. Assess for symptoms of active disease—productive cough, night sweats, afternoon temperature elevation, unintentional weight loss, and pleuritic chest pain.
3. Auscultate lungs for crackles.
4. During drug therapy, assess for liver dysfunction.

a. Question the patient about loss of appetite, fatigue, joint pain, fever, tenderness in liver region, clay-colored stools, dark urine, and vision changes.
b. Monitor for fever, right upper quadrant abdominal tenderness, nausea, vomiting, rash, and persistent paresthesia of hands and feet.
c. Monitor results of periodic liver function studies.

Nursing Diagnoses

- Ineffective Breathing Pattern related to pulmonary infection and potential for long-term scarring with decreased lung capacity.
- Risk for infection of staff and other patients related to nature of the disease and patient's symptoms.
- Imbalanced Nutrition: Less Than Body Requirements related to poor appetite, fatigue, and productive cough.
- Noncompliance related to lack of motivation particularly in LTBI and long-term treatment associated with health risk to patient, close contacts, and public health.

Nursing Interventions

Improving Breathing Pattern

1. Administer and teach self-administration of medications as ordered.
2. Encourage rest and avoidance of exertion if acutely ill.
3. Monitor breath sounds, respiratory rate, sputum production, dyspnea, and urine and stool color.
4. Provide supplemental oxygen as ordered.

Preventing Transmission of Infection

1. Be aware that TB is transmitted by respiratory droplets.
2. Provide care for hospitalized patient in a negative pressure room to prevent respiratory droplets from escaping when door is opened.
3. Enforce rule that all staff and visitors use well-fitted standard N-95 particulate masks for contact with patient.
4. Use high-efficiency particulate masks, such as high-efficiency particulate air (HEPA) filter masks or positive air pressure respirators, for high-risk procedures, including suctioning, bronchoscopy, or pentamidine treatments.
5. Use standard precautions for additional protection: gowns and gloves for direct contact with patient, linens or articles in room, and meticulous hand hygiene.
6. Educate the patient to control spread of infection through secretions.
   a. Cover mouth and nose with double-ply tissue when coughing or sneezing. Do not sneeze into bare hand.
   b. Wash hands after coughing or sneezing.
   c. Dispose of tissues promptly into closed plastic bag.
   d. Limit contact with others while infectious.

Improving Nutritional Status

1. Explain the importance of eating a nutritious diet to promote healing and improve defense against infection.
2. Provide small, frequent meals and liquid supplements during symptomatic period.
3. Monitor weight.
4. Administer vitamin supplements, as ordered, particularly pyridoxine (vitamin B_6), to prevent peripheral neuropathy in patients taking INH.

Improving Compliance

1. Educate the patient about the etiology, transmission, and effects of TB. Stress the importance of continuing to take medicine for the prescribed time because bacilli multiply slowly and thus can only be eradicated over a long period.
2. Review adverse effects of the drug therapy (see page 207). Question the patient specifically about common toxicities of drugs being used and emphasize immediate reporting should these occur.
3. Participate in observation of medication taking, weekly pill counts, or other programs designed to increase compliance with treatment for TB.

 NURSING ALERT Patient compliance remains a major problem in eradicating TB. Directly observed therapy (DOT) can be helpful (taking medication in an observed setting) and is especially critical for patients with drug-resistant TB, HIV-infected patients, a history of nonadherence to treatment, and those on intermittent treatment regimens (ie, two or three times weekly). Coordinate with case manager, local health department, and home health agency to ensure needed follow-up.

Community and Home Care Considerations

1. Improve ventilation in the home by opening windows in room of affected person and keeping bedroom door closed as much as possible.
2. Instruct patient to cover mouth with fresh tissue when coughing or sneezing and to dispose of tissues promptly in plastic bags.
3. Discuss TB testing of people residing with patient.
4. Investigate living conditions, availability of transportation, financial status, alcohol and drug abuse, and motivation, which may affect compliance with follow-up and treatment. Initiate referrals to a social worker for interventions in these areas.
5. Report new cases of TB to local or state public health department for screening of close contacts and monitoring.

Patient Education and Health Maintenance

1. Review possible complications: hemorrhage, pleurisy, and symptoms of recurrence (persistent cough, fever, or hemoptysis).
2. Instruct patient on avoidance of job-related exposure to excessive amounts of silicone (working in foundry, rock quarry, sand blasting), which increases risk of reactivation.
3. Encourage patient to report at specified intervals for bacteriologic (smear) examination of sputum to monitor therapeutic response and compliance.
4. Instruct patient in basic hygiene practices and investigate living conditions. Crowded, poorly ventilated conditions contribute to development and spread of TB.
5. Encourage regular symptom screening. Follow-up chest x-ray is recommended if an individual with LTBI chooses not to be treated. A single posteroanterior chest x-ray annually for 2 years is sufficient. Any individual with a history of positive TB test who develops symptoms suggestive of TB (fever, night sweats, weight loss, productive cough, or hemoptysis) should be screened with chest x-ray as part of the clinical evaluation for possible recurrent TB disease.
6. Instruct patient on prophylaxis with INH for people with LTBI or for children or patients infected with HIV who are close household contacts of patients with active TB because these individuals are at high risk of becoming infected.
7. Educate asymptomatic people about PPD testing and treatment of latent TB for positive results, based on risk grouping.

Evaluation: Expected Outcomes

- Afebrile; dyspnea relieved.
- Standard precautions observed; disposes of respiratory secretions properly.
- Maintains body weight.
- Takes medications as prescribed.

Pleurisy

Pleurisy or *pleuritis* is inflammation of the parietal and visceral pleura of the lung.

Pathophysiology and Etiology

1. Inflammation may occur in the course of pulmonary infectious, vascular, or neoplastic disorders:
   a. Pneumonia (bacterial, viral), TB, abscess, and some upper respiratory infections.
   b. Pulmonary embolism or infarction.
   c. Lung cancer.
2. Inflammation of the pleura stimulates nerve endings, causing pain.
3. Additional fluid may develop in pleural space, causing pleural effusion.

Clinical Manifestations

1. Chest pain—becomes severe, sharp, and knifelike on inspiration (pleuritic pain).
   a. May become minimal or absent when breath is held.
   b. May be localized or radiate to the shoulder or abdomen.
2. Intercostal tenderness on palpation.
3. Pleural friction rub—grating or leathery sounds heard in both phases of respiration; heard low in the axilla or over the lung base posteriorly; may be heard for only a day or so.
4. Evidence of infection: fever, malaise, and increased white blood cell count.

Diagnostic Evaluation

1. Chest x-ray may show pleural thickening.
2. Sputum examination may indicate infectious organism.
3. Examination of pleural fluid obtained by thoracentesis for smear and culture.
4. Pleural biopsy may be necessary to rule out other conditions.

Management

1. Treatment for the underlying primary disease (pneumonia, infarction); inflammation usually resolves when the primary disease subsides.
2. Pain relief, using pharmacologic and nonpharmacologic methods.
3. Intercostal nerve block may be necessary when pain causes hypoventilation.

Complications

1. Severe pleural effusion.
2. Atelectasis because of shallow breathing to avoid pain.

Nursing Assessment

1. Assess patient's level of pain.
2. Evaluate for pleural effusion (dyspnea, decreased breath sound, and dullness to percussion on affected side).
3. Auscultate lungs for pleural friction rub.

Nursing Diagnosis

- Ineffective Breathing Pattern related to stabbing chest pain.

Nursing Interventions

Easing Painful Respiration

1. Assist patient to find comfortable position that will promote aeration; lying on affected side decreases stretching of the pleura and, therefore, the pain decreases.
2. Instruct patient in splinting chest while taking a deep breath or coughing.
3. Administer or teach self-administration of pain medications, as ordered.
4. Employ nonpharmacologic interventions for pain relief, such as application of heat, muscle relaxation, and imagery.
5. Assist with intercostal nerve block if indicated.
6. Evaluate patient for signs of hypoxia (with SpO_2 or ABG) when anxiety, restlessness, and agitation of new onset are noted, before administering as-needed sedatives. Consider evaluation by a health care provider when these signs are present, especially if accompanied by cyanotic nail beds, circumoral pallor, and increased respiratory rate.

Patient Education and Health Maintenance

1. Instruct patient to seek early intervention for pulmonary diseases so pleurisy can be avoided.
2. Reassure and encourage patience because pain will subside.
3. Advise patient on reporting shortness of breath, which could indicate pleural effusion.

Evaluation: Expected Outcomes

- Respirations deep without pain.

Pleural Effusion

Pleural effusion refers to a collection of fluid in the pleural space. It is almost always secondary to other diseases.

Pathophysiology and Etiology

1. May be either transudative or exudative.
2. Transudative effusions occur primarily in noninflammatory conditions such as congestive heart failure; it is an accumulation of low-protein, low-cell-count fluid.
3. Exudative effusions occur in an area of inflammation caused by pneumonia, TB, or malignancy; it is an accumulation of high-protein fluid.
4. Occurs as a complication of:
   a. Disseminated cancer (particularly lung and breast) and lymphoma.
   b. Pleuropulmonary infections (pneumonia).
   c. Heart failure, cirrhosis, and nephrosis.
   d. Other conditions—sarcoidosis, lupus, and peritoneal dialysis.
   e. Medications such as procainamide, hydralazine, quinidine, nitrofurantoin, dantrolene, methysergide, procarbazine, and methotrexate.

Clinical Manifestations

1. Dyspnea, pleuritic chest pain, and cough.
2. Dullness or flatness to percussion (over areas of fluid) with decreased or absent breath sounds.

Diagnostic Evaluation

1. Chest x-ray or ultrasound detects the presence of fluid.
2. Thoracentesis—biochemical, bacteriologic, and cytologic studies of pleural fluid indicate cause.

Management

General

1. Transudative effusions are normally managed by treating the underlying cause (congestive heart failure, fluid overload) with diuretics and other medications; however, thoracentesis may be necessary for refractory effusion.
2. Thoracentesis is done to remove fluid that is impeding lung expansion and relieve dyspnea.
   a. Chest x-ray, ultrasound, or fluoroscopy may assist in localization.
   b. Repeated thoracentesis may be necessary until underlying cause is resolved, as fluid redevelops.

For Malignant Effusions

1. Video-assisted thoracoscopy, chest tube drainage, radiation, and/or chemotherapy.
2. In malignant conditions, pleurodesis may be required. Thoracentesis may provide only transient benefits because effusion may reaccumulate within a few days.
3. Pleurodesis—production of adhesions between the parietal and visceral pleura accomplished by tube thoracostomy, pleural space drainage, and intrapleural instillation of a sclerosing agent (tetracycline, doxycycline, or minocycline).
   a. Drug introduced through tube into pleural space; tube clamped.
   b. Patient is assisted into various positions for 3 to 5 minutes each to allow drug to spread to all pleural surfaces.
   c. Tube is unclamped, when directed, and chest drainage is facilitated for 24 hours or longer.
   d. Resulting pleural irritation, inflammation, and fibrosis cause adhesion of the visceral and parietal surfaces when they are brought together by the negative pressure caused by chest suction.

Complications

1. Large effusion could lead to respiratory failure.

Nursing Assessment

1. Obtain history of previous pulmonary condition.
2. Assess patient for dyspnea, tachypnea, and signs of fluid overload.
3. Auscultate and percuss lungs for abnormalities.

Nursing Diagnosis

- Ineffective Breathing Pattern related to collection of fluid in pleural space.

Nursing Interventions

Maintaining Normal Breathing Pattern

1. Institute treatments to resolve the underlying cause, as ordered.
2. Assist with thoracentesis, if indicated (may be done at bedside or in interventional radiology suite).
3. Maintain chest drainage, as needed (see page 187).
4. Provide care after pleurodesis.
   a. Monitor for excessive pain from the sclerosing agent, which may cause hypoventilation.
   b. Administer prescribed analgesic.
   c. Report uncontrolled pain, which may necessitate intrapleural lidocaine instillation.
   d. Administer oxygen as indicated by dyspnea and hypoxemia.
   e. Observe patient's breathing pattern, oxygen saturation, and other vital signs for evidence of improvement or deterioration.

Patient Education and Health Maintenance

1. Instruct patient to seek early intervention for unusual shortness of breath, along with signs of worsening heart or lung disease.

Evaluation: Expected Outcomes

- Reports absence of shortness of breath.

Lung Abscess

A *lung abscess* is a localized, pus-containing, necrotic lesion in the lung characterized by cavity formation.

Pathophysiology and Etiology

1. Most commonly occurs due to aspiration of vomitus or infected material from upper respiratory tract.
2. Secondary causes include:
   a. Aspiration of foreign body into the lung.
   b. Pulmonary embolus.
   c. Trauma.
   d. TB and necrotizing pneumonia.
   e. Bronchial obstruction (usually a tumor) causes obstruction to bronchus, leading to infection distal to the growth.
3. The right lung is involved more frequently than the left because of dependent position of the right bronchus, the less acute angle that the right main bronchus forms within the trachea, and its larger size.
4. In the initial stages, the cavity in the lung may communicate with the bronchus.
5. Eventually, the cavity becomes surrounded or encapsulated by a wall of fibrous tissue, except at one or two points where the necrotic process extends until it reaches the lumen of some bronchus or pleural space and establishes a communication with the respiratory tract, the pleural cavity (bronchopleural fistula), or both.
6. The organisms typically seen are *Klebsiella pneumoniae* and *Staphylococcus aureus*.

Clinical Manifestations

1. Cough, fever, and malaise from segmental pneumonitis and atelectasis.
2. Headache, anemia, weight loss, dyspnea, and weakness.
3. Pleuritic chest pain from extension of suppurative pneumonitis to pleural surface.
4. Production of mucopurulent sputum, usually foul-smelling; blood streaking common; may become profuse after abscess ruptures into bronchial tree.
5. The chest may be dull to percussion, with decreased or absent breath sounds and intermittent pleural friction rub.

Diagnostic Evaluation

1. Chest x-ray to help diagnose and locate lesion.
2. Chest CT to locate and identify if lesion is singular or multiple areas of involvement.
3. Direct bronchoscopic visualization to exclude possibility of tumor or foreign body; bronchial washings and brush biopsy may be done for cytopathologic study.

4. Sputum culture and sensitivity tests to determine causative organisms and antimicrobial sensitivity.

Management

1. Administration of appropriate antimicrobial agent, usually by IV route, until clinical condition improves, and then oral administration.
2. Percutaneous drainage by interventional radiology.
3. Bronchoscopy to drain abscess is controversial.
4. Surgical intervention only if patient fails to respond to medical management, sustains a hemorrhage, or has a suspected tumor.
5. Nutritional management is usually a high-calorie, high-protein diet.

Complications

1. Hemoptysis from erosion of a vessel.
2. Empyema and bronchopleural fistula.
3. Entrapment of the lung.
4. Hemoptysis.
5. Further expansion of abscess.
6. Lung necrosis.

Nursing Assessment

1. Examine the oral cavity because poor condition of teeth and gums increases the number of anaerobes in the oral cavity and could be a source for infection. Promote frequent oral care.
2. Perform chest examination for abnormalities.
3. Monitor temperature to evaluate effectiveness of therapy.

Nursing Diagnoses

- Ineffective Breathing Pattern related to the presence of suppurative lung disease.
- Acute or Chronic Pain related to infection.
- Imbalanced Nutrition: Less Than Body Requirements related to catabolic state from chronic infection.

Nursing Interventions

Minimizing Respiratory Dysfunction

1. Monitor patient's response to antimicrobial therapy by vital signs, energy level, and appetite.
2. Evaluate patient thoroughly for signs of hypoxia, including SpO_2, when anxiety, restlessness, and agitation of new onset are noted before administering as-needed sedatives. Notify health care provider for evaluation when these signs are present, especially if accompanied by cyanotic nail beds, circumoral pallor, and increased respiratory rate.
3. Perform postural drainage as directed (positions to be assumed depend on location of abscess) and encourage coughing and breathing exercises.
   a. Measure and record the volume of sputum to follow patient's clinical course (may be of limited use because of patient swallowing of sputum).
   b. Give adequate fluids to enhance liquefying of secretions.

Attaining Comfort

1. Use nursing measures to combat generalized discomfort: oral hygiene, positions of comfort, and relaxing massage.
2. Encourage rest and limitation of physical activity during febrile periods.
3. Monitor chest tube functioning.

4. Administer analgesics as directed. Use caution with opioids that might depress respirations.

Improving Nutritional Status

1. Provide a high-protein, high-calorie diet.
2. Offer liquid supplements for additional nutritional support when anorexia limits patient's intake. Monitor weight weekly.
3. Obtain nutritional consult and consider medication side effects causing anorexia.

Patient Education and Health Maintenance

1. Teach the patient that an extended course of antimicrobial therapy (4 to 8 weeks) is usually necessary; mixed infections are common and may require multiple antibiotics.
2. Encourage patient to have periodontal care, especially in the presence of gingival lesions.
3. Stress importance of follow-up x-rays to monitor abscess cavity closure.
4. Remind family that patient may aspirate if weakness, confusion, alcoholism, seizures, and swallowing difficulties are present. Train in aspiration precautions.
5. Encourage patient to assume responsibility for attaining and maintaining an optimal state of health through a planned program of nutrition, rest, and exercise.

Evaluation: Expected Outcomes

- Respirations unlabored; temperature in normal range; less purulent sputum expectorated.
- Appears more comfortable; verbalizes less pain.
- Eats better; weight stable.

Cancer of the Lung (Bronchogenic Carcinoma)

Bronchogenic carcinoma is the most common cause of cancer deaths worldwide. It is classified according to cell type:

- Non–small cell lung cancer (NSCLC) (80%) includes epidermoid (squamous cell) carcinoma, adenocarcinoma, and bronchoalveolar carcinoma. This requires careful staging that will determine prognosis and treatment. Surgery may be an option for stage I-II and offers that best chance of survival but is only appropriate for approximately 20% to 25% of patients.
- Small cell lung cancer (about 20%) is almost always metastatic and is commonly treated with combination chemotherapy. The overall 5-year survival rate is low because of initial presentation with locally advanced or metastatic disease. Approximately 65% to 80% of patients present with unresectable disease.

Pathophysiology and Etiology

Predisposing Factors

1. Cigarette, pipe, cigar smoking, and secondhand smoke exposure—amount, frequency, and duration of smoking have positive relationship to cancer of the lung.
2. Occupational exposure to radon, asbestos, air pollution, polycyclic aromatic hydrocarbons (from incomplete combustion of carbon-based fuels, such as wood, coal, diesel, fat, tobacco, incense, or tar), arsenic, chromium, nickel, iron, radioactive substances, isopropyl oil, and petroleum oil mists alone or in combination with tobacco smoke.
3. History of lung cancer.
4. Age greater than 65 years.

NURSING ALERT Suspect lung cancer in patients who belong to a susceptible, high-risk group and who have repeated unresolved respiratory infections. The National Cancer Institute has found that low-dose spiral chest CT provides a decided benefit in screening and management of lung cancer.

Staging and Classification

1. Staging refers to anatomic extent of tumor, lymph node involvement, atelectasis, bronchus involvement, and metastatic spread, including malignant pleural effusions. Classification refers to criteria that classify pathologic type of lung cancer.
2. Staging done by the tumor, node, metastasis staging system for NSCLC is an internationally accepted system used to determine the disease stage and extent of disease and is used to guide management (particularly surgical) and determine prognosis.
   a. Imaging including chest CT and PET scan.
   b. Pathology including biopsy (mediastinoscopy, tissue).
3. The International Association for the Study of Lung Cancer (IASLC) has developed a classification system using standardized criteria and terminology for the pathologic diagnosis of lung cancer in small biopsies and cytology. NSCLC can be further classified into a more specific type, such as adenocarcinoma or squamous cell carcinoma, based on this system. This classification system is important because 70% of lung cancer patients present with advanced stages that are potentially unresectable.

 EVIDENCE BASE Nicholson, A. G., Chansky, K., Crowley, J., et al. (2016). The International Association for the Study of Lung Cancer Lung Cancer Staging Project: Proposals for the revision of the clinical and pathologic staging of small cell lung cancer in the forthcoming eighth edition of the TNM Classification for Lung Cancer. *Journal of Thoracic Oncology, 11*(3), 300–311.

Clinical Manifestations

Symptoms are related to size and location of tumor, extent of spread, and involvement of other structures.

1. Cough, especially a new type or changing cough, results from bronchial irritation.
2. Dyspnea and wheezing (suggests partial bronchial obstruction).
3. Chest pain (poorly localized and aching).
4. Excessive sputum production and repeated upper respiratory infections.
5. Hemoptysis.
6. Malaise, fever, weight loss, fatigue, and anorexia.
7. Paraneoplastic syndrome—metabolic or neurologic disturbances related to the secretion of substances by the neoplasm.
8. Symptoms of metastasis—bone pain; abdominal discomfort, nausea, and vomiting from liver involvement; pancytopenia from bone marrow involvement; and headache from CNS metastasis.
9. Usual sites of metastasis—lymph nodes, bones, liver, and CNS.

Diagnostic Evaluation

1. Abnormal findings seen on chest x-ray are typically followed with chest CT. If suggestive of possible cancer, a needle biopsy or bronchoscopy is typically performed to establish diagnosis, followed by a positron emission tomography (PET) scan for staging and consideration of surgical options.
2. CT scan of the chest and abdomen and whole-body PET scan are indicated in most candidates for surgical resection.
3. Cytologic examination of sputum/chest fluids for malignant cells for pleural effusion.
4. Fiberoptic bronchoscopy for observation of location and extent of tumor and for biopsy or surgery.
5. PET scan—sensitive in detecting small nodules and metastatic lesions.
6. Lymph node biopsy; mediastinoscopy to establish lymphatic spread; to plan treatment.
7. Pulmonary function tests (PFTs)—to determine if patient will have adequate pulmonary reserve to withstand surgical procedure.
8. Laboratory testing, including complete blood count, metabolic panel, calcium level, and liver function tests.

Management

Treatment depends on the cell type, the stage of disease, and the physiologic status of the patient. It includes a multidisciplinary approach that may be used separately or in combination, including surgical resection, radiation, chemotherapy, and biotherapy.

Complications

1. Hypercoagulable state.
2. Complications of treatment including pancytopenia, rash, and hair loss.
3. Superior vena cava syndrome—oncologic complication caused by obstruction of major blood vessels draining the head, neck, and upper torso.
4. Pleural effusion and pulmonary scarring.
5. Infectious complications, especially upper respiratory infections.
6. Brain metastasis.
7. With advanced lung cancer—massive hemoptysis, central airway obstruction, malignant pleural effusion, venous thrombosis, spinal cord compression, hypercalcemia, and SIADH.

Nursing Assessment

1. Determine onset and duration of coughing, sputum production (purulent vs. bloody), and degree of dyspnea. Auscultate breath sounds. Observe symmetry of the chest during respirations.
2. Take anthropometric measurements: weigh patient, review laboratory tests, and conduct appraisal of 24-hour food intake.
3. Ask about pain, including location, intensity, and factors influencing pain.
4. Monitor vital signs including oximetry.

Nursing Diagnoses

- Ineffective Breathing Pattern related to obstructive and restrictive respiratory processes associated with lung cancer.
- Imbalanced Nutrition: Less Than Body Requirements related to hypermetabolic state, taste aversion, and anorexia secondary to radiotherapy/chemotherapy.
- Acute or Chronic Pain related to tumor effects, invasion of adjacent structures, and toxicities associated with radiotherapy/chemotherapy.
- Anxiety and/or depression related to treatment-related side effects, uncertain outcome, and fear of recurrence.

Nursing Interventions

See also Chapter 8, page 107, for interventions related to cancer treatment.

Improving Breathing Patterns

1. Teach breathing retraining exercises to increase diaphragmatic excursion with resultant reduction in work of breathing.
2. Give prescribed treatment for productive cough (expectorant, antimicrobial agent) and mobilize patient, as tolerated, to potentially control thickened or retained secretions and subsequent dyspnea.
3. Augment the patient's ability to cough effectively.
   a. Splint chest manually with hands.
   b. Instruct patient to inspire fully and cough two to three times in one exhalation.
   c. Provide humidifier/vaporizer to provide moisture to loosen secretions.
4. Support patient undergoing removal of pleural fluid (by thoracentesis or tube thoracostomy) and instillation of sclerosing agent to obliterate pleural space and prevent fluid recurrence.
5. Administer oxygen by way of nasal cannula as prescribed.
6. Encourage energy conservation through pacing of activities and sitting for tasks.
7. Allow patient to sleep in a reclining chair or with head of bed elevated if severely dyspneic.
8. Recognize the anxiety associated with dyspnea; teach relaxation techniques.

Improving Nutritional Status

1. Emphasize that nutrition is an important part of the treatment of lung cancer.
   a. Encourage small amounts of high-calorie, high-protein foods frequently, rather than three daily meals.
   b. Ensure adequate protein intake—milk, eggs, chicken, fowl, fish, cheese, and oral nutritional supplements if patient cannot tolerate meats or other protein sources.
2. Administer or encourage prescribed vitamin supplement to avoid deficiency states, glossitis, and cheilosis.
3. Change consistency of diet to soft or liquid if patient has esophagitis from radiation therapy.
4. Give enteral or total parenteral nutrition for malnourished patient who is unable or unwilling to eat.
5. Obtain nutritional consultation.

Controlling Pain

1. Take thorough history of pain; assess presence/absence of support system.
2. Administer prescribed drug, usually starting with nonsteroidal anti-inflammatory drugs (NSAIDs) and progressing to adjuvant analgesic and short- and long-acting opioids.
   a. Administer regularly to control pain.
   b. Titrate to achieve pain control.
3. Consider alternative methods, such as cognitive and behavioral training, biofeedback, and relaxation, to increase patient's sense of control. Mind–body modalities (meditation, hypnosis, relaxation techniques, cognitive–behavioral therapy, biofeedback, and guided imagery) and massage therapy may be helpful for mood disorders and chronic pain. Acupuncture may improve pain control.
4. Evaluate problems of insomnia, depression, anxiety, and so forth that may be contributing to patient's pain.
5. Initiate bowel training program because constipation is an adverse effect of some analgesic/opioid agents.
6. Facilitate referral to pain clinic/specialist if pain becomes refractory (unyielding) to usual methods of control.
7. Radiation therapy may be used to treat pain caused by bone metastasis.

Minimizing Anxiety

1. Realize that shock, disbelief, denial, anger, and depression are all normal reactions to the diagnosis of lung cancer.
2. Try to have the patient express concerns; share these concerns with health professionals. Link patient and family with cancer support groups.
3. Encourage the patient to communicate feelings to significant people in his or her life.
4. Prepare patient physically, emotionally, and intellectually for prescribed therapeutic program.
5. Expect some feelings of anxiety and depression to recur during illness.
6. Encourage the patient to keep active and remain in the mainstream. Continue with usual activities (work, recreation, sexual) as much as possible.
7. Administer antidepressants that may be used to treat depression; however, therapeutic effect is delayed 3 to 4 weeks.

Patient Education and Health Maintenance

1. Teach patient to use NSAIDs or other prescribed medication, as necessary, for pain without being overly concerned about addiction.
2. Help the patient realize that not every ache and pain is caused by lung cancer; some patients do not experience pain.
3. Radiation therapy may be used for pain control if tumor has spread to bone, control of hemoptysis, bronchial obstruction, or brain metastasis.
4. Advise the patient to report new or persistent pain; it may be due to some other cause such as arthritis.
5. Suggest talking to a social worker about financial assistance or other services that may be needed.
6. For additional information, contact the American Cancer Society, 1-800-ACS-2345, *www.cancer.org*; National Comprehensive Cancer Network, *www.nccn.org*.
7. Facilitate referral to cancer support group or mental health professional.
8. Support patient and family to make decisions regarding long-term care, possibly pulmonary rehabilitation.

Evaluation: Expected Outcomes

- Performs self-care without dyspnea.
- Eats small meals four to five times per day; weight stable.
- Reports pain decreased from level 6 to level 2 or a level that patient reports as tolerable for completing activities of daily living (ADLs) when treated with medication.
- Verbalizes emotions and concerns associated with cancer diagnosis; practices relaxation techniques.

CHRONIC DISORDERS

 See additional online content: Patient Education Guidelines 11-1.

Bronchiectasis

Bronchiectasis is a chronic inflammation and dilatation of the bronchi caused by immune defects, cystic fibrosis, aspiration, and lung infections.

Pathophysiology and Etiology

1. May be a complication of respiratory infections including pneumonia, mycobacterium, and other organisms leading to

damage to the bronchial wall, and buildup of thick sputum, causing obstruction.
2. Causes chronic coughing and excess mucus production, which is often purulent.
3. May involve a single lobe or segment or one or both lungs more diffusely.
4. As the condition progresses, there may be atelectasis and fibrosis, which lead to respiratory insufficiency.
5. Other causes include pulmonary infections; obstruction of bronchi; aspiration of foreign bodies, vomitus, chemicals, or material from upper respiratory tract; cilial dysmotility syndrome; alpha$_1$-antitrypsin deficiency; and immunodeficiency.

Clinical Manifestations

1. Persistent cough with production of increased amounts of sputum that may be purulent.
2. Intermittent hemoptysis; dyspnea.
3. Recurrent fever and pulmonary infections.
4. Crackles and rhonchi heard over involved lobes.
5. Finger clubbing.

Diagnostic Evaluation

Early diagnosis is essential to prevent complications.
1. High-resolution CT is necessary for diagnosis of bronchiectasis.
2. Chest x-ray may reveal areas of atelectasis with widespread dilation of bronchi.
3. Sputum examination may detect offending pathogens.
4. PFT to evaluate airflow obstruction and impairment.

Management

The goal is to prevent progression of the disease, thereby improving symptoms, limiting exacerbations, decreasing complications, and reducing morbidity and mortality.
1. Infection controlled by:
    a. Smoking cessation.
    b. Prompt antimicrobial treatment of exacerbations of infection.
    c. Immunization against potential pulmonary pathogens (influenza and pneumococcal vaccine).
2. Secretion clearance techniques may be helpful, such as postural drainage, devices that provide PEP and/or oscillations to lung walls including PEP valve, flutter valve, Acapella device, vest therapy, and, possibly, percussion and vibration or other methods.
3. Bronchodilators for bronchodilation and improved secretion clearance.
4. Mobilization and exercise such as in a pulmonary rehabilitation program.
5. Early management of acute exacerbations, including antibiotics, corticosteroids, and oxygen for hypoxemia. Severe exacerbation is normally managed with hospitalization, IV antibiotics, bronchodilators, and secretion clearance.
6. Surgical resection (segmental resection) when conservative management fails.

Complications

1. Progressive excess mucus production or suppuration.
2. Hemoptysis, major pulmonary hemorrhage.
3. COPD, emphysema, chronic respiratory failure, pulmonary hypertension, cor pulmonale.

Nursing Assessment

1. Obtain history regarding amount and characteristics of sputum produced, including hemoptysis.
2. Auscultate lungs for diffuse rhonchi and crackles.

Nursing Diagnosis

• Ineffective Secretion Clearance related to tenacious and copious secretions.

Nursing Interventions

Maintaining Airway Clearance

1. Encourage use of secretion clearance therapy techniques to empty the bronchi of accumulated secretions (see page 165).
    a. Assist with postural drainage positioning for involved lung segments to drain the bronchiectatic areas by gravity, thus reducing the degree of infection and symptoms. Contraindicated with increased intracranial pressure, uncontrolled hypertension, recent face or head surgery.
    b. Vibratory vest therapy and PEP devices (such as PEP valve, flutter valve, Acapella device) for enhanced secretion clearance.
    c. Chest percussion and vibration may be used to assist in mobilizing secretions (use after bronchodilators and before meals). Contraindicated with osteoporosis, known rib or vertebral fractures.
    d. Encourage effective coughing to help clear secretions.
2. Encourage increased mobilization and intake of fluids to reduce viscosity of sputum and make expectoration easier.
3. Consider vaporizer to provide humidification and keep secretions thin.

Patient Education and Health Maintenance

1. Instruct the patient to avoid smoking, noxious fumes, dust, smoke, and other pulmonary irritants.
2. Teach the patient to monitor sputum. Report if untoward change in quantity or character occurs.
3. Instruct the patient and family about importance of pulmonary drainage.
    a. Teach drainage exercises, use of secretion clearance device(s), and chest physical therapy techniques.
    b. Encourage AM postural drainage to address nocturnal accumulation of secretions.
    c. Encourage patient to engage in physical activity throughout the day to help mobilize mucus.
4. Encourage regular oral hygiene and dental care.
5. Emphasize the importance of influenza and pneumococcal immunizations and prompt evaluation of treatment of respiratory infections.

Evaluation: Expected Outcomes

• Decreased sputum and pulmonary infections; lungs clear after chest physical therapy.

Chronic Obstructive Pulmonary Disease

 EVIDENCE BASE Global Strategy for the Diagnosis, Management and Prevention of COPD. (2018). Global Initiative for Chronic Obstructive Lung Disease (GOLD) 2018. Available: http://goldcopd.org.

Chronic obstructive pulmonary disease (*COPD*) is a common, preventable, and treatable disease characterized by persistent respiratory symptoms and airflow limitation because of airway and/or alveolar abnormalities usually caused by significant exposure to noxious particles or gases, which cause an abnormal inflammatory response in the airways. Airflow limitation is not fully reversible. Emphysema or destruction of the gas-exchanging surfaces of the lungs describes one component of COPD. Chronic bronchitis is another component

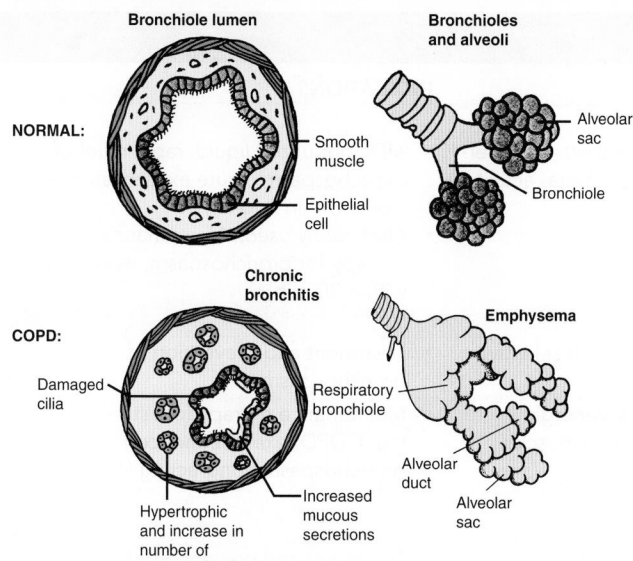

Figure 11-3. Airway changes in chronic obstructive pulmonary disease compared with normal.

occurring in some patients. Asthma is not considered part of COPD because of reversibility seen on spirometry (see Chapter 28).

Pathophysiology and Etiology

1. Irritants from cigarette smoke and pollutants deposited in the lower respiratory tract cause inflammation and a cellular response that leads to alveolar wall destruction causing hyperinflation of the terminal bronchioles (emphysema) and increased size and number of mucus glands in bronchiole walls, which increases mucus production (chronic bronchitis). See Figure 11-3.
   a. In chronic bronchitis, the diameter of the bronchiole lumen is reduced, cilia are damaged, and mucus obstructs the bronchioles.
   b. In emphysema, hyperinflation causes trapped air to remain in the terminal bronchioles and alveoli, reducing oxygenation.
2. Risk factors for COPD include the following:
   a. Cigarette smoking (primary risk factor).
   b. Environmental air pollution
   c. Indoor air pollution from heating and cooking with biomass (energy sources from organic material).
   d. Host factors including genetic predisposition, abnormal lung development, and accelerated aging.
3. Alpha$_1$-antitrypsin deficiency is a genetically determined cause of emphysema and liver disease. Alpha$_1$-antitrypsin is the most common protease inhibitor in the blood and inhibits neutrophil elastase, an elastin and basement membrane–degrading protease released by neutrophils. When alveolar structures are left unprotected from exposure to elastase, progressive destruction of elastin tissues results in the development of emphysema.

Clinical Manifestations

Chronic Bronchitis and Emphysema
Usually insidious, gradual in onset, and steadily progressive.
1. Dyspnea (particularly with stairs or inclines) and decreased exercise tolerance occur in all cases. Skeletal muscle dysfunction is common.
2. Cough, which may be productive. Chronic bronchitis is characterized by cough and increased sputum production for at least 3 months during 2 consecutive years.
3. Increased anteroposterior diameter of the chest (barrel chest) because of air trapping, causing hyperinflation and diaphragmatic flattening in emphysema.
4. Wheezing, decreased breath sounds, and chest tightness may be present.

Exacerbation of COPD
Episodic and often recurrent, contributing to disease worsening because of increased inflammatory airway response.
1. Acute change in the patient's baseline dyspnea, cough, and sputum amount and color, which requires a change in treatment (typically oral steroids and/or antibiotics).
2. Triggers may include viral and/or bacterial infection or environmental pollutants or irritants. One third of exacerbations have no identifiable cause.
3. Exacerbations are associated with increased hyperinflation and air trapping with decreased expiratory flow contributing to worsening dyspnea as well as worsening ventilation/perfusion abnormalities, which may lead to hypoxemia.
4. Because exacerbations have increased risk of mortality and morbidity and decreased quality of life, prevention and early detection and management are important.

Diagnostic Evaluation

1. Spirometry or PFTs are necessary to accurately diagnose COPD. Airflow obstruction based on spirometry or pulmonary function including a postbronchodilator FEV$_1$/FVC of less than 70% of predicted for age, height, and gender. FEV$_1$ percent predicted is used to stage severity of COPD.
   a. Stage I (mild)—FEV$_1$/FVC < 0.7; FEV$_1$ ≥ 80% predicted.
   b. Stage II (moderate)—FEV$_1$/FVC < 0.7; FEV$_1$ 50% to 80% predicted.
   c. Stage III (severe)—FEV$_1$/FVC < 0.7; FEV$_1$ 30% to 50% predicted.
   d. Stage IV (very severe)—FEV$_1$/FVC < 0.7; FEV$_1$ < 30% predicted, or FEV$_1$ < 50% predicted plus chronic respiratory failure.
2. The GOLD COPD guidelines also emphasize exacerbation history and COPD Assessment Test (CAT) and modified Medical Research Council Dyspnea Scale (mMRC) scores to further characterize COPD.
3. ABG or oximetry can be used to detect hypoxemia (SaO$_2$ or SpO$_2$ less than 92%). ABG can additionally detect respiratory failure (PaO$_2$ less than 60 mm Hg with or without PCO$_2$ greater than 50 mm Hg on room air).
4. Chest x-ray—for diagnosis of pneumonia and pneumothorax.
5. Alpha$_1$-antitrypsin assay is useful in identifying genetically determined deficiency in emphysema (helpful when COPD occurs at young age or nonsmoker).

Management

The goals of COPD management are to relieve symptoms, prevent disease progression, reduce mortality, improve exercise tolerance, improve health status/quality of life, and prevent and treat complications and exacerbations. The goal of acute care is to improve airflow obstruction. Treatment regimens are based on severity.
1. Smoking cessation is essential to reduce disease progression and improve survival.
2. Inhaled bronchodilators (see Table 11-4, pages 216–220) reduce dyspnea and bronchospasm and improve secretion

text continues on page 220

Table 11-4   Commonly Used Pulmonary Drugs

DRUGS/ADMINISTRATION	PHARMACOLOGIC EFFECTS	INDICATIONS
Bronchodilators		
Albuterol (metered-dose inhaler [MDI], nebulized solution, oral)	• Short-acting sympathomimetic (beta$_2$-adrenergic agonist) with highly selective beta$_2$ activity	• MDI, nebulized liquid: rapid relief of bronchospasm, acute exacerbation—works within 3 to 5 min • *Oral (rarely used):* Maintenance therapy for bronchospasm, works within 30 min
Levalbuterol (HFA and nebulized solution)	• Short-acting sympathomimetic with selective beta$_2$ activity	• Treatment and prevention of bronchospasm
Salmeterol xinafoate (dry powder inhaler [DPI])	• Selectively stimulates beta-2 adrenergic receptors, relaxing airway smooth muscle; long-acting	• Maintenance therapy for asthma, COPD, exercise-induced bronchospasm; long-acting (12 hr)
Formoterol (DPI)	• Selectively stimulates beta-2 adrenergic receptors, relaxing airway smooth muscle; long-acting	• Treatment and prevention of bronchospasm; long-acting
Indacaterol (DPI)	• Selectively stimulates beta-2 adrenergic receptors, relaxing airway smooth muscle; long-acting	• Treatment and prevention of bronchospasm; long-acting
Arformoterol (nebulized solution)	• Selectively stimulates beta-2 adrenergic receptors, relaxing airway smooth muscle	• Maintenance therapy for COPD; long-acting
Ipratropium bromide (MDI, nebulized liquid)	• Anticholinergic	• Maintenance therapy for COPD, asthma, bronchospasm • Acts within 15 min
Tiotropium (DPI)	• Long-acting anticholinergic	• Maintenance therapy for COPD
Aclidinium bromide (dry powder inhaler)	• Long-acting anticholinergic	• Maintenance therapy for COPD
Aminophylline (IV injection)	• Methylxanthine compound—relaxes smooth muscle by increasing level of cyclic adenosine monophosphate	• Acute exacerbation of asthma or bronchitis
Theophylline preparations (oral)	• Methylxanthine compound—relaxes muscle by increasing cyclic adenosine monophosphate	• Mild bronchodilator, maintenance therapy for bronchospasm, asthma, COPD maintenance
Albuterol + ipratropium combination (MDI nebulized solution)	• Sympathomimetic with selective beta$_2$ and anticholinergic activity	• Fast-acting and maintenance therapy for bronchospasm; exacerbation of COPD
Tiotropium bromide and olodaterol	• Long-acting selective beta$_2$ and anticholinergic activity	• Long-acting control of COPD
Umeclidinium	• Long-acting anticholinergic activity	• Long-acting control of COPD
Umeclidinium and vilanterol	• Long-acting selective beta$_2$ and anticholinergic activity	• Long-acting control of COPD
Fluticasone furoate and vilanterol trifenatate	• See fluticasone and vilanterol	• See fluticasone and vilanterol

ADVERSE EFFECTS	NURSING CONSIDERATIONS
• Throat irritation, URI symptoms, cough, tremor, dizziness, nervousness, tachycardia, headache, nausea, tremors, hypokalemia, tachyphylaxis • Continuous nebulization may cause hypokalemia	• Observe inhalation by patient to be certain that correct technique is used. • Caution patient not to exceed prescribed dose. Adverse effects may be associated with excessive use. Does not reduce inflammation. • HFA MDIs must be primed for four puffs before initial use and after not using for long periods.
• Tachycardia, hypertension, nervousness	• Administered every 4 to 6 hr.
• Headache, throat irritation, nasal congestion, rhinitis, palpitations, tachycardia, tremor, hypertension, bronchospasm • Possible increased risk of asthma-related deaths	• Observe inhalation by patient to make sure that correct technique is used. • Instruct patient that it is not for immediate relief of bronchospasm and dyspnea. • Maximum dose two puffs every 12 hr.
• URI, dyspepsia, chest pain, back pain, fever, diarrhea, nausea, vomiting, dry mouth, dizziness, insomnia, nervousness, tremor, palpitations, bronchospasm; possible increased risk of asthma-related deaths	• Train patient for proper use of aerolizer. • Instruct patient that it is not for immediate relief of bronchospasm and dyspnea. • Administer twice daily or 15 min before exercise.
• Cough, throat irritation, headache, tremor, palpitations	• Once-daily dosing.
• Pain, chest pain, back pain, diarrhea, sinusitis, leg cramps, dyspnea, rash, flulike symptoms, bronchospasm • Possible increased risk of asthma-related deaths	• Not indicated for acute bronchospasm.
• Bronchitis, dyspnea, URI, cough, COPD exacerbation, nausea, dry mouth, flulike symptoms Rare: Can cause blurring of vision if sprayed into the eyes (atropine derivative) • Voice hoarseness • Urinary retention	• Instruct patient to use spacer device with MDI or close lips around inhaler mouthpiece; close eyes during inhalation.
• Dry mouth, pharyngitis, constipation, increased heart rate, blurred vision, urinary retention, URI symptoms, chest pain, UTI, dyspepsia, rhinitis, abdominal pain, angioedema	• Not indicated for acute bronchospasm. • Eye discomfort and visual changes require prompt ophthalmology evaluation.
• Urinary retention • Increased interocular pressures • Headache, URI, cough	• Acute dyspnea, avoid in severe allergies to milk proteins. • Rash, hives, facial swelling, itching.
• CNS: irritability, restlessness, insomnia • CV: palpitations, tachycardia, hypotension • GI: nausea, vomiting, diarrhea	• Too rapid administration can cause hypotension, extra systoles, and muscle tremors. Administer at prescribed rate with an IV infusion pump. • Requires monitoring of blood levels, associated with frequent drug interactions.
• CNS: irritability, restlessness, insomnia, seizures in toxic ranges • CV: palpitations, tachycardia, hypotension • GI: nausea, vomiting, diarrhea	• Teach patients to take at equal intervals throughout the day. • To decrease GI irritation, take with milk or crackers. • Monitor theophylline blood level periodically as directed to ensure therapeutic range and prevent toxicity. • Be alert for drug interactions.
• See albuterol and ipratropium	• See albuterol and ipratropium. • One puff of Combivent equals one puff of albuterol and one puff of ipratropium.
• See tiotropium and formoterol	• See tiotropium and formoterol.
• Nasal and throat irritation, URI, cough, muscle aches urinary retention	• Bronchospasm. • Narrow-angle glaucoma closure.
• Increase in heart rate, BP, EKG changes, hyperglycemia • Nasal and throat irritation, URI, cough, muscle aches urinary retention	• See salmeterol and umeclidinium.
• See fluticasone and vilanterol	• See fluticasone and vilanterol.

(continued)

Table 11-4   Commonly Used Pulmonary Drugs (*Continued*)

DRUGS/ADMINISTRATION	PHARMACOLOGIC EFFECTS	INDICATIONS
Corticosteroids		
Prednisone, prednisolone (IV injection, oral preparation)	• Potent anti-inflammatory activity	• Acute exacerbation of asthma or bronchitis (IV preparation) • Acute exacerbation (oral preparation) of asthma or COPD
Beclomethasone (MDI)	• Synthetic corticosteroid with potent anti-inflammatory activity; effective only by inhalation • Not effective in acute attack; must be used for 2 to 4 wk to show effectiveness	• Asthma • Severe COPD with frequent exacerbations
Mometasone (DPI)	• Anti-inflammatory steroid; effective only by inhalation • Not effective in acute attack; must be used for up to 2 to 4 wk to show effectiveness	• Asthma maintenance • COPD (severe COPD with frequent exacerbations)
Ciclesonide (MDI)	• Anti-inflammatory steroid; effective only by inhalation • Not effective in acute attack; must be used for up to 2 to 4 wk to show effectiveness	• Asthma maintenance
Fluticasone (MDI, DPI)	• Anti-inflammatory steroid; effective only by inhalation • Not effective in acute attack; must be used for 2 to 4 wk to show effectiveness	• Asthma • COPD (severe COPD with frequent exacerbations)
Budesonide (DPI, nebulized liquid)	• Anti-inflammatory steroid; effective only by inhalation • Not effective in acute attack; must be used for 2 to 4 wk to show effectiveness	• Asthma • COPD (severe COPD with frequent exacerbations)
Fluticasone and salmeterol (MDI, DPI)	• Combination inhaled corticosteroid and long-acting beta-agonist bronchodilator	• Asthma maintenance • COPD maintenance • Maintenance therapy for controlled bronchospasm
Budesonide and formoterol (MDI)	• Combination inhaled corticosteroid and long-acting beta agonist	• Asthma maintenance • COPD maintenance
Mometasone and formoterol (MDI)	• Combination inhaled corticosteroid and long-acting beta agonist	• Asthma maintenance • COPD maintenance
Mast Cell Stabilizers		
Cromolyn (solution for inhalation, powder used with special inhaler)	• Inhibits activation of a variety of inflammatory cells associated with asthma, prevents bronchospasm • Not effective in acute attack; must be used for 2 to 4 wk to show effectiveness	• Maintenance therapy for asthma

ADVERSE EFFECTS	NURSING CONSIDERATIONS
• CNS: depression, euphoria, mood changes, insomnia • GI: gastric irritation, peptic ulcer • Metabolic: hypernatremia, hypokalemia, hyperglycemia, water retention, and weight gain • Long-term, high-dose: adrenal insufficiency, osteoporosis, muscle weakness, cataracts, glaucoma, fragile and easily bruised skin, immunosuppression	• Long-term use: Do not stop abruptly because of adrenal suppression. • Take oral form with food. • Usually given as taper from higher dose to lowest possible dose that achieves desired effect. Alternatively, short course may be recommended. Long-term use should be avoided if possible. • Advise patient of possible increased appetite and weight gain risk; advise to eat small, frequent meals high in protein, fruits, and vegetables, and low in simple carbohydrates.
• Oral candidiasis, dysphonia, cough, pharyngitis, bronchospasm, headache, sinusitis, URI, rhinitis, pain, back pain, bronchospasm • May experience skin bruising in high doses	• Bronchospasm, glaucoma, cataracts, osteoporosis. • Not used with status asthmaticus or acute asthma episodes • Use a spacer device with MDI • Gargle, rinse, and spit after use to prevent oral candidiasis.
• Oral candidiasis, dysphonia • Risk for systemic adverse effects associated with oral steroids is low • May experience skin bruising in high doses • Headache, rhinitis, URI, sinusitis, bronchospasm	• Use water gargle, rinse, and spit after use to prevent oral yeast growth.
• Oral candidiasis, dysphonia • Risk for systemic adverse effects associated with oral steroids is low • May experience skin bruising in high doses • Headache, rhinitis, URI, sinusitis, bronchospasm	• Use water gargle, rinse, and spit after use to prevent oral yeast growth; avoid eyes.
• Oral candidiasis, dysphonia • Risk for systemic adverse effects associated with oral steroids is low • May experience skin bruising in high doses • URI, headache, sinusitis, bronchospasm	• Longer acting. • Use a spacer device with MDI; use water gargle, rinse, and spit after use to prevent oral candidiasis.
• Oral candidiasis • Risk for systemic adverse effects associated with oral steroids is low. • May experience skin bruising in high doses • Nasopharyngitis, rhinitis, nausea, bronchospasm	• Longer acting. • Use water gargle, rinse, and spit after use to prevent oral candidiasis.
• See fluticasone and salmeterol	• See fluticasone and salmeterol.
• See budesonide and formoterol	• See budesonide and formoterol.
• See mometasone and formoterol	• See mometasone and formoterol
• Cough, bronchospasm	• Should not be used with status asthmaticus or acute asthma episodes. May be given in combination with bronchodilator if administration causes bronchospasm.

(continued)

Table 11-4 Commonly Used Pulmonary Drugs (*Continued*)

DRUGS/ADMINISTRATION	PHARMACOLOGIC EFFECTS	INDICATIONS
Leukotriene Receptor Antagonists		
Zafirlukast	• Blocks leukotriene receptors	• Prophylaxis and chronic treatment of mild to moderate asthma for persons older than age 4
Zileuton	• Blocks leukotriene receptors	• Prophylaxis and chronic treatment of mild to moderate asthma for persons older than age 12
Montelukast	• Blocks leukotriene receptors	• Prophylaxis and chronic treatment of mild to moderate asthma for persons older than age 5 • Exercise-induced bronchospasm
Antifibrotics		
Nintedanib	• Treatment of idiopathic pulmonary fibrosis, binds to multiple tyrosine kinases, inhibiting intracellular signaling of fibroblasts	• Reduce progression of idiopathic pulmonary fibrosis
Pirfenidone	• Treatment of idiopathic pulmonary fibrosis, mechanism unknown	• Reduce progression of idiopathic pulmonary fibrosis
Other		
Roflumilast	• Inhibits phosphodiesterase type 4 leading to increased intracellular cAMP	• Chronic bronchitis and frequent exacerbations
Omalizumab	• Inhibits IgE binding to mast cells and basophils, decreasing mediator release	• Asthma prophylaxis, aeroallergen associated

clearance; these are delivered by metered-dose inhalers (MDIs), dry powder inhalers, or nebulizer devices. One or more long-acting agents are normally used for daily control, with short-acting "rescue" agents used as needed prior to exertion or when symptoms worsen.

   a. Anticholinergics such as tiotropium (a long-acting agent) and ipratropium (a short-acting agent).

   b. Short-acting beta-adrenergic agonists such as albuterol and levalbuterol.

   c. Long-acting beta-adrenergic agonists such as salmeterol, formoterol, and arformoterol.

3. Methylxanthines, such as theophylline, are oral bronchodilators, but are not considered first-line treatment because of suboptimal effectiveness, side effects, and drug interactions.

4. Inhaled corticosteroids are recommended for patients with symptomatic COPD with FEV_1 that is less than 50% of the predicted value and repeated exacerbations and asthma COPD overlap syndrome (ACOS).

5. Oral corticosteroids are used in acute exacerbations for antiinflammatory effect and may also be given an IV line in severe cases. Long-term treatment with systemic corticosteroids is not recommended due to significant adverse effects (see page 702).

6. For retained secretions, mobilizing the patient, bronchodilators, and for some, use of chest physical therapy, including postural drainage for secretion clearance, and breathing retraining, may be used for improved ventilation and control of dyspnea.

7. Supplemental oxygen therapy for patients with hypoxemia. Use caution in increasing oxygen flow rates in patients with CO_2 retention.

8. Pulmonary rehabilitation to improve function, strength, symptom control, disease self-management techniques, independence, mood, and quality of life and reduce health care utilization.

9. Antimicrobial agents for pneumonia, exacerbations, or bronchitis suspected or known to be because of bacterial infections.

10. Lung volume reduction surgery is a potential option for treatment of upper lobe emphysema in patients with poor exercise capacity.

11. Influenza (annual) and pneumococcal vaccination.

12. Lung transplantation may be considered for people with advanced COPD.

13. Self-management strategies such as prevention and management of exacerbations. Disease self-management strategies include the use of action plans, frequent hand hygiene, physical activity, and regular medical follow-up.

14. Treatment for alpha₁-antitrypsin deficiency:

   a. Regular IV infusions (normally every week) of human alpha₁-antitrypsin as replacement therapy to correct the antiprotease imbalance in the lungs.

   b. Smoking cessation.

   c. Lung transplantation may be considered.

 DRUG ALERT Long-acting inhaled bronchodilators are the gold standard of COPD management because of their effectiveness and safety.

 DRUG ALERT High-dose or long-term prednisone therapy is associated with significant side effects including hypertension, edema, muscle weakness, increased risk of cataracts and glaucoma, weight gain, hyperglycemia, depression, insomnia, gastric and esophageal ulcer, osteoporosis, skin frailty, and bruising. Ensure that a plan is implemented for tapering steroid dose after an exacerbation, prescription is written, instructions are communicated to patient and family, and follow-up can be scheduled with health care provider.

ADVERSE EFFECTS	NURSING CONSIDERATIONS
• Potential drug interactions, particularly warfarin, cisapride • Headache, infection, nausea, diarrhea	• Will not reverse acute bronchospasm.
• Potential drug interactions • Headache, sinusitis, nausea	• Will not reverse acute bronchospasm.
• Potential drug interactions, particularly phenobarbital, amiodarone • Headache, flu, abdominal pain	• Will not reverse acute bronchospasm.
• Diarrhea, nausea, abdominal pain, vomiting, decreased appetite, headache, weight loss	Arterial thromboembolism, MI, HTN, GI perforation, bleeding Monitor LFTs at baseline, monthly × 6 months, and then every 3 months thereafter.
• Nausea, rash, abdominal pain, URI, diarrhea, fatigue • Photosensitivity: patient must wear sunscreen when outdoors	Angioedema Agranulocytosis Monitor LFTs at baseline, monthly × 6 months, and then every 3 months thereafter.
• Diarrhea, weight loss, nausea, headache, suicidality	
• Injection site reaction, viral infection, URI, sinusitis, anaphylaxis	

Complications

1. Respiratory failure.
2. Pneumonia, overwhelming respiratory infection.
3. Right-sided heart failure, pulmonary hypertension, dysrhythmias.
4. Depression, anxiety disorder.
5. Skeletal muscle dysfunction.

Nursing Assessment

1. Determine smoking pack per year history, exposure history, positive family history of respiratory disease, onset and triggers of dyspnea.
2. Determine level of dyspnea, how it compares to patient's baseline.
3. Note amount, color, and consistency of sputum.
4. Inspect for use of accessory muscles during respiration and use of abdominal muscles during exhalation; note increase of anteroposterior diameter of the chest.
5. Auscultate for decreased/absent breath sounds, crackles, decreased heart sounds.
6. Determine oxygen saturation, pulse, and respiratory rate at rest and with activity.

Nursing Diagnoses

• Ineffective Breathing Pattern related to chronic airflow limitation.
• Ineffective Airway Clearance related to bronchoconstriction, increased mucus production, ineffective cough, possible pulmonary infection, immobility, and weakness.
• Risk for Infection related to compromised pulmonary function, retained secretions, and compromised defense mechanisms.

• Impaired Gas Exchange related to chronic airflow obstruction and V/Q abnormalities because of destruction of alveolar–capillary membrane.
• Imbalanced Nutrition: Less Than Body Requirements related to increased work of breathing, hyperinflation, drug effect on body mass index (less than 21 or greater than 30), and skeletal muscle dysfunction.
• Activity Intolerance related to airflow limitation, dynamic hyperinflation, resulting in shortness of breath and fatigue, skeletal muscle dysfunction.
• Disturbed Sleep Pattern related to hypoxemia and hypercapnia, dyspnea, cough, and wheezing.
• Ineffective Coping related to the stress of living with chronic disease, loss of independence, depression, anxiety disorder, panic of breathlessness.

 NURSING ALERT If disease is moderately advanced, issues of an advance directive and resuscitation status need to be addressed. Although effective treatment and prevention and management of exacerbations and comorbidities often stabilize disease, COPD is progressive. It is better to have these discussions with the patient before a crisis situation.

Nursing Interventions

Improving Airway Clearance

1. Eliminate pulmonary irritants, particularly cigarette smoking.
   a. Cessation of smoking is a top priority, improving survival, slowing progression of COPD, and reducing pulmonary irritation, sputum production, and cough.
   b. Keep patient's room as free from pulmonary irritants as possible.

2. Administer bronchodilators to improve dyspnea, reduce hyperinflation at rest and with activity, control bronchospasm and dyspnea, and assist with raising sputum.
   a. Train, teach back, and monitor patient's inhaler technique.
   b. Assess for adverse effects—tremors, tachycardia, cardiac dysrhythmias, CNS stimulation, hypertension.
   c. Auscultate the chest after administration of aerosol bronchodilators to assess for improvement of aeration and reduction of adventitious breath sounds.
   d. Observe if patient has reduction in dyspnea.
   e. Monitor serum theophylline level, as ordered, to ensure therapeutic level and prevent toxicity.
3. Use controlled coughing (see page 177).
4. Mobilize the patient when stable. Use pursed-lip breathing, controlled cough, and possibly postural drainage positions to aid in clearance of secretions, particularly if secretions are tenacious, excessive, and/or mucopurulent (see page 176).
5. Keep secretions thin.
   a. Encourage fluid intake within level of cardiac reserve.
   b. If appropriate, give continuous aerosolized sterile water or nebulized normal saline to humidify bronchial tree and liquefy sputum.

Improving Breathing Pattern

1. Teach and supervise breathing retraining exercises to improve dyspnea and decrease work of breathing (see page 176). Use pursed-lip breathing at intervals and during periods of dyspnea especially associated with activity and/or panic to reduce hyperinflation, control rate and depth of respiration, and improve respiratory muscle coordination. Pursed-lip breathing should be practiced for 10 breaths four times daily before meals and before sleep. Inspiratory-to-expiratory ratio should be 1:≥2. Evidence for effectiveness of diaphragmatic breathing is less robust, particularly given flattened diaphragm in COPD.
2. Discuss and demonstrate relaxation exercises to reduce stress, tension, and anxiety.
3. Encourage patient to assume position of comfort to decrease dyspnea. Positions might include leaning the trunk forward with arms supported on a fixed object, sleeping with two or three pillows, or sitting upright.

Controlling Infection

1. Recognize early manifestations of respiratory infection—increased dyspnea; change in color, amount, and character of sputum including purulence; cough; wheeze; and possibly irritability and low-grade fever. Promptly report findings to physician for possible workup and treatment.
2. If ordered, obtain sputum for Gram stain and culture and sensitivity.
3. Administer prescribed antimicrobials to control bacterial infections in the bronchial tree, thus clearing the airways. Administer bronchodilators to improve ventilation.

Improving Gas Exchange

1. Monitor for hypoxemia with a typical goal of SaO_2 or SpO_2 of 92% to 93%. Watch for and report excessive somnolence, restlessness, anxiety, headaches, irritability or confusion, central cyanosis, and dyspnea at rest, which is caused by acute respiratory insufficiency and may signal respiratory failure.
2. Review ABG levels; document for evaluation and comparisons by clinical team.
3. Give supplemental oxygen, as ordered, to correct hypoxemia in a controlled manner. Monitor and minimize CO_2 reten-

tion. Patients that experience CO_2 retention may need lower oxygen flow rates.
4. Be prepared to assist with noninvasive ventilation *or* intubation and mechanical ventilation if acute respiratory failure and significant CO_2 retention occur.

 NURSING ALERT Normally, CO_2 levels in the blood provide a stimulus for respiration. However, in some patients with COPD, chronically elevated CO_2 may impair this mechanism and low oxygen levels may act as stimulus for respiration. Giving a high flow rate or percent of supplemental oxygen to people who retain CO_2 may suppress the hypoxic drive, leading to worsening hypoventilation, respiratory depression and decompensation, and the development of a worsening respiratory acidosis.

Improving Nutrition

1. Take nutritional history, weight, and height and calculate BMI. Patients are at risk for cachexia (survival is decreased with BMI less than 21) and obesity because of poor nutritional intake, work of breathing, and inactivity.
2. Encourage frequent, small meals if patient is dyspneic and/or underweight; even a small increase in abdominal contents may press on the diaphragm and impede breathing and decrease interest in eating. Encourage snacking on nutritious, calorie-appropriate, and high-protein snacks, such as nuts, avocados, and dairy if tolerated.
3. Offer liquid nutritional supplements, if needed, to improve nutrient intake and provide appropriate calorie intake.
4. Encourage foods high in potassium (including bananas, dried fruits, dates, figs, orange juice, grape juice, milk, peaches, potatoes, tomatoes), and monitor for low potassium, which may occur with COPD, corticosteroid use, and diuretic use.
5. Restrict sodium, as directed, if fluid retention is a problem or comorbidity of CHF, HTN, or heart disease.
6. Avoid foods producing gas and abdominal distention and/or discomfort.
7. Employ good oral hygiene before meals to sharpen taste sensations.
8. Avoid hurrying and encourage pursed-lip breathing between bites if patient is short of breath; rest after meals.
9. Give supplemental oxygen while patient is eating to relieve dyspnea if ordered.
10. Monitor body weight and evaluate body mass index.

Increasing Activity Tolerance

1. Reemphasize the importance of exercise and physical conditioning programs (may reverse skeletal muscle dysfunction, improve dyspnea, improve muscle utilization of oxygen, and improve independence). This is part of pulmonary rehabilitation and may be included as part of physical therapy.
   a. Discuss walking, stationary bicycling, swimming, and "sit and be fit"-type videos.
   b. Encourage use of portable lightweight oxygen system for ambulation for patients with hypoxemia.
2. Encourage patient to carry out regular exercise program 3 to 7 days per week to increase physical endurance, but to discuss with physician before beginning program.
3. Train patient in energy conservation techniques and pacing of activities.

Improving Sleep Patterns

1. Use nocturnal oxygen therapy, when ordered.
2. Avoid the use of high-dose sedatives and hypnotics that may cause respiratory depression.
3. Administer long- or short-acting inhaled anticholinergics, as directed (have been found to improve nocturnal respiratory symptoms in COPD).
4. Sleep with head of bed elevated based on patient's preference to improve pulmonary mechanics.

Enhancing Coping

1. Recognize signs of depression and anxiety disorders or use validated questionnaires to screen for mood disorders, which are common and often undiagnosed and untreated in COPD. Contributing factors include persistent dyspnea, fatigue, loss of independence, personal identity, social isolation, and quality of life that may make the patient irritable, apprehensive, anxious, and depressed, with feelings of helplessness and hopelessness.
2. Assess the patient for thoughts of suicide or self-harm and intentions. Communicate any positive findings promptly to the patient's MD, social worker, and appropriate resources, if needed.
3. Demonstrate a sincere, supportive, and open approach to the patient.
   a. Be a good listener and show that you care.
   b. Be sensitive to patient's fears, anxiety, and depression; provide emotional support.
   c. Provide patient with control of as many aspects of care as possible.
4. Administer antidepressants and antianxiety agents as directed, but avoid oversedation.
5. Support and encourage the patient to discuss concerns about disease, symptoms, and impact on the patient.
6. Be aware that dyspnea, fatigue, and altered self-image may lead to discomfort with sexuality and intimacy in patients with COPD. Encourage discussion of concerns and fears, and discuss adaptations and clarify misunderstandings. Encourage patient to use a bronchodilator and secretion clearance techniques before sexual activity, plan for sexual relations at time of day when patient has highest level of energy, use supplemental oxygen, if needed, and consider alternative displays of affection to loved one.
7. Support patient and spouse/family members. Refer to local or national support groups (American Lung Association: *www.lungusa.org* 1-800-LUNGUSA).

Community and Home Care Considerations

1. Help to relax and pace activities. Obtain occupational therapy consult to help employ work simplification techniques, such as sitting for tasks, pacing activities, and using dressing aids (grabber, sock aid, long-handled shoe horn), shower bench, and handheld shower head.
2. Encourage enrollment in a pulmonary rehabilitation program where available and Better Breathers club or other support group found through the American Association for Cardiovascular and Pulmonary Rehabilitation at (312) 321-5146 or *www.aacvpr.org*. Components of pulmonary rehabilitation include supervised exercise training, breathing retraining techniques, proper use of medications and inhalers, secretion clearance techniques, prevention and management of respiratory infection, panic control, controlling dyspnea with ADLs and stair climbing, control of pulmonary irritants, monitored and supervised exercise, proper use of oxygen systems, and group support.

3. Suggest vocational counseling to help patient maintain gainful employment within physical limits for as long as possible.
4. Warn patient to avoid excessive fatigue, which is a factor in producing respiratory distress. Advise to adjust activities per individual fatigue patterns.
5. Advise in strategies and mechanisms to cope with emotional stress and mood disorders. Stress may trigger worsening dyspnea and panic. Teach coping strategies, such as pursed-lip breathing, relaxation techniques, meditation, and guided imagery.
6. Stress that progression of worsening lung function may be slowed through smoking cessation and prevention of exacerbations. Long-term ongoing medical follow-up is a key aspect of disease self-management.
7. For patients who use oxygen or who are hypoxic, coordinate with oxygen supplier and patient to promote safe adherence to oxygen prescription and use of appropriate oxygen system so patient can maintain activities and control hypoxemia.
8. Use community resources, such as Meals on Wheels or a home care aide, if energy level is low.

Patient Education and Health Maintenance

General Education

1. Give the patient a clear explanation of the disease, what to expect, and how to treat and live with it. Reinforce by frequent explanations, reading material, demonstrations, and question-and-answer sessions.
2. Review with the patient the objectives of treatment and nursing management.
3. Work with the patient to set goals (eg, stair climbing, return to work).
4. Encourage patient involvement in disease self-management techniques, such as identification and prompt reporting of respiratory infection or respiratory deterioration and physical activity. Encourage patient to have open communication, partnership, and regular follow-up with primary care provider.

Avoid Exposure to Respiratory Irritants

1. Advise patient to stop smoking and avoid exposure to secondhand smoke. Offer strategies to promote long-term cessation including the use of medications, support groups, and counseling.
2. Advise patient to avoid exposure to indoor and outdoor pulmonary irritants and particulates, including dust, smog, and other respiratory irritants.
3. Advise patient to keep entire house well ventilated.
4. Warn patient to avoid extremely hot/cold weather if exposure causes bronchospasm and dyspnea. Use a scarf over the nose and mouth and drink warm beverages in cold weather.
5. Stay indoors and exercise indoors with air conditioning when air pollution level is high.
6. Shower with warm (*not hot*) water to avoid excess exposure to steam.
7. If sensitive to dry air, instruct patient to humidify indoor air in winter; maintain 30% to 50% humidity for optimal mucociliary function. Clean and dry humidifier frequently to avoid mold and bacterial growth
8. If the patient is sensitive to dust, pollen, and other particles, consider the use of a HEPA air cleaner to remove particles from air. Advise regular replacement.

Improve Airflow

1. Teach the proper technique for inhalation of medication to maximize aerosol deposition in the bronchial tree. See page 806 for patient education on inhaler use.

a. Use spacer device if unable to use MDI effectively.

b. If using a dried powder inhaler, instruct in proper use according to manufacturer's instructions. Spacer devices are not necessary.

2. MDIs with HFA propellants require priming (spray four puffs of medication before first use and if not used for several days). Rinse plastic cartridge holder well daily and air-dry to prevent blockage.

3. Inhalers have built-in counters. Advise patient to refill inhaler well in advance of running out of medication.

 DRUG ALERT To prevent oral candidiasis with use of inhaled corticosteroids, instruct patient on use of a spacer device and to rinse mouth after use.

Evaluation: Expected Outcomes

- Coughs up secretions easily; decreased wheezing and crackles.
- Reports less dyspnea; effectively using pursed-lip breathing.
- No fever or change in sputum.
- ABG levels and/or SpO_2 improved.
- Tolerates small, frequent meals; weight stable.
- Reports walking longer distances without tiring.
- Sleeping in 4- to 6-hour intervals; uses low-flow oxygen at night as prescribed.
- Demonstrates more effective coping; expresses feelings; seeks support group.

Cor Pulmonale

Pulmonary heart disease (cor pulmonale) is typically due to right heart strain caused by excessively high pressures in pulmonary circulation. This alteration in the structure or function of the right ventricle results from disease of lung structure or function or its vasculature, such as pulmonary hypertension (except when this alteration results from disease of the left side of the heart or from congenital heart disease). It is heart disease caused by lung disease.

Pathophysiology and Etiology

1. Chronic lung disease or alteration of the pulmonary vasculature causes increased pressure in pulmonary circuit producing strain on the right ventricle, leading to right-sided heart failure.

2. Often chronic (associated with right ventricular hypertrophy), but may develop acutely because of pulmonary embolism and, less commonly, ARDS associated with right ventricular dilatation.

3. May develop due to pulmonary vasoconstriction because of alveolar hypoxia or acidosis and anatomic compromise of the pulmonary vascular bed.

4. Causes include:
   a. Pulmonary vascular disease (acute or chronic).
   b. Idiopathic pulmonary hypertension.
   c. Underlying lung disease such as COPD, cystic fibrosis, interstitial lung disease.
   d. Polycythemia vera, sickle cell disease, macroglobulinemia.
   e. Significant kyphoscoliosis.
   f. Obstructive sleep apnea.

Clinical Manifestations

1. Fatigue, tachypnea, exertional dyspnea, and cough.
2. Anterior chest pain and hemoptysis.
3. Distended jugular veins, peripheral edema (often associated with hypercapnia), and possible cyanosis.

4. In advanced stages, right upper abdominal discomfort, jaundice, and syncope with exertion.
5. Split second heart sound on auscultation of the chest.

Diagnostic Evaluation

1. Chest x-ray shows right-sided heart enlargement and enlargement of central pulmonary arteries.
2. ECG changes are consistent with right-sided heart hypertrophy and/or right heart strain.
3. Echocardiogram shows right-sided heart enlargement.
4. Right heart catheter examination to confirm diagnosis and evaluate for pulmonary hypertension and underlying disease.
5. ABG levels—decreased PaO_2 and pH and increased $PaCO_2$.
6. PFTs to confirm underlying lung disease such as obstruction.
7. V/Q scanning or chest CT if history and physical examination suggest pulmonary thromboembolism as the cause or if other diagnostic tests do not suggest other etiologies. If interstitial lung disease is suspected, chest CT will aid in diagnosis.
8. Hematocrit for polycythemia, serum alpha$_1$-antitrypsin if deficiency is suspected, antinuclear antibody level for collagen vascular disease, such as scleroderma, coagulation studies to evaluate hypercoagulability states.

Management

The goal is the treatment of underlying lung disease and management of heart disease.

1. In cases of hypoxemia, supplemental oxygen to improve oxygen delivery to peripheral tissues, thus decreasing cardiac work and lessening sympathetic vasoconstriction. Liter flow individualized during activities, rest, and sleep.

2. Targeted therapy such as prostacyclin analogues and endothelin receptor antagonists may be used in primary pulmonary hypertension (PPH).
   a. Epoprostenol, treprostinil, and iloprost are prostacyclin (PGI2) analogues and have potent vasodilatory properties. Epoprostenol and treprostinil are administered via the IV route and iloprost is inhaled.
   b. Bosentan is a mixed endothelin-A and endothelin-B receptor antagonist indicated for pulmonary arterial hypertension, including PPH. In clinical trials, bosentan improved exercise capacity, decreased rate of clinical deterioration, and improved hemodynamics.
   c. The PDE5 inhibitors sildenafil and tadalafil promote selective smooth muscle relaxation in lung vasculature. Their use in secondary pulmonary hypertension, such as in patients with COPD, is unclear.

3. The use of the cardiac glycoside digoxin is somewhat controversial; it can improve RV function but must be used with caution and should be avoided during acute hypoxia.

4. Oral anticoagulants in underlying thromboembolic event or primary PAH.

5. Diuretics are used if RV filling volume is markedly elevated and to manage peripheral edema.
   a. Used cautiously because of hemodynamic adverse effects with excessive volume depletion.
   b. Can lead to a decline in cardiac output as well as hypokalemic metabolic alkalosis.

6. Vasodilators including calcium channel blockers, particularly oral sustained-release nifedipine and diltiazem, can lower pulmonary pressures, although these agents appear more effective in primary rather than secondary pulmonary hypertension.

7. Bronchodilators to improve lung function.

8. Mechanical ventilation, if patient in respiratory failure.
9. Sodium restriction to reduce edema.

Complications

1. Respiratory failure.
2. Dysrhythmias.

Nursing Assessment

1. Determine if patient has long-standing history of lung disease.
2. Assess degree of dyspnea, fatigue, and hypoxemia.
3. Inspect for jugular vein distention and peripheral edema.

Nursing Diagnoses

- Impaired Gas Exchange related to excess fluid in lungs and increased pulmonary vascular resistance.
- Excess Fluid Volume related to right-sided heart failure.

Nursing Interventions

Improving Gas Exchange

1. Monitor ABG values and/or oxygen saturation as a guide in assessing adequacy of ventilation.
2. Use continuous low-flow oxygen as directed to reduce pulmonary artery pressure.
3. Avoid CNS depressants (opioids, hypnotics). They have depressant action on respiratory centers and mask symptoms of hypercapnia.
4. Monitor for signs of respiratory infection because infection causes CO_2 retention and hypoxemia.

Attaining Fluid Balance

1. Watch alterations in electrolyte levels, especially potassium, which can lead to disturbances of cardiac rhythm.
2. Employ ECG monitoring when necessary and monitor closely for dysrhythmias.
3. Limit physical activity until improvement is seen.
4. Restrict sodium intake based on evidence of fluid retention.

Patient Education and Health Maintenance

1. Emphasize the importance of stopping cigarette smoking; cigarette smoking is a major cause of pulmonary heart disease.
   a. Ask patient about smoking habits.
   b. Inform patient of risks of smoking and benefits to be gained when smoking is stopped.
   c. Discuss the use of behavior modification techniques and smoking cessation aids.
2. Teach patient to recognize and treat infections immediately.
3. Advise patient to avoid environments with poor air quality, have good ventilation, but keep windows closed and use air conditioning, if necessary.
4. Explain to patient and family that restlessness, depression, and poor sleeping as well as irritable and angry behavior may be characteristic; patient should improve with rise in oxygen and fall in CO_2 levels.
5. Explain the use of supplemental oxygen, which will reduce further workload on the right side of the heart.

Evaluation: Expected Outcomes

- Less dyspneic; ABG levels improved, oxygen saturation.
- Edema reduced; no dysrhythmias.

INTERSTITIAL LUNG DISEASE (PULMONARY FIBROSIS)

Interstitial lung disease (*ILD*) is a general term that refers to a variety of chronic lung disorders, such as *idiopathic pulmonary fibrosis, sarcoidosis, asbestosis, silicosis, scleroderma, hypersensitivity pneumonitis,* and *coal worker's pneumoconiosis* (*CWP*). There are estimated to be 130 types of interstitial lung disease; only about one third have known causes. Causes include abnormal immune response or abnormal healing in response to a variety of causes, including connective tissue diseases, occupational and environmental exposure, drugs and poisons, radiation, and infections. The most common ILD is idiopathic pulmonary fibrosis.

Overview

Unknown etiology such as idiopathic pulmonary fibrosis.

1. Connective tissue diseases including scleroderma, rheumatoid arthritis, Sjogren syndrome, systemic lupus erythematosus (SLE), polymyositis, dermatomyositis, and mixed connective tissue disease. Sarcoidosis is considered a multisystem disorder, although it may resemble a connective tissue disorder.
2. Hypersensitivity pneumonitis (acute or chronic) may be due to repeated inhalation of certain fungal, bacterial, animal protein, or reactive antigens from occupational or environmental exposure. Susceptible persons develop immune reactions leading to pulmonary inflammation and possible scarring.
3. Occupational exposure may include asbestosis (increased risk for lung cancer), silicosis, and CWP.
4. Environmental exposure may include:
   a. Hard metal disease (cobalt, tungsten, carbide).
   b. Gas, fumes, vapors, and aerosols.
   c. Poison exposure.
   d. Cancer drugs (nitrofurantoin, methotrexate, busulfan, bleomycin).
   e. Anti-inflammatory drugs (aspirin, gold, penicillamine).
   f. Cardiac drugs (amiodarone).
   g. IV use of heroin, methadone, propoxyphene, and talc used in IV drug abuse.
   h. Exposure to radiation.
   i. Infections.
5. Chronic changes include lung tissue damage, inflammation of alveoli with scarring, and fibrosis and stiffening of the interstitium tissue.
6. The damage limits oxygen transport through scarred alveolar–capillary membranes into the bloodstream.

Presentation

Additional information follows on idiopathic pulmonary fibrosis, interstitial lung disease because of sarcoidosis and other connective tissue diseases, and occupational lung diseases. A generalized nursing process appears on pages 227 to 228.

1. The most prevalent symptom is dyspnea, particularly with exercise, along with dry cough and fatigue.
2. Bibasilar crackles are heard on auscultation.
3. Connective tissue diseases may be associated with joint pain and swelling, rash, dry eyes, and dry mouth.
4. Symptoms may vary in severity and the course of the disease may be unpredictable.

Idiopathic Pulmonary Fibrosis

 EVIDENCE BASE Raghu, G., Rochwerg, B., Zhang, Y. et al. (2015). An official ATS/ERS/JRS/ALAT clinical practice guideline: Treatment of idiopathic pulmonary fibrosis. An update of the 2011 clinical practice guideline. *American Journal of Respiratory Critical Care Medicine, 192*(2), e3–e19.

Pathophysiology and Etiology

1. *Idiopathic pulmonary fibrosis* is a chronic, progressive fibrosing interstitial pneumonia of unknown cause, occurring primarily in older adults and limited to the lungs. It is characterized by progressive worsening of dyspnea and lung function and associated with a poor prognosis.
2. Lung function may worsen gradually or more rapidly, worsen due to acute exacerbation of IPF or remain stable based on pulmonary function testing (usually measurement of FVC and/or diffusion capacity of oxygen or DLCO) or findings on chest CAT scan.
3. Incidence is approximately 7 to 16 cases per 100,000 people, although this number is believed to be much higher than reported.
4. It is generally diagnosed between ages 50 and 70 with increased incidence with age.

Clinical Manifestations

1. Dyspnea and hypoxemia are common with exertion and may be present at rest.
2. Chronic, dry cough.
3. Breath sounds commonly include bibasilar inspiratory crackles.
4. Finger clubbing may be present.
5. Patients may have pulmonary hypertension and gastroesophageal reflux disorder.
6. History of smoking is common.

Diagnostic Evaluation

1. A multidisciplinary diagnosis that includes pulmonology, radiology and pathology is recommended. Exclusion of other causes of interstitial lung disease is important.
2. High-resolution chest CT shows usual interstitial pneumonia, basilar honeycombing, traction bronchiectasis with predominant subpleural reticular distribution, and absence of other features that would be inconsistent with IPF.
3. PFTs show decreased FVC with decreased diffusion capacity.
4. ABG may show low arterial oxygen level.
5. Exercise test shows hypoxemia.
6. Chest x-ray may demonstrate patchy, nonuniform infiltrates, ground-glass pattern, reticular nodular pattern, and small lung volume.
7. Right-sided heart catheterization may be performed if pulmonary hypertension is suspected or if elevated PA pressures seen on echocardiogram.

Management

1. Two medications (pirfenidone and nintedanib) have been found to reduce loss of lung function.
2. Other agents such as prednisone, azathioprine, *N*-acetylcysteine, and warfarin do not provide clinical benefit when used specifically to treat IPF. They may be used for other non-IPF disorders or appropriate comorbidities.
3. Several promising clinical trials are developing. Patients should be informed of the National Institutes of Health registry of clinical trials at *www.clinicaltrials.gov*. The database includes information about a trial's purpose, who may participate, locations, and study contacts.
4. Supportive measures include oxygen for hypoxemia and pulmonary hypertension.
5. Options for cough include management of comorbidities (GERD, rhinitis, asthma), cough lozenges, and possibly prednisone (controversial).
6. Treatment of dyspnea includes pulmonary rehabilitation, which also works to improve endurance.
7. Lung transplantation may offer improved symptoms, function, and survival for some patients.

Sarcoidosis and Other Connective Tissue Diseases

For comprehensive management of connective tissue disorders, see Chapter 30.

General Considerations

1. *Sarcoidosis* is an inflammatory, multisystem disorder of unknown cause that affects the connective tissue and lungs.
   a. Granulomatous disease in which clumps of inflammatory epithelial cells (nodules) occur in many organs, primarily in lungs.
   b. Nodules in the lungs can lead to narrowing of the airways, inflammation, and fibrosis of lung tissue.
   c. Other tissues including the skin, eyes, nose, muscles, heart, liver, spleen, bowel, kidney, testes, nerves, lymph nodes, and brain.
2. Rheumatoid arthritis is an inflammatory connective tissue disorder that causes interstitial lung disease because of pleural inflammation in about 20% of cases, mostly females between ages 50 and 60.
3. SLE is a multisystem autoimmune disease that causes pleural inflammation and pneumonitis.
4. Scleroderma is a connective tissue disorder that causes hardening of the skin and fibrotic changes, resulting in interstitial fibrosis.
5. Ankylosing spondylitis is a seronegative arthropathy causing back pain and possible pulmonary manifestations.

Occupational Lung Diseases

Pathophysiology and Etiology

1. *Asbestosis*: Asbestos fibers are inhaled and enter alveoli, which, in time, are obliterated by fibrous tissue that surrounds the asbestos particles.
   a. Fibrous pleural thickening and pleural plaque formation produce restrictive lung disease, decrease in lung volume, diminished gas transfer, and hypoxemia with subsequent development of cor pulmonale.
   b. Found in workers involved in manufacture, cutting, and demolition of asbestos-containing materials; there are more than 4,000 known sources of asbestos fiber (asbestos mining and manufacturing, construction, roofing, demolition work, brake linings, floor tiles, paints, plastics, shipyards, insulation).

2. *Silicosis*: When silica particles (which have fibrogenic properties) are inhaled, nodular lesions are produced throughout the lungs. These nodules undergo fibrosis, enlarge, and fuse.
   a. Dense masses form in the upper portion of the lungs; restrictive and obstructive lung disease results.
   b. Exposure to silica dust is encountered in almost any form of mining because the earth's crust is composed of silica and silicates (gold, coal, tin, copper mining); also stone cutting, quarrying, manufacture of abrasives, ceramics, pottery, and foundry work.
3. *CWP* ("black lung") is a variety of respiratory diseases found in coal workers in which there is an accumulation of coal dust in the lungs, causing a tissue reaction in its presence.
   a. Dusts (coal, kaolin, mica, silica) are inhaled and deposited in the alveoli and respiratory bronchioles.
   b. There is an increase of macrophages that engulf the particles and transport them to terminal bronchioles.
   c. When normal clearance mechanisms can no longer handle the excessive dust load, the respiratory bronchioles and alveoli become clogged with coal dust, dying macrophages, and fibroblasts, which lead to the formation of the coal macule, the primary lesion of CWP.
   d. As macules enlarge, there is dilation of the weakening bronchiole, with subsequent development of focal or centrilobular emphysema.
4. Hypersensitivity pneumonitis is considered a disease of exposures to various agents including mold and birds (feathers and related products such as down). Diagnosis can be difficult and requires good history taking about exposure to potential occupational and environmental antigens and detailed home and work history.
   a. Effects of inhaling organic dust (moldy hay, mushroom compost, malt, moldy maple bark, pigeon or parrot droppings, feathers, microwave popcorn fumes, hot tub exposure, or contaminated grain), noxious particles, gases, or fumes. Development of disease depends on composition of inhaled substance, its antigenic (precipitating an immune response) or irritating properties, the dose inhaled, the length of time inhaled, and the host's response.
   b. Exposure to inorganic dusts stimulates pulmonary interstitial fibroblasts, resulting in pulmonary interstitial fibrosis.
   c. Acute symptoms of fever, cough, and chills may occur 4 to 12 hours after exposure and recur with repeated exposure. Chronic disease develops years later.
   d. Noxious fumes may cause acute injury to alveolar wall with increasing capillary permeability and pulmonary edema.

 NURSING ALERT Asbestosis is strongly associated with bronchogenic cancer and mesotheliomas of the pleura and peritoneal surfaces. Smoking increases the risk of lung cancer 50 to 100 times.

Clinical Manifestations

Occupational lung diseases may develop slowly (over 20 to 30 years) and may be asymptomatic in the early stages.
1. Chronic cough; productive in silicosis and CWP.
2. Dyspnea on exertion; progressive and irreversible in asbestosis and CWP.
3. Susceptibility to lower respiratory tract infections.
4. Bibasilar crackles in asbestosis.
5. Expectoration of varying amounts of black fluid in CWP.

Diagnostic Evaluation

1. Chest x-ray—nodules of upper lobes in silicosis and CWP; diffuse parenchymal fibrosis, especially of lower lobes, in asbestosis.
2. High-resolution chest CT to evaluate and characterize fibrosis.
3. PFTs primarily show restrictive pattern.
4. Bronchoscopy with lavage to identify specific exposure.
5. Lung tissue biopsy may be needed to rule out other disorders.

Management

1. Pulmonary rehabilitation may be considered for patients with chronic, disabling symptoms.
2. For hypersensitivity pneumonitis, anti-inflammatory medications may be recommended if the condition is worsening, including prednisone and possibly azathioprine, mycophenolate, or cyclophosphamide.
3. For most other occupational lung diseases, there is no specific treatment; exposure is eliminated and the patient is treated symptomatically.
4. Silicosis is associated with high risk of TB; patients should receive evaluation and appropriate treatment for TB.
5. Smoking cessation measures for people who have been exposed to asbestos to decrease risk of lung cancer.
6. Keep asbestos worker under cancer surveillance; watch for changing cough, hemoptysis, weight loss, and melena.
7. Bronchodilators may be of some benefit if any degree of airway obstruction is present.

Complications

1. Respiratory failure.
2. Lung cancer in asbestosis.
3. Hypoxemia.

Nursing Care of the Patient with Interstitial Lung Disease

Nursing Assessment

1. Obtain occupational and environmental exposure history. Determine length and degree of exposure.
2. Obtain full medical history and family history for connective tissue disorders.
3. Obtain medication history and allergies.
4. Obtain history of smoking, respiratory infections, and other chronic lung disease.
5. Evaluate symptoms and functional capacity, and auscultate lungs for crackles.

Nursing Diagnoses

- Ineffective Breathing Pattern related to fibrotic lung tissue causing restriction.
- Impaired Gas Exchange related to fibrotic lung tissue and secretions.

Nursing Interventions

Improving Breathing Pattern

1. Administer oxygen therapy, as required.
2. If ordered, administer or teach self-administration of bronchodilators.
3. Encourage smoking cessation.

Promoting Gas Exchange

1. Encourage mobilization of secretions through hydration and breathing and coughing exercises.
2. Advise patient on pacing activities to prevent excess dyspnea or fatigue.

Patient Education and Health Maintenance

1. Provide information about the importance of smoking cessation as well as methods and resources for smoking cessation.
2. Instruct patient in health maintenance, such as adequate nutrition and exercise and immunizations, so additional medical problems can be avoided.
3. Encourage participation in pulmonary rehabilitation.
4. Advise patient that compensation may be obtained for impairment related to occupational lung disease through the Worker's Compensation Act.
5. Provide information to healthy workers on prevention of occupational lung disease.
   a. Enclose toxic substances to reduce their concentration in the air.
   b. Employ engineering controls to reduce exposure.
   c. Monitor air samples.
   d. Use standards established by NIOSH and USDPH to eliminate exposure to asbestos and other pulmonary toxins. These may include the use of appropriate masks, respirators, and hoods depending on the toxin.

Evaluation: Expected Outcomes

- Reports less dyspnea.
- Reports improved quality of life.

TRANSITIONAL CARE ALERT Patients and family members require clear understanding of their diagnosis, treatment options, and expectations regarding the course of the disease. Those with hypoxemia require linkage with durable medical equipment companies to provide both stationary oxygen concentrators and lightweight portable oxygen that supports ambulation and independence. Once oxygen needs are determined, the patient should be trained in monitoring SpO_2 and goals of therapy. Patients and family members require linkage to community organizations for support.

TRAUMATIC DISORDERS

Pneumothorax

A *pneumothorax* is air in the pleural space occurring spontaneously or from trauma (see Figure 11-4). In patients with chest trauma, it is usually the result of a laceration to the lung parenchyma, tracheobronchial tree, or esophagus. The patient's clinical status depends on the rate of air leakage and size of wound. Pneumothorax is classified as:

Spontaneous pneumothorax—sudden onset of air in the pleural space with deflation of the affected lung in the absence of trauma.

Tension pneumothorax—buildup of air under pressure in the pleural space resulting in interference with filling of both the heart and lungs.

Open pneumothorax (sucking wound of the chest)—implies an opening in the chest wall large enough to allow air to pass freely in and out of thoracic cavity with each attempted respiration.

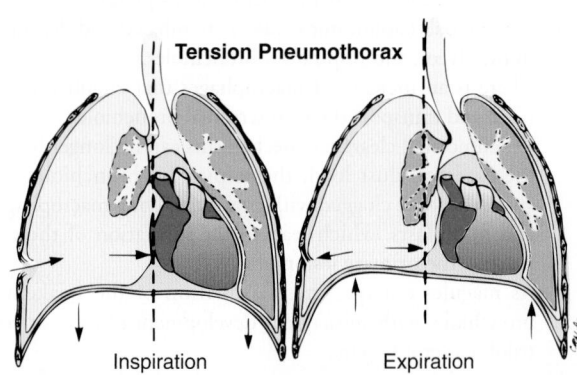

Figure 11-4. Open pneumothorax and tension pneumothorax. In open pneumothorax, air enters the chest during inspiration and exits during expiration. There may be slight inflation of the affected lung because of a decrease in pressure as air moves out of the chest. In tension pneumothorax, air can enter but not leave the chest. As the pressure in the chest increases, the heart and great vessels are compressed and the mediastinal structures are shifted toward the opposite side of the chest. The trachea is pushed from its normal midline position toward the opposite side of the chest, and the unaffected lung is compressed.

Pathophysiology and Etiology

1. When there is a large, open hole in the chest wall, the patient will have a "steal" in ventilation of the other lung.
2. A portion of the V_T will move back and forth through the hole in the chest wall, rather than the trachea as it normally does.
3. Spontaneous pneumothorax is usually due to rupture of a subpleural bleb.
   a. May occur secondary to chronic respiratory diseases or idiopathically.
   b. May occur in healthy people, particularly in thin, white males and those with family history of pneumothorax.

Clinical Manifestations

1. Moderate to very severe dyspnea and often severe chest discomfort radiating to the back.
2. Hyperresonance and diminished breath sounds on the affected side.
3. Reduced mobility of affected half of the thorax.
4. Tracheal deviation away from the affected side in tension pneumothorax.
5. Clinical picture of open or tension pneumothorax is one of air hunger, agitation, hypotension, and cyanosis.

Diagnostic Evaluation

- Chest x-ray confirms the presence of air in the pleural space.

Management

Spontaneous Pneumothorax

1. Observe and allow for spontaneous resolution for less than 50% pneumothorax in otherwise healthy person.
2. Needle aspiration or chest tube if greater than 50% pneumothorax.
3. Pleurodesis may be done to prevent recurrence. Chemical pleurodesis uses various solutions inserted through chest tube to irritate and thereby cause adhesion of parietal and visceral pleura. Surgical pleurodesis uses mechanical irritation to achieve adhesion, with possible removal of parietal pleura.
4. Thoracotomy to remove apical blebs in some cases.

Tension Pneumothorax

1. Immediate decompression to prevent cardiovascular collapse by chest tube insertion to let air escape.
2. Chest tube drainage with underwater seal suction to allow for full lung expansion and healing.

Open Pneumothorax

1. Close the chest wound immediately to restore adequate ventilation and respiration.
   a. Patient is instructed to inhale and exhale gently against a closed glottis (Valsalva maneuver) as a pressure dressing (petroleum gauze secured with elastic adhesive) is applied.
   b. This maneuver helps to expand collapsed lung.
2. Chest tube is inserted and water seal drainage set up to permit evacuation of fluid/air and produce reexpansion of the lung.
3. Surgical intervention may be necessary to repair trauma.

Complications

1. Acute respiratory failure.
2. Cardiovascular collapse with tension pneumothorax.

Nursing Assessment

1. Obtain history for chronic respiratory disease, trauma, and onset of symptoms.
2. Inspect the chest for reduced mobility and tracheal deviation.
3. Auscultate the chest for diminished breath sounds and percuss for hyperresonance.

Nursing Diagnoses

- Ineffective Breathing Pattern related to air in the pleural space.
- Impaired Gas Exchange related to atelectasis and collapse of the lung.

Nursing Interventions

Achieving Effective Breathing Pattern

1. Provide emergency care as indicated.
   a. Apply petroleum gauze to sucking chest wound (see "Management").
   b. Assist with emergency thoracentesis or thoracostomy.
   c. Be prepared to perform cardiopulmonary resuscitation or administer medications if cardiovascular collapse occurs.
2. Maintain patent airway; suction as needed.
3. Position patient upright if condition permits to allow greater chest expansion.
4. Maintain patency of chest tubes.
5. Assist patient to splint chest while turning or coughing and administer pain medications, as needed.

Resolving Impaired Gas Exchange

1. Encourage patient in the use of incentive spirometer.
2. Monitor oximetry and ABG levels to determine oxygenation.
3. Provide oxygen as needed.

Patient Education and Health Maintenance

1. Instruct patient to continue use of the incentive spirometer at home.
2. For patients with spontaneous pneumothorax, there is an increased risk for recurrence; therefore, encourage these patients to report sudden dyspnea immediately.

Evaluation: Expected Outcomes

- Breath sounds equal bilaterally; less dyspneic.
- ABG levels improved.

Chest Injuries

Chest injuries are potentially life-threatening because of immediate disturbances of cardiorespiratory physiology and hemorrhage and later developments of infection, damaged lung, and thoracic cage. Traumatic chest injuries include *rib fracture or contusion, hemothorax, flail chest, pulmonary contusion,* and *cardiac tamponade or contusion.* Patients with chest trauma may have injuries to multiple organ systems. The patient should be examined for intra-abdominal injuries, which must be treated aggressively.

Pathophysiology and Clinical Manifestations

Rib Fracture

1. Most common chest injury may be severe if several ribs are fractured, especially unstable fractures or in the presence of other morbidities.
2. May interfere with ventilation and may lacerate the underlying lung.
3. Causes pain at fracture site; painful, shallow respirations; and localized tenderness and crepitus (crackling) over fracture site.

Hemothorax

1. Blood in pleural space as a result of penetrating or blunt chest trauma.
2. Accompanies a high percentage of chest injuries.
3. Can result in hidden blood loss and increased risk of empyema.
4. Patient may be asymptomatic, dyspneic, hypoxemic, hypotensive, apprehensive, or in shock.
5. Diminished or absent breath sounds of the affected side, tracheal deviation to the unaffected side.

Flail Chest

1. Loss of stability of chest wall as a result of multiple rib fractures or combined rib and sternum fractures.
   a. When this occurs, one portion of the chest has lost its bony connection to the rest of the rib cage.
   b. During respiration, the detached part of the chest will be pulled in on inspiration and moved outward on expiration (paradoxical movement).
2. Normal mechanics of breathing are impaired to a degree that seriously jeopardizes ventilation, causing dyspnea, hypoxemia, cyanosis, and risk of acute respiratory failure.
3. Generally associated with other serious chest injuries: lung contusion, lung laceration, and diffuse alveolar damage. Also associated with tracheal damage, ARDS, and pneumonia.

Pulmonary Contusion

1. Injury of the lung parenchyma that results in leakage of blood and edema fluid into the alveolar and interstitial spaces of the lung. May occur with rib fracture or chest trauma.
2. May not be fully developed for 24 to 72 hours.
3. Signs and symptoms include:
   a. Tachypnea, tachycardia, and hypoxemia.
   b. Crackles on auscultation.
   c. Pleuritic chest pain.
   d. Secretions may be copious.
   e. Cough—constant, loose, rattling.

Cardiac Tamponade

1. Compression of the heart as a result of accumulation of fluid within the pericardial space.
2. Caused by penetrating injuries, metastasis, cardiac rupture, cardiac surgery, pericarditis, and other disorders.
3. Signs and symptoms include:
   a. Tachycardia.
   b. Muffled heart sounds.
   c. Falling BP.
   d. Distended jugular veins, elevated central venous pressure (CVP).
   e. Pulsus paradoxus (audible BP fluctuation with respiration).
   f. Dyspnea, cyanosis, shock.

 NURSING ALERT A rapidly developing tamponade interferes with ventricular filling and causes impairment of circulation. Thus, there is a reduced cardiac output and poor venous return to the heart. Cardiac collapse can result. In the patient with hypovolemia caused by associated injuries, the CVP may not rise, thus masking the signs of cardiac tamponade.

Management and Nursing Interventions

The goal is to restore normal cardiorespiratory function as quickly as possible. This is accomplished by performing effective resuscitation if required while simultaneously assessing the patient, restoring chest wall integrity when possible, and reexpanding the lung. The order of priority is determined by the clinical status of the patient.

Rib Fracture

1. Give analgesics (usually nonopioid) to assist in effective coughing and deep breathing.
2. Encourage deep breathing with slow, full inspiration; give local support to injured area by splinting with pillow or hands.
3. Assist with intercostal nerve block to relieve pain so coughing and deep breathing may be accomplished. An intercostal nerve block is the injection of a local anesthetic into the area around the intercostal nerves to relieve pain temporarily after rib fractures, chest wall injury, or thoracotomy.
4. For multiple rib fractures, epidural anesthesia may be used.

Hemothorax

1. Assist with chest tube insertion and set up drainage system for complete and continuous removal of blood and air.
   a. Auscultate lungs and monitor for relief of dyspnea.
   b. Monitor amount of blood loss in drainage.
2. Assist with thoracentesis to aspirate blood from pleural space, if being done before a chest tube insertion.
3. Replace volume with IV fluids or blood products.
4. Trauma patients with pulmonary contusion and flail chest should receive adequate IV fluids to maintain adequate tissue perfusion. Once adequately resuscitated, unnecessary fluid

administration should be meticulously avoided. A pulmonary artery catheter may be useful to avoid fluid overload.

5. The use of optimal analgesia and chest physiotherapy should be applied to minimize the likelihood of respiratory failure and ensuing ventilatory support.
6. Patients may require noninvasive positive pressure ventilation or mechanical ventilation with PEEP.
7. Steroids should not be used in therapy for pulmonary contusion.
8. Diuretics may be used in the setting of hydrostatic fluid overload as evidenced by elevated pulmonary capillary wedge pressures in hemodynamically stable patients or in the setting of known concurrent heart failure.

Flail Chest

1. Analgesia for pain management. Thoracic epidural analgesia may be used for some patients to relieve pain and improve ventilation.
2. Stabilize cardiopulmonary status. If respiratory compromise or failure is present, prepare for immediate ET intubation and mechanical ventilation—treats underlying pulmonary contusion and serves to stabilize the thoracic cage for healing of fractures, improves alveolar ventilation, and restores thoracic cage stability and intrathoracic volume by decreasing work of breathing.
3. Prepare for operative stabilization of chest wall in select patients. Surgical fixation may be considered in severe unilateral flail chest or in patients requiring mechanical ventilation when thoracotomy is otherwise required.

Pulmonary Contusion

For moderate lung contusion:
1. Employ mechanical ventilation to keep lungs inflated.
2. Administer diuretics for pulmonary edema.
3. Use PAP monitoring.
4. Monitor for development of pneumonia, ARDS.

Cardiac Tamponade

For penetrating injuries:
1. Assist with pericardiocentesis (see page 255) to provide emergency relief and improve hemodynamic function until surgery can be undertaken.
2. Prepare for emergency thoracotomy to control bleeding and to repair cardiac injury.

Additional Responsibilities

1. Secure and support the airway as indicated. ET intubation or tracheostomy may be needed.
2. Assist with noninvasive continuous positive airway pressure (CPAP) or mechanical ventilation to help to clear tracheobronchial tree, help the patient breathe with less effort, and reduce paradoxical motion.
3. Secure one or more IV lines for fluid replacement and obtain blood for baseline studies, such as hemoglobin level and hematocrit.
4. Monitor serial CVP readings to prevent hypovolemia and circulatory overload.
5. Monitor ABG/SpO$_2$ results to determine requirements for supplemental oxygen and mechanical ventilation.
6. Obtain urinary output hourly to evaluate tissue perfusion.
7. Continue to monitor thoracic drainage to provide information about rate of blood loss, whether bleeding has stopped, and whether surgical intervention is necessary.
8. Institute ECG monitoring for early detection and treatment of cardiac dysrhythmias (dysrhythmias are a frequent cause of death in chest trauma).

9. Maintain ongoing surveillance for complications:
   a. Aspiration.
   b. Atelectasis.
   c. Pneumonia.
   d. Mediastinal/subcutaneous emphysema.
   e. ARDS.
   f. Respiratory failure.

Patient Education and Health Maintenance

1. Instruct patient in splinting techniques.
2. Make sure patient is aware of importance of seat belt use to reduce serious chest injuries caused by automobile accidents.
3. Teach patient to report signs of complications—increasing dyspnea, fever, and cough.

SELECTED REFERENCES

Broaddus, V. C., Mason, R. J., Ernst, J. D., et al. (2016). *Murray & Nadel's textbook of respiratory medicine* (6th ed.). Toronto: Elsevier Canada.

Center for Disease Control and Prevention. (2016). Prevention and Control of Seasonal Influenza with Vaccines: Recommendations of the Advisory Committee on Immunization Practices—United States, 2016–17 Influenza Season. *MMWR, 65*(5), 1–54. Available: *www.cdc.gov/flu/professionals/acip/index.htm*

Centers for Disease Control and Prevention. (2016). Treatment options for latent tuberculosis infection (LTBI). Available: *www.cdc.gov/tb/publications/factsheets/treatment/LTBItreatmentoptions.htm*

Centers for Disease Control and Prevention. (2016). Tuberculin skin testing. Available: *www.cdc.gov/tb/publications/factsheets/testing/skintesting.htm*

Du, W., Liu, J., Zhou, J., et al. (2018). Obstructive sleep apnea COPD the overlap syndrome and mortality results from the 2005 2008 National Health and Nutrition Examination Survey. *International Journal of COPD*, 13, 665–674. DOI *https://doi.org/10.2147/COPD.S148735*

Ezer, N., Kale, M., Sigel, K., et al. (2018). Outcomes after video-assisted thoracoscopic lobectomy versus open lobectomy for early-stage lung cancer in older adults. *Annals of the American Thoracic Society, 15*(1), 76–82.

Garcia, D. A., & Crowther, M. A. (2012). Reversal of warfarin: Case-based practice recommendations. *Circulation, 125*, 2944–2947.

Global Strategy for the Diagnosis, Management and Prevention of COPD. (2018). Global Initiative for Chronic Obstructive Lung Disease (GOLD) 2018. Available: *http://goldcopd.org*

Herchline, T., & Bronzem M. (2016). Tuberculosis workup. Medscape Drugs and Diseases. Available: *www.medscape.com/viewarticle/872992*

Jacobs, S., Lindell, K. O., Collins, E. G., et al. (2018). Patient perceptions of the adequacy of supplemental oxygen therapy: results of the American Thoracic Society Nursing Assembly Oxygen Working Group Survey. *Annals of the American Thoracic Society, 15*(1): 24–32.

Kaynar, A., & Pinsky, M. (2016). Respiratory Failure, Medscape Drugs and Diseases. Available: *http://emedicine.medscape.com/article/167981*

Kobayashi, M., Bennett, N. M., Gierke, R., et al. (2015). Intervals between PCV13 and PPSV23 vaccines: Recommendations of the Advisory Committee on Immunization Practices (ACIP). *MMWR, 64*(34), 944–947.

Nicholson, A. G., Chansky, K., Crowley, J., et al. (2016). The International Association for the Study of Lung Cancer Lung Cancer Staging Project: Proposals for the Revision of the Clinical and Pathologic Staging of Small Cell Lung Cancer in the Forthcoming Eighth Edition of the TNM Classification for Lung Cancer. *Journal of Thoracic Oncology, 11*(3), 300–311.

Poterucha, T. J., Bergmark, B., Aranki, S., et al. (2015). Surgical pulmonary embolectomy. *Circulation, 132*, 1146–1151.

Raghu, G., Rochwerg, B., Zhang, Y., et al. (2015). An official ATS/ERS/JRS/ALAT clinical practice guideline: Treatment of idiopathic pulmonary fibrosis. An update of the 2011 clinical practice guideline. *American Journal of Respiratory Critical Care Medicine, 192*(2), e3–e19.

Rubins, J., & Soo Hoo, G. (2016). Pleural effusion treatment & management. Medscape Drugs and Diseases. Available: *http://emedicine.medscape.com/article/299959-treatment*

Storre, J. H., Callegari, J., Magnet, F. S., et al. (2018). Home noninvasive ventilatory support for patients with chronic obstructive pulmonary disease patient selection and perspectives. *International Journal of COPD*, 13, 753–760. DOI *https://doi.org/10.2147/COPD.S154718*

Swaminathan, A., & Byrd, P. (2016). Aspiration pneumonia. Medscape Drugs and Diseases. Available: *http://emedicine.medscape.com/article/296198*

Yusen, R., Criner, G., Stemberg, A., et al. (2018). The long-term oxygen treatment trial for chronic obstructive pulmonary disease: Rationale, design, and lessons learned. *Annals of the American Thoracic Society, 15*(1), 89–101.

12

Cardiovascular Function and Therapy

OVERVIEW AND ASSESSMENT
Common Manifestations of Heart Disease

In patients with cardiac disease, chest pain is the most common manifestation and is the second most common chief complaint presenting to emergency departments. Heart disease may also be characterized by shortness of breath, palpitations, weakness, fatigue, dizziness, syncope, diaphoresis, edema or swelling, or GI complaints.

 NURSING ALERT Older, diabetic, and female patients may not present with typical symptoms of acute coronary syndrome (ACS). Consider the diagnosis of ACS in these patients when they present with other complaints, such as back pain, nausea, fatigue, dyspnea, light-headedness, cold sweats, jaw pain, and right arm pain (without chest pain).

Chest Pain
Characterization
1. How does the patient describe chest pain? Is it mild or severe, transient or constant? What activity or other factors make it worse, or better? Can it be characterized as tightness, discomfort, fullness, pressure-like, crushing, or searing? Does it radiate to the jaw, neck, back, or arm (particularly left)?
2. Assess chest pain systematically. See Box 12-1. Most pain management scales (visual analogues or numerical scales) are fast and easy to use but can only be used to measure the intensity of the pain; these scales do not measure the other essential elements for describing chest pain. In your assessment, ascertain the character and quality of the pain; location and radiation of the pain; factors that precipitate, aggravate, or relieve the pain; the duration of the pain; and any associated symptoms.
3. Use one of two popular and similar assessment mnemonics—OLDCARTS or the PQRST assessment (see Chapter 5, page 41) to evaluate chest pain.

Significance
1. Ischemia caused by an increase in demand for coronary blood flow and oxygen delivery, which exceeds available blood supply, may result from coronary artery disease (CAD) or a decreased supply without an increased demand because of coronary artery spasm or thrombus.
2. Pain that is brought on by exertion and relieved by rest suggests angina pectoris or psychogenic pain. Psychogenic pain differs from angina in that it is usually associated with other symptoms, such as headache, back pain, stomach pain, and hyperventilation. Angina is usually caused by three Es: exercise, emotion, and eating.
3. Chest pain that worsens on deep inspiration or cough is suggestive of pleural, pericardial, or chest wall type pain.
4. Chest wall tenderness and pain on inspiration are suggestive of costochondritis.
5. Chest pain that is relieved by leaning forward and aggravated by lying down suggests pericarditis.

BOX 12-1 Chest Pain Assessment Tips

Consider all chest pain and associated symptoms to be signs of myocardial ischemia (angina pectoris or MI) until it is ruled out.

The severity of the chest pain does not correlate with the cause of the pain. Indigestion and vague symptoms in a female patient, for example, may indicate myocardial ischemia or infarction. Diabetic and older patients may present with noncardiac symptoms that, with further testing, are found to be related to ischemia.

The patient's perception of pain should also be considered, including such factors as gender, response to pain, cultural beliefs, and level of stress.

Location of perceived pain may be misleading. Referred pain occurs with many diseases—that is, pain is perceived by the patient to be in one area, but its source is actually located in another area.

The patient may present with one problem but have multiple coexisting problems. Older patients, for example, may have several health problems in addition to the reason for the present visit. Likewise, patients who delay seeking medical attention sometimes present with multisystem problems.

The patient may experience no symptoms at all.

6. Sudden onset of chest pain accompanied by dyspnea is suggestive of pulmonary emboli or pneumothorax.
7. Dissecting aortic aneurysm is likely in the hypertensive patient who complains of a sudden onset of tearing, ripping pain.
8. If the patient reports chest pain while eating, this suggests angina or esophageal spasm or biliary (cholecystitis), pancreatic (pancreatitis), or gastric disease (gastroesophageal reflux disease or ulcers).
9. A panic attack may imitate a heart attack but is more common in younger individuals and in women more than in men.

Shortness of Breath (Dyspnea)

Characterization
1. What precipitates or relieves dyspnea?
2. How many pillows does patient sleep with at night?
3. How far can patient walk or how many flights of stairs can patient climb before becoming dyspneic?
4. Determine the type of dyspnea.
   a. Exertional—breathlessness on moderate exertion that is relieved by rest.
   b. Paroxysmal nocturnal—sudden dyspnea at night; awakens patient with feeling of suffocation; sitting up relieves breathlessness.
   c. Orthopnea—shortness of breath when lying down. Patient must keep head elevated with more than one pillow to minimize dyspnea.

Significance
1. Exertional dyspnea occurs as a result of an elevated pulmonary artery pressure (PAP) because of left ventricular dysfunction.
2. Paroxysmal (nocturnal) dyspnea, also known as cardiac asthma, is precipitated by stimuli that aggravate previously existing pulmonary congestion, resulting in shortness of breath that generally occurs at night and usually awakens the patient.

3. Orthopnea (dyspnea in the supine position) is caused by alterations in gravitational forces resulting in an elevation in pulmonary venous pressure and PAP. These, in turn, increase the pulmonary closing volume and reduce vital capacity. Orthopnea indicates advanced heart failure.

 NURSING ALERT Patients with cardiac dyspnea tend to take short, shallow breaths, and patients with pulmonary dyspnea will likely breathe slower and deeper.

Palpitations

Characterization
1. Does patient feel heart pounding, fluttering, beating too fast, or skipping beats?
2. Does patient experience dizziness, pain, or dyspnea with palpitations?
3. What brings on this sensation?
4. How long does it last?
5. What does patient do to relieve these sensations?

Significance
1. Pounding, jumping, fluttering sensations occur in the chest because of a change in the patient's heart rate or rhythm or an increase in the force of its contraction.
2. Palpitations can occur as a result of cardiac arrhythmia as well as many other cardiac and noncardiac conditions.
3. Palpitations can be a manifestation of anxiety and panic disorders.
4. Palpitations can be intermittent, sustained and regular, or irregular.
5. Palpitations are most significant if dizziness and difficulty breathing occur simultaneously.
6. Palpitations that have a gradual onset and terminate in a pounding heartbeat may indicate sinus tachycardia.
7. Palpitations may be caused by noncardiac causes, such as thyrotoxicosis, hypoglycemia, pheochromocytoma, and fever.
8. Certain substances, such as tobacco, coffee, tea, unregulated synthetic cannabinoid, and alcohol, as well as certain drugs, including epinephrine, ephedrine, aminophylline, and atropine, may also precipitate arrhythmias and palpitations.

Weakness and Fatigue

Characterization
1. What activities can you perform without becoming tired?
2. What activities cause you to become tired, weak, or fatigued?
3. Is the fatigue relieved by rest?
4. Is leg weakness accompanied by pain or swelling?

Significance
1. Fatigue can be produced by low cardiac output (CO) because of right- or left-sided heart failure. The heart can't provide sufficient blood to meet the increased metabolic needs of cells.
2. As heart disease advances, fatigue is precipitated by less effort.
3. Weakness or tiring of the legs may be caused by peripheral arterial or venous disease.
4. Weakness and tiredness may be related to electrolyte imbalances, such as hypokalemia, hyperkalemia, hypercalcemia, hypernatremia, hyponatremia, hypophosphatemia, and hypermagnesemia.

5. Other disorders, such as chronic fatigue syndrome, multiple sclerosis, fibromyalgia, influenza, and Lyme disease, may also cause weakness and fatigue.

Dizziness and Syncope

Characterization

1. Is the dizziness characterized as light-headedness, feeling faint, off balance, vertigo, or spinning?
   a. How long does the dizziness last and what relieves it?
2. How many episodes of syncope or near syncope have been experienced?
3. Did a hot room, hunger, sudden position change, defecation, or pressure on your neck precipitate the episode?

Significance

1. Patients who experience anxiety attacks and hyperventilation syndrome frequently experience faintness and dizziness.
2. Patients who suffer repeated bouts of unconsciousness may be experiencing seizures rather than syncope.
3. Syncope can be a result of hypoglycemia, anemia, or hemorrhage.
4. Vasovagal (vasodepressor or neurocardiogenic) syncope can be precipitated by a hot or crowded environment, alcohol, extreme fatigue, severe pain, hunger, prolonged standing, and emotional or stressful situations. Vasovagal syncope is caused by temporary slowing of the heart and reduction of brain perfusion.
5. Orthostatic or postural hypotension, another cause of dizziness, occurs when the patient stands up suddenly.
6. Cardiac syncope results from a sudden reduction in CO because of bradyarrhythmias and/or tachyarrhythmias.
7. Cerebrovascular disease such as carotid stenosis can cause dizziness and syncope because of reduced cerebral blood flow.

Nursing History

History of Present Illness

1. The patient's history is the single most important aspect in evaluating chest discomfort. The quality, location, duration, and modifying (ie, aggravating and relieving) factors are essential to making a correct diagnosis.
2. How long has the patient been ill? What has the course of the illness been, including current management? Obtain a characterization and review of systems (see Chapter 5).

Past Medical History

Medical and Surgical History

1. Assess childhood and adult illnesses, hospitalizations, accidents, and injuries.
   a. Does the patient have hypertension, diabetes mellitus, hyperlipidemia, chronic obstructive pulmonary disease (COPD), or other chronic illnesses (bleeding disorders or acquired immunodeficiency syndrome)? These may increase the risk of cardiac disease or aggravate disease.
   b. Review the patient's past illnesses and hospitalizations: trauma to the chest (possible myocardial contusion), sore throat and dental extractions (possible endocarditis), rheumatic fever (valvular dysfunction, endocarditis), and thromboembolism (MI, pulmonary embolism).

Review of Allergies

1. Ask if the patient is allergic to any drugs, foods, environmental agents, or animals and what reaction occurred.
   a. Allergies to penicillin or other commonly used emergency drugs, such as lidocaine or morphine, may influence the choice of drug treatments, if needed.
   b. Allergies to shellfish indicate iodine allergy; many contrast dyes used in radiologic procedures contain iodine.
   c. Does the patient have allergies to aspirin or nonsteroidal anti-inflammatory drugs, such as naproxen and ibuprofen? (An upset stomach or indigestion from aspirin is not an allergy—rather, it is sensitivity; the patient may still be able to take an enteric-coated aspirin.)

Medications

1. Assess the patient's prescription drugs, if any. Many cardiac drugs must be tapered to prevent a "rebound effect," whereas other drugs affect heart rate and may cause orthostatic hypotension. Estrogen preparations may lead to thromboembolism.
2. Assess the patient's use of over-the-counter medications, which may cause an increase in heart rate and blood pressure.
3. Assess the patient's use of herbal preparations, vitamin and mineral supplements, and other alternative or complementary therapies. Herbal preparations can interact with other drugs and anesthesia and interfere with normal blood clotting.

Family History

1. Note the ages and health status of patient's family members (parents, grandparents, siblings, and other blood relatives).
2. A family history of CAD, MI, sudden death, hypertension, hyperlipidemia, hypercholesterolemia, or diabetes could place the patient at an increased risk for heart disease.

Personal and Social History

1. Assess the patient's health habits, such as alcohol or drug use (cocaine may cause MI), tobacco use, nutrition, obesity, pattern of recurrent weight gain after dieting, occupation, stress, sleeping patterns, and physical activity (sedentary lifestyle) (see Chapter 5 for additional information).
2. Many lifestyle choices increase the risk of acute and chronic cardiovascular disease.

Physical Examination

General Appearance

1. Is the patient awake and alert or lethargic, stuporous, or comatose?
2. Does the patient appear to be in acute distress, for example, clenching the chest (Levine sign)? Focus the physical assessment on what is essential when examining a patient in acute distress.
3. Observe the patient's general build (eg, thin, emaciated, or obese) and skin color (eg, pink, pale, ruddy, flushed, or cyanotic).
4. Assess the patient for shortness of breath and distention of jugular veins.

Vital Signs

1. Obtain temperature and note route.
2. Determine heart rate and rhythm.
   a. Assess pulse rate and rhythm using the radial artery.
   b. Time for 1 full minute; note regularity.
   c. Compare apical and radial heart rate (pulse deficit).
   d. Rhythm should be noted as regular, regularly irregular, or irregularly irregular.

3. Monitor blood pressure.
   a. Blood pressure can be measured indirectly using a sphygmomanometer and a stethoscope and electronic devices (dynamo) or directly by way of an arterial catheter. Be sure to use the right cuff size. Small cuff will result in overestimated BP.
   b. Avoid taking blood pressure in an arm with an arteriovenous shunt or fistula or on the same side as a mastectomy site or any type of lymphedema.
   c. If possible, take pressure in both arms and note differences (5 to 10 mm Hg difference is normal). Differences of more than 10 mm Hg may indicate subclavian steal syndrome or dissecting aortic aneurysm.
   d. Determine pulse pressure (systolic pressure minus diastolic pressure), which reflects stroke volume, ejection velocity, and systemic resistance and is a noninvasive indicator of CO (30 to 40 mm Hg, normal; less than 30 mm Hg, decreased CO).
   e. Note presence of pulsus alternans—loud sounds alternate with soft sounds with each auscultatory beat (hallmark of left-sided heart failure).
   f. Note presence of pulsus paradoxus—abnormal fall in blood pressure more than 10 mm Hg during inspirations (cardinal sign of cardiac tamponade).
4. Assess for orthostatic hypotension.
   a. Orthostatic hypotension occurs when a patient's blood pressure drops 15 to 20 mm Hg or more (with or without an increase in heart rate of at least 20 beats/minute) when rising from a supine to sitting or standing position.
   b. Autonomic compensatory factors for upright posture are inadequate because of volume depletion; bed rest; drugs, such as beta-or alpha-adrenergic blockers; or neurologic disease; prompt hypotension occurs with assumption of the upright position.
   c. Note changes in heart rate and blood pressure in at least two of three positions: lying, sitting, and standing; allow at least 3 minutes between position changes before obtaining rate and pressure.

 DRUG ALERT Note that patients taking beta-adrenergic blockers may not exhibit a compensatory increase in heart rate when changing to upright position.

 NURSING ALERT Vital signs are dependent on age, gender, weight, exercise tolerance, and medical conditions, so note patient's baseline for future comparison.

Head, Neck, and Skin

1. Examination of the head includes assessment of facial characteristics and facial expressions and color of skin and eyes, any of which can reveal underlying cardiac disease.
   a. Earlobe creases in a patient younger than age 45 may indicate a genetic tendency toward CAD.
   b. Facial color: look for a malar flush, cyanotic lips, or slightly jaundiced skin (rheumatic heart disease).
   c. de Musset sign (head bobbing with each heartbeat) may indicate severe aortic insufficiency.
   d. Facial edema may be noted with constrictive pericarditis and associated tricuspid valve disease.
2. Examine the neck for jugular venous pulse. Jugular vein distention is characteristic of heart failure and other cardiovascular disorders, such as constrictive pericarditis, tricuspid stenosis, and obstruction of the superior vena cava.
3. Examine the skin for temperature, diaphoresis, cyanosis, pallor, and jaundice.
   a. Warm, dry skin indicates adequate CO; cool, clammy skin indicates compensatory vasoconstriction because of low CO.
   b. Cyanosis may be central (noted on the tongue, buccal mucosa, and lips) because of bronchiectasis, COPD, heart failure, lung cancer, pneumothorax, polycythemia vera, pulmonary edema, pulmonary emboli, shock, and sleep apnea or peripheral (noted on distal aspects of extremities, tip of the nose, and earlobes) because of chronic arteriosclerotic occlusive disease, Buerger disease, deep vein thrombosis (DVT), heart failure, acute peripheral occlusions, and Raynaud disease and cold exposure.
   c. Jaundice may be a sign of right-sided heart failure or chronic hemolysis from prosthetic heart valve.
   d. Xanthelasmas are yellow plaque (fatty deposits) evident on the skin, commonly seen along the nasal side of one or both eyelids, palms, and tendons. Xanthelasmas are associated with hyperlipidemia and CAD and may occur normally in the absence of hyperlipidemia.
   e. Pallor indicates decreased peripheral oxyhemoglobin or decreased total oxyhemoglobin. Onset may be sudden or gradual and extent may be generalized (most apparent on the face, conjunctiva, oral mucosa, and nail beds) or local (seen only in the affected limb).

Chest

See page 54.

Extremities

1. Inspect nail beds for color, splinter hemorrhages, clubbing, and capillary refill.
   a. Color—pale nail beds may be indicative of anemia, whereas cyanosis may be indicative of decreased oxygenation.
   b. Splinter hemorrhages are thin brown lines in nail bed and are associated with endocarditis. Janeway lesions (nontender, small erythematous, or hemorrhagic macular or nodular lesions on the palm and soles) are indicative of infective endocarditis.
   c. Clubbing (swollen nail base and loss of normal angle) is associated with chronic pulmonary or cardiovascular disease.
   d. Capillary refill indicates an estimate of the rate of peripheral blood low.
2. Inspect and palpate for edema—if pitting edema, describe degree of edema in terms of depth of pitting that occurs with slight pressure: 1+ or mild, 0 to ¼ inch (0 to 0.6 cm); 2+ or moderate, ½ inch (1.3 cm); and 3+ to 4+ or severe, ¾ to 1 inch (2 to 2.5 cm).
3. Inspect hands and feet for tenderness. Tender nodes (Osler nodes) may be associated with infective endocarditis.
4. Palpate arterial pulses (see page 59).

Laboratory Studies

Cardiovascular function and disease are evaluated by blood tests that indirectly monitor heart function and structural damage.

Enzymes and Isoenzymes

The diagnostic utilization of cardiac markers has evolved dramatically over the past 50 years. When myocardial tissue is damaged (eg, because of MI), cellular injury results in the release of

Table 12-1 Cardiac Markers—Normal Values, Rise, Peak, Advantages, and Disadvantages

ENZYME	RISE (HR)	PEAK (HR)	NORMALIZATION	ADVANTAGES	DISADVANTAGES
CK	3–12	10–36	3–4 d	• Rises fairly early	• Lacks cardiac specificity • Increases only after severe damage
CK-MB	3–8	9–30	2–3 d	• Can detect reinfarction • Low cost	• Lacks cardiac specificity • False-positive results • Increases only after severe damage
CK Isoforms	2–6	6–12	1 d	• Highly sensitive in early stages of AMI	• Elevates slowly • Lacks cardiac specificity • False-positive results
TnT	3–12	12–96	5–14 d	• Cardiac specific and sensitivity in late AMI	• Low sensitivity in early AMI • Inability to diagnose subsequent myocardial infarction (MI)
TnI	3–12	12–24	5–10 d	• Cardiac specific and sensitivity in late AMI	• Low sensitivity in early AMI • Inability to diagnose subsequent MIs
Myoglobin	1–4	6–12	1 d	• Extremely sensitive • Shows in blood before CK-MB	• Low cardiac specificity • Not beneficial in late AMIs • False-positive results

intracellular enzymes and proteins (cardiac enzymes, isoenzymes, and biochemical markers) into the bloodstream, which, in turn, causes elevated peripheral blood enzyme levels (see Table 12-1).

1. The troponin complex is located on the thin filament of the contractile apparatus of striated and skeletal muscle and consists of three subunits: troponin C (TnC), troponin T (TnT), and troponin I (TnI). In the presence of myocardial damage, the troponin complex on the myofibril breaks down, and the subunits of troponin are slowly released into the bloodstream.
   a. TnC is not sensitive or specific for myocardial injury.
   b. TnT has a sensitivity of approximately 50% within 4 hours of the onset of chest pain, but increases to approximately 75% sensitivity after 6 hours of onset and approximately 100% sensitivity in 12 hours. However, its specificity for myocardial injury is lower.
   c. TnI has been found to be the most sensitive and specific for myocardial injury. It has little sensitivity within 4 hours of the onset of chest pain, but increases to 96% sensitivity after 6 hours of the onset of symptoms.
   d. Troponins are the preferred test for the diagnosis of acute myocardial infarction (AMI).

2. High sensitivity troponin (hs-cTnT and hs-cTnI) testing detects troponins at much lower levels, increasing sensitivity and reducing diagnostic time. Also detects circulating troponins in stable CAD in the absence of myocardial necrosis. Potentially can be used to monitor therapeutic response in patients with CAD.

3. Creatine kinase (CK) has a 98% sensitivity for AMI 72 hours after infarction. CK is a catalyst for energy production and is found in the brain, myocardium, and skeletal muscle. CK is sensitive but not specific for myocardial injury.

4. CK isoenzymes are more specific than CK. Three CK isoenzymes have been identified: CK-MM, CK-MB, and CK-BB, with only CK-MB related to the heart. The specificity of CK-MB is greater than 85% and in some cases as high as 100%, but false positives do occur. Two types of CK-MB assays (CK-MB mass and CK-MB activity) are presently used.
   a. CK-MB mass assays are found to be more sensitive than CK-MB activity assays.
   b. CK-MB mass increases about 3 hours after onset of chest pain, whereas CK-MB activity requires another hour to elevate.
   c. CK-MB index is the ratio of CK-MB to the total CK and is considered abnormal when it exceeds 3% to 5%.
   d. CK-MB is no longer recommended for most patients being evaluated for an ACS.

5. Eventually, electrophoresis further breaks down CK-MB into its isoforms or subforms (CK-MB$_1$ and CK-MB$_2$). Normally, the ratio of CK-MB$_2$ to CK-MB$_1$ is 1:1. In myocardial injury, the CK-MB$_2$/MB$_1$ ratio increases to greater than 1.5 within 1 to 1½ hours. CK-MB isoforms have 56% sensitivity for patients presenting within 4 hours of the onset of symptoms.

6. Myoglobin is a small, oxygen-binding protein found in cardiac and skeletal muscles and is rapidly released into the bloodstream. Myoglobin is sensitive very early after injury, but has poor sensitivity over time and can generate many false-positive results. When myoglobin levels are assessed with CK-MB results, sensitivity increases (as high as 96%), but specificity can drop to as low as 81%.
   a. Myoglobin is directly related to muscle mass and is affected by age (levels increase with age), race (blacks have higher levels), gender (women have higher levels), and physical activity.
   b. Myoglobins can be elevated in the presence of reinfarction, skeletal muscle or neuromuscular disorders, trauma, severe burns, electrical shock, alcohol withdrawal delirium, metabolic disorders, systemic lupus erythematosus, strenuous exercise, renal failure, IM injections, cardiac bypass surgery, seizures, and heart failure.

Other Biochemical Markers

1. Homocysteine is a toxic by-product of the metabolism of the amino acid methionine into cysteine. Homocysteine exerts a direct cytotoxic effect on the endothelium of blood vessels by blocking the production of nitrous oxide, resulting in decreased pliability of vessels and development of atherosclerotic plaque. Increased homocysteine levels ultimately result in atherosclerosis, CAD, MI, stroke, thromboembolism, and peripheral vascular disease.
   a. Hyperhomocysteinemia (increased homocysteine levels) is related to gender (male), advanced age, smoking, hypertension, elevated cholesterol, decreased folate, decreased levels of vitamin B$_6$ and B$_{12}$, and lack of exercise.

b. Homocysteine can also be elevated in the presence of other diseases, drug use, and caffeine intake.

2. B-type natriuretic peptide (BNP) is synthesized in the ventricular myocardium and released as a response to increased wall stress. BNP is used for diagnosis and prognosis of suspected heart failure. Plasma levels of BNP increase in the presence of left ventricular systolic and diastolic dysfunction, particularly in the presence of decompensating heart failure.

   a. An increased BNP level identifies patients at the highest risk of developing sudden cardiac death and those who are in need of heart transplant. It is also associated with heart failure readmissions.

   b. BNP is considered a useful marker of myocardial function and is used to guide therapy.

3. C-reactive protein (CRP) is an inflammatory marker that may be an important risk factor for atherosclerosis and ischemic heart disease. CRP is produced by the liver in response to systemic cytokinesis. Elevated CRP is associated with AMI, stroke, and the progression of peripheral vascular disease. However, it can also be elevated with any inflammatory process. In addition to revealing events associated with CAD, CRP can also be used to identify patients at risk for developing CAD.

4. Lipoprotein(a) is a molecule that is similar to low-density lipoprotein cholesterol (LDL-C). It increases cholesterol deposits in the arterial wall, enhances oxidation of LDL-C, and inhibits fibrinolysis, resulting in the formation of atherosclerotic plaque and thrombosis. Treatment of elevated lipoprotein(a) is suggested only for patients with a history of premature vascular disease without other risk factors.

5. Factor I, or fibrinogen, is directly linked to increased cardiovascular risk. It is involved in the coagulation cascade (converting fibrinogen to fibrin by thrombin), stimulates smooth muscle cell migration and proliferation, and promotes platelet aggregation, which increases blood viscosity.

6. D-dimer may be done to evaluate for aortic dissection when chest pain is present. It is a degradation product of cross-linked fibrin and reflects activation of the extrinsic pathway of the coagulation cascade by tissue factor exposed in the aortic media by the intimal tear. It is also used to evaluate for the presence of thrombus or embolus (see page 323).

 NURSING ALERT When measured at first contact or during the hospital stay, the natriuretic peptides are strong predictors of both short- and long-term mortality in patients with STEMI and UA/NSTEMI.

Nursing and Patient Care Considerations

1. A single set of negative cardiac biomarkers is not sufficient to rule out myocardial infarction. Make sure that enzymes are drawn in a serial pattern, usually on admission and every 3 to 6 hours until three samples are obtained; enzyme activity is then correlated with the extent of heart muscle damage.

2. Maintain standard precautions while obtaining blood specimens and properly dispose of all equipment.

3. Advise patient that results of blood tests will be interpreted based on time and within the context of risk factors and other diagnostic tests.

 NURSING ALERT Greater peaks in enzyme activity and the length of time an enzyme remains at its peak level are correlated with serious damage to the heart muscle and, thus, a poorer prognosis.

Radiology and Imaging

Chest X-Ray

Chest x-rays can be used to assess heart size, contour, and position and may also reveal cardiac and pericardial calcification as well as physiologic alterations in pulmonary circulation. For further description and nursing considerations, see page 166.

Myocardial Imaging

Description

With the use of radionuclides and scintillation cameras, radionuclide angiograms can be used to assess left ventricular performance.

1. Thallium 201 is a radionuclide (an unstable atom that produces a small amount of energy) that behaves like potassium in the body and is distributed throughout the myocardium in proportion to blood flow.

   a. Negative result of "cold spot" imaging with thallium 201 rules out MI.

   b. A positive result, on the other hand, is inconclusive because it cannot differentiate between old and new infarction or areas of ischemia versus infarction.

2. Technetium-99m–labeled sestamibi is a myocardial perfusion marker used to assess cell membrane and mitochondrial integrity and to reveal myocardial perfusion.

   a. Sestamibi is not taken up by acute or chronic infarct tissue, and the amount of uptake of the radionuclide by other tissue correlates with the size of the infarction, the amount of CK released in the blood, and the postinfarction left ventricular ejection fraction (LVEF).

   b. "Hot spot" or positive imaging with technetium-99m is used when diagnosis of MI is unclear.

3. Radionuclide ventriculogram with technetium-99m is used to evaluate valve structure and ventricular function.

   a. Contrast medium is injected through a catheter, opacifying the ventricular cavity to enable measuring of right and LVEF.

   b. Also distinguishes regional from global ventricular wall motion and allows subjective analysis of cardiac anatomy to detect intracardiac shunts as well as valvular or congenital abnormalities.

   c. Complications include arrhythmias, intramyocardial or pericardial injection of contrast medium, and, possibly, development of emboli because of injection of air or a thrombosis through the catheter.

4. Dual single-photon emission computed tomography with simultaneous imaging using two isotopes improves the accuracy of assessing the infarcted area. The overlap of two isotopes may reflect the presence of salvaged myocardium adjacent to necrotic tissue.

Nursing and Patient Care Considerations

1. Advise patient that a radionuclide will be injected through a central venous, Swan-Ganz, or IV catheter or into an antecubital vein.

2. Reassure patient that the radionuclide will not cause radiation injury or affect heart function.

3. Explain to patient that hot flashes and nausea or vomiting may occur. A test dose will be administered before the dose required for contrast to assess patient's tolerance of radionuclide.

4. Results of the study will be discussed by the patient's health care provider after the study is interpreted by the radiologist.

Treadmill Stress Testing

Description

1. In treadmill stress testing, the patient walks a treadmill or rides a stationary bicycle until reaching a target heart rate, typically 70% to 80% of the maximum predicted heart rate. Treadmill stress testing has 70% sensitivity and specificity among the general population.
2. Indications for stress testing have been adapted from the American Heart Association (AHA) and the American College of Cardiology (see Box 12-2).
3. Reasons for terminating a stress test include:
   a. ST-segment elevations of 2 mm or more.
   b. 20 mm Hg drop in systolic blood pressure.
   c. Drop in heart rate or the development of heart block.
   d. Progressively increasing angina.
   e. ST-segment depression of 2 mm or greater.
   f. Three or more premature ventricular contractions (PVCs).
   g. Supraventricular arrhythmias.
   h. Severe hypertension.
   i. ST-segment depression at baseline that progresses during the test.
   j. Claudication.
   k. Fatigue, dyspnea, or feelings of light-headedness.
   l. Equipment malfunction.
   m. Sustained ventricular tachycardia.
4. Complications of stress testing include supraventricular tachyarrhythmias, bradycardias, heart failure, hypotension, ventricular ectopy (because of ventricular tachycardia), ventricular fibrillation, stroke, MI, and death.
5. Contraindications for performing a stress test include:
   a. AMI within 2 days.
   b. Unstable coronary syndrome.
   c. Wolff-Parkinson-White syndrome.

BOX 12-2   Indications for Stress Test

CLASS I INDICATIONS
(Clear indications for stress testing)
- Suspected or proven coronary artery disease (CAD).
- Male patients who present with atypical chest pain.
- Evaluation of functional capacity and assessment of prognosis in patients with CAD.
- Patients with exercise-related palpitations, dizziness, or syncope.
- Evaluation of recurrent exercise-induced arrhythmias.

CLASS II INDICATIONS
(Stress testing may be indicated)
- Evaluation of typical or atypical symptoms in women.
- Evaluation of variant angina.
- Evaluation of patients who are on digoxin preparations or who have a right bundle-branch block.

CLASS III INDICATIONS
(Stress testing is probably not necessary)
- Young or middle-age asymptomatic patients who have no risk factors for CAD.
- Young or middle-age asymptomatic patients who present with noncardiac chest pain.
- Evaluation of patients for CAD who have complete left bundle-branch block.
- Evaluation of patients for CAD who have preexcitation syndrome.

---

   d. Uncontrolled arrhythmias.
   e. High-degree atrioventricular (AV) blocks.
   f. Acute myocarditis.
   g. Acute pericarditis.
   h. Severe aortic stenosis.
   i. Uncontrolled hypertension.
   j. Acute aortic dissection.
   k. Acute pulmonary embolism or pulmonary infarct.

Nursing and Patient Care Considerations

1. Explain to patient how the procedure will be done and screen for contraindications.
2. Advise patient to abstain from eating, smoking, and consuming caffeine for 2 hours before the test.
3. Inform patient that monitoring will occur throughout the test for signs of complications.
4. Advise patient to inform you of how he or she is feeling during the test.
5. Monitor patient throughout testing for color, respirations, ECG changes, and blood pressure.

Echocardiography (Ultrasound Cardiography)

Description

1. *Echocardiography* is used to visualize and assess cardiac function, structure, and hemodynamic abnormalities. It is the most commonly used noninvasive cardiac imaging tool.
2. It records high-frequency sound vibrations that are sent into the heart through the chest wall. The cardiac structures return the echoes derived from the ultrasound. The motions of the echoes are traced on an oscilloscope and recorded on film, CD, or DVD.
3. Clinical usefulness includes demonstration of valvular and other structural deformities, detection of pericardial effusion, evaluation of prosthetic valve function, and diagnosis of cardiac tumors of asymmetric thickening of interventricular septum, cardiomegaly (heart enlargement), clots, vegetations on valves, and wall motion abnormalities.
4. Types include two-dimensional (2-D), M-mode, and Doppler mode. The methods are complementary and are commonly used in conjunction.
   a. 2-D echocardiography—provides a wider view of the heart and its structures because it involves a planar ultrasound beam.
   b. M-mode—utilizes a single ultrasound beam and provides a narrow segmental view.
   c. Doppler mode—evaluates pressures and blood flow across the valves; also assesses for atrial and ventricular septal defects.

Nursing and Patient Care Considerations

1. Advise patient that traditional echocardiography is noninvasive and that no preparation is necessary.
2. Position patient on left side, if tolerated, to bring the heart closer to the chest wall. Assist patient to clean the chest of transducer gel after the test.

Transesophageal Echocardiography

Description

1. In *transesophageal echocardiography* (*TEE*), an ultrasound transmitter located at the end of a catheter is passed through the esophagus to the stomach, where flexion of the tip permits imaging of the heart through the stomach wall and the diaphragm, thus allowing clearer and more accurate diagnostic evaluation. It is particularly useful in evaluating valvular disease.

2. As the catheter is slowly withdrawn, views of cardiac structures are obtained at several levels in various 2-D planes.
3. TEE can be used for continuous monitoring of cardiac and noncardiac patients during surgery.
4. Atrial fibrillation is the most common indication for performing a TEE, used to evaluate for thromboembolism.

Nursing and Patient Care Considerations
1. Explain procedure to patient and provide written information, if possible.
2. This is an invasive procedure; patient will require mild sedation and must be kept on nothing-by-mouth status (NPO) for a specified time—usually 4 to 6 hours—before the procedure.
3. The entire procedure takes less than 30 minutes.
4. Results of the study will be discussed with patient by the patient's health care provider after it is interpreted by the radiologist.

Stress Echocardiography

Description
1. *Stress (treadmill) echocardiography* has been found to have better sensitivity and specificity than treadmill stress testing alone.
2. Stress echocardiography is used to evaluate changes in wall motion when the patient is at rest and under stress.
3. Stress echocardiography can be coupled with pharmacologic stress testing. Myocardial perfusion imaging with dobutamine, adenosine, and dipyridamole is an alternative for patients who cannot exercise because of degenerative joint disease, physical deconditioning, neurologic disorders, COPD, or peripheral vascular disease.

Nursing and Patient Care Considerations
1. Explain procedure to patient and provide written information, if possible.
2. Withhold caffeine-containing products for 24 hours before adenosine and dipyridamole stress testing.
3. Discuss with cardiologist which medications should be withheld before test.
4. Maintain NPO status before testing for 2 hours or according to facility policy.
5. Establish a patent IV access.
6. Results of the study will be discussed with patient by the patient's health care provider after fully interpreted.

 DRUG ALERT Theophylline-containing products should be discontinued 48 to 72 hours before an adenosine or dipyridamole stress test. Patients receiving oral dipyridamole should not be given IV adenosine because of potential for precipitating severe heart block. If possible, beta-adrenergic blockers should be withheld for 48 to 72 hours before a dobutamine stress test.

Cardiac MRI

Magnetic resonance imaging (*MRI*) is used to evaluate diseased heart muscle. Currently, three techniques are being used. Resting MRI can assess end-diastolic wall thickness and contractile function. Dobutamine MRI is used to evaluate contractile reserve. Contrast-enhanced MRI allows for the visualization of the *in vivo* regions of microvascular obstruction. The extent of microvascular obstruction determines the magnitude of myocardial scarring. Once determined, the extent of microvascular obstruction is a strong predictor of myocardial remodeling and outcome after revascularization. It may eventually replace cardiac catheterization. Safety has been demonstrated in patients with permanent pacemakers and implantable cardioverter–defibrillators. For further description and nursing considerations, see page 166.

Phlebography (Venography)

Description
An x-ray visualization of the vascular tree after the injection of a contrast medium to detect venous occlusion.

Nursing and Patient Care Considerations
1. Inform patient that an intense burning sensation in the vessel where the solution is injected may be experienced. This will last for only a few seconds.
2. Note evidence of allergic reaction to the contrast medium; this may occur as soon as the contrast medium is injected, or it may occur after the test.
   a. Perspiring, dyspnea, nausea, and vomiting.
   b. Rapid heart rate and numbness of extremities.
   c. Hives.
3. Advise patient to notify health care provider of signs of allergic reaction.
4. Observe injection site for redness, swelling, bleeding, and thrombosis.

Positron Emission Tomography

Description
1. Considered the most sensitive modality for detecting hibernating viable myocardium and predicting left ventricular recovery after coronary revascularization.
2. F-FDG, a glucose analog that is transported into cells through glucose membrane transporter, is injected. It does not undergo any further metabolism (unlike glucose) and essentially is trapped within the cell.
3. Trapped F-FDG accumulates and becomes an index of cellular glucose utilization signifying ongoing cellular metabolism. Reduced FDG uptake (reduced or absent glucose metabolism) signifies myocardial scar. Also see page 167.
4. Used to determine blood flow to the heart muscle and viability of areas with decreased function because of previous MI.
5. Allows for the differentiation of nonfunctioning heart muscle from heart muscle that would benefit from a procedure.

Nursing and Patient Care Considerations
1. Inform patient not to eat for 4 hours prior to the scan.
2. Check blood glucose prior to test for diabetic patients; if greater than 200, may need to reschedule test.
3. Encourage patient to drink water following the scan to assist excretion of contrast medium.

Other Diagnostic Tests

Electrocardiogram

Basic Principles
1. Despite its limited sensitivity and specificity, the 12-lead ECG is still the standard for the evaluation of myocardial ischemia.
2. Electrical activity is generated by the cells of the heart as ions are exchanged across cell membranes.
3. Electrodes that are capable of conducting electrical activity from the heart to the ECG machine are placed at strategic positions on the extremities and chest precordium (see Figure 12-1).

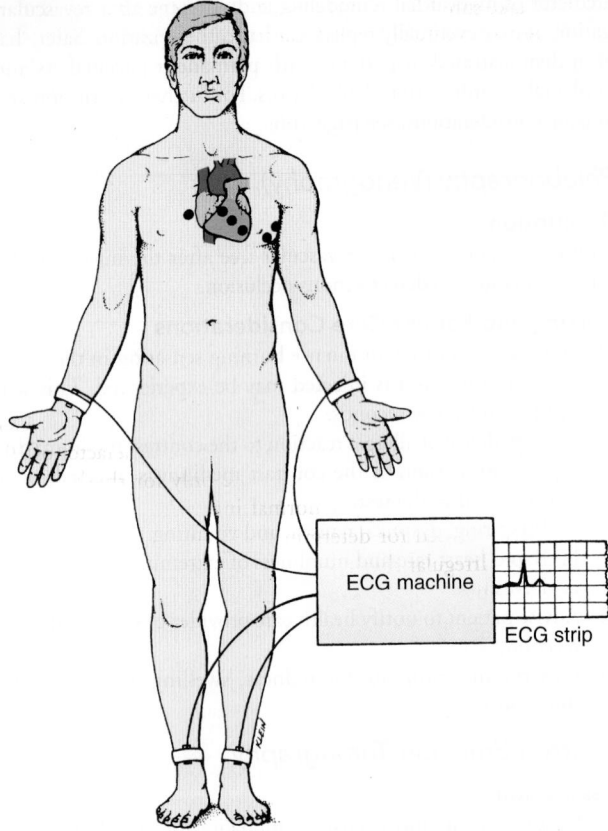

Figure 12-1. Transmission of the heart's impulse to a graphic display by ECG machine. The electrodes, which conduct electrical activity from the heart to the ECG machine, are placed at strategic positions on the extremities and chest precordium.

4. The electrical energy sensed is then converted to a graphic display by the ECG machine. This display is referred to as the ECG.
5. Each ECG lead consists of a positive and negative pole; each lead also has an axis that represents the direction in which current flows.
6. Each lead takes a different view of the heart; therefore, the tracing will be different with each view obtained.
7. The direction in which electrical current flows determines how the waveform will appear.
8. There are three sets of leads:
   a. Standard limb or bipolar leads (I, II, III) utilize three electrodes; these leads form a triangle known as Einthoven triangle.
   b. Augmented unipolar leads (AVR, AVL, AVF).
   c. Precordial unipolar leads (V_1, V_2, V_3, V_4, V_5, V_6).
9. A heart contraction is represented on the ECG graph paper by the designated P wave, QRS complex, and T waves.
   a. The P wave is the first positive deflection and represents atrial depolarization or atrial contraction.
   b. The PR interval represents the time it takes for the electrical impulse to travel from the sinoatrial node to the AV node and down the bundle of His to the right and left bundle branches.
   c. The Q wave is the first negative deflection after the P wave; the R wave is the first positive deflection after the P wave.
   d. The S wave is the negative deflection after the R wave.

e. The QRS waveform is generally regarded as a unit and represents ventricular depolarization. Atrial repolarization (relaxation) occurs during the QRS complex, but cannot be seen.
f. The T wave follows the S wave and is joined to the QRS complex by the ST segment. The ST segment represents ventricular repolarization or relaxation. The point that represents the end of the QRS complex and the beginning of the ST segment is known as the J point.
g. The T wave represents the return of ions to the appropriate side of the cell membrane. This signifies relaxation of the muscle fibers and is referred to as *repolarization* of the ventricles.
h. The QT interval is the time between the Q wave and the T wave; it represents ventricular depolarization (contraction) and repolarization (relaxation).

Indications
1. The ECG is a useful tool in the diagnosis of conditions that may cause aberrations in the electrical activity of the heart. Examples of these conditions include:
   a. MI and other types of CAD such as angina.
   b. Cardiac dysrhythmias.
   c. Cardiac enlargement.
   d. Electrolyte disturbances (calcium, potassium, magnesium, and phosphorous).
   e. Inflammatory diseases of the heart.
   f. Effects on the heart by drugs, such as antiarrhythmics and tricyclic antidepressants.
2. Despite its many advantages, however, the ECG also has several shortcomings:
   a. Fifty percent of all patients with AMI have no ECG changes.
   b. A patient may have a normal ECG, present pain-free, and still have significant risk for myocardial ischemia.
   c. Several disease processes can mimic that of an AMI, including left bundle-branch blocks, ventricular paced rhythms, and left ventricular hypertrophy.

ECG Leads and Normal Waveform Interpretation
See Figure 12-2.
1. The normal amplitude of the P wave is 3 mm or less; the normal duration of the P wave is 0.04 to 0.11 second. P waves that exceed these measurements are considered to deviate from normal.

Figure 12-2. Waveform analysis.

2. The PR interval is measured from the upstroke of the P wave to the QR junction and is normally between 0.12 and 0.20 second. There is a built-in delay in time at the AV node to allow for adequate ventricular filling to maintain normal stroke volume.

3. The QRS complex contains separate waves and segments, which should be evaluated separately. Normal QRS complex should be between 0.06 and 0.10 second.
   a. The Q wave, or first downward stroke after the P wave, is usually less than 3 mm in depth. A Q wave of significant deflection is not normally present in the healthy heart. A pathologic Q wave usually indicates a completed MI.
   b. The R wave is the first positive deflection after the P wave, normally 5 to 10 mm in height. Increases and decreases in amplitude become significant in certain disease states. Ventricular hypertrophy produces very high R waves because the hypertrophied muscle requires a stronger electrical current to depolarize.

4. The ST segment begins at the end of the S wave, the first negative deflection after the R wave, and terminates at the upstroke of the T wave.

5. The T wave represents the repolarization of myocardial fibers or provides the resting state of myocardial work; the T wave should always be present.
   a. Normally, the T wave should not exceed a 5-mm amplitude in all leads except the precordial (V_1 to V_6) leads, where it may be as high as 10 mm.

6. The P, Q, R, S, and T waves all appear differently depending on which lead you are viewing.

Nursing and Patient Care Considerations

1. Perform ECG or begin continuous ECG monitoring as indicated.
   a. Provide privacy and ask patient to undress, exposing the chest, wrists, and ankles. Assist with draping as appropriate. Remove large jewelry or metal from upper body to avoid interference.
   b. Place leads on the chest and extremities as labeled, using self-adhesive electrodes or water-soluble gel or other conductive material.
   c. Instruct patient to lie still, avoiding movement, coughing, or talking, while ECG is recording to avoid artifact.
   d. Make sure ECG machine is plugged in and grounded and operate according to manufacturer's directions.
   e. If continuous cardiac monitoring is being done, advise patient on the parameters of mobility as movement may trigger alarms and false readings.

2. Interpret the rhythm strip (see Figure 12-3). Develop a systematic approach to assist in accurate interpretation.
   a. Determine the rhythm—is it regular, irregular, regularly irregular, or irregularly irregular? Use calipers, count blocks between QRS complexes, or measure the distance between R waves to determine regularity.
   b. Determine the rate—is it fast, slow, or normal?
      i. A gross determination of rate can be accomplished by counting the number of QRS complexes within a 6-second time interval (use the superior margin of ECG paper) and multiplying the complexes by a factor of 10. *Note:* This method is accurate only for rhythms that are occurring at normal intervals and should not be used for determining rate in irregular rhythms. Irregular rhythms are always counted for 1 full minute for accuracy.
      ii. Another means of obtaining rate is to divide the number of large 5-square blocks between each two QRS complexes into 300. Five large 5-square blocks represent 1 minute on the ECG paper. For example, in Figure 12-3, the number of large square blocks between complexes no. 5 and no. 6 equals 5, and 300 divided by 5 equals 60, or a rate of 60.
   c. Evaluate the P wave—are P waves present? Is there a P for every QRS complex? If there is not a P for every QRS, do the P waves have a normal configuration?
   d. Measure and evaluate the PR interval.
   e. Evaluate the QRS complex—measure the QRS complex and examine its configuration.
   f. Evaluate the ST segment—an elevated ST segment heralds a pattern of injury and usually occurs as an initial change in acute MI. ST depression occurs in ischemic states. Calcium and potassium changes also affect the ST segment.
   g. Evaluate the T wave—are T waves present? Do all T waves have a normal shape? Could a P wave be hidden in the T wave, indicating a junctional rhythm or third-degree heart

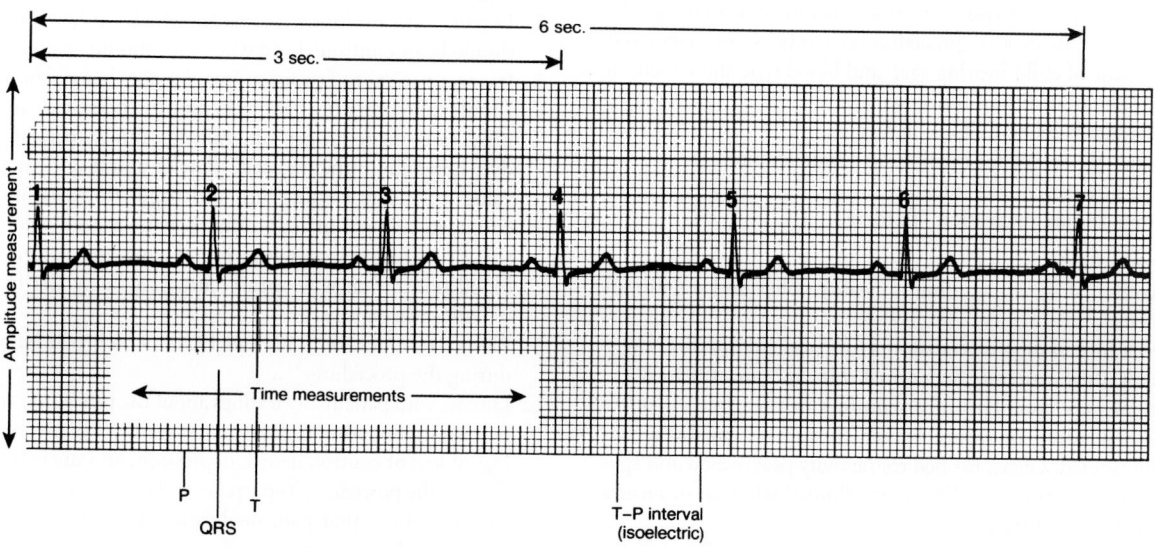

Figure 12-3. Lead II shows normal sinus rhythm on ECG paper.

block? Is it positively or negatively deflected (inverted T waves indicate ischemia) or peaked (indicative of hyperkalemia)?

h. Evaluate the QT interval—should be less than one half the R-R interval. Prolonged QT interval may indicate digoxin toxicity, long-term quinidine or procainamide therapy, or hypomagnesemia.

See Chapter 13 for common cardiac dysrhythmias.

Angiography

Description

1. Invasive imaging procedure that enables visualization of blood vessels for their patency of blood flow versus blockage through the insertion of a catheter into an artery or vein followed by injection of contrast dye.
2. Various types include coronary, aortic, renal, peripheral, cerebral, and pulmonary angiography, lymphangiogram, ventriculography, and fluorescein angiography.
3. Provide information that may direct assessment and management of cardiovascular and cerebrovascular disease, peripheral blockage (arterial and venous), aneurysms, arterial and venous malformations, thrombosis (deep vein or pulmonary embolus), and fistulae, guide mapping prior to interventional procedures, and diagnose internal bleeding.

Nursing and Patient Care Considerations
Preprocedure

1. Question patient for known allergies, particularly to iodine (shellfish). If so, notify health care provider, who may want to prepare patient with oral corticosteroids and diphenhydramine before the study.
2. Make sure there is a signed consent and that patient/family questions have been answered.
3. Make sure fasting guidelines have been followed, varying from NPO to liquid or light diet. Follow facility policy; should be in accordance with American Society of Anesthesiologists guidelines (minimum fasting 6 hours from light meal, 2 hours from clear liquids) to minimize risk of pulmonary aspiration should emesis occur.
4. Make sure laboratory testing has been ordered and results have been reviewed, including blood urea nitrogen (BUN) and creatinine, to evaluate kidney function for ability to clear contrast dye; hemoglobin/hematocrit, platelet count, and coagulation values, to ensure clotting and anticoagulation baseline; white blood cell (WBC) count, to rule out infection that may be exacerbated by invasive procedure; electrolytes; pregnancy test (in female of child-bearing age); and blood type and screen, in case blood transfusion is necessary.
5. Make sure baseline ECG is on file.
6. Ensure IV patency for medication administration.
7. Make sure patient has voided.
8. Administer premedication, if ordered.

Postprocedure

1. Record vital signs according to facility policy and stability of patient.
2. Check for bleeding or hematoma formation at insertion site.
3. Check distal extremity for normal color and intact pulses.
4. Patient may complain of discomfort in the groin or other site depending on route by which contrast medium was administered. Check for bed rest/activity progression and special fluid instructions. Encourage fluids/hydration to ensure clearance of contrast dye.
5. Provide patient with discharge instructions, including follow-up care, medications, and driving and activity restrictions.

Diagnostic Electrophysiology Studies

Description

Electrophysiology studies (EPS) are a complex invasive procedure in which flexible catheters (with 2 to 10 electrodes) are placed percutaneously in the right or left femoral vein, the subclavian vein, the internal jugular vein, or the median cephalic veins. EPS assesses pacing thresholds and measures conduction intervals in the high right atrium, the right ventricular apex, the right ventricular outflow tract, the coronary sinuses, the bundle of His, and, occasionally, the left ventricle. The test is followed by programmed stimulation protocols to evaluate the heart's conduction system.

Indications for EPS

1. Definite indications for EPS include:
   a. Sustained ventricular tachycardia.
   b. Cardiac arrest in the absence of AMI, antiarrhythmic drug toxicity, or electrolyte imbalance.
   c. Syncope of uncertain origin (for which noncardiac causes have been ruled out).
   d. Wide QRS tachycardia of uncertain etiology.
   e. To evaluate the effectiveness of a device for the detection and electrical termination of tachycardias (pacemakers or implanted defibrillators).
   f. Symptomatic Wolff-Parkinson-White syndrome.
   g. Frequent symptomatic regular supraventricular tachycardia unresponsive to medications.
2. Possible indications for EPS include:
   a. Asymptomatic Wolff-Parkinson-White syndrome.
   b. Post–myocardial infarction.
   c. Nonsustained ventricular tachycardia.
   d. Cardiomyopathy.
   e. Frequent ventricular ectopy.
   f. Supraventricular tachycardia.
3. Contraindications for EPS include:
   a. Asymptomatic sinus bradycardia.
   b. Asymptomatic bundle-branch blocks.
   c. Palpitation.
   d. Atrial fibrillation or flutter.
   e. Third-degree AV blocks.
   f. Second-degree Mobitz type II AV blocks.

Nursing and Patient Care Considerations

1. Anticoagulants (warfarin) should be discontinued at least 3 days before EPS.
2. Discuss with health care provider which cardiac medications should be discontinued and when they should be discontinued.
3. Instruct patient to fast for at least 6 hours before the study.
4. Ensure laboratory tests are sent; may include BUN and creatinine, to evaluate kidney function for ability to clear contrast dye; hemoglobin/hematocrit, platelet count and coagulation values to ensure clotting and anticoagulation baseline; WBC count, to rule out infection that may be exacerbated by invasive procedure; electrolytes; blood type and screen, in case blood transfusion is necessary; and pregnancy test in females of child-bearing age.
5. Place electrodes for a 12-lead ECG, which will be recorded during the procedure.
6. Discuss with patient any feelings about the procedure and his or her physical condition. Patients frequently experience anxiety, fear of loss of control, denial, depression, and uncertainty.
7. Explain the procedure, its purpose, and the preparation involved.
8. Inform patient that pain medication and conscious sedation will be used during the procedure.
9. Postprocedure care includes:

a. Keeping extremity used for IV straight, restraining if necessary.
b. Monitoring patient's groin for bleeding or hematoma formation.
c. Monitoring vital signs as ordered.
d. Providing emotional support to patient and family.

Cardiac Catheterization

Description

1. *Cardiac catheterization* is a diagnostic procedure in which a catheter is introduced into the heart and blood vessels to provide physiologic data to guide treatment; measure cardiovascular hemodynamics; acquire radiographic images of coronary arteries, cardiac chambers, and aorta; collect blood from various chambers for analysis; and evaluate pulmonary blood flow and shunts.
2. The radial approach is becoming the preferred access site especially when there is peripheral vascular disease or morbid obesity. The femoral vein is another frequently used site. The catheter is directed up the aorta and into the coronary vasculature to visualize coronary anatomy (right or left) and measure hemodynamics. In rare instances of aortic disease, a transseptal approach may be used.
3. Right-sided heart catheterization—right side of the heart is accessed to evaluate pulmonary shunts, cardiac anomalies, and valvular disease. A radiopaque catheter is passed from the femoral vein and through the inferior vena cava or from the basilic vein and through the superior vena cava into the right atrium, right ventricle, and pulmonary vasculature under direct visualization with a fluoroscope.
   a. Right atrium and right ventricle pressures are measured; blood samples are taken for hematocrit and oxygen saturation.
   b. After entering the right atrium, the catheter is then passed through the tricuspid valve and similar tests are performed on blood within the right ventricle.
   c. Finally, the catheter is passed through the pulmonic valve, and as far as possible beyond that point, capillary samples are obtained, capillary wedge pressure is recorded, and CO can be determined.
   d. Complications include cardiac dysrhythmias, venous spasm, thrombophlebitis, infection at insertion site, cardiac perforation, and cardiac tamponade.
4. Left-sided heart catheterization—primarily done to diagnose coronary artery disease; usually done by retrograde approach by advancing the catheter up the aorta into the coronary anatomy.
   a. Retrograde approach—catheter may be introduced percutaneously by puncture of the femoral artery or by direct radial or brachial approach and advanced under fluoroscopic control into the ascending aorta and into the left ventricle.
   b. Transseptal approach—catheter is passed from the right femoral vein (percutaneously or by saphenous vein cut down) upward into the right atrium. A long needle is passed up through the catheter and is used to puncture the septum separating the right and left atria; needle is withdrawn and the catheter is advanced under fluoroscopic control into the left ventricle.
   c. The catheter tip is placed at the coronary sinus, and contrast medium is injected directly into one or both of the coronary arteries to evaluate patency.
   d. Gives hemodynamic data—permits flow and pressure measurements of left side of the heart.
   e. Usually performed to evaluate the patency of coronary arteries and function of the left ventricular muscle and mitral and aortic valves; may also be done to evaluate patients before surgery.
   f. Ventriculography—study of the left ventricle; catheter is passed into the left ventricle, and dye is injected with a rapid, uniform rate via an injector machine to measure ejection fraction or function of the left ventricle.
   g. Complications of left-sided heart catheterization and implications for nursing assessment include dysrhythmias (ventricular fibrillation), syncope, vasospasm, pericardial tamponade, MI, pulmonary edema, allergic reaction to contrast medium, perforation of great vessels of the heart, systemic embolization (stroke, MI), loss of pulse distal to arteriotomy, and possible ischemia of the lower arm and hand.
5. Angiography is usually combined with heart catheterization for coronary artery visualization.
6. Contraindications for cardiac catheterization include uncontrolled ventricular irritability, electrolyte imbalance, medication toxicity (digitalis), uncontrolled heart failure, renal failure, recent stroke (within past 3 months), active GI bleeding, active infection, uncontrolled hypertension, patient's refusal, and pregnancy. Some of these conditions can be reversed or improved prior to catheterization.

Nursing and Patient Care Considerations
Preprocedure

1. Question patient for known allergies, particularly iodine (shellfish), and make health care provider aware so that premedication with corticosteroid and antihistamine may be considered.
2. Make sure that there is a signed consent form and that patient and family questions have been answered.
3. Make sure that fasting guidelines have been followed, varying from NPO to liquid or light diet. Follow facility policy; should be in accordance with American Society of Anesthesiologists guidelines (minimum fasting 6 hours from light meal, 2 hours from clear liquids).
4. Make sure laboratory testing has been ordered and results reviewed (see page 242). Make sure baseline ECG is on file.
5. Ensure IV patency for administration of medications.
6. Mark distal pulses.
7. Explain to patient that he or she will be lying on an examination table for a prolonged period and may experience certain sensations:
   a. Occasional thudding sensations in the chest—from extrasystoles, particularly when the catheter is manipulated in ventricular chambers.
   b. Strong desire to cough, which may occur during contrast medium injection into right side of heart during angiography.
   c. Transient feeling of hot flashes or nausea as the contrast medium is injected.
8. Evaluate patient's emotional status before catheterization, dispel myths, and provide factual information.
9. Have patient void before the procedure.
10. Allow for premedication (if any) to take effect prior to procedure.

Postprocedure

1. Record vital signs according to facility protocol and patient's condition.
2. Check for bleeding or hematoma formation at insertion site.
3. Check distal extremity for normal color and intact pulses, and evaluate complaints of pain, numbness, or tingling sensation to determine signs of arterial insufficiency.
4. Assess for complaints of chest pain and respond immediately.
5. Follow activity restriction/progression directions, which are based on coagulation status and whether a vascular closure method was employed.

6. Evaluate complaints of back, thigh, or groin pain (may indicate retroperitoneal bleeding).
7. Obtain postprocedure ECG and labs according to facility protocol.
8. Be alert for signs and symptoms of vagal reaction (nausea, diaphoresis, hypotension, bradycardia); treat as directed with atropine and fluids.
9. Assess neurologic status if receiving IIB/IIIA platelet inhibitors or thrombolytics according to facility protocol.
10. Provide discharge instructions, including follow-up care, medications, driving and activity restrictions, and the need to report any pain or above-listed problems.

GENERAL PROCEDURES AND TREATMENT MODALITIES

 See additional online content: Procedure Guidelines 10-1–10-8.

Hemodynamic Monitoring

Hemodynamic monitoring is the assessment of the patient's circulatory status; it includes measurements of heart rate (HR), precise measurements of intra-arterial pressure, CO, central venous pressure (CVP), PAP, pulmonary artery wedge pressure, mixed venous oxygenation data, and blood volume. It describes the intravascular pressure and flow of blood that occurs when the heart muscle contracts and pumps blood throughout the body.

The primary purpose is the early detection, identification, and treatment of life-threatening conditions, such as AMI, heart failure, cardiac tamponade, and all types of shock (septic, cardiogenic, neurogenic, anaphylactic). It is also useful in determining fluid and vasoactive therapy during the acute phase of patient's care, especially patients with multiorgan dysfunctions. It is also indicated for pre-, peri-, and postoperative surgery as well as for research studies.

Central Venous Pressure Monitoring

1. Refers to the measurement of right atrial pressure or the pressure of the great veins within the thorax (normal range: 5 to 10 cm H_2O or 2 to 8 mm Hg).
   a. Right-sided cardiac function is assessed through the evaluation of CVP.
   b. Left-sided heart function is less accurately reflected by the evaluation of CVP, but may be useful in assessing chronic right- and left-sided heart failure and differentiating right and left ventricular infarctions.
2. Requires the threading of a catheter into a large central vein (subclavian, internal, or external jugular, median basilic, or femoral). The catheter tip is then positioned in the right atrium, upper portion of the superior vena cava, or the inferior vena cava (femoral approach only). See Figure 12-4.
   a. To obtain venous access when peripheral vein sites are inadequate.
   b. To obtain central venous blood samples.
   c. To administer blood products, total parenteral nutrition, and some drug therapies contraindicated for peripheral infusion.
   d. To insert a temporary pacemaker.

Cardiac Output

Cardiac output (CO) is the amount (volume) of blood ejected by the left ventricle into the aorta in 1 minute. Normal CO is 4 to 8 L/minute.

Figure 12-4. CVP monitoring.

Underlying Considerations

1. CO is determined by stroke volume (SV) and HR. Thus, CO = SV × HR. CO must be maintained to adequately oxygenate the body.
   a. HR = number of cardiac contractions per minute. The integrity of the conduction system and nervous system innervation of the heart influence functioning of this determinant.
   b. SV = amount of blood ejected from ventricle per beat (normal SV is 50 to 100 mL/beat). The amount of blood returning to the heart (preload), venous tone, resistance imposed on the ventricle before ejection (afterload), and the integrity of the cardiac muscle (contractility) influence the functioning of this determinant.
2. The body alters CO through increases or decreases in one or both of these parameters. CO is maintained if the HR falls by an increase in SV. Likewise, a decrease in SV produces a compensatory rise in HR to keep the CO normal.
3. CO will decrease if either of the determinants cannot inversely compensate for the other.
4. CO measurements are adjusted to patient size by calculating the cardiac index (CI). CI equals CO divided by body surface area (BSA); BSA is determined through standard charts based on individual height and weight. Normal CI is 2.5 to 4 L/minute/m².

Assessment of Cardiac Output

Signs of low CO include:
1. Changes in mental status.
2. An increase in HR.
3. Shortness of breath.
4. Cyanosis or duskiness of buccal mucosa, nail beds, and earlobes.
5. Falling blood pressure.
6. Low urine output.
7. Cool, moist skin.
8. Decreased or no appetite.

Methods

1. CO is measured by various techniques. In the clinical setting, it is usually measured by the thermodilution technique in conjunction with a flow-directed balloon-tipped pulmonary artery catheter (commonly known as Swan-Ganz catheter after the inventors).
2. The Swan-Ganz catheter is positioned in its final position in a branch of the pulmonary artery; it has a thermistor (external sensing device) situated 1½ inches (4 cm) from the tip of the catheter, which measures the temperature of the blood that flows by it.

Pulmonary Artery Pressure Monitoring

Purposes

1. To monitor pressures in the right atrium (CVP), right ventricle, pulmonary artery, and distal branches of the pulmonary artery (known as *pulmonary artery occlusion pressure* or *pulmonary artery wedge pressure*). The latter reflects the level of the pressure in the left atrium (or filling pressure in the left ventricle); thus, pressures on the left side of the heart are inferred from pressure measurement obtained on the right side of the circulation. Provides estimation of diastolic filling of the left side of the heart.
2. To measure CO through thermodilution.
3. To obtain blood for central venous oxygen saturation.
4. To continuously monitor mixed venous oxygen saturation (SvO_2); available on special catheters.
5. To provide for temporary atrial/ventricular pacing and intra-atrial ECG (available only on special catheters).
6. To evaluate the hemodynamic response to fluid therapy, medications, and other treatments.

Underlying Considerations

1. Left atrial pressure is closely related to left ventricular end diastolic pressure (LVEDP—filling pressure of the left ventricle) and is therefore an indicator of left ventricular function. Because there are no valves in the pulmonary arterial system when the Swan-Ganz catheter is wedged, it reflects an uninterrupted flow of blood to the left atrium.
2. The pulmonary artery diastolic pressure (PADP) reflects the LVEDP in patients with normal lungs and mitral valve. The PADP can be continuously monitored as an approximation of LVEDP (limits excessive balloon inflation to obtain a PAOP and subsequent risk of balloon rupture or damage to the pulmonary artery).
3. SaO_2 is affected by four factors: CO, hemoglobin, arterial oxygen saturation (SaO_2), and tissue oxygen consumption.
4. Changes in SaO_2 alert the clinician to changes in these factors. More rapid detection of change facilitates interventions to correct problems before significant deterioration in patient's condition occurs.
5. If the amount of oxygen supplied to the tissues is inadequate to meet demands, more oxygen will be extracted from venous blood and SaO_2 will decrease. If oxygen supply exceeds demand, SaO_2 will increase.
6. Pulmonary artery (PA) catheters are associated with significant risk and disadvantages, including increased cost and mortality. Placement of a PA catheter is invasive and does not directly impact patient outcomes.

Methods

1. The Swan-Ganz catheter is a flow-directed (1.5 mL), balloon-tipped, 4- to 5-lumen catheter that is percutaneously inserted at the bedside and allows for continuous PAP monitoring as well as periodic measurement of PAOP and other parameters.

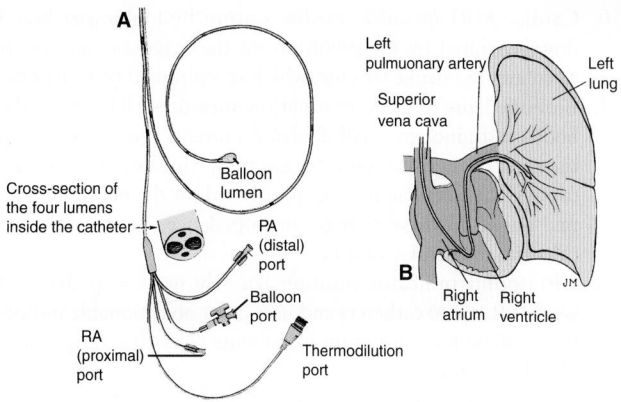

Figure 12-5. Swan-Ganz catheter showing **(A)** multiple lumens and **(B)** location within the heart.

2. The catheter is 110 cm long, marked at increments of 10 cm, and is available in varying diameters. See Figure 12-5.
3. Most catheters in use incorporate thermodilution for determination of CO.
4. If monitoring of SvO_2 is desired, a PA catheter incorporating fiberoptics is used.
5. If temporary cardiac pacing capability is desired, a catheter with a lumen for a pacing wire may be used.
6. Catheter may be inserted under fluoroscopy or at the bedside using the hemodynamic waveform as a guide to correct position.

Newer Technology for Hemodynamic Monitoring

Complications associated with insertion of invasive pulmonary artery catheters have led to the development of newer noninvasive or minimally invasive methods of hemodynamic monitoring.

1. Indirect Fick method—modification of the original Fick principle first developed in 1870.
2. Thoracic electrical bioimpedance (TEB)—noninvasive measurement of the electrical resistance of the thorax to a high-frequency, very-low-magnitude current. As thoracic fluid in the chest increases, TEB decreases; changes in CO correspond to changes in aortic blood flow.
3. Pulse contour devices—measure CO by assessing the contours of arterial pressure waveforms in relationship to the patient's stroke volume.
4. Continuous SvO_2 monitoring—measures mixed venous oxygen by means of a modified PA catheter to assess oxygen-carrying hemoglobin (oxyhemoglobin) and non–oxygen-carrying hemoglobin (deoxyhemoglobin).
5. Continuous CO monitoring—utilizes a modified PA catheter.
6. Right ventricular ejection fraction measurement—assesses the amount of blood forced from the ventricle during systole; it is an indication of the strength or contractility of the heart as determined by a special type of arterial catheter.
7. Esophageal Doppler CO monitoring—utilizes sound waves to measure aortic blood flow and thereby determine SV.
8. Exhaled CO_2 monitoring—completely noninvasive technique based on the Fick equation that measures CO.
9. Lithium dilution CO is another thermodilution method that assesses CO through injection of lithium chloride into a central or peripheral venous catheter and measurement of the concentration of lithium chloride over time using lithium-sensitive electrodes.

10. Cardiac MRI measures cardiac output by looking at blood flow generated by the picture from the magnetic current. It calculates the stroke volume, which is multiplied by heart rate.

11. Bioimpedance CO determination measures changes in the body's resistance to small electrical current. Blood volume in the chest changes during every ejection, which can be detected using eight electrical patches positioned on the neck and thorax. Based on these changes in impedance, a computer can calculate the cardiac output.

12. Ultrasound indicator dilution (mostly used in pediatrics) works off *in situ* catheters and uses an unobjectionable indicator to allow for routine measurements of cardiac output and blood volumes.

Cardiac Pacing

 EVIDENCE BASE Wiegand, D. L. (Ed.). (2017). *AACN procedure manual for critical care* (7th ed.). St. Louis, MO: Saunders.

A *cardiac pacemaker* is an electronic device that delivers direct electrical stimulation to stimulate the myocardium to depolarize, initiating a mechanical contraction. The pacemaker initiates and maintains the heart rate when the heart's natural pacemaker is unable to do so. Pacemakers can be used to correct bradycardias, tachycardias, sick sinus syndrome, and second- and third-degree heart blocks and for prophylaxis. Pacing may be accomplished through a permanent implantable system, a temporary system with an external pulse generator and percutaneously threaded leads, or a transcutaneous external system with electrode pads placed over the chest. A recent development is the leadless pacemaker.

Clinical Indications

1. Symptomatic bradydysrhythmias.
2. Symptomatic sinus bradycardia that results from required drug therapy.
3. Symptomatic heart block.
   a. Mobitz II second-degree heart block.
   b. Complete heart block.
   c. Bifascicular and trifascicular bundle-branch blocks.
4. Hypersensitive carotid sinus syndrome and neurocardiogenic syncope.
5. Prophylaxis.
   a. After acute MI: dysrhythmia and conduction defects.
   b. Before or after cardiac surgery.
   c. During cardiac resynchronization therapy in patients with severe systolic heart failure.
   d. During diagnostic and therapeutic procedures such as cardiac catheterization, EPS, percutaneous transluminal coronary angioplasty (PTCA), stress testing, before permanent pacing, and during transcatheter aortic valve replacement (TAVR).
6. Tachydysrhythmias (supraventricular tachycardia, ventricular tachycardia); to override rapid rhythm disturbances.

Types of Pacing

Permanent Pacemakers

There are two types of permanent pacers; the standard pacer that paces one side of the heart causing uncoordinated contraction of the left and right ventricle or biventricular that coordinates the contraction of the left and right ventricle

Standard Pacemakers

1. Used to treat chronic heart conditions; surgically placed utilizing a local anesthetic, the leads are placed transvenously in the appropriate chamber of the heart and then anchored to the endocardium.
2. The pulse generator is placed in a surgically made pocket in subcutaneous tissue under the clavicle or in the abdomen. Choices for types of generators include single- or dual-chamber devices, biventricular devices, unipolar or bipolar pacing/sensing configuration, and various types of sensors for rate response.
3. Once placed, it can be programmed externally as needed.
4. Implantable cardioverter–defibrillators can also have standard pacing functionality.

Biventricular Pacemakers

1. Biventricular pacemakers are also referred to as cardiac resynchronization therapy.
2. Biventricular pacing is used to treat moderate to severe heart failure as a result of left ventricular dyssynchrony.
3. Intraventricular conduction defects result in an uncoordinated contraction of the left and right ventricle, which causes a wide QRS complex and is associated with worsening heart failure and increased mortality.
4. Biventricular pacemakers utilize three leads (one in the right atrium, one in the right ventricle, and one in the left ventricle via the coronary sinus) to coordinate ventricular contraction and improve CO.
5. Biventricular pacemakers can incorporate implantable cardioverter–defibrillators or be used alone.

Leadless Pacemakers

1. Self contained, single chamber, implanted directly through femoral vein into right ventricle.
2. Fixated into the myocardium by a screw helix or nitinol tines.
3. Developed to eliminate complications of pocket or lead related problems.
4. 10 year estimated battery life; retrievable if necessary.

Temporary Pacemakers

1. Temporary pacemakers are usually placed during an emergency, such as when a patient demonstrates signs of decreased CO.
2. Indicated for patients with high-grade AV blocks, bradycardia, or low CO. They serve as a bridge until the patient becomes stable enough for placement of a permanent pacemaker.
3. Can be placed transvenously, epicardially, transcutaneously, and transthoracically.
   a. Transvenous pacemakers are inserted transvenously (into a vein, usually the subclavian, internal jugular, antecubital, or femoral) into the right ventricle (or right atrium and right ventricle for dual-chamber pacing) and then attached to an external pulse generator. This procedure may be done at the bedside or under fluoroscopy.
   b. Epicardial pacemaker wires are attached to the endocardium, brought out through a surgical incision in the thorax. These wires are then connected to an external pulse generator. This is commonly seen after cardiac surgery.
   c. With transcutaneous pacing, noninvasive multifunction electrode pads are placed either anterior-posteriorly (anterior chest wall under the left nipple, slightly midaxillary, and on the patient's back directly behind anterior pad) or anterior-laterally (anterior chest wall under the left nipple, slightly midaxillary, and on patient's upper right chest wall below the clavicle). The multifunction electrode pads are

connected to an external energy source (defibrillator with pacing capability). The electrical impulses flow through the multifunction electrode pads and subcutaneous skin to the heart, thereby pacing the heart. Note: transcutaneous pacing should not be utilized continuously for more than 2 hours. Transvenous pacing should then be initiated.

   d. The transthoracic pacemaker is a type of temporary pacemaker that is placed only in an emergency via a long needle, using a subxiphoid approach. The pacer wire is then placed directly into the right ventricle.

4. Monitor for evidence of lead migration and perforation of the heart.
   a. Observe for muscle twitching and/or cough (may indicate chest wall or diaphragmatic pacing).
   b. Evaluate patient's complaints of chest pain (may indicate perforation of pericardial sac).
   c. Auscultate for pericardial friction rub.
   d. Observe for signs and symptoms of cardiac tamponade: distant heart sounds, distended jugular veins, pulsus paradoxus, and hypotension.

5. Provide an electrically safe environment for patient. Stray electrical current can enter the heart through temporary pacemaker lead system and induce dysrhythmias.
   a. Protect exposed parts of the electrode lead terminal in temporary pacing systems per manufacturer's recommendations.
   b. Wear rubber gloves when touching temporary pacing leads. Static electricity from your hands can enter the patient's body through the lead system.
   c. Make sure all equipment is grounded with three-prong plugs inserted into a proper outlet when using an external pacing system.
   d. Epicardial pacing wires should have the terminal needle protected by a plastic tube; place tube in rubber glove to protect it from fluids or electrical current when disconnected from generator.

 NURSING ALERT Transport patient to other parts of facility with portable ECG monitoring and nurse. Patients with temporary pacemakers should never be placed in unmonitored areas.

6. Use sedation, if BP is stable, when transcutaneous pacing a patient. The mA used to overcome the impedance to reach the heart through the skin is high and can be quite painful to the patient.
7. Monitor for infection by checking temperature every 4 hours; report elevations and assess central IV site (where temporary pacing wire is inserted) for signs and symptoms of infection, such as redness and drainage.
8. Prevent accidental pacemaker malfunctions.
   a. Use clear plastic covering over external temporary generators at all times (eliminates potential manipulation of programmed settings).
   b. Secure temporary pacemaker generator to patient's chest or waist; never hang it on an IV pole.
   c. Transfer of patient from bed to stretcher should only be attempted with an adequate number of personnel so that patient can remain passive; caution personnel to avoid underarm lifts.
   d. Evaluate transcutaneous pacing electrode pads every 2 hours for secure contact to chest wall; change electrode pads every 24 hours or if pads do not have complete contact with the skin.

Pacemaker Design

Pulse Generator

Contains the circuitry and batteries to generate the electrical signal.
1. The pulse generator in a permanent pacemaker is encapsulated in a metal box that is embedded under the skin. The box protects the generator from electromagnetic interferences and trauma.
2. In the leadless pacemaker the pulse generator is self contained in the device implanted in the right ventricle.
3. A temporary pacing generator is an external system that either utilized the defibrillator with pacing capability or contained in a small box with dials for programming. It is an external system.
   a. Transcutaneous pacing systems utilize an external energy source such as a defibrillator with pacing ability. Dials for programming the unit are on the device.
   b. Electromechanical interference is more likely to occur with temporary systems.
   c. Temporary pacing systems use batteries, which need replacement based on use of device. The transcutaneous system has rechargeable battery circuitry but should be plugged into an electrical outlet most of the time to ensure adequate battery life for transport.
4. Permanent pacing systems use reliable power sources such as lithium batteries. Lithium batteries have a projected life span of 8 to 12 years.

Pacemaker Lead

Transmits the electrical signal from the pulse generator to the heart. One, two, or three leads may be placed in the heart.
1. "Single-chamber" pacemaker.
   a. "Single-chamber" pacemakers have one lead in either the atrial or ventricular chamber.
   b. The sensing and pacing capabilities of the pacemaker are confined to the chamber where the lead is placed.
2. "Dual-chamber" pacemaker.
   a. A "dual-chamber" pacemaker has two leads.
   b. One lead is in the right atrium and the other lead is located in the right ventricle.
   c. Pacing and sensing can occur in both heart chambers, closely "mimicking" normal heart function (physiologic pacing).
3. Biventricular pacemaker.
   a. One lead is in the right atrium, one is in the right ventricle, and one is in the left ventricle via the coronary sinus.
   b. In single right ventricle (traditional) pacing, there is slight delay of the left ventricle contracting as the electrical impulse begins in the right ventricle and moves to the left ventricle, giving the characteristic left bundle-branch block appearance. By pacing both right and left ventricle at the same time, the pacemaker can resynchronize a heart whose opposing walls do not contract in synchrony.
4. Pacemaker leads may be threaded through a vein into the right atrium and/or right ventricle (endocardial/transvenous approach) or introduced by direct penetration of the chest wall and attached to the left ventricle or right atrium (see Figure 12-6).
5. Fixation devices located at the end of the pacemaker lead allow for secure attachment of the lead to the heart, reducing the possibility of lead dislodgement.
6. Temporary leads protrude from the incision and are connected to the external pulse generator. Permanent leads are connected to the pulse generator implanted underneath the skin.

Pacemaker Function

Cardiac pacing refers to the ability of the pacemaker to stimulate the atrium, the ventricle, or both heart chambers in sequence and

Figure 12-6. Permanent pacemaker insertion with **(A)** unipolar lead (threaded through central vein into the right ventricle) and **(B)** bipolar leads (passed through the chest wall and sutured to external surface of the left ventricle).

initiate electrical depolarization and cardiac contraction. Cardiac pacing is evidenced on the ECG by the presence of a "spike" or "pacing artifact."

Pacing Functions

1. Atrial pacing—direct stimulation of the right atrium producing a "spike" on the ECG preceding a P wave.
2. Ventricular pacing—direct stimulation of the right or left ventricle producing a "spike" on the ECG preceding a QRS complex causing a widen QRS complex (bundle-branch block appearance).
3. AV pacing—direct stimulation of the right atrium and either ventricle in sequence; mimics normal cardiac conduction, allowing the atria to contract before the ventricles. ("Atrial kick" received by the ventricles allows for an increase in CO.)

Sensing Functions

Cardiac pacemakers have the ability to "see" intrinsic cardiac activity when it occurs (sensing).

1. Demand—ability to "sense" intrinsic cardiac activity and deliver a pacing stimulus only if the heart rate falls below a preset rate limit.
2. Fixed—no ability to "sense" intrinsic cardiac activity; the pacemaker can't "synchronize" with the heart's natural activity and consistently delivers a pacing stimulus at a preset rate.
3. Triggered—ability to deliver pacing stimuli in response to "sensing" a cardiac event.
   a. "Sees" atrial activity (P waves) and delivers a pacing spike to the ventricle after an appropriate delay (usually 0.16 second, similar to PR interval).
   b. Maintains AV synchrony and increases heart rate based on increases in the body demands that occur with exercise or during stress.
   c. "Physiologic" sensors are being developed as alternatives to "trigger" a ventricular response because many patients have atrial dysfunction.
   d. "Sensor-driven" rate-responsive pacemakers do not sense atrial activity; a triggered ventricular beat occurs when the pacemaker senses either increases in muscle activity, temperature, and oxygen utilization or changes in blood pH.

Capture Functions

1. The pacemaker's ability to generate a response from the heart (contraction) after electrical stimulation is referred to as capture. Capture is determined by the strength of the electrical stimulus, measured in milliamperes (mA), the amount

of time the stimulus is applied to the heart (pulse width), and by contact of the distal tip of the pacing lead to healthy myocardial tissue.
   a. "Electrical" capture is indicated by a pacer spike followed by a corresponding P wave or QRS complex.
   b. "Mechanical" capture of the ventricles is determined by a palpable pulse corresponding to the electrical event.

Pacemaker Codes

The Intersociety Commission for Heart Disease (ICHD) has established a five-letter code to describe the normal functioning of today's sophisticated pacemakers. Each letter indicates the particular characteristic of the pacer (see Table 12-2).

Nursing Process for Permanent Pacemaker Implantation

Nursing Assessment and Preprocedure Care

1. Assess patient's knowledge level of procedure.
2. Instruct patient that he or she may have nothing by mouth before the procedure.
3. Facilitate IV line insertion.
4. Explain to patient that pacemaker insertion will be performed in an operating or special procedures room with fluoroscopically and continuous ECG monitoring.
5. Describe local anesthetic that will be used to minimize discomfort; sedation.
6. Explain to patient that the usual placement for a permanent pacemaker is in the left upper chest.
7. If the patient had a recent infection, ensure that blood cultures are taken and are negative according to hospital policy, before any implantable device procedure so that implant or leads do not become infected.
8. Advise the patient that the incision will be closed with Steri-Strips (suture or staples may also be used).

Nursing Diagnoses

- Decreased Cardiac Output related to potential pacemaker malfunction and dysrhythmias.
- Risk for Injury related to pneumothorax, hemothorax, bleeding, microshock, and accidental malfunction.
- Risk for Infection related to surgical implantation of pacemaker generator and/or leads.

Table 12-2	Five-Letter Code for Pacemakers	
LETTER OR POSITION	**CHARACTERISTIC**	**CODE KEY**
I	Chamber paced (Where is the pacing taking place?)	V = Ventricle A = Atrium D = Dual (Both atrium and ventricle) O = None
II	Chamber sensed (Which chamber is being sensed?)	V = Ventricle A = Atrium D = Dual (Both atrium and ventricle) O = None
III	Mode of response (Response to the sensed events)	T = Triggers pacing I = Inhibits firing in response to a sensed intrinsic event D = Dual (triggers and inhibits at the same time) O = None; asynchronous pacemaker
IV	Programmability (Program functions)	P = Single programmability M = Multiple programmability C = Communication function (telemetry) O = Absence of rate modulation or programmability
V	Antitachyarrhythmia function	P = Overdrive pacing S = Shock intervention for cardioversion or defibrillation D = Dual (Pacing and shocking capabilities) O = Absence of pacing and shocking capabilities

- Anxiety related to pacemaker insertion, fear of death, lack of knowledge, and role change.
- Impaired Physical Mobility related to imposed restrictions of arm movement.
- Acute Pain related to surgical incision and transcutaneous external pacing stimuli.
- Disturbed Body Image related to pacemaker implantation.

Nursing Interventions

Maintaining Adequate Cardiac Output

1. Record the following information after insertion of the pacemaker:
   a. Pacemaker manufacturer, model, and lead type.
   b. Operating mode (based on ICHD code).
   c. Programmed settings: lower rate limit, upper rate limit, AV delay, and pacing thresholds.
   d. Patient's underlying rhythm.
   e. Patient's response to procedure.
2. Attach ECG electrodes for continuous monitoring of heart rate and rhythm.
   a. Set alarm limits 5 beats below lower rate limit and 5 to 10 beats above upper rate limits (ensures immediate detection of pacemaker malfunction or failure).
   b. Keep alarms on at all times.
3. Analyze rhythm strips per facility protocol and as necessary.
   a. Identify presence or absence of pacing artifact.
   b. Differentiate paced P waves and paced QRS complexes from spontaneous beats.
   c. Measure AV delay (if pacemaker has dual chamber functions).
   d. Determine the paced rate.
   e. Analyze the paced rhythm for presence and consistency of capture (every pacing spike is followed by atrial and/or ventricular depolarization).
   f. Analyze the rhythm for presence and consistency of proper sensing. (After a spontaneous beat, the pacemaker should not fire unless the interval between the spontaneous beat

and the paced beat equals the lower pacing rate and/or the paced beat follows the programmed AV delay.)
4. Monitor vital signs as per facility protocol and as necessary.
5. Monitor urine output and level of consciousness—ensures adequate cardiac output achieved with paced rhythm.
6. Observe for dysrhythmias (ventricular ectopic activity can occur because of irritation of ventricular wall by lead wire).
   a. Monitor for competitive rhythms, such as runs of atrial fibrillation or flutter, accelerated junctional, or idioventricular or ventricular tachycardia.
   b. Report dysrhythmias.
   c. Administer antidysrhythmic therapy, as directed.
7. Obtain 12-lead ECG, as ordered.

Avoiding Injury

1. Note that a postpacemaker insertion chest x-ray has been taken to ensure correct lead wire position and that no fluid is in lungs.
2. Monitor for signs and symptoms of hemothorax—inadvertent punctures of the subclavian vein or artery, which can cause fatal hemorrhage; observe for diaphoresis, hypotension, shortness of breath, chest deviation, and restlessness; immediate surgical intervention may be necessary.
3. Monitor for signs and symptoms of pneumothorax—inadvertent puncture of the lung; observe for acute onset of dyspnea, cyanosis, chest pain, absent breath sounds over involved lung, acute anxiety, and hypotension. Prepare for chest tube insertion.
4. Evaluate continually for evidence of bleeding/hematoma.
   a. Check incision site frequently for bleeding/hematoma.
   b. Apply manual pressure carefully without pushing against pacemaker generator box.
   c. Palpate for pulses distal to insertion site. (Swelling of tissues from bleeding may impede arterial flow.)
5. Be aware of hazards in the facility that can interfere with pacemaker function or cause pacemaker failure and permanent pacemaker damage.
   a. Avoid use of electric razors.
   b. Avoid direct placement of defibrillator paddles over pacemaker generator; anterior placement of paddles should

be 4 to 5 inches (10 to 12.5 cm) away from pacemaker; always evaluate pacemaker function after defibrillation.

c. Electrocautery devices and transcutaneous electrical nerve stimulator (TENS) units pose a risk.

d. Recent studies have shown that patients may safely have an MRI with a permanent pacemaker. Check with the cardiologist.

e. Caution must be used if patient will receive radiation therapy; the pacemaker should be repositioned if the unit lies directly in the radiation field.

6. Monitor for electrolyte imbalances, hypoxia, and myocardial ischemia. (The amount of energy the pacemaker needs to stimulate depolarization may need adjustment if any of these are present.)

Preventing Infection

1. Take temperature every 4 hours; report elevations. (Suspect permanent pacemaker as infection source if temperature elevation occurs.)

2. Observe incision site for signs and symptoms of local infection: redness, purulent drainage, warmth, and soreness.

3. Be alert to manifestations of bacteremia. (Patients with endocardial leads are at risk for endocarditis; see page 287.)

4. Clean incision site, as directed, using sterile technique.

5. Instruct patient to keep incision site dry, which means no showers for 24 hours.

6. Evaluate patient's complaints of increasing tenderness and discomfort at incision site.

7. Administer antibiotic therapy, as prescribed, after permanent pacemaker insertion.

Relieving Anxiety

1. Offer careful explanations regarding anticipated procedures and treatments, and answer the patient's questions with concise explanations.

2. Encourage patient and family to use coping mechanisms to overcome anxieties—talking, crying, and walking.

3. Encourage patient to accept responsibility for care.
   a. Review care plan with patient and family.
   b. Encourage patient to make decisions regarding a daily schedule of self-care activities.
   c. Engage patient in goal setting. Establish with patient priorities of care and time frames to accomplish goals up until discharge.

4. Monitor for unwarranted fears expressed by patient and family (commonly, pacemaker failure) and provide explanations to alleviate fear. Explain to patient life expectancy of batteries and the measures taken to check for failure (see "Patient Education").

Minimizing the Effects of Immobility

1. Encourage patient to take deep breaths frequently each hour (promotes pulmonary function); however, caution against vigorous coughing because this could cause lead dislodgement.

2. Instruct patient in dorsiflexion exercises of ankles and tightening of calf muscles. This promotes venous return and prevents venous stasis. Exercises should be done hourly.

3. Restrict movement of affected extremity (no restriction for leadless pacemaker).
   a. Place arm nearest to permanent pacemaker implant in sling as directed. Sling use can range from 6 to 24 hours, according to prescribed order.
   b. Instruct patient to gradually resume range of motion (ROM) of extremity as directed (usually 24 hours for permanent implants); avoid over-the-head motions for approximately 5 days and limit the weight of carried items to less than 3 pounds.
   c. Evaluate patient's arm movements to ensure normal ROM progression; assist patient with passive ROM of extremity as necessary (prevents development of shoulder stiffness caused by prolonged joint immobility); consult physical therapy as directed if stiffness and pain occur.

4. Assist patient with activities of daily living (ADLs) as appropriate.

Relieving Pain

1. Prepare patient for the discomfort he or she may experience after pacemaker implant.
   a. Explain to patient that incisional pain will occur after procedure; pain will subside after the first week, but he or she may have some soreness for up to 4 weeks.

2. Administer analgesics as directed; attempt to coincide peak analgesic effect with performance of ROM exercises and ADLs.

3. Offer back rubs to promote relaxation.

4. Provide patient with diversional activities.

5. Evaluate effectiveness of pain-relieving modalities.

6. Explain to the patient about the potential for discomfort during transcutaneous pacing; however, assure patient that the lowest energy possible will be used and analgesics/anxiolytics will be given.

Maintaining a Positive Body Image

1. Encourage patient and family to express concerns regarding self-image and pacemaker implant.

2. Reassure patient and significant other that sexual activity and modes of dressing will not be altered by pacemaker implantation.

3. Offer pacemaker support group information to the patient.

4. Encourage spouse or significant other to discuss concerns of self-image with patient.

Patient Education and Health Maintenance

Anatomy and Physiology of the Heart

Use diagrams to identify heart structure, conduction system, area where pacemaker is inserted, and why the pacemaker is needed.

Pacemaker Function

1. Give patient the manufacturer's instructions (for particular pacemaker) and help familiarize patient with pacemaker.

2. If available, give patient a pacemaker to hold and identify unique features of patient's pacemaker, or show patient picture of pacemaker.

3. Explain to patient the purpose and function of the component parts of the pacemaker: generator and lead system.

Activity

1. Reassure patient that normal activities will be able to be resumed.

2. Explain to patient that it takes about 2 months to develop full ROM of arm (fibrosis occurs around the lead and stabilizes it in the heart).

3. Specific instructions include the following:
   a. Instruct patient not to lift items over 3 pounds (1.4 kg) or perform difficult arm maneuvers.
   b. Tell patient to avoid activities that involve rough contact around pacemaker site.
   c. Caution patient not to fire a rifle with it resting over pacemaker implant.

d. Sexual activity may be resumed when desired.

e. Instruct patient not to rub or massage around pacemaker site.

4. Instruct patient to gauge activities according to sensations of moderate pain in the arm or site of implant and stretching sensation in and around implant site.

Pacemaker Failure

1. Teach patient to check own pulse rate daily for 1 full minute and to keep a chart for physician visit. This pulse check should be done at rest. (Patients may check pulse daily to ensure all is well and promote a sense of control.)

2. Teach patient to:

    a. Immediately report slowing of pulse lower than set rate, or greater than 100.

    b. Report signs and symptoms of dizziness, fainting, palpitation, prolonged hiccups, and chest pain to health care provider immediately. These signs are indicative of pacemaker failure.

    c. Take pulse while these feelings are being experienced.

3. Encourage patient to wear identification bracelet and carry pacemaker identification card that lists pacemaker type, rate, health care provider's name, and facility where the pacemaker was inserted; encourage significant other to also keep a card with patient's pacemaker information.

Electromagnetic Interference

1. Advise patient that improvements in pacemaker design have reduced problems of electromechanical interference (EMI).

2. Caution patient that EMI could interfere with pacemaker function.

    a. Inappropriate inhibition or triggering of pacemaker stimuli causing light-headedness, syncope, or death.

    b. Atrial oversensing may cause inappropriate pacemaker acceleration and can cause palpitations, hypotension, or angina in patients.

    c. Rapid pacing can also result in ventricular fibrillation.

    d. Reversion to a synchronous pacing mode. A common response to transient reversion is asynchrony pacing, which can cause irregular heartbeats and/or a decrease in CO, and that may stimulate ventricular tachyarrhythmias.

    e. Reprogramming of the pacemaker or permanent damage to the pacemaker's circuitry or the electrode–tissue interface is less frequent in occurrence.

    f. Teach patient to move 4 to 6 feet away from source and to check pulse if dizziness or palpitations occur. Pulse should return to normal after moving away from interference.

3. Explain that high-energy radiation, linear power amplifiers, antennas, industrial arc welders, electrocautery equipment, TENS, unshielded motors (cars, boats), MRI equipment found in facilities, and junkyards may affect pacemaker function.

4. Tell patient that metal detectors or handheld wands may affect pacemaker function and that pacemakers will set off the alarm at metal detector gates. Therefore, patient should show pacemaker identification card and request a hand search.

5. Antitheft devices may interfere with pacemaker function if the patient remains stationary for an extended period of time near the device. Walking by the device should not interfere with pacemaker function.

6. Tell patient that household and kitchen appliances will not affect pacemaker function. Microwave ovens are no longer a threat to pacemaker operation (however, old warning signs may still be near microwave ovens). Cell phones are safe as long as they are 6 inches away from pacemaker site. Encourage patient to use the ear on the opposite side of the pacemaker site.

Care of Pacemaker Site

1. Advise patient to wear loose-fitting clothing around the area of pacemaker implantation until it has healed.

2. Watch for signs and symptoms of infection around generator and leads—fever, heat, pain, and skin breakdown at implant site.

3. Advise patient to keep incision clean and dry. Encourage tub baths rather than showers for the first 10 days after pacemaker implantation.

    a. Instruct patient not to scrub incision site or clean site with bath water.

    b. Teach patient to clean incision site with antiseptic, as directed.

4. Explain to patient that healing will take approximately 3 months.

    a. Instruct patient to maintain a well-balanced diet to promote healing.

5. Inform patient that there is no increased risk of endocarditis with dental cleaning or procedures, so antibiotic prophylaxis is not necessary.

 GERONTOLOGIC ALERT Older patients may experience delayed wound healing because of poor nutritional status. Evaluate nutritional intake carefully and offer a balanced diet including vitamin C to ensure proper healing.

Follow-Up

1. Make sure that the patient has a copy of ECG tracing (according to facility policy) for future comparisons. Encourage patient to have regular pacemaker checkups for monitoring function and integrity of pacemaker.

2. Inform patient that transtelephonic evaluation of implanted cardiac pacemakers for battery and electrode failure is available.

3. Review medications with patient before discharge.

4. Inform patient that the pulse generator will have to be surgically removed to replace battery and that it is a relatively simple procedure performed under local anesthesia.

Evaluation: Expected Outcomes

- Vital signs stable; pacing spikes rated on ECG tracing.
- Breath sounds noted throughout; respirations unlabored.
- Incision without drainage.
- Asks questions and participates in care.
- Affected arm and pacer site show decreased edema.
- Reports pain relief.
- Verbalizes acceptance of pacemaker.

Defibrillation and Cardioversion

Defibrillation is the use of electrical energy, delivered over a brief period, to temporarily depolarize the heart, so that when it repolarizes, it has a better chance of resuming normal electrical activity. It is used to treat ventricular fibrillation and ventricular tachycardia without a pulse, with the goal of converting to normal sinus rhythm.

Synchronized cardioversion is the use of electrical energy that is synchronized to the QRS complex so as not to hit the T wave during the cardiac cycle, which may cause ventricular fibrillation. It is used to treat atrial fibrillation, atrial flutter, supraventricular tachycardia, and ventricular tachycardia with a pulse.

Concepts

1. Types of defibrillators:
   a. Direct current defibrillators contain a transformer, an alternating-current–direct current converter, a capacitor to store direct current, a charge switch, and a discharge switch to the electrodes to complete the circuit.
   b. Portable defibrillators have a battery as a power source and must be plugged in at all times when not in use.
   c. Automatic external defibrillator (AED) may be used inside the facility or in the community to deliver electric shock to the heart before trained personnel arrive with a manual defibrillator. AEDs are accurate to be used by less trained individuals because the device has a detection system that analyzes the person's rhythm, detects the presence of ventricular fibrillation or tachycardia, and instructs the operator to discharge a shock.

2. Steps in defibrillation:
   a. Immediately implement CPR until the defibrillator is available.
   b. Expose the patient's bare chest and apply defibrillator paddles or pads according to manufacturer's instructions. See Figure 12-7.
   c. Turn the defibrillator to recommended setting, usually 200 joules, and charge paddles.
   d. Once the defibrillator is charged, give the "all-clear" warning, and ensure that no one is touching the patient. Shock the patient by doing the following:
      i. Paddles: Push the discharge buttons (shock) on the paddles while exerting 25 pounds of pressure on the patient's chest.
      ii. Pads: Push the discharge buttons (shock) on the defibrillator device.
   e. Continue CPR for 2 minutes and repeat defibrillation process unless return of spontaneous circulation (ROSC) has occurred.
   f. Once ROSC is restored, continue supportive care of the patient.

3. Steps in cardioversion:
   a. Ensure that laboratory results are available, serum potassium level is normal, digoxin has not been given, and oxygen is available. The procedure is usually elective; therefore, fasting may be ordered.
   b. Have emergency equipment available in the room, such as oxygen and suction.
   c. Apply paddles or multifunctional pads according to manufacturer's instructions; for cardioversion, pads are preferred.

   d. Turn defibrillator to synchronize setting and charge to the ordered level. Ensure that the synchronized marking is visible.
   e. Once the machine is charged, give the "all-clear" warning and ensure that no one is touching the patient. Shock the patient by doing the following:
      i. Paddles: Push the discharge buttons (shock) on the paddles while exerting 25 pounds of pressure on the patient's chest.
      ii. Pads: Push the discharge buttons (shock) on the defibrillator device.
   f. Be aware that when the shock button is pressed, there may be a delay while synchronizing with the R wave until the shock is delivered.

 NURSING ALERT Synchronized cardioversion is generally contraindicated when a patient has been taking a significant amount of digoxin because more lethal dysrhythmias may occur after electric discharge.

Implantable Cardioverter–Defibrillator

The *implantable cardioverter–defibrillator (ICD)* is a device that delivers electric shocks directly to the heart muscle (defibrillation) to terminate lethal dysrhythmias: ventricular fibrillation and ventricular tachycardia. The ICD is surgically placed by one of four approaches: lateral thoracotomy, median sternotomy (in conjunction with cardiac surgery), subxiphoid, or subintercostal. All ICDs have a pacing function, if needed. See Figure 12-8.

Concepts

1. Sudden cardiac death as a result of ventricular tachycardia or fibrillation remains the leading cause of death in the United States.
2. ICDs terminate ventricular fibrillation and tachycardia automatically, thereby preventing sudden death.
3. Currently, ICDs can deliver high-energy or low-energy shocks, can be programmed for demand and rate-response

Figure 12-7. Paddle placement for ventricular fibrillation.

Figure 12-8. Implantable cardioverter–defibrillator.

pacing, can be programmed for antitachycardic pacing, provide noninvasive electrical stimulation to conduct EPS, can be programmed for tiered therapy, and have the ability to record and store ECGs of tachycardic episodes.

Indications

1. Cardiac arrest because of ventricular fibrillation or tachycardia not because of transient or reversible causes.
2. Spontaneous sustained ventricular tachycardia with structural heart disease.
3. Syncope of undetermined origin with clinically relevant, hemodynamically significant ventricular tachycardia or ventricular fibrillation induced by EPS when drug therapy is not effective or tolerated.
4. Nonsustained ventricular tachycardia in patients with CAD, prior MI, left ventricular dysfunction, and inducible ventricular fibrillation or sustained ventricular tachycardia at EPS that is not suppressed by class I antiarrhythmic drugs.
5. Spontaneous sustained ventricular tachycardia in patients without structural disease not amenable to other treatment.
6. Nonischemic dilated cardiomyopathy with LVEF less than or equal to 35% and who are in the NYHA functional class II or III.

Design

The ICD is slightly larger than a pacemaker and consists of two parts:
1. Pulse generator—contains the circuitry and battery to detect dysrhythmias and generate the electric shock. The generator is usually placed in the left pectoral region and is commonly referred to as the active can or hot-can.
   a. Battery life depends on amount of shocks and pacing and is usually 5 to 6 years.
   b. The direct-current electric shock delivered is 25 to 35 joules. Depending on the device, it can be programmed up to 41 joules.
2. Lead system—consists of two components.
   a. Pace–sense component: monitors the heart rhythm and can deliver pacing output.
   b. Shocking coils: deliver the electrical shocks needed for defibrillation.
3. Most ICDs (but not all) can be noninvasively deactivated by a doughnut-shaped magnet. This will disable the ICD therapies of ATP and electrical cardioversion–defibrillation but will not turn off the pacemaker function. However, the magnet may initiate asynchronous pacing.

Function

Electric shocks are delivered in a programmed sequence:
1. The device detects a lethal dysrhythmia, charges and reconfirms that the lethal dysrhythmia is still present, and then "defibrillates" the heart. The lethal dysrhythmia must meet two programmed criteria (rate and amount of time spent from the isoelectric line) to trigger the device to emit an initial electric shock. The number of joules necessary to convert each patient is determined during insertion and testing of the device; it is usually 15 to 25 joules.
2. Nontermination of the lethal dysrhythmia by the initial shock triggers the device to continue the sequence (detect, charge, and defibrillate) until a total of four or five shocks have been delivered (the number of shocks depends on device model implanted).
   a. Subsequent shocks are slightly higher, at 30 to 32 joules.
   b. The total sequence lasts approximately 2 minutes.

3. Termination of the lethal dysrhythmia after the shock sequence signals the device to revert to the "detection" mode of operation and not to reinitiate the shocking sequence. The device will reinitiate the shocking sequence only if a rhythm other than the lethal dysrhythmia is detected and maintained for at least 35 seconds. If this criterion is met and another lethal dysrhythmia is detected, the device will cycle through the shocking sequence again.
4. Termination of a lethal dysrhythmia at any time during the shocking sequence signals the device to interrupt the sequence, return to a detection mode, and reinitiate the shocking sequence if another lethal dysrhythmia is detected.

Complications

1. Many complications that occurred previously with ICDs have been decreased by the use of the transvenous technique for implantation that is similar to that of permanent pacemaker insertion.
2. Complications associated with implantation of the ICD include:
   a. Acceleration of arrhythmias.
   b. Air emboli.
   c. Bleeding.
   d. Perforation of the myocardium.
   e. Pneumothorax.
   f. Puncture of the subclavian vein.
   g. Thromboemboli.
   h. Venous occlusion.
3. Complications that can occur after placement of an ICD:
   a. Chronic nerve damage.
   b. Diaphragmatic stimulation.
   c. Erosion of pulse generator.
   d. Formation of pocket hematoma.
   e. Fluid accumulation/seroma.
   f. Infection of pocket/system.
   g. Keloid formation.
   h. Lead dislodgement.
   i. Lead fracture and insulation breaks.
   j. Venous thrombosis.

Nursing Diagnoses

- Anxiety related to invasive procedure and fear of death.
- Risk for Infection related to invasive procedure and implanted device.
- Decreased Cardiac Output related to surgical procedure, hypotension, cardiac tamponade, and/or dysrhythmias.
- Ineffective Breathing Pattern related to surgical procedure and discomfort.

Nursing Interventions

Reducing Anxiety

1. Explain to patient and family reason for implant, surgical procedure, and preprocedure and postprocedure management:
   a. Performed in the operating room or in an electrophysiology laboratory.
   b. Incision location.
   c. May need endotracheal (ET) intubation if unable to sedate.
   d. IV line; continuous ECG monitoring.
   e. Early mobilization after procedure.
   f. Coughing and deep breathing exercises.
   g. Management of incisional pain.
   h. Device turned on once implanted.

2. Provide emotional support to patient and family.
   a. Assess patient's and family's knowledge level, support systems, and usual coping mechanisms.
   b. Psychiatric counseling may be beneficial because patient is facing life-threatening issues.
   c. Encourage patient and family to verbalize fears and/or expectations of hospitalization, lifestyle adjustments, self-concept, body image, and device malfunction (misfiring or failure to fire).
   d. Reinforce to patient that daily activities will not increase the risk of the device misfiring.
   e. Explain the sensation that might be felt if the device fires and the patient is conscious. (Many patients will become unconscious before the device fires and therefore feel no sensations.) Sensations experienced in conscious patients vary, but are commonly described as a severe chest blow.
3. Allow patient to participate in care as much as possible.
   a. Encourage patient to dress in street clothes during hospitalization. (Loose-fitting clothes are recommended to prevent chafing and irritation at implant site.)
   b. Allow patient to look at incision site.
   c. Give patient instructional booklets about the device.

Preventing Infection

1. Check temperature every 4 hours; report elevations. (Early postoperative fever may be due to atelectasis; defibrillator system as infection source commonly occurs within 5 to 10 days of implantation.)
2. Evaluate incision site every 4 hours for signs of infection.
3. Culture drainage from incision.
4. Evaluate incision for tissue erosion.
5. Monitor WBC count and differential.
6. Clean incision and change dressing as directed, using aseptic technique.
7. Administer antibiotics, as ordered, before and after the procedure.

 GERONTOLOGIC ALERT Older patients may not demonstrate abnormal temperature elevations with infections and experience prolonged wound healing.

Maintaining Adequate Cardiac Output

1. Monitor vital signs frequently until stable.
2. Evaluate incision site for evidence of bleeding or hematoma.
3. Evaluate urine output.
4. Be alert to risk for dysrhythmias postoperatively. (Manipulation of the heart and swelling may induce dysrhythmias 24 to 48 hours after implant.)
5. Monitor for changes in blood pressure as a sudden drop may indicate cardiac tamponade.
6. Evaluate carefully all complaints of chest pain (noncardiac pain may be due to lead fracture or dislodgement; pain may be noted along wire pathways).
7. Auscultate heart sounds every 4 hours for presence of friction rub or muffled heart sounds.

NURSING ALERT Cardiopulmonary resuscitation (CPR) should be started immediately on any patient with an implantable defibrillator who becomes unconscious and has no pulse. A slight "buzz" sensation will be felt if the implanted device delivers a shock, but it is not harmful. Gloves may be worn to minimize the sensation.

Promoting Effective Breathing Pattern

1. Ask patient to take several deep breaths every hour to expand lung fields.
2. Encourage coughing and deep breathing exercises frequently; medicate with analgesics before exercises and provide a pillow for splinting.
3. Monitor use of incentive spirometer.
4. Elevate head of bed to promote adequate ventilation.
5. Auscultate lung fields every 4 hours.
6. Assist with position changes every 2 hours while on bed rest.
7. Encourage early ambulation.
8. Administer analgesics, as ordered.

Patient Education and Health Maintenance

Introduction to Implantable Defibrillator

1. Review anatomy of the heart with emphasis on the conduction system, using a diagram of the heart.
2. Give accurate explanations, using correct medical terminology (allows patient to interact with the health care team more effectively), regarding reason for device implantation, components of system, and function of device.
   a. Use manufacturer's instructional booklet and video presentation about the device.
   b. Encourage family members to participate in education process.

Living with the Implantable Defibrillator

1. Instruct patient and family on actions to be taken if the device fires.
   a. Explain signs and symptoms that may be experienced if a lethal dysrhythmia occurs: palpitations, dizziness, shortness of breath, and chest pain.
   b. If signs and symptoms occur, lie down and try to call 911 for help if alone.
   c. Family members should check for a pulse if patient becomes unconscious. CPR should be started immediately if no pulse is present and 911 has been called.
   d. Reinforce that shocks emitted from device are not harmful, and CPR should never be delayed to wait for device to complete the shocking sequence.
   e. If patient remains conscious or is unconscious with a pulse, family members should monitor patient during episode, continually assessing for a pulse during shocking sequence. After the episode, follow health care provider's instructions as directed.
   f. Notify health care provider immediately.
2. Explore with patient and family fears about failure of device, sensation associated with a shock, and injury to others if a shock occurs.
   a. Sensations experienced vary but are most commonly described as a severe blow to the chest.
   b. No injury will occur to others if in contact with patient during a shock; a slight shock may be felt by your partner if the device fires during sexual intercourse.
   c. Battery life depends on frequency of use. The device is evaluated in 4 to 6 weeks after implantation and then every 3 months. Newer devices may allow for checks from home.
3. Review sources of EMI that should be avoided (see page 251).
4. Advise patient that there is no increased risk of endocarditis, so antibiotic prophylaxis before dental work is not necessary.
5. Review with health care provider resumption of activities, such as lifting, driving, sports, and sexual activity.

Other Instructions

1. Review care of incision site (see page 251).
2. Loose-fitting clothing should be worn until healing takes place.
3. Provide MedicAlert card; encourage carrying card at all times and obtaining a corresponding MedicAlert bracelet.
4. Explain how to keep diary of episodes and record dates of 4- to 6-month follow-up appointments.
5. Provide information to family members regarding CPR training courses.
6. Encourage use of support groups.
7. Always carry a list of current medications and name and number of physician and emergency contacts.

Evaluation: Expected Outcomes

- Verbalizes understanding of device and surgical procedure.
- Afebrile; incision without drainage.
- Vital signs stable; no dysrhythmias.
- Respirations unlabored; lungs clear.

Pericardiocentesis

Pericardiocentesis is an invasive procedure, which involves the puncture of the pericardial sac to aspirate fluid. The pericardium typically contains 10 to 50 mL of sterile fluid. Excessive fluid within the pericardial sac can cause compression of the heart chambers, resulting in an acute decrease in CO (cardiac tamponade). Fluid accumulation (pericardial effusion) can occur rapidly (acute) or slowly (subacute). The amount of excess fluid the pericardium is able to accommodate is individually based on the ability of the pericardium to stretch. Once the stretch has been maximized, intrapericardial pressure rises, possibly causing circulatory compromise.

Acute—a rapid increase of fluid into pericardial space (as little as 200 mL) causes a marked rise in intrapericardial pressure. Emergency intervention is required to prevent severe circulatory compromise.

Subacute—slow accumulation of fluid into pericardial sac over weeks or months, causing the pericardium to stretch and accommodate up to 2 L of fluid without severe increases in intrapericardial pressure.

Both of these situations require intervention to remove the pericardial fluid. Pericardiocentesis is frequently performed in the cardiac catheterization laboratory under fluoroscopy or assisted by echocardiographic imaging. In the case of severely decompensated cardiac tamponade, pericardiocentesis can be safely performed at the bedside with echocardiography.

Purposes

1. To remove fluid from the pericardial sac caused by:
   a. Infection.
   b. Malignant neoplasm or lymphoma.
   c. Trauma (blunt or penetrating wounds or from cardiac surgery or procedure).
   d. Drugs and toxins.
   e. Radiation.
   f. MI.
   g. Collagen vascular disease.
   h. Aortic dissection extending to the pericardium.
   i. Metabolic disorders, especially uremia, dialysis, and hypothyroidism.
   j. Cardiac diagnostic or interventional procedures.
   k. An idiopathic condition.

2. To obtain fluid for diagnosis.
3. To instill certain therapeutic drugs.

Sites for Pericardiocentesis

1. Subxiphoid—needle inserted in the angle between left costal margin and xiphoid.
2. Near cardiac apex, three-fourth inch (2 cm) inside left border of cardiac dullness.
3. To the left of the fifth or sixth interspace at the sternal margin.
4. Right side of fourth intercostal space just inside border of dullness.

Nursing Considerations

1. Administer sedation as prescribed to reduce anxiety.
2. If performed at bedside, ensure that patient is monitored and that emergency resuscitation equipment, defibrillator, and pacemaker are immediately available.
3. During and following the procedure, monitor for complications including dysrhythmias and bloody drainage (hemopericardium).
4. Following the procedure, report the presence of pericardial friction rub and distant heart sounds, indicating reaccumulation of fluid causing cardiac tamponade.

Percutaneous Coronary Intervention

 EVIDENCE BASE Mitchell, J., & Brown, D. (2016). Update on percutaneous coronary intervention in stable coronary artery disease. *JAMA Internal Medicine, 176*(12), 1855–1856.

Percutaneous coronary intervention (PCI) is a broad term used to describe all invasive coronary interventions. Initially, PCI was limited to balloon angioplasty; however, it now includes intracoronary stenting and a wide spectrum of percutaneous procedures utilized to treat coronary disease. PCI has also replaced coronary artery bypass grafting (CABG) as the preferred treatment for CAD. Commonly performed PCIs include percutaneous transluminal coronary angioplasty (PTCA) with intracoronary stenting, laser-assisted PTCA, and direct coronary atherectomy (DCA). Radial vascular access is recommended over femoral access for PCI, because of lower vascular complication rate and comparable efficacy and safety in relation to the primary outcome of death.

Types of Procedures

Percutaneous Transluminal Coronary Angioplasty

Percutaneous transluminal coronary angioplasty (PTCA) accesses the femoral, brachial, or radial artery, with the right femoral artery being the most common access site. The site is anesthetized and an arterial sheath is placed into the vessel. Under fluoroscopy, a catheter is advanced through the arterial sheath and directed to the coronary lesion. To visualize the coronary anatomy, specific radiographic projections are used with the fluoroscopy tube through the use of an injection of contrast dye. Once a coronary lesion or narrowing is identified, a balloon-tipped catheter is advanced through wire to the lesion. The balloon is then inflated to displace coronary plaque against the vessel wall (see Figure 12-9). Balloon inflation and deflation may be repeated until optimal flow is achieved in the affected vessel.

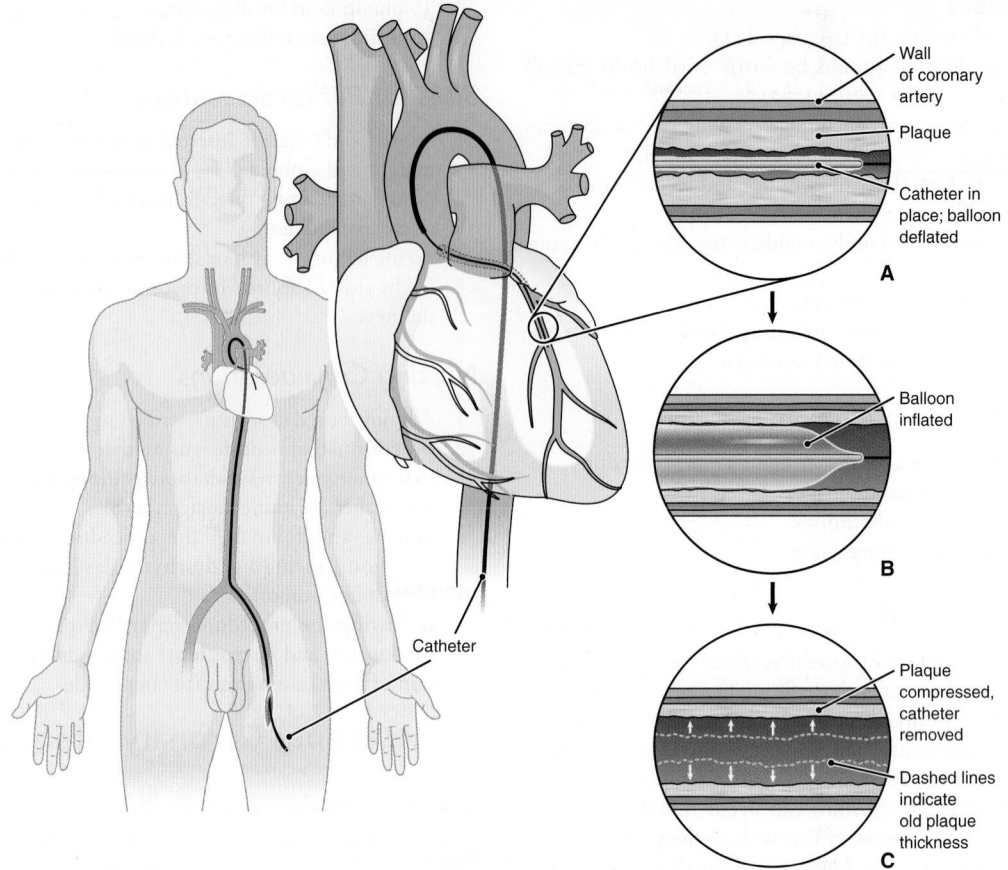

Figure 12-9. Percutaneous transluminal coronary angioplasty. **(A)** The balloon-tipped catheter is passed into the affected coronary artery. **(B)** The balloon is then rapidly inflated and deflated with controlled pressure. **(C)** The balloon disrupts the intima and causes changes in the atheroma, resulting in an increase in the diameter of the lumen of the vessel and improvement of blood flow. (Redrawn from Purcell, J.A., and Giffin, P.A. (1981). Percutaneous transluminal coronary angioplasty. *American Journal of Nursing* 9:1620–1626.)

Intracoronary Stenting

Intracoronary stents are small meshed metal tubes that are mounted onto a balloon angioplasty catheter. Once initial angioplasty is performed, the angioplasty catheter is removed and replaced with a stent catheter. When the balloon is inflated, the stent is deployed and pressed into the intima of the artery where the occlusion existed. The balloon is deflated and the catheter is removed; however, the stent remains. The intracoronary stent acts as a scaffold helping to hold the artery open, thereby improving blood flow and relieving symptoms once caused by the blockage. Stents may be uncoated, called bare metal stents, or coated, called drug-eluting stents (DESs). DESs are intended and are preferred over bare metal stents to limit the overgrowth of normal tissue following implantation.

Laser-Assisted Balloon Angioplasty

A laser light is directed by a percutaneously inserted flexible fiberoptic catheter and can "vaporize" atheromatous lesions in the coronary vessels. Balloon angioplasty of the vessel may then be performed. This technique may minimize damage to the intimal lining, open diseased vessels more effectively, prevent early and long-term restenosis, and expand the use of angioplasty to calcified, unusual lesions and total occlusions. The most important complication of laser-assisted balloon angioplasty involves minor to major coronary dissection of the treated lesion.

Direct Coronary Atherectomy

Direct coronary atherectomy (DCA) permits more controlled vascular injury and decreases the degree of arterial mural stretch that can occur with PTCA and balloon angioplasty. To remove plaque, DCA works by changing plaque into microscopic debris, thereby opening the diseased vessel more effectively, especially in patients who have coronary lesions not amenable to standard angioplasty. Complications associated with DCA include vascular spasm at the site of plaque removal or distal to the treated site; possible myocardial necrosis, evidenced by elevations of CK-MB; vessel perforation (infrequent but devastating); and groin complications and groin bleeding (more common with atherectomy procedures because of the size of the catheters involved).

Indications

Indications for PCI include the following (only after a comprehensive risk–benefit analysis has been reviewed): recurrent ischemia despite anti-ischemia therapy, elevated troponin levels, new ST-segment depression, symptoms of heart failure or new or worsening mitral insufficiency, depressed left ventricular systolic function, hemodynamic instability, sustained ventricular tachycardia, PCI within 6 months, prior CABG, and high-risk findings from noninvasive testing, including unprotected left main artery disease.

Contraindications

1. PCI is not indicated for patients who have no evidence of high-risk findings associated with single-vessel or multivessel CAD.
2. Procedure-related morbidity or mortality may be linked to the following relative contraindications, many of which may be avoided or reversed prior to PCI:
   a. Allergy (severe) to radiographic contrast dye.
   b. Anticoagulated state.
   c. Decompensated heart failure (eg, acute pulmonary edema).
   d. Digoxin toxicity.
   e. Febrile state.
   f. Severe renal insufficiency.
   g. Uncorrected hypertension.
   h. Uncorrected hypokalemia.
   i. Ventricular irritability, uncontrolled.

Complications

1. Major complications or adverse outcomes include death, post-procedure MI, or need for emergent cardiac bypass surgery.
2. Other complications include:
   a. Anaphylaxis.
   b. Arrhythmias.
   c. Arterial dissection/coronary artery dissection.
   d. Bleeding.
   e. Cardiac perforation.
   f. Coronary occlusion, total.
   g. Hematoma at access site.
   h. Renal failure.
   i. Restenosis—occurs in 30% to 50% of PTCA and 10% to 30% of intracoronary stenting procedures.
   j. Stroke.
   k. Tamponade.

 NURSING ALERT Although the occurrence of complications from PCI has declined, immediate CABG surgery must be available with a cardiac surgical team on standby.

 DRUG ALERT Missed doses of anticoagulants following intracoronary stenting procedures are clearly linked to restenosis. The patient's ability to adhere to strict anticoagulation protocol will impact on the success of the procedure.

Nursing Diagnoses

- Anxiety related to impending invasive procedure.
- Decreased Cardiac Output related to dysrhythmias, vessel restenosis, or spasm.
- Risk for Injury (bleeding) related to femoral catheter and effect of anticoagulant and/or thrombolytic therapy.
- Acute Pain related to invasive procedure or myocardial ischemia.

Nursing Interventions

Reducing Anxiety

1. Reinforce the reasons for the procedure.
   a. Describe the location of the coronary vessels using a diagram of the heart.
   b. Describe/draw the location of the patient's lesion using heart diagram.
2. Explain the events that will occur before, during, and after the procedure. Preparation minimizes anxiety and increases compliance with care regimen.
   a. Performed in the cardiac catheterization laboratory; similar to the cardiac catheterization procedure (see page 243).
   b. Mild sedation given; patient remains awake throughout the procedure to report any chest pain (indicates myocardial ischemia).
   c. Assure patient that chest pain will be taken care of during the procedure.
3. Prepare patient for complications of procedure. Provide preoperative teaching to patient and family regarding procedure, potential complications, and risks associated with heart surgery (see page 260).
4. Explain the necessity of the IV, ECG monitoring, frequent vital sign and groin checks, and remaining NPO before the procedure.

Maintaining Adequate Cardiac Output

1. Check vital signs according to facility policy, typically every 15 minutes for 1 hour, then every 30 minutes for 2 hours, and subsequently every 1 to 2 hours.
2. Continually evaluate for signs and symptoms of restenosis.
   a. Emphasize importance of reporting any chest discomfort or jaw, back, or arm pain and/or nausea and abdominal distress.
   b. Perform ECG for all complaints suspicious of possible myocardial ischemia.
   c. Administer oxygen and vasodilator therapy for pain, as directed.
   d. Obtain CK and isoenzymes as directed.
   e. Keep patient NPO if prolonged chest pain occurs (patient may return to catheterization laboratory).
3. Administer medications to maintain vessel patency.
   a. Antiplatelet or antithrombin agents may be given during and after procedure to prevent reocclusion (eg, cangrelor, tirofiban, bivalirudin, eptifibatide, abciximab). Clopidogrel, or prasugrel, or ticagrelor may be given prior to PCI after STEMI.
   b. Low-dose heparin or low molecular weight heparin (enoxaparin) may also be used.
   c. Many patients are then maintained on medications such as clopidogrel, ticagrelor, or prasugrel. Aspirin and statins are also used. Reinforce compliance with drug therapy.
4. Evaluate fluid and electrolyte balance.
   a. Record intake and output.
   b. Encourage fluid intake or maintain IV fluids pre- and post-procedure to ensure adequate hydration to prevent contrast medium–induced nephropathy.
   c. Observe for dysrhythmias possibly related to potassium imbalance. Excessive diuresis causes potassium depletion.
   d. Administer potassium supplement, as prescribed.
5. Be alert to the risk of vasovagal reaction during removal of groin catheter if closure device is not employed.
   a. Observe for bradycardia, hypotension, diaphoresis, or nausea.
   b. Administer IV atropine, as directed.
   c. Place patient in Trendelenburg position to promote blood return to the heart and improve hypotension.
   d. Give fluid challenge as directed.

Preventing Bleeding

1. Refer to facility policy for activity progression regimen, usually gradual head elevation with ambulation within 4 to 6 hours after sheath removal. Maintain bed rest with affected extremity immobilized and head of bed elevated no more than 30 degrees (in the event the catheter remains) to prevent catheter dislodgement and bleeding.
2. Mark peripheral pulses before procedure with indelible ink.
3. Check peripheral pulse of affected extremity and insertion site with each vital sign check.
4. Observe color, temperature, and sensation of affected extremity with each vital sign check.
5. Report if extremities become cool and pale and pulses become significantly diminished or absent.
6. Look for presence of hematoma and mark hematoma to note change in size. Report if hematoma continues to enlarge.
7. Note petechiae, hematuria, and complaints of flank pain (vessel patency is maintained by not reversing intraprocedure heparinization; chance of bleeding is increased).
8. Apply direct pressure over insertion site if bleeding is observed and report immediately.
9. Check bed linen under patient frequently for blood.
10. Ask patient to report sensation of warmth at groin area.

Relieving Pain

1. Administer analgesics and anxiolytic medication, as directed.
2. Ensure a restful environment.
   a. Provide back rubs for muscle relaxation.
   b. Minimize noise and interruptions.
   c. Offer sleep medication, as indicated.
3. Progress patient's diet as tolerated (clear liquids/full liquid diet until catheters removed); assist patient with meals.

Patient Education and Health Maintenance

Instruct patient as follows:
1. Modification of cardiac risk factors as means of controlling progression of CAD.
2. Name of medications, action, dosage, and adverse effects.
   a. Common medications to prevent clot formation.
   b. Medications to increase blood flow to the heart.
   c. Medications to slow heart rate and reduce chest pain.
   d. Medications to increase blood flow and prevent coronary artery spasm.
3. Dates and importance of any follow-up tests.
4. Symptoms for which patient should seek medical attention, such as adverse effects of medication and chest pain—especially chest pain unrelieved by nitroglycerin.
5. Restenosis (with or without stent) can occur; the patient typically presents with the previous same symptoms; however, the symptoms may vary if a different lesion is involved.

Evaluation: Expected Outcomes

- Verbalizes understanding of procedure.
- Vital signs stable; urine output adequate.
- No bleeding or hematoma at insertion site.
- Verbalizes relief of pain.

Intra-Aortic Balloon Pump Counterpulsation

Counterpulsation is a method of assisting the failing heart and circulation by mechanical support when the myocardium is unable to generate adequate CO. The mechanism of counterpulsation therapy is opposite to the normal pumping action of the heart; counterpulsation devices pump while the heart muscle relaxes (diastole) and relax when the heart muscle contracts (systole).

Indications

1. Postcardiotomy support; low cardiac output after cardiopulmonary bypass.
2. Severe unstable angina that is refractory to pharmacologic therapy.
3. Cardiogenic shock/left-sided heart failure after MI, myocarditis, cardiomyopathy, myocardial contusion, and refractory heart failure.
4. Postinfarction ventricular septal defects or mitral insufficiency resulting in shock.
5. Emergency support following PTCA or high-risk percutaneous coronary interventions.
6. Hemodynamic deterioration in patients awaiting heart transplant.
7. Refractory ventricular arrhythmias.
8. Patients with severe left main coronary arterial stenosis whom surgery is pending.
9. Adjunctive therapy after fibrinolysis in patients at high-risk restenosis.

Function

1. A balloon catheter is introduced into the femoral artery percutaneously or surgically, threaded to the proximal descending thoracic aorta, and positioned 1 to 2 cm distal to the origin of the left subclavian artery (see Figure 12-10).
2. In patients with severe peripheral arterial disease, axillary artery approach should be considered, especially if longer support is needed (see Figure 12-10). This allows for early mobilization and reduces the risk of infection.
3. The balloon catheter is attached to an external console, allowing for inflation and deflation of the balloon with gas such as He (helium). Helium has low viscosity that allows quick travel through the long connecting tubes, and it has low potential for gas embolization should the balloon rupture.
4. The external console integrates the inflation and deflation sequence with the mechanical events of the cardiac cycle (systole–diastole) by "triggering" gas delivery in synchronization with the patient's ECG, the patient's arterial waveform, atrial/ventricular paced rhythm, or intrinsic pump rate.
   a. The most common method of "triggering" or signaling the intra-aortic balloon pump (IABP) is from the R wave of the patient's ECG signal.
   b. The balloon is automatically set to inflate in the middle of the T wave or at the dicrotic notch of the arterial waveform. This occurs immediately after aortic valve closure.
5. Eases the workload of a damaged heart by increasing coronary blood flow (diastolic augmentation) and decreasing the resistance in the arterial tree against which the heart must pump (afterload reduction).
6. This results in an increase in CO and a reduction in myocardial oxygen requirements.
7. The balloon is inflated at the onset of diastole; this results in an increase in diastolic aortic pressure (diastolic augmentation), which increases blood flow through the coronary arteries.
8. The balloon is deflated just before the onset of systole (just before aortic valve opening), facilitating the emptying of blood from the left ventricle and decreasing pressure within the aorta. This action results in less work for the left ventricle.

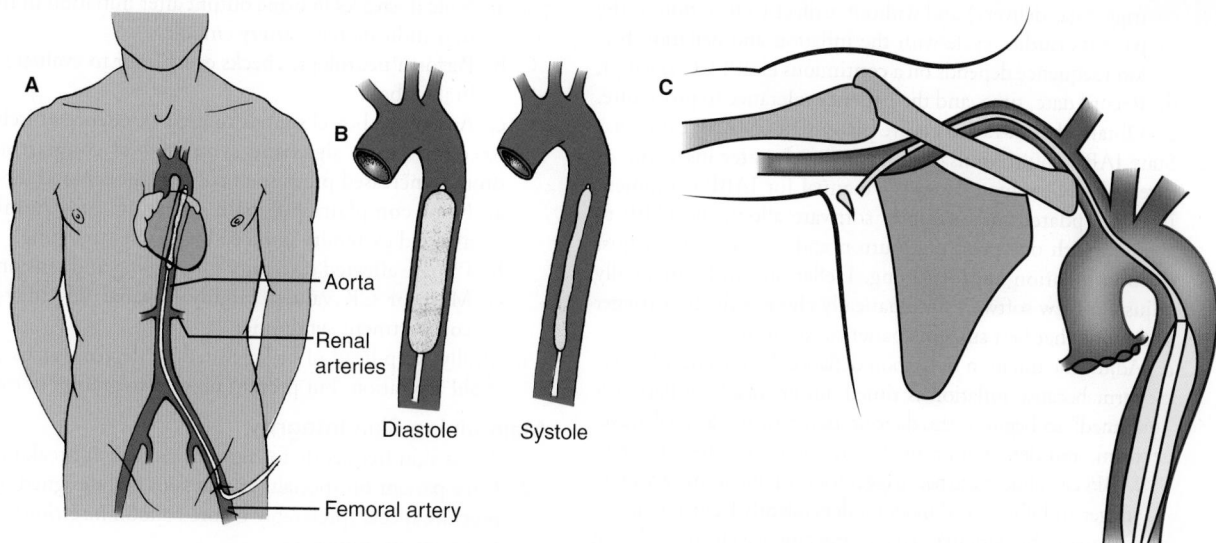

Figure 12-10. Counterpulsation. **(A)** Introduction of the intra-aortic balloon catheter via the femoral artery. **(B)** The intra-aortic balloon pump augments diastole, resulting in increased perfusion of the coronary arteries and myocardium and a decrease in the left ventricular workload. **(C)** Axillary approach.

Contraindications

1. Aortic insufficiency—IABP will increase aortic insufficiency.
2. Aortic aneurysm or aortic dissection—IABP catheter may perforate a weakened vessel wall leading to thrombus formation, and inflation and deflation of the catheter may cause a thrombus to break off to become an embolus.
3. Peripheral vascular disease—femoral or iliac artery insertion may be impossible in a patient with severe vascular disease.
4. Terminal illness—outcome will not be affected, unless the patient meets the criteria for heart transplantation.
5. Prosthetic graft in thoracic aorta—may disrupt graft.
6. Coagulopathy—increases the risk of bleeding.
7. Uncontrolled sepsis.

Complications

1. Vascular injuries that may occur from IABP are:
    a. Plaque dislodging.
    b. Dissection of the aorta.
    c. Laceration of the aorta.
    d. Ischemia of the limb distal to the insertion site.
    e. Arterial perforation.
2. Peripheral nerve damage can occur from IABP if a cut down was used to insert the catheter.
3. Impairment of cerebral circulation because of balloon migration occluding the subclavian artery or by embolus and impairment of renal circulation because of balloon malposition or embolus. (Impaired circulation occurs more frequently in patients with peripheral vascular occlusive disease, in women with small vessels, and in patients with insulin-dependent diabetes.)
4. Infection at the insertion site and septicemia occur in 0.2% of patients with IABP.
5. Thrombocytopenia.
6. Hemorrhage because of anticoagulation.
7. Aortic dissection.

Nursing Diagnoses

- Anxiety related to invasive procedure, critical illness, and environment.
- Decreased Cardiac Output related to myocardial ischemia and/or mechanical intervention.
- Impaired Tissue Perfusion related to foreign body in the aorta.
- Impaired Skin Integrity related to decreased mobility.

Nursing Interventions

Relieving Anxiety

1. Explain IABP therapy to patient and family geared to their level of understanding.
    a. Review purpose of therapy and how the IABP functions.
    b. Reinforce mobility restrictions: supine position with head of bed elevated 15 to 30 degrees and no movement or flexing of leg with IABP catheter.
    c. Explain the need for frequent monitoring of vital signs, rhythm, insertion site of affected extremity, and pulses.
    d. Discuss the sounds associated with functioning external console: balloon inflation and deflation and alarms.
2. Encourage family members to participate in patient's care.
    a. Allow family to visit patient frequently.
    b. Solicit family members' assistance in reinforcing mobility restrictions to patient and notifying nursing staff of patient comfort needs.
    c. Encourage family members to ask questions.
3. Allow patient to verbalize fears regarding therapy and illness.
4. Make sure that informed consent is obtained.
5. Administer anxiolytic medications as prescribed and indicated.
6. Keep the family informed of changes in the patient's condition.
7. Encourage realistic hope based on the patient's condition and discuss the patient's progress with the family.
8. Determine the family's previous coping mechanism to stressful situations.

Maintaining Adequate Cardiac Output

1. Assist during insertion of IABP catheter.
    a. Offer patient reassurance and comfort measures (patient is only mildly sedated).
    b. Ensure strict aseptic environment during insertion.
    c. Establish ECG monitoring, choosing the lead with the largest R wave (external console senses R wave of ECG to

trigger gas delivery) and without artifact (integration of the patient's cardiac cycle with the inflation and deflation balloon sequence depends on a continuous clear ECG tracing).

   d. Record date, time, and the patient's tolerance to procedure.

   e. Obtain chest x-ray to ensure placement of IABP catheter.

2. Start IABP counterpulsation immediately after insertion, as directed; review manufacturer's manual for IABP equipment in use. Updated manufacturer software allows the IABP to start up with one press of a button and automatically adjust balloon inflation and/or timing. Deflation can be manually adjusted. New software automatically chooses the best trigger and mode that best suits the patient's condition.

   a. Adjust the duration of balloon deflation by the arterial waveform because inflation is timed automatically; inflation is "timed" to begin at the dicrotic notch of the arterial waveform, and deflation occurs before the next systole. Current IABPs can choose the best trigger for the patient (mostly ECG trigger and if in "auto" mode) independently from a user.

   b. Compare the patient's arterial pressure waveform with and without balloon augmentation to evaluate effectiveness of therapy. Note difference in patient's end-diastolic pressure and balloon-assisted end-diastolic pressure (the balloon-assisted end-diastolic pressure should be lower, indicating a reduction in afterload).

   c. Monitor hemodynamic parameters with Swan-Ganz catheter (see page 245). Record mean arterial pressure (MAP), CVP, PAP, pulmonary capillary wedge pressure (PCWP), and CO to evaluate overall effectiveness of therapy. Perform hemodynamic calculations to evaluate systemic vascular resistance and left ventricular stroke work. Use IABP MAP when titrating vasoactive medications.

   d. Assess capillary refill, pedal, and left radial pulses every 15 minutes for the first hour and then hourly. The balloon catheter or a thrombus can obstruct flow to the distal extremities. If the catheter migrates too high, it can obstruct flow of the left subclavian artery.

3. Monitor vital signs every 15 to 30 minutes for 4 to 6 hours and then hourly, if stable.

4. Monitor the IABP catheter site with vital signs and check for distal pulses to prevent limb ischemia.

5. Monitor neurologic status at least every 2 to 4 hours.

6. Monitor urine output from indwelling catheter every hour.

7. Maintain accurate intake and output and weigh patient daily (preferably at the same time every day).

8. Report chest pain immediately.

9. Treat dysrhythmias as directed.

10. Check for blood oozing around IABP catheter every hour for 8 hours and then every 4 hours (anticoagulation therapy is used to prevent thrombus formation); apply direct pressure and report bleeding.

Maintaining Adequate Tissue Perfusion

1. Evaluate for ischemia of extremity with IABP catheter.

   a. Mark pulses with indelible ink to facilitate checks.

   b. Monitor peripheral pulses (dorsalis pedis, posterior tibial, popliteal, and left radial) for rhythm, character, and pulse quality every 15 minutes for 1 hour, then every 30 minutes for 1 hour, and then hourly.

   c. Use Doppler device for pulses difficult to palpate and to auscultate for bruits and hums.

   d. Observe skin temperature, color, sensation, and movement of affected extremity. (Dusky, cool, mottled, painful, numb/tingling extremity indicates ischemia.)

2. Observe for possible indications of thromboemboli.

   a. Note decreases in urine output after initiation of therapy—may indicate renal artery emboli.

   b. Perform neurologic checks every hour to evaluate for cerebral emboli.

   c. Auscultate bowel sounds to detect evidence of ischemia.

3. Recognize early signs and symptoms of compartment syndrome. Increased pressure in tissue reduces blood flow.

   a. Note complaints of pain, pressure, and numbness of affected extremity induced by passive stretching.

   b. Palpate affected extremity for swelling and tension.

   c. Monitor CK values. Highly elevated CK may indicate compartment syndrome.

4. Ideally, keep head of bed elevated 30 degrees versus supine to avoid aspiration, but prevent upward migration of catheter.

Maintaining Skin Integrity

1. Assess skin frequently for signs of redness or breakdown.

2. Place patient on specialty mattress or bed designed to prevent pressure ulcers (preferably before balloon insertion).

3. Pad bony prominences.

4. Implement passive ROM exercises with exception of extremity with IABP catheter.

5. Turn patient from side to side as a unit every 2 hours. Patients are usually debilitated and prone to pressure ulcers.

Evaluation: Expected Outcomes

1. States activity restrictions and rationale.

2. Blood pressure and CO readings improved.

3. Peripheral pulses strong; extremities warm and nail beds pink.

4. No skin redness or breakdown.

Heart Surgery

Open-heart surgery is most commonly performed for CAD, valvular dysfunction, and congenital heart defects. The procedure may require temporary cardiopulmonary bypass (blood is diverted from the heart and the lungs and mechanically oxygenated and circulated) to provide a bloodless field that leads to increased visibility of cardiac structures during the operation.

   Newer and less invasive procedures include *minimally invasive direct coronary artery bypass (MIDCAB)* and *robotic-assisted bypass and valve surgeries.* An estimated 405,000 coronary bypass graft surgeries occur yearly in the United States. Heart transplant will not be discussed. For information on percutaneous ventricular assist devices, see Box 12-3.

Types of Procedures

Coronary Artery Bypass Graft

 EVIDENCE BASE Fudulu, D., Benedetto, U., Pecchinenda, G. G., et al. (2016). Current outcomes of off-pump versus on-pump coronary artery bypass grafting: evidence from randomized controlled trials. *Journal of Thoracic Disease, 8*(S10), S758–S771.

Parasca, C. A., Head, S. J., Milojevic, M., et al. (2016). Incidence, characteristics, predictors, and outcomes of repeat revascularization after percutaneous coronary intervention and coronary artery bypass grafting. *JACC Cardiovascular Intervention, 9*(24), 2493–2507.

Benedetto, U., Gaudino, M., Ng, C., et al. (2016). Coronary surgery is superior to drug eluting stents in multivessel disease. Systematic review and meta-analysis of contemporary randomized controlled trials. *International Journal of Cardiology, 210,* 19–24.

| BOX 12-3 | **Percutaneous Ventricular Assist Device Therapy** |

The use of the percutaneous left ventricular assist device (LVAD) constitutes important advances in management of patients with severe cardiogenic shock and may serve as a bridge to recovery or heart transplantation for some patients. The immediate therapeutic benefit of the percutaneous LVAD in patients with cardiogenic shock is the restoration of normal hemodynamics and vital organ perfusion. Although the intra-aortic balloon pump (IABP) decreases preload and afterload, the percutaneous LVAD augments cardiac output and may even completely replace left ventricular function. In severe cases of cardiogenic shock, the IABP and percutaneous LVAD may be used at the same time. For the high-risk percutaneous coronary intervention patient, short-term hemodynamic stability can be provided, and the device can be implanted rapidly and percutaneously in a prophylactic or emergency setting.

There are three principal indications for percutaneous LVAD support:

- Reversible, severe left-sided heart failure (providing temporary circulatory support until recovery has ensued or revascularization has been performed).
- Large ischemic area at risk (temporary circulatory support during high-risk percutaneous or surgical revascularization procedures).

- Bridging therapy (temporary circulatory support as bridge to a permanent surgical assist device or heart transplantation).

The percutaneous LVAD works by creating a left ventricular bypass in one of two ways. One approach is to enter the left atrium transseptally by placing a catheter that pulls oxygenated blood into a centrifugal pump and then flows it back into the femoral artery, thus creating a left atrial-to-femoral bypass. The second technique is retrograde placement of a "caged" blood flow inlet in the left ventricle, which pulls oxygenated blood via catheter to a microaxial pump into the ascending aorta, thereby creating a left ventricular-to-aortic bypass. There are advantages to both systems, and selection should be patient specific.

Historically, surgically implanted right ventricular assist devices (RVADs) have been used mostly for support of cardiac surgical patients. In several reported cases, percutaneous RVADs have successfully supported patients with right ventricular infarct complicated by shock. However, further investigation of this newer therapy is warranted to determine patient outcomes and potential benefits for patients requiring RV support.

1. Coronary artery bypass graft (CABG) surgery involves anastomosis of a graft (vein or artery) with distal portion bypassing the blocked coronary vessel restoring adequate blood supply to the heart muscle. The proximal end, in some cases, is anastomosed to the aorta (when the internal mammary artery is chosen as conduit, the proximal end remains attached in its normal circulation pattern). The choice of conduit is often multifactorial. Arterial conduit has been shown to have a longer patency rate. For this reason, the internal mammary artery is often chosen if time allows for its dissection from the chest wall and the length is adequate to bypass the blocked vessel. The saphenous vein remains the most commonly used because it is easily accessed and does not require extra prepping to prevent spasm (as is the case with a radial graft). Several studies suggest poor graft vein patency and increased revascularization rate for patients undergoing off-pump CABG compared to on-pump CABG
   a. Multiple grafts can be placed to bypass multiple lesions.
   b. Traditional procedure is done through sternotomy, whereas newer procedures are less invasive.
2. The heart is stopped (in some cases) and the patient is placed on a cardiopulmonary bypass machine (on-pump CABG). In other situations, CABG is performed while the heart is beating using a stabilizer to decrease movement (off-pump CABG). Compared to CABG, PCI with drug-eluding stents has been shown to increase relative risk of death, risk of myocardial infarction, and revascularization rates at 3.4 years after initial treatment. Primarily done to alleviate anginal symptoms and improve survival and quality of life.
3. Indications for CABG include:
   a. Left main coronary artery stenosis of 70% or greater.
   b. Proximal vessel disease greater than 50% to 70% stenosis of three main coronary arteries.

   c. Multivessel disease and decreased left ventricular function.
   d. Unstable angina (UA).
   e. Chronic stable angina that is lifestyle-limiting and unresponsive to medical therapies or PTCA and stenting cannot be achieved.
4. Relative contraindications for CABG include:
   a. Small coronary arteries distal to the stenosis.
   b. Severe aortic stenosis.
   c. Severe left ventricular failure with coexisting pulmonary, renal, carotid, and peripheral vascular disease.

Valvular Surgery

1. Prosthetic or biologic valves are placed in the heart as definitive therapy for incompetent heart valves. Mechanical valves are of man-made material and require a lifetime of anticoagulation therapy. Biologic valves are general either porcine or bovine derivatives. The decision for mechanic or biologic valve is a shared decision between the patient and provider.
2. Valve repair or replacement can be done in conjunction with CABG surgery.
3. Usually done as an open-heart procedure through sternotomy incision or minithoracotomy. A selected group of patients may need a transcutaneous valvular replacement (ie, TAVR).
4. Postoperative care of a patient with either a mitral valve or an aortic valve is similar to that of a patient who has undergone post-CABG surgery. Patients who have mechanical valve need lifetime anticoagulation therapy regardless of the position of the valve replaced. Generally, MVR need higher INR goals (ie, INR = 3 or greater) than AVR (ie, INR = 2.5 or lower in cases of increased risk of bleeding), which is partially influenced by the pressure gradient. In the immediate postoperative period, heparin infusion can be used as a bridge anticoagulation until warfarin can be institute to the therapeutic INR goal. It is important to educate patients to not stop the anticoagulation and to always seek medical advice prior to doing so.

Congenital Heart Surgery

1. Defects of the heart can be surgically repaired and reconstructed.
2. Temporary cardiopulmonary bypass is not always required.

Minimally Invasive Direct Coronary Artery Bypass (MIDCAB)

1. Done through a left anterior small thoracotomy, a short parasternal incision, or a small incision using a port access and video-assisted technology.
2. Cardiopulmonary bypass machine is not needed because the heart remains beating.
3. The procedure is limited to proximal disease of the left anterior descending or right coronary artery.
4. With this procedure, there is less blood transfusion, less pain and discomfort, less infection, and less time under anesthesia; therefore, intensive care unit (ICU) length of stay is significantly shorter.

Off-Pump CABG (Beating-Heart Bypass Surgery)

1. CABG surgery is done using a median sternotomy without the use of cardiopulmonary bypass machine; preferred method in high-risk patients (eg, patients with poor ventricular function or with severe aortic atherosclerosis).
2. Postaccess procedures are performed through a small anterior thoracotomy incision and a few 1-cm lateral port incisions that allow direct access to the heart and good visualization through a thoracoscope.
   a. Multiple vessel bypass can be performed as well as mitral valve surgery and repair of atrial septal defect.
   b. In emergency, if the heart stops, cardiopulmonary bypass can be used during surgery.
   c. Reduces postoperative length of stay to 1 to 3 days.
   d. Contraindicated in patients with occlusion in posterior and lateral arteries, severe atherosclerosis, and aortic aneurysms.
3. Transmyocardial laser revascularization (TMLR) provides relief to patients having refractory angina that is not amendable to conventional revascularization. Indications for TMLR include severe coronary heart disease, viable myocardium with reversible ischemia, LVEF of more than 20%, and target vessels that are too small for catheter revascularization.

Preoperative Management

1. Review of patient's condition to determine status of vascular, pulmonary, renal, hepatic, hematologic, and metabolic systems.
   a. Cardiac history; circulatory studies.
   b. Pulmonary health—patients with COPD may require prolonged postoperative respiratory support. Chest computed tomography scans, baseline arterial blood gas, or pulmonary function tests should be ordered and used as reliable predictors of long-term pulmonary outcomes. (Vital capacity greater than 2.5 L and forced expiratory volume in 1 second greater than 1.5 L are ideal for favorable outcomes.)
   c. Depression—can produce a serious postoperative depressive state and can affect postoperative morbidity and mortality.
   d. Present alcohol intake; smoking history.
2. Preoperative laboratory studies.
   a. Complete blood count, serum electrolytes, lipid profile, and hemoglobin A1C, if diabetic.
   b. Ensure active blood type and cross with the correct number of packed red blood cells (PRBCs) and other blood products on hold at the blood bank.
   c. Antibody screen, urine, and other cultures.
   d. Preoperative coagulation survey (platelet count, prothrombin time, partial thromboplastin time)—extracorporeal circulation will affect certain coagulation factors.
   e. Renal and hepatic function tests.
3. Evaluation of medication regimen. These patients are usually taking multiple drugs.
   a. Digoxin—may be receiving large doses to improve myocardial contractility; may be stopped several days before surgery to avoid digitoxic dysrhythmias from cardiopulmonary bypass.
   b. Diuretics—assess for potassium depletion and volume depletion; give potassium supplement to replenish body stores.
   c. Beta-adrenergic blockers such as metoprolol and propranolol—usually continued.
   d. Psychotropic drugs such as benzodiazepines (diazepam, alprazolam)—postoperative withdrawal may cause extreme agitation.
   e. Alcohol—sudden withdrawal may produce delirium.
   f. Anticoagulant/antiplatelet aggregate drugs, such as warfarin and clopidogrel—discontinued several days before operation to allow coagulation mechanism to return to normal.
   g. Corticosteroids—if taken within the year before surgery, may lead to adrenal crisis. It is essential that these patients be dosed adequately to prevent hypotension or death.
   h. Prophylactic antibiotics—may be given preoperatively.
   i. Drug sensitivities or allergies are noted.
   j. If patients are taking herbal supplements, they should be discontinued as far in advance as possible to prevent interactions with certain types of anesthesia.
4. If patient is taking any antihyperglycemic agents (ie, insulin, metformin), discuss with provider the need to reduce basal insulin doses and holding metformin before surgery. Ensure that basal insulin is not completely withheld, because this may result in diabetic ketoacidosis or hyperosmolar hyperglycemia state.
5. Improvement of underlying pulmonary disease and respiratory function to reduce risk of complications.
   a. Encourage patient to stop smoking.
   b. Treat infection and pulmonary vascular congestion.
6. Preparation for events in the postoperative period.
   a. Take the patient and family on tour of ICU. This lessens anxiety about being in ICU.
      i. Introduce the patient to staff personnel who will be caring for him or her.
      ii. Give family a schedule of visiting hours and times for phone contact.
   b. Teach chest physical therapy procedures to optimize pulmonary function.
      i. Have the patient practice with incentive spirometer.
      ii. Show and practice diaphragmatic breathing techniques.
      iii. Have the patient practice effective coughing and leg exercises.
   c. Prepare patient for presence of monitors, chest tubes, IV lines, blood transfusion, ET tube, nasogastric (NG) tube, pacing wires, arterial line, and indwelling catheter.
      i. Explain to the patient that chest tubes will be inserted below incision into the chest cavity for drainage and maintenance of negative pressure.
      ii. Explain to the patient that ET tube will prevent speaking, but communication will be possible through writing until tube is removed (usually within 6 hours when the patient is awake and able to maintain own airway).
      iii. Explain to the patient that diet will consist of liquids until 24 hours after surgery.

iv. Explain that monitoring equipment and IV lines will restrict movement and nursing staff will position the patient comfortably every 2 hours and as necessary.

d. Discuss with the patient the need to monitor vital signs frequently and the likelihood of frequent disturbances of the patient's rest.

e. Discuss pain management with the patient; assure the patient that analgesics will be administered as necessary to control pain. Discuss the use of the patient control analgesia (PCA) machine.

f. Tell the patient that both hands may be loosely restrained for a few hours after surgery to eliminate possibility of pulling out tubes and IV lines inadvertently.

g. Discuss with the patient the importance of physical and occupational therapy to increase mobility and decrease hospital stay. Patient will be assisted from the bed to chair by the morning of postoperative day 1.

7. Evaluation of emotional state to reduce anxieties.

a. Patients undergoing heart surgery are more anxious and fearful than other surgical patients. (Moderate anxiety assists patient to cope with stresses of surgery. Low anxiety level may indicate that the patient is in denial. High anxiety may impair the patient's ability to learn and listen.)

b. Offer support and help patient and family mobilize positive coping mechanisms.

c. Answer questions and alleviates fears and misconceptions.

8. Surgical preparation.

a. Shave anterior and lateral surfaces of the trunk and neck; shave entire body down to ankles (for coronary bypass).

b. Shower or bathe per facility policy. Assist patient with antiseptic scrubs used on their chest prior to surgery.

c. Give sedative and/or antibiotics before going to the operating room, as ordered.

d. Ensure removable dental work, jewelry, and nail polish removed.

 GERONTOLOGIC ALERT Older patients with underlying respiratory problems (ie, smoking, COPD, asthma) and debilitated patients are at greater risk for postoperative respiratory complications.

Complications

Complications following cardiac surgery can be divided into early complications (cardiovascular, pulmonary, renal, GI, and neuropsychologic) and late postoperative complications.

Early Complications

 EVIDENCE BASE Sheth, K. N., & Nourollahzadeh, E. (2017). Neurologic complications of cardiac and vascular surgery. *Handbook of Clinical Neurology*, 141, 573–592.

Ha, A. C. T., Mazer, C. D., Verma, S., et al. (2016). Management of postoperative atrial fibrillation after cardiac surgery. *Current Opinion in Cardiology*, 31(2), 183–190.

1. Cardiovascular dysfunction or low output syndrome can occur as a result of decreased preload (from bleeding or volume loss), increased afterload, arrhythmias, cardiac tamponade, or myocardial depression with or without myocardial necrosis.

2. Postoperative bleeding can occur secondary to coagulopathy, uncontrolled hypertension, or inadequate hemostasis.

3. Cardiac tamponade results from bleeding into the pericardial sac or accumulation of fluids in the sac, which compresses the heart and prevents adequate filling of the ventricles. Cardiac tamponade should be suspected when there is low CO, hypotension, tachycardia, increased CVP, narrow pulse pressure, or sharp drop in chest tube output postoperatively.

4. Myocardial depression (impaired myocardial contractility), which can be reversible, occurs secondary as a result of myocardial necrosis in 15% of all CABG surgeries.

5. Perioperative MI continues to be a serious problem that can occur in 5% of patients with stable angina and up to 10% of patients with unstable angina postoperatively as a result of the surgical procedure.

6. Cardiac dysrhythmias commonly occur after heart surgery. Ischemia, hypoxia, electrolyte imbalances, alterations in autonomic nervous system, hypertension, and increased catecholamine levels, among others, may attribute to dysrhythmia development.

a. Atrial arrhythmias may occur after CABG or after valvular surgery; can occur anytime during the first 2 to 3 weeks postoperatively, but peak incidence is 3 to 5 days. Studies suggest perioperative beta-blockade is an effective therapy for prevention.

b. PVCs occur in 8.9% to 24% of patients, most frequently after aortic valve replacement and CABG.

7. Hypotension may be caused by inadequate cardiac contractility and reduction in blood volume or by mechanical ventilation (when the patient "fights" the ventilator or positive end-expiratory pressure is used), all of which can produce a reduction in CO.

8. Pulmonary complications occur as a result of intubation and coronary pulmonary bypass.

a. Continuous pulse oximetry, arterial blood gas (ABG) studies, and chest x-ray are done frequently to monitor pulmonary function of a patient after heart surgery.

b. Noncardiac pulmonary edema can occur immediately after surgery and can occur the first several days after surgery as a result of increased pulmonary capillary permeability.

c. Pneumothorax can occur anytime postoperatively, especially when chest tubes are removed.

d. Phrenic nerve damage can occur, resulting in diaphragmatic paralysis.

e. Pulmonary emboli, although uncommon, can result from atrial fibrillation, heart failure, obesity, hypercoagulability, and immobilization.

f. Older patients are at increased risk of developing pneumonia, atelectasis, and pulmonary effusions.

g. Be vigilant and report copious amounts of secretion or any changes in patient's secretion.

9. Renal insufficiency or failure can occur as a result of deficient perfusion (can be due to heart–lung machine), hemolysis, low CO before and after open-heart surgery, hypotension, and by use of vasopressor agents to increase blood pressure.

10. GI postoperative complications can include abdominal distention, ileus, gastroduodenal bleeding, cholecystitis, hepatic dysfunction, "shock liver syndrome," pancreatitis, mesenteric ischemia, diarrhea, or constipation.

11. Neuropsychologic complications postoperatively include ischemic stroke, neuropsychologic dysfunction, postcardiotomy delirium, and peripheral neurologic deficits.

GERONTOLOGIC ALERT Older patients postoperatively are more sensitive to hypovolemia, excessive bleeding, and cardiac tamponade, which affect preload and result in a decrease in CO.

 GERONTOLOGIC ALERT Atrial fibrillation occurs in 35% of elderly patients postoperatively and may need to be treated with antiarrhythmics, cardioversion, and anticoagulants.

 GERONTOLOGIC ALERT Neurologic complications increase disproportionate to cardiac risk in elderly patients.

Late Complications

1. Late complications of cardiac surgery usually occur after the 4th day of surgery and include postpericardiotomy syndrome, cardiac tamponade, and incisional wound infections.
2. Postpericardiotomy syndrome is a group of symptoms occurring in 10% to 40% of patients several days after cardiac surgery.
   a. The cause of postpericardiotomy syndrome is not certain, but it may result from anticardiac antibodies, viral etiology (such as cytomegalovirus), or other causes.
   b. Postpericardiotomy syndrome occurs as the result of tissue trauma, which triggers an autoimmune response and inflammation of the pericardial cavity, resulting in pericardial and severe pleural pain.
   c. Manifestations—fever, malaise, arthralgias, dyspnea, pericardial effusion, pleural effusion and friction rub, and pleural/pericardial pain.
   d. Treatment regimen may include corticosteroids, aspirin, or colchicine. Pericardiocentesis or thoracentesis may be needed for persistent effusion.
3. Cardiac tamponade can occur in 1% to 2% of patients and is commonly associated with administration of anticoagulants or antiplatelet therapy, usually occurring after 72 hours following surgery.
4. Wound infections, including sternal wound infections and mediastinitis, occur in 0.4% to 5% of all patients having cardiac surgery. Mortality rate associated with sternal wound infection and mediastinitis can vary between 8% and 45%.
   a. Wound infections usually appear 4 to 14 days postoperatively with symptoms of fever, leukocytosis, inflammation, and purulent drainage.
   b. *Staphylococcus epidermidis* and *Staphylococcus aureus* organisms are the most common causative organism, but the infection can be caused by a number of pathogens ranging from gram positives, gram negatives, or even fungi.
5. MIs (postoperative) can occur at a rate of 1.34% because of bypass time greater than 100 minutes and presence of unstable angina.
6. Constrictive pericarditis has an incidence of 0.2% to 2.0%. Risk factors reveal normal left ventricular function, warfarin administration, and inadequate drainage of early postoperative pericardial effusion as the significant causes.
7. Respiratory complications—chest wall pain and prolonged ventilation—more than 14 days of ventilatory support (morbidity rate of 9.9%).
8. Renal dysfunction—up to 40% developed transient oliguria, with 2% progressing to renal failure requiring dialysis.

Postoperative renal dysfunction results from postoperative hypovolemia, anemia, hypotension, low output syndrome, sepsis, and pericardial tamponade.

Other Complications

1. Postperfusion syndrome—diffuse syndrome characterized by systemic inflammatory response syndrome.
2. Febrile complications—probably from body's reaction to tissue trauma or accumulation of blood and serum in pleural and pericardial spaces.
3. In older patients, decreased kidney function can increase the risk of developing drug toxicities, adverse reactions, oliguria, and renal failure.
4. Failure to wean from the ventilator because of underlying pulmonary disease or postoperative pulmonary complications.

Postoperative Management

1. Adequate oxygenation is ensured; respiratory insufficiency is common after open-heart surgery.
   a. Patients require intubation during cardiac surgery, and the majority of them continued to require mechanical ventilation after being transported to the cardiac surgery ICU.
   b. Chest x-ray taken immediately after surgery and daily thereafter to evaluate state of lung expansion and to detect atelectasis or pneumothorax and to demonstrate heart size and contour and confirm placement of central line, ET tube, and chest drains.
2. Hemodynamic monitoring during the immediate postoperative period for cardiovascular and respiratory status and fluid and electrolyte balance to prevent or recognize complications.
3. Drainage of mediastinal and pleural chest tubes is monitored.
4. Fluid and electrolyte balance is monitored closely with daily weight.
5. Hypokalemia may be caused by inadequate intake, diuretics, vomiting, excessive NG drainage, and stress from surgery.
   a. Hyperkalemia may be caused by increased intake, red cell breakdown (from the pump, bleeding, or transfusion), acidosis, renal insufficiency, tissue necrosis, and adrenal cortical insufficiency.
   b. Hyponatremia may be due to reduction of total body sodium or to an increased water intake, causing a dilution of body sodium.
   c. Hypocalcemia may be due to alkalosis (which reduces the amount of calcium in the extracellular fluid) because hydrogen ions dissociate from serum albumin and more calcium binds to albumin, reducing ionized calcium level in the blood) and multiple blood transfusions.
   d. Hypercalcemia may cause dysrhythmias imitating those caused by digoxin toxicity.
6. Postoperative medications include:
   a. Aspirin daily as MI prophylaxis.
   b. Analgesics.
   c. Antihypertensives or antiarrhythmics, if needed.
   d. Beta-blockers.
   e. ACE inhibitors for patients with ejection fraction less than 30%.
   f. Antibiotics, if indicated.
7. Monitoring for complications.
8. Cardiac pacing, if indicated, by way of temporary pacing wires from the incision.

Nursing Diagnoses

- Anxiety related to fear of unknown, fear of death, and fear of pain.
- Impaired Gas Exchange related to alveolar capillary membrane changes, immobility, and altered blood flow.
- Decreased Cardiac Output related to mechanical factors: decreased preload and impaired contractility.
- Risk for Deficient Fluid Volume related to physiologic effects of heart–lung machine.
- Acute Pain related to sternotomy and leg incisions.
- Sleep Deprivation related to intensive care environment.
- Risk for Injury related to postoperative complications.

Nursing Interventions

Minimizing Anxiety

1. Orient to surroundings as soon as patient awakens from surgical procedure. Tell patient that the surgery is over and orient to location, time of day, and your name.
2. Allow family members to visit patient as soon as condition stabilizes. Encourage family members to talk to and touch patient. (Family members may be overwhelmed by intensive care environment.)
3. As patient becomes more alert, explain purpose of all equipment in environment. Continually orient patient to time and place. Make sure patient has glasses and hearing aids, if needed.
4. Administer anxiolytics, as directed.
5. Remove lines and tubing once medically appropriate.

Promoting Adequate Gas Exchange

1. Frequently check function of mechanical ventilator, patient's respiratory effort, and ABG levels.
2. Check ET tube placement (note location and measurement).
3. Auscultate chest for breath sounds. Crackles indicate pulmonary congestion; decreased or absent breath sounds indicate pneumothorax; rales may indicate pulmonary edema.
4. Sedate patient adequately to help tolerate ET tube and cope with ventilatory sensations. Implement ventilator care bundle (ie, routine mouth care with chlorhexidine, keep HOB at 30 degrees) to prevent ventilator-associated pneumonia.
5. Use chest physiotherapy for patients with lung congestion to prevent retention of secretions and atelectasis.
6. Promote coughing, deep breathing, and turning to keep airway patent, prevent atelectasis, and facilitate lung expansion. Have patient sit at least 30 degrees unless medically contraindicated.
7. Suction tracheobronchial secretions carefully. Prolonged suctioning leads to hypoxia and possible cardiac arrest.
8. Administer diuretics, as prescribed.
9. Institute ventilatory weaning protocol when patient is awake and can initiate own breaths and assist with extubation (see page 183), when indicated.

Maintaining Adequate Cardiac Output

1. Monitor cardiovascular status to determine effectiveness of CO. Continuous monitoring of blood pressure by way of intra-arterial line, heart rate, CVP, left atrial or PAP, and PCWP from monitor modules is observed, correlated with the patient's condition, and recorded.
2. Monitor and record urine output every hour (normal urinary output 0.5 to 1 mL/kg/hr).

3. Observe buccal mucosa, nail beds, lips, earlobes, and extremities for duskiness, cyanosis—late signs of low CO.
4. Feel the skin; cool, moist skin or weak pulses reveal lowered CO. Note temperature and color of extremities.
5. Monitor neurologic status.
   a. Observe for symptoms of hypoxia—restlessness, headache, confusion, dyspnea, hypotension, and cyanosis. Obtain ABG values and core temperature.
   b. Note the patient's neurologic status hourly in terms of level of responsiveness, response to verbal commands and painful stimuli, pupillary size and reaction to light, and movement of extremities, handgrasp ability.
   c. Monitor for and treat postoperative seizures.

Maintaining Adequate Fluid Volume

1. Administer IV fluids as ordered, but limit if signs of fluid overloading occur.
2. Keep intake and output flow sheets as a method of determining positive or negative fluid balance and the patient's fluid requirements.
   a. IV fluids (including flush solutions through arterial and venous lines) are considered intake.
   b. Measure postoperative chest drainage—should not exceed 200 mL/hr for first 4 to 6 hours.
3. Be alert to changes in serum electrolyte levels.
   a. Hypokalemia may cause dysrhythmias, digoxin toxicity, metabolic alkalosis, weakened myocardium, and cardiac arrest.
      i. Watch for specific ECG changes.
      ii. Replace electrolytes, as needed.
   b. Hyperkalemia may cause mental confusion, restlessness, nausea, weakness, and paresthesia of extremities. Treatment may include administering an ion-exchange resin and sodium polystyrene sulfonate, which binds the potassium or hemodialysis. Temporary treatment includes sodium bicarbonate, insulin (with dextrose), albuterol, and calcium.
   c. Hyponatremia may cause weakness, fatigue, confusion, seizures, and coma.
   d. Hypocalcemia may cause numbness and tingling in the fingertips, toes, ears, and nose, carpopedal spasm, muscle cramps, and tetany. Give replacement therapy, as needed.
   e. Hypercalcemia may cause digoxin toxicity.
      i. Treatment may include fluids, diuretics, calcitonin, or hemodialysis.
      ii. This condition may lead to asystole and death.
4. Monitor hematocrit and hemoglobin (frequency depends on hemodynamics and evidence of bleeding) and report any significant change in findings.
   a. Ensure that patient has current blood type and screen. Transfuse blood products, as ordered.
   b. Check coagulation tests, including prothrombin time, international normalized ratio, and partial thromboplastin time, if patient is coagulopathic, bleeding, or anticoagulated for mechanical device.

Relieving Pain

1. Examine surgical incision sites.
2. Record nature, type, location, duration of pain, and contributing factors.
3. Differentiate between incisional pain and anginal pain. Obtain ECG and have provider confirm if there are any changes.
4. Report restlessness and apprehension not corrected by analgesics—may be from hypoxia or a low output state.

5. Administer medications as prescribed, or monitor constant infusion to reduce amount of pain and to aid the patient in performing deep breathing and coughing exercises more effectively.
6. Assist patient to position of comfort.
7. Encourage early mobilization.

Promoting Sleep and Recovery

1. Watch for symptoms of postcardiotomy delirium (may appear after brief lucid period).
   a. Signs and symptoms include delirium (impairment of orientation, memory, intellectual function, judgment), transient perceptual distortions, visual and auditory hallucinations, disorientation, and paranoid delusions.
   b. Symptoms may be related to sleep deprivation, increased sensory output, disorientation to night and day, prolonged inability to speak because of ET intubation, age, and preoperative cardiac status.
2. Keep the patient oriented to time and place; notify the patient of procedures and expectations of cooperation.
3. Encourage family to visit at regular times—helps patient regain sense of reality.
4. Plan care to allow rest periods, day–night pattern, and uninterrupted sleep.
5. Encourage mobility as soon as possible.
   a. Keep environment as free as possible of excessive auditory and sensory input.
   b. Prevent bodily injury.
   c. Have physical therapy work with patient and provide analgesics prior to therapy.
6. Reassure patient and family that psychiatric disorders after cardiac surgery are usually transient.
7. Remove patient from the ICU as soon as possible. Allow patient to talk about psychotic episode—helps deal with and assimilate experience.

Avoiding Complications

1. Monitor ECG continuously for arrhythmias.
   a. Evaluate possible cause of dysrhythmias—inadequate oxygenation, electrolyte imbalance, MI, mechanical irritation (eg, pacing wires, invasive lines, chest tubes), and any vasopressor or inotropic medications.
   b. Treat dysrhythmias immediately because they may lead to decreased CO. Atrial or AV pacing is used to treat sinus bradycardia or junctional rhythm with heart rates less than 70 beats/minute.
2. Assess for signs of cardiac tamponade—arterial hypotension; rising CVP; rising left atrial pressure; muffled heart sounds; weak, thready pulse; jugular vein distention; and falling urine output.
   a. Check for diminished amount of drainage in the chest collection bottle; may indicate that fluid is accumulating elsewhere, reposition as needed to facilitate fluid drainage.
   b. Prepare for pericardiocentesis.
   c. Assist with echocardiogram to evaluate tamponade.
3. Check cardiac enzyme levels daily. Elevations may indicate MI. (Symptoms may be masked by the usual postoperative discomfort.)
   a. Watch for decreased CO in the presence of normal circulating volume and filling pressure.
   b. Obtain serial ECGs and isoenzymes to determine extent of myocardial injury.
   c. Assess pain to differentiate myocardial pain from incisional pain.

4. Monitor for hypertension or hypotension.
   a. Mild systolic hypertension occurs in 48% to 55% of all CABG patients within the first 6 hours postoperatively.
   b. Hypotension may be caused by bleeding, hypovolemia, decreased systemic vascular resistance (eg, systemic inflammatory response syndrome), cardiogenic shock, tamponade, medications, or arrhythmias.
   c. Blood pressure goal following cardiac surgery is dependent on the patient's conditions (eg, carotid disease, renal disease, bleeding).
5. Initiate measures to prevent embolization such as antiembolic stockings, not putting pressure on popliteal space (leg crossing, raising knee gatch), and starting passive and active exercises.
   a. Assess for signs of DVT and pulmonary embolism.
   b. Maintain integrity of all invasive lines.
6. Monitor for bleeding.
   a. Watch for steady and continuous drainage of blood.
   b. Assess for arterial hypotension, low CVP, increasing pulse rate, and low left atrial pressure and PCWP.
   c. Prepare to administer blood products, IV solutions, or protamine sulfate, antifibrinolytics, DDAVP, or vitamin K.
   d. Prepare for potential return to surgery if bleeding persists (over 300 mL/hr) for 2 hours.
   e. Monitor hemoglobin levels; if the patient's hemoglobin drops below 8 g/dL, transfusions of red blood cells or platelets may be necessary.
   f. During the first 4 to 12 hours, blood recovered from mediastinal tubes can be autotransfused to the patient.
7. Be alert for fever and signs of infection. Check blood glucose levels as ordered.
   a. Administer prophylactic antibiotics, if ordered, for the first 48 hours.
   b. Control higher degrees of fever through use of hypothermia mattress.
   c. Evaluate for atelectasis, pleural effusion, or pneumonia if fever persists. (The most common cause of early postoperative fever [within 24 hours] is atelectasis.)
   d. Evaluate for urinary tract infection and wound infection.
   e. Draw blood cultures to rule out infectious cause if fever persists.
8. Measure urine volume; less than 0.5 to 1 mL/kg/hr can indicate decreased renal function.
   a. Monitor BUN and serum creatinine levels as well as urine and serum electrolyte levels.
   b. Give rapid-acting diuretics and/or inotropic drugs (dopamine, dobutamine) to increase CO and renal blood flow.
   c. Prepare the patient for peritoneal dialysis or hemodialysis if indicated. (Renal insufficiency may produce serious cardiac dysrhythmias.)

Community and Home Care Considerations

Preparing the patient with cardiovascular disease or after cardiac surgery for the return home and optimizing the patient's health status in the home are important nursing functions. The key areas on which to focus include assessment, education, and evaluating responses.

1. Perform a thorough assessment of the patient's clinical condition, functional status, and home safety and support systems. Based on assessment, determine the patient's need for supportive services.
2. Coordinate services such as home health aides.

3. Refer patients to area meal delivery service as appropriate. These services provide special diets in most cases (eg, low sodium or low cholesterol).
4. Coordinate outpatient cardiac rehabilitation services as appropriate.
5. Establish outpatient or home-based physical and occupational therapy as appropriate for graduated exercise and energy conservation techniques.
6. If therapist recommends inpatient rehabilitation, coordinate with facility social worker/discharge planner to find a rehabilitation facility suited for patient as well as his or her family.
7. Educate patient, family, and caregivers about potential complications and medication regimen.

 TRANSITIONAL CARE ALERT Medication management is a key issue when a cardiac surgery patient is leaving the hospital. Ensure that patient is discharged with an accurate medication list, and clear instructions on what has changed compared to previous home medications. Ensure that prescriptions are given to the patient or transmitted to chosen pharmacy and that insurance coverage of medications and cost of all medications have been determined.

Patient Education and Health Maintenance

Note: Specific guidelines will vary slightly among facilities and health care providers. Check facility policy and orders.
1. Instruct about activities.
   a. Increase activities gradually within limits. (Avoid strenuous activities until after exercise stress testing.)
   b. Take short rest periods.
   c. Avoid lifting more than 20 pound (9.1 kg).
   d. Participate in activities that do not cause pain or discomfort.
   e. Increase walking time and distance each day.
   f. Stairs (one to two times daily) the first week; increase as tolerated.
   g. Avoid large crowds at first.
   h. Avoid driving until after first postoperative checkup.
   i. Resumption of sexual relations parallels ability to participate in other activities.
      i. Usually may resume sexual activity 2 weeks after surgery.
      ii. Avoid sexual activity if tired or after heavy meal.
      iii. Consult health care provider if chest discomfort, difficult breathing, or palpitations occur and last longer than 15 minutes after intercourse.
   j. Return to work after first postoperative checkup, as advised by health care provider.
2. Expect some chest discomfort.
3. Advise about diet.
   a. Some patients are placed on minimum salt restriction (eg, no salt added at table); cholesterol may be limited. Have a dietitian talk to the patient and family regarding diet.
   b. Weigh daily and report weight gain of more than 5 pound (2.3 kg) per week.
   c. If the patient is taking warfarin, advise patient not to change normal dietary habits, but to maintain similar intake pattern each day to prevent changes in INR.

4. Tight blood glucose control is recommended (keeping blood sugars 80 to 110 mg/dL) to prevent sternal wound infection.
5. Teach patient and family about wound care and how to avoid infections.
6. Teach about medications.
   a. Label all medications; give purposes and adverse effects.
   b. Patients with mechanical valves may continue warfarin regimen indefinitely. Explain bleeding precautions and need for periodic laboratory studies.
7. Advise patients with prosthetic valves:
   a. Pregnancy is usually discouraged because of anticoagulation therapy.
   b. Need for antibiotic coverage before dental and surgical procedures.
   c. Patients taking anticoagulants should watch for bleeding and should avoid use of aspirin (and many other drugs)—interferes with action of warfarin.
8. Advise the patient to carry an identification card stating cardiac condition and medications being taken.
9. Encourage compliance with rehabilitation and exercise program after exercise stress testing.
10. Inform the patient whom to contact (and how) in case of an emergency.
11. See also section on patient education after MI, page 280, and patient education about infective endocarditis, page 289.
12. Explore community support groups such as AHA (*www.americanheart.org*).
13. Be diligent in providing older patients with education and discharge instructions that they will be able to follow because of sensory impairments, immobility, and transportation barriers.

 GERONTOLOGIC ALERT Older patients are extremely vulnerable to complications because of decreased functional ability and the normal process of aging.

Evaluation: Expected Outcomes

- Verbalizes understanding of surgical procedure, reduction of fear.
- Extubated 24 hours postoperative; spontaneous unlabored respirations 14 to 18 per minute.
- Blood pressure and heart rate stable; adequate urine output.
- Serum electrolytes within normal range.
- Verbalizes reduced pain.
- Sleeps for 2- to 3-hour intervals during night; oriented to time and place; no hallucinations.
- No bleeding noted; afebrile; ECG shows normal sinus rhythm.

SELECTED REFERENCES
Benedetto, U., Gaudino, M., Ng, C., et al. (2016). Coronary surgery is superior to drug eluting stents in multivessel disease. Systematic review and meta-analysis of contemporary randomized controlled trials. *International Journal of Cardiology, 210*, 19–24.

Bessman, E. S. (2014). Chapter 15: Emergency cardiac pacing. In J. R. Roberts, et al. (Eds.), *Roberts & Hedges' clinical procedures in emergency medicine* (6th ed., pp. 277–297). Philadelphia, PA: Saunders.

Dwivedi, A., Huffman, C., & Shah, B. (2015). An analysis of the 2015 ACC/AHA/SCAI focused update on primary PCI for patients with STEMI. American College of Cardiology. Available: *http://www.acc.org/latest-in-cardiology/articles/2015/11/11/16/44/an-analysis-of-the-2015-acc-aha-scai-focused-update-on-primary-pci-for-patients-with-stemi*

Fudulu, D., Benedetto, U., Pecchinenda, G. G., et al. (2016). Current outcomes of off-pump versus on-pump coronary artery bypass grafting: evidence from randomized controlled trials. *Journal of Thoracic Disease, 8*(S10), S758–S771.

Ha, A. C. T., Mazer, C. D., Verma, S., et al. (2016). Management of postoperative atrial fibrillation after cardiac surgery. *Current Opinion in Cardiology, 31*(2), 183–190.

Hollander, J., Than, M., & Mueller, C. (2016). State-of-the-art evaluation of emergency department patients presenting with potential acute coronary syndromes. *Circulation, 134,* 547–556.

Levine, G. N., Bates, E. R., Bittl, J. A., et al. (2016). 2016 ACC/AHA guideline focused update on duration of dual antiplatelet therapy in patients with coronary artery disease: a report of the American College of Cardiology/American Heart Association Task Force on Clinical Practice Guidelines. *Circulation, 134*(10), e123–e155.

Levine, G., O'Gara, P., Bates, E., et al. (2016). 2015 ACC/AHA/SCAI focused update on primary percutaneous coronary intervention for patients with ST-elevation myocardial infarction: an update of the 2011 ACCF/AHA/SCAI guideline for percutaneous coronary intervention and the 2013 ACCF/AHA guideline for the management of ST-elevation myocardial infarction: a report of the American College of Cardiology/American Heart Association Task Force on Clinical Practice Guidelines and the Society for Cardiovascular Angiography and Interventions. *Journal of the American College of Cardiology, 67,* 1235–1250.

Mitchell, J., & Brown, D. (2016). Update on percutaneous coronary intervention in stable coronary artery disease. *JAMA Internal Medicine, 176*(12), 1855–1856.

O'Connor, R., Al Ali, A., Brady, W., et al. (2015). Part 9: Acute Coronary Syndromes: 2015 American Heart Association guidelines update for cardiopulmonary resuscitation and emergency cardiovascular care. *Circulation, 132,* s483–s500.

Parasca, C. A., Head, S. J., Milojevic, M., et al. (2016). Incidence, characteristics, predictors, and outcomes of repeat revascularization after percutaneous coronary intervention and coronary artery bypass grafting. *JACC Cardiovascular Interventions, 9*(24), 2493–2507.

Ramanathan, K., Farkouh, M., Cosmi, J., et al. (2011). Rapid complete reversal of systemic hypoperfusion after intra-aortic balloon pump counterpulsation and survival in cardiogenic shock complicating an acute myocardial infarction. *American Heart Journal, 162*(2), 268–275.

Roffi, M., Patrono, C., Collet, J., et al. (2015). 2015 ESC Guidelines for the management of acute coronary syndromes in patients presenting without persistent ST-segment elevation: Task force for the management of acute coronary syndromes in patients presenting without persistent ST-segment elevation of the European Society of Cardiology. *European Heart Journal, 37*(3), 267–315.

Samii, S. M. (2015). Indications for pacemakers, implantable cardioverter-defibrillator and cardiac resynchronization devices. *Medical Clinics of North America, 99*(4), 795–804.

Sheth, K. N., & Nourollahzadeh, E. (2017). Neurologic complications of cardiac and vascular surgery. *Handbook of Clinical Neurology, 141,* 573–592.

Siontis, G. C. M., Juni, P., Pigrim, T., et al. (2014). Predictors of permanent pacemaker implantation in patients with severe aortic stenosis undergoing TAVR. *Journal of the American College of Cardiology, 64*(2), 129–140.

Smith, J., Negrelli, J., Manek, M., et al. (2015). Diagnosis and management of acute coronary syndrome: An evidence-based update. *Journal of the American Board of Family Medicine, 28*(2), 283–293.

Unverzagt, S., Buerke, M., de Waha, A., et al. (2015). Intra-aortic balloon pump counterpulsation (IABP) for myocardial infarction complicated by cardiogenic shock. *Cochrane Database Systematic Review,* (3), 1–72.

Wiegand, D. L. (Ed.). (2017). *AACN procedure manual for critical care* (7th ed.). St. Louis, MO: Saunders.

13
Cardiac Disorders

CARDIAC DISORDERS

 See additional online content:
Nursing Care Plan 13.1

Coronary Artery Disease

 EVIDENCE BASE Smith, J., Negrelli, J., Manek, M., et al. (2015). Diagnosis and management of acute coronary syndrome: An evidence-based update. *Journal of the American Board of Family Medicine, 28*(2), 283–293.

Fihn, S. D., Blankenship, J. C., Alexander, K. P., et al. (2014). 2014 ACC/AHA/AATS/PCNA/SCAI/STS focused update of the guideline for the diagnosis and management of patients with stable ischemic heart disease: A report of the American College of Cardiology/American Heart Association Task Force on Practice Cardiovascular Guidelines, and the American Association for Thoracic Surgery, Preventive Cardiovascular Nurses Association, Society for Cardiovascular Angiography and Interventions, and Society of Thoracic Surgeons. *Circulation, 130*, 1749–1767.

Coronary artery disease (CAD) is the leading cause of death worldwide. CAD is characterized by the accumulation of plaque within the layers of the coronary arteries. The plaques progressively enlarge, thicken, and calcify, causing a critical narrowing (greater than 70% occlusion) of the coronary artery lumen, resulting in a decrease in coronary blood flow and an inadequate supply of oxygen to the heart muscle.

Acute coronary syndrome (ACS) is an umbrella term that is used to describe many of the complications associated with CAD. These include unstable angina, non–ST-elevation myocardial infarction (NSTEMI), and ST-elevation myocardial infarction (STEMI).

Pathophysiology and Etiology

1. The most widely accepted cause of CAD is atherosclerosis (see Figure 13-1), which is the gradual accumulation of plaque within an artery forming an atheroma. Plaque consists of lipid-filled macrophages (foam cells), fibrin, cellular waste products, and plasma proteins, covered by a fibrous outer layer (smooth muscle cells and dense connective tissue).
   a. When the endothelium is injured by being exposed to low-density lipoproteins, by-products of cigarette smoke, hypertension, hyperglycemia, infection, and increased homocysteine, hyperfibrinogenemia, and lipoprotein(a), an inflammatory response occurs, making the endothelium sticky and thereby attracting adhesion molecules.
   b. Over time, the plaque thickens, extends, and calcifies, causing narrowing of the lumen.
   c. Eventual hemorrhage and ulceration of the plaque may cause significant coronary obstruction.
2. Angina pectoris, caused by inadequate blood flow to the myocardium, is the most common manifestation of CAD.
   a. Angina is usually precipitated by physical exertion or emotional stress, which puts an increased demand on the heart to circulate more blood and oxygen.
   b. The ability of the coronary artery to deliver blood to the myocardium is impaired because of obstruction by a significant coronary lesion (greater than 70% narrowing of the vessel).
   c. Angina can also occur in other cardiac problems, such as arterial spasm, aortic stenosis, cardiomyopathy, or uncontrolled hypertension.
   d. Noncardiac causes include anemia, fever, thyrotoxicosis, and anxiety/panic attacks.
3. ACS is caused by a decrease in the oxygen available to the myocardium because of:
   a. Unstable or ruptured atherosclerotic plaque.
   b. Coronary vasospasm.
   c. Atherosclerotic obstruction without clot or vasospasm.
   d. Inflammation or infection.
   e. Unstable angina because of a noncardiac cause.
   f. Thrombus formation with subsequent coronary artery occlusion (the most common cause) (see "Myocardial Infarction," page 274).
4. Risk factors for the development of CAD include:
   a. Nonmodifiable: age (risk increases with age), male sex (women typically suffer from heart disease 10 years later than men because of the postmenopausal decrease in cardiac-protective estrogen), race (nonwhite populations have increased risk), and family history.
   b. Modifiable: elevated lipid levels, hypertension, obesity, tobacco use, metabolic syndrome (obesity, hypertension, and diabetes mellitus), sedentary lifestyle, and stress.

Figure 13-1. The pathogenesis of atherosclerosis.

c. Recent studies have shown that there are new risk factors associated with the development of CAD. These include increased levels of homocysteine, fibrin, and lipoprotein(a) and infection or inflammation (measured by C-reactive protein [CRP]).

d. The American Heart Association (AHA) also lists left ventricular hypertrophy (LVH) as a risk factor.

5. An atherosclerotic cardiovascular disease (ASCVD) risk assessment every 4 to 6 years is promoted for short-term and long-term prediction of the development of cardiovascular disease based on age, sex, race, lipid panel, systolic blood pressure, blood pressure medication use, smoking status, and diabetes status. Additional risk markers are diastolic blood pressure, chronic kidney disease, body mass index (BMI), and family history.

 EVIDENCE BASE Goff, D., Lloyd-Jones, D., D'Agostino, R. Sr., et al. (2014). Assessing cardiovascular risk: Systematic evidence review from the Risk Assessment Work Group. *Journal of the American College of Cardiology, 63*(25), 2935–2959.

STANDARDS OF CARE GUIDELINES 13-1
Chest Pain

- Thoroughly evaluate any complaint of chest pain.
- Be alert to those at highest risk for myocardial infarction (MI)—smokers, those with hypertension, diabetes, or hyperlipidemia—but do not discount that MI may occur in those without risk factors.
- Be alert to common alternative presentation of coronary artery disease and MI in women, diabetics, and older patients (nausea, indigestion, fatigue).
- Notify health care provider and obtain electrocardiogram for complaint of chest pain.
- For chest pain not relieved by rest or nitroglycerin, assist and advise patient to obtain emergency care immediately. Call 911 for emergency response team if pain is consistent with MI.

This information should serve as a general guideline only. Each patient situation presents a unique set of clinical factors and requires nursing judgment to guide care, which may include additional or alternative measures and approaches.

Clinical Manifestations

See Standards of Care Guidelines 13-1

Chronic Stable Angina Pectoris
Chest pain or discomfort that is provoked by exertion or emotional stress and relieved by rest and nitroglycerin.

1. Character—substernal chest pain, pressure, heaviness, or discomfort. Other sensations include a squeezing, aching, burning, choking, strangling, and/or cramping pain.
   a. Pain may be mild or severe and typically presents with a gradual buildup of discomfort and subsequent gradual fading.
   b. May produce numbness or weakness in the arms, wrists, or hands.
   c. Associated symptoms include diaphoresis, nausea, indigestion, dyspnea, tachycardia, and increase in blood pressure.
   d. Women may experience atypical symptoms of chest pain, such as jaw pain, shortness of breath, or indigestion. Patients with diabetes or history of heart transplant may not experience chest pain.
2. Location—behind middle or upper third of the sternum; the patient will generally make a fist over the site of the pain (positive Levine sign, indicating diffuse deep visceral pain) rather than point to it with his or her finger.
3. Radiation—usually radiates to the neck, jaw, shoulders, arms, hands, and posterior intrascapular area. Pain occurs more commonly on the left side than the right.
4. Duration—usually lasts 2 to 15 minutes after stopping activity; nitroglycerin relieves pain within 1 minute.
5. Other precipitating factors—exposure to weather extremes, eating a heavy meal, and sexual intercourse all increase the workload of the heart, thus increasing oxygen demand.

Unstable (Preinfarction) Angina Pectoris
Chest pain occurring at rest; no increase in oxygen demand is placed on the heart, but an acute lack of blood flow to the heart occurs because of coronary artery spasm or the presence of an enlarged plaque or hemorrhage/ulceration of a complicated lesion. Critical narrowing of the vessel lumen occurs abruptly in either instance.

1. A change in frequency, duration, and intensity of stable angina symptoms is indicative of progression to unstable angina.
2. Unstable angina pain lasts longer than 10 minutes, is unrelieved by rest or sublingual nitroglycerin, and mimics signs and symptoms of impending MI.

 NURSING ALERT Unstable angina can cause sudden death or result in MI. Early recognition and treatment are imperative to prevent complications.

Silent Ischemia
The absence of chest pain with documented evidence of an imbalance between myocardial oxygen supply and demand (ST depression of 1 mm or more) as determined by electrocardiography (ECG), exercise stress test, or ambulatory (Holter) ECG monitoring.

1. Silent ischemia most commonly occurs during the first few hours after awakening (circadian event) because of an increase in sympathetic nervous system activity, causing an increase in heart rate, blood pressure, coronary vessel tone, and blood viscosity.

Diagnostic Evaluation

1. Characteristic chest pain and clinical history.
2. Nitroglycerin test—relief of pain with nitroglycerin.

3. Blood tests.
   a. Cardiac markers, creatine kinase (CK) and its isoenzyme CK-MB, and troponin-I to determine the presence and severity if acute cardiac insult is suspected.
   b. HbA_{1C} and fasting lipid panel to rule out modifiable risk factors for CAD.
   c. Coagulation studies, CRP, homocysteine, and lipoprotein(a) (increased levels are associated with a twofold risk in developing CAD).
   d. Hemoglobin to rule out anemia, which may reduce myocardial oxygen supply.
4. Twelve-lead ECG—may show LVH, ST- and T-wave changes (2 mm or greater ST elevation in contiguous leads for male and 1.5 mm or greater in female diagnostics for myocardial infarction), arrhythmias, and Q waves.
5. ECG stress testing—progressive increases of speed and elevation while walking on a treadmill increase the workload of the heart. ST- and T-wave changes occur if myocardial ischemia is induced.
6. Radionuclide imaging—a radioisotope, thallium-201, injected during exercise is imaged by camera. Low uptake of the isotope by heart muscle indicates regions of ischemia induced by exercise. Images taken during rest show a reversal of ischemia in those regions affected.
7. Radionuclide ventriculography (gated blood pool scanning)—red blood cells tagged with a radioisotope are imaged by camera during exercise and at rest. Wall motion abnormalities of the heart can be detected and ejection fraction estimated.
8. Cardiac catheterization—coronary angiography performed during the procedure determines the presence, location, and extent of coronary lesions.
9. Positron emission tomography (PET)—cardiac perfusion imaging with high resolution to detect very small perfusion differences caused by stenotic arteries. Not available in all settings.
10. Coronary computed tomography angiography (CTA)—scans the coronary arteries that supply blood to the heart and determines whether they are narrowed by plaques. Three-dimensional images can be created. Recommended for low- to intermediate-risk patients with chest pain.

Management

Drug Therapy

Antianginal medications (nitrates, beta-adrenergic blockers, calcium channel blockers, and angiotensin-converting enzyme [ACE] inhibitors) are used to maintain a balance between oxygen supply and demand. Coronary vessel relaxation promotes blood flow to the heart, thereby increasing oxygen supply. Reduction of the workload of the heart decreases oxygen demand and consumption. The goal of drug therapy is to maintain a balance between oxygen supply and demand.

1. Nitrates—caused by generalized vasodilation throughout the body. Nitrates can be administered via oral, sublingual, transdermal, intravenous (IV), or intracoronary (IC) route and may provide short- or long-acting effects.
   a. Short-acting nitrates (sublingual) provide immediate relief of acute anginal attacks or prophylaxis if taken before activity.
   b. Long-acting nitrates prevent anginal episodes and/or reduce severity and frequency of attacks.
2. Beta-adrenergic blockers—inhibit sympathetic stimulation of receptors that are located in the conduction system of the heart and in heart muscle.

   a. Some beta-adrenergic blockers inhibit sympathetic stimulation of receptors in the lungs as well as the heart ("nonselective" beta-adrenergic blockers); vasoconstriction of the large airways in the lung occurs; generally contraindicated for patients with chronic obstructive lung disease or asthma.
   b. "Cardioselective" beta-adrenergic blockers (in recommended dose ranges) affect only the heart and can be used safely in patients with lung disease.
3. Calcium channel blockers—inhibit movement of calcium within the heart muscle and coronary vessels; promote vasodilation and prevent/control coronary artery spasm.
4. ACE inhibitors—have therapeutic effects by remodeling the vascular endothelium and have been shown to reduce the risk of worsening angina.
5. Antilipid agents—reduce total cholesterol and triglyceride levels and have been shown to assist in the stabilization of plaque.
6. Antiplatelet agents—decrease platelet aggregation to inhibit thrombus formation.
7. Folic acid and B complex vitamins—treat increased homocysteine levels.

Percutaneous Coronary Interventions

1. Percutaneous transluminal angioplasty.
   a. A balloon-tipped catheter is placed in a coronary vessel narrowed by plaque.
   b. The balloon is inflated and deflated to stretch the vessel wall and flatten the plaque (see page 255).
   c. Blood flows freely through the unclogged vessel to the heart.
2. IC atherectomy.
   a. A blade-tipped catheter is guided into a coronary vessel to the site of the plaque.
   b. Depending on the type of blade, the plaque is cut, shaved, or pulverized and then removed.
   c. Requires a larger catheter introduction sheath, so its use is limited to larger vessels.
3. IC stent.
   a. A diamond mesh tubular device is placed in the coronary vessel.
   b. Prevents restenosis by providing a "skeletal" support.
   c. Drug-eluting stents contain an anti-inflammatory drug, which decreases the inflammatory response within the artery.

Other Interventional Strategies

1. Coronary artery bypass graft (CABG) surgery.
   a. A graft is surgically attached to the aorta, and the other end of the graft is attached to a distal portion of a coronary vessel.
   b. Bypasses obstructive lesions in the vessel and returns adequate blood flow to the heart muscle supplied by the artery (see page 260).
   c. Recommended for patients with diabetes mellitus, multivessel CAD, and acceptable surgical risk instead of PCI.
2. Transmyocardial revascularization—by means of a laser beam, small channels are formed in the myocardium to encourage new blood flow.

Secondary Prevention

EVIDENCE BASE Eckel, R., Jakicic, J., Ard, J., et al. (2014). 2013 AHA/ACC guideline on lifestyle management to reduce cardiovascular risk: A report of the American College of Cardiology American/Heart Association Task Force on Practice Guidelines. *Circulation*, *129*(25 Suppl 2), S76–S99.

1. Cessation of smoking.
2. Control of high blood pressure (below 130/85 mm Hg in those with renal insufficiency or heart failure; below 130/80 mm Hg in those with diabetes; below 140/90 mm Hg in all others).
3. Diet low in saturated fat (less than 7% of calories), cholesterol (less than 200 mg/day), trans fatty acids, sodium (less than 2 g/day), alcohol (2 or fewer drinks/day in men, 1 or fewer in women).
4. Low-dose aspirin daily for those at high risk.
5. Physical exercise (at least 30 to 60 minutes of moderate-intensity exercise most days).
6. Weight control (ideal body mass index 18.5 to 24.9 kg/m^2); waist circumference less than 40 inches for men and less than 35 inches for women.
7. Control of diabetes mellitus (fasting glucose less than 110 mg/dL and HbA$_{1C}$ less than 7%).
8. Control of blood lipids with low-density lipoprotein (LDL) goal less than 100 mg/dL (less than 70 mg/dL in high-risk patients).

Complications

1. Sudden death because of lethal dysrhythmias.
2. Heart failure.
3. MI.

Nursing Assessment

1. Ask patient to describe anginal attacks.
   a. When do attacks tend to occur? After a meal? After engaging in certain activities? After physical activities in general? After visits of family/others?
   b. Where is the pain located? Does it radiate?
   c. Was the onset of pain sudden? Gradual?
   d. How long did it last—Seconds? Minutes? Hours?
   e. Was the pain steady and unwavering in quality?
   f. Is the discomfort accompanied by other symptoms? Sweating? Light-headedness? Nausea? Palpitations? Shortness of breath?
   g. Is there anything that makes it worse (such as moving, deep breathing, food)?
   h. How is the pain relieved? How long does it take for pain relief?
2. Obtain a baseline 12-lead ECG.
3. Assess patient's and family's knowledge of disease.
4. Identify patient's and family's level of anxiety and use of appropriate coping mechanisms.
5. Gather information about the patient's cardiac risk factors. Use the patient's age, total cholesterol level, LDL and HDL levels, systolic BP, and smoking status to determine the patient's 10-year risk for development of CHD according to the Framingham Risk Scoring Method.
6. Evaluate patient's medical history for such conditions as diabetes, heart failure, previous MI, or obstructive lung disease that may influence choice of drug therapy.
7. Identify factors that may contribute to noncompliance with prescribed drug therapy.
8. Review renal and hepatic studies and complete blood count (CBC).
9. Discuss with patient current activity levels. (Effectiveness of antianginal drug therapy is evaluated by patient's ability to attain higher activity levels.)
10. Discuss patient's beliefs about modification of risk factors and willingness to change.

Nursing Diagnoses

- Acute Pain related to an imbalance in oxygen supply and demand.
- Decreased Cardiac Output related to reduced preload, afterload, contractility, and heart rate secondary to hemodynamic effects of drug therapy.
- Anxiety related to chest pain, uncertain prognosis, and threatening environment.

Nursing Interventions

Relieving Pain

1. Determine intensity of patient's angina.
   a. Ask patient to compare the pain with other pain experienced in the past and, on a scale of 0 (no pain) to 10 (worst pain), rate current pain.
   b. Observe for associated signs and symptoms, including diaphoresis, shortness of breath, protective body posture, dusky facial color, and/or changes in level of consciousness (LOC).
2. Position patient for comfort; Fowler position promotes ventilation.
3. Administer oxygen, if appropriate.
4. Obtain BP, apical heart rate, and respiratory rate.
5. Obtain a 12-lead ECG.
6. Administer antianginal drug(s), as prescribed.
7. Report findings to health care providers.
8. Monitor for relief of pain and note duration of anginal episode.
9. Take vital signs every 5 to 10 minutes until angina pain subsides.
10. Monitor for progression of stable angina to unstable angina: increase in frequency and intensity of pain, pain occurring at rest or at low levels of exertion, pain lasting longer than 5 minutes.
11. Determine level of activity that precipitated anginal episode.
12. Identify specific activities patient may engage in that are below the level at which anginal pain occurs.
13. Reinforce the importance of notifying nursing staff when angina pain is experienced.

Maintaining Cardiac Output

1. Carefully monitor the patient's response to drug therapy.
   a. Take BP and heart rate in a sitting and a lying position on initiation of long-term therapy (provides baseline data to evaluate for orthostatic hypotension that may occur with drug therapy).
   b. Recheck vital signs as indicated by onset of action of drug and at the time of drug's peak effect.
   c. Note changes in BP of more than 10 mm Hg and changes in heart rate of more than 10 beats/minute.
   d. Note patient complaints of headache (especially with use of nitrates) and dizziness (more common with ACE inhibitors).
      i. Administer or teach self-administration of analgesics, as directed, for headache.
      ii. Encourage supine position to relieve dizziness (usually associated with a decrease in BP; preload is enhanced by lying supine, thereby providing a temporary increase in BP).
   e. Institute continuous ECG monitoring or obtain 12-lead ECG as directed. Interpret rhythm strip every 4 hours and as needed for patients on continuous monitoring

(beta-adrenergic blockers and calcium channel blockers can cause significant bradycardia and varying degrees of heart block).

f. Evaluate for development of heart failure (beta-adrenergic blockers and some calcium channel blockers have negative inotropic properties).

i. Obtain daily weight and intake and output.

ii. Auscultate lung fields for crackles and assess for shortness of breath and decrease in oxygen saturation.

iii. Monitor for the presence of edema.

iv. Monitor central venous pressure (CVP), if applicable.

v. Assess jugular vein distention.

vi. Assess liver engorgement and check liver function studies.

g. Monitor laboratory tests as indicated (cardiac markers).

2. Monitor for poor perfusion.

a. Decreasing blood pressure.

b. Weak pulses.

c. Dizziness.

d. Shortness of breath.

e. Cool extremities.

f. Pale.

g. Diaphoretic.

3. Be sure to remove previous nitrate patch or paste before applying new paste or patch (prevents hypotension) and to reapply on different body site. To decrease nitrate tolerance, transdermal nitroglycerin may be worn only in the daytime hours and taken off at night when physical exertion is decreased.

4. Be alert to adverse reaction related to abrupt discontinuation of beta-adrenergic blocker and calcium channel blocker therapy. These drugs must be tapered to prevent a "rebound phenomenon": tachycardia, increase in chest pain, hypertension.

5. Discuss use of chromotherapeutic therapy with health care provider (tailoring of antianginal drug therapy to the timing of circadian events).

6. Report adverse drug effects to health care provider.

Decreasing Anxiety

1. Rule out physiologic etiologies for increasing or new-onset anxiety before administering as-needed sedatives. Physiologic causes must be identified and treated in a timely fashion to prevent irreversible adverse or even fatal outcomes; sedatives may mask symptoms delaying timely identification and diagnosis and treatment.

2. Assess patient for signs of hypoperfusion, auscultate heart and lung sounds, obtain a rhythm strip, and administer oxygen, as prescribed. Notify the health care provider immediately.

3. Document all assessment findings, health care provider notification and response, and interventions and response.

4. Explain to patient and family reasons for hospitalization, diagnostic tests, and therapies administered.

5. Encourage patient to verbalize fears and concerns about illness through frequent conversations—conveys to patient a willingness to listen.

6. Answer patient's questions with concise explanations.

7. Administer medications to relieve patient's anxiety as directed. Sedatives and tranquilizers may be used to prevent attacks precipitated by aggravation, excitement, or tension.

8. Explain to patient the importance of anxiety reduction to assist in control of angina. (Anxiety and fear put increased stress on the heart, requiring the heart to use more oxygen.) Teach relaxation techniques.

9. Discuss measures to be taken when an anginal episode occurs. (Preparing patient decreases anxiety and allows patient to describe angina accurately.)

a. Review the questions that will be asked during anginal episodes.

b. Review the interventions that will be employed to relieve anginal attacks.

Patient Education and Health Maintenance

Instruct Patient and Family about CAD

1. Assess readiness to learn (pain free, shows interest, and comfortable), learning style, cognition, and education level.

2. Review the chambers of the heart and the coronary artery system, using a diagram of the heart.

3. Show patient a diagram of a clogged artery; explain how the blockage occurs; point out on the diagram the location of patient's lesions.

4. Explain what angina is (a warning sign from the heart that there is not enough blood and oxygen because of the blocked artery or spasm).

5. Review specific risk factors that affect CAD development and progression; highlight those risk factors that can be modified and controlled to reduce risk.

6. Discuss the signs and symptoms of angina, precipitating factors, and treatment for attacks. Stress to patient the importance of treating angina symptoms at once.

7. Distinguish for patient the different signs and symptoms associated with stable angina versus preinfarction angina.

8. Give patient and family handouts to review and encourage questions for a later teaching session.

Identify Suitable Activity Level to Prevent Angina

Advise the patient about the following:

1. Participate in a normal daily program of activities that do not produce chest discomfort, shortness of breath, and undue fatigue. Spread daily activities out over the course of the day; avoid doing everything at one time. Begin regular exercise regimen, as directed by health care provider.

2. Avoid activities known to cause anginal pain—sudden exertion, walking against the wind, extremes of temperature, high altitude, and emotionally stressful situations, which my accelerate heart rate, raise BP, and increase cardiac workload.

3. Refrain from engaging in physical activity for 2 hours after meals. Rest after each meal, if possible.

4. Do not perform activities requiring heavy effort (eg, carrying heavy objects).

5. Try to avoid cold weather, if possible; dress warmly and walk more slowly. Wear scarf over the nose and mouth when in cold air.

6. Lose weight, if necessary, to reduce cardiac load.

7. Instruct patient that sexual activity is not prohibited and should be discussed with health care provider.

Instruct about Appropriate Use of Medications and Adverse Effects

1. Carry nitroglycerin at all times.

a. Nitroglycerin is volatile and is inactivated by heat, moisture, air, light, and time.

b. Keep nitroglycerin in original dark glass container, tightly closed to prevent absorption of drug by other pills or pillbox.

c. Nitroglycerin should cause a slight burning or stinging sensation under the tongue when it is potent.

2. Place nitroglycerin under the tongue at first sign of chest discomfort.
   a. Stop all effort or activity, sit, and take nitroglycerin tablet—relief should be obtained in a few minutes.
   b. Repeat dosage in 5 minutes for total of three tablets if relief is not obtained.
   c. Keep a record of the number of tablets taken to evaluate change in anginal pattern.
   d. Take nitroglycerin prophylactically to avoid pain known to occur with certain activities.
3. Demonstrate for patient how to administer nitroglycerin paste correctly.
   a. Place paste on calibrated strip.
   b. Remove previous paste on the skin by wiping gently with tissue. Be careful to avoid touching paste to fingertips as this will lead to increased dosing from absorption.
   c. Rotate site of administration to avoid skin irritation.
   d. Apply paste to the skin; use plastic wrap to protect clothing if not provided on strip.
   e. Have patient return demonstration.
4. Instruct patient on administration of transdermal nitroglycerin patches.
   a. Remove previous patch; fold in half so that medication does not touch fingertips and will not be accessible in trash. Wipe area with tissue to remove any residual medication.
   b. Apply patch to a clean, dry, nonhairy area of the body.
   c. Rotate administration sites.
   d. Instruct patient not to remove patch for swimming or bathing.
   e. If patch loosens and part of it becomes nonadherent, it should be folded in half and discarded. A new patch should be applied.
5. Teach patient about potential adverse effects of other medications. Instruct patient not to stop taking any of these without discussing with health care provider.
   a. Constipation—verapamil.
   b. Ankle edema—nifedipine.
   c. Heart failure (shortness of breath, weight gain, edema)—beta-adrenergic blockers or calcium channel blockers.
   d. Dizziness—vasodilators, antihypertensives.
   e. Impotence–decreased libido and sexual functioning—beta-adrenergic blockers.
6. Ensure that patient has enough medication until next follow-up appointment or trip to the pharmacy. Warn against abrupt withdrawal of beta-adrenergic blockers or calcium channel blockers to prevent rebound effect.

 NURSING ALERT Instruct patient to call 911 if chest pain persists or has worsened after the first sublingual nitroglycerin tablet was administered (5 minutes). Furthermore, instruct patient to continue to take other sublingual nitroglycerin tablets every 5 minutes until emergency medical services have arrived (instruct patient not drive self to the hospital).

Counsel on Risk Factors and Lifestyle Changes

1. Inform patient of methods of stress reduction, such as biofeedback and relaxation techniques.
2. Review low-fat and low-cholesterol diet. Explain AHA guidelines (see *www.heart.org*), which recommend eating fish at least twice per week, especially fish high in omega-3 oils.
   a. Omega-3 oils have been shown to improve arterial health and decrease BP, triglycerides, and the growth of atherosclerotic plaque.
   b. Omega-3 oils can be found in fatty fish, such as mackerel, salmon, sardines, herring, and albacore tuna.
   c. Suggest available cookbooks (AHA) that may assist in planning and preparing foods.
   d. Have patient meet with dietitian to design a menu plan.
3. Inform patient of available cardiac rehabilitation programs that offer structured classes on exercise, smoking cessation, and weight control.
4. Instruct patient to avoid excessive caffeine intake (coffee, cola drinks), which can increase the heart rate and produce angina.
5. Tell patient not to use "diet pills," nasal decongestants, or any over-the-counter (OTC) medications that can increase heart rate or stimulate high BP.
6. Encourage patient to avoid alcohol or drink only in moderation (alcohol can increase hypotensive adverse effects of drugs).
7. Encourage follow-up visits for control of diabetes, hypertension, and hyperlipidemia.
8. Have patient discuss supplement therapy (ie, vitamins B_6, B_{12}, C, E, folic acid, and L-arginine) with health care provider.
9. For additional information, refer patient to the AHA (*www.americanheart.org*).
10. Refer patient to health care provider to discuss the use of phosphodiesterase inhibitors (PDE5) for erectile dysfunction.

 DRUG ALERT Patient should not take PDE5, such as sildenafil, concurrently with nitrates or alpha-adrenergic blockers because severe hypotension and cardiac event may occur.

Evaluation: Expected Outcomes

- Verbalizes relief of pain.
- BP and heart rate stable.
- Verbalizes lessening anxiety, ability to cope.

Myocardial Infarction

 EVIDENCE BASE Gara, P. T., Kushner, F. G., Ascheim, D. D., et al. (2013). ACCF/AHA guideline for the management of ST elevation myocardial infarction. *Circulation, 127*, 529–555.

Myocardial infarction (MI) is one of the manifestations of acute coronary syndrome (ACS) and refers to a dynamic process by which one or more regions of the heart experience a prolonged decrease or cessation in oxygen supply because of insufficient coronary blood flow; subsequently, necrosis or "death" to the affected myocardial tissue occurs. The onset of the MI process may be sudden or gradual, and the progression of the event to cell death takes approximately 3 to 6 hours.

Pathophysiology and Etiology

1. Acute coronary thrombosis (partial or total)—associated with 90% of MIs.
   a. Severe atherosclerosis (greater than 70% narrowing of the artery) precipitates thrombus.
   b. Thrombus formation begins with plaque rupture and platelets' adhesion to the damaged area.
   c. Activation of the exposed platelets causes expression of glycoprotein IIb/IIIa receptors that bind fibrinogen.
   d. Further platelet aggregation and adhesion occurs, enlarging the thrombus and occluding blood supply.

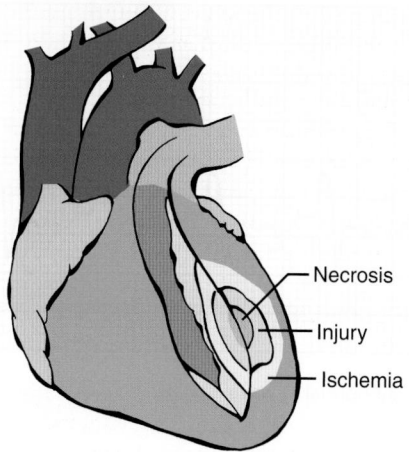

Figure 13-2. Different degrees of damage occur to the heart muscle after a myocardial infarction. This diagram shows the zones of necrosis, injury, and ischemia.

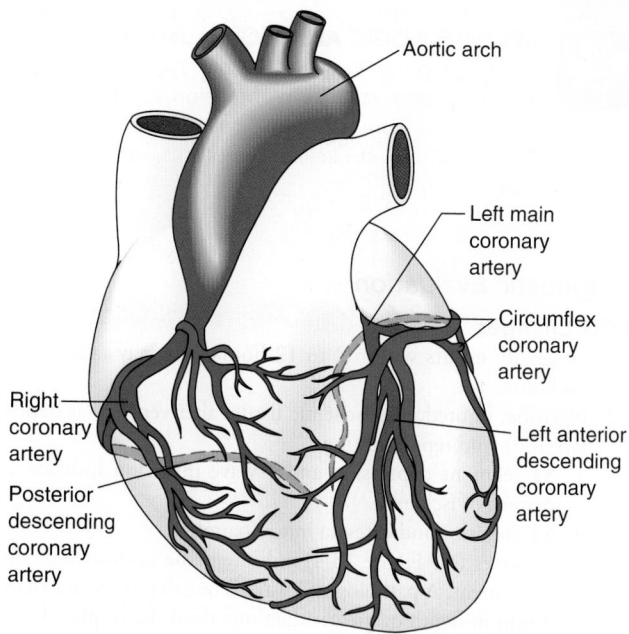

Figure 13-3. Diagram of the coronary arteries arising from the aorta and encircling the heart. Some of the coronary veins are also shown. (Smeltzer, S., and Bare, B. [2000]. Brunner and Suddarth's textbook of medical-surgical nursing [9th ed.]. Philadelphia: Lippincott Williams & Wilkins.)

2. Other etiologic factors include coronary artery spasm, coronary artery embolism, infectious diseases causing arterial inflammation, hypoxia, anemia, and severe exertion or stress on the heart in the presence of significant CAD (ie, surgical procedures, shoveling snow).
3. Different degrees of damage occur to the heart muscle (see Figure 13-2):
   a. Zone of necrosis—death to the heart muscle caused by extensive and complete oxygen deprivation; irreversible damage.
   b. Zone of injury—region of the heart muscle surrounding the area of necrosis; inflamed and injured, but still viable if adequate oxygenation can be restored.
   c. Zone of ischemia—region of the heart muscle surrounding the area of injury, which is ischemic and viable; not endangered unless extension of the infarction occurs.
4. Classification of MI:
   a. STEMI—whereby ST-segment elevations are seen on ECG. The area of necrosis may or may not occur through the entire wall of heart muscle.
   b. NSTEMI—no ST-segment elevations can be seen on ECG. ST depressions may be noted as well as positive cardiac markers, T-wave inversions, and clinical equivalents (chest pain). Area of necrosis may or may not occur through the entire myocardium.
5. The region(s) of the heart muscle that becomes affected depends on which coronary artery(ies) is/are obstructed (see Figure 13-3).
   a. The left ventricle is a common and dangerous location for an MI because it is the main pumping chamber of the heart. The left anterior descending artery supplies oxygen to this part of the heart.
   b. Right ventricular infarctions commonly occur with damage to the inferior and/or posterior wall of the left ventricle. Occlusion in the right coronary or circumflex arteries can lead to this type of infarct.
6. The severity and location of the MI determine prognosis.

NURSING ALERT Early reperfusion and revascularization (ie, within 24 hours) are recommended for NSTEMI. Although revascularization can be delayed in low-risk patients, studies show this can increase length of stay and cost. Reperfusion can occur via femoral or radial approach. Radial approach is associated with reduced complications and mortality.

Clinical Manifestations

1. Chest pain.
   a. Severe, diffuse, steady substernal pain; may be described as crushing, squeezing, or dull.
   b. Not relieved by rest or sublingual vasodilator therapy such as nitroglycerine, but requires opioids (ie, morphine).
   c. May radiate to the arms (usually the left), shoulders, neck, back, and/or jaw.
   d. Continues for more than 15 minutes.
   e. May produce anxiety and fear, resulting in increased heart rate, blood pressure, and respiratory rate.
   f. Some patients, women or diabetics, may exhibit no complaints of pain (silent MI).
2. Diaphoresis; cool, clammy skin; facial pallor.
3. Hypertension or hypotension.
4. Bradycardia or tachycardia.
5. Premature ventricular and/or atrial beats.
6. Palpitations, severe anxiety, dyspnea.
7. Disorientation, confusion, restlessness.
8. Fainting, marked weakness.
9. Nausea, vomiting, hiccups.
10. Atypical symptoms: epigastric or abdominal distress, dull aching or tingling sensations, shortness of breath, extreme fatigue.

NURSING ALERT Many patients do not have symptoms; these are "silent MIs." Nevertheless, there is still resultant damage to the heart. Women and diabetics usually present with atypical and/or vague complaints (eg, indigestion, fatigue). These patients are at higher risk of death during hospitalization. This is influenced by delay in seeking medical attention, and they are less likely to receive therapies that have been shown to be effective in MI treatment (ie, fibrinolytics or primary PCI, aspirin, beta-blockers, or heparin).

GERONTOLOGIC ALERT Older patients are more likely to experience silent MIs or have atypical signs and symptoms, such as hypotension, low body temperature, shortness of breath, vague complaints of discomfort, mild perspiration, strokelike symptoms, dizziness, or change in sensorium.

Diagnostic Evaluation

ECG Changes
1. Generally occurs within 2 to 12 hours, but may take 72 to 96 hours.
2. Necrotic, injured, and ischemic tissues alter ventricular depolarization and repolarization.
   a. ST-segment depression and T-wave inversion indicate a pattern of ischemia.
   b. ST elevation indicates an injury pattern.
   c. Q waves (see Figure 13-4) indicate tissue necrosis and are permanent. A pathologic Q wave is one that is greater than 3 mm in depth or greater than one third the height of the R wave.
3. Location of the infarction (anterior, anteroseptal, inferior, posterior, lateral) is determined by the leads in which the ST changes (elevation vs. depression) are seen. Of note, the changes must be in two contiguous or related leads to be diagnostic.

NURSING ALERT A normal ECG does not rule out the possibility of infarction because ECG changes can be subtle and obscured by underlying conditions (bundle-branch blocks, electrolyte disturbances).

Cardiac Markers
1. Cardiac enzymes (biochemical markers) are not diagnostic of an acute MI with a single elevation; serial markers are drawn (see page 236).
   a. Marker elevation is then correlated to the extent of heart muscle damage.

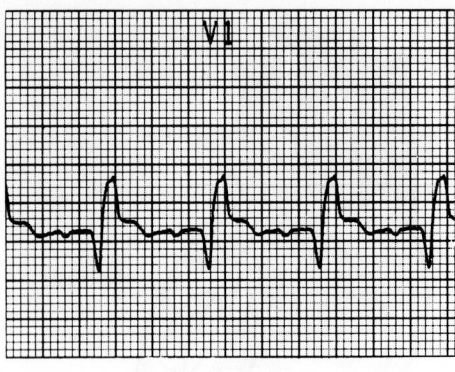

Figure 13-4. Abnormal Q wave.

b. Characteristic elevation over several hours confirms an MI (see Figure 13-5).

Other Findings
1. Elevated CRP and lipoprotein(s) because of inflammation in the coronary arteries.
2. Abnormal coagulation studies (prothrombin time [PT], partial thromboplastin time [PTT]).
3. Elevated white blood cell (WBC) count and sedimentation rate because of the inflammatory process involved in heart muscle cell damage.
4. Radionuclide imaging allows recognition of areas of decreased perfusion.
5. PET scan determines the presence of reversible heart muscle injury and irreversible or necrotic tissue; extent to which the injured heart muscle has responded to treatment can also be determined.
6. Cardiac muscle dysfunction can be noted on echocardiography or cardiac magnetic resonance imaging (MRI).

Management

The goals for UA/NSTEMI therapy are immediate relief of ischemia and prevention of severe outcomes such as death or myocardial infarction or reinfarction. To achieve this requires administration of anti-ischemic therapy (ie, rest, supplemental oxygen, nitroglycerin,

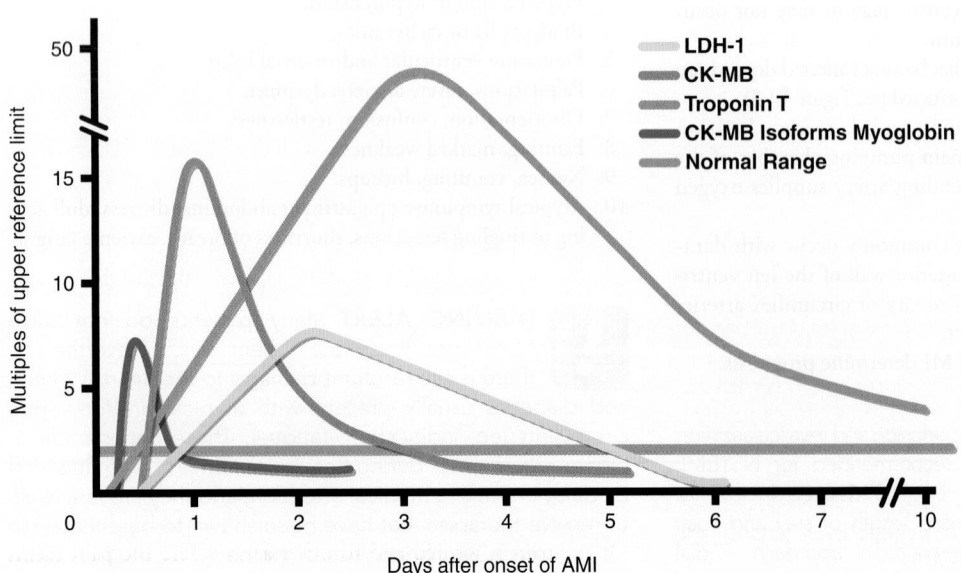

Figure 13-5. Release of cardiac markers after acute myocardial infarction (AMI). Following AMI, myoglobin and CK-MB levels rise, but the increases last only a few days. Levels of troponin T can be sustained for 4 to 10 days following AMI, allowing for more accurate diagnosis. All results are normalized to the upper reference limit. (Wu, A. H. B. [1995]. Cardiac troponins T and I in coronary artery diseases. *Endocrinology and Metabolism In-Service Training and Continuing Education.* 13, 81. © American Association for Clinical Chemistry, Inc.)

beta-blockers, ACE inhibitors) and antithrombotic therapy (ie, aspirin, clopidogrel, ticlopidine) and ongoing risk stratification and use of invasive procedure (ie, cardiac catheterization) to provide early restoration of coronary blood flow. Growing evidence suggest the use of supplemental oxygen in the absence of hypoxia may lead to increase infarct size. Caution should be exercised when administering oxygen to patients experiencing STEMI.

 EVIDENCE BASE Nehme, Z., Stub, D., Bernard, S., et al. (2016). Effect of supplemental oxygen exposure on myocardial injury in ST elevation myocardial infarction. *Heart, 2016,* 444–451.

Pharmacologic Therapy

The pharmacologic therapy for MI is standard (see Table 13-1, page 278). Use the MONA acronym to outline immediate pharmacologic interventions.

1. M (morphine)—IV rather than intramuscular (IM) is used to treat chest pain. Endogenous catecholamine release during pain imposes an increase in the workload on the heart, thus causing an increase in oxygen demand. Morphine's analgesic effects decrease the pain, relieve anxiety, and improve cardiac output by reducing preload and afterload.
2. O (oxygen)—given via nasal cannula or face mask. Increases oxygenation to ischemic heart muscle.
3. N (nitrates)—given sublingually via spray or through IV administration. Vasodilator therapy reduces preload by decreasing blood return to the heart and decreasing oxygen demand.
4. A (aspirin)—immediate dosing by mouth (chewed) is recommended to halt platelet aggregation.

Other Medications

1. Fibrinolytic agents such as tissue plasma activator, streptokinase, and reteplase are given IV to reestablish blood flow in coronary vessels by dissolving thrombus.
   a. Contraindicated in the management of unstable angina or NSTEMI or posterior wall MI. Studies have shown no clinical benefits in the absence of ST elevation MI or bundle-branch block.
   b. No effect on the underlying stenosis that precipitated the thrombus to form.
2. Antiarrhythmics, such as amiodarone to decrease the ventricular irritability that occurs after MI.
   a. Bolus of amiodarone is given via IV line over 10 minutes; then, an infusion is given in varying doses over 24 hours (1 mg/minute for 6 hours then 0.5 mg/minute for 18 hours).
   b. Correction of electrolyte imbalances such as hyperkalemia that also causes ventricular irritability.

Percutaneous Coronary Interventions

 EVIDENCE BASE Tricoci, P., Lokhnygina, Y., Berdan, L. G., et al. (2016). ACC/AHA/SCAI focused update on primary percutaneous coronary intervention for patients with ST elevation myocardial infarction : An update of the 2011 ACCF/AHA/SCAI guideline for percutaneous coronary intervention and the 2013 ACCF/AHA guideline for the management of ST-elevation myocardial infarction: A report of the American College of Cardiology/American Heart Association Task Force on Clinical Practice Guidelines and the Society for Cardiovascular Angiography and Interventions. *Journal of the American College of Cardiology, 67*(10).

1. Mechanical opening of the coronary vessel can be performed during an evolving infarction.
2. Percutaneous coronary interventions (PCIs), including percutaneous transluminal coronary angioplasty, coronary stenting, and atherectomy, can be used instead of, or as an adjunct to, fibrinolytic therapy (see page 255).
3. Fibrinolytic therapy is considered in STEMI patients if PCI is not able to be performed within 90 minutes. The guidelines suggest patients presenting to non–PCI capacity facilities should be transferred to PCI-capable facility within 120 minutes of presentation for immediate PCI. However, if delays are anticipated (ie, transfer delay by greater than 120 minutes), then fibrinolytic therapy should be considered within 30 minutes of presentation to facility.

GERONTOLOGIC ALERT Older patients are extremely susceptible to respiratory depression in response to opioids. Titrate dose carefully and monitor respiratory status.

Surgical Revascularization

1. Cardiac surgery (ie, CABG) following STEMI is associated with high mortality in the first 3 to 7 days; thus, the benefit of revascularization must be weighed against the risk of cardiac surgery. However, newer surgical approaches such as off-pump CABG have mitigated this risk for some patients.
2. Benefits of this therapy include definitive treatment of the stenosis and less scar formation on the heart.

Complications

1. Dysrhythmias.
2. Sudden cardiac death because of ventricular arrhythmias.
3. Infarct expansion (thinning and dilation of the necrotic zone).
4. Infarct extension (additional heart muscle necrosis occurring after 24 hours of acute infarction).
5. Heart failure (with 20% to 35% left ventricle damage).
6. Cardiogenic shock.
7. Reinfarction.
8. Ischemic cardiomyopathy.
9. Cardiac rupture.
10. Papillary muscle rupture.
11. Ventricular mural thrombus.
12. Ischemic stroke.
13. Thromboemboli (deep vein thrombosis and pulmonary embolism).
14. Ventricular aneurysm.
15. Cardiac tamponade.
16. Pericarditis (2 to 3 days after MI).
17. Dissection of coronary arteries during angioplasty.
18. Psychiatric problems—depression, personality changes.

Nursing Assessment

1. Gather information regarding the patient's chest pain:
   a. Nature and intensity—describe the pain in patient's own words and compare it with pain previously experienced.
   b. Onset and duration—exact time pain occurred as well as the time pain relieved or diminished (if applicable).
   c. Location and radiation—point to the area where the pain is located and to other areas where the pain seems to travel.

Table 13-1   ACS Medications at a Glance

DRUG AND ACTION	CLINICAL CONSIDERATIONS
Aspirin Antiplatelet drug that blocks prostaglandin synthesis and thromboxane A_2 formation	• Administer as soon as acute coronary syndrome (ACS) is suspected. • Give patient 160 to 325 mg; if not already taking aspirin, patient should chew this dose. • If patient is allergic to aspirin, give clopidogrel or ticlopidine instead.
Clopidogrel, ticagrelor Antiplatelet drugs that inhibit platelet aggregation Note: Restenosis is possible after PCI in those patients with the CYP2C19 gene, which causes significantly lower levels of the active metabolite of clopidogrel	• Alternatives for patients who cannot use aspirin. • Recent research indicates that using clopidogrel and aspirin concurrently reduces risk of myocardial infarction (MI), stroke, and death.
Unfractionated heparin, low molecular weight heparin (dalteparin, enoxaparin) Potentiate antithrombin III activity, inactivate thrombin, prevent conversion of fibrinogen to fibrin	**Unfractionated heparin** • Weight-adjusted dosage is given to achieve therapeutic partial thromboplastin time (PTT) and activated clotting time. • Reversible with protamine sulfate. **Low molecular weight heparin** • PTT is not monitored. • Give by subcutaneous injection. • Effects are not reversible.
Glycoprotein (GP) IIb/IIIa inhibitors (abciximab, tirofiban, eptifibatide) Block GP sites on platelets, preventing platelet aggregation	• Indicated for intermediate- or high-risk ACS or with percutaneous coronary intervention. • Each drug has specific indications and dosage ranges. Consult package insert for specifics.
Fibrinolytics (alteplase, tenecteplase, streptokinase, reteplase) Break up the fibrin meshwork in clots	• Indicated in ST-segment elevation ACS only. • Certain agents require weight-adjusted dose. See package inserts for details.
Beta-adrenergic blockers (metoprolol, atenolol) Reduce cardiac output and heart rate, reduce ventricular remodeling, and decrease endothelial dysfunction	• Start all ACS patients on a beta-adrenergic blocker as tolerated. • As ordered, titrate dosage to meet therapeutic goals: heart rate, 60 beats/minute; blood pressure (BP), >90 mm Hg systolic.
Angiotensin-converting enzyme inhibitors (captopril, enalapril) Decrease endothelial dysfunction and prevent conversion of angiotensin I to angiotensin II	• Indicated for patients with heart failure, those with a heart rate above 100 beats/minute, and those with an anterior MI, hypertension, or diabetes. • Start with a drug with a short half-life, such as captopril, within 24 hours to treat acute MI; on discharge, switch to a longer-acting drug, such as lisinopril or enalapril.
Nitroglycerin Dilates peripheral vessels, relaxes vascular smooth muscle, and decreases preload	• Can be given sublingually, orally, or via IV line spray in an acute care setting • Do not allow BP to drop below 90 mm Hg systolic. • Switch the patient to a topical patch or an oral form for long-term use.
Morphine Acts as an analgesic and sedative	• Indicated in acute care setting only; not for prolonged use. • Give until patient is free from chest pain or to relieve pulmonary congestion. • Monitor BP, level of consciousness, and respiratory rate.

Granger, B., & Miller, C. (2001). Acute coronary syndromes: Putting the new guidelines to work. Nursing 2001, 31(11), 42.

d. Precipitating and aggravating factors—describe the activity performed just before the onset of pain and if any maneuvers and/or medications alleviated the pain.

2. Question patient about other symptoms experienced associated with the pain. Observe patient for diaphoresis, facial pallor, dyspnea, guarding behaviors, rigid body posture, extreme weakness, and confusion.

3. Evaluate cognitive, behavioral, and emotional status.

4. Question patient about prior health status with emphasis on current medications, allergies (opiate analgesics, iodine, shellfish), recent trauma or surgery, nonsteroidal anti-inflammatory drug (NSAID) ingestion, peptic ulcers, fainting spells, drug and alcohol use.

5. Analyze information for contraindications for fibrinolytic therapy and PCI.

6. Gather information about presence or absence of cardiac risk factors.

7. Identify patient's social support system and potential caregivers.

8. Identify significant others' reaction to the crisis situation.

Nursing Diagnoses

• Anxiety related to chest pain, fear of death, threatening environment.

• Activity Intolerance related to insufficient oxygenation to perform activities of daily living, deconditioning effects of bed rest.

- Risk for Bleeding related to dissolution of protective clots.
- Risk for Decreased Cardiac Tissue Perfusion related to coronary restenosis, extension of infarction.
- Ineffective Coping related to threats to self-esteem, disruption of sleep–rest pattern, lack of significant support system, loss of control, and change in lifestyle.

Nursing Interventions

Alleviating Anxiety

1. Rule out physiologic etiologies for increasing or new-onset anxiety before administering as-needed sedatives. Physiologic causes must be identified and treated in a timely fashion to prevent irreversible adverse or even fatal outcomes; sedatives may mask symptoms, delaying timely identification, diagnosis, and treatment.
   a. Autonomic signs of anxiety are increases in heart rate, BP, respiratory rate, and tremulousness, but they may also be signs of physiologic complications.
   b. Anxiety with dyspnea, tachypnea, and tachycardia may indicate pulmonary embolism; frothy pink sputum and orthopnea indicate pulmonary edema.
   c. Appearance of heart murmurs or friction rub indicates valvular dysfunction, possible intraventricular septal rupture, and pericarditis.
2. Whenever anxiety increases, assess patient for signs of hypoperfusion, auscultate heart and lung sounds, obtain a rhythm strip, and administer oxygen, as prescribed. Notify the health care provider immediately.
3. Assess and document emotional status frequently. Document all assessment findings, health care provider notification and response, and interventions and response.
4. Explain to patient and family reasons for hospitalization, diagnostic tests, and therapies administered.
5. Explain equipment, procedures, and need for frequent assessment to patient and significant others.
6. Discuss with patient and family the anticipated nursing and medical regimen.
   a. Explain visiting hours and need to limit number of visitors per facility policy.
   b. Offer family preferred times to phone unit to check on patient's status.
7. Administer antianxiety agents, as prescribed.
   a. Explain to patient the reason for sedation: undue anxiety can make the heart more irritable and require more oxygen.
   b. Assure patient that the goal of sedation is to promote comfort and, therefore, should be requested if anxious, excitable, or "jittery" feelings occur.
   c. Observe for adverse effects of sedation, such as lethargy, confusion, and/or increased agitation.
8. Maintain consistency of care with one or two nurses regularly assisting patient, especially if severe anxiety is present.
9. Offer massage, imagery, and progressive muscle relaxation to promote relaxation, reduce muscle tension, and reduce workload on the heart.

Increasing Activity Tolerance

1. Promote activity tolerance with early gradual increase in mobilization—prevents deconditioning, which occurs with bed rest.
   a. Minimize environmental noise.
   b. Provide a comfortable environmental temperature.
   c. Avoid unnecessary interruptions and procedures.
   d. Structure routine care measures to include rest periods after activity.
   e. Discuss with patient and family the purpose of limited activity and visitors—to help the heart heal by lowering heart rate and BP, maintaining cardiac workload at lowest level, and decreasing oxygen consumption.
   f. Promote restful diversional activities for patient (reading, listening to music, drawing, crossword puzzles, crafts).
   g. Encourage frequent position changes while in bed.
2. Assist patient with prescribed activities.
   a. Assist patient to rise slowly from a supine position to minimize orthostatic hypotension related to medications.
   b. Encourage passive and active range-of-motion (ROM) exercise as directed while on bed rest.
   c. Measure the length and width of the unit so patients can gradually increase their activity levels with specific guidelines (walk one width [150 feet] of the unit).
   d. Elevate patient's feet when out of bed in chair to promote venous return.
   e. Implement a step-by-step program for progressive activity, as directed. Typically can progress to the next step if they are free from chest pain and ECG changes during the activity.

Preventing Bleeding

1. Take vital signs every 15 minutes during infusion of fibrinolytic agent and then hourly.
2. Observe for hematomas or skin breakdown, especially in potential pressure areas such as the sacrum, back, elbows, ankles.
3. Be alert to verbal complaints of back pain indicative of possible retroperitoneal bleeding.
4. Observe all puncture sites every 15 minutes during infusion of fibrinolytic therapy and then hourly for bleeding.
5. Apply manual pressure to venous or arterial sites if bleeding occurs. Use pressure dressings for coverage of all access sites.
6. Observe for blood in stool, emesis, urine, and sputum.
7. Minimize venipunctures and arterial punctures; use heparin lock for blood sampling and medication administration.
8. Avoid IM injections.
9. Caution patient about vigorous tooth brushing or shaving.
10. Avoid trauma to patient by minimizing frequent handling of patient.
11. Monitor laboratory values: PT, international normalized ratio, PTT, hematocrit (HCT), and hemoglobin.
12. Check for current blood type and crossmatch.
13. Administer antacids or GI prophylaxis, as directed, to prevent stress ulcers.
14. Implement emergency interventions, as directed, in the event of bleeding: fluid, volume expanders, blood products.
15. Monitor for changes in mental status and headache.
16. Avoid vigorous oral suctioning.
17. Avoid use of automatic BP device above puncture sites or hematoma. Use care in taking BP; use arm not being used for fibrinolytic therapy.

Maintaining Cardiac Tissue Perfusion

1. Observe for persistent and/or recurrence of signs and symptoms of ischemia, including chest pain, diaphoresis, hypotension—may indicate extension of MI and/or reocclusion of coronary vessel.
2. Report immediately.

3. Administer oxygen, as directed.
4. Record a 12-lead ECG.
5. Prepare patient for possible emergency procedures: cardiac catheterization, bypass surgery, PCI, fibrinolytic therapy, intra-aortic balloon pump.

Strengthening Coping Abilities

1. Listen carefully to patient and family to ascertain their cognitive appraisals of stressors and threats.
2. Assist patient to establish a positive attitude toward illness and progress adaptively through the grieving process.
3. Manipulate environment to promote restful sleep by maintaining patient's usual sleep patterns.
4. Be alert to signs and symptoms of sleep deprivation—irritability, disorientation, hallucinations, diminished pain tolerance, aggressiveness.
5. Minimize possible adverse emotional response to transfer from the intensive care unit to the intermediate care unit:
   a. Introduce the admitting nurse from the intermediate care unit to the patient before transfer.
   b. Plan for the intermediate care nurse to answer questions the patient may have and to inform patient what to expect relative to physical layout of unit, nursing routines, and visiting hours.

Patient Education and Health Maintenance

Goals are to restore patient to optimal physiologic, psychological, social, and work level; to aid in restoring confidence and self-esteem; to develop patient's self-monitoring skills; to assist in managing cardiac problems; and to modify risk factors.

1. Inform the patient and family about what has happened to patient's heart.
   a. Explain basic cardiac anatomy and physiology.
   b. Identify the difference between angina and MI.
   c. Describe how the heart heals and that healing will not be complete for 6 to 8 weeks after infarction.
   d. Discuss what the patient can do to assist in the recovery process and reduce the chance of future heart attacks.
2. Instruct patient on how to judge the body's response to activity.
   a. Introduce the concept that different activities require varying expenditures of oxygen.
   b. Emphasize the importance of rest and relaxation alternating with activity.
   c. Instruct patient how to take pulse before and after activity as well as guidelines for the acceptable increases in heart rate that should occur.
   d. Review signs and symptoms indicative of a poor response to increased activity levels: chest pain, extreme fatigue, shortness of breath.
3. Design an individualized activity progression program for patient as directed.
   a. Determine activity levels appropriate for patient, as prescribed, and by predischarge low-level exercise stress test.
   b. Encourage patient to list activities he or she enjoys and would like to resume.
   c. Establish the energy expenditure of each activity (ie, which are most demanding on the heart) and rank activities from lowest to highest.
   d. Instruct patient to move from one activity to another after the heart has been able to manage the previous workload as determined by signs and symptoms and pulse rate.

4. Give patient specific activity guidelines and explain that activity guidelines will be reevaluated after the heart heals.
   a. Walk daily, gradually increasing distance and time, as prescribed.
   b. Avoid activities that tense muscles, such as weight lifting, lifting heavy objects, isometric exercises, pushing and/or pulling heavy loads, all of which can cause vagal stimulation.
   c. Avoid working with arms overhead.
   d. Gradually return to work.
   e. Avoid extremes in temperature.
   f. Do not rush; avoid tension.
   g. Advise getting at least 7 hours of sleep each night and taking 20- to 30-minute rest periods twice per day.
   h. Advise limiting visitors to three to four daily for 15 to 30 minutes and shorten phone conversations.
5. Tell patient that sexual relations may be resumed on advice of health care provider, usually after exercise tolerance is assessed.
   a. If patient can walk briskly or climb two flights of stairs, he or she can usually resume sexual activity; resumption of sexual activity parallels resumption of usual activities.
   b. Sexual activity should be avoided after eating a heavy meal, after drinking alcohol, or when tired.
   c. Discuss impotence as an adverse effect of drug therapy and phosphodiesterase contraindications.
6. Advise eating three to four small meals per day rather than large, heavy meals. Rest for 1 hour after meals.
7. Advise limiting caffeine and alcohol intake.
8. Driving a car must be cleared with health care provider at a follow-up visit.
9. Teach patient about medication regimen and adverse effects.
10. Instruct the patient to call 911 when chest pressure or pain not relieved in 5 minutes by nitroglycerin or rest.
11. Instruct the patient to notify health care provider when the following symptoms appear:
    a. Shortness of breath.
    b. Unusual fatigue.
    c. Swelling of feet and ankles.
    d. Fainting, dizziness.
    e. Very slow or rapid heartbeat.
12. Assist patient to reduce risk of another MI by risk factor modification.
    a. Explain to patient the major risk factors that can increase chances for having another MI.
    b. Instruct patient in strategies to modify risk factors.
13. For additional information and support, refer patient to AHA (www.americanheart.org) and the ACC (www.acc.org).

Evaluation: Expected Outcomes

- No signs of anxiety or agitation.
- Activity slowly progressing and tolerated well.
- No signs of bleeding.
- No recurrent chest pain.
- Sleeps well; emotionally stable.

Hyperlipidemia

Hyperlipidemia is a group of metabolic abnormalities resulting in combinations of elevated serum cholesterol. Total cholesterol (TC) and triglycerides (TG) are two of the major lipids in the body. The liver serves as the key organ for cholesterol metabolism and regulation. Lipids are transported through the bloodstream by lipoproteins. Lipoproteins are made up of a phospholipid and specific proteins called *apoproteins* or *apolipoproteins*. There are five main classes of lipoproteins:

- Chylomicrons.
- Very-low-density lipoproteins (VLDLs).
- Intermediate-density lipoproteins (IDLs).
- Low-density lipoproteins (LDLs).
- High-density lipoproteins (HDLs).

Pathophysiology and Etiology

Primary Hyperlipidemias
1. Genetic metabolic abnormalities resulting in the overproduction or underproduction of specific lipoproteins or enzymes. They tend to be familial, autosomal codominant genetic disorders characterized by raised serum LDL-C levels resulting from defects in hepatic uptake.
2. Primary hyperlipidemias include hypercholesterolemia, defective apolipoproteinemia, hypertriglyceridemia, combined hyperlipidemia, dysbetalipoproteinemia, polygenic hypercholesterolemia, lipoprotein lipase deficiency, apoprotein C-II deficiency, lethicin cholesterol acetyltransferase deficiency.

Secondary Hyperlipidemias
1. Very common and are multifactorial.
2. Etiologic factors include chronic diseases, such as diabetes, hypothyroidism, nephrotic syndrome, and liver disease.
3. Other etiologic factors are obesity, dietary intake, pregnancy, alcoholism.
4. Medications include beta-adrenergic blockers, alpha-adrenergic blockers, diuretics, glucocorticoid and anabolic steroids, and estrogen preparations.

Consequences
1. Atherosclerotic plaque formation in blood vessels.
2. Causes narrowing and possible ischemia and may lead to thromboembolus formation.
3. Result in cardiovascular, cerebrovascular, and peripheral vascular disease.
4. Familial genetic hyperlipidemia increases the risk of early onset of cardiovascular disease.

Clinical Manifestations
1. Usually asymptomatic until significant target organ damage is done.
2. May be metabolic signs, such as corneal arcus, xanthoma, xanthelasma, pancreatitis.
3. Chest pain, MI.
4. Carotid bruit, transient ischemic attacks, stroke.
5. Intermittent claudication, arterial occlusion of lower extremities, loss of pulses.

Diagnostic Evaluation and Management

Diagnosis and management of hyperlipidemia begin with serum lipoprotein evaluation and review of history to determine which of four statin benefit groups the individual falls within and then focuses on tailoring statin therapy in those most likely to benefit in terms of primary and secondary risk reduction. Heart-healthy lifestyle habits should be encouraged for all individuals (Table 13-2 and Box 13-1).

Table 13-2 Classification of Serum Lipids

TOTAL CHOLESTEROL (TC) mg/dL (mmol/L)	CATEGORY
<200 (<5.2)	Normal
200–239 (5.2–6.1)	Borderline high
≥240 (≥6.2)	High
LDL-Cholesterol mg/dL (mmol/L)	
<100 (<2.6)	Normal
100–129 (2.6–3.3)	Above, near optimal
130–159 (3.4–4.0)	Borderline high
160–189 (4.1–4.8)	High
≥190 (≥4.9)	Very high
HDL-Cholesterol mg/dL (mmol/L)	
<40 (<1.0)	Low
≥60 (≥1.6)	High
Triglycerides (TG) mg/dL (mmol/L)	
<150 (<1.7)	Normal
150–199 (1.7–2.2)	Borderline high
200–499 (2.3–5.6)	High
≥500 (≥5.6)	Very high

Management of Dyslipidemia Working Group. (2006). VA/DoD clinical practice guideline for the management of dyslipidemia. Washington, DC: Department of Veterans Affairs, Department of Defense, p. 140.

EVIDENCE BASE Stone, N. J., Robinson, J. G., Lichtenstein, A. H., et al. (2014). 2013 ACC/AHA guideline on the treatment of blood cholesterol to reduce atherosclerotic cardiovascular risk in adults: A report of the American College of Cardiology/American Heart Association Task Force on Practice Guidelines. *Journal of American College of Cardiology, 63*(25), 2889–2934.

1. The appropriate intensity of statin therapy should be initiated or continued:
   a. Clinical ASCVD (history of MI, unstable or stable angina, coronary artery procedures, or evidence or clinically significant MI or other revascularization, stroke, TIA and peripheral arterial disease presumed to be of atherosclerotic origin)
      i. Age ≤ 75 years and no safety concerns: high-intensity statin.
      ii. Age greater than 75 years or safety concerns: moderate-intensity statin.
   b. Primary prevention—primary LDL-C ≥190 mg/dL.
      i. Rule out secondary causes of hyperlipidemia.
      ii. Age ≥ 21 years: high-intensity statin.
      iii. Achieve at least a 50% reduction in LDL-C.
      iv. LDL-C–lowering nonstatin therapy may be considered to further reduce LDL-C.
   c. Primary prevention—Diabetes 40 to 75 years of age and LDL-C 70 to 189 mg/dL.
      i. Moderate-intensity statin.
      ii. Consider high-intensity statin when ≥7.5% 10-year ASCVD risk using the Pooled Cohort Equations (defined as nonfatal MI, CHD death, or nonfatal and fatal stroke).

BOX 13-1	LDL Goal-Directed Hyperlipidemia Treatment

LDL goal <70 mg/dL: Considered an optional goal for high-risk patients with coronary heart disease or a risk equivalent (peripheral artery disease, carotid artery disease, diabetes, aortic aneurysm). Treatment recommendation: therapeutic lifestyle changes; optional drug therapy if LDL < 100 mg/dL.

LDL goal <100 mg/dL: Goal for high-risk patients who have coronary heart disease or a risk equivalent and 10-year risk >20%. Treatment recommendations: therapeutic lifestyle changes and drug therapy if LDL ≥ 100 mg/dL; optional drug therapy if LDL < 100 mg/dL.

LDL goal <130 mg/dL: Goal for moderately high-risk patients with two or more risk factors and 10-year risk 10% to 20%. Treatment recommendations: therapeutic lifestyle changes initiated if LDL ≥ 130 mg/dL; drug therapy if LDL ≥ 130 mg/dL; optional drug therapy if LDL is 100 to 129 mg/dL.

LDL goal <130 mg/dL: Goal for moderate-risk patients with two or more risk factors and 10-year risk <10%. Treatment recommendation: therapeutic lifestyle changes initiated if LDL ≥ 130 mg/dL; drug therapy initiated if LDL ≥ 160 mg/dL.

LDL goal <160 mg/dL: Goal for lower-risk patients with 0 to 1 risk factors. Treatment recommendations: therapeutic lifestyle changes initiated if LDL ≥ 160 mg/dL; drug therapy initiated if LDL ≥ 190 mg/dL; optional drug therapy if LDL is 160 to 189 mg/dL.

   d. Primary prevention—no diabetes 40 to 75 years of age and LDL-C 70 to 189 mg/dL.
      i. Estimate 10-year ASCVD risk using the Risk Calculator based on the Pooled Cohort Equations in those NOT receiving a statin; estimate risk every 4 to 6 years.
      ii. To determine whether to initiate a statin, engage in a clinician–patient discussion of the potential ASCVD risk reduction, adverse effects, drug–drug interaction, and patient preferences.
      iii. Re-emphasize heart-healthy lifestyle habits and address other risk factors.
      iv. ≥7.5% 10-year ASCVD risk: consider moderate- or high-intensity statin.
      v. 5 to less than 7.5% 10-year ASCVD risk: consider moderate-intensity statin.
      vi. Other factors may be considered: LDL-C ≥160 mg/dL, family history of premature ASCVD, hs-CRP ≥2.0 mg/L, CAC score ≥300 Agatston units, ABI less than 0.9, or lifetime ASCVD risk.
   e. Primary prevention when LDL-C less than 190 mg/dL and age less than 40 or greater than 75 years or less than 5% 10-year ASCVD risk.
      i. Statin therapy may be considered in selected individuals.
   f. Statin therapy is not routinely recommended for individuals with NYHA class II to IV heart failure or who are receiving maintenance hemodialysis.

2. Regularly monitor adherence to lifestyle and drug therapy with lipid and safety assessments, and assess adherence, response to therapy, and adverse effects with 4 to 12 weeks following statin initiation or change in therapy.
   a. Measure a fasting lipid panel.
   b. Do not routinely monitor ALT or CK unless symptomatic.
   c. Screen and treat type 2 diabetes according to current practice guidelines. Heart-healthy lifestyle habits should be encouraged to prevent progression to diabetes.
   d. Anticipate therapeutic response: approximately ≥50% reduction in LDL-C from baseline for high-intensity statin and 30% to less than 50% for moderate-intensity statin.
      i. Insufficient evidence for LDL-C or non–HDL-C treatment targets from RCTs.
      ii. For those with unknown baseline LDL-C, and LDL-C, 100 mg/dL was observed in RCTs of high-intensity statin therapy.
   e. Less than anticipated therapeutic response:
      i. Reinforce improved adherence to lifestyle and drug therapy.
      ii. Evaluate for secondary causes of hyperlipidemia if indicated.
      iii. Increase statin intensity or if on maximally tolerated statin, consider addition of nonstatin therapy in selected high-risk individuals.
   f. Regularly monitor adherence to lifestyle and drug therapy every 3 to 12 month once adherence has been established. Continue assessment of adherence for optimal ASCVD risk reduction and safety.
3. In individuals intolerant of the recommended intensity of statin therapy, use the maximally tolerated intensity of statin. If there are muscle or other symptoms, establish that they are related to the statin.

Drug Classifications
See Table 13-3.
1. HMG-CoA reductase inhibitors (statins) are the most effective way to lower elevated LDL and TC, as a result of lower intrahepatic cholesterol and an uptake of hepatic cell surface LDL receptors. They also raise levels of HDL, lower levels of CRP, and may lower TGs. They can be used alone or in combination with other lipid-lowering drugs.
   a. Require periodic liver function monitoring.
   b. Should not be taken with large volume of grapefruit juice; can increase risk of myopathy.
   c. Should not be taken by women who are pregnant, lactating, or plan to get pregnant.
   d. Musculoskeletal side effects include myalgia, rhabdomyolysis, elevated creatine kinase.
2. Cholesterol absorption inhibitors—the newest class of lipid-lowering drugs; inhibit intestinal absorption of phytosterols and cholesterol and reduce LDL. Do not require liver function testing if given as monotherapy.
3. Bile acid sequestrants bind to cholesterol in the gut, decreasing absorption. Contraindicated in those with history of bile obstruction and phenylketonuria (aspartame-containing agent only).
4. Nicotinic acid (vitamin B$_3$)—works by inhibiting VLDL secretion, thus decreasing production of LDL. The main adverse effect is severe flushing; however, taking 81 to 325 mg of

Table 13-3 Drugs Affecting Lipoprotein Metabolism

DRUG CLASS	AGENTS AND DAILY DOSES	LIPID/LIPOPROTEIN EFFECTS		ADVERSE EFFECTS	CONTRAINDICATIONS
HMG-CoA reductase inhibitors (statins)	• Lovastatin (20–80 mg) • Pravastatin (20–40 mg) • Simvastatin (20–80 mg) • Fluvastatin (20–80 mg) • Atorvastatin (10–80 mg) • Rosuvastatin (5–40 mg) • Pitavastatin (1–4 mg)	LDL HDL TG	↓ 18%–55% ↑ 5%–15% ↓ 7%–30%	• Myopathy • Increased liver enzymes	*Absolute:* • Active or chronic liver disease *Relative:* • Concomitant use of certain drugs*
Bile acid sequestrants	• Cholestyramine (4–16 g) • Colestipol (5–20 g) • Colesevelam (2.6–3.8 g)	LDL HDL TG	↓ 15%–30% ↑ 3%–5% No change or increase	• GI distress • Constipation	*Absolute:* • Bowel obstruction • Biliary obstruction
Nicotinic acid	• Immediate-release (crystalline) nicotinic acid (1.5–3 g) • Extended-release nicotinic acid (Niaspan®) (1–2 g); sustained-release nicotinic acid (1–2 g)	LDL HDL TG	↓ 5%–25% ↑ 15%–35% ↓ 20%–50%	• Flushing (may be reduced by taking with aspirin and food) • Hyperglycemia • Hyperuricemia, gout • Upper GI distress • Hepatotoxicity • New onset of atrial fibrillation • Weight loss	*Absolute:* • Hepatic dysfunction • Active peptic ulcer disease *Relative:* • Diabetes • Hyperphosphatemia • Gout • Unstable angina, MI
Fibric acids	• Gemfibrozil (600 mg BID) • Fenofibrate (200 mg) • Clofibrate (1,000 mg BID)	LDL (*may be increased in patients with high TG*) HDL TG	↓ 5%–20% ↑ 10%–20% ↓ 20%–50%	• Dyspepsia • Gallstones • Myopathy • Pancreatitis • Rhabdomyolysis in conjunction with statin use • Muscle symptoms	*Absolute:* • Severe renal disease • Severe hepatic disease
Cholesterol absorption inhibitors	• Ezetimibe (10 mg)	LDL Apoprotein B	↓ (additional 25% over a statin when used in combination; also a TG reduction) ↓	• Back pain • Arthralgia • Diarrhea • Abdominal pain • Sinusitis	• Contraindicated in active liver disease if combined with a statin
PCSK9 inhibitors	• Alirocumab (75–150 mg SQ every 2 weeks) • Evolocumab (140 mg SQ every 2 weeks or 420 mg SQ monthly in the abdomen, thigh, or upper arm)	LDL-C	↓29.9%–67%	• Nasopharyngitis • Injection site reaction • Influenza-like symptoms • Bruising	

*Cyclosporine, macrolide antibiotics, various antifungal agents, and cytochrome P-450 inhibitors (fibrates and niacin) should be used with appropriate caution.
Adapted from ATP III guidelines at a glance quick desk reference. National Cholesterol Education Program [Electronic]. Available: https://www.nhlbi.nih.gov/files/docs/guidelines/atglance.pdf.

aspirin beforehand may help. Newer sustained-release forms have fewer adverse effects. Niacin should be avoided in patients with severe peptic disease.

5. Fibric acid derivatives—inhibit synthesis of VLDL, decrease TG, increase HDL. Contraindicated in liver, biliary, or kidney disease.
6. PCSK9 inhibitors are monoclonal antibodies. They target and inactivate a specific protein in the liver called proprotein convertase subtilisin/kexin 9. This protein binds to the LDL receptor and acts as an enzyme to break down the receptor so it can no longer remove LDL from the bloodstream. By inhibiting this protein, a dramatic reduction of LDL is seen in the bloodstream.

Other Treatment Considerations

1. TLC should be considered immediately for all patients with hyperlipidemia and is an important adjunct therapy for patients who receive medications.
2. Children and adolescents should be considered for screening and treatment of hyperlipidemia if they have positive family history and a family history of obesity. Other indications for screening (in these populations) include being overweight and

exhibiting features of metabolic syndrome (hypertension, type 2 diabetes, central adiposity).
3. Drug therapy is recommended for boys at or older than age 10 and after the onset of menses in girls following a 6- to 12-month dietary trial. HMG-CoA reductase inhibitors are the drug class of choice.
4. Some dietary products may serve as adjunct therapy, such as omega-3 fatty acids, soy protein, plant stanols, and fiber.

Complications

1. Disability from MI, stroke, and lower extremity ischemia.

Nursing Interventions and Patient Education

1. Teach diet basics and obtain nutritional consult.
2. Teach patient to engage in exercise.
3. Engage patient in smoking cessation program.
4. Tell patients that for every 1% increase in HDL, there is a 2% to 3% decrease in risk for CHD.
5. Explain the goal of recommended cholesterol levels. Encourage patients to keep a log of lipid results.
6. Encourage follow-up laboratory work—repeat lipoprotein analysis and liver function test monitoring every 3 months for those on HMG-CoA reductase inhibitors.
7. Teach patient taking bile acid sequestrants not to take other medications for 1 hour before or 2 hours after because it prevents absorption of many medications.
8. For more information on hyperlipidemia and TLC, refer patient to AHA (www.heart.org) or the National Heart, Lung, and Blood Institute diseases and conditions index (www.nhlbi.nih.gov/health/dci).

Cardiogenic Shock

Cardiogenic shock is the failure of the heart to pump blood adequately to meet the oxygenation needs of the body. It occurs when the heart muscle loses its contractile power. It most commonly occurs as a result of acute myocardial infarction (AMI), and left ventricular pump failure is the primary insult. It is the most common cause of death in the post-AMI patient (about 5% to 10% of AMI patients develop cardiogenic shock), with a resulting mortality of 50% to 60%.

Pathophysiology and Etiology

1. Persistent hypotension with a marked systolic of less than 80 to 90 mm Hg or mean arterial pressure 30 mm Hg lower than baseline because of left ventricular failure.
2. Impaired contractility causes a marked reduction in CO and ejection fraction.
3. Decreased CO results in a lack of blood and oxygen to the heart as well as other vital organs (brain and kidneys).
4. Lack of blood and oxygen to the heart muscle results in continued damage to the muscle, a further decline in contractile power, and a continued inability of the heart to provide blood and oxygen to vital organs.
5. MI causing extensive damage (40% or greater) to the left ventricular myocardium is the most common cause.
6. Mechanical complications such as ventricular septal rupture, contained free wall rupture, and papillary muscle rupture are strongly suspected in patients with shock, particularly a first MI.
7. In addition to MI with or without complications, common causes of cardiogenic shock include:
   a. Aortic dissection—complicated by acute severe aortic insufficiency or MI.
   b. Acute decompensation of heart failure.
   c. Acute myocarditis.
   d. Takotsubo stress-induced cardiomyopathy.
   e. Postcardiotomy.
   f. Cardiac tamponade.
   g. Peripartum cardiomyopathy.
   h. Hypertrophic cardiomyopathy with severe outflow obstruction.
   i. Massive pulmonary embolism.

Clinical Manifestations

1. Confusion, restlessness, mental lethargy (because of poor perfusion of the brain or metabolic encephalopathy).
2. Low systolic blood pressure (90 mm Hg or 30 mm Hg less than previous levels) or MAP <65 mm Hg.
3. Oliguria—urine output less than 30 mL/hour for at least 2 hours (because of decreased perfusion of kidneys).
4. Cold, clammy skin (blood is shunted from the peripheral circulation to perfuse vital organs); profoundly diaphoretic with mottled extremities.
5. Weak, thready peripheral pulses, fatigue, hypotension (because of inadequate CO).
6. Dyspnea, tachypnea, cyanosis (increased left ventricular pressures result in elevation of left atrial and pulmonary pressures, causing pulmonary congestion).
7. Dysrhythmias (because of lack of oxygen to heart muscle) and sinus tachycardia (as a compensatory mechanism for a decreased CO).
8. Chest pain (because of lack of oxygen and blood to heart muscle).
9. Decreased bowel sounds, nausea, or abdominal pain (because of paralytic ileus from decreased perfusion to GI tract).
10. Metabolic acidosis because of increased lactate production and reduced clearance (caused by anaerobic metabolism and liver dysfunction).
11. Hypoperfusion causes release of catecholamines, which increase contractility and peripheral blood flow but also may increase myocardial oxygen demand and have proarrhythmic effects.

Diagnostic Evaluation

1. Altered hemodynamic parameters (pulmonary artery wedge pressure 15 mm Hg or greater, cardiac index (CI) less than 2.0, elevated systemic vascular resistance [SVR], high right ventricular end-diastolic pressure (RVEDP) greater than 20 mm Hg and decreased mixed venous oxygen saturation).
2. Chest x-ray—pulmonary vascular congestion.
3. Abnormal laboratory values—elevated blood urea nitrogen (BUN) and creatinine, elevated liver enzymes, increased PTT and PT, elevated serum lactate, elevated brain natriuretic peptide (BNP). BNP may be useful as an indicator of heart failure and as an independent prognostic indicator of survival. Abnormally elevated cardiac enzymes.
4. ECG—acute injury pattern consistent with an AMI.
5. Doppler echocardiogram—reveals any ventricular wall motion or surgically correctable cause, such as valvular dysfunction and tamponade.
6. Pulmonary artery catheterization for severely hypotensive patient.

Management

Recent studies have suggested that treatment for cardiogenic shock resulting from an AMI should focus on revascularization and thrombolytics. Reduction in mortality related to early revascularization in patients with STEMI is supported by research. Augmenting

CO with devices (intra-aortic balloon pump [IABP] is a method of choice) is crucial until revascularization is established. Mechanical ventilation is supportive and left ventricular assist device and extra-corporeal membrane oxygenation may be used.

The standard treatment of beta-adrenergic blockers, ACE inhibitors, analgesics, and nitrates after acute MI does little to treat cardiogenic shock and may exacerbate systolic hypotension.

Pharmacologic Therapy

Pharmacologic therapy may need to be discontinued or its use decreased when a patient has gone into cardiogenic shock. Standard therapy for a failing heart includes:

1. Positive inotropic drugs (epinephrine, dopamine, dobutamine, amrinone, milrinone) stimulate cardiac contractility. Dobutamine, amrinone, and milrinone may lower BP because of vasodilatory effect.
2. Vasodilator therapy.
   a. Decreases the workload of the heart by reducing venous return and lessening the resistance against which the heart pumps (preload and afterload reduction).
   b. CO improves, left ventricular pressures and pulmonary congestion decrease, and myocardial oxygen consumption is reduced.
3. Vasopressor therapy may be needed to maintain adequate perfusion pressure (MAP 70 mm Hg or greater). These medications are norepinephrine, epinephrine, vasopressin, and phenylephrine. These should be used in the lowest possible dose. Higher vasopressor doses are associated with poor survival.
4. Diuretic therapy is used to reduce plasma volume and peripheral edema. The reduction in extracellular fluid and plasma volume associated with diuresis may initially decrease cardiac output and, consequently, blood pressure, with a compensatory increase in peripheral vascular resistance. Continuous renal replacement therapy has been considered for patients in cardiogenic shock if unable to diurese because of low renal perfusion.

 DRUG ALERT Use vasoactive drugs with extreme caution in the presence of cardiogenic shock. They require constant vigilance and astute observation to maintain an adequate perfusion pressure while achieving afterload reduction.

Reperfusion Therapy

Revascularization in cardiogenic shock patient may increase the patient's survival rate. See pages 255–260.

1. Percutaneous cardiac interventions (PCI)—prompt restoration of blood flow can lead to improved left ventricular function, thus salvaged ischemic myocardium. Timing of revascularization less than 90 minutes of door-to-door angioplasty after onset of symptoms provides better survival rates of CS patients. Antithrombotic therapy such as antiplatelets and anticoagulation is a mainspring during PCI. They showed to reduce mortality of cardiogenic shock patients following an acute MI.
2. Thrombolytics—use of fibrinolytic drugs lead to improved left ventricular systolic function and survival in patients with myocardial infarction associated with either ST-segment elevation or left bundle-branch block. Limitation to its use due to contraindication generally because of allergy and bleeding concerns such as recent hemorrhagic stroke.

Counterpulsation Therapy

See page 258.

1. Improves blood flow to the heart muscle and reduces myocardial oxygen needs.
2. Results in improved CO (1.5 L/minute increase) and preservation of viable heart tissue.
3. Should be instituted as quickly as possible to increase survival because of its overall benefits.

Total Circulatory and Mechanical Support

1. Left ventricular assist device (LVAD) or right ventricular assist device may be used as bridge to recovery in some patients.
2. Extracorporeal life support (ECMO)- circulates blood using a membrane oxygenator which relieves both left and right heart and the lungs of part of their workload.

Emergency Cardiac Surgery

1. Bypass graft (see page 260).
2. Heart transplantation.

Complications

1. Neurologic impairment/stroke.
2. Acute respiratory distress syndrome.
3. Renal failure.
4. Cardiopulmonary arrest.
5. Dysrhythmia.
6. Ventricular aneurysm.
7. Multiorgan dysfunction syndrome.
8. Bowel ischemia.
9. Limb ischemia.
10. Death.

Nursing Assessment

Clinical assessment begins with attention to the airway/breathing/circulation and vital signs.

1. Identify patients at risk for development of cardiogenic shock.
2. Assess for early signs and symptoms indicative of shock:
   a. Restlessness, confusion, or change in mental status.
   b. Increasing heart rate and decreasing blood pressure.
   c. Decreasing pulse pressure (indicates impaired CO).
   d. Presence of pulsus alternans (indicates left-sided heart failure).
   e. Decreasing urine output, weakness, fatigue.
3. Observe for presence of central and peripheral cyanosis.
4. Observe for development of edema and cool extremities.
5. Identify signs and symptoms indicative of extension of MI—recurrence of chest pain, diaphoresis.
6. Identify patient's and significant other's reaction to crisis situation.

 NURSING ALERT Cardiogenic shock carries an extremely high mortality (above 50% to 60% in hospital). Astute assessments and immediate actions are essential to prevent death.

Nursing Diagnoses

- Decreased Cardiac Output related to impaired contractility because of extensive heart muscle damage.
- Impaired Gas Exchange related to pulmonary congestion because of elevated left ventricular pressures.
- Ineffective Tissue Perfusion (renal, cerebral, cardiopulmonary, GI, and peripheral) related to decreased blood flow.
- Anxiety related to intensive care environment and threat of death.

Nursing Interventions

1. Administer oxygen by face mask or artificial airway to ensure adequate oxygenation of tissues and adjust oxygen flow rate as blood gas measurement indicates.
2. Administer diuretic with caution if ordered to increase renal blood flow and urine output.
3. Monitor and record blood pressure, pulse, respiratory rate, and peripheral pulse every 1 to 5 minutes until the patient stabilizes. Record hemodynamic pressure readings according to hospital protocol.
4. Monitor ABG values, complete blood count, and electrolyte levels.
5. To ease emotional stress, allow frequent rest periods as possible.
6. Allow family members to visit and comfort the patient as much as possible.
7. During therapy, assess skin color and temperature and note any changes. Cold and clammy skin may be a sign of continuing peripheral vascular constriction, indicating progressive shock.

Improving Cardiac Output

1. Establish continuous ECG monitoring to detect dysrhythmias, which increase myocardial oxygen consumption.
2. Monitor hemodynamic parameters continually with pulmonary artery catheter (see page 245) to evaluate effectiveness of implemented therapy.
   a. Obtain pulmonary artery pressure (PAP), pulmonary artery wedge pressure, and CO readings, as indicated.
   b. Calculate the CI (CO relative to body size) and SVR (estimation of afterload).
   c. Cautiously titrate vasoactive drug therapy according to hemodynamic parameters.
3. Be alert to adverse responses to drug therapy.
   a. Dopamine may cause an increase in heart rate, which may result in ischemia.
   b. Vasodilators, such as nitroglycerin and nitroprusside, may worsen hypotension.
   c. Dobutamine may result in dysrhythmias.
   d. Diuretics may cause hyponatremia, hypokalemia, and hypovolemia.
4. Administer vasoactive drug therapy through central venous access (peripheral tissue necrosis can occur if peripheral IV access infiltrates and peripheral drug distribution may be lessened from vasoconstriction).
5. Monitor blood pressure and MAP with intra-arterial line continuously during active titration of vasoactive drug therapy.
6. Maintain MAP greater than 65 mm Hg (blood flow through coronary vessels is inadequate with MAP less than 65 mm Hg).
7. Measure and record urine output every hour from indwelling catheter and fluid intake.
8. Obtain daily weight.
9. Evaluate serum electrolytes for hyponatremia, hypomagnesemia, and hypokalemia.
10. Be alert to incidence of chest pain (indicates myocardial ischemia and may further extend heart damage).
    a. Report immediately.
    b. Obtain a 12-lead ECG; check cardiac enzymes—CK, CK-MB, myoglobin, and troponin.
    c. Anticipate use of counterpulsation therapy.
11. Anticipate pump failure; evaluate need for surgical intervention (ie, ventricular assist device, extracorporeal membrane oxygenation).

Improving Oxygenation

1. Monitor rate and rhythm of respirations every hour.
2. Auscultate lung fields for abnormal sounds (coarse crackles indicate severe pulmonary congestion) every hour; notify health care provider.
3. Evaluate arterial blood gas (ABG) levels and correlate with oxygen saturation.
4. Administer oxygen therapy to increase oxygen tension and improve hypoxia.
5. Elevate head of bed 20 to 30 degrees, as tolerated (may worsen hypotension), to facilitate lung expansion.
6. Reposition patient frequently to promote ventilation and maintain skin integrity.
7. Observe for frothy pink sputum and cough (may indicate pulmonary edema); report immediately.

Maintaining Tissue Perfusion

1. Perform a neurologic check every hour using the Glasgow Coma Scale.
2. Report changes immediately.
3. Obtain BUN and creatinine blood levels and monitor urine output to evaluate renal function.
4. Auscultate for bowel sounds every 2 hours.
5. Evaluate character, rate, rhythm, and quality of arterial pulses every 2 hours.
6. Monitor temperature every 2 to 4 hours.
7. Use sheepskin foot and elbow protectors to prevent skin breakdown.
8. Obtain serum lactate to evaluate tissue perfusion and acidosis.

Relieving Anxiety

1. As with the above, always evaluate signs of increasing anxiety and/or new-onset anxiety for a physiologic cause before treating with anxiolytics.
2. Explain equipment and rationale for therapy to patient and family. Increasing knowledge assists in alleviating fear and anxiety.
3. Encourage patient to verbalize fears about diagnosis and prognosis.
4. Explain sensations patient will experience before procedures and routine care measures.
5. Offer reassurance and encouragement.
6. Utilize social worker or pastoral care for support.
7. Provide for periods of uninterrupted rest and sleep.
8. Assist patient to maintain as much control as possible over environment and care.
   a. Develop a schedule for routine care measures and rest periods with patient.
   b. Make sure that a calendar and clock are in view of patient.

Patient Education and Health Maintenance

1. Assess patient's readiness to learn.
2. Teach patients taking digoxin the importance of taking their medication as prescribed, taking pulse before daily dose, and reporting for periodic blood levels.
3. Teach signs of impending heart failure—increasing edema, shortness of breath, decreasing urine output, decreasing BP, increasing pulse—and tell patient to notify health care provider immediately.
4. See specific measures for MI (see page 280), cardiomyopathy (see page 296), and valvular disease (see page 307).
5. Teach patient importance of keeping follow-up appointments with his or her primary care physician and cardiologist.

6. Have dietitian teach patient and family about a low-sodium, low-fat diet, and reiterate the importance of adhering to this diet.

7. Explain to the patient the need to work with a physical and occupational therapist—especially if the patient has low ejection fraction—for energy conservation.

Evaluation: Expected Outcomes

- CO greater than 4 L/minute; CI greater than 2.2; PCWP less than 18 mm Hg.
- Respirations unlabored and regular; normal breath sounds throughout lung fields.
- Normal sensorium; urine output adequate; skin warm and dry.
- Verbalizes lessened anxiety and fear.

Infective Endocarditis

Infective endocarditis (IE; bacterial endocarditis) is an infection of the inner lining of the heart caused by direct invasion of bacteria or other organisms that could potentially result in myocardial abscess or heart failure and other complications.

Pathophysiology and Etiology

1. When the inner lining of the heart (endocardium) becomes inflamed, a fibrin clot (vegetation) forms.

2. The fibrin clot may become colonized by pathogens during transient episodes of bacteremia resulting from invasive procedures (venous and arterial cannulation, dental work causing gingival bleeding, GI tract surgery, liver biopsy, sigmoidoscopy), indwelling catheters, urinary tract infections, and wound and skin infections.

3. Platelets and fibrin surround the invading microorganisms, forming a protective covering and causing the infected vegetation to enlarge.

   a. The enlarged vegetation (the basic lesion of endocarditis) can deform, thicken, stiffen, and scar the free margins of valve leaflets as well as the fibrous ring (annulus) supporting the valve.

   b. The vegetations may also travel to various organs and tissues (spleen, kidney, coronary artery, brain, and lungs) and obstruct blood flow.

   c. The "protective covering" surrounding the vegetation makes it difficult for WBCs and antimicrobial agents to infiltrate and destroy the infected lesion.

4. Some of the bacterial causes include:

   a. *Streptococcus viridans*—bacteremia occurs after dental work or upper respiratory infection.

   b. *Staphylococcus aureus*—most common cause of IE; bacteremia occurs after cardiac surgery or parenteral drug abuse.

   c. *Staphylococcus epidermidis*—bacteremia occurs due to prosthetic heart valves and IV access procedures.

   d. Enterococci (penicillin-resistant group *D. streptococci*)—bacteremia usually occurs in older patients (over age 60) with genitourinary tract infection.

   e. Gram-negative bacteria such as *Pseudomonas aeruginosa*, *Actinobacter*, and HACEK group bacteria. The HACEK group consists of *Haemophilus* species, *Aggregatibacter* species, *Cardiobacterium hominis*, *Eikenella corrodens*, and *Kingella* species.

   f. Facultative intracellular parasites such as *Bartonella* and other opportunistic pathogens such as *Salmonella* and *Brucella* can cause infective endocarditis.

5. Fungi (*Candida albicans*, *Aspergillus*) and rickettsiae are additional causes.

6. IE may develop on a heart valve already injured by rheumatic fever, congenital defects, on abnormally vascularized valves, normal heart valves, and mechanical and biological heart valves.

7. IE may be acute or subacute, depending on the microorganisms involved. Acute IE manifests rapidly with danger of intractable heart failure and occurs more commonly on normal heart valves.

8. Subacute IE manifests as a prolonged chronic course with a lesser risk of complications and occurs more commonly on damaged or defective valves.

9. IE may follow cardiac surgery, especially when prosthetic heart valves are used. Foreign bodies, such as pacemakers, patches, grafts, and dialysis shunts, predispose to infection.

10. High incidence among drug abusers, in whom the disease mainly affects normal valves, usually the tricuspid.

11. Hospitalized patients with indwelling catheters, those on prolonged IV therapy or prolonged antibiotic therapy, those with burns, and those on immunosuppressive drugs or steroids may develop fungal endocarditis.

12. Relapse because of metastatic infection is possible, usually within the first 2 months after completion of antibiotic regimen.

13. Genitourinary disorders, infection, and manipulations, which includes pregnancy, delivery, and abortion, may predispose to infection as well.

 NURSING ALERT The incidence of nosocomial bacteremias is commonly associated with intravascular lines, and wound care may result in infective endocarditis.

Clinical Manifestations

Severity of manifestations depends on invading microorganism.

General Manifestations

1. Fever, chills, sweats (fever may be absent in older patients or those with uremia).
2. Anorexia, weight loss, weakness.
3. Cough and back and joint pain (especially in patients over age 60).
4. Splenomegaly.

Skin and Nail Manifestations

1. Janeway lesions—light pink macules on palms or soles, nontender, may change to light tan within several days or fade in 1 to 2 weeks; usually an early sign of endocardial infection.
2. Petechiae—conjunctiva and mucous membranes.
3. Splinter hemorrhages in nail beds.
4. Osler nodes—painful red nodes on pads of fingers and toes; usually late sign of infection and found with a subacute infection.
5. Clubbing of fingers and toes—primarily occurs in patients who have an extended course of untreated infective endocarditis.

Heart Manifestations

1. New pathologic or changing murmur—no murmur with other signs and symptoms may indicate right-sided heart infection.
2. Tachycardia—related to decreased CO.
3. Symptoms consistent of heart failure, pericardial friction rub.
4. New heart block or arrhythmia.

Central Nervous System Manifestations

1. Localized headaches, stiff neck.
2. Transient cerebral ischemia or other neurological symptoms.
3. Altered mental status, aphasia.

4. Hemiplegia.
5. Cortical sensory loss.
6. Roth spots on fundi (retinal hemorrhages).

Pulmonary Manifestations
1. Pneumonitis, pleuritis, pulmonary edema, infiltrates, effusions (causing friction rub)—occur with right heart involvement.

Embolic Phenomena
1. Lung—hemoptysis, chest pain, shortness of breath.
2. Kidney—hematuria, abnormal urine color.
3. Spleen—pain in the left upper quadrant of the abdomen radiating to left shoulder.
4. Heart—MI, aortic insufficiency, heart failure.
5. Brain—sudden blindness, paralysis, brain abscess, meningitis, CVA.
6. Blood vessels—mycotic aneurysms.
7. Abdomen—melena, acute pain.

Diagnostic Evaluation

Varied clinical manifestations and similarities to other diseases make early diagnosis of IE difficult. Accurate diagnosis is essential to guide therapy. A definitive clinical diagnosis can be made based on the finding of 2 major criteria, 5 minor criteria, or 1 major and 3 minor criteria.

Major Criteria (Based on Modified Duke Criteria)
1. Blood cultures—at least two positive serial blood cultures (90% of IE patients have positive blood cultures).
2. Endocardial involvement (diagnosed with transesophageal echocardiogram)—identification of vegetations and assessment of location and size of lesions.
3. New valvular insufficiency/regurgitation.
4. Development of abscess or new partial dehiscence of prosthetic valve or new valvular regurgitation.

Minor Criteria
1. Predisposing cardiac condition or IV drug use.
2. Fever higher than 100.4°F (38°C).
3. Vascular factors—pulmonary complication, arterial emboli, Janeway lesions, mycotic aneurysm, intracranial hemorrhage.
4. Immunologic factors—Osler nodes, Roth spots, rheumatoid factor, glomerulonephritis.
5. Microbiology—positive cultures, but not meeting major criteria.

Management

1. IV antimicrobial therapy, based on sensitivity of causative agent. Six weeks of therapy is recommended for most patients except uncomplicated right-sided IE in whom 2 weeks of therapy is recommended.
2. Combination antibiotic therapy is highly effective and can be given for 2 weeks, depending on what group of pathogens identified. Bactericidal serum levels of selected antibiotics are monitored by serial titers; if serum lacks adequate bactericidal activity, higher dosage or a different antibiotic is needed.
3. Supplemental nutrition.
4. Surgical intervention for specific complications but surgery should be delayed for at least a month in patients who suffered a hemorrhagic CVA. Surgery should not be delayed in patients following silent embolic event or transient ischemic attack, associated heart failure, abscess, or high embolic risk patients.
   a. Acute destructive valvular lesion—excision of infected valves or removal of prosthetic valve.

b. Hemodynamic impairment, severe heart failure.
c. Recurrent emboli.
d. Resistant infection.
e. Drainage of abscess or empyema.
f. Repair of peripheral or cerebral mycotic aneurysm.

Complications

1. Severe heart failure because of valvular insufficiency.
2. Uncontrolled/refractory infection.
3. Embolic episodes (brain ischemia or necrosis of extremities and organs).
4. Conduction disturbances.
5. Organ dysfunction resulting from immunological process (kidneys, eyes, skin).
6. Tissue destruction by microorganism, valvular damage, mycotic aneurysms, hemorrhage, and abscess formation.

Nursing Assessment

1. Identify factors that may predispose to endocarditis, such as rheumatic heart disease, congenital heart defects, idiopathic hypertrophic subaortic stenosis, IV drug abuse, prosthetic heart valves, aortic or mitral stenosis, previous history of endocarditis, recent genitourinary surgery, as well as homelessness or squalid living conditions.
2. Determine onset of signs and symptoms of endocarditis (early treatment of infection improves prognosis).
3. Identify potential incidents that may have precipitated a transient bacteremia capable of causing endocarditis.
4. Obtain blood cultures, CBC, sedimentation rate, C-reactive protein, renal and hepatic studies, and a baseline 12-lead ECG.
5. Assess patient for allergies, with special emphasis on adverse reactions to antibiotic therapy.
6. Note if patient is currently on antibiotic therapy (may affect blood culture results).
7. Identify patient's and family's level of anxiety and use of appropriate coping mechanisms.

Nursing Diagnoses

- Decreased Cardiac Output related to structural factors (incompetent valves).
- Ineffective Tissue Perfusion (renal, cerebral, cardiopulmonary, GI, and peripheral) related to interruption of blood flow.
- Hyperthermia related to illness, potential dehydration, and aggressive antibiotic therapy.
- Imbalanced Nutrition: Less Than Body Requirements related to anorexia.
- Anxiety related to acute illness and hospitalization.

Nursing Interventions

Maintaining Adequate Cardiac Output
1. Auscultate heart to detect new murmur or change in existing murmur; presence of gallop.
2. Monitor BP and pulse.
   a. Note presence of pulsus alternans (indicative of left-sided heart failure).
   b. Evaluate pulse pressure (30 to 40 mm Hg indicates adequate CO).
3. Evaluate jugular vein distention.
4. Record intake and output.
5. Record daily weight.
6. Auscultate lung fields for evidence of crackles (rales).

7. Monitor liver function studies (elevated with liver engorgement related to right heart failure).

8. Assess skin color and temperature.

Maintaining Tissue Perfusion

1. Observe patient for altered mentation, hemoptysis, hematuria, aphasia, loss of muscle strength, and complaints of pain.
2. Monitor vital signs.
3. Monitor urine output.
4. Observe for splinter hemorrhages of nail beds, Osler nodes, and Janeway lesions.
5. Notify health care provider of observed changes in the patient's status.
6. Assess skin color and temperature.
7. Reposition patient frequently to prevent skin breakdown and pulmonary complications associated with bed rest.

Maintaining Normothermia

1. Observe basic principles of asepsis, good handwashing techniques, and continuity of patient care by primary nurse.
2. Employ meticulous IV care for long-term antibiotic therapy.
   a. Note the date of needle or cannula insertion on nursing care plan.
   b. If a peripheral site is used, rotate the site every 72 hours or if site becomes tender, reddened, infiltrated, or has purulent drainage.
   c. Change gauze or transparent dressing every 24 hours to prevent infection.
   d. If a continuous venous access device is used, follow facility policy for site care and dressing changes and flushing procedures.
3. For IM antibiotic therapy, develop chart for rotation of sites.
4. Note that missed doses of antibiotic may have irreversible deleterious consequences, so scheduling is essential to prevent the patient being off the unit when antibiotic is due.
5. Observe for allergic reaction to antibiotic therapy (severe respiratory distress, rash, itching, fever), stop the antibiotic, and notify health care provider promptly so a substitute can be ordered.
6. Obtain audiogram before potentially ototoxic antibiotic is started, and observe for adverse effects such as ototoxicity and renal failure.
7. Assess effectiveness of therapy by obtaining urine culture after 48 hours of drug therapy, and blood cultures after 24 to 48 hours of therapy.
8. Monitor temperature every 4 hours.
   a. Document results on a graph.
   b. Note increases in heart rate and/or respirations with elevated temperatures.
   c. Provide blankets and temperature-controlled comfortable environment if patient has shaking chills; change bed linens, as necessary.
   d. Administer antipyretic or analgesic medications, as directed.
9. Observe patient for a general "sense of well-being" within 5 to 7 days after initiation of therapy.
10. Promote adequate hydration because diaphoresis and increased metabolic rate may cause dehydration.
11. Encourage oral fluid intake.
12. Administer IV fluids as directed.
13. Observe skin turgor and mucous membranes.

 DRUG ALERT Rapid infusion of vancomycin (less than 1 hour) may cause red neck syndrome (intense red rash over the upper half of the body) because of histamine release. Slow the rate of infusion and the rash will clear.

Improving Nutritional Status

1. Assess patient's daily caloric intake and monitor weight.
2. Discuss food preferences with patient.
3. Consult with a dietitian about nutritional needs of patient and food preferences.
4. Encourage small meals and snacks throughout the day.
5. Educate family about the patient's caloric needs.
6. Encourage family to assist the patient with meals and bring in patient's favorite foods.

Reducing Anxiety

1. Rule out physiologic etiologies for increasing or new-onset anxiety before administering as-needed sedatives. Physiologic causes must be identified and treated in a timely fashion to prevent irreversible adverse or even fatal outcomes; sedatives may mask symptoms, delaying timely identification, diagnosis, and treatment.
2. Assess patient for signs of hypoperfusion, auscultate heart and lung sounds, obtain a rhythm strip, and administer oxygen, as prescribed. Notify the health care provider immediately.
3. Document assessment findings, health care provider notification and response, and interventions and response.
4. Explain to patient and family reasons for hospitalization, diagnostic tests, and therapies administered.
5. Encourage patient to verbalize fears about illness and hospitalization.
6. Explain procedures to patient before initiation.
7. Encourage diversional activities for patient, such as television, reading, and interaction with other patients.

Patient Education and Health Maintenance

For Patients at Risk for Infective Endocarditis

1. Discuss anatomy of the heart and changes that occur during endocarditis, using diagrams of the heart.
2. Give patient written literature on early signs and symptoms of disease; review these with patient.
3. Discuss with patient the mode of entry of infection.
4. Indicate that antibiotic prophylaxis is recommended prior to dental procedures that manipulate the gingival and some respiratory procedures (see Table 13-4), for patients with the following conditions:
   a. Congenital heart disease (particularly unrepaired cyanotic defects) repaired with prosthetic material (for 6 months following repair) or repaired with residual defect.
   b. Prosthetic cardiac valve.
   c. Previous IE.
   d. Heart transplantation recipient with cardiac valvular disease.
5. Identify individual steps necessary to prevent infection.
   a. Practice good oral hygiene, regular tooth brushing, and flossing. See dentist regularly.
   b. Notify health care personnel of any history of congenital heart disease or valvular disease.
   c. Discuss importance of carrying emergency identification with information of medical history at all times.
   d. Take temperature if infection is suspected, and notify health care provider of elevation.
   e. Educate patients at risk to look for and treat signs and symptoms of illness indicating bacteremia—injuries, sore throats, furuncles, and so forth.
6. Encourage at-risk individuals to receive pneumococcal and influenza vaccines.

Table 13-4   Preventing Endocarditis: Regimens for a Dental Procedure

SITUATION	AGENT	REGIMEN: SINGLE DOSE 30–60 MINUTES BEFORE PROCEDURE	
		ADULTS	CHILDREN
Oral	Amoxicillin	2 g	50 mg/kg
Unable to take oral medication	Ampicillin OR	2 g IM or IV	50 mg/kg IM or IV
	Cefazolin or ceftriaxone	1 g IM or IV	50 mg/kg IM or IV
Allergic to penicillins or ampicillin—oral	Cephalexin*,† OR	2 g	50 mg/kg
	Clindamycin OR	600 mg	20 mg/kg
	Azithromycin or clarithromycin	500 mg	15 mg/kg IM or IV
Allergic to penicillins or ampicillin and unable to take oral medication	Cefazolin or ceftriaxone† OR	1 g IM or IV	50 mg/kg IM or IV
	Clindamycin	600 mg IM or IV	20 mg/kg IM or IV

*Or other first- or second-generation oral cephalosporin in equivalent adult or pediatric dosage.
†Cephalosporins should not be used in individuals with a history of anaphylaxis, angioedema, or urticaria with penicillins or ampicillin.
IM, intramuscular; IV, intravenous.

For Individuals Who Have Had Endocarditis Regarding Possible Relapse

1. Discuss importance of keeping follow-up appointments after discharge (infection can recur in 1 to 2 months).
2. Review the tests that will be performed after discharge—blood cultures, physical examination, echocardiography.
3. Teach patient to inspect soles for Janeway lesions (indicative of possible relapse).
4. Contact social worker or case manager to assist patient with financial planning and home discharge arrangements, if applicable.

Evaluation: Expected Outcomes

- BP stable; no change in murmur; no gallop noted.
- No change in LOC, strength, or neurologic function.
- Normal temperature; negative blood cultures; no hearing impairment.
- Tolerates increased daily caloric intake well.
- Verbalizes decrease in anxiety.

Rheumatic Endocarditis (Rheumatic Heart Disease)

Rheumatic endocarditis is an acute, recurrent inflammatory disease that causes damage to the heart as a sequela to group A beta-hemolytic streptococcal infection, particularly the valves, resulting in valve leakage (insufficiency) and/or obstruction (narrowing or stenosis). There are associated compensatory changes in the size of the heart's chambers and the thickness of chamber walls. It is a major burden in developing countries where it causes most of the cardiovascular morbidity and mortality in young people, leading to about 250,000 deaths per year worldwide.

See discussion of rheumatic fever in children in Chapter 45, page 1220.

Pathophysiology and Etiology

1. Rheumatic fever is a sequela to group A beta-hemolytic streptococcal infection that occurs in about 3% of untreated infections. It is a preventable disease through detection and adequate treatment of streptococcal pharyngitis.
2. Connective tissue of the heart, blood vessels, joints, and subcutaneous tissues can be affected.
3. Lesions in connective tissue are known as Aschoff bodies, which are localized areas of tissue necrosis surrounded by immune cells.
4. Heart valves, mainly the mitral valve, are affected, resulting in valve leakage and narrowing.
5. Compensatory changes in the chamber sizes and thickness of chamber walls occur.
6. Heart involvement (pancarditis) also includes pericarditis, myocarditis, epicarditis, and endocarditis.

Clinical Manifestations

1. Symptoms of streptococcal pharyngitis may precede rheumatic symptoms.
   a. Sudden onset of sore throat; throat reddened with exudates.
   b. Swollen, tender lymph nodes at angle of the jaw.
   c. Headache and fever 101°F to 104°F (38.3°C to 40°C).
   d. Abdominal pain (children).
   e. Some cases of streptococcal throat infection relatively asymptomatic.
2. Warm and swollen joints (polyarthritis), beginning in the lower extremities (knees and ankles) and may include the large joints in the upper extremities (elbows, wrists). Pain in joints.
3. Sydenham chorea (irregular, jerky, involuntary, unpredictable muscular movements).
4. Erythema marginatum (transient mesh-like macular rash on the trunk and extremities, never on the face, in about 5% to 13% of patients).
5. Subcutaneous nodules (hard, painless nodules over extensor surfaces of extremities; rare).
6. Fever.
7. Prolonged PR interval as shown on ECG.
8. Heart murmurs; pleural and pericardial rubs.
9. History of previous rheumatic fever or rheumatic heart disease.

Diagnostic Evaluation

1. Throat culture—streptococcal organisms.
2. Sedimentation rate, WBC count and differential, and CRP—increased during acute phase of infection.
3. Elevated antistreptolysin-O (ASO)/streptococcal antibody titer.
4. ECG—prolonged PR interval or heart block.
5. Echocardiography and Doppler study.
6. Cardiac catheterization to evaluate valvular damage and left ventricular function in those with severe cardiac dysfunction.

Management

1. Antimicrobial therapy—penicillin, erythromycin, or cephalosporin. Early treatment is key to survival.
2. Rest—to maintain optimal cardiac function.
3. Salicylates or NSAIDs—fever and pain; should be used with caution, especially in the elderly, due to risk of renal failure and gastrointestinal bleeding.
4. Steroids—during acute inflammatory phase.
5. Prevention of recurrent episodes through long-term penicillin therapy for 5 years or until 21 years old, whichever is longer, if patient does not have carditis, or 10 years if with carditis; periodic prophylaxis throughout life.
6. Beta-blockers, ACE inhibitors, digoxin, other afterload reduction medications, diuretics, supplemental oxygen, rest, sodium and fluid restrictions—to manage heart failure.
7. Though chorea is self-limiting, phenobarbital and diazepam may relieve the symptom.
8. Percutaneous mitral balloon valvuloplasty (PMBV) is recommended for patients with rheumatic mitral stenosis.

Complications

1. Valvular heart disease.
2. Cardiomyopathy.
3. Heart failure.
4. Atrial arrhythmias.
5. Pulmonary and systemic embolism.

Nursing Assessment

1. Ask patient about symptoms of fever or throat or joint pain.
2. Ask patient about chest pain, dyspnea, fatigue.
3. Observe for skin lesions or rash on the trunk and extremities.
4. Palpate for firm, nontender movable nodules near tendons or joints.
5. Auscultate heart sounds for murmurs and/or rubs.

Nursing Diagnoses

- Hyperthermia related to disease process.
- Decreased Cardiac Output related to decreased cardiac contractility.
- Activity Intolerance related to joint pain and easy fatigability.

Nursing Interventions

Reducing Fever

1. Administer penicillin therapy, as prescribed, to eradicate hemolytic streptococcus; an alternative drug may be prescribed if patient is allergic to penicillin or sensitivity testing and desensitization may be done.
   a. Coordinate schedule to prevent missed or delayed dose of antibiotic because of patient being off unit to prevent deleterious effects.
2. Give salicylates or NSAIDs, as prescribed, to suppress rheumatic activity by controlling toxic manifestations, to reduce fever, and to relieve joint pain.
3. Assess for effectiveness of drug therapy.
   a. Take and record temperature every 3 hours.
   b. Evaluate patient's comfort level every 3 hours.

Maintaining Adequate Cardiac Output

1. Assess for signs and symptoms of acute rheumatic carditis.
   a. Be alert to patient's complaints of chest pain, palpitations, and/or precordial "tightness."
   b. Monitor for tachycardia (usually persistent when patient sleeps) or bradycardia.
   c. Be alert to development of second-degree heart block or Wenckebach disease (acute rheumatic carditis causes PR-interval prolongation).
2. Auscultate heart sounds every 4 hours.
   a. Document presence of murmur or pericardial friction rub.
   b. Document extra heart sounds (S_3 gallop, S_4 gallop).
3. Monitor for development of chronic rheumatic endocarditis, which may include valvular disease and heart failure.

Maintaining Activity

1. Maintain bed rest for duration of fever or if signs of active carditis are present.
2. Provide ROM exercise program.
3. Provide diversional activities that prevent exertion.
4. Discuss the need for tutorial services with parents to help child keep up with schoolwork.

Patient Education and Health Maintenance

1. Counsel patient to maintain good nutrition.
2. Counsel patient on hygienic practices.
   a. Discuss proper handwashing, disposal of tissues, laundering of handkerchiefs (decrease risk of exposure to microbes).
   b. Discuss importance of using patient's own toothbrush, soap, and washcloths when living in group situations.
3. Counsel patient on importance of receiving adequate rest.
4. Instruct patient to seek treatment immediately should sore throat or fever occur.
5. Support patients in long-term antibiotic therapy to prevent relapse (5 years for most adults).
6. Instruct patient with valvular disease to use prophylactic antibiotic therapy an hour before certain procedures and surgery (see page 289).
7. Discuss patient's ability to pay for medical treatment. If appropriate, contact social services for patient. (Financial difficulties may inhibit patient from seeking early treatment of symptoms.)

Evaluation: Expected Outcomes

- Afebrile.
- Denies chest pain; normal sinus rhythm.
- Maintains bed rest while febrile.

Myocarditis

Myocarditis is an inflammatory process involving the myocardium, thus damaging the heart muscle. Although the exact cause of myocarditis is still unknown, it is thought to attack otherwise healthy individuals. It is thought the cause of sudden death among young adults and cause acute or chronic dilated cardiomyopathy.

Pathophysiology and Etiology

1. Focal or diffuse inflammation of the myocardium; may be acute or chronic.
2. May follow infectious process—viral or "idiopathic" (particularly coxsackie group B and may develop after influenza A or B, herpes simplex, parvovirus, cytomegalovirus, adenovirus, enterovirus, Epstein-Barr, rubella, and human immunodeficiency virus [HIV]), bacterial, parasitic, protozoal, rickettsial, spirochetal, and fungal (*Candida*, *Aspergillus*, and *Histoplasma*).
3. Hepatitis C virus has been associated with myocarditis by identification of HCV antibodies.
4. May be associated with chemotherapy (especially doxorubicin), immunosuppressive therapy, or vaccinia virus inoculation for protection against smallpox infection.
5. Systemic disorders such as sarcoidosis and celiac disease, autoimmune conditions such as systemic lupus, and other collagen diseases may cause myocarditis.
6. May be associated with exposures to certain chemicals (arsenic and hydrocarbons); allergic or toxic reactions to penicillin or sulfonamides; insect/snake bites; cocaine use.
7. Radiation exposure—most cases are the result of therapy for Hodgkin lymphoma or breast or lung cancer. Less common is exposure to a nuclear reactor or after detonation of a nuclear device.

Clinical Manifestations

1. Symptoms depend on type of infection, degree of myocardial damage, capacity of the myocardium to recover, and host resistance. Can be acute or chronic and can occur at any age. Symptoms may be minor and go unnoticed.
   a. Fatigue and dyspnea.
   b. Palpitations.
   c. Occasional precordial discomfort/vague chest pain.
2. Cardiac enlargement.
3. Abnormal heart sounds: murmur, S_3 or S_4, or friction rubs.
4. Signs of heart failure (eg, pulsus alternans, dyspnea, crackles, lower extremity edema, low urine output).
5. Fever with tachycardia or other signs of viral infection, such as headache, joint pain, and sore throat.
6. Joint pain or swelling; leg swelling

Diagnostic Evaluation

1. Transient ECG changes—ST segment flattened, T-wave inversion, conduction defects, extrasystoles, supraventricular and ventricular ectopic beats, brady- or tachyarrhythmias.
2. Elevated WBC count, C-reactive protein, and sedimentation rate.
3. Measurement of serum cardiac biomarkers such as CPK and troponin—may be elevated.
4. Chest x-ray—may show heart enlargement and lung congestion.
5. Elevated antibody titers (ASO titer as in rheumatic fever).
6. Stool and throat cultures isolating bacteria or a virus.
7. Endomyocardial biopsy for definitive diagnosis. This is the gold standard for establishing the diagnosis.
8. Echocardiogram—defines size, structure, and function of the heart.
9. Cardiovascular MRI—may be helpful to determine structural alterations; can provide accurate tissue characterization
10. Nuclear imaging using *gallium* (detects the extent of myocardial inflammation) or *indium* (antimyosin antibodies—shows the extent of myocyte necrosis)

Management

Treatment objectives are targeted toward management of complications. Supportive care is the first line of treatment.

1. Elevated ventricular filling pressures should be treated with intravenous diuretics and vasodilators (when feasible) such as nitroprusside.
2. Antidysrhythmic therapy (usually amiodarone).
3. Strict bed rest to promote healing of damaged myocardium.
4. Antimicrobial therapy if causative bacteria are isolated.
5. Anticoagulation therapy.
6. ACE inhibitor or beta-adrenergic blocker (should be used with caution; may cause hypotension)—to strengthen the heart's pumping ability and to reduce its workload, thus improving left ventricular systolic dysfunction.
7. In severe cases, aggressive therapy may be necessary: inotropes, such as dobutamine and dopamine; IABP counterpulsation therapy.
8. A ventricular assist device or extracorporeal membrane oxygenation may rarely be required to sustain patients with refractory cardiogenic shock as well as consideration of urgent heart transplantation.
9. IV immunoglobulin has antiviral effects; interferon-α and interferon-β; immunosuppressive regimen of steroids and cyclosporine or azathioprine improves systolic function.

Complications

1. Heart failure, pericarditis.
2. Cardiomyopathy.
3. Arrhythmias.
4. Sudden cardiac death.

Nursing Assessment

1. Assess for fatigue, palpitations, fever, dyspnea, and chest pain.
2. Auscultate heart sounds.
3. Assess limbs for swelling, discoloration of the skin, and temperature of the skin.
4. Evaluate history for precipitating factors.
5. Pay special attention to variation in blood pressure, increased heart rate with ectopies, and tachypnea.

Nursing Diagnoses

- Hyperthermia related to inflammatory/infectious process.
- Decreased Cardiac Output related to decreased cardiac contractility and dysrhythmias.
- Activity Intolerance related to impaired cardiac performance and febrile illness.
- Acute Pain related to disease process

Nursing Interventions

Reducing Fever
1. Administer antipyretics as directed.
2. Check temperature every 4 hours.
3. Administer antibiotics as directed.

Maintaining Cardiac Output

1. Evaluate for clinical evidence that disease is subsiding—monitor pulse, auscultate for abnormal heart sounds (murmur or change in existing murmur), check temperature, auscultate lung fields, monitor respirations.
2. Record daily intake and output.
3. Record daily weight.
4. Check for peripheral edema.
5. Elevate head of bed, if necessary, to enhance respiration. Encourage use of incentive spirometry.
6. Treat the symptoms of heart failure as prescribed (see page 298).
7. Evaluate patient's pulse and apical rate for signs of tachycardia and gallop rhythm—indications that heart failure is recurring.
8. Evaluate for evidence of dysrhythmias—patients with myocarditis are prone to develop dysrhythmias.
   a. Institute continuous cardiac monitoring if evidence of a dysrhythmia develops.
   b. Have equipment for resuscitation, defibrillation, and cardiac pacing available in case of life-threatening dysrhythmia.

 DRUG ALERT Digoxin should not be considered for patients with myocarditis. High doses of digoxin may increase production of proinflammatory cytokines and may worsen myocardial injury. If digoxin was given, assess for toxic signs and symptoms, such as anorexia, nausea, fatigue, weakness, yellow-green halos around visual images, or prolonged PR interval.

Reducing Fatigue

1. Ensure bed rest to reduce heart rate, stroke volume, BP, and heart contractility; also helps to decrease residual damage and complications of myocarditis and promotes healing.
   a. Prolonged bed rest may be required until there is reduction in heart size and improvement of function.
2. Provide diversional activities for patient.
3. Allow patient to use bedside commode rather than bed pan (reduces cardiovascular workload).
4. Discuss with patient activities that can be continued after discharge.
   a. Discuss the need to modify activities in the immediate future.
   b. Explore patient's feelings and concerns about role fulfillment.

Reducing Chest Pain

1. Assess for chest pain; provide pain medication if not contraindicated.
2. Provide a quiet environment and comfort measures such as change in position, back rub, emotional support.
3. Provide supplemental oxygen as indicated.

Patient Education and Health Maintenance

Instruct patient as follows:
1. There is usually some residual heart enlargement; physical activity may be slowly increased; begin with chair rest for increasing periods; follow with walking in the room and then outdoors.
2. Report any symptom involving rapid heartbeat.
3. Avoid competitive sports, cigarettes, illicit drugs, and alcohol. Myocardial toxic medications such as doxorubicin cannot be used.

4. Pregnancy is not advisable for women with cardiomyopathies associated with myocarditis.
5. Prevent infectious diseases with appropriate immunizations (pneumococcal and influenza vaccines).
6. Refer patient to cardiac phase II rehabilitation—a safe, monitored environment to increase patient's exercise work capacity.

Evaluation: Expected Outcomes

- Afebrile.
- BP and heart rate stable; no dysrhythmias noted.
- Maintains bed rest.
- Pain reported at 2 on a scale of 0 to 10.

Pericarditis

Pericarditis is an inflammation of the pericardium, the membranous sac enveloping the heart. It is usually a manifestation of a more generalized disease. In healthy individuals, the pericardial cavity contains about 15 to 50 mL of an ultrafiltrate of plasma. Diseases of the pericardium present clinically in four ways:

Acute and recurrent pericarditis. Pericardial effusion is an abnormal accumulation of fluid in the pericardial cavity.

Cardiac tamponade is an acute type of pericardial effusion in which the heart is compressed, either by blood or by a penetrating injury, so that its normal function is impeded.

Constrictive pericarditis is a condition in which a chronic inflammatory thickening of the pericardium compresses the heart so it is unable to fill normally during diastole.

Pathophysiology and Etiology

1. Acute idiopathic pericarditis is the most common and typical form; etiology unknown.
2. Infection.
   a. Viral—Coxsackievirus; Herpes viruses; adenovirus; parvovirus B19, HIV.
   b. Bacterial—*Staphylococcus*, meningococcus, *Streptococcus*, pneumococcus, gonococcus, *Mycobacterium tuberculosis*.
   c. Fungal (rare)—Histoplasma, Aspergillus, Blastomyces and Candida species.
   d. Parasitic (rare)—Echinococcus and Toxoplasma.
3. Connective tissue disorders (lupus erythematosus, periarteritis nodosa) and gastrointestinal diseases (ulcerative colitis, Crohn and Whipple disease).
4. MI; early, 24 to 72 hours; or late, 1 week to 2 years after MI (Dressler syndrome).
5. Malignant disease; thoracic irradiation (primary or metastatic pericardial tumors).
6. Chest trauma, heart surgery, pacemaker insertion, coronary percutaneous interventions and radiofrequency ablation.
7. Drug-induced—procainamide, phenytoin, hydralazine, methyldopa, and isoniazid.
8. Asbestosis (may induce pericardial as well as lung lesions).
9. Metabolic disorders such as uremia; hypothyroidism may cause pericardial effusion, not necessarily pericarditis.

Clinical Manifestations

1. Pain in anterior chest, aggravated by thoracic motion—may vary from mild to sharp and severe; located in precordial area (may be felt beneath the clavicle, neck, scapular region); may be relieved by leaning forward.
2. Pericardial friction rub—scratchy, grating, or creaking sound occurring in the presence of pericardial inflammation.

3. Edema, ascites, and dyspnea—from pericardial effusion and cardiac tamponade.
4. Fever, sweating, chills—because of inflammation of the pericardium.
5. Dysrhythmias.

Diagnostic Evaluation

1. Echocardiogram—most sensitive method for detecting pericardial effusion.
2. Chest x-ray—may show enlarged cardiac silhouette with clear lung fields.
3. ECG—to evaluate for MI (acute stage of pericarditis, ST elevation is found in several or all leads).
4. WBC count and differential indicating infection.
5. Antinuclear antibody serologic tests elevated in lupus erythematosus.
6. Purified protein derivative test positive in tuberculosis.
7. ASO titers—elevated if rheumatic fever is present.
8. BUN—to evaluate for uremia.
9. Elevated erythrocyte sedimentation rate and serum C-reactive protein levels.
10. Elevated cardiac biomarkers—troponin and MB fraction of creatinine kinase.
11. Pericardiocentesis—for examination of pericardial fluid for etiologic diagnosis and relief from cardiac tamponade.
12. Cardiac MRI or CT.

Management

The objectives of treatment are targeted toward determining the etiology of the problem; administering pharmacologic therapy for specified etiology, when known; and being alert to the possible complication of cardiac tamponade.

1. Bacterial pericarditis—penicillin or other antimicrobials.
2. Rheumatic fever—penicillin G and other antimicrobials (see page 291).
3. Tuberculosis—antituberculosis chemotherapy (see page 206).
4. Fungal pericarditis—amphotericin B and fluconazole.
5. Systemic lupus erythematosus—corticosteroids.
6. Renal pericarditis—dialysis biochemical control of end-stage renal disease.
7. Neoplastic pericarditis—intrapericardial instillation of chemotherapy; radiotherapy.
8. Post-MI syndrome—bed rest, aspirin, prednisone.
9. Postpericardiotomy syndrome (after open heart surgery)—treat symptomatically.
10. Emergency pericardiocentesis if cardiac tamponade develops.
11. Partial pericardiectomy (pericardial "window") or total pericardiectomy for recurrent constrictive pericarditis.
12. NSAIDs are recommended for symptom relief of acute pericarditis; colchicine and steroid regimen are used as adjunct to NSAID therapy.

Complications

1. Cardiac tamponade.
2. Heart failure.
3. Hemopericardium (especially patients receiving anticoagulants after MI).

Nursing Assessment

1. Assess chest pain.
   a. Ask the patient if pain is aggravated by breathing, turning in bed, twisting body, coughing, yawning, or swallowing.

b. Assess for relief with sitting up and/or leaning forward.
   c. Be alert to the patient's medical diagnoses when assessing pain. Post-MI patients may experience a dull, crushing pain radiating to the neck, arm, and shoulders, mimicking an extension of infarction. Report change in character of chest pain or worsening pain.
2. Auscultate heart sounds.
   a. Listen for pericardial friction rub by asking patient to hold breath briefly.
   b. Listen to the heart with patient in different positions.
   c. Assess for pulsus paradoxus.
3. Evaluate history for precipitating factors.

Nursing Diagnoses

- Acute Pain related to pericardial inflammation.
- Decreased Cardiac Output related to impaired ventricular expansion.

Nursing Interventions

Reducing Discomfort

1. Give prescribed drug regimen for pain and symptomatic relief.
2. Relieve anxiety of patient and family by explaining the difference between pain of pericarditis and pain of recurrent MI. (Patients may fear extension of myocardial tissue damage.)
3. Explain to patient and family that pericarditis does not indicate further heart damage.
4. Encourage patient to remain on bed rest when chest pain, fever, and friction rub occur.
5. Assist patient to position of comfort.

Maintaining Cardiac Output

 NURSING ALERT Normal pericardial sac contains less than 30 mL of fluid; pericardial fluid may accumulate slowly without noticeable symptoms. However, a rapidly developing effusion can produce serious hemodynamic alterations.

1. Assess heart rate, rhythm, BP, respirations at least hourly in the acute phase; continuously if hemodynamically unstable.
2. Assess for signs of cardiac tamponade—increased heart rate, decreased BP, presence of paradoxical pulse, distended jugular veins, restlessness, muffled heart sounds.
3. Prepare for emergency pericardiocentesis or surgery. Keep pericardiocentesis tray at bedside (see page 253).
4. Assess for signs of heart failure (see page 298).
5. Monitor closely for the development of dysrhythmias.

Patient Education and Health Maintenance

1. Advise restriction of activity until biomarkers are normal.
2. Instruct patient about signs and symptoms of pericarditis and the need for long-term medication therapy to help relieve symptoms.
3. Review all medications with the patient—purpose, adverse effects, dosage, and special precautions.

Evaluation: Expected Outcomes

- Verbalizes relief of pain.
- Pulse and heart rate stable, no dysrhythmias, no friction rub.

Cardiomyopathy

Cardiomyopathy refers to disease of the heart muscle or electrical dysfunction. Causes of cardiomyopathy are classified as primary or secondary. Primary cardiomyopathies have genetic, mixed, or acquired etiologies, whereas secondary cardiomyopathies have infiltrative, toxic, or inflammatory causes. The four main types are dilated, hypertrophic, restrictive (less common), and arrhythmogenic right ventricular cardiomyopathy.

Pathophysiology and Etiology

Dilated Cardiomyopathy

Dilated cardiomyopathy is the most common form of cardiomyopathy. It can be divided into ischemic and nonischemic cardiomyopathy.

1. Ischemic cardiomyopathy.
   a. It is caused by inadequate oxygen supply because of obstruction in coronary arteries.
   b. The lack of oxygen interrupts both mechanical and electrical functions of the cells, decreases contractility, and causes dysrhythmia.
   c. The scar formed from MI leads to systolic dysfunction.
2. Nonischemic cardiomyopathy.
   a. Cause is idiopathic (unknown).
   b. 10% to 50% of cases are identified by genetic mutation.
3. Both the right and left ventricles dilate (enlarge) significantly, causing a decrease in the ability of the heart to pump blood efficiently to the body.
4. Blood remaining in the ventricles after contraction causes increases in ventricular, atrial, and pulmonary pressures.
5. Increased pressures continue to diminish the ability of the heart to pump blood to the body, and heart failure symptoms occur after all compensatory mechanisms are exhausted.
6. Alcohol abuse, chemotherapy, chemical agents, myocarditis, pregnancy (third trimester, postpartum), valve disease, endocrine disorders such as thyroid disease, and infections, such as HIV, can cause dilated cardiomyopathy.

Hypertrophic Cardiomyopathy

1. Hypertrophic cardiomyopathy is primarily due to the abnormal thickening of the ventricular septum of the heart.
2. The thickening of the heart muscle commonly occurs asymmetrically (septum is proportionately thicker than the other ventricular walls), but may also occur symmetrically (septum and the ventricular free wall both become equally thickened).
3. The ultrastructure of the heart is also disrupted by patches of myocardial fibrosis, disorganization of myocardial fibers, and abnormalities of the coronary microvasculature.
4. The thickened heart muscle and ultrastructure disruption change the shape, size, and distensibility of the ventricular cavity and alter the normal thickness and functioning of the mitral valve; as a result, the heart's ability to relax and contract normally is impaired.
   a. Muscle stiffness impairs the filling of the ventricle with blood during relaxation.
   b. Forceful contractions eject blood from the heart too rapidly, causing abnormal pressure gradients; mechanical narrowing of the passage by which the blood leaves the heart also may occur, acutely obstructing blood flow to the body.
5. Some forms of hypertrophic cardiomyopathy have familial presentation suggestive of genetic mutations.

Restrictive Cardiomyopathy

1. The heart muscle becomes infiltrated by various substances, resulting in severe fibrosis.
2. The heart muscle becomes stiff and nondistensible, impairing the ability of the ventricle to fill with blood adequately.

3. Amyloidosis and hemochromatosis (excess iron deposition) may cause restrictive cardiomyopathy.

Arrhythmogenic Right Ventricular Cardiomyopathy

1. Autosomal genetic disorder; affects 1 in 2,000 to 5,000; more common among men.
   a. Characterized by placement of the right ventricular myocytes by fibrofatty tissue, right ventricular dysfunction, and ventricular dysrhythmias.

Clinical Manifestations

1. Exertional dyspnea.
2. Chest pain.
3. Signs of heart failure (see page 298).
4. Pulmonary edema (see page 304).
5. Dysrhythmias (frequent atrial/ventricular ectopic beats; sinus, atrial, and ventricular tachycardia).
6. Pericardial effusions (with restrictive cardiomyopathy).
7. Cardiac murmur.
8. Syncope.
9. Sudden cardiac death may be the first sign with arrhythmogenic right ventricular cardiomyopathy.

Diagnostic Evaluation

1. Chest x-ray (cardiomegaly).
2. ECG—may show dysrhythmia, LV hypertrophy.
3. Echocardiogram to detect abnormalities of heart wall movements.
4. Twenty-four–hour Holter monitoring to detect dysrhythmias.
5. Radionuclide imaging to assess ventricular function.
6. Cardiac catheterization to help determine cause (ischemic or nonischemic).
7. Pulmonary artery catheter for hemodynamic monitoring.

Management

The goal of therapy is to maximize ventricular function and prevent complications.

Dilated Cardiomyopathy

1. Effective management of heart failure by conventional therapy (see page 298).
2. Oral anticoagulants may be instituted to prevent thrombus and pulmonary embolus.
3. Heart transplantation may be considered in eligible patients.
4. Mechanical circulatory support device (ie, LVAD or BiVAD) may also be considered.

 DRUG ALERT Patients with dilated cardiomyopathy and other forms of heart failure (HF) are susceptible to digoxin toxicity, especially with the concomitant use of amiodarone, furosemide, or verapamil and in patients with renal impairment. Monitor patient carefully for evidence of nausea, vomiting, yellow vision, and dysrhythmias.

Hypertrophic Cardiomyopathy

1. Guidelines for the management of cardiomyopathy and heart failure in general center around the measurement of ejection fraction (EF). Patients with EF greater than 50 are considered to have heart failure with preserved ejection fraction (HF*p*EF).

Those with EF less than or equal to 40 are considered to have heart failure with reduced ejection fraction (HF*r*EF). Beta-adrenergic blockers—reduce the force of the heart muscle's contraction, diminish obstructive pressure gradients, and decrease oxygen requirements. Three beta-blockers have been shown to be effective in reducing mortality in patients with chronic HF*r*EF; these include metoprolol sustained release, bisoprolol, and carvedilol.

2. Antidysrhythmic therapy—digoxin is most commonly used to slow ventricular response and increase myocardial contractility in patients with HF, although beta-blockers have been shown to be more effective than digoxin during exercise. Combination of beta-blockers and digoxin is more effective than either drug alone. If contraindicated, amiodarone may be an alternative.
3. Myotomy and myectomy—surgical resection of a portion of the septum to reduce muscle thickness and provide symptom relief.
4. Device implantation—pacemakers and automatic internal defibrillators may be implanted to prevent sudden death.

 DRUG ALERT Verapamil and diltiazem should be avoided in heart failure treatment because they depress myocardial function with increasing heart failure.

 DRUG ALERT Chest pain experienced by patients with hypertrophic cardiomyopathy is managed by rest and elevation of the feet (improves venous return to the heart). Vasodilator therapy (nitroglycerin) may worsen chest pain by decreasing venous return to the heart and further increasing obstruction of blood flow from the heart; agents that increase contractility of the heart muscle (dopamine, dobutamine) should also be avoided or used with extreme caution.

Restrictive Cardiomyopathy

1. Therapy is palliative unless specific underlying process is established.
2. Heart failure can be controlled with fluid restriction and diuretic therapy.
3. Digoxin is beneficial for controlling atrial fibrillation.
4. Oral anticoagulants are instituted to prevent emboli.

Arrhythmogenic Right Ventricular Cardiomyopathy

Antidysrhythmic agents such as carvedilol, sotalol, amiodarone.
1. Implantable cardioverter–defibrillator.
2. Myocardial ablation or transplantation.

Complications

1. Mural thrombus (because of blood stasis in ventricles with dilated cardiomyopathy).
2. Severe heart failure.
3. Sudden cardiac death.
4. Pulmonary embolism.

Nursing Assessment

1. Evaluate patient's chief complaint, which may include fever, syncope, general aches, fatigue, palpitations, dyspnea.
2. Evaluate etiologic factors, such as alcohol abuse, pregnancy, recent infection, or history of endocrine disorders.
3. Assess for positive family history.
4. Auscultate lung sounds for crackles (pulmonary edema) or decreased sounds (pleural effusion).
5. Assess heart size through palpation of the chest for point of maximal impulse (PMI) and auscultate for abnormal sounds.
6. Evaluate cardiac rhythm and ECG for evidence of atrial or ventricular enlargement and infarction.

Nursing Diagnoses

• Decreased Cardiac Output related to decreased ventricular function and/or dysrhythmias.
• Anxiety related to fear of death and hospitalization.
• Fatigue related to disease process.

Nursing Interventions

Improving Cardiac Output

1. Monitor heart rate, rhythm, temperature, and respiratory rate at least every 4 hours.
2. Evaluate CVP, pulmonary artery wedge pressure, and PCWP by pulmonary artery catheter to assess progress and effect of drug therapy.
3. Calculate CO, CI, and SVR.
4. Observe for changes in CO, such as decreased BP, change in mental status, decreased urine output.
5. Administer pharmacologic support, as directed, and observe for changes in hemodynamic and clinical status.
6. Administer medications to control or eradicate dysrhythmias, as directed.
7. Administer anticoagulants as directed, especially for patients in atrial fibrillation.
   a. Monitor coagulation studies.
   b. Observe for evidence of bleeding.

Relieving Anxiety

1. Always evaluate increasing and/or new-onset anxiety for a physiologic cause and report to the health care provider before administration of anxiolytics.
2. Explain all procedures and treatments.
3. Inform patient and visitors of visiting hours and policy and whom to contact for information.
4. Orient patient to unit, purpose of equipment, and care plan.
5. Encourage questions and voicing of fears and concerns.

Reducing Fatigue

1. Make sure that patient and visitors understand the importance of rest.
2. Assist patient in identifying stressors and reducing their effect (important for patients with hypertrophic cardiomyopathy because stress worsens the outflow obstruction).
3. Provide uninterrupted periods and assist with ambulation, as ordered.
4. Teach the use of diversional activities and relaxation techniques to relieve tension.

Patient Education and Health Maintenance

1. Medication education such as digoxin.
   a. Take daily only after taking pulse; notify health care provider if pulse is below 60 beats/minute (or other specified rate).

b. Report signs of digoxin toxicity—anorexia, nausea, vomiting, yellow vision.

c. Follow-up for periodic blood levels.

2. Advise low-sodium diet (less than 1,500 g daily). Teach how to read labels.

3. Advise reporting signs of heart failure—weight gain, edema, shortness of breath, increased fatigue.

4. Make sure that family members know cardiopulmonary resuscitation (CPR) because sudden cardiac arrest is possible.

Evaluation: Expected Outcomes

- Blood pressure and hemodynamic parameters stable; urine output adequate; baseline mental status.
- Asks questions and cooperates with care.
- Rests at intervals.

Heart Failure

 EVIDENCE BASE Yancy, C. W., Jessup, M., Bozkurt, B., et al. (2016). 2016 ACC/AHA/HFSA focused update on new pharmacological therapy for heart failure: An update of the 2013 ACCF/AHA guideline for the management of heart failure: A report of the American College of Cardiology/American Heart Association Task Force on Clinical Practice Guidelines and the Society for Cardiovascular Angiography and Interventions. *American Journal of Cardiology, 68*(13).

Heart failure is a clinical syndrome that results from the progressive process of remodeling, in which mechanical and biochemical forces alter the size, shape, and function of the ventricle's ability to fill with or pump enough oxygenated blood to meet the metabolic demands of the body.

Pathophysiology and Etiology

1. Cardiac compensatory mechanisms (increased heart rate, vasoconstriction, heart enlargement) initially occur to assist the struggling heart.

   a. These mechanisms are able to "compensate" for the heart's inability to pump effectively and maintain sufficient blood flow to organs and tissue at rest.

   b. Physiologic stressors that increase the workload of the heart (exercise, infection) may cause these mechanisms to fail and precipitate the "clinical syndrome" associated with a failing heart (elevated ventricular/atrial pressures, sodium and water retention, decreased CO, circulatory and pulmonary congestion).

   c. The compensatory mechanisms may hasten the onset of failure because they increase afterload and cardiac work.

2. Caused by disorders of heart muscle resulting in decreased contractile properties of the heart, such as coronary artery disease, hypertension, dilated cardiomyopathy, and valvular heart disease.

3. Risk factors include:

   a. Hypertension.

   b. Hyperlipidemia.

   c. Diabetes.

   d. CAD.

   e. Family history.

   f. Smoking.

   g. Alcohol consumption.

   h. Use of cardiotoxic drugs.

   i. Ventricular dysrhythmias.

   j. Atrial dysrhythmias.

Systolic versus Diastolic Failure

Heart failure (HF) is classified as either HFpEF or HFrEF. Systolic and/or diastolic dysfunction may exist in either HF types (see Figure 13-6).

1. Systolic failure—poor contractility of the myocardium results in decreased CO and an elevated SVR.

2. Diastolic failure—stiff myocardium, which impairs the ability of the left ventricle to fill up with blood. This causes an increase in pressure in the left atrium and pulmonary vasculature, causing the pulmonary signs of heart failure.

Acute versus Chronic Heart Failure

1. Acute failure—sudden onset of symptoms such as acute pulmonary edema and decreased CO; requires intervention and medical attention.

2. Chronic failure—long-term process with accompanying compensatory mechanism; can progress to acute phase in the setting of dysrhythmias, ischemia, or sudden illness.

3. Acute on chronic HF—patients with established history of HF who presents with exacerbation.

Neurohormonal Compensatory Mechanisms in Heart Failure

1. Sympathetic Nervous System

   a. Increased catecholamines to compensate for low CO.

   b. Shunting of blood from nonvital to vital organs.

   c. Increased oxygen demand, decreased coronary artery perfusion, and decreased diastolic filling.

2. Renin–Angiotensin–Aldosterone System

   a. Increased fluid retention in response to decreased CO.

   b. Increased vasoconstriction (action of angiotensin II).

   c. Increased SVR.

   d. Increased workload of the heart.

   e. Further decreased CO over time.

3. Ventricular Hypertrophy

   a. Compensatory mechanism to overcome the increased afterload.

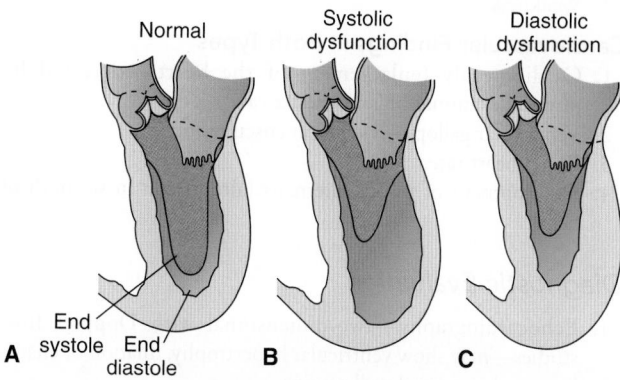

Figure 13-6. Heart failure because of systolic and diastolic dysfunction. The ejection fraction represents the difference between end-diastolic function and end-systolic volume. **(A)** Normal systolic and diastolic function with normal ejection fraction; **(B)** systolic dysfunction with decreased ejection fraction because of impaired systolic function; **(C)** diastolic dysfunction with decreased ejection fraction because of decreased diastolic filling. (Porth, C. M. [2005]. *Pathophysiology: Concepts of altered health states* [7th ed.]. Philadelphia: Lippincott Williams & Wilkins.)

4. Ventricular Remodeling
   a. Change of round bowl shape of the heart as a result of compensation.

Clinical Manifestations

Initially, there may be isolated left-sided heart failure, but eventually, the right ventricle fails because of the additional workload. Combined left- and right-sided heart failure is common. Heart failure may be classified according to physical activity (New York Heart Association Functional Classification) or disease progression (ACC/AHA Guidelines); see page 299.

Signs of Left-Sided Heart Failure (Forward Failure)
Altering the filling and pumping function of left ventricle, congestion occurs mainly in the lungs from blood backing up into pulmonary veins and capillaries.
1. Shortness of breath, dyspnea on exertion, tachypnea, paroxysmal nocturnal dyspnea (because of reabsorption of dependent edema that has developed during the day), orthopnea, cyanosis, pulmonary edema, and hemoptysis.
2. Cough—may be dry, unproductive; usually occurs at night.
3. Fatigability—from low CO, nocturia, insomnia, dyspnea, catabolic effect of chronic failure.
4. Insomnia, restlessness.
5. Tachycardia—ventricular gallop (S_3 and S_4).

Signs of Right-Sided Heart Failure (Backward Failure)
Altering the pumping function of right ventricle, there are signs and symptoms of elevated pressures and congestion in systemic veins and capillaries.
1. Edema of ankles; unexplained weight gain (pitting edema is obvious only after retention of at least 10 pound [4.5 kg] of fluid).
2. Liver congestion—may produce upper abdominal pain.
3. Distended jugular veins, increased CVP, pulmonary hypertension (increased PCWP).
4. Abnormal fluid in body cavities (pleural space, abdominal cavity), splenomegaly
5. Anorexia and nausea—from hepatic and visceral engorgement.
6. Nocturia—diuresis occurs at night with supine position and improved CO.
7. Weakness.

Cardiovascular Findings in Both Types
1. Cardiomegaly (enlargement of the heart)—detected by physical examination and chest x-ray.
2. Ventricular gallop—evident on auscultation.
3. Rapid heart rate.
4. Development of pulsus alternans (alternation in strength of beat).

Diagnostic Evaluation

1. Echocardiography—two-dimensional with Doppler flow studies—may show ventricular hypertrophy, dilation of chambers, and abnormal wall motion.
2. ECG (resting and exercise)—may show ventricular hypertrophy and ischemia.
3. Chest x-ray may show cardiomegaly, pleural effusion, and vascular congestion.
4. Cardiac catheterization—(left heart catheterization to rule out CAD).
   a. Right-sided heart catheterization—to measure pulmonary pressure and left ventricular function.

5. ABG studies may show hypoxemia because of pulmonary vascular congestion.
6. Bloodwork: CBC, electrolytes, Ca, Mg, renal function, glycohemoglobin, lipid profile, thyroid function, and liver function studies to fully assess patient condition that may impact heart failure.
7. Human B-type natriuretic peptide (BNP, triage BNP, N-terminal prohormone brain NP, or proBNP).
   a. As volume and pressure in the cardiac chambers rise, cardiac cells produce and release more BNP. This test aids in the differentiation of heart failure from other pulmonary diseases (ie, chronic obstructive pulmonary disease) and establish acute exacerbation of HF.
   b. A level greater than 100/mL is diagnostic for heart failure. In addition, the higher the BNP, the more severe the heart failure. BNP has inverse relationship with BMI so severity or degree of volume retention cannot be determined by the BNP values in obese patients.
   c. BNP is used in emergency departments to quickly diagnose and start treatment.
8. Radionuclide ventriculogram.
9. Thallium scan to rule out underlying causes.

Management

Overview Based on ACC/AHA Stage
See Table 13-5.
1. Stage A—focuses on eliminating risk factors by initiating therapeutic lifestyle changes, such as smoking cessation, increasing physical activity, and decreasing alcohol consumption. This stage also focuses on controlling chronic diseases, such as hypertension, high cholesterol, and diabetes. Beta-adrenergic blockers, ACE inhibitors, and diuretics are useful in treating this stage.
2. Stage B—treatment similar to stage A, with emphasis on use of ACE inhibitors and beta-adrenergic blockers.
3. Stage C—same as A and B, but with closer surveillance and follow-up.
   a. Digoxin is typically added to the treatment plan in this stage.
   b. Use of diuretic, hydralazine, nitrate, aldosterone antagonist, as indicated.
   c. Drug classes to be avoided due to worsening of heart failure symptoms include antiarrhythmic agents, calcium channel blockers, and NSAIDs.
   d. Patients post-MI (ie, 40 days post MI) with EF 35 or less who have New York State Heart Association class II or III symptoms and on guideline-supported medical therapies are recommended for implantable cardioverter–defibrillator placement.
4. Stage D—may need mechanical circulatory support, continuous inotropic therapy, cardiac transplantation, or palliative care.
   a. Treatment aimed at decreasing excess body fluid.
   b. May not tolerate other classes of drugs used in previous stages.
5. Unlike NYHA functional class, once a patient progresses to stage C, for example, they cannot go back to stage B.

Drug Classes
1. Diuretics (preload reduction).
   a. Eliminate excess body water and decrease ventricular pressures.
   b. A low-sodium diet and fluid restriction complement this therapy.
   c. Some diuretics may have slight venodilator properties.

Table 13-5	Heart Failure Guidelines and Recommendations	
NEW YORK HEART ASSOCIATION CLASSIFICATION	**AMERICAN COLLEGE OF CARDIOLOGY/AMERICAN HEART ASSOCIATION GUIDELINES**	**RECOMMENDATIONS**
—	**Stage A.** People at high risk of developing heart failure but without structural heart disease or symptoms of heart failure.	• Treat hypertension, lipid disorders, diabetes • Encourage patient to stop smoking and to exercise regularly • Discourage use of alcohol , illicit drugs • Angiotensin-converting enzyme (ACE) inhibitor, if indicated
Class I. Patients with cardiac disease without limitations of physical activity. Ordinary physical activity does not cause undue fatigue, palpitations, dyspnea, or anginal pain.	**Stage B.** People who have structural heart disease but no symptoms of heart failure.	• All stage A therapies • ACE inhibitor unless contraindicated • Beta-adrenergic blocker unless contraindicated
Class II. Patients with cardiac disease who have slight limitations of physical activity. They are comfortable at rest. Ordinary physical activity results in fatigue, palpitations, dyspnea, or anginal pain. **Class III.** Patients with cardiac disease who have marked limitation of physical activity. They are comfortable at rest. Less than ordinary physical activity causes fatigue, palpitations, dyspnea, or anginal pain.	**Stage C.** People who have structural heart disease with current or prior symptoms of heart failure.	• All stage A and B therapies • Sodium-restricted diet • Diuretics • Digoxin • Avoid or withdraw antiarrhythmic agents, most calcium channel blockers, and nonsteroidal anti-inflammatories • Consider aldosterone antagonists, angiotensin receptor blockers, hydralazine, and nitrates
Class IV. Patients with cardiac disease who cannot carry out any physical activity without discomfort. Symptoms of cardiac insufficiency or of anginal syndrome may be present even at rest. Any physical activity increases discomfort.	**Stage D.** People with refractory heart failure who require specialized interventions.	• All therapies for stages A, B, and C • Mechanical assist device, such as biventricular pacemaker or left ventricular assist device • Continuous inotropic therapy • Hospice care

Caboral, M., & Mitchell, J. (2003). New guidelines for heart failure: Focus on prevention. Nurse Practitioner, 28(1), 13–16, 22–23.

2. Positive inotropic agents—increase the heart's ability to pump more effectively by improving the contractile force of the muscle.
   a. Digoxin may be initiated at any time to reduce symptoms of HF, prevent hospitalizations, control rhythm, and improve exercise tolerance.
   b. Dopamine improves blood flow and urine output.
   c. Dobutamine.
   d. Milrinone and amrinone are potent vasodilators and increase contractility.
3. Vasodilator therapy—decreases the workload of the heart by dilating peripheral vessels. By relaxing capacitance vessels (veins and venules), vasodilators reduce ventricular filling pressures (preload) and volumes. By relaxing resistance vessels (arterioles), vasodilators can reduce impedance to left ventricular ejection and improve stroke volume.
   a. Nitrates (preload reducers), such as nitroglycerin, isosorbide, nitroglycerin ointment—predominantly dilate systemic veins.
   b. Hydralazine—predominantly affects arterioles; reduces arteriolar tone.
   c. Prazosin—balanced effects on both arterial and venous circulation.
   d. Sodium nitroprusside—afterload reducer; predominantly affects arterioles.
   e. Morphine—analgesic of choice because it enhances peripheral dilation, decreases venous return, and decreases anxiety, thus decreasing workload of the heart.

4. ACE inhibitors (decrease left ventricle dilation and remodeling)—inhibit the formation of angiotensin II. In doing so, produce vasodilation. Also prevent ventricular remodeling with chronic use.
   a. Studies have shown ACE inhibitors can alleviate HF symptoms and improve clinical status as well as overall sense of well-being among HF patients.
   b. The following ACE inhibitors have been shown to reduce morbidity and mortality: captopril, enalapril, lisinopril, perindopril, ramipril, and trandolapril.
5. Beta-adrenergic blockers—negative inotropes that decrease myocardial workload and protect against fatal dysrhythmias by blocking norepinephrine effects of the sympathetic nervous system.
   a. Metoprolol or metoprolol sustained release is commonly used.
   b. Carvedilol is a nonselective beta- and alpha-adrenergic blocker. Patients may actually experience increase in general malaise for a 2- to 3-week period while they adjust to the medication. To reduce the risk of orthostatic hypotension, instruct patient to take medicine with food.
6. Angiotensin II-receptor blockers—similar effects as ACE inhibitors, although mechanism of action is different. Used in patients who cannot tolerate ACE inhibitors because of cough or angioedema.
7. Aldosterone antagonists—decrease sodium retention, sympathetic nervous system activation, and cardiac remodeling.

a. Spironolactone is most commonly used.

b. May cause hyperkalemia, especially in those with impaired renal function, in those taking high doses of ACE inhibitors, or in those who use potassium supplements.

8. Nesiritide (decreases pulmonary artery pressure)—used in patients with decompensated heart failure. It produces smooth muscle cell relaxation and diuresis and a reduction in afterload and dyspnea.

9. Amiodarone—to treat arrhythmias.

 DRUG ALERT Assess patient's risk for hyperkalemia when administering aldosterone antagonists, such as their use of ACE inhibitors, prescription or OTC potassium supplements, and NSAIDs; monitor serum creatinine and potassium levels closely.

Diet Therapy

1. Restricted sodium.
2. Restricted fluids.

Mechanical Circulatory Support

May be used in stage D heart failure and acute exacerbation of heart failure.

1. IABP; see page 256, helps decrease afterload.
2. Cardiac resynchronization therapy or biventricular pacing—helps to restore synchronous ventricular contractions, improves ventricular left ventricle filling, and improves CO.
3. Total artificial heart or left, right, or biventricular assist device.
4. Partial left ventriculectomy (reduction ventriculoplasty or Batista procedure)—a triangular section of the weakened heart muscle is removed to reduce ventricular wall tension. This procedure is not commonly used.
5. Endoventricular circular patch plasty or the Dor procedure—removal of diseased portion of septum or left ventricle with a synthetic or autologous tissue patch, thus providing a more normal shape and size of the heart, which improves hemodynamics.
6. Acorn cardiac support device—a polyester mesh, custom-fitted jacket is surgically placed on the epicardial surface, providing diastolic support. Over time, it decreases or halts remodeling.
7. Intubation—for pulmonary edema or respiratory distress.
8. ICD—for patients with previous cardiac arrest, sustained ventricular arrhythmias, and in those post-MI with ejection fraction less than 30%.
9. Heart transplant.

Complications

1. Intractable or refractory heart failure—becomes progressively refractory to therapy (does not yield to treatment).
2. Cardiac arrhythmias.
3. Myocardial failure and cardiac arrest.
4. Digoxin toxicity—from decreased renal function and potassium depletion.
5. Pulmonary infarction, pneumonia, and emboli.

Nursing Assessment

1. Obtain history of symptoms, onset and duration of the symptoms, limits of activity, response to rest, and history of response to drug therapy. Determine neurologic status during the history.

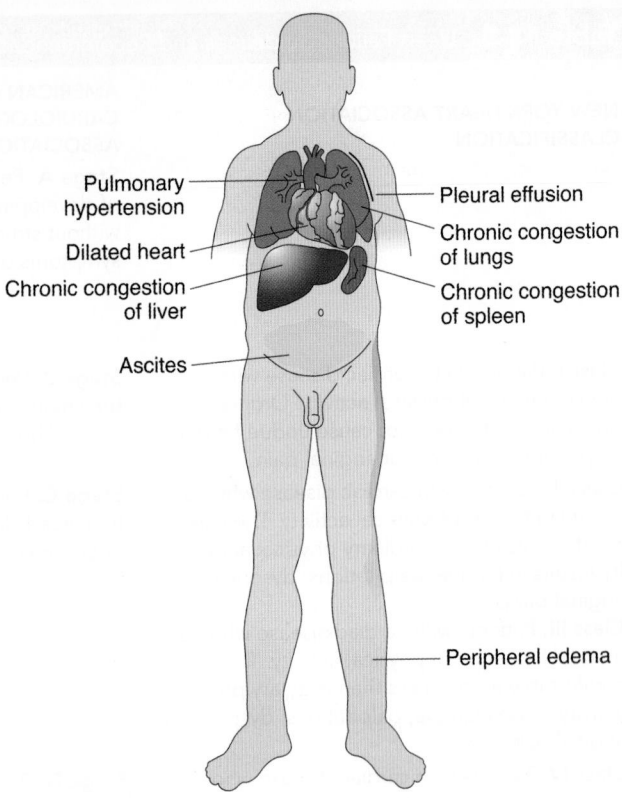

Figure 13-7. Consequences of heart failure.

2. Assess heart sounds, rhythm, PMI, and blood pressure. Assess peripheral vascular system, particularly for edema (see Figure 13-7). Assess respiratory effort, auscultate chest for breath sounds and presence of wheezes and crackles, and percuss for possible pleural effusion.
3. Inspect for jugular vein distention and obtain hemodynamic measurements, as indicated, and note change from baseline.
4. Assess abdomen for ascites and determine weight and change from baseline weight.
5. Note results of serum electrolyte levels and other laboratory tests.
6. Identify sleep problems and signs of depression that is often present in patients with heart failure.

Nursing Diagnoses

- Decreased Cardiac Output related to impaired contractility and increased preload and afterload.
- Impaired Gas Exchange related to alveolar edema because of elevated ventricular pressures.
- Excess Fluid Volume related to sodium and water retention.
- Activity Intolerance related to oxygen supply and demand imbalance.
- Deficient Knowledge related to lack of previous exposure to information.

Nursing Interventions

Maintaining Adequate Cardiac Output

1. Place patient at physical and emotional rest to reduce work of the heart.
   a. Provide rest in semirecumbent position or in armchair in air-conditioned environment—reduces work of the heart, increases heart reserve, reduces BP, decreases work of

respiratory muscles and oxygen utilization, and improves efficiency of heart contraction; recumbency promotes diuresis by improving renal perfusion.

b. Provide bedside commode—to reduce work of getting to bathroom and for defecation.

c. Provide for psychological rest—emotional stress produces vasoconstriction, elevates arterial pressure, and speeds the heart.
   i. Promote physical comfort.
   ii. Avoid situations that tend to promote anxiety and agitation.
   iii. Offer careful explanations and answers to the patient's questions.

2. Evaluate frequently for progression of left-sided heart failure. Take frequent blood pressure readings.
   a. Watch for decreasing mean arterial pressure.
   b. Note narrowing of pulse pressure.
   c. Note alternating strong and weak pulsations (pulsus alternans).

3. Auscultate heart sounds frequently and monitor cardiac rhythm.
   a. Note presence of S_3 or S_4 gallop (S_3 gallop is a significant indicator of heart failure).
   b. Monitor for premature ventricular beats.
   c. Assess chest pain.
   d. Measure CVP or JVP.

4. Observe for signs and symptoms of reduced peripheral tissue perfusion: cool temperature of the skin, facial pallor, poor capillary refill of nail beds.

5. Administer pharmacotherapy as directed.
   a. Monitor for adverse effects and effect of drug therapy.

6. Monitor clinical response of patient with respect to relief of symptoms (lessening dyspnea and orthopnea, decrease in crackles, relief of peripheral edema).

 NURSING ALERT Watch for sudden unexpected hypotension, which can cause myocardial ischemia and decrease perfusion to vital organs.

Improving Oxygenation

1. Raise head of bed 8 to 10 inches (20 to 25 cm)—reduces venous return to heart and lungs; alleviates pulmonary congestion.
   a. Support lower arms with pillows—eliminates pull of patient's weight on shoulder muscles.
   b. Sit orthopneic patient on side of bed with feet supported by a chair, head and arms resting on an over-the-bed table, and lumbosacral area supported with pillows.

2. Auscultate lung fields at least every 4 hours for crackles and wheezes in dependent lung fields (fluid accumulates in areas affected by gravity).
   a. Mark with indelible ink the level on the patient's back where adventitious breath sounds are heard.
   b. Use markings for comparative assessment over time and among different care providers.

3. Observe for increased rate of respirations (could be indicative of falling arterial pH).

4. Observe for Cheyne-Stokes respirations (may occur in older patients because of a decrease in cerebral perfusion stimulating a neurogenic response).

5. Reposition the patient every 2 hours (or encourage the patient to change position frequently)—to help prevent atelectasis and pneumonia.

6. Encourage deep breathing exercises every 1 to 2 hours—to avoid atelectasis. The use of incentive spirometry can be beneficial.

7. Offer small, frequent feedings—to avoid excessive gastric filling and abdominal distention with subsequent elevation of diaphragm that causes decrease in lung capacity.

8. Administer oxygen, as directed.

Restoring Fluid Balance

1. Administer prescribed diuretic, as ordered.

2. Give diuretic early in the morning—nighttime diuresis disturbs sleep.

3. Keep input and output record—patient may lose large volume of fluid after a single dose of diuretic. Watch fluid intake. Monitor urinary output; it should be 0.5 to 1 mL/kg/hour.

4. Weigh patient daily—to determine if edema is being controlled; weight loss should not exceed 1 to 2 pound (0.5 to 1 kg/day).

5. Assess for signs of hypovolemia caused by diuretic therapy—thirst; decreased urine output; orthostatic hypotension; weak, thready pulse; increased serum osmolality; and increased urine specific gravity.

6. Be alert for signs of hypokalemia, which may cause weakening of cardiac contractions and may precipitate digoxin toxicity in the form of dysrhythmias, anorexia, nausea, vomiting, abdominal distention, paralytic ileus, paresthesias, muscle weakness and cramps, confusion. Check electrolytes frequently.

7. Give potassium supplements, as prescribed.

8. Be aware of disorders that may be worsened by diuretic therapy, including hyperuricemia, gout, volume depletion, hyponatremia, magnesium depletion, hyperglycemia, and diabetes mellitus. There is no evidence to support that patients who are allergic to sulfa drugs are also allergic to thiazide diuretics.

9. Watch for signs of bladder distention in older male patients with prostatic hyperplasia.

10. Administer IV fluids carefully through an intermittent access device to prevent fluid overload.

11. Monitor for pitting edema of lower extremities and sacral area. Use convoluted foam mattress and sheepskin to prevent pressure ulcers (poor blood flow and edema increase susceptibility).

12. Observe for the complications of bed rest—pressure ulcers (especially in edematous patients), phlebothrombosis, pulmonary embolism.

13. Be alert to complaints of right upper quadrant abdominal pain, poor appetite, nausea, and abdominal distention (may indicate hepatic and visceral engorgement).

14. Monitor patient's diet. Diet may be limited in sodium—to prevent, control, or eliminate edema; may also be limited in calories.

15. Caution patients to avoid adding salt to food and foods with high-sodium content.

Improving Activity Tolerance

1. Increase patient's activities gradually. Alter or modify patient's activities to keep within the limits of his or her cardiac reserve.
   a. Assist patient with self-care activities early in the day (fatigue sets in as day progresses).
   b. Be alert to complaints of chest pain or skeletal pain during or after activities.

2. Observe the pulse, symptoms, and behavioral response to increased activity.
   a. Monitor patient's heart rate during self-care activities.
   b. Allow heart rate to decrease to preactivity level before initiating a new activity.

i. Note time lapse between cessation of activity and decrease in heart rate (decreased stroke volume causes immediate rise in heart rate).

ii. Document time lapse and revise patient care plan as appropriate (progressive increase in time lapse may be indicative of increased left-sided heart failure).

3. Relieve nighttime anxiety and provide for rest and sleep—patients with heart failure have a tendency to be restless at night because of cerebral hypoxia with superimposed nitrogen retention. Give appropriate sedation to relieve insomnia and restlessness.

Improving Knowledge

1. Explain the disease process; note that the term "failure" may be terrifying.
   a. Explain the pumping action of the heart: to move blood through the body to provide nutrients and aid in the removal of waste.
   b. Explain the difference between heart failure and heart attack.
2. Provide teaching about the signs and symptoms of recurrence.
   a. Watch for weight gain and report a gain or loss of more than 2 to 3 pound (1 to 1.4 kg) in a few days.
   b. Weigh patient at same time daily to detect any tendency toward fluid retention: swelling of ankles, feet, abdomen; persistent cough; tiredness; loss of appetite; frequent urination at night.
3. Review medication regimen.
   a. Medications recommended for patients with ejection fraction less than 40% include preload reductors, such as diuretics, and afterload reductors, such as ACE inhibitors.
   b. Medications to control heart rate include digoxin or beta-adrenergic blockers.
   c. Anticoagulation, if indicated.

TRANSITIONAL CARE ALERT To reduce readmission for heart failure, ensure that the patient and caregiver understand how each medication works to optimize heart function and that they will be able to obtain all prescriptions; that they understand who to notify for increase in daily weight; that salt and fluid restriction are clear; and that follow-up for up for lab work and office visit is arranged.

Patient Education and Health Maintenance

1. Advise patient of symptoms that need to be reported to health care provider.
   a. Sudden weight gain.
   b. Increased shortness of breath, inability to lie down, wheezing, increased cough.
   c. Increased swelling of feet, legs, abdomen.
2. Help patient understand all medications.
   a. Give written instructions.
   b. Make sure the patient has a pill organizer or check-off system to show that medications have been taken.
   c. Inform the patient of adverse drug effects.
   d. If the patient is taking oral potassium solution, it may be diluted with juice and taken after a meal.
   e. Tell the patient to weigh self daily at same time and log weight if on diuretic therapy.
   f. Ask whether patient is taking coenzyme Q10 or other supplements; should discuss with health care provider.

3. Review activity program instructions:
   a. Increase walking and other activities gradually, provided they do not cause fatigue and dyspnea.
   b. In general, continue at whatever activity level can be maintained without the appearance of symptoms.
   c. Avoid excesses in eating and drinking.
   d. Undertake a weight reduction program until optimal weight is reached.
   e. Avoid extremes in heat and cold, which increase the work of the heart; air conditioning may be essential in a hot, humid environment.
   f. Keep *regular* appointment with health care provider or clinic.
4. Restrict sodium as directed.
   a. Teach restricted sodium diet (less than 1,500 mg/day) and the DASH diet; see page 342.
   b. Give patient a written diet plan with lists of permitted and restricted foods.
   c. Advise patient to look at all labels to ascertain sodium content. Take into account serving size.
   d. Teach the patient to rinse the mouth well after using tooth cleansers and mouthwashes—some of these contain large amounts of sodium. Water softeners should be checked for salt content.
   e. Teach the patient that sodium is often hidden in foods, such as bread, and in medications such as antacids, cough remedies, pain relievers, estrogens, and other drugs.
   f. Encourage use of flavorings, spices, herbs, and lemon juice.
   g. Avoid salt substitutes with renal disease.
5. Instruct patient to buy frozen foods over canned foods.
6. Make sure patient sets up follow-up appointments.
7. Advise patient on smoking cessation; provide information, if indicated.

Evaluation: Expected Outcomes

- Normal BP and heart rate.
- Respiratory rate, 16 to 20 breaths/minute; ABG levels within normal limits; no signs of crackles or wheezes in lung fields.
- Weight decrease of 2.2 pound (1 kg) every 2 days; no pitting edema of lower extremities and sacral area.
- Heart rate within normal limits; rests between activities.
- States recurrent symptoms to watch for and knows medications and doses.

Acute Pulmonary Edema

Acute pulmonary edema refers to excess fluid in the lung, either in the interstitial spaces or in the alveoli.

Pathophysiology and Etiology

1. The presence of fluid in the alveoli impedes gas exchange, especially oxygen movement into pulmonary capillaries (see Figure 13-8).
2. May be caused by:
   a. Heart disease—acute left-sided heart failure, MI, aortic stenosis, severe mitral valve disease, hypertension, heart failure.
   b. Circulatory overload—transfusions and infusions.
   c. Drug hypersensitivity, allergy, poisoning.
   d. Lung injuries—smoke inhalation, shock lung, pulmonary embolism, or infarct.
   e. Central nervous system injuries—stroke, head trauma.

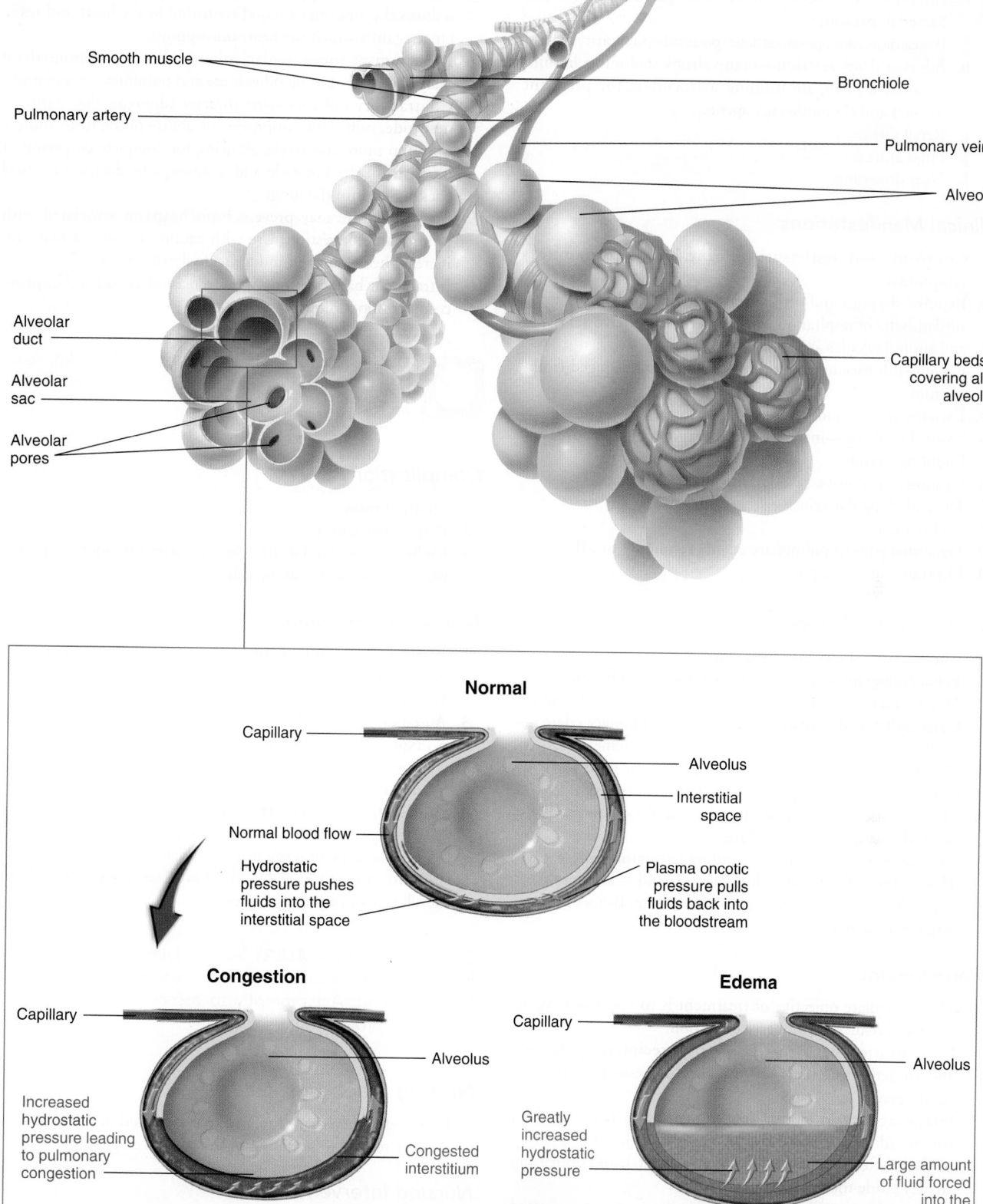

Figure 13-8. Normal alveoli and how pulmonary edema develops.

f. Infection and fever—infectious pneumonia (viral, bacterial, parasitic).

g. Postcardioversion, postanesthesia, postcardiopulmonary bypass.

h. Adverse drug reaction—many drugs including heroin, cocaine, aspirin, nicardipine as tocolytic for pregnant women and chemotherapy agents.

i. Renal disease.

j. High altitude

k. Near drowning.

Clinical Manifestations

1. Coughing and restlessness during sleep (premonitory symptoms).
2. Extreme dyspnea and orthopnea—patient usually uses accessory muscles of respiration with retraction of intercostal spaces and supraclavicular areas.
3. Cough with varying amounts of white- or pink-tinged frothy sputum.
4. Extreme anxiety and panic.
5. Noisy breathing—inspiratory and expiratory wheezing and bubbling sounds.
6. Cyanosis with profuse cold, clammy perspiration.
7. Distended jugular veins.
8. Tachycardia.
9. Precordial pain (if pulmonary edema secondary to MI).
10. Decreased urine output.

Diagnostic Evaluation

1. Chest x-ray—shows interstitial edema.
2. Echocardiogram—evaluates valves and ejection fraction.
3. Measurement of pulmonary artery wedge pressure by Swan-Ganz catheter (differentiates etiology of pulmonary edema—cardiogenic or altered alveolar–capillary membrane).
4. Blood cultures in suspected infection—may be positive.
5. Cardiac markers in suspected MI—may be elevated.
6. BUN, creatinine, serum electrolytes, and blood counts.
7. proBNP elevated in heart failure.
8. ABG analysis—may show impending respiratory failure.
9. Thoracentesis-fluid sample for diagnosis and treatment.
10. Lung ultrasound—valuable in early detection; B-lines indicate interstitial edema.

Management

1. The immediate objective of treatment is to improve oxygenation and reduce pulmonary congestion.
2. Identification and correction of precipitating factors and underlying conditions are then necessary to prevent recurrence.
3. Increasing oxygen tension (oxygen therapy), reducing fluid volume (diuretics, vasodilators), improving the heart's ability to pump effectively (glycosides, beta agonists), and decreasing anxiety guide therapeutic interventions.
4. Oxygen therapy—high concentrations of oxygen are used to combat hypoxemia. Intubation and/or ventilatory support may be necessary to improve hypoxemia and prevent hypercarbia. Noninvasive ventilation (NIV) is the first line of intervention.
5. Morphine—reduces anxiety, promotes venous pooling of blood in the periphery, and reduces resistance against which the heart must pump.

6. Vasodilator therapy (nitroglycerin and nitroprusside)—reduces the amount of blood returning to the heart and resistance against which the heart must pump.
7. Reduction of intravascular volume (diuresis or immediate dialysis)—decreases blood volume and pulmonary congestion.
8. Contractility enhancement therapy (digoxin, dobutamine, nesiritide, milrinone) improves the ability of the heart muscle to pump more effectively, allowing for complete emptying of blood from the ventricle and a subsequent decrease in fluid backing up into the lungs.
9. Aminophylline may prevent bronchospasm associated with pulmonary congestion. Use with caution because it may also increase heart rate and induce tachydysrhythmias.
10. Intra-aortic balloon pump—to decrease afterload and improve coronary blood flow.

DRUG ALERT Use extreme caution in administering nitroglycerin to patients with aortic stenosis who are preload dependent.

Complications

1. Dysrhythmias.
2. Respiratory failure.
3. Right ventricular failure—lower extremity edema, ascites, pleural effusion, hepatomegaly.

Nursing Assessment

1. Be alert to development of a new nonproductive cough.
2. Assess for signs and symptoms of hypoxia—restlessness, confusion, headache.
3. Auscultate lung fields frequently.
   a. Note inspiratory and expiratory wheezes, rhonchi, moist fine crackles appearing initially in lung bases and extending upward.
4. Auscultate for extra heart sounds.
   a. Note presence of third heart sound (may be difficult to hear because of respiratory sounds).
5. Identify precipitating factors that place patient at risk for development of pulmonary edema.

NURSING ALERT Acute pulmonary edema is a true medical emergency; it is a life-threatening condition. Act promptly to assess patient and notify health care provider of findings.

Nursing Diagnoses

- Impaired Gas Exchange related to excess fluid in the lungs.
- Anxiety related to sensation of suffocation and fear.

Nursing Interventions

Improving Oxygenation

1. Give oxygen in high concentration to relieve hypoxia and dyspnea and to keep oxygen saturation greater than 94% or patient's baseline.
2. Position the patient to reduce venous return to the heart—upright position, head and shoulders up, and feet and legs hanging down to favor pooling of blood in dependent

portions of body by gravitational forces and to decrease venous return.

3. Give morphine in small, titrated intermittent doses (IV) as directed.
   a. Morphine usually is not given if pulmonary edema is caused by stroke or occurs with chronic pulmonary disease or cardiogenic shock.
   b. Watch for excessive respiratory depression.
   c. Monitor BP because morphine may intensify hypotension.
   d. Have morphine antagonist available—naloxone.
4. Give diuretics IV or monitor during dialysis.
   a. Insert an indwelling catheter—large urinary volume will accumulate rapidly.
   b. Watch for falling BP, increasing heart rate, and decreasing urinary output—indications that the total circulation is not tolerating diuresis and that hypovolemia may develop.
   c. Check electrolyte levels because potassium loss may be significant.
   d. Watch for signs of urinary obstruction in men with prostatic hyperplasia.
5. Administer vasodilator if patient fails to respond to therapy.
   a. Monitor by measuring BP, PAP, and CO.
6. Assist with insertion of IABP, if needed, and monitor patient according to facility's protocol.
7. Administer aminophylline, if ordered.
   a. Monitor blood levels of drug.
   b. Evaluate for adverse effects of drug—ventricular dysrhythmias, hypotension, headache.
8. Administer cardiac glycosides as ordered.
9. Assist with cardioversion, if indicated (pulmonary edema may precipitate tachycardias).
10. Give appropriate drugs for severe, sustained hypertension.
11. Continually evaluate the patient's response to therapy. Reevaluate lung fields and cardiac assessment and monitor urine output and laboratory values.

Decreasing Anxiety

1. Stay with patient and display a confident attitude—the presence of another person is therapeutic because the acute anxiety of the patient may tend to intensify the severity of patient's condition. (Arterial vasoconstriction diminishes as anxiety is relieved.)
2. Explain to patient in a calm manner all therapies administered and the reason for their use. Explain to patient the importance of wearing oxygen mask. Assure patient that mask will not increase sensation of suffocation.
3. Inform patient and family of progress toward resolution of pulmonary edema.
4. Allow time for patient and family to voice concerns and fears.

Patient Education and Health Maintenance

During convalescence, instruct patient as follows to prevent recurrence of pulmonary edema:
1. Remind patient of early symptoms before onset of acute pulmonary edema; these should be reported promptly.
2. If coughing develops (a wet cough), sit with legs dangling over side of bed.
3. See "Patient Education, Heart Failure," page 302.

Evaluation: Expected Outcomes

- Unlabored respirations at 12 to 20 breaths/minute, lungs clear on auscultation, pulse oximetry greater than 94%.
- Appears calm and rests comfortably.

Acquired Valvular Disease of the Heart

 EVIDENCE BASE Nishimura, R., Otto, C., Bonow, R., et al. (2014). 2014 AHA/ACC guideline for the management of patients with valvular heart disease: Executive summary: A report of the American College of Cardiology/American Heart Association Task Force on Practice Guidelines. *Circulation, 129*, 2440–2492.

The function of normal heart valves is to maintain the forward flow of blood from the atria to the ventricles and from the ventricles to the great vessels.

Valvular damage may interfere with valvular function by stenosis (obstruction) or by impaired closure that allows backward leakage of blood (valvular insufficiency, regurgitation, or incompetence).

Pathophysiology and Etiology

Mitral Stenosis

1. Mitral stenosis is the progressive thickening and contracture of valve cusps with narrowing of the orifice and progressive obstruction to blood flow. Rheumatic fever is the most common cause of mitral stenosis in adults. Calcium deposit around the valves is rare with mitral stenosis. In children, the cause may be congenital.
2. Acute rheumatic valvulitis has "glued" the mitral valve flaps (commissures) together, thus shortening the chordae tendineae, so that the flap edges are pulled down, greatly narrowing the mitral orifice.
3. The left atrium has difficulty emptying itself through the narrow orifice into the left ventricle; therefore, it dilates and hypertrophies. Pulmonary circulation becomes congested.
4. As a result of the abnormally high PAP that must be maintained, the right ventricle is subjected to a pressure overload and may eventually fail.

Mitral Insufficiency

1. Mitral insufficiency (regurgitation or incompetence) is incomplete closure of the mitral valve during systole, allowing blood to flow back into the left atrium.
2. Left atrial pressures increase, reflected by increases in PAP and PCWP.
3. LVH may develop due to inefficient emptying.
4. May be due to myxomatous (connective tissue) degeneration, which causes stretching of leaflets and chordae tendineae; chronic rheumatic heart disease, ischemic heart disease, CAD, and infective endocarditis may also result due to medications and penetrating and nonpenetrating trauma.

Aortic Stenosis

1. Aortic stenosis is a narrowing of the orifice between the left ventricle and the aorta.
2. The obstruction to the aortic outflow places a pressure load on the left ventricle that results in hypertrophy and failure.
3. Left atrial pressure increases.
4. Pulmonary vascular pressure increases, which may eventually lead to right-sided heart failure.
5. May be caused by congenital anomalies (bicuspid aortic valve), calcification, or acute rheumatic fever.

Aortic Insufficiency

1. Because of abnormalities of aortic valve or aortic root.
2. Valve flaps fail to completely seal the aortic orifice during diastole and thus permit backflow of blood from the aorta into the left ventricle.

3. The left ventricle increases the force of contraction to maintain an adequate CO, usually resulting in hypertrophy.
4. The low aortic diastolic pressures result in decreased coronary artery perfusion.
5. May be caused by rheumatic or infective endocarditis, congenital malformation, aortic root dilation, Marfan syndrome, Ehlers-Danlos syndrome, Reiter syndrome, hypertension, systemic lupus erythematosus, or diseases that cause dilation or tearing of the ascending aorta (syphilitic disease, rheumatoid spondylitis, dissecting aneurysm).

Tricuspid Stenosis

1. Tricuspid stenosis is restriction or narrowing of the tricuspid valve orifice because of commissural fusion and fibrosis.
2. Usually follows rheumatic fever and is commonly associated with diseases of the mitral valve. Could be congenital in origin.

Tricuspid Insufficiency

1. Tricuspid insufficiency (regurgitation) allows the regurgitation of blood from the right ventricle into the right atrium during ventricular systole.
2. Common causes include dilation of right ventricle, rheumatic fever, and congenital anomalies.

Clinical Manifestations

1. Fatigue, weakness.
2. Dyspnea, cough, orthopnea, nocturnal dyspnea.
3. Characteristic murmur (see "Nursing Assessment").
4. Dysrhythmias, palpitations.
5. Hemoptysis (from pulmonary hypertension) and hoarseness (from compression of left recurrent laryngeal nerve by dilated left atrium) in mitral stenosis.
6. Low BP, dizziness, syncope, angina, and symptoms of heart failure in aortic stenosis.
7. Arterial pulsations visible and palpable over the precordium and visible in the neck, widened pulse pressure, and water-hammer (Corrigan) pulse (pulse strikes palpating finger with a quick, sharp stroke and then suddenly collapses) in aortic insufficiency.
8. Symptoms of right-sided heart failure—edema, ascites, hepatomegaly—in tricuspid stenosis and insufficiency.

Diagnostic Evaluation

1. ECG may show dysrhythmias.
2. Echocardiography (including 3D) may show abnormalities of valve structure and function and chamber size and thickness.
3. Chest x-ray may show cardiomegaly and pulmonary vascular congestion.
4. Cardiac catheterization and angiocardiography confirm diagnosis and determine severity.
5. Cardiac MRI provides more information and confirms diagnosis.
6. Exercise testing for patients with severe valvular disease to determine prognosis.

Management

Medical Therapy

1. Antibiotic prophylaxis for endocarditis before invasive procedures—indicated in most cases; see page 289.
2. Treatment of heart failure—diuretics, sodium restriction, vasodilators, cardiac glycosides, as indicated.

Surgical Intervention

See page 260 for care of the patient undergoing heart surgery.

1. For mitral stenosis:
   a. Closed mitral valvotomy—introduction of a dilator through the mitral valve to split its commissures.
   b. Open mitral valvotomy—direct incision of the commissures.
   c. Mitral valve replacement.
   d. Balloon valvuloplasty—a balloon-tipped catheter is percutaneously inserted, threaded to the affected valve, and positioned across the narrowed orifice. The balloon is inflated and deflated, causing a "cracking" of the calcified commissures and enlargement of the valve orifice.
2. For mitral insufficiency—mitral valve replacement or annuloplasty (retailoring of the valve ring).
3. For aortic stenosis or insufficiency:
   a. Replacement of aortic valve with prosthetic or tissue valves.
   b. Balloon valvuloplasty (aortic stenosis).
4. For tricuspid stenosis or insufficiency—valvuloplasty or replacement may be done at the time of surgical intervention for associated rheumatic mitral or aortic disease.
5. Transcatheter aortic valve implantation or replacement (TAVR)—a less invasive procedure where a bioprosthetic valve is used. Mostly for patients with severe symptomatic AS aged 75 years or older with surgical risk but expected to survive.
6. Percutaneous pulmonary valve implantation (PPVI)—for patients with pulmonary valve and right ventricular outflow tract defects.

Complications

1. Left-sided heart failure.
2. Possible, right-sided heart failure.
3. Dysrhythmias.
4. Pulmonary edema.

Nursing Assessment

Mitral Stenosis

1. Auscultate for accentuated first heart sound, usually accompanied by an "opening snap" (because of sudden tensing of valve leaflets) at the apex with diaphragm of stethoscope.
2. Place the patient in left lateral recumbent position. With bell of stethoscope at the apex, auscultate for a low-pitched diastolic murmur (rumbling murmur). Note duration of murmur (long duration is indicative of significant stenosis).

Mitral Insufficiency

1. Auscultate for diminished first heart sound.
2. Auscultate for systolic murmur (prominent finding), commencing immediately after first heart sound at apex, and note radiation of sound to the axilla and left intrascapular area.
3. Mild insufficiency may produce a pansystolic murmur (little connection between severity of mitral insufficiency and intensity of murmur auscultated).

Aortic Stenosis

1. Auscultate for prominent fourth heart sound and possible paradoxical splitting of second heart sound (suggestive of associated left ventricular dysfunction). First heart sound is normal.
2. Auscultate for a midsystolic murmur at the base of the heart (right upper sternal border) and at the apex of the heart. Note harsh and rasping quality at the base of the heart and a higher pitch at the apex of the heart.
3. There may be a palpable thrill.

Aortic Insufficiency

1. Auscultate for soft first heart sound.
2. Place the patient in sitting position, leaning forward.

3. Place diaphragm of stethoscope along left sternal border at the third and fourth intercostal space and then along the right sternal border. Auscultate for a high-pitched decrescendo diastolic murmur. To increase audibility of murmur, ask the patient to hold breath at end of deep expiration. Reauscultate for murmur.

Tricuspid Stenosis
1. Auscultate for a rumbling or blowing middiastolic murmur at the left sternal border (increases with inspiration).

Tricuspid Insufficiency
1. Auscultate for a third heart sound (may be accentuated by inspiration).
2. Auscultate for a pansystolic murmur in the parasternal region at the fourth intercostal space. Murmur is usually high-pitched.

Nursing Diagnoses
- Decreased Cardiac Output related to altered preload, afterload, or contractility.
- Activity Intolerance related to reduced oxygen supply.
- Ineffective Coping related to acute or chronic illness.

Nursing Interventions

Maintaining Adequate Cardiac Output
1. Assess frequently for change in existing murmur or new murmur.
2. Assess for signs of left- or right-sided heart failure; see page 298.
3. Assess for pulmonary edema.
4. Monitor and treat dysrhythmias, as ordered.
5. Prepare the patient for surgical intervention (see page 260).

Improving Tolerance
1. Maintain bed rest while symptoms of heart failure are present.
2. Allow patient to rest between interventions.
3. Begin activities gradually (eg, chair sitting for brief periods).
4. Assist with or perform hygiene needs for patient to reserve strength for ambulation.

Strengthening Coping Abilities
1. Instruct the patient about specific valvular dysfunction, possible etiology, and therapies implemented to relieve symptoms.
   a. Include family members in discussions with the patient.
   b. Stress the importance of adapting lifestyle to cope with illness.
2. Discuss with patient surgical intervention as the treatment modality, if applicable.
3. Assess the patient's use of appropriate coping mechanisms.

4. Refer the patient to appropriate counseling services, if indicated (vocational, social work, cardiac rehabilitation, substance abuse).

Patient Education and Health Maintenance
1. Review activity restriction and schedule with patient and family.
2. Instruct patient to report signs of impending or worsening heart failure—dyspnea, cough, increased fatigue, ankle swelling.
3. Review sodium and fluid restrictions.
4. Review medications—purpose, action, schedule, and adverse effects.
5. See "Patient Education, Heart Failure," page 302; "Infective Endocarditis," page 289; and "Rheumatic Endocarditis," page 291.

Evaluation: Expected Outcomes
- Blood pressure and heart rate within normal limits.
- Tolerates chair sitting for 15 minutes every 2 hours.
- Discusses ways to cope with lifestyle and activity changes.

Cardiac Dysrhythmias

Cardiac dysrhythmias are disturbances in regular heart rate and/or rhythm because of change in electrical conduction or automaticity. Dysrhythmias may arise from the sinoatrial (SA) node (sinus bradycardia or tachycardia) or anywhere within the atria or ventricles (known as ectopy or ectopic beats). Some may be benign and asymptomatic, whereas other dysrhythmias are life-threatening.

Dysrhythmias may be detected by change in pulse, abnormality on auscultation of heart rate, or ECG abnormality. Continuous cardiac monitoring is indicated for potentially life-threatening dysrhythmias.

Sinus Tachycardia

See Figure 13-9.

Etiology
1. Sympathetic nerve fibers, which act to speed up excitation of the SA node, are stimulated by underlying causes, such as anxiety, exercise, fever, shock, drugs, altered metabolic states (such as hyperthyroidism), or electrolyte disturbances.
2. The wave of impulse is transmitted through the normal conduction pathways; the rate of sinus stimulation is simply greater than normal (rate exceeds 100 beats/minute).

Figure 13-9. Sinus tachycardia.

Figure 13-10. Sinus bradycardia.

Analysis

Rate: 100 to 150 beats/minute.

Rhythm: R–R intervals are regular.

P wave: present for each QRS complex, normal configuration, and each P wave is identical or may be buried in previous T wave.

PR interval: falls between 0.12 and 0.20, or 0.16 second. P wave may be hidden in preceding T wave in rapid rates.

QRS complex: normal in appearance; one follows each P wave.

QRS interval: less than 0.11 seconds.

T wave: follows each QRS complex and is positively conducted.

QT interval: less than 0.48 seconds. This is usually corrected for heart rate and gender.

Management

1. Treatment is directed toward elimination of the cause rather than the dysrhythmia. Sometime, this is a compensatory mechanism for decreased cardiac output; thus, correction is not needed.
2. Urgency is dependent on the effect of rapid heart rate on coronary artery filling time to prevent cardiac ischemia.
3. Administration of oxygen and normal saline solution should be considered as initial treatment.

Sinus Bradycardia

See Figure 13-10.

Etiology

1. The parasympathetic fibers (vagal tone) are stimulated and cause the sinus node to slow.
2. Underlying causes:
   a. Drugs.
   b. Altered metabolic states such as hypothyroidism.

c. The process of aging, which causes increasing fibrotic tissue and scarring of the SA node.
d. Certain cardiac diseases such as acute MI (especially inferior wall MI).

3. The wave of impulse is transmitted through the normal conduction pathways; the rate of sinus stimulation is simply less than normal (less than 60 beats/minute).

Analysis

Rate: less than 60 beats/minute.

Rhythm: R–R interval is regular.

P wave: present for each QRS complex, normal configuration, and each P wave is identical.

PR interval: falls between 0.12 and 0.18 second.

QRS complex: normal in appearance; one follows each P wave.

QRS interval: 0.04 to 0.11 second.

T wave: follows each QRS and is positively conducted.

Management

1. The urgency of treatment depends on the effect of the slow rate on maintenance of CO.
2. Atropine 0.5 mg IV push blocks vagal stimulation to the SA node and therefore accelerates heart rate. Dopamine and epinephrine are alternatives if atropine is ineffective.
3. If bradycardia persists, a pacemaker may be required.
4. Sinus bradycardia is common in athletic individuals and does not require treatment.

Premature Atrial Contraction

See Figure 13-11.

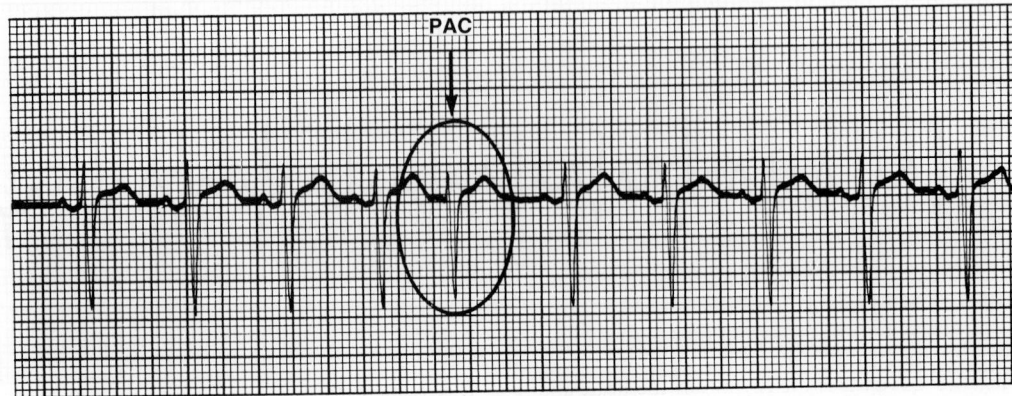

Figure 13-11. Normal sinus rhythm with premature atrial contraction.

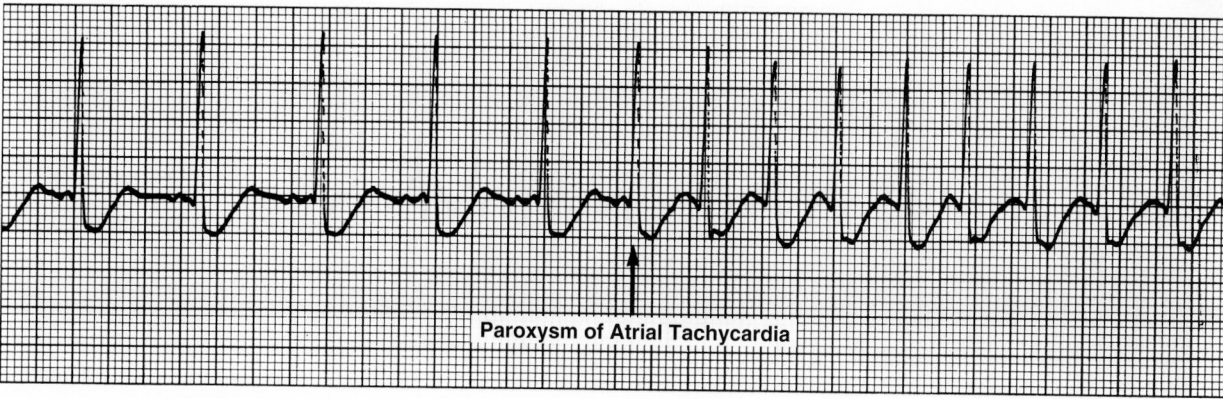

Paroxysm of Atrial Tachycardia

Figure 13-12. Paroxysmal atrial tachycardia.

Etiology

1. May occur in the healthy heart where they are idiopathic and benign.
2. In the diseased heart, premature atrial contractions (PACs) may represent ischemia and a resultant irritability in the atria. They may increase in frequency and be the precursor of more serious dysrhythmias.
3. May be caused by electrolyte abnormalities, hypoxia, MI, heart failure, and acid–base disturbances.
4. The wave of impulse of the PAC originates within the atria and outside the sinus node. Because the impulse originates within the atria, the P wave will be present, but it will be different in appearance as compared with those beats originating within the sinus node. The impulse traverses the remainder of the conduction system in a normal pattern; thus, the QRS complex is identical in configuration to the normal sinus beats.

Analysis

Rate: may be slow or fast.

Rhythm: will be irregular; caused by the early occurrence of the PAC.

P wave: will be present for each normal QRS complex; the P wave of the premature contraction will be distorted in shape.

PR interval: may be normal but can also be shortened, depending on where in the atria the impulse originated. (The closer the site of atrial impulse formation to the atrioventricular [AV] node, the shorter the PR interval will be.)

QRS complex: within normal limits because all conduction below the atria is normal.

T wave: normally conducted.

Management

1. Generally requires no treatment if laboratory values are normal.
2. PACs should be monitored for increasing frequency.

Paroxysmal Atrial Tachycardia

See Figure 13-12.

Etiology

1. Causes include:
   a. Syndromes of accelerated pathways (eg, Wolff-Parkinson-White syndrome).
   b. Syndrome of mitral valve prolapse.
   c. Ischemic CAD.
   d. Excessive use of alcohol, cigarettes, caffeine.
   e. Drugs—digoxin is a frequent cause.
2. An ectopic atrial focus captures the rhythm of the heart and is stimulated at a very rapid rate; the impulse is conducted

normally through the conduction system so the QRS complex usually appears within normal limits.

3. The rate is often so rapid that P waves are not obvious but may be "buried" in the preceding T wave.

Analysis

Rate: between 150 and 250 beats/minute.

Rhythm: regular.

P wave: present before each QRS complex; however, the faster the rate, the more difficult it becomes to visualize P waves. (The P waves can frequently be measured with calipers by observing the varying configuration of the preceding T waves.)

PR interval: usually not measurable.

QRS complex: will appear normal in configuration and within 0.06 to 0.10 second.

T wave: will be distorted in appearance as a result of P waves being buried in them.

Management

1. Treatment is directed first to slowing the rate and, second, to reverting the dysrhythmia to a normal sinus rhythm.
2. Reducing the rate may be accomplished by having the patient perform a Valsalva maneuver. This stimulates the vagus nerve to slow the heart.
   a. A Valsalva maneuver may be done by having the patient gag or "bear down" as though attempting to have a bowel movement.
   b. The health care provider may choose to perform carotid massage.
3. Adenosine is the drug of choice for paroxysmal atrial tachycardia associated with hypotension, chest pain, or shortness of breath.
   a. The initial dose is 6 mg rapid IV push followed by a fast normal saline flush. If there is no response in 1 to 2 minutes, a second and third bolus of 12 mg may be given, each followed by fast normal saline flushes.
   b. Has a very short half-life and is therefore eliminated quickly.
4. IV beta-adrenergic blockers, such as esmolol, may be used.
5. Calcium channel blockers (eg, verapamil) are effective in reverting this dysrhythmia. Beware of hypotension, however, especially in the volume-depleted patient.
6. If drug therapy is ineffective, elective cardioversion can be used.

Atrial Flutter

See Figure 13-13.

Etiology

1. Occurs with atrial stretching or enlargement (as in AV valvular disease), MI, and heart failure.

Figure 13-13. Atrial flutter.

2. An ectopic atrial focus captures the rhythm in atrial flutter and fires at an extremely rapid rate (200 to 400 beats/minute) with regularity.
3. Conduction of the impulse through the conduction system is normal; thus, the QRS complex is unaffected.
4. An important feature of this dysrhythmia is that the AV node sets up a therapeutic block, which disallows some impulse transmission.
   a. This can produce a varying block or a fixed block (ie, sometimes the AV node will transmit every second flutter wave, producing a 2:1 block, or the rhythm can be 3:1 or 4:1).
   b. If the AV node conducted 1:1, then the outcome would be a ventricular rate of about 300 beats/minute. The patient would rapidly deteriorate.

Analysis

Rate: atrial rate between 250 and 400 beats/minute; ventricular rate will depend on degree of block.

Rhythm: regular or irregular, depending on kind of block (eg, 2:1, 3:1, or a combination).

P wave: not present; instead, it is replaced by a saw-toothed pattern that is produced by the rapid. firing of the atrial focus. These waves are also referred to as "F" waves.

PR interval: not measurable.

QRS complex: normal configuration and normal conduction time.

T wave: present but may be obscured by flutter waves.

Management

1. The urgency of treatment depends on the ventricular response rate and resultant symptoms. Too rapid or slow a rate will decrease CO.
2. A calcium channel blocker, such as diltiazem, may be used to slow AV nodal conduction. Use with caution in the patient with heart failure, hypotension, or concomitant beta-adrenergic blocker therapy.
3. Digoxin may be used.
4. An IV beta-adrenergic blocker, such as esmolol, may also be used.
5. If drug therapy is unsuccessful, atrial flutter will typically respond to cardioversion. Small doses of biphasic electrical current (50 to 100 joules) are usually successful.
6. Electrophysiologic studies and subsequent ablation therapy are highly effective because the ectopic focus is usually readily identified.

Atrial Fibrillation

See Figure 13-14.

Etiology

1. Fibrotic changes associated with the aging process, acute MI, valvular diseases, and digoxin preparations may cause atrial fibrillation.
2. Fluid shifts in the body (ie, after hemodialysis or surgery).
3. Multiple atrial foci fire impulses at rapid and disorganized rates.
4. The atria are not depolarized effectively; thus, there are no well-formed P waves.
5. Instead, the baseline between QRS complexes is filled with a "wiggly" line that is described as fine or coarse.
6. If the atrial rate is rapid enough, the line will appear almost flat. The atria are said to be firing at rates of between 300 and 500 times per minute.
7. The conduction of a QRS complex is so random that the rhythm is extremely irregular.
8. Atrial fibrillation may be described as controlled if the ventricular response is 100 beats/minute or less; the dysrhythmia is uncontrolled if the rate is above 100 beats/minute.

Figure 13-14. Atrial fibrillation with slow ventricular response (controlled).

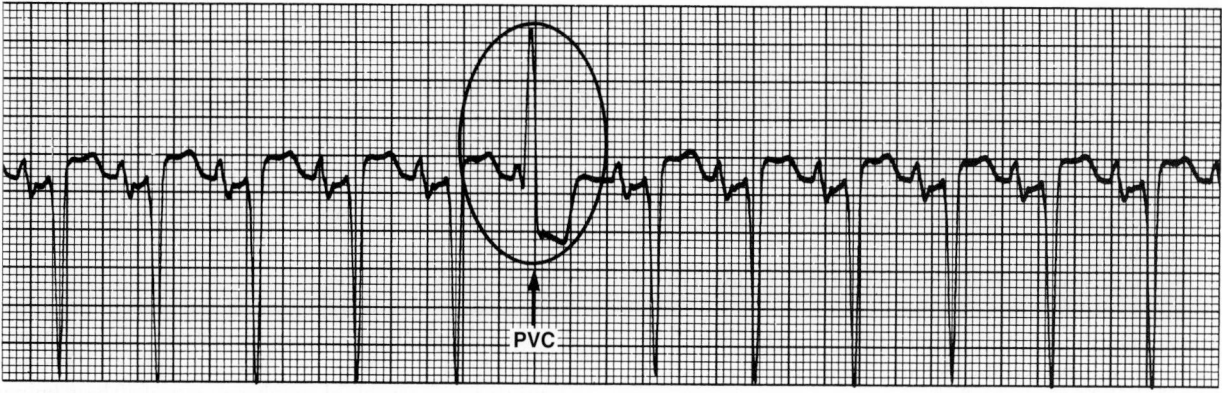

Figure 13-15. Normal sinus rhythm with premature ventricular contraction.

Analysis

Rate: atrial fibrillation is usually immeasurable because fibrillatory waves replace P waves; ventricular rate may vary from bradycardia to tachycardia.

Rhythm: classically described as an "irregular irregularity."

P wave: replaced by fibrillatory waves, sometimes called "little f" waves.

PR interval: not measurable.

QRS complex: a normally conducted complex.

T wave: normally conducted.

Management

1. Controlled atrial fibrillation of long-standing duration requires no treatment as long as the patient is experiencing no untoward effects. Most cardiologists agree that reversion of long-standing atrial fibrillation is hazardous because of the potential for a thrombus to be dislodged from the atria at the time of reversion.

2. Uncontrolled atrial fibrillation (ventricular responses of 100 beats/minute or greater) is treated with beta-adrenergic blocker or calcium channel blockers to control rate at rest and activity. If the atrial fibrillation is of recent onset, the cardiologist may choose to revert the rhythm to a sinus rhythm.

3. Digoxin is a second-line drug for rate control because it only controls rate at rest.

4. Cardioversion (electrical or pharmacologic) for recent-onset atrial fibrillation may be required starting with low amounts of biphasic electrical current (100 to 200 joules).

5. Chronic anticoagulation therapy may be warranted to prevent microemboli.

Premature Ventricular Contraction

See Figure 13-15.

Etiology

1. May be caused by acute MI, other forms of heart disease, pulmonary diseases, electrolyte disturbances, metabolic instability, and drug abuse.

2. The wave of impulse originates from an ectopic focus (foci) within the ventricles at a rate faster than the next normally occurring beat.

3. Because the normal conduction pathway is bypassed, the configuration of the premature ventricular contraction (PVC) is wider than normal and is distorted in appearance. PVCs may occur in regular sequence with normal rhythm—every other beat (bigeminy), every third beat (trigeminy), and so forth (see Figure 13-16).

Analysis

Rate: may be slow or fast.

Rhythm: will be irregular because of the premature firing of the ventricular ectopic focus.

P wave: will be absent because the impulse originates in the ventricle, bypassing the atria and AV node.

PR interval: not measurable.

QRS complex: will be widened greater than 0.12 second, bizarre in appearance when compared with normal QRS complex. (The QRS of a PVC is commonly referred to as having a "sore thumb" appearance.)

T wave: the T wave of the PVC is usually deflected opposite to the QRS.

Figure 13-16. Ventricular bigeminy.

Management

1. PVCs are usually the precursors of more serious ventricular dysrhythmias. The following conditions involving PVCs require prompt and vigorous treatment, especially if the patient is symptomatic or unstable:
   a. PVCs occurring at a rate exceeding six per minute.
   b. Occur as two or more consecutively.
   c. PVCs fall on the peak or down slope of the T wave (period of vulnerability).
   d. Are of varying configurations, indicating a multiplicity of foci.
2. Historically, the standard treatment for PVCs has been lidocaine. Today, however, amiodarone IV is the preferred method because of lidocaine's risk for toxicity.
   a. Can be given by bolus of 150 mg IV over 10 minutes.
   b. IV infusion consists of a loading dose of 1 mg/minute for 6 hours, followed by a maintenance rate of 0.5 mg/minute for 18 hours.
   c. After IV load, patient may require oral dosing.
3. Lidocaine toxicities include confusion and slurred speech. It should be used with caution in older adults and in those with liver disease.
4. Amiodarone toxicities include pulmonary fibrotic changes, hypothyroidism, and liver dysfunction.
5. If ventricular premature beats occur in conjunction with a bradydysrhythmia, atropine may be chosen to accelerate the heart rate and eliminate ectopic beats.
6. Atropine should be used with caution with acute MI. The injured myocardium may not be able to tolerate the accelerated rate.
7. Electrolyte infusions may also be needed to treat PVCs. Magnesium sulfate may be used, especially in patients with acute MI. It may be given as 1 g IV over 1 hour or according to facility policy. Potassium infusions can be given at 10 mmol/hour and should be diluted accordingly to route of IV administration.

 DRUG ALERT Be alert to the development of confusion, slurring of speech, and diminished mentation because lidocaine toxicity affects the central nervous system. Should these symptoms appear, slowing the lidocaine may cause them to abate.

Ventricular Tachycardia

See Figure 13-17.

Etiology

1. Occurs with:
   a. Acute MI, cardiomyopathy.
   b. Syndromes of accelerated rhythm that deteriorate (eg, Wolff-Parkinson-White syndrome).
   c. Metabolic acidosis, especially lactic acidosis.
   d. Electrolyte disturbance.
   e. Toxicity to certain drugs, such as digoxin or isoproterenol.
2. A life-threatening dysrhythmia that originates from an irritable focus within the ventricle at a rapid rate. Because the ventricles are capable of an inherent rate of 40 beats/minute or less, a ventricular rhythm at a rate of 100 beats/minute may be considered tachycardia.

Analysis

Rate: usually between 100 and 220 beats/minute.
Rhythm: usually regular but may be irregular.
P wave: not present.
PR interval: not measurable.
QRS complex: broad, bizarre in configuration, widened greater than 0.12 second.
T wave: usually deflected opposite to the QRS complex.

Management

1. Ventricular tachycardia (VT) less than 30 seconds is called nonsustained VT. VT more than 30 seconds is sustained VT and requires immediate treatment.
2. If the patient has a pulse and is hemodynamically stable, medications are the initial treatments. Amiodarone IV bolus can be given to halt the dysrhythmia. Other potential medications that may be used (if amiodarone fails) include lidocaine and procainamide. If patient becomes hemodynamically unstable, prepare for synchronized cardioversion with 200 joules of biphasic electrical current.
3. If the patient is pulseless, defibrillation is recommended with 200 joules of biphasic electrical current.
4. The purpose of cardioversion–defibrillation is to abolish all abnormal electrical activity and allow the intrinsic cardiac rhythm the opportunity to restart.
5. In some cases, VT may be refractory to drug therapy. Nonpharmacologic treatments, such as endocardial resection,

Figure 13-17. Ventricular tachycardia.

aneurysmectomy, antitachycardia pacemakers, cryoablation, automatic internal defibrillators, and catheter ablation, are alternative treatment modalities.

6. An atypical form of VT, referred to as polymorphous VT or *torsades de pointes* (twisting of the points), can result as a consequence of drug therapy (eg, quinidine therapy) or electrolyte imbalance such as hypomagnesemia. It is important to diagnose polymorphous VT as the treatment differs from monomorphic VT.
   a. *Torsades de pointes* is characterized by a QT interval prolonged to greater than 0.60 second, varying R–R intervals, and polymorphous QRS complexes.
   b. The treatment of choice is administration of magnesium sulfate 1 g IV over 5 to 60 minutes.
   c. If the patient loses consciousness and pulse, defibrillate with 120 to 200 joules of biphasic electrical current.
   d. Ventricular pacing to override the ventricular rate and, thus, capture the rhythm is also an acceptable treatment.
   e. Procainamide should be avoided because its effect is to prolong the QT interval.

 NURSING ALERT VT is life-threatening and its presentation calls for immediate intervention by the nurse.

Ventricular Fibrillation

See Figure 13-18.

Etiology
1. Occurs in acute MI, acidosis, electrolyte disturbances, and other deteriorating ventricular rhythms.
2. The ventricles are firing chaotically at rates that exceed 300 beats/minute, resulting in ineffective impulse conduction. CO ceases, and the patient loses pulse, BP, and consciousness.
3. Must be reversed immediately or the patient will die.

Analysis
Rate: not measurable because of absence of well-formed QRS complexes.
Rhythm: chaotic.
P wave: not present.
QRS complex: bizarre, chaotic, no definite contour.
T wave: not apparent.

Management
1. The only treatment for ventricular fibrillation is immediate defibrillation. Defibrillate at 120 to 200 joules with a biphasic defibrillator. Current advanced cardiac life support guidelines no longer recommend three stacked shocks before initiating CPR and medication administration. Epinephrine and vasopressin are first-line drugs after defibrillation because these drugs may make the fibrillation more vulnerable to defibrillation.
2. Unsuccessful defibrillation may be a result of lactic acidosis (treatable with sodium bicarbonate).
3. Check adequacy of the high-quality CPR being performed: 100 compressions/minute at a 2 to 2½-inch depth.

Atrioventricular Block

Etiology
1. May be caused by ischemia or inferior wall MI, digoxin toxicity, hypothyroidism, or Stokes-Adams syndrome.
2. Impaired tissue at the level of the AV node prevents the timely passage of the wave of impulse through the conduction system.
3. In first-degree AV block, the impulse is transmitted normally, but it is delayed at the level of the AV node. The PR interval exceeds 0.20 second.
4. In second-degree AV block, two or more atrial impulses occur before the ventricles are stimulated.
   a. Second-degree type 1 (Mobitz 1 Wenckebach)—block occurs above the AV node. There is an increase in delay of electrical impulse (increasing PR interval) with every beat until one P wave fails to conduct and is not followed by a QRS complex (beat is dropped). Mobitz type 1 is usually a temporary and benign dysrhythmia and seldom requires intervention (pacing) unless ventricular rate is slow and the patient is unstable.
   b. Second-degree type 2 (Mobitz 2)—block occurs below the AV node in the bundle of His or bundle-branch system. The atria and ventricles are discharging impulses, but the activity bears no relationship to each other. There is a sudden failure to conduct an atrial impulse to the ventricles without a delay of the PR interval.
5. In third-degree AV block, or complete heart block, the electrical impulse is completely blocked from the SA node to the AV node. An independent pacemaker in the ventricles takes over at a much slower rate than the atria and are firing independently of each other.

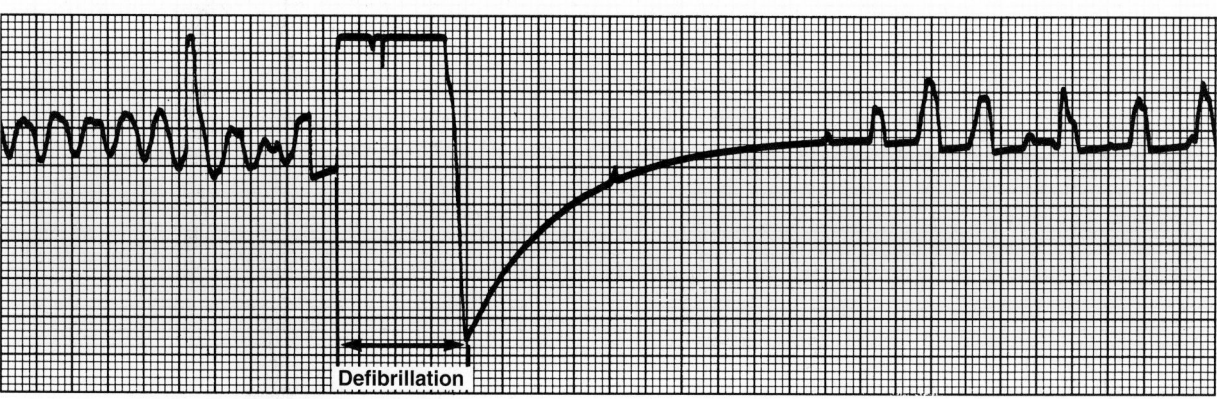

Figure 13-18. Ventricular fibrillation with defibrillation.

Figure 13-19. First-degree AV block.

Analysis

1. First-degree AV block (see Figure 13-19).
   Rate: usually normal but may be slow.
   Rhythm: regular.
   P wave: present for each QRS complex, identical in configuration.
   PR interval: prolonged to greater than 0.20 second.
   QRS complex: normal in appearance and between 0.06 and 0.10 second.
   T wave: normally conducted.
2. Second-degree AV block (see Figure 13-20).
   Rate: usually normal.
   Rhythm: may be regular or irregular.
   P wave: present but some may not be followed by a QRS complex. A ratio of two, three, or four P waves to one QRS complex may exist.
   PR interval: varies in Mobitz I (Wenckebach), usually lengthens until one is not conducted; constant in Mobitz II, but not all P waves conducted.
   T wave: normally conducted.
3. Third-degree AV block (complete heart block) (see Figure 13-21).
   Rate: atrial rate is measured independently of the ventricular rate; the ventricular rate is usually very slow.
   Rhythm: each independent rhythm will be regular, but they will bear no relationship to each other.

P wave: present but no consistent relationship with the QRS.
PR interval: not really measurable.
QRS complex: depends on the escape mechanism (ie, AV node will have normal QRS, ventricular will be wide, and the rate will be slower).
T wave: normally conducted.

Management

Like that of other dysrhythmias, the treatment of heart blocks depends on the effect the rate is having on CO.

1. First-degree AV block usually requires no treatment.
2. Second-degree AV block, type 1 and type 2, may require treatment if the ventricular rate falls too low to maintain effective CO. Mobitz type 2 is more serious than Mobitz type 1.
3. Third-degree AV block usually requires intervention. However, some patients may be able to tolerate third-degree block for a length of time.
4. Transcutaneous pacing should be employed in the emergent situation while transvenous pacing is being set up.
5. Atropine may be given while awaiting the pacemaker, but it must be remembered that the effect of atropine is to block vagal tone, and the vagus acts on the sinus node. Because the AV node is the culprit in heart block, atropine may not be helpful.

Figure 13-20. Second-degree AV block (Mobitz I).

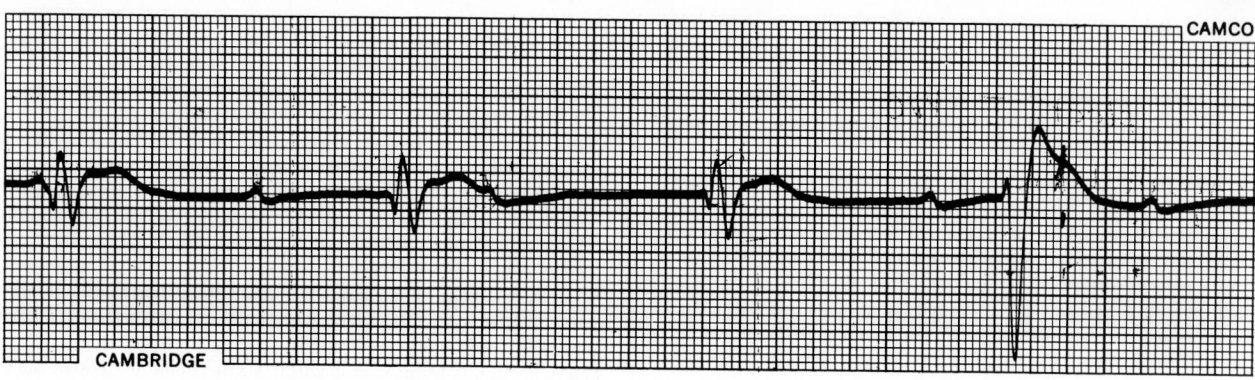

Figure 13-21. Third-degree AV block.

SELECTED REFERENCES

Albert, N. M. (2016). A systematic review of transitional-care strategies to reduce rehospitalization in patients with heart failure. *Heart & Lung: The Journal of Acute and Critical Care, 45*(2), 100–113.

Alkashkari, W., Alsubei, A., and Hijazi, Z. M. (2018). Transcatheter pulmonary valve replacement: current state of art. *Current Cardiology Reports,* 20, 27. Available: *https://doi-org.ezp.welch.jhmi.edu/10.1007/s11886-018-0966-y*

Ambrosioni, J., Hernandez-Meneses, M., Téllez, A., et al. (2017). The changing epidemiology of infective endocarditis in the twenty-first century. *Current Infectious Disease Report, 19*(5), 21.

Baddour, L. M., Wilson, W. R., Bayer, A. S., Fowler, V. G., & Tleyjeh, I. M. (2015). Infective endocarditis in adults: Diagnosis, antimicrobial therapy, and management of complications: A scientific statement for healthcare professionals from the American Heart Association. *Circulation, 132*(1524–4539), 1–53.

Berndt, N. C., Bolman, C., de Vries, H., et al. (2013). Smoking cessation treatment practices: Recommendations for improved adoption on cardiology wards. *Journal of Cardiovascular Nursing, 28*(1), 35–47.

Catapano A.L., Graham I., De Backer G., et al. (2016). 2016 ESC/EAS Guidelines for the Management of Dyslipidaemias. *European Heart Journal*, 37, 2999.

Chou, R., Dana, T., Blazina, I., et al. (2016). Statins for prevention of cardiovascular Ddsease in adults: Evidence report and systematic Rrview for the US Preventive Services Task Force. *JAMA,* 316, 2008.

Coffey, S., Cairns, B., & Iung, B. (2016). The modern epidemiology of heart valve. *Heart, 102,* 75–85.

Eckel, R., Jakicic, J., Ard, J., et al. (2014). 2013 AHA/ACC guideline on lifestyle management to reduce cardiovascular risk: A report of the American College of Cardiology American/Heart Association Task Force on Practice Guidelines. *Circulation, 129*(25 Suppl 2), S76–S99.

Erdmann, J., Kessler, T., Munoz Venegas, L., & Schunkert, H. (2018). A decade of genome-wide association studies for coronary artery disease: The challenges ahead. Cardiovascular Research, cvy084, Available: *https://doi-org.ezp.welch.jhmi.edu/10.1093/cvr/cvy084*

Fihn, S. D., Blankenship, J. C., Alexander, K. P., et al. (2014). 2014 ACC/AHA/AATS/PCNA/SCAI/STS focused update of the guideline for the diagnosis and management of patients with stable ischemic heart disease: A report of the American College of Cardiology/American Heart Association Task Force on Practice Cardiovascular Guidelines, and the American Association for Thoracic Surgery, Preventive Cardiovascular Nurses Association, Society for Cardiovascular Angiography and Interventions, and Society of Thoracic Surgeons. *Circulation, 130,* 1749–1767.

Fox, C. S. (2013). Weighty matters: Balancing weight gain with cardiovascular risk among patients with type 1 diabetes mellitus on intensive insulin therapy. *Circulation, 127,* 157–159.

Gara, P. T., Kushner, F. G., Ascheim, D. D., et al. (2013). 2013 ACCF/AHA guideline for the management of ST-elevation myocardial infarction. *Circulation, 127,* 529–555.

Gersh, B. J., Maron, B. J., Bonow, R. O., et al. (2011). ACCF/AHA guideline: 2011 ACCF/AHA guideline for the diagnosis and treatment of hypertrophic cardiomyopathy: A report of the American College of Cardiology Foundation/American Heart Association Task Force on Practice Guidelines. *Circulation, 124,* e783–e831.

Goff, D., Lloyd-Jones, D., D'Agostino, R. Sr., et al. (2014). Assessing cardiovascular risk: Systematic evidence review from the risk assessment work group. *Journal of the American College of Cardiology, 63*(25), 2935–2959.

Haas, N., Giacomo Carere, R., Kretschmar, O., et al. (2018). Early outcomes of percutaneous pulmonary valve implantation using the Edwards SAPIEN XT transcatheter heart valve system. *International Journal of Cardiology,* 250, 86–91.

Hadjiiphilippou, S., & Ray, K. (2018). Lipids and Lipoproteins in Risk Prediction. *Cardiology Clinics, 36*(2), 213–220.

Hoerr, V., Franz, M., Pletz, M. W., et al. (2018). S. aureus endocarditis: Clinical aspects and experimental approaches. International Journal of Medical Microbiology (in press). Available: *https://doi.org/10.1016/j.ijmm.2018.02.004*

Ito, M. K., & Santos, R. D. (2017). PCSK9 inhibition with monoclonal antibodies: Modern management of hypercholesterolemia. *The Journal of Clinical Pharmacology, 57*(1), 7–32.

Levine, G., Bates, E., Bittl, J., et al. (2016). 2016 ACC/AHA guideline focused update on duration of dual antiplatelet therapy in patients with coronary artery disease: A report of the American College of Cardiology/American Heart Association Task Force on Clinical Practice Guidelines: An update of the 2011 ACCF/AHA/SCAI guideline for percutaneous coronary intervention, 2011 ACCF/AHA guideline for coronary artery bypass graft surgery, 2012 ACC/AHA/ACP/AATS/PCNA/SCAI/STS guideline for the diagnosis and management of patients with stable ischemic heart disease, 2013 ACCF/AHA guideline for the management of ST-elevation myocardial infarction, 2014 ACC/AHA guideline for the management of patients with non–ST-elevation acute coronary syndromes, and 2014 ACC/AHA guideline on perioperative cardiovascular evaluation and management of patients undergoing noncardiac surgery. *Circulation, 134,* e123–e155.

McGivery, K., Atkinson, P., Lewis, D., et al. (2018). Emergency department ultrasound for the detection of B-lines in the early diagnosis of acute decompensated heart failure: A systematic review and meta-analysis. Clinical Journal of Emergency Medicine, 1–10. Available: doi:10.1017/cem.2018.27. [Epub ahead of print]

Melis, M., Cupelli, A., Sottosanti, L., et al. (2015). Off-label use of nicardipine as tocolytic and acute pulmonary oedema: A post-marketing analysis of adverse drug reaction reports in EudraVigilance. *Pharmacoepidemiology and Drug Safety,* 24, 1220–1224.

Nadeau-Routhier, C., Marsit, O. & Beaudoin, J. (2017). Current Management of Patients with Severe Aortic Regurgitation. *Current Treatment Options in Cardiovascular Medicine,* 19, 9. Available: *https://doi-org.ezp.welch.jhmi.edu/10.1007/s11936-017-0508-8*

Nehme, Z., Stub, D., Bernard, S., et al. (2016). Effect of supplemental oxygen exposure on myocardial injury in ST-elevation myocardial infarction. *Heart, 2016,* 444–451.

Nishimura, R., Otto, C., Bonow, R., et al. (2017). 2017 AHA/ACC focused update of the 2014 AHA/ACC guideline for the management of patients with valvular heart disease: A report of the American college of Cardiology/American heart association task force on clinical practice guidelines. *Journal of American Medical Association, 70*(2), 252–289.

Nunes, P. M., Guimaraes, M., Pinto, M. P., et al. (2018). Outcomes of infective endocarditis in the current era: Early predictors of a poor prognosis. *International Journal of Infectious Diseases,* 68, 102–107.

O'Gara, P. T., Kushner, F. G., Ascheim, D. D., et al. (2013). 2013 ACCF/AHA guideline for the management of ST-elevation myocardial infarction: A report of the American College of Cardiology Foundation/American Heart Association Task Force on Practice Guidelines. *Journal of the American College of Cardiology, 61*(4), 78–140.

Pac-Kozuchowska, E., Krawiec, P., and Grywalska, E. (2018). Selected risk factors for atherosclerosis in children and their parents with positive family history of premature cardiovascular diseases: a prospective study. *BMC Pediatrics, 18*(1), 1. Available: *https://doi-org.ezp.welch.jhmi.edu/10.1186/s12887-018-1102-2*

Palazzuoli, A., Ruocco, G., Beltrami, M., et al. (2018). Combined use of lung ultrasound, B-type natriuretic peptide, and echocardiography for outcome prediction in patients with acute HFrEF and HFpEF. *Clinical Research in Cardiology.* Available: *https://doi.org/10.1007/s00392-018-1221-7.* [Epub ahead of print]

Picano, E., & Scali, M. C. (2017). The lung water cascade in heart failure. *Echocardiography*, 34, 1503–1507.

Reed, G. W., Rossi, J. E., Cannon, C. P. (2016). Myocardial infarction. *The Lancet*, 389(10065), 197–210.

Silverman, M. G., Ference, B. A., Im, K., et al. (2016). Association between lowering LDL-C and cardiovascular risk reduction among different therapeutic interventions: A systematic review and meta-analysis. *JAMA*, 316, 1289.

Smith, J., Negrelli, J., Manek, M., et al. (2015). Diagnosis and management of acute coronary syndrome: An evidence-based update. *Journal of the American Board of Family Medicine*, 28(2), 283–293.

Staniute, M., Brozaitiene, J., Bunevicius, R. (2013). Effects of social support and stressful life events on health-related quality of life in coronary artery disease. *Journal of Cardiovascular Nursing*, 28(1), 83–89.

Stone, N. J., Robinson, J. G., Lichtenstein, A. H., et al. (2014). 2013 ACC/AHA guideline on the treatment of blood cholesterol to reduce atherosclerotic cardiovascular risk in adults: A report of the American College of Cardiology/American Heart Association Task Force on Practice Guidelines. *Journal of American College of Cardiology*, 63(25), 2889–2934.

Suzuki, T., Mawatari, M., Iizuka, T., et al. (2017). An Ineffective Differential Diagnosis of Infective Endocarditis and Rheumatic Heart Disease after Streptococcal Skin and Soft Tissue Infection. *Intern Med*, 56(17), 2361–2365.

Thornhill, M. H., Dayer, M., Lockhart, P. B., et al. (2016). Guidelines on prophylaxis to prevent infective endocarditis. *British Dental Journal*, 220(2), 51–56.

Tricoci, P., Lokhnygina, Y., Berdan, L. G., et al. (2016). ACC/AHA/SCAI focused update on primary percutaneous coronary intervention for patients with ST-elevation myocardial infarction : An update of the 2011 ACCF/AHA/SCAI guideline for percutaneous coronary intervention and the 2013 ACCF/AHA guideline for the management of ST-elevation myocardial infarction: A report of the American College of Cardiology/American Heart Association Task Force on Clinical Practice Guidelines and the Society for Cardiovascular Angiography and Interventions. *Journal of the American College of Cardiology*, 67(10).

Vallejo-Vaz, A.J., Robertson, M., Catapano, A.L., et al. (2017). Low-density lipoprotein cholesterol lowering for the primary prevention of cardiovascular disease among men with primary elevations of low-density lipoprotein cholesterol levels of 190 mg/dL or above: Analyses from the WOSCOPS (West of Scotland Coronary Prevention Study) 5-year randomized trial and 20-year observational follow-up. *Circulation*, 136, 1878.

Wakefield, B. J., Boren, S. A., Groves, P. S., et al. (2013). Heart failure care management programs: A review of study interventions and meta-analysis of outcomes. *Journal of Cardiovascular Nursing*, 28(1), 8–19.

Wessler, J., Stant, J., Duru, S., et al. (2015). Updates to the ACCF/AHA and ESC STEMI and NSTEMI Guidelines: Putting guidelines into clinical practice. *The American Journal of Cardiology*, 115(5s), 24a–28a.

Wang, Y., Shen, Z., Lu, X., et al. (2018). Sensitivity and specificity of ultrasound for the diagnosis of acute pulmonary edema: a systematic review and meta-analysis. *Medical Ultrasonography*, 20(1), 32–36.

Yancy, C. W., Jessup, M., Bozkurt, B., et al. (2016). 2016 ACC/AHA/HFSA focused update on new pharmacological therapy for heart failure: An update of the 2013 ACCF/AHA guideline for the management of heart failure: A report of the American College of Cardiology/American Heart Association Task Force on Clinical Practice Guidelines and the Society for Cardiovascular Angiography and Interventions. *American Journal of Cardiology*, 68(13).

Yanagawa, B., Butany, J., & Verma, S. (2016). Update on rheumatic heart disease. *Current Opinion in Cardiology*, 31(2), 162–168.

Yu, H., Lim, S., Kim, M., et al. (2018). Urine Cotinine level with smoking history predicts a risk of coronary artery calcification. *Environmental Toxicology and Pharmacology*, 59, 146–151.

14
Vascular Disorders

GENERAL PROCEDURES AND TREATMENT MODALITIES

See additional online content: Procedure Guidelines 14-1

Anticoagulant Therapy

EVIDENCE BASE Guyatt, G., Akl, E., Crowther, M., et al. (2012). Executive summary: Antithrombotic therapy and prevention of thrombosis, 9th ed: American College of Chest Physicians Evidence-Based Clinical Practice Guidelines. *Chest, 141*(2 Suppl), 7S–47S.

Anticoagulant therapy is the administration of medications to achieve the following:

- Disrupt the blood's natural clotting mechanism when there is a risk of pathologic clotting.
- Prevent formation of a thrombus in immobile and/or postoperative patients.
- Intercept the extension of a thrombus once it has formed.
- Agents are used in the acute treatment of thromboembolic disorders, for long-term prevention of recurrent thromboembolism, or for short-term prevention following surgery for some orthopedic conditions.

Types of anticoagulants include Coumadin derivatives, such as warfarin given orally; unfractionated heparin (UFH) given subcutaneously (SC) or intravenously (IV); Coumadin or low molecular weight heparin (LMWH) given SC, particularly dalteparin and enoxaparin; factor Xa inhibitors, particularly fondaparinux given SC and rivaroxaban, apixaban, edoxaban given orally; direct thrombin inhibitors, such as dabigatran given orally, and argatroban, bivalirudin, or hirudin given through IV administration.

NURSING ALERT Anticoagulants may be contraindicated or used with extreme caution in conditions that may lead to bleeding, in patients who may have poor follow-up, and in patients with hepatic and renal insufficiency.

Anticoagulant Indications

1. LMWH (dalteparin, enoxaparin) may be given prophylactically pre- and postoperatively in specific patient populations with high-risk procedures, such as active malignancy with an abdominal surgery; following some orthopedic surgical procedures such as total hip replacement, knee replacement, or arthroscopic procedures; and for long surgical procedures or periods of immobility in high-risk patients. They are also used for the acute treatment of deep vein thrombosis (DVT) (often while warfarin is being started). Dalteparin is indicated for prevention of unstable angina or non-Q-wave infarction. The benefits over heparin include:
   a. Steady bioavailability.
   b. Longer half-life.
   c. Less platelet inhibition (than UFH).
   d. More mobility for the patient (it may be given at home).
   e. Does not cause paradoxical thrombotic events.
2. Factor Xa inhibitor fondaparinux is given prophylactically before and after some orthopedic procedures or abdominal surgery in high-risk patients and for the acute treatment of DVT (with warfarin). Edoxaban, rivaroxaban, and apixaban are indicated for treatment of acute DVT and pulmonary embolus, for prevention of DVT after hip and knee surgery, and for reducing risk of stroke in patients with nonvalvular atrial fibrillation.
3. Warfarin is used following DVT and pulmonary emboli and for long-term prophylaxis, such as prevention of thromboembolic complications of atrial fibrillation, cardiac valve replacement, or recurrent myocardial infarctions (MIs) and lower-extremity arterial bypass surgeries.
4. Direct thrombin inhibitors are the newest class of anticoagulant.
   a. Dabigatran is indicated for prevention of thromboembolic complications/stroke in patients with nonvalvular atrial fibrillation.
   b. Argatroban, bivalirudin, and hirudin are administered via IV line, so they are used on a shorter-term basis. They are indicated for patients who have a history of heparin-induced thrombocytopenia (HIT).

317

5. Perioperative considerations include discontinuing oral anticoagulants.
   a. IV UFH may be prescribed preoperatively because its half-life is short; thus, the anticoagulant effects are reversed within 30 minutes to 1 hour after discontinuation.
   b. LMWH may be given preoperatively several hours before surgery and 4 to 8 hours after surgery.
   c. It is recommended that the initial dose of fondaparinux be given 6 to 8 hours following surgery.
   d. Rivaroxaban and apixaban may be given as soon as postoperative hemostasis occurs.

 DRUG ALERT Oral anticoagulants should be discontinued preoperatively according to manufacturer guidelines to reduce the risk of hemorrhage in the intraoperative phase.

Nursing and Patient Care Considerations

Administering Unfractionated Heparin
1. Obtain baseline coagulation and hematologic studies before initiating anticoagulation therapy to ensure that the patient does not have an underlying bleeding or clotting disorder.
2. Weigh patient before initiating therapy because UFH, as well as some forms of LMWH, are calculated based on weight.
3. Administer subcutaneously into lower abdomen.
4. For IV administration, begin continuous infusion.
   a. Use continuous infusion pump.
   b. Assess frequently to make sure the pump is functioning properly, that there are no kinks or leaks in IV tubing, and that the IV site is without signs or symptoms of infiltration.
5. Double-check concentration and dose of heparin, especially when giving high dosages.
6. Be aware that heparin may be continued for 4 to 5 days after oral anticoagulant is initiated due to the delayed onset of therapeutic effectiveness with some oral anticoagulants.

 NURSING ALERT Active life-threatening bleeding is a contraindication to antithrombotic therapy. The decision for treatment in each patient should be weighed against the individual risk of bleeding.

Administering Other Anticoagulants
1. Administer low molecular weight heparin SC; dosage varies with drug and its intended purpose.
   a. Usually begun 1 to 24 hours before surgery or once or twice daily after surgery, limited to 7 to 14 days.
   b. If warfarin is started, continue LMWH until warfarin becomes therapeutic.
2. Administer fondaparinux once daily; dosage depends on whether it is prophylactic or treatment for thrombosis.
   a. Must be continued for at least 5 days or until warfarin level is therapeutic. May be given for longer following orthopedic procedures.
   b. Provided in preloaded syringes. (*Note:* Do not expel the air bubble from the syringe. Must not be given intramuscularly.)
3. Give rivaroxaban orally at the same time every day, such as with the evening meal.
   a. Obtain a baseline creatinine level, as dosage may be decreased in patients with renal insufficiency.

b. Usually given for 35 days post hip replacement; 12 days post knee replacement.
c. Give twice daily first 21 days then once daily in treatment of acute PE or DVT.
4. Give warfarin orally at the same time every day, usually in the afternoon or at dinnertime.
   a. Therapeutic range is monitored by international normalized ratio (INR), usually drawn at least 16 hours after last dose.
   b. Monitor frequently until stable, with any medication changes, and then every 12 weeks when consistently stable INR.
5. Give dabigatran orally twice daily. Instruct patient to swallow capsules whole; do not open, crush, or chew.
6. Give apixaban orally twice daily.
   a. Decrease dose in patients with at least two of the following: 80 years or older, weight less than 60 kg, or Cr greater than 1.5.
   b. For DVT prophylaxis in hip replacement 2.5 mg orally twice daily for 35 days.
   c. For DVT prophylaxis in knee replacement 2.5 mg orally twice daily for 12 days.
   d. For DVT/PE treatment start 10 mg orally twice daily for 7 days and then reduce to 5 mg dose.

 DRUG ALERT Be aware that dabigatran has a 60-day shelf life.

Monitoring Clotting Profiles
1. Partial thromboplastin time (PTT) is the coagulation test used to monitor the anticoagulation effects of UFH.
   a. The patient's PTT should be 2 to 2½ times the control.
   b. Obtain PTT levels daily or as ordered. Heparin dose will be adjusted to achieve the desired level of anticoagulation.
2. Prothrombin time (PT) and INR are the coagulation tests used to monitor the anticoagulation effects of warfarin.
   a. The patient's INR should be 2 to 3½ times the control. *Note:* The desired levels of INR are determined by protocol for condition and risk factors being followed or by the health care provider.
   b. Obtain PT/INR levels daily or as ordered. Warfarin dose will be adjusted to achieve the desired level of anticoagulation.
3. Other laboratory studies to monitor as ordered or if bleeding is suspected:
   a. Platelet count—HIT may occur, particularly with UFH; 50% decrease in platelet count causing local bleeding or systemic reaction with IV.
   b. Hemoglobin and hematocrit—baseline and periodically.
   c. Fibrinogen—if abnormal bleeding while on UFH.
4. Be aware of drug–drug (including over-the-counter [OTC] and herbal supplements) and food–drug interactions that may alter the effects of warfarin. This occurs because of alterations in the clearance of the drug or the rate of intestinal absorption. The patient is encouraged to eat a consistent diet and to notify health care provider of any new drugs, so that INR can be tested more frequently, if indicated. Consult a pharmacist, drug reference book, or online list for information on specific foods and drugs.
5. No monitoring of PTT or other coagulation tests is required for LMWH, factor Xa inhibitors, or direct thrombin inhibitors; however, PTT may be monitored for LMWH therapy in patients with renal disease and patients weighing less than 110.2 pound (50 kg) or more than 176.4 pound (80 kg).

DRUG ALERT Drug and food interactions can alter the effect of some anticoagulants. A change in intake should prompt more frequent monitoring and, possibly, a change in dose.

Preventing Bleeding

1. Follow precautions to prevent bleeding.
   a. Handle patient carefully while turning and positioning.
   b. Maintain pressure on IV and venipuncture sites for at least 5 minutes. Apply ice if patient is prone to bleeding.
   c. Assist with ambulation and keep walkways/hallways free from clutter to prevent falls.
2. Observe carefully for any possible signs of bleeding and report immediately so that anticoagulant dosage may be reviewed and altered, if necessary:
   a. Hematuria—frank blood in urine or microhematuria as detected on the test strip.
   b. Melena—assess for dark/tarry stools; use test cards for occult blood.
   c. Hemoptysis—assess for frank blood in emesis; use test cards for occult blood.
   d. Bleeding gums—note any pink saliva or frank bleeding with dental hygiene.
   e. Epistaxis—frequent/persistent nosebleeds.
   f. Bruising/hematomas—inspect skin carefully.
3. Have on hand the antidotes to reverse anticoagulants being used (see Table 14-1, page 320).
   a. Heparin—protamine sulfate, by IV injection.
   b. Warfarin—phytonadione (vitamin K_1, AquaMEPHYTON); oral or IV and dose is dependent on the INR level and the degree or risk of patient bleeding
   c. Dabigatran—idarucizumab by IV injection

 DRUG ALERT When epidural anesthesia or spinal puncture is employed, anticoagulants increase the risk of epidural or spinal hematoma, which may result in paralysis. Monitor these patients closely for sensory and motor dysfunction.

 DRUG ALERT Vitamin K ingestion can lead to warfarin resistance and subsequently increased risk of thromboembolism.

 NURSING ALERT There is a risk of bleeding in any patient receiving anticoagulants. Risk of bleeding is patient and treatment dependent. Recent updates for labeling on warfarin include genetic variations that may produce resistance to drug therapeutic levels. Advanced age and hypertension add an increased risk for intracerebral hemorrhage.

Patient Education and Health Maintenance

1. Instruct patient about taking anticoagulants.
   a. Follow instructions carefully and take medications exactly as prescribed; if a dose is missed, do NOT double up dose; rather, notify the health care provider.
   b. Notify all health care providers, including dentist, that you are taking anticoagulants.
   c. Avoid foods that may alter the effects of anticoagulants or, if used, should be used in the same quantity every day: green, leafy vegetables, fish, liver, green tea, and tomatoes.
   d. Take medications at the same time each day and do not stop taking them unless directed by health care provider, even if symptoms of thrombus/embolus are not present.
   e. Wear a medical identification bracelet or carry a card indicating that you are taking anticoagulants; include name, address, and telephone number of health care provider.
2. Advise the patient to notify the health care provider of the following:
   a. All medications both prescribed and OTC (including vitamins and herbal supplements) that patient is currently taking.
   b. Accidents, infections, excessive diarrhea, and other significant illnesses that may affect blood clotting.
   c. Scheduled invasive procedures by other health care providers, including routine dental examinations and other dental procedures or cardiac catheterizations. If surgical care by another health care provider or dentist is needed, inform other provider that anticoagulants are being taken.
3. Advise the patient to avoid:
   a. Taking any other medications without first checking with health care provider, particularly:
      i. Vitamins, especially if they contain vitamin K.
      ii. Herbal supplements.
      iii. Aspirin or nonsteroidal anti-inflammatory drugs (NSAIDs).
      iv. Mineral oil.
      v. Cold medicines, antibiotics.
      vi. Oral contraceptives and hormones.
      vii. Antireflux medicines.
      viii. Oral antifungals.
   b. Excessive use of alcohol; may affect clotting ability; check on acceptable limits for social drinking.
   c. Participation in activities in which there is high risk of injury.
   d. Foods that may cause diarrhea or upset stomach; rapid changes in diet.
   e. Shaving with a sharp razor.
4. Instruct the patient to be alert for these warning signs:
   a. Excessive bleeding that does not stop quickly (such as following shaving, a small cut, tooth brushing with gum injury, nosebleed).
   b. Excessive menstrual bleeding.
   c. Skin discoloration or bruises that appear suddenly—particularly on the fingers and toes or deep purple spots anywhere on the body ("blue toe syndrome").
   d. Black or bloody stools; for questionable stool discoloration, test for occult blood.
   e. Blood in urine.
   f. Faintness, dizziness, or unusual weakness.
5. Stress the importance of close follow-up and compliance with periodic laboratory work for blood clotting profiles, need to notify health care provider if unable to keep scheduled appointments, and contact provider with questions about dosage.

Thrombolytic Therapy

Thrombolytic therapy is the administration of thrombolytic agents to dissolve any formed thrombus and to inhibit the body's hemostatic function. Thrombolytic agents are available for parenteral use only. Commonly used thrombolytics include streptokinase, tissue plasminogen activator, and urokinase.

Table 14-1 Guide to Anticoagulants

DRUG	CONTRAINDICATIONS	MONITORING	ANTIDOTE	OTHER CONSIDERATIONS
Unfractionated heparin (UFH)	• Allergy • Acute major bleeding • Thrombolytic therapy given within past 24 hr in stroke victim • HIT most frequently develops 1–2 wk after starting therapy	• Get baseline complete blood count, platelet count, prothrombin time/INR, and creatinine before starting therapy; liver function tests and albumin with suspected liver disease • Daily partial thromboplastin time or heparin assay • Monitor platelet count every other day (for HIT).	• Protamine sulfate IV over 10 min • Risk for anaphylaxis is 1%	• Generally safe in pregnancy unless patient has mechanical heart valve. • Safe in the breastfeeding patient. • Monitor for HIT: reaction at injection site, systemic reaction after bolus injection, 50% decrease in platelets
Low molecular weight heparins (LMWH)	• Allergy • Acute major bleeding • Thrombolytic therapy given within past 24 hr in stroke victim • HIT • Renal failure	• Same baseline as UFH • Monitor platelet count every 2–3 d if also receiving UFH	• No agent for complete reversal • Protamine sulfate provides for 60%–75% reversal.	• Generally safe in pregnancy unless patient has mechanical heart valve. • Generally safe in the breastfeeding patient • Monitor for HIT
Factor Xa inhibitors	• Allergy • Acute major bleeding • Thrombolytic therapy given within past 24 hr in stroke victim • Renal failure	• Same baseline as UFH • No routine monitoring of PTT or INR • Fondaparinux: monitor heparin assay regularly in those with renal insufficiency, body weight <50 kg, or those who are obese.	• No antidote for apixaban, edoxaban • Idarucizumab is the reversal agent for dabigatran; 5 g dose (2–50 mL vials of 2.5 g) given IV • Fondaparinux: possible partial reversal with recombinant factor VIIa. • Rivaroxaban: activated charcoal to reduce absorption in overdose	• Safety unknown in the pregnant or breastfeeding patient. • Use cautiously in bacterial endocarditis, uncontrolled hypertension, and other conditions. • Increased risk of bleeding in renal or hepatic impairment. • Risk of spinal or epidural hematoma with spinal procedures
Warfarin sodium	• Allergy • Hemorrhage • Pregnancy	• Same baseline as UFH • Monitor INR daily to every few days until stable and then monthly (best time is at least 16 hr after last dose). • If starting medication that can affect warfarin, check INR in 3–4 d.	• Vitamin K orally or IV over 60 min. • May lead to warfarin resistance and thromboembolism • Transfusion of fresh frozen plasma may be given.	• Only small amount secreted in breast milk • Hold for 4 d prior to surgery. • Increased risk of thromboembolism if INR < 1.7; increased risk of bleeding if INR > 4.0. • Purple toe syndrome may occur 3–10 wk after starting therapy. • Numerous drug and food interactions
Direct thrombin inhibitors	• Allergy • Active bleeding	• Assess baseline renal function, and annually if creatinine clearance <50 mL/min or age >75 yr	• No known antidote • About 60% of drug may be cleared with dialysis over 3–4 hr • Transfusion of fresh frozen plasma or packed red cells may be given.	• Safety not known in pregnancy or breastfeeding • Risk of bleeding increases with age • Consult medication reference for drug interactions.

Thrombolytic therapy is contraindicated in conditions that may lead to bleeding and should be given only in a controlled setting, such as a cardiac catheterization laboratory, endovascular OR, or an intensive care unit (ICU). Thrombolytic therapy for deep vein or peripheral arterial thrombosis, however, may be given on stepdown units or medical–surgical floors in some facilities with appropriate staff education.

Clinical Indications

1. Acute MI from coronary thrombosis
2. Pulmonary embolus
3. Acute occlusion of peripheral arteries/prosthetic grafts
4. Iliofemoral DVT

Nursing and Patient Care Considerations

1. Monitor clotting profiles every 2 to 4 hours; these are essential before the initiation of treatment to disclose any bleeding tendencies and to serve as a baseline for assessment of drug efficacy. UFH will generally be given parenterally at the same time.
2. Observe for signs of bleeding and report immediately.
   a. Have typed and crossmatched blood on hold in case bleeding is severe.
   b. Have aminocaproic acid on hand to treat bleeding.
3. Monitor for allergic reaction. A small number of patients (less than 5%) may experience an allergic reaction.
   a. Observe patient for onset of a new rash, fever, and chills.
   b. Report any suspected allergic reaction immediately.
   c. Administer corticosteroids, if ordered, to treat reaction.
4. Monitor electrocardiogram (ECG) for dysrhythmias after reperfusion if thrombolytic therapy is being used for coronary thrombus.
5. Frequently assess color, warmth, and sensation of extremity if therapy is being used for peripheral arterial occlusion.
6. Move patient as little as possible.
7. Minimize phlebotomy.
8. Observe for changes in level of consciousness or other signs of intracranial bleeding.

Care of the Patient Undergoing Vascular Surgery

Vascular surgery may involve operations of the arteries, veins, or lymphatic system. Surgery may be performed on an urgent basis, as in *embolectomy* for acute arterial embolism, or electively for *vein ligation and stripping* for varicose veins after conservative management fails. Other vascular procedures include *thrombectomy* and *vena cava filter insertion* for venous problems and *arterial bypass grafting* (aortoiliac, aortofemoral, femoral–femoral, femoropopliteal, and femoral–distal), *endarterectomy, endovascular grafting*, and *percutaneous transluminal angioplasty (PTA)* for arterial problems with or without placement of an intraluminal stent.

Preoperative Management

1. Additional health conditions, such as heart disease, hypertension, diabetes mellitus, and chronic lung disease, are fully evaluated, and management is adjusted to decrease operative risks.
2. Chronic skin and tissue changes are assessed preoperatively, and impairment is minimized through protection of the affected parts, treatment with antibiotics, and proper positioning to enhance circulation (elevated for venous and lymphatic problems, level or slightly dependent for arterial problems).
3. Nutritional status is assessed and improved preoperatively to aid in wound healing postoperatively.
4. Risk factors for vascular disease, such as smoking, obesity, and sedentary lifestyle, are reviewed, and patient teaching is initiated to prevent recurrence or progression of vascular disorder.
5. The patient is prepared emotionally and physically for surgery, with teaching focusing on positioning in bed; expected exercises and activity to be followed postoperatively; frequent checking of circulation and wound; and prevention of complications, such as bleeding, infection, and neurovascular compromise.

Postoperative Management

1. Bed rest may be maintained for 24 hours in some cases to reduce swelling and the risk of bleeding.
2. If surgery involved revascularization, peripheral pulses are assessed distal from operative site to ensure adequate tissue perfusion. (Use portable Doppler, if necessary.)
3. If surgery involved use of bypass graft, the graft site is protected and assessed for patency as well.
4. Extremity is positioned with the popliteal space supported to prevent trauma and promote circulation.
5. Anticoagulation may be continued, but it increases chance of bleeding following surgery.
6. Hydration, nutrition, and oxygenation are promoted to ensure wound healing.
7. Surgical incisions are assessed for redness, drainage, and approximation and may be covered with dry dressings, and possible incisional wound vacuum devices.
8. Endovascular and PTA procedures are less invasive, but incision site of catheter is carefully monitored for bleeding and peripheral circulation is assessed.
9. Breathing exercises using an incentive spirometer are performed every 2 hours while patient is awake to prevent postoperative pulmonary complications if the patient is immobilized.

Nursing Diagnoses

- Ineffective Peripheral Tissue Perfusion related to underlying vascular disorder, postoperative swelling.
- Risk for Infection related to surgical incision and impaired circulation.
- Acute Pain related to surgical incision and swelling.
- Impaired Physical Mobility related to pain and imposed restrictions.

Nursing Interventions

Promoting Tissue Perfusion

1. Maintain dressing or compression bandages, as directed.
2. Monitor for bleeding through dressing—reinforce and notify surgeon, as indicated.
3. Monitor for hematoma formation beneath skin—increased pain and swelling. Apply pressure and notify surgeon.
4. Measure vital signs frequently for tachycardia and hypotension, which may indicate hemorrhage.

5. Perform frequent neurovascular checks to involved extremity. Check warmth, color, capillary refill, sensation, movement, and pulses; compare with other side.
6. Position as directed—usually legs elevated and fully supported.

Preventing Infection

1. Maintain IV infusion or heparin lock for antibiotic administration, as ordered, and assess daily for signs of infiltration and infection.
2. Check incision site for drainage, warmth, and erythema, which indicate infection.
3. Change incision dressing, as ordered and as needed, for drainage or soiling.
4. Monitor temperature for elevation.
5. Monitor hematologic profiles for elevation in white blood cell (WBC) count.

Relieving Pain

1. Assess pain level and administer analgesic as ordered.
2. If patient-controlled anesthesia is being used, instruct patient on use and make sure the pump is functioning properly.
3. Position for comfort, using pillows for support.
4. Watch for adverse effects of opioids, such as hypotension, respiratory depression, nausea and vomiting, and constipation.
5. Administer pain medication before activity.
6. Instruct patient in alternative coping methods such as visualization.

Minimizing Immobility

1. Encourage isometric and range-of-motion (ROM) exercises while on bed rest.
   a. Exercise affected extremity by pushing foot into footboard, making a fist, or simply contracting muscles without movement if approved by surgeon.
   b. Perform full ROM of other extremities.
2. Encourage ambulation as soon as allowed.
   a. Avoid dangling legs because of possible compression against the back of bed or chair.
   b. Avoid long periods of sitting or standing.
   c. Encourage short periods of walking every 2 hours.

Patient Education and Health Maintenance

1. Instruct patient and significant other in care of incision and wound at home. Make sure that patient has proper resources available.
2. Instruct patient about wearing elastic stockings or applying ace wrap, if ordered. Have patient perform return demonstration.
3. Instruct patient and significant other in signs of infection, graft failure, or worsening circulatory problem that should be reported.
4. Refer patient to vascular rehabilitation (if available), physical therapy, and occupational therapy as indicated.
5. Refer for additional support for risk factor modification, such as supervised weight loss programs, nutritional counseling, and smoking cessation.
6. Instruct patient to avoid restrictive clothing (including socks, hose, shoes), especially over areas of revascularization.
7. Instruct patient to inspect feet (using a mirror, if necessary), including plantar aspect and between toes, daily and to inspect shoes for foreign objects, such as small stones, before putting them on.
8. Instruct patient to wear thick socks and well-fitting shoes with wide toe box to avoid development of breakdown/ulceration on pressure points. Instruct patient not to wear sandals.
9. Instruct patient never to walk barefoot.
10. Review any medications, especially anticoagulants.
11. Make sure that the patient knows when and where to follow up.

Evaluation: Expected Outcomes

- Affected extremity with good color, capillary refill, and pulses; warm and sensitive to touch; moving adequately.
- Incision site is well approximated and without signs and symptoms of infection.
- Reports adequate pain control on current regimen.
- Ambulates for 10 minutes every 2 hours without difficulty or shows signs of progressing independence with the assistance of physical or occupational therapy.

CONDITIONS OF VEINS

See additional online content: Procedure Guidelines 14-2, 14-3

Venous Thrombus

 EVIDENCE BASE Dupras, D., Bluhm, J., Felty, C., et al. (2013). Institute for Clinical Systems Improvement. *Venous thromboembolism diagnosis and treatment.* Available: www.icsi.org/guidelines__more/catalog_guidelines_and_more/catalog_guidelines/catalog_cardiovascular_guidelines/vte_treatment/

See Table 14-2.

There are several types of venous thrombosis:

Phlebitis is an inflammation in the wall of a vein. The term is used clinically to indicate a superficial and localized condition that can be treated with application of heat.

Superficial thrombophlebitis is a condition in which a clot forms in a vein secondary to phlebitis or because of partial obstruction of the vein. It is more commonly seen in the greater or lesser saphenous veins of the lower extremities but may also be seen in the upper extremities, most commonly at IV sites.

Phlebothrombosis is the formation of a thrombus or thrombi in a vein; in general, the clotting is related to (1) stasis, (2) abnormality of the walls of the vein, and (3) abnormality of the

Table 14-2	Comparison of Arterial and Venous Obstruction	
FACTOR	**ARTERIAL OBSTRUCTION**	**VENOUS OBSTRUCTION**
Onset	May be sudden	Gradual
Color	Pale later—mottled, cyanotic	Slightly cyanotic rubescent
Skin temperature	Cold	Warm
Leg size	May be reduced	Enlarged
Leg hair and nails	Decreased hair; thick, brittle nails	No change
Edema	None to mild	Typically calf to foot
Sensation	Sensory changes	Normal sensation
Arterial pulses	Pulse deficit	Normal
Effect of elevating leg	Condition worsens	Slight improvement

clotting mechanism. Superficial or deep veins may be affected; however, deep veins of the lower extremities are most commonly involved.

DVT is thrombosis of deep rather than superficial veins. Two serious complications are pulmonary embolism and postphlebitic syndrome.

Note: Although phlebothrombosis and DVT do not necessarily represent identical pathologies, for clinical purposes, they are used interchangeably when discussing the same process.

Pathophysiology and Etiology

General Points
1. Three antecedent factors are believed to play a significant role in the development of venous thromboses: (1) stasis of blood, (2) injury to the vessel wall, and (3) altered blood coagulation (Virchow triad). Thrombosis does not occur with stasis alone.
2. Usually two of the three factors occur before thrombosis develops.

Thrombosis-Related Situations
1. Venous stasis—following operations, childbirth, or bed rest for any prolonged illness.
2. Prolonged sitting or as a complication of varicose veins.
3. Injury (bruise) to a vein; may result from direct trauma or internal trauma such as from IV catheters, infusion of medications, and/or infiltration of medications.
4. Extension of an infection of tissues surrounding the vessel.
5. Continuous pressure of a tumor, aneurysm, or excessive weight gain in pregnancy.
6. Unusual activity in a person who has been sedentary (particularly heavy lifting or prolonged holding of heavy objects) increases risk of upper-extremity thromboses.
7. Hypercoagulability associated with malignant disease and blood dyscrasias.

High-Risk Factors
1. Malignancy.
2. Previous venous insufficiency.
3. Conditions causing prolonged bed rest—MI, heart failure, sepsis, traction, end-stage cancer, and human immunodeficiency virus/acquired immunodeficiency syndrome.
4. Leg trauma—fractures, cast, joint replacements.
5. General surgery—over age 40.
6. Obesity, smoking.
7. Inherited coagulopathy (eg, antithrombin III deficiency, protein C&S deficiency, factor V Leiden thrombophilia, and others).

Clinical Manifestations

Clinical features vary with site and length of affected vein.
1. DVT may occur asymptomatically or may produce severe pain, fevers, chills, malaise, and swelling and cyanosis of affected arm or leg. The chief symptom is unilateral limb edema in which the onset is sudden.
2. Superficial thrombophlebitis produces visible and palpable signs, such as heat, pain, swelling, erythema, tenderness, and induration, along the length of the affected vein.
3. Extensive vein involvement may cause lymphadenitis or arterial compromise if the swelling is extensive enough.

Diagnostic Evaluation

1. Venous duplex/color duplex ultrasound—this commonly done, noninvasive test allows for visualization of the thrombus, including any free-floating or unstable thrombi that may cause emboli. It is to detect thrombi of the upper and lower extremities.
2. Impedance plethysmography—a noninvasive measurement of changes in calf volume corresponding to changes in blood volume brought about by temporary venous occlusion with a high-pneumatic cuff. Electrodes measure electrical impedance as cuff is deflated. Slow decrease in impedance indicates diminished blood flow associated with thrombus.
3. Venography—IV injection of a radiocontrast agent. The vascular tree is visualized and obstruction is identified.
4. Intravascular ultrasound (IVUS)—a catheter-based intervention for VTE, 360-degree ultrasound imaging of a vein.
5. Coagulation profiles—PTT, PT/INR, circulating fibrin, monomer complexes, fibrinopeptide A, serum fibrin, D-dimer, proteins C and S, antithrombin III levels, factor V Leiden, and prothrombin gene mutation. Detect intravascular coagulation or coagulopathies.

Management

Goals of management are to prevent propagation of the thrombus, prevent recurrent thrombus formation, prevent pulmonary emboli, and limit venous valvular damage.

Anticoagulation
For documented cases of DVT to prevent embolization.
1. UFH may be given IV administration initially, followed by 3 to 6 months of oral anticoagulant therapy.
2. Oral anticoagulants, rivaroxaban and apixaban, may also be initiated for acute treatment; no IV medication dosing is needed. Dabigatran requires parental anticoagulation for 5 to 10 days prior to oral dosing.
3. LMWH is safely given in isolated DVT and/or pulmonary embolism; when the patient is taught the proper technique, it may be safely used at home. It is followed by 3 to 6 months of oral anticoagulation.
4. Dabigatran, rivaroxaban, and apixaban may be given as surgical prophylaxis in elective hip or knee surgery.
5. UFH and LMWH may also be given SC as prophylaxis for the prevention of DVT, especially in postoperative and immobile patients.
6. Fondaparinux may be used for treatment and is given SC. It is beneficial for patients with sensitivity to heparins or HIT.

Thrombolytic Therapy
1. May be used in life- or limb-threatening situations.
2. Most effective in dissolving existing clots within the first 24 hours of thromboembolic event and may be considered up to 14 days.
3. Ultrasound-assisted delivery of thrombolytic works faster and with less risk of bleeding than regular infusion.

Nonpharmacologic Therapies
For superficial thrombophlebitis and as an adjunct to anticoagulation with DVT.
1. Ambulation is encouraged unless there is mobile thrombus in a proximal deep vein
2. Elevation of effected extremity: at least 10 to 20 degrees above the level of the heart to enhance venous return and decrease swelling (see Figure 14-1).
   a. The popliteal space should be supported but not constricted.
   b. If the upper extremity is affected, a sling or stockinette attached to an IV pole may be used.

Figure 14-1. Elevation of entire legs above the level of the heart using a foam wedge.

3. Compression: promotes venous return and reduces swelling
   a. Electrically or pneumatically controlled stockings, boots, or sleeve.
   b. Gradient compression stockings or garments after the acute phase to prevent postphlebitic syndrome or to prevent DVT during periods of immobility for high-risk patients. Level of compression ordered according to condition and severity.
      i. 8 to 15 mm Hg (light)—tired, achy legs; mild fatigue; prevention.
      ii. 15 to 20 mm Hg (therapeutic)—spider veins, minor swelling, aching, pregnancy.
      iii. 20 to 30 mm Hg (medical grade)—fatigue, low-grade varicosities, postsclerotherapy.
      iv. 30 to 40 mm Hg (medical grade)—heaviness, fatigue, postsurgery/sclerotherapy, thrombosis, complications of varicose veins, postphlebitic syndrome, treatment of edema, venous ulcers, varices with pregnancy, stasis dermatitis, and lymphedema.
      v. 40 to 50 mm Hg (medical grade)—severe edema for above causes, severe chronic venous insufficiency.
4. Dry heat
   a. Warm water bottles, heating pad.
   b. Ultrasound (acoustic vibration with frequencies beyond human ear perception).
5. Moist heat
   a. Hydrotherapy.
   b. Whirlpool bath.
   c. Warm compresses.

Surgery

1. Placement of a filter into the inferior vena cava to prevent fatal pulmonary embolism in a patient who cannot tolerate prolonged anticoagulant therapy or who has recurrent emboli in the presence of adequate anticoagulation.
2. Thrombectomy may be necessary for severely compromised venous drainage of the extremity.
3. Endovascular thrombolysis with direct catheter infused lytic therapy to the affected limb
4. See page 321 for surgical care.

Complications

1. Pulmonary embolism.
2. Postphlebitic syndrome.

Nursing Assessment

1. Obtain history of risk factors for thrombophlebitis.
2. Note symmetry or asymmetry of legs. Measure and record leg circumferences daily. Acute, unilateral edema may be first sign of a DVT.

3. Observe for evidence of venous distention or edema, puffiness, stretched skin, and hardness to touch.
4. Examine for signs of obstruction because of occluding thrombus—swelling, particularly in loose connective tissue or popliteal space, ankle, or suprapubic area.
5. Monitor for signs of pulmonary embolus, including shortness of breath, chest pain, and tachycardia.
6. Hand-test extremities for temperature variations—use dorsum (back) of same hand; first compare ankles, then move to the calf and up to the knee.
7. Assess for calf pain, which may be aggravated when foot is dorsiflexed with the knee flexed. Unfortunately, this sign is nonspecific and has a low sensitivity for detecting thrombophlebitis.
8. Assess all IV catheter insertion sites for signs and symptoms of infection and infiltration. Rotate peripheral IV sites every 72 hours or as needed.

Nursing Diagnoses

- Acute Pain related to decreased venous blood flow.
- Risk for Bleeding related to anticoagulant therapy.
- Impaired Physical Mobility related to pain and imposed treatment.

Nursing Interventions

1. Elevate legs as directed to promote venous drainage and reduce swelling.
2. Apply warm compresses or heating pad as directed to promote circulation and reduce pain.
   a. Make sure that water temperature is not too hot.
   b. Cover plastic water bottle or heating pad with towel before applying to skin.
3. Administer acetaminophen, codeine, or other analgesic, as prescribed and as needed. Avoid the use of aspirin (or aspirin-containing drugs) and NSAIDs during anticoagulant therapy to prevent further risk of bleeding.

 NURSING ALERT Avoid massaging or rubbing calf because of the danger of breaking up the clot, which can then circulate as an embolus.

Preventing Bleeding

See page 319 for nursing interventions for patients on anticoagulant therapy.

Preventing Other Hazards of Immobility

1. Prevent venous stasis by proper positioning in bed.
   a. Support full length of legs when they are to be elevated.
   b. Prevent pressure ulcers that may occur over bony prominences, such as sacrum, hips, knees, and heels. Be aware of bony prominence of one leg pressing on soft tissue of other leg (in side-lying position, place a soft pillow between legs).
   c. Avoid hyperflexion at knee as in jackknife position (head up, knees up, pelvis, and legs down); this promotes stasis in pelvis and extremities.
2. Initiate active exercises unless contraindicated, in which case, use passive exercises.
   a. If the patient is on bed rest:
      i. Simulate walking if lying on back—5 minutes every 2 hours.
      ii. Simulate bicycle pedaling if lying on side—5 minutes every 2 hours.

b. If contraindicated, resort to passive exercises—5 minutes every 2 hours.

3. Encourage adequate fluid intake, frequent changes of position, and effective coughing and deep-breathing exercises.

4. Be alert for signs of pulmonary embolism—chest pain, dyspnea, anxiety, and apprehension—and report immediately.

5. After the acute phase (48 hours), apply compression stockings as directed. Check color, warmth, and capillary refill through opening at toe if using open-toe stocking and remove at least once per day to look for skin changes, pressure points, and calf tenderness. Educate patient about continued use of compression stockings at home as directed.

6. Encourage walking when allowed.

a. If permissible, have the patient sit up and move to side of bed in sitting position. Provide a foot support (stool or chair)—dangling of feet is not desirable because pressure may be exerted against popliteal vessels and may obstruct blood flow.

b. If the patient is permitted out of bed, encourage walking 10 minutes each hour.

c. Discourage crossing of legs and long periods of sitting because compression of vessels can restrict blood flow.

 EVIDENCE BASE National Collaborating Center for Acute Care. (2015). *Venous thromboembolism: Reducing the risk.* NICE Clinical Guideline 92. Update 2015. Available: www.nice.org.uk/guidance/CG092.

Community and Home Care Considerations

Practice preventive measures for bedridden patients who are prone to develop thrombosis:

1. Have the patient lie in bed in the slightly reversed Trendelenburg position because it is better for the veins to be full of blood than empty.

2. Place a padded footboard across the foot of the bed.

a. Instruct the patient to press the balls of the feet against the footboard, as if rising up on toes.

b. Have the patient relax the foot.

c. Request that the patient do this 5 to 10 times per hour.

3. Make sure the patient wears prescription compression stockings at all times when legs are dependent or as ordered by the provider. If having difficulty applying stockings, the patient can use a plastic sandwich bag over forefoot while sliding on foot of stocking and then pull it out the open toe. There are also devices available from various manufacturers to assist with applying stockings

Patient Education and Health Maintenance

1. Teach patient signs of recurrent thrombophlebitis and pulmonary embolism to report immediately.

2. Provide thorough instructions about anticoagulant therapy (see page 319).

3. Teach patient to promote circulation and prevent stasis by applying compression stockings at home.

4. Advise against straining or any maneuver that increases venous pressure in the leg. Eliminate the necessity to strain at bowel movement by increasing fiber and fluids in the diet.

5. Warn patient of hazards of smoking and obesity: nicotine constricts veins, decreasing venous blood flow. Extra pounds increase pressure on leg veins. Make appropriate referrals to nutritionist, smoking-cessation classes, etc., as needed.

6. Advise patient to avoid prolonged periods of sitting or standing. If necessary, perform exercises to encourage venous return.

 NURSING ALERT Prescription compression stockings have no role in the management of the acute phase of DVT, the first 48 hours, but are of value after ambulation has begun. Their use will minimize or delay the development of postphlebitic syndrome.

Evaluation: Expected Outcomes

- Patient verbalizes reduced pain.
- No bleeding is observed.
- Normal respiratory status is maintained.

Chronic Venous Insufficiency

Chronic venous insufficiency may be a residual effect of phlebitis, or thrombosis, also called *postphlebitic syndrome.* It may also occur as a result of heredity. It results from chronic occlusion of the veins, destruction of the valves, congenitally weak or absent valves, or weakness in the calf muscle pump of the lower extremity.

Pathophysiology and Etiology

1. In the case of venous thrombosis, smaller vessels dilate because the main channel for returning blood from the leg to the heart is blocked by a thrombus.

2. Valves of diseased connecting veins (perforators) that serve to keep blood flowing from the superficial system into the deep system can no longer prevent backflow. The result is chronic venous stasis, resulting in swelling and edema, as well as superficial varicose veins.

3. The lower leg becomes discolored because of venous stasis, which leads to edema and pigmentation changes because of hemosiderin buildup in the skin resulting in a brownish discoloration. Uncontrolled edema may lead to dermatitis and ulceration.

4. Most commonly involved deep veins are the iliac and femoral veins. The saphenous vein is the most common superficial vein affected.

Clinical Manifestations

1. Chronic edema; worse while legs are dependent.

2. Intractable induration, discoloration, pain, and ulceration; area surrounding medial malleolus is the most common site.

Diagnostic Evaluation and Management

1. Doppler, plethysmography—noninvasive screening that shows obstruction and valve incompetency.

2. Best treatment is prevention of phlebitis and constant use of compression if phlebitis has occurred.

3. After this syndrome has developed, only palliative and symptomatic treatment is possible because the damage is irreparable.

Complications

1. Stasis ulcers.
2. Cellulitis.
3. Recurrent thrombosis.

Nursing Interventions and Patient Education

Instruct the patient as follows:

1. Wear prescription compression stockings to prevent edema.
2. Avoid sitting or standing for long periods or sitting with legs crossed.
3. Elevate legs on a chair for 5 minutes every 2 hours.
4. Elevate legs above level of head by lying down two or three times daily.
5. Raise foot of bed 6 to 8 inches (15 to 20 cm) at night to allow venous drainage by gravity.
6. Apply bland, oily lotions to prevent scaling and dryness of the skin.
7. Avoid constricting bandages.
8. Prevent injury, bruising, scratching, or other trauma to the skin of the leg and foot.
9. Be alert for signs of ulceration, drainage, warmth, erythema, and pain, indicating infection.
10. Ambulate several times a day, as tolerated, to improve blood flow by contraction of the calf muscle pump of the lower leg.

Stasis Ulcers

Stasis ulcer is an excavation of the skin surface produced by sloughing of inflammatory necrotic tissue, usually caused by venous insufficiency in the lower extremity.

Pathophysiology and Etiology

1. Stasis ulcer results from inadequate oxygen and other nutrients to the tissues because of edema and decreased circulation.
2. Secondary bacterial infection occurs because of decreased microcirculation that limits the body's response to infection.
3. Postphlebitic syndrome and stasis with uncontrolled edema are responsible for most leg ulcers.

Clinical Manifestations

Severity of symptoms depends on the extent and duration of venous insufficiency.

1. Open sore that is inflamed (see Figure 14-2) (beefy red base) and has irregular edges. The ulcers are most often found in the ankle area.
2. Drainage may be present or the area may be covered by a dark crust.
3. Patient may complain of swelling, heaviness, aching, and fatigue.

Figure 14-2. Venous ulcer.

4. Edema and pigmentation around ulcer.
5. Crusting of the skin around ulcer.

 GERONTOLOGIC ALERT Most venous ulcers occur in people older than age 65.

Diagnostic Evaluation

1. Noninvasive tests, such as plethysmography and venous Doppler, may show impeded blood flow and incompetent valves.
2. Wound cultures will identify microorganisms, if infected.

Management

Removing Devitalized Tissue

1. Necrotic material is flushed out with cleaning agents to dissolve slough. These agents are chemically or naturally derived enzymes that are proteolytic or fibrinolytic.
2. Surgical excision of slough—if necrotic tissue is loose, this procedure can be done without anesthesia; if the tissue is adherent, anesthesia will be required. Some debridements may be done at the bedside or in the clinic with topical anesthetic.

Stimulating Formation of Granulation Tissue

1. Dressing of choice:
   a. Nonadherent so that removal is painless and does not damage newly forming tissue.
   b. Highly absorbent.
   c. Safe, nontoxic.
   d. Sterile, accessible, and inexpensive.
2. Application of compression over dressings, generally through the use of bandages or elastic stockings. In some circumstances, inflatable pneumatic leggings may be appropriate.
3. Unna's boot or other layered compression bandage, an effective treatment of choice, is an example of a combined dressing and compression bandage.
4. The use of human growth factor ointment to the ulcer may be appropriate to stimulate tissue growth.
5. Bed rest with leg elevation.
6. Diuretic therapy for edema reduction may improve capillary circulation.
7. Application of skin grafts.
   a. Skin grafts are used for ulcers that will not heal.
   b. They are not recommended for first-line treatment.
   c. Skin-equivalent grafts may be used particularly if skin grafts fail.

Preventing Recurrence

1. Ligation of the saphenofemoral or saphenopopliteal vessels with stripping.
2. Laser or radiofrequency ablation of the saphenofemoral or greater saphenous vein and saphenofemoral junction.
3. Ligation of the lower leg communicating veins (usually endoscopic).
4. Deep vein bypass or reconstruction.
5. Injection compression sclerotherapy.
6. See page 321 for surgical care.

Complications

1. Infection.
2. Sepsis.

Nursing Assessment

1. Observe appearance and temperature of the skin.
2. Note location and appearance of ulcer.
3. Determine presence and quality of all peripheral pulses. Use Doppler, if needed.
4. Observe for drainage and signs of infection.

Nursing Diagnoses

- Impaired Tissue Integrity related to stasis ulcer.
- Acute Pain related to stasis ulcer.

Nursing Interventions

Restoring Tissue Integrity

1. Elevate affected extremity to decrease edema.
2. Place lamb's wool between toes to prevent pressure on a toe.
3. Provide overbed cradle to protect leg from pressure of bed linens.
4. Consider air-fluidized bed to provide pressure relief.
5. Administer prescribed antibiotics.
6. Apply wet-to-moist dressings, chemical beads or ointments, and topical antibiotics, as ordered. Wounds should not be allowed to completely dry out. Slight moisture aids the healing process.
7. Apply Unna's boot or other compression system to lower extremity, as ordered.
8. Ensure adequate nutritional intake to enhance wound healing.

Reducing Pain

1. Administer prescribed analgesics, such as NSAIDs, to reduce pain and inflammation.
2. Medicate 30 to 45 minutes before a dressing change.
3. Encourage short periods of ambulation after pain medication is given.

Community and Home Care Considerations

1. Make sure that all supplies are obtained for home care. Utilize social services and other resources to help with financial arrangements, as needed.
2. Assess the patient's ability to perform dressing changes at home. Include significant others in teaching to assist patient.
3. Make home visits several times per week to assess healing of ulcer, assess for infection, and assist family in carrying out dressing changes and other measures.

Patient Education and Health Maintenance

1. Stress the importance of following explicitly the recommendations of the health care provider.
2. Explain the hazards of trying other remedies without professional advice.
3. Indicate that the treatment may be long but that patience is an important aspect.
4. Encourage maintenance of healthy tissue when the ulcer has healed by continuing with the safeguards practiced before because breakdown of healed tissue frequently occurs.
5. Encourage participation in physical therapy and a regular exercise program.
6. Encourage weight control and proper dietary intake to ensure adequate amounts of protein, vitamins (A, C, E), zinc, and a reduced sodium intake.
7. Teach patient the correct method of dressing changes.
8. Instruct patient on injury prevention, including keeping hallways and walkways clear of obstacles and using a nightlight to avoid injury if awakened at night.
9. Encourage use of compression stockings when ordered.

Evaluation: Expected Outcomes

- Skin is of normal color and temperature, nontender and nonswollen, and demonstrates new epithelium.
- Verbalizes only minimal discomfort with dressing changes.

Varicose Veins

Primary varicose veins are unilateral or bilateral dilation and elongation of saphenous veins; deeper veins are normal. As the condition progresses, because of hydrostatic pressure and vein weakness, the vein walls become distended, with asymmetric dilation, and some of the valves become incompetent. The process is irreversible. *Secondary varicose veins* result from obstruction of deep veins.

Telangiectasias (spider veins) are dilated superficial capillaries, arterioles, and venules. They may be cosmetically unattractive but do not pose a threat to circulation.

Pathophysiology and Etiology

1. Dilation of the vein prevents the valve cusps from meeting; this results in increased backup pressure, which is passed into the next lower segment of the vein. The combination of vein dilation and valve incompetence produces the varicosity (see Figure 14-3).
2. Varicosities may occur elsewhere in the body (esophageal and hemorrhoidal veins) when flow or pressure is abnormally high.
3. Predisposing factors:
   a. Hereditary weakness of vein wall or valves.
   b. Long-standing distention of veins brought about by pregnancy, obesity, or prolonged standing.
   c. Advanced age—loss of tissue elasticity.

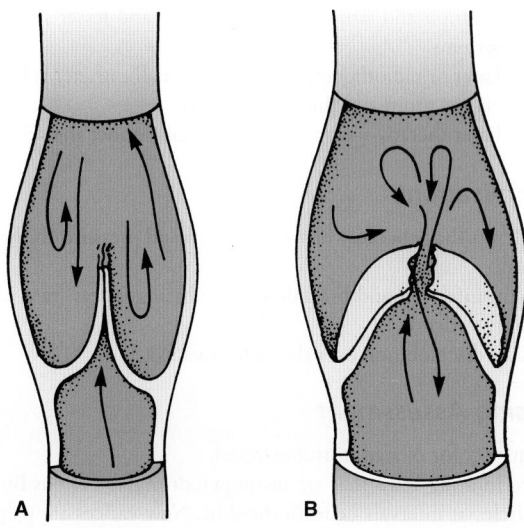

Figure 14-3. Valve incompetence develops as dilation of a vessel prevents effective approximation of valve cusps. **(A)** Closed venous valve. **(B)** Incompetent venous valve.

Clinical Manifestations

1. Disfigurement because of large, discolored, tortuous leg veins.
2. Easy leg fatigue, cramps in leg, heavy feeling, increased pain during menstruation, and nocturnal muscle cramps.

Diagnostic Evaluation

1. Photoplethysmography—a noninvasive technique to observe venous flow hemodynamics by noting changes in the blood content of the skin; used to detect incompetence in valves located inside the vein.
2. Doppler ultrasound and duplex imaging—can detect accurately and rapidly the presence or absence of venous reflux in deep or superficial vessels.
3. Venous outflow and reflux plethysmography—able to detect deep venous occlusion.
4. Ascending and descending venography—an invasive technique that can also demonstrate venous occlusion and patterns of collateral flow. This test is expensive and may not be required if a careful history, physical examination, and laboratory testing are done.

Management

1. Conservative therapies, such as encouraging weight loss if appropriate and avoiding activities that cause venous stasis by obstructing venous flow.
2. Surgery may be considered for ulceration, bleeding, and cosmetic purposes in selected patients if patency of deep veins is ensured.
3. Surgical procedures—a single method or combination of methods is tailored to meet the needs of the individual:
   a. Sclerosing injection—may be combined with ligation or limited to treatment of isolated varicosities. The affected vessel may be sclerosed by injecting sodium tetradecyl sulfate or similar sclerosing agent. Compression bandage is then applied without interruption for 2 to 6 weeks; inflamed endothelial surfaces adhere by direct contact.
   b. Multiple vein ligation—either by multiple incisions or ambulatory phlebectomy (veins are removed using tiny incisions and hooks to grasp the veins).
   c. Ligation and stripping of the greater and lesser saphenous systems.
   d. Laser or radiotherapy treatment—small catheter is inserted via the groin and the veins ablated.
   e. Laser therapy—eliminates small veins under the skin.

Complications

1. Hemorrhage because of weakening of and pressure on the vein wall.
2. Skin infection and breakdown, producing ulcers (rare in primary varices).
3. Skin discoloration over the veins injected.

Nursing Assessment

1. Inspect for dilated, tortuous vessel.
2. Perforating veins that are incompetent may be felt as bulging circles at intervals beneath the skin. New varices are palpated along the surface of the muscle or bone. Chronic varices create deep pockets and may feel "boggy" with deep palpation.
3. Assess for any ulceration, chronic venous insufficiency, or signs of infection.

Nursing Diagnoses

- Impaired Tissue Integrity related to chronic changes and postoperative inflammation.
- Acute Pain related to surgical incisions, inflammation.

Nursing Interventions

Promoting Tissue Integrity Postoperatively

1. Maintain compression bandages from toes to groin. Monitor neurovascular status of feet (color, warmth, capillary refill, sensation, and pulses) to prevent compromise from swelling.
2. Elevate legs about 30 degrees, providing support for the entire leg. Make sure that knee gatch of the bed is positioned for straight incline. Encourage early ambulation.
3. Monitor for signs of bleeding, especially during the first 24 hours.
   a. Blood soaked through bandages.
   b. Increased pain, hematoma formation.
   c. Hypotension and tachycardia.
4. If incisional bleeding occurs, elevate the leg above the level of the heart, apply pressure over the site, and notify the surgeon.
5. Be alert for complaints of pain over bony prominences of the foot and ankle; if the elastic bandage is too tight, loosen it.
6. Maintain IV for fluids and antibiotics, as ordered.
7. After removal of compression bandages (about 7 days postoperatively), observe or teach patient to observe for signs of cellulitis or incisional infection.
8. Encourage use of prescription compression stockings for several weeks to months following surgery.

Relieving Pain

1. Administer analgesics, as prescribed.
2. Encourage early and frequent ambulation with legs elevated when not walking.
3. When ambulatory, advise patient to avoid prolonged standing, sitting, or crossing or dangling legs to prevent obstruction.

Patient Education and Health Maintenance

Postoperative Instructions

Instruct the patient to:

1. Wear pressure bandages or compression stockings as prescribed—usually for 3 to 4 weeks after surgery.
2. Elevate legs about 30 degrees and provide adequate support for entire leg.
3. Take analgesics for pain, as ordered.
4. Report such signs as sensory loss, calf pain, or fever to the health care provider.
5. Avoid dangling of legs.
6. Walk frequently.
7. Be aware that patchy numbness can be expected but should disappear in less than 1 year.
8. Follow conservative management instructions (below) to prevent recurrence.

Conservative Management

Instruct the patient to:

1. Avoid activities that cause venous stasis by obstructing venous flow:
   a. Wearing tight garters, tight girdle, compression around popliteal area.
   b. Sitting or standing for prolonged periods of time.
   c. Crossing the legs at knees for prolonged periods while sitting (reduces circulation by 15%).

2. Control excessive weight gain.
3. Wear firm elastic support, as prescribed, from toe to knee when in upright position.
   a. Put compression stockings on in bed before getting up.
   b. Thigh-high compression may be ordered presenting a compliance challenge.
4. Elevate foot of bed 6 to 8 inches (15 to 20 cm) or use a wedge for night sleeping.
5. Avoid injuring legs.

Evaluation: Expected Outcomes

- Skin is of normal color and temperature, nontender and nonswollen, and intact.
- Actively moves extremity; verbalizes reduced pain.

CONDITIONS OF THE ARTERIES
Arteriosclerosis and Atherosclerosis

Arteriosclerosis is an arterial disease manifested by a loss of elasticity and a hardening of the vessel wall. More commonly known as "hardening of the arteries," it is a normal part of the aging process and generally occurs uniformly throughout the arterial system.

Atherosclerosis is the most common type of arteriosclerosis, manifested by the formation of atheromas (patchy lipoidal degeneration of the intima). Lesions, or plaques, form throughout the arterial wall, reducing the size of the vessel and limiting the flow of blood. Over time, atherosclerotic lesions can completely occlude the lumen by buildup of the plaque material and may contribute to thrombus formation.

Pathophysiology and Etiology

1. Etiology thought to be a reaction to injury:
   a. Endothelial cell injury causes increased platelet and monocyte aggregation to site of injury.
   b. Smooth muscle cells migrate and proliferate.
   c. Matrix of collagen and elastic fibers forms.
2. There are two types of atherosclerotic lesions: fatty streaks and fibrous plaques (see Figure 14-4).

3. Risk factors include heredity, increasing age, male gender, cigarette smoking, hypertension, dyslipidemia, diabetes mellitus, renal disease, obesity, physical inactivity, and stress.

 NURSING ALERT Smoking is the number one risk factor for atherosclerosis.

Clinical Manifestations

1. May affect entire vascular system or one segment of the vascular tree.
2. Symptoms and signs are based on area affected:
   a. Brain (cerebroarteriosclerosis)—transient ischemic attacks (TIA); stroke; vision disturbances, such as amaurosis fugax (one type of TIA), which is described by patients as a shade over a portion of eye (see Chapter 15).
   b. Heart (coronary artery disease [CAD])—angina, MI, and heart failure (see Chapter 13).
   c. GI tract (aortic occlusive disease, aortic aneurysm, and mesenteric ischemia)—abdominal pain, unintentional weight loss, and lower back pain.
   d. Kidneys (renal artery stenosis)—renal insufficiency and poorly controlled hypertension.
   e. Extremities (peripheral arterial disease [PAD])—intermittent claudication (pain in a muscle associated with exercise caused by lack of oxygen to the muscle), pain at rest, tissue loss (with or without presence of infection or gangrene), and embolic events.
      i. PAD is often undiagnosed because pain is attributed to arthritis or accepted as a normal change because of aging.
      ii. It affects approximately 8 to 12 million Americans and approximately 800,000 Canadians.
3. Decreased or absent pulses; bruits of major vessels.

 GERONTOLOGIC ALERT Atherosclerotic cardiovascular disease afflicts 80% of the population older than age 65 and is the most common condition of the arterial system in older adults.

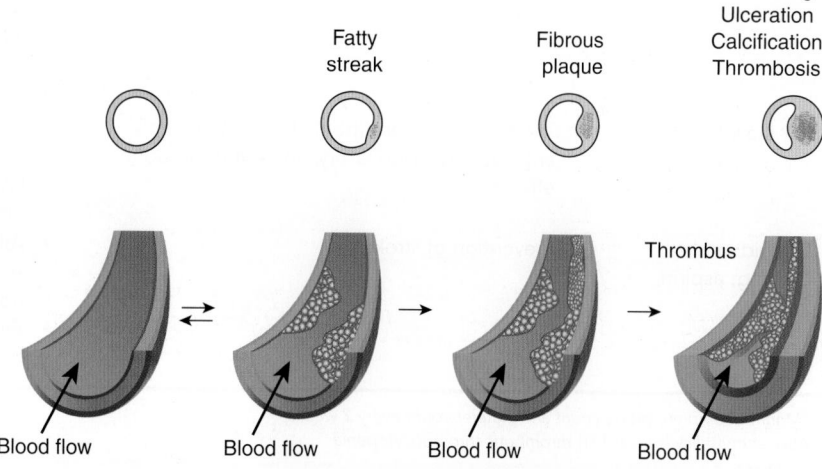

Figure 14-4. Atherosclerosis is a progressive process that occurs over decades. The earliest lesion is a fatty streak, which may regress or progress to a fibrous plaque. Irreversible fibrous plaques may eventually develop into atheroma, which may be complicated by hemorrhage, ulceration, calcification, and thrombus. Target organ disease includes myocardial infarction, stoke, and peripheral arterial occlusion.

Fatty streak

Fibrous plaque

Complicated lesion: Hemorrhage Ulceration Calcification Thrombosis

Thrombus

Blood flow Blood flow Blood flow Blood flow

Diagnostic Evaluation

Specific to body system affected:

1. Arteriography of involved area may show stenosis and increased collateral circulation.
2. Computed tomography (CT) scan.
3. Magnetic resonance imaging (MRI)/magnetic resonance angiography (MRA).
4. Noninvasive testing of the vascular system: duplex studies, sequential Doppler studies, pulse volume resistance, and ankle–brachial index (ABI).
   a. For ABI, systolic pressure of the posterior tibial and dorsalis pedis arteries are determined by Doppler for each side as measures of ankle pressure.
   b. The greater ankle systolic pressure for each side is divided by the brachial systolic pressure of the same side. Normally, the systolic pressures are equal. In presence of atherosclerotic disease, the pressure below an occluded area is less than the arm pressure.
   c. Normal ABI is 1.00 to 1.40.
   d. Result below 0.90 indicates obstruction of the lower-extremity arteries.
   e. Result greater than 1.40 indicates noncompressible vessels because of calcification, so ABI cannot be interpreted.

5. ECG, Holter monitoring, exercise stress testing, myocardial imaging, and cardiac catheterization may be done to evaluate CAD.

Management

Medical Management

1. Modification of risk factors—stress, weight loss, exercise, dietary changes, and monitoring for type 2 diabetes.
2. Prescriptive management—anticoagulants, antiplatelet therapy (see Table 14-3), lipid-lowering agents, and antihypertensives.
3. Specific treatment for end-organ dysfunction—see cerebrovascular insufficiency (page 365), CAD (page 269), peripheral arterial occlusive disease (page 331).
4. Vascular rehabilitation/exercise (if available).

Surgical Management

1. Endovascular procedures:
   a. PTA with or without placement of intraluminal stent—to relieve arterial stenosis when lesions are accessible, as in superficial femoral and iliac arteries, through the use of special inflatable balloon catheters and metal stents.
   b. Endovascular grafting—placement of prosthetic graft via a transluminal approach. Graft material covers a metallic

Table 14-3 Antiplatelet Therapy

Antiplatelet therapy is used to prevent platelet aggregation and thrombus formation. It is used in the treatment of cerebrovascular disease, coronary artery disease, and intermittent claudication. This table lists some common antiplatelet medications, their indications, and potential contraindications/precautions.

MEDICATION	USE	CONTRAINDICATIONS/PRECAUTIONS
Aspirin	Prevention of myocardial infarction, transient ischemic attack, stroke	• Allergy to ASA • Active gastric ulcers
Ticlopidine	Prevention of stroke	• Sensitivity to drug • Neutropenia, thrombocytopenia, history of TTP, active bleeding disorders* • Liver and renal impairment • See drug–drug interactions
Ticagrelor	Decreased platelet aggregation Prevention of MI/coronary artery stent thrombosis	• Sensitivity to drug • GI and Intracranial bleeding • Liver impairment
Pentoxifylline	Treatment of intermittent claudication	• Sensitivity to drug • Recent cerebral or retinal hemorrhage • Caffeine or theophylline intolerance
Clopidogrel	Reduction of atherosclerotic events	• Sensitivity to drug • Active pathologic bleeding (eg, peptic ulcer, intracranial hemorrhage) • Severe hepatic or renal disease • See drug–drug interactions
Cilostazol	Treatment of intermittent claudication—has antiplatelet, vasodilatory, and antithrombotic effects	• Sensitivity to drug • Heart failure, liver impairment • Liver impairment • See drug–drug interactions
Dipyridamole, 200 mg; aspirin, 25 mg	Prevention of stroke	• Allergy to ASA • Active ulcer disease • Renal and hepatic impairment • Bleeding disorders • See drug–drug interactions

*Monitor complete blood count and platelet count every 2 weeks.
ASA, acetylsalicylic acid; TTP, thrombotic thrombocytopenia.

stent, which may or may not be impregnated with medication to decrease failure. The stent is placed via femoral artery or radial artery and is deployed. This is commonly used for abdominal aortic aneurysms, renal arteries, and mesenteric and iliac arteries.

   c. Rotational atherectomy—high-speed rotary cutter that removes lesions by abrading plaque. Benefits of this therapy are minimal damage to the normal endothelium and low incidence of complications.

   d. Laser angioplasty—amplified light waves are transmitted by fiberoptic catheters. Laser beam heats the tip of a percutaneous catheter and vaporizes the atherosclerotic plaque.

2. Surgical revascularization of the affected vessels, including:
   a. Embolectomy—removal of blood clot from the artery.
   b. Thrombectomy—removal of thrombus from the artery.
   c. Endarterectomy—removal of atherosclerotic plaque from the artery.
   d. Bypass—use of a graft, either vein graft or prosthetic material, to route blood flow around blocked area.

Complications

Long-term complications of atherosclerosis are related to the specific body system affected:

1. Brain—long- and short-term disabilities associated with stroke.
2. Heart—stable or unstable angina, MI, and heart failure.
3. Aorta—ischemic bowel, aneurysms, impotence, renal failure, and nephrectomy.
4. Lower extremities—intermittent claudication, nonhealing ulcers, infections or gangrene, and amputation.

Nursing Interventions and Patient Education

See "Care of the Patient Undergoing Vascular Surgery," page 321. In addition, attention is directed at reducing risk factors by smoking cessation (page 24), stress reduction (page 25), weight reduction (page 23), adequate control of diabetes (Chapter 25) and/or hypertension (page 338), adjusting diet to reduce cholesterol intake (page 274), and taking lipid-lowering medications. Encourage active lifestyle to promote cardiovascular health and empower patients to manage their care.

Peripheral Arterial Occlusive Disease (Aorta and Distal Arteries)

Peripheral arterial occlusive disease (PAOD) (also known as peripheral artery disease or PAD) is a form of arteriosclerosis in which the peripheral arteries become blocked. Chronic occlusive arterial disease occurs much more frequently than does acute (which is the sudden and complete blocking of a vessel by a thrombus or embolus). Patients at increased risk for PAD include patients aged 65 or older and those with other risk factors for atherosclerosis, such as diabetes, smoking history, hyperlipidemia, hypertension, family history of PAD or other forms of atherosclerotic disease such as renal or mesenteric atherosclerosis, or abdominal aortic aneurysms, CAD, or carotid atherosclerosis.

 EVIDENCE BASE Gerhard-Herman, M., Gornik, H., Barrett, C., et al. (2017). AHA/ACC guideline on the management of patients with lower extremity peripheral artery disease. A report of the American College of Cardiology/American Heart Association Task Force on Clinical Practice Guidelines. *Journal of the American College of Cardiology, 69*(11), e71–e126.

Pathophysiology and Etiology

Arteriosclerosis Obliterans

1. Most commonly caused by atherosclerosis with contributing factors as discussed in previous section.
2. May involve the following vessels in isolation or combination:
   a. Aortoiliac system.
   b. Femoral arteries—superficial femoral, profunda femoris.
   c. Popliteal artery.
   d. Trifurcating vessels—anterior tibial (AT), posterior tibial (PT), and peroneal arteries.
   e. Dorsalis pedis (DP) artery.
   f. Pedal arch.
3. Lesions tend to form at areas of bifurcation of the vessels.
4. Pattern of disease differs in nondiabetics and diabetics:
   a. Nondiabetics—disease usually involves macrocirculation (larger vessels [eg, aorta, iliac, femoral arteries]) and is more common in isolated segments.
   b. Diabetics—disease usually involves microcirculation (smaller vessels [eg, popliteal, tibial, peroneal, and small vessels in the foot/digits]) and occurs in more diffuse segments.

Thromboangiitis Obliterans (Buerger Disease)

Inflammatory process of arterial wall, which is followed by thrombosis. Also affects adjacent veins and nerves. Associated with heavy cigarette smoking.

Clinical Manifestations

Symptoms appear gradually and are specific to the area affected.

Aortoiliac

1. Mesenteric ischemia, pain after eating that increases as disease progresses.
2. Unintentional weight loss.
3. Renal insufficiency.
4. Poorly controlled hypertension.
5. Impotence.
6. Intermittent claudication (including gluteal claudication).

Femoral, Popliteal, and Distal Arteries

1. Intermittent claudication (calf, thigh, and foot).
2. Pain at rest—associated with severe arterial ischemia. Severe pain in feet aggravated by elevation of lower extremity. Pain is relieved by placing foot in dependent position.
3. Dependent rubor—dusky purple color of extremity when in dependent position; changes to pallor when elevated.
4. Numbness or tingling of feet or toes.
5. Trophic changes associated with tissue malnutrition:
   a. Hair loss.
   b. Thick toenails.
   c. Thin, shiny skin.
   d. Cool temperature of extremity.
6. Tissue loss or nonhealing ulcers, which may develop wet or dry gangrene (see Figure 14-5). Arterial ulcers are usually painful, pale, and have well-demarcated (punched-out) edges.

Diagnostic Evaluation

Noninvasive

1. Vascular physical examination.
2. ABI—see page 330; may be done before and after exercise.
   a. A toe brachial index (TBI) should be measured in patients that have suspected PAD when the resting ABI is greater than 1.40.

Figure 14-5. Arterial ulcer.

b. This is particularly useful in diabetic patients as the associated increased calcification of the distal arteries may artificially elevate the ABI result.

3. Doppler ultrasound—decreased velocity of flow through a stenotic vessel or no flow with total occlusion.

4. Segmental plethysmography—decreased pressure distal to region of occlusion.

Invasive

1. Angiography—to confirm occlusion.
2. MRA—to confirm occlusion.
3. Spiral CT—to obtain a three-dimensional view of artery and occlusion.

Management

1. Goals:
   a. Reestablish blood flow to areas of critical ischemia.
   b. Preserve the extremity.
   c. Relieve pain associated with intermittent claudication or pain at rest.
   d. Provide sufficient blood flow for wound healing.

2. Aggressive risk factor management to prevent progression, including walking, weight reduction, smoking cessation, and control of other conditions such as hypertension, dyslipidemia, and diabetes mellitus.

3. Pharmacologic treatment with antiplatelet agents or anticoagulants to improve blood flow by increasing erythrocyte flexibility and lowering blood viscosity.

4. When conservative measures clearly are not enough, revascularization surgery (endarterectomy, arterial bypass grafting, or a combination) may be required.

5. Endovascular procedures, such as PTA with stenting, may be used alone or with revascularization surgery for dilatation of localized noncalcified segments of narrowed arteries with or without intraluminal stenting.

6. Hyperbaric oxygen therapy may be used for nonhealing wounds and gas gangrene. This is limited to centers that have a hyperbaric oxygen chamber (most commonly used for diving accidents).

a. Increased atmospheric pressure inside the chamber combined with 100% oxygen delivery allows for greater concentration of oxygen to be delivered to all parts of the body.
b. Typical treatment programs last 2 hours, five or six times per week for 4 weeks or more.
c. Adverse effects include pressure or popping in ears, slight light-headedness at the end of treatment sessions, and possible temporary change in vision.

7. Amputation of affected extremity in cases of severe infection and gangrene, failed attempts at revascularization, or when revascularization is not considered a viable option.

8. See page 321 for surgical care.

Complications

1. Ulceration with slow healing.
2. Gangrene, sepsis.
3. Severe occlusion may necessitate limb or partial limb amputation.

Nursing Assessment

1. Auscultate abdomen and listen for presence of bruits.
2. Observe lower extremities for color, sensation, and temperature. Compare bilaterally for differences.
3. Palpate pulses (see Figure 14-6) and record. If pulses are nonpalpable, attempt to locate pulse with a handheld Doppler. About 10% of people have absent DP artery from birth.

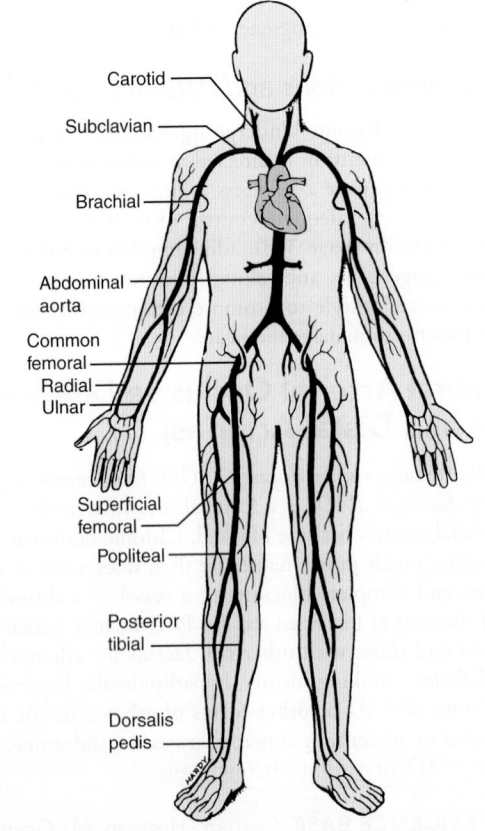

Figure 14-6. Salient points in evaluating peripheral arterial insufficiency. Reduced or absent femoral pulses indicate aortoiliac disease. Absent popliteal pulses indicate superficial femoral occlusion. Pulse deficits in one extremity, with normal pulses in the contralateral extremity, may suggest acute arterial embolus. Absent pedal pulses indicate tibioperoneal artery involvement.

4. Inspect nails for thickening and opacity; inspect skin for shiny, atrophic, hairless, and dry appearance—reflect chronic changes.
5. Assess for pain:
   a. Severe abdominal pain after eating.
   b. Pain in legs with exercise.
   c. Pain in feet at rest.
6. Assess for ulcers of toes and feet.

Nursing Diagnoses

- Ineffective Peripheral Tissue Perfusion related to decreased arterial blood flow.
- Risk for Peripheral Neurovascular Dysfunction of lower extremities.
- Risk for Infection related to decreased arterial flow.

Nursing Interventions

Promoting Tissue Perfusion

1. Perform frequent neurovascular checks of affected extremity.
2. Inspect lower extremity and feet for new areas of ulceration or extension of existing ulceration.
3. Provide and encourage well-balanced diet to enhance wound healing.
4. Encourage walking or performance of ROM exercises to increase blood flow, which will increase collateral circulation.
5. Administer or teach self-administration of pain medication to achieve comfort level conducive to ambulation.

Protecting Lower Extremities

1. Encourage patient to wear protective footwear, such as rubber-soled slippers or shoes with closed, wide toe box when out of bed.
2. Instruct patient and family to keep hallways and walkways free of clutter to avoid injury.
3. Avoid tight-fitting socks and shoes.
4. Instruct patient to avoid sitting with legs crossed.
5. Avoid using adhesive tape and harsh soaps on the affected skin.
6. Instruct patient to check temperature of bath water with forearm before entering tub.
7. Perform and teach foot care, including washing and carefully drying and inspecting feet daily.

Preventing Infection

1. Apply moisturizing lotion to intact skin of lower extremities to prevent drying and cracking of the skin.
2. Encourage patient to wear clean hose or socks daily: woolen socks for winter and cotton for summer.
3. Teach patient to:
   a. Trim toenails straight across after soaking the feet in warm water.
   b. Place wisps of cotton under corner of great toenail if there is a tendency toward ingrown toenails.
   c. Have a podiatrist cut corns and calluses; do not use corn pads or strong medications.
4. Teach patient signs to report:
   a. Redness, swelling, irritation, blistering, and foul odor.
   b. Itching, burning, and rashes.
   c. Bruises, cuts, and unusual appearance of the skin.
   d. New areas of ulceration.
5. Instruct patient to check with physician before using any OTC or topical lotions or creams on wound.
6. Administer antibiotics postoperatively to prevent infection around prosthetic graft material.

Patient Education and Health Maintenance

1. Instruct patient on the importance of walking to improve circulation; set up a plan for incremental increase in distance.
2. Instruct patient not to sit or stand in one position for long periods.
3. Instruct patient, when sitting, to keep knees below the level of the hips to avoid hip flexion.
4. Instruct patient to avoid tight-fitting clothing (eg, elastic-topped socks or clothing made out of Lycra/Spandex), especially over area of graft placement.
5. Instruct patient not to cross legs when sitting or lying down.
6. Instruct patient on methods to promote vasodilation by keeping extremity warm and stopping use of other vasoconstricting substances such as caffeine.
7. Instruct patient on the importance of daily foot care.
8. Encourage patient to stop smoking.
9. Encourage follow-up for control of chronic conditions and ongoing risk factor management.

Evaluation: Expected Outcomes

- No new ulcer formation.
- Verbalizes importance of wearing protective shoes and washing and inspecting feet daily.
- No signs of infection of lower extremities.

Aneurysm

An *aneurysm* is a distention of an artery brought about by a weakening/destruction of the arterial wall. They are lined with intraluminal debris, such as plaque and thrombi. Because of the high pressure in the arterial system, aneurysms can enlarge, producing complications by compressing surrounding structures; left untreated, and they may rupture, causing a fatal hemorrhage. A dissection occurs when the layers of the artery become separated. Blood flows between the layers, causing further disruption of the arterial wall. Additionally, the intraluminal thrombus may totally occlude the artery, leading to acute ischemia to all arteries distal to the area of thrombosis, or they may embolize clot and/or plaque to the arteries distal to the aneurysm.

The *aorta* is the most common site for aneurysms; however, they may form in any vessel. Peripheral vessel aneurysms may involve the renal artery, subclavian artery, popliteal artery (knee), or any major artery. These produce a pulsating mass and may cause pain or pressure on surrounding structures.

Pathophysiology and Etiology

1. Aneurysms may form as the result of:
   a. Atherosclerosis.
   b. Heredity.
   c. Infection.
   d. Trauma.
   e. Immunologic conditions.
2. False aneurysms (pseudoaneurysm) are associated with trauma to the arterial wall, as in blunt trauma or trauma associated with arterial punctures for angiography and/or cardiac catheterization.
3. The ascending aorta and the aortic arch are the sites of greatest hemodynamic stress and also are the most common sites of arterial dissection.
4. Contributing factors include:
   a. Hypertension.
   b. Arteriosclerosis.

c. Local infection, pyogenic or fungal (mycotic aneurysm).
d. Congenital weakness of vessels.
e. Syphilis.
f. Trauma.
5. Morphologically, aneurysms may be classified as follows:
   a. Saccular—distention of a vessel projecting from one side.
   b. Fusiform—distention of the whole artery (ie, entire circumference is involved).
   c. Dissecting—hemorrhagic or intramural hematoma, separating the medial layers of the aortic wall.
6. Abdominal aortic aneurysms are described as infrarenal, when the "neck" of the aneurysm is located below the level of the renal arteries, juxtarenal, when the aneurysm involves the renal arteries, or suprarenal, when the aneurysm is located above the level of the renal arteries or involves the renal arteries.

Clinical Manifestations

Aneurysm of the Thoracoabdominal Aorta
From the aortic arch to the level of the diaphragm. At first, no symptoms; later, symptoms may come from heart failure or a pulsating tumor mass in the chest.
1. Pulse and BP difference in upper extremities if aneurysm interferes with circulation in the left subclavian artery.
2. Pain and pressure symptoms.
3. Constant, boring pain because of pressure.
4. Intermittent and neuralgic pain because of impingement on nerves.
5. Dyspnea, causing pressure against trachea.
6. Cough, often paroxysmal and brassy in sound.
7. Hoarseness, voice weakness, or complete aphonia, resulting from pressure against recurrent laryngeal nerve.
8. Dysphagia because of impingement on esophagus.
9. Edema of chest wall—infrequent.
10. Dilated superficial veins on chest.
11. Cyanosis because of vein compression of chest vessels.
12. Ipsilateral dilation of pupils because of pressure against cervical sympathetic chain.
13. Abnormal pulsation apparent on chest wall, because of erosion of aneurysm through rib cage—in syphilis.

Abdominal Aneurysm
1. Many of these patients asymptomatic.
2. Abdominal pain most common, either persistent or intermittent—often localized in middle or lower abdomen to the left of midline.
3. Lower back pain caused by pressure on the spine from enlarging aneurysm.
4. Feeling of an abdominal pulsating mass, palpated as a thrill, auscultated as a bruit.
5. Hypertension.
6. Distal variability of BP; pressure in arm greater than thigh.
7. Upon rupture, will present with hypotension and/or hypovolemic shock.

 GERONTOLOGIC ALERT Most abdominal aneurysms occur between ages 60 and 90. Rupture of the aneurysm is likely if there is coexistent hypertension or if the aneurysm is larger than 2.4 inches (5.5 to 6 cm).

Diagnostic Evaluation
1. Abdominal or chest x-ray may show calcification that outlines aneurysm.
2. CT scanning and ultrasonography are used to detect and monitor size of aneurysm.
3. MRI/MRA.
4. Spiral CT gives three-dimensional view of the aneurysm and any attendant atherosclerosis.
5. Arteriography allows visualization of aneurysm and vessel.

Management
1. May follow small aneurysms (1.6 inches [4 cm] or less) with CT scanning or ultrasound every 6 months and aggressively control BP.
2. The prognosis is poor for untreated patients as aneurysm enlarges. It is especially true if it enlarges 5 mm in 3 months or in patients with chronic obstructive pulmonary disease.
3. Surgery:
   a. Resection of the aneurysm via abdominal incision and placement of a prosthetic graft to restore vascular continuity.
   b. Endovascular grafting involves repair of aneurysm using a stent graft, which is deployed via the femoral artery. It attaches above and below the aneurysm and provides a new channel for the blood.
   c. Thoracic aneurysms are the most difficult to treat, endovascular grafting is possible, and some require the use of atrial–femoral circulatory bypass intraoperatively.

Complications
1. Fatal hemorrhage.
2. Myocardial ischemia.
3. Stroke.
4. Paraplegia because of interruption of anterior spinal artery.
5. Abdominal ischemia.
6. Ileus.
7. Graft occlusion.
8. Graft infections.
9. Acute renal failure.
10. Impotence.
11. Lower-extremity ischemia.
12. "Trash toes"—results from distal embolization of plaque and blood clots.

Nursing Assessment
1. In patient with thoracoabdominal aortic aneurysm, be alert for sudden onset of sharp, ripping, or tearing pain located in the anterior chest, epigastric area, shoulders, or back, indicating acute dissection or rupture.
2. In patients with abdominal aortic aneurysm, assess for abdominal (particularly left lower quadrant) pain and intense lower back pain caused by rapid expansion. Be alert for syncope, tachycardia, and hypotension, which may be followed by fatal hemorrhage because of rupture.

Nursing Diagnoses
• Risk for Ineffective Gastrointestinal, Renal, Cardiac, Cerebral Tissue Perfusion (vital organs) related to aneurysm or aneurysm rupture or dissection.

e. Rigidity of extremity.

f. Pulselessness.

Diagnostic Evaluation

1. Neurovascular assessment of affected area.
2. Doppler ultrasonography, segmental limb pressure, and pulse volume recordings—may indicate decreased flow.
3. Arteriography—confirms diagnosis.
4. MRA or spiral CT—to confirm diagnosis and give a three-dimensional view of the area.
5. Digital subtraction angiography, MRA, and MRI may be done for cerebral embolization.

Management

1. Drug therapy—anticoagulants (see page 317) and thrombo-lytics (see page 319).
2. Surgery:
   a. Embolectomy (see Figure 14-7) must be performed within 6 to 10 hours to prevent muscle necrosis and loss of extremity.
   b. Fasciotomy—incisions made over leg compartments to aid expansion of edematous tissue and relief of pressure on the arterial system.
   c. Amputation of the affected limb if revascularization is inappropriate due to metabolic complications.
3. Treatment of shock.
4. Bed rest.

 NURSING ALERT Arterial embolization of a large artery, such as the iliac, is life-threatening and requires emergency operative intervention.

Complications

1. Irreversible ischemia and loss of extremity.
2. Metabolic complications:
   a. Acidosis.
   b. Hyperkalemia.
   c. Renal failure.
3. Shock.

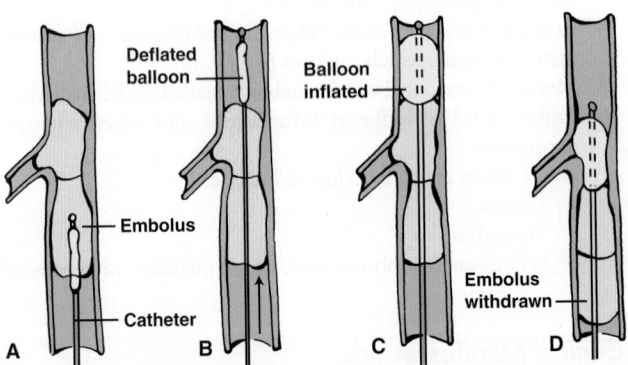

Figure 14-7. Extracting an embolus from a vessel can be done with the use of a Fogarty embolectomy catheter. The catheter, with a soft, deflated balloon near the tip, is threaded through the artery via an arteriotomy. **(A,B)** It is passed through the embolus and its throm-bus; **(C)** it is then inflated. **(D)** A steady pull downward withdraws the embolus along with the catheter.

Nursing Assessment

1. Assess for acute, severe pain.
2. Assess for gradual or acute loss of sensory and motor function.
3. Check for aggravation of pain by movement of and pressure on the extremity.
4. Palpate for loss of distal pulses.
5. Inspect for pale, mottled, and numb extremity.
6. Inspect for collapse of superficial veins because of decreased blood flow to the extremity.
7. Inspect for sharp line of color and temperature demarcation. This may occur distal to the site of occlusion as a result of ischemia.
8. Assess for edema.

Nursing Diagnoses

- Impaired Comfort related to impaired blood supply.
- Ineffective Peripheral Tissue Perfusion related to lack of blood flow by clot.
- Risk for Infection related to surgery.

Nursing Interventions

Protecting the Extremity

1. Protect extremity by keeping it at or below the body's hori-zontal plane.
2. Protect leg from hard surfaces, tight or heavy surfaces, and tight or heavy overlying bed linens.
3. Handle extremity gently and prevent pressure or friction while repositioning.
4. Administer pain medications, as ordered.

Promoting Tissue Perfusion

1. Administer UFH IV line to reduce tendency of emboli to form or expand (useful in smaller arteries).
2. Monitor thrombolytic therapy IV line to dissolve clot, as ordered.
3. Monitor patient for signs of bleeding (gums, urine, and stool).
4. Monitor coagulation, hematology, and electrolyte studies.
5. Prepare the patient for surgery (see page 321).
6. Postoperatively, promote movement of extremity to stimulate circulation and prevent stasis.

Preventing Infection

1. Postoperatively, check surgical wound for bleeding, swelling, erythema, and discharge.
2. Maintain IV infusion or venous access device to administer IV antibiotics, if indicated.
3. Continue to monitor the patient for tachycardia, fever, pain, erythema, warmth, swelling, and drainage at incision site.

Patient Education and Health Maintenance

1. Teach prevention techniques, such as daily aerobic activity, observation for skin breakdown, and prevention of injury.
2. Teach patient the medical regimen and importance of taking prescribed medications, such as oral anticoagulants, to prevent reembolization.
3. Encourage patient to report symptoms of arterial occlusion: paralysis, numbness, tingling, pallor, and coldness of extremity.

Evaluation: Expected Outcomes

- Patient reports no pain; no injury noted.
- Limb has normal color, sensation, movement, and temperature.
- No signs of infection.

Vasospastic Disorder (Raynaud Phenomenon)

Raynaud phenomenon is a vasospastic disorder that is brought on by an unusual sensitivity to cold, emotional stress, or autoimmune disorders. It is termed primary Raynaud disease when it is idiopathic, unaccompanied by other systemic manifestations. It is termed secondary Raynaud syndrome when it is associated with autoimmune disorders.

Pathophysiology and Etiology

1. The condition is a form of intermittent arteriolar vasoconstriction that results in coldness, pain, and pallor of fingertips, toes, or tip of the nose and a rebound circulation with redness and pain.
2. The cause is unknown, although it may be secondary to connective tissue and other immunologic disorders such as scleroderma, systemic lupus, polymyositis, and Sjögren syndrome.
3. Episodes may be triggered by emotional factors or by unusual sensitivity to cold.
4. Most common in women between ages 16 and 40 and seen much more commonly in cold climates and during the winter months.

Clinical Manifestations

1. Intermittent arteriolar vasoconstriction resulting in coldness, pain, and pallor.
2. Involvement of the fingers appears to be asymmetric; thumbs are less often involved.
3. Characteristic color changes: white–blue–red.
   a. White—blanching, dead-white appearance if spasm is severe.
   b. Blue—cyanotic, relatively stagnant blood flow.
   c. Red—a reactive hyperemia on rewarming.
4. Occasionally, there is ulceration of the fingertips (most common in autoimmune disorders).

Diagnostic Evaluation

1. Clinical symptoms must last at least 2 years to confirm the diagnosis.
2. Tests may be done to rule out secondary disease processes, such as chronic arterial occlusive or connective tissue disease.
3. Noninvasive blood flow tests for finger pressures and arterial waveforms.

Management

1. Avoidance of trigger and aggravating factors.
2. Protection of the fingers and toes with warm mittens (not gloves) and warm boots in cold weather.
3. Longer-acting calcium channel blockers are frequently used to prevent or reduce vasospasm.
4. Nitroglycerin or sympatholytics, such as reserpine, guanethidine, or prazosin, may be helpful for some. Adverse effects, such as headache, dizziness, and orthostatic hypotension, may be prohibitive.
5. Antiplatelet agents, such as aspirin or dipyridamole, may be given to prevent total occlusion.
6. Sympathectomy—removal of the sympathetic ganglia or division of their branches; may offer some improvement (extremely rare).

Complications

1. Chronic disease may cause atrophy of the skin and muscles.
2. Ulceration and gangrene (rare).

Nursing Assessment

1. Perform thorough history and review of systems for clues to underlying disorder.
2. Assess for blanching of digits when exposed to cold. Color turns cyanotic and then red with normal temperature.
3. Note whether warmth brings about symptom relief.

Nursing Diagnoses

- Risk for Peripheral Neurovascular Dysfunction related to vasospastic process.
- Acute Pain related to hyperemic stage.

Nursing Interventions

Minimizing Sensory Alteration

1. Assist patient in avoiding exposure to cold; for example, use mittens to handle cold items (water pitcher, refrigerated items). Always wear mittens outside in the cold. Teach patient rewarming techniques—warm water, putting fingers in axillary or groin area.
2. Encourage patient to stop smoking.
3. Help patient to understand the need to avoid stressful situations.
4. Offer patient options for stress management.
5. Administer and teach patient about drug therapy.
6. Instruct patient about the need to take drugs every day to prevent or minimize symptoms.
7. Monitor for orthostatic hypotension precaution if taking sympatholytics.
8. Advise patient that episode may be terminated by placing hands (or feet) in warm water.

Relieving Pain

1. Explain to patient that pain may be experienced when spasm is relieved—hyperemic phase.
2. Administer or teach self-administration of analgesics.
3. Reassure patient that pain is temporary; persistent pain, ulceration, or signs of infection should be reported.

Patient Education and Health Maintenance

1. Avoid whatever provokes vasoconstriction of vessels of hands.
2. Prevent injury to hands, which can aggravate vasoconstriction and lead to ulceration.
3. Minimize exposure to cold because this precipitates a reaction. Avoid wet and windy environments.
4. Wear warm clothing—boots, mittens, and hooded jackets—when going out in cold weather and waterproof clothing when raining or snowing.
5. Avoid placing hands in cold water, the freezer, or the refrigerator unless protective mittens are worn.
6. Use extra precautions to avoid injuries to fingers and hands from needlesticks and knife cuts.

Evaluation: Expected Outcomes

- Follows medication regimen, avoiding triggers.
- Reports decreased length of painful phase with episodes.

HYPERTENSIVE DISORDERS
Hypertension

EVIDENCE BASE James, P., Oparil, S., Carter, B., et al. (2014). Evidence based guidelines for the management of high blood pressure in adults (JNC 8). *JAMA, 311*(5), 507–520.

The American Heart Association defines *blood pressure* (BP) as the force of blood pushing against the arterial wall as it relates to blood viscosity (thickness) and resistance of blood vessel. Systolic blood pressure (SBP) is the highest arterial pressure when the heart contracts and empties. Diastolic blood pressure (DBP) is the lowest arterial pressure when the heart relaxes to fill with blood. *Hypertension* (high BP) is a disease of vascular regulation in which the mechanisms that control arterial pressure within the normal range are altered. The predominant mechanisms of blood pressure control are the central nervous system (CNS), the renin–angiotensin–aldosterone system, and extracellular fluid volume. Why these mechanisms fail is not known.

Pathophysiology and Etiology

Elevated diastolic pressure leads to strain on the arterial wall, which over time causes thickening and calcification of the arterial media (a condition called sclerosis) and eventually narrowing of the blood vessel lumen. Elevated blood pressure is seen when there is increased cardiac output and increased peripheral resistance.

Primary or Essential Hypertension

(Approximately 95% of patients with hypertension.)

1. When the diastolic pressure is 90 mm Hg and/or the systolic pressure is 140 mm Hg or higher and other causes of hypertension are absent, the condition is said to be primary hypertension. More specifically, an individual is considered hypertensive when the average of two or more properly measured, seated BP readings taken at rest on each of two or more office visits exceeds the upper limits of normal (see Box 14-1).
2. Cause of essential hypertension is unknown; however, there are several areas of investigation:
   a. Hyperactivity of sympathetic vasoconstricting nerves.
   b. Presence of vasoactive substance released from the arterial endothelial cells, which acts on smooth muscle, sensitizing it to vasoconstriction.
   c. Increased cardiac output, followed by arteriole constriction.
   d. Excessive dietary sodium intake, sodium retention, insulin resistance, and hyperinsulinemia play roles that are not clear. There is a growing body of evidence implicating excess sodium intake in the pathogenesis of elevated BP.
   e. Familial (genetic) tendency.
3. Systolic BP elevation in the absence of elevated diastolic BP is termed isolated systolic hypertension and is treated in the same manner.

Secondary Hypertension

1. Occurs in approximately 5% of patients with hypertension secondary to other pathology.

BOX 14-1 | **Hypertension Classification for Adults**

- <120 systolic and <80 diastolic—normal
- 120–139 systolic or 80–89 diastolic—prehypertension
- 140–159 systolic or 90–99 diastolic—stage 1 hypertension
- ≥160 systolic or ≥100 diastolic—stage 2 hypertension

---

2. Renal pathology:
   a. Chronic kidney disease, congenital anomalies, pyelonephritis, renal artery stenosis, acute and chronic glomerulonephritis, and obstructive uropathy (hydronephrosis).
   b. Reduced blood flow to kidney causes release of renin. Renin reacts with a serum protein to form angiotensin I, which is converted to angiotensin II through the action of angiotensin-converting enzyme in the lungs, leading to vasoconstriction and increased salt and water retention.
3. Coarctation of the aorta (stenosis of the aorta)—blood flow to upper extremities is greater than flow to the kidneys. The kidneys release renin when they sense hypotension.
4. Endocrine disturbances:
   a. Pheochromocytoma—a tumor of the adrenal gland that causes release of epinephrine and norepinephrine and a rise in BP (extremely rare).
   b. Adrenal cortex tumors lead to an increase in aldosterone secretion (hyperaldosteronism) and an elevated BP (rare).
   c. Cushing syndrome leads to an increase in adrenocortical steroids (causing sodium and fluid retention) and hypertension.
   d. Hyperthyroidism causes increased cardiac output.
5. Obstructive sleep apnea causes nocturnal hypertension, which leads to sustained daytime hypertension.
6. Prescription medications such as estrogens and steroids (cause fluid retention), sympathomimetics (cause vasoconstriction and tachycardia), antidepressants (prevent the breakdown of epinephrine), appetite suppressants (cause tachycardia and vasoconstriction), and NSAIDs (cause fluid retention and can lead to renal insufficiency).
7. Nonprescription drugs and substances such as cocaine (cause vasoconstriction and tachycardia); NSAIDs; herbal agents such as St. John's wort, ginseng, ephedra (unclear etiology of hypertension); antihistamines (cause vasoconstriction and tachycardia); and nicotine (causes vasoconstriction).
8. Food substrates such as sodium chloride, ethanol, licorice, and glucose, all of which can cause increased fluid retention.

Consequences of Hypertension

1. Hypertension can cause intimal wall injury in the arteries, which can lead to arteriosclerosis in which smooth muscle cell proliferation, lipid infiltration, and calcium accumulation occur in the vascular endothelium.
2. Prolonged hypertension damages small blood vessels in the brain, eyes, heart, and kidneys.
3. The major objective in patients with high BP is to prevent target organ damage of the heart (left ventricular hypertrophy, angina, myocardial infarction, heart failure), brain (stroke, transient ischemic attack, dementia), kidneys (chronic kidney disease), eyes (retinopathy, blindness), or vasculature (aneurysm, PAD).
4. The Heart Disease and Stroke Statistics 2016 Update reported that compared to individuals with normal BP (120/80 mm Hg), those patients with prehypertension have a 1.5- to 2-fold risk for major cardiovascular events between the ages 60 to 80 years.

Prevalence and Risk Factors

EVIDENCE BASE Mozaffarian, D., Benjamin, E., Go, A., et al. (2015). Heart disease and stroke statistics-2015 update: A report from the American Heart Association. *Circulation, 131*(4), e29–e322.

1. Hypertension affects approximately 1 billion people worldwide and is the most common modifiable risk factor for arteriosclerosis.

2. There are an estimated 80 million Americans with hypertension (about 32.6% of the adult population), and this number is expected to increase due to the aging of the population. Only a fraction of these people are aware of their hypertension and are treated for it, and even fewer have gained adequate control of their BP.

3. The National Health and Nutrition Examination Surveys (NHANES), designed to monitor the health and nutritional status of the civilian US population, showed that among US adults with high blood pressure, the percentage of individuals with hypertension who were aware of their condition increased from 69.6% in 1999–2000 to 80.6% in 2007–2008. The number of individuals who take antihypertensive medications and attained control of their blood pressure also increased during this period.

4. Risk factors include age between 30 and 70, African American race, overweight or obese, sleep apnea, family history, tobacco use, sedentary lifestyle, diabetes mellitus, metabolic syndrome, lower education/socioeconomic status, psychological stressors, and dietary factors (increased consumption of fats, sodium, and alcohol, with lower intake of potassium-rich foods).

 NURSING ALERT There is a higher incidence of hypertension in the African American population, along with higher mortality rate and risk for complications such as stroke, left ventricular hypertrophy, heart failure, and kidney disease.

Clinical Manifestations

1. Usually asymptomatic; known as the silent killer.
2. May cause headache, dizziness, blurred vision, chest pain, and shortness of breath when greatly elevated.
3. Elevated BP readings taken in a seated position on at least two occasions.

Diagnostic Evaluation

1. ECG—to determine effects of hypertension on the heart (left ventricular hypertrophy, ischemia) or presence of underlying heart disease.
2. Chest x-ray—may show cardiomegaly or aortic dilation by the presence of a widened mediastinum.
3. Proteinuria, elevated serum blood urea nitrogen (BUN), and elevated creatinine levels—indicate kidney disease as a cause or effect of hypertension; first voided urine microalbumin or spot urine for albumin–creatinine ratio are early indicators.
4. Serum potassium—decreased in primary hyperaldosteronism; elevated in Cushing syndrome; both are causes of secondary hypertension.
5. Urine (24-hour) for catecholamines—increased in pheochromocytoma.
6. Renal ultrasound to detect renal vascular diseases.
7. Renal artery duplex imaging to identify renal artery stenosis.
8. Outpatient ambulatory BP measurements.
9. Tests for causes of secondary hypertension are done if hypertension is resistant to treatment or specific signs and symptoms of secondary hypertension are present.

Management

Blood Pressure Target Goals

1. Blood pressure (BP) goals are based on research and published guidelines and/or consensus statements. Clinicians must be aware of their patients' target BP goals.
2. Guidelines from the 8th Report of the Joint National Commission (JNC-8):
   a. BP goals for all patients are less than 150/90 mm Hg.

b. BP goals for patients with diabetes and chronic kidney disease are less than 140/90 mm Hg.
3. Guidelines from the American Heart Association:
   a. Individuals with ischemic heart disease, CAD equivalents, and high risk for CAD have a target BP goal of less than 130/80 mm Hg.
   b. If the patient has LV dysfunction, the target BP is less than 120/80 mm Hg.
4. Guidelines from the American Diabetes Association indicate that individuals with diabetes should have a target BP of less than 140/90 mm Hg.

Lifestyle Modifications

Lifestyle modifications reduce BP, prevent or delay the incidence of hypertension, enhance antihypertensive drug therapy, and decrease cardiovascular risk (see Box 14-2).

If, despite lifestyle changes, BP remains at or above 140/90 mm Hg (or is not at optimal level in the presence of other cardiovascular risk factors) over 3 to 6 months, drug therapy should be initiated. If BP is extremely elevated or in presence of cardiovascular risk factors, single-drug therapy may be initiated.

Drug Therapy

See Table 14-4.

1. Considerations in selecting therapy include:
   a. Race—African Americans respond well to calcium channel blockers and thiazide diuretics, if compelling conditions are not noted. A renin–angiotensin system (RAS) blocker is first line for African Americans with kidney disease, diabetes, or heart failure. Caucasians respond well to angiotensin converting enzyme (ACE) inhibitors.
   b. Age—some adverse effects such as fatigue and light-headedness may not be tolerated well by older adults. Diuretics are typically the first drug prescribed.
   c. Concomitant diseases and therapies—some agents also treat migraines, benign prostatic hyperplasia, heart failure; have beneficial effects on conditions such as renal insufficiency; or have adverse effects on such conditions as diabetes or asthma.
   d. Quality-of-life impact—tolerance of adverse effects.
   e. Cost considerations—newer and brand name agents usually more expensive.
   f. Dosing—multiple doses may reduce adherence.

BOX 14-2	Lifestyle Therapy for Blood Pressure Control

- Weight control—may reduce BP 5–20 mm Hg per 10 kg (22 pound) weight loss; goal is to maintain normal BMI of 18.5–24.9 kg/m².
- DASH eating plan—may reduce systolic BP 8–14 mm Hg; diet is rich in fruits, vegetables, and low-fat dairy products; reduced intake of saturated and total fat.
- Reduced sodium intake—may reduce systolic BP 2–8 mm Hg; salt intake is limited to no more than 2,400 mg sodium per day.
- Physical activity—may reduce systolic BP 4–9 mm Hg; regular aerobic physical activity (such as brisk walking) should occur at least 30 minutes most days per week.
- Moderate alcohol intake—may reduce systolic BP 2–4 mm Hg; alcohol intake is limited to no more than two drinks per day for most men and no more than one drink per day for women and lighter-weight persons. One drink is equivalent to 12 ounce beer, 5 ounce wine, or 1 ounce 80-proof whiskey.

Table 14-4 Evidence-Based Dosing for Antihypertensive Drugs

ANTIHYPERTENSIVE MEDICATION	INITIAL DAILY DOSE/NO. OF DOSES PER DAY	TARGET DOSE IN RCTs REVIEWED (mg)
ACE inhibitor		
Captopril	50 (2)	150–200
Enalapril	5 (1–2)	20
Lisinopril	10 (1)	40
Angiotensin receptor blockers		
Eprosartan	400 (1–2)	600–800
Candesartan	4 (1)	12–32
Losartan	50 (1–2)	100
Valsartan	40–80 (1)	160–320
Irbesartan	75 (1)	300
Beta-blockers		
Atenolol	25–50 (1)	100
Metoprolol	50 (1–2)	100–200
Calcium channel blockers		
Amlodipine	2.5 (1)	10
Diltiazem extended release	120–180 (1)	360
Nitrendipine	10 (1–2)	20
Thiazide-type diuretics		
Bendroflumethiazide	5 (1)	10
Chlorthalidone	12.5 (1)	12.5–25
Hydrochlorothiazide	12.5–25 (1–2)	25–100
Indapamide	1.25 (1)	1.25–2.5

These dosages may vary from those listed in the Physicians' Desk Reference. Please review current medication reference materials for most current dosing. Many antihypertensive agents are combination medications. RCT, randomized controlled trial.

2. Medications available:
   a. Diuretics—lower BP by promoting urinary excretion of water and sodium to lower blood volume.
   b. Beta-adrenergic blockers—lower BP by slowing the heart and reducing cardiac output by blocking beta-adrenergic receptors that produce epinephrine.
   c. Alpha-receptor blockers—lower BP by dilating peripheral blood vessels and lowering peripheral vascular resistance. Research has indicated these medications provide little protection against heart failure but are effective in improving benign prosthetic hypertrophy.
   d. Central alpha agonists—lower BP by diminishing sympathetic outflow from the CNS, thereby lowering peripheral resistance.
   e. Peripheral adrenergic agents—inhibit peripheral adrenergic release of vasoconstricting catecholamines such as norepinephrine.
   f. Combined alpha and beta-adrenergic blockers—work through alpha- and beta-receptors.
   g. ACE inhibitors—lower BP by blocking the enzyme that converts angiotensin I to the potent vasoconstrictor angiotensin II and reducing sympathetic nervous system activity; also raise the level of bradykinin, a potent vasodilator, and lower aldosterone levels.
   h. Angiotensin receptor blockers—similar in action to ACE inhibitors.
   i. Calcium antagonists (calcium channel blockers, or CCB)—stop the movement of calcium into the cells; relax smooth muscle, which causes vasodilation; and inhibit reabsorption of sodium in the renal tubules. Nondihydropyridine CCB (verapamil and diltiazem) have a negative inotropic effect and may worsen heart failure.
   j. Direct vasodilators—smooth muscle relaxants that primarily dilate arteries and arterioles.
   k. Aldosterone inhibitors—antagonize aldosterone receptors and inhibit sodium reabsorption in the collecting duct of the nephron in the kidneys.
   l. Direct renin inhibitors—inhibits renin within the renin–angiotensin system (RAS).
3. If hypertension is not controlled with the first drug within 1 to 3 months, three options can be considered:
   a. If the patient has faithfully taken the drug and not developed adverse effects, the dose of the drug may be increased.
   b. If the patient has had adverse effects, another class of drugs can be substituted.
   c. A second drug from another class could be added. If adding the second agent lowers the pressure, the first agent can be slowly withdrawn or, if necessary, combination therapy can be continued.
   d. Some patients require two medications at the time of diagnosis. This should be considered for patients who are 20 mm Hg above their systolic goal or 10 mm Hg above their diastolic goal.
4. The best management of hypertension is to use the fewest drugs at the lowest doses while encouraging the patient to maintain lifestyle changes. After BP has been under control for at least 1 year, a slow, progressive decline in drug therapy can be attempted. However, most patients need to resume medication within 1 year.
5. If the desired BP is still not achieved with the addition of a second drug, a third agent or a diuretic or both (if not already prescribed) could be added. 75% of individuals with hypertension require two or more antihypertensive agents to reach their BP goal.

6. Resistant hypertension is defined as an individual that requires three or more antihypertensive agents to control blood pressure.

 DRUG ALERT ACE inhibitors are a drug of choice for diabetics as they delay progression to end-stage renal disease. However, they may worsen renal function in the presence of renal artery stenosis.

Complications

See Figure 14-8.
1. Angina pectoris or MI because of decreased coronary perfusion.
2. Left ventricular hypertrophy and heart failure because of consistently elevated aortic pressure.
3. Renal failure because of diminished perfusion to the glomerulus.
4. TIAs, stroke, or cerebral hemorrhage because of cerebral ischemia and arteriosclerosis.
5. Retinopathy.
6. Accelerated hypertension (see page 343).

Nursing Assessment

Nursing History
Query the patient about the following:
1. Family history of high BP.
2. Previous episodes of high BP.
3. Dietary habits and salt intake.
4. Target organ disease or other disease processes that may place the patient in a high-risk group—diabetes, CAD, kidney disease.
5. Tobacco use.
6. Episodes of headache, weakness, muscle cramps, tingling, palpitations, sweating, and vision disturbances.
7. Medication that could elevate BP (refer to "Secondary Hypertension," above):
   a. Hormonal contraceptives, corticosteroids.
   b. NSAIDs.
   c. Nasal decongestants, appetite suppressants, and tricyclic antidepressants.

8. Other disease processes, such as gout, migraines, asthma, heart failure, and benign prostatic hyperplasia, which may be helped or worsened by particular antihypertensive drugs.

Physical Examination
1. Auscultate heart rate and heart sounds for the presence of an S4, indicating stiffening of the walls of the left ventricle, which may occur in hypertension.
2. If skilled in doing so, perform funduscopic examination of the eyes for the purpose of noting vascular changes. Look for edema, spasm, and hemorrhage of the eye vessels. Refer to ophthalmologist for definitive diagnosis.
3. Palpate the chest wall for a shift of the point of maximal impulse to the left, which occurs in heart enlargement. Palpate peripheral pulses for possible PAD.
4. Auscultate for bruit over the aorta, renal arteries, and peripheral arteries to determine the presence of atherosclerosis.
5. Determine mental status by asking patient about memory, ability to concentrate, and ability to perform simple mathematical calculations.

Blood Pressure Determination
1. Measure BP in both arms to determine whether there is a difference. If the SBP is greater than 15 mm Hg in one arm than the other, this may indicate the presence of subclavian stenosis in the arm with the lower SBP. If this BP differential is found, BP should be monitored in the arm with the highest SBP.
2. Avoid taking BP readings immediately after stressful or taxing situations. Wait 30 minutes after patient has smoked.
3. Have the patient assume position of comfort and remain silent. Make sure feet are on the floor or otherwise supported. The patient should be seated and relaxed for at least 5 minutes, and the blood pressure should be taken around the same time each day it is taken to observe for trends in BP.
4. Support the bared arm; avoid constriction of arm by a rolled sleeve.
5. Use a BP cuff of the correct size.
   a. The bladder within the cuff should encircle at least 80% of the patient's arm.
   b. Many adults will require a large cuff.
   c. Two or more readings separated by 2 minutes should be averaged.

Figure 14-8. Determinants and clinical effects of high blood pressure. GFR, glomerular filtration rate; TIA, transient ischemic attack.

6. Be aware that falsely elevated BPs may be obtained with a cuff that is too narrow; falsely low readings may be obtained with a cuff that is too wide.
7. Auscultate and record precisely the systolic and diastolic pressures.
   a. Systolic—the pressure within the cuff indicated by the level of the mercury column at the moment when the first clear, rhythmic pulsatile sound is heard (phase 1).
   b. Diastolic—the pressure within the cuff just as the sound disappears (ie, the onset of silence).

 NURSING ALERT The finding of an isolated elevated BP does not necessarily indicate hypertension. However, the patient should be regarded as at risk for high BP until further assessment—through history taking, repeat BP measurements, and diagnostic testing—either confirms or refutes the diagnosis.

 GERONTOLOGIC ALERT Elderly patients are more likely to have hypertension and isolated systolic hypertension because of age-related changes of decreased arterial compliance and arterial stenosis. Another age-related change, autonomic dysregulation, may cause orthostatic hypotension—a risk factor for syncope and falls.

Nursing Diagnoses

- Noncompliance with medication regimen and lifestyle changes.
- Readiness for Enhanced Self-health Management related to control of hypertension and prevention of target organ disease.

Nursing Interventions/Patient Education

Enlisting Cooperation and Compliance

1. Enlist the patient's cooperation in redirecting lifestyle in keeping with the guidelines of therapy, acknowledge the difficulty, and provide support and encouragement.
2. Develop a plan of instruction for medication self-management.
   a. Plan the patient's medication schedule so that they are given at proper and convenient times (once daily, if possible); set up a daily checklist on which the patient can record the medication taken or provide pill sorter.
   b. Be sure the patient knows the generic and brand names for all medications and throws away old medications and dosages so they will not be mixed up with current medications.
   c. Explore the cost of medications and ability for the patient to pay for prescriptions each month. Encourage the patient to discuss generic equivalents, mail-order drugs, or prescription assistance programs with the health care provider. Refer patient to Partnership for Prescription Assistance (*www.pparx.org*).
3. Stress the fact that there may be no correlation between high BP and symptoms; the patient cannot tell by the way he or she feels whether BP is normal or elevated. Because hypertension is chronic, regular follow-up is important to prevent complications and reduce more serious health care interventions in the future.
4. Assess for and try to eliminate side effects of medication regimen.
   a. Explain that antihypertensive drugs affect people differently, and side effects such as anorexia, fatigue, nausea, or lightheadedness often occur during the first few days or weeks of therapy until the body develops tolerance to them.
   b. Warn the patient of the possibility that orthostatic hypotension may occur initially with some drug therapy, but

it can be minimized by being cautious in hot, humid environments; getting up slowly; or sitting or lying down briefly if feeling faint.
   c. If constipation occurs, encourage high-fiber diet.
   d. If ankle swelling occurs, elevate legs periodically.
   e. If dry cough develops, dosage or drug may need to be changed.
   f. Advise the patient to notify the health care provider if side effects are significant, dosage may be lowered or a substitute medication may be ordered. However, the patient should not discontinue medication without notifying the health care provider.
5. Educate the patient to be aware of serious adverse effects (fainting, palpitations, shortness of breath) and report them immediately so that adjustments can be made in individual pharmacotherapy.

 GERONTOLOGIC ALERT Polypharmacy, cognitive changes, and sensory deficits in older adults may make dosage adjustment and control of BP difficult. Work with the patient, family, and home care nurse to devise a simple method for the patient to take the proper medications. Older patients are also more sensitive to therapeutic levels of drugs and may demonstrate adverse effects while on an otherwise average dosage. Monitor closely for safety and efficacy of therapy. They may be more sensitive to postural hypotension and should be cautioned to change positions with great care.

Encouraging Self-Management

1. Explain the meaning of high BP, risk factors, and their influences on the cardiovascular, cerebral, and renal systems.
2. Stress that there can never be total cure, only control, of essential hypertension; emphasize the consequences of uncontrolled hypertension.
3. Instruct the patient regarding proper method of taking BP at home and at work if health care provider so desires. Inform patient of desired range and the readings that are to be reported.
4. Determine recommended dietary plans and provide dietary education, as appropriate.
   a. Print out copy of the DASH Eating Plan and review with patient. Help patient suggest food preferences that include whole grains, fruits, vegetables, low-fat dairy, and nuts in quantities outlined in plan. Available at *www.nhlbi.nih. gov/health/health-topics/topics/dash*.
   b. Teach patient and family members how to read food labels to monitor sodium intake.
   c. Refer to dietitian for thorough dietary education and planning, as needed.
5. Educate patient about factors that may affect BP, such as dehydration, diarrhea, and other illnesses, so BP should be monitored closely and treatment adjusted.
6. Encourage the patient to keep follow-up appointments as directed by health care provider, have blood work drawn to monitor serum creatinine and electrolytes, and schedule eye exam by an ophthalmologist yearly.

Evaluation: Expected Outcomes

- Takes medications regularly; keeps follow-up appointments.
- Monitors BP correctly at home; able to identify sodium content on food labels.

Malignant Hypertension

Malignant hypertension, also called *accelerated hypertension*, occurs when the BP elevates extremely rapidly, threatening one or more of the target organs: brain, kidneys, or heart. Malignant hypertension is defined as blood pressure ≥180/120 mm Hg or isolated diastolic BP greater than 130 mm Hg and is a medical emergency.

Pathophysiology and Etiology

1. When rapid hypertension occurs, the normal autoregulation of the artery eventually fails.
2. The rise in pressure in the arterioles and capillaries leads to damage to the vascular wall, which disrupts the endothelium and allows fibrinous material to enter the vascular wall, thereby narrowing or obliterating the vascular lumen.
3. For example, within the brain, the breakthrough vasodilation from failure of autoregulation leads to the development of cerebral edema and symptoms of hypertensive encephalopathy.
4. Etiology includes collagen vascular disorders, renal failure, renal artery stenosis, and toxemia of pregnancy.

Clinical Manifestations

1. Brain effects:
   a. Encephalopathy.
   b. Stroke.
   c. Progressive headache, stupor, and seizures.
2. Kidney effects:
   a. Decreased blood flow and vasoconstriction.
   b. Elevated BUN.
   c. Increased plasma renin activity.
   d. Lowered urine-specific gravity.
   e. Proteinuria.
   f. Renal failure.
3. Cardiac effects:
   a. Left-sided heart failure.
   b. Acute MI.
   c. Right-sided heart failure.

Management

Goal is to lower BP to reduce the probability of permanent damage to target organs.

1. If diastolic BP exceeds 115 to 130 mm Hg, clinical condition is assessed very carefully.
2. Immediate hospitalization and treatment if the following are present:
   a. Seizures.
   b. Abnormal neurologic signs.
   c. Severe occipital headache.
   d. Pulmonary edema.
3. The patient is hemodynamically monitored in the ICU.
4. Antihypertensive agents are administered parenterally. Agents include:
   a. Nitroprusside—a rapidly acting arteriolar and venous dilator, given as an IV infusion. Initial dose: 0.25 to 0.5 mcg/kg/minute; maximum dose: 8 to 10 mcg/kg/minute. Avoid in neurologic emergencies. Preferred in perioperative HTN.
   b. Nitroglycerin—a rapidly acting venous and, to a lesser degree, arteriolar dilator, given as an IV infusion. Initial dose: 5 mcg/minute; maximum dose: 200 mcg/minute. Preferred perioperative.
   c. Labetalol—an alpha- and β-adrenergic blocker, given as an IV bolus or infusion. Bolus: 20 mg initially, followed by 20 to 80 mg every 10 minutes to a total dose of 300 mg. Infusion: 0.5 to 2 mg/minute. Preferred in acute ischemic stroke.
   d. Esmolol—antagonizes beta-1 adrenergic receptors, given as bolus 1,000 mcg/kg IV, then 150 mcg/kg/minute IV prn, max 300 mcg/kg/minute, may continue 50 mcg/kg/minute IV q4min prn, taper to d/c.
   e. Nicardipine—a calcium channel blocker, given as an IV infusion. Initial dose: 5 mg/hour; maximum dose: 15 mg/hour. Preferred in acute ischemic stroke.
   f. Clevidipine—a calcium channel blocker. Initial dose: 1 to 2 mg/hour; 32 mg/hour maximum dose: 16 mg/hour.
   g. Fenoldopam—a peripheral dopamine-1 receptor agonist, given as an IV infusion. Initial dose: 0.01 mcg/kg/minute; the dose is titrated at 15-minute intervals, depending on the blood pressure response normal dosing: 0.01 to 1.6 mcg/kg/minute.
   h. Hydralazine—an arteriolar dilator, given as an IV bolus. Initial dose: 10 mg given every 20 to 30 minutes; maximum dose: 20 mg. Avoid in neurologic emergencies.
   i. Propranolol—a β-adrenergic blocker, given as an IV infusion and then followed by oral therapy. Dose: 1 to 10 mg load, followed by 3 mg/hour.
   j. Phentolamine—an alpha-adrenergic blocker, given as an IV bolus. Dose: 5 to 10 mg every 5 to 15 minutes.
   k. Enalaprilat—an ACE inhibitor, given as an IV bolus. Dose: 1.25 to 5 mg every 6 hours.
5. Diuretics may be administered to maintain a sodium diuresis when the arterial pressure falls.
6. Vasopressor agents should be available if the BP responds too vigorously to antihypertensive agents.

Nursing Interventions

1. Record BP frequently or monitor BP via an intra-arterial line or electronically controlled cuff. Some drugs necessitate the taking of BP readings every 5 minutes or more frequently while titrating drug therapies.
2. Monitor for adverse effects of medications—headache, tachycardia, and orthostatic hypotension.
3. Measure urine output accurately.
4. Observe for hypokalemia, especially if patient is placed on diuretic therapy. Monitor for ventricular dysrhythmias.
5. Observe for CNS complications.
   a. Note signs of confusion, irritability, lethargy, and disorientation.
   b. Listen for complaints of headache, difficulty with vision.
   c. Check for evidence of nausea or vomiting.
   d. Be alert for signs of seizure activity. Provide a safe environment—padded side rails. Keep bed in lowest position.
6. Reduce activity and provide quiet environment.
7. Monitor ECG continuously.
8. Maintain constant vigilance until BP is decreased and stable and then begin a hypertension teaching program.

 NURSING ALERT BP should be reduced gradually and wide pressure variations avoided because lowered BP may not be adequate to perfuse vital organs.

LYMPHATIC DISORDERS

The lymphatic system is a network of vessels and nodes that are interrelated with the circulatory system. It removes tissue fluid from intercellular spaces and protects the body from bacterial invasion. Lymph nodes are located along the course of the lymphatic vessels and filter lymph before it is returned to the bloodstream.

Lymphedema and Lymphangitis

Lymphedema is a swelling of the tissues (particularly in the dependent position) produced by an obstruction to the lymph flow in an extremity. This results in excessive accumulation of fluid in the interstitial space, which is composed of high molecular weight proteins.

Lymphangitis is an acute inflammation of lymphatic channels, which most commonly arises from a focus of infection in an extremity.

Pathophysiology and Etiology

Lymphedema

1. Classified as primary (congenital malformations) or secondary (acquired obstruction).
2. Swelling in the extremities occurs due to an increased quantity of lymph fluid that results from an obstruction of lymphatics.
3. Obstruction may be in both the lymph nodes and the lymphatic vessels. Eventually, subcutaneous tissue becomes fibrotic, impairing vascular flow and oxygen transfer to tissues.
4. It may be caused or aggravated by radiation therapy, trauma, cancer, morbid obesity, or surgery involving the lymph tissue (particularly radical mastectomy). It may be associated with varicose veins and chronic phlebitis.

Lymphangitis

1. Most commonly caused by infection in an extremity. The pooled protein-rich lymph fluid creates a good medium for growth of bacteria and fungi.
2. The characteristic red streak extending up an arm or leg from the infected wound outlines the course of the lymphatics as they drain.
3. Recurrent lymphangitis is typically associated with lymphedema.

Clinical Manifestations

1. Lymphedema: edema may be massive and is usually firm.
2. Lymphangitis:
   a. Displays characteristic red streaks that extend up an arm or leg from an infection that is not localized and that can lead to septicemia.
   b. Produces general symptoms—high fever and chills.
   c. Produces local symptoms—local pain, tenderness, and swelling along involved lymphatics.
   d. Produces local lymph node symptoms—enlarged, red, and tender (acute lymphadenitis).
   e. Produces an abscess—necrotic and pus-producing (suppurative lymphadenitis)

Diagnostic Evaluation

1. Duplex ultrasound-easy noninvasive study
2. Lymphoscintigraphy—reliable alternative to lymphangiography using radioactive colloid material; detects obstruction or inflammation.
3. CT or MRI.
4. Lymphangiography—outlines lymphatic system.
5. Check feet for tinea pedis (athlete's foot), which is a common cause of bacterial entry into the skin and lymphatics.

Management

Lymphedema

1. Self-monitoring-monitor lymphedema, including serial measurement of limb circumference.
2. Leg elevation to reduce swelling.
3. Diet and exercise and maintenance of ideal body weight. Exercise and weight training.
4. Lymphedema therapy.
   a. Compression garments to help squeeze the fluid out of tissues. This may be in the form of medical-grade stockings or pneumatic compression, which provides intermittent pumping to squeeze fluid from the extremity. These may be used in upper or lower extremities.
   b. Manual lymphatic drainage, massage to help move fluid and myofascial release to break up fibrotic tissue.
   c. Complete decongestive therapy; see Table 14-5.
5. Diuretics are usually not effective and can worsen edema and promote volume depletion.
6. Experimental therapies: low lever laser therapy and gene therapy.
7. Surgery:
   a. Lymphatic bypass procedures.
   b. Excision of affected subcutaneous tissue and fascia with skin grafting.
   c. Transfer of superficial lymphatics to deep lymphatic system by buried dermal flap.
   d. Liposuction of lower-extremity lymphedema—limited; more common for upper extremity.

Lymphangitis

1. Administer empiric antibiotics.
2. Treat affected extremity by rest, elevation, and the application of hot, moist dressings.
3. Incise and drain if necrosis and abscess formation occur.
4. Treat tinea pedis, if present.

Complications

1. Abscess formation (rare with lymphangitis).
2. Firm, nonpitting lymphedema unresponsive to treatment (congenital lymphedema, called lymphedema praecox).
3. Elephantiasis secondary to parasite (*Filaria*)—chronic fibrosis of subcutaneous tissue and chronic swelling of the extremity (rare in the United States).
4. Septicemia.
5. Complications of surgery include flap necrosis, hematoma, abscess under flap, and cellulitis.

Table 14-5	Complete Decongestive Therapy
PHASE/TIME FRAME	**COMPONENTS**
Phase 1: Treatment 2–4 wk	Meticulous skin and nail care to prevent infection Therapeutic exercise Manual lymphatic drainage and compression using multilayer dressings
Phase 2: Maintenance ongoing (to conserve and optimize benefit of phase 1)	Compression garments during active awake hours Self-compression bandaging at night Skin care and continue exercise as needed Self-manual lymphatic drainage

Nursing Assessment

1. Assess extremity for edema and inflammation.
   a. Palpate edema to evaluate its quality (soft and pitting or firm and nonpitting).
   b. Note any areas of abscess formation (suppurative lymphadenitis).
2. Watch for signs of fever and chills.

Nursing Diagnoses

- Risk for Impaired Skin Integrity related to edema and/or inflammation.
- Acute Pain related to incision and/or surgery.

Nursing Interventions

Maintaining Skin Integrity

1. Apply elastic bandages or prescription compression stockings (after acute attack with lymphangitis).
2. Advise the patient to rest frequently with affected part elevated—each joint higher than the preceding one.
3. Make sure the patient washes and dries thoroughly the crevices of the skin if edema has caused skin folds.
4. Administer diuretics as prescribed to control excess fluid.
5. Give antibiotics or antifungals, as prescribed.
6. Recommend isometric exercises with extremity elevated.
7. Suggest moderate sodium restriction in diet.
8. Observe postoperatively for signs of infection.

Relieving Pain Postoperatively

1. Encourage comfortable positioning and immobilization of affected area.
2. Administer or teach patient to administer analgesics, as prescribed; monitor for adverse effects.
3. The use bed cradle to relieve pressure from bed covers.

Patient Education and Health Maintenance

1. Instruct patient on proper application of compression garments.
2. Encourage compliance with therapy, which often involves frequent rewrapping of compression bandages, exercise, and massage for several months.
3. Advise patient to avoid trauma to extremity.
4. Instruct patient to use lotions that are free of perfumes, which may irritate skin.
5. Advise patient to practice good hygiene to avoid superimposed infections.
6. Instruct patient about the signs and symptoms of infection to report to health care providers.
7. Instruct patient to inspect feet and legs daily for evidence of skin breakdown, particularly between toes, and to look for tinea pedis.

Evaluation: Expected Outcomes

- Skin is normal color and temperature, nontender, nonswollen, and intact.
- Verbalizes no pain on actively moving extremity.

SELECTED REFERENCES

American Diabetes Association. (2017). Standards of medical care in diabetes 2017. *Diabetes Care, 40*(Suppl 1), S1–S129.

Benjamin, E. J., Blaha, M. J., Chiuve, S. E., et al. (2017). Heart disease and stroke statistics-2017 update: A report from the American Heart Association. *Circulation, 135*, e146–e603. Available: *www.circ.ahajournals.org/content/early/2017/01/25/CIR.0000000000000485 www.nice.org.uk/guidance/CG092*

Branas, A., & Cohn, J. (2016). Treatment of lymphedema: Complete decongestive therapy. *OncoLink*. Philadelphia, PA: Trustees of the University of Pennsylvania. Available: *www.oncolink.org/support/side-effects/lymphedema/lymphedema-what-you-need-to-know/treatment-for-lymphedema-complete-decongestive-therapy-cdt*

Dupras, D., Bluhm, J., Felty, C., et al. (2013). Institute for Clinical Systems Improvement. *Venous thromboembolism diagnosis and treatment.* Available: *www.icsi.org/guidelines__more/catalog_guidelines_and_more/catalog_guidelines/catalog_cardiovascular_guidelines/vte_treatment/*

Elliott, W., & Varon, J. (2016). Drugs used for the treatment of hypertensive emergencies. *UpToDate.* Available: *www.uptodate.com/contents/drug-treatment-of-hypertensive-emergencies*

Gerhard-Herman, M., Gornik, H., Barrett, C., et al. (2017). AHA/ACC guideline on the management of patients with lower extremity peripheral artery disease. A report of the American College of Cardiology/American Heart Association Task Force on Clinical Practice Guidelines. *Journal of the American College of Cardiology, 69*(11), e71–e126.

Go, A., Bauman, M., King, S., et al. (2014). An effective approach to high blood pressure control. *Journal of the American College of Cardiology, 63*(12), 1230–1238.

Guyatt, G., Akl, E., Crowther, M., et al. (2012). Executive summary: Antithrombotic therapy and prevention of thrombosis, 9th ed: American College of Chest Physicians Evidence-Based Clinical Practice Guidelines. *Chest, 141*(2 Suppl), 7S–47S.

Hering, D., Lambert, E. A., Marusic, P., et al. (2013). Substantial reduction in single sympathetic nerve firing after renal denervation in patients with resistant hypertension. *Hypertension, 61*, 457–464.

Hinkle, J., & Cheever, K. (2016). *Brunner and Suddarth's textbook of medical-surgical nursing* (13th ed.). Philadelphia, PA: Lippincott Williams & Wilkins.

Holbrook, A., Schulman, S., Witt, D. M., et al. (2012). Evidence-Based management of anticoagulant therapy: Antithrombotic therapy and prevention of thrombosis, 9th ed: American College of Chest Physicians Evidence-Based Clinical Practice Guidelines. *Chest, 141*(2 Suppl), e152S–e184S.

James, P. A., Oparil, S., Carter, B., et al. (2014). Evidence based guidelines for the management of high blood pressure in adults (JNC 8). *JAMA, 311*(5), 507–520.

Johnson, M. P. (2013). Transitions to care in patients receiving oral anticoagulants: General principles, procedures and impact of new oral anticoagulants. *Journal of Cardiovascular Nursing, 28*(1), 54–65.

Kearon, C., Ake, E., Ornelas, J., et al. (2016). Antithrombotic therapy for VTE disease. *Chest, 149*(2), 315–352.

Marston, W. (2015). Efficacy of endovenous ablation of the Saphenous veins for prevention and healing of venous ulcers. *Journal of Vascular Surgery Venous and Lymphatic Disorders, 3*(1), 113–116.

Mozaffarian, D., Benjamin, E., Go, A., et al. (2015). Heart disease and stroke statistics-2015 update: A report from the American Heart Association. *Circulation, 131*, e29–e322.

O'Donnell, T., Rasmussen, J., & Sevick-Muraca, E. (2016). New diagnostic modalities in the evaluation of lymphedema. *Journal of Vascular Surgery Venous and Lymphatic Disorders, 5*(2), 261–273.

Prins, M. H., Lensing, A. W. A., Bauersachs, R., et al. on behalf of the EINSTEIN investigators. (2013). Oral rivaroxaban versus standard therapy for the treatment of symptomatic venous thromboembolism. *Thrombosis Journal, 11*(1), 21.

Ridner, S., Fu, M., Wanshai, A., et al. (2012). Self-management of lymphedema: A systematic review of the literature form 2004–2011. *Nursing Research, 61*(4), 291–299.

Solomon, J., & Hume, A. (2016). Direct oral anticoagulants: A patient-centered review. *Journal of Nurse Practitioners, 12*(8), 523–529.

The EINSTEIN-PE Investigators. (2012). Oral rivaroxaban for the treatment of symptomatic pulmonary embolism. *New England Journal of Medicine, 366*(14), 1287–1297.

U.S. Preventive Services Task Force. (2014). *Guide to preventive services: Screening for abdominal aortic aneurysm.* Available: *www.uspreventiveservicestaskforce.org/*

Vedantham, S., Sista, A., Klein, S., et al. (2014). Quality improvement guidelines for the treatment of lower extremity deep vein thrombosis with use of endovascular thrombus removal. *Journal of Interventional Radiology, 25*(9), 1317–1325.

15
Neurologic Disorders

OVERVIEW AND ASSESSMENT

See additional online content: Procedure Guidelines 15-1

A baseline neurologic assessment is needed to detect changes in neurologic function and includes a patient history, general physical examination, and thorough neurologic examination. An important goal of the neurologic assessment is to identify the minimum amount of stimulation required to elicit maximum response. Common manifestations of neurologic dysfunction include motor, sensory, autonomic, and cognitive deficits. By exploring these symptoms, obtaining a pertinent history, and performing a thorough neurologic examination, the reader will gain an understanding of the underlying disorder and become skilled in planning care for patients with neurologic disorders (see Standards of Care Guidelines 15-1, page 347). See Chapter 5, page 65, for neurologic examination techniques. Documentation using appropriate terminology and comparison of right to left for asymmetrical findings is important. See Box 15-1, page 347, for definitions of findings.

Radiology and Imaging

Structural and functional imaging techniques have evolved to facilitate the rapid diagnosis and treatment of neurologic disorders. Brain mapping describes the process of translating the brain into a functionally useful group of dynamic maps or patterns. The diagnosis and evaluation of neurologic disorders is increasingly guided by functional brain mapping techniques that detect changes in brain patterns associated with neuropathology. Structural or anatomic imaging reveals information about the structure of the nervous system, including the brain and spinal cord. Functional or physiologic imaging focuses on the function of the brain and biochemical and metabolic processes in brain cells.

Computed Tomography

Description
1. Computed tomography (CT) is a structural imaging study that uses a computer-based x-ray to provide a cross-sectional image of the brain. A computer calculates differences in tissue absorption of the x-ray beams. The CT scan produces a three-dimensional view of structures in the brain and

STANDARDS OF CARE GUIDELINES 15-1
Neurologic Disorders

When caring for patients with neurologic disorders, consider the following assessments and interventions:

- Use age-appropriate assessment and examination techniques.
- Be aware of the status of the patient when assuming care, so comparison can be made with subsequent assessments.
- Perform a thorough systematic assessment, including mental status, vital signs, and cardiovascular status.
- Document the patient's condition to provide a record for continuity of care.
- Provide translation services for patients who have difficulty understanding or speaking English because this may impact the interpretation of the neurologic examination.
- Evaluate for signs of worsening neurologic condition through a systematic examination. Follow the institutional guidelines and clinician's orders regarding the frequency of assessments. If the patient shows signs of neurologic deterioration, more frequent assessment and/or interventions may be necessary.
- Be cautious in the administration of sedatives, opiates, or other medications that affect neurologic functioning because these may mask signs of neurologic deterioration.
- Notify appropriate health care provider of new or worsening neurologic symptoms, such as a change in behavior or level of consciousness; a change in functioning of the cranial nerves; motor, sensory, or neurovascular deficits; or alterations in the pattern of breathing or vital signs. Implement appropriate interventions for acute changes in neurologic status.
- Institute safety precautions for patients with neurologic deficits because they may be especially prone to falls. Follow institutional guidelines for patients with seizure disorder.
- Assess the patient's level of functioning in his or her activities of daily living. For those with cranial nerve or motor deficits, assess for difficulty swallowing prior to eating. For patients with difficulty swallowing, implement appropriate institutional protocols to prevent aspiration. This may include contacting the primary clinician to obtain an evaluation from a speech therapist or changing the diet.
- Use a multidisciplinary approach to care when indicated, including medical and surgical specialists, pharmacists, dietitian/nutritional therapist, physical/occupational/speech therapists, and rehabilitation specialists.
- Be aware that families or caretakers of patients with cognitive impairment or who are nonverbal may be able to provide assistance in the interpretation of behavioral cues.
- Assess family support and coping throughout the trajectory of the disease. Social issues (such as financial, community support systems, etc.) may require the expertise of a social worker or other clinical resource support personnel.

BOX 15-1 Definitions of Neurologic Findings

Acalculia—inability to do mathematical calculations.
Agnosia—inability to recognize sensory input.
Amaurosis fugax—sudden, temporary, or fleeting blindness, not caused by disease of the eye.
Anisocoria—inequality in size of the pupils.
Apraxia—inability to perform coordinated movements.
Confabulation—fluent, nonsensical speech.
Decerebrate rigidity (extensor posturing)—dysfunction of vestibulospinal tract and the RAS of the upper brain stem; jaw clenched, neck extended, elbows extended, forearms pronated, wrists flexed, knees extended, and feet plantar flexed.
Decorticate rigidity (flexor posturing)—dysfunction of corticospinal tract above the brain stem; arms adducted, elbows and wrists flexed, legs extended and internally rotated, and feet plantar flexed.
Dyslexia—visual aphasia.
Dysarthria—difficulty speaking.
Dyspraxia—partial loss of ability to perform coordinated movements.
Fluent aphasia (Wernicke's, sensory)—comprehension is poor but speech is fluent and nonsensical.
Homonymous hemianopsia—corresponding visual field deficits in half of the visual field bilaterally.
Micrographia—change in handwriting with the script becoming smaller and more cramped.
Nonfluent aphasia (Broca's, motor)—comprehension intact but has poor expression through speech.
Nystagmus—involuntary oscillation of the eyeball, vertical, horizontal, or rotary.
Paratonia—progressively increasing and irregular resistance to passive movements.

distinguishes between soft tissues and water. Intravenous (IV) contrast dye may be used to examine the integrity of the blood–brain barrier. New multidetector scanners allow for rapid imaging.

2. CT of the brain is primarily used to detect cerebral hemorrhage, whereas CT of the brain with contrast is used to detect tumors and inflammatory disorders.
3. Spinal CT may be used to evaluate lower back pain due to bony lesions or degenerative changes. CT myelography is typically reserved for those who have had previous spinal surgery or a questionable diagnosis.
4. May be used when magnetic resonance imaging (MRI) is contraindicated (metallic or electronic implants) or not tolerated (claustrophobia).
5. *Advantages of CT*: Widespread availability, short imaging time, excellent images of bone, and 100% sensitivity for detection of cerebral hemorrhage.
6. *Disadvantages of CT*: Does not provide information about function of tissues; exposes the patient to ionizing radiation at higher doses than traditional x-rays; imposes a weight restriction of 300 pounds; if contrast is used, there is the risk of contrast-induced nephropathy.

Nursing and Patient Care Considerations

1. Instruct the patient to remove metal items, such as earrings, eyeglasses, and hair clips.
2. Ask whether the patient has an allergy to iodine or history of previous allergy to IV dye to determine if the patient needs to be premedicated.
3. Evaluate for adequate renal function if contrast will be used.
4. Tell the patient to expect a sensation of feeling flushed if contrast dye is injected through the IV catheter.
5. Inform the patient that the procedure usually takes less than 5 minutes.

6. Request that the patient remain as immobile as possible during the examination.
7. Tell the patient to resume usual activities after the procedure.
8. Encourage increased fluid intake for the rest of the day to assist in expelling the contrast dye.

Magnetic Resonance Imaging

Description

1. Conventional MRI is a noninvasive structural imaging procedure that uses powerful magnetic field and radiofrequency waves to create an image. When tissue is placed in a strong magnetic field, hydrogen atoms in the tissue line up within the field. In MRI, pulsating radiofrequency waves are applied to the magnetic field to alter the tissue magnetization, creating a clear image of the tissue.
2. MRI is the imaging procedure of choice for most neurologic diseases (eg, detection of demyelinating diseases, nonacute hemorrhage, and cerebral tumors; evaluation of spinal cord injury (SCI), acute herniated disks, and cerebral infarction) and has largely replaced myelography, a more invasive procedure. See Table 15-1 for comparison to CT.
3. Specific protocols have been developed for trauma, stroke, and epilepsy.
4. MRI may be ordered with or without contrast. The contrast (gadolinium) alters the magnetic properties of tissue to differentiate tissue types. Contrast may be administered via IV line, by mouth, or through insertion into the rectum.
5. Closed MRI uses scanning equipment that resembles a tunnel-like chamber. Open MRI uses more sophisticated equipment that does not involve a closed chamber. During open MRI, the patient can comfortably see the surroundings from all views while the scan is in progress. This is ideal for patients who are claustrophobic or anxious, children, older adults, and the very obese.
6. Imaging orientation:

   a. Axial—slice dividing the head into upper and lower halves.
   b. Coronal—slice dividing the head into front and back halves.
   c. Sagittal—slice dividing the head into left and right halves.
7. Imaging sequences:
   a. T1—excellent tissue discrimination that provides anatomic images.
   b. T2—sensitive to the presence of increased water and visualization of edema for differentiation of normal tissue and pathologic changes.
   c. MRI with gadolinium—improves specificity of normal/abnormal tissue. With blood–brain barrier disruption, there is leakage of contrast medium. The pattern of contrast uptake into brain tissue helps differentiate such conditions as central nervous system (CNS) infections, neoplasms, meningeal diseases, and noninfectious inflammatory processes.
   d. Fluid-attenuated inversion recovery—evaluates edema within white matter; also used to identify subarachnoid disease.
   e. Diffusion-weighted imaging (DWI)—helps to evaluate the extent of a stroke and demyelinating disease and differentiates tumors from abscesses; shows increased enhancement with cytotoxic edema.
   f. Apparent diffusion coefficient (ADC)—shows decreased attenuation associated with acute stroke.
   g. DWI/ADC mismatch—increased enhancement on DWI in conjunction with decreased enhancement on ADC indicates acute stroke.
   h. Perfusion-weighted imaging (PWI)—evaluates cerebral blood flow, transit time, and blood volume. Useful in the evaluation of the extent of the ischemia stroke and determining whether there is salvageable tissue or a penumbra.
   i. DWI/PWI mismatch—increased enhancement on DWI with flow deficit on PWI indicates acute stroke.
   j. MRI single-photon emission computed tomography (SPECT)—provides assessment of neurochemicals (choline, lactate, *N*-acetylaspartate, glutamine/glutamate) for differentiation of brain tumors, abscess, demyelinating disease, and postradiation necrosis
   k. Swan—useful in the evaluation microscopic bleeds and small blood vessels
   l. GRE—useful in the evaluation of small lesions.
8. *Advantages of MRI*: No ionizing radiation, sensitivity to blood flow, imaging in several planes, and superior visualization of soft tissues. An important advantage is its ability to distinguish water, iron, fat, and blood. Sensitive to detection of white matter changes and valuable in detecting changes associated with Alzheimer disease and multiple sclerosis.
9. *Disadvantages of MRI*: Contraindicated for patients with pacemakers, nontitanium aneurysm clips, or other implanted objects that could be dislodged by the magnetic field. Dental amalgam, gold, and stainless steel are generally considered safe but may distort the image. If contrast is used, there is the risk of contrast-induced nephropathy. MRI scanner has the appearance of a tunnel-like chamber, and its constricted opening prevents its use for extremely obese people. Because of its narrow dimensions, MRI may induce claustrophobic and anxiety reactions, so antianxiety medication may be necessary before the procedure or an open MRI may be used.

Table 15-1 Comparison of CT and MRI		
CONSIDERATIONS	**CT**	**MRI**
Radiation exposure	• Minimal	• None
Imaging planes	• Axial, coronal, and sagittal	• Axial, coronal, and sagittal
Cost	• Several hundred dollars	• Several thousand dollars, but dependent on protocol being used
Advantages	• Rapid evaluation for intracranial hemorrhage and subarachnoid hemorrhage	• Detection of stroke, multiple sclerosis, epilepsy, tumors
Disadvantages	• Poor visualization of anatomic structures; radiation exposure	• May result in claustrophobia • May need prior x-rays if metallic fragments are suspected—if identified, cannot complete study

BOX 15-2	Contrast-Induced Nephropathy

When IV contrast medium is to be used in any radiologic study, renal function must be adequate to clear the substance. Check for risk factors for contrast-induced nephropathy:

- Renal insufficiency (creatinine level greater than 1.5 or a glomerular filtration rate of less than 60 mL/minute).
- Diabetic nephropathy and other conditions that cause reduced renal perfusion.
- High total dose of contrast (less than 5 mL/kg or greater than 100 mL).

If risk factors are present, hydration with normal saline starting 1 hour prior to the procedure and for 6 hours following the procedure is recommended.

Metformin should be held for 24 hours before any procedure and for 48 hours after the procedure if IV contrast is utilized.

Nursing and Patient Care Considerations

1. Encourage the patient to use the bathroom before the procedure because it may take from 20 to 60 minutes, though the scan time is dependent on the protocol requested and number of scans performed.
2. Instruct the patient to remove metal items, including eyeglasses, jewelry, hair clips, hearing aids, dentures, and clothing with zippers, buckles, or metal buttons.
3. Evaluate for adequate renal function if contrast will be used (see Box 15-2, above).
4. Encourage the patient to remain as still as possible during the procedure.
5. Describe the tunnel-like narrow chamber of the closed MRI scanner and inform the patient that it sometimes causes feelings of anxiety or claustrophobia. Evaluate the need for sedation.
6. Inform the patient the scanner will make a dull, thumping noise throughout the procedure.
7. Tell the patient to resume usual activities after the procedure.

Functional MRI

Description

1. Functional MRI (fMRI) is an imaging study that aids in identifying regions of the brain activated by particular stimuli and tasks. Imaging is performed during presentation of a stimulus or performance of a specific task and during rest periods. A statistical comparison is performed with images obtained during the stimulus/task periods compared with those performed during the rest periods by evaluating the conversion of oxyhemoglobin to deoxyhemoglobin and utilization of glucose, which occurs during normal brain activity. Involves IV administration of contrast material that lowers signal intensity on MRI in relation to blood flow as the material passes through the brain.
2. *Advantages of fMRI*: Does not use ionizing radiation and can be applied repeatedly in the same patient without risk. Offers potential in early detection of patients with prodromal dementia. It is also useful in preoperative evaluation of patients with lesions (tumors, seizure foci) adjacent to eloquent areas of the brain (speech center, premotor and motor cortex, and memory centers).
3. *Disadvantages of fMRI*: Same as MRI.

Nursing and Patient Care Considerations

1. Instruct the patient as for MRI. Full cooperation of the patient is vital for head motion and task performance reasons. Global cognitive impairment, aphasia, neglect, substantial sensory disturbances, and severe depression are usually exclusion criteria. The performance of motor tasks during imaging should be monitored.
2. Medications that may interfere with performance of tasks during the procedure should be avoided, if possible, including benzodiazepines, sedatives, and opioids.

Positron Emission Tomography

Description

1. Positron emission tomography (PET) is a computer-based imaging technique that permits study of the brain's function by evaluating the metabolism, blood flow, and chemical processes within the brain. PET measures emissions of particles of injected radioisotopes—called positrons—and converts them to an image of the brain.
2. PET scanners are not frequently used or widely available because of their high cost, and PET requires sophisticated equipment to produce its radioisotopes, or positron emitter.
3. A glucose-like solution and mildly radioactive tracers are combined for injection or inhalation. After injection into the arterial bloodstream or inhalation of this radioactive compound, pairs of gamma rays are emitted into adjacent tissue during radioactive decay. The PET scanner measures the gamma rays to determine how quickly the tissues absorb the radioactive isotopes. A computer processes the data into an image that shows where the radioactive material is located, corresponding to cellular metabolism.
4. *Advantages of PET*: Provides information on patterns of glucose and oxygen metabolism. Areas of decreased metabolism indicate dysfunction. PET is useful for early detection of Alzheimer disease and other dementias, Parkinson disease, amyotrophic lateral sclerosis (ALS), Huntington disease, multiple sclerosis, and psychiatric disorders, such as depression or schizophrenia. PET can also help locate/identify abnormal brain activity, such as seizure foci, and assess brain function after stroke.
5. *Disadvantages of PET*: Ionizing radiation, high initial cost.

Nursing and Patient Care Considerations

1. Inform the patient that this procedure requires injection or inhalation of a radioactive substance that emits positively charged particles. Explain that the image is created when the negative particles found in the body combine with the positive particles of the imaging substance.
2. Explain that, after injection of the radioisotope, the patient will be asked to rest quietly on a stretcher for about 45 minutes to allow the substance to circulate.
3. Reassure the patient that radiation exposure is minimal.
4. Encourage the patient to void before the test because the scan and associated procedures may take several hours.
5. Advise the patient to increase fluid intake after the procedure to flush out the radioisotope and to resume meals.
6. Tell the patient that it may take a few days to get results of the PET scan because it requires processing before it is available for interpretation.

Single Photon Emission Computed Tomography

Description

1. SPECT is a widely available noninvasive functional imaging technique that evaluates cerebral vascular supply. A radioactive tracer is administered by inhalation or injection into the bloodstream; the tracer then decays to emit only a single photon. It uses a rotating camera to track the single photons emitted from radioactive decay and collects information from multiple views. Evaluation of the radioactive tracers creates images that show cerebral blood flow in various regions of the brain.
2. The radioactive tracer compounds used are commercially prepared and do not require the specialized equipment used in PET scanning.
3. SPECT is typically used to evaluate cerebral blood flow in patients with ischemic stroke, subarachnoid hemorrhage (SAH), migraine, dementia (including Alzheimer disease), epilepsy, and other degenerative diseases.
4. *Advantages of SPECT*: Can perform hemodynamic, chemical, and functional imaging; widely available.
5. *Disadvantages of SPECT*: Ionizing radiation, provides only relative measurements.

Nursing and Patient Care Considerations

1. Inform the patient that this is a noninvasive procedure that should cause minimal discomfort.
2. Tell the patient that results of the scan are typically available for interpretation by a specialist immediately after the procedure.

Transcranial Doppler Studies

Description

1. Transcranial Doppler (TCD) ultrasonography involves noninvasive testing to measure flow changes in the form of velocities of the cerebral arteries. It helps evaluate vasospasm post-SAH, occlusion, or flow abnormalities as with stroke.
2. Bone windows (temporal, transorbital, or foramen magnum) are accessed using a fiberoptic probe after application of ultrasound gel. The fiberoptic probe is directed at a specific artery, and the velocities are then recorded.
3. Specific criteria are utilized for identification of each cerebral vessel prior to assessment of the vessel (specific bone window, depth, flow direction, and waveform).
4. *Advantages of TCD studies*: Low cost; can be performed at bedside and repeated as needed (useful in monitoring trends).
5. *Disadvantages of TCD studies*: Results are operator dependent; inability to obtain signal; limited data on sensitivity and specificity.

Nursing and Patient Care Considerations

1. Explain that the study will be done with patient in a reclining position.
2. Inform the patient that the test normally takes less than 1 hour, depending on the number of arteries that are to be studied.

CT Perfusion

Description

1. CT perfusion involves rapid injection (5 to 10 mL/second) of 40 mL of iodine contrast during continuous scanning. Computer analysis of "wash-in" and "wash-out" of the contrast generates a single-slice acquisition blood flow map.
2. The test requires a 20 gauge catheter or larger for injection of the contrast. Contrast is cleared through the kidneys; therefore, renal function should be evaluated prior to study to reduce the risk of contrast-induced nephropathy (see page 349).
3. CT scan is programmed to analyze specific area of concern. Three 1-cm thick computer-generated images are produced that reflect relative cerebral blood flow, relative blood volume, and mean transit time.
4. *Advantages of CT perfusion*: 90% sensitivity and 100% specificity for cerebral ischemia; can be performed in conjunction with CT angiogram. Can be used in evaluating cerebral vasospasm in aneurysmal SAH, though the sensitivity and specificity is unknown.
5. *Disadvantages of CT perfusion*: Limited anatomic assessment; radiation exposure; if contrast is used, there is the risk of contrast-induced nephropathy; requires large-bore catheter.

Nursing and Patient Care Considerations

1. Instruct the patient about the rationale for placement of large-bore catheter.
2. Assess the patient for contrast allergy and premedicate, if indicated.
3. Inform the patient that radiation exposure, although present, is minimal.

Cerebral Angiography

Description

1. Following local anesthesia, a radiopaque dye is injected through a catheter in the femoral artery (or brachial artery if femoral is inaccessible) and passed through one of the major cervical blood vessels to assess cerebral circulation. Serial x-rays are taken after contrast dye illuminates the cerebral arterial and venous systems. The structure and patency of cerebral arteries are examined. Contrast is cleared through the kidneys. The test is frequently performed on an outpatient basis, unless the patient is already hospitalized.
2. Three-dimensional imaging is available for more thorough evaluation of vascular abnormalities.
3. *Advantages of cerebral angiography*: Useful in detection of stenosis or occlusion, aneurysms, and vessel displacement due to pathologic processes (eg, tumor, abscess, hematoma).
4. *Disadvantages of cerebral angiography*: Involves considerable exposure to radiation. Contraindicated in patients with a stroke in evolution. Potential complications: temporary or permanent neurologic deficit, including stroke, anaphylaxis, bleeding or hematoma at the IV site, and impaired circulation in the extremity distal to the injection site, usually the femoral artery. There is risk of contrast-induced nephropathy.

Nursing and Patient Care Considerations

1. Omit the meal before the test, although clear liquids may be taken.
2. Evaluate for adequate renal function; should have recent normal serum creatinine.
3. Ask the patient about allergies and specifically rule out presence of iodine allergy, which requires pretest preparation. Commonly, patients with allergy to iodine also have allergies to radiopaque contrast media that may cause severe reaction.
4. Options for pretest allergy prevention include the following:
   a. Elective procedure: Give prednisone 50 mg orally 13, 7, and 1 hour prior to contrast and diphenhydramine 50 mg orally 1 hour prior to contrast.

b. Urgent procedure: Give methylprednisolone IV and diphenhydramine 50 mg orally, IM, or IV 1 hour prior to contrast.

5. Mark pedal peripheral pulses.

6. Explain that a local anesthetic will be used to insert a catheter into the femoral artery (brachial artery may be used) and threaded into the required cerebral vessel.

7. Tell the patient to expect some discomfort when the catheter is inserted into the artery. Additionally, the sensation of a warm, flushed feeling and metallic taste should be expected when the dye is injected.

8. Caution the patient that he or she will need to lie still during the procedure and that he or she will be asked to hold breath intermittently during scanning.

9. After angiography:
   a. Maintain bed rest and do not flex lower extremities, as ordered, and monitor vital signs. Instruct the patient to maintain bed rest for up to 6 hours. If a closing device is utilized, the time can be reduced to 2 to 3 hours.
   b. Check the patient frequently for neurologic symptoms, such as motor or sensory alterations, reduced level of consciousness (LOC), speech disturbances, dysrhythmias, or blood pressure (BP) fluctuations.
   c. Monitor puncture site for bleeding, hematoma, and pulses, as ordered. Apply pressure if bleeding or hematoma is noted and inform physician.
   d. Evaluate renal function and monitor for adverse reaction to contrast medium (eg, restlessness, respiratory distress, tachycardia, facial flushing, nausea, and vomiting).
   e. Assess skin color, temperature, and peripheral pulses of the extremity distal to the IV site—change may indicate impaired circulation due to occlusion. Inform physician, if noted.

Computed Tomographic Angiography

Description

1. CT angiography is a minimally invasive three-dimensional (3-D) imaging technique that uses multisectional spiral CT imaging in conjunction with rapid power injection of contrast (50 mL) into a large antecubital vein. Multiple, thin slices are reconstructed to provide 3-D imaging of cerebral vasculature.

2. Proper timing of contrast injection with initialization of CT scans is essential to optimize intravascular enhancement.

3. *Advantages of CT angiography*: Speed of scanning allows for unstable patients to be evaluated; increasing in availability.

4. *Disadvantages of CT angiography*: Exposure to radiation; need for large-bore (18 to 20 gauge) catheter; potential for anaphylaxis; contraindicated for patients with acute/chronic renal failure.

Nursing and Patient Care Considerations

1. Restrict food for 4 to 6 hours before procedure.

2. Assess for contrast allergy and premedicate, if indicated.

3. Evaluate renal function as contrast is cleared through kidneys. Elevated creatinine may preclude the individual from obtaining the study.

Magnetic Resonance Angiography/Venography of the Brain

1. Magnetic resonance angiography/venography (MRA/MRV) is a 3-D phase contrast technique. The test focuses on high signal or blood flow while suppressing background nonactive tissue.

2. Two flow-opposing acquisitions are obtained, and the computer subtracts the background signal to construct the cerebral vasculature.

3. *Advantages of MRA/MRV*: No exposure to radiation.

4. *Disadvantages of MRA/MRV*: Less sensitivity than CT angiography (sensitivity increases in aneurysms larger than 5 mm).

Nursing and Patient Care Considerations

1. Same as those for MRI, page 349.

Dynamic Volume Computed Tomography

Description

1. This scanning technique can include entire organs, such as the heart or brain, in a single rotation and enables dynamic processes, such as blood volume and time to peak, to be observed.

2. The scanning process takes less time and requires a smaller dose of iodinated contrast and less radiation than does conventional CT, making it an ideal diagnostic test in emergency situations (heart attack or stroke) or for those who cannot tolerate large doses of iodine contrast (renal disease).

Nursing and Patient Care Considerations

1. The general considerations for conventional CT are the same.

2. Inform the patient about lying flat on the table while the tube revolves around the area to be scanned.

3. If contrast will be used, the patient will most likely have an IV catheter placed for the injection of dye. A sensation of warmth or metallic taste in the mouth may be experienced after the dye injection.

Other Diagnostic Tests

Other diagnostic tests include lumbar puncture, which provides information about the CNS through direct contact with the cerebrospinal fluid (CSF); a variety of tests that measure electrical impulses in portions of the nervous system; and neuropsychological evaluation.

Lumbar Puncture

Description

1. A needle is inserted into the lumbar subarachnoid space, usually between the third and fourth lumbar vertebrae, and CSF is withdrawn for diagnostic and therapeutic purposes.

2. Purposes include the following:
   a. Obtaining CSF for examination (microbiologic, serologic, cytologic, or chemical analysis).
   b. Measuring cerebrospinal pressure and assisting in detection of obstruction of CSF circulation.
   c. Determining the presence or absence of blood in the spinal fluid.
   d. Aiding in the diagnosis of viral or bacterial meningitis, subarachnoid or intracranial hemorrhage, tumors, and brain abscesses.
   e. Administering antibiotics and cancer chemotherapy intrathecally in certain cases.
   f. Determining levels of tau protein and beta-amyloid in the CSF—a new test that may be used to assist in the diagnosis of Alzheimer disease. Elevated levels of tau protein and decreased levels of beta-amyloid are associated with Alzheimer disease.

Nursing and Patient Care Considerations

1. Assist the patient to side-lying position with small pillow under head and a pillow between legs with back arched and knees drawn up toward abdomen. Alternately a sitting position, leaning forward, may be used, particularly for obese persons.
2. Assist in sending CSF sample tubes for evaluation.
3. After the procedure, support the patient in lying flat for 2 hours, ensuring hydration, and monitor for a spinal headache and CSF leak.

Electroencephalography

Description

1. EEG measures electrical activity of the brain cells. Electrodes are attached to multiple sites on the scalp to provide a recording of electrical activity that is generated in the cerebral cortex. Electrical impulses are transmitted to an electroencephalograph, which magnifies and records these impulses as brain waves on a strip of paper. New devices allow for continuous EEG monitoring of selective areas of the brain; thus limited data are collected. It is useful in the intensive care unit (ICU) setting for continuous monitoring to evaluate for seizure activation.
2. Provides physiologic assessment of cerebral activity for diagnosis of epilepsy, alterations in brain activity in coma, and organic brain syndrome and sleep disorders. Particularly helpful in the investigation of patients with seizures.
3. Usually performed in a room designed to eliminate electrical interference; however, in the case of a comatose patient, it may be performed at bedside using a portable unit.
4. Restlessness and fatigue can alter brain wave patterns.
5. For a baseline recording, the patient is instructed to lie still and relax with eyes closed. After a baseline recording in a resting phase, the patient may be tested in various stress situations (eg, asked to hyperventilate for 3 minutes, look at a flashing strobe light) to elicit abnormal electrical patterns.
6. In patients with epilepsy, continuous monitoring is performed with video monitoring. This is useful for interpretation and correlation of physiologic seizure activity and clinical seizures.
   a. Grids or strips are placed intraoperatively for more accurate assessment of seizure foci.
   b. Mapping of seizure activity is performed to determine precise location of seizure foci.
   c. Once foci are located, the site is evaluated for possible surgical resection.

Nursing and Patient Care Considerations

1. For routine EEG, tranquilizers, anticonvulsants, sedatives, and stimulants should be held for 24 to 48 hours before the study.
2. Thoroughly wash and dry patient's hair to remove hair sprays, creams, or oils.
3. Explain that the electrodes will be attached to the patient's skull with a special paste.
4. Assure the patient that the electrodes will not cause shock, and encourage the patient to relax during the procedure because anxiety can affect brain wave patterns.
5. Meals should be taken as usual to avoid sudden changes in blood glucose levels.

Evoked Potential Studies

Description

1. These tests measure the brain's electrical responses to visual, somatosensory, or auditory stimuli.
   a. Visual evoked potentials—produced by asking the patient to look at rapidly reversing checkerboard patterns. These assist in evaluating multiple sclerosis and traumatic injury. EEG electrodes are placed over the occiput and record the transmission time from the retina to the occiput.
   b. Somatosensory evoked potentials—generated by stimulating a peripheral sensory nerve and useful in diagnosing peripheral nerve disease and injury. These measure transmission time up the spinal cord to the sensory cortex.
   c. Auditory evoked potentials—produced by applying sound, such as clicks, to help locate auditory lesions and evaluate integrity of the brain stem. The transmission time up the brain stem into the cortex is measured.
2. Can be performed intraoperatively or during interventional procedures in which the patient is under general anesthesia. Acute changes may indicate potential for deficits.

Nursing and Patient Care Considerations

1. Explain that the electrodes will be attached to the patient's scalp to measure the electrical activity of the nervous system. Placement of the electrodes will depend on the type of evoked potentials being measured.
2. Ask the patient to remove all jewelry.
3. Assure the patient that the procedure is not painful and does not cause any electric shock.
4. Inform the patient that the test usually takes 45 to 60 minutes.

Needle Electromyography

Description

1. In combination with nerve conduction studies, needle electromyography (EMG) is the gold standard for assessing the neurophysiologic characteristics of neuromuscular diseases. Because it is invasive and painful, its use is limited when activity from several muscles needs to be monitored simultaneously. It is the recording of a muscle's electrical impulses at rest and during contraction. A needle is attached to an electrode and inserted into a muscle. A mild electrical charge is delivered to stimulate the muscle at rest and during voluntary contraction. The response of the muscle is measured on an oscilloscope screen.
2. Useful in distinguishing lower motor neuron (LMN) disorders from muscle disorders (eg, ALS from muscular dystrophy).
3. Nerve conduction time, another diagnostic test, is often measured simultaneously.

Nursing and Patient Care Considerations

1. Explain that this test measures the electrical activity of muscles.
2. Advise the patient to avoid caffeine and tobacco products for 3 hours before the test, as these substances can affect test results.
3. Inform the patient that the procedure normally takes at least 1 hour.
4. Tell the patient a needle will be inserted through the skin into select muscles and to expect some degree of discomfort when the needle is inserted.
5. Inform the patient that, after the test, a mild analgesic or warm compresses may be needed to relieve muscle soreness.
6. Inform the patient to observe the needle insertion sites for bleeding, hematoma, redness, or other signs of infection and to notify the health care provider if any of these are observed.

Nerve Conduction Studies (Electroneurography)

Description

1. A peripheral nerve is stimulated electrically through the skin and underlying tissues. A recording electrode detects the response from the stimulated nerve. The time between the stimulation of the nerve and the response is measured on an oscilloscope, and speed of conduction along the nerve is calculated.
2. Used to determine LMN dysfunction, differentiating disease or injury in peripheral nerves, spinal nerve roots, or the anterior horn of the spinal cord by measuring nerve conduction velocity.

Nursing and Patient Care Considerations

1. Explain that surface-stimulating electrodes with special paste are applied and taped to the nerve site (leg, arm, or face).
2. Advise the patient that an electric current is passed through the electrode and that a mild sensation or slight discomfort may be experienced while the current is applied.

Neuropsychological Testing

Description

1. A series of tests that evaluate effects of neurologic disorders on cognitive functioning and behavior.
2. A neuropsychologist selects appropriate tests to determine the extent and type of functional deficits.
3. Paper-and-pencil tests, puzzles, and word and recall games are commonly used. Testing may assess the following:
   a. Intelligence, attention span, memory, judgment.
   b. Motor, speech, and sensory function.
   c. Affect, coping, and adaptation.
   d. Language quality, abstraction, distractibility.
   e. Ability to sequence learned behaviors.
   f. Used in diagnosis of organic brain dysfunction and dementia.
   g. Valuable in determining vocational rehabilitation training needs.
4. Utilized in some facilities to determine competency of a patient with regard to instituting durable power of attorney or need for guardianship.

Nursing and Patient Care Considerations

1. Assure the patient that these tests are not intended to evaluate mental illness.
2. Explain that testing evaluates the ability to remember, calculate numbers, and perform abstract reasoning.
3. The patient should be well rested because testing is mentally tiring and lengthy. A complete examination is a 4- to 6-hour process, depending on the patient's ability to concentrate.
4. Anticipate fatigue and frustration after the examination.

Polysomnography

Description

1. Polysomnography is a noninvasive, all-night sleep study that measures character of sleep, simultaneously monitoring EEG, cardiac and respiratory function, and movements during sleep. It is used to confirm fragmented sleep patterns in narcolepsy and sleep-related epilepsy.
2. Testing is time-consuming and labor-intensive. Procedures typically include multiple physiologic measures, such as EEG, EMG, electrocardiogram [ECG]), heart rate, respiratory effort, air flow, and oxygen saturation.

Nursing and Patient Care Considerations

1. Explain that the electrodes placed on the scalp, chest, extremities, and face will be uncomfortable but do not deliver electrical current.
2. Reassure the patient that a technician will be in the next room.
3. Advise the patient to wear comfortable nightwear.

Multisleep Latency Test

Description

1. Multisleep latency test (MSLT) is a sleep study performed during the day. It is the most widely objective assessment of daytime sleepiness and is commonly used to confirm a diagnosis of narcolepsy.
2. Testing consists of four "napping" periods of 20 to 35 minutes, during which time the patient lies down on a bed in a darkened room and is allowed to fall asleep. The multiple short sleep periods during the MSLT increase the observation of rapid-eye-movement (REM) periods.

Nursing and Patient Care Considerations

1. Explain the time and duration of the naps.
2. Reassure the patient of freedom to move about between naps.
3. Tell the patient to wear comfortable clothing and to bring reading or other materials for use between naps.

GENERAL PROCEDURES AND TREATMENT MODALITIES

See additional online content: Procedure Guidelines 15-2

Nursing Management of the Patient with an Altered State of Consciousness

Unconsciousness is a condition in which there is a depression of cerebral function ranging from stupor to coma. Coma results from impairment in both the arousal and the awareness of consciousness. The arousal of consciousness is mediated by the reticular activating system (RAS) in the brain stem, whereas the awareness component is mediated by cortical activity within the cerebral hemispheres.

Both arousal and awareness are assessed when using the Glasgow Coma Scale (GCS) as a measure of LOC (see Table 15-2).

When using the GCS, *coma* may be defined as no eye opening on stimulation, absence of comprehensible speech, and failure to obey commands. The GCS is designed to provide a rapid assessment of LOC and does not provide a means to monitor or localize neurologic dysfunction. Facility-generated neurologic assessment tools may be used in combination with the GCS to assess, monitor, and trend neurologic function.

An altered state of consciousness may be caused by many factors, including hypoxemia; trauma; neoplasms; vascular, degenerative, and infectious disorders; as well as a variety of metabolic disorders and structural neurologic lesions. Diagnostic evaluation and management depend on the underlying cause, overall intracranial dynamics, age, comorbidities, and general state of health.

Nursing Assessment

1. Assess eye opening (level of responsiveness).
   Eye opening = arousal
   Tracking = awareness
2. Assess neurologic function using the GCS. The GCS addresses eye opening, verbal responses, and motor responses. If the patient's eyes do not open spontaneously or to your voice,

Table 15-2 Glasgow Coma Scale

PARAMETER	FINDING	SCORE
Eye opening	Spontaneously	4
	To speech	3
	To pain	2
	Do not open	1
Best verbal response	Oriented	5
	Confused	4
	Inappropriate speech	3
	Incomprehensible sounds	2
	No verbalization	1
Best motor response	Obeys command	6
	Localizes pain	5
	Withdraws from pain	4
	Abnormal flexion	3
	Abnormal extension	2
	No motor response	1

Interpretation: Best score = 15; worst score = 3; 7 or less generally indicates coma; changes from baseline are most important.

then assess responses using painful stimuli by applying pressure against the nail bed, trapezius/axillary pinch, or sternum. Use the least amount of pain for the best response.

3. Assess cognitive function.
   a. Orientation.
      i. Person, place, and time.
      ii. Where are you, why are you here.
      iii. General information—national and local current events.
   b. Speech—aphasia and other problems (see Table 15-3).
      i. Expressive aphasia (motor/Broca's)—inability to express self.
      ii. Receptive aphasia (sensory/Wernicke's)—inability to understand the spoken language.
      iii. Global aphasia—inability to speak or understand spoken language.
      iv. Other aphasia syndromes—amnesia, conduction.
   c. Other alterations include the following:
      i. Confabulation—fluent, nonsensical speech.
      ii. Perseveration—continuation of thought process with inability to change train of thought without direction or repetition.

4. Assess motor function—voluntary versus reflexive:
   a. Voluntary movement.
      i. Normal complex movement—strength and symmetry in the upper extremities (UE), pronator drift proximally and grip strength distally; in the lower extremities (LE), leg lifts proximally and dorsi/plantar flexion distally.
      ii. Localization—ability to determine location of stimuli; patient localizes area of painful stimuli.
      iii. Withdrawal—abduction of the upper extremity; moving away from the stimuli.
   b. Reflexive movement.
      i. Abnormal flexor posturing (decorticate)—dysfunction of corticospinal tracts above the brain stem. Abnormal flexion of the UE with adduction of the UE, internal rotation of the upper extremity, wrist and extension, and internal rotation and plantar flexion of the LE.
      ii. Abnormal extension posturing (decerebrate)—dysfunction of vestibulospinal tract and the RAS of the upper brain stem. Abnormal extension, hyperpronation, and adduction of the UE and wrist flexion; abnormal extension and internal rotation of the LE with plantar flexion of the feet and toes.
      iii. Mixed posturing—varied extensor and flexor tone in UE.
      iv. Flaccid—medullary compression with complete loss of motor tone.

5. Test cranial nerve (CN) reflexes to assess for brain stem dysfunction.
   a. Assess pupil size, symmetry, and reaction to light.
   b. Assess extraocular movements (CNs III, IV, VI) and reflex eye movements elicited by head turning (oculocephalic response). This should not be performed on patients with suspected cervical spine injury, patients in a cervical collar, or patients known to have cervical spine injuries.
   c. The oculovestibular (caloric) response (CNs III, IV, VI, VIII) is tested by medical staff when the patient is comatose, as part of the brain death examination.
   d. Assess CNs V and VII together to evaluate facial pain, blink, eye closure, and grimace.
   e. Assess CNs IX, X, XII to evaluate gag, swallowing reflex, tongue protrusion, and patient's ability to handle own secretions.

6. Assess respiratory rate and pattern (normal, Kussmaul, Cheyne-Stokes, apneic).

Table 15-3 Differentiating Aphasia

APHASIA	FLUENCY	RATE	COMPREHENSION	GRAMMAR	REPETITION
Fluent (Wernicke/receptive aphasia)	Intact, although speech is nonsensical	Normal	Absent to poor	Intact	Intact
Nonfluent (Broca/expressive aphasia)	Poor	Slow, halting	Intact	Absent	Poor
Global	Poor	Slow	Absent	Absent	Poor
Conduction	Intact, although there is functional transposition of sounds with phonetic paraphrases	Normal	Intact	Intact	Poor
Anomic or amnesiac aphasia	Difficulty naming and finding words	Halting	Intact	Intact	Intact

7. Assess deep tendon reflexes; evaluate tone for spasticity, rigidity, and paratonia (abnormal resistance increasing throughout flexion and extension, indicating frontal lobe dysfunction).
8. Examine head for signs of trauma, and mouth, nose, and ears for evidence of edema, blood, and CSF (may indicate basilar skull fracture).
9. Monitor any change in neurologic status over time and report changes to health care provider, as indicated.

 KEY DECISION POINT A critical indicator of neurologic function is the LOC. A change in GCS of two or more points may be significant. If patient demonstrates deterioration, as evidenced by a change in neurologic examination, notify the health care provider without delay and reevaluate the neurologic status more often than required by orders based on nursing judgment.

Nursing Diagnoses

- Decreased Intracranial Adaptive Capacity.
- Ineffective Airway Clearance related to upper airway obstruction by tongue and soft tissues, inability to clear respiratory secretions.
- Risk for Imbalanced Fluid Volume related to inability to ingest fluids, dehydration from osmotic therapy (when used to reduce intracranial pressure [ICP]).
- Impaired Oral Mucous Membranes related to mouth breathing, absence of pharyngeal reflex, inability to ingest fluid.
- Risk for Impaired Skin Integrity related to immobility or restlessness.
- Impaired Tissue Integrity of cornea related to diminished/absent corneal reflex.
- Hyperthermia related to infectious process; damage to hypothalamic center.
- Impaired Urinary Elimination related to unconscious state.
- Bowel Incontinence related to unconscious state.

Nursing Interventions

Minimizing Secondary Brain Injury

1. Monitor for change in neurologic status, decreased LOC, onset of CN deficits.
2. Identify trends in neurologic function and communicate findings to medical staff.
3. Monitor response to pharmacologic therapy, including drug levels, as indicated.
4. Monitor laboratory data, CSF cultures, and Gram stain, if applicable, and communicate findings to medical staff.
5. Assess neurologic drains and dressings for patency and characteristics of drainage.
6. Institute measures to minimize risk for increased ICP, cerebral edema, seizures, or neurovascular compromise.
7. Adjust care to reduce risk of increasing ICP: body positioning in a neutral position (head aligned with shoulders) without flexing head, reduce hip flexion, distribute care throughout 24-hour period sufficiently for ICP to return to baseline.
8. Monitor temperature status; maintain normothermia. Institute cooling procedure as ordered.

Maintaining an Effective Airway

1. Position the patient to prevent the tongue from obstructing the airway, encourage drainage of respiratory secretions, and promote adequate exchange of oxygen and carbon dioxide.

2. Keep the airway free from secretions with suctioning. In the absence of cough and swallowing reflexes, secretions rapidly accumulate in the posterior pharynx and upper trachea and can lead to respiratory complications (eg, aspiration).
   a. Insert oral airway if tongue is paralyzed or is obstructing the airway. An obstructed airway increases ICP. This is considered a short-term measure.
   b. Prepare for insertion of cuffed endotracheal tube to protect the airway from aspiration and to allow efficient removal of tracheobronchial secretions.
   c. See page 176 for technique of tracheal suctioning.
   d. Use oxygen therapy as prescribed to deliver oxygenated blood to the CNS.
   e. Before suctioning, pretreat with sedative, opioid, or endotracheal lidocaine, if indicated.

Attaining and Maintaining Fluid and Electrolyte Balance

1. Monitor prescribed IV fluids carefully, maintaining euvolemia and minimizing large volumes of "free water," which may aggravate cerebral edema.
2. Maintain hydration and enhance nutritional status with use of enteral or parenteral fluids.
3. Measure urine output.
4. Evaluate pulses (radial, carotid, apical, and pedal) and measure BP; these parameters are a measure of circulatory adequacy/inadequacy.
5. Maintain circulation; support the BP and treat life-threatening cardiac dysrhythmias.

Maintaining Healthy Oral Mucous Membranes

1. Remove dentures. Inspect the patient's mouth for dryness, inflammation, and the presence of crusting.
2. Provide mouth care by brushing teeth and cleansing the mouth with appropriate solution every 2 to 4 hours to prevent parotitis (inflammation of parotid gland).
3. Apply lip emollient to maintain hydration and prevent dryness.

Skin Integrity

1. Keep the skin clean, dry, well lubricated, and free from pressure because comatose patients are susceptible to the formation of pressure ulcers.
2. Turn the patient from side to side on a regular schedule to relieve pressure areas and help clear lungs by mobilizing secretions; turning also provides kinesthetic (sensation of movement), proprioceptive (awareness of position), and vestibular (equilibrium) stimulation.
3. Reposition carefully after turning to prevent ischemia and shearing over pressure areas.
4. Position extremities in functional position, and monitor the skin underneath splints/orthosis to prevent skin breakdown and pressure neuropathies.
5. Perform range-of-motion (ROM) exercises of extremities at least four times daily; contracture deformities develop early in unconscious patients.

Maintaining Corneal Integrity

1. Protect the eyes from corneal irritation as the cornea functions as a shield. If the eyes remain open for long periods, corneal drying, irritation, and ulceration are likely to result.
2. Make sure the patient's eye is not rubbing against bedding if blinking and corneal reflexes are absent.
3. Inspect the condition of the eyes with a penlight.
4. Ensure that contact lenses have been removed.

5. Irrigate eyes with sterile saline or prescribed solution to remove discharge and debris.
6. Instill prescribed ophthalmic ointment in each eye to prevent glazing and corneal ulceration.
7. Apply eye patches, when indicated, ensuring that eyes remain closed under patch.

Reducing Fever

1. Look for possible sites of infections (respiratory, CNS, urinary tract, wound) when fever is present in an unconscious patient.
2. Monitor temperature frequently or continuously.
3. Control persistent elevations of temperature. Fever increases metabolic demands of the brain, decreases circulation and oxygenation, and results in cerebral deterioration.
   a. Monitor core temperature continuously and treat hyperthermia promptly. Hyperthermia increases the brain's metabolic rate and increases the risk of secondary injury. A body core temperature is 4 to 5 degrees lower than brain temperature.
   b. Maintain a cool ambient temperature. Anticipate potential for overcooling and make environmental adjustments accordingly (eg, operating room environment).
   c. Minimize excess covering on bed.
   d. Administer prescribed antipyretics.
   e. Use cool-water sponging and an electric fan blowing over the patient to increase surface cooling for hyperthermia resistant to antipyretics.
   f. Use an external cooling device to maintain normothermia, but avoid rapid overcooling. Intravascular cooling devices may also be used.

Promoting Urinary Elimination

1. An indwelling or external urethral catheter may be used for short-term management.
2. Use intermittent bladder catheterization for distention as soon as possible to minimize risk of infection. Palpate over the patient's bladder at intervals or use a bladder scan to detect urine retention and an overdistended bladder.
3. Monitor for fever and cloudy urine.
4. Initiate a bladder-training program as soon as consciousness is regained.

Promoting Bowel Function

1. Auscultate for bowel sounds; palpate lower abdomen for distention.
2. Observe for constipation due to immobility and lack of dietary fiber. Stool softener or laxative, scheduled or as needed, may be prescribed to promote bowel elimination. The goal is bowel movement every other day.
3. Monitor for diarrhea resulting from infection, antibiotics, enteric feedings, hyperosmolar fluids, and fecal impaction.
   a. Perform a rectal examination if fecal impaction is suspected.
   b. Use fecal collection bags and provide meticulous skin care if the patient has fecal incontinence.

Family Education and Support

1. Develop a supportive and trusting relationship with the family or significant other.
2. Provide information and frequent updates on the patient's condition and progress.
3. Involve them in routine care and teach procedures that they can perform at home.

4. Demonstrate and teach methods of sensory stimulation to be used frequently.
   a. Use physical touch and reassuring voice.
   b. Talk to the patient in a meaningful way even when the patient does not seem to respond. Assume the patient is able to hear even if unresponsive.
   c. Orient the patient periodically to person, time, and place.
5. Demonstrate and teach methods frequently used to manage restlessness/agitation.
   a. Eliminate distractions.
   b. Reduce environmental stimuli (turn off television and radio, close door).
   c. Use one-to-one communication.
   d. Talk slowly and simplify information without talking down to the person.
6. Teach the family to recognize and report unusual restlessness, which could indicate cerebral hypoxia, metabolic imbalance, or pain.
7. Enlist the help of the social worker, home health agency, or other resources to assist family with such issues as financial concerns, guardianship, need for additional follow-up care (rehabilitation, long-term care facility), need for medical equipment in home, and/or respite care.

Evaluation: Expected Outcomes

- Neurologic status remains at baseline or improved.
- Maintains clear airway; coughs up secretions.
- Absence of signs of dehydration.
- Intact, pink mucous membranes.
- No skin breakdown or erythema.
- Absence of trauma to cornea.
- Core temperature within normal limits.
- Absence of urinary tract infection (UTI); maintenance of normal bladder emptying.
- Bowel movement on regular basis in response to bowel regimen.

Nursing Management of the Patient with Increased Intracranial Pressure

Intracranial pressure (ICP) is the pressure exerted by the contents inside the cranial vault—the brain tissue (gray and white matter), CSF, and the blood volume. A pressure reading at or greater than 20 mm Hg is defined as increased ICP.

 EVIDENCE BASE American Association of Neuroscience Nurses. (2016). *AANN core curriculum for neuroscience nursing* (6th ed.). Glenview, IL: Author.

Pathophysiology and Etiology

1. ICP is composed of the following components and volume ratio: brain tissue, 80%; CSF, 10%; blood volume, 10%.
2. The Monro-Kellie doctrine states that the intracranial vault is a closed structure with a fixed intracranial volume. The intracranial contents must be kept in equilibrium and the ratio between volume and pressure must remain constant. Any increase in the volume of one component must be accompanied by a reciprocal decrease in one of the other components. When this volume–pressure relationship becomes unbalanced, ICP increases.

3. The brain attempts to compensate for rises in ICP by:
   a. Displacement/shunting of CSF from the intracranial compartment to the lumbar subarachnoid space (SAS). Normally, about 500 mL of CSF are produced and absorbed in 24 hours. About 125 to 150 mL circulates throughout the ventricular system and the SAS in the following ratio: 25 mL in the ventricles, 90 mL in the lumbar SAS, and 35 mL in the cisterns and surrounding SAS.
   b. Increased CSF absorption.
   c. Decreased cerebral blood volume by displacement of cerebral venous blood into the venous sinuses. Compensatory measures are finite. Increased ICP will ultimately occur if the volume of the intracranial mass exceeds the volume compensated.
4. Intracranial compliance is "tightness" of the brain. Compliance is the relationship between intracranial volume and ICP. It is a nonlinear relationship; as ICP increases, compliance decreases. With functional compensatory mechanisms, an increase in volume causes a small, transient increase in ICP. As compliance decreases, small increases in volume result in moderate increases in pressure. When compensatory mechanisms are exhausted, very slight increases in volume will produce large increases in pressure. The patient's response to changes in ICP will depend on where the patient is on the volume–pressure curve.
5. Factors that influence the ability of the body to achieve this steady state include the following:
   a. Systemic BP.
   b. Ventilation and oxygenation.
   c. Metabolic rate and oxygen consumption (fever, shivering, physical activity).
   d. Regional cerebral vasospasm.
   e. Oxygen saturation and hematocrit.
6. Inability to maintain a steady state results in increased ICP. Traumatic brain injury (TBI), cerebral edema, intracerebral hemorrhage, ischemic stroke, abscess and infection, lesions, intracranial surgery, and radiation therapy can be potential etiologies of increased ICP.
7. Increased ICP constitutes an emergency and requires prompt treatment. ICP can be monitored by means of an intraventricular catheter, a subarachnoid screw or bolt, or an epidural pressure recording device.
8. Alterations or compromise in cerebral blood flow can be measured noninvasively by a TCD study. Increased velocities indicate vasospasm, diminished velocities indicate low blood flow, and absent velocities are consistent with no flow or brain death.

Nursing Assessment

Change in LOC
Caused by increased ICP. Assess for the following:
1. Change in LOC (awareness): drowsiness, lethargy.
2. Early behavioral changes: restlessness, irritability, confusion, and apathy.
3. Falling score on the GCS (see page 354).
   a. Change in orientation: disorientation to time, place, or person.
   b. Difficulty or inability to follow commands.
   c. Difficulty or inability in verbalization or in responsiveness to auditory stimuli.
   d. Change in response to painful stimuli (eg, purposeful to inappropriate or absent responses).
   e. Posturing (abnormal flexion or extension).

Changes in Vital Signs
Caused by pressure on brain stem. Assess for the following:
1. Rising BP or widening pulse pressure (the difference between systolic and diastolic BP). This may be followed by hypotension and labile vital signs, indicating further brain stem compromise.
2. Pulse changes with bradycardia changing to tachycardia as ICP rises.
3. Respiratory irregularities: tachypnea (early sign of increased ICP); slowing of rate with lengthening periods of apnea; Cheyne-Stokes (rhythmic pattern of increasing and decreasing depth of respirations with periods of apnea) or Kussmaul (paroxysms of difficult breathing) breathing; central neurogenic hyperventilation (prolonged, deep breathing); apneustic (sustained inspiratory effort) breathing; and ataxic (incoordinated and spasmodic) breathing.
4. Hyperthermia followed by hypothermia.

 KEY DECISION POINT Watch for Cushing triad—bradycardia, hypertension (with widening pulse pressure), and irregular respirations; this is classic symptomatology related to uncompensated increased ICP and is considered a neurologic medical emergency. Alert health care provider and prepare for therapeutic intervention.

 NURSING ALERT Respiratory irregularities may not be apparent if the patient is mechanically ventilated.

Pupillary Changes
1. Caused by increased pressure on optic and oculomotor nerves. Fundoscopic exam may reveal changes.
2. Inspect the pupils with a penlight to evaluate size, configuration, and reaction to light.
3. Compare both eyes for similarities or differences, particularly pupillary changes related to location and progression of brain stem herniation.
   a. Midbrain involvement—fixed and dilated.
   b. Pontine involvement—pinpoint pupils.
   c. Uncal herniation.
      i. Unilaterally dilating pupil ipsilateral to lesion.
      ii. Anisocoria (unequal) with sluggish light reaction in dilated pupil.
      iii. If treatment is delayed or unsuccessful, contralateral pupil becomes dilated and fixed to light.
      iv. When herniation of the brain stem occurs, both pupils assume midposition and remain fixed to light.
   d. Central transtentorial herniation.
      i. Pupils are small bilaterally (1 to 3 mm).
      ii. Reaction to light is brisk but with small range of constriction.
      iii. If treatment is delayed or unsuccessful, small pupils dilate moderately (3 to 5 mm) and fix irregularly at midposition.
      iv. When herniation of the brain stem occurs, both pupils dilate widely and remain fixed to light.
4. Pupillometer can be used to measure pupillary size and reactivity, detecting subtle change by utilizing infrared light.

Extraocular Movements

1. Evaluate gaze to determine if it is conjugate (paired, working together) or dysconjugate (eye deviates or movement is asymmetric).
2. Evaluate movement of eyes.
   a. Inability to abduct or adduct: deviation of one or both eyes.
   b. Alteration in vision (eg, blurred vision, diplopia, field cut).
   c. Spontaneous roving, random eye movements.
   d. Nystagmus on horizontal/vertical gaze.
3. Oculocephalic reflex (doll's eyes): brisk turning of the head left, right, up, or down with observation of eye movements in response to the stimulus. Tests brain stem pathways between CNs III, IV, VI, and VIII. This should not be performed on patients with suspected cervical spine injury, patients in a cervical collar, or patients with known cervical spine injuries unless part of the brain death examination.
4. Oculovestibular reflex (cold calorics): 30 to 60 mL of ice water instilled into the ear with the head of the bed elevated to 30 degrees. Tests brain stem pathways between CNs III, IV, VI, and VIII. Response preserved longer than the doll's eyes maneuver. Performed by health care provider as part of brain death examination.

Other Changes

Be alert for the following:
1. Headache increasing in intensity and aggravated by movement and straining.
2. Vomiting recurrent with little or no nausea, especially in early morning; may be projectile.
3. Papilledema from optic nerve compression.
4. Subtle changes, such as restlessness, headache, forced breathing, purposeless movements, and mental cloudiness.
5. Motor and sensory dysfunctions (proximal muscle weakness, presence of pronator drift).
6. Contralateral hemiparesis progressing to complete hemiplegia.
7. Speech impairment (expressive, receptive, or global aphasia) when dominant hemisphere involved.
8. Seizure activity: focal or generalized.
9. Decreased brain stem function (CN deficits, such as loss of corneal reflex, gag reflex, and ability to swallow).
10. Pathologic reflexes: Babinski, grasp, chewing, sucking.

Nursing Diagnosis

• Decreased Intracranial Adaptive Capacity.

Nursing Interventions

Decreasing ICP

 NURSING ALERT Increased ICP is a true life-threatening medical emergency that requires immediate recognition and prompt therapeutic intervention.

1. Establish and maintain airway, breathing, and circulation.
2. Promote normal Pco_2. Hyperventilation is not recommended for prophylactic treatment of increased ICP as cerebral circulation is reduced by 50% the first 24 hours after injury. Hyperventilation causes cerebral vasoconstriction and decreases cerebral blood flow to decrease ICP; this can potentiate secondary injury to the brain. Hyperventilation should be used only after all other treatment options have been exhausted or in an acute crisis.

3. Avoid hypoxia. Decreased Po_2 (less than 60 mm Hg) causes cerebral vasodilation, thus increasing ICP.
4. Maintain cerebral perfusion pressure (CPP) greater than 50 mm Hg. CPP is determined by subtracting the ICP from the MAP: CPP = MAP – ICP.
5. Administer mannitol (0.25 to 1 g/kg), an osmotic diuretic, if ordered. Osmotic diuretics act by establishing an osmotic gradient across the blood–brain barrier that depletes the intracellular and extracellular fluid volume within the brain and throughout the body. Mannitol will be ineffective if the blood–brain barrier is not intact.
6. Administer hypertonic saline (2% or 3%), if ordered. It creates an osmotic gradient that pulls extra fluid from the brain with an intact blood–brain barrier, lowers ICP, improves cerebral blood flow by reducing viscosity, and improves oxygen carrying capacity. Saline (23.4%) is used as a bolus to treat acute increases in ICP in conjunction with or in place of mannitol; requires central access for administration and should be given over 5 minutes.
7. Insert an indwelling urinary catheter for management of diuresis.
8. Administer corticosteroids, such as dexamethasone, as ordered, to reduce vasogenic edema associated with brain tumors. Corticosteroids are not recommended in the treatment of cytoxic (intracellular) cerebral edema related to trauma or stroke.
9. Maintain balanced fluids and electrolytes. Watch for increased or decreased serum sodium due to the following conditions that may occur with increased ICP.
   a. Diabetes insipidus (DI) results from the absence of antidiuretic hormone (ADH); this is reflected by increased urine output with elevation of serum osmolarity and sodium.
   b. The syndrome of inappropriate antidiuretic hormone (SIADH) results from the secretion of ADH in the absence of changes in serum osmolality. This is a hypervolemic state reflected by decreased urine output with decreased serum sodium and increased free water.
   c. Cerebral salt wasting is associated with abnormal release of aldosterone resulting in increased elimination of sodium and decreased interstitial volume (hypovolemic state) (see Table 15-4).

Table 15-4	Differentiating Etiology of Hyponatremia	
	CEREBRAL SALT WASTING	**SIADH**
Volume		
Plasma	Decreased CVP < 6	Increased
Urine output	Marked increase	Normal or decreased
Sodium		
Serum	Decreased	<135 mEq/L
Urine	Marked increase	>20 mEq/L
Osmolality		
Serum	Increased or no change	Decreased (<280 mmol/L)
Urine	Increased or no change	Increased (>100 mmol/kg)
Serum K⁺	Increased	Decreased or no change
Hematocrit	Increased	Decreased or no change
Treatment	Fludrocortisone	Fluid restriction Oral: Salt replacement IV: 3% saline

10. Monitor effects of anesthetic agents, such as propofol, and sedatives, such as midazolam or dexmedetomidine hydrochloride, which may be given to prevent sudden changes in ICP due to coughing, straining, or "fighting" the ventilator. Short-acting medications are preferred to allow for intermittent neurologic assessment.

11. High-dose barbiturates, such as pentobarbital, may be used in patients with refractory increased ICP. (*Note*: Prophylactic use is not recommended. It is utilized when all other treatments have failed.) Dosing: 10 mg/kg over 30 minutes; then 5 mg/kg every hour for 3 hours followed by maintenance dose of 1 mg/kg/hr. (Goal serum barbiturate level of 3 to 4 mg/dL.)

   a. High-dose barbiturates induce a comatose state and suppress brain metabolism, which, in turn, reduces cerebral blood flow and ICP. Only pupillary response is assessed.

   b. Be alert to the high level of nursing support required. All responses to environmental and noxious stimuli (suctioning, turning) are abolished as well as all protective reflexes.

   c. Cough or gag reflex will be absent and the patient will be unable to protect the airway, increasing susceptibility to pneumonia.

   d. Monitor ICP, arterial pressure, and serum barbiturate levels, as indicated. Perform continuous EEG monitoring to document burst suppression (suppression of cortical activity) and ensure adequate dosing of barbiturates, if used.

   e. Monitor temperature because barbiturate coma causes hypothermia.

   f. Diminished GI motility and high risk for ileus.

12. Maintain normothermia and treat fever aggressively. Fever increases cerebral blood flow and cerebral blood volume; acute increases in ICP occur with fever spikes. Cerebral temperature is 4 to 5 degrees higher then body core temperature; therefore, small increases in body core temperature can create drastic increases in the core temperature of the brain. Infection is a common complication of ICP, and in the presence of fever, an infectious workup should be completed.

13. Avoid positions or activities that may increase ICP. Keep head in alignment with shoulders; neck flexion or rotation increases ICP by impeding venous return. Keep head of bed elevated 30 degrees to reduce jugular venous pressure and decrease ICP.

   a. Minimize suctioning, keep procedure less than 15 seconds, and, if ordered, instill lidocaine via endotracheal (ET) tube before suctioning. Coughing and suctioning are associated with increased intrathoracic pressure, which is associated with ICP spikes. Inject 5 to 10 mL of lidocaine into ET tube before suctioning to dampen the cough response.

   b. Minimize other stimuli, such as alarms, television, radio, and bedside conversations, which may precipitously increase ICP (stimuli that create elevation in ICP are patient-dependent).

14. Maintain normal blood sugar levels. Treat with sliding scale insulin or insulin drip as ordered.

15. Initiate treatment modalities, as ordered, for increased ICP (above 20 mm Hg or if there is a significant shift in pressure).

16. Pretreat prior to known activities that raise ICP and avoid taking pressure readings immediately after a procedure. Allow patient to rest for approximately 5 minutes.

17. Record ICP readings every hour and correlate with significant clinical events or treatments (suctioning, turning).

Evaluation: Expected Outcomes

- ICP and vital signs stable; alert and responsive.

Intracranial Monitoring

 EVIDENCE BASE Kawoos, U., McCarron, R. M., Auker, C. R., & Chavko, M. (2015). Advances in intracranial pressure monitoring and its significance in managing traumatic brain injury. *International Journal of Molecular Sciences, 16*(12), 28979–28997. Available: *http://doi.org/10.3390/ijms161226146*.

Intracranial monitoring, including ICP monitoring, is a technology that helps the nurse assess, plan, intervene, and evaluate patient responses to care. ICP monitoring is widely used. See Figure 15-1.

1. External ventricular drain (EVD): catheter is inserted into lateral ventricle (right is preferred) through a drilled burr hole opening; connected to fluid-filled transducer, which converts mechanical pressure to electrical impulses and waveform; allows ventricular drainage. EVD is the most accurate method to measure ICP.

2. Subarachnoid (bolt) hollow screw inserted into SAS beneath the skull and dura through drill hole; also connected to pressure transducer system.

3. Epidural sensor inserted beneath skull but not through dura, so does not measure pressure directly; fiberoptic cable is connected directly to monitor.

4. Parenchymal device is inserted directly into brain tissue.

ICP Waveforms

ICP pulse waveforms are generated from a pressure wave transmitted through the cardiovascular system into the tissues within the intracranial cavity. See Figure 15-2.

1. The normal pulse waveform consists of three identifiable components: P-1, P-2, and P-3.

Figure 15-1. Intracranial pressure monitoring system. (*A*) Intraventricular; (*B*) subarachnoid; (*C*) subdural; (*D*) parenchymal; (*E*) epidural. (Redrawn from Diepenbrock, N.H. [2015]. Quick reference to critical care [5th ed.]. Philadelphia: Lippincott Williams & Wilkins.)

Figure 15-2. Intracranial pressure waves. (A) Normal ICP waveform. **(B)** A waves (plateau waves) are pathologic. B and C waves have little clinical significance.

A waves are clinically significant as elevation in ICP is related to compromise in autoregulation secondary to increased cerebral blood volume and decreased cerebral blood flow.

3. B and C wave patterns are related to respiration and are of little clinical significance. B wave patterns are of shorter duration and smaller amplitude than A wave patterns and may precede A wave patterns. C wave patterns are small, rhythmic oscillations that fluctuate with changes in respiration and BP.

Other Monitoring Systems

1. Licox Brain Oxygen Monitoring System—placed in the brain tissue through a burr hole and monitors brain tissue partial pressure of oxygen (PbrO$_2$), cerebral temperature, and indirect ICP. Continual monitoring of the cerebral temperature and oxygenation levels provides direct information on the acute changes in the intracranial tissue that can potentiate secondary brain injury.
2. Microdialysis—catheter is placed into the brain tissue through a burr hole for monitoring of cerebral oxygen, glucose, lactate, lactate–pyruvate, glutamate, and glycerol. The catheter is connected to a 2.5-mL syringe and into a microinfusion pump. The pump is perfused with Ringer solution. Samples are obtained periodically for analysis.
3. Jugular venous oximetry—A fiberoptic oximetric catheter is placed into the jugular bulb of the internal jugular vein for measurement of jugular venous oxygen saturation (SjvO$_2$). SjvO$_2$ is helpful in evaluating arterial saturation, cerebral metabolic rate for oxygen, and cerebral blood flow. The normal range is between 54% and 75%. A low SjvO$_2$ is suggestive of increased brain extraction of oxygen related to systemic arterial hypoxia, decreased cerebral blood flow from hypotension or vasospasm, or an elevated ICP with a low CPP. Desaturation is thought to be associated with ischemic events and directly related to increased morbidity.

Nursing Interventions

1. Note the pattern of waveforms and any sustained elevation of pressure above 20 mm Hg.
2. Avoid overstimulation of the patient.
   a. Note the stimuli that cause increased pressure, such as bathing, suctioning, repositioning, or visitors. Adjust care, as indicated.
   b. Premedicate, as indicated.
   c. Provide rest periods between periods of care.
   d. Limit visitors as status indicates.
   e. Limit unnecessary conversation at patient's bedside.
   f. Eliminate external environmental stimuli. Close doors, turn off suction equipment when not in use, limit television or radio as status indicates.
3. Watch for developing or increasing P-2 waves and frequency of A (plateau) waves. Report these, and begin measures to lower increased ICP.

> **! NURSING ALERT** Sustained elevation in ICP greater than 20 mm Hg and CPP less than 50 mm Hg correlates with worsening outcomes following traumatic brain injury. Measures to reduce increased ICP should be performed immediately and the health care provider notified when the ICP remains elevated for more than 5 minutes.

a. P-1, the percussive wave, reflects pulsations of the choroid plexus, where CSF is produced, as transmitted from the cardiovascular system at systole. It is the highest of the three waveform components under normal conditions.
b. P-2, the tidal wave, has a more variable shape and reflects relative brain volume. P-2 can become elevated in response to a mass lesion or when brain compliance is decreased.
c. P-3, the dicrotic wave, follows the dicrotic notch on the downslope of the individual ICP pulse waveform and is usually the lowest waveform segment.
2. Plateau or A wave patterns are pathological, reflecting a rapid rise in ICP up to 50 to 100 mm Hg, and may be followed by a variable period during which the ICP remains elevated and then falls to baseline. Truncated patterns that do not exceed an elevation of 50 mm Hg are early indicators of neurologic deterioration.

Nursing Management of the Patient Undergoing Intracranial Surgery

Craniotomy is the surgical opening of the skull to gain access to intracranial structures to perform a biopsy, remove a tumor, relieve increased ICP, evacuate a blood clot, evaluate and treat the cause of intracranial hemorrhage, or remove epileptogenic tissue. Surgical approach is based on location of the lesion and may be supratentorial (above the tentorium or dural covering that divides the cerebrum from cerebellum) or infratentorial (below the tentorium, including the brain stem). Craniotomy may be performed by means of burr holes (made with a drill or hand tools) or by making a bony flap. *Craniectomy* is excision and removal of a portion of the skull. *Cranioplasty* is repair of a cranial defect by means of a plastic or metal plate. *Transsphenoidal surgery* is an approach that gains access to the pituitary gland through the nasal cavity and sphenoidal sinus (see Chapter 24).

Preoperative Management

1. Diagnostic findings, surgical procedure, and expectations are reviewed with the patient.
2. Presurgical shampoo with an antimicrobial agent may be ordered. Skull preparation is performed in the operating room.
3. Depending on primary diagnosis, corticosteroids may be ordered preoperatively to reduce vasogenic cerebral edema.
4. Depending on the type and location of lesion, anticonvulsants may be ordered to reduce risk of seizures.
5. The patient is prepared for the use of intraoperative antibiotics to reduce risk of infection.
6. Urinary catheterization is performed to assess urinary volume during operative period.
7. If cerebral edema develops, intraoperative or postoperative osmotic diuretic (mannitol) or corticosteroids may be ordered for its treatment.
8. Neurologic assessment is performed to evaluate and record the patient's neurologic baseline and vital signs for postoperative comparison.
9. Family and patient are made aware of the immediate postoperative care and where the physician will contact the family after surgery.
10. Supportive care is given, as needed, for neurologic deficits.

Postoperative Management

1. Respiratory status is assessed by monitoring rate, depth, and pattern of respirations. A patent airway is maintained.
2. Vital signs and neurologic status are monitored using a facility-based neurologic assessment tool; findings are documented. Arterial line may be used for blood pressure monitoring.
3. Pharmacologic agents may be prescribed to control increased ICP.
4. Incisional and headache pain may be controlled with analgesic such as an opioid or acetaminophen, as prescribed. Monitor response to medications.
5. Position head of bed at 15 to 30 degrees, or per clinical status of the patient, to promote venous drainage. Determining appropriate position of head of bed is patient-dependent and should be adjusted based on observed changes in the patient's clinical response and ICP to positioning.
6. Turn side to side every 2 hours; positioning restrictions will be ordered by the health care provider (craniectomy patients should not be turned on the side of the cranial defect).
7. CT scan of the brain is performed if the patient's status deteriorates.
8. Oral fluids are provided when the patient is alert and swallow reflex has returned. Intake and output are monitored. Speech therapy may be ordered for bedside swallow study or radiographic swallow study.
9. Signs of infection are monitored by checking craniotomy site, ventricular drainage, nuchal rigidity, or presence of CSF (fluid collection at surgical site).
10. Periorbital edema is controlled by such measures as elevation of head of bed and cold compresses. Removal of surgical dressing and increase in activity will assist in the resolution of periorbital edema.

Potential Complications

1. Intracranial hemorrhage/hematoma.
2. Cerebral edema.
3. Infections (eg, postoperative meningitis, pulmonary, wound).
4. Seizures.
5. CN dysfunction.
6. Decreased CPP causing cerebral ischemia.

Nursing Diagnoses

- Risk for Ineffective Cerebral Tissue Perfusion related to increased ICP.
- Risk for Aspiration related to decreased swallow reflex and postoperative positioning.
- Risk for Infection related to invasive procedure.
- Acute Pain related to surgical wound.
- Constipation related to use of opioids and immobility.

Nursing Interventions

Maintaining ICP within Normal Range

1. Closely monitor LOC, vital signs, pupillary response, and ICP, if indicated. Notify health care provider if ICP is greater than 20 mm Hg or CPP is less than 50 mm Hg.
2. Teach the patient to avoid activities that can raise ICP, such as excessive flexion or rotation of the head and Valsalva maneuver (coughing, straining with defecation).
3. Administer medications, as prescribed, to reduce ICP.
4. Check ICP waveform before nursing interventions that create noxious tactile stimuli, such as suctioning, prolonged physical assessment, turning, and ROM exercises and delay interventions based on patient response.

Preventing Aspiration

1. Offer fluids only when the patient is alert and swallow reflexes have returned.
2. Have suction equipment available at bedside. Suction only if indicated. Pretreat with sedation or endotracheal lidocaine to prevent elevation of ICP.
3. Elevate head of bed to maximum of order, or per clinical status, and patient comfort.

Preventing Nosocomial Infections

1. Use sterile technique for dressing changes, catheter care, and ventricular drain management.
2. Be aware of patients at higher risk of infection—those undergoing lengthy operations, those with ventricular drains left in

longer than 72 hours, and those with operations of the third ventricle.

3. Assess surgical site for redness, tenderness, and drainage.
4. Watch for leakage of CSF, which increases the danger of meningitis.
   a. Watch for sudden discharge of fluid from wound; a large leak usually requires surgical repair.
   b. Warn against coughing, sneezing, or nose blowing, which may aggravate CSF leakage.
   c. Assess for elevation of temperature and neck rigidity.
   d. Note patency of ventricular catheter system.
   e. Early removal of Foley catheter.
5. Institute measures to prevent respiratory or UTI postoperatively.

Relieving Pain

1. Medicate patient as prescribed and according to assessment findings.
2. Elevate head of bed per protocol to relieve headache.
3. Provide distractive measures for pain management.
4. Darken room if patient is photophobic.

Avoiding Constipation

1. Encourage fluids when the patient is able to manage liquids.
2. Ambulate as soon as possible.
3. Change to nonopioid agents for pain control as soon as possible.
4. Avoid Valsalva-like maneuvers.
5. Use stool softeners and laxatives, as ordered.

Family Education and Support

1. Keep the patient and family aware of progress and plans to transfer to step-down unit, general nursing unit, subacute care, or rehabilitation facility.
2. Encourage frequent visiting and interaction of family for stimulation of patient as care allows.
3. Begin discharge planning early, and obtain referral for home care nursing, social work, or physical and occupational therapy, as needed.

Evaluation: Expected Outcomes

- Normal ICP and CPP maintained between 50 and 70 mm Hg.
- Gag reflex present; breath sounds clear.
- Afebrile without signs of infection.
- Verbalizes decreased pain.
- Passed soft stool.

CRANIAL NERVE DISORDERS

Bell Palsy

Idiopathic *Bell palsy* is an acute peripheral facial paralysis of the infratemporal portion of CN VII (facial nerve) that most often occurs unilaterally. The annual incidence of Bell palsy is approximately 25 to 30 cases per 100,000 persons. It is typically a self-limiting process that improves in 3 to 6 months.

Pathophysiology and Etiology

1. Cause is unknown. Possible etiologies include sensory ganglionitis of the CNS with secondary muscle palsy, caused by inflammation, vascular ischemia, and autoimmune demyelination.

2. Most patients experience a viral prodrome (eg, upper respiratory infection, herpes simplex virus) 1 to 3 weeks before onset of symptoms.
3. Can affect anyone at any age; however, it disproportionately affects pregnant women and those who have diabetes, hypertension, or influenza.
4. Generally self-limiting. With or without treatment, most patients improve significantly within 2 weeks and about 80% recover completely within 3 months. In rare cases, the symptoms may never completely resolve or may recur. Risk factors thought to be associated with a poor outcome include (1) over age 60 years, (2) complete paralysis, and (3) decreased taste or salivary flow on the side of paralysis.

Clinical Manifestations

1. Acute onset of unilateral upper and lower facial paralysis (over a 48-hour period and reaches its peak within 72 hours). Paralysis of the ipsilateral side of the face from vertex of scalp to chin; facial muscles weak throughout the forehead, cheek, and chin; can affect speech and taste, distort face, decrease tearing, and cause posterior auricular pain.
2. Involvement of all branches of facial nerve: facial weakness, diminished taste from anterior two thirds of the tongue, decreased blink reflex, decreased lacrimation, inability to close eye, painful eye sensations, photophobia, drooling.
3. Patients may experience neck, mastoid, or ear pain or hyperacusis on the affected side.

Diagnostic Evaluation

1. History to determine previous illness, onset of paralysis, and associated symptoms.
2. Exclusion of lesions that mimic Bell palsy, such as tumor, infection (Lyme disease, meningitis), trauma, stroke, or other conditions (sarcoidosis, multiple sclerosis, Guillain-Barré syndrome) through thorough neurologic examination and CT scan or brain MRI imaging with contrast media.
3. Electrophysiologic testing, specifically action potentials, EMGs, and nerve conduction velocities, to evaluate nerve function.
4. Lyme disease serological testing history of tick bite or bilateral weakness. About 5% to 10% of untreated Lyme disease patients may develop Bell palsy.

 NURSING ALERT A rapid neurologic examination should be performed to differentiate Bell palsy from other conditions that could be causing facial droop. The patient with Bell palsy should have normal LOC, motor strength (except in the area of facial nerve), sensation, and reflexes. Depending on the clinical concern a head CT scan or brain MRI may be indicated for abnormal neurologic findings beyond the facial nerve.

Management

1. Corticosteroid therapy should be initiated within 72 hours of onset to decrease inflammation (eg, prednisone 50 to 60 mg for the first 5 days, followed by a tapering dose). Acyclovir combined with prednisone may improve facial function. When using corticosteroids for the treatment of Bell palsy, caution should be used in patients with tuberculosis, peptic

ulcer disease, diabetes mellitus, renal or hepatic dysfunction, or malignant hypertension. For patients who have a contraindication to steroid therapy, acyclovir alone may be given.
2. Eye care to maintain lubrication and moisture if unable to close. May need to be patched during sleep.
3. Physical therapy, electrical stimulation to maintain muscle tone.
4. Biofeedback as adjunct therapy.
5. Surgical treatment of Bell palsy may include to anastomose facial nerve to other cranial nerve (CN VII to XI or CN VII to XII, surgical closure of eyelid to protect cornea (tarsorrhaphy), facial nerve decompression, placement of gold weights into the eyelid and facial lifts. Bell palsy is usually self-limiting and therefore generally does not require surgical treatment.

Complications

1. Corneal ulceration.
2. Impairment of vision.
3. Synkinesis (an abnormal, involuntary facial muscle contraction during normal facial muscle movements).
4. Psychosocial adjustment to prolonged paralysis.

 NURSING ALERT Keratitis (inflammation of the cornea), ulceration, and vision loss are major threats to a patient with Bell palsy. Protect the cornea if the eye does not close.

Nursing Assessment

1. Test motor components of facial nerve (VII) by assessing patient's smile and ability to whistle, purse lips, wrinkle forehead, and close eyes. Observe for facial asymmetry.
2. Observe patient's ability to handle secretions, food, and fluids; observe for drooling.
3. Assess patient's ability to blink and speak clearly.
4. Assess effect of altered appearance on body image.

Nursing Diagnoses

- Risk for Dry Eye related to loss of protective eye closure.
- Disturbed Body Image related to facial nerve paralysis.

Nursing Interventions

Preventing Eye Dryness and Maintaining Corneal Integrity
1. Administer and teach the patient to administer artificial tears and ophthalmic ointment as prescribed.
2. Patch eye to keep shut at night, as directed.
3. Inspect eye for redness or discharge.
4. Advise the patient to report eye pain immediately.

Enhancing Body Image
1. Encourage the patient to express feelings related to body image disturbance.
2. Encourage the patient to use mirror as means to obtain feedback about actual versus perceived appearance.
3. Perform and teach the patient to perform facial massage to alleviate feelings of stiffness and enhance recovery.

Patient Education and Health Maintenance

1. Instruct the patient to wear wraparound sunglasses to decrease normal evaporation from the eye from sun and wind, to avoid eye irritants, and to increase environmental humidity.

2. Instruct the patient in use of ophthalmic drops and ointment, proper methods of lid closure, and patching of the eye.
3. Demonstrate facial exercises (eg, raise eyebrows, squeeze eyes shut, purse lips) and stress their importance to prevent muscle atrophy.
4. For further information, refer the patient to Bell's Palsy Research Foundation (*www.bellspalsyresearch.com*).

Evaluation: Expected Outcomes

- Cornea without redness, pain, or discharge.
- Verbalizes adjustment to body image disturbance.

Trigeminal Neuralgia (Tic Douloureux)

Trigeminal neuralgia (tic douloureux) is an intensely painful neurologic condition that affects one or more branches of the fifth cranial (trigeminal) nerve. Patients experience sudden paroxysms of "lancinating" or electric shock–like facial pain localized to one or more branches of the nerve (see Figure 15-3). The pain is often precipitated by trigger points that "fire" when the patient talks, shaves, eats, touches the face, brushes the teeth, or is exposed to cold wind. Approximately 40,000 patients in the United States suffer from this condition at any particular time. The incidence is 4 to 5 cases per 100,000. Patients who present with the disease between ages 20 and 40 are more likely to suffer from a demyelinating lesion in the pons secondary to multiple sclerosis (MS).

Pathophysiology and Etiology

1. Unknown cause, but degenerative or viral origin suspected.
2. Any of the three trigeminal nerve branches can be affected:
   a. V_1: ophthalmic branch; pain involves the eye and forehead.
   b. V_2: maxillary branch; pain involves the cheek, upper teeth, upper gums, and nose.
   c. V_3: mandibular branch; pain involves the lower jaw, side of the tongue, lower teeth, and lower gum and extends to the ear.

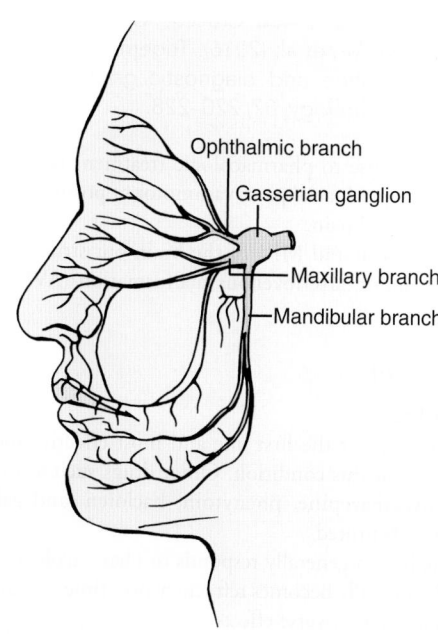

Figure 15-3. The main divisions of the trigeminal nerve are the ophthalmic, maxillary, and mandibular. Sensory root fibers arise in the gasserian ganglion.

3. Compression from artery adjacent to the nerve strips myelin from the nerve when it pulsates. Loss of myelin acts like an uninsulated wire that "fires" abnormally in response to stimuli.

 GERONTOLOGIC ALERT Trigeminal neuralgia is commonly seen in older adults. Pain typically appears to be localized to one or more teeth. Patients may seek dental care for pain relief, resulting in one or more tooth extractions without alleviation of pain.

Clinical Manifestations

1. Sudden, severe episodes of intense facial pain localized to one or more of the branches of the nerve, lasting less than 30 to 60 seconds and ending abruptly.
2. Pain may occur spontaneously or be precipitated by activation of trigger points, such as touching the face, talking, chewing, yawning, and brushing the teeth, that place pressure on the terminal end of the branch affected.
3. Pain is always unilateral and does not cross the midline. Bilateral pain is sometimes seen in patients with MS and should result in a high index of suspicion for this condition. MS and hypertension are the two risk factors found in epidemiologic studies.
4. Some patients experience numbness, particularly around the mouth.

Diagnostic Evaluation

1. History of characteristic symptoms and pattern; neurologic examination is normal. In contrast to migraine pain, persons with trigeminal neuralgia rarely suffer attacks during sleep, which is a key point in the history.
2. New classification and diagnostic grading system to make diagnosis of classic TN, secondary TN due to identifiable neurologic disorder, or idiopathic TN.

 EVIDENCE BASE Cruccu, G., Finnerup, N. B., Sindou, M., et al. (2016). Trigeminal neuralgia: New classification and diagnostic grading for practice and research. *Neurology, 87*, 220–228.

3. Quick response to pharmacologic treatment is important to rule out atypical facial pain, vasomotor or postherpetic neuralgia, and dental pain.
4. Head CT scan and MRI of the brain out structural lesions, such as tumor, arteriovenous malformation (AVM), MS, or other disorders.

Management

Pharmacologic

1. Levetiracetam is the first line and most effective medication used to treat this condition. Other drugs such as carbamazepine, oxcarbazepine, phenytoin, baclofen, and gabapentin may be substituted.
2. Although pain generally responds to pharmacologic intervention, it gradually becomes refractory over time, or patients suffer undesirable adverse effects.

Surgical

Operative procedure selected is one that will provide the greatest chance of long-term pain relief with the fewest complications.

1. Alcohol, phenol block, or glycerol injection for pain may last several months after injection.
2. Percutaneous radiofrequency trigeminal gangliolysis directs low-voltage stimulation of nerve by electrode inserted through foramen ovale; sensory function is destroyed with goal to preserve motor function; may cause decreased corneal sensation if V1 affected; paresthesias, jaw weakness, or undesirable, painful numbness (anesthesia dolorosa). Pain may recur as nerve regenerates, necessitating repeat procedure.
3. Rhizotomy (transection of nerve root at Gasserian ganglion) causes complete loss of sensation; other complications include burning, stinging, discomfort in and around eye, herpetic lesions of face, keratitis, and corneal ulceration. Pain may recur as nerve regenerates.
4. Percutaneous balloon microcompression for selective destruction of nerve fibers that mediate light touch and trigger pain. Relieves pain in ophthalmic branch while sparing corneal sensation.
5. Microvascular decompression of trigeminal nerve. Most effective form of therapy, with 75% to 80% of patients pain-free without need for long-term medication after procedure. Treatment of choice for younger patients who are low anesthesia risk, do not want facial numbness, and are willing to accept craniotomy.
6. Gamma knife surgery is less invasive than the percutaneous procedures. It is about as effective as the percutaneous procedures; however, relief may not come for weeks to months and it is a bit more expensive.

Complications

1. Anorexia and weight loss.
2. Dehydration.
3. Anxiety, fear.
4. Depression, social isolation, and suicidal ideations in extreme cases.

Nursing Assessment

1. Take history of the pain, including duration, severity, and aggravating factors.
2. Assess nutritional status and hydration.
3. Assess for anxiety and depression, including problems with sleep, social interaction, and coping ability/skills.

Nursing Diagnoses

- Chronic Pain related to physiologic changes of the disorder.
- Imbalanced Nutrition: Less Than Body Requirements related to fear of eating.
- Powerlessness related to lack of control over painful episodes.

Nursing Interventions

Relieving Pain

1. To minimize painful episodes, review with patient potential trigger factors, and develop individualized methods of coping with identified triggers.
2. Encourage the patient to take medication regularly, including "rescue" medication for breakthrough periods.
3. Help the patient maintain a method of communication without causing pain from talking.

Maintaining Adequate Nutrition

1. To maximize nutritional intake, instruct the patient to take foods and fluids at room temperature and to chew on the unaffected side.
2. Have the patient consult with the dietitian for appropriate meal texture and composition.
3. Encourage small, frequent meals to avoid fatigue and pain.
4. Advise about use of nutritional supplements, if indicated.

Increasing Control

1. Support the patient through treatment trials.
2. Teach relaxation exercises, such as relaxation breathing, progressive muscle relaxation, and guided imagery, to relieve tension (see page 25).
3. Encourage participation in support groups (eg, Trigeminal Neuralgia Association) and facilitate a therapeutic relationship with the health care provider.

Patient Education and Health Maintenance

1. Educate the surgical patient regarding self-care after denervation procedures.
   a. Instruct the patient to inspect the eye for redness and foreign bodies three to four times per day if corneal sensation is impaired.
   b. Instruct the patient to instill lubricating eye drops every 4 hours if corneal sensation is impaired.
   c. Instruct the patient to avoid drinking hot or very cold liquids.
   d. Instruct the patient to chew on unaffected side to avoid biting tongue, lips, and inside of mouth.
   e. Instruct the patient who wears dentures that jaw muscle will regenerate over time; avoid having dentures refitted, but maintain regular dental checkups because pain will not be felt.
   f. Instruct the patient to report any change in sensation.
2. Refer patient to the Facial Pain Association for education and support network (*www.fpa-support.org*) or the National Institute of Neurological Disorders and Stroke (*www.ninds.nih.gov*).

Evaluation: Expected Outcomes

- Verbalizes reduced pain.
- Maintains weight.
- Verbalizes decreased anxiety and depression.

CEREBROVASCULAR DISEASE
Cerebrovascular Insufficiency

EVIDENCE BASE Kernan, W. N., Ovbiagele, B., Black, H. R., et al. (2014) Guidelines for the prevention of stroke in patients with stroke and transient ischemic attack: A guideline for healthcare professionals from the American heart association/American stroke association. *Stroke, 45*(7), 2160–2236.

Cerebrovascular insufficiency is an interruption or inadequate blood flow to a focal area of the brain, resulting in transient or permanent neurologic dysfunction. *Transient ischemic attack* (TIA) lasts less than 24 hours. *Ischemic stroke* is similar to myocardial infarction, in that the pathogenesis is loss of blood supply to the tissue, which can result in irreversible damage if blood flow is not restored quickly.

Pathophysiology and Etiology

1. Cerebrovascular insufficiency can be caused by atherosclerotic plaque or thrombosis, resulting in increased P_{CO_2}, decreased P_{O_2}, decreased blood viscosity, hyperthermia/hypothermia, and increased ICP.
2. Carotid arteries, vertebral arteries, major intracranial vessels, or microcirculation may be affected.
3. Cardiac causes of emboli include atrial fibrillation, mitral valve prolapse, infectious endocarditis, and prosthetic heart valve.
4. Event may be classified as TIA—transient episode of cerebral dysfunction with associated clinical manifestations lasting usually minutes to an hour, possibly up to 24 hours.
5. Symptoms persisting longer than 24 hours are classified as stroke (also known as *brain attack*).

Risk Factors for Stroke
Medical Conditions

1. Diabetes mellitus (44% risk reduction in hypertensive diabetics with controlled BP).
2. Hypertension (30% to 40% risk reduction with treatment): goal BP is lower than 140/90; if renal insufficiency or heart failure, less than 130/85; if diabetic, less than 130/80.
3. Hyperlipidemia (20% to 30% risk reduction in patients with known coronary artery disease.
4. Coronary artery disease and cardiac disorders, such as congenital heart disease, valvular conditions, endocarditis, atrial fibrillation (68% risk reduction with oral anticoagulation; 21% with aspirin).
5. History of TIA or stroke.
6. Rare: Endothelial damage (inflammation or infection, drug-induced, fibromuscular dysplasia, carotid or vertebral artery dissections).

Behaviors

1. Cigarette smoking (smoking cessation results in a 50% risk reduction in 1 year; return to baseline in 5 years).
2. Alcohol abuse.
3. Physical inactivity.
4. Cocaine use (hemorrhagic stroke).

Nonmodifiable Factors

1. Increasing age—risk doubles for each decade over age 50.
2. Gender—men are at greater risk than women.
3. Heredity—increased risk with family history of stroke.
4. Ethnic background—blacks and Hispanics at higher risk than whites.

Other

There have been reports in the literature of increased risk due to childbirth, hormone replacement therapy or contraceptive use, and migraine headaches. Chiropractic manipulation has been associated with ischemic stroke related to dissection.

DRUG ALERT Increased stroke risk has been noted in women who smoke and take oral contraceptives and who have a history of migraines.

Clinical Manifestations of Transient Ischemic Attacks

1. History of intermittent neurologic deficit, sudden in onset, with maximal deficit within 5 minutes and lasting less than 24 hours.

2. Carotid system involvement: amaurosis fugax, homonymous hemianopsia, unilateral weakness, unilateral numbness or paresthesias, aphasia, dysarthria.
3. Vertebrobasilar system involvement: vertigo, homonymous hemianopsia, diplopia, weakness that is bilateral or alternates sides, dysarthria, dysphagia, ataxia, perioral numbness.
4. Carotid bruit.
5. History of headaches lasting days before ischemia.

Diagnostic Evaluation

1. Cerebral angiography, digital subtraction angiography, CT angiography, MRA, Doppler ultrasound—all provide information about carotid arteries, vertebral arteries, and intracranial circulation.
2. Anticoagulation monitoring: partial prothrombin time (PTT) or heparin anti-Xa test to determine heparin dose, or International Normalized Ratio (INR) to monitor warfarin therapy.
3. MRI stroke protocol: consists of a standard MRI in conjunction with DWI and ADC or PWI scan (see page 348).
4. Transesophageal echocardiography to rule out emboli from heart.

Management

1. Platelet aggregation inhibitors, such as aspirin, or clopidogrel to reduce risk of stroke.
2. Surgical or endovascular intervention to increase blood flow to the brain—carotid endarterectomy, extracranial/intracranial anastomosis, transarterial stenting, or angioplasty.
3. Reduction of other risk factors to prevent stroke, such as control of hypertension, diabetes, and hyperlipidemia, and smoking cessation.
4. Treatment of arrhythmias.
5. Treatment of isolated systolic hypertension.
6. Anticoagulation agents for patients who continue to have symptoms despite antiplatelet therapy (this remains controversial) and those with major source of cardiac emboli.

Complications

1. Complete ischemic stroke (30% of TIAs will progress to stroke within 5 years of initial TIA).
2. Hemorrhagic conversion of ischemic stroke.
3. Cerebral edema.

Nursing Assessment

1. Obtain history of possible TIA; hypertensive and diabetic control; hyperlipidemia; cardiovascular disease or dysrhythmias, such as atrial fibrillation; smoking.
2. Perform physical examination, including neurologic, cardiac, and circulatory systems; be sure to listen for carotid bruit.
3. Assess the patient for history of headache and, if positive, for duration of headache.

Nursing Diagnoses

- Risk for Ineffective Cerebral Tissue Perfusion related to underlying arteriosclerosis.
- Risk for Injury related to surgical procedure.
- Readiness for Enhanced Therapeutic Regimen Management regarding therapeutic lifestyle changes.

Nursing Interventions
Improving Cerebral Perfusion

1. Teach the patient signs and symptoms of TIA and need to notify health care provider immediately. Use the acronym FAST to know what to look for: F, face weakness; A, arm weakness; S, speech difficulties; T, time—immediately seek medical assistance.
2. Administer or teach self-administration of anticoagulants, antiplatelet agents, antihypertensives, and other medication; also teach about monitoring for adverse effects and therapeutic effect.
3. Prepare the patient for surgical or endovascular intervention as indicated (see page 361).

Providing Care and Preventing Complications After Surgical Procedure

Also see "Nursing Management of the Patient Undergoing Intracranial Surgery," page 361, and "Cerebral Angiography," page 350.

1. After surgical procedure, closely monitor vital signs and administer medication as prescribed to avoid hypotension (which can cause cerebral ischemia) or hypertension (which can precipitate cerebral hemorrhage).
2. Perform frequent neurologic checks, including pupil size, equality, and reaction; handgrip and plantar flexion strength; sensation; mental status; and speech. Notify the health care provider of any deficits immediately.
3. Observe operative area closely for swelling. Mild swelling is expected, but if hematoma formation is suspected, prepare the patient for immediate surgery.
4. Medicate for pain and avoid agitation or sudden changes in position, which could affect BP.
5. Elevate head of bed when vital signs are stable.
6. Following carotid endarterectomy:
   a. Monitor for hoarseness, impaired gag reflex, or difficulty swallowing and facial weakness, which indicate CN injury.
   b. Keep head in neutral position to relieve stress on surgical site; monitor drainage.
   c. Keep tracheostomy tube at bedside and assess for stridor; hematoma formation can cause airway obstruction.
7. Following extracranial–intracranial anastomosis, avoid pressure over the anastomosis of the superior temporal artery (extracranial) and the middle cerebral artery (intracranial) to prevent rupture or ischemia of the site. If the patient wears glasses, remove the eyeglass arm on the operative side to avoid this possible pressure point.
8. Following transcranial stenting, administer medications, as directed.
   a. Heparin—bolus given intraprocedure, then possible continuous IV drip postprocedure to maintain PTT within ordered range; monitor PTT every 6 hours.
   b. Clopidogrel before procedure, as ordered. Can be given as a loading dose of 150 mg the evening before procedure, 300-mg loading dose before procedure, 75 mg daily 48 hours before procedure, or 75 mg daily 1 week before procedure. Dosing is according to surgeon preference.
   c. Daily dosing of 75 mg clopidogrel for 30 to 90 days (specific duration varies), as directed.
   d. Aspirin 81 mg daily, as directed.
9. Monitor puncture site for bleeding, hematoma, and pulse, as ordered. Apply pressure if bleeding or hematoma is noted and inform physician.

NURSING ALERT In the event of an acute neurologic deficit, the heparin drip should be stopped until an acute intracerebral bleed has been ruled out.

DRUG ALERT Loading dose of clopidogrel, intraprocedure heparin bolus, postprocedure heparin drip, and postprocedure clopidogrel daily dosing minimize the risk of thromboembolic complications following transarterial carotid stenting while increasing the risk of hemorrhagic complications. Close monitoring of neurologic status and PTT is warranted. Inform health care provider of any changes in neurologic status, PTT levels out of ordered range, and signs of bleeding.

Encouraging Lifestyle Changes to Reduce Risk

1. Help the patient begin to formulate a plan for smoking cessation.
2. Teach the patient and family members the basics of nutrition, how to read labels, and how to follow a low-fat diet (particularly one low in saturated fats).
3. Obtain a referral to a nutritionist for help with weight management and low-fat, low-sodium diet, as indicated.
4. Encourage daily activity for 30 minutes, if possible. Obtain physical therapy referral for endurance training and monitoring, as indicated.
5. Monitor INR if warfarin is prescribed, and educate the patient about the risk of bleeding.

Patient Education and Health Maintenance

1. Encourage the patient receiving long-term oral anticoagulants to comply with follow-up monitoring of INR and to report any signs of bleeding.
2. Encourage patients receiving antiplatelet agents to report any signs of bleeding.
3. Encourage the use of electric razors and toothbrushes to prevent bleeding.
4. Reinforce with patient and family the importance of accessing the medical system, by calling 911, when symptoms first occur.
5. Refer the patient to the American Stroke Association (*www.strokeassociation.org*) or the National Institute of Neurologic Disorders and Stroke (*www.ninds.nih.gov*) for additional information and support.

Evaluation: Expected Outcomes

- Alert without neurologic deficits.
- Respirations unlabored, vital signs stable, no swelling of neck; reports relief of pain.
- Expresses readiness to quit smoking and adhere to a low-fat diet.

Cerebrovascular Accident (Stroke, Brain Attack)

Stroke, cerebrovascular accident (CVA), or *brain attack* is the onset and persistence of neurologic dysfunction resulting from disruption of blood supply to the brain and indicates infarction rather than ischemia. Strokes are classified as ischemic (more than 70% of strokes) or hemorrhagic (associated with greater morbidity and mortality). About 14% of strokes in the United States are of cardiac origin. About 60% of hemorrhagic strokes are the result of hypertension. Stroke is the leading cause of long-term disability and the third leading cause of death in the United States, with an annual incidence of 700,000.

Pathophysiology and Etiology

Ischemic Stroke

1. Partial or complete occlusion of a cerebral blood flow to an area of the brain due to the following:
   a. Thrombus (most common)—due to arteriosclerotic plaque in a cerebral artery, usually at bifurcation of larger arteries; occurs over several days.
   b. Embolus—a moving clot of cardiac origin (frequently due to atrial fibrillation) or from a carotid artery that travels quickly to the brain and lodges in a small artery; occurs suddenly with immediate maximum deficits.
2. Area of brain affected is related to the vascular territory that was occluded. Subtle decrease in blood flow may allow brain cells to maintain minimal function, but as blood flow decreases, focal areas of ischemia occur, followed by infarction to the vascular territory. See Figure 15-4 for cerebral circulation.
3. An area of injury includes edema, tissue breakdown, and small arterial vessel damage. The small arterial vessel damage poses a risk of hemorrhage. The larger the area of infarction, the greater the risk of hemorrhagic conversion.
4. Ischemic strokes are not activity-dependent; may occur at rest.

NURSING ALERT Early detection of warning signs promotes early diagnosis and intervention aimed at lessening stroke mortality and morbidity.

Hemorrhagic Stroke

1. Leakage of blood from a blood vessel and hemorrhage into brain tissue, causing edema, compression of brain tissue, and spasm of adjacent blood vessels.

Circle of Willis

Figure 15-4. The circle of Willis as seen at the base of a brain removed from the skull. (Anatomical Chart Company.)

2. May occur outside the dura (extradural), beneath the dura mater (subdural), in the SAS, or within the brain substance (intracerebral).
3. Causal mechanisms include the following:
   a. Increased pressure due to hypertension.
   b. Head trauma causing dissection or rupture of vessel.
   c. Deterioration of vessel wall from chronic hypertension, diabetes mellitus, or cocaine use.
   d. Congenital weakening of blood vessel wall with aneurysm or AVM.
4. The intracranial hemorrhage becomes a space-occupying lesion within the skull and compromises brain function.
   a. The mass effect causes pressure on brain tissue.
   b. The hemorrhage irritates local brain tissue, leading to surrounding focal edema.
   c. SAH or hemorrhage into a ventricle can block normal CSF flow, leading to hydrocephalus.
5. Hemorrhage commonly occurs suddenly while a person is active.

Clinical Manifestations

1. Clinical manifestations vary depending on the vessel affected and the cerebral territories it perfuses. Symptoms are usually multifocal. Headache may be a sign of impending cerebral hemorrhage or infarction; however, it is not always present.
2. Common clinical manifestations related to vascular territory (see Table 15-5).
   a. Numbness (paresthesia), weakness (paresis), or loss of motor ability (plegia) on one side of the body.
   b. Difficulty in swallowing (dysphagia).
   c. Aphasia (nonfluent, fluent, global).
   d. Visual difficulties of inattention or neglect (lack of acknowledgment of one side of the sensory field), loss of half of a visual field (hemianopsia), double vision, photophobia.
   e. Altered cognitive abilities and psychological affect.
   f. Self-care deficits.

Diagnostic Evaluation

1. CT scan—to determine cause and location of stroke and type of stroke, ischemic versus hemorrhagic.
2. MRA or CT angiogram—noninvasive evaluation of cerebrovascular structures in ischemic stroke.
3. Carotid ultrasound—to detect carotid stenosis in ischemic stroke.
4. Cerebral angiography—invasive evaluation of cerebrovasculature to determine the extent of cerebrovascular injury/insufficiency and to evaluate for structural abnormalities.
5. PET, MRI with DWI—to localize ischemic damage in ischemic stroke.
6. CT perfusion/MR perfusion—provides evaluation of cerebral blood flow, cerebral blood volume, and mean transient time to determine the extent of ischemic changes.
7. TCD—noninvasive method used to evaluate cerebral perfusion. Useful in the bedside evaluation and to provide a means for ongoing monitoring of cerebral blood flow to document changes and trends.

Management

Acute Treatment: Ischemic Stroke

1. Support of vital functions—maintain airway, breathing, oxygenation, circulation.
   a. Maintain pulse oximetry greater than 92%. Utilize oxygen therapy, as needed.
   b. Arrhythmias are common. Telemetry may be indicated to monitor. Atrial fibrillation is the most common arrhythmia in stroke population.
2. Astute neurologic assessment utilizing the National Institute of Health Stroke Scale (www.strokecenter.org/wp-content/uploads/2011/08/NIH_stroke_scale.pdf) and management of increased ICP.
3. IV fluids (normal saline) at maintenance until able to tolerate oral diet. Colloids may be used for reperfusion and hemodilution.

Table 15-5 Stroke Deficits Related to Vascular Territory

CEREBRAL ARTERY	BRAIN AREA INVOLVED	SIGNS AND SYMPTOMS*
Anterior cerebral	Infarction of the medial aspect of one frontal lobe if lesion is distal to communicating artery; bilateral frontal infarction if flow in other anterior cerebral artery is inadequate	Paralysis of contralateral foot or leg; impaired gait; paresis of contralateral arm; contralateral sensory loss over toes, foot, and leg; problems making decisions or performing acts voluntarily; lack of spontaneity, easily distracted; slowness of thought; urinary incontinence; cognitive and affective disorders
Middle cerebral	Massive infarction of most of lateral hemisphere and deeper structures of the frontal, parietal, and temporal lobes; internal capsule; basal ganglia	Contralateral hemiplegia (face and arm); contralateral sensory impairment; aphasia; homonymous hemiplegia; altered consciousness (confusion to coma); inability to turn eyes toward paralyzed side; denial of paralyzed side or limb (hemiattention); possible acalculia, alexia (visual aphasia), finger agnosia, and left–right confusion; vasomotor paresis and instability
Posterior cerebral	Occipital lobe; anterior and medial portion of temporal lobe	Homonymous hemianopia and other visual defects, such as color blindness, loss of central vision, and visual hallucinations; memory deficits; perseveration (repeated performance of same verbal or motor response)
	Thalamus involvement	Loss of all sensory modalities; spontaneous pain; intentional tremor; mild hemiparesis; aphasia
	Cerebral peduncle involvement	Oculomotor nerve palsy with contralateral hemiplegia
Basilar and vertebral	Cerebellum and brain stem	Visual disturbance such as diplopia, dystaxia, vertigo, dysphagia, dysphonia

*Dependent on hemisphere involved and adequacy of collaterals.

4. Maintain BP within prescribed parameters. Limit BP fluctuations.
   a. Management of systemic hypertension with labetalol, nicardipine, or alternative IV antihypertensive agents to keep systolic BP (SBP) less than 200 mm Hg. Goal is to promote adequate cerebral perfusion to prevent further ischemia. Avoid lowering BP greater than 25% within the first 24 hours. Hemorrhagic conversion/transformation can occur and is associated with degree of necrotic tissue and vascular injury. Hyperglycemia and BP fluctuations or rapid increases in BP increase the risk of hemorrhagic conversion.
   b. Management of hypotension—SBP goal greater than 100. Vasopressor agents to maintain SBP within prescribed range. Sustained hypotensive episodes are associated with poor outcome.
   c. Pretreatment with tissue plasminogen activator (tPA)—unable to receive tPA if SBP greater than 185 mm Hg or diastolic BP greater than 110 mm Hg.
   d. Post-tPA—maintain SBP less than 180 mm Hg or diastolic BP less than 105 mm Hg for first 24 hours post tPA.
5. Thrombolytic therapy (see Box 15-3, below).
   a. Recombinant tPA administered IV is the only Food and Drug Administration (FDA)–approved medical treatment for acute ischemic stroke. Dosing: IV 0.9 mg/kg within 3 hours of onset of symptoms.
   b. Transarterial tPA within 6 hours of onset of symptoms. Benefits have been demonstrated in acute ischemic stroke related to occlusion of middle cerebral artery. Advantages include the following:
      i. Higher concentration delivered to clot.
      ii. Can be performed in conjunction with mechanical disruption of clot.
      iii. Provides precise imaging of pathology and evaluation of collateral circulation.
      iv. Defines extent of injury and recanalization.
   c. Disadvantages include the following:
      i. Risk of hemorrhage related to catheter manipulation.
      ii. Dislodgement of clot.
      iii. Delay in thrombolytic therapy due to access delays.
      iv. Limited facility-based accessibility.
   d. Additional treatment options (transarterial or endovascular):
      i. Abciximab—antiplatelet agent delivered intra-arterially (IA).
      ii. Verapamil—potent vasodilator injected into intracranial vessel to treat acute spasm.
      iii. Clot retrieval or manipulation of clot.
      iv. Angioplasty and stenting have been utilized in acute dissection, though data are limited.
6. Maintain normal glucose levels because hypoglycemia and hyperglycemia are associated with a poor outcome. Sliding scale insulin or insulin drip should be given to maintain normoglycemia.
7. Maintain normothermia because hyperthermia is associated with a poor neurologic outcome.
8. Deep vein thrombosis (DVT) prophylaxis—sequential stockings and low-dose heparin or low molecular weight heparin (LMWH) should be utilized. Data do not suggest any increased risk of hemorrhage in this population.
9. Focus on early rehabilitation.

Acute Treatment: Hemorrhagic Stroke

1. Support of vital functions—maintain airway, breathing, oxygenation, circulation.
   a. Maintain pulse oximetry greater than 92%. Utilize oxygen therapy, as needed.
   b. Arrhythmias are common. Telemetry may be indicated to monitor.
   c. IV fluids (normal saline) at maintenance until able to tolerate oral diet.
2. Neurologic assessment—Facility-based neurologic assessment tool should be used. Notify the health care provider of clinical deterioration. Deterioration can be related to rebleed or development of cerebral edema.
3. Reversal of coagulopathies:
   a. Obtain patient's medication history. Medications to be concerned about include warfarin, aspirin, clopidogrel, ticlopidine, and dipyridamole/aspirin.
   b. Obtain INR and platelet function analyzer (PFA-100), as ordered. Elevated INR is associated with warfarin use. PFA epinephrine greater than 164 denotes platelet dysfunction related to aspirin use and PFA adenosine diphosphate greater than 116 denotes nonaspirin platelet dysfunction and has been used to determine the effectiveness of clopidogrel or ticlopidine or the presence of von Willebrand disease.
   c. As ordered, treat with platelets, cryoprecipitate, or vitamin K to reverse coagulopathy. Prothrombin complex concentrate may be used for rapid reversal.
4. Management of BP within prescribed parameters—maintain SBP less than 160 to reduce vessel wall stressors. Goal is to

---

BOX 15-3	Inclusion and Exclusion Criteria for tPA Therapy

INCLUSION

- Onset of symptoms
  - Within 4.5 hours IV tPA.
  - Within 6 hours IA tPA.
- Ischemic stroke with measurable deficits using the NIH Stroke Scale (see page 368).
- No hemorrhage noted on CT scan of brain.
- Clearly defined time of symptom onset.

EXCLUSION

- Head CT demonstrates early signs of infarction or hemorrhage.
- Uncontrolled hypertensive nonresponsive to IV or oral agent (systolic greater than 185 or diastolic greater than 110 mm Hg).
- Glucose level greater than 400 mg/dL.
- Coagulopathy.
  - Heparin within past 48 hours.
  - Patient on warfarin.
  - Elevated PTT or prothrombin time.
  - Platelet count less than 100,000.
- History of previous intracranial hemorrhage, head trauma, or stroke within past 3 months.
- GI or genitourinary tract hemorrhage in the past 3 weeks.
- History of major surgery in the past 2 weeks.

prevent rebleeding while promoting adequate cerebral perfusion. Labetalol, hydralazine, nicardipine, or alternative IV antihypertensive agents may be used.

5. Neurosurgical consultation for possible evacuation of intracerebral hemorrhage may be explored.

6. Treatment of clinical seizures with phenytoin or levetiracetam. Seizures commonly occur within the first 24 hours of intracerebral hemorrhage.

7. Maintain normal glucose level because hypoglycemia/hyperglycemia is associated with a poor outcome. Sliding scale insulin or insulin drip should be given to maintain normoglycemia.

8. Maintain normothermia because hyperthermia is associated with a poor neurologic outcome. Current data do not support the use of therapeutic, or induced, hypothermia in patients with ischemic stroke; however, research is ongoing to determine potential applications.

9. DVT prophylaxis—sequential stockings and low-dose heparin or LMWH should be utilized. Data do not suggest any increased risk of hemorrhage in this population.

10. Focus on early rehabilitation.

Subsequent Treatment

1. Aspirin is the only antiplatelet agent that has been evaluated in acute ischemic stroke. Aspirin is recommended within 24 hours poststroke. (In tPA patients, aspirin should not be given until 24 hours post tPA.) Alternative antiplatelet agents include ticlopidine, dipyridamole/aspirin 200/25, and clopidogrel.

2. Antispasmodic agents can be used for spastic paralysis.

3. Early initiation of a rehabilitation program, including physical therapy, occupational therapy, and speech therapy, and counseling, as needed.

4. Depression is common; therefore, early initiation of antidepressants can be beneficial, such as selective serotonin reuptake inhibitors.

Complications

1. Aspiration pneumonia.
2. Dysphagia in 25% to 50% of patients after stroke.
3. Spasticity, contractures.
4. DVT, pulmonary embolism.
5. Brain stem herniation.
6. Poststroke depression.

Nursing Assessment

1. Maintain neurologic flow sheet (National Institutes of Health (NIH) Stroke Scale for ischemic stroke and facility-based neurologic assessment tool for hemorrhagic stroke).

2. Assess for voluntary or involuntary movements, tone of muscles, presence of deep tendon reflexes (reflex return signals end of flaccid period and return of muscle tone).

3. Also assess mental status, CN function, sensation/proprioception.

4. Monitor bowel and bladder function/control.

5. Monitor effectiveness of anticoagulation therapy.

6. Frequently assess level of function and psychosocial response to condition.

7. Assess for skin breakdown, contractures, and other complications of immobility.

 DRUG ALERT Oral anticoagulants are adjusted to maintain an INR at 2 to 3 to prevent stroke associated with atrial fibrillation. Monitor for potential complications of intracranial and subdural hemorrhage. Report INRs that are elevated to reduce the risk of bleeding or decreased levels to adjust therapy to be more effective.

Nursing Diagnoses

• Risk for Injury related to neurologic deficits.
• Impaired Physical Mobility related to motor deficits.
• Impaired Environmental Interpretation Syndrome related to brain injury.
• Impaired Verbal Communication related to brain injury.
• Bathing, Dressing, Toileting Self-Care Deficit related to hemiparesis/paralysis.
• Imbalanced Nutrition: Less Than Body Requirements related to impaired self-feeding, chewing, swallowing.
• Impaired Urinary Elimination related to motor/sensory deficits.
• Disabled Family Coping related to catastrophic illness, cognitive and behavioral sequelae of stroke, and caregiving burden.

 NURSING ALERT Use of clinical pathways maximizes stroke patient outcomes across the care continuum. Case management models of care foster interdisciplinary utilization, timeliness of referrals, patient education, patient satisfaction, and efficient use of health care resources. The specific role of the nurse in stroke recovery integrates therapeutic aspects of coordinating, maintaining, and training.

Nursing Interventions

Preventing Falls and Other Injuries

1. Maintain bed rest during acute phase (24 to 48 hours after onset of stroke) with head of bed slightly elevated and side rails in place.

2. Administer oxygen, as ordered, during acute phase to maximize cerebral oxygenation.

3. Frequently assess respiratory status, vital signs, heart rate and rhythm, and urine output to maintain and support vital functions.

4. When patient becomes more alert after acute phase, maintain frequent vigilance and interactions aimed at orienting, assessing, and meeting the needs of the patient.

5. Try to allay confusion and agitation with calm reassurance and presence.

6. Assess the patient for risk for fall status.

Preventing Complications of Immobility

Interventions to improve functional recovery require active participation of the patient and repetitive training. Functional demand and intensive training are believed to trigger CNS reorganization—responsible for late functional recovery after stroke.

1. Maintain functional position of all extremities.
   a. Apply a trochanter roll from the crest of the ilium to the midthigh to prevent external rotation of the hip.
   b. Place a pillow in the axilla of the affected side when there is limited external rotation to keep arm away from chest and prevent adduction of the affected shoulder.

c. Place the affected upper extremity slightly flexed on pillow supports with each joint positioned higher than the preceding one to prevent edema and resultant fibrosis; alternate elbow extension.

d. Place the hand in slight supination with fingers slightly in flexion.

e. Avoid excessive pressure on ball of foot after spasticity develops.

f. Do not allow top bedding to pull affected foot into plantar flexion; may use tennis shoes in bed.

g. Place the patient in a prone position for 15 to 30 minutes daily, and avoid sitting up in chair for long periods to prevent knee and hip flexion contractures.

h. Encourage neutral positioning of affected limbs to promote relaxation and to limit abnormal increases in muscular tone to enhance functional recovery (reflex-inhibiting positioning).

i. "Forced use" is an experimental treatment designed to overcome nonuse of the hemiparetic upper extremity in regaining functional use of the affected arm with selected chronic hemiparetic patients.

j. "Constraint-induced movement therapy" restricts the contralateral upper extremity in effort to force use of the affected arm.

2. Apply splints and braces, as indicated, to support flaccid extremities or on spastic extremities to decrease stretch stimulation and reduce spasticity.

a. Volar splint to support functional position of wrist.

b. Sling to prevent shoulder subluxation of flaccid arm.

c. High-top sneaker for ankle and foot support.

3. Exercise the affected extremities passively through ROM four to five times daily to maintain joint mobility and enhance circulation; encourage active ROM exercise as able (see page 141).

4. Teach the patient to use the unaffected extremity to move the affected one.

5. Assist with ambulation, as needed, with help of physical therapy, as indicated.

a. Check for orthostatic hypotension when dangling and standing.

b. Gradually position the patient from a reclining position to head elevated, and dangle legs at the bedside before transferring out of bed or ambulating; assess sitting balance in bed.

c. Assess the patient for excessive exertion.

d. Have the patient wear walking shoes or tennis shoes.

e. Assess standing balance and have the patient practice standing.

f. Help the patient begin ambulating as soon as standing balance is achieved; ensure safety with a patient waist belt.

g. Provide rest periods as patient will tire easily.

Optimizing Orientation and Awareness

1. Be aware of the patient's cognitive alterations and adjust interaction and environment accordingly.

2. Participate in cognitive retraining program—reality orientation, visual imagery, cueing procedures—as outlined by rehabilitation nurse or therapist.

3. In patients with increased awareness, use pictures of family members, clock, calendar; post schedule of daily activities where patient can see it.

4. Focus on the patient's strengths and give positive feedback.

5. Be aware that depression is common and therapy should include psychotherapy and early initiation of antidepressants.

Facilitating Communication

1. Speak slowly, using visual cues and gestures; be consistent and repeat as necessary.

2. Speak directly to the patient while facing him or her.

3. Give plenty of time for response and reinforce attempts as well as correct responses.

4. Minimize distractions.

5. Use alternative methods of communication other than verbal, such as written words, gestures, or pictures.

Fostering Independence

1. Teach the patient to use nonaffected side for activities of daily living (ADL) but not to neglect affected side.

2. Adjust the environment (eg, call light, tray) to side of awareness if spatial neglect or visual field cuts are present; approach the patient from the uninvolved side.

3. Teach the patient to scan environment if visual deficits are present.

4. Encourage the family to provide clothing a size larger than patient wears, with front closures, Velcro, and stretch fabric; teach the patient to dress while sitting to maintain balance.

5. Make sure personal care items, urinal, and commode are nearby and that patient obtains assistance with transfers and other activities, as needed.

6. Be aware that ADL require anticipatory (automatic coordination of multiple muscle groups in anticipation of a specific movement) and reactive (adjustment of posture to stimuli) postural adjustments.

7. Be aware that patients usually have clear goals in relation to functional abilities, against which all success and forward progress will be measured; help them set realistic short- and long-term goals.

Promoting Adequate Oral Intake

1. Perform a bedside swallow screen. Follow institutional protocol. If any coughing or difficulties are noted, contact speech therapy for official consult.

2. Initiate referral for a speech therapist for individuals with compromised LOC, dyspraxic speech, or speech difficulties to evaluate swallowing function at bedside or radiographically to demonstrate safe and functional swallowing mechanisms before initiation of oral diet.

3. Help the patient relearn swallowing sequence using compensatory techniques (see page 369).

a. Place ice on tongue and encourage sucking.

b. Progress to ice pops and soft foods.

c. Make sure mechanical soft or pureed diet is provided, based on ability to chew.

4. Encourage small, frequent meals and allow plenty of time to chew and swallow. Dietary consults can be helpful for selection of food preferences.

5. Remind the patient to chew on the unaffected side.

6. Encourage the patient to drink small sips from a straw with chin tucked to the chest, strengthening effort to swallow while chin is tucked down.

7. Inspect mouth for food collection and pocketing before entry of each new bolus of food.

8. Inspect oral mucosa for injury from biting tongue or cheek.

9. Encourage frequent oral hygiene.

10. Teach the family how to assist the patient with meals to facilitate chewing and swallowing.

a. Reduce environmental distractions to improve patient concentration.

b. Provide oral care before eating to improve aesthetics and afterward to remove food debris.

c. Position the patient so he or she is sitting with 90 degrees of flexion at the hips and 45 degrees of flexion at the neck. Use pillows to achieve correct position.

d. Maintain position for 30 to 45 minutes after meals to prevent regurgitation and aspiration.

Attaining Bladder Control

1. Insert indwelling bladder catheterization during acute stage for accurate fluid management; remove as soon as status stabilizes.

2. Establish regular voiding schedule—every 2 to 3 hours, correlated with fluid intake—when bladder tone returns. If the patient is unable to void, intermittent catheterization can be used to empty bladder and prevent overstretching of bladder. The bladder scan device is useful in monitoring bladder capacity and identifying individuals at risk.

3. Assist with standing or sitting to void (especially males).

4. See page 148 for bladder retraining program details.

Strengthening Family Coping

1. Consult a social worker for assistance with patient/family support, to obtain copy of durable power of attorney, address guardianship, and long-term care decisions, as needed.

2. Encourage the family to maintain outside interests.

3. Teach stress management techniques, such as relaxation exercises, use of community and faith-based support networks.

4. Encourage participation in support group for family respite program for caregivers or other available resources in area.

5. Involve as many family and friends in care as possible.

6. Provide information about stroke and expected outcome.

7. Teach the family that stroke survivors may show depression in the first 3 months of recovery.

Community and Home Care Considerations

1. Hemiplegic complications resulting from stroke commonly include "frozen" shoulder; adduction and internal rotation of arm with flexion of elbow, wrist, and fingers; external rotation of the hip with flexion of the knee and plantar flexion of the ankle.

2. Perform ROM exercises and instruct the patient and family on these as well as on proper positioning.

3. Reinforce that these muscle and ligament deformities resulting from stroke can be prevented with daily stretching and strengthening exercises.

4. Depression after stroke is a major problem because it can increase morbidity. Monitor for signs of depression, such as difficulty sleeping, frequent crying, anorexia, feelings of guilt, or sadness. Notify the health care provider for possible medication therapy.

5. Continue to support family who may be caring for a hemiplegic or aphasic person at home or in long-term care for a long time. Six months after stroke, around 9% to 21% of survivors are severely disabled, fully dependent, and live in institutions.

Patient Education and Health Maintenance

1. Teach the patient and family to adapt home environment for safety and ease of use.

2. Instruct the patient of the need for rest periods throughout day.

3. Reassure the family that it is common for poststroke patients to experience emotional lability and depression; treatment can be given.

4. Encourage consistency in the environment without distraction.

5. Assist the family to obtain self-help aids for the patient.

6. Instruct the family in management of aphasia (see Box 15-4, below).

BOX 15-4   Management of Aphasia

Aphasia is an acquired disorder of communication resulting from brain damage due to stroke, head injury, brain tumors, or brain cysts. It may involve impairment of the ability to speak, to understand speech of others, and to read, write, calculate, and understand gestures. Most aphasic individuals have difficulty with expression and comprehension to varying degrees. Fatigue has adverse effect on speech.

To enhance your communication with the patient with aphasia, keep the environment simple and relaxed, minimize distractions, and use multiple sensory channels.

Refer the family to:
American Speech-Language-Hearing Association
10801 Rockville Pike
Rockville, MD 20852
301-897-5700
www.asha.org

APHASIA SYNDROMES

- Fluent aphasia (Wernicke or receptive aphasia): Patient retains verbal fluency but may have difficulty in understanding speech. Speech is effortless and lacks clear content, information, and direction (nonsensical).
- Nonfluent aphasia (Broca or expressive aphasia): Varied degrees of difficulty in initiation of speech, difficulty in formation of words with poor articulation, and difficulty in finding appropriate words. Speech is slow and laborious. Auditory comprehension is preserved.
- Anomic or amnesiac aphasia: Characteristic feature is difficulty naming and finding words. However, grammar, comprehension, and repetition remain intact.
- Conduction aphasia: Major difficulty is with sequencing phonemes resulting in literal paraphrasic errors. Auditory comprehension remains intact; however, patient has difficulty repeating spoken language.
- Global aphasia: Severe disruption of communication (verbal speech, written, reading, and auditory comprehension).

NURSING INTERVENTIONS

- Speak at your normal rate and volume: The patient is not hard of hearing.
- Allow plenty of time to answer.
- Do not ask questions that require complex answers.
- Rote phrases can be spontaneous.
- Provide pad and pen if the patient prefers and is able to write.
- Avoid forcing speech.
- Watch the patient for clues and gestures if his or her speech is jargon; make neutral statements.
- Allow plenty of time for response.
- Ask for minimal word response.
- Encourage the patient to speak slowly.
- Expect frustration and anger at inability to communicate.
- Keep environment simple.
- Use gestures as well as language.
- Allow the patient to manipulate objects for additional sensory input.

7. Educate those at risk for stroke about lifestyle modifications and medication therapy that can lower risk.
8. Refer the patient and family for more information and support to such agencies as the National Stroke Association (*www.stroke.org*).

Evaluation: Expected Outcomes

- No falls, vital signs stable.
- Maintains body alignment, no contractures.
- Oriented to person, place, and time.
- Communicates appropriately.
- Brushes teeth, puts on shirt and pants independently.
- Feeds self two thirds of meal.
- Voids on commode at 2-hour intervals.
- Family seeks help and assistance from others.

Rupture of Intracranial Aneurysm

 EVIDENCE BASE Connolly, E. S., Rabinstein, A. A., Carhuapoma, R., et al. (2012). Guidelines for the management of aneurysmal subarachnoid hemorrhage: A guideline for healthcare professionals from the American Heart Association/American Stroke Association. *Stroke, 43,* 1711–1737.
Grasso, G., Alafaci, C., & Macdonald, R. L. (2017). Management of aneurysmal subarachnoid hemorrhage: State of the art and future perspectives. *Surgical Neurology International.* 8, 11.

An *intracranial aneurysm* is an abnormal localized dilation of the wall of a cerebral artery due to congenital absence of the muscle layer of the vessel. Constant blood flow against the weakened area results in growth of the aneurysm and thinning of the vessel wall. Aneurysms usually occur at a bifurcation of an artery or major branches of the circle of Willis. They may be of congenital, traumatic, arteriosclerotic, or infectious origin. Most are saccular and asymptomatic until rupture; other types are fusiform and berry (see Figure 15-5). When an aneurysm ruptures, sudden bleeding occurs in the SAS between the arachnoid and the pia, causing SAH, which produces symptoms related to meningeal irritation. Hemorrhage can extend into the ventricular system, causing obstruction of CSF flow (hydrocephalus) or into the brain tissue (intracerebral bleed), causing further neurologic compromise. Depending on the extent of SAH, cerebral vasospasm (transient thickening of intralumen of a vessel) can occur, producing decreased cerebral blood flow, ischemia, and potential infarction or delayed cerebral ischemia (DCI). Transient thickening of the vessel is believed to be in response to

the circulating blood and/or its breakdown products in the CSF. Vasospasm commonly occurs 3 to 14 days after SAH and peaks on day 5. Aneurysmal SAH account for 5% of all strokes.

Grading of Aneurysms

Hunt-Hess Scale is used to determine prognosis and timing of surgical or endovascular intervention.

0, Unruptured; asymptomatic discovery.

I, Asymptomatic or minimal headache with slight nuchal rigidity.

II, Moderate to severe headache, nuchal rigidity; no neurologic deficit other than CN deficit.

III, Drowsiness, confusion, or mild focal deficit (eg, hemiparesis), or combination of these findings.

IV, Stupor, moderate to severe deficit, possibly early decerebrate rigidity and vegetative disturbances.

V, Deep coma, decerebrate rigidity, moribund appearance.

Pathophysiology and Etiology

1. Etiology is believed to be multifactorial and includes structural abnormality of the cerebral vessel wall, atherosclerotic changes, hypertension, and environment. It is believed that inflammation has a role in the growth of the aneurysm.
2. Associated conditions: Polycystic disease, Ehlers-Danlos syndrome, Marfan's, Osler-Weber-Rendu syndrome, fibromuscular dysplasia, moyamoya syndrome, sickle cell anemia, collagen type III disorder, bacterial endocarditis (mycotic aneurysms), trauma (dissecting aneurysms), and familial incidence (less than 2%).
3. Risk factors for rupture
   a. Modifiable: HTN, smoking, alcohol abuse, and cocaine
   b. Nonmodifiable: sex (female), known aneurysm, size greater than 7 mm, history of previous aneurysm rupture and saccular aneurysms.
4. May become symptomatic because of pressure of enlarging aneurysm on nearby CNs or brain tissue.
5. Rupture and hemorrhage into SAS may cause increased ICP, hydrocephalus, and ischemia.
6. Vasospasm may occur within 3 to 14 days, peak day 5 days after rupture, causing ischemia (DCI) and infarction.
7. Rebleeding may occur because of lysis of clot with greatest risk for rebleeding in the first 6 to 72 hours after initial bleed (5% to 10%). Risk is greater in Hunt-Hess grades III to IV, large aneurysms, and sentinel bleed. Immediate repair of the aneurysm reduces the risk of rebleed. Seventy percent mortality after rebleed.
8. DCI is an independent variable for poor outcome.

Incidence

1. 12/100,000 incidence of aneurysms with 30,000 annual cases of SAH in the United States.
2. Age: Women 55 to 85 and men 25 to 45 and over 85.
3. 10% to 15% have multiple aneurysms.
4. Familial tendency less than 2%.

Clinical Manifestations

1. Sudden onset of severe headache, often accompanied by nausea and vomiting, but no neurologic deficits; leaking of aneurysm or AVM may cause a warning bleed.
2. Sudden, severe headache (commonly described as the "worst headache of my life"), meningeal signs (nuchal rigidity,

Figure 15-5. Types of aneurysms. **(A)** Saccular aneurysm; **(B)** berry aneurysm; **(C)** fusiform aneurysm.

photophobia, irritability), and neurologic dysfunction (related to vascular territory) are commonly related to SAH secondary to ruptured intracranial aneurysm, which can be catastrophic.

3. Neurologic deficit related to vascular territory (see page 372); progressive CN III, IV, VI deficits due to mass effect.
4. Sentinel bleeds—10% to 20% of patients with SAH experience an acute, sudden headache that appears days or weeks before admission for SAH. Etiology of sentinel bleed is unclear. Theories include leakage of blood from the aneurysm or expansion of the aneurysm.

Diagnostic Evaluation

1. History and physical examination.
2. CT scan—to determine presence of blood in SAS, rule out other lesions, and evaluate mass effect. Modified Fischer grade—estimates blood volume and location on CT. Assists in predicting risk for vasospasm. The Modified Fisher scale was adapted from the Fisher scale and adjusted based on clinical analysis of the occurrence of vasospasm.
   a. Grade 0: no SAH; no intraventricular hemorrhage (IVH), 0% risk of vasospasm
   b. Grade 1: focal or diffuse, thin SAH, no IVH; 24% risk of vasospasm
   c. Grade 2: thin focal (less than 1 mm) or diffuse SAH, IVH present; 33% risk of vasospasm
   d. Grade 3: thick focal (greater than 1 mm) or diffuse SAH, no IVH; 33% risk of vasospasm
   e. Grade 4: thick focal (greater than 1 mm) or diffuse SAH; 40% risk of vasospasm
3. Lumbar puncture (if no mass effect on CT)—grossly bloody CSF with more than 25,000 red blood cells (RBCs), CSF will not clear with subsequent taps as a traumatic tap would.
4. MRA or CT angiogram—noninvasive evaluation of cerebral vascular structures. Can be useful in the workup of suspected aneurysms (individuals with persistent headaches or unexplained neurologic deficits such as CN palsies). CT angiogram is the preferred study, though renal function must assessed secondary to use of contrast dye.
5. Cerebral angiogram—gold standard test; provides definitive evaluation of aneurysm etiology, presence, location, and configuration. Useful in determining the presence of vasospasm, extent of vasospasm, and collateral circulation.
6. TCD—noninvasive method to evaluate cerebral perfusion. Useful in the bedside evaluation and to provide a means for ongoing monitoring of cerebral blood flow to document changes and trends. Results are operator dependent.

Management

Unruptured

1. Evaluation of diagnostic studies is key to determine need for intervention, scheduling of elective surgical clipping, or endovascular embolization, if indicated.
2. Normalize BP if hypertensive (SBP goal 120 to 140).
3. Smoking cessation.

After Rupture

1. Intracranial aneurysm precautions to minimize the risk of rebleeding and control BP—bed rest with the head elevated, decreased environmental stimuli, avoidance of Valsalva maneuver and neck flexion, no caffeine, physical care as condition indicates.
2. Rapid repair of aneurysm should be performed by surgical clipping or endovascular embolization.

3. Management of systemic hypertension with labetalol, nicardipine, vasotec, hydralazine, or alternative IV antihypertensive agent can be used to maintain SBP less than 160 mm Hg (physician dependent), prior to definitive treatment. Debate continues on the precise SBP goal to be utilized. Close blood pressure monitoring should be maintained to prevent precipitous drop in BP.
4. Fluid goal is euvolemia. Prophylactic hypervolemia is not recommended. Fluid boluses should be considered prior to initiating vasopressor therapy. Close monitoring of intake and output (I&O), including running total I&O, and daily weights should be obtained to accurately assess fluid status. Routine use of central venous access for central venous pressure (CVP) monitoring is not recommended.
5. Neuroprotective agents.
   a. Nimodipine, a calcium channel blocker, has demonstrated reduced incidence of delayed neurologic deficits and is felt to be neuroprotective during SAH and vasospasm. The medication is administered on admission and continues for 21 consecutive days. Dosing: 60 mg orally q4h for SBP greater than 140 mm Hg and 30 mg orally q4h for SBP 120 to 140 mm Hg, or per physician orders.
      i. Nimodipine has cerebral specificity to block the influx of calcium at the intracellular space. It is the only drug approved by the FDA for treatment of vasospasm.
      ii. For optimal effect, the nimodipine should be started within 96 hours of SAH.
   b. Plasma expanders and hypervolemia to increase cerebral perfusion.
   c. The data on the neuroprotective benefits of statins, specifically simvastatin, remain controversial, though patients on statins should have the drug continued. Statins may be considered in individuals not previously on statins. Dosing: 80mg daily started within 48 hours for 14 days. Lipid panel should be performed prior to institution and a liver function panel should be obtained on day 7.
   d. Maintenance of magnesium level within normal limits. Hypomagnesium should be avoided.
6. Induced hypertension can be used in symptomatic vasospasm to prevent DCI. Colloids should be used initially with use of vasopressors as a secondary measure. Common vasopressor agents utilized are phenylephrine and norepinephrine. Fludrocortisone can be used as an oral agent to maintain SBP goal. No data exist on the specific SBP goal to be utilized. Neurologic examination should be utilized to determine specific SBP or MAP goal.
7. Management of acute obstructive hydrocephalus related to IVH by placement of ventriculostomy or EVD.
   a. Adjustment of drain to promote drainage of CSF.
   b. Intraventricular tPA-clot lysis may be used to promote CSF drainage. Current studies indicate low risk for intracranial bleeding with reduced risk for vasospasm.
   c. Surgical placement of ventricular-peritoneal shunt may be necessary.
8. Witnessed seizures: Phenytoin, fosphenytoin, or levetiracetam are the preferred medications. Duration of drug therapy is variable and levels are monitored for accurate dosing. Prophylactic use of antiepileptics is not recommended, although it may be considered. If prophylactic antiepileptics are utilized, a 3- to 7-day course or discontinuing after the aneurysm is secured is recommended.

9. Cardiopulmonary complications are common. Baseline electrocardiography should be obtained on admission. Cardiac enzymes and echocardiogram are recommended if cardiopulmonary dysfunction is suspected.

10. Maintain normal glucose level because hypoglycemia and hyperglycemia is associated with a poor outcome. Sliding scale insulin or insulin drip should be utilized to maintain blood sugar at 80 to 180. Glucose level less than 80 and greater than 200 should be avoided.

11. Maintain normothermia. Hyperthermia is associated with a poor neurologic outcome. Antipyretic agents are first-line treatment for the management of fever. External surface cooling devices or intravascular cooling devices should be employed when antipyretics are ineffective. Fever workup should be performed to evaluate for potential infectious etiology of fever.

12. DVT prophylaxis—sequential stockings and low-dose heparin or LMWH should be utilized, although remains physician-dependent. Data do not suggest any increased risk of hemorrhage in this population. Low-dose heparin or LMWH should be held prior to and after any intracranial procedure for 24 hours.

Surgical Intervention

1. Surgical obliteration of aneurysm by clipping, ligation, or IA technique.
2. Assessment of Hunt-Hess grade and medical stability assist in determining the timing of intervention, usually within 24 to 72 hours.
3. Method of treatment is determined by evaluating aneurysm size, location, neck width, condition of the patient, and associated medical conditions.
4. Surgical methods:
   a. Craniotomy is performed to access the aneurysm. Placement of titanium clips across the neck of the aneurysm or wrapping of fusiform aneurysm. Multiple-size titanium clips are available to secure aneurysm.
   b. *Advantages*: removal of intracerebral hemorrhagic/subarachnoid blood; low rate of aneurysm recurrence.
   c. *Disadvantage*: open procedure.
5. IA techniques:
   a. Superselective angiography with placement of microcatheter into the aneurysm for evaluation.
   b. Obliteration of the aneurysm.
      i. Multiple types of coils are available. Type and length of coil utilized are dependent on configuration of aneurysm. Coils fill the aneurysm and are detached using electronic heating. Multiple coils are placed until there is no blood flow noted on angiography to the aneurysm.
      ii. Coil embolization with aid of microstent—the microstent is used to form a bridge across the neck of the aneurysm and in fusiform aneurysms, allowing for placement of coils.
      iii. *Advantages*: minimally invasive treatment; shorter duration of anesthesia.
      iv. *Disadvantage*: potential for recurrence if aneurysm not completely occluded.
   c. Interventional treatment of vasospasm.
      i. Balloon angioplasty—dilation of vessel by expansion of a transarterial balloon to treat vasospasm.
      ii. IA injection or verapamil or papaverine for temporary local vasodilation.

 DRUG ALERT Heparin can be used intraprocedurally and postprocedurally, as directed, to minimize risk of thromboembolic events. Risks include thromboembolic complications and rupture of aneurysm with extension of SAH.

Complications

 NURSING ALERT Mortality ranges from 20% to 50% (12% to 15% die before reaching the hospital, 25% die within 24 hours post SAH, and 45% to 50% die within 30 days). Survivors are left with a 50% chance of functional disability. Rebleed and DCI secondary to vasospasm is directly related to mortality and morbidity.

1. Aneurysm rebleed—risk is 4% on day 1, then 1.5% per day on days 2 to 13, 20% within 14 days, and 50% within 6 months; highest risk within first 6 hours. Seventy percent mortality in rebleed.
2. Delayed ischemic neurologic deficit occur secondary to diminished cerebral blood flow. Cerebral vasospasm and DCI are the most common cause. Greatest risk: 3 to 14 days after SAH. Current theory is that cerebral vasospasm is a reversible thickening of medial wall and smooth muscle proliferation, causing narrowing of the vessel lumen. Seventy percent to 80% of patients have radiographic vasospasm, with 30% being symptomatic or demonstrating the effects of DCI.
3. Obstructive hydrocephalus—20% to 30% of patients develop obstructive hydrocephalus. EVD placement allows for temporary CSF drainage; 18% to 26% will require placement of a ventricular-peritoneal shunt.
4. Seizures—1% to 7% at presentation. Witnessed seizures are treated with AEDs, although specific duration of treatment remains controversial. Prophylactic use of AEDs is not recommended, although it may be considered. If prophylactic AEDs are used, a 3- to 7-day course or discontinuing after the aneurysm is secured is recommended.
5. Hypernatremia related to alterations in ADH secretion or imbalance in fluid status. Close monitoring of sodium level may be indicated.
6. Hyponatremia—differentiate between SIADH and cerebral salt wasting to ensure appropriate treatment (see page 358).
7. Cardiopulmonary complications: (related to abnormal catecholamine release).
   a. Cardiovascular changes ranging from atrial fibrillation, bradycardia, and T-wave abnormalities to left ventricular dysfunction with or without myocardial failure and myocardial injury in severe cases.
   b. Neurogenic pulmonary edema.

Nursing Assessment

1. Perform and document neurologic assessment with vital signs and as patient condition warrants.
2. Monitor for changes in or decreasing LOC, CN dysfunction, pupillary abnormality, and motor deficit, which signify increased ICP, cerebral vasospasm, DCI, or expanding lesion.
3. Assess for increasing headache, which could signal rebleeding.
4. Monitor for focal neurologic deficits, which may indicate vasospasm.

Nursing Diagnoses

- Risk for Ineffective Cerebral Tissue Perfusion related to potential rebleeding, vasospasm, and IICP.
- Ineffective Tissue Perfusion (cerebral) related to disease process and vasospasm.
- Acute Pain secondary to cerebral hemorrhage, meningeal irritation, and surgical procedure.
- Anxiety of patient/family related to treatment, intracranial surgery or endovascular treatment, and uncertainty of patient outcome.

Nursing Interventions

Modifying Activity to Prevent Complications

1. Prior to treatment reduce environmental stimuli, limit stress, and decrease the risk of rebleed and/or increased ICP.
   a. Maintain complete bed rest with head elevated 30 degrees to reduce cerebral edema.
   b. Maintain quiet environment with low lighting, noise control, and limit activity to prevent photophobia, agitation, and pain.
   c. Encourage the awake patient to avoid activities that increase BP or ICP: straining, sneezing, acute flexion/rotation of the neck; assist the patient with position changes.
   d. Avoid Valsalva maneuver, which may increase ICP, by administering stool softeners to prevent straining; avoiding rectal temperatures, enemas, and suppositories; and teaching the awake patient to exhale through mouth during defecation.
   e. Avoid caffeinated beverages and extremes of temperatures.
   f. Provide physical care, such as bathing and feeding, as needed.
2. Implement nursing interventions to minimize ICP and cerebral swelling (eg, elevate head of bed 30 degrees, maintain proper head and neck alignment to avoid jugular vein compression, avoid prolonged suctioning procedures, keep procedure less than 15 seconds, collaborate with physicians to use lidocaine before suctioning if intubated).
3. Medicate the patient, as ordered, during periods of extreme agitation.
4. Perform and document neurologic assessment with vital signs and as patient condition warrants, which includes monitoring LOC, CN function, pupillary function, and motor function. Insidious onset of confusion, disorientation, and decreased LOC or focal deficit associated with vascular territory associated with aneurysm bleed may indicate vasospasm (peak occurrence is 5 days after bleed, up 14 days after bleed). Speech slurring or onset of pronator drift may be first signs of deterioration.
5. Assess for signs of increased ICP, including agitation, change in LOC, bradycardia, and widening pulse pressure, and changes in respiratory pattern (Cheyne-Stokes pattern, apneustic, ataxic).
6. Monitor arterial blood gas (ABG) values for hypoxia and hypercapnia, which aggravate ICP.
7. Monitor ventriculostomy, if present, for patency, amount, and character of drainage, and correct height level every 4 hours.
8. Recognize need for maintenance of BP parameters based on status of treated versus untreated aneurysm (ie, treated, SBP 120–180 or as directed; untreated, SBP 120–160). (BP goal posttreatment remains controversial. BP goal may vary related to physician preference or be based on clinical examination.)

9. Evaluate effectiveness of antihypertensive or vasopressor therapy.
10. Perform ongoing physical assessment, including respiratory, cardiac, GI, and genitourinary (GU) function to detect potential complications.

 NURSING ALERT There are no evidence-based data to support daily sampling of CSF. If CSF is cloudy or purulent, notify the health care provider. If ordered, obtain CSF samples from EVD using sterile technique and send for culture and Gram stains, white blood cell (WBC) count, RBC count, glucose, and protein analysis.

Maintaining Safety

1. Frequently monitor neurologic status based on condition, including LOC, pupillary reaction, motor and sensory function, CN function, speech, and presence of headache.
2. Administer crystalloid to maintain euvolemia.
3. Monitor BP, hemodynamic monitoring, neurologic status, and input and output status at least every hour, or as status indicates, while in the ICU.
4. Maintain safety factors based on neurologic deficits; prevent physical injury related to vision, hearing, and body awareness deficits.
5. Monitor for seizure activity and administer antiepileptic drugs (AEDs) as directed.
6. See "Nursing Management of the Patient with an Altered State of Consciousness," page 505.

Reducing Pain

1. Assess level of pain and pain relief; report any increase in headache.
2. Administer analgesics, as prescribed; if opioid is being given with sedative, monitor for CNS depression, decreased respirations, and decreased BP. Stool softeners should be given if analgesics are utilized.
3. Administer dexamethasone, as prescribed, for headache control. May be useful for headaches as a result of inflammatory changes secondary to coils.
4. Encourage distraction and relaxation techniques to promote calming effect.
5. Explain to the patient/significant other the limited use of opioids secondary to need to assess the patient's LOC at all times.
6. Encourage elevated head of bed to minimize cerebral swelling.
7. Provide cool compresses to head.
8. Assess the patient for experiences of unrelieved or increased pain; assess for any changes in neurologic signs, nuchal rigidity, photophobia, and/or changes in vision, which could signal hemorrhage, hydrocephalus, or meningeal irritation.

Reducing Anxiety

1. Provide ongoing assessment of psychosocial issues (sexuality, anxiety, fear, depression, frustration, emotional lability).
2. Be attuned to verbal and nonverbal cues from the patient/family that signal problems with coping.
3. Inform the patient regarding all treatment modalities.
4. Encourage discussion of risks/benefits with the surgeon/interventional neuroradiologist.
5. Use reassurance and therapeutic conversation to relieve fear and anxiety.
6. Provide support to the patient/family in dealing with the stress and uncertainty of hospitalization.

7. Consult social services for assistance with patient/family support to obtain copy of advance directives, including durable power of attorney, address guardianship, and long-term care decisions, as needed.
8. Prepare the patient and family for surgery or endovascular treatment.

Community and Home Care Considerations

1. Assess the level of knowledge and ability of the patient/significant other to retain information.
2. Assess ongoing home care needs.
3. Assess the need for skilled nursing or rehabilitation center placement and obtain social service referral to help with planning.
4. Provide teaching to the family and caregivers and act as liaison between health care team and family.
5. Teach the patient and family how to deal with permanent neurologic deficits, and make sure that they obtain needed supplies and services.

Patient Education and Health Maintenance

1. Instruct the patient/family on purpose and frequency of neurologic radiologic procedures.
2. Explain what an aneurysm is, signs/symptoms of rupture, and possible threats of rupture.
3. Educate the patient about activities to avoid to prevent sudden increased pressure, such as heavy lifting and straining prior to definitive treatment.
4. Encourage lifelong medical follow-up and immediate attention if severe headache develops.
5. Instruct the patient/family on need for and use of invasive monitoring and drainage systems.
6. Reinforce the need for head of bed not to be adjusted.
7. Provide educational material for procedures.
8. Set mutual goals for discharge and communicate discharge preparations with other disciplines (registered nurse, physician, physical therapist, discharge coordinator).
9. Explain medications to the patient/significant other and potential adverse effects. Explain the importance of continued nimodipine therapy and correct usage.
10. Have the patient verbalize discharge instructions regarding wound care, activity restrictions, medications, and reportable signs/symptoms.

Evaluation: Expected Outcomes

- No signs of rebleeding, increased ICP, vasospasm; vital signs and neurologic signs stable.
- Safety maintained; no seizure activity.
- Verbalizes decreased pain or control of pain to an intensity that is acceptable.
- The patient and family able to state reason for surgery/endovascular intervention, possible risks; openly discuss fears and uncertainties.

Rupture of Intracranial Arteriovenous Malformation

EVIDENCE BASE Ajiboye, N., Chalouhi, N., Starke, R. M., et al. (2014). Cerebral arteriovenous malformations: Evaluation and management. *Scientific World Journal, 2014,* Article ID 649036.

An *arteriovenous malformation (AVM)* is a system of dilated arteries and veins with dysplastic vessels. The normal capillary beds are absent, and the arterial blood flows directly into the draining veins (fistula). AVMs are congenital lesions that can enlarge over the patient's life span; these lesions are often asymptomatic until rupture. The lifetime risk of bleed in an unruptured AVM is 2% to 4% per year throughout the patient's life span, depending on size and structural configuration of the lesion.

Pathophysiology and Etiology

1. AVMs generally contain a nidus (central core) and "red" engorged veins (oxygenated veins) and have been described as a tangled mass of discolored vessels that have the appearance of a cluster of grapes.
2. The artery to venous connection, or fistula, creates increased pressure within the venous system, resulting in vascular dilation, congestion, and hypoperfusion.
3. AVMs are generally low-pressure abnormalities at birth and can progress to a high-flow, high-pressure abnormality in adulthood.
4. Parenchymal AVMs can be located in the pia matter, subcortical tissue, paraventricular region, or a combination of these regions.
5. Approximately 50% of patients with AVMs present with hemorrhage. Other signs of AVM rupture include seizures and signs of mass effect.
6. Intracerebral bleeding in a ruptured AVM tends to be superficial; cerebral vasospasm rarely occurs. The Spetzler-Martin grading system is used as a prognostic indicator as well as a tool to define risks associated with treating AVMs. Grading scale of 1 to 5: 1 = lowest risk, 5 = greatest risk for treatment (see Table 15-6).

Clinical Manifestations

1. Sudden onset of severe headache, often accompanied by nausea and vomiting, but without neurologic deficits, may be an early sign of a ruptured AVM.
2. Progressively worsening headache, as well as new onset of seizure activity due to spontaneous superficial intracerebral hemorrhage, are commonly related to a ruptured AVM.
3. May present with loss of consciousness and severe deficits if massive bleed. Focal signs or deficits are dependent on the location of the bleed and compression of adjacent brain structures (visual disturbances, CN deficits, hemiparesis, etc.).

Table 15-6 Spetzler-Martin Grading System	
	POINTS
Size of Nidus	
Small	1
Medium	2
Large	3
Eloquence of Brain Tissue	
No	0
Yes	1
Deep Vascular Component	
No	0
Yes	1

Grading scale of 1 to 5: 1 = lowest risk, 5 = greatest risk for treatment.

Diagnostic Evaluation

1. History and physical examination.
2. CT scan—to determine presence of blood, rule out other lesions; increased density if blood present, may also show increased ICP or mass effect.
3. MRI and MRA or CT angiogram—noninvasive evaluation of cerebral vascular structures. Useful in the diagnosis of AVM, but does not define vascular changes and flow patterns.
4. Cerebral angiogram—gold standard test and the only diagnostic tool that provides definitive evaluation of AVM presence, location, and vascular structure. Will also evaluate flow patterns, pressure gradients, and collateral circulation and identify intranidal aneurysms and feeding vessels.

Management

Unruptured

1. Aimed at diagnostic evaluation of AVM to determine appropriate intervention—surgical, endovascular, radiosurgery, or a combination.
2. Surgical resection—dependent on location, eloquence of brain tissue, and size.
3. Endovascular management with *N*-butyl cyanoacrylate liquid polymer, polyvinyl alcohol particles, detachable coils, and balloon occlusion.
   a. Staged embolization is generally performed on larger AVMs to reduce flow patterns gradually.
   b. Initial embolization is aimed at protecting area at risk for rupture, reducing the nidus, or controlling the area at highest risk for bleeding.
   c. Can be used as primary treatment modality or as an adjunct to surgical resection and radiosurgery.
4. Radiosurgery (gamma knife/linear accelerator)—lesions less than or equal to 2.5 to 3 cm in size. Radiation creates vessel wall injury, initiating clot formation that leads to eventual blockage of vessel (this can take 1 to 3 years to occur). During this time, the AVM remains at risk for rupture.
5. AEDs for seizures as presenting symptom—fosphenytoin, phenytoin, or levetiracetam may be given initially via IV for rapid loading. Levels should be monitored for accurate dosing.
6. Normalize BP if hypertensive.
7. Smoking cessation.

After Rupture

1. Maintenance and close monitoring of SBP within prescribed limits to prevent rebleed from hypertension and ischemia from decreased cerebral perfusion with nicardipine, labetalol, vasotec, apresoline, or alternative IV antihypertensive agents.
2. Vasopressor agents may be needed to maintain SBP within prescribed range.
3. Antiepileptics for seizures as presenting symptom—phenytoin, fosphenytoin, and levetiracetam; duration based on provider preference and location and extent of bleed.
4. Surgical intervention.
   a. Evacuation of hematoma with or without resection of AVM.
   b. Endovascular management—partial embolization of AVM, specifically area of suspected rupture.

Complications

1. Bleed or rebleed.
2. Hydrocephalus; obstructive initially requiring ventriculostomy, nonobstructive long term, may require shunt.
3. Seizures.
4. Permanent deficit or deterioration and death.

Nursing Assessment

1. Perform and document neurologic assessment with vital signs and as patient condition warrants.
2. Monitor for changes in or decreasing LOC, CN function, pupillary function, and motor function, including drift (inability to maintain unsupported position).
3. Assess for increasing headache or focal neurologic deficits, which could signal rebleeding.
4. Assess vital signs and pupillary changes frequently for development of increased ICP.

Nursing Diagnoses

- Risk for Ineffective Cerebral Tissue Perfusion related to potential rebleeding, hydrocephalus, and seizures.
- Acute Pain secondary to cerebral hemorrhage, meningeal irritation, surgical procedure.
- Anxiety of patient/family related to treatment, intracranial surgery or endovascular treatment, and uncertainty of patient outcome.

Nursing Interventions

Maintaining Cerebral Perfusion and Preventing Complications

1. Medicate the patient as ordered during periods of extreme agitation.
2. Institute seizure precautions by providing padded side rails, suction equipment, and oral airway at the bedside.
3. Perform and document neurologic assessment with vital signs and as patient condition warrants, which includes monitoring LOC, CN function, pupillary function, and motor function.
   a. Assess for signs of increased ICP, including bradycardia and widening pulse pressure, changes in respiratory pattern (Cheyne-Stokes pattern, apneustic, ataxic).
   b. Assess for subjective neurologic complaints specific to decreased perfusion (eg, diplopia, headache, blurred vision).
   c. Assess for signs and symptoms of rebleed: insidious onset of confusion, disorientation, and decreased LOC, or focal deficit associated with area of bleed.
   d. Document findings and report any changes such as drowsiness and speech slurring or onset of pronator drift, which may be first sign of deterioration.
4. Implement nursing interventions to minimize ICP and cerebral swelling (eg, elevate head of bed 30 degrees, maintain proper head and neck alignment to avoid jugular vein compression, avoid prolonged suctioning procedures, keep procedure less than 15 seconds, collaborate with physicians to use lidocaine presuctioning if intubated).
5. Monitor ABG values for hypoxia and hypercapnia, which aggravate ICP.
6. Monitor ventriculostomy, if present, to manage acute hydrocephalus, for patency, amount, and character of drainage, and correct height level every 4 hours.
   a. If CSF is cloudy or purulent or other signs of potential infection are present, contact the health care provider.
   b. Obtain CSF samples from the external ventricular device using sterile technique and send for culture and Gram stain, WBC count, glucose, and protein, as directed.

c. Monitor results and report abnormal values.

d. Administer prophylactic antibiotics, as ordered. Use of prophylactic antibiotics is controversial and provider dependent.

7. Recognize need for maintenance of BP parameters and evaluate effectiveness of antihypertensive or vasopressor therapy.

8. Maintain fluid volume status, evaluate electrolytes, evaluate hemoglobin and hematocrit, and monitor input and output status at least every hour, or as status indicates

9. Maintain safety factors for neurologic deficits (eg, prevent sensory overload, physical injury related to vision, or hearing, body awareness deficits).

10. Also see "Nursing Management of the Patient with an Altered State of Consciousness," page 353.

Reducing Pain

1. Assess level of pain and pain relief; report any increase in headache.

2. Administer analgesics as prescribed; if opioid is being given with sedative, monitor for CNS depression, decreased respirations, and decreased BP.

3. Encourage distraction and relaxation techniques to promote calming effect.

4. Explain to the patient/significant other the limited use of opioids secondary to need to assess patient's LOC at all times.

5. Encourage elevated head of bed to minimize cerebral swelling.

6. Provide cool compresses to head.

7. Assess the patient for experiences of unrelieved or increased pain; assess for any changes in neurologic signs, which could signal hemorrhage, hydrocephalus, or meningeal irritation.

Reducing Anxiety

1. Provide ongoing assessment of psychosocial issues (anxiety, fear, depression, frustration, emotional lability).

2. Be attuned to verbal and nonverbal cues from the patient/family that signal problems with coping.

3. Inform the patient regarding all treatment modalities.

4. Encourage discussion of risks/benefits with the surgeon/interventional neuroradiologist.

5. Use reassurance and therapeutic conversation to relieve fear and anxiety.

6. Provide support to the patient/family in dealing with the stress and uncertainty of hospitalization.

7. Consult social services for assistance with the patient/family support and long-term care decisions, as needed.

8. Prepare the patient and family for surgery or endovascular treatment.

Community and Home Care Considerations

1. Assess level of knowledge and ability of the patient/significant other to retain information.

2. Assess ongoing home care needs.

3. Assess need for nursing home or rehabilitation center placement and obtain social service referral to help with planning.

4. Provide teaching to family and caregivers and act as liaison between health care team and family.

5. Teach the patient and family how to deal with permanent neurologic deficits and make sure that they obtain needed supplies and services.

Patient Education and Health Maintenance

1. Instruct the patient/family on purpose and frequency of neurologic/radiologic procedures.

2. Explain what an AVM is, signs/symptoms of rupture, and possible threats of rupture.

3. Educate the patient to the risk of rebleed, which is 50% within 6 months if untreated, and remains for rest of life if not definitively treated.

4. Encourage lifelong medical follow-up and immediate attention if severe headache develops.

5. Explain the need for follow-up angiograms to verify complete eradication of AVM or to define extent of eradication to facilitate treatment planning.

6. Provide educational material for procedures.

7. Set mutual goals for discharge, and communicate discharge preparations with other disciplines (registered nurse, physician, physical therapist, discharge coordinator).

8. Explain medications to the patient/significant other and potential adverse effects.

9. Have patient verbalize discharge instructions regarding wound care, activity restrictions, medications, and reportable signs/symptoms.

Evaluation: Expected Outcomes

- No signs of rebleeding, increased ICP, decreased cerebral perfusion, or seizures; vital signs stable; neurologic parameters stable.
- Verbalizes decreased pain or control of pain to an intensity that is acceptable.
- Decrease in anxiety sufficient to allow the completion of necessary procedures and to promote recovery.

INFECTIOUS DISORDERS
Meningitis

Meningitis is an inflammation of the pia mater and arachnoid membranes that surround the brain and the spinal cord. The subarachnoid space between these two meninges contains CSF that may reflect the signs and symptoms of meningitis.

Pathophysiology and Etiology

1. Viral meningitis is the most common form. More than 10,000 cases are reported annually, but the actual incidence may be as high as 75,000. It is usually self-limiting; management is supportive. It is usually caused by a nonpolio enterovirus (90%). The incidence of viral meningitis drops with age. As a general rule, the younger the patient, the greater the risk of viral meningitis. This organism is spread by the fecal–oral route and through sewage.

2. In the United States, the incidence of acute, bacterial meningitis is approximately three cases per 100,000 per year. The mortality is 10% to 30% and many who recover are left with long-term problems (eg, hearing deficit).

3. Bacterial meningitis may cause damage to the CNS from the inflammatory process rather than the pathogen. The organisms causing these infections seem to vary depending on the age and immune status of the patient. Bacterial meningitis is usually more serious than viral meningitis. It is typically caused by *Streptococcus pneumoniae* (pneumococcal meningitis), which is a gram-positive diplococcus, and *Neisseria meningitidis* (meningococcal meningitis), which is a gram-negative diplococcus.

a. Most bacteria that cause meningitis begin by colonizing the nasopharynx and then invade the circulation and CSF, causing an inflammatory response mediated by cytokines.

b. Bacterial meningitis can result in brain damage due to chemicals released by bacteria that kill or damage neurons, purulent exudates that may result in vasculitis and vasospasm, and increased ICP that causes cerebral edema.

4. Fungal meningitis, particularly *Cryptococcus neoformans*, affects immunosuppressed patients (eg, human immunodeficiency virus [HIV]–positive) through soil contaminated with excrement from pigeons and chickens. Cryptococcal antigen, or culture, is found in the CSF, but meningeal signs may be minimal. In HIV-positive patients, tuberculous meningitis, tuberculomas, and atypical mycobacterial infections of the brain may be noted.

5. Parasitic meningitis is usually cause by flukes, worms, or amoeba.

6. Hospital-acquired postcraniotomy meningitis, caused predominantly by gram-negative bacilli, can result in mortalities of 30%; multiple craniotomy operations place the patient at even higher risk. It develops approximately 7 to 8 days postoperatively.

7. Neoplastic meningitis affects approximately 3% to 8% of patients who have systemic cancers. The mean survival time is approximately 5 to 8 months. In neoplastic meningitis, malignant cells infiltrate the leptomeninges as a complication of breast cancer, lung cancer, malignant melanoma, non-Hodgkin lymphoma, and acute leukemia.

8. Meningitis is the primary intracranial complication of acute and chronic sinusitis (sphenoid sinusitis most common). *S. pneumonia* and *Staphylococcus aureus* are the most common organisms.

9. *Listeria monocytogenes*, a gram-positive bacilli, may cause meningitis through contaminated hot dogs, cold meats, and unpasteurized dairy products.

10. The incidence of *Haemophilus influenzae* meningitis has decreased because of the haemophilus b conjugate vaccine.

Clinical Manifestations

1. Classic symptoms are fever, headache, and nuchal rigidity. Constitutional symptoms of vomiting, diarrhea, cough, and myalgias appear in more than 50% of patients. History of temperature elevation occurs in 76% to 100% of patients who seek medical attention. A common pattern is low-grade fever in the prodromal stage and higher temperature elevations at the onset of neurologic signs.

2. Altered mental status; confusion in older patients.

3. Petechial (appears like "rug" burn) or purpuric rash from coagulopathy, especially with *N. meningitidis*.

4. Photophobia.

5. Neck tenderness or a bulging anterior fontanel in infants.

6. Children may exhibit behavioral changes, arching of the back and neck, a blank stare, refusal to feed, and seizures. Viral meningitis can cause a red, maculopapular rash in children.

7. Positive Brudzinski and Kernig signs (see Figure 15-6).

8. Neonates may exhibit poor feeding, altered breathing patterns, or listlessness.

9. Onset may be over several hours or several days depending on the infectious agent, the patient's age, immune status, comorbidities, and other variables. Some viruses cause rapid onset of symptoms, whereas others may involve prodromal nonspecific flulike symptoms, such as malaise, myalgia, and upper respiratory symptoms. In many cases, symptoms have a biphasic pattern; the nonspecific flulike symptoms and low-grade fever precede neurologic symptoms by approximately 48 hours. With the onset of neck stiffness and headache, the fever usually returns.

 KEY DECISION POINT If the patient presents with meningitis-like symptoms and appears very ill, evaluation and treatment for bacterial meningitis must be urgently initiated. Patients with bacterial meningitis are typically sicker than patients with a viral etiology, with high fever, severe headache +/– photophobia, and mental status changes. Blood and CSF cultures should be taken as soon as possible as the goal of treatment is to administer appropriate IV antibiotics within 30 minutes of presentation.

Diagnostic Evaluation

1. Complete blood count (CBC) with differential is indicated to detect an elevated leukocyte count in bacterial and viral meningitis, with a greater percentage of polymorphonuclear leukocytes (90%) in bacterial and (less than 50%) in viral meningitis (normal 0% to 15%).

2. Blood cultures are obtained to indicate the organism.

A Brudzinski's sign

B Kernig's sign

Figure 15-6. **Signs of meningeal irritation include nuchal rigidity and positive Brudzinski and Kernig signs. (A)** To elicit Brudzinski sign, place the patient supine and flex the head upward. Resulting flexion of both hips, knees, and ankles with neck flexion indicates meningeal irritation. **(B)** To test for Kernig sign, once again place the patient supine. Keeping the bottom leg straight, flex the other hip and knee to form a 90-degree angle. Slowly extend the upper leg. This places a stretch on the meninges, resulting in pain and spasm of the hamstring muscle. Resistance to further extension can be felt.

3. CSF evaluation for pressure, leukocytes, protein, glucose—CSF normally has five or fewer lymphocytes or mononuclear cells/mm³.
   a. In acute bacterial meningitis, the CSF may indicate elevated pressure, elevated leukocytes (several thousand), elevated protein, and low glucose. A culture and smear will identify the organism. WBC differential should be done by a stained smear of sediment.
   b. In viral encephalitis, the CSF may indicate normal/moderately elevated pressure, few/elevated leukocytes (fewer than 1,000), normal or slightly elevated protein, and normal glucose.
4. MRI/CT with and without contrast rules out other disorders. A CT scan with contrast must be obtained to detect abscesses.
5. Latex agglutination may be positive for antigens in meningitis.
6. Low CD4+ counts indicate immunosuppression in HIV-positive patients and other patients with immunosuppressive disorders.
7. In patients with acquired immunodeficiency syndrome (AIDS), MRI is used to detect meningeal irritation, evidence of a sinus infection, or brain abscess.

Management

1. The assessment and management of meningitis should be approached through a team effort with nursing, infectious disease and otolaryngology specialists, neurology, internal medicine, and laboratory and diagnostic staff. Droplet precautions are warranted for suspected *N. meningitidis* and *H. influenzae* meningitis.
2. Most patients are given IV antibiotics as soon as possible until the laboratory findings determine the type of meningitis (eg, viral, bacterial). However, cultures should be taken before initiating antibiotics.
3. To manage inflammation, dexamethasone or another corticosteroid is given via IV line.
   a. This may result in GI bleeding and mask clinical responses to treatments (eg, resolved fever).
   b. This steroid should be used before or with the first dose of antibiotics (IV 0.6 mg/kg/day in four divided doses for the first 4 days of antibiotics) and should be confined to patients older than age 6 weeks.
   c. Plasmapheresis may be used experimentally to remove cytokines in some cases.
4. Temozolomide, a second-generation alkylating agent, is effective against many cancers that result in neoplastic meningitis. External beam radiation may be used in conjunction with chemotherapy (eg, intrathecal thiotepa or methotrexate).
5. Cochlear implantation rehabilitation due to deafness caused by meningitis should be considered. Realistic goals must be set because the patient may develop only environmental sound awareness and still have to deal with learning disabilities.
6. If meningitis is suspected after neurosurgical procedures, consider potential IV line bacteremia, CSF leak, or immunosuppression.
7. Antifungal agents, such as amphotericin B and the triazoles, fluconazole, and itraconazole, are indicated for cryptococcal meningitis. Relapse is common if the patient does not have chronic suppressive therapy with fluconazole or another antifungal agent.
8. Empiric antituberculosis drugs must be initiated if infection by *Mycobacterium tuberculosis* is suspected.

 NURSING ALERT Be aware that bacterial resistance to antibiotics has been increasing, making meningitis very difficult to treat in some instances.

Complications

1. Bacterial meningitis, particularly in children, may result in deafness, learning difficulties, spasticity, paresis, or CN disorders.
2. Increased ICP in AIDS patients with cryptococcal meningitis can result in severe visual losses.
3. Seizures occur in 20% to 30% of patients.
4. Increased ICP may result in cerebral edema, decreased perfusion, and tissue damage.
5. Severe brain edema may result in herniation or compression of the brain stem.
6. Purpura may be associated with disseminated intravascular coagulation.

Nursing Assessment

1. Obtain a history of recent infections such as upper respiratory infection and exposure to causative agents. Meticulous history taking is essential and must include evaluation of exposure to ill contacts, mosquitoes, ticks, and outdoor activities in areas of endemic Lyme disease, travel history with possible exposure to tuberculosis, as well as history of medication use, IV drug use, and sexually transmitted disease risk. Another important part of history is prior antibiotic use, which may alter the clinical picture of bacterial meningitis.
2. Assess neurologic status and vital signs.
3. Evaluate for signs of meningeal irritation.
4. Assess sensorineural hearing loss (vision and hearing), CN damage (eg, facial nerve palsy), and diminished cognitive function.

Nursing Diagnoses

- Hyperthermia related to the infectious process and cerebral edema.
- Risk for Imbalanced Fluid Volume related to fever and decreased intake.
- Ineffective Cerebral Tissue Perfusion related to infectious process and cerebral edema.
- Acute Pain related to meningeal irritation.
- Impaired Physical Mobility related to prolonged bed rest.

Nursing Interventions

Reducing Fever
1. Administer antimicrobial agents on time to maintain optimal blood levels.
2. Monitor temperature frequently or continuously and administer antipyretics, as ordered.
3. Institute other cooling measures, such as a hypothermia blanket, as indicated.

Maintaining Fluid Balance
1. Prevent IV fluid overload, which may worsen cerebral edema.
2. Monitor intake and output closely.
3. Monitor CVP frequently.

Enhancing Cerebral Perfusion
1. Assess LOC, vital signs, and neurologic parameters frequently. Observe for signs and symptoms of increased ICP (eg, decreased LOC, dilated pupils, widening pulse pressure).

2. Maintain a quiet, calm environment to prevent agitation, which may cause an increased ICP.
3. Prepare the patient for a lumbar puncture for CSF evaluation and repeat spinal tap, if indicated. Evaluate the patient for ICP prior to lumbar puncture.
4. Notify the health care provider of signs of deterioration: increasing temperature, decreasing LOC, seizure activity, or altered respirations.

Reducing Pain

1. Administer analgesics, as ordered; monitor for response and adverse reactions. Avoid opioids, which may mask a decrease in LOC.
2. Darken the room if photophobia is present.
3. Assist with position of comfort for neck stiffness, and turn the patient slowly and carefully with head and neck in alignment.
4. Elevate the head of the bed to decrease ICP and reduce pain.

Promoting Mobility

1. Frequently turn and reposition the patient to prevent skin breakdown.
2. Progress from passive to active exercises based on the patient's neurologic status.
3. Suggest early physical and occupational therapy referrals to promote return to optimal level of functioning.

 DRUG ALERT Note and report any missed doses of antibiotics, osmotic diuretics, and steroids; administer necessary doses as soon as possible to avert deleterious consequences due to missed doses.

Community and Home Care Considerations

1. Prevent bacterial meningitis by eliminating colonization and infection with the offending organism.
   a. Administer vaccines against *H. influenzae* type B for children; *N. meningitidis* serogroups A, C, Y, and W135 for patients at high risk (especially college students, those without spleens, those who are immunodeficient); and *S. pneumoniae* for patients with chronic illnesses and older adults.
   b. Administer vaccines for travelers to countries with a high incidence of meningococcal disease and household contacts of someone who has had meningitis.
   c. Chemoprophylaxis for meningococcal disease, most commonly with rifampin, may be necessary for health care workers, household contacts in the community, day care centers, and other highly susceptible populations.
2. If maintenance antifungal prophylaxis is initiated for patients with low CD4+ counts, as seen in some patients with AIDS, the patient must understand the importance of long-term pharmacologic therapy.

Patient Education and Health Maintenance

1. Advise close contacts of the patient with meningitis that prophylactic treatment may be indicated; they should check with their health care providers or the local public health department.
2. Encourage the patient to follow medication regimen as directed to eradicate the infectious agent completely.

3. Encourage follow-up and prompt attention to infections in future.
4. Direct the patient and family to the Centers for Disease Control and Prevention. (*www.cdc.gov/meningitis/index.html*) for support and additional information.

Evaluation: Expected Outcomes

- Afebrile.
- Adequate urine output; CVP in normal range.
- Alert LOC; normal vital signs.
- Pain controlled.
- Optimal level of functioning after resolution.

Encephalitis

Encephalitis is an inflammation of cerebral tissue, typically accompanied by meningeal inflammation. Meningoencephalitis is most commonly caused by a viral infection. Like meningitis, encephalitis can be infectious or noninfectious and acute, subacute, or chronic.

Pathophysiology and Etiology

1. In primary encephalitis, the brain or spinal cord is the predominant foci of the toxin or pathogen. Secondary encephalitis is a less serious form of encephalitis; it is caused by an infection that is spread from another part of the body.
2. Acute viral encephalitis, accounting for the vast majority of cases, is caused by a direct infection of the gray matter containing neural cells. It results in perivascular inflammation and neuronal destruction. It is more common in children and is most commonly caused by the herpes simplex virus and, to a lesser degree, by the arboviruses.
3. Brain stem encephalitis targets the basal ganglia or CNS.
4. Postischemic inflammatory encephalitis occurs because of brain inflammation following a CVA. In patients with cerebral ischemia, inflammation can result in secondary brain injury and microvascular occlusion can be caused by activated leukocytes or a microvascular thrombus. This edema can result in increased ICP and compromised cerebral perfusion.
5. West Nile virus (WNV) is an arthropod virus (arbovirus). The mosquito is the primary vector and birds are the primary hosts. Mortality can be as high as 30%.
6. *Herpes simplex encephalitis* may result from reactivation of the virus that has been dormant in the cranial and other ganglia or to reinfection. Direct spread to the brain by the olfactory or trigeminal nerve is suspected with herpes simplex virus type 1, which is responsible for almost all cases of herpes simplex encephalitis in children and adults. Mortality is as high as 75%. Herpes simplex type 2 is more common in neonates who are born to mothers with this infection during pregnancy.
7. Herpes zoster virus (varicella) is a rare cause of encephalitis.
8. Postinfectious encephalomyelitis follows a viral or bacterial infection process, but organisms do not directly affect the neural tissue in the white matter; however, perivascular inflammation and demyelination do occur in the cerebral tissue.
   a. The incidence of postinfectious encephalomyelitis has decreased considerably with immunization against measles, mumps, and rubella and because of the eradication of smallpox. It is rare in infancy.
   b. The most common cause is respiratory or GI infection 1 to 3 weeks before the acute onset of encephalomyelitis symptoms.

c. May be caused by specific species of mosquitoes and ticks (arthropods), which may be seasonal and geographic hosts (eg, California encephalitis, St. Louis equine encephalitis).

9. *Cytomegalovirus encephalitis* should be considered in patients who have advanced HIV infection, have evidence of the cytomegalovirus in other sites, and have progressive neurologic deterioration.

10. *Toxoplasma* encephalitis is also common in patients with AIDS.

Clinical Manifestations

1. Signs and symptoms may develop hours or weeks after exposure.
2. Classic symptoms include fever, headache, and altered mental status (eg, disorientation, neurologic deficits, seizures).
3. Increased ICP may result in alteration in consciousness, nausea, and vomiting.
4. Motor weakness, such as hemiparesis, may be detected.
5. Increased deep tendon reflexes and extensor plantar response are noted.
6. Bizarre behavior and personality changes may present at onset.
7. Hypothalamic–pituitary involvement may result in hypothermia, diabetes insipidus, SIADH (see page 358).
8. Neurologic symptoms may include superior quadrant visual field defects, aphasia, dysphagia, ataxia, and paresthesias.
9. The patient with brain stem encephalitis may present with nystagmus, decreased extraocular movements, hearing loss, dysphagia, dysarthria, respiratory abnormalities, and motor involvement.
10. Limbic encephalitis may cause mood and personality changes that progress to severe memory loss and delirium.
11. In WNV, about two thirds of symptomatic patients have encephalitis with signs and symptoms of fever, vomiting, headache, nuchal rigidity, decreased LOC, CN dysfunction, and an erythematous rash. Seizures are uncommon.

Diagnostic Evaluation

1. Lumbar puncture, with evaluation of CSF, is performed to detect leukocytosis, increased mononuclear cell pleocytosis, increased proteins, and normal or slightly lowered glucose.
2. Polymerase chain reaction analysis of the virus deoxyribonucleic acid (DNA) and the detection of intrathecally produced viral antibodies are essential in diagnosing the specific virus (eg, herpes simplex virus, cytomegalovirus). Arbovirus-specific immunoglobulin (Ig)M in CSF and a fourfold change in specific IgG antibody are diagnostic for arboviral encephalitis.
3. EEG may demonstrate slow brain wave complexes in encephalitis.
4. Gadolinium-enhanced MRI differentiates postinfectious encephalomyelitis from acute viral encephalitis.
   a. Enhanced multifocal white matter lesions are seen in encephalomyelitis, which may remain for months after clinical recovery.
   b. Herpes simplex virus encephalitis typically causes medial–temporal and orbital–frontal lobe inflammation and necrosis; low-density abnormalities may be present in the temporal lobes. An MRI is preferred over a CT scan.
   c. Cytomegalovirus, seen in patients who have advanced HIV disease, may have enhanced periventricular areas.
5. Brain tissue biopsy indicates presence of infectious organisms.
6. WNV can have pleocytosis and may be seen on an MRI with enhancement of the meninges and periventricular areas. The enzyme-linked immunosorbent assay, WNV ELISA, can be done from blood or CSF; a cell culture can also be diagnostic.

Management

1. Differentiate acute viral encephalitis from noninfectious diseases, such as sarcoidosis, vasculitis, systemic lupus erythematosus, and others.
2. In patients who are immunosuppressed, such as HIV-positive patients, differentiate acute viral encephalitis from cytomegalovirus encephalitis, toxoplasmic encephalitis, and fungal infections.
   a. Patients with cytomegalovirus may be treated with ganciclovir and foscarnet, commonly used to treat cytomegalovirus retinitis in HIV-positive patients.
   b. Pyrimethamine and sulfadoxine are commonly used to treat *Toxoplasma* encephalitis.
   c. When encephalomyelitis develops, supportive care is indicated because there is no known treatment; corticosteroids may be used.
3. IV acyclovir over 10 to 21 days is indicated for herpes simplex virus. Mothers who have genital herpes simplex may be treated with acyclovir during the third trimester to avoid shedding the virus to their babies.
4. Anticonvulsants are used to manage seizures.

 DRUG ALERT Acyclovir, indicated for acute viral encephalitis caused by herpes simplex type 1, inhibits replication of the virus DNA. Acyclovir should be infused over 1 hour because crystalluria and renal failure may result if administration is too rapid.

Complications

1. Sequelae of the herpes simplex virus may cause temporal lobe swelling, which can result in compression of the brain stem. This virus may also cause aphasia, major motor and sensory deficits, and Korsakoff psychosis (amnestic syndrome).
2. Relapse of encephalitis may be seen after initial improvement and completion of antiviral therapy.
3. Mortality and morbidity depend on the infectious agent, host status, and other considerations.

Nursing Assessment

1. Obtain patient history of recent infection, animal exposure, tick or mosquito bite, recent travel, and exposure to ill contacts.
2. Perform a complete physical assessment.
3. Before delivery, women should be questioned regarding a history of congenital herpes simplex virus and examined for evidence of this virus; a cesarean delivery should be explored with the physician.
4. Vesicular lesions or rashes on neonates should be reported immediately because these could indicate active herpes simplex type 2 infection.

 NURSING ALERT Although most cases of viral encephalitis only require universal precautions to prevent infection, patients that present with open lesions to the skin, as occurs in herpes simplex or herpes zoster, should have contact isolation procedures implemented.

Nursing Diagnoses

- Risk for Injury related to seizures and cerebral edema.
- Ineffective Cerebral Tissue Perfusion related to disease process.
- Hyperthermia related to infectious process.
- Impaired Environmental Interpretation Syndrome related to disease process.

Nursing Interventions

Preventing Injury

1. Maintain a quiet environment and provide care gently, avoiding overactivity and agitation, which may cause increased ICP.
2. Maintain seizure precautions with side rails padded, airway, and suction equipment at bedside.
3. Administer medications, as ordered; monitor response and adverse reactions.

Promoting Cerebral Perfusion

1. Monitor neurologic status closely. Observe for subtle changes, such as behavior or personality changes, weakness, or CN involvement, and notify the health care provider.
2. In arbovirus encephalitis, restrict fluids as directed to passively dehydrate the brain.
3. Reorient the patient frequently.
4. Provide supportive care if coma develops; may last several weeks.
5. Encourage significant others to interact with the patient and participate in the patient's rehabilitation, even while the patient is in a coma.

Relieving Fever

1. Monitor temperature and vital signs frequently.
2. Administer antipyretics and other cooling measures, as indicated.
3. Monitor fluid intake and output and provide fluid replacement through IV lines as needed. Be alert to signs of other coexisting infections, such as urinary tract infection or pneumonia, and notify health care provider so cultures can be obtained and treatment started.
4. Maintain standard precautions to prevent transmission of infection, and contact precautions may be indicated if skin lesions are present.

Managing Safe Behavior in the Environment

1. Frequently orient to person, place, time, and purpose.
2. Provide simple instructions and frequent cues to perform required activities.
3. Maintain consistency in care and avoid overstimulation.
4. Maintain constant surveillance and safety precautions.

Community and Home Care Considerations

1. Promote vaccination of patient, family, and significant others for measles, mumps, and rubella.
2. Pregnant women who have a history of genital herpes simplex, or their partners, should inform their physician of this history.
3. Contacts of rabies-infected patients should be offered rabies prophylaxis.
4. Direct the patient and family to the Encephalitis Society (*www. encephalitis.info*) for support and additional information.

Patient Education and Health Maintenance

1. Explain the effects of the disease process and the rationale for care.
2. Reassure significant others based on patient's prognosis.

3. Encourage follow-up for evaluation of deficits and rehabilitation progress.
4. Educate others about the signs and symptoms of encephalitis if epidemic is suspected.
5. To prevent WNV, advise the use of repellants when outdoors and removal of standing water that acts as a breeding ground for mosquitoes.

Evaluation: Expected Outcomes

- No seizures or signs of increased ICP.
- Alert with no neurologic deficits.
- Afebrile.
- Participating safely in ADL

Brain and Spinal Abscesses

A *brain abscess* is a free or encapsulated collection of infectious material of brain parenchyma, between the dura and the arachnoid linings (subdural abscess) or between the dura and the skull (epidural abscess). Spinal abscesses typically occur in the epidural region.

Pathophysiology and Etiology

1. Intracranial subdural abscesses, usually due to a streptococcus organism, are caused by purulent drainage between the dura and arachnoid. It can result from pus from the meninges, middle ear or mastoid, sinuses, septicemia, or skull fracture. It occurs most frequently in children and young adults.
2. Intracranial epidural abscesses, typically involving an infection of the cranium, commonly occur because of chronic mastoiditis or sinusitis, head trauma, or craniotomy. Abscesses may be related to a subdural empyema (collection of purulent drainage originating from nasal sinuses, meninges, middle ear, or skull osteomyelitis), meningitis, or intraparenchymal abscess.
3. Spinal epidural abscesses occur in the spinal canal external to the dura. Epidural penetration may seed through the blood and occur from infected adjacent tissue (eg, infected pressure ulcer), from another infected site (eg, skin), or contamination from spinal surgery or spinal instrumentation (eg, lumbar puncture). *S. aureus* is a frequent causative agent and the midthoracic vertebrae are most commonly affected.
4. Intramedullary abscesses are more common in the pediatric population and are associated with lumbosacral dermal sinuses. Approximately 20% to 30% are "cryptic" abscesses with no apparent source of infectious seeding.
5. In the initial inoculation period, organisms invade the brain parenchyma, resulting in local inflammation and edema. The resulting cerebritis develops into a necrotic lesion and then becomes encapsulated.
6. Fungal brain abscesses are commonly seen in HIV-positive patients and other populations that are immunosuppressed. Diffuse microabscesses may occur with infections caused by *Candida* species.
7. *M. tuberculosis* may cause abscesses of pus containing acid-fast bacilli (AFB) surrounded by a dense capsule. These abscesses are also found in patients who are HIV positive or have other immunosuppressive diseases.

Clinical Manifestations

1. Headache is poorly localized with a dull ache.
2. Increased ICP may result in nausea, vomiting, and decreased LOC.

3. Fever is found in less than 50% of cases.
4. Neurologic findings, such as hemisensory and paresis deficits, aphasia, and ataxia, may be present.
5. Seizures are frequently present.
6. Dental abscess, sinusitis, and otitis media may be present.
7. Signs and symptoms of a cerebral subdural empyema include severe headache, fever, nuchal rigidity, and signs of meningeal irritation (Kernig and Brudzinski sign; see page 380).
8. Patients with intracranial epidural abscess commonly present with fever, lethargy, and severe headache.
9. Spinal epidural abscesses may be evidenced by severe back pain, fever, headache, lower-extremity weakness or paralysis, nuchal rigidity, Kernig sign, and local tenderness.

Diagnostic Evaluation

1. CT scan and MRI with contrast locate the sites of abscess and follow evolution and resolution of the suppurative process.
   a. In the inflammatory stage of cerebritis, imaging reveals high signal intensity centrally (inflammation) and peripherally (edema). When an abscess develops, the capsule becomes isointense.
   b. There may be decreased ring enhancement with patients who are immunosuppressed, which may be due to a lack of inflammatory response.
   c. Microabscesses may not be detected by the CT scan or MRI.
   d. MRI with gadolinium enhancement should be considered to detect spinal epidural abscesses.
2. Blood cultures are obtained to identify the organism; positive Gram stain, leukocytosis, and elevated erythrocyte sedimentation rate (ESR) will be found.
3. Cultures are obtained from the suspected source of infection, using stereotaxic needle aspiration or brain surgery, to identify the organism and sensitivity to antimicrobials.
4. A metastatic brain abscess may be differentiated from a metastatic tumor by CT scan or MRI. Abscesses have hypodense centers with a smooth surrounding capsule, whereas tumors may have irregular borders and diffuse enhancement.
5. EEG detects seizure disorders.
6. Findings in cerebral subdural empyema include increased WBC count and increased pressure of the CSF.
7. In intracranial epidural abscesses, CT or MRI scans are useful; MRIs are usually more sensitive. Findings from the CSF may not be definitive. To avoid transtentorial herniation, lumbar puncture is not indicated until large cranial masses are ruled out.
8. Diagnostic findings in spinal epidural abscesses may include increased WBC count and ESR. The CSF may be cloudy.

Management

1. With cerebral subdural empyema or intracranial epidural abscesses, management consists of trephining (drilling through skull to evacuate purulent material), systemic antibiotics, and treatment of cerebral edema.
2. Closed stereotaxic needle biopsy, under CT guidance, may be used for drainage evacuation instead of craniotomy.
3. Spinal epidural abscesses may be managed with a laminectomy and surgical drainage, with antibiotics before and after the procedure. The abscess site is thoroughly irrigated with antibiotic solution and aerobic and anaerobic cultures are taken.
4. Radical surgical debridement, especially with fungal infections, may be indicated with antimicrobial therapy.

5. Initiation of empiric antimicrobial therapy is based on Gram stain and the suspected site of origin. Because brain abscesses are frequently caused by multiple organisms, antimicrobial therapy is directed toward the most common etiologic agents: streptococci, anaerobic bacteria (eg, *Bacteroides* species).
   a. *S. aureus* may be suspected if surgical procedures have been performed.
   b. Gram-negative bacteria (eg, *Clostridium* species) should be suspected if a cranial wound has been contaminated with soil.
   c. A 6- to 8-week course of parenteral antibiotics is typical, followed by a 2- to 3-month course of oral antimicrobial therapy.
   d. Penicillin G, metronidazole, and third-generation cephalosporins are common therapeutic agents.
6. Antifungal therapy, such as amphotericin B, is initiated for candidiasis and other fungal infections.
7. Antituberculosis pharmacotherapy, such as rifampin, isoniazid, and pyrazinamide, should be used to treat abscesses containing AFB.
8. Adjunctive therapy includes corticosteroids and osmotic diuretics to reduce cerebral edema and anticonvulsants to manage seizures.

 NURSING ALERT If a subdural drain is used to provide continuous drainage of the abscess, the patient should be placed in a supine position to prevent rapid fluid shifts into the drainage device.

Complications

1. The brain abscess can rupture into the ventricular space, causing a sudden increase in the severity of the patient's headache. This complication is often fatal.
2. Papilledema may occur in less than 25% of cases, indicating intracranial hypertension.
3. Lumbar puncture may be contraindicated if there is a spinal epidural abscess because pus may be transferred into the subarachnoid space.
4. Permanent neurologic deficits, such as seizure disorders, visual defects, hemiparesis, and CN palsies, may be present.
5. There is greater mortality if the patient has acute onset of symptoms with severe mental status changes and has rapid progression of neurologic impairment.
6. Delayed treatment of a spinal epidural abscess may result in transection syndrome, in which flaccid paraplegia with sensory loss occurs at the level of the abscess.
7. In chronic otitis media, intracranial and intratemporal complications frequently result from progressive bony erosion, which may expose the dura, labyrinth, and facial nerves.

Nursing Assessment

1. Obtain history of previous infection, immunosuppression, headache, and related symptoms.
2. Perform neurologic assessment, including CN evaluation, motor, and cognitive status.

Nursing Diagnoses

- Acute Pain related to cerebral mass.
- Impaired Environmental Interpretation Syndrome related to disease process.

- Risk for Injury related to neurologic deficits.
- Anxiety related to surgery, prognosis, and relapse.

Nursing Interventions

Relieving Pain
1. Administer pain medications, as ordered.
2. Provide comfort measures, such as quiet environment, positioning with head slightly elevated, and assistance with hygiene needs.
3. Provide passive relaxation techniques, such as soft music and back rubs.

Promoting Thought Processes
1. Frequently monitor vital signs, LOC, orientation, and seizure activity.
2. Report acute changes, which can signal increased ICP, to health care provider.
3. Administer medications, as ordered, noting response and adverse reactions.
4. Prepare the patient for repeated diagnostic tests to evaluate response to therapy and surgery.

Minimizing Neurologic Deficits
1. Maintain a safe environment with side rails up, call light within reach, and frequent observation.
2. Evaluate other CN function and report changes.
3. Refer to occupational therapist, speech therapist, or other rehabilitation specialist to provide adjunct to nursing rehabilitation.

Reducing Anxiety
1. Prepare the patient and family for surgery when indicated. Encourage discussion with surgeon to understand risks and benefits of the procedure.
2. Explain postoperative progression and nursing care (see page 361).

Community and Home Care Considerations
1. Patient follow-up is essential for sinusitis, otitis media, respiratory infections, and other infectious processes that may result in a brain abscess.
2. Continue with rehabilitation to regain or compensate for neurologic deficits.
3. Continue with pharmacologic regimen in community setting.
4. Observe for recurrence of brain and spinal abscesses.

Patient Education and Health Maintenance
1. Maintain wellness with vaccinations, immunizations, and overall health.
2. Reinforce need for dental procedure prophylaxis to avoid dental abscesses.
3. Instruct on need for immediate assessment of head wounds.

Evaluation: Expected Outcomes
- Verbalizes reduced pain.
- Oriented to person, place, and time; follows simple commands.
- No injury related to neurologic deficits.
- Reduced anxiety regarding disease process and procedures.

DEGENERATIVE DISORDERS
Parkinson Disease

Parkinson disease is a chronic, progressive neurologic disease affecting the brain centers responsible for control and regulation of movement. It is characterized by tremor, bradykinesia, rigidity, and postural abnormalities. Parkinson can complicate the diagnosis, clinical course, and recovery from other illness. Approximately 1% of the total US population older than age 60 is affected by idiopathic Parkinson disease, and it less commonly affects people of younger ages. It is the second most common neurodegenerative disease.

Pathophysiology and Etiology
1. A deficiency of dopamine, due to degenerative changes in the substantia nigra of the brain, is thought to be responsible for the symptoms of Parkinson disease.
2. Underlying etiology may be related to a virus; genetic susceptibility; toxicity from pesticides, herbicides, methyl-phenyl-tetrahydropyridine, or welding fumes; repeated head injuries; or other unknown cause.
3. The clinical diagnosis of Parkinson disease may be difficult because older patients may have other causes of rigidity, bradykinesia, and tremor.

Clinical Manifestations
1. Bradykinesia (slowness of movement), loss of spontaneous movement, and delay in initiating movements.
2. Resting ("pill-rolling") tremor of 4 to 5 Hz. The tremor may be worse on one side of the body, affecting the limbs and sometimes involving the head, neck, face, and jaw.
3. Rigidity in performance of all movements. Rigidity is always present but increases during movement. May lead to sensations of pain, especially in the arms and shoulders.
4. Poor balance when moving abruptly or suddenly changing body position. May lead to falls.
5. Autonomic disorders—sleeplessness, salivation, sweating, orthostatic hypotension, dizziness.
6. Depression, dementia.
7. Masklike facies secondary to rigidity.
8. Gait difficulties characterized by a decreased or nonexistent arm swing; short, shuffling steps (festination); difficulty in negotiating turns; and sudden freezing spells (inability to take the next step).
9. Verbal fluency may be impaired.
10. Finger-tapping responses are slowed.
11. Micrographia (change in handwriting, with the script becoming smaller).
12. Problems with speech, breathing, swallowing, and sexual function.

Diagnostic Evaluation
1. Observation of clinical symptoms; may perform imaging studies to rule out other disorders.
2. Physical examination of upper-extremity elbow flexion/extension reveals rigidity on extension.
3. Sensorimotor assessment of grip reveals abnormally high grip forces and longer than normal to complete object lift, particularly with lighter loads.
4. Favorable response to a single dose of levodopa or apomorphine helps confirm the diagnosis.

Management

Pharmacologic

1. Anticholinergics, including trihexyphenidyl, benztropine, and procyclidine, to reduce transmission of cholinergic pathways, which are thought to be overactive when dopamine is deficient. These medications are most effective in controlling tremor but are known to cause confusion and hallucinations.
2. Amantadine, originally an antiflu medication, blocks the reuptake of dopamine or increases the release of dopamine by neurons in the brain, thereby increasing the supply of dopamine in the synapses. Widely used as an early monotherapy, its effect may be augmented by drug-free days.
3. Levodopa, a dopamine precursor, combined with carbidopa, a decarboxylase inhibitor, to inhibit destruction of L-dopa in the bloodstream, making more available to the brain. The addition of carbidopa prevents levodopa from being metabolized in the gut, liver, and other tissues and allows more to get to the brain. Therefore, a smaller dose of levodopa is required to treat symptoms and the unpleasant adverse effects are greatly reduced.
4. Bromocriptine, pramipexole, and ropinirole are dopaminergic agonists that activate dopamine receptors in the brain. Can be taken alone or in combination with levodopa–carbidopa.
5. Use of the monoamine oxidase inhibitor selegiline or deprenyl boosts the effect of levodopa–carbidopa when levodopa becomes less effective.
6. Tolcapone and entacapone are catechol-*O*-methyltransferase inhibitors for adjunct treatment. They prolong the duration of symptom relief by blocking the action of an enzyme that breaks down levodopa before it reaches the brain. Must be taken with levodopa.
7. Other medications that include levodopa include
   a. Combination formula of carbidopa/levodopa with entacapone (Stalevo), which is usseful in patients stable on both medications.
   b. An enteral suspension of carbidopa/levodopa infused directly into the small intestine, for those with advanced PD who experience unpredictable gastric emptying (requires jejunostomy tube).
   c. An extended-release capsule (Rytary) used as a secondary drug in those patients who experience early wearing off of levodopa therapy.
8. Apomorphine is an injectable, long-acting dopamine agonist, beneficial in patients experiencing early wearing off of levodopa therapy

 DRUG ALERT History of melanoma and angle-closure glaucoma are contraindications to levodopa therapy; patients should have suspicious skin lesions removed before initiating therapy, as it may activate a malignant melanoma.

 GERONTOLOGIC ALERT Older patients may have reduced tolerance to anti-Parkinson drugs and may require smaller doses. Watch for and report psychiatric reactions, such as anxiety, confusion, and hallucinations; cardiac effects, such as dizziness, orthostatic hypotension, and pulse irregularity; and blepharospasm (twitching of the eyelid), an early sign of toxicity. Other adverse effects may include dry mouth, nausea, drowsiness, and insomnia.

Surgery

1. New surgical treatments for Parkinson disease and essential tremor are promising.
2. Medial pallidotomy (electrode destroys cells in the globus pallidus) often improves long-standing symptoms, such as dyskinesia, akinesia, rigidity, and tremor, and for patients who have developed dyskinetic movements in reaction to their medications.
3. Deep brain stimulation of the thalamus decreases tremor and uncontrollable movements unresponsive to medication. Electrodes are implanted in the thalamus or globus pallidus and connected to a pacemaker-like device, which are programmed by a provider trained in DBS programming. Patients are provided the ability to adjust programs if deemed appropriate by the provider.
4. Gamma knife surgery provides concentrated gamma rays and destroys cells within the thalamus; beneficial in patients with essential tremor and who are unable to tolerate surgery
5. Brain tissue transplants are still in the experimental stages but have produced encouraging results using stem cells and genetically engineered animal cells that can be made to produce dopamine.

Complications

1. Dementia.
2. Aspiration.
3. Injury from falls.

Nursing Assessment

1. Obtain history of symptoms and their effect on functioning. Mobility, feeding, communication, and self-care difficulties will have many nursing implications (see Figure 15-7).
2. Assess CNs, cerebellar function (coordination), motor function.
3. Observe gait and performance of activities.
4. Assess speech for clarity and pace.
5. Assess for signs of depression.
6. Assess family dynamics, support systems, and access to social services.

Nursing Diagnoses

- Impaired Physical Mobility related to bradykinesia, rigidity, and tremor.
- Imbalanced Nutrition: Less Than Body Requirements related to motor difficulties with feeding, chewing, and swallowing.
- Impaired Verbal Communication related to decreased speech volume and facial muscle involvement.
- Constipation related to diminished motor function, inactivity, and medications.
- Ineffective Coping related to physical limitations and loss of independence.

Nursing Interventions

Improving Mobility and Reducing Risk of Falls

1. Encourage the patient to participate in daily exercise, such as walking, riding a stationary bike, swimming, or gardening.
2. Advise the patient to do stretching and postural exercises as outlined by a physical therapist.
3. Encourage the patient to take warm baths and receive massages to help relax muscles.

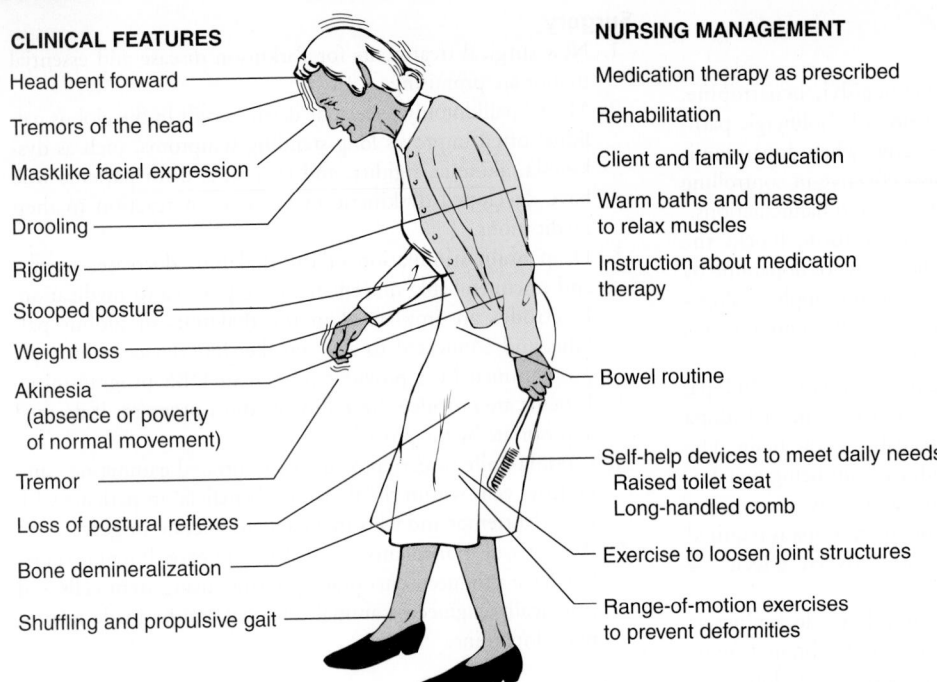

CLINICAL FEATURES

Head bent forward

Tremors of the head

Masklike facial expression

Drooling

Rigidity

Stooped posture

Weight loss

Akinesia
(absence or poverty
of normal movement)

Tremor

Loss of postural reflexes

Bone demineralization

Shuffling and propulsive gait

NURSING MANAGEMENT

Medication therapy as prescribed

Rehabilitation

Client and family education

Warm baths and massage
to relax muscles

Instruction about medication
therapy

Bowel routine

Self-help devices to meet daily needs:
  Raised toilet seat
  Long-handled comb

Exercise to loosen joint structures

Range-of-motion exercises
to prevent deformities

Figure 15-7. Appearance of woman with Parkinson disease. (LifeART image, 2004.)

4. Instruct the patient to take frequent rest periods to overcome fatigue and frustration.
5. Teach postural exercises and walking techniques to offset shuffling gait and tendency to lean forward.
   a. Instruct the patient to use a broad-based gait.
   b. Have the patient make a conscious effort to swing arms, raise the feet while walking, use a heel-toe gait, and increase the width of stride.
   c. Tell the patient to practice walking to marching music or sound of ticking metronome to provide sensory reinforcement.
6. Assess for proper supportive footwear and safe use of mobility aid such as walker or cane.

Optimizing Nutritional Status

1. Teach the patient to think through the sequence of swallowing—close lips with teeth together lift tongue up with food on it; then move tongue back and swallow while tilting head forward.
2. Instruct the patient to chew deliberately and slowly, using both sides of mouth.
3. Tell the patient to make conscious effort to control accumulation of saliva by holding head upright and swallowing periodically.
4. Have the patient use secure, stabilized dishes and eating utensils.
5. Suggest smaller meals and additional snacks.
6. Monitor weight.
7. Suggest nutritionist and speech therapist referrals to improve oral intake and nutritional status.

Maximizing Communication Ability

1. Encourage compliance with medication regimen.
2. Suggest referral to speech therapist.
3. Teach the patient facial exercises and breathing methods to obtain appropriate pronunciation, volume, and intonation.
   a. Take a deep breath before speaking to increase the volume of sound and number of words spoken with each breath.
   b. Exaggerate pronunciation and speak in short sentences; read aloud in front of a mirror or into a tape recorder to monitor progress.

   c. Exercise facial muscles by smiling, frowning, grimacing, and puckering.

Preventing Constipation

1. Encourage foods with moderate fiber content—whole grains, fruits, and vegetables.
2. Increase water intake.
3. Obtain a raised toilet seat to encourage normal position.
4. Encourage the patient to follow regular bowel regimen that may include stool softener and other mild medications for constipation.

Strengthening Coping Ability

1. Help the patient establish realistic goals and outline ways to achieve goals.
2. Provide emotional support and encouragement.
3. Encourage use of all resources, such as therapists, primary care provider, social worker, and social support network.
4. Encourage open communication, discussion of feelings, and exchange of information about Parkinson disease.
5. Have the patient take an active role in activity planning and evaluation of treatment plan.
6. Observe for changes in depression to determine if the patient is responding to antidepressants.

Community and Home Care Considerations

1. Recommend interdisciplinary home health care program. Requires skilled assessment of needs of patient, professional nursing and therapeutic services, patient and family education, and case management to optimize patient outcomes.
2. Encourage use of soothing music to reduce pain and depression.
3. Assess safety in environment to reduce risk of falls.
4. Utilize physical therapy services to encourage safe ambulation and reduce fear of falls.
5. Encourage use of social services, respite care and health visitors, mental health counselors, and support groups to prevent caregiver strain.

6. Use occupational therapy aids to ensure mobility and safety, such as grab rails in the tub or shower, raised toilet seat, hand rails on both sides of the stairway, rope secured to foot of bed to achieve sitting position, and straight-backed wooden chairs with armrests.

 NURSING ALERT Bowel and bladder management is an extremely important factor in the decision to keep the patient at home. Techniques to reduce incontinence episodes, such as having frequently scheduled toileting time, and to handle episodes of incontinence, such as having cleaning supplies and a change of clothes/briefs in the bathroom, should be taught to decrease caregiver burden.

Patient Education and Health Maintenance

1. Instruct the patient to avoid sedatives, unless specifically prescribed, which have additive effect with other medications.
2. Instruct the patient in medication regimen, signs of toxicity, and adverse reactions, such as orthostatic hypotension, dry mouth, dystonia, muscle twitching, urine retention, impaired glucose tolerance, anemia, and elevated liver function tests.
3. Encourage follow-up and monitoring for diabetes, glaucoma, hepatotoxicity, and anemia while undergoing drug therapy. Increasing episodes of freezing should be reported.
4. Teach the patient ambulation cues to avoid "freezing" in place and possibly avoid falls by doing one of the following:
   a. Raise head, raise toes, and then rock from one foot to another while bending knees slightly.
   b. Raise arms in a sudden short motion.
   c. Take a small step backward and then start forward.
   d. Step sideways and then start forward.
5. Instruct the family not to pull patient during episodes of "freezing," which increases the problem and may cause falling.
6. Refer the patient/family for more information and support to such agencies as National Parkinson's Foundation (*www.parkinson.org*) and National Institute of Neurologic Disorders and Stroke (*www.ninds.nih.gov*).

Evaluation: Expected Outcomes

- Attends physical therapy sessions; does facial exercises 10 minutes twice per day.
- Eats three small meals and two snacks; no weight loss.
- Enunciation clear; speaking in four to five words per breath.
- Passes soft stool every day.
- Asks questions about Parkinson's; obtains help from family and/or friends.

Multiple Sclerosis

Multiple sclerosis (MS) is a chronic, frequently progressive neurologic disease of the CNS of unknown etiology and uncertain trajectory. MS is characterized by the occurrence of small patches of demyelination of the white matter of the optic nerve, brain, and spinal cord. MS is distinguished by exacerbations and remissions of symptoms over the course of the illness. MS is the most common CNS disease among young adults and the third leading cause of disability in the United States. It is estimated that 400,000 Americans have this disorder of the brain and spinal cord, causing disruption of electrical messages from the brain to the peripheral nervous system.

Pathophysiology and Etiology

1. *Demyelination* refers to the destruction of the myelin, the fatty and protein material that covers certain nerve fibers in the brain and spinal cord (see Figure 15-8).
2. Demyelination results in disordered transmission of nerve impulses.
3. Inflammatory changes lead to scarring of the affected nerve fibers.
4. Cause is unknown but may possibly be related to autoimmune dysfunction, genetic susceptibility, or an infectious process.
5. More prevalent in the northern latitudes and among whites.

Classification

The National Multiple Sclerosis Advisory Committee recognizes four clinical forms of MS:

1. Relapsing remitting (RR)—clearly defined acute attacks evolve over days to weeks. Partial recovery of function occurs over weeks to months. Average frequency of attacks is once every 2 years and neurologic stability remains between attacks without disease progression. (At the time of onset, 90% of cases of MS are diagnosed as RR.)
2. Secondary progressive (SP)—always begins as RR, but clinical course changes with increasing relapse rate, with a steady deterioration in neurologic function unrelated to the original attack. (Fifty percent of those with RR will progress to SP within 10 years; 90% will progress within 25 years.)

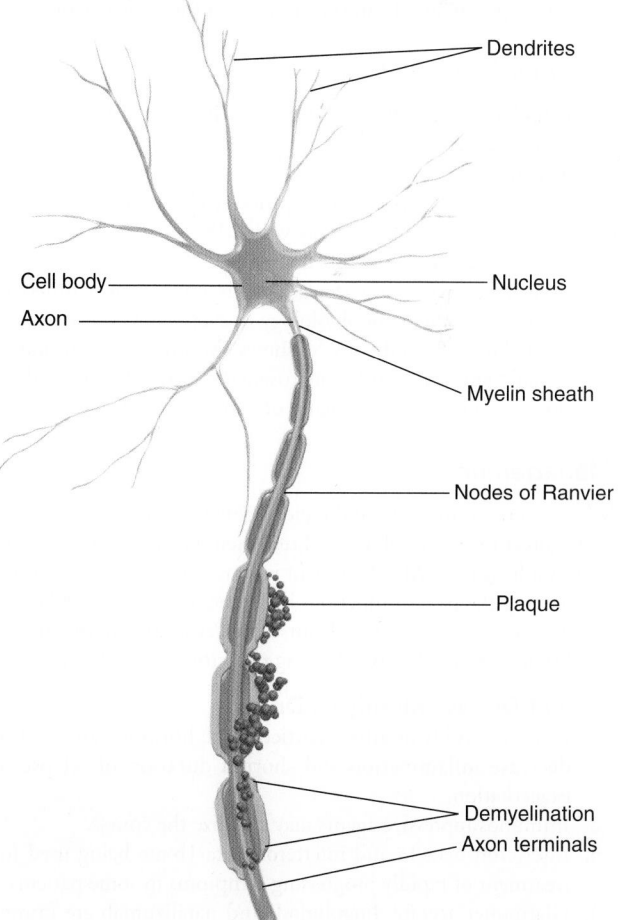

Figure 15-8. Myelin destruction of the nerve cell axon in multiple sclerosis. (Hickey, J. [2013]. Clinical Practice of Neurological & Neurosurgical Nursing [7th ed.]. Philadelphia: Lippincott Williams & Wilkins.)

3. Primary progressive (PP)—characterized by steady progression of disability from onset without exacerbations and remissions. More prevalent among males and older individuals. Worst prognosis for neurologic disability. (Ten percent of cases of MS are diagnosed as PP.)

4. Progressive relapsing (PR)—the same as PP except that patients experience acute exacerbations along with a steadily progressive course (rarest form).

Clinical Manifestations

Lesions can occur anywhere within the white matter of the CNS. Symptoms reflect the location of the area of demyelination.

1. Fatigue and weakness.
2. Abnormal reflexes—absent or exaggerated.
3. Vision disturbances—impaired and double vision, nystagmus.
4. Motor dysfunction—weakness, tremor, incoordination.
5. Sensory disturbances—paresthesias, impaired deep sensation, impaired vibratory and position sense.
6. Impaired speech—slurring, scanning (dysarthria).
7. Urinary dysfunction—hesitancy, frequency, urgency, retention, incontinence; upper UTI. Urinary dysfunction affects about 90% of patients with MS and may exacerbate relapse of MS.
8. Neurobehavioral syndromes—depression, cognitive impairment, emotional lability.
9. Symptoms of MS are often unpredictable, varying from person to person and from time to time in the same person.

Diagnostic Evaluation

1. Establishing a definitive diagnosis is often difficult, with much uncertainty concerning prognosis once the diagnosis is made.
2. Serial brain MRI studies have proved to be useful for diagnosing and monitoring patients with MS—show small plaques scattered throughout white matter of CNS.
3. Magnetic resonance spectroscopy is now being studied to monitor specific pathophysiology of evolving MS plaques.
4. Electrophoresis study of CSF shows abnormal IgG antibody.
5. Visual, auditory, and somatosensory evoked potentials—slowed conduction is evidence of demyelination.

Management

MS treatment is dynamic and rapidly evolving, covering two main areas: direct treatment of MS and treatment of the effects or symptoms resulting from MS. Treatment is aimed at relieving symptoms and helping the patient function. However, a therapeutic relationship between the patient and nurse creates a critical and strong bond that is essential across the long trajectory of the illness.

Current Disease-Modifying Drugs

1. Corticosteroids or adrenocorticotropic hormone are used to decrease inflammation and shorten duration of relapse or exacerbation.
2. Immunosuppressive agents may stabilize the course.
3. Interferon beta-1a and interferon beta-1b are being used for treatment of rapidly progressing symptoms in some patients.
4. Glatiramer acetate, fingolimod, and natalizumab are immunomodulators used in RR disease.
5. Mitoxantrone, a chemotherapeutic agent used for the treatment of SP (chronic), PR, or worsening RR MS not responding to other disease-modifying drugs.

Treating Exacerbations

1. A true exacerbation of MS is caused by an area of inflammation in the CNS.
2. The treatment most commonly used to control exacerbations is IV, high-dose corticosteroids. Methylprednisolone is one of the most commonly used corticosteroids in MS.
3. Plasmapheresis (plasma exchange) is only considered for the 10% who do not respond well to standard corticosteroid treatment.

Chronic Symptom Management

1. Treatment of spasticity with such agents as baclofen, dantrolene, diazepam; physical therapy; nerve blocks and surgical intervention.
2. Control of fatigue with amantadine and lifestyle changes.
3. Treatment of depression with antidepressant drugs and counseling.
4. Bladder management with anticholinergics, intermittent catheterization for drainage, prophylactic antibiotics.
5. Bowel management with stool softeners, bulk laxative, suppositories.
6. Multidisciplinary rehabilitation management with physical therapy, occupational therapy, speech therapy, cognitive therapy, vocational rehabilitation, and complementary and alternative medicine, as indicated, to restore or maintain functions essential to daily living in individuals who have lost these capacities through the disease process.
7. Control of dystonia with carbamazepine.
8. Management of pain syndromes with carbamazepine, phenytoin, perphenazine/amitriptyline, and nonpharmacologic modalities.

Complications

1. Dysphagia and respiratory dysfunction.
2. Infections: bladder, respiratory, sepsis.
3. Complications from immobility.
4. Speech, voice, and language disorders such as dysarthria.

Nursing Assessment

1. Observe motor strength, coordination, and gait.
2. Perform CN assessment.
3. Evaluate elimination function.
4. Explore coping, effect on activity and sexual function, emotional adjustment.
5. Assess patient and family coping, support systems, and available resources.
6. Assess for anxiety, depression, sleep disturbances, cognitive impairment, and pain, which commonly occur in patients with MS.

Nursing Diagnoses

- Impaired Physical Mobility related to muscle weakness, spasticity, and incoordination.
- Fatigue related to disease process and stress of coping.
- Risk for Injury related to motor and sensory deficits.
- Risk for Aspiration related to dysphagia.
- Impaired Urinary Elimination related to the disease process.
- Interrupted Family Processes related to inability to fulfill expected roles.
- Sexual Dysfunction related to disease process.

Nursing Interventions

Promoting Motor Function

1. Perform muscle-stretching and muscle-strengthening exercises daily, or teach the patient or family to perform, using a stretch–hold–relax routine to minimize spasticity and prevent contractures.
2. Apply ice packs before stretching to reduce spasticity.
3. Tell the patient to avoid muscle fatigue by stopping activity just short of fatigue and to take frequent rest periods.
4. Encourage walking and activity and teach the patient how to use such devices as braces, canes, and walkers, when necessary.
5. Inform the patient to avoid sudden changes in position, which may cause falls due to loss of position sense, and to walk with a wide-based gait.
6. Encourage frequent change in position while immobilized to prevent contractures; sleeping prone will minimize flexor spasm of hips and knees.

Minimizing Fatigue

1. Help the patient and family understand that fatigue is an integral part of MS.
2. Plan ahead and prioritize activities. Take brief rest periods throughout the day.
3. Avoid overheating, overexertion, and infection.
4. Encourage energy-conservation techniques, such as sitting to perform activity, limiting trips up and down stairs, pulling, or pushing rather than lifting.
5. Help the patient develop a healthy lifestyle with balanced diet, rest, exercise, and relaxation.

Preventing Injury

1. Suggest use of an eye patch or frosted lens (alternate eyes) for patients with double vision.
2. Encourage regular ophthalmologic consultation to maximize vision and be aware of potential for hearing changes and assess as needed.
3. Provide a safe environment for patient with any sensory alteration.
   a. Orient the patient to the environment and keep arrangement of furniture and personal articles constant.
   b. Make sure floor is free from obstacles, loose rugs, or slippery areas.
   c. Teach the use of all senses to maintain awareness of environment.

Managing Dysphagia

1. Initiate referrals to speech/language pathologist and dietician for evaluation and treatment of swallowing problems.
2. Ensure that the patient is alert and distractions are minimized at mealtimes; provide supervision, as indicated.
3. Use safe swallowing practices, including proper positioning, double swallow, and chin tuck.
4. Monitor the patient for signs and symptoms of choking or aspiration; use suctioning as indicated.
5. Educate and counsel patients and care partners about feeding options as disease progresses.

Maintaining Urinary Elimination

1. Ensure adequate fluid intake to help prevent infection and stone formation.
2. Assess for urine retention and catheterize for residual urine, as indicated.
3. Teach the patient to report signs of UTI immediately.
4. Set up bladder-training program to reduce incontinence.
   a. Encourage fluids every 2 hours.
   b. Follow regular schedule of voiding, every 1 to 2 hours, lengthening as tolerated.
   c. Restrict fluid volume and salty foods 1 to 2 hours before bedtime.
5. See pages 148 to 149 for more information on urine retention and incontinence.

Normalizing Family Processes

1. Encourage verbalization of feelings of each family member.
2. Encourage counseling and use of church or community resources.
3. Suggest dividing up household duties and childcare responsibilities to prevent strain on one person.
4. Explore adaptation of some roles so the patient can still function in family unit.
5. Expand treatment efforts to include the whole family.
6. Support mothers with MS who often face fatigue and episodic exacerbations during their childrearing years.

Promoting Sexual Function

1. Encourage open communication between partners.
2. Discuss birth control options, if appropriate.
3. Suggest sexual activity when the patient is most rested.
4. Suggest consultation with sexual therapist to help obtain greater sexual satisfaction.

Community and Home Care Considerations

1. The nurse case manager functions as care provider, facilitator, advocate, educator, counselor, and innovator aimed at intervening in a wide variety of settings to improve patient function and mobility.
2. Teach the patient receiving interferon beta-1a and interferon beta-1b to expect adverse effects of flulike symptoms, fever, asthenia, chills, myalgias, sweating, and local reaction at the injection site. Liver function test elevation and neutropenia may also occur. Adverse effects may persist for up to 6 months of treatment before subsiding.
3. Instruct the patient receiving interferon beta-1a and interferon beta-1b in self-injection technique.
4. Teach the patient and family to use their own judgment, knowledge, and ingenuity to control MS symptoms.
5. Teach the patient and family how to conduct periodic self-assessment of daily functioning so that home care team can continue to make modifications in treatment plan.

 DRUG ALERT Ensure rotation of subcutaneous injection site of disease-modifying drugs to prevent skin reactions. Avoid injections into an area of skin that is sore, reddened, infected, or damaged. Injection sites include the inner thigh, outer surface of the upper arm, stomach, or buttocks. If the patient is thin, thigh and arm sites are preferred. Use a diagram or log of the date and site location for each injection.

Patient Education and Health Maintenance

1. Encourage the patient to maintain previous activities, although at a lowered level of intensity, and reinforce appropriate and safe use of adaptive equipment and aides.

2. Teach the patient to respect fatigue and avoid physical over-exertion and emotional stress; remind the patient that activity tolerance may vary from day to day.
3. Advise the patient to avoid exposure to heat and cold or infectious agents.
4. Encourage a nutritious diet that is high in fiber to promote health and good bowel elimination.
5. Advise the patient that some medications may accentuate weakness, such as some antibiotics, muscle relaxants, antiarrhythmics and antihypertensives, antipsychotics, oral contraceptives, and antihistamines; check with health care provider or pharmacist before taking any new medications.
6. Try to include children in the education of MS and the relationship of fatigue and functional status.
7. Refer the patient/family for more information and support to such agencies as the National Multiple Sclerosis Society (*www.nmss.org*).

Evaluation: Expected Outcomes

- Performs exercises correctly without spasm.
- Rests at intervals; tolerates activity well.
- Moves about in environment without injury.
- No episodes of aspiration.
- Voids every 2 hours with no incontinent episodes.
- Family sharing care, discussing feelings.
- Reports satisfaction with sexual activity.

Amyotrophic Lateral Sclerosis

Amyotrophic lateral sclerosis (ALS), also known as Lou Gehrig disease, is an incapacitating, fatal neuromuscular disease that affects as many as 20,000 Americans, with 5,000 new cases occurring in the United States each year. ALS results in progressive muscle weakness and progressive wasting and paralysis of the muscles. It is accompanied by other LMN signs, such as atrophy or fasciculations. Approximately 80% of cases begin between ages 40 and 70. The life expectancy of an ALS patient averages 2 to 5 years.

Pathophysiology and Etiology

1. Degeneration of upper motor neurons (nerves leading from the brain to medulla or spinal cord) and LMNs (nerves leading from the spinal cord to the muscles of the body).
2. Results in progressive loss of voluntary muscle contraction and functional capacity, involving the legs, feet, arms, and hands, and those that control swallowing and breathing. Patients develop variable hyperreflexia, clonus, spasticity, extensor plantar responses, and limb or tongue fasciculations. Extraocular muscles and bladder and anal sphincter muscles typically are spared. ALS rarely affects cognitive functions.
3. Cause is unknown. Usually affects men in the fifth or sixth decade of life.
4. Nearly 10% of ALS cases are familial; the disease is transmitted in an autosomal dominant fashion. The copper/zinc SOD1 gene is mutated in 10% to 20% of these familial cases. Although the primary mechanism of SOD1-mediated neural injury is currently unknown, apoptosis, excitotoxicity, and oxidative stress are thought to play major roles in pathogenesis. Sporadic ALS shares clinical features with familial ALS. However, no SOD1 mutations or polymorphisms have been identified in these patients. Common pathways of disease pathogenesis may play a role, with different molecular abnormalities that lead to similar phenotypes.
5. Several studies have shown an inflammatory component to the affected spinal cord regions, with the presence of activated microglia, reactive astrocytes, and IgG deposition. Whether this reaction precedes or accompanies the molecular events that promote neuronal cell death is unknown.

Clinical Manifestations

1. Progressive weakness and wasting of muscles of arms, trunk, and legs.
2. Fasciculations and signs of spasticity.
3. Progressive difficulty swallowing with drooling (sialorrhea) and regurgitation of liquids through the nose, speaking (nasal and unintelligible sounds), and, ultimately, breathing.
4. CN deficits (bulbar symptoms) are present in 20% of cases (prevalence increases with age), along with dysarthria, voice deterioration, and dysphagia. (Patients with bulbar presentation have poorer prognosis; these symptoms also have a profound impact on quality of life because of nutritional risk factors, aspiration, and respiratory complications.)

Diagnostic Evaluation

1. Electromyography to evaluate denervation and muscle atrophy.
2. Nerve conduction study to evaluate nerve pathways.
3. Pulmonary function tests to evaluate respiratory function.
4. Barium swallow to evaluate ability to achieve various phases of swallowing mechanisms.
5. MRI, CT to rule out other disorders.
6. Laboratory tests: creatine kinase, heavy metal screen, thyroid function tests, CSF evaluation to rule out other causes of muscle weakness.

Management

1. There is no cure for ALS, nor is there a proven therapy that will prevent or reverse the course of the disorder.
2. Riluzole has been shown to prolong the survival of ALS patients by 2 to 3 months.

 EVIDENCE BASE Miller, R. G., Mitchell, J. D., Moore, D. H. (2012). Riluzole for amyotrophic lateral sclerosis (ALS)/motor neuron disease (MND). *Cochrane Database of Systematic Reviews*, (3), CD001447.

3. Most treatment is palliative and symptomatic.
4. Botulinum toxin B injections into the parotid and submandibular glands, amitriptyline therapy, or low-dose radiation therapy to the salivary glands may be used to treat drooling.
5. There are insufficient data to support or refute any specific intervention for the treatment of cramps, spasticity, depression, anxiety, insomnia, pain, dyspnea, or cognitive/behavioral impairments in ALS.
6. Neuropsychological screening may be conducted to assess for cognitive and behavioral impairments.
7. Feeding gastrostomy.
8. Tracheostomy and mechanical ventilation eventually become necessary and should be discussed prior to need to ascertain the patient's wishes regarding these measures.

NURSING ALERT Although no formal research has been conducted addressing the best time to discuss care preferences and end-of-life care in ALS, it is important to elicit this information to guide the selection of various therapeutics, such as intubation, tube feeding, treatment of infection, and management of changes in LOC. Having the family or significant other present when these discussions occur can help to alleviate miscommunication or disagreements in the plan of care.

Complications

1. Respiratory failure.
2. Aspiration pneumonia.
3. Cardiopulmonary arrest.
4. Locked-in syndrome—fully conscious but unable to respond in any way.

Nursing Assessment

1. Evaluate respiratory function: rate, depth, tidal volume.
2. Perform CN assessment, particularly gag reflex and swallowing.
3. Assess voluntary motor function and strength.

Nursing Diagnoses

- Ineffective Breathing Pattern related to respiratory muscle weakness.
- Impaired Physical Mobility related to disease process.
- Imbalanced Nutrition: Less Than Body Requirements related to inability to swallow.
- Fatigue related to denervation of muscles.
- Social Isolation related to fatigability and decreased communication skills.
- Risk for Infection related to inability to clear airway.

Nursing Interventions

Maintaining Respiration

1. Monitor vital capacity frequently. Document pattern and report any decrease below patient's baseline.
2. Position patient upright, suction upper airway, and perform chest physical therapy to enhance respiratory function.
3. Encourage use of incentive spirometer to exercise respiratory muscles.
4. Assess for signs of hypoxia, such as tachypnea, hypopnea, restlessness, poor sleep, and excessive fatigue.
5. Obtain ABG values as ordered.
6. Establish the wishes of the patient in terms of life-support measures; obtain copy of advance directive for chart, if applicable.
7. Assist with intubation, tracheostomy, and mechanical ventilation when indicated (see Chapter 10).
8. Provide suctioning and routine care of a patient with artificial airway and mechanical ventilation.

Optimizing Mobility

1. Encourage the patient to continue usual activities as long as possible but modify exertion to avoid fatigue.
2. Encourage physical therapy exercises to strengthen unaffected muscles and perform ROM exercises to prevent contractures.
3. Encourage energy-conservation techniques.

4. Obtain assistive devices, as needed, to help the patient maintain independence, such as special feeding devices, remote controls, and a motorized wheelchair.

Meeting Nutritional Requirements

1. Provide high-calorie, small, frequent feedings.
2. Provide meals that are of a texture the patient can handle; semisolid food is usually easiest to swallow.
   a. Avoid easily aspirated, pureed, and mucus-producing foods (eg, milk).
   b. Try warm or cold foods that stimulate temperature receptors in mouth and may help in swallowing.
   c. Do not wash down solids with fluids—may cause choking and aspiration.
3. Allow the patient to make his or her own food selection.
4. Provide assistive devices for self-feeding when possible.
5. Make mealtimes a pleasant experience in a bright room, with quiet company so the patient may concentrate on eating and avoid undue embarrassment.
6. Examine oral cavity for food debris before and after meals, and assess swallowing function and buildup of saliva.
7. Encourage rest periods before meals to alleviate muscle fatigue.
8. Place the patient upright for meals with neck flexed to partially protect the airway.
9. Instruct the patient to take a breath before swallowing, hold breath to swallow, exhale or cough after swallow, and swallow again.
10. Tell the patient to avoid talking while eating.
11. Prepare the patient for gastrostomy or other alternate feeding methods when appropriate and desired by patient.

Minimizing Fatigue

1. Encourage activity alternating with frequent naps.
2. Encourage the patient to accomplish most important activities early in day.
3. Consult with occupational therapist about energy-conservation techniques in performing ADL.

Maintaining Social Interaction

1. Use mechanical speech aids or communication board.
2. Use an environmental control board.
3. Eye movements/blinks may be the last voluntary movement; develop a code system to serve as a communication method.
4. Because standard call lights cannot be activated by the severely debilitated ALS patient, provide adaptive call light (environmental control unit) and/or some type of constant monitoring and surveillance to meet patient's needs.
5. Allow the patient to select which social activities are meaningful.
6. Refer to counselor or psychologist for coping with communication barriers and inevitability of losses.

Preventing Aspiration and Infection

1. Consult with a speech therapist for techniques and devices to assist swallowing.
2. Discourage bed rest to prevent pulmonary stasis.
3. Perform chest physiotherapy, as tolerated.
4. Monitor for fever and tachycardia and obtain sputum, urine, and other cultures, as indicated.

Community and Home Care Considerations

1. Teach caregivers how to perform suctioning, tracheostomy care, and ventilator care in the home, as indicated. Clean technique will be used rather than sterile.
2. Teach caregivers how to perform gastrostomy feedings and care of tube.

3. Assess for adequate supplies for care and ability of caregivers to carry out procedures.
4. Encourage cleanliness in home environment and avoidance of contact with anyone with respiratory infection. Give influenza and pneumonia vaccines, as indicated.

Patient Education and Health Maintenance

1. Stress the importance of maintaining physical exercise.
2. Review with the patient and family proper eating mechanics to avoid fatigue and aspiration.
3. Inform the patient of right to make decisions early in the disease process regarding an advance directive and life-sustaining treatment.
4. Encourage the family to seek support and respite care.
5. Remind the family that the patient with ALS maintains full alertness, sensory function, and intelligence. Encourage them to maintain interaction, socialization, and stimulation and to seek out technology such as mind-activated computer-driven communication devices.
6. Refer the patient/family for more information and support to such agencies as the ALS Association (*www.alsa.org*).

Evaluation: Expected Outcomes

- Normal respiratory rate and rhythm, shallow, unlabored at rest.
- Does active ROM exercises for 15 minutes twice per day; uses assistive utensils to feed self.
- Tolerates small, frequent feedings without aspiration.
- Naps twice per day for 1 to 2 hours.
- Communicates needs effectively to staff and family.
- No signs of respiratory or urinary infection.

NEUROMUSCULAR DISORDERS

Guillain-Barré Syndrome (Polyradiculoneuritis)

Guillain-Barré syndrome (GBS) is an acute, rapidly progressing, ascending inflammatory demyelinating polyneuropathy of the peripheral sensory and motor nerves and nerve roots. GBS is most often, but not always, characterized by muscular weakness and distal sensory loss or dysesthesias. GBS is the most frequently acquired demyelinating neuropathy. It affects 1 in 100,000 people and must be identified quickly to initiate treatment and decrease life-threatening complications. Usually, GBS occurs a few days or weeks following symptoms of a respiratory or GI viral infection. Occasionally, surgery or vaccinations will trigger the syndrome. The disorder can develop over the course of hours, days, or weeks. Maximum weakness usually occurs within the first 2 weeks after symptoms appear, and by the 3rd week of the illness, 90% of all patients are at their weakest. About 30% of those with GBS have residual weakness after 3 years and the recurrence rate is approximately 3%.

Mortality results from respiratory failure, autonomic disturbances, sepsis, and complications of immobility and occurs at a rate of about 5% despite intensive medical care.

Pathophysiology and Etiology

1. Believed to be an autoimmune disorder that causes acute neuromuscular paralysis due to destruction of the myelin sheath surrounding peripheral nerve axons and subsequent slowing of transmission.
2. Viral infection, immunization, or other event may trigger the autoimmune response.
3. About 30% to 40% of cases are preceded by *Campylobacter* infection, an acute infectious diarrheal illness.
4. Cell-mediated immune reaction is aimed at peripheral nerves, causing demyelination and, possibly, axonal degeneration.

Clinical Manifestations

1. Paresthesias and, possibly, dysesthesias.
2. Acute onset of symmetric progressive muscle weakness, most often beginning in the legs and ascending to involve the trunk, upper extremities, and facial muscles; paralysis may develop.
3. Difficulty with swallowing, speech, and chewing due to CN involvement.
4. Decreased or absent deep tendon reflexes, position, and vibratory perception.
5. Autonomic dysfunction (increased heart rate and postural hypotension).
6. Decreased vital capacity, depth of respirations, and breath sounds.
7. Occasionally spasm and fasciculations of muscles.

Diagnostic Evaluation

1. History and neurologic examination. Progressive weakness, decreased sensation, decreased deep tendon reflexes.
2. Lumbar puncture for CSF examination—reveals low blood cell count, high protein.
3. Electrophysiologic studies—nerve conduction velocity shows decreased conduction velocity of peripheral nerves.

Management

1. Plasmapheresis produces temporary reduction of circulating antibodies to reduce the severity and duration of the GBS episode.
2. High-dose Ig therapy and corticosteroids are used to reduce the severity of the episode.
3. ECG monitoring and treatment of cardiac dysrhythmias.
4. Analgesics and muscle relaxants, as needed.
5. Intubation and mechanical ventilation if respiratory paralysis develops.

Complications

1. Respiratory failure.
2. Cardiac dysrhythmias.
3. Complications of immobility and paralysis.
4. Anxiety and depression.

Nursing Assessment

1. Assess pain level due to muscle spasms and dysesthesias.
2. Assess cardiovascular function including orthostatic BPs.
3. Assess respiratory status closely to determine hypoventilation due to weakness.
4. Perform CN assessment, especially CN IX for gag reflex.
5. Assess motor strength.

Nursing Diagnoses

- Ineffective Breathing Pattern related to weakness/paralysis of respiratory muscles.
- Impaired Physical Mobility related to paralysis.
- Imbalanced Nutrition: Less Than Body Requirements, related to CN dysfunction.

- Impaired Verbal Communication related to intubation, CN dysfunction.
- Chronic Pain related to disease pathology.
- Anxiety related to communication difficulties and deteriorating physical condition.

Nursing Interventions

Maintaining Respiration

1. Monitor respiratory status through vital capacity measurements, rate and depth of respirations, breath sounds.
2. Monitor level of weakness as it ascends toward respiratory muscles.
3. Watch for breathlessness while talking, a sign of respiratory fatigue.
4. Maintain calm environment and position the patient with head of bed elevated to provide for maximum chest excursion.
5. As much as possible, avoid opioids and sedatives that may depress respirations.
6. Monitor the patient for signs of impending respiratory failure; heart rate above 120 or below 70 beats/minute; respiratory rate above 30 breaths/minute; prepare to intubate.
7. Long-term respiratory management may be necessary with placement of a tracheostomy.

Avoiding Complications of Immobility

1. Position the patient correctly and provide ROM exercises.
2. Encourage physical and occupational therapy exercises to regain strength during the rehabilitative period.
3. Assess for complications, such as contractures, pressure ulcers, edema of lower extremities, and constipation.
4. Provide assistive devices, as needed, such as cane or wheelchair, for patient to take home.
5. Recommend referral to rehabilitation services or physical therapy for evaluation and treatment.

Promoting Adequate Nutrition

1. Assess chewing and swallowing ability by testing CN V, IX, and X; if function is inadequate, provide alternate nutrition through enteral or parenteral methods.
2. During rehabilitation period, encourage a well-balanced, nutritious diet in small, frequent feedings with vitamin supplement, if indicated.
3. Recommend referral to dietitian for evaluation and proper diet therapy.

Maintaining Communication

1. Develop a communication system with the patient who cannot speak.
2. Have frequent contact with the patient and provide explanation and reassurance, remembering that the patient is fully conscious.
3. Provide some type of patient call system. Because standard call lights cannot be activated by the severely weak patient, provide adaptive call light and/or some type of constant monitoring and surveillance to meet patient's needs.
4. Recommend referral to speech therapy for evaluation and treatment.
5. Refer to counselor, social worker, or psychologist to develop/enhance coping skills and regain sense of control.

Relieving Pain

1. Administer analgesics, as required; monitor for adverse reactions, such as hypotension, nausea and vomiting, and respiratory depression.

2. Provide adjunct pain management therapies, such as therapeutic touch, massage, diversion, and guided imagery.
3. Provide explanations to relieve anxiety, which augments pain.
4. Turn the patient frequently to relieve painful pressure areas.

Reducing Anxiety

1. Get to know the patient and build a trusting relationship.
2. Discuss fears and concerns while verbal communication is possible.
3. Reassure the patient that recovery is probable.
4. Use relaxation techniques such as listening to soft music.
5. Provide choices in care and give the patient a sense of control.
6. Enlist the support of significant others.

Community and Home Care Considerations

1. Be aware that GBS is a significant cause of new long-term disability for at least 1,000 people per year in the United States, necessitating long-term rehabilitation and community reintegration. Outcome can range from mild paresthesias to death. The chance of recovery is significantly affected by age, antecedent gastroenteritis, disability, electrophysiologic signs of axonal degeneration, latency to nadir, and duration of active disease.
2. Given the young age at which GBS sometimes occurs, the patient and family must be treated as an integral unit, assessing family communication, knowledge, adjustment, and use of support systems.
3. Include in caregiver training strategies the need for exercise, positioning, and activity to prevent secondary complications, such as contractures, DVT, hypercalcemia, and pressure ulcers.

Patient Education and Health Maintenance

1. Advise the patient and family that acute phase lasts 1 to 4 weeks, then the patient stabilizes and rehabilitation can begin; however, convalescence may be lengthy, from 3 months to 2 years.
2. Instruct the patient in breathing exercises or use of incentive spirometer to re-establish normal patterns.
3. Teach the patient to wear good supportive and protective shoes while out of bed to prevent injuries due to weakness and paresthesia.
4. Instruct the patient to check feet routinely for injuries because trauma may go unnoticed because of sensory changes.
5. Reinforce maintenance of normal weight; additional weight will further stress motor abilities.
6. Encourage the use of scheduled rest periods to avoid overfatigue.
7. Refer the patient/family for more information and support to such agencies as Guillain-Barré Syndrome Foundation International (*www.gbsfi.com*).

Evaluation: Expected Outcomes

- Normal respiratory rate and rhythm, shallow, unlabored.
- Performs assistive ROM exercises every 2 hours; no pressure ulcers or edema present.
- Gag reflex present; eating small meals without aspiration.
- Uses short phrases and head nodding to communicate effectively.
- Verbalizes decreased pain.
- Verbalizes reduced anxiety.

Myasthenia Gravis

Myasthenia gravis (MG) is a chronic autoimmune disorder affecting the neuromuscular transmission of impulses in the voluntary muscles of the body. MG is characterized by fluctuating weakness increased by exertion. Weakness increases during the day and improves with rest. Presentation and progression vary because of an antibody-mediated attack against acetylcholine receptors at the neuromuscular junction. Loss of acetylcholine receptors leads to a defect in neuromuscular transmission. Cardinal features are muscle weakness and fatigue. Evidence suggests that the frequency and recognition of MG is increasing.

Pathophysiology and Etiology

1. MG is idiopathic in most patients. Penicillamine is known to induce various autoimmune disorders, including MG.
2. Depletion of acetylcholine receptors at neuromuscular junctions brought about by an autoimmune attack (see Figure 15-9). In about 90% of patients, no specific cause can be identified, but genetic makeup is a predisposing factor, suggesting environmental factors may be involved in development of this disorder.
3. The reduced number of acetylcholine receptors results in diminished amplitude of end-plate potentials. Failed transmission of nerve impulses to skeletal muscle at the myoneural junction results in decreased muscle power, clinically manifested as extreme fatigue and weakness. The pattern of muscle involvement varies among individuals.
4. About 80% to 90% of patients with MG have serum antibodies to acetylcholine.
5. Thyroid gland abnormalities are present in 80% of patients. Thymic tumor is the most important known cause; 10% of patients with MG have a thymoma.
6. *Cholinergic crisis* can result from overmedication with anticholinergic drugs, which release too much acetylcholine at the neuromuscular junction.
7. *Brittle crisis* occurs when the receptors at the neuromuscular junction become insensitive to anticholinesterase medication.
8. Women are three times more susceptible to developing MG than men.
9. Spontaneous remissions are rare. Long and complete remissions are even less common. Most remissions (with treatment) occur during the first 3 years of disease.

Clinical Manifestations

1. Extreme muscular weakness and easy fatigability.
2. Vision disturbances—diplopia and ptosis from ocular weakness. Extraocular muscle weakness or ptosis is present initially in 50% of patients and occurs during the course of illness in 90%. Bulbar muscle weakness is also common, along with weakness of head extension and flexion.
3. Facial muscle weakness causes a masklike facial expression. Patients may present a snarling appearance when attempting to smile.
4. Dysarthria and dysphagia from weakness of laryngeal and pharyngeal muscles.
5. Proximal limb weakness, with specific weakness in the small muscles of the hands. Patients progress from mild to more severe disease over weeks to months. Weakness tends to spread from the ocular to facial to bulbar muscles and then to truncal and limb muscles. The disease remains ocular in only 16% of patients. About 87% of patients generalize within 13 months after onset.
6. Respiratory muscle weakness can be life-threatening. Intercurrent illness or medication can exacerbate weakness, quickly precipitating a myasthenic crisis and rapid respiratory compromise.
7. Impending myasthenic crisis may be triggered by respiratory infection, aspiration, physical/emotional stress, and changes in medications. Symptoms include:
   a. Sudden respiratory distress.
   b. Signs of dysphagia, dysarthria, ptosis, and diplopia.
   c. Tachycardia, anxiety.
   d. Rapidly increasing weakness of extremities and trunk.

Diagnostic Evaluation

1. Serum test for acetylcholine receptor antibodies—positive in up to 90% of patients.
2. Electrophysiologic testing, such as EMG, shows decreased response to repetative nerve stimulation.
3. Edrophonium (Tensilon) test—IV injection of this short-acting anticholinesterase relieves symptoms temporarily. After injection, a marked but temporary improvement in muscle strength identified by performance of repetitive movements or EMG testing suggests MG. It also differentiates myasthenic crisis from cholinergic crisis.
4. Thyroid function tests should be done to evaluate for coexistent thyroid disease and CT scan to assess enlargement of thymus gland. Chest CT scan is mandatory to identify thymoma in all cases of MG. This is especially true in older individuals.

Management

1. With treatment, most patients can lead fairly normal lives.
2. Oral anticholinesterase drugs, such as neostigmine and pyridostigmine, are first-line treatments for mild MG, enhancing neuromuscular transmission.
3. Immunosuppressive drugs, such as prednisone, are the mainstay of treatment when weakness is not adequately controlled by anticholinergic medication. Azathioprine may be added as a steroid-sparing agent. Immunosuppressant treatment is often permanent.

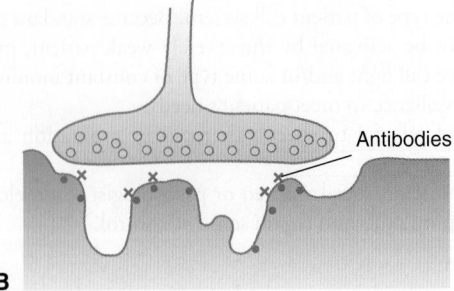

Figure 15-9. Myasthenia gravis. **(A)** Normal acetylcholine receptor site; **(B)** acetylcholine receptor site in myasthenia gravis. (Smeltzer, S., & Bare, B. [2000]. *Brunner and Suddarth's textbook of medical-surgical nursing* [9th ed.]. Philadelphia, PA: Lippincott Williams & Wilkins.)

4. Plasmapheresis removes antibodies from the blood and is used for patients in myasthenic crisis or for short-term treatment of patients undergoing thymectomy. IV Ig is also an option and has less side effects.
5. Thymectomy is indicated for patients with tumor or hyperplasia of the thymus gland (thymectomy is not usually beneficial in late-onset patients).
6. Interventions for myasthenic crisis:
    a. Immediate hospitalization and may require intensive care.
    b. Edrophonium to differentiate crisis and treat myasthenic crisis; temporarily worsens cholinergic crisis; unpredictable results with brittle crisis.
    c. Airway management—mechanical ventilation, vigorous suctioning, oxygen therapy, postural drainage with percussion and vibration. Tracheostomy may be required, depending on duration of intubation. Maintain semi-Fowler's position, especially in obese patients.
    d. Plasmapheresis, IV Ig, and high-dose parenterally administered corticosteroids are used to reduce symptoms.
    e. Neostigmine IV for myasthenic crisis.
    f. Discontinuation of anticholinergic medications until respiratory function improves; atropine to reduce excessive secretions for cholinergic crisis.

 DRUG ALERT Plasmapheresis must be carried out before IV Ig therapy because plasmapheresis will remove the IV Ig proteins that are effective in symptom reduction.

Complications

1. Aspiration.
2. Complications of decreased physical mobility.
3. Respiratory failure.

Nursing Assessment

1. Expect the patient to complain of extreme muscle weakness and fatigue.
2. Assess CN function, motor fatigability with repetitive activity, and speech. Observe eye muscles (usually affected first) for ptosis, ocular palsy, and diplopia.
3. Assess respiratory status—breathlessness, respiratory weakness, tidal volume, and vital capacity measurements.
4. Assess complications secondary to drug treatment—long-term immunomodulating therapies may predispose patients with MG to various complications.
    a. Long-term steroid use may lead to or aggravate many conditions, such as osteoporosis, cataracts, hyperglycemia, weight gain, avascular necrosis of hip, hypertension, and gastritis or peptic ulcer disease. To decrease the risk of ulcer, patients should take an H2 blocker or antacid.
    b. Increased risk for infection from immunomodulating therapy, especially if the patient is on more than one agent. Such infections include tuberculosis, systemic fungal infections, and *Pneumocystis carinii* pneumonia.
    c. Risk of lymphoproliferative malignancies may be increased with chronic immunosuppression.
    d. Immunosuppressive drugs may have teratogenic effects. In addition, risk of congenital deformity (arthrogryposis multiplex) is increased in offspring of women with severe MG.

 DRUG ALERT Neonates born to women with MG need to be monitored for respiratory failure for 1 to 2 weeks after birth. Discuss these aspects with women in reproductive years prior to beginning therapy with these drugs.

Nursing Diagnoses

- Fatigue related to disease process.
- Risk for Aspiration related to muscle weakness of face and tongue.
- Impaired Social Interaction related to diminished speech capabilities and increased secretions.

Nursing Interventions

Minimizing Fatigue

1. Plan exercise, meals, and other ADL during energy peaks. Time administration of medications 30 minutes before meals to facilitate chewing and swallowing.
2. Assist the patient in developing realistic activity schedule.
3. Provide an eye patch and alternate eyes for the patient with diplopia to allow safe participation in activity.
4. Allow for rest periods throughout the day.
5. Obtain assistive devices to help the patient perform ADL.

 DRUG ALERT Many medications can accentuate the weakness experienced by the patient with MG, including some antibiotics (such as ciprofloxacin, aminoglycosides, chloroquine, and procaine penicillin), antiarrhythmics (such as procainamide, beta-adrenergic blockers, and quinidine), local and general anesthetics, muscle relaxants, and analgesics such as nonsteroidal anti-inflammatory drugs (NSAIDs). Assess function after administering any new drug, and report deterioration in condition.

Preventing Aspiration

1. Assess the patient's oral motor strength before each meal.
2. Teach the patient to position his or her head in a slightly flexed position to protect airway during eating.
3. Modify diet, as needed, to minimize risk of aspiration; for instance, soft, solid foods instead of liquids. Teach the patient that eating warm foods (not hot foods) can ease swallowing difficulties.
4. Have suction available that the patient can operate.
5. Administer IV fluids and nasogastric tube feedings to the patient in crisis or with impaired swallowing; elevate head of bed after feeding.
6. Suction the patient frequently if on a mechanical ventilator; assess breath sounds and check chest x-ray reports because aspiration is a common problem.

Maintaining Social Interactions

1. Encourage the patient to use an alternate communication method, such as flash cards or a letter board, if speech is affected.
2. Instruct the patient to speak in a slow manner to avoid voice strain; refer to speech therapy, as needed.
3. Show the patient how to cup chin in hands during speech to support lower jaw and assist with speech.

4. Teach the patient to tilt head and to carry a handkerchief to manage secretions in public.
5. Encourage family participation in care.
6. Refer the patient to the Myasthenia Gravis Foundation of America (*www.myasthenia.org*) to meet other patients with the disease who lead productive lives.

Community and Home Care Considerations

1. Assess the home environment for physical and emotional stressors, such as uncomfortable temperature, draft, or loud noises.
2. Emphasize continued follow-up and compliance with treatment regimen.
3. Identify the need for additional home care services such as respiratory therapy, physical therapy, and nutritional services.
4. Assess the patient frequently for fluctuation in condition and inform caregivers that this is common.
5. Teach the patient and family how to use home suction in case of aspiration. Make sure everyone in household knows the Heimlich maneuver.

Patient Education and Health Maintenance

1. Instruct the patient and family regarding the symptoms of crisis. Intercurrent infection or treatment with certain drugs may worsen symptoms of MG temporarily. Mild exacerbation of weakness is possible in hot weather.
2. Review the peak times of medications and how to schedule activity for best results. For patients on anticholinesterase therapy:
   a. Stress accurate dosage and times; take anticholinesterase drugs 30 to 45 minutes before meals.
   b. Tell the patient not to skip medication.
   c. Instruct the patient to avoid taking medication with fruit, coffee, tomato juice, or other medications.
   d. Inform the patient of adverse effects such as GI distress.
3. Stress the importance of activity with scheduled rest periods before fatigue develops.
4. Teach the patient ways to prevent crisis and aggravation of symptoms.
   a. Avoid exposure to colds and other infections.
   b. Avoid excessive heat and cold.
   c. Inform the dentist of condition because use of procaine is not well tolerated.
   d. Avoid emotional upset; plan ahead to minimize stress.
5. Encourage the patient to wear a MedicAlert bracelet.
6. Stress the importance of adequate nutrition; instruct to chew food thoroughly and eat slowly.
7. Advise the patient to avoid alcohol, tonic water.
8. Refer the patient/family for more information to the Myasthenia Gravis Foundation of America (*www.myasthenia. org*).

Evaluation: Expected Outcomes

- Demonstrates optimal self-care in bathing, eating, toileting, and dressing without fatigue.
- Breathes effectively; cough is effective; suctioning own secretions; lungs clear.
- Visits with friends, participates in social activities, uses alternative method of communications.

TRAUMA
Traumatic Brain Injury

EVIDENCE BASE Carney, N., Totten, A. M., O'Reilly, C., et al. (2016). *Guidelines for the management of severe traumatic brain injury* (4th ed.). Campbell, CA: Brain Injury Foundation. 1–244. Available: https://braintrauma.org/uploads/03/12/Guidelines_for_Management_of_Severe_TBI_4th_Edition.pdf
Kinoshita, K. (2016). Traumatic brain injury: pathophysiology for neurocritical care. *Journal of Intensive Care*, 4(29), 2–10.

Traumatic brain injury (TBI) is the disruption of normal brain function due to trauma-related injury. TBI produces compromised neurologic function, resulting in focal or diffuse symptoms. Falls are the most common etiology of injury, followed by motor vehicle accidents. TBI is the leading cause of trauma-related deaths and accounts for 40% of trauma-related injuries. The goal of treatment is to prevent secondary brain injury by providing supportive care (see Chapter 35 for emergency management of TBI). There are limited evidence-based data to direct medical management. Current practice is based on clinical experience, as the only class I evidence is that steroids should not be used

Pathophysiology and Etiology

Types of Traumatic Brain Injury

1. Concussion—transient interruption in brain activity; no structural injury noted on radiographic studies.
2. Cerebral contusion—bruising of the brain with associated swelling. Coup injury is the site of initial trauma; the contrecoup injury is the site of rebound injury. Temporal and frontal lobes are common sites.
3. Intracerebral hematoma—bleeding into the brain tissue commonly associated with edema.
4. Epidural hematoma (EDH)—blood between the inner table of the skull and dura. Frequently associated with injury or laceration of the middle meningeal artery secondary to a temporal bone fracture. EDH is commonly associated with a lucid interval, followed by unresponsiveness.
5. Subdural hematoma—blood between the dura and arachnoid caused by venous bleeding; commonly associated with additional cerebral injuries: contusion or intracerebral hematoma.
6. Diffuse axonal injury (DAI) or shear injury—axonal tears within the white matter of the brain. Frequently occurs within the corpus callosum or brain stem and at the junction of the frontal/temporal poles. Associated with prolonged coma and poor prognosis.

Mechanism of Injury and Effects

1. Mechanism of injury is related to acceleration and deceleration of the brain (soft gelatin matter) within the skull (hard external surface with sharply edged internal surface). May be caused by blunt or penetrating injury.
2. The initial insult is the primary injury and the injury related to the sequela is the secondary injury. Cellular changes (release of oxygen-free radicals and neurotransmitters, calcium loss, and increase in lactate acid) and systemic instability (hypotension, anemia, hypoxia, hypercarbia, hypovolemia) potentiate secondary injury.
3. Neurologic deficits result from primary brain injury (contusion, hematoma, DAI, or shearing of white matter) or

secondary injury (ischemia and mass effect from hemorrhage and cerebral edema of surrounding brain tissue).

4. Second impact syndrome (SIS) occurs in repetitive concussion when there is insufficient time for the brain to recover from the previous injury. SIS is common in sports-related injuries and is associated with cerebral injury and cerebral edema, which can be severe.

5. Studies have shown that mild TBI with a positive CT scan is more indicative of moderate injury, resulting in a more pronounced neurobehavioral presentation and extended neurologic recovery time beyond the typical 3 months.

6. Coagulopathy may result from increased release of intracranial thromboplastin, causing elevation in PTT and fibrinogen levels, which in turn results in clotting dysfunction, from mild bleeding to disseminated intravascular coagulation.

7. Paroxysmal sympathetic hyperactivity (PSH) or sympathetic storming may result from uncontrolled release of sympathetic hormones spontaneously or in response to some stressor. PSH results in tachycardia, tachypnea, hyperthermia, diaphoresis, agitation, and dystonia.

8. DI—reduced secretion of ADH with excessive fluid and electrolyte loss through the kidneys due to edema or compression of the pituitary/hypothalamic region; may cause severe dehydration.

9. SIADH—oversecretion of ADH with normal to increased intravascular volume (hypervolemic state) and dilutional hyponatremia (see page 358).

10. Cerebral salt wasting—increase in urinary secretion of sodium accompanied by volume depletion (hypovolemic state) (see page 358).

Classification

See page 354 for GCS.

1. Mild (GCS 13 to 15, with loss of consciousness to 15 minutes).
2. Moderate (GCS 9 to 12, with loss of consciousness for up to 6 hours).
3. Severe (GCS 3 to 8, with loss of consciousness greater than 6 hours).

Associated Injuries: Extracranial Trauma

1. Facial trauma and skull fractures—occur in 20% of major TBI. Temporal skull is thinnest; frontal and occipital bones are the thickest.
   a. Linear fracture—fracture through entire thickness of bone that runs in linear pattern.
   b. Basilar skull fracture.
      i. Anterior fossa results in contusions around the eyes (raccoon eyes) and risk of rhinorrhea.
      ii. Posterior fossa results in contusions around the ears (Battle sign) and risk of otorrhea.
   c. Depressed fracture—displacement of fracture past the inner table of the skull; risk of dural tear, CSF leak, and intracranial injury; may be closed or open.
   d. Facial fractures—orbital (LeForte I to II), mandible, zygoma, maxillary, nasal fractures.
2. Vascular injuries—vertebral or carotid artery dissection.
3. Spine fracture with or without SCI.
4. Soft tissue injuries.

Clinical Manifestations

1. Disturbances in consciousness: confusion to coma.
2. Headache, vertigo.
3. Agitation, restlessness.
4. Respiratory irregularities.
5. Cognitive deficits (confusion, aphasia, reading difficulties, writing difficulties, acalculi [inability to perform simple arithmetic] and memory deficits such as retrograde and antegrade amnesia and difficulty learning new information).
6. Pupillary abnormalities.
7. Sudden onset of neurologic deficit.
8. Coma and coma syndromes.
9. Otorrhea may indicate leakage of CSF from ear (otorrhea) due to posterior fossa skull fracture; rhinorrhea may indicate leakage of CSF from nares (rhinorrhea) due to anterior fossa skull fracture.
10. Raccoon eyes and Battle sign indicate skull base fractures.
11. Episodes of altered LOC, tachycardia, tachypnea, hyperthermia, agitation due to sympathetic storming (aggravated stress response).
12. Abnormal bleeding due to coagulopathy.
13. Cardiac arrhythmias due to increased release of catecholamines in stress response.

Diagnostic Evaluation

1. CT scan to identify and localize lesions, edema, bleeding.
2. Skull and cervical spine films to identify fracture, displacement.
3. Neuropsychological tests during rehabilitation phase to determine extent of cognitive deficits.
4. MRI to identify and diagnose DAI (rarely performed because it does not alter medical management).
5. CBC, coagulation profile, electrolyte levels, serum osmolarity, ABG values, and other laboratory tests to monitor for complications and guide treatment.

Management

1. Airway—assess and maintain patent airway.
   a. Intubate for GCS less than 8 (comatose) or clinical signs of respiratory failure.
   b. Placement of nasogastric tube with intubation to prevent aspiration.
2. Breathing—all intubated patients should have ventilatory support.
   a. Oxygen, as needed, to maintain PaO_2 greater than 100 mm Hg.
   b. Maintain $PaCO_2$ 35 to 45 mm Hg.
   c. Avoid use of hyperventilation.
   d. Consider early tracheostomy if anticipate intubation greater than 2 weeks.
3. Circulation—prevent hypotension.
   a. Maintain SBP above 90 mm Hg. This may be maintained with use of fluid or vasopressors.
   b. Maintain normovolemia.
   c. Treat symptomatic anemia with packed RBC.
   d. Treat symptomatic arrhythmias.
4. Management of increased ICP and cerebral edema.
5. Management of PSH with medications, such as oxycodone (opiate), propranolol (beta-adrenergic blocker), clonidine (alpha-adrenergic antagonist), dantrolene (muscle relaxant), and bromocriptine or amantadine (dopamine-receptor agonists). Response to medications varies.
6. Supportive care—rehabilitation services, skin care.
7. Nutritional support should be initiated within 3 to 5 days; 25 kcal/kg via nasogastric feeding tube. Conversion to gastrostomy tube if anticipated need for alternative feeds is greater than 1 to 2 weeks.

8. Antibiotics, as ordered, to prevent infection with open skull fractures or penetrating wounds.
9. Surgery to evacuate intracranial hematomas, debridement of penetrating wounds, elevation of skull fractures, or repair of CSF leaks.
10. Treatment of hypernatremia (due to DI, dehydration, diaphoresis) with fluid replacement, vasopressin therapy.
11. Treatment of hyponatremia.
    a. Cerebral salt wasting: monitor daily fluid status, fluid administration, oral salt replacement, and IV saline 0.9% or 3% (250 to 500 mL over 3 to 5 hours).
    b. SIADH: monitor daily fluid status, fluid restriction, oral salt replacement, IV saline 2% or 3% bolus over 3 to 5 hours.
12. Seizure prophylaxis is not recommended to prevent posttraumatic seizures, as it has been shown to inhibit cognitive recovery; however, prophylactic antiepileptics are ordered in some cases; duration is 7 days.
    a. If seizure activity is witnessed and there is associated temporal lobe injury or penetrating injuries, antiepileptics are recommended.
    b. Given IV for rapid loading and should be converted to enteric route. Phenytoin, fosphenytoin sodium, and levetiracetam are commonly used. Dilantin levels should be monitored for accurate dosing. (Note: there are no evidence-based data to support the use of levetiracetam for prophylaxis.)

Complications

1. Infections: systemic (respiratory, urinary), neurologic (meningitis, ventriculitis).
2. Increased ICP, hydrocephalus, brain herniation.
3. Posttraumatic seizures and seizure disorder.
4. Permanent neurologic deficits: cognitive, motor, sensory, speech.
5. Neurobehavioral alterations: impulsivity, uninhibited aggression, emotional lability.
6. Persistent PSH.
7. Disseminated intravascular coagulation.
8. DI, SIADH, cerebral salt wasting.
9. Death.

Nursing Assessment

1. Monitor for signs of increased ICP—altered LOC, abnormal pupil responses, vomiting, increased pulse pressure, bradycardia, hyperthermia.
2. Monitor for signs of PSH—altered LOC, diaphoresis, tachycardia, tachypnea, hypertension, hyperthermia, agitation, and dystonia. PSH is generally seen in severe TBI (GCS 3 to 8) or minimally responsive patients.
3. Monitor cardiac status for hypotension and arrhythmias (bradycardia, elevated T waves, premature ventricular contractions, premature atrial contractions, and sinus arrhythmias)—common and frequently asymptomatic. Tachycardia with hypotension is indicative of hypovolemia; patient should be evaluated for additional source of blood loss.
4. Be alert for DI—excessive urine output, dilute urine (specific gravity less than 1.005), hypernatremia.
5. Be alert for hyponatremia and assess etiology (SIADH or cerebral salt wasting); see page 358.
6. Monitor laboratory findings and report abnormal values:
    a. Abnormal PTT, PT, and fibrinogen levels indicating coagulopathy.

b. Electrolyte imbalance—alterations in serum potassium (hypokalemia) and sodium (hypernatremia/hyponatremia) levels are common.
c. Anemia—related to additional trauma or may be dilutional.
d. Elevated WBC count—indicating infection related to trauma or invasive procedures.
e. Hypoxia or hypercarbia.
7. Perform CN, motor, sensory, and reflex assessment.
8. Assess for behavior that warrants potential for injury to self or others.

 NURSING ALERT Regard every patient who is unresponsive with a brain injury as having a potential spinal cord injury. Cervical collar and spine precautions should be maintained until spinal fracture has been ruled out. A significant number of patients are under the influence of alcohol at the time of injury, which may mask the nature and severity of the injury.

Nursing Diagnoses

- Ineffective Cerebral Tissue Perfusion related to increased ICP.
- Ineffective Breathing Pattern related to increased ICP or brain stem injury.
- Imbalanced Nutrition: Less Than Body Requirements related to compromised neurologic function and stress of injury.
- Impaired Environmental Interpretation Syndrome related to physiology of brain injury.
- Risk for Injury related to altered thought processes.
- Compromised Family Coping related to unpredictability of outcome.

Nursing Interventions

Maintaining Adequate Cerebral Perfusion

1. Maintain a patent airway.
2. Monitor ICP, as ordered (see page 359).
3. Monitor cerebral oxygenation, temperature, or neurochemicals, as ordered. Provide oxygen therapy to maintain Pao_2 above 100 and carbon dioxide within normal range.
4. Maintain SBP above 90 to enhance cerebral perfusion and administer treatment for arrhythmias if the patient is symptomatic. Evaluate for source of blood loss if the patient is tachycardic and hypotensive.
5. Monitor LOC, CN function, and motor and sensory function as per GCS or neurologic flow sheet; identify emerging trends in neurologic function; and communicate findings to medical staff.
6. If the patient has severe TBI, monitor for signs of PSH (abnormal stress response) and identify triggers and effective treatment modalities. Institute nursing measures that have been found to be helpful, such as maintaining normothermia, pretreating before known trigger, applying cool compress to forehead, and providing relaxing music.
7. Monitor response to pharmacologic therapy, including antiepileptic levels, as directed.
8. Monitor laboratory data, CSF cultures, and Gram stains, if applicable, and institute prompt antibiotic therapy, as directed.
9. Monitor for hypernatremia and administer fluid replacement, as directed. If due to DI, vasopressin may be utilized.

10. Monitor for hyponatremia. Determine if hyponatremia is related to SIADH or cerebral salt wasting. Administer fluids/ restrict fluids and administer oral or IV salt replacement, as directed. Administer 250 to 500 mL 2% or 3% saline solution over 3 to 5 hours. Central venous access is required for 3% saline to prevent damage to peripheral vein wall.

11. Monitor coagulation panel and replace clotting factors at room temperature, as directed.

12. Assess dressings and drainage tubes after surgery for patency, security, and characteristics of drainage.

13. Institute measures to minimize increased ICP, ischemic changes, cerebral edema, seizures, or neurovascular compromise, such as careful positioning, to avoid flexing head, reducing hip flexion (can reduce venous drainage, causing congestion), and spreading out care evenly over 24-hour period.

> **NURSING ALERT** PSH places the patient at high risk for secondary brain injury, cardiac abnormalities, weight loss, skin breakdown, and infection. Be alert to triggers (suctioning, turning, hyperthermia, infection, auditory stimuli) and treat promptly to control symptoms.

> **NURSING ALERT** Severe states of hypernatremia and hyponatremia can cause further neurologic compromise (seizures, nausea, confusion, irritability/agitation, coma). Close monitoring of laboratory values is indicated to evaluate trends and maintain normal range. Hypernatremia and hyponatremia should not be reversed quickly because the rapid change can create rebound cerebral edema and be detrimental to the patient. Rapid increase in serum sodium level can cause central pontine myelinolysis and results in severe damage of myelin sheath of white matter in pons.

Maintaining Respiration

1. Monitor respiratory rate, depth, and pattern of respirations; report any abnormal pattern, such as Cheyne-Stokes respirations or periods of apnea.

2. Assist with intubation and ventilatory assistance, if needed.

3. Obtain frequent ABG values to maintain Pao_2 greater than 100 mm Hg and $Paco_2$ 35 to 45 mm Hg.

4. Positive end-expiratory pressure (PEEP) (5 to 8 cm) is felt to be physiological and not detrimental; however, excessive PEEP can create increases in intrathoracic pressure, diminish venous drainage, reduce mean arterial pressure (MAP), and increase ICP.

5. Turn the patient every 2 hours and assist with coughing and deep breathing.

6. Suction the patient, as needed.

Meeting Nutritional Needs

1. Nutritional support should be initiated by day 5 and should provide 140% of energy requirements (100% in paralyzed patient), with 15% in the form of protein. Supplements should provide 25 kcal/kg.
   a. Continuous enteric feedings.
      i. Elevate the head of the bed during feedings.
      ii. Check residuals to prevent aspiration.
      iii. Monitor for diarrhea.
      iv. Transgastric jejunal feedings reduce the risk of ventilator associate pneumonia.

   b. Consider IV hyperalimentation—for patients unable to tolerate nasogastric feedings.
   c. Oral feeding—started when adequate swallowing mechanism is demonstrated.

2. Administer H_2-blocking agents to prevent gastric ulceration and hemorrhage from gastric acid hypersecretion.

3. Consult with dietitian to provide adequate calories and nitrogen supplement.

4. Monitor glucose levels frequently, utilizing fingerstick samples and glucometer. Insulin (IV drip/sliding scale) may be required to regulate serum glucose levels within a normal range to avoid hypoglycemia and hyperglycemia, which worsens the effects of secondary brain injury.

5. Perform bedside dysphagia screen to evaluate swallow function before initiation of oral foods. Consult speech therapist for bedside or radiographic swallow study if patient fails swallow screen or appears at risk for dysphagia. Assessment of swallowing function decreases risk of aspiration. Speech therapy is essential for retraining and developing adaptive techniques.

> **NURSING ALERT** Caloric needs of a patient with a head injury increase by 100% to 200%. Consult your dietitian to institute nutritional support within the first 5 days after injury to support the recovery process. Weight loss is generally in the form of muscle loss and can be as much as 25 to 30 pounds (11.3 to 13.6 kg).

Promoting Cognitive Function

1. Periodically assess the patient's LOC and compare to baseline.

2. Be aware of the patient's cognitive alteration and adjust interaction and environment accordingly.

3. Provide meaningful stimulation using all senses—visual, olfactory, gustatory, acoustic, and tactile.

4. Observe the patient for fatigue or restlessness from overstimulation.

5. Involve the family in sensory stimulation program to maximize its effectiveness.

6. Decrease environmental stimuli when the patient is in agitated state.

7. Reorient to surroundings using repetition, verbal and visual cues, and memory aids; routinely orient the patient after awakening.

8. Use pictures of family members, clock, and calendar as outlined by occupational and speech therapist.

9. Encourage the family to provide items from home to increase sense of identity and security.

10. Anticipate the need for additional help with toileting, eating, and performing ADL due to cognitive impairment.

11. Break down ADL into simple steps that patient can progressively take part in.

12. Structure the environment and care activities to minimize distraction and provide consistency.

13. Identify and maintain usual patterns of behavior—sleep, medication use, elimination, food intake, and self-care routine.

14. Refer the patient for cognitive retraining, if appropriate.

Preventing Injury

1. Instruct the family regarding the behavioral phases of recovery from brain injury, such as restlessness and combativeness.

2. Investigate for physical sources of restlessness, such as uncomfortable position, signs of UTI, or pressure ulcer development.

3. Reassure the patient and family during periods of agitation and irrational behavior.
4. Pad side rails and wrap hands in mitts if patient is agitated. Maintain constant vigilance and avoid restraints, if possible.
5. Keep environmental stimuli to a minimum to avoid confusion and agitation. Veil beds can be useful in reducing injury in the agitated patient.
6. Provide adequate light if the patient is hallucinating.
7. Avoid sedatives to avoid medication-induced confusion and altered states of cognition.

Strengthening Family Coping

1. Refer the family to community support services, such as respite care, faith-based groups, city and state social services, and resources on the Internet. Suggest the Brain Injury Association of America (*www.biausa.org*) for further information.
2. Assist the family members to establish stress management techniques that can be integrated into their lifestyle, such as ventilation of feelings, use of respite care, relaxation techniques.
3. Consult with social worker or psychologist to assist the family in adjusting to patient's permanent neurologic deficits.
4. Help the family assist the patient to recognize current progress and not focus on limitations.

Community and Home Care Considerations

1. Observe for signs of postconcussion syndrome (PCS), which include headache, decreased concentration, irritability, dizziness, insomnia, restlessness, diminished memory, anxiety, easy fatigability, and alcohol intolerance.
2. Be aware that persistence of these symptoms can interfere with relationships and employability of the patient.
3. Encourage the patient and family to report these symptoms and obtain additional support and counseling, as needed. PCS may persist as long as 2 years.
4. Act as liaison to coordinate all home care services the patient will need while keeping in touch with the patient's primary care provider, neurologist, and neurosurgeon.

5. Provide the necessary education to caregivers in tube feedings, positioning, ROM exercises, and so forth.
6. Make sure that coaches and parents from community recreation programs and schools are familiar with and follow guidelines for sports-related concussion (see Table 15-7).

Patient Education and Health Maintenance

1. Review the signs of increased ICP with the family.
2. Reinforce the lability of cognitive, language, and physical functioning of the person with brain injury and the lengthy recovery period.
3. Teach the family techniques to calm the agitated patient.
   a. Therapeutic use of touch, massage, and music.
   b. Elimination of distractions (television, radio, alarms, crowds).
   c. Provide one-on-one communication.
   d. Distract patients.

Evaluation: Expected Outcomes

- No signs of increased ICP.
- Respirations—24 breaths/minute, regular.
- Tube feedings tolerated well without residual.
- Oriented to person, place, and time.
- Less agitated; side rails maintained.
- Family reports using respite care.

Spinal Cord Injury

 EVIDENCE BASE Fehlings, M. G., Tetreault, L. A., Wilson, J. R., et al. (2017). A Clinical Practice Guideline for the Management of Acute Spinal Cord Injury: Introduction, Rationale, and Scope. *Global Spine Journal, 7*(3S), 84S–94S.

Spinal cord injury (SCI) is a traumatic injury to the spinal cord that may vary from a mild cord concussion with transient numbness to immediate and complete tetraplegia. The most common

SEVERITY	RECOMMENDATIONS
Table 15-7 American Academy of Neurology Guidelines for Sports-Related Concussion	
Grade 1 Transient confusion without loss of consciousness and resolution of symptoms within 15 minutes	• Removal from game and only returned to the game if remaining asymptomatic after 15 minutes • If second grade 1 concussion occurs, removal from sports activity until asymptomatic for 1 week
Grade 2 Transient confusion without loss of consciousness and symptoms persisting longer than 15 minutes	• Removal from sporting event and further workup if symptoms do not resolve in 1 week • No sporting activity for 1 week • If grade 2 occurs after a grade 1 concussion, removal from sporting event and no sporting activities for 2 weeks
Grade 3 Loss of consciousness	• Removal from sporting event • Return to sporting activities if asymptomatic for 1 week (brief loss of consciousness) • Return to sporting activities if asymptomatic for 2 weeks (prolonged loss of consciousness) • Unconsciousness with neurologic findings should be transported to nearest emergency for full evaluation • Removal from sporting activity for 1 year and discouraged from future participation in contact sports if any structural findings on computed tomography scan or magnetic resonance imaging

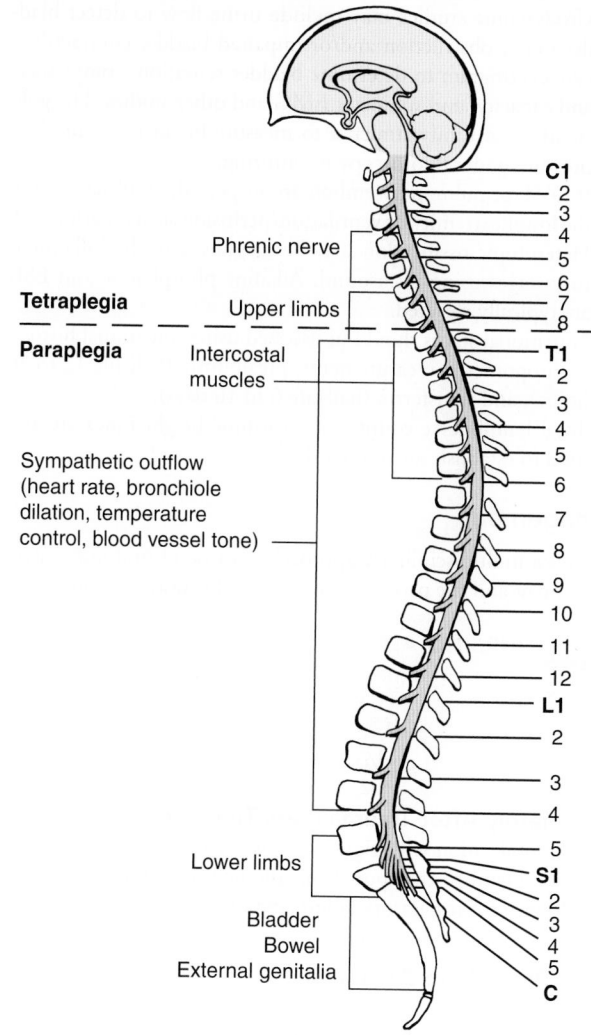

Phrenic nerve

Tetraplegia

Upper limbs

Paraplegia

Intercostal
muscles

Sympathetic outflow
(heart rate, bronchiole
dilation, temperature
control, blood vessel tone)

Lower limbs

Bladder
Bowel
External genitalia

C1
2
3
4
5
6
7
8
T1
2
3
4
5
6
7
8
9
10
11
12
L1
2
3
4
5
S1
2
3
4
5
C

Figure 15-10. Levels of spinal cord innervation.

sites are the cervical areas C5, C6, and C7, and the junction of the thoracic and lumbar vertebrae, T12 and L1. Injury to the spinal cord may result in loss of function below the level of cord injury (see Figure 15-10). SCI requires comprehensive and specialized care. The Model Spinal Cord Injury System is a network of comprehensive, federally funded, regional SCI centers in the United States. The Department of Veterans Affairs operates 23 SCI centers. (Also see Chapter 35 for emergency management of SCI.)

Pathophysiology and Etiology

1. The estimated annual incidence of SCI is about 11,000 new cases per year, and the prevalence is approximately 35 cases per million people in the United States. The mean age is 33 and approximately 80% are males. The primary etiologies are vehicular crashes (39%), falls (29.5%), violence (14.4%), and sports-related injuries (8.4%). Most injuries result in tetraplegia; 50% are complete. (A complete SCI is absence of motor and sensory function at the lowest sacral segment affected; see below for a description of incomplete SCI.) About 90% of these patients are discharged to noninstitutional settings.

2. The life expectancy for an individual with SCI is lower (80% to 85%) than that of a person without SCI. The leading causes of death are pneumonia, emboli, and septicemia.

3. SCI may result from trauma, vascular disorders, infectious conditions, tumor, and other insults.

4. SCI can affect upper motor neurons (UMNs) or LMNs. UMNs extend from the motor strip in the cerebral cortex of the brain through the corticospinal tract in the spinal cord, where they synapse with interneurons in the ventral horn. LMNs originate in the ventral horn, exit the spinal cord at each segment, and extend to the neuromuscular junction. Each LMN innervates 10 to 2,000 muscle fibers.
    a. Spasticity results from injury above T12 or a UMN lesion (intact reflex arch below level of inury).
    b. Flaccidity/reflex loss results from injury at L1 or a LMN injury.

 GERONTOLOGIC ALERT Older patients are at greater risk for altered glucose metabolism, loss of bone minerals leading to fractures, musculoskeletal pain and weakness, and greater loss of function with spinal cord injury.

Clinical Manifestations

1. Patients with tetraplegia have damage to the cervical segments of nerves (C1–C8) in the spinal canal. Function may be impaired in the upper extremities, trunk, pelvic organs, and lower extremities.

2. Patients with paraplegia have damage to the thoracic, lumbar, or sacral segments of nerves in the spinal cord. The arms are unaffected, but function may be impaired in the trunk, pelvic organs, and lower extremities.

3. The International Standards for Neurological Classification of Spinal Cord Injury, promoted by the American Spinal Injury Association (ASIA), are used (available: *http://asia-spinalinjury. org/wp-ontent/uploads/2016/02/International_Stds_Diagram_ Worksheet.pdf*). The ASIA Impairment Scale is based on completeness of injury and motor/sensory function.
    ASIA A—complete; absent sensory and motor function in the sacral segments S4–S5.
    ASIA B—incomplete; intact sensory but absent motor function below the neurologic level of injury (LOI) and includes level S4–S5.
    ASIA C—incomplete; intact motor function distal to neurologic LOI, and more than half of key muscles distal to LOI have muscle grade less than 3.
    ASIA D—incomplete; intact motor function distal to neurologic LOI, and more than half of key muscles distal to LOI have muscle grade greater than or equal to 3.
    ASIA E—normal; intact motor and sensory function.

4. Sacral sensation is intact if there is deep sensation and sensation at the anal mucocutaneous junction; sacral motor is intact if the patient has voluntary contraction of the external anal sphincter with digital stimulation.

5. The zone of partial preservation (ZPP) indicates areas of partial sensory/motor innervation below the LOI; the ZPP is applicable only to complete injuries.

6. The neurologic level of injury is the lowest neural level with normal sensory and motor function on both sides of the body. When describing the LOI, the neurologic level is noted unless stated specifically that the skeletal LOI, which is the level of greatest vertebral damage, is being discussed.

7. Various syndromes (incomplete injuries) may characterize the clinical presentation (see Table 15-8).

8. Sensation function (eg, sensitivity of pinprick/light touch) is tested on each of the 28 dermatomes on both sides of the body. The following grading is suggested: 0 = Absent; 1 = Impaired; 2 = Normal. The external anal sphincter should also be tested (sensory incomplete if sensate).

9. Motor function is tested on each of the 10 paired myotomes on both sides of the body. The following grading is suggested: 0 = Total paralysis; 1 = Contraction visible or palpable; 2 = Active movements and full ROM without gravity; 3 = Active movement and full ROM against gravity; 4 = Active movement and full ROM with moderate resistance; 5 = Normal motor with active movement and full ROM against full resistance. The external anal sphincter tone should also be tested (motor incomplete if contraction).

10. Most recovery occurs within 6 months of injury; patients with incomplete injuries have greater recovery than patients with complete injuries.

11. Instability exists when ligamentous structures and vertebra cannot protect the vulnerable spinal cord and movement can further damage the injured spinal cord; stability exists when ligamentous structures and vertebra can protect the spinal cord from further neurologic injury.

12. Vertebral fractures may be simple, compressed or wedge, dislocated (vertebra overrides another vertebra), subluxed (vertebra partially dislocated over another vertebrae), comminuted (vertebrae shattered), or teardrop (vertebrae chipped). Jefferson fractures, which may occur with head injuries, involve the C1 level.

Diagnostic Evaluation

1. CT of spine—to detect boney injury and dislocation

2. MRI of spine—to detect soft tissue injury, hemorrhage, edema, bony injury; syringomyelia (cystic degeneration in spinal cord) may present as cord compression, syrinx (cavity) at the fracture site, and kyphosis at fracture site.

3. Electrophysiologic monitoring to determine function of neural pathways.

4. Urodynamic studies may include urine flow to detect bladder outlet obstruction and/or impaired bladder contractility; cystometrogram to determine bladder sensation, compliance, and capacity; and sphincter EMG and other studies. The gold standard in urodynamics is to measure bladder and urethral pressure under fluoroscopy monitoring.

5. If DVT or pulmonary emboli are suspected, an ultrasound of the lower extremity or ventilation/perfusion scan is performed.

6. Heterotopic ossification may be diagnosed in the inflammatory stages using ultrasound. Alkaline phosphatase and ESR are typically elevated.

7. Nutritional status should be assessed using nutritional history, anthropometric measurements, prealbumin (half-life 12 to 36 hours), and transferrin (half-life 6 to 10 days).

8. Total lymphocyte count and creatinine height index are also used to establish nutritional risk.

Management

Requires a multidisciplinary approach because of multiple-system involvement and the psychosocial aspects of catastrophic injuries.

 NURSING ALERT Patients sustaining an SCI have better outcomes when treated by a multidisciplinary SCI team. Once the patient is stabilized, the option of transferring the patient to an SCI facility should be provided to the patient and/or family.

Immediately After Trauma (Less Than 1 Hour)

1. Immobilization with rigid cervical collar, sandbags, and rigid spine board to transport from the field to acute care facility. Monitor for respiratory failure, hypotension, and/or bradycardia and treat appropriately.

Acute Phase (1 to 24 Hours)

1. Maintenance of pulmonary and cardiovascular stability.
   a. Intubation and mechanical ventilation, if needed.
   b. Vasopressors to maintain adequate perfusion to sustain mean MAP greater than 85 mm Hg.
   c. Medical stabilization before spinal stabilization and decompression.

Table 15-8 Incomplete Spinal Cord Clinical Syndromes

SYNDROME	AFFECTED SITE	DEFICIT	PRESERVATION
Central cord	Central cervical spinal cord	More motor deficit in upper extremities than lower extremities caused by medial damage of corticospinal tract	Sacral sensory; lower extremities have better motor function than upper extremities because of lateral sparing of corticospinal tract
Brown-Sequard	Hemisection of spinal cord	Ipsilateral motor function and fine touch, vibration, and proprioception (posterior tract); contralateral sensory function pain and temperature (spinothalamic tract)	Ipsilateral sensory function of pain and temperature (spinothalamic tract); contralateral motor function, fine touch, vibration, and proprioception (posterior tract)
Anterior cord	Main anterior spinal artery of anterior spinal cord affecting anterior two thirds of spinal cord	Variable motor deficit; variable sensory deficit of pain and temperature (spinothalamic tract)	Posterior one third of spinal cord (posterior spinal artery); sensory function of proprioception, light touch, vibration (posterior tract)
Conus medullaris	Conus and lumbar nerve roots in spinal cord	Variable motor deficit; bowel, bladder, and lower-extremity reflexes (flaccid)	Lesions of proximal conus may be reflexic (eg, butocavernosa, micturition)
	Lumbosacral nerve roots in spinal cord (distal from conus medullaris)	Variable motor deficit; bowel, bladder, and lower-extremity reflexes (flaccid)	Lesions proximal to level of injury may be reflexic (eg, bulbocavernosus, micturition)

2. Spinal cord immobilization—use of skeletal tongs.
   a. Crutchfield and Vinke tongs require predrilled holes in the skull under local anesthesia; Gardner-Wells and Heifitz tongs do not.
   b. Weight is added to traction gradually to reduce the vertebral fracture; weight maintained at a level to ensure vertebral alignment. Lateral spine films are taken after the addition of weight to assess spinal alignment.
3. Rigid kinetic turning bed can be used to immobilize patients with thoracic and lumbar injuries.
4. Surgical interventions are considered when the patient has vertebral instability that may result in further neurologic damage; an injury that is incomplete at onset may become complete if instability exists. The objectives are to remove all of the bony and soft tissues that are compressing the spinal cord, thereby minimizing the possibility of deteriorating neurologic status, and stabilize the vertebra surrounding the spinal cord so that rehabilitation may begin as soon as possible. Goals of treatment of the spinal fractures are aimed at protecting the neural elements and preventing deformity and instability.
   a. Surgical Timing: current practice is early surgical intervention (less than 24 hours), though there is no class I evidence that clearly defines the timing of surgery. STATSCIS (Surgical Treatment of Acute Spinal Cord Injury Study), a prospective, nonrandomized clinical trial, revealed that early surgical decompression (within 24 hours) is safe, with 19.8% demonstrating neurologic improvement (greater than 2 grade improvement AIS) compared to 8.8% in the late decompressive group (2012).

 EVIDENCE BASE Fehlings M. G., Vaccaro, A., Wilson, J., Singh, A., Cadotte, D. W., Harrop, J. S., …Rampersaud, R. (2012). Early versus delayed decompression for traumatic cervical spinal cord injury: Results of the Surgical Timing in Acute Spinal Cord Injury Study (STASCIS). *PLoS One, 7*(2), e32037. Available: http://dx.doi.org/10.1371/journal.pone.0032037

   b. Decompression, typically using the anterior approach in cervical instances, may be accomplished by removing the bony structures and soft tissues (eg, fusion, decompression laminectomy). Realignment of the soft tissues and vertebral column is required.
   c. Stabilization, typically done using the posterior approach, involves the use of wires, bone grafts, plates, screws, and other fixation devices to prevent movement at the damaged bony site.
5. Methylprednisolone sodium. (Solu-Medrol) is not recommended (class I evidence) in SCI related to high rate of significant complications
   a. Higher rate of hyperglycemia, GI hemorrhage, wound infections, and higher mortality in concomitant TBI (class I evidence).
   b. Higher rate of pneumonia, steroid-induced myelopathy (class II evidence).
6. Management of neurogenic bladder—Foley catheter.
7. Pressure ulcer prevention—pressure reduction mattress or kinetic turning frame.
8. Prevention of DVT and its sequelae is an important aspect of the treatment of patients who have sustained SCI because of the high risk of thromboembolic complications.
   a. Class I, II, and III evidence support the utilization of external device in conjunction with LMWH/adjusted-dose heparin within 1 to 2 days post injury.

 EVIDENCE BASE Hadley, M. N., Walters, B. C., Aarabi, B., Dhall, S. S., Gelb, D. E., Harrigan, M. R., et al. (2013). Guidelines for the management of acute cervical spine and spinal cord injuries. *Neurosurgery, 72*(2), 1–94.

Subacute Phase (within 1 Week)

1. Stiff orthosis is utilized for external stabilization of cervical fractures. Devices include the Halo brace, Minerva collar, extended Philadelphia collar, and fabricated orthosis. Device is selected based on the type of fracture and extent of instability. Average length of time in a halo brace is 12 weeks, followed by a Philadelphia collar for 4 weeks. Halo brace is used for cervical injuries (see Figure 15-11).
   a. Graphite rings are MRI compatible, lightweight, and radiolucent.
   b. Some halos are now open posteriorly, which reduces the incidence of cervical fracture displacement.
   c. The ring is attached to stainless steel pins (two anterior pins, two posterior pins) and attached to a vest by four connecting rods (also MRI compatible and radiolucent).
   d. Torque wrenches connect the rods to the ring and vest; pressures are typically 8 inches/pound for pins (2 to 5 inches/pound in children) and locking bolts are 28 inches/pound.
   e. Pins and locking bolts must be retightened approximately 24 to 48 hours after placement and periodically thereafter.
   f. Pin sites should be cleaned daily with half-strength hydrogen peroxide or soap and water.
2. H_2-receptor blockers to prevent gastric irritation and hemorrhage.
3. Early mobilization and passive exercise as soon as patient is surgically and medically stable.
4. Hyperalimentation, if unable to tolerate enteric feeds, to retard negative nitrogen balance.
5. Interventions to help prevent thromboembolism include compression hose, compression boots, range of motion, adjusted-dose heparin, or LMWH.

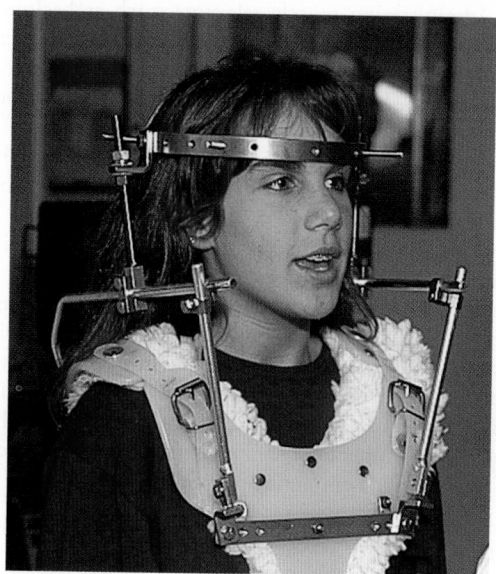

Figure 15-11. Halo brace. (Smeltzer, S., & Bare, B. [2000]. *Brunner and Suddarth's textbook of medical-surgical nursing* [9th ed.]. Philadelphia, PA: Lippincott Williams & Wilkins.)

a. Prior to applying mechanical compression, tests to exclude the presence of lower-extremity DVT should be performed if thromboprophylaxis has been delayed for more than 72 hours after injury.

b. Vena cava filters are not recommended, though may be utilized in patients who have not achieved success with anticoagulant prophylaxis or who have a contraindication to anticoagulation. They are not a substitute for thromboprophylaxis due to morbidity related to DVT (eg, postphlebitic syndrome) and propagation of vena caval embolism.

Chronic Phase (Beyond 1 Week)

1. Segmental instrumentation systems are used in conjunction with a body jacket and are used for patients with thoracolumbar injuries.
2. To prevent thrombophlebitis in the chronic phase, compression boots should be continued for 2 weeks; anticoagulants should also be continued based on risk category.
   a. Minimum of 8 weeks from time of injury for those with incomplete or complete motor injury with no additional risk factors.
   b. For those with complete motor injury with additional risk factors, anticoagulants should be continued for 12 weeks.
3. Management of complications may include treatment of infections with antibiotics; treatment of respiratory compromise with phrenic nerve pacing, mechanical ventilation, and other methods; pressure ulcer treatment; management of heterotopic ossification with calcium chelators and antiinflammatory agents; drainage of syringomyelia; management of spasticity with oral or intrathecal antispasmodics, surgical procedure, or spinal cord stimulation; and management of central neuropathic pain with antiepileptics, minor sedatives, antidepressants, nerve block, or surgical procedure.
4. Spasticity should be managed by
   a. Maintaining calm, stress-free environment.
   b. Allowing ample time for activities such as positioning and transferring.
   c. Performing joint ROM exercises with slow, smooth movements.
   d. Avoiding temperature extremes.
   e. Administering muscle relaxants, such as baclofen (via pump or orally), diazepam, and dantrolene, as prescribed.
   f. Botulism toxin injections can be utilized.
   g. Clonidine has been used to manage spasticity and facilitate walking in patients with incomplete injuries.
5. External sphincterotomy may be used for detrusor–sphincter dyssynergia. Other options include urethral stents and balloon dilatation.
6. Resistive inspiratory muscle training shows promise in promoting respiratory muscle strength and reducing sleep-induced breathing disturbances in patients with tetraplegia. Resistive training devices are used to perform respiratory maneuvers at scheduled times during the day.
7. Rehabilitation includes medical and psychosocial support, physical therapy, urologic evaluation, occupational therapy, and multiple other interventions to facilitate an increased level of function and community participation.

Complications

1. Spinal shock lasting a few hours to a few weeks noted by loss of all reflex, motor, sensory, and autonomic activity below the level of the lesion.
2. Respiratory arrest, pneumonia, atelectasis requiring mechanical ventilation with cervical injury.
3. Cardiac arrest may result from initial trauma, worsening of initial injury from edema, concomitant injuries, and other illnesses.
4. Thromboembolic complications—in 15% of patients.
5. Infections—respiratory, urinary, pressure ulcers, sepsis.
6. Autonomic dysreflexia—exaggerated autonomic response to stimuli below the level of the lesion in patients with lesions at or above T_6 is a medical emergency and can result in dangerous elevation of BP.
7. Autonomic dysfunction resulting in orthostatic hypotension, thermodysregulation, and vasomotor abnormalities.
8. Urologic—bladder storage pressure greater than 35 to 40 cm due to neurogenic bladder may result in renal deterioration; SCI patients who have indwelling urinary catheters are at increased risk of bladder cancer.
9. Paralytic ileus—common in subacute and acute stage.
10. Heterotopic ossification—bony overgrowth that occurs below the level of injury any time after SCI.
11. Syringomyelia—cystic formation in the spinal cord may occur any time after SCI.
12. Depression—occurs in 25% of men and 47% of women with SCI.
13. Pressure ulcers may occur in up to 35% of patients with SCI.
14. Spasticity may result in contractures.
15. Amenorrhea occurs in 60% of women with SCI, usually temporary.
16. Neuropathic pain occurs in 34% to 94% of patients with SCI.
17. Complications can arise from the halo apparatus in persons with cervical injuries.
    a. Pin/ring loosening—can result from bone reabsorption. Signs and symptoms include increased pain, altered pin position, and drainage.
    b. Infection—can result from bacterial infections. Signs and symptoms include drainage and erythema.
    c. Skull/dural penetration—can result from inner table penetration, usually due to a fall. Signs and symptoms include a headache, visual disturbances, and CSF leak from the pin site.
    d. Dysphagia and respiratory problems—can result from halo or vest positioning. Signs and symptoms include difficulty swallowing and respiratory distress.

Nursing Assessment

1. Assess cardiopulmonary status and vital signs to help determine degree of autonomic dysfunction, especially in patients with tetraplegia.
2. Determine LOC and cognitive function indicating TBI or other pathology.
3. Perform frequent motor and sensory assessment of trunk and extremities—extent of deficits may increase because of edema and hemorrhage. Later, increasing neurologic deficits and pain may indicate development of syringomyelia.
4. Note signs and symptoms of spinal shock, such as flaccid paralysis, urine retention, absent reflexes.
5. Assess bowel and bladder function.
6. Assess quality, location, and severity of pain.
7. Perform psychosocial assessment to evaluate motivation, support network, financial, or other problems.
8. Assess for indicators of powerlessness, including verbal expression of no control over situation, depression, nonparticipation, dependence on others, passivity.

Nursing Diagnoses

- Ineffective Breathing Pattern related to paralysis of respiratory muscles or diaphragm.
- Impaired Physical Mobility related to motor dysfunction.
- Risk for Impaired Skin Integrity related to immobility and sensory deficit.
- Urinary Retention related to neurogenic bladder.
- Constipation or Bowel Incontinence related to neurogenic bowel.
- Risk for Injury related to autonomic dysreflexia and orthostatic hypotension.
- Powerlessness related to loss of function, long rehabilitation, depression.
- Sexual Dysfunction related to erectile dysfunction and fertility changes.
- Chronic Pain related to neurogenic changes.

Nursing Interventions

Attaining an Adequate Breathing Pattern

1. For patients with high-level lesions, continuously monitor respirations and maintain a patent airway. Be prepared to intubate if respiratory fatigue or arrest occurs.
2. Frequently assess cough and vital capacity. Teach effective coughing, if patient is able (see Box 15-5).
3. Provide adequate fluids and humidification of inspired air to loosen secretions.
4. Suction, as needed; observe vagal response (bradycardia—should be temporary).
5. When appropriate, implement chest physiotherapy regimen to assist pulmonary drainage and prevent infection.
6. Monitor results of ABG values, chest x-ray, and sputum cultures.
7. Tape halo wrench to body jacket or halo traction in the event the jacket must be removed for basic or advanced life support or respiratory distress.

BOX 15-5   Assisted Coughing

Many patients with tetraplegia have an impairment of the diaphragmatic and intercostal muscles. The result is a weak or ineffective cough. To increase the mechanical effectiveness of the patient's cough, perform or teach the assisted cough technique.

1. Place the patient in supine, low semi-Fowler's position.
2. Place the heels of your hands on the costophrenic angle of the patient's rib cage.
3. With the patient's head turned away, ask the patient to hyperventilate and exhale once or twice. Allow your hands to move with the patient.
4. During the next breath, ask the patient to take a deep breath and cough while exhaling.
5. As the patient coughs, thrust your hands down and in (inferiorly and medially) to add power to the diaphragm during exhalation.
6. Allow one or two normal breaths and repeat the procedure.

 NURSING ALERT Incorrect hand placement may cause injury to the internal organs, ribs, and xiphoid process.

Promoting Mobility

1. Place the patient on firm bed until spinal cord stabilization. After stabilization, turn every 2 hours on a pressure reduction surface, ensuring good alignment. Specialized beds, such as a kinetic turning bed, may be used.
2. Logroll the patient with unstable SCI.
3. Perform ROM exercises to prevent contractures and maintain rehabilitation potential.
4. Monitor BP with position change in the patient with lesions above midthoracic area to prevent orthostatic hypotension.
5. Encourage physical therapy and practicing of exercises as tolerated. Functional electrical stimulation may facilitate independent standing and walking.
6. Encourage weight-bearing activity to prevent osteoporosis and risk of kidney stones.

 NURSING ALERT Never attempt to reposition the patient by grasping a halo or any other stabilization device. This may result in severe damage to the brain, head, or vertebra.

Protecting Skin Integrity

1. Pay special attention to pressure points when repositioning patient. Seating and mobility requirements must be determined.
2. Obtain pressure relief mattress and appropriate wheelchair and cushion.
3. Inspect for pressure ulcer development daily over bony prominences, including the back of the head, ears, trunk, heels, and elbows. Observe under stabilization devices for pressure areas, particularly on the scapulae. Use a risk assessment tool to determine risk of developing pressure ulcer.
4. Keep the skin clean, dry, and well lubricated.
5. Turn the patient a minimum of every 2 hours and instruct him to perform wheelchair weight shifts every 15 minutes. Place the patient in prone position at intervals, unless contraindicated.
6. Institute treatment for pressure ulcers immediately and relieve pressure to promote healing.

Promoting Urinary Elimination

1. Consider use of intermittent catheterization, typically beginning every 4 hours, as an alternative to an indwelling catheter.
2. If the patient has an upper motor neuron lesion (above L1) and no indwelling catheter, promote reflex voiding by tapping the bladder, gently pulling the patient's pubic hair, or stroking the patient's inner thigh.
3. If the patient has a lower motor neuron lesion (L1 or below) and no indwelling catheter, promote voiding by using a bladder Crede method by gently compressing the suprapubic area to promote voiding.
4. Encourage fluid intake of 3,000 to 4,000 mL of fluid per day (2,000 mL/day if intermittent catheterization is used) to prevent infection and urinary calculi. Space fluids out over 24-hour period to avoid bladder overdistention. Juices should be encouraged to help decrease urinary pH (inhibiting stone production) and bacterial adherence to a catheter.
5. Monitor for urine retention by percussing the suprapubic area for dullness, catheterizing for residual urine after voiding, or using noninvasive devices such as the .
6. Prophylactic antibiotics for prevention of recurrent UTIs are not supported because of the increase in resistant organisms.
7. The use of biofilms and other materials that inhibit adhesion of pathogens to catheters is being explored.

Promoting Bowel Elimination

1. Assess bowel sounds and note abdominal distention. Paralytic ileus is common immediately after injury.
2. Encourage intake of high-calorie, high-protein, and high-fiber (15 g) diet when food is tolerated.
3. Assess for loose stool oozing from rectum and perform rectal examination to check for fecal impaction; remove fecal matter, if necessary.
4. Institute a bowel program as early as possible.
   a. Schedule bowel care at the same time of day to develop a predictable outcome.
   b. Stimulate the gastrocolic reflex 30 minutes before bowel care with food or liquid intake.
   c. Perform bowel care with the patient in a bowel chair or in left side-lying position; the procedure should not take more than 2 hours.
   d. Use abdominal massage, deep breathing, warm fluids, and leaning forward in the chair to enhance success.
5. For patients with upper motor neuron lesions, perform reflexic bowel care.
   a. Insert a glycerin or bisacodyl suppository or mini-enema (4 mL).
   b. Alternatively, use digital stimulation with gloved, lubricated finger—perform a semicircular motion against posterior rectal wall. Repeat every 5 to 10 minutes until evacuation is complete.
   c. For patients with lower motor neuron lesions, perform areflexic bowel care, by perform manual stool elimination.
6. Have the patient perform Valsalva maneuver (after urinary elimination to prevent vesicoureteral reflux of urine).
7. For chronic constipation without relief from more conservative approaches, consider a bulk-forming agent or laxative 8 hours before bowel care.

Preventing Autonomic Dysfunction and Orthostatic Hypotension

1. Be alert to signs of autonomic dysreflexia (see Box 15-6), try to avoid triggers, assess for causes, and treat, as directed.
2. Be alert for, prevent, and manage orthostatic hypotension, especially in patients with cervical SCI.
3. Use tilt table, as ordered, to gradually increase the patient's ability to tolerate sitting after acute SCI.
4. Other conservative strategies consist of use of embolic hose, abdominal binder, and high-salt diet.
5. Administer a sympathomimetic, such as ephedrine or pseudoephedrine, as ordered, before the patient is transferred to wheelchair.

 DRUG ALERT Caution should be exercised for patients with SCI who are taking tricyclic antidepressants because of autonomic dysfunction. SCI patients are more vulnerable to anticholinergic adverse effects and orthostatic hypotension. In addition, numerous potential drug reactions are associated with monoamine oxidase inhibitors and SCI.

Empowering the Patient

1. Explain all procedures to the patient. Answer questions.
2. Make sure that the patient plays an integral part in decision-making about care plan. Allow the patient to make modifications to treatment plan when possible.
3. Schedule procedures and planning sessions when the patient is rested and experiencing decreased anxiety.
4. Praise the patient for incremental gains in function or participation.
5. Discuss stress management techniques, such as relaxation therapy, counseling, and problem solving.

BOX 15-6 | Autonomic Dysreflexia

Be aware of and try to prevent common causes of autonomic dysreflexia whenever possible:
- Bladder distention, UTI, bladder or kidney stones.
- Urinary abnormalities or procedures.
- Bowel distention, bowel impaction.
- Constrictive clothing, shoes, or apparatus.
- Noxious stimuli such as pain, strong smells, pressure.

Be alert for signs and symptoms of autonomic dysreflexia:
- Sudden and significant increase in systolic and diastolic BP 20–40 mm Hg above the patient's baseline. (Normal SBP for a person with tetraplegia is 90–110 mm Hg.) In children and adolescents, a systolic increase of greater than 15–20 mm Hg above baseline is significant.
- Pounding headache.
- Bradycardia and/or cardiac arrhythmias.
- Profuse sweating, piloerection, and flushing above the level of injury (LOI).
- Blurred vision and spots in visual field.
- Nasal congestion.
- Apprehension and anxiety.

Take the following actions if autonomic dysreflexia occurs:
- Check BP; if elevated, call health care provider immediately.
- Immediately sit the patient up.
- Loosen clothing and other constrictive apparatus.
- Monitor BP every 2 to 5 minutes.

- Check the urinary system—catheterize patient (use 2% lidocaine jelly and wait 2 minutes); if catheter in place, check for kinks in tubing obstructing drainage; if catheter blockage suspected, gently irrigate with 10–15 mL normal saline (use 5–10 mL in children younger than age 2); replace catheter if not draining adequately.
- If BP remains greater than 150 mm Hg systolic, check for impaction (use 2% lidocaine jelly and wait 2 minutes). Remove stool.
- If BP remains greater than 150 mm Hg systolic, administer immediate-release nifedipine 10 mg (bite and swallow), nitroglycerin ointment 2% 1 inch (2.5 cm) above the LOI, or another antihypertensive agent.
- If autonomic dysreflexia is still unresolved, check for additional causes (eg, pressure ulcer, ingrown toenail).

After the episode of autonomic dysreflexia, document the following:
- Monitor BP for at least 2 hours for recurrent hypertension or symptomatic hypotension. Notify the health care provider as indicated.
- Provide patient teaching for prevention and treatment of complication.
- Make sure all caregivers understand autonomic dysreflexia and that the patient carries an identification card indicating LOI and emergency information.

6. Refer to vocational training program if the patient expresses an interest.
7. Use peer counseling for patient to gain support from others with SCI.
8. Be alert for signs of depression (problems with sleep, loss of interest, guilt, loss of energy, lack of concentration, change in appetite, feeling sad) or risk for suicide and refer to mental health counselor. Administer antidepressant medications, as directed.
9. Explore the use of hands-free environmental control units to control environment (eg, turn on television).

Minimizing Alteration in Sexuality and Fertility
1. Encourage the patient to discuss alternate expression of feelings with partner.
2. Advise bowel care and urinary elimination before intercourse.
3. Advise women that 90% regain regular menstrual cycles by 1 year. Pregnancy can occur and delivery occurs in 40% before 37 weeks' gestation. Autonomic dysreflexia may occur as a complication of delivery.
4. Refer the patient to a urologist or other health care provider to explore sexuality options.
   a. Women with SCI experience little sensation during sexual intercourse, but fertility and ability to bear children are usually not affected.
   b. Men with SCI may consider implantation of a penile prosthesis or an assistive device to obtain an erection. Sildenafil has been used to manage erectile dysfunction in men with SCI. Ejaculation is more common with lower motor neuron or incomplete injuries; men with injuries at T_{10} and above may ejaculate with vibrostimulation.

Reducing Pain
1. Assess pain using consistent pain scale. Report changes from baseline or new location or type of pain.
2. Manage neurogenic pain with pharmacologic agents, as directed.
3. Help the patient assess the effects of nonpharmacologic treatment such as acupuncture.

Community and Home Care Considerations

Promoting Optimal Function
1. Determine short- and long-term functional goals. Expected outcomes should relate to motor recovery, level of functional independence, social integration, and quality of life.
2. Monitor neurologic status, including functional outcomes, periodically throughout the patient's life span. Functional outcomes may relate to
   a. Respiratory, bowel, bladder, and skin.
   b. Bed/wheelchair mobility, transfers, positioning.
   c. Standing and ambulation.
   d. Independent ADL, such as eating, grooming, bathing, and dressing.
   e. Communication, including speech, computer skills, handwriting, telephone.
   f. Transportation, including driving, adapted vehicle use, public transportation.
   g. Homemaking, including meal planning and preparation and chores.
3. Periodically evaluate the need for an increased level of assistance and equipment as the patient with an SCI ages.

4. Assist the patient in arranging modifications necessary to his or her home and in obtaining financial assistance for modifications to the environment.
5. Coordinate continued rehabilitation effort to ensure social support, ongoing pharmacologic treatment, and monitoring for long-term complications, such as depression; vocational training; and adaptation to home and work environments. Use Functional Independence Measure or other instrument to set and achieve goals with the patient in ADL, transferring, locomotion, and other functional aspects.
6. Teach bowel care and urinary elimination procedures to the patient and all caregivers to ensure continuity.
7. Teach care of traction and immobilization devices.
8. Enlist help of occupational therapist, physical therapist, vocational therapist, recreational therapist, and other specialists, as needed.
9. Alert caregivers that autonomic dysreflexia is a complication that may occur up to several years after SCI involving T6 and above. Teach the patient and caregivers preventive and emergency treatment measures.

Patient Education and Health Maintenance
1. Teach the patient and family about the physiology of nerve transmission and how the SCI has affected normal function, including mobility, sensation, and bowel and bladder function.
2. Reinforce that rehabilitation is lengthy and involves compliance with therapy to increase function.
3. Explain that spasticity may develop 2 weeks to 3 months after injury and may interfere with routine care and ADL.
4. Teach the patient to protect skin from pressure ulcer development by frequent repositioning while in bed, weight-shifting and liftoffs every 15 minutes while in a wheelchair, and avoiding shear forces and friction.
5. Teach inspection of skin daily for development of pressure ulcers, using a mirror, if necessary.
6. Encourage sexual counseling, if indicated, to promote satisfaction in personal relationships.
7. Teach importance of seat belts.

Evaluation: Expected Outcomes
- Respirations adequate, ABG values within normal limits.
- Repositioning hourly, no orthostatic changes.
- No evidence of pressure ulcers or DVT.
- Reflex (or areflexic) voiding without retention.
- Bowel evacuation controlled.
- No episodes of autonomic dysreflexia.
- Verbalizes feeling of control over condition.
- Patient and partner exploring sexuality and sexual options.
- Reports pain at or lower than 2 to 3 level on a scale of 1 to 10.

Vertebral Compression Fractures

Vertebral fractures commonly occur with trauma but can also be associated with osteoporosis or cancer.

Pathophysiology and Etiology
1. The vertebral body is made up of cancellous (soft) and outer cortical (hard) bone. The fracture creates an area of weakness within the vertebral column.

2. This weakness is further stressed and compressed with normal biomechanical stresses (weight-bearing activities from standing, sitting, and lifting). Over time, the fracture loses height, compressing the vertebral body.
3. The periosteum layer of the bone contains many pain receptors and, with weight-bearing activities that apply pressure on the fractured bone, stimulates the nerve endings, thereby producing pain.
4. Risk factors include:
   a. Osteoporosis—women over age 50; men over age 70; prolonged use of steroids.
   b. Metastatic cancer—breast, lung, renal, prostrate, melanoma, multiple myeloma.
5. Other risk factors include the following:
   a. Smoking.
   b. Inactivity.
   c. Poor nutrition.

Clinical Manifestations

General Considerations
1. A vertebral body may fracture without causing debilitating pain.
2. Symptoms depend on location, extent of fracture, progression of fracture, and effect on surrounding structures.
3. Most symptomatic fractures result in pain, although the development of instability can result in sensory changes, loss of reflex, and muscle weakness from canal compromise.

Cervical
1. Pain and stiffness in the neck, top of shoulders, and region of the scapula.
2. Pain with rotation, flexion, and extension.
3. Paresthesias and numbness of upper extremities.
4. Weakness of upper extremities.

Thoracic/Lumbar
1. Middle to lower back pain at site of fracture.
2. Pain aggravated with activity and relieved with rest and flexion.
3. Progressive kyphosis or postural deformity of the lumbar spine. Progressive thoracic kyphosis decreases lung capacity and can compromise pulmonary function.
4. Point tenderness to palpation on clinical examination.

Diagnostic Evaluation

1. Plain x-rays (anteroposterior and lateral views)—evaluate vertebral structure, height loss, and alignment.
2. CT scan—evaluation of extent of fracture and canal involvement.
3. MRI—differential diagnosis includes infectious process or metastatic lesion. MRI has greater sensitivity for soft tissue abnormalities.
4. Bone scan—evaluation of microscopic changes within the bone. Identification of additional metastatic lesions, infectious process, microscopic fractures.

Management

Conservative Treatment
1. Orthosis/brace; heat or ice to affected area.
2. Physical therapy.
3. Anti-inflammatory drugs.
4. Analgesics, opioids may be necessary during acute phase.
5. Treatment and prevention of osteoporosis.

Surgical/Invasive Intervention
1. Surgical intervention—spinal instrumentation is not considered an option in patients with advanced osteoporosis secondary to the risk of nonfusion and hardware failure.
2. Vertebroplasty—injection of methyl methacrylate (bone cement) with barium (radiopaque) into vertebral body aimed at providing stabilization of vertebral body.
3. Kyphoplasty—partial restoration of vertebral height using percutaneous placement of a balloon into vertebral body, inflation of the balloon with radiopaque solution (creates a cavity), and deflation and removal of the balloon followed by insertion of methyl methacrylate with barium. May be done under moderate sedation or general anesthesia. Reduced risk of glue leakage secondary to creation of the cavity.

Complications
1. Pulmonary embolus due to leakage of cement into venous system following vertebroplasty or kyphoplasty.
2. Spinal cord or nerve root compromise due to leakage of cement following vertebroplasty or kyphoplasty.
3. Muscular spasms related to preprocedure deconditioning and postprocedure change in posture.

Nursing Assessment
1. Perform repeated assessments of motor function and sensation.
2. Assess for localized tenderness.
3. Assess pain level on scale of 1 to 10.

Nursing Diagnoses
- Acute Pain related to area of compression.
- Risk for impaired breathing pattern related to invasive procedure and complications.

Nursing Interventions

Minimizing Pain
1. Administer or teach self-administration of analgesics as prescribed; inform patient about potential adverse effects (sedation, constipation, GI upset). Advise use of over-the-counter stool softeners.
2. Administer or teach self-administration of anti-inflammatories, as prescribed; advise taking with food or antacid to prevent GI upset.
3. Teach self-administration of muscle relaxants, as prescribed; inform patient about potential adverse effects of sedation.
4. Instruct in proper application and use of orthosis, if ordered.
5. Apply moist ice or heat to affected area of back, per patient-defined relief of pain.
6. Inspect skin several times a day, especially under stabilization devices, for redness and evidence of pressure sore development. Pressure ulcers can cause severe pain.
7. Educate the patient about vertebroplasty or kyphoplasty, as indicated.
   a. One to two small punctures with a large-bore needle will be made at site of vertebral body to be treated. Level will be verified using fluoroscopy before insertion of bone cement.
   b. Routine postprocedure care will include assessment of vital signs and neurologic function, pain control, and ambulation, as ordered. Assess movement and sensation of extremities. Report any new deficit. CT of spine may be ordered if encroachment on spinal cord or nerve root is suspected.
8. Encourage compliance with physical therapy treatments, as ordered.

Preventing Respiratory Complications Postoperatively

1. Monitor vital signs and assess respiratory status and report any breathing difficulties. Chest x-ray or CT of chest (PE protocol) may be ordered if pulmonary embolus is suspected.
2. Administer analgesics and NSAIDs to control pain from incision and muscular inflammation due to procedure. Differentiate increased respiratory rate due to pain and anxiety rather than hypoxemia.
3. Enforce bed rest for 2 to 3 hours; patient may turn side to side, as directed; gradually increase activity, as tolerated.
4. Position for comfort. May apply heat or ice to affected muscles if spasm occurs and administer muscle relaxant, as indicated.
5. Report any increasing pain, weakness, or breathing difficulties. Auscultate lungs and report abnormalities.

Patient Education and Health Maintenance

1. Advise the patient of 10- to 25-pound lifting restriction for 1 week after vertebroplasty/kyphoplasty, as ordered, and to avoid strenuous activities; level of activity may be increased gradually as status indicates.
2. Demonstrate proper body mechanics to be used for bending, reaching, and lifting in all activities.
3. Alternate ice and heat for 20-minute intervals five to six times per day, as needed.
4. No soaking baths for 1 week to enhance wound healing of puncture sites.
5. Encourage the patient to do stretching and strengthening exercises for back and aerobic exercise for endurance on a daily basis.
6. Physical therapy may be indicated for reconditioning, heat therapy, and massage.
7. Instruct the patient to report any changes in neurologic function or recurrence of pain.

Evaluation: Expected Outcomes

- Verbalizes reduced pain.
- Vital signs stable, respirations unlabored, out of bed without difficulty.

Peripheral Nerve Injury

Peripheral nerve injury (PNI) is an injury to nerves in the upper extremity (eg, radial, ulnar, median) or lower extremity (eg, peroneal, sciatic, femoral, tibial). PNI may include damage to major nerves, the nerve root, the plexus (eg, brachial or lumbar), and other peripheral sites.

Pathophysiology and Etiology

1. The incidence of PNI is approximately 2% to 3% in populations with multiple injuries. Males have higher incidence than females.
2. PNI damage may occur by congenital, traumatic, chemical, pathologic, thermal, or mechanical means. Focal trauma is the most common of all PNI. Injuries can be direct (eg, gunshot) or indirect (eg, casting).
3. The most frequently injured site is the upper extremity, specifically the upper arm. Childhood PNIs occur predominantly in the lower extremities.
4. Injury to the nerve causes impairment in axonal function and, possibly, disruption of myelination. Approximately 50% of motor nerves and 75% of cutaneous nerves are myelinated.

Schwann cells contain multiple axons. Myelinated axons enhance conduction between nodes, accelerating transmission compared to nonmyelinated axons. Fibers are classified according to diameter, conduction speed, myelination, and target.

5. Sensory regeneration, as opposed to motor regeneration, may take years following a PNI.
6. Nerve injuries are classified according to the Sunderland system, which establishes grades of nerve function on which to base recovery and need for surgery.
   a. First-degree PNI (neurapraxia)—there is a conduction impairment, but the anatomy is intact. Complete recovery is anticipated in 3 months.
   b. Second-degree PNI (axonotmesis)—wallerian degeneration occurs distal to the PNI site and axons disintegrate. Complete recovery is anticipated.
   c. Third-degree PNI—scarring occurs in the endoneural tube. Axons recover 1 inch (2.5 cm) per month. Incomplete recovery is anticipated.
   d. Fourth-degree PNI (eg, crush injury)—axonal regeneration is blocked by scar tissue. Surgical repair is typically required.
   e. Fifth-degree PNI (eg, penetrating trauma)—the peripheral nerve is severed. Surgical intervention is required.
7. Compression neuropathy depends on the amount and extent of compression force. Edema, connective tissue thickening, and segmental demyelization of large fibers occur.
8. Useful function can be achieved when up to 75% of axons are damaged.

Clinical Manifestations

1. Flaccid paralysis.
2. Absent deep tendon reflexes.
3. Atonic/hypotonic muscles.
4. Progressive muscle atrophy.
5. Fasciculations peak 2 to 3 weeks after injury.
6. Trophic changes: skin is warm and dry 3 weeks after injury and then becomes cold and cyanotic with loss of hair, brittle fingernails, and ulceration.
7. Causalgia (chronic pain syndrome): Neuropathic pain may be crawling, electric, tingling, or burning. (It typically follows the cutaneous sensory nerve distribution of the PNI.)
8. Specifics to area affected:
   a. Radial nerve injury—weakness in extension, possible wrist drop, inability to grasp objects/make a fist, impaired sensation over posterior forearm and dorsum of the hand.
   b. Brachial plexus—difficulty in abduction of shoulder, weakness with supination and flexion of the forearm (upper trunk) or extension of the forearm (middle trunk), or paralysis and atrophy of small muscles of the hand (lower trunk).
   c. Median and ulnar nerve injuries—sensory (median nerve) and motor (ulnar) loss of function in the hand (pronation, opposition of thumb, paralysis of finer flexor muscles).
   d. Femoral—weakness of knee and hip extension, atrophy of quadriceps, absence of knee jerk, loss of sensation of anterior aspect of the thigh.
   e. Common peroneal—footdrop, sensory loss on dorsum of foot, difficulty with eversion.
   f. Sciatic—footdrop, pain across gluteus and thigh, loss of knee flexion, weakness/paralysis of muscles below knee.

9. Chronic nerve compression may begin with intermittent signs and symptoms; these may only occur in specific maneuvers such as digital pressure or position. For example, damage to the brachial plexus, entrapped at the supra/infraclavicular junction, may elicit symptoms following arm elevation for 1 minute. In carpal tunnel syndrome (compression of the median nerve), wrist flexion or external pressure applied proximally to the carpal tunnel may evoke symptoms.

Diagnostic Evaluation

1. The electrodiagnostic examination consists of nerve conduction studies (sensory, motor, mixed) and needle electrode examination.
   a. The electrodiagnostic examination tests only large myelinated axons; it does not assess pain, temperature, or paresthesia.
   b. It can confirm PNI occurrence and determine the type of axon, pathophysiology, severity, location, and injury prognosis.
2. Muscle ultrasonography evaluates the extent of muscle involvement and assesses acute nerve injuries.
3. MRI and electrophysiologic studies such as electroneurography and EMG detect the site and degree of nerve injury.
4. Muscle imaging may detect atrophy and mesenchymal alteration of skeletal muscles.
5. Tinel sign (tapping the axons of the regenerating nerve produces a paresthesia in the normal distribution of the nerve) reveals the rate of axonal regeneration.

Management

1. Microsurgery reapproximates the severed peripheral nerve endings. The sooner the repair is performed, the better the chance of recovery. Microsurgical repair can be done with tension-free coaptation using technology such as carbon dioxide laser welding, fibrin gluing, and ring coupling. Autogenous nerve grafts are the gold standard.
2. Primary nerve repair (neurorrhaphy) may be done within 1 week of injury (eg, open wounds—except gunshots). Secondary nerve repair is performed after 1 week (eg, crush injury with soft tissue damage). In partially transected nerves, surgery may be delayed 2 to 3 months to determine whether regeneration will take place.
   a. Nerve grafting—Two neurorrhaphy sites are used. Thin, cutaneous nerve grafts with large fascicles and minimal connective tissue are optimal. Common donor sites include the sacral nerve (lateral aspect of the foot), lateral antebrachial cutaneous nerve (lateral forearm), and the median antebrachial cutaneous nerve (medial arm and elbow). Small segments of nerve grafts may be placed to create a bridge to facilitate axonal and Schwann cell growth. Nerve "conduits," connectors of nerve sites, may be composed of bone, vein, artery, silicone, or other material.
   b. End-to-side neurorrhaphy—the severed nerve's distal end is attached to the side of a healthy nerve.
   c. Nerve transfer—Ideally, the donor nerve fascicles are in close proximity to the target muscle motor end plate or target sensory nerve. If the patient has multiple nerve injuries, such as a complete brachial plexus injury, nerve transfer priority is given to promoting elbow flexion, shoulder abduction, and external rotation, respectively. Sensory nerve priorities are given to the ulnar thumb and radial index finger.

3. Tissue expansion is used to compensate for tissue deficit.
4. Insulin-like growth factor and acidic fibroblast growth factor have enhanced regeneration when administered systemically or topically and other factors are being investigated.
5. Corticosteroids may be used to decrease edema.
6. Occupational therapy may be consulted to splint or cast the patient. Splinting (eg, hands) or casting may be indicated to reduce tension on the PNI site and facilitate healing. Day splints are typically functional splints; night splints are positioning splints. Splint material depends on the amount of resistance to be exerted by the orthosis, the splint size, and the patient's compensatory movements.
   a. Radial nerve splint—volar or dorsal cock-up splints are indicated if wrist extension is impaired.
   b. Median nerve splint—a thumb opposition splint preserves the function of the hand grip.
   c. Ulnar nerve splint—this functional and positioning splint prevents "claw hand" deformity and contractures of fingers four and five.
7. Flexibility is primarily due to connective tissues stretching as opposed to muscle contraction. Passive and active ROM exercises are essential to provide stretch and prevent contractions. Ultrasound diathermy may be used on deep muscles, and topical heat may be used for superficial muscles to promote stretching. Progressive resistance and strengthening, including isometric activities, are used to restore function. Functional electrical stimulation may also be used.
8. Fibrosis, caused by edema, may be minimized by elevating the affected limb. Using static graduated compression devices (eg, sleeves, gloves, hose) or sequential compression devices, distal to proximal wrapping, may also minimize edema. Likewise, massage may reduce edema.
9. Desensitization techniques (eg, scheduled exposure to irritating textures, vibration) may be used to manage hyperesthesia. Sensory reeducation may be protective (compensatory). Sensory restoration is progressive, with temperature and pain returning first, followed by transient light touch and vibration.
10. Neuropathic pain may be managed by traditional analgesics, antidepressants (eg, tricyclic), anticonvulsants (eg, gabapentin), topical and transdermal agents (eg, capsaicin), NSAIDs, alpha-adrenergic agonists (eg, clonidine), calcium channel blockers (eg, nicardipine), or transcutaneous electrical stimulation.
11. Carpal tunnel syndrome management may include activity modification, NSAIDs, serial steroid injections, vitamin B_6, diuretics, and a wrist splint for 6 months. Endoscopic surgical release of the ligament may also be an option.
12. Complex peripheral injuries, such as injury to the brachial plexus, may require multimodal treatment, including surgery, pain management, and functional rehabilitation. A multidisciplinary team approach is most effective in maximizing outcomes.

Complications

1. Infection, if injury is penetrating and site becomes contaminated.
2. Compartment syndrome due to edema or positioning.
3. Muscle atrophy/flaccid paralysis; disuse syndrome.
4. Sensory deficit.
5. Contractures.
6. Chronic pain.
7. Nerve damage resulting from surgical repair.

Nursing Assessment

1. Perform frequent neurovascular checks of the affected extremity (pressure, vibration, and two-point discrimination sensation; motor function, strength; pulses; temperature; capillary refill; degree of swelling).
2. Assess degree of pain on a scale of 0 to 10.
3. Test reflexes of affected extremity.
4. Observe for signs of infection if there is an open wound.
5. Assess for concomitant injuries such as head or skeletal trauma.

Nursing Diagnoses

- Risk for Peripheral Neurovascular Dysfunction.
- Chronic Pain related to injury.
- Risk for Infection secondary to tissue disruption, surgery.

Nursing Interventions

Protecting Neurovascular Function

1. Administer corticosteroids and diuretics, as ordered, to decrease swelling and development of compartment syndrome.
2. Keep extremity elevated to promote venous drainage.
3. Perform neurovascular check to evaluate status of injury.
   a. Incorporate Tinel sign into assessment.
   b. Report any changes in condition.
4. Postoperatively assist rehabilitation team in reeducating nerves and muscles to achieve function.
5. Observe for paresthesias, pain, or altered skin integrity in areas of splinting and casting.

Promoting Comfort

1. Administer and teach self-administration of analgesics, as ordered.
2. Elevate extremity.
3. Avoid exposing denervated areas to temperature extremes.
4. Apply such devices as splints and slings, as ordered.
5. Maintain mobility with ROM exercises. Perform gently, following administration of analgesics.

Preventing Infection

1. Assess wound and dressing frequently for erythema, warmth, swelling, odor, and drainage.
2. Monitor temperature with vital signs for hyperthermia and tachycardia, indicating infection.
3. Encourage deep-breathing exercises and ambulation to prevent pulmonary complications.

Patient Education and Health Maintenance

1. Teach management of wound and dressing and casts or splints.
2. Review analgesia schedule and need for elevation of injured area.
3. Teach exercises for involved area.
4. Suggest assistive devices to promote independence.
5. Stress the importance of complying with long-term rehabilitation, physical therapy, and follow-up evaluations.
6. Support a community accident prevention program, including the use of seat belts, industrial regulations, and sports and recreational safety measures.

Evaluation: Expected Outcomes

- Stable neurovascular status; functional use of extremity.
- Patient reports adequate relief of pain.
- Wound/surgical site free of erythema, drainage, odor.

CENTRAL NERVOUS SYSTEM TUMORS
Brain Tumors

 EVIDENCE BASE Hayat, M. A. (2015). *Tumors of the central nervous system glioma, meningioma, neuroblastoma, and spinal tumors (Vol. 14).* New York: Springer.

Stupp, R., Brada, M., van den Bent, M. J., Tonn, J. C., & Pentheroudakis, G. (2014). High-grade glioma: ESMO clinical practice guidelines for diagnosis, treatment and follow-up. *Annuals of Oncology, 25*(suppl 3), ii93–iii101.

Intracranial neoplasms are the result of abnormal proliferation of cells within the CNS. A *tumor* is a mass of cancerous cells within the brain. It is believed that there is a 2- to 3-cm surrounding area of cancer cells with the potential to develop into a tumor. Tumors require blood to grow and recruit a vascular supply to support the metabolic needs of the tumor. Intracranial tumors are primary or metastatic tumors and malignancy depends on cell type and location. Primary tumors include tumors of the brain itself, the skull or meninges, the pituitary gland, and the blood vessels. Metastatic tumors spread from the primary site of cancer (breast, lung, prostate, kidney) through the vascular supply and lymphatic systems. Defining primary cancer cell type determines the treatment modality and influences the overall prognosis.

Primary CNS tumor etiology remains unknown. Glioma research has identified a genetic mutation of p53 on chromosome 17 occurs in 50% of all cancers. Loss of heterozygosity of chromosome arm 10q also has been reported in gliomas, although research continues into potential genetic mutation and growth factors, as well as attempting to identify a tumor marker. No known environmental risks have been identified. Primary CNS tumors rarely metastasize outside the CNS.

Pathophysiology and Etiology

Tumors may originate in the CNS or metastasize from elsewhere in the body (50% of all brain tumors) and may be benign or malignant; all tumors produce effects of space-occupying lesion (edema, increased ICP). Malignancy may be related not only to cell type and invasiveness but also to location and operative accessibility (ie, the tumor is located in an area of the brain that will not tolerate compression of the brain structures or is not surgically accessible). The World Health Organization grading scale is currently used to classify gliomas, although other grading scales are available. The grading system evaluates the probability of tumor recurrence and malignancy from low (Grades I to II) to high (Grades III to IV). Tumors arise from any tissue of the CNS. See Figure 15-12.

1. Gliomas—tumors of the neuroepithelial/glial cells (supportive tissue of the brain; account for 40% to 50% of intracranial neoplasms):
   a. Astrocytoma—overgrowth of the astrocyte cells (connective tissue) of the brain. Tumors are graded on a scale from I to IV that defines growth pattern, invasiveness, infiltration, cell differentiation, margination, and necrosis.
      i. Grade I (polycystic astrocytoma)—slow-growing tumor with well-defined cells and minimal infiltration
      ii. Grade II (astrocytoma)—some atypical cells with higher rate of recurrence and risk of advancing to Grade III or IV with recurrence

Corpus callosum
astrocytoma
oligodendroglioma
lipoma

Third ventricle and area
ependymoma

Lateral ventricle
ependymoma
glioblastoma multiforme

Cerebrum
astrocytoma
oligodendroglioma
primitive
neuroectodermal
tumor lymphoma
metastatic tumors

Pineal area
pineocytoma
pineoblastoma

Optic chiasm
astrocytoma

Pituitary area
craniopharyngioma
pituitary adenoma
epidermoid cyst

Acoustic nerve
neuroma

Brain stem
astrocytoma
glioblastoma multiforme
metastatic tumors

Fourth ventricle
ependymoma

Cerebellum
medulloblastoma
astrocytoma
hemangioblastoma
metastatic tumors

Figure 15-12. Common brain tumor sites.

iii. Grade III (anaplastic astrocytoma) that is highly invasive and infiltrative, with poorly marginated borders and a rapid growth pattern and risk of advancing to Grade IV with recurrence

iv. Grade IV (glioblastoma multiforme)—a malignant tumor that is highly invasive, infiltrative, and poorly marginated, with necrosis and a very rapid growth pattern (accounts for 55% of gliomas).

b. Oligodendroglioma—overgrowth of oligodendroglial cells with calcification. Begins as a less invasive tumor but demonstrates malignancy as it progresses. The frontal and temporal lobes of the cerebrum are common locations. Rare in children.

c. Ependymoma (5% to 6% of intracranial gliomas)—overgrowth of the ependymal cells of the brain. Slow growing; commonly occurs in the floor of the 4th ventricle; presents with signs and symptoms of increased ICP and hydrocephalus; 69% of cases occur in children.

d. Mixed gliomas—two or more cell types within a tumor.

e. Medulloblastoma—most common pediatric malignant tumor. Commonly located in the 4th ventricle/cerebellar vermis; rapid growth pattern, highly invasive; high risk for metastasis within CSF.

f. Hemangioblastoma—rare, benign tumor commonly located in the posterior fossa; von Hippel-Lindau disease is multiple hemangiomas within CNS.

g. Colloid cyst—a rare cyst that contains neuroepithelial cells; occurs in the third ventricle.

2. Meningioma—arises from meningeal lining of the brain. Can involve the skull; accounts for 20% of primary brain tumors (90% are benign; 10% are atypical or anaplastic). Higher incidence in females ages 40 to 70. Rare in children.

a. Grade I meningiomas are benign, slow-growing, encapsulated lesions without brain tissue infiltration—but may have a dural tail.

b. Grade II (atypical meningiomas), rapid-growing tumors with increased miotic activity and higher risk of recurrence after resection; risk of advancing to anaplastic tumor.

c. Grade III (anaplastic meningioma), which has malignant features and invasion of brain tissue.

3. Peripheral nerve tumors—generally benign tumors that occur secondary to nerve sheath overgrowth.

a. Acoustic neuroma/schwannoma, located on CN VIII.

b. Neurofibromatosis type 1 (von Recklinghausen).

c. Neurofibromatosis type 2.

4. Pituitary tumors.

a. Pituitary adenoma, occurs primarily in the anterior of the pituitary and can be

i. Secreting tumor—prolactin (causes amenorrhea/galactorhhea in women, impotence in men, and infertility in both genders) adrenocorticotrophic hormone (causes Cushing syndrome) or growth hormone (causes acromegaly).

ii. Nonsecreting tumor.

b. Craniopharyngioma (considered a developmental tumor)—a benign cystic lesion with calcification, occurring in the anterior pituitary margin. Fifty percent occur in children.

5. Germ cell tumors and tumor-like cysts.

a. Dermoid cysts—occur in the ectodermal layer and contain hair and sebaceous glands.

b. Epidermoid cysts containing cell debris and keratin.

c. Pineal tumor—overgrowth of germ cells, pineal cells, or mixed germ types (includes teratomas) within the pineal region (more common in children and males).

d. Cordoma—rare neoplasm that contains embryonic remnant occurring along the neuraxis.

6. Hematopoietic tumors—include primary malignant lymphoma (rare, diffusely infiltrating tumor of the brain, occurs in adults, high rate of recurrence) and secondary lymphoma associated with AIDS.

7. Secondary CNS tumors/metastatic lesions—commonly from lung cancer (40% to 50%), breast cancer (14% to 20%), melanoma (10%), renal (5%), and undetermined primary sites (10% to 15%). Single lesions common with lung and breast cancer, can have multiple lesions that are unresectable. Indicate systemic spread of primary cancer.

Clinical Manifestations

Manifestations depend on the location and biologic nature of the tumor. If the tumor is in a noneloquent area of the brain or is slow growing, specific symptoms may not develop until the late stages of the process. Instead, the tumor may produce generalized symptoms related to the increasing size of the tumor and the expanding area of cerebral edema surrounding the margins of the tumor. This is referred to as the "mass" effect of the tumor.

1. Generalized symptoms (due to increased ICP)—headache (especially in the morning), vomiting, papilledema, malaise, altered cognition, and consciousness.

2. Focal neurologic deficits (related to region of tumor):
   a. Parietal area—sensory alterations, speech and memory disturbances, neglect, visuospatial deficits, right–left confusion, depression.
   b. Frontal lobe—personality, behavior, and memory changes; contralateral motor weakness; expressive aphasia.
   c. Temporal area—memory disturbances, auditory hallucinations, receptive aphasia, complex partial seizures, visual field deficits.
   d. Occipital area—visual agnosia and visual field deficits.
   e. Cerebellar area—coordination, gait, and balance disturbances, dysarthria.
   f. Brain stem—dysphagia, incontinence, cardiovascular instability, respiratory depression, coma, CN dysfunction.
   g. Hypothalamus—loss of temperature control, diabetes insipidus, SIADH.
   h. Pituitary/sella turcica—visual field deficits, amenorrhea, galactorrhea, impotence, cushingoid symptoms, elevated growth hormone, panhypopituitarism.

3. Referred symptoms (related to the vasogenic [extracellular] edema surrounding the tumor).

4. Seizures.

Diagnostic Evaluation

1. CT—with and without contrast to visualize tumor, hemorrhage, shift of midline, cerebral edema.
2. MRI—to visualize tumor; more useful than CT.
3. EEG—to detect locus of irritability, if seizures are present.
4. Angiography—to detect and evaluate the vascular supply of the tumor.
5. MR spectroscopy—evaluates the neurochemicals located within a core segment of the lesion; useful in differentiating tumors from infectious lesions.

6. Functional MRI—evaluates the functional eloquence of the brain tissue affected by the tumor, and the tissue at risk, for mass effect.
7. Skull radiography—to determine bone involvement, identify pineal shift, helpful in children.
8. Stealth-guided surgery or stereotactic biopsy surgery—needed for definitive diagnosis, cell type.

Management

Effectiveness of treatment depends on tumor type and location, capsulation, or infiltrative status. Tumors in vital areas, such as the brain stem, or nonencapsulated and infiltrating tumors, may not be surgically accessible and treatment may produce severe neurologic deficits (blindness, paralysis, mental impairment). Treatment is usually multimodal.

 NURSING ALERT Treatment of high-grade gliomas is palliative. There is no current treatment modality that provides a definitive cure. Treatment is aimed at improving duration of survival.

1. Surgery—removal/debulking by way of craniotomy, stealth guidance, laser resection, or ultrasonic aspiration.
   a. Craniotomy: goal is gross total resection of the tumor for maximum removal of tumor cells. Biopsy may be performed on tumors in eloquent locations; whereas surgery may not be an option for some tumors secondary to location. Gross total resection is associated with longer survival compared with subtotal resection in glioblastoma multiforme; 10% are inoperable based on location of the tumor.
   b. Awake craniotomy—allows intraoperative brain mapping.
   c. Image-guided surgery—computer-generated intraoperative localization of lesion.
   d. Laser resection or ultrasonic aspiration—may augment surgical resection.
   e. Endovascular treatment—useful in embolization of the arterial feeders to the meningiomas to reduce surgical risk related to blood loss.

2. Radiation therapy—external radiation to tumor bed with 2- to 3-cm border.
   a. Conventional therapy daily for 6 weeks; shorter to brain stem.
   b. Prophylactic radiation to brain stem for other brain tumors with high risk of metastasis.
   c. Brachytherapy—can use radioisotopes implanted through interstitial catheters to permit high doses for high-grade malignant tumors.

3. Radiosurgery—stereotactic radiosurgery by way of linear accelerator scalpel, proton beam, or gamma knife delivers a single, high dose of radiation to a precisely targeted tumor area. Destroys only targeted abnormal tissue, limiting damage to surrounding brain tissue.

4. Chemotherapy (the blood–brain barrier limits the effectiveness of chemotherapy agents).
   a. Metastatic tumors—single or combination drug therapy; may require autologous bone marrow transplantation (aspirated before chemotherapy and reinfused afterward to treat bone marrow depression).
   b. Primary glioma—may be used as adjunct to surgery and radiation.

i. Temozolomide (Temodar), an oral agent, is considered first line in chemotherapy for glioblastoma multiforme.

ii. Carmustine (BCNU) wafers are biodegradable chemotherapy wafers that are surgically placed into the tumor bed during tumor debulking. Up to 8 wafers are placed in the space where the tumor was located and they slowly break down over time.

iii. Bevacizumab (Avastin), has been approved by the FDA for the treatment of recurrent glioblastoma multiforme. Studies demonstrate a reduction in cerebral edema though there is no change in length of survival

iv. Immunotherapy (epidermal growth factor receptor variant III) remains investigational, though has shown promising results in phase II studies.

5. Shunting procedure—to manage hydrocephalus, which may be obstructive or nonobstructive depending on location, tumor type, degree of necrosis, and associated edema and inflammation.

6. Supportive therapy and medications.
   a. Antiepileptics for treatment of seizure activity; may be utilized for prophylaxis.
   b. Dexamethasone to reduce swelling and reduce radiation edema; also given during end stage to enhance quality of life.
   c. The presence of tumors creates a hypercoaguable state. Prophylactic use of anticoagulant may or may not be ordered, though may be required in the presence of DVT or PE.

7. Investigational therapies currently in progress:
   a. Currently, there are over 50 ongoing trials evaluating the effectiveness of immunotherapy.
   b. Use of combination therapy of bevacizumab and lomustine is currently in phase III of evaluation.

Complications

1. Increased ICP and brain herniation; death.
2. Neurologic deficits from expanding tumor or treatment.

Nursing Assessment

1. Assess vital signs and signs of increased ICP (see page 357).
2. Assess CN function, LOC, mental status, affect, and behavior.
3. Monitor for seizures.
4. Assess level of pain using visual analogue scale (0 to 10) or face scale, as indicated.
5. Assess level of anxiety.
6. Assess patient and family patterns of coping, support systems, and resources.
7. If treated with chemotherapy, assess bone marrow function by monitoring neutrophil and platelet counts.

Nursing Diagnoses

- Acute Pain related to brain mass, surgical intervention.
- Risk for Decreased Cerebral Tissue Perfusion related to physiologic effects of tumor, altered LOC, possible seizures, increased ICP, and sensory and motor deficits.
- Anxiety related to diagnosis, surgery, radiation, and/or chemotherapy.
- Imbalanced Nutrition: Less Than Body Requirements related to compromised neurologic function and stress of injury.
- Disabled Family Coping related to changes in roles and structure.

Nursing Interventions

Also see care of the undergoing chemotherapy (page 112), radiation (page 122), and craniotomy (page 361).

Relieving Pain

1. Provide analgesics around the clock at regular intervals that will not mask neurologic changes.
2. Maintain the head of the bed at 15 to 30 degrees to reduce cerebral venous congestion.
3. Provide a darkened room or sunglasses if the patient is photophobic.
4. Maintain a quiet environment to increase patient's pain tolerance.
5. Provide scheduled rest periods to help the patient recuperate from stress of pain.
6. Instruct the patient to lie with the operative side up.
7. Alter diet, as tolerated, if the patient has pain on chewing.
8. Collaborate with the patient on alternative ways to reduce pain such as use of music therapy.

Preventing Injury

1. Report any signs of increased ICP or worsening neurologic condition to health care provider immediately.
2. Adjust care to reduce risk of increased ICP; body positioning without flexion of head, reduce hip flexion, distribute care throughout the 24-hour period to allow ICP to return to baseline.
3. Monitor laboratory data, CSF cultures, and Gram stains, and communicate results to medical staff.
4. Monitor intake and output, osmolality studies, and electrolytes; prevent overhydration, which can worsen cerebral edema.
5. Monitor response to pharmacologic therapy, including drug levels.
6. Initiate seizure precautions; pad the side rails of the bed to prevent injury if seizures occur; have suction equipment available.
7. Maintain availability of medications for management of status epilepticus (see page 424).
8. Initiate fall precautions; side rails up at all times, call light within reach at bedside, assist with toileting on a regular basis.
9. Gradually progress patient to ambulation with assistance as tolerated, enlist help from physical therapist, occupational therapist early, as indicated, to prevent falls.
10. If the patient is dysphagic or unconscious, initiate aspiration precautions: elevate head of the bed 30 degrees and position the patient's head to the side to prevent aspiration.
11. If dysphagic, position the patient upright and instruct in sequenced swallowing to maintain feeding function (see page 505).
12. Maintain oxygen and suction at the bedside in case of aspiration.
13. For the patient with visual field deficits, place materials in visual field.

Minimizing Anxiety

1. Provide a safe environment in which the patient may verbalize anxieties.
2. Help the patient to express feelings related to fear and anxiety.
3. Answer questions and provide written information.
4. Include the patient/family in all treatment options and scheduling.
5. Introduce stress management techniques.

6. Provide consistency in care and continually provide emotional support.
7. Assess the patient's usual coping behaviors and provide support in these areas.
8. Consult with social worker for community resources.

> **NURSING ALERT** Anxiety and depression prior to and following surgery are associated with shorter postsurgical survival in patients with glioblastoma multiforme. Screening assessments can be performed with standard instruments and levels indicating a high risk of anxiety or depression should be reported to the health care provider.

Optimizing Nutrition
1. Medicate for nausea before position changes, radiation, or chemotherapy, and as needed.
2. Maintain adequate hydration within guidelines for cerebral edema.
3. Offer small, frequent meals as tolerated.
4. Consult with dietitian to evaluate food choices and provide adequate caloric needs through enteral or parenteral nourishment if unable to take oral nutrition.
5. Alter consistency of diet, as necessary, to enhance intake.

Strengthening Family Coping
1. Recognize stages of grief.
2. Foster a trusting relationship.
3. Provide clear, consistent explanations of procedures and treatments.
4. Encourage family involvement in care from the beginning.
5. Establish a means of communication for family with patient when verbal responses are not possible.
6. Consult with social worker and mental health provider if the family needs assistance in adjusting to neurologic deficits.
7. Assist the family to use stress management techniques and community resources such as respite care.
8. Encourage discussion with health care provider about prognosis and functional outcome.
9. Discuss development of advance directive and durable power of attorney (DPA). Maintain positive attitude and define that rationale as a way to allow for patient-defined extent of care in the advent of deterioration.

Patient Education and Health Maintenance
1. Explain the adverse effects of treatment.
2. Encourage close follow-up after diagnosis and treatment.
3. Explain the importance of continuing corticosteroids and how to manage adverse effects, such as weight gain and hyperglycemia.
4. Encourage the use of community resources for physical and psychological support, such as transportation to medical appointments, financial assistance, and respite care.
5. Refer the patient/family for more information and support to such agencies as the National Institute of Neurologic Disorders and Stroke (*www.ninds.nih.gov*) and the National Brain Tumor Foundation (*www.braintumor.org*).

Evaluation: Expected Outcomes
- Reports satisfactory comfort level.
- No new neurologic deficits, seizures, falls, or other complications.
- Expresses decreased anxiety.
- Nutritional intake meeting metabolic demands.
- Patient and family verbalize understanding of treatment and available resources.

Tumors of the Spinal Cord and Canal

Tumors of the spinal cord and canal may be extradural (existing outside the dural membranes), including chordoma and osteoblastoma; intradural–extramedullary (within the SAS), including meningiomas, neurofibromas, and schwannomas; or intramedullary (within the spinal cord), including astrocytomas, ependymomas, and neurofibromatosis "dumbbell tumors." Vascular tumors can affect any part of the spinal cord or canal.

Pathophysiology and Etiology
1. Astrocytomas, characterized by asymmetrical expansion in the spinal cord, are more common in children than adults. Ependymomas, usually with a cyst, are the most common intramedullary tumor in the adult but are rare in children. These tumors are central in the spinal cord.
2. Vascular tumors can affect the spinal cord in various ways. Hemangioblastomas often cause edema and syrinx (fluid-filled cavity) formation. Cavernomas are located on the dorsal surface of the spinal cord.
3. Approximately 85% of all patients with cancer develop bony metastasis, with the spinal column as the primary site. Spinal cord compression due to cancer typically presents with incomplete paraplegia involving the thoracic spine.
4. Cause for abnormal cell growth is unknown.
5. Extradural tumors spread to the vertebral bodies.
6. Spinal cord and/or nerve compression can result.

Clinical Manifestations
Depends on location and type of tumor and extent of spinal cord compression.
1. Back pain that is localized or radiates; may be absent in more than 50% of patients.
2. Weakness of extremity with abnormal reflexes.
3. Sensory changes.
4. Bladder, bowel, or sexual dysfunction.

Diagnostic Evaluation
1. A plain x-ray or CT scan can detect a pathologic fracture, collapse, or destruction resulting from a mass.
2. MRI is sensitive to tumor detection.

Management
1. Two surgical approaches may be used to manage spinal cord tumors:
   a. Anterior decompression is typically indicated because most spinal cord tumors are anterior.
   b. The posterolateral approach may be used for excision of thoracic tumors. Endoscopy, or other surgical techniques using instrumentation, can be used to visualize the anterior part of the cord. In thoracic tumors above T_5, posterolateral decompression negates the need for an anterior thoracotomy or sternotomy.
2. Intraoperative somatosensory-evoked potentials and motor-evoked potentials can be used to "map" the optimal spinal

cord site for incision and identify sensory and motor tracts within the spinal cord. This mapping reduces the neurologic deficits that are frequently associated with tumor incisions.

3. Various techniques are used to remove spinal cord tumors, including the following:
   a. Intramedullary tumors are totally resected. Corticosteroids are administered before and after surgery. MRI verifies tumor characteristics preoperatively (eg, exact level). Microsurgical laser techniques, ultrasound, and x-rays may be used intraoperatively. In surgery, every effort must be made to keep the anterior spinal artery intact.
   b. Vascular tumors may be managed in different ways. Hemangioblastomas are usually removed from the outside inward by exterior coagulation and progressive tumor shrinkage before removal. Cavernomas are usually removed by exterior coagulation and progressive tumor shrinkage before removal but from the inside outward.
   c. Neoplastic tumors may be treated with radiation or surgically excised using an anterior approach because these tumors typically cause anterior cord compression.

4. Radiation therapy may be used over 2 to 4 weeks; dosing protocols vary. Spinal radiation before surgical decompression may adversely affect wound healing. In patients who have a good functional status, radiotherapy to a malignant spinal cord tumor can significantly improve survival time.

5. Corticosteroids, such as dexamethasone and prednisone in moderate to high doses, are indicated for use before radiation therapy to improve the ambulation rate in the paretic patient.
   a. Corticosteroids are not typically used in nonparetic ambulatory patients.
   b. They are tapered over 2 weeks before discontinuing.

6. Chemotherapy is considered experimental.

7. When compared to patients with traumatic SCI, the rehabilitation of patients with spinal cord tumors is shorter; however, cancer patients have more limited functional improvement than SCI patients.

Complications

1. Spinal cord infarction secondary to compression.
2. Nerve or spinal compression from tumor expansion.
3. Tetraplegia or paraplegia due to spinal cord compression.

Nursing Assessment

1. Perform motor and sensory components of the neurologic examination.
2. Assess pain using scale of 0 to 10, as indicated.
3. Assess autonomic nervous system relative to level of lesion—pupillary responses, vital signs, bowel, and bladder function.
4. Assess for spinal or nerve compression—progressive increase in pain, paralysis or paresis, sensory loss, loss of rectal sphincter tone, and sexual dysfunction.

Nursing Diagnoses

- Anxiety related to surgery and outcome.
- Pain related to nerve compression.
- Risk for Peripheral Neurovascular Dysfunction related to nerve compression.
- Impaired Urinary Elimination related to spinal cord compression.
- Risk for Infection and Risk for Injury related to surgery.

Nursing Interventions

Relieving Anxiety

1. Provide an accepting environment for patient to verbalize anxieties.
2. Provide explanations regarding all procedures. Answer questions or refer the patient to someone who can answer questions.
3. Refer to cancer and SCI support groups, as needed.
4. Provide the patient/family with written information regarding disease process and medical interventions.
5. Reduce environmental stimulation.
6. Promote periods of rest to enhance coping skills.
7. Involve the family in distraction techniques.
8. Provide options in care when possible.

Relieving Pain

1. Administer analgesics, as indicated, and evaluate for pain control.
2. Instruct the patient in the use of patient-controlled analgesia, if available.
3. Instruct the patient in relaxation techniques, such as deep breathing, distraction, and imagery.
4. Position patient off surgical site postoperatively.

Compensating for Sensory Alterations

1. Reassure the patient that the degree of sensory/motor impairment may decrease during the postoperative recovery period as the amount of surgical edema decreases.
2. Instruct the patient with sensory loss to visually scan the extremity during use to avoid injury related to lack of tactile input.
3. Instruct the patient with painful paresthesias in appropriate use of ice, exercise, and rest.
4. Assess the patient with sensory and motor alterations and refer to physical therapy for assistance with ADL, ambulation.

Achieving Urinary Continence

1. Assess the urinary elimination pattern of the patient.
2. Instruct the patient in the therapeutic intake of fluid volume and relationship to elimination.
3. Instruct the patient in an appropriate means of urinary elimination and bowel management (see page 356).

Preventing Postoperative Complications

1. Provide routine postoperative care to prevent complications.
2. Monitor surgical site for bleeding, CSF drainage, signs of infection.
3. Keep surgical dressing clean and dry.
4. Clean surgical site, as ordered.
5. Pad the bed rails and chair if the patient experiences numbness or paresthesias to prevent injury.
6. Support the weak/paralytic extremity in a functional position.

Patient Education and Health Maintenance

1. Encourage the patient with motor impairment to use adaptive devices.
2. Demonstrate proper positioning and transfer techniques.
3. Instruct the patient with sensory losses about dangers of extreme temperatures and the need for adequate foot protection at all times.
4. If the patient has suspected or confirmed neurofibromatosis, suggest referral to genetic counselor. Also, encourage follow-up for MRI every 12 months to monitor disease progression.
5. Refer to cancer and SCI support groups, as needed.

Evaluation: Expected Outcomes

- Asks questions and discusses care options.
- Reports that pain is relieved.
- Reports decreased paresthesias; ambulatory postoperatively.
- Voids at intervals without residual urine.
- Incision healing, skin intact.

OTHER DISORDERS
Seizure Disorders

Seizures (also known as *epileptic seizures* and, if recurrent, *epilepsy*) are defined as a sudden alteration in normal brain activity that causes distinct changes in behavior and body function. Seizures are thought to result from disturbances in the cells of the brain that cause cells to give off abnormal, recurrent, uncontrolled electrical discharges.

Pathophysiology and Etiology

Altered Physiology

1. The pathophysiology of seizures is unknown. It is known, however, that the brain has certain metabolic needs for oxygen and glucose. Neurons also have certain permeability gradients and voltage gradients that are affected by changes in the chemical and humoral environment.
2. Factors that change the permeability of the cell population (ischemia, hemorrhage) and ion concentration (Na^+, K^+) can produce neurons that are hyperexcitable and demonstrate hypersynchrony, producing an abnormal discharge.
3. A seizure may manifest itself as an altered behavior, motor, or sensory function relating to any anatomic location in the brain.

Classification

The International League Against Epilepsy developed an international classification of epileptic seizures that divides seizures into two major classes: partial-onset seizures and generalized-onset seizures. Partial-onset seizures begin in one focal area of the cerebral cortex, whereas generalized-onset seizures have an onset recorded simultaneously in both cerebral hemispheres.

1. *Simple-partial seizures* can have motor, somatosensory, psychic, or autonomic symptoms *without impairment* of consciousness.
2. *Complex-partial seizures* have an *impairment* (but not a loss) of consciousness with simple-partial features, automatisms, or impairment of consciousness only.
3. *Generalized seizures* have a loss of consciousness with convulsive or nonconvulsive behaviors.
4. Simple-partial seizures can progress to complex-partial seizures and complex-partial seizures can secondarily become generalized.

Etiology

The etiology may be unknown or due to one of the following:

1. Trauma to head or brain resulting in scar tissue or cerebral atrophy.
2. Tumors.
3. Cranial surgery.
4. Metabolic disorders (hypocalcemia, hypoglycemia/hyperglycemia, hyponatremia, anoxia).
5. Drug toxicity, such as theophylline, lidocaine, penicillin.
6. CNS infection.
7. Circulatory disorders.
8. Drug withdrawal states (alcohol, barbiturates).
9. Congenital neurodegenerative disorders.
10. Nonepileptogenic behaviors, which can emulate seizures but have a psychogenic, rather than an organic, origin.

Clinical Manifestations

Manifestations are related to the area of the brain involved in the seizure activity and may range from single abnormal sensations, aberrant motor activity, altered consciousness or personality to loss of consciousness, and convulsive movements.

1. Impaired consciousness.
2. Disturbed muscle tone or movement.
3. Disturbances of behavior, mood, sensation, or perception.
4. Disturbances of autonomic functions.

Diagnostic Evaluation

1. EEG with or without video monitoring—locates epileptic focus, spread, intensity, and duration; helps classify seizure type.
2. MRI, CT scan—to identify lesion that may be cause of seizure.
3. SPECT or PET scan—additional tests to identify seizure foci.
4. Neuropsychological studies—to evaluate for behavioral disturbances.
5. Serum laboratory studies or lumbar puncture—to evaluate for infectious, hormonal, or metabolic etiology.

Management

1. Pharmacotherapy—antiepileptic drugs (AEDs) selected according to seizure type (see Table 15-9, pages 420 to 423).
2. Biofeedback—useful in the patient with reliable auras.
3. Surgery considered in patients who are refractory to antiepileptic medications or require the use of more than two AEDs. Standardized surgical procedures include anteromesial temporal resection, corpus callosotomy, hemispherectomy.
4. Stimulation surgery—in those who are refractory to medication and not candidates for traditional surgery.
   a. Vagal nerve stimulation—sends regular electrical impulses to the brain via the Vagus nerve to reduce seizures.
   b. Intracranial neurostimulator—new procedure that monitors electrical activity of the brain and is programmed to deliver impulses at a certain rate and pulse width to reduce seizures.

Complications

1. Status epilepticus (see Box 15-7).
2. Injuries due to falls, especially head injuries.
3. SUDEP: Sudden unexplained death in epilepsy patients.

Nursing Assessment

1. Obtain seizure history, including prodromal signs and symptoms, seizure behavior, postictal state, history of status epilepticus.
2. Document the following about seizure activity:
   a. Circumstances before attack, such as visual, auditory, olfactory, or tactile stimuli; emotional or psychological disturbances; sleep; hyperventilation.
   b. Description of movement, including where movement or stiffness started; type of movement and parts involved; progression of movement; whether beginning of seizure was witnessed.

text continues on page 424

Table 15-9 Antiepileptic Drugs

GENERIC NAME	DOSAGE FORMS	USUAL DOSES	HALF-LIFE
Carbamazepine	• Suspension 100 mg/5 mL • Tablet 200 mg • Chewtab 100 mg • Extended-release tablets 100, 200, 400 mg • Extended-release sprinkle capsules 200, 300 mg	• 10–40 mg/kg/day divided bid for extended-release; tid to qid for immediate-release	Initial 20–50, then 5–14 hr; induces own metabolism over first 2 wk
Clonazepam	• Tablets 0.5, 1, 2 mg	• 0.01–0.3 mg/kg/day divided tid or given QHS • 0.5 mg PO tid—adults maximum 20 mg/day	20–40 hr
Diazepam (rectal)	• Pediatric rectal gel 2.5, 5, 10 mg • Adult rectal gel 10, 15, 20 mg	• 2–5 y/o—0.5 mg/kg • 6–11 y/o—0.3 mg/kg • >12 y/o—0.2 mg/kg	30–60 hr
Ethosuximide	• Capsule 250 mg • Solution 250 mg/5 mL	• 15–40 mg/kg/day divided bid	30–60 hr
Felbamate	• Tablets 400, 600 mg • Suspension 600 mg/5 mL	• 15–45 mg/kg/day (or 1,200–3,600 mg) divided tid to qid; usual maximum 60 mg/kg/day	14–23 hr
Gabapentin	• Capsule 100, 300, 400 mg • Tablets 600, 800 mg • Solution 250 mg/5 mL	• Initially 10–20 mg/kg/day divided tid to qid; titrate up to 40–60 mg/kg/day; usual maximum 90 mg/kg/day	5–9 hr
Lamotrigine	• Tablets 25, 100, 150, 200 mg • Chew tablets 2, 5, 25 mg	• 200–500 mg/day divided bid • 2–15 mg/kg/day; start dose slowly	12–50 hr up to 70 hr with VPA
Lacosimide	• 50, 100, 150, 200 mg tablets. Oral solution 10 mg/mL; Injection solution 10 mg/mL	• 200–400 mg/d in two divided doses.	12–16 hr
Levetiracetam	• Tablets 250, 500, 750 mg	• Initially 10 mg/kg PO divided bid or 500 mg PO bid; increase every 2 wks to 40–60 mg/kg/day	Adults 7 hr
Lorazepam	• Tablets 0.5, 1, 2 mg • Solution 2 mg/mL • Injection 2, 4 mg/mL	• 0.05–0.1 mg/kg/dose; 4 mg/dose maximum may repeat in 10–15 min	10–20 h
Oxcarbazepine	• Tablets 150, 300, 600 mg	• Adult initially 300 mg PO bid, increase weekly to a usual maintenance dose of 1,200–2,400 mg/day • Child initially 10 mg/kg/day; titrate to a dose of 30–60 mg/kg/day	Parent 1–2½ hr; Metabolite 8–15 hr

USUAL TARGET RANGE	MECHANISM OF ACTION	INDICATIONS	DOSE-RELATED ADVERSE EFFECTS
4–12 mcg/mL	Modulates sodium channels	• Simple-partial • Complex partial • Generalized tonic/clonic seizures	Double or blurred vision, lethargy (reduced by slow-dose titration)
20–70 mcg/mL	Enhances GABA	• Myoclonic • Lennox-Gastaut syndrome • Atonic • Absence	Drowsiness (50%), ataxia (30%), behavioral disturbances (25%), movement disorders, slurred speech, hypersecretion
Not applicable	Enhances GABA	• Acute repetitive seizures	Sedation
40–100 mcg/mL	Reduces current in the T-type calcium channel	• Absence	GI distress, drowsiness, hiccups, sedation
30–100 mcg/mL	Blocks glycine binding to the NMDA receptors, modulates sodium channel, enhances GABA	• Lennox-Gastaut syndrome • Complex partial seizures	Anorexia, weight loss, vomiting, insomnia, headache, somnolence; rare cases of aplastic anemia (25 cases per 100,000) and liver failure (8 cases per 100,000) have also been seen
4–20 mcg/mL	Not known	• Partial seizures with or without secondary generalized tonic/clonic seizures	Somnolence, dizziness, ataxia, nystagmus, weight gain, nausea, vomiting, blurred vision, tremor, slurred speech, peripheral edema, dyspepsia, hiccups
3–20 mcg/mL	Blocks sodium channels and blocks release of glutamate	• Simple-partial seizures • Complex partial seizures • Generalized tonic/clonic seizures • Lennox-Gastaut syndrome • Absence	Fatigue, drowsiness, ataxia, dizziness, headache, nausea, vomiting, double or blurred vision, nystagmus
10–20 mcg/mL	Modulates Na⁺ channels	• Adjunctive treatment focal seizures with or without secondary generalization in patients 16 yr and older in age.	Dizziness, ataxia, fatigue, headache. Tremor, somnolence, balance disorder, memory impairment, vertigo, asthenia, gait disturbance, depression and bradycardia. Blurred vision, diplopia, nystagmus. Nausea, vomiting, and diarrhea
5–50 mcg/mL	Inhibits propagation of seizure by unknown mechanism	• Partial-onset seizures	Somnolence (14.8%), asthenia (14.7%), coordination difficulties (3.4%), dizziness, nervousness, behavioral problems, decreased blood counts
50–240 mcg/mL	Enhances GABA	• Status epilepticus	Sedation with risk of respiratory depression, amnesia, abnormal behavior, withdrawal reactions
10–35 mcg/mL for the monohydroxy derivative	Modulates sodium channels	• Partial-onset seizures	Headache, drowsiness, fatigue, nausea, dizziness, hyponatremia (hematologic toxicity not observed to date); dermatological reactions (rash)

(continued)

Table 15-9   Antiepileptic Drugs (*Continued*)

GENERIC NAME	DOSAGE FORMS	USUAL DOSES	HALF-LIFE
Phenobarbital C-IV	• Capsule 16 mg • Elixir 15 mg/5 mL, 20 mg/5 mL • Tablet 8, 15, 16, 30, 32, 60, 65, 100 mg • Injection 30, 60, 65, 130 mg/mL	• 2–6 mg/kg/day divided qid to bid (high end of range for infants/young children)	40–140 hr
Phenytoin, Fosphenytoin	• Injection 50 mg/mL (Fosphe-nytoin is 50 mg/mL phenytoin equivalent) • Suspension 125 mg/5 mL, 30 mg/5 mL • Chew tablets 50 mg • Capsules 30, 100 mg	• 4–12 mg/kg/day divided bid to tid for children getting PO; qid to bid for adults getting PO; divided q6h for IV dosing	5–34 hr
Primidone	• Suspension 250 mg/5 mL • Tablets 50, 250 mg	• 10–25 mg/kg/day divided bid to tid; maximum 2 mg/day	4–20 hr (PEMA ½ 30–36 hr)
Rufinamide	200 and 400 mg film-coated tablets. Oral suspension: 40 mg/mL	1,800–3,200 mg twice a day. Children: 45 mg/kg/d.	6–10 h
Tiagabine	• Tablets 2, 4, 12, 16, 20 mg	• Adult 32–56 mg/day divided bid to qid (start with a 4 mg PO qid, adjust weekly) • Child 0.1 mg/kg/day divide tid, increase to 0.6 mg/kg/day (1 mg/kg/day with enzyme inducers)	2–9 hr
Topiramate	• Tablets 25, 100, 200 mg • Sprinkle capsules 15, 25 mg	• Children initiate at 0.5–1 mg/kg/day divided bid; usual dose is 6–12 mg/kg/day divided bid to tid • Adult: 200–800 mg/day divided bid; initiate slowly with 25 mg qh, increase weekly	12–30 hr
VPA/divalproex sodium	• Solution 250 mg/5 mL • Capsule 250 mg • Sprinkle 125 mg • Extended-release 500 mg • Tablet 125, 200, 500 mg	• 15–60 mg/kg/day divided bid to tid	7–20 hours
Vigabatrin	• Tablet 500 mg scored	• Adult: 2–4 mg/day divided bid • Children: 1–2 mg/day or 40–100 mg/kg/day	5–7 hr
Zonisamide	• Capsule 100 mg	• Adult 200–400 mg/day PO bid (max 600 mg), initially 100 mg PO qid and adjust every 2 wk • Children initially 1 mg/kg/day, adjust every 2 wk (maximum 15 mg/kg/day)	27–60 hr

GABA, gamma-aminobutyric acid; NMDA, N-methyl-D-aspartate; PEMA, phenylethylmalonamide; VPA, valproic acid.

USUAL TARGET RANGE	MECHANISM OF ACTION	INDICATIONS	DOSE-RELATED ADVERSE EFFECTS
15–40 mcg/mL	Enhances GABA	• Generalized tonic/clonic seizures • Simple-partial seizures • Complex partial seizures	Sedation, mental dullness, cognitive impairment, hyperactivity, ataxia
10–20 mcg/mL total 1–2 mcg/mL free (for patients with protein binding)	Modulates sodium channels	• Generalized tonic/clonic seizures • Complex partial seizures • Simple-partial seizures	Nystagmus, ataxia, lethargy, propylene glycol in IV preparation can cause myocardial depression, bradycardias, other electrocardiogram changes, hypotension, rash
5–20 mcg/mL	Enhances GABA	• Generalized tonic/clonic seizures • Simple-partial seizures • Complex partial seizures	Same as phenobarbital
10–25 mcg/mL	Modulates Na⁺ Channel	Adjunctive treatment focal seizures with or without secondary generalization. In children >4 yrs. used as adjunctive treatment of seizures associated with Lennox-Gastaut syndrome	Somnolence, coordination abnormalities. Dizziness, gait disturbances, and ataxia. Vomiting, rash, headache, increased risk of suicide thoughts or behavior. Contraindicated in patients with familial short QT syndrome
5–70 mcg/mL	Inhibits neuronal and glial uptake of GABA	• Partial-onset seizures	Sedation, dizziness, memory impairment, inattention, emotional lability, headache, abdominal pain, anorexia, tremor
2–25 mcg/mL	Modulates sodium channels, enhances GABA activity, and modulates NMDA receptor	• Partial-onset seizures • Lennox-Gastaut syndrome • Generalized tonic/clonic • Juvenile myoclonic epilepsy	Speech and language problems, difficulty with concentration and attention, confusion, fatigue, paresthesias, weight loss
50–150 mcg/mL	Unknown (may modulate sodium channel, enhance GABA)	• Generalized tonic/clonic seizures • Absence • Myoclonic • Partial-onset seizures • Lennox-Gastaut syndrome	GI upset, lethargy, changes in menstrual cycle, thrombocytopenia
Not known	Inhibits GABA-transaminase (preventing GABA metabolism)	• Infantile spasms due to tuberous sclerosis	Drowsiness, fatigue, ataxia, behavioral changes, weight gain, psychosis (in predisposed patients and upon abrupt withdrawal), hematologic, visual field problems
15–40 mcg/mL	Modulates sodium and T-type calcium channels	• Partial-onset seizures • Generalized seizures • Absence • Myoclonic • Lennox-Gastaut • Infantile spasms	Drowsiness, psychosis (2%)

BOX 15-7 Emergency Management of Status Epilepticus

Status epilepticus (acute, prolonged, repetitive seizure activity) is a series of generalized seizures without return to consciousness between attacks. The term has been broadened to include continuous clinical and/or electrical seizures lasting at least 5 minutes, even without impairment of consciousness. Status epilepticus is considered a serious neurologic emergency. It has high mortality and morbidity (permanent brain damage, severe neurologic deficits). Factors that precipitate status epilepticus in patients with pre-existing seizure disorder include medication withdrawal, fever, metabolic or environmental stresses, alcohol or drug withdrawal, and sleep deprivation.

NURSING INTERVENTIONS
- Establish airway and maintain blood pressure (BP).
- Obtain blood studies for glucose blood urea nitrogen, electrolytes, and anticonvulsant drug levels to determine metabolic abnormalities and serve as a guide for maintenance of biochemical homeostasis.
- Administer oxygen—there is some respiratory depression associated with each seizure, which may produce venous congestion and hypoxia of the brain.

- Establish IV lines and keep open for blood sampling, drug administration, and infusion of fluids.
- Administer IV anticonvulsant (lorazepam, phenytoin, diazepam) *slowly* to ensure effective brain tissue and serum concentrations.
  - Give additional anticonvulsants, as directed—effects of lorazepam are of short duration.
  - Monitor anticonvulsant drug levels regularly.
- Monitor the patient continuously; depression of respiration and BP induced by drug therapy may be delayed.
- Use mechanical ventilation, as needed.
- If initial treatment is unsuccessful, general anesthesia may be required.
- Assist with search for precipitating factors.
  - Monitor vital and neurologic signs on a continuous basis.
  - Use electroencephalographic monitoring to determine nature and abolition (after diazepam administration) of epileptic activity.
  - Determine (from family member) if there is a history of epilepsy, alcohol/drug use, trauma, recent infection.

c. Position of the eyes and head; size of pupils.
d. Presence of automatisms, such as lip smacking or repeated swallowing.
e. Incontinence of urine or feces.
f. Duration of each phase of the attack.
g. Presence of unconsciousness and its duration.
h. Behavior after attack, including inability to speak, any weakness or paralysis (Todd paralysis), sleep.
3. Investigate the psychosocial effect of seizures.
4. Obtain history of drug or alcohol abuse.
5. Assess compliance and medication-taking strategies.

 DRUG ALERT Nonadherence to medication regimen as well as toxicity of antiepileptic medications can increase seizure frequency. Obtain drug levels before implementing medication changes.

Nursing Diagnoses

- Ineffective Cerebral Tissue Perfusion related to seizure activity.
- Risk for Injury related to seizure activity.
- Ineffective Coping related to psychosocial and economic consequences of epilepsy.

Nursing Interventions

Maintaining Cerebral Tissue Perfusion
1. Maintain a patent airway until the patient is fully awake after a seizure.
2. Provide oxygen during the seizure if color change occurs.
3. Stress the importance of taking medications regularly.
4. Monitor serum levels for therapeutic range of medications.
5. Monitor the patient for toxic adverse effects of medications.
6. Monitor platelet and liver functions for toxicity due to medications.

Preventing Injury
1. Provide a safe environment by padding side rails and removing clutter.
2. Place the bed in a low position.
3. Do not restrain the patient during a seizure.
4. Do not put anything in the patient's mouth during a seizure.
5. Place the patient on his or her side during a seizure to prevent aspiration.
6. Protect the patient's head during a seizure. If seizure occurs while ambulating or from chair, cradle head or provide cushion/support for protection against head injury.
7. Stay with the patient who is ambulating or who is in a confused state during seizure.
8. Provide a helmet to the patient who falls during seizure.
9. Manage the patient in status epilepticus.

Strengthening Coping
1. Consult with social worker for community resources for vocational rehabilitation, counselors, support groups.
2. Teach stress-reduction techniques that will fit into the patient's lifestyle.
3. Initiate appropriate consultation for management of behaviors related to personality disorders, brain damage secondary to chronic epilepsy.
4. Answer questions related to use of computerized video EEG monitoring and surgery for epilepsy management.

Community and Home Care Considerations

1. Counsel patients with uncontrolled seizures about driving or operating dangerous equipment. Be familiar with state laws regarding driving while on or tapering AEDs.
2. Assess home environment for safety hazards in case the patient falls, such as crowded furniture arrangement, sharp edges on tables, and glass. Soft flooring and furniture and padded surfaces may be necessary.

3. Provide instructions on safety precautions while performing activities alone to prevent injury, drowning, or choking.
4. Support the patient in discussion about seizures with employer, school, and so forth.

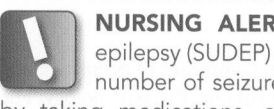 **NURSING ALERT** Sudden unexpected death in epilepsy (SUDEP) can be reduced by decreasing the number of seizures that a patient experiences and by taking medications, as prescribed. Although multiple medications may be required to reduce seizure frequency, it should be considered within the context of quality of life and risk reduction.

Patient Education and Health Maintenance

1. Encourage the patient to determine existence of trigger factors for seizures (eg, skipped meals, lack of sleep, emotional stress, menstrual cycle).
2. Remind the patient of the importance of following medication regimen.
3. Tell the patient to avoid alcohol because it interferes with metabolism of antiepileptic medications.
4. Encourage the patient and family to discuss feelings and attitudes about epilepsy.
5. Encourage the patient to carry or wear a MedicAlert card or bracelet.
6. Encourage a moderate lifestyle that includes exercise, mental activity, and nutritional diet.
7. For the surgical candidate, reinforce instructions related to surgical outcome of the specific surgical approach (temporal lobectomy, corpus callosotomy, hemispherectomy, and extratemporal resection).
8. Refer the patient/family for more information and support to such agencies as the Epilepsy Foundation of America (*www.efa.org*).

Evaluation: Expected Outcomes

- Takes medication as ordered, drug level within normal range.
- No injuries observed.
- Reports using support services and stress-management techniques.

Narcolepsy

Narcolepsy is a neurologic disorder characterized by abnormalities of REM sleep, some abnormalities of non-REM sleep, and excessive daytime sleepiness.

Pathophysiology and Etiology

1. Recent advances suggest that this common sleep disorder may be a neurodegenerative or autoimmune disorder resulting in the loss of hypothalamic neurons that contain a peptide, hypocretin (orexin). Hypocretin plays a central role in the timing of sleep and wakefulness and inhibits REM sleep. The deficiency in hypocretin contributes to the abnormalities of sleep and wakefulness in narcolepsy.
2. Genetic susceptibility—associated with class II human leukocyte antigens.
3. Although considered a hypersomnia disorder, the person does not experience excessive amounts of sleep in a 24-hour period. Typically, patients with narcolepsy have a normal amount of sleep over 24 hours. They have abnormal REM sleep that intrudes into wakefulness.
4. Onset is usually between ages 15 and 25.

Clinical Manifestations

1. Four classic symptoms (all symptoms not present in all patients):
    a. Excessive daytime sleepiness is usually the first symptom.
    b. Cataplexy (abrupt loss of muscle tone after emotional stimulation such as laughter, anger).
    c. Sleep paralysis (powerless to move limbs, speak, open eyes, or breathe deeply while fully aware of condition).
    d. Hypnagogic hallucinations (drowsiness before sleep, usually visual or auditory).
2. Symptoms enhanced by high temperature, indoor activity, and idleness.
3. Clinical manifestations may abate, but never phase out completely.
4. Patient may complain of inability to focus vision or thought process rather than have a feeling of sleepiness.
5. Nocturnal sleep disturbance—occurs 2½ to 3 hours after falling asleep.
    a. After being awake for 45 to 60 minutes, the patient will fall back to sleep for another 2½ to 3 hours and then awaken again.
    b. This is believed to be the source of the daytime somnolence.

Diagnostic Evaluation

1. An overnight polysomnogram in a sleep disorders lab is included in the evaluation to assess nighttime sleep—indicates the underlying cause for the complaint of sleepiness. The polysomnogram helps evaluate sleep quality and excludes other disorders, such as sleep apnea.
2. The polysomnogram is followed the next day by a multiple sleep latency test to assess daytime sleepiness—indicates severity of the problem. Patients are given four or five opportunities to nap every 2 hours. Patients with narcolepsy typically fall asleep more rapidly than the norm of 10 to 15 minutes.

Management

1. Long-term treatment is required. Mutual goal-setting is imperative because not everyone derives benefit from treatment. Even with medication, patients may never attain normal levels of alertness.
2. Nonpharmacologic therapy includes support groups, short naps (10 to 20 minutes, three times daily), caffeinated beverages, exercise, sleep hygiene techniques, and avoidance of heavy meals.
3. Stimulants prescribed may include pemoline, methylphenidate, dextroamphetamine, and methamphetamine.
4. Antidepressants for cataplexy; protriptyline, desipramine, fluoxetine.

Complications

1. Injury related to falling asleep.
2. Psychosocial problems such as disturbed relationships, loss of employment, and depression.

Nursing Assessment

1. Obtain history of sleep and activity pattern.
2. Assess emotional status and social interactions.
3. Assess response to medication and lifestyle treatment.

Nursing Diagnoses

- Disturbed Sleep Pattern related to disease process.
- Fatigue related to disrupted nighttime sleep.
- Ineffective Coping related to interference with activity.

Nursing Interventions

Promoting Normal Sleep–Wake Cycle

1. Review daily schedule to determine periods of sleep and cataplexy. Advise to wake at the same time daily.
2. Help the patient establish nondrug therapies (exercise, diet) that will fit into lifestyle.
3. Make sure that the bedroom is dark, cool, and quiet to facilitate sleep.
4. Administer or teach self-administration of prescribed medications.
   a. Advise of adverse effects of amphetamines, such as nervousness, irritability, tremors, and GI upset.
   b. Warn the patient to take only as prescribed and not to increase dosage because of tolerance and drug dependence.

Reducing Fatigue

1. Schedule 10- to 20-minute rest periods two or three times per day. Help the patient incorporate naps into lifestyle.
2. Encourage the patient to incorporate small amounts of caffeinated beverages at intervals and smaller, more frequent meals rather than large, heavy meals during the day to maintain energy.
3. Plan diversional activities and relaxation during fatigued periods.

Strengthening Coping

1. Encourage active participation in selection of treatment modalities.
2. Assist the patient in identifying trigger factors of worsening symptoms.
3. Teach problem solving strategy to promote sense of control over activities and symptoms during the day.
4. Review patient coping mechanisms and reinforce positive ones.
5. Assist the patient to discuss information about narcolepsy with friends, family, school, and employers to help reduce anxiety and/or embarrassment about his or her condition.
6. Encourage the use of support groups and community resources, such as the American Sleep Association (*www.sleepassociation.org*).

Patient Education and Health Maintenance

1. Review the normal sleep cycle and the pathophysiology of narcolepsy.
2. Stress the importance of nonpharmacologic measures as an adjunct to treatment.
3. Inform the patient of rights of employment conditions under the Americans with Disabilities Act (see page 160).
4. Advise caution with using alcohol, working with machinery, or using dangerous equipment to prevent injury to self or others during sleepiness or cataplexy.
5. If the patient drives, advise using caution and avoiding lengthy trips.
6. Encourage the patient to wear a MedicAlert bracelet.
7. Encourage follow-up with health care provider, specialist, and mental health counselor, as needed.

Evaluation: Expected Outcomes

- Complies with medication regimen.
- Reports working without undue fatigue.
- Identifies trigger factors.

Headache Syndromes

Headaches are one of the most common complaints of people seeking health care. Pain in the head is a symptom of underlying pathology. The International Headache Society instituted a classification system that is the standard for defining various types of headaches. It divides headaches into two categories: primary headache disorders, which include migraine, tension-type headache, and cluster headache, and secondary headache disorders. Identifying the etiology of headaches requires an understanding of the characteristics of each type of headache.

 EVIDENCE BASE Tepper, S. J., & Tepper, D. E. (2014). *The cleveland clinic manual of headache therapy*. New York: Springer.

Pathophysiology and Etiology

Primary Headaches

Diagnosis is generally based on the characteristic clinical history and elimination of other pathology such as stroke, intracranial bleed, AVM, or brain tumor.

1. Migraine headache—consists of initial vasospasm followed by dilation of intracranial and extracranial arteries; occurs in about 10% of the population.
   a. Caused by hyperactivity to the neurotransmitter serotonin; familial predisposition.
   b. Attack may consist of any of five phases: prodrome, aura, headache, resolution, and postdrome.
   c. Classified with or without aura (usually visual); aura is due to reduced cortical neuronal activity.
2. Tension headache—due to irritation of sensitive nerve endings in the head, jaw, and neck from prolonged muscle contraction in the face, head, and neck; mild or moderate intensity that does not prohibit activity.
   a. Precipitating factors include fatigue, stress, and poor posture.
   b. Characterized by hatband distribution.
3. Cluster headache—release of increased histamine results in vasodilation.
   a. Usually unilateral, recurring.
   b. Occurs more often in men.

Secondary Headaches

Headache due to a neurologic or systemic disease.

1. Mass lesion (tumor, abscess, AVM, subdural or EDH).
2. Intracranial infection (bacterial/viral/fungal meningitis or encephalitis).
3. Inflammation (giant cell arteritis, vasculitis).
4. Cerebrovascular disease (SAH, intracranial hemorrhage, occlusive vascular disease).
5. Increased ICP.
6. Low-pressure headache (postlumbar puncture, trauma-induced).
7. Sinus infection, viral infection such as influenza, systemic illness.

Clinical Manifestations

1. Migraine: sensory, motor, or mood alterations precede headache; gradual onset of severe unilateral, throbbing headache; may become bilateral.

a. Migraine with aura (classic migraine), characteristic aura may include scintillating scotoma (area of decreased vision surrounded by area of less abnormal or normal vision with zigzag appearance), hemianopsia (loss of half of field of vision), and paresthesias; headache follows aura in less than 1 hour; usually lasts less than a day.

b. Migraine without aura (common migraine), nausea, vomiting, and photophobia may accompany moderate to severe headache; worsened by activity; may last 4 to 72 hours and greatly impair activities.

c. Either type of migraine may be triggered in women by hormonal fluctuations (menses, pregnancy), excess or lack of sleep, change in eating habits, and certain food additives.

2. Tension/muscle contraction: dull, bandlike, constricting, persistent pain and pressure in the back of the head and neck, across forehead, bitemporal areas; may be tender points of head or neck.

a. Not aggravated by activity, but may be worsened by noise and light.

b. No nausea and vomiting, but may be associated with anorexia.

3. Cluster headache: sudden, sharp, burning, excruciating, unilateral pain; always involving facial area from neck to temple and often occurs during the evening or night; more frequent in men.

a. Occurs in clusters of 2 to 8 weeks followed by headache-free periods.

b. Associated with unilateral excessive tearing, redness of the eye, stuffiness of nostril on affected side, facial swelling, flushing, and sweating.

c. Attacks last several minutes to several days. Multiple attacks may occur in 1 day.

Diagnostic Evaluation

1. Skull/sinus films to rule out lesions, sinusitis.
2. CT scan/MRI to rule out lesions, hemorrhage, chronic sinusitis.
3. ESR and other blood studies to help determine inflammatory process with temporal arteritis.

 NURSING ALERT "Red flags" for possible serious cause of headache (hemorrhage, stroke, tumor, infection) include altered level of consciousness; neurologic findings such as weakness, facial droop, dysarthria, or aphasia; nausea and vomiting; new onset of or change in characteristic headaches; and patient reporting that it is "the worst headache of my life." These patients should be evaluated with a brain CT scan.

Management

Pharmacologic Treatment

Medications are intended to reduce the frequency, severity, and duration of the headache. Effectiveness of medication is individualized. Some persons may need a combination of medications.

1. Aspirin, acetaminophen, and NSAIDs for mild to moderate pain of tension, sinus, or mild vascular headaches.
2. Some drugs may abort vascular headaches if taken at the onset, including methysergide, a serotonin antagonist; ergotamine, a vasoconstrictor; or 5HT-agonists such as sumatriptan.

3. Sumatriptan is available in subcutaneous injection and nasal inhalation, as well as in oral form.
4. Other oral 5HT-agonists include zolmitriptan, naratriptan, and rizatriptan.
5. Inhalation of 100% oxygen may abort a cluster headache.
6. Some drugs may be used continuously as prophylactic treatment for recurrent migraines, including beta-adrenergic blockers, calcium channel blockers, and antidepressants.
7. Antihistamines and decongestants may be effective for sinus headaches.
8. Corticosteroids may be used for temporal arteritis.
9. Occasionally, opioid analgesics, muscle relaxants, and anti-anxiety agents may be needed for severe pain.
10. Vitamin supplements including magnesium and Vitamin B_2 may be beneficial in preventing headache episodes.

 DRUG ALERT Vasoconstrictors and 5HT-agonists used to abort vascular headaches are contraindicated in patients with uncontrolled hypertension, coronary artery disease, and peripheral vascular disease.

Nonpharmacologic Management

1. Relaxation techniques, guided imagery, paced breathing.
2. Biofeedback, cognitive therapy.
3. Trigger identification and control of such factors as intake of alcohol (red wine), skipped meals, oversleeping, or undersleeping. Anticipatory guidance in proper sleep hygiene
4. To prevent migraine: avoidance of monosodium glutamate, mixed spices such as "seasoned salt," nitrates and nitrites commonly contained in bacon, hot dogs, or deli meats.
5. Rest in a quiet, dark room at onset of headache.
6. If caffeine user, spread caffeine intake evenly over the day.
7. Routine exercise program.

Complications

1. Usually none from primary headaches.

Nursing Assessment

1. Obtain a history of related symptoms, triggering factors, degree of pain, and medications used.
2. Perform a complete neurologic examination to detect any focal deficits or signs of increased ICP that indicate tumor or hemorrhage.
3. Assess coping mechanisms and emotional status.

Nursing Diagnoses

- Acute Pain related to headache.
- Ineffective Coping related to chronic and/or disabling pain.

Nursing Interventions

Controlling Pain

1. Reduce environmental stimuli: light, noise, and movement to decrease severity of pain.
2. Suggest light massage for tight muscles in neck, scalp, or back for tension headaches.
3. Apply warm, moist heat to areas of muscle tension.
4. Encourage patient to lie down and attempt to sleep.
5. Teach progressive muscle relaxation to treat and prevent tension headaches.

a. Alternately tense and relax each group of muscles for a count of five, starting with the forehead and working downward to the feet.
b. Try to maintain a state of relaxation of each muscle group until the whole body feels relaxed.
c. Relaxation of just head and neck may also be helpful if time is limited.
6. Teach patient the cause of headache and proper use of medication.
7. Encourage adequate rest once headache is relieved to recover from fatigue of the pain.

Promoting Positive Coping
1. Encourage patient to become aware of triggering factors and early symptoms of headache, so it can be prevented or promptly treated. Hunger, lack of exercise, and erratic sleep schedules may trigger headaches.
2. Encourage adequate nutrition, rest and relaxation, and avoidance of stress and overexertion to better cope with headaches.
3. Implement problem solving to help patient manage problems that arise in social or work situations related to headaches.
4. Review coping mechanisms and strengthen positive ones.
5. Promote use of headache diary.

Patient Education and Health Maintenance
1. Teach proper administration of medication.
   a. Self-injection of sumatriptan given subcutaneously with autoinjector.
   b. Oral inhalation technique of ergotamine through metered-dose inhaler.
   c. Nasal spray dosing of sumatriptan.
2. Teach about adverse effects of medications.
   a. GI upset, gastritis, and possible ulcer formation with NSAIDs—take with food.
   b. Numbness, coldness, paresthesias, and pain of extremities with ergot derivatives—report to health care provider.
   c. Chest pain, wheezing, flushing with sumatriptan—report to health care provider.
   d. Hypotension with beta-adrenergic blockers and calcium channel blockers—arise slowly, do not exceed prescribed dosage, do not discontinue beta-adrenergic blockers abruptly.
3. Advise avoidance of alcohol, which can worsen headaches.
4. Teach about foods that are high in tyramine, which may trigger migraines—aged cheese, red wine, some processed meats. Some food additives such as nitrates may also trigger migraines, and many people identify their own individual triggers.
5. Teach patient how to perform relaxation techniques to reduce stress and promote inner well-being.
6. Refer patient for more information to the International Headache Society (*http://www.ihs-headache.org/*).

Evaluation: Expected Outcomes
- Reports fewer, less-severe headaches.
- Describes use of positive coping mechanisms.

Herniated Intervertebral Disk

Herniation of the intervertebral disk (ruptured disc) is a protrusion of the nucleus of the disk into the annulus (fibrous ring around the disk) with subsequent nerve compression. The herniation may occur in any portion of the vertebral column (see Figure 15-13).

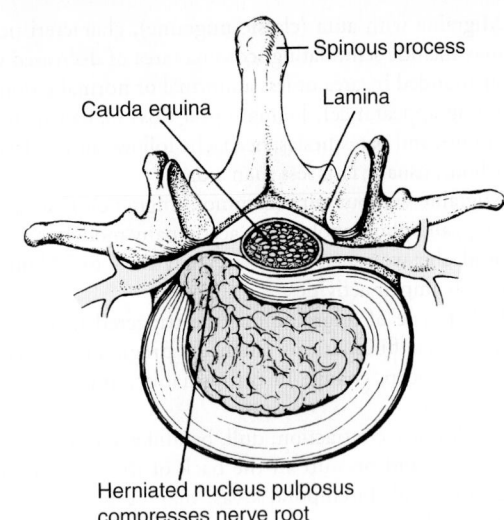

Figure 15-13. Ruptured vertebral disk. (Smeltzer, S., and Bare, B. [2000]. Brunner and Suddarth's textbook of medical-surgical nursing [9th ed.]. Philadelphia: Lippincott Williams & Wilkins.)

The pressure on spinal nerve roots or the spinal cord causes severe, chronic, or recurrent back and leg pain.

Pathophysiology and Etiology
1. The intervertebral disk is a cartilaginous plate made up of gelatinous material in the center, known as the nucleus pulposus, and is encapsulated in the fibrous annulus.
2. About 90% of herniated disks involve the lumbar and lumbosacral spine. The most common site is the L4–L5 disk space. The cause of a herniated lumbar disk is usually a flexion injury, but many patients do not recall experiencing a traumatic event. Cervical herniation is less common; but when it does occur, it is usually in individuals age 45 or older.
3. Risk factors for herniation include
   a. Degeneration (aging), trauma, and congenital predisposition.
   b. Biomechanical factors, such as twisting and repetitive motions in occupational settings.
   c. Sedentary occupations.
   d. Obesity.
   e. Smoking.
4. The herniation compresses the spinal nerve root, usually restricted to one side and, with further degeneration of the disk, may eventually produce pressure on the spinal cord.
5. This sequence may take months to years, producing acute and chronic symptoms.

Clinical Manifestations
General Considerations
1. An intervertebral disk may herniate without causing symptoms.
2. Symptoms depend on location, size, rate of development, and effect on surrounding structures.
3. Most symptomatic disk herniations result in pain, sensory changes, loss of reflex, and muscle weakness that resolve without surgery.

Cervical
1. Pain and stiffness in the neck, top of shoulders, and region of the scapula.
2. Pain in upper extremities and head.
3. Paresthesias and numbness of upper extremities.
4. Weakness of upper extremities.

Lumbar

1. Lower back pain with varying degrees of sensory and motor dysfunction.
2. Pain radiating from the lower back into the buttocks and down the leg, referred to as sciatica.
3. A stiff or unnatural posture.
4. Some combination of paresthesias, weakness, and reflex impairment.
5. Positive straight-leg raise test: pain occurs in leg below the knee when leg is raised from a supine position.

 NURSING ALERT Cauda equina syndrome is an urgent condition caused by an acute compression of the cauda equina area of the spinal cord by massive disk extrusion. Symptoms include progressive sensory and motor loss of lower extremities, saddle anesthesia (loss of sensation around perineum), bowel and/or bladder incontinence, or sexual dysfunction. It must be recognized early and compression must be relieved to prevent permanent loss of these functions. If patients report such symptoms, emergent assessment and intervention is indicated.

Diagnostic Evaluation

1. CT scan or MRI—demonstrates herniation; MRI has greater sensitivity.
2. Electromyography—localizes specific spinal nerve involvement.
3. Myelogram—rarely done, but demonstrates herniation and pressure on spinal cord or nerve roots.

Management

Nonpharmacologic Measures

1. Bed rest on a firm mattress (2 days usually sufficient) usually results in improvement in 80% of patients.
2. Heat or ice massage to affected area.
3. Cervical collar or possibly cervical traction is widely used, although efficacy is not proven.
4. Physical therapy may be prescribed to maximize function and assist the patient in recovery.
5. Epidural steroid injection may be administered by interventional radiologist, particularly with the presence of radiculopathy, radiating/shooting pain down the extremity, to relieve symptoms.
6. Nonpharmacologic and pharmacologic measures may be used together for 4 to 6 weeks as conservative management if there is no progressive neurologic deficit.
   a. More than 90% of low back pain episodes resolve completely by 4 to 6 weeks and those with herniated disc may experience spontaneous remission of pain.
   b. Surgical intervention is reserved for those with neurologic deficits or persistent symptoms over 6 weeks and is designed to relieve radicular (sciatic) pain.

Pharmacotherapy

1. Anti-inflammatory drugs, such as ibuprofen or prednisone.
2. Muscle relaxants, such as diazepam or cyclobenzaprine.
3. Analgesics; opioids may be necessary for several days during acute phase.

Surgical Intervention

1. May be done if there is progression of neurologic deficit or failure to improve with conservative management.

2. Surgical procedures include discectomy (decompression of nerve root), laminectomy, spinal fusion, microdiscectomy, and percutaneous discectomy.
3. Hemilaminectomy with excision of the involved disk is the surgical procedure most often indicated for lumbar disk disease.

Chemonucleolysis

1. Less common invasive treatment for lumbar disk herniation.
2. Injection of chymopapain into herniated disk that produces loss of water and proteoglycans from the disk, reducing the size of the disk and subsequent pressure on the nerve root.
3. May cause severe complications, such as transverse myelitis, allergic reactions, and persistent muscle spasm.

Alternative and Complementary Measures

1. Acupuncture.
2. Manipulative therapy.
3. Massage therapy for adjunct pain relief.
4. Homeopathic remedies.
5. Various nutritional supplements.

Complications

1. Permanent neurologic dysfunction (weakness, numbness).
2. Chronic pain with associated psychosocial issues.
3. Cauda equina syndrome.

Nursing Assessment

1. Perform repeated assessments of motor function, sensation, and reflexes to determine progression of condition.
2. Assess level at which straight-leg raise test is positive; generally, radiation of pain below knee at 45 degrees of elevation is considered positive for nerve root involvement; positive at lesser elevation may indicate worsening condition.
3. Assess pain level on scale of 0 to 10.

Nursing Diagnoses

- Acute Pain related to area of compression.
- Impaired Physical Mobility related to pain and disease physiology.
- Deficient Knowledge related to impending surgery.
- Risk for Infection and other complications of surgical procedure.

Nursing Interventions

Minimizing Pain

1. Administer or teach self-administration of anti-inflammatory drugs, as prescribed, and with food or antacid to prevent GI upset.
2. Administer or teach self-administration of prescribed muscle relaxant; observe safety because drowsiness may result.
3. Administer or teach self-administration of analgesics, as prescribed; be prepared for sedation.
4. Encourage regular activity with limits of pain.
5. Apply dry or moist heat to affected area of back, as desired.
6. Encourage relaxation techniques, such as imagery and progressive muscle relaxation.

Maintaining Mobility

1. Encourage ROM exercises while in bed.
2. Properly fit and use a cervical collar (if appropriate to level of injury).

3. Apply a back brace or cervical skin traction, if ordered.
4. Inspect skin several times a day, especially under stabilization devices, for redness and evidence of pressure ulcer development.
5. Provide good skin care to pressure-prone areas.
6. Assist the patient with activities at bedside and discourage lifting or straining of any kind.
7. Encourage compliance with physical therapy treatments and activity restrictions, as ordered.

Preparing the Patient for Surgery

1. Educate the patient about surgical procedure.
   a. Procedure is generally short.
   b. Small incision will be made on front or back of neck for cervical herniation; second incision may be on hip if a bone graft is taken from iliac crest for spinal fusion.
   c. Routine postoperative care will include frequent assessment of vital signs and neurologic function, frequent turning and deep breathing, pain control, and ambulation on the first postoperative day.
2. Document baseline neurologic assessment to compare with after surgery.
3. Explain your actions to the patient as you prepare the operative area, administer preoperative medications, and perform any other preoperative order.

Preventing Complications Postoperatively

1. Monitor vital signs and surgical dressing frequently because hemorrhage is a possible complication.
2. If the patient has a wound drainage system, check tubing frequently for patency and secure vacuum seal.
3. Assess movement and sensation of extremities regularly, report new deficit.
4. Administer analgesics and steroid medications to control pain from incision and swelling around nerve roots and spinal cord due to surgery.
5. Maintain cervical collar, if ordered.
6. Logroll the patient to reposition frequently and encourage coughing and deep breathing.
7. Position the patient for comfort with a small pillow under his or her head (but avoid extreme neck flexion) and pillow under knees to take pressure off lower back.
8. Provide fluids as soon as gag reflex and bowel sounds are noted.
9. Assess for hoarseness, which suggests that cervical surgery resulted in a recurrent laryngeal nerve injury; this injury may cause an ineffective cough.
10. Watch for dysphagia due to edema of the esophagus and provide dietary modifications, as necessary.
11. Make sure that the patient voids after surgery; report urine retention.
12. Encourage ambulation as soon as possible by having the patient lie on the side close to the edge of the bed and push up with arms while swinging legs toward floor in one motion; alternate walking with bed rest, discourage sitting.
13. Report any sudden reappearance of radicular pain (may indicate nerve root compression from slipping of bone graft or collapsing of disk space) or burning back pain radiating to buttocks (may indicate arachnoiditis).

Community and Home Care Considerations

1. Demonstrate and encourage back strengthening, aerobic exercise (walking, biking, swimming), and endurance exercises.
2. Make sure that the patient avoids heavy lifting and bending/twisting from the waist and uses proper body mechanics in all activities.
3. Discourage prolonged bed rest and inactivity.
4. Refer for vocational counseling, if indicated.
5. If cervical skin traction is ordered for home use, teach the patient how to apply the chinstrap and head halter. The weight should hang freely over the back of a chair or doorknob near the head of the bed. Make sure the patient maintains proper alignment of the neck and removes traction before moving the head.

Patient Education and Health Maintenance

1. Educate the patient regarding lifestyle changes—smoking cessation, increased activity, weight loss.
2. Provide instructions regarding back anatomy and back care to reduce symptoms.
3. Teach the patient the importance of cervical collar use and other conservative measures to try to reduce inflammation and heal disk herniation.
4. Tell the patient who has had a cervical disk herniation to avoid extreme flexion, extension, or rotation of the neck and to keep the head in neutral position during sleep.
5. Encourage the patient with a lumbar disk herniation to maintain ADL within pain limits, but lifting and sitting for prolonged periods are discouraged.
6. Encourage the patient to do stretching and strengthening exercises of extremities and abdomen after acute symptoms have subsided. The back can be gently stretched by lying on the back and bringing the knees up toward the chest.
7. Teach the patient about proper body mechanics and the use of leg and abdominal muscles rather than the back. Knees should be bent on lifting and load should be carried close to midtrunk.
8. Encourage follow-up with physical therapy, as indicated, for reconditioning and work hardening.
9. Tell the patient to avoid the prone position, long car rides, and sitting in a soft chair.
10. Instruct the patient to report any changes in neurologic function or recurrence of radicular pain.
11. Encourage good nutrition, avoidance of obesity, and proper rest to reduce risk of recurrence.

Evaluation: Expected Outcomes

- Verbalizes reduced pain.
- Maintains mobility with active lifestyle.
- Expresses understanding of preoperative preparation and postoperative care.
- Incision healing without signs of infection; patient ambulating with minimal pain.

SELECTED REFERENCES

Aiaz, M., Jefferies, S., Brazil, L., et al. (2014). Current and investigational drug strategies for glioblastoma. *Clinical Oncology, 26*, 419–430.

Ajiboye, N., Chalouhi, N., Starke, R. M., et al. (2014). Cerebral arteriovenous malformations: Evaluation and management. *Scientific World Journal, 2014*, 649036.

American Association of Neuroscience Nurses. (2014). *Care of the adult patient with a brain tumor.* Glenview, IL: Author.

American Association of Neuroscience Nurses. (2016). *AANN Core Curriculum for neuroscience nursing* (6th ed.). Glenview, IL: Author.

American Association of Nurses and American Association of Neuroscience Nurses. (2013). *Neuroscience nursing: Scope and standards of practice.* Glenview, IL: Author.

Bonner, S. & Smith, C. (2013). Initial management of acute spinal cord injury. *Continuing Education in Anaesthesia, Critical Care & Pain, 13*(6), 224–231.

Brettler, S., & Merchant, K. (2016). Movement disorders. In M. K. Bader, L. R. Littlejohns, & D. M. Olson (Eds.), *AANN core curriculum for neuroscience nursing* (pp. 527–534). Glenview, IL: AANN.

Britton, P. N., Eastwood, K., Brew, B. J., et al. (2015). Consensus guidelines for the investigation and management of encephalitis. *Medical Journal of Australia, 202,* 576–577.

Carney, N., Totten, A. M., O'Reilly, C., et al. (2016). *Guidelines for the management of severe traumatic brain injury* (4th ed.). Campbell, CA: Brain Injury Foundation, 1–244.

Chin, L. (2016). Spinal Cord Injuries Treatment & Management. *Medscape Drugs and Diseases.* Available: *http://emedicine.medscape.com/article/793582*

Connolly, E. S., Rabinstein, A. A., Carhuapoma, R., et al. (2012). Guidelines for the management of aneurysmal subarachnoid hemorrhage: a guideline for healthcare professionals from the American Heart Association/American Stroke Association. *Stroke, 43,* 1711–1737.

Cruccu, G., Finnerup, N. B., Sindou, M., et al. (2016). Trigeminal neuralgia: New classification and diagnostic grading for practice and research

deGroot, J. F. (2015). High grade gliomas. *Continuum.* 21(2), 332–344. *Neurology, 87,* 220–228. e, 31(4), 403–479.

Derdeyn, C. P., Zipfel, G. J., F., Albuquerque, F. C., et al. (2017). Management of brain arteriovenous malformations: A scientific statement for healthcare professionals from the American Heart Association/American Stroke Association. *Stroke, 48,* e00–e00.

De Oliveira Manoel, A. E., Goffi, A., Marotta, T. R., et al. (2016). The critical care management of poor-grade subarachnoid haemorrhage. *Critical Care, 20,* 21. Available: *https://ccforum.biomedcentral.com/articles/10.1186/s13054-016-1193-9*

D'Souza, S. (2015). Aneurysmal subarachnoid hemorrhage. *Journal of Neurosurgical Anesthesiology, 27*(3), 222–240.

Eviston, T. J., Croxson, G. R., Kennedy, P. G. E., et al. (2015). Bell's palsy: Aetiology, clinical features and multidisciplinary care. *Journal of Neurology Neurosurgery Psychiatry, 86,* 1356–1361.

Fehlings M. G., Vaccaro, A., Wilson, J., Singh, A., Cadotte, D. W., Harrop, J. S., … Rampersaud, R. (2012). Early versus delayed decompression for traumatic cervical spinal cord injury: Results of the Surgical Timing in Acute Spinal Cord Injury Study (STASCIS). *PLOS ONE, 7*(2), e32037. Available: *http://dx.doi. org/10.1371/journal.pone.0032037*

Fehlings, M. G., Tetreault, L. A., Wilson, J. R., et al. (2017). A Clinical Practice Guideline for the Management of Acute Spinal Cord Injury: Introduction, Rationale, and Scope. *Global Spine Journal, 7*(3S), 84S–94S.

Fowler, S. B., Herrington, J. B., Koopman, W. J., & Ricci, M. M. (2014). Care of the patient with Myasthenia Gravis. *AANN Clinical Practice Guideline Series.* Chicago, IL: AANN.

Grasso, G., Alafaci, C., & Macdonald, R. L. (2017). Management of aneurysmal subarachnoid hemorrhage: State of the art and future perspectives. *Surgical Neurology International.* 8, 11.

Greenberg, M. (2016). *Handbook of neurosurgery* (8th ed.). New York: Thieme Medical Publishers.

Gupta., P, Noskho, M. G., & Miller, J. P. (2015). Intracranial pressure monitoring. *eMedicine.* Available: *http://emedicine.medscape.com/article/1829950*

Hadley, M. N., Walters, B. C., Aarabi, B., et al. (2013). Guidelines for the management of acute cervical spine and spinal cord injuries. *Neurosurgery, 72*(2), 1–94.

Harary, M., Dolmans, R. G. F., & Gormely, W. B. (2018). Intracranial pressure monitoring-Review and areas for development. *Sensors,* 18, 465.

Harrop, J. S. (2016). Spinal cord tumors—management of intradural intramedullary neoplasms. Treatment and management. *Medscape Drugs and Diseases.* Available: *http://emedicine.medscape.com/article/249306*

Hauser, S., & Josephson, S. (2017). *Harrison's neurology in clinical medicine* (4th ed.). New York: McGraw-Hill.

Hayat, M. A. (2015). *Tumors of the central nervous system glioma, meningioma, neuroblastoma, and spinal tumors* (Vol. 14). New York: Springer.

Hemphill, J. C., Greenberg, S. M. Anderson, C. S., et al. (2015). Guidelines for the management of spontaneous intracerebral hemorrhage. *Stroke, 46*(7), 2032–2060.

Hinkle, J. L., Morrison, K., & Siewert, L. (2016). Ischemic stroke. In M. K. Bader, L. Littlejohns, & D. M. Oldson (Eds.), *AANN core curriculum for neuroscience nursing* (6th ed., pp. 229–246). Glenview, IL: AANN.

Hutchinson, P. J., Kolias, A. G., Timofeev I. S., et al.; for the RESCUEicp Trial Collaborators. (2016) Trial of decompressive craniectomy for traumatic intracranial hypertension. *New England Journal of Medicine, 375,* 1119–1130.

Jeong, H. W., Seo, J. H., Kim, S. T., Jung, C. K., & Suh, S. (2014). Clinical practice guideline for the management of intracranial aneurysms. *Neurointervention, 9*(2), 63–71. Available: *http://doi.org/10.5469/neuroint.2014.9.2.63*

Kawoos, U., McCarron, R. M., Auker, C. R., & Chavko, M. (2015). Advances in intracranial pressure monitoring and its significance in managing traumatic brain injury. *International Journal of Molecular Sciences, 16*(12), 28979–28997.

Khoo, T. K., Yarnall, A. J., Duncan, G. W., et al. (2013). The spectrum of nonmotor symptoms in early Parkinson disease. *Neurology, 80,* 276–281.

Kinoshita, K. (2016). Traumatic brain injury: pathophysiology for neurocritical care. *Journal of Intensive Care, 4*(29), 2–10.

Koopman, W. J., & Ricci, M. M. (2016). Neuromuscular disorders. In M. K. Bader, L. R. Littlejohns, & D. M. Olson (Eds.), *AANN core curriculum for neuroscience nursing* (pp. 574–577). Glenview, IL: AANN.

Kriebel-Gasparro, A. (2016). Parkinson's disease: update on medication management. *Journal for Nurse Practitioners, 12,* e81–e89.

Layon, A. J., Gabriella, A., & Friedman, W. (2014). *Textbook of neurointensive care.* London: Springer-Verlag.

Liebeskind, D. S., Kirshner, H. S., & Lutsep, H. L. (2016). Cerebral aneurysms. medscape drugs and diseases. Available: *http://emedicine.medscape.com/article/1161518-overview*

Magennis, B., & Corry, M. (2013). Parkinson's disease: making the diagnosis and monitoring progression. *British Journal of Neuroscience Nursing, 9,* 167–171.

Maloni, H., & Remington, G. (2016). Degenerative disorders. In M. K. Bader, L. Littlejohns, & D. M. Oldson (Eds.). *AANN core curriculum for neuroscience nursing* (6th ed., pp. 511–525). Glenview, IL: AANN.

Maloni, H. (2018). Cognitive impairment in multiple sclerosis. *Jounral for Nurse Practitioners,* 14(3), 172–177.

Marupudi, N. I. & Mittal, S. (2015). Diagnosis and management of hyponatremia in patients with aneurysmal subarachnoid hemorrhage. *Journal of Clinical Medicine, 4*(4), 756–767.

Ovbiagele, B., Black, H. R., Bravata, D. M., et al. (2014). Guidelines for the prevention of stroke in patients with stroke and transient ischemic attack. *Stroke, 45,* 2160–2236.

Powers, W. J., Rabinstein, A. A., Ackerson, T., et al. (2018). 2018 Guidelines for the early management of patients with acute ischemic stroke: A guideline for healthcare professionals from the American Heart Association/American Stroke Association. *Stroke, 49,* e46–e99.

Roth, P., & Weller, M. (2015). Management of neoplastic meningitis. *Chinese Clinical Oncology, 4,* 1–8.

Sahrakar, K. (2015). Lumbar disc disease. *Medscape Drugs and Diseases.* Available: *http://emedicine.medscape.com/article/249113-overview*

Sieb, J. P. (2013). Myasthenia gravis: an update for the clinician. *Clinical and Experimental Immunology, 175,* 408–418.

Smith, M. (2016). Critical care management of severe head injury. *Intensive Care Medicine, 15*(4), 164–167.

Solomon, R. A. & Connolly, E. S. (2017). Arteriovenous malformations of the brain. *New England Journal of Medicine, 376,* 1859–1866.

Stocchetti, N., & Zanier, E. R. (2016). Chronic impact of traumatic brain injury on outcome and quality of life: A narrative review. *Critical Care, 20*(148), 1–10.

Stupp, R., Brada, M., van den Bent, M. J., et al. (2014). High-grade glioma: ESMO clinical practice guidelines for diagnosis, treatment and follow-up. *Annuals of Oncology, 25*(suppl 3), ii93–iii101.

Stone, N. J., Robinson, J. G., Lichtenstein, A. H., et al. (2013). 2013 ACC/AHA guidelines on the treatment of blood cholesterol to reduce atherosclerotic cardiovascular risks in adults. *Stroke, 129* (suppl 2), S1–S45.

Sudulagunta, S. R., Sodalagunta, M. B., Khorram, H., et al. (2015). Guillian-Barre syndrome: Clinical profile and management. *German Medical Science, 13,* 1–15.

Tepper, S. J. & Tepper, D. E. (2014). *The cleveland clinic manual of headache therapy.* New York: Springer.

Thompson, B. G., Brown, R. D., Amin-Hanjani, S., et al. (2015). Guidelines for the management of patients with unruptured intracranial aneurysms: a guideline for healthcare professionals from the American Heart Association/American Stroke Association. *Stroke, 46,* 2368–2400.

Vakharia, K., & Vakharia, K. (2016). Bell's palsy. *Facial Plastic Surgery Clinics of North America, 24,* 1–10.

van Es, M. A., Hardiman, O., Chio, A., et al. (2017). Amyotrophic lateral sclerosis. *The Lancet, 390,* 2084–2098.

Wong, C. C., & McGirt, M. J. (2013). Vertebral compression fractures: A review of current management and multimodal therapy. *Journal of Multidisciplinary Healthcare, 6,* 205–214.

Yousem, D. M., & Grossman, R. I. (2017). *Neuroradiology: The requisites* (4th ed.). Philadelphia, PA: Elsevier.

Zasler, N. D., Katz, D. I., & Zafontw, R. D. (2013). *Brain injury medicine; principles and practice.* New York: Demos Medical.

16
Eye Disorders

INTRODUCTION
Terms and Abbreviations

Definitions of Terms

1. *Accommodation:* Focusing apparatus of the eye that adjusts to objects at different distances by means of increasing the convexity of the lens (brought about by contraction of the ciliary muscles).
2. *Ametropia:* Abnormal vision.
   a. *Myopia:* Nearsightedness: rays of light coming from an object at a distance of 20 feet or more are brought to a focus in front of the retina.
   b. *Hyperopia:* Farsightedness: rays of light coming from an object at a distance of 20 feet or more are brought to a focus in back of the retina.
3. *Astigmatism:* Uneven curvature of the cornea causing the patient to be unable to focus horizontal and vertical rays of light on the retina at the same time.
4. *Emmetropia:* Normal vision: rays of light coming from an object at a distance of 20 feet (6 m) or more are brought to focus on the retina by the lens (see Figure 16-1).
5. *Presbyopia:* The elasticity of the lens decreases with increasing age; an emmetropic person with presbyopia will read the paper at arm's length and will require prescription lenses to correct the problem.
6. *Strabismus:* Deviation of the eye so that the visual axes are not physiologically coordinated.
7. *Vision:* Passage of rays of light from an object through the cornea, aqueous humor, lens, and vitreous humor to the retina and its appreciation in the cerebral cortex.
8. *Visual acuity:* Measurement of a person's ability to see at a distance or near (reading distance) and is measured against a standard of a normal person's visual ability.

Common Abbreviations

OD (oculus dexter) or RE—right eye.
OS (oculus sinister) or LE—left eye.

OU (oculus unitas)—both eyes.
IOP—intraocular pressure.
IOL—intraocular lens.
EOL—extraocular lens.
VA—visual acuity.

Eye Care Specialists

1. **Ophthalmologist:** Physician specializing in diagnosis, surgery, and treatment of the eye; may specialize in a specific part of the eye or disorder, such as a cornea specialist or glaucoma specialist.
2. **Optometrist:** Doctor of optometry who can examine, diagnose, and manage visual problems and diseases of the eye but does not perform surgery.
3. **Optician:** Technician who fits, adjusts, and gives eyeglasses or other devices on the written prescription of an ophthalmologist or optometrist.
4. **Ocularist:** Technician who makes ophthalmic prostheses.

Subjective Data

EVIDENCE BASE American Society of Ophthalmologic Registered Nurses. (2014). *Essentials of ophthalmic nursing. Book 1* (2nd ed.). San Francisco, CA: Author.

Subjective data for eye assessment include complaints of altered vision or other symptoms, associated lifestyle and other factors, and recent and past health history.

Presenting Symptoms

1. Explore the chief complaint from patient by asking the following questions:
   a. Is there pain, foreign body sensation (scratchy, something in the eye), photophobia, dryness, redness, itchiness, lacrimation, or drainage?

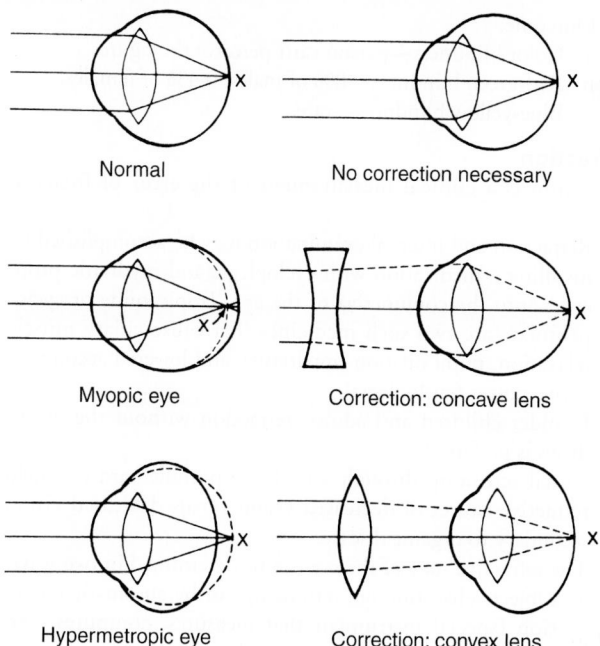

Figure 16-1. Normal vision and refractory errors.

b. Is there blurred vision, double vision, loss of vision, or change in vision in a portion of the visual field?
c. Are there other visual symptoms such as glare, halos, floaters?
d. Is there difficulty in functioning, such as driving or reading, because of visual problem?
2. Review related systems.
  a. Neurologic: Are there scintillations, scotomas, transient ischemic attacks, headache, sensory or motor dysfunction?
  b. Ear, nose, and throat: Any nasal congestion, rhinitis, sinus pain, dry mouth?
  c. Integumentary: Are there changes in skin and mucous membranes?
  d. Endocrine: Any complaints of polyuria, polydipsia; signs of hyperthyroidism (see page 709)?
  e. Musculoskeletal: Is there joint pain or swelling?

History

1. Review ocular history.
  a. Have there been previous eye injuries, surgeries, and ocular procedures?
  b. Is patient using glasses or contact lenses?
  c. Was there childhood poor vision or patching of the eye?
  d. Are there current visual problems such as glaucoma, cataracts, macular degeneration, or diabetic retinopathy?
2. Obtain medication history, including nonprescription, herbal, topical, and inhalant products.
3. Determine allergies to medications; note type of reaction.
4. Determine history of systemic conditions such as diabetes, cardiovascular disease, arthritis, Marfan syndrome, albinism, sickle cell anemia.
5. Obtain family history of ocular conditions such as glaucoma, cataracts, macular degeneration, color blindness, retinitis pigmentosa, retinoblastoma, nystagmus, keratoconus, choroideremia, corneal dystrophies, and other chronic diseases.

6. Perform functional assessment.
  a. Depending on the patient's circumstance, administer the National Eye Institute Visual Function Questionnaire (VFQ-25) available at *www.rand.org/health/surveys_tools/vfq.html*, or other valid visual functioning questionnaires such as the VF-14.
  b. This helps determine the need for surgery based on the extent to which the eye disorder interferes with the patient's ability to carry out a visually dependent activity of daily living such as driving and reading.

GERONTOLOGIC ALERT Question older patients about driving. Change in driving pattern, such as avoidance of night driving and less rush-hour driving, may indicate visual dysfunction as well as impaired reflexes and ability to concentrate in complex situations. A common complaint is not being able to read road signs in time to respond to them.

Ocular Examination

See Figure 16-2. Also see "Adult Physical Assessment," page 45.

NURSING ALERT Every patient who seeks medical attention for an eye complaint should have visual acuity tested.

External Examination

Includes examination of the eye and accessory organs without the aid of special apparatus.

Visual Acuity at Distance (Snellen Chart and Other Methods)
1. Letters and objects are of different sizes that can be seen by the normal eye at a distance of 20 feet (6 m) from the chart.
2. Letters appear in rows and are arranged, so the normal eye can see them at distances of 30, 40, and 50 feet (9, 12, and 15 m), and so forth.

Figure 16-2. Three-dimensional cross-section of the eye. (Smeltzer, S., and Bare, B. [2000]. *Brunner and Suddarth's textbook of medical-surgical nursing* [9th ed.]. Philadelphia: Lippincott Williams & Wilkins.)

3. Each eye is tested separately, with and without correction (glasses or contact lenses), whereas the nontesting eye is completely occluded.
4. Test the right eye (OD) first and then the left eye (OS).
5. A person who can identify letters of the size 20 at 20 feet (6 at 6 m) is said to have 20/20 (6/6) vision.
6. If vision is less than 20/200 (6/60), additional tests may be recorded as:
   a. Counting fingers (CF)—at feet (meters).
   b. Hand motion (HM)—ability to detect hand movement at a certain distance.
   c. Light perception and projection (LP).
   d. Light perception only.
   e. No light perception.

Visual Acuity at Near (Jaeger Chart and Other Methods)

1. Letters and objects are of different sizes that can be seen by the normal eye at a reading distance of 14 inches from the chart.
2. Letters appear in rows and are arranged, so the normal eye can read them at different levels on the Jaeger chart.
3. Each eye is tested separately, with and without correction (glasses or contact lenses), whereas the nontesting eye is completely occluded.
4. Test the right eye (OD) first and then the left eye (OS).
5. The vision is documented in Jaeger or Snellen notation where J1+ is equivalent to 20/20, J2 equivalent to 20/30, and so forth.

Visual Fields

Determines function of optic pathways and identifies loss of visual field and functional capacity.
1. Equipment—light source and test objects. May be performed manually or as automated visual fields.
2. Peripheral field—useful in detecting decreased peripheral vision in one or both eyes.
   a. Patient is seated 18 to 24 inches (45.5 to 61 cm) in front of the examiner.
   b. The left eye is covered, whereas the patient focuses with the right eye on a spot about 12 inches (30.5 cm) from the eye.
   c. A test object is brought in from the side at 15-degree intervals through a complete 360 degrees.
   d. The patient signals when he or she sees the test object and again when the object disappears through the 360 degrees.

Color Vision Tests

These tests are done to determine the person's ability to perceive primary colors and shades of colors. It is particularly significant for people whose occupation requires discerning colors, such as artists, interior decorators, transportation workers, surgeons, and nurses. (Useful in diagnosing diffuse retinal dysfunction and various types of optic neuropathies.)
1. Equipment.
   a. Polychromatic plates—dots of primary colors printed on a background of similar dots in a confusion of colors.
   b. Individual colored disks—each disk is matched to its next closest color.
2. Procedure.
   a. Various polychromatic plates are presented to the patient under specified illumination.
   b. The patterns may be letters or numbers that the normal eye can perceive instantly, but that are confusing to the person with a perception defect.

3. Outcome.
   a. Color blindness—person can't perceive the figures.
   b. Red-green blindness—8% of males, 0.4% of females.
   c. Blue-yellow blindness—rare.

Refraction

Refraction is a clinical measurement of the error of focus in an eye.
1. Refraction and internal examination may be accomplished by instilling a medication with cycloplegic and mydriatic properties into the conjunctiva of the eye. Tropicamide or cyclopentolate are two such medicines that cause ciliary muscle relaxation, pupil dilation (mydriasis), and lowered accommodative power (cycloplegia).
2. In older children and adults, refraction without the use of drugs is preferred.
3. Visual screening through a multiple pinhole card can help refractive causes of decreased vision versus decreased vision secondary to organic disease.
4. The refractive state of the eye can be determined in two ways:
   a. Objectively—through retinoscopy or by automatic refraction (special instrument that measures, computes, and prints out refraction errors of each eye).
   b. Subjectively—trial of lenses to arrive at the best visual image.

Internal Examination

Ophthalmoscopic Examination

1. Direct ophthalmoscopy—uses a strong light reflected into the interior of the eye through an instrument called an ophthalmoscope.
2. Indirect ophthalmoscopy—allows the examiner to obtain a stereoscopic view of the retina. Light source is from a head-mounted light. The examiner views the retina through a convex lens held in front of the eye and a viewing device on the head mount. The image appears inverted. This method of examination allows the examiner to use binocular vision with depth perception and a wider viewing field.
3. Clinical significance:
   a. Detection of cataracts, vitreous opacities, corneal scars.
   b. Close examination for the pathologic changes in retinal blood vessels that may occur with diabetes or hypertension.
   c. Examination of the choroid for tumors or inflammation.
   d. Examination of the retina for retinal detachment, scars, or exudates and hemorrhages.

Slit-Lamp Examination

1. Special equipment that magnifies the cornea, sclera, and anterior chamber and provides oblique views into the trabeculum for examination by the ophthalmologist.
2. Helps detect disorders of the anterior portion of the eye.
3. The room is generally darkened and the pupils are dilated.
4. The patient sits with chin and forehead resting against equipment supports.

Tonometry

1. Measures IOP, which depends on the amount of aqueous humor secreted into the eye and ease by which it leaves.
2. Tonometry is indicated as one of the measurements to screen for glaucoma, assess the development of glaucoma if suspected, evaluate glaucoma therapy, and diagnose phthisis and drug-induced IOP increase.
3. Normal tension is considered less than or equal to 20 mm Hg.

Figure 16-3. Example of an applanation tonometer.

4. Tonometry techniques.
   a. Goldmann applanation tonometry (see Figure 16-3).
      i. This is the most effective measuring method for determining IOP; however, it requires a biomicroscope and a trained interpreter. May be part of the slit-lamp examination or done by hand-held device.
      ii. After instillation of topical anesthesia, the cornea is flattened by a known amount (3.14 mm).
      iii. The pressure necessary to produce this flattening is equal to the IOP, counterbalancing the tonometer.
   b. Schiotz tonometry (rarely used at present).
   c. Electronic tonometer that provides a digital reading of IOP, such as the Tono-Pen.
   d. Pneumatonometer or air applanation tonometry—requires no topical anesthesia and measures tension by sensing deformation of the cornea in reaction to a puff of pressurized air.
   e. Perkins hand-held tonometer.
   f. Finger tension—pressure determined by use of digital pressure.

Radiology and Imaging

Several imaging studies beyond the basic eye examination may be done to further evaluate eye disease.

Fluorescein Angiography

Description

1. Provides information concerning vascular obstructions, microaneurysms, abnormal capillary permeability, and defects in retinal pigment permeability.

2. Introduction of sodium fluorescein IV administration over several minutes, usually through a brachial vein.
3. Indirect ophthalmoscopy using a blue filter may be done and photographs of the ocular fundus are obtained.

Nursing and Patient Care Considerations

1. Advise the patient that a series of eye drops will be given to dilate the pupil for better visualization of the retina. The patient will be positioned in a special chair with head immobilized.
2. Dye will be injected into the arm over several minutes. Photographs will be taken during injection and up to 1 hour after injection.
3. Adverse effects include nausea because of dye injection, burning in eye from eye drop instillation, blurred vision and photophobia for 4 to 8 hours because of pupil dilation, and possible yellow skin and urine discoloration for up to 48 hours after dye injection.

 DRUG ALERT Serious reactions, such as hoarseness, respiratory obstruction, tachycardia, and anaphylactic reaction leading to death may result from sodium fluorescein IV administration.

Eye and Orbit Sonography

Description

1. Sound waves are used in the diagnosis of intraocular and orbital lesions. Three types of ultrasonography are used in ophthalmoscopy:
   a. A-scan—uses stationary transducers to measure the distance between changes in acoustic density. This is used to differentiate between benign and malignant tumors and to measure the length of the eye to determine the power of an IOL.
   b. B-scan—moves linearly across the eye; increases in acoustic density are shown as an intensification on the line of the scan that presents a picture of the eye and the orbit.
   c. IOL Master technology—evaluates the length of the eye, surface curvature, and IOL power; has increased the accuracy of biometry by fivefold. It is also less technician-dependent for accuracy.
2. Abnormal patterns are seen in alkali burns, detached retina, keratoprosthesis, thyroid ophthalmopathy, foreign bodies, vascular malformations, benign and malignant tumors, and a variety of other conditions.

Nursing and Patient Care Considerations

1. Advise the patient that topical anesthetic drops are applied to the eye before the procedure so the patient will not feel the transducer contacting the eye.
2. The procedure may take as little as 8 to 10 minutes or 30 minutes or longer, if a lesion is detected, to locate the lesion.
3. Warn patient not to rub eyes until the anesthetic has worn off to avoid trauma to the eye.

Electroretinography

Description

Used to evaluate hereditary and acquired disorders of the retina; an electrode is placed over the eye to evaluate the electrical response to light.

Nursing and Patient Care Considerations

1. Advise the patient that the eyes are propped open and patient will be positioned lying or sitting down.

2. Topical anesthetic drops are instilled.
3. A cotton wick electrode saturated in saline is applied to the cornea.
4. Various intensities of light are produced and the electrical potential is measured.
5. Caution the patient not to rub eyes for up to 1 hour after procedure to avoid trauma while eyes are anesthetized.

GENERAL PROCEDURES AND TREATMENT MODALITIES

 See additional online content: Procedure Guidelines 16-1–16-5.

Common Eye Procedures

Instillation of Medications

1. Ophthalmic medications may be used for diagnostic and therapeutic purposes:
   a. To dilate or contract the pupil.
   b. To relieve pain, discomfort, itching, and inflammation.
   c. To act as an antiseptic in cleansing the eye.
   d. To combat infection.
2. Solution or ointment is administered using clean technique.
   a. Use one finger to pull downward on skin of lower lid.
   b. Drop solution or squeeze out 1/8 inch ribbon of ointment into center of conjunctival sac.
   c. Instruct the patient to close eye slowly but do not squeeze lids tightly or rub them.

See Figure 16-4 and Table 16-1.

Irrigation of the Eye

1. Ocular irrigation is often necessary for the following:
   a. To irrigate chemicals or foreign bodies from the eyes.
   b. To remove secretions from the conjunctival sac.
   c. To treat infections or relieve itching.
   d. To provide moisture on the surface of the eyes of an unconscious patient.
2. Use prescribed solution or 1,000 mL of normal saline solution with IV tubing.
3. Test pH with litmus paper before flushing if chemical injury is suspected and after irrigation until pH is 7.
4. Evert the lower conjunctival sac and have the patient look up, and then direct the irrigating solution from the inner canthus toward the outer canthus along the lower conjunctival sac.

Application of Dressing or Patch

1. One or both eyes may need shielding for the following:
   a. To keep an eye at rest, thereby promoting healing.
   b. To prevent the patient from touching eye.

Figure 16-4. Instilling eye medication: **(A)** solution (drops) and **(B)** ointment.

c. To absorb secretions.
d. To protect the eye.
e. To control or lessen edema.
2. Instill ointment if directed and make sure that eye is closed before securing gauze patch or eye shield with tape strips placed diagonally from midforehead to outer cheek.

Removing a Particle from the Eye

1. Typically, removing a foreign body from the eye is an uncomplicated first-aid measure.
   a. As the patient looks upward, place your finger below the lower lid and pull downward to expose the conjunctival sac.
   b. Inspect for particles using a light and magnifying lens.
   c. Remove particle with cotton-tipped applicator moistened in saline by gently wiping across the conjunctival sac.
2. If no offending particle is found, proceed to the upper lid.
   a. As the patient looks downward, place the cotton applicator horizontally on the upper lid and gently pull the lid outward and upward over the applicator (see Figure 16-5).
   b. Remove particle if found and return eyelid to neutral position.
3. If a particle appears to be embedded, medical intervention is required, that is, local anesthetic, antibiotic therapy, and clinical expertise in using other instruments.
4. The cornea should be evaluated for abrasion from the foreign body by use of fluorescein staining, even if a foreign body cannot be found.

Removing Contact Lenses

1. Because contact lenses need regular cleaning and changing, if a person is injured and incapacitated because of an accident, sickness, or other cause, the lenses should be removed.
2. Determine the type of lens from the patient or family.
   a. Soft corneal lenses are widely used. The diameter covers the cornea plus a portion of the sclera of the eye. Extended- and daily-wear soft lenses are available.
   b. Rigid or gas-permeable lenses are usually smaller than the cornea of the eye, although some are made to extend beyond the cornea onto the sclera of the eye. These lenses need to be removed promptly.
3. Do not remove lenses if the iris is not visible on opening the eyelids; await the arrival of an ophthalmologist. If patient is to be transported, note that contacts are in the eyes. (Write out the message and tape it to the patient or send with transporter.)
4. To remove soft lenses, retract the lower lid and attempt to slide the lens off the cornea using your index finger, and then pinch the lens between 2 fingers and gently remove it.

Ocular Surgery

Common types of ocular surgery are described, followed by a nursing process overview for any patient having ocular surgery. Also see the following entries for specific surgical care: conditions of the eyelids, page 441; cataract, page 442; retinal detachment, page 448; and acute glaucoma and chronic glaucoma, page 446.

Corneal Transplantation (Keratoplasty)

Description
1. The transplantation of a donor cornea, usually obtained at autopsy, to repair a corneal scar, burn, deformity, or dystrophy.

Table 16-1 Ophthalmic Pharmacologic Agents*

PHARMACOLOGY	ACTION	PRODUCTS
Sympathomimetics	Given topically for the treatment of glaucoma. Immediate effect is decrease in production of aqueous humor. Long-term effect is an increase in outflow of aqueous humor. May be used in combination with miotics, beta-adrenergic blockers, carbonic anhydrase inhibitors, or hyperosmotic agents.	• Epinephrine • Dipivefrin • Phenylephrine
Miotics, direct-acting	Cholinergic agents given topically that affect the muscarinic receptors of the eye; results include miosis and contraction of the ciliary muscle. In narrow-angle glaucoma, miosis opens the angle to improve aqueous outflow. Contraction of the ciliary muscle enhances the outflow of aqueous humor by indirect action of the trabecular network—the exact mechanism is unknown. Primary use of miotics is in glaucoma but can be used to counter the effects of cycloplegics/mydriatics.	• Acetylcholine • Carbachol • Pilocarpine
Miotics, cholinesterase inhibitors	Topical agents that inhibit the enzyme cholinesterase, causing an increase in the activity of the acetylcholine already present in the body. Causes intense miosis and contraction of the ciliary muscle. Decrease in IOP that is seen as a result of increased outflow of aqueous humor. Used for treatment of open-angle glaucoma, conditions where the outflow of aqueous is obstructed; post iridectomy problems; and accommodative esotropia (inward deviation of one eye).	• Demecarium bromide • Isoflurophate • Physostigmine
Beta-adrenergic blockers	Act on the beta receptors of the adrenergic nervous system. Two types of beta sites: B_1 and B_2. The B_1 site is primarily the myocardium resulting in decreased heart rate and cardiac output. B_2 primarily bronchial and vascular smooth muscle resulting in bronchoconstriction, decreased blood pressure. There are two types of ophthalmic beta-adrenergic blockers: cardioselective blocker (betaxolol) acts only on B_1 sites and may on rare occasions cause cardiac effects if absorbed systemically. All other nonselective blockers act on B_1 and B_2 sites and cause significant cardiac and pulmonary effects if absorbed systemically. Used for treatment of increased IOP by decreasing the formation of aqueous humor and causing a slight increase in the outflow facility.	• Betaxolol • Levobunolol • Timolol • Carteolol
Carbonic anhydrase inhibitors	Oral agents that act to inhibit the action of carbonic anhydrase. Suppression of this enzyme results in a decreased production of aqueous humor. Used in combination regimen to treat glaucoma and postoperative rise in IOP.	• Acetazolamide • Methazolamide
Osmotic diuretics	Osmotic agents given intravenously used for reduction of IOP in acute attack of glaucoma or before ocular surgery where preoperative reduction of IOP is indicated.	• Mannitol • Glycerin
Prostaglandin analogues	Newer agents used in the lowering of IOP presumably by increasing uvealscleral flow or filtration of aqueous. Used in open-angle glaucoma resistant to other agents.	• Latanoprost • Travoprost • Bimatoprost • Unoprostone
Mydriatics	Topical agents that result in dilation of the pupil, vasoconstriction, and an increase in the outflow of aqueous humor. Used for pupillary dilatation for surgery and examination.	• Phenylephrine
Cycloplegic mydriatics	Topical agents that block the reaction of the sphincter muscle of the iris and the muscle of the ciliary body to cholinergic stimulation, resulting in dilatation of the pupil (mydriasis) and paralysis of accommodation (cycloplegia). Used in conditions requiring pupil to be dilated and kept from accommodation.	• Atropine • Homatropine • Scopolamine • Cyclopentolate • Tropicamide
Ophthalmic anti-infectives	Topical agents used for treatment of ophthalmic infections. Commercial products are intended for treatment of superficial ocular problems, such as conjunctivitis and blepharitis. Extemporaneous (compounded) drops are used for more serious topical infections (ie, corneal ulcer, endophthalmitis [intraocular infection]).	*Antibiotics* • Bacitracin • Chloramphenicol • Ciprofloxacin • Erythromycin • Gentamicin • Gatifloxacin • Levofloxacin • Moxifloxacin

(continued)

Table 16-1   Ophthalmic Pharmacologic Agents* *(Continued)*

PHARMACOLOGY	ACTION	PRODUCTS
		• Neomycin/polymyxin/ bacitracin • Norfloxacin • Sulfacetamide • Tobramycin *Antifungal* • Amphotericin B • Fluconazole • Natamycin *Antiviral* • Trifluridine • Vidarabine
Local anesthetics	Block the transmission of nerve impulses. Used topically to provide local anesthetic for tests, such as tonometry, and for procedures of short duration. Injections used in ophthalmology for retrobulbar blocks.	*Topical* • Proparacaine • Tetracaine injection • Lidocaine
Ophthalmic steroid anti-inflammatories	Mostly corticosteroids. Used topically to relieve pain and photophobia as well as suppress other inflammatory processes of the conjunctiva, cornea, lid, and interior segment of the globe.	• Dexamethasone • Fluorometholone • Loteprednol • Prednisolone acetate
Nonsteroidal anti-inflammatory drugs (NSAIDs)	Act by inhibiting an enzyme involved in the synthesis of prostaglandins, which are key in the body's response to inflammation. These drugs, given topically, are analgesics and anti-inflammatories.	• Diclofenac sodium • Flurbiprofen • Ketorolac • Suprofen
Anti-allergy medications	There are a number of different types of drugs, given topically, in this category, including antihistamine, mast cell stabilizers, NSAID anesthetic, and astringents (some in combination).	*Antihistamines* • Emedastine • Levocabastine • Olopatadine • Pheniramine *Mast cell stabilizers* • Cromolyn • Lodoxamide *Astringent* • Zinc sulfate
Vasoconstrictors	Topical agents that contract local blood vessels, resulting in less redness and irritation.	• Naphazoline
Alpha-selective adrenergic agonist agents	Topical agents that mimic the effects of endogenous adrenergic compounds by selectively binding to alpha-2 receptors, resulting in aqueous formation, pupil diameter, and ocular flow. Commonly used for lowering elevated IOP.	• Apraclonidine hydrochloride • Brimonidine tartrate
Anti-VEGF agents	Slow growth of abnormal blood vessels under the retina by blocking the effects of VEGF to slow vision loss and possibly improve vision in wet age-related macular degeneration.	• Bevacizumab • Pegaptanib • Ranibizumab

*All pharmacologic agents should be reviewed from manufacturer's information or drug reference source before administration for contraindications, adverse reactions, and cautions.
IOP, intraocular pressure; VEGF, vascular endothelial growth factor.

Figure 16-5. Removing a particle from the eye.

2. Types of grafts.
  a. Full thickness (6.5 to 8 mm)—most common.
  b. Partial-thickness lamellar.
3. Fresh cornea is the preferred tissue; it is removed from the donor within 12 hours after death and used within 24 hours.
4. Special solutions for storage of fresh cornea are available, which may extend storage up to 3 days.
5. *Cryopreservation* is the care and handling of a corneal graft by freezing to retain its transparency.

Complications

1. Hemorrhage.
2. Graft dislocation.
3. Infection.
4. Postoperative glaucoma.
5. Graft rejection—may occur 10 to 14 days postoperatively; signs and symptoms include decreased vision, ocular irritation, corneal edema, and red sclera.

Refractive Surgery

Description

1. A variety of procedures used to correct nearsightedness, farsightedness, and astigmatism; may eliminate need for glasses or contact lenses, especially with aging.
2. May not be appropriate with corneal disease, retinal disease, glaucoma, severe diabetes, uncontrolled vascular disease, autoimmune disease, or pregnancy.
3. There is no guarantee on desired effect, but complication rate is extremely low.
4. Procedures are quick, performed in physician's office or clinic, and most people are back to full activity in 1 to 3 days.
5. Specific procedures are used to correct nearsightedness, farsightedness, or astigmatism.
6. May eliminate need for glasses, especially with aging.

Types of Procedures

1. Radial keratotomy.
   a. Procedure designed to provide correction of myopia (nearsightedness).
   b. The cornea is anesthetized topically, and under a microscope, the surgeon marks the visual axis.
   c. Eight to sixteen radial incisions are made into the corneal surface to flatten it. This permits images to fall on the retina instead of in front of it.
   d. Time to optimal correction is about 3 months. (Procedure is being performed much less frequently now with the development of laser surgery for refraction.)
2. Excimer photorefractive keratectomy.
   a. Limited to correcting myopia and some astigmatism.
   b. The front surface of the corneal epithelium is removed (by laser, manual scraping, or both).
   c. The laser is then used to change the corneal curvature by vaporizing the tissue (reshaping or sculpting the cornea).
   d. Optimal visual recovery about 6 months.
3. Laser-assisted in situ keratomileusis (LASIK); also laser-automated lamellar keratoplasty (laser ALK).
   a. Procedure is designed to treat a wider range of prescriptions than the other refractive procedures.
   b. Microsurgical instrument (microkeratome) is used to create a corneal flap.
   c. A cool laser beam (using an excimer laser) reshapes the cornea and the flap is then closed.
   d. The excimer laser can remove corneal tissue with an accuracy of up to 0.25 microns.
   e. Only about 50 microns of tissue are removed to achieve the desired correction.
   f. Refractive recovery about 3 months.
4. Holmium laser thermokeratoplasty (Holmium LTK).
   a. Tissue is heated, not vaporized.
   b. Cornea is marked to pinpoint where to aim the laser.
   c. The laser heats only selected portions of the cornea to shrink collagen fibers around the cornea edges.

Vitrectomy

1. This procedure is performed for conditions such as unresolved hemorrhage with diabetic retinopathy, intraocular foreign body, and vitreoretinal adhesions.
2. It involves the removal of all or part of the vitreous humor, the transparent, gelatin-like substance behind the lens.
3. As the vitreous is removed, saline is infused to replace the vitreous. At the end of the procedure, gas, air, or silicone oil may be introduced into the eye to act as a tamponade to keep the retina in place.
   a. If gas is used, the patient may be restricted to prone position (for at least 50 minutes of each hour) for 1 to 6 weeks until the SF6 gas is absorbed.
   b. If air or oil is used, a semi-Fowler's position is allowed.
4. Precautions should be taken to prevent increased IOP, which would disrupt healing.
   a. Avoid straining to have bowel movement or bend over.
   b. Avoid coughing or sneezing or sudden movements of the head.
   c. Monitor for headache, which may be a sign of increased IOP.

Enucleation

1. Complete removal of the eyeball, usually performed due to trauma, infection, tumor such as melanoma, or prevention of sympathetic ophthalmia.
2. At surgery, the eye is removed by opening the conjunctiva and extraocular muscles, severing the optic nerve, and removing the eyeball.
3. A ball implant is then covered by the muscles and maintains the contour of the eye. The conjunctiva is then closed and a plastic conformer is placed to maintain the integrity of the eyelid.
4. An individualized prosthesis can be fitted 4 to 6 weeks later and a second procedure may be done to improve ocular motility.
5. Care considerations include acceptance of body image, adjustment to mononuclear vision, and care of the enucleated socket and prosthesis, including the following:
   a. Inspecting eye and lid.
   b. Instilling medication.
   c. Irrigating site to remove mucus.
   d. Removing the prosthesis.
   e. Using aseptic technique when performing care.
6. Complications include hemorrhage, infection, and implant extrusion.

Nursing Assessment

1. Collect subjective and objective data about patient's general state of health.
2. Ascertain what symptoms the patient has been having (eye pain, visual loss, drainage, history of trauma) and how that has impacted usual activity.
3. Assess the patient's mobility and self-care ability.
4. Assess visual, as well as other sensory impairments, which may impact safety and independence.
5. Gather data regarding usual support systems used by the patient. Is family near? Do friends visit regularly? Is increased supervision required after surgery because of visual impairment?

6. Review patient's medications and determine if anticoagulants have been taken. They are usually stopped just prior to retinal surgery; however, they are usually continued for patients undergoing cataract surgery.

Nursing Diagnoses

- Deficient Knowledge of postoperative expectations and continuing care.
- Risk for Injury related to increased IOP and altered vision.
- Impaired Environmental Interpretation Syndrome related to visual disturbance.
- Fear of blindness related to invasive procedure to eye.
- Bathing, Dressing, Feeding Self-Care Deficit related to reduced or altered vision.

Nursing Interventions

Preparing for Surgery

1. Explain to the patient preoperative orders as well as postoperative expectations. (These will be specific for each type of surgery and particular health care provider.)
   a. Eye surgery is usually performed under local anesthesia and that he or she will be awake but sedated and must remain still during procedure.
   b. Postoperatively, a specific position in bed may be maintained for a few hours.
      i. The patient may be required to lie on the unoperated side
      ii. Following vitrectomy, the patient may be required to lie prone for at least 50 minutes of every hour. Advise the patient that he or she stand up to use bathroom and shower but must keep nose pointing to the ground. Although this is a difficult restriction to follow, it's the only way to improve visual outcome with this procedure.
      iii. Following some surgeries, supine position may be required with only a small pillow.
2. Instruct the patient to wash hair the evening before surgery; long hair of female patients should be arranged so it is off the face. There may be restrictions on using makeup to prevent makeup flakes from entering the operative site, thereby increasing the risk for infection and inflammation.
3. Check agency surgical policy regarding skin preparation. Patients may be requested to shower with antibacterial soap the evening before or morning of surgery.
4. Check that operative permit is correct and signed with specified eye having surgery noted. Ask patient which eye (do not suggest an eye). Verification can prevent two thirds of wrong site incidents.
5. Remove dentures, contact lenses, or eye prosthesis and metal objects before patient goes to the operating room based on facility policy and type of anesthesia. (Wedding band can usually be taped in place.)
6. Inform the patient if eye bandages are necessary postoperatively.
   a. Eye patch used following keratoplasty.
   b. Pressure patch used after vitrectomy. Drainage is expected for 2 days postoperatively.
   c. Pressure dressing and ice used after enucleation.
7. Administer preoperative medications, including eye drops, as prescribed.
8. Position bed side rails (up) after administering medications and place the call bell next to the patient.
9. Be available to answer questions the patient may have relating to the surgery or postoperative period.

 NURSING ALERT For patients requiring bed rest (ie, after keratoplasty, eye injury, retinal detachment surgery), measures should be taken to prevent pulmonary and/or circulatory complications. This may include range-of-motion exercises, anti-embolism stockings, and pneumatic compression devices.

Preventing Injury Postoperatively

1. Position the patient, as permitted, for specific surgery.
   a. Prone if vitrectomy was done with gas to hold retina in place.
   b. Semi-Fowlers for vitrectomy with air or oil was used.
2. Position side rails (up) to offer the patient a sense of security.
3. Place the call bell next to the patient; have the patient call the nurse rather than risk increased IOP from the stress and strain of attempting to be self-sufficient.
4. Advise the patient to avoid bending over, quick movements of the head, or straining that may cause increase in IOP. Medicate, if indicated, for excessive coughing or sneezing. (May not be a concern for current, small-incision cataract surgery.)
5. Monitor for headache, which may be a sign of IOP.
6. Instruct caregivers to tell the patient when they enter and leave the room.
7. Avoid activities such as combing hair that may cause tension on sutures or operative site.
8. Apply cold compresses to control edema and associated discomfort following vitrectomy.

Compensating for Altered Vision

1. Orient the patient to any new environment—room arrangement and people.
2. Encourage self-care within the patient's limits.
3. Supervise attempts of the patient to feed himself or herself and in other self-care activities.

 GERONTOLOGIC ALERT Be aware that older people may have additional sensory/perceptual alterations, such as hearing loss and decreased position sense, which increases their risk of falls and feeling of isolation.

Reducing Fear

1. Be aware that dependence on sight is recognized when one faces diminishment or loss of sight.
2. Recognize that patients' concern of surgical outcome may be manifested differently, for example, fear, depression, tension, resentment, anger, or rejection.
3. Encourage the patient to express feelings.
4. Demonstrate interest, empathy, and understanding.
5. Reassure the patient that rehabilitative programs and personnel are available.
6. Refer patient to the local blind or low-vision association for training and adaptive equipment.

Increasing Self-Care Activities

1. Provide diversional and occupational therapy to keep the patient occupied mentally within the limits of decreased vision.
2. Encourage rest periods, as necessary.
3. Provide adequate diet and fluids to promote proper elimination and decreased straining.

4. Discourage the patient from smoking, shaving with a straight edge, and use of pointed objects near eyes for safety reasons.

5. Caution the patient against rubbing eyes or wiping them with soiled tissues.

6. Instruct the patient to wear dark glasses if eyes are light sensitive.

7. Maintain safe environment—doors should be completely open or closed, floors kept clear of articles.

Patient Education and Health Maintenance

1. Advise the patient to consult ophthalmologist before undertaking diversional or recreational therapy that may be fatiguing to the eyes—such as reading, working on computer, and craft work.

2. Emphasize that lights should not be too bright or glaring.

3. Before the patient leaves the hospital, provide discharge instructions about medications, including topical antibiotics, corticosteroids, and pain medications.

4. Instruct the patient and family on instillation of eye medications, proper cleansing of the eyelids and lashes, and application of an eye shield or patch.

5. Provide instructions on massaging the eyelid in the postoperative period following eyelid surgery.

6. Assure patient of temporary bruising and swelling of eyelids.

7. Ensure that patient has follow-up information about eyeglasses, prosthesis fitting, and follow-up visits. Advise patient that improved vision may not occur quickly following keratoplasty.

8. Advise watching for signs of graft rejection 10 to 14 days following keratoplasty: decreased vision, irritation, corneal edema, and redness of sclera.

9. Educate the patient about talking books, records, tapes, and audio machines available from most public libraries without charge.

 TRANSITIONAL CARE ALERT Confirm the following with the patient and family before discharge: Is a return appointment date with health care provider confirmed?

Are prescriptions for patient's medications in hand or have been sent to pharmacy?

Do the patient and family member know how to use the prescribed medications?

Does the patient understand the restrictions placed on him or her and the reasons for them (positioning, straining, return to usual activities)?

Does the patient understand visual limitation and expected outcome?

Do the patient and family know what signs and symptoms to report to health care provider between appointments (ie, pain, temperature above 101°F [38.3°C], discharge from surgical area)?

Evaluation: Expected Outcomes

- Complies with preoperative routine; asks appropriate questions.
- Describes precautions that must be taken as safety measures, carries cane to prevent possible falls.

- Demonstrates improved vision in accordance with expectations of the surgery.
- Appears relaxed and positive concerning outcome of surgery.
- Manages self-care with minimal assistance.

COMMON EYE DISORDERS
Conditions of the Conjunctiva and Eyelids

The *eyelids* are the outermost defense mechanisms of the eyes, functioning as a physical barrier as well as to maintain moisture and disperse tears. The *palpebral conjunctiva* lines the upper and lower lids and the bulbar conjunctiva forms a protective coating over the sclera. The conjunctiva responds to infections, inflammatory disorders, and environmental irritants. Blood vessels in the conjunctiva dilate readily, causing redness, and pain receptors respond to inflammatory changes. Inflammatory disorders are outlined in Table 16-2. Structural disorders that may be amenable to surgery include:

- Entropion—inward turning of the eyelid margin.
- Ectropion—outward turning of the eyelid margin.
- Ptosis (blepharoptosis)—drooping of the upper eyelid.
- Lagophthalmos—inadequate closure of the eyelids.
- Pinguecula—overgrowth of tissue on the conjunctiva.
- Ptergium—overgrowth of tissue on the cornea

Pathophysiology and Etiology

1. Entropion and ectropion are classified as congenital, involutional, paralytic (CN VII palsy), cicatricial, or mechanic. Caused by severe eye disease, trauma, surgery, chemical burn.

2. Ptosis is classified according to the underlying cause and timing of onset described as acquired or congenital. General causes include neurologic, muscular, and autoimmune disorders; eye socket tumors may also cause ptosis.

3. Pinguecula is a degenerative lesion and ptergium is a fibrovascular lesion; both typically result from ultraviolet light exposure.

Clinical Manifestations

1. Sagging and/or irritation of eyelid.
2. Redness, tearing, burning of the eye.
3. Superficial punctate keratitis (inflammation of cornea).
4. Yellowish nodules in bulbar conjunctiva (pinguecula); wing shaped folds of tissue across limbus of the cornea (pinguecula).
5. Loss of superior field of vision with ptosis or reduce visual acuity may be seen with pinguecula.
6. Lashes roll back against the ocular surface after eye lid is released—positive digital inversion test (entropion).

Diagnostic Evaluation

1. External examination detecting appearance and function of eyelids.
2. Inspection of the conjunctiva, sclera, and cornea, followed by slit-lamp examination.
3. Lid position measurements—margin-reflex distance (MRD), palpebral fissure, levator function, and distance between upper lid crease to lid margin.
4. Cranial nerve (CN) testing for extraocular movements (3rd, 4th, 6th CN) and visual fields (2nd CN).

Table 16-2   Conditions of the Eyelids and Conjunctiva

CONDITION	TREATMENT AND NURSING CONSIDERATIONS
Blepharitis An inflammatory reaction of the eyelid margin caused by bacteria (usually *Staphylococcus aureus*) or seborrheic skin condition, resulting in flaking, redness, irritation, and possibly recurrent styes of the upper or lower lid, or both.	Diagnostic culture usually not necessary. Mild cases treated with eyelid margin scrub at least once daily (baby shampoo may be used). If *S. aureus* is likely, antibiotic ointment is prescribed one to four times per day to eyelid margin. Teach patient to scrub eyelid margin with cotton swab to remove flaking and then apply ointment with cotton swab, as directed.
Hordeolum (Stye)/Chalazion The term "stye" refers to an inflammation or infection of the glands and follicles of the eyelid margin. External hordeolum involves the hair follicles of the eyelashes; chalazion is a granulomatous (chronic) infection of the meibomian glands. Bacteria, usually *Staphylococcus*, and seborrhea are the causes. Pain, redness, foreign body sensation, and a pustule may be present.	Treatment usually consists of warm soaks to help promote drainage, good handwashing and eyelid hygiene, and possible application of antibiotic ointment. In some cases, incision and drainage in the office with local anesthetic may be necessary. Teach patient how to clean eyelid margins and not to squeeze the stye.
Conjunctivitis Inflammation or infection of the bulbar (covering the sclera and cornea) or palpebral (covering inside lids) conjunctiva. May be allergic; bacterial (*S. aureus*, *Streptococcus pneumoniae*, *Haemophilus influenzae*, and others); gonococcal; viral (adenovirus, herpes simplex, coxsackievirus, and others); or irritative (topical medication, chemicals, wind, smoke, contact lenses, ultraviolet light) causes. Trachoma is caused by *Chlamydia trachomatis* and is a major cause of blindness worldwide, but is rare in North America. Symptoms of conjunctivitis vary from mild pruritus and tearing to severe drainage, burning, hyperemia, and chemosis (edema). The term "pink eye" usually refers to infectious conjunctivitis.	Fluorescein staining may be done to rule out ulceration or keratitis (involvement of cornea). Culture if purulent exudate; special culture for *Neisseria gonorrhoeae*. Warm soaks (10 minutes four times per day) used when crusting and drainage present; cold compresses helpful for allergic and irritative causes. If topical antibiotic ordered, teach patient instillation technique. Urge good handwashing to prevent spread. Allergic conjunctivitis treated with topical or oral antihistamines, vasoconstrictors, and mast cell stabilizers.

5. Pharmacologic testing—phenylephrine or cocaine test to rule out Horner syndrome and edrophonium (Tensilon) test to rule out myasthenia gravis as causes of ptosis.

Management

1. Lubricating agents to treat inflammation of the cornea.
2. Massaging of eyelid, especially with cicatricial ectropion to help stretch scarring and improve anatomical position.
3. Manual inversion of eyelid margin for entropion.
4. Treatment of trichiasis by removing lashes with fine forceps.
5. Taping upper eyelid in ptosis.
6. Surgical management for ectropion and entropion.
   a. Ectropion and entropion repair—involves a horizontal tightening technique of the lower lid.
   b. Lateral canthoplasty (elongation of the eye opening).
   c. Lower lid retractor insertion.
7. Surgical management for ptosis.
   a. Approach depends of the cause and degree of ptosis and considers the object of the surgery, which is to balance the lid position in primary gaze.
   b. Complications of surgery include overcorrection and undercorrection of the eyelids, corneal or conjunctival irritation, abnormal contour of the eyelids, lagophthalmos.
8. Surgical excision of pterygium may be necessary due to large size. Other options include stontium beta-irradiation or mitomycin-C administration.

9. Surgery for pinguecula is indicated when tissue growth passes the limbus and invades the Bowman's layer of the cornea.

For nursing management see page 439.

Disorders of the Cornea and Uveal Tract

The *cornea* is the outermost tissue that functions in vision. It must remain clear and smooth to admit light to the retina. Blood vessels are contained in the *limbus* (periphery). Epithelial layers of the cornea repair rapidly, but if they are penetrated, infection can rapidly spread inward and vision may be lost.

The *uveal tract* is made up of the iris, which controls pupil size; ciliary body, which secretes aqueous humor and controls accommodation; and choroid layer, which provides vasculature to the anterior uveal tract. Disorders of the uveal tract may cause pupil changes, problems with accommodation, clouding of the anterior chamber or vitreous, and more serious problems because of adhesions (see Table 16-3).

Cataract

Clouding or opacity of the crystalline lens that impairs vision.

Pathophysiology and Etiology

1. Senile cataract—commonly occurs with aging.
2. Congenital cataract—occurs at birth.

Table 16-3 Conditions of the Cornea and Uveal Tract

CONDITION	TREATMENT AND NURSING CONSIDERATIONS
Corneal Abrasion and Ulceration (Keratitis)	
Loss of epithelial layers of cornea because of some type of trauma—contact with fingernail, tree branch, spark or other projectile, or overwearing contact lens. May lead to corneal ulceration and secondary infection into cornea (keratitis), which may lead to blindness. Symptoms are pain, redness, foreign body sensation, photophobia, increased tearing, and difficulty opening eye.	Treatment is urgent. Fluorescein staining and examination with Woods lamp or slit lamp to identify the abrasion or ulceration. Antibiotic ointment may be instilled and eye patched for 24 hr. No benefit to patching has been found for simple abrasions, however. Cycloplegic drops may also be used in large abrasions or ulcers. Abrasion heals in 24–48 hr. Ulceration should be followed by an ophthalmologist. Make sure that patch is secure enough so patient cannot open eyelid, but not so tight that patient "sees stars." Teach patient to use topical antibiotic (or antiviral in cases of herpes simplex dendritic keratitis) after patch is removed, and follow-up as directed. Review safety practices, such as wearing protective eye shields, not rubbing eyes, using contact lenses properly, and washing hands frequently.
Iritis/Uveitis	
Uveitis is an inflammation of the intraocular structures. It is classified by involved structures (1) anterior uveitis—iris (iritis) or iris and ciliary body (iridocyclitis), (2) intermediate uveitis—structures posterior to the lens (pars plantis or peripheral uveitis), and (3) posterior uveitis—choroid (choroiditis), retina (retinitis), or vitreous near the optic nerve and macula. Anterior uveitis is most common and is usually unilateral. Posterior uveitis is usually bilateral. Causes of uveitis are infections; immune-mediated disorders, such as ankylosing spondylitis, Crohn disease, Reiter syndrome, and lupus; and trauma, or it may be idiopathic. Onset is acute with deep eye pain, photophobia, conjunctival redness, small pupil that does not react briskly, ciliary flush (redness around limbus), and decreased visual acuity.	Urgent ophthalmology evaluation is needed. Inflammation is treated with a topical corticosteroid and a cycloplegic agent. Teach patient how to instill medications and adhere to dosing schedule to prevent permanent eye damage. Suggest sunglasses to decrease pain from photophobia. Encourage follow-up for IOP measurements because corticosteroids can increase IOP.

3. Traumatic cataract—occurs after injury.
4. Aphakia—absence of crystalline lens.
5. Additional risk factors for cataract formation include diabetes; ultraviolet light exposure; high-dose radiation; and drugs such as corticosteroids, phenothiazines, and some chemotherapy agents.

Clinical Manifestations

1. Blurred or distorted vision.
2. Glare from bright lights.
3. Gradual and painless loss of vision.
4. Previously dark pupil may appear milky or white.

Diagnostic Evaluation

1. Slit-lamp examination—to provide magnification and visualize opacity of lens.
2. Tonometry—to determine IOP and rule out other conditions.
3. Direct and indirect ophthalmoscopy to rule out retinal disease.
4. Perimetry—to determine the scope of the visual field (normal with cataract).

Management

General
1. Surgical removal of the lens is indicated.
   a. When a cataract interferes with activities, the patient is a candidate for cataract surgery.
   b. Because cataract often occurs in both eyes, surgery is recommended when vision in the better eye causes problems in daily activities. Surgery is done on only one eye at a time.

2. Cataract surgery is usually done under either regional block or topical anesthesia, with or without IV sedation, and on an outpatient basis.
3. Oral medications may be given to reduce IOP.
4. IOL implants are usually implanted at the time of cataract extraction, replacing thick glasses that may provide suboptimal refraction.
5. In the rare instance that intraocular lens implant is not used, the patient will be fitted with appropriate eyeglasses or a contact lens to correct refraction after the healing process.

Surgical Procedures
1. There are two types of extractions:
   a. Intracapsular extraction—the lens as well as the capsule are removed through a small incision. (This technique is rarely used in the United States.)
   b. Extracapsular extraction—the lens capsule is incised and the nucleus, cortex, and anterior capsule are extracted.
      i. The posterior capsule is left in place and is usually the base to which an IOL is implanted.
      ii. A conservative procedure of choice, simple to perform, is usually done under local anesthesia.
2. Phacoemulsification is usually used to remove the lens.
   a. A hollow needle vibrating at ultrasonic speed is used to emulsify the lens.
   b. Then the emulsified particles are irrigated and aspirated from the anterior chamber.
3. Cryosurgery is rarely used to remove the lens. A pencil-like instrument with a metal tip is supercooled (−35°C) and then touched to the exposed lens, freezing it so the lens is easily lifted out.

Intraocular Lens Implantation

1. The implantation of a synthetic lens (IOL) is designed for distance vision; the patient may wear prescription glasses for reading and near vision. Intraocular lens implant restores binocular vision.
2. Previously, most IOLs were spherical with the front surface curved. Aspheric IOLs increase contrast sensitivity.
   a. In 2003, the FDA approved the use of the multifocal IOL. The lens incorporates more than one optical power to permit focusing at different distances.
   b. In 2004, the FDA approved an aspheric IOL. The lens can reduce postoperative spherical aberrations and, therefore, improve the ability to see in varying light conditions, such as rain, snow, fog, twilight, and nighttime darkness.
   c. In 2005, the FDA approved the first toric IOL, which is designed to correct astigmatism.
   d. Sophisticated calculations are required to determine the prescription for the lens.
   e. Numerous types of IOLs are available. Designs and materials change as new developments occur.
3. Advantages of the IOL include:
   a. Provides an alternative for the person who cannot wear contact lenses.
   b. Cannot be lost or misplaced like conventional glasses.
   c. Provides superior vision correction and better depth perception than glasses.
4. Complications (specific to implantation):
   a. Pain from inflammation of various eye structures—usually controlled by nonsteroidal anti-inflammatories, but systemic antibiotics and immunosuppression may be required.
   b. Rosy vision (glare) because of keeping pupil from full constriction; excessive light enters pupil, causing a dazzling of macula (minute corneal opacity).
   c. Degeneration of the cornea.
   d. Malpositioning or dislocation of lens.
5. Implants may not be advisable for patients with severe myopia, history of chronic iritis, retinal detachment, diabetic retinopathy, glaucoma, and complications during surgery.

Contact Lens

Extended-wear contact lens is an option for those who do not receive IOL implants. They restore binocular vision and result in magnification of images in the range of 7% to 10%.

The patient will need to take the lens out for cleaning periodically or, if the patient is an older adult or debilitated, will need to follow-up at intervals for cleaning at the ophthalmologist's office.

Complications

1. Blindness.

Nursing Assessment

Preoperative
1. Assess knowledge level regarding procedure.
2. Determine visual limitations and effect on daily living.
3. Assess anxiety and fears about loss of vision and surgery.

Postoperative
1. Assess pain level.
   a. Sudden onset—may be due to ruptured vessel or suture and may lead to hemorrhage.
   b. Severe pain—accompanied by nausea and vomiting; may be caused by increased IOP and may require immediate treatment.

2. Assess visual acuity in unoperated eye.
3. Assess for signs of infection—fever, inflammation, pain, drainage.
4. Assess the patient's functional level and ability to be independent.

Nursing Diagnoses

- Deficient Knowledge of operative course.
- Delayed Surgical Recovery related to complications.

Nursing Interventions

Preparing the Patient for Surgery
1. Orient the patient and explain procedures and plan of care to decrease anxiety.
2. Instruct the patient not to touch eyes to decrease contamination.
3. Obtain conjunctival cultures, if requested, using aseptic technique.
4. Administer preoperative eye drops—antibiotic, mydriatic–cycloplegic, and other medications—mannitol solution IV, sedative, antiemetic, and opioid, as directed. Explain medication actions to patient.

Preventing Complications Postoperatively
1. Medicate for pain, as prescribed, to promote comfort.
2. Administer medication to prevent nausea and vomiting, as needed.
3. Notify the health care provider of sudden pain associated with restlessness and increased pulse, which may indicate increased IOP, or fever, which may indicate infection.
4. Caution the patient against coughing or sneezing to prevent increased IOP.
5. Advise the patient against rapid movement or bending from the waist to minimize IOP. The patient may be more comfortable with head elevated 30 degrees and lying on the unaffected side.
6. Allow the patient to ambulate as soon as possible and to resume independent activities.
7. Assist the patient in maneuvering through environment with the use of one eye while eye patch is on (1 to 2 days).
8. Encourage the patient to wear eye shield at night to protect operated eye from injury while sleeping.

Patient Education and Health Maintenance

Promoting Independence
1. Advice the patient to increase activities, as tolerated, unless given restrictions by the surgeon.
2. Caution against activities that cause patient to strain (eg, lifting heavy objects, straining at defecation, and strenuous activity) for up to 6 weeks, as directed.
3. Instruct the patient and family about proper eye drop or ointment instillation.
4. Advise the patient to bring all medications to follow-up visits to permit dosage adjustments by ophthalmologist. Discontinued medications can then be discarded to prevent confusion.

Adjusting to Visual Change
1. Inform the patient receiving corrective lenses that fitting for temporary corrective lenses for the first 6 weeks will occur several days after surgery.
   a. Prescription for permanent lenses will be determined 6 to 12 weeks after surgery.

b. Prescription for a permanent contact lens will be determined about 3 to 6 weeks after surgery.

2. Encourage the patient to wear dark glasses after eye dressings are removed to provide comfort from photophobia because of lack of pupil constriction from mydriatic–cycloplegic drops.

Adjusting to the Eyeglasses

1. Stress the importance of patience in the coming weeks of adjustment—it is easy to become frustrated.
2. Tell the patient that if glasses are to be worn, they will cause the perceived image to be about one third larger than normal. Glasses cannot restore binocular vision as an intraocular lens implant or contact lens will because of the discrepancy of image size between the treated eye and untreated eye.
3. If glass is used in the prescription, it is heavier and thicker than the more expensive plastic cataract eyeglass lenses.
4. Instruct the patient to look through the center of corrective glasses and to turn head when looking to the side because peripheral vision is markedly distorted.
5. It is necessary to relearn space judgment—walking, using stairs, reaching for articles on the table (such as a cup of coffee), and pouring liquids—because of loss of binocular vision and peripheral distortion.
6. Advise patients to use handrails while walking and doing steps and to reach out slowly for objects to be picked up.

Becoming Familiar with Contact Lenses

Teach the patient that:

1. With contact lenses, magnification is only about 7% to 10%; peripheral vision is not distorted so binocular vision is achieved and spatial distortion is usually not an issue.
2. Patients do need to learn how to remove daily-wear and extended-wear lenses or return to the ophthalmologist's office for replacement of extended-wear lens periodically.

Becoming Familiar with Intraocular Lens

1. Teach the patient that with an intraocular lens, magnification problems are negligible. Both the operated eye and the unoperated eye can work together after cataract surgery with lens implantation, and the preoperative glasses can usually be worn in the recuperative period.
2. Advise the patient that eyeglasses may not be required for distance but may be needed for reading and writing.
3. Caution the patient against straining of any type. Bend knees only if necessary to reach for something on the floor.
4. Recommend sponge bathing. Avoid getting soap in the eyes.
5. Advice avoidance of tilting head forward when washing hair; tilt head slightly backward. Vigorous shaking of the head is to be avoided.

Evaluation: Expected Outcomes

- Vision maximized and distortions or limitations in vision described by patient.
- Independent activities demonstrated, denies discomfort.

Acute (Angle-Closure) Glaucoma

A condition in which an obstruction occurs at the access to the trabecular meshwork and the canal of Schlemm. IOP is normal when the anterior chamber angle is open, and glaucoma occurs when a significant portion of that angle is closed. Glaucoma is associated with progressive visual field loss and eventual blindness if allowed to progress. This is most commonly an acute painful condition (about 10% of glaucoma cases), not to be confused with chronic open-angle glaucoma (about 90% of cases).

Pathophysiology and Etiology

1. Mechanical blockage of anterior chamber angle results in accumulation of aqueous humor (fluid).
2. Anterior chamber is anatomically shallow in most cases.
3. The shallow chamber with narrow anterior angles is more prone to physiologic events that result in closure.
4. Angle closure occurs because of pupillary dilation or forward displacement of the iris.
5. Angle closure can occur in subacute, acute, or chronic forms.
6. Episodes of subacute closure may precede an acute attack and cause transient blurred vision and pain but no increased IOP.
7. Acute angle closure causes a dramatic response with sudden elevation of IOP and permanent eye damage within several hours if not treated.
8. Within several days, scar tissue forms between the iris and cornea, closing the angle. The iris and ciliary body begin to atrophy, the cornea degenerates because of edema, and the optic nerve begins to atrophy.

Clinical Manifestations

1. Pain in and around eyes because of increased ocular pressure; may be transitory attacks.
2. Rainbow of color (halos) around lights.
3. Vision becomes cloudy and blurred.
4. Pupil mid-dilated and fixed.
5. Nausea and vomiting may occur.
6. Hazy-appearing cornea because of corneal edema.
7. Although onset may have initial subclinical symptoms, severity of symptoms may progress to cause acute symptoms of increased IOP—nausea and vomiting, sudden onset of blurred vision, severe pain, profuse lacrimation, and ciliary injection.

 NURSING ALERT Acute angle-closure glaucoma is a medical emergency and requires immediate treatment. Untreated, it can result in blindness in less than 1 week.

Diagnostic Evaluation

1. Tonometry—elevated IOP, usually greater than 50 mm Hg.
2. Ocular examination may reveal a pale optic disk.
3. Gonioscopy (using special instrument called gonioscope) to study the angle of the anterior chamber of the eye.

 NURSING ALERT Dilatation of pupils is avoided if the anterior chamber is shallow. This is determined by oblique illumination of the anterior segment of the eye. A flashlight is shined across the iris from the temporal side. If the iris is bulging (with a shallow anterior chamber), a crescent shadow appears on the nasal side of the iris.

Management
Pharmacologic
1. Emergency pharmacotherapy is initiated to decrease eye pressure before surgery.
2. Medications are based on the patient's condition but may include:
   a. Parasympathomimetic drugs used as miotic drugs—pupil contracts; iris is drawn away from cornea; aqueous humor may drain through lymph spaces (meshwork) into canal of Schlemm.
   b. Carbonic anhydrase inhibitor—restricts action of enzyme that is necessary to produce aqueous humor.
   c. Beta-adrenergic blockers—nonselective—may reduce production of aqueous humor or may facilitate outflow of aqueous humor.
   d. Hyperosmotic agents—to reduce IOP by promoting diuresis.

Surgery
1. Surgery is indicated if:
   a. IOP is not maintained within normal limits by medical regimen.
   b. There is progressive visual field loss with optic nerve damage.
2. Types of surgery include:
   a. Peripheral iridectomy—excision of a small portion of the iris whereby aqueous humor can bypass pupil; treatment of choice. Typically a laser procedure.
   b. Trabeculectomy—partial-thickness scleral resection with small part of trabecular meshwork removed and iridectomy. Necessary if peripheral anterior adhesions (synechiae) have developed due to repeated glaucoma attacks.
   c. Laser iridotomy—multiple tiny laser incisions to iris to create openings for aqueous flow; may be repeated.
3. Other eye is usually operated on eventually as a preventive measure.

Complications
Uncontrolled IOP that can lead to optic atrophy and total blindness.

Nursing Assessment
1. Evaluate the patient for severe pain, nausea, and vomiting and signs of increased IOP.
2. Assess visual symptoms and effect on daily activity.
3. Establish history of onset of attack and previous attacks.
4. Assess the patient's level of anxiety and knowledge base of glaucoma and treatment.

Nursing Diagnoses
- Acute Pain related to increased IOP.
- Fear related to pain and potential loss of vision.

Nursing Interventions
Relieving Pain
1. Notify the health care provider immediately of the patient's condition.
2. Administer opioids and other medications, as directed. Medications that may cause nausea and vomiting are avoided. The patient may be medicated with antiemetic if nausea occurs.

3. Explain to the patient that the goal of treatment is to reduce IOP as quickly as possible.
4. Explain procedures to the patient.
5. Reassure the patient that, with reduction in IOP, pain and other signs and symptoms should subside.
6. Explain adverse effects of medications:
   a. Mannitol (IV)—transient blurred vision, rhinitis, thirst, nausea, transient circulatory overload, and headache.
   b. Acetazolamide or methazolamide (oral)—drowsiness, anorexia, paresthesia, stomach upset, tinnitus, fluid and electrolyte imbalance, rare kidney, or liver dysfunction.
   c. Pilocarpine (topical)—burning and redness of eye, headache, constricted pupil, poor vision in dim light, retinal detachment, and rare lens opacity.

Relieving Fear
1. Provide reassurance and calm presence to reduce anxiety and fear.
2. Prepare the patient for surgery, if necessary.
3. Describe procedure to the patient; surgery will likely be done on outpatient basis.
   a. Patch will be worn for several hours and sunglasses may help with photophobia.
   b. Vision will be blurred for first few days after the procedure.
   c. Frequent initial follow-up will be necessary for tonometry to make sure control of IOP.

Patient Education and Health Maintenance
1. Instruct the patient in use of medications. Stress the importance of long-term medication use to control this chronic disease. Patients commonly forget that eye drops are medications and that glaucoma is a chronic illness.
2. Remind the patient to keep follow-up appointments.
3. Instruct the patient to seek immediate medical attention if signs and symptoms of increased IOP return—severe eye pain, photophobia, and excessive lacrimation.
4. Advise the patient to notify all health care providers of condition and medications and to avoid use of medications that may increase IOP, such as corticosteroids and anticholinergics (such as antihistamines), unless the benefit outweighs the risk (see Table 16-4).

Evaluation: Expected Outcomes
- Pain is decreased.
- Describes treatment regimen and verbalizes reduced fear.

Chronic (Open-Angle) Glaucoma

Glaucoma is characterized as a disorder of increased IOP, degeneration of the optic nerve, and visual field loss. Incidence increases with age—2% at age 40, 7% at age 70, and 8% at age 80.

Pathophysiology and Etiology
1. Degenerative changes occur in the trabecular meshwork and canal of Schlemm, causing microscopic obstruction.
2. Aqueous fluid cannot be emptied from the anterior chamber, increasing IOP.
3. IOP varies with activity and some people tolerate elevated IOP without optic damage (ocular hypertension), whereas others exhibit visual field defects and optic damage with minimal or transient IOP elevation.
4. The risk of eye damage increases with age, family history of glaucoma, diabetes, and hypertension.

Table 16-4 Drugs That Elevate Intraocular Pressure

MEDICATION	ROUTE	EFFECT
Corticosteroids	Oral, inhalant, intravenous, intravitreal, periocular topical solutions (creams and drops)	Elevates IOP
Viscoelastic agents	Intraocular	Elevates IOP
Alpha-chymotrypsin	Intraocular	Transient elevation of IOP
Topamax (anticonvulsant)	Oral	Elevates IOP
Anticholinergics	Topical	Causes angle-closure glaucoma
Sulfonamides	Oral	Causes angle-closure glaucoma
Tricyclic antidepressants	Oral	Causes acute angle-closure glaucoma
Monoamine oxidase inhibitors	Oral	Causes acute angle-closure glaucoma
Antihistamines	Oral	Causes acute angle-closure glaucoma
Antiparkinsonian	Oral	Causes acute angle-closure glaucoma
Antipsychotics	Oral	Causes acute angle-closure glaucoma
Antispasmolytic	Oral	Causes acute angle-closure glaucoma
Cycloplegic agents	Topical	Contraindicated in narrow-angle glaucoma
Mydriatic agents	Topical	Contraindicated in narrow-angle glaucoma
Sympathomimetic agents	Topical	Contraindicated in narrow-angle glaucoma

Clinical Manifestations

1. Mild, bilateral discomfort (tired feeling in eyes, foggy vision).
2. Slowly developing impairment of peripheral vision—central vision unimpaired.
3. Progressive loss of visual field.
4. Halos may be present around lights with increased ocular pressure.

Diagnostic Evaluation

1. Tonometry—IOP usually greater than 24 mm Hg but may be within normal limits.
2. Ocular examination—to check for clipping and atrophy of the optic disk.
3. Visual fields testing for deficits.

 NURSING ALERT Because of the relative ease of developing chronic glaucoma asymptomatically, encourage people of all ages to have an eye examination that includes measurement of eye pressure (tonometry) periodically to facilitate early detection and treatment to prevent loss of eyesight.

Management

1. Commonly treated with a combination of topical miotic agents (increase the outflow of aqueous humor by enlarging the area around trabecular meshwork) and oral carbonic anhydrase inhibitors and beta-adrenergic blockers (decrease aqueous production).
2. Remission may occur; however, there is no cure. The patient should continue to see health care provider at 3- to 6-month intervals for control of IOP.
3. If medical treatment is not successful, surgery may be required, but is delayed as long as possible.
4. Types of surgery include:
   a. Laser trabeculoplasty.
      i. An outpatient procedure, treatment of choice if increased ocular pressure unresponsive to medical regimen only.
      ii. As many as 100 superficial surface burns are placed evenly at junction of pigmented and nonpigmented trabeculum meshwork for 360 degrees in anesthetized eye, which allows increased outflow of aqueous humor.
      iii. Maximum decrease in IOP is achieved in 2 to 3 months, but IOP may rise again in 1 to 2 years.
   b. Iridencleisis—an opening is created between anterior chamber and space beneath the conjunctiva; this bypasses the blocked meshwork and aqueous humor is absorbed into conjunctival tissues.
   c. Cyclodiathermy or cyclocryotherapy—the ciliary body's function of secreting aqueous humor is decreased by damaging the body with high-frequency electrical current or supercooled probe applied to the surface of the eye over the ciliary body.
   d. Corneoscleral trephine (rarely done)—a permanent opening at the junction of the cornea and sclera is made through the anterior chamber so aqueous humor can drain.

DRUG ALERT Using beta-adrenergic blocker eye drops in the treatment of glaucoma can cause an adverse reaction in patients taking oral beta-adrenergic blockers for cardiovascular disease. Monitor vital signs because the risk for bradycardia exists.

Nursing Assessment

1. Assess frequency, duration, and severity of visual symptoms.
2. Assess the patient's knowledge of disease process and anxiety about the diagnosis.
3. Assess the patient's motivation to participate in long-term treatment.

Nursing Diagnosis

- Deficient Knowledge about glaucoma and surgical procedure.

Nursing Interventions

Providing Information about Glaucoma

1. Review the normal anatomy and physiology of the eye as well as the changes that occur in the drainage of aqueous humor with glaucoma.
2. Make sure that the patient understands that, although asymptomatic, IOP could still be elevated and damage to the eye could be occurring. Therefore, ongoing use of medication and follow-up are essential.
3. Teach the patient the action, dosage, and adverse effects of all medications. Make sure of adequate administration of eye drops by watching the patient give return demonstration.
   a. Timolol and betaxolol—adverse effects include headache, eye irritation, decreased corneal sensitivity, blurred vision, bradycardia, palpitations, bronchospasm, hypotension, and heart failure.
   b. Pilocarpine—adverse effects include eye irritation, blurring, and redness; headache; pupil constriction; poor vision in dim light; possible hypertension and tachycardia; and rare retinal detachment and lens opacity.
   c. Acetazolamide and methazolamide—adverse effects include drowsiness, anorexia, paresthesia, stomach upset, tinnitus, fluid and electrolyte imbalance, and rare kidney and liver dysfunction.
4. Discuss visual defects with the patient and ways to compensate. Vision loss is permanent and treatment is aimed at stopping the process.
5. Inform the patient that surgery is done on an outpatient basis and recovery is quick. Prolonged restrictions are not required.
   a. After surgery, elevation of head 30 degrees will promote aqueous humor drainage after a trabeculectomy.
   b. Additional medications after surgery include topical steroids and cycloplegics to decrease inflammation and to dilate the pupil.

Patient Education and Health Maintenance

1. Patient must remember that glaucoma cannot be cured, but it can be controlled.
2. Remind the patient that periodic eye checkups are essential because pressure changes may occur.
3. Alert the patient to avoid, if possible, circumstances that may increase IOP:
   a. Upper respiratory infections.
   b. Emotional upsets—worry, fear, anger.
   c. Exertion, such as snow shoveling, pushing, and heavy lifting.
4. Recommend the following:
   a. Continuous daily use of eye medications as prescribed.
   b. Moderate use of the eyes.
   c. Exercise in moderation to maintain general well-being.
   d. Unrestricted fluid intake: alcohol and coffee may be permitted unless they are noted to cause increased IOP in the particular patient.
   e. Maintenance of regular bowel habits to decrease straining.
   f. Wearing a medical identification tag indicating the patient has glaucoma

Evaluation: Expected Outcomes

- Verbalizes understanding of glaucoma as a chronic disease; demonstrates proper instillation of ophthalmic medications.

Retinal Detachment

Retinal detachment is defined as detachment of the sensory area of the retina (rods and cones) from the pigmented epithelium of the retina. A break in the continuity of the retina may first occur from small degenerative holes and tears, which may lead to detachment.

Pathophysiology and Etiology

1. Spontaneous detachment may occur due to degenerative changes in the retina or vitreous.
2. Trauma, inflammation, or tumor causes detachment by forming a mass that mechanically separates the retinal layers.
3. Diabetic retinopathy commonly leads to retinal degeneration and tears disrupting the integrity of the retina.
4. Myopia and loss of a lens from a cataract (aphakia) also predisposes to retinal tears and detachment because the posterior chamber is enlarged, leading to vitreous pull.
5. After detachment occurs, that portion of the retina cannot perceive light because the blood and oxygen supply is cut off; hence, part of visual field is lost.
6. Detachment occurs most commonly in patients over age 40.

Clinical Manifestations

1. Retinal detachment may occur slowly or rapidly, but without pain.
2. The patient complains of flashes of light or blurred, "sooty" vision because of stimulation of the retina by vitreous pull.
3. The patient notes sensation of particles moving in line of vision (more so than usual—"floaters" that a person can see floating across field of vision when looking at a light background).
4. Delineated areas of vision may be blank.
5. A sensation of a veillike coating coming down, coming up, or coming sideways in front of the eye may be present if detachment develops rapidly.
   a. This veillike coating, or shadow, is commonly misinterpreted as a drooping eyelid or elevated cheek.
   b. Straight-ahead vision may remain good in early stages.
6. Unless the retinal holes are sealed, the retina will progressively detach; ultimately, there will be a loss of central vision as well as peripheral vision, leading to legal blindness.

Diagnostic Evaluation

Indirect ophthalmoscopy shows gray or opaque retina. The retina is normally transparent. Slit-lamp examination and three-mirror gonioscopy magnify the lesion.

Management

General

1. Sedation, bed rest, and eye patch may be used to restrict eye movements.
2. Surgical intervention may be indicated.
3. Return of visual acuity with a reattached retina depends on:
   a. Amount of retina detached before surgery.
   b. Whether the macula (area of central vision) was detached.
   c. Length of time the retina was detached.
   d. Amount of external distortion caused by the scleral buckle.
   e. Possible macular damage as a result of diathermy of cryocoagulation.
4. Surgical reattachment is successful approximately 90% to 95% of the time. If the retina remains attached 2 months postoperatively, the condition is likely to be corrected and is unlikely to recur.

Surgical Procedures

1. Photocoagulation—a light beam (either laser or xenon arc) is passed through the pupil, causing a small burn and producing an exudate between the pigment epithelium and retina.
2. Electrodiathermy—an electrode needle is passed through the sclera to allow subretinal fluid to escape. An exudate forms from the pigment epithelium and adheres to the retina.
3. Cryosurgery or retinal cryopexy—a supercooled probe is touched to the sclera, causing minimal damage; as a result of scarring, the pigment epithelium adheres to the retina.
4. Scleral buckling—a technique whereby the sclera is shortened to allow a buckling to occur, which forces the pigment epithelium closer to the retina (often accompanied by vitrectomy).

Complications

1. Glaucoma.
2. Infection.

Nursing Assessment

Preoperative

1. Assess for history of trauma or other risk factors.
2. Assess level of anxiety and knowledge level regarding procedures.
3. Determine visual limitations and obtain visual description from patient to determine assistance needed.

Postoperative

1. Assess pain level.
2. Assess visual acuity if unoperated eye not patched.
3. Determine the patient's ability to ambulate and assume independent activities, as tolerated.

Nursing Diagnoses

- Anxiety related to visual deficit and surgical outcome.
- Delayed Surgical Recovery related to complications.

Nursing Interventions

Reducing Anxiety Before Surgery

1. Instruct the patient to remain quiet in prescribed position. (Detached area of retina remains in dependent position.) Assist with all activities and offer frequent reassurance.
2. Patch both eyes. Make sure that the patient is oriented to surroundings and can call for assistance.
3. Describe preoperative procedures before carrying them out.
4. Wash the patient's face with antibacterial solution.
5. Administer preoperative medications, as ordered.
6. Instruct the patient not to touch eyes.

Preventing Postoperative Complications

1. Caution the patient to avoid bumping head.
2. Encourage the patient not to cough or sneeze or to perform activities that will increase IOP.
3. Assist the patient with activities, as needed.
4. Encourage ambulation and independence.
5. Administer medications for pain, nausea, and vomiting, as prescribed.
6. Provide sedate, diversional activities such as radio, audio books.
7. If the patient's anticoagulation therapy has been stopped, provide preventative measures such as compression stockings, leg exercises, and carefully monitor for signs and symptoms of thrombosis and embolism..

Patient Education and Health Maintenance

1. Encourage self-care at discharge, if done in an unhurried manner. (Avoid falls, jerks, bumps, or accidental injury.)
2. Instruct the patient about the following:
   a. Rapid eye movements should be avoided for several weeks.
   b. Driving is restricted.
   c. Within 3 weeks, light activities may be pursued.
   d. Within 6 weeks, heavier activities and athletics are possible. Define such activities for the patient.
   e. Avoid straining and bending head below the waist.
   f. Use meticulous cleanliness when instilling eye medications.
   g. Apply a clean, warm, moist washcloth to eyes and eyelids several times a day for 10 minutes to provide soothing and relaxing comfort.
   h. Symptoms that indicate a recurrence of the detachment: floating spots, flashing light, and progressive shadows. Recommend that the patient contact health care provider if they occur.
3. Advise on follow-up. The first follow-up visit to the ophthalmologist should occur in 2 weeks, with other visits scheduled thereafter.

Evaluation: Expected Outcomes

- Verbalizes understanding of treatment.
- Follows activity restrictions.

Other Problems of the Retina and Vitreous

The retina is a multilayered structure that receives images and transmits them to the brain. It is nourished by retinal arteries and veins. Problems result from inflammation, trauma, vascular changes, congenital defects, and aging. Central lesions affect the macula, impairing central vision, near vision, and color discrimination. Peripheral lesions impair peripheral vision, causing blind spots, night blindness, and eventual tunnel vision. See Table 16-5 for treatment of individual disorders.

 NURSING ALERT Central retinal artery occlusion is a medical emergency. Vision may be salvaged if treated within 24 hours of onset.

Nursing Assessment

1. Take history of eye problems, general health, and family history of eye disease.
2. Obtain functional history of how eye problem may be impairing work, recreation, and other activities.
3. Assess bilateral visual acuity, peripheral vision, and color discrimination.
4. Assist with pupil dilation and ophthalmoscopy, as directed.

Nursing Diagnoses

- Risk for Injury related to sudden visual loss.
- Readiness for Enhanced Self-Care related to gradual visual loss.
- Risk for Injury related to visual impairment.
- Anxiety related to fear of further visual loss.

Table 16-5 Other Conditions of the Retina and Vitreous

CONDITION	TREATMENT AND NURSING CONSIDERATIONS
Vitreous Hemorrhage Bleeding into the vitreous may occur due to trauma, sickle cell disease, hypertension, diabetic retinopathy, retinal tear or detachment, intraocular lens displacement, and clotting abnormalities. It causes decrease or loss of vision in affected eye.	The underlying cause is treated and surgery to repair the retina may include photocoagulation, cryotherapy, scleral buckle, or vitrectomy. (See "Retinal Detachment," page 448.) Assist the patient with visual deficit and activity and position restrictions before surgery. Maintain eye patches, activity restriction, and medication administration after surgery.
Central Retinal Artery Occlusion Sudden occlusion of the central retinal artery causes painless loss of vision in one eye with loss of light perception. It may have been preceded by episodes of transient blindness (amaurosis fugax) for 10–15 min. It is caused by an embolus, usually from the ipsilateral carotid artery.	Treatment consists of massaging the globe in an attempt to break up the embolus or move it distally, inhalation of a mixture of 95% oxygen and 5% CO_2 to get the retinal vessels to dilate, and IV infusion of acetazolamide to lower IOP. Place the patient in Trendelenburg position and monitor vital signs, as directed. Offer reassurance and assist with additional testing and treatment, as indicated.
Central Retinal Vein Occlusion Occlusion of the central retinal vein or a branch causes sudden (over several hours), painless decrease in visual acuity. Usually occurs in people with hypertension or other vascular disorders.	Urgent ophthalmologic evaluation is needed. Photocoagulation may be used to prevent local hemorrhage and promote neovascularization. Corticosteroids are used to treat retinal edema and an aspirin or anticoagulant may be used to prevent further occlusive disease. Encourage regular screening for glaucoma in follow-up as a complication from scar tissue formation after photocoagulation.
Macular Degeneration Age-related changes in the choroid deprive the fovea centralis of blood supply, causing a dry (atrophic) form (onset over several years) or wet (exudative) form (onset over several days to weeks with neovascularization and hemorrhaging). Central and near vision are affected, but some peripheral vision remains bilateral.	Support patient and family. Be realistic about prognosis—there is no cure but treatment may include laser, anti-VEGF therapy, diet, and vitamins (AREDS formulation) to slow the progression of the disease. Anti-VEGF therapy involves intraocular injection of medication every few weeks; can be painful and may raise the risk of infection. Refer patient to the local chapter of The Lions Club or other agencies for vision rehabilitation in order to assist with adaptive devices for low vision.
Retinitis Inflammation of the retina, usually caused by cytomegalovirus as a complication of human immunodeficiency virus disease. Symptoms include blurred vision, floaters and/or flashes in the eye, and loss of peripheral vision and eventually blindness. Determination of the progression of the disease is made by direct and indirect ophthalmoscopy and intravenous fluorescein angiography.	Antiviral medications can help control the symptoms and slow the progression of retinitis. Other treatment modalities include vitrectomy, silicone oil injection, and retinal detachment repair. Nursing interventions focus on patient education of drug side effects, care of central venous lines for intravenous medication, and monitoring blood count and for signs of kidney damage. Patient may be referred to community resources for low-vision assistance.
Diabetic Retinopathy A vascular disorder of the retina that leads to diminished vision as a complication of diabetes mellitus. Classified as nonproliferative or proliferative and typically occurs in four stages.	See page 740. Untreated diabetic retinopathy may cause complications such as retinal detachment, vitreous hemorrhage, clinically significant macular edema, glaucoma, and blindness.

AREDS, Age-Related Eye Disease Study; IOP, intraocular pressure; VEGF, vascular endothelial growth factor.

Nursing Interventions

Ensuring Safety following Sudden Loss of Vision

1. Orient the patient to the layout of the facility and explain procedures.
2. Assist with self-care activities and educate patient on how to call for assistance.
3. Have personal articles placed nearby and take care not to move things without alerting the patient.
4. Ensure clear path for patient to move and ambulate; remove obstacles; provide ambulation aide as needed.
5. Help the patient understand visual weaknesses, such as where blind spots are and how to compensate by turning head to scan environment, using magnifying glass, having environment brightly lit.
6. Use side rails and direct visual supervision, if needed.
7. Assist the patient on stairs, make sure wearing good footwear, and obtain occupational therapy referral if needed.

Compensating for Gradual Loss of Vision

1. Discuss strategies/modifications to carry out usual activities.
2. Engage support people in assistance with patient activity.

3. Refer patients with vision less than 20/70 to the Blind Association or other resource for education and assistive devices.
4. Advise patient to memorize environment while some vision is intact, and then do not rearrange furniture or change environment.

Relieving Anxiety

1. Keep the patient informed during the diagnostic process.
2. Educate about resources such as local blind association.
3. Encourage participation in support groups.

Patient Education and Health Maintenance

1. Encourage frequent follow-up with ophthalmologist.
2. Advise the patient to use corrective lenses as directed and keep lens prescription up to date and to have a spare pair of glasses available.
3. Warn the patient against straining eyes by excessive exposure to the sun, reading, or computer work.
4. Rest eyes, as needed.
5. Report sudden deterioration in vision or other changes: sudden loss of vision, increase in floaters, flashes of light, sharp pain.

Evaluation: Expected Outcomes

- Performs daily activities without injury.
- Increasing independence with self-care activities.
- Reports understanding of disease and acceptance of treatment plan.

Eye Trauma

Trauma to the eye may be caused by blunt or sharp injury or chemical or thermal burns. The eyelids, protective layers, surrounding soft tissue, or the globe itself may be injured. Vision may be impaired by direct injury or latent scarring. See Table 16-6 for specific conditions.

Nursing Assessment

1. Obtain history of mechanism of injury as well as extent of other injuries.
2. Assess level of pain and visual symptoms.
3. Perform neurologic assessment and assess vital signs.
4. Assess visual acuity.

Table 16-6 Eye Trauma		
CONDITION	**CLINICAL MANIFESTATIONS**	**MEDICAL MANAGEMENT**
Blunt Contusion		
Bruising of periorbital soft tissue	• Swelling and discoloration of the tissue • Bleeding into the tissue and structures of the eye • Pain • Diagnosis: Tests must determine if injury to parts of eye and systemic trauma	• Treatment to reduce swelling • Pain management dependent on structures involved *Note:* If there is any possibility of a ruptured globe, a loose patch and shield should be placed and ocular manipulation discouraged until ophthalmologist assessment completed.
Hyphema		
Presence of blood in the anterior chamber	• Pain • Blood in anterior chamber • Increased intraocular pressure	• Usually spontaneous recovery • If severe, bed rest or chair rest with bathroom privileges, eye shield, interior chamber paracentesis, topical steroids, and cycloplegics
Orbital Fracture		
Fracture and dislocation of walls of the orbit, orbital margins, or both	• May be accompanied by other signs of head injury • Rhinorrhea • Contusion • Diplopia • Diagnosis: x-ray, computed tomography	• May heal on own if no displacement or impingement on other structures • Surgery (repair the orbital floor with plate freeing entrapped orbital tissue)
Foreign Body		
On cornea (25% all ocular injuries), conjunctiva Intraocular particles penetrate sclera, cornea, globe	• Severe pain • Lacrimation • Foreign body sensation • Photophobia • Redness • Swelling *Note:* Wood and plant foreign body may cause severe infection within hours.	• Medical emergency • Removal of foreign body through irrigation, cotton-tipped applicator, or magnet • Treatment of intraocular foreign body depends on size, magnetic properties, tissue reaction, location • Surgical removal
Laceration/Perforation		
Cutting or penetration of soft tissue or globe	• Pain • Bleeding • Lacrimation • Photophobia	• Medical emergency • Surgical repair—method of repair depends on severity of injury • Antibiotics—topically and systemically

(continued)

Table 16-6 Eye Trauma (*Continued*)

CONDITION	CLINICAL MANIFESTATIONS	MEDICAL MANAGEMENT
Ruptured Globe Concussive injury to globe with tears in the ocular coats, usually the sclera	• Pain • Altered intraocular pressure • Limitation of gaze in field of rupture • Hyphema • Hemorrhage (poor prognostic sign) • Diagnosis: computed tomography, ultrasound	• Medical emergency • Surgical repair • Vitrectomy • Scleral buckle • Antibiotics • Steroids • Enucleation
Burns Chemical—caused by alkali or acid agent	• Pain • Burning • Lacrimation • Photophobia	• Medical emergency • Copious irrigation until pH is 7 • Severe scarring may require keratoplasty • Antibiotics
Thermal—usually burn to eyelids—may be first-, second-, or third-degree	• Pain • Burned skin • Blisters	• First aid—apply sterile dressings • Pain control • Leave fluid blebs intact • Suture eyelids together to protect eye—if perforation a possibility • Skin grafting with severe second- and third-degree burns
Ultraviolet—excessive exposure to sunlight, sunlamp, snow blindness, welding	• Pain—delayed several hours after exposure • Foreign body sensation • Lacrimation • Photophobia *Note:* Symptoms occur sometime after exposure.	• Pain relief • Condition self-limiting • Bilateral patching with antibiotic ointment and cycloplegics

Nursing Diagnoses

- Acute Pain from tissue trauma.
- Fear related to loss of vision.

Nursing Interventions

Relieving Pain

1. Medicate for pain, as directed; however, monitor for respiratory depression, hypotension, and decreased level of consciousness if opioid analgesic is used.

    Note: Medications that depress the central nervous system may be contraindicated if head injury is suspected.
2. Provide ice and cool compresses to relieve swelling and pain.
3. Provide additional comfort measures, such as positioning, dimmed lights, and quiet environment.
4. Irrigate and patch eye, as directed.
5. Monitor vital signs and neurologic status, as indicated.
6. Watch for and report signs of infection, such as fever, drainage, increased pain, warmth, and redness.

Reducing Fear

1. Provide psychological support and assist with self-care activities, as needed.
2. Describe procedures and treatments to the patient and family.
3. Maintain safe environment.
4. Prepare the patient for surgery, as indicated (see page 440).

Patient Education and Health Maintenance

1. Teach the patient how to administer medications such as topical antibiotics.
2. Instruct on use of patch or shield.
3. Advise the patient to report increase in pain, decrease in vision, redness, and fever.
4. Teach safety measures with decreased visual acuity.
5. Advise the use of corrective lenses, as prescribed.
6. Stress follow-up care.
7. Attempt to prevent future trauma with protective eyewear.

Evaluation: Expected Outcomes

- Rests comfortably, reports less pain.
- Cooperates with procedures.

Resources

For further information regarding eye disorders and resources, contact:

- American Council of the Blind (*www.acb.org*).
- American Macular Degeneration Foundation (*www.macular.org*).
- Wilmer Eye Institute at Johns Hopkins (*www.wilmer.jhu.edu*).
- National Eye Institute, Eye Health Information (*www.nei.nih.gov/health*).
- Common Eye Problems & Conditions (*www.eyecaresource.com*).
- Royal National Institute of Blind People (*www.rnib.org.uk*).
- American Academy of Ophthalmology (*www.geteyesmart.org*, *www.eyecareamerica.org*).

SELECTED REFERENCES

American Foundation for the Blind. (2017). Home modifications for people who are blind or have low vision. Vision Aware. Available: *www.visionaware.org/home_modifications*

American Society of Ophthalmologic Registered Nurses. (2011). *Ophthalmic procedures in the office and clinic* (3rd ed.). San Francisco, CA: Author.

Cakiner-Egilmez, T. (2015). Glaucoma Medications Update: How to Improve Compliance and Adherence. *Insight, 40*(3), 5–10.

Ching, D. W., Agarwal, A., Lee, C. S., et al. (2016). A Review of the Role of Intravitreal Corticosteroids as an Adjuvant to Antibiotics in Infectious Endophthalmitis. *Ocular Immunology and Inflammation, 2016*, 1–8. Available: *www.tandfonline.com/doi/full/10.1080/09273948.2016.1245758.*

Dansby-Kelly, A. (Ed.). (2016). *Ophthalmic procedures in the operating room and ambulatory surgery center* (4th ed.). San Francisco, CA: American Society of Ophthalmologic Registered Nurses.

Dean, E. C., Gomez, J. L., & Welch, R. M. (2014). *Essentials of ophthalmic nursing. Book 1.* San Francisco, CA: American Society of Ophthalmologic Registered Nurses.

Dobrzynski, J. M., & Kostis, J. B. (2015). Statins and cataract—A visual insight. *Current Atherosclerosis Reports, 17*(2), 477.

Kong, K. L., & Khan, J.. (2015) Ophthalmic patients on antithrombotic drugs: A review and guide to perioperative management. *British Journal of Ophthalmology, 99*(8), 1025–1030.

Lara-Smalling, A., & Cakiner-Egilmez, T. (2014). Diabetes and cataract surgery: Preoperative risk factors and positive nursing intervention. *Insight, 39*(2), 18–20.

Mangione, C. M., Lee, P. P., Gutierrez, P. R., et al. (2001). Development of the 25-item National Eye Institute Visual Function Questionnaire (VFQ-25). *Archives of Ophthalmology, 119*, 1050–1058.

Melillo, P., Orrico, A., Attanasio, M., et al. (2015). A pilot study for development of a novel tool for clinical decision making to identify fallers among ophthalmic patients. *BMC Medical Informatics and Decision Making, 15*(Suppl. 3), S6.

Onkar, A., Samdariya, S., Pareek, P., & Suwarna, S. (2017). Strontium Beta-Irradiation: Can it Prove Strong Enough in Curbing the Ophthalmic Hydra Called Pterygium. *Surgery Current Research, 7*(4), 298.

Pacheco, L. (Ed.). (2017). *Care and handling of ophthalmic microsurgical instruments* (4th ed.). San Francisco, CA: American Society of Ophthalmologic Registered Nurses.

Spaeth, G. L., Danish-Meyer, H., Goldberg, I., & Kampik, A. (2012). Ophthalmic Surgery: Principles and Practice. Philadelphia: Saunders.

U.S. Food and Drug Administration. (2014). LASIK. Available: *www.fda.gov/MedicalDevices/ProductsandMedicalProcedures/SurgeryandLifeSupport/LASIK/*

Welch, R. M., Waldo, M. N., Gomez, J. L., & Dean, E. C. (2015). *Essentials of ophthalmic nursing. Book 2.* San Francisco, CA: American Society of Ophthalmologic Registered Nurses.

Welch, R. M., Waldo, M. N., Gomez, J. L., & Dean, E. C. (2015). *Essentials of ophthalmic nursing. Book 3.* San Francisco, CA: American Society of Ophthalmologic Registered Nurses.

Welch, R. M., Waldo, M. N., Gomez, J. L., & Dean, E. C. (2015). *Essentials of ophthalmic nursing. Book 4.* San Francisco, CA: American Society of Ophthalmologic Registered Nurses.

Wells, J. A., Glassman, A. R., Ayala, A. R., et al. (2015). Aflibercept, bevacizumab, or ranibizumab for diabetic macular edema. *New England Journal of Medicine, 372*(13), 1193–1203.

Yanoff, M., Berry J., Crandall A., et al. (2017). Advances in Ophthalmology and Optometry. New York: Elsevier.

Zeng, W., Liu, Z., Dai, H., et al. (2017). Anti-fibrotic, anti-VEGF or radiotherapy treatments as adjuvants for pterygium excision: a systematic review and network meta-analysis. *BMC Ophthalmology, 17*, 211.

17

Ear, Nose, and Throat Disorders

OVERVIEW AND ASSESSMENT

History

Obtaining a history, including the patient's signs and symptoms, current health patterns, and previous past medical history, will help in identifying ear, nose, and throat (ENT) problems and developing an individualized plan of care.

Key Signs and Symptoms

1. Epistaxis.
   a. When did the bleeding first begin? Did it occur spontaneously or occur after facial or nasal trauma, nose blowing, digital manipulation, or recent nasal or sinus surgery? In many cases, anterior bleeding commonly flows from the nasal vestibule and, in reclining position, will drip into the throat. Posterior bleeding commonly causes dripping into the oropharynx when upright or supine. Nasal endoscopy or examination via anterior rhinoscopy is performed to confirm the site of bleeding.
   b. Unilateral or bilateral? What side of the nose is the bleeding coming from, and, if bilateral, on what side did it begin? Ask the patient about measures employed to control the bleeding thus far.
   c. Assess current medication history: Is the patient taking acetylsalicylic acid (ASA/aspirin), nonsteroidal anti-inflammatory drugs (NSAIDs), antiplatelet agents, or anticoagulants? When was the last dose taken?
   d. Is there a history of current oxygen therapy? Is there a history of chronic bleeding disorders? Obtain results of recent blood work: complete blood count (CBC), prothrombin

time (PT), international normalized ratio (INR), or partial prothrombin time (PTT).

2. Headache.
   a. Exactly what parts of the head or face hurt? Is it pain or a pressure sensation? Use the PQRST Method of Pain Assessment with emphasis on location, duration, and symptom onset.
   b. Assess for associated neck, dental, or jaw pain; nausea; vomiting; visual changes; and/or sensitivity to light or sound. Assess for associated nasal congestion, postnasal drip, or clear or purulent rhinorrhea. Assess for history of migraine disease.

3. Sore throat—Assess onset and duration of symptoms, previous medical treatment, and symptom response.
   a. Is it accompanied by swollen glands, high fever, nasal congestion, and postnasal drip? Assess for associated weight loss; head, neck, or ear pain; voice changes; neck mass; trismus; or difficulty breathing. Has the patient been able to eat or drink?
   b. Is it acute or chronic? Was there any exposure to others with throat infection?

4. Nasal congestion.
   a. Is it acute or chronic? Accompanied by fever and purulent drainage? Assess severity and duration of symptoms, associated purulent or clear rhinorrhea, fever, facial pain or sinus tenderness, itchy eyes, sneezing, or postnasal drip. If symptoms are chronic, assess if worsened with changes in barometric pressure, vary with seasons, or brought on by odors or allergen exposure.
   b. Assess for current/chronic history of use of nasal sprays containing oxymetazoline or if the patient is experiencing

anosmia/microsmia (loss of sense of smell or diminished sensitivity). Ask if the patient has had previous history of nasal polyps, previous nasal or sinus surgery, or nasal fracture.

5. Hoarseness.
   a. Assess history of recent surgical procedures involving the head or neck, recent endotracheal intubation, radiation treatment to the head/neck, history of tobacco/alcohol use, occupation as vocal performer, or history of lung disease with use of inhaled steroids, chronic or recent antibiotic therapy, and symptoms of gastroesophageal reflux.
   b. Is it acute (less than 2 weeks), recurrent, or chronic (more than 2 weeks)? Assess onset and duration of symptoms, subjective impairment in communication, or voice-related quality.
   c. Assess for recent URI symptoms, associated dysphagia, odynophagia (pain with swallowing), globus sensation (sensation of something in the throat), throat pain, weight loss, ear pain, neck mass or enlarged lymph nodes in neck, hemoptysis, or shortness of breath.

6. Earache (otalgia).
   a. Is it worsened by manipulation of the auricle or is it a deep, throbbing pain? Is there otorrhea? Assess onset and duration of pain using the PQRST Pain Scale. Assess for associated erythema or edema of the external ear canal or external auricle, pruritus, hearing loss, or otorrhea. Is the pain intermittent or constant?
   b. Were there preceding upper respiratory infection symptoms? Is the pain associated with hearing loss, aural fullness, vertigo, headache, or fluctuation of hearing? Have there been any recent dental procedures?
   c. Assess history for nighttime bruxism (grinding teeth), clenching of the jaw or teeth, malocclusion, or pain worsened with movement of the jaw, dental pain, or swelling of the muscles of mastication.
   d. Assess for ear pain that occurs with swallowing and associated symptoms of head and neck cancer.

7. Hearing loss.
   a. Was it sudden or gradual in onset? Assess subjective onset of hearing loss. Did the patient experience sudden or gradual onset of the hearing loss? Is there associated tinnitus, vertigo, aural fullness, or ear pain?
   b. Unilateral or bilateral? Assess for history of noise exposure; recreational shooting; occupational, acoustic trauma; or history of chronic otitis media. Assess for history of familial/hereditary hearing loss.

8. Dizziness.
   a. Is the patient light-headed or experiencing vertigo (as if the room or self is spinning)? Assess for subjective light-headedness, room spinning, or imbalance. Are symptoms acute or chronic and associated with symptoms of fluctuation of hearing, aural fullness, or tinnitus (symptoms of Ménière disease).
   b. Is the dizziness associated with a change in head or body position? Do symptoms occur with rolling over in bed, looking up or bending over, or when going from sitting to standing? Are there feelings of presyncope, history of syncopal episode when rising from sitting to standing? Are there changes in blood pressure associated with lying, sitting, and standing?
   c. Assess for duration of symptoms and associated nausea, vomiting, headache, or focal neurological symptoms.

 NURSING ALERT Hoarseness for longer than 4 weeks, or earlier if serious cause is suspected, is an indication for ENT evaluation and laryngoscopy.

Current Health Patterns

1. Inquire about nutrition; dental care; normal mouth care habits; dental caries; use of partial or full dentures; and stress-related grinding, clenching, or clamping of teeth.
2. Ask about history of alcohol, smoking, use of a pipe, and smokeless tobacco. Is there a personal history of human immunodeficiency virus (HIV), sexually transmitted disease, recreational drug use, or human papillomavirus (HPV)?
3. Determine personal hygiene about ears. Are cotton swabs or other objects used for cleaning or to relieve itching? Does the patient wear hearing aids or ear plugs?
4. Is there any loud noise exposure? Is there history of noise exposure via recreational shooting or in the patient's occupation? Ask about use of noise protection when exposed to prolonged and loud noise. Is there family history of hearing loss?
5. Does the patient frequently strain voice through talking, singing, or shouting? Is the patient a singer?
6. What medications is the patient taking? Have antibiotics been used? For how long?

Past Medical History

1. Is there a history of allergic rhinitis, other allergy symptoms, immunotherapy, chronic or recurrent sinusitis, previous nasal surgery, chronic otitis media, chronic pharyngitis, history of snoring, or obstructive sleep apnea?
2. Is there any immunosuppressive illness, such as diabetes mellitus, cancer, HIV infection, autoimmune disease, recent radiation, or chemotherapy?
3. Is there a history of previous thyroid, carotid artery, or other surgery involving the laryngeal nerve?
4. Any history of previous or recent head, facial, or nasal trauma?

See Chapter 5, page 47, for physical assessment of the ears, nose, throat, and neck.

Diagnostic Tests

Audiometry

Description

1. Audiometry is the most basic and accurate testing to determine and measure hearing ability. The results are plotted on a graph known as an audiogram. Testing is performed by an audiologist. The following points below describe aspects of audiometry:
   a. Pure tone threshold audiometry is the lowest level at which sound is heard across various sound frequencies. This is compared to normative data to measure hearing loss and used to monitor hearing sensitivity over time.
   b. Speech audiometry provides information about the patient's communication ability. Speech reception threshold is defined as the softest level at which the patient can repeat a word. Speech recognition or speech discrimination is the percentage of words that a patient can repeat accurately at the comfortable listening level. This helps to determine ability to understand conversational speech.
   c. Pure tone testing is performed by presenting pure tones via air and bone conduction. Air conduction testing is done by presenting pure tones at various octave levels from

250 to 8,000 Hz through a transducer, such as insert earphone or cushion headphone. The patient sits in a soundproof booth, and the audiologist presents tones and the patient is asked to indicate when the sound is heard. Testing by bone conduction is done with use of a bone oscillator, which is placed on the mastoid of the test ear, and pure tones are presented at 500, 1,000, 2,000, and 4,000 Hz.

d. Immittance testing includes tympanometry and acoustic reflex testing.

   i. Acoustic reflex testing measures the response of the stapedius muscle in response to auditory signals. It provides information about the acoustic and the facial nerves, as well as information about a conductive or sensorineural hearing loss.

   ii. Tympanometry measures the changes that occur to the tympanic membrane and middle ear when changes in air pressure are introduced into the ear canal. It can provide information about eustachian tube dysfunction, middle ear fluid, tympanic membrane perforation, patency of pressure-equalizing tubes, and middle ear disease such as otosclerosis.

Nursing and Patient Care Considerations

1. The patient wears earphones and signals upon hearing a tone.
2. A soundproof room is used to increase accuracy.
3. No special patient preparation or participation is necessary for tympanometry.

Cineradiography

Description

1. This motion study is performed to study the functional dynamics of the pharynx and esophagus.
2. It provides a more physiologic examination than esophagram (barium swallow). Mucosal detail is seen better with cineradiography, whereas video capture allows more dynamic evaluation with less radiation.
3. "Modified barium swallow" evaluates laryngotracheal aspiration while a speech pathologist provides various consistencies of food and swallowing techniques. An esophagram evaluates the pharyngeal and esophageal mucosa.

Nursing and Patient Care Considerations

1. The patient is usually kept NPO the night before surgery.
2. The patient will be given radioprotective gear to prevent radiation from reaching other parts of the body.

Electronystagmography

Description

1. *Electronystagmography* is the recording of eye movements, specifically nystagmus, during various oculomotor and vestibular testing. Videonystagmography is the recording of eye movements using infrared video image analysis in three dimensions. The pattern of nystagmus, in conjunction with the patient's neurotological examination and clinical history, may provide information about the underlying etiology of the patient's symptoms.
2. Used to establish the diagnosis of Ménière disease, vestibular neuronitis or labyrinthitis, benign paroxysmal positional vertigo (BPPV), or migraine-associated vertigo and to assist in ruling out vestibular pathology in a patient with symptoms of dizziness.
3. The test takes place in a dimly lit room, with the patient on an examination table, and lasts for 60 to 90 minutes.
4. Electrodes are placed on the forehead and lateral to each eye in electronystagmography (ENG) testing. Video goggles are used in videonystagmography. Eye movements are recorded in response to various position changes and visual stimuli, with eyes open and eyes closed.

5. Caloric testing is the evaluation of nystagmus induced by warm or cold water irrigation into the external ear canals. Caloric testing can also be obtained by instilling cool and warm air into the ear canal. Caloric testing is used to measure the degree of vestibular dysfunction. Testing of patients with a normally functioning vestibular system will induce vertigo.
6. The audiologist may perform the vertebral artery test with older adults, patients who have history of neck trauma, or patients in whom vertebral artery disease is suspected. Patients who elicit symptoms when the head is hyperextended may not be able to have portions of the positional testing completed.

Nursing and Patient Care Considerations

1. Patient preparation includes avoiding a heavy meal before the procedure and avoiding caffeine and alcohol for 48 hours before the procedure.
2. Medications that may affect the vestibular system, such as sedatives, antianxiety agents, narcotics, and medications ordered for dizziness, may be held for several days before the procedure.
3. The patient will receive instructions from the facility/provider who will be administering the test for specific medications that will need to be held and for how long before testing is performed. The patient should be counseled in the importance of following these preprocedure instructions, as they may affect the accuracy of the testing.

GENERAL PROCEDURES AND TREATMENT MODALITIES

Nasal Surgery

Types of Surgery and Indications

Facial Trauma and Nasal Fractures

1. Nasal bone fractures are common after blows to the nose during sports activities, interpersonal altercations, motor vehicle accidents, or falls. These can be diagnosed via physical examination or nasal/facial images, including high-resolution CT scans (3-D reconstuction can be generated).
2. Nasal fractures are treated with observation, closed reduction, closed reduction with septoplasty, or open reduction with or without internal stabilization, based on the severity of the injury. The best time to perform surgery is within the first few hours after injury or after 7 to 10 days when acute edema begins to resolve. Closed reduction should be performed before fibrosis of fracture lines, usually within 2 weeks after injury but up to 3 weeks after is diagnosed.
   a. Observation should be performed 7 to 10 days after the injury, especially when the swelling has subsided, to prevent missing a deformity.
   b. Closed reduction is effective for noncomminuted and mild nasal fractures with or without dorsal septal disruption.
3. Repair and stabilization of other maxillofacial fractures usually require an operating room procedure for wiring or plating.

Nasal Septal Surgery

1. Septoplasty is an intranasal procedure performed under general anesthesia to remove portions of, straighten, or trim the septal bone and/or cartilage. Silastic splints are sutured on either side of the septum to stabilize the repositioned septum. The splints are removed several days postoperatively. This surgery is performed to treat chronic nasal obstruction and may be done in conjunction with sinus surgery to promote a clear nasal airway.

2. Submucosal turbinate reduction or excision of middle turbinate concha bullosa is an intranasal procedure performed under local or general anesthesia in the operating room to surgically trim, excise, or reduce tissue in the nasal cavity that contributes to nasal obstruction. May be done in conjunction with septoplasty.

Rhinoplasty

1. Involves changing the nose's external appearance. Grafted cartilage or bone harvested from other parts of the body may be used.
2. A septorhinoplasty may be done when there are external and internal nasal deformities.

Sinus Surgery

1. Functional endoscopic sinus surgery (FESS) is corrective sinus surgery performed under general anesthesia in the operating room using direct visualization via a rigid nasal endoscope or, more recently, with assistance of image-guided systems. Image-guided systems utilize CT scans to provide surgeon with intraoperative landmarks and map.
2. Diseased mucosa is removed and the natural sinus ostia are widened to facilitate the normal sinus drainage patterns.
3. In addition to nasal and sinus conditions, surgery may also be used to treat traumatic optic neuropathy, fluid (CSF) leaks, nasolacrimal duct obstruction, dysthyroid orbitopathy, posterior orbital lesions, and choanal atresia.
4. Packing may be placed intraoperatively depending on surgeon's preference and amount of bleeding. Packing is usually very small, filling only the area adjacent to the sinus ostia, so is not visible except for a retrieval string extending outside the nasal ala.
5. Balloon catheter sinuplasty: The procedure uses a small balloon catheter to open blocked sinus passageways. The procedure is done to widen and restructure the blocked passageways without surgical removal of bone and tissue (see Figure 17-1).
6. Other approaches to the sinuses, such as the Caldwell-Luc procedure (opening under lip to enter maxillary sinus and strip out diseased mucosa), may be performed but newer techniques are more often utilized. A nasoantral window (creating an opening between the maxillary sinus and the anterior inferior nose), and anterior/posterior ethmoidectomies may be performed, as well as opening and draining the frontal or sphenoid sinuses. The patient with historically extensive postoperative nasal and sinus packing is rarely seen, and this is now used only in selected complicated cases with extensive bleeding.

Preoperative Management

1. The head of the bed should be raised to promote drainage, lessen edema, and make the patient more comfortable.
2. Intermittent cold compresses and pain medications should be utilized, as ordered.
3. Antibiotics may be used preoperatively to reduce bacterial colonization of nose and sinuses.
4. The patient should be advised that a sensation of pressure may be felt in the nasal area during surgery performed under local anesthetic.
5. The patient should be counseled about the possible use of packing with some surgeries, which may be removed several days postoperatively.
6. Instructions for stopping aspirin, NSAIDs, and antiplatelet and anticoagulant medications will be provided by the surgeon and individualized after collaboration with the patient's cardiologist or primary care provider.

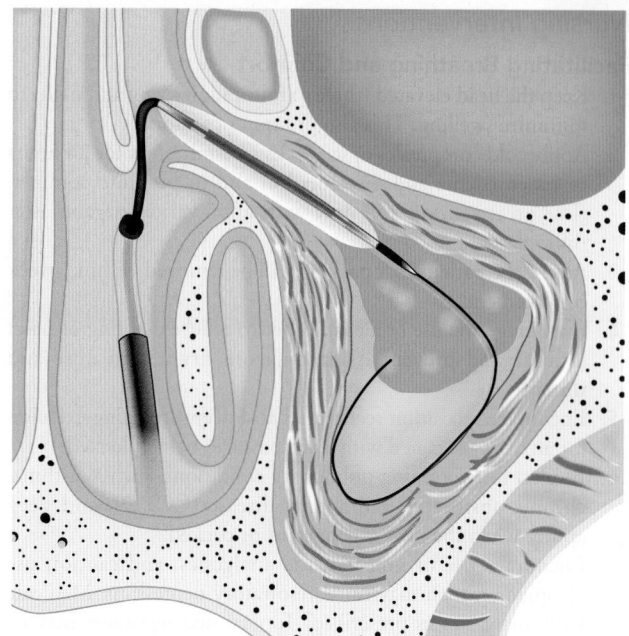

Figure 17-1. Balloon catheter sinus surgery. A catheter is introduced through the nose and into the sinus ostia, where the balloon is inflated to enlarge the sinus opening and promote drainage.

 NURSING ALERT In most cases, the patient should avoid use of aspirin, nonsteroidal anti-inflammatory drugs, anticoagulants, antiplatelet agents, and herbal medications such as *Ginkgo biloba*, garlic, green tea, and any other drugs that may affect platelet function before surgery. If the patient has taken these medications within a week of surgery, make sure the surgeon is notified.

Complications

1. Hematoma/hemorrhage: septal hematoma or postoperative bleeding. A septal hematoma will need to be drained by the surgeon immediately if this should occur.
2. Local infection—contaminated nasal packing is an excellent culture medium for pathogens. Most patients are treated postoperatively with antibiotics, but this is surgeon-specific.
3. Aspiration.
4. Pressure necrosis (from packing) may occur, but the current trend is toward less packing.
5. Blindness from orbital hematoma or unintended orbital involvement in endoscopic sinus surgery.
6. CSF rhinorrhea from unintended or traumatic violation of the cribriform plate. This is commonly referred to as a CSF leak.
7. Pulmonary decompensation.

Nursing Diagnoses

• Ineffective Breathing Pattern (nasal airway clearance) related to nasal packing and swelling.
• Risk for Aspiration related to bleeding, inability to blow nose.
• Deficient Knowledge related to performance of nasal hygiene.
• Impaired Oral Mucous Membrane related to mouth breathing.
• Risk for Infection related to alterations in nasal/sinus mucous membranes and drainage patterns.

Nursing Interventions

Facilitating Breathing and Comfort

1. Keep the head elevated (three to four pillows) day and night to minimize swelling. This also promotes comfort.
2. Apply cold compresses or ice packs intermittently for 24 hours to lessen edema and discoloration and to promote comfort. (Use great caution and only with approval of surgeon after rhinoplasty.)
3. Advise the patient that packing will be removed within 1 week of placement.
4. Encourage the use of a humidifier to relieve crusting of nasal mucosa and prevent irritation from dryness in nose and throat.
5. Encourage relaxation techniques and deep-breathing exercises for anxiety associated with nasal passages being blocked.
6. Be alert for worsening pulmonary conditions, such as asthma, chronic obstructive pulmonary disease (COPD), and sleep apnea, when the nose is congested or packed.
7. Encourage use of non-narcotic analgesics, and caution use of opioids, which may cause respiratory depression. Medicate with analgesics as prescribed. Topical decongestants may be prescribed to relieve nasal congestion in the first few days postoperatively. Pain after nasal surgery is usually mild to moderate.

Preventing Bleeding and Aspiration

1. Monitor closely for bleeding; check for increased swallowing, blood dripping down back of throat (use flashlight and tongue blade), and expectoration of large amounts of clots and blood.
2. Change the 4 × 4 gauze pad under the nose as it becomes soaked with blood; bleeding should gradually decrease.

Teach family and patient that blood will be bright red at first and will gradually lessen over the next several days.
3. Notify the surgeon if bleeding increases. Expect a temporary minor increase in bleeding with vomiting, sneezing, ambulation, or crying in the first 48 hours.
4. Teach the patient that mild nausea is normal postoperatively and may be from anesthesia, pain medications, or swallowing of blood; however, be alert for continuous trickle of blood postnasally.
5. Instruct the patient not to blow the nose but to blot secretions with tissue and spit out any secretions collecting in oropharynx.
6. Regularly observe and document visible packing retrieval strings external to nose, taped to cheek, if present. Postoperative instructions should be given upon discharge with appointments for postoperative splint removal or sinus debridement, if indicated. The surgeon will discuss activity and work restrictions specific to the patient.

Ensuring Proper Nasal Hygiene

1. Encourage the patient to use a vaporizer to help relieve crusting of nasal mucosa from dryness.
2. Remind the patient that sneezing, straining, and nose blowing increase venous pressure and can result in bleeding/hematoma.
3. Advise the patient to keep the mouth open while sneezing if unable to control sneezing.
4. Teach the patient an appropriate method of nasal hygiene as approved by surgeon. After FESS, the patient will need regular appointments for sinus debridement by the surgeon. Advise the patient that sinus irrigation will need to be done to control nasal crusting and to facilitate healing

---

PATIENT EDUCATION GUIDELINES 17-1

Nasal Saline Irrigation

This procedure will help clear nasal passages of crusted drainage that may be blocking the sinus opening. Perform this once or twice per day to feel less nasal congestion and to help sinuses drain.

1. Prepare saline solution right before irrigation. *Commercially prepared sinus irrigation kits are readily available that contain packets and sinus rinse bottle.*
2. Mix ½ tsp table salt and ¼ tsp baking soda with 8 ounce warm distilled or sterilized water until well dissolved. Do not use tap water.
3. Lean forward from the waist over a sink.
4. Fill a bulb syringe (1 ounce infant ear or nasal bulb) or rinse bottle with the saline solution by squeezing it in the solution and letting it fill by suction. If using sinus rinse kit, follow instructions.
5. Insert the tip of the filled syringe into one nostril, aimed toward the eye away from the nasal septum.
6. Squeeze the syringe gently and feel the solution run backward in the nose and out the other nostril and possibly down the back of the throat and out of the mouth.
7. When comfortable with this procedure, you may be able to rotate head forward, backward, and from side to side to irrigate the sinuses as well as the nose.

Nose irrigation with bulb syringe or sinus irrigation kit.

5. In general, the patient may gently clean the nasal ala area with saline and/or peroxide for comfort, but large crusts should be removed by surgeon or allowed to work themselves free.

6. Instruct the patient to avoid environmental irritants, especially smoke.

Protecting Oral Mucous Membranes

1. Administer frequent mouth care because the patient is forced to breathe through the mouth.
2. Use flexible straw to sip mouthwash for rinsing purposes.
3. Encourage fluid intake and use of lip protectant.

Preventing Infection

1. Be alert for uncontrolled postoperative pain, fever, foul odor or taste in mouth, or unusual drainage.
2. Administer or encourage prophylactic antibiotics on time, if ordered.
3. Advise patient to keep follow-up appointment for splint removal, packing removal, and sinus debridement.

Patient Education and Health Maintenance

1. Tell the patient to notify the surgeon immediately for uncontrolled postoperative pain, any visual changes postoperatively, fever, unilateral clear nasal discharge with leaning the head forward, uncontrolled excessive nasal bleeding, dyspnea, or blanching or necrosis of the external nasal tissues or the palate while packing is in place.
2. After Caldwell-Luc procedure or rhinoplasty, advise the patient that numbness in operative area may be present for several weeks to months.
3. Instruct the patient to avoid strenuous activity, lifting, and trauma to nose.
4. After splint removal, avoid trauma to nose and sleep in supine position. The operating surgeon will provide more specific postoperative instructions.
5. Excessive sun exposure should also be avoided after rhinoplasty for 1 year because of a tendency for hyperpigmentation.
6. If a nasal splint is present, tell the patient to avoid getting it wet; do not attempt to remove it.

7. Advise the patient that postoperative follow-up may need to continue for several weeks to months to monitor for excess scar formation or cosmetic deformity.

Evaluation: Expected Outcomes

- Mouth breathing without difficulty.
- No excessive bleeding; protects airway without aspiration.
- Nasal and palatal tissues free from blanching or darkening.
- Oral mucous membranes dry, but pink and intact.
- Afebrile; no signs of infection.

Ear Surgery

Ear surgery may involve the tympanic membrane, the middle ear cavity, the mastoid, or the inner ear. It may be done for perforation of the eardrum to facilitate drainage and remove diseased tissue in cases of infection or cholesteatoma, to relieve vertigo, or to treat hearing loss.

Types of Surgery

1. Myringotomy—creating a surgical opening into tympanic membrane (with knife or laser) for possible drainage tube insertion.
2. Tympanoplasty—reconstruction of diseased or deformed middle ear components (see Table 17-1).
   a. Type I (myringoplasty)—purpose is to close perforation by placing a graft over it to create a closed middle ear to improve hearing and decrease risk of infection and cholesteatoma. Perforation is closed using one of the following:
      i. Fascia from temporalis muscle (this is the most commonly used material).
      ii. Vein grafts from hand or forearm.
      iii. Epithelium from auditory canal (eustachian tube).
   b. Type II to V—suitable replacement (polyethylene, Teflon or titanium prosthesis, bone, cartilage) is used to maintain continuity of conduction sound pathway. The necessity of a two-stage procedure is determined.

Table 17-1 Types of Tympanoplasty

| Type | MIDDLE EAR DAMAGE | | REPAIR PROCESS |
	Tympanic Membrane	Ossicles	
I	Perforated	Normal	• Close perforation—myringoplasty
II	Perforated	Erosion of malleus and/or incus	• Close perforation; graft against incus or whatever remains of malleus
III	Tympanic membrane destroyed or widely perforated	Rest of ossicular chain destroyed but stapes are intact and mobile.	• Grafts implanted to contact the normal stapes • Tympanostapedopexy
IV	Tympanic membrane destroyed or widely perforated	Ossicular chain destroyed. Head, neck, and crura of stapes destroyed. Stapes footplate mobile.	• Expose mobile stapes footplate—graft implanted. Air pocket between graft and round window provides protection. • The cavum minor operation
V	Tympanic membrane destroyed or widely perforated	Ossicular chain destroyed. Head, neck, and crura of stapes destroyed. Stapes footplate fixed.	• Make opening in horizontal semicircular canal; graft seals off middle ear to give sound protection for round window. • Tympanoplasty and fenestration of lateral semicircular canal

     i. First stage—eradication of all diseased tissues; area is cleaned out to achieve a dry, healed middle ear.

     ii. Second stage—performed 4 to 6 months after first stage; reconstruction, using grafts.

3. Mastoidectomy—removal of mastoid process of temporal bone.

   a. Simple or cortical mastoidectomy is done via a postauricular approach, but the bony ear canal is left intact.

   b. Modified radical mastoidectomy or canal wall down mastoidectomy is done with a meatoplasty for the best results. A wide excision of the mastoid and diseased middle ear contents through a postauricular incision is performed with the bony canal being drilled out. A new larger ear canal is created that gives better access to the areas where cholesteatoma usually occurs (the attic and antrum).

4. Stapedectomy—removal of footplate of stapes and insertion of a graft or prosthesis.

5. Stapedotomy—removal of the stapes suprastructure, allowing a hole to be created with a laser in the stapes footplate. The base of the prosthesis will be inserted into the opening, and the other end will be crimped around the incus.

6. Labyrinthectomy—destruction of the labyrinth (inner ear) through the middle ear and aspiration of the endolabyrinth.

7. Endolymphatic decompression and shunt—release of pressure on the endolymphatic system in the labyrinth and creation of a shunt for fluid to the subarachnoid space or the mastoid.

8. Cochlear implant—implantation of electronic device that bypasses the damaged cochlea and stimulates auditory nerve.

9. Osseointegrated implantation for placement of a hearing implant for single-sided deafness or for conductive hearing loss (Baha system or Oticon implantable hearing system).

Preoperative Management

1. Hearing function is fully evaluated.
2. Antibiotics are given to treat infection.
3. The patient is prepared emotionally for the effects of surgery.
4. Careful assessment for signs of acute infection is performed, which may delay surgery.

Postoperative Management

1. Antibiotics may be continued to prevent local and central nervous system (CNS) infection.
2. Patients are advised to have limited activity for the first 24 hours to decrease symptoms of nausea and vertigo (if the inner ear was disturbed) or to prevent disruption of prosthesis.
3. Analgesics, antiemetics, and antihistamines are given, as needed.
4. The patient is positioned to promote drainage but maintain some immobility. Using two extra pillows to elevate the head, thereby preventing edema for 2 weeks, is a good idea.
5. The patient is often seen 7 to 10 days after surgery to remove any metal stent placed. Additional packing may be removed up to 6 weeks postoperatively if prosthesis or graft procedure was performed. Often, an eardrop will be used to slowly dissolve remaining packing over a period of 6 to 8 weeks to give some weight to the grafted tympanic membrane.
6. Hearing will be reevaluated after edema has subsided and healing has occurred. The time frame for this varies by procedure but may be as long as 3 to 4 months after surgery to allow for healing.
7. With an osseointegrated implant, a fitting of the outer processor is usually delayed by 2 to 3 months to allow the bone to osseointegrate around the implant. In children, or in radiated bone, this may be done in two stages separated by 6 months to allow for a slower rate of bone growth.
8. Cochlear implant activation and placement of the outer speech processor and external transmitter occurs approximately 4 weeks after surgery to allow for healing.

Complications

1. Infection: local, CNS (meningitis, brain abscess).
2. Hearing loss.
3. Facial nerve paralysis—rare.
4. Dizziness—usually temporary.

Nursing Diagnoses

• Acute Pain related to surgical incision and swelling.
• Risk for Infection related to invasive procedure.
• Risk for Injury related to vertigo.

Nursing Interventions

Relieving Pain

1. Administer or teach self-administration of analgesic, as indicated, postoperatively.
2. Tell the patient to expect pain to subside within first few hours with simple procedures or within first day or 2 with major procedures.
3. Position the patient for comfort following the instructions from the surgeon.
   a. On side with surgical ear upward to maintain graft position and immobility.
   b. Lying on side with surgical ear down to promote drainage from ear canal.
   c. Position of patient preference.
4. Elevate the head of bed to reduce swelling and pressure.
5. Advise the patient to avoid sudden movement. Use pillows for support.

Preventing Infection

1. Reinforce external dressings, as needed, until after first changed by surgeon, then change when saturated to prevent bacterial growth in damp dressings.
2. Loosely pack cotton or gauze in ear canal, as indicated, without causing increased pressure.
3. Do not probe or insert anything into ear canal.
4. Administer or teach self-administration of antibiotics, as prescribed. Do not use eardrops unless specifically ordered postoperatively.
5. Wash hands before ear care and instruct the patient not to touch ear.
6. Take care not to get the dressing or ear wet.
7. Advise the patient not to blow the nose, which could cause nasopharyngeal secretions to be forced up the eustachian tube into the middle ear.
8. Instruct the patient to report any increased pain, fever, ear inflammation, or drainage, indicating local infection.
9. Be alert for headache, fever, stiff neck, or altered level of consciousness, which may indicate CNS infection.

Ensuring Safety

1. Be aware that dizziness or vertigo may occur for the first several days postoperatively.
2. Maintain side rails up while the patient is in bed.
3. Assist the patient with ambulation for the first time after surgery and as needed thereafter.
4. Encourage the patient to move slowly because sudden movements may exacerbate vertigo.

5. Administer or teach self-administration of antiemetics and antihistamines, as ordered and as needed; watch for sedation.
6. Instruct the patient not to blow nose, cough, lean forward, or perform Valsalva maneuver to avoid disrupting graft or prosthesis, aggravating vertigo, or forcing bacteria up the eustachian tube. If coughing or blowing nose is necessary, do so with open mouth to relieve pressure.

Patient Education and Health Maintenance

1. Advise the patient that there may be a temporary hearing loss for a few weeks after surgery because of tissue edema, packing, and so forth. The effects of a hearing restoration operation will not be known for several weeks and additional rehabilitation may be necessary to optimize results.
2. Advise the patient to protect the ear, perform dressing changes, or place loose cotton in outer ear, as indicated. Replace cotton twice daily or sooner if saturated by drainage.
3. Encourage follow-up for packing removal, as directed.
4. Instruct the patient to avoid sudden pressure changes in the ear.
   a. Do not blow the nose.
   b. Do not fly in a small plane. The date for which a patient may fly is individualized by their surgery and surgeon's preference.
   c. Do not dive.
5. Advise against smoking.
6. Tell the patient to protect ears when going outdoors for the 1st week. A cotton ball is all that is needed.
7. Tell the patient to avoid getting the ear wet until completely healed.
8. Tell the patient to avoid crowds or exposure to colds so upper respiratory infection is prevented.
9. Instruct the patient about signs and symptoms of complications to report.
   a. Return of tinnitus.
   b. Vertigo.
   c. Fluctuations of hearing ability.
   d. Fever, headache, ear inflammation, increased pain, stiff neck.
   e. Facial drooping or numbness.
10. Advise the patient that facial nerve paralysis may be temporary and to increase fluid intake through a straw during this time.

Evaluation: Expected Outcomes

- Verbalizes relief of pain.
- No signs of infection.
- Ambulates without difficulty.

CONDITIONS OF THE MOUTH AND JAW
Candidiasis

EVIDENCE BASE Sawant, B. & Khan, T. (2017). Recent advances in delivery of antifungal agents for therapeutic management of candidiasis. *Biomedicine and Pharmacotherapy*, 96, 1478–1490.

Candidiasis is an opportunistic fungal infection commonly caused by *Candida albicans*. It may be localized in the mouth and pharynx but may also occur in the esophagus. Candidiasis can become a source of systemic dissemination, particularly in high-risk persons.

Pathophysiology and Etiology

1. Commonly seen in individuals with immunosuppression from disease states or treatment regimens such as diabetes, cancer, or HIV and those receiving radiation therapy and/or chemotherapy.
2. May be caused by altered oral environment from xerostomia, use of inhaled steroids for asthma and COPD, or chronic antibiotic therapy, preexisting infections, poor oral hygiene or nutritional status, or wearing dentures.

Clinical Manifestations

1. Oral examination reveals diffuse, white, painless plaques. Underlying mucosa may be erythematous.
2. May be asymptomatic but may result in mild oral discomfort, burning, or alterations in taste.
3. Patients with disease spread beyond the oral cavity may present with chest pain, pain and difficulty with swallowing, or hoarseness.

Diagnostic Evaluation

1. Microscopic smear of plaques shows characteristic hyphae.
2. Oral fungal culture positive for *C. albicans*.
3. Occasionally, biopsy of lesions may be necessary to rule out leukoplakia (premalignant plaques).

Management

1. Topical antifungal medications such as nystatin suspension or clotrimazole troches are most often used.
2. Systemic treatment is indicated if topical agents fail or for esophageal cases with fluconazole, ketoconazole (used cautiously in immunosuppressed patients), or amphotericin B.
3. Topical oral rinses or preparations containing combinations of hydrocortisone, diphenhydramine, antifungals, or antibiotics may be used to enhance healing and to lessen discomfort.
4. Viscous lidocaine may be used topically to coat the oral mucosa before meals to lessen pain and enhance oral intake.
5. Oral prostheses may also be treated to avoid harboring and reintroducing infection.

Complications

1. Candidal infection throughout the GI tract.
2. Candidal sepsis in patients who are immunocompromised.

Nursing Assessment

1. Carefully examine oral cavity daily to monitor lesions as well as response to prescribed antifungal therapy.
2. Assess level of pain; administer analgesics, as prescribed; and monitor response to analgesics.
3. Assess nutritional status and effect of pain on oral intake. Monitor oral intake, nutritional and hydration status, weight loss/gain, and signs of dehydration.
4. Teach patients that are prescribed inhaled steroid therapy for asthma/COPD to rinse mouth after each use to prevent oropharyngeal candidiasis.

Nursing Diagnoses

- Imbalanced Nutrition: Less Than Body Requirements related to oral discomfort.
- Deficient Knowledge related to antifungal therapy.

Nursing Interventions

Attaining Adequate Nutrition

1. Administer analgesics, as prescribed, 30 to 60 minutes before meals.
2. Provide soft foods, soothing liquids; avoid temperature extremes.
3. Provide gentle suctioning if pain becomes so severe that patient cannot handle secretions and provide intravenous (IV) fluids.

Ensuring Adequate Therapy

1. Administer antifungal agents, as prescribed. Observe the patient for proper use of topical preparation.
   a. Make sure that mouth is clean and free of food debris before administering drug.
   b. For swish-and-swallow preparations, tell the patient to swish and hold in the mouth for at least 10 minutes before swallowing.
   c. For troches, have the patient suck until dissolved.
2. Observe for signs and symptoms of systemic drug adverse effects: nausea, vomiting, diarrhea. Renal, bone marrow, cardiovascular, hepatic, or neurologic toxicities may occur in patients receiving systemic therapy with underlying chronic disease states.
3. Explain the importance of continuing therapy for duration prescribed.

Patient Education and Health Maintenance

1. Instruct high-risk patients about daily oral examination and signs and symptoms to observe.
2. Teach the patient to avoid highly seasoned foods, extremes in temperature, alcoholic beverages, and smoking, all of which irritate the oral mucosa.
3. Encourage good oral hygiene.
4. May need to refrain from wearing dentures because of oral discomfort.
5. Encourage the patient on long-term systemic antifungal therapy to follow up for liver function test monitoring, as directed.

Evaluation: Expected Outcomes

- Adequate intake of liquids and soft foods as evidenced by stable body weight and signs of dehydration.
- Swishes oral suspension for 10 minutes before spitting or swallowing.

Herpes Simplex Infection (Type 1)

Also known as *cold sores* or *fever blisters*, herpes simplex virus (HSV; usually type 1) is commonly associated with lip and oral lesions 80% of the time. HSV1 causes genital outbreaks in 20% of the cases.

Pathophysiology and Etiology

1. After a primary infection and the patient produces antibodies, the virus remains latent in the sensory ganglia.
2. Recurrent herpes labialis may be precipitated by sun exposure, fever, oral trauma, fatigue, emotional upset, hormonal changes, and other factors.
3. The spread of HSV1 is through respiratory droplets or exposure to infected saliva via a break in the skin or mucous membranes.
4. HSV type 2 (and rarely HSV type 1) is associated with genital lesions and is sexually transmitted.

Clinical Manifestations

1. Prodromal period—tingling, soreness, and burning in area where lesion will develop.
2. Small vesicles appear on erythematous, edematous base, frequently near the mucocutaneous junction of the lips and oral mucosa. Lesions may be spread to genitalia during oral sex.
3. Lesions may be quite severe in the immunosuppressed.
4. Vesicles rupture, causing painful ulcerations.
5. Lesions heal spontaneously in 7 to 14 days, but reoccur.

Diagnosis and Management

1. No diagnostic tests are necessary but serologic testing may be done. The diagnoses of herpes simplex is made from viral culture from skin vesicles, serology, or monoclonal antibody testing.
2. Treatment may not be necessary if cases are mild and are usually short lived.
3. Comfort measures, such as mild oral or topical analgesics.
4. Good hygiene to prevent spread to self and others.
5. Antiviral agents, including acyclovir, famiciclovir, and valacyclovir, are available to decrease the duration of symptoms.
6. Penciclovir 1% cream—FDA approved; applied every 2 hours while awake at earliest sign. If used within 1 hour of outbreak, will decrease duration of viral shedding.
7. Acyclovir 5% cream may be used on topical lesions. Oral or IV antivirals may also be used if clinically indicated.

Nursing Interventions and Patient Education

1. Advise adequate rest and nutrition and avoidance of identified triggers.
2. Advise that virus is transmitted through close contact, such as kissing and sharing food and cups, so avoid these from prodromal period until well healed.
3. Recommend good hand washing and hygiene.
4. Apthous ulcers or canker sores—not caused by HSV1.

Temporomandibular Disorders

Temporomandibular disorders are conditions affecting the jaw joint that consist of one or more of the following:
1. Myofascial pain—pain in the muscles serving the jaw (temporalis, masseter, medial and lateral pterygoids), neck, and shoulder.
2. Internal derangement of the jaw joint (dislocated or displaced joint disk or injured condyle).
3. Degenerative joint disease (eg, arthritis).

Pathophysiology and Etiology

1. Causes include rheumatoid or osteoarthritis; scleroderma; ankylosing spondylitis; trauma; teeth clenching or bruxism (teeth grinding). Neoplasms and acute infections such as parotitis, dental infections, and peritonsillar abscesses cause referred ear pain and should be differentiated from temporomandibular disorders.
2. Any mental and physical stresses can induce or exacerbate symptoms.
3. Above factors result in inflammation and muscle spasm of temporomandibular joint (TMJ).

Clinical Manifestations

1. Pain at the joint, temples, mandible, or masticatory muscles may worsen with jaw movement. Referred muscle spasm of the neck, trapezius, and sternocleidomastoid muscle causes discomfort.

2. Clicking or crepitus from opening and closing of the jaw or popping of the joint.
3. Limitation of movement, dislocation, or jaw locking.
4. May be associated with headaches, earaches, or tinnitus.
5. Change in the bite where the upper and lower teeth do not match in the normal comfortable way.
6. May experience deteriorating oral hygiene or halitosis from limited oral opening (trismus), making dental hygiene difficult.
7. May experience difficulty chewing because of limited jaw excursion, resulting in altered diet and weight loss.
8. Jaw clicking alone is common and requires no workup or intervention if asymptomatic.

Diagnostic Evaluation

1. Diagnosis can usually be achieved by history and physical examination without extensive testing. Provocative maneuvers performed on physical examination that reproduce pain with opening and closing of the jaw are generally suggestive of TMJ arthralgia.
2. Dental and TMJ x-rays may or may not be helpful.
3. Occlusal analysis evaluates for malocclusion of the jaw and teeth in a bite position.
4. CT scan and magnetic resonance imaging (MRI) are usually normal unless there is underlying degenerative changes, fracture, or neoplasm of jaw or cervical spine.
5. Arthrography (joint x-rays using dye).
6. Arthroscopy (endoscopic invasive joint examination).

Management

1. Initial management employs jaw rest (soft, no-chew diet for 2 weeks, plus avoiding extreme jaw movements, such as wide yawning and gum chewing).
2. Anti-inflammatory/analgesic medications such as ibuprofen.
3. Application of warm, moist heat or ice packs.
4. Muscle relaxants may be prescribed.
5. Therapeutic night guard or splint—to realign malocclusion or joint disk and to optimize muscle relaxation.
6. Physical therapy for gentle stretching and relaxing exercises with or without ultrasound (deep-heat) therapy—to enhance analgesia and muscle relaxation and to promote local tissue metabolism.
7. Transcutaneous electrical nerve stimulation reduces muscle spasm of head, neck, and back and reduces pain.
8. In general, conservative reversible measures above are employed as long as possible before progressing to invasive/surgical management.
   a. Arthroscopy—investigational procedure to visualize joint, reposition disk, lyse adhesions, or debride joint.
      i. Reserved for conditions not improved by medical management.
      ii. Complications include cranial nerve (CN) VII damage with facial paralysis and paresis, perforation of the external auditory canal, and piercing of the middle cranial fossa.
   b. Surgery—to remove the disk or reshape bony prominences.
9. Complications include malocclusion, CN VII damage, and infection.

Nursing Interventions and Patient Education

1. Assess the character, frequency, location, and duration of pain. Evaluate what triggers and relieves the pain. Determine how effective previous treatments have been.
2. Explore the effect of the disorder on the patient's lifestyle, especially eating habits. Assist the patient to alter methods of oral hygiene and eating if severe trismus is present.
3. Instruct the patient on the indications, dosages, and adverse effects of analgesics and anti-inflammatory medications.
4. Teach the patient proper use of heat therapies. Cold applications may be preferred by some patients to reduce pain and spasm.
5. Encourage the patient to perform active mouth opening, protrusion, and lateral movement exercises of the jaw for 5 minutes, four to five times per day, as prescribed, to stretch muscles and reduce spasm.
6. Encourage the use of soft food and liquid supplements during times of acute pain exacerbated by eating. Advise reduction of foods that require excessive chewing, such as raw vegetables, tough meat, nuts. Discourage gum chewing.
7. Explore tension-reducing modalities with the patient, especially progressive muscle relaxation to reduce muscle tension and spasm.
8. Encourage follow-up with dentist, oral surgeon, ENT specialist, or other caregiver, as indicated.
9. Encourage proper use of the night guard or dental splint, including periodic appointments to assess fit.
10. May need MedicAlert bracelet and preoperative anesthesia consultation for elective surgeries if maximum jaw opening is less than 30 mm, limiting access for airway intubation.

Maxillofacial and Mandibular Fractures

Fractures of the maxillofacial bones or mandible may occur as the result of industrial, athletic, and vehicular accidents; violent acts; and falls.

Pathophysiology and Etiology

1. Maxillofacial fractures usually occur due to blow to the cheek or face.
2. Mandibular fractures frequently occur due to blow to the chin.
3. May be nondisplaced or displaced, usually closed, and includes soft tissue injury.
4. May also occur as part of planned surgical reconstruction for jaw problems.
5. Injuries sustained in altercations or motor vehicle accidents may be associated with alcohol intoxication or recreational drug use.

Clinical Manifestations

1. Malocclusion, asymmetry, abnormal mobility, crepitus (grating sound with movement), pain, or tenderness.
2. Tissue injury: swelling, ecchymosis, bleeding, and pain.

Diagnostic Evaluation

1. CT is the gold standard for evaluating the extent of injuries.
2. Panorex can also be used is CT is not available.

Management

1. Maintenance of adequate respiratory functioning—may include oxygen support, endotracheal intubation, or tracheostomy. See Chapter 35, page 936.
2. Control of bleeding—usually accomplished with direct pressure.
3. Reduction of the fracture—usually closed reduction.

4. Immobilization—depends on location, type, and severity of the fracture.
   a. Barton bandage with a Kling or stockinette bandage.
   b. Interdental fixation with rubber bands or wiring.
   c. Intermaxillary fixation with rubber bands or wiring.
   d. Interosseous fixation with open reduction.
5. Maintenance of adequate nutritional intake with liquid or soft diet—to maintain immobilization of fracture site.
6. Pain control—to promote comfort.
7. Control of infection with antibiotics in the presence of positive cultures.

Complications

1. Airway obstruction, aspiration.
2. Hemorrhage, infection.
3. Disfigurement.
4. Extraocular muscle entrapment/orbital globe displacement with resultant visual disturbance.
5. Acute drug or alcohol withdrawal.

Nursing Assessment

1. Obtain description of injury and review chart and diagnostic tests for extent of injury.
2. Continually assess respiratory status.
3. Assess level of pain.
4. Assess visual acuity and extraocular movement.
5. Assess for tremors, delirium or hallucinations, anxiety, and seizure activity related to alcohol or drug withdrawal.

Nursing Diagnoses

- Risk for Aspiration related to immobilization of jaw.
- Imbalanced Nutrition: Less Than Body Requirements related to pain, injury, and immobilization.
- Acute Pain related to injury and surgical intervention.
- Disturbed Body Image related to disfigurement of injury or surgical repair.
- Risk for Infection related to surgery.

Nursing Interventions

Preventing Aspiration

1. Maintain effective airway.
   a. Elevate head of bed 30 to 45 degrees or position leaning over a bedside stand to reduce edema and improve handling of secretions.
   b. Make sure suctioning equipment is readily accessible; teach patient oral and nasal suctioning; position on side or upright during suctioning.
   c. Administer antiemetic, as prescribed, for nausea and vomiting to prevent aspiration.
   d. Make sure wire cutters or scissors are present for immediate removal of the wires or rubber bands if the airway becomes obstructed. (Vertical rubber bands or wires should be cut.)
   e. Make sure that a method for calling the nurse (call bell) is within easy access for the patient at all times in case of emergency.
2. Monitor blood pressure, pulse, respirations, and temperature to note early onset of infection or aspiration.

Maintaining Nutritional Status

1. Administer liquid diet, as prescribed; place straw against teeth or through any gaps in the teeth. Teeth may initially be sensitive to hot and cold.
2. Position in upright position before, during, and for 45 to 60 minutes after all feedings.
3. Evaluate ongoing nutritional and hydration status; weight; intake, output, and specific gravity; laboratory values—24-hour urea nitrogen, transferrin level, electrolytes, and albumin.
4. Advance to blenderized diet, as tolerated.
5. Make environment as pleasant as possible to enhance appetite—remove all sources of odor, decrease interruptions, position comfortably.

Increasing Comfort

1. Administer liquid or a suspension of analgesics, as prescribed—avoid opioids on an empty stomach, which may cause nausea and vomiting.
2. Administer diazepam as prescribed to reduce anxiety and control reflex muscle spasm.
3. Apply paraffin wax to the ends of wire fixation devices to decrease irritation to the gums and oral mucosa.
4. Apply petroleum jelly to the lips to decrease dryness and prevent cracking.

Strengthening Body Image

1. Provide firm reassurance regarding progress to reduce anxiety and allay fears.
2. Avoid unrealistic promises in relation to scars or disfigurement.
3. Allow the patient to choose the first time for looking in the mirror.
4. Provide privacy, as requested. The patient may be sensitive to appearance.
5. Provide alternative form of communication, such as magic slate or picture board, because maxillomandibular fixation limits articulating ability, making speech difficult to understand.

Preventing Infection

1. Provide mouth care every 2 hours while awake for the first several days, then four to six times per day.
2. Initially, provide mouth care with warm normal saline mouth swishes.
3. As diet is progressed, remove collected debris with a pressurized water stream cleaner and encourage the patient to brush teeth with a soft, child-size toothbrush.
4. Observe facial injuries for swelling, erythema, pain, or warmth to detect onset of infection.
5. Change facial dressings as needed to prevent soiling with secretions, food, or drainage, which may promote bacterial growth.

Patient Education and Health Maintenance

1. Encourage adequate nutrition—inform the patient and family that foods can be blenderized and thinned with juices or broths to a consistency that can be taken through a straw.
2. Explore with the patient options for maintaining proper oral care; encourage the patient to practice the options of choice.
3. Discuss the use of antiemetic medications to prevent nausea and vomiting, stressing the complications this could cause.
4. Make sure the patient has wire cutters or scissors at all times and knows how to use them should airway obstruction occur.
5. Encourage follow-up health care visits, including counseling for alcohol or drug abuse.

Evaluation: Expected Outcomes

- No evidence of aspiration.
- Tolerates fluids through straw; maintains adequate body weight.
- Expresses relief of pain.
- Views self in mirror; notices improvement in appearance.
- No signs of infection; oral hygiene maintained.

PROBLEMS OF THE NOSE, THROAT, AND SINUSES

Rhinopathies

Rhinopathies are disorders of the nose that interrupt its normal functions of olfaction and warming, filtering, and humidifying inspired air. These include *allergic rhinitis, nonallergic rhinitis, vasomotor rhinitis*, and other conditions.

Pathophysiology and Etiology

1. Allergic rhinitis—immunoglobulin E (IgE)-mediated response causing release of vasoactive substances from mast cells (see page 791).
2. Non–IgE-mediated allergy/sensitivity—exposure to irritants such as tobacco smoke, perfumes, soaps, hair sprays, air pollution, or certain foods may produce symptoms of nasal congestion, postnasal drip, or rhinorrhea but are not caused by inhalant allergy.
3. Nonallergic rhinitis includes infectious rhinitis, rhinitis medicamentosa, rhinitis of pregnancy, or vasomotor rhinitis.
   a. Infectious—viral (common cold), bacterial (purulent rhinitis).
   b. Drug-induced (rebound rhinitis; rhinitis medicamentosa)—caused by excessive use of topical nasal decongestants. These products include oxymetazoline and phenylephrine. Many systemic medications may induce nasal congestion and stuffiness and include specific beta-blockers, antihypertensives, and antidepressants.
   c. Vasomotor rhinitis—consists of symptoms caused by autonomic instability with disruption of the normal balance of sympathetic and parasympathetic innervation. This produces nasal congestion, rhinorrhea, and postnasal drip. Symptoms may be manifested on exposure to cold weather or eating spicy, hot, or cold foods (gustatory rhinitis).
   d. Rhinitis of pregnancy—nasal congestion resulting from estrogen-mediated mucosal engorgement, especially in the last trimesters of pregnancy, may also occur with oral contraceptive use, postmenopausal estrogen therapy, and during the last portion of the menstrual cycle. Edema of the nasal mucosa and turbinate congestion occur.

   e. Nonallergic rhinitis with eosinophilia syndrome—patients have symptoms of rhinitis, negative allergy testing, but large number of eosinophils in nasal secretions. Treatment is similar to those with vasomotor rhinitis.

Manifestations of Allergic Rhinitis

1. Hypersecretion—wet, running/dripping nose or postnasal drip.
2. Eyes—edema of the conjunctivae, tearing and itching of the eyes, increase in vascularity, fine allergic shiners, or dark staining under eyes.
3. Nasal cavity—congestion, pressure, or stuffiness (see Figure 17-2). Chronic nasal crusting and erythema around outer nares and turbinates are often swollen, edematous with pale or bluish hue. Allergic salute often seen in children caused by upward lifting of the tip of the nose with the hand.
4. Oral cavity—chronic mouth breathing, enlarged lymph tissue in the oropharynx, prominent vascularity, or cobblestoning in posterior pharynx.

Management

1. Treatment of underlying cause.
   a. Allergy—antihistamines (see Chapter 28).
   b. Nonallergic rhinitis—treatment modalities can include avoidance if caused by chemical, food, or other irritants.
2. Topical decongestants (for short-term use); systemic decongestants—topical or systemic decongestants may be used for short-term usage only, no more than 2 to 3 days, in patients with various forms of nonallergic rhinitis.
3. Intranasal corticosteroids—used in the treatment of allergic and nonallergic rhinitis because of their antiinflammatory effects.
4. Vasomotor rhinitis—treated with ipratropium, which blocks vagally mediated reflexes that cause congestion.

 DRUG ALERT Severe rebound nasal obstruction may occur with overuse of topical decongestants. Stress the importance of only using for 2 to 3 days, as directed.

A. Rhinitis

Edematous conchae; polyps may develop

Occluded sinus openings

Enlarged nasal mucosa

B. Sinusitis

Thick mucus occludes sinus cavity and prevents drainage

Discharging mucus

Figure 17-2. Rhinitis and sinusitis. **(A)** The mucous membranes lining the nasal passages become inflamed, congested, and edematous, blocking sinus openings and obstructing air passage. **(B)** The sinus cavity mucous membranes are also marked by inflammation and congestion, with thickened mucous secretions filling the sinus cavities and further occluding the openings. (From Smeltzer, S., & Bare, B. [2000]. *Brunner and Suddarth's textbook of medical-surgical nursing* [9th ed.]. Philadelphia, PA: Lippincott Williams & Wilkins.)

Nursing Interventions and Patient Education

1. Educate patients about avoidance measures for known or suspected allergens or irritants such as smoke.
2. Do not overuse topical nasal sprays and drops.
3. Advise about adverse effect of systemic decongestants is stimulation of sympathetic nervous system—insomnia, nervousness, palpitations.
4. Be aware that intranasal corticosteroids do not cause significant systemic absorption in usual doses but occasionally may cause nasal fungal infections and in rare cases cause nasal septal perforation and epistaxis.
5. Educate patients about correct administration technique for nasal sprays, particularly to direct the tip of the spray bottle away from the septum, toward the outward corner of the eye or toward the ear.

Epistaxis

Epistaxis refers to nosebleed or hemorrhage from the nose. It most commonly originates in the anterior portion of the nasal cavity.

Pathophysiology and Etiology

1. Local causes:
   a. Dryness leading to crust formation—bleeding occurs with removal of crusts by nose picking, rubbing, or blowing.
   b. Trauma—direct blows.
2. Systemic causes are less common—hypertension, arteriosclerosis, renal disease, bleeding disorders. Episodic epistaxis is mostly commonly seen with patients on antiplatelet, anticoagulant, and antithrombolytic agents. Osler-Weber-Rendu syndrome or hereditary hemorrhagic telangiectasia, hemophilia, von Willebrand disease, and liver disease are examples of bleeding disorders that can predispose patients to frequent episodes of epistaxis.
3. Most nosebleeds are anterior; posterior bleeds are more difficult to control.

Diagnostic Evaluation

1. Inspection with nasal speculum to determine site of bleeding or nasal endoscopy by otolaryngologist. Important to determine which side bled first.
2. Laboratory evaluation to exclude blood dyscrasias and coagulopathy.

Management

Depends on severity and source of bleeding in nasal cavity.
1. The patient is placed in an upright posture, leaning forward to reduce venous pressure, and instructed to breathe gently through the mouth to prevent swallowing of blood. The patient is asked to sit on a 90-degree angle, while the nasal ala, or the soft part of the anterior nose, is pinched and pressure is applied for 10 to 15 minutes, or as needed to control the bleeding.
2. With anterior bleeds, the patient is instructed to compress the soft part of nose with index finger and thumb for 5 to 10 minutes to maintain pressure on the nasal septum.
3. A cotton pledget soaked with a vasoconstricting agent may be inserted into each nostril and pressure is applied if bleeding is not controlled. After 5 to 10 minutes, the cotton is removed and the site of bleeding is identified. Oxymetazoline, in combination with a topical anesthetic agent such as lidocaine, may

be sprayed directly into the nasal cavity or applied on pledgets or cotton balls. Suction may be used to evacuate the bloody contents of the nasal cavity to visualize the source of bleeding.
4. The blood vessel may be cauterized with use of silver nitrate sticks or with electrocautery.
5. If bleeding continues despite use of pressure or cautery, anterior or posterior packing may be placed into the nasal cavity or nasopharynx. Packing is usually kept in for 72 hours or more. Balloon tamponade may be required to apply pressure over a larger area.
6. Surgical ligation of vessels may be required if bleeding is unable to be controlled with above measures.

 NURSING ALERT Monitor the patient for a vasovagal episode during insertion and with removal of nasal packing. This is best prevented with reclining the patient back when symptoms first occur.

Complications

1. Rhinitis; maxillary and frontal sinusitis.
2. Orthostatic hypotension from sudden blood loss.

Nursing Interventions and Patient Education

1. Monitor vital signs and assist with control of bleeding. Assess for changes in blood pressure and pulse indicative of hypovolemia.
2. Be aware that packing is uncomfortable and painful and may be in place for 48 to 72 hours. Antibiotics may be prescribed to prevent secondary infection from packing.
3. Nosebleed precautions and postprocedure instructions should be given to the patient. Instructions for holding specific antiplatelet and anticoagulant medications will be coordinated in conjunction with the patients' clinical history. The patient should be advised to avoid sneezing with mouth closed, blowing nose, removing the packing, and avoiding any strenuous activity.
4. Monitor patient with posterior packing for hypoxia (from aspiration of blood, sedation, and preexisting pulmonary dysfunction). Patients who require posterior balloon packing are admitted for observation and monitoring. These patients are at risk for soft palate necrosis and airway obstruction. If coagulopathies are found on blood work, these are corrected while the patient is hospitalized. Monitor PT, INR, and PTT, if ordered.
5. Instruct the patient as follows for self-management of minor bleeding episodes:
   a. Sit up and lean forward while compressing the soft part (lower half) of nose between index finger and thumb.
   b. If bleeding continues, moisten a small piece of cotton with vasoconstricting nose drops (phenylephrine or oxymetazoline) and place inside the nose.
   c. Apply pressure to the bleeding site 5 to 10 minutes.
6. Instruct the patient to avoid blowing or picking nose after a nosebleed.
7. Advise patients prone to nosebleeds to:
   a. Apply a lubricant to nasal septum twice daily to reduce dryness. Nasal saline spray may also be advised a few days after nasal cautery is performed and on a regular basis if patient has recurrent episodes.
   b. A bedside humidifier is recommended, especially if the environmental air is dry.
   c. If the patient uses chronic oxygen therapy or CPAP, a humidifier may be recommended on the oxygen delivery or CPAP delivery system.

Sinusitis

Rhinosinusitis is defined as a symptomatic inflammation of the sinuses and nasal cavity. It may be precipitated by congestion from viral upper respiratory infection and/or nasal allergy. A patient with chronic allergic disease may be prone to recurrent episodes of sinusitis or chronic rhinosinusitis. Obstruction of the sinus ostia (resulting from mucosal swelling and/or mechanical obstruction) leads to retention of secretions and is the usual precursor to sinusitis.

Rhinosinusitis is classified by duration as acute (less than 4 weeks), subacute (4 to 12 weeks), or chronic (more than 12 weeks). Acute rhinosinusitis can be classified as bacterial or viral.

Clinical Manifestations

Acute Sinusitis

1. Defined as up to 4 weeks of purulent, nonclear nasal drainage with nasal congestion and/or facial pain/pressure/fullness (see Figure 17-3). There may be both symptoms of nasal congestion and facial pain, and symptoms are present for 10 days or more. There may be chronic exacerbations of symptoms within the 4 weeks.
2. Nasal congestion or obstruction is defined as subjective symptoms of difficulty breathing through nose and/or red and edematous nasal mucosa visualized on physical examination.
3. Anosmia (lack of smell) may be reported.
4. Other symptoms that may be present include fever, cough, ear pressure, maxillary dental pain, and fatigue.
5. Viral rhinosinusitis is differentiated from bacterial by duration—symptoms for 10 days or less without worsening symptoms. Bacterial rhinosinusitis manifests for 10 days with worsening symptoms.

Chronic Rhinosinusitis

1. Mucopurulent nasal drainage, nasal obstruction, facial pain/pressure/fullness and/or decreased sense of smell. May also have malaise and ear pain or pressure and cough. Patients may have recurrent episodes or continued symptoms for 12 weeks or more.
2. Symptoms may or may not be present but are nondiagnostic of chronic rhinosinusitis.

Diagnostic Evaluation

1. Sinus plain film consisting of Caldwell, Waters, and lateral views may be obtained but not routinely recommended for acute, isolated, or noncomplicated cases. X-rays may reveal air–fluid level, mucosal thickening, or opacification of one or more sinus cavities.
2. CT scanning recommended when complication is suspected or in patients with chronic sinus disease.
3. Nasal endoscopy, performed by an ENT specialist, is used to evaluate the nasal and sinus cavity and to obtain cultures of material for the purpose of directing appropriate antibiotic therapy.
4. CT with contrast or MRI with gadolinium may be obtained if cranial extension suspected.

Management

1. Topical decongestant spray or drops or systemic decongestants may be used to treat the nasal congestion associated with rhinosinusitis. Topical therapy should be limited to no more than 3 successive days of use as increased use beyond 3 days may cause rebound nasal congestion (rhinitis medicamentosa).
2. Topical nasal corticosteroids are frequently used in chronic sinusitis and may be used in acute cases. Nasal corticosteroids have been shown to decrease severity of symptoms when used with appropriate antibiotic therapy.
3. Antibiotics—amoxicillin is the initial drug of choice in adults with acute rhinosinusitis. For penicillin-allergic patients, sulfamethoxazole–trimethoprim or macrolide antibiotics may also be used as first-line therapy. The most common organisms identified in patients with acute bacterial rhinosinusitis are *Streptococcus pneumoniae*, *Haemophilus influenzae*, and *Moraxella catarrhalis*. Other less common organisms include *Staphyloccocus aureus* and anaerobes.
4. Usually 10- to 14-day course for acute sinusitis; azithromycin or fluoroquinolones may be prescribed for 3 to 5 days.
5. Prolonged therapy for chronic sinusitis (up to several months).
6. Analgesics—pain may be significant.
7. Warm compresses; cool vapor humidity for comfort and to promote drainage; nasal saline irrigation.
8. Surgical interventions (for chronic sinusitis when conservative treatment is unsuccessful).
   a. Endoscopic sinus surgery—endoscopic removal of diseased tissue from affected sinus; used to treat chronic sinusitis of maxillary, ethmoid, and frontal sinuses.
   b. Nasal antrostomy (nasal–antral window)—surgical placement of an opening under inferior turbinate to provide aeration of the antrum and to permit exit for purulent materials.
   c. For nursing care, see page 458.

Complications

1. Extension of infection to the orbital contents and eyelids.
2. Bone infection (osteomyelitis) may spread by direct extension or through blood vessels. Frontal bone commonly affected.
3. CNS complications include meningitis, subdural and epidural purulent drainage, brain abscess, and cavernous sinus thrombosis (acute thrombophlebitis originating from an infection in an area having venous drainage to cavernous sinus).

Figure 17-3. Referred pain from the paranasal sinuses. (From Galen, B. [1997]. Chronic recurrent sinusitis: Recognition and treatment. *Lippincott's Primary Care Practice*, 1[2], 183–197.)

NURSING ALERT Watch for lid edema, edema of ocular conjunctiva, drooping lid, limitation of extra-ocular motion, vision loss; may indicate orbital cellulitis, which necessitates immediate treatment.

Nursing Interventions and Patient Education

1. Teach the patient signs and symptoms of acute, bacterial rhinosinusitis versus signs and symptoms of rhinitis. Educate the patient in regard to symptoms that prompt medical attention.
2. Advise the patients about adverse reactions of antibiotic therapy including side effects, drug interactions, and symptoms that prompt medical attention.
3. Stress the importance of complying with antibiotic therapy for complete duration and following up for recurrence.
4. Teach the patient with recurrent sinusitis how to irrigate nasal passages with saline to remove crusted mucus near the sinus openings and enhance drainage (page 458).

Pharyngitis

Pharyngitis is an inflammation of the pharynx, including palate, tonsils, and posterior wall of the pharynx, most commonly caused by acute infection, usually transmitted through respiratory secretions. Streptococcal pharyngitis (*strep throat*) and rhinoviruses (the common cold) are frequent causes. Pharyngitis is diagnosed in 11 million emergency rooms and outpatient office visits per year.

Pathophysiology and Etiology

1. Acute bacterial pharyngitis is usually caused by group A beta-hemolytic streptococci.
2. Other bacterial causes include *H. influenzae*, *M. catarrhalis*, *Corynebacterium diphtheriae* (diphtheria), *Neisseria gonorrhoeae* (gonorrhea), and other groups of streptococcus. Transmission of *N. gonorrhoeae* is through oral contact with genital secretions; it is a sexually transmitted disease.
3. Viral pharyngitis is common and causes include rhinovirus, adenovirus, parainfluenza virus, coxsackievirus, coronavirus, and others.
4. More chronic causes are irritation from postnasal drip of allergic rhinitis and chronic sinusitis, chemical irritation, and systemic diseases.

Clinical Manifestations

1. For acute bacterial infections, abrupt onset of sore throat and fever, usually above 100.4°F (38.0°C), and exposure to *Streptococcus* within the preceding 2 weeks is suggestive of streptococcal pharyngitis.
   a. Throat pain is aggravated by swallowing.
   b. Pharynx appears reddened with edema of uvula; tonsils enlarged and reddened; pharynx and tonsils may be covered with exudate (see Figure 17-4).
   c. Palatal petechiae and a scarlatiniform rash are highly specific but uncommonly seen.
2. Varying degrees of sore throat, nasal congestion, fatigue, and fever with other bacterial and viral causes.

Figure 17-4. Assessment of pharyngitis. **(A)** Normal throat. **(B)** Normal large tonsils without redness. **(C)** Mild redness without exudate. **(D)** Intense redness without exudate. **(E)** Redness with exudate on tonsils (probably indicates group A streptococcal infection). (**A:** Smeltzer, S., and Bare, B. [2000]. Brunner and Suddarth's textbook of medical-surgical nursing [9th ed.]. Philadelphia: Lippincott Williams & Wilkins; **B–E:** The Wellcome Collection, National Medical Slide Bank, London, UK.)

3. Cough, conjunctivitis, and diarrhea are common with viral causes.
4. Swollen, palpable, and tender cervical lymph nodes in most cases. Anterior cervical lymph node swelling and enlargement are common.

Diagnostic Evaluation

1. Throat culture or rapid streptococcal antigen detection test to rule out streptococci. Rapid strep tests provide results within 5 minutes; false-negative rate is higher than with culture method.
2. Gonococcal antigen detection test to rule out gonococcal pharyngitis, if genital gonococcal infection or positive sexual contact is suspected.
3. Viral testing is not practical, and viral causes are self-limiting.

Management

1. For streptococcal pharyngitis, penicillin V 250 mg four times a day orally for 10 days or penicillin G benzathine in a single intramuscular (IM) dose of 2.4 million units appears to shorten duration of symptoms and prevents rheumatic fever.
2. Amoxicillen, amoxicillen-clavulanate, macrolides, erythromycin and cephalosporins are used for bacterial pharyngitis.

Complications

1. Acute rheumatic fever.
2. Peritonsillar abscess/cellulitis.
3. Acute glomerulonephritis.
4. Scarlet fever.
5. Sinusitis, otitis media, and mastoiditis.

 NURSING ALERT Acute rheumatic fever, a complication of streptococcal pharyngitis, can be prevented if patient is treated adequately with penicillin and, possibly, another antibiotic. Unfortunately, there is no evidence that antibiotic therapy will prevent acute glomerulonephritis.

Nursing Interventions and Patient Education

1. Advise the patient to have any sore throat with fever evaluated, especially in the absence of cold symptoms.
2. Encourage compliance with full course of antibiotic therapy, despite feeling better in several days, to prevent complications.
3. Advise lukewarm saline gargles and use of antipyretic/analgesics, as directed, to promote comfort.
4. Encourage bed rest with increased fluid intake during fever.

EAR DISORDERS

See additional online content: Procedure Guidelines 17-1

Hearing Loss

Hearing loss ranks high as a health disability. There are multiple causes, and the range of hearing loss varies from mild hearing loss to profound hearing loss with complete inability to understand the spoken word. Two major types of hearing loss are conductive and sensorineural. There are 37.5 million Americans with hearing loss.

Classification of Hearing Loss

1. Conductive loss—any condition interfering with sound transmission through the external auditory canal or transmission of tympanic membrane vibrations through the middle ear ossicles to the inner ear.
2. Sensorineural (perceptive) loss—hearing loss due to disease of the inner ear or nerve pathways; sensitivity to and discrimination of sounds are impaired. Hearing aids usually are helpful.
3. Combined or mixed hearing loss—combination of the above.
4. Sudden sensorineural hearing loss—30-dB hearing loss in one or both ears in three contiguous frequencies that occurs within 3 days or less. It can be caused by an acute viral infection or vascular event.

See Table 17-2 for tuning fork tests that assist in differentiating conductive from sensorineural hearing loss.

Presbycusis

A progressive, bilaterally perceptive hearing loss of older adults, usually involving high frequencies, that occurs with the aging process.
1. An audiogram should be obtained by a professional audiologist to evaluate the degree of hearing loss, word discrimination ability, and identification of any hearing loss suggestive of a retrocochlear etiology.
2. The patient should be counseled by an otolaryngologist in collaboration with an audiologist, who can make recommendations for hearing amplification.
3. Helpful aids should be considered, such as a telephone amplifier, radio and television earphone attachments, and a buzzer instead of a doorbell.
4. Understanding and help from family members are important.

Otosclerosis

Otosclerosis is defined as an abnormal growth of bone of the middle ear that prevents the ossicles, or middle ear bones, from working properly and impeding movement of the stapes. Causes progressive hearing loss in one or both ears, vertigo, and tinnitus.

The cause is unknown, but there is a familial tendency, and women are affected more often than men.

Clinical Manifestations

1. Young adults present with a history of slow, progressive hearing loss of soft-spoken tones, with no signs of middle ear infection. In women of childbearing age, often progresses during pregnancy.
2. Audiometry findings substantiate conductive or mixed hearing loss.

Table 17-2	Tuning Fork Tests	
EAR CONDITION	**WEBER TEST**	**RINNE TEST**
Normal, no hearing loss	No shifting of sounds laterally	Sound perceived longer by *air* conduction
Conductive loss	Shifting of sounds to poorer ear	Sound perceived as long or longer by *bone* conduction
Sensorineural loss	Shifting of sounds to better ear	Sound perceived longer by *air* conduction

Management

1. No known medical treatment exists for this form of deafness, but amplification with a hearing aid may be helpful.
2. Surgery—stapedotomy or stapedectomy.
   a. The removal of otosclerotic lesions at the footplate of stapes or complete removal of the stapes and the creation of a tissue implant with prosthesis to maintain suitable conduction.
   b. To perform such delicate surgery, an otologic binocular microscope is used.

Cochlear Implant

A *cochlear implant* is a device that emits auditory signals for profoundly deaf people (see Figure 17-5). The single-electrode system bypasses the damaged cochlear system and stimulates the remaining auditory nerve fibers. This results in the perception of sound.

Description

1. Purpose is for the patient to detect louder environmental sounds but will not restore normal hearing. Many recipients continue to rely on lip-reading to make sense of the sound input being received. Some patients are able to rely entirely on

Figure 17-5. Nucleus 24 cochlear implant system. Sounds are picked up by the small, directional microphone located in the headset at the ear. A thin cord carries the sound from the microphone to the speech processor, a powerful miniaturized computer. The speech processor filters, analyzes, and digitizes the sound into coded signals that are sent from the speech processor to the transmitting coil. The transmitting coil sends the coded signals as FM radio signals to the cochlear implant under the skin. The cochlear implant delivers the appropriate electrical energy to the array of electrodes, which have been inserted into the cochlea. The electrodes along the array stimulate the remaining auditory nerve fibers in the cochlea. The resulting electrical sound information is sent through the auditory system to the brain for interpretation. The entire process takes microseconds.

hearing with their cochlear implant device and may even be able to use the telephone.

2. The microphone and sound processor are positioned externally; the electrode array is implanted internally and inserts into the cochlea. The receiver–stimulator is inserted into a bony well created in the mastoid behind the ear.
3. Electrical stimuli converted from the sound processor are sent inside the body to the implanted electrode. These electrical signals stimulate the auditory nerve fibers, which are interpreted by the brain.
4. Success rate is highly variable, which has made the cochlear implant controversial. As of 2012, over 324,000 devices have been implanted and registered worldwide.

Patient Criteria

There are no standardized criteria for patient selection. Some data that are considered include the following:

1. Severe to profound sensorineural hearing loss in both ears.
2. Little to no benefit with hearing aids.
3. No medical contraindications.
4. Physically healthy adult or child as young as age 8 months.
5. No evidence of brain impairment that would prevent useful processing of the information delivered. Some would argue that implantation in those with mental impairment would still allow more awareness of environmental sounds, making them safer.
6. Reasonable expectations and optimism; motivation must be present.

Nursing Interventions

1. Encourage the prospective patient to visit with someone who is currently using an implant to learn its positive and negative results.
2. Explain the rehabilitation process; usually begins 2 months after surgery. Included are:
   a. Adjustment of controls.
   b. Operation and maintenance of stimulator unit.
   c. Listening critically and learning lip-reading.
   d. Learning discrimination of sounds through cochlear implant. Understanding speech through cochlear implant is not possible with this device alone.
   e. Many people trained with such an implant can lip-read more easily and can distinguish voices and environmental sounds.
3. Pneumococcal vaccination is important for all cochlear implant candidates and recipients. This should be given at least 2 weeks prior to surgery.
4. For care after surgery, see page 460.

Other Implantable Devices

1. Osseointegrated devices transmit sound from an external device, worn above the ear, through the skin and into the skull to the inner ear. This device is indicated in those with conductive hearing loss when a hearing aid is contraindicated such as chronic ear infection, those with aural atresia or microtia without the normal ear canal needed to carry sound to the middle ear, and those with single-sided deafness.
2. Semi-implantable hearing aids are being tested for conductive and mixed hearing loss.

Maximizing Communication with the Person Who is Hearing Impaired

When hearing loss is permanent or not amenable to medical or surgical intervention, aural rehabilitation is necessary for the patient to maintain communication and prevent isolation. Aural rehabilitation is a multifaceted process that includes auditory training (listening skills), speech reading (formerly called lip-reading), and the use of hearing aids. Nurses strive to maintain effective communication with patients. These suggestions promote better communication.

When the Person Is Hearing Impaired and Able to Lip-Read

1. Face the person as directly as possible when speaking.
2. Place yourself in good light so the person can see your mouth.
3. Do not chew, smoke, or have anything in your mouth when speaking.
4. Speak slowly and enunciate distinctly.
5. Provide contextual clues that will assist the person in following your speech. For example, point to a tray if you are talking about the food on it.
6. To verify that the patient understands your message, write it for him or her to read (ie, if you doubt that the patient is understanding you).

When the Person is Hearing Impaired and Difficult to Understand

1. Pay attention when the person speaks; facial and physical gestures may help you understand what person is saying.
2. Exchange conversation with person when it is possible to anticipate replies. This is particularly helpful in your initial contact with person and may help you become familiar with speech peculiarities.
3. Anticipate context of speech to assist in interpreting what the person is saying.
4. If unable to understand the person, resort to writing or include in your conversation someone who does understand; request that the person repeat that which is not understood.

Organizations That Help the Hearing Impaired

- Alexander Graham Bell Association for the Deaf (*www.agbell.org*)
- American Speech-Language-Hearing Association (*www.asha.org*)
- National Association of the Deaf (*www.nad.org*)

Community and Home Care Considerations

1. Prevention of hearing loss should be discussed in the community—in schools, the workplace, and community gatherings.
2. Preventable hearing loss includes
   a. Noise-induced hearing loss—long periods of exposure to loud noise from machinery or engines.
   b. Acoustic trauma—single exposure to intense noise such as an explosion or amplified music.
3. Prevention involves avoidance of both types of noise, generally noise above 85 or 90 dB.
4. Teach people to be aware of their surroundings and avoid noisy places or turn off sources of noise in the environment whenever possible.
5. Teach proper use of ear protection including earplugs and headsets both in the workplace and elsewhere.
6. Advise people that the Occupational Safety and Health Administration requires ear protection when noise exposure is above the legal limits, so workers have a right to protective equipment.

Otitis Externa

Otitis externa is an inflammation/infection of the external ear, pinna, and/or ear canal.

Pathophysiology and Etiology

1. Bacterial causes: Most common causes are *Pseudomonas aeruginosa*, *Proteus mirabilis*, and *S. aureus*.
2. May be caused by fungal source: *Aspergillus niger, C. albicans.*
3. Commonly caused by chronic dermatologic conditions, such as seborrhea, psoriasis, eczema, or contact dermatitis. Allergic reaction to topical otic such as neomycin/polymyxin preparations may also occur in some patients.
4. Trauma to the ear canal, usually from cleaning the canal.
5. Stagnant water in ear canal after swimming or from water irrigation for cerumen removal is a common etiology.
6. Necrotizing malignant otitis externa is a serious infection into deeper tissue adjacent to the ear canal, including cellulitis and osteomyelitis. It is usually caused by *Pseudomonas* and may be seen in diabetic patients, older patients, debilitated patients, or patients with compromised immune systems.
7. Methicillin-resistant *S. aureus* otorrhea has been a common cause of chronic ear drainage. Treatment is based on culture and sensitivity of the ear drainage.

Clinical Manifestations

1. Otalgia or ear pain, increased by manipulation of auricle or tragus; hearing loss and aural fullness. Itching may also be present.
2. Periauricular lymphadenopathy.
3. Foul-smelling white to purulent drainage otorrhea. Drainage may be thick and purulent or thin and white, depending on the causative organism.
4. Red, swollen ear canal with discharge on otoscopic examination; ear canal can be swollen shut.

Management

1. Instillation of isopropyl alcohol drops (dries moisture), acetic acid solution (restores acidity), or topical antibiotics (curbs infection). A combination of these treatments may be used depending on the cause. Antifungal agents, in ointment, powder, or drop form, may be used.
   a. Prophylactic use of alcohol drops or acetic acid solution by swimmers or those prone to otitis externa may be indicated.
   b. Antibiotic drops include combination products containing polymyxin, neomycin, and hydrocortisone; ciprofloxacin; and ofloxacin. Tobramycin preparations may be used with methicillin-resistant infections (confirmed by culture and sensitivity).
   c. A 10-day course of treatment is usually indicated.
   d. Parenteral antibiotics will be used for necrotizing otitis externa.
2. If canal is swollen and tender, an antibiotic solution containing a corticosteroid is chosen to reduce inflammation and swelling. If acute inflammation and closure of the ear canal prevent drops from saturating canal, a wick may need to be inserted by an ENT specialist so drops will gain access to walls of entire ear canal.
3. Burow solution (aluminum acetate solution) or topical corticosteroid cream or lotion may be used in otitis externa caused by dermatitis.
4. Fungal infections may be treated with a topical antifungal such as nystatin or ketoconazole.
5. In chronic otitis externa, debris from ear canal may need to be removed through suction after pain and swelling have subsided. Avoid water irrigation, as this promotes bacterial and fungal growth from stagnant moisture.
6. Warm compresses and analgesics may be needed.

Nursing Interventions and Patient Education

1. Demonstrate proper application of eardrops.
2. Advise the patient that otitis externa can be prevented or minimized by thoroughly drying the ear canal after coming into contact with water or moist environment.
3. Teach the patient to use prophylactic eardrops after swimming to assist in preventing swimmer's ear, as directed by health care provider.
4. Advise the use of properly fitting earplugs for recurrent cases.
5. Teach proper ear hygiene: clean auricle and outer canal with washcloth only; do not insert anything smaller than finger wrapped in washcloth in ear canal. Avoid inserting cotton swabs or sharp objects into ear canal because:
   a. Cerumen may be forced against the tympanic membrane, causing impaction.
   b. The canal lining may be abraded, making it more susceptible to infection.
   c. The tympanic membrane may be injured.

Impacted Cerumen and Foreign Bodies

Cerumen impaction is defined as accumulation of cerumen, or "ear wax," that causes symptoms of ear pain, fullness, or hearing loss and/or prevents visualization of the tympanic membrane.

Etiology and Clinical Manifestations

1. Cerumen is a mixture of glandular secretions from the ear canal mixed with squamous epithelium. Cerumen builds up over a period of time, causing a decrease in hearing acuity and a feeling that the ear is plugged.
   a. May be underlying seborrhea or other dermatologic condition that causes flaking of skin that mixes with cerumen and becomes obstructive.
   b. Cerumen may be pushed back into external canal and cover tympanic membrane by action of cotton swab.
2. Insect may fly or crawl into the ear, causing initial low rumbling sound; later, feeling that ear is plugged and decreased hearing acuity. Foreign bodies may be placed into the ear canal, especially by children, and include food particles, small objects, or tips of cotton swabs.
3. The patient often seeks treatment for symptoms related to the foreign body or impacted cerumen.

Management

1. Accumulated cerumen does not have to be removed unless it causes symptoms, interferes with examination of the ear drum, or interferes with hearing. May be removed by curette or by irrigation with a syringe or electronic irrigation device (see Figure 17-6).

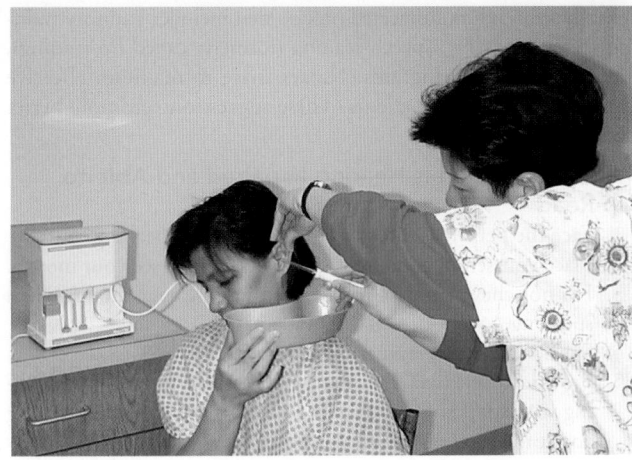

Figure 17-6. Using an electronic irrigation device to irrigate the external auditory cavity.

   a. Avoid directing irrigation stream directly at tympanic membrane, rather direct stream at wall of canal.
   b. Use warm water at approximately body temperature.
2. Foreign bodies may be removed by instrumentation or irrigation by health care provider.
   a. Insects—treat by instilling oil drops to smother insect, which then can be removed with ear spatula or irrigation.
   b. Vegetable foreign bodies (eg, peas)—irrigation is contraindicated because vegetable matter absorbs water, which would further wedge it in the canal.
   c. Only a skilled person should attempt to remove foreign body to prevent tympanic membrane perforation and trauma to canal.
   d. General anesthesia may be required to remove foreign bodies from young children, if they are unable to cooperate.

 NURSING ALERT Do not attempt to irrigate ear or instill anything into external canal if eardrum may be perforated; otoscopic examination should be done to rule out tympanic membrane rupture or acute infection. If the tympanic membrane is unable to be visualized and perforation is suspected, or acute infection is suspected, do not irrigate and refer to ENT specialist. Some antibiotic eardrops are contraindicated if the tympanic membrane is not intact.

Nursing Interventions and Patient Education

1. Teach proper ear hygiene, especially not putting anything in ears.
2. Explain the normal protective function of cerumen.

PATIENT EDUCATION GUIDELINES 17-2

Instilling Ear Drops

1. Hold the medication bottle between your hands for 1 to 2 minutes to warm drops before administering.
2. Lie on side with affected ear facing upward. Shake drops. Pull ear up and back, and then, instill drops by squeezing the bulb the ordered number of times.
3. Pump tragus by pushing on the flap of skin protecting the ear canal five to six times to ensure drops reach eardrum.
4. Remain on side for 1 to 2 minutes. Repeat, if necessary, on opposite ear.

3. If patient has a problem with cerumen buildup and has been advised by health care provider to use a ceruminolytic periodically, make sure that the patient is getting cerumen out of the ear before more medication is instilled. A bulb syringe may be used by the patient at home to help remove softened cerumen.
4. Advise the patient to report persistent fever, pain, drainage, or hearing impairment.

Acute Otitis Media

Acute otitis media is an inflammation and infection of the middle ear caused by the entrance of pathogenic organisms, with rapid onset of signs and symptoms. Acute otitis media or acute suppurative otitis media is infection of the middle ear caused by contamination from bacteria from the middle ear fluid through the eustachian tube.

Pathophysiology and Etiology

1. Pathogenic organisms gain entry into the normally sterile middle ear, usually through a dysfunctional eustachian tube.
2. Organisms include *S. pneumoniae, H. influenzae, M. catarrhalis,* and *S. aureus.*
3. In serous (secretory) otitis media, no purulent infection occurs, but blockage of the eustachian tube causes negative pressure and transudation of fluid from blood vessels and development of effusion in the middle ear.

Clinical Manifestations

1. Pain is usually the first symptom.
2. Fever may rise to 104°F to 105°F (40°C to 40.6°C).
3. Purulent drainage (otorrhea) is present if tympanic membrane is perforated.
4. Irritability may be noted in the young person.
5. Headache, hearing loss, anorexia, nausea, and vomiting may be present.
6. Purulent effusion may be visible behind tympanic membrane or tympanic membrane may be reddened and bulging on otoscopic examination.
7. History may reveal previous upper respiratory infection, allergic rhinitis, eustachian tube dysfunction, history of reflux, adenoid hypertrophy, history of cleft palate, smoking in household, sibling otitis media in children, or child in daycare. Patients who have received radiation therapy of the head and neck or experienced barotrauma or those with nasopharyngeal tumor may develop middle ear effusions.

Diagnostic Evaluation

1. Pneumatic otoscopy shows a tympanic membrane that is full, bulging, and opaque with impaired mobility (or retracted with impaired mobility).
2. Cultures of discharge through ruptured tympanic membrane may suggest causative organism.

Management

1. Antibiotic treatment—amoxicillin is first-line treatment; cephalosporins, macrolides, or trimethoprim–sulfamethoxazole may be used in patients with penicillin allergy.
2. Amoxicillin/clavulanate and cephalosporins are used for treatment failure due to increasing rate of beta-lactamase–producing bacteria that inactivate penicillin and other antibiotics.
3. Usual treatment course is 10 days.
4. Follow-up is indicated to determine effectiveness of therapy.

5. Nasal or topical decongestants and antihistamines have a limited role in promoting eustachian tube drainage.
6. Surgery—myringotomy with placement of pressure-equalizing tubes.
   a. An incision is made into the posterior inferior aspect of the tympanic membrane for relief of persistent effusion. A pressure-equalizing tube may be inserted to prevent recurrent episodes.
   b. Performed in selected patients to prevent recurrent episodes or in patients with middle ear effusion for 3 months or more.
   c. May be done because of failure of patient to respond to antimicrobial therapy; for severe, persistent pain; and for persistent conductive hearing loss.

Complications

1. Perforation of tympanic membrane.
2. Chronic otitis media and mastoiditis.
3. Conductive hearing loss.
4. Meningitis and brain abscess.

Nursing Assessment

1. Obtain history of upper respiratory infection, previous ear infections, allergies, and progression of symptoms.
2. Assess fever and level of pain.
3. Obtain baseline hearing evaluation, if indicated.

Nursing Diagnosis

- Acute Pain related to inflammation and increased middle ear pressure.

Nursing Interventions

Relieving Pain
1. Administer or teach self-administration of anti-inflammatories and other analgesics, as prescribed.
2. Administer or teach self-administration of antibiotics, as prescribed. Oral corticosteroids may be prescribed, as well as nasal steroids.
3. Encourage the use of local warm compresses or heating pad to promote comfort and help resolve infectious process.
4. Be alert for such symptoms as headache, slow pulse, vomiting, and vertigo, which may be significant for sequelae that involve the mastoid or the brain.

Patient Education and Health Maintenance

1. Encourage follow-up after treatment to ensure resolution.
2. Advise the patient that sudden relief of pain may indicate tympanic membrane rupture. Do not instill anything in ear and call health care provider.
3. Instruct the patient to follow up for recurrence of symptoms, such as pain, fever, and ear congestion.

Evaluation: Expected Outcomes

- Verbalizes relief of pain at follow-up visit.

Chronic Otitis Media and Mastoiditis

Chronic otitis media is a chronic inflammation of the middle ear with tissue damage, usually caused by repeated episodes of acute otitis media. It may be caused by an antibiotic-resistant organism or a particularly virulent strain of organism. It may be associated with tympanic membrane perforation. *Mastoiditis* is inflammation of the mastoid air cells of the temporal bone adjacent to the ear.

Pathophysiology and Etiology

1. The accumulation of pus inflammatory exudate under pressure in the middle ear cavity may result in necrosis of tissue, with damage to the tympanic membrane and possibly the ossicles.
   a. The most common organisms are *S. pneumoniae, H. influenzae,* and *Moraxella catarrhalis.*
   b. Other organisms may be present, such as *Pseudomonas, Proteus,* and *Bacteroides* species.
2. Persistent rupture of the tympanic membrane and damage to the ossicles lead to conductive hearing loss.
3. Extension of infection may occur into the mastoid cells (mastoiditis).
4. Cholesteatoma may form (mass of squamous epithelium and desquamated debris in the middle ear), which may cause erosion of the ossicles or inner ear.

Clinical Manifestations

1. Painless or dull ache, decreased hearing, tendernss of mastoid.
2. Otorrhea may be odorless or foul smelling.
3. Vertigo and pain may be present if CNS complications have occurred.
4. History will indicate several episodes of acute otitis media and possible rupture of tympanic membrane.
5. Fever and postauricular erythema and edema.

Diagnostic Evaluation

1. Conductive hearing loss is present through audiometric tests.
2. CT of temporal bone may show mastoid pathology, for example, cholesteatoma or opacification of mastoid cells.
3. Culture of exudate from middle ear (through ruptured tympanic membrane or at time of surgery).

Management

Note: If advanced chronic ear disease is left untreated, inner ear and life-threatening CNS complications may develop because of erosion of surrounding structures.

Medical Therapy
1. Antibiotic and steroid eardrops may control middle ear infection and inflammation, but when mastoiditis develops, parenteral antibiotic therapy is necessary.
2. Eardrops containing neomycin, garamycin, tobramycin, and quinolones, such as ciprofloxacin, are instilled into the middle ear when the tympanic membrane is ruptured. Otic drops containing antibiotics or antibiotic powder preparations may be used for infection and otorrhea. Local cleaning using microscope and instrumentation is mainstay of treatment and done by ENT specialist.
3. IV antibiotics must cover beta-lactamase–producing organisms—ampicillin–sulbactam, cefuroxime—based on culture results.

Surgical Interventions
1. Indicated when cholesteatoma is present.
2. Indicated when there is pain, profound deafness, dizziness, sudden facial paralysis, or stiff neck (may lead to meningitis or brain abscess).
3. Types of procedures:

   a. Simple mastoidectomy—removal of diseased bone and insertion of a drain; indicated when there is persistent infection and signs of intracranial complications.
   b. Radical mastoidectomy—removal of posterior wall of ear canal, remnants of the tympanic membrane, and the malleolus and incus.
   c. Posteroanterior mastoidectomy—combines simple mastoidectomy with tympanoplasty (reconstruction of middle ear structures).

Complications

1. Acute and chronic mastoiditis.
2. Cholesteatoma.
3. CNS infection (meningitis, intracranial abscess).
4. Postoperatively—facial nerve paralysis, bleeding, vertigo.

Nursing Assessment

1. Assess for history of ear infection and treatment compliance. Identify factors that may prevent compliance with treatment in the future—lack of money/prescription coverage, lack of transportation, lack of knowledge on severity of infection, and so forth.
2. Assess for ear drainage and patency of tympanic membrane.
3. Assess for hearing loss.
4. Palpate for mastoid tenderness.

For nursing process related to patients undergoing surgical treatment, see "Care Related to Ear Surgery," page 460.

Patient Education and Health Maintenance

1. Teach the patient to keep the ear dry—use ENT-approved or molded ear plugs during showering, washing hair, and swimming—to prevent any water from gaining access to middle ear.
2. Encourage the patient to follow up for frequent ear cleaning.
3. Stress the importance of adhering to antibiotic schedule and to notify the home care nurse or health care provider if there is any problem with venous access or a dose is missed for any reason.
4. Advise of complications and to report headache, change in mental status or arousal, or increased ear pain.
5. Stress the importance of follow-up hearing evaluations and early intervention for any signs of ear infection in the future.

Ménière Disease

Ménière disease (or *endolymphatic hydrops*) is a chronic inner ear disease characterized by spontaneous episodes of vertigo, fluctuating hearing loss, aural fullness, and tinnitus.

Pathophysiology and Etiology

1. Cause is unknown.
2. Fluid distention of the endolymphatic spaces of the labyrinth destroys cochlear hair cells. Pathology of the disease is endolymphatic hydrops, which is thought to be caused by overaccumulation of endolymphatic fluid and distention of the endolymphatic-containing areas in the cochlea and vestibular organs.
3. Usually unilateral, later may become bilateral. Diagnoses primarily based on clinical symptoms but audiometry and ENG are traditionally obtained.
4. Occurs most frequently between ages 30 and 60.
5. Severity of attacks may diminish over the years, but hearing loss increases.

Clinical Manifestations

1. Sudden attacks occur, in which the patient feels that the room is spinning (vertigo); may last 30 minutes to several hours or days.
2. Aural fullness, tinnitus, and reduced hearing or fluctuating hearing loss occurs on involved side.
3. Headache, nausea, vomiting, and disequilibrium may be present.
4. The most comfortable position for the patient is lying down.
5. After multiple attacks, tinnitus and impaired hearing may be continuous.

Diagnostic Evaluation

1. ENG or EcOG (see page 456), along with the patients' history and neurotologic exam, is used to establish diagnosis of Ménière disease.
2. Audiogram may reveal low-frequency sensorineural hearing loss in affected ear.
3. CT scan and MRI to rule out acoustic neuroma. Only MRI of internal auditory canal with gadolinium can differentiate Ménière disease symptoms from the symptoms of an intracranial lesion.

Management
Medical

1. The patient can be asked to keep a diary noting presence of aural symptoms (eg, tinnitus, distorted hearing) when episodes of vertigo occur.
2. Administration of a vestibular suppressant to control symptoms.
   a. Meclizine up to 25 mg four times a day.
   b. Diphenhydramine 25 to 50 mg three or four times a day.
   c. Lorazepam may be helpful as vestibular suppressant.
3. Intratympanic injections of aminoglycosides and corticosteroids can improve vertigo control.
4. Streptomycin (IM) or gentamicin (transtympanic injection) may be given to selectively destroy vestibular apparatus if vertigo is uncontrollable.
5. An antiemetic, such as promethazine, may be needed to reduce nausea, vomiting, and resistant vertigo.

 DRUG ALERT In general, meclizine is not recommended on a long-term basis, as it prevents central nervous system compensation. Meclizine may be used for symptomatic relief on a short-term basis.

Surgical

1. Conservative—endolymphatic subarachnoid or mastoid shunt to relieve symptoms without destroying function.
2. Destructive surgery.
   a. Labyrinthectomy—recommended if the patient experiences progressive hearing loss and severe vertigo attacks so normal tasks cannot be performed; results in total deafness of affected ear.
   b. Vestibular nerve section—neurosurgical suboccipital approach to the cerebellopontine angle for intracranial vestibular nerve neurectomy.

Complications

1. Irreversible hearing loss.
2. Disability and social isolation due to vertigo and hearing loss.
3. Injury due to falls.

Nursing Assessment

1. Assess for frequency and severity of attacks.
2. Provide screening hearing tests.
3. Evaluate effect on the patient's activities and potential for fall or injury.

Nursing Diagnoses

- Risk for Injury related to sudden attacks of vertigo.
- Social Isolation related to fear of attack and hearing loss.

Nursing Interventions

For care related to labyrinth surgery, see page 460.

Ensuring Safety

1. Help the patient recognize an aura so that he or she has time to prepare for an attack.
2. Encourage the patient to lie down during attack, in safe place, and lie still.
3. Put side rails up on bed if in hospital.
4. Have the patient close eyes if this lessens symptoms.
5. Inform the patient that the dizziness may last for varying lengths of time. Maintain safety precautions until attack is complete.

Minimizing Feelings of Isolation

1. Provide encouragement and understanding. Show the patient that you understand the seriousness of this disorder, even though there is little that can be done to ease the discomfort.
2. Assist the patient to identify specific triggers to control attacks.
   a. Remind the patient to move slowly because jerking or making sudden movements may precipitate an attack.
   b. Avoid noises and glaring, bright lights, which may initiate an attack.
   c. Control environmental factors and personal habits that may cause stress or fatigue.
   d. If there is a tendency to allergic reactions to foods, eliminate those foods from the diet.
3. Avoid oversedation of the patient through polypharmacy with sedatives, anticholinergics, and opioids that may increase risk of falling if attack occurs.
4. Teach the patient to be aware of other sensory cues from the environment, visual, olfactory, and tactile, if hearing is affected.

Patient Education and Health Maintenance

1. Teach about medication therapy, including adverse effects of vestibular suppressants—drowsiness, dry mouth.
2. Advise sodium restriction as adjunct to vestibular suppressant therapy.
3. Advise the patient to keep a log of attacks, triggers, and severity of symptoms.
4. Encourage follow-up hearing evaluations and provide information about surgical care if planned.
5. Teach the patient hearing-conservation methods—avoid loud noises, wear earplugs if necessary, avoid smoking, and avoid use of ototoxic drugs, such as aspirin, quinine, and some antibiotics.

Evaluation: Expected Outcomes

- Lays down with side rails up and eyes closed during attack; resolves without injury.
- Identifies dietary triggers and follows treatment plan.

Vestibular Labyrinthitis

Labyrinthitis is an inflammation of the inner ear caused by a viral or bacterial infection. It is characterized by hearing loss, vertigo, and usually nausea and vomiting.

See Box 17-1, for other causes of vertigo, including BPPV.

Pathophysiology and Etiology

1. Bacterial labyrinthitis is usually associated with acute otitis media or cholesteatoma. Infectious organisms may enter the inner ear through the oval or round window. Bacterial meningitis can cause labyrinthitis by spread of the bacterial infection via the cochlear aqueduct and internal auditory canal.
2. Viral labyrinthitis can occur as a result of viral illnesses of the respiratory tract system and may include measles, mumps, rubella, or herpetic infections of the facial or acoustic nerve. This may be seen in Ramsey-Hunt syndrome.

BOX 17-1 | **Vertigo**

Vertigo is a type of dizziness characterized by the illusion of movement: a perception either that the surroundings are moving while the body remains still or that one's body is moving while the surroundings remain still. It is caused by vestibular dysfunction—in either the peripheral vestibular system (inner ear) or the central vestibular system (brain stem and cerebellum).

- Common causes of vertigo of peripheral origin include Ménière disease, labyrinthitis, acoustic neuroma, and benign paroxysmal positional vertigo (BPPV).
- Causes of central vertigo include multiple sclerosis, basilar migraine, transient ischemic attack or stroke of the basilar artery, brain tumor, trauma, and cerebral hemorrhage.
- Other causes of dizziness are vasovagal syncope, hypovolemia, autonomic neuropathy of diabetes, severe anemia, aortic stenosis, hypoglycemia, hypoxia, hypocarbia, multiple sensory deficits, adverse drug effects, and emotional illness.

BPPV is the most common cause of vertigo. Its onset is sudden, it can be severe in intensity, and it is always related to change in position of the head. It can be diagnosed by thorough history and physical examination, including some provocative maneuvers such as the Dix-Hallpike maneuver. Diagnostic tests are required only to rule out central vestibular dysfunction and dizziness caused by other disorders. Patients with BPPV may be very concerned about their symptoms and are at risk for injury due to imbalance.

NURSING CONSIDERATIONS

- Ensure safety by creating an uncluttered environment, using side rails and handrails as necessary, using proper footwear, and encouraging the patient to call for help.
- Teach patient to avoid sudden position changes, including simple head movements, such as looking up or turning over in bed.
- Discourage use of alcohol and sedating drugs, which may further impair safe ambulation.
- Most episodes of BPPV last seconds to minutes and completely resolve within 3 months; however, if severe or prolonged, suggest referral to a physical therapist for vestibular rehabilitation.

---

3. Vestibular neuronitis or neuritis is a disorder of the vestibular nerve (CN XII) characterized by severe, sudden onset of vertigo with normal hearing. Etiology most commonly from viral illness but may be attributed to other causes. The course is usually self-limiting. The patient may have an unsteady gait but is able to walk. (This is differentiated by cerebellar disease, in which the patient has vertigo and nystagmus and is usually unable to walk.) Treatment is supportive with meclizine, benzodiazepines, antiemetics, or vestibular rehabilitation.

Clinical Manifestations

1. Sudden onset of incapacitating vertigo, with varying degrees of nausea and vomiting, hearing loss, and tinnitus.
2. Persists; does not occur in episodic attacks like Ménière disease.

Management

1. The rare cases of bacterial labyrinthitis are treated with antibiotics, as with the suspected predisposing infection.
   a. Bacterial labyrinthitis is treated by antibiotics, antiemetics, vestibular suppressants, and vestibular rehabilitation.
   b. Diagnostic imaging may include CT of temporal bone, MRI of internal auditory canal with gadolinium, and lumbar puncture, if bacterial meningitis is suspected.
2. Viral and physiologic causes are treated with symptomatic support. In patients with viral labyrinthitis, management may include antiviral therapy, antiemetics, vestibular suppressants, and, later in illness, vestibular rehabilitation.
3. A vestibular suppressant and antiemetic medication such as meclizine, diazepam, or promethazine may be needed, as with Ménière disease.
4. Audiometric evaluation should be obtained with all patients with vertigo to differentiate between vestibular labyrinthitis and vestibular neuronitis. MRI of brain and internal auditory canal is obtained when asymmetrical hearing loss is present to rule out acoustic neuroma.

Complications

1. Permanent hearing loss.
2. Injury from fall.

Nursing Assessment

1. Assess frequency and severity of attacks and how patient handles them.
2. Assess for fever related to bacterial infection.
3. Assess for additional neurologic symptoms—visual changes, change in mental status, sensory and motor deficits—that may indicate CNS pathology.
4. Assess for effectiveness of vestibular stimulants and antiemetics.
5. If fall occurs, assess for injury.

Nursing Diagnoses

- Risk for Injury related to gait disturbance secondary to vertigo.
- Anxiety related to sudden onset of symptoms.
- Risk for Deficient Fluid Volume related to vomiting and impaired intake.
- Bathing and Hygiene Self-Care Deficit related to vertigo.

Nursing Interventions

Preventing Injury

1. At onset of attack, have the patient lie still in darkened room with eyes closed or fixed on stationary object until the vertigo passes.

2. Make sure that the patient can obtain help at all times through use of call system, close proximity to staff, or companion.
3. Remove obstacles in the patient's environment.
4. Make sure that sensory aids are available—glasses, hearing aid, proper lighting.
5. Use side rails while the patient is in bed.
6. Administer medications, as directed; assess for and avoid oversedation.

Minimizing Anxiety
1. Explain the physiology behind vertigo and the possible triggers.
2. Support patient and family through the diagnostic process.
3. Assist the patient to adjust activities to minimize the impact.
4. Teach stress-reduction techniques, such as deep breathing, talking and asking questions, and distraction.

Ensuring Adequate Fluid
1. Keep diet light while vertigo is present.
2. Administer antiemetics, as directed.
3. Assess intake and output, as indicated.
4. Encourage fluids and small feedings while patient is feeling better.

Encouraging Safe Self-Care
1. Encourage activity while vertigo is minimal; rest during attacks.
2. Set up environment for the patient's safety and convenience—chair near sink, walker to hold on to while walking, if necessary, and so forth.
3. Assist the patient with hygiene and other care, as needed.

Patient Education and Health Maintenance
1. Teach patients with viral labyrinthitis that attacks are self-limiting, will become less severe, and should leave no permanent disability.
2. Teach safety measures during vertigo attacks.
3. Tell the patient that vertigo is best tolerated while lying flat in bed in a darkened room, with eyes closed or looking at stable object.
4. Teach patients how to take medications and to avoid other CNS depressants such as alcohol.
5. Encourage follow-up.

Evaluation: Expected Outcomes
- Rests in bed during attack with side rails up.
- Verbalizes feelings and questions about treatment.
- Takes fluids, light diet every 4 hours, after medication administration.
- Performs appropriate hygiene and dressing by him- or herself at bedside.

MALIGNANT DISORDERS

 See additional online content: Procedure Guidelines 17-2

Cancer of the Oral Cavity, Oropharynx, Nasopharynx, and Paranasal Sinuses

Cancer of the oral cavity may arise from the lips, buccal mucosa, gums, retromolar trigone, hard palate, floor of the mouth, salivary glands, and anterior two thirds of the tongue. Cancer of the oropharynx may arise from the tonsillar fossa, pharyngeal wall, and palatal arch (soft palate, uvula, and anterior border of the anterior tonsillar pillar). Cancer of the nasopharynx may arise from the fossa of Rosenmuller. Cancer of the paranasal sinuses may arise from the maxillary sinuses (80%) or, less commonly, in the ethmoid, frontal, and sphenoid sinuses.

Pathophysiology and Etiology

 EVIDENCE BASE National Cancer Institute. (2017). Cancer Stat Fact: Oral Cavity and Pharynx Cancer. *Surveillance, epidemiology and end results program (SEER)*. Bethesda, MD: Author. Available: *https://seer.cancer.gov/statfacts/html/oralcav.html*.

1. Oral and oropharyngeal cancer accounts for approximately 3% of all cancers diagnosed annually in the United States. About 48,000 people will be diagnosed with oral cavity and pharynx cancer and about 9,500 will have died from this disease in 2016. Prevalence is greater in men and between the ages of 55 to 64. Approximately 90% are squamous cell carcinoma.
   a. High-risk factors include use of tobacco and excessive alcohol (particularly in combination), use of smokeless tobacco (snuff), pipe smoking, marijuana use, exposure to HPV (causes greater than 60% of all oropharyngeal cancers in the United States), poor oral hygiene, and genetic factors.
   b. Overall survival rate depends on the primary location of the tumor and the stage of the disease at diagnosis. On average, 64% of those with this disease will survive more than 5 years.
2. Nasopharyngeal carcinoma is most prevalent in persons from Chinese or Asian ancestry because of a diet high in preservation (eg, salted fish). These types of cancers have a high genetic predisposition.
   a. Strong association with the Epstein-Barr virus.
   b. The most common presentation is neck mass. Blood-stained saliva or sputum is the second-most common presentation.
   c. Occurs 75% of the time in males, usually between ages 30 and 60. Overall survival rate is 50% to 90%, depending on the stage of disease at diagnosis.
3. Malignant paranasal sinus tumors are rare and have relatively poor survival outcomes. They are usually squamous cell in origin.
   a. The majority of cancer occurs in the maxillary sinus (50% to 70%), in the nasal cavity (15% to 30%), and ethmoid sinus (10% to 20%).
   b. Pathology is classified into epithelial and nonepithelial categories, with many subsets being attributable to environmental or occupational toxins.
   c. Overall survival rate is 27% to 94%, with the higher stage of cancer contributing to poorer prognosis.

Clinical Manifestations
1. Commonly asymptomatic in early stages.
2. Oral cancer—nonhealing, nonpainful crusting and ulcerated leukoplakic and erythemic lesions.
3. Cancer of the lip—presence of a lesion that fails to heal.
4. Cancer of the tongue—swelling, ulceration, areas of tenderness or pain, bleeding, abnormal texture, or limited movement of the tongue.
5. Floor of the mouth cancer—red, slightly elevated, mucosal lesion with ill-defined borders, leukoplakia, indurated, ulceration, or wartlike growth.
6. Cancer of the tonsil—swelling, neck mass, wartlike growth, odynophagia, otalgia.

7. Cancer of the retromolar trigone area—trismus, otalgia, dysphagia, odynophagia.
8. Cancer of the pharyngeal wall—dysphagia, odynophagia, otalgia, neck mass.
9. Cancer of the nasopharynx—epistaxis, unilateral serous otitis, unilateral nasal blockage, loss of sense of smell (CN I), eye movement abnormalities (CN III, IV, and V), and tongue movement impairment and dysphagia (CN IX, X, and XII).
10. More advanced stages characterized by ulceration, bleeding, pain, induration, CN impairments, dysphagia, odynophagia, weight loss, and/or cervical lymphadenopathy (neck mass).

Diagnostic Evaluation

1. Careful inspection of the oral cavity with indirect mirror examination of pharynx.
2. Flexible or rigid nasopharyngoscopy to directly examine the nasopharynx and pharynx.
3. Excisional biopsy of suspected tissue is the gold standard.
4. Radiologic studies: CT, with or without contrast as clinically indicated, MRI and possibly FDG-PET/CT for stage III-IV disease.

Management

EVIDENCE BASE National Comprehensive Cancer Network. (2017). *NCCN guidelines: Head and neck cancers.* Fort Washington, PA: Author. Available: www.nccn.org.

Selection of treatment depends on the size and site of lesion and how extensively surrounding tissues are involved.
1. Oral cavity cancer treatment consists of the following:
    a. Surgery to remove the primary disease plus any neck lymph nodes, or definitive radiotherapy.
    b. For more advanced cancer, surgery followed by chemoradiation or multimodal clinical trials is recommended.
2. Surgical resection of nasopharyngeal cancer may be difficult because of the location and the relationship to many important structures.
    a. Radiation therapy is the treatment of choice in early-stage cancers of these areas.
    b. For more advanced nasopharyngeal cancer, the recommendation is to perform multimodal clinical trials, or concurrent chemoradiation, or induction chemotherapy followed by chemoradiation.
    c. If metastasis is present, clinical trials are recommended, or concurrent platinum-based combination chemotherapy, or concurrent chemoradiation.
3. Oropharynx cancer (base of tongue cancer, tonsil, posterior pharyngeal wall and soft palate) cancer should be tested for human papillomavirus (HPV) status to determine prognosis; however, this does not affect the treatment recommendations.
    a. For low-grade cancer, the treatment choice is definitive radiation, or transoral or open resection of the primary tumor with neck dissection followed by chemoradiation, or multimodal clinical trials.
    b. For high-grade cancers, the treatment choices remain the same as above except for the addition of induction chemotherapy with radiation or systemic chemotherapy and radiation therapy.
4. Paranasal sinus cancer treatment usually consists of minimally invasive or open surgery followed by radiation; chemotherapy may also be utilized.

Complications

1. Second primary cancers of the larynx, hypopharynx, esophagus, and lungs.
2. Secondary to treatment:
    a. Surgery—transient salivary outflow obstruction, infection, voice changes, fistula formation, loss of swallowing, cosmetic defects.
    b. Radiation (early effects)—taste alterations, mucositis, xerostomia, dysphagia, odynophagia, anorexia, dermatitis, fatigue, pain.
    c. Radiation (late effects)—thyroid dysfunction, radiation caries, osteoradionecrosis, xerostomia, trismus, nasopharyngeal stenosis, CSF leak and other neurologic complications, tissue fibrosis, trismus, laryngeal edema, vascular complications.
    d. Chemotherapy—nausea, vomiting, dehydration, skin reaction, mucositis, hyperuremia, liver abnormalities, weight loss, anorexia, myelosuppression, peripheral neuropathy, hypomagnesemia, ototoxicity, nephrotoxicity, alopecia, and cognitive effects.

Nursing Assessment

1. Obtain complete history, noting risk factors such as smoking and alcohol use, exposure to Epstein-Barr virus, diet, high-risk sexual behavior, and exposure to environmental toxins.
2. Question the patient regarding changes in swallowing, smell or taste, salivation, discomfort when eating, sore throat, foul breath odor, weight loss, epistaxis, unilateral nasal obstruction, changes in hearing, neck mass, changes in tongue movement, and changes in vision.
3. Note the quality of voice patterns and odor of breath.
4. Inspect the oral cavity: erythema, red velvety areas; white patches; crusting, bleeding; swelling; record the size, location, and description.
5. Use nasal speculum to inspect the nares for obstruction.
6. Palpate the cervical lymph nodes for size, firmness, or tenderness.

Nursing Diagnoses

- Acute Pain related to malignant infiltration, lesions, difficulty swallowing, surgery, radiation therapy.
- Imbalanced Nutrition: Less Than Body Requirements related to pain, difficulty in chewing or swallowing, history of alcohol abuse, dysphagia, xerostomia.
- Disturbed Body Image related to changes in facial contour, cosmetic defect from surgery, CN deficits.

Nursing Interventions

Also see page 480 if radical neck dissection has been performed.

Achieving an Acceptable Level of Comfort
1. Provide systemic analgesics or analgesic gargles, as prescribed.
2. If ordered by the provider, perform mouth care with soft toothbrush and flossing between teeth.
3. If the patient cannot tolerate brushing and flossing:
    a. Gently lavage oral cavity with a catheter inserted between the patient's cheek and gums with warm water or salt water rinses.
4. Provide management of excessive salivation and mouth odors.
    a. Insert a gauze wick in corner of mouth; place basin conveniently to catch drooling; replace frequently to absorb and direct excess saliva.
    b. Suction secretions with a soft rubber catheter, if not allergic to latex, as needed; instruct the patient on suctioning methods.

5. Provide management of decreased salivation, if necessary.
   a. Encourage intake of fluids, particularly water, if not contraindicated.
   b. Instruct the patient to avoid dry, bulky, and irritating foods.
   c. Offer lemon lozenges or chewing gum to stimulate salivation.
   d. Encourage use of humidifier.
   e. Suggest foods with sauces and gravies to make them moist and easier to swallow.
6. Maintain a clean and odor-free environment by removing soiled dressings, tissues, and gauzes and providing room deodorants.

Improving Nutritional Status

1. Handle feeding problems in one or a combination of the following ways, as ordered:
   a. IV fluid to prevent dehydration.
   b. Nasogastric (NG) tube feedings or prophylactic placement of gastrostomy tube for feedings.
   c. Orally—serve meals high in protein and vitamin content and low in acidity and salt.
2. Provide mouth care before and after eating.
3. Allow the patient to have meals in privacy, if desired.
4. Offer easily chewed foods; mash or blenderize, if necessary.
5. Add herbs or sweeteners to enhance flavor.
6. Provide methods to compensate for decreased salvation by offering the following:
   a. Sip fluids, especially water, and carry water bottle throughout day.
   b. Avoid dry, bulky, and irritating foods.
   c. Use lemon lozenges or chewing gum to stimulate salivation.
   d. Use cholinergic stimulants or saliva substitutes as prescribed.
   e. Use a humidifier.
   f. Add gravy and sauces to food.
7. Encourage daily fluoride treatment as prescribed while undergoing radiation.
8. Have patient remove dentures if mucositis is present.
9. If swallowing difficulties persist, consult the speech–language pathologist.
10. Monitor weight, intake and output, and laboratory tests, such as 24-hour urine for urea nitrogen, C-reactive protein, albumin, prealbumin, transferrin level, and electrolytes.
11. Maintain a clean and odor-free environment by removing soiled material and using room deodorizer.

 EVIDENCE BASE Buglione M., Cavagnini R., Di Rosario F., et al. (2016). Oral toxicity management in head and neck cancer patients treated with chemotherapy and radiation: Dental pathologies and osteoradionecrosis (Part 1) literature review and consensus statement. *Critical Reviews in Oncology/Hematology, 97*, 131–142.
Buglione M., Cavagnini R., Di Rosario F., et al. (2016). Oral toxicity management in head and neck cancer patients treated with chemotherapy and radiation: Xerostomia and trismus (Part 2). Literature review and consensus statement. *Critical Reviews in Oncology/Hematology, 102*, 47–54.

Strengthening Body Image

1. Assess the patient's reaction to condition.
   a. Evaluate the patient's apprehension and offer emotional support.
   b. Correct misinformation.

   c. Determine therapeutic care plan for the patient's rehabilitation.
2. Recognize that face and neck surgery can be disfiguring and the patient often is embarrassed, withdrawn, and depressed.
3. Assist the patient in caring for personal appearance.
4. Observe closely for indications of the patient's needs, which may be communicated in other ways, such as acting out or withdrawn behavior.
5. Allow verbalization of fears, anger, and distaste with body changes in a nondefensive manner.
6. Communicate acceptance of appearance in an honest manner.
7. Encourage the patient's family and friends to visit so patient is aware that others care about him or her.
8. Provide diversional activities.

Community and Home Care Considerations

1. Teach mouth care procedure and dressing care to maintain cleanliness and prevent odor.
2. Emphasize adequate nutrition—proper consistency, proper seasoning, and right temperature. Show the family how to prepare food in blender or food processor, as necessary. Teach tube-feeding procedure, if applicable.
3. If suctioning is required, instruct as to method, use, and care of equipment and obtain supplies for family.
4. Provide detailed instructions and demonstration to the patient and caregiver on incisional care.
5. Assess for signs of obstruction, hemorrhage, infection, and depression and teach caregivers what to do about them if they occur.
6. If the patient is undergoing radiation therapy, encourage them to perform appropriate skin care, avoid exposure to potential chemical irritants, limit direct sun exposure, and avoid application of lotions, ointments, or fragrances to the head and neck region, which might alter the depth at which the maximum radiation dose is delivered.
7. Encourage the radiated patient to use sialogogues such as hard candy to stimulate saliva flow. Pilocarpine may be prescribed to prevent xerostomia for patients who have completed radiation therapy.

Patient Education and Health Maintenance

1. Encourage cessation of high-risk behaviors to all—smoking, alcohol consumption, use of smokeless tobacco, pipe smoking.
2. Emphasize the need for routine follow-up examinations with specialists, dentist (for the use of fluoride trays during radiation), and speech pathologist, if indicated.

Evaluation: Expected Outcome

- Reports adequate comfort levels, is pain-free, and handles secretions adequately.
- Achieves adequate nutritional status, able to eat prescribed diet.
- Verbalizes acceptance of body image, demonstrates behaviors that reflect positive self-esteem (eg, shaves, dresses, applies makeup).

Neck Dissection for Head and Neck Malignancy

Systematic removal of lymph nodes with their surrounding fibrofatty tissue from the various compartments of the neck. The goal of neck dissection is to eradicate metastases involving the cervical lymph nodes. Metastases originate from primary lesions involving the oral cavity, pharynx, and larynx. The cervical lymph nodes are grouped into six major levels (I to VI) with additional division into two sublevels (A and B) of levels I, II, and V.

Surgical Procedures

1. Resection of lesion is the primary intervention.
2. Radical neck dissection—removal of lymph nodes in levels I through V and internal jugular vein (IJ), sternocleidomastoid muscle (SCM), and the spinal accessory nerve (CN XI).
3. Modified radical neck dissection—removal of lymph nodes in levels I through V, and preservation of one or more of IJ, SCM, CN XI.
4. Selective neck dissection—en bloc removal of one or more lymph node (LN) groups that are at greatest risk for harboring metastasis.
5. Commonly followed by postoperative radiation therapy. In some instances where resection is impossible, radiation therapy is the sole treatment for head and neck malignancy.
6. Surgical reconstruction may be performed with a rotational flap, skin graft, or free flap to promote healing and improve aesthetics.

Preoperative Management

1. Interventions to improve nutritional status preoperatively include nutritional supplements, hyperalimentation, alcohol withdrawal, and counseling.
2. The patient's general health status is evaluated and underlying conditions, such as cirrhosis, diabetes mellitus, pulmonary, and cardiovascular disease, are identified and treated, if possible.
3. The patient is evaluated for level of understanding of disease process, treatment regimen, and follow-up care.
4. Emotional preparation for major surgery, long rehabilitation, and change in body image is provided.

Postoperative Management

1. A major goal of postoperative management is protection of the airway. After the patient has fully recovered from anesthesia, the endotracheal tube is removed (unless respiratory compromise occurs).
2. The patient is closely monitored for hemorrhage. Wound drainage is facilitated with a negative pressure drain. The drain is removed when output is less than 25 mL in a 24-hour period.
3. Prophylactic antibiotics are given to prevent infection because of extensive incision, lymph node resection, and close proximity to oral secretions.
4. Oral nutritional supplements, enteral feedings, or hyperalimentation is provided until oral intake is adequate and nutritional status is improved.
5. Provide adequate pain control with analgesics, in addition to narcotics as needed. When the patient is taking narcotics, provide stool softeners and/or laxatives to prevent narcotic-induced constipation.
6. Shoulder range of motion assessment is performed to determine if cranial nerve XI (spinal accessory) has been weakened during surgery. Physical therapy will provide strengthening exercises.

Complications

1. Surgery—air leaks, bleeding, chylous fistula, facial or cerebral edema, blindness, carotid artery rupture, and damage to nerves such as the phrenic, vagus, brachial plexus, spinal accessory, and cutaneous nerves and the mandibular branch of the facial, hypoglossal, or lingual nerves.

2. Radiation.
   a. Early—radiation mucositis, xerostomia erythema, desquamation, dysphagia, secondary infection, oral pain.
   b. Long-term—atrophy, fibrosis, salivary dryness, hoarseness, difficulty swallowing, bone pain, osteonecrosis, pathologic fractures, limitation of movement, poor wound healing.

Nursing Diagnoses

- Ineffective Breathing Pattern related to laryngeal edema, secretions, presence of a tracheostomy.
- Risk for Infection related to surgery, proximity of secretions to suture line, radiation.
- Imbalanced Nutrition: Less Than Body Requirements related to anorexia, inability to swallow, pain on swallowing.
- Disturbed Body Image related to surgical scarring, radiation changes.

Nursing Interventions

Maintaining Effective Breathing Pattern

1. Place the patient in Fowler position.
2. Observe for signs of respiratory embarrassment, such as dyspnea, cyanosis, edema, hoarseness, or dysphagia.
3. Provide supplemental oxygen by face mask, if necessary; if tracheostomy is present, provide humidified air or oxygen by tracheostomy collar or adequate ambient humidification.
4. Auscultate for decreased breath sounds, crackles, or wheezes; auscultate over the trachea in the immediate postoperative period to assess for stridor indicative of edema.
5. Encourage deep breathing and coughing.
6. Assist the patient in assuming a sitting position to bring up secretions.
7. Suction secretions orally or aseptically through a tracheostomy if patient is unable to cough them up.

Preventing Infection

1. Assess vital signs for indication of infection—increased heart rate, elevation of temperature.
2. Inspect wound for hemorrhage, drainage, or tracheal constriction; reinforce dressings, as needed.
3. Inspect incision for signs of infection—increased pain and tenderness, redness, warmth, swelling, drainage.
4. If a drain is used, expect approximately 80 to 120 mL of serosanguineous secretions to be drawn off during the first postoperative day; this diminishes with each day. Ensure that the drain is stripped at the insertion site at least three times per day to prevent clotting. Assess for color and amount of drainage.
   a. The initial output will be serosanguineous and eventually will turn serous. If the fluid appears milky, the surgeon should be notified right away as this may be indicative of a chyle leak.
   b. A high output of several hundred milliliters or more per day may also indicate chyle leak. If the output is less than 600 mL of chyle per day, the leak is initially managed conservatively with closed-wound drainage, pressure dressings, and zero-fat nutritional support. Parenteral alimentation through a central line may also be utilized to further reduce chylous output.
5. Aseptically clean skin area around drain exit, using saline or prescribed solution.
6. Make sure that the incision site remains clean and dry; remove secretions immediately.

Improving Nutritional Status

1. Postoperatively provide IV fluids and hyperalimentation, tube feedings through NG tube or gastrostomy tube, or oral feedings as soon as swallowing is established.
2. Provide mouth care before and after meals.
3. Assess for excessive or decreased salivation, which may impair swallowing.
4. Make sure that emergency suctioning and airway equipment is available at the bedside during meals in the event of choking or aspiration. Utilize speech–language therapist to evaluate dysphagia.
5. Position the patient in an upright position, supporting shoulders and neck with pillows, if necessary.
6. Ask whether the patient would prefer privacy during meals.
7. Provide an environment that is clean and free from interruptions and odor.
8. Assist with oral intake, providing easily chewed foods. Mash or blenderize meals, if necessary.

Strengthening Body Image

1. Respect the patient's desire for privacy during treatments, dressing changes, and feedings.
2. Prepare visitors for the patient's change in appearance.
3. If the patient has difficulty speaking, assist with alternate communication methods and allow adequate time for communication.
4. Observe for lower facial paralysis; this may indicate facial nerve injury.
5. Watch for shoulder dysfunction, which may follow resection of spinal accessory nerves.
   a. Use muscle exercises provided by the physical therapist and muscle reeducation postoperatively.
   b. Work with the patient to obtain good functional range of motion.
6. Encourage the patient to verbalize concerns and feelings.
   a. Consult the health care provider to determine the nature and extent of explanation and prognosis that has been given to the patient.
   b. Encourage the patient to seek confirmation of personal philosophy and religious beliefs because this may provide answers.
   c. Accentuate the positive.
   d. Encourage the patient to participate in the plan of care.
   e. Recognize that a great effort has to be made in behavior modification to change a lifestyle that included alcohol consumption and cigarette smoking. Provide educational material and support.

Community and Home Care Considerations

1. Determine if the patient requires home care for drain care and/or home physical therapy.
2. If the patient has a permanent tracheostomy, instruct the patient and caregivers about the following:
   a. Need for increased humidification in the home environment.
   b. Avoiding activities that may cause aspiration (eg. swimming).
3. Referral for speech-language pathologist to meet ongoing communication needs.

Patient Education and Health Maintenance

Exercises

1. Instruct the patient and family regarding exercises to prevent limited range of shoulder motion and discomfort (see Figure 17-7).

2. Perform exercises morning and evening. Initially, exercises are done only once; the number is increased by one each day until each exercise is done 10 times.
3. After each exercise, the patient is instructed to relax.

Follow-Up Visits

1. Emphasize the need for frequent follow-up visits and completion of radiation therapy, if prescribed.
2. Recommend a dental follow-up to ensure good oral hygiene and dental rehabilitation, if indicated.

Evaluation: Expected Outcomes

- Maintains adequate breathing pattern; absence of dyspnea, shortness of breath; is able to handle secretions.
- Is free from signs and symptoms of infection; vital signs stable; incision is clean, dry, without redness or drainage.
- Is adequately hydrated; maintains stable nutrition and weight; can tolerate diet without choking or aspiration.
- Discusses concerns about condition; verbalizes positive aspects of self.

Cancer of the Larynx

Cancer of the larynx is a malignant growth of the vocal cords. It accounts for 0.8% of all cancers. The supraglottic larynx refers to the area above the vocal cords including the epiglottis. The subglottic larynx refers to the area below the vocal cords to about the first tracheal ring. When treated early, the likelihood of cure is great. The National Cancer Institute at the National Institutes of Health estimated that in 2017, there were approximately 13,360 new cases diagnosed in the United States and 3,660 persons were estimated to die from the disease. The 5-year survival rate is estimated to be 61%.

 EVIDENCE BASE National Cancer Institute. (2017). Cancer Stat Facts: Larynx Cancer. *Surveillance, epidemiology and end results program.* Bethesda, MD: Author. Available: *https://seer.cancer.gov/statfacts/html/laryn.html.*

Pathophysiology and Etiology

1. Occurs predominantly in men older than age 60.
2. Most patients have a history of smoking and heavy alcohol intake. Other risk factors include laryngopharyngeal reflux; industrial exposure to diesel exhaust, asbestos, organic solvents, sulfuric acid, mustard gas, certain mineral oils, metal dust, asphalt, wood dust, stone dust, mineral wool, and cement dust; genetic susceptibility; and diet.
3. In North America, about two thirds of carcinomas of the larynx arise in the glottis, almost one third arise in the supraglottic region, and about 3% arise in the subglottic region of the larynx.
4. When limited to the vocal cords, spread is slow because of lessened blood supply.
5. When cancer involves the supraglottis, cancer spreads more rapidly to the lymph nodes of the neck than does glottis cancer.

Clinical Manifestations

Depend on tumor location; sequence in appearance related to pattern and extent of tumor growth.

1A. Gently turn head to each side and look as far as possible.

1B. Gently tip right ear toward right shoulder as far as possible. Repeat on left side.

1C. Move chin to chest and then lift head up and back.

2A. Place hands in front with elbows at right angles away from body.

2B. Rotate shoulders back, bringing elbows to side.

2C. Relax whole body.

3A. Lean or hold on to low table or chair with hand on the unoperated side. Bend body slightly at waist, and swing shoulder and arm from left to right.

3B. Swing shoulder and arm from front to back.

3C. Swing shoulder and arm in a wide circle, gradually bringing arm above head.

Figure 17-7. Rehabilitation exercises after head and neck surgery to regain maximum shoulder function and neck motion.

Supraglottic Cancer
1. Tickling sensation in throat.
2. Dryness and fullness (lump) in throat.
3. Painful swallowing (odynophagia) associated with invasion of extralaryngeal musculature.
4. Coughing on swallowing.
5. Pain radiating to ear (late symptom).

Glottic Cancer (Cancer of the Vocal Cord)
1. Most common cancer of the larynx.
2. Hoarseness or aphonia (loss of voice).
3. Aspiration.
4. Dyspnea.
5. Pain (in later stages).

Subglottic Cancer (Uncommon)
1. Coughing.
2. Short periods of difficulty in breathing.

3. Hemoptysis; fetid odor, which results from ulceration and disintegration of tumor.

Diagnostic Evaluation
1. Indirect mirror examination of larynx may indicate lesion.
2. Direct laryngoscopy and biopsy to identify lesion.
3. CT scan and other special radiologic tests to detect tumor.
4. The T, N, M classification system is used for staging (see page 112). In larynx cancer, prognosis can be predicted by the tumor size and nodal involvement. If lymph nodes are involved, the prognosis is usually poorer than when no lymph nodes are involved.

Management

General Considerations
Depends on sites and stages of cancer. Early malignancy may be removed endoscopically.

1. Early glottic squamous cell carcinoma (SCC, defined as stage I or II disease) may be treated with either radiation therapy or surgery, with or without neck dissection. Surgical treatment goal of early glottic SCC is to preserve the larynx and is referred to as conservation laryngeal surgery or partial laryngectomy.

2. Advanced glottic SCC (stage III or IV disease) is associated with poor prognosis. T3 glottic carcinomas have a low risk of nodal metastasis. T3 tumors may be treated with concurrent chemotherapy and radiation therapy, surgery, induction chemotherapy, or multimodal clinical trials. T4 glottic carcinoma is treated with total laryngectomy and usually postoperative radiation therapy, with or without chemotherapy.

3. According to the National Comprehensive Cancer Network, the patient should be examined every 1 to 3 months for the first year after treatment, every 2 to 6 months in the 2nd year, every 4 to 8 months in the 3rd, 4th, and 5th years, and every 12 months thereafter.

EVIDENCE BASE National Comprehensive Cancer Network. (2017). *NCCN guidelines: Head and neck cancers.* Fort Washington, PA: Author. Available: *www.nccn.org/professionals/physician_gls/pdf/head-and-neck.pdf.*

Surgery

1. Laser excision for early-stage disease.
2. Partial laryngectomy—removal of small lesion on true cord, along with a substantial margin of healthy tissue.
3. Supraglottic laryngectomy—removal of all laryngeal structures superior to the floor of the ventricle, maintaining both true vocal cords, both arytenoids, the base of the tongue, and the hyoid bone. Is performed for T1, T2, or selected T3 supraglottic tumors. An acceptable alternative to supraglottic laryngectomy is transoral laser microsurgery for T1–T2 and selected T3 tumors.
4. Hemilaryngectomy—removal of one true vocal cord, false cord, one half of thyroid cartilage, arytenoid cartilage.
5. Total laryngectomy—removal of entire larynx (epiglottis, false or true cords, cricoid cartilage, hyoid bone; two or three tracheal rings are usually removed when there is extrinsic cancer of the larynx [extension beyond the vocal cords]). A radical neck dissection may also be performed because of metastasis to cervical lymph nodes.
6. Total laryngectomy with tracheoesophageal puncture (TEP). During surgery, a puncture is made in the posterior wall of the trachea, which is also the anterior wall of the esophagus. A voice prosthesis or a red rubber catheter is inserted into the puncture. The red rubber catheter serves two purposes: to mature the track until a voice prosthesis is inserted and to provide enteral feedings until the patient is allowed to swallow. If a voice prosthesis is inserted at the time of surgery, the patient is fed through either a nasogastric or gastrostomy tube.

Complications

1. Pharyngocutaneous fistula may develop after any surgical procedure that involves entering the pharynx or esophagus.
   a. Monitor for saliva collecting beneath the skin flaps or leaking through suture line into neck drains.
   b. Management—NG tube or gastrostomy feeding, meticulous local wound care with frequent dressing changes, promotion of drainage.

2. Hemorrhage (carotid artery rupture) or hematoma formation.
   a. A major postoperative complication (eg, skin necrosis or salivary fistula) usually precedes carotid artery rupture.
   b. Management—immediate wound exploration in operating room.
3. Drain failure.
4. Infection.
5. Wound dehiscence—patients who have been radiated prior to surgery and/or who are malnourished are more at risk for wound dehiscence.
6. Complications of radiation—edema of the larynx, soft tissue and cartilage necrosis, skin reaction, chondritis.
7. Long-term complications:
   a. Stomal stenosis.
   b. Pharyngoesophageal stenosis and stricture.
   c. Hypothyroidism.

Nursing Assessment

1. Ask about alcohol intake, smoking and drug history, and chronic illnesses.
2. Take a nutrition history and 24-hour food intake recall. Review results of laboratory test. Weigh the patient.
3. Observe ability to swallow.
4. Review recommendations of speech–language pathologist for communication.
5. Assess for independence, self-assuredness, and willingness to try new things; these are strengths on which to build.
6. Assess reality of the patient's expectations.
7. Assess patient's ability to care for self, particularly concerning stomal care.
8. Assess the patient's social support system. Who will be home with the patient after discharge?

Nursing Diagnoses

- Readiness for Enhanced Knowledge about laryngectomy.
- Ineffective Breathing Pattern related to artificial airway, accumulation of secretions, inability to cough secondary to surgical procedure.
- Imbalanced Nutrition: Less Than Body Requirements related to impaired swallowing secondary to surgical alteration of pharynx and larynx; laryngeal edema and pain; radiation-induced mucositis.
- Impaired Verbal Communication related to surgery or absence of larynx; presence of artificial airway.
- Deficient Knowledge related to stoma care and living with effects of laryngectomy.

Nursing Interventions

Preparing for Total Laryngectomy
1. Collaborate with the surgeon in preparing the patient; interpret and reiterate what surgeon and speech–language pathologist have explained.
   a. Inform the patient that breathing will occur through an opening (tracheostoma) in the neck.
   b. Advise the patient that speech will be altered by surgery.
2. Expect reactions of anxiety and depression because the psychosocial effects of voice loss are substantial.
3. Practice a means of communication (pad and pencil, sign language, pictures, word cards, artificial larynx) that can be used until speech therapy begins.
4. Arrange for the patient to be visited by laryngectomee (one who has had larynx removed) for support.

5. Provide portable battery-operated suction machine, suction catheter kits, and other supplies from a home care company and educate patient on suctioning procedure prior to the patient's discharge. Initiate referral for home care nursing and other community services.
6. Provide information about other community support services such as the International Association of Laryngectomees or Supporting Patients with Oral Head and Neck Cancer.
7. Reinforce information about alternative modes of communication.
   a. Artificial larynx, using either neck or intraoral placement: Electrolarynx provides communication assistance in early postoperative period or later to those unable to learn alternative method.
   b. TEP with voice prosthesis: A one-way valved voice prosthesis is inserted through TEP to allow the patient to shunt pulmonary air into esophagus for voice production (see Figure 17-8).
   c. Esophageal speech is accomplished by training the patient to force air down the esophagus and release it in a controlled manner.

Improving Breathing Pattern

1. Monitor for signs of difficulty breathing—suprasternal and intercostal retractions, tachypnea, dyspnea, tachycardia, and changes in sensorium.
2. Auscultate trachea/chest for evidence of stridor or wheezing and for absence of breath sounds.
3. Make sure the patient uses a specific signal to indicate need for suctioning; enter on nursing care plan.
4. Suction secretions according to the prescriber's orders to prevent accumulation of mucus which may lead to mucus pluging.
   a. Also suction nasal secretions because the patient is unable to blow nose.
   b. Remove crusts from stoma at least three times daily to prevent webbing of mucus across the stoma.
5. Use chest physical therapy, as necessary, to remove secretions.
6. Assist the patient in secretion removal.
   a. Teach the patient to bend forward until stoma is below lung level and to exhale rapidly. This aids in secretion removal from lungs.

Figure 17-8. Schematic representation of tracheoesophageal puncture speech. When the patient plugs the stomal opening, air is forced from the lungs through a one-way valve voice prosthesis. Air travels into the esophagus and out the mouth, creating speech.

Voice prosthesis
Tracheostoma valve

   b. Teach the patient to wipe resultant secretions away from tracheostoma with a handkerchief.
7. Encourage breathing exercises because most patients have been heavy smokers.
8. Supply constant humidification to moisten tracheostoma and avoid viscous secretions; tracheal air will require additional warmth and moisture.
9. Keep calm and maintain sense of security.
   a. Reassure the patient that someone is always near to assist.
   b. Have call bell within reach.
10. Remind patient that they are now a neck breather and can no longer breathe out of their nose or mouth.
11. In the event of airway obstruction, clear the stoma and ventilate through stoma.

Facilitating Adequate Nutrition

1. Monitor IV fluids during first few postoperative days.
2. Administer fluids and nutrients by NG or gastrostomy tube.
   a. Tube feedings may be started after bowel sounds are heard and continued until sufficient healing of pharynx has occurred (approximately 7 to 14 days) and patient is ready to resume oral feedings.
   b. Avoid manipulating NG tube as it is resting on or near suture line.
   c. Clean nostrils and lubricate with water-soluble lubricant.
   d. Clean crust on outside of tube.
   e. Pay attention to oral hygiene, with regular toothbrushing and prescribed antiseptic mouthwashes.
3. Assure the patient that swallowing is safe and may feel differently than before surgery. Some structures and muscles removed during surgery may cause the patient to "work harder" to swallow.
   a. Patients may need more liquids to wash down foods.
   b. It may be easier to eat smaller, more frequent meals.
   c. A modified barium swallow may be ordered several days after surgery to be sure adequate healing has occurred and that there are no leaks or fistulas opening into the airway.
   d. After a total laryngectomy, there is a separation of the airway (trachea) from the esophagus; and theoretically, there is no risk for aspiration. However, if a TEP is present and occupied by either a voice prosthesis or red rubber catheter, leakage around the TEP site could occur.
4. The speech–language pathologist will educate the patient and family about the presence, care, and maintenance of the TEP and any potential problems.

Providing Alternative Communication

1. Advise the patient to communicate by writing or with artificial larynx until voice work can begin with speech–language pathologist.
2. Discourage forced whispering, which increases pharyngeal tension.
3. Encourage the patient to join local laryngectomy support group (eg, Lost Chord Club, New Voice Club, International Association of Laryngectomees), which gives opportunity to practice new speech and serves as a bridge between therapy and return to social life.
4. Inform the patient of the various communication methods:
   a. An electrolarynx, which is placed against the neck, cheek, or in the mouth for a monotone, mechanical sound, can be used immediately after surgery. The speech–language pathologist will provide instruction on the use of the device.

b. Esophageal speech is the act of air charging, which is achieved by thrusting the tongue back and forcing a bolus through the cricopharyngeus. The air bolus then is regurgitated through the pharyngoesophageal segment, which vibrates to produce sound.

c. Tracheoesophageal speech, which is the most common voice restoration option, involves placing a one-way valve voice prosthesis into the TEP. The patient takes a breath and occludes the stoma with either a finger or stoma button. This air is forced through the voice prosthesis into the pharynx, which vibrates and produces sound.

Providing Information about Laryngectomy

1. Inform the patient that it is very important to keep the stoma clear of mucus. This is accomplished through regular tracheal suctioning and by cleaning mucus from the stoma several times per day.
2. A laryngectomy or tracheostomy tube may be worn if there is neck edema and narrowing of the stoma. The tube is not always permanent. The type of tube used is determined by the provider or speech–language pathologist.
3. Demonstrate procedure for cleaning and changing tube.
   a. See page 173 for tracheostomy tube care. A laryngectomy tube is cleaned the same way as an inner cannula.
   b. Place gauze dressing under tube to absorb secretions, as prescribed. Change when it becomes soiled to prevent skin irritation and odor.
   c. Encourage the patient to change the laryngectomy or tracheostomy fastener when soiled.
4. Tracheostoma care—teach the patient to:
   a. Wash hands before touching stoma to prevent infection.
   b. Wet washcloth with warm water; wring dry and gently wipe stoma. Do not use soap, tissues, or cotton balls because these may enter airway.
   c. Apply petroleum around exterior of stoma to prevent skin irritation.
   d. Report excessive redness, swelling, purulent secretions, or bleeding.
5. Stoma cover.
   a. Stoma cover is necessary to filter air and increase humidity of air; also necessary for hygienic purposes.
   b. Stoma cover can be crocheted, made of cotton cloth, or commercially available as foam filters.
   c. For men: ascot or turtleneck sweaters may be worn. When a regular shirt is worn, the second button from the top can be sewed over the buttonhole as though it were fastened. This leaves a wide opening through which a handkerchief can be inserted when coughing.
   d. For women: a variety of fashionable scarves, jewelry, high-neck dresses, and turtleneck sweaters can be worn.
6. Bowel care: discuss high-fiber diet and use of stool softener because patient with tracheostoma is usually not able to hold breath to "bear down" for bowel movement.
7. If the patient snored before surgery, he or she will no longer snore after laryngectomy because air no longer passes through the nose and mouth. For the same reason, the patient may have difficulty sniffing and blowing his or her nose. The speech–language pathologist can provide techniques for briefly sniffing through the nose.
8. Swallowing after laryngectomy will resume no sooner than 5 days after surgery. A barium swallow may be ordered to detect a leak in the internal incision line. Swallowing may be a little slower and/or more difficult. The speech–language pathologist will provide swallowing therapy.

Community and Home Care Considerations

1. Provide humidification in the home; use heat-moisture exchanger, a humidifier, or cool mist vaporizer, especially in bedroom and when dry heat is used.
2. Tell the patient to avoid cold air; cover tracheostoma with thin layer of foam or other cover to warm and humidify air.
3. Encourage the patient to drink fluids liberally (2 to 3 quarts [2 to 3 L]) to help liquefy secretions.
4. Have the patient always keep stoma covered for hygienic management of secretions and to keep dust and foreign matter from entering trachea.
5. Place a protective shield over stoma before bathing, showering, or shampooing hair and while getting a haircut or shaving. Use an electric razor instead of blade because shaving cream can irritate.
6. Swimming is to be avoided as there is no way to prevent water from entering the stoma.
7. Ensure working smoke detectors are available in the home as the sense of smell is decreased.

Patient Education and Health Maintenance

1. Tell the patient to expect some loss of smell and taste sensation.
2. Advise the patient to check with health care provider before taking medication because many drugs (such as antihistamines and cold products) tend to dry the mucous membranes of the stoma.
3. Warn the patient to seek immediate attention for pain, difficulty breathing or swallowing, appearance of pus or blood-streaked sputum.

Evaluation: Expected Outcomes

- Verbalizes understanding of tracheostoma and communication options.
- Breathes quietly; no evidence of noisy secretions.
- Swallows soft foods; maintains weight.
- Makes needs known; speech therapy has started.
- Manages tracheostomal care; has made provisions for home humidification and tracheostomal supplies.

SELECTED REFERENCES

Andrews, B. (2013). *Pharmacological management of otitis externa and the draining tympanostomy tube.* Available: http://sohnnurse.com/wp-content/uploads/122-Andrews-Revised-Pharmacologic-Management-of-Otitis-Externa....pdf

Armstrong, W. B., Vokes, D. E., & Sunil, P. V. (2015). Malignant tumors of the larynx. In P. W. Flint, B. H. Haughey, V. J. Lund, et al. (Eds.), *Cummings otolaryngology head and neck surgery* (6th ed., pp. 1601–1633). Philadelphia, PA: Elsevier.

Beckera, S. D., Becker, D. G., Becker, S. D. (2018). Review and update on postoperative opioid use after nasal and sinus surgery. *Current Opinion in Otolaryngology & Head & Neck Surgery, 26*(1), 41–45.

Branstetter, B. (2015). Diagnostic imaging of the pharynx and esophagus. In P. W. Flint, B. H. Haughey, V. J. Lund, et al. (Eds.), *Cummings otolaryngology head and neck surgery* (6th ed., pp. 1507–1536). Philadelphia, PA: Elsevier.

Buglione, M., Cavagnini, R., Di Rosario F., et al. (2016). Oral toxicity management in head and neck cancer patients treated with chemotherapy and radiation: Dental pathologies and osteoradionecrosis (Part 1) literature review and consensus statement. *Critical Reviews in Oncology/Hematology, 97,* 131–142.

Cannon, R. B., Houlton, J. J., Mendez, E., & Futran, N. D. (2017). Methods to reduce postoperative surgical site infections after head and neck oncology surgery. *Lancet Oncol, 18*(7), e405–e413.

Cheraghlou, S., Otremba, M., Kuo, Y. P., Agogo, G. O., Hersey D., & Judson, B. L. (2018). Prognostic Value of Lymph Node Yield and Density in Head and Neck Malignancies. *Otolaryngol Head Neck Surg, 1,* 194599818756830.

Chong, L, Head, K., Hopkins, C., et al. (2016). Saline irrigation for chronic rhino-sinusitis. *Cochrane Database of Systemic Reviews*, (4), CD011995. Available: *www.cochrane.org/CD011995/ENT_saline-irrigation-chronic-rhinosinusitis*

Donaldson, J. D. (2017) *Acute Otitis Media Guidelines*. Medscape Drugs and Diseases. New York. Available: https://emedicine.medscape/com/article/859316-guidelines.

Dort, J. C., Farwell, G., Findlay, M., et al. (2017). Optimal perioperative care in major head and neck cancer surgery with free flap reconstruction: a consensus review and recommendations from the enhanced recovery after surgery society. *JAMA Otolaryngology—Head & Neck Surgery*, *143*(3), 292–303.

Fakhry, C., & Gourin, C. G. (2015). Human papillomavirus and the epidemiology of head and neck cancer. In P. W. Flint, B. H. Haughey, V. J. Lund, et al. (Eds.), *Cummings otolaryngology head and neck surgery* (6th ed., pp. 1083–1087). Philadelphia, PA: Elsevier.

Hain, T. C. (2017). Vestibular neuritis and labyrinthitis. *Dizziness-and-Balance.com*. Available: *www.dizziness-and-balance.com/disorders/unilat/vneurit.html*

Ho, A. S., Zanation, A. M., & Ganly, I. (2015). Malignancies of the paranasal sinuses. In P. W. Flint, B. H. Haughey, V. J. Lund, et al. (Eds.), *Cummings otolaryngology head and neck surgery* (6th ed., pp. 1176–1201). Philadelphia, PA: Elsevier.

Katz, A. (2017). Human Papillomavirus-Related Oral Cancers: The Nurse's Role in Mitigating Stigma and Dispelling Myths. *Am J Nurs*, *117*(1):34–39.

Kellman, R. M. (2015). Maxillofacial trauma. In P. W. Flint, B. H. Haughey, V. J. Lund, et al. (Eds.), *Cummings otolaryngology head and neck surgery* (6th ed., pp. 325–350). Philadelphia, PA: Elsevier.

Lewis, A., Kang, R., Levine, A., & Maghami, E. (2015). The new face of head and neck cancer: The HPV epidemic. *Oncology Journal, Head and Neck Cancer*, *29*(9), 616–626. Available: *www.cancernetwork.com/oncology-journal/new-face-head-and-neck-cancer-hpv-epidemic*

Lewis, M. A. O. & Williams, D. W. (2017). Diagnosis and management of oral candidosis. *BDJ*, *223*, 675–681.

McGregor, S. P., Huang, W. W. (2018). Dermatologic Manifestations of Herpes Simplex and Management. https://emedicine.medscape.com/article/1132351-treatment#d7.

National Cancer Institute. (2017). Cancer stat facts: larynx cancer. *Surveillance, epidemiology and end results program*. Bethesda, MD: Author. Available: *https://seer.cancer.gov/statfacts/html/laryn.html*

National Cancer Institute. (2017). Surveillance cancer stat: Oral cavity and pharynx cancer. *Surveillance, epidemiology and end results program (SEER)*. Bethesda, MD: Author. Available: *https://seer.cancer.gov/statfacts/html/oralcav.html*

National Comprehensive Cancer Network. (2017). *NCCN guidelines: Head and neck cancers*. Fort Washington, PA: Author. Available: *www.nccn.org/professionals/physician_gls/pdf/head-and-neck.pdf*

National Comprehensive Cancer Network. (2017). *NCCN Clinical Practice Guidelines in Oncology: Head and Neck Cancers*, Version 2.2017.

Pappas, P., Kauffman, C. A., & Andes, D., et al. (2016). Clinical management guidelines for the management of candidiasis: 2016 update by the Infectious Disease Society of America. *Clinical Infectious Diseases*, *62*, 409–417.

Pichichero, M. E., Sexton, D., & Edwards, M. (2017). Treatment and prevention of streptococcal tonsillopharyngitis. *UpToDate*. New York: Wolters Kluwer. Available: *www.uptodate.com/contents/treatment-and-prevention-of-streptococcal-tonsillopharyngitis*

Popovtzer, A., & Eisbruch, A. (2015). Radiotherapy for head and neck cancer: Radiation physics, radiobiology and clinical principles. In P. W. Flint, B. H. Haughey, V. J. Lund, et al. (Eds.), *Cummings otolaryngology head and neck surgery* (6th ed., pp. 1088–1109). Philadelphia, PA: Elsevier.

Prichard, D., Norton, C., & Bharucha, A. E. (2016). Management of opioid-induced constipation. *British Journal of Nursing*, *25*(10), S4–S11.

Ramakrishnan, V. R., Meyers, A. (2015). *Pharmacology for nonallergic rhinitis. Medscape drugs and diseases*. New York: WebMD. Available: emedicine.medscape.com/article/874171/overview

Rassekh, C. H., & Haughey, B. H. (2015). Total laryngectomy and laryngopharyngectomy. In P. W. Flint, B. H. Haughey, V. J. Lund, et al. (Eds.), *Cummings otolaryngology head and neck surgery* (6th ed., pp. 1699–1713). Philadelphia, PA: Elsevier.

Robbins, K. T., Samant, S., & Ronen, O. (2015). Neck dissection. In P. W. Flint, B. H. Haughey, V. J. Lund, et al. (Eds.), *Cummings otolaryngology head and neck surgery* (6th ed., pp. 1837–1861). Philadelphia, PA: Elsevier.

Rosenfield, R. M., Piccirillo, J. F., Chandrasekhar, S. S., et al. (2015). Clinical practice guideline (Update): Adult sinusitis. *Otolaryngology—Head and Neck Surgery*, *152*(2 suppl), S1–S39.

Rosenfield, R. M., Shin, J. J., Schwartz, S. R., et al. (2016). Clinical practice guideline: Otitis media with effusion. *Otolaryngology—Head and Neck Surgery*, *154* (1 suppl), S1–S41.

Rotter, B. E. (2015). Temporomandibular joint disorders. In P. W. Flint, B. H. Haughey, V. J. Lund, et al. (Eds.), *Cummings otolaryngology head and neck surgery* (6th ed., pp. 1345–1352). Philadelphia, PA: Elsevier.

Schwartz, S. R., Magit, A. E., Rosenfield, R. M., et al. (2017). Clinical Practice guideline (Update): Earwax (Cerumen impaction). *Otolaryngology—Head and Neck Surgery*, *156*(1 suppl), S1–S29.

Schoo, D. P., Tan, G. X., Ehrenburg, M. R., et al. (2017). Intratympanic (IT) therapies for Menière's Disease: Some consensus among the confusion. *Curr Otorhinolaryngol Rep*, *5*(2), 132–141.

Sheikh, J., Kaliner, M. A. (2017). Allergic rhinitis treatment and management. *Medscape Drugs and Diseases*. New York: WebMD. Available: emedicine.medscape.com/article/134825-overview

Sinha, P., & Harreus, U. (2015). Malignant neoplasms of the oropharynx. In P. W. Flint, et al., *Cummings otolaryngology head and neck surgery* (6th ed., pp.1432–1453). Philadelphia, PA: Elsevier.

Stachler, R. H., Francis, D. D., Schwartz, S. R., (2018). Clinical practice guideline (Update): Hoarseness. *Otolaryngology-Head and Neck Surgery*, 158, 8.

Tan, L., & Loh, T. (2015). Benign and malignant tumors of the nasopharynx. In P. W. Flint, B. H. Haughey, V. J. Lund, et al. (Eds.), *Cummings otolaryngology head and neck surgery* (6th ed., pp. 1420–1431). Philadelphia, PA: Elsevier.

Tardy, M. E., Thomas, J. R., & Sclafani, A. P. (2015). Rhinoplasty. In P. W. Flint, B. H. Haughey, V. J. Lund, et al. (Eds.), *Cummings otolaryngology head and neck surgery* (6th ed., pp. 506–542). Philadelphia, PA: Elsevier.

Tewfik, T. L.(2018) Medical Treatment for Guidelines for Adult Sinusitis. https://emedicine.medscape.com/article/861646-guidelines.

Tsai, V., Diamond, H. (2016). Temporomandibular Joint Syndrome. *Medscape drugs and diseases*. New York: WebMD. Available: *http://emedicine.medscape.com/article/809598-treatment*

Turner, M. D. (2015) Oral manifestations of systemic disease. In P. W. Flint, B. H. Haughey, V. J. Lund, et al. (Eds.), *Cummings otolaryngology head and neck surgery* (6th ed., pp. 214–226). Philadelphia, PA: Elsevier.

Waltman, A. A.(2018) Otitis Externa Treatment and Management. https://emedicine.medscape.com/article/994550-treatment.

18
Gastrointestinal Disorders

OVERVIEW AND ASSESSMENT

The gastrointestinal (GI) system is composed of the alimentary canal and its accessory organs. The alimentary canal begins at the mouth and extends through the pharynx, esophagus, stomach, small intestine, colon, and rectum and ends at the anus. The accessory organs include the tongue, salivary glands, liver, gallbladder, and pancreas.

The functions of the GI system include ingestion and propulsion of food; mechanical and chemical digestion of food; synthesis of nutrients, such as vitamin K; absorption of nutrients into the bloodstream; and the storage and elimination of nondigestible waste products from the body through feces.

Subjective Data

A comprehensive health history should be obtained to elicit subjective data related to major manifestations of GI problems. Common manifestations include nutritional problems, abdominal pain, indigestion, nausea, vomiting, diarrhea, constipation, bloody bowel movements, change in bowel habits, weight loss, and dysphagia. See Standards of Care Guidelines 18-1, page 488.

Nutritional Problems

1. Characteristics: What is your typical 24-hour food intake? What is your usual weight? Has there been a recent weight gain or loss? If a recent weight change, how many pounds and over what time period? How is your appetite?
2. Associated factors: Explore other factors that may influence weight changes—food preferences; family/individual routines associated with eating; cultural and religious values; psychological factors, such as depression, anxiety, stress; physical factors, such as activity level, health status, dental problems, allergies; access/transportation to grocery stores; eating habits, self-imposed dietary restrictions; body image; nutritional knowledge; and finances.
3. History: Any history of eating disorders? Any family history of ulcer, GI cancer, inflammatory bowel disease, obesity?

Abdominal Pain

1. Characteristics: Can you describe the pain (sharp, dull, superficial, or deep)? Is the pain intermittent or continuous? Was the onset sudden or gradual? Can you point to where the pain is located? What makes the pain better, worse?

STANDARDS OF CARE GUIDELINES 18-1
Gastrointestinal Dysfunction

When caring for a patient after abdominal surgery or with any type of GI disorder:

- Make sure that adequate bowel sounds are present before allowing anything by mouth. Periodically reassess for bowel sounds, bloating, nausea, vomiting, and abdominal distension or tenderness.
- Monitor food/fluid intake and output as indicated.
- Periodically monitor weight, and watch for trend in weight loss or weight gain.
- Assess stools for frequency, consistency, color, and amount.
- Report increase in pain, fever, nausea, vomiting, bloating, change in stools, or signs of wound infection to health care provider promptly.
- Monitor complete blood count, electrolytes, albumin, and protein as directed.

This information should serve as a general guideline only. Each patient situation presents a unique set of clinical factors and requires nursing judgment to guide care, which may include additional or alternative measures and approaches.

Table 18-1 Nature of Vomitus

COLOR/TASTE/CONSISTENCY	POSSIBLE SOURCE
Yellowish or greenish	• May contain bile • Medication—senna
Bright red (arterial)	• Hemorrhage, peptic ulcer
Dark red (venous)	• Hemorrhage, esophageal or gastric varices
"Coffee grounds"	• Digested blood from slowly bleeding gastric or duodenal ulcer
Undigested food	• Gastric tumor • Ulcer, obstruction • Gastric paresis
"Bitter" taste	• Bile
"Sour" or "acid"	• Gastric contents
Fecal components	• Intestinal obstruction

2. Associated factors: Are there other symptoms associated with the pain—fever, chills, night sweats, nausea, vomiting, diarrhea, constipation, anorexia, weight loss, dyspepsia, black tarry stools or blood in the stool?
3. History: Any family history of GI cancer, ulcer disease, inflammatory bowel disease? Any previous history of tumors, malignancy, ulcers?

Indigestion (Dyspepsia)

1. Characteristics: Have you experienced any of the following symptoms—a feeling of fullness, heartburn, excessive belching, flatus, nausea, a bad taste, mild or severe pain? How is your appetite? If pain or tenderness, where is it located? Does the pain radiate to any other areas? What precipitating factors are associated with the pain? What makes the symptoms better, worse? Are the symptoms associated with food intake? If associated with food, the amount and type?
2. Associated factors: Is there nausea, vomiting, dysphagia, blood in bowel movements, or diarrhea? Is there a history of alcohol, nonsteroidal anti-inflammatory drug (NSAID), bisphosphonate, or aspirin use?
3. History: Any family history of cancer or inflammatory bowel disease? Any history of bowel obstruction? Any previous abdominal surgeries?

Nausea and Vomiting

1. Characteristics: Is the nausea or vomiting associated with certain stimuli, such as specific foods, odors, activity, or a certain time of day? Does it occur before or after food intake? How many times per day does vomiting occur? What specific fluids/foods can be tolerated when vomiting occurs? What is the amount, color, odor, and consistency of the vomitus (see Table 18-1)?

2. Associated factors: Is there fever, headache, dizziness, weakness, or diarrhea? Missed menstrual period? Any weight loss? Any new medications? Any psychological stress, depression, or emotional problems?
3. History: Any history of gallbladder disease? Ulcer disease? GI cancer? Unprotected intercourse?

Diarrhea

1. Characteristics: How long has the diarrhea been present? Determine the frequency, consistency, color, quantity, and odor of stools. Are there blood, mucus, pus, or food particles in the stools? Does this represent a change in bowel habits? Any nocturnal diarrhea? What makes the diarrhea worse, better? Any associated weight loss? (see Box 18-1 on page 489).
2. Associated factors: Any fever, nausea, vomiting, abdominal pain, abdominal distention, flatus, cramping, urgency with straining? Is the patient taking antibiotics? Has there been any recent travel to foreign countries? (Mexico, South America, Africa, and Asia are countries with the highest risk of traveler's diarrhea.) Is the patient experiencing emotional stress or anxiety? Are there any recently prescribed medications?
3. History: Is there a history of celiac disease, colon cancer, ulcerative colitis, Crohn disease, malabsorption syndrome? Has the patient undergone surgery recently (eg, bariatric surgery)?

 DRUG ALERT Obtain history of over-the-counter (OTC), herbal, or "natural" products the patient may be taking. Ginger is commonly used as an antiemetic and, although generally safe, it can cause heartburn. Licorice root is used for upset stomach and to soothe ulcers but can cause sodium and fluid retention and loss of potassium. Goldenseal is used as an antidiarrheal but can cause a number of adverse reactions, including skin and mucous membrane irritation, interference with anticoagulation, and cardiac and nervous system excitability. Also, many herbs can impair absorption of other medicines. Remind patients that herbal products are not found naturally in the body or in significant amounts in the daily diet, so should be treated like drugs.

BOX 18-1 Causes of Diarrhea and Constipation

CAUSES OF DIARRHEA

- Infectious agents (*Escherichia coli*, *Salmonella*, *Shigella*, *Campylobacter*, *Giardia*, *Amoeba*, *Clostridium difficile*, *Yersinia*, *Cyclospora*, *Cryptosporidium*, *Rotavirus*).
- Drugs (antibiotics, magnesium).
- Fecal impaction.
- Bowel disease (irritable bowel syndrome [IBS], ulcerative colitis, Crohn disease).
- Malabsorption syndromes (lactose intolerance, celiac sprue, fat malabsorption).
- Short bowel syndrome.
- Malignant syndromes (Zollinger-Ellison syndrome, carcinoid syndrome).

CAUSES OF CONSTIPATION

- Inadequate fluid intake.
- Psychological factors.
- Electrolyte imbalances.
- Hormonal abnormalities, such as hypothyroidism.
- Mechanical bowel obstruction, such as ileus.
- Drugs (laxative abuse, anticholinergic agents, calcium channel blockers, opiates).
- Loss of innervation (Hirschsprung disease).
- Neuromuscular (paralysis, spinal cord injury or sacral lesion, multiple sclerosis).
- Anorectal disorders (hemorrhoids, fecal impaction, cancer, abscess, fissures).
- Sedentary lifestyle.

Constipation

1. Characteristics: What is the frequency, consistency, color of the stools? Is there a change in bowel habits? If a change, has this been gradual or sudden? What is the size of the stools? Have there been dietary changes? Is there blood or mucus in the stools? Any laxative use?
2. Associated factors: Are there periods of diarrhea? Is there abdominal pain or distention? Is the patient experiencing stress? Is there a change in activity level? Does the patient have a regular time for defecation? Does the patient use antacids containing calcium or an anticholinergic? Have there been any fevers, chills, night sweats, or weight loss?
3. History: Any family history of colorectal cancer? Any history of depression or metabolic disorders, such as hypothyroidism or hypercalcemia?

Dysphagia

1. Characteristics: Is the onset acute or gradual? Is the problem with swallowing intermittent or continuous? Is this associated with solid foods, liquids, or both? Has there been any nasal regurgitation? Where does the food stick: neck (cricopharyngeal), midesophagus, or sternal xiphoid process?
2. Associated factors: Is there any regurgitation, heartburn, chest or back pain, weight loss? Any hoarseness, voice change, or sore throat? Have there been any fevers, chills, night sweats, or weight loss?
3. History: Is there a family history of esophageal cancer? Is there a history of stroke, palsy, or any other neurologic conditions? Is there a history of alcohol or tobacco intake?

Physical Examination

When performing a physical examination of the abdomen, include the following: inspection of the abdomen, auscultation of all four abdominal quadrants, percussion for tympany or dullness, light and deep palpation.

 NURSING ALERT Auscultation should be performed before percussion and palpation, which may stimulate bowel sounds. Deep palpation in noted areas of tenderness or pain should be performed last.

Key Findings

1. Tenting of the skin when the skin is rolled between the thumb and index finger. Tenting may indicate dehydration.
2. Mouth lesions, missing teeth, and swollen or bleeding gums may contribute to weight loss and nutritional deficiencies.
3. Body weight may indicate obesity or such problems as anorexia nervosa or malignancy.
4. Palpable mass may indicate an enlarged organ, inflammation, malignancy, hernia.
5. Rebound tenderness, guarding, and rigidity may indicate appendicitis, cholecystitis, peritonitis, pancreatitis, duodenal ulcer.
6. Protuberant or bulging abdomen or flanks can indicate ascites. Two physical assessment skills that may help to confirm the presence of ascites are testing for shifting dullness and testing for a fluid wave.
7. Distention and absence of bowel sounds may indicate intestinal obstruction.

Characteristics of Stool

1. The appearance of blood in the stool may be characteristic of its source.
   a. Upper GI bleeding—tarry black (melena).
   b. Lower GI bleeding—bright red blood.
   c. Lower rectal or anal bleeding—blood streaking on the surface of stool or on toilet paper.
2. Other characteristics of stool may indicate a particular GI problem.
   a. Bulky, greasy, foamy, foul smelling, gray with silvery sheen—steatorrhea (fatty stool).
   b. Light gray "clay-colored" (because of the absence of bile pigments, acholic)—biliary obstruction.
   c. Mucus or pus visible—chronic ulcerative colitis, shigellosis.
   d. Small, dry, rocky-hard masses—constipation, obstruction.
   e. Marble-size stool pellets—IBS.

Laboratory Tests

Laboratory tests for GI disorders include a variety of stool studies and blood tests.

 EVIDENCE BASE Rex, D., Boland, C., Dominitz, J., et al. (2017). Colorectal cancer screening: Recommendations for physicians and patients from the U.S. Multi- Society Task Force on Colorectal Cancer. *The American Journal of Gastroenterology*, 112, 1016–1030.

Fecal Immunochemical Test (FIT) for Occult Blood Detection

Description

An immunochemical test card has antibodies that detect human hemoglobin in stool. This test is used to screen for colon cancer when colonoscopy is not an option. FIT is preferred over the stool guaiac tests because of higher sensitivity and ease of use (eg, no dietary restrictions).

Nursing and Patient Care Considerations

1. Advise patient not to collect specimen during menstruation or if hemorrhoidal bleeding is present. Usually, at least two stool specimens need to be collected, on separate occasions.
2. Collect specimen or advise patient regarding proper collection of specimen.
   a. Check expiration date of collection kit.
   b. Sit on toilet and proceed with bowel movement so that stool will be on top of collection paper. Do not put toilet paper in specimen.
   c. Use the sample probe and brush across the stool sample so that the groove of probe is filled with stool (obtain sample from several different locations within the stool).
   d. Insert probe back into the sample container and tighten the lid of the container, or place stool on the card depending on the type of collection kit being used.
   e. Write the date on sample container label.
3. Follow manufacturer instructions for processing.

Stool Guaiac Tests for Occult Blood

Description

Commercially available guaiac-impregnated slides or wipes test feces for blood. May be used as another option for colon cancer screening.

Nursing and Patient Care Considerations

1. Advise patient about the test preparation procedure. Common practices are listed below. For 3 days before the test and during the stool collection period:
   a. Diet should have a high-fiber content.
   b. Avoid red meat in the diet.
   c. Avoid foods with a high peroxidase content, such as turnips, cauliflower, broccoli, horseradish, and melon.
   d. Avoid iron preparations, iodides, bromides, aspirin, NSAIDs, or vitamin C supplements greater than 250 mg/day.
   e. Avoid enemas or laxatives before stool specimen collection.
2. Collect sample or advise patient on collection procedure.
   a. A wooden applicator is used to apply a stool specimen to the slide or a special wipe is used and placed in the packet.
   b. Avoid urine or toilet tissue contamination.
3. When hydrogen peroxide (denatured alcohol–stabilizing mixture) is added to samples, any blood cells present liberate their hemoglobin, and a bluish ring appears on the electrophoretic paper. Read precisely at 30 seconds.
4. Three stool samples are taken because of the possibility of intermittent bleeding and false-negative results.
   a. A single positive test is an indication for further diagnostic evaluation for GI lesions.
   b. False-positive results occur in about 10% of tests.
   c. Test may become false negative in 10% of specimens tested 4 or more days after streaking on paper.

Stool DNA Test

Description

This test detects DNA associated with colon cancer. Cells are shed from the tumor into the intestinal lumen as stool passes through. The procedure is similar to guaiac tests. The specificity of this type of testing is inferior to the FIT and colonoscopy so is not used as commonly.

Other Common Stool Studies

Description

There are multiple types of stool analyses that are helpful in detecting conditions affecting the GI tract, liver, and pancreas. Basic stool examination is for amount, consistency, and color. Normal color varies from light to dark brown, but various foods and medications may affect stool color. Additional testing may include tests for ova and parasites; stool cultures that can identify viruses and bacteria; fecal leukocytes; fecal fat, which can help in the diagnosis of malabsorption syndromes; and stool for *Helicobacter pylori*, which is performed at least 4 weeks after treatment to confirm eradication.

Nursing and Patient Care Considerations

1. Use a tongue blade to place a small amount of fresh stool in a container. The container may be sterile or may have a preservative depending on which test has been ordered. Remind patient not to mix urine or toilet paper in the specimen.
2. Save a sample of fecal material if unusual in appearance, contains worms or blood, blood streaked, unusual in color, or has excess mucus; show to health care provider.
3. For accurate specimen results, the vials must be sent to the laboratory as soon as possible. Certain stool studies allow for refrigeration of the sample, but this is test dependent.
4. Send specimens to be examined for parasites to the laboratory immediately, so the parasites may be observed under a microscope while viable, fresh, and warm.
5. Consider that barium, bismuth, mineral oil, and antibiotics may alter the results.

Hydrogen Breath Test

Description

1. The hydrogen breath test is used to evaluate carbohydrate malabsorption and maldigestion, to detect the presence of excess bacteria in the small intestine, and to estimate small bowel transit time.
2. A substance, such as lactulose, lactose, or another carbohydrate, is ingested and, after a certain time period, exhaled gases are measured.
3. The test measures the amount of hydrogen, methane, and carbon dioxide produced in the colon, absorbed in the blood, and then exhaled in the breath. The levels of hydrogen and methane are indicators of bacterial metabolism in the small intestine.
4. This test is diagnostic for lactose intolerance, other carbohydrate malabsorption syndromes, and small intestine bacterial overgrowth (SIBO).

Nursing and Patient Care Considerations

1. Patient should have nothing by mouth (NPO) for 12 hours before the procedure.
2. Patient should not smoke after midnight before the test.
3. Antibiotics should not be used for 4 weeks, and laxatives/enemas should not be used for 1 week before the test. These products may alter the laboratory results.
4. Appropriate diet instructions should be given before discharge if the test is positive.

Helicobacter pylori Testing

Description

1. Diagnostic tests for *H. pylori* include a serum antibody test, urea breath test, and fecal antigen test. Alternatively, if an endoscopy is being performed, then biopsies of the gastric mucosa can be evaluated for *H. pylori* with rapid urea testing; histology review by a pathologist, or culture; or polymerase chain reaction testing.
2. A positive serum antibody test may not differentiate between current and past disease.

3. The urea breath test and fecal antigen test are useful in detecting active *H. pylori* prior to treatment with antibiotics. Both of these tests can be used to confirm eradication after antibiotic therapy has been completed.

Nursing and Patient Care Considerations

1. Symptomatic patients and patients with an active or past history of ulcer disease or with gastric MALT lymphoma should be tested for *H. pylori*. Endoscopy may be necessary for patients with symptoms of weight loss, anemia, or occult blood loss and for patients older than 50.
2. It is recommended that negative *H. pylori* test results in a patient with ulcer-related complications be confirmed by a second test.
3. Describe the procedure for urea breath testing to the patient.
    a. Antibiotics, proton pump inhibitors, and bismuth preparations must be held for 2 weeks prior to testing.
    b. Foods and fluids should be held for at least 1 hour prior to testing.
    c. A baseline breath sample will be taken by having the patient breathe into a container, then patient will ingest a carbon-labeled urea substance, and a final breath sample will be taken shortly after ingestion.
    d. The whole process takes about 40 minutes.
4. When confirming eradication of *H. pylori*, testing should not be done earlier than 4 weeks posttreatment.
5. False-positive results from *H. pylori* breath testing may be caused by achlorhydria or urease production associated with other GI disorders.

 EVIDENCE BASE Chey, W. D., Leontiadis, G. I., Howden, C. W., et al. (2017). Treatment of H. pylori infection. *American Journal of Gastroenterology*, *112*, 212–238.

Radiology and Imaging Studies

Upper GI Series and Small Bowel Series

Description

1. Upper GI series and small bowel series are fluoroscopic x-ray examinations of the esophagus, stomach, and small intestine after the patient ingests barium sulfate.
2. As the barium passes through the GI tract, fluoroscopy outlines the GI mucosa and organs.
3. Spot films record significant findings.
4. Double-contrast studies administer barium first, followed by a radiolucent substance, such as air, to produce a thin layer of barium to coat the mucosa. This allows for better visualization of any type of lesion.

Nursing and Patient Care Considerations

1. Explain the procedure to patient.
2. Instruct patient to maintain low-residue diet for 2 to 3 days before test and a clear liquid dinner the night before the procedure.
3. Emphasize NPO after midnight before the test.
4. Encourage patient to avoid smoking before the test.
5. Explain that the health care provider may prescribe all opioids and anticholinergics to be withheld 24 hours before the test because they interfere with small intestine motility. Other medications may be taken with sips of water, if ordered.

6. Explain that the patient will be instructed at various times throughout the procedure to drink the barium (480 to 600 mL).
7. Explain that a cathartic will be prescribed after the procedure to facilitate expulsion of barium.
8. Instruct patient that stool will be light in color for the next 2 to 3 days from the barium.
9. Instruct patient to notify health care provider if he has not passed the barium in 2 to 3 days because retention of the barium may cause obstruction or fecal impaction.
10. Note that a water-soluble iodinated contrast agent (eg, Gastrografin) may be used for a patient with a suspected perforation or colonic obstruction. Barium is toxic to the body if it leaks into the peritoneum with perforation. It can also worsen an obstruction; thus, it is not used if an obstruction is suspected.

Barium Enema

Description

1. Fluoroscopic x-ray examination visualizing the entire large intestine is administered after the patient is given an enema of barium sulfate.
2. Can visualize structural changes, such as tumors, polyps, diverticula, fistulas, obstructions, and ulcerative colitis.
3. Air may be introduced after the barium to provide a double-contrast study.

Nursing and Patient Care Considerations

1. Explain to patient:
    a. What the x-ray procedure involves.
    b. That proper preparation provides a more accurate view of the tract and that preparations may vary.
    c. That it is important to retain the barium so all surfaces of the tract are coated with opaque solution.
2. Instruct patient on the objective of having the large intestine as clear of fecal material as possible:
    a. Patient may be given a low-fiber, low-fat diet 1 to 3 days before the examination.
    b. The day before the examination, intake may be limited to clear liquids (no drinks with red dye).
    c. The day before the examination, an oral laxative, suppository, and/or cleansing enema may be prescribed.
3. Patient will be NPO after midnight the day of the procedure.
4. An enema or cathartic may be ordered after the barium enema to cleanse bowel of barium and prevent impaction.
5. Inform patient that barium may cause light-colored stools for several days after the procedure.

 NURSING ALERT If barium enema and upper GI series are both ordered, the upper GI series is done last so that barium traveling down the digestive tract does not interfere with the results of the barium enema.

Ultrasonography (Ultrasound)

Description

1. A noninvasive test that focuses high-frequency sound waves over an abdominal organ to obtain an image of the structure.
2. Ultrasound can detect small abdominal masses, fluid-filled cysts, gallstones, dilated bile ducts, ascites, and vascular abnormalities.
3. Doppler ultrasonography may be ordered for vascular assessment.

Nursing and Patient Care Considerations

1. An ultrasound should be done prior to barium studies or at least 24 hours after barium administration because it may interfere with the images.
2. Abdominal ultrasound usually requires patient to be NPO for at least 6 hours before the procedure.
3. Change position of patient, as indicated, for better visualization of certain organs.

Computed Tomography

Description

1. Computed tomography (CT) is an x-ray technique that provides excellent anatomic definition and is used to detect tumors, cysts, and abscesses.
2. The CT scan can also reveal masses, dilated bile ducts, pancreatic inflammation, and some gallstones.
3. It identifies changes in intestinal wall thickness and mesenteric abnormalities.
4. Ultrasound and CT can be used to perform guided needle aspiration of fluid or cells from lesions anywhere in the abdomen. The fluid or cells are then sent for laboratory tests (eg, cytology or culture).

Nursing and Patient Care Considerations

1. Instruct patient to fast for 4 hours before the procedure. Patient can take usual medications with a sip of water, but should hold diabetic medications.
2. A pregnancy test should be obtained on females of childbearing potential. If pregnant, do not proceed with scan and notify health care provider.
3. Ask if there are known allergies to iodine or contrast media. Intravenous (IV) administration of contrast medium may be performed to provide better visualization of body parts. If allergic, notify the technician and health care provider immediately.
4. Instruct patient to report symptoms of itching or shortness of breath if receiving contrast media, and observe patient closely.

Endoscopic Procedures

 EVIDENCE BASE Society of Gastroenterology Nurses and Associates, Inc. (2014). *Standards of clinical nursing practice and role delineations.* Chicago, IL: Author. Available: www.sgna.org/Portals/0/Education/PDF/Standards-Guidelines/SGNA_StandardsofClinicalNursingPractice_2014_Final.pdf.

Endoscopy is the use of a flexible tube (the fiberoptic endoscope) to visualize the GI tract and to perform certain diagnostic and therapeutic procedures. Images are produced through a video screen or telescopic eyepiece. The tip of the endoscope moves in four directions, allowing for wide-angle visualization. The endoscope can be inserted through the rectum or mouth, depending on which portion of the GI tract is to be viewed. Capsule endoscopy utilizes an ingestible camera device rather than an endoscope.

Endoscopes contain multipurpose channels that allow for air insufflation, irrigation, fluid aspiration, and the passage of special instruments. These instruments include biopsy forceps, cytology brushes, needles, wire baskets, laser probes, and electrocautery snares.

Endoscopic functions other than visualization include biopsy or cytology of lesions, removal of foreign objects or polyps, control of internal bleeding, and opening of strictures.

Capsule Endoscopy

Description

1. Adjunctive diagnostic tool used to detect abnormalities of the small bowel (angiodysplasias, areas of active bleeding, polyps, ulcerations, tumors or causes of diarrhea, and nutritional malabsorption).
2. The procedure involves swallowing a capsule (camera device), which passes through the digestive system while taking pictures of the intestine.
3. Images are transmitted to sensor array abdominal leads, which are attached to a Walkman-like recording device belted to the patient's waist.
4. After approximately 8 hours, the recording device is removed and is connected to a computer to download the images for review. The capsule will be excreted naturally through the digestive tract.

 NURSING ALERT Capsule endoscopy is contraindicated for patients with small bowel obstruction, dysphagia, fistulas, severe delayed gastric emptying, gastrectomy with gastrojejunostomy, or GI stricture. There is a risk of trapping the capsule, delayed passage, or impaired peristalsis. Pacemakers or implanted defibrillators may alter the quality and quantity of study information.

Nursing and Patient Care Considerations

1. Give patient instructions on bowel prep. Inform patient that a good bowel prep allows for better pictures. Patient will be NPO for about 12 hours before swallowing the camera.
2. Oral medications are discontinued 2 hours before the study. Antispasmodics, bismuth preparations, and antidiarrheal medications should be held for 24 hours before the study. Iron preparations and Carafate should be held 5 days before the study to prevent mucosal staining.
3. Instruct patient not to smoke 24 hours before the procedure to prevent mucosal staining.
4. Instruct patient to avoid strenuous activity, heavy lifting, bending or stooping, or immersion in water while wearing the leads and recorder. This is to prevent detachment of the leads or damage of the recorder.
5. After ingesting the capsule, patient is instructed not to eat or drink for at least 2 hours and then can advance to clear liquids. After 4 hours, patient can have a light snack and medications. When the procedure is completed, patient can resume a normal diet.
6. During the capsule endoscopy procedure, instruct the patient to check the blinking light on the top of the data recorder every 15 minutes. Avoid radio equipment (ham radio or broadcasting towers), which may interfere with the capsule's signal.
7. The capsule is naturally excreted within 1 to 3 days. Patient should be instructed to call the physician for the following symptoms: abdominal bloating or pain, chest pain, vomiting, or fever. These symptoms may indicate that the capsule has obstructed the GI tract.

 NURSING ALERT The patient should verify excretion of the capsule before undergoing MRI.

Esophagogastroduodenoscopy

Description

1. Allows for visualization of the esophagus, stomach, and duodenum.
2. Esophagogastroduodenoscopy (EGD) can be used to diagnose acute or chronic upper GI bleeding, esophageal or gastric varices, polyps, malignancy, ulcers, gastritis, esophagitis, esophageal stenosis, and gastroesophageal reflux.
3. Instruments passed through the scope can be used to perform a biopsy or cytologic study, remove polyps or foreign bodies, control bleeding, or open strictures.

Nursing and Patient Care Considerations

1. Ensure that patient is NPO for 6 to 12 hours before the procedure to prevent aspiration and allow for complete visualization of the stomach.
2. Remove dentures and partial plates to facilitate passing the scope and preventing injury.
3. As an outpatient, advise that someone must accompany the patient to drive home because of the patient being sedated.
4. Inform the health care provider of any known allergies and current medications. Medications may be held until after the test is completed.
5. Obtain prior x-rays, and send with patient.
6. Describe what will occur during and after the procedure:
   a. The throat will be anesthetized with a spray or gargle.
   b. An IV sedative will be administered.
   c. Patient will be positioned on the left side with a towel or basin at the mouth to catch secretions.
   d. A plastic mouthpiece will be used to help relax the jaw and protect the endoscope. Emphasize that this will not interfere with breathing.
   e. Patient may be asked to swallow once while the endoscope is being advanced. Then, the patient should not swallow, talk, or move the tongue. Secretions should drain from the side of the mouth, and the mouth may be suctioned.
   f. Air is inserted during the procedure to permit better visualization of the GI tract. Most of the air is removed at the end of the procedure. Patient may feel bloated, burp, or pass flatus from remaining air.
   g. Keep patient NPO according to protocol until patient is alert and gag reflex has returned.
   h. May resume regular diet after gag reflex returns and fluids are tolerated.
   i. May experience a sore throat for 24 to 36 hours after the procedure. When the gag reflex has returned, throat lozenges or warm saline gargles may be prescribed for comfort.
7. Monitor vital signs every 30 minutes for 3 to 4 hours, and keep the side rails up until patient is fully alert.
8. Monitor patient for abdominal or chest pain, cervical pain, dyspnea, fever, hematemesis, melena, dysphagia, light-headedness, or a firm distended abdomen. These may indicate complications.
9. Instruct patient on the above listed signs and symptoms and advise to report immediately should any occur, even after discharge.
10. Possible complications include perforation of the esophagus or stomach, pulmonary aspiration, hemorrhage, respiratory depression or arrest, infection, cardiac arrhythmias or arrest.

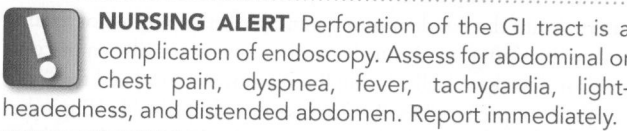 **NURSING ALERT** Perforation of the GI tract is a complication of endoscopy. Assess for abdominal or chest pain, dyspnea, fever, tachycardia, light-headedness, and distended abdomen. Report immediately.

Flexible Sigmoidoscopy and Colonoscopy

1. Sigmoidoscopy is the visualization of the anal canal, rectum, sigmoid colon, and proximal colon through a fiberoptic sigmoidoscope.
2. Colonoscopy is the visualization of the entire large intestine, sigmoid colon, rectum, and anal canal. It is used as a screening test for colon cancer because it can be used to identify and remove potentially precancerous and cancerous polyps.
3. Sigmoidoscopy or colonoscopy can be used to diagnose malignancy, polyps, inflammation, or strictures.
4. Colonoscopy is used for surveillance in patients with a history of chronic ulcerative colitis, previous colon cancer, or colon polyps.
5. Lower GI endoscopy can be used to perform biopsy, remove foreign objects, or obtain diagnostic specimens.
6. Colonoscopy requires bowel preparation for a couple of days before the procedure and use of conscious sedation during the procedure. The bowel preparation usually includes approximately 1 gallon of an iso-osmolar electrolyte solution (Colyte, GoLYTELY, or NuLYTELY) to consume over a 3- to 4-hour period the day before the procedure, a clear liquid diet the day before, and an oral laxative the night before (protocols vary). Alternate prep may also be used.
7. CT colonography, also known as virtual colonoscopy, is evolving as a noninvasive screening method.

 DRUG ALERT Sodium phosphate preps should be avoided in people with congestive heart failure, renal impairment, and in others that may be more sensitive to electrolyte imbalances.

Endoscopic Ultrasound

Description

1. This procedure is a combination of endoscopy and ultrasonography to visualize the GI tract and can be used to evaluate the upper GI tract or the lower GI tract.
2. An ultrasonic transducer is built into the distal end of the endoscope.
3. This procedure allows for high-quality resolution and imaging of the walls of the esophagus, stomach, duodenum, small intestines, and colon. Adjacent abdominal structures can also be studied.
4. Endoscopic ultrasound (EUS) is also indicated to evaluate and stage lesions of the GI tract.

Nursing and Patient Care Considerations

1. Verify patient's compliance with the pretest bowel preparation the day before the procedure, usually an oral laxative (such as magnesium citrate) and a clear liquid diet.
2. Patient must be NPO after midnight.
3. Explain to patient that a feeling of fullness will occur when water is introduced into the GI tract. This eliminates airspace and provides for high resolution.
4. If an upper EUS is performed, maintain the NPO status until the gag reflex returns. A lower EUS can be performed using a rectal approach.
5. Observe patient for a change in vital signs, bleeding, pain, vomiting, and abdominal distention or rigidity.
6. Make sure that patients who have had endoscopic procedures requiring sedation have a caregiver to drive them home after the procedure.

GENERAL PROCEDURES AND TREATMENT MODALITIES

 See additional online content: Procedure Guidelines 18-1–18-5

Relieving Constipation and Fecal Impaction

One method of evacuating the lower bowel is an enema, the installation of a solution into the rectum and sigmoid colon. If fecal impaction is discovered on exam, manual disimpaction may be performed to remove stool and promote bowel elimination (see Figure 18-1). However, it is best to try to prevent constipation by using fiber, laxatives, or stool softeners so that enemas and manual disimpaction are not needed.

Purposes of Enema Administration

1. Bowel preparation for diagnostic tests or surgery to empty the bowel of fecal content.
2. Delivery of medication into the colon (such as enemas containing steroids to treat ulcerative proctitis or a sodium polystyrene sulfonate enema to decrease the serum potassium level).
3. To soften the stool (oil-retention enemas).
4. To relieve gas (tidal, milk and molasses, or Fleet enemas).
5. To promote defecation and evacuate feces from the colon for patients with constipation or an impaction (not a first-line therapy).

Figure 18-1. Fecal impaction. **(A)** Note shaded area inside rectal sphincter, which indicates fecal impaction. **(B)** By gently stimulating the rectal wall with a gloved index finger and using a circular motion, it is possible to loosen fecal material. **(C)** It may be necessary to gently insert two fingers in an attempt to crush the fecal mass. A scissor-like motion is used.

Nursing and Patient Care Considerations

1. Consider manual removal of fecal impaction in the following patients at risk:
   a. Older adults with chronic constipation or insufficient hydration or who are inactive.
   b. Orthopedic patients who have been in traction or in body casts.
   c. When barium has not been adequately removed after radiologic examination.
   d. Patients with neurologic or psychotic disorders.
2. Fecal impaction can occur with a descending/sigmoid colostomy. The fingers may be used to break up feces through the stoma, followed by cleansing irrigation.
3. Contraindications of manual removal of fecal impaction include:
   a. Pregnancy.
   b. After genitourinary, rectal, perineal, abdominal, or gynecologic surgery.
   c. Myocardial infarction, coronary insufficiency, pulmonary embolus, heart failure, heart block.
   d. GI or vaginal bleeding.
   e. Blood dyscrasias, bleeding disorders.
   f. Hemorrhoids, fissures, and rectal polyps.
4. Prepare for enema administration by helping the patient to lying position on left side with knees bent. Lubricate 3 to 4 inches (7.5 to 10 cm) of the tip of enema tubing with water-soluble lubricant, even if prelubricated.
5. Insert enema tip 3 to 4 inches into the rectum and instill slowly, to avoid cramping and rectal spasm. When completely instilled, ask the patient to hold the enema solution as long as possible, before gently withdrawing the tubing.
6. Ensure that patient can safely transfer to bathroom, commode, or bed pan when the overwhelming urge to defecate is felt.

 NURSING ALERT Be aware that manual removal of fecal impaction may cause syncope because of stimulation of the vagus nerve.

Nasogastric and Nasointestinal Intubation

 EVIDENCE BASE Emergency Nurses Association. (2015). *Clinical practice guideline: Gastric tube placement verification.* Des Plaines, IL: Author. Available: *www.ena.org/practice-research/research/CPG/Documents/GastricTubeCPG.pdf.*

Nasogastric (NG) intubation refers to the insertion of a tube through the nasopharynx into the stomach. NG intubation has multiple purposes including stomach decompression, stomach lavage (irrigation because of active bleeding or poisoning), medication administration, and short-term feeding. Extended-use NG tubes are made of a flexible, soft plastic material with manufacturer's recommendations that may include leaving the tube in place for up to 30 days before changing the tube.

Nasointestinal (NI) intubation is performed by a health care provider and may be assisted by a nurse. A small-bore tube is inserted into the duodenum or jejunum for the purpose of feeding and maintaining nutrition. It can be done manually, endoscopically, or fluoroscopically. Using fluoroscopy is considered the "gold standard" or preferred method of insertion. Intestinal feeding tubes are soft, flexible, small-diameter (8 or 12 French) tubes with a longer length than gastric feeding tubes (measuring up to 47 inches [120 cm] as compared with approximately 30 inches [76 cm] for a gastric feeding tube). Some tubes are weighted at the distal end of the tube, so they will be carried by peristalsis. All tubes should be routinely pretested for patency and function before passage.

Nursing and Patient Care Considerations

1. Before inserting the tube, ensure unobstructed nasal passage, then approximate the distance to the stomach by measuring from the tip of the patient's nose to the earlobe and down to the xiphoid process, and then mark this point on the tube with tape (see Figure 18-2). Lubricate the first 2 to 3 inches of the tube with water-soluble lubricant.
2. With the patient's head in neutral position, insert the tube into the nostril and slowly direct the tube backward and downward. The patient may gag as the tube passes the pharynx, allow the patient to rest, tilt the head slightly forward, and take a sip of water. Turn the tube 180 degrees and continue to advance the tube slowly to predetermined mark.
3. If patient is unconscious, advance the tube between respirations to make sure it does not enter the trachea.
   a. You will need to stroke the unconscious patient's neck to facilitate passage of the tube down the esophagus.
   b. Watch for cyanosis while passing the tube in an unconscious patient. Cyanosis indicates the tube has entered the trachea.
4. If patient has a nasal condition that prevents insertion through the nose, the tube is passed through the mouth.
   a. Remove dentures, slide the distal end of the tube over the tongue, and proceed the same way as a nasal intubation.
   b. Make sure to coil the end of the tube and direct it downward at the pharynx.
5. Be aware that pain or vomiting after the tube is inserted indicates tube obstruction or incorrect placement; may need to be pulled back or removed.
6. If the NG tube is not draining, reposition tube by advancing or withdrawing it slightly (with a physician's order). After repositioning, always check for placement.
7. Recognize the complications when the tube is in for prolonged periods: nasal erosion, sinusitis, esophagitis, esophagotracheal fistula, gastric ulceration, and pulmonary and oral infections.
8. Assess the color, consistency, and odor of gastric contents. Coffee ground–like contents may indicate GI bleeding. Report findings immediately.
9. The tube should be irrigated before and after medication administration through the tube.

Figure 18-2. Measuring NG tube length.

   a. Medications should be given in liquid form, if possible.
   b. Clamp the tube for 30 to 45 minutes to ensure medication absorption before reconnecting to suction, if ordered.
10. Check GI function by auscultating for bowel sounds on a regular basis after the tube has been clamped for 30 minutes.
11. When discontinuing an NG tube, remove all tape and have the patient take a deep breath, hold it, and pull steady and slowly (covering it with a towel as it emerges) and then more quickly when it reaches the pharynx.

Caring for the Patient Undergoing Gastrointestinal Surgery

Types of Procedures

Gastric Surgeries

1. Total gastrectomy—complete excision of the stomach with esophageal–jejunal anastomosis.
2. Subtotal or partial gastrectomy—a portion of the stomach excised:
   a. Billroth I procedure—gastric remnant anastomosed to the duodenum.
   b. Billroth II procedure—gastric remnant anastomosed to the jejunum.
3. Gastrostomy (Janeway or Spivak)—rectangular stomach flap created into abdominal stoma, used for intermittent tube feedings.

Hernia Surgeries

1. Herniorrhaphy—surgical repair of a hernia with suturing of the abdominal wall.
2. Hernioplasty—reconstructive hernia repair with mesh sewn over the defect for reinforcement.

Bowel Surgeries

1. Appendectomy—excision of the vermiform appendix.
2. Bowel resection—segmental excision of small and/or large bowels with varied approaches:
   a. Anastomosis of proximal and distal ends of the bowel.
   b. Anastomosis of proximal and distal ends of the bowel with temporary diverting loop ostomy.
   c. Both ends of bowel exteriorized to the abdominal wall with proximal ostomy and distal mucous fistula.
   d. Hartmann procedure—proximal large bowel as ostomy; distal end of large bowel oversewn inside abdomen as Hartmann pouch.
3. Low anterior resection—subtotal resection of the rectum with colorectal or coloanal anastomosis.
4. Abdominoperineal resection—a combined abdominal and perineal approach for removal of the rectum and anus with permanent colostomy.
5. Subtotal colectomy—partial removal of the large bowel or colon.
6. Total colectomy—complete removal of the large bowel or colon with varied approaches:
   a. Ileorectal anastomosis—colon removal with the ileum anastomosed to the rectum.
   b. Proctocolectomy—colon removal including the rectum and anus with permanent ileostomy.
   c. Ileal reservoir—anal anastomosis. (Colon removal, subtotal proctectomy, possible distal rectal mucosectomy, creation of pelvic reservoir from two, three, or four loops of the ileum with anastomosis at anal canal. Usually, a temporary

loop ileostomy is performed as fecal diversion to protect the reservoir and the ileal–anal anastomosis. After take-down of temporary loop ileostomy [2 to 3 months postoperatively], the reservoir stores feces and patient eliminates under voluntary control through the anus [see page 525].)

   d. Kock or Barnett continent internal reservoir (BCIR) procedures—proctocolectomy, creation of a continent small bowel reservoir with nipple valve abdominal stoma used for stool removal through routine intubation. (Continence is provided through the nipple valve.)

7. Roux-en-Y jejunostomy—the jejunum severed with distal end exteriorized as permanent stoma for intermittent tube feedings; proximal end reanastomosed to GI tract distal to stoma to reestablish pathway.

Laparoscopic Surgery

1. GI surgical procedures are increasingly being assisted by the use of a laparoscope, either partially or totally. The laparoscope is usually inserted through a 1-cm umbilical incision with additional trocars used for visualization and assistance. Dissection is performed with endocautery, scissors, or laser.

2. Advantages may include reduction in postoperative pain, shorter hospital and recuperative periods, decreased risk of infection, and improved cosmetic outcome. The direct cost of a laparoscopic procedure may be greater than an open procedure; however, the overall cost of the procedure and recuperative period may be lower due to a more rapid recovery.

3. Contraindications may include obesity, internal adhesions, and bowel obstruction with distention.

4. Cholecystectomies and appendectomies are routinely done through laparoscopy; hernia repairs can be done using the laparoscope. Other GI surgeries, including ostomies and bowel resections (may include select cancer patients), are increasingly being done through this surgical approach.

Preoperative Management

1. All diagnostic tests and procedures are explained to promote cooperation and relaxation.

2. The patient is prepared for the type of surgical procedure as well as postoperative care (IV, patient-controlled analgesia pump, NG tube, surgical drains, incision care, possibility of ostomy).

3. Measures to prevent postoperative complications are taught, including coughing, turning, and deep breathing; using the incentive spirometer; and splinting the incision.

4. IV fluids or total parenteral nutrition (TPN) before surgery may be ordered to improve fluid and electrolyte balance and nutritional status.

5. Intake and output is monitored.

6. Preoperative laboratory studies are obtained.

7. Bowel cleansing will be initiated 1 to 2 days before surgery for better visualization. Preparation may include diet modifications, such as liquid or low residue, oral laxatives, suppositories, enemas, or polyethylene glycoelectrolyte solution (Colyte, GoLYTELY).

8. Antibiotics are ordered to decrease the bacterial growth in the colon.

9. An ostomy specialty nurse is consulted if patient is scheduled for an ostomy to initiate early understanding and management of postoperative care.

10. Patient may not have anything by mouth after midnight the night before surgery. Medications may be withheld, if ordered. This will keep the GI tract clear.

Postoperative Management and Nursing Care

1. Physical assessment is completed at least once per shift, or more frequently, as indicated.
   a. Monitor vital signs for signs of infection and shock—fever, hypotension, tachycardia.
   b. Monitor intake and output for signs of imbalance, dehydration, and shock. Include all drains in evaluating intake and output.
   c. Assess the abdomen for increased pain, distention, rigidity, and rebound tenderness because these may indicate postoperative complications. Report abnormal findings.
   d. Expect diminished or absent bowel sounds in the immediate postoperative phase.
   e. Evaluate dressing and incision. Check for purulent or bloody drainage, odor, and unusual tenderness or redness at incision site, which may indicate bleeding or infection.
   f. Evaluate for passing of flatus or feces.
   g. Monitor for nausea and vomiting. Note the presence of fecal smell or material in vomitus because it may indicate an obstruction.
   h. Check NG aspirate, vomitus, and stools for signs of bleeding. Record and report findings if present.

2. Laboratory values are monitored and patient is evaluated for signs and symptoms of electrolyte imbalance.

3. Wound drains, IV lines, and all other catheters are monitored and evaluated for signs of infection or infiltration.

4. To maintain patency of NG tube, the tube may be irrigated with 30 mL of normal saline solution every 2 hours and as needed. If there are large amounts of NG output, IV replacement may be necessary.

5. Subcutaneous heparin may also be ordered to prevent embolus. Antiembolism stockings may be used.

6. Turning, coughing, deep breathing, and incentive spirometry are performed every 2 hours. Dangling at bedside is encouraged the night of surgery, and an attempt at ambulation the first postoperative day is made, unless ordered otherwise.

7. Patient-controlled analgesia for pain control or other analgesics, as ordered, are administered to promote comfort.

8. Wound dressing is changed every day or as needed, maintaining aseptic technique.

9. Diet is advanced, as ordered, after presence of bowel sounds indicates GI tract has regained motility. After 1 to 2 days of NPO postoperatively, the usual diet progression is ice chips, sips of water, clear liquids, full liquids, soft or regular diet.

10. Dietary education includes fiber, avoiding gas-producing foods, and maintaining adequate fluid intake.

11. Reinforcement of teaching and assistance with ostomy care, if indicated.

12. Administration of medications, as ordered, which may include a stool softener or laxative when bowel function has returned.

 NURSING ALERT Because of the type of abdominal surgery and location of the suture line, the health care provider may order not to irrigate or manipulate the NG tube.

Complications

1. Paralytic ileus or obstruction.
2. Peritonitis or sepsis.
3. Anastomotic leakage, which may result in peritonitis.

Nursing Diagnoses

- Acute Pain related to surgical incision.
- Imbalanced Nutrition: Less Than Body Requirements related to dietary modifications after surgery.
- Impaired Skin Integrity related to surgical incision.
- Constipation related to surgery.
- Risk for Infection related to surgical incision.
- Deficient Fluid Volume related to surgical procedure.

Nursing Interventions

Promoting Comfort

1. Assess pain location, intensity, and characteristics, and make sure they are appropriate for postoperative stage.
2. Administer prescribed pain medications, and provide instructions if using a patient-controlled analgesia pump, to keep patient comfortable.
3. Assess the effectiveness of the pain medications. If ordered, promethazine can potentiate the effectiveness of pain medication.
4. Encourage the patient to change positions frequently and to splint incision when turning, coughing, or deep breathing to minimize discomfort.

Improving Nutritional Status

1. Monitor intake and output each shift, or more frequently if indicated, to maintain fluid balance.
2. Advance diet as tolerated.
3. Weigh the patient daily to ensure adequate calorie intake.
4. Provide snacks or high-protein, high-calorie supplements and assist in menu selection, if needed.
5. Instruct the patient to avoid gas-producing foods, and encourage ambulation.

Improving Skin Integrity

1. Assess wound for signs of erythema, swelling, and purulent drainage, which may indicate infection.
2. Change surgical dressing every 24 hours, and as needed, to protect the skin from drainage and decrease risk of infection.
3. Apply dressings around drains and tubes to protect the skin from leakage, if indicated.
4. Turn the patient frequently or encourage position changes to prevent skin breakdown over bony prominences.

Promoting Bowel Elimination

1. Assess for presence of bowel sounds to evaluate return of bowel function.
2. Ask the patient if passing flatus rectally or through an ostomy—also indicative of return of bowel function.
3. Evaluate for abdominal distention, nausea, or vomiting, which may indicate obstruction.
4. Monitor stool for frequency, amount, and consistency.
5. Administer stool softener or laxative, as ordered, to promote comfort with elimination.
6. Encourage diet with adequate fiber and fluid content for natural laxative effect.
7. Encourage and assist with ambulation to promote peristalsis.

Preventing Infection

1. Monitor temperature every shift or as ordered, and review previous readings to recognize early increases.
2. Change surgical dressings every 24 hours, or more frequently, as indicated. Maintain aseptic technique to avoid contamination.
3. Monitor wound for signs and symptoms of infection, such as redness, swelling, purulent drainage, odor, and pain.
4. Obtain a wound culture, as ordered.
5. Monitor the patient with a Foley catheter for signs and symptoms of urinary tract infection (UTI), such as concentrated, cloudy urine; hematuria; fever. If Foley is discontinued, monitor for the above plus complaints of burning and frequency.
6. Assist the patient in washing perineum daily, and as needed if incontinence is present, for increased comfort and hygiene.
7. Assess breath sounds and monitor for crackles.
8. Instruct the patient to turn, cough, deep-breathe, and use incentive spirometer every 2 hours to minimize complications.
9. Encourage early ambulation to initiate bowel function and reduce risk of embolus.
10. Administer antibiotics, as ordered, to maintain constant blood level.

Maintaining Fluid Volume

1. Monitor intake and output every 8 hours, or more frequently, if ordered, to assess recent status. Include amount of wound drainage from dressing changes and drains that may be in place.
2. Assess the patient for signs of dehydration—flushed, dry skin; tenting of the skin; oliguria; tachycardia, hypotension, and rapid respirations; increase in hematocrit, blood urea nitrogen (BUN), and electrolytes; fever; weight loss.
3. Monitor laboratory results and report abnormal findings.
4. Assess the patient for signs of electrolyte imbalance—nausea or vomiting, cardiac dysrhythmia, tremor, seizures, anorexia, malaise, weakness, irregular pulse; changes in behavior, mental status.
5. Weigh the patient daily to ensure adequate caloric intake.
6. Administer parenteral fluids, enteral feedings, and blood products, as ordered, to maintain volume during period of decreased oral intake.

Community and Home Care Considerations

1. Reinforce discharge instructions and the importance of postoperative regimen to include health provider follow-up appointments and laboratory and other scheduled tests or therapies.
2. A person who has undergone a total gastrectomy needs lifelong parenteral administration of vitamin B_{12} to prevent pernicious anemia. This may also apply to people with the terminal ileum removed and sometimes for those with ileostomies.
3. Change dressing and reinforce ostomy care as directed by health care provider. Report any signs of infection—unusual drainage, redness, warmth, increased pain, swelling.
4. Instruct to gradually increase activities of daily living (ADLs). No heavy lifting (more than 10 pounds), pushing, pulling, or driving for 6 to 8 weeks postoperatively.
5. Referral to additional community resources if applicable (support groups, meal programs, social services).

Patient Education and Health Maintenance

1. Review signs and symptoms of wound infection so early intervention may be instituted.
2. Explain signs and symptoms of other postoperative complications to report—elevated temperature, nausea or vomiting, abdominal distention, changes in bowel function and stool consistency or color.

3. Instruct the patient to report promptly blood in the stool or the coughing up of blood.
4. Teach the patient regarding wound and/or ostomy care, if applicable, to promote healing and self-confidence.
5. Encourage the patient to turn, cough, deep-breathe; use incentive spirometer; and ambulate. Discuss the importance of these functions during the recovery period.
6. Review dietary changes, such as increased fiber content and fluid intake, and their importance in improving bowel function.
7. Review actions and adverse effects of prescribed medications to encourage compliance and understanding of management.
8. Assess the need for home health follow-up and initiate appropriate referrals if indicated.

Evaluation: Expected Outcomes

- Verbalizes increased comfort (using a 0 to 10 pain scale, with 0 being no pain and 10 being the highest score to measure pain).
- Consumes 50% to 75% of each meal; no weight loss.
- Incisional flaps approximated and healing ridge present.
- Passing flatus and stool.
- No signs and symptoms of infection.
- Vital signs stable; fluid and electrolytes in balance.

Caring for the Patient Undergoing Ostomy Surgery

See Standards of Care Guidelines 18-2.

Types of Fecal Ostomies

Colostomy

See Figure 18-3.
1. A surgically created opening between the colon and the abdominal wall to allow fecal elimination. It may be a temporary or permanent diversion.
2. A colostomy may be placed in any segment of the large intestine (colon), which will influence the nature of fecal discharge. The more right-sided the colostomy, the looser the stool. Transverse and descending/sigmoid colostomies are the most common types.
3. A colostomy may be performed as part of an abdominoperineal resection for rectal cancer, a fecal diversion for unresectable cancer, a temporary measure to protect an anastomosis, or a surgical treatment for inflammatory bowel diseases, trauma, perforated diverticulitis, ischemic bowel, cancer, and congenital conditions.

Ileostomy

1. A surgically created opening between the ileum of the small intestine and the abdominal wall to allow elimination of small bowel effluent.
2. An ileostomy is usually formed at the terminal ileum of the small bowel and is usually placed in the right lower quadrant of the abdomen. Stool from an ileostomy drains frequently (average four to five times per day) and contains proteolytic enzymes, which can be harmful to the skin.
3. Diagnoses that may require a temporary or permanent ileostomy include ulcerative colitis, Crohn disease, familial polyposis, cancer, congenital defects, and trauma.

Characteristics of Stomas

1. A stoma is the part of the intestine (small or large) that is brought above the abdominal wall to become the outlet for

---

STANDARDS OF CARE GUIDELINES 18-2
Care of the Patient with an Ostomy

- Prepare patient and patient's family preoperatively by explaining the surgical procedure, stoma characteristics, and ostomy management with a pouching system.
- Have ostomy specialty nurse mark an optimal stoma site.
- Postoperatively, monitor the stoma color and amount and color of stomal output every shift; document and report any abnormalities.
- Periodically change a properly fitting pouching system over the ostomy to avoid leakage and protect the peristomal skin. Use this time as an opportunity for teaching.
- Assess peristomal skin with each pouching system change, document findings, and treat any abnormalities (skin breakdown because of leakage, allergy, or infection) as indicated.
- Teach patient and/or caregiver self-care skills of routine pouch emptying, cleansing skin and stoma, and changing of the pouching system until independence is achieved.
- Instruct patient and family in lifestyle adjustments regarding gas and odor control, procurement of ostomy supplies, and bathing, clothing, and travel tips.
- Encourage patient to verbalize feelings regarding the ostomy, body image changes, and sexual issues.
- Inform patient of community resources, such as United Ostomy Association, local and mail-order ostomy supply dealers, ostomy specialty nurses, American Cancer Society, and Crohn's & Colitis Foundation.

This information should serve as a general guideline only. Each patient situation presents a unique set of clinical factors and requires nursing judgment to guide care, which may include additional or alternative measures and approaches.

---

discharge of intestinal waste. Stoma is often used interchangeably with "ostomy."
2. Normal stomal characteristics: pink-red, moist, bleeds slightly when rubbed, no feeling to touch, stool functions

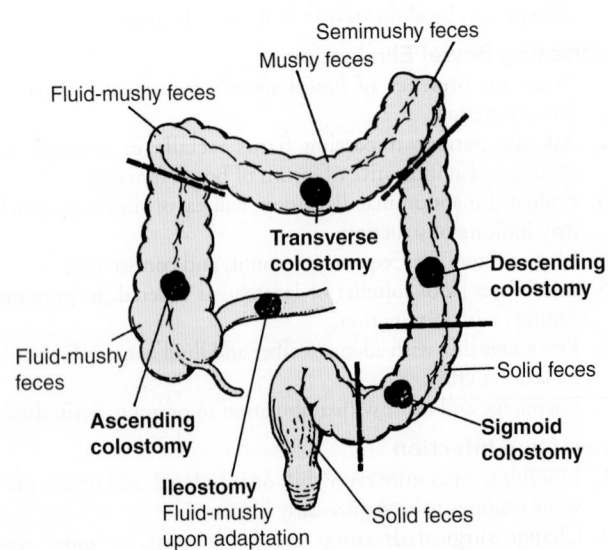

Figure 18-3. A diagrammatic representation of the placement of fecal ostomies and nature of discharge at these sites.

involuntary, and postoperative swelling gradually decreases over several months.
3. Stoma classifications:
   a. End stoma: After the bowel is divided, the proximal bowel is exteriorized to abdominal wall, everted (which exposes mucosal lining), and sutured to the dermis or subcutaneous tissue. There is only one opening that drains stool. The distal bowel is either surgically removed or sutured closed within abdominal cavity.
   b. Double-barrel stoma: After the bowel is divided, the proximal and distal ends of the bowel are exteriorized to abdominal wall, everted, and sutured to the dermis or subcutaneous tissue. If the stomas are brought up next to each other requiring them to be pouched together, they are referred to as a double-barrel stoma; if the stomas are apart to be pouched separately, they may be referred to as an end stoma (proximal), which drains stool, and a mucous fistula (distal), which drains mucus. This type of stoma is usually temporary.
   c. Loop stoma: A bowel loop is brought to the abdominal wall through an incision and stabilized temporarily with a rod, catheter, or a skin or fascial bridge. The anterior wall of the bowel is opened surgically or by electrocautery to expose the proximal and distal openings. The posterior wall of the bowel remains intact and separates the functioning proximal opening and the nonfunctioning distal opening. This type of stoma is usually temporary.

Preoperative Management and Nursing Care

1. Prepare the patient for general abdominal surgery (see page 496). Have the patient see an ostomy specialty nurse.
   a. An ostomy specialty nurse has the title of certified ostomy care nurse or certified wound, ostomy, and continence nurse (CWOCN, previously known as a certified enterostomal therapy nurse). These nurses play a vital role in the rehabilitation of patients with ostomies and related problems.
   b. The Wound Ostomy and Continence Nurses Society has an official publication called the *Journal of Wound, Ostomy, and Continence Nursing* (*www.wocn.org*).
2. Administer replacement fluid, as ordered, before surgery because of possible increased output during the postoperative phase.
3. Provide low-residue diet before NPO status.
4. Explain that the abdomen may be marked by the ostomy specialty nurse or surgeon to ensure proper positioning of the stoma. *Note:* The abdominal location of the stoma is usually determined by anatomical location of the bowel segment (eg, a sigmoid colostomy is ideally located in left lower abdominal quadrant).
5. Other considerations when selecting a stoma include:
   a. Positioning within rectus muscle.
   b. Avoidance of bony prominences, such as iliac crest and costal margin.
   c. Clearance from umbilicus, scars, and deep creases, observed in lying, sitting, and standing positions.
   d. Positioning on a flat pouching surface.
   e. Avoidance of beltline when possible.
   f. Positioning within patient's visibility to optimize independent ostomy care.
6. Support the patient and family with the many psychosocial considerations of ostomy surgery.

Postoperative Management and Nursing Care

1. Administer general abdominal surgery care (see page 496).
2. Assess stoma every shift for color and record findings:
   a. Normal color: pink-red.
   b. Dusky: dark red; purplish hue (ischemic sign).
   c. Necrotic: brown or black; may be dry (notify health care provider to determine extent of necrosis).
3. Apply pouching system as close to stoma as possible without it being rubbed. It is acceptable to have a 1/16- to 1/8-inch clearance to prevent constriction, which can contribute to edema (see Figure 18-4).
4. Check for abdominal distention, which reduces blood flow to stoma through mesenteric tension.
5. Evaluate and empty drains and ostomy pouch frequently to promote patency and maintain seal.
6. Monitor intake and output with extreme accuracy because output may remain high during early postoperative period.
7. Suction and irrigate NG tube frequently, as ordered, to relieve pressure and decrease gastric contents.
8. Offer continued support to patient and family.

Complications

1. Mucocutaneous separation (between the skin and stoma).
2. Stomal ischemia.
3. Stomal stricture or stenosis (usually a long-term complication).
4. Stomal prolapse.
5. Peristomal hernia.
6. Stomal laceration.
7. Stomal retraction.
8. Peristomal skin breakdown from exposure to fecal output, allergic reaction to products, or infection, such as candidiasis.

Nursing Diagnoses

- Deficient Knowledge related to surgical procedures and ostomy management.
- Disturbed Body Image related to change in structure, function, and appearance.
- Impaired Skin Integrity related to irritation of peristomal skin by drainage and equipment.
- Imbalanced Nutrition: Less Than Body Requirements related to increased output and inadequate intake.
- Sexual Dysfunction related to altered body structure.

Nursing Interventions

Educating the Patient

1. Review the surgical procedure with the patient and discuss the information that the surgeon and other providers have given. Clarify any misunderstandings.
2. Avoid overwhelming the patient with information.
3. Include family in discussions, when appropriate.
4. Use available educational materials, including pictures and drawings, if the patient is receptive.
5. Involve the ostomy specialty nurse (CWOCN) in ostomy teaching and reinforce information, including lifestyle modifications.
6. Use a team approach; the need for information may come from many disciplines.
7. Assess the patient's response to teaching. If the patient is not interested, provide alternative times for teaching and review.

Figure 18-4. Changing a two-piece pouching system. Pouching systems are varied by manufacturer and chosen according to patient needs. Systems are one-piece or two-piece and disposable or reusable. A disposable, one-piece pouch is commonly used with backing as adhesive tape, skin barrier, or both. A disposable two-piece system consists of a skin barrier wafer with or without a tape border and a pouch. Reusable systems consist of double-backed adhesive disks, cement, or belt to provide a seal and can be used for weeks to months. **(A)** A wafer with flange (1.5 to 4 inch) is applied after cleaning and drying of peristomal skin. **(B)** A transparent or opaque drainable pouch is positioned over stoma at desired angle. **(C)** Pouch may be removed without removal of wafer. **(D)** Stoma may be assessed without removing wafer.

8. Introduce gradual steps toward achieving independent ostomy management. The patient may progress through the following steps:
   a. Observe stoma, pouch change, and emptying procedure.
   b. Learn tail closure application and removal.
   c. Empty and rinse pouch.
   d. Assist with pouching system change until independent.
9. Consider the psychosocial issues of the patient and their effect on learning.

Promoting a Positive Self-Image
1. Encourage the patient to verbalize feelings about the surgical outcome. Acknowledge that it is normal to have negative feelings toward ostomy surgery; empathize with the patient.
2. Describe behaviors to attain a sense of control such as resuming ADLs.
3. Provide support during initial viewing of the stoma and encourage the patient to touch the area.
4. Encourage spouse or significant other to view the stoma.
5. Arrange a visit by a United Ostomy Association ostomy visitor if the patient desires. This is preferably done preoperatively.
6. Offer counseling, as necessary, and encourage the patient to use normal support systems, such as family, church, and community groups.

Maintaining Skin Integrity
1. Select pouching system based on type of ostomy and condition of stoma and skin (see Figure 18-3).
2. Empty pouch when one-third to one-half full to avoid overfilling, which interferes with pouch seal.
   a. Remove tail closure from pouch tail.
   b. Cuff bottom of pouch tail.

   c. Drain stool from pouch.
   d. Clean pouch tail with toilet tissue or wipe (may rinse pouch if desired).
   e. Uncuff pouch and reapply tail closure.
3. Treat peristomal skin breakdown as needed.
   a. Dust skin breakdown with skin barrier powder (eg, Stomahesive powder).
   b. Seal powder with water or skin sealant (eg, Skin-Prep). May be applied one to three times per day, depending on the severity of the skin breakdown.
   c. Allow skin to dry before applying pouching system.

> **! NURSING ALERT** When peristomal skin is exposed to excess moisture, candidiasis can occur. It presents as an erythematous rash, which may include papules, pustules, or white patches. Patients may complain of pruritus. The treatment procedure is the same as for skin breakdown, using a prescribed antifungal powder (nystatin) in place of the skin barrier powder. The antifungal powder should be used at each pouching system change and continued 2 weeks after the condition has cleared. Positive identification of *Candida albicans* can be done through a culture or microscopic visualization. Treatment is usually initiated without culture or scraping if the signs and symptoms are classic.

Maximizing Nutritional Intake
1. Review dietary habits with the patient to determine patterns, preferences, and bowel irritants.
2. Advise the patient to avoid foods that stimulate elimination, such as nuts, seeds, and certain fruits.

3. Recommend consistency in dietary habits as well as moderation.
4. Coordinate consult with nutritionist, as needed.
5. Weigh daily; monitor vital signs and electrolytes to determine patient's nutritional status.

Achieving Sexual Well-Being

1. Encourage the patient and significant other to express feelings about the ostomy.
2. Discuss ways to conceal pouch during intimacy, if desired: pouch covers, special ostomy underwear. May briefly use small-capacity pouch (minipouch or cap).
3. Recommend different positions for sexual activity to decrease stoma friction and skin irritation.
4. Review, when appropriate, that an ostomy in a woman does not prevent a successful pregnancy.
5. Recommend counseling as needed.

Patient Education and Health Maintenance

Skin Care

1. Instruct the patient to inspect peristomal skin with each pouching system change.
2. Review techniques for treating peristomal skin problems.
3. Recommend alternative products if patient develops allergic reaction to an ostomy product.
4. Teach the patient to notify health care provider when skin care problems do not resolve by usual methods.

Colostomy Irrigation

1. Teach colostomy irrigation procedure, to patients with a descending or sigmoid colostomy. Reinforce its purposes of cleansing the colon and stimulating the colon to move at a desired time regularly to regain control of fecal elimination.
   a. Irrigation may occur every day or every other day depending on bowel pattern.
   b. It usually takes 1 to 2 months to establish control.
   c. Patients with a preoperative history of regular, formed bowel movements are more likely to realize success.
2. Set up patient in front of commode with irrigation sleeve directed into the commode, and lubricate tip of the enema before gently inserting no more than 3 inches into stoma.
3. Allow solution to flow in slowly, over 5 to 10 minutes, and slower if cramping occurs.
4. Remove tubing and allow fecal matter to drain for 10 to 15 minutes before closing sleeve, which should be left in place for 20 more minutes before cleansing stoma and applying usual colostomy bag.

Odor Control

1. Encourage pouch hygiene through rinsing, keeping pouch tail free of stool, airing of reusable pouches, discarding odor-impregnated pouches.
2. Recommend the use of pouch deodorants, room deodorizers, and oral deodorizers, such as bismuth subgallate or parsley.
3. Avoid use of pinholes in pouch.

Gas Control

1. Suggest avoidance of straws, excessive talking while eating, chewing gum, and smoking to reduce swallowed air.
2. Instruct about gas-forming foods, such as beans and cabbage, and eliminate when appropriate. It takes about 6 hours for gas to travel from the mouth to colostomy.
3. Recommend using the arm over stoma to muffle gas sounds when appropriate.

ADLs

Educate the patient about the following:

1. Resumption of normal bathing habits (tub or shower) with or without pouching system.
2. Picture framing the edges of the pouching system with water-proof tape, if needed, for bathing or swimming.
3. Clothing modifications are usually minimal. Girdles without stays and panty hose are acceptable.
4. Carrying an ostomy supply kit during work or travel in case of an emergency.
5. Participating in sports as desired. Caution must be exercised with contact sports. During vigorous activities, a belt or binder may provide extra security.
6. For additional information and support, refer to the United Ostomy Association, a self-help group for ostomates and other interested people, at *www.uoa.org*. The official membership publication is the *Ostomy Quarterly*. Encourage ostomy patients to participate in a local chapter. Chapters usually publish a local newsletter, conduct monthly meetings, and provide trained ostomy visitors on request by health care providers.
7. Ostomy manufacturers offer literature covering a wide variety of ostomy-related topics.
8. Encourage the patient to maintain contact with health care providers.

Evaluation: Expected Outcomes

- Verbalizes knowledge regarding ostomy surgery and general care of ostomy.
- Can view ostomy.
- No skin breakdown around ostomy.
- Plans menus with nutritionist; weight stable.
- Discusses intimacy concerns with partner.

ESOPHAGEAL DISORDERS

Esophageal varices are covered in Chapter 19, page 536.

Gastroesophageal Reflux Disease and Esophagitis

Gastric contents flow back into the esophagus, and sometimes further back into the mouth and lungs, in gastroesophageal reflux disease (GERD) because of incompetent lower esophageal sphincter (LES). Esophagitis, or inflammation of the esophageal mucosa, may result.

Pathophysiology and Etiology

1. Gastroesophageal reflux associated with an incompetent LES—gastric contents reflux (flow backward) through the LES into the esophagus.
2. Can be the result of impaired gastric emptying from gastroparesis or partial gastric outlet obstruction.
3. The acidity of gastric content and amount of time in contact with esophageal mucosa are related to the degree of mucosal damage.
4. Inflammation and ulceration of the esophagus may result, causing esophagitis.
5. May be caused by motility disorders (scleroderma, esophageal spasm).

Clinical Manifestations

GERD

1. The most common symptom is heartburn (pyrosis), typically occurring 30 to 60 minutes after meals and in reclining

positions. May have complaints of spontaneous reflux (regurgitation) of sour or bitter gastric contents into the mouth.
2. Other typical symptoms include globus (sensation of something in the throat), mild epigastric pain, dyspepsia, and nausea and/or vomiting.
3. Dysphagia is a less common symptom.
4. Atypical symptoms include chest pain, hoarseness, recurrent sore throat, frequent throat clearing, chronic cough, dental enamel loss, bronchospasm (asthma/wheezing), and odynophagia (sharp substernal pain on swallowing).
5. Symptoms that may suggest other disease etiologies need further evaluation: atypical chest pain (rule out possible cardiac causes), dysphagia, odynophagia, GI bleeding, shortness of breath, or weight loss (rule out cancer or esophageal stricture).

Esophagitis
1. Esophagitis is an acute or chronic inflammation of the esophagus. Severity of symptoms may be unrelated to the degree of esophageal tissue damage.
2. Symptoms vary according to etiology of esophagitis. Symptoms include dysphagia, odynophagia, severe burning, chest pain.
3. Causes of esophagitis other than GERD:
   a. Infectious—*Candida*, herpes, human immunodeficiency virus, cytomegalovirus.
   b. Chemical (alkali or acid) or radiation therapy.
   c. Medication-induced—may include doxycycline, ascorbic acid, quinidine, potassium chloride, bisphosphonates, tetracycline.

Diagnostic Evaluation

1. Uncomplicated GERD may be diagnosed on patient history of typical symptoms.
2. Endoscopy can visualize inflammation, lesions, or erosions. Biopsy can confirm diagnosis.
3. Esophageal manometry measures LES pressure and determines if esophageal peristalsis is adequate. This study should be used before patients undergo surgical treatment for reflux. This test is also done before a pH probe for determination of correct catheter placement.
4. Acid perfusion (Bernstein test)—onset of symptoms after ingestion of dilute hydrochloric acid and saline is considered positive. This test differentiates between cardiac and noncardiac chest pain.
5. Ambulatory 24-hour pH monitoring is performed when GERD is suspected but not responding to standard therapies, prior to antireflux surgery, or when the patient's symptoms may not be typical. It determines the amount of gastroesophageal acid reflux and has a 70% to 90% specificity rate.
   a. The Bravo pH capsule system is a catheter-free system in which a capsule containing a radiotelemetry pH sensor is inserted into the esophagus. This sensor transmits signals to an external pager-size receiver, allowing the patient to be catheter-free during the 24 hours of pH testing.
   b. The Bravo pH capsule system is contraindicated for patients with pacemakers, implantable defibrillators, or neurostimulators. It is also contraindicated for patients with a history of severe esophagitis, varices, obstructions, bleeding diatheses, or strictures.
6. Barium esophagography—use of barium with radiographic studies to diagnose mechanical and motility disorders. This test is not recommended in diagnosing GERD.

 NURSING ALERT The patient should not undergo MRI within 30 days of Bravo capsule pH monitoring.

Management

Treatment goals include eliminating symptom, healing esophageal damage (if present), and preventing complications and relapse.

Lifestyle Modifications
1. Head of bed raised 6 to 8 inches (15 to 20 cm).
2. Do not lie down for 2 to 3 hours after eating—time frame for greatest reflux.
3. Bland diet—avoid garlic, onion, peppermint, fatty foods, chocolate, coffee (including decaffeinated), citrus juices, colas, and tomato products.
4. Avoid overeating—causes LES relaxation.
5. No tight-fitting clothes.
6. Weight loss.
7. Smoking cessation.
8. Reduce alcohol.

Pharmacologic Treatment
1. Antacids—reduce gastric acidity. Use on an as-needed basis. Provide symptomatic relief, but do not heal esophageal lesions.
2. Histamine-2 (H_2)-receptor antagonists, such as ranitidine, cimetidine, famotidine, nizatidine—decrease gastric acid secretions. Provide symptomatic relief. May require lifelong therapy.
3. If symptoms do not respond to H_2-receptor antagonist, change to a once-per-day proton pump inhibitor (PPI), such as omeprazole, esomeprazole, pantoprazole, rabeprazole, or lansoprazole, to block gastric acid secretion.
4. PPIs have been shown to be more effective than H_2-receptor antagonists in achieving faster healing rates for erosive esophagitis.
5. Drug maintenance therapy may be needed depending on the severity of disease and recurrence of symptoms after initial drug therapy is stopped.
6. Use the lowest effective drug dose of H_2-receptor blocker or PPI.

 DRUG ALERT Patients with renal insufficiency and older patients may need decreased dosing of H_2-receptor antagonists.

 DRUG ALERT PPIs should be taken 30 minutes before a meal for optimal control of gastric acidity. Impaired absorption of calcium may occur with PPI use, leading to fracture risk. Calcium citrate is recommended because it is not dependent on an acid environment for absorption.

Endoscopic and Surgical Treatment
1. Nissen fundoplication and bariatric surgery (for the obese patient) are the most common surgical therapies for long-term management of GERD. Surgery is not recommended for those who do not respond to PPI therapy.
   a. Upper portion of the stomach is wrapped around the distal esophagus and sutured, creating a tight LES.
   b. This procedure can be performed laparoscopically.

c. Combined with vagotomy–pyloroplasty if associated with gastroduodenal ulcer.

d. Antireflux surgery may not eliminate the need for future pharmacologic treatment.

2. Many endoscopic therapies for the treatment of GERD have not been efficacious and are no longer used. In the United States, there are only two endoscopic therapies being used:

a. The Stretta procedure is a radiofrequency energy delivery system used to provide a thermal burn to the gastroesophageal junction.

b. Transoral incisionless fundoplication (TIF) is done using the EsophyX device on an endoscope to tighten the GE valve, thereby reducing reflux.

Complications

1. Esophageal stricture formation.
2. Ulceration of the esophagus, with or without fistula formation.
3. Aspiration may be complicated by pneumonia.
4. Development of Barrett esophagus—presence of columnar epithelium above the gastroesophageal junction associated with adenocarcinoma of the esophagus.

Nursing Interventions and Patient Education

1. Teach the patient about prescribed medications, adverse effects, and when to notify the health care provider. PPIs may interact with carbamazepine, cyclosporine, diazepam, diclofenac, digoxin, iron, ketoconazole, lidocaine, methotrexate, metoprolol, nifedipine, phenytoin, propranolol, quinidine, theophylline, and warfarin.

2. Inform the patient about medications that may exacerbate symptoms. Anticholinergics may further impair functioning of the LES, allowing reflux; antihistamines, antidepressants, antihypertensives, antispasmodics, and some neuroleptics and antiparkinsonian drugs decrease saliva production, which may decrease acid clearance from the esophagus.

3. Advise the patient to sit or stand when taking any solid medication (pills, capsules): emphasize the need to follow the drug with at least 100 mL of liquid.

4. Familiarize the patient and family with foods and activities to avoid, such as fatty foods, garlic, onions, alcohol, coffee, chocolate, and peppermint.

5. Caution the patient against straining, bending over, tight-fitting clothes, and smoking.

6. Encourage the patient to sleep with the head of the bed elevated (not pillow elevation).

7. Encourage a weight reduction program, if the patient is overweight, to decrease intra-abdominal pressure.

Hiatal Hernia

A hiatal hernia is a protrusion of a portion of the stomach through the hiatus of the diaphragm and into the thoracic cavity.

Pathophysiology and Etiology

1. There are two types of hiatal hernias (see Figure 18-5):

a. Sliding hernia: The stomach and gastroesophageal junction slip up into the chest (most common).

b. Paraesophageal hernia (rolling hernia): Part of the greater curvature of the stomach rolls through the diaphragmatic defect.

2. Caused by muscle weakening because of aging or other conditions, such as esophageal carcinoma or trauma, or following certain surgical procedures.

Clinical Manifestations

1. May be asymptomatic.
2. Heartburn (with or without regurgitation of gastric contents into the mouth).
3. Dysphagia, chest pain.

Diagnostic Evaluation

1. Barium study of the esophagus outlines hernia.
2. Endoscopic examination visualizes defect.

Management

1. Elevation of the head of the bed (6 to 8 inches [15 to 20 cm]) to reduce nighttime reflux.
2. Antacid therapy to neutralize gastric acid.
3. H_2-receptor antagonist (cimetidine, ranitidine) if patient has esophagitis.
4. Surgical repair of hernia if symptoms are severe.

Complications

1. Aspiration of reflux contents.
2. Ulceration, hemorrhage.
3. Gastritis.
4. Stricture.
5. Incarceration of the portion of the stomach in the chest.

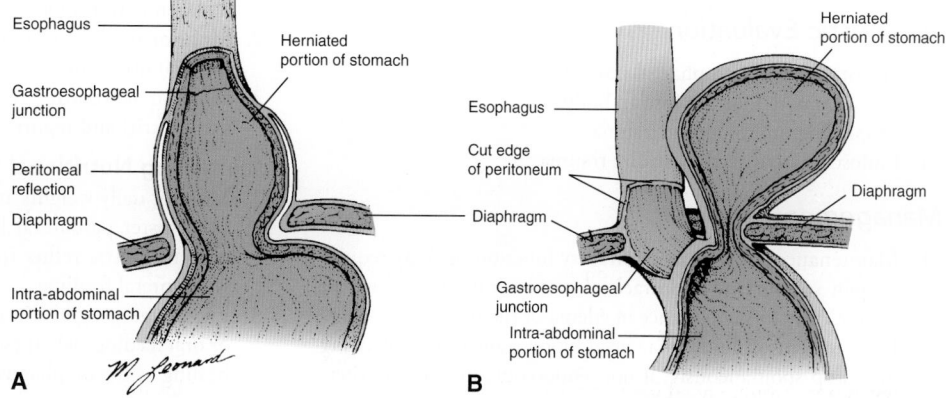

Figure 18-5. Hiatal hernia. **(A)** Sliding hernia. **(B)** Paraesophageal hernia. **A** **B**

Nursing Interventions and Patient Education

1. Instruct the patient on the prevention of reflux of gastric contents into the esophagus by:
   a. Eating smaller meals.
   b. Avoiding stimulation of gastric secretions by omitting caffeine and alcohol.
   c. Refraining from smoking.
   d. Avoiding fatty foods: promote reflux and delay gastric emptying.
   e. Refraining from lying down for at least 1 hour after meals.
   f. Losing weight, if obese.
   g. Avoiding bending from the waist and/or wearing tight-fitting clothes.
2. Advise the patient to report to health care facility immediately for the onset of acute chest pain, which may indicate incarceration of a large paraesophageal hernia.

Esophageal Trauma and Perforations

Esophageal trauma or perforations are injuries to the esophagus caused by external or internal insult.

Pathophysiology and Etiology

1. External: Stab or bullet wounds, crush injuries, blunt trauma.
2. Internal:
   a. Swallowed foreign objects (coins, pins, bones, dental appliances, caustic poisons).
   b. Spontaneous or postemetic rupture—usually in the presence of underlying esophageal disease (reflux, hiatal hernia).
   c. Mallory-Weiss syndrome—nonpenetrating mucosal tear at the gastroesophageal junction. Caused by an increase in transabdominal pressure from lifting, vomiting, or retching. Alcoholism is a predisposing condition.

Clinical Manifestations

1. Pain at the site of injury or impaction, aggravated by swallowing—chest pain, may be severe.
2. Dysphagia or odynophagia.
3. Persistent foreign object sensation.
4. Subcutaneous emphysema and crepitus of the face, neck, or upper thorax—noted in cervical, thoracic, and esophageal perforations.
5. Temperature elevation occurring within 24 hours of trauma.
6. Blood-stained saliva or excessive salivation.
7. Hematemesis; previous history of vomiting or retching—Mallory-Weiss syndrome.
8. Respiratory difficulty if there is pressure on the tracheobronchial tree from injury or edema.

Diagnostic Evaluation

1. History of recent esophageal trauma.
2. Chest x-ray to look for foreign body.
3. Esophagogram to outline trauma.
4. Endoscopy to directly visualize trauma.

Management

1. Maintenance of adequate respiratory functioning; may require oxygen support or endotracheal intubation—to ensure an open airway in the presence of edema of the neck.
2. Replacement of fluids. May need blood transfusion. Bleeding may stop spontaneously; if not, endoscopic hemostatic therapy or surgery is indicated.
3. Restoration of the continuity of the esophagus by removing the cause.
4. For external wound injury, emergency first aid wound care and surgical repair may be indicated.
5. For swallowed foreign bodies:
   a. Barium swallow determines location of foreign body; usually removed through endoscopy.
   b. Some patients with a history of food impaction may be treated with a spasmolytic such as IV glucagon.
6. For chemical ingestion:
   a. If lye or other caustic or organic solvent was swallowed, do not try to induce vomiting.
   b. Treat with IV fluids and analgesics.
   c. A gastrostomy may be performed, either as a temporary or a permanent means of feeding the patient.
   d. Resulting strictures may be relieved by dilating the narrow esophagus.
   e. Reconstructive surgery may be necessary to create a new passageway for food between the pharynx and stomach.

Complications

1. Airway occlusion.
2. Shock.
3. Perforation with mediastinitis or pleural effusion.
4. Stricture formation.
5. Abscess or fistula formation.

Nursing Assessment

1. Assess the following to determine status of patient:
   a. Vital signs.
   b. Respiratory status.
   c. Bleeding.
   d. Ability to swallow—choking, gagging.
2. Monitor the patient for hypovolemic shock.

Nursing Diagnoses

- Deficient Fluid Volume related to blood loss from injury.
- Imbalanced Nutrition: Less Than Body Requirements related to esophageal injury.
- Ineffective Breathing Pattern related to pain and trauma.
- Acute Pain related to injury.

Nursing Interventions

Maintaining Fluid Volume

1. Administer IV fluids and blood transfusion for volume replacement, if indicated.
2. Monitor intake and output. Urine output should be greater than 30 mL/hour.
3. Monitor laboratory results (electrolytes, hemoglobin, and hematocrit) and report abnormal findings.

Maintaining Nutritional Status

1. Monitor daily weights and skin turgor.
2. Administer parenteral hyperalimentation as prescribed—to prevent gastric reflux into the esophagus, which may occur with enteral feedings.
3. Encourage progression of diet through NG, esophagostomy, or oral feedings when esophagoscopy or esophagogram reveals healing of the esophagus.
4. Continue to monitor intake and output.

Maintaining Respiratory Function

1. Auscultate the lungs and trachea for stridor, crackles, or wheezes. Assess respiratory rate, depth, use of accessory muscles, and skin color.
2. Position the patient in semi-Fowler position to facilitate breathing and reduce neck edema.
3. Monitor vital signs frequently for signs and symptoms of shock and infection.
4. Administer oxygen as prescribed.
5. Have emergency airway equipment at bedside.

Reducing Pain

1. Administer analgesics as prescribed—IV analgesia may be required to control pain and allow the esophagus to rest.
2. Provide reassurance and support.
3. Assess and record pain relief.
4. Evaluate for symptoms that may indicate spillage of digestive contents into the mediastinum, pleura, or abdominal cavity—sudden onset of acute pain.

Patient Education and Health Maintenance

1. Instruct the patient on the indications and adverse effects of analgesics.
2. Inform the patient on the signs and symptoms to report on possible complications: increase in severity or nature of pain and difficulty breathing or swallowing.
3. Teach patient with dysphagia how to swallow (see Box 18-2). This assists the patient who has difficulty swallowing after injury or surgical correction of the oropharynx or upper esophagus (also helpful with neurologic deficit or stroke).

BOX 18-2	Teaching a Patient with Dysphagia How to Swallow

1. Sit the patient upright and the head in midline and forward position, chin pointed toward the chest.
2. Instruct the patient to smell the food before each bite; hold each bite for a few seconds; hold lips together firmly; concentrate on swallowing; then, swallow.
3. If the patient has an increase in saliva during the meal, instruct the patient to collect the saliva with the tongue and consciously swallow it between bites throughout the meal.
4. If the patient complains of a dry mouth during meals, instruct him to move tongue in a circular fashion against the insides of the cheeks to stimulate salivation.
5. Caution the patient against talking during the meal or with the mouth full of food.
6. Advise the following tips about food and fluid intake:
   a. Try foods that hold some shape and are moist enough to prevent crumbling but dry enough to hold a bolus shape—casseroles, custards, scrambled eggs.
   b. Use mugs and glasses with spouts or use a straw.
   c. Avoid sticky foods—peanut butter, chocolate, milk, ice cream.
   d. Moisten dry foods with margarine, gravy, or broths.
   e. Liquids such as juices can be thickened with sherbet.
   f. Safely try warm and cold foods and fluids, which are thought to maximally stimulate receptors that activate swallowing mechanism.

4. Teach the patient about tests or surgical procedures that may be performed.

Evaluation: Expected Outcomes

- Urine output greater than 30 mL/hour; electrolytes stable.
- No further weight loss, tolerating parenteral feedings well.
- Lungs clear; respirations unlabored.
- States pain decreased to level of 2 or 3 on 0 to 10 scale.

Motility Disorders of the Esophagus

Primary motility disorders include achalasia, diffuse esophageal spasm, and those of nonspecific origin. Secondary motility disorders may be caused by neuromuscular, GI, endocrine, or connective tissue disorders.

Pathophysiology and Etiology

Primary Motility Disorders

1. Achalasia refers to excessive resting tone of the LES, incomplete relaxation of the LES with swallowing, and failure of normal peristalsis in the lower two thirds of the esophagus. The pathology is related to defective innervation of the myenteric plexus innervating the involuntary muscles of the esophagus.
2. Diffuse esophageal spasm is a motor disorder in which high-amplitude, nonpropulsive, nonperistaltic tertiary contractions (a form of aperistalsis) are present. LES functioning is frequently normal.

Secondary Motility Disorders

1. Neuromuscular dysfunction includes myasthenia gravis, Parkinson disease, muscular dystrophy, amyotrophic lateral sclerosis, and cerebral palsy.
2. Connective tissue disorders include scleroderma.
3. GI causes include GERD.
4. Other secondary causes include the autonomic neuropathy of diabetes mellitus.

Clinical Manifestations

Achalasia

1. Gradual onset of dysphagia with solids and liquids.
2. Substernal discomfort or a feeling of fullness.
3. Regurgitation of undigested food during a meal or within several hours after a meal.
4. Weight loss.

Diffuse Esophageal Spasm

1. Intermittent dysphagia for solids or liquids—does not progress to continuous dysphagia.
2. Aggravation of symptoms (large volume of food and hot or cold liquids).
3. Anterior chest pain.

Secondary Motility Disorders

Symptoms of esophagitis from gastroesophageal reflux.

Diagnostic Evaluation

Achalasia

1. Chest x-ray, which may show an enlarged, fluid-filled esophagus.
2. Barium esophagography showing dilation, decreased or absence of peristalsis, decreased emptying, and a "bird beak" narrowing of the distal esophagus.
3. Esophageal manometry to confirm the diagnoses suspected.
4. EUS or a chest CT for suspected tumor.

Diffuse Esophageal Spasm

1. Barium esophagography showing simultaneous contractions of the esophagus having a "corkscrew" or "rosary bead" appearance.
2. Esophageal manometry showing intermittent contractions with episodes of normal peristalsis.

Secondary Motility Disorders

Diagnostic workup may include barium esophagography or manometry.

Management

Achalasia

1. Drug therapy using calcium channel blockers such as nifedipine to reduce LES pressure. This type of treatment is usually best for patients presenting with mild symptoms and a non-dilated esophagus or patients who are medically unstable to undergo invasive therapies.
2. Esophageal dilation using a balloon-tipped catheter is the preferred treatment for most patients.
3. Surgical therapy (Heller myotomy of the LES) may be used on patients who do not respond to balloon dilation. This surgery requires a laparotomy or thoracotomy or may be done through a thoracoscope.

Diffuse Esophageal Spasm

1. Drug therapy using nitrates and calcium channel blockers is the primary treatment.
2. Dilation may provide some symptom relief.
3. Surgical myotomy is used rarely for patients with a debilitating disorder who are able to withstand a surgical procedure.

Other Motility Disorders

1. Treatment of the gastroesophageal reflux.
2. Dilation may be required for peptic stricture.

Complications

1. Malnutrition.
2. Pneumonia, lung abscess, bronchiectasis from nocturnal regurgitation causing aspiration.
3. Esophagitis and esophageal diverticula.
4. Perforation from dilation procedure.
5. Peptic stricture or Barrett esophagus from severe erosive esophagitis.

Nursing Assessment

1. Assess for difficulty with swallowing, vomiting, weight loss, chest pain associated with eating.
2. Inquire as to what facilitates passage of food, such as position changes, use of liquids.

Nursing Diagnoses

- Imbalanced Nutrition: Less Than Body Requirements related to dysphagia.
- Acute Pain related to heartburn or surgical procedure.

Nursing Interventions

Improving Nutritional Status

1. Direct the patient to eat sitting in an upright position; eat slowly and chew food thoroughly.
2. Avoid food and beverages that precipitate symptoms.
3. Suggest that the patient sleep with head elevated to avoid reflux or aspiration.

4. Provide a bland diet and tell the patient to avoid alcohol as well as spicy, very hot, and very cold foods, to minimize symptoms.
5. Eliminate sources of tension as a precipitating factor producing stress during mealtimes.
6. Administer pharmacologic agents as prescribed.

Promoting Comfort

1. Assess the patient for discomfort, chest pain, regurgitation, and cough. If a surgical procedure was performed, assess for incisional pain.
2. Provide appropriate postoperative care. Incisional approach determines the nature of postoperative care (eg, an incision through the chest implies nursing care similar to that given to a patient with a thoracotomy [see page 184]).
3. Administer analgesics as ordered.
4. Assess for effectiveness of pain medication.

Patient Education and Health Maintenance

1. Encourage lifestyle activity changes similar to those for patients with reflux (see page 503).
2. See Box 18-2 on page 505 to help the patient with dysphasia with swallowing.
3. Provide information on all diagnostic procedures or surgery performed.

Evaluation: Expected Outcomes

- Demonstrates proper positioning for eating; describes dietary habits that minimize symptoms; compliant with medications regimen.
- States pain decreased to 2 or 3 on 0 to 10 scale.

Esophageal Diverticulum

An esophageal diverticulum is an outpouching of the esophageal wall, usually in the cervical posterior side, secondary to an obstructive or inflammatory process.

Pathophysiology and Etiology

1. *Zenker diverticulum*—protrusion of pharyngeal mucosa at the pharyngoesophageal junction between the interior pharyngeal constrictor and cricopharyngeal muscle.
2. Mid or distal esophageal diverticula may develop above strictures or may be secondary to motility disorders.

Clinical Manifestations

Zenker Diverticulum

1. Difficulty in swallowing, fullness in the neck, throat discomfort, a feeling that food stops before it reaches the stomach, and regurgitation of undigested food.
2. Belching, gurgling, or nocturnal coughing brought about by diverticulum becoming filled with food or liquid, which is regurgitated and may irritate the trachea.
3. Halitosis and foul taste in the mouth caused by food decomposing in a pouch (diverticulum).
4. Weight loss because of nutritional depletion.

 GERONTOLOGIC ALERT Hoarseness, asthma, and pneumonitis may be the only signs of esophageal diverticula in older adults.

Mid or Distal Esophageal Diverticula

Generally no symptoms.

Diagnostic Evaluation

1. Barium esophagogram outlines diverticulum.
2. Endoscopy is not indicated and may be dangerous because of the possibility of rupture.

Management

Zenker Diverticulum

1. Small Zenker diverticula may not be treated, but the underlying cause is treated with dilation or myotomy.
2. For larger Zenker diverticula, transverse cervical diverticulectomy or diverticulopexy with suspension and cricopharyngeal myotomy may be done.
   a. Caution is taken to avoid injury to common carotid artery and internal jugular vein.
   b. The sac is dissected free and then excised flush with esophageal wall.
3. For mid or distal esophageal diverticula, underlying primary condition must be treated.

Complications

1. Aspiration pneumonia.
2. Malnutrition.
3. Lung abscess.

Nursing Assessment

1. Obtain history of dysphagia, coughing, throat discomfort, choking, and regurgitation of food.
2. Evaluate for halitosis.
3. Determine what measures assist the patient with food intake and what foods and fluids the patient can tolerate.
4. Evaluate weight loss and dietary habits.

Nursing Diagnoses

- Imbalanced Nutrition: Less Than Body Requirements related to dysphagia.
- Acute Pain related to symptoms and surgical procedure.

Nursing Interventions

Improving Nutritional Status

1. Provide frequent, small meals, which are better tolerated.
2. Elevate head of bed for 2 hours after eating.
3. Monitor intake and output.
4. Weigh daily.

Maintaining Comfort and Preventing Complications

1. Preoperatively, or if the condition is nonoperative, implement nursing interventions similar to those for esophagitis.
2. Postoperatively, wound care is similar to that of other surgical incisions of the same anatomical position (eg, thoracotomy [see page 184].
3. Administer appropriate pain medications and assess effectiveness.
4. Patient may need oral suctioning to control drooling.
5. Maintain NG tube if in place.
   a. Irrigate the tube as ordered.
   b. Do not manipulate NG tube because of location of the tube and suture line.

Patient Education and Health Maintenance

1. Instruct patient regarding treatment of esophagitis caused by gastroesophageal reflux (see page 502).
2. Instruct patient on importance of good oral hygiene.

Evaluation: Expected Outcomes

- Tolerates oral feedings; maintains weight.
- States pain decreased to 2 or 3 on 0 to 10 scale.

Cancer of the Esophagus

Malignant lesions of the esophagus occur in two main types that are defined histologically: squamous cell and adenocarcinoma.

Pathophysiology and Etiology

1. Adenocarcinoma is the most common type of esophageal cancer in the United States comprising 60% of all cases.
2. Squamous cell carcinoma cases have decreased significantly in the United States because of changes in lifestyle such as reduction of smoking and alcohol use.
3. Highest rate in the United States occurs in Caucasian men who are usually older than age 60.
4. Cause is unknown but has been associated with:
   a. Barrett esophagus.
   b. Achalasia.
   c. GERD.
   d. Chronic use of alcohol and tobacco (squamous cell carcinoma).
   e. Other head and neck cancers.

Clinical Manifestations

1. Dysphagia is the usual presenting symptom, although it is a late sign, by which time there often is regional or systemic involvement.
2. Mild, atypical chest pain associated with eating precedes dysphagia but is rarely significant enough for the patient to seek health care.
3. Pain on swallowing (odynophagia).
4. Progressive weight loss.
5. Hoarseness (if laryngeal involvement).
6. Lymphadenopathy (supraclavicular or cervical) or hepatomegaly with metastatic involvement.
7. Later symptoms—hiccups, respiratory difficulty, foul breath, and regurgitation of food and saliva.

Diagnostic Evaluation

1. Chest x-ray may show adenopathy, mediastinal widening, metastasis, or a tracheoesophageal fistula.
2. Endoscopy with cytology and biopsy.
3. Surveillance endoscopy of Barrett esophagus is beneficial for early detection of malignant changes.
4. Barium esophagram may show polypoid, infiltrative, or ulcerative lesion requiring biopsy.
5. CT scanning may be helpful in delineating the extent of the tumor as well as in identifying presence of adjacent tissue invasion and metastases.

Management

1. The goal of treatment may be cure or palliation, depending on the staging of the tumor and the patient's overall condition in relation to nutritional, cardiovascular, pulmonary, and functional status.
2. The wide variability in treatment reflects the overall poor results from any one approach.
3. Surgery.

a. Lesions of the middle and lower esophagus are excised with use of the thoracotomy approach with esophagogastrectomy or colon interposition (section of the colon is used to replace the excised portion of the esophagus).

b. Lesions of the cervical esophagus are excised with a bilateral neck dissection and esophagogastrectomy; laryngectomy and thyroidectomy may be necessary.

c. A two-step approach may be selected when resection with a cervical esophagostomy and feeding gastrostomy are performed initially; subsequent reconstructive surgery is performed.

4. Radiation, chemotherapy, or their combination; combination therapy appears to have better results.

5. Palliative treatment of dysphagia through dilation done by endoscopy or laser therapy.

6. The goal of palliative treatment is to reduce the complications of the tumor to improve quality of life. Any one or a combination of the aforementioned therapies can be used for palliative treatment.

Complications

1. Preoperatively: Malnutrition, aspiration pneumonitis, hemorrhage, sepsis, and tracheoesophageal fistula.

2. Postoperatively: Pneumonia, dumping syndrome, nutritional deficiencies, reflux esophagitis, and anastomosis leakage.

Nursing Assessment

1. Obtain history of symptoms, such as dysphagia, pain, cough, and hoarseness.

2. Evaluate for dietary changes and weight loss.

3. Assess support system and personal coping mechanisms.

Nursing Diagnoses

- Imbalanced Nutrition: Less Than Body Requirements related to disease process and treatment.

- Risk for Infection related to chronic disease, invasive procedures, and treatment.

- Ineffective Coping related to dealing with cancer.

Nursing Interventions

Improving Nutritional and Fluid Status

1. Provide the preoperative patient with a high-protein, high-calorie diet as tolerated. Nutritional supplements may be indicated. TPN may be ordered if unable to take food or fluids orally.

2. Postoperatively, administer IV fluids as prescribed. Initially, the patient may require large volumes if extensive excision of lymph nodes was performed. TPN may be ordered.

3. Assess for bowel sounds; administer fluids per NG tube and liquid feedings through jejunostomy, as prescribed.

4. Encourage patient in advancing diet from liquids to soft foods.

5. Remind patient to remain in upright position for approximately 2 hours after eating to avoid reflux.

6. Provide mouth care for patient comfort and hygiene.

Monitoring for Complications

1. Monitor blood pressure (BP), pulse, respiration, and temperature to note early onset of hemorrhage, infection, dysrhythmias, aspiration, or anastomosis leakage.

2. Observe drainage from incision and/or chest tube for bleeding or purulence.

3. Monitor arterial blood gas (ABG) levels, manage pain, suction, provide chest physiotherapy, and provide oxygen as indicated.

Strengthening Individual Coping

1. Encourage patient to utilize support system during treatment and recovery process.

2. Provide information about laryngectomy, gastrostomy, and other procedures related to surgery, as indicated.

3. Provide training in relaxation techniques and diversional therapy for anxiety and pain control after surgery.

4. Refer to the American Cancer Society (*www.acs.org*) for additional information and sources of support.

Patient Education and Health Maintenance

1. Encourage the patient to avoid overeating, take small bites, chew food well, and avoid chunks of meat and stringy raw vegetables and fruit.

2. Depending on type of surgery, small, frequent meals may be better tolerated.

3. Encourage rest postoperatively and advancing activities as tolerated.

4. Instruct the patient regarding signs and symptoms of complications to report: nausea, vomiting, elevated temperature, cough, and difficulty swallowing.

Evaluation: Expected Outcomes

- Good skin turgor; eating small, frequent meals; gaining weight.
- Vital signs stable; incision without drainage.
- Performing self-care with the help of support people.

GASTRODUODENAL DISORDERS
Gastrointestinal Bleeding

GI bleeding is not just a gastroduodenal disorder but may occur anywhere along the alimentary tract. Bleeding is a symptom of an upper or lower GI disorder. It may be obvious in emesis or stool, or it may be occult (hidden).

Pathophysiology and Etiology

1. Trauma anywhere along the GI tract.

2. Erosions or ulcers.

3. Rupture of an enlarged vein such as a varicosity (esophageal or gastric varices).

4. Inflammation, such as esophagitis (caused by acid or bile), gastritis, inflammatory bowel disease (chronic ulcerative colitis, Crohn disease), and bacterial infection.

5. Alcohol and drugs (aspirin-containing compounds, NSAIDs, anticoagulants, corticosteroids).

6. Diverticular disease.

7. Cancers.

8. Vascular lesions or disorders, such as bowel ischemia, aortoenteric fistula, and arteriovenous malformations.

9. Mallory-Weiss tear.

10. Anal disorders, such as hemorrhoids or fissures.

Clinical Manifestations

Characteristics of Blood

1. Bright red: vomited from high in the esophagus (hematemesis); passed from the rectum or distal colon (coating stool).

2. Dark red: higher up in the colon and small intestine; mixed with stool.
3. Shades of black ("coffee ground"): vomited from the esophagus, stomach, and duodenum.
4. Tarry stool (melena): occurs in patient who accumulates excessive blood in the stomach.

Signs and Symptoms of Bleeding

1. Massive bleeding.
   a. Acute, bright red hematemesis or large amount of melena with clots in the stool.
   b. Rapid pulse, drop in BP, hypovolemia, and shock.
2. Subacute bleeding.
   a. Intermittent melena or coffee-ground emesis.
   b. Hypotension.
   c. Weakness and dizziness.
3. Chronic bleeding.
   a. Intermittent appearance of blood.
   b. Increased weakness, paleness, or shortness of breath.
   c. Occult blood.
   d. Iron deficiency anemia.

Diagnostic Evaluation

1. It is not difficult to diagnose bleeding, but it may be difficult to locate the source of bleeding.
2. History: change in bowel pattern, presence of pain or tenderness, recent intake of food and what kind (eg, red beets), alcohol consumption, and drugs (eg, aspirin or steroids).
3. Complete blood count (CBC) (hemoglobin, hematocrit, platelets) and coagulation studies (partial thromboplastin time, prothrombin time with international normalized ratio) may show abnormalities.
4. An NG tube may be used to determine if bleeding is occurring in the upper GI tract; however, there is not good evidence to support this practice and its utility is falling by the wayside.
5. Endoscopy: identifies source of bleeding, determines risk of rebleeding, and provides endoscopic therapy, if needed.
6. Colonoscopy: identifies source of lower GI bleeding and allows for therapy if needed.
7. Imaging may detect cause of bleeding.
8. Test of stool for occult blood.

Management

Based on Etiology

1. If aspirin or NSAIDs are the cause, discontinue medication and treat bleeding.
2. If ulcer is the cause, assess medications, dietary and lifestyle modifications, and for *Helicobacter pylori*.
3. Therapeutic endoscopic procedure (cautery, injection).
4. Surgery may be indicated for cancers, inflammatory diseases, and vascular disorders.

Emergency Intervention

1. Patient remains on NPO status.
2. IV lines and oxygen therapy initiated.
3. If life-threatening bleeding occurs, treat shock; administer blood replacement, intra-arterial vasopressin or embolization.
4. Surgical therapy, if indicated.

Other Measures

1. Electrocoagulation using a heater probe.
2. Injection of sclerosant or epinephrine.
3. Banding or clips.

4. Intravenous PPIs are sometimes used to reduce risk of rebleeding.
5. IV antibiotics may be given to reduce risk for secondary infections, which can occur after GI bleeding, and thereby reduce risk for mortality.
6. Beta-blockers may be given to reduce rebleeding risk in those with esophageal/gastric varices.
7. Surgery is indicated when more conservative measures fail.

Complications

1. Hemorrhage.
2. Shock.
3. Death.
4. Infection.

Nursing Assessment

1. Obtain history regarding:
   a. Change in bowel patterns or hemorrhoids.
   b. Change in color of stools (dark black, red, or streaked with blood).
   c. Alcohol consumption.
   d. Medications, such as aspirin, NSAIDs, antibiotics, anticoagulants, and corticosteroids.
   e. Hematemesis.
   f. Other medical conditions.
2. Evaluate for presence of abdominal pain or tenderness.
3. Monitor vital signs and laboratory tests for changes that indicate bleeding (hemoglobin, hematocrit, platelet count, coagulation studies).
4. Test for occult blood, if indicated.
5. Assess output as renal perfusion may be affected.

Nursing Diagnoses

- Deficient Fluid Volume related to blood loss.
- Imbalanced Nutrition: Less Than Body Requirements related to nausea, vomiting, and diarrhea.

Nursing Interventions

Attaining Normal Fluid Volume

1. Maintain NG tube and NPO status to rest GI tract and evaluate bleeding.
2. Monitor intake and output, as ordered, to evaluate fluid status.
3. Monitor vital signs, as ordered.
4. Observe for changes indicating shock, such as tachycardia, hypotension, increased respirations, decreased urine output, and change in mental status.
5. Administer IV fluids and blood products, as ordered, to maintain volume.

Attaining Balanced Nutritional Status

1. Weigh daily to monitor caloric status.
2. Administer IV fluids, TPN, if ordered, to promote hydration and nutrition while on oral restrictions.
3. Begin liquids when patient is no longer NPO. Advance diet as tolerated. Diet should be high-calorie and high-protein. Small, frequent feedings may be indicated.
4. Offer snacks; high-protein supplements.

Patient Education and Health Maintenance

1. Discuss the cause and treatment of GI bleeding with patient.

2. Instruct patient on reporting signs and symptoms of GI bleeding: melena, emesis that is bright red or "coffee-ground" color, rectal bleeding, weakness, fatigue, and shortness of breath.

3. Instruct patient on how to test stool or emesis for occult blood, if applicable.

Evaluation: Expected Outcomes

• Intake and output equal; vital signs stable.
• Tolerates small feedings; weight stable.

Peptic Ulcer Disease

Peptic ulcer disease refers to ulcerations in the mucosa of the lower esophagus, stomach, or duodenum (see Figure 18-6).

Pathophysiology and Etiology

1. Etiology of peptic ulcer disease is multifactorial.
   a. *H. pylori* infection—present in most patients with peptic ulcer disease.
   b. NSAID-induced injury—presents as a chemical gastropathy.
   c. Acid secretory abnormalities (especially in duodenal ulcers).
   d. Zollinger-Ellison syndrome (hypersecretory syndrome) should be considered in refractory ulcers.
2. Risk factors may include drugs (NSAIDs, prolonged high-dose corticosteroids), family history, Zollinger-Ellison syndrome, cigarettes, stress, O blood type, and lower socioeconomic status.
3. Studies are inconclusive in determining an association between ulcer formation and diet or the intake of alcohol and caffeine.

Clinical Manifestations

1. Gnawing or burning epigastric pain occurring 1½ to 3 hours after a meal.
2. Nocturnal epigastric, abdominal pain or burning; may awaken patient at night, usually around midnight to 3 A.M.
3. Epigastric tenderness on examination.
4. Early satiety, anorexia, weight loss, heartburn, and belching (may indicate reflux disease).

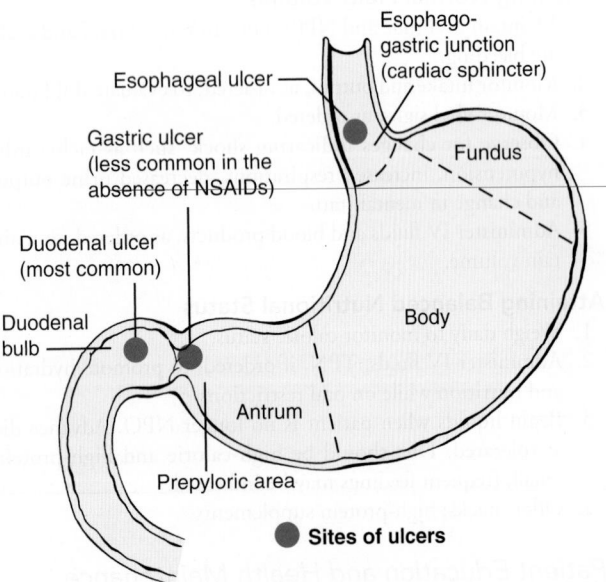

Figure 18-6. Esophageal, gastric, and duodenal ulcer sites.

5. Dizziness, syncope, hematemesis, or melena (may indicate hemorrhage).
6. Anemia.

 NURSING ALERT Sudden, intense midepigastric pain radiating to the right shoulder may indicate ulcer perforation.

Diagnostic Evaluation

1. Upper GI endoscopy with possible tissue biopsy and cytology.
   a. PyloriTek, a biopsy urea test, is up to greater than 97% specific and greater than 96% sensitive for detection of *H. pylori*.
   b. Point-of-service test with results within 1 hour.

 EVIDENCE BASE Serim Research Corporation. (2012). PyloriTek for *H. pylori*. Available: *www.serim.com/products_overview.aspx?fid=2*.

2. Upper GI radiographic examination (barium study).
3. Serial stool specimens to detect occult blood.
4. Gastric secretory studies (gastric acid secretion test and fasting serum gastrin level)—elevated in Zollinger-Ellison syndrome.
5. Serology to test for *H. pylori* antibodies or stool test to assess for *H. pylori* antigen.
6. C-urea breath test to detect *H. pylori*.

 DRUG ALERT Stop antisecretory PPI at least 2 weeks before the C-urea breath test. It can cause false-negative test result.

Management

General Measures

1. Eliminate use of NSAIDs or other causative drugs.
2. Eliminate cigarette smoking (impairs healing).
3. A well-balanced diet with meals at regular intervals. Avoid dietary irritants.

Drug Therapy

Multiple drug regimens are used to treat *H. pylori* (see Table 18-2, page 511), usually involving triple therapy with two antibiotics and a proton pump inhibitor for 10 to 14 days to eradicate the bacteria.

 DRUG ALERT Antibiotic resistance is a problem that has led to longer therapy and research into alternative drug regimens.

Surgery

1. Surgical interventions may be indicated for hemorrhage, obstruction, perforation, and acid reduction (see Figure 18-7, page 511). Surgery may also be indicated with ulcer disease of long duration or severity or difficulty with medical regimen compliance.
2. Gastroduodenostomy (Billroth I).
   a. Partial gastrectomy with removal of antrum and pylorus of the stomach.
   b. The gastric stump is anastomosed with the duodenum.
3. Gastrojejunostomy (Billroth II).
   a. Partial gastrectomy with removal of antrum and pylorus of the stomach.
   b. The gastric stump is anastomosed with the jejunum.

Table 18-2 Medication Considerations for *H. pylori* Therapy

COMMON DRUG REGIMEN	DOSING	NURSING CONSIDERATIONS
Omeprazole 20 mg	bid × 14 d	• Antibiotics: Metronidazole and clarithromycin may cause unpleasant metallic taste, nausea, and vomiting; it may help to eat small, frequent meals, suck on sugar-free candy, take with food.
Amoxicillin 1,000 mg	bid × 14 d	
Clarithromycin 500 mg	bid × 14 d	
PPI (standard dose)	bid × 10 to 14 d	Avoid alcohol within 72 hours of taking metronidazole; can cause severe reaction. Clarithromycin may interact with lovastatin, salmeterol, phenytoin, and other medications; do not drink grapefruit juice during therapy.
Bismuth subsalicylate 300 mg	qid × 10 to 14 d	
Metronidazole 250 mg	qid × 10 to 14 d	
Tetracycline 500 mg	qid × 10 to 14 d	Tetracycline may increase sensitivity to sun; food and dairy products decrease absorption.

Report inability to take antibiotic or vomiting doses.

Report watery or bloody diarrhea, which may indicate pseudomembranous colitis.

• Proton pump inhibitors: may cause dizziness, headache, and stomach upset.

Best taken before meals.

Do not take with certain drugs such as antiepileptics and warfarin.

• Bismuth subsalicylate: Interacts with many drugs such as antiepileptics, salicylates, corticosteroids.

May turn stool black.

May interfere with radiologic testing of the GI tract.

Report ringing in the ears may indicate salicylate toxicity.

DRUG ALERT Avoid treatment if patient may be pregnant.

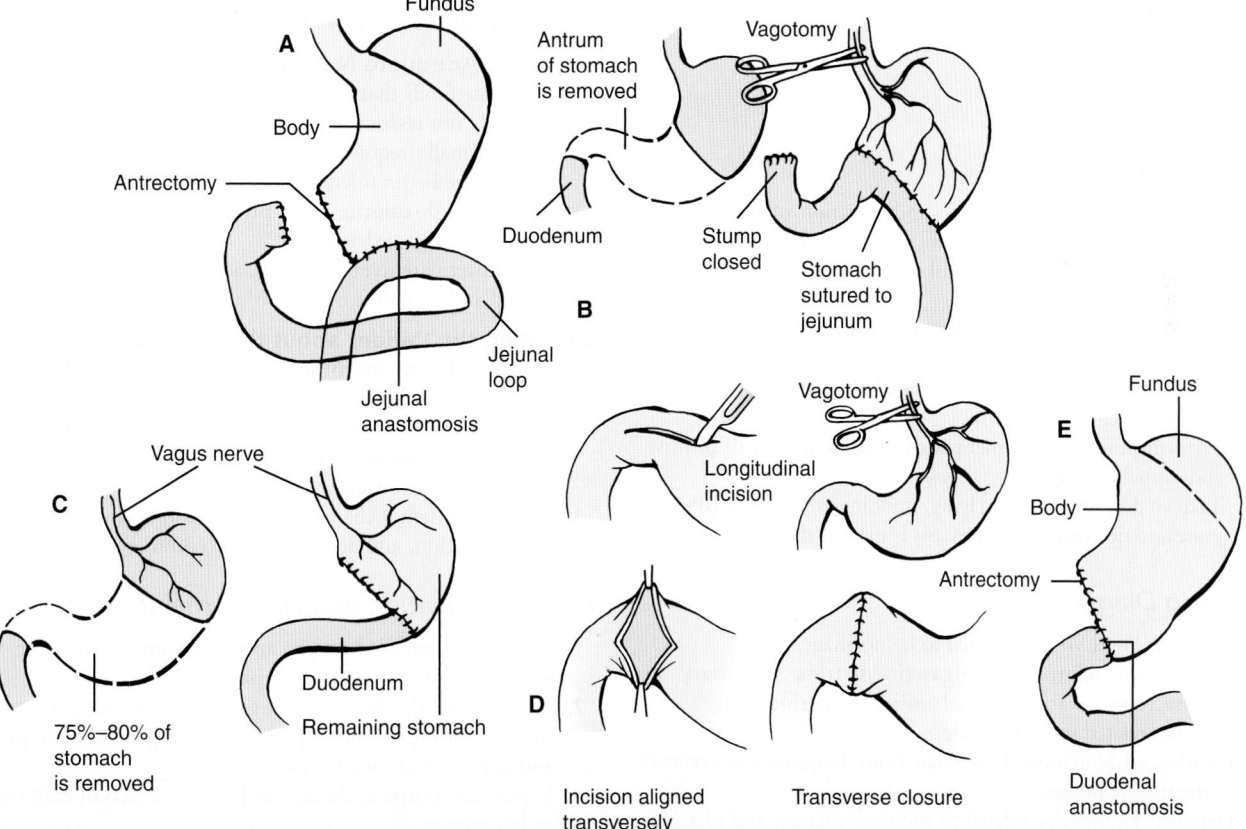

Figure 18-7. Surgical procedures for peptic ulcer. **(A)** Gastrojejunostomy (Billroth II). The jejunum is anastomosed to the gastric stump after a partial gastrectomy (removal of antrum and pylorus). **(B)** Antrectomy and vagotomy. The resected portion includes a small cuff of the duodenum, the pylorus, and the antrum (about one half of the stomach). The stump of the duodenum is closed by suture, and the side of the jejunum is anastomosed to the cut end of the stomach. **(C)** Subtotal gastrectomy. The resected portion includes a small cuff of the duodenum, the pylorus, and from two thirds to three quarters of the stomach. The duodenum or side of the jejunum is anastomosed to the remaining portion of the stomach. **(D)** Vagotomy and pyloroplasty. A longitudinal incision is made in the pylorus, and it is closed transversely to permit the muscle to relax and to establish an enlarged outlet. This compensates for the impaired gastric emptying produced by vagotomy. **(E)** Gastroduodenostomy (Billroth I). The duodenum is anastomosed to the gastric stump after removal of the antrum and pylorus (partial gastrectomy).

4. Antrectomy.
   a. Gastric resection includes a small cuff of duodenum, the pylorus, and the antrum (lower half of the stomach).
   b. The duodenal stump is closed and the jejunum is anastomosed to the stomach.
5. Total gastrectomy.
   a. Also called an esophagojejunostomy.
   b. Removal of the stomach with attachment of the esophagus to the jejunum or duodenum.
6. Pyloroplasty.
   a. A longitudinal incision is made in the pylorus, and it is closed transversely to permit the muscle to relax and to establish an enlarged outlet.
   b. Often, a vagotomy is performed at the same time.
7. Vagotomy.
   a. The surgical division of the vagus nerve to eliminate the impulses that stimulate HCL secretion.
   b. There are three types: *selective vagotomy*, which severs only the branches that interrupt acid secretion; *truncal vagotomy*, which severs the anterior and posterior trunks to decrease acid secretion and gastric motility; and *parietal vagotomy*, which severs only the part of vagus that innervates the parietal acid–secreting cells.
   c. Traditionally performed by laparotomy, the vagotomy procedure can also be done using a laparoscope.

Complications

1. GI hemorrhage.
2. Ulcer perforation.
3. Gastric outlet obstruction.

Nursing Assessment

1. Determine location, character, and radiation of pain, factors aggravating or relieving pain, how long it lasts, and when it occurs.
2. Ask about eating patterns, regularity, types of food, and eating circumstances.
3. Ask about medications (especially aspirin, steroids, or anti-inflammatory drugs).
4. Inquire about a history of illnesses, including previous GI bleeds.
5. Obtain psychosocial history.
6. Perform physical assessment with documentation of positive abdominal findings.
7. Take vital signs, including lying, standing, and sitting BPs and pulses, to determine if orthostasis is present due to bleeding.

Nursing Diagnoses

- Deficient Fluid Volume related to hemorrhage.
- Acute Pain related to epigastric distress secondary to hypersecretion of acid, mucosal erosion, or perforation.
- Diarrhea related to GI bleeding.
- Imbalanced Nutrition: Less Than Body Requirements related to the disease process.
- Deficient Knowledge related to physical, dietary, and pharmacologic treatment of disease.

Nursing Interventions

Avoiding Fluid Volume Deficit

1. Monitor intake and output continuously to determine fluid volume status.

2. Monitor stools for blood and emesis.
3. Monitor hemoglobin and hematocrit and electrolytes.
4. Administer prescribed IV fluids and blood replacement, as prescribed.
5. Insert NG tube as prescribed, and monitor the tube drainage for signs of visible and occult blood.
6. Administer medications through the NG tube to neutralize acidity, as prescribed.
7. Prepare the patient for saline lavage, as ordered.
8. Observe the patient for an increase in pulse and a decrease in BP (signs of shock).
9. Prepare the patient for diagnostic procedure or surgery to determine or stop the source of bleeding.

Achieving Pain Relief

1. Administer prescribed medication.
2. Provide small, frequent meals to prevent gastric distention if not NPO.
3. Advise the patient about the irritating effects of certain drugs and foods.

Decreasing Diarrhea

1. Monitor the patient's elimination patterns to determine effects of medications.
2. Monitor vital signs and watch for signs of hypovolemia.
3. Administer antidiarrheal medication as prescribed.
4. Watch for signs and symptoms of impaired skin integrity (erythema, pain, pruritus) around the anus to promote comfort and decrease risk of infection.

Achieving Adequate Nutrition

1. Eliminate foods that cause pain or distress; otherwise, the diet is usually not restricted.
2. Provide small, frequent meals that neutralize gastric secretions and may be better tolerated.
3. Provide high-calorie, high-protein diet with nutritional supplements, as ordered.
4. Administer parenteral nutrition, as ordered, if bleeding is prolonged and patient is malnourished.

Educating the Patient about the Treatment Regimen

1. Explain all tests and procedures to increase knowledge and cooperation and minimize anxiety.
2. Review the health care provider's recommendations for diet, activity, medication, and treatment. Allow time for questions and clarify any misunderstandings.
3. Give the patient a chart listing medications, dosages, times of administration, and desired effects to promote compliance.

Patient Education and Health Maintenance

1. Teach the patient the signs and symptoms of bleeding and when to notify the health care provider.
2. Promote healthy lifestyle changes to include adequate nutrition, cessation of smoking, decreased alcohol consumption, and stress reduction strategies.
3. Explain the purpose, dosage, and adverse effects of each medication prescribed.

Evaluation: Expected Outcomes

- Vital signs stable; fluid volume maintained.
- Pain free.
- No more than two to three loose stools per day.
- Eats small, frequent meals each day; reports no loss of weight.

- Describes peptic ulcer disease, its treatment, and complications; complies with treatment regimen.

Gastric Cancer

Malignant tumor of the stomach.

Pathophysiology and Etiology

1. Risk factors include:
   a. Chronic atrophic gastritis with intestinal metaplasia.
   b. Pernicious anemia or having had gastric resections (more than 15 years).
   c. Gastric adenomatous polyps (more common in men).
   d. Incidence increases with age.
   e. Cigarette smoking.
   f. Family history of gastric cancer.

Clinical Manifestations

1. Typically, patient presents with same symptoms as gastric ulcer; later, on evaluation, the lesion is found to be malignant.
2. Progressive loss of appetite, noticeable change in or appearance of common GI symptoms—gastric fullness (early satiety) and dyspepsia lasting longer than 4 weeks.
3. Blood (usually occult) in the stools.
4. Vomiting—may indicate pyloric obstruction or cardiac–orifice obstruction. Occasionally, vomiting has a coffee-ground appearance because of slow leaks of blood from ulceration of the cancer.
5. Later manifestations include the following:
   a. Pain, usually induced by eating and relieved by vomiting.
   b. Weight loss, loss of strength, anemia, metastasis (usually to the liver), hemorrhage, and obstruction.
   c. Abdominal or epigastric mass.

Diagnostic Evaluation

1. History—weight loss and fatigue over several months.
2. Upper GI radiography and endoscopy—afford visualization and provide means for obtaining tissue samples for histologic and cytologic review.
3. Imaging, such as bone or liver scan—may determine extent of disease.

Management

1. The only successful treatment of gastric cancer is surgical removal. Gastric resection is surgical removal of part of the stomach.
2. If tumor has spread beyond the area that can be excised surgically, cure is not possible.
   a. Palliative surgery, such as subtotal gastrectomy with or without gastroenterostomy, may be performed to maintain continuity of the GI tract.
   b. Surgery may be combined with chemotherapy to provide palliation and prolong life.

Complications

1. If surgery is performed, possible risk of hemorrhage or infection.
2. Dumping syndrome following gastrectomy.
3. Metastasis and death.

Nursing Assessment

1. Assess for anorexia, weight loss, and GI symptoms (gastric fullness, dyspepsia, vomiting).
2. Evaluate for pain, noting characteristics/location.
3. Check stool for occult blood.
4. Monitor CBC to assess for anemia.

Nursing Diagnoses

- Pain related to disease process or surgery.
- Risk for Injury, Shock, and Other Complications related to surgery and impaired gastric tissue function.
- Imbalanced Nutrition: Less Than Body Requirements related to malignancy and treatment.

Nursing Interventions

Promoting Comfort and Wound Healing

1. Turning, coughing, and deep breathing every 2 hours to prevent vascular and pulmonary complications and promote comfort.
2. Institute NG suction, if ordered, to remove fluids and gas in the stomach and prevent painful distention.
3. Administer parenteral antibiotics, as ordered, to prevent infection.
4. Administer analgesics, as ordered.

Preventing Shock and Other Complications

1. Shock and hemorrhage.
   a. Monitor changes in BP, pulse, and respiration.
   b. Observe the patient for evidence of changes in mental status, pallor, clammy skin, and dizziness.
   c. Check the dressings and suction canister frequently for evidence of bleeding.
   d. Administer IV infusions and blood replacement, as prescribed.
2. Cardiopulmonary complications.
   a. Encourage the patient to cough and take deep breaths to promote ventilatory exchange and enhance circulation.
   b. Assist the patient to turn and move, thereby mobilizing secretions.
   c. Promote ambulation, as prescribed, to increase respiratory exchange.
3. Thrombosis and embolism.
   a. Initiate a plan of self-care activities to promote circulation.
   b. Encourage early ambulation to stimulate circulation.
   c. Prevent venous stasis by use of elastic stockings, if indicated.
   d. Check for tight dressings or binder that might restrict circulation.
4. Dumping syndrome—a complex reaction that may occur because of excessively rapid emptying of gastric contents. Manifestations include nausea, weakness, perspiration, palpitation, some syncope, and possibly diarrhea. Instruct the patient as follows:
   a. Eat small, frequent meals rather than three large meals.
   b. Suggest a diet high in protein and fat and low in carbohydrates, and avoid meals high in sugars, milk, chocolate, and salt.
   c. Reduce fluids with meals, but take them between meals.
   d. Take anticholinergic medication before meals (if prescribed) to lessen GI activity.
   e. Relax when eating; eat slowly and regularly.
   f. Take a rest after meals.

5. Phytobezoar formation (formation of gastric concretion composed of vegetable matter) can be seen with partial gastrectomy and vagotomy. After a gastric resection, the remaining gastric tissue is not able to disintegrate and digest fibrous foods. This undigested fiber congeals to form masses that become coated by mucus secretions of the stomach.
   a. Avoid fibrous foods, such as citrus fruits (skins and seeds), because they tend to form phytobezoars.
   b. Stress the importance of adequate chewing.

Attaining Adequate Nutritional Status
1. Administer parenteral nutrition, if ordered.
2. Follow prescribed diet progressions.
   a. Give fluids by mouth when audible bowel signs are present.
   b. Increase fluids according to the patient's tolerance.
   c. Offer a diet with vitamin supplements when the patient's condition permits.
   d. Avoid high-carbohydrate foods, such as milk, which may trigger dumping syndrome.
   e. Offer diet, as prescribed—usually high in protein and calories to promote wound healing.

Patient Education and Health Maintenance

1. Emphasize the importance of coping with stressful situations. Provide information about support groups.
2. Review nutritional requirements with the patient.
3. Stress the importance of IM vitamin B_{12} supplements after gastrectomy to prevent surgically induced pernicious anemia.
4. Encourage follow-up visits with the health care provider.
5. Recommend annual blood studies and medical checkups for any evidence of pernicious anemia or other problems.
6. Instruct on measures to prevent dumping syndrome.

Evaluation: Expected Outcomes

- States pain decreased to 2 or 3 on 0 to 10 scale.
- Vital signs stable; no evidence of complications.
- Tolerating small, frequent meals.

Intestinal Conditions

Abdominal Hernias

An abdominal hernia occurs when the contents of the abdomen, usually the small intestine, push through a weak point in the muscular wall of the abdomen. The weakness of the abdominal wall can be congenital in nature, because of acquired weakness (eg, aging or trauma) or because of increased intra-abdominal pressure (eg, because of heavy lifting, obesity, pregnancy, straining, coughing, ascites, or proximity to tumor).

Pathophysiology and Etiology

Classification by Site
1. Inguinal—a hernia into the inguinal canal that is more common in males (see Figure 18-8). This type of hernia is further differentiated based on the causative factor.
   a. Indirect inguinal—congenital hernia that occurs when the entrance of the inguinal canal does not close after birth, causing a weakness in the abdominal wall. Through this weakened area, the hernia extends down the inguinal canal and often into the scrotum or labia.

Figure 18-8. Direct and indirect inguinal hernia. (Bickley, L. [2003]. *Bates' guide to physical examination and history taking* [8th ed.]. Philadelphia, PA: Lippincott Williams & Wilkins.)

   b. Direct inguinal—caused by degeneration of the abdominal muscles allowing the small intestine to pass through the posterior inguinal wall into the groin.
2. Femoral—hernia follows the tract below the inguinal ligament through the femoral canal.
3. Umbilical—intestinal protrusion at the umbilicus because of failure of umbilical orifice to close. Occurs most often in obese women, in children, and in patients with increased intra-abdominal pressure from cirrhosis and ascites.
4. Ventral or incisional—intestinal protrusion because of weakness at the abdominal wall; may occur after impaired incisional healing because of infection or drainage.
5. Peristomal—hernia through the fascial defect around a stoma and into the subcutaneous tissue.

Classification by Severity
1. Reducible—the protruding mass can be placed back into the abdominal cavity.
2. Irreducible—the protruding mass cannot be moved back into the abdomen.
3. Incarcerated—an irreducible hernia in which the intestinal flow is completely obstructed.
4. Strangulated—an irreducible hernia in which the blood and intestinal flow are completely obstructed; develops when the loop of the intestine in the sac becomes twisted or swollen and a constriction is produced at the neck of the sac.

Clinical Manifestations

1. Bulging over herniated area appears when the patient stands or strains and disappears when supine.
2. Hernia tends to increase in size and recurs with intra-abdominal pressure.
3. Strangulated hernia presents with pain, vomiting, swelling of hernial sac, lower abdominal signs of peritoneal irritation, and fever.

Diagnostic Evaluation

1. Usually diagnosed by clinical manifestations:
2. Abdominal x-rays—reveal abnormally high levels of gas in the bowel.
3. Laboratory studies (complete blood count, electrolytes)—may show hemoconcentration (increased hematocrit), dehydration (increased or decreased sodium), and elevated white blood cell (WBC) count, if strangulated.

Management

1. Mechanical (reducible hernia only).
   a. A truss is an appliance with a pad and belt that is held snugly over a hernia to prevent abdominal contents from entering the hernial sac. A truss provides external compression over the defect and should be removed at night and reapplied in the morning before patient arises. This nonsurgical approach may be used only when a patient is not a surgical candidate.
   b. Peristomal hernia is often managed with a hernia support belt with Velcro, which is placed around an ostomy pouching system (similar to a truss).
   c. Conservative measures—no heavy lifting, straining at stool, or other measures that would increase intra-abdominal pressure.
2. Surgical—recommended to correct hernia before strangulation occurs, which then becomes an emergency situation.
   a. Herniorrhaphy—removal of hernial sac; contents replaced into the abdomen; layers of muscle and fascia sutured. Laparoscopic herniorrhaphy is a possibility and often performed as outpatient procedure.
   b. Hernioplasty involves reinforcement of suturing (often with mesh) for extensive hernia repair.
   c. Strangulated hernia requires resection of ischemic bowel in addition to repair of hernia.

Complications

1. Bowel obstruction.
2. Recurrence of hernia.

Nursing Assessment

1. Ask the patient if hernia is enlarging and uncomfortable, reducible or irreducible; determine relationship to exertion and activities.
2. Assess bowel sounds and determine bowel pattern.
3. Determine if the patient is exhibiting signs and symptoms of strangulation, such as distention, fever, nausea, and vomiting.

Nursing Diagnoses

- Chronic Pain related to bulging hernia (mechanical).
- Acute Pain related to surgical procedure.
- Risk for Infection related to emergency procedure for strangulated or incarcerated hernia.

Nursing Interventions

Achieving Comfort

1. Fit the patient with truss or belt when hernia is reduced, if ordered.
2. Trendelenburg position may reduce pressure on hernia, when appropriate.
3. Emphasize to the patient to wear truss under clothing and to apply before getting out of bed when hernia is reduced.
4. Give stool softeners, as directed.
5. Evaluate for signs and symptoms of hernial incarceration or strangulation.
6. Insert NG tube for incarcerated hernia, if ordered, to relieve intra-abdominal pressure on herniated sac.

Relieving Pain Postoperatively

1. Have the patient splint the incision site with hand or pillow when coughing to lessen pain and protect site from increased intra-abdominal pressure.
2. Administer analgesics, as ordered.
3. Teach about bed rest, intermittent ice packs, and scrotal elevation as measures used to reduce scrotal edema or swelling after repair of an inguinal hernia.
4. Encourage ambulation as soon as permitted.
5. Advise the patient that difficulty in urinating is common after surgery; promote elimination to avoid discomfort, and catheterize if necessary.

Preventing Infection

1. Check dressing for drainage and incision for redness and swelling.
2. Monitor for other signs and symptoms of infection: fever, chills, malaise, and diaphoresis.
3. Administer antibiotics, if appropriate.

Patient Education and Health Maintenance

1. Advise that pain and scrotal swelling may be present for 24 to 48 hours after repair of an inguinal hernia.
   a. Apply ice intermittently.
   b. Elevate scrotum and use scrotal support.
   c. Take medication prescribed to relieve discomfort.
2. Teach to monitor self for signs of infection: pain, drainage from incision, and temperature elevation. Also, report continued difficulty in voiding.
3. Inform that heavy lifting should be avoided for 4 to 6 weeks. Athletics and extremes of exertion are to be avoided for 8 to 12 weeks postoperatively, per provider instructions.

Evaluation: Expected Outcomes

- Hernia effectively reduced with truss or belt; patient comfortable.
- Verbalizes pain decreased to 2 or 3 on 0 to 10 scale.
- No swelling present; afebrile and no drainage from incision.

Intestinal Obstruction

Intestinal obstruction is an interruption in the normal flow of intestinal contents along the intestinal tract. The block may occur in the small or large intestine, may be complete or incomplete, may be mechanical or paralytic, and may or may not compromise the vascular supply. Obstruction most frequently occurs in the young and the old.

Pathophysiology and Etiology

Types and Causes

1. Mechanical obstruction—a physical block to passage of intestinal contents without disturbing blood supply of the bowel. High small bowel (jejunal) or low small bowel (ileal) obstruction occurs four times more frequently than colonic obstruction (see Figure 18-9). Causes include:
   a. Extrinsic—adhesions from surgery, hernia, wound dehiscence, masses, volvulus (twisted loop of the intestine). Up to 70% of small bowel obstructions are caused by adhesions.
   b. Intrinsic—hematoma, tumor, intussusception (telescoping of intestinal wall into itself), stricture or stenosis, congenital conditions (atresia, imperforate anus), trauma, inflammatory diseases (Crohn, diverticulitis, ulcerative colitis).
   c. Intraluminal—foreign body, fecal or barium impaction, polyp, gallstones, meconium in infants.

Figure 18-9. Three causes of intestinal obstruction. **(A)** Intussusception. Note shortening of the colon by the movement of one segment of the bowel into another. **(B)** Volvulus of the sigmoid colon. The twist is counterclockwise in most cases of sigmoid volvulus. **(C)** Hernia (inguinal). Note that the sac of the hernia is a continuation of the peritoneum of the abdomen and that the hernial contents are the intestine, omentum, or other abdominal contents that pass through the hernial opening into the hernial sac.

Labels on figure C:
- Small intestine
- Peritoneum
- Hernial sac
- Testicle

  d. In postoperative patients, approximately 90% of mechanical obstructions are due to adhesions. In nonsurgical patients, hernia (most often inguinal) is the most common cause of mechanical obstruction.
2. Paralytic (adynamic, neurogenic) ileus.
  a. Peristalsis is ineffective (diminished motor activity perhaps because of toxic or traumatic disturbance of the autonomic nervous system).
  b. There is no physical obstruction and no interrupted blood supply.
  c. Disappears spontaneously after 2 to 3 days.
  d. Causes include:
    i. Spinal cord injuries; vertebral fractures.
    ii. Postoperatively after any abdominal surgery.
    iii. Peritonitis, pneumonia.
    iv. Wound dehiscence (breakdown).
    v. GI tract surgery.
3. Strangulation—obstruction compromises blood supply, leading to gangrene of the intestinal wall. Caused by prolonged mechanical obstruction.

Altered Physiology

1. Increased peristalsis, distention by fluid and gas, and increased bacterial growth proximal to obstruction. The intestine empties distally.
2. Increased secretions into the intestine are associated with diminution in the bowel's absorptive capacity.
3. The accumulation of gases, secretions, and oral intake above the obstruction causes increasing intraluminal pressure.
4. Venous pressure in the affected area increases and circulatory stasis and edema result.
5. Bowel necrosis may occur because of anoxia and compression of the terminal branches of the mesenteric artery.
6. Bacteria and toxins pass across the intestinal membranes into the abdominal cavity, thereby leading to peritonitis.
7. "Closed loop" obstruction is a condition in which the intestinal segment is occluded at both ends, preventing either the downward passage or the regurgitation of intestinal contents.

Clinical Manifestations

Fever, peritoneal irritation, increased WBC count, toxicity, and shock may develop with all types of intestinal obstruction.
1. Simple mechanical—high small bowel: colic (cramps); mid- to upper abdomen, some distention, early bilious vomiting, increased bowel sounds (high-pitched tinkling heard at brief intervals), minimal diffuse tenderness.
2. Simple mechanical—low small bowel: significant colic (cramps), midabdominal, considerable distention, vomiting slight or absent, later feculent, increased bowel sounds and "hush" sounds, minimal diffuse tenderness.
3. Simple mechanical—colon: cramps (mid- to lower abdomen), later-appearing distention, and then vomiting may develop (feculent); increase in bowel sounds; minimal diffuse tenderness.
4. Partial chronic mechanical—may occur with granulomatous bowel in Crohn disease. Symptoms are cramping, abdominal pain, mild distention, and diarrhea.
5. Strangulation symptoms are initially those of mechanical obstruction, but progress rapidly—pain is severe, continuous, and localized. There is moderate distention, persistent vomiting, usually decreased bowel sounds, and marked localized tenderness. Stools or vomitus becomes bloody or contains occult blood.

Diagnostic Evaluation

1. Fecal material aspiration from NG tube.
2. Abdominal and chest x-rays.
  a. May show presence and location of small or large intestinal distention, gas, or fluid.
  b. "Bird beak" lesion in colonic volvulus.
  c. Foreign body visualization.
3. Contrast studies—small bowel follow-through with water-soluble contrast (eg, Gastrografin) can be both diagnostic and therapeutic.
4. Laboratory tests.
  a. Electrolytes, BUN, and creatinine may be abnormal because of hypovolemia and vomiting.
  b. Elevated WBC counts because of inflammation; marked increase with necrosis, strangulation, or peritonitis.
  c. Lactate level may be increased if ischemia of small bowel is present.
5. Flexible sigmoidoscopy or colonoscopy may identify the source of the obstruction such as tumor or stricture.

Management

Nonsurgical Management

1. Correction of fluid and electrolyte imbalances with normal saline or Ringer solution with potassium as required.
2. NG suction to decompress bowel and decrease risk of perforation.
3. Treatment of shock and peritonitis.
4. TPN may be necessary to correct protein deficiency from chronic obstruction, paralytic ileus, or infection.
5. Analgesics and sedatives, avoiding opiates because of GI motility inhibition.
6. Antibiotics to prevent or treat infection.
7. Ambulation for patients with paralytic ileus to encourage return of peristalsis.

Surgery

Consists of relieving obstruction. Options include:
1. Closed bowel procedures: lysis of adhesions, reduction of volvulus, intussusception, or incarcerated hernia.
2. Enterotomy for removal of foreign bodies or bezoars.

3. Resection of the bowel for obstructing lesions or strangulated bowel with end-to-end anastomosis.
4. Intestinal bypass around obstruction.
5. Temporary ostomy may be indicated (see "Caring for the Patient Undergoing Ostomy Surgery," page 498).

Complications

1. Dehydration because of loss of water, sodium, and chloride.
2. Peritonitis.
3. Shock because of loss of electrolytes and dehydration.
4. Death because of shock.

Nursing Assessment

1. Assess the nature and location of the patient's pain and the presence or absence of distention, flatus, defecation, emesis, and obstipation.
2. Listen for high-pitched bowel sounds, peristaltic rushes, or absence of bowel sounds.
3. Assess vital signs.

GERONTOLOGIC ALERT Watch for air–fluid lock syndrome in older patients, who typically remain in the recumbent position for extended periods. Fluid collects in dependent bowel loops and peristalsis is too weak to push fluid "uphill." Conduct frequent checks of the patient's level of responsiveness; decreasing responsiveness may offer a clue to an increasing electrolyte imbalance or impending shock.

Nursing Diagnoses

- Acute Pain related to obstruction, distention, and strangulation.
- Risk for Deficient Fluid Volume related to impaired fluid intake, vomiting, and diarrhea from intestinal obstruction.
- Ineffective Breathing Pattern related to abdominal distention, interfering with normal lung expansion.
- Risk for Ineffective Gastrointestinal Perfusion.

Nursing Interventions

Achieving Pain Relief

1. Administer prescribed analgesics.
2. Provide supportive care during NG intubation to assist with discomfort.
3. To relieve air–fluid lock syndrome, turn the patient from supine to prone position every 10 minutes until enough flatus is passed to decompress the abdomen. A rectal tube may be indicated.
4. To reduce fear and anxiety associated with pain, recognize the patient's concerns and initiate measures to provide emotional support. Encourage presence of support person.

Maintaining Electrolyte and Fluid Balance

1. Measure and record all intake and output.
2. Administer IV fluids and parenteral nutrition as prescribed.
3. Monitor electrolytes, urinalysis, hemoglobin, and blood cell counts, and report any abnormalities. Collect stool samples to test for occult blood, if ordered.
4. Monitor urine output to assess renal function and to detect urine retention because of bladder compressions by the distended intestine.
5. Monitor vital signs; a drop in BP may indicate decreased circulatory volume because of blood loss from strangulated hernia.
6. Record amount and consistency of stools.

Maintaining Proper Lung Ventilation

1. Keep the patient in Fowler position to promote ventilation and relieve abdominal distention.
2. Maintain NG tube as prescribed to decompress bowel.
3. Monitor ABG levels for oxygenation levels, if ordered.

Ensuring Gastrointestinal Perfusion to Prevent Complications

1. Prevent infarction by carefully assessing the patient's status; pain that increases in intensity or becomes localized or continuous may herald strangulation.
2. Detect early signs of peritonitis, such as rigidity and tenderness, in an effort to minimize this complication.
3. Avoid enemas, which may distort an x-ray or make a partial obstruction worse.
4. Observe for signs of shock—pallor, tachycardia, hypotension.
5. Watch for signs of:
   a. Metabolic alkalosis (slow, shallow respirations; changes in sensorium; tetany).
   b. Metabolic acidosis (disorientation; deep, rapid breathing; weakness; and shortness of breath on exertion).

Patient Education and Health Maintenance

1. Explain the rationale for NG suction, NPO status, and IV fluids initially. Advise the patient to progress diet slowly as tolerated once home.
2. Advise plenty of rest and slow progression of activity as directed by surgeon or other health care provider.
3. Teach wound care, if indicated.
4. Encourage the patient to follow-up as directed and to call surgeon or health care provider if increasing abdominal pain, vomiting, or fever occurs prior to follow-up.

Evaluation: Expected Outcomes

- Maintains position of comfort; states pain decreased to 3 or 4 on 0 to 10 scale.
- Urine output greater than 30 mL/hour; vital signs stable.
- Respirations 24 breaths/minute and unlabored with head of bed elevated 45 degrees.
- Alert, lucid, vital signs stable, abdomen firm, not rigid.

Appendicitis

Appendicitis is inflammation of the vermiform appendix caused by an obstruction of the intestinal lumen from infection, stricture, fecal mass, foreign body, or tumor.

Pathophysiology and Etiology

1. Obstruction is followed by edema, infection, and ischemia.
2. As intraluminal tension develops, necrosis and perforation usually occur.
3. Appendicitis can affect any age group; most common in adolescents/young adults, especially males.

Clinical Manifestations

1. Generalized or localized abdominal pain in the epigastric or periumbilical areas and upper right abdomen. Within 2 to 12 hours, the pain localizes in the right lower quadrant and intensity increases.
2. Anorexia, moderate malaise, mild fever, nausea, and vomiting.
3. Usually, constipation occurs, occasionally diarrhea.
4. Rebound tenderness, involuntary guarding, generalized abdominal rigidity.

Diagnostic Evaluation

1. Physical examination consistent with clinical manifestations.
2. WBC count reveals moderate leukocytosis (10,000 to 16,000/mm³) with shift to the left (increased immature neutrophils).
3. Urinalysis to rule out urinary disorders.
4. Abdominal x-ray may visualize shadow consistent with fecalith in appendix; perforation will reveal free air.
5. Abdominal ultrasound or CT scan can visualize the appendix and rule out other conditions, such as diverticulitis and Crohn disease. Focused appendiceal CT can quickly evaluate for appendicitis.

 GERONTOLOGIC ALERT In older adults, be aware of vague symptoms: milder pain, less pronounced fever, and leukocytosis with shift to the left on differential.

Management

1. Surgery (appendectomy) is indicated.
   a. Simple appendectomy or laparoscopic appendectomy in absence of rupture or peritonitis.
   b. An incisional drain may be placed if an abscess or rupture occurs.
2. Preoperatively maintain bed rest, NPO status, IV hydration, possible antibiotic prophylaxis, and analgesia.

Complications

1. Perforation (in 95% of cases).
2. Abscess.
3. Peritonitis.

Nursing Assessment

1. Obtain history for location and extent of pain.
2. Auscultate for presence of bowel sounds; peristalsis may be absent or diminished.
3. On palpation of the abdomen, assess for tenderness anywhere in the right lower quadrant, but usually localized over McBurney point (point just below midpoint of line between the umbilicus and iliac crest on the right side). Assess for rebound tenderness in the right lower quadrant as well as referred rebound when palpating the left lower quadrant.
4. Assess for positive psoas sign by having the patient attempt to raise the right thigh against the pressure of your hand placed over the right knee. Inflammation of the psoas muscle in acute appendicitis will increase abdominal pain with this maneuver.
5. Assess for positive obturator sign by flexing the patient's right hip and knee and rotating the leg internally. Hypogastric pain with this maneuver indicates inflammation of the obturator muscle.

Nursing Diagnoses

- Acute Pain related to inflamed appendix.
- Risk for Infection related to perforation.

Nursing Interventions

Preoperative nursing care is listed; for postoperative care, see "Caring for the Patient Undergoing Gastrointestinal Surgery," page 496.

Relieving Pain

1. Monitor pain level, including location, intensity, pattern.
2. Assist patient to comfortable positions, such as semi-Fowler and knees up.
3. Restrict activity that may aggravate pain, such as coughing and ambulation.
4. Apply ice bag to the abdomen for comfort.
5. Give antiemetics and analgesics, as ordered, and evaluate response.
6. Avoid indiscriminate palpation of the abdomen to avoid increasing the patient's discomfort.

 DRUG ALERT Do not give analgesics/antipyretics to mask fever, and do not administer cathartics because they may cause rupture.

Preventing Infection

1. Monitor frequently for signs and symptoms of worsening condition indicating perforation, abscess, or peritonitis: increasing severity of pain, tenderness, rigidity, distention, ileus, fever, malaise, and tachycardia.
2. Administer antibiotics, as ordered.
3. Promptly prepare the patient for surgery.

Patient Education and Health Maintenance

1. Instruct the patient to avoid heavy lifting for 4 to 6 weeks after surgery.
2. Instruct the patient to report symptoms of anorexia, nausea, vomiting, fever, abdominal pain, incisional redness, or drainage postoperatively.

Evaluation: Expected Outcomes

- Verbalizes decreased pain to 2 or 3 on 0 to 10 scale with positioning and analgesics.
- Afebrile; no rigidity or distention.

Diverticular Disease

 EVIDENCE BASE Stollman, N., Smalley, W., Hirano, I., et al. (2015). American Gastroenterology Association Institute guidelines on the management of acute diverticulitis. *Gastroenterology, 149,* 2944–1949.

Diverticular disease is a wide-spectrum disease encompassing all problems that can be caused by diverticula. A *diverticulum* is a pouch or saccular dilation of the colon wall. *Diverticulosis* is a condition exhibiting multiple diverticula without inflammation. *Diverticulitis* is inflammation and infection of one or more diverticula. Diverticular disease is usually categorized into complicated or uncomplicated disease.

Pathophysiology and Etiology

Diverticulosis

1. Marks the formation of diverticula, which are herniations of the mucosal and submucosal layers of the colon developing at weak points where nutrient blood vessels penetrate the colon wall (see Figure 18-10).
2. Causes for diverticular disease are unclear, but data suggest excessive intraluminal pressure plays a key role. A contributing factor may be a low-residue diet, which reduces fecal residue,

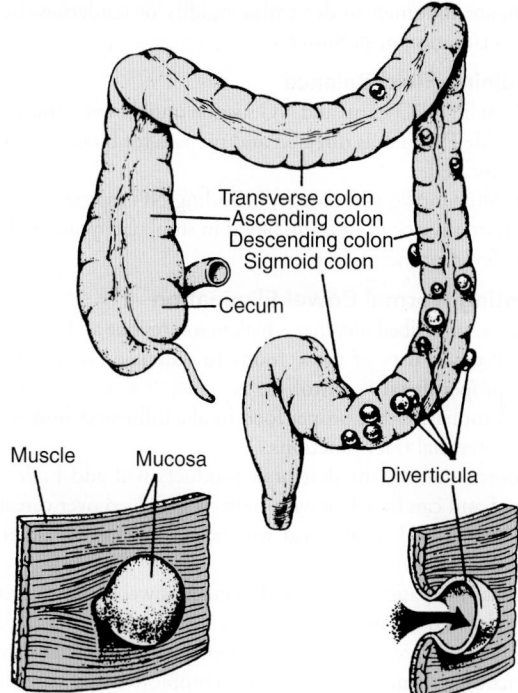

Figure 18-10. Diverticula are most common in the sigmoid colon; they diminish in number and size as the colon approaches the cecum. Diverticula are rarely found in the rectum.

narrows the bowel lumen, and leads to higher pressure intra-abdominally during defecation.

3. The risk of developing diverticulosis is about 40% by age 60 and more than 60% of those 80 years and older.

Diverticulitis

1. Results when one or more diverticula become inflamed and usually perforate the thin diverticular wall, which consists of mucosal and serosal layers. The exact cause is unknown, but postulated to be caused by stasis or obstruction of the diverticula leading to bacterial overgrowth, inflammation, and ischemia.
2. Complicated diverticulitis refers to diverticular disease that has led to abscess, perforation, fistula, stricture, or obstruction.
3. Uninflamed or minimally inflamed diverticula may erode adjacent arterial branches causing acute massive rectal bleeding.
4. It is estimated that 10% to 25% of people with diverticulosis will develop diverticulitis.

Clinical Manifestations

Diverticulosis

1. May be asymptomatic.
2. Crampy abdominal pain.
3. Bowel irregularity—constipation or diarrhea.
4. Periodic abdominal distention.
5. Sudden massive hemorrhage may be the first symptom.

Diverticulitis

1. Left lower quadrant pain.
2. Low-grade fever, chills, leukocytosis.
3. Sometimes, an abdominal mass is palpable.
4. Urinary frequency and dysuria are associated with bladder involvement in the inflammatory process.

5. Ruptured diverticula produce abscesses or peritonitis with abdominal rigidity; signs of shock and sepsis (hypotension, chills, high fever). Near a blood vessel, a rupture may cause massive hemorrhage.
   a. Sepsis may spread through the portal vein to the liver, causing liver abscesses.
   b. Sometimes, fistulae form with the bladder, the adjacent small bowel, the vagina, and the perianal area or skin.
   c. Chronic diverticulitis may cause adhesions that narrow the bowel's opening and can cause partial or complete bowel obstruction.

Diagnostic Evaluation

1. Laboratory studies: WBC may show leukocytosis with shift to the left; hemoglobin/hematocrit may be low with chronic or acute bleeding.
2. CT scan is the preferred imaging study because it is the most accurate in correctly identifying diverticulitis and in staging its severity. CT guidance can also be used if an abscess needs to be drained.
3. Sigmoidoscopy/colonoscopy—to rule out carcinoma and confirm diagnosis. These studies should not be done during an acute attack. A waiting period of 6 weeks after resolution of symptoms is preferred.
4. Barium enema (after infection subsides)—may visualize diverticular sacs, narrowing of colonic lumen, partial or complete obstruction, or fistulae.

 NURSING ALERT In patients with acute diverticulitis, a barium enema may rupture the bowel.

Management

Diverticulosis

1. High-fiber diet with possible avoidance of large seeds or nuts, which may obstruct diverticular sac.
2. Bran therapy, psyllium preparation, or stool softeners, such as docusate sodium (Colace), to avoid constipation.
3. Encourage adequate fluid intake.
4. Intestinal diverticulosis with pain usually responds to a liquid or low-residue diet and stool softeners to relieve symptoms, minimize irritation, and reduce progression to diverticulitis.

Uncomplicated Diverticulitis

1. Medical management.
   a. If symptoms are mild, treatment can occur as an outpatient. Usually, a broad-spectrum antibiotic is given for 7 to 14 days.
   b. If fever or systemic symptoms, patient should be treated in the hospital with intravenous broad-spectrum antibiotic.
2. Surgical management.
   a. Elective resection may be considered, but this is dependent on severity of disease, risk of subsequent attacks, age, comorbidities, and complications of the disease.

Complicated Diverticulitis

Treatment is dependent upon the associated complication that has occurred.

1. Abscess—may be managed with bowel rest and antibiotics while under close observation; however, percutaneous drainage may be needed if patient becomes septic. Sigmoid resection may also be recommended.

2. Perforation—surgical resection of the diseased area with colostomy (Hartmann procedure) is the most widely accepted treatment. Surgical resection with primary anastomosis may be done if patient is a good candidate. Recent studies show that laparoscopic lavage may be an alternative to resection, but further studies are needed.
3. Fistulae—usually require surgical resection depending on type of fistula and its associated symptoms.
4. Stricture/obstruction—if the obstruction is complete, surgery is required. If a partial obstruction has occurred, bowel rest, intravenous hydration, and antibiotics may successfully treat symptoms; however, surgery may be required later.
5. Hemorrhage—NPO, IV therapy, blood transfusion as necessary, and NG tube placement. Colonoscopy to identify source of bleeding.
   a. If colonoscopy is not successful in identifying source of bleeding, a technetium 99–labeled red blood cell scan will be done.
   b. Mesenteric angiography is an alternative study that may be used and has potential to be therapeutic, because the bleeding source can be thrombosed if identified.
   c. Surgical resection is not typical, because this type of hemorrhage is usually self-limited.

Complications

1. Hemorrhage from colonic diverticula, usually in the right colon.
2. Bowel obstruction.
3. Fistula formation (colovesical fistula is the most common).
4. Septicemia.

Nursing Assessment

1. Have the patient describe the amount of fiber and fluid intake per day and past and present bowel patterns. Any constipation, diarrhea, or alternating of both?
2. Ask if experiencing abdominal cramping or pain, bloody stools, or stool/gas passage from the vagina or in urine.
3. Watch for signs and symptoms of peritonitis: increasing abdominal pain, guarding, rebound tenderness, abdominal distention, and nausea/vomiting.
4. Monitor vital signs: temperature may be elevated; tachycardia and hypotension may indicate peritonitis/massive bleeding.

Nursing Diagnoses

- Acute Pain related to intestinal discomfort, diarrhea, and/or constipation.
- Risk for Deficient Fluid Volume related to diarrhea, fluid and electrolyte loss, nausea, and vomiting.
- Constipation or Diarrhea related to the disease process.
- Deficient Knowledge of the relationship between diet and diverticular disease.

Nursing Interventions

Achieving Pain Relief
1. Observe for signs and location of pain, type, and severity, and intervene when appropriate.
   a. Administer nonopiate analgesics as prescribed (opiates may mask signs of perforation).
   b. Administer anticholinergics, as prescribed, to decrease colon spasm.
2. Auscultate bowel sounds to monitor bowel motility.

3. Palpate abdomen to determine rigidity or tenderness because of perforation or peritonitis.

Maintaining Fluid Balance
1. Maintain NPO status and NG suction until bowel sounds return.
2. Provide IV fluid as directed and prepare for blood transfusion if indicated.
3. Monitor intake and output, including NG aspirate.
4. Report any occult or frank blood in stool, tachycardia, drop in BP, fever, or increased pain.

Promoting Normal Bowel Elimination
1. Follow prescribed diet that is high in soft residue and low in sugar.
   a. Provide lists of these foods to enhance familiarity with proper dietary control.
   b. Emphasize that proper food intake influences how well the intestinal tract functions.
2. Inform the patient that bran products will add bulk to the stool and can be taken with milk or sprinkled over cereal.
3. Monitor food intake and weight periodically to determine caloric status.
4. Advise the patient to establish regular bowel habits to promote regular and complete evacuation.
5. Observe and record color, consistency, and frequency of stools.
6. Encourage fluids if constipated to promote bowel stimulation.

Increasing Understanding of Disease
1. Explain the disease process to the patient and its relationship to diet.
2. Have the patient continue periodic medical supervision and follow-up; report problems and untoward symptoms.
3. Refer to nutritionist, as needed.

Patient Education and Health Maintenance

1. Instruct on high-residue diet choices.
2. Emphasize the importance of establishing regular bowel habits.
3. Advise the patient to report left lower quadrant pain, generalized abdominal tenderness, and fever.

Evaluation: Expected Outcomes

- Expresses relief of pain and has a decrease in symptoms.
- No change in vital signs; stool negative for occult blood.
- Reports near-normal bowel function; no diarrhea or constipation.
- Delineates the general nature of diverticulosis and can list dietary regimen that helps or aggravates the condition.

Peritonitis

Peritonitis occurs when bacteria or other microorganisms cause a generalized or localized inflammation of the peritoneum, the membrane lining the abdominal cavity and abdominal organs (see Figure 18-11).

Pathophysiology and Etiology

1. Primary peritonitis, also known as spontaneous bacterial peritonitis (SBP), occurs when bacteria cross through the intestinal wall into the peritoneum, causing infection. SBP can occur in patients with cirrhosis, nephrotic syndrome, and ovarian diseases (eg, cancer).
2. Secondary peritonitis is due to perforation, rupture of an organ, trauma, or peritoneal dialysis.

Figure 18-11. Pathophysiology of peritonitis.

Clinical Manifestations

1. Initially, local type of abdominal pain tends to become constant, diffuse, and more intense.
2. The abdomen becomes extremely tender and muscles become rigid; rebound tenderness and ileus may be present; the patient lies very still, usually with legs drawn up.
3. Percussion: Resonance and tympany because of paralytic ileus; loss of liver dullness may indicate free air in the abdomen.
4. Auscultation: Decreased bowel sounds.
5. Nausea and vomiting often occur; peristalsis diminishes; anorexia is present.
6. Elevation of temperature and pulse as well as leukocytosis.
7. Fever; thirst; oliguria; dry, swollen tongue; signs of dehydration.
8. Weakness, pallor, diaphoresis, and cold skin are the results of the loss of fluid, electrolytes, and protein into the abdomen.
9. Hypotension, tachycardia, and hypokalemia may occur.
10. With generalized peritonitis, large volumes of fluid may be lost into abdominal cavity (ascites). Shallow respirations may result from abdominal distention and upward displacement of the diaphragm.

Diagnostic Evaluation

1. WBC count to determine if leukocytosis is present (leukopenia if severe).
2. ABG levels may show hypoxemia or metabolic acidosis with respiratory compensation.
3. Urinalysis may indicate urinary tract problems as primary source.
4. Peritoneal aspiration (paracentesis) to demonstrate blood, pus, bile, bacteria (Gram stain), amylase.
5. Abdominal x-rays may show free air in the peritoneal cavity, gas and fluid collection in small and large intestines, generalized bowel dilation, intestinal wall edema.

6. CT scan of the abdomen or sonography may reveal intra-abdominal mass, abscess, ascites.
7. Radionuclide scans (gallium, hepatobiliary iminodiacetic acid, and liver/spleen scan) may identify an intra-abdominal abscess.
8. Chest x-ray may show elevated diaphragm.
9. Exploratory laparotomy may be performed to identify the underlying cause.

Management

1. Treatment of inflammatory conditions preoperatively and postoperatively with antibiotic therapy may prevent peritonitis. Broad-spectrum antibiotic therapy to cover aerobic and anaerobic organisms is the initial treatment, followed by specific antibiotic therapy after culture and sensitivity results.
2. Bed rest, NPO status, and respiratory support, if needed.
3. IV fluids and electrolytes, possibly TPN.
4. Analgesics for pain; antiemetics for nausea and vomiting.
5. NG intubation to decompress the bowel.
6. Possibly rectal tube to facilitate passage of gas.
7. Operative procedures to close perforations, remove infection source (ie, inflamed organ, necrotic tissue), drain abscesses, and lavage peritoneal cavity.
8. Abdominal paracentesis may be done to remove accumulating fluid.
9. Blood transfusions, if appropriate.
10. Oral feedings after return of bowel sounds and passage of gas and/or feces.

Complications

1. Intra-abdominal abscess formation (ie, pelvic subphrenic space).
2. Septicemia.
3. Hypovolemic problems.
4. Renal or liver failure.
5. Respiratory insufficiency.

Nursing Assessment

1. Assess for abdominal distention and tenderness, guarding, rebound, hypoactive or absent bowel sounds to determine bowel function.
2. Observe for signs of shock—tachycardia and hypotension.
3. Monitor vital signs, ABG levels, CBC, electrolytes, and central venous pressure to monitor hemodynamic status and assess for complications.

Nursing Diagnoses

- Acute Pain related to peritoneal inflammation.
- Deficient Fluid Volume related to vomiting and interstitial fluid shift.
- Imbalanced Nutrition: Less Than Body Requirements related to GI symptomatology.

Nursing Interventions

Achieving Pain Relief

1. Place the patient in semi-Fowler position before surgery to enable less painful breathing.
2. After surgery, place the patient in Fowler position to promote drainage by gravity.
3. Provide analgesics as prescribed.

Maintaining Fluid and Electrolyte Volume

1. Keep the patient NPO to reduce peristalsis.
2. Provide IV fluids to establish adequate fluid intake and to promote adequate urine output, as prescribed.
3. Record accurately intake and output, including the measurement of vomitus and NG drainage.
4. Minimize nausea, vomiting, and distention by use of NG suction, antiemetics.
5. Monitor for signs of hypovolemia: dry mucous membranes, oliguria, postural hypotension, tachycardia, diminished skin turgor.

Achieving Adequate Nutrition

1. Administer TPN, as ordered, to maintain positive nitrogen balance until patient can resume oral diet.
2. Reduce parenteral fluids and give oral food and fluids per order when the following occur:
   a. Temperature and pulse return to normal.
   b. Abdomen becomes soft.
   c. Peristaltic sounds return (determined by abdominal auscultation).
   d. Flatus is passed and patient has bowel movements.

Patient Education and Health Maintenance

1. Teach the patient and family how to care for open wounds and drain sites, if appropriate.
2. Assess the need for home care nursing to assist with wound care and assess healing; refer as necessary.
3. Encourage follow-up as directed and reporting of increased pain, fever, and anorexia.

Evaluation: Expected Outcomes

- Minimal analgesics needed; abdomen soft, nontender, and no distention.
- Balanced intake and output; no evidence of dehydration or electrolyte imbalances.
- Bowel sounds present; tolerating soft diet.

Irritable Bowel Syndrome

Irritable bowel syndrome is a functional bowel disorder characterized by abdominal pain and altered bowel function. It is the most common functional GI disorder and is estimated to affect 20% of Americans.

Pathophysiology and Etiology

The exact etiology of IBS is unknown. Pathophysiologic processes include abnormal GI motility, heightened visceral hypersensitivity, and abnormal central nervous system processing. IBS is not a life-threatening disorder, and surgery is not necessary. It does not transform into inflammatory bowel disease and does not increase the risk for colorectal cancer and occurs in 70% of females, with greatest prevalence in youth and middle age.

Clinical Manifestations

1. Functional abnormalities vary and may come and go, leading to a chronic problem.
2. Symptoms may include:
   a. Lower abdominal pain.
   b. Diarrhea, constipation, or alternating of both.
   c. Bloating, distention.
   d. Mucous drainage.
   e. Fecal urgency, feeling of incomplete evacuation.
3. Patients usually have a characteristic pain pattern ranging from pain in the postprandial period, occurring before or at the time of bowel movement, or arising during times of stress or anxiety.
4. Symptoms that occur after eating may be associated with certain foods.

Diagnostic Evaluation

Overview

Diagnosis can be made based on symptom criteria alone.
1. Careful medical history.
2. Rectal examination—normal or tenderness at left lower quadrant abdomen, which may reflect a spasm in the sigmoid colon.
3. If patient fulfills the Rome III diagnostic criteria for IBS (see below), and there are no warning signs of other disease processes, the diagnosis is confirmed.
4. Traditional warning signs, which could signal other organic diseases include fever, chills, night sweats, bleeding, obvious anemia, weight loss, and onset occurring in patients older than age 50.

Rome III Diagnostic Criteria

1. Recurrent abdominal pain or discomfort at least 3 days per month in the past 3 months associated with two or more of the following:
   a. Improvement with defecation.
   b. Onset associated with a change in frequency of stool.
   c. Onset associated with a change in form (appearance) of stool.
2. Symptoms described above for the past 3 months with symptom onset at least 6 months prior to diagnosis.
3. Discomfort means an uncomfortable sensation not described as pain. In pathophysiology research and clinical trials, a pain/discomfort frequency of at least 2 days a week during screening evaluation for subject eligibility.

 EVIDENCE BASE Hayee, B. (2015). Managing irritable bowel syndrome in primary care: A clinical update. *Nursing In Practice*, 83.

Tests to Rule Out Other Disease Processes

1. CBC to test for anemia.
2. Sedimentation rate and C-reactive protein to detect inflammation.
3. Stool testing for ova and parasites; fecal occult blood testing.
4. Serology testing for celiac disease.
5. Barium enema—should be done when warning signs are present.
6. Flexible sigmoidoscopy/colonoscopy—should be done when warning signs are present.

Management

Treatment is focused on relieving symptoms. Treating the patient's most predominant symptoms determines the most successful therapy.
1. Pain—predominant symptom:
   a. Anticholinergic drugs: dicyclomine or hyoscyamine taken before meals; should be used only for limited periods such as during a flareup.
   b. Combination agents: phenobarbital, hyoscyamine, atropine, and scopolamine or chlordiazepoxide and clidinium bromide are second-line agents.

c. Nonopioid agents: acetaminophen, tramadol, gabapentin, carbamazepine, and anti-inflammatory agents.

d. Tricyclic antidepressants: desipramine, doxepin, and amitriptyline.

2. Constipation—predominant symptom:
   a. Fiber: psyllium, ispaghula husk, and polycarbophil.
   b. Osmotic laxatives: lactulose, sorbitol, and lubiprostone.
3. Diarrhea—predominant symptom:
   a. Loperamide—reduces stool consistency and improves stool consistency.
   b. Cholestyramine—binds bile salts.
4. Eliminate irritating dietary substances, such as caffeine, fatty foods, fructose, or lactose, which may cause such symptoms as spasms, cramps, bloating, and/or diarrhea.
5. A regular exercise routine can improve gastric emptying and relieve constipation and stress.

 DRUG ALERT Opioids should not be used to treat abdominal pain in patients with IBS because of possibility of drug interaction or dependency leading to addiction.

Complications

1. This disorder is associated with:
   a. Psychological distress.
   b. Sexual dysfunction.
   c. Interference with work and sleep.
   d. Decreased quality of life.
2. Unnecessary surgery because of misdiagnosis (such as cholecystectomy, appendectomy, or partial colectomy).

Nursing Assessment

1. Assess the patient for contributing factors that may affect symptoms, such as diet, emotions, professional and personal relationships, fears, concerns, financial stressors, and problems at home or work.
2. Record specific symptoms that the patient is experiencing to determine best treatment options.
3. Explore pain characteristics: frequency, duration, location, timing, and intensity.

Nursing Diagnoses

- Chronic Pain related to functional disorder.
- Constipation or Diarrhea related to change in bowel motility.
- Ineffective Coping related to anxiety, stress, and depression.

Nursing Interventions

Minimizing Pain or Discomfort

1. Assess and evaluate abdominal pain using a pain scale.
2. Review pain medications for proper usage and possibility of adverse effects—drowsiness and dry mouth with anticholinergics, combination agents, and tricyclic antidepressants; bloating, abdominal pain, gas, diarrhea, or constipation with other medications.

Decreasing Diarrhea or Constipation

1. Monitor amount, consistency, and frequency of stool.
2. Encourage exercise and adequate fluid/fiber intake to promote bowel motility for constipation.

3. Encourage adequate fluid intake to prevent fluid volume deficit and electrolyte imbalance for diarrhea.

Providing Supportive Care

1. Validate the patient's complaints and express interest in diagnosis.
2. Follow-up and reassess the patient's complaints and status of treatment goals.
3. Refer the patient for pain management, psychological counseling, or behavior management therapy if indicated.

Patient Education and Health Maintenance

1. Educate the patient on the diagnosis and the natural course of IBS.
2. Instruct the patient about all prescribed medications, including purpose, dosage, and adverse effects.
3. Encourage the patient to participate in stress-reducing activities, such as exercise, relaxation techniques, and music therapy.
4. Encourage participation in counseling sessions to deal with anxiety and depression.
5. Suggest ways for the patient to learn coping skills and stress management.

Evaluation: Expected Outcomes

- Expresses pain is controlled for ADLs.
- Relates that bowel symptoms are manageable with treatment plan.
- Verbalizes strategies to deal with the psychological components of disorder.

Ulcerative Colitis

 EVIDENCE BASE Bressler, B., Marshall, J., Bernstein, C., et al. (2015). Clinical practice guidelines for the medical management of nonhospitalized ulcerative colitis: The Toronto consensus. *Gastroenterology, 148,* 1035–1058.

Ulcerative colitis is a chronic, idiopathic, diffuse inflammatory disease of the mucosa and, less frequently, the submucosa of the colon and rectum. If only the rectum is involved, it may be called ulcerative proctitis.

Pathophysiology and Etiology

1. The exact cause of ulcerative colitis is unknown. Possible theories include:
   a. Genetic predisposition.
   b. Environmental factors (viral or bacterial pathogens, dietary).
   c. Immunologic imbalance or disturbances.
   d. Defect in intestinal barrier causing hypersensitive mucosa and increased permeability.
   e. Defect in repair of mucosal injury, which may develop into a chronic condition.
2. Multiple crypt abscesses develop in intestinal mucosa that may become necrotic and lead to ulceration and perforation.
3. May manifest as a systemic disease with inflammatory changes of connective tissue (see Figure 18-12). Most common in young adulthood and middle age, with peak incidence at ages 20 to 40.
4. Incidence greatest in whites of Jewish descent.

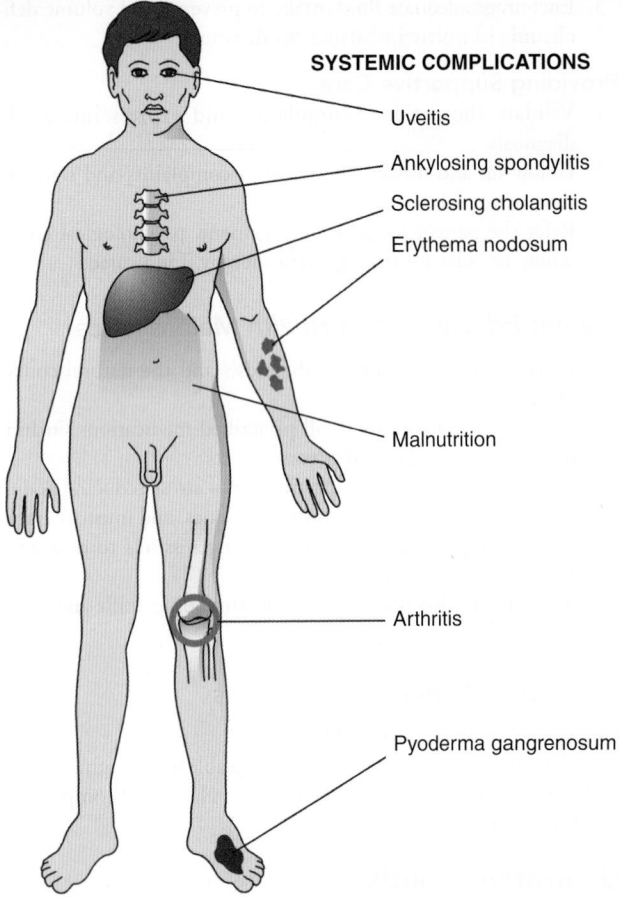

SYSTEMIC COMPLICATIONS

Uveitis

Ankylosing spondylitis

Sclerosing cholangitis

Erythema nodosum

Malnutrition

Arthritis

Pyoderma gangrenosum

Figure 18-12. GI and systemic complications of ulcerative colitis. (Rubin, R., & Strayer, D.S. [2011]. Rubin's Pathology: Clinicopathologic Foundations of Medicine [6th ed.]. Philadelphia: Lippincott Williams & Wilkins.)

Clinical Manifestations

1. Bloody diarrhea is a key symptom.
2. Tenesmus (painful straining), sense of urgency, and frequency.
3. Increased bowel sounds; the abdomen may appear flat, but, as condition continues, the abdomen may appear distended.
4. There often is weight loss, fever, dehydration, hypokalemia, anorexia, nausea and vomiting, iron deficiency anemia, and cachexia (general lack of nutrition and wasting with chronic disease).
5. Crampy abdominal pain.
6. The disease usually begins in the rectum and sigmoid and spreads proximally, at times, involving the entire colon. Anal area may be irritated and reddened; left lower abdomen may be tender on palpation.
7. There is a tendency for the patient to experience remissions and exacerbations.
8. Increased risk of developing colorectal cancer.
9. May exhibit extracolonic manifestations of eye (iritis, uveitis), joint (polyarthritis), and skin complaints (erythema nodosum, pyoderma gangrenosum).

Diagnostic Evaluation

Diagnosis is based on a combination of laboratory, radiologic, endoscopic, and histologic findings.

Laboratory Tests

1. Stool examination to rule out enteral pathogens; fecal analysis positive for blood during active disease.
2. CBC—hemoglobin and hematocrit may be low because of bleeding; WBC may be increased.
3. Elevated erythrocyte sedimentation rate (ESR).
4. Decreased serum levels of potassium, magnesium, and albumin may be present.

Other Diagnostic Tests

1. Barium enema to assess extent of disease and detect pseudopolyps, carcinoma, and strictures. May show absence of haustral markings; narrow, lead-pipe appearance; superficial ulcerations.
2. Flexible proctosigmoidoscopy/colonoscopy findings reveal mucosal erythema and edema, ulcers, and inflammation that begins distally in the rectum and spreads proximally for variable distances. Pseudopolyps and friable tissue may be present.
3. Histological findings from biopsies of the colon include changes in crypt height, loss of crypts, and neutrophils infiltrates in the crypts.
4. CT scan can identify complications such as toxic megacolon.
5. Rectal biopsy—differentiates from other inflammatory diseases or cancer.

Management

General Measures

1. Bed rest, IV fluid replacement, clear liquid diet.
2. For patients with severe dehydration and excessive diarrhea, TPN may be recommended to rest the intestinal tract and restore nitrogen balance.
3. Treatment of anemia—iron supplements for chronic bleeding and blood replacement for massive bleeding.

Drug Therapy

1. Aminosalicylates (5-ASA)—first-line therapy for acute and maintenance therapy. Oral and rectal formulations are available. Dose-related adverse effects include vomiting, anorexia, headache, fever, rash, dyspepsia, and lowered sperm count (sulfasalazine).
2. Corticosteroids—initial agent used in the management of moderate to severe ulcerative colitis. Used to induce remission of symptoms and can be used concomitantly with 5-aminosalicylic acid preparations. Not used for maintenance therapy because of potential side effects. Enema available for proctitis and left-sided colitis.
3. Immunosuppressive drugs—purine analogues, azathioprine, and 6-mercaptopurine may be indicated when the patient is refractory or dependent on corticosteroids.
4. Anti-TNF therapy—when other agents are not effective, these drugs (eg, infliximab, adalimumab) can be used to induce and maintain remission of symptoms. Side effects can include opportunistic infections, headache, rash, and arthralgias.

Surgical Measures

1. Surgery is recommended when patients fail to respond to medical therapy, if clinical status is worsening, for uncontrollable adverse effects of medications, severe hemorrhage, perforation, toxic megacolon, dysplasia, or cancer.
2. Noncurative approaches (possible curative, reconstructive procedure at later date):
   a. Temporary loop colostomy for decompression if toxic megacolon present without perforation.
   b. Subtotal colectomy, ileostomy, and Hartmann pouch.
   c. Colectomy with ileorectal anastomosis.

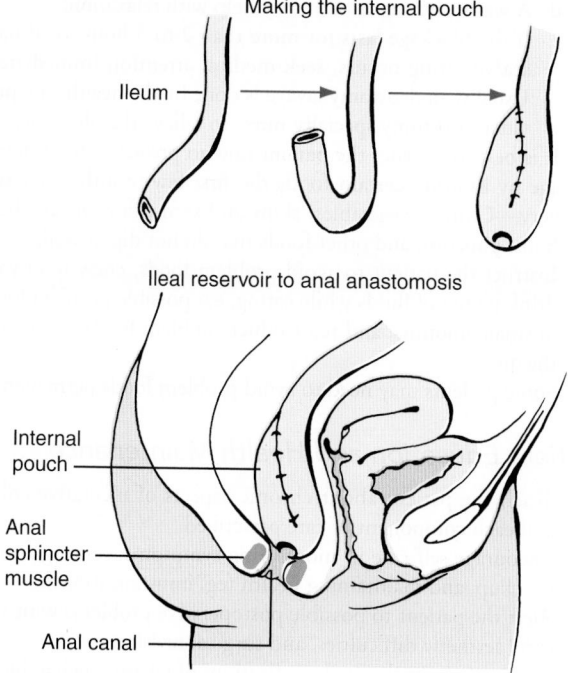

Making the internal pouch

Ileum

Ileal reservoir to anal anastomosis

Internal pouch

Anal sphincter muscle

Anal canal

Figure 18-13. Ileal reservoir–anal anastomosis. This reservoir is constructed of two loops of the small intestine forming a J configuration (J pouch).

3. Reconstructive procedures—curative:
   a. Total proctocolectomy with permanent end ileostomy.
   b. Total proctocolectomy with continent ileostomy (Kock or BCIR).
   c. Total colectomy with ileal reservoir—anal (or ileal reservoir–distal rectal) anastomosis—procedure of choice. Multiple reservoir shapes can be surgically created; however, the J-shaped pouch (reservoir) is the easiest to construct (see Figure 18-13).
   d. The ultimate surgical goal is to remove the entire colon and rectum to cure patient of ulcerative colitis.

Complications

1. Perforation, hemorrhage.
2. Toxic megacolon (life-threatening)—fever, tachycardia, abdominal distention, peritonitis, leukocytosis, dilated colon on abdominal x-ray.
3. Abscess formation, stricture, anal fistula.
4. Malnutrition, anemia, electrolyte imbalance.
5. Skin lesions (erythema nodosum, pyoderma gangrenosum).
6. Arthritis, ankylosing spondylitis.
7. Colon malignancy.
8. Liver disease (sclerosing cholangitis).
9. Eye lesions (uveitis, conjunctivitis).
10. Growth retardation in prepubertal children.
11. Possible infertility in females.

Nursing Assessment

1. Review nursing history for patterns of fatigue and overwork, tension, family problems that may exacerbate symptoms.
2. Assess food habits and use of any dietary or herbal supplements used as alternative therapies that may have a bearing on triggering symptoms (milk intake may be a problem). Many patients use vitamins, herbs, and homeopathic remedies without realizing the effect on bowel function.
3. Determine the number and consistency of bowel movements and any rectal bleeding present.
4. Listen for hyperactive bowel sounds; assess weight.

Nursing Diagnoses

- Chronic Pain related to disease process.
- Imbalanced Nutrition: Less Than Body Requirements related to diarrhea, nausea, and vomiting.
- Deficient Fluid Volume related to diarrhea and loss of fluid and electrolytes.
- Risk for Infection related to disease process and surgical procedures.
- Ineffective Coping related to fatigue, feeling of helplessness, and lack of support system.

Nursing Interventions

Promoting Comfort

1. Follow prescribed treatment of reducing or eliminating food and fluid and instituting parenteral feeding or low-residue diets to rest the intestinal tract.
2. Give sedatives and tranquilizers, as prescribed, not only to provide general rest but also to slow peristalsis.
3. Be aware of skin breakdown around the anus, which causes discomfort.
   a. Cleanse the skin gently after each bowel movement.
   b. Apply a protective emollient, such as petroleum jelly, skin sealant, or moisture barrier ointment.
4. Relieve painful rectal spasms (produced by frequent diarrheal stools) with anodyne suppositories, as prescribed.
5. Report any evidence of sudden abdominal distention—may indicate toxic megacolon.
6. Reduce physical activity to a minimum, or provide frequent rest periods.
7. Provide commode or bathroom next to bed because urgency of movements may be a problem.

Achieving Nutritional Requirements

1. Maintain an acutely ill patient on parenteral replacement of vitamins, fluids, and electrolytes (potassium), as prescribed.
2. When resuming oral fluids and foods, select those that are nonirritating to the mucosa (mechanically, thermally, and chemically). If this fails, an elemental diet may be prescribed to provide low residue to rest the lower intestinal tract.
3. Avoid dairy products if the patient is lactose intolerant.
4. Provide a well-balanced, low-residue, high-protein diet to correct malnutrition.
5. Determine which foods the patient can tolerate and modify diet plan accordingly.
6. Bolster with supplemental vitamin therapy, including vitamins C, B complex, and K, as prescribed.
7. Possibly avoid cold fluids, which may increase intestinal motility.
8. Administer prescribed medications for symptomatic relief of diarrhea.

Maintaining Fluid Balance

1. Maintain accurate intake and output records.
2. Weigh daily; rapid increase or decrease may relate to fluid imbalance.
3. Monitor serum electrolytes and report abnormalities.

4. Observe for decreased skin turgor, dry skin, oliguria, decreased temperature, weakness, and increased hemoglobin, hematocrit, BUN, and specific gravity, all of which are signs of fluid loss leading to dehydration.

Minimizing Infection and Complications

1. Give antibacterial drugs as prescribed.
2. Administer corticosteroids as prescribed.
3. Provide conscientious skin care after severe diarrhea.
4. For severe proctitis, instill rectal steroids, as prescribed, to produce a remission of symptoms.
5. Administer prescribed therapy to correct existing anemia.
6. Observe for signs of colonic perforation and hemorrhage—abdominal rigidity, distention, hypotension, and tachycardia.

Providing Supportive Care

1. Recognize psychological needs of the patient.
   a. Fear, anxiety, and discouragement.
   b. Hypersensitivity may be evident.
2. Acknowledge the patient's complaints.
3. Encourage the patient to talk; listen and offer psychological support.
4. Answer questions about the permanent or temporary ostomy, if appropriate.
5. Initiate patient education about living with chronic disease.
6. Include the patient as part of the health care team to provide continuity of care, communication, and periodic evaluation.
7. Offer educational and emotional support to family members.
8. Refer for psychological counseling, as needed.

Community and Home Care Considerations

Pouchitis

1. Patients undergoing one of the continent restorative procedures (Kock, BCIR, or ileal reservoir–anal anastomosis) must be alert for a common late postoperative complication called pouchitis.
2. The symptoms include increased stool output, cramps, and malaise.
3. It is thought to be related to stasis within the pouch/reservoir and usually responds to metronidazole.
4. Assess for these symptoms and notify health care provider.

Food Blockage

1. Patients with a temporary or permanent ileostomy must be alert for signs and symptoms of a food blockage.
   a. This is a mechanical blockage of undigested foodstuffs at the level of the fascia.
   b. It is most likely to occur in the first 6 weeks postoperatively when the bowel is edematous; however, patients with an ileostomy must be aware that it can occur at any time if precautions are not taken.
2. Symptoms may include spurty, watery stool with strong odor, decreased or no stool output, abdominal discomfort, cramping or bloating, and stomal swelling. Nausea and vomiting are late symptoms and require immediate attention.
3. Treatment includes:
   a. Avoiding solid foods and drinking clear liquids when symptoms occur. Patients with ileostomies must never take laxatives.
   b. Applying a pouching system with a larger opening to allow for stomal swelling.
   c. Gently massaging the abdomen around the stoma and/or pulling the knees to the chest and rocking the body back and forth.

d. A warm shower or bath may help with relaxation.
e. If the blockage lasts for more than 2 to 3 hours or if nausea/vomiting occurs, seek medical attention immediately. Usually, an ileostomy lavage is done by the health care provider or ostomy specialty nurse to relieve the blockage.
4. It is best to instruct the patient how to prevent a food blockage by limiting certain foods the first few months after surgery—Chinese vegetables, skins and seeds, fatty meats, bean hulls, popcorn, and other foods that do not digest well.
5. Instruct the patient to avoid problem foods, chew food well, drink plenty of fluids while eating, eat possible problem foods in small amounts, and reintroduce problem foods slowly into the diet.
6. Some patients may need to avoid problem foods permanently.

Patient Education and Health Maintenance

1. Teach the patient about chronic aspects of ulcerative colitis and each component of care prescribed.
2. Encourage self-care in monitoring symptoms, seeking annual checkup, and maintaining health (eg, immunizations).
3. Alert the patient to possible postoperative problems with skin care, aesthetic difficulties, and surgical revisions.
4. Inform patients that early indications of relapse, such as bleeding or increased diarrhea, should be reported immediately so treatment may be initiated.
5. If the patient has an ileostomy, provide information about the local chapter of the United Ostomy Association (*www.uoa.org*).
6. Encourage the patient to share experiences with others undergoing similar procedures.
7. For further information and support, refer to the Crohn and Colitis Foundation of America at *www.ccfa.org*.

Evaluation: Expected Outcomes

- Reports lessening of pain; functions well with minimal analgesics.
- Demonstrates improved food and fluid intake; avoids roughage intake.
- Controls diarrhea; maintains fluid and electrolyte balance.
- Afebrile, no skin breakdown, vital signs stable, no abdominal rigidity.
- Shows improved psychological outlook; participates in counseling, if desired; uses support systems.

Crohn Disease

Crohn disease is a chronic, idiopathic inflammatory disease that can affect any part of the GI tract. It is predominantly a transmural disease of the bowel wall. Other names for this disease include *regional enteritis, granulomatous colitis, transmural colitis, ileitis,* and *ileocolitis.*

Pathophysiology and Etiology

1. The exact etiology is unknown for this disease. It is thought to be multifactorial with the following theories:
   a. Genetic predisposition.
   b. Environmental agents, such as infections (viral or bacterial overload) or dietary factors, may trigger the disease.
   c. Immunologic imbalance or disturbances.
   d. Defect in the intestinal barrier that increases the permeability of the bowel.
   e. Defect in the repair of mucosal injury, leading to chronic condition.
   f. Cigarette smoking is a risk factor in developing disease and increases exacerbations. In contrast, cigarette smoking seems to have a protective effect with ulcerative colitis.

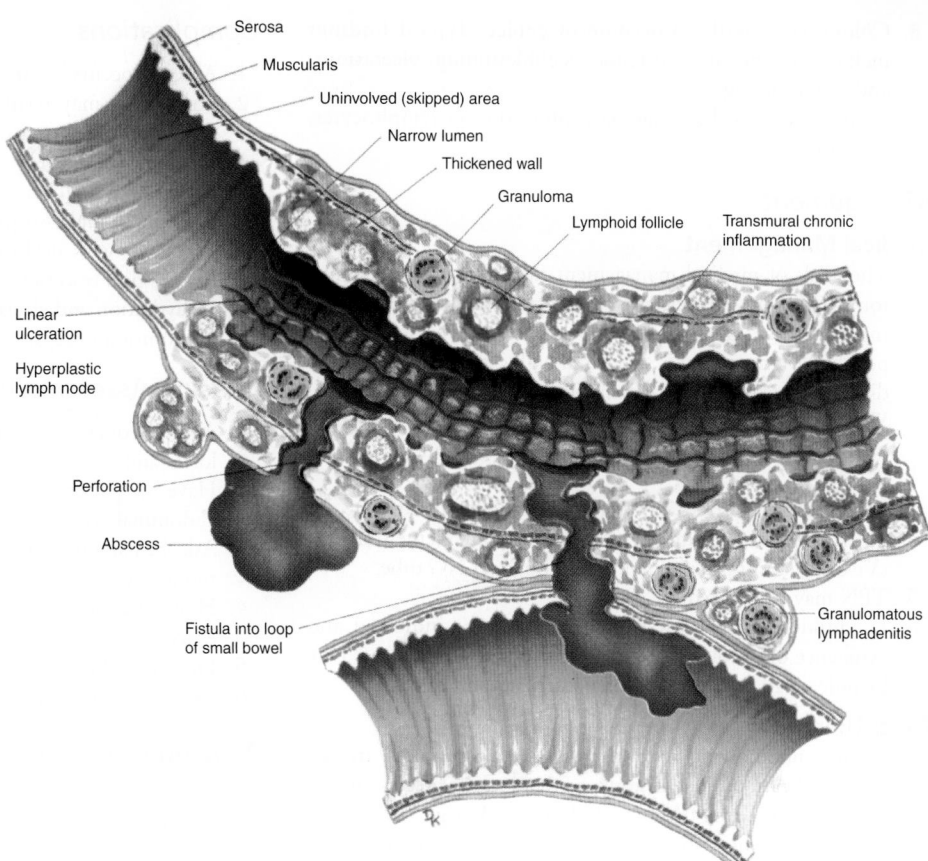

Serosa
Muscularis
Uninvolved (skipped) area
Narrow lumen
Thickened wall
Granuloma
Lymphoid follicle
Transmural chronic inflammation
Linear ulceration
Hyperplastic lymph node
Perforation
Abscess
Fistula into loop of small bowel
Granulomatous lymphadenitis

Figure 18-14. Transmural intestinal changes in Crohn disease. (Rubin, R., & Strayer, D.S. [2011]. Rubin's Pathology: Clinicopathologic Foundations of Medicine [6th ed.]. Philadelphia: Lippincott Williams & Wilkins.)

2. Intestinal tissue is thickened and edematous; ulcers enlarge, deepen, and form transverse and longitudinal linear ulcers that intersect, resembling a cobblestone appearance. The deep penetration of these ulcers may form fissures, abscesses, and fistulae. The healing and fibrosis of these lesions may lead to stricture (see Figure 18-14).

3. The rectum is typically spared from disease, and "skip lesions" are discontinuous areas of diseased bowel.

4. Transmural inflammation is a characteristic finding of this disease as well as granulomas.

5. Involvement of the upper GI tract (mouth, esophagus, stomach, and duodenum) is rare, and, if present, there is usually disease elsewhere.

6. May occur at any age; however, peak incidence is in the third decade, with a smaller peak in the fifth decade.

7. Most common in whites and those of Jewish descent.

8. The clinical presentation can be divided into three patterns:
   a. Inflammatory.
   b. Fibrostenotic (stricturing).
   c. Perforating (fistulizing).

9. Recurrences tend to fall into the same pattern for each individual patient and may provide an approach to treatment.

Clinical Manifestations

These are characterized by exacerbations and remissions—may be abrupt or insidious.

1. Crampy intermittent pain.

2. Chronic diarrhea—usual consistency is soft or semiliquid. Bloody stools or steatorrhea (because of malabsorption) may occur.

3. Fever may indicate infectious complication such as abscess.

4. Fecal urgency and tenesmus.

5. Other symptoms include anorexia, weight loss, malaise, nausea, arthralgias, and hematochezia.

6. Rectal examination may reveal a perirectal abscess, fistula, fissure, or skin tags (which represent healed perianal lesions).

7. The *inflammatory pattern* may display malabsorption, weight loss, and less abdominal pain; *fibrostenotic pattern* may display a partial small bowel obstruction, diffuse abdominal pain, nausea, vomiting, and bloating; *perforating pattern* may display a sudden profuse diarrhea because of enteroenteric fistula, fever, and localized tenderness because of abscess, or other fistulizing symptoms, such as pneumaturia and recurrent UTIs.

Diagnostic Evaluation

1. The diagnosis is based on a combination of laboratory, radiologic, endoscopic, and histologic findings.

2. CBC may show mild leukocytosis, thrombocytosis, anemia.

3. Elevated ESR, hypoalbuminemia.

4. Stool analysis may reveal leukocytes but no enteric pathogens; guaiac-positive stool. Fecal calprotectin to assess amount of inflammation (disease activity).

5. Upper GI and small bowel follow-through barium studies may show the classic "string sign" at the terminal ileum, which suggests a constriction of an intestinal segment.

6. A barium enema may permit visualization of lesions in the large intestine and terminal ileum.

7. CT of the abdomen and pelvis is helpful with diagnosis but is more often used to evaluate complications, such as abscess or fistulae.

8. Colonoscopy is the procedure of choice. Typical findings include presence of skip lesions, cobblestoning, ulcerations, and rectal sparing.
9. Biopsy may reveal granulomas, infiltration of lymphocytes, and monocytes.

Management

Medical Management

1. The goals of medical management include managing symptoms, reducing complications, inducing remissions, improving nutrition, and avoiding surgical interventions when possible. Management is also based on location and severity of disease and extraintestinal complications.
2. Weight loss, water and electrolyte imbalances, and iron, vitamin, mineral, and protein deficiencies occur in 80% of patients.
3. During acute episodes, bowel rest is usually required.
4. Nutritional replacements may include an elemental diet (Vivonex) administered orally or through an NG tube.
5. TPN may be ordered.
6. For milder cases, a low-residue diet may be indicated and avoidance of untolerated foods. Nutritional supplements may be ordered to provide additional nutrients and calories.

Drug Therapy

1. There is no known cure for this disease; it is primarily treated with medications. The disease severity and the area of the GI tract influence drug therapy (see Table 18-3, page 529).
2. 5-Aminosalicylic acid (5-ASA)—can be used in mild disease but poor evidence to support use.
3. Corticosteroids—to reduce inflammation; given orally, by IV line, or by suppository, retention enema, or foam, depending on the severity of disease. Steroids should be tapered off whenever possible.
4. Immunomodulators (6-mercaptopurine, azathioprine, methotrexate, cyclosporine, and tacrolimus)—used in patients who are steroid-dependent or steroid-refractory. Assists with fistula improvement or healing.
5. Antidiarrheals (loperamide, cholestyramine, or codeine [but try to avoid])—decrease stool frequency in mild to moderate disease; use with caution.
6. Miscellaneous drugs—antispasmodics (dicyclomine), bulking agents (psyllium), or tricyclic antidepressants (amitriptyline) for treatment of abdominal pain.
7. Infliximab and adalimumab—monoclonal antibodies that block the activity of the inflammatory agent and tumor necrosis factor. They are indicated for moderate to severe disease not responding to traditional therapies and for patients with draining fistulae.

Surgery

Indicated only for the complications of Crohn disease. Approximately 70% of Crohn disease patients will eventually require one or more operations to relieve obstruction, close fistulae, drain abscesses, repair perforations, manage hemorrhage, or widen strictures. Depending on the patient, surgical options include:

1. Segmental bowel resection with anastomosis.
2. Subtotal colectomy with ileorectal anastomosis.
3. Total colectomy with ileostomy for severe disease in the colon and rectum (see page 498 for care of the ostomy patient).
4. Kock pouch and ileal reservoir–anal anastomosis are contraindicated in Crohn patients. These procedures require the use of the small intestine in which Crohn disease may develop.

Complications

1. Abscess (occurs in 20%) and fistulae (occur in 40%).
2. Strictures—may result from inflammation, edema, abscess, and adhesions, but usually from fibrostenosis.
3. Hemorrhage, bowel perforation, intestinal obstruction.
4. Nutritional deficiencies: poor caloric intake because of food avoidance, malabsorption of bile salts and fat, vitamin B_{12} deficiency with ileal disease, short-gut syndrome after extensive surgical resections.
5. Dehydration and electrolyte disturbances.
6. Peritonitis and sepsis.

Nursing Assessment

1. Assess frequency and consistency of stools to evaluate volume losses and effectiveness of therapy.
2. Have the patient describe the location, severity, and onset of abdominal cramping or pain.
3. Ask the patient about weight loss and anorexia; weigh daily to monitor changes.
4. Have the patient describe foods eaten to elicit dietary exacerbations.
5. Determine if the patient smokes, including duration and amount.
6. Ask about family history of GI diseases.

Nursing Diagnoses

- Imbalanced Nutrition: Less Than Body Requirements related to pain, nausea.
- Deficient Fluid Volume related to diarrhea.
- Chronic Pain related to the inflammatory disease of the small intestine.
- Ineffective Coping related to feelings of rejection and embarrassment.

Nursing Interventions

Achieving Adequate Nutritional Balance

1. Encourage a diet that is low in residue, fiber, and fat and high in calories, protein, and carbohydrates, with vitamin and mineral supplements.
2. Monitor weight daily.
3. Provide small, frequent feedings to prevent distention.
4. Have the patient participate in meal planning to encourage compliance and increase knowledge.
5. Prepare the patient for elemental diet or TPN if the patient is debilitated.

Maintaining Fluid and Electrolyte Balance

1. Monitor intake and output.
2. Provide fluids, as prescribed, to maintain hydration (1,000 mL/24 hours is minimum intake to meet body fluid needs).
3. Monitor stool frequency and consistency.
4. Monitor electrolytes (especially potassium) and acid–base balance because diarrhea can lead to metabolic acidosis.
5. Watch for cardiac dysrhythmias and muscle weakness because of loss of electrolytes.

Controlling Pain

1. Administer medications for control of inflammatory process, as prescribed.
2. Observe and record changes in pain—frequency, location, characteristics, precipitating events, and duration.
3. Monitor for distention, increased temperature, hypotension, and rectal bleeding—all signs of obstruction because of the inflammation.

Table 18-3 Drugs Used to Treat Inflammatory Bowel Disease

CATEGORY	ROUTE	DRUG	ADVERSE EFFECTS	CONSIDERATIONS
5-ASA drugs	Oral	Sulfasalazine	Headache, diarrhea, abdominal pain, abdominal cramping, malaise, hair loss, rash, orange discoloration of urine, bone marrow suppression, photosensitivity, and decreased sperm motility in men.	• Monitor CBC for signs of bone marrow suppression. • Recommend daily sunscreen use. • Decreased sperm motility is reversible upon drug discontinuation. • Urine discoloration is harmless.
	Oral	Olsalazine	Headache, diarrhea, abdominal pain, abdominal cramping, malaise, rash, joint pain, and nephrotoxicity. Rare cases of hepatitis have been reported to the FDA.	• Use with caution in patients with renal insufficiency
	Oral	Mesalamine and balsalazide	Headache, diarrhea, abdominal pain, abdominal cramping, malaise, rash, arthralgias, and nephrotoxicity	• Use mesalamine with caution in patients with renal insufficiency. Researchers have yet to determine the safety of balsalazide in patients with renal impairment. • Asacol tablets may be excreted whole in stool. Ask patients to report frequent passage of whole tablets.
	Rectal	Mesalamine	Abdominal pain, cramping, rectal bleeding, fever, and nephrotoxicity.	• Effective for distal disease (inflammation in the rectum and sigmoid colon). • Most adverse effects are mild and transient. • Available in both enema and suppository form for topical treatment of distal disease. The enema form allows coverage from the rectum to the sigmoid colon; suppositories suppress rectal inflammation.
Corticosteroids	Oral	Prednisone, methylprednisolone, and budesonide	Cushingoid appearance, hypertension, acne, water retention, weight gain, hair loss, increased appetite, hypokalemia, gastric irritation, ulcer formation, adrenal suppression, decreased resistance to infection. Complications associated with prolonged use include osteoporosis, cataract development, growth retardation, peptic ulceration, hyperglycemia, hypertension, aseptic joint necrosis, and glaucoma.	• May be administered in IV form when the gastrointestinal tract isn't able to absorb drugs properly. • Budesonide is approved for treating mild to moderately active Crohn disease of the terminal ileum. Because of budesonide's first-pass metabolism, systemic adverse effects are less common than those that occur with conventional steroids. • Corticosteroids aren't indicated for maintenance therapy in treating IBD secondary to associated long-term adverse effects.
	IV	Hydrocortisone and methylprednisolone		
	Rectal	Hydrocortisone/pramoxine and hydrocortisone		
Immune-modulating agents	Oral	6-Mercaptopurine and azathioprine	Bone marrow suppression, increased vulnerability to infection, rash, fever, malaise, arthralgias, hepatic dysfunction, nausea, vomiting, diarrhea, pancreatitis, hair loss, and neoplasm development.	• Monitor for bone marrow suppression. • Pregnancy category D. • Testing available that evaluates the patient's ability to metabolize the drug, determines therapeutic levels, and monitors for hepatotoxicity.
Biologic agents	IV	Infliximab	Infusion-related reactions: pruritus, rash, chest pain, hypotension, hypertension, dyspnea, headache, nausea, vomiting, fatigue, and fever.	• Infusion reactions usually resolve with decreasing the rate of infusion.
	SQ	Adalimumab	Other potential adverse effects (rare): autoantibody development (lupus-like syndrome) and increased susceptibility to infection.	• Perform tuberculosis (TB) skin test prior to first dose because of the drug's ability to allow latent TB to become active; a positive skin test (>5-mm induration) indicates the need for treatment for latent TB, before initiation of infliximab therapy. • Do not administer to patients with an active infection.

Adapted with permission from Rayhorn, N., & Rayhorn, D. (2002). Inflammatory bowel disease: Symptoms in the bowel and beyond. The Nurse Practitioner, 27(11), 24–25.

4. Clean rectal area and apply ointments, as necessary, to decrease discomfort from skin breakdown.
5. Prepare the patient for surgery if response to medical and drug therapy is unsatisfactory.
6. Surgery is determined specifically for each patient.
7. Recurrence of the disease is possible after surgery.

Providing Psychosocial Support

1. Offer understanding, concern, and encouragement—this person is often embarrassed about frequent and malodorous stools and often is fearful of eating.
2. Facilitate supportive psychological counseling, if appropriate.
3. Encourage the patient's usual support people to be involved in management of the disease and seek additional support groups as needed.
4. Encourage health-promoting behavior.

Patient Education and Health Maintenance

1. Provide comprehensive education about anatomy and physiology of the GI system, the chronic disease process, drug therapy, potential complications, and potential surgery.
2. Instruct patient about all prescribed medications, including the purpose, dosage, and adverse effects as well as to discuss use of any OTC drugs with health care provider.
3. Encourage regular follow-up and to report signs of complications: increasing abdominal distention, cramping pain, diarrhea, malaise, anorexia, fever, and passing stool through the urethra or vagina.
4. Explain the importance of adequate hydration and nutrition (based on individual tolerance) and monitoring weight.
5. Encourage the patient to participate in stress-reducing activities, such as exercise, relaxation techniques, music therapy.
6. For further information and support, refer to Crohn's & Colitis Foundation at *www.ccfa.org*.

Evaluation: Expected Outcomes

- Improved nutritional intake; weight stable.
- Adequate fluid intake; no evidence of dehydration; electrolyte levels within normal limits.
- Demonstrates relief of pain and manageable symptoms.
- Verbalizes improved attitude toward ways to live with the disease.

Colorectal Cancer

Colorectal cancer refers to malignancies of the colon and rectum. This type is the third leading cause of death in the United States. Colorectal tumors are nearly all adenocarcinomas. Lymphoma, carcinoid, melanoma, and sarcomas account for only 5% of colorectal lesions.

Pathophysiology and Etiology

1. Risk factors include:
   a. Age: Risk increases sharply after age 45 in African Americans, 50 in others.
   b. Previous history of resected colorectal cancer or adenomatous polyps.
   c. Family history of colorectal cancer or adenomatous polyps, especially if one first-degree relative diagnosed before age 60 or two first-degree relatives diagnosed at any age.
   d. Familial adenomatous polyposis (FAP; also a variant called Gardner syndrome) is an inherited condition characterized by multiple adenomatous polyps of the colon, in which cancer will inevitably develop in all affected individuals.
   e. Hereditary nonpolyposis colorectal cancer (HNPCC)—hereditary condition with a markedly increased risk of developing colorectal cancer as well as other cancers, such as endometrial, ovarian, renal, pancreatic, gastric, and small intestinal. There are few or no adenomatous polyps, and the bowel may undergo rapid change from normal tissue to polyp to cancer.
   f. Chronic ulcerative colitis—increasing risk after 10-year history.
   g. Incidence is higher in industrialized countries and lower in underdeveloped countries. Reason unclear but may be related to diet. The Western diet, which is high in refined grains, processed and red meats, high-fat dairy products, desserts, and fried foods, has been shown to increase risk of colorectal cancer.
   h. Immunodeficiency disease.
2. Colorectal lesions occur most frequently in the rectum and sigmoid areas; however, it appears there is a trend toward increasing frequency of right-sided lesions.
3. Most adenocarcinomas are ulcerative in appearance. A left-sided lesion tends to be annular and scarlike; a right-sided lesion tends to be a cauliflower-like mass that protrudes into the bowel lumen.
4. A lesion starts in the mucosal layers of the colonic wall and eventually penetrates the wall and invades surrounding structures and organs (bladder, prostate, ureters, vagina). Cancer spreads by direct invasion, lymphatic spread, and through the bloodstream. The liver and lungs are the most common metastatic sites.

 EVIDENCE BASE Kahi, C. J., Boland, C. R., Bominitz, J. A., et al. (2016). Colonoscopy surveillance after colorectal cancer resection: Recommendations of the US multi-society task force on colorectal cancer. *American Journal of Gastroenterology, 111*(3), 337–346.

Clinical Manifestations

Colorectal cancer is often asymptomatic. If present, symptomatology varies according to the location of the lesion and the extent of involvement.

1. Right-sided lesions—change in bowel habits, usually diarrhea; vague abdominal discomfort; black, tarry stools; anemia; weakness; weight loss; palpable mass in right lower quadrant.
2. Left-sided lesions—change in bowel habits, often increasing constipation with bouts of diarrhea because of partial obstruction; bright, streaked red blood in stool; cramping pain; weight loss; anemia; palpable mass.
3. Rectal lesions—change in bowel habits with possible urgent need to defecate, alternating constipation and diarrhea, and narrowed caliber of stool; bright red blood in stool; feeling of incomplete evacuation; rectal fullness progressing to dull constant ache.

Diagnostic Evaluation

1. Fecal immunochemical test—replaces the older guaiac-based tests.
2. Flexible sigmoidoscopy—can be used if colonoscopy is declined.

3. Colonoscopy with biopsy—diagnostic procedure of choice after strong suspicious clinical history or abnormal barium enema. CT colonography, also known as virtual colonoscopy, may be used for screening.
4. Pelvic MRI and endorectal ultrasonography—provide information about cancer penetration and pararectal lymph nodes.
5. Carcinoembryonic antigen (CEA)—70% of patients have elevated CEA levels. The CEA level monitors possible recurrence or metastasis.
6. CT scan of the abdomen, liver, lungs, and brain—may reveal metastatic disease.

Management

Surgical Resection

Treatment of choice for those with resectable lesions. Regional lymph node dissection determines staging and guides decisions regarding adjuvant therapy. Surgical options include:

1. Laparotomy with wide segmental bowel resection of tumor, including regional lymph nodes and blood vessels (right hemicolectomy, transverse colectomy, left hemicolectomy, or sigmoid resection).
2. Transanal excision—select people with tumors less than 1¼ inches (3 cm) and well differentiated less than 3 inches (7.5 cm) from the anal verge and localized to the rectal wall may avoid laparotomy.
3. Low anterior resection for upper rectal lesions—may include temporary loop colostomy to protect anastomosis with second procedure for takedown of colostomy.
4. Colonic J pouch—may be offered as a new surgical technique for rectal cancer (see page 525).
5. Select patients may be offered laparoscopic cancer surgery, although this remains controversial.
6. Abdominoperineal resection with permanent end colostomy for lower rectal lesions when adequate margins cannot be obtained, or there is involvement of anal sphincters. Because of improved stapling devices used deep in the pelvis, abdominoperineal resection accounts for fewer than 5% of colorectal resections.
7. Temporary loop colostomy to decompress bowel and divert fecal stream, followed by later bowel resection, anastomosis, and takedown of colostomy.
8. More extensive surgery involving the removal of other organs if cancer has spread, such as liver wedge, bladder, uterus, and/or small intestine, may be performed.
9. Unresectable colorectal cancer—diverting colostomy or ileostomy as palliation for obstructing tumor, laser fulguration, or the placement of an expandable wire stent.
10. Total proctocolectomy or ileal reservoir–anal anastomosis procedure for patients with FAP and chronic ulcerative colitis before colorectal cancer develops.

Other Therapy

1. Radiation therapy may be used preoperatively to improve resectability of the tumor and may be used postoperatively as adjuvant therapy to treat residual disease.
2. Chemotherapy may be used as adjuvant therapy to improve survival time.
   a. Used for residual disease, recurrence of disease, unresectable tumors, and metastatic disease.
   b. Drug combinations may include 5-fluorouracil plus levamisole or 5-fluorouracil plus leucovorin.
   c. A newer drug, irinotecan, is being used in protocols for advanced colorectal cancer.

3. Blood replacement of whole blood or packed red blood cells if severe anemia exists.

Complications

1. Obstruction.
2. Hemorrhage.
3. Anemia.
4. Metastasis.

Nursing Assessment

1. Interview patient regarding dietary habits and family and medical history to identify risk factors.
2. Question the patient regarding symptomatology of colorectal cancer, changes in bowel habits, rectal bleeding, tarry stools, abdominal discomfort, weight loss, weakness, and anemia.
3. Palpate the abdomen for tenderness (usually not tender), presence of mass.
4. Test stool for occult blood.

Nursing Diagnoses

- Imbalanced Nutrition: Less Than Body Requirements related to malignancy effects and weight loss.
- Constipation and/or Diarrhea related to change in bowel lumen.
- Chronic pain related to malignancy, inflammation, and possible intestinal obstruction.
- Fatigue related to anemia, radiation, chemotherapy, and metastatic disease.
- Fear related to diagnosis, prognosis, potential for complications.

Nursing Interventions

Achieving Adequate Nutrition

1. Meet the patient's nutritional needs by serving a high-calorie, low-residue diet for several days before surgery, if condition permits.
2. Observe and record fluid losses, such as may be sustained by vomiting and diarrhea.
3. Maintain hydration through IV therapy and record urine output. Metabolic tissue needs are increased, and more fluids are needed to eliminate waste products.
4. Serve smaller meals spaced throughout the day to maintain adequate calorie and protein intake if not NPO.
5. Encourage the patient to participate in meal planning to promote compliance.
6. Adjust diet before and after treatments, such as chemotherapy or radiation. Serve clear liquids, bland diet, or NPO, as prescribed.
7. Instruct the patient to take prescribed antiemetic, as needed, especially if receiving chemotherapy.

Relieving Constipation or Diarrhea

1. Monitor amount, consistency, frequency, and color of stool.
2. For constipation, use laxatives or enemas, as needed, and encourage exercise and adequate fluid/fiber intake to promote bowel motility.
3. For diarrhea, encourage adequate fluid intake to prevent fluid volume deficit and electrolyte imbalance.
4. For diarrhea related to radiation or chemotherapy, administer antidiarrheal medications and discuss foods that may slow transit time of bowel, such as bananas, rice, peanut butter, and pasta.

NURSING ALERT Antidiarrheal medications and foods to control diarrhea are contraindicated for the patient with an obstructing lesion. Use these measures only postoperatively after lesion resection for control of diarrhea related to cancer therapy.

Relieving Pain

1. Assess type and severity of pain and administer analgesics, as needed.
2. Evaluate effectiveness of analgesic regimen.
3. Investigate different approaches, such as relaxation techniques, repositioning, imaging, laughter, music, reading, and touch, for control or relief of pain.

Maintaining Energy Level

1. Institute an individualized activity plan after assessing the patient's activity level and tolerance, noting shortness of breath or tachycardia.
2. Allow for frequent rest periods to regain energy.
3. Administer blood products or recombinant human erythropoietin, as ordered, if fatigue is related to severe anemia.

Minimizing Fear

1. Encourage the patient and family to express feelings and fears together and separately.
2. Acknowledge that it is normal to have negative feelings toward cancer, surgery, colostomy, and treatment options.
3. Provide information and answer questions regarding disease process, treatment modalities, and complications. Offer diverse educational materials, such as brochures and videotapes.
4. Refer for counseling, if desired.
5. Genetic testing can confirm a hereditary diagnosis such as FAP or HNPCC.

Patient Education and Health Maintenance

1. Provide detailed information or resources about treatment modalities of radiation and chemotherapy.
2. Teach and demonstrate to the patient and/or family the skills necessary for colostomy management, which may include colostomy irrigation. The ostomy specialty nurse can provide formal education in this area.
3. Initiate a home care nursing referral to assist with wound care, to manage treatment adverse effects, and to continue teaching colostomy care.

4. Become an advocate for colon cancer prevention by educating the public about screening. Beginning at age 45 for African Americans and age 50 for others, men and women should follow one of the following American Cancer Society guidelines for early detection of colon cancer.
   a. Flexible sigmoidoscopy every 5 years.
   b. Colonoscopy every 10 years.
   c. Double-contrast barium enema every 5 years.
   d. Computed tomographic colonography (CTC) every 5 years.
   e. Alternately, stool-based testing can be done annually, but if positive, a colonoscopy must follow. Tests include guaiac-based fecal occult blood test (gFOBT) with high sensitivity for cancer, FIT with high sensitivity for cancer, and stool DNA (sDNA) with high sensitivity for cancer (interval uncertain pending further research).
5. For additional information and support, refer to the American Cancer Society at *www.cancer.org*.

 EVIDENCE BASE Smith, R. A., Manassram-Baptiste, D., Brooks, D., et al. (2015). Cancer screening in the United States, 2015: A review of current American Cancer Society guidelines and issues in cancer screening. *CA—Cancer Journal for Clinicians, 65*, 30–54.

Evaluation: Expected Outcomes

- Exhibits weight gain and improves nutritional status by adequate dietary intake.
- Has regular soft bowel movements.
- Minimal pain, controlled with analgesics or other techniques.
- Able to perform ADLs with adequate amounts of energy; no shortness of breath on exertion.
- Sleeping well; able to discuss feelings and fears related to surgery, prognosis, and treatment options.

ANORECTAL CONDITIONS
Hemorrhoids

Hemorrhoids are vascular masses in the lower rectum or anus. External hemorrhoids appear outside the external sphincter, whereas internal hemorrhoids appear above the internal sphincter (see Figure 18-15). When blood within the hemorrhoids becomes clotted because of obstruction, the hemorrhoids are referred to as thrombosed.

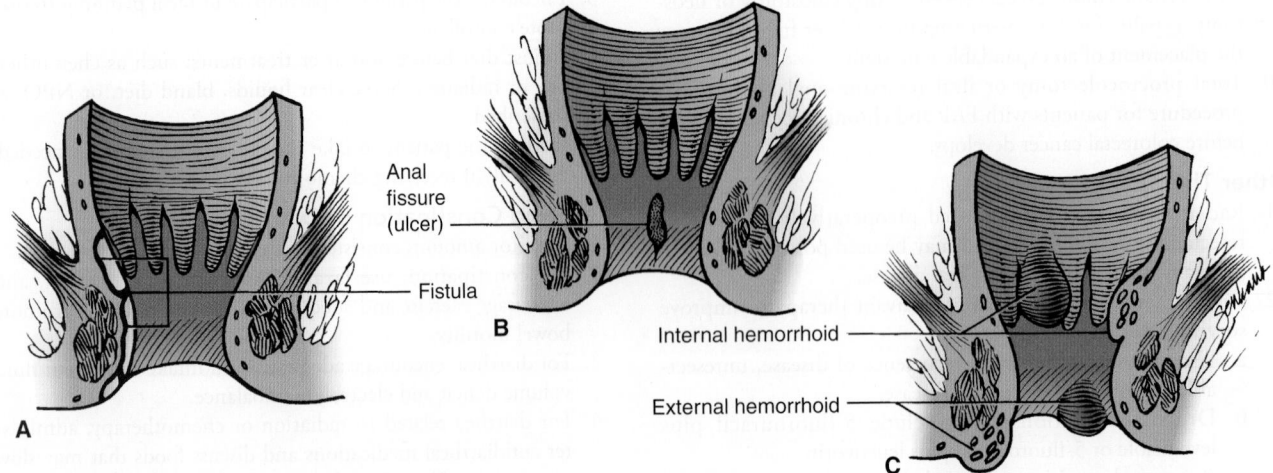

Figure 18-15. Various types of anal lesions. **(A)** Fistula. **(B)** Fissure. **(C)** External and internal hemorrhoids. (Smeltzer, S., & Bare, B. [2003]. Brunner and Suddarth's textbook of medical-surgical nursing [10th ed.]. Philadelphia: Lippincott Williams & Wilkins.)

Pathophysiology and Etiology

1. The exact pathogenesis remains controversial. Theories include:
   a. Abnormal dilation of veins of internal hemorrhoidal venous plexus.
   b. Abnormal distention of the arteriovenous anastomoses.
   c. Downward displacement or prolapse of anal cushions.
   d. Destruction of the anchoring connective tissue system.
2. Predisposing factors include:
   a. Pregnancy, prolonged sitting/standing.
   b. Straining at stool, chronic constipation/diarrhea.
   c. Anal infection, rectal surgery, or episiotomy.
   d. Hereditary factor.
   e. Exercise.
   f. Coughing, sneezing, vomiting.
   g. Loss of muscle tone because of age.
   h. Anal intercourse.
3. Increased intra-abdominal pressure causes engorgement in the vascular tissue lining the anal canal.
4. Loosening of vessels from surrounding connective tissue occurs with protrusion or prolapse into anal canal.

Clinical Manifestations

1. Bleeding during or after defecation, bright red blood on stool because of injury of mucosa covering hemorrhoid (most common).
2. Visible (if external) and palpable mass.
3. Constipation and anal itching.
4. Sensation of incomplete fecal evacuation.
5. Infection or ulceration, mucus discharge.
6. Pain noted more in external hemorrhoids.
7. Sudden rectal pain because of thrombosis in external hemorrhoids.

Diagnostic Evaluation

1. History and visualization by external examination through anoscopy or proctosigmoidoscopy.
2. Barium enema or colonoscopy to rule out more serious colonic lesions causing rectal bleeding.

Management

Asymptomatic hemorrhoids require no treatment.

Medical

1. Bowel habits should be regulated with nonirritating stool softeners and high-fiber diet to keep stools soft.
2. Frequent, warm sitz baths to ease pain and combat swelling.
3. Analgesics as needed.
4. Topical creams, lotions, pads, and suppositories containing such active ingredients as witch hazel, zinc monohydrate, pramoxine hydrochloride, glycerol stearate, phenylephrine, and hydrocortisone, to reduce swelling and provide comfort.
5. Control of itching by improved anal hygiene measures and control of moisture.
6. Avoid prolonged use of topical anesthetics on hemorrhoids or fissures because they often produce hypersensitive (allergic) perianal skin rashes with severe itching.
7. Manual reduction of external hemorrhoids if prolapsed.

8. Injection of sclerosing solutions (phenol 5%) to produce scar tissue and decrease prolapse.
9. Cryodestruction (cryosurgery)—freezing of hemorrhoids.
   a. Profuse drainage and swelling occur.
   b. Foul-smelling discharge may last for 7 to 10 days after cryosurgery.
10. Other procedures include infrared coagulation (infrared radiation) and bipolar diathermy (heat).

Surgical

1. Surgery may be indicated when the following conditions exist:
   a. Prolonged bleeding.
   b. Disabling pain.
   c. Intolerable itching.
   d. Prolapse.
2. Rubber ring ligation is the treatment of choice.
   a. During anoscopy, the apex of the hemorrhoid is grasped and drawn through a drum.
   b. A trigger device expels two rubber bands, which encircle the base of the hemorrhoid.
   c. After a period of time, the hemorrhoid sloughs away.
3. Dilation of the anal canal and lower rectum under general anesthesia is another treatment.
   a. This procedure is not advocated for patients whose main complaints are prolapse or incontinence.
   b. It also is not recommended for aging patients with weak sphincters.
4. Incision and removal of clot from acutely thrombosed hemorrhoid.
5. Hemorrhoidectomy—excision of internal/external hemorrhoids.

Complications

1. Hemorrhage, anemia.
2. Incontinence.
3. Prolapse and strangulation.

Nursing Interventions and Patient Education

1. After thrombosis or surgery, assist with frequent positioning, using pillow support for comfort.
2. Provide analgesics, warm sitz baths, or warm compresses to reduce pain and inflammation.
3. Apply anal pads, creams, or suppositories, as ordered, to relieve discomfort.
4. Observe anal area postoperatively for drainage and bleeding; report if excessive.
5. Administer stool softener/laxative to assist with bowel movements soon after surgery to reduce risk of stricture.
6. Encourage regular exercise, high-fiber diet, and adequate fluid intake (8 to 10 glasses/day) to avoid straining and constipation.
7. Discourage regular use of laxatives—firm, soft stools dilate the anal canal, decreasing stricture formation.
8. Determine the patient's normal bowel habits, and identify predisposing factors to educate patient about changes necessary to prevent recurrence of symptoms.

Other Conditions of the Anorectum

See Table 18-4, pages 534 to 535.

Table 18-4   Anorectal Disorders

CONDITION	ETIOLOGY	CLINICAL MANIFESTATIONS
Fissure Linear laceration of anal epithelium; typically located in the posterior midline	• Constipated stools may tear anal lining • Perineum strain during childbirth • Tuberculosis, syphilis, and Crohn disease are less common causes	• Tearing acute pain during and after bowel movement; discomfort may continue several hours after bowel movement • Spotting of bright red blood with stool; spasm of anal canal; burning
Abscess Localized area of pus from inflammation of anorectal tissue	• Infection develops from abrasion from foreign object, such as enema tip or fishbone • Acute phase of anal fistula, suspect Crohn disease • Tuberculosis or actinomycosis	• Painful, reddened bulge or swelling near the anus; pain increases with sitting; moderate to severe pain • Purulent drainage
Fistula Abnormal tubelike passage from the skin near the anus into anal canal	• Often preceded by anal abscess • May be associated with inflammatory bowel disease, cancer, or foreign body • Hidradenitis suppurativa	• Purulent drainage from opening • Itching and pain
Anal condylomas; venereal warts	• Infectious cauliflower-like papillomas; probably sexually transmitted papillomavirus • Differentiate from syphilitic warts, hemorrhoids, and anal/skin cancers	• Thrive in moist, macerated surfaces, as with purulent drainage • Often recur • Rarely invade the urethra, bladder, or rectum
Proctitis Acute or chronic inflammation of rectal mucosa	• Common infecting organisms: *Neisseria gonorrhoeae*, *Chlamydia*, herpes simplex virus, *Treponema pallidum* (syphilis) • Radiation	• Anorectal pain; purulent, mucoid, or bloody discharge; pruritus; tenesmus • Diarrhea and/or constipation
Stricture Narrowing of the anorectal lumen, preventing dilation of sphincter	• Usually results from scarring after anorectal surgery (hemorrhoidectomy) or inflammation • Congenital anomalies	• Constipation, ribbon stools, may not completely evacuate stools • Pain with bowel movement; itching
Rectal Prolapse Mucosal membrane protrudes through the anus	• The support structures are weakened (sphincters and muscles), leading to rectal intussusception • Conditions may include neurologic disorders, chronic diseases, aging	• Associated with constipation and straining; rectal fullness • Bloody diarrhea; rectal ulcer secondary to intussusception

SELECTED REFERENCES

ASGE Standards of Practice Committee; Muthusamy, V., Lightdale, J., et al. (2015). The role of endoscopy in the management of GERD. *Gastrointestinal Endoscopy, 81*(6), 1305–1310.

Bharucha, A. E., Pemberton, J. H., & Locke, G. R. (2013). American Gastroenterological Association technical review on constipation. *Gastroenterology, 144,* 218–238.

Cabebe, E., Espat, N., & Cloutier, M. (2016). *Esophageal cancer guidelines.* Available: www.emedicine.medscape.com/article/2500007-overview

Caraballo, H. L. (2013). Guidelines for the evaluation and management of upper gastrointestinal bleeding. *Evidence Based Medicine, 5*(6). Available: www.ebmedicine.net/index.php

Chey, W., Leontiadis, G., Howden, C. W., et al. (2017). Treatment of H. pylori infection. *American Journal of Gastroenterology, 112,* 212–238.

Di Saverio, S., Coccolini, F., Galati, M., et al. (2013). Bologna guidelines for diagnosis and management of adhesive small bowel obstruction (ASBO): 2013 update of the evidence-based guidelines from the world society of emergency surgery ASBO working group. *World Journal of Emergency Surgery, 8,* 42.

Emergency Nurses Association. (2015). *Clinical practice guideline: Gastric tube placement verification.* Des Plaines, IL: Author. Available: www.ena.org/practice-research/research/CPG/documents/gastrictubeCPG.pdf

Fujishiro, M., Iguchi, M., Kakushima, N., et al. (2016). Guidelines for endoscopic management of non-variceal upper gastrointestinal bleeding. *Digestive Endoscopy, 28,* 363–378.

Kahi, C. J., Boland, C. R., Bominitz, J. A., et al. (2016). Colonoscopy surveillance after colorectal cancer resection: Recommendations of the US multi-society task force on colorectal cancer. *American Journal of Gastroenterology, 111*(3), 337–346.

Kamm, M. (2017). Rapid changes in epidemiology of inflammatory bowel disease. *Lancet, 390* (10114): 2741–2742.

Katz, P., Gerson, L., & Vela, M. (2013). Guidelines for the diagnosis and management of gastroesophageal reflux disease. *American Journal of Gastroenterology, 108,* 308–328.

Kirkland-Kyhn, H., Martin, S., Zaratkiewicz, S., et al. (2018). Ostomy Care at Home: Educating family caregivers on stoma management and potential complications. *American Journal of Nursing, 118*(4), 63–68.

MANAGEMENT	NURSING CONSIDERATIONS
• Promotion of regular, soft bowel movements through stool softeners, suppositories, high-fiber diet, bulking agents • Topical creams • Fissurectomy; sphincterotomy	• Assist with warm sitz baths and local application of anesthetic ointment to reduce pain • Instruct to eat high-fiber foods and drink fluids to prevent constipation
• Incision and drainage of purulent exudate • Placement of drainage catheter for 7 to 10 days; possible packing dressing • Warm sitz baths; pulsed lavage	• Wound assessment • Pain medications as needed • Alert for passage of bowel movements, postoperatively
• Fistulotomy • Fistulectomy • Bowel rest to allow fistula to heal; possible fecal diversion temporarily	• Wound assessment • Pain medications as needed • Alert for passage of bowel movements, postoperatively
• Application of podophyllum resin (may be painful) • Electrofulguration • Alpha-interferon injections/synergistic with podophyllum resin • Fluorouracil	• Encourage good anal hygiene and frequent use of talc dusting powder • Schedule follow-up visits to assess area periodically for recurrence
• Treatment specific to isolated organism—antibiotics, antivirals • Bulking agents, antispasmodics	• Review medications • Assist with examination and treatment
• Treatment of inflammatory cause • Dilation by digital, instrumentation, or balloon methods • If stenosis severe, may need plastic surgery to anal canal	• Prevention of stenosis after anal surgery facilitated by anal hygiene, warm sitz baths, and dilation • Postoperative care includes stool softeners, warm sitz baths, and wound care
• Treatment depends on underlying cause • Sclerosing agent injection may fix the rectum in place • Surgery may include sphincter repair or resection of prolapsed tissue	• Diet/fluid instructions to avoid constipation • Teach perineum-strengthening exercises

Kohn, G., Price, R., Demeester, S., et al; Society of American Gastrointestinal and Endoscopic Surgeons. (2013). Guidelines for the management of hiatal hernia. *Surgical Endoscopy, 27*(12), 4409–4428.

Leiberman, D., Rex, D., Winawer, S., et al. (2012). American College of Gastroenterology guidelines for colonoscopy surveillance after screening and polypectomy: A consensus update by the US multi-society task force on colorectal cancer. *Gastroenterology, 143,* 844–857.

National Cancer Institute. (2016). *Colorectal cancer screening (PDQ)- Health professional version.* Available: *www.cancer.gov/types/colorectal/hp/colorectal-screening-pdq*

Osman, D., Djibré, M., Da Silva, D., & Goulenok, C. (2012). Management by the intensivist of gastrointestinal bleeding in adults and children. *Annals of Intensive Care, 2,* 46.

Queen, T., & Adler, D. (2014). Esophageal cancer: Current diagnosis and management. *Journal of Clinical Outcomes Management, 21*(8). Available: *www.jcomjournal.com/esophageal-cancer-current-diagnosis-and-management/*

Rex, D., Boland, C., Dominitz, J., et al. (2017). Colorectal cancer screening: Recommendations for physicians and patients from the U.S. Multi- Society Task Force on Colorectal Cancer. *The American Journal of Gastroenterology,* 112, 1016–1030.

Sanchez-Velazquez, P., Grande, L., and Pera, M. (2016). Outpatient treatment of uncomplicated diverticulitis: a systematic review. *European Journal of Gastroenterology and Hepatology, 28*(6);622–627.

Smyth, E., Verheij, M., Allum, W., et al. (2016). Gastric cancer: ESMO clinical practice guidelines. *Annals of Oncology, 27*(5), v38–v49.

Society of Gastroenterology Nurses and Assoc., Inc. (2014). *Standards of clinical nursing practice and role delineations.* Chicago, IL: Author. Available: *www.sgna.org/Portals/0/Education/PDF/Standards-Guidelines/SGNA_StandardsofClinicalNursingPractice_2014_Final.pdf*

Wound, Ostomy and Continence Nurses Society. (2014). *Stoma complications: Best practice for Clinicians.* Mt. Laurel, NJ: Author.

19
Hepatic, Biliary, and Pancreatic Disorders

OVERVIEW AND ASSESSMENT
Assessment of Accessory Organ Dysfunction

The liver and its bile ducts, the gallbladder, and the pancreas are called accessory glands in the GI system. Their function is to aid digestion through the delivery of bile and enzymes to the small intestine. The liver plays additional roles in detoxification of chemicals and synthesis and storage of important nutrients. The pancreas also functions as an endocrine gland, as discussed in Chapter 24.

Effects of Aging on Liver and Gallbladder

Liver function tests generally remain within normal range, but a number of other physiologic changes occur within the hepatic and biliary systems with aging.

1. Decline in liver volume and size.
2. Decrease in blood flow.
3. Reduced drug metabolism.
4. Decline in capability of drug clearance.
5. Slower repair of damaged liver cells after injury.
6. Decreased production and flow of bile with decline in gallbladder contraction after meals.
7. Atypical clinical presentation of gallbladder and bile duct disorders.
8. Increased cholesterol secretion in bile leading to increased occurrence of gallstones.
9. Slower clearance of hepatitis B surface antigen, if infected.
10. Rapid progression of hepatitis C infection with lower response rate to therapy.

 GERONTOLOGIC ALERT Use caution with administering potentially hepatotoxic drugs, such as acetaminophen, to older adults.

History

1. Was the patient born between the years of 1945 and 1965?
2. Have there been blood transfusions (before 1992)? Are there known blood disorders? GI bleeding?
3. Has there been contact with a person who has an infection such as hepatitis? Any unprotected sexual activity or ingestion of potentially contaminated food?
4. Has there been drug or chemical toxicity, such as carbon tetrachloride, chloroform, phosphorus, arsenicals, ethanol, halothane, isoniazid, or acetaminophen? Have amanita mushrooms been ingested recently? Are certain medications being taken, such as phenothiazine derivatives, sulfonamides, antidiabetic drugs, propylthiouracil, monoamine oxidase inhibitors, methyldopa, azathioprine, corticosteroids, thiazide diuretics, estrogens, and valproic acid? Any antiviral medications taken for Aquired Immune Deficiency Syndrome such as didanosine or antineoplastic agents, as many of these drugs can cause hepatic, biliary, and pancreatic gastrointestinal symptoms?
5. Is there a history of nonsterile needle puncture, as in subcutaneous ("skin popping"), intramuscular ("muscling"), or intravenous (IV) drug use? Tattoos?
6. Does medical history include gallstones, hepatitis, pancreatitis, Wilson disease, Budd-Chiari syndrome, biliary cirrhosis, liver surgery, or transplantation?
7. Any family history of gallstones, pancreatitis, gallbladder, or pancreatic cancer or related cancers such as breast or ovarian cancer?
8. Is there a history of organ transplantation (before 1992)?
9. How much alcohol is or has been ingested during the patient's life and what specific type of alcohol (i.e., beer, wine, liquor)?

Common Manifestations

1. Any jaundice—yellow color of sclera and skin, pruritus, dark tea-colored urine, light gray or clay-colored (acholic) stool?
2. Any dyspepsia, anorexia, nausea, vomiting, right upper quadrant or epigastric pain, or pain radiating to the back or shoulder blade? What is the relationship of pain to eating or to position?

3. Has there been fatigue, malaise, loss of vigor and strength, easy bruising, or weight loss?
4. Any fever, chills, headache, myalgias, arthralgias, photophobia?
5. Any steatorrhea—stools that are loose, greasy, foamy, orange in color, and foul smelling and that float?

Physical Examination Findings

1. Skin—yellow sclera or skin? Rashes or scratches on body from severe scratching because of pruritus? Any signs of bruising or petechiae on body, palmar erythema, or overt bleeding?
2. Neurologic—what is the level of consciousness (LOC)? Any asterixis (flapping tremor elicited when the arms are extended and wrists dorsiflexed)?
3. Abdomen—any tenderness or liver enlargement in the right upper quadrant? Any ascites? Any palpable masses in the abdomen? Any fluid wave?
4. Peripheral vascular—any edema, anasarca, or telangiectasia?

Laboratory Tests

See Table 19-1, page 538.

CA 19-9

Description
A tumor antigen found in serum; used as a marker to assess the efficacy of treatment in pancreatic cancer, surgical outcomes, and survival.

Nursing and Patient Care Considerations
1. Tell patient a blood test will be taken and the results will be ready in 1 to 2 days.
2. Not a screening test for pancreatic cancer, this is an adjunct with other tests to provide support for a diagnosis of pancreatic cancer and to better measure the recurrence of pancreatic cancer after treatment.
3. Antigen level may be elevated with benign conditions including biliary tract obstruction, thyroid disease, inflammatory bowel disease, and acute or chronic pancreatitis.

Alpha-fetoprotein

Description
An oncofetal antigen found in serum that appears when a tumor returns to a more primitive state. Alpha-fetoprotein (AFP) is elevated in 70% to 95% of hepatocellular carcinomas (primary liver cancer).

Nursing and Patient Care Considerations
1. Tell patient a blood test will be taken and the results will be ready in 1 to 3 days.
2. Not a screening test for primary liver cancer, this is an adjunct with other tests to provide support for a diagnosis of primary liver cancer and to detect/ predict liver metastasis.
3. AFP may also be elevated in certain tumors of the gonads (testes and ovaries), retroperitoneum, and mediastinum.

Radiology and Imaging Studies

Ultrasonography

Description
1. A noninvasive test that focuses high-frequency sound waves over an area in the abdomen to generate an image of the structure.
2. Ultrasound of the abdomen can detect gallstones, dilated bile duct, fluid-filled cysts, ascites, and small abdominal masses.
3. This test is the preferred diagnostic procedure. It is rapid and accurate, and does not expose the patient to radiation. It can be used safely in patients with liver dysfunction and jaundice.
4. It is reported to be able to detect gallstones with 95% accuracy.
5. Ultrasound with Doppler can assess the patency of the portal vein, hepatic artery, hepatic vein, and direction of blood flow. It can be used to diagnose patients with Budd-Chiari syndrome or vessel thrombosis after major liver surgery or liver transplant.

Nursing and Patient Care Considerations
1. The patient should have nothing to eat or drink for 4 to 8 hours prior to the exam, and a fat-free meal is preferred the evening before the test, in order to minimize air in the stomach and bowel, which would obscure images of the gallbladder, liver, pancreas, and spleen. Medications may be taken with small sips of water.
2. Explain to the patient that a gel is applied to the skin over the selected area and a wandlike transducer is swept across the area of interest.
3. Ultrasound pictures will be obtained.

Hepatobiliary Scan

Description
1. A noninvasive nuclear medicine study (also referred to as a hepatobiliary iminodiacetic acid [HIDA] scan) using radioactive materials to evaluate gallbladder function and aid in the diagnosis of hepatobiliary disorders, such as common bile duct obstruction, acute and chronic cholecystitis, bile leaks, bile reflux, and hepatocellular dysfunction after liver transplantation.
2. A radioactive agent is administered in an IV line. It is taken up by the hepatocytes and excreted rapidly through the biliary tract.
3. The biliary tract is scanned, and images of the gallbladder and biliary tract are obtained.

Nursing and Patient Care Considerations
1. Patient should have nothing by mouth (NPO) for at least 4 hours before the procedure to optimize emptying of gallbladder.
2. If possible, no opiates should be administered for at least 8 hours before the procedure because of opiate effects on smooth muscle motility of biliary tree and gallbladder.
3. Inform the patient that the scan takes approximately 2 to 4 hours and additional images may need to be taken up to 24 hours later.

Endoscopic Retrograde Cholangiopancreatography

Description
1. Endoscopic retrograde cholangiopancreatography (ERCP) involves visualization of the common bile, pancreatic, and hepatic ducts with a flexible fiber-optic endoscope inserted into the esophagus, passed through the stomach, and into the duodenum.
2. The common bile duct and the pancreatic duct are cannulated, and contrast medium is injected into the ducts, permitting visualization and radiographic evaluation.

Table 19-1 Liver Diagnostic Studies

TEST AND PURPOSE	NORMAL	NURSING CONSIDERATIONS
Bile Formation and Secretion		
Serum Bilirubin Measures bilirubin in the blood; this determines the ability of the liver to take up, conjugate, and excrete bilirubin. Bilirubin is a product of the breakdown of hemoglobin.		
Direct (conjugated)—soluble in water	0–0.3 mg/dL	• Abnormal in biliary and liver disease, causing jaundice clinically.
Indirect (unconjugated)—insoluble in water	0–1 mg/dL	• Abnormal in hemolysis and in functional disorders of uptake or conjugation.
Total serum bilirubin	0.1–1.2 mg/dL	• Used as screening test for liver or biliary dysfunction.
Urine Bilirubin Not normally found in urine, but if direct serum bilirubin is elevated, some spills into urine.	None (0)	• Tea-colored urine; when specimen is shaken, yellow-green tinted foam can be observed. • If the patient is receiving phenazopyridine, mark the laboratory slip to this effect because there may be a false- positive bilirubin result.
Urobilinogen Formed in small intestine by action of bacteria on bilirubin. Related to amount of bilirubin excreted into bile.	Urine urobilinogen <1 mg in 2-hr specimen or 0.5 to 4 mg/dL in 24-hr specimen Fecal urobilinogen 50 to 300 mg/24 hr	• Random urine specimen is collected over 2-hr after lunch, or a total level is collected over a 24-hr period. • Place specimen in dark brown container and send it to laboratory immediately or refrigerate to prevent decomposition. • If the patient is receiving antimicrobials, mark laboratory slip to this effect because production of urobilinogen can be falsely reduced.
Protein Studies		
Albumin and Globulin Measurement Is of greater significance than total protein measurement.		• As one increases, the other decreases.
Albumin—produced by liver cells	3.5–5.5 g/dL	• Albumin ↓ (decrease) in cirrhosis, chronic hepatitis
Globulin—produced in lymph nodes, spleen, bone marrow, and Kupffer cells of liver	2.5–5.9 g/dL	• Globulin ↑ (increase) in cirrhosis, chronic obstructive jaundice, viral hepatitis
Coagulation		
Prothrombin Time (PT) Prothrombin and other clotting factors are manufactured in the liver; its rate is influenced by the supply of vitamin K.	9.6–12.5 sec	• PT may be prolonged in liver disease, in which case it will not return to normal with vitamin K. It may also be prolonged in malabsorption of fat and fat-soluble vitamins, in which case it will return to normal with vitamin K.
Calculated from PT International Normalized Ratio (INR)	0.8–1.2	• Used to monitor warfarin therapy.
Fat Metabolism		
Cholesterol Measures lipid metabolism by determining serum cholesterol levels.	140–200 mg/dL	• Serum cholesterol level is decreased in parenchymal liver disease. • Serum lipid level is increased in biliary obstruction.
Liver Detoxification		
Serum Alkaline Phosphatase Because bile disposes this enzyme, any impairment of liver cell excretory function will cause an elevation. In cholestasis or obstruction, increased synthesis of enzyme causes very high levels in blood.	30–120 IU/L	• Elevated to more than three times normal in extrahepatic obstructive jaundice, intrahepatic cholestasis, liver metastasis, or granulomas. Also elevated in osteoblastic diseases, Paget disease, and hyperparathyroidism.

Table 19-1 Liver Diagnostic Studies (Continued)

TEST AND PURPOSE	NORMAL	NURSING CONSIDERATIONS
Enzyme Production		
These enzymes are found in high concentration in the liver as well as some other tissues. Liver injury results in enzyme release into blood.		
Aspartate aminotransferase (AST)	0–37 IU/L	• An elevation in these enzymes indicates liver cell damage.
Alanine aminotransferase (ALT)	0–40 IU/L	• Some drugs such as opioids may also cause a rise in AST and ALT.
Lactate dehydrogenase (LDH)	105–333 IU/L	• LDH is found in liver, heart, kidney, muscle, and blood cells.
Gamma glutamyl transpeptidase (GGT)	0–51 IU/L	• GGT is also found in the kidneys, pancreas, and bile ducts but is most sensitive to alcohol-induced liver damage.
Ammonia (NH_3), serum	0–32 mmol/L	• Ammonia levels rise when the liver is unable to convert ammonia to urea.

3. Done to detect extrahepatic biliary obstruction, such as calculi, tumors of the bile duct, strictures or injuries to the bile duct; intrahepatic biliary obstruction caused by stones or tumor; and pancreatic disease, such as chronic pancreatitis, pseudocyst, pancreatic duct anomalies, or tumor.

4. May be combined with a therapeutic biliary or pancreatic procedure, such as endoscopic sphincterotomy, placement of biliary or pancreatic stents, tissue biopsy, removal of fluid for cytology, or retrieval of retained gallstones from the common bile duct.

Nursing and Patient Care Considerations
Preprocedure

1. Assess for allergies to iodine, seafood, or contrast media to determine the need for premedication with antihistamines or steroids (per facility protocol) to prevent a reaction.

2. Patient must be NPO for at least 6 hours before the procedure. Withhold medications according to provider order.

3. Any patient receiving heparin should have the infusion stopped for 4 to 6 hours before the procedure. If patient is receiving warfarin, aspirin, clopidogrel, or other platelet-inhibiting or blood-thinning medication, a recent international normalized ratio (INR)/partial prothrombin time (PTT) must be available.

4. Make sure that dentures are removed; instruct the patient to gargle and swallow topical anesthetic to decrease gag reflex, as ordered.

5. Verify that the patient has a signed consent form before sedation is given.

6. Establish baseline vital signs.

7. Establish IV access.

8. Administer antibiotic prophylaxis, as ordered.

9. If outpatient procedure, the patient must have a responsible adult to drive him or her home as patient is not allowed to drive or operate machinery for 24 hours because of the effects of mild sedation.

Postprocedure

1. Monitor and document vital signs.

2. Observe for and report abdominal distention and signs of perforation, GI bleeding, or possible pancreatitis, including

chills, fever, pain, vomiting, hypotension, and tachycardia. Notify the health care provider immediately.

3. Maintain NPO status until the patient is alert and gag reflex returns. Check for gag reflex by applying gentle pressure with a tongue depressor placed on the back of the tongue.

Endoscopic Ultrasound
Description

1. In endoscopic ultrasound (EUS), a high-frequency ultrasound probe is placed at the tip of an endoscope to assess the pancreas through the GI lumen. This helps to provide images of the pancreas and adjacent organs.

2. It is useful in staging pancreatic tumors and establishing the size of the tumor, its extension into adjacent structures, local and regional nodal involvement, and any blood vessels that may be involved.

3. Tissue may also be obtained by fine needle aspiration through EUS guidance to confirm the diagnosis of a pancreatic malignancy.

Nursing and Patient Care Considerations

1. Instruct the patient that tissue may be obtained for analysis.

2. Verify that the patient has a signed consent form for the procedure and tissue aspiration before sedation is given.

3. Preprocedure and postprocedure care is the same as for ERCP.

Magnetic Resonance Cholangiopancreatography
Description

1. A noninvasive, nonradiation radiologic technique that produces images of the pancreatic ducts and biliary tree similar in appearance to those obtained from an ERCP with the advantage of providing images of the surrounding parenchyma.

2. Magnetic resonance cholangiopancreatography (MRCP) can detect the level and presence of biliary obstruction, but cannot offer therapeutic intervention.

3. MRCP does not require the administration of contrast material and provides ideal imaging for patients with allergies to iodine-based contrast materials or kidney disease. Noniodine contrast agent may be given to enhance the picture of the biliary anatomy or secretin may be given as it stimulates exocrine

secretion of the pancreas and improves visualization of the pancreatic duct by increasing its caliber.

Nursing and Patient Care Considerations
Preprocedure

1. Confirm that the patient does not have a pacemaker or internal defibrillator because the magnetic field could cause malfunction.
2. Confirm that the patient does not have any metal hardware in or on the body, such as intracranial aneurysm clips, intraocular metal fragments, cochlear ear devices, metal joint replacements, retained bullets or shrapnel, or steel sutures, because this may cause artifact and a distorted picture from the magnetic pull by the metal.
3. Remove all metal attachments from the patient, such as watch, jewelry, piercings, cell phone, IV poles, and infusion devices.
4. Confirm that the patient does not have a fear of enclosed spaces (claustrophobia) or anxiety as the patient may not be able to undergo the procedure or may require a sedative.
5. The patient must be NPO for at least 4 hours before the procedure.
6. Inform the patient that the test takes about 10 to 30 minutes.

Postprocedure

1. The patient may resume usual activities.
2. The health care provider will notify the patient of the results when available, usually in 1 to 3 days.

Positron Emission Tomographic (PET) Scan

Description

1. Positron emission tomography (PET) is an imaging technique that uses positively charged radioactive particles to detect subtle changes in the body's metabolism and chemical activities.
2. Fluorodeoxyglucose 18F (18F-FDG) is injected via IV line as a radiotracer and has a short half-life of 110 minutes and is cleared rapidly from the body.
3. The radiotracer used most often for PET scan has a glucose component; because malignant tumors use glucose and grow at a faster rate than normal tissue, PET scans are able to locate areas of high tracer uptake, which represents tumor growth.
4. A PET scan provides a black-and-white or color-coded image of the function of a particular area of the body, rather than its structure. Functional change precedes structural change in tissues and organs; therefore, PET scans can detect abnormalities earlier than a computed tomography (CT) scan or magnetic resonance imaging (MRI).
5. PET scan application in hepatic, biliary, and pancreatic disease includes the detection of cancer—particularly when other conventional imaging findings are negative—and response to cancer treatment. PET scan can also be used to evaluate the physiology of the heart and brain at baseline or following an event to determine remaining function.

Nursing and Patient Care Considerations
Preprocedure

1. The patient should begin a limited carbohydrate diet 24 hours prior to the procedure. The test provides images showing where certain molecules are in the body, including where glucose is located. This is greatly affected by the level of sugar in the blood; therefore, the diet the day before the scan impacts the quality of pictures.
2. The patient must be NPO, except for plain water, for at least 6 hours before the procedure.

3. Patients with diabetes or patients with glucose intolerance may require adjustments in diet and oral hypoglycemic or insulin dosage on the day of the test as blood glucose levels must be no higher than 200 mg/dL. Adjustments should be made on an individual basis.
4. Patients are not to do exercise of any sort for the 48 hours prior to the exam. This includes even nominal exercise such as golf and gardening.
5. Advise the patient to remove jewelry or other items containing metal.
6. Inform the patient that scanning time varies from 15 minutes to 2 hours, depending on the areas to be scanned, but the total time in the imaging center is longer (2 to 3 hours).
7. Caution the patient that it is essential to arrive on time for this test because the FDG tracer is radioactive only for a short time. Some centers order the tracer on a per case basis, scheduling delivery of the radiotracer to coincide with the patient's time of arrival.
8. Inform the patient that an IV line will be used to inject the radiotracer. To allow the radiotracer to disperse throughout the body, the scan will be performed 30 to 60 minutes after the injection.
9. Make sure that a bowel preparation has been carried out, if ordered. A urinary catheter may be inserted for a pelvic PET scan.
10. Inform the patient that the radiotracer is rapidly cleared from the body and that the test has no adverse effects.

Postprocedure

1. The patient may resume usual activities.
2. The patient may be encouraged to increase fluid intake to assist in flushing out the radiotracer.

Percutaneous Transhepatic Cholangiography

Description

1. Percutaneous transhepatic cholangiography (PTC) is a fluoroscopic examination of the intrahepatic and extrahepatic biliary ducts after injection of contrast medium into the biliary tree through percutaneous needle injection.
2. Helps to distinguish obstructive jaundice caused by liver disease from jaundice caused by biliary obstruction, such as from a tumor, injury to the common bile duct, stones within the bile ducts, or sclerosing cholangitis.
3. A biliary catheter may be placed during the procedure to drain the biliary tree, called percutaneous transhepatic biliary drainage (PTBD). This relieves jaundice, decreases pruritus, improves nutritional status, allows easy access into the biliary tree for further procedures, and can be used as an anatomic landmark and stent of a surgical anastomosis to allow for healing.

Nursing and Patient Care Considerations
Preprocedure

1. Assess for allergies to iodine, seafood, or contrast media to determine need to be premedicated with antihistamines or steroids (per facility protocol) to prevent reaction.
2. The patient must be NPO for at least 4 hours before the procedure.
3. Verify that the patient has had all questions answered and has a signed consent form before sedatives are given.
4. Inform the patient that the procedure takes 30 to 60 minutes.
5. Establish baseline hemoglobin, hematocrit, and platelet count.

6. Make sure prothrombin time (PT) and INR are within normal limits.
7. Establish baseline vital signs.
8. Establish an IV line.
9. Administer antibiotic prophylaxis, as ordered.

Postprocedure

1. Monitor and document vital signs and assess puncture site for bleeding, hematoma, or bile leakage.
2. Assess for and report signs of peritonitis from bile leaking into the abdomen (fever, chills, diffuse abdominal pain, tenderness, distention), or cholangitis (infection in the biliary tree) from bacteria in the bile being released into the GI tract and then into the bloodstream.
3. Continue antibiotic prophylaxis per facility protocol.
4. If the patient has PTBD, monitor the catheter exit site for bleeding or bile drainage and monitor drainage in bile bag for color, amount, and consistency. The drainage initially may have some blood mixed with bile but should clear within a few hours. The liver makes 700 to 1,000 mL of bile in 24 hours, and there should be adequate drainage when bile is draining into a bile bag (called external drainage).
   a. Report frank blood and blood clots that appear in the bile bag.
   b. Large amounts of bile drainage may require fluid replacement.
   c. Maintain patency and security of biliary catheter; perform routine care and dressing at catheter exit site.
   d. Perform routine flushing of biliary catheter per order.
   e. Cap off the end of the biliary catheter to allow internal drainage of bile, if indicated. Teach the patient the care and flushing of biliary catheter and signs of complications, if indicated.
5. Signs of complications include fever, chills, persistent jaundice, inability to flush the catheter, bleeding from the catheter, redness or discharge from the catheter site, leakage around the exit site of the catheter, and dislodgment of the catheter.
6. Notify the health care provider immediately if the patient complains of abdominal bloating and exquisite abdominal tenderness as the patient may be bleeding into the abdomen.

NURSING ALERT Do not aspirate from a PTBD catheter because this draws bacteria from the bowel back through the liver and may cause cholangitis. Gently push solution into the PTBD catheter to prevent increased pressure within the biliary tree.

Other Diagnostic Tests

Transient Elastography

Description

1. Noninvasive measure superior to traditional ultrasound in evaluating the liver. The probe measures the velocity as this wave passes through the liver.
2. Can replace biopsy to evaluate fibrosis and cirrhosis.
3. Used for initial assessment of liver scarring, as well as follow-up for progression of disease.

Nursing and Patient Care Considerations

1. Technical limitations of the test preclude its use in patients who have ascites, individuals who are morbidly obese, and/or patients who have large amounts of chest wall fat.
2. Ensure that the patient has NPO for at least 2 hours before the procedure.

3. Inform the patient that the test takes about 10 minutes and causes no discomfort.
4. Following the procedure, the patient may resume normal activity and diet.

Liver Biopsy

 EVIDENCE BASE Dohan, A., Guerrache, Y., Boudiaf, M., Gavini, J. P., Kaci, R., & Soyer, P. (2014). Transjugular liver biopsy: Indications, technique and results. *Diagnostic and Interventional Imaging, 95*(1), 11–15.

Description

Liver biopsy is the gold standard for diagnosis of cirrhosis or cancer. Sampling of liver tissue through needle aspiration establishes a diagnosis of liver disease through histologic review. The sample may be taken from the liver directly (percutaneous) or through the internal jugular vein (transjugular). Both forms of biopsy include the risks of an invasive procedure: pain, risk for bleeding, and requires close monitoring and observation. The transjugular liver biopsy utilizes fluoroscopy and is a safer option for patients with diffuse liver disease and severe alteration in coagulation or massive ascites.

Nursing and Patient Care Considerations
Preprocedure

1. Establish baseline hemoglobin level, hematocrit, and platelet count.
2. Any patient receiving heparin should have the infusion stopped for 4 to 6 hours before the procedure. If the patient is receiving warfarin, aspirin, clopidogrel, or other platelet-inhibiting or blood-thinning medication, a recent INR, PTT and PT must be available and within normal limits.
3. Verify informed consent.
4. Establish baseline vital signs.
5. Inform the patient that cooperation in holding breath for about 10 seconds during the procedure is important to obtain biopsy without damaging the diaphragm.
6. An IV may be inserted for sedation, as needed.

Postprocedure

1. Position the patient on right side with pillow supporting lower rib cage for several hours following transcutaneous biopsy to prevent bleeding
2. Neck discomfort is common following transjugular liver biopsy. Utilize positioning and nonpharmacologic methods to promote comfort.
3. Check vital signs and observe biopsy site frequently for bleeding or drainage.
4. Report increasing pulse, decreasing blood pressure (BP), increasing pain, and apprehension, which may indicate hemorrhage.

Fine Needle Aspiration

Description

1. The removal of fluid from a cyst or the removal of cells from a mass to establish a diagnosis through histologic review.
2. A fine needle is inserted into the suspicious area, and a small sample is withdrawn.
3. The needle is guided by fluoroscopy, CT scan, or ultrasound and can usually reach most internal organs with minimal risk to the patient.

Nursing and Patient Care Considerations

Preprocedure

1. Establish baseline hemoglobin, hematocrit, and platelet count.
2. Verify informed consent.
3. Establish baseline vital signs.
4. Tell the patient that a mild sedative may be given and a pain block may be performed in the area where the needle will be placed.
5. Encourage the patient to cooperate with body position to obtain the necessary cells.
6. An IV may be inserted for sedation, as needed. If performed as an outpatient procedure, the patient must have a responsible adult to drive him or her home as the patient is not allowed to drive or operate machinery for 24 hours after procedure because of the effects of sedation.

Postprocedure

1. Monitor vital signs per facility protocol.
2. Assess the patient for any signs of complications, including pain, hypotension, tachycardia, and abdominal distention or hematoma at the biopsy site.
3. Inform the patient that bruising or some discomfort may be experienced at the biopsy site.
4. Instruct the patient on resuming anticoagulants based on health care provider directions.

HEPATIC DISORDERS

See additional online content: Procedure Guidelines 19-1, 19-2

Hepatic disorders may disrupt normal liver function, which include the following:

- Storage of vitamins A, B, D; iron; and copper.
- Synthesis of plasma proteins, including albumin and globulins.
- Synthesis of the clotting factors vitamin K and prothrombin.
- Storage of glycogen and synthesis of glucose from other nutrients (gluconeogenesis).
- Breakdown of fatty acids for energy.
- Production of bile.
- Detoxification and excretion of waste products.

Hepatitis

EVIDENCE BASE Eastern Association for the Study of the liver (2017). Clinical Practice Guidelines on the management of Hepatitis B virus infection. *Journal of Hepatology, 67,* 270–298.

Hepatitis is defined as inflammation of the liver. Viral infection is the most common cause associated with a broad spectrum of clinical manifestation from non-symptom producing infection, through icteric hepatitis, to hepatic necrosis. Five types of viral hepatitis have been identified.

Pathophysiology and Etiology

Type A Hepatitis

1. Hepatitis A (HAV) is caused by a ribonucleic acid (RNA) virus of the enterovirus family.
2. Mode of transmission is primarily fecal–oral, usually through the ingestion of food or liquids contaminated with the virus.
   a. Prevalent in underdeveloped countries or in instances of overcrowding and poor sanitation.
   b. Infected food handler can spread the disease, and people can contract it by consuming water or shellfish from contaminated waters.
   c. Commonly spread by person-to-person contact and, rarely, by blood transfusion. Vaccines are available.
3. Incubation period is 15 to 28 days, with the average being 28 days.
4. Occurrence is worldwide, usually among children and young adults.
5. Mortality is 0% to 1%, with recovery as the rule.

Type B Hepatitis

1. Hepatitis B (HBV) is a double-shelled particle containing deoxyribonucleic acid. This particle is composed of the following:
   a. HBcAg—hepatitis B core antigen (antigenic material in an inner core).
   b. HBsAg—hepatitis B surface antigen (antigenic material in an outer coat).
   c. HBeAg—hepatitis B envelop antigen (an independent protein circulating in the blood).
2. Each antigen stimulates a specific antibody:
   a. Anti-HBc—hepatitis B core antibodies (persists during the acute phase of illness; may indicate continuing HBV in the liver).
   b. Anti-HBs— hepatitis B surface antibodies (detected during late convalescence; usually indicates recovery and development of immunity).
   c. Anti-HBe—hepatitis B envelop antibodies (usually signifies reduced infectivity).
3. Significance:
   a. HBsAg—usually detected transiently in blood of 80% to 90% of infected people; may be noted in blood for months or years, indicating that the patient has acute or chronic hepatitis B or is a carrier.
   b. HBeAg—if absent, the patient is an asymptomatic carrier. If present, it indicates highly infectious period of acute, active hepatitis. If it persists, it indicates progression to chronic state.
4. Mode of transmission is primarily through blood (percutaneous and mucosal route).
   a. Oral route through saliva or through breast-feeding.
   b. Sexual activity through blood, semen, saliva, or vaginal secretions. Hepatitis B is recognized as a sexually transmitted infection.
   c. Homosexual men and those with HIV are at high risk.
5. Incubation period is 45 to 160 days (average of 120 days).
6. Occurrence is for all ages, but it mostly affects young adults worldwide. Vaccines are available.
7. Fifteen to twenty-five percent of chronically infected persons develop chronic liver disease, including cirrhosis, liver failure, or liver cancer. It causes 1,800 deaths per year in the U.S. and is the main cause of cirrhosis and hepatocellular carcinoma worldwide.

Type C Hepatitis

1. Hepatitis C (HCV) is RNA virus of the enterovirus family.
2. Mode of transmission is through blood and body fluids. Previously was transmitted though blood products but since 1992, the commercial blood supply has been tested; now, the rate of transmission through blood transfusions is less than 1%.
   a. Current transmission through sharing of needles with IV drug use or from accidental needle sticks in the health care setting.
   b. Vertical transition from mother to fetus.
   c. Less common causes include hemodialysis; sharing personal care items that may have come in contact with another person's blood, such as razors or toothbrushes; or sexual intercourse with an infected person.

3. Incubation period varies from 14 to 180 days (average 45 days).
4. Occurs in all age groups.
   a. May occur sporadically or in epidemic proportions.
   b. Increasing number of cases diagnosed in Baby Boomer generation, born between the years of 1945 and 1965; 75% to 85% of newly infected persons develop chronic hepatitis.
   c. There is currently no vaccine available.
   d. As many as 20% of those infected with HCV will develop cirrhosis or liver cancer.

Type D Hepatitis (Delta Hepatitis)

 EVIDENCE BASE Kushner, T., Serper, M., & Kaplan, D. E. (2015). Delta hepatitis within the Veterans Affairs medical system in the United States: Prevalence, risk factors, and outcomes. *Journal of Hepatology, 63*(3), 586–592.

1. Hepatitis D virus (HDV) is a defective RNA agent that appears to replicate only with the hepatitis B virus. It requires HBsAg to replicate.
   a. Occurs along with HBV or may superinfect a chronic HBV carrier.
   b. Cannot outlast a hepatitis B infection.
   c. May be acute or chronic.
2. Mode of transmission and incubation are the same as for HBV.
3. Rarely seen in the United States because of high rates of hepatitis B vaccination beginning in infancy. Occurrence in the United States is primarily in IV drug users, veterans who have served in high-infection areas, or patients requiring multiple transfusions.
4. The highest incidence exists in the Mediterranean, the Middle East, and South America. Prevalence is low in North America and Northern Europe, South Africa, and Eastern Asia.
5. Mortality—accounts for 50% of fulminant hepatitis, which has a high mortality.

Type E Hepatitis

1. Nonenveloped, single-strand RNA virus.
2. Mode of transmission is fecal–oral.
3. Incubation is 15 to 60 days (mean 40 days).
4. Occurrence is primarily in India, Africa, Asia, and Central America, but may be found in recent travelers to these areas and is more common in young adults. More severe cases occur in pregnant women (third trimester) and those with preexisting chronic liver disease.
5. Most people recover completely. In those with severe cases, mortality rates can be as high as 30%.

Autoimmune Hepatitis

1. In addition to viral hepatitis, autoimmune hepatitis (AIH) has also been identified. It is a chronic form of hepatitis that is progressive and fluctuates with degree of liver damage.
2. Although the cause of AIH is unknown, it is thought to be self-antigen mediated.
3. Treatment usually consists of anti-inflammatory or immunosuppressive agents, which may need to be taken throughout the patient's life.
4. AIH may lead to chronic or fulminant liver failure and transplantation.

Clinical Manifestations

Type A Hepatitis

1. May have no symptoms.
2. Prodromal symptoms: fatigue, anorexia, malaise, headache, low-grade fever, nausea, and vomiting.

3. Highly contagious during this period, usually 2 weeks before the onset of jaundice.
4. Icteric phase: jaundice, tea-colored urine, clay-colored stool, and right upper quadrant tenderness.
5. Symptoms may be mild in children; adults are more likely to have severe symptoms and a prolonged course of disease.

Type B Hepatitis

1. An estimated 30% of the world's population shows serological evidence of HBV current or past infection. Symptom onset usually more insidious and prolonged compared with HAV but may be asymptomatic.
2. Prodromal symptoms: fatigue, anorexia, transient fever, abdominal discomfort, nausea and vomiting, headache; can last 1 week to 2 months.
3. Extrahepatic manifestations may include myalgias, photophobia, arthritis, angioedema, urticaria, maculopapular eruptions, skin rashes, and vasculitis.
4. Icteric phase: Jaundice.
5. In rare cases, it may progress to abrupt and severe hepatic failure, also called fulminant hepatitis.
6. May become chronic active or chronic persistent (asymptomatic) hepatitis.

Type C Hepatitis

1. Similar to those associated with HBV but usually less severe.
2. Symptoms usually occur 6 to 7 weeks after exposure but may be attributed to another viral infection and not diagnosed as hepatitis.
3. Genotype 1 HCV is the most common infection, accounting for approximately 70% to 75% of all hepatitis C infections.
4. Approximately 60% to 85% of people infected with HCV go on to develop a chronic infection. (Complications of chronic HCV include cirrhosis, decompensated liver disease, and hepatocellular carcinoma.)
5. In patients with HCV who do not receive treatment, the estimated risk of developing hepatocellular carcinoma after 20 years is 1% to 3%.
6. It is recommended that high-risk individuals be tested for HCV because many may remain asymptomatic for approximately 20 years.

Type D Hepatitis

1. Similar to HBV but more severe.
2. With superinfection of chronic HBV carriers, causes sudden worsening of condition and rapid progression of cirrhosis.

Diagnostic Evaluation

1. Elevated serum transferase levels (aspartate transaminase [AST], alanine transaminase [ALT]) for all forms of hepatitis.
2. Radioimmunoassays that reveal immunoglobulin (Ig) M antibodies to hepatitis virus in the acute phase of HAV.
3. Radioimmunoassays to include HBsAg, anti-HBc, and anti-HBsAg detected in various stages of HBV (see Figure 19-1).
4. Hepatitis C antibody—may not be detected for 6 weeks after exposure; antibody test used for screening purposes for past exposure of current infection. Positive results should be confirmed by nucleic acid testing for HCV RNA, which indicates active infection.
5. Antidelta antibodies of HBsAg for HDV or the detection of IgM in acute disease and IgG in chronic disease.
6. Hepatitis E IgM.
7. Liver biopsy to detect chronic active disease, progression, and response to therapy.

Figure 19-1. Time course for clinical, laboratory, and virologic features of acute hepatitis B infection. ALT, alanine aminotransferase; anti-HBc, antibody to hepatitis B core antigen; anti-HBe, antibody to hepatitis Be antigen; anti-HBs, antibody to hepatitis B surface antigen; HBeAg, hepatitis Be antigen; HBsAg, hepatitis B surface antigen. (Betts, R.F., Chapman, S.W., Penn, R.L. [2003]. Reese and Betts' a practical approach to infectious diseases [5th ed.]. Philadelphia: Lippincott Williams & Wilkins.)

Management

All Types of Hepatitis
1. Rest according to the patient's level of fatigue.
2. Therapeutic measures to control dyspeptic symptoms and malaise.
3. Hospitalization for protracted nausea and vomiting or life-threatening complications; enteral feedings may be necessary.
4. Small, frequent feedings of a high-calorie, low-fat foods.
5. Vitamin K is administered if INR/PT is prolonged.
6. IV fluid and electrolyte replacement, as indicated.
7. Administration of antiemetic for nausea.
8. After jaundice has cleared, gradual increase in physical activity. This may require many months.

Patients with HBV
1. First-line therapy is nucleoside analogs (NA) with high barrier to drug resistance, such as entecavir, or tenofovir. NAs with a low barrier to resistance, including lamivudine, adefovir, or telbivudine, can lead to drug resistance and are not recommended.
2. All patients should be vaccinated for hepatitis A.

 EVIDENCE BASE Terrault, N. A., Lok, A. S. F., McMahon, B. J., & Chang, K. M. (2018). Update on prevention, diagnosis, and treatment of chronic hepatitis B: AASLD 2018 hepatitis B guidance. *Hepatology, 67*(4), 1560–1599.

Patients with HCV

 EVIDENCE BASE AASLD/IDSA HCV Guidance Panel. (2015). Hepatitis C Guidance: AASLD-IDSA recommendations for testing, managing, and treating adults infected with Hepatitis C virus. *Hepatology, 62*(3), 932–954.

1. HCV infection will clear spontaneously clear in 20% to 50% of patients. In at least two thirds of patients, this will occur within 6 months of the estimated time of infection (median, 16.5 weeks).
2. Antiviral treatment is recommended for all patients with chronic HCV infection, except those with limited life expectancy due to nonhepatic causes.
3. First-line treatment no longer includes pegylated interferon and ribavirin, as the flulike side effects and treatment course of 48 weeks were intolerable to most patients.
4. Treatment of the virus is guided by genotype and presence or absence of cirrhosis. A 12-week course of multiple direct acting antivirals includes elbasvir/grazoprevir, ledipasvir/sofosbuvir, or simeprevir/sofosbuvir. Ninety percent of all patients who complete treatment achieve sustained virologic response (SVR).
5. Close monitoring including complete blood count, liver function tests, and HCV viral load during the treatment period is imperative.
6. Patients should be vaccinated against hepatitis A and B if they do not have immunity. Patients who complete treatment can still recontract the disease, making education on prevention important.

Complications
1. Dehydration, hypokalemia.
2. Chronic "carrier" hepatitis or chronic active hepatitis.
3. Cholestatic hepatitis.
4. Fulminant hepatitis (liver transplantation may be necessary).
5. HBV and HCV chronic infections have a higher risk of developing hepatocellular carcinoma.

Nursing Assessment
1. Assess for systemic and liver-related symptoms.
2. Obtain history on risk factors, such as IV drug use, sexual activity, travel to endemic countries, and ingestion of possible contaminated food or water to assess for any mode of transmission of the virus.
3. Assess size and texture of liver to detect enlargement or characteristics of cirrhosis.
4. Obtain vital signs, including temperature.

Nursing Diagnoses

All Types of Hepatitis
- Imbalanced Nutrition: Less Than Body Requirements related to effects of liver dysfunction.
- Deficient Fluid Volume related to nausea and vomiting.
- Activity Intolerance related to anorexia and liver dysfunction.
- Deficient Knowledge related to transmission.

Patients with HBV
- Risk for Bleeding related to coagulopathy because of impaired liver function.
- Acute Confusion related to encephalopathy because of impaired liver function.

Nursing Interventions

Maintaining Adequate Nutrition
1. Encourage frequent small feedings of high-calorie, low-fat diet. Avoid large quantities of protein during acute phase of illness as the body is unable to metabolize protein by-products.
2. Encourage eating meals in an upright sitting position to decrease pressure on the liver.
3. Encourage taking pleasing meals in an environment with minimal noxious stimuli (i.e., odors, noise, interruptions).
4. Administer or teach self-administration of antiemetics, as prescribed.

DRUG ALERT Avoid the use of phenothiazines as an antiemetic in patients with liver dysfunction, such as prochlorperazine, which have a cholestatic effect and may cause or worsen jaundice. Metoclopramide is preferred.

Maintaining Adequate Fluid Intake
1. Provide frequent oral fluids, as tolerated.
2. Administer IV fluids for patients with inability to maintain oral fluids, as prescribed.
3. Monitor intake and output.

Maintaining Adequate Rest and Activity
1. Promote periods of rest during symptom-producing phase, according to level of fatigue.
2. Promote comfort by administering or teaching self-administration of analgesics as prescribed.
3. Provide emotional support and diversional activities when recovery and convalescence are prolonged.
4. Encourage gradual resumption of activities and mild exercise during convalescent period.

Ensuring Prevention of Disease Transmission
1. Educate the patient about disease and about disease transmission.
2. Emphasize the self-limiting nature of most forms of hepatitis and the need for follow-up of liver function tests.
3. Stress importance of proper public and home sanitation and of proper preparation and dispensation of foods.
4. Encourage specific protection for close contacts.
   a. Immunoglobulin or vaccine should be administered as soon as possible (within 2 weeks) to household contacts of HAV patients.
   b. Hepatitis B immune globulin as soon as possible to blood or body fluid contacts of HBV patients, followed by HBV vaccine series.
5. Explain precautions to the patient and family about transmission and prevention of transmission to others.
   a. Good hand washing and hygiene after using the bathroom.
   b. Avoidance of sexual activity (especially for HBV) until free of HBsAg.
   c. Avoidance of sharing needles, drug paraphernalia, eating utensils, and toothbrushes to prevent blood or body fluid contact (especially for HBV and HCV).
6. Report all cases of hepatitis to public health officials.

Preventing and Controlling Bleeding
1. Monitor and teach the patient to monitor and report signs of bleeding.
2. Monitor PT/INR and administer vitamin K, as ordered.
3. Avoid trauma that may cause bruising, limit invasive procedures, if possible, and maintain adequate pressure on needle-stick sites.

Monitoring Thought Processes
1. Monitor for signs of encephalopathy—lethargy and somnolence with mild confusion and personality changes, such as excessive sexual or aggressive activity and loss of usual inhibitions. Lethargy may alternate with excitability, euphoria, or unruly behavior.
2. Monitor for worsening of condition, from stupor to coma; assess for asterixis.

3. Maintain calm, quiet environment and reorient the patient, as needed.

Patient Education and Health Maintenance
1. Identify persons at high risk for each type of hepatitis and advise prevention and screening.
2. Educate adolescents about the risk of piercing and tattooing in transmission of HCV.
3. Encourage vaccination for HBV with series of three injections (at birth, 1 month, and 6 months) for high-risk patients, such as health care workers or institutionalized persons, as well as vaccination of all children at birth or in adolescence.
4. Instruct all patients who have received a blood transfusion to refrain from donating blood for 12 months. Anyone testing positive for hepatitis B or C is ineligible to donate blood.
5. Stress the need to follow precautions with blood and secretions until the patient is deemed free of HBsAg.
6. Explain to HBV carriers that their blood and secretions will remain infectious.
7. For additional information, refer to the local public health department, American Red Cross, or the Centers for Disease Control and Prevention (*www.cdc.gov*).

Evaluation: Expected Outcomes
- Tolerates small carbohydrate feedings.
- No vomiting, tolerates fluids.
- Maintains self-care and light ambulation.
- Family members seek active immunization.
- No signs of bleeding.
- Lethargic but oriented, no tremor.

Hepatic Cirrhosis

 EVIDENCE BASE National Institute for Health and Care Excellence. (2016). NICE guideline: Cirrhosis in over 16s: Assessment and management. Available: *http://nice.org.uk/guidance/ng50.*

It is a chronic disease with diffuse destruction and fibrotic regeneration of hepatic cells. (see Figure 19-2). As necrotic tissue is replaced by fibrotic tissue, normal liver structure and vasculature are altered, impairing blood and lymph flow, resulting in hepatic insufficiency and portal hypertension.

Pathophysiology and Etiology
1. Laënnec cirrhosis (macronodular), also known as alcoholic cirrhosis.
   a. Fibrosis—mainly around central veins and portal areas.
   b. Usually due to chronic alcohol toxicity and malnutrition.
2. Postnecrotic cirrhosis (micronodular).
   a. Broad bands of scar tissue.
   b. Because of previous acute viral hepatitis or drug-induced massive hepatic necrosis.
3. Biliary cirrhosis.
   a. Scarring around bile ducts and lobes of the liver.
   b. Results from chronic biliary injury and obstruction of the intrahepatic or extrahepatic biliary system.
   c. Partial or total obstruction of the bile ducts can lead to infectious cholangitis and cirrhosis, which is much rarer with Laennec's or postnecrotic cirrhosis.

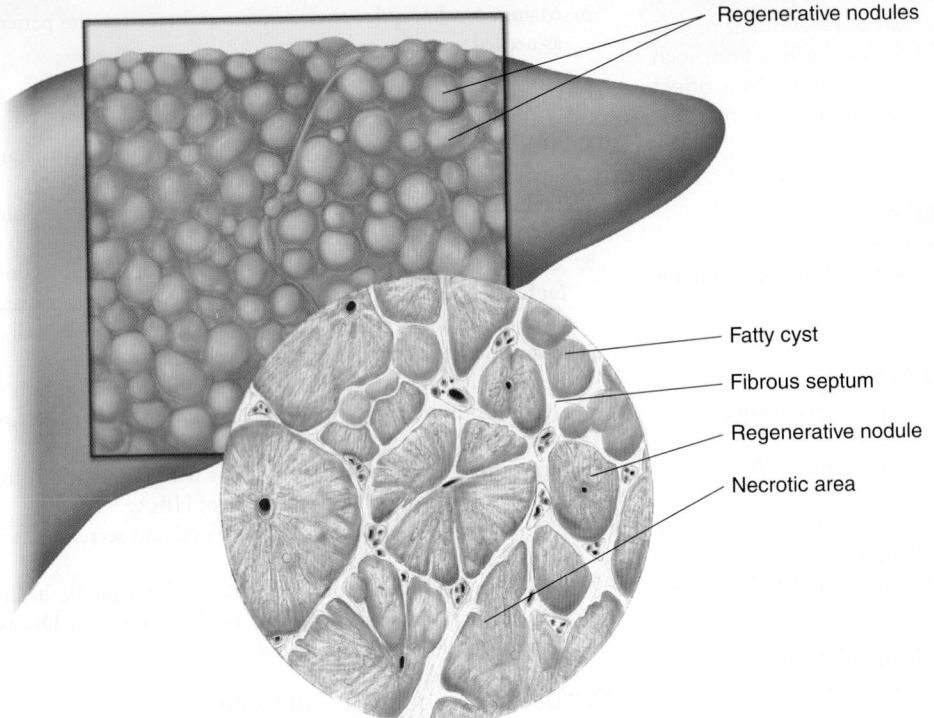

Regenerative nodules

Fatty cyst

Fibrous septum

Regenerative nodule

Necrotic area

Figure 19-2. Fibrotic changes to liver tissue in cirrhosis. (Anatomical Chart Company.)

Clinical Manifestations

1. Onset is insidious; may take years to develop.
2. Early symptoms include fatigue, anorexia, ankle edema in the evening, epistaxis and bleeding gums, and weight loss.
3. Later signs and symptoms because of chronic failure of the liver and obstruction of portal circulation.
   a. Chronic dyspepsia, constipation, or diarrhea.
   b. Esophageal varices, dilated cutaneous veins around the umbilicus (caput medusa), internal hemorrhoids, ascites, splenomegaly, and pancytopenia.
   c. Plasma albumin is reduced, leading to edema and contributing to ascites.
   d. Anemia and poor nutrition lead to fatigue and weakness, wasting, and depression.
   e. Deterioration of mental function from lethargy to delirium to coma and eventual death.
   f. Estrogen–androgen imbalance causes spider angiomata and palmar erythema; menstrual irregularities in females; testicular and prostatic atrophy, gynecomastia, loss of libido, and impotence in males.
4. Bleeding tendencies, such as nosebleeds, easy bruising, hematemesis, occult blood in stool, or profuse hemorrhage from stomach and esophageal varices.

Diagnostic Evaluation

1. CT scan is helpful to determine the size of the liver and its irregularities and in detection of a mass.
2. Transient elastography to diagnose cirrhosis.
3. Liver biopsy detects degree of destruction and fibrosis of hepatic tissue in those who are not candidates for transient elastography.
4. Gastrointestinal endoscopy to determine esophageal varices.
5. Paracentesis to examine ascitic fluid for cell, protein, and bacterial counts.
6. PTC differentiates extrahepatic from intrahepatic obstructive jaundice.
7. Laparoscopy allows direct visualization of the liver.
8. Serum liver function test results may be elevated, but normal enzymes do not rule out cirrhosis.

Management

1. Minimize further deterioration of liver function through the withdrawal of toxic substances, alcohol, and medications.
2. Correction of nutritional deficiencies with vitamins and nutritional supplements and a high-calorie and moderate- to high-protein diet.
3. Treatment of ascites and fluid and electrolyte imbalances.
   a. Restrict sodium and water intake, depending on amount of fluid retention.
   b. Diuretic therapy, frequently with spironolactone, a potassium-sparing diuretic that inhibits the action of aldosterone on the kidneys. Furosemide or toresemide, loop diuretics, may also be used in conjunction with spironolactone to help balance potassium depletion.
   c. Abdominal paracentesis to remove fluid and relieve symptoms. A tunneled cuffed catheter with a one-way valve and a closed drainage system may be placed for chronic symptom management.
   d. Administration of albumin to maintain osmotic pressure.
4. Transjugular intrahepatic portosystemic shunt (TIPS), an interventional radiologic procedure, may be performed in patients whose ascites is resistant to other forms of treatment. TIPS is a percutaneously created connection within the liver between the portal and systemic circulations.
   a. Used for patients with complications related to portal hypertension.
   b. Complications include bacterial infections, shunt obstruction, encephalopathy, and increase in coagulopathies.
5. Symptomatic relief measures such as analgesics, antipruritic, and antiemetic medications.

6. Treatment of other problems associated with liver failure. Administer lactulose, rifaximin, or neomycin for hepatic encephalopathy.
7. Liver transplantation may be necessary.

Complications

1. Hyponatremia and water retention.
2. Bleeding esophageal varices.
3. Coagulopathies.
4. Spontaneous bacterial peritonitis (SBP).
5. Hepatic encephalopathy, which may be precipitated by the use of sedatives, sepsis, or electrolyte imbalance.

Nursing Assessment

1. Obtain history of precipitating factors, such as alcohol use, hepatitis, or biliary disease. Establish present pattern of alcohol intake.
2. Assess mental status through interview and interaction with the patient.
3. Perform abdominal examination, assessing for ascites (see Figure 19-3).
4. Observe for bleeding.
5. Assess daily weight first thing in the morning and abdominal girth measurements.

Nursing Diagnoses

- Activity Intolerance related to fatigue, general debility, and discomfort.
- Imbalanced Nutrition: Less Than Body Requirements related to anorexia and GI disturbances.
- Impaired Skin Integrity related to edema, jaundice, and compromised immunologic status.
- Risk for Bleeding related to altered clotting mechanisms.
- Acute Confusion related to deterioration of liver function and increased serum ammonia level.

Nursing Interventions

Promoting Activity Tolerance

1. Encourage alternating periods of rest and ambulation.
2. Maintain some periods of bed rest with legs elevated to mobilize edema and ascites.
3. Encourage and assist with gradually increasing periods of exercise.

Improving Nutritional Status

1. Encourage the patient to eat multiple, small, frequent high-calorie, moderate-protein meals.
2. Suggest small, frequent feedings and attractive meals in an aesthetically pleasing setting at mealtimes.
3. Encourage oral hygiene before meals.
4. Administer or teach self-administration of medication for nausea, vomiting, diarrhea, or constipation.

Protecting Skin Integrity

1. Note and record degree of jaundice of skin and sclera and scratches on the body.
2. Encourage frequent skin care, bathing without soap, and massage with emollient lotions.
3. Advise the patient to keep fingernails short.
4. Administer antipruritic medications as ordered.

Preventing Bleeding

1. Observe stools and emesis for color, consistency, and amount; test for occult blood.
2. Be alert for symptoms of anxiety, epigastric fullness, weakness, and restlessness, which may indicate GI bleeding.
3. Observe for external bleeding: ecchymosis, leaking needlestick sites, epistaxis, petechiae, and bleeding gums.
4. Keep the patient quiet and limit activity if signs of bleeding are exhibited.
5. Administer vitamin K, as prescribed.
6. Stay in constant attendance during episodes of bleeding.
7. Institute and teach measures to prevent trauma:
   a. Maintain safe environment.
   b. Gentle blowing of nose.
   c. Use of soft toothbrush.
8. Use small-gauge needles for injections and maintain pressure over site until bleeding stops.
9. Management of bleeding from esophageal varices can include endoscopic variceal ligation (banding) or injection sclerotherapy.

Promoting Improved Thought Processes

1. Limit sedatives and promote sleep/wake cycles to prevent delirium.
2. Protect from sepsis through good hand washing and prompt recognition and management of infection.
3. Monitor fluid intake and output and serum electrolyte levels to prevent dehydration and hypokalemia (may occur with the use of diuretics), which may precipitate hepatic coma.

Figure 19-3. Assessing for ascites. **(A)** To percuss for shifting dullness, each flank is percussed with the patient in a supine position. If fluid is present, dullness is noted at each flank. The most medial limits of the dullness should be marked as indicated in *a*. The patient should then be shifted to the side. **(B)** Note what happens to the area of dullness if fluid is present; the area of dullness begins at *b*. **(C)** To detect the presence of a fluid wave, the examiner places one hand alongside each flank. A second person then places a hand, ulnar side down, along the patient's midline and applies light pressure. The examiner then strikes one flank sharply with one hand, while the other hand remains in place to detect any signs of a fluid impulse. The assistant's hand should dampen any wave impulses traveling through the abdominal wall, unless fluid is present.

4. Keep environment warm.
5. Pad the side rails of the bed, keep the bed in the lowest position, and provide careful nursing surveillance to ensure the patient's safety.
6. Assess LOC and frequently reorient, as needed.
7. Administer lactulose or neomycin through a retention enema or nasogastric (NG) tube, as ordered, for elevated ammonia levels and decreasing LOC.

 DRUG ALERT Opioids, sedatives, and barbiturates are used cautiously in the restless patient with cirrhosis to prevent precipitation of hepatic coma.

 TRANSITIONAL CARE ALERT Patients with cirrhosis should be monitored closely to prevent readmission. Patient education must include daily weights, good nutrition, and avoiding liver toxic medications, herbal supplements, and alcohol. The support of community health nursing and the family are vital.

Patient Education and Health Maintenance

1. Advise the patient to avoid substances (over-the-counter medications, herbs, illicit drugs, toxins) that may affect liver function.
2. Stress the necessity of giving up alcohol completely.
3. Urge acceptance of assistance from a substance use program.
4. Involve the person closest to the patient because recovery usually is not easy and relapses are common.
5. Provide written dietary instructions.
6. Encourage daily weighing for self-monitoring of fluid retention or depletion.
7. Discuss adverse effects of diuretic therapy.
8. Emphasize the importance of rest, a sensible lifestyle, and an adequate, well-balanced diet.
9. Stress the importance of continued follow-up for laboratory tests and evaluation by a health care provider.

Evaluation: Expected Outcomes

- Ambulates three times daily.
- Tolerates small, frequent meals.
- Skin without breakdown or scratches.
- No bleeding or bruising; results of stool tests are negative for occult blood.
- Drowsy but easily aroused and oriented.

Bleeding Esophageal Varices

Esophageal varices are dilated tortuous veins usually found in the submucosa of the lower esophagus; however, they may develop higher in the esophagus or extend into the stomach.

Pathophysiology and Etiology

1. Nearly always because of portal hypertension, which may result from obstruction of the portal venous circulation and cirrhosis of the liver.
   a. Because of increased obstruction of the portal vein, venous blood from the intestinal tract and spleen seeks an outlet through collateral circulation, which creates new pathways of return to the right atrium and causes an increased strain on the vessels in the submucosal layer of the lower esophagus and upper part of the stomach.
   b. These collateral vessels are tortuous and fragile and bleed easily.
2. Other causes of varices are abnormalities of the circulation in the splenic vein or superior vena cava and hepatic venothrombosis.
3. Mortality is high because of further deterioration of liver function to hepatic coma and complications, such as aspiration pneumonia, sepsis, and renal failure.

Clinical Manifestations

1. Hematemesis—vomiting of bright red blood.
2. Melena—passage of black, tarry stools, which indicates that blood has been in the GI tract for at least 14 hours.
3. Bright red rectal bleeding from hypermotility of the bowel or rectal varices.
4. Blood loss may be sudden and massive, causing shock.

Diagnostic Evaluation

1. Upper GI endoscopy for patients with a suspected upper GI source of bleeding.
2. Hemoglobin and hematocrit may be decreasing, and liver function tests can be abnormal.

Management

 EVIDENCE BASE Tulachan S. S., Bhagatwala J., & Sridhar S. (2018). Endoscopic Management of Esophageal Varices and Variceal Hemorrhage. In: Sridhar S., Wu G. (Eds.), *Diagnostic and Therapeutic Procedures in Gastroenterology* (pp. 165–178). Clinical Gastroenterology. Totowa, N.J.: Humana Press.

1. Restoration of circulating blood volume with blood transfusions and IV fluids.
2. Use of IV vasoconstrictors, such as octreotide or vasopressin to control bleeding. These medications may be used to reduce portal pressure by decreasing splanchnic blood flow and to increase clotting and hemostasis. Vasopressin has a significant vasoconstrictive effect on other organs, such as the heart and intestine.
3. Gastric lavage to remove blood from the GI tract and to enhance visualization for endoscopic examination.
4. Endoscopic esophageal ligation (variceal banding) may be urgent or nonurgent and is usually the first-line treatment to control acute bleeding. The procedure may need to be repeated until all varices are obliterated. The goal is to achieve rapid hemostasis and prevent early rebleeding.
5. Esophageal balloon tamponade, whereby balloons are inflated in the distal esophagus and the proximal stomach to collapse the varices and induce hemostasis. This procedure should be reserved for patients who are known, without a doubt, to be bleeding from esophageal varices and in whom all forms of conservative therapy have failed.
   a. Complications include esophageal necrosis, perforation, aspiration, asphyxiation, and stricture.
   b. If hemostasis is not achieved within 2 hours, another treatment should be immediately considered. Tamponade should not be used for more than 24 hours.
   c. Patients must be continuously monitored in intensive care setting.

6. Endoscopic sclerotherapy—during endoscopy, a sclerosing agent is injected directly into the varix to promote thrombosis and sclerosis of bleeding sites.
   a. To control bleeding and reduce the frequency of subsequent variceal hemorrhages, but repeated treatments may be required.
   b. Complications include esophageal ulceration, stricture, and perforation.
7. Portal systemic shunt (portocaval or portorenal) done through TIPS procedure or surgically, to treat portal hypertension and bleeding.
8. Evaluation for liver transplantation if TIPS or surgical shunt do not control portal hypertension.
9. Beta-adrenergic blocker therapy to reduce the resting pulse.
10. High-dose proton pump inhibitor (PPI) therapy for long-term management of erosive gastropathy.
11. Antibiotics, as patients with variceal hemorrhage are at high risk for SBP.

 NURSING ALERT Precaution must be taken during balloon tamponade therapy to ensure that the patient does not pull or inadvertently displace the tube. Keep scissors taped to the head of the bed. In the event of *acute respiratory distress*, use the scissors to cut across tubing (to deflate both balloons) and remove tubing.

Complications

1. Exsanguination or recurrent hemorrhage.
2. Portal systemic encephalopathy.
3. Spontaneous bacterial peritonitis.

Nursing Assessment

1. Monitor vital signs and respiratory status.
2. Assess LOC and impending signs of liver failure.

Nursing Diagnoses

- Ineffective Tissue Perfusion related to GI bleeding.
- Risk for Aspiration related to GI bleeding and intubation.
- Anxiety related to fear of unknown procedures and consequences of GI bleeding.

Nursing Interventions

Maintaining Adequate Tissue Perfusion

1. Assess BP, heart rate, skin condition, and urine output for signs of hypovolemia and shock.
2. Monitor frequently the patient receiving vasopressin infusion for complications: hypertension, bradycardia, abdominal cramps, chest pain, or water intoxication.
3. Observe the patient for straining, gagging, or vomiting; these increase pressure in the portal system and increase risk of further bleeding.
4. Check all GI secretions and stool for occult and frank blood.
5. Administer infusion of blood products, as prescribed.
6. Administer vitamin K and fresh frozen plasma (FFP), as prescribed.

Preventing Aspiration

1. Assess respirations and monitor oxygen saturation of blood.
2. Note and report occurrence of signs of obstructed airway or ruptured esophagus from the esophageal balloon: changes in skin color, respirations, breath sounds, LOC, or vital signs; chest pain.
3. Check location and inflation of esophageal balloon; maintain traction on tubes, if applicable.
4. Have scissors readily available. Cut tubing and remove esophageal balloon immediately if the patient develops acute respiratory distress.
5. Keep head of bed elevated to avoid gastric regurgitation and aspiration of gastric contents.
6. When using the Sengstaken-Blakemore esophageal balloon tube, ensure removal of secretions above the esophageal balloon: position NG tube in the esophagus for suctioning purposes; provide intermittent oropharyngeal suctioning.
7. Inspect nares for skin irritation; clean and lubricate frequently to prevent bleeding.

Reducing Anxiety and Fear

1. Explain all procedures to the patient.
2. Provide care in a concerned, nonjudgmental manner.
3. Remain with the patient or maintain close observation and place call bell within the patient's reach.
4. Work swiftly and confidently, not hurriedly and anxiously.
5. Provide alternate means of communication if tubes or other equipment interfere with the patient's ability to talk.
6. Use touch and other tactile stimuli to provide reassurance to the patient.
7. Use protective restraints to prevent dislodging of tubes in a confused, combative patient.

Patient Education and Health Maintenance

1. Discuss signs and symptoms of recurrent bleeding and the need to seek emergency medical treatment if these occur.
2. Instruct the patient to avoid behaviors that increase portal system pressure: straining, gagging, and Valsalva maneuver.
3. Explain to the patient that alcohol consumption can cause further complications.
4. Encourage the patient to abstain from alcohol consumption; discuss support organizations such as Alcoholics Anonymous.

Evaluation: Expected Outcomes

- BP stable; urine output adequate.
- Airway maintained without aspiration.
- Cooperates and indicates understanding of treatment.

Liver Cancer

 EVIDENCE BASE Yu, S. J. (2016). A concise review of updated guidelines regarding the management of hepatocellular carcinoma around the world: 2010–2016. *Clinical and Molecular Hepatology, 22*(1), 7–17.

Cancer of the liver, or *hepatocellular carcinoma* (HCC), is a primary cancer of the liver and is relatively uncommon in the United States. It is the 5th most common malignancy and second leading cause of cancer-associated death around the world, with more than 600,000 deaths reported internationally each year.

Cholangiocarcinoma is a primary malignant tumor of the bile ducts, which can be intrahepatic or extrahepatic. This type of cancer is uncommon in the United States but is more commonly seen in Asia.

Liver metastasis may occur from a primary site, which is found in about one half of all late cancer cases. Neoadjuvant therapy is given to shrink metastatic liver tumor to make them more amenable to resection.

Pathophysiology and Etiology

1. Incidence of primary cancer of the liver is increasing in the United States.
2. Alcoholic cirrhosis, HBV, HCV, biliary cirrhosis, and chronic liver injury have been implicated in its etiology.
3. Rarer associated causes are metabolic syndrome; hemochromatosis; alpha$_1$-antitrypsin deficiency; aflatoxins; chemical toxins, such as vinyl chloride and Thorotrast; carcinogens in herbal medicines; nitrosamines; and ingestion of hormones, as in oral contraceptives.
4. Arises in normal tissue as a discrete tumor or in end-stage cirrhosis in a multinodular pattern.
5. Liver metastasis reaches the liver by way of the portal system, lymphatic channels, or by direct extension from an abdominal tumor.

Clinical Manifestations

1. Depends on the state of the liver in which it arises; without cirrhosis and with good liver function, carcinoma of the liver may grow to huge proportions before becoming symptomatic, but in a cirrhotic patient, the lack of hepatic reserve usually leads to a more rapid course.
2. The most common presenting symptom is right upper quadrant abdominal pain, usually dull or aching, and may radiate to the right shoulder.
3. A right upper quadrant mass, weight loss, abdominal distention with ascites, fatigue, anorexia, malaise, and unexplained fever.
4. Jaundice is present only in a minority of patients at diagnosis in primary cancer of the liver. In cholangiocarcinoma, the presenting symptom is usually painless obstructive jaundice.
5. With portal vein obstruction, ascites and esophageal varices occurs.

Diagnostic Evaluation

1. Increased levels of serum bilirubin, alkaline phosphatase, and liver enzymes.
2. AFP is the principal tumor marker for hepatocellular carcinoma and is elevated in 70% to 95% of patients with the disease.
3. Ultrasonography and CT along with MRI are the most useful noninvasive tests to detect liver cancer and assess if the tumor can be surgically resected.
4. PET scan to look for recurrent or metastatic disease.
5. Percutaneous needle biopsy or biopsy assisted by ultrasonography or CT scan.
6. Laparoscopy with liver biopsy may be performed.

Management

EVIDENCE BASE National Comprehensive Cancer Network. (2016). Clinical practice guidelines in oncology: Hepatobiliary cancers. Available: *www.nccn.org/professionals/physician_gls/f_guidelines.asp.*

Nonsurgical Treatment

Varying degrees of success with nonsurgical management. These therapies may prolong survival and improve the patient's quality of life by reducing pain, but the overall effect is palliative.

1. Indicated in patients who are not surgical candidates because of inadequate hepatic reserve or tumor location. Regional therapies are used to reduce the size of the tumor and make surgical excision possible.
2. Radiofrequency ablation uses heat produced by a radiofrequency electrode to kill tumors. This can be performed by the percutaneous or laparoscopic approach and is used for relatively small tumors.
3. Hepatic artery occlusion and embolization with the use of chemotherapeutic agents or radiofrequency to treat nonresectable liver tumors.
4. Radiation therapy can help reduce pain and discomfort of large unresectable tumors.
5. Systemic treatment with a multikinase inhibitor, sorafenib is able to improve the median overall survival by approximately 3 months.
6. Clinical trials on chemotherapy administered systemically or intra-arterially, to the site of the tumor, continue to show low efficacy in liver cancer.
7. Percutaneous alcohol injection direct into the tumor is an ablative procedure that is safe for treating small liver tumors, but efficacy is limited.
8. PTBD is used to drain obstructed biliary ducts in patients with inoperable tumors or in patients considered poor surgical risks.
9. Percutaneous or endoscopic placement of internal stents may also palliate a patient with obstructed bile ducts with a terminal diagnosis.

Surgical Treatment

EVIDENCE BASE Zheng, J., Kuk, D., Gönen, M. et al. (2017). Actual 10-Year survivors after resection of hepatocellular carcinoma. *Ann Surg Oncol, 24*(5), 1358–1366.

1. Surgery is the best treatment for patients who meet the following criteria: tumor size is less than 5 cm, lack of macrovascular involvement, and confined to the liver with no extrahepatic disease.
   a. The 5-year survival rate is 50%; recurrence and metastasis are frequent.
   b. Surgery is an option only after the extent of the tumor and hepatic reserve have been considered.
2. Surgical resection may be along anatomic divisions of the liver or nonanatomic resections.
3. Percutaneous portal vein embolization may be performed prior to surgery of large liver tumors. Cutting off blood supply to the diseased portion of the liver allows enlargement of the nondiseased portion of the liver. An adequate amount of liver is needed to sustain a patient and prevent postoperative complications.
4. Liver transplantation is an accepted treatment for liver cancer, especially if hepatic reserve is low and the patient meets the surgical criteria.
   a. The Model for End-stage Liver Disease (MELD) is a severity scoring system for chronic liver disease that uses a patient's laboratory values for serum bilirubin, serum creatinine, and the INR to predict 3-month survival.
   b. MELD is used by the United Network for Organ Sharing (UNOS) for prioritization of patients awaiting liver transplantation in the United States.
   c. Patients may be treated with nonsurgical therapies including embolization or radiation while waiting for a liver transplant.

Complications

1. Malnutrition, biliary obstruction with jaundice.
2. Sepsis, liver abscesses.
3. Acute blood loss.
4. Fulminant liver failure, metastasis.

Nursing Assessment

1. Obtain history of hepatitis, alcoholic liver disease and cirrhosis, exposure to toxins, or other potential causes.
2. Assess for signs and symptoms of malnutrition, including recent weight loss, loss of strength, anorexia, and anemia.
3. Assess for abdominal pain, any right shoulder pain, and enlargement of the liver.
4. Assess for fever, jaundice, ascites, or bleeding.
5. Note any change in mental status as a sign of hepatic encephalopathy.

Nursing Diagnoses

- Acute and Chronic Pain related to growth of tumor.
- Imbalanced Nutrition: Less Than Body Requirements related to anorexia.
- Excess Fluid Volume related to ascites and edema.
- Altered Mental Status related to metabolic imbalance.

Nursing Interventions

Care of the patient after liver surgery is similar to general abdominal surgery (see page 496).

Controlling Pain

1. Administer pharmacologic agents, as ordered, to control pain, considering metabolism through a liver with decreased function.
   a. Titrate drugs carefully, using lowest dose that is effective.
   b. Monitor for signs of drug toxicity, particularly respiratory depression and decreased LOC.
2. Provide nonpharmacologic methods of pain relief, such as massage, heat/cold, and guided imagery.
3. Position the patient for comfort, usually in semi-Fowler position.
4. Assess the patient's response to pain-control measures.

Improving Nutritional Status

1. Encourage the patient to eat small meals and take liquid supplements as able.
2. Assess and report changes in factors affecting nutritional needs: increased body temperature, pain, signs of infection, stress level. Encourage additional calories, as tolerated.
3. Monitor daily weight.

Relieving Excess Fluid Volume

1. Monitor vital signs and record accurate fluid intake and output.
2. Restrict sodium and fluid intake, as prescribed.
3. Administer diuretics and replacement potassium and phosphate, as prescribed.
4. Administer albumin and protein supplements, as prescribed, to draw fluid from interstitial to intravascular space.
5. Measure and record abdominal girth daily at the level of the umbilicus.
6. Weigh daily, watching for increases that indicate increased fluid retention such as abdominal and lower-extremity edema.
7. Monitor laboratory tests as directed, and report abnormal values.

Improving Mental Status

1. Assess the patient's LOC and changes in behavior.
2. Limit noise and environmental stimuli.
3. Frequently reorient to person, place, and time.
4. Speak slowly and clearly while allowing the patient to respond.
5. Provide for precautions to prevent falls and promote safety.

Patient Education and Health Maintenance

1. Instruct the patient and family on preparation for surgery, reinforce and clarify surgical procedure proposed, and review postoperative instructions.
2. Instruct the patient and family on nonsurgical treatment, if appropriate.
3. Explore pain management options.
4. Inform the patient of signs and symptoms of complications.
5. Instruct the patient in continued surveillance for recurrence.
6. Instruct the patient and family in care of tubes or drains.

Evaluation: Expected Outcomes

- Verbalizes reduced pain.
- Tolerates small feedings; no weight loss.
- Abdominal girth decreased; urine output greater than intake.
- Patient safety maintained.

Fulminant Liver Failure

Fulminant liver failure is acute necrosis of the liver cells without preexisting liver disease, resulting in the inability of the liver to perform its many functions.

Pathophysiology and Etiology

1. Drug-related hepatotoxicity accounts for more than 50% of acute liver failure cases, including acetaminophen toxicity (42%) and idiosyncratic drug reactions (12%). Idiosyncratic reactions to poisons, chemicals, and such medications as, tetracycline, isoniazid, halogenated anesthetics, monoamine oxidase inhibitors, valproate, amiodarone, methyldopa, and amanita mushrooms.
2. HBV is the most common cause worldwide.
3. Ischemia and hypoxia because of hepatic vascular occlusion, hypovolemic shock, acute circulatory failure, septic shock, or heat stroke may be causes.
4. Miscellaneous causes include hepatic vein obstruction, Budd-Chiari syndrome, acute fatty liver of pregnancy, AIH, partial hepatectomy, complication of liver transplantation.
5. Progression of hepatocellular injury and necrosis is rapid, with development of hepatic encephalopathy within 8 weeks of onset of disease. In contrast, subfulminant hepatic failure indicates patients with liver disease for up to 26 weeks before the development of hepatic encephalopathy.
6. Survival rate has improved to approximately 60%.

Clinical Manifestations

1. Right upper quadrant tenderness.
2. Malaise, anorexia, nausea, vomiting, fatigue.
3. Jaundice.
4. Tea-colored urine that is frothy when shaken.
5. Pruritus caused by bile salts deposited on skin.
6. Steatorrhea and diarrhea because of decreased fat absorption.
7. Peripheral edema or ascites as the fluid moves from the intravascular to the interstitial spaces, secondary to hypoproteinemia or portal hypertension.

8. Easy bruising, petechiae, melena or hematemesis caused by clotting deficiency.
9. Hypotension, tachycardia due to reduced systemic vascular resistance.
10. Altered LOC, ranging from irritability and confusion to stupor, somnolence, and coma.
11. Change in deep tendon reflexes—initially hyperactive, become flaccid, asterixis.
12. Fetor hepaticus—breath odor of acetone.
13. Portal systemic encephalopathy, also known as hepatic coma or hepatic encephalopathy, can occur in conjunction with cerebral edema.
14. Cerebral edema may lead to signs of increased intracranial pressure (ICP) (eg, papilledema, hypertension, and bradycardia). This is commonly the cause of death because of brain stem herniation and/or respiratory arrest.

Diagnostic Evaluation

1. Prolonged PT/INR; sensitive markers of hepatic failure.
2. Decreased platelet count.
3. Elevated AST and ALT result from hepatocellular necrosis.
4. Elevated ammonia and bilirubin levels.
5. Hypoglycemia due to impaired glycogen production and gluconeogenesis.
6. Dilutional hyponatremia or hypernatremia, hypokalemia, hypocalcemia, and hypomagnesemia.

Management

 EVIDENCE BASE Stine, J. G., Lewis, J. H. (2015). Current and future directions in the treatment and prevention of drug-induced liver injury: A systematic review. *Expert Review of Gastroenterology and Hepatology, 25,* 1–20.

1. Acetaminophen overdose treated with *N*-acetylcysteine (NAC).
2. Airway protection as encephalopathy worsens and coma ensues. May require intubation and mechanical ventilation.
3. Oral or rectal administration of lactulose to minimize formation of ammonia and other nitrogenous by-products in the bowel.
4. Rectal administration of neomycin to suppress urea-splitting enteric bacteria in the bowel and decrease ammonia formation.
5. Cerebral edema management may include head of bed elevated to 30 degrees, ICP monitoring, administration of an osmotic diuretic such as mannitol, or barbiturates.
6. Careful hemodynamic monitoring and administration of vasopressors as ordered.
7. Low-molecular-weight dextran or albumin followed by a potassium-sparing diuretic (spironolactone) to enhance fluid shift from interstitial back to intravascular spaces.
8. Pancreatic enzymes, if diarrhea and steatorrhea are present, to permit better tolerance of fats in the diet.
9. Cholestyramine to promote fecal excretion of bile salts to decrease itching.
10. Antacids, PPIs, and histamine-2 (H$_2$) antagonists to reduce the risk of bleeding from stress ulcers.
11. Restriction of sodium while maintaining adequate caloric intake with hypertonic intravenous dextrose solution, enteral tube feedings, or total parenteral nutrition.
12. Supplemental vitamins (A, B complex, C, and K) and folate.
13. Infusion of FFP to maintain PT/INR; cryoprecipitate, as needed to manage coagulopathy.
14. Additional medical interventions, depending on the patient's condition, may include hemodialysis, hemofiltration, hemoperfusion, or plasmapheresis.
15. Liver transplantation has become the treatment of choice.
16. Current research under way regarding use of liver support dialysis.

Complications

1. Acute respiratory failure.
2. Infections and sepsis.
3. Cardiac dysfunction, hypotension.
4. Hepatorenal failure.
5. Hemorrhage.

Nursing Assessment

1. Obtain history of exposure to medications, chemicals, or toxins; exposure to infectious hepatitis; and course of illness.
2. Assess respiratory status, LOC, and vital signs.
3. Assess for ascites, edema, jaundice, bleeding, asterixis, and presence or absence of reflexes.
4. Assess results of arterial blood gas (ABG) tests, electrolytes, INR, hemoglobin level, and hematocrit.

Nursing Diagnoses

• Deficient Fluid Volume related to hypoproteinemia, peripheral edema, ascites.
• Ineffective Breathing Pattern related to anemia and decreased lung expansion from ascites.
• Imbalanced Nutrition: Less Than Body Requirements related to GI adverse effects and decreased absorption, storage, and metabolism of nutrients.
• Risk for Impaired Skin Integrity related to malnutrition, deposition of bile salts, peripheral edema, decreased activity.
• Risk for Infection related to altered immune response.
• Risk for Injury related to encephalopathy.

Nursing Interventions

Maintaining Adequate Fluid Volume

1. Monitor vital signs frequently.
2. Weigh the patient daily and keep an accurate intake and output record; record frequency and characteristics of stool.
3. Measure and record abdominal girth at the level of the umbilicus daily.
4. Assess and record peripheral edema.
5. Restrict sodium and fluids; replace electrolytes, as directed.
6. Administer low-molecular-weight dextran or albumin and diuretics, as prescribed.
7. Assess for signs and symptoms of hemorrhage or bleeding.

Improving Respiratory Status

1. Monitor respiratory rate, depth, use of accessory muscles, nasal flaring, and breath sounds.
2. Monitor ABG values, hemoglobin level, and hematocrit, report abnormalities.
3. Elevate head of the bed to lower diaphragm and decrease respiratory effort.
4. Turn the patient frequently to prevent stasis of secretions.
5. Administer oxygen therapy, as directed.

Improving Nutritional Status

1. Enlist a nutrition specialist to help evaluate nutritional status and needs.
2. Encourage the patient to eat in an upright sitting position to decrease abdominal tenderness and feeling of fullness.
3. Provide small, frequent meals or dietary supplements.
4. Provide mouth care if the patient has bleeding gums or fetor hepaticus.
5. Restrict intake of sodium.
6. Provide enteral and parenteral feedings, as needed.

Maintaining Skin Integrity

1. Inspect skin for alteration in integrity.
2. Provide good skin care.
3. Bathe with mild soap and apply soothing lotions.
4. Keep the patient's fingernails short to prevent scratching from pruritus. Mitts can be applied for those with confusion.
5. Administer medications, as prescribed, for pruritus.
6. Assess for signs of bleeding from broken areas on the skin.
7. Turn and position the patient frequently to prevent pressure ulcers.
8. Avoid trauma and friction to the skin.

Preventing Infection

1. Be alert for signs of infection, such as fever, cloudy urine, abnormal breath sounds.
2. Use good hand washing and aseptic technique when caring for a break in the skin or mucous membranes.
3. Restrict visits with anyone who may have an infection.
4. Encourage the patient not to scratch the skin.

Preventing Injury

1. Maintain close observation, bed side rails up, and nurse call system within reach.
2. Assist with ambulation, as needed, and avoid obstructions to prevent falls.
3. Have a well-lit room and frequently reorient the patient.
4. Observe for subtle changes in behavior or change in sleeping pattern to detect increasing encephalopathy.

Patient Education and Health Maintenance

1. Teach the patient and family to notify health care provider of increased abdominal discomfort, bleeding, increased edema or ascites, hallucinations, or lapses in consciousness.
2. Instruct the patient to avoid activities that increase the risk of bleeding: scratching, falling, forceful nose blowing, aggressive tooth brushing, and use of straight-edged razor.
3. Advise limiting activities when fatigued and encourage use of frequent rest periods.
4. Maintain close follow-up for laboratory testing and evaluation by health care provider.

Evaluation: Expected Outcomes

- BP stable, urine output adequate.
- Respirations unlabored.
- Tolerates multiple small feedings per day.
- Skin intact without abrasions.
- No fever or signs of infection.
- No falls.

BILIARY DISORDERS

The gallbladder and bile ducts constitute the biliary system. The gallbladder stores and concentrates bile produced by the liver. The hormone cholecystokinin, secreted by the small intestine, stimulates contraction of the gallbladder and relaxation of the sphincter of Oddi for delivery of bile into the small intestine.

Bile assists in the emulsification (breakdown) of fat; absorption of fatty acids, cholesterol, and other lipids from the small intestine; and excretion of conjugated bilirubin from the liver.

Common terms related to the gallbladder and bile ducts are as follows:

Cholecyst—gallbladder.
Cholecystitis—inflammation of the gallbladder.
Cholelithiasis—presence or formation of gallstones in the gallbladder.
Cholecystectomy—removal of the gallbladder.
Cholecystostomy—drainage of the gallbladder through a tube.
Choledocho—common bile duct.
Choledochotomy—incision into the common bile duct.
Choledocholithiasis—presence of stones in the common bile duct.
Choledocholithotomy—incision of the common bile duct for the extraction of an impacted gallstone.
Choledochoduodenostomy—surgical formation of a communication between the common bile duct and the duodenum.
Choledochojejunostomy—surgical formation of a communication between the common bile duct and the jejunum.

Cholelithiasis, Cholecystitis, Choledocholithiasis

These conditions refer to stones or inflammation of the biliary system (see Figure 19-4). Cholecystitis may be acute or chronic.

Pathophysiology and Etiology

Cholelithiasis

1. Cholesterol stones occur when cholesterol supersaturates the bile in the gallbladder and precipitates out of the bile. The cholesterol-saturated bile predisposes to the formation of gallstones and acts as an irritant, producing inflammatory changes in the gallbladder.
   a. Cholesterol stones make up 80% of gallstones in the United States.
   b. Four times more women than men develop cholesterol stones.
   c. Women are usually older than age 40, and obese.
   d. Stone formation increases in users of contraceptives, estrogens, and cholesterol-lowering drugs, which are known to increase biliary cholesterol saturation.
   e. Gallstones are associated with high-calorie diets, type 2 diabetes mellitus, dyslipidemia, hyperinsulinism, obesity, and metabolic syndrome.
   f. Bile acid malabsorption, genetic predisposition, and rapid weight loss are also risk factors for cholesterol gallstones.
2. Pigment stones occur when free bilirubin combines with calcium.
   a. Found in patients with cirrhosis, hemolysis, and infections in the biliary tree.
   b. These stones cannot be dissolved.
3. An estimated 10% to 15% of adults in the United States have gallstones, with 1 million new cases discovered each year.
   a. Incidence of stone formation increases with age because of increased hepatic secretion of cholesterol and decreased bile acid synthesis.
   b. Increased risk in patients with malabsorption of bile salts with GI disease, post gastric bypass, with bile fistula, with gallstone ileus, with carcinoma of the gallbladder, or in those who have had ileal resection or ileal bypass.

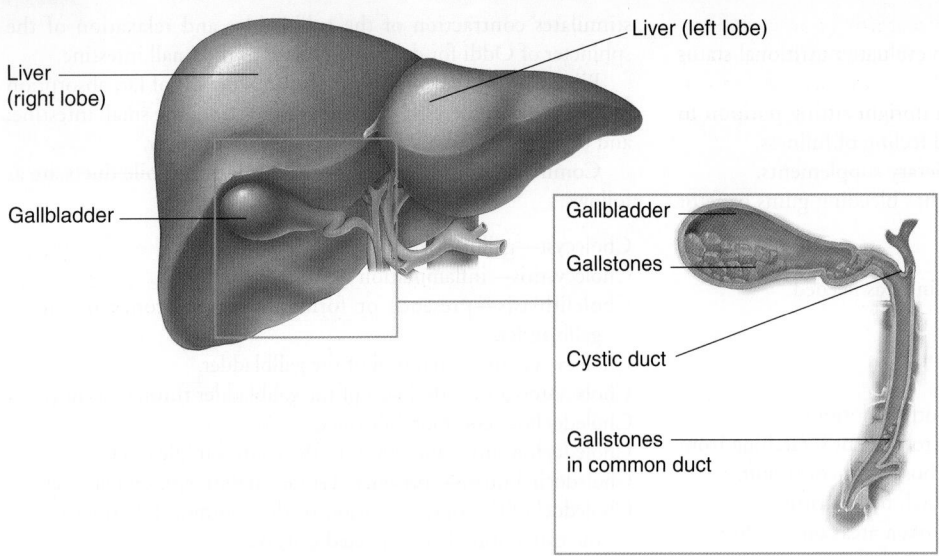

Figure 19-4. Cholelithiasis and choledocholithiasis. (Anatomical Chart Company.)

Cholecystitis

1. Acute cholecystitis, an acute inflammation of the gallbladder, is most commonly caused by gallstone obstruction.
   a. Secondary bacterial infection may occur and progress to empyema (purulent effusion of the gallbladder).
2. Acalculous cholecystitis is acute gallbladder inflammation without obstruction by gallstones.
   a. Occurs after major surgical procedures, severe trauma, or severe burns.
3. Chronic cholecystitis occurs when the gallbladder becomes thickened, rigid, and fibrotic and functions poorly. Results from repeated attacks of cholecystitis, calculi, or chronic irritation.

Choledocholithiasis

1. Small gallstones can pass from the gallbladder into the common bile duct and travel to the duodenum. More commonly, they remain in the common bile duct and can cause obstruction, resulting in jaundice and pruritus.
2. Common bile duct stones are frequently associated with infected bile and can lead to cholangitis (inflammation/infection in the biliary system).
3. Patients experience biliary pain in the upper abdomen, jaundice, chills and fever, mild hepatomegaly, abdominal tenderness, and, occasionally, rebound tenderness.

Clinical Manifestations

1. Gallstones that remain in the gallbladder are usually asymptomatic.
2. Biliary colic can be caused by gallstones.
   a. Steady, severe, aching pain or sensation of pressure in the epigastrium or right upper quadrant, which may radiate to the right scapular area or right shoulder.
   b. Begins suddenly and persists for 1 to 3 hours until the stone falls back into the gallbladder or passes through the cystic duct.
3. Acute cholecystitis causes biliary colic pain that persists more than 4 hours and increases with movement, including respirations.
   a. Also causes nausea and vomiting, low-grade fever, and jaundice (with stones or inflammation in the common bile duct).
   b. Right upper quadrant guarding and Murphy sign (inability to take a deep inspiration when examiner's fingers are pressed below the hepatic margin) are present.

4. Chronic cholecystitis causes heartburn, flatulence, and indigestion. Repeated attacks of symptoms may occur resembling acute cholecystitis.

Diagnostic Evaluation

1. Ultrasonography, CT scan, and HIDA scan may show stones or inflammation.
2. MRCP is a noninvasive exam that can identify gallstones anywhere in the biliary tract.
3. ERCP or PTC to visualize location of stones and extent of obstruction.
4. Elevated conjugated bilirubin and alkaline phosphatase because of obstruction.
5. Elevated amylase and lipase levels, with gallstone pancreatitis.
6. White blood cell count and blood cultures if sepsis.

Management

1. Supportive management may include IV fluids, NG suction, pain management with nonsteroidal anti-inflammatory drugs (NSAIDs) or oral antispasmodics, and antibiotics.
2. A cholecystostomy tube may be placed percutaneously into the gallbladder to decompress the organ in preparation for future surgery. This may be placed by interventional radiology.
3. Oral therapy with chenodeoxycholic acid, ursodeoxycholic acid, or a combination of both to decrease the size of existing cholesterol stones or to dissolve small ones.
   a. Indicated for patients at high risk for surgery because of comorbid conditions.
   b. Major adverse effects include diarrhea, abnormal liver function tests, and increases in serum cholesterol.
   c. Six to twelve months of therapy, may eventually result in dissolution of small gallstones, but with a recurrence rate of more than 50%.
4. Surgical management.
   a. Cholecystectomy, open or laparoscopic.
   b. Intraoperative cholangiography and choledochoscopy for common bile duct exploration.
   c. Placement of a T tube in the common bile duct to decompress the biliary tree and allow access into the biliary tree postoperatively.
5. After cholecystectomy, intracorporeal lithotripsy may be used to fragment retained stones in the common bile duct by pulsed

laser or hydraulic lithotripsy applied through an endoscope directly to the stones. The stone fragments are removed by irrigation or aspiration. Retained stones may also be removed by basket retrieval through the endoscopic or percutaneous transhepatic biliary approach.

Complications

1. Cholangitis.
2. Gangrene, empyema, or perforation of the gallbladder.
3. Biliary fistula through the duodenum or jejunum.
4. Gallstone ileus.
5. Adenocarcinoma of the gallbladder.

Nursing Assessment

1. Obtain history and demographic data that may indicate risk factors for biliary disease.
2. Assess the patient's pain for location, description, intensity, and relieving and exacerbating factors.
3. Assess for signs of dehydration: dry mucous membranes, poor skin turgor, and low urine output with elevated specific gravity.
4. Assess sclera and skin for jaundice.
5. Monitor temperature and WBC count for indications of infection.

Nursing Diagnoses

- Acute Pain related to biliary colic or stone obstruction.
- Deficient Fluid Volume related to nausea and vomiting and decreased intake.

Nursing Interventions

Also see Care of the Patient Undergoing Cholecystectomy.

Relieving Pain

1. Assess pain location, severity, and characteristics.
2. Administer medications or monitor patient-controlled analgesia (PCA) to control pain.
3. Assist in attaining position of comfort.

Restoring Normal Fluid Volume

1. Administer IV fluids and electrolytes, as prescribed.
2. Administer antiemetics, as prescribed, to decrease nausea and vomiting.
3. Maintain NG decompression, if needed.
4. Begin food and fluids, as tolerated, after acute symptoms subside or postoperatively.
5. Observe and record amount of biliary tube drainage, if applicable.

Patient Education and Health Maintenance

1. Instruct the patient in care of tubes or catheters that may be in place at discharge.
   a. Observe for bleeding or drainage around insertion site.
   b. Replace dressing per facility protocol.
   c. Report change or decrease in drainage.
2. Review discharge instructions for activity, diet, medications, and follow-up.
3. Emphasize symptoms of complications to be reported, such as increased or persistent pain, fever, abdominal distention, nausea, anorexia, jaundice, unusual drainage.
4. Encourage follow-up, as indicated.

Evaluation: Expected Outcomes

- Verbalizes reduced pain level.
- Tolerates oral fluids and solid food; adequate urine output.

Care of the Patient Undergoing Cholecystectomy

 EVIDENCE BASE Benner, P., & Kautz, D. (2015). Postoperative care of patients undergoing same-day laparoscopic cholecystectomy. *AORN Journal*, *102*(1), 15–32.

Cholecystectomy is surgical removal of the gallbladder for acute and chronic cholecystitis. Laparoscopic cholecystectomy is the most commonly performed abdominal surgery in industrialized countries, with almost 900,000 procedures performed annually.

Procedure

1. Open laparotomy—gallbladder removed after making an abdominal incision.
2. Laparoscopy—gallbladder removed from a small opening just above the umbilicus through the use of a laparoscope for viewing (see Figure 19-5).
   a. Three other small punctures are made in the abdomen to place other special instruments used to assist in the manipulation and removal of the gallbladder.
   b. The organs in the abdomen can be viewed through the laparoscope and via a television monitor through a camera attached to the laparoscope.
3. If the patient is scheduled for a laparoscopic cholecystectomy, consent is also obtained for a traditional open cholecystectomy

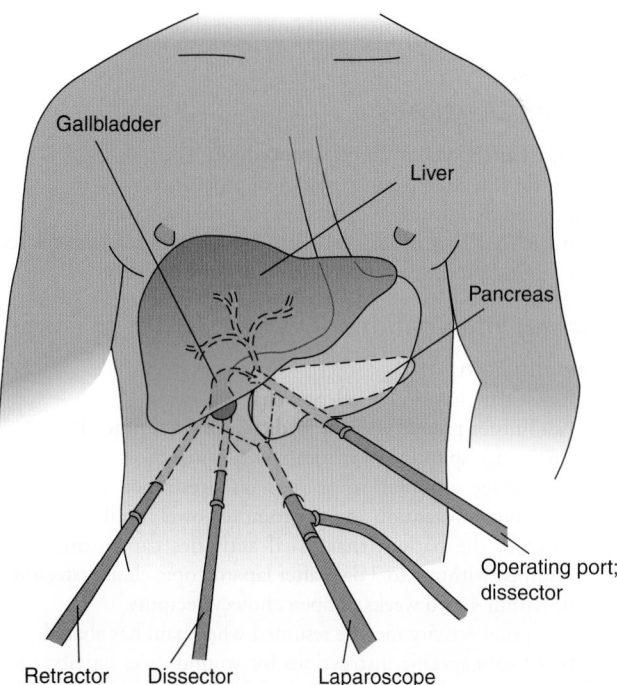

Figure 19-5. Laparoscopic cholecystectomy. The surgeon makes four small incisions (less than ½ inch each) in the abdomen and inserts a laparoscope with a miniature camera into the opening. The camera apparatus displays the gallbladder and adjacent tissues on a screen allowing the surgeon to visualize the organ for removal.

in case the gallbladder is not accessible through the laparoscopic technique.

4. After cholecystectomy, bile ducts will eventually dilate to accommodate the volume of bile once held by the gallbladder to aid in the digestion of fats.

Preoperative Management

1. IV fluids are given before surgery to improve hydration status if the patient has been vomiting.
2. Antibiotics are ordered for acute cholecystitis.
3. Educate the patient about the procedure and what to expect postoperatively.
4. The patient must remain NPO from midnight the night before surgery and must void before surgery.

Postoperative Management

1. Postoperatively, the patient is evaluated for the following:
   a. Vital signs, LOC.
   b. Level of pain.
   c. Appearance of wound or puncture sites: wound drain or T-tube patency (if common bile duct exploration also performed), security and drainage (if present).
   d. Intake and output.
   e. Postoperative nausea and vomiting
2. Early ambulation is encouraged to prevent thromboembolism, to facilitate voiding, and to stimulate peristalsis.
3. Monitor for complications including: incisional infection, hemorrhage, and bile duct injury (persistent pain, fever, abdominal distention, nausea, anorexia, or jaundice).

Potential Complications

1. Infection, hemorrhage, or bile duct injury.
2. Pneumonia or atelectasis.
3. Deep vein thrombosis or pulmonary embolism.
4. Impaired wound healing.

Nursing Diagnoses

- Acute Pain related to surgical procedure.
- Risk for Infection related to surgical procedure.
- Impaired Skin Integrity related to surgical procedure.
- Imbalanced Nutrition: Less Than Body Requirements related to surgical procedure, wound pain, or tube drainage.

Nursing Interventions

Relieving Pain

1. Assess pain location, level, and characteristics.
2. Administer prescribed pain medications or monitor PCA.
3. Encourage splinting of incision when moving.
4. Encourage ambulation as soon as prescribed to decrease abdominal distention and to promote bowel motility.
5. Instruct the patient that usual activities can normally be resumed within 5 to 7 days after laparoscopic cholecystectomy or within 4 to 6 weeks of open cholecystectomy.
   a. Sexual activity may be resumed when pain has abated.
   b. Obtain specific instructions for wound care; activity, such as heavy lifting; strenuous activity; showers and tub baths; and driving per surgeon's protocol.

Preventing Infection

1. Assess wound dressings for any increased or purulent drainage.
2. Assess wound drain or T-tube site for drainage, and note amount, color, and odor.

3. Assess bile drainage from T tube into bile bag:
   a. Report decrease in drainage.
   b. Maintain T-tube patency and security.
4. Report right upper quadrant pain, abdominal distention, fever, chills, or jaundice, as these may indicate a bile duct injury.
5. Administer antibiotics, as prescribed.
6. Encourage use of incentive spirometer, coughing and deep breathing, and ambulation to decrease risk of pulmonary infection.

Maintaining Skin Integrity

1. Assess wounds for healing.
2. Perform wound care as prescribed.
3. Assess for adequate hydration.
4. Assess and report any signs of redness, swelling, pain, or drainage from the wounds.

Providing Adequate Nutrition

1. Assess for nausea and vomiting and administer antiemetics, as prescribed.
2. Encourage fluid intake and advance to regular diet, as tolerated.
3. Administer replacement fluids for bile drainage from T tube, if indicated.
4. Clamp T tube, when indicated, and assess tolerance of food and color of stools.

Patient Education and Health Maintenance

1. Teach the patient and family that rapid postoperative recovery should be expected.
2. Advise the patient and family to notify the surgeon immediately of any subtle change in the patient's postoperative course or persistent symptoms. A bile duct injury should be suspected after a laparoscopic cholecystectomy in patients who do not show the expected recovery during the early postoperative period.
3. Advise the patient to advance diet, as tolerated. Fats can be taken *as tolerated* because the bile ducts dilate to accommodate storage of bile, as needed.

Evaluation: Expected Outcomes

- Verbalizes decreased pain.
- No fever or signs of infection.
- Wound healing without drainage.
- Tolerates fluids and small solid feedings.

PANCREATIC DISORDERS

The pancreas secretes enzymes, including amylase and lipase, through the pancreatic duct when stimulated by cholecystokinin and secretin to aid in digestion of carbohydrates and fat in the small intestine. The pancreas also secretes hormones, such as insulin and glucagon, which help to regulate and maintain normal serum glucose.

Acute Pancreatitis

Acute pancreatitis is an inflammation of the pancreas, ranging from mild edema to extensive hemorrhage, resulting from various insults to the pancreas. It is defined by a discrete episode of abdominal pain and serum pancreatic enzyme elevations. The structure and function of the pancreas usually return to normal after an acute attack. Chronic pancreatitis occurs when there is persistent cellular damage to the pancreas (see Table 19-2 for comparison).

Table 19-2 Acute Versus Chronic Pancreatitis: Comparing Findings

	ACUTE PANCREATITIS	CHRONIC PANCREATITIS
Definition	• Inflammation that leads to swelling of the pancreas • Autodigestion—enzymes normally secreted by the pancreas become activated inside the pancreas and start to digest the pancreatic tissue	• Associated with widespread scarring and destruction of pancreatic tissue • Affects more men than women
Etiology	• Gallstones passing through the common bile duct • Alcohol misuse • Viral infection, hereditary conditions, traumatic injury, certain medications (especially estrogens, corticosteroids, thiazide diuretics, and azathioprine), pancreatic or common bile duct surgical procedures, or ERCP • Underlying pancreatic tumor • Hypercalcemia • Hypertriglyceridemia • Idiopathic	• Alcohol misuse (70% of patients) • Hereditary pancreatitis • Ductal destruction (from trauma, stones, tumors) • Tropical pancreatitis • Systemic diseases (cystic fibrosis, systemic lupus erythematosus, hyperparathyroidism) • Congenital conditions such as pancreas divisum • Hypercalcemia • Hypertriglyceridemia • Idiopathic
Symptoms	• Sudden attack of constant, severe upper abdominal pain that may radiate to the back • Pain that is sudden and steady • Pain that may be aggravated by walking or lying down and relieved by sitting or leaning forward (proning) • Other possible symptoms: nausea, vomiting, diarrhea, bloating, fever, diaphoresis, and jaundice	• Constant, dull mid to upper abdominal pain; may also have back pain • Pain that worsens with eating food or drinking alcohol; lessens with sitting or leaning forward (proning) • As disease progresses, attacks of pain that last longer and occur more frequently • May have nausea, vomiting • Weight loss
Course	• Mild disease in 85% of patients with rapid recovery within a few days of onset of illness	• Destruction of pancreatic tissue that slowly progresses from chronic inflammatory damage
Diagnosis	• Medical history • Social history • Serum amylase and lipase • Serum triglycerides • Ultrasound, CT scan, MRI	• Medical history • Social history • Liver function tests • Fecal elastase test • Abdominal x-ray that may reveal calcium deposits in the pancreas • Imaging studies, such as ultrasound, CT scan, ERCP, EUS, MRI/MRCP • CEA and CA 19-9 to assess for pancreatic cancer
Treatment	• Depends on severity as acute pancreatitis may be mild, moderate, or severe • IV fluids • Pain medication • Diet advancement based on pain and nausea • Surgery for such complications as necrosis, infection, bleeding	• Pain management • Nutritional support and diet modification with smaller, frequent, low-fat meals • Pancreatic enzymes • Diabetes control • Pancreatic duct drainage procedures or excision of damage of all or part of the pancreas • Alcohol abstinence

Complications	• Severe acute pancreatitis may lead to:
	  • Multiple organ system failure, such as lung, liver, kidney, and heart
	  • Infected pancreatic necrosis
	  • Pancreatic abscess
	  • Pancreatic pseudocysts
	  • Pancreatic fistula
	  • Pancreatic ascites
	  • Damage to surrounding organs, such as small bowel, colon, and duodenum (due to inflammation)
		• Malnutrition from poor absorption of nutrients, especially fats
		• Frequent bowel movements that are loose, greasy, foul-smelling (steatorrhea)
		• Insulin-dependent diabetes
		• Increased risk of pancreatic cancer
		• Pseudocyst
		• Bleeding from the stomach
		• Increased risk of venous thrombobembolism
		• Possible bouts of acute pancreatitis

Prognosis	• Can usually fully recover without recurrence if cause is removed	• Can maintain quality of life with supportive care and adherence to medical regimen

Pathophysiology and Etiology

1. Excessive alcohol consumption is the most common cause in the United States.
2. Also commonly caused by biliary tract disease, such as cholelithiasis and acute and chronic cholecystitis.
3. Less common causes are bacterial or viral infection, blunt abdominal trauma, peptic ulcer disease, ischemic vascular disease, hypertriglyceridemia (greater than 1,000 g/dL), hypercalcemia; the use of corticosteroids, thiazide diuretics, and oral contraceptives; surgery on or near the pancreas or after instrumentation of the pancreatic duct by ERCP; tumors of the pancreas or ampulla; and (rarely) hereditary pancreatitis.
4. Mortality is high (10%) because of shock, anoxia, hypotension, or multiple organ dysfunction.
5. Attacks may resolve with complete recovery, may recur without permanent damage, or may progress to chronic pancreatitis.
6. Autodigestion of all or part of the pancreas is involved, but the exact mechanism is not completely understood.

Clinical Manifestations

(Depends on severity of pancreatic damage.)

1. Abdominal pain, usually constant, midepigastric or periumbilical, radiating to the back or flank. The patient assumes a fetal position or leans forward while sitting (known as "proning") to relieve pressure of the inflamed pancreas on celiac plexus nerves. Pain can be mild to incapacitating.
2. Nausea and vomiting.
3. Fever.
4. Involuntary abdominal guarding, epigastric tenderness to deep palpation, and reduced or absent bowel sounds.
5. Dry mucous membranes; hypotension; cold, clammy skin; cyanosis; and tachycardia, which may reflect mild to moderate dehydration from vomiting or capillary leak syndrome (third space loss).
6. Shock may be the presenting manifestation in severe episodes, with respiratory distress and acute renal failure.
7. Purplish discoloration of the flanks (Turner sign) or of the periumbilical area (Cullen sign) occurs in extensive hemorrhagic necrosis of the pancreas.

Diagnostic Evaluation

1. A minimum of 2 out of 3 criteria must be met to diagnose acute pancreatitis: Abdominal pain; elevated serum lipase (or amylase) at least 3 times greater than the upper limit of normal; characteristic findings of acute pancreatitis on CT scan or MRI.
2. Serum glucose, bilirubin, alkaline phosphatase, lactate dehydrogenase, AST, ALT, potassium, and cholesterol may be elevated.
3. Serum albumin, calcium, sodium, magnesium, and, possibly, potassium may be low because of dehydration, vomiting, and the binding of calcium in areas of fat necrosis.
4. Elevated C-reactive protein (CRP) level in the first 72 hours is suggestive of severe acute pancreatitis and is predictive of a worse clinical course.
5. Abdominal x-ray to detect an ileus or isolated loop of small bowel overlying pancreas. Pancreatic calcifications or gallstones may suggest an alcohol or biliary etiology.
6. Abdominal ultrasound to determine if the patient has gallstones or obstruction in the common bile duct.
7. Chest x-ray for detection of pulmonary complications. Pleural effusions are common, especially on the left, but may be bilateral.

Management

 EVIDENCE BASE Crockett, S. D, Wani, S., Gardner, T. B., et al. (2018). American Gastroenterological Association Institute guideline on initial management of acute pancreatitis. *Gastroenterology, 154*(4), 1096–1101.

Depending on severity of the episode, management focuses on alleviation of symptoms and support of the patient to prevent complications.

1. Aggressive hydration, defined as 250 to 500 mL/hour of isotonic crystalloid solution should be provided to all patients, unless contraindicated, for the first 24 to 48 hours.
2. Adequate oxygenation, which is often reduced by pain, anxiety, acidosis, abdominal pressure, or pleural effusions.
3. Pain control to alleviate pain and anxiety, which increases pancreatic secretions.
4. NG intubation and suction to relieve gastric stasis, distention, and ileus, if needed. Maintenance of alkaline gastric pH with PPIs or H_2-receptor antagonists and antacids to suppress acid drive of pancreatic secretions and to prevent stress ulcers.
5. Begin oral or enteral nutrition within 24 hours. This may help to protect the gut mucosal barrier and limit bacterial movement, reducing the risk for complications of acute pancreatitis.
6. Supportive pharmacotherapy.
   a. Electrolyte replacements, as needed.
   b. Sodium bicarbonate to treat metabolic acidosis.
   c. Insulin to treat hyperglycemia.
   d. Antibiotic therapy for documented infection or sepsis.
7. Cholecystectomy is indicated during the hospital admission for acute gallstone pancreatitis.
8. Surgical intervention if complications occur.
   a. Incision and drainage of abscess and infected pseudocysts.
   b. Debridement or pancreatectomy to remove necrotic pancreatic tissue.

Complications

1. Pancreatic ascites, abscess, or pseudocyst.
2. Acute necrotic collections or walled-off pancreatic necrosis.
3. Pulmonary infiltrates, pleural effusion, acute respiratory distress syndrome.
4. Hemorrhage with hypovolemic shock.
5. Acute renal failure.
6. Sepsis and multiple-organ dysfunction syndrome.

Nursing Assessment

1. Obtain history of gallbladder disease, alcohol use, hypertriglyceridemia, or precipitating factors.
2. Assess GI symptoms, including nausea and vomiting, diarrhea, and passage of stools containing fat.

3. Assess characteristics of abdominal pain.
4. Assess nutritional and fluid status.
5. Assess respiratory rate and pattern and breath sounds.

 GERONTOLOGIC ALERT The incidence of severe, systemic complications of pancreatitis increases with age. Assess for any changes in mental status in an older person with pancreatitis as an indicator of an underlying complication. Acute pancreatitis in an older person without other precipitating factors may indicate an underlying pancreatic tumor obstructing the pancreatic duct.

Nursing Diagnoses

- Acute Pain related to disease process.
- Deficient Fluid Volume related to vomiting, self-restricted intake, fever, and fluid shifts.
- Ineffective Breathing Pattern related to severe pain and pulmonary complications.
- Imbalanced Nutrition: Less Than Body Requirements related to fear of eating, malabsorption, and glucose intolerance.

Nursing Interventions

Controlling Pain
1. Administer opioid analgesics, as ordered, to control pain.
2. Assist the patient to a comfortable position.
3. Maintain patency of NG suction to remove gastric secretions and to relieve abdominal distention, if indicated.
4. Provide frequent oral hygiene and care.
5. Administer antacids, PPIs, or H_2-receptor antagonists, as prescribed.
6. Report increase in severity of pain, which may indicate hemorrhage of the pancreas, rupture of a pseudocyst, or inadequate dosage of the analgesic.

Restoring Adequate Fluid Balance
1. Monitor and record vital signs, skin color, and temperature.
2. Monitor intake and output and weigh daily.
3. Evaluate laboratory data for hemoglobin, hematocrit, albumin, calcium, potassium, sodium, and magnesium levels and administer replacements, as prescribed.
4. Observe and measure abdominal girth if pancreatic ascites is suspected.
5. Report trends in falling BP or urine output or rising pulse because this may indicate hypovolemia and shock or renal failure.

Improving Respiratory Function
1. Assess respiratory rate and rhythm, effort, oxygen saturation, and breath sounds frequently.
2. Position in upright or semi-Fowler position to enhance diaphragmatic excursion.
3. Administer oxygen supplementation, as prescribed, to maintain adequate oxygen levels.
4. Report signs of respiratory distress immediately.
5. Instruct the patient in coughing and deep breathing to improve respiratory function.

Nutrition
1. Assess nutritional status, history of weight loss, and dietary habits, including alcohol intake.
2. Administer antacids or H_2-receptor antagonists to prevent neutralization of enzyme supplements, as indicated.
3. Monitor intake and output and daily weight.
4. Assess for GI discomfort with meals and character of stools.
5. Monitor blood glucose levels and teach balanced, low concentrated carbohydrate diet and insulin therapy as indicated.
6. Identify foods that aggravate symptoms, and teach low-fat diet.

 TRANSITIONAL CARE ALERT Patients with acute pancreatitis are often critically ill with long hospitalization, requiring extended rehabilitation. Assess the need for supportive services such as subacute care, home care, and outpatient rehabilitation. Identify risk factors for readmission such as lack of supportive caregiver, insurance, transportation, education, and financial resources, as well as the presence of alcohol or drug addiction. Engage social worker as well as community agencies for follow-up and ongoing problem solving after the patient leaves the hospital.

Patient Education and Health Maintenance

1. Instruct the patient to gradually resume a low-fat diet.
2. Instruct the patient to increase activity gradually, providing for daily rest periods.
3. Reinforce information about the disease process and precipitating factors. Stress that subsequent bouts of acute pancreatitis may destroy the pancreas, cause additional complications, and lead to chronic pancreatitis.
4. If pancreatitis is a result of alcohol use, the patient needs to be reminded of the importance of eliminating all alcohol; advise about Alcoholics Anonymous or other substance use counseling.

Evaluation: Expected Outcomes

- Verbalizes reduced pain level.
- BP stable; urine output adequate.
- Respirations unlabored; breath sounds clear.

Chronic Pancreatitis

Chronic pancreatitis is defined as the persistence of pancreatic cellular damage after acute inflammation and decreased pancreatic endocrine and exocrine function. Prevalence of chronic pancreatitis is 50 per 100,000 people.

Pathophysiology and Etiology

1. Chronic pancreatitis often develops in patients between the ages of 30 and 40, and is more common in men.
2. Alcohol misuse is the most common cause; less common causes are hyperparathyroidism, hereditary pancreatitis, malnutrition, and trauma to the pancreas.
3. With chronic inflammation, destruction of the secreting cells of the pancreas causes maldigestion and malabsorption of protein and fat and possibly diabetes mellitus if islet cells of the pancreas have been affected.
4. As cells are replaced by fibrous tissue, obstruction of the pancreatic and common bile ducts and duodenum may result.

Clinical Manifestations

1. Pain is usually located in the epigastrium or left upper quadrant, frequently radiating to the back; similar to that observed in acute pancreatitis, but more constant and occurring at unpredictable intervals. As the disease progresses, recurring attacks of pain will be more severe, more frequent, and of longer duration.

2. Weight loss, nausea, vomiting, and anorexia.
3. Malabsorption and steatorrhea occur late in the course of the disease.
4. Glucose intolerance.

Diagnostic Evaluation

1. Serum amylase and lipase may be normal to low because of decreased pancreatic exocrine function.
2. Fecal fat analysis determines need for pancreatic enzyme replacement.
3. Bilirubin and alkaline phosphatase may be elevated if biliary obstruction occurs.
4. Secretin and cholecystokinin stimulatory test results are abnormal.
5. Plain abdominal x-ray to determine diffuse calcification of the pancreas.
6. CT scan identifies pancreatic structural changes, such as calcifications, masses, ductal irregularities, enlargement, and pseudocysts.
7. ERCP defines ductal anatomy and localizes complications, such as pancreatic pseudocysts and ductal disruptions.

Management

1. Alcohol abstinence and tobacco cessation.
2. Pain management, including supportive behavioral therapy.
3. Small meals and hydration with correction of nutritional deficiencies.
4. Pancreatic enzyme replacement.
5. Treatment of diabetes mellitus.
6. Endoscopic placement of pancreatic stent allowing free flow of pancreatic juices through distorted and irregular/narrowed pancreatic duct.
7. Surgical interventions to reduce pain, restore drainage of pancreatic secretions, correct structural abnormalities, and manage complications.
   a. Pancreatojejunostomy—side-to-side anastomosis of pancreatic duct to jejunum to drain pancreatic secretions into jejunum.
   b. Revision of sphincter of ampulla of Vater by a sphincteroplasty, in which the sphincter is sewn open to allow free flow of pancreatic juices.
   c. Drainage of pancreatic pseudocyst into nearby structures or by external drain.
   d. Resection of part of pancreas (Whipple procedure, distal pancreatectomy) or removal of entire pancreas (total pancreatectomy).
   e. Autotransplantation of islet cells.

Complications

1. Pancreatic pseudocyst formation.
2. Pancreatic ascites and pleural effusions.
3. GI hemorrhage.
4. Biliary tract obstruction.
5. Pancreatic fistula.
6. Splenic vein thrombosis.
7. Pancreatic cancer.
8. Diabetes mellitus.

Nursing Assessment

1. Assess level of abdominal pain.
2. Assess nutritional status.
3. Assess for steatorrhea and malabsorption.
4. Assess for signs and symptoms of diabetes mellitus.
5. Assess current level of alcohol intake and motivation and resources available to abstain from drinking such as Alcoholics Anonymous.

Nursing Diagnoses

For surgical care, see "Care of the Patient Undergoing Gastrointestinal Surgery" (page 495).

- Acute and Chronic Pain related to chronic and unrelenting insult to pancreas.
- Imbalanced Nutrition: Less Than Body Requirements related to fear of eating, malabsorption, and glucose intolerance.
- Anxiety related to surgical intervention or not knowing when pain may recur.

Nursing Interventions

Controlling Pain

1. Assess and record the character, location, frequency, and duration of pain.
2. Determine precipitating and alleviating factors of the patient's pain.
3. Explore the effect of pain on the patient's lifestyle and eating habits.
4. Administer or teach self-administration of analgesics, as ordered, to control pain.
5. Use nonpharmacologic methods to promote relaxation, such as distraction, imagery, and progressive muscle relaxation.
6. Assess response to pain-control measures and refer to pain management clinic, if indicated.

Improving Nutritional Status

1. Assess nutritional status, history of weight loss, and dietary habits, including alcohol intake.
2. Administer pancreatic enzyme replacement with meals, as prescribed.
3. Administer antacids, PPIs, or H_2-receptor antagonists to prevent neutralization of enzyme supplements, as indicated.
4. Monitor intake and output and daily weight.
5. Assess for GI discomfort with meals and character of stools.
6. Monitor blood glucose levels and teach balanced, low–concentrated carbohydrate diet and insulin therapy, as indicated.
7. Identify foods that aggravate symptoms and teach low-fat diet.

 DRUG ALERT Warn the patient that dangerous hypoglycemic reaction may result from use of insulin while drinking alcohol and skipping meals.

Relieving Anxiety about Surgical Intervention

1. Describe planned surgical intervention and the expected results.
   a. Decreased pain.
   b. Ability to eat better and improve general condition.
2. Prepare the patient for adverse effects and complications of surgery.
   a. Total pancreatectomy will cause permanent diabetes mellitus, dependence on insulin, severe malabsorption, and the need for lifelong pancreatic enzyme replacement. Consultation and close monitoring by endocrinologist and diabetic educator.
   b. Malnutrition and debility increase the patient's risk for poor healing and complications of surgery.

3. Assist the patient to prepare for surgery by encouraging abstinence of alcohol and intake of nutritional and vitamin supplements.
4. Encourage the patient to enlist the help of support network and strengthen appropriate coping mechanisms.
5. After surgery, provide meticulous care to prevent infection, promote wound healing, and prevent routine complications of surgery.

Patient Education and Health Maintenance

1. Instruct the patient regarding correct use of analgesics.
2. Instruct in proper administration of pancreatic enzyme replacement.
   a. Take just before or during meals.
   b. May be enteric coated. Do not crush or chew tablets; powder may be sprinkled on food if swallowing tablets is difficult.
   c. Take with antacid, PPI, or H_2-receptor antagonist, as directed, to prevent pancreatic enzyme from being destroyed by gastric acid secretions.
3. Advise the patient to monitor number and characteristics of stools; report increased stools or food intolerance.
4. Diabetic teaching with follow-up to monitor progression of condition, if applicable.
5. Stress that treatment will be ineffective if alcohol consumption is continued.

Evaluation: Expected Outcomes

- Verbalizes reduced pain level.
- Weight stabilized or weight gain noted.
- Verbalizes understanding of effects of surgical procedure.

Pancreatic Cancer

Cancer of the pancreas is a highly lethal malignancy that may arise in the head (about 70% of cases) or body and tail of the pancreas. Adenocarcinoma of the cells that line the ducts of the pancreas is the most common (85%) type. Pancreatic cancer is the fourth leading cause of cancer deaths in the United States because 90% of tumors are not resectable at the time of diagnosis.

Pathophysiology and Etiology

1. Incidence is increasing with 50,000 cases diagnosed each year in the United States.
2. Occurs more commonly in males than females, in blacks than in whites.
3. Usually occurs between ages 60 and 80 but can be found in younger patients.
4. Smoking, prolonged exposure to industrial chemicals, high-fat diet, diabetes mellitus, and chronic pancreatitis are considered risk factors. A small percentage of pancreatic cancer is inherited.
5. Obesity and physical inactivity are now considered risk factors for pancreatic cancer.
6. Obstruction of bile flow may occur with tumors in the head of the pancreas because of compression of the distal common bile duct.
7. Obstruction of pancreatic duct produces pain and exocrine dysfunction.

Clinical Manifestations

1. Symptoms are commonly vague and nonspecific, preventing early detection.
2. Weakness, weight loss, anorexia, nausea, vomiting, and abdominal pain may occur.

3. Pain usually occurs in the upper abdomen and is gnawing or boring and may radiate around the flank to the back.
   a. Pain is usually worse at night, and patients tend to lie with knees to chest position or may lean forward when seated (proning) to relieve pain.
   b. Pain may become more localized, severe, and unremitting as the disease progresses.
4. Early satiety and a feeling of bloating after eating may occur.
5. Hepatomegaly.
6. Biliary obstruction produces jaundice, dark tea-colored urine, clay-colored stools, and pruritus.
7. Depression and lethargy may be present.

Diagnostic Evaluation

1. Liver function tests elevated; coagulation studies may be prolonged.
2. Carcinoembryonic antigen (CEA) and CA 19-9—may be elevated.
3. Transabdominal ultrasonography detects tumors larger than 1 cm.
4. ERCP defines anatomy and allows placement of biliary stent for unobstructed flow of bile by tumor in the head of the pancreas prior to surgery or as palliation in patients not deemed surgical candidates.
5. MRCP—defines anatomy without contrast dye.
6. Abdominal CT scan to assess resectability.
7. PET scan to differentiate cancer from cyst as well as to assess for recurrence or metastatic disease.
8. Biopsy through percutaneous fine needle aspiration or EUS for cytology and to confirm malignancy.

Management

The goal of treatment may be cure or palliation, depending on the staging of the tumor. Despite advances in treatment, the 5-year survival rate is 5% in nonoperative cases and 20% to 30% in those who undergo surgery.

Surgery

Surgical resection is the only potentially curative treatment. Unfortunately, because of the late presentation of the disease, only 15% to 20% of patients are candidates for pancreatectomy.

1. Whipple procedure (pancreaticoduodenectomy) is the removal of the head of the pancreas and distal portion of the common bile duct including the gallbladder, duodenum, and the distal stomach with anastomosis of the remaining pancreas, stomach, and common bile duct to the jejunum (see Figure 19-6). If the gallbladder is present, it is also removed. Modifications of the conventional pancreaticoduodenectomy procedure have been developed in an attempt to improve outcomes or minimize the morbidity associated with the operation.
   a. Stomach and pylorus may be preserved—pylorus-preserving pancreaticoduodenectomy This procedure may decrease the incidence of postoperative dumping, marginal ulceration, and bile reflux gastritis.
   b. Subtotal stomach-preserving pancreaticoduodenectomy—preserve as much stomach as possible while minimizing problems related to delayed gastric emptying.
2. Total pancreatectomy, including a splenectomy, may be performed for diffuse tumor throughout the pancreas.
3. Distal pancreatectomy is the removal of the distal pancreas and spleen for tumors localized in the body and tail.

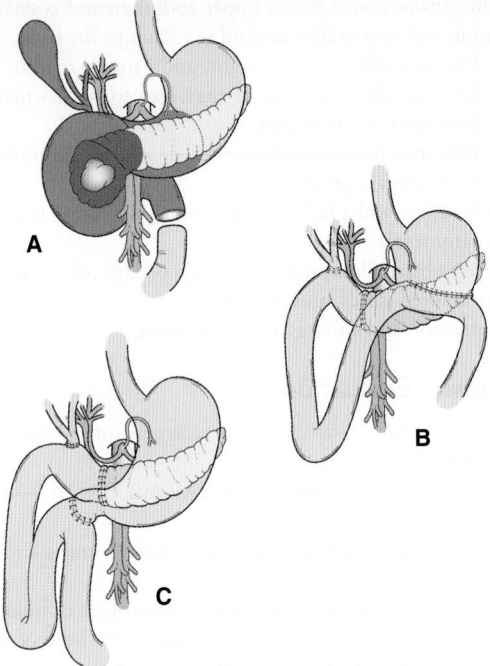

Figure 19-6. Pancreaticoduodenectomy. **(A)** The standard pancreaticoduodenectomy (Whipple procedure) involves a wide area of resection around the tumor, including the gallbladder, distal stomach including the pyloric region, duodenum, and head of the pancreas, as indicated. **(B)** Anastomoses of the common bile duct, fundus of the stomach, and body and tail of the pancreas to the jejunum. **(C)** Pylorus-preserving variant involves conservation of the stomach, including the pyloric valve anastomosed to the jejunum.

4. Palliative bypass for nonresectable tumors: choledochojejunostomy or cholecystojejunostomy for obstructive jaundice or gastrojejunostomy for gastric outlet obstruction.

Other Measures

1. Chemotherapy alone or in combination with radiation therapy may be given before surgery to shrink tumors that involve major blood vessels.
2. Chemotherapy combined with radiation therapy may be given for resectable tumors after surgery for microscopic or undetectable disease left behind.
3. Chemotherapy and radiation therapy may be given for tumors deemed unresectable at the time of surgery and after palliative bowel bypass surgery.
4. Chemotherapy may be given alone for treatment of unresectable or metastatic disease.
5. Radiation therapy may be used alone.
   a. External beam irradiation for local control, to reduce pain, and to palliate obstruction.
   b. Intraoperative radiation therapy given after the pancreas resection has also been used in some centers.
6. Endoscopic or percutaneous stent placement for relief of biliary or duodenal obstruction.
7. Chemical splanchnicectomy, injection of alcohol into the celiac plexus, numbs the nerves in the area of the pancreas to provide temporary pain relief.
   a. May be performed intraoperatively by the surgeon or percutaneously under CT guidance as an outpatient procedure by an anesthesia pain service.

8. Immunotherapies under investigation that show promising results include immune modulators, therapeutic vaccines, monoclonal antibodies, oncolytic viruses, adjuvant immunotherapies, and cytokines.

EVIDENCE BASE National Cancer Institute Physician Data Query (PDQ), American Cancer Society Facts & Figures 2016, National Comprehensive Cancer Network (NCCN) Guidelines for Patients, *ClinicalTrials.gov*, CRI grantee progress reports.

TRANSITIONAL CARE ALERT With the high mortality rate associated with pancreatic cancer, it is suggested to involve the palliative care specialists early in the course of treatment. Palliative care includes pain and symptom management as well as goals of care discussion regarding end of life care and hospice when appropriate. Earlier involvement has been shown to improve patients' symptom management, prevent unnecessary admissions to the hospital, and provide support to the patient and family.

Complications

1. Biliary, gastric, and duodenal obstruction.
2. Metastasis and liver failure/ ascites secondary to metastasis.
3. Portal hypertension and pain because of encasement of major blood vessels and celiac nerve plexus in the area of the pancreas.
4. Venous thromboembolism: incidence of VTE is four- to sevenfold higher in pancreatic cancer as in other common adenocarcinomas.
5. Malnutrition, weight loss, anorexia, and cachexia.

Nursing Assessment

1. Obtain history for risk factors, pain, and symptoms of pancreatic dysfunction.
2. Assess nutritional status, including diet history, anorexia, weight loss, nausea and vomiting, steatorrhea, skin turgor.
3. Evaluate laboratory results for alterations in glucose, pancreatic enzymes, liver function, and coagulation studies.
4. Assess psychosocial status to determine depression, usual coping strategies, support systems, and experience with past serious illness.
5. Assess use of alternative therapies or over-the-counter medications.

DRUG ALERT The efficacy of herbal medications to treat or cure pancreatic cancer has not been proven. Little is known about the interaction of herbal medications with conventional medications or treatments. Herbal medications may interact with chemotherapy drugs and compromise treatment. If a patient is using alternative treatments or herbal medications, this must be known to all health care providers.

Nursing Diagnoses

• Acute Pain related to pancreatic tumor or surgical incision.
• Imbalanced Nutrition: Less Than Body Requirements related to disease process and surgical intervention.

- Deficient Fluid Volume related to hypoproteinemia, surgical alterations.
- Impaired Tissue Integrity related to malnutrition, surgical incisions, and altered pancreatic or bile drainage.

Nursing Interventions

For surgical care, see "Care of the Patient Undergoing Gastrointestinal Surgery" (page 495).

Controlling Pain

1. Administer opioids, as ordered, or monitor PCA.
2. Teach relaxation techniques, such as relaxation breathing, progressive muscle relaxation, and imagery, as adjuncts for pain relief.
3. Assist with frequent turning and comfortable positioning.
4. Administer adjuvant medications, such as antidepressants and anxiolytics, as prescribed.
5. Assess the patient's response to pain and symptom-control measures.
6. Consider palliative care or hospice services for symptom management if the patient no longer benefits from therapy.

Improving Nutritional Status

1. Administer parenteral nutrition, as prescribed, preoperatively and postoperatively, if indicated.
2. Monitor serum glucose level for hyperglycemia or hypoglycemia.
3. Progress diet slowly when oral intake is tolerated; observe for nausea, vomiting, and gastric distention.
4. Administer high-protein, high-carbohydrate diet with vitamin supplements and pancreatic enzymes, as prescribed.
5. Encourage use of spices to stimulate taste buds, provide cool foods to decrease odor, use plastic utensils if the patient complains of metallic taste from treatments, and offer small, frequent meals.
6. Provide appetite stimulant, such as megestrol, as needed.
7. Monitor serum albumin.
8. Weekly weights.
9. Assess for fat and protein malabsorption: stools that float, have greasy appearance, are orange in color, and are foul smelling.

Attaining Adequate Fluid Volume

1. Monitor vital signs and record accurate intake and output.
2. Monitor wound drain output.
3. Evaluate laboratory values for hypoalbuminemia, hyponatremia, hypochloremia, and metabolic alkalosis; replace electrolytes, as prescribed.
4. Administer fluid replacement, as indicated.
5. Report change in vital signs or increased pain: may indicate hemorrhage, leak from anastomosis, or tumor progression.

Maintaining Tissue Integrity

1. Observe skin for jaundice, breakdown, irritation, or excoriation.
2. Administer antipruritic medication, provide frequent skin care with mild soap and with thorough rinsing, apply emollient lotions, trim fingernails short to prevent scratching.
3. Inspect skin around drains for irritation and protect skin from leakage of fluids from drains or tubes.
4. Inspect surgical dressings and incision for bleeding, drainage, or signs of infection.
5. Prevent tension on anastomoses by monitoring for abdominal distention and maintaining patency of surgically placed tubes and drains.

6. Maintain aseptic technique in handling wound dressings and drainage of all secretions.

Community and Home Care Considerations

1. Educate the patient and family about course of disease and support them through the process.
2. Provide assistive devices and direct care to help with energy conservation. Patients who die of pancreatic cancer may have progressive weight loss from anorexia leading to severe cachexia, fatigue, and muscle wasting, which is refractory to any intervention.
3. Assess for bowel obstruction, which may also deplete energy and lower nutritional status. Notify health care provider of reduced bowel activity, increased pain, or abdominal distention.
4. Emphasize to the patient and family that pain can always be managed and patients need not die in pain. The plan for pain management should be aggressive and should provide the patient an optimal quality of life.
5. Encourage the family to take advantage of palliative care or hospice services.

Patient Education and Health Maintenance

1. Instruct the patient and family on self-care measures for pancreatic insufficiency.
   a. Glucose monitoring, insulin administration, signs and symptoms of hypoglycemia and hyperglycemia.
   b. Pancreatic enzyme replacement; high-protein, high-carbohydrate diet.
2. Teach wound and drain care, as needed.
3. Explore options for pain management.
4. Coordinate referral for home care for any wound or drain care, new diabetic management, new medications, change in diet, or referral for palliative care or hospice services.

Evaluation: Expected Outcomes

- Verbalizes reduced pain.
- Weight stable.
- Vital signs stable; urine output adequate.
- Incision intact without drainage or bleeding.

SELECTED REFERENCES

Abraham, S., Rivero, H. G., Erlikh, I. V., et al. (2014). Surgical and nonsurgical management of gallstones. *American Family Physician, 89*(10), 795–802.

Adler, D. G., Lieb, J. G., Cohen, J., et al. (2015). Quality indicators for ERCP. *American Journal of Gastroenterology, 110*, 91–101.

American Cancer Society. (2017). *Cancer facts and figures 2017.* Atlanta, GA: Author.

ASGE Training Committee, Jorgensen, J., Kubiliun, N., et al. (2016). Endoscopic retrograde cholangiopancreatography (ERCP): Core curriculum. *Gastrointestinal Endoscopy, 83*, 279.

Balaban, E. P., Mangu, P. B., Khorana, A. A., et al. (2016). Locally advanced, unresectable pancreatic cancer: American Society of Clinical Oncology clinical practice guideline. *Journal of Clinical Oncology, 34*(22), 2654–2668.

Benner, P., & Kautz, D. (2015). Postoperative care of patients undergoing same-day laparoscopic cholecystectomy. *AORN Journal, 102*(1), 15–32.

Boyum, J. H., Atwell, T. D., Schmit, G. D., et al. (2016). Incidence and risk factors for adverse events related to image-guided liver biopsy. *Mayo Clinic Proceedings, 91*(3), 329–335.

Buch, P. (2016). What you need to know about chronic pancreatitis. *Gastroenterology Nursing, 39*(2), 145.

Chalasani, N. P., Hayashi, P. H., Bonkovsky, H. L., et al. (2014). ACG clinical guideline: The diagnosis and management of idiosyncratic drug-induced liver injury. *American Journal of Gastroenterology, 109*, 950–966.

Chinnakotla, S., Radosevich, D. M., Dunn, T. B., et al. (2014). Long-term outcomes of total pancreatectomy and islet auto transplantation for hereditary/genetic pancreatitis. *Journal of the American College of Surgeons, 218*(4), 530–543.

Costi, R., Gnocchi, A., Di Mario, F., & Sarli, L. (2014). Diagnosis and management of choledocholithiasis in the golden age of imaging, endoscopy and laparoscopy. *World Journal of Gastroenterology, 20*(37), 13382–13401.

Crockett, S. D., Wani, S., Gardner, T. B., et al. (2018). American Gastroenterological Association Institute guideline on initial management of acute pancreatitis. *Gastroenterology, 154*(4), 1096–1101.

Dick, J. F., Gardner, T. B., & Merrens, E. J. (2016). Acute pancreatitis: New developments and strategies for the hospitalist. *Journal of Hospital Medicine, 11*(10), 724–729.

Dohan, A., Guerrache, Y., Boudiaf, M., et al. (2014). Transjugular liver biopsy: Indications, technique and results. *Diagnostic and Interventional Imaging, 95*(1), 11–15.

Dugum, M., & McCullough, A. (2015). Diagnosis and management of alcoholic liver disease. *Journal of Clinical and Translational Hepatology, 3*(2), 109–116.

Eastern Association for the Study of the liver (2017). Clinical Practice Guidelines on the management of Hepatitis B virus infection. *Journal of Hepatology, 67,* 270–298.

Fan, J., Huang, T., Jane, S., & Chen, M. (2015). Prevention of liver cancer through the early detection of risk-related behavior among Hepatitis B or C carriers. *Cancer Nursing, 38*(3), 169–176.

Fontana, R. J., Ellerbe, C., Durkalski, V. E., et al.; for the US Acute Liver Failure Study Group. (2015). Two-year outcomes in initial survivors with acute liver failure: results from a prospective, multicentre study. *Liver International, 35*(2), 370–380.

Fragomeli, V., & Weltman, M. (2015). Addressing viral hepatitis in the opiate substitution setting: An integrated nursing model of care. *Journal of Hepatology and Gastroenterology, 30*(S2), 6–11.

Gargya, V., Smolarek, S., & Walsh, T. N. (2015). Concerns about acute cholecystitis: Early versus delayed cholecystectomy: A multicenter randomized trial. *Annals of Surgery, 262*(2), e63–e64.

Geng, X., Huang, R., Lin, J., et al. (2016). Transient elastography in clinical detection of liver cirrhosis: A systematic review and meta-analysis. *Saudi Journal of Gastroenterology, 22*(4), 294–303.

Greenberg, J. A., Hsu, J., Bawazeer, M., et al. (2016). Clinical practice guideline: management of acute pancreatitis. *Canadian Journal of Surgery, 59*(2), 128–140.

Gurusamy, K. (2016). Early laparoscopic cholecystectomy appears better than delayed laparoscopic cholecystectomy for patients with acute cholecystitis. *BMJ Evidence-Based Medicine, 21,* 28. Available: *http://ebm.bmj.com/content/21/1/28*

Hoyer, D. P., Munteanu, M., Canbay, A., et al. (2014). Liver transplantation for acute liver failure: Are there thresholds not to be crossed? *Transplant International, 27*(6), 625–633.

Jaffee, E. (Ed.). (2016). *Immunotherapy for pancreatic cancer.* New York: Cancer Research Institute. Available: *www.cancerresearch.org/we-are-cri/home/cancer-types/pancreatic-cancer*

Johnston, P. C., Lin, Y. K., Walsh, R. M., et al. (2014). Factors associated with islet yield and insulin independence after total pancreatectomy and islet cell autotransplantation in patients with chronic pancreatitis utilizing off-site islet isolation: Cleveland Clinic experience. *Journal of Clinical Endocrinology and Metabolism, 100*(5), 1765–1770.

Johnstone, C. C. (2016). An overview of the management of patients with chronic pancreatitis. *Nursing Standard, 31*(13), 54–63.

Kachaamy, T., Harrison, E., Pannala, R., et al. (2015). Measures of patient radiation exposure during endoscopic retrograde cholangiography: Beyond fluoroscopy time. *World Journal of Gastroenterology, 21*(6), 1900–1906.

Kesseli, S. J., Sith, K. A., & Gardner, T. B. (2015). Total pancreatectomy with islet autologous transplantation: The cure for chronic pancreatitis? *Clinical and Translational Gastroenterology, 6*(1), e73.

Khorana, A. A., Mangu, P. B., Berlin, J., et al. (2016). Potentially curable pancreatic cancer: American Society of Clinical Oncology clinical practice guideline. *Journal of Clinical Oncology, 34*(21), 2541–2556.

Kwo, P. Y., Cohen, S. M., & Lim, J. K. (2017). ACG clinical guideline: Evaluation of abnormal liver chemistries. *American Journal of Gastroenterology, 112*, 18–35.

Lo Re, V., Haynes, K., Forde, K. A., et al. (2015). Risk of acute liver failure in patients with drug-induced liver injury: Evaluation of Hy's law and a new prognostic model. *Clinical Gastroenterology and Hepatology, 13*(13), 2360–2368.

National Cancer Institute. (2016). Physician Data Query (PDQ) Cancer Information Summary. Available: *www.cancer.gov*

National Comprehensive Cancer Network Foundation. (2014). *NCCN Guidelines for patients: Pancreatic cancer.* Available: *www.nccn.org*

National Institute for Health and Care Excellence (NICE). (2016). *Cirrhosis in over 16s: Assessment and management.* NICE 2016 Jul: NG50 PDF.

Oettle, H., Riess, H., Stieler, J. M., et al. (2014). Second-line oxaliplatin, folinic acid, and fluorouracil versus folinic acid and fluorouracil alone for gemcitabine-refractory pancreatic cancer: Outcomes from the CONKO-003 trial. *Journal of Clinical Oncology, 32,* 2423–2429.

Peck-Radosavljevic, M. (2014). Drug therapy for advanced-stage liver cancer. *Liver Cancer, 3,* 125–131.

Rahib, L., Smith, B. D., Aizenberg, R., et al. (2014). Projecting cancer incidence and deaths to 2030: The unexpected burden of thyroid, liver, and pancreas cancers in the United States. *Cancer Research, 74,* 2913–2921.

Raigani, S., Ammori, J., Kim, J., & Hardacre, J. M. (2014). Trends in the treatment of resectable pancreatic adenocarcinoma. *Journal of Gastrointestinal Surgery, 18,* 113–123.

Randial Pérez, L. J., Fernando Parra, J., & Aldana Dimas, G. (2014). The safety of early laparoscopic cholecystectomy (<48 hours) for patients with mild gallstone pancreatitis: A systematic review of the literature and meta-analysis. *Cirugía Española, 92,* 107–113.

Roulin, D., Saadi, A., Di Mare, L., et al. (2016). Early versus delayed cholecystectomy for acute cholecystitis, are the 72 hours still the rule?: A randomized trial. *Annals of Surgery, 264*(5), 717–722.

Satter, N., Forrest, E., & Preiss, D. (2014). Non-alcoholic fatty liver disease. *BMJ, 349,* g4596.

Sherman, D. W., & McMilllan, S. C. (2015). The physical health of patients with advanced pancreatic cancer and the psychological health of their family caregivers when newly enrolled in hospice. *Journal of Hospice and Palliative Nursing, 17*(3), 235–241.

Shimada, H., Noie, T., Ohashi, M., et al. (2014). Clinical significance of serum tumor markers for gastric cancer: A systematic review of literature by the Task Force of the Japanese Gastric Cancer Association. *Gastric Cancer, 17*(26), 26–33.

Sohal, D. P., Mangu, P. B., Khorana, A. A., et al. (2016). Metastatic pancreatic cancer: American Society of Clinical Oncology clinical practice guideline. *Journal of Clinical Oncology, 34*(23), 2784–2796.

Stine, J. G., & Lewis, J. H. (2015). Current and future directions in the treatment and prevention of drug-induced liver injury: A systematic review. *Expert Review of Gastroenterology and Hepatology, 25,* 1–20.

Sun, V., Chung, V., Singh, G., Leong, L., Fakih, M., Fong, Y., & Ferrell, B. (2016). Pilot study of an interdisciplinary supportive care planning intervention in pancreatic cancer. *Supportive Care in Cancer, 24*(8), 3417–3424.

Sun, H., Ma, H., Hong, G., et al. (2014). Survival improvement in patients with pancreatic cancer by decade: A period analysis of the SEER database, 1981–2010. *Scientific Reports, 4,* 6747.

Tang, C., Von Ah, D., & Fulton, J. (2018). The symptom experience of patients with advanced pancreatic cancer: An integrative review. *Cancer Nursing, 41*(1), 33–44. Available: *http://journals.lww.com/cancernursingonline/toc/9000/00000*

Terrault N. A., Ghany M., Kang C., et al. for the Hepatitis B Research Network (HBRN). (2015). Seroprevalence and clinical features of hepatitis D virus (HDV) infection in a North American cohort. *Hepatology, 62,* 989A–990A.

Terrault, N. A., Lok, A. S. F., McMahon, B. J., & Chang, K. M. (2018). Update on prevention, diagnosis, and treatment of chronic hepatitis B: AASLD 2018 hepatitis B guidance. *Hepatology, 67*(4), 1560–1599.

Trepo, C., Chan, H. L. Y., & Lok, A. (2014). Hepatitis B virus infection. *The Lancet, 384*(9959), 2053–2063.

Tsai, H., Hsiehb, M., Tsaic, Y., et al. (2014). Liver function tests may be useful tools for advanced cancer patient care: A preliminary single-center result. *The Kaohsiung Journal of Medical Sciences, 30*(3), 146–152.

Tsochatzis, E. A., Bosch, J., & Burroughs, A. K. (2014). Liver cirrhosis. *Lancet, 383*(9930), 1749–1761.

Tulachan S. S., Bhagwatwala J., & Sridhar S. (2018). Endoscopic Management of Esophageal Varices and Variceal Hemorrhage. In: Sridhar S., Wu G. (Eds.), *Diagnostic and Therapeutic Procedures in Gastroenterology* (pp. 165–178). Clinical Gastroenterology. Totowa, N.J.: Humana Press.

Woreta, T. A., & Alqahtani, S. A. (2014). Evaluation of abnormal liver tests. *Medical Clinics of North America, 98*(1), 1–16.

Younossi, M., Bacon, B., Dieterich, D., et al. (2016). Disparate access to treatment regimens in chronic hepatitis C patients: Data from the TRIO network. *Journal of Viral Hepatitis, 23*(6), 447–454.

Yu, S. J. (2016). A concise review of updated guidelines regarding the management of hepatocellular carcinoma around the world: 2010–2016. *Clinical and Molecular Hepatology, 22*(1), 7–17.

Yu, Z., Wu, S., & Wan, G. (2016). Study on the nursing effect on complications of severe acute pancreatitis. *International Journal of Clinical and Experimental Medicine, 9*(2), 5228–5232.

Zheng, J., Kuk, D., Gönen, M. et al. (2017). Actual 10-Year survivors after resection of hepatocellular carcinoma. *Ann Surg Oncol, 24*(5), 1358–1366.

20
Nutritional Problems

OVERVIEW AND ASSESSMENT

 See additional online content: Procedure Guidelines 20-1–20-3

Nutrition Overview

Knowledge of nutrients and the basic principles of nutrition is important in the role of patient teaching for disease prevention and health promotion. The principles also help to provide an understanding and background to diseases affected by a person's nutritional status. The basic food groups and their placement on a plate help to serve as a guide to basic, healthy nutrition.

Key Principles

1. Nutrients, including carbohydrates, fats, proteins, vitamins, and minerals, have specific functions within the body. They work together to provide energy, regulate metabolic processes, and synthesize tissues.
2. Nutrition influences all body systems favorably and unfavorably. Examples of unfavorable effects include the link between cholesterol and heart disease or salt intake and high blood pressure (BP). Favorable effects are many, such as the association of fiber intake with improved GI function and the role of folic acid in preventing neural tube defects.
3. Nutritional needs vary in response to metabolic changes, age, sex, growth periods, stress (trauma, disease, pregnancy, lactation), and physical condition.
4. Nutritional supplements may be needed depending on disease states, dietary intake, and other factors.
5. The types of foods eaten and eating patterns are developed during a lifetime and are determined by psychosocial, cultural, religious, and economic influences.
6. The nurse works with the registered dietitian to promote optimum nutrition for each patient.

MyPlate and the Dietary Guidelines for Americans

1. Dietary guidelines were first developed in 1958 and were based on four basic food groups: grains, vegetables and fruits, meat, and milk. In 2010, the Department of Health and Human Services and U.S. Department of Agriculture (USDA) Dietary Guidelines for Americans were restructured and divided the four basic food groups into five food groups, which now consist of grains, fruits, vegetables, protein, and dairy. Although the guidelines have been reformatted, it still holds true that a well-balanced diet consists of foods from each of these groups and is composed of foods low in fat, cholesterol, and sodium and high in fiber (*www.dietaryguidelines. gov*). See Chapter 3, page 23, for more specific information about the guidelines.
2. In response to growing scientific knowledge regarding the linkage of diet and disease, the USDA developed the MyPlate Plan (see Figure 20-1). It reflects making food choices for a healthy lifestyle and includes basic information on how to build a healthy plate by cutting back on foods high in solid fats, added sugars, and salt; eating the right amount of calories; and being physically active. Additionally, the 2015–2020 *Dietary Guidelines* have added five overarching Guidelines to encourage healthy eating patterns such that individuals can enjoy foods that meet their personal, cultural, and traditional preferences and fit within their budget:
   a. Follow a healthy eating pattern across the life span.
   b. Focus on variety, nutrient density, and amount.
   c. Limit calories from added sugars and saturated fats and reduce sodium intake.
   d. Shift to healthier food and beverage choices.
   e. Support healthy eating patterns for all.

Nutritional Assessment

Nutrition assessment is an ongoing process designed to identify a person's nutritional status and the significance on the person's well-being. Although there are many methods and tools for assessing nutritional status, there is no universal method or "gold standard." Weight loss is perhaps the most validated parameter of nutritional status. However, multiple factors must be evaluated and considered to determine risk for or degree of malnutrition. One such factor is determining nutritional intake.

There are many methods to assess the nutritional status including the type and amount of food consumed. Techniques to capture nutritional intake may include a 24-hour recall of foods eaten, a food diary kept by the patient for several days, or a food frequency questionnaire that reflects food-intake patterns. In addition to these specific tools, the following information is useful to determine nutritional patterns and status.

Figure 20-1. MyPlate illustrates healthy eating. (U.S. Department of Agriculture.)

Key History Points

1. General background information—name, age, sex, family composition, socioeconomic status, occupation.
2. General health status and any chronic conditions, including diabetes and associated dietary restrictions as well as any hospitalizations.
3. Cultural and religious factors influencing dietary patterns.
4. Family history of diseases, including diabetes and obesity.
5. Current medications, over-the-counter products, and herbal supplements.
6. Food habits.
   a. Typical daily intake, including meal frequency, meal timing, and meal location.
   b. Snacking patterns.
   c. Food intolerance or dislikes.
   d. Nutritional supplements, including vitamins, minerals, fortified beverages, and foods.
   e. Alcohol consumption.
   f. Use of specific diets or dietary restrictions.
7. Food purchase and preparation.
   a. Who purchases and prepares food and where food is purchased.
   b. Facilities for food storage and preparation.
   c. Factors influencing the types of food purchased.
8. Nutritionally related problems.
   a. General well-being, energy level.
   b. Changes in appetite.
   c. Weight change during the past 6 months.
   d. Difficulty chewing or swallowing, use of dentures.
   e. Change in sense of taste or smell.
   f. Eructation, flatulence, nausea, vomiting, diarrhea, constipation, or abdominal pain or swelling in relation to food intake.
   g. Bowel habits.

Physical Examination and Anthropometrics

1. Perform a systematic physical examination, observing for a wide variety of physical findings associated with nutritional status.
   a. Listlessness, apathy.
   b. Cognitive and sensory deficits.
   c. Poor muscle tone or wasting of muscle.
   d. Dull, brittle hair; hair may be thin or sparse, easily plucked.
   e. Rough, dry, and scaly skin or dermatitis.
   f. Ecchymosis.
   g. Premature whitening of hair.
   h. Cheilosis (fissures at angles of mouth).
   i. Stomatitis (inflammation of mouth).
   j. Inflammation and easy bleeding of gums.
   k. Glossitis (inflammation of tongue).
   l. Dental caries and poor dentition.
   m. Spoon-shaped, brittle, ridged nails.
   n. Skeletal deformities such as bowlegs.
2. Perform anthropometry, as indicated. (Anthropometry comes from the word *anthropology* and is the science that studies the size, weight, and proportions of the human body to determine body fat mass, lean mass, and nutritional status.) Types of anthropometric measurements include height and weight, skin-fold thickness, and circumferential tests.
3. Height and weight are determined on patient admission and are later used as a baseline for comparisons in nutritional status.
   a. Height should be measured with a stadiometer.
   b. Weight should be measured using a consistent and reliable scale and at a consistent time, standing with shoes and overgarments removed.
   c. Unintended weight loss of more than 10% of body weight during 6 months is considered clinically significant and may be associated with physiologic abnormalities and increased morbidity and mortality.
4. Body mass index (BMI) is weight in kilograms divided by height in meters squared (see Table 20-1).
   a. BMI of less than 18.5 is classified as underweight.
   b. BMI of 18.5 to 24.9 is classified as normal weight.
   c. BMI of 25 to 29.9 is classified as overweight.
   d. BMI of 30 to 39.9 is classified as obese.
   e. BMI greater than 40 is classified as extremely obese.
5. Metabolism is generally faster in younger people, and for this reason, babies and children have higher energy requirement needs than do adults. Requirement needs are based on many

Table 20-1	Body Mass Index (BMI)*					
WEIGHT	5'	5'3"	5'6"	5'9"	6'	6'3"
140	27	25	23	21	19	18
150	29	27	24	22	20	19
160	31	28	26	24	22	20
170	33	30	28	25	23	21
180	35	32	29	27	25	23
190	37	34	31	28	26	24
200	39	36	32	30	27	25
210	41	37	34	31	29	26
220	43	39	36	33	30	28
230	45	41	37	34	31	29
240	47	43	39	36	33	30
250	49	44	40	37	34	31

*Body mass index = weight (kg)/height (m²).

Figure 20-2. Anthropometric measurements. **(A and A1)** Marking the midpoint of the upper arm. **(B)** Obtaining the mid–upper arm circumference. **(C)** Measuring triceps skin-fold thickness.

factors including age, gender, activity level, and disease state. Exact measurements of caloric requirements for infants can be obtained by using charts; these estimate the body surface area by height and weight and the standard basal metabolic rate for a given weight (see Appendix B, page 1502).

6. Skin-fold thickness provides an estimate of body fat based on the amount of fat in subcutaneous tissue using calibrated calipers to measure the thickness of the skin at designated sites (see Figure 20-2).
    a. Grasp skin and subcutaneous fat, pulling it away from the underlying muscle, and place the caliper jaws over the skin-fold flap.
    b. Take the reading within 2 to 3 seconds and without using excessive pressure.
    c. Repeat the reading twice and take an average of the three readings to increase accuracy.
7. Skin-fold sites include the following:
    a. Vertical measurements:
        i. Triceps: On the posterior midline of the upper arm, midpoint between the acromion and olecranon processes.
        ii. Abdomen: Two cm to the right of the umbilicus.
        iii. Thigh: On the anterior midline of the thigh, midway between the proximal border of the patella the inguinal crease (hip).
    b. Diagonal measurements:
        i. Subscapular: Just below the inferior border of the left scapula.
        ii. Chest/Pectoral: One half the distance between the anterior axillary line and the nipple (in men); or one third the distance between the anterior axillary line and the nipple (in women).
        iii. Suprailiac: In line with the natural angle of the iliac crest taken in the anterior axillary line immediately superior to the iliac crest.
8. Circumferential tests provide information on the amount of skeletal muscle and adipose tissue. Mid-upper arm circumference (MAC)—an indirect estimate of the body's muscle mass:
    a. Place a tape measure around the midpoint of the nondominant upper arm and secure it snugly.
    b. To calculate, multiply the triceps skin fold by 3.14 and subtract the product from the MAC.
    c. Adult standards are 16.5 mm for women and 12.5 mm for men.

9. Advanced body composition analysis is a set of advanced techniques that provide various measurements including total body fat, muscle mass percentages, bone weight, and visceral adipose tissue (VAT) score among other measurements of body composition. Methods may include the following:
    a. Dual-energy X-ray absorptiometry (DEXA).
    b. Underwater (hydrostatic) weighing.
    c. Air displacement plethysmography (ADP).
    d. Bioelectrical impedance analysis (BIA).

Laboratory Tests

1. Serum albumin, prealbumin.
    a. Albumin is a protein made by the liver and is responsible for maintaining blood volume and serum electrolyte balance. The half-life of albumin is about 21 days. A decrease in nutritional status may result in a drop in albumin synthesis. However, in chronic malnutrition, serum albumin levels are typically normal or high.
    b. Prealbumin is also made by the liver and is a more sensitive but expensive test that measures more recent nutritional status. Its half-life is 2 to 3 days.
2. Hemoglobin—made by the liver; decreased amounts are related to iron deficiency anemia or other defect in hemoglobin synthesis or dilution of the blood such as during pregnancy.
3. Serum transferrin—another transport protein made by the liver; responsible for binding iron to plasma and transporting it to the bone marrow. Reduced levels are found in catabolic states and some chronic diseases.
4. Twenty-four-hour urine creatinine—an increase in this measure indicates increased tissue breakdown.
5. Twenty-four-hour urine urea nitrogen or total urinary nitrogen—this test can be used to determine nitrogen balance.

 NURSING ALERT Serum albumin, prealbumin, and transferrin levels measure visceral proteins that inversely correlate with metabolic stress, such as inadequate nutrition, but do not directly measure nutritional status.

GENERAL PROCEDURES AND TREATMENT MODALITIES

The inability to take nutrients through the oral route either totally or in part may require alternative means to enhance and maintain nutritional status. Alternative methods of nutritional support include enteral feeding and parental nutrition. The decision as to which method is used will depend on many factors including the patient's acuity and nutritional status.

Enteral Feeding

Administration of nutrients directly into the stomach, duodenum, or jejunum through a tube is more physiologically beneficial and cost-effective than is parenteral feeding. Enteral feeding carries less risk of infection than does parenteral feeding and maintains a functional GI tract by preventing mucosal atrophy and biliary and hepatic dysfunction. Enteral therapy is appropriate for patients with at least a minimally functional GI tract who cannot take adequate nutrition by mouth.

Enteral therapy has become utilized more frequently as more commercially available enteral formulas have been developed and long-term enteral feeding tubes have become safer and more easily inserted.

Clinical Indications

1. Increased metabolic needs and inability to take adequate oral diet—trauma, burns, cancer, sepsis.
2. Coma or mechanical ventilation.
3. Head/neck surgery.
4. Malabsorption.
5. Obstruction of esophagus or oropharynx.
6. Severe anorexia nervosa.
7. Dysphagia.

Sites of Tube Insertion

Short-Term Nutritional Support (<30 days)

1. Nasogastric (NG) feeding—tubes are passed through the nose or mouth (orogastric) into the stomach and secured in place.
   a. Tube placement must be verified by x-ray before use. Aspiration of contents for pH or auscultation of air injected through tube has been shown to be of limited value. New techniques that are available include colorimetric carbon dioxide detectors and electronic capnographics, both of which measure end-tidal carbon dioxide to determine if the tube has gone into the trachea.
   b. If there is a question about tube placement in the respiratory tract, the tube should be removed.
2. Nasoenteric feeding (ie, nasoduodenal or nasojejunal)—tube is passed through the nose into duodenum or jejunum and secured in place. X-ray is usually needed to verify correct tube placement.

Long-Term Nutritional Support (>30 days)

1. Gastrostomy—insertion of a tube surgically, radiologically, or by a percutaneous endoscopic procedure into the stomach.
2. Gastrostomy button—small device inserted through gastrostomy stoma to allow for long-term feeding with minimal effect on body image.
3. Jejunostomy—insertion of a tube directly into the jejunum either surgically or by a percutaneous endoscopic procedure. Jejunostomy feedings are generally by continuous infusion using a feeding pump.

Types of Tubes

1. Large-bore NG polyurethane tube—size 12 to 18F, used very short term (eg, Salem Sump).
2. Small-bore NG tube—made of polyurethane, silicone, or polyvinyl chloride with a tungsten-weighted tip or non-weighted tip, size 8 to 12F and 30 to 36 inches (76 to 91.5 cm) long.

3. Nasointestinal tube—made of silicone, polyurethane, or polyvinyl chloride with a tungsten-weighted tip or nonweighted tip, size 8 to 12F and 40 to 60 inches (101.5 to 152.5 cm) long.
4. Gastrostomy tube—catheter made of silicone, polyurethane, polyvinyl chloride, or latex; a balloon on the distal end to stabilize tube may be used and ranges from 5 to 30 mL capacity, size 14 to 28F. Adults usually have 20F tubes, and children usually start with 14F.
5. Gastrostomy button—silicone; ranging from 18 to 28F and 1 inch (2.5 cm) long; useful for person wanting minimal alteration in body image.
6. Jejunostomy tube—size ranging from 5 to 14F with or without a balloon (a balloon may obstruct lumen of jejunum). A plain red rubber catheter is occasionally used as a short-term jejunostomy tube, and some gastrostomy tubes may be used for jejunostomy.

Delivery Systems for Feeding Solution

1. Intermittent or continuous infusion of feeding solution by gravity is accomplished by hanging container of feeding solution from an intravenous (IV) pole and adjusting delivery rate by a flow regulator.
2. Continuous feeding by controller feeding pump allows uniform flow, particularly of viscous solutions.
3. Bolus feeding involves enteral formula poured into barrel of a large (60 mL) syringe attached to a feeding tube and allowed to infuse by gravity.

 NURSING ALERT Bolus feeding may precipitate dumping syndrome, particularly if given into the small intestine. Dumping syndrome occurs when hyperosmolar substances enter the intestine quickly, causing an influx of water into the GI tract that can result in nausea, vomiting, bloating, cramping, and diarrhea. Dumping syndrome may also cause dizziness, nervousness, and nausea.

Community and Home Care Considerations

Teach patient and family:
1. Technique for administration of tube feeding (intermittent, continuous, bolus).
2. Signs and symptoms of potential complications.
3. Need to assess tube placement and residual before each feeding (for gastric feedings only).
4. Principles of medical asepsis, including careful hand washing, refrigeration of formula, cleaning of equipment with soap and water, and thorough drying between feedings.
5. When the gastrostomy or jejunostomy tube insertion site is well healed, surrounding skin can be cleaned with soap and water.
6. Gauze dressing can be applied, as needed.
7. Leakage around tube or signs of peristomal skin irritation should be reported.

Complications

See Table 20-2.

Parenteral Nutrition

Parenteral nutrition is the introduction of nutrients, including amino acids, lipids, dextrose, vitamins, minerals, and water, through a venous access device (VAD) directly into the intravascular fluid to provide nutrients required for metabolic functioning of the body.

Table 20-2 Complications of Enteral Feeding and Treatment

COMPLICATIONS	CAUSES	INTERVENTIONS
Tube displacement	Tube migration into the esophagus	• Observe for eructation of air when injecting air to test for tube placement in the stomach. • Aspirate gastric contents; if none is obtained, suspect esophageal placement.
	Tube placement into the respiratory tract	• Observe for gagging, dyspnea, inability to speak, coughing when tube insertion attempted. • Obtain chest x-ray.* • Withdraw tube and attempt reinsertion with the patient's head flexed forward.*
Tube obstruction	Tube kinking	• Obtain chest x-ray to confirm and withdraw and reinsert new tube.*
	Tube clogging	• Flush tube every 4 hr with 30 mL of water and after administration of intermittent feeding and medication administration. • Administer medications in liquid form if possible. Crush medications finely (if crushable). • Attempt to declog by administering water first. If unsuccessful, then administer pancreatic enzyme/bicarbonate mixture.
Aspiration	Patient lying flat	• Elevate HOB 30 to 45 degrees during continuous feedings or for 30 to 60 min after bolus feeds.
	Absent or depressed gag reflex	• Elevate HOB 30 to 45 degrees during continuous feedings or for 30 to 60 min after bolus feeds.
	Reflux	• Elevate HOB 30 to 45 degrees during continuous feedings or for 30 to 60 min after bolus feeds. • Administer proton pump inhibitor per provider orders.
	Improper tube placement	• Confirm proper placement with x-ray imaging. • Tape tube in place.
Vomiting	Tube migration into the esophagus	• See interventions for tube displacement above.
	Decreased absorption	• Auscultate for decreased bowel sounds, observe for abdominal distention. • Consider decreasing amount of tube feeding.* • Consider administration on a continuous basis.* • Consider placement of a small-bore, weighted-tip nasointestinal tube.*
	Rapid rate of infusion	• Administer no faster than 200 to 300 mL during 10 to 20 min. • Consider administration on a continuous basis.*
	Excessive infusion of air	• If giving a bolus feeding, pinch tubing off when refilling syringe with formula. • If giving continuous feeding, make certain bag does not empty before closing off tubing.
	Patient position	• Maintain the patient at 30- to 45-degree angle of head elevation during and 30 to 60 min after feeding. If administering continuous feeding, maintain head elevation at all times.
	Nausea	• Antiemetics.
	Obstruction	• Assess for distention and decreased bowel sounds; obtain x-ray.
	Constipation	• Assess for impaction and review frequency of bowel movements.
Diarrhea	Drug therapy	• Evaluate drug regimen for possible causes of drug-induced diarrhea from antibiotics, elixirs with high osmolarity, elixirs with sorbitol, magnesium-containing antacids.
	High osmolarity of formula	• Begin administration of formula at slow rate.* • Consider continuous feeding rather than intermittent.*
	Lactose intolerance	• Administer lactose-free formula. (Few commercial formulas contain lactose.)
	Bacterial contamination of formula	• Change administration set daily or per facility protocol. • Maintain strict medical asepsis, including careful hand washing before administration of formula. • Allow formula to hang no longer than 8 hr (unless it is a "ready-to-hang" container that can hang for 24 to 48 hr).
	Rapid infusion rate	• Administer slowly; consider continuous rather than intermittent infusion.*
	Fecal impaction	• Manually clear the impaction.
	Clostridium difficile	• Administer antibiotics.

(continued)

Table 20-2 Complications of Enteral Feeding and Treatment (*Continued*)

COMPLICATIONS	CAUSES	INTERVENTIONS
Constipation	Lack of fiber	• Ensure that the patient is not impacted and administer formula with fiber.*
	Decreased fluid intake	• Increase intake of water.*
	Drug therapy	• Evaluate drug regimen for possible cause, including aluminum-containing antacids or lack of stool softener.
Hyperglycemia	Diabetes, impaired metabolism	• Monitor serum glucose, assess for dehydration caused by hyperosmotic diuresis; observe for symptoms of hyperglycemia, including polyuria, polydipsia. • Administer insulin.* • Observe for hypercapnia (increased respirations, elevated P_{CO_2}).
Hypernatremia	Dehydration	• Assess for signs and symptoms of dehydration (I&O, daily weight, skin turgor, blood urea nitrogen, CVP, tachycardia, hypotension). • Rehydrate with extra water via the feeding tube or, if the patient is severely hypernatremic, use IV route. • Rehydrate with D5W or hypotonic saline solutions.*
Hyponatremia	Overhydration, excessive sodium loss (diaphoresis, nasogastric suction)	• Observe for signs and symptoms of hypervolemia (shortness of breath, rales, I&O, daily weight, peripheral edema, elevated CVP). • Observe for signs and symptoms of hyponatremia (lethargy, headaches, mental status change, nausea, vomiting, abdominal cramping). • Replace sodium, administer diuretics, or, depending on the cause of hypernatremia, restrict fluids.*
Hyperkalemia	Metabolic acidosis/renal insufficiency	• Observe for signs and symptoms of hyperkalemia (dysrhythmias, nausea, diarrhea, muscle weakness). • Treat underlying cause. • Administer exchange resin, glucose, and insulin.* • Choose lower potassium formula.
Hypokalemia	Diarrhea, refeeding syndrome	• See interventions for diarrhea. • If severe, replace potassium.*

*Obtain orders from health care provider.
CVP, central venous pressure; H_2, histamine; HOB, head of bed; I&O, intake & output.

Clinical Indications

1. Patient cannot tolerate enteral nutrition because of:
   a. Paralytic ileus.
   b. Intestinal obstruction.
   c. Acute pancreatitis and enteral feedings not possible.
   d. Severe malabsorption.
   e. Persistent vomiting and jejunal route not possible.
   f. Enterocutaneous fistula and enteric feeding not possible.
   g. Inflammatory bowel disease.
   h. Short-bowel syndrome.
2. Hypermetabolic states for which enteral therapy is either not possible or inadequate, such as burns, trauma, or sepsis.
3. In these situations, additional components are added to the enteral therapy, or individualized solutions are developed to meet the nutritional needs of the patient.

Methods of Parenteral Nutrition

Total Nutrient Admixture

1. Given through a central vein, commonly into the superior vena cava, total nutrient admixture (TNA) is a parenteral formula that combines carbohydrates in the form of a concentrated (20% to 70%) dextrose solution; proteins in the form of amino acids (3% to 15%); lipids in the form of an emulsion (10% to 30%), including triglycerides, egg phospholipids, glycerol, and water; and vitamins and minerals.

2. Central TNA is indicated for patients requiring parenteral feeding for 7 or more days.

Peripheral Parenteral Nutrition

1. Given through a peripheral vein, this parenteral formula combines a less concentrated dextrose solution with amino acids, vitamins, minerals, and lipids.
2. Unlike TNA given centrally, peripheral parenteral nutrition provides fewer calories and, occasionally, a larger percentage of calories is supplied by lipids rather than by carbohydrates.
3. Indicated for patients requiring parenteral nutrition for fewer than 7 days who do not already have enteral access.

Total Parenteral Nutrition

1. Total parenteral nutrition (TPN) combines dextrose, amino acids, vitamins, and minerals and is given through a central IV line.
2. If lipids are needed, they are given intermittently or mixed with the TPN solution through a central IV line.

Fat Emulsion (Lipids)

1. Ten percent, twenty percent, or thirty percent emulsion composed of triglycerides, egg phospholipids, glycerol, and water. It also contains vitamin K.
2. May be given centrally or peripherally.

Complications

See Table 20-3 on page 571.

Table 20-3 Complications of Total Parenteral Nutrition and Treatment

COMPLICATIONS	CAUSES	INTERVENTIONS
Sepsis	• High glucose content of fluid • Venous access device contamination	• Monitor temperature, white blood cell count, insertion site for signs and symptoms of infection. • Maintain strict surgical asepsis when changing dressing and tubing. • Consider removal of venous access device with replacement in alternate site.* • If blood cultures positive, consider institution of antibiotic therapy.*
Electrolyte imbalance	• Iatrogenic • Effect of underlying diseases (ie, fistula, diarrhea, vomiting) • Blood sample contaminated by parenteral nutrition	• Monitor electrolyte levels at least daily initially. • Monitor signs and symptoms of electrolyte imbalance. • Treat underlying cause.* • Change concentration of electrolytes in total parenteral nutrition (TPN) as necessary to address blood levels.*
Hyperglycemia	• Insufficient insulin secretion • High glucose content of fluid • Blood sample contaminated by parenteral nutrition	• Monitor blood glucose frequently. • Administer exogenous insulin per addition to TPN, subcutaneously or through a separate IV drip.* • Decrease glucose content of fluid if warranted.*
Hypoglycemia	• Abrupt discontinuation of parenteral nutrition administered through a central vessel	• Reduce rate of parenteral nutrition by 50% × 2 hr, then discontinue. • If TPN/peripheral parenteral nutrition must be stopped abruptly, hang a separate dextrose solution if insulin has been administered.
Hypervolemia	• Iatrogenic • Underlying disease (ie, heart failure, renal failure)	• Monitor intake and output, daily weights, central venous pressure (CVP), breath sounds, peripheral edema. • Consider administering more concentrated solution.*
Hyperosmolar diuresis	• High osmolarity of parenteral nutrition	• Monitor intake and output, daily weights, CVP. • Consider decreasing concentration or increasing amount of fluid administered.*
Hepatic dysfunction	• IV nutrition	• Monitor liver function tests, triglyceride levels, presence of jaundice. • Consider alteration in macronutrients.*
Hypercapnia	• Excessive calorie delivery	• Consider reducing total calories.*
Lipid intolerance	• Low birth weight or premature neonate • History of liver disease • History of elevated triglycerides	• Monitor for bleeding (check stools for occult blood, coagulation studies, platelet levels). • Monitor oxygen levels for impaired oxygenation. • Monitor for fat overload syndrome: monitor triglyceride levels and liver function tests, hepatosplenomegaly, decreased coagulation, cyanosis, dyspnea. • Monitor allergic reaction: nausea, vomiting, headache, chest pain, back pain, fever. • Administer lipid-containing solutions slowly initially, while observing for symptoms.
Lipid particulate aggregation	• Unstable mixture of dextrose solution with lipid emulsion	• Observe for cracking or creaming of fluid and discontinue use of fluid with these characteristics.

Obtain orders from health care provider.

Delivery Systems for Parenteral Nutrition

1. Central VADs:
   a. Insertion of long-term VADs, such as Hickman, Broviac, or Groshong catheters.
   b. Peripherally inserted central catheters (peripherally inserted central catheter lines) may be used.
   c. Multilumen, central VADs can allow concomitant administration of TNA and other solutions, including medications or blood, each running through a separate lumen.
2. Peripheral IV access:
   a. Insertion of an angiocatheter into a vein in the arm or leg.
   b. Midline catheters of longer length and with the ability to remain in place for more than 3 days.
3. Delivery of parenteral nutrition should be controlled by a volume control infuser.
4. Filters should be used whenever possible.
   a. A 0.22-micron filter may be used for TPN (without added fat emulsion).
   b. A 1.2-micron filter may be used for TNA or fat emulsion.

Nursing Interventions and Patient Education

1. Use strict sterile technique to attach IV tubing (with filter) to parenteral nutrition bag, purge air, make sure all clamps are closed, and then close clamp on VAD before attaching IV tubing to VAD. If central VAD is being used, have the patient bear down and hold breath to perform the Valsalva maneuver, which prevents air from being sucked into tubing.
2. Regulate flow and monitor administration hourly for patient tolerance and development of complications.

3. Change central VAD dressing according to facility protocol, maintaining sterility.
   a. The patient should be in supine position with head turned away from dressing.
   b. Clean the skin first with alcohol, then povidone iodine, starting at the insertion site and moving outward in a circular pattern.
   c. Apply a transparent dressing over the insertion site when skin is thoroughly dry.
   d. Loop and tape tubing outside of dressing.

NUTRITIONAL DISORDERS

Nutritional disorders can have a negative impact on the health and well-being of a person. In addition, some nutritional disorders may in turn lead to the development of other diseases or health issues. If not identified and treated in a timely fashion, these disorders can have a devastating effect.

Obesity

Obesity is a local, national, and global epidemic that impacts all ages, races, and socioeconomic classes and both genders. *Obesity* is an overabundance of body fat and is typically measured by a person's BMI (weight in kilograms divided by height in meters squared). A BMI greater than 30 is considered obese. Obesity has become a global health issue affecting both rich and poor countries. Current global estimates find that nearly 500 million adults are obese, with a projected increase to 1 billion obese adults by 2030. According to the Centers for Disease Control, the prevalence of obesity among US adults was 36.5% during the time period 2011–2014, with an overall higher incidence noted among women (38.3%) as compared to men (34.3%). During the same time period, there was a 17% prevalence rate among youth ages 2 to 19 years.

 EVIDENCE BASE Ogden, C. L., Carroll, M. D., Fryar, C. D., & Flegal, K. M. (2015). Prevalence of obesity among adults and youths, United States 2011–2014. *NHCS Data Brief*, (219), 1–8.

Pathophysiology and Etiology

Increasing evidence reveals that obesity is a multifactorial disease and may be the result of several different factors. Such factors may include the following:

1. Heredity and genetic factors.
   a. Identical twins raised separately are more likely to have similar amounts of body fat than are fraternal twins raised separately.
   b. Genetic defects in certain disorders such as Bardet-Biedl syndrome and Prader-Willi syndrome can directly cause obesity.
2. Environmental factors.
   a. Some evidence shows that children reared by parents with obesity have an increased tendency toward obesity.
   b. Increased availability of high-fat, high-calorie foods.
   c. Reduction in physical activity.
   d. Modern-day conveniences (ie, riding lawnmowers, escalators, elevators, etc.).
3. Psychological factors.
   a. Depression.
   b. Anxiety.
   c. Anger.
   d. Posttraumatic stress.
   e. Boredom.

4. Physiologic factors.
   a. Endocrine abnormalities (rare causes of obesity)—Cushing syndrome, polycystic ovary syndrome, hypothyroidism, hypogonadism, or hypothalamic lesions.
   b. Age—advancing age may be associated with obesity, usually due to changes in activity level and metabolic rate, or in women because of hormonal changes; early childhood and the start of puberty may also be associated with obesity.
5. Pharmacologic factors.
   a. Corticosteroids.
   b. Antidepressants.
   c. Hormones and other medications.

Clinical Manifestations

1. BMI greater than 30, depending on body composition.
2. Increased weight is correlated with increased incidence of comorbid conditions.
   a. Cardiovascular disease.
   b. Type 2 diabetes mellitus.
   c. Hypertension.
   d. Obstructive sleep apnea.
   e. Osteoarthritis.
   f. Gastroesophageal reflux disease.
   g. Gallbladder disease.
   h. Cancer of the breast, endometrium, prostate, and colon.
   i. Stroke.
   j. Dyslipidemia.
   k. Stress urinary incontinence.
   l. Infertility.
   m. Depression (may be a cause of obesity as well as caused by obesity).
3. Metabolic syndrome (insulin resistance syndrome)—a group of characteristics that when co-occuring increase the risk of coronary artery disease, stroke, and type 2 diabetes.
   a. Obesity.
   b. Hypertension.
   c. Insulin resistance.
   d. High triglycerides.

Diagnostic Evaluation

1. Nutritional assessment—a systematic method for obtaining, verifying, and interpreting data needed to identify nutrition-related problems and their causes and significance.
2. Anthropometric and physical assessment—to evaluate increased body fat and effects of obesity on body.
3. Selected hormonal studies (thyroid, adrenal)—to assess for potential underlying cause.

Management

Conservative Measures

1. Diet therapy—has been controversial, but a well-balanced diet containing all the major food groups is still advised and recommended as a first-step therapy.
   a. A 1,000-calorie deficit per day is required to lose 2.2 pounds (1 kg) of body weight per week.
   b. Diet therapy should be individualized to the patient; however, the overall goal is to create a calorie deficit through reduced calorie intake or increased calorie expenditure.
   c. A balance of food groups is essential to maintain vitamin and nutrient balance. Nutrient supplementation may be necessary (calcium, vitamin D, iron, B_{12}, zinc, and folate).

d. Food preparation should include seasoning with herbs, onion, garlic, and pepper, and foods should be baked, broiled, steamed, or sautéed using minimal oil.

e. Food attractively arranged on smaller plates, using whole rather than processed foods and eaten slowly, will assist the overall process.

f. Eliminating entire food groups from the diet, such as carbohydrates (in many popular protein- and fat-based diets), will eventually result in craving of those foods eliminated, disruption of normal metabolic processes, and quick weight gain when the food is added to the diet.

2. Exercise—Regular physical activity is an important component in weight loss and weight maintenance along with reduced caloric intake. The most recent recommendations from the American College of Sports Medicine (2011) are to incorporate moderate aerobic physical activity to include a minimum of 150 minutes per week and goal of 300 minutes per week, including strength training 2 to 3 times per week. Physical activity may also add other health benefits if done on a regular basis such as improved cardiovascular status and emotional well-being.

 EVIDENCE BASE Garber, C. E., Blissmer, B., Deschenes, M., et al. (2011). Quantity and quality of exercise for developing and maintaining cardiorespiratory, musculoskeletal, and neuromotor fitness in apparently healthy adults: Guidance for prescribing exercise. *Medicine and Science in Sports and Exercise, 43*(7), 1334–1359.

3. Behavior modification is a cornerstone of any successful diet.
a. Identify and eliminate situations or cues leading to overeating or high-calorie foods with use of a food diary.
b. Provide positive reinforcement of proper dietary habits.
c. Should a lapse in diet habits occur, focus on a prompt and positive return to appropriate dietary habits.
d. Stress-reduction techniques, such as visual imagery or progressive muscle relaxation; peer support may be helpful.

Pharmacotherapy

1. Anorexia medications include amphetamines, sympathomimetics, and norepinephrine-releasing agents or reuptake inhibitors; reduce appetite and stimulate weight loss initially.
a. However, tolerance may develop and weight may be regained when the drugs are discontinued.
b. Numerous long-term studies have failed to show long-term success with these agents.

2. Phentermine products are available in prescription form and primarily act on chemicals in the brain to decrease appetite. Phentermine products also have a stimulant component and should not be used in uncontrolled hypertension, advanced heart disease, history of drug abuse, or with monoamine oxidase (MAO) inhibitors.

3. Phentermine–topiramate extended release is an FDA-approved drug available in prescription form. This drug combines the effects of phentermine with the weight loss effects of topiramate (a medication used to treat seizures).

4. Naltrexone hydrochloride and bupropion hydrochloride, branded as Contrave, is a combination of two medications, naltrexone (used to treat narcotic and alcohol dependency) and bupropion (an antidepressant), to help decrease appetite and control eating.

5. Liraglutide was FDA approved in 2014 and is an injectable medication used for the management of diabetes. Liraglutide decreases the production of glucagon, which in turn slows down the emptying of the stomach. It also works in the brain to reduce the amount of food consumed.

6. Lorcaserin is a serotonin 2C receptor agonist that works on chemicals in the brain to decrease appetite. It is available in short and long acting forms.

7. Orlistat, a pancreatic lipase inhibitor, blocks the breakdown of fat in the GI system; about 30% of dietary fat is eliminated.
a. Adverse effects include oily or fatty stool, flatulence, and GI distress.
b. Long-term safety of the drug has not been determined, but addition of a fat-soluble vitamin supplement (vitamins A, D, E, and K and beta carotene) taken 1 hour before or 2 hours after orlistat will prevent a theoretical vitamin deficiency.
c. Should not be used in cases of cholestasis or malabsorption.
d. Orlistat is available over the counter in a lower dosage than originally prescribed.
e. These medications are only adjunct to diet and exercise therapy.

8. Several other medications used to treat depression, seizures, and/or diabetes have been prescribed off-label to help promote weight loss. These medications have not been approved by the FDA for the treatment of obesity:
a. Bupropion—an antidepressant medication.
b. Topiramate—an anticonvulsant medication.
c. Zonisamide—an anticonvulsant medication.
d. Metformin—an oral medication used to treat diabetes.

9. Sibutramine is no longer available in the United States because of studies that identified an increased risk of developing cardiovascular events such as heart attack or stroke.

Metabolic and Bariatric Surgery

Numerous surgical procedures have been used to help treat obesity and metabolic disorders. Although gastric bypass has been considered the gold standard for years, many new surgical treatment options have emerged, lending to a greater availability of treatment options (see Figure 20-3). These surgical therapies are generally reserved for patients with severe obesity (i.e., BMI > 35 with comorbid conditions or BMI > 40) who cannot lose weight and maintain weight loss through the above therapies. Bariatric surgery has proven to be a safe and effective means for weight loss when performed by an experienced surgeon within a multidisciplinary center. In addition to the anatomical and mechanical changes created by the various procedures, there is increasing evidence of metabolic or hormonal changes that lead to weight loss. Metabolic/hormonal changes associated with these surgeries include a decrease in the hormone ghrelin, which produces a decrease in hunger, and an increase in PYY and GLP-1 creating an increase in satiety.

1. Roux-en-Y gastric bypass—a restrictive and malabsorptive procedure in which a small 1- to 2-ounce pouch/stomach (normal size = 30 to 50 ounces) is created by stapling and completely separating the smaller proximal stomach pouch from the larger distal stomach pouch. To this proximal pouch, a portion of the jejunum or Roux limb is attached, thus bypassing the distal stomach pouch and allowing the new pouch to empty food contents into the bowel. The biliopancreatic limb is then anastomosed to the Roux limb, thus creating a "Y" configuration and a method of elimination of digestive juices from the distal stomach and duodenum.

2. Adjustable gastric banding—a silicone band or "belt" is placed at the gastroesophageal junction, creating a small upper segment of the stomach. An access port or reservoir, which is connected to the band by tubing, is placed midabdomen just under the skin, which allows for band adjustments to create a narrower passage into the larger remaining stomach. This in turn slows the emptying process from the upper segment into the lower segment of the stomach thus causing satiety with a smaller amount of food. Hormonal changes with this surgery initially increase ghrelin production, which increases hunger.

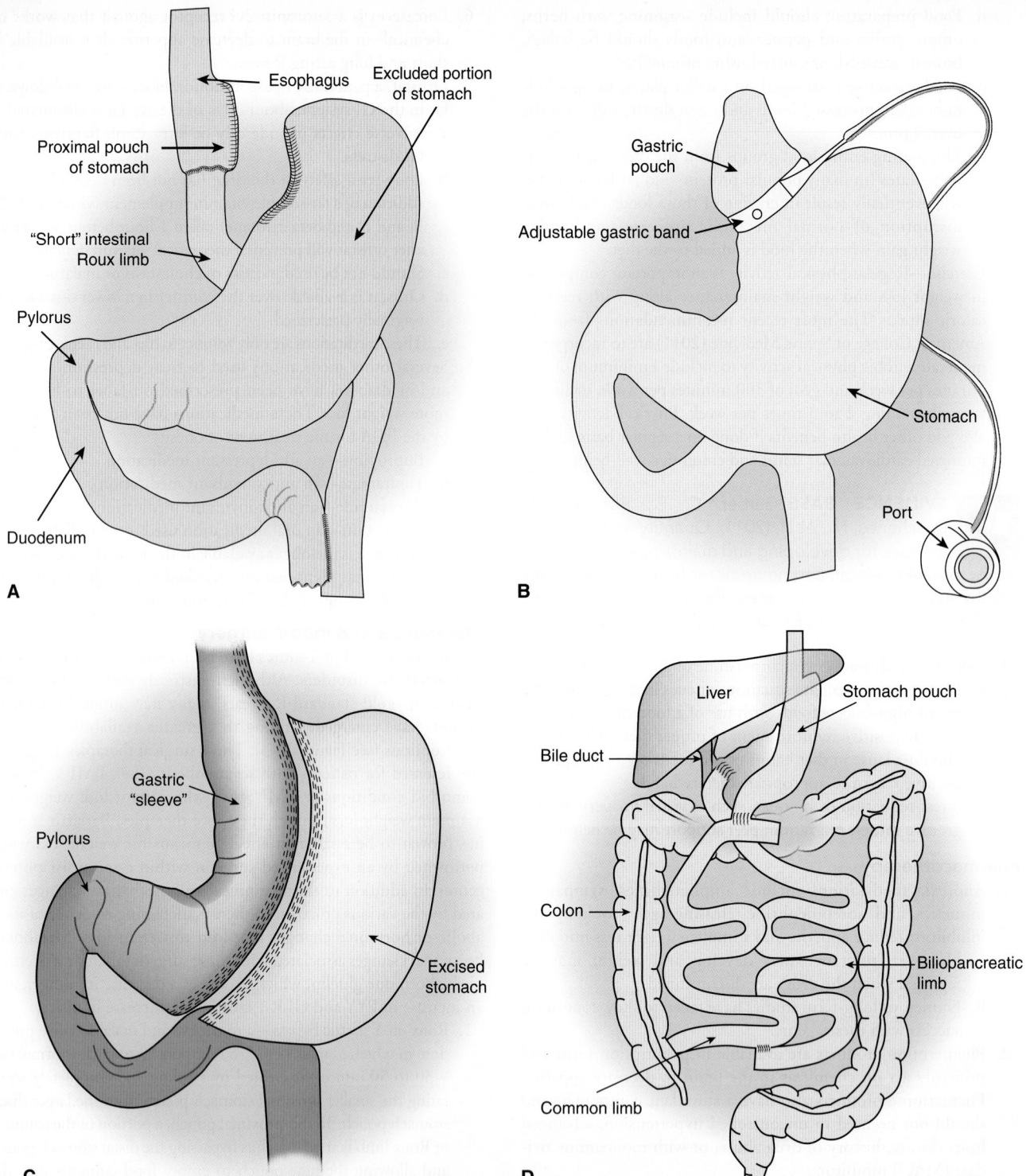

Figure 20-3. Bariatric procedures. **(A)** Adjustable gastric band. **(B)** Gastric bypass with Roux-en-Y anastomosis. **(C)** Sleeve gastrectomy. **(D)** Biliopancreatic diversion with duodenal switch.

3. Sleeve gastrectomy—a restrictive procedure in which a "sleeve" is created by stapling the stomach into a long tube from the esophagus to the duodenum. The remnant stomach is removed, whereas the pylorus remains intact and allows for normal emptying of stomach contents.

4. Biliopancreatic diversion with duodenal switch (BPD/DS)—a primarily malabsorptive procedure with some restrictive qualities. The BPD/DS is a complex surgical procedure in which

a partial gastrectomy is performed along with the division and rerouting of the small intestine (ie, duodenum—hence duodenal switch). This inhibits the absorption of calories and some nutrients, but allows for normal absorption of other key nutrients such as protein, calcium, iron, and vitamin B_{12}. In contrast to the gastric bypass, the BPD/DS maintains the pyloric valve, which prevents complications such as dumping syndrome, marginal ulcers, and/or stomal stenosis from occurring.

5. Other—there are several investigational procedures for severe obesity on the horizon that may add viable options for weight loss in the future but are not recognized as of yet.

Medical Devices

1. vBloc Neuromodulation is a medical device implanted surgically on the lower stomach. The device functions by blocking the vagus nerve and hence creating a sensation of fullness and decreased hunger. vBloc is currently approved by the FDA for a BMI 40 to 45 or 35 to 39.9 with comorbid conditions.
2. Intragastric balloons are available as single or double balloons that are inserted endoscopically into the stomach for no longer than 6 months. The balloon(s) mimic a sleeve gastrectomy by filling a portion of the stomach to reinforce proper portion control and a sensation of fullness. Both single (Orbera) and double (ReShape Dual Balloon) balloons are FDA approved but are not typically covered by insurance. Prior history of metabolic and bariatric surgery may be a contraindication for these products.
3. AspireAssist is an FDA-approved endoluminal device in which a modified PEG tube is placed endoscopically into the stomach and then connected to a small handheld device. The device is activated approximately 20 to 30 minutes postprandial by a discreet button enabling the emptying of up to 30% of the meal into the toilet. The AspireAssist is for patients with a BMI 35 to 55.

Complications

1. Obesity is a risk factor for many comorbid conditions including diabetes, gallbladder disease, osteoarthritis of weight-bearing joints, hypertension, CAD, obstructive sleep apnea, metabolic syndrome, as well as several other conditions.
2. Vitamin and mineral deficiencies because of surgical intervention, severely restricted diet, or noncompliance with recommended regimen.
   a. A moderate, well-balanced weight reduction diet will generally not cause deficiencies, although a multiple vitamin/mineral supplement may be used.
   b. A low-calorie diet (fewer than 800 to 1,000 calories per day) will require careful monitoring and vitamin/mineral supplements.
   c. Complications of bariatric surgery may include marginal ulcers, anastomotic leaks, fistulas, infection, pulmonary emboli, chronic nausea and vomiting, vitamin D and B_{12} deficiency, thiamine, copper, and iron deficiency. A daily vitamin and mineral supplement is necessary.

Nursing Assessment

1. Obtain a complete nutritional assessment (may be in collaboration with a registered dietitian).
2. Assess behavioral and emotional components of eating, coping mechanisms, and past successes and failures with dieting.

Nursing Diagnoses

- Imbalanced Nutrition: More Than Body Requirements related to high-calorie, high-fat diet, and limited exercise.
- Deficient Fluid Volume related to weight loss surgery.
- Readiness for Enhanced Self-Concept related to appearance and weight.

Nursing Interventions

Modifying Nutritional Intake

1. Assist the patient in assessing current dietary habits and identifying poor dietary habits.
2. Assist the patient in developing appropriate diet plan based on likes and dislikes, activity level, and lifestyle.
3. Suggest behavior modification strategies, such as exercise (ie, walking) during lunch break, preventing access to quick snacks, eating only at mealtimes at the table.
4. Provide emotional support to the patient during weight-reduction efforts through positive reinforcement and creative problem solving.
5. Provide the patient with alternative coping mechanisms, including stress-reduction techniques such as progressive relaxation and guided imagery.
6. Assess the patient's ability to tolerate exercise through measurement of vital signs before, during, and after exercise and ask about symptoms of shortness of breath and chest pain.
7. Discourage fad dieting.

Preventing Complications Postoperatively

1. Provide initial postoperative care as for gastrointestinal surgery (see page 494).
2. Administer IV fluids, as directed. Record intake and output.
3. Start oral fluids per surgeon's protocol (this will vary from facility to facility and surgeon to surgeon). General progression for most patients will be to start with small sips and gradually advance to larger sips of clear liquids.
4. Advance diet as per surgeon's protocol. Confirmation of the bariatric diet stages with the facility's bariatric program and/or surgeon is crucial, as this will vary from facility to facility and surgeon to surgeon.
5. Observe for and report increased abdominal pain, distention, or alteration in abdominal drain output (if utilized), which may indicate leakage or bleeding at anastomosis or staple sites or obstruction.
6. Monitor vital signs, breath sounds, and wounds for signs of infection, pneumonia or other potential complications.
7. Watch for and report signs of dehydration (thirst, oliguria, dry mucous membranes) and hypokalemia (muscle weakness, anorexia, nausea, decreased bowel sounds, and dysrhythmias).
8. Warn the patient that overeating may cause vomiting or painful esophageal distention. Dumping syndrome may occur especially in the postoperative roux-en-y gastric bypass patient with food products that are high in fat or high in sugar.
9. Stress the importance of good dietary habits and behavior modification to lose weight because metabolic and bariatric surgery is only an adjunct to treatment.
10. Encourage close, long-term follow-up for monitoring of weight loss and nutritional status. Additional long-term complications may include marginal ulcers, hernias, strictures, and/or malnutrition.

TRANSITIONAL CARE ALERT Following bariatric surgery, educate the patient on the importance of strict adherence to diet protocol and to avoid premature advancement to the another stage without discussing with the surgeon, dietitian, or other staff member. Encourage the patient to meet fluid (48 to 64 oz fluid/day) and protein (individualized) goals. Advise the patient to notify the surgeon for fever (greater than 101°F); tachycardia (heart rate greater than 100); severe abdominal pain; nausea or vomiting; difficulty breathing or ability to catch breath; or any redness, drainage, or swelling from incisions. Prevention and prompt attention to signs of complications can prevent readmission and adverse outcomes.

Strengthening Self-Concept

1. Direct patient education and conversation in a nonjudgmental manner.
2. Get to know the patient and point out the positive aspects of patient's health and well-being.
3. Encourage the patient to make change in weight for the positive health aspects, not just for cosmetic reasons.
4. Make referral to behavioral health professional and support groups as needed.
5. Be a good role model—show a healthy attitude toward sensible eating, exercise, and other healthy practices.
6. Be sensitive to discrimination, behaviors, and attitudes toward people with obesity.

Patient Education and Health Maintenance

1. Discuss fat, carbohydrate, and protein, their inclusion in common foods, and their calories per gram.
2. Describe the five basic food groups and their placement in the MyPlate plan.
3. Explain the purpose of a balanced diet and the need for vitamins and minerals from food sources; supplement needed following bariatric surgery.
4. Review the health hazards of obesity.
5. Advise the patient of plateau period that may occur without weight loss for some time, but advise the patient not to get discouraged.
6. Tell the patient to keep a food diary to show to nutritionist and to weigh self no more than once per week.
7. If the patient is interested in liquid diets or herbal supplements to lose weight, encourage discussion with health care provider. Some preparations may contain ephedra, a powerful stimulant that may cause increased BP, significant adverse effects, and many drug interactions.
8. Refer to such organizations as Obesity Action Coalition (*www. obesityaction.org*) and the National Institutes of Diabetes and Digestive and Kidney Disease: Weight-control Information Network (*http://win.niddk.nih.gov/publications/gastric.htm*) for further information on weight loss options.

Evaluation: Expected Outcomes

- Loses 10% to 15% excess body weight during the first month.
- No abdominal distention, nausea or vomiting, or wound infection.
- Verbalizes feeling good about self, secondary to change in diet and exercise habits.

Eating Disorders

Disordered eating can run the full gamut from starvation as noted in anorexia nervosa, to overeating behaviors such as binge-eating disorder—or may include a combination of both as seen in bulimia nervosa. Eating disorders can affect both genders but are generally more prevalent among women than among men. Lifetime prevalence is estimated at 0.3% for anorexia, 0.9% for bulimia, and 1.6% for binge-eating disorder. The disordered eating may develop during childhood or later in life, but is more common during teens or young adulthood, and may be chronic or intermittent during many years. There are multiple causes that may be attributable to the eating disorder including genetic, biological, hormonal, environmental, behavioral, psychological, and social etiologies. See Table 20-4 on page 577 for comparison of the three most common eating disorders.

Although this section focuses on anorexia nervosa, bulimia nervosa, and binge-eating disorder, there are other disordered or maladaptive eating behaviors, including pica, orthorexia, and Prader-Willi Syndrome. Pica is a disorder of eating objects with no nutritional value, such as dirt, paper, or ice. Orthorexia is the unhealthy obsession of consuming healthy foods. Prader-Willi Syndrome is a genetic disorder that produces hormonal symptoms such as a constant hunger, leading to obesity. Another category of eating disorders on the rise is OSFED or other specified feeding or eating disorder and includes subtypes such as atypical anorexia nervosa, purging disorder, and night eating syndrome.

Diagnostic Evaluation

1. Serum chemistry for electrolytes, blood urea nitrogen (BUN), and creatinine and bicarbonate—may be abnormal, indicating fluid and electrolyte imbalances.
2. Hormonal tests may include thyroid function tests, luteinizing hormone (LH), follicle-stimulating hormone (FSH), estrogen, and testosterone.
3. Serum glucose and lipid testing to determine body's response to dietary intake.
4. Electrocardiogram to determine arrhythmias caused by electrolyte imbalance.

Management

Although pathophysiology, etiology, and symptoms may differ somewhat between each eating disorder, the assessment, diagnosis, and treatment and therapies are very similar. Paramount to the entire process, however, is the multidisciplinary clinical approach that should include nurses, nutritionists, behavioral health providers, advanced practice providers, physicians, and other health care providers who specialize in treating patients with eating disorders.

1. Dietary modification and nutritional counseling to achieve gradual weight gain and/or normal eating habits.
   a. Balanced diet with incremental inclusion of foods previously perceived as restricted by the patient.
   b. Increased activity, exercise gradually.
2. Enteral or parenteral feeding as needed if prescribed diet cannot be maintained by the patient and physical status warrants. Enteral feeding is preferred and is used more frequently.
3. Individual counseling focuses on patient's need to control weight, alteration in body image, and associated diagnoses, including depression and suicidal ideation.
4. Psychological counseling and support, such as talk therapy or behavioral therapy.
   a. Assist the patient to develop insight into behavior and a more realistic body image.
   b. Assist the patient to develop effective coping strategies and problem-solving mechanisms.
5. Antidepressants, antianxiety, and other pharmacologic agents for associated psychiatric problems may be tried.
   a. Selective serotonin uptake inhibitor (SSRI) such as fluoxetine to treat bulimia nervosa.
   b. Stimulant such as lisdexamfetamine (Vyvanse) to treat binge-eating disorder.
6. Inpatient treatment (preferably on specialized eating disorder unit) is recommended if weight is less than 75% ideal; marked orthostatic hypotension; bradycardia less than 40; sustained tachycardia greater than 100; inability to maintain core body temperature of 98.6°F (37°C); suicidal or no response to outpatient therapy.

Table 20-4 Comparison of Eating Disorders

DISORDER/DESCRIPTION	PATHOPHYSIOLOGY/ETIOLOGY	CLINICAL MANIFESTATIONS
Anorexia nervosa: characterized by self-induced weight loss >15% of normal weight for age and height and is associated with high morbidity and mortality. Anorexia is characterized by periods of starvation and may be mixed with episodes of binging and purging.	• Semistarvation state with glucose and protein sparing, fat utilization, endocrine changes, and fluid and electrolyte disturbances. Results in: • Loss of fat stores • Decreased protein synthesis • Decrease in thyroid hormone • Hypothalamic or pituitary dysfunction—decrease in follicle-stimulating hormone (FSH), luteinizing hormone (LH), and estrogen	• Extremely restricted eating • Extreme thinness (emaciation) • Relentless pursuit of thinness and unwillingness to maintain a normal or health weight • Intense fear of gaining weight • Distorted body image, a self-esteem that is heavily influenced by perceptions of body weight and shape, or a denial of the seriousness of low body weight • Amenorrhea, bradycardia, hypotension, cold intolerance
Bulimia nervosa: characterized by recurrent episodes of binge eating and feeling of loss of control ever eating behavior during these episodes. The binging episodes lead to self-disgust and are typically followed by inappropriate methods to prevent weight gain, including self-induced vomiting, excessive use of laxatives, diuretics, fasting, or excessive exercise.	• Onset of illness typically occurs in late adolescence or early 20s • Ten times more common in young women than in young men • May be associated with a personal or family history of obesity, substance abuse, depression, anxiety, or mood disorders • Self-induced vomiting • Starvation may be as evident as in anorexia nervosa • Eating binges may occur as often as several timers per day and be present for many months	• Physical signs may include calluses or skin changes on hand and fingers, loss of dental enamel, swollen lymph nodes, and bad breath or mouthwash smell on breath because of self-induced vomiting • Endocrine changes, such as amenorrhea, may be present
Binge-eating disorder (BED): disordered eating that results in a loss-of-control eating episode(s). BED is not associated with inappropriate compensatory behaviors, however, is often associated with some type of psychopathology.	• Presence of comorbid psychopathology: specific phobia, social phobia, unipolar major depression, posttraumatic stress disorder, alcohol abuse, or dependence • Increased risk for developing chronic pain, diabetes mellitus, and hypertension • More likely to be obese • Binge episodes at least once a week for 3 mo	• Eating unusually large amounts of food in a specific amount of time • Eating even when full or not hungry • Eating fast during binge episodes • Eating until uncomfortably full • Eating alone or in secret to avoid embarrassment • Feeling distressed, ashamed, or guilty about eating • Frequently dieting, possibly without weight loss

Complications

1. Fluid and electrolyte imbalance.
   a. Hypokalemia, hyponatremia, hypochloremia.
   b. Hyperkalemia.
   c. Metabolic alkalosis.
   d. Dehydration.
2. Cardiac disturbances.
   a. Dysrhythmias, bradycardia, tachycardia.
   b. Hypotension.
   c. Cardiac arrest.
3. Nutritional imbalance.
   a. Obesity.
   b. Cachexia.
4. Seizures due to hyponatremia.
5. Increased risk of infection related to a decrease in white blood cells.
6. Endocrine dysfunction.
   a. Amenorrhea, decreased estrogen in females.
   b. Decreased testosterone in males, decreased libido.
   c. Decreased thyroid hormone.
7. Esophageal tear or gastric rupture.
8. Dental erosion.
9. Comorbid psychiatric conditions.
   a. Depression.
   b. Anxiety disorders.
   c. High risk for suicide.

Nursing Assessment

1. Perform a complete nutritional assessment. Obtain a detailed dietary history and complete review of systems, including psychological, gynecologic, endocrine, GI systems, activities of daily living, and exercise history.
2. Perform physical examination, including vital signs, height and weight, heart rate and rhythm, bowel sounds, and observation for hematemesis and dental caries (which may indicate self-induced vomiting).
3. Evaluate fluid and electrolyte status and manifestations of associated problems.
4. Assess for signs and symptoms of depression, anxiety, personality disorder, and associated eating behaviors and history of family dysfunction.

Nursing Diagnoses

- Imbalanced Nutrition: More or Less Then Body Requirements related to binge/purge behavior and/or self-restricted intake.
- Disturbed Body Image related to weight.
- Ineffective Coping related to lack of control over eating habits.
- Risk for Suicide related to psychological distress.

Nursing Interventions

Attaining Appropriate Weight

1. Assist the patient to select well-balanced diet and maintain appropriate eating habits.
2. Encourage small, frequent meals or snacks of high-calorie foods and beverages. Liquid nutritional supplements may be best tolerated.
3. Monitor and assess daily intake and output, weight (before breakfast), urine for ketones, and serum electrolytes to determine physical response to nutritional interventions.
4. Provide positive reinforcement for appropriate eating behaviors.
5. Provide positive reinforcement for improved intake and weight gain or stabilization of weight.
6. Assess bowel function. Promote fluids and activity to prevent constipation if the patient cannot tolerate food high in fiber.
7. Teach the patient risks associated with abnormal eating behavior and the benefits of maintaining healthful nutritional and exercise habits.

Fostering a Healthy Body Image

1. Establish a trusting relationship and provide for patient's safety and security needs.
2. Encourage the patient to verbalize feelings about body image, self-concept, fears, and frustrations.
3. Emphasize the importance of counseling, stress management, assertiveness training, and other therapies over a long term to strengthen body image and acceptance.

Improving Coping

1. Encourage the patient to set realistic goals for weight and appearance. Involve the patient in treatment plan, offering choices to increase sense of control.
2. Assist the patient to identify and implement alternative coping strategies in times of stress, including expression and exploration of feelings, problem solving, appropriate use of exercise, and relaxation techniques.
3. Set limits so that the patient will fell in control of self. Be alert for lying and manipulation that the patient may display to preserve control.
4. Include family in counseling and teaching sessions, as appropriate.

Preventing Suicide

1. Assess level of risk by obtaining the history of past suicide attempts, recent suicidal thoughts, and current ideation, plan, and possible method.
2. Maintain level of observance called for by situation.
3. Make sure that access to sharp objects is prohibited.
4. Make sure that a crisis intervention team is on call, if needed.

Patient Education and Health Maintenance

1. Teach principles of nutrition and healthful diet and eating habits. Discuss food matter-of-factly to avoid reinforcing patient's preoccupation with food.
2. Teach the effect of starvation on both physiologic and psychological functioning.

3. Involve patient's family and significant others in the treatment plan, as appropriate.
4. Describe the dangers of using laxatives and diuretics in weight control, such as electrolyte imbalances, dehydration, and bowel atony.
5. Stress the importance of maintaining follow-up visits and counseling.
6. Refer to such agencies as American Anorexia-Bulimia Association (*www.aaba.org*), Eating Disorder Information Center (*www.nedic.ca*), Eating Disorders Awareness and Prevention (*www.edap.org*), National Association of Anorexia Nervosa and Associated Disorders (*www.anad.org*), and National Eating Disorder Association (*www.nationaleatingdisorders.org*).

Evaluation: Expected Outcomes

- Well-balanced dietary intake without evidence of vomiting. Gain of 1 pound (0.5 kg) during first week (anorexia nervosa).
- Verbalizes satisfaction with body image and weight.
- Verbalizes appropriate problem-solving approach.
- Denies suicidal ideation and thoughts.

Malabsorption Syndrome

Malabsorption syndrome is a group of symptoms and physical signs that occur because of poor nutrient absorption in the small intestine, particularly fat absorption, with a resultant decrease in absorption of fat-soluble vitamins A, D, E, and K. Poor absorption of other nutrients, including carbohydrates, minerals, and other vitamins and proteins, may also occur. *Celiac sprue*, and *lactose intolerance* are common types of malabsorption syndromes.

Pathophysiology and Etiology

Malabsorption has multiple etiologies, including gallbladder, liver, or pancreatic disease, lymphatic obstruction, vascular impairment, and bowel resection. Two common causes:

1. Celiac sprue—malabsorption of nutrients resulting from atrophy of villi and microvilli of the small intestine because of an intolerance to gluten found in common grains, such as wheat, rye, oats, and barley (see Chapter 48).
2. Lactose intolerance—typically of genetic origin, this digestive enzyme deficiency prevents the digestion of lactose found in milk, causing osmosis of water into the lumen of the intestine.

Clinical Manifestations

1. Steatorrhea.
2. Abdominal distention and pain.
3. Flatulence.
4. Anorexia, weight loss, edema.
5. Vitamin deficiency—fat soluble (A, D, E, K).
6. Protein deficiency and negative nitrogen balance.
7. Anemia, weakness, and fatigue due to poor absorption of iron, folic acid, and vitamin B_{12}.

Diagnostic Evaluation

1. Fecal fat analysis—72-hour stool collection; fecal fat may be increased.
2. M2A Imaging System—a device that provides images via a receiver and recorder tracing the transit of a capsule that is

swallowed by the patient. Used to evaluate and diagnose malabsorption syndromes as well as other gastrointestinal diseases.
3. Lower GI series (barium enema)—may be used to evaluate the colon.
4. Serum measurement of vitamin levels, total protein, and albumin may be decreased.
5. Prothrombin time may be prolonged because of vitamin K deficiency.

Management

1. Treatment of the underlying cause, if possible, by eliminating causative agents, such as grains or milk.
2. Promotion of adequate nutritional intake through a carefully designed diet that substitutes alternatives to the offending agent and that ensures replacement of deficient nutrients through oral, enteral, or parenteral therapy.
3. Medications such as pancreatic enzymes.

Complications

1. Dehydration.
2. Electrolyte imbalance with possible cardiac dysrhythmias.
3. Protein deficiency with muscle atrophy and edema.
4. Vitamin deficiency with tetany, bleeding, anemia, and osteoporosis.
5. Skin breakdown.

Nursing Assessment

1. Assess fluid and electrolyte status through careful monitoring of intake and output, daily weight, serum electrolytes, vital signs, and other signs and symptoms of dehydration and electrolyte imbalance.
2. Assess GI function through observation of frequency and characteristics of stool, bowel sounds, and distention, pain, and other associated symptoms.
3. Assess nutritional status.

Nursing Diagnoses

- Imbalanced Nutrition: Less Than Body Requirements related to malabsorption of nutrients.
- Deficient Fluid Volume related to loss of fluid through stool.
- Acute Pain related to abdominal distention and cramps.
- Risk for Impaired Skin Integrity related to irritation of anal area by stool.

Nursing Interventions

Improving Nutritional Status

1. Ensure that diet is free from causative agents, such as dairy or wheat products.
2. Provide diet high in missing nutrients, including proteins, carbohydrates, fats, vitamins, and minerals.
3. Teach the patient to use substitute products for causative agents, such as gluten-free flour, corn, soybean, and lactose-free milk substitutes.
4. Monitor weight and characteristics of stool closely.

Restoring Fluid Balance

1. Monitor intake and output and urine-specific gravity.
   a. Include watery stool in output.
   b. Be aware that edema is caused by low serum proteins, not fluid overload.

2. Monitor vital signs frequently, based on condition.
3. Be alert for dehydration—orthostatic hypotension, tachycardia, decreased skin turgor, dry mucous membranes, thirst, oliguria.
4. Observe for signs and symptoms of potential electrolyte disturbances—nausea, vomiting, dysrhythmias, tremors, seizures, anorexia, weakness—and report abnormal results of serum electrolytes.
5. Administer IV fluids or parenteral or enteral nutrition, as ordered.

Relieving Pain

1. Assess timing, frequency, and character of pain and its relationship to food.
2. Encourage Fowler position and frequent change in position for comfort.
3. Administer analgesics, antidiarrheals, and antiflatulents, as ordered.

Maintaining Tissue Integrity

1. Provide meticulous perineal care after each stool with application of hydrophobic ointments, if necessary, to prevent skin breakdown.
2. Give careful attention to general skin condition, assessing for redness, breakdown, and poor turgor, and maintain general skin integrity through cleanliness, lubrication, padding of bony prominences, frequent turning, and adequate hydration and nutrition.

Patient Education and Health Maintenance

1. Provide nutritional counseling for the patient and family, particularly if symptoms are secondary to food intolerance; stress which foods to avoid and the importance of carefully reading all food labels, recommend appropriate food substitutions, and necessary nutritional supplements.
2. Advise regarding signs and symptoms that indicate worsening of disease—increased frequency of stool, diarrhea or steatorrhea, increased pain.
3. Suggest such support groups as the Celiac Sprue Association (*www.csaceliacs.org*) and the Crohn's and Colitis Foundation of America (*www.ccfa.org*).

Evaluation: Expected Outcomes

- Maintains weight and energy level.
- Vital signs stable; urinary output adequate.
- Verbalizes decreased pain after meals.
- No skin breakdown noted.

Vitamin and Mineral Deficiencies

Vitamins are organic compounds found in food needed for growth, reproduction, good health, and resistance to infection. Minerals are inorganic compounds found in nature and serve a variety of physiologic functions. Specific requirements depend on age, activity, metabolic rate (increased fever), and special processes, such as pregnancy, lactation, and disease processes.

See Table 20-5 on pages 580 to 585 for vitamin and mineral needs for healthy adults age 19 or older. Needs are different for children and pregnant or lactating women.

Dietary reference intake tables have been developed by the Food and Nutrition Board at the Institute of Medicine of the National Academies and include the following:

Table 20-5 Vitamin and Mineral Requirements and Imbalances

VITAMIN, RDA, AND EAR	FUNCTION	CLINICAL MANIFESTATIONS OF IMBALANCE
Vitamin A (Retinol) RDA: 700–900 mcg EAR: 500–625 mcg fat soluble	• Tissue maintenance via antioxidant ability • Helps regulate the immune system • Skeletal and soft tissue growth and development • Visual adaptation to light and dark • Supports reproductive function	*Deficiency:* Night blindness, xerophthalmia, keratinization, generalized mucosa dryness/damage, vomiting, diarrhea, weight loss, urinary and vaginal infections, tooth decay, follicular hyperkeratosis, fatigue *Toxicity:* Hair loss, joint pain, dry skin, mouth soreness, anorexia, vomiting, liver damage
Vitamin B_1 (Thiamine) RDA: 1.1–1.2 mg EAR: 0.9–1.0 mg water soluble	• Carbohydrate metabolism • Necessary for neurologic, gastric, cardiac, and musculoskeletal function	*Deficiency:* Appetite loss, constipation, dyspnea, fatigue, irritability, nervousness, memory loss, paresthesias, muscle pain, beriberi, blurred or double vision, difficulty swallowing, nausea, vomiting *Toxicity:* Large doses may be given generally without difficulty, although anaphylaxis has been reported
Vitamin B_2 (Riboflavin) RDA: 1.1–1.3 mg EAR: 0.9–1.1 mg water soluble	• Carbohydrate metabolism • Promotes growth, red blood cell formation, and healthy eyes and skin	*Deficiency:* Sore throat, cheilosis, dermatitis, burning and itching of eyes, tearing and vascularization of corneas; late-stage symptoms include neuropathy and growth retardation *Toxicity:* None known
Vitamin B_6 (Pyridoxine) RDA: 1.3–1.7 mg EAR: 1.1–1.4 mg water soluble	• Required for protein metabolism • Maintains neurologic function and RBC production	*Deficiency:* Anemia, weakness, glossitis, cheilosis, irritability, seizures *Toxicity:* Neuromuscular damage, peripheral neuropathy
Vitamin B_{12} (Cobalamin) RDA: 2.4 mcg EAR: 2.0 mcg water soluble	• Maintains neurologic function and RBC development via hemoglobin synthesis	*Deficiency:* Megaloblastic anemia, memory impairment, confusion, depression, fatigue, nervousness, decreased reflex response, balance impairment, speech difficulties, demyelination of the large fibers of the spinal cord, anorexia, vomiting, weight loss, yellowing of skin, abdominal pain, dyspnea, diarrhea, glossitis, burning of lips or mouth, palpitations, tachycardia, sore tongue, weakness *Toxicity:* None
Biotin RDA: 30 mcg EAR: Not established water soluble	• Metabolism of proteins, fats, and carbohydrates	*Deficiency:* Dry skin, fatigue, grayish skin discoloration, muscle pain, depression, insomnia, anorexia *Toxicity:* None
Folate (Folic Acid) RDA: 400 mcg EAR: 320 mcg water soluble	• RBC formation • DNA and RNA synthesis and support of cell growth and reproduction • Prevention of birth defects	*Deficiency:* Glossitis, diarrhea, megaloblastic anemia, digestive problems, fatigue, palpitations, restless leg syndrome *Toxicity:* Inactivation of anticonvulsants, masking of vitamin B_{12} deficiency
Niacin RDA: 14–16 mg EAR: 11–12 mg water soluble	• Metabolism of carbohydrates, fats, and proteins • Works with thiamine and riboflavin for the production of cellular energy • Promotes skin, neurologic, and GI function	*Deficiency:* Apathy, fatigue, appetite loss, headaches, indigestion, muscle weakness, nausea, insomnia, dermatitis, diarrhea, confusion, disorientation, memory impairment, glossitis, stomatitis, pellagra *Toxicity:* Liver damage, flushing
Pantothenic Acid RDA: 5 mg EAR: Not established water soluble	• Vital for overall metabolism • Aids in formation of carbohydrates, proteins, and fats • Aids in cortisone production, ATP production, stress tolerance, vitamin utilization, hemoglobin synthesis	*Deficiency:* Diarrhea, hair loss, respiratory infections, nervousness, muscle cramps, premature aging, intestinal disorders, eczema, kidney disorders *Toxicity:* None
Vitamin C RDA: 75–90 mg EAR: 60–75 mg water soluble	• Antioxidant action decreases cellular dysfunction • Promotes wound healing • Aids in connective tissue, bone, tooth, and cartilage formation • Promotes capillary integrity • Promotes nonheme iron absorption	*Deficiency:* Bleeding gums, tooth decay, nosebleeds, low infection resistance, bruising, anemia, delayed wound healing, anorexia, joint pain, lethargy, perifollicular hemorrhage *Toxicity:* GI distress

DIAGNOSTIC EVALUATION	MANAGEMENT
Deficiency: • History and physical findings are helpful in diagnosis of most vitamin imbalances • Serum level <35 mg/dL suggests vitamin deficiency	*Deficiency:* • Replacement therapy of 30,000 international units to treat night blindness. • Good dietary sources of vitamin A are green and yellow fruits and vegetables and liver • In patients with malabsorption of fat-soluble vitamins and patients with low dietary intake of vitamin A, IV supplements are required
Deficiency: • Erythrocyte transketolase activity <15% to 20%	*Deficiency:* • Treat underlying cause • High-protein diet with supplemental B complex vitamins • Food sources rich in thiamine are brewer's yeast, meat, wheat germ, enriched grains and beans • Parenteral therapy with 50 to 100 mg/day followed by 5 to 10 mg/day PO
Deficiency: • Erythrocyte glutathione activity >1.2 to 1.3 • Decreased urinary riboflavin levels	*Deficiency:* • Good dietary sources of B_2 are dairy products, vegetables, enriched grains, eggs, nuts, liver • Oral supplements of 5 to 15 mg/day
Deficiency: • Pyridoxal phosphate levels <50 ng/mL	*Deficiency:* • Oral supplementation: 10 to 20 mg • Good dietary sources of B_6 are bananas, brewer's yeast, fish, meat, whole grains, liver. • Individuals taking oral contraceptives or isoniazid may need to supplement their diets with pyridoxine • Pregnancy also increases need
Deficiency: • Serum levels of <100 pg/mL • Decreased hematocrit with elevation of MCV • Schilling test also measures absorption of radioactive B_{12}	*Deficiency:* • B_{12} 200 mcg/day IM for 1 wk, then every month for life if deficiency is due to pernicious anemia • Oral vitamin B_{12} may be necessary for strict vegetarians • Good dietary sources of B_{12} are eggs, fish, organ meats, lean meat, dairy products
—	*Deficiency:* • Good sources of biotin are egg yolks, vegetables, yeast, milk, grains
Deficiency: • Serum level <3 ng/mL	*Deficiency:* • Nutritional supplementation: 1 mg/day PO • Avoid alcohol • Good sources of folate are citrus fruits, eggs, milk, green leafy vegetables, dairy products, organ meats, seafood, whole grains, yeast
Deficiency: • Serum levels <30 mcg/100 mL • Diminished or absent metabolites in urine	*Deficiency:* • Good sources of niacin are eggs, lean meats, organ meats, poultry, seafood, fish, dairy products, nuts, whole and enriched grains, brewer's yeast • Nutritional supplementation: 10 to 150 mg • Supplemental niacin may also be necessary when taking oral contraceptives
—	*Deficiency:* • This vitamin is widely available in foods, especially organ meats, legumes, vegetables, fruits
Deficiency: • Serum levels <0.2 mg/100 dL	*Deficiency:* • Nutritional supplementation: 100 to 1,000 mg/day of vitamin C • Good sources of vitamin C are citrus fruits, green leafy vegetables, broccoli, tomatoes, peppers, potatoes, strawberries • Avoid smoking

(continued)

Table 20-5 Vitamin and Mineral Requirements and Imbalances (*Continued*)

VITAMIN, RDA, AND EAR	FUNCTION	CLINICAL MANIFESTATIONS OF IMBALANCE
Vitamin D RDA: 15 mcg EAR: 10 mcg fat soluble	• Regulates calcium and phosphate absorption and metabolism and bone formation • Aids in renal phosphate clearance, myocardial function, nervous system maintenance, and normal blood clotting	*Deficiency:* Rickets, osteomalacia, weakness, spasm/twitching of eyes, burning in mouth, sweating *Toxicity:* Hypercalcemia, bone pain, nausea, vomiting, itching, thirst, agitation, weakness. Calcifications in soft tissue can be fatal
Vitamin E (Tocopherol) RDA: 15 mg EAR: 12 mg fat soluble	• Antioxidant action decreases cellular dysfunction • Aids in RBC formation	*Deficiency:* Neuromuscular disturbances, including decreased reflexes, vibratory and position sense, ataxia, night blindness, fatigue, leg weakness or cramps, dry skin *Toxicity:* Iinterference with vitamin K
Vitamin K RDA: 90–120 mcg EAR: Not established fat soluble	• Promotes coagulation through the formation of prothrombin and other clotting factors	*Deficiency:* Abnormal bleeding times, hemorrhage, epistaxis, hematemesis, and bleeding at any orifice or puncture site are possible *Toxicity:* No tolerable upper limit has been established
Minerals		
Calcium AI: 1,000–1,200 mg EAR: 800–1,000 mg	• Aids in bone and tooth formation, muscle contraction, blood coagulation, nerve impulse transmission, cardiac function, cell membrane permeability, enzyme activation	*Deficiency:* Tooth decay, muscle cramps, tetany, nervousness and delusion, cardiac palpitations, heart failure, and paresthesias *Toxicity:* Constipation, loss of appetite, nausea, vomiting, dry mouth, renal calculi
Chloride AI: 2,000–2,300 mg	• Helps keep the body's acid–base balance • Helps with metabolism	*Deficiency:* Extremely rare but can cause loss of appetite, weakness, and lethargy *Toxicity:* May result in fluid retention
Chromium AI: 20–35 mcg EAR: Not established	• Maintains serum glucose levels • Maintains fat metabolism	*Deficiency:* Glucose intolerance, vertigo, abdominal pain, shock, convulsions, anuria, dermatitis *Toxicity:* Unknown
Copper RDA: 900 mcg EAR: 700 mcg	• Hemoglobin synthesis • Maintenance of hemostasis • Energy production	*Deficiency:* Hypochromic anemia, bone disease, weakness, skin lesions, altered respiratory status *Toxicity:* Nausea, vomiting, diarrhea, abdominal pain, malaise
Iodine RDA: 150 mcg EAR: 95 mcg	• Thyroid hormone synthesis	*Deficiency:* Hypothyroidism or goiter, nervousness, irritability, obesity, cold hands and feet, chills, brittle hair, fatigue, bradycardia, decreased cardiac output, thick tongue, hoarseness, poor memory, hearing loss, anorexia *Toxicity:* Goiter
Iron RDA: 8–18 mg EAR: 5–8.1 mg	• Hemoglobin synthesis • Cellular oxidation • Transportation of oxygen	*Deficiency:* Iron deficiency anemia, fatigue, tachycardia, palpitations, dyspnea, susceptibility to infection, brittle nails *Toxicity:* Iron poisoning; nausea, vomiting, gastrointestinal irritation, constipation, diarrhea
Magnesium RDA: 310–420 mg EAR: 265–350 mg	• Parathyroid hormone regulation • Acid–base balance • Enzyme activation • Smooth muscle regulation • Metabolism of carbohydrates and protein • Cell growth and reproduction	*Deficiency:* Tetany, tremors, confusion, depression, tachycardia, dysrhythmias, seizures *Toxicity:* Nausea, vomiting, drowsiness, muscle weakness, decreased deep tendon reflexes, hypotension, respiratory depression

DIAGNOSTIC EVALUATION	MANAGEMENT
Deficiency: • Low levels of vitamin D (serum 25 [OH] D) • Radiographic bone deformities • Abnormal bone densitometry	*Deficiency:* • Nutritional supplementation: ergocalciferol, 25 mcg/day PO • Good sources of vitamin D are egg yolks, yeast, enriched milk, fish liver oils • Exposure to sunlight
Deficiency: • Serum levels <0.5 mg/dL	*Deficiency:* • Nutritional supplementation: 100 to 400 international units/day PO • Parenteral therapy may be necessary to treat neurologic symptoms • Good sources of vitamin E are vegetable oils, milk, eggs, meat, fish, green leafy vegetables
Deficiency: • Prothrombin time extended longer than PTT	*Deficiency:* • Administration of vitamin K 15 mg subcutaneously • Good sources of vitamin K are green leafy vegetables, liver, wheat germ, cheeses, egg yolks, soybean oil
Deficiency: • Dual-energy x-ray absorptiometry (DEXA) for bone mineral density *Toxicity:* • Serum level >10.5 mg/dL	*Deficiency:* • Oral supplements of 1 to 2 g/day of elemental calcium • In severe hypocalcemia, 10 mL of 10% calcium gluconate IV administered no faster than 2 mL/min • Good sources of calcium are milk products, green leafy vegetables, legumes, tofu processed with calcium *Toxicity:* • Force fluids, diuretics, and limit dietary intake; administration of phosphate salts and glucocorticoids may also be necessary
Deficiency: • Serum levels <98 *Toxicity:* • Serum levels >108	• No specific treatment.
Deficiency: • Serum levels <0.3 mg/mL	*Deficiency:* • Nutritional supplementation: 50 to 200 mg/day • Good sources of chromium are brewer's yeast, whole grains, cereals
Deficiency: • In addition to diminished serum levels, 24-hour urine samples showing levels of urinary excretion of copper below 15 to 60 mcg/24 hr	*Deficiency:* • Nutritional supplementation: 0.1 mg/kg/day PO • IV supplementation: 1 to 2 mg/day • Good sources of copper are nuts, seeds, organ meats, seafood
Deficiency: • Low T_3 and T_4 levels • Thyroid scan	*Deficiency:* • Nutritional supplementation: 50 to 100 mg daily PO • Good sources of iodine are iodized salt, seafood
Deficiency: • Decreased hemoglobin, hematocrit, iron, and ferritin levels and increased total iron-binding capacity	*Deficiency:* • Nutritional supplementation: ferrous sulfate 325 mg PO tid; Imferon 250 mg/day IM for each gram of hemoglobin below normal • IV supplementation: 1.5 to 2 g over 4 to 6 hr • Good sources of iron are egg yolks, fish, organ meats, wheat germ, beef, peas, chicken, turkey, legumes, spinach
Deficiency: • Serum levels <1.3 mEq/L *Toxicity:* • Serum levels >2.1 mEq/L	*Deficiency:* • Nutritional supplementation: 1 to 2 g IV during 15 min • Good sources of magnesium are nuts, meat, whole grains, green vegetables, seafood, dairy products *Toxicity:* • Supportive measures

(continued)

Table 20-5 Vitamin and Mineral Requirements and Imbalances (*Continued*)

VITAMIN, RDA, AND EAR	FUNCTION	CLINICAL MANIFESTATIONS OF IMBALANCE
Minerals (*Continued*)		
Phosphorus RDA: 700 mg EAR: 580 mg	• Nerve and muscle activity • Vitamin utilization • Kidney function • Metabolism of carbohydrates, proteins, and fats • Cell growth and repair • Myocardial contraction • Energy production • Bone and tooth formation • Acid–base balance • Red blood cell function	*Deficiency:* Anorexia, weakness, tremor, paresthesias, anemia, mental status change, hypoxia, osteomalacia *Toxicity:* Tetany, soft tissue calcification, seizures, renal damage
Potassium AI: 4,700 mg	• Muscle contraction • Cardiac function • Protein synthesis • Nerve impulse transmission • Carbohydrate metabolism • Acid–base balance • Major intracellular cation	*Deficiency:* Muscle weakness, fatigue, malaise, flaccidity, mental confusion, irritability, depression, dysrhythmias, hypotension, nausea, vomiting, anorexia, decreased GI motility, muscle cramps, paresthesias, hyperglycemia, polyuria, metabolic alkalosis *Toxicity:* Muscle weakness, paralysis, paresthesias, nausea, vomiting, diarrhea, metabolic acidosis, prolonged cardiac conduction, ventricular dysrhythmias
Sodium AI: 1,300–1,500 mg	• Maintains fluid balance • Cell membrane permeability and absorption of glucose • Bioelectric potential of tissues • Cardiac function • Acid–base balance • Regulation of neuromuscular function	*Deficiency:* Muscle weakness, irritability, headache, seizures, nausea, vomiting, malaise, abdominal cramping, hypotension, tachycardia *Toxicity:* Flushed skin, oliguria, agitation, thirst, dry mucous membranes, seizures
Zinc RDA: 8–11 mg EAR: 6.8–9.4 mg	• Cellular metabolism • Maintenance of taste and smell • Burn and wound healing • Gonadal function • Maintenance of serum vitamin A concentration • Acid–base balance • Protein digestion • Promotion of growth	*Deficiency:* Fatigue, hair loss, poor wound healing, impaired growth, bone deformities, loss of taste, anorexia, iron deficiency anemia, hypogonadism, hyperpigmentation *Toxicity:* Diminished deep tendon reflexes, malaise, decreased level of consciousness, diarrhea, leukopenia

ADH, antidiuretic hormone; AI, adequate intake; ATP, adenosine triphosphate; DRI, dietary reference intake; EAR, estimated average requirement; IM, intramuscular; IV, intravenous; MCV, mean corpuscular volume; PO, by mouth; PTT, partial thromboplastin time; RBC, red blood cell; RDA, recommended daily allowance; tid, three times per day.

DIAGNOSTIC EVALUATION	MANAGEMENT
Deficiency: • Serum levels <2.5 mg/dL *Toxicity:* • Serum levels >4.5 mg/dL	*Deficiency:* • Nutritional supplementation: PO or IV phosphate • Good sources of phosphate are dairy products, eggs, fish, grains, meat, poultry, cheeses, beans, cocoa, chocolate, liver, milk, peas, nuts *Toxicity:* • Administration of phosphate-binding agents • Hemodialysis or peritoneal dialysis
Deficiency: • Serum levels <3.5 mEq/L *Toxicity:* • Serum levels >5 mEq/L.	*Deficiency:* • Nutritional supplementation: PO or IV, IV replacement generally at a rate of 10 mEq/hr with careful cardiac monitoring and frequent measurements of serum potassium levels • Good sources of potassium are bananas, oranges, beef, prunes, beans, seafood, raisins *Toxicity:* • Infuse calcium gluconate 10% (10 mL) • Sodium bicarbonate infusion • Insulin and glucose infusion • Oral or rectal exchange resins • Hemodialysis or peritoneal dialysis
Deficiency: • Serum levels <135 mEq/L *Toxicity:* • Serum levels >145 mEq/L	*Deficiency:* • Restrict free water intake • Infuse 0.9% saline solution if the patient is hypovolemic • Infuse 3% saline and administer diuretic if sodium levels significantly low • Demeclocycline may be used to block ADH in the renal tubules to promote water excretion *Toxicity:* • Administer salt-free solutions such as D5W followed by 0.45% saline solution • Low-sodium diet • Administer vasopressin if diminished ADH is the cause
Deficiency: • Serum levels <75 mcg/dL	*Deficiency:* • Nutritional supplementation: zinc sulfate 200 mg PO tid • Good sources of zinc are liver, seafood, beans, lentils, oatmeal, wheat bran, egg yolks, peas, chicken, and milk *Toxicity:* • Supportive measures

Recommended dietary allowance—the average daily dietary intake level sufficient to meet the nutrient requirements of nearly all (97% to 98%) healthy individuals in a group.

Adequate intake—amount believed to cover the needs of all healthy individuals in the groups, but lack of data or uncertainty in the data prevents being able to specify with confidence the percentage of individuals covered by this intake.

Estimated average requirement—average daily nutrient intake level estimated to meet the requirements of half of the healthy individuals in a group.

SELECTED REFERENCES

Blumenstein, I., Shastri, Y., & Stein, J. (2014). Gastroenteric tube feeding: Techniques, problems and Solutions. *World Journal of Gastroenterology, 20*(26), 8505–8524.

Campbell, S. M. (2015). *Best practices for managing tube feeding. A Nurse's Pocket Manual*. Abbott Nutrition. Available: *http://static.abbottnutrition.com/cms-prod/abbottnutrition.com/img/M4619.005%20Tube%20Feeding%20manual.pdf*

Espie, J., & Wisler, I. (2015). Focus on anorexia nervosa: modern psychological treatment and guidelines for the adolescent patient. *Dovepress, 6*, 9–16. Available: *www.dovepress.com/focus-on-anorexia-nervosa-modern-psychological-treatment-and-guideline-peer-reviewed-fulltext-article-AHMT*

Forman, S. (2016). Eating disorders: Overview of epidemiology, clinical features, and diagnosis. *UpToDate*. New York: Wolters Kluwer.

Garber, C. E., Blissmer, B., Deschenes, M., et al. (2011). Quantity and quality of exercise for developing and maintaining cardiorespiratory, musculoskeletal, and neuromotor fitness in apparently healthy adults: Guidance for Prescribing Exercise. *Medicine and Science in Sports and Exercise, 43*(7), 1334–1359.

Harrington, B. C., Jimerson, M., Haxton, C., & Jimerson, D. C. (2015). Initial evaluation, diagnosis, and treatment of anorexia nervosa and bulimia nervosa. *American Family Physician, 91*(1), 46–52.

Hudson, J. I., McElroy, S. L., Ferreira-Cornwell, M. C., et al. (2017). Efficacy of lisdexamfetamine in adults with moderate to severe binge-eating disorder. *JAMA Psychiatry, 74*(9), 903–910.

Keller, J., & Layer, P. (2014). The pathophysiology of malabsorption. *Visceral Medicine, 30*, 150–154. Available: *www.ncbi.nlm.nih.gov/pmc/articles/PMC4513829/*

Kim, Y., Jung, A. D., Dhar, V. K., et al. (2018). Laparoscopic sleeve gastrectomy improves renal transplant candidacy and posttransplant outcomes in morbidly obese patients. *Am J Transplant, 18*(2), 410–416.

Kowalski, K., Mulak, A., Jasinska, M., & Paradowski L. (2017). Diagnostic challenges in celiac disease. *Adv Clin Exp Med, 23*(4), 729–737.

McClave, S. A., DiBaise, J. K., Mullin, G. E., & Martindale, R. G. (2016). Nutrition therapy in the adult hospitalized patient. *American Journal of Gastroenterology, 111*, 315–334.

McLawhorn, A. S., Levack, A. E., Lee, Y. Y., et al. (2017). Bariatric surgery improves outcomes after lower extremity arthroplasty in the morbidly obese: A propensity score-matched analysis of a New York Stateide database. *Surgery for Obesity and Related Disorders, 13*(3), 457–462.

Mechanick, J. I., Youdim, A., Jones, D. B., et al. (2013). AACE/TOS/ASMBS guidelines: Clinical practice guidelines for the perioperative nutritional, metabolic, and nonsurgical support of the bariatric surgery patient-2013 update. *Endocrine Practice, 19*(2), e1–e36.

Mehler, P. S., & Brown, C. (2015). Anorexia nervosa—Medical complications. *Journal of Eating Disorders, 3*(11), 1–8. Available: *https://jeatdisord.biomedcentral.com/articles/10.1186/s40337-015-0040-8*

Mehler, P. S., & Rylander, M. (2015). Bulimia nervosa—Medical complications. *Journal of Eating Disorders, 3*(12), 1–5. Available: *https://jeatdisord.biomedcentral.com/articles/10.1186/s40337-015-0044-4*

National Institute of Diabetes, Gastrointestinal, and Kidney Disease. (2016). Prescription medicine to treat overweight and obesity. Available: *www.niddk.nih.gov/health-information/health-topics/weight-control/prescription-medications-treat-overweight-obesity/Pages/facts.aspx*

National Institutes of Health Office of Dietary Supplements. (2017). Nutrient recommendations: Dietary reference intakes (DRI). Available: *https://ods.od.nih.gov/Health_Information/Dietary_Reference_Intakes.aspx/*

Nearing, E. E., Santos, T. M., Topolski, M. S., et al. (2017). Benefits of bariatric surgery before elective joint arthroplasty: is there a role for weight loss optimization? *Surg Obes Relat Dis, 13*(3), 457–462.

Nordqvist, C. (2014). What is bulimia nervosa. *Medical News Today*. Available: *www.medicalnewstoday.com/articles/105102.php*

Nordqvist, C. (2015). Anorexia nervosa: Causes, symptoms and treatments. *Medical News Today*. Available: *www.medicalnewstoday.com/articles/267432.php*

Obera weight loss system. (2017). Apollo Endosurgery, Inc. Available: *www.orbera.com/*

Ogden, C. L., Carroll, M. D., Fryar, C. D., & Flegal, K. M. (2015). Prevalence of obesity among adults and youths, United States 2011–2014. *NHCS Data Brief.* (219), 1–8.

Parrott, J., Frank, L., Rabena, R., et al. (2017). American Society for Metabolic and Bariatric Surgery Integrated Health Nutritional Guidelines for the Surgical Weight Loss Patient 2016 Update: Micronutrients. *Surgery for Obesity And Related Disorders, 13*(5), 727–741.

ReShape: The nonsurgical weight loss procedure. (2017). ReShape Medical, Inc. Available: *https://reshapeready.com/reshape-cc/*

Romagnolo, D. F., & Selmin, O. I. (2017) Mediterranean diet and prevention of chronic diseases. *Nutr Today, 52*(5), 208–222.

Swanson, S., Crow, S., Le Grange, D., et al. (2011). Prevalence and correlates of eating disorders in adolescents. *Archives of General Psychiatry, 22*, E1–E10.

The Aspire Assist: A new approach to weight loss. (2016). Aspire Bariatrics. Available: *www.aspirebariatrics.com/about-the-aspireassist/*

The U.S. Food and Drug Administration expanded the approved uses of Vyvanse to treat binge-eating disorder in adults to help curb episodes of binge eating. (2015). *Evidence base*. Available: *https://ohsonline.com/articles/2015/02/03/fda-expands-uses-of-vyvanse-to-treat-binge.aspx?admgarea=ht.BehavioralSafety*

U.S. Department of Health and Human Services and U.S. Department of Agriculture. (2015). 2015–2020 Dietary guidelines for Americans (8th ed.). Available: *http://health.gov/dietaryguidelines/2015/guidelines/*

Vargas, E. J., Rizk, M., Bazerbachi, F., & Abu Dayyeh, B. K. (2018). Medical devices for obesity treatment: endoscopic bariatric therapies. *Med Clin North Am, 102*(1), 149–163.

Velazquez, A., & Apovian, C. M. (2018). Update on obesity pharmacotherapy. *Ann N Y Acad Sci, 1411*(1), 106–119.

Watts, C. D., Martin, J. R., Houdek, M. T., et al. (2016). Prior bariatric surgery may decrease the rate of reoperation and revision following total hip arthroplasty. *Bone Joint J, 98-B*(9), 1180–1184.

UNIT VI

RENAL, GENITOURINARY, AND REPRODUCTIVE HEALTH

21
Renal and Urinary Disorders

OVERVIEW AND ASSESSMENT

 See additional online content: Procedure Guidelines 21-1

Subjective Data

Subjective data include characterization of symptoms, history of present illness, past medical and surgical history, demographic data, and lifestyle factors. Signs and symptoms involving the urinary tract may be due to disorders of the kidneys, ureters, or bladder; surrounding structures; or disorders of other body systems. See Standards of Care Guidelines 21-1.

Changes in Micturition (Voiding)

Changes in the Amount or Color of Urine

1. Hematuria—blood in the urine, may be gross (visible by color change) or microscopic.
   a. Considered a serious sign and requires evaluation.
   b. Color of bloody urine depends on several factors including the amount of blood present and the anatomical source of the bleeding.

c. Microscopic hematuria is the presence of red blood cells (RBCs) in urine, which can be seen only under a microscope; urine appears normal.
   d. Hematuria may be due to a systemic cause, such as blood dyscrasias, anticoagulant therapy, or extreme exercise.
   e. Painless hematuria may indicate neoplasm in the urinary tract.
   f. Hematuria is common in patients with urinary tract stone disease, malignancy, acute infection, glomerulonephritis, trauma to the kidneys or urinary tract, thrombosis and embolism involving renal artery or vein, and polycystic kidney disease.
2. Polyuria—large volume of urine voided in a given time.
   a. Volume is out of proportion to usual voiding pattern and fluid intake.
   b. Demonstrated in diabetes mellitus, diabetes insipidus, chronic renal disease, use of diuretics.
3. Oliguria—small volume of urine.
   a. Output between 50 and 500 mL/24 hours.
   b. May result from acute renal failure, CKD stage V, shock, dehydration, fluid and electrolyte imbalance, or obstruction.
4. Anuria—absence of urine output.
   a. Output less than 50 mL/24 hours.
   b. Indicates serious renal dysfunction requiring immediate medical or surgical intervention, or CKD stage V.

STANDARDS OF CARE GUIDELINES 21-1
Renal Impairment

- Be aware that systemic factors, urologic status, and renal function affect urine output. Notify health care provider of decreased urine output.
- Patients at risk for renal impairment include those with cardiovascular disease, diabetes, and hypertension; postoperative patients; hypotensive patients; and those with prostate and other diseases of the urinary tract.
- Thorough assessment of the urinary tract includes:
  - Hourly intake and output measurement.
  - Assessment of color, clarity, and specific gravity of the urine.
  - Palpation of the abdomen for suprapubic tenderness.
  - Percussion of the flanks for costovertebral angle tenderness.
  - Prostate examination.
  - Subjective assessment for symptoms, such as urgency, frequency, nocturia, hesitancy, dribbling, decreased force of stream, hematuria, and incontinence.
- Be alert to drugs or agents that may impair urinary and renal function, such as nonsteroidal anti-inflammatory drugs, anticholinergics, sympathomimetics, aminoglycoside antibiotics, antifungals, calcineurin inhibitors, angiotensin-converting enzyme inhibitors, angiotensin receptor blockers, chemotherapeutic agents, and contrast media.
- Report abnormal urinalysis, urine culture, and renal function test results to health care provider promptly.

This information should serve as a general guideline only. Each patient situation presents a unique set of clinical factors and requires nursing judgment to guide care, which may include additional or alternative measures and approaches.

Symptoms Related to Irritation of the Lower Urinary Tract

1. Dysuria—painful or uncomfortable urination.
   a. Burning sensation seen in a wide variety of inflammatory and infectious urinary tract conditions.
2. Frequency—voiding occurs more frequently than usual when compared with patient's usual pattern or with a generally accepted norm of once every 3 to 6 hours.
   a. Determine if habits governing fluid intake have been altered—it is essential to know normal voiding pattern to evaluate frequency.
   b. Increasing frequency can result from a variety of conditions, such as infection and diseases of the urinary tract, metabolic disease, hypertension, medications (diuretics).
3. Urgency—strong desire to urinate that is difficult to postpone.
   a. Because of inflammatory conditions of the bladder, prostate, or urethra; acute or chronic bacterial infections; neurogenic voiding dysfunctions; chronic prostatitis or bladder outlet obstruction in men; overactive bladder; and urogenital atrophy in postmenopausal women.
4. Nocturia—urination at night that interrupts sleep.
   a. Causes include urologic conditions affecting bladder function, poor bladder emptying, bladder outlet obstruction, or overactive bladder.
   b. Metabolic causes include decreased renal concentrating ability or heart failure, hyperglycemia, and remobilization of dependent edema.
5. Strangury—slow and painful urination; only small amounts of urine voided. Wrenching sensation at end of urination produced by spasmodic muscular contraction of the urethra and bladder.
   a. Blood staining may be noted.
   b. Seen in numerous urological conditions, including severe cystitis, interstitial cystitis, urinary calculus, and bladder cancer.

Symptoms Related to Obstruction of the Lower Urinary Tract

1. Weak stream—decreased force of stream when compared to usual stream of urine when voiding.
2. Hesitancy—undue delay and difficulty in initiating voiding.
   a. May indicate compression of the urethra, outlet obstruction, neurogenic bladder.
3. Terminal dribbling—prolonged dribbling or urine from the meatus after urination is complete. May be caused by bladder outlet obstruction.
4. Incomplete emptying—feeling that the bladder is still full even after urination. Indicates urinary retention, overactive bladder, or a condition that prevents the bladder from emptying well; may lead to infection.
5. Urinary retention—inability to void.

Involuntary Voiding

1. Urinary incontinence—involuntary loss of urine; may be due to pathologic, anatomical, or physiologic factors affecting the urinary tract (see page 148).
2. Nocturnal enuresis—involuntary voiding during sleep. May be physiologic during early childhood; thereafter, may be functional or symptomatic of obstructive or neurogenic disease (usually of the lower urinary tract) or dysfunctional voiding.

Urinary Tract Pain

1. Kidney pain—may be felt as a dull ache in costovertebral angle or may be a sharp, colicky pain felt in the flank area that radiates to the groin or testicle. Because of distention of the renal capsule; severity related to how quickly it develops.
2. Ureteral pain—felt in the back and/or abdomen and can radiate to the groin, urethra, penis, scrotum, or testicle.
3. Bladder pain (lower abdominal pain or pain over suprapubic area)—may be due to bladder infection, overdistended bladder, or bladder spasms.
4. Urethral pain—from irritation of the bladder neck, from foreign body in canal, or from urethritis because of infection or trauma; pain increases when voiding.
5. Pain in scrotal area—because of inflammatory swelling of the epididymis or testicle, torsion of the testicle, testicular mass, or scrotal infection. May also be referred pain from neurological, renal, or gastrointestinal (GI) source.
6. Testicular pain—because of injury, mumps, orchitis, torsion of the spermatic cord, testes, or testes appendix.
7. Perineal or rectal discomfort—because of acute or chronic prostatitis, prostatic abscess, or trauma.
8. Pain in glans penis—usually from prostatitis; penile shaft pain results from urethral problems; may also be referred pain from ureteral calculus.

Related Symptoms

1. GI symptoms related to urologic conditions include nausea, vomiting, diarrhea, abdominal discomfort, paralytic ileus.
2. Occur with urologic conditions because the GI and urinary tracts have common autonomic and sensory innervation and because of renointestinal reflexes.
3. Fever and chills may also occur with infectious processes.

History

Seek the following historical data related to urinary and renal function:

1. What are patient's present and past occupations? Look for occupational hazards related to the urinary tract—contact with chemicals, plastics, tar, rubber; also truck or school bus drivers, dry cleaners, farmers.
2. What is patient's smoking history?
3. What is the past medical and surgical history, especially in relation to urinary problem?
4. Is there any family history of renal disease?
5. What childhood diseases did patient have?
6. Is there a history of urinary tract infections (UTIs)? Did any occur before age 12?
7. Did enuresis continue beyond the age when most children gain control?
8. Any history of genital lesions or sexually transmitted diseases (STDs)?
9. For the female patient: Number of children? Vaginal or cesarean delivery? Any forceps deliveries? When? Any signs of vaginal discharge? Vaginal/vulvar itch or irritation? Family history of pelvic organ prolapse ("dropped" bladder or uterus) or urinary incontinence?
10. Does patient have diabetes mellitus? Hypertension? Allergies? Neurologic disease or dysfunction? Vascular disease?
11. Has patient ever been hospitalized for a UTI? What diagnostic tests were performed? Cystoscopy? Urodynamics? Kidney x-ray procedures? Was patient catheterized for a time? Were antibiotics administered via intravenous (IV) or oral route?
12. Has patient ever had surgery for bladder or prostate problems or traumatic injuries involving the pelvis?
13. Is patient taking any prescription or over-the-counter (OTC) drugs or herbal preparations that may affect renal or urinary function? Have any drugs been prescribed for renal or urinary problems?
14. Is patient at risk for UTI?

Objective Data

Objective data should focus on physical examination of the abdomen, the genitalia, and rectal exam in some cases. Complete body system assessment may be indicated in some conditions such as renal failure. See Chapter 5.

Laboratory Tests

Common laboratory studies pertaining to renal and urologic disorders include blood and urinary excretion tests for renal function, prostate-specific antigen, and urinalysis.

Tests of Renal Function

Description

1. Renal function tests are used to determine effectiveness of the kidneys' excretory functioning, to evaluate the severity of kidney disease, and to follow patient's progress.

2. There is no single test of renal function; rather, optimal results are obtained by combining a number of clinical tests.

Nursing and Patient Care Considerations

Renal function may be within normal limits until about 50% of renal function has been lost (see Table 21-1).

Prostate-Specific Antigen

Description

1. Prostate-specific antigen (PSA) is an amino acid glycoprotein that is measured in the serum by a simple blood test.
2. An elevated PSA indicates the presence of prostate disease but is not exclusive to prostate cancer.
3. Level rises continuously with the growth of prostate cancer.
4. Normal serum PSA level is less than 4 ng/mL.
5. Patients who have undergone surgical treatment for prostate cancer are monitored every 6 to 12 months with PSA levels for recurrence. Cancer recurrence is suspected with PSA greater than 0.2 ng/mL on two occasions (test is repeated for possible lab error).

Nursing and Patient Care Considerations

1. No patient preparation is necessary.
2. Current or recent UTI, prostatitis, digital rectal exam, or urethral instrumentation can cause an artificial elevation of PSA.
3. Clinical laboratories may differ slightly in methods used for determining PSA; patients having serial PSA should be sent to the same laboratory.

Urinalysis

Description

Involves examination of the urine for overall characteristics, including appearance, pH, specific gravity, and osmolality as well as microscopic evaluation for the presence of normal and abnormal cells.

1. Appearance—normal urine is clear. Foamy urine can be seen with proteinuria. Cloudy urine may or may not be pathologic.
   a. Nonpathologic causes: normal urine may develop cloudiness on refrigeration, from standing at room temperature, or from precipitation of phosphates in alkaline urine (phosphaturia).
   b. Pathologic causes: because of pus (pyuria), blood, epithelial cells, bacteria, fat, colloidal particles, phosphate, or lymph fluid (chyluria).
2. Odor—normal urine has a faint aromatic odor.
   a. Characteristic odors produced by ingestion of asparagus.
   b. Cloudy urine with ammonia odor: urea-splitting bacteria such as *Proteus*, causing UTIs.
   c. Offensive odor: may be due to bacterial action in the presence of pus.
   d. Acetone scent can be detected in diabetic ketoacidosis.
3. Color—varies with urine concentration and is affected by metabolites, medications, and certain foods.
   a. Normal urine is clear yellow or amber because of the pigment urochrome.
   b. Dilute urine is pale yellow or clear.
   c. Concentrated urine is tea-colored and may be a sign of insufficient fluid intake.
   d. Blue, blue-green: medication, namely amitriptyline, propofol, indomethacin, and methenamine; pseudomonas infection.
   e. Red or red-brown: because of blood pigments, porphyria, bleeding lesions in urogenital tract, some drugs such as phenazopyridine and foods (beets).

Table 21-1 Tests of Renal Function

There is no single test of renal function because this function is subject to variation. The rate of change of renal function is more important than the result of a single test.

TEST	PURPOSE/RATIONALE	TEST PROTOCOL
Renal concentration test • Specific gravity • Osmolality of urine	• Both tests evaluate the ability of the kidney to dilute or concentrate urine. • Values are elevated in prerenal states, including dehydration. Concentration ability is lost (resulting in low values) in CKD and some types of AKI despite changes in volume status.	• Fluids may be withheld 12 to 24 hours to evaluate the concentrating ability of the tubules under controlled conditions. Specific gravity measurements of urine are taken at specific times to determine urine concentration.
Creatinine clearance	• Provides a reasonable approximation of rate of glomerular filtration. • Measures volume of blood in mL cleared of creatinine in 1 min. • Most sensitive indication of early renal disease.	• Collect all urine over 24-hour period. • Draw one sample of blood within the period.
Serum creatinine	• A test of renal function reflecting the balance between production and filtration by renal glomerulus. • Most sensitive test of renal function.	• Obtain sample of blood serum.
Serum urea nitrogen (blood urea nitrogen [BUN])	• Serves as index of renal excretory capacity. • Serum urea nitrogen depends on the body's urea production and on urine flow. (Urea is the nitrogenous end product of protein metabolism.) • Affected by protein intake, hydration status, and catabolism.	• Obtain sample of blood serum.
Protein	• Random specimen may be affected by dietary protein intake. Proteinuria >300 mg/24 hours may indicate renal disease.	• Collect all urine over 24-hour period.
Microalbumin/creatinine ratio	• Sensitive test for the subsequent development of proteinuria; >25 mg/g for females and >17 mg/g for males predicts early nephropathy.	• Collect random urine specimen.
Urine casts	• Mucoproteins and other substances present in renal inflammation; help to identify type of renal disease (eg, red cell casts present in glomerulonephritis, fatty casts in nephrotic syndrome, white cell casts in pyelonephritis).	• Collect random urine specimen.

f. Yellow-brown, green-brown, or tea colored: may reveal obstructive lesion of bile duct system, obstructive jaundice, or hepatitis.

g. Dark brown or black: because of malignant melanoma, leukemia, methemoglobin or medications, namely methyldopa, levodopa.

4. pH of urine—reflects the ability of the kidney to maintain normal hydrogen ion concentration in plasma and extracellular fluid; indicates *acidity* or *alkalinity* of urine.
   a. pH should be measured in fresh urine because the breakdown of urine to ammonia causes urine to become alkaline.
   b. Normal pH is 4.5 to 8.0.
   c. Urine acidity (pH less than 4.5) or alkalinity (pH greater than 8.0) has relatively little clinical significance unless the patient is being treated for renal calculus disease or being evaluated for renal tubular acidosis.

5. Specific gravity (SG)—reflects the kidney's ability to concentrate or dilute urine; may reflect degree of hydration or dehydration.
   a. Normal specific gravity ranges from 1.005 to 1.030.
   b. Specific gravity is low and matches the specific gravity of plasma at 1.010 (isosthenuria) in late stages of chronic kidney disease (CKD).
   c. Volume depletion will cause the SG to be elevated, and volume overload will result in a low SG.

6. Osmolality—indication of the amount of osmotically active particles in urine (number of particles per unit volume of water). It is similar to specific gravity but is considered a more precise test and only 1 to 2 mL of urine are required. Osmolality can range from 50 to 1200 mOsm/kg.

Nursing and Patient Care Considerations

1. Freshly voided urine provides the best results for routine urinalysis; some tests may require a first morning specimen.
2. The urine should be refrigerated to ensure accurate results if urine sample cannot be delivered to lab immediately.
3. Obtain sample of about 30 mL.
4. Urine culture and sensitivity tests are typically performed using the same specimen obtained for urinalysis; therefore, use clean-catch or catheterization technique.
5. Patients with urinary diversions, especially ileal conduit diversions, require catheterized urine specimen. The urinalysis will normally demonstrate bacteria if the specimen is collected from intestinal diversion.

Radiology and Imaging Studies

These tests include simple x-rays, x-rays with the use of contrast media, ultrasound, nuclear scans, and imaging via computed tomography (CT) and magnetic resonance imaging (MRI). Patient age and pregnancy status help dictate imaging choice.

EVIDENCE BASE McCarthy, C., Baliyan, V., Kordbacheh, H., et al. (2016). Radiology of renal stone disease. *International Journal of Surgery, 36,* 638–646.

X-Ray of Kidneys, Ureters, and Bladder

Description
1. Consists of plain film of the abdomen.
2. Delineates size, shape, and position of the kidneys.
3. Reveals deviations, such as radiopaque calcifications (stones), tumors, or kidney displacement.
4. Not reliable as sole imaging modality to diagnose stones as it will not show radiolucent stones.

Nursing and Patient Care Considerations
1. No preparation is needed.
2. Usually done before other testing.
3. Patient will be asked to wear a gown and remove all metal from the x-ray field.

Pyelogram

Description
1. Antegrade pyelogram: Injection of small amount of radiopaque contrast directly into the renal pelvis, usually via an existing nephrostomy tube.
2. Retrograde pyelogram: Injection of radiopaque contrast material through ureteral catheters, which have been passed into ureters by means of cystoscopic manipulation.
3. The radiopaque solution is introduced by syringe injection. May require sedation.
4. Mostly used to determine location and severity of an obstruction in the urinary system.
5. Used in place of previously used intravenous pyelogram (IVP) for visualization of the collecting system.

Nursing and Patient Care Considerations
1. Contraindicated in patients with UTI.
2. May require sedation.
3. Allergic reactions are rare as only a small amount of dye is absorbed into the body.

Cystourethrogram

Description
1. Visualization of the urethra and bladder by x-ray after retrograde instillation of contrast material through a catheter. An examination of only the bladder is a *cystogram* and of only the urethra is a *urethrogram*.
2. Used to identify injuries, vesicoureteral reflux, tumors, or structural abnormalities of the urethra or bladder or to evaluate emptying problems or incontinence (voiding cystourethrogram).

Nursing and Patient Care Considerations
1. Carries risk of infection because of instrumentation.
2. Allergy to contrast material is a contraindication.
3. Additional x-rays may be taken after the catheter is removed and patient voids (voiding cystourethrogram).
4. Provide reassurance to allay patient's embarrassment.

Renal Angiography

Description
1. IV catheter is threaded through the femoral and iliac arteries into the aorta or renal artery.
2. Contrast material is injected to visualize the renal arterial supply.

3. Evaluates blood flow dynamics, demonstrates abnormal vasculature, and differentiates renal cysts from renal tumors.
4. May be done prior to renal transplant or to embolize a kidney before nephrectomy for renal tumor.

Nursing and Patient Care Considerations
1. NPO after midnight before the examination; clear liquids permitted up to 2 hours before exam. Adequate hydration is essential.
2. Continue oral medications (special orders needed for diabetic patients).
3. IV access required.
4. May not be done on the same day as other studies requiring barium or contrast material.
5. Maintain bed rest for approximately 4 hours after the examination, with the leg kept straight on the side used for groin access.
6. Observe frequently for hematoma or bleeding at access site. Keep sandbag at bedside for use if bleeding occurs.

Renal Scan

Description
1. Radiopharmaceuticals (also called radiotracers or isotopes) are injected intravenously.
   a. Tc-DTPA, Tc^{99m}-DMSA is used for anatomical or MAG3 visualization and evaluation of glomerular filtration.
   b. Other radiopharmaceuticals may also be used depending on the purpose of the scan.
2. Assesses renal function and not used to assess for renal anatomy, mass, or stones.
3. Studies are obtained with a scintillation camera placed posterior to the kidney with patient in a supine, prone, or sitting position.

Nursing and Patient Care Considerations
1. Patient should be well hydrated. Give several glasses of water or IV fluids, as ordered, before scan.
2. Furosemide or captopril may be administered in conjunction with the scan to determine their effects.

Ultrasound

Description
1. Uses high-frequency sound waves passed into the body and reflected back in varying frequencies based on the composition of soft tissues. Organs in the urinary system create characteristic ultrasonic images that are electronically processed and displayed as an image.
2. Abnormalities, such as masses, malformations, stones, or obstructions, can be identified; useful in differentiating between solid and fluid-filled masses.
3. A noninvasive technique without the use of radiation.

Nursing and Patient Care Considerations
1. Ultrasound examination of the prostate is performed using a rectal probe. A laxative or enema may be ordered to be given within hours of the examination.
2. Ultrasound examination of the bladder requires that the bladder be full.
3. Patient should not have had any studies using barium for 2 days before ultrasound of the kidney or bladder.

Computed Tomography and Magnetic Resonance Imaging

CT urogram has replaced IVP and is now the radiographic modality of choice to visualize the kidneys, ureter, and bladder. Noncontrast CT known as "stone survey" is the preferred method for evaluating urolithiasis. MRI may be ordered to evaluate for tumors.

See descriptions on page 166.

Other Tests

Other tests that may be done to evaluate disorders of the renal and urologic systems include cystoscopy, urodynamic testing, and needle biopsy of the kidney.

Cystoscopy

Description

1. *Cystoscopy* is a method of direct visualization of the urethra and bladder by means of a cystoscope that is inserted through the urethra into the bladder. It has a self-contained optical lens system that provides a magnified, illuminated view of the bladder.
2. Uses include:
   a. To inspect the bladder wall directly for tumor, stone, or ulcer and to inspect the urethra for abnormalities or to assess degree of prostatic obstruction.
   b. To allow insertion of ureteral catheters for radiographic studies or before abdominal or GU surgery.
   c. To see configuration and position of ureteral orifices.
   d. To remove calculi from the urethra, bladder, and ureter.
   e. To diagnose and treat lesions of the bladder, urethra, and prostate.
   f. To perform endoscopic prostate surgeries including transurethral resection of the prostate (TURP) (see page 601).

Nursing and Patient Care Considerations

1. Simple cystoscopy is usually performed in an office setting. More complicated cystoscopies, involving resections or ureteral catheter insertions, are done in the operating room suite, where IV sedation or spinal or general anesthesia may be used.
2. Patient's genitalia are cleaned with an antiseptic solution just before the examination. A local topical anesthetic (lidocaine gel) is instilled into the urethra before insertion of cystoscope.
3. Because fluid flows continuously through the cystoscope, patient may feel an urge to urinate during the examination.
4. Contraindicated in patients with known UTI.
5. Nursing interventions after cystoscopic examination:
   a. Monitor for complications: urinary retention, urinary tract hemorrhage, infection within the prostate or bladder.
   b. Expect patient to have some burning on voiding, blood-tinged urine, and urinary frequency from trauma to mucous membrane of the urethra.
   c. Administer or teach self-administration of antibiotics prophylactically, as ordered, to prevent UTI.
   d. Advise warm sitz baths or analgesics, such as ibuprofen or acetaminophen, to relieve discomfort after cystoscopy. Increase hydration.
   e. Provide routine catheter care if urine retention persists and an indwelling catheter is ordered.

Urodynamics

Description

Urodynamics is a term that refers to any of the following tests that provide physiologic and functional information about the lower urinary tract. They measure the ability of the bladder to store and empty urine. Most urodynamic equipment uses computer technology with results visible in real time on a monitor.

1. Uroflowmetry (flow rate)—a record of the volume of urine passing through the urethra per unit of time (mL/s). It is shown on graph paper and gives information about the rate and flow pattern of urination. It is used to evaluate obstructive voiding. Minimum volume of urine needed for accurate test is 150 mL.
2. Cystometrography—recording of the pressures exerted during filling and emptying of the urinary bladder to assess its function. Data about the ability of the bladder to store urine at low pressure and the ability of the bladder to contract appropriately to empty urine are obtained.
   a. A small catheter is placed through the urethra (or suprapubic area) into the bladder. The residual volume is measured if patient recently voided, and the catheter is left in place.
   b. The catheters are connected to urodynamic equipment designed to measure pressure at the distal end of the catheter.
   c. Water, saline, or contrast material is infused at a slow rate into the bladder.
   d. When the bladder feels full, patient is asked to "void." A normal detrusor contraction of the bladder appears as a sharp rise in bladder pressure on the graph. If the patient is unable to void, the test may be considered normal because it is difficult to void normally with catheters in place.
3. Sphincter electromyography (EMG)—measures the activity of the pelvic floor muscles during bladder filling and emptying. EMG activity may be measured using surface (patch) electrodes placed around the anus or with percutaneous wire or needle electrodes.
4. Pressure-flow studies—involve all of the above components, along with the simultaneous measurement of intra-abdominal pressure by way of a small tube with a fluid-filled balloon that is placed in the rectum. This permits better interpretation of actual bladder pressures without the influence of intra-abdominal pressure.
5. Video urodynamics—use all of the above components. The fluid used to fill the bladder is contrast material, and the entire study is performed under fluoroscopy, providing radiographic pictures in combination with the recording of bladder and intra-abdominal pressures. Video urodynamics are reserved for patients with complicated voiding dysfunction.

Nursing and Patient Care Considerations

1. Contraindicated in patients with UTI.
2. Frequently performed by nurses; essential to provide information and support throughout the test to ensure clinically significant results.
3. Patients may have burning on urination afterward (because of instrumentation); encourage fluids.
4. Short-term antibiotics are commonly given to prevent infection.

Needle Biopsy of the Kidney

Description

Performed by percutaneous needle biopsy through renal tissue with ultrasound guidance or by open biopsy through a small flank incision; useful in securing specimens for electron and immunofluorescent microscopy to determine diagnosis, treatment, and prognosis of renal disease.

Nursing and Patient Care Considerations

1. Prebiopsy nursing management.
   a. Ensure that coagulation studies, platelet count, and hematocrit results are reported to provide baseline values and to identify patients at risk for postbiopsy bleeding.
   b. Establish an IV line, as ordered.
   c. Ensure that patient is NPO for several hours before the procedure, as ordered.
   d. Describe the procedure to patient, including holding breath (to prevent movement of the thorax) during insertion of the biopsy needle.
   e. Instruct patient to urinate before the procedure.

2. Postbiopsy nursing management.
   a. Place patient in a supine position immediately after biopsy and on bed rest for 8 to 24 hours to minimize bleeding.
   b. Take vital signs every 5 to 15 minutes for the first hour and then with decreasing frequency if stable to assess for hemorrhage, which is a major complication.
   c. Watch for rise or fall in blood pressure (BP), anorexia, vomiting, or development of dull, aching discomfort in the abdomen.
   d. Assess for flank pain (usually represents bleeding into the muscle) or colicky pain (clot in the ureter).
   e. Assess for backache, shoulder pain, or dysuria.
   f. Persistent bleeding may be suspected when an enlarging hematoma is palpable through the abdomen.
   g. If perirenal bleeding develops, avoid palpating or manipulating the abdomen after the first examination has determined that a hematoma exists.
   h. Collect serial urine specimens to evaluate for hematuria.
   i. Assess for any patient complaints, especially frequency and urgency on urination.
   j. Keep fluid intake at 3,000 mL daily, if tolerated, unless patient has renal insufficiency.
   k. Hematocrit and hemoglobin may be ordered to assess for anemia prior to discharge.
3. Instruct patient on the following after biopsy:
   a. Avoid strenuous activity, strenuous sports, and heavy lifting for at least 2 weeks.
   b. Notify health care provider if any of the following occur: flank pain, hematuria, light-headedness and fainting, rapid pulse, or any other signs and symptoms of bleeding.
   c. Report for follow-up 1 to 2 months after biopsy; will be checked for hypertension and the biopsy area is auscultated for a bruit.

GENERAL PROCEDURES AND TREATMENT MODALITIES

 See additional online content: Procedure Guidelines 21-2–21-4

Catheterization

Catheterization may be done to relieve acute or chronic urinary retention, to drain urine preoperatively and postoperatively, to determine the amount of residual urine after voiding, or to determine accurate measurement of urinary drainage in critically ill patients.

Catheterization of Female

1. Engage assistance if needed for positioning patient with knees bent and legs spread with light directed onto the vulva. Maintain strict sterile technique using prepackaged indwelling catheter tray, or sterile straight catheter, sterile gloves, lubricant, and cleansing components set up on sterile field as indicated. Nondominant hand usually used for spreading labia and dominant hand remains sterile. See Figure 21-1.
2. Cleanse urethral meatus with povidone–iodine or other cleansing solution via cotton balls manipulated with sterile forceps.
3. Introduce well-lubricated catheter 2 to 3 inches (5 to 7.5 cm) into the urethral meatus using sterile gloved hand, watching for flow of urine.
4. Obtain specimen and secure the catheter and drainage bag as indicated. Note the amount of urine drained.

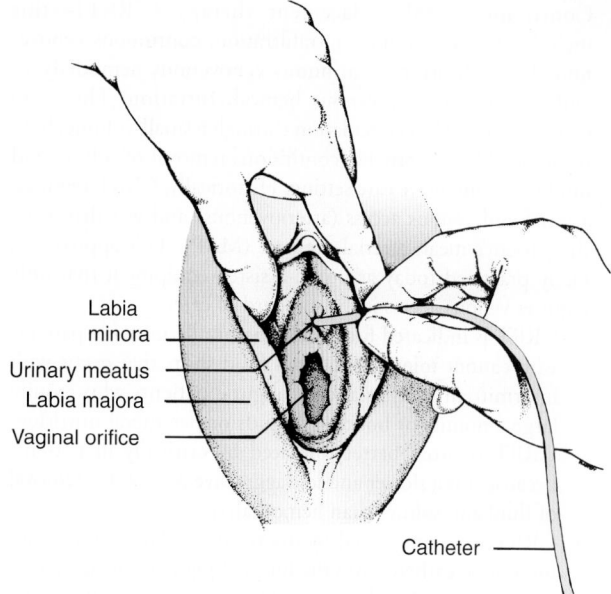

Figure 21-1. Urethral catheterization of the female patient.

Catheterization of Male

1. Grasp the shaft of the penis with nondominant hand; elevate it, retracting the foreskin, if present.
2. Cleanse with downward motion from urethral meatus, using a new sterile cotton ball with each stroke.
3. Apply gentle traction as you insert the well-lubricated catheter 6 to 10 inches (15 to 25 cm) with your sterile hand. Watch for urine flow and advance the catheter another 1 inch (2.5 cm).
4. Obtain specimen and secure the catheter and drainage bag as indicated. Note the amount of urine drained.

Suprapubic Catheterization

1. Establishes drainage from the bladder by introducing a catheter percutaneously through the anterior abdominal wall into the bladder.
2. May be done for acute urinary retention when urethral catheterization is not possible; for urethral trauma, stricture, or fistula to divert flow of urine from the urethra; or for obtaining an uncontaminated urine specimen for culture.
3. Once the surgical tract is healed, the catheter may be changed by the nurse monthly.

Dialysis

Dialysis refers to the diffusion of solute molecules through a semipermeable membrane, passing from the side of higher concentration to that of lower concentration. The purpose of dialysis is to maintain fluid, electrolyte, and acid–base balance and to remove endogenous and exogenous toxins. It is a substitute for some kidney excretory functions but does not replace the kidneys' endocrine functions. Methods of dialysis include:

1. Peritoneal dialysis.
   a. Continuous ambulatory peritoneal dialysis (CAPD).
   b. Automated peritoneal dialysis (APD)/continuous cycling peritoneal dialysis—uses APD machine to do multiple exchanges overnight, with or without a prolonged dwell time during the day.
2. Hemodialysis (see page 595).

3. Continuous renal replacement therapy (CRRT)—this includes slow continuous ultrafiltration, continuous venovenous hemofiltration, continuous venovenous hemodialysis, and continuous venovenous hemodiafiltration. These use extracorporeal blood circulation through a small-volume, low-resistance filter to provide continuous removal of solutes and fluid in the intensive care setting. Historically, CRRT required arterial and venous access (arteriovenous) and was driven by the patient's mean arterial pressure (MAP). This approach is rarely practiced today as pump-assisted equipment that only requires venous access is the standard of care.

   a. CRRT is indicated for hemodynamically unstable patients who cannot tolerate the rapid fluid shifts that occur with intermittent dialysis and in oliguric patients who require large amounts of hourly IV fluids or parenteral nutrition. CRRT is often better tolerated by critically ill patients because it is a slower and less aggressive process for removal of fluid and solutes than hemodialysis.

   b. CRRT is accomplished by insertion of a large-gauge double-lumen catheter into the internal jugular, subclavian, or femoral vein. A roller-type pump is used to propel blood through the system and anticoagulation may be used to prevent clotting. This is the current standard of care because of consistent blood flow rates.

   c. Care for the patient on CRRT is provided in an intensive care setting, with special attention given to assessing and calculating fluid and electrolyte balance, aggressively managing hypotension, preventing hemorrhage, monitoring for heat loss through the extracorporeal circulation, assessing for infection, and preventing clotting.

Continuous Ambulatory Peritoneal Dialysis

Continuous ambulatory peritoneal dialysis (CAPD) is a form of intracorporeal dialysis that uses the peritoneum as the semipermeable membrane (see Figure 21-2).

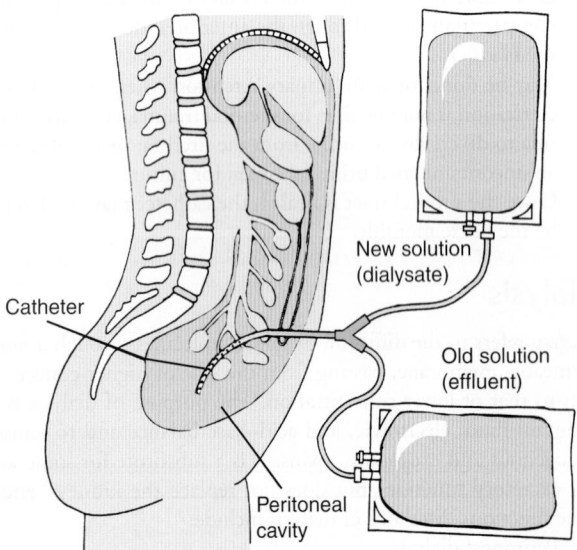

Figure 21-2. Continuous ambulatory peritoneal dialysis. The peritoneal catheter is implanted through the abdominal wall. Fluid infuses into the peritoneal cavity and drains after a prescribed time. (Porth, C. [1998]. *Pathophysiology: Concepts of altered health states* [5th ed.]. Philadelphia, PA: Lippincott-Raven Publishers.)

Procedure

1. A permanent indwelling catheter is implanted into the peritoneum; the internal cuff of the catheter becomes embedded by fibrous ingrowth, which stabilizes it and minimizes leakage.

2. A tube for connecting the catheter to an administration set is attached via a locking mechanism to the distal end of the peritoneal catheter, called the transfer set. It remains with the patient (attached to the catheter tubing) and must be changed at regular intervals per manufacturer recommendations without contamination. Specific transfer sets may only fit administration tubing from the same manufacturer, but there are devices available to make the transfer set compatible with other PD systems.

3. There are many types of administration sets, the most common being the double bag system. The double bag system has a preattached bag of dialysate solution and drainage, which has been shown to reduce peritonitis rates.

4. In CAPD, a patient is prescribed a set number of exchanges (fill, drain, and dwell) throughout the day.

5. During the fill, the dialysate bag is raised to shoulder level and infused by gravity into the peritoneal cavity (approximately 10 minutes for a 2-L volume).

6. During the dwell time, diffusion and osmosis occur. The typical dwell time is 4 to 6 hours.

7. At the end of the dwell time, the dialysate fluid is drained from the peritoneal cavity by gravity. Drainage of 2 L plus ultrafiltration takes about 10 to 20 minutes if the catheter is functioning optimally.

8. After the dialysate is drained, a fresh bag of dialysate solution is infused using aseptic technique and the procedure is repeated.

9. Patient performs four to five exchanges daily, 7 days per week, with an overnight dwell time allowing uninterrupted sleep; most patients become unaware of fluid in the peritoneal cavity.

Advantages Over Hemodialysis

1. Physical and psychological freedom and independence.
2. More liberal diet and fluid intake.
3. Relatively simple and easy to use.
4. Satisfactory biochemical control of uremia.

Complications

1. Infectious peritonitis, exit-site and tunnel infections.
2. Noninfectious catheter malfunction, obstruction, dialysate leak.
3. Peritoneal–pleural communication; hernia formation.
4. GI bloating, distention, nausea.
5. Hypervolemia, hypovolemia.
6. Bleeding at catheter site.
7. Bloody effluent secondary to internal bleeding. In female patients, this may occur during menstruation.
8. Obstruction may occur if the omentum becomes wrapped around the catheter or the catheter becomes caught in a loop of bowel.

Patient Education

1. The use of CAPD as a long-term treatment depends on prevention of recurring peritonitis.

   a. Use strict aseptic technique when performing bag exchanges. All persons in the room, including patient, must wear a mask any time connecting or disconnecting the transfer set to or from another system.

   b. Perform bag exchanges in clean, closed-off area without pets and other activities.

   c. Wash hands before touching bag.

   d. Inspect bag and tubing for defects and leaks.

2. Do not omit bag changes—this will cause inadequate control of renal failure.
3. Some weight gain may accompany CAPD—the dialysate fluid contains a significant amount of dextrose, which adds calories to daily intake.
4. Report signs and symptoms of peritonitis—cloudy peritoneal fluid, abdominal pain or tenderness, malaise, fever.

Hemodialysis

Hemodialysis is a process of cleansing the blood of accumulated waste products. It is used for patients with end-stage renal failure or for acutely ill patients who require short-term dialysis.

Procedure

1. Patient's access is prepared and cannulated.
2. Heparin may be administered to prevent circuit clotting.
3. Blood flows through a semipermeable dialyzer in one direction, and dialysis solution surrounds the membranes and flows in the opposite direction.
4. Dialysis solution consists of highly purified water to which sodium, potassium, calcium, magnesium, chloride, and dextrose have been added. Bicarbonate is added to achieve the proper pH balance.
5. Through the process of diffusion, solutes in the form of electrolytes, metabolic waste products, and acid–base components can be removed or added to the blood.
6. Excess water is removed from the blood (ultrafiltration).
7. The blood is then returned to the body through patient's access.

Requirements for Hemodialysis

1. Access to patient's circulation.
2. Dialysis machine and dialyzer with semipermeable membrane.
3. Appropriate dialysate bath.
4. Time—approximately 4 hours, three times weekly.
5. Place—dialysis center or home (if feasible).

Methods of Circulatory Access

1. Arteriovenous fistula (AVF)—creation of a vascular communication by suturing a vein directly to an artery (see Figure 21-3).
   a. Usually, radial artery and cephalic vein are anastomosed in nondominant arm; vessels in the upper arm may also be used. Leg vessels are used if unable to place in UE.
   b. Over time, the venous limb of the fistula system dilates. By means of two large-bore needles inserted into the dilated venous limb, blood may be obtained and passed through the dialyzer. The arterial end is used for arterial flow and the distal end for reinfusion of dialyzed blood.
   c. Maturation of AVF requires at least 6 to 8 weeks; a central vein catheter is used in the interim.
2. Arteriovenous graft—arteriovenous connection consisting of a tube graft usually made from an autologous saphenous vein or from polytetrafluoroethylene. Ready to use in 3 to 4 weeks.
3. Central vein catheters (CVC)—direct cannulation of veins (subclavian, internal jugular, or femoral) is used for temporary dialysis access. Tunneled catheters may be placed for permanent dialysis access in patients who refuse or are not candidates for AVF/AVG placement. CVC access is the least preferred permanent access because of increased risk of clotting and infection.

Complications of Vascular Access

1. Infection.
2. Clotting.

Figure 21-3. An internal arteriovenous fistula *(top)* is created by a side-to-side anastomosis of the artery and vein. A graft *(bottom)* can also be established between the artery and vein. (Smeltzer, S., & Bare, B. [2000]. *Brunner and Suddarth's textbook of medical-surgical nursing* [9th ed.]. Philadelphia, PA: Lippincott Williams & Wilkins.)

3. Central vein thrombosis or stenosis.
4. Stenosis or thrombosis of AVF/AVG.
5. Ischemia distal to the vascular access (steal syndrome).
6. Aneurysm or pseudoaneurysm.
7. Hemorrhage.

Monitoring During Hemodialysis

1. Involves constant monitoring of dialysis access, hemodynamic status, electrolyte, and acid–base balance as well as maintenance of sterility and a closed system.
2. Performed by specially trained nurses and dialysis technicians who are familiar with the protocol and equipment being used.

Chronic Hemodialysis Management

1. Dietary management involves restriction or adjustment of protein, sodium, potassium, phosphorous, or fluid intake. Ongoing consultation with a dietician is standard.
2. Careful adjustment of medications that are normally excreted by the kidney or are dialyzable. Certain medications are contraindicated.
3. Surveillance for complications:
   a. Arteriosclerotic cardiovascular disease, heart failure, disturbance of lipid metabolism (hypertriglyceridemia), coronary heart disease, stroke.
   b. Infections, systemic, or localized.
   c. Anemia.
   d. GI complications: Gastric ulcers, GI bleeding, constipation, and diarrhea.
   e. Bone problems (renal osteodystrophy)—from alterations in mineral metabolism.
   f. Electrolyte imbalances.
   g. Hypertension.
   h. Hypervolemia/pulmonary edema.
   i. Psychosocial problems: depression, anxiety, suicide, alteration in body image, and sexual dysfunction.
4. Hepatitis B and hepatitis C surveillance. All patients are encouraged to be vaccinated against hepatitis B.

5. Support agencies are American Association of Kidney Patients (*www.aakp.org*), National Kidney Foundation (*www.kidney.org*), National Kidney and Urologic Diseases Information Clearing House (*www.niddk.nih.gov*).

Kidney Surgery

Kidney surgery may include partial or total nephrectomy (removal of the kidney), kidney transplantation for end-stage renal disease (ESRD), procedures to remove stones or tumors, and procedures to insert drainage tubes (nephrostomy). Incisional approaches vary but may involve the flank, thoracic, and abdominal regions. Nephrectomy is most commonly performed for malignant tumors of the kidney but may also be indicated for trauma and kidneys that no longer function because of obstructive disorders and other renal disease. Nephrectomy is also the procedure of choice to remove a healthy kidney for donation to a transplant recipient. The absence of one kidney does not result in impaired renal function when the remaining kidney is normal and healthy.

Many surgical procedures were previously performed as "open" procedures, but are now being done with laparoscopic "keyhole" surgeries. An endoscope is introduced and the abdomen is inflated with carbon dioxide. Instruments are passed through other sites or a sleeve may be used, which allows a hand to be introduced at the operative site. Advantages are decreased postoperative pain, decreased blood loss, and, in some cases, decreased length of hospital stay.

Preoperative Management

1. Patient is prepared for surgery, and consent is witnessed. Preoperative antibiotics and bowel cleansing regimen may be prescribed.
2. Risk factors for thromboembolism are identified (smoking, oral contraceptive use, varicosities of lower extremities), and antiembolism stockings may be applied. Leg exercises are taught, and the patient is prepared for pneumatic/sequential compression stockings that will be used postoperatively.
3. Pulmonary status is assessed (presence of dyspnea, productive cough, other related cardiac symptoms), and deep breathing exercises, effective coughing, and use of incentive spirometer are taught.
4. If embolization of the renal artery is being done preoperatively for patients with renal cell carcinoma, the following symptoms of postinfarction syndrome are observed for (may last up to 3 days):
   a. Flank pain.
   b. Fever.
   c. Leukocytosis.
   d. Hypertension.

Postoperative Management

1. Vital signs are monitored and incisional area is assessed for evidence of bleeding or hemorrhage.
2. Possible pulmonary complications of atelectasis, pneumonia, and pneumothorax are observed. Pulmonary clearance through deep breathing, percussion, and vibration is maintained. Chest tube drainage may be used in patients who have an open procedure (the proximity of the thoracic cavity to the operative area may result in the need for chest tube drainage postoperatively).
3. Patency of urinary drainage tubes is maintained (nephrostomy, suprapubic, or urethral catheter). Ureteral stents may be used.
4. Respiratory status and lower extremities are assessed for thromboembolic complications.

5. Bowel sounds, abdominal distention, and pain are monitored, which may indicate paralytic ileus and need for nasogastric decompression.
6. For kidney transplantation patients, immunosuppressant drugs are ordered.
   a. A combination of medications is used, including a corticosteroid; calcineurin inhibitor, such as tacrolimus or cyclosporine; and mycophenolate mofetil.
   b. Early signs of rejection include temperature greater than 100.4°F (38°C), decreased urine output, weight gain of 3 pound (1.5 kg) or more overnight, pain or tenderness over the graft site, hypertension, increased serum creatinine.

 NURSING ALERT Use frequent and close observation of BP, pulse, and respiration to recognize hemorrhage (and shock)—chief danger after renal surgery. Watch for pain, sanguineous drainage from drain sites, or expanding pulsatile flank mass. Prepare for rapid blood and fluid replacement and reoperation.

Nursing Diagnoses

- Acute Pain related to surgical incision.
- Impaired Urinary Elimination related to urinary drainage tubes or catheters.
- Risk for Infection related to incision, potential pulmonary complications, and possibly immunosuppression.
- Risk for Imbalanced Fluid Volume related to fluid replacement needs and transplanted/remaining kidney function.

Nursing Interventions

Relieving Pain

1. Assess pain location, level, and characteristics. Transient renal colic-like pain may be caused by passage of blood clots down the ureter; however, report any persistent increasing or unrelievable pain, which may indicate obstruction of urinary drainage or hemorrhage.
2. Administer pain medications; evaluate effectiveness of patient-controlled analgesia (PCA).
3. Encourage patient to ambulate; splint incision to move or cough.

Promoting Urinary Elimination

1. Maintain patency of urinary drainage tubes and catheters while in place. Prevent kinking or pulling.
2. Use handwashing and asepsis when providing care and handling urinary drainage system (especially important for patient taking immunosuppressants).
3. Make sure indwelling catheter is dependent and draining.
   a. Report decrease in output or excessive clots.
   b. Be alert for signs of urinary infection, such as cloudy urine, fever, or bladder or flank ache.
4. Intervene to encourage removal of catheter when patient becomes ambulatory.
5. Maintain adequate fluid intake, IV or oral, when allowed.

Preventing Infection

1. Monitor for fever, elevated leukocyte count, abnormal breath sounds.
2. Administer antibiotics, as prescribed.
3. Assist patient with use of incentive spirometer, coughing and deep breathing, and ambulation to decrease risk of pulmonary infection. Provide meticulous care to chest tube sites.

4. Change dressings promptly if drainage is present—drainage is an excellent culture medium for bacteria.

5. Obtain specimens for bacteriologic testing of urine, wounds, sputum, and discontinued catheters, drains, and IV lines as indicated. Before removing catheters or urinary drains, disinfect skin around entry site, then remove. Using aseptic technique, cut off tip of catheter or drain and place in sterile container for laboratory culture.

6. Monitor vascular access to hemodialysis to ensure patency and watch for evidence of infection.

7. For kidney transplantation patients, provide antimicrobial therapy.
   a. Oral antifungals to prevent mucosal candidiasis, which commonly occurs due to immunosuppression.
   b. Antiviral medications are routinely used to prevent cytomegalovirus infection.

8. Provide regular skin care and assist with hygiene.

Maintaining Fluid Balance

1. Closely monitor intake and output, especially after kidney transplantation.
   a. Expect normal urine output to be 30 to 100 mL/hour.
   b. Report oliguria with less than 30 mL/hour or polyuria of 100 to 500 mL/hour.

2. Monitor serum electrolyte results and electrocardiogram (ECG) for changes associated with electrolyte imbalance.
   a. T-wave inversion and U waves with hypokalemia; tall peaked T waves with hyperkalemia.
   b. Report arrhythmias or other cardiac symptoms immediately.

3. Monitor BP and heart rate, central venous pressure (CVP), and pulmonary artery pressure (if indicated) to anticipate adjustment of fluid replacement.

4. Avoid using dialysis access extremity for IV lines, intra-arterial monitoring, or restraints.

5. Although rare, hemodialysis may be required in the postoperative period if the transplanted kidney does not function immediately.

Patient Education and Health Maintenance

After Nephrectomy

1. Provide information about continued recovery from surgery, including engaging in regular exercise, refraining from heavy lifting or strenuous activities, and resuming normal dietary intake.

2. Promote wearing a MedicAlert bracelet and inform all health care providers of solitary kidney status.

3. Encourage close follow-up and need to seek medical attention for any signs of urinary infection, urinary obstruction, or urinary tract disease if there is only one kidney present to prevent damage to that kidney.

After Kidney Transplantation

1. Explain and reinforce symptoms of rejection—fever, chills, sweating, lassitude, hypertension, weight gain, peripheral edema, decrease in urine output.
   a. Hyperacute rejection—occurs within minutes or hours of transplantation and is rarely treatable.
   b. Accelerated rejection—occurs 24 hours to 5 days after transplantation and is treated by plasmapheresis and IV immunoglobulin G.
   c. Acute T-cell–mediated rejection (90% of all rejection episodes)—occurs days to weeks after transplantation and is treated by IV steroids or additional immunosuppression.

d. Chronic rejection—occurs months to years after transplantation and results in slowly declining function of the allograft.

2. Observe for symptoms of urine leak, such as sudden loss of kidney function, pain over transplant site, and copious drainage of yellow fluid from the wound.

3. Explain continued protection of vascular access graft, which may still be enlarged, tender to palpation, and associated with edema of overlying tissues.

4. Encourage compliance with laboratory tests (blood urea nitrogen [BUN], creatinine, serum chemistry, hematology, bacteriology, cyclosporine, or tacrolimus levels) to monitor patient's immune status and detect early signs of rejection.

5. Instruct patient and family about prescribed immunosuppressant and complications of therapy—infection or incomplete control of rejection.
   a. Review immunosuppressive medications in detail, including color identification of pills, dose schedules, adverse effects, and the necessity for taking the medication.
   b. Review other medications, such as histamine-2 (H_2) blockers or proton pump inhibitors (PPIs), to prevent stress ulcers and prophylaxis for *Candida* and community-acquired infections.

6. Review in detail postoperative self-care regimen (may be inpatient or outpatient), including adequate fluid intake, daily weight, measurement of urine, stool test for occult blood, prevention of infection, exercise.

7. Instruct to report immediately:
   a. Decrease in urinary output.
   b. Weight gain, edema.
   c. Malaise, fever.
   d. Graft swelling and tenderness (visible and palpable below the skin).
   e. Changes in BP readings.
   f. Respiratory distress.
   g. Anxiety, depression, change in appetite or sleep.

8. Discuss with health care provider the feasibility of participating in contact sports because of the risk of trauma to the transplanted kidney.

9. Stress that follow-up care after transplantation is a lifelong necessity.

10. For additional support and information, refer to American Association of Kidney Patients (*www.aakp.org*) and the United Network for Organ Sharing (*https://unos.org*).

Evaluation: Expected Outcomes

- Verbalizes relief of pain.
- Urinary drainage clear without clots.
- Absence of fever or signs of infection.
- Vital signs stable; urine output 50 mL/hour.

Urinary Diversion

EVIDENCE BASE Wein, A. J., Kavoussi, L. R., Partin, A. W., et al. (Eds.). (2017). *Campbell-Walsh urology* (11th ed., Vols. 1–4). Philadelphia, PA: W.B. Saunders.

Urinary diversion refers to diverting the urinary stream from the bladder so that it exits by way of a new avenue. A number of operative procedures may be performed to achieve this (see Figure 21-4). Methods of urinary diversion include:

1. Ileal conduit (or "Bricker loop")—most common; transplants the ureters into an isolated section of the terminal

Types of Cutaneous Diversions

A

Conventional ileal conduit. The surgeon transplants the ureters to an isolated section of the terminal ileum (ileal conduit), bringing one end to the abdominal wall. The ureter may also be transplanted into the transverse sigmoid colon (colon conduit) or proximal jejunum (jejunal conduit).

B

Cutaneous ureterostomy. The surgeon brings the detached ureter through the abdominal wall and attaches it to an opening in the skin.

C

Vesicostomy. The surgeon sutures the bladder to the abdominal wall and creates an opening (stoma) through the abdominal and bladder walls for urinary drainage.

D

Nephrostomy. The surgeon inserts a catheter into the renal pelvis via an incision into the flank or by percutaneous catheter placement, into the kidney.

Types of Continent Urinary Diversions

A
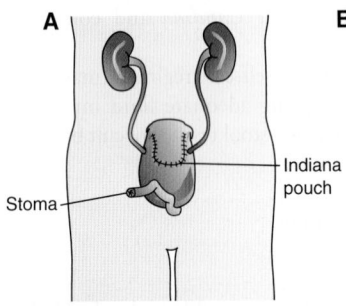

Indiana pouch. The surgeon introduces the ureters into a segment of ileum and cecum. Urine is drained periodically by inserting a catheter into the stoma.

B
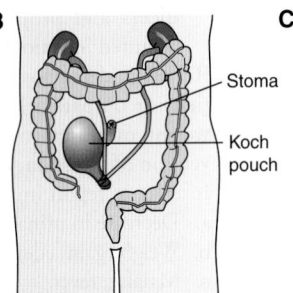

Continent ileal urinary diversions (Koch pouch). The surgeon transplants the ureters to an isolated segment of small bowel, ascending colon, or ileocolonic segment and develops an effective continence mechanism or valve. Urine is drained by inserting a catheter into the stoma.

C

In male patients, the Koch pouch can be modified by attaching one end of the pouch to the urethra, allowing more normal voiding. The female urethra is too short for this modification.

D
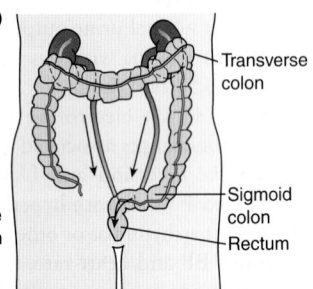

Ureterosigmoidostomy. The surgeon introduces the ureters into the sigmoid, thereby allowing urine to flow through the colon and out of the rectum.

Figure 21-4. Methods of urinary diversion. (Smeltzer, S., & Bare, B. [2000]. *Brunner and Suddarth's textbook of medical-surgical nursing* [9th ed.]. Philadelphia, PA: Lippincott Williams & Wilkins.)

ileum, bringing one end through the abdominal wall to create a stoma. Urine flows from the kidney into the ureters, then through the ileal conduit, and exits through urinary stoma. The ureters may also be transplanted into a segment of the transverse colon (colon conduit).

2. Nephrostomy—insertion of a catheter into the renal pelvis by way of an incision into the flank or by percutaneous catheter placement into the kidney. They are rarely placed for long periods of time; they are a short-term method of diverting urine away from an obstruction or lesion below the level of the renal pelvis.

3. Continent urinary diversion procedures—create a urinary reservoir from an intestinal segment that is either brought to the skin using a valve mechanism that permits catheterization or is anastomosed directly to the proximal urethra.
   a. Continent urinary reservoir (Kock pouch, Indiana pouch, Mainz pouch, and others)—transplants the ureters into a pouch created from small bowel or large and small bowel. Mechanisms to discourage ureteral reflux are used to implant the ureters into the pouch, including an intussuscepted nipple valve or tunneling the ureters through the teniae of the bowel. The existing ileocecal valve, or a surgically created intussuscepted nipple valve, provides the continence mechanism. Patient does not have to wear an external appliance, but the procedure does require intermittent self-catheterization of the pouch.
   b. Orthotopic bladder replacement (hemi-Kock pouch, neobladder, and others)—pouch created from small or large and small bowel is anastomosed to urethral stump; voiding is through the urethra. Patient usually has nocturnal incontinence; not all patients are candidates for this procedure.

Preoperative Management

1. Functional assessment should be performed including degree of manual dexterity and visual acuity along with cognitive function—essential for stoma care or self-catheterization postoperatively.

2. Patient's psychosocial resources are evaluated, including available support persons, education, occupation, and economic resources (including insurance coverage of ostomy supplies, if needed), coping strengths, attitudes toward urinary diversion.

3. Bowel preparation is performed to prevent fecal contamination during surgery and the potential complication of infection.

a. Clear liquids only and prescribed laxatives for mechanical cleansing of the bowel.

b. Antibiotics, as prescribed (nonabsorbable; active against enteric organisms), to reduce bacterial count in the bowel lumen.

4. Adequate hydration is ensured, including IV infusions, to ensure urine flow during surgery and to prevent hypovolemia.

5. The procedure is explained by the surgeon and the WOCN (wound, ostomy, continence nurse) before surgery.

a. For ileal or colon conduit, the stoma site is planned preoperatively with patient standing, sitting, and lying—to place the stoma away from bony prominences, skin creases, and scars and where the patient can see it.

b. Stoma site may also be marked even though continent urinary diversion procedure is planned, in case findings during surgery prevent continent procedure and standard ileal or colon conduit is necessary.

Postoperative Management

1. Patient is assessed for immediate postoperative complications: wound or UTI, urinary or fecal anastomotic leakage, small bowel obstruction, paralytic ileus, deep vein thrombosis, pulmonary embolism, and necrosis of stoma.

2. Intake and output are monitored including amount of urinary output, patency of drainage catheters, and degree of hematuria.

3. Pelvic gravity or suction drains are evaluated—sudden increase in drainage suggests an anastomotic leak; send specimen of drainage for creatinine, if ordered. (Presence of measurable creatinine in the drainage indicates urine in drainage, confirming a urine leak.)

4. Ureteral stents are used to protect ureterointestinal anastomoses; stents will emerge from stoma or through separate wound (stents are not visible in orthotopic bladder replacement patients). They are removed in 3 weeks.

Nursing Diagnoses

- Impaired Urinary Elimination related to urinary diversion.
- Acute Pain related to surgery.
- Disturbed Body Image related to urinary diversion.
- Sexual Dysfunction related to reconstructive surgery and impotence (in men).

Nursing Interventions

Achieving Urinary Elimination

For ileal or colon conduit patients:

1. Maintain a transparent urostomy pouch over the stoma postoperatively to allow for easy assessment.

2. Inspect the stoma for color and size; whether it is flush, nippled, or retracted; and the condition of the skin around the stoma. Document baseline information for subsequent comparison.

a. Stoma should be red, wet with mucus, soft, and slightly rubbery to the touch (stoma lacks nerve ending, so feeling in stoma is absent).

b. Cyanotic stoma indicates poor circulation.

c. Necrotic stoma is blue-black or tan-brown.

3. Report bleeding, necrosis, sloughing, suture separation.

4. Check patency of ureteral stents.

5. Keep the pouch on at all times, and observe normal urine (but not fecal) drainage at all times.

a. Connect pouches to drainage bag when patient is in bed and record urine volume hourly.

b. Initial urostomy pouch remains in place for several days postoperatively; it is changed every 3 to 4 days when patient teaching begins.

For continent urinary diversion patients:

1. Maintain patency of drainage catheters placed into internal urinary pouch during surgery; irrigate with 30 mL saline every 2 to 4 hours to prevent obstruction from mucous accumulation.

2. Assess stoma—should be very small and flush.

3. Record urine output and character of urine.

4. Monitor output of pelvic drain (on gentle suction or gravity drainage) every 8 hours.

5. Advise patient that approximately 3 weeks after surgery, the drainage catheter is removed from the pouch after a radiographic study ("pouch-o-gram") confirms healing of all anastomoses.

Controlling Pain

1. Administer analgesic medications or teach use of and monitor PCA (IV or epidural).

2. Assess response to pain control.

3. Provide positioning for comfort, alternating with ambulation, as able.

Resolving Body Image Issues

1. Assess patient's reaction to looking at new urinary stoma, if applicable; provide reassurance and support.

2. Be on the alert for difficulty coping, which may be manifested in irritability or lack of motivation to learn.

a. Give extra support until patient can cope.

b. Reinforce the concept that the stoma will be manageable.

c. Acknowledge feelings of fear and anxiety as normal.

3. Encourage patient to participate gradually in care of stoma or catheters.

4. Encourage verbalization of feelings and concerns related to urinary diversion.

5. If possible, arrange for patient to speak with another patient who has undergone the same surgery; this provides realistic expectations and support for a positive outcome.

6. Help patient and family to gain independence through learning to manage the ostomy. Provide for demonstrations, supervised practice, written instructions, and return demonstrations until patient is independent in self-care.

Coping with Sexual Dysfunction

1. Be aware that many men experience impotence as a result of surgery; provide information or referrals about options including medications, pharmacologic erection programs, and penile prostheses.

2. Allow patient to express feelings related to loss of sexual function and encourage discussion with partner.

3. Tell women that they may usually resume sexual activity after healing is complete.

Patient Education and Health Maintenance

For Ileal or Colon Conduit Patients

1. Obtain and familiarize patient with the appropriate equipment. Most urostomy pouching systems are disposable. The choice of pouch is determined by location of stoma, patient activity, body build, and economic status.

a. Two-piece pouches consist of a skin barrier (or wafer) that fits around the stoma and adheres to the skin and a pouch that snaps onto the skin barrier.

b. One-piece pouches may be precut for the correct stoma size and include the adhesive; the pouch is applied directly to the peristomal skin.

2. Assist patient to determine stoma size (for ordering correct appliance). The stoma will shrink considerably as edema subsides and the size is recalibrated several times during the first 3 to 6 weeks postoperatively.

a. Measuring guides are included with most urostomy pouches.

b. The inside diameter of the skin barrier should not be more than 1/16 inch larger than the diameter of the stoma.

3. Teach how to change the pouch.

a. Change pouch early in the morning before taking fluids or before evening meal—urine output is lower at these times.

b. Prepare the new pouching system according to manufacturer's directions.

c. Wash the peristomal skin with non–cream-based soap and water. Rinse and pat dry. *The skin must be dry or appliance will not adhere.*

d. A gauze or tissue wick may be applied over the stoma to absorb urine while the appliance is being changed. Keep the skin free from direct contact with urine. Suggest the use of tampons to soak up urine from stoma while changing pouch at home, if desired; however, do not insert into stoma.

e. Center the skin barrier directly over the stoma and apply it carefully. Apply gentle pressure around appliance for secure adherence.

f. Apply a belt to keep pouch in place, if desired; it is especially useful in patients with soft abdomens.

4. Advise that additional adhesives, such as pastes or cements, are not usually necessary with a well-fitting pouch.

5. Tell patient that frequency of pouch changes depends on the type of pouch used—generally pouches should be changed every 3 to 4 days.

6. Advise emptying the pouch when it is one third to one-half full to prevent weight of urine from loosening adhesive seal—open drain valve (spigot) for periodic emptying.

7. Teach how to attach outlet on pouch to a bedside urinary drainage container with plastic tubing (at least 5 feet to allow turning) and how to secure tubing to the leg to prevent twisting or kinking.

a. Position the drainage bottle lower than the level of the bed to enhance flow by gravity.

b. Clean nighttime drainage equipment with vinegar and water. Rinse well.

8. Advise patient to drink liberal amounts of fluids to flush the conduit free of mucus and reduce possibility of urinary infection.

9. Teach that the stoma may bleed if it is bumped or rubbed; report bleeding that continues for several hours.

10. Advise carrying spare pouches in handbag or pocket and bringing an extra pouch to every visit with health care provider.

11. Advise wearing cotton (rather than nylon) underwear or the use of specially made underwear for ostomy patients that prevents contact between plastic pouch and skin. Heavy girdles are not allowed because they may cause chafing of the stoma and prevent free flow of urine.

12. Advise reporting problems with peristomal skin or with leakage from the pouch or the development of fever, chills, pain, change in color of urine (cloudy, bloody), and diminishing urine output.

13. For additional information and support, refer to United Ostomy Associations of America (*www.ostomy.org*).

For Continent Ileal Urinary Reservoir Patients

1. Teach irrigation of catheter; this must be done every 4 to 6 hours at home.

2. Teach how to change stoma dressing.

3. Instruct in use of leg bag or bedside urinary drainage bag while catheter remains in place.

4. Teach how to catheterize continent urinary diversion when healing is verified:

a. Red rubber or plastic, straight, or coudé catheters are used.

b. Apply a small amount of water-soluble lubricant to the tip of the catheter.

c. Use clean technique; wash hands before each catheterization.

d. Maintain schedule of catheterizations during initial "training" period to allow the pouch to adapt gradually to holding larger amounts of urine (every 2 hours during day and every 3 hours at night; increase by 1 hour each week for 5 weeks).

e. After training period, catheterize four to five times per day; pouch should not hold more than 400 to 500 mL.

f. Irrigate pouch with saline through catheter once per day to clear it of accumulated mucus.

5. Teach patient to report problems such as leakage of urine from stoma between catheterizations.

6. Tell patient to shower or bathe normally, wear normal clothing; only a small dressing or an adhesive bandage needs to be worn over the stoma.

7. Advise patient to drink 8 to 10 glasses of water daily.

For Orthotopic Bladder Replacement

1. Teach patient to irrigate Foley catheter that will stay in place for 3 weeks after surgery; irrigate with 30 mL saline every 4 to 6 hours.

2. Instruct in use of leg bag or bedside drainage bag while catheter remains in place.

3. Instruct on how to change dressing.

4. After healing of pouch is confirmed and catheter is removed, teach patient to "void."

a. Voiding is accomplished by abdominal straining; mucus is expected in voided urine.

b. Voiding schedule must be maintained for the first 5 to 6 weeks (every 2 hours during day and every 3 hours at night; increase by 1 hour each week).

c. Incontinence is anticipated after catheter is removed; usually more pronounced when patient is asleep and muscles are relaxed.

5. Teach patient to perform pelvic floor exercises, which must be done faithfully for the rest of his or her life; as pelvic floor sphincter muscles strengthen, incontinence subsides. Most patients continue to have small amounts of nocturnal incontinence.

a. Contract pelvic floor muscles (as if stopping stream of urine or flatus) for 5 seconds; then, relax for 5 to 10 seconds.

b. Repeat approximately 15 to 20 times for one set, and do three sets per day.

c. May require referral to physical therapist to assist in the process.

6. Provide information about absorbent products that may be used temporarily; also, teach about preventive skin care.

7. Instruct in clean self-catheterization, which may be needed if the urethra becomes obstructed with mucus; pouch should be irrigated with saline if catheterization is necessary.

8. Reassure patient that time, patience, and continued adherence to voiding and exercise schedule will result in continence.

Evaluation: Expected Outcomes

- Urine draining by way of urinary diversion.
- Verbalizes good pain control.
- Discusses feelings about change in body image; seeks support through family.
- Verbalizes reasonable expectations about sexual function.

Prostatic Surgery

Prostatic surgery may be done for benign prostatic hyperplasia (BPH) or prostate cancer. Surgical approach depends on size of the gland, severity of obstruction, age, underlying health, and prostatic disease.

Surgical Procedures

 EVIDENCE BASE Wein, A. J., Kavoussi, L. R., Partin, A. W., et al. (Eds.). (2017). *Campbell-Walsh urology* (11th ed., Vols. 1–4). Philadelphia, PA: W.B. Saunders.

1. TURP (formerly the most common procedure) is done without an incision by means of endoscopic instrument.
2. Photovaporization of the prostate (PVP) is starting to replace TURP; it is done through a cystoscope, using a laser to vaporize diseased prostatic tissue.
3. Transurethral microwave thermotherapy (TUMT) of the prostate and transurethral needle ablation (TUNA) of the prostate are both office-based procedures that use heat to destroy diseased prostatic tissue.
4. Indigo interstitial laser therapy of the prostate is another procedure that is done on an outpatient basis.
5. Open prostatectomy.
   a. Suprapubic—incision into suprapubic area and through bladder wall; commonly done for BPH.
   b. Perineal—incision between the scrotum and rectal area; may be done for poor surgical risk patients, but causes highest incidence of urinary incontinence and impotence.
   c. Radical retropubic—incision at the level of symphysis pubis; may preserve nerves responsible for sexual function; done for prostate cancer.
6. Robotic radical prostatectomy uses a laparoscopic approach for removal of cancerous prostate.

Preoperative Management

1. Information about the procedure and the expected postoperative care, including catheter drainage, irrigation, and monitoring of hematuria, is discussed.
2. Complications of surgery are discussed.
   a. For radical and laparoscopic prostatectomy, incontinence or dribbling of urine may occur for up to 1 year after surgery; pelvic floor (Kegel) exercises help regain urinary control.
   b. For TURP and PVP, retrograde ejaculation—seminal fluid released into the bladder and eliminated in the urine rather than through the urethra during intercourse occurs in 75% or patients; impotence is usually not a complication but occurs in 5% to 10% of TURP and PVP patients

and can be as high as 75% in those undergoing radical prostatectomy.
3. Bowel preparation is given or patient is instructed in home administration and fasting after midnight.
4. Optimal cardiac, respiratory, and circulatory status should be achieved to decrease risk of complications.
5. Prophylactic antibiotics are ordered.

Postoperative Management

1. Urinary drainage is maintained and observed for signs of hemorrhage.
2. Wound care is provided to prevent infection.
3. Pain is controlled and early ambulation is promoted.
4. Surveillance is maintained for complications.
   a. Wound infection and dehiscence.
   b. Urinary obstruction or infection.
   c. Hemorrhage.
   d. Thrombophlebitis, deep vein thrombosis, and pulmonary embolism.
   e. Urinary incontinence, sexual dysfunction.

Nursing Diagnoses

- Impaired Urinary Elimination related to surgical procedure and urinary catheter.
- Risk for Infection related to surgical incision, immobility, and urinary catheter.
- Acute Pain related to surgical procedure.
- Anxiety related to urinary incontinence, difficulty voiding, and erectile dysfunction.

Nursing Interventions

Facilitating Urinary Drainage

1. Maintain patency of urethral catheter placed after surgery.
   a. For TURP and open prostatectomy for BPH, monitor flow of three-way closed irrigation and drainage system (see Figure 21-5) if used. Continuous irrigation helps prevent clot formation, which can obstruct catheter, cause painful bladder spasms, and lead to infection.
   b. If Foley is obstructed and with a health care provider order, manually irrigate with 50 to 60 mL irrigating fluid using aseptic technique.
   c. Avoid overdistention of the bladder, which could lead to hemorrhage.
   d. Administer anticholinergic medications to reduce bladder spasms, as ordered.
2. Assess degree of hematuria and any clot formation; drainage should become light pink within 24 hours.
   a. Report bright red bleeding with increased viscosity (arterial)—may require surgical intervention.
   b. Report increase in dark red bleeding (venous)—may require traction of the catheter so the inflated balloon applies pressure to prostatic fossa.
   c. Prepare for blood transfusion if bleeding persists.
3. Administer IV fluids, as ordered, and encourage oral fluids when tolerated to ensure hydration and urine output.

 DRUG ALERT Anticholinergic medications are contraindicated in patients with narrow angle-closure glaucoma.

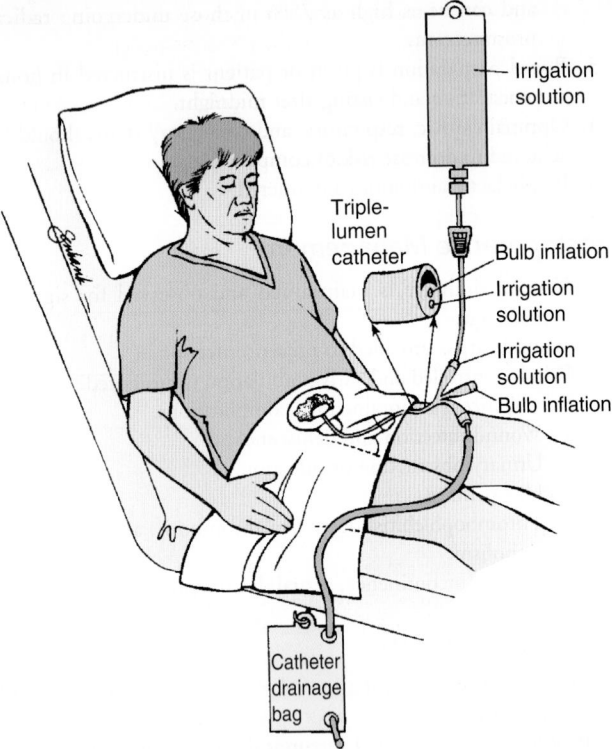

Figure 21-5. A three-way system for bladder irrigation. (Smeltzer, S., & Bare, B. [2000]. *Brunner and Suddarth's textbook of medical-surgical nursing* [9th ed.]. Philadelphia, PA: Lippincott Williams & Wilkins.)

Preventing Infection

1. After open prostatectomy, provide frequent monitoring of vital signs, intake and output, and observation of incisional dressing, if present.
2. Encourage ambulation to prevent venous thrombosis, pulmonary embolism, and pneumonia.
3. Observe urine for cloudiness or odor and obtain urine for evaluation of infection, as ordered.
4. Administer antibiotics, as prescribed.
5. Report testicular pain, swelling, and tenderness, which could indicate epididymitis from spreading infection.
6. Assist with perineal care if perineal incision is present to prevent contamination by feces.

Relieving Pain

1. Administer pain medication or monitor PCA, as directed.
2. Position patient for comfort and tell him or her to avoid straining, which will increase pelvic venous congestion and may cause hemorrhage.
3. Administer stool softeners to prevent discomfort from constipation.
4. Make sure catheter is secured to patient's thigh and tubing is not creating traction on catheter, which will cause pain and potential hemorrhage.

 NURSING ALERT Avoid rectal temperatures, enemas, or rectal tubes postoperatively to prevent hemorrhage or disruption of healing.

Reducing Anxiety

1. Provide realistic expectations about postoperative discomfort and overall progress.

a. Tell patient to avoid sexual intercourse, straining at stool, heavy lifting, and long periods of sitting for 6 to 8 weeks after surgery.
b. Advise follow-up visits after treatment because urethral stricture or bladder neck contracture may occur.
2. Reassure patient that urinary incontinence and frequency, urgency, and dysuria are expected after removal of catheter and should gradually subside.
3. Reassure patient that there may be measures to help.
4. Reinforce the risks for impotence as told by the surgeon. Remind patient that erectile function may not return for 12 months.
5. Encourage patient to express fears and anxieties related to potential loss of sexual function and to discuss concerns with partner.
6. Advise that options are available to restore sexual function if impotence persists.

Patient Education and Health Maintenance

1. Advise patient that PVP is commonly done on an outpatient basis; patient may go home the evening of surgery.
2. Reinforce instructions provided on catheter care, maintaining patency, and catheter irrigation.
   a. For open, radical, and laparoscopic prostatectomy patients, the catheter will be removed in 2 to 3 weeks. A cystogram may be performed to confirm healing of anastomosis prior to removing catheter.
   b. Advise that stress incontinence may occur after catheter is removed and is more pronounced when abdominal pressure is increased, such as with coughing, laughing, straining.
   c. For patients who experience urgency before surgery, caution that they may have urge incontinence for several weeks postoperatively.
   d. Discuss the use of absorbent products to contain urine leakage around catheter and after catheter is removed.
3. Teach measures to regain urinary control. Teach patient to perform pelvic floor exercises correctly. Have patient squeeze the pelvic floor muscles (as if stopping stream of urine or flatus) for 5 seconds and then relax for 5 to 10 seconds. This should be done 15 to 20 times, three times per day. Caution against using abdominal muscles (straining or Valsalva maneuver), which increases incontinence.
4. Reinforce availability of options such as medications for urinary urgency and oral medicine such as sildenafil, vacuum erectile device, penile injections, and penile prosthesis to restore sexual function.
5. Encourage prostate cancer patients to have a PSA blood test 3 months after surgery and yearly thereafter.

Evaluation: Expected Outcomes

- Clear yellow drainage by way of catheter.
- Incision without drainage; afebrile.
- Verbalizes good pain relief.
- Verbalizes realistic expectations for urinary and sexual functioning.

RENAL AND UROLOGIC DISORDERS
Acute Kidney Injury

Acute kidney injury (AKI) is a clinical syndrome in which there is a sudden decline in renal function. This results in disturbances in fluid and electrolyte balance, acid–base homeostasis, blood pressure regulation, erythropoiesis, and mineral metabolism. It is frequently associated with an increase in BUN and creatinine, oliguria, hyperkalemia, and sodium and fluid retention.

Pathophysiology and Etiology

Causes

See Figure 21-6.

1. Prerenal causes—result from conditions that decrease renal blood flow (hypovolemia, shock, hemorrhage, burns, impaired cardiac output, diuretic therapy, and renal artery disorders).
2. Intrarenal causes—result from injury to renal tissue and are usually associated with intrarenal ischemia, toxins, immunologic processes, systemic disorders, trauma, and vascular disorders.
3. Postrenal causes—arise from obstruction or disruption to urine flow anywhere along the urinary tract.

Clinical Course

1. Onset: begins when the kidney is injured and lasts from hours to days.
2. Oliguric–anuric phase: urine volume less than 400 to 500 mL/24 hours.
   a. Accompanied by rise in serum concentration of elements usually excreted by the kidney (urea, creatinine, organic acids, and the intracellular cations—potassium and magnesium).
   b. In approximately 50% patients with AKI, urine output remains greater than 500 cc/day. This is called nonoliguric

AKI. These patients often have less complications and better prognosis for recovery than oliguric patient.
3. Diuretic phase
   a. Characterized by high urine output because of the kidney's inability to concentrate urine.
   b. Close monitoring of fluid volume and electrolytes is essential.
4. Recovery phase.
   a. Usually lasts several months to 1 year.
   b. Complete recovery of renal function may occur or they may be some residual deficits because of scarring of kidney tissue.
   c. Avoiding secondary insults to the kidney, such as nephrotoxic drugs, contrast dye, hypotension, and infection, is important to minimize permanent kidney damage.

Clinical Manifestations

1. Prerenal—signs and symptoms consistent with hypovolemia may be present such as decreased tissue turgor, dryness of mucous membranes, weight loss, hypotension, oliguria or anuria, reduced jugular venous distention, and tachycardia. However, if the prerenal cause is related to vasodilation, third spacing of fluid, or cardiovascular disease, signs/symptoms of increased extracellular fluid may be present.
2. Intrarenal—presentation based on the cause; edema usually present.

Prerenal
- Dehydration
- Shock
- Heart failure
- Burns
- Sepsis

Intrarenal
- Acute tubular necrosis
- Acute glomerulonephritis
- Diabetes
- Interstitial nephritis

Postrenal
- Urolithiasis
- Tumor
- Benign prostatic hyperplasia
- Ureteral stricture
- Neurogenic bladder
- Bladder outlet obstruction

Figure 21-6. Causes of acute renal failure.

3. Postrenal—findings may include a distended bladder, an abdominal mass, and an enlarged prostate. Renal colic may be present with nephrolithiasis.

Diagnostic Evaluation

1. Urinalysis—reveals proteinuria, hematuria, casts, increased WBC and nitrate (possible infection), glycosuria, and pH. Also can give clues of hydration status (specific gravity).
2. Rising serum creatinine and BUN levels.
3. Urine chemistry examinations to help distinguish various forms of acute renal failure.
4. Renal ultrasonography—for estimate of renal size, to evaluate for masses, and to exclude a treatable obstructive uropathy.
5. CT/MRI to evaluate for masses or vascular disorders and renal angiography to evaluate for renal artery stenosis.
6. Renal biopsy in selected cases of unexplained proteinuria.

Management

Preventive Measures

1. Identify patients with preexisting renal disease.
2. Initiate adequate hydration before, during, and after any procedure requiring NPO status.
3. Avoid exposure to nephrotoxins. Be aware that many drugs or their metabolites are excreted by the kidneys.
4. Prevent and treat shock with blood and fluid replacement. Prevent prolonged periods of hypotension.
5. Close monitoring of urinary output and hydration status (CVP, edema, pulmonary exam) in critically ill patients.
6. Ensure adequate hydration if contrast dye studies are indicated and attempt to avoid scheduling consecutive dye studies. Patients at most risk for contrast-induced nephropathy (CIN) are those with baseline renal impairment, diabetes, elderly patients, and patients with heart failure.
7. Avoid infections; give meticulous care to patients with indwelling catheters and IV lines.
8. Take every precaution to make sure that the right person receives the right blood to avoid severe transfusion reactions, which can precipitate renal complications.

 DRUG ALERT Nonsteroidal anti-inflammatory drugs (NSAIDs) may reduce glomerular filtration rate in people at risk for renal insufficiency, causing renal failure.

Corrective and Supportive Measures

1. Correct reversible cause of acute renal failure (eg, improve renal perfusion, maximize cardiac output, surgical relief of obstruction).
2. Be alert for and correct underlying fluid excesses or deficits.
3. Correct and control acid/base and electrolyte imbalances: hyperkalemia, hypocalcemia, hyperphosphatemia, and metabolic acidosis.
4. Restore and maintain MAP greater than 65.
5. Support nutrition.
6. Adjust renally excreted medication dosages/frequency. Timing of medications may also be adjusted in patient receiving intermittent hemodialysis.
7. Initiate hemodialysis, peritoneal dialysis, or CRRT if indicated.

Complications

1. Infection.
2. Metabolic acidosis.
3. Anemia.

4. Arrhythmias because of electrolyte imbalances including hyperkalemia, hypocalcemia, and metabolic acidosis.
5. Electrolyte and mineral (sodium, potassium, calcium, phosphorus, magnesium) abnormalities.
6. Hypervolemic complications: pulmonary edema and HTN.
7. GI bleeding because of stress ulcers and platelet abnormalities.
8. Multiple organ system failure.

Nursing Assessment

1. Determine if there is a history of cardiac disease, hypovolemia, trauma, malignancy, sepsis, benign prostatic hypertrophy, abdominal tumors, kidney stones, or intercurrent illness.
2. Determine if patient has been exposed to potentially nephrotoxic drugs (antibiotics, NSAIDs, contrast agents, solvents).
3. Conduct an ongoing physical examination for tissue turgor, pallor, alterations in mucous membranes, BP, heart rate changes, pulmonary edema, and peripheral edema.
4. Monitor intake and output.

Nursing Diagnoses

- Risk for Imbalanced Fluid Volume.
- Risk for Electrolyte Imbalance related to kidney injury.
- Risk for Infection related to alterations in the immune system and host defenses.
- Imbalanced Nutrition: Less Than Body Requirements related to catabolic state, anorexia, and malnutrition associated with acute kidney injury.
- Risk for Bleeding related to GI mucosal irritation and altered platelet function.
- Acute Confusion related to the effects of uremic toxins on the central nervous system (CNS).
- Knowledge deficit of disease, treatment, prognosis, and monitoring.

Nursing Interventions

Monitoring and Maintaining Fluid Balance

See Table 21-2.

1. Monitor for signs and symptoms of hypervolemia.
   a. Crackles on auscultation of lungs; engorged neck veins (jugular venous distention); periorbital edema; ascites; edema of extremities/sacrum.
   b. Elevated blood pressure.
   c. Elevated CVP.
2. Assess for evidence of hypovolemia.
   a. Dry mucous membranes; poor skin turgor.
   b. Hypotension; orthostatic blood pressure changes.
3. Monitor urinary output and urine specific gravity, as ordered; measure and record intake and output including urine, gastric suction, stool, and wound drainage.
4. Monitor serum and urine electrolyte concentrations.
5. Weigh patient daily to provide an index of fluid balance.
6. Adjust fluid intake to avoid volume overload and volume depletion.
   a. Fluid restriction is usually initiated in oliguric patients.
   b. During oliguric–anuric phase, give only enough fluids to replace losses (usually 400 to 500 mL/24 hours plus measured fluid losses).
   c. Fluid allowance should be distributed throughout the day.
   d. Restrict salt and water intake if there is evidence of extracellular excess.
7. Provide patient education on fluid and sodium restriction, if indicated.

Table 21-2 Signs and Symptoms of Fluid and Electrolyte Imbalances

	DEFICIT	EXCESS
Volume	Acute weight loss (>5%), drop in body temperature, dry skin and mucous membranes, postural hypotension, longitudinal wrinkles or furrows of tongue, oliguria or anuria	Acute weight gain (>5%), edema, hypertension, distended neck veins, dyspnea, rales
Sodium	Abdominal cramps, muscle weakness, apprehension, convulsions, hypotension and tachycardia, oliguria or anuria	Agitation, muscle irritability, dry, sticky mucous membranes, HTN, tachycardia, edema, dyspnea, thirst, rough and dry tongue, increased viscosity of saliva
Potassium	Anorexia, abdominal distention, intestinal ileus, muscle weakness, tenderness, and cramps; dizziness, hypotension, cardiac arrhythmias	Diarrhea, intestinal colic, irritability, nausea, muscle weakness, flaccid paralysis, cardiac arrhythmias and arrest
Calcium	Irritability, laryngospasm, positive Chvostek and Trousseau signs, tingling of extremities, tetany	Lethargy, mental confusion, anorexia, nausea, vomiting, abdominal pain and distention, constipation, bone pain
Bicarbonate	Deep, rapid breathing (Kussmaul), shortness of breath on exertion, stupor, weakness (metabolic acidosis)	Depressed respirations, muscle hypertonicity, tetany (metabolic alkalosis)
Magnesium	Positive Chvostek sign, seizures, disorientation, seizures, hyperactive deep tendon reflexes, dysrhythmias	Hypotension, bradycardia, lethargy, hypoactive deep tendon reflexes, respiratory depression

Maintaining Electrolyte and Acid–Base Balance

1. Monitor and replace serum electrolytes ordered.
   a. Evaluate for signs and symptoms of hyperkalemia (see table above).
   b. Notify health care provider of value above 5.5 mg/L.
   c. Watch for ECG changes—tall, tented T waves; depressed ST segment; wide QRS complex.
   d. Administer sodium bicarbonate or glucose and insulin to shift potassium into the cells, as ordered.
   e. Administer cation exchange resin (sodium polystyrene sulfonate) orally or rectally to provide more prolonged correction of elevated potassium, as ordered.
   f. Instruct patient about the importance of following prescribed diet, avoiding foods high in potassium.
   g. Prepare for dialysis when rapid lowering of potassium is needed.
   h. Administer blood transfusions *during* dialysis to prevent hyperkalemia from stored blood.
2. Monitor acid–base status as directed.
   a. Arterial blood gas (ABG) or venous blood gas.
   b. CO_2 on chemistry panel approximates ABG bicarbonate level.
3. Prepare for ventilator therapy if severe acidosis is present.
4. Administer oral alkalizing medications or IV sodium bicarbonate as ordered.
5. Be prepared to implement dialysis for uncontrolled acidosis.

Preventing and Monitoring for Infection

1. Monitor for signs of infection.
2. Remove bladder catheter as soon as possible; monitor for UTI.
3. Use intensive pulmonary hygiene—high incidence of lung edema and infection.
4. Carry out meticulous wound care.
5. If antibiotics are administered, care must be taken to adjust the dosage for renal impairment.

Maintaining Adequate Nutrition

1. Work collaboratively with dietitian to direct nutritional support.
2. Protein sources should be of high biologic value—rich in essential amino acids (fish, eggs, meat)—so that the patient does not rely on tissue catabolism for essential amino acids.
3. Encourage small frequent meals if the patient is experiencing nausea or reflux symptoms.

4. Weigh patient daily.
5. Monitor BUN, creatinine, electrolytes, serum albumin, prealbumin, total protein, and transferrin.
6. Be aware that food and fluids containing large amounts of sodium, potassium, and phosphorus may need to be restricted.

Monitoring For and Preventing GI Bleeding

1. Examine all stools and emesis for gross and occult blood.
2. Administer H_2-receptor antagonist or PPIs, as directed as prophylaxis for gastric stress ulcers. If an H_2-receptor antagonist is used, care must be taken to adjust the dose for the degree of renal impairment.
3. Prepare for endoscopy when GI bleeding occurs.

Monitoring Cognition and Orientation

1. Speak to the patient in simple orienting statements, using repetition when necessary.
2. Monitor for and report mental status changes—somnolence, lassitude, lethargy, and fatigue progressing to irritability, disorientation, twitching, seizures.
3. Use seizure precautions—padded side rails and airway and suction equipment at bedside, if indicated.
4. Prepare for dialysis, which may help prevent confusion related to uremia.

Patient Education and Health Maintenance

1. Explain to patient that he/she may have residual defects in kidney function and that AKI puts him/her at increased risk for CKD.
2. Educate patient on importance of follow-up with their provider for ongoing monitoring of renal function.
3. Advise avoidance of any medications unless specifically prescribed.
4. Provide education on means to slow the progression of kidney disease in patient with residual deficits in kidney function.
   a. Avoid or minimize exposure to nephrotoxins such as NSAIDs, radiocontrast dye, some antibiotics, some chemotherapeutic agents, and some anticonvulsants.
   b. Maintain good blood pressure control (target HgbA1c of 7).
   c. Monitor for and aggressively treat UTIs.
   d. Avoid intravascular volume depletion.
   e. Smoking cessation.
   f. Low-sodium diet.
   g. Maintain healthy BMI (20 to 25 kg/m^2).

Evaluation: Expected Outcomes

- BP stable; no edema or shortness of breath.
- Serum electrolytes and arterial blood gas values within normal range.
- No signs of infection.
- Adequate caloric intake, stable weight, and normal total protein and albumin level.
- Stool negative for occult; Hgb level stable.
- Alert and oriented × 3.

Chronic Kidney Disease

Chronic kidney disease (CKD) is a progressive deterioration of renal function, which, if left untreated, eventually results in death because of uremia (an excess of urea and other nitrogenous wastes in the blood) and its complications. The treatment for end-stage renal disease (ESRD) is dialysis or kidney transplantation. According to the National Kidney Foundation, approximately 30 million Americans have some type of CKD. Most cases are asymptomatic until later stages and most people die from other comorbidities (ie, cardiac disease, DM) before reaching ESRD.

Pathophysiology and Etiology

Causes

1. Hypertension.
2. Diabetes mellitus.
3. Glomerulopathies (from lupus or other disorders).
4. Interstitial nephritis.
5. Hereditary renal disease, polycystic disease.
6. Obstructive uropathy.
7. Developmental or congenital disorder.

Clinical Course and Consequences of Decreasing Renal Function

1. Rate of progression varies based on underlying cause and severity of that condition.
2. Stages 1 to 5 based on glomerular filtration rate (GFR); stage 5 is most severe: end-stage renal disease.
3. Retention of sodium and water causes volume overload, which can lead to edema, heart failure, hypertension, and HTN.
4. Metabolic acidosis results from the kidney's inability to excrete hydrogen ions, produce ammonia, and conserve bicarbonate.
5. Decreased GFR causes increase in serum phosphate with reciprocal decrease in serum calcium, which can lead to bone demineralization.
6. Erythropoietin production by the kidney decreases, causing anemia.
7. Uremia affects the CNS, which, if left untreated, can cause altered cognitive function, personality changes, seizures, and coma.

Clinical Manifestations

1. GI—anorexia, metallic taste in the mouth, nausea, vomiting, diarrhea, constipation, ulceration of GI tract, and hemorrhage.
2. Cardiovascular—hyperkalemic ECG changes, hypertension, pericarditis, pericardial effusion, pericardial tamponade.
3. Respiratory—pulmonary edema, pleural effusions, pleural rub.
4. Neuromuscular—fatigue, sleep disorders, headache, lethargy, muscular irritability, peripheral neuropathy, seizures, coma.
5. Metabolic and endocrine—changes in insulin metabolism, decreased vitamin D_3 levels (resulting in decreased calcium absorption), secondary hyperparathyroidism (high parathyroid hormone levels), hyperlipidemia, sex hormone disturbances causing decreased libido, impotence, amenorrhea.
6. Electrolyte and acid–base disturbances—metabolic acidosis, hyperkalemia, hypermagnesemia, hypocalcemia (see page 605).
7. Dermatologic—pallor, hyperpigmentation, pruritus, ecchymosis, uremic frost (deposits of urate crystals on the skin from untreated ESRD).
8. Skeletal abnormalities—bone demineralization from metabolic acidosis and renal osteodystrophy.
9. Hematologic—anemia, impaired platelet function causing increased bleeding tendencies, and white blood cell dysfunction, resulting in a state of immunosuppression.
10. Psychosocial functions—personality and behavior changes, alteration in cognitive processes.

Diagnostic Evaluation

1. CBC for anemia.
2. Elevated serum creatinine, BUN, phosphorus, potassium.
3. Decreased serum calcium, bicarbonate, and proteins, especially albumin.
4. ABG levels—metabolic acidosis: low blood pH, low carbon dioxide, low bicarbonate.
5. Spot urine for protein/creatinine ratio. Findings can be validated with 24-hour urine collection.

Management

The goal is to conserve renal function as long as possible and prevent complications.

1. Detection and treatment of underlying causes of renal failure (eg, glycemic control, optimal blood pressure management).
2. Dietary regulation—protein restriction may be beneficial prior to initiation of dialysis to minimize uremic symptoms. Other dietary restrictions include sodium, potassium, and phosphorus restrictions and possible fluid restriction (ESRD).
3. Treatment of associated conditions:
   a. Anemia—erythropoiesis-stimulating agents, such as epoetin alfa and darbepoetin; PO or IV iron administration.
   b. Acidosis—replacement of bicarbonate stores by oral administration of sodium bicarbonate.
   c. Hyperkalemia—restriction of dietary potassium; administration of cation exchange resin.
   d. Phosphate retention and hypocalcemia—dietary PO_4 restriction, administration of phosphate-binding agents; IV or PO vitamin D_3 or vitamin D_3 analogs.
4. Prevent fluid overload through sodium and fluid restriction. May give diuretics pre-ESRD.
5. Maintenance dialysis or kidney transplantation when symptoms can no longer be controlled with conservative management.
6. Provide patient education on lifestyle measures to help slow progression of CKD (see AKI, page 602).

Complications

1. Cardiovascular events (ie, myocardial infarction, heart failure, cerebral vascular accident)—leading cause of death in patients with CKD.
2. Bleeding: GI bleeding; vascular access bleeding in ESRD.
3. Infection: pulmonary, urinary, and systemic; access related.

Nursing Assessment

1. Obtain history of chronic disorders and underlying health status.
2. Assess degree of renal impairment and involvement of other body systems by obtaining a review of systems and reviewing laboratory results.

3. Perform a thorough physical examination, including vital signs, cardiovascular, pulmonary, GI, neurologic, dermatologic, and musculoskeletal systems.
4. Assess psychosocial response to disease process including availability of resources and support network.

Nursing Diagnoses

- Excess Fluid Volume related to disease process.
- Imbalanced Nutrition: Less Than Body Requirements related to anorexia, nausea, vomiting, and restricted diet.
- Impaired Skin Integrity related to changes in oil and sweat glands and retained skin pigments.
- Constipation related to fluid restriction and ingestion of phosphate-binding agents.
- Risk for Injury because of hemodynamic instability, increased bleeding tendency, muscle cramps, and altered cognition.
- Ineffective Therapeutic Regimen Management related to difficulty making lifestyle changes related to diet, medication regimen, and dialysis treatment schedule or medical appointments.

Nursing Interventions

Maintaining Fluid and Electrolyte Balance
See interventions related to AKI, page 604.

Maintaining Adequate Nutritional Status
See interventions related to AKI, page 605.

Maintaining Skin Integrity
1. Keep skin clean while relieving itching and dryness.
   a. Soap for sensitive skin.
   b. Oatmeal baths.
   c. Bath oil added to bathwater.
2. Apply ointments or creams for comfort and to relieve itching.
3. Keep nails short and trimmed to prevent excoriation.
4. Keep hair clean and moisturized.
5. Administer antihistamines for relief of itching, if indicated, but discourage patient from taking any OTC drugs without discussing with health care provider.

Preventing Constipation
1. Encourage high-fiber diet, bearing in mind the potassium content of some fruits and vegetables, such as apricots, dried fruit, and potato skins.
2. Medications.
   a. Commercial fiber supplements may be prescribed.
   b. Use stool softeners, as prescribed.
   c. Avoid laxatives and cathartics that cause electrolyte toxicities (compounds containing magnesium or phosphorus).
3. Increase activity as tolerated.

Prevent Injury
1. Inspect patient's gait, range of motion, and muscle strength.
2. Administer analgesics, as ordered, and provide massage/heat/IV fluid for severe muscle cramps.
3. Increase activity as tolerated—avoid immobilization because it increases bone demineralization.
4. Check orthostatic blood pressures. Alert provider to orthostatic BP changes and tachycardia.
5. Monitor for signs and symptoms of bleeding.

Increasing Understanding of and Compliance with Treatment Regimen
1. Prepare patient for dialysis or kidney transplantation.
2. Offer hope while providing realistic expectations.
3. Assess patient's understanding of treatment regimen as well as concerns and fears.
4. Explore alternatives that may reduce or eliminate adverse effects of treatment.
   a. Adjust schedule so rest can be achieved after dialysis.
   b. Offer smaller, more frequent meals to reduce nausea and facilitate taking medication.
5. Encourage strengthening of social support system and coping mechanisms to lessen the impact of the stress of CKD.
6. Provide social work and nutritionist referral.
7. Contract with patient for behavioral changes if noncompliant with therapy.
8. Discuss option of supportive psychotherapy for depression or anxiety.
9. Promote decision-making by patient.
10. Refer patients and family members to renal support agencies.

Patient Education and Health Maintenance

1. To promote adherence to the therapeutic program, teach the following:
   a. Weigh self every morning to monitor for fluid overload.
   b. Fluid restriction requirements.
   c. Methods to adhere to fluid restrictions: measure allotted fluids and save some for ice cubes. Thirst-quenching strategies: sucking on ice; sugarless candy or gum; frozen grapes; rinsing mouth with water; avoiding high-sodium intake.
2. For further information and support, refer to the National Kidney Foundation (*www.kidney.org*).
3. Encourage all people in the following at-risk patient groups to obtain screening for CKD: older adults, Native Americans, African Americans, Latinos, people with diabetes, people with hypertension, those with autoimmune disease, and those with family history of kidney disease. More information on the National Kidney Foundation's Clinical Practice Guidelines for Chronic Kidney Disease can be obtained from *www.kidney. org/professionals/kdoqi/index.cfm*.

Evaluation: Expected Outcomes

- BP stable; no excessive weight gain.
- Tolerates small meals and adheres to protein restriction.
- No skin excoriation; reports relief of itching.
- Regular soft bowel movements.
- Ambulates without falls.
- Asks questions and reads education materials about CKD and its treatment.

Acute Glomerulonephritis

Acute *glomerulonephritis* (GN) refers to a group of kidney diseases in which there is an inflammatory reaction in the glomeruli because of an immunologic mechanism.

Pathophysiology and Etiology

1. Occurs after an infection elsewhere in the body or may develop secondary to systemic disorders.
2. An antigen–antibody reaction produces immune complexes that lodge in the glomeruli, producing thickening of and damage to the glomerular basement membrane; the renal vasculature, interstitium, and tubular epithelium may also be affected.

3. Immune complexes activate a variety of secondary mediators, such as complement pathways, neutrophils, macrophages, prostaglandins, and leukotrienes. These affect vascular tone and permeability, resulting in tissue injury.
4. Eventual scarring and loss of filtering surface may lead to renal failure.

Clinical Manifestations

1. Mild disease is frequently discovered accidentally through a routine urinalysis.
2. Pharyngitis or impetigo from group A streptococcus (if postinfectious GN).
3. Tea-colored urine, oliguria.
4. Periorbital edema, edema of extremities.
5. Fatigue and anorexia.
6. Hypertension, headache.

Diagnostic Evaluation

1. Urinalysis for hematuria (microscopic or gross), proteinuria, cellular elements, and various casts.
2. Twenty-four–hour urine for protein (increased) and creatinine clearance (may be reduced) outline the degree of renal function.
3. Elevated BUN and serum creatinine levels, low albumin level, increased antistreptolysin titer (increased in postinfectious GN from reaction to streptococcal organism) and, in some cases, decreased serum complement.
4. Needle biopsy of the kidney reveals obstruction of glomerular capillaries from proliferation of endothelial cells.

Management

1. Management is symptomatic and includes antihypertensives, diuretics, drugs for management of hyperkalemia, H_2 blockers, and phosphate-binding agents.
2. Antibiotic therapy is initiated to eliminate infection (if still present).
3. Fluid intake is restricted.
4. Potassium and sodium intake is restricted in presence of hyperkalemia, edema, or signs of heart failure.

Complications

1. Hypertension and heart failure.
2. Endocarditis can occur in postinfectious GN.
3. Fluid and electrolyte imbalances: hyperkalemia, hyperphosphatemia, hypocalcemia, hypervolemia.
4. Malnutrition.
5. Hypertensive encephalopathy and seizures.
6. ESRD.

Nursing Assessment

1. Obtain medical history; focus on recent infections or symptoms of chronic immunologic disorders (systemic lupus erythematosus, scleroderma).
2. Assess urine specimen for blood, protein, color, and amount.
3. Perform physical examination, specifically looking for signs of edema, hypertension, and hypervolemia (engorged neck veins, elevated jugular venous pressure, adventitious lung sounds, gallop rhythm).
4. Evaluate ECG and serum laboratory values for electrolyte imbalance.

Nursing Diagnoses

- Imbalanced Nutrition: Less Than Body Requirements related catabolic state, anorexia, and malnutrition related to acute glomerulonephritis.
- Excess Fluid Volume related to sodium retention and decreased glomerular filtration rate.

Nursing Interventions

Maintaining Adequate Nutritional Status
See interventions related to AKI, page 605.

Improving Fluid Balance
1. Carefully monitor fluid balance: strict intake and output and replace fluids according to patient's fluid losses (urine, feces, other drainage, and take into account insensible loss if rapid breathing or sweating) and record daily body weight, as prescribed.
2. Monitor pulmonary artery pressure and CVP during acute hospitalizations.
3. Monitor for signs and symptoms of heart failure: distended neck veins, tachycardia, gallop rhythm, enlarged and tender liver, crackles at bases of lungs.
4. Monitor for hypertension; observe for hypertensive encephalopathy and any evidence of seizure activity.

 NURSING ALERT Hypertensive encephalopathy is a medical emergency, and treatment is aimed at reducing BP without impairing renal function.

Patient Education and Health Maintenance

1. Explain that patient must have follow-up evaluations of BP, urinary protein, and creatinine and serum electrolyte concentrations to determine if there is exacerbation of disease activity.
2. Encourage patient to treat any infection promptly.
3. Tell patient to notify health care provider of signs of fluid accumulation or uremia (nausea, vomiting, decreased appetite, difficulty concentrating, pruritus).

Evaluation: Expected Outcomes

- Urine output adequate; vital signs stable.
- No edema, shortness of breath, or adventitious heart or lung sounds.

Nephrotic Syndrome

Nephrotic syndrome is a clinical disorder characterized by marked increase of protein in the urine (proteinuria), decrease in albumin in the blood (hypoalbuminemia), edema, and excess lipids in the blood (hyperlipidemia). These occur as a consequence of excessive leakage of plasma proteins into the urine because of increased permeability of the glomerular capillary membrane.

Pathophysiology and Etiology

1. Seen in any condition that seriously damages the glomerular capillary membrane.
   a. Chronic glomerulonephritis.
   b. Diabetes mellitus with intercapillary glomerulosclerosis.
   c. Amyloidosis of the kidney.
   d. Systemic lupus erythematosus.

e. Preeclampsia.
f. Viral infections (hepatitis B, hepatitis C, or human immunodeficiency).
2. Hypoalbuminemia results in decreased oncotic pressure, causing generalized edema as fluid moves out of the vascular space (see Figure 21-7).
3. Decreased circulating volume then activates the renin–angiotensin system, causing retention of sodium and further edema.
4. Decreased plasma oncotic pressure stimulates synthesis of proteins (including lipoproteins) resulting in hypercholesterolemia. Impaired metabolism and clearance of lipids may also play a role in nephrotic syndrome hyperlipidemia.

Clinical Manifestations

1. Insidious onset of pitting dependent edema, periorbital edema, and ascites; weight gain.
2. Fatigue, headache, malaise, irritability.
3. Marked proteinuria—leading to depletion of body proteins.

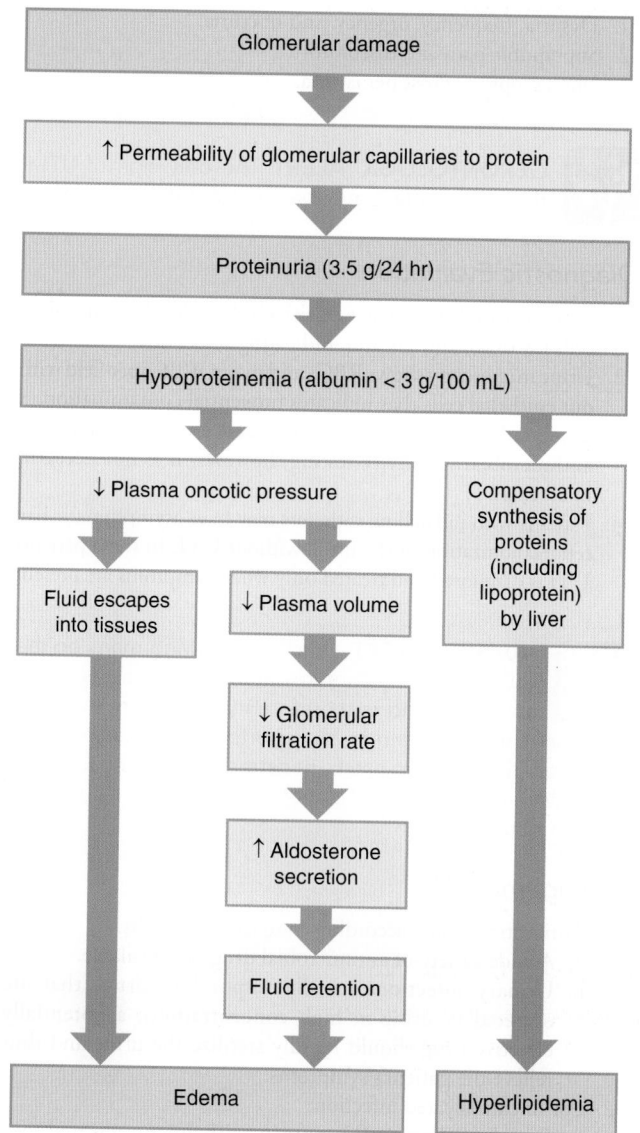

Figure 21-7. Pathophysiology of the nephrotic syndrome. (Rubin, E., & Farber, J.L. [1999]. *Pathology* [3rd ed.]. Philadelphia, PA: Lippincott Williams & Wilkins.)

4. Hyperlipidemia (increased cholesterol and triglycerides)—may lead to accelerated atherosclerosis.

Diagnostic Evaluation

1. Urinalysis—marked proteinuria, microscopic hematuria, urinary casts, appears "foamy."
2. Twenty-four–hour urine for protein (increased) and creatinine clearance (may be decreased).
3. Protein electrophoresis and immunoelectrophoresis of the urine to categorize the proteinuria.
4. Needle biopsy of the kidney—for histologic examination of renal tissue to confirm diagnosis.
5. Serum chemistry—decreased total protein and albumin, normal or increased creatinine, increased triglycerides, and altered lipid profile.

Management

1. Treatment of causative glomerular disease.
2. Diuretics (used cautiously) and angiotensin-converting enzyme inhibitors (ACEI) to control proteinuria (ACEI used only in chronic disease).
3. Corticosteroids or immunosuppressive agents to decrease proteinuria.
4. General management of edema.
   a. Sodium and fluid restriction.
   b. Infusion of salt-poor albumin.
   c. Dietary protein supplements if indicated.
5. Diet low in saturated fats.
6. Lipid-lowering agents.

Complications

1. Hypovolemia.
2. Thromboembolic complications—renal vein thrombosis, venous and arterial thrombosis in extremities, pulmonary embolism, coronary artery thrombosis, and cerebral artery thrombosis secondary to loss of hemostasis control proteins such as antithrombin III, protein S, and protein C.
3. Altered drug metabolism because of decrease in plasma proteins.
4. Progression to CKD and possibly ESRD.

Nursing Assessment

1. Obtain history of onset of symptoms including changes in characteristics of urine and onset of edema.
2. Perform physical examination looking for evidence of edema and hypovolemia.
3. Assess vital signs, daily weights, intake and output, and laboratory values.

Nursing Diagnoses

- Risk for Deficient Fluid Volume intravascularly related to disease process.
- Risk for Infection related to treatment with immunosuppressive agents.

Nursing Interventions

Increasing Circulating Volume and Decreasing Edema

1. Monitor daily weight, intake and output, and urine specific gravity.
2. Monitor CVP (if indicated), vital signs, orthostatic BP, and heart rate to detect hypovolemia.

3. Monitor serum BUN and creatinine to assess renal function.
4. Administer diuretics or immunosuppressive agents, as prescribed, and evaluate patient's response.
5. Infuse IV albumin, as ordered.
6. Enforce mild to moderate sodium and fluid restriction if edema is severe.

Preventing Infection

1. Monitor for signs and symptoms of infection.
2. Monitor temperature routinely.
3. Monitor CBC with diff as ordered.
4. Use aseptic technique for all invasive procedures and educate patient on the importance of strict handwashing.

Patient Education and Health Maintenance

1. Teach patient signs and symptoms of nephrotic syndrome; also, review causes, purpose of prescribed treatments, and importance of long-term therapy to prevent ESRD.
2. Instruct patient in adverse effects of prescribed medications and methods of preventing infection if taking immunosuppressive agents.
3. Carefully review with patient and family dietary and fluid restrictions; consult dietitian for assistance in meal planning.
4. Discuss the importance of maintaining exercise, decreasing cholesterol and fat intake, and changing other risk factors, such as smoking, obesity, and stress, to reduce risk of severe thromboembolic complications.
5. In patients with severe disease, prepare for dialysis and possible transplantation.

Evaluation: Expected Outcomes

- Vital signs remain stable; edema decreased.
- No signs of infection.

URINARY DISORDERS
Lower Urinary Tract Infections

EVIDENCE BASE National Institute for Clinical Excellence. (2015). Urinary tract infections in adults. Available: *www.nice.org.uk/guidance/qs90.*

A *urinary tract infection* (UTI) is caused by the presence of pathogenic microorganisms in the urinary tract with or without signs and symptoms. Lower UTIs may predominate at the bladder (cystitis) or urethra (urethritis).

Bacteriuria refers to the presence of bacteria in the urine (10^3 bacteria/mL of urine or greater generally indicates infection).

In *asymptomatic bacteriuria*, organisms are found in urine, but patient has no symptoms.

Recurrent UTIs may indicate the following:
Unresolved—bacteria fails to respond to antimicrobial therapy.
Recurrent—reinfection after eradication of pathogens.

Pathophysiology and Etiology

1. Ascending infection after entry by way of the urinary meatus.
   a. Women are more susceptible to developing acute cystitis because of shorter length of urethra; anatomical proximity to the vagina, periurethral glands, and rectum (fecal contamination); and the mechanical effect of coitus.
   b. Women with recurrent UTIs typically have gram-negative organisms at the vaginal introitus; there may be some defect of the mucosa of the urethra, vagina, or external genitalia of these patients that allows enteric organisms to invade the bladder.
   c. Poor voiding habits may result in incomplete bladder emptying, increasing the risk of recurrent infection.
   d. Acute infection in women most commonly arises from organisms of the patient's own intestinal flora (*Escherichia coli*).
2. Although *E. coli* causes 86% of UTIs, other pathogens, such as *Klebsiella* species, *Proteus* species, and *Staphylococcus saprophyticus*, may also cause these infections.
3. In men, obstructive abnormalities (strictures, prostatic hyperplasia) are the most frequent cause.
4. UTI is a considerable source of nosocomial infection and sepsis in older adults.
5. Upper urinary tract disease may occasionally cause recurrent bladder infection.

Clinical Manifestations

1. Dysuria, frequency, urgency, and nocturia.
2. Suprapubic pain and discomfort.
3. Microscopic or gross hematuria.

GERONTOLOGIC ALERT The only sign of UTI in the older patient may be mental status changes.

Diagnostic Evaluation

1. Urine dipstick may react positively for blood, white blood cells (WBCs), and nitrates, indicating infection.
2. Urine microscopy shows RBCs and many WBCs per field without epithelial cells that indicates urogential contamination.
3. Urine culture is used to detect presence of bacteria and for antimicrobial sensitivity testing; however, it is not necessary in all cases.
4. Patients with indwelling catheters may have asymptomatic bacterial colonization of the urine without UTI. In these patients, UTI is diagnosed and treated only when symptoms are present.

NURSING ALERT Urinalysis showing many epithelial cells is likely contaminated by vaginal secretions in women and is therefore inaccurate in indicating infection. Urine culture may be reported as contaminated as well. Obtaining a clean-catch, midstream specimen is essential for accurate results, and catheterization may be necessary in some patients.

Management

1. Antibiotic therapy according to sensitivity results.
   a. A wide variety of antimicrobial drugs are available.
   b. Urinary infections usually respond to drugs that are excreted in urine in high concentrations; a potentially effective drug should rapidly sterilize the urine and thus relieve the patient's symptoms.
2. For uncomplicated infection:
   a. First-line therapy for women with uncomplicated cystitis includes a 5-day course of nitrofurantoin or a 3-day course of co-trimoxazole or a fluoroquinolone such as ciprofloxacin, although fluoroquinolones are often reserved

for serious infections. A single dose of fosfomycin has also shown effectiveness in women.

    b. Seven to ten days of therapy is recommended for women over age 65.

    c. Men are treated with 7 to 10 days of antibiotic therapy.

    d. Follow-up culture to prove treatment effectiveness may be indicated.

    e. Adverse effects include nausea, diarrhea, drug-related rash, and vaginal candidiasis.

3. Pregnant women are usually treated for 7 to 10 days.

4. Women with recurrent infections may be treated longer, undergo diagnostic testing to rule out a structural abnormality, or be maintained on a daily dose of antibiotic as prophylaxis.

5. For complicated infection, see treatment of pyelonephritis (see page 613).

6. For severe discomfort with voiding, phenazopyridine may be ordered to reduce bladder irritation three times per day for 2 days.

Complications

1. Pyelonephritis.
2. Hematogenous spread resulting in sepsis.

Nursing Assessment

1. Determine if patient has a history of UTIs in childhood or during pregnancy or has had recurrent infections.

2. Question about voiding habits, personal hygiene practices, and methods of contraception (use of diaphragm or spermicides is associated with development of cystitis).

3. Ask if patient has any associated symptoms of vaginal discharge, itching, or irritation—dysuria may be a prominent symptom of vaginitis or infection from sexually transmitted pathogens, rather than UTI.

4. Examine for suprapubic tenderness, as well as abdominal tenderness, guarding, rebound, or masses that may indicate more serious process.

Nursing Diagnoses

1. Acute Pain related to inflammation of the bladder mucosa.
2. Deficient Knowledge related to prevention of recurrent UTI.

Nursing Interventions

Relieving Pain

1. Administer or teach self-administration of antibiotic—eradication of infection is usually accompanied by rapid resolution of symptoms.

2. Encourage patient to take prescribed analgesics and antispasmodics, if ordered.

3. Encourage rest during the acute phase if symptoms are severe.

4. Encourage plenty of fluids to promote urinary output and to flush out bacteria from urinary tract.

Increasing Understanding and Practice of Preventive Measures

1. For women with recurrent UTIs, give the following instructions:

    a. Reduce vaginal introital concentration of pathogens by hygienic measures.

    b. Wash genitalia in shower or while standing in bathtub—bacteria in bath water may gain entrance into the urethra.

    c. Cleanse around the perineum and urethral meatus after each bowel movement, with front-to-back cleansing to minimize fecal contamination of periurethral area.

2. Drink liberal amounts of water to lower bacterial concentrations in the urine.

3. Avoid bladder irritants—coffee, tea, alcohol, cola drinks, and aspartame.

4. Decrease the entry of microorganisms into the bladder during intercourse.

    a. Void immediately after sexual intercourse.

    b. A single dose of an oral antimicrobial agent may be prescribed after sexual intercourse.

5. Avoid external irritants such as bubble baths, talcum powders, perfumed vaginal cleansers, or deodorants.

6. Patients with persistent bacteria may require long-term antimicrobial therapy to prevent colonization of periurethral area and recurrence of UTI.

    a. Take antibiotic at bedtime after emptying the bladder to ensure adequate concentration of drug overnight because low rates of urine flow and infrequent bladder emptying predispose to multiplication of bacteria.

    b. Use self-monitoring tests (dipsticks) at home to monitor for UTI.

Patient Education and Health Maintenance

1. Advise women with simple, uncomplicated cystitis that they do not require follow-up as long as symptoms are completely resolved with antibiotic therapy. Men usually need follow-up cultures and possibly additional testing if more than one episode of infection.

2. Instruct patient to void frequently (every 2 to 3 hours) and to empty bladder completely because this enhances bacterial clearance, reduces urine stasis, and prevents reinfection. Infrequent voiding distends the bladder wall, leading to hypoxia of bladder mucosa, which is then more susceptible to bacterial invasion.

3. Instruct patients who have had UTIs during pregnancy to have follow-up studies.

4. Female patients with uncomplicated but recurrent cystitis may self-administer a 2- or 3-day course of antibiotics when symptoms begin, if prescribed.

5. Cranberry juice or capsules may help to prevent cystitis by altering the bladder mucosa so that the bacteria cannot attach. Acidophilus and cranberry capsules are available in health food and vitamin stores.

Evaluation: Expected Outcomes

- Verbalizes relief of symptoms.
- Verbalizes self-care measures to prevent recurrence.

Interstitial Cystitis/Bladder Pain Syndrome

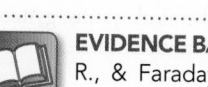 **EVIDENCE BASE** Hanno, P. M., Erickson, D., Moldwin, R., & Faraday, M. M. (2015). American Urological Association. Diagnosis and treatment of interstitial cystitis/bladder pain syndrome: AUA guideline amendment. *The Journal of Urology*, 193(5), 1545–1553.

Interstitial cystitis (also called *painful bladder syndrome*) is a syndrome of chronic, cystitis-like symptoms in the absence of bacterial infection. It is a diagnosis of exclusion.

Pathophysiology and Etiology

1. The etiology of interstitial cystitis is unknown. However, theories include an inflammatory or autoimmune process that alters the normal configuration of cells in the bladder epithelium, although infectious, neurological, psychological, and vascular origins are also considered possible.
   a. One plausible theory is a neurogenic origin, in which an initial peripheral inflammatory response later activates the sacral nerves to continue to respond without evidence of continued inflammation.
   b. Mast cell involvement in the inflammatory response also seems a plausible etiology, with many patients having a concomitant history of allergies.
2. The bladder is normally lined with a gel-like substance composed of glycosaminoglycans (heparin, hyaluronic acid, and chondroitin) that acts as an impermeable barrier to irritating solutes such as potassium.
3. Disruption to the bladder epithelium leads to irritant seepage, which produces the symptoms.
4. The bladder wall is chronically inflamed with no evidence of bacterial infection.
5. Occurs far more frequently in women than in men.

Clinical Manifestations

1. History of slow, progressive increase in urinary frequency and urgency. Urgency may be extreme; frequency (as many as 16 times per day) and nocturia increase with duration of symptoms.
2. Symptoms of suprapubic pain and pressure occurring for at least 3 to 6 months.
   a. Bladder pain may be continuous, may increase prior to voiding when the bladder is full, or may present as diffuse perineal, vaginal, suprapubic, or lower back pain.
   b. Pain is usually relieved by voiding.
3. Symptoms are exacerbated by sexual intercourse and at the time of menstruation.
4. Symptoms may be present for 5 to 7 years before diagnosis is made.

Diagnostic Evaluation

1. Tender bladder base during pelvic examination, assessed by palpation of the anterior vaginal wall.
2. Urinalysis and urine culture to rule out infection.
3. Cystoscopy under anesthesia with bladder biopsies and bladder distention; presence of bleeding or ulcerations on bladder distention is characteristic of some cases of interstitial cystitis.
4. Urodynamic tests commonly reveal a small bladder capacity with early sensation of urgency and, in some cases, poor detrusor function with incomplete bladder emptying.
5. In potassium sensitivity testing, symptoms are produced when potassium is placed in the bladder; however, the use of this test is controversial as inflammation also produces a positive test.
6. Diagnosis is usually made by ruling out other potential causes of symptoms, including radiation or chemical cystitis, gynecologic or urologic malignancies, STD, and urolithiasis.

Management

1. Treatment is individualized and focused on symptom control.
2. Dietary modification to identify foods that act as triggers can be accomplished through an elimination diet. Possible triggers are citrus fruits, tomatoes, caffeinated beverages, carbonated beverages, chocolate, and spicy foods.
3. Bladder retraining (increasing intervals between voiding) is commonly necessary to increase bladder capacity that has been diminished by frequent voiding; pelvic floor strengthening with Kegel exercises can help with urgency and frequency.
4. Oral administration of pentosan polysulfate relieves symptoms in some patients, with maximal effect seen after 3 to 6 months; many continue this therapy for years. If no improvement after 3 to 6 months, the drug is discontinued.
5. Antihistamines may be beneficial for patients who have allergies. Hydroxyzine has been beneficial in patients.
6. Tricyclic antidepressants such as amitriptyline may be helpful for their analgesic, anticholinergic, and antihistaminic effects. Gabapentin is also used for chronic pain.
7. Bladder distention during cystoscopy under general anesthesia relieves symptoms in 30% to 50% of patients, especially those with small bladder capacity. Relapse commonly occurs 3 months' posttreatment, however, and the effectiveness of this treatment diminishes with repeated use.
8. Intravesical therapy with various substances, including silver nitrate and dimethyl sulfoxide, may be used.
9. Transcutaneous electrical nerve stimulation has demonstrated some relief for the pain syndrome associated with interstitial cystitis.
10. Stress management techniques such as yoga and meditation.

 DRUG ALERT Pentosan polysulfate has anticoagulant properties; therefore, it should not be used by patients taking other anticoagulant drugs or in conditions associated with increased risk for bleeding. Reversible alopecia may occur as well but resolves once the drug is discontinued.

Complications

1. Psychosocial problems related to pain, urgency, and frequency.
2. Secondary bacteriuria.

Nursing Assessment

1. Assess voiding patterns including frequency, nocturia, and urgency (a voiding diary is helpful). Determine if symptoms increase in relation to certain foods, menstrual cycle, or sexual intercourse.
2. Assess level of pain using a scale of 1 to 10; determine if pain increases during or after voiding and if bladder spasms occur. Some practitioners may use a symptom questionnaire such as the O'Leary-Sant Interstitial Cystitis Symptom and Problem Index or the Pelvic Pain and Urgency/Frequency questionnaire.
3. Perform abdominal examination and assist with pelvic examination, if indicated, to rule out gynecologic causes and to identify location of pain on palpation.
4. Assess impact on relationships and quality of life.

Nursing Diagnoses

- Chronic Pain related to disease process.
- Impaired Urinary Elimination related to frequency, urgency, dysuria, and nocturia.
- Ineffective Coping related to interruption of lifestyle and chronic, unrelenting symptoms.

Nursing Interventions

Controlling Pain

1. Administer pharmacologic agents, as ordered, to relieve pain and other symptoms. Counsel patient on adverse effects, such as drowsiness, with antihistamines and tricyclic antidepressants.
2. Instruct patient in comfort and preventive measures, such as application of heating pad, avoidance of bladder irritants (caffeine, alcohol, chocolate, and acidic or spicy foods), and avoidance of known allergens.
3. If prescribed, teach patient self-catheterization and the self-administration of intravesical medications.

Improving Urinary Elimination

1. Encourage patient to use a voiding diary as well as a dietary record to make associations between intake of certain foods or fluids and increase in symptoms.
2. Set up bladder retraining program to increase bladder capacity and reduce symptoms.
   a. Have patient start with every 10- to 15-minute voiding intervals during the day.
   b. Instruct patient to gradually (every week or two) increase intervals by 15 minutes.
   c. The ultimate goal (over a period of about 3 months) should be voiding intervals of 3½ hours during the day.
   d. Teach Kegel exercises to help strengthen supporting muscles. Warm baths and perineal massage may help with relaxation before exercises.
   e. Make a referral for biofeedback training, if needed, to enhance Kegel exercises.
3. Advise patient to restrict fluids only when necessary because of impending limited access to toilet facilities; normal fluid intake should be encouraged otherwise.
4. Assess patient's response to pharmacologic therapy.

Strengthening Coping

1. Inquire about patient's ability to work and carry on roles as spouse, parent, etc., based on frequency and discomfort.
2. Explore with patient positive coping strategies for self and family in dealing with chronic illness.
3. Encourage counseling, as needed.

Patient Education and Health Maintenance

1. Teach patient mechanism of action and adverse effects of pharmacologic therapies.
2. Teach self-catheterization using clean technique, if needed, to self-administer medications or accomplish complete bladder emptying.
3. Provide information about food and fluids known to be bladder irritants.
4. Refer for additional information and support to agencies such as Interstitial Cystitis Association (*www.ichelp.org*).

Evaluation: Expected Outcomes

- Verbalizes some relief of pain.
- Verbalizes less urgency, frequency, and nocturia.
- Identifies coping strategies.

Acute Bacterial Pyelonephritis

Bacterial pyelonephritis is an acute infection and inflammatory disease of the kidney and renal pelvis involving one or both kidneys.

Pathophysiology and Etiology

1. Enteric bacteria, such as *E. coli*, are the most common pathogen; other gram-negative pathogens include *Proteus* species, *Klebsiella*, and *Pseudomonas*. Gram-positive bacteria are less common, but include *Enterococcus* and *Staphylococcus aureus*.
2. Bacterial infection usually ascends from the lower urinary tract; however, hematogenous migration is possible (particularly with *S. aureus*).
3. Pyelonephritis can result from urinary obstruction such as vesicoureteral reflux (incompetence of ureterovesical valve, which allows urine to regurgitate into ureters, usually at the time of voiding), other renal disease, trauma, or pregnancy.
4. Low-grade inflammation with interstitial infiltrations of inflammatory cells may lead to tubular destruction and abscess formation.
5. Chronic pyelonephritis may result in scarred, atrophic, and nonfunctioning kidneys.

Clinical Manifestations

1. Fever, chills.
2. Flank pain (with or without radiation to the groin).
3. Nausea, vomiting, anorexia, abdominal pain, diarrhea.
4. Costovertebral angle tenderness (unilateral or bilateral).
5. Urgency, frequency, and dysuria may be present.

 GERONTOLOGIC ALERT Older patients may not exhibit the usual febrile response to pyelonephritis, but have nonspecific GI or pulmonary symptoms instead.

Diagnostic Evaluation

1. Urinalysis (dipstick or microscopic) to identify leukocytes, bacteria, nitrites, and RBCs and WBCs in urine; white cell casts may also be seen.
2. Urine culture to identify causative bacteria.
3. CBC shows elevated WBC count consisting of neutrophils and bands.
4. CT scan of the abdomen—with contrast—is the imaging study of choice. Other studies include intravenous urography (IVU) or renal ultrasound to evaluate for urinary tract obstruction; other radiologic or urinary tests may be conducted, as necessary.
5. Blood cultures may be drawn, if indicated.

Management

1. For severe infections (dehydrated, cannot tolerate oral intake) or complicating factors (suspected obstruction, pregnancy, advanced age, immunocompromised), inpatient antibiotic therapy is recommended.
   a. Usually, immediate treatment is started with an IV fluoroquinolone, aminoglycoside, or extended-spectrum cephalosporin to cover the prevalent gram-negative pathogens; may be subsequently adjusted according to culture results.
   b. An oral antibiotic may be started 24 hours after fever has resolved and oral therapy continued for 2 weeks.
2. Oral antibiotic therapy is acceptable for outpatient treatment.
   a. A fluoroquinolone or co-trimoxazole is used—10 to 14 days is the usual length of treatment.
3. Repeat urine cultures should be performed after the completion of therapy.
4. Supportive therapy is given for fever and pain control and hydration.

Complications

1. Bacteremia with sepsis.
2. Papillary necrosis leading to renal failure.
3. Renal abscess requiring treatment by percutaneous drainage or prolonged antibiotic therapy.
4. Perinephric abscess.
5. Paralytic ileus.

Nursing Assessment

1. Monitor symptoms and assess ability to tolerate oral fluids and food.
2. Obtain urologic history that could suggest recurrent infections or urinary tract obstruction.
3. Obtain vital signs; monitor for impending sepsis.
4. Assess bowel sounds for possible paralytic ileus.

Nursing Diagnoses

- Hyperthermia because of infection.
- Acute Pain related to renal swelling and edema.

Nursing Interventions

Reducing Body Temperature

1. Administer or teach self-administration of antibiotics, as prescribed, and monitor for effectiveness and adverse effects.
2. Assess vital signs frequently and monitor intake and output; administer antiemetic medications to control nausea and vomiting.
3. Administer antipyretic medications, as prescribed and according to temperature.
4. Report fever that persists beyond 72 hours after initiating antibiotic therapy; further testing for complicating factors will be ordered.
5. Use measures to decrease body temperature, if indicated: cooling blanket, application of ice to armpits and groins, and so forth.
6. Correct dehydration by replacing fluids, orally if possible, or via IV administration.
7. Monitor CBC, blood cultures, and urine studies for resolving infection.

Relieving Pain

1. Administer or teach self-administration of analgesics and monitor their effectiveness.
2. Use comfort measures, such as positioning, for local relief of flank pain.
3. Assess patient's response to pain control measures.

Patient Education and Health Maintenance

1. Explain to patient possible causes of pyelonephritis and its signs and symptoms; also, review signs and symptoms of lower UTI.
2. Review antibiotic therapy and importance of completing prescribed course of treatment and having follow-up urine cultures.
3. Explain preventive measures, including good fluid intake, personal hygiene measures, and healthy voiding habits.

Evaluation: Expected Outcomes

- Afebrile within 48 hours.
- Verbalizes reduced pain.

Nephrolithiasis and Urolithiasis

Nephrolithiasis refers to renal stone disease; *urolithiasis* refers to the presence of stones in the urinary system. Stones, or calculi, are formed in the urinary tract from the kidney to bladder by the crystallization of substances excreted in the urine.

 EVIDENCE BASE Turk, C., Knoll, T., Petrik, A., et al. (2015). Guidelines on urolithiasis. European Association of Urology. Available: *http://uroweb.org/wp-content/uploads/22-Urolithiasis_LR_full.pdf*

Pathophysiology and Etiology

1. Most stones (75%) are composed mainly of calcium oxalate crystals; the rest are composed of calcium phosphate salts, uric acid, struvite (magnesium, ammonium, and phosphate), or the amino acid cysteine.
2. Causes and predisposing factors:
   a. Hypercalcemia and hypercalciuria caused by hyperparathyroidism, renal tubular acidosis, multiple myeloma, and excessive intake of vitamin D, milk, and alkali.
   b. Chronic dehydration, poor fluid intake, and immobility.
   c. Diet high in purines and abnormal purine metabolism (hyperuricemia and gout).
   d. Genetic predisposition for urolithiasis or genetic disorders (cystinuria).
   e. Chronic infection with urea-splitting bacteria (*Proteus vulgaris* and *mirabilis*).
   f. Chronic obstruction with stasis of urine and foreign bodies within the urinary tract.
   g. Excessive oxalate absorption in inflammatory bowel disease and bowel resection or ileostomy.
   h. Living in mountainous, desert, or tropical areas.
3. Stones may be found anywhere in the urinary system and vary in size from mere granular deposits (called sand or gravel) to bladder stones the size of an orange.
4. One of three patients with stones are men; in both sexes, the peak age of onset is 40 to 60 years.
5. Most stones migrate downward (causing severe colicky pain when the stone obstructs the ureter) and are discovered in the lower ureter. Spontaneous stone passage can be anticipated in 80% to 90% of patients with calculus less than 5 mm in size.
6. Some stones may lodge in the renal pelvis, ureters, or bladder neck, causing obstruction, edema, secondary infection, and, in some cases, nephron damage.
7. Those with stones for the first time have a 50% risk of recurrence within the next 7 to 10 years.

Clinical Manifestations

1. Pain pattern depends on site of obstruction (see Figure 21-8).
   a. Renal stones produce an increase in hydrostatic pressure and distention of the renal pelvis and proximal ureter causing renal colic. Pain relief is immediate after stone passage.
   b. Ureteral stones produce symptoms because of obstruction as they pass down the ureter (ureteral colic).
   c. Bladder stones may be asymptomatic or produce symptoms similar to cystitis.
2. Obstruction—stones blocking the flow of urine will produce symptoms of colic, chills, and fever.
3. GI symptoms include nausea, vomiting, diarrhea, and abdominal discomfort—because of renointestinal reflexes and shared nerve supply (celiac ganglion) between the ureters and intestine.

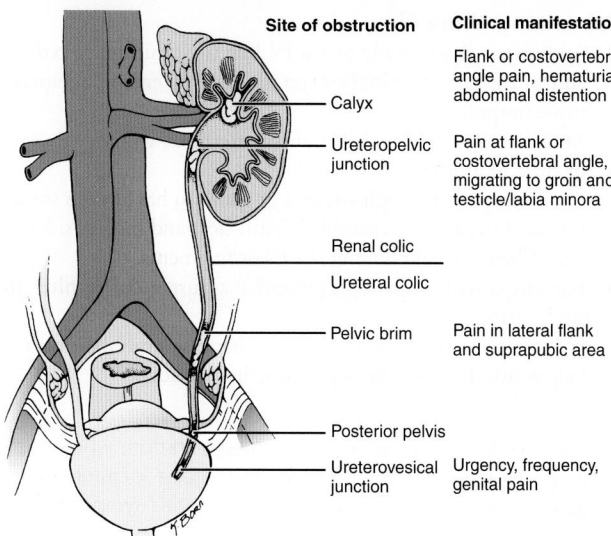

Site of obstruction	Clinical manifestations
Calyx	Flank or costovertebral angle pain, hematuria, abdominal distention
Ureteropelvic junction	Pain at flank or costovertebral angle, migrating to groin and testicle/labia minora
Renal colic	
Ureteral colic	
Pelvic brim	Pain in lateral flank and suprapubic area
Posterior pelvis	
Ureterovesical junction	Urgency, frequency, genital pain

Figure 21-8. Areas where calculi may obstruct the urinary system. The ensuing clinical manifestations depend on the site of obstruction. Stones that have broken loose may obstruct the flow of urine, cause severe pain, and injure the kidney. (Creason, C. [2010]. *Stedman's medical terminology: steps to success in medical language.* Philadelphia, PA: Lippincott Williams & Wilkins.).

Diagnostic Evaluation

1. Kidney, ureters, and bladder radiography may show stone.
2. IVU—to determine site and evaluate degree of obstruction.
3. Regular ultrasound may be as sensitive with good technique; however, it won't show radiolucent stones.
4. Spiral CT scan stone study—special noncontrast CT technique to assess for stone in the ureter; it is the study of choice and will show all stones.
   a. Requires no preparation and is noninvasive.
   b. Takes only 10 minutes.
5. Analysis of available stone material—crystals can be identified by polarization microscopy, x-ray diffraction, and infrared spectroscopy.
6. Urinalysis—hematuria and pyuria; pH less than 5.5 may indicate uric acid stone; more than 7.5 may indicate struvite stone; urine culture and drug sensitivity studies to detect infection.
7. Serum kidney function tests; electrolytes, calcium, phosphorus, uric acid, and magnesium levels; serum parathyroid hormone may also be evaluated.

Management

General Principles

1. If it is a small stone (less than 5 mm) and able to treat as outpatient, 80% to 90% of patients will pass stone spontaneously with hydration, pain control, and reassurance.

2. Patient may be hospitalized for intractable pain, persistent vomiting, high-grade fever, obstruction with infection, bilateral ureteral calculi, and solitary kidney with obstruction.

Extracorporeal Shock Wave Lithotripsy (ESWL)

1. Noninvasive procedure used for both renal and ureteral radiopaque stones less than 2 cm and greater than 4 mm.
2. High-energy shock waves are directed at the kidney stone, disintegrating it into minute particles that pass in the urine. (A shock wave is a large, condensed wave of energy produced by high-speed motion.)
3. Patient is placed on specially designed table and immersed in a water bath or placed on an adjustable stretcher positioned over a cushion of water.
   a. In water bath model, shock waves travel through water surrounding the patient.
   b. In cushion model, a layer of gel lies between the stretcher and water; shock waves move through the cushion and gel.
4. Position of the kidney stone is located by fluoroscopy and the shock waves are targeted directly at the stone. The shock waves do not affect soft tissue.
5. Eliminates need for surgery in majority of patients and can be repeated for recurrent stones with no apparent risk to kidney structure or function. Long-term adverse effects may include increased risk of hypertension or diabetes.
6. Complications include pain from both the procedure and passing stone fragments, urinary infection, and perirenal hematoma (bleeding around the kidney).
7. Contraindications to ESWL include pregnancy and uncorrected bleeding disorders.

Percutaneous Nephrolithotomy

For stones in renal collecting system or upper portion of ureter and larger than 2 cm in diameter (see Figure 21-9).

1. Under fluoroscopic guidance, a needle is advanced into collecting system; guide wire is advanced into renal pelvis or ureter.
2. Tract is dilated with mechanical dilators or high-pressure balloon dilator until nephroscope can be inserted up against stone.
3. Stones can be broken apart with hydraulic shock waves or a laser beam administered by way of nephroscope; fragments are removed using forceps, graspers, or basket.
4. May be combined with ESWL.
5. Complications include hemorrhage, infection, and extravasation of urine.

Ureteroscopy

1. Used for distal ureteral calculi; may be used for midureteral calculi.

Figure 21-9. **(A)** Extracorporeal shock wave lithotripsy for renal calculi dissolution. **(B)** A percutaneous nephrostomy tract permits access to the collecting system of the kidney for removal of renal calculi under direct vision via a nephroscope. (Smeltzer, S., & Bare, B. [2003]. *Brunner and Suddarth's textbook of medical-surgical nursing* [10th ed.]. Philadelphia, PA: Lippincott Williams & Wilkins.)

2. Flexible or rigid ureteroscopes are used in conjunction with baskets or graspers.
3. Electrohydraulic, ultrasonic, or laser equipment may also be used to fragment stone.
4. A stent may be inserted and left in place after surgery to maintain patency of the ureter.

Open Surgical Procedures

Indicated for only 1% to 2% of all stones; rarely performed, most likely to be done percutaneously or laparoscopically, if indicated.
1. Pyelolithotomy—removal of stones from kidney pelvis.
2. Nephrolithotomy—incision into the kidney for removal of stone.
3. Nephrectomy—removal of the kidney; indicated when the kidney is extensively and irreparably damaged and is no longer a functioning organ; partial nephrectomy sometimes done.
4. Ureterolithotomy—removal of stone in the ureter.
5. Cystolithotomy—removal of stone from the bladder.

Complications

1. Obstruction—from remaining stone fragments.
2. Infection—from dissemination of infected stone particles or bacteria resulting from obstruction.
3. Impaired renal function—from prolonged obstruction before treatment and removal.
4. Perirenal hematoma—from bleeding around the kidney caused by trauma of shock waves or laser treatments.

Nursing Assessment

1. Obtain history, focusing on history of calculi, family history of calculi, episodes of dehydration, prolonged immobility, UTI, dietary, bleeding history, and medication history.
2. Assess pain location and radiation; assess level of pain using a scale of 1 to 10. Observe for presence of associated symptoms: nausea, vomiting, diarrhea, abdominal distention.
3. Monitor for signs and symptoms of UTI, such as chills, fever, dysuria, frequency. Examine urine for hematuria.
4. Observe for signs and symptoms of obstruction, such as frequent urination of small amounts, oliguria, anuria.

Nursing Diagnoses

- Acute Pain related to inflammation, obstruction, and abrasion of urinary tract by migration of stones.
- Impaired Urinary Elimination related to blockage of urine flow by stones.
- Risk for Infection related to obstruction of urine flow and instrumentation during treatment.

Nursing Interventions

Controlling Pain

1. Give prescribed NSAID or opioid analgesic (orally or via IV patient-controlled analgesia) until cause of pain can be removed.
   a. Monitor patient closely for increasing pain; may indicate inadequate analgesia.
   b. Large doses of opioids are typically required to relieve pain; so, monitor for respiratory depression and drop in BP.
2. Encourage patient to assume position that brings some relief.
3. Reassess pain frequently using pain scale.
4. Administer antiemetics (usually given orally IV, but rectal suppository may be given), as indicated, for nausea.

Maintaining Urine Flow

1. Administer fluids orally or via IV line (if vomiting) to reduce concentration of urinary crystalloids and ensure adequate urine output.
2. Monitor total urine output and patterns of voiding. Report oliguria or anuria.
3. Strain all urine through strainer or gauze to harvest the stone; uric acid stones may crumble. Crush clots and inspect sides of urinal/bed pan for clinging stones or fragments.
4. For outpatient treatment, patient may use a coffee filter to strain urine.
5. Help patient to walk, if possible, because ambulation may help move the stone through the urinary tract.

 NURSING ALERT Avoid overhydration, which may result in increased distention at stone location, causing an increase in pain and associated symptoms.

Controlling Infection

1. Administer parenteral or oral antibiotics, as prescribed during treatment, and monitor for adverse effects.
2. Assess urine for color, cloudiness, and odor.
3. Obtain vital signs and monitor for fever and symptoms of impending sepsis (tachycardia, hypotension).

Patient Education and Health Maintenance

Recovery from Surgical Interventions for Stone Disease

1. Encourage fluids to accelerate passing of stone particles.
2. Teach about analgesics that still may be necessary for colicky pain, which may accompany passage of stone debris.
3. Warn that some blood may appear in urine for several weeks.
4. Encourage frequent walking to assist in passage of stone fragments.
5. Teach patient to strain urine through a coffee filter or stone strainer and to save stone for analysis.
6. Teach patient to take alpha-adrenergic blockers to help dilate the ureter, thus improving stone passage.

Prevention of Recurrent Stone Formation

1. For patients with calcium oxalate stones:
   a. Instruct on diet—avoid excesses of calcium and phosphorus; maintain a low-sodium diet (sodium restriction decreases amount of calcium absorbed in the intestine). (*Note:* Patient should not decrease calcium intake; rather, he or she should maintain regular intake.)
   b. Teach purpose of drug therapy—thiazide diuretics to reduce urine calcium excretion through the kidneys.
2. For patients with uric acid stones:
   a. Teach methods to alkalinize urine to enhance urate solubility.
   b. Instruct on testing urine pH.
   c. Teach purpose of taking allopurinol—to lower uric acid concentration.
   d. Provide information about reduction of dietary purine intake (reduce red meat, fish, and fowl intake).
3. For patients with infected (struvite) stones:
   a. Teach signs and symptoms of urinary infection (in patients with neurologic or spinal cord disease, teach use of dipsticks to evaluate urine for nitrites and leukocytes); encourage patient to report infection immediately; must be treated vigorously.
   b. Try to avoid prolonged periods of recumbency—slows renal drainage and alters calcium metabolism.

4. For patients with cystine stones (occur in *cystinuria*, a hereditary disorder of amino acid transport):
   a. Teach patient to alkalinize urine by taking sodium bicarbonate tablets to increase cystine solubility; instruct patient how to test urine pH with a pH indicator.
   b. Teach patient about drug therapy with D-penicillamine—to lower cystine concentration or dissolution by direct irrigation with thiol derivatives.
   c. Explain importance of maintaining drug therapy consistently.
5. For all patients with stone disease:
   a. Explain the need for consistently increased fluid intake (24-hour urinary output greater than 2 L)—lowers the concentration of substances involved in stone formation.
      i. Drink enough fluids to achieve a urinary volume of 2,000 to 3,000 mL or more every 24 hours.
      ii. Drink larger amounts during periods of strenuous exercise and in hot, humid weather because of perspiration.
   b. Encourage a diet low in sugar and animal proteins—refined carbohydrates appear to lead to hypercalciuria and urolithiasis; animal proteins increase urine excretion of calcium, uric acid, and oxalate.
   c. Increase consumption of fiber—inhibits calcium and oxalate absorption.
   d. Save any stone passed for analysis. (Only patients with more than one episode of urolithiasis are advised to have a metabolic evaluation.)
   e. Can discontinue urine straining once stone is passed.

Evaluation: Expected Outcomes

- Verbalizes reduced pain level.
- Urine output adequate with low specific gravity.
- Afebrile; urine clear.

Renal Cell Carcinoma

Renal cell carcinoma accounts for 85% of primary malignant renal tumors, occurring twice as more frequently in men than in women. Most renal cell tumors are found in the renal parenchyma and develop with few (if any) symptoms.

Pathophysiology and Etiology

1. Unknown etiology; tobacco exposure, through use of cigarettes or chew, causes a twofold increase in risk. Obesity and hypertension are additional risk factors for developing renal cell cancer. Exposure to asbestos, solvents, and cadmium also increases risk.
2. Occurs most frequently in persons between ages 50 and 70.
3. Early-stage renal cancer usually diagnosed incidentally during CT scan or sonogram for an unrelated health problem.
4. Incidence is 10% to 20% higher in African American men.

Clinical Manifestations

1. Many renal tumors produce no symptoms.
2. Weight loss, fever, and night sweats—from systemic effects of renal cancer.
3. Classic triad (late symptoms, occurs in only 7% to 10% of patients):
   a. Hematuria—intermittent or continuous, microscopic or gross.
   b. Flank pain—from distention of renal capsule, invasion of surrounding structures.
   c. Palpable mass in the flank or abdomen.
4. Hematuria, dyspnea, cough, and bone pain with advanced disease.

Diagnostic Evaluation

1. Ultrasonography—helpful in differentiating renal cyst from renal tumor.
2. Three-phase CT scan with and without IV contrast—primary technique for detecting, diagnosing, categorizing, and staging a renal mass.
3. IVP—used as a screening procedure and rarely performed, IVP alone may fail to detect some renal tumors.
4. MRI—determines if thrombosis is in renal vein and evaluates for vascular extension.

Management

The goal is to eradicate the tumor and prevent metastasis.

Radical Nephrectomy

Removal of the kidney and associated tumor, adrenal gland, surrounding perirenal fat, Gerota fascia, and possibly regional lymph nodes—provides maximum opportunity for disease control.

1. Performed through a vertical midline, subcostal, thoracoabdominal, or flank incision.
2. See page 596 for care of patient after renal surgery.
3. Increasingly done laparoscopically.
4. Partial nephrectomy is done for localized tumors as nephron sparing.

Renal Artery Embolization

Preoperative occlusion of renal artery followed by nephrectomy—limited to patient with large vascular tumor in which the renal artery may be difficult to reach early in procedure.

1. Catheter is advanced into renal artery.
2. Embolizing material (Gelfoam, steel coils) is injected into artery and carried with arterial blood flow to occlude the tumor vessels.
3. Monitor for postinfarction syndrome (lasts 2 to 3 days)—severe abdominal pain, nausea, vomiting, diarrhea, fever.
4. Complications — arterial obstruction, bleeding, diminution of renal function.

Chemotherapy and Immunotherapy

Renal cell carcinomas are generally refractory to chemotherapeutic agents, radiation, and hormonal manipulation.

1. Interleukin-2—lymphokine that stimulates growth of T lymphocytes—may offer some benefit to patients with metastatic renal cancer, although toxicity is severe.
2. Sunitinib and sorafenib inhibit vascular endothelial growth factor and platelet-derived growth factors.
   a. Main adverse effects include rash, diarrhea, and hand–foot skin rash.
   b. Possible 3- to 5-month increase in survival.

Cryoablation

1. Freezing of tumor with liquid nitrogen or argon gas through percutaneous needles placed into tumors, using ultrasound guidance.
2. Appropriate for tumors 3.5 cm or less in size.

Thermal Ablation

1. Use of heat through percutaneous needles to cause tissue necrosis, thus killing tumor cells.
2. Appropriate for tumors 3.5 cm or less in size.

Complications

Metastasis to the lung, bone, liver, brain, and other areas.

Nursing Assessment

1. Assess for clinical manifestations of systemic disease—fatigue, anorexia, weight loss, pallor, fever, and bone pain—as well as evidence of metastasis.
2. Assess cardiopulmonary and nutritional status before surgery.
3. Monitor for adverse effects and complications of diagnostic tests and treatment.
4. Assess pain control and coping ability.

Nursing Diagnoses

- Anxiety related to diagnosis of cancer and possibility of metastatic disease.
- Acute Pain and Hyperthermia related to postinfarction syndrome.

Also see page 596 for nursing diagnoses and interventions related to renal surgery.

Nursing Interventions

Reducing Anxiety

1. Explain each diagnostic test, its purpose, and possible adverse reactions. Ensure that informed consent has been obtained, as indicated.
2. Assess patient's understanding about diagnosis and treatment options. Answer questions, and encourage a more thorough discussion with health care provider, as needed.
3. Encourage patient to discuss fears and feelings; involve family and significant others in teaching.

Controlling Symptoms of Postinfarction Syndrome

1. Administer analgesics, as prescribed, to control flank and abdominal pain.
2. Encourage rest and assist with positioning for 2 to 3 days until syndrome subsides.
3. Obtain temperature every 4 hours and administer antipyretics, as indicated.
4. Restrict oral intake and provide IV fluids while patient is nauseated.
5. Administer antiemetics, as ordered.

Patient Education and Health Maintenance

1. Ensure that patient understands where and when to go for follow-up (surgeon, primary care provider, oncologist, and radiologist for metastatic workup and treatment).
2. Explain the importance of follow-up for hypertension and renal function, even if patient feels well.
3. Advise patient with one kidney to wear a MedicAlert bracelet and notify all health care providers because potentially nephrotoxic medications and procedures must be avoided.

Evaluation: Expected Outcomes

- Asks questions and verbalizes fears.
- Afebrile; states reduced pain.

Injuries to the Kidney

Trauma to the abdomen, flank, or back may produce renal injury. Suspicion is high in a patient with multiple injuries.

Pathophysiology and Etiology

1. *Blunt trauma* (falls, sporting accidents, motor vehicle accidents) can suddenly move the kidney out of position and in contact with a rib or lumbar vertebral transverse process, resulting in injury. This is the most common injury to the kidney, accounting for 80% to 85% of all renal injuries.
2. *Penetrating trauma* (gunshot and stab wounds) can injure the kidney if it lies in the path of the wound.
3. Renal trauma is classified according to severity of injury (see Figure 21-10):
   a. Grade I (most common): renal contusion or bruising with normal radiographic imaging.
   b. Grade II: perirenal hematoma or laceration that extends into renal cortex.
   c. Grade III: laceration extends into renal cortex and renal medulla.
   d. Grade IV: laceration extends into collecting system, urine extravasation; requires surgical management.
   e. Grade V: shattered kidney or avulsion of renal artery or renal vein/artery injury; requires surgical management.
4. Eighty percent of patients with renal trauma will have injuries to other organ systems also necessitating treatment.

Clinical Manifestations

1. Hematuria is common but not indicative of severity of injury.
2. Flank pain; perirenal hematoma.
3. Nausea, vomiting, abdominal rigidity—from ileus (seen when there is retroperitoneal bleeding).
4. Shock—from severe or multiple injuries.

Diagnostic Evaluation

1. History of injury—determine if injury was caused by blunt or penetrating trauma.
2. IVU with nephrotomograms—to define extent of injury to the involved kidney and the function of contralateral kidney.
3. CT scan with IV contrast—differentiates between major and minor injuries.
4. Arteriography—to evaluate the renal artery, if necessary.

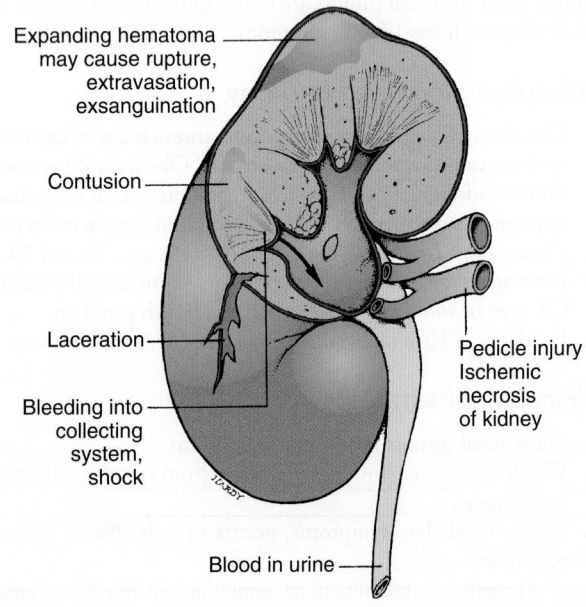

Figure 21-10. Types and physiologic effects of renal injuries: contusion, laceration, rupture, and pedicle injury. (Smeltzer, S., & Bare, B. [2000]. *Brunner and Suddarth's textbook of medical–surgical nursing* [9th ed.]. Philadelphia, PA: Lippincott Williams & Wilkins.)

Management

1. Contusions and minor lacerations are managed conservatively with bed rest, IV fluids, and monitoring of serial urines for clearing of hematuria.
2. Major lacerations (grades IV and V) are surgically repaired.
3. Ruptures are surgically repaired, usually by partial nephrectomy.
4. Renal pedicle injury is a hemorrhagic emergency and requires immediate surgical repair and possible nephrectomy.

 NURSING ALERT If there is a history consistent with renal injury and patient presents in shock, suspect a renal pedicle injury. This is a hemorrhagic emergency, requiring immediate treatment of shock and preparation for surgery.

Complications

1. Hemorrhage, shock with cardiovascular collapse.
2. Hematoma or urinoma formation, abscess formation.
3. Hypertension.
4. Pyelonephritis.
5. Nephrolithiasis.
6. Hydronephrosis.
7. Arteriovenous fistula.

Nursing Assessment

1. Obtain history of traumatic event and any history of renal disease.
2. Inspect for any abrasions, lacerations, or entrance and exit wounds to upper abdomen or lower thorax.
3. Monitor BP and pulse to assess for bleeding and impending shock; perirenal hemorrhage may cause rapid exsanguination.
4. Assess for presence and degree of hematuria.

 NURSING ALERT Watch for any *sudden* change in patient's condition—drop in BP, increasing flank or abdominal pain and tenderness, or palpable mass in the flank. May indicate hemorrhage, which requires surgical intervention.

Nursing Diagnoses

- Risk for Ineffective Renal Perfusion related to injury.
- Impaired Urinary Elimination related to injury.
- Acute Pain related to injury.

Nursing Interventions

Restoring and Maintaining Renal Perfusion

1. Assess vital signs frequently, including BP, heart rate, and CVP to monitor for hemorrhage and impending shock.
2. Assess abdomen and back for local tenderness and palpable mass, swelling, and ecchymosis, indicating hemorrhage or urine extravasation.
3. Outline original mass with marking pen for future comparison of size.
4. Establish IV access for support of BP with fluids or vasopressors, replacement of blood, and perfusion of kidneys.
5. Monitor serial hematocrit determinations to be sure that bleeding has stopped.

Preserving Urinary Elimination

1. Save, inspect, and compare each urine specimen—to follow the course and degree of hematuria.
   a. Label each specimen with date and time.
   b. If specimen is not grossly bloody, dipstick for blood or send to laboratory for microscopic examination.
2. Monitor intake and output carefully.
3. Give antibiotics, as directed, to discourage infection from perirenal hematoma or urinoma or severely contaminated wounds.
4. Monitor for paralytic ileus (lack of bowel sounds) caused by retroperitoneal bleeding.
   a. Keep patient NPO until bowel sounds return.
   b. Administer IV fluids to maintain urine output.

Controlling Pain

1. Administer analgesic medication, as prescribed; exercise caution with drugs that may aggravate hypotension or mask complications of hemorrhage.
2. Encourage bed rest and positioning of comfort until hematuria clears to facilitate healing of minor injuries.
3. Expect a low-grade fever with retroperitoneal hematomas as absorption of the clot occurs; administer antipyretics, as ordered, for comfort.

Patient Education and Health Maintenance

1. Instruct patient not to engage in strenuous activity for at least 1 month after blunt trauma to minimize incidence of delayed or secondary bleeding.
2. Teach patient signs and symptoms of late complications—infection and nephrolithiasis.
3. Advise patient to have BP measured frequently and consistently to monitor for hypertension.
4. Review safety precautions to prevent future injuries.

Evaluation: Expected Outcomes

- Vital signs stable.
- Serial urines clearing.
- Reports decreased pain.

Injuries to the Bladder and Urethra

Injuries to the bladder and urethra commonly occur along with pelvic fracture or may be due to surgical interventions.

Pathophysiology and Etiology

1. Bladder injuries are classified as follows:
   a. Contusion of the bladder.
   b. Intraperitoneal rupture.
   c. Extraperitoneal rupture.
   d. Combination intraperitoneal and extraperitoneal bladder rupture.
2. Urethral injuries (occurring almost exclusively in men) are classified as follows:
   a. Partial or complete rupture.
   b. Anterior or posterior urethral rupture.
3. Injuries to the bladder and urethra are commonly associated with pelvic fractures and multiple trauma.
4. Certain surgical procedures (endoscopic urologic procedures, gynecologic surgery, surgery of the lower colon and rectum) also carry a risk of trauma to the bladder and urethra.

5. Intraperitoneal bladder rupture occurs when the bladder is full of urine and the lower abdomen sustains blunt trauma. The bladder ruptures at its weakest point, the dome. Urine and blood extravasate into the peritoneal cavity.
6. Extraperitoneal bladder rupture occurs when the lower bladder is perforated by a bony fragment during pelvic fracture or with a sharp instrument during surgery. Urine and blood extravasate into the pelvic cavity.
7. Urethral rupture occurs during pelvic fracture (posterior) or when the urethra or penis is manipulated accidentally during surgery or injury (anterior).

Clinical Manifestations

1. Inability to void.
2. Gross hematuria; presence of blood at urinary meatus may indicate ruptured urethra.
3. Shock and hemorrhage—pallor, rapid and increasing pulse rate.
4. Suprapubic pain and tenderness.
5. Rigid abdomen—indicates intraperitoneal rupture.
6. Absence of prostate on rectal examination in posterior urethral rupture.
7. Swelling or discoloration of the penis, scrotum, and anterior perineum in anterior urethral rupture.

Diagnostic Evaluation

1. Retrograde urethrogram—to detect rupture of the urethra.
2. Cystogram—to detect and localize perforation/rupture of the bladder.
3. Plain film of the abdomen—may show associated pelvic fracture.
4. Abdominal CT with contrast—best study to evaluate extent of kidney injury.
5. Excretory urogram—to survey the kidneys and ureters for injury.

 NURSING ALERT If ruptured urethra is suspected and/or blood at meatus observed, do not catheterize because doing so may complete a partial urethral rupture. A urethrogram must be obtained first to determine patency of the urethra.

Management

Bladder Injury
1. Treatment instituted for shock and hemorrhage.
2. Surgical intervention carried out for intraperitoneal bladder rupture. Extravasated blood and urine will first be drained and urine diverted with suprapubic cystostomy or indwelling catheter.
3. Small extraperitoneal bladder ruptures will heal spontaneously with indwelling suprapubic or urethral catheter drainage.
4. Large extraperitoneal bladder ruptures are repaired surgically.

Urethral Injury Management—Controversial
1. Immediate repair—the urethra is manipulated into its correct anatomical position with reanastomosis after evacuation of hematoma.
2. Delayed repair—suprapubic cystostomy drainage for 6 to 12 weeks allows the urethra to realign itself while hematoma and edema resolve; then, surgical reanastomosis.
3. Two-stage urethroplasty—reconstruction of the urethra occurs in two separate surgeries with urinary elimination diverted until final procedure.

Complications
1. Shock, hemorrhage, peritonitis.
2. UTI.
3. Urethral stricture disease.
4. Impotence.
5. Incontinence.

Nursing Assessment
1. Obtain vital signs; assess for evidence of shock.
2. Obtain detailed history of injury, if possible.
3. Inspect urinary meatus for evidence of bleeding. If present, do not insert Foley until retrograde urethrogram verifies patent urethra.
4. Perform physical examination for symptoms of bladder rupture, dullness to palpation, and rebound tenderness or rigidity.

Nursing Diagnoses
- Risk for Deficient Fluid Volume related to trauma and resulting hemorrhage.
- Impaired Urinary Elimination related to disruption of intact lower urinary tract.
- Acute Pain related to traumatic injury.
- Fear related to traumatic injury and uncertain prognosis.

Nursing Interventions

Stabilizing Circulatory Volume
1. Monitor vital signs and CVP frequently, as indicated by condition.
2. Establish IV access and replace blood and fluids, as ordered.

Facilitating Urinary Elimination
1. Inspect urethral meatus for blood and, if present, do not catheterize but prepare for diagnostic evaluation and suprapubic cystostomy.
2. Obtain urine specimen, if possible, and assess for degree of hematuria and presence of infection.
3. Prepare patient for surgical repair by assisting with preoperative workup and describing postoperative experiences.
4. Postoperatively, maintain patency and flow of indwelling urinary catheters.
5. Inspect suprapubic incision and Penrose drains from perivesical areas for bleeding, extravasation of urine, or signs of infection.

Controlling Pain
1. Administer analgesics, as ordered (when patient's vital signs are stable).
2. Assess patient's response to pain control medications.
3. Position for comfort (usually semi-Fowler position), if not contraindicated by other injuries, and prevent pulling of catheter tubing.

Relieving Fear
1. Provide information to the conscious patient throughout the stabilization and evaluation phase; prepare for surgery, if impending.
2. Keep patient's family or significant others informed of condition and progress.
3. Provide information on long-term outcome of treatment.

Patient Education and Health Maintenance
1. Teach patient to care for indwelling catheters that will remain in place during healing or after surgery.
   a. Empty catheter frequently.
   b. Clean catheter and insertion area with soap and water.

c. Inspect urine for blood, cloudiness, or concentration.

d. Drink plenty of fluids to keep urine flowing.

2. Teach patient to report signs and symptoms of UTI.

3. Instruct patient (after surgical repair of bladder rupture) that bladder capacity may be temporarily decreased, causing frequency and nocturia; this resolves over time.

4. Explain possibility of recurrent urethral stricture disease to patients with urethral injury; instruct in daily self-catheterization to dilate the urethra, if prescribed.

5. Support patient (after severe urethral injury) if there is a chance of impotence or incontinence.

Evaluation: Expected Outcomes

- Vital signs stable.
- Adequate urine output by way of catheter.
- Verbalizes relief of pain.
- Verbalizes reduction in fear.

Cancer of the Bladder

Cancer of the bladder is the second most common urologic malignancy. Approximately 90% of all bladder cancers are transitional cell carcinomas, which arise from the epithelial lining of the urinary tract; transitional cell tumors can also occur in the ureters, renal pelvis, and urethra. The remaining 10% of bladder cancers are adenocarcinoma, squamous cell carcinoma, or sarcoma.

Pathophysiology and Etiology

1. Many bladder tumors are diagnosed when the lesions are superficial; papillary tumors are easily resected.

2. One fourth of patients with bladder cancer present with non-papillary, muscle invasive disease.

3. Bladder tumors tend to be either low-grade superficial tumors or high-grade invasive cancers.

4. Metastasis occurs in the bladder wall and pelvis, para-aortic or supraclavicular nodes, liver, lungs, and bone.

5. Although the specific etiology is unknown, it appears that multiple agents are linked to the development of cancer of the bladder, including:

   a. Cigarette smoking—the risk of developing bladder cancer is up to four times higher in smokers.

   b. Prolonged exposure to aromatic amines or their metabolites—generally dyes manufactured by the chemical industry and used by other industries.

   c. Exposure to cyclophosphamide, radiation therapy to the pelvis, chronic irritation of the bladder (as in long-term indwelling catheterization), and excessive use of the analgesic drug phenacetin, which has been taken off the market.

6. Bladder cancer is the fourth most common cancer in men; it occurs four times more frequently in men than in women; peak incidence occurs in the sixth to eighth decades.

Clinical Manifestations

1. Painless hematuria, either gross or microscopic—most characteristic sign.

2. Dysuria, frequency, urgency—bladder irritability.

3. Pelvic or flank pain—obstruction or distant metastases.

4. Leg edema—from invasion of pelvic lymph nodes.

Diagnostic Evaluation

1. Cystoscopy for visualization of number, location, and appearance of tumors; for biopsy.

2. Urine and bladder washing for cytologic study.

3. Urine for flow cytometry—uses a computer-controlled fluorescence microscope to scan and image the nucleus of each cell on a slide; based on the fact that cancer cells contain abnormally large amounts of deoxyribonucleic acid.

4. IVU—may reveal filling defect indicative of bladder tumor; also determines status of upper tracts.

5. CT urography (three-phase CT scan)—replacing IVU or IVP as the test of choice to evaluate kidneys, ureter, and bladder.

6. To evaluate for metastatic disease:

   a. CT scan or MRI—to evaluate extent of disease and tumor responsiveness.

   b. Chest x-ray—to evaluate for pulmonary metastases.

   c. Pelvic lymphadenectomy (during cystectomy)—most accurate for staging.

Management

Surgery

1. Transurethral resection and fulguration—endoscopic resection for superficial tumors.

   a. May be followed by intravesical chemotherapy to prevent tumor recurrence.

   b. Complications include hemorrhage, infection, bladder perforation, and temporary irritative voiding.

   c. Laser irradiation of bladder tumors is also used to destroy tumors; however, it does not allow for tumor specimen collection for pathologic analysis.

2. Partial cystectomy when lesions are located only in the dome of the bladder, away from the ureteral orifices.

3. Radical cystectomy (removal of the bladder) for invasive or poorly differentiated tumors.

   a. Requires diversion of the urinary stream (see page 596).

   b. In men, includes removal of the bladder, prostate and seminal vesicles, proximal vas deferens, and part of proximal urethra.

   c. Men may be impotent.

   d. In women, consists of anterior exenteration with removal of the bladder, urethra, uterus, fallopian tubes, ovaries, and segment of anterior wall of the vagina.

   e. May be combined with chemotherapy and radiation.

Intravesical (within the Bladder) Chemotherapy and Immunotherapy

1. Instillation of immunotherapeutic agent bacillus Calmette-Guerin (BCG) stimulates immune response to prevent recurrence of transitional cell bladder tumors. BCG is attenuated mycobacterium initially developed as a vaccine for tuberculosis and has demonstrated antitumor activity in selected cancers.

2. Instillation of antineoplastic agents, such as thiotepa, mitomycin-C, and doxorubicin, allows a high concentration of drug to come in contact with the tumor and urothelium with minimal systemic toxicity.

3. Patient is instructed as follows:

   a. Minimize fluid intake and avoid taking diuretic medications for several hours before the instillation period to maximize concentration of drug treatment period.

   b. Change position, as directed during instillation, in an effort to have drug contact as much of urothelial surface as possible.

   c. Wash hands and perineal area after voiding the medication to prevent contact dermatitis.

   d. Do not void for 2 hours after instillation; then, increase fluid intake and void frequently.

e. When using BCG, place two cups of bleach into toilet with each void for 6 hours after starting voiding to neutralize the chemotherapeutic agent and prevent possible contamination to others.

f. Course of treatment involves weekly instillations for 6 weeks followed by monthly instillations.

4. Complications from intravesical chemotherapy and immunotherapy include UTI, irritative voiding symptoms, allergic reaction, bone marrow suppression, or systemic BCG reaction. A systemic BCG reaction occurs when fever higher than 100°F (37.8°C) persists for more than 24 hours; it is treated with antituberculosis agents.

Systemic Chemotherapy

Metastatic bladder cancer is a chemotherapeutically responsive disease; gemcitabine and cisplatin have lower toxicity, improved tolerability, and similar overall survival to the MVDC combination (methotrexate, vinblastine, doxorubicin, and cisplatin), which had been in wide use.

Radiation Therapy

External beam radiation therapy is commonly used in combination with chemotherapy.

Complications

Regional metastasis through the pelvis as well as metastasis to the lung, liver, and bone.

Nursing Assessment

1. Assess for hematuria, irritative voiding symptoms, risk factors (especially smoking history), weight loss, fatigue, and signs of metastasis.
2. Assess coping ability and knowledge of the disease and explore feelings about impotence.

Nursing Diagnoses

• Impaired Urinary Elimination related to hematuria and transurethral surgery.
• Acute Pain related to irritative voiding symptoms and catheter-related discomfort.
• Anxiety related to diagnosis of cancer.

Nursing Interventions

Maintaining Urinary Elimination after Transurethral Surgery

1. Maintain patency of indwelling urinary drainage catheter; manual irrigation is not recommended due to dangers of bladder perforation; continuous bladder irrigation may be used, if necessary.
2. Ensure adequate hydration either orally or via IV line.
3. Monitor intake and output, including irrigation solution.
4. Monitor urine output for clearing of hematuria.

Controlling Pain

1. Administer analgesic medication for pelvic discomfort.
2. Administer anticholinergic medications or belladonna and opium suppositories to relieve bladder spasms.
3. Ensure patency of catheter drainage; do not irrigate unless specifically ordered.
4. Remove indwelling catheter as soon as possible after procedure.

Relieving Anxiety

1. Allow patient to verbalize fears and concerns about altered sexuality.

2. Provide realistic information about diagnostic studies, surgery, and treatments.

Patient Education and Health Maintenance

1. Advise patient that irritative voiding symptoms and intermittent hematuria are possible for several weeks after transurethral resection of bladder tumors.
2. Teach patient with superficial bladder cancer importance of vigilant adherence to follow-up schedule: after initial 6-week induction course of BCG, they need cystoscopy and three weekly instillations of BCG at 3 and 6 months and then every 6 months thereafter for 3 years. Yearly cystoscopy is required as 70% of superficial tumors will recur.
3. Review purpose and adverse effects of intravesical chemotherapy treatments (usually not given until after recurrence).

Evaluation: Expected Outcomes

• Urine output adequate and clear.
• Verbalizes relief of pain and bladder spasms.
• Verbalizes lessened anxiety.

CONDITIONS OF THE MALE REPRODUCTIVE TRACT

Urethritis

EVIDENCE BASE Centers for Disease Control and Prevention. (2015). Sexually transmitted disease treatment guidelines 2015. *MMWR, 64*(3), 1–137.

Urethritis is inflammation of the urethra. It is usually an ascending infection in men. In women, it is usually associated with cystitis (see page 610) or vaginitis (see page 655).

Pathophysiology and Etiology

1. Nongonococcal urethritis—urethritis not caused by gonococcus; may be sexually transmitted:
   a. *Chlamydia trachomatis*—most clinically significant of the pathogens, three cases of chlamydia diagnosed for every one case of gonorrhea. Usually asymptomatic.
   b. *Ureaplasma urealyticum* and *Mycoplasma genitalium*—responsible for up to one third of cases.
   c. *Trichomonas vaginalis* and herpes simplex virus are other sexually transmitted organisms causing urethritis in men and women.
   d. Incubation period of 1 to 5 weeks depending on the organism; in some cases, infection may be subclinical for a period of time, particularly in men.
2. Gonococcal urethritis—caused by *Neisseria gonorrhoeae*, sexually transmitted; usually most virulent and destructive.
   a. Incubation period usually 3 to 10 days.
   b. Urethritis in homosexual men is more commonly gonococcal than nongonococcal.
3. Gonococcal and nongonococcal urethritis can both be present.
4. Nonsexually transmitted.
   a. Bacterial urethritis—may be associated with UTI.
   b. From trauma—secondary to passage of urethral sounds, repeated cystoscopy, indwelling catheter.

Clinical Manifestations

1. Can be asymptomatic.
2. Itching and burning around area of the urethra.
3. Urethral discharge: may be scant or profuse; thin, clear, or mucoid; or thick and purulent (gonococcal).
4. Dysuria and frequency.
5. Penile discomfort.

Diagnostic Evaluation

1. Gram stain—*N. gonorrhoeae* is detected as gram-positive diplococci on microscopic examination of urethral discharge or urine.
2. Culture of urethral discharge on selective medium.
3. Deoxyribonucleic acid (DNA) amplification tests on urethral voided specimen or other DNA/antibody tests of urethral discharge (currently, primary test)—to detect *C. trachomatis* and *N. gonorrhoeae*.
4. Wet mount microscopic examination of fresh urethral discharge—trichomonads may be visible and motile.
5. First voided urine for screening—either positive leukocyte esterase test by dipstick or greater than 10 WBC per high-power field by microscopy indicates urethritis.
6. In rare cases, urethroscopy may be necessary to isolate a lesion such as warts caused by human papillomavirus (HPV).

Management

1. Gonococcal urethritis: one dose oral antibiotic of cefixime 400 mg or one dose IM treatment with ceftriaxone 125 mg.
2. Chlamydial urethritis: single dose of oral antibiotic azithromycin 1 g or doxycycline 100 mg orally twice per day for 7 days.
3. Unless proven otherwise by negative testing, treatment for chlamydia is given along with treatment for gonorrhea.
4. Recurrent urethritis despite appropriate treatment for nongonococcal urethritis or confirmed presence of *T. vaginalis* treatment is one dose oral metronidazole 2 g.

 DRUG ALERT Fluoroquinolones are now avoided in the treatment of gonococcal infections because of drug resistance.

Complications

Depends on cause, but may include:
1. Prostatitis, epididymitis, urethral stricture, sterility because of vas epididymal duct obstruction.
2. Rectal infection, pharyngitis, conjunctivitis, skin lesions, arthritis with gonococcal infection.
3. Long-term complications of these infections in women include pelvic inflammatory disease and infertility.

Nursing Assessment

1. Obtain history of unprotected sexual contact and assess patient's understanding of risk.
2. Assess for signs and symptoms involving urinary and reproductive tracts.
3. Perform genital and abdominal examination to assess for extent of infection.

Nursing Diagnoses

- Risk for Infection related to ascending or systemic spread of pathogens.
- Risk for Infection related to high-risk sexual activity.

Nursing Interventions

Resolving Infection and Preventing Complications
1. Collect urethral swab of discharge, urine, and blood, as ordered, for laboratory examination.
2. Use standard precautions when handling specimens.
3. Administer antibiotics, as prescribed.
   a. Usually ordered based on presumptive diagnosis before test results are obtained.
   b. Monitor for and advise patient of adverse effects or allergic reactions.

Preventing Spread of Infection
1. Encourage compliance with antimicrobial regimen for the prescribed time period.
2. Advise abstinence from sexual activity until treatment is complete and cure is established (usually 7 to 10 days).
3. Instruct the patient to avoid sexual activity with previous sexual partner until that person has been tested and treated for infection as well.
4. The use of condoms may prevent transmission, but depends on technique.

Patient Education and Health Maintenance

1. Advise safer sex practices, such as abstinence, mutual monogamy, and use of male or female condom to prevent transmission of sexually transmitted organisms as well as unintended pregnancy.
2. Emphasize the need for follow-up care if symptoms persist or return.
3. Advise patient that reporting of gonorrhea to the public health department is required by law in all of the United States and Canada.
4. Tell patient that he or she will be called on to name all sexual partners within the past 60 days and that the process will be confidential.
5. Provide written information about all STDs and ensure that patient understands the dangers of high-risk sexual behavior.

Evaluation: Expected Outcomes

- Signs of infection resolved.
- Reports sexual contacts have been treated.

Benign Prostatic Hyperplasia

Benign prostatic hyperplasia (BPH) is enlargement of the prostate that constricts the urethra, causing urinary symptoms. One in four men who reach age 80 will require treatment for BPH.

Pathophysiology and Etiology

1. The process of aging and the presence of circulating androgens are required for the development of BPH.
2. The prostatic tissue forms nodules as enlargement occurs.
3. The normally thin and fibrous outer capsule of the prostate becomes spongy and thick as enlargement progresses.

4. The prostatic urethra becomes compressed and narrowed, requiring the bladder musculature to work harder to empty urine.

5. Effects of prolonged obstruction cause trabeculation (formation of cords) of the bladder wall, decreasing its elasticity.

Clinical Manifestations

1. In early or gradual prostatic enlargement, there may be no symptoms because the bladder musculature can initially compensate for increased urethral resistance.

2. Obstructive symptoms—hesitancy, diminution in size and force of urinary stream, terminal dribbling, sensation of incomplete emptying of the bladder, urinary retention.

3. Irritative voiding symptoms—urgency, frequency, nocturia.

Diagnostic Evaluation

1. American Urologic Association Symptom Index score greater than 7 (uses rating of questions about the obstructive and irritative symptoms): 0 to 7, mild; 8 to 19, moderate; and 20 to 35, severe.

2. Rectal examination—smooth, firm, symmetric, or asymmetric enlargement of the prostate.

3. Urinalysis—to rule out hematuria and infection.

4. Serum creatinine and BUN—to evaluate renal function.

5. Serum PSA—may be elevated in patients with BPH.

6. Optional diagnostic studies for further evaluation:
   a. Urodynamics—measures peak urine flow rate, voiding time and volume, and status of the bladder's ability to effectively contract.
   b. Measurement of postvoid residual urine; by ultrasound or catheterization.
   c. Cystourethroscopy—to inspect the urethra and bladder and evaluate prostatic size.
   d. Uroflow—graphically demonstrates voiding pattern and can help characterize the severity of obstruction.

Management

1. Patients with mild symptoms (in the absence of significant bladder or renal impairment) are followed annually; BPH does not necessarily worsen in all men.

2. Pharmacologic management.
   a. Alpha-adrenergic blockers, such as doxazosin, tamsulosin, terazosin, and alfuzosin—relax smooth muscle of bladder neck and prostate to facilitate voiding.
   b. 5-Alpha-reductase inhibitors such as finasteride and dutasteride—exert antiandrogen effect on prostatic cells and can reverse or prevent hyperplasia. These drugs decrease the size of the prostate and improve urinary symptoms. Effect of drug may take up to 6 months. Women should not handle drug because it can be absorbed through the skin and is pregnancy category X. In addition, patients taking dutasteride cannot donate blood.

3. Surgery (also see page 601)—options include TURP (formerly most common procedure), transurethral incision of the prostate, or open prostatectomy for very large prostates, usually by suprapubic approach.

4. PVP is starting to replace TURP; it is done through a cystoscope, using a laser to vaporize diseased prostatic tissue.

5. TUMT and TUNA are both office-based procedures that use heat to destroy diseased prostatic tissue.

6. Indigo interstitial laser therapy of the prostate is another procedure that is done on an outpatient basis.

 DRUG ALERT Although prescribed for their effect on prostatic smooth muscle, alpha-adrenergic blockers (except for tamsulosin and alfuzosin) also have an antihypertensive effect. Dosage is usually titrated up from an initial small dose. It is commonly recommended that the first dose, or all once per day doses, be taken at bedtime.

 DRUG ALERT Finasteride is present in semen and may have deleterious fetal effects.

Complications

1. Acute urinary retention, involuntary bladder contractions, bladder diverticula, and cystolithiasis.

2. Vesicoureteral reflux, hydroureter, hydronephrosis.

3. Gross hematuria, UTI.

Nursing Assessment

1. Obtain history of voiding symptoms, including onset, frequency of day and nighttime urination, presence of urgency, dysuria, sensation of incomplete bladder emptying, and decreased force of stream. Determine impact on quality of life.

2. Perform rectal (palpate size, shape, and consistency) and abdominal examination to detect distended bladder, degree of prostatic enlargement.

3. Perform simple urodynamic measures—uroflowmetry and measurement of postvoid residual, if indicated.

Nursing Diagnosis

- Impaired Urinary Elimination related to obstruction of the urethra.

Also see page 601 for care of the patient undergoing prostatic surgery.

Nursing Interventions

Facilitating Urinary Elimination

1. Provide privacy and time for patient to void.

2. Assist with catheter introduction with guide wire or by way of suprapubic cystotomy, as indicated.
   a. Monitor intake and output.
   b. Maintain patency of catheter.

3. Administer medications, as ordered, and monitor for and teach patient about adverse effects.
   a. Alpha-adrenergic blockers—hypotension, orthostatic hypotension, syncope (especially after first dose), potential impotence, potential retrograde ejaculation, blurred vision, rebound hypertension if discontinued abruptly.
   b. Finasteride and dutasteride—hepatic dysfunction, potential impotence, interference with PSA testing, presence in semen with potential adverse effect on fetus of pregnant woman.

4. Assess for and teach patient to report hematuria and signs of infection.

 DRUG ALERT Treatment with finasteride and dutasteride decreases the PSA by half, so this should be taken into account when obtaining PSA to monitor for prostate cancer.

Patient Education and Health Maintenance

1. Explain to patient symptoms and complications of BPH—urinary retention, hydronephrosis, cystitis, increase in irritative voiding symptoms. Encourage reporting these problems and maintaining close follow-up.
2. Advise patients with BPH to avoid certain drugs that may impair voiding (see Table 21-3), particularly OTC cold medicines containing sympathomimetics such as phenylpropanolamine.
3. Advise patient that irritative voiding symptoms do not immediately resolve after relief of obstruction; symptoms diminish over time.
4. Tell patient postoperatively to avoid sexual intercourse, straining at stool, heavy lifting, and long periods of sitting for 6 to 8 weeks after surgery, until prostatic fossa is healed.
5. Advise follow-up visits after treatment because urethral stricture may occur and regrowth of prostate is possible after TURP.
6. Be aware of herbal or "natural" products marketed for "prostate health."
   a. Advise patients that saw palmetto has shown some efficacy in reducing symptoms of BPH in a number of clinical trials.
   b. The active ingredient in commercial preparations is lipidosterolic extract of *Serenoa repens*; dosage is 160 mg twice per day.
   c. It should be taken with breakfast and an evening meal to minimize GI adverse effects.
   d. Although it appears safe and there are no known drug interactions, tell patients they must discuss use of saw palmetto with their health care providers.
7. Advise patient to notify all health care providers of medications. If cataract surgery is being planned, the ophthalmologist should be aware of tamsulosin use, which may increase risk of floppy iris syndrome.

Evaluation: Expected Outcomes

- Voiding adequate without residual urine.

Prostatitis

Prostatitis is an inflammation of the prostate gland. It is classified as bacterial prostatitis (acute or chronic) or chronic pelvic pain syndrome (without presence of bacterial invasion).

Pathophysiology and Etiology

Acute and Chronic Bacterial Invasion of the Prostate

1. From reflux of infected urine into ejaculatory and prostatic ducts.
2. From hematogenous (bloodstream) origin, lymphogenous spread, or direct extension from the rectum.
3. Secondary to urethritis—from ascent of bacteria from the urethra.
4. May be stimulated by urethral instrumentation or rectal examination of the prostate when bacteria are present.
5. May be caused by gram-negative enteric bacteria, such as *Pseudomonas aeruginosa*, *E. coli*, and *Klebsiella pneumonia*, and gram-positive cocci, such as *Streptococcus* and *Staphylococcus*; may also be caused by *C. trachomatis*.

Chronic Pelvic Pain Syndrome

Pain or discomfort without other signs of infection and no known etiologic cause; difficult to diagnose and manage.

Table 21-3 Bladder Function and Drug Actions

FUNCTION	DRUG GROUPS	EXAMPLES
Detrusor Muscle		
Increased tone and contraction	Cholinergic drugs (stimulate parasympathetic receptors that cause detrusor muscle contraction)	• Bethanechol • Neostigmine
Decreased tone, possible retention	Anticholinergic drugs (block parasympathetic receptors that cause detrusor muscle contraction)	• Methantheline • Propantheline • Oxybutynin • Darifenacin • Solifenacin • Trospium
Relaxes bladder tone	Calcium channel–blocking drugs (may interfere with influx of calcium to support detrusor muscle tone)	• Nifedipine • Verapamil • Diltiazem • Tolterodine tartrate
Internal Sphincter		
Increased tone, possible retention	Alpha$_1$-adrenergic agonists (activate alpha receptors that cause contraction of muscles of the internal sphincter)	• Phenylephrine • Ephedrine • Phenylpropanolamine
Decreased tone	Alpha$_1$-adrenergic blockers	• Alfuzosin • Prazosin • Doxazosin • Terazosin • Tamsulosin
External Sphincter		
Decreased tone, possible retention	Skeletal muscle relaxants	• Baclofen • Dantrolene • Diazepam

Clinical Manifestations

1. Sudden chills and fever (moderate to high fever) and body aches with acute prostatitis.
2. Symptoms are more subtle with chronic prostatitis and chronic pelvic pain syndrome.
3. Bladder irritability—frequency, dysuria, nocturia, urgency, hematuria to varying degrees.
4. Pain in the perineum, rectum, lower back, lower abdomen, and tip of the penis.
5. Pain after ejaculation, symptoms of urethral obstruction.

Diagnostic Evaluation

1. Urinalysis.
2. Urine culture and sensitivity tests.
   a. Prostate massage is inadvisable because it can precipitate frank sepsis or bacteremia.
   b. In acute bacterial prostatitis, there are numerous WBCs and a positive culture; in chronic bacterial prostatitis, there is a lower bacterial colony count; in chronic pelvic pain syndrome, there may be WBCs but a negative culture.
3. Rectal examination commonly reveals exquisitely tender, painful, swollen (boggy) prostate that is warm to the touch (with acute bacterial prostatitis).
4. Serum WBC count is elevated in acute bacterial prostatitis.
5. Bladder scan for postvoid residual evaluates bladder emptying.
6. Transrectal ultrasound detects prostate abscess.

Management

Acute Bacterial Prostatitis

1. Antimicrobial therapy generally for 2 to 4 weeks based on drug sensitivity; commonly a fluoroquinolone or sulfamethoxazole–trimethoprim.
2. IV therapy with ampicillin or an aminoglycoside in the hospitalized patient. Patients are hospitalized if there is suspected abscess, urosepsis, or immunocompromise.
3. Urinary retention is managed with suprapubic cystostomy; urethral catheterization usually is avoided.
4. Antipyretics, analgesics, hydration, stool softeners, and sitz baths for symptom relief.

Chronic Bacterial Prostatitis

1. Usually 4 to 6 weeks of oral antibiotic therapy with ability to diffuse into prostate.
   a. Quinolones such as ciprofloxacin, levofloxacin, ofloxacin, or norfloxacin.
   b. Sulfonamide such as sulfamethoxazole–trimethoprim.
2. Oral antispasmodic agents may provide relief from urinary frequency and urgency.
3. Alpha-adrenergic blockers may help with urination.

Chronic Pelvic Pain Syndrome

1. Usually requires multiple modalities.
2. Alpha-adrenergic blockers and skeletal muscle relaxants may provide some relief of symptoms.
3. Aggressive diagnostic intervention should take place to rule out other conditions, such as cancer of the prostate or interstitial cystitis.
4. Anti-inflammatory medications such as NSAIDs are helpful.
5. Tricyclic antidepressants may be helpful for pain control.
6. Pentosan may be helpful to relieve discomfort.
7. Quinoline antibiotics may be taken for 4 to 6 weeks.
8. Pelvic floor massage and biofeedback may help relieve perineal muscle spasms.

Complications

1. Bacteriuria, urethritis, epididymitis, prostatic abscess, bacteremia, septicemia.
2. Acute urinary retention.
3. Constipation.

Nursing Assessment

1. Obtain history of previous lower UTIs or STDs and recent voiding patterns.
2. Perform examination of genitalia for urethral discharge; rectal examination (except in acute bacterial prostatitis because of tenderness and possibility of disseminating infection) to assess tenderness of the prostate.
3. Collect specimens: urine for culture and expressed prostatic secretions. To help distinguish urethral, bladder, and prostate infections, have the patient collect the first 10 mL of urine and label this voided bladder-1. This will be a urethral specimen. Next, have the patient collect a midstream urine specimen and label this voided bladder-2. This is a bladder specimen. Have the patient urinate after a prostatic massage and label this voided bladder-3. This is a prostatic specimen.

Nursing Diagnoses

- Hyperthermia related to infectious process.
- Acute Pain related to prostatic inflammation.
- Chronic Pain related to chronic prostatitis, chronic pelvic pain syndrome.

Nursing Interventions

Reducing Fever

1. Start antibiotic therapy as soon as specimens are obtained for culture.
2. Administer antipyretic medications; use cooling measures, if necessary.
3. Keep patient well hydrated, via IV administration or orally, because of fluid loss through fever; however, avoid overhydration, which increases urine volume and reduces antibiotic concentration in urine.

Relieving Pain

1. Administer analgesic or anti-inflammatory medication, as ordered.
2. Maintain bed rest in acute prostatitis to relieve perineal and suprapubic pain.
3. Maintain high-fiber diet and give stool softeners, as needed, to prevent constipation, which increases pain.

Controlling Chronic Pain

1. Administer or teach self-administration of analgesics, anti-inflammatory agents, alpha-adrenergic blockers, or skeletal muscle relaxants as ordered.
2. Advise warm sitz baths to relieve pain and promote muscular relaxation of pelvic floor and reduce potential for urinary retention.
3. Assess patient's response to supportive measures and coping with chronic pain.

Patient Education and Health Maintenance

1. Instruct patient to take antibiotic, as prescribed; emphasize importance of completing long course of therapy to prevent recurrence and resistance of organisms.

2. Teach patient symptoms of recurrence and of disseminated spread of infection.
3. Instruct patient in comfort measures: sitz baths (10 to 20 minutes) several times daily, continued use of stool softeners, and not sitting for long periods.
4. Advise patient to avoid sexual arousal and intercourse during period of acute inflammation; sexual intercourse may be beneficial in the treatment of chronic prostatitis to stimulate the secretion of prostatic fluid and relieve prostate congestion; chronic prostatic infection is not sexually transmittable.
5. Encourage prescribed follow-up because recurrence is possible.

Evaluation: Expected Outcomes

- Afebrile.
- Verbalizes relief of pain after analgesic.
- Verbalizes reduction of chronic pain.

Cancer of the Prostate

Cancer of the prostate is the leading cause of cancer and second leading cause of cancer death among American men and is the most common carcinoma in men older than 65.

Pathophysiology and Etiology

1. The incidence of prostate cancer is 30% higher in African American men.
2. The majority of prostate cancers arise from the peripheral zone of the gland.
3. Prostate cancer can spread by local extension, by lymphatics, or by way of the bloodstream.
4. The etiology of prostate cancer is unknown; however, there is an increased risk for persons with a family history of the disease.
5. The influences of dietary fat intake, serum testosterone levels, and industrial exposure to carcinogens are under investigation.

Clinical Manifestations

1. Most early-stage prostate cancers are asymptomatic.
2. Symptoms because of obstruction of urinary flow:
   a. Hesitancy and straining on voiding, frequency, and nocturia.
   b. Diminution in size and force of urinary stream.
3. Symptoms because of metastasis:
   a. Pain in lumbosacral area radiating to hips and down legs (from bone metastases).
   b. Perineal and rectal discomfort.
   c. Anemia, weight loss, weakness, nausea, oliguria (from uremia).
   d. Hematuria (from urethral or bladder invasion, or both).
   e. Lower extremity edema—occurs when pelvic node metastases compromise venous return.

Diagnostic Evaluation

1. Digital rectal examination—the prostate can be felt through the wall of the rectum; hard nodule may be felt (see Figure 21-11).
2. Transrectal ultrasound–guided needle biopsy (through anterior rectal wall or through the perineum) for histologic study of biopsied tissue includes Gleason tumor grade if carcinoma is present.
3. Transrectal ultrasonography—sonar probe placed in the rectum.

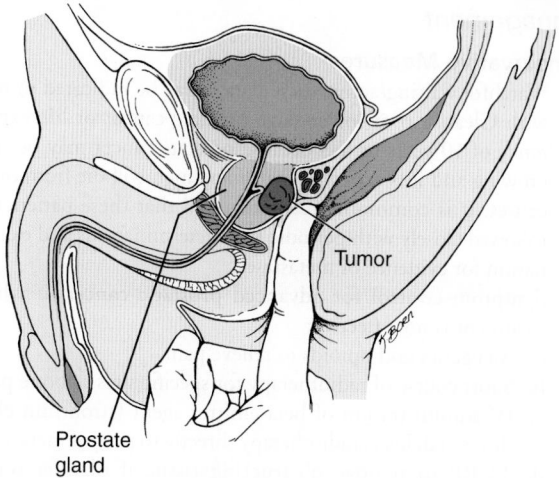

Figure 21-11. The prostate gland can be felt through the wall of the rectum. The size of the gland, overall consistency, and the presence of any firm areas and nodules are noted.

4. PSA—a protease produced by both benign and malignant prostate tissues. An elevated PSA may be due to BPH, prostatitis, or prostate cancer.
   a. Prostate cancer is suspected if PSA is above 4; however, prostate cancer may also occur at levels under 4.0.
   b. A free PSA level can be used to help stratify the risk of an elevated PSA. The lower the free PSA level, the higher the risk for prostate cancer.
   c. PSA velocity: PSA increases of 0.75 ng in 1 year could indicate prostate cancer.
   d. Age-specific PSA can help stratify risk for prostate cancer as well.
5. Guidelines among various cancer, urologic, and prevention organizations such as United States Preventive Services Task Force (USPSTF) and the American Urological Association (AUA) regarding prostate cancer screening vary. The USPSTF states that there is insufficient evidence to recommend screening. ACS is not in favor of routine screening until an informed discussion with those patients wanting to be screened takes place. The National Comprehensive Cancer Network (NCCN) recommends baseline DRE/PSA at 40 years of age and annual screening at age 50. AUA recommends baseline DRE/PSA at 40 years of age. All recommend informed discussion with patients.
6. Staging evaluation—skeletal x-rays, CT scan, MRI, bone scan, analysis of pelvic lymph nodes provide accurate staging information.
7. Newer imaging study called the ProstaScint scan uses an IV infusion of monoclonal antibody to prostate-specific membrane antigen.
   a. Immediate and delayed images at 48 and 72 hours may identify soft tissue and bone metastasis for staging.
   b. Radiation is excreted through urine and feces and body fluids but is very low and not a risk to others.
   c. Patient is monitored for signs of allergic reactions following test.
8. Research is being conducted on numerous genetic and chromosomal abnormalities. Overexpression of the *AMACR* gene was found in 90% of prostate cancer patients. Testing for this gene could result in identifying prostate cancer at an earlier stage.

Management
Conservative Measures
1. Watchful waiting/active surveillance may be indicated in men with Gleason 6 or lower-stage prostate cancer or life expectancy of 10 years or less because prostate cancer may be slow growing and it is expected that many men will die from other causes. It is commonly recommended that these patients be followed closely with periodic PSA determinations and examination for evidence of metastases.
2. Symptom control for advanced prostatic cancer in which treatment is not effective:
   a. Analgesics and opioids to relieve pain.
   b. Short course of radiotherapy for specific sites of bone pain.
   c. IV administration of beta-emitter agent (strontium chloride 89) delivers radiotherapy directly to sites of metastasis.
   d. TURP to remove obstructing tissue if bladder outlet obstruction occurs.
   e. Suprapubic catheter placement.
   f. Zoledronic acid is given intravenously for bone metastasis pain.

Surgical Interventions
1. Radical prostatectomy—removal of entire prostate gland, prostatic capsule, and seminal vesicles; may include pelvic lymphadenectomy.
   a. Procedure is used to treat stage T_1 and T_2 prostate cancers.
   b. Complications may include urinary incontinence and impotence and possible rectal injury.
   c. Newer nerve-sparing techniques may preserve sexual potency and continence.
2. Cryosurgery of the prostate freezes prostate tissue, killing tumor cells without removing the gland.

Radiation
1. External beam radiation or intensity-modulated radiotherapy focused on the prostate—to deliver maximum radiation dose to tumor and minimal dose to surrounding tissues.
2. Brachytherapy—interstitial implantation of radioactive substances into the prostate, which delivers doses of radiation directly to tumor while sparing uninvolved tissue.
3. Used to treat stages T_1, T_2, and T_3, especially if patient is not a good surgical candidate. Both forms of radiation are used in some patients; external beam followed by brachytherapy.
4. Complications include radiation cystitis (urinary frequency, urgency, nocturia), urethral injury (stricture), radiation enteritis (diarrhea, anorexia, nausea), radiation proctitis (diarrhea, rectal bleeding), impotence, skin reaction, and fatigue.

Hormone Manipulation (Palliative)
1. Prostate cancer is a hormone-sensitive cancer. The aim of hormonal treatment is to deprive tumor cells of androgens or their by-products and thereby alleviate symptoms and retard progress of disease.
2. Bilateral orchiectomy (removal of testes) results in reduction of the major circulating androgen, testosterone. A small amount of androgen is still produced by adrenal glands.
3. Pharmacologic methods of achieving androgen deprivation—also used to reduce tumor volume before surgery or radiation therapy.
   a. Luteinizing hormone–releasing hormone (LHRH) agonists (such as leuprolide and goserelin acetate) reduce testosterone levels as effectively as orchiectomy.
   b. Antiandrogen drugs (flutamide, bicalutamide, nilutamide) block androgen action directly at the target tissues (testes and adrenals) and block androgen synthesis within the prostate gland and adrenal glands.
   c. Combination therapy with LHRH agonist and an antiandrogen blocks the action of all circulating androgen.
4. Complications of hormonal manipulation include hot flashes, nausea and vomiting, gynecomastia, sexual dysfunction, and osteoporosis.

Complications
1. Bone metastasis—vertebral collapse and spinal cord compression, pathologic fractures.
2. Complications of treatment.

Nursing Assessment
1. Obtain history of current symptoms; assess for family history of prostate cancer.
2. Palpate lymph nodes, especially in supraclavicular and inguinal regions (may be first sign of metastatic spread); assess for flank pain and distended bladder.
3. Assess comorbidities, nutritional status, and coping before treatment.

Nursing Diagnoses
- Anxiety related to fear of disease progression and treatment options.
- Sexual Dysfunction related to effects of therapy.
- Chronic Pain related to bone metastasis.

Also see page 601 for care of the patient after prostatectomy.

Nursing Interventions
Reducing Anxiety
1. Help patient assess the impact of the disease and treatment options on quality of life.
2. Give repeated explanations of diagnostic tests and treatment options; help patient gain some feeling of control over disease and decisions.
3. Help patient and family set achievable goals.
4. Convey a sense of caring and reassurance in your physical care.

Achieving Optimal Sexual Function
1. Although patient may be ill while experiencing the effects of therapy, he may wonder about sexual function. Give him the opportunity to communicate his concerns and sexual needs.
2. Let patient know that decreased libido is expected after hormonal manipulation therapy and impotence may result from some surgical procedures and radiation.
3. Expect patient's behavior to reflect depression, anxiety, anger, and regression. Encourage expression of feelings and communication with partner.
4. Suggest such options as sexual counseling, learning other methods of sexual expression, and consideration of implant, pharmacologic agents, and other options for treatment of erectile dysfunction.
5. Have patient ask urologist about penile rehabilitation after radical open or laparoscopic prostatectomy. The early incorporation of PDE5 inhibitors, vacuum erectile device, or intracavernosal injections may increase the return of postprostatectomy erections.

DRUG ALERT Yohimbine is an herbal preparation sold OTC as an aphrodisiac and treatment for male erectile dysfunction. Caution patients that it is considered an unsafe herb by the U.S. Department of Agriculture because of its many drug and food interactions and adverse effects, including hypertension, tachycardia, and tremor.

Controlling Pain

1. Administer and teach self-administration of opioid analgesics, as ordered; oral sustained-release opioids, sustained-release transdermal patches, and subcutaneous or epidural patient–controlled infusion pumps are among the many options.
2. Encourage patient to take prescribed aspirin, acetaminophen, or NSAIDs for reduction of mild pain or to supplement opioid pain control regimen.
3. Make sure that patient is not undermedicated; help patient and family understand that addiction is not a concern in hormonally refractory or metastatic prostate cancer.
4. Teach relaxation techniques, such as imagery, music therapy, progressive muscle relaxation.
5. Use safety measures to prevent pathologic fractures from falls.
6. Encourage follow-up and palliative treatment such as radiation therapy to bony lesions for pain improvement.

Community and Home Care Considerations

EVIDENCE BASE Smith, R. A., Manassram-Baptiste, D., Brooks, D., et al. (2015). Cancer screening in the United States, 2015: A review of current American Cancer Society guidelines and issues in cancer screening. *CA—Cancer Journal for Clinicians, 65,* 30–54.

Encourage awareness of prostate cancer in the community.
1. Risks include being African American, over age 50, and having a first-degree relative with prostate cancer. High-fat diet has also been linked to prostate cancer.
2. Asymptomatic men with at least a 10-year life expectancy should have the opportunity to make an informed decision about screening.
3. If screening is desired after a detailed discussion between patient and health care provider, digital rectal examination and PSA blood testing begin at age 50 for men at average risk, at age 45 for African American men and those with a first-degree relative with history of prostate cancer, or at age 40 if a man has multiple relatives diagnosed with prostate cancer before age 65.
4. There is insufficient and conflicting evidence whether prostate cancer screening saves lives.
5. PSA less than 2.5 ng/mL indicates low risk for prostate cancer; therefore, recommendation is to repeat in 2 years.
6. If any urinary obstructions symptoms develop, patient should seek evaluation.

Patient Education and Health Maintenance

1. Teach patient importance of follow-up for check of PSA levels (every 6 to 12 months depending on pathology and recommendation of urologist) and evaluation for disease progression through periodic bone scan or CT scan. Cancer recurrence is suspected with PSA greater than 0.2 on two occasions.

2. Teach IM or subcutaneous administration of hormonal agents, as indicated.
3. If bone metastasis has occurred, encourage safety measures around the home to prevent pathologic fractures such as removal of throw rugs, use of handrail on stairs, use of night-lights.
4. Advise reporting symptoms of worsening urethral obstruction, such as increased frequency, urgency, hesitancy, and urinary retention.
5. Advise patient to monitor for signs of metastasis, such as fatigue, weight loss, weakness, pain, and bowel and bladder dysfunction.
6. For additional information and support, refer to agencies such as Us TOO International (*www.ustoo.com*); Man to Man, a program of the American Cancer Society (*www.cancer.org*); and American Urological Association Foundation (*www.urologyhealth.org*).

Evaluation: Expected Outcomes

- Discusses treatment options; asks questions.
- Verbalizes understanding of sexual dysfunction and interest in seeking sexual counseling.
- Reports pain relief after opioid administration.

Testicular Cancer

Testicular cancer is a disease that occurs in younger men between age 15 and 35. It is relatively uncommon, affecting 9 of 100,000 men annually. It is the most treatable form of urologic cancer.

Pathophysiology and Etiology

1. The majority of testicular cancers are of germ cell origin; the most common germinal tumors in adults are seminoma, embryonal carcinoma, teratoma, and choriocarcinoma (the latter three are also called *nonseminomas*).
2. The etiology of testicular tumors is unknown, but there is a relationship between cryptorchidism (failure of the testes to descend into the scrotum) and tumor occurrence.
3. Testicular tumors metastasize in a stepwise fashion to the retroperitoneal lymph nodes with subsequent involvement of the mediastinal lymph nodes, lungs, and liver.
4. Testicular germ cell tumors are considered potentially curable; seminomas are extremely responsive to radiation therapy; nonseminomas are sensitive to platinum-based chemotherapy.

Clinical Manifestations

1. Painless swelling or enlargement of the testis; accompanied by sensation of heaviness in the scrotum.
2. Pain in the testis (if patient has epididymitis or bleeding into tumor).
3. Symptoms of metastatic disease: cough or dyspnea, lymphadenopathy, back pain, GI symptoms, lower extremity edema, or bone pain.

Diagnostic Evaluation

1. Elevated serum markers of human chorionic gonadotropin, lactic acid dehydrogenate, and alpha-fetoprotein; assay of tumor markers also used for diagnosis, detection of early recurrence, staging, and monitoring response to therapy.
2. Scrotal ultrasonography—to identify location of lesion and differentiate between solid and cystic lesion.

3. Chest x-ray—to seek pulmonary or mediastinal metastasis.
4. CT scanning of the chest, abdomen, and pelvis—to evaluate retroperitoneal lymph nodes and to follow progress of therapy.

Management

Choice of treatment depends on tumor histology and stage of disease.

Surgery

1. Inguinal orchiectomy—removal of the testis and its tunica and spermatic cord.
2. Retroperitoneal lymph node dissection (RPLND) may be performed after orchiectomy in nonseminomas for staging and therapeutic purposes.
3. Complications of surgery:
   a. RPLND causes infertility because of ejaculatory dysfunction.
   b. Modified nerve-sparing unilateral lymphadenectomy can be done on selected patients, thus preserving ejaculation.
   c. Unilateral orchiectomy eliminates half of germinal cells, thus reducing sperm count.
   d. Libido and ability to attain an erection are preserved.

Radiation Therapy

1. Radiation therapy to lymphatic drainage pathways (after orchiectomy in seminomas); cure rate is close to 99%.
2. Other testicle is shielded, usually preserving fertility.

Chemotherapy

1. Cisplatin combination therapy is used in treatment of nonseminomatous primary tumor and regional lymphatic metastases and in managing distant metastatic disease.
2. Discomforts of chemotherapy include significant nausea and vomiting, alopecia, myalgia, GI cramping, and mucositis.

Complications

1. Infertility; loss of testicle.
2. Retrograde ejaculation after retroperitoneal lymphadenectomy.
3. Death from metastatic disease.

Nursing Assessment

1. Examine testicular mass; ascertain when it was discovered and if it has changed or enlarged since initial discovery.
2. Examine supraclavicular and inguinal lymph nodes for enlargement.
3. Assess for symptoms of metastatic disease.

Nursing Diagnoses

- Anxiety related to diagnosis of cancer and impending treatments.
- Disturbed Body Image related to loss of testicle and fertility.
- Risk for Injury related to complications of treatment.

Nursing Interventions

Reducing Anxiety

1. Provide realistic information about impending surgery or treatment; dispel myths associated with testicular disease; emphasize positive cure rates.
2. Refer patient to educational and support services through the American Cancer Society and local cancer support groups.

Preserving Body Image

1. Reassure patient that orchiectomy will not diminish virility and RPLND will alter fertility and ejaculation but not libido, erection, and sensation.
2. Advise patient that testicular prosthesis can preserve look and feel of the scrotum.
3. Refer the patient for counseling, as needed, for problems and concerns with relationships, peers, or work life.
4. Discuss possible donation of sperm because of infertility issues.

Preventing Complications of Treatment

1. Provide routine postoperative care, including early ambulation, respiratory care, and administration of pain medication.
2. After RPLND, monitor for paralytic ileus, which is common after extensive resection.
   a. Auscultate bowel sounds frequently and observe for abdominal distention.
   b. Withhold oral fluids until bowel sounds have returned.
   c. Report complaints of nausea and vomiting.
   d. Begin nasogastric decompression, if indicated.
3. For nursing care involving radiation and chemotherapy, see pages 122 and 112.

Patient Education and Health Maintenance

1. Teach all young men to perform monthly testicular self-examination; after orchiectomy, patient should examine remaining testicle monthly.
2. Review schedule for radiation treatments or chemotherapy; teach patient and family possible adverse effects; discuss expectations for treatment period.
3. Provide information about retrograde ejaculation after RPLND and alternatives for fertility.

Evaluation: Expected Outcomes

- Verbalizes understanding of treatment and complications.
- No abdominal distention noted.
- Discusses concerns about sexual function with staff and partner.

Epididymitis

Epididymitis is an infection of the epididymis that usually spreads from the urethra or bladder to the epididymis by way of the ejaculatory duct and vas deferens.

Pathophysiology and Etiology

1. Occurs as a complication of UTI, urethral stricture disease, bacterial prostatitis, gonococcal or nongonococcal bacterial urethritis.
2. In men under age 35, sexually transmitted organisms are the main etiologic agents, usually *C. trachomatis* and *N. gonorrhoeae*.
3. In homosexual men, *E. coli* is a common cause.
4. In older men, the main causes are bladder outlet obstruction and urinary bacteria (*E. coli*, *P. aeruginosa*).

Clinical Manifestations

1. Unilateral scrotal pain and tenderness.
2. Edema, redness, and tenderness of the scrotum.

3. Dysuria, frequency.
4. Fever, nausea, vomiting.
5. Pyuria, bacteriuria, leukocytosis.

Diagnostic Evaluation

1. Urine culture and sensitivity.
2. Examination (Gram stain, culture, gonorrhea, and *Chlamydia* testing) of urethral discharge and expressed prostatic secretions to establish causative organism.
3. Ultrasound with Doppler to rule out testicular torsion.

Management

1. Antimicrobial therapy after collection of specimens.
   a. Treatment of choice for presumed sexually transmitted infections is combination ceftriaxone 250 mg IM in a single dose with doxycycline 100 mg orally twice per day for 10 days.
   b. For presumed *E. coli* and other infections, a quinolone, such as ciprofloxacin 500 mg orally twice a day for 10 days or co-trimoxazole for 10 days, is recommended.
2. Analgesics for pain relief.
3. Bed rest with the scrotum elevated on a towel to allow for lymphatic drainage.
4. In some cases, the spermatic cord is injected with a local anesthetic to relieve pain.

Complications

1. Spread of infection to testicle—epididymo-orchitis.
2. Infertility; risk is greater when infection is bilateral.

Nursing Assessment

1. Obtain history of STDs (or symptoms), UTI, or prostatitis; recent urologic instrumentation or surgery.
2. Assess for elevated temperature, pain level, and swollen and tender scrotum.
3. Assess for sexual behavior risk—multiple partners, nonuse of condoms, history of STDs.

Nursing Diagnosis

- Acute Pain related to scrotal inflammation.

Nursing Interventions

Relieving Pain

1. Administer or teach self-administration of analgesics, as ordered—commonly NSAIDs or acetaminophen. Assess patient's response.
2. Encourage bed rest during the acute phase.
3. Apply scrotal support to relieve edema and discomfort, to improve lymphatic drainage, and to take tension off the spermatic cord.
   a. Use rolled towel under the scrotum or scrotal bridge.
   b. Suggest a cotton-lined athletic supporter for ambulation.

Patient Education and Health Maintenance

Instruct the patient as follows:
1. Avoid straining (lifting, straining at stool, and sexual activity) until infection is under control.
2. Sexual partners within the past 60 days of patients with chlamydial or gonorrheal urethritis or epididymitis should be examined and treated.

PATIENT EDUCATION GUIDELINES 21-1

Testicular Self-Examination

1. Examine for testicular tumor once per month, at a convenient time such as the first of the month or your birth date every month, preferably while showering or bathing.
2. Use both hands to feel the testes through the scrotal tissue.
3. Locate the epididymis; this is, the irregular cordlike structure on the top and at the back of the testicle that stores and transports sperm. The spermatic cord (and vas) extends upward from the epididymis.
4. Feel each testis between the thumb and first two fingers of each hand. The testes lie freely in the scrotum, are oval shaped, and measure 4 to 5 cm in length, 3 cm in width, and about 2 cm in thickness.
5. Note size, shape, and abnormal tenderness. An abnormality may be felt as a firm area on the front or side of the testicle.
6. Stand in front of mirror and look for changes in size/shape of the scrotum. It is normal to find one testis larger than the other.
7. Report any evidence of a small, pea-sized lump or other abnormality.

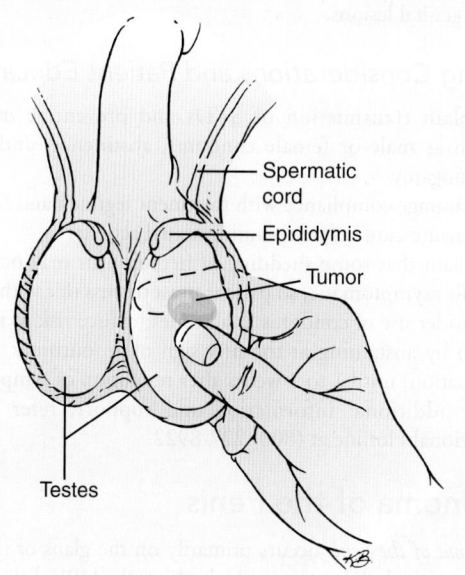

Using the fingertips and thumb, the epididymis, testes, and spermatic cord are located bilaterally.

3. Follow-up with health care provider, as directed—it may take 2 to 4 weeks or longer for epididymitis to resolve completely.
4. Report signs of infection in the reproductive tract immediately to obtain treatment and prevent spread.
5. Obtain follow-up care to ensure complete resolution of infection; uncontrolled infection may impair fertility.
6. Use safer sex practices, such as abstinence, mutual monogamy, and condoms, to prevent further infection associated with sexual activity.

Evaluation: Expected Outcomes

- Verbalizes relief of pain.

Genital Lesions Caused by Sexually Transmitted Diseases

 EVIDENCE BASE Centers for Disease Control and Prevention. (2015). Sexually transmitted treatment guidelines, 2015. *MMWR, 64*(3), 1–137.

Genital lesions are ulcerations or other skin or mucous membrane lesions that indicate infection with an STD and may actively shed the infecting organism.

Pathophysiology and Etiology

Causes include:
1. Syphilis—*Treponema pallidum.*
2. Chancroid—*Haemophilus ducreyi.*
3. Lymphogranuloma venereum—specific subtypes of *C. trachomatis.*
4. Genital herpes—herpes simplex virus.
5. Condylomata acuminata (genital warts)—specific subtypes of HPV.

Clinical Manifestations

See Table 21-4, for clinical manifestations, diagnosis, and treatment of genital lesions.

Nursing Considerations and Patient Education

1. Explain transmission of STDs and preventive measures, such as male or female condoms, abstinence, and mutual monogamy.
2. Encourage compliance with treatment regimen and follow-up to ensure cure before resuming sexual activity.
3. Explain that some shedding of herpes virus may occur even while asymptomatic, so patient must discuss this with partner; consider use of condoms at all times; reduce risk of transmission by abstaining at the first sign of an outbreak (tingling sensation) until 1 to 2 weeks after resolution of symptoms.
4. For additional information and support, refer to STD National Hotline at (800) 227-8922.

Carcinoma of the Penis

Carcinoma of the penis occurs primarily on the glans of the penis. Risk factors include uncircumcised, phimosis, HPV, lichen sclerosus, balanitis xerotica obliterans, increasing age, smoking, poor personal hygiene, and the accumulation of smegma under the skin of an uncircumcised penis. It primarily occurs in men older than age 50 and represents 0.5% of malignancies in men in the United States.

Pathophysiology and Etiology

1. Several types of penile lesions are potentially premalignant.
   a. Condylomata acuminata.
   b. Giant condylomata acuminata (Buschke-Löwenstein tumor).
   c. Kaposi sarcoma.
   d. Leukoplakia.
2. Erythroplasia of the glans (erythroplasia of Queyrat) is a carcinoma *in situ* of the penis and may involve the glans, prepuce, or penile shaft or may spread to the remainder of the genitalia and perineal region. It appears as a red, velvety lesion with ulcerations.
3. Bowen disease is a squamous cell carcinoma *in situ* resembling a red plague. Commonly involving the shaft of the penis.
4. Malignant lesions that ulcerate metastasize quickly to the regional femoral and iliac lymph nodes.
5. Distant metastasis occurs in the inguinal lymph nodes; in rare cases to lungs, liver, bone, or brain.

Clinical Manifestations

1. Can present as a painless, wartlike growth or ulcer on the glans or prepuce or with painful, bleeding, or exudative lesion.
2. Phimosis (constriction of foreskin with inability to retract over glans) may obscure a lesion, preventing detection until advanced stages.
3. Lymphadenopathy; secondary infection of lesions or metastatic disease.
4. Malodorous and persistent discharge from the penis is a late symptom.

Diagnostic Evaluation

1. Biopsy of penile lesion and lymph nodes.
2. Ultrasonography and MRI of inguinal lymph nodes.
3. Chest x-ray, CT or MRI scan, bone scan to assess for distant nodal metastases.
4. Positron emission tomography (PET) scans assist in primary staging or to assess for lymph node metastases.
5. Sentinel node biopsy to determine whether nonenlarged inguinal lymph nodes contain cancer.

Management

1. Localized lesions are surgically removed by partial penectomy, laser or cryotherapy, or Mohs micrographic surgery; total penectomy with perineal urethrostomy is necessary for more involved tumors.
2. Because inguinal lymphadenopathy may be due to inflammation and not malignancy, patients are prescribed a 4- to 6-week course of antibiotics after partial or total penectomy and are reassessed. If lymphadenopathy remains, then a bilateral lymphadenectomy is performed for cancer control.
3. Radiation therapy to small superficial tumors and lymph nodes may control the disease.

Complications

1. Disfigurement because of ulceration or treatment.
2. Complications of lymphadenectomy—necrosis and infection of skin flap, chronic edema of lower extremities.

Table 21-4 Characteristics and Management of Genital Lesions Caused by STDs

DISORDER AND INCUBATION	CLINICAL MANIFESTATIONS	DIAGNOSIS AND TREATMENT
Herpes Genitalis 2–20 days	Clustered vesicles on erythematous, edematous base that rupture, leaving shallow, painful ulcer that eventually crusts; mild regional lymphadenopathy; recurrent and may be brought on by stress, infection, pregnancy, sunburn.	• Diagnostic tests include Tzanck smear, viral culture, antigen test of tissue or exudate from lesion, or serum antibody tests. • No cure, but symptomatic period is diminished by acyclovir or other antiherpetic started with each recurrence; or recurrences greatly reduced or prevented by continuous treatment. • Analgesics and sitz baths promote comfort.
Syphilis 10–90 days for primary; up to 6 months following lesion (chancre) for secondary	*Primary:* Nontender, shallow, indurated, clean ulcer; mild regional lymphadenopathy. *Secondary:* Maculopapular rash including palms and soles, mucous patches, and condylomatous lesions; fever, generalized lymphadenopathy.	• VDRL test or RPR blood test with confirmation by specific treponemal antibody tests. • Preferred treatment is benzathine penicillin G 2.4 million units IM in a single dose; erythromycin or ceftriaxone may be used in penicillin allergy.
Chancroid 3–14 days	Bacterial disease caused by *H. ducreyi.* Vesiculopustule that erodes, leaving a tender, painful, shallow or deep, well-circumscribed ulcer with ragged, undermined borders and a friable base covered by purulent exudate; unilateral or bilateral large, tender inguinal lymph nodes (buboes) in 50% of patients.	• Identification of *H. ducreyi* on special culture media. • Treated with azithromycin, ciprofloxacin, erythromycin, or ceftriaxone IM. Single-dose regimens are available. • Apply warm soaks to buboes.
Lymphogranuloma Venereum 3–30 days	Small, transient, nontender papule or superficial ulcer precedes firm, adherent unilateral inguinal and femoral lymph nodes (buboes) with characteristic groove in between (groove sign); may suppurate.	• Microimmunofluorescence testing of bubo aspirate, if possible. Clinical diagnosis after ruling out other causes for genital lesions and lymphadenopathy. • Treatment of choice is doxycycline, but erythromycin may be effective. • Incision and excision of buboes should be avoided: aspiration may be helpful.
Condyloma Acuminatum 3 weeks to 3 months, possibly years before grossly visible	Single or multiple, soft, fleshy, flat or vegetating growths may occur on the penis, anal area, urethra; no lymphadenopathy.	• Diagnosed by inspection or biopsy. • Topical therapy with podofilox 0.5% for external warts, podophyllin 10% to 25% solution, or trichloroacetic acid 80% to 90% imiquimod. May require multiple applications. • Cryotherapy, electrodissection, electrocautery, carbon dioxide laser, and surgical excision may also be done. • Recurrence is common.

IM, intramuscular; HPV, human papillomavirus; RPR, rapid plasma reagin; VDRL, Venereal Disease Research Laboratory.

Nursing Assessment

1. Obtain history of current lesion, history of STDs, and hygiene.
2. Perform genital examination for characteristics of lesion, phimosis, inguinal lymph node enlargement.
3. Assess support system and personal coping mechanisms.

Nursing Diagnoses

- Fear related to diagnosis of cancer.
- Disturbed Body Image related to partial or total penectomy.

Nursing Interventions

Resolving Fears

1. Provide patient with opportunity to acquire information about causes and prognosis of disease.
2. Interpret diagnostic and staging results to patient.
3. Encourage realistic expectations regarding outcome of treatment.

Enhancing Coping with Body Image Changes

1. Maintain a nonjudgmental approach; allow patient to ventilate feelings about loss of part or all of the penis.

2. Provide routine postoperative care confidently, watching for bleeding, monitoring urination, and anticipating pain.
3. Provide opportunity for patient to discuss alternative methods of sexual expression with knowledgeable professional.
   a. About 40% of patients are able to participate in sexual activity and stand erect to void after partial penectomy.
4. Monitor patient for symptoms of depression requiring intervention.

Patient Education and Health Maintenance

1. Instruct the uncircumcised patient about proper hygiene—importance of daily removal of all retained smegma.
2. Explain expected postoperative function of the penis in patient undergoing partial penectomy.
3. Describe how voiding will occur to patient undergoing perineal urethroplasty.
4. Provide information about follow-up and monitoring for recurrences or radiation and chemotherapy, as appropriate.

Evaluation: Expected Outcomes

- Verbalizes understanding and acceptance of diagnosis and treatment plan.
- Discusses feelings and interest in seeking counseling.

SELECTED REFERENCES

Badalto, G., & Kaufmann, M. (2016). Adult UTI. American Urological Association. Available: *www.auanet.org/education/adult-uti.cfm*

Bellomo, R., Kellum, J. A., & Ronco, C. (2012). Acute kidney injury. *The Lancet, 380,* 756–766.

Brusch, J. L., & Bronze, M. S. (2017). Urinary tract infection (UTI) and cystitis (bladder infection) in females. *Medscape Drugs and Diseases.* Available: *https://emedicine.medscape.com/article/233101-overview.*

Brusch, J. L., & Bronze, M. S. (2017). Urinary tract infection (UTI) in males. *Medscape Drugs and Diseases.* Available: *https://emedicine.medscape.com/article/231574-overview.*

Centers for Disease Control and Prevention. (2015). Sexually transmitted diseases treatment guidelines, 2015. *MMWR, 64*(3), 1–137.

Chirag, D., & Schwartz, B. F. (2017). *Nephrolithiasis. Medscape Drugs and Diseases. http://emedicine.medscape.com/article/437096-overview.*

Counts, C. S. (Ed.). (2015). *Core curriculum for nephrology nursing* (6th ed.). Pitman, NJ: Anthony Janetti.

Cox, A., Golda, N., Nadeau, G., et al. (2016). CUA guideline: Diagnosis and treatment of interstitial cystitis/bladder pain syndrome. *Canadian Urological Association Journal, 10*(5–6), E136–E155.

Cupples, S., Lerret, S., McCalmont, V., & Ohler, L. (2016). *Core curriculum for transplant nurses* (2nd ed.). St. Louis, MO: Mosby.

Dave, C., & Schwartz, B. F. (2016). Nephrolithiasis. *Medscape drugs and diseases.* New York: WebMD. Available: *https://emedicine.medscape.com/article/437096-overview*

Escudier, B., Porta, C., Schmidinger, M., Rioux-Leclercq, N., et al. (2016). Renal cell carcinoma: ESMO Clinical Practice Guidelines for diagnosis, treatment and follow-up. *Annals of Oncology, 27*(suppl 5):v58–v68.

Fulop, T., & Batuman, V. (2016). Acute pyelonephritis. *Medscape drugs and diseases.* New York: WebMD. Available: *https://emedicine.medscape.com/article/245559-overview*

Fulop, T. & Batuman, V. (2017). Acute pyelonephritis. *Medscape Drugs and Diseases.* Available: *https://emedicine.medscape.com/article/245559-overview.*

Gilbert, S.J. & Weiner, D.E. (2018). *National Kidney Foundation Primer on Kidney Disease,* 7th edition. New York: Elsevier, 2018.

Girardeau, R. (2017). Acute kidney injury: An overview of renal failure and considerations for treatment. *Journal of Emergency Medical Services,* 42(12): 53–57.

Hanno, P. M., Erickson, D., Moldwin, R., Faraday, M. M.; American Urological Association. (2015). Diagnosis and treatment of interstitial cystitis/bladder pain syndrome: AUA guideline amendment. *Journal of Urology, 193*(5), 1545–1553.

Honicker, T., & Holt, K. (2016). Contrast-induced acute kidney injury: Comparison of preventative therapies. *Nephrology Nursing Journal, 43*(2), 109–117.

Jerauld, A., Wormuth, L., & Carlson, B. (2016). New approaches in managing interstitial cystitis/bladder pain syndrome. *US Pharmacist, 41*(9), 29–33.

Juliao, A., Plata, M., Kazzazi, A., et al. (2012). American urological association and European association of urology guidelines in the management of benign prostatic hypertrophy: Revisited. *Current Opinion in Urology, 22,* 34–39.

Kalantar-Zadeh, K. & Fouque, D. (2017). Nutritional management of chronic kidney disease. *New England Journal of Medicine, 377,* 1765–1776.

Lambert, P., Chaisson, K., Horton, S. et al. (2017). Reducing acute kidney injury due to contrast material: How nurses can improve patient safety. *Critical Care Nurse, 37*(11): 13–26.

Lameire, N. H., Bagga, A., Cruz, D., et al. (2013). Acute kidney injury: an increasing global concern. *The Lancet, 382,* 170–179.

Levey, A. S., & Coresh, J. (2012). Chronic kidney disease. *The Lancet, 379,* 165–180.

Levin, A., Tonelli, M., Bonventre, J., et al. (2017). Global kidney health 2017 and beyond: a roadmap for closing gaps in care, research, and policy. *Lancet, 390,* 1888–1917.

Maxson, R. (2017). Medications in kidney disease. *The Journal for Nurse Practitioners, 13* (10): 687–692.

National Kidney Foundation. (2012). KDIGO Clinical Practice Guideline for AKI. *Kidney International Supplements, 2*(1), 1–138.

National Kidney Foundation. (2012). KDOQI Clinical Practice Guidelines for Diabetes and CKD: 2012 update. *American Journal of Kidney Diseases, 60*(5), 850–886.

Norton, J., Newman, E., Romancito, G., et al. (2017). Improving outcomes for patients with chronic kidney disease Part 1. *American Journal of Nursing, 117*(2), 22–32.

Norton, J., Newman, E., Romancito, G., et al. (2017). Improving outcomes for patients with chronic kidney disease Part 2. *American Journal of Nursing, 117*(3), 26–35.

Ostermann, M., & Joannidis, M. (2016). Acute kidney injury 2016: diagnosis and diagnostic workup. *Critical Care, 20,* 299.

Rosner, M. H. (2018). Prevention of contrast-associated acute kidney injury. *New England Journal of Medicine, 378,* 671–672.

Rovner, E. S., & Kim, E. D. (2017). Interstitial cystitis. *Medscape Drugs and Diseases.* Available: *https://emedicine.medscape.com/article/2055505-overview.*

Sachdeva, K., & Abel, J. E. (2017). *Renal cell carcinoma. Medscape drugs and diseases.* New York: WebMD. Available: *https://emedicine.medscape.com/article/281340-overview*

Smith, R. A., Manassram-Baptiste, D., Brooks, D., et al. (2015). Cancer screening in the United States, 2015: A review of current American Cancer Society guidelines and issues in cancer screening. *CA: A Cancer Journal for Clinicians, 65,* 30–54.

Smith, C. A. (2016). Evidence-based treatment of chronic kidney disease. *The Nurse Practitioner, 41*(11), 42–48.

Stevens, P., & Levin, A. (2013). Evaluation and management of chronic kidney disease: Synopsis of the kidney disease improving global outcomes 2012 clinical practice guideline. *Annals of Internal Medicine, 158,* 825–830.

Turk, C., Knoll, T., Petrik, A., et al. (2015). Guidelines on urolithiasis. European Association of Urology. Available: *uroweb.org/wp-content/uploads/22-Urolithiasis_LR_full.pdf*

Vaziri, N. (2016). Disorders of lipid metabolism in nephrotic syndrome: Mechanism and consequences. *Kidney International, 90*(1), 41–52.

Velez, R., Richmond, E., & Dudley-Brown, S. (2017). Antibiogram, clinical practice guidelines, and treatment of urinary tract infection. *The Journal for Nurse Practitoners, 13,* 617–622.

Webster, A. C., Nagler, E.V., Morton, R. L., et al. (2017). Chronic kidney disease. *Lancet, 389,* 1238–1252.

Wein, A. J., Kavoussi, L. R., Partin, A. W., et al. (Eds.). (2017). *Campbell-Walsh urology* (11th ed., Vols. 1–4). Philadelphia, PA: W.B. Saunders.

Workeneh, B. T., & Batumen, V. (2017). Acute kidney injury. *Medscape drugs and diseases.* Available: *https://emedicine.medscape.com/article/243492-overview*

22
Gynecologic Disorders

OVERVIEW AND ASSESSMENT
The Menstrual Cycle

The *menstrual cycle* is the cyclical pattern of ovarian hormone secretion (estrogen and progesterone) under the control of pituitary hormones (luteinizing hormone [LH] and follicle-stimulating hormone [FSH]) that results in thickening of the uterine endometrium, ovulation, and menstruation. Cycle length varies among women.

Phases of the Menstrual Cycle

The menstrual cycle is generally divided into two phases: follicular (or proliferative) and luteal (or secretory). See Figure 22-1. Further subdivisions of the cycle are:

1. Menstrual or bleeding phase (or early follicular phase): starts day 1 of the cycle and lasts approximately 5 days; endometrial sloughing and discharge occur because of low levels of estrogen and progesterone.
2. Postmenstrual phase (or early follicular phase); approximately days 5 to 8—thin endometrium. Ovarian follicles grow.
3. Proliferative phase (or mid to late follicular phase): approximately days 8 to 15; estrogen starts to increase the thickness of the endometrium. A selected ovarian follicle continues to grow. A surge in LH occurs. Transition from proliferative phase to secretory phase occurs with ovulation, the expulsion of a mature follicle (or ovum) from the ovary.
4. Secretory phase (or luteal phase, which lasts 14 days after LH surge in most women): approximately days 16 to 23; endometrium thickens because of increased progesterone; after ovulation, a corpus luteum forms and then regresses unless pregnancy occurs.
5. Premenstrual phase (or late luteal phase): days 24 to 28; levels of estrogen and progesterone begin to fall.

Characteristics of Menstruation

See Table 22-1.

Subjective Data

Explore patient's gynecologic history, current symptoms, and general history to elicit important data. Provide a private and comfortable setting for history taking before the patient undresses. Reassure the patient about confidentiality and rationale for history taking (see Chapter 5).

Gynecologic Review of Systems

1. Menstrual history: date of start of last menstrual period (LMP) or age at last menses. Documented in this manner: age at menarche × cycle length × number of days of bleeding (eg, 13 × 28 × 4). Symptoms of dysmenorrhea? Symptoms of premenstrual syndrome? Intermenstrual spotting/bleeding, postcoital bleeding, or postmenopausal bleeding?
2. Obstetric history: gravida (number of pregnancies) and para (number of term births, preterm births, miscarriages/abortions, living children) (eg, G2P1102). Difficulty conceiving or assisted reproduction? For each pregnancy, list date; gestational age at delivery; mode of delivery; maternal

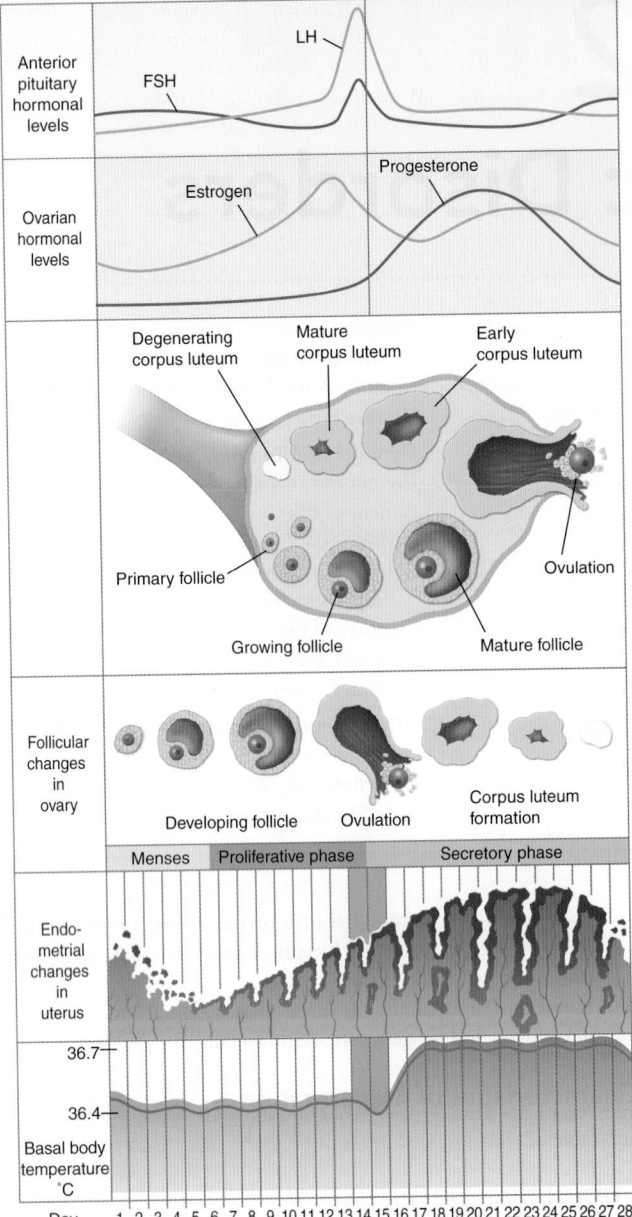

Figure 22-1. The menstrual cycle. (Premkumar, K. [2011]. *Anatomy & physiology: the massage connection* [3rd ed.]. Baltimore, MD: Lippincott Williams & Wilkins.)

Table 22-1	Characteristics of Menstruation	
CHARACTERISTIC	**RANGE**	**AVERAGE**
Menarche (age at onset)	9 to 17 yr	12.5 yr
Cycle length	21 to 35 days	28 days
Flow—duration	2 to 8 days	3 to 5 days
Flow—amount	10 to 80 mL	35 mL
Menopause (age at onset)	45 to 55 yr	51 yr

Irregular Bleeding

1. Characteristics: date of LMP? Frequency, duration, and amount of flow for most recent several cycles? Previous menstrual pattern and change? What is the color and consistency of blood? What are the sizes of the clots? Significant change in quantity or quality of menstrual flow? Bleeding or spotting between periods, postcoital bleeding, or postmenopausal bleeding? Pain with bleeding? Age at menarche? Age at menopause?
2. Associated factors: pregnancy and childbirth history? Is the patient sexually active? What method of contraception is used? Is the patient taking hormone replacement or hormonal contraceptives? Any other medications? Is the patient obese or underweight? Does the patient have acne and hirsutism? History of amenorrhea? Coagulation disorders?
3. Significance: may indicate infection of the vagina or cervix; malignancy of the vulva, vagina, cervix, or uterus; benign tumor of the uterus; ovarian cyst; polyps; fibroids; adenomyosis; pregnancy; endometriosis; polycystic ovarian syndrome; thyroid, hypothalamic, or pituitary disorder; coagulopathy; endometrial hyperplasia; or perimenopausal phase.

Vaginal Discharge

1. Characteristics: color, amount, and duration of the discharge? Any odor, itching, burning, urinary symptoms, or pain? Fever? Dyspareunia (painful intercourse—vulvar, vaginal, or internal pain with intercourse)? Onset related to menses or to intercourse?
2. Associated factors: LMP? What is the sexual history, such as number of partners or new partner within the past 6 months, type of sexual activity, and symptoms in partner? Is barrier method of contraception used? Is the patient menopausal or postmenopausal? Environmental factor changes? Vaginal dryness? Does the patient take estrogen replacement? Recent use of antibiotics? Recent douching? Recent over-the-counter product use or herbal/natural remedies? History of sexually transmitted diseases?
3. Significance: may indicate normal or pathologic discharge, bacterial vaginosis, candidal vaginitis, cervicitis, gonorrhea, chlamydia, trichomoniasis, pelvic inflammatory disease (PID), or genital malignancy.

Pelvic Pain

1. Characteristics: frequency, duration, severity, and location of pain? Does the pain radiate? Was the onset sudden or gradual? What aggravates and what relieves it? Relationship to menstrual cycle, eating, physical exercise, bowel, or bladder function? Any dyspareunia? Does it feel like heaviness in the pelvis? Intensity and effect on daily activities?
2. Associated factors: LMP? Fever, nausea, vomiting, dizziness, abnormal bleeding? Urinary symptoms? Back pain? Recent

complications (gestational diabetes, hypertension); and fetal, delivery, or neonatal complications.
3. Cervical cytology/Papanicolaou (Pap) test history: date and result of most recent test? Diagnosis and follow-up of abnormal Pap tests? History of HPV vaccination (as age-appropriate)?
4. Sexual history: age of first sexual activity? Partner preference (men, women, or both)? Activity type? Satisfaction? Frequency? Number of partners in past year and during lifetime?
5. Methods of contraception and sexually transmitted disease (STD) prevention: desire for pregnancy testing or STD screening? Desire for other methods? Desire for preconceptual counseling? Use of condoms?
6. Screening for intimate partner violence and previous emotional, physical, or sexual abuse or assault.

significant weight loss or gain? Use of estrogen preparations? Difficulty conceiving? Did the patient perform a home pregnancy test? Use of an intrauterine device (IUD)? Any change in bowel habits or diarrhea? History of sexual abuse? Use of pain medications and home remedies?

3. Significance: may indicate condition arising from relaxed pelvic muscles, PID, endometriosis, interstitial cystitis, urinary tract infection, irritable bowel syndrome, history of sexual abuse (posttraumatic stress disorder), ectopic pregnancy, miscarriage, uterine fibroids, or cervical or uterine cancer.

Physical Examination

Physical examination for a patient with a gynecologic disorder should focus on the abdomen and genitalia. Palpate the abdomen for masses or tenderness. Request verbal permission before starting the pelvic examination. Consider using a chaperone during the examination. If the patient has presented as a victim of sexual assault, then do not ask the patient to undress nor examine the patient but ensure immediate transfer to a local emergency department with sexual assault nurse examiners or other professionals with expertise in forensic evidence collection and supportive services after assault. See Chapter 35, page 962.

The nurse in a gynecologic or obstetric setting may perform a vaginal examination to obtain specimens for diagnostic studies and assess the patient's condition.

Laboratory Tests

CA 125

Description
Tumor antigen used as a marker for ovarian cancer.

Nursing and Patient Care Considerations
1. Tell the patient a blood test will be performed and the results will be ready in 1 to 3 days.
2. Not a specific or definitive screening test for ovarian cancer; rather, it is better used as a measure of response to treatment.
3. Level may be elevated in benign gynecologic disease, in hepatic cirrhosis, and in healthy women.
4. Should not be used as an independent screening tool.

Cervical Cytology

Description
A Pap smear of the cervix is obtained during pelvic examination to screen for cervical dysplasia or cancer. May also help to detect human papillomavirus (HPV), endometrial cancer, or infections. Classification by Bethesda system indicates any cellular abnormalities.

Bethesda System 2001
1. Specimen type—conventional smear (slide) versus liquid based.
2. Specimen adequacy.
   a. Satisfactory for evaluation—result is given but presence of other factors, such as absence of transformation zone, is also listed.
   b. Unsatisfactory for evaluation—result may not be given; lists reason, such as inadequate number of cells or obscured by blood or inflammation.
3. Interpretation of results—only a screening tool, not diagnostic.
   a. Negative for intraepithelial lesion or malignancy: no cell abnormalities.

   i. Presence of an organism (*Trichomonas*, fungal elements, shift in flora) and cellular changes consistent with HSV may also be listed.
   ii. Other nonneoplastic findings (reactive reparative changes, glandular cells, atrophy) may be described.
   b. Epithelial cell abnormalities—atypical squamous cells are common.
      i. Atypical squamous cells of undetermined significance—management options based on population and can include HPV testing, repeat Pap test in 1 year intervals, and/or colposcopy.
      ii. Atypical squamous cells, cannot exclude high-grade intraepithelial lesion—potentially more serious; do immediate colposcopy and endocervical sampling for further evaluation.
      iii. Low-grade squamous intraepithelial lesion—management options based on population and can include repeat Pap test in 6-month intervals, HPV testing, and/or colposcopy.
      iv. High-grade squamous intraepithelial lesion—management options based on population and can include colposcopy with biopsy and endocervical curettage.
      v. Squamous cell carcinoma—colposcopy and biopsy.
   c. Glandular cell abnormalities—atypical, not otherwise specified (NOS) or atypical, favor neoplastic (require further evaluation); colposcopy, and HPV testing. Endometrial biopsy is performed if over 35 years of age and on younger women with risk factors for endometrial neoplasia such as unexplained uterine bleeding, chronic anovulation, or in obese women.
   d. Endocervical adenocarcinoma *in situ*; colposcopy, cervical biopsy, conization, and possible referral to oncologist. Hysterectomy may be performed for women who do not desire to preserve fertility.
   e. Adenocarcinoma—endocervical, endometrial, extrauterine, and NOS—biopsy and conization; consider referral to gynecologic oncologist.

Nursing and Patient Care Considerations

 EVIDENCE BASE American College of Obstetricians and Gynecologists. (2012). Cervical cytology screening. *Obstetrics and Gynecology, 120,* 1222–1230.
Saslow, D., Solomon, D., Lawson, H. W., et al. (2012). American Cancer Society, American Society for Colposcopy and Cervical Pathology, and American Society for Clinical Pathology screening guidelines for the prevention and early detection of cervical cancer. *CA—Cancer Journal for Clinicians, 62,* 147–172.

1. Pap test should not be performed during menses, unless the liquid-based system is used.
2. Instruct the patient not to use douche, medication, tampon, or cream in the vagina and to avoid sexual intercourse for 48 hours before the examination.
3. Recommend regular screening based on established guidelines set forth by the American Cancer Society, U.S. Preventive Services Task Force, and American College of Obstetricians and Gynecologists (ACOG). The same screening guidelines apply to all women whether vaccinated against HPV or not. More frequent testing is recommended if the woman has human immunodeficiency virus (HIV), is immunosuppressed, was exposed to diethylstilbestrol in utero, or has been

treated for cervical intraepithelial neoplasia (CIN) 2, CIN 3, or cervical cancer.

    a. Recommend starting Pap testing at age 21.

    b. Recommend testing every 3 years from ages 21 to 65 for women without risk factors such as DES exposure.

    c. For those aged 30 to 65 wanting to extend the screening interval, screen with a combination of HPV testing and cytology every 5 years.

    d. Discontinue screening after age 65 if adequate negative prior screening and no history of CIN 2 or greater within the last 20 years.

    e. Discontinue after total hysterectomy if no dysplasia or cancer.

4. Make sure that the patient obtains results. If the patient has an abnormal smear, explain that this is not always conclusive but requires further testing based on age, such as repeat Pap test, HPV testing, colposcopy, biopsy, or conization. Encourage the patient to return for further testing.

5. Yearly examination for breast cancer screening; detection of other genital cancers, infections, and reproductive problems; and contraception management may be indicated.

Tests for Gonorrhea and Chlamydia

 EVIDENCE BASE Centers for Disease Control and Prevention. (2015). Sexually transmitted diseases treatment guidelines, 2015. Atlanta, GA: Author. Available: *https://www.cdc.gov/std/tg2015/default.htm.*

Description

1. Commonly known as deoxyribonucleic acid (DNA) probe or antigen detection tests, a single specimen can detect both STD-causing organisms. Will detect even subclinical infection; can be used as screening test.

2. Can also be done by culture method, but takes longer and requires separate specimens and special processing for each.

3. Screening for chlamydia and gonorrhea can also be done on urine specimen using amplified DNA technology. This method is more expensive, but saves time in specimen collection (especially for women) in screening centers.

Nursing and Patient Care Considerations

1. Explain the procedure to the patient before taking the specimen.

2. Specimens should be taken from the cervix without douching for 24 hours or from the male urethra before urinating.

3. Obtain specimen with cotton-tipped swab inserted and rotated in the cervical os for 10 seconds or urethral meatus in a male patient. Small-tipped swabs are available for the urethra. Send swab to laboratory in provided container with preservative.

4. For urine testing, ask the patient to provide the first 10 to 20 mL of voided urine in a specimen container (this represents a urethral specimen, ie, more likely to contain the organism, if present, without being diluted by a larger amount of urine from the bladder).

5. May also use ThinPrep as a testing vehicle.

Radiology and Imaging Studies

Hysterosalpingography

Description

1. This fluoroscopic x-ray study of the uterus and fallopian tubes is used to determine tubal patency, detect pathology in the uterine cavity, identify peritoneal adhesions, and to treat unexplained fertility.

2. A bivalve speculum is introduced while the patient is in the lithotomy position and contrast medium is injected into the uterine cavity; the medium will enter the peritoneum in 10 to 15 minutes if tubes are patent.

Nursing and Patient Care Considerations

1. Determine the date of last menstrual period; the test is done a few days after menses ends, before ovulation. Obtain pregnancy test if patient is within childbearing years, as indicated.

2. Verify that the patient does not have a history of allergy to contrast media or iodine.

3. Administer prescribed antibiotic and analgesic.

4. After procedure, apply a perineal pad for drainage of excess contrast medium or blood, and instruct the patient to notify the health care provider if bloody drainage continues after 3 days or if signs of infection are present.

5. Inform the patient that pain medication may be necessary for shoulder discomfort because of dye irritation of the phrenic nerve.

Pelvic Ultrasonography

 EVIDENCE BASE American College of Radiology. (2014). ACR–ACOG–AIUM–SRU practice guideline for the performance of pelvic ultrasound. Available: *www.acr.org/~/media/ACR/Documents/PGTS/guidelines/US_Pelvic.pdf.*

Description

A noninvasive test that uses high-frequency sound waves to form images of the interior pelvic cavity; used to detect uterine, tubal, ovarian, and pelvic cavity pathology, to measure organ size, and to evaluate pregnancy.

Nursing and Patient Care Considerations

1. Inform patient that a full bladder may be necessary to make the uterus easier to visualize.

2. Instruct patient to drink 16 to 32 ounces of water (may differ among facilities) before the procedure and not to void. If transvaginal ultrasound will be performed, inform patient that a vaginal probe will be inserted to obtain more accurate measurements from internal organs. Have the patient empty her bladder prior to insertion of probe. (Probe is not used if patient is virginal.)

3. After the procedure, help the patient wipe off ultrasound gel from abdomen and allow her to empty her bladder.

4. Abnormalities are represented as different densities that differentiate solid from cystic masses and can help make a diagnosis; however, explain to the patient that further testing may be necessary.

Other Diagnostic Procedures

See Standards of Care Guidelines 22-1, page 639.

Colposcopy

Description

Examination of the cervix with a bright light and magnification of 10 to 40 times; done to determine distribution of abnormal squamous epithelium and to pinpoint areas from which biopsy tissue can be taken; may be done with cervicography (photographing the cervix).

STANDARDS OF CARE GUIDELINES 22-1
Caring for a Patient
Undergoing Gynecologic Surgery

When caring for a patient undergoing gynecologic surgery, the following care is essential to prevent complications and to promote healthy adaptation:

- Discuss procedure with patient before surgery—does she know why surgery is being done? Does she know which organs will be removed or altered? Does she understand the implications for childbearing, sexuality, menopause? Answer questions and contact surgeon, if necessary.
- After the procedure, assess vital signs as frequently as indicated for signs of shock, infection, fluid overload, and atelectasis.
- Assess incision for drainage and signs of infection? (redness, oozing, warmth, increased pain).
- Assess vaginal area for excessive bleeding or foul-smelling drainage.
- Monitor intake and output.
- If patient has an indwelling catheter, ensure that it is draining clear urine greater than 30 to 50 mL/hour.
- After catheter has been removed, ensure that patient voids in adequate amounts and monitor for urinary retention or signs of infection.
- Ensure adequate IV and then oral fluids, but monitor for edema and shortness of breath, signs of fluid overload.
- Monitor level of pain and relief with analgesics, but watch for oversedation, hypotension, and decreased bowel sounds as adverse effects of opioids.
- Provide comfort measures, such as positioning, splinting incision during position changing, or coughing, applying ice pack to the perineum.
- Auscultate bowel sounds for return, signaling progression of diet. Report nausea, vomiting, and loss of or decrease in bowel sounds immediately; intervention for bowel obstruction may be needed.
- Institute thromboembolism prevention, as ordered, and monitor for calf tenderness.
- Encourage ambulation as early as possible, but encourage gradual resumption of activities, according to surgeon instructions.
- Notify surgeon of fever, shortness of breath, increased pain, excessive bleeding or drainage, foul odor, change in vital signs, urinary retention, decreased urine output, nausea and vomiting, or tender, swollen calf.

This information should serve as a general guideline only. Each patient situation presents a unique set of clinical factors and requires nursing judgment to guide care, which may include additional or alternative measures and approaches.

Nursing and Patient Care Considerations
1. The procedure is preferably done when the cervix is least vascular (usually 1 week after the end of the menstrual flow). Obtain pregnancy test if the patient is within childbearing years, as indicated.
2. Explain that a vaginal speculum will be inserted and that a biopsy may be taken, causing only slight discomfort.
3. Help the patient into lithotomy position, drape her appropriately, and provide emotional support throughout the procedure. Provide distraction techniques, such as music and posters (hung on the ceiling), as appropriate.
4. After the cervix and vagina are swabbed with acetic acid solution and inspected through the colposcope, biopsies may be taken. Biopsy tissue is preserved in 10% formalin, labeled, and sent to the laboratory. Saline may be used to rinse the area, and bleeding may be stopped with silver nitrate or ferric subsulfate (Monsel solution).
5. After the procedure, assist the patient to rise slowly and give the following discharge instructions:
   a. Avoid heavy lifting for 24 hours.
   b. There may be some bleeding and cramping; however, more than that of a normal period must be reported to the health care provider.
   c. Obtain the health care provider's instructions regarding douching and sexual intercourse.

Conization

Description
Excision of a cone-shaped piece of tissue from the cervix, including the area where the squamous and columnar epithelial tissue meet (transformation zone) for diagnostic and therapeutic purposes. The transformation zone is the area of most cervical cancers. The procedure can be done via scalpel, laser, or electrosurgery techniques.

Nursing and Patient Care Considerations
1. Explain to the patient that this test can be a minor surgical procedure that requires local or general anesthesia. Obtain pregnancy test if patient is within childbearing years, as indicated.
2. After excision, bleeding is controlled by cauterization or suturing and packing.
3. The patient should be observed for several hours after the procedure for excessive bleeding.
4. Instruct the patient to avoid tampons, douching, and intercourse as well as not to immerse herself in water (no swimming, hot tub, tub bath) for 2 weeks, or as directed by health care provider, to allow healing.

Hysteroscopy

Description
Endoscopic visualization of the uterine cavity used to evaluate endometrial cancer, check tubal patency, determine the cause of uterine bleeding, remove polyps or fibroids, and observe the placement and appearance of IUDs.

Nursing and Patient Care Considerations
1. Obtain pregnancy test prior to the procedure if the patient is within childbearing years, as indicated.
2. Administer prescribed sedative before the procedure, and explain that a local anesthetic will also be injected into the cervix in the operating room.
3. The patient will be assisted into the lithotomy position, and the perineum and vagina will be cleaned immediately before sterile draping.
4. Explain that instruments called sounds are inserted into the cervical canal for dilation before insertion of the hysteroscope. With the scope in place, normal saline or CO_2 gas is slowly infused into the endometrial cavity to distend it and allow for viewing.
5. Observe patient for several hours and give discharge instructions.
   a. Over-the-counter analgesics may be needed for minor discomfort if analgesic has not been prescribed.
   b. Notify the health care provider of severe cramping or bleeding, fever, or unusual discharge.

Endometrial Biopsy

Description

1. The procedure is done with or without local anesthesia to obtain cells from the uterine lining to assist in the diagnosis of endometrial cancer, menstrual disorders, and infertility.
2. During speculum examination, a uterine sound is placed, followed by a curette or Pipelle suction device to withdraw specimen (may be done several times).

Nursing and Patient Care Considerations

1. Obtain pregnancy test if patient is within childbearing years, as indicated.
2. Administer prostaglandin inhibitor to decrease postoperative uterine cramping.
3. Assist patient into the dorsal lithotomy position and explain procedure.
4. Label the specimen, place in formalin, and send to the laboratory.
5. Inform the patient that she may experience light bleeding and occasional cramping for a few days.
6. Instruct the patient to report fever, chills, and increased bleeding; no tampons, douching, or intercourse for 2 to 3 days.

GENERAL PROCEDURES AND TREATMENT MODALITIES

Fertility Control

Nurses who work with women in the gynecologic setting or in any setting may be involved in contraceptive counseling.

Basic Principles

1. *Contraception* is the prevention of fertility on a temporary basis.
2. *Sterilization* is the permanent prevention of fertility. Female and male sterilization procedures can be performed. Some procedures can be reversed but with possible complications and variable success rates.
3. Contraception effectiveness depends on motivation, which is a result of education, culture, religious beliefs, and personal situation. It is best to include both partners in any contraception decision.
4. Nurses should be familiar with contraceptive methods and educate patients without moral judgment.
5. Failure rate (pregnancy) is determined by experience of 100 women for 1 year and is expressed as pregnancies per 100 woman-years.

Contraceptive Methods

See Table 22-2.

Sterilization Procedures

Tubal sterilization is frequently performed for birth control. Hysterectomy and oophorectomy, performed for other reasons, also result in sterility. Male sterilization by vasectomy is another option.

General Considerations

1. Approaches.
   a. Abdominal is most frequently used: may be postpartum laparotomy, minilaparotomy, or laparoscopy. Laparoscopy

with electrocoagulation is frequently performed. It is a safe and effective procedure.
   b. Uterine approach utilizing hysteroscopy to visualize the tubal ostia and insert coils or plugs.
2. Techniques vary by surgeon preference.
   a. Electrocoagulation: burn section of tube with or without excision; low reversal rate.
   b. Pomeroy: the tube is tied in midsection and section removed; may be reversed.
   c. Fimbriectomy: the fimbriated end removed and end tied; irreversible.
   d. Cornual resection: removal of the section of the tube nearest to the uterus and suture cornual opening closed.
   e. Silastic bands: plastic or metal clips to occlude tube; may be reversed, although rare.
   f. Coils or plugs inserted in the tubal ostia through hysteroscopy.

Complications

a. Failure to successfully block the tubes—pregnancy or tubal pregnancy.
b. Hemorrhage, infection, uterine perforation, and damage to the bowel, bladder, or aorta.

Nursing and Patient Care Considerations

1. Assess motivation for sterilization and level of knowledge about the procedure. Informed consent is needed. The couple should be thoroughly counseled about the permanence of the procedure.
   a. Teach the patient that there is no effect on hormones and menstruation will continue.
   b. Teach patient there should not be any adverse effect on sexual response.
2. Birth control should be used prior to sterilization unless performed during the menstrual period, during a Cesarean section, immediately postpartum, or after an abortion procedure.
3. Prepare the patient to expect some abdominal soreness for several days; instruct her to report any bleeding, increasing pain, or fever.
4. Sexual intercourse and strenuous activity should be avoided for 2 weeks.

Dilation and Curettage

Dilation and curettage is a common gynecologic surgery for diagnostic and therapeutic purposes, which consists of widening the cervical canal with a dilator and scraping the uterine cavity with a curette. Performed to control uterine bleeding, secure endometrial and endocervical tissue for cytologic examination, and treat missed, incomplete, or induced abortion.

Nursing and Patient Care Considerations

1. Prepare patient for the procedure—answer questions; request that she void; administer an enema, if ordered; and administer nonsteroidal anti-inflammatory drug (NSAID) or a sedative, as directed.
2. Immediately postoperatively, monitor vital signs at frequent intervals; potential for hemorrhage exists.
3. Monitor perineal pads and the bed for amount of bleeding; report excessive amounts.

Table 22-2 Contraceptive Methods

METHODS	DEFINITION	PROCEDURE	ADVANTAGES	DISADVANTAGES
Natural Methods				
Periodic abstinence	• Abstain from inter-course during fertile period of each cycle.	• Determine fertile period by: • Calendar method—ovulation occurs 14 days before the next menstrual period. • Cervical mucus method—increase in mucus at the time of ovulation; clear and stringy. • Basal body temperature—drops immediately before ovulation and rises 24 to 72 hr after ovulation. • Symptothermal method—combines mucus and temperature.	• No health hazards. • Inexpensive. • May be religiously acceptable. • Increased knowledge of cycles.	• 20% failure rate. • Requires consistent record-keeping. • Decrease in spontaneity.
Coitus interruptus (withdrawal method)	• Withdrawal of the penis from the vagina when ejaculation is imminent.	• Must withdraw before ejaculation so that ejaculation occurs away from female genitalia.	• No cost. • No health hazards. • Always available.	• Failure rate of 19%; pre-ejaculatory fluid may contain sperm. • Interruption of sexual act.
Lactation amenor-rhea method	• Breast-feeding has a contraceptive effect due to prolactin's inhibition of luteinizing hormone, which maintains menstrual cycle.	• Three requirements: Baby is < 6 months old and is breast-fed on demand, around the clock, without formula or food supplementation, and the woman has not had her menses.	• No health hazards. • No cost.	• Need to use other method such as spermicide or barrier, which has no effect on breast milk if the three conditions are not met.
Barrier Methods				

! **NURSING ALERT** Warn patients who use condoms, diaphragms, and the cervical cap that latex sensitivity may be a problem—watch for itching, swelling, and generalized reactions.

METHODS	DEFINITION	PROCEDURE	ADVANTAGES	DISADVANTAGES
Condom—male and female	• Latex or polyurethane or processed collagenous tissue sheaths, placed over an erect penis to prevent semen from entering the vagina. • Female condom is placed in the vagina.	• Place condom over an erect penis. • Leave dead space at the tip of condom (from which air has been expelled) to allow room for ejaculate. • Use spermicide on exterior for added protection. • Grasp ring around condom at withdrawal to avoid leaving condom in the vagina.	• Failure rate is low with proper use (2% to 3%). • Prevention of STD • Inexpensive • No health hazard • May help premature ejaculation by decreasing sensitivity • Increases male involvement in contraception	• Decreased sensitivity • Interruption of sexual act • Sensitivity to latex may be a problem • Failure rate with typical use is 12%. • Female condoms are more expensive and made of polyurethane.
Diaphragm	• Rubber cap shaped like a dome with a flexible rim.	• Check for holes. • Place spermicide inside dome. • Place diaphragm against and covering cervical opening, behind lower edge of pubic bone. • Leave in place for 6 to 8 hr after intercourse.	• Failure rate with perfect use is 6% and 12% with typical use. • May reduce the risk of developing cervical cancer. • May place in the vagina several hours before intercourse. • Can use while breast-feeding.	• Occasional toxic shock or allergic reactions. • May experience pelvic discomfort. • Possible increase in urinary tract infections (UTIs) • Must be properly cleaned with soap and water, dried and stored to preserve integrity of rubber.

(continued)

Table 22-2 Contraceptive Methods (*Continued*)

METHODS	DEFINITION	PROCEDURE	ADVANTAGES	DISADVANTAGES
Cervical cap	• Rubber cap, shaped like a cup with a tall dome and flexible rim.	• Place spermicide inside cap and place cap over cervical opening prior to intercourse.	• Failure rate 14% to 29%. • Can be left in place for up to 48 hr. • Can use while breast-feeding.	• Must be properly cleaned with soap and water, dried, and stored. • Can be difficult to insert and remove.
Spermicides Nonoxynol 9 or octoxynol 9	• Available in a variety of forms: foam, jelly, cream, suppository, tablet.	• Place next to the cervix before intercourse; better if used with a barrier method.	• Available in a variety of forms. • Sold over the counter.	• Less effective if not used with barrier method; generally, 28% failure rate. • Some patients are allergic. • Increases risk of UTI. • Frequent use may cause genital lesions, increasing risk of HIV transmission.
Intrauterine Devices	• Small device made of plastic with exposed copper or progesterone release system; acts to inhibit implantation.	• Health care provider inserts device, usually at the time of menses. • Check intrauterine device string regularly—at least once per month—or after each intercourse when it is first inserted.	• Failure rate low, 1% or less. • Convenient; permits spontaneous intercourse. • Replace every 3 to 12 yr, depending on the type.	• Risk of PID for the first month and resultant tubal damage and infertility. • May cause spotting, bleeding, or pain. • Risk of spontaneous abortion. • Risk of uterine rupture (rare).
Hormones Combination oral contraceptives	• Tablets containing estrogen to inhibit ovulation and progestin to make cervical mucus impenetrable to sperm; lowest effective doses are used.	• Take daily in a cyclical or continuous manner.	• <1% failure rate in the first year with correct use. • Decreased pelvic pain due to endometriosis, decreased risk of ovarian and endometrial cancer, decreased bleeding due to uterine fibroids. • Aids in menstrual disorders. • Improves acne.	• Serious adverse reactions include thromboembolism, stroke, myocardial infarction, and cerebral embolism, especially for those who smoke cigarettes or are overweight. • Questionable risk of breast, cervical cancer. • May experience nausea, vomiting, headache, bloating. • Must remember to take at same time daily.
Progestin-only oral contraceptive (minipill)	• Smaller doses of progestins than in combined oral contraceptives.	• Take daily.	• As low as <1% failure rate during the first year with correct use. • Avoids estrogen-related adverse effects and possibly cardiovascular risks. • The thickened cervical mucus may reduce the risk of ascending infection with development of PID. • Safe in breast-feeding.	• May cause irregular menses, spotting, amenorrhea. • Must be taken at the same time daily (no more than 3 hr late) or protection is lost.

Table 22-2 Contraceptive Methods (*Continued*)

METHODS	DEFINITION	PROCEDURE	ADVANTAGES	DISADVANTAGES
Hormones (*Continued*)				
Combination trans-dermal contraceptive patch	• Estrogen and progesterone are absorbed systemically, as efficacious as oral hormones.	• Apply weekly to buttocks, inner aspect of upper arms, or abdomen for 3 weeks and then off for 1 week for menses.	• Same as oral hormones but administered weekly. • Avoids first-pass metabolism through the liver.	• Same as oral hormones. • May become loose or cause minor skin reaction. • Increased risk of DVT compared to oral method. • Women >190 pounds should not use.
Hormonal vaginal contraceptive	• Vaginal ring containing estrogen and progesterone, as effective as oral contraceptive.	• Insert ring into the vagina; remove after 3 weeks for 1 week for menses.	• Same as oral contraceptives except it is administered monthly. • Avoids first-pass metabolism through the liver.	• Same as oral contraceptives. • Requires vaginal insertion and retrieval. • May cause vaginitis, leukorrhea.
Postcoital contraception (morning-after pill)	• May be combined estrogen and progestin, high-dose estrogen, or progestin.	• More effective if started within 24 to 72 hr after intercourse, may be used up to 5 days after intercourse.	• Very effective.	• May be religiously opposed. • Can cause nausea.
Progesterone implant	• Progesterone release system made up of Silastic rod.	• Implanted in subcutaneous fat of the upper arm.	• Long term (up to 3 yr). • Convenient. • Only 0.4% failure rate.	• May cause irregular bleeding, spotting, amenorrhea, acne, headaches. • May be difficult to remove. • High initial expense.
Progesterone injection	• IM injection of long-acting progesterone.	• Injections should be every 11 to 13 weeks.	• Convenient. • <1% failure rate with correct use.	• Requires every 3-month follow-up. • May cause irregular bleeding, spotting, amenorrhea, weight gain. • Long-term effects still unknown. • High discontinuation rate in adolescents due to adverse effects and missed appointments. • Need calcium supplementation.
Progesterone Antagonist				
RU-486; mifepristone	• Drug that prevents implantation and leads to menses (medical abortion).	• Given orally within 10 days of a missed period; may be combined with prostaglandin suppository.	• Causes abortion in 95% of users up to 5 weeks after conception.	• Is an abortifacient; not a contraceptive in most cases. • May cause nausea, bleeding, incomplete abortion.

STD, sexually transmitted disease.

4. Offer prescribed analgesics for lower back and pelvic pain; cramping may occur for 2 to 3 days because of dilation of the cervix.
5. Instruct patient to maintain decreased activity for remainder of day to decrease cramping and bleeding.
6. Instruct patient to use perineal pads at home and to report fever (more than 100.4°F), heavy bleeding (saturating a pad within 1 hour more than once), cramps lasting longer than 48 hours, increasing pain, and prolonged or a foul-smelling vaginal discharge.

7. Instruct patient to avoid strenuous activity until bleeding stops.
8. Inform patient that the procedure does not affect sexual functioning, but that she should refrain from sexual intercourse, douching, and tampons for at least 2 weeks, according to preference of health care provider.

Laparoscopy

Laparoscopy is the endoscopic visualization of the pelvic and abdominal cavities through a small incision below the umbilicus. It is used to diagnose pelvic pain and infertility; differentiate between ovarian, tubal, and uterine masses; evaluate genital anomalies; treat endometriosis, ectopic pregnancy, and adhesions; perform tubal sterilizations; and as a major surgical tool to treat a multitude of gynecologic indications including laparoscopically assisted hysterectomy.

Nursing and Patient Care Considerations

1. Obtain pregnancy test if the patient is within childbearing years, as indicated.
2. Prepare patient by ensuring that she has taken nothing by mouth (NPO), answering questions about the procedure, and administering a sedative and enema, if ordered.
3. Inform the patient that she may experience shoulder or abdominal discomfort after the procedure from the infusion of carbon dioxide given to separate the intestines from pelvic organs. Elevation of feet higher than shoulders after the procedure helps relieve this.
4. The patient will receive local, general, or regional anesthesia and will be placed in Trendelenburg position to displace the intestines for better visualization.
5. After the procedure, monitor bleeding and vital signs and administer analgesics, as indicated.
6. Inform patient that passing gas and bowel movements may be difficult initially because of the manipulation of the intestines; ambulation and fluids will be helpful.
7. Advise patient to report bleeding, cramping, or fever; avoid strenuous activity for 2 to 3 days; and not to have intercourse for 1 week. Additional restrictions may be advised for complex procedures.

Hysterectomy

Hysterectomy is the surgical removal of the uterus. It is the second most common operation in the United States among reproductive-age women.

Types of Hysterectomy

1. Abdominal.
   a. Subtotal/supracervical hysterectomy—corpus of the uterus is removed, but cervical stump remains.
   b. Total hysterectomy—entire uterus is removed, including the cervix; tubes and ovaries remain.
   c. Total hysterectomy with bilateral salpingo-oophorectomy—entire uterus, tubes, and ovaries are removed.
2. Vaginal—removal of the uterus and cervix through the vagina.
3. Laparoscopically assisted vaginal hysterectomy—allows for the removal of pelvic adhesions that would otherwise prevent vaginal hysterectomy.
4. Laparoscopic supracervical hysterectomy—laparoscopic removal of the uterus that spares the cervix.
5. Laparoscopic total hysterectomy—laparoscopic removal of the entire uterus and cervix.

Indications

1. Uterine fibroids, endometriosis and adenomyosis, and dysfunctional uterine bleeding—most common.
2. Uterine prolapse and chronic pelvic pain.
3. Cancer of the vagina, cervix, uterus, ovaries, or fallopian tubes.
4. Obstetric complications—rare.

Preoperative Management

1. Procedure and reason for hysterectomy, what the procedure involves, and what to expect postoperatively are explained.
2. Patient must remain NPO from midnight the night before surgery and must void before surgery.
3. An enema may be administered before surgery to evacuate the bowel and prevent contamination and trauma during surgery.
4. Vaginal irrigation is performed before surgery and skin preparation is done, if ordered.
5. Implement the Universal Protocol for Preventing Wrong Site, Wrong Procedure, and Wrong Person Surgery (see Chapter 7).
6. Preoperative medication is given to help the patient relax.

Postoperative Management

1. Postoperatively, the following assessments are made:
   a. Wound appearance and drainage.
   b. Vital signs and level of consciousness.
   c. Level of pain and comfort to include nausea and vomiting.
   d. Vaginal drainage (serous, bloody).
   e. Intake and output.
   f. Urge to void, bladder distention, and residual urine (if appropriate).
   g. Clarity, color, and sediment of urine.
   h. Homans sign or impaired circulation.
   i. Return of bowel sounds, passage of flatus, and first bowel movement.
2. Exercise and ambulation are encouraged to prevent thromboembolus, facilitate voiding, and stimulate peristalsis.

Complications

1. Incisional/pelvic infection.
2. Hemorrhage.
3. Urinary tract injury.
4. Bowel obstruction.
5. Thrombophlebitis/venous thromboemboli.

Nursing Diagnoses

- Acute Pain related to surgical procedure.
- Impaired Urinary Elimination related to decreased sensation and stimulation.
- Risk for Infection related to surgical procedure.
- Disturbed Body Image related to alteration in female organs and hormones.
- Sexual Dysfunction related to alteration in reproductive organs and function.

Nursing Interventions

Relieving Pain

1. Assess pain location, level, and characteristics.
2. Administer prescribed pain medications. Ensure that patient knows how to use patient-controlled analgesia pump and is using it properly.
3. Encourage patient to splint incision when moving.

4. Encourage patient to ambulate as soon as possible to decrease flatus and abdominal distention.
5. Institute sitz baths or ice packs, as prescribed, to alleviate perineal discomfort.
6. Monitor level of sedation related to opioid administration—may interfere with ambulation and elimination.

Promoting Urinary Elimination
1. Monitor intake and output, bladder distention, and signs and symptoms of bladder infection.
2. Maintain patency of indwelling catheter if one is in place.
3. Catheterize patient intermittently if uncomfortable or if she has not voided in 8 hours.
4. Catheterize to check for residual urine after patient voids; should be less than 100 mL. Continue to check if more than 100 mL or bladder infection may develop.
5. Encourage patient to empty bladder around the clock, not only when feeling the urge, because of loss of sensation of bladder fullness.
6. Encourage fluid intake to decrease risk of urinary infection.

Preventing Infection
1. Assess vaginal drainage amount, color, and odor, incision site, and temperature.
2. Administer antibiotics, as prescribed.
3. Assist use of incentive spirometer, coughing and deep breathing, and ambulation to decrease risk of pulmonary infection. Monitor respirations and breath sounds for compromise.

Strengthening Body Image
1. Allow the patient to discuss her feelings about herself as a woman.
2. Encourage the patient to discuss her feelings with her spouse or significant other.
3. Reassure the patient that she will not go through premature menopause if her ovaries were not removed.

Regaining Sexual Function
1. Discuss changes regarding sexual functioning, such as shortened vagina and possible dyspareunia because of dryness.
2. Offer suggestions to improve sexual functioning.
   a. Use of water-soluble lubricants.
   b. Change position—female-dominant position offers more control of depth of penetration.

Patient Education and Health Maintenance
1. Advise patient that a total hysterectomy with bilateral salpingo-oophorectomy produces a surgical menopause. Patient may experience hot flashes, vaginal dryness, and mood swings unless short-term hormonal replacement therapy is instituted.
2. Advise patient against sitting too long at one time, as in driving long distances, because of the possibility of blood pooling in the lower extremities, which increases the risk of thromboembolism.
3. Suggest that patient delay driving a car until the third postoperative week because even pressing the brake pedal puts stress on the lower abdomen. Avoid hazardous activities when taking opioid analgesics.
4. Tell patient to expect a tired feeling for the first few days at home and not to plan too many activities for the first week. She can perform most of her usual daily activities within 4 to 6 weeks or per provider instruction. Teach patient that the recovery period differs for each individual and is dependent on medical history and any complications that may have occurred. Inform her that it may be 2 to 3 months or even a year "to feel like herself again."
5. Tell patient not to feel discouraged if, at times during convalescence, she experiences depression, feels like crying, and

seems unusually nervous. This is common but will not last. Tell patient to call her provider if the feelings persist.
6. Remind patient to ask her surgeon about strenuous or lifting activities, which are usually restricted for 4 to 6 weeks.
7. Reinforce instructions given by the surgeon on intercourse, douching, and use of tampons, which are usually discouraged for 6 to 8 weeks. Sexual intercourse should be resumed cautiously to prevent injury and discomfort. Showers are permitted, but tub baths are deferred until healing is sufficient.
8. Instruct patient to report fever higher than 100°F (37.8°C), heavy vaginal bleeding, drainage, increased pain or cramping, foul odor of discharge, and bleeding or increased drainage from incision site.
9. Emphasize the importance of follow-up visits and routine physical and gynecologic examinations.

Evaluation: Expected Outcomes
- Verbalizes decreased pain.
- Voids every 4 to 6 hours of sufficient quantity.
- No fever or signs of infection.
- Verbalizes positive statements about self and positive outlook on recovery.
- Verbalizes understanding of possible changes in sexual functioning and what to do about it.

MENSTRUAL CONDITIONS
Dysmenorrhea

Dysmenorrhea is painful menstruation; most common of gynecologic dysfunctions.

Pathophysiology and Etiology
Primary Dysmenorrhea
1. No pelvic lesion; usually intrinsic to the uterus.
2. Current research supports increased prostaglandin production by the endometrium as the chief cause.
3. May also be because of hormonal, obstructive, and psychological factors.

Secondary Dysmenorrhea
1. Caused by lesion, such as endometriosis, pelvic infection, congenital abnormality, uterine fibroids, or ovarian cyst, or may be caused by passage of a clot through undilated cervix.

Clinical Manifestations
1. Pain may be caused by increased uterine contractility and uterine hypoxia.
2. Characteristics of pain—recurrent, crampy, colicky or dull, usually in lower midabdominal region, and spasmodic or constant.
3. Nausea, vomiting, diarrhea, headache, chills, tiredness, nervousness, and lower backache may be experienced.
4. Usually self-limiting without complications.

Diagnostic Evaluation
Tests to rule out underlying cause:
1. Chlamydia and gonorrhea tests—may show infection.
2. Pelvic ultrasound—may detect tumor, endometriosis, and cysts.
3. Serum or urine pregnancy test—to rule out ectopic pregnancy.
4. Possibly, hysteroscopy and laparoscopy—primarily to detect endometriosis.

Management

The following measures are for primary dysmenorrhea; treatment of secondary dysmenorrhea is aimed at underlying pathology.

1. Nonsteroidal anti-inflammatory agents, such as ibuprofen or naproxen sodium for their antiprostaglandin action. Most effective with loading dose 1 to 2 days before onset of menses and taken on a regular schedule for 2 to 3 days.
2. Local heat, such as heating pad, to increase blood flow and decrease spasms, for 20-minute intervals with increased effectiveness with other therapies.
3. Hormonal contraceptives to decrease contractility and menstrual flow. Evidence supports decreased dysmenorrhea symptoms with monthly oral contraceptives, extended-cycle oral contraceptives, intravaginal hormonal devices, and intrauterine hormonal systems.
4. Exercise to increase endorphin release, which decreases pain perception, and to suppress prostaglandin release.

Nursing Assessment

1. Obtain menstrual and gynecologic history that could suggest underlying pathology.
2. Assess level of pain using scale of 1 to 10; assess the patient's emotional response to pain, coping mechanisms, and ability to carry out activities.
3. Obtain vital signs, including temperature, to rule out infection.
4. Perform abdominal and pelvic examination (if indicated) to obtain specimens.

Nursing Diagnoses

- Acute Pain related to uterine contractions.
- Risk for Activity Intolerance related to pain severity and associated symptoms.
- Readiness for Enhanced Coping related to chronic, recurrent condition.

Nursing Interventions

Controlling Pain

1. Administer pharmacologic agents, as ordered, to control pain and menstrual flow.
2. Apply heating pad to lower back or abdomen, as indicated, for 20-minute intervals.
3. Assess the patient's response to pain-control measures.
4. Encourage verbalization of feelings and reassure patient through the evaluation process.
5. Encourage activity and exercise, as tolerated.

Decreasing Risk for Activity Intolerance

Instruct the patient that tolerance will increase with increased activity. The more active she is, the better she will feel.

Enhancing Coping Skills

Instruct the patient in stress-reduction techniques, breathing techniques, and lifestyle changes that may improve symptoms such as exercise, healthy eating habits, adequate sleep, and smoking cessation.

Patient Education and Health Maintenance

1. Explain to the patient possible causes of dysmenorrhea.
2. Teach the patient nonpharmacologic methods to reduce pain.
   a. Apply a heating pad to the lower midabdomen or back or take warm tub baths for 20-minute intervals.
   b. Exercise regularly (30 minutes, five or more times per week).
   c. Healthy eating habits; see *www.myplate.gov.*
   d. Smoking cessation.

3. Teach the patient to use prescribed medications effectively by taking medication at the beginning of discomfort and repeating as necessary, especially on the first day of menses.
4. Teach the patient adverse effects of medications.
5. Encourage patient to reduce stress through adequate sleep, good nutrition, exercise, smoking cessation, and coping with stressors.
6. Discuss patient's feelings toward menstruation (hygienic issues, inconvenience, female identity).

Evaluation: Expected Outcomes

- Verbalizes reduced pain level.
- Demonstrates participation in functional activities of daily living without intolerance.
- Describes methods to reduce pain and to increase coping skills.

Premenstrual Syndrome and Premenstrual Dysphoric Disorder

 EVIDENCE BASE Hofmeister, S., & Bodden, S. (2016). Premenstrual syndrome and premenstrual dysphoric disorder. *American Family Physician,* 94(3), 236–240.

Premenstrual syndrome (PMS) is a group of behavioral, psychological, and physical symptoms that include headache, irritability, depressed mood, breast tenderness, and abdominal bloating that are clearly related to onset of menstruation.

Premenstrual dysphoric disorder (PMDD) is a severe form of PMS.

Pathophysiology and Etiology

1. Etiologic theories include hormonal imbalances, such as ovarian steroid interaction; dysfunction of neurotransmitters (such as serotonin), prostaglandins, or endorphins; psychological factors, such as attitudes and beliefs related to menstruation; and environmental factors, such as nutrition and pollution.
2. Most common in women in their thirties.
3. May occur in 20% to 32% of menstruating women. Up to 80% of women experience one or more of the symptoms during the luteal phase of their menstrual cycle.

Clinical Manifestations

1. Symptoms may begin 7 to 14 days before onset of menstrual flow; may diminish 1 to 2 days after menses begins.
2. Physical—edema of extremities, abdominal fullness, breast swelling and tenderness, headache, vertigo, palpitations, acne, backache, constipation, thirst, and weight gain.
3. Psychological and behavioral—labile mood, irritability, fatigue, lethargy, depressed mood, anxiety, crying spells, changes in appetite, and decreased concentration.
4. Diagnosis based on clinical manifestations; usually neither diagnostic laboratory nor radiological evaluation is necessary.
5. Usually self-limiting without complications.

Management

1. First-line pharmacological therapy for severe PMS or PMDD includes selective serotonin reuptake inhibitors (SSRIs) such as citalopram, escitalopram, fluoxetine, and sertraline and serotonin–norepinephrine reuptake inhibitors such as venlafaxine.
2. Drospirenone (a spironolactone derivative diuretic) combined with low-dose estrogen in oral contraceptives helps symptoms. Theoretically, longer cycles of oral contraceptives with shorter

inactive phases would ameliorate symptoms by suppressing natural hormones.

3. Calcium supplementation of 1,200 mg elemental calcium per day has good evidence that supports decreased mood swings, irritability, depression, and anxiety.
4. Vitamin B_6 supplements of 50 to 100 mg daily (should not exceed 100 mg/day).
5. Cognitive–behavioral therapy has some limited evidence supporting relief of symptoms.
6. Healthy lifestyle changes, such as restriction of sodium, caffeine, tobacco, alcohol, and refined sweets, and inclusion of aerobic exercise, although often recommended, have insufficient evidence to support their efficacy in treatment of PMS symptoms.
7. High-dose daily vitamin D intake is supported by some evidence.
8. Prostaglandin inhibitors such as ibuprofen will decrease dysmenorrhea-related symptoms.
9. Spironolactone, a diuretic with androgenic effect, may decrease fluid retention and weight gain.
10. With great caution because of abuse potential, anxiolytic agents may be prescribed for use during the luteal phase for patients with anxiety symptoms.
11. Herbal supplements, for example, chasteberry, also known as *Vitex agnus-castus*, were found to be effective in one randomized controlled trial, but more studies are needed.

 DRUG ALERT Paroxetine should be avoided in women of childbearing age because of increased risk of congenital abnormalities.

Nursing Assessment

1. Ask the patient to describe symptoms, their onset, and means of relief.
2. Assess the patient's diet, activity, and rest habits.
3. Assess the patient's emotional response to symptoms and methods of coping.

Nursing Diagnoses

- Deficient Knowledge related to self-care measures.
- Anxiety related to symptoms and difficulty coping with condition.

Nursing Interventions

Increasing Knowledge and Coping Skills
Use patient education as a tool to help patient increase control over symptoms.

Reducing Anxiety
1. Administer medications, as ordered; warn patient that diuretics will cause increased urination and anxiolytics may cause drowsiness or cognitive impairment.
2. Provide emotional support for patient and significant others.
3. Teach stress management and relaxation measures such as imagery and progressive muscle relaxation (see Chapter 3).
4. Suggest counseling, as indicated.

Patient Education and Health Maintenance

1. Encourage patient to keep a diary for several consecutive months, which includes dates, cycle days, stressors, symptoms, and their severity, to determine if therapy is effective.
2. Instruct patient in the use and adverse effects of prescribed medications.

3. Teach patient possible causes of syndrome and nonprescription methods to alleviate distress, such as calcium and vitamin B_6 intake.
4. Refer for further resources and support to such groups as the National Association for Premenstrual Syndrome (UK) (*http://pms.org.uk*) or womenshealth.gov, a project of the U.S. Department of Health and Human Services Office on Women's Health (*www.womenshealth.gov*).

Evaluation: Expected Outcomes

- Verbalizes increased knowledge and sense of control over condition.
- Reduced signs and symptoms of anxiety.

Amenorrhea

Amenorrhea is the absence of menstrual flow.

Pathophysiology and Etiology

Primary Amenorrhea
1. Menarche does not occur by age 16 with pubertal development or by age 14 with absence of secondary sex characteristics.
2. May be caused by chromosomal disorders, such as Turner syndrome, agenesis of the uterus, or constitutional delay of growth and puberty.
3. Transverse vaginal septum or imperforate hymen.

Secondary Amenorrhea
1. Menstruation stops for 3 months in women with previously established regular menstrual cycles or 9 months in a woman with previously established oligomenorrhea (infrequent or longer menstrual cycles).
2. May be caused by pregnancy, lactation, menopause, or corpus luteal ovarian cysts.
3. Excessive exercise, inadequate nutrition with decreased body fat stores, and excessive weight loss may cause amenorrhea in young athletes (included in the female athlete triad: an eating disorder, amenorrhea, and osteoporosis).
4. Amenorrhea and anovulation secondary to polycystic ovary syndrome (PCOS) commonly occur in obese women but may be seen in women with normal body mass index (BMI).
5. Ovarian, adrenal, or pituitary tumors and thyroid disorders are hormonal causes.
6. Some medications, such as antipsychotics (phenothiazines), antidepressants, antihypertensives, histamine H2 blockers, opiates, chemotherapy, and hormonal contraceptives, may also induce amenorrhea.
7. It may be a result of severe depression, severe psychological trauma, physical trauma, or radiation.

Diagnostic Evaluation

1. Pregnancy test.
2. Prolactin level (elevated) with pituitary tumor.
3. Thyroid-stimulating hormone (TSH).
4. Progesterone challenge test in secondary amenorrhea if both prolactin and TSH are normal and pregnancy test is negative.
   a. Positive result—bleeding occurs; chronic anovulation is most likely.
   b. Negative result—no bleeding occurs; may indicate ovarian failure; other tests are needed.
5. Hormonal levels—LH and FSH—to determine type of hypogonadism in primary amenorrhea or to detect ovarian failure in secondary amenorrhea.

6. Genetic karyotyping to detect chromosome abnormalities in primary amenorrhea.
7. Ultrasound to identify presence of the uterus and/or outflow obstruction.

Management

Treatment is based on causative factor.
1. Discontinue causative medications if benefit of discontinuance outweighs risk.
2. Nutritional, exercise, or psychological counseling, as indicated.
   a. Recommend decreased exercise in athletes to increase body fat stores and restore normal BMI.
   b. Recommend weight reduction if obese.
3. Low-dose hormonal contraceptives to regulate cycle after underlying cause has been determined.
4. In polycystic ovarian syndrome, insulin-sensitizing agents decrease androgen levels, improve ovulation rate, and improve glucose tolerance. Clomiphene citrate is first-line for ovulation induction. Laser treatment plus eflornithine is indicated for hirsutism in PCOS.
5. Treatment of tumor or other underlying cause. Surgery, as indicated.

Complications

1. Amenorrhea increases risk for osteoporosis and endometrial hyperplasia, which may lead to atypia and cancer of the endometrium.
2. PCOS conveys risk of metabolic syndrome, type 2 diabetes, and cardiovascular disease. Improvement in ovulation rate increases the risk of pregnancy.

Nursing Assessment

1. Assess for signs of chromosomal disorders, such as abnormal genitalia, masculinization, short stature, and characteristic facies.
2. Assess for signs of pituitary tumor, such as headache, vision disturbances, dizziness, and galactorrhea.
3. Assess weight and body build, BMI, change in weight, and nutritional and exercise habits that may indicate anorexia or loss of body fat because of exercise.
4. Assess for signs of PCOS: elevated blood pressure, elevated BMI, waist circumference, stigmata of insulin resistance, and hirsutism.
5. Assess emotional status, areas of stress, and coping ability.

Nursing Diagnoses

- Imbalanced Nutrition: Less Than Body Requirements related to inadequate nutritional intake and/or rigorous exercise.
- Imbalanced Nutrition: More Than Body Requirements related to obesity or PCOS.
- Disturbed Body Image related to lack of menses and perception of inappropriate weight.

Nursing Interventions

Meeting Nutritional Requirements
1. Explore knowledge of the food groups, behavior regarding meals, and exercise routine; point out misconceptions, dangerous behavior, and ideas for improvement.
2. Monitor weight and BMI and return of menstrual cycles.
3. Refer for individual or group nutritional counseling as needed.

Improving Body Image
1. Explore patient's body image and coping strategies. Provide emotional support for patient and family.
2. Describe diagnostic tests and who will give results to patient.
3. Point out ineffective coping mechanisms and teach more positive coping mechanisms such as assertiveness. Instruct in relaxation techniques.

Patient Education and Health Maintenance

1. Teach patient the physiology of the normal menstrual cycle and possible causes in diagnostic workup for amenorrhea.
2. Teach proper use and adverse effects of prescribed medications.
3. Teach the patient to chart menstrual periods on a calendar and maintain regular gynecologic and medical follow-up visits.
4. Teach patients with PCOS that they should be screened for type 2 diabetes and cardiovascular risk factors such as fasting lipid levels and BMI.

Evaluation: Expected Outcomes

- Verbalizes adequate dietary intake and appropriate exercise regimen.
- Achieves normal BMI with restoration of menses.
- Verbalizes understanding of diagnostic tests and improved body image.

Abnormal Uterine Bleeding

 EVIDENCE BASE American College of Obstetrics and Gynecology. (2013). Management of abnormal uterine bleeding associated with ovulatory dysfunction. *Obstetrics and Gynecology, 122,* 176–185.

Abnormal uterine bleeding (AUB) is irregular or excessively heavy menstrual bleeding. It may be acute or chronic and is abnormal in regularity, volume, frequency, or duration, and it occurs in the absence of pregnancy.

Pathophysiology and Etiology

Causes of AUB are subdivided into anovulatory and ovulatory patterns.

Anovulatory AUB
1. Common causes of anovulatory AUB include polycystic ovarian syndrome (PCOS), uncontrolled diabetes mellitus, thyroid disorders (hypo- and hyperthyroidism), hyperprolactinemia, or medications (such as antipsychotics and antiepileptics).
2. In adolescents, AUB is frequently caused by immature hypothalamic–pituitary–ovarian axis.
3. Ovarian failure in perimenopausal women frequently causes DUB. Recurrent irregular menstrual cycles are considered abnormal if they occur 8 years before menopause.
4. Anovulation may be related to hypothalamic or pituitary dysfunction, impaired follicular formation or rupture, or corpus luteum dysfunction.
5. Temporary estrogen withdrawal at ovulation may cause mid-cycle ovulatory bleeding.

Ovulatory AUB
1. Excessive bleeding or duration may be related to hypothyroidism, late-stage liver disease, or bleeding disorders (such von Willebrand disease).

2. Structural abnormalities, such as submucosal fibroids or endometrial fibroids, may cause AUB.
3. Approximately one half of women with ovulatory AUB have no identifiable cause.

Clinical Manifestations

Anovulatory AUB Patterns/Dysfunctional Bleeding
1. Amenorrhea—no bleeding for three cycles or more.
2. Oligomenorrhea—significantly diminished menstrual flow; infrequent intervals (greater than 35 days) or irregular intervals.
3. Metrorrhagia—bleeding from the uterus between regular menstrual periods; significant because it is usually a symptom of disease.
4. Menometrorrhagia—excessive bleeding at the usual time of menstruation and at other irregular intervals.

Ovulatory Patterns
1. Menorrhagia—excessive bleeding during regular menstruation cycles; can be increased in duration or amount.
2. Polymenorrhea—frequent menstruation occurring at intervals of less than 21 days.
3. Menometrorrhagia—excessive bleeding at the usual time of menstruation and at other irregular intervals.

Diagnostic Evaluation

Tests to rule out pathologic causes of abnormal bleeding include:
1. Pregnancy test.
2. Complete blood count (CBC) to detect anemia and platelet count.
3. TSH to rule out thyroid disorder; prolactin to rule out pituitary adenoma.
4. Thorough history and examination to look for anovulatory medical conditions (such as obesity and hirsutism—signs of PCOS) and to rule out enlarged uterus, trauma, or foreign body.
5. Other tests that may be done during physical exam include a Pap smear to rule out cervical dysplasia or malignancy; chlamydia and gonorrhea tests to rule out PID.
6. Endometrial biopsy to determine hormonal effect on the uterus and rule out malignancy.
7. Transvaginal ultrasound to rule out ovarian or uterine pathology or structural abnormality. Saline infusion sonohysterography is more sensitive and specific than transvaginal ultrasound.
8. Coagulation screen to rule out blood dyscrasias in adolescents with menorrhagia. Iron studies are not first-line, but are recommended if hematocrit and hemoglobin are low.
9. If cause is still undetermined, then hysteroscopy is recommended to detect uterine fibroids, polyps, and other lesions.

Management

Treatment is based on underlying cause.
1. Hormonal contraceptives (birth control pills or hormone-releasing IUD) to control chronic bleeding or induce regular withdrawal bleeding. Endometrial biopsy should be repeated after 3 to 6 months of treatment to monitor endometrial hyperplasia. Combination estrogen–progesterone oral contraceptives, although commonly prescribed first-line, lack adequate evidence for treatment of AUB.
2. In women who cannot take estrogen because of an increased thrombotic risk, progesterone-only administration can be effective. Cyclical oral progesterone for 21 days significantly reduces menorrhagia. For patients with menorrhagia,

levonorgestrel-releasing intrauterine system is superior to oral contraceptives. Long-acting progestin injections may reduce bleeding but cause irregular spotting.
3. In emergencies, parenteral conjugated estrogen may be used to stop acute bleeding. Because of increased risk of thromboembolism, concomitant use of low molecular weight heparin may be considered.
4. Treat underlying anemia with iron, possible transfusions.
5. NSAIDs are useful to decrease menstrual flow volume in menorrhagia.
6. Tranexamic acid, an antifibrinolytic agent, has demonstrated efficacy in decreasing menorrhagia. In an underlying bleeding disorder (such as von Willebrand disease), intranasal desmopressin may be indicated.
7. Androgen therapy with a gonadotropin-releasing hormone, such as leuprolide acetate, to reduce menstrual blood loss in perimenopausal women or to reduce the size of uterine fibroids before surgery.
8. Surgical procedures, such as hysteroscopic polypectomy or resection of uterine submucosal fibroids.
9. Hysteroscopic endometrial resection (removal of diseased or abnormal tissue) or endometrial ablation (application of heat to endometrium to induce scarring) when above methods are not helpful.
   a. By 5 years postablation, one third of patients require another surgery.
   b. The uterus is preserved, but it results in infertility.
10. Hysterectomy in refractory cases.

Complications

1. Recurrent anovulation in anovulatory AUB increases the risk of endometrial cancer because of the impact of unopposed estrogen on the endometrium. Women with regular ovulation and AUB have no greater risk of endometrial cancer because the endometrium regularly sloughs.
2. Severe anemia may result from menorrhagia or menometrorrhagia.

Nursing Assessment

1. Ask patient for menstrual and gynecologic history, sexual activity, and possibility of pregnancy.
2. Assess frequency, duration, and amount of menstrual flow.
3. Assess for other symptoms of underlying pathology, such as systemic hormonal conditions, pelvic pain, fever, and abdominal masses or tenderness.
4. Assess for signs and symptoms of anemia—fatigue, shortness of breath, pallor, and tachycardia.

Nursing Diagnoses

- Fatigue related to excessive blood loss.
- Fear of bleeding through clothing related to excessive or unpredictable bleeding.

Nursing Interventions

Increasing Energy Level
1. Administer medications, as ordered. Teach patient indications and side effects.
2. Encourage good dietary intake with increased sources of iron-fortified cereals and breads, meat (especially red meat), and green, leafy vegetables.

3. Administer oral iron preparations with meals to prevent nausea and with vitamin C–rich foods or drinks to enhance absorption. Treat constipation, as necessary.
4. Monitor hemoglobin and infuse packed red blood cells, as ordered.
5. Encourage activity, as tolerated.

Relieving Fear

1. Review pattern of menstrual flow with patient and help her plan for excessive bleeding.
2. Suggest wearing double tampons (if able) and double sanitary pads.
3. Tell the patient to expect heavy gush of blood on arising from lying or reclining position.
4. Prepare the patient to carry an adequate supply of sanitary products and a change of clothing until bleeding is under control.

Patient Education and Health Maintenance

1. Teach patient the causes of AUB and about the diagnostic process to rule out pathologic causes of abnormal bleeding.
2. Teach patient to prevent anemia by eating a diet high in iron and by consuming vitamin C or citrus fruit to enhance absorption of iron.
3. Teach about hormonal therapy, related adverse effects, and what adverse effects to expect and what to expect of bleeding. Bleeding should stop within first week of hormonal contraceptives but should start again in fourth week as regular menstrual period would with cyclical contraceptives.
4. Advise the patient to keep a calendar or log of menses.

Evaluation: Expected Outcomes

- Verbalizes adequate energy to perform activities.
- Verbalizes more confidence in ability to conceal bleeding.

Menopause

 EVIDENCE BASE National Collaborating Centre for Women's and Children's Health. (2015). Menopause: Diagnosis and Management. (NG23). London (UK): National Institute for Health and Care Excellence (NICE). Available: www.nice.org.uk/guidance/ng23?un lid=9768812920161027O835.

Menopause is described as the physiologic cessation of menses. Climacteric or perimenopause is the period during which there is decline in ovarian function and the woman experiences symptoms of estrogen deficiency and, possibly, irregular cycles. Menopause has occurred if menses has not occurred for 12 months.

Pathophysiology and Etiology

1. Menopause is caused by the cessation of ovarian function and decreased estrogen production by the ovary; average age range is 45 to 55, with the average age of 51.
2. Anovulation may occur during perimenopause, disrupting menstrual cycles.
3. Artificial or surgical menopause may occur secondary to surgery or radiation involving the ovaries. Some chemotherapeutic agents also cause a chemical menopause.
4. Hysterectomy without ovary removal may result in earlier menopause because of disruption of the blood supply to the ovaries.

Clinical Manifestations

1. Genitalia—atrophy of the vulva, vagina, and urethra results in dryness, bleeding, itching, burning, dysuria, thinning of pubic hair, loss of labia minora, and decreased secretions during intercourse.
2. Sexual function—vaginal dryness, discomfort, dyspareunia, and decreased intensity and duration of sexual response, but can still have active and satisfactory function.
3. Vasomotor—60% to 75% of women experience "hot flashes," which may be preceded by an anxious feeling and accompanied by sweating. These may occur at night, causing "night sweats."
   a. Psychological—insomnia, irritability, anxiety, memory loss, fear, and depression may be experienced.
   b. Some women experience palpitations.
   c. Symptoms, severity, and personal/cultural meanings vary with each individual.

Diagnostic Evaluation

1. Levels of LH and FSH will increase, and estradiol will decrease; however, levels may fluctuate often during perimenopause, so diagnosis is based on symptoms.
2. FSH greater than 30 to 40 IU/L indicates menopause; greater than 100 IU/L indicates complete ovarian failure.
3. Laboratory studies of FSH are not necessary to diagnose the perimenopausal phase or menopause itself.

Management

Menopausal Hormone Therapy/Estrogen Replacement Therapy

1. Indicated at the smallest possible dose for the shortest time period (less than 5 years) to reduce vasomotor symptoms (with the added benefit to prevent osteoporosis). Common systemic routes of administration include oral and transdermal.
2. Progesterone cotherapy preparations (oral, transdermal; or in combination products with estrogen) are required in a cyclical dosage pattern if the uterus is intact to prevent endometrial hyperplasia and possible cancer. Continuous progesterone therapy is no longer recommended because of association with adverse breast outcomes.
3. Vaginal preparations are most effective for atrophic vaginitis. Concomitant progesterone is not indicated with vaginal estrogen because of minimal systemic absorption of estrogen.
4. Available as synthetic, animal based, and natural (plant source) products.
5. Menopausal hormone therapy is contraindicated with the following conditions:
   a. Increased risk of thromboembolic disease, previous or current idiopathic deep vein thrombosis, or pulmonary embolism.
   b. Past, current, or suspected breast cancer.
   c. Estrogen-sensitive cancers (uterine, ovarian), untreated endometrial hyperplasia, and undiagnosed genital bleeding.
   d. Active or recent angina or myocardial infarction.
   e. Untreated hypertension.
   f. Active liver disease.
   g. Hypersensitivity to active substances in menopausal hormone therapy.
   h. Porphyria cutanea tarda (absolute contraindication).
6. Data are lacking to support progesterone or progestin alone for treatment of hot flashes.

Other Measures

1. Vaginal lubricants to decrease vaginal dryness and dyspareunia.
2. Calcium and vitamin D supplements to prevent bone loss.
3. Nonhormonal treatment of menopausal symptoms that may be considered includes SSRIs for depressive symptoms, clonidine (central alpha-blocker) or gabapentin for vasomotor symptoms. These therapies are supported by evidence.
4. Dietary supplements (considered natural products by consumers)—limited data are available on efficacy and safety. The patient should discuss potential benefits and risks with a health care provider.
   a. Soy products (isoflavones)—inconsistent relief of hot flashes. May cause headache and oily skin. Contraindicated as a phytoestrogen in women with strong personal or family history of hormone-dependent cancers (breast, uterine, ovarian), thromboembolic events, or cardiovascular events.
   b. Black cohosh—has demonstrated some relief of hot flashes, but has contraindications (as above) as a phytoestrogen. Nausea, hypotension, and spontaneous abortion are adverse effects. No safety studies were conducted beyond 6 months; thus, recommended use should not exceed 6 months.
   c. Vitamin E—400 IU daily has demonstrated minimal relief of hot flashes.

 DRUG ALERT Clinical trial data on the following commonly used herbal supplements have not demonstrated improved symptom relief over placebo: evening primrose, ginseng, dong quai, and red clover.

Complications

1. Osteoporosis has been clearly linked to estrogen depletion in menopause.
2. Coronary artery disease (CAD) rarely develops in women before menopause and may be associated with the effects of estrogen depletion on blood vessels.
3. Vaginal atrophy related to a dry, estrogen-depleted epithelium increases the risk for dyspareunia, recurrent vulvovaginitis, and urinary tract infections. More research is required related to the etiology and treatment of postmenopausal stress and urge urinary incontinence.
4. Psychosocial issues of menopause: risk of depression increases.

Nursing Assessment

1. Obtain history of the patient's current symptoms and menstrual cycle.
2. Obtain history for other risk factors for CAD, osteoporosis, stroke, depression, breast cancer, and uterine cancer.
3. Assess genitalia for atrophy, dryness, and elasticity.
4. Assess the patient's emotional response to menopause.

Nursing Diagnoses

- (Risk for) Sexual Dysfunction related to menopausal symptoms and psychological impact of menopause.
- Readiness for Enhanced Self-Health Management.

Nursing Interventions

Maintaining Sexuality Patterns

1. Explore with patient her feelings about menopause, clear up misconceptions about sexual functioning, and encourage her to discuss her feelings with her partner.
2. Tell the patient that sexual functioning may decrease during menopause but may even increase because of loss of fear of pregnancy and increased time if children are grown.
3. Instruct the patient how to use a water-based lubricant for intercourse to decrease dryness or discuss vaginal estrogen replacement therapy.

Increasing Self-Health Management

1. Provide patient with information related to estrogen replacement therapy, including dosage schedule, route, adverse effects, and what to expect of menstrual bleeding.
   a. Women who still have a uterus can expect a period at the end of every month if they take hormones cyclically. Progesterone cyclical cotherapy is indicated to prevent endometrial hyperplasia.
   b. Systemic preparations (oral, transdermal) are indicated for systemic symptoms, such as hot flashes and mood swings.
   c. Vaginal preparations are indicated for vaginal atrophy and may help to reduce recurrent UTIs.
2. Help patient to understand the risks versus benefits of menopausal hormone therapy, formulate questions, and initiate discussion with her health care provider about treatment options for vasomotor symptoms. Refer patient to clinical trial results from the Women's Health Initiative (*www.nhlbi.nih.gov/whi*).

Patient Education and Health Maintenance

1. Teach the patient about foods that are high in calcium and vitamin D—dairy products, dark green vegetables, salmon, and fortified foods. Encourage her to maintain weight-bearing activities several times weekly to prevent osteoporosis.
2. Counsel patient on reducing risk factors for CAD, including smoking cessation.
3. Encourage patient to keep regular medical and gynecologic follow-up visits, including all age-appropriate screenings, such as mammography, pelvic exam, dual-energy x-ray absorptiometry (DEXA) scan for osteoporosis, lipid panel, and colonoscopy.
4. Advise patient that vulvovaginal infection and trauma are possible because of the dryness of the tissue and to seek prompt evaluation if pain and discharge occur or increases.
5. Encourage patients to talk to their health care providers about concerns such as breast cancer with hormonal therapy. Also, refer the patient for information on postmenopausal hormone therapy to *https://www.nhlbi.nih.gov/files/docs/pht_facts.pdf.*
6. Encourage patients to report all use of supplements to their health care providers so they can use these preparations appropriately and safely.

 GERONTOLOGIC ALERT In the postmenopausal woman, if vaginal bleeding not associated with hormone replacement occurs, encourage the patient to see her health care provider immediately because cancer may be suspected.

Evaluation: Expected Outcomes

- Verbalizes confidence in sexual function and identity.
- Verbalizes satisfactory coping with menopausal symptoms and appropriate self-health management behaviors.

INFECTIONS AND INFLAMMATION OF THE VULVA, VAGINA, AND CERVIX

Some conditions are considered sexually transmitted, others are caused by inflammation or non–sexually transmitted infections. For syphilis, see page 632.

 EVIDENCE BASE Centers for Disease Control and Prevention. (2015). Sexually transmitted diseases treatment guidelines. Available: www.cdc.gov/std/treatment.

Vulvitis

Vulvitis is inflammation of the vulva.

Pathophysiology and Etiology

Causative Factors

1. Infections—*Trichomonas*, molluscum contagiosum, bacteria, fungi, herpes simplex virus (HSV), and human papillomavirus (HPV; genital warts). Also, see pages 658–661.
2. Irritants.
    a. Urine, feces, and vaginal discharge.
    b. Close-fitting, synthetic fabrics.
    c. Chemicals, such as laundry detergents, vaginal sprays, deodorants, perfumes, some soaps, chlorine, dryer sheets, and bubble bath.
3. Carcinoma.
4. Chronic dermatologic conditions, such as psoriasis or eczema.

Predisposing Factors

1. Illnesses, such as diabetes mellitus and dermatologic disorders.
2. Atrophy due to menopause.

Clinical Manifestations

1. Pruritus—more acute at night, aggravated by warmth, often associated with candidal infections.
2. Reddened, edematous tissue, possible ulceration.
3. Pain, burning, and dyspareunia.
4. Exudate—possibly profuse and purulent—involving vaginitis.
5. Lesions of molluscum contagiosum are multiple, from 1 mm to 1 cm in size, and filled with white caseous material.
6. Lesions of HSV are vesicles with an erythematous base, clustered in a somewhat linear pattern.
7. Lesions of HPV are flesh-colored, irregular, raised, soft warty-like growths.

Diagnostic Evaluation

1. Vulvar smears and cultures—may show infectious organism.
2. Biopsy of vulvar tissue—may be necessary to rule out malignancy and chronic dermatologic conditions.

Management

1. Oral or topical anti-infectives (antibiotics, antifungals, antivirals) to treat infectious agents.
2. Extremely low-dose topical steroids to treat inflammation in some cases.
3. Vaginal estrogen to treat vaginal atrophy associated with menopause.

4. Treatment of underlying disorder.
5. Molluscum contagiosum may be treated by scalpel excision, silver nitrate, electrical cautery, or curette or may be left untreated, allowing spontaneous resolution.

Complications

1. Scarring and chronic discomfort.
2. Transmission of STD to partner.

Nursing Assessment

1. Question the patient about medical history, symptoms, and sexual activity.
2. Determine use of chemical-containing products on undergarments or directly on the vulva.
3. Examine the genitalia and lymph nodes.

Nursing Diagnosis

- Acute Pain related to vulvar inflammation.

Nursing Interventions

Relieving Pain

1. Administer prescribed medications and instruct the patient on their use, method of application, and adverse effects.
2. Instruct use of sitz baths, sitting in or over warm water for 15 to 20 minutes, three to four times daily. May also use cool compresses to soothe and clean vulva.
3. Instruct the patient about the nature of the condition (eg, chronic recurrent or curable) and expectations for symptoms after treatment.

Patient Education and Health Maintenance

1. Teach the patient hygienic principles.
    a. Wipe from front to back after voiding.
    b. Use cotton with warm water and bland soap for cleansing, rinse, and pat dry. May also use fragrance-free hypoallergenic wet wipes.
2. Teach the patient to avoid chemical irritants, such as sprays, perfumed and deodorant soaps, new laundry detergents, static-control dryer sheets, and bubble bath.
3. Teach the patient to avoid mechanical irritants, such as tight clothing, synthetic fabrics, and undergarments; replace these with loose-fitting cotton undergarments. Avoid chronic moisture; change bathing suit after swimming.
4. Teach the patient how to use sitz bath and cool compresses at home and to avoid scratching.
5. Teach the patient that some infections, such as *Trichomonas*, molluscum contagiosum, and HSV, are sexually transmitted; so the partner needs to seek treatment before intercourse is resumed. Assist the patient with health communication techniques to inform partner.
6. Educate about STD prevention and encourage screening (see Box 22-1).

Evaluation: Expected Outcomes

- Verbalizes increased comfort level and control of symptoms.

Bartholin Cyst or Abscess

Bartholin cyst or *abscess*, also called *bartholinitis*, is an infection of the greater vestibular gland, causing cyst or abscess formation.

Sexually Transmitted Disease Prevention Counseling

Sexually transmitted diseases can be prevented through interactive, client-centered counseling approaches that address personal risk. Key techniques to facilitate rapport include use of open-ended questions and understandable language. Most effective strategies are performed in nonjudgmental and empathetic ways, incorporating the patient's culture, language, gender, sexual orientation, age, and developmental level. Motivational interviewing techniques and assessing for readiness to change are also helpful.

The first step in counseling is taking a sexual history, including:

- Type and number of partners.
- Methods for prevention of pregnancy.
- Methods for prevention of STDs.
- Past history of STDs.
- Exposure to intravenous drug use or sex workers.

An individualized prevention plan may incorporate one or more of the following specific methods of prevention:

- Abstinence from oral, vaginal, and anal sex. Encourage abstinence until beginning a mutually monogamous lifetime relationship.
- Monogamy: to be in a long-term, mutually monogamous relationship with an uninfected person. Before starting a mutually monogamous sexual relationship, individuals may consider screening for STDs.
- Reduce the number of lifetime sexual partners.

- Pre-exposure vaccination:
  - HPV vaccine (ages 9 to 26).
  - Hepatitis B vaccine (plus hepatitis A vaccine for men who have sex with men and IV drug users).
- Proper use of male condoms (latex or polyurethane; not "natural" or "lambskin" condoms, which do not protect against viral transmission) with correct use:
  - A new condom with each new sex act.
  - Carefully handle the condom so as not to puncture it.
  - Put condom on after penis is erect.
  - Ensure adequate lubrication.
  - Use only water-based lubricants; oil-based lubricants (petroleum jelly, massage oil, cooking oils) will weaken condom.
  - Hold condom firmly at base during withdrawal to avoid slipping off.
  - Condoms with spermicidal lubricants are not recommended to prevent STDs.
- Proper use of female condoms (lubricated polyurethane or nitrile sheath with a ring on each end, ie, inserted into the vagina): Use as a protective barrier before intimate contact.
- Adolescents and women who use nonbarrier methods of contraception (hormones, IUDs, surgery) should be counseled about barrier methods to prevent STDs because they may incorrectly perceive that they are not at risk for STDs.
- Spermicides do not prevent STD/HIV transmission; they may increase it by disrupting normal epithelium.

 EVIDENCE BASE Centers for Disease Control and Prevention. (2015). Sexually transmitted diseases (STDs). Atlanta, GA: Author. Available: *www.cdc.gov/std/treatment.*

Pathophysiology and Etiology

1. These glands lie on both sides of the vagina at the base of the labia minora; they lubricate the vagina.
2. If they become obstructed secondary to infection, abscess or cyst formation may occur (see Figure 22-2).
3. Abscess or cyst may spontaneously rupture or enlarge and become painful.
4. Most are sterile or abscess/cellulitis caused by mixed vaginal flora.
5. May also be caused by sexual transmission of infection (gonorrhea or chlamydia).

Figure 22-2. Site and infection of vestibular gland.

Clinical Manifestations

1. Asymptomatic cyst.
2. Pain, erythema, tenderness, swelling.
3. Edema, cellulitis, possible abscess formation.

Diagnostic Evaluation

1. Culture, if draining or upon excision, to identify infectious organisms.
2. If older than age 40, or recurrent, carcinoma must be ruled out by biopsy.

Management

1. May be treated conservatively with warm soaks or sitz baths if small or asymptomatic; antibiotics used if cellulitis is present.
2. May need incision and drainage; provides immediate relief, but may recur. Procedures are generally done under local anesthesia and take about 20 minutes in an outpatient office.
   a. Contents are opened and drained; culture sent. Then, sutures are closed.
      i. As an alternative, a Word catheter, Foley catheter, or Jacobi ring is inserted to keep cavity open (called fistulization).
      ii. Healing occurs around catheter and it is removed 2 to 4 weeks later to provide a new opening to the gland.
3. Marsupialization, for recurrent abscesses.
   a. Cyst is incised and sutured open to incision edges.
   b. Healing occurs from within the area of the abscess.

4. Other acceptable methods of treatment include silver nitrate gland ablation, cyst or abscess ablation or excision with a carbon dioxide laser, and needle aspiration with or without alcohol sclerotherapy.

5. Complete excision under general anesthesia if carcinoma is suspected.

6. All treatment methods heal within 2 weeks or less. Recurrence may occur in up to 20% of patients with all treatment methods. No method has been demonstrated to be superior in healing rate or recurrence rate.

Complications

Scarring from recurrent infection and rupture.

Nursing Assessment

1. Obtain history of sexual activity, including new partners and history of STDs. Risk for Bartholin gland cyst or abscess is similar to risk for STDs.
2. Inspect the labia minora for warmth, erythema, and swelling.
3. Assess for signs of other STDs—rash, genital ulcers, and vaginal discharge.

Nursing Diagnoses

• Acute Pain related to infection and enlargement of gland.

Nursing Interventions

Relieving Pain

1. Administer pain medications and antibiotics, as ordered; explain adverse effects to patient.
2. Instruct patient to apply warm soaks or to use sitz bath three to four times per day for 15 to 20 minutes to promote comfort and drainage.
3. Encourage patient to limit activity as much as possible because pain is exacerbated by activity.
4. Prepare patient for incision and drainage, if indicated. Gather supplies for procedure; assist during procedure, as necessary.
5. For marsupialization: apply ice packs intermittently for 24 hours to reduce edema and provide comfort; thereafter, warm sitz baths, a perineal heat pack, or a lamp provides comfort.

Patient Education and Health Maintenance

1. If STD is the suspected cause of infection, advise patient to instruct her partner to be tested and treated prophylactically.
2. Advise patient to abstain from intercourse until cyst or abscess has resolved, partner has been examined and treated, and patient has completed all her antibiotics (approximately 2 weeks).
3. Review principles of perineal hygiene with patient.
4. Discuss STDs and methods of prevention—abstinence, monogamy, and proper use of female or male condoms. See page 653.
5. Encourage patient to follow-up for recurrent abscess to rule out malignant lesions. Surgical treatment is commonly necessary for recurrences.

Evaluation: Expected Outcomes

• Verbalizes relief of pain.

Vaginal Fistula

A *vaginal fistula* is an abnormal, tortuous opening between the vagina and another hollow organ (see Figure 22-3).

Figure 22-3. Sites of vaginal fistulas. (Smeltzer, S., & Bare, B. [2007]. *Brunner and Suddarth's textbook of medical-surgical nursing* [9th ed.]. Philadelphia, PA: Lippincott Williams & Wilkins.)

Pathophysiology and Etiology

Causes

1. Obstetric injury, especially in long labors and in countries with inadequate obstetric care (rarely occurs in developed nations).
2. Pelvic surgery (rare)—hysterectomy or vaginal reconstructive procedures.
3. Carcinoma (rare)—extensive disease or complication of treatment such as radiation therapy.

Types

1. *Vesicovaginal* fistula is an opening between the bladder and vagina.
2. *Rectovaginal* fistula is an opening between the rectum and vagina.
3. *Ureterovaginal* fistula is an opening between the ureter and vagina.
4. *Urethrovaginal* fistula is an opening between the urethra and vagina.
5. *Vaginoperineal* fistula is an opening between the vagina and perineum.

Clinical Manifestations

1. Vesicovaginal—the most common type of fistula.
   a. Constant trickling of urine into the vagina.
   b. Loss of urge to void because the bladder is continuously emptying.
   c. May cause excoriation and inflammation of the vulva.
2. Rectovaginal.
   a. Fecal incontinence and flatus through the vagina; malodorous.
   b. May present as vulvar cancer.
3. Ureterovaginal fistula—rare.
   a. Urine in the vagina but the patient still voids regularly.
   b. May cause severe UTIs.
4. Urethrovaginal fistula.
   a. Dysuria.
   b. Urine in the vagina on voiding.
5. Vaginoperineal fistula—pain and inflammation of the perineum.

Diagnostic Evaluation

1. Methylene blue test—after instillation of this dye in the bladder via catheter, place tampon in the vagina. Remove after the woman has ambulated.
   a. Methylene blue appears in the vagina in vesicovaginal fistula.
   b. Methylene blue does not appear in the vagina in uterovaginal fistula.
2. Indigo–carmine test—after a methylene blue test shows negative results, indigo carmine is injected intravenously (IV). If dye appears in the vagina, this indicates ureterovaginal fistula.
3. Cystoscopy with retrograde pyelography.
4. Intravenous pyelography (IVP)—helps to detect ureteral fistulas.

Management

1. Fistulas recognized at the time of delivery should be corrected immediately.
2. Historically, surgeries were delayed for 8 to 12 weeks to allow recovery from infection or inflammation. However, early excision and repair within 1 to 2 weeks of urine leakage have become common.
3. Surgical closure of opening via vaginal route is most common in developing nations. In developed nations, laparoscopic, vaginal, or abdominal or robot-assisted routes may be used.
4. Fecal or urinary diversion procedure may be required for large fistulas.
5. Rarely, a fistula may heal without surgical intervention.
6. Medical approach.
   a. Prosthesis to prevent incontinence and allow tissue to heal; done for patients who are not surgical candidates.
   b. Prosthesis is inserted into the vagina; it is connected to drainage tubing leading to a leg bag.

Complications

1. Hydronephrosis, pyelonephritis, and possible renal failure with ureterovaginal fistula.
2. Risk for vaginal infection and pelvic organ infection from rectovaginal fistula.

Nursing Assessment

1. Obtain obstetric, gynecologic, and surgical history.
2. Monitor intake and output and voiding pattern.
3. Assess drainage on perineal pads.
4. Watch for signs of infection (fever, chills, flank pain).

Nursing Diagnoses

- Risk for Infection related to contamination of urinary tract by vaginal flora or contamination of the vagina by rectal organisms.
- Impaired Urinary Elimination related to fistula.

Nursing Interventions

Preventing Infection

1. Encourage frequent sitz baths.
2. Perform vaginal irrigation, as ordered, and teach patient the procedure.
3. Before repair surgery, administer prescribed antibiotics to reduce pathogenic flora in the intestinal tract. A single injectable dose of gentamicin before surgery is as effective as extended use of amoxicillin, chloramphenicol, or cotrimoxazole.
4. After rectovaginal repair:

   a. Maintain patient on clear liquids, as prescribed, to limit bowel activity for several days.
   b. Encourage rest.
   c. Administer warm perineal irrigations to decrease healing time and increase comfort.

Maintaining Urinary Drainage

1. Suggest the use of perineal pads or incontinence products preoperatively.
2. After vesicovaginal repair:
   a. Maintain proper drainage from indwelling catheter (intermittent flushing with sterile normal saline) to prevent pressure on newly sutured tissue (usually for about 7 days postoperatively).
   b. Administer vaginal or bladder irrigations gently because of tenderness at operative site.
   c. Maintain strict intake and output records. IV fluids or copious oral fluid intake may be recommended to maintain good bladder flow.
   d. Prophylactic antibiotics to prevent infection may be recommended.
3. If medical management is indicated, teach patient the use of prosthetic device.
4. Encourage patient to express feelings about her altered route of elimination and share them with a significant other.

Patient Education and Health Maintenance

1. Teach patient to report signs of infection early.
2. Teach the patient to clean the perineum gently and to follow surgeon's instructions on when to resume sexual intercourse and strenuous activity.
3. Advise patient to keep regular follow-up appointments.

Evaluation: Expected Outcomes

- No signs of infection—afebrile and no complaints of flank pain or difficulty voiding.
- Clear urine flows from catheter postoperatively; voids without difficulty after catheter removal.

Vaginitis

Vaginitis is inflammation of the vagina caused by infectious pathogens.

Pathophysiology and Etiology

1. May be caused by sexually transmitted organisms or overgrowth of vaginal flora.
2. Normal vaginal secretions because of estrogen secretion and acidity inhibit the growth of pathogens.
3. Such conditions as diabetes, pregnancy, stress, coitus, and menopause alter normal vaginal environment.
4. Types of vaginitis (see Table 22-3).
   a. Simple (contact).
   b. Bacterial vaginosis (most often caused by *Gardnerella*).
   c. *Trichomonas*.
   d. *Candida albicans*.
   e. Atrophic.

Clinical Manifestations

Signs and symptoms vary with etiology or causative organism.
1. Vaginal itching, irritation, burning.
2. Odor and increased or unusual vaginal discharge.

Table 22-3 Types of Vaginitis

DESCRIPTION	MANIFESTATIONS	MANAGEMENT
Simple Vaginitis (Contact Vaginitis)		
• An inflammation of the vagina, with discharge; due to mechanical, chemical, allergic, or other noninfectious irritation, poor hygiene, imbalance in vaginal flora. • Urethritis commonly accompanies vaginitis because of the proximity of the urethra to the vagina. • Predisposing factors: contact allergens, excessive perspiration, synthetic underclothing, poor hygiene, foreign bodies (tampons, condoms, spermicides, condoms with spermicides, diaphragms that have been left in too long).	• Increased (yet minimal) vaginal discharge with itching, redness, burning, and edema. • Voiding and defecation aggravate the above symptoms.	• Stimulate the growth of lactobacilli (Doderlein bacilli) through consumption of yogurt with live active cultures. • Current evidence does not support douching. • Foster cleanliness by meticulous care after voiding and defecation. • Discontinue use of causative agent.
Bacterial Vaginosis		
• An inflammation of the vagina commonly referred to as nonspecific vaginitis because it is *not* caused by *Trichomonas*, *Candida*, or gonorrhea. It is not considered an STD. • Increased levels of *Gardnerella vaginalis* are usually responsible for symptoms.	• Vaginal discharge with odor. • Itching and burning may suggest concomitant organisms present. • It is benign in that when the discharge is wiped away, underlying tissue is healthy and pink. • Vaginal pH is >4.5. • May be asymptomatic. • Presence of "clue" cells on microscopic examination of saline slide • Positive KOH "whiff" test (fishy odor).	• Treatment only recommended for symptomatic women. • Metronidazole taken orally for 7 days or topical clindamycin or metronidazole. • Alcohol intake should be avoided during metronidazole treatment and for 24 hr after completion to avoid nausea and vertigo. Studies have demonstrated that metronidazole is not teratogenic. • Treating partners is not recommended. • Clindamycin cream weakens latex condoms. • Data do not support douching.
Trichomonas vaginalis		
• STD. A condition produced by a protozoan (pear-shaped and motile) that thrives in an alkaline environment. Recurrence may occur because of low levels of antimicrobial resistance.	• Copious malodorous discharge; may be frothy and yellow-green in color. • May have pruritus, dyspareunia, and spotting. • Red, speckled (strawberry) punctate hemorrhages on the cervix. • May also have vulvar edema, dysuria, and hyperemia secondary to irritation of discharge. • Motile organisms visible on saline microscopy. • Point of care rapid test and cultures are available.	• Destroy infective protozoa by taking oral metronidazole 2 g or tinidazole 2 g. • *Note:* Treatment during pregnancy is acceptable after the first trimester for tinidazole and throughout pregnancy for metronidazole. • Prevent reinfection by treating partner concurrently, even though male may be asymptomatic. • Avoid alcohol during treatment. • Rescreen after 3 months because of possibility of low-level antimicrobial resistance.
Candida albicans		

• A fungal infection caused by *Candida albicans*. Associated factors include:
  • Steroid therapy
  • Obesity
  • Pregnancy
  • Antibiotic therapy
  • Diabetes mellitus
  • Oral contraceptives
  • Frequent douching
  • Chronic debilitative diseases
• Characteristics
  • *C. albicans* is a normal inhabitant of the intestinal tract and therefore a frequent contaminant of the vagina.
  • Because this fungus thrives in an environment rich in carbohydrates, it is seen commonly in patients with poorly controlled diabetes.
  • This infection is observed in patients who have been on antibiotic or steroid therapy for a while (reduces natural protective organisms in the vagina).
	• Vaginal discharge is thick and irritating; white or yellow patchy, cheese-like particles adhere to vaginal walls.
	• Itching is the most common complaint.
	• May also experience burning, soreness, vulvar edema, excoriations, fissures, dyspareunia, frequency, and dysuria.
	• Microscopic examination will reveal hyphae, buds, and pseudohyphae.
	• Vaginal pH is normal (<4.5).
		• Eradicate the fungus by applying antifungal vaginal cream (clotrimazole, miconazole, or ketoconazole), suppository, or tablet for 1 to 14 nights, as ordered; or, take oral fluconazole in single dose.
		• Oral fluconazole is contraindicated in pregnancy; topical creams may be used.
		• Side effects of topical vaginal creams include burning and irritation. Systemic fluconazole is associated with GI intolerance, headaches, and rare and transitory elevations in liver function tests.
		• Azole antifungals have clinically important interactions with many medications.
		• Incorporate live culture yogurt into diet to enhance lactobacillus colonization and improve microorganism balance in the vagina.
		• Treat the symptomatic or uncircumcised partner with balanitis by applying antifungal cream under the foreskin nightly for 7 nights.
		• For severe or recurrent cases, use systemic antifungal, such as weekly fluconazole for suppression therapy.

Table 22-3 Types of Vaginitis (*Continued*)

DESCRIPTION	MANIFESTATIONS	MANAGEMENT
Atrophic Vaginitis		
• A common postmenopausal occurrence due to atrophy of the vaginal mucosa secondary to decreased estrogen levels; more susceptible to infection.	• Vaginal itching, dryness, burning, dyspareunia, and vulvar irritation. • May also have vaginal bleeding. • Vaginal mucosa appears dry and slightly paler. **NURSING ALERT** In the postmenopausal woman, if vaginal bleeding occurs, encourage patient to see her health care provider immediately because bleeding is a warning sign of cancer.	• Vaginal estrogen treatment is most effective. • The condition reverses itself under treatment, which must be maintained. • If infection is also present, this is treated. • If the uterus is intact and systemic estrogen therapy is used to treat additional menopausal symptoms, progesterone must be added to prevent endometrial hyperplasia due to unopposed estrogen.

STD, sexually transmitted disease.

3. Dyspareunia, pelvic pain, dysuria.
4. Asymptomatic.

Diagnostic Evaluation

1. History and physical examination.
2. Wet smear for microscopic examination.
   a. Saline slide: discharge mixed with saline; useful in detecting *Gardnerella* and *Trichomonas* organisms.
   b. Potassium hydroxide (KOH): useful in detecting *C. albicans*. Whiff test: if fishy odor is noted when KOH is applied, suspect *Gardnerella* organisms causing bacterial vaginosis.
3. Vaginal pH (not diagnostic, but may indicate infection)—use Nitrazine paper.
   a. Normal pH: 4.0 to 4.5.
   b. Bacterial vaginosis: greater than 4.5.
   c. *Trichomonas*: greater than 4.5.
4. Chlamydia and gonorrhea cultures or DNA probe—to rule out chlamydia or gonorrhea cervicitis.
5. Pap smear—not considered a diagnostic tool for vaginitis: it has low sensitivity and specificity to detect bacterial vaginosis and *Trichomonas*.

Management

1. Anti-infectives (oral or vaginal preparations).
2. Estrogen replacement (systemic or vaginal preparation) for atrophic vaginitis.
3. Evaluation and treatment of sexual partners for STDs, such as *Trichomonas*.
4. Vaginal recolonization with lactobacilli through ingestion of yogurt with active cultures.

Nursing Assessment

1. Obtain a health history including questions specific to the condition.
   a. Nature of discharge: cheeselike, frothy, puslike, thick or thin, or scant? Onset? Color? Odor? Other symptoms: dysuria, itching, and dyspareunia?
   b. Menstrual history.
   c. Disease history: diabetes mellitus and its control? Previous vaginal infections? STDs?
   d. Obstetric history.
   e. Sexual history: age of onset of sexual activity? New partner? Numbers of current and lifetime partners? Frequency of sexual activity? Its nature? Urogenital symptoms or infections in partner? Current barrier use?
   f. Medications and allergies. Current contraceptive use?
   g. Vaginal hygiene: use of douches, deodorants, sprays, and ointments; types of tampons, bubble bath, shower/bath soap, and nature of clothing (tight-fitting)?
2. Perform a physical examination, including a vaginal examination, and obtain vaginal and/or cervical discharge specimens, as indicated.

Nursing Diagnoses

• Acute or Chronic Pain related to vaginal irritation.
• Impaired Tissue Integrity related to vaginal infection.
• Risk-Prone Health Behavior related to sexual activity and transmission of infection.

Nursing Interventions

Relieving Pain

1. Instruct patient to discontinue use of irritating agents, such as bubble baths and vaginal douches.
2. Suggest that the patient take cool baths or sitz baths and pat dry or dry with hair dryer on low setting.
3. Encourage the patient to wear loose cotton undergarments.
4. Encourage the patient to take analgesics.
5. Provide emotional support.

Restoring Tissue Integrity

1. Teach the patient to clean the perineum and pat dry before applying medication.
2. Demonstrate application of prescribed medication.
3. Emphasize importance of taking prescribed medication for full length of therapy and as directed; teach patient adverse effects.
4. Stress importance of follow-up visits.

Reducing Risk

1. Emphasize importance of sexual abstinence and vaginal rest (nothing in the vagina) until therapy is complete and sexual partner has been treated, if indicated.
2. Tell patient use of condoms may be protective but may produce irritation.

3. Instruct the patient in the use of water-soluble lubricant if the vagina is dry and atrophic.
4. Instruct the patient that some oil-based vaginal medications may decrease the efficacy of condoms to protect against STDs and pregnancy.

Patient Education and Health Maintenance

1. Teach causes of vaginitis and its symptoms so patient can seek treatment promptly.
2. Discuss STDs and methods of prevention—abstinence, monogamy, and proper use of female or male condoms. See page 653.
3. Teach measures to prevent vaginitis.
   a. Wipe from front to back after toilet use.
   b. Keep area clean and dry.
   c. Wear loose cotton clothing to absorb moisture and provide good circulation.
   d. Change sanitary pads and tampons frequently so they do not become saturated.
   e. Avoid bubble baths, vaginal deodorants, sprays, and douches.
   f. If the patient insists on using douches (not recommended), use a mild vinegar solution (2 teaspoons white vinegar to 1 quart water) at the end of a menstrual cycle. Teach proper technique: to infuse gently to lightly bathe tissues and to avoid using a forceful stream that could push bacteria higher inside the pelvis.
4. For recurrent *Candida* infections, encourage good control if the patient has diabetes or encourage the patient to be tested for diabetes. Teach all patients to eliminate concentrated carbohydrates from diet to prevent recurrence.

Evaluation: Expected Outcomes

- Verbalizes relief of pain.
- Vaginal mucosa pink, with normal amount and color of secretions.
- Reports practice of prevention methods.

Human Papillomavirus Infection

EVIDENCE BASE Centers for Disease Control and Prevention. (2015). *Sexually transmitted diseases treatment guidelines*. Available: *www.cdc.gov/std/treatment.*

Human papillomavirus (HPV) infection may be asymptomatic but frequently causes *condyloma acuminatum* or genital warts.

Pathophysiology and Etiology

1. Sexually transmitted; highly contagious.
2. More than 40 types of HPV can infect the genital tract, many are asymptomatic, and multiple types may coexist.
3. Ninety percent of visible genital warts are caused by HPV types 6 and 11. Up to 70% of cervical cancer and precancerous lesions are caused by types 16 and 18. Types 31, 33, 45, 52, 58, and others have been strongly associated with cervical dysplasia.
4. Incubation period of up to 8 months.

Clinical Manifestations

1. Single or multiple soft, fleshy painless growths of the vulva, vagina, cervix, urethra, or anal area that may be irritating or uncomfortable (see Figure 22-4).
2. May be subclinical infection and still contagious.
3. Occasional vaginal bleeding, discharge, odor, and dyspareunia.

Figure 22-4. Genital lesions. **(A)** Condyloma acuminatum. **(B)** Genital herpes.

Diagnostic Evaluation

1. Pap smear—shows characteristic cellular changes (koilocytosis).
2. Acetic acid swabbing on vaginal examination will whiten lesions and make them more identifiable in genital mucosa. However, this test is not specific to HPV and is not recommended for screening.
3. Viral DNA tests to detect subclinical cases; however, the significance of positive and negative results has not been determined. HPV testing can be done from a liquid Pap smear cervical cancer screening for women older than 30 years, if the Pap smear is abnormal (known as reflex testing), to confirm the presence of HPV causing cellular changes on the cervix. HPV testing is not recommended for genital wart diagnosis.
4. Colposcopy is also used to diagnose subclinical HPV infection.
5. Anoscopy or urethroscopy may be necessary to identify anal and urethral lesions.
6. Genital warts are usually diagnosed on physical exam through visual inspection.

Management

Therapies are likely to reduce HPV infectivity but do not eradicate HPV. Treatment method is guided by provider and patient preferences.

1. External lesions may be treated by the patient with multiple applications of a topical preparation.
   a. Podofilox—applied with cotton swab or finger to visible warts twice per day for 3 days and then no treatment for 4 days; may be repeated for up to four cycles of therapy.
   b. Imiquimod—applied by finger three times per week for up to 16 weeks; may be washed off 6 to 10 hours after application.
   c. Sinecatechins ointment—applied by finger three times daily for up to 16 weeks; not washed off after use.
   d. Safety of these products during pregnancy is unknown and therefore is not recommended.
2. Noncervical lesions may be treated by health care provider with topical preparations, such as podophyllin resin, trichloroacetic acid, or bichloroacetic acid.
   a. Requires multiple visits for repeat treatments.
   b. May require washing off several hours later.
3. Cryotherapy with liquid nitrogen or cryoprobe, electrocautery, laser treatment, or local excision of large warts or cervical lesions.

4. Highly recurrent, particularly in first 3 months—may require retreatment.
5. Subclinical genital HPV infection typically clears spontaneously and treatment is not recommended.
6. Three vaccines for HPV are available in the United States.
   a. Bivalent human papillomavirus vaccine types 16 and 18; recombinant.
   b. Quadrivalent vaccine human papillomavirus vaccine types 6, 11, 16, and 18; recombinant.
   c. 9-valent vaccine types 6, 11, 16, 18, 31, 33, 45, 52, and 58.
7. Vaccine schedule: ACIP recommends anyone starting the series before age 15 receives two doses of vaccine at least 6 months apart. If the two doses are received less than 5 months apart, a third dose of vaccine is recommended.
   a. The Centers for Disease Control and Prevention (CDC) recommends all vaccines for females aged 11 or 12 to 26 (licensed for ages 9 to 26).
   b. The quadrivalent vaccine is recommended for males aged 11 or 12 to 26 (licensed for ages 9 to 26).
   c. They are most effective when all doses are administered before the onset of sexual activity.

Complications

1. Implicated in cervical intraepithelial neoplasia.
2. May cause neonatal laryngeal papillomatosis if infant born through infected birth canal.
3. Obstruction of anal canal and vagina by enlarging lesions.
4. Scarring and pigment changes if treatment not employed properly.

Nursing Assessment

1. Obtain history of STDs, Pap test results, and sexual partners.
2. Inspect external genitalia for lesions; assist with vaginal examination.

Nursing Diagnosis

• Disturbed Body Image related to genital warts.

Nursing Interventions

Improving Body Image

1. Explain to the patient that the goal of therapy is to remove visible lesions; however, HPV will not be cured or eliminated. Genital warts are not life-threatening.
2. Encourage the patient to comply with treatment schedule and inspect areas for resolution of lesions or redevelopment of new lesions.
3. Advise the patient of high recurrence rate; 3-month follow-up visit is advisable; if lesions redevelop, the patient should follow up for retreatment.
4. Advise patient about proper use of male or female condoms to reduce the risk of transmission, although not fully because HPV can infect areas not covered by the condom. Condom use, abstinence, and monogamy will protect against other STDs.
5. Encourage female patients to follow up regularly for Pap tests because HPV has been associated with cervical neoplasia.
6. Advise patient of risk to neonate during delivery; patient should receive close prenatal care if pregnant.

Patient Education and Health Maintenance

1. Advise patient to discuss HPV with her partner. He should receive treatment for visible lesions. Screening for other STDs in both patient and partner is recommended.

2. Make sure patient realizes that even though lesions may be gone, she may still transmit HPV to new sexual partners. Abstinence, monogamy, and condoms are advisable to prevent transmission of all STDs. See page 653.

Evaluation: Expected Outcomes

• Presents with no visible lesions at follow-up visit.

Herpes Genitalis

 EVIDENCE BASE Centers for Disease Control and Prevention. (2015). Sexually transmitted diseases treatment guidelines. Available: *www.cdc.gov/std/treatment.*

Herpes genitalis is a viral infection that causes lesions of the cervix, vagina, and external genitalia.

Pathophysiology and Etiology

1. Caused by HSV, usually type 2, but may be type 1.
2. Sexually transmitted.
3. An estimated 50 million people are infected in the United States.
4. Recurrent infection; virus lies dormant in dorsal root ganglia of spinal nerves between outbreaks.

Clinical Manifestations

1. Lesions occur 2 to 30 days after initial exposure, sometimes with fever, malaise, lymphadenopathy, and headache for primary infection (see Figure 22-4, page 658).
2. Lesions are preceded by sensation of tingling; proceed from vesicles on erythematous, edematous base to painful ulcers that crust and heal without scars.
3. Internal lesions may cause watery discharge and dyspareunia.
4. Recurrent lesions may be stimulated by fever, stress, illness, local trauma, menses, and sunburn.
5. Infection can be asymptomatic.

Diagnostic Evaluation

1. PCR assay for HSV DNA and viral culture are preferred tests. Failure to detect HSV by PCR or culture does not rule out HSV infection because viral shedding is intermittent.
2. Pap smear and Tzanck smear are neither sensitive nor specific for HSV and therefore not recommended.
3. Type-specific glycoprotein G (gG) serological tests—to detect HSV-1 or HSV-2 antibodies in the following cases: recurrent or atypical genital symptoms with negative viral culture, clinical diagnosis of genital herpes without laboratory confirmation, partner with genital herpes, persons presenting for STD evaluation, and persons with HIV.
4. Screening in the general population for HSV1 and HSV2 is not recommended.

Management

1. Systemic antivirals, such as acyclovir, famciclovir, and valacyclovir, suppress virus and decrease length, severity, and shedding of infection.
   a. Oral therapy may be episodic—started as soon as the first episode is diagnosed and whenever the first signs of a recurrence are recognized (within 24 hours of onset of prodromal symptoms or lesion onset).

b. Oral therapy may be given continuously to suppress recurrences and viral shedding, which reduces transmission, especially within the first 12 months of disease onset.

c. IV administration (acyclovir) may be necessary for severe infections (disseminated infections, pneumonitis, hepatitis, meningoencephalitis) or for immunocompromised patients.

d. Topical treatment (acyclovir) is the least effective and not recommended.

2. Pain medication—ranges from acetaminophen and NSAID drugs to oral opioids.

3. Local comfort measures, such as lidocaine gel, sitz baths, compresses, and use of a hair dryer to area on cool setting.

4. Immunization has been under investigation. See *www.clinicaltrials.gov*.

Complications

1. Disseminated infection, meningitis, pneumonitis, and hepatitis.

2. Neonatal infection if neonate born through infected canal.

Nursing Assessment

1. Question the patient about frequency and type of sexual activity and discomfort noted.

2. Question the patient about pruritus, burning, tenderness, urinary symptoms, and unusual discharge.

3. Assess the patient's view of herpes, transmission, stigmas, misconceptions, and fears.

4. Inspect genitalia for lesions, erythema, and edema. Use a speculum to examine the vagina and cervix, as indicated.

Nursing Diagnoses

- Acute Pain related to HSV outbreak.
- Impaired Skin Integrity related to herpetic lesions.
- Anxiety related to stigma attached to herpes.
- Sexual Dysfunction related to potential transmission of herpes.

Nursing Interventions

Relieving Pain

1. Demonstrate and encourage the use of warm sitz baths to increase blood supply to the areas and facilitate healing.

2. Instruct patient to keep the area clean and dry. Pat dry with a clean towel or use blow dryer on cool setting. Wear loose cotton undergarments and loose clothing.

3. Encourage bed rest if case is severe.

4. Administer pain medications, as prescribed.

5. Encourage the patient to void in a warm sitz bath if urination is painful.

6. Insert indwelling catheter if urination is extremely painful or if retention occurs.

7. Encourage fluid intake.

Restoring Skin Integrity

1. Administer an antiviral agent and teach the patient proper use and adverse effects.

2. Keep lesions clean and dry.

3. Teach the patient not to rub or to scratch lesions.

Relieving Anxiety

1. Explore with the patient her feelings about herpes and its effects on relationships.

2. Reiterate that when the patient is feeling better physically, her feelings about herself will improve.

3. Encourage the patient to discuss antiviral suppressive therapy to reduce the risk of transmission and to reduce frequency and duration of recurrent outbreaks.

4. Discuss effects of stress on future outbreaks. Assist the patient to identify stressors in her life and how to cope with them. Review stress-reduction methods, such as relaxation, breathing, and imagery.

5. Encourage the patient to discuss her feelings with family and significant others.

Restoring Satisfying Sexual Function

1. Teach the patient to avoid intercourse from first sign of active outbreak (often a tingling sensation) to resolution of lesions (at least 2 weeks after primary infection, approximately 1 week after recurrent outbreaks).

2. Teach the patient that shedding of virus through genital secretions is possible even during asymptomatic period, so the partner must be notified.

3. Inform the patient that she and her partner should use condoms for intercourse, but condoms may not be fully protective. Encourage the patient to discuss suppressive antiviral therapy with her health care provider.

4. Explore possibility of noncoital aspects of sexual relationship.

5. Teach patient that virus may be spread through the genital–oral route.

Patient Education and Health Maintenance

1. Inform the patient that initial outbreak is usually more painful than recurrent outbreaks and that outbreaks vary from monthly to only a few times per year.

2. Teach the patient to recognize precipitating factors and change lifestyle to prevent potential triggers, if possible.

3. Remind the patient of the effects on a neonate and the importance of notifying her health care provider if she becomes pregnant.

4. Instruct the patient in methods to decrease risk of sexual transmission: abstinence, monogamy, male or female condom use, and antiviral suppressive therapy. See patient page 653. The patient must inform partner of the risk of transmission to a potential sexual partner before any intimate contact. Viral shedding is highest during the prodromal and active lesion stages.

5. Tell the patient that oral lesions can occur with HSV2 because of transmission by oral intercourse, but that most oral cold sores are caused by HSV-1 infection.

6. Refer the patient to support groups, such as the American Social Health Association (*www.ashastd.org* or 800-227-8922).

Evaluation: Expected Outcomes

- Verbalizes decreased pain.
- Skin intact, without signs of secondary infection and scarring.
- Verbalizes reduced anxiety and more confidence.
- Reports satisfying sexual activity.

Chlamydial Infection

 EVIDENCE BASE Centers for Disease Control and Prevention. (2015). Sexually transmitted diseases treatment guidelines. Available: *www.cdc.gov/std/treatment*.

Chlamydia infection is the most common STD that occurs in women and men, particularly in adolescents and young adults. Women are asymptomatic or present with cervicitis; men are commonly asymptomatic but may present with urethritis.

Pathophysiology and Etiology

1. Chlamydia infection in women is the result of sexual intercourse, with infection entering the vagina, infecting the cervix and, possibly, spreading up through the endometrium and fallopian tubes.
2. Adolescents and young women ages 15 to 24 are at highest risk for infection, possibly because of susceptibility of cervical tissue to the organism and higher-risk sexual behaviors in this age group.
3. *C. trachomatis* is the most common sexually transmitted pathogen in men and women in the United States, with an incidence of more than 456.1 cases per 100,000 people.

Clinical Manifestations

1. May be asymptomatic or have vaginal discharge—may be clear mucoid to creamy discharge.
2. May have dysuria and mild pelvic discomfort.
3. May have intermenstrual spotting.
4. The cervix may be covered by thick mucopurulent discharge and be tender, erythematous, edematous, and friable.

Diagnostic Evaluation

1. DNA testing (or nucleic acid hybridization tests or NAATs) of cervical swab, vaginal swab, urine, or male urethral swab—most sensitive and specific; can be done simultaneously for gonorrhea.
2. Chlamydia culture from cervical exudate and cervical mucosa.
3. The CDC recommends annual screening for all sexually active women younger than age 25 and for older women at high risk (multiple sex partners or new partner).

Management

1. Antibiotic regimens include:
   a. Azithromycin 1 g orally in a single dose.
   b. Doxycycline 100 mg orally twice per day for 7 days.
   c. Alternatives include erythromycin, levofloxacin, or ofloxacin.
2. Current and/or most recent sexual partners (during 60 days or more preceding onset) should be tested and treated despite test results.

 NURSING ALERT Because chlamydia infection and gonorrhea frequently coexist, especially in adolescents and young adults, treatment of both STDs is recommended.

Complications

1. PID.
2. Ectopic pregnancy or infertility secondary to untreated or recurrent PID.
3. Transmission to neonate born through infected birth canal.

Nursing Assessment

1. Obtain history of sexual activity and symptoms or infections in partner.
2. Perform abdominal and pelvic examination for tenderness caused by possible spread to pelvic organs.

Nursing Diagnosis

• Risk for Infection related to sexual activity.

Nursing Interventions

Preventing Infection Transmission

1. Advise abstinence from sexual intercourse until 7 days after treatment has been completed.
2. Ensure that partner is treated at the same time; recent partners should receive treatment despite lack of symptoms and negative chlamydia test result. Abstinence should continue until 7 days after partners have completed treatment.
3. Report case to local public health department (chlamydia is a reportable infectious disease in most of the United States).
4. Ensure that patient begins treatment and will have access to prescription and transportation for follow-up. Single-dose azithromycin as directly observed therapy is often a good choice for patients with limited access to health care resources.
5. Retesting for chlamydia is recommended 3 months after treatment to detect reinfection, particularly in adolescents and young women.

Patient Education and Health Maintenance

1. Teach about all STDs, mode of transmission, symptoms, and complications. Clarify misconceptions.
2. Explain the treatment regimen to the patient, and advise her of adverse effects and the importance of informing her partner about the need for treatment.
3. Discuss STDs and methods of prevention—abstinence, monogamy, and proper use of female or male condoms. See page 653.
4. Stress the importance of follow-up examination and retesting. Recurrence rates are highest in younger patients.
5. Encourage screening periodically for at-risk women.
6. For further information on STDs, refer patients to such agencies as the American Social Health Association (*www.ashastd.org* or 800-227-8922).

Evaluation: Expected Outcomes

• Returns for follow-up; states complied with abstinence during treatment of self and partner; verbalizes use of measures to prevent STD transmission.

Gonorrhea

 EVIDENCE BASE Centers for Disease Control and Prevention. (2015). Sexually transmitted diseases treatment guidelines. Available: *www.cdc.gov/std/treatment.*

Gonorrhea is a common STD that affects men and women, causing cervicitis in women and urethritis in men. In women, it can easily ascend to the uterus and fallopian tubes, if untreated.

Pathophysiology and Etiology

1. Gonorrhea is caused by the gram-positive diplococci *Neisseria gonorrhoeae*.
2. Infection occurs through sexual transmission, causing cervicitis in women and possible conjunctivitis, pharyngitis, and proctitis.

3. Untreated infection may lead to PID, generalized dissemination, or gonococcal arthritis.
4. Gonorrhea has an incidence of 110.7 cases per 100,000 population in the United States each year; teens and young adults are most commonly affected.

Clinical Manifestations

1. Frequently asymptomatic in women.
2. May cause mucopurulent vaginal discharge or a painful burning sensation when urinating.
3. Vaginal speculum examination may reveal cervical discharge and inflammation.
4. Cervical motion tenderness and tender pelvic organs on bimanual examination if infection has begun to ascend.

Diagnostic Evaluation

1. DNA testing (or nucleic acid hybridization tests or NAATs) of cervical swab, vaginal swab, urine, or male urethral swab (most sensitive and specific; can be done simultaneously for chlamydia).
2. Endocervical culture should be performed to provide antimicrobial susceptibility results.
3. Pharyngeal or conjunctival secretions can be tested if pharyngitis or conjunctivitis is suspected. Follow laboratory specifications for these tests.
4. Joint aspiration and blood cultures may be necessary if disseminated infection is suspected.

Management

1. Uncomplicated gonococcal infection of the cervix, urethra (in men), or rectum (in men or women) can be treated with a single-dose antibiotic, such as the following (plus treatment for coinfection with chlamydia):
   a. Cefixime 400 mg orally.
   b. Ceftriaxone 250 mg IM.
   c. Alternative regimens involving other cephalosporins are also approved.
2. Pharyngeal infections should be treated for coinfection with chlamydia with the following:
   a. Ceftriaxone 250 mg IM single dose *plus.*
   b. Azithromycin 1 g orally single dose or doxycycline 100 mg orally twice daily × 7 days.
3. Gonococcal conjunctivitis should be treated with ceftriaxone 1 g IM single dose plus concomitant chlamydial treatment.
4. Disseminated infections require IV or IM therapy, such as:
   a. Ceftriaxone 1 g IM or IV every 24 hours.
   b. Cefotaxime 1 g IV every 8 hours.
   c. Ceftizoxime 1 g IV every 8 hours.
5. For IV or IM therapy, patient is switched to oral therapy 24 to 48 hours after improvement and then takes cefixime 400 mg orally twice daily to complete 7 days of antimicrobial therapy.
6. In all cases of suspected gonorrhea, concomitant treatment of chlamydia is recommended with appropriate second antibiotic agent.

 DRUG ALERT Fluoroquinolone therapy is no longer recommended for treatment of gonorrhea in the United States because of resistance.

Complications

1. PID, ectopic pregnancy, and infertility.

2. Disseminated infection.
3. Ophthalmia neonatorum and sepsis (rare) caused by infant born through infected birth canal.

Nursing Assessment

1. Question the patient on history of STDs, STD protection, sexual activity, and usual women's health self-care practices.
2. Obtain history of symptoms in patient and partner—incubation period is usually 3 to 7 days in men, but symptoms are typically overlooked in women.
3. Assess for ability to change lifestyle practices that may have led to STD.

Nursing Diagnosis

• Risk for Infection related to sexual activity.

Nursing Interventions

Stopping Transmission of STD
1. Administer antibiotics, as prescribed, explaining adverse effects to patient.
2. Make sure that patient can obtain prescription medication at discharge.
3. Monitor for relief of pain, discharge, and other symptoms.
4. Explain importance of sexual abstinence until symptoms are resolved completely and until 7 days after therapy is complete in patient and partner.
5. Report to public health department and tell patient that information will be obtained to ensure testing of sexual contacts.

Patient Education and Health Maintenance

1. Teach patient about all possible STDs, their prevalence, and their mode of transmission. Clarify misconceptions.
2. Advise patient of complications of gonorrhea and chlamydia.
3. Discuss STDs and methods of prevention—abstinence, monogamy, and proper use of female or male condoms. See page 653.
4. Stress the importance of follow-up examination and testing to ensure eradication of infection. Encourage follow-up for routine women's health care and periodic STD screening.
5. For additional information, refer to the American Social Health Association (*www.ashastd.org*) or Centers for Disease Control and Prevention (*www.cdc.gov/std/default.htm*).

Evaluation: Expected Outcomes

• Reports resolution of symptoms and use of condoms, abstinence, or other prevention measures at follow-up visit.

PROBLEMS RESULTING FROM RELAXED PELVIC MUSCLES

Cystocele is a downward displacement (protrusion) of the bladder into the vagina (see Figure 22-5). *Urethrocele* is downward displacement of the urethra into the vagina.

Pathophysiology and Etiology

1. Associated with obstetric trauma to fascia, muscle, and ligaments during childbirth (results in poor support).
2. Typically becomes apparent years later, when genital atrophy associated with aging occurs.
3. May also be caused by congenital defect or may appear after hysterectomy.

Figure 22-5. Pelvic support disorders. **(A)** Cystocele. **(B)** Rectocele. **(C)** Enterocele. (Smeltzer, S., & Bare, B. [2000]. *Brunner and Suddarth's textbook of medical-surgical nursing* [9th ed.]. Philadelphia, PA: Lippincott Williams & Wilkins.)

Clinical Manifestations

1. May be asymptomatic in early stages.
2. Pelvic pressure or heaviness, backache, nervousness, and fatigue.
3. Urinary symptoms—urgency, frequency, incontinence, and incomplete emptying.
4. Aggravated by coughing, sneezing, standing for long periods, and obesity, which increase intra-abdominal pressure.
5. Relieved by resting or by lying down.

Diagnostic Evaluation

1. Pelvic examination identifies condition.
2. Urinalysis and culture are done to rule out infection.

Management

1. Vaginal pessary—silicone (can be latex or polycarbonate) device inserted into the vagina as temporary treatment to support pelvic organs.
   a. Prolonged use may lead to necrosis and ulceration.
   b. Should be removed and cleaned at least once weekly.
2. Estrogen therapy after menopause to decrease genital atrophy.
3. Pelvic floor muscle exercises to improve symptoms.
4. Surgery—if cystocele is large and interferes with bladder functioning.
   a. May do anterior vaginal colporrhaphy (repair of anterior vaginal wall).
   b. Complications of surgery include urinary retention and bleeding (requires vaginal packing).

Complications

Urinary incontinence and infection.

Nursing Assessment

1. Obtain history of obstetric trauma, abdominal surgery, menopause, and use of estrogen.
2. Ask about urinary symptoms and pain.
3. Observe the perineum while the patient bears down or is in upright position for bulge from the vagina.

Nursing Diagnoses

- Acute Pain related to pelvic pressure.
- Stress Urinary Incontinence related to relaxed pelvic muscles and displaced organs.
- Urinary Retention related to displaced organs.

Nursing Interventions

Relieving Pain

1. Encourage periods of rest with legs elevated to relieve strain on the pelvis.
2. Advise use of mild analgesics, as necessary.
3. Provide postoperative care.
   a. Encourage voiding every 4 to 8 hours to reduce pressure so that no more than 150 mL will accumulate in the bladder—intermittent catheterization or use of an indwelling catheter may be required.
   b. Administer perineal care to patient after each voiding and defecation.
   c. Use available sprays for anesthetic and antiseptic effects.
   d. Apply an ice pack locally to relieve congestion and discomfort.
   e. Administer analgesics, as prescribed, for relief of pain.

Controlling Incontinence

1. Teach the patient Kegel pelvic floor exercises to regain muscle tone.
   a. Practice while voiding by stopping the flow of urine for 3 to 5 seconds and then releasing for 5 seconds.
   b. Patient can tighten pelvic floor muscle at any time, repeat 10 times, three times per day, and increase as able.
2. Encourage the patient to void frequently and respond to the urge to void promptly.
3. Warn the patient to avoid straining to prevent incontinence.

Preventing Urinary Retention

1. Encourage fluids to decrease bacterial flora in the bladder.
2. Catheterize patient if retention is suspected.
3. Obtain urine specimen for culture and sensitivity if infection is suspected.

Patient Education and Health Maintenance

1. Teach women to avoid straining, remain active, avoid obesity, and perform Kegel exercises to minimize pelvic relaxation in their older years.
2. Encourage prompt attention to symptoms of UTI—dysuria urgency, frequency, and foul-smelling urine.

Evaluation: Expected Outcomes

- Verbalizes reduced pain.
- Reports decreased frequency of incontinence.
- Voids regularly without symptoms of infection.

Rectocele and Enterocele

Rectocele is displacement (protrusion) of the rectum into the vagina. *Enterocele* is displacement of the intestine into the vagina (see Figure 22-5).

Pathophysiology and Etiology

1. Posterior vaginal wall becomes weakened, allowing displacement.
2. Weakening caused by obstetric trauma, childbirth, pelvic surgery, and aging.

Clinical Manifestations

1. Pelvic pressure or heaviness, backache, and perineal burning.
2. Constipation—may have difficulty in fecal evacuation; the patient may use fingers in the vagina to push feces up so defecation may occur.
3. Incontinence of feces and flatus—if tear between the rectum and vagina.
4. Visible protrusion into the vagina.
5. Symptoms are aggravated by standing for long periods.

Diagnostic Evaluation

1. Vaginal examination reveals condition.
2. May use Sims speculum to uplift the cervix and fully evaluate condition.

Management

1. Pessary—plastic device inserted into the vagina to aid pelvic support.
2. Estrogen replacement vaginally to prevent atrophy.
3. Pelvic floor muscle exercises to improve symptoms.
4. Surgery, if rectocele is large enough to interfere with bowel functioning: posterior colpoplasty (perineorrhaphy)—repair of posterior vaginal wall.

Complications

Total fecal incontinence.

Nursing Assessment

1. Obtain history of childbirth, pelvic surgery, and symptoms of bowel function.
2. Observe for bulge into the vagina while the patient bears down or is in upright position.
3. Monitor bowel movements.

Nursing Diagnoses

- Acute Pain related to pelvic pressure.
- Constipation related to displaced rectum or bowel.

Nursing Interventions

Relieving Pain

1. Encourage periods of rest with legs elevated to relieve pelvic strain.
2. Encourage use of mild analgesics, as needed; avoid opioids, which may worsen constipation.
3. Postoperative care:
   a. Suggest low Fowler position to reduce edema and discomfort.
   b. Administer perineal care to patient after each voiding and defecation.
   c. Heat may enhance the healing process, but use cautiously to avoid burns.
   d. Use ice packs locally to relieve congestion and discomfort.
   e. Administer analgesics and stool softeners, as ordered.

Relieving Constipation

1. Teach the patient to increase fluid and fiber in diet.
2. Encourage use of stool softeners or bulk laxatives to make passage of stool easier.

Patient Education and Health Maintenance

1. Advise the patient to follow surgeon's instructions for resuming activity and to avoid heavy lifting, straining, and intercourse until cleared.
2. Educate the patient for the future to avoid straining and obesity, which may cause return of rectocele or enterocele.

Evaluation: Expected Outcomes

- Verbalizes reduced pain.
- Passes soft stool daily.

Uterine Prolapse

Uterine prolapse is an abnormal position of the uterus in which the uterus protrudes downward.

Pathophysiology and Etiology

1. The uterus herniates through pelvic floor and protrudes into the vagina (prolapse) and possibly beyond the introitus (procidentia).
2. Usually caused by obstetric trauma and overstretching of musculofascial supports.
3. Degrees (see Figure 22-6).
   a. First degree—the cervix prolapses into vaginal canal.
   b. Second degree—the cervix is at the introitus.
   c. Third degree—the cervix extends over the perineum.
   d. Marked procidentia—the entire uterus protrudes outside vaginal cavity.

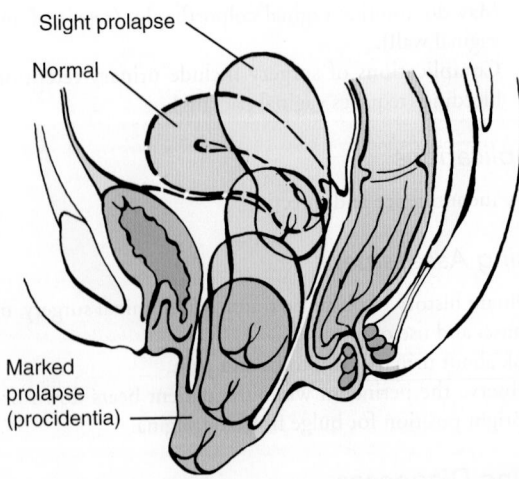

Figure 22-6. Degrees of uterine prolapse. (Reeder, S., Martin, L., & Koniak-Griffin, D. [1997]. *Maternity nursing: Family, newborn, and women's health care* [18th ed.]. Philadelphia, PA: Lippincott-Raven Publishers.)

Clinical Manifestations

1. Low backache or dyspareunia.
2. Pressure and heaviness in pelvic region.
3. Bloody discharge because of the cervix rubbing against clothing or inner thighs.
4. Urinary frequency, urgency, or repeated bladder infections.
5. Symptoms are aggravated by obesity, standing, straining, coughing, or lifting a heavy object because of increased intra-abdominal pressure.

Diagnostic Evaluation

Pelvic examination identifies condition.

Management

1. Hysterectomy or surgical correction.
2. Vaginal pessary—plastic device inserted into the vagina as temporary or palliative measure if surgery cannot be done.
3. Pelvic floor muscle exercises to improve symptoms.
4. Estrogen cream— decrease genital atrophy.

Complications

1. Necrosis of the cervix and uterus.
2. Infection.

Nursing Assessment

1. Obtain history of childbirth and surgery.
2. Ask about symptoms and aggravating factors.
3. Examine patient in lying or standing position; if the cervix not readily visible, spread labia gently; do not attempt to insert speculum.

Nursing Diagnoses

- Acute Pain related to downward pressure and exposed tissue.
- Impaired Tissue Integrity related to exposed cervix and uterus.
- Sexual Dysfunction related to loss of vaginal cavity.

Nursing Interventions

Relieving Pain
1. Administer sitz baths and explain procedure to patient.
2. Provide heating pad for lower back or lower abdomen.
3. Administer pain medications, as ordered.
4. Check for proper placement of pessary.
5. Increase fluid intake and encourage patient to void frequently to prevent bladder infection.

Maintaining Cervical and Uterine Mucosal Integrity
1. For second- and third-degree prolapse, apply saline compresses frequently.
2. Provide postoperative care.
   a. Administer perineal care to patient after each voiding and defecation.
   b. If urinary retention occurs, catheterize or use indwelling catheter until bladder tone is regained.
   c. Apply an ice pack locally to relieve congestion.
   d. Promote ambulation but prevent straining to reduce pelvic pressure.

Restoring Sexual Function
1. Discuss with patient noncoital sexual activity before treatment is instituted.

2. Explain to patient that sexual intercourse is possible with pessary; however, vaginal canal may be shortened.
3. Reinforce surgeon's instructions postoperatively about waiting to have vaginal penetration.
4. Encourage the patient to explore with partner ways to engage in sexual activity without strain and with greatest comfort.

Patient Education and Health Maintenance

1. Encourage the patient with pessary to follow up, as directed, for removal and cleaning of pessary and evaluation of any vaginal irritation or trauma.
2. Encourage all patients to report vaginal discharge, pain, or bleeding before or after treatment.

Evaluation: Expected Outcomes

- Verbalizes reduced pain.
- Cervix and uterus without ulceration.
- Verbalizes satisfying sexual activity.

GYNECOLOGIC TUMORS
Cancer of the Vulva

Cancer of the vulva is most commonly carcinoma of the labia majora, labia minora, or clitoris; it may also originate as a urethral tumor.

Pathophysiology and Etiology

1. Most common in postmenopausal women, with an average age of 65. Although there has recently been increased incidence in women aged 40 to 50 (which may be related to HPV screening), many new cases have been diagnosed because of increase in older population.
2. Represents 4% of gynecologic cancers.
3. The cause is unknown, but HPV has been shown to be responsible for 60% of vulvar cancers.
4. Spreads primarily through local, direct extension and lymphatic system; distant metastasis can occur late in the disease process.

Clinical Manifestations

1. Lump or mass present for several months—first is leukoplakic (white plaque or mild ulceration); becomes reddened, pigmented, and ulcerated.
2. Vulvar pruritus is a common complaint,
3. Discharge or bleeding; may be foul-smelling because of secondary infection.
4. Dysuria because of invasion of urethra with bacteria.
5. Edema of tissues.
6. Lymphadenopathy.
7. Pain or dyspareunia.

Diagnostic Evaluation

Biopsy of lesion and lymph nodes. If small, lesion may be excised at the time of biopsy. Most lesions are squamous cell carcinoma.

Management

 EVIDENCE BASE National Cancer Institute. (2017). Vulvar cancer treatment (PDQ). Bethesda, MD: Author. Available: *http://cancer.gov/cancertopics/pdq/treatment/vulvar/HealthProfessional.*

Choice of surgical methods depends on the site and extent of the primary lesion and the risk of lymph node involvement. The most conservative operation that is consistent with cure of disease is chosen.

1. Precancerous lesions—vulvar intraepithelial neoplasia.
   a. Simple vulvectomy is seldom indicated.
   b. Skinning vulvectomy with possible grafting.
   c. Local excision or laser therapy or a combination.
   d. Fluorouracil cream 5% (response rate 50% to 60%).
2. Carcinoma *in situ*—noninvasive.
   a. Simple vulvectomy is seldom indicated.
   b. Skinning vulvectomy with possible grafting.
   c. Local excision or laser therapy or a combination.
   d. Fluorouracil cream 5% (response rate 50% to 60%).
3. Invasive carcinoma—radical or modified radical vulvectomy with bilateral groin lymph node resection.
   a. Pelvic nodes may also be removed if involvement is suspected.
   b. If cancer is confined to the vulva, there is a 70% to 93% 5-year survival rate after surgery (for patients with negative nodes).
4. Advanced carcinoma—pelvic exenteration or surgery and radiation as a palliative measure.
   a. Radiation therapy has an increased role in the preoperative and postoperative management.
   b. Preoperative radiation therapy can decrease the volume of disease and decrease the need for radical surgery.
   c. Postoperative radiation therapy is used for patients with positive lymph nodes and close surgical margins.
   d. Long-term outcomes of treatment compared to morbidity associated with treatment are being studied.
5. Chemotherapy alone or in combination with radiation may shrink lesion so surgery can be less extensive.
6. Cisplatin and/or 5-FU used as radiation sensitizers has been shown to increase efficacy of radiation treatment.

Complications

1. Lymphatic spread.
2. Complications after vulvectomy are common—wound infection, wound breakdown, lymphedema, leg cellulitis, and introital stenosis.

Nursing Assessment

1. Obtain history of lesion, including when the patient first noticed it and any change in appearance.
2. Obtain gynecologic history, especially about past infections.
3. Assess overall health for tolerance of treatment.
4. Assess support systems and personal coping skills.

Nursing Diagnoses

- Fear related to cancer and radical surgery.
- Impaired Tissue Integrity related to surgery.
- Sexual Dysfunction related to vulvectomy.

Nursing Interventions

Relieving Fear Preoperatively

1. Have patient describe what her understanding is about the problem; answer questions and clear up misconceptions.
2. Emphasize the positive outcomes of the prescribed treatment plan; reinforce what the surgeon has already described to her.
3. Prepare the patient for surgery and describe to her the postoperative appearance of the wound and use of drains and urinary catheter (see Figure 22-7).

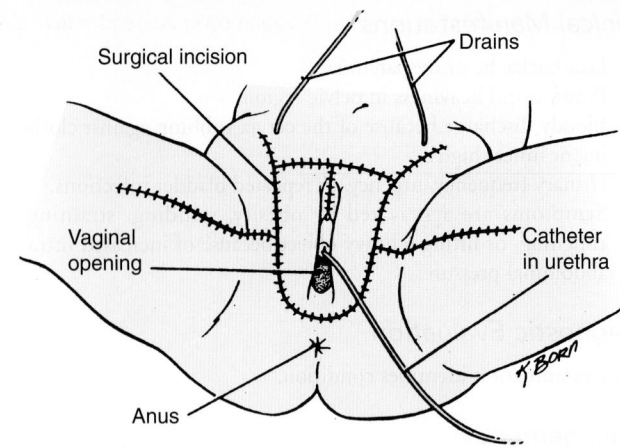

Figure 22-7. Postoperative appearance after radical vulvectomy.

a. Provide skin preparation as directed and cleanse the vulva via a chlorhexidine shower the night before surgery; 2% chlorhexidine gluconate antiseptic solution may also be ordered.
b. Administer bowel preparation, as ordered, to evacuate intestinal tract before surgery; there will be no bowel movement for 2 to 3 days postoperatively.

Promoting Tissue Healing Postoperatively

1. Maintain drainage and compression of tissues to remove fluid that could cause edema and prevent wound healing. Empty drains, as needed (at least every 8 hours).
2. Keep wound clean and dry.
   a. Perform sterile dressing changes, as prescribed.
   b. Apply heat lamp, if prescribed, to decrease moisture and increase circulation and healing.
   c. Perform perineal care or sitz baths after each bowel movement or voiding (after catheter is removed).
   d. Maintain patency of urinary catheter, as ordered, to prevent wound contamination with urine.
   e. Encourage low Fowler position to promote comfort and reduce tension on sutures.
   f. Prevent straining with defecation by providing a low-residue diet initially and stool softeners later, as ordered.
   g. Provide deep vein thrombosis prophylaxis (anticoagulant or sequential compression device), as prescribed, and encourage leg exercises to prevent thrombus/embolus formation. Encourage careful ambulation when allowed while preventing perineal tension.

Restoring Sexual Function

1. Encourage the patient to ventilate feelings about sexual mutilation and altered functioning.
2. Tell the patient that if the vagina is still intact, vaginal intercourse is still possible.
3. Inform the patient of changes that may occur because of surgery—loss of sexual arousal if the clitoris is removed, shortening of the vagina, and decreased lubrication.
4. Help the patient explore alternate methods of sexual intimacy and encourage her to discuss feelings with her partner.

Patient Education and Health Maintenance

1. Encourage follow-up visits for additional therapy, if required.
2. Encourage regular health checkups and screening for cancer and other age-related illnesses.
3. Encourage early evaluation of any suspicious lesions, bleeding, or discharge.

Carcinoma in situ   **Squamous cell carcinoma**

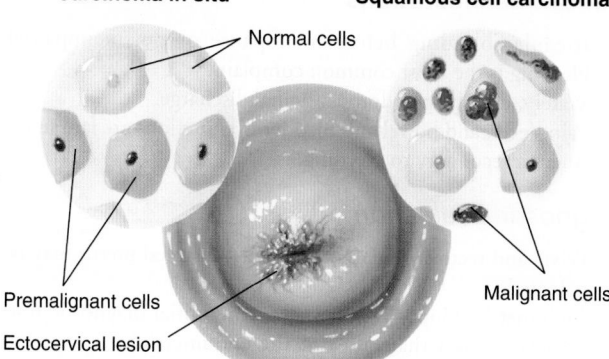

Normal cells

Premalignant cells

Ectocervical lesion

Malignant cells

Figure 22-8. Cervical cancer. (Anatomical Chart Company.)

Evaluation: Expected Outcomes

- Verbalizes reduced fear.
- Perineum healed without complications.
- Verbalizes understanding of anatomic changes and sexual function.

Cancer of the Cervix

Cancer of the cervix is the fourth most common gynecologic malignancy. There are about 13,000 new cases and 4,000 deaths each year in the United States.

Pathophysiology and Etiology

1. Early sexual activity, multiple sexual partners, a high-risk sexual partner, history of HIV and other STDs—especially HPV—and a history of vulvar or vaginal squamous intraepithelial neoplasia or cancer, and immunosuppression are major risk factors. There also appears to be an increased risk of cervical cancer associated with the use of oral contraceptives.
2. Incidence is higher in lower socioeconomic status and in Hispanics, African Americans, American Indians, and Alaska Natives—presumably related to decreased access to health care and screening.
3. Decreased mortality in United States, but most frequent malignancy among women in developing countries.
4. Types (see Figure 22-8):
   a. Dysplasia (precancer)—atypical cells with some degree of surface maturation.
   b. Carcinoma *in situ*—cytology similar to invasive carcinoma, but confined to the epithelium.
   c. Invasive carcinoma—stroma is involved; 69% are of the squamous cell type. Spreads by local invasion and lymphatics to the vagina and beyond.

Clinical Manifestations

1. Early disease is usually asymptomatic, although patient may notice watery, vaginal discharge.
2. Initial symptoms include postcoital bleeding, irregular vaginal bleeding or spotting between periods or after menopause, and malodorous discharge.
3. As disease progresses, bleeding becomes more constant and is accompanied by pain that radiates to buttocks and legs as well as urinary and rectal symptoms that may be due to invasion of these organs.
4. Weight loss, anemia, edema of lower extremities, and fever signal advanced disease.

Diagnostic Evaluation

1. Pap smear—routine screening measure; abnormal results warrant further diagnostic tests, such as colposcopy and biopsy or conization.
2. Staging is done clinically rather than surgically as with other cancers. Based on physical findings on abdominal and pelvic examination.
3. Supplemental imaging can include chest x-ray, IVP, urography, colposcopy, cystoscopy, proctosigmoidoscopy, computed tomography (CT) scan with IV contrast, and barium studies of the lower colon and rectum.

Management

 EVIDENCE BASE National Cancer Institute. (2017). Cervical cancer Treatment (PDQ). Bethesda, MD: Author. Available: *www.cancer.gov/cancertopics/pdq/treatment/cervical/HealthProfessional.*

Dysplasia to Carcinoma *In Situ*

1. Techniques to destroy abnormal cells in the cervical transformation zone.
2. Cryosurgery, laser therapy, electrocautery (loop electrosurgical excision procedure), or conization may be performed on outpatient basis.
3. Vaginal discharge, bleeding, pain, and cramping result from these procedures in various degrees, but postoperative convalescence is minimal.

Microinvasive Stage

1. Surgical conization—large excision of cervical tissue, may be done under local or general anesthesia.
2. Invasive cervical cancer—extent is staged and treated with hysterectomy, radiotherapy, or chemotherapy.

Other Management

1. Radiotherapy.
   a. Intracavitary (localized for earlier stage) or external (more generalized dosage to the pelvis for stages IIB through IVB).
   b. Cisplatin, a radiation sensitizer, is used to improve survival.
2. Chemotherapy—cisplatin may be used in combination with radiation for locally advanced disease or for metastatic disease in which recurrence is common. Other agents that may be used include ifosfamide, carboplatin, and topotecan.
3. Surgery.
   a. Total hysterectomy, conization, modified radical hysterectomy, and intracavitary radiation therapy may be performed for stage IA with or without oophorectomy and/or lymph node dissection.
   b. Radical hysterectomy and bilateral lymph node resections for stages IB and IIA. Radiation and chemotherapy may also be considered for these stages after hysterectomy.
   c. Pelvic exenteration for advanced cases if the patient is a candidate. Usually done for patients with isolated central recurrence.
      i. Removal of the vagina, uterus, uterine tubes, ovaries, bladder, rectum, and supporting structures and the creation of an ileal conduit and fecal stoma.
      ii. Performed for pelvic recurrence after radiation or chemotherapy.

Complications

1. Spread to the bladder and rectum; metastasis to lungs, mediastinum, bones, and liver.
2. Complications of intracavitary radiotherapy include cystitis, proctitis, vaginal stenosis, and uterine perforation.
3. Complications of external radiation include bone marrow depression, bowel obstruction, and fistula.

Nursing Assessment

1. Obtain history of Pap tests, sexual activity, and past STDs.
2. Obtain history of symptoms.
3. Assess understanding of disease and responses, such as guilt, fear, denial, and anxiety.

Nursing Diagnoses

- Anxiety related to cancer and treatment.
- Disturbed Body Image related to surgical treatment.

Nursing Interventions

Relieving Anxiety

1. Assist the patient to seek information on stage of cancer and treatment options.
2. Prepare the patient for hysterectomy or other surgery (see page 644 for nursing interventions for hysterectomy).
3. Prepare the patient for radiation therapy to the uterus (see page 669 for nursing interventions for radiation therapy).

Enhancing Body Image

1. Provide emotional support during treatment.
2. Encourage the patient to take pride in appearance by dressing and putting on makeup as able.
3. Encourage activity and socialization when the patient is able.

Patient Education and Health Maintenance

1. Explain the importance of lifelong follow-up, regardless of treatments, to determine the response to treatment and detect spread of cancer.
2. Refer to cancer support group in community.
3. Encourage all women to discuss cervical cancer screening guidelines with their health care providers (see page 637).

Evaluation: Expected Outcomes

- Reports decreased anxiety and increased decision-making ability.
- Reports continued interest in appearance and femininity.

Endometrial Cancer

Cancer of the uterus is usually adenocarcinoma of the endometrium of the fundus or body of the uterus. Most common gynecologic cancer in the United States.

Pathophysiology and Etiology

1. Most patients are postmenopausal with an average age of early 60s at the time of diagnosis.
2. Cause is unknown but associated with increased estrogen exposure as in tamoxifen use and unopposed estrogen replacement, obesity, anovulation, or estrogen-secreting tumors.
3. Hypertension and diabetes mellitus are also risk factors.

Clinical Manifestations

1. Irregular bleeding before menopause or postmenopausal bleeding is the most common complaint.
2. Watery, usually malodorous vaginal discharge.
3. Pain, fever, and bowel and bladder dysfunctions are late signs.
4. Anemia secondary to bleeding.

Diagnostic Evaluation

1. Pelvic and rectovaginal examination—enlarged uterus may be palpated.
2. Endometrial biopsy is preferred as the initial diagnostic test; however, if less than 50% of the endometrium is affected, malignancy can be missed.
3. Transvaginal ultrasound to measure endometrial thickness.
4. Dilation and curettage—if endometrial sampling cannot be performed in office, hysteroscopy may also be helpful.
5. Atypical glandular cells may be found on cervical cytology.
6. Metastatic workup—includes CA 125 (which may be elevated, especially in papillary serous carcinomas), x-ray studies, and cystoscopy.

Management

 EVIDENCE BASE National Cancer Institute. (2017). Endometrial cancer treatment (PDQ). Bethesda, MD: Author. Available: *www.cancer.gov/cancertopics/pdq/treatment/endometrial/HealthProfessional*.

1. Staging for endometrial cancer is based on surgical aspects versus clinical staging.
   a. Emphasis is placed on histologic grade, depth of myometrial invasion, and cervical involvement.
   b. These parameters assist in prediction of lymph node involvement and help determine need for lymph node dissection.
2. Early stage I requires total abdominal hysterectomy with bilateral salpingo-oophorectomy (TAH/BSO).
3. Advanced stage I and stage II require TAH/BSO and selective lymph node dissection.
4. Radiation therapy (intracavitary or external) may be added after surgery or chosen instead of surgery for more advanced stages or for patients who are high-risk surgical candidates.
   a. Acute complications include hemorrhagic cystitis, vaginitis, enteritis, and proctitis.
   b. Chronic complications include vaginal dryness, vaginal stenosis, cystitis, bladder dysfunction, proctitis, small bowel obstruction, fistulas, strictures, and leg edema.
5. Hormonal therapy—progestational agents may alter receptor sites in the endometrium for estrogen and thus decrease growth (for metastatic disease); may provide stabilization of disease.
6. Chemotherapy—for metastatic and recurrent disease; using cisplatin, doxorubicin, and possibly paclitaxel.

Complications

Spread throughout the pelvis; metastasis to lungs, liver, bone, and brain.

Nursing Assessment

1. Obtain history of menses, pregnancy, and estrogen replacement.
2. Ask about irregular or postmenopausal bleeding and other symptoms.
3. Assess the patient's response to possible diagnosis of cancer—fear, guilt, and denial.

Nursing Diagnoses

- Fear related to cancer and treatment options.
- Acute Pain related to disease process and surgical treatment.

Nursing Interventions

Relieving Fear

1. Support patient through the diagnostic process, and reinforce information given by health care provider about treatment options.
2. Prepare patient for radiation therapy, if indicated (see below).
3. Prepare patient for hysterectomy, if indicated (see page 644).
4. Provide complete and concise explanations for all care you provide; emphasize the positive aspects of patient's recovery.

Relieving Pain

1. Administer pain medications, as prescribed, and monitor the patient's response.
2. Encourage use of relaxation techniques, such as deep breathing, imagery, and distraction, to help promote comfort.

Patient Education and Health Maintenance

1. Explain importance of reporting postmenopausal bleeding.
2. Encourage keeping follow-up visits.
3. Explain that surgery or radiation treatment does not prevent satisfying sexual activity.
4. Refer to local cancer support group or American Cancer Society (*www.acs.org*).

Evaluation: Expected Outcomes

- Verbalizes understanding of diagnosis and treatment chosen.
- Verbalizes decreased pain.

Care of the Patient Receiving Intracavitary Radiation Therapy

Procedural Considerations

1. An applicator (tandems and ovoids are most common) is positioned in the endocervical canal and vagina in the operating room with the patient under anesthesia. (High-dose remote brachytherapy is also used. This is an outpatient procedure and the treatment takes just minutes. The radioactive source is removed between treatments.)
2. After recovery from anesthesia, x-rays are taken to check correct placement.
3. Radiologist inserts radioactive material (radium or cesium) into applicator, which remains in place 24 to 72 hours. Therapy is individualized according to the stage of disease and patient's response to and tolerance of radiation.
4. External radiation over the pelvis may be supplemented to eliminate cancer spread via lymphatic system.

Nursing Interventions

Patient Preparation

1. Patients require a thorough medical evaluation before treatment to evaluate risks and precautions related to pre-existing medical problems or special needs.
2. An indwelling catheter is placed in the operating room.
3. Encourage patient to bring diversional activities because she will remain on bed rest during radiation treatment.
4. Instruct patient on radiation safety measures:
   a. Neither patient nor her secretions are radioactive, but the applicator is.

   b. Do not touch source of radiation.
   c. Notify someone immediately if source is dislodged.
   d. When applicators are removed, no radioactivity remains.
   e. Radioactivity is monitored by specially trained personnel.
   f. No pregnant women or children younger than age 18 are allowed to visit.
   g. Lead shields may be used to decrease radiation that emanates from the patient.
5. Reinforce that help is readily available.

During Radiation Treatment

1. Maintain patient on strict bed rest on her back with head of bed elevated 15 to 30 degrees. Patient may be logrolled three or four times per day. Use convoluted foam mattress.
2. Have patient bathe upper body. Perineal care and linen changes are done by the nursing staff.
3. Maintain the patient on a low-residue diet to prevent bowel movements, which could dislodge the apparatus. Encourage the patient to eat several small portions rather than few large servings. Medication to induce constipation is given.
4. Inspect indwelling catheter frequently to ensure proper drainage. A distended bladder may cause severe radiation burns.
5. Encourage fluids to prevent bladder infection.
6. Observe for signs and symptoms of radiation sickness—nausea, vomiting, fever, diarrhea, and abdominal cramping.
7. Check applicator position every 8 hours and monitor amount of bleeding and drainage (a small amount is normal).
8. Check the patient frequently to minimize anxiety, but minimize time spent at bedside to reduce radiation exposure.
9. Mild sedatives or pain medication may be given for patient comfort.

 NURSING ALERT Long-handled forceps and a lead-lined container are left in the room after loading in the event the radioactive sources are dislodged. Maintain cardinal rules of time, distance, and shielding when caring for the patient.

During Radiation Removal

1. Before removal of the applicator, the patient is medicated with appropriate analgesic.
2. The radioactive sources are removed by radiation personnel and safely stored for transport.
3. The indwelling catheter is removed, and then the applicator is removed.
4. The patient is given an enema or suppository to reverse the induced constipation.
5. The patient should be evaluated for safe ambulation because of prolonged bed rest before discharge.

 NURSING ALERT Rules and regulations regarding radiation safety are strictly enforced to protect patients and health care workers.

Myomas of the Uterus

Myomas (fibroids, leiomyomas, fibromyomas) are benign tumors of the uterine myometrium (smooth muscle).

Pathophysiology and Etiology

1. The most common pelvic tumor in women. Approximately 80% of women have fibroids, but many are not symptomatic.

2. May spontaneously regress after menopause.
3. Unknown cause; increased incidence in black women.

Clinical Manifestations

1. Small myomas do not cause symptoms.
2. First indication may be palpable mass.
3. Irregular bleeding—usually menorrhagia.
4. Pain may come from pressure on adjacent organs—possible heavy feeling in the pelvis or degeneration associated with vascular occlusion.
5. Secondary symptoms include fatigue because of anemia, urinary disturbances, and constipation.

Diagnostic Evaluation

1. Transvaginal ultrasound or hysteroscopy—to identify size and location of myomas.
2. Magnetic resonance imaging (MRI) may be helpful in clarifying anatomy and myoma location; however, it is expensive and best reserved for surgical planning of difficult procedures.

Management

1. Myomectomy may be done for small or accessible tumor and may be done through hysteroscopy, laparoscopy, or laparotomy. If fertility preservation is desired, abdominal myomectomy is preferred for symptomatic women.
2. Hysterectomy for large or numerous tumors.
3. Medical therapies for management of symptoms include gonadotropin-releasing hormone antagonist therapy to create hypoestrogenic environment and to try to shrink tumors. Hormonal birth control, NSAIDs, or antifibrinolytic agents are used for heavy menstrual bleeding.
4. Frequently resolve on their own postmenopausally.
5. Uterine artery embolization—transvenous procedure in which the blood supply to the myoma is obstructed and the myoma degenerates.

Complications

1. Infertility with hysterectomy.
2. Habitual abortion.

Nursing Assessment

1. Ask about pain, menstrual irregularity, possible urinary symptoms, and constipation.
2. Assess the patient's understanding of condition as benign.

Nursing Diagnosis

- Acute and Chronic Pain related to tumor growth.

Nursing Interventions

Relieving Pain

1. Teach patient proper use and adverse effects of analgesics and use of heating pad, as desired.
2. Encourage the patient to avoid long periods of standing; rest with the pelvis in dependent position periodically to achieve comfort.
3. Encourage patient to void frequently to avoid increased pressure from distended bladder.
4. Advise a high-fiber diet to prevent constipation.
5. Prepare the patient for surgery, if indicated.

Patient Education and Health Maintenance

1. Tell the patient to report increased symptoms and worsening bleeding because myomas may be enlarging and treatment may be indicated.
2. Reassure the patient that myomas do not become malignant, but she should keep regular follow-up visits for cancer screening.

Evaluation: Expected Outcomes

- Verbalizes control of pain.

Ovarian Cysts

Ovarian cysts are growths arising from ovarian components, usually benign.

Pathophysiology and Etiology

1. Commonly arise from functional changes in the ovary—from graafian follicle or from persistent corpus luteum.
2. Dermoid cysts may develop from abnormal embryonic epithelium.
3. Frequently found during childbearing years.

Clinical Manifestations

1. May be asymptomatic or cause minor pelvic pain.
2. Possible menstrual irregularity.
3. Tender, palpable mass.
4. Rupture causes acute unilateral lower abdominal pain and tenderness; may mimic mittelschmerz, PID, appendicitis, or ectopic pregnancy.
5. Discomfort during bowel movement or pressure on the bowel.

Diagnostic Evaluation

1. Pelvic sonogram to determine size and characteristics.
2. Pregnancy test to rule out ectopic pregnancy.
3. Biopsy (at the time of surgery) is done for suspicious cysts.
4. Other tests that may be ordered: CBC with diff. and CA 125.

Management

1. Cysts without malignant characteristics and cysts that measure less than 10 cm in diameter can be observed with repeat ultrasound in 2 to 3 months.
2. Surgery for large, complex, or leaking cyst by laparoscopy or laparotomy.

Complications

Rupture may cause peritoneal inflammation.

Nursing Assessment

1. Obtain history of sexual activity, use of contraception, and past episodes of PID to rule out ectopic pregnancy.
2. Obtain history of recent menses—irregular bleeding and spotting commonly signal follicular cyst; delayed menses and prolonged bleeding signal corpus luteal cyst.
3. Perform vital signs and abdominal examination for tenderness, guarding, and rebound, which may indicate rupture.

Nursing Diagnoses

- Acute Pain related to abnormal growth.
- Risk for Deficient Fluid Volume related to rupture of cyst or postoperative change in intra-abdominal pressure.

Nursing Interventions

Relieving Pain

1. Encourage the use of analgesics, as prescribed, and of heating pad, if desired.
2. Teach the patient the proper use of hormonal contraceptives, if prescribed, with adverse effects; encourage monthly follow-up visits to determine if cyst is resolving.
3. Tell the patient that heavy lifting, strenuous exercise, and sexual intercourse may increase pain.

Maintaining Fluid Volume

1. Monitor for nausea, vomiting, rigid abdomen, and change in vital signs related to rupture of cyst. Administer IV fluids, as directed, and maintain NPO status until abdominal rigidity resolves.
2. Reassure the patient that symptoms will resolve.
3. Prepare the patient with large or nonresponsive cyst for surgery, as indicated.
4. Postoperatively monitor vital signs frequently and maintain IV infusion while NPO.
5. Assess frequently for abdominal distention because of fluid and gas pooling in abdominal cavity.
6. Place the patient in semi-Fowler position for greatest comfort, and encourage early ambulation to reduce distention (help patient arise slowly to prevent orthostatic hypotension).
7. Administer antiemetics and insert a nasogastric tube, as ordered, to prevent vomiting.
8. As distention resolves, assess bowel sounds and advance oral intake slowly.

Patient Education and Health Maintenance

1. Reassure patient that in most cases ovarian function remains and she remains fertile.
2. Reassure patient about low malignancy rate of cysts.
3. Encourage the patient to report recurrent symptoms or worsening of pain if cyst is being treated medically.

Evaluation: Expected Outcomes

- Verbalizes reduced pain.
- Vital signs stable; no orthostasis.

Ovarian Cancer

Ovarian cancer is a gynecologic malignancy with high mortality because of advanced disease by the time of diagnosis. It is the leading cause of morbidity of gynecologic cancers.

Pathophysiology and Etiology

1. Median age is 60 years. One of 70 women will develop ovarian cancer.
2. Cause is unknown, but about 10% of cases are associated with family history of breast, endometrial, colon, or ovarian cancer.
3. Smoking and personal history of breast, colon, or endometrial cancer are also risk factors.
4. There is also higher incidence in nulliparous women.

Clinical Manifestations

1. No early manifestations.
2. First manifestations—(vague) bloating, increased abdominal size, urinary urgency or frequency, difficulty eating or feeling full, and abdominal or pelvic pain, which may occur with other symptoms, almost daily, and are more severe than expected.
3. Late manifestations—abdominal pain, ascites, pleural effusion, and intestinal obstruction.

Diagnostic Evaluation

1. Pelvic examination to detect enlargement, nodularity, and immobility of the ovaries.
2. Pelvic sonography (transabdominal and transvaginal) is the most useful diagnostic test and CT scan is done to determine metastatic spread.
3. Color Doppler imaging may be used to detect vascular changes within the ovaries.
4. Paracentesis or thoracentesis if ascites or pleural effusion is present.
5. Laparotomy to stage the disease and determine effectiveness of treatment.
6. Increase of CA 125 signifies progression, but not as useful as diagnostic or screening tool because level can be elevated because of inflammation and other causes.

Management

1. TAH/BSO and omentectomy is usual treatment because of delayed diagnosis. Optimal debulking to less than 1 cm is the goal.
2. Chemotherapy is more effective if tumor is optimally debulked (less than 1-cm residual disease); usually follows surgery because of frequency of advanced disease; may be given IV or intraperitoneal.
3. Radiation therapy is not usually valuable.
4. Second-look laparotomy may be done after adjunct therapies to take multiple biopsies and determine effectiveness of therapy. Practice is controversial because it does not affect survival.
5. Immunotherapy is being investigated in clinical trials as stand-alone treatment or in conjunction with other modalities.

Complications

Direct intra-abdominal or lymphatic spread and peritoneal seeding

Nursing Assessment

1. Obtain history of irregular menses, pain, and postmenopausal bleeding.
2. Ask about vague GI-related complaints.
3. Ask about history of other malignancy and family history of breast or ovarian cancer.
4. Assess the patient's general health status in terms of tolerating surgical and adjuvant therapy.

 NURSING ALERT A combination of a long history of ovarian dysfunction and persistent undiagnosed GI complaints raises the suspicion for ovarian cancer. A palpable ovary in a postmenopausal woman is abnormal and should be evaluated as soon as possible.

Nursing Diagnoses

- Ineffective Coping related to advanced stage of cancer.
- Imbalanced Nutrition: Less Than Body Requirements related to nausea and vomiting from chemotherapy.
- Disturbed Body Image related to hair loss from chemotherapy.
- Acute Pain related to surgery.

Nursing Interventions

Strengthening Coping

1. Provide emotional support through diagnostic process; allow patient to express feelings and encourage positive coping mechanisms.
2. Administer anxiolytic and analgesic medications, as prescribed, and teach patient and caregivers the potential adverse effects.
3. Refer patient to cancer support group locally or American Cancer Society (*www.acs.org*) or National Cancer Institute (*www.cancer.org*).

Maintaining Adequate Nutrition

1. Administer or teach the patient or caregiver to administer antiemetics, as needed, for nausea and vomiting.
2. Encourage small, frequent, bland meals or liquid nutritional supplements as able.
3. Assess the need for IV fluids if the patient is vomiting.
4. Monitor for passage of gas and bowel movements after surgery. Bowel dysfunction related to surgery may cause nausea and anorexia.

Maintaining Body Image

1. Prepare the patient for body image changes with chemotherapy (ie, hair loss).
2. Encourage the patient to prepare ahead of time with turbans, wigs, and hats.
3. Encourage the patient to enhance her appearance with makeup, clothing, and jewelry as she is used to doing.
4. Stress the positive effects of the patient's treatment plan.

Relieving Pain

1. Prepare the patient for surgery, as indicated; explain the extent of incision, IV, catheter, packing, and drain tubes expected (see page 644 for a discussion of hysterectomy).
2. Postoperatively, administer analgesics, as needed, and explain to the patient that she may be drowsy.
3. Reposition frequently and encourage early ambulation to promote comfort and prevent adverse effects.

Patient Education and Health Maintenance

1. Explain to the patient the onset of menopausal symptoms with ovary removal.
2. Tell the patient that disease progression will be monitored closely by laboratory tests and second-look laparoscopy may be necessary.
3. Female relatives of patient should notify their physicians; biannual pelvic examinations may be necessary.

Evaluation: Expected Outcomes

- Openly discusses prognosis, asks appropriate questions, and makes plans for short-term future.
- Maintains weight.
- Verbalizes satisfaction in appearance with wig.
- Verbalizes good control over pain.

OTHER GYNECOLOGIC CONDITIONS

 See additional online content: Nursing Care Plan 22-1

Pelvic Inflammatory Disease

 EVIDENCE BASE Centers for Disease Control and Prevention. (2015). *Sexually transmitted diseases treatment guidelines.* Available: *www.cdc.gov/std/treatment.*

Pelvic inflammatory disease (PID) includes several inflammatory disorders of the upper female genital tract, often with infection that may involve the fallopian tubes, ovaries, uterus, or peritoneum.

Pathophysiology and Etiology

1. Incidence has been increasing; high recurrence rate because of reinfections.
2. Commonly polymicrobial; causative agents include *N. gonorrhoeae*, *C. trachomatis*, anaerobes (*Gardnerella vaginalis*), gram-negative bacteria, and *streptococci*. Cervical infection ascends through the endometrium, into the fallopian tubes, and possibly into the peritoneal cavity.
3. Predisposing factors include multiple sexual partners, early onset of sexual activity, use of IUDs (the wick promotes ascension of bacteria), and procedures such as therapeutic abortion, cesarean sections, and hysterosalpingograms.

Clinical Manifestations

1. Pelvic pain—most common presenting symptom; usually dull and bilateral.
2. Fever greater than 101°F—especially with gonococcal infections.
3. Cervical discharge—mucopurulent.
4. Irregular bleeding.
5. GI symptoms—nausea, vomiting, and acute abdomen usually signify abscess.
6. Urinary symptoms—dysuria and frequency.
7. Presentation with chlamydia may be mild.

> **NURSING ALERT** Localized right or left lower quadrant tenderness with guarding, rebound, or palpable mass signifies tuboovarian abscess with peritoneal inflammation. Immediate evaluation and surgical intervention are necessary to prevent rupture and widespread peritonitis. Other significant causes include acute appendicitis and ectopic pregnancy.

Diagnostic Evaluation

1. Diagnostic criteria for empiric treatment of PID in women at risk for STDs are warranted if no cause for pelvic pain can be identified or if any of the following three minimum criteria are present:
   a. Cervical motion tenderness.
   b. Uterine tenderness.
   c. Adnexal tenderness.
2. In addition to the presence of the minimum criteria, signs/symptoms of lower genital tract infection (such as cervical exudate, a friable cervix, and white blood cells on microscopic examination of cervical secretions) improve the specificity of the diagnosis.
3. Endocervical DNA testing or culture to identify organisms (*Gonorrhea* or *chlamydia*).

4. CBC may show elevated leukocytes.
5. Elevated C-reactive protein or elevated erythrocyte sedimentation rate shows inflammation.
6. Some cases may warrant endometrial biopsy, hysterosalpingostomy, transvaginal ultrasound, MRI, or laparoscopic visualization of the fallopian tubes.

Management

1. Patients with mild to moderate symptoms can be treated on an outpatient basis with oral antimicrobial regimens and timely follow-up at 48 to 72 hours after initiation of antibiotic and at completion of 2-week antibiotic course.
2. Inpatient treatment is required for surgical emergencies; abscess; pregnancy; severe infection with nausea, vomiting, and high fever; cannot take oral fluids; immunodeficient patient; or more aggressive antibiotics required to preserve fertility.
3. Parenteral antimicrobial regimens recommended by the CDC during hospitalization include the following:
   a. Cefotetan 2 g IV every 12 hours or cefoxitin 2 g IV every 6 hours *plus* doxycycline 100 mg IV or orally every 12 hours. *Note:* Doxycycline is contraindicated during pregnancy and IV infusion is painful; oral administration is preferred when possible.
   b. Clindamycin 900 mg IV every 8 hours *plus* gentamicin 2 mg/kg of body weight IV or IM as loading dose, followed by 1.5 mg/kg every 8 hours as maintenance dosage. (A single daily dose [3 to 5 mg/kg] of gentamicin may be substituted.)
4. Outpatient, oral antimicrobial regimens recommended by the CDC include:
   a. Ceftriaxone 250 mg IM single dose *plus* doxycycline 100 mg orally twice per day for 14 days, with or without metronidazole 500 mg orally twice per day for 14 days.
   b. Cefoxitin 2 g IM single dose *and* probenecid 1 g orally administered concurrently as a single dose *plus* doxycycline 100 mg orally twice daily for 14 days, with or without metronidazole 500 mg orally twice daily for 14 days.
   c. Other IM third-generation cephalosporin (ceftizoxime or cefotaxime) *plus* doxycycline 100 mg orally twice a day for 14 days, with or without metronidazole 500 mg twice a day for 14 days.
5. Parenteral therapy can be switched to oral therapy 24 to 48 hours after improvement is shown (reduced fever, decreased pain, resolution of nausea and vomiting). Ongoing oral therapy after parenteral therapy may be one of the following regimens:
   a. Doxycycline 100 mg orally twice per day to complete a total of 14 days.
   b. Clindamycin 450 mg orally four times per day to complete a total of 14 days.
   c. With or without addition of metronidazole 500 mg orally twice per day to complete 14 days.
6. Surgical treatment or interventional drain placement may be necessary to drain abscess or later to treat adhesions or tubal damage.

↺ **TRANSITIONAL CARE ALERT** If patient with PID is to be treated at home, stress the importance of follow-up, usually in 48 hours, to determine if oral antibiotic treatment is effective. Advise patient to report worsening of symptoms immediately to avoid hospitalization and further complications.

Complications

1. Abscess rupture and sepsis.
2. Infertility because of adhesions to fallopian tubes and ovaries.
3. Ectopic pregnancy caused by inability of fertilized egg to pass stricture.
4. Dyspareunia because of adhesions.

Nursing Assessment

1. Obtain history of menstruation, contraception, sexual activity (including number of partners and new partner), STD history, and symptoms in sexual partner.
2. Assess level of pain and fever; evaluate vital signs for hypotension and increased pulse, indicating hypovolemia.
3. Perform abdominal and pelvic examinations, if indicated; be alert for abdominal tenderness, rebound, guarding, or a mass.
4. Assess the patient's feelings about having an STD.

Nursing Diagnoses

- Acute Pain related to pelvic inflammation and infection.
- Deficient Fluid Volume related to fever and decreased oral intake.
- Risk for Infection related to STDs.

Nursing Interventions

Relieving Pain

1. Administer or teach the patient to self-administer analgesics as prescribed; monitor for adverse effect of drowsiness and constipation.
2. Assist to comfortable position of pelvic dependence, with upper body and legs slightly elevated.
3. Suggest heating pad to lower abdomen or low back.

Restoring Fluid Balance

1. Administer antiemetics as needed for nausea and vomiting impairing fluid intake.
2. Monitor intake and output.
3. Restart oral intake with ice chips and sips of water when vomiting has ceased for 2 hours.

Resolving Infection and Further Transmission

1. Administer or teach self-administration of antibiotics as prescribed.
2. Report sexually transmitted infection such as gonorrhea to state or local health department, and advise that patient's partners in past 60 days should be treated.
3. Review STD prevention guidelines.

Patient Education and Health Maintenance

1. Encourage compliance with antibiotic therapy for full length of prescription.
2. Stress the need for sexual abstinence and pelvic rest (nothing in the vagina, including no douching or tampons) until completion of the patient's and partner's antimicrobial regimens, resolution of the patient's and partner's symptoms, and follow-up visit.
3. Advise testing and empiric treatment of gonorrhea and chlamydia for all sexual partners (within past 60 days or more). Tell patient that diagnosis of chlamydia or gonorrhea necessitates reporting to public health department and partners will be traced.
4. Repeat patient and partner testing for gonorrhea and chlamydia is recommended 3 to 6 months after treatment completion.
5. Discuss STDs and methods of prevention—abstinence, monogamy, and proper use of female or male condoms. See page 653.

Evaluation: Expected Outcomes

- Verbalizes relief of pain.
- Vital signs stable; intake equals output.
- Reports abstinence during treatment period for self and partner and continued plan to prevent STDs.

Endometriosis

EVIDENCE BASE Dunselman, G. A., Vermeulen, N., Becker, C., et al. (2014). European Society for Human Reproduction and Embryology guideline: Management of women with endometriosis. *Human Reproduction, 29*, 400–412.

Endometriosis is the abnormal proliferation of uterine endometrial tissue outside the uterus.

Pathophysiology and Etiology

1. May also be found outside the pelvic cavity; an intact uterus is not needed to have endometriosis (see Figure 22-9).
2. Peaks in women ages 25 to 45; may occur at any age. Increased risk in siblings, women with shorter menstrual cycles, and longer duration of flow. More common in white women than black women, in women who do not exercise, and in obese women.
3. Responds to ovarian hormonal stimulation—estrogen increases it; progestins decrease it.
   a. Bleeds during uterine menstruation, resulting in accumulated blood and inflammation and subsequent adhesions and pain.
   b. Regresses during amenorrhea (ie, pregnancy and menopause) and hormonal contraceptive and androgen use.
4. Theories of origin:
   a. May be embryonic tissue remnants that differentiate as a result of hormonal stimulation and spread via lymphatic or venous channels.
   b. May be transferred via surgical instruments.
   c. May be caused by retrograde menstruation through fallopian tubes into peritoneal cavity (but this theory does not account for some types of endometriosis)

Figure 22-9. Common sites of endometriosis. Ectopic endometrial tissue can implant almost anywhere in the pelvic peritoneum. It can even invade distant sites such as the lungs. (Anatomical Chart Company.)

d. Genetic predisposition may increase the likelihood in women with a first-degree relative with endometriosis.
e. Lymphatic or vascular distribution of endometrial tissue.

Clinical Manifestations

1. Depends on sites of implantation; may be asymptomatic.
2. Pelvic pain—especially during or before menstruation.
3. Dyspareunia.
4. Painful defecation—if implants are on the sigmoid colon or rectum.
5. Abnormal uterine bleeding.
6. Persistent infertility (in 30% to 40% of women with endometriosis).
7. Hematuria, dysuria, and flank pain—if bladder involved.

Diagnostic Evaluation

1. Pelvic and rectal examinations—tender, fixed nodules or ovarian mass or uterine retrodisplacement; nodules may not be palpable.
2. Transvaginal ultrasound—diagnostic tool of choice to first assess for endometriosis. MRI and CT are reserved for inconclusive ultrasound results.
3. Laparoscopy—for definitive diagnosis to view implants, obtain tissue for histologic analysis, and determine extent of disease.

Management

Medical

The goal of medical suppressive therapy is to decrease pain. However, if therapy is stopped, pain recurs. Medical therapies are ineffective for infertility associated with endometriosis.

1. Hormonal contraceptives—such as combination oral contraceptives (OCs); use small amount of estrogen and maximum amount of progestin and androgen effect to decrease implant size. OC use for more than 24 months effectively decreases endometrioma recurrence and decreases the frequency and intensity of dysmenorrhea.
2. Progestins—such as depot medroxyprogesterone acetate; create a hypoestrogenic environment. Efficacy is equivalent to OCs.
3. Nonsteroidal anti-inflammatory drugs—such as ibuprofen and naproxen sodium—decrease dysmenorrhea with antiprostaglandin action
4. If after 3 months of OCs and NSAIDs treatment has not provided adequate pain relief, then gonadotropin-releasing hormone (GnRH) agonist (leuprolide) injections may be administered during a 6-month period—create hypoestrogenic environment. Menopausal-like side effects, such as hot flashes and vaginal dryness, may not be tolerable to some women. If GnRH therapy will continue later, then norethindrone acetate add-back therapy will be added to prevent bone mineral loss and alleviate some symptoms. Calcium, vitamin D, and bisphosphonates may be added also.
5. Aromatase inhibitors, such as letrozole—inhibits the action of aromatase, which converts androgens to estrogen, thereby reducing estrogen levels in all tissues including the endometriosis. More RCTs are needed to determine its efficacy.
6. Danazol—synthetic androgen suppresses endometrial growth. Rarely used secondary to intolerable adverse effects (increased facial hair, acne, weight gain, vasomotor symptoms) and other drugs are available with better side effect profiles. Contraindicated in pregnancy.

Surgical

1. Laparoscopic surgery—preferred procedure to remove implants and lyse adhesions by excision; not curative; high recurrence rate.
2. Carbon dioxide laser laparoscopy—for minimal to moderate disease; vaporizes tissue; may be done at same time as diagnosis; good pregnancy rate.
3. Laparotomy—rarely performed; involves a larger abdominal incision than laparoscopy; for severe endometriosis or persistent symptoms.
4. Presacral neurectomy—rarely performed; to decrease central pelvic pain; preserves fertility; limited efficacy in relieving pain; severe constipation results.
5. Hysterectomy—if fertility is not desired and symptoms are severe; greater pain relief is achieved when ovaries are also removed.

Complications

1. Infertility.
2. Rupture of cyst—mimics ruptured appendix.
3. Chronic pelvic pain.
4. Dyspareunia.
5. Bowel or ureter obstruction.

Nursing Assessment

1. Obtain history of symptoms to determine spread and severity of disease.
2. Assess pain—level, location, frequency, duration, characteristics, and impact on functioning.
3. Perform abdominal examination to assess for areas of tenderness and nodules.
4. Assess for impact of endometriosis and/or infertility on patient and her relationship with significant other.

Nursing Diagnoses

- Acute and Chronic Pain related to hormonal stimulation and adhesions.
- Readiness for Enhanced Self-Care related to difficult management of disease and infertility.

Nursing Interventions

Reducing Pain

1. Teach use of analgesics and other prescribed medication, with adverse effects.
2. Encourage use of heating pad to painful areas, as needed.
3. Teach patient relaxation techniques to control pain, such as deep breathing, imagery, and progressive muscle relaxation.
4. Encourage patient to try position changes for sexual intercourse if experiencing dyspareunia.

Fostering Enhanced Self-Care

1. Include patient in treatment planning; answer questions about drug and surgical treatment so she can make informed choices.
2. Encourage adequate rest and nutrition.
3. Provide emotional support and encourage patient to discuss treatment of infertility with her physician.
4. Prepare the patient for surgery, as indicated.

Patient Education and Health Maintenance

1. Instruct the patient in the adverse effects of prescribed medication.
2. Refer patient to support groups such as Endometriosis Association (*www.endometriosisassn.org*) and reliable resources for information such as *Endometriosis.org* (*http://endometriosis.org*).

Evaluation: Expected Outcomes

- Verbalizes reduced pain.
- Verbalizes increased self-care measures.

Toxic Shock Syndrome

Toxic shock syndrome (TSS) is a rare condition caused by a bacterial toxin from Staphylococcus aureus or sometimes by group A Streptococcus pyogenes in the bloodstream; it can be life-threatening.

Pathophysiology and Etiology

1. Cause is uncertain, but 70% of cases historically were associated with menstruation and superabsorbent tampon use. Menstrual cases have declined since the withdrawal of superabsorbent tampons from the market around 1986. Now, half of TSS cases are not menstrually related.
2. TSS does occur in nonmenstruating or postmenopausal females, males, and children with conditions such as cellulitis, surgical wound infections, subcutaneous abscesses, vaginal infections, after childbirth, and with the use of contraceptive sponge or diaphragm.
3. See Figure 22-10 for pathophysiology.

Clinical Manifestations

1. Patients may initially present with fever, hypotension, and diffuse rash.
2. May have sudden onset of fever greater than 102°F (38.9°C), often with flulike symptoms (myalgias, headache, sore throat).

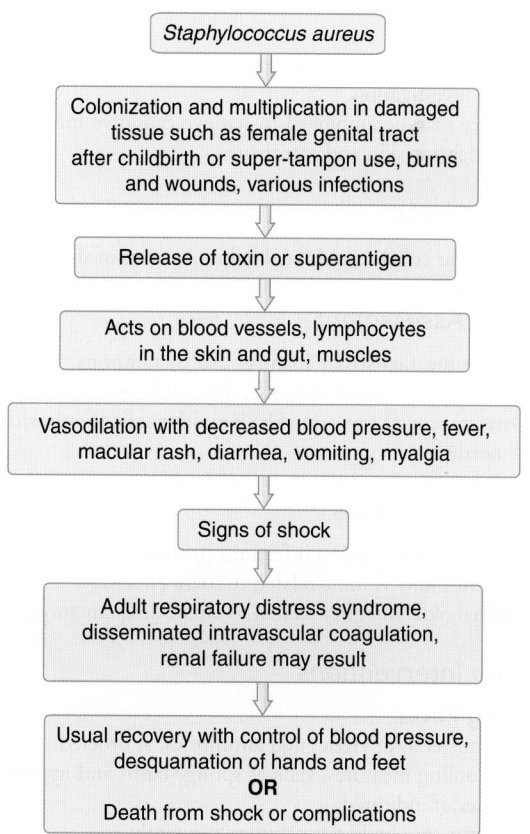

Figure 22-10. Pathophysiology of toxic shock syndrome.

3. Hypotension and rapid progression to shock within 72 hours of onset.
4. Rash (similar to sunburn) that is diffuse, red, and macular; followed by desquamation, particularly of the palms and soles, 1 to 2 weeks after illness onset.
5. Mucous membrane hyperemia.
6. Vomiting and profuse watery diarrhea.
7. Rapid progression to multisystem involvement.

Diagnostic Evaluation

1. Blood, urine, throat, and vaginal or cervical cultures; possibly cerebrospinal fluid culture to detect or rule out infectious organism.
2. Tests to rule out other febrile illnesses—Rocky Mountain spotted fever, Lyme disease, meningitis, and Epstein-Barr or coxsackie virus.
3. CBC, electrolytes, blood urea nitrogen, creatinine, coagulation studies, and other tests to monitor condition.

Management

Management will be achieved in an intensive care unit because of the nature of the rapidly progressing shock, circulatory compromise, impending potential acute renal failure, and multisystem organ failure.

1. Fluid and electrolyte replacement to increase blood pressure and prevent renal failure.
2. Inotropes and vasopressor medications (ie, dopamine), as needed.
3. Intravenous antibiotics (ie, penicillins, cephalosporins, vancomycin); methicillin-resistant *Staphylococcus aureus* has been reported in some cases of TSS.
4. Mechanical ventilation in acute respiratory distress and lactic acidosis.
5. The use of steroids and immunoglobulins is controversial and under investigation.
6. Surgery may be employed to remove causative infectious site or to debride skin and soft tissue.

Complications

Cardiovascular collapse and renal failure because of shock.

Nursing Assessment

1. Determine menstrual history, use of tampons, or whether there has been recent skin infection, childbirth, or surgery.
2. Determine vital signs quickly; hemodynamic monitoring may be needed.

Nursing Diagnoses

- Hyperthermia related to infectious process.
- Deficient Fluid Volume related to toxin effects.
- Impaired Skin Integrity related to latent desquamation.

Nursing Interventions

Reducing Fever

1. Administer antipyretics and antibiotics, as ordered.
2. Use cooling measures, such as sponge baths and hypothermia blanket, if indicated.
3. Monitor core body temperature frequently.

Restoring Fluid Volume

1. Perform hemodynamic monitoring, as indicated (ie, arterial line, central venous pressure, or pulmonary artery pressure).
2. Maintain strict intake and output measurement.
3. Insert indwelling catheter to monitor urine output.
4. Administer IV fluids and vasopressors, as ordered, to control hypotension.
5. Monitor respiratory status for pulmonary edema and respiratory distress syndrome because of fluid overload from increased fluid replacement or from lactic acidosis from acute renal failure. Mechanical ventilation may be required.
6. Administer diuretics, as ordered, if edema results.

Restoring Skin Integrity

1. Tell the patient to expect desquamation of the skin, as in peeling sunburn.
2. Protect skin and avoid use of harsh soaps and alcohol that cause drying.
3. Tell the patient to apply mild moisturizer and avoid direct sunlight until healed.
4. Advise the patient that reversible hair loss may occur 1 to 2 months after TSS.

Patient Education and Health Maintenance

1. Tell the patient to expect fatigue for weeks to months after TSS.
2. Tell the patient not to use tampons in future to reduce risk of recurrence.
3. Encourage follow-up examination and cultures.
4. Teach prevention of TSS.
   a. Avoid use of tampons if menstrual flow is light. Use pads whenever possible.
   b. Alternate use of pads with tampons; avoid superabsorbent tampons.
   c. Change tampons frequently and do not wear one longer than 8 hours—4 hours maximum in heavy discharge time.
   d. Be careful of vaginal abrasions that can be caused by some applicators.
   e. Be alert to symptoms of TSS.

Evaluation: Expected Outcomes

- Afebrile.
- Normotensive and good urine output.
- Skin heals without scar.

SELECTED REFERENCES

American College of Radiology. (2014). ACR–ACOG–AIUM–SRU practice guideline for the performance of pelvic ultrasound. Available: *www.acr.org/-/media/ACR/Documents/PGTS/guidelines/us/us_pelvic.pdf.*

Bedsider. (2017). Birth control methods. Available: *www.bedsider.org/methods.*

Behara, M., & Lucidi, R. (2016). Abnormal (dysfunctional) uterine bleeding medication. Medscape drugs and diseases. Available: *http://emedicine.medscape.com/article/257007-medication.*

Centers for Disease Control and Prevention. (2015). *Sexually transmitted diseases treatment guidelines.* Atlanta, GA: author. Available: *www.cdc.gov/std/tg2015/default.htm.*

Columbo, N., Czeutzby, C., Amant, F., Bosse, T., González-Martín, A., Ledermann, J., ... Sessa, C. (2016). ESMO-ESGO-ESTRO consensus guidelines: ESMO-ESGO-ESTRO consensus conference on endometrial cancer: Diagnosis, treatment and follow-up. *International Journal of Gynecological Cancer, 26*(1), 2–30.

Crull, J., Mayer, D., & Jessup, A. (2014). Early detection of ovarian cancer. *Women's Healthcare: A Clinical Journal for Nurse Practitioners, 2*(1), 8–31.

Dunselman, G. A., Vermeulen, N., Becker, C., Calhaz-Jorge, C., D'Hooghe, T., De Bie, B., … Nelen W.. (2014). European Society for Human Reproduction and Embryology: Management of women with endometriosis. *Human Reproduction, 29*, 400–412.

Hofmeister, S. & Bodden, S. (2016). Premenstrual syndrome and premenstrual dysphoric disorder. *American Family Physician, 94*(3), 236–240.

Khan, A., Fortier, M., Reid, R., & Menopause and Osteoporosis Working Group. (2014). Society of Obstetricians and Gynaecolgoists of Canada Clinical practice guideline: Osteoporosis in menopause. *Journal of Obstetrics and Gynaecology Canada, 36*(9), 839–840.

Lein, D. A. & Poth, M. A. (2013). Amenorrhea: An approach to diagnosis and management. *American Family Physician, 87*(11), 781–787.

Meites, E., Kempe, A., & Markowitz, L. E. (2016). Use of a 2-dose schedule for human papillomavirus vaccination—Updated recommendations of the Advisory Committee on Immunization Practices. *Morbidity and Mortality Weekly Report, 65*, 1405–1408.

Nanette, S., Epperson, N., & Matthews, S. (2015). Menopausal symptoms and their management. *Postmenopausal Endocrinology, Endocrinology and Metabolism Clinics of North America, 44*(3), 497–515.

National Cancer Institute. (2017). *Vulvar cancer treatment (PDQ).* Bethesda, MD: Author. Available: *http://cancer.gov/cancertopics/pdq/treatment/vulvar/HealthProfessional.*

National Cancer Institute. (2017). *PDQ cervical cancer treatment.* Bethesda, MD: Author. Available: *www.cancer.gov/cancertopics/pdq/treatment/cervical/HealthProfessional.*

National Cancer Institute. (2017). *Endometrial cancer treatment (PDQ).* Bethesda, MD: Author. Available: *www.cancer.gov/cancertopics/pdq/treatment/endometrial/HealthProfessional.*

National Center for Complimentary and Integrative Health. (2016). *Herbs at a glance.* Bethesda, MD: Author. Available: *nccih.nih.gov/health/herbsataglance.htm.*

National Collaborating Centre for Women's and Children's Health. (2015). *Menopause: diagnosis and management.* London (UK): National Institute for Health and Care Excellence (NICE); 2015 Nov 12. 29 p. (NICE guideline; no. 23).

National Collaborating Centre for Women's and Children's Health. (2016). *Heavy menstrual bleeding.* London (UK): National Institute for Health and Care Excellence (NICE). NICE Clinical Guideline 44. Available: *https://pathways.nice.org.uk/pathways/heavy-menstrual-bleeding.*

North American Menopause Society. (2017). The 2017 hormone therapy position statement of the North American Menopause Society. *Menopause, 24*(7), 728–753.

Nyirjesy, I. (2015). *Conization of cervix treatment and management. Medscape Drugs and Diseases.* New York: WebMD. Available: *http://emedicine.medscape.com/article/270156-treatment#a1133.*

Saslow, D., Solomon, D., Lawson, H. W., Killackey, M., Kulasingam, S. L., Cain, J., … Myers, E. R. (2012). American Cancer Society, American Society for Colposcopy and Cervical Pathology, and American Society for Clinical Pathology screening guidelines for the prevention and early detection of cervical cancer. *CA—Cancer Journal for Clinicians, 62*, 147–172.

Smith, R. & Kaunitz, A. (2016). *Treatment of primary dysmenorrhea in adult women. Up to Date.* New York: Wolters Kluwer. Available: *www.uptodate.com/contents/treatment-of-primary-dysmenorrhea-in-adult-women.*

Stevens, D. (2016). *Treatment of streptococcal toxic shock syndrome. Up to Date.* New York: Wolters Kluwer. Available: *www.uptodate.com/contents/treatment-of-streptococcal-toxic-shock-syndrome.*

U.S. Preventive Services Task Force. (2016). *U.S. Preventive Services Task Force Issues New Cervical Cancer Screening Recommendations.* Rockville, MD: Author. Available: *www.uspreventiveservicestaskforce.org/Page/Name/us-preventive-services-task-force-issues-new-cervical-cancer-screening-recommendations.*

U.S. Preventive Services Task Force. (2017). Hormone Therapy for the Primary Prevention of Chronic Conditions in Postmenopausal Women. U.S. Preventive Services Task Force Recommendation Statement. *JAMA, 318*, 2224–2233.

Welt, C. (2015). *Physiology of the normal menstrual cycle. UpToDate.* New York: Wolters Kluwer. Available: *www.uptodate.com.*

23
Breast Conditions

OVERVIEW AND ASSESSMENT

 See additional online content: Procedure Guidelines 23-1

Subjective Data

Obtain a nursing history about specific breast complaints and general health information from the patient to plan care and appropriate patient teaching.

Breast Manifestations

1. Palpable lumps—date noted; affected by menstruation; changes noted since detection.
2. Nipple discharge—date of onset, color, unilateral or bilateral, spontaneous or provoked.
3. Pain or tenderness—localized or diffuse, cyclic or constant, unilateral or bilateral.
4. Date of last mammogram and result.
5. Patient's practice of breast self-examination (BSE).

History

General Information
1. Age.
2. Past medical–surgical history; injuries; bleeding tendencies.
3. Medications, including current or prior use of hormonal contraceptives and hormones, over-the-counter (OTC) products, vitamins, and herbal supplements.

Gynecologic and Obstetric History
1. Menarche.
2. Date of last menses.
3. Pregnancies, miscarriages, abortions, deliveries.
4. Lactation history.
5. Prior breast history, including previous history of irradiation involving breast region.
6. Family history of breast cancer.

Examination and Screening

Perform a breast examination for any breast complaint and teach patient how to examine breasts, if desired. Although research has not

shown that screening breast exams by a health professional or self-breast exams are effective in reducing mortality, examination should be done for any breast complaint. Screening breast exam may also allow women to become more comfortable and familiar with their own bodies. Mammography is the primary breast cancer screening method.

1. If a woman chooses to examine breasts once per month, exam is best done just after the menstrual period, because breasts are less engorged and a tumor is easier to detect, and at regular monthly intervals after the cessation of menses.
2. Compare inspection and palpation findings with the opposite breast.
3. Remind patient that 90% of breast lumps are not cancerous.
4. Do not neglect men when there is a breast complaint—1% of breast cancers occur in men.
5. It is acceptable for women to choose not to do BSE or to do BSE irregularly.

 GERONTOLOGIC ALERT Normal breast changes in older patients include drooping, flaccid breasts caused by decreased subcutaneous tissue from decreased estrogen levels. Nipple size and erection are also reduced.

Guidelines for Early Detection

 EVIDENCE BASE Smith, R., Andrews, K., Brooks, D., et al. (2017). Cancer screening in the United States, 2017: A review of current American Cancer Society guidelines and issues in cancer screening. *CA—A Cancer Journal for Clinicians*, 67, 100–121.

Meneses, K. (2016). When should I have a mammogram? Recent changes in ACS mammography guidelines: Implications for practice. *Journal of the Advanced Practitioner in Oncology*, 7, 567–570.

Women at Average Risk
1. Recommendations vary by organization.
2. American Cancer Society recommends women begin annual mammography at age 45, biennial at age 55, but should be available to women at age 40, and continue as long as life

expectancy is projected to be 10 years or longer. Because of lack of evidence, clinical breast exam and breast self-exam are no longer recommended.

3. National Comprehensive Cancer Network, American College of Obstetricians and Gynecologists, and the American College of Radiology recommend women should have annual mammographic screening beginning at age 40.

4. U.S. Preventive Services recommends women aged 50 to 74 undergo biennial screening mammography and end screening at age 75. Clinical breast exam is not recommended after age 40.

Older Women

1. Screening decisions in older women should be individualized by considering the potential benefits and risks of mammography in the context of current health status and estimated life expectancy. As long as a woman is in reasonably good health and would be a candidate for treatment, she should continue to be screened with mammography.

 GERONTOLOGIC ALERT Many older women may not be aware of newer treatments for breast cancer and may fear radical mastectomy, therefore avoiding breast cancer screening. Provide information about incidence, screening, and treatment and encourage discussion with a health care provider.

Women at Increased Risk

 EVIDENCE BASE Himes, D. O., Root, A. E., Gammon, A., et al. (2016). Breast cancer assessment: Calculating lifetime risk using the Tyrer-Cuzick model. *Journal for Nurse Practitioners, 12,* 581–592.

1. Women at increased risk for breast cancer might benefit from additional screening strategies beyond those offered to women of average risk, such as earlier initiation of screening, shorter screening intervals, or the addition of screening modalities other than mammography and physical examination, such as ultrasound or magnetic resonance imaging (MRI).

2. Screening MRI is recommended for women with an approximately 20% to 25% or greater lifetime risk of developing breast cancer, including women with a strong family history of breast or ovarian cancer, women who were treated for Hodgkin disease, women with a history of LCIS or atypical hyperplasia, and those with a prior history of breast cancer. Annual MRI should be considered in these women. Several models exist that attempt to calculate lifetime risk of breast cancer for women with identifiable factors associated with the disease. The Gail model, the Tyrer-Cuzick model, and the Claus model are examples of risk prevention models that estimate risk of breast cancer based on family history and other characteristics. These and a variety of other evidence based studies and risk calculators can be found on the National Institutes of Health, Division of Cancer Control and Population Sciences webpage *https://epi.grants.cancer.gov/cancer_risk_prediction/breast.html.*

Laboratory Tests

Nipple Discharge Cytology

Description

Secretions are smeared on a slide, fixed, and submitted for cytologic examination. There is a high rate of false-negative test results with this method.

Nursing and Patient Care Considerations

1. Wash nipple area with water and pat dry before obtaining specimen if crusting of drainage is present.

2. Gently milk breast or ask woman to express fluid to obtain a large drop on nipple.

3. Carefully touch slide to drop and draw slide across nipple to obtain smear. Spray with fixative or drop into container with fixative.

4. Inform patient of results promptly to reduce anxiety and explain that other tests may be needed.

Ductal Lavage

Description

A procedure that targets asymptomatic women at increased risk for breast cancer. Breast duct epithelial cells are collected from the nipple for cytological analysis.

Nursing and Patient Care Considerations

Advise patient to discuss questions with health care provider. This test is not widely used, and there are insufficient data at this time to recommend its use for screening.

Tumor-Specific Tests

Tests to evaluate the characteristics of a tumor and/or its potential to regrow.

1. Estrogen and progesterone receptors identify patients most likely to benefit from hormonal forms of therapy. Approximately 75% are estrogen receptor positive. A negative result is associated with a less favorable prognosis.

2. HER2—human epidermal growth factor receptor that has been demonstrated in 15% to 30% of breast cancers. Found by many investigators to be associated with poorer survival, regardless of clinical stage. May affect treatment decisions.

3. Histologic grade is reported using an Elston-Ellis modification of the Scarff-Bloom-Richardson Scale. It is a combination of nuclear grade, mitotic rate, and tubule formation with scores given for each. A low score equates to a low grade (grade I), and a higher score to a higher grade (grade III). In general, high-grade tumors are more likely to recur when compared to low-grade tumors.

4. Multiparameter gene assays (eg, Oncotype DX and MammaPrint) quantify the likelihood of distant breast cancer recurrence and measure how chemotherapy may assist with planning treatment. The Oncotype DX assay is included in the National Comprehensive Cancer Network guideline treatment decision pathway. Breast cancer diagnostic and treatment guidelines are available at *www.nccn.org.* A similar assay for ductal carcinoma in situ (DCIS) continues under investigation. Results provide estimates of local recurrence risk and may help to select patients who are candidates for minimal therapy and may change radiotherapy recommendations. There is currently controversy regarding the overtreatment of DCIS.

5. Cancer subtyping—as determined by gene expression profiling—is currently under investigation.

6. Pathologists may use other special stains to aid in diagnosis.

Tests to Detect Metastasis

1. Increased values on liver function tests may indicate possible liver metastasis.

2. Increased calcium and alkaline phosphatase levels may indicate possible bony metastasis.

3. Additional metastatic workup may include chest x-ray, bone scan, computed tomography (CT) scan, and positron emission tomography (PET) scan.
4. Biological markers (ie, CA15.3 and CA27.29) may be used for monitoring patients with metastatic disease in conjunction with diagnostic imaging, history, and physical examination. Present data are insufficient to recommend their use alone for screening, diagnosis, or staging. However, they may be used to indicate treatment failure.

Radiology and Imaging

Mammography

Description

1. Low-dose x-ray of breast used to screen for breast abnormalities or may be used when a lump is found on physical examination. Can detect patients with clustered microcalcifications.
2. Compression of the breast is used to reduce the amount of radiation absorbed by the breast tissue and separate overlapping tissue.
3. Two views are taken routinely: craniocaudal and mediolateral; other views are done as necessary.
4. Best performed at a facility that is accredited by the American College of Radiology. The machines and staff at these facilities have met specific criteria. Computer-aided detection has been developed to aid radiologists in detecting abnormalities. Assessment categories have been developed to describe the results and provide follow-up recommendations. A category 0 is incomplete and needs additional images.
   a. Category 1 is a negative result (normal mammogram) with nothing on which to comment.
   b. Category 2 is a normal mammogram, but there is a benign finding on which to comment.
   c. Category 3 is probably benign, but short-interval follow-up may be recommended to determine stability of the finding.
   d. Category 4 describes a suspicious abnormality, and biopsy should be considered.
   e. Category 5 is highly suggestive of malignancy; appropriate action should be taken.
   f. Category 6 describes a known, biopsy-proven malignancy requiring appropriate action.
5. Mammography is not routinely done if a woman is pregnant.
6. The breasts of young women tend to be extremely dense and are poorly suited to mammography.
7. False-negative results occur even in the best facilities; figure may reach 10%.
8. Both screen film and digital mammography use x-rays to obtain images. With digital mammography, a film image is replaced with an electronic image similar to digital photography. For younger women under age 50, women with radiographically dense breasts, and premenopausal and perimenopausal women, digital mammography is more accurate than film mammography and thus has supplanted film mammography as the technology of choice. Digital tomosynthesis creates a three-dimensional picture of the breasts that may make breast cancers easier to see, and adding tomosynthesis has increased breast cancer detection and decreased false-positive results.

 EVIDENCE BASE American College of Radiology. (2013). *BI-RAD Atlas* (5th ed.). Reston, VA: Author. Available: *www.acr.org*.

Nursing and Patient Care Considerations

1. Recommend regular screening based on established guidelines (see page 678). Tell patients that routine screening mammography has been shown to reduce mortality from breast cancer. Procedure takes approximately 15 minutes.
2. Remind patients not to apply deodorant, cream, or powder to breast, nipple, or underarm areas on examination day.
3. Advise that some discomfort may be felt from compressing the breast.
4. Patients should have an opportunity to become informed about the benefits, limitations, and potential harms associated with regular screening. Overdiagnosis of clinically insignificant disease is possible. Benefits are thought to outweigh the exposure to low dose of radiation.
5. Alert patient that extra views do not imply that the patient has breast cancer.

 NURSING ALERT Because health teaching is an important nursing role, nurses should educate women about the importance of routine screening. Because of differences in screening guidelines, women may also need advice regarding the timing of mammograms.

Community Health Education

Implement patient teaching of importance of screening on a community level by:

1. Reinforcing that early detection is associated with decreased mortality.
2. Helping patients and families establish and maintain support networks.
3. Tailoring patient education messages to patients of different cultures.
4. Knowing the resources available and making people aware of them.
   a. National Cancer Institute—answers questions and provides booklets about cancer. Call 800-4-CANCER or go to *www.cancer.gov*.
   b. American Cancer Society—offers many services to patients and their families. Call 800-ACS-2345 for local chapter or go to *www.cancer.org*.
   c. Susan G. Komen Foundation at *www.komen.org*.

Ultrasonography

Description

1. Uses high-frequency sound waves to get an image of the breast.
2. Helps determine if a lump is a cyst or a solid mass.
3. May be used if patient is pregnant or is younger than age 35.

Nursing and Patient Care Considerations

1. Advise that this test is painless and noninvasive.
2. No preparation is necessary.

Galactography/Ductogram

1. A contrast mammogram is obtained by injection of water-soluble contrast medium into a duct for patient with persistent bloody nipple discharge. It is a time-consuming procedure that is not routinely used.
2. It may outline an intraductal papilloma.
3. Its ability to differentiate benign from malignant lesions is limited.
4. Thermography, infrared imaging of the breasts, cannot locate small, deep cancers and remains under investigation.

Magnetic Resonance Imaging

1. Produces images from the combination of a magnetic field, radio waves, and computer processing.
2. May be used in newly diagnosed breast cancer patients for presurgical planning. May help in determining extent of disease, multifocality, and unsuspected disease in the contralateral breast, and after neoadjuvant chemotherapy, may help to downstage a patient and possibly decrease the magnitude of the planned procedure.
3. Useful in high-risk women, those with dense breasts, and in those with silicone implants.
4. Because MRI is less accessible and more expensive than mammography, it is not useful for generalized screening. There may be increased false-positive results.
5. See page 166 for description of MRI.

Other Tests

In addition to laboratory tests and imaging studies, biopsy methods are commonly used to evaluate breast conditions. A biopsy is the only certain way to learn whether a breast lump or suspicious area seen on a mammogram is cancerous.

Fine Needle Aspiration

Description

1. Uses a thin needle and syringe to collect tissue or to drain lump after using a local anesthetic. If it is a cyst, removing the fluid will collapse it; no other treatment may be needed. Ultrasound may be used to locate a nonpalpable cyst.
2. Normal cyst fluid appears straw-colored or greenish. Fluid should be sent for cytology if it appears suspicious (clear or bloody); otherwise, it is discarded.
3. This office procedure uses local anesthetic with results usually within 24 hours.
4. It has limited sensitivity, possibly because of insufficient acquisition of cytologic material.

Nursing and Patient Care Considerations

1. Inform patient of small risk of hematoma and infection.
2. Adhesive bandage applied after procedure; usually no discomfort.
3. Solid lesions may warrant an excisional biopsy.

Needle Biopsy

Description

1. Office procedure uses local anesthetic and removes a small piece of breast tissue using a needle with a special cutting edge.
2. For palpable lesions with a high suspicion of malignancy. May provide a tissue diagnosis quickly—usually approximately 24 hours—without doing an excisional biopsy to plan definitive surgery.
3. Ultrasound guidance may be used for nonpalpable lesions.

Nursing and Patient Care Considerations

1. Inform patient of small risk of hematoma and infection.
2. Tell patient that several passes may be necessary to obtain specimen, with minor discomfort.
3. Pressure dressing applied after procedure.
4. Recommend use of acetaminophen or ibuprofen for postprocedure discomfort—usually minimal, if any.

Stereotactic Core Needle Biopsy

Description

1. An x-ray–guided method for localizing and sampling nonpalpable lesions detected on mammography with 90% to 95% sensitivity in detecting breast cancer.

2. Performed as an outpatient procedure with the patient lying prone on a special table using an automated biopsy gun with a vacuum system to draw tissue into a sampling chamber and rotate cutter to excise tissue. There may be a weight limit for this table.
3. After local anesthetic is administered, a needle is placed in the lesion with confirmation of its position on stereotactic x-ray views. Multiple samples are taken from different portions of the lesion. Allows harvesting of larger quantities of tissue with a single needle insertion. A tiny clip may be left in place at the end of the procedure to mark the area.
4. The procedure is quicker and less expensive than mammographically guided needle localization followed by surgical excisional biopsy and is an alternative to surgical excisional biopsy to make a diagnosis.

Nursing and Patient Care Considerations

1. Inform patient that it is a 1-hour outpatient procedure that requires no special preparation.
2. The patient should dress comfortably and will need to remain still during the procedure.
3. Complications may include minor bleeding, hematoma, and infection.
4. Explain that nonspecific, suspicious, or atypical findings may result in proceeding to excisional biopsy.
5. Remind patient that area in question will not be removed, only sampled.

Note: Many nonpalpable abnormalities that require breast biopsy are being identified because of increased use of screening mammography.

Excisional Biopsy

Description

1. Surgical removal of a palpable or nonpalpable lesion. A frozen section may be done for immediate tissue diagnosis.
2. Excisional biopsy or lumpectomy entails entire removal of a mass; incisional biopsy entails partial removal of a mass.
3. This outpatient procedure may be performed under local or general anesthesia.
4. Curvilinear incision is usually made directly over the mass, which is excised en bloc including a 1-cm grossly free margin of tissue.
5. Tumor ablation with insertion of a probe percutaneously that destroys cancer cells by freezing, heating, or with radiofrequency has been attempted; however, existing evidence is inadequate to recommend ablation as an alternative to surgical excision.

Nursing and Patient Care Considerations

1. Pressure dressing is placed, which can be removed in 24 to 48 hours.
2. Inform patient to watch for bleeding, hematoma, and signs of infection.
3. Recommend analgesics for discomfort and a support bra for comfort.
4. May take several days to get results, a stressful time for patients.

Needle Localization with Biopsy

Description

1. Performed when there is a nonpalpable mammographic finding.
2. Mammogram is used as a guide for placing a needle at the site of the breast change after injecting some local anesthetic.

3. A wire may be left in place for the surgeon, and dye may be injected to mark the site.
4. Excisional biopsy is then done (see above) removing the area around the tip of the wire.

Nursing and Patient Care Considerations

Inform patient that this may be a tedious procedure because she must remain immobile as the breast is compressed in the mammogram machine or stereotactic table and views are obtained.

Sentinel Lymph Node Biopsy

Description

1. A diagnostic surgical procedure utilizing selective lymph node sampling.
2. Pathologic study of the first (sentinel) axillary lymph node to receive drainage from a tumor; predicts the status of the remainder of the lymph nodes in the axilla.
3. Localization accomplished by injection of a blue dye and/or radioactive particles around a tumor to identify lymph nodes with afferent drainage.
4. The excised sentinel lymph nodes are subjected to routine pathologic examination and, possibly, immunohistochemical staining to detect micrometastasis.
5. The status of the sentinel lymph node is used to determine whether to proceed with full axillary dissection and/or determine treatment modalities.
6. If the sentinel lymph node tests negative, no further axillary surgery is indicated.
7. If test result is positive, further axillary dissection may be needed. However, in women undergoing breast-conserving surgery and having fewer than three involved lymph nodes, completion axillary lymph node dissection may be omitted per American Society of Clinical Oncology guidelines with no difference in overall survival.

 EVIDENCE BASE Morrow, M. (2018). Management of the node-positive axilla in breast cancer in 2017: selecting the right option. *JAMA Oncology, 4*(2), 250–251.

Nursing and Patient Care Considerations

1. This is a reliable procedure, which is usually performed at the same time as definitive surgery—in conjunction with a breast-preserving procedure or mastectomy.
2. There is less morbidity and cost than with axillary dissection.

GENERAL PROCEDURES AND TREATMENT MODALITIES

 See additional online content: Patient Education Guidelines 23-1: Breast Self Exam

Surgery for Breast Cancer

Surgery for breast cancer may involve *mastectomy* or a *breast-preserving procedure*. The objective of breast-preserving procedures is a cosmetically acceptable breast after complete excision of the tumor. Research studies that compare breast conservation with mastectomy have demonstrated equivalent patient survival. Contraindications to breast conservation include multifocal disease; diffuse, extensive DCIS; inability to tolerate radiation therapy; and persistent positive margins. The evolving field of oncoplastic surgery uses techniques to allow the removal of large volumes of breast tissue while avoiding deformity. Although mastectomy rates have remained stable, risk-reducing contralateral prophylactic mastectomy has risen. See Table 23-1 for the surgical approach options that are available. The following discussion covers mastectomy and axillary node dissection.

Table 23-1	Types of Surgery for Breast Cancer	
PROCEDURE	**DESCRIPTION**	**INDICATIONS**
Lumpectomy (excisional biopsy)	Removal of tumor and surrounding tissue	For diagnosis of an abnormal mammographic finding or palpable breast lump if needle biopsy not performed. Further surgery may be needed.
Quadrantectomy (partial mastectomy)	Removal of a breast quadrant that includes the tumor area and possibly overlying skin	Normal- to large-sized breasts. Usually done at the same time as axillary surgery.
Sentinel lymph node biopsy	Removal of only a few gatekeeper lymph nodes	Performed to predict status of lymph nodes—if negative for tumor, axillary dissection is not performed. May be done in conjunction with quadrantectomy or mastectomy.
Axillary dissection	Surgical removal of the axillary lymph nodes	Performed when lymph node is positive for tumor, mainly for prognosis, staging, and locoregional disease control.
Simple mastectomy*	Surgical removal of the entire breast	Large or multifocal tumors; women with very small breasts in whom local excision of tumor will be cosmetically unacceptable; ineligibility for radiation therapy; patient preference; prophylaxis.
Modified radical mastectomy*	Surgical removal of the entire breast and the axillary lymph nodes (simple mastectomy plus axillary dissection)	Positive lymph nodes; advanced disease.
Radical mastectomy*	Removal of entire breast, pectoral muscles, axillary nodes	Rarely done today—may be performed for advanced disease.

*Mastectomy may be followed by immediate or delayed reconstruction.

Preoperative Management

See Chapter 7 for routine preoperative care. In addition:
1. The nature of the procedure is explained, along with expected postoperative care that includes drain care, location of the incision, and mobility of the arm.
2. Information is clarified about diagnosis and possibility of further therapy.
3. Measures are taken to recognize the extreme anxiety and fear that the patient, family, and significant others experience.
   a. Discuss patient's concerns and usual coping mechanisms.
   b. Explore support systems with patient.
   c. Discuss concerns regarding body image changes.
4. Evaluate the patient's overall medical condition to guide preoperative care, help determine how well the patient will tolerate surgery, and help prepare for complications that may occur postoperatively.

 GERONTOLOGIC ALERT Assessment of preoperative mental status of the older patient will help determine if a cognitive change occurs postoperatively.

Potential Complications

1. Infection.
2. Hematoma, seroma.
3. Lymphedema.
4. Paresthesia, pain of axilla and arm.
5. Impaired mobility of arm.

Postoperative Management and Nursing Care

See Chapter 7 for routine postoperative care. In addition:
1. Dressing is removed and the wound is assessed for erythema, hematoma (fluid under incision), edema, tenderness, odor, and drainage. Report suspected hematoma promptly.
   a. Initial dressing may consist of gauze held in place by elastic, tape, or clear occlusive dressing wrap.
   b. Usually removed within 24 hours.
   c. Incision may remain open to air or elastic wrap may be replaced if patient prefers.
2. Suction drain from wound is maintained.
   a. May have 100 to 200 mL serous to serosanguineous drainage in the first 24 hours.
   b. Report if grossly bloody or excessive in amount.
3. Arm on affected side is observed for edema, erythema, and pain.
4. Patient teaching about drain care, exercises, and surgical outcome occurs.
5. Breast cancer surveillance of female relatives, especially sisters, daughters, and mother, is discussed.

 NURSING ALERT Mastectomy patients may have an elastic wrap bandage that should fit snugly but not so tightly that it hinders respiration. It should fit comfortably and support unaffected breast.

Nursing Diagnoses

- Impaired Physical Mobility related to impaired movement of arm on operative side.
- Deficient Knowledge related to care of incision, drain, and arm.
- Ineffective Tissue Perfusion of affected arm related to lymphedema.
- Disturbed Body Image related to loss of breast (for mastectomy patient).
- Anxiety related to diagnosis of cancer.
- Sexual Dysfunction related to loss of breast and diagnosis of breast cancer.
- Compromised Family Coping related to diagnosis of cancer.

Nursing Interventions

In addition to routine postoperative interventions, provide the following care.

Mobilizing Affected Arm
1. Assess patient's ability to perform self-care and factors impeding performance.
2. Encourage wrist and elbow flexion and extension initially. Encourage use of arm for washing face, combing hair, applying lipstick, and brushing teeth. Encourage patient to gradually increase use of arm.
3. Encourage patient to avoid abduction initially to help prevent seroma formation.
4. Support arm in sling, if prescribed, to prevent abduction of the arm.
5. Instruct and provide patient with exercises to do when permitted (see Table 23-2).

Increasing Knowledge
1. Explain how wound will gradually change and that the newly healed wound may have less sensation because of severed nerves.
2. Instruct patient on signs of infection, hematoma, or seroma formation to be reported.
3. Teach patient to bathe incision gently and to blot carefully to dry, and later, with approval, massage the healed incision gently with cocoa butter to encourage circulation and increase skin elasticity.
4. Teach care of drains, if appropriate; empty contents, measure, and record.
5. Teach importance of BSE, mammograms, and regular follow-up visits.
6. Encourage discussion with health care provider about pregnancy after breast cancer, if indicated.

 GERONTOLOGIC ALERT Signs and symptoms of infection may not be obvious in older patients. Assess patients for mental status changes or urinary incontinence.

Promoting Lymphatic Drainage
1. Instruct patient in potential problem of lymphedema of the arm, when lymph fluid collects in the arm. At particular risk are patients who undergo axillary node dissection in combination with radiation therapy to axilla. There is decreased risk when sentinel lymph node biopsy only is performed. Explain that lymphedema may occur years postoperatively. May present as arm heaviness, decreased flexibility, aching, or swelling.
2. Do not take blood pressure, draw blood, inject medications, or start intravenous lines in affected arm. Post sign over bed.
3. Elevate affected arm on pillows, above level of heart, and hand above elbow to promote gravity drainage of fluid.
4. Teach patient to massage affected arm, if prescribed, which will increase circulation and decrease edema. Treatment for

Table 23-2	Exercises for the Rehabilitation of the Patient Following Mastectomy

EXERCISE	EQUIVALENT DAILY ACTIVITIES
1. Stand erect. • Lean forward at waist. • Allow arms to hang. • Swing arms from side to side together, then in opposite direction. • Next, swing arms from front to back together, then in opposite direction.	• Broom sweeping • Vacuum cleaning • Mopping floor • Pulling out and pushing in drawers • Weaving • Playing golf
2. Stand erect facing wall with palms flat against wall, arms extended. • Relax arms and shoulders and allow upper part of body to lean forward against hands. • Push away to original position; repeat.	• Pushing self out of bath tub • Kneading bread • Breaststroke—swimming • Sawing or cutting types of crafts
3. Stand erect facing wall with palms flat against wall. • Climb the wall with the fingers; descend, repeat.	• Raising windows • Washing windows • Hanging clothes on line • Reaching to an upper shelf
4. Stand erect and clasp hands at small of back; raise hands; lower; repeat. • Clasp hands back of neck; reach downward; upward; repeat.	• Fastening brassiere • Buttoning blouse or dress • Pulling up a dress zipper • Fastening beads • Washing the back
5. Toss a rope over a shower curtain rod. • Hold the ends of the rope (knotted) in each hand and alternately pull on each end. • Using a seesaw motion and with arms outstretched, slide the rope up and down over the rod.	• Drying the back with a bath towel • Raising and lowering a window blind • Closing and opening window drapes
6. Flex and extend each finger in turn.	• Sewing, knitting, crocheting • Typing, painting, playing piano or other musical instrument

severe lymphedema may also include the application of elastic bandages and/or intermittent pneumatic compression. Compressive sleeves and exercises may be recommended to prevent lymphedema.

5. Teach patient care of the affected arm to prevent lymphedema and infection.

 EVIDENCE BASE American Cancer Society. (2018). Lymphedema. Available: *www.cancer.org/treatment/ treatments-and-side-effects/physical-side-effects/ lymphedema.html.*

Enhancing Body Image

1. Assess mastectomy patient's knowledge of prosthesis and reconstruction options and provide information, as needed.
2. Discuss patient's views on her altered body image.
3. Suggest clothing adjustments to camouflage loss of breast.
4. Assist patient to obtain a temporary prosthesis (may be provided by Reach to Recovery [see below]). First prosthesis should be light and soft to allow incision to heal. She may wear heavier type usually 4 to 8 weeks after surgeon's approval has been secured. Provide information regarding where to obtain permanent prosthesis and bras.
5. Encourage patient to discuss feelings with partner.
6. Encourage patient to allow herself to experience the grief process over the loss of her breast and to learn to cope with these feelings.

Reducing Anxiety

1. Familiarize patient with Reach to Recovery (*www.cancer.org*, then click on Support Programs), an American Cancer Society program that consists of volunteers who have had mastectomies or breast-preserving procedures and who make postoperative hospital visits to provide support and information. Clear first with patient's care provider.
2. Discuss patient's usual coping mechanisms.
3. Encourage and assist family to support patient.
4. Assist patient to maintain control by planning care with her and incorporating her usual routines.
5. Refer patient for postmastectomy support group, as needed and desired.
6. Offer list of community resources.
7. Remind patient that stress related to breast cancer and mastectomy may persist for a year or more and to seek help.
8. Include family in supportive interventions and measures to increase coping skills.

Maintaining Sexual Activity

1. Discuss effect of diagnosis and surgery on view of self as a woman.
2. Explore alternative means of sexual activity, such as changing position during intercourse, to decrease pressure on incision.
3. Encourage patient to discuss concerns with partner.
4. Assist patient and partner to look at incision when ready.

Facilitating Family Coping

1. Allow family members to acknowledge their feelings.
2. Approach family with warmth, respect, and support.
3. Acknowledge family strengths.
4. Involve family in care of patient.
5. Discuss stresses.
6. Direct family to community agencies, as indicated.

Community and Home Care Considerations

Because of short stays (1 to 2 days) after mastectomy, many patients can achieve the following benefits from home care:

1. Assess incision and drain tubes for proper healing and no signs of infection.
2. Teach patient drain tube and dressing care.
3. Support patient with adjustment back into home and community.
4. Monitor for lymphedema and reinforce teaching about arm care and exercises.
5. Goals of home care for these patients are to provide assessment of cardiovascular status and to ensure return of energy and proper healing.

PATIENT EDUCATION GUIDELINES 23-1

Prevention of Lymphedema

To reduce the risk of lymphedema of your arm after the removal of lymph nodes, follow these general guidelines to prevent infection and obstruction of blood and lymph fluid.

- Take care of your skin to prevent dryness, cracking, and irritation that may lead to infection.
- Keep your arm clean and cover any open areas.
- Take care of your fingernails to avoid ripped cuticles and nails.
- Avoid using a razor for underarm hair removal.
- Protect hands and fingers from injury while gardening, sewing, cooking, and other chores.
- Avoid constricting clothing around arms.
- Avoid having blood drawn or needles inserted into affected arm.
- Avoid having blood pressure taken on affected arm.
- Prevent insect bites and stings through use of repellent and protective clothing.

For more information, refer to American Cancer Society (*www.cancer.org*).

TRANSITIONAL CARE ALERT Help identify those patients who may require longer hospitalizations and, possibly, a short stay in a subacute unit for rehabilitation to avoid readmission to the hospital. Factors that may be related to a delay in recovery include increased age, comorbid conditions, reduced nutritional status, infection, limited mobility, and limited support system or lack of presence of a caregiver.

Patient Education and Health Maintenance

1. Advise patient to call surgeon for signs of infection, increased pain, or edema of arm.
2. Make sure that patient knows schedule for follow-up with surgeon.
3. Provide resources for patient for ongoing information and support: The American Cancer Society (800-ACS-2345 or *www.cancer.org*) has numerous pages of information about surgery, nutrition and cancer, lymphedema, psychosocial issues, and other concerns.
4. Stress the importance of continued yearly mammogram.

Evaluation: Expected Outcomes

- Moves affected arm within prescribed limits.
- States care of incision, drains, and follow-up guidelines.
- No infection or swelling in affected arm.
- Expresses positive body image.
- Exhibits minimal anxiety.
- Reports satisfactory sexual activity and sexuality.
- Maintains a functional support system.

Breast Reconstruction After Mastectomy

Breast reconstruction (mammoplasty) may be performed at the same time as mastectomy (immediate) or as long after surgery as desired (delayed). Benefits include improved psychological coping because of improved body image and self-esteem. Cost is usually covered by insurance. Reconstruction selection is based on an assessment of cancer treatment, patient body type, smoking history, comorbidities, and patient concerns. An advantage of immediate reconstruction is a smaller scar through the use of a skin-sparing mastectomy. In general, the nipple–areolar complex is sacrificed with skin-sparing mastectomy. Nipple-sparing mastectomy may be an option for some women as well, especially those undergoing prophylactic mastectomy or those with a low nipple involvement rate. It appears to be a safe procedure for properly selected patients. Trials are warranted to determine the best incision and reconstruction methods. Reconstruction does not interfere with the detection of tumors.

 NURSING ALERT Because breast reconstruction does not affect disease recurrence or survival, the expectations and desires of the patient are paramount in the decision-making process. Collaboration among members of the breast cancer team is essential.

Implants

Indicated for patients with inadequate breast tissue and skin of good quality.

Description

1. Uses prosthetic implants placed in pocket under the skin or pectoralis muscle. A variety of implants are available that contain saline, silicone gel, or a combination of both.
2. If opposite breast is ptotic (protruding downward), mastopexy may be necessary for symmetry.
3. A dermal matrix may be used at surgery to help provide a foundation for the tissue expander and/or implant.
4. Complications include capsular contracture resulting in firmness; may be painful and cause infection.
5. Tissue expanders may be necessary before implants are inserted.
   a. Inflatable envelope is placed under muscle or skin and is filled with saline when incision is healed (about 4 weeks).
   b. Saline is instilled every 1 to 3 weeks until the expander is beyond desired size.
   c. Later, expander is removed and a permanent implant is placed.
   d. Some types of expanders may be left in permanently.
6. Advantages of implant reconstruction over other methods: only one incision; less fibrosis.
7. Disadvantages may take months and may not be as cosmetically pleasing as other methods.

Nursing and Patient Care Considerations
1. Teach signs and symptoms of infection, hematoma, migration, and deflation.
2. Teach patient to massage breast to decrease capsule formation around implant.
3. Teach patient she may feel discomfort with expanders, if used.

Flap Grafts

Description
1. Transfer of skin, muscle, and subcutaneous tissue from another part of the body to the mastectomy site.
2. Types:
   a. Latissimus dorsi—skin, fat, and muscles of back between shoulder blades—are tunneled under the skin to front of chest. Usually, an implant is also needed.
   b. Transverse rectus abdominis myocutaneous flap—muscle, fat, skin, and blood supply are tunneled to breast area.
   c. Perforator flap reconstruction, that is, deep inferior epigastric perforator (DIEP) or superior gluteal artery perforator (SGAP), uses tissue as above without using muscle. Because of its complexity, offered by few breast centers.
3. Disadvantages include cost, slow process (done in stages), and increased morbidity.
4. Complications include flap loss, hematoma, infection, seroma, and abdominal hernia.

 NURSING ALERT Smoking increases the risk of complications for all types of reconstruction. Patients who smoke should be made aware of increased rates of wound infections and healing complications.

Nursing and Patient Care Considerations
1. Assess flap and donor site for color, temperature, and wound drainage.
2. Control pain.
3. Provide support with bra or abdominal binder to maintain position of prosthesis.
4. Teach patient to perform BSE monthly and that she may have some asymmetry.

Nipple–Areolar Reconstruction
1. Usually done at a separate time from breast reconstruction.
2. Uses skin and fat from reconstructed breast for nipple and upper thigh for areola; tanning or tattoo done to obtain appropriate color.

Other Surgeries of the Breast

Reduction mammoplasty may be done for cosmetic purposes or to relieve uncomfortable symptoms. Augmentation mammoplasty is considered a cosmetic procedure.

Reduction Mammoplasty

Description
1. Removal of excess breast tissue, which also involves a reduction in skin and possible transposition of nipple–areolar complex.
2. Used for alleviation of symptoms that may include back and neck pain, muscle spasm, and grooving at the shoulders secondary to bra straps.

3. Complications include hematoma, infection, necrosis of skin flap, and nipple inversion.

Nursing and Patient Care Considerations
1. Explore reasons patient may desire surgery.
2. Discuss postoperative expectations with patient.
3. Nursing interventions are similar to those in patient undergoing reconstruction.

Augmentation Mammoplasty

Description
1. Enlarging of the breasts with the use of implants.
2. Implants may be made of silicone or saline. In most cases, this is a self-pay procedure if for cosmetic purpose.
3. Complications include hematoma, wound infection, diminished sensation of the nipple, and capsular contracture, resulting in firmness of the breast.
4. Breast implants are not associated with an increased incidence of breast cancer.

Nursing and Patient Care Considerations
1. Discuss patient's expectations preoperatively.
2. Nursing interventions are similar to those in the patient undergoing reconstruction with implants.

DISORDERS OF THE BREAST

See Standard of Care Guidelines 23-1, page 687.

Fissure of the Nipple

A *fissure* is a type of ulcer that develops in the nipple of a nursing mother.

Etiology and Clinical Manifestations
1. May be caused by lack of preparation of nipples in the prenatal period.
2. Condition aggravated by sucking infant.
3. Nipple appears sore and irritated.
4. Nipple bleeds.
5. Infection may result.

Management and Nursing Interventions
1. Wash nipples with sterile saline solution.
2. Use artificial nipple for nursing.
3. If above does not initiate healing process, stop nursing and use breast pump.
4. Teach proper breastfeeding techniques to prevent fissures.
   a. Wash, dry, and lubricate nipples in prenatal period in preparation for nursing.
   b. Make sure infant's mouth covers areola.
   c. Keep nipple clean by washing and drying after each nursing period.
   d. Use lanolin cream to prevent cracking; must remove before breastfeeding.

Nipple Discharge

Nipple discharge may be serous, serosanguineous, bloody, purulent, or multicolored. It is commonly associated with benign conditions; rarely, malignancy is responsible. It may be spontaneous or nonspontaneous (occurs only when breast is compressed), and it is important to differentiate between the two.

STANDARD OF CARE GUIDELINES 23-1
Problems of the Breast

When caring for any patient undergoing evaluation, diagnostic testing, treatment, or counseling for a breast-related problem, ensure optimal outcome by adhering to the following guidelines:

- Explain the mammogram procedure or other diagnostic test and make sure patient knows when and how she will obtain results.
- Perform breast examination according to American Cancer Society guidelines.
- Inform health care provider and patient of any suspicious findings on breast examination—asymmetry of breasts, dimpling, skin changes, nipple discharge, fixed or hard mass.
- Inform health care provider and patient of abnormal mammogram or other test result and make sure that follow-up is arranged.

After Surgery for Breast Cancer
- Assess for evidence of bleeding from the incision or flaps, including increase in pain, and notify surgeon promptly for increased pain or bleeding.
- Assess drainage from suction drain for amount, color, and odor. Report if grossly bloody, purulent, or excessive in amount (may have 100 to 200 mL in the first 24 hours).
- Assess newly reconstructed breast flaps for viability by color, warmth, and wound drainage. Notify surgeon promptly for increased warmth, change in color, purulent or excessive drainage.
- Maintain proper protective positioning (avoid abduction to prevent edema) of arm and follow precautions for lymphedema.
- Assess patient's emotional response and provide support throughout the diagnostic and treatment process.

This information should serve as a general guideline only. Each patient situation presents a unique set of clinical factors and requires nursing judgment to guide care, which may include additional or alternative measures and approaches.

Etiology and Clinical Manifestations

1. Galactorrhea—bilateral, nonspontaneous, multiple ducts, milky gray or green discharge usually seen in patients in childbearing years.
   a. Commonly seen after pregnancy and can last for 1 to 2 years.
   b. May also be secondary to excessive breast manipulation, increased production of prolactin, medication, an endocrine anovulatory syndrome, or pituitary adenoma.
2. Mastitis—usually unilateral, purulent (see below).
3. Discharge containing blood—usually caused by intraductal papilloma (wart) or other benign lesion but, in rare cases, may be malignant.

Diagnostic Evaluation

1. Evaluate a spontaneous nipple discharge with clinical examination, test for occult blood, mammography, and/or ultrasonography. MRI is not usually helpful.
   a. Use of a Hemoccult card gently pressed against the nipple when expressing discharge will help determine if the discharge is bloody, which warrants further workup.
   b. May get prolactin level; if elevated, may indicate pituitary adenoma.
2. Nonspontaneous milky gray or green discharge generally is not of pathologic significance and may not require workup.

Management and Nursing Interventions

1. Nursing interventions are aimed at alleviating anxiety and providing support to patient undergoing diagnostic testing. Reassure woman that nipple discharge rarely indicates cancer.
2. Bromocriptine may be given to suppress galactorrhea.
3. Treat for mastitis if purulent (see below).
4. Surgery may be indicated to treat cause of bloody and some other discharges caused by breast lesions.
   a. Most commonly because of wartlike intraductal papilloma in one of larger collecting ducts at edge of areola. May be secondary to fibrocystic changes or duct ectasia.
   b. Excisional biopsy and histologic examination may be done to rule out cancer.
   c. Ductoscopy, an image-guided excision using direct visualization of the ductal system and an intraductal biopsy, is being investigated at some larger centers.
5. Pituitary surgery for excision of adenoma (see page 707).

Acute Mastitis

Acute mastitis is inflammation of the breast secondary to infection. Breast infections may be lactational or nonlactational.

Pathophysiology and Etiology

1. Lactational infections usually occur at beginning of lactation in first-time, breastfeeding mothers. May also occur later in chronic lactation mastitis and central duct abscesses.
2. Milk stasis may lead to obstruction, followed by noninfectious inflammation, then infectious mastitis.
3. Source of infection may be from hands of patient, personnel caring for patient, baby's nose or throat, or blood-borne.
4. Nonlactational infections usually present with central subareolar inflammation.
5. Most common pathogens: *Staphylococcus aureus*, *Escherichia coli*, and *Streptococcus*.

Clinical Manifestations

1. Redness, warmth, edema; breast may feel doughy and tough. Fever may be present.
2. Patient may complain of dull pain in affected area and may have nipple discharge.
3. Complication is mammary abscess (see below).

Management and Nursing Interventions

1. Diagnosis is usually made by characteristic manifestations.
2. Antibiotics are given—10- to 14-day course of penicillinase-resistant antibiotic.
   a. Dicloxacillin—250 to 500 mg every 6 hours.
   b. Clindamycin—150 to 300 mg every 6 hours.
   c. Amoxicillin clavulanate 500 mg three times daily or 875 mg twice daily.
3. May have patient stop breastfeeding (controversial).

4. Apply heat to resolve tissue reaction; may cause increased milk production and worsen symptoms.
5. May apply cold to decrease tissue metabolism and milk production.
6. Have the patient wear firm breast support.
7. Encourage the breastfeeding patient to practice meticulous personal hygiene to prevent mastitis.
8. Consider lactation consult.

Mammary Abscess

Mammary abscess is a localized collection of pus in a cavity of breast tissue. About 3% of patients with mastitis may develop a breast abscess.

Etiology and Clinical Manifestations

1. May follow acute mastitis if untreated. Some patients may develop a chronic subareolar abscess thought to be caused by a plugging of major mammary ducts in the nipple with infection of obstructed secretions. This usually occurs in smokers.
2. Patient may have fever, chills, and malaise.
3. Affected area is sensitive and erythematous; may have palpable mass.
4. Pus may be expressed from nipple.

Management and Nursing Interventions

1. May perform needle aspiration if superficial mass.
2. Incision and drainage may be done, if deep.
3. A biopsy of the cavity wall may be done at time of incision and drainage to rule out breast carcinoma associated with abscess.
4. Administer antibiotics and analgesics, if ordered.
5. Apply hot, wet dressings to increase drainage and hasten resolution. Pack wound, as directed.
6. A diagnostic mammogram and sonogram may be ordered after resolution of the abscess to rule out cancer.

Fibrocystic Change/Breast Pain

Fibrocystic change is a general term that includes various changes in the breast, namely, fibrosis and cystic dilation of the ducts. May be present in up to 50% of women.

Pathophysiology and Etiology

1. Pathogenesis is not known but is related to the cyclic stimulation of the breast by estrogen and represents a change from the normal stimulation and regression pattern of this process.
2. Occurs usually in women between ages 35 and 50 and is a source of considerable discomfort in a sizable percentage of women.
3. Hormone replacement therapy (HRT) may be associated with fibrocystic changes in a woman who has never experienced this previously.

Clinical Manifestations

1. Increased generalized breast lumpiness or excessive nodularity with tenderness, pain, and breast swelling. Symptoms may decrease after menses.
2. Lumps or cysts—soft or firm; single or multiple; smooth, round, and movable. Cysts may enlarge and become tender and painful. There may be many cysts of different sizes; some may be palpable.
3. Possible nipple discharge—may be milky, yellow, or greenish.

Diagnostic Evaluation

1. Physical examination detects changes.
2. Mammography or ultrasound.
3. Aspiration—if a palpable, symptomatic mass exists or the cyst is complex.
4. Cytology of cyst fluid is not cost-effective and rarely of clinical value in fibrocystic breast changes.

Management

There is no satisfactory treatment and management is usually geared toward relief of symptoms.

Surgical Management

1. Needle aspiration and conservative medical follow-up if:
   a. The aspirate appears like normal cyst fluid and is not blood-stained.
   b. Cyst completely resolves after aspiration.
   c. No indication of an underlying neoplasm.
2. Surgical excision—indicated if a cyst keeps recurring after several aspirations or if a single solid discrete lump is present.

Medical Management

1. Sporadic discomfort may be relieved by OTC analgesics, including topical nonsteroidal anti-inflammatory drugs (ie, diclofenac).
2. Bromocriptine, a dopamine agonist.
   a. May help with mastalgia by decreasing serum prolactin levels.
   b. Adverse effects include nausea, vomiting, headache, dizziness, and fatigue; used rarely because of intolerable adverse effects.
3. Contraceptives or supplemental progestins during the secretory phase of the menstrual cycle may help with pain control.
   a. Mastalgia that begins after initiating hormonal contraceptive pills may resolve after a few cycles.
   b. Switching to a lower estrogen/higher progesterone ratio may help.
4. Danazol, a synthetic androgen used for severe fibrocystic changes to decrease hormonal stimulation of the breast by suppressing gonadotropins.
   a. Adverse effects include a deepening of the voice, which may be permanent, menstrual irregularity, weight gain, depression, bloating, and acne.
   b. Tamoxifen is currently being investigated.

Other Measures

1. Diet modifications.
   a. Eliminating caffeine (coffee, tea, cola drinks, and chocolate) from the diet may help reduce symptoms in some women.
   b. Decreasing fat intake may improve swelling, tenderness, and nodularity.
2. Stopping tobacco use has been suggested to relieve symptoms.
3. Prophylactic lumpectomy—rarely indicated for intractable pain not relieved with medical therapy in women with multiple previous biopsies or biopsy evidence of a precancerous lesion.

Nursing Interventions and Patient Teaching

1. Suggest monthly BSE if the patient is interested—cysts may mask underlying cancer.
2. Reinforce patient's confidence in BSE by rechecking her findings.
3. Offer suggestions for alternative methods if BSE is difficult to do (ie, tender breasts).
4. Encourage patient to see health care provider regularly for examinations.

5. Recommend that patient wear a well-fitted support bra.
6. Offer emotional support for her anxiety and fear of cancer.
7. Reassure that discomfort is common to many women and that it is rarely the only presenting sign of cancer.

Benign Tumors of the Breast

Benign tumors of the breast are characterized clinically as benign lesions that are distinct and persistent over time. Approximately 90% of breast lumps are benign.

Pathophysiology and Etiology

1. Fibrocystic changes—solid lumps may be fatty or fibrous tissue or fluid-filled cysts (see above).
2. Galactocele—a milk-filled cyst.
3. Fibroadenoma—a benign breast tumor composed of epithelial and stromal components.
   a. Common in young women.
   b. A slight increase in the risk of breast cancer among women with fibroadenomas.
4. Other benign tumors include adenosis, intraductal papillomas, lipomas, and neurofibromatosis that may produce a palpable mass.

Clinical Manifestations

1. Gross cysts—may be tender or nontender. Consistency depends on pressure of fluid within cyst and breast tissue around them; may be soft and fluctuant or may feel like a solid tumor if dense.
2. Galactocele—firm, nontender mass.
3. Fibroadenoma—may be a firm, smooth, movable lump that is usually painless. Size does not usually fluctuate with menstrual cycle changes but tends to enlarge over time.

Diagnostic Evaluation

1. Physical examination, mammography, and ultrasound identify and characterize lesion.
2. Cyst aspiration—diagnostic aspiration is usually curative in a galactocele or breast cyst.
3. If a lump does not respond to cyst aspiration, excisional biopsy remains the "gold standard" to rule out cancer.

Management and Nursing Interventions

1. Nonsuspicious or indeterminate masses in young women may be observed through one or two menstrual cycles for resolution of the mass.
2. In general, any distinct and persistent solid lump should have biopsy and possibly excision.
3. Nursing care is directed toward support as woman goes through diagnostic process.

Disorders of the Male Breast

Disorders of the male breast include gynecomastia (benign) and malignant breast cancer.

Clinical Features

Gynecomastia
1. Overdevelopment of breast tissue, usually bilateral.
2. Common in infants, adolescents, and men older than age 50.

3. Usually results from hormonal alterations—idiopathic systemic disorders, such as endocrine disorders, disease of the liver, pituitary adenoma, and chronic renal failure; such drugs as cimetidine, thiazides, spironolactone, omeprazole, phenytoin, reserpine, nifedipine, and theophylline; such neoplasms as testicular tumors and in association with lung and prostate cancer (may be related to therapy).
4. Pubertal gynecomastia has an onset in boys ages 10 to 12 and generally regresses within 18 months. Need to rule out illicit drugs in teens. Marijuana, alcohol, amphetamines, heroin, LSD, and methadone can cause gynecomastia.
5. Asymptomatic and pubertal gynecomastia does not require further tests but should be reevaluated in 6 months. There is no evidence that links gynecomastia with male breast cancer.
6. Investigation is warranted if the drugs used by the patient do not explain the gynecomastia and the breast is tender or the diameter of the breast tissue is more than 4 cm.
7. Reduction subcutaneous nipple-sparing mammoplasty is considered for patients with long-standing gynecomastia for cosmetic and accompanying psychosocial reasons.

 DRUG ALERT Question teenage boys presenting with gynecomastia about illicit drug use.

Breast Cancer
1. Resembles cancer of the breast in women.
2. Less than 1% of all breast cancers—incidence greatest in men in their 60s.
3. Carries poor prognosis because men may delay seeking treatment until disease is advanced.
4. Risk factors: family history (20% of men with breast cancer have a first-degree relative with the disease), estrogen exposure, occupation, and some genetic syndromes, such as Cowden and Klinefelter's. Men chronically exposed to hot environments, such as steel mills, have been shown to be at increased risk as well those employed in the soap and perfume industry and those exposed to petroleum and exhaust fumes.
5. There are no specific screening recommendations for men.
6. Nursing care and treatment is essentially the same as for postmenopausal female breast cancer, including tamoxifen, chemotherapy, and/or radiation therapy.

Cancer of the Breast

Breast cancer is the most common cancer in women in the United States and is second only to lung cancer as a cause of cancer death.

 EVIDENCE BASE National Comprehensive Cancer Network. (2017). *Clinical practice guidelines in oncology: Breast cancer.* Version 4.2017. Fort Washington, PA: Author. Available: www.nccn.org.

Pathophysiology and Etiology

1. Most breast cancer (85% to 90%) begins in the lining of the milk ducts, sometimes in the lobule. Eventually, it grows through the wall of the duct and into the fatty tissue. (See Table 23-3 for types of breast cancer.)
2. Family history accounts for approximately 7% of all breast cancers.

Table 23-3 Types of Breast Cancer

CELL TYPE	DESCRIPTION	INCIDENCE*	COMMENTS
In situ			
DCIS	Abnormal cells in duct	28% Frequently found in combination with invasive cancer	A noninvasive breast cancer; the majority found by mammogram
Invasive			
Ductal	Classified on basis of microscopic appearance as ductal or lobular	85%–90%	Characterized by stony hardness on palpation
Lobular	As above	5%–10%	Relatively uncommon; tends to be more infiltrative
Others			
Tubular Medullary Mucinous Papillary Sarcoma	Types frequently associated with above; cell type must dominate to be assigned.	<10% of all breast cancers	Axillary metastasis uncommon in tubular; medullary associated with fast growth rate and favorable prognosis
Inflammatory	Applies to distinctive inflamed appearance of skin; no consistent histologic type	1%–4%	Presents with erythema, warmth, tenderness, and edema; may be treated with chemotherapy or radiation therapy first
Paget disease of nipple	Usually associated with underlying intraductal or invasive carcinoma	2%	Presents as scaly, erythematous, periareolar eruption

*Percent greater than 100—infiltrating carcinoma frequently includes small areas containing other special types or a combination of in situ and infiltrating carcinoma is seen.
DCIS, ductal carcinoma in situ.*

a. Current genetic models attribute 5% to 10% of all breast cancer to dominantly inherited breast cancer susceptibility genes.
b. Two breast/ovarian susceptibility genes have been identified as BRCA1 and BRCA2. Testing may be performed on those patients with an increased likelihood of breast and ovarian cancer based on personal and family history. The NCCN has outlined criteria for this testing. See their guidelines for these criteria. Women of Ashkenazi Jewish descent have an increased likelihood of BRCA mutations. Knowledge of a mutation can help patients make informed decisions to manage their risk for future breast cancers. It is important to have genetic counseling before the test because of its implications. Screening is not warranted for general population.
3. Present knowledge does not indicate that carcinogens play an important role in the development of breast cancer.

Epidemiology of Breast Cancer

EVIDENCE BASE Siegel, R. L., Miller, K. D., & Jemal, A. (2018). Cancer statistics, 2018. *CA—A Cancer Journal for Clinicians, 67,* 7–30.

Incidence

1. The American Cancer Society estimates that 252,710 to 268,390 (2550 male) new cases of invasive breast cancer will be diagnosed in 2018 in the United States, with 41,070 to 41,400 deaths. This accounts for 30% of all new cancer diagnoses in women.

2. There are expected to be 63,410 to 63,960 cases of DCIS are expected in 2018.

Survival Rates
1. Five-year overall survival rates:
Localized: 97%.
Regional: 78.7%.
Distant: 23.3%.

2. In the general population, the relative survival rate is lower among black women than white women.
3. Lymph node status is the most important prognostic indicator of disease-free survival.
4. Age, comorbidity, staging (tumor size, lymph node status, and distant metastasis), nuclear grade, histologic differentiation, possibly HER2 status, and treatment are important prognostic factors for survival (see Table 23-4). These factors can be used to estimate overall 10-year survival.
5. There has been a decline in the death rate in the United States from breast cancer. This may be related to:
a. Change in lifestyle such as diet.
b. Early diagnosis—increased use and improvement in screening mammography.
c. Improved treatment.

NURSING ALERT Black women are more likely than white women to be diagnosed with large tumors and distant-stage disease. This is true with black males as well. Learn about the demographics of your patient population.

Table 23-4   Staging of Breast Cancer

STAGE	DESCRIPTION
0	Carcinoma in situ
I	Tumor 2 cm or less in greatest dimension; no axillary lymph node metastasis other than micrometastasis; no evidence of distant metastasis.
II	Tumor < 2 cm in greatest dimension but with one to three positive lymph nodes, a tumor 2 -5 cm with or without axillary lymph node metastasis, or a tumor >5 cm without spread to lymph nodes; no evidence of distant metastasis.
III	Any size tumor with four or more positive axillary lymph nodes or with direct extension to the chest wall or skin; inflammatory breast cancer; no evidence of distant metastasis.
IV	Any of the above plus distant metastasis (ie, liver, lungs, bone, brain).

Based on information from the National Cancer Institute and the American Joint Committee on Cancer (2010).

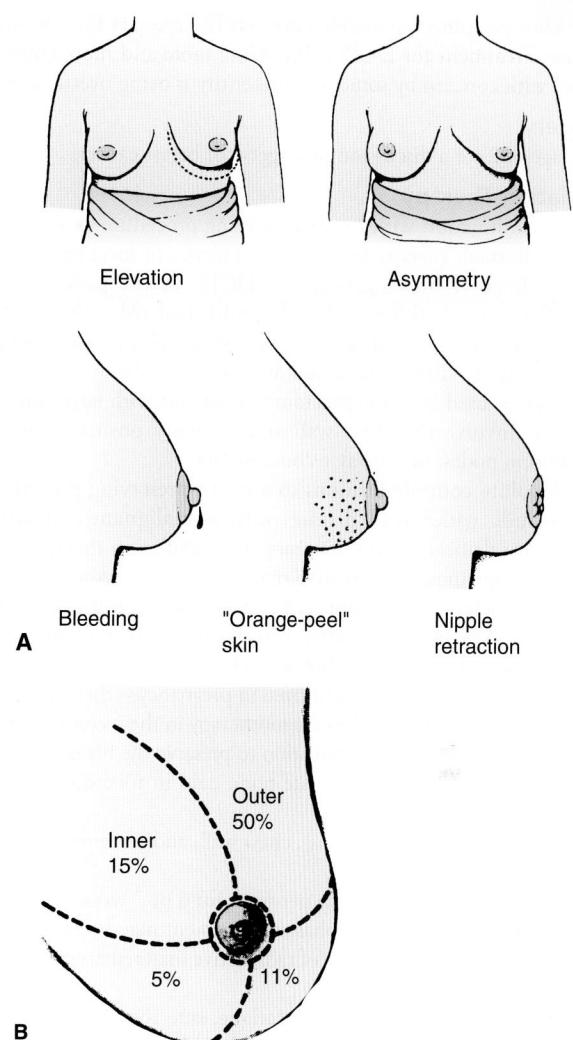

Figure 23-1. **(A)** Signs of cancer of the breast. **(B)** Distribution of carcinomas in different areas of breast.

Risk Factors

A woman's lifetime risk of developing breast cancer is 12.5% based on a life span of 80 years.

1. Major—female gender, increased age, a diagnosis of lobular carcinoma in situ, a prior history of breast or ovarian cancer, and family history (especially mother, sisters). Approximate twofold risk in women with affected sister or mother; this increases if more relatives were affected or if affected close relatives developed breast cancer before menopause.
2. Probable—nulliparity, older age at first live childbirth, late menopause, early menarche, benign proliferative breast disease, diagnosis of atypical ductal or lobular hyperplasia on biopsy, long-term use of estrogen replacement therapy that increases with duration of use, and previous exposure to chest wall irradiation.
3. Controversial—hormonal contraceptive use (estrogen and progestin may stimulate tumor growth with long-term use), multiple breast biopsies, decreased physical activity, alcohol use, obesity, and increased dietary fat intake.
4. Results of breast cancer prevention trials have shown a reduction in incidence of breast cancer in high-risk women treated with tamoxifen, exemestane, or raloxifene.

 GERONTOLOGIC ALERT Age is the greatest single risk factor for the development of cancer. Cancer warning signals may be unheeded in older women, so thorough history-taking and physical examination are essential.

Clinical Manifestations

See Figure 23-1.

1. A firm lump or thickening in breast, usually painless; 50% located in upper outer quadrant of breast. Enlargement of axillary or supraclavicular lymph nodes may indicate metastasis.
2. Nipple discharge—spontaneous, may be bloody, clear, or serous.
3. Breast asymmetry—a change in the size or shape of the breast or abnormal contours. As woman changes positions, compare one breast to other.

4. Nipple retraction or scaliness, especially in Paget disease.
5. Late signs—pain, ulceration, edema, orange-peel skin (peau d'orange) from interference of lymphatic drainage.
6. Inflammatory breast cancer may present with erythema.
7. Many small invasive breast cancers as well as noninvasive breast cancer (DCIS) do not present with a palpable mass but are found on mammography.

 NURSING ALERT Pain is not usually an early warning sign of breast cancer.

Diagnostic Evaluation

See page 679.

Management

Based on type and stage of breast cancer, receptors, and menopausal status. For women with localized invasive breast cancer, information from clinical trials indicates that treatment with a breast-preserving procedure has similar survival rates as mastectomy. Surgery for DCIS (noninvasive breast cancer) may involve only a lumpectomy, but mastectomy may be necessary for extensive disease. Treatment for DCIS is becoming more and more controversial with concern by some that this entity is being overtreated.

Surgery
See page 682 for a discussion of surgery for breast cancer.

Radiation Therapy
1. In conjunction with breast-preserving procedure as adjuvant (additional) therapy to decrease incidence of local recurrence for invasive breast cancer and DCIS. In the patient with DCIS, if it is thought that the individual risk is low, some patients may be treated by excision alone. May be used preoperatively to shrink a large tumor to operable size.
2. May be used after a mastectomy in patients with large tumors that involve the chest wall and/or many positive axillary lymph nodes; may delay reconstruction.
3. Absolute contraindications to a breast-preserving procedure include widespread disease, diffuse malignant-appearing microcalcifications on mammography, radiation therapy during pregnancy, and positive margins. Relative contraindications include active connective tissue disease, tumors greater than 5 cm in size, positive BRCA, and history of previous radiation therapy to the breast or chest wall.
4. Treatment may be individualized in pregnancy—that is, appropriate surgery followed by chemotherapy in the second or third trimester and delayed irradiation to preserve the breast.
5. May also be used to alleviate bone pain in metastatic breast cancer.
6. Radiation directed to breast, chest wall, and remaining lymph nodes.
   a. Usually five treatments per week for 6 or 7 weeks.
   b. A booster or second phase of treatment may be given.
   c. May include implants of radioactive material after external treatment completed.
7. Adverse effects include mild fatigue, sore throat, dry cough, nausea, and anorexia; later, skin will look and feel sunburned. Eventually, the breast may become firmer. Complications include increased arm edema, decreased arm mobility, pneumonitis, and brachial nerve damage. See page 122 for care of patient undergoing radiation therapy.
8. Accelerated partial breast irradiation through a balloon temporarily surgically implanted in the breast treats only the lumpectomy bed. Treatment is twice per day for 5 days. Early data suggest acceptable locoregional disease control with this approach; however, long-term follow-up studies are needed.
9. A one-time dose of radiation intraoperatively is also under investigation and shows promise. Both of these methods of partial breast irradiation should be performed only as part of a prospective trial. Whole breast radiotherapy remains the gold standard.

Chemotherapy
1. Major use is in adjuvant systemic treatment postoperatively; usually begins 4 weeks after surgery (stressful for patient who just finished major surgery).
2. Treatments are given every 2 to 4 weeks for 6 to 9 months. Because the drugs differ in their mechanisms of action, combinations of agents are used to treat cancer.
3. Main drugs used for breast cancer include doxorubicin, cyclophosphamide, paclitaxel, 5-fluorouracil (5-FU), gemcitabine, and methotrexate. For advanced cancer, docetaxel, vinorelbine, capecitabine, mitoxantrone, and fluorouracil by continuous infusion and oral forms of fluorouracil are used.
4. Indications for chemotherapy include:
   a. Large tumors, positive lymph nodes, premenopausal women, and poor prognostic factors. Currently, adjuvant chemotherapy and/or hormonal therapy are recommended for all patients with invasive breast cancers 1 cm wide or larger although the benefit in some patients may be relatively small.
   b. Patients who score high on gene assay as well as those tumors that are shown to be "triple negative"—ER/PR as well as HER2 negative.
   c. Data are insufficient to make definitive recommendations for patients older than 80 years.
5. Other agents that may be used include:
   a. Trastuzumab—a member of the epithelial growth receptor family; increased survival when added to chemotherapy in metastatic breast cancer. Treatment is expensive; may be given to patients who express this gene (HER2).
6. Pertuzumab—another monoclonal antibody that may be used prior to surgery (neoadjuvant) in early-stage or locally advanced HER2 positive breast cancer patients.
   a. Bevacizumab—binds to vascular endothelial growth factor and blocks tumor blood vessel growth. Used in advanced breast cancer.
   b. Pamidronate, zoledronic acid, or denosumab may be added if bone metastasis present to help reduce pain. Patients should undergo dental exam prior to initiation of this therapy for preventive maintenance and to correct dental problems, as osteonecrosis of the jaw is more common in those with poor oral hygiene.
   c. Poly ADP ribose polymerase inhibitors, such as olaparib, are enzymes that help repair DNA and may be helpful in triple-negative cancers.
7. Adverse effects include bone marrow suppression, cardiotoxicity, nausea and vomiting, diarrhea, alopecia, weight gain or loss, fatigue, stomatitis, anxiety, depression, and premature menopause (see page 112 for nursing care of patient undergoing chemotherapy). Childbearing after treatment of invasive breast cancer does not increase rates of breast cancer recurrence or death.
8. Chemotherapy may also be used as primary treatment in inflammatory breast cancer and occasionally in large tumors.
9. Hope for the future is the development of specific targeted biologic therapies and more individualized treatment.

Endocrine Therapy
1. Selective estrogen receptor modulators, such as tamoxifen and raloxifene, bind estrogen receptors, thereby blocking effects of estrogen.
   a. Adjuvant systemic therapy after surgery.
   b. Benefits estrogen receptor–positive patients, regardless of menopausal status.
   c. Given for at least 5 years; oral administration once or twice per day.
   d. Adverse effects include hot flashes, irregular periods, vaginal irritation, nausea and vomiting, headaches, increased risk of endometrial cancer, and thromboembolic events.
   e. Women on tamoxifen should have an annual gynecologic assessment if uterus present.
2. Aromatase inhibitors, such as anastrozole, exemestane, and letrozole, block conversion of androgen, which is secreted by the adrenal glands, into estrogen. Large clinical trials report more favorable outcomes with aromatase inhibitors, and treatment has shifted from 5 years of tamoxifen therapy to initial treatment with an aromatase inhibitor in postmenopausal women.

a. Anastrozole as well as fulvestrant, an estrogen receptor agonist, may be used as a second-line therapy after tamoxifen in patients whose cancer has returned or progressed.
b. Aromatase inhibitors are ineffective in premenopausal women.
c. Adverse effects include hot flashes, vaginal dryness, musculoskeletal symptoms, osteoporosis, and increased rate of bone fracture. Therefore, women on aromatase inhibitors should have monitoring of bone health.
3. Hormones may be used in advanced disease. Remissions may last months to several years. Agents commonly used include:
a. Estrogens, such as diethylstilbestrol or ethinyl estradiol, in high doses to suppress follicle-stimulating hormone (FSH) and luteinizing hormone and may decrease endogenous estrogen production.
b. Progestins may decrease estrogen receptors.
c. Androgens may suppress FSH and estrogen production.
d. Aminoglutethimide suppresses estrogen production by blocking adrenal steroids; "medical adrenalectomy," especially useful for women with bone and soft tissue metastasis.
4. Corticosteroids suppress estrogen and progesterone secretion from the adrenals.

 DRUG ALERT Traditionally, breast cancer survivors have not been considered candidates for estrogen. However, debates and studies continue to be conducted regarding the safety of estrogen in this population.

Bone Marrow Transplant
1. Autologous method after high-dose chemotherapy.
2. Clinical trials have shown it to be ineffective for breast cancer.

Oophorectomy
Removal of ovaries.
1. Treatment for recurrent or metastatic disease in estrogen receptor–positive premenopausal women.
2. Deprives tumor of primary estrogen source—remissions of 3 months to several years.
3. Medical ablation with tamoxifen has been compared to surgical oophorectomy in estrogen receptor–positive postmenopausal women and response rates are similar.
4. Surgical ablation is now considered second choice because of its increased risks.
5. The benefits of tamoxifen in combination with oophorectomy are the subject of ongoing research.

Adrenalectomy
Removal of adrenal glands to eliminate androgen production (which converts to estrogen).
1. Rarely done because of need for long-term steroid replacement therapy.
2. Remissions may last 6 months to several years.
3. Medical ablation with drugs being studied.

Complications
1. Metastasis—most common sites: lymph nodes, lung, bone, liver, and brain.
2. Signs and symptoms of metastasis may include bone pain, neurologic changes, weight loss, anemia, cough, shortness of breath, pleuritic pain, and vague chest discomfort.

Nursing Assessment
1. Assess general health status and underlying chronic illnesses that may have an impact on patient's response to treatment.
2. Identify what the patient and family need to know regarding breast cancer and its treatment and take measures to decrease their impact. Base education on patient and family needs.
3. Determine level of anxiety, fears, and concerns.
4. Identify coping ability and availability of support systems.

 NURSING ALERT Evidence suggests that active lifestyle and achieving and maintaining an ideal body weight (20 to 25 body mass index) may lead to optimal breast cancer outcomes.

Nursing Diagnoses
Also see page 682 for breast surgery care and Chapter 8, Cancer nursing.

- Anxiety related to diagnosis of cancer.
- Deficient Knowledge related to disease process and treatment options.
- Ineffective Coping by patient or family related to diagnosis, prognosis, financial stress, or inadequate support.

Nursing Interventions

 EVIDENCE BASE Greenlee, H., Dupont-Reyes, M., Balneaves, L., et al. (2017). Clinical practice guidelines on the evidence-based use of integrative therapies during and after breast cancer treatment. *CA-A Cancer Journal for Clinicians, 67*, 194–232.

Reducing Anxiety
1. Realize that diagnosis of breast cancer is a devastating emotional shock to patient. Support patient through the diagnostic process. Many women must make challenging decisions in a brief period of time. Some communities have developed nursing navigators as a way of assisting and supporting individuals through the process. Check if there is a nurse navigator in your community.
2. Interpret the results of each test in language patient can understand.
3. Stress the advances made in earlier diagnosis and treatment options.

Providing Information about Treatment
1. Involve patient in treatment planning.
2. Describe surgical procedures.
3. Prepare patient for the effects of chemotherapy; encourage patient to plan ahead for the common adverse effects of chemotherapy.
4. Educate patient about the effects of radiation therapy.
5. Teach patient about hormonal therapy. Patient may develop hot flashes with the start of hormonal therapy or with the discontinuation of HRT at the time of diagnosis of breast cancer (see Chapter 22 for information on menopausal symptoms). Measures that may help with symptoms of hot flashes include:
a. Clonidine, belladonna/ergotamine/phenobarbital, antidepressant medications.
b. Various supplements and herbs have been used but have not been rigorously tested. Soy has been suggested, but

there is no compelling evidence that phytoestrogens help menopausal symptoms. Indeed, concerns have been raised regarding stimulating breast cancer cell growth and, therefore, should not be used.

c. Progesterone may be helpful, but the possible effect on breast cancer needs further study.

Strengthening Coping

1. Repeat information and speak in calm, clear manner.
2. Display empathy and acceptance of patient's emotions.
3. Explore coping mechanisms.
4. Evaluate where patient is in stages of acceptance.
5. Help patient identify and use support persons.
6. Obtain visit from support group member.
7. Refer for counseling, financial aid, and so forth.
8. Resources include American Cancer Society (800-ACS-2345 or *www.cancer.org*), National Cancer Institute (*www.cancer.gov*), National Alliance of Breast Cancer Organizations (*www.nabco.org*), and the Susan G. Komen Breast Cancer Foundation (*www.komen.org*).

Patient Education and Health Maintenance

1. Encourage patient to continue close follow-up and to report any new symptoms. Most women will be seen every 3 months for the first 2 years, every 6 months for the next 3 years, and once per year after 5 years.
2. Stress importance of continued yearly mammogram.
3. Inform patient that yearly laboratory work, bone scan, and chest x-ray may be performed when clinically indicated.
4. Suggest to patient that psychological intervention may be necessary for anxiety, depression, or sexual problems.

Evaluation: Expected Outcomes

- Verbalizes less anxiety.
- Verbalizes understanding of all treatment options and their adverse effects.
- Identifies appropriate coping mechanisms and support systems.

SELECTED REFERENCES

American Cancer Society. (2012). Lymphedema: What every woman with breast cancer should know. Available: *www.cancer.org/treatment/treatmentsandsideeffects/physicalsideeffects/lymphedema/whateverywomanwithbreastcancershouldknow-toc*

American College of Radiology. (Revised 2017). ACR practice parameter for the performance of screening and diagnostic mammography. *www.acr.org*

American College of Radiology. (2013). BI-RAD Atlas (5th ed.). *www.acr.org*

American Joint Committee on Cancer. (2016). *AJCC cancer staging manual* (8th ed.). New York: Springer.

Greenlee, H., Dupont-Reyes, M., Balneaves, L., et al. (2017). Clinical practice guidelines on the evidence-based use of integrative therapies during and after breast cancer treatment. *CA-A Cancer Journal for Clinicians, 67,* 194–232.

Guiano, A., Connolly, J., Edge, S., et al. (2017). Major changes in the American Joint Committee on cancer eighth edition cancer staging. *CA-A Cancer Journal for Clinicians, 67,* 290–303.

Himes, D. O., Root, A. E., Gammon, A., et al. (2016). Breast cancer assessment: Calculating lifetime risk using the Tyrer-Cuzick model. *Journal for Nurse Practitioners, 12,* 581–592.

Manders, J. B., Kuerer, H. M., Smith, B. D., et al. (2017). Clinical utility of the 12-gene DCIS score assay: Impact on radiotherapy recommendations for patients with ductal carcinoma in situ. *Annals of Surgical Oncology, 24,* 660–668.

Mayden, K. D. (2016). Understanding biomarkers in early-stage invasive breast cancer: Tools from the ASCO clinical guideline. *Journal of the Advanced Practitioner in Oncology, 7,* 666–671.

Meneses, K. (2016). When should I have a mammogram? Recent changes in ACS mammography guidelines: Implications for practice. *Journal of the Advanced Practitioner in Oncology, 7,* 567–570.

Monticciolo, D., Newell, M., Hendrick, R., et al. (2017). Breast cancer screening for average-risk women: Recommendations from the ACR Commission on breast imaging. *Journal of the American College of Radiology, 14*(9), 1137–1143.

Morrow, M. (2018). Management of the node-positive axilla in breast cancer in 2017: selecting the right option. *JAMA Oncology, 4*(2), 250–251.

National Comprehensive Cancer Network. (2017). Clinical practice guidelines in oncology breast cancer Version 4.2017. Available: *www.nccn.org*

Rafferty, E., Durand, M., Conant, E., et al. (2016). Breast cancer screening using tomosynthesis and digital mammography in dense and non-dense breasts. *JAMA, 315*(16), 1784–1786.

Siegel, R. L., Miller, K. D., & Jemal, A. (2018). Cancer statistics, 2017. *CA—A Cancer Journal for Clinicians, 68,* 7–30.

Smith, R., Andrews, K., Brooks, D., et al. (2017). Cancer screening in the United States, 2017: A review of current American Cancer Society guidelines and issues in cancer screening. *CA—A Cancer Journal for Clinicians, 67,* 100–121.

24

Endocrine Disorders

OVERVIEW AND ASSESSMENT
The Function of Hormones

The endocrine system and the nervous system maintain homeostasis. The endocrine glands produce hormones, chemical substances that are secreted into the bloodstream and that exert a stimulatory or inhibitory effect on target tissues or on glands. Hormones achieve their effect by binding with specific receptors located on the membrane on the target cell (eg, catecholamines) or by penetrating the cell membrane and forming a complex that influences cellular metabolism (eg, steroids). The target cell response may be reflected through the production and secretion of a second hormone or through a change in cell metabolism that alters the concentration of electrolytes or other substances in the bloodstream.

General Effects of Hormone Action

1. Regulate the overall metabolic rate and the storage, conversion, and release of energy.
2. Regulate fluid and electrolyte balance.
3. Initiate coping responses to stressors.
4. Regulate growth and development.
5. Regulate reproduction processes.

Regulation of Hormones

1. Hormone secretion is typically controlled through a negative feedback system.
   a. Fall in blood concentration of hormone leads to activation of the regulator endocrine gland and to release of its stimulator hormones.
   b. Elevations in blood concentration of target cell hormones or changes in blood composition resulting from target cell activity can cause inhibition of hormone secretion.
2. Endocrine disorders are manifested as states of hormone deficiency or hormone excess. The underlying pathophysiology may be expressed as:
   a. *Primary*—the secreting gland releases inappropriate hormone because of disease of the gland itself.
   b. *Secondary*—the secreting gland releases abnormal amounts of hormone because of disease in a regulator gland (eg, pituitary).
   c. *Tertiary*—the secreting gland releases inappropriate hormone because of hypothalamic dysfunction, resulting in abnormal stimulation by the pituitary.
3. Abnormal hormone concentrations may also be caused by hormone-producing tumors (adenomas) located at a remote site.

History

Patients with diseases of the endocrine system commonly report nonspecific complaints. Commonly, symptoms may reflect changes in general well-being, such as fatigue, weakness, weight change, appetite, sleep patterns, or emotional status. A thorough review of systems is necessary to detect changes in various body systems caused by an endocrine disorder (see Table 24-1).

Physical Examination

Objective findings may be obvious and related to the patient's complaints or may be "silent signs" of which the patient is completely unaware. Thorough physical examination of all body systems, particularly the integumentary, cardiovascular, and neurologic systems, may reveal key findings for endocrine dysfunction (see Chapter 5).

Tests of Thyroid Function

Total Thyroxine

Description
1. This is a direct measurement of the concentration of total thyroxine (T_4) in the blood, using a radioimmunoassay technique.
2. It is an accurate index of thyroid function when T_4-binding globulin (TBG) is normal.
3. Low plasma-binding protein states (malnutrition, liver disease) may give low values.
4. High plasma-binding protein values (pregnancy, estrogen therapy) may give high values.
5. It can be used to diagnose hypofunction and hyperfunction of the thyroid and to guide and evaluate thyroid hormone replacement therapy.

Nursing and Patient Care Considerations
1. The test to monitor thyroid hormone therapy may be performed 6 to 8 weeks after dosage adjustment because of the time required for thyroid-stimulating hormone (TSH) to reflect the body's response to the new dose.
2. Interpretation of test results:
   a. Hypothyroidism—below normal.
   b. Hyperthyroidism—above normal.

Free Thyroxine

Description
1. Direct measurement of free T_4 concentration in the blood using a two-step radioimmunoassay method.
2. Accurate measure of thyroid function independent of the variable influence of thyroid-binding globulin levels.
3. Used to aid in the diagnosis of hyperthyroidism and hypothyroidism.
4. Used to monitor and guide thyroid hormone replacement therapy.

Nursing and Patient Care Considerations
1. Interpretation of test results:
   a. Hyperthyroidism—above normal.
   b. Hypothyroidism—below normal.
2. Results best interpreted in conjunction with TSH levels for diagnostic purposes.
3. Often used to monitor thyroid hormone replacement therapy, levels meaningful only after 6 to 8 weeks of therapy to evaluate adequacy of dosage because of long half-life of T_4.

Thyroid-Binding Globulin

Description
1. This measures the concentration of the carrier protein for T_4 in the blood.
2. Because most T_4 is protein bound, changes in TBG will influence values of T_4.
3. Helpful in distinguishing between true thyroid disease and T_4 test abnormalities caused by TBG excess or deficit.

Nursing and Patient Care Considerations
Determine if patient is taking estrogen or is pregnant, both of which can elevate TBG; results may be depressed by malnutrition or by liver disease.

Triiodothyronine

Description
1. Directly measures concentration of triiodothyronine (T_3) in the blood using a radioimmunoassay technique.
2. T_3 is less influenced by alterations in thyroid-binding proteins; it binds to albumin.
3. T_3 has a shorter half-life than T_4 and occurs in minute quantities in the active form.
4. Useful to rule out T_3 thyrotoxicosis, hyperthyroidism when T_4 is normal, and to evaluate effects of thyroid replacement therapy.

Nursing and Patient Care Considerations
1. T_3 can be transiently depressed in the acutely ill patient.
2. Interpretation of test results:
   a. Hypothyroidism—below normal.
   b. Hyperthyroidism—above normal.

T_3 Resin Uptake

Description
1. This is an indirect measure of thyroid function, based on the available protein-binding sites in a serum sample that can bind to radioactive T_3.
2. The radioactive T_3 is added to the serum sample in the test tube and will bind with available protein-binding sites. The unbound T_3 binds to resin for T_3 uptake, reflecting the amount of T_3 left over because of lack of binding sites.
3. Estrogen and pregnancy produce an increase in binding sites, thus causing a lowered T_3 resin uptake.

Nursing and Patient Care Considerations
1. Results may be altered if patient has been taking estrogens, androgens, salicylates, or phenytoin.
2. Interpretation of test results:
   a. Hypothyroidism—below normal.
   b. Hyperthyroidism—above normal.

Free Thyroid Index

Description
The free thyroid index is a laboratory estimate of free T_4 concentration with calculated adjustment for variations in patient's TBG concentration.

Nursing and Patient Care Considerations
Interpretation of test results:
1. Below normal—hypothyroidism.
2. Above normal—hyperthyroidism.

Table 24-1   Clinical Manifestations of Endocrine Dysfunction

SIGN OR SYMPTOM	POSSIBLE CAUSES	SIGN OR SYMPTOM	POSSIBLE CAUSES
Cardiovascular		Pathologic fractures	• Hyperparathyroidism
Tachycardia or tachyarrhythmia	• Hyperthyroidism • Pheochromocytoma • Adrenal insufficiency	Joint pain	• Hypothyroidism • Acromegaly
Bradycardia	• Hypothyroidism	Bone pain	• Hyperparathyroidism
Orthostatic hypotension	• Adrenal insufficiency	Bone thickening	• Acromegaly
Hypertension	• Pheochromocytoma • Hyperaldosteronism • Cushing syndrome • Hyperparathyroidism • Hypothyroidism	**Urologic**	
		Polyuria	• Diabetes insipidus • Diabetes mellitus
		Kidney stones	• Hyperparathyroidism • Acromegaly • Cushing syndrome
Heart failure	• Hyperthyroidism • Hypothyroidism • Cushing syndrome	**Integumentary**	
Neurologic		Hirsutism	• Adrenal hyperfunction • Acromegaly
Fatigue	• Adrenal insufficiency • Hypothyroidism • Hyperparathyroidism	Hair loss	• Hypoparathyroidism • Hypothyroidism • Cushing syndrome
Nervousness, tremor	• Pheochromocytoma • Hyperthyroidism	Sparse body hair	• Pituitary insufficiency • Adrenal insufficiency • Hypogonadism
Confusion, lethargy, or coma	• Diabetic ketoacidosis • Hypothyroidism • Syndrome of inappropriate antidiuretic hormone	Hyperpigmentation	• Addison disease • Hyperthyroidism • Ectopic corticotropin production
Paresthesia	• Hypothyroidism • Hypoparathyroidism • Diabetes mellitus	Profuse diaphoresis	• Hyperthyroidism • Pheochromocytoma
Headache	• Acromegaly • Pituitary tumor • Pheochromocytoma	Thin skin	• Cushing syndrome
		Coarse hair	• Hypothyroidism
		Fine hair	• Hyperthyroidism
Psychosis	• Hyperaldosteronism • Hypothyroidism • Hyperthyroidism • Cushing syndrome • Adrenal insufficiency • Hyperparathyroidism	Edema	• Cushing syndrome
		Reproductive	
		Amenorrhea	• Hyperthyroidism • Hypogonadism • Cushing syndrome • Acromegaly • Pituitary tumor
Chvostek sign, Trousseau sign	• Hypoparathyroidism		
Increased reflexes	• Hyperthyroidism		
Decreased reflexes	• Hypothyroidism	Gynecomastia	• Hypogonadism • Pituitary tumor
Peptic ulcer	• Cushing syndrome	Loss of libido, impotence	• Hypogonadism • Hypothyroidism • Adrenal insufficiency • Diabetes mellitus
Diarrhea	• Adrenal insufficiency		
Constipation	• Hypothyroidism • Hyperparathyroidism • Pheochromocytoma		
Weight loss	• Hyperthyroidism • Hyperparathyroidism • Pheochromocytoma	**Ophthalmic/Visual**	
		Exophthalmos	• Graves disease
		Diplopia	• Graves disease • Pituitary tumor
Hyperdefecation	• Hyperthyroidism	Visual field deficit	• Pituitary tumor
Abdominal pain	• Addisonian crisis • Hyperparathyroidism	Periorbital swelling	• Hypothyroidism • Graves disease
Musculoskeletal		**Body Habitus**	
Weakness	• Hyperthyroidism • Hypothyroidism • Cushing syndrome • Adrenal insufficiency • Hyperparathyroidism • Hypoparathyroidism • Hyperaldosteronism	Round face, "buffalo hump"	• Cushing syndrome
		Abnormally tall stature	• Prepubertal growth • Acromegaly

Thyrotropin, Thyroid-Stimulating Hormone

Description

1. Direct measure of TSH, the hormone secreted by the anterior pituitary gland that regulates the production and secretion of T_4 by the thyroid gland.
2. Third-generation TSH chemiluminometric assays are most commonly utilized.
3. Preferred test differentiates between thyroid disorders caused by disease of the thyroid gland itself and disorders caused by disease of the pituitary or hypothalamus. Also useful to detect early stages of hypothyroidism (subclinical hypothyroidism) and to monitor hormone replacement therapy (HRT). Patient must be on a stable dose of thyroxine for 6 to 8 weeks for TSH levels to accurately reflect adequacy of treatment.
4. Morning samples are preferred.

Nursing and Patient Care Considerations

1. Interpretation:
   a. In primary hypothyroidism, TSH levels are elevated.
   b. In secondary hypothyroidism (failure of the pituitary gland), TSH levels are low.
   c. In hyperthyroidism, TSH levels are low.

Thyrotropin-Releasing Hormone Stimulation Test

Description

1. The thyrotropin-releasing hormone (TRH) stimulation test evaluates the patency of the pituitary–hypothalamic axis. Once used primarily to distinguish between primary and central hypothyroidism (secondary or tertiary), this test is rarely used for that purpose with the advent of more sensitive TSH assays. Now, its primary use is to distinguish between secondary and tertiary hypothyroidism and evaluate acromegaly.
2. A baseline sample is drawn, then TRH is administered via intravenous (IV) injection and blood samples are drawn to determine TSH levels at 30, 90, and 120 minutes.

Nursing and Patient Care Considerations

1. Interpretation:
   a. Increased TSH should be seen within 30 minutes.
   b. No rise in secondary hypothyroidism.
   c. Blunted rise in hyperthyroidism.
   d. Delayed rise (90-minute sample) associated with tertiary hypothyroidism.
   e. Elevated growth hormone levels associated with acromegaly.
2. A subnormal response can occur in patients taking L-dopa or cortisol.

Thyroid Autoantibodies

Description

Used to detect selected autoantibodies associated with some thyroid diseases and the levels of those autoantibodies.

1. Thyroid-stimulating immunoglobulin (TSI)—autoantibodies that stimulate the TSH receptor on the thyroid gland, causing hyperfunction of the thyroid. Helpful in the diagnosis of Graves disease.
2. Thyroid peroxidase antibodies (TPO)—associated with Hashimoto thyroiditis and Graves disease.
3. Thyroglobulin antibodies—elevated with Hashimoto thyroiditis and Graves disease.

Tests of Parathyroid Function

Parathyroid Hormone

Description

1. Test is either an intact PTH (second-generation assay) or PTH 1-84 assay (third generation), which should be measured concurrently with serum calcium level.
2. Range of normal values may vary by laboratory and method.

Nursing and Patient Care Considerations

Elevated PTH in hyperparathyroidism; decreased PTH in hypoparathyroidism.

Serum Calcium, Total

Description

1. This is a direct measurement of protein-bound and "free" ionized calcium.
2. Ionized calcium fraction is the best indicator of changes in calcium metabolism.
3. Results can be affected by changes in serum albumin, the primary protein carrier.
4. Used to detect alterations in calcium metabolism caused by parathyroid disease or malignancy.

Nursing and Patient Care Considerations

1. Sample may be obtained from fasting patient and should be collected in tube with heparin as anticoagulant.
2. Test should be repeated to confirm parathyroid disease.
3. Elevations in serum calcium can be caused by dehydration, vitamin D intoxication, thiazide diuretics, immobilization, hyperthyroidism, or lithium therapy.
4. Low values may be seen in renal failure, chronic disease states, malabsorption syndrome, and vitamin D deficiency.
5. Interpretation of test results:
   a. Hyperparathyroidism, malignancy—elevated.
   b. Hypoparathyroidism—below normal.

Serum Calcium, Ionized

Description

1. Approximately 45% to 50% of total serum calcium is in biologically active ionized form.
2. This is the preferred method of testing changes in calcium metabolism caused by parathyroid disease, malignancy, or thyroid surgery.

Nursing and Patient Care Considerations

1. Sample should be collected in tube with heparin as anticoagulant.
2. Test should be repeated on three different occasions to confirm parathyroid disease.
   a. Hyperparathyroidism, malignancy—elevated.
   b. Hypoparathyroidism—below normal.

 NURSING ALERT Tourniquet use during blood sample collection for calcium studies should be kept to a minimum. Prolonged constriction will cause migration of plasma proteins into the bloodstream locally; this results in spuriously high serum calcium values and pseudohypercalcemia.

Serum Phosphate

Description

1. Test measures the level of inorganic phosphorus in the blood.
2. Alteration in parathyroid function tends to have opposite effects on calcium and phosphorus metabolism.
3. Used to confirm metabolic abnormalities that affect calcium metabolism.

Nursing and Patient Care Considerations

Elevated in hypoparathyroidism; low values in hyperparathyroidism.

Tests of Adrenal Function

Plasma Cortisol

Description

1. This is a direct measure of the primary secretory product of the adrenal cortex by radioimmunoassay technique.
2. Serum concentration varies with circadian cycle, so normal values vary with time of day and stress level of patient (8:00 A.M. levels typically double that of 8:00 P.M. levels).
3. Useful as an initial step to assess adrenal dysfunction, but further workup is usually necessary.

Nursing and Patient Care Considerations

1. A fasting sample is preferred.
2. Blood samples should coincide with circadian rhythm with draw time indicated on laboratory slip.
3. Interpretation of test results:
   a. Decreased values seen in Addison disease, anterior pituitary hyposecretion, and secondary hypothyroidism.
   b. Increased values seen in hyperthyroidism, stress (eg, trauma, surgery), carcinoma, Cushing syndrome, hypersecretion of corticotropin by tumors (oat cell cancer), adrenal adenoma, and obesity.

Salivary Cortisol

Description

1. Because cortisol-binding globulin (CBG) is normally absent from saliva, it does not interfere with cortisol levels. Therefore, salivary cortisol can be more reliably measured without variation because of fluctuating CBG levels.

Nursing and Patient Care Considerations

1. A mouth swab is collected from patient in the evening and can be done at home after rinsing the mouth before brushing teeth.

Twenty-Four–Hour Urinary Free Cortisol Test

Description

1. Test measures cortisol production during a 24-hour period.
2. Useful to establish diagnosis of hypercortisolism.
3. Less influenced by diurnal variations in cortisol.

Nursing and Patient Care Considerations

1. Instruct patient in appropriate collection technique.
2. Collection jug should be kept on ice and sent to laboratory promptly when collection completed.
3. Interfering factors:
   a. Elevated values—pregnancy, hormonal contraceptives, spironolactone, and stress.
   b. Recent radioisotope scans can interfere with test results.

Dexamethasone Suppression Tests

Description

1. The dexamethasone suppression test (DST) is a valuable method to evaluate adrenal hyperfunction.
2. Adrenal production and secretion of cortisol is stimulated by adrenocorticotropic hormone (ACTH; corticotropin) from the pituitary gland.
3. Dexamethasone is a synthetic steroid effective in suppressing corticotropin secretion.
4. In a healthy patient, the administration of dexamethasone will inhibit corticotropin secretion and will cause cortisol levels to fall below normal.
5. Certain drugs (rifampin, phenytoin) increase metabolic clearance of dexamethasone and may contribute to false-positive test results.
6. Those on estrogen-containing drugs should stop 6 weeks prior to test, and this test is not reliable in pregnancy.

Nursing and Patient Care Considerations

Explain the procedure to patient.

1. Overnight low-dose (1 mg) DST (used primarily to identify those *without* Cushing syndrome).
   a. Administer dexamethasone 1 mg orally at 11:00 P.M.
   b. Draw cortisol level at 8:00 A.M. before patient rises.
   c. Expect suppressed cortisol levels (less than 5 mcg/dL). Test is highly sensitive when a 2-mg cutoff is used for diagnosis.
2. Forty-eight–hour low-dose (2 mg) DST.
   a. Patient is instructed to take 0.5 mg of dexamethasone every 6 hours for a 2-day period.
   b. Plasma cortisol sample is collected 9 hours after first dose is administered and again at 48 hours.
   c. It is essential that patient have clearly written instructions for compliance with dosing and blood sampling schedule for test to be valid.
3. High-dose overnight DST (helpful to distinguish Cushing disease from other forms of Cushing syndrome).
   a. Give patient dexamethasone 8 mg orally at 11:00 P.M.
   b. Draw cortisol level at 8:00 A.M. before patient rises.
   c. Suppressed cortisol levels (less than 50% of baseline value) indicative of patient with corticotropin-secreting pituitary adenoma (Cushing disease).
   d. Unsuppressed cortisol levels are associated with ectopic corticotropin secretion (malignancy) or adrenal tumors.
4. Encourage patient to take dexamethasone with milk because it may cause gastric irritation.

Adrenocorticotropic Stimulation Test

Description

1. ACTH stimulates the production and secretion of cortisol by the adrenal cortex.
2. Demonstrates the ability of the adrenal cortex to respond appropriately to ACTH.
3. This is an important test to evaluate adrenal insufficiency but may not distinguish primary insufficiency from secondary insufficiency.

Nursing and Patient Care Considerations

1. Obtain baseline cortisol level.
2. Administer 0.25 mg ACTH (cosyntropin IV or intramuscularly [IM]).
3. Collect cortisol levels at times ordered (usually at 30 and 60 minutes).

4. Interpretation of test results:
   a. Range of normal responses may vary; however, typically a rise in cortisol of double baseline value is considered normal.
   b. Diminished response—adrenal insufficiency with low cortisol values.

 DRUG ALERT Infusion of cosyntropin can cause flushing or slight reduction in blood pressure (BP). Warn patients about these effects, monitor BP, and ensure safety.

Corticotropin-Releasing Hormone Stimulation Test

Description

1. Test measures responsiveness of the pituitary gland to corticotropin-releasing hormone (CRH)—a hypothalamic hormone that regulates pituitary secretion of ACTH.
2. Useful to differentiate the cause of excess cortisol secretion when ectopic source of ACTH is suspected.
3. In general, CRH will stimulate ACTH secretion in the pituitary but not in nonpituitary corticotropin-secreting tissues.

Nursing and Patient Care Considerations

1. Describe procedure to patient.
   a. Fasting patient is given CRH (1 mcg/kg or 100 mcg) via IV line.
   b. Catheters are advanced through the femoral veins to areas near the adrenal glands, so sampling can take place near ACTH secretion.
   c. Blood samples for ACTH test are collected at 5, 10, 15, 30, 45, 60, 90, and 120 minutes.
2. Normal response is a rise in ACTH to at least double the baseline value.
3. Interpretation of test results:
   a. Brisk rise in ACTH double baseline value—Cushing disease.
   b. No response in ACTH—corticotropin-independent Cushing syndrome (adrenal tumor) or ectopic source of corticotropin secretion (ectopic tumor).
   c. Test can produce false-negative response.

Urine Vanillylmandelic Acid and Metanephrine

Description

1. Direct measure of metabolites of catecholamines secreted by the adrenal medulla.
2. Metanephrine is a more reliable measure of catecholamine secretion.
3. Preferred method to diagnose pheochromocytoma, neuroblastoma, and other neural crest tumors.

Nursing and Patient Care Considerations

1. Obtain proper urine collection jug with hydrochloride preservative, and explain 24-hour urine collection to patient.
2. A wide range of medications and foods may alter test performed by some laboratories. Verify with the laboratory and health care provider the need to hold some medications, such as sympathomimetics and methyldopa, and such foods as coffee, tea, vanilla extract, and bananas before and during urine collection.
3. Interpretation—pheochromocytoma: vanillylmandelic acid greater than 10 mcg/mg of creatinine or greater than 10 mg/24 hours; metanephrine greater than 0.7 mcg/mg of creatinine or greater than 0.7 mg/24 hours.

Plasma Catecholamines

Description

Direct measure of circulating catecholamines using radioimmunoassay technique; more sensitive test than urine test, but more prone to false-positive results.

Nursing and Patient Care Considerations

1. Collect sample from IV catheter 20 to 30 minutes after venipuncture, if possible, to reduce the rise in catecholamine levels from pain and anxiety.
2. Collect the sample in a heparinized tube.
3. Interpretation—levels higher than 2,000 ng/L diagnostic for pheochromocytoma.

Clonidine Suppression Test

Description

1. Based on the principle that catecholamine production by pheochromocytomas is autonomous, as opposed to other causes of excess catecholamines, which are regulated by the sympathetic nervous system.
2. Clonidine, as a central alpha-adrenergic agonist, suppresses production of catecholamines.
3. Useful to differentiate pheochromocytoma from essential hypertension when test results are inconclusive.
4. Corticosteroids should be avoided prior to testing.

Nursing and Patient Care Considerations

1. Collect baseline catecholamine sample from IV catheter 20 to 30 minutes after venipuncture, if possible, to reduce the rise in catecholamine levels from pain and anxiety.
2. Give clonidine 0.3 mg orally.
3. After 3 hours, collect second catecholamine sample.
4. Interpretation—in patients without pheochromocytoma, a significant drop in catecholamines should be seen at 3 hours (less than 500 pg/mL or reduction of total catecholamines by 50%), whereas in patients with pheochromocytoma, no drop in catecholamines will be evident.

 DRUG ALERT Warn patients not to rise quickly and monitor for orthostatic hypotension after clonidine administration.

Aldosterone (Urine or Blood)

Description

1. Direct measure, using radioimmunoassay technique, of aldosterone, a hormone secreted by the adrenal cortex that regulates renal control of sodium and potassium.
2. May be measured in the blood or in 24-hour urine collection specimen.
3. Urine test is more reliable because it is less influenced by short-term fluctuations in the bloodstream.
4. Useful to diagnose primary aldosteronism.

Nursing and Patient Care Considerations

1. Test results can be elevated by stress, strenuous exercise, upright posture, and medications such as diazoxide, hydralazine, and nitroprusside.
2. Test results may be decreased by excessive licorice ingestion and the medications, fludrocortisone and propranolol.

Tests of Pituitary Function

Serum Growth Hormone

Description

1. Direct radioimmunoassay measurement of human growth hormone (GH), secreted by the anterior pituitary gland; useful to diagnose acromegaly, gigantism, pituitary tumors, pituitary-related growth failure in children, or GH deficiency in adults.
2. Because GH secretion is episodic, single fasting samples may not be reliable to detect GH excess or deficiency.
3. These conditions are best evaluated by using a stimulation test (for deficiency states) or a suppression test (for hormone excess conditions).

Nursing and Patient Care Considerations

1. Blood sample is taken after an overnight fast (caloric intake will lower GH blood levels).
2. Patient should be restful and calm before blood sample collection.
3. Normal range: males—less than 5 ng/mL; females—less than 8 ng/mL.
4. May be elevated by the following medications: alcohol, L-dopa, hormonal contraceptives, alpha-antagonists, and beta-adrenergic blockers.

Serum Prolactin

Description

Direct radioimmunoassay measurement of prolactin, secreted by the anterior pituitary gland; helps diagnose pituitary tumors.

Nursing and Patient Care Considerations

1. Blood sample is taken after an overnight fast.
2. Normal values: men—1 to 20 ng/mL; women—1 to 25 ng/mL.
3. Values above 300 ng/mL highly suggestive of pituitary tumor.
4. Elevated values may be caused by exercise or by breast stimulation, such as from friction.
5. Medications that will elevate test results include phenothiazines, reserpine, estrogens, tricyclic antidepressants, methyldopa, antihypertensive medications, and selective serotonin reuptake inhibitors.

Adrenocorticotropic Hormone

Description

1. Direct measurement of ACTH concentration in the bloodstream by radioimmunoassay technique.
2. One measure of pituitary gland function useful to provide important information regarding adrenal gland dysfunction.
3. Useful to identify cause of adrenal abnormalities when compared with serum cortisol levels.

Nursing and Patient Care Considerations

1. Because ACTH is rapidly degraded, blood samples should be centrifuged and frozen promptly to avoid falsely low results.
2. High stress levels in patient can invalidate results.
3. Interpretation of test results:
   a. Elevated levels with elevated cortisol—Cushing disease or ectopic production of ACTH.
   b. Elevated levels with low cortisol—Addison disease.
   c. Low levels with elevated cortisol—adrenal tumor.
   d. Low levels with low cortisol—hypopituitarism.

Insulin Tolerance Test

Description

1. Dynamic test measures pituitary response to induced hypoglycemia, particularly GH secretion and ACTH-stimulated cortisol production by the adrenal gland.
2. Useful to diagnose functional hypopituitarism that is caused by pituitary disease or that appears after pituitary surgery.
3. Considered the "gold standard" for diagnosis of GH deficiency.

Nursing and Patient Care Considerations

1. After overnight fast, insulin 0.15 unit/kg (usual dose but may vary) body weight is given via IV line.
2. Blood samples are collected, usually at baseline, every 15 minutes after insulin dose.
3. The test is considered valid if blood glucose falls to half of baseline or less than 35 mg/dL.
4. Peak response is seen at 60 to 100 minutes.
5. For adrenal response, a rise in cortisol by a factor of at least 1.5 is necessary to show normal response.
6. GH deficiency is present if growth hormone levels fail to rise above 3 mcg/L.
7. This test is contraindicated in people with epilepsy or heart disease. In people with suspected adrenal insufficiency, ACTH stimulation test should be done first.
8. For people in whom the insulin tolerance test is contraindicated, other agents may be used, such as clonidine, arginine, glucagon, L-dopa, or GH-releasing hormone, to stimulate GH secretion.

 NURSING ALERT Test should be performed with health care provider present. Dextrose 50% solution should be available at bedside to treat hypoglycemia, and test stopped if blood sugar falls below 35mg/dL.

Glucose Suppression Test

Description

Postprandial elevations of glucose inhibit the secretion of GH by the pituitary gland. Failure to suppress GH levels after ingestion of glucose suggests a GH-secreting tumor.

Nursing and Patient Care Considerations

1. Patient should fast for this test.
2. Seventy-five to hundred grams of concentrated glucose is administered by mouth.
3. Blood samples are collected at baseline, 30, and 60 minutes.
4. Interpretation of test results:
   a. GH levels less than 2 mcg/L are considered normal.
   b. GH levels that are not suppressed are suggestive of acromegaly.
5. Failure of GH suppression may also be caused by starvation or protein calorie restriction.
6. Patients may complain of nausea after ingesting Glucola.

Water Deprivation Test

Description

1. Functional test of the adequacy of posterior pituitary secretion of antidiuretic hormone (ADH) and its ability to concentrate urine and to maintain serum osmolality in the face of water deprivation.
2. Useful to determine the diagnosis and etiology of diabetes insipidus (DI).

Nursing and Patient Care Considerations

1. The test is begun by obtaining patient's weight, serum, and urine osmolality at time 0.
2. Patient weight, urine output volume, and osmolality are determined hourly.
3. Deprivation is continued until urine osmolality "plateaus," as evidenced by a change of less than 10% in urine osmolality between consecutive measurements and a 2% reduction in patient's body weight. At this time, samples are collected for serum sodium, osmolality, and vasopressin.
4. The test may be stopped if patient loses more than 3% of his or her body weight or if cardiac instability occurs.
5. If urine osmolality remains below that of serum (usually 300 mOsm/kg), the diagnosis of DI is confirmed and the second stage of the test, which distinguishes central and nephrogenic DI, is begun.
6. Artificial ADH (desmopressin acetate [DDAVP]) 2 mcg is given SubQ or IM to determine changes in urine osmolality at 30, 60, and 120 minutes in response to the injected hormone.
7. If the highest urine osmolality value obtained after injection is more than 50% higher than the preinjection value, DI is caused by pituitary failure. If the osmolality value is less than 50% of preinjection value, then DI is caused by renal disease.

 NURSING ALERT Patients with suspected DI who undergo the water deprivation test must be monitored closely because dehydration may occur rapidly in people with severe disease.

Radiology and Imaging

Radioactive ^{131}I Uptake

Description

1. Measures thyroid uptake patterns of iodine as a whole or within specified areas of the gland. A solution of sodium iodide-131 (^{131}I) is administered orally to fasting patient.
2. After a prescribed interval, usually 24 hours, measurements of radioactive counts per minute are taken with a scintillator.
3. Normal thyroid will remove 15% to 50% of the iodine from the bloodstream.
4. Hyperthyroidism may result in the removal of as much as 90% of the iodine from the bloodstream (eg, Graves disease); it may also cause a low uptake with some forms of thyroiditis.
5. Hypothyroidism is reflected in low uptake.

Nursing and Patient Care Considerations

After the test, radioactive iodine is eliminated through urine. The following measures are recommended from 1 to 21 days (depending on dose given, most average 3 days):

1. Drink lots of fluids.
2. Flush toilet two to three times after use.
3. Avoid close contact with other—6 feet distance.
4. Avoid contact with infants, children, and pregnant women.
5. Do not share a bed.
6. Avoid public areas.
7. Do not share utensils and/or prepare foods for others.

Thyroid Scan

Description

1. Rapid imaging of thyroid tissue, particularly suspicious nodules, as contrast imaging agent is rapidly taken up by functioning tissue.

2. Useful to diagnose thyroid carcinoma.
3. Contrast media is usually administered via IV line.
   a. Technetium (^{99m}Tc) pertechnetate or ^{123}I is used for best images.
4. Images can be obtained from gamma counter within 20 to 60 minutes.

Nursing and Patient Care Considerations

1. May interfere with serum radioimmunoassay tests; contact laboratory to determine when blood test can be done.
2. Benign adenomas may be visualized as "hot" nodules, indicating increased uptake of iodine, or as "cold" nodules, indicating decreased uptake.
3. Malignant nodules usually take the form of "cold" nodules.
4. No specific measures need to be taken after the test.

GENERAL PROCEDURES AND TREATMENT MODALITIES

See Standards of Care Guidelines 24-1, page 703.

Steroid Therapy

Steroid therapy is a treatment used in some endocrine disorders and in various other conditions. Steroids are hormones that affect metabolism and many body processes.

Classification of Steroids

(By major metabolic effects on the body.)

Mineralocorticoids

1. Concerned with sodium and water retention and potassium excretion.
2. Example—aldosterone and 11-desoxycorticosterone.

Glucocorticoids (Corticosteroids, Steroids)

1. Concerned with metabolic effects, including carbohydrate metabolism.
2. Example—cortisol.

Sex Hormones

1. Important when secreted in large amounts or when the growth of hormone-sensitive cancers is stimulated.
2. Examples:
   a. Androgens—testosterone.
   b. Estrogens—estradiol.
   c. Progestins—progesterone.

Effects of Glucocorticoids

1. Antagonize action of insulin; promote gluconeogenesis, which provides glucose.
2. Increase breakdown of protein (inhibit protein synthesis).
3. Increase breakdown of fatty acids.
4. Suppress inflammation, inhibit scar formation, block allergic responses.
5. Decrease number of circulating eosinophils and leukocytes; decrease size of lymphatic tissue.
6. Exert a permissive action (allow the full effects) on catecholamines.
7. Exert a permissive action on functioning of central nervous system (CNS).
8. Inhibit release of adrenocorticotropin.
9. In summary, glucocorticoids are necessary to resist noxious stimuli and environmental change.

STANDARDS OF CARE GUIDELINES 24-1
Endocrine Disorders

When caring for a patient with an endocrine disorder, remember that important metabolic functions may be disrupted, such as fluid and electrolyte balance, glucose and protein metabolism, energy production, calcium ionization, blood pressure (BP) control, thermoregulation, cardiac contractility, intestinal peristalsis, and ability of the body to react to stress.

- Monitor closely for electrolyte imbalance—sodium, potassium, chloride, bicarbonate—by checking laboratory test results, changes in the electrocardiogram pattern, and signs of particular excess or deficit (see Chapter 21, page 605).

- Check fingerstick or serum glucose periodically for patients on corticosteroids or for patients with adrenal disease; watch for signs of hyperglycemia (polydipsia, polyphagia, polyuria, blurred vision) or hypoglycemia (nervousness, tremor, difficulty concentrating, lethargy).

- Monitor for hypocalcemia after thyroidectomy, parathyroidectomy, or with hypoparathyroidism by checking serum calcium and phosphorus levels; watch for muscular twitching, anxiety, apprehension, spasms, and tetany. Check Chvostek sign and Trousseau sign.

- Monitor vital signs for heart rate, BP, and presence of arrhythmias.

- Monitor temperature and respiratory rate changes in thyroid and adrenal disease.

- Monitor intake and output, weight changes, and edema.

- Maintain a calm, quiet environment and provide meticulous care to prevent infection or dehydration in patients with adrenal hypofunction or patients on corticosteroid replacement.

- After surgery, check for bleeding, signs of infection, changes in vital signs. Monitor respiratory status carefully after thyroidectomy.

- Report worsening condition or development of suspicious signs and symptoms promptly to prevent serious complications, such as myxedema coma, thyroid storm, hypocalcemic tetany, adrenal crisis.

- Provide support, and explain care slowly and repeatedly because patient may have mental slowness, confusion, or lethargy because of his or her condition. Ask patient to restate important information to verify understanding.

This information should serve as a general guideline only. Each patient situation presents a unique set of clinical factors and requires nursing judgment to guide care, which may include additional or alternative measures and approaches.

Uses of Steroids

1. Physiologically—to correct deficiencies or malfunction of a particular endocrine organ or system (eg, Addison disease).
2. Diagnostically—to determine proper functioning of the endocrine system.
3. Pharmacologically—to treat the following:
   a. Asthma and obstructive lung disease.
   b. Acute rheumatic fever.
   c. Blood conditions, such as idiopathic thrombocytopenic purpura, leukemia, hemolytic anemia.
   d. Allergic conditions—allergic rhinitis, anaphylaxis (after epinephrine).
   e. Dermatologic problems—drug rashes, contact dermatitis, atopic dermatitis.
   f. Ocular diseases—conjunctivitis, uveitis.
   g. Connective tissue disorders—systemic lupus erythematosus, rheumatoid arthritis.
   h. GI problems—ulcerative colitis.
   i. Organ transplant recipients—as an immunosuppressive agent.
   j. Neurologic conditions—cerebral edema, multiple sclerosis.

Preparing the Patient to Receive Steroid Therapy

1. Determine contraindications/precautions for such therapy.
   a. Peptic ulcer.
   b. Diabetes mellitus.
   c. Viral infections.
2. Administer a tuberculin test, if indicated, before therapy because steroids may suppress response to the test.
3. Assess the patient's own level of steroid secretion, if possible.
4. Explain the nature of the therapy, what is required of the patient, how long therapy will last, adverse effects to watch for, and answer any questions.

Choice of Steroid and Method of Administration

1. May be given by various methods—orally, parenterally, sublingually, rectally, by inhalation, or by direct application to skin or mucous membrane.
2. Combinations of steroids with other drugs should be avoided.
3. To help avoid steroid adverse effects, alternate-day therapy may be used; dose is taken in the morning.
4. May be given in initial high doses, then reduced; if the patient has been taking steroids for several weeks, doses must be tapered gradually to prevent addisonian crisis.

Nursing Interventions

Preventing Infection

1. Steroids may affect the circulating blood, resulting in decreased eosinophils and lymphocytes, increased red cells, and increased incidence of thrombophlebitis and infection.
2. Encourage the patient to avoid crowds and the possibility of exposure to infection.
3. Encourage exercise to prevent venous stasis.
4. Be aware that signs of infection/inflammation may be masked—fever, redness, swelling.
5. Practice and encourage good handwashing technique and asepsis.

Preventing Nutritional and Metabolism Complications

1. Determine whether the patient needs assistance in dietary control. Steroids may cause weight gain and an increase in appetite.
2. Encourage a high-protein diet. Because steroids affect protein metabolism, there may be negative nitrogen balance.
3. Encourage the patient to take steroids with milk or with food. Because steroids increase secretion of gastric acid and have an inhibiting effect on secretion of mucus in the stomach, they may cause peptic ulcer.

4. Be on guard for early evidence of gastric hemorrhage, such as melena, blood in vomitus.
5. Check fasting blood glucose levels.
   a. Steroids precipitate gluconeogenesis and insulin antagonism, which results in hyperglycemia, glucosuria, decreased carbohydrate tolerance.
   b. Temporary insulin injections may be necessary.

Observing for Bone Complications

1. Be on the alert for the possibility of pathologic fractures. Stress safety measures to prevent injury.
   a. Steroids affect the musculoskeletal system, causing potassium depletion and muscular weakness.
   b. Steroids cause increased output of calcium and phosphorus, which may lead to osteoporosis.
2. Administer a diet high in calcium and protein.
3. Recommend activities of daily living (ADLs) and weight-bearing program; recommend normal range of motion and safe repositioning for those who are bedridden.
4. Obtain baseline DXA scan, if on long-term steroid use.

Avoiding Electrolyte Disturbance

1. Restrict sodium intake and increase potassium intake.
   a. Mineralocorticoids differ from other steroids, resulting in sodium retention and potassium depletion; edema, weight gain.
   b. Lemon juice is high in potassium and low in sodium.
   c. Avoid saline as a diluent in preparing injectable medications.
2. Check BP frequently, and weigh the patient daily.
3. Observe for edema.

Monitoring Behavioral Reactions

1. Watch for convulsive seizures (especially in children). Steroids may alter behavior patterns, increase excitability, and may affect the CNS.
2. Avoid overstimulating situations.
3. Recognize and report any mood that deviates from the usual behavior patterns.
4. Report unusual behavior, haunting dreams, withdrawal, or suicidal tendencies.

Preventing Stress Reactions

1. Recommend that the patient carry an identification card that indicates steroid therapy and name of health care provider.
2. Be aware that steroids affect the hypothalamic–pituitary–adrenal system, which affects the patient's ability to respond to stress.
3. Advise the patient to avoid extremes of temperature, infections, and upsetting situations.

Preventing Injury and Promoting Healing

1. Instruct the patient to avoid injury; stress safety precautions. Because steroids interfere with fibroblasts and granulation tissue, altered response to injury results in impaired growth and delayed healing.
2. Observe daily the healing process of wounds, particularly surgical wounds, to recognize the potential for wound dehiscence.

Patient Education and Health Maintenance

1. Teach patient that steroids are valuable and useful medications, but that if taken for longer than 2 weeks, they may produce certain adverse effects.
   a. Acceptable adverse effects may include weight gain (because of increased appetite and water retention), acne, headaches, fatigue, and increased urinary frequency.

b. Unacceptable adverse effects that are to be reported to the health care provider include dizziness when rising from chair or bed (orthostatic hypotension indicative of adrenal insufficiency), nausea, vomiting, thirst, abdominal pain, or pain of any type.
   c. Additional reportable adverse effects include convulsive seizures, feelings of depression or nervousness, or development of an infection.
2. Advise patient that a fall or an automobile accident may precipitate adrenal failure. This requires an immediate injection of hydrocortisone phosphate.
3. Tell patients on long-term therapy that they should wear a MedicAlert bracelet and carry a kit with hydrocortisone, as prescribed.
4. Instruct patient to inform any physician, dentist, or nurse about steroid therapy.
5. Tell patient that regular follow-up visits to health care provider are required.

Care of the Patient Undergoing Fine Needle Aspiration Biopsy

 EVIDENCE BASE Haugen, B. R., Alexander, E. K., Bible, K. C., et al. (2016). American Thyroid Association Management Guidelines for Adult Patients with Thyroid Nodules and Differentiated Thyroid Cancer: The American Thyroid Association Guidelines Task Force on Thyroid Nodules and Differentiated Thyroid Cancer. *Thyroid, 26*(1), 1–133.
Jonklaas, J., Bianco, A. C., Bauer, A. J., et al. (2014). Guidelines for the Treatment of Hypothyroidism: Prepared by the American Thyroid Association Task Force on Thyroid Hormone Replacement. *Thyroid, 24*(12), 1670–1751.

Fine needle aspiration (FNA) *biopsy* is a procedure by which tissue from within a thyroid nodule is removed to detect malignancy. This procedure can easily be performed on an outpatient basis and requires no special patient preparation. Complications are uncommon but may include hematoma, tracheal perforation, and infection.

Preparation and Procedure

1. No special patient preparation activities are necessary for this procedure.
2. The procedure is explained to patient, and consent is obtained.
3. Patient is positioned comfortably on an examination table in the supine position with the neck fully exposed.
4. A rolled towel or sheet is placed beneath the patient's shoulder to hyperextend the neck, allowing ease of access to the biopsy site.
5. The biopsy site area is cleaned with alcohol and/or an antibacterial cleaning agent.
6. One percent lidocaine may be injected intracutaneously for local anesthetic to promote patient comfort.
7. A 25-G needle is inserted into the thyroid nodule and manipulated by the physician until a small amount of bloody material is seen on the hub of the needle.
8. The needle is removed and attached to a syringe. The contents of the needle are expressed onto a clean glass slide. A second slide is placed on top of the first slide and then pulled apart quickly to create a thin smear.

9. The slides are placed in a fixative and transported to a cytologist for interpretation.

Postprocedure Management

1. The biopsy site may be dressed with an adhesive bandage or other small dressing.
2. Follow-up visit for patient should be arranged to discuss results.

Nursing Considerations

1. Prevent infection by making sure that biopsy area is prepped appropriately before procedure.
2. Employ comfort measures during procedure, as necessary.
3. Assure patient that most thyroid nodules are determined to be benign and that most thyroid malignancies have a high cure rate.
4. Advise patient that some soreness at the biopsy site should be expected for a brief time.
5. Make sure that patient follows up for results and definitive treatment.

Care of the Patient Undergoing Thyroidectomy

Thyroidectomy involves the partial or complete removal of the thyroid gland to treat thyroid tumors, hyperthyroidism, or hyperparathyroidism.

Types of Procedures

1. Thyroidectomy can be total (removal of the entire thyroid gland); subtotal (95% of gland removed)—to prevent damage to the parathyroid glands; and partial (one lobe or isthmus removed)—to treat nodular disease.
2. The parathyroid glands are usually spared to prevent hypocalcemia.
3. Indications for thyroidectomy include Graves disease refractory to ^{131}I therapy, large goiters, adenoma (thyroid cancer), and some nodules.

Preoperative Management

1. The patient must be euthyroid at time of surgery, so thioamides are administered to control hyperthyroidism.
2. Iodide is given to increase firmness of the thyroid gland and to reduce its vascularity and blood loss.
3. An attempt is made to counteract the effects of hypermetabolism by maintaining a restful and therapeutic environment and by providing a nutritious diet.
4. The patient is prepared for surgery physically and emotionally in the following ways:
   a. Make a special effort to ensure that patient has a good night's rest preceding surgery.
   b. Explain to patient that speaking is to be minimized immediately postoperatively and that oxygen may be administered to facilitate breathing.
   c. Explain that postoperatively, fluids may be given via IV line to maintain fluid, electrolyte, and nutritional needs; IV glucose may also be given in the hours before the administration of anesthetic agents.

Postoperative Management

1. The patient is monitored for bleeding and respiratory distress that indicates laryngeal edema, secondary to swelling in the area of surgery.

2. Signs of hypocalcemia are watched for—irritability, twitching, spasms of the hands and feet.
   a. Calcium levels are monitored. If in 48 hours level falls below 7 mg/100 mL (3 mEq), IV calcium (gluconate, lactate) replacement is given.
   b. IV calcium is used cautiously in patients who have renal disease or who are taking digoxin.
3. Thyroid function is monitored after surgery.

Complications

1. Hemorrhage, edema of the glottis, damage to laryngeal nerve.
2. Hypothyroidism following subtotal thyroidectomy occurs in 5% of patients in first postoperative year; increases at rate of 2% to 3% per year.
3. Hypoparathyroidism occurs in about 4% of patients and is usually mild and transient; requires calcium supplements via IV administration and orally when more severe.

Nursing Diagnoses

- Risk for Bleeding related to invasive procedure of the neck.
- Risk for Injury related to possible removal of parathyroid glands.

Nursing Interventions

Observing for Hemorrhage and Airway Edema

1. Administer humidified oxygen, as prescribed, to reduce irritation of airway and to prevent edema.
2. Move patient carefully; provide adequate support to the head so that no tension is placed on the sutures.
3. Place patient in semi-Fowler position, with the head elevated and supported by pillows; avoid flexion of the neck.
4. Monitor vital signs frequently, watching for tachycardia and hypotension that indicates hemorrhage (most likely between 12 and 24 hours postoperatively).
5. Observe for bleeding at sides and back of the neck, and anteriorly, when patient is in dorsal position.
6. Watch for repeated clearing of the throat or for complaint of smothering or difficulty swallowing, which may be early signs of hemorrhage.
7. Watch for irregular breathing, swelling of the neck, and choking—other signs pointing to the possibility of hemorrhage and tracheal compression.
8. Reinforce dressing, if indicated.
9. Be alert for voice changes, which may indicate damage to laryngeal nerve.
10. Keep a tracheostomy set in patient's room for 48 hours for emergency use.

Preventing Tetany

1. Watch for the development of tetany caused by removal or disturbance of parathyroid glands through a progression of signs:
   a. Tingling of toes and fingers and around the mouth; apprehension.
   b. Positive Chvostek sign—spasm of facial muscles caused by tapping on the cheek over the facial nerve; causes a twitch of the lip or side of the face (see Figure 24-1A, page 706).
   c. Positive Trousseau sign—carpopedal spasm induced by occluding circulation in the arm or lower leg with a BP cuff (20 mm Hg above systolic pressure); within

Figure 24-1. (A) Chvostek sign. **(B)** Trousseau sign.

3 minutes, flexion of the hands at the wrists and of the fingers at the metacarpophalangeal joints and extension of the fingers at the phalangeal joints or the feet are dorsiflexed at the ankles and the toes plantar flexed (see Figure 24-1B).
2. Be prepared to treat hypocalcemic tetany.
   a. Position patient for optimal ventilation; remove pillow to prevent head from bending forward and compressing trachea.
   b. Keep side rails padded and elevated, and position the patient to prevent injury if a seizure occurs; do not use restraints because they only aggravate the patient and may result in muscle strain or fractures.
   c. Have equipment available to treat respiratory difficulties that includes airway suction equipment, tracheostomy, and cardiac arrest equipment.
3. Administer IV calcium, as directed.

Patient Education and Health Maintenance

1. Teach patient about complications to look for if discharge occurs within a day or two of surgery.
2. Advise patient to rest at home and to prevent any strain on suture line, as directed by surgeon.
3. Advise nutritious diet; report difficulty swallowing.
4. Encourage follow-up for monitoring and thyroid hormone replacement after surgery.

Evaluation: Expected Outcomes

- No signs of hemorrhage or edema.
- No signs of hypocalcemia.

Care of the Patient Undergoing Adrenalectomy

Adrenalectomy may be unilateral or bilateral to treat adrenal tumors, Cushing syndrome, or hyperaldosteronism. It is accomplished through abdominal or flank incision. Careful manipulation of the gland is necessary—if surgery is indicated for pheochromocytoma—to prevent excessive release of epinephrine causing hypertensive crisis.

Preoperative Management

1. BP and fluid volume are optimized.
2. Surgical and nursing care is explained to patient. Patient is shown where adrenal glands lie on the top of the kidneys and where incision may be on the abdomen or loin area.
3. BP will be checked frequently before and after surgery, and glucocorticoids will be given to cover period of stress (surgery) because at least one adrenal gland will be removed.
4. Patient is prepared as for major abdominal surgery (see page 495).

Complications

Hemorrhage, adrenal crisis.

Postoperative Management

1. Usual postoperative care for abdominal surgery includes frequent check of vital signs; assessment for hemorrhage; turning, coughing, and deep breathing; early ambulation; slow progression of diet when bowel sounds return; and control of pain with scheduled opioid administration or patient-controlled analgesia (see page 1509).
2. IV hydrocortisone is given, as directed, to prevent adrenal crisis.
3. Nonstressful environment is maintained, rest is promoted, and meticulous care is given to protect patient from infection and from other complications that could cause adrenal crisis.
4. Serum sodium, potassium, and glucose are monitored for abnormality.
   a. Sodium and potassium may normalize, or potassium may become elevated (because of transient adrenal insufficiency after surgery).
   b. Electrolyte imbalances may persist for 4 to 18 months after surgery.
   c. Hypertension may persist for 3 to 6 months after surgery.
5. Hydrocortisone treatment causes glucose to rise and worsens control in patients with diabetes; may require additional treatment.

Nursing Diagnoses

- Risk for Infection related to nature of surgery.
- Readiness for Enhanced Knowledge about corticosteroid replacement.

Nursing Interventions

Ensuring Healing

1. Assess dressing for leakage initially, and after it has been changed, assess wound for signs of infection.
2. Perform dressing changes, wound care, and teach family how to do wound care at home.

Providing Patient Education

1. Teach patient with bilateral adrenalectomy that glucocorticoid and mineralocorticoid replacement is necessary for rest of life.
2. Administer additional doses IM in times of stress.
3. Administer oral glucocorticoids after unilateral adrenalectomy, and teach patient that this treatment will be needed for 6 months to 2 years after surgery until remaining adrenal gland can compensate.

4. Encourage wearing or carrying a medical alert tag containing this information at all times so that proper treatment can be instituted if patient becomes unconscious.
5. Encourage follow-up to monitor for signs of adrenal insufficiency.

Care of the Patient Undergoing Transsphenoidal Hypophysectomy

Procedure

1. Transsphenoidal approach to pituitary removal is carried out through the nasal cavity, sphenoid sinus, and into the sella turcica (see Figure 24-2).
2. Advantages over intracranial approach to hypophysectomy include:
   a. No need to shave the head.
   b. No visible scar.
   c. Low blood loss, less need for transfusions.
   d. Lower infection rate.
   e. Well tolerated by frail and older patients.
   f. Good visualization of tumor field.
3. Disadvantages include:
   a. Restricted field of surgery.
   b. Potential cerebrospinal fluid (CSF) leak.

Preoperative Management

1. Sinus infection is assessed and treated, if necessary.
2. Hydrocortisone may be given preoperatively because the source of ACTH is being removed.
3. The patient is prepared physically and emotionally for surgery.
   a. Deep-breathing exercises.
   b. Avoid coughing and sneezing postoperatively to prevent CSF leak.

Complications

1. CSF leak, meningitis.
2. Transient DI.
3. Syndrome of inappropriate antidiuretic hormone (SIADH).

Figure 24-2. Transsphenoidal approach to the pituitary. A special nasal speculum is used to view the sinus cavity. After the dura is opened, the tumor is removed using microcurettes or other specially designed instruments.

Postoperative Management

1. Vital signs, visual acuity, and neurologic status are monitored.
2. Urine output and specific gravity and serum electrolytes and osmolality are monitored for development of DI or SIADH.
3. Drainage from nose is monitored for signs of infection or CSF leak (clear fluid).

Nursing Diagnoses

• Delayed Surgical Recovery related to potential complications.
• Risk for Infection secondary to invasive procedure.

Nursing Interventions

Protecting Against Complications

1. Monitor vital signs, visual acuity, and neurologic status frequently for signs of increasing intracranial pressure (see page 357).
2. Monitor fluid intake and output, and report any increase in output and decrease in specific gravity, which may indicate DI.
3. Report persistent clear fluid from nose and increasing headache; could signal CSF leak.
4. Teach patient signs of complications and to report them immediately and to follow up as scheduled.
5. Assess level of pain, and administer analgesic or supervise patient-controlled analgesia.

Preventing Infection

1. Observe for signs of infection. Check incision within inner aspect of upper lip for drainage or bleeding.
2. Note frequency of nasal dressing changes and character of drainage. Prepare patient for packing removal one to several days postoperatively.
3. Encourage the use of a humidifier to prevent drying from mouth breathing.

Evaluation: Expected Outcomes

• Vital signs stable, urine specific gravity 1.010, no clear drainage from nose.
• No purulent drainage noted.

DISORDERS OF THE THYROID GLAND

See additional online content: Nursing Care Plan 24-1

The thyroid gland affects the basal metabolic rate of all tissues, including the speed of chemical reactions, the volume of oxygen consumed, and the amount of heat produced. The stimulating effect is through the production and distribution of two hormones:

1. Levothyroxine (T_4)—contains four iodine atoms; maintains body's metabolism in a steady state; T_4 serves as a precursor of T_3.
2. Triiodothyronine (T_3)—contains three iodine atoms; approximately five times as potent as T_4; has a more rapid metabolic action and utilization than T_4 does. T_3 affects the protein

synthesis and substrate by modifying gene transcription in most tissue.

3. Most conversion of T_4 to T_3 occurs at the cellular level in the periphery. Some T_3 is produced in the thyroid gland.

Hypothyroidism

Hypothyroidism is a condition that arises from a deficiency in endogenous production of thyroid hormone in the bloodstream.

Pathophysiology and Etiology

1. Primary hypothyroidism is the most common form of this condition and is generally caused by:
   a. Autoimmune disease—chronic lymphocytic thyroiditis (also known as Hashimoto's thyroiditis).
   b. Postpartum thyroiditis.
   c. Use of radioactive iodine.
   d. Destruction, suppression, or removal of all or some of the thyroid tissue by thyroidectomy.
   e. Dietary iodide deficiency.
   f. Subacute granulomatous thyroiditis.
   g. Drug-induced iatrogenic hypothyroidism.
   h. Genetic causes.
2. Secondary hypothyroidism is caused when damage occurs to the hypothalamic–pituitary axis (ie, tumor, necrosis, head trauma, certain drugs, brain/pituitary irradiation).
3. Inadequate secretion of thyroid hormone leads to a general slowing of all physical and mental processes.
4. General depression of most cellular enzyme systems and oxidative processes occurs.
5. The metabolic activity of all cells of the body decreases, reducing oxygen consumption, decreasing oxidation of nutrients for energy, and producing less body heat.
6. The signs and symptoms of the disorder range from vague, nonspecific complaints that make diagnosis difficult to severe symptoms that may be life threatening if unrecognized and untreated.

Clinical Manifestations

1. Fatigue and lethargy, decreased energy, exhaustion.
2. Weight gain-despite possible decreased appetite.
3. Complaints of cold hands and feet, cold intolerant
4. Increased blood pressure, decreased pulse.
5. Reduced attention span; impaired short-term memory.
6. Constipation; decreased peristalsis.
7. Generalized appearance of "doughy" thick, puffy skin; subcutaneous swelling in the hands, feet, and eyelids.
8. Thinning hair; loss of the lateral one third of the eyebrow.
9. Dry skin.
10. Enlarged tongue.
11. Depression, other psychological problems.
12. Menorrhagia or amenorrhea; may have difficulty conceiving or may experience spontaneous abortion; decreased libido, erectile dysfunction.
13. Neurologic signs include polyneuropathy, cerebellar ataxia, muscle aches or weakness, clumsiness, prolonged deep tendon reflexes (especially ankle jerk).
14. Hyperlipoproteinemia and hypercholesterolemia.
15. Enlarged heart on chest x-ray.
16. Increased susceptibility to all hypnotic and sedative drugs and anesthetic agents.
17. Syndrome of subclinical hypothyroidism: state in which the patient is asymptomatic and the free T_4 level is within the normal range; however, the TSH level is elevated, suggesting impending thyroid gland failure. Therefore, many clinicians may elect to treat this condition as if the patient were symptomatic.

Diagnostic Evaluation

1. Low T_3 and T_4 levels.
2. Elevated TSH levels in primary hypothyroidism.
3. Elevation of serum cholesterol.
4. Electrocardiogram (ECG)—sinus bradycardia, low voltage of QRS complexes, and flat or inverted T waves.
5. Elevation of thyroid peroxidase antibodies and antithyroglobulin antibodies.

Management

Approach

1. Depends on severity of symptoms; may necessitate replacement therapy in mild cases or lifesaving support and treatment in severe hypothyroidism and myxedema coma.
2. As thyroid hormone levels gradually return to normal, the patient is monitored closely to prevent complications resulting from sudden increases in metabolic rate and oxygen requirements.

Restoration of Normal Metabolic State (Euthyroid)

1. Thyroid hormone: T_4, levothyroxine; T_3, liothyronine; T_3 and T_4 mixed. T_4 replacement therapy is typically the treatment of choice.
   a. In myxedema coma, a loading dose of levothyroxine is administered parenterally (until consciousness is restored) to restore T_4 level. Use of T_3 is controversial, may increase adverse cardiac events.
   b. Later, patient is continued on oral thyroid hormone therapy.
   c. With rapid administration of thyroid hormone, plasma T_4 levels may initiate adrenal insufficiency; hence, steroid therapy may be started.
   d. Mild symptoms in alert patient or asymptomatic cases (with abnormal laboratory results only) require only initiation of low-dose thyroid hormone given orally.
2. Monitoring to anticipate treatment effects.
   a. Diuresis, decreased puffiness.
   b. Improved reflexes and muscle tone.
   c. Accelerated pulse rate.
   d. A slightly higher level of total serum T_4.
   e. All signs of hypothyroidism should disappear in 3 to 12 weeks.
   f. Decreasing TSH level.
   g. Patients on T_4 can have an increase of dose every 4 to 6 weeks until TSH is therapeutic.

 GERONTOLOGIC ALERT When starting thyroid hormone replacement, care must be taken with older patients and with those who have coronary ischemia disease, because of increased oxygen demands of the heart. It is preferable to start with much lower doses 25% to 50% lower than needed.

Complications

1. Myxedema coma—hypotension, unresponsiveness, bradycardia, hypoventilation, hyponatremia, (possibly) convulsions, hypothermia, cerebral hypoxia.
2. High mortality in myxedema coma.

Nursing Assessment

1. Obtain history of symptoms, medication program, and past history of thyroid disease, surgery, or treatment.
2. Perform multisystem assessment, including cardiac, respiratory, neurologic, and GI systems.

Nursing Diagnoses

- Decreased Cardiac Output related to decreased metabolic rate and decreased cardiac conduction.
- Constipation related to decreased bowel motility.
- Activity Intolerance related to reduced metabolic rate.

Nursing Interventions

Increasing Cardiac Output

1. Monitor vital signs frequently to detect changes in cardiovascular status and ability to respond to stress.
2. Monitor ECG tracings to detect arrhythmias and deterioration of cardiovascular status.
3. Prevent chilling to avoid increasing metabolic rate, which, in turn, places strain on the heart. Provide bed socks, bed jacket, warm environment.
4. Avoid rapid rewarming techniques (warmed IV fluids, hypothermia blanket) because the resulting increased oxygen requirements and peripheral vasodilation may worsen cardiac failure.
5. Administer fluids cautiously, even though hyponatremia is present.
6. Administer all prescribed drugs with caution before and after thyroid replacement begins.
   a. Monitor the effects of sedatives, opioids, and anesthetics closely because patient is more sensitive to these agents.
   b. After thyroid replacement is initiated, the thyroid hormones may increase the effects of digoxin (monitor pulse) and anticoagulants (watch for signs of bleeding).
7. Report occurrence of angina and be alert for signs and symptoms of myocardial infarction and cardiac failure.
8. Monitor arterial blood gas levels to assess cardiopulmonary function.

Promoting Normal Bowel Movements

1. Encourage too fluid intake of at least 64 ounces daily, unless contraindicated.
2. Recommend high-fiber food intake, including fresh or frozen fruit and vegetables lightly cooked, whole grains, and beans.
3. Advise patient to increase activity as tolerated and paying attention to the body's natural urge to evacuate the bowel.

Increasing Exercise Tolerance

1. Provide for uninterrupted rest periods between activities to assist with reconditioning.
2. Encourage exercise and walking goals based on patient's age and previous physical conditioning, in consultation with a physical therapist if required.

3. Recommend gradually increasing exercise and activity but stop if short of breath, chest pain, dizziness, or weakness. Report these symptoms if they do not resolve quickly with rest.

Patient Education and Health Maintenance

Instruct the patient about the following:
1. The need to receive lifelong thyroid hormone replacement therapy.
2. How and when to take medications.
3. Signs and symptoms of insufficient and excessive medication; reinforce teaching by providing written instructions.
4. The necessity of having blood evaluations periodically to determine thyroid levels.
5. Energy conservation techniques and the need to increase activity gradually.
6. Fluid intake and use of fiber to prevent constipation.
7. Control of dietary intake to limit calories and reduce weight.
8. Assist patient in identifying sources of information (see Box 24-1) and support available in the community such as local Office on Aging.

Evaluation: Expected Outcomes

- BP and pulse rate stable.
- Soft bowel movement without straining daily.
- Walking 15 minutes three times a day.

Hyperthyroidism

 EVIDENCE BASE Ross D. S., Burch H. B., Cooper D. S., et al. (2016). American Thyroid Association Guidelines for Diagnosis and Management of Hyperthyroidism and Other Causes of Thyrotoxicosis. *Thyroid, 26*(10), 1343–1421.

Hyperthyroidism, a hypermetabolic condition, is characterized by excessive amounts of thyroid hormone in the bloodstream.

Pathophysiology and Etiology

1. More common in women than in men.
2. Graves disease (most prevalent)—diffuse hyperfunction of the thyroid gland with autoimmune etiology and associated with ophthalmopathy.
   a. TSI, an immunoglobulin found in the blood of patients with Graves disease, is capable of reacting with the receptor for TSH on the thyroid plasma membrane and of stimulating thyroid hormone production and secretion.
   b. Most common in younger women; may subside spontaneously.
3. Toxic nodular goiter (single or multiple)—more common preexisting goiter.
4. Toxic adenoma—present in 3% to 5% of thyrotoxicosis cases.
5. Hyperthyroidism is characterized by hypertrophy and hyperplasia of the thyroid gland, which is accompanied by increased vascularity and blood flow and enlargement of the gland.
6. Most of the clinical manifestations result from increased metabolic rate, excessive heat production, increased neuromuscular and cardiovascular activity, and hyperactivity of the sympathetic nervous system.
7. Hyperthyroidism ranges from a mild increase in metabolic rate to the severe hyperactivity known as thyrotoxicosis, thyroid storm, or thyroid crisis.
8. Hyperthyroidism can also be the result of ingestion of excessive amounts of thyroid hormone medication (factitious hyperthyroidism).

Clinical Manifestations

1. Nervousness, emotional lability, irritability, apprehension.
2. Difficulty sitting quietly; anxiety, hyperactivity.
3. Rapid pulse at rest and on exertion (ranges between 90 and 160); palpitations.
4. Heat intolerance; profuse perspiration; flushed skin (eg, hands may be warm, soft, moist).
5. Fine tremor of hands; change in bowel habits—constipation or diarrhea.
6. Increased appetite and progressive weight loss; frequent stools.
7. Muscle fatigability and weakness; amenorrhea.
8. Atrial fibrillation possible (cardiac decompensation common in older patients).
9. Exophthalmos, periorbital edema, chemosis, diplopia, proptosis suggestive of Graves disease.
10. Thyroid gland may be palpable, and a bruit may be auscultated over gland.
11. Course may be mild, characterized by remissions and exacerbations.
12. May progress to emaciation, extreme nervousness, delirium, disorientation, thyroid storm or crisis, and death.
13. Thyroid storm or crisis, an extreme form of hyperthyroidism, is characterized by hyperpyrexia, diarrhea, dehydration, tachycardia, arrhythmias, extreme irritation, delirium, coma, shock, and death if not adequately treated.
14. Thyroid storm may be precipitated by stress (surgery, infection) or inadequate preparation for surgery in a patient with known hyperthyroidism.

Diagnostic Evaluation

1. Elevated T_3 and T_4.
2. Elevated serum T_3 resin uptake and free thyroid index.
3. Low TSH levels.
4. Presence of TSI antibodies (if Graves disease is the cause).
5. ^{131}I uptake scan may be elevated or below normal depending on the underlying cause of the hyperthyroidism.

Management

Approach to Management

1. Treatment depends on causes, age of patient, severity of disease, and complications.
2. Remission of hyperthyroidism (Graves disease) occurs spontaneously within 1 to 2 years; however, relapse can be expected in half the patients. Antithyroid drugs, radiation, or surgery may be used for treatment.
3. Nodular toxic goiter—surgery or use of radioiodine is preferred.
4. Thyroid carcinoma—surgery or radiation is used.
5. Goal of therapy is to bring the metabolic rate to normal as soon as possible and to maintain it at this level.

Pharmacotherapy

1. Drugs that inhibit hormone formation:
   a. Thioamides—propylthiouracil and methimazole.
   b. Act by depressing the synthesis of thyroid hormone by inhibiting thyroid peroxidase.
   c. Propylthiouracil given in divided daily doses; methimazole may be given in a single daily dose.
   d. Duration of treatment is determined by clinical criteria.
      i. Thyroid gland becomes smaller.
      ii. Treatment continued until patient becomes clinically euthyroid; this varies from 3 months to 2 years; if euthyroidism cannot be maintained without therapy, then radiation or surgery is recommended.
      iii. Therapy is withdrawn gradually to prevent exacerbation.
2. Drugs to control peripheral manifestations of hyperthyroidism:
   a. Propranolol, a beta-adrenergic blocking agent.
      i. Inhibits peripheral conversion of T_4 to T_3.
      ii. Abolishes tachycardia, tremor, excess sweating, nervousness.
      iii. Controls hyperthyroid symptoms until antithyroid drugs or radioiodine can take effect.
   b. Glucocorticoids—decrease the peripheral conversion of T_4 to T_3, a more potent thyroid hormone.

Radioactive Iodine

1. Action—limits secretion of thyroid hormone by destroying thyroid tissue.
2. Dosage is calculated to help prevent hypothyroidism.
3. Chief advantage over thioamides is that a lasting remission can be achieved.
4. Chief disadvantage is that permanent hypothyroidism can be produced.

Surgery

1. Used for those with large goiters or for those for whom the use of radioiodine or thioamides is contraindicated.
2. Subtotal thyroidectomy involves removal of most of the thyroid gland (see page 705).

 DRUG ALERT Observe the patient for evidence of iodine toxicity: swelling of buccal mucosa, excessive salivation, coryza, skin eruptions. If these occur, iodides are discontinued.

Emergency Management of Thyroid Storm

1. Inhibition of new hormone synthesis with thioamides (PTU and methimazole).
2. Inhibition of thyroid hormone release using a solution of potassium iodine.
3. Inhibition of peripheral effects of thyroid hormones with propranolol, corticosteroids, and propylthiouracil (PTU).
4. Treatment aimed at systemic effects of thyroid hormones and prevention of decompensation.
   a. Hyperthermia—cooling blanket, acetaminophen.
   b. Dehydration—administration of IV fluids and electrolytes.
5. Treatment of precipitating event.

Complications

1. Thioamide toxicity—agranulocytosis may occur suddenly.
2. Hypothyroidism if overtreated with antithyroid medication or if radiation treatment is used.
3. Radiation thyroiditis (a transient exacerbation of hyperthyroidism) may occur as a result of leakage of thyroid hormone into the circulation from damaged follicles.
4. Infiltrative ophthalmopathy.
   a. Occurs in 50% of patients with Graves disease.
   b. Features include exophthalmos, weakness of extraocular muscles, lid edema, lid lag.

Nursing Assessment

1. Obtain history of symptoms, family history of thyroid disease, medications, any recent physical stress, particularly infection.
2. Perform multisystem assessment that includes cardiac, respiratory, neurologic, and GI systems.
3. Closely monitor patient's temperature for thyroid storm.

Nursing Diagnoses

- Imbalanced Nutrition: Less Than Body Requirements related to hypermetabolic state and fluid loss through diaphoresis.
- Risk for Impaired Skin Integrity related to diaphoresis, hyperpyrexia, restlessness, and rapid weight loss.
- Disturbed Thought Processes related to insomnia, decreased attention span, and irritability.
- Anxiety related to condition and concern about upcoming surgery/radioiodine treatment.

Nursing Interventions

Providing Adequate Nutrition

1. Determine patient's food and fluid preferences.
2. Provide high-calorie foods and fluids consistent with the patient's requirements.
3. Provide a quiet, calm environment at meals.
4. Restrict stimulants (tea, coffee, alcohol); explain rationale of requirements and restrictions to patient.
5. Encourage and permit patient to eat alone if embarrassed or if otherwise disturbed by voracious appetite.
6. Monitor IV infusion when prescribed to maintain fluid and electrolyte balance.
7. Monitor fluid and nutritional status by weighing patient daily and by keeping accurate intake and output records.
8. Monitor vital signs to detect changes in fluid volume status.
9. Assess skin turgor, mucous membranes, and neck veins for signs of increased or decreased fluid volume.

Maintaining Skin Integrity

1. Assess skin frequently to detect diaphoresis.
2. Bathe frequently with cool water; change linens when damp.
3. Avoid soap to prevent drying and apply lubricant skin lotions to pressure points.
4. Protect and relieve pressure from bony prominences while immobilized or while hypothermia blanket is used.

Promoting Normal Thought Processes

1. Explain procedures to patient in an unhurried, calm manner.
2. Limit visitors; avoid stimulating conversations or television programs.
3. Reduce stressors in the environment; reduce noise and lights.
4. Promote sleep and relaxation through use of prescribed medications, massage, and relaxation exercises.
5. Minimize disruption of patient's sleep or rest by clustering nursing activities.
6. Use safety measures to reduce risk of trauma or falls (padded side rails, bed in low position).

Relieving Anxiety

1. Encourage patient to verbalize concerns and fears about illness and treatment.
2. Support patient who is undergoing various diagnostic tests.
   a. Explain the purpose and requirements of each prescribed test.
   b. Explain results of tests if unclear to the patient or if questions arise.
3. Clear up misconceptions about treatment options.

Patient Education and Health Maintenance

1. Instruct patient as follows:
   a. When to take medications.
   b. Signs and symptoms of insufficient and excessive medication.
   c. Necessity of having blood evaluations periodically to determine thyroid levels.
   d. Signs of agranulocytosis (fever, sore throat, upper respiratory infection) or rash, fever, urticaria, or enlarged salivary glands caused by thioamide toxicity.
   e. Signs and symptoms of thyroid storm (ie, tachycardia, hyperpyrexia, extreme irritation) and predisposing factors to thyroid storm (ie, infection, surgery, stress, abrupt withdrawal of antithyroid medications and adrenergic blockers).
2. Reinforce teaching by providing written instructions as well.
3. Assist patient in identifying sources of information and support available in the community (see Box 24-1, page 709).

Evaluation: Expected Outcomes

- Food and fluid intake adequate, gaining weight.
- Skin cool, dry, and intact.
- Maintains concentration, follows conversation, and responds appropriately.
- Verbalizes concerns and questions about illness, treatment, and surgery.

Subacute Thyroiditis

Subacute thyroiditis is a self-limiting, painful inflammation of the thyroid gland, usually associated with viral infections.

Pathophysiology and Etiology

1. Affects younger women predominantly.
2. Acute inflammation results in sudden release of preformed T₃ and T₄, commonly causing symptoms of hyperthyroidism initially.
3. A clinical variant of this disorder, "silent thyroiditis," has been described as similar to subacute thyroiditis; however, the symptoms may be milder and, the thyroid gland is not painful.
4. Subacute thyroiditis has been associated with onset within 6 months of the postpartum period in women.

Clinical Manifestations

1. Pain, swelling, thyroid tenderness lasts several weeks or months and then disappears.
2. Sore throat.
3. Pain referred to the ear, making swallowing difficult and uncomfortable.
4. Fever, malaise, chills, fatigue, anorexia, and/or myalgia.
5. May develop clinical manifestations of hyperthyroidism (irritability, nervousness, insomnia, and weight loss) or hypothyroidism, depending on the point of time in the natural course of the disease when patient presents.

Diagnostic Evaluation

1. TSH level is low.
2. ¹³¹I uptake is low.
3. Serum T₃ and T₄ levels are elevated.
4. Erythrocyte sedimentation rate is increased, usually greater than 50 m/hour.
5. C-reactive protein may also be elevated.

Management

1. Analgesics and mild sedatives.
2. The patient may be placed on beta-adrenergic blockers to reduce the symptoms of thyrotoxicosis.
3. Steroids may be administered for inflammation, pain, fever, and malaise.
4. Aspirin or nonsteroidal anti-inflammatory drugs may be used in mild cases to treat the symptoms of inflammation.

 DRUG ALERT Aspirin should be avoided if the patient exhibits signs of hyperthyroidism because it displaces thyroid hormone from its binding site and may increase the amount of free circulating hormone, resulting in exacerbation of the symptoms of hyperthyroidism.

Complications

In about 10% of patients, permanent hypothyroidism occurs and long-term T₄ therapy is needed.

Nursing Assessment

1. Assess for signs and symptoms of hyperthyroidism (see page 710).
2. Assess for level of discomfort.
3. Evaluate patient's coping skills regarding pain.

Nursing Diagnosis

• Pain related to inflammation of the thyroid gland.

Nursing Interventions

Reducing Pain

1. Administer or teach self-administration of pain relief medication, as prescribed.
2. Provide a restful environment and explain all tests and procedures to patient/family.
3. Assess for degree of pain relief.
4. Notify health care provider if pain relief medications are inadequate for acceptable pain control.

Patient Education and Health Maintenance

1. Explain all medications patient is to continue at home.
2. Reassure patient that subacute thyroiditis usually resolves spontaneously during weeks to months.
3. Teach patient signs and symptoms of hypothyroidism (ie, fatigue and lethargy, weight gain, cold intolerance) that may be experienced. These should be reported as inflammation of the gland subsides.
4. Assist patient in identifying sources of information and support available in the community (see Box 24-1, page 709).

Evaluation: Expected Outcomes

• Verbalizes acceptable pain relief.

Hashimoto Thyroiditis (Lymphocytic Thyroiditis)

Hashimoto thyroiditis is a chronic progressive disease of the thyroid gland caused by infiltration of lymphocytes; it results in progressive destruction of the parenchyma and hypothyroidism if untreated.

Pathophysiology and Etiology

1. Cause is unknown; believed to be an autoimmune disease, because of genetic susceptibility and environmental factors and perhaps related to Graves disease.
2. Ninety-five percent of cases occur in women in their 40s or 50s.
3. Possibly the most common cause of adult hypothyroidism.
4. Appears to be increasing in incidence.

Clinical Manifestations

1. Marked by a slowly developing, firm enlargement of the thyroid gland.
2. Usually no gross nodules.
3. Basal metabolic rate is usually low.
4. Periods of hyperthyroidism caused by large amounts of T₃ and T₄ being released into bloodstream.

Diagnostic Evaluation

1. T₃ and T₄ may be normal but usually become subnormal as the disease progresses.
2. TSH level is usually elevated.
3. Antithyroglobulin antibodies and antimicrosomal antibodies are virtually always present.
4. Normal or high concentration of thyroglobulin-binding protein.

Management

1. Thyroid medications to maintain a normal level of circulating thyroid hormone; this is done to suppress production of

TSH, to prevent enlargement of the thyroid, and to maintain a euthyroid state.
2. Surgical resection of goiter if tracheal compression, cough, or hoarseness occurs.
3. Careful follow-up to detect and treat hypothyroidism.

Complications
1. Progressive hypothyroidism.
2. Without treatment, Hashimoto thyroiditis may progress from goiter and hypothyroidism to myxedema.

Nursing Assessment
1. Assess for signs and symptoms of hyperthyroidism and hypothyroidism.
2. Assess size of the thyroid gland and symptoms of compression—neck tightness, cough, hoarseness.

Nursing Diagnosis
- Anxiety related to enlargement of the neck/thyroid gland.

Nursing Interventions

Reducing Anxiety
1. Explain physiology of the disorder and the reason for enlarging gland. Show anatomic pictures of the thyroid gland, if possible.
2. Administer or teach self-administration of thyroid hormone to suppress stimulation on gland and possibly reduce size.
3. Reassure regarding slow progression of gland enlargement (during months) and the option of surgical resection, if necessary.
4. Suggest wearing loose-necked clothing, avoiding jewelry or scarves around the neck, and avoiding excessive neck flexion or hyperextension, which may aggravate feeling of compression.

Patient Education and Health Maintenance
1. Teach signs of tracheal compression that should be reported to health care provider as soon as possible—difficulty breathing, cough, hoarseness.
2. Explain outcome of hypothyroidism and necessity of taking thyroid hormones every day for life.
3. Explain the need for regular medical follow-up visits to monitor thyroid hormone and TSH levels.
4. Assist patient in identifying sources of information and support available in the community (see Box 24-1, page 709).

 GERONTOLOGIC ALERT Careful and regular follow-up of older patients with Hashimoto thyroiditis is especially important because the progression to hypothyroidism is usually subtle in older people and is unlikely to be recognized promptly.

Evaluation: Expected Outcomes
- Verbalizes reduced anxiety, appears more relaxed, sleeps better.

Cancer of the Thyroid

Cancer of the thyroid is a malignant neoplasm of the gland.

Pathophysiology and Etiology
1. Incidence is more common with women. Usually diagnosed 30 to 50 years of age but also increasing with girls ages 15 to 19 years of age.
2. Exposure to radiation increases risk of thyroid carcinoma significantly. Exposure to Agent Orange also has been associated with higher risk.
3. Papillary and well-differentiated adenocarcinoma (most common, approximately 80%).
   a. Growth is slow, and spread is confined to lymph nodes that surround thyroid area.
   b. Cure rate is excellent after removal of involved areas.
4. Follicular (rapidly growing, widely metastasizing type, approximately 10%).
   a. Occurs predominantly in middle-aged and older persons.
   b. Brief encouraging response may occur with irradiation.
   c. Progression of disease is rapid; high mortality.
5. Parafollicular–medullary thyroid carcinoma.
   a. Rare, inheritable type of thyroid malignancy, which can be detected early by a radioimmunoassay for calcitonin.
6. Undifferentiated anaplastic carcinoma (approximately less than 3%).
   a. The most aggressive and lethal solid tumor found in humans.
   b. Least common of all thyroid cancers.
   c. Usually fatal within months of diagnosis.

Clinical Manifestations
1. On palpation of the thyroid, there may be a firm, irregular, fixed, painless mass or nodule.
2. The occurrence of signs and symptoms of hyperthyroidism is rare.

Diagnostic Evaluation
1. A thyroid uptake and scintigraphy using ^{99m}Tc will detect a "cold" nodule indicating a nonfunctional thyroid area.
2. Ultrasound-guided FNA biopsy for diagnostics.
3. Surgical exploration.

Management
1. Surgical removal is extensive, as required.
   a. Postoperative radiation therapy is commonly done to reduce chances of recurrence.
   b. Follow-up includes periodic ^{131}I uptake scan to detect evidence of recurrence along with following other laboratory tests.
2. Thyroid replacement.
   a. Thyroid hormone is administered to suppress secretion of TSH.
   b. Such treatment is continued indefinitely and requires annual checkups.
3. For unresectable cancer, patient is referred for treatment with ^{131}I, chemotherapy, or radiation therapy.

Complications
1. Untreated thyroid carcinoma can be fatal.
2. Removal of the thyroid can disrupt the parathyroid function; calcium levels need to be monitored.

Nursing Assessment

1. Explore risk factors such as exposure to radiation and family history.
2. Explore patient's feelings and concerns regarding the diagnosis, treatment, and prognosis.

Nursing Diagnosis

- Anxiety related to concern about cancer, upcoming surgery.

Nursing Interventions

Also see "Care of the Patient Undergoing Thyroidectomy," page 705.

Allaying Anxiety

1. Provide all explanations in a simple, concise manner and repeat important information, as necessary, because anxiety may interfere with patient's processing of information.
2. Stress the positive aspects of treatment and high cure rate, as outlined by health care provider.
3. Encourage support by significant other, clergy, social worker, nursing staff, as available.

Patient Education and Health Maintenance

1. Instruct the patient on thyroid hormone replacement and follow-up blood tests.
2. Stress the need for periodic evaluation for recurrence of malignancy.
3. Supply additional information or suggest community resources dealing with cancer prevention and treatment.
4. Assist patient in identifying sources of information and support available in the community (see Box 24-1, page 709).

Evaluation: Expected Outcomes

- Discusses concerns with family, hospital, clergy.

DISORDERS OF THE PARATHYROID GLANDS

The *parathyroid glands* are small, pea-size glands embedded in the posterior section of the thyroid gland. Functions include the production, storage, and release of PTH in response to the serum level of ionized calcium. PTH increases serum calcium by decreasing elimination of calcium ions in the urine by the kidney, increasing absorption of calcium ions from the gut, and increasing bone contribution of calcium ions to the plasma.

Hyperparathyroidism

Hyperparathyroidism is hypersecretion of PTH.

Pathophysiology and Etiology

1. Disorder is most common among post-menopausal women older than age 50.
2. Primary hyperparathyroidism.
   a. Single parathyroid adenoma is the most common cause (approximately 85% of cases).
   b. Parathyroid hyperplasia accounts for approximately 14% of cases.
   c. Parathyroid carcinoma accounts for less than 1% of cases.
   d. May present asymptomatic, but can affect central nervous, cardiac, renal and gastrointestinal systems.
3. Secondary hyperparathyroidism.
   a. Primarily the result of chronic kidney disease and renal failure.

Figure 24-3. Pathogenesis of hyperparathyroidism. (Stewart, J.G. [2017]. *Anatomical Chart Company atlas of pathophysiology* [4th ed.]. Philadelphia: Lippincott Williams & Wilkins.)

4. Excess secretion of PTH results in increased serum calcium levels (see Figure 24-3).

Clinical Manifestations

1. May be asymptomatic with incidental elevated calcium and PTH.
2. Decalcification of bones.
   a. Skeletal pain, backache, pain on weight bearing, pathologic fractures, deformities, formation of bony cysts.
   b. Formation of bone tumors—overgrowth of osteoclasts.
   c. Formation of calcium-containing renal calculi.
3. Depression of neuromuscular function.
   a. The patient may trip, drop objects, show general fatigue, lose memory for recent events, experience emotional instability, have changes in level of consciousness, with stupor and coma.
   b. Cardiac arrhythmias, hypertension, cardiac standstill, palpations, bradycarida, changes in PR and QT intervals on ECG, fatigue, irritability.
4. Other signs and symptoms
   a. Anorexia, nausea, constipation, polydipsia, polyuria, depression, acute pancreatitis, and proximal myopathy weakness.

Diagnostic Evaluation

1. Persistently elevated serum calcium (11 mg/100 mL); test is performed on at least two occasions to determine consistency of results and albumin level also obtained. If change in serum albumin or pH, ionized calcium is more accurate.
2. Exclusion of other causes of hypercalcemia—malignancy (usually bone or breast), vitamin D excess, multiple myeloma, sarcoidosis, milk-alkali syndrome, such drugs as thiazides, Cushing disease, hyperthyroidism.
3. PTH increased and alkaline phosphatase increased; phosphorus decreased.
4. 24-hour urine collection to evaluate kidney function

5. Skeletal changes are revealed by x-ray or dual-energy x-ray absorptiometry (DEXA) test.
6. Cine computed tomography (CT) will disclose parathyroid tumors more readily than x-ray.
7. Sestamibi scan is used to evaluate location of the tumor prior to surgery.

Management

Treatment of Hypercalcemia

1. Hydration with IV saline, loop diuretics such as furosemide and ethacrynic acid—to increase urinary excretion of calcium in patients not in renal failure.
2. Oral phosphate may be used as an antihypercalcemic agent.
3. In patients developing osteoporosis, pamidronate, calcitonin, or etidronate disodium are effective in treating hypercalcemia by inhibiting bone resorption.
4. Dietary calcium is restricted, and all drugs that might cause hypercalcemia (thiazides, lithium, vitamin A&D, canagliflozin, hormone therapy, antacids) may be discontinued.
5. Dialysis may be necessary in patients with resistant hypercalcemia or those with renal failure.
6. Digoxin is reduced because the patient with hypercalcemia is more sensitive to toxic effects of this drug.
7. Monitoring of daily serum calcium, blood urea nitrogen (BUN), potassium, and magnesium levels.
8. Removal of underlying cause.
9. Calcimimetics are a new class of medications that can decrease PTH secretion.

Treatment of Primary Hyperparathyroidism

Surgery for removal of abnormal parathyroid tissue.

Complications

1. Formation of renal calculi, calcification of kidney parenchyma, renal shutdown.
2. Ulceration of upper GI tract leading to hemorrhage and perforation.
3. Demineralization of bones, cysts, and fibrosis of marrow leads to fractures, especially of vertebral bodies and ribs.
4. Hypoparathyroidism after surgery.

Nursing Assessment

1. Obtain review of systems and perform multisystem examination to detect signs and symptoms of hyperparathyroidism.
2. Closely monitor patient's input and output and serum electrolytes, especially calcium level.
3. Monitor ECG to detect changes secondary to hypercalcemia. (During moderate elevations of serum calcium, QT interval is shortened; with extreme hypercalcemia, widening of the T wave is seen.)

Nursing Diagnoses

- Deficient Fluid Volume related to effects of elevated serum calcium levels.
- Impaired Urinary Elimination related to renal calculi and calcium deposits in the kidneys.
- Impaired Physical Mobility related to weakness, bone pain, and pathologic fractures.
- Anxiety related to surgery.

Nursing Interventions

Achieving Fluid and Electrolyte Balance

1. Monitor fluid intake and output.

2. Provide adequate hydration—administer water, glucose, and electrolytes orally or via IV line, as prescribed.
3. Prevent or promptly treat dehydration by reporting vomiting or other sources of fluid loss.
4. Help patient understand why and how to avoid dietary sources of calcium—dairy products, broccoli, calcium-containing antacids.

Promoting Urinary Elimination

1. Strain all urine to observe for calculi.
2. Increase fluid intake to 3,000 mL/day to maintain hydration and prevent precipitation of calcium and formation of calculi.
3. Instruct patient about dietary recommendations for restriction of calcium.
4. Observe for signs of urinary tract infection (UTI), hematuria, and renal colic.
5. Assess renal function through serum creatinine and BUN levels.

Increasing Physical Mobility

1. Assist patient in hygiene and activities if bone pain is severe or if patient experiences musculoskeletal weakness.
2. Protect patient from falls or injury.
3. Turn patient cautiously and handle extremities gently to avoid fractures.
4. Administer analgesia, as prescribed.
5. Assess level of pain and patient's response to analgesia.
6. Encourage patient to participate in mild exercise gradually as symptoms subside.
7. Instruct and demonstrate correct body mechanics to reduce strain, backache, and injury.

Relieving Anxiety

1. Encourage patient to verbalize fears and feelings about upcoming surgery.
2. Explain tests and procedures to patient.
3. Reassure patient about skeletal recovery.
   a. Bone pain diminishes fairly quickly.
   b. Fractures are treated by orthopedic procedures.
4. Prepare patient for surgery as for thyroidectomy (see page 705).

Patient Education and Health Maintenance

1. Instruct patient about calcium-reducing medications.
   a. Calcitonin is given subcutaneously—teach proper technique.
   b. Etidronate disodium—calcium-rich foods should be avoided within 2 hours of dose; therapeutic response may take 1 to 3 months.
   c. Pamidronate—monitor hypercalcemia-related parameters when treatment begins. Adequate intake of calcium and vitamin D is necessary to prevent hypocalcemia. Bisphosphonates should be used with caution in patients with active upper GI problems.
2. Teach signs and symptoms of tetany that patient may experience postoperatively and should report to health care provider (numbness and tingling in extremities or around mouth).
3. Assist patient in identifying sources of information and support available in the community (see Box 24-1, page 709).

Evaluation: Expected Outcomes

- Output equals intake, normal skin turgor, moist mucous membranes.

- No signs and symptoms of renal calculi or UTI; serum creatinine and BUN levels normal.
- Reports less bone and joint pain; uses correct body mechanics, avoid immobilization.
- Verbalizes concerns and fears about surgery; appears less anxious.

Hypoparathyroidism

Hypoparathyroidism results from a deficiency of PTH and is characterized by hypocalcemia and neuromuscular hyperexcitability.

Pathophysiology and Etiology

1. The most common cause is accidental removal or destruction of parathyroid tissue or its blood supply during thyroidectomy or radical neck dissection for malignancy.
2. Decrease in gland function (idiopathic hypoparathyroidism); may be autoimmune or familial in origin.
3. Malignancy or metastasis from a cancer to the parathyroid glands.
4. Resistance to PTH action.
5. With inadequate PTH secretion, there is decreased resorption of calcium from the renal tubules, decreased absorption of calcium in the GI tract, and decreased resorption of calcium from bone.
6. Blood calcium falls to a low level, causing symptoms of muscular hyperirritability, uncontrolled spasms, and hypocalcemic tetany.
7. In response to decreased serum calcium levels and lack of PTH, the serum phosphate level rises and phosphate excretion by the kidneys decreases.

Clinical Manifestations

1. Neuromuscular irritability: laryngeal spasm, bronchospasm, muscle cramps, paresthesias, seizures.
2. Tetany—general muscular hypertonia; attempts at voluntary movement result in tremors and spasmodic or uncoordinated movements; fingers assume classic tetanic position; Chvostek and Trousseau signs (see page 706).
3. Neurological signs and symptoms such as extrapyramidal signs, personality disturbances, irritability, parkinsonism, dystonic spasms.
4. Mental status changes: confusion, psychosis, fatigue, anxiety, poor memory.
5. Ectodermal changes: dry skin, brittle nails, course hair, atopic eczema, psoriasis.
6. Cardiac changes: ECG with prolong QT interval, congestive heart failure, cardiomyopathy.
7. Ophthalmologic changes: subcapsular cataracts, papilledema.

Diagnostic Evaluation

1. Decrease in serum calcium level to a low level (7.5 mg/100 mL or less).
2. Phosphorus level in blood is elevated.
3. May have concurrent hypomagnesemia and/or vitamin D deficiency.
4. Pseudohypocalcemia—total serum calcium level is low, but serum ionized calcium is normal. This is due to calcium binding to protein.
5. PTH levels are low in most cases; may be normal or elevated in pseudohypoparathyroidism.
6. In chronic hypoparathyroidism, bone density may be increased as seen on radiography.

Management

IV Calcium Administration

1. A syringe and an ampule of a calcium solution (calcium chloride, calcium glucceptate, calcium gluconate) are to be kept at the bedside at all times.
2. Most rapidly effective calcium solution is ionized calcium chloride (10%).
3. For rapid use to relieve severe tetany, infusion carried out every 10 minutes.
   a. All IV calcium preparations are administered slowly. It is highly irritating, stings, and causes thrombosis; patient experiences unpleasant burning flush of skin and tongue.
   b. Typical doses are as follows:
      i. Calcium chloride—500 mg to 1 g (5 to 10 mL) as indicated by serum calcium; administer at rate of less than 1 mL/minute of 10% solution.
      ii. Calcium gluconate—500 mg to 2 g (10 to 20 mL) at a rate of less than 0.5 mL/minute of a 10% solution.
      iii. Calcium glucceptate—1 to 2 g (5 to 10 mL) at a rate of less than 1 mL/minute.
4. A slow drip of IV saline containing calcium gluconate is given until control of tetany is ensured; then, IM or oral administration of calcium is prescribed.
5. Later, vitamin D is added to calcium intake—increases absorption of calcium and also induces a high level of calcium in the bloodstream. Thiazide diuretics may also be added because of their calcium-retaining effect on the kidney; doses of calcium and vitamin D may be lowered.
6. Administration of IV calcium seems to cause rapid relief of anxiety.

 DRUG ALERT Too-rapid calcium administration may cause cardiac arrest.

Other Measures

1. Treat renal calculi.
2. Monitor patient for hypercalciuria.
3. Monitor blood calcium level periodically; variations in vitamin D may affect calcium levels.

Complications

1. Acute complications related to hypocalcemia include seizures, tetany, and mental disorders, all of which can be reversed with calcium therapy.
2. If onset of hypocalcemia is acute, the major concerns are laryngeal spasm, acute airway obstruction, and cardiovascular failure.
3. Long-term complications include subcapsular cataracts, calcification of the basal ganglia, and papilledema (caused by precipitation of calcium out of serum and deposition in tissue); shortening of the fingers and toes; and bowing of the long bones (caused by inadequate PTH and additional genetic abnormalities). Of these complications, only papilledema is reversible.

Nursing Assessment

1. Perform multisystem assessment, focusing on neuromuscular system.
2. Closely monitor patient's input and output and serum electrolytes, especially calcium level.
3. Assess anxiety.

Nursing Diagnosis

- Risk for electrolyte imbalance related to impaired calcium regulation.

Nursing Interventions

Maintaining Normal Serum Calcium Levels

1. Assess neuromuscular status frequently in patients with hypoparathyroidism and in those at risk for hypocalcemia (patients in the immediate postoperative period after thyroidectomy, parathyroidectomy, radical neck dissection).
2. Check for Trousseau and Chvostek signs, and notify health care provider if test results are positive.
3. Assess respiratory status frequently in acute hypocalcemia and postoperatively.
4. Monitor serum calcium and phosphorus levels.
5. Promote high-calcium diet, if prescribed—dairy products; green, leafy vegetables.
6. Instruct the patient about signs and symptoms of hypo- and hypercalcemia that should be reported.
7. Use caution in administering other drugs to the patient with hypocalcemia.
   a. The hypocalcemic patient is sensitive to digoxin; as hypocalcemia is reversed, the patient may rapidly develop digoxin toxicity.
   b. Cimetidine interferes with normal parathyroid function, especially with renal failure, which increases the risk of hypocalcemia.

Patient Education and Health Maintenance

1. Explain to patient and family the function of PTH and the roles of vitamin D and calcium in maintaining good health.
2. Discuss the importance of each medication prescribed for the control of hypocalcemia including vitamin D, calcium, and thiazide diuretic.
   a. Take medications, as prescribed.
   b. Do not substitute with over-the-counter preparations without the advice and supervision of the health care provider.
3. Provide patient with a written list about hypercalcemia and hypocalcemia, and advise the patient to contact the health care provider immediately should signs of either condition develop.
4. Advise patient to wear a medical alert tag.
5. Explain the need for periodic medical follow-up for life.

Evaluation: Expected Outcome

- Verbalizes understanding of diet and medications; calcium level within normal limits.

DISORDERS OF THE ADRENAL GLANDS

The *adrenal medulla*, or inner portion of the gland, is not necessary to maintain life but enables a person to cope with stress. It secretes two hormones:

- *Epinephrine* (adrenalin) acts on alpha and beta receptors to increase contractility and excitability of heart muscle, leading to increased cardiac output; facilitates blood flow to muscles, brain, and viscera; enhances blood sugar by stimulating conversion of glycogen to glucose in the liver; and inhibits smooth muscle contraction.
- *Norepinephrine* (noradrenaline) acts primarily on alpha receptors to increase peripheral vascular resistance, leading to increases in diastolic and systolic BP.
  - The adrenal cortex, or outer portion of the gland, is essential to life. It secretes adrenocortical hormones—synthesized from cholesterol.
- *Glucocorticoids* (cortisone and hydrocortisone) enhance protein catabolism and inhibit protein synthesis; antagonize action of insulin and increase blood sugar; increase synthesis of glucose by the liver; influence defense mechanism of the body and its reaction to stress; and influence emotional reaction.
- *Mineralocorticoids* (aldosterone and desoxycorticosterone) regulate reabsorption of sodium; regulate excretion of potassium by renal tubules.
- *Adrenosterones* (adrenal androgens) exert minimal effect on sex characteristics and function.

Primary Aldosteronism

Primary aldosteronism refers to excessive secretion of aldosterone by the adrenal cortex.

Pathophysiology and Etiology

1. Excessive secretion of aldosterone results in the conservation of sodium and excretion of potassium primarily not only in the renal tubules but also in the sweat glands, salivary glands, and GI tract.
2. Caused primarily by a cortical adenoma, bilateral adrenal hyperplasia, or genetic–familial primary aldosteronism.
3. Secondary aldosteronism occurs in conjunction with heart failure, renal dysfunction, or cirrhosis of the liver.
4. Women constitute 70% of patients with aldosterone-secreting adenomas, and the incidence of primary aldosteronism is four times higher among African Americans than among the general population.

Clinical Manifestations

1. Hypertension (5% to 15% of cases of hypertension are a result of primary aldosteronism, which usually can be treated successfully by surgical removal of the adenoma).
2. A profound decline in blood levels of potassium (hypokalemia) and hydrogen ions (alkalosis) results in muscle weakness and inability of kidneys to acidify or concentrate urine, leading to excess volume of urine (polyuria).
3. A decline in hydrogen ions (alkalosis) results in tetany, paresthesia.
4. An elevation in blood sodium (hypernatremia) results in excessive thirst (polydipsia) and arterial hypertension.

Diagnostic Evaluation

1. Suspected in all hypertensive patients with spontaneous hypokalemia; also if hypokalemia develops concurrently with start of diuretics and remains after diuretics are discontinued.
2. The screening test of choice is the aldosterone/renin ratio, which is suggestive of primary aldosteronism if the ratio is greater than 20:1.
3. Salt loading may be used as a confirmatory test—ingestion of at least 200 mEq/day (approximately 12 g salt) for 4 days does

not influence the serum potassium level without aldosteronism but will cause a decrease of serum potassium to less than 3.5 mEq/L in a patient with aldosteronism.
4. CT scanning to determine and localize cortical adenoma.

Management

1. Removal of adrenal tumor if the tumor is localized to one side—unilateral adrenalectomy.
2. If the cause is bilateral adrenal hyperplasia—spironolactone is used to treat both hypertension and potassium-depleted stages; therapy is needed 4 to 6 weeks before the full effect on BP is seen.
   a. Adverse effects include reduced testosterone in men (decreased libido, impotence, gynecomastia) and GI discomfort.
   b. Amiloride may be used instead in sexually active men or in cases of GI intolerance.
   c. Sodium restriction is necessary—no saline infusions, low-sodium diet.
   d. Potassium supplementation is usually necessary, based on severity of deficit.
3. Addition of antihypertensive agent—thiazide diuretic such as triamterene.
4. Management of underlying causes of secondary aldosteronism.

Complications

Long-term effects of untreated hypertension—stroke, renal failure, heart failure.

Nursing Assessment

1. Obtain history of symptoms, such as muscle weakness, paresthesia, thirst, and polyuria.
2. Perform multisystem physical examination.
3. Evaluate BP.

Nursing Diagnosis

• Excess Fluid Volume related to sodium retention.

Nursing Interventions

Also see "Care of the Patient Undergoing Adrenalectomy," page 706.

Maintaining Normal Fluid and Sodium Balance
1. Monitor fluid intake and output, daily weight, ECG changes for hypokalemia.
2. Teach low-sodium diet, administration of potassium supplements, as ordered; evaluate serum sodium and potassium results.
3. Monitor BP; administer or teach self-administration of antihypertensives, as ordered.
4. Assess for dependent edema; encourage activity, frequent repositioning, and elevation of feet periodically.

Patient Education and Health Maintenance

1. Instruct patient about the nature of illness, the necessary treatment, and the need for continued medical care after discharge.
2. Instruct patient on the importance of following prescribed medical treatments.
   a. For medical management, patient must remain on spironolactone for life.

b. Patient should report significant adverse effects that interfere with sexual performance and quality of life.
c. Glucocorticoid administration may be temporary after subtotal or unilateral adrenalectomy, chronic for bilateral adrenalectomy; dose may need to be increased during times of illness or stress.
3. Teach patient and family members how to take BP readings, if indicated.

Evaluation: Expected Outcomes

• Intake equals urine output, daily weight stable.

Cushing Syndrome

Cushing syndrome is a condition in which the plasma cortisol levels are elevated, causing signs and symptoms of hypercortisolism.

Pathophysiology and Etiology

1. Is more common in women than in men.
2. The normal feedback mechanisms that control adrenocortical function are ineffective, resulting in secretion of adrenal cortical hormones despite adequate amounts of these hormones in the circulation.
3. The manifestations of Cushing syndrome are the result of excess hormones (glucocorticoids).
4. Excess of one hormone or all the hormones can occur; the predominant hormone secreted in excess (usually glucocorticoids) determines the predominant symptoms.
5. Pituitary Cushing syndrome (Cushing disease)—hyperplasia of both adrenal glands caused by overstimulation of the adrenal cortex by ACTH, usually from a pituitary adenoma or hyperplasia.
   a. Most common cause of Cushing syndrome.
   b. Affects mostly women between ages 20 and 40.
6. Adrenal Cushing syndrome.
   a. Associated with tumors of the adrenal cortex—adenoma or carcinoma.
7. Ectopic—results from autonomous ACTH secretion by extra-pituitary neoplasms (such as lung).
8. Iatrogenic Cushing syndrome caused by exogenous glucocorticoid administration.

Clinical Manifestations

Manifestations Caused by Excess Glucocorticoids
1. Weight gain or obesity (see Figure 24-4).
2. Heavy trunk; thin extremities.
3. "Buffalo hump" (fat pad) in neck and supraclavicular area.
4. Rounded face (moon face); plethoric, oily.
5. Fragile and thin skin, striae and ecchymosis, acne.
6. Muscles wasted because of excessive catabolism.
7. Osteoporosis—characteristic kyphosis, backache.
8. Mental disturbances—mood changes, psychosis.
9. Increased susceptibility to infections.

Manifestations Caused by Excess Mineralocorticoids
1. Hypertension.
2. Hypernatremia, hypokalemia.
3. Weight gain.
4. Expanded blood volume.
5. Edema.

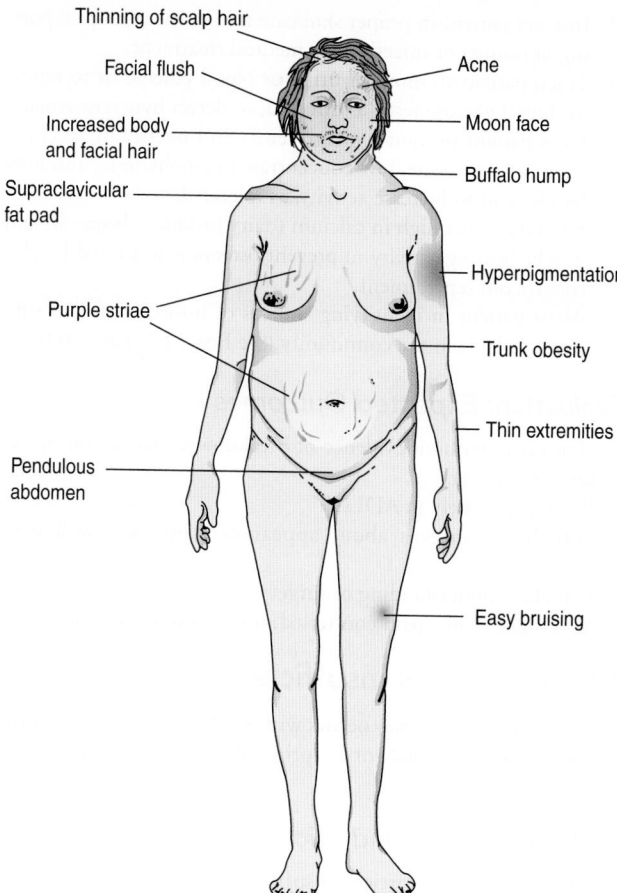

Thinning of scalp hair
Facial flush
Increased body and facial hair
Supraclavicular fat pad
Purple striae
Pendulous abdomen
Acne
Moon face
Buffalo hump
Hyperpigmentation
Trunk obesity
Thin extremities
Easy bruising

Figure 24-4. Clinical manifestations of Cushing syndrome. (Smeltzer, S., & Bare, B. [2000]. *Brunner and Suddarth's textbook of medical–surgical nursing* [9th ed.]. Philadelphia, PA: Lippincott Williams & Wilkins.)

Manifestations Caused by Excess Androgens
1. Women experience virilism (masculinization).
   a. Hirsutism—excessive growth of hair on the face and midline of the trunk.
   b. Breasts—atrophy.
   c. Clitoris—enlargement.
   d. Voice—masculine.
   e. Loss of libido.
2. If exposed *in utero*—possible hermaphrodite.
3. Males—loss of libido.

Diagnostic Evaluation
1. Excessive plasma cortisol levels.
2. An increase in blood glucose levels and glucose intolerance.
3. Decreased serum potassium level.
4. Reduced eosinophils.
5. Elevated urinary 17-hydroxycorticoid and 17-ketogenic steroid levels.
6. Elevation of plasma ACTH in patients with pituitary tumors.
7. Low plasma ACTH levels with adrenal tumor.
8. Loss of diurnal variation of cortisol secretion.
9. X-rays of the skull may detect erosion of the sella turcica by a pituitary tumor.
10. Overnight DST or 48-hour low-dose DST, possibly with cortisol urinary excretion measurement.
11. Elevated levels of cortisol measured in saliva are significant.
12. CT scan, MRI, and ultrasonography detect location of tumor.

Management
Surgery and Radiation
Tumor (adrenal or pituitary) is removed or treated with irradiation.
1. An important development in the management of pituitary Cushing syndrome in adults is transsphenoidal adenomectomy or hypophysectomy (pituitary removal) (see page 707).
2. Transfrontal craniotomy may be necessary when pituitary tumor has enlarged beyond sella turcica (see page 361).
3. Hyperplasia of adrenals—bilateral adrenalectomy.

Replacement Therapy Postoperatively
1. Adrenalectomy patients require lifelong replacement therapy with the following:
   a. A glucocorticoid—cortisone.
   b. A mineralocorticoid—fludrocortisone.
2. After pituitary irradiation or hypophysectomy, patient may require adrenal replacement, plus thyroid, posterior pituitary, and gonadal replacement therapy.
3. After transsphenoidal adenomectomy, patient requires hydrocortisone replacement therapy for periods of 12 to 18 months and additional hormones if excessive loss of pituitary function has occurred.
4. Protein anabolic steroids may be given to facilitate protein replacement; potassium replacement is usually required.

Medical Treatment
1. If patients cannot undergo surgery, cortisol synthesis–inhibiting medications may be used.
   a. Mitotane, an agent toxic to the adrenal cortex (dichlorodiphenyltrichloroethane derivative)—known as medical adrenalectomy. Nausea, vomiting, diarrhea, somnolence, and depression may occur with use of this drug.
   b. Metyrapone to control steroid hypersecretion in patients who do not respond to mitotane therapy.
   c. Aminoglutethimide blocks cholesterol conversion to pregnenolone, effectively blocking cortisol production. Adverse effects include GI disturbances, somnolence, and skin rashes.

Complications
Possibility of recurrence in patients with adrenal carcinoma.

Nursing Assessment
1. Observe patient for signs and symptoms of Cushing disease.
2. Perform multisystem physical examination.
3. Monitor intake and output, daily weights, and serum electrolytes.

Nursing Diagnoses
- Impaired Skin Integrity related to altered healing, thin and fragile skin, and edema.
- Dressing, Grooming, Toileting Self-Care Deficit related to muscle wasting, osteoporosis, weakness, and fatigue.
- Disturbed Body Image related to altered physical appearance and emotional instability.
- Anxiety related to surgery.
- Delayed Surgical Recovery related to potential complications.

Nursing Interventions
Maintaining Skin Integrity
1. Assess skin frequently to detect reddened areas, breakdown or tearing of skin, excoriation, infection, or edema.

2. Handle skin and extremities gently to prevent trauma; protect from falls by use of side rails.
3. Avoid use of adhesive tape to reduce risk of trauma to skin on its removal.
4. Encourage patient to turn in bed frequently or to ambulate to reduce pressure on bony prominences and areas of edema.
5. Use meticulous skin care to reduce injury and breakdown.
6. Provide foods low in sodium to minimize edema formation.
7. Assess intake and output and daily weight to evaluate fluid retention.

Encouraging Active Participation in Self-Care
1. Assist patient with ambulation and hygiene when weak and fatigued.
2. Assist patient in planning schedule to permit exercise and rest.
3. Encourage patient to rest when fatigued.
4. Encourage gradual resumption of activities as patient gains strength.
5. Identify for patient the signs and symptoms indicating excessive exertion.
6. Instruct patient in correct body mechanics to avoid pain or injury during activities.
7. Use assistive devices during ambulation to prevent falls and fractures.
8. Encourage foods high in potassium (bananas, orange juice, tomatoes), and administer potassium supplement, as prescribed, to counteract weakness related to hypokalemia.

Strengthening Body Image
1. Encourage patient to verbalize concerns about illness, changes in appearance, and altered role functions.
2. Identify situations that are disturbing to patient, and explore with patient ways to avoid or modify those situations.
3. Be alert for evidence of depression; in some instances, this has progressed to suicide; alert health care provider of mood changes, sleep disturbance, change in activity level, change in appetite, or loss of interest in visitors or other experiences.
4. Refer for counseling, if indicated.
5. Explain to patient who has benign adenoma or hyperplasia that, with proper treatment, evidence of masculinization can be reversed.

Reducing Anxiety
1. Answer questions about surgery and encourage thorough discussion with health care provider if patient is not well informed.
2. Describe nursing care to expect in postoperative period.
3. Prepare the patient for abdominal surgery (see page 495) or hypophysectomy (see page 707) as indicated.

Providing Postoperative Care
1. Provide routine postoperative care for patient with abdominal surgery (see page 495) or hypophysectomy (see page 707).
2. Monitor closely for infection because glucocorticoid administration interferes with immune function; maintain sterile technique, clean environment, and good handwashing.
3. Monitor thyroid function tests and provide HRT, as ordered, after hypophysectomy.
4. Monitor fluid intake and output and urine specific gravity to detect DI caused by ADH deficiency after hypophysectomy.

Patient Education and Health Maintenance
1. Instruct patient on lifetime HRT and the need to follow up at regular intervals to determine if dosage is appropriate or to detect adverse effects.
2. Instruct patient in proper skin care and in the prompt reporting of trauma or infection for medical treatment.
3. Teach patient to monitor urine or blood glucose or to report for blood glucose tests, as directed, to detect hyperglycemia.
4. Help patient prevent hyperglycemia and obesity by teaching about a low-calorie, low-concentrated carbohydrate, and low-fat diet and to increase activity, as tolerated.
5. Encourage diet high in calcium (dairy products, broccoli) and weight-bearing activity to prevent osteoporosis caused by glucocorticoid replacement.
6. Assist patient in identifying sources of information and support available in the community (see Box 24-1, page 709).

Evaluation: Expected Outcomes
• Skin intact without evidence of breakdown, excoriation, infection, or trauma.
• Participates safely in ADLs.
• Verbalizes concerns about appearance, interacts well with visitors.
• Verbalizes understanding of surgery.
• Vital signs stable, pain controlled, no signs of infection.

Adrenocortical Insufficiency

Adrenocortical insufficiency occurs with inadequate secretion of the hormones of the adrenal cortex, primarily the glucocorticoids and mineralocorticoids.

Pathophysiology and Etiology
1. Primary adrenocortical insufficiency (Addison disease)—destruction and subsequent hypofunction of the adrenal cortex, usually caused by autoimmune process.
2. Secondary adrenocortical insufficiency—ACTH deficiency from pituitary disease or suppression of hypothalamic–pituitary axis by corticosteroid treatment for nonendocrine disorders causes atrophy of the adrenal cortex.
3. Inadequate aldosterone produces disturbances of sodium, potassium, and water metabolism.
4. Cortisol deficiency produces abnormal fat, protein, and carbohydrate metabolism; no cortisol during a period of stress can precipitate addisonian crisis, an exaggerated state of adrenal cortical insufficiency, and can lead to death.

Clinical Manifestations
1. Hyponatremia, hyperkalemia, and some have anemia.
2. Water loss, dehydration, and hypovolemia.
3. Muscular weakness, fatigue, weight loss.
4. GI problems—anorexia, nausea, vomiting, diarrhea, constipation, abdominal pain.
5. Hypotension, hypoglycemia, low basal metabolic rate, increased insulin sensitivity.
6. Mental changes—depression, irritability, anxiety, apprehension caused by hypoglycemia and hypovolemia.
7. Normal responses to stress lacking.
8. Hyperpigmentation.

Diagnostic Evaluation
1. Blood chemistry—decreased glucose and sodium; increased potassium, calcium, and BUN levels.
2. Increased lymphocytes on complete blood count.
3. Low fasting plasma cortisol levels; low aldosterone levels.

4. Twenty-four–hour urine studies—decreased 17-ketosteroid, 17-hydroxycorticoid, and 17-ketogenic steroid levels.
5. ACTH stimulation test—no rise or minimal rise in plasma cortisol and urinary 17-ketosteroid levels.

Management

1. Restoration of normal fluid and electrolyte balance: high-sodium, low-potassium diet and fluids.
2. Treatment of glucocorticoid deficiency with such agents as hydrocortisone or prednisone. Patients with chronic obstructive pulmonary disease and heart failure may require preparations with low mineralocorticoid activity, such as methylprednisolone, to prevent fluid retention.
3. Mineralocorticoid deficiency is treated with fludrocortisone.
4. Cardiovascular support, if indicated.
5. Immediate treatment if addisonian (adrenal) crisis or circulatory collapse is imminent:
   a. IV sodium chloride solution to replace sodium ions.
   b. Hydrocortisone.
   c. Injection of circulatory stimulants, such as atropine sulfate, calcium chloride, epinephrine.
6. Diagnosis and treatment of underlying cause of adrenocortical insufficiency or addisonian crisis (eg, antibiotic therapy to treat infection if this is a factor in crisis).

 NURSING ALERT Overtreatment may be manifested by hypertension, edema from sodium and water retention, and weakness caused by potassium loss.

Complications

1. Adrenal crisis—hypotension, nausea, vomiting, weakness, lethargy, fever, confusion, acute abdomen, and possibly coma.
2. May be precipitated by physiologic stress, such as surgery, infection, trauma, dehydration.

Nursing Assessment

1. Obtain recent or past history of corticosteroid therapy, including length of treatment, dosage, and compliance.
2. Review history for sources of stress, such as surgical procedures, infection, or development of other illness.
3. Perform thorough physical examination for manifestations of adrenocortical insufficiency or contributing factors.

Nursing Diagnoses

- Deficient Fluid Volume related to renal losses of sodium and water.
- Risk for Infection related to ineffective stress response.
- Activity Intolerance related to decreased cortisol production and fatigue.

Nursing Interventions

Achieving Normal Fluid and Electrolyte Balance

1. Assess fluid intake and output and serial daily weights.
2. Monitor vital signs frequently; a drop in BP may suggest an impending crisis.
3. Monitor results of serum sodium and potassium.
4. Assess skin turgor and mucous membranes for dehydration.

5. Encourage diet high in sodium and fluid content; administer or teach self-administration of potassium supplements, if prescribed.
6. Administer or teach self-administration of prescribed glucocorticoids and mineralocorticoids; document response.
7. Administer IV infusions of sodium, water, and glucose, as indicated.

Protecting Well-Being

1. Minimize stressful situations.
2. Protect patient from infection.
   a. Control patient's contacts so that infectious organisms are not transmitted.
   b. Protect patient from drafts, dampness, exposure to cold.
   c. Prevent overexertion.
   d. Use meticulous handwashing and sterile techniques.
3. Assess comfort and emotional status of patient.
   a. Control the temperature of the room to avoid sharp deviations in patient's temperature.
   b. Maintain a quiet, peaceful environment; avoid loud talking and noisy radios.
4. Observe and report early signs of addisonian crisis (sudden drop in BP, nausea and vomiting, fever).

Increasing Activity Tolerance

1. Assist the patient with ADLs.
2. Provide for periods of rest and activity to avoid overexertion.
3. Provide for high-calorie, high-protein diet.

Patient Education and Health Maintenance

1. Instruct patient about the necessity for long-term therapy for adrenocortical insufficiency and medical follow-up visits.
   a. Inform patient that therapy must be continued throughout his or her life.
   b. Emphasize the importance of taking more hormones when under stress.
   c. Suggest that patient carry an identification card that indicates the type of medication being taken and health care provider's telephone number.
2. Educate patient about manifestations of excessive use of medications and reportable symptoms.
3. Identify actions to take to avoid factors that may precipitate addisonian crisis (infection, extremes of temperature, trauma).
4. Assist patient in identifying sources of information and support available in the community (see Box 24-1, page 709).

Evaluation: Expected Outcomes

- Normal skin turgor, moist mucous membranes, stable vital signs.
- No signs of infection or stress.
- Completes daily activities with minimal assistance.

Pheochromocytoma

Pheochromocytoma is a catecholamine-secreting neoplasm associated with hyperfunction of the adrenal medulla. It may appear wherever chromaffin cells are located; however, most are found in the adrenal medulla.

Pathophysiology and Etiology

1. Pheochromocytoma can occur at any age but is most common between the ages of 30 and 60; it is uncommon in people older than age 65.

2. Most pheochromocytoma tumors are benign; 10% are malignant with metastasis into bone, liver, and lymph nodes.
3. 35% of extra-adrenal pheochromocytomas are malignant.
4. Tumors located in the adrenal medulla produce both increased epinephrine and norepinephrine; those located outside the adrenal gland tend to produce epinephrine only.
5. May occur as component of multiple endocrine neoplasia IIA, an autosomal dominant syndrome characterized by pheochromocytoma, thyroid cancer, and hyperparathyroidism.

Clinical Manifestations

1. Variation in signs and symptoms depends on the predominance of norepinephrine or epinephrine secretion and on whether secretion is continuous or intermittent.
2. Excess secretion of norepinephrine and epinephrine produces hypertension, hypermetabolism, and hyperglycemia.
3. Hypertension may be paroxysmal (intermittent) or persistent (chronic).
   a. Chronic form mimics essential hypertension; however, antihypertensives are not effective.
   b. Headaches and vision disturbances are common.
4. The hypermetabolic and hyperglycemic effects produce excessive perspiration, tremor, pallor or face flushing, nervousness, elevated blood glucose levels, polyuria, nausea, vomiting, diarrhea, abdominal pain, and paresthesia.
5. Emotional changes, including psychotic behavior, may occur.
6. Symptoms may be triggered by allergic reactions, physical exertion, emotional upset, or may occur without identifiable stimulus.

Diagnostic Evaluation

1. Metanephrine (metabolites of epinephrine and norepinephrine) are elevated in 24-hour urine specimen.
2. Epinephrine and norepinephrine in urine and blood are elevated while patient is symptomatic.
3. CT scan and magnetic resonance imaging (MRI) of the adrenal glands or of the entire abdomen are done to identify tumor.

Management

Medical Control of BP and Preparation for Surgery
1. Alpha-adrenergic blocking agents, such as phentolamine or phenoxybenzamine, inhibit the effects of catecholamines on BP.
   a. Effective control of BP and blood volume may take 1 or 2 weeks.
   b. Surgery is delayed until BP is controlled and blood volume has been expanded.
2. Catecholamine synthesis inhibitors, such as metyrosine, may be used preoperatively or for long-term management of inoperable tumors.
   a. Adverse effects include sedation and crystalluria.

Surgery
Unilateral or bilateral adrenalectomy or other tumor removal.

Complications

Metastasis of tumor.

Nursing Assessment

1. Obtain history of signs and symptoms patient has been experiencing.

2. Assess for predisposing factors that may be triggering signs and symptoms (ie, physical exertion, emotional upset, allergies).
3. Perform thorough physical examination to determine effects of hypertension.

Nursing Diagnoses

• Anxiety related to the systemic effects of epinephrine and norepinephrine.
• Ineffective Tissue Perfusion related to hypotension during the postoperative period.

Nursing Interventions

Reducing Anxiety
1. Remain with patient during acute episodes of hypertension.
2. Ensure bed rest and elevate the head of bed 45 degrees during severe hypertension.
3. Carry out tasks and procedures in calm, unhurried manner when with patient.
4. Instruct patient about use of relaxation exercises.
5. Reduce environmental stressors by providing calm, quiet environment. Restrict visitors.
6. Eliminate stimulants (coffee, tea, cola) from the diet.
7. Reduce events that precipitate episodes of severe hypertension—palpation of the tumor, physical exertion, emotional upset.
8. Administer sedatives, as prescribed, to promote relaxation and rest.
9. Monitor for orthostatic hypotension after administration of phentolamine.
10. Encourage oral fluids and maintain IV infusion preoperatively to ensure adequate volume expansion going into surgery.

Maintaining Tissue Perfusion Postoperatively
1. Monitor vital signs, ECG, arterial BP, neurologic status, and urine output closely postoperatively.
2. Assess for and report complications of hypertension, hypotension, and hyperglycemia.
3. Maintain adequate hydration with IV infusion to prevent hypotension. (Because reduction of catecholamines immediately postoperatively causes vasodilation and enlargement of vascular space, hypotension may occur.)
4. Monitor intake and output and laboratory results for BUN, creatinine, and glucose levels.

Patient Education and Health Maintenance

1. Instruct patient how and when to take medications. Warn patients who take metyrosine of sedation and need to avoid taking other CNS depressants and participating in activities that require alertness; need to increase fluid intake to at least 2,000 mL/day to prevent renal calculi.
2. Inform patient regarding the need for continued follow-up for:
   a. Recurrence of pheochromocytoma.
   b. Assessment of any residual renal or cardiovascular injury related to preoperative hypertension.
   c. Documentation that catecholamine levels are normal 1 to 3 months postoperatively (by 24-hour urine test).
3. Help patient identify sources of information and support available in the community (see Box 24-1, page 709).

Evaluation: Expected Outcomes

• Reports less anxiety during hypertensive episodes.
• BP stable, adequate urine output.

DISORDERS OF THE PITUITARY GLAND

The pituitary gland (hypophysis) exerts prime control over the body's hormonal functions. It is located in the sella turcica at the base of the brain. Its function is regulated by the hypothalamus. The pituitary consists of two parts that are structurally and functionally separate: the anterior pituitary and the posterior pituitary. Hypothalamic control of the anterior pituitary is mediated by releasing factors secreted by the hypothalamus; the posterior pituitary is regulated through direct neural stimulation. See Table 24-2 for hormones of the pituitary gland.

Diabetes Insipidus

Diabetes insipidus (DI) is a disorder of water metabolism caused by deficiency of ADH, also called vasopressin, secreted by the posterior pituitary (central DI) or by inability of the kidneys to respond to ADH (nephrogenic DI).

Pathophysiology and Etiology

1. Primary: idiopathic.
2. Secondary: head trauma, neurosurgery, tumors (intracranial or metastatic), vascular disease (aneurysms, infarct), infection (meningitis, encephalitis).
3. Nephrogenic DI: long-standing renal disease, hypokalemia, some medications.
4. Deficiency of ADH results in decreased renal water reabsorption; it may be partial or complete (see Figure 24-5).
5. DI may be transient or permanent.

Clinical Manifestations

1. Marked polyuria—daily output of greater than 3 L for adults, 2 L for children of dilute urine; corresponding to a urine osmolality of less than 250 mOsm/kg.
2. Polydipsia (intense thirst)—drinks 4 to 40 L of fluid daily; has craving for cold water.
3. High serum osmolality (above 295 mOsm) and high serum sodium level (greater than 142 mEq/L).

Diagnostic Evaluation

1. Serum osmolality—high; urine osmolality—low.
2. Water deprivation test determines central and nephrogenic DI.
3. Measurements of serum and urine ADH—decreased to absent.

Table 24-2	Hormones of the Pituitary Gland
HORMONE	**TARGET TISSUE**
Anterior Pituitary	
Growth hormone	Multiple sites
Thyroid-stimulating hormone	Thyroid gland
Adrenocorticotropic hormone	Adrenal glands
Prolactin	Breasts
Luteinizing hormone	Ovaries, testes
Follicle-stimulating hormone	Ovaries, testes
Melanocyte-stimulating hormone	Melanocytes (skin)
Posterior Pituitary	
Oxytocin	Uterus, breasts
Antidiuretic hormone	Kidneys

Figure 24-5. The mechanisms of diabetes insipidus. (Rubin, R., & Strayer, D.S. [2011]. *Rubin's pathology: clinicopathologic foundations of medicine* [6th ed.]. Philadelphia: Lippincott Williams & Wilkins.)

Management

1. Administration of ADH or its derivative.
   a. DDAVP—vasopressin derivative administered intravenously, into the nose through a soft, flexible nasal tube, by nasal spray, or orally in tablet form. Potency varies by form of preparation (eg, IV form almost 10 times more potent than nasal spray).
      i. Duration of action 8 to 12 hours.
      ii. For patients who have some residual hypothalamic ADH (determined by low levels of circulating ADH).
      iii. Dosage may be reduced in older adults and in individuals with renal impairment.
   b. Chlorpropamide—potentiates action of vasopressin on renal concentrating mechanism.
   c. Tricyclic antidepressants and selective serotonin reuptake inhibitor antidepressants may potentiate the action of DDAVP.
   d. Carbamazepine—potentiates action of endogenous vasopressin (rarely used).
2. For patients with nephrogenic DI—chlorpropamide or thiazide diuretics may be of value. Reversible by discontinuing causative medication if cause is drug related.

Complications

1. If untreated, may result in death.
2. Overtreatment of DDAVP may cause hyponatremia and water intoxication.

 GERONTOLOGIC ALERT Older patients are more sensitive to the effects of DDAVP, so make sure that overdosage does not occur and watch for early signs of hyponatremia and water intoxication—drowsiness, confusion, headache, anuria, weight gain—to prevent seizures, coma, and death.

Nursing Assessment

1. Obtain complete health history to determine possible cause of DI.
2. Assess hydration status.

Nursing Diagnosis

- Risk for Deficient Fluid Volume related to disease process.

Nursing Interventions

Maintaining Adequate Fluid Volume

1. Measure fluid intake and output accurately.
2. Obtain daily weights.
3. Monitor hemodynamic status, as indicated, via frequent BP, heart rate, central venous pressure, and other measurements.
4. Provide patient with ample water to drink and administer IV fluids as indicated.
5. Monitor results of serum and urine osmolality and serum sodium tests.
6. Administer or teach self-administration of medication, as prescribed, and document patient response.

Patient Education and Health Maintenance

1. Inform patient that metabolic status must be monitored on a long-term basis because the severity of DI changes from time to time.
2. Advise patient to avoid limiting fluids to decrease urine output; thirst is a protective function.
3. Advise patient to wear a medical alert tag stating that the wearer has DI.
4. Teach patient to be alert for signs of dehydration—decreased weight, decreased urine output, increased thirst, dry skin and mucous membranes; and overhydration—increased weight and edema; report these to the health care provider.

5. Tell patient to consider eliminating coffee and tea from diet—may have an exaggerated diuretic effect.
6. Give written instruction on vasopressin administration. Have patient demonstrate intranasal and injection technique.

Evaluation: Expected Outcomes

- Fluid intake equals output, weight stable.

Pituitary Tumors

Pituitary tumors represent various cell types. Symptoms reflect tumor effects on target tissues or on local structures surrounding the pituitary gland.

Pathophysiology and Etiology

1. Multiple oncogene abnormalities are thought to be involved with pituitary tumorigenesis.
2. Typically, pituitary tumors are characterized by size and by what hormones, if any, are secreted.
   a. Size.
      i. Microadenoma—less than 10 mm wide.
      ii. Macroadenoma—greater than 10 mm wide.
   b. Functional status.
      i. Hormone secreting—exaggerated hormone activity; may secrete multiple hormones.
      ii. Nonsecreting—usually diminished hormone activity.
3. Malignancy in pituitary tumors is rare.

Clinical Manifestations

1. Mass effects—effects of tumor on surrounding structures.
   a. Nonspecific headache.
   b. Impairment of cranial nerves II, III, IV, and VI on testing because of bilateral hemianopsia, which results from pressure on the optic chiasm.
   c. Vision disturbances, such as visual field defects and diplopia.
2. Endocrine effects—effects of hormone imbalances caused by tumor (see Table 24-3).

Diagnostic Evaluation

1. MRI of the brain and sellar region; CT can also be done but is inferior.
2. Serum hormone levels to identify suspected abnormalities based on clinical evaluation.
3. Provocative testing to detect hormone secretion abnormalities of the pituitary, such as glucose tolerance test and DST.

Table 24-3 Clinical Manifestations Associated with Hormone Effects of Pituitary Tumors

HORMONE	HYPERPITUITARISM (INCREASED SECRETION)	HYPOPITUITARISM (DIMINISHED SECRETION)
Growth hormone	• Gigantism (child) • Acromegaly (adult)	• Shortness of stature (child) • Silent (adult)
Prolactin	• Infertility and galactorrhea (female)	• Postpartum lactation failure
Adrenocorticotropic hormone	• Cushing disease	• Adrenocortical insufficiency
Thyroid-stimulating hormone	• Hyperthyroidism	• Hypothyroidism
Luteinizing hormone and follicle-stimulating hormone	• Gonadal dysfunction	• Hypogonadism

Management

Hypophysectomy

1. Surgical removal of the pituitary; considered first line of treatment for pituitary adenomas.
2. Transsphenoidal hypophysectomy—direct approach through the sinus and nasal cavity to sella turcica (see page 707).
3. Frontal craniotomy—uncommon approach except where tumor occupies broad area (see page 361).

Other Methods of Pituitary Ablation

1. Cryogenic destruction or stereotaxic radiofrequency coagulation (may be used in conjunction with surgery or drug therapy).
2. Radiation therapy.
3. Drug therapy.
   a. Bromocriptine for prolactinomas and, in some instances, GH-secreting tumors is given daily.
   b. Cabergoline, a dopamine agonist, is administered twice per week for the treatment of acromegaly.
   c. Somatostatin analogues (octreotide, lanreotide) used in the treatment of acromegaly.
   d. GH antagonist (pegvisomant) used in the treatment of acromegaly.
   e. HRT for hypopituitarism.

Complications

1. Hypothyroidism and adrenocortical insufficiency after ablation, requiring hormone replacement.
2. Menstruation ceases and infertility occurs almost always after total or nearly total ablation.
3. Transient or permanent DI after surgery.
4. Without treatment—death or severe disability caused by stroke, blindness, or imbalances of ACTH, TSH, or ADH.

Nursing Assessment

1. Obtain history of signs and symptoms.
2. Perform thorough neurologic examination and general physical examination to identify signs of hormone deficiency or excess.
3. Assess patient's understanding of the management plan, coping with the diagnosis, and support from others.

Nursing Diagnoses

- Anxiety related to ablation treatment.
- Readiness for Enhanced Management of Therapeutic Regimen.

Nursing Interventions

Also see "Care of the Patient Undergoing Transsphenoidal Hypophysectomy," page 707.

Reducing Anxiety

1. Provide emotional support through the diagnostic process and answer questions about treatment options.
2. Prepare patient for surgery or other treatment by describing nursing care thoroughly.
3. Stress likelihood of positive outcome with ablation therapy.

Promoting Management of the Therapeutic Regimen

1. Teach patient the nature of hormonal deficiencies after treatment and the purpose of replacement therapy.
2. Instruct patient about the early signs and symptoms of cortisol or thyroid hormone deficiency or excess and the need to report them.

3. Describe and demonstrate the correct method of administering prescribed medications.
4. Encourage patient in assuming active role in self-care through information seeking and problem solving.

Patient Education and Health Maintenance

1. Advise patient on temporary limitations in activities.
2. Teach patient the need for frequent initial follow-up visits and lifelong medical management when on hormonal therapy.
3. If applicable, advise patient on the need for postsurgery radiation therapy and periodic follow-up MRI and visual field testing.
4. Teach patient to notify health care provider if signs of thyroid or cortisol imbalance become evident.
5. Advise patient to wear medical alert tag.
6. Help patient identify sources of information and support available in the community (see Box 24-1, page 709).

Evaluation: Expected Outcomes

- States rationale for treatment, asks appropriate questions.
- Demonstrates correct medication administration.

SELECTED REFERENCES

Bilezikian, J.P., Brandi, M.L., Eastell, R., et al. (2014). Guidelines for the Management of Asymptomatic Primary Hyperparathyroidism: Summary Statement from the Fourth International Workshop, *The Journal of Clinical Endocrinology & Metabolism*, 99(10), 3561–3569.

Bornstien, S., Allilio, B., Arlt, W., et al. (2016). Diagnosis and treatment of primary adrenal insufficiency: An Endocrine Society Clinical Practice Guideline. *Journal of Clinical Endocrinology Metabolism*, 101(2), 364–389.

Brandi, M.L., Bilezikian, J.P., Shoback, D., et al. (2016) Management of Hypoparathyroidism: Summary Statement and Guidelines, *The Journal of Clinical Endocrinology & Metabolism*, 101(6), 2273–2283.

Funder, J.W., Carey, R.M., Mantero, F., et al. (2016). The Management of Primary Aldosteronism: Case Detection, Diagnosis, and Treatment: An Endocrine Society Clinical Practice Guideline, *The Journal of Clinical Endocrinology & Metabolism*, 101(5), 1889–1916.

Garber, J.R., Cobin, R.H., Gharib, H., et al. (2012). Clinical Practice Guidelines for Hypothyroidism in Adults: Cosponsored by the American Association of Clinic Endocrinologists and the American Thyroid Association. *Endocrine Practice*, 18(6):e1-e45.

Gharib, H, Papini, E, Garber, J.R.,et al. (2016). American Association of Clinical Endocrinologists, American College of Endocrinology, and Associazione Medici Endocrinolgi Medical Guidelines for Clinical Practice for the Diagnosis and Management of Thyroid Nodules-2016 Update. *Endocrine Practice*, 22(suppl 1), 1–60.

Haugen, B. R., Alexander, E. K., Bible, K. C., et al. (2016). American Thyroid Association Management Guidelines for Adult Patients with Thyroid Nodules and Differentiated Thyroid Cancer: The American Thyroid Association Guidelines Task Force on Thyroid Nodules and Differentiated Thyroid Cancer. *Thyroid*, 26(1), 1–133.

Jonklaas, J., Bianco, A. C., Bauer, A. J., et al. (2014). Guidelines for the Treatment of Hypothyroidism: Prepared by the American Thyroid Association Task Force on Thyroid Hormone Replacement. *Thyroid*, 24(12), 1670–1751.

Katznelson, L., Laws, E.R, Melmed, S. et al. (2014). Acromegaly: An Endocrine Society Clinical Practice Guideline, *The Journal of Clinical Endocrinology & Metabolism*, 99(11), 3933–3951.

Key, M., & Heering, H. (2017). Thyroidectomy: Providing Postoperative Care of the Patient Undergoing. *CINAHL Nursing Guide*. Retrieved from *http://web.b.ebscohost.com.libpublic3.library.isu.edu/nrc/detail?vid=72&sid=e793c8c0-8be2-4ee5-8f2e-36e76686386fd%40pdc-v-sessmgr01&bdata=JnNpdGU9bnJjLWxpdmU%3d#AN=T707697&db=nrc*

Lenders, J. W. M., Duh, Q., Eisenhofer, G., et al. (2014). Pheochromocytoma and paraganglioma: An Endocrine Society Clinical Practice Guideline. *Journal of Clinical Endocrinology Metabolism*, 99(6), 1915–1942.

Lewis, T. III. (2016), Overview of disorders of calcium concentrations. Merck Manual Professional Version. Available: *www.merckmanuals.com/professional/endocrine-and-metabolic-disorders/electrolyte-disorders/overview-of-disorders-of-calcium-concentration*.

March, P., & Schub, T. (2017). Diabetes Insipidus. *CINAHL Nursing Guide*. Retrieved from *http://web.b.ebscohost.com.libpublic3.library.isu.edu/nrc/detail?vid=81&sid=e793c8c0-8be2-4ee5-8f2e-36e7686386fd%40pdc-v-sessmgr01&bdata=JnNpdGU9bnJjLWxpdmU%3d#AN=T700381&db=nrc*

McKay, O. (2017). Less Than Total Thyroidectomy for Goiter: When and How?. *Gland Surgery, 6*(suppl 1), S49–58.

National Institute of Diabetes and Digestive and Kidney Disease. (2014). *Adrenal insufficiency and Addison's disease. (DHHS Publication No. 14-3054)*. Washington, DC: US Government Printing Office.

National Institute of Diabetes and Digestive and Kidney Disease. (2012). *Cushing's syndrome. (DHHS Publication No. 08-3007)*. Washington, DC: US Government Printing Office.

National Institute of Diabetes and Digestive and Kidney Disease. (2012). *Primary hyperparathyroidism. (DHHS Publication No. 12-3425)*. Washington, DC: US Government Printing Office.

Nieman, L.K., Beverly M. K. Biller, Findling, J.W., et al. (2015), Treatment of Cushing's Syndrome: An Endocrine Society Clinical Practice Guideline, *The Journal of Clinical Endocrinology & Metabolism, 100*(8), 2807–2831.

Raverot, G., Burman, P., McCormack, A., et al. (2018). European Society of Endocrinolgy Clinical Practice Guideline for Management of Aggressive Pituitary Tumors and Carcinomas. *European Journal of Endocrinology, 178*(1): G1–G24.

Ross, D. S., Burch, H. B., Cooper, D. S., et al. (2016). American Thyroid Association Guidelines for Diagnosis and Management of Hyperthyroidism and Other Causes of Thyrotoxicosis. *Thyroid*, 26(10), 1343–1421.

Shugart, K. (2017). Cushing's Syndrome. *CINAHL Nursing Guide*. Retrieved from *http://web.b.ebscohost.com.libpublic3.library.isu.edu/nrc/detail?vid=76&sid=e793c8c0-8be2-4ee5-8f2e-36e7686386fd%40pdc-v-sessmgr01&bdata=JnNpdGU9bnJjLWxpd mU%3d#AN=T700379&db=nrc*

Stack, B.C., Brimston, D.N, Bodenner, D.L., et al. (2015). American Association of Clinical Endocrinologist and American College of Endocrinology Clinical Review: Post Operative Hypoparathyroid definition and Management. *Endocrine Practice, 21*(6), 674–685.

Stayer, D., Schub, T. (2016). Acromeglay. *CINAHL Nursing Guide* Retrieved from *http://search.ebscohost.com.libpublic3.library.isu.edu/login.aspx?direct=true&db=nrc &AN=T701802&site=nrc-live*

Swearmgen, B. (2015). Transsphenoidal Surgery for Pituitary Adenomas and Other Sellar Masses. In UpToDate. Retrieved from *https://www.uptodate.com/contents/transsphenoidal-surgery-for-pituitary-adenomas-and-other-sellar-masses?source=search_result&search=pituitary%20 tumor&selectedTitle=3-150*

Terris, D.J., Snyder, S., Carneiro-Pla, D., et al. (2013). American Thyroid Association Surgical Affairs Committee Writing Task Force. American Thyroid Association Statement on Outpatient Thyroidecomy. *Thyroid, 23*(10), 1193–1202.

Uribe, L.M., KaraKushian, A.L. (2017) Addison Disease. *CINAHL Nursing Guide*. Retrieved from: *http://search.ebscohost.com.libpublic3.library.isu.edu/login.aspx?dire ct=true&db=nrc&AN=T703739&site=nrc-live*

Wells, S.A., Sylvia, A. L., Henning, D., et al. (2015). Revised American Thyroid Association Guidelines, for the Management of Medullary Thyroid Carcinoma. *Thyroid, 25*(6), 567–610.

Velez, R.P., Donnelly-Strozzo, M., and Stanik-Hutt, J. (2016). Simplifying the Complexity of Primary Hyperparathyroidsm. *The Journal for Nurse Practitioners, 12*(5), 346–352.

OVERVIEW AND ASSESSMENT

 EVIDENCE BASE Centers for Disease Control and Prevention (CDC). (2017) National Diabetes Statistics Report: Estimates of Diabetes and Its Burden in the United States, 2017. Available: *https://www.cdc.gov/diabetes/pdfs/data/statistics/national-diabetes-statistics-report.pdf*.

In 2015, diabetes mellitus (DM) was estimated to affect more than 30 million Americans. This is more than 9% of the US population and yet almost 24% of those with DM are unaware that they have it. Unfortunately, if current trends continue and in the absence of major lifestyle changes and an overhaul of our current health care delivery system, the number of Americans diagnosed with DM is expected to increase by 64% by 2025. This translates to roughly 1 in every 3 Americans.

It is thought that the factors contributing to the explosion of diabetes are an aging population, increased prevalence of type 2 diabetes mellitus in youth, growing numbers of ethnic minorities, and the increasing trend of obesity. In 2013-2014 the National Center for Health Statistics estimated that more than 70% of American adults were classified as being overweight or obese.

Additionally, the cost of caring for people with diabetes is staggering. In 2016, Rowley and colleagues found that, the United States spent over $407 billion on diabetes care alone. This is more than two times the health care costs of those without diabetes. By 2025, they estimate that the cost will exceed $560 billion.

Diabetes mellitus is the leading cause of blindness, kidney failure, and lower limb amputations. People with diabetes are two to four times more likely to be diagnosed with heart disease, three times more likely to have dental disease, and twice as more likely to suffer from depression.

This is a very serious disease with even more serious consequences. All nurses must stay current on the latest care recommendations. Screening for this disease is essential because early treatment leads to a reduction of morbidity and mortality.

Insulin Secretion and Function

1. Insulin is a hormone secreted by the beta cells of the islet of Langerhans in the pancreas.

2. Small amounts of insulin are released into the bloodstream in response to changes in blood glucose levels throughout the day (basal secretion).
3. Increased secretion or a bolus of insulin, released during meals, helps maintain euglycemia.
4. Through an internal feedback mechanism that involves the pancreas and the liver, circulating blood glucose levels are maintained at a normal range of 60 to 100 mg/dL.
5. Insulin is essential for the utilization of glucose for cellular metabolism as well as for the proper metabolism of protein and fat.
   a. Carbohydrate metabolism—insulin affects the conversion of glucose into glycogen for storage in the liver and skeletal muscles and allows for the immediate release and utilization of glucose by the cells.
   b. Protein metabolism—amino acid conversion occurs in the presence of insulin to replace muscle tissue or to provide needed glucose (gluconeogenesis).
   c. Fat metabolism—storage of fat in adipose tissue and conversion of fatty acids from excess glucose occurs only in the presence of insulin.
6. Glucose can be used in the endothelial and nerve cells without the aid of insulin.
7. Without insulin, plasma glucose concentration rises and glycosuria results.
   a. Absolute deficits in insulin result from decreased production of endogenous insulin by the beta cell of the pancreas.
   b. Relative deficits in insulin are caused by inadequate utilization of insulin by the cell.

Classification of Diabetes

 EVIDENCE BASE American Association of Clinical Endocrinologists (AACE) and American College of Endocrinology (ACE). (2015). Clinical practice guidelines for developing a diabetes mellitus comprehensive care plan—2015. *Endocrine Practice, 21*(Suppl. 1).
    American Diabetes Association (ADA). (2018). Standards of medical care in diabetes—2018. *Diabetes Care, 41*(Suppl. 1).

Type 1 Diabetes Mellitus

Type 1 diabetes mellitus (T1DM), formerly known as insulin-dependent diabetes mellitus or juvenile diabetes mellitus.

1. Little or no endogenous insulin, requiring injections of insulin to control diabetes, prevent ketoacidosis, and sustain life.
2. Only 5% to 10% of all people with diabetes have T1DM.
3. Etiology is not well understood: includes autoimmune, viral, and certain histocompatibility antigens as well as genetic components.
4. Clinical manifestation is abrupt with classic symptoms of polydipsia, polyphagia, polyuria, and weight loss.
5. Most commonly seen in patients under age 30 but can be seen in older adults.

Type 2 Diabetes Mellitus

Type 2 diabetes mellitus (T2DM), formerly known as non–insulin-dependent diabetes mellitus or adult-onset diabetes mellitus.

1. Caused by a combination of insulin resistance and relative insulin deficiency—some individuals have predominantly insulin resistance, whereas others have predominantly deficient insulin secretion, with little insulin resistance.
2. Approximately 90% to 95% of people with diabetes have T2DM.
3. Etiology: strong hereditary component, commonly associated with obesity.
4. Usual presentation is slow and typically insidious with symptoms of fatigue, weight loss, poor wound healing, and recurrent infection.
5. Found primarily in adults over age 30; however, it is now more frequently seen in younger adults and adolescents who are overweight.
6. People with this type of diabetes may be treated with insulin but are still referred to as having T2DM.

Gestational Diabetes Mellitus

Gestational diabetes mellitus (GDM) is defined as the onset of carbohydrate intolerance that initially presents during pregnancy and resolves upon delivery.

1. Affects approximately 2% to 10% of pregnancies; however, the new diagnostic criteria may yield that as many as 18% of pregnancies are affected by GDM.
2. Women with GDM have a 35% to 60% chance of developing T2DM diabetes in the next 10 to 20 years. They should be screened for diabetes 6 to 12 weeks postpartum and continue to have lifelong screening at least every 3 years.
3. GDM is associated with significant risk of maternal and fetal complications.
4. Because of the worldwide increases of both obesity and diabetes rates, both the AACE/ACE and the ADA recommend that all pregnant women with risk factors (Box 25-1) for T2DM be screened for the presence of T2DM at the initial prenatal visit using the standard diagnostic criteria. Women who screen positive in the 1st trimester should be classified as having preexisting pregestational diabetes, not GDM.
5. Pregnant women who screen negative for T2DM in the 1st trimester should then be screened for GDM at 24 to 28 weeks of gestation. AACE/ACE recommends using the one-step strategy; the American College of Obstetricians and Gynecologists (ACOG) supports using the two-step

---

BOX 25-1	**Risk Factors and Screening for Type 2 Diabetes**

ADULTS

Begin screening at any age if overweight (BMI ≥ 25 kg/m²) *plus* any *one* of the following risk factors; otherwise begin screening all adults at age 45.

Screening should occur at least every 3 years.

- Family history of diabetes (first-degree relative).
- Sedentary lifestyle/habitual inactivity.
- Race/ethnicity (ie, black, Hispanic American, Native American, Alaskan American, and Pacific Islander).
- Previous diagnosis of prediabetes (IFG or IGT or A1C ≥ 5.7%).
- History of GDM.
- HTN ≥ 140/90 mm Hg.
- HDL cholesterol less than 35 mg/dL and/or triglyceride level greater than 250 mg/dL.
- History of insulin resistance (ie, polycystic ovary disease, acanthosis nigricans, severe obesity).
- History of cardiovascular disease.

CHILDREN

Begin screening at age 10 or onset of puberty (whichever first) and continuing at least every 3 years if:

Overweight (BMI greater than 85th percentile for age, gender, OR weight for height greater than 85th percentile, OR weight greater than 120% of ideal height) *plus* any *two* of the following risk factors:

- Family history of type 2 diabetes in first- or second-degree relative.
- Race/ethnicity (ie, Native American, black, Latino, Asian American, Pacific Islander).
- Signs of insulin resistance or conditions associated with insulin resistance (ie, acanthosis nigricans, hypertension, dyslipidemia, PCOS, or small-for-gestational age birth weight).
- Maternal history of DM or GDM during child's gestation.

---

strategy and following the diagnostic criteria established by either Carpenter and Coustan or the National Diabetes Data Group. The ADA states that either screening method is appropriate (Box 25-1).

Diabetes Because of Other Causes

1. Genetic defects of insulin secretion and/or insulin action.
2. Pancreatic diseases (such as cystic fibrosis, pancreatitis, and pheochromocytoma).
3. Drug-induced (such as corticosteroids and medications used to treat HIV/AIDS).

Prediabetes

1. *Prediabetes* is an abnormality in glucose values intermediate between normal and overt diabetes.
2. Associated with obesity, dyslipidemia, and hypertension; prediabetes is a potent risk factor for developing T2DM and cardiovascular disease.
3. Every effort should be made to assist the patient with aggressive lifestyle modifications (diet, exercise, and weight

loss) to prevent the progression from prediabetes to overt T2DM.

4. There are two forms of prediabetes, based on when glucose is elevated. Patients that simultaneously have both forms of prediabetes have a very high risk of developing T2DM.
   a. Impaired fasting glucose (IFG)—defined as having fasting blood glucose levels of 100 to 125 mg/dL.
   b. Impaired glucose tolerance (IGT)—defined as blood glucose measurement of 140 to 199 mg/dL using a 2-hour 75-g OGTT.

Laboratory Tests

 EVIDENCE BASE AACE/ACE. (2015). Clinical practice guidelines for developing a diabetes mellitus comprehensive care plan—2015. *Endocrine Practice*, 21(Suppl. 1).

ADA. (2018). Standards of medical care in diabetes—2018. *Diabetes Care, 41*(Suppl. 1).

International Society for Pediatric and Adolescent Diabetes (ISPAD). (2014). Clinical practice guidelines 2014. *Pediatric Diabetes, 15*(Suppl. 20).

This section includes the laboratory tests used to diagnose and monitor short- and long-term glucose control as well as the recommended glucose treatment goals for different population groups. See Box 25-1 for details pertaining to the screening criteria for T2DM in nonpregnant adults, adolescents, children, and older adults.

Blood Glucose

Description
1. Fasting blood sugar (FBS), drawn after at least an 8-hour fast, to evaluate circulating amounts of glucose.
2. Postprandial test, drawn usually 2 hours after a well-balanced meal, to evaluate glucose metabolism.
3. Random glucose, drawn at any time, without regard to the time of last caloric intake.

Nursing and Patient Care Considerations
1. For fasting glucose, make sure that patient has maintained 8-hour fast overnight; sips of water are allowed.
2. Advise patient to refrain from smoking before the glucose sampling because this affects the test results.
3. For postprandial glucose, advise patient that no additional food or caloric beverages should be consumed during the 2-hour interval.
4. For random blood glucose, note the time and content of the last meal.

Blood Glucose Values: Diagnostic Criteria and Treatment Goals
1. Diagnostic blood glucose values for diabetes mellitus all ages (ADA, AACE/ACE, and ISPAD):
   a. Fasting blood glucose ≥126 mg/dL, confirmed with a repeat test on another day.
   b. Random blood sugar (regardless of time of last caloric intake) ≥ 200 mg/dL *and* presence of classic symptoms of diabetes (polyuria, polydipsia, polyphagia, and weight loss). This test, when patients present symptomatic as described above, does not need to be repeated nor does the diagnosis need to be confirmed with another test.
   c. Fasting blood glucose result of 100 to 125 mg/dL is prediabetes (IFG) and demands close follow-up and repeat monitoring at least every 3 years.

2. Blood glucose treatment goals for many nonpregnant adults with diabetes mellitus:
   a. Premeal: 80 to 130 mg/dL (ADA) or less than 110 mg/dL (AACE/ACE).
   b. 1 to 2 hours postmeal: less than 180 mg/dL (ADA) or less than 140 mg/dL (AACE/ACE).

3. Blood glucose treatment goals for children and adolescents:
   a. Fasting and premeal: 70 to 145 mg/dL (ISPAD) or 90 to 130 mg/dL (ADA).
   b. Postmeal: 90 to 180 mg/dL (ISPAD).
   c. Bedtime: 120 to 180 mg/dL (ISPAD) or 90 to 150 mg/dL (ADA).
   d. Nocturnal (overnight): 80 to 162 mg/dL (ISPAD) or 90 to 150 mg/dL (ADA).

4. Blood glucose treatment goals for pregnant women with gestational diabetes (ADA and AACE/ACE):
   a. Premeal: ≤95 mg/dL.
   b. 1 hour postmeal: ≤140 mg/dL.
   c. 2 hours postmeal: ≤120 mg/dL.

5. Blood glucose treatment goals for pregnant women with preexisting diabetes:
   a. Premeal, bedtime: 60 to 99 mg/dL (AACE/ACE) or ≤95 mg/dL (ADA).
   b. 1 hour postmeal: 100 to 129 mg/dL (AACE/ACE) or ≤140 mg/dL (ADA).
   c. 2 hours postmeal: ≤120 mg/dL (ADA).

6. Blood glucose treatment goals for older adults (ADA):
   a. Healthy, few complications: 90 to 130 mg/dL fasting; 90 to 150 mg/dL bedtime.
   b. Complex with multiple coexisting chronic conditions: 90 to 150 mg/dL fasting; 100 to 180 mg/dL bedtime.
   c. Very complex/frail: 100 to 180 mg/dL fasting; 110 to 200 mg/dL bedtime.

7. Blood glucose treatment goals for hospitalized patients (critically and noncritically ill).
   a. 140 to 180 mg/dL (ADA and AACE/ACE).

 NURSING ALERT Capillary blood glucose values obtained by fingerstick samples tend to be higher than values in venous samples. Diagnostic tests are always to be conducted in a laboratory using venous samples.

Oral Glucose Tolerance Test

Description
The *oral glucose tolerance test (OGTT)* evaluates insulin response to glucose loading. FBS is obtained before the ingestion of a glucose load and blood samples are drawn at timed intervals.

Nursing and Patient Care Considerations
1. Advise patient that for accuracy in results, certain instructions must be followed:
   a. Usual diet and exercise pattern must be followed for 3 days before OGTT.
   b. During OGTT, patient must refrain from smoking and remain seated.
   c. Hormonal contraceptives, salicylates, diuretics, phenytoin, and nicotinic acid can impair results and may be withheld before testing based on the advice of the health care provider.

Diagnostic Criteria Using the 75-g 2-hour OGTT (Nonpregnant Adults, Children, Adolescents)

1. ADA and AACE/ACE diagnostic OGTT values when screening for diabetes mellitus in children, adolescents, and nonpregnant adults:
   a. 200 mg/dL or higher at the 2-hour interval.
   b. 140 to 199 mg/dL at the 2-hour interval is prediabetes (IGT) and demands close follow-up and repeat monitoring at least every 3 years.
   c. See Box 25-2, page 733 for diagnostic criteria using OGTT for gestational Diabetes.

Glycated Hemoglobin (Glycohemoglobin, HbA₁ᶜ, A1c)

HbA$_{1c}$, A1c)

Description

Measures glycemic control over a 60- to 120-day period by measuring the irreversible reaction of glucose to hemoglobin through freely permeable erythrocytes during their 120-day life cycle. Currently used to screen for diabetes as well as to monitor control.

Nursing and Patient Care Considerations

1. No prior preparation, such as fasting or withholding insulin/medications, is necessary.
2. Test results can be affected by red blood cell disorders (eg, thalassemia, sickle cell anemia), room temperature, ionic charges, and ambient blood glucose values.
3. Many methods exist for performing the test, making it necessary to consult the laboratory for normal values.
4. Should be performed at least twice yearly in patients whose diabetes is stable and well controlled. Quarterly (every 3 months) testing is recommended for patients who have had treatment changes/adjustments or whose diabetes is not well controlled.

Diagnostic Criteria and Treatment Goals for A1c Values

1. ADA and AACE/ACE diagnostic A1c values when screening for diabetes mellitus in children, adolescents, and nonpregnant adults.
   a. 6.5% or higher (diagnosis should be confirmed with repeat A1c or a fasting glucose or OGTT).
   b. 5.7% to 6.4% (ADA) or 5.5% to 6.4% (AACE/ACE) is considered prediabetes and demands close follow-up and repeat monitoring at least every 3 years.
2. The joint position statement (2009) of the ADA, the American College of Cardiology Foundation, and the American Heart Association asserts that in general, the A1c goal for nonpregnant adults is less than 7%, but that this must be individualized based on life expectancy, duration of diabetes, history of hypoglycemia, presence of microvascular complications, and presence of cardiovascular disease.
3. The ISPAD and ADA treatment A1c goal for children and adolescents is less than 7.5% across all age groups.
4. The ADA and AACE/ACE treatment A1c goal of pregnant women with pre-existing type 1 or type 2 diabetes is less than 6% (if without excessive hypoglycemia).
5. Because GDM is diagnosed late in pregnancy, the A1c is not a reliable marker of control (3-month average) and the fructosamine assay (2- to 3-week average) may be more meaningful.

EVIDENCE BASE Skyler, J., Bergenstal, R., Bonow, R. O., et al. (2009). Intensive glycemic control and the prevention of cardiovascular events: Implications of the ACCORD, ADVANCE, and VA Diabetes trials: A position statement of the American Diabetes Association and a scientific statement of the American College of Cardiology Foundation and the American Heart Association. *Diabetes Care, 32*(1), 187–192.

Fructosamine Assay

Description

Glycated protein with a much shorter half-life than glycated hemoglobin, reflecting control over a shorter period, approximately 14 to 21 days. May be advantageous in patients with hemoglobin variants that interfere with the accuracy of glycated hemoglobin tests.

Nursing and Patient Care Considerations

1. Note if patient has hypoalbuminemia or elevated globulins because test may not be reliable.
2. Should not be used as a diagnostic test for diabetes mellitus.
3. No special preparation or fasting is necessary.

C-Peptide Assay (Connecting Peptide Assay)

Description

Cleaved from the proinsulin molecule during its conversion to insulin, C-peptide acts as a marker for endogenous insulin production.

Nursing and Patient Care Considerations

1. Test can be performed after an overnight fast or after stimulation with Sustacal, intravenous (IV) glucose, or 1 mg of glucagon SubQ.
2. Absence of C-peptide indicates no beta cell function, reflecting possible T1DM or insulinopenia in T2DM.

Autoantibody Testing

Description

An *autoantibody* is an antibody (a type of protein) manufactured by the immune system that is directed against one or more of the individual's own proteins. Islet cell autoantibodies cause destruction to the pancreatic β-cells and are strongly associated with the development of T1DM. The appearance of autoantibodies to one or several of the autoantigens—GAD65, tyrosine phosphates (IA-2, IA-2β), ZnT8, or insulin—signals an autoimmune pathogenesis of β-cell destruction. The positivity of any of these autoantibodies in the presence of hyperglycemia is used to confirm the diagnosis of T1DM. Because T1DM affects such a small number of the population, screening is only recommended for 1st-degree family members of people diagnosed with T1DM. Generalized screening would be costly and therefore is not recommended.

Nursing and Patient Care Considerations

1. No special preparation or fasting is necessary.
2. Screen patients with T1DM for other autoimmune disorders such as hypothyroidism and celiac disease.

GENERAL PROCEDURES AND TREATMENT MODALITIES

See additional online content: Procedure Guidelines 25-1, 25-2

Glucose Monitoring

EVIDENCE BASE AACE/ACE. (2016). Outpatient glucose monitoring consensus statement. *Endocrine Practice, 22*(2), 231–261.
ADA. (2018). Standards of medical care in diabetes—2018. *Diabetes Care, 41*(Suppl. 1).

Accurate determination of capillary blood glucose assists patients in the control and daily management of diabetes mellitus. Blood glucose monitoring helps evaluate effectiveness of medication, reflects glucose excursion after meals, assesses glucose response to exercise regimen, and assists in the evaluation of episodes of hypoglycemia and hyperglycemia to determine appropriate treatment.

Procedure

1. The most appropriate schedule for glucose monitoring is determined by the patient and health care provider.
   a. Medication regimens and meal timing are considered to set the most effective monitoring schedule.
   b. Scheduling of glucose tests should reflect cost-effectiveness for the patient. Glucose meter test strips may cost greater than $1 per strip. Medicare restricts frequency of testing to once a day for those not taking insulin and up to three times a day for those who are.
   c. Glucose monitoring is intensified during times of stress or illness or when changes in therapy are prescribed.
2. Patients with T2DM who are not being treated with insulin or other medications that increase the risk of hypoglycemia (ie, sulfonylureas) should be testing blood glucose using a structured format where information obtained is used to guide treatment.
3. Patients with T1DM as well as those with T2DM who are using a multiple-dose insulin regimen should test blood sugar at least three times a day. Those times should include before/after meals, at bedtime, and occasionally at 2:00 to 3:00 A.M.
4. Alternate-site testing has been recommended by some clinicians for patients who complain of painful fingers and for individuals such as musicians, who use their fingertips for occupational activities. However, testing in such sites as the forearm, palm, thigh, and calf have not proved as accurate as fingertip testing in most studies.
   a. If alternate site is used, the area should be rubbed until it is warm before testing.
   b. Do not use an alternate site when:
      i. Glucose levels are rapidly changing (postprandial, hypoglycemia, reaction to exercise/activity).
      ii. Accuracy is critical (hypoglycemia is suspected, before exercise, or before driving).
   c. Check with the glucometer manufacturer to see if it is approved for alternate-site testing.
5. Continuous glucose monitoring (CGM) is a supplemental tool for use in selected patients, such as those with T1DM experiencing frequent hypoglycemia episodes, severe hypoglycemia, and/or hypoglycemia unawareness. CGM measures glucose in the interstitial fluid. Ongoing advances in technology have rendered these readings highly reliable and correlate closely with plasma glucose.
   a. CGM systems currently available in the US will vary as to whether or not calibration is required by the user or as to whether or not confirmatory fingerstick testing is required to confirm CGM readings. As this technology continues to advance in accuracy, less input will be required by the user.
   b. CGM also detect changes in glucose patterns and will alert the user of potentially dangerous rises and falls. This enables the user to be proactive and avert harmful events.
   c. Current CGM are available for either a professional use (by experienced clinicians as a diagnostic tool) or for personal use (as either stand-alone devices or in an integrated insulin pump/CGM system).
6. In 2016, the FDA approved the 1st hybrid closed loop system (insulin delivery via an insulin pump that will adjust basal rates based on CGM data). It will not be long before a fully automated, closed loop system (bionic pancreas) will be available.

Insulin Therapy

EVIDENCE BASE AACE/ACE. (2018). Consensus statement by the AACE and ACE on the comprehensive type 2 diabetes management algorithm—2018 Executive Summary. *Endocrine Practice, 24*(1), 91–120.
ADA. (2018). Standards of medical care in diabetes—2018. *Diabetes Care, 41*(Suppl. 1).

Insulin therapy involves the subcutaneous injection of rapid-, short-, intermediate-, or long-acting insulin at various times to achieve the desired effect (see Table 25-1). Short-acting regular human insulin as well as some of the rapid-acting analogs can also be administered intravenously. As of this publication, there are 10 different types of insulin available in the United States. They are available in different concentrations (u-100, u-200, u-300, u-500) and premixed combinations. Most of the available insulin products are human insulin manufactured synthetically (analogs). Beef and pork insulins are no longer available in the United States.

DRUG ALERT The following insulin types can be used during pregnancy (category B): human regular, human NPH, aspart, lispro, and detemir. All others, to include Afrezza inhaled insulin, remain category C and should not be used during pregnancy if other alternatives are available.

Self-Injection of Insulin

1. Teaching of self-injection of insulin should begin as soon as the need for insulin has been established.
2. Teach the patient and another family member or significant other.
3. Use written and verbal instructions and demonstration techniques.
4. Teach injection first because this is the patient's primary concern; then, teach loading the syringe.
5. Almost all insulin preparations are available in prefilled pen devices. These are much easier and safer for the patients to learn and use. It is recommended that pen devices be used whenever possible. These are most appropriate for patients with dexterity or vision limitation.

Community and Home Care Considerations

1. Assist the patient in deciding whether to reuse insulin syringe at home. The patient may decide to do so because of cost; however, reuse has become controversial because the newer, finer needles may become dull or bent after one or two injections, causing tearing of tissue, which can lead to lipodystrophy.
   a. Needles should not be reused if painful injection or irritated site results.

Table 25-1 Insulin Products Available in the United States and Their Onset, Peak, Duration, Route, and Pregnancy Category

TYPE	ONSET	PEAK	DURATION	ROUTE
Rapid-Acting Analogs				
Insulin aspart (Fiasp)	<5 min	<1 hr	<3 hr	SQ, IV
Insulin aspart (Novolog)	<15 min	1–2 hr	3–4 hr	SQ, pump, IV
Insulin glulisine (Apidra)	<15 min	1–2 hr	3–4 hr	SQ, pump, IV
Insulin lispro (Humalog)	<15 min	1–2 hr	3–4 hr	SQ, pump
Afrezza human insulin	<15 to 30 min	53 min	2 hr	Inhaled
Short-Acting Human Insulin				
Humulin R	0.5–1 hr	2–4 hr	5–7 hr	SQ, IV
Novolin R	0.5–1 hr	2–4 hr	5–7 hr	SQ, IV
Intermediate-Acting Basal				
Insulin isophane susp. (NPH)	2–4 hr	4–10 hr	10–16 hr	SQ
Humulin N	2–4 hr	4–10 hr	10–16 hr	SQ
Novolin N				
Long-Acting Basal Analogs				
Insulin detemir (Levemir)	3–4 hr	None	6–24 hr	SQ
Insulin glargine (Lantus)	3–4 hr	None	<24 hr	SQ
Ultra–Long-Acting Basal Analogs				
Insulin glargine u-300 (Toujeo)	6 hr	None	>24 hr	SQ
Insulin degludec u-100 and u-200 (Tresiba)	30–90 min	None	>40 hr	SQ
Premixed Insulin				
Analog Preparations				
Novolog Mix 70/30 (aspart)	<15 min	2–4 hr	24 hr	SQ
Humalog Mix 75/25 (lispro)	<15 min	0½–1.5 hr	24 hr	SQ
Humalog Mix 50/50 (lispro)	<15 min	1 hr	16 hr	SQ
Ryzodeg 70/30 (degludec + aspart)	<15 min	72 min	>24 hr	SQ
NPH and Regular Suspensions				
Humulin 70/30	30 min	2–12 hr	24 hr	SQ
Novolin 70/30	30 min	2–12 hr	24 hr	SQ

Notes: No FDA-approved insulins derived from beef are available in the United States. They were discontinued in 1998 because of concerns about bovine spongiform encephalopathy (BSE; "mad cow disease").
Iletin II Regular (Pork), Iletin II NPH (Pork), Humulin Lente, and Humulin Ultralente were all discontinued by the manufacturer (Lilly) in 2005 because of reduced demand and high cost.
Exubera (inhaled insulin) was discontinued by Pfizer in late 2007 because of poor sales.

b. Needle should be recapped by patient and stored in a clean place if it is going to be reused.

2. Assist the patient in obtaining the appropriate syringe size and needle length for injections.

   a. Determine if there are visual or dexterity issues that make a syringe with gradations farther apart more desirable.

   b. There is no medical reason to use needles greater than 8 mm in length, even in obese patients. Needle lengths of 4, 5, and 6 mm are reliable to deliver medication into the subcutaneous space. To prevent inadvertent intramuscular injection in patients who are thin, the needle can be inserted at a 45-degree angle (rather than at a 90-degree angle) and/or the skin should be folded prior to needle insertion.

   c. There are now insulin syringes available specifically for the use of u-500 regular insulin that are to be prescribed and dispensed with each vial of u-500 regular insulin. U-500 insulin is also now available in prefilled pen devices. Both the new u-500–specific syringes and the prefilled pens make the administration of this insulin much safer.

 NURSING ALERT Using a u-100 syringe or tuberculin syringe to dose u-500 regular insulin is not safe and is not recommended.

3. Advise the patient that it is not necessary to use alcohol to wipe off the top of the vial or prepare the skin before injection. It has not proved to result in lower rate of infection and adds cost and time to the procedure. The patient should maintain good hygiene (handwashing using soap and water).

4. Instruct the patient to store insulin currently in use in a clean, secure place away from direct sunlight and heat. In-use insulin does not require refrigeration. Check manufacturer recommendations for when to discard insulin vials and pens; recommendations may vary from 10 to 56 days after initial use. All unopened vials/pens must be stored in the refrigerator until initial use.

5. Check manufacturer's recommendations before teaching the patient how to mix insulin; for example, the patient should know that insulin glargine and insulin detemir must never be mixed with any other insulin. Other manufacturers' Web sites containing recommendations are Aventis (*www.aventis.com*), Eli Lilly (*www.lilly.com*), and Novo Nordisk (*www.novonordisk.com*).

Screening and Diagnosing Parameters for Gestational Diabetes

ONE-STEP STRATEGY

WHEN: 24–28 weeks' gestation
HOW: 75-g 2-hr OGTT performed in the morning following 8-hr fast the night before
WHAT is diagnostic for GDM (any ONE of the results):
  Fasting glucose: ≥92 mg/dL
  1-hr interval: ≥180 mg/dL
  2-hr interval: ≥153 mg/dL

TWO-STEP STRATEGY

WHEN: 24–28 weeks' gestation
HOW:
  Step 1: nonfasting, 50-g glucose load test; PROCEED to Step 2 if 1-hr result: ≥135 mg/dL **or** ≥140 mg/dL (determined by the provider and patient risk factors).
  Step 2: 100-g 3-hr OGTT performed in the morning following an 8-hr fast the night before.
WHAT is diagnostic for GDM (**2 positive results; choose 1 set of criteria to follow**):

GLUCOSE VALUE:	CARPENTER/ COUSTAN	NATIONAL DIABETES DATA GROUP
Fasting:	≥95 mg/dL	≥105 mg/dL
1-hr interval:	≥180 mg/dL	≥190 mg/dL
2-hr interval:	≥155 mg/dL	≥165 mg/dL
3-hr interval:	≥140 mg/dL	≥145 mg/dL

6. Avoid prefilling syringes if possible because manufacturers have no data on the stability of insulin stored in syringes for long periods. If prefilling is the only option, store in refrigerator or suggest an insulin pen injection device.

7. Help the patient develop a plan for the disposal of needles. There are no federal regulations for discarding needles used at home; however, needles and lancets can pose a risk for injury. The rules and regulations regarding sharps disposal are different in towns and counties around the country, so advise the patient to check with local sanitation or health departments.

   a. Sharps can be placed in a hard plastic or metal container with a tightly secured lid after use.

   b. More information on disposal can be obtained from the Environmental Protection Agency (*www.epa.gov/osw/ nonhaz/industrial/medical/med-home.pdf*) or by contacting the Coalition for Safe Community Needle Disposal (800-643-1643 or *www.safeneedledisposal.org*).

Insulin Regimens

See Figure 25-1.

Basal Insulin Only (Figure 25-1A)

1. Either NPH or long-acting analogs may be used as monotherapy only in T2DM as a supplement for better glucose control when patients are still capable of producing some exogenous insulin. Patients with T1DM will always require mealtime coverage in addition to basal insulin.

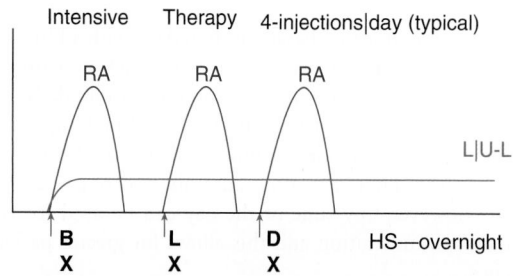

KEY: B = Breakfast
      L = Lunch
      D = Dinner
      HS: Sleep/Bedtime

* = CAN BE GIVEN ANYTIME OF DAY
** = ONLY TAKEN IF THAT MEAL IS EATEN
X = ATE MEAL
↑ = INJECTION ADMINISTERED

Figure 25-1. Insulin regimens.

2. NPH is not used as frequently as a basal insulin because of the availability of the newer analog basal insulins that are more reliable, longer acting, and associated with less hypoglycemia. However, NPH is available without a prescription and may also be the most affordable option for some patients.

3. Basal insulin is traditionally administered at bedtime to assist with controlling early-morning hyperglycemia. Patients may take NPH in addition to a mealtime insulin before dinner and can be mixed in the same syringe. If NPH is taken before dinner, a snack before bed is usually necessary to prevent nocturnal hypoglycemia because of the onset of the peaking action several hours later. Bedtime dosing of NPH typically eliminates the need for a bedtime snack and will better address dawn phenomenon (elevated glucose values upon awakening the following morning).

4. The longer-acting insulin analogs typically allow for once-daily dosing and can be administered at various times of the day, and eating snacks between meals to prevent hypoglycemia is usually not required.

5. When used as basal insulin, NPH is typically administered twice daily—in the morning to address afternoon hyperglycemia and again at bedtime to provide overnight coverage. Typically, $^{2}/_{3}$ to $^{3}/_{4}$ of the daily dosage is given before breakfast and $^{1}/_{3}$ to $^{1}/_{4}$ is given at bedtime.

Basal Plus Prandial Insulin (Figure 25-1B, 2 Mixed Injections/Day)

1. Short-acting regular insulin or rapid-acting lispro, glulisine, or aspart insulin is added to NPH to promote postprandial glucose control.

2. Short- or rapid-acting insulin added to morning NPH controls glucose elevations after breakfast.

3. Increased blood glucose levels after supper can be controlled by the addition of short- or rapid-acting insulin before supper.

4. NPH and regular, lispro, glulisine, or aspart insulin given before breakfast and before supper is termed a "split-mix" regimen, providing 24-hour insulin coverage. However, there is an increased risk of nocturnal hypoglycemia (2:00 to 3:00 A.M.) when NPH is given before supper. Therefore, an alternative is to administer the prandial insulin alone before the evening meal and the NPH at bedtime (see Figure 25-1C).

Intensive Insulin Therapy (Figure 25-1D)

1. Designed to mimic the body's normal insulin responses to glucose.

2. Characterized by at least 1 basal injection daily with additional mealtime injections for every meal and snack consumed. Typically consists of four to five injections of insulin daily.

3. Long-acting (detemir or glargine insulin) or ultra–long-acting (glargine u-300 or degludec insulin) analog is used for basal insulin control. These are often administered once daily at bedtime; however, any time of the day can be used for the once-daily administration and this allows for greater patient adherence.

4. Regular insulin acts as a premeal bolus given 30 minutes before each meal. However, analog rapid-acting insulin (lispro, glulisine, or aspart) are used more frequently instead of regular. The rapid-acting insulin is taken within 1 to 15 minutes before eating. As with NPH, regular human insulin is available without a prescription and is often a more affordable choice for some patients.

5. Twenty-four–hour insulin coverage designed in this way can be flexible to accommodate mealtimes and physical activity.

Sliding Scale versus Algorithm Therapy

1. Sliding scale therapy uses short- or rapid-acting insulin to retrospectively correct hyperglycemia. Sliding scale dosing is not recommended because it fails to prevent and adequately address hyperglycemia and places patients at significant risk for hypoglycemia hours later.

2. Algorithm therapy prospectively determines short- or rapid-acting insulin dosages, considering meal content, premeal blood glucose level, and physical activity.

3. Individualization of insulin dosages is the most important aspect of sliding scale and algorithm therapy.
   a. The patient is encouraged to test blood glucoses to analyze insulin dose response.
   b. A pattern of increased blood glucose associated with certain foods (eg, pasta, pizza) can help determine the appropriate regimen of insulin dosage.
   c. Physical activity, which enhances insulin activity and decreases serum glucose, may indicate the need to reduce the dosage of premeal insulin.

Continuous Subcutaneous Insulin Infusion (Insulin Pump Therapy)

Pump therapy is more commonly considered for treatment of T1DM, but it is becoming more common in the treatment of T2DM when multiple daily injections/intensive insulin management is required.

1. Continuous subcutaneous insulin infusion (CSII) or insulin pump therapy provides continuous infusion of regular, lispro, glulisine, or aspart insulin via subcutaneous catheter.

2. There are several different pumps available. The type of insulin pump used by the patient is determined by the patient with the guidance of an expert clinician.

3. The catheter should be replaced every 72 hours or sooner if the site becomes painful or inflamed.
   a. Usually, the insulin pump is removed for bathing and tubing and catheter are changed at that time. Several pumps are waterproof and do not need to be disconnected with bathing, showering, or even swimming.
   b. To reduce tubing and catheter blockage, diluted insulin may be used. However, this is less of a problem with the newer insulin analogs (lispro, glulisine, and aspart).
   c. A tube-free pump is available. The patient wears a "pod" filled with enough insulin to last 2 to 3 days. The pod is discarded and a new pod placed every 2 to 3 days. The delivery of insulin is remotely controlled via a handheld device.

4. Intensive insulin management by pump therapy requires patient motivation.
   a. Blood glucose monitoring must be done at least four to six times per day. Most insulin pumps are now available as integrated systems, which utilize CGM. (See Glucose Monitoring.)
   b. Frequent contact with health care team is necessary to adjust insulin dosage.
   c. Careful recordings of diet, insulin, and activity are required to evaluate adjustments.
   d. Increased cost of insulin pump and infusion set compared to usual syringe method.
   e. Heightened risk of hypoglycemia with tighter glucose control.
   f. Danger of hyperglycemia exists should insulin catheter become kinked or dislodged, and patient then fails to receive appropriate insulin dosage.
   g. Increased visibility of diabetes by use of an external device, although newer pumps are smaller and more discreet.

5. Advantages of CSII in improving blood glucose control:
   a. Insulin pump can deliver basal insulin at individualized programmed rates throughout a 24-hour period.
   b. Bolus injections of short-acting insulin given 30 minutes before eating or rapid-acting insulin no more than 15 minutes before a meal allow for flexibility in meal content and timing.
   c. Correction supplements of short- or rapid-acting insulin are easily given to rapidly correct elevated glucose levels.

Combination Noninsulin Agents and Insulin Therapy

1. Except for using pramlintide in addition to insulin, all other combinations of insulin with noninsulin agents are only FDA-approved to be used for patients with T2DM.
2. Always refer to the full prescribing information for each non-insulin agent to determine if and how they are FDA-approved for use with insulin therapy.
3. Because of the increased risk for hypoglycemia, concomitant use of insulin and sulfonylureas is not recommended.

DIABETES MELLITUS AND RELATED DISORDERS

 See additional online content: Procedure Guidelines 25-3

Diabetes Mellitus

Diabetes mellitus is a metabolic disorder characterized by hyperglycemia and results from defective insulin production, secretion, or utilization. T1DM in children is covered in Chapter 50.

Pathophysiology and Etiology

1. There is an absolute or relative lack of insulin produced by beta cells, resulting in hyperglycemia.
2. Defects at the cell level, impaired secretory response of insulin to rises in glucose, and increased nocturnal hepatic glucose production (gluconeogenesis) are seen in type 2 diabetes.
3. Etiology of type 1 diabetes is not well understood; viral, autoimmune, and environmental theories are under review.
4. Etiology of type 2 diabetes involves heredity, genetics, and obesity.
5. Risk factors for type 2 diabetes in adults and children include family history and ethnicity and a variety of other factors (see page 728).

Clinical Manifestations

1. Onset is usually abrupt with T1DM and insidious with T2DM.
2. Classic symptoms of hyperglycemia include polyuria, polydipsia, polyphagia, weight loss, fatigue, and blurred vision.
3. Chronic hyperglycemia often presents as disorders of altered tissue response, evidenced by poor wound healing and recurrent infections of the skin and genitourinary tract.

Diagnostic Evaluation

See page 729.

Management

 EVIDENCE BASE AACE/ACE. (2018). Consensus statement by the AACE and ACE on the comprehensive type 2 diabetes management algorithm—2018 Executive Summary. *Endocrine Practice, 24*(1), 91–120.
ADA. (2018). Standards of medical care in diabetes—2018. *Diabetes Care, 41*(Suppl. 1).

A multidisciplinary approach, which combines diet, exercise, behavioral/psychosocial therapy, and pharmacological agents, is required to optimally manage glucose control and the comorbid conditions of hypertension, dyslipidemia, and obesity.

Diet

1. The goal of meal planning is to meet nutritional requirements essential for healthy growth/development, achieve/maintain healthy weight, and control blood glucose and lipid levels (see Table 25-2).
2. Weight reduction is a primary treatment for T2DM. A target of greater than 5% weight loss is desired.
3. Medical nutrition therapy should be conducted by a registered dietitian, preferably one who is also a certified diabetes educator.

Exercise

Regularly scheduled, moderate exercise performed 30 to 60 minutes at least every other day promotes the utilization of carbohydrates, assists with weight control, enhances the action of insulin, and improves cardiovascular fitness.

Psychosocial Care

1. Psychosocial care should be an integrated component of comprehensive diabetes management for all patients with diabetes.
2. Assess for symptoms of diabetes distress, depression, anxiety, disordered eating, and cognitive capacity.
3. Assess for life circumstances that impact patient ability to perform self-care management. Include input from family members/caregivers.
4. Promptly refer to behavioral health specialist when problems are identified.

 EVIDENCE BASE Young-Hyman, D., de Groot, M., Hill-Briggs, F., Gonzalez, J. S., et al. (2016). Psychosocial care for people with diabetes: A position statement of the ADA. *Diabetes Care, 39*(12), 2126–2140.

Medication

Both the ADA and AACE/ACE treatment algorithms place emphasis on individualizing pharmacological treatment based on effectiveness, risk of hypoglycemia, risk of weight gain, cost, and patient preferences. Lifestyle management (diet and exercise) will always remain the cornerstone of management even when medications are required. Insulin is always an appropriate therapy for glucose management and should be discussed with the patient early in the disease process to alleviate fears and other stigma associated with its use.

Only insulin and amylin analogs are approved for use in patients with T1DM.

1. Oral and injectable antidiabetic agents for patients with T2DM who do not achieve glucose control with diet and exercise only (see Table 25-3, pages 736 to 737).
2. Insulin therapy is essential for patients with T1DM who require replacement (see pages 731 to 735). Insulin therapy may also be used for T2DM when glucose management is unresponsive to diet, exercise, and noninsulin therapy as well as when β-cell failure progresses or they are unable to tolerate/safely use other diabetes medications.

 DRUG ALERT Hypoglycemia may result from insulin therapy as well as rebound hyperglycemia (Somogyi effect). Insulin therapy commonly results in increased appetite and weight gain.

Table 25-2   Meal Planning Guidelines

PRINCIPLE	ACTION
Each meal should consist of a balance of carbohydrates, proteins, and fats.	• Carbohydrates should be varied to include fruits, starches, and vegetables. • Protein selections that are lean will help reduce fat and cholesterol intake. • Fats should be used sparingly with <10% of total calories derived from saturated fats. High in calories, fats contribute to weight gain in type 2 diabetes mellitus (DM).
Consistency in timing of meals and amounts of food eaten on a day-to-day basis help regulate blood glucose levels.	• Avoid skipping or delaying meals. • Measure portion sizes using a scale or measuring cups. • Know the equivalent amounts of commonly used foods within a food group (eg, 1 slice of bread = ½ cup cooked pasta).
Increase the intake of soluble and insoluble fiber.	• Substitute foods high in fiber for processed foods when possible (eg, whole-grain bread in place of white bread). • Eat fresh fruits and vegetables in place of juices.
Avoid salt whenever possible.	• Do not season foods with salt or salt-containing spices. • Limit use of foods with "hidden" sodium content (eg, crackers, pickled foods, cheese, processed meats). • Use salt-containing condiments sparingly (ketchup, soy sauce, gravies, bouillon).
Prepare foods to retain vitamins and minerals and reduce fats.	• Do not fry foods. • Bake, broil, or boil foods and discard fat. • Eat raw fruits and vegetables or steam vegetables to retain fiber. • Avoid adding calories with butter or cream sauces, fatback, and bacon. • Trim all visible fat from meat; skim off fat from stews or other prepared dishes.
Distribute snacks in the meal plan depending on insulin/medication regimens, physical activity, and lifestyle.	• Smaller, more frequent meals may enhance glucose control in type 2 DM. • Unplanned activity may call for an additional snack to avoid hypoglycemia.
Use alcohol only in moderation.	• Always consume alcohol with food to avoid hypoglycemia. • Do not omit food from meal plan in exchange for alcohol. • Limit intake to 1 to 2 drinks/wk (4 oz. dry wine, 12 oz. beer, or 1.5 oz. distilled liquor = 1 alcohol serving).
Use alternative nonnutritive, noncaloric sweeteners in moderation.	• Limit "diet" soda intake to 2 L/day. • Avoid frequent use of foods and beverages with concentrated sucrose.

Table 25-3   Antidiabetic Medications (Noninsulin)

AGENT	HOW GIVEN
Insulin-Secreting Agents	
Second-Generation Sulfonylureas	
• Glyburide	1.25–20 mg PO in single or divided doses with meals
• Glyburide, micronized	0.75–12 mg PO in single or divided dose
• Glipizide	2.5–40 mg PO in single or divided doses with meals
• Glipizide, long-acting	2.5–20 mg PO in single dose, usually before breakfast
• Glimepiride	1–8 mg PO in single dose with first main meal
Meglitinide Analog	
• Repaglinide	0.5–16 mg PO in 2–4 divided doses, 1–30 min before meals Do not take if meal is skipped.
Amino Acid Derivative	
• Nateglinide	120–360 mg PO in 3 divided doses, 1–30 min before meals Do not take if meal is skipped.
Insulin-Sensitizing Agents	
Biguanides	
• Metformin	500–2,550 mg PO in 2–3 divided doses
• Metformin, long-acting	500–2,000 mg PO in single or two divided doses
Thiazolidinediones	
• Pioglitazone	15–45 mg PO once daily
• Rosiglitazone	4–8 mg PO in single or two divided doses
Glucose Absorption–Delaying Agents	
Alpha Glucosidase Inhibitors	
• Acarbose	50–300 mg PO in 3 divided doses before meals
• Miglitol	50–300 mg PO in 3 divided doses before meals

Table 25-3 Antidiabetic Medications (Noninsulin) (Continued)

AGENT	HOW GIVEN
Incretin Agents	
DPP-4 Inhibitors	
• Sitagliptin	25–100 mg PO once daily
• Linagliptin	5 mg PO once daily
• Saxagliptin	2.5–5 mg PO once daily
• Alogliptin	6.25–25 mg PO once daily
GLP-1 Receptor Agonists	
• Exenatide	5–10 mcg subcutaneously twice daily 1–60 min before meals
• Liraglutide	1.2–1.8 mg subcutaneously once daily
• Lixisenatide	10–20 mcg subcutaneously once daily
• Exenatide, extended release	2 mg subcutaneously every 7 days
• Albiglutide	20–50 mg subcutaneously every 7 days
• Dulaglutide	0.75–1.5 mg subcutaneously every 7 days
• Semaglutide	0.5–1 mg subcutaneously every 7 days
Glucose-Excreting Agents	
SGLT2 Inhibitors	
• Canagliflozin	100–300 mg PO once daily
• Empagliflozin	10–25 mg PO once daily
• Dapagliflozin	5–10 mg PO once daily
• Ertugliflozin	5–15 mg PO once daily
Amylin Analog	
• Pramlintide	Type 1: 15–60 mcg subcutaneously with each main meal Type 2: 60–120 mcg subcutaneously with each main meal
Other Agents	
Bile Acid Sequestrant	
• Colesevelam	625 mg tablets: 3 tabs PO twice daily or 6 tabs PO once daily
Dopamine Agonist	
• Bromocriptine	0.8–4.8 mg PO once daily in the morning

Combination Agents with Brand Names

- Actoplus Met, Actoplus Met XR (pioglitazone + metformin)
- Amaryl M (glimepiride + metformin)
- Avandamet (rosiglitazone + metformin)
- Avandaryl (rosiglitazone + glimepiride)
- Duetact (pioglitazone + glimepiride)
- Glucovance (glyburide + metformin)
- Glyxambi (linagliptin + empagliflozin)
- Invokamet, Invokamet XR (canagliflozin + metformin)
- Janumet, Janumet XR (sitagliptin + metformin)
- Jentadueto (linagliptin + metformin)

- Kazano (alogliptin + metformin)
- Kombiglyze XR (saxagliptin + metformin)
- Metaglip (glipizide + metformin)
- Oseni (alogliptin + pioglitazone)
- PrandiMet (repaglinide + metformin)
- Qtern (dapagliflozin + saxagliptin)
- Soliqua 100/33 (lixisenatide + insulin glargine)
- Steglatro (ertugliflozin + metformin)
- Steglujan (ertugliflozin + sitagliptin)
- Synjardy (empagliflozin + metformin)
- Xigduo, Xigduo XR (dapagliflozin + metformin)
- Xultophy 100/3.6 (liraglutide + insulin degludec)

DPP-4, dipeptidyl peptidase 4; GLP-1 RA, glucagon-like peptide-1 receptor agonist; PO, by mouth; XR, extended release.

3. Sulfonylurea compounds promote the increased secretion of insulin by the pancreas and partially normalize both receptor and postreceptor defects.
   a. Many drug interactions exist, so patient should alert all health care providers of use.
   b. Potential adverse reactions include hypoglycemia, photosensitivity, GI upset, allergic reaction, reaction to alcohol, cholestatic jaundice, and blood dyscrasias.
4. Metformin, a biguanide compound, appears to diminish insulin resistance. It decreases hepatic glucose production and intestinal reabsorption of glucose and increases insulin reception and glucose transport in cells.
   a. Many drug interactions exist, so patient should alert all health care providers of its use.

   b. Metformin must be used cautiously in renal insufficiency, conditions that may cause dehydration, and hepatic impairment.
   c. Potential adverse reactions include GI disturbances, metallic taste, and lactic acidosis (rare). Riomet is the only formulation available as an oral solution.

 DRUG ALERT Lactic acidosis is a rare complication of metformin that prompts caution when dehydration, vomiting, diarrhea, fasting states, hemodynamic instability, heavy alcholol use, and use of iodinated contrast media occur.

5. Alpha glucosidase inhibitors (AGI) (acarbose and miglitol) delay the digestion and absorption of complex carbohydrates

(including sucrose or table sugar) into simple sugars, such as glucose and fructose, thereby lowering postprandial and fasting glucose levels.

   a. Contraindicated in inflammatory bowel disease and other conditions of the intestinal tract. They are used cautiously in renal insufficiency and with several other drugs.

   b. Flatulence, abdominal pain, and diarrhea are common.

   c. If these medications are taken in conjunction with insulin secretagogues (ie, sulfonylureas) and hypoglycemia occurs, patient must use a monosaccharide (glucose tablets) or milk to treat hypoglycemia because sucrose will not be broken down to an absorbable sugar. Juice will not be effective.

6. Thiazolidinedione (TZD) derivatives (rosiglitazone and pioglitazone) primarily decrease resistance to insulin in skeletal muscle and adipose tissue without increasing insulin secretion. Secondarily, they reduce hepatic glucose production.

   a. They should be used cautiously in liver disease and heart failure. Liver function tests should be monitored periodically.

   b. Ovulation may occur in anovulatory premenopausal women.

   c. Adverse reactions include edema, weight gain, anemia, elevation in serum transaminases, and increased incidence of bone fracture.

   d. Pioglitazone is associated with increased risk of bladder cancer; therefore, it should not be used in patients with a history of bladder cancer.

   e. Thiazolidinediones themselves do not cause hypoglycemia; however, when administered with insulin or oral medications that increase the secretion of insulin, the risk for hypoglycemia is increased. Be aware that insulin requirements will reduce with TZD therapy, so glucose monitoring and insulin adjustments should be done regularly.

 DRUG ALERT Both pioglitazone and rosiglitazone can cause or worsen heart failure and are contraindicated for use in patients with New York Heart Association class III or class IV heart failure.

7. Meglitinide analogues (repaglinide) and amino acid derivatives (nateglinide) stimulate pancreatic release of insulin in response to a meal. They have a more rapid onset and shorter duration than sulfonylureas.

   a. Should not be taken when a meal is skipped or missed.

   b. Should be used cautiously in patients with renal and hepatic dysfunction and may cause hypoglycemia.

8. Dipeptidyl peptidase 4 inhibitors (DPP-4i) (sitagliptin, linagliptin, saxagliptin, alogliptin) inhibit the breakdown of glucagon-like peptide-1 (GLP-1). GLP-1 stimulates insulin release from the pancreas and decreases glucagon secretion, which inhibits glycogenolysis and gluconeogenesis. These agents are most effective at controlling postprandial blood glucose and, when used alone or in combination with metformin or TZD, do not cause hypoglycemia.

   a. Dose is based on renal function.

   b. Generally well tolerated and weight-neutral. Adverse reactions include upper respiratory infections, nasopharyngitis, and headaches.

   c. Can be combined with all other diabetes medication except for those in the GLP-1 RA class.

 NURSING ALERT Patients with a history of pancreatitis should not be prescribed either DPP4-i or GLP-1 RA.

9. Sodium glucose cotransporter 2 inhibitors (SGLT2i) (canagliflozin, empagliflozin, dapagliflozin, ertugliflozin) block glucose absorption in the proximal renal tubule by inhibiting SGLT2 receptors. Glucose is excreted in the urine, which leads to modest weight loss and some improvement in systolic blood pressure.

   a. Dose is based on renal function.

   b. These have been known to cause ketoacidosis in the absence of significant glucose elevations (euglycemic diabetic ketoacidosis), especially in patients who are ill, suffer trauma, or require surgery. These should be stopped and resumed only when patient is stable. Patients should be advised to stop these medications and seek medical assistance immediately if they experience any symptoms consistent with DKA (nausea/vomiting, abdominal pain).

   c. Adverse reactions include urinary tract infections (cystitis and mycotic infection of the genital tract) in both men and women.

10. Bile acid sequestrant (colesevelam) is traditionally a cholesterol-lowering agent that has now been indicated for the treatment of T2DM. The exact mechanism of action is unclear but may have effect on sensitizing the liver to insulin, reducing hepatic glucose production. May also work by reducing intestinal absorption of glucose.

   a. Side effects include nausea, bloating, and constipation.

 DRUG ALERT Bile acid sequestrant cause triglyceride levels to rise and therefore should not be used in patients with baseline elevation of triglyceride levels.

11. Dopamine agonist (bromocriptine) is another agent in which the mechanism of action is unclear and its role in diabetes management ill defined. It is believed it acts to reduce glucose levels by reducing the effects of insulin resistance on the central nervous system.

   a. Side effects include hypotension and syncope, especially with dose titrations. Proceed slowly and cautiously, especially in older patients.

12. GLP-1 receptor agonists (GLP-1 RA) (exenatide, liraglutide, exenatide long-acting, albiglutide, dulaglutide, lixisenatide, semaglutide) work to lower blood glucose by enhancing first-phase insulin secretion by the pancreas, slowing gastric emptying, suppressing glucagon secretion, and reducing appetite, which can facilitate weight loss.

   a. Exenatide is injected twice daily within 1 to 60 minutes before breakfast and dinner.

   b. Liraglutide is injected once daily without regard to meals.

   c. Lixisenatide is also injected once daily but recommended before breakfast.

   d. Exanatide long-acting, albiglutide, dulaglutide and semaglutide are all injected once-weekly. They differ in the preparation involved prior to administration. These tend to be better tolerated than the agents requiring more frequent administration.

   e. These are used as add-on therapy to all other diabetes medication with the exception of DPP-4; all but long-acting exenatide are approved for use with insulin. Please refer to full prescribing information available with each product. They are not to be used as a substitute for insulin.

   f. Most common adverse effects are nausea and vomiting. Other adverse reactions include GI upset, headache, and pancreatitis.

   g. All are available in a disposable pen device.

h. Lixisenatide and liraglutide are each available as daily fixed ratio combination therapies with long-acting insulin (lixisenatide plus insulin glargine; liraglutide plus insulin degludec).

DRUG ALERT GLP-1 RA can cause hypoglycemia when used with sulfonylureas or insulin. They should not be used in patients with severe GI disorders, such as gastroparesis, and used cautiously when renal impairment is present. They have also been associated with medullary thyroid cancer in rodents.

13. Amylin analog (pramlintide). Amylin is cosecreted by the B cells of the pancreas to assist with postprandial glucose control. Its actions are like GLP-1 incretin mimetics (reduced gastric emptying, suppression of glucagon, increased satiety, and weight loss). It is indicated for patients with either type 1 or type 2 diabetes who require a mealtime insulin bolus.

a. It is not a substitute for insulin but must be administered immediately prior to meals that must consist of at least 250 kcal or at least 30 g of carbohydrates.

b. If used with insulin, mealtime dose of insulin must be reduced by 50%. Pramlintide cannot be mixed with insulin and must be injected at least 1 inch (2.5 cm) away from insulin injection site.

c. It is contraindicated in patients with confirmed gastroparesis and should be used with caution in patients who require the use of drugs to stimulate gastric motility.

d. The most common adverse effects are GI related (nausea/vomiting). It is available in a disposable pen device.

DRUG ALERT Pramlintide may cause severe insulin-induced hypoglycemia and is contraindicated in patients with hypoglycemia unawareness.

General Health

In addition to the glycemic and A1C goals discussed previously, prevention and management guidelines have been established for blood pressure (BP), lipid values, and kidney function to prevent complications. Patients with diabetes are at a much higher risk for cardiovascular disease than the general population; therefore, cardiovascular risk factors must be monitored and aggressively treated. Several authoritative groups recommend the following goals of treatment for nonpregnant adults, adolescents, and children with diabetes mellitus.

EVIDENCE BASE AACE/ACE. (2018). Consensus statement by the AACE and ACE on the comprehensive type 2 diabetes management algorithm—2018 Executive Summary, *Endocrine Practice*, 24(1), 91–120.

Adults:
1. BP < 140/90 mm Hg (all ages) (ADA); <130/80 mm Hg (AACE/ACE; Whelton, et al.); pregnant women: 120 to 160/80 to105 mm Hg
   a. Measure at every visit; goal may be individualized.
2. Lipid control (all ages)
   a. Low-density lipoprotein less than 100 mg/dL.
   b. High-density lipoprotein greater than 40 mg/dL; greater than 50 mg/dL women.
   c. Triglycerides less than 150 mg/dL.

d. Diabetes is considered an independent risk factor for cardiovascular disease; therefore, according to the ACA/AHA guidelines, all patients with diabetes between the ages of 45 and 75 years should be prescribed a moderate-intensity statin (without regard to the above parameters). More aggressive treatment is recommended if additional cardiovascular risk factors are present. Use careful consideration of benefit/risk ratio when prescribing statin therapy in adults younger than 45 and older than 75 years of age.

e. Statins are contraindicated during pregnancy; use with extreme caution in all women of child-bearing age.

3. Microalbumin (spot urine) less than 30 mg/g creatinine (monitor at least annually).

4. Aspirin (75 to 162 mg/day) for most men and women ≥50 years with at least one additional major cardiovascular risk factor.

Children and adolescents:
1. BP below the 90th percentile for sex, age, and height.
2. Lipid control:
   a. Low-density lipoprotein less than 100 mg/dL. Statin may be required if LDL greater than 160 despite lifestyle modifications

Complications

Acute

1. Hypoglycemia (blood glucose ≤70 mg/dL) occurs because of an imbalance in food, activity, and insulin/oral antidiabetic agent. Blood glucose less than 54 mg/dL is considered serious, clinically important hypoglycemia.
2. Diabetic ketoacidosis (DKA) occurs primarily in type 1 diabetes during times of severe insulin deficiency or illness, producing severe hyperglycemia, ketonuria, dehydration, and acidosis (see page 748).
3. Hyperosmolar hyperglycemic state (HHS) primarily affects patients with type 2 diabetes, causing severe dehydration, hyperglycemia, hyperosmolarity, and stupor (see page 749).

Chronic

See Table 25-4.
1. In type 1 diabetes, chronic complications usually appear about 5 years after the initial diagnosis.
2. The prevalence of microvascular complications (retinopathy, nephropathy, and neuropathy) is higher in type 1 diabetes.
3. Because of its insidious onset, chronic complications can appear at any point in type 2 diabetes. Approximately 50% will have at least one complication at time of diagnosis.
4. Macrovascular complications (ie, cardiovascular disease)—occurring in type 1 and type 2 diabetes—are the leading cause of morbidity and mortality among persons with diabetes.

Nursing Assessment

1. Obtain a history of current problems, family history, and general health history.
   a. Has the patient experienced polyuria, polydipsia, polyphagia, and any other symptoms?
   b. Number of years since initial diagnosis of diabetes.
   c. Family members diagnosed with diabetes, their subsequent treatment, and complications.

text continues on page 744

Table 25-4   Chronic Complications of Diabetes Mellitus

CONDITION	ASSESSMENT
Macrovascular Complications	
Cerebrovascular Disease	
• *Incidence*: Two to four times more likely in diabetes. • Hypertension, increased lipids, smoking, uncontrolled blood glucose, increase risk of stroke and transient ischemic attack	• Increased BP • Change in mental status • Hemiparesis • Aphasia • Clinical presentation mimics that of nondiabetic patient.
Coronary Artery Disease	
• *Incidence*: Increased vessel disease with more vessels affected in diabetes. Higher incidence of "silent" myocardial infarctions (MIs). • Hyperglycemia contributes to atherosclerosis and vessel deterioration.	• Severe CAD is commonly asymptomatic, seen only in ECG changes. ECG changes may indicate silent MI. • Symptoms can also present as pain in the jaw, neck, or epigastric area.
Peripheral Vascular Disease	
• *Incidence*: 60% of nontraumatic amputations are related to diabetes. • Intermittent claudication, absent pedal pulses, and ischemic gangrene are increased in diabetes.	• Physical examination of the lower extremities may reveal changes in skin integrity associated with diminished circulation. • Decreased lower leg hair, absent or decreased anterior tibial or dorsal pedis pulses, poor capillary refill of toenails may occur. The extremity may appear pale/cool. Further examination for neurologic changes is indicated.
Microvascular Complications	
Retinopathy	
• *Incidence*: Type 1—Will develop after 3–5 yr of diagnosis and by 15–20 yr of diabetes duration. Almost all patients will have some degree of retinopathy. Type 2—Approximately 7% present with retinopathy at diagnosis, which increases to 50%–80% after 20 yr. DM is the leading cause of preventable blindness in the United States. • Appearance of hard exudates, blot hemorrhages, and microaneurysms on the retina in background retinopathy. Progresses to neovascularization in proliferative diabetic retinopathy.	• Usually asymptomatic in the early stages. Symptoms occurring with acute visual problems—"floaters," flashing lights, blurred vision—may indicate hemorrhage or retinal detachment. Funduscopic examination should be done by an ophthalmologist for full retinal visualization.
Nephropathy	
• *Incidence*: Type 1—20% to 30% will have renal impairment after 15-yr duration of diabetes; 4%–17% will progress to end-stage renal disease (ESRD) after 20 yr. Type 2—25% will have at least mild renal impairment and another 5% will have ESRD after 10 yr of diabetes duration. The incidence is higher in Native Americans, Hispanics, and blacks. DM is the leading cause of kidney failure in the United States. • Thickening of the glomerular basement membrane, mesangial expansion, and renal vessel sclerosis are caused by diabetes. • Subsequently, diffuse and nodular intercapillary glomerulosclerosis diminishes renal function.	• Evidence of increased glomerular filtration rate. • Microalbuminuria is the first clinical sign of renal disease. • Elevation in blood urea nitrogen and creatinine levels indicates advanced renal disease. • Gross proteinuria is a further indication of renal deterioration.
Peripheral Neuropathy	
• In general, neuropathy affects 60%–70% of persons with diabetes, with nearly 50% asymptomatic. • It can affect almost every organ system with varying specific symptoms. • Distal symmetrical polyneuropathy involving the lower extremities is most commonly seen. • In conjunction with peripheral vascular disease, neuropathy to the feet increases susceptibility to trauma and infection. The more severe forms of peripheral neuropathy are a major contributing cause of lower extremity amputations. • Three clinical syndromes of distal symmetrical polyneuropathy are seen: acute painful, small-fiber, and large-fiber neuropathy.	• Decreased light touch, vibratory, temperature sensation. Loss of foot proprioception, followed by ataxia, gait disturbances. • Diminished ankle jerk response. • Formation of "hammertoes," Charcot joint disease, which predispose patient to new pressure point areas. • Hypersensitivity or other dysesthetic symptoms are experienced, followed by hypnoanesthesia or anesthesia, which is not reversible.

INTERVENTION	PREVENTION/TEACHING
• Check blood glucose level to differentiate signs and symptoms of stroke versus hypoglycemia. Monitor for bleeding if aspirin or other antiplatelet/anticoagulant medication is used.	• Maintain target goals of blood glucose, avoiding severe hypoglycemia and hyperglycemia, which predispose the patient to stroke. In hypoglycemia, increased levels of adrenalin and catecholamines can produce cardiac arrhythmias. • Hyperglycemia can lead to dehydration, which affects platelet aggregation.
• Usual medical treatment for angina prevails—sublingual nitroglycerin, oral nitrates. Beta-adrenergic blockers and calcium channel blockers can also be used.	• Emphasis must be placed on reducing cardiac risk factors (eg, cigarette smoking, hypertension, hyperlipidemia). Avoid wide fluctuations in blood glucose. Patients with autonomic neuropathy, which can cause orthostatic hypotension, should be carefully monitored when cardiac drug therapies are introduced. Beta-adrenergic blockers can blunt or eliminate the clinical signs and symptoms of hypoglycemia.
• Any lesion, decrease in peripheral pulses, or change in skin color, temperature, or sensation should be evaluated within 24–48 hr. To ensure proper healing and prevent infection, treatment should begin as soon as possible and be carefully monitored. Mild antiseptics/antibiotic preparations are used to avoid further damage to the surrounding skin. Avoid the use of surgical tape to skin. Rest affected leg to promote circulation and wound healing.	• Foot care guidelines and smoking cessation must be stressed. Safe exercise guidelines and weight reduction, as appropriate, will further reduce risk of foot injury.
• Laser therapy (photocoagulation) can be helpful in macular edema (focal laser) and proliferative retinopathy (panretinal laser). Reduction of active neovascularization by laser therapy reduces the risk of vitreous hemorrhage. Vitrectomy may be needed to treat retinal detachment or remove vitreous hemorrhage. • During the acute phase, before laser therapy, patients must avoid activities that increase the chances of vitreous hemorrhage (eg, weight lifting, high-impact aerobics).	• Stress importance of annual eye examination with an ophthalmologist (preferably retina specialist). Optimal glucose control can prevent or slow the progression of retinopathy. Maintaining normal BP also reduces the risk of retinopathy.
• Hypertension control, blood glucose control, and reduction of protein and sodium are essential. Angiotensin-converting enzyme inhibitors are the drugs of choice to control BP. Calcium channel blockers may also be used. In end-stage renal disease, dialysis or transplantation may be necessary.	• Frequent hypertension screening, noting any deviation from patient's normal reading. Early initiation of BP control to prevent kidney damage. Excellent glucose control with insulin/oral agent adjustment to compensate for reduced kidney function, which predisposes the patient to hypoglycemia. Avoidance of nephrotoxic drugs, dyes, or renal procedures that may cause infection. Immediate treatment for any urinary tract infections.
• All foot wounds or injuries are immediately evaluated. Culture and sensitivity tests ordered for any drainage present. Affected foot is elevated—avoid weightbearing. Wet-to-dry dressings applied as ordered. Avoid use of caustic chemicals, dressing tapes. • Use of systemic antibiotics, as needed. • Medication for painful neuropathy may include use of the tricyclic antidepressant drugs (amitriptyline), a serotonin and epinephrine reuptake inhibitor (duloxetine), or topical application of capsaicin ointment.	• In general, blood glucose control is recommended, avoiding wide fluctuations. In patients who are poorly controlled, care must be taken to correct glucoses slowly to avoid increasing symptoms of neuropathy. • Foot care guidelines. • Smoking cessation. • Frequent evaluation by podiatrist for modified footwear (eg, orthotics, extra-depth shoes). • Safe exercise guidelines. • Weight reduction, as necessary.

(continued)

Table 25-4   Chronic Complications of Diabetes Mellitus (*Continued*)

CONDITION	ASSESSMENT
Autonomic Neuropathy	
Cardiac Autonomic Neuropathy • Affects 30% of patients with T1DM after 20 yr and 60% of patients with T2DM after 15 yr. • Asymptomatic in early stages. Loss of heart rate variability detected on ECG. • Late stages: resting tachycardia, orthostatic hypotension, exercise intolerance. • >3-fold mortality; 38% "silent" MI	• Patients may report episodes of syncope, weakness, or visual impairment, particularly with positional changes. Evaluate BP and pulse in lying and standing position at each visit. BP changes that indicate neuropathic involvement: fall in systolic pressure of >30 mm Hg or fall in diastolic pressure of >10 mm Hg with change from lying to standing position.
Gastroparesis • *Incidence*: Occurs in 50% of people with long-standing diabetes. • *Characteristics*: Delayed gastric emptying, prolonged pylorospasms, and loss of the powerful contractions of the distal stomach to grind and mix foods.	• Typical symptoms may include nausea/vomiting, early satiety, abdominal bloating, epigastric pain, change in appetite. Wide fluctuations in blood glucoses and postmeal hypoglycemia caused by poor glucose absorption. Visualization of the gut by upper GI barium series may show retained food after an 8- to 12-hr fast.
Diarrhea • *Incidence*: Approximately 20% of patients with diabetes. • *Characteristics*: Frequent, watery movements. • Mild steatorrhea. • Can be intermittent, persistent, or alternate with constipation.	• Diarrhea occurs without warning, frequently at night or after meals. Fecal incontinence may be caused by loss of internal sphincter control and anorectal sensation. Other causes, such as celiac sprue, pancreatic insufficiency, and lactose intolerance, must be investigated. Bacterial overgrowth in the bowel is also suspected.
Sexual Dysfunction • Affects 35%–75% men and 46% women with diabetes. • Sexual dysfunction in both men and women can involve changes in libido, ability to achieve orgasm, and sexual satisfaction.	• *Men*: History of poor erectile function despite stimulation. Absence of early-morning erection in response to increased hormonal levels. • *Women*: May experience decreased vaginal lubrication and dyspareunia. • Screening for use of ethanol or other medications associated with impotence (eg, antidepressants, antihypertensives).
Bladder Dysfunction • *Incidence*: Affects 37%–50% of people with diabetes, W > M. • Inability to sense a full bladder, incomplete void/overflow incontinence. Increased frequency of UTI and pyelonephritis leading to or exacerbating renal failure.	• Overflow incontinence is common problem for women. Inquire about use of pads in undergarments, which may be clue. • Distended bladder • Burning/pain with voiding; straining to empty bladder. Nocturia.
Hypoglycemia Unawareness • *Incidence*: Severe hypoglycemia occurs most frequently in patients with T1DM (30%–40% annual prevalence); however, it will also occur in patients with T2DM who are treated with insulin, sulfonylureas, and/or glinides. • Occurs in ~17% of type 1 diabetic patients and at a rate of two to three times more frequently than those with T2DM. • Condition in which the usual warning signs of hypoglycemia are no longer experienced. The symptoms may be different (and therefore not recognized), less pronounced, or even absent. • Can eventually lead to hypoglycemia-associated autonomic failure, which includes both hypoglycemia unawareness and defective glucose counterregulatory hormones.	• Patients may exhibit irrational thought; unprovoked anger or irritability; insisting that they "feel fine" in the midst of very unusual behavior; inappropriate laughing/silliness/giddiness/crying.

INTERVENTION	PREVENTION/TEACHING
• Improvement in blood glucose control to prevent fluid loss from glycosuria. Moderate amounts of sodium may be used in the diet to encourage fluid retention during hot weather or strenuous exercise. Mechanical devices such as support stockings (full hose to waist) may decrease venous pooling. Drugs to enhance volume expansion may be used (eg, fludrocortisone).	• Encourage increased fluid intake to maintain hydration. • Caution should be used in changing position from lying to standing. Sitting on side of bed with feet dangling is recommended until BP stabilizes. • Avoid standing in one position, which may increase venous pooling. • Observe exercise programs.
• Excellent glucose control to avoid hyperglycemia, which interferes with gut contractility. Avoidance of severe postmeal hypoglycemia by small, frequent meals, low fat, and low fiber. This diet is also helpful in bloating/early satiety. Medication to improve gut motility is metoclopramide.	• Maintenance of excellent glucose control. Regular exercise improves/maintains GI motility. Avoid use of laxatives. Small, frequent meals may help.
• Dietary changes may include increased fiber, elimination of milk products. Sphincter-strengthening exercises may help. Medications: For diarrhea, hydrophilic fiber supplement, cholestyramine, or synthetic opiates are used. • Tetracycline and ampicillin are used for bacterial overgrowth.	• Routine bowel elimination habits. • Maintenance of adequate hydration. • Excellent blood glucose control reduces dehydration. • Inclusion of dietary fiber in the daily diet. • Daily exercise program that includes walking or swimming has been effective in encouraging bowel regularity.
• *Men*: Referral to urologist for full examination is indicated. Treatment options may include injection of alprostadil (a prostaglandin), inflatable penile prosthesis, or oral medications. • *Women*: Increase lubrication with use of water-based lubricant or estrogen creams, which may also help thicken the vaginal mucosa, affecting dyspareunia.	• Reduce consumption of alcohol, which may hasten or contribute to neuropathy. • Maintain target ranges of blood glucose control to reduce likelihood of vaginal infections. • Discuss alternative ways of maintaining intimacy.
• Crede maneuver every 4 hr • Bethanechol (10–30 mg three times daily) • Doxazosin • Intermittent self-catheterization	• Avoid caloric beverages, which lead to significant hyperglycemia and glucosuria. • Avoid caffeine and other bladder irritants (nicotine). • Establish a scheduled routine for attempting to empty bladder to avoid overflow incontinence
• Can be reversed by avoiding frequent low blood sugars. Raising target blood sugar (ie, 140 mg/dL) by easing up on aggressive/intensive insulin treatment for a few weeks will allow the counterregulatory hormone response to return to normal.	• Increase frequency of blood glucose monitoring and stay alert to physical warning signs for 48 hr following low blood sugar. Keeping a glucose log will help patients predict when lows are more likely to occur. An occasional 2:00 A.M. blood glucose test can help with identifying unrecognized nocturnal hypoglycemia.

(continued)

Table 25-4 Chronic Complications of Diabetes Mellitus (*Continued*)

CONDITION	ASSESSMENT
Hypoglycemia Unawareness (*Continued*)	
• *Causes*: Long-standing diabetes, reduced glucagon excretion, frequent low blood sugars, alcohol consumption within the previous 12 hr, previous low blood sugar within the last 24–48 hr, certain medications (ie, beta-adrenergic blockers) • Women more susceptible because of reduced counterregulatory response and reduced symptoms. • More likely to occur in patients with other types of autonomic neuropathy.	• Grand mal seizures can occur if hypoglycemia is not recognized and treated.

BP, blood pressure; CAD, coronary artery disease; ECG, electrocardiography.

2. Perform a review of systems and physical examination to assess for signs and symptoms of diabetes, general health of patient, and presence of complications.
   a. General: recent weight loss or gain, increased fatigue, tiredness, anxiety.
   b. Skin: skin lesions, infections, dehydration, evidence of poor wound healing.
   c. Eyes: changes in vision—floaters, halos, blurred vision, dry or burning eyes, cataracts, glaucoma.
   d. Mouth: gingivitis, periodontal disease.
   e. Cardiovascular: orthostatic hypotension, cold extremities, weak pedal pulses, leg claudication.
   f. GI: diarrhea, constipation, early satiety, bloating, increased flatulence, hunger, or thirst.
   g. GU: increased urination, nocturia, impotence, vaginal discharge.
   h. Neurologic: numbness and tingling of the extremities, decreased pain and temperature perception, changes in gait and balance.

Nursing Diagnoses

• Imbalanced Nutrition: More than Body Requirements related to intake in excess of activity expenditures.
• Fear related to medication injection.
• Risk for Unstable Blood Glucose Level related to effects of insulin, inability to eat.
• Activity Intolerance related to poor glucose control.
• Deficient Knowledge related to use of oral hypoglycemic agents and injectable agents.
• Risk for Impaired Skin Integrity related to decreased sensation and circulation to lower extremities.
• Readiness for Enhanced Self-Health Management related to shared goal of avoiding readmission.

Nursing Interventions

See Standards of Care Guidelines 25-1.

Improving Nutrition
1. Assess current timing and content of meals.
2. Advise patient on the importance of an individualized meal plan in meeting weight-loss goals. Reducing intake of carbohydrates may benefit some patients; however, fad diets or diet plans that stress one food group and eliminate another are generally not recommended.

STANDARDS OF CARE GUIDELINES 25-1
Caring for Patients with Diabetes Mellitus

When caring for patients with diabetes mellitus:
• Assess level of knowledge of disease and ability to care for self.
• Assess adherence to diet therapy, monitoring procedures, medication treatment, and exercise regimen.
• Assess resources/support system available to patient; involve behavioral health, social work services, and case management as needed.
• Assess for signs of hyperglycemia: polyuria, polydipsia, polyphagia, weight loss, fatigue, blurred vision.
• Assess for signs of hypoglycemia: sweating, tremor, nervousness, tachycardia, light-headedness, confusion.
• Perform thorough skin and extremity assessment for peripheral neuropathy or peripheral vascular disease and any injury to the feet or lower extremities.
• Assess for trends in blood glucose and other laboratory results.
• Reinforce appropriate insulin dosage is given at the right time and in relation to meals and exercise.
• Assess adequate knowledge of diet, exercise, and medication treatment and cognitive skills to safely adhere to prescribed regimen.
• Immediately report to health care provider any signs of skin or soft tissue infection (redness, swelling, warmth, tenderness, drainage).
• Get help immediately for signs of hypoglycemia that do not respond to usual glucose replacement.
• Get help immediately for patient presenting with signs of either ketoacidosis (nausea and vomiting, Kussmaul respirations, fruity breath odor, hypotension, and altered level of consciousness) or hyperosmolar hyperglycemic nonketotic syndrome (nausea and vomiting, hypothermia, muscle weakness, seizures, stupor, coma).

This information should serve as a general guideline only. Each patient situation presents a unique set of clinical factors and requires nursing judgment to guide care, which may include additional or alternative measures and approaches.

INTERVENTION	PREVENTION/TEACHING
• Injected glucagon is the best treatment when the patient resists treatment, becomes unconscious, or has seizures because of hypoglycemia.	• Carry glucose tablets/gel at all times to quickly and appropriately raise blood sugar levels. • All patients using intensive insulin management should have glucagon emergency kits and their family members must know how and when to administer. • Patients will need to closely match insulin doses to diet and exercise. They may need to reduce their insulin doses during and for several hours following increased physical activity. • Avoid alcohol or limit to no more than 1 to 2 drinks per day and never drink on an empty stomach. • Patients should wear a MedicAlert ID at all times to facilitate appropriate treatment by emergency personnel.

3. Discuss the goals of dietary therapy for the patient. Setting a goal of greater than 5% weight loss over several months is usually achievable and effective in reducing blood sugar and other metabolic parameters.
4. Assist patient to identify problems that may have an impact on dietary adherence and possible solutions to these problems. Emphasize that lifestyle changes should be maintainable for life.
5. Explain the importance of exercise in maintaining/reducing body weight.
   a. Caloric expenditure for energy in exercise.
   b. Carryover of enhanced metabolic rate and efficient food utilization.
6. Assist patient to establish goals for weekly weight loss and incentives to assist in achieving them.
7. Strategize with patient to address the potential social pitfalls of weight reduction.

Teaching About Insulin

1. Assist patient to reduce fear of injection by encouraging verbalization of fears regarding insulin injection, conveying a sense of empathy, and identifying supportive coping techniques.
2. Demonstrate and explain thoroughly the procedure for insulin self-injection.
3. Help patient to master technique by taking a step-by-step approach.
   a. Allow patient time to handle insulin and syringe/pen to become familiar with the equipment.
   b. Teach self-injection first to alleviate fear of pain from injection.
   c. Instruct patient in filling syringe when he or she expresses confidence in self-injection procedure.
4. Review dosage and time of injections in relation to meals, activity, and bedtime based on patient's individualized insulin regimen.

 GERONTOLOGIC ALERT Assess older patients for sensory deficits; such as impaired vision, hearing, fine touch, and tremors that may have an impact on learning and ability to self-administer insulin. Suggest use of an insulin pen or magnifying glass to assist with drawing up insulin. Pen must be inverted 10 times to ensure mixing.

Preventing Injury Secondary to Hypoglycemia

1. Closely monitor blood glucose levels to detect hypoglycemia (blood glucose ≤70 mg/dL).
2. Instruct patient in the importance of accuracy in insulin preparation, administration, and meal timing to avoid hypoglycemia.
3. Assess patient for the signs and symptoms of hypoglycemia.
   a. Adrenergic (early symptoms)—sweating, tremor, pallor, tachycardia, palpitations, nervousness from the release of adrenalin when blood glucose falls rapidly.
   b. Neurologic (later symptoms)—light-headedness, headache, confusion, irritability, slurred speech, lack of coordination, staggering gait from depression of central nervous system as glucose level progressively falls.
4. Treat hypoglycemia promptly using the 15-g/15-minute rule according to the ADA with 15-g of rapidly absorbed carbohydrates.
   a. One-half cup (4 oz.) juice, 1 cup skim milk, 4 glucose tablets, 1 tablespoon of sugar/honey, or five to six pieces of hard candy may be taken orally.
   b. Wait 15 minutes.
   c. Repeat blood glucose; if less than 70 mg/dL, repeat the treatment.
   d. If greater than 70 mg/dL and more than 3 hours since last dose of rapid-acting insulin, no further treatment required.
   e. If greater than 70 mg/dL but less than 3 hours since last dose of rapid-acting insulin, follow with a snack of 75 to 100 calories.
   f. If using a "split-mix" or REG/NPH insulins and more than 30 minutes before next planned meal/snack, have meal/snack now.
   g. Nutrition bar specially designed for diabetics—supplies glucose from sucrose, starch, and protein sources with some fat to delay gastric emptying and prolong effect; may prevent relapse. Used after hypoglycemia treated with fast-acting carbohydrate.
   h. Glucagon 1 mg (SubQ or IM) is given if the patient cannot safely ingest a treatment. Family member or staff must administer injection.
   i. IV bolus of 50 mL of 50% dextrose solution can be given if the patient fails to respond to glucagon within 15 minutes.
5. Encourage patient to carry a portable treatment for hypoglycemia at all times.

6. Assess patient for cognitive or physical impairments that may interfere with ability to accurately administer insulin.
7. Between-meal snacks as well as extra food taken before exercise should be encouraged to prevent hypoglycemia.
8. Encourage patients to wear an identification bracelet or card that may assist in prompt treatment in a hypoglycemic emergency.
   a. Identification bracelet can be obtained from MedicAlert Foundation International (*www.medicalert.org*).
   b. Identification card may be requested from the ADA (*www.diabetes.org*).
9. If hypoglycemia occurs frequently, please discuss with health care provider. Dose adjustments of insulin and/or oral medications may be necessary.
10. Address safety issues if patient has hypoglycemic attacks—driving, operating machinery, and exertional activity. Cognitive recovery takes 45 to 75 minutes following blood glucose levels of less than 50 mg/dL.

 DRUG ALERT If the patient is taking an alpha glucosidase inhibitor, he or she must use a monosaccharide (glucose tablets) to treat hypoglycemia because sucrose will not be broken down to an absorbable sugar.

Improving Activity Tolerance

1. Advise patient to assess blood glucose level before and after strenuous exercise.
2. Instruct patient to plan exercises on a regular basis each day.
3. Encourage patient to eat a carbohydrate snack before exercising to avoid hypoglycemia.
4. Advise patient that prolonged strenuous exercise may require increased food at bedtime to avoid nocturnal hypoglycemia.
5. Instruct patient to avoid exercise whenever blood glucose levels exceed 250 mg/day and urine ketones are present. Patient should contact health care provider if levels remain elevated.

6. Counsel patient to inject insulin into the abdominal site on days when arms or legs are exercised.

Providing Information About Noninsulin Agents

1. Identify barriers to learning, such as visual or hearing impairments, low literacy, and distractive environment.
2. Encourage active participation of the patient and family in the educational process.
3. Teach the action, use, and adverse effects of noninsulin agents (see pages 735 to 739).
4. Identify financial barriers to accessing medications and follow-up care. Offer resources such as Partnership for Prescription Assistance (*www.PPARx.org*).

Maintaining Skin Integrity

1. Assess feet and legs for skin temperature, sensation, soft tissue injuries, corns, calluses, dryness, hammertoe or bunion deformation, hair distribution, pulses, deep tendon reflexes.
   a. Use a monofilament to test sensation of the feet and detect early signs of peripheral neuropathy (see Figure 25-2).
   b. Test vibratory sense over interphalangeal joints of the feet using a low-frequency (128 Hz) tuning fork. Vibratory sense is typically lost before tactile sensation. The test is considered abnormal if the vibratory sensation is felt for less than 10 seconds.
2. Protect skin from dryness and breakdown.
   a. Use heel protectors, special mattresses, and foot cradles for patients on bed rest.
   b. Avoid applying drying agents to skin (eg, alcohol).
   c. Apply skin moisturizers (preferably creams) to maintain suppleness and prevent cracking and fissures.
3. Instruct patient in foot care.
4. Advise the patient who smokes to stop smoking, or reduce if possible to reduce vasoconstriction and enhance peripheral blood flow. Help patient to establish behavior modification techniques to eliminate smoking in the hospital and to continue them at home for smoking cessation program.

Figure 25-2. The Semmes-Weinstein 5.07 (10-g) monofilament test. (From Cameron, B. L. [2002]. Making diabetes management routine. *American Journal of Nursing, 102*[2], 27.)

Focusing on Transitional Care

Some strategies that nursing staff can employ to facilitate safer transition out of the hospital and reduce the chance for readmission are:

1. Promote diabetes education at the bedside. This should start as early as possible during the inpatient stay, as soon as the patient is able to participate.
   a. Use routine blood glucose monitoring, insulin administration, and meal selection as teaching moments—allow the patient to actively participate in these activities.
   b. Provide clear instructions and printed materials.
   c. Assess patient technique for insulin administration and glucose testing.
2. Ensure patients are being discharged with all medications with correct dose and adequate supplies.
   a. Insulin pens must have pen needles ordered.
   b. Make certain that the glucose test strips are compatible with the patient's glucose meter.
   c. Assess patient understanding of all medications prescribed, including timing with meals.
   d. Ensure that all chronic medications were not inadvertently stopped; all changes in medications must be made very clear to patient to prevent medication errors.
3. Ensure a 7-day follow-up appointment with the patient's primary care or specialist provider is scheduled prior to discharge and that the patient has a secured means of transportation.
4. Provide patient with written discharge summary and instructions with symptoms to report and phone number to call.
5. Establish a transitional care team who can provide 3-day postdischarge follow-up phone call and coordination with home health care professionals.

TRANSITIONAL CARE ALERT People with diabetes are involved in almost 22% of all inpatient hospitalizations, and 13% will have diabetes as the primary reason for admission. Unfortunately, the 30-day readmission rates can be as high as 21% for patients with diabetes mellitus. The risk increases based on comorbidities, if admitted via emergency department, low socioeconomic status, and/or lack of health insurance. Discharge planning must begin upon admission and updated as the patient's needs change or are more clearly understood. A1c levels should be obtained on all patients known to have diabetes—even if diabetes was not the primary reason for hospitalization. Patients with an A1c greater than 9% upon admission are very high risk for poor outcomes and readmission.

Community and Home Care Considerations

1. A home care or visiting nurse referral can be initiated to follow up on patient education initiated in the hospital or clinic and ensure that the patient has the resources to care for self at home.
2. Patient should be checking fingerstick glucose at home, and glucometer should be checked by home care or clinic nurse periodically to make sure it is properly calibrated and correlates with meter used at clinic or hospital.
3. As long as the home is clean and the patient uses reasonable hygiene, procedures for glucose self-monitoring and insulin injection do not need to be sterile. No alcohol preparation of the skin or insulin vial is needed.

4. Assist patients with choosing the diabetes self-care products and devices that best meet their needs/circumstances. An annual update is available at *www.forecast.diabetes.org/consumerguide*.
5. Insulin syringes may be reused, so long as the needle is kept clean and no pain or signs of skin irritation develop after multiple uses.
6. Insulin pens should be used when possible.
7. Although urine glucose testing is no longer used to monitor diabetes control, the patient may benefit from urine ketone testing, especially when ill. Teach the patient how to test urine with ketone test strip and to notify health care provider if ketosis persists.
8. Make sure that all patients have a handy source of glucose for hypoglycemic episodes. A small tube of glossy decorating gel for cakes or 3 sugar packets, easily carried in a pocket or purse, contains about 15 g glucose and can be used to treat hypoglycemia.
9. Draw blood for analysis or ensure that patients attend laboratory appointments.
   a. For patients taking a thiazolidinedione, baseline serum transaminases (aspartate aminotransferase and alanine aminotransferase) should be obtained prior to initiation and repeated anytime the patient is suspected of liver injury (fatigue, anorexia, RUQ pain, dark urine).
   b. Renal function tests (serum creatinine and estimated glomerular filtration rate) and urine for microalbuminuria or microalbumin/creatinine ratio will be monitored at least yearly.
   c. Glycated hemoglobin is followed every 3 to 6 months and does not require fasting.
   d. Fasting lipid panel (12 to 14 hours fasting) is done at least annually.

Patient Education and Health Maintenance

1. Ongoing education of patient to include advanced skills and rationales for treatment, prevention, and management of complications.
2. Educational focus—lifestyle management issues, to include sick day management.
3. For additional information and support, refer to drug manufacturers' Web sites for special programs for people with diabetes and to agencies, such as ADA (*www.diabetes.org*) and American Dietetic Association (*www.eatright.org*). Travel recommendations can be found at *www.joslin.org/info/diabetes_and_travel_10_tips_for_a_safe_trip.html*.

Evaluation: Expected Outcomes

- Maintains appropriate weight with minimal to no gain.
- Demonstrates correct technique for self-injection of insulin.
- Signs and symptoms of hypoglycemia identified and treated appropriately.
- Exercises daily.
- Verbalizes appropriate use and action of noninsulin agents.
- No skin breakdown.
- Patient verbalizes understanding of discharge instructions and has medications and injection supplies before leaving hospital.

PATIENT EDUCATION GUIDELINES 25-1

Diabetes Sick-Day Guidelines

- Never omit insulin dosage. Check with health care provider about noninsulin medication. For instance, metformin, GLP-1 RA, and SGLT2i should be withheld if vomiting or in danger of becoming dehydrated.
    - Take at least the usual dosage of insulin.
    - Keep regular insulin on hand for supplemental doses, as prescribed by health care provider.
- Monitor blood glucose and urine ketones every 2 to 4 hours.
    - Whenever blood glucose is greater than 240 mg/dL, test urine ketones.
    - Record all test results.
- Drink plenty of fluids.
    - Six to eight ounce of fluid every hour is recommended; every 3rd hour, the fluid should include sodium (i.e., broth).

- If unable to eat, drink fluids that contain carbohydrates (e.g., fruit juices, regular soda); patient must consume 150 to 200 g of carbohydrates/day.
- Contact health care provider or report to nearest ER if illness becomes severe or unmanageable.
    - Fever, nausea, vomiting (greater than 1 episode), and diarrhea (greater than 5 episodes or for longer than 6 hours) increase risk of dehydration.
    - Signs and symptoms of infection—redness, swelling, drainage—need immediate attention.
- Large amount of urine ketones or other signs and symptoms of diabetic ketoacidosis: call health care provider immediately.

Diabetic Ketoacidosis

 EVIDENCE BASE Gosmanov, A. R., Gosmonova, E. O., & Kitabchi, A. E. (2015). Hyperglycemic crises: Diabetic ketoacidosis (DKA) and hyperglycemic hyperosmolar state (HHS). In K. Dungan (Ed.), *Endotext*. Available: *www.endotext.org/chapter/diabetic-complications/hyperglycemic-crises-diabetic-ketoacidosis-dka-and-hyperglycemic*.

Wolfsdorf, J. I., Allgrove, J., Craig, M. E., Edge, J., et al. (2014). Diabetic ketoacidosis and hyperglycemic hyperosmolar state. *Pediatric Diabetes, 15*(Suppl. 20), 154–179.

Diabetic ketoacidosis (DKA) is an acute complication of diabetes mellitus (usually type 1 diabetes) characterized by hyperglycemia, ketonuria, acidosis, and dehydration. Underlying infection is the most common cause of this acute complication.

Pathophysiology and Etiology

1. Insulin deficiency prevents glucose from being used for energy, forcing the body to metabolize fat for fuel.
2. Free fatty acids, released from the metabolism of fat, are converted to ketone bodies in the liver.
3. Ketone bodies are organic acids that cause metabolic acidosis.
4. Increase in the secretion of glucagon, catecholamines, growth hormone, and cortisol, in response to the hyperglycemia caused by insulin deficiency, accelerates the development of DKA.
5. Osmotic diuresis caused by hyperglycemia creates a shift in electrolytes, with losses in potassium, sodium, phosphate, and water.
6. Caused by inadequate amounts of endogenous or exogenous insulin.
    a. Commonly occurs due to failure to increase the dose of insulin during periods of stress (eg, infection, surgery, pregnancy).
    b. May occur in previously undiagnosed or untreated diabetics.

Clinical Manifestations

Early

1. Polydipsia, polyuria.
2. Fatigue, malaise, drowsiness.
3. Anorexia, nausea, vomiting.
4. Abdominal pain, muscle cramps.

Later

1. Kussmaul respirations (deep respirations).
2. Fruity, sweet breath.
3. Hypotension, weak pulse.
4. Stupor and coma.

Diagnostic Evaluation

1. Serum glucose level is elevated over 250 mg/dL.
2. Serum and urine ketone bodies are present.
3. Serum bicarbonate and pH are decreased because of metabolic acidosis, and partial pressure of carbon dioxide is decreased as a respiratory compensation mechanism.
4. Serum sodium and potassium levels may be low, normal, or high because of fluid shifts and dehydration, despite total body depletion.
5. BUN, creatinine, hemoglobin, and hematocrit are elevated because of dehydration.
6. Urine glucose is present in high concentration and specific gravity is increased, reflecting osmotic diuresis and dehydration.

 NURSING ALERT Severity of DKA is not determined by serum glucose levels; the degree of acidosis determines severity of DKA.

Management

1. IV fluids to replace losses from osmotic diuresis, vomiting.
2. IV insulin drip to increase glucose utilization and decrease lipolysis. Only use insulin preparations approved for IV administration. Should not be started until serum potassium is greater than 3.3 mEq/L.
3. Electrolyte replacement—sodium chloride and phosphate as required and potassium chloride and bicarbonate based on laboratory results.

Complications

1. Premature discontinuation of IV insulin or the failure to initiate subcutaneous insulin injections prior to discontinuing IV insulin will result in rebound of DKA.
2. Too-rapid infusion of IV fluids in cases of severe dehydration can cause cerebral edema and death.

Nursing Assessment

1. Assess skin for dehydration—poor turgor, flushing, dry mucous membranes.
2. Observe for cardiac changes reflecting dehydration, metabolic acidosis, and electrolyte imbalance—hypotension; tachycardia; weak pulse; electrocardiographic changes, including elevated P wave, flattened T wave, or inverted, prolonged QT interval.
3. Assess respiratory status—Kussmaul respirations, acetone breath characteristic of metabolic acidosis.
4. Perform GI assessment—nausea, vomiting, extreme thirst, abdominal bloating and cramping, diarrhea.
5. Determine GU symptoms—nocturia, polyuria.
6. Observe for neurologic signs—crying, restlessness, twitching, tremors, drowsiness, lethargy, headache, decreased reflexes.
7. Interview family or significant other regarding precipitating events to episode of DKA.
   a. Patient self-care management before hospitalization.
   b. Unusual events that may have precipitated episode (eg, chest pain, trauma, illness).

Nursing Diagnoses

- Deficient Fluid Volume related to hyperglycemia.
- Ineffective Therapeutic Regimen Management related to failure to increase insulin during illness.

Nursing Interventions

Restoring Fluid and Electrolyte Balance

1. Assess BP and heart rate frequently, depending on patient's condition; assess skin turgor and temperature.
2. Monitor intake and output every hour.
3. Replace fluids, as ordered, through peripheral IV line.
4. Monitor urine specific gravity to assess fluid changes.
5. Monitor blood glucose frequently.
6. Assess for symptoms of hypokalemia—fatigue, anorexia, nausea, vomiting, muscle weakness, decreased bowel sounds, paresthesia, arrhythmias, flat T waves, ST-segment depression.
7. Administer replacement electrolytes and insulin, as ordered. Flush the entire IV infusion set with solution containing insulin and discard the first 50 mL because plastic bags and tubing may absorb some insulin and the initial solution may contain decreased concentration of insulin.
8. Monitor serum glucose, bicarbonate, and pH levels periodically.
9. Provide reassurance about improvement of condition and that correction of fluid imbalance will help reduce discomfort.

 NURSING ALERT Electrolyte levels may not reflect the total body deficit of potassium (primarily) and sodium (to a lesser extent) because of compartment shifts and fluid volume loss. Replacement is necessary despite normal to high values.

 DRUG ALERT Premature interruption of IV insulin administration may result in reaccumulation of ketone bodies and worsening acidosis. Glucose will normalize before acidosis resolves, so IV insulin is continued until bicarbonate levels normalize, subcutaneous insulin takes effect, and the patient tolerates oral caloric intake.

Preventing Further Episodes of DKA

1. Review with patients precipitating events and causes of DKA.
2. Assist patient in identifying warning signs and symptoms of DKA.
3. Instruct patient on sick-day guidelines (see page 748).

Patient Education and Health Maintenance

1. Make sure that patient and caretakers can demonstrate drawing up and administering insulin in the proper dose, blood glucose monitoring, and urine ketone testing.
2. Make sure that patient and caretakers know whom to notify in the event of hyperglycemia, stressful situation, or symptoms of DKA.

Evaluation: Expected Outcomes

- BP and heart rate stable; glucose and bicarbonate levels improving.
- Verbalizes sick-day guidelines correctly.

Hyperosmolar Hyperglycemic State

 EVIDENCE BASE Gosmanov, A. R., Gosmonova, E. O., & Kitabchi, A. E. (2015). Hyperglycemic crises: Diabetic ketoacidosis (DKA) and hyperglycemic hyperosmolar state (HHS). In K. Dungan (Ed.), *Endotext*. Available: www.endotext.org/chapter/diabetic-complications/hyperglycemic-crises-diabetic-ketoacidosis-dka-and-hyperglycemic.
Wolfsdorf, J. I., Allgrove, J., Craig, M. E., Edge, J., et al. (2014). Diabetic ketoacidosis and hyperglycemic hyperosmolar state. *Pediatric Diabetes, 15*(Suppl. 20), 154–179.

Hyperosmolar hyperglycemic state (HHS) is an acute complication of diabetes mellitus (particularly type 2 diabetes) characterized by hyperglycemia, dehydration, and hyperosmolarity, with little or no ketosis. Underlying infection is the most common cause of this acute complication.

Pathophysiology and Etiology

1. Prolonged hyperglycemia with glucosuria produces osmotic diuresis.
2. Loss of water, sodium, and potassium results in severe dehydration, causing hypovolemia and hemoconcentration.
3. Hyperosmolarity is a result of excessive blood sugar and increasing sodium concentration in dehydration.
4. Insulin continues to be produced at a level that prevents ketosis.
5. Increased blood viscosity decreases blood flow to the organs, creating tissue hypoxia.
6. Intracellular fluid and electrolyte shifts produce neurologic signs and symptoms.
7. Caused by inadequate amounts of endogenous/exogenous insulin to control hyperglycemia.
   a. Precipitating event may occur, such as cardiac failure, burn, or chronic illness that increases need for insulin.
   b. Use of therapeutic agents that increase blood glucose levels (eg, glucocorticoids, immunosuppressive agents).
   c. Use of therapeutic procedures that cause stress or increase blood glucose levels (eg, hyperosmolar hyperalimentation, peritoneal dialysis).

Clinical Manifestations

Early

1. Polyuria, dehydration.
2. Fatigue, malaise.
3. Nausea, vomiting.

Later

1. Hypothermia.
2. Muscle weakness.
3. Seizures, stupor, coma.

Diagnostic Evaluation

1. Serum glucose and osmolality are greatly elevated, with glucose values usually greater than 600 mg/dL.
2. Serum and urine ketone bodies are minimal to absent.
3. Serum sodium and potassium levels may be elevated, depending on degree of dehydration, despite total body losses.
4. BUN and creatinine may be elevated because of dehydration.
5. Urine specific gravity is elevated because of dehydration.

Management

1. Correct fluid and electrolyte imbalances with IV fluids.
2. Provide insulin via IV drip to lower plasma glucose.
3. Evaluate complications, such as stupor, seizures, or shock, and treat appropriately.
4. Identify and treat underlying illnesses or events that precipitated HHS.

Complications

1. Too rapid infusion of IV fluids can cause cerebral edema and death.
2. HHS is a medical emergency that, if not treated properly, can cause death (10% to 50% mortality).
3. Patients who become comatose will need nasogastric (NG) tubes to prevent aspiration.

Nursing Assessment

1. Assess level of consciousness (LOC).
2. Assess for dehydration—poor turgor, flushing, dry mucous membranes.
3. Assess cardiovascular status for shock—rapid, thready pulse, cool extremities, hypotension, electrocardiogram changes.
4. Interview family or significant other regarding precipitating events to episode of HHS.
   a. Evaluate patient's self-care regimen before hospitalization.
   b. Determine events, treatments, or drugs that may have caused the event.

Nursing Diagnoses

- Deficient Fluid Volume related to severe dehydration.
- Risk for Aspiration related to reduced LOC and vomiting.

Nursing Interventions

Restoring Fluid Balance

1. Assess patient for increasing signs and symptoms of dehydration, hyperglycemia, or electrolyte imbalance.
2. Institute fluid replacement therapy, as ordered (usually normal or half-strength saline initially), maintaining patent IV line.
3. Assess patient for signs and symptoms of fluid overload and cerebral edema as IV therapy progresses.
4. Administer regular insulin IV, as ordered, and add dextrose to IV infusion as blood glucose falls below 300 mg/dL, to prevent hypoglycemia.
5. Monitor hydration status by monitoring hourly intake and output and urine specific gravity.

Preventing Aspiration

1. Assess patient's LOC and ability to handle oral secretions.
   a. Cough and gag reflex.
   b. Ability to swallow.
2. Properly position patient to reduce possibility of aspiration.
   a. Elevate head of bed unless contraindicated.
   b. If nausea is present, use sidelying position.
3. Suction as frequently as needed to maintain patent airway.
4. Withhold oral intake until patient is no longer in danger of aspiration.
5. Insert NG tube as indicated for gastric decompression.
6. Monitor respiratory rate and breath sounds for signs of aspiration pneumonia.
7. Provide mouth care to maintain adequate mucosal hydration.

Patient Education and Health Maintenance

1. Advise patient and family that it may take 3 to 5 days for symptoms to resolve.
2. Instruct patient and family in signs and symptoms of hyperglycemia and use of sick-day guidelines (see page 748).
3. Explain possible causes of HHS.
4. Review changes in medication, activity, meal plan, or glucose monitoring for home care. It may not be necessary to continue insulin therapy following HHS; many patients can be treated with diet and oral agents.

Evaluation: Expected Outcomes

- BP stable, dehydration resolved.
- No evidence of aspiration.

Metabolic Syndrome

Metabolic syndrome (also known as syndrome X, insulin resistance syndrome, and dysmetabolic syndrome) is a term that has been used to characterize a constellation of related risk factors that increase the risk of developing several significant health problems to include T2DM and cardiovascular disease. There has been much discussion and debate in the literature as to whether or not metabolic syndrome is an actual diagnosis and if so, which diagnostic criteria should be included when screening. To improve consistency, a "harmonized definition" was set forth in 2009 by the International Diabetes Federation Task Force on Epidemiology and Prevention; National Heart, Lung, and Blood Institute; American Heart Association; World Heart Federation; International Atherosclerosis Society; and International Association for the Study of Obesity.

Three of the following five criteria must be met:

- Increased waist circumference (population-specific and country-specific criteria) (in the United States, greater than 35 inches for women and greater than 40 inches for men).
- Hypertriglyceridemia: ≥150 mg/dL*.
- Low HDL cholesterol: less than 40 mg/dL in men and less than 50 mg/dL in women*.

- Elevated BP: systolic BP ≥ 130 mm Hg or diastolic BP ≥ 85 mm Hg*.
- Elevated fasting glucose: ≥100 mg/dL*.

*= or taking medications to address.

 EVIDENCE BASE Alberti, K. G., Eckel, R. H., Grundy, S. M., Zimmet, P. Z., et al. (2009). Harmonizing the metabolic syndrome: A joint interim statement of the International Diabetes Federation Task Force on Epidemiology and Prevention; National Heart, Lung, and Blood Institute; American Heart Association; World Heart Federation; International Atherosclerosis Society; and International Association for the Study of Obesity. *Circulation, 120*(16), 1640–1645.

Pathophysiology and Etiology

1. The central feature of this metabolic disorder is the diminished responsiveness of peripheral tissues to circulating insulin (insulin resistance).
2. The typical physiological response of the body to this condition is the increased production and secretion of insulin, leading to a state of compensatory hyperinsulinemia to maintain glucose homeostasis.
3. Although this response is beneficial from the standpoint of glucose metabolism, it is now understood that the state of hyperinsulinemia necessary to prevent glucose intolerance gives rise to other abnormalities that have significant health consequences.
4. In addition to increased risk of type 2 diabetes associated with insulin resistance, hyperinsulinemia has also been associated with the development of hypertension, dyslipidemia, atherosclerotic cardiovascular disease, cerebrovascular disease, polycystic ovarian syndrome (PCOS), nonalcoholic fatty liver disease (NAFLD), and obstructive sleep apnea (OSA).
5. Because these clinical features are associated with insulin resistance, the term "syndrome" has been applied to signify that these conditions are linked to a common problem.
6. Although the pathogenesis of insulin resistance is not fully understood, genetic factors, lifestyle (diet, physical activity), and obesity play an important role in the development and natural course of this condition.

Risk Factors

1. Prediabetes, cardiovascular disease, PCOS, hypertension, hyperlipidemia, or acanthosis nigricans.
2. History of glucose intolerance or gestational diabetes.
3. Family history of type 2 diabetes, cardiovascular disease, or hypertension.
4. Sedentary lifestyle.
5. Obesity.

Management

1. Treatment of metabolic syndrome involves measures that are directed at treating any diagnosed disease resulting from insulin resistance (diabetes, hypertension, hypercholesterolemia) as well as the underlying insulin resistance. This is accomplished by interventions that improve insulin sensitivity.
2. Nonpharmacological interventions effective in reducing insulin resistance include lifestyle changes that can have a direct impact on insulin sensitivity and include regular physical activity and nutritional management designed to reduce body weight. Smoking cessation and reduced alcohol intake are also important lifestyle changes.
3. No pharmacologic agents have been FDA-approved for use in the treatment of metabolic syndrome or prediabetes. However, metformin is being used more frequently, especially if the risk for developing T2DM is very high. Other agents currently available with known insulin-sensitizing effects (ie, thiazolidinedione compounds) have shown effectiveness in treating individuals with PCOS and prediabetes. The potential role of these agents in the management of metabolic syndrome is under investigation.
4. Antiobesity medications are available to treat patients struggling with obesity (BMI greater than 30 kg/m²). Surgical interventions (ie, bariatric surgery) are recommended for morbidly obese patients (BMI greater than 40 kg/m² or greater than 35 kg/m² with comorbid conditions).

SELECTED REFERENCES

ACCORD (Action to Control Cardiovascular Risk in Diabetes) Study Group. (2008). Effects of intensive glucose lowering in type 2 diabetes. *New England Journal of Medicine, 358*(24), 2545–2559.

ADVANCE (Action in Diabetes and Vascular Disease: Preterax and Diamicron Modified Release Controlled Evaluation) Collaborative Group. (2008). Intensive blood glucose control and vascular outcomes in patients with type 2 diabetes. *New England Journal of Medicine, 358*(24), 2560–2572.

Alberti, K. G., Eckel, R. H., Grundy, S. M., et al. (2009). Harmonizing the metabolic syndrome: A joint interim statement of the International Diabetes Federation Task Force on Epidemiology and Prevention; National Heart, Lung, and Blood Institute; American Heart Association; World Heart Federation; International Atherosclerosis Society; and International Association for the Study of Obesity. *Circulation, 120*(16), 1640–1645.

American Association of Clinical Endocrinologists (AACE) and American College of Endocrinology (ACE). (2018). Consensus statement by the AACE and ACE on the comprehensive type 2 diabetes management algorithm—2018 Executive Summary. *Endocrine Practice, 24*(1), 91–120.

American Association of Clinical Endocrinologists (AACE) and American College of Endocrinology (ACE). (2015). Clinical practice guidelines for developing a diabetes mellitus comprehensive care plan—2015. *Endocrine Practice, 21*(Suppl. 1).

American Association of Clinical Endocrinologists (AACE) and American College of Endocrinology (ACE). (2016). Outpatient glucose monitoring consensus statement. *Endocrine Practice, 22*(2), 231–261.

American Association of Diabetes Educators (AADE). (October 12, 2015). Diabetes and physical activity. Practice synopsis. Available: *www.diabeteseducator.org/docs/default-source/default-document-library/diabetes-and-physical-activity2f6fd636a05f-68739c53ff0000b8561d.pdf:sfvrsn=0.*

American College of Obstetricians and Gynecologists (ACOG). (2018). Practice bulletin No. 190: Gestational diabetes mellitus. *Obstetrics & Gynecology, 131*(2), E49–E64.

American Diabetes Association (ADA). (2018). Standards of medical care in diabetes—2018. *Diabetes Care, 41*(Suppl. 1).

Camilleri, M., Parkman, H. P., Shafi, M. A., Abell, T. L., & Gerson, L. (2013). American College of Gastroenterology clinical guideline: Management of gastroparesis. *American Journal of Gastroenterology, 108*(1), 18–37.

Centers for Disease Control and Prevention. (2017). National chronic kidney disease fact sheet, 2017. Available *https://www.cdc.gov/kidneydisease/pdf/kidney_factsheet.pdf.*

Centers for Disease Control and Prevention (CDC). (2017) National Diabetes Statistics Report: Estimates of Diabetes and Its Burden in the United States, 2017. Available: *https://www.cdc.gov/diabetes/pdfs/data/statistics/national-diabetes-statistics-report.pdf.*

Colberg, S. R., Sigal, R. J., Yardley, J. E., Riddell, M. C., et al. (2016). Physical activity/exercise and diabetes: A position statement of the American Diabetes Association. *Diabetes Care, 39*(11), 2065–2079.

Corsino, L., Dhatariya, K., & Umpierrez, G. (2015). Management of diabetes and hyperglycemia in hospitalized patients. In K. Dungan (Ed.), *Endotext.* Available: *www.endotext.org/chapter/diabetes-treatment-strategies/management-of-the-hospitalized-diabetic-patient/*

Danne, T., Nimri, R., Battelino, T., et al. (2017). International consensus on use of continuous glucose monitoring. *Diabetes Care, 40*(12), 1631–1640.

de Ferranti, S. D., de Boer, I. H., Fonseca, V., et al. (2014). Type 1 diabetes mellitus and cardiovascular disease: A scientific statement from the American

Heart Association and American Diabetes Association. *Diabetes Care, 37*(10), 2843–2863.

Diabetes Costs and Prevalence Forecasts Diabetes 2025—State and Metropolitan Trends. (n.d.). Institute for Alternative Futures. Retrieved January 23, 2012, from *http://altfutures.org/diabetes2025/.*

Diabetes Prevention Program Research Group. (2002). Reduction in the incidence of type 2 diabetes with lifestyle intervention of metformin. *New England Journal of Medicine, 346*(6), 393–403.

Ducat, L., Philipson, L. H., & Anderson, B. J. (2014). The mental health comorbidities of diabetes. *JAMA, 312*(7), 691–692.

Duckworth, W., Abraira, C., Moritz, T., et al. (2009). Glucose control and vascular complicationsin veterans with type 2 diabetes. *New England Journal of Medicine, 360*(2), 129–139.

Dungan, K. (2015). Diabetes mellitus and carbohydrate metabolism—DiabetesManager. In A. J. M. Boulton, G. Chrousos, L. J. De Groot, K. Dungan, et al. (Eds.). *Endotext.* Available: *www.endotext.org/section/diabetes/*

Evert, A. B., Boucher, J. L., Cypress, M., Dunbar, S. A., et al. (2013). Nutrition therapy recommendations for the management of adults with diabetes. *Diabetes Care, 36*(11), 3821–3842.

Fox, C. S., Hill Golden, S., Anderson, C., Bray, G. A., et al. (2015). Update on prevention of cardiovascular disease in adults with type 2 diabetes mellitus in light of recent evidence: A scientific statement from the American Heart Association and the American Diabetes Association. *Diabetes Care, 38*(9), 1777–1803.

Frid, A. H., Kreugel, G., Grassi, G., et al. (2016). New insulin delivery recommendations. *Mayo Clinic Proceedings, 91*(9), 1231–1255.

Fryar, C. D., Carroll, M. D., & Ogden, C. L. (July 2016). Prevalence of overweight, obesity, and extreme obesity among adults aged 20 and over: United States, 1960-1962 through 2013-2014. National Center for Health Statistics. Available: *https://www.cdc.gov/nchs/data/hestat/obesity_adult_13_14/obesity_adult_13_14.pdf*

Goncalves-Bradley, D., Lannin, N. A., Clemson, L. M., Cameron, I. D., et al. (2016). Discharge planning from hospital (Review). *Cochrane Database of Systematic Reviews, 1,* CD000313. Available: *www.onlinelibrary.wiley.com/doi/10.1002/14651858.CD000313.pub5/full*

Gosmanov, A. R., Gosmonova, E. O., & Kitabchi, A. E. (2015). Hyperglycemic crises: Diabetic ketoacidosis (DKA) and hyperglycemic hyperosmolar state (HHS). In K. Dungan (Ed.), *Endotext.* Available: *www.endotext.org/chapter/diabetic-complications/hyperglycemic-crises-diabetic-ketoacidosis-dka-and-hyperglycemic/*

Gregg, E. W., Li, Y., Wang, J., et al. (2014). Changes in diabetes-related complications in the United States, 1990–2010. *New England Journal of Medicine, 370*(16), 1514–1523.

Healthy People 2020 [Internet]. (2017). Washington, DC: U.S. Department of Health and Human Services, Office of Disease Prevention and Health Promotion. Available: *www.healthypeople.gov/2020/topics-objectives/topic/diabetes*

Hirschman, K. B., & Bixby, M. B. (2014). Transitions in care from the hospital to home for patients with diabetes. *Diabetes Spectrum, 27*(3), 192–195.

International Society for Pediatric and Adolescent Diabetes (ISPAD). (2014). Clinical practice consensus guidelines 2014 compendium. *Pediatric Diabetes, 15*(Suppl. 20). Available: *www.ispad.org/?page=ISPADClinicalPract*

Kruger, D. (2016). The utility and interpretation of ambulatory glucose profiles. *Clinician Reviews, 26*(Suppl. 1), S1-S8.

Lam, D. W., & LeRoith, D. (2015). Metabolic syndrome. In K. Dungan (Ed.), *Endotext.* Available: *www.endotext.org/chapter/pathogenesis-of-diabetes/metabolic-syndrome/.*

Lane, W. (2016). When and how to use U500 (or other concentrated) insulin. 2016 Meet-The-Professor: Endocrine Case Management. Endocrine Society. Available: *press.endocrine.org/doi/pdf/10.1210/MTP5.9781943550043.ch18.*

Maahs, D., Daniels, S. R., de Ferranti, S. D., et al. (2014). Cardiovascular disease risk factors in youth with diabetes mellitus: A scientific statement from the American Heart Association. *Circulation, 130*(17), 1532–1558.

Munshi, M. N., Florez, H., Huang, E. S., et al. (2016). Management of diabetes in long-term care and skilled nursing facilities: A position statement of the American Diabetes Association. *Diabetes Care, 39*(2), 308–318.

National Center for Health Statistics. (2016). Health, United States, 2016 with Chartbook on Long-term Trends in Health. Available: *https://www.cdc.gov/nchs/data/hus/hus16.pdf.*

National Kidney Foundation. KDOQI™. (2012). Clinical practice guidelines for diabetes and CKD: 2012 update. *American Journal of Kidney Disease, 60*(5), 850–886. Available: *www.ajkd.org/article/S0272-6386(12)00957-2/pdf*

Nadeau, K. J., Anderson, B. J., Berg, E. G., et al. (2016). Youth-onset type 2 diabetes consensus report: Current status, challenges, and priorities. *Diabetes Care, 39*(9), 1635–1642.

Pop-Busui, R., Boulton, A. J. M., Feldman, E. L., et al. (2017). Diabetic neuropathy: A position statement by the American Diabetes Association. *Diabetes Care, 40*(1), 136–154.

Rowley, W. R., Bezold, C., Arikan, Y., Byrne, E., et al. (2016). Diabetes 2030: Insights from yesterday, today, and future trends. *Population Health Management.* Available *http://altfutures.org/wp-content/uploads/2016/04/Diabetes-2030-Population-Health-Management-2016-pop.2015.0181.pdf.*

Rubin, D. J. (2015). Hospital readmission of patients with diabetes. *Current Diabetes Reports, 15*(4), 1–9.

Seaquist, E. R., Anderson, J., Childs, B., Cryer, P., et al. (2013). Hypoglycemia and diabetes: A report of a Workgroup of the American Diabetes association and the Endocrine Society. *Diabetes Care, 36*(5), 1384–1395.

Sesti, G., Incalzi, R. A., Bonora, E., et al. (2018). Management of diabetes in older adults. *Nutrition, Metabolism & Cardiovascular Disease, 28*(3), 206–218.

Skyler, J., Bergenstal, R., Bonow, R. O., et al. (2009). Intensive glycemic control and the prevention of cardiovascular events: Implications of the ACCORD, ADVANCE, and VA Diabetes trials: A position statement of the American Diabetes Association and a scientific statement of the American College of Cardiology Foundation and the American Heart Association. *Diabetes Care, 32*(1), 187–192.

Solomon, S. D., Chew, E., Duh, E. J., et al. (2017). Diabetic retinopathy: A position statement of the American Diabetes Association. *Diabetes Care, 40*(3), 412–418.

Tuttle, K. R., Bakris, G. L., Bilous, R. W., et al. (2014). Diabetic kidney disease: A report from an ADA Consensus Conference. *Diabetes Care, 37*(10), 2864–2883.

UK Prospective Diabetes Study Group. (1998). Intensive blood-glucose control with sulfonylureas or insulin compared with conventional treatment and risk of complications in patients with type 2 diabetes (UKPDS 33). *Lancet, 352,* 837–853.

Valencia, W. M., & Florez, H. (2014). Pharmacological treatment of diabetes in older people. *Diabetes, Obesity and Metabolism, 16*(12), 1192–1203.

Walsh, J., & Roberts, R. (2016). *Pumping insulin: Everything for success on an insulin pump and CGM* (6th ed.). San Diego, CA: Torey Pines Press.

Whelton, P. K., Carey, R. M., Aronow, W. S., et al. (2017). 2017 ACC/AHA/AAPA/ABC/ACPM/AGS/APhA/ASH/ASPC/NMA/PCNA Guideline for the prevention, detection, evaluation, and management of high blood pressure in adults. *Journal of the American College of Cardiology.* Available *https://doi.org/10.1016/j.jacc.2017.11.006*

Wolfsdorf, J. I., Allgrove, J., Craig, M. E., Edge, J., et al. (2014). Diabetic ketoacidosis and hyperglycemic hyperosmolar state. *Pediatric Diabetes, 15*(Suppl. 20), 154–179. Available: *www.c.ymcdn.com/sites/www.ispad.org/resource/resmgr/Docs/CPCG_2014_CHAP_11.pdf*

Yilmaz, Z., Piracha, F., Anderson, L., et al. (2017). Supplements for diabetes mellitus: A review of the literature. *Journal of Pharmacy Practice, 30*(6), 631–638.

Young-Hyman, D., de Groot, M., Hill-Briggs, F., Gonzalez, J. S., et al. (2016). Psychosocial care for people with diabetes: A position statement of the ADA. *Diabetes Care, 39*(12), 2126–2140.

Ziegler, D., & Fonseca, V. (2015). From guideline to patient: A review of recent recommendations for pharmacotherapy of painful diabetic neuropathy. *Journal of Diabetes Complications, 29*(1), 146–156.

26

Hematologic Disorders

OVERVIEW AND ASSESSMENT

 See additional online content: Procedure Guidelines 26-1

Blood, the body fluid circulating through the heart, arteries, capillaries, and veins, consists of plasma and cellular components. The average male adult has about 5.5 L of blood and the average female 4.5 L. Plasma, the fluid portion, accounts for 55% of the blood volume and is composed of 92% water, 7% protein, and 1% inorganic salts; nonprotein organic substances such as urea; dissolved gases; hormones; and enzymes. Plasma proteins include albumin, fibrinogen, and globulins. Cellular components include erythrocytes (red blood cells [RBCs]), leukocytes and lymphocytes (white blood cells [WBCs]), and platelets. These cells are derived from pluripotent stem cells in the bone marrow, a process known as hematopoiesis (see Figure 26-1). Under normal conditions, only mature cells are found in circulating blood. The cellular components of blood account for 45% of the blood volume.

Characteristics of Cellular Components

Blood has multiple functions that are carried out by plasma or the cellular components (see Table 26-1, page 754).

Erythrocytes (RBCs)

1. Enucleated, biconcave disc.
2. Approximately 5 million erythrocytes per cubic millimeter of blood.
3. Cell contents consist primarily of hemoglobin, essential for oxygen transport. Whole blood contains 14 to 15 g of hemoglobin per 100 mL of blood.
4. Circulate about 115 to 130 days before elimination by reticuloendothelial system, primarily in the spleen and liver.

Leukocytes (WBCs)

See Table 26-2, page 754.
1. Approximately 5,000 to 10,000 leukocytes (WBCs) per cubic millimeter of blood.
2. Classified as granulocytes or mononuclear leukocytes.
   a. Granulocytes account for about 70% of all WBCs; have abundant granules in cytoplasm; include neutrophils, basophils, and eosinophils.
   b. Mononuclear leukocytes have single-lobed nucleus and granule-free cytoplasm; include monocytes and lymphocytes.

Platelets (Thrombocytes)

1. Approximately 150,000 to 450,000 platelets per cubic millimeter of blood.

Figure 26-1. Steps in differentiation of blood cells.

2. Small particles without nuclei arise as a result of budding from giant cells (megakaryocytes) in bone marrow.
3. Primary function is to control bleeding through hemostasis.

Subjective and Objective Data

The patient who presents with a hematologic disorder may have a disruption of the hematologic, immune, or coagulation system, producing a diverse array of symptoms and physical examination findings. Patients commonly present with vague complaints of fatigue, frequent infections, swollen glands, and bleeding tendencies. Characterize these complaints and obtain a review of systems, concentrating on the neurologic, respiratory, cardiovascular, GI, genitourinary (GU), and integumentary systems to look for more clues of hematologic dysfunction. Perform a systematic physical examination, paying careful attention to the cardiovascular, respiratory, and integumentary systems.

Review of Systems

1. Skin and mucous membranes: Any bruises, infections, drainage, or bleeding from wound sites?
2. Neurologic: Any dizziness, tingling or numbness (paresthesia), headache, forgetfulness or confusion, difficulty walking (disturbance in gait), tiredness (fatigue), or weakness?
3. Respiratory: Experiencing shortness of breath, especially on exertion?

Table 26-1   Functions of Blood

METHOD	INVOLVED	CELLS AND SUBSTANCES FUNCTION
Oxygen and carbon dioxide transport	Binding to hemoglobin; dissolved in plasma	• Erythrocyte • Hemoglobin • Plasma
Nutrient and metabolite transport	Bound to plasma proteins; dissolved in plasma	• Plasma proteins • Plasma
Hormone transport	In plasma	• Plasma
Transport of waste products to kidneys and liver	In plasma	• Plasma
Transport of cells and substances involved in immune reactions	In plasma to site of infection or foreign body	• Granulocytes • Monocytes • Lymphocytes • Immunoglobulins • Other substances
Clotting at breaks in blood vessels	Hemostasis	• Platelets • Clotting factors
Maintenance of fluid balance	Blood volume regulation	• Water • Electrolytes
Body temperature regulation	Peripheral vasoconstriction or dilation	—
Maintenance of acid–base balance	Acid–base regulation	• Electrolytes

Table 26-2   Characteristics of White Blood Cells

CELL	MAJOR FUNCTION	PHYSICAL CHARACTERISTICS
Neutrophil	Ingest and destroy microorganisms (phagocytosis)	Small cell, multilobed nucleus, most plentiful leukocyte
Eosinophil	Host resistance to helminthic infections; also allergic response	Bilobed nucleus; red-staining granules
Basophil	Allergic response	Bilobed nucleus; granules containing heparin and histamine
Monocyte	Phagocytosis	Large cell, kidney-shaped nucleus
B lymphocyte	Produce antibodies (immunoglobulins); humoral immunity	Small, agranular
T lymphocyte	Regulation of immune response; cellular immunity	Small, agranular; include cytotoxic, helper (T4) and suppressor (T8) T cells; identified by surface markers

4. Cardiovascular: Chest pain or feelings of funny heartbeats (palpitations)?
5. GI: Any bleeding from gums, abdominal pain, black stools, or blood-streaked vomit (emesis)? Any mouth sores, rectal pain, or diarrhea?
6. GU: Excessive menstrual flow? Any blood in urine or discomfort on urination?

Key History Questions

1. What are your present medications? Do you take over-the-counter (OTC) medications, vitamins, herbals, or nutritional supplements? What else have you taken in the past several months?
2. What medical problems have you had in the past? Any surgeries? Ask specifically about partial or total gastrectomy, splenic injury or splenectomy, tendency to bleed (eg, with dental procedures), infectious diseases, human immunodeficiency virus (HIV) infection, and cancer.
3. What is your occupation? Ask about exposure to substances such as benzene, pesticides, and ionizing radiation.
4. Do you have a family history of hematologic or malignant disorder?
5. Determine the social history and lifestyle. Do you use illicit drugs or alcohol? What is your pattern of sexual activity?

Key Examination Findings

1. Dyspnea; shiny smooth tongue; ataxia; and pallor of conjunctivae, nail beds, lips, and oral mucosa—suggest anemia.
2. Decreased blood pressure (BP), tachycardia, and possibly altered level of consciousness (LOC)—suggest anemia or altered blood clotting.
3. Hematuria, tarry stools, petechiae, and bleeding sites—suggest altered clotting.
4. Fever; tachycardia; abnormal breath sounds; delirium; oral lesions; and erythema, swelling, tenderness, and drainage of the skin—suggest infection.

Laboratory Studies

Laboratory studies routinely done for patients with hematologic disorders include complete blood count (CBC), blood smear, and iron profile.

Complete Blood Count

Description

1. Generally includes absolute numbers or percentages of erythrocytes, leukocytes, platelets, hemoglobin, and hematocrit in blood sample.
   a. Erythrocyte (RBC) indices—can be done to provide information on the size, hemoglobin concentration, and hemoglobin weight of an average RBC; aids in diagnosis and classification of anemias.
   b. Leukocyte (WBC) differential—can be done to determine the percentage of each type of granulocyte (neutrophils, eosinophils, and basophils) and nongranulocytes (lymphocytes and monocytes).
2. Absolute value of each is determined by multiplying the percentage by the total number of WBCs.
3. Used to evaluate infection or potential for infection and identify various types of leukemia.

Nursing and Patient Care Considerations

Blood sample can be drawn at any time without fasting or patient preparation.

Blood Smear

Description

Blood sample prepared for microscopic viewing using appropriate stains, allowing visual analysis of numbers and characteristics of cells; can identify abnormal cells of certain anemias, leukemias, and other disorders that affect the bloodstream.

Nursing and Patient Care Considerations

Can be done from blood sample drawn for CBC; no additional sample or patient preparation is necessary.

Iron Profile

Description

Test completed on blood sample that generally includes levels of serum ferritin, iron, total iron-binding capacity, folate, and vitamin B_{12}; used to determine type and severity of anemia.

Nursing and Patient Care Considerations

Recent administration of chloramphenicol, hormonal contraceptives, iron supplements, and corticotropin may affect results of serum iron and iron-binding capacity. No patient preparation needed.

Other Diagnostic Procedures

Bone Marrow Aspiration and Biopsy

Description

1. Aspiration and biopsy of bone marrow from the iliac crest or (rarely) sternum to obtain specimen to examine microscopically. Special needles are inserted into the bone to collect the specimens directly from the bone marrow.
2. Purposes include diagnosis of hematologic disorders; monitoring of course of illness and response to treatment; diagnosis of other disorders, such as primary and metastatic tumors, infectious diseases, and certain granulomas; and isolation of bacteria and other pathogens by culture.

Nursing and Patient Care Considerations

1. Give medication for pain and anxiety before or after the procedure, as ordered. A bone marrow aspiration with biopsy is more painful and may require use of mild to moderate sedation with appropriate monitoring.
2. Watch for bleeding and hematoma formation after procedure.

Lymph Node Biopsy

Description

1. Surgical excision or needle aspiration usually of a superficial lymph node in the cervical, supraclavicular, axillary, or inguinal region.
2. Performed to determine the cause of lymph node enlargement, to distinguish between benign and malignant lymph node tumors, and to stage metastatic carcinoma.

Nursing and Patient Care Considerations

1. Local anesthetic is usually given.
2. Specimen is placed in normal saline or 10% formaldehyde solution for transportation to the laboratory for cytologic and histologic evaluation.

GENERAL PROCEDURES AND TREATMENT MODALITIES

 See additional online content: Procedure Guidelines 26-2

Splenectomy

The *spleen* is a fist-size organ located in the upper left quadrant of the abdomen. It includes a central "white pulp" where storage and some proliferation of lymphocytes and other leukocytes occurs and a peripheral "red pulp" involved in fetal erythropoiesis, and later in erythrocyte destruction and the conversion of hemoglobin to bilirubin. It may be surgically removed because of trauma or to treat certain hemolytic or malignant disorders with accompanying splenomegaly. A laparoscopic technique, usually with a lateral approach, is preferred to remove a normal to slightly enlarged spleen in benign conditions, such as idiopathic thrombocytopenic purpura, hemolytic anemia, or sickle cell disease. Compared with open surgery, laparoscopic splenectomies have a shortened hospital stay, decreased postoperative pain, and decreased risk of wound complications such as adhesions and infections.

Preoperative Management

1. For general aspects of preoperative nursing management, see Chapter 7.
2. Stabilization of preexisting condition:
   a. For trauma: volume replacement with intravenous (IV) fluids, evacuation of stomach contents via nasogastric tube to prevent aspiration, urinary catheterization to monitor urine output, assessment for pneumothorax or hemothorax, and possible chest tube placement.
   b. For hemolytic or malignant disorder with accompanying thrombocytopenia: coagulation studies, administration of coagulation factors (eg, vitamin K, fresh-frozen plasma, cryoprecipitate), and platelet and red cell transfusions.
3. Preoperative pulmonary evaluation and teaching.
4. For patients undergoing elective splenectomy, vaccination against pneumococcus, *Haemophilus influenzae* type b, and meningococcus are given at least 2 weeks before surgery.

Postoperative Management

1. For general aspects of postoperative nursing management, see Chapter 7.
2. Prevention of respiratory complications: hypoventilation and limited diaphragmatic movement, atelectasis of left lower lobe, pneumonia, and left pleural effusion.
3. Monitoring for hemorrhage.
4. Pharmacologic deep vein thrombosis (DVT) prophylaxis, begun in the operating room or if the patient is at increased bleeding risk, as soon as bleeding risk subsides.
5. Administration of opioids for pain and observance for adverse effects.
6. Monitoring for fever.
   a. Postsplenectomy fever—mild, transient fever is expected.
   b. Persistent fever may indicate subphrenic abscess or hematoma.
7. Monitoring daily platelet count: thrombocytosis (elevation of platelet count) may appear a few days after splenectomy and may persist during first 2 weeks.

Potential Complications

1. Pancreatitis and fistula formation: tail of pancreas is anatomically close to splenic hilum.
2. Hemorrhage.
3. Atelectasis and pneumonia.
4. Overwhelming postsplenectomy infection (OPSI)—increased risk of developing a life-threatening bacterial infection with encapsulated organisms, such as *Streptococcus pneumoniae*, *Neisseria meningitidis*, or *H. influenzae* type b. The incidence of OPSI is 0.23% to 0.42% per year with a lifetime risk of 5%. An OPSI is a medical emergency and requires immediate IV antibiotics in an intensive care setting. IV immunoglobulins are also used.

 NURSING ALERT The risk of OPSI is highest soon after splenectomy and in patients whose splenectomy occurred during childhood or for a malignant disease. Early symptoms include fever and malaise; the infection may progress within hours to sepsis and death, with mortality as high as 50% to 70%. Patient education before and after splenectomy is imperative. The nurse should include the risks of OPSI; recognition of early symptoms and prompt medical attention; use of medical alert identification; immunization against *S. pneumoniae*, *H. influenzae* type b, and *N. meningitidis*; and, in some cases, prophylactic and standby antibiotics.

Nursing Diagnoses

- Ineffective Breathing Pattern related to pain and guarding of surgical incision.
- Risk for Deficient Fluid Volume related to hemorrhage caused by surgery of highly vascular organ.
- Risk for Injury (thromboembolism) related to thrombocytosis.
- Risk for Infection related to surgical incision and removal of the spleen.
- Acute Pain related to surgical incision.

Nursing Interventions

Maintaining Effective Breathing

1. Assess breath sounds and report absent, diminished, or adventitious sounds.
2. Assist with aggressive chest physiotherapy and incentive spirometry.
3. Encourage early and progressive mobilization.

Monitoring for Hemorrhage

1. Monitor vital signs frequently and as condition warrants.
2. Measure abdominal girth and report abdominal distention.
3. Assess for pain and report increasing pain.
4. Prepare the patient for surgical re-exploration if bleeding is suspected.

Avoiding Thromboembolic Complications

1. Monitor platelet count daily; report abnormal result promptly.
2. Administer DVT prophylaxis, as ordered.
3. Assess for possible thromboembolism.
   a. Assess skin color, temperature, tenderness, and swelling.
   b. Advise the patient to report chest pain, shortness of breath, pain, or weakness.
4. Report signs of thromboembolism immediately.

Preventing Infection

1. Assess surgical incision daily or if increased pain, fever, or foul smell.

2. Maintain meticulous hand washing and change dressings using sterile technique.
3. Teach the patient to report signs of infection (fever, malaise) immediately.
4. Educate the patient and family regarding OPSI, including plan for postsplenectomy immunizations, recognition of symptoms, and use of prophylactic and standby antibiotics.

Relieving Pain

1. Administer opioids or teach self-administration, as prescribed and as necessary, to maintain level of comfort.
2. Warn the patient of adverse effects, such as nausea and drowsiness; watch for hypotension and decreased respirations.
3. Teach the use of nonpharmacologic methods, such as music, relaxation breathing, progressive muscle relaxation, distraction, and imagery to help manage pain.
4. Document dosage of medications and response to medication.
5. Make sure the patient has analgesics for use postdischarge.

Patient Education and Health Maintenance

1. Teach care of incision.
2. Encourage to gradually increase activity according to guidelines given by the surgeon.
3. Advise proper rest, nutrition, and stress avoidance while recovering from surgery.
4. Encourage follow-up as directed by the surgeon and primary care provider to maintain immunizations.
5. Encourage the patient to seek prompt medical attention for any infections and to contact health care provider immediately for high fever.

Evaluation: Expected Outcomes

- Respirations unlabored, breath sounds clear.
- Vital signs stable, abdominal girth unchanged.
- No warmth, redness, swelling, or tenderness of extremity.
- Afebrile, no purulent drainage from incision.
- Verbalizes decreased pain.

ANEMIAS

Anemia is the lack of sufficient circulating hemoglobin to deliver oxygen to tissues. Anemia has multiple causes and is commonly associated with other diseases and disorders (eg, renal disease, cancer, Crohn disease, alcoholism). Anemia may be caused by inadequate production of RBCs, abnormal hemolysis and sequestration of RBCs, or blood loss. Iron deficiency anemia, pernicious anemia, folic acid deficiency anemia, and aplastic anemia are the anemias most commonly seen in adults. Hereditary hemolytic disorders include spherocytosis, hemoglobinopathies (eg, sickle cell), and enzymatic deficiencies such as glucose 6-phosphate dehydrogenase (G6PD). Treatments for anemia include nutritional counseling, supplements, RBC transfusions, and, for some patients, administration of exogenous erythropoietin (epoetin alfa or darbepoetin alfa), a growth factor stimulating production and maturation of erythrocytes. New erythropoiesis-stimulating agents are under development. Erythropoietin is used to stimulate RBC production in anemias associated with chronic renal failure, chemotherapy treatment, and HIV.

 DRUG ALERT Erythropoietic-stimulating agents, such as epoetin alfa and darbepoetin alfa, have been associated with increased risk of death and serious cardiovascular events. Use the lowest possible dose and monitor for such potential problems as hypertension—particularly in patients with chronic kidney disease—and deep venous thrombosis.

Iron Deficiency Anemia (Microcytic, Hypochromic)

Iron deficiency anemia is a condition in which the total body iron content is decreased below a normal level, affecting hemoglobin synthesis. RBCs appear pale and are small.

Pathophysiology and Etiology

1. The most common cause is chronic blood loss (GI bleeding including occult colorectal cancers, excessive menstrual bleeding, and hookworm infestation), but anemia may also be caused by insufficient intake of iron (weight loss, inadequate diet), iron malabsorption (end-stage renal disease, small-bowel disease, gastroenterostomy), or increased requirements (pregnancy, periods of rapid growth).
2. Decreased hemoglobin may result in insufficient oxygen delivery to body tissues.
3. The incidence of iron deficiency anemia, the most common type of anemia, varies widely by age, sex, and race. In the United States, it is more than twice as common in women as compared to men, affecting 10% of non-Hispanic white women and 20% of black and Hispanic women. It is a major health problem in developing countries.
4. Symptoms generally develop when hemoglobin has fallen to less than 11 g/100 mL.

Clinical Manifestations

1. Headache, dizziness, fatigue, and tinnitus.
2. Palpitations, dyspnea on exertion, and pallor of skin and mucous membranes.
3. In developing world: smooth, sore tongue; cheilosis (lesions at corners of mouth), koilonychia (spoon-shaped fingernails), and pica (craving to eat unusual substances).

Diagnostic Evaluation

1. CBC and iron profile—decreased hemoglobin, hematocrit, serum iron, and ferritin; elevated red cell distribution width and normal or elevated total iron-binding capacity (transferrin).
2. Determination of source of chronic blood loss may include sigmoidoscopy, colonoscopy, upper and lower GI studies, and stools and urine for occult blood examination.

Management

1. Diagnosis and correction of chronic blood loss.
2. Oral or parenteral iron therapy.
   a. Oral ferrous sulfate preferred and least expensive; treatment continues until hemoglobin level is normalized and iron stores replaced (up to 6 months).
   b. Parenteral therapy may be used when the patient cannot tolerate or is noncompliant with oral therapy. May use sodium ferric gluconate, iron sucrose, or iron dextran.

Complications

1. Severe compromise of the oxygen-carrying capacity of the blood may predispose to ischemic organ damage, such as myocardial infarction or stroke.
2. Anaphylaxis to parenteral iron therapy, especially with iron dextran.

Nursing Assessment

1. Obtain history of symptoms, dietary intake, past history of anemia, and possible sources of blood loss.
2. Examine for tachycardia, pallor, dyspnea, and signs of GI or other bleeding.

Nursing Diagnoses

• Imbalanced Nutrition: Less Than Body Requirements related to inadequate intake of iron.
• Activity Intolerance related to decreased oxygen-carrying capacity of the blood.
• Ineffective Tissue Perfusion related to decreased oxygen-carrying capacity of the blood.

Nursing Interventions

Promoting Iron Intake

1. Assess diet for inclusion of foods rich in iron. Arrange nutritionist referral, as appropriate.
2. Administer iron replacement, as ordered. Monitor iron levels of patients on chronic therapy.

 DRUG ALERT Anaphylactic reactions may occur after parenteral iron administration. Monitor the patient closely for hypotension, angioedema, and stridor after injection. Do not administer with oral iron.

Increasing Activity Tolerance

1. Assess level of fatigue and normal sleep pattern; determine activities that cause fatigue.
2. Assist in developing a schedule of activity, rest periods, and sleep.
3. Encourage conditioning exercises to increase strength and endurance.

Maximizing Tissue Perfusion

1. Assess the patient for palpitations, chest pain, dizziness, and shortness of breath; minimize activities that cause these symptoms.
2. Elevate head of bed and provide supplemental oxygen, as ordered.
3. Monitor vital signs and fluid balance.

Patient Education and Health Maintenance

1. Educate the patient on proper nutrition and good sources of iron: select a well-balanced diet that includes animal proteins, iron-fortified cereals and bread, beans, dried fruits, legumes, and tofu (see Table 26-3). The daily requirement of iron for adult females age 19 to 50 is 18 mg, for men 8 mg; however, more is needed to build iron stores in those who have been anemic and for those who are at risk for anemia.
2. Teach the patient about iron supplementation.
   a. Take iron on empty stomach, with full glass of water or fruit juice.

Table 26-3 Dietary Sources of Iron

FOOD	SERVING SIZE	MG PER SERVING
Cereal (fortified)	1 oz	1.8–21
Chicken liver	3.5 oz	12.8
Oatmeal (fortified)	1 cup	10
Soybeans	1 cup	8.8
Beef liver	3 oz	7.5
Lentils	1 cup	6.6
Beans (kidney, lima, navy, pinto)	1 cup	3.6–5.2
Oysters	6 pieces	4.5
Pumpkin seeds, roasted	1 oz	4.2
Beef (various cuts)	3–3.5 oz	2–3.9
Molasses	1 tbsp	3.5
Tofu	1/2 cup	3.4
Spinach, cooked	1/2 cup	3.2
Clams	3/4 cup	3.0
Sardines	3 oz	2.5
Turkey	3.5 oz	1.6–2.3
Macaroni (enriched, cooked)	1 cup	1.9
Bread (enriched)	2 slices	1.8
Rice (cooked)	1 cup	1.8
Apricots (dried)	10 pieces	1.7
Raisins	1/2 cup	1.5
Prune juice	1/2 cup	1.5
Pork	3–3.5 oz	1.2–1.5
Peas	1/2 cup	1.3
Chicken	3–3.5 oz	1.1–1.3

   b. Liquid forms may stain teeth; mix well with water or fruit juice and use a straw.
   c. Anticipate some epigastric discomfort, change in color of stools to green or black, and, in some cases, nausea, constipation, or diarrhea. Prevent and treat constipation with increased fiber, fluids, and exercise. Report GI intolerance to health care provider.
   d. Keep iron medications away from children as overdose may be fatal.
3. Encourage follow-up laboratory studies and visits to health care provider.

Evaluation: Expected Outcomes

• Incorporates several foods high in iron into diet; takes prescribed iron supplementation, as ordered.
• Tolerates increased activity; obtains sufficient rest.
• Vital signs stable without complaints of chest pain, palpitations, or shortness of breath.

Megaloblastic Anemia: Pernicious (Macrocytic, Normochromic)

A *megaloblast* is a large, nucleated erythrocyte with delayed and abnormal nuclear maturation. *Pernicious anemia* is a type of megaloblastic anemia associated with vitamin B12 deficiency.

Pathophysiology and Etiology

1. Vitamin B_{12} is necessary for normal deoxyribonucleic acid synthesis in maturing RBCs.
2. Pernicious anemia demonstrates familial incidence related to autoimmune gastric mucosal atrophy.
3. Normal gastric mucosa secretes a substance called intrinsic factor, necessary for absorption of vitamin B_{12} in ileum. If a defect exists in gastric mucosa, or after gastrectomy or small-bowel disease, intrinsic factor may not be secreted and orally ingested B_{12} may not be absorbed.
4. Some drugs interfere with B_{12} absorption, notably ascorbic acid, cholestyramine, colchicine, neomycin, cimetidine, and hormonal contraceptives.
5. Lower serum vitamin B_{12} concentrations are associated with aging, but the evidence linking subnormal vitamin B_{12} to anemia in older people remains limited and inconclusive.

Clinical Manifestations

1. Of anemia—pallor, fatigue, dyspnea on exertion, and palpitations. May be angina pectoris and heart failure in older adults or those predisposed to heart disease.
2. Of underlying GI dysfunction—sore mouth, glossitis, anorexia, nausea, vomiting, loss of weight, indigestion, epigastric discomfort, recurring diarrhea, or constipation.
3. Of neuropathy (occurs in high percentage of untreated patients)—paresthesia that involves hands and feet, gait disturbance, bladder and bowel dysfunction, and psychiatric symptoms caused by cerebral dysfunction.

Diagnostic Evaluation

1. CBC and blood smear—decreased hemoglobin and hematocrit; marked variation in size and shape of RBCs with a variable number of unusually large cells.
2. Folic acid (normal) and B_{12} levels (decreased).
3. Gastric analysis—volume and acidity of gastric juice diminished.
4. Schilling test for absorption of vitamin B_{12} uses small amount of radioactive B_{12} orally and 24-hour urine collection to measure uptake—decreased.

Management

Parenteral replacement with hydroxocobalamin or cyanocobalamin (B_{12}) is necessary by intramuscular (IM) injection from health care provider, generally every month.

Complications

Neurologic: paresthesia, gait disturbances, bowel and bladder dysfunction, and cerebral dysfunction may be persistent.

Nursing Assessment

1. Assess for pallor, tachycardia, dyspnea on exertion, and exercise intolerance to determine the patient's response to anemia.
2. Assess for paresthesia, gait disturbances, changes in bladder or bowel function, and altered thought processes indicating neurologic involvement.
3. Obtain history of gastric surgery or GI disease.

Nursing Diagnoses

- Chronic Confusion related to neurologic dysfunction in absence of vitamin B_{12}.
- Impaired Comfort related to neurologic dysfunction in absence of vitamin B_{12}.

Nursing Interventions

Improving Thought Processes
1. Administer parenteral vitamin B_{12}, as prescribed.
2. Provide the patient with quiet, supportive environment; reorient to time, place, and person, if needed; give instructions and information in short, simple sentences and reinforce frequently.

Minimizing the Effects of Paresthesia
1. Assess extent and severity of paresthesia, imbalance, or other sensory alterations.
2. Refer the patient for physical therapy and occupational therapy, as appropriate.
3. Provide safe, uncluttered environment; make sure personal belongings are within reach; provide assistance with activities, as needed.

Patient Education and Health Maintenance

1. Advise the patient that monthly vitamin B_{12} administration should be continued for life.
2. Instruct the patient to see health care provider approximately every 6 months for hematologic studies and GI evaluation; may develop hematologic or neurologic relapse if therapy inadequate.

 TRANSITIONAL CARE ALERT Patients with pernicious anemia have higher incidence of gastric cancer and thyroid dysfunction; therefore, periodic stool examinations for occult blood, gastric cytology, and thyroid function tests should be done. It is important to ensure that patient has access to a primary care provider and that patient records with follow up recommendations are communicated. Patients should also be educated on the signs and symptoms to report.

Evaluation: Expected Outcomes

- Oriented, cooperative, and follows instructions.
- Carries out activities without injury.

Megaloblastic Anemia: Folic Acid Deficiency

Chronic *megaloblastic anemia* is caused by folic acid (folate) deficiency.

Pathophysiology and Etiology

1. Dietary deficiency, malnutrition, marginal diets, excessive cooking of foods; commonly associated with alcoholism.
2. Impaired absorption in jejunum (eg, with small-bowel disease).
3. Increased requirements (eg, with chronic hemolytic anemia, exfoliative dermatitis, pregnancy).
4. Impaired utilization from folic acid antagonists (methotrexate) and other drugs (phenytoin, broad-spectrum antibiotics, sulfamethoxazole, alcohol, hormonal contraceptives).

Clinical Manifestations

1. Of anemia: fatigue, weakness, pallor, dizziness, headache, tachycardia.
2. Of folic acid deficiency: sore tongue, cracked lips.

Diagnostic Evaluation

1. Vitamin B_{12} and folic acid level—folic acid will be decreased.
2. CBC will show decreased RBC, hemoglobin, and hematocrit with increased mean corpuscular volume and mean corpuscular hemoglobin concentration.

Management

Oral folic acid (folate) replacement on daily basis.

Complications

Folic acid deficiency has been implicated in the etiology of congenitally acquired neural tube defects.

Nursing Assessment

1. Obtain nutritional history.
2. Monitor level of dyspnea, tachycardia, and development of chest pain or shortness of breath for worsening of condition.

Nursing Diagnosis

• Imbalanced Nutrition: Less Than Body Requirements related to inadequate intake of folic acid.

Nursing Interventions

Improving Folic Acid Intake
1. Assess diet for inclusion of foods rich in folic acid: beef liver, peanut butter, red beans, oatmeal, broccoli, and asparagus.
2. Arrange nutritionist referral, as appropriate.
3. Administer folic acid (folate) supplement.
4. Assist alcoholic patient to obtain counseling and additional medical care, as needed.

Community and Home Care Considerations

1. Encourage pregnant patient to maintain prenatal care and to take folic acid supplement.
2. Provide alcoholic patient with information about treatment programs and Alcoholics Anonymous meetings in the community.

Patient Education and Health Maintenance

1. Teach the patient to select balanced diet that includes green vegetables (asparagus, broccoli, spinach), yeast, liver and other organ meats, and some fresh fruits; avoid overcooking vegetables.
2. Encourage the patient to follow up periodically to monitor CBC.

Evaluation: Expected Outcomes

• Eats appropriate and nutritious diet; takes folic acid supplements, as prescribed.

Aplastic Anemia

Aplastic anemia is a rare disorder characterized by bone marrow hypoplasia or aplasia resulting in pancytopenia (insufficient numbers of RBCs, WBCs, and platelets).

Pathophysiology and Etiology

Destruction of hematopoietic stem cells is thought to be through an immune-mediated mechanism.

1. Most often (70% to 80% of patients) characterized as idiopathic because no cause is found.
2. May be caused by exposure to chemical toxins (eg, benzene); ionizing radiation; viral infections, particularly hepatitis; certain drugs (eg, chloramphenicol).
3. May be congenital (eg, Fanconi anemia, Diamond-Blackfan anemia, and Shwachman-Diamond syndrome).
4. Clinical course is variable and dependent on degree of bone marrow failure; severe aplastic anemia is almost always fatal if untreated.

Clinical Manifestations

1. From anemia: pallor, weakness, fatigue, exertional dyspnea, palpitations.
2. From infections associated with neutropenia: fever, headache, and malaise; adventitious breath sounds; abdominal pain, diarrhea; erythema, pain, exudate at wounds, or sites of invasive procedures.
3. From thrombocytopenia: bleeding from gums, nose, GI or GU tracts; purpura, petechiae, ecchymoses.

Diagnostic Evaluation

1. CBC and peripheral blood smear show decreased RBC, WBC, and platelets (pancytopenia).
2. Bone marrow aspiration and biopsy: bone marrow is hypocellular or empty with greatly reduced or absent hematopoiesis.

Management

1. Removal of causative agent or toxin.
2. Allogeneic bone marrow transplantation (BMT)—treatment of choice for patients with severe aplastic anemia (see page 784). This treatment option provides long-term survival for 75% to 90% of patients, depending on the age of the patient, history of prior blood transfusions, and source of marrow.
3. Immunosuppressive treatment with cyclosporine and antithymocyte globulin or cyclophosphamide. This treatment option provides long-term survival for 60% to 70% of patients.
4. Androgens (oxymetholone or testosterone enanthate) may stimulate bone marrow regeneration; significant toxicity encountered. They may be used when other treatments have failed.
5. Supportive treatment includes platelet and RBC transfusions, antibiotics, and antifungals. Blood components should be irradiated for patients eligible for BMT, and this approach is also recommended for patients receiving immunosuppressive therapy.

Complications

1. Untreated severe aplastic anemia is almost always fatal, generally because of overwhelming infection. Even with treatment, morbidity and mortality caused by infections and bleeding are high.
2. Late complications, even after successful treatment, include clonal hematologic diseases such as paroxysmal nocturnal hemoglobinuria, myelodysplasia, and acute myelogenous leukemia (AML).

Nursing Assessment

1. Obtain a thorough history that includes medications, past medical history, occupation, and hobbies.
2. Monitor for signs of bleeding and infection.

Nursing Diagnoses

- Risk for Infection related to granulocytopenia secondary to bone marrow aplasia.
- Risk for Bleeding related to disease process.

Nursing Interventions

Minimizing Risk of Infection

1. Care for patient in protective environment while hospitalized (eg, private room with strict hand washing and avoidance of any contaminants).
2. Encourage good personal hygiene, including daily shower or bath with mild soap, mouth care, and perirectal care after using the toilet.
3. Monitor vital signs, including temperature, frequently; notify health care provider of oral temperature of 101°F (38.3°C) or higher.
4. Minimize invasive procedures or possible trauma to skin or mucous membranes.
5. Obtain cultures of suspected infected sites or body fluids.

Minimizing Risk of Bleeding

1. Use only soft toothbrush or toothette for mouth care and electric razor for shaving; keep nails short by filing.
2. Avoid IM injections and other invasive procedures.
3. Prevent constipation with stool softeners, as prescribed.
4. Restrict activity based on platelet count and active bleeding.
5. Monitor pad count for menstruating patient; avoid use of vaginal tampons.
6. Control bleeding by applying pressure to site, using ice packs and prescribed topical hemostatic agents.
7. Administer blood product replacement, as ordered; monitor for allergic reaction, anaphylaxis, and volume overload.

Patient Education and Health Maintenance

1. Teach the patient how to minimize risk of infection.
   a. Wash hands after contact with possible source of infection.
   b. Immediately clean any abrasion or wound of mucous membranes or skin.
   c. Monitor temperature and report fever or other sign of infection immediately.
   d. Avoid crowds and people with illnesses.
   e. Avoid raw or undercooked foods.
   f. Use condoms and other safe-sex practices.
2. Teach the patient how to minimize risk of bleeding.
   a. Avoid falls or other injury.
   b. Use electric razor rather than plain razor.
   c. Use nail clippers or file rather than scissors.
   d. Avoid blowing nose.
   e. Use soft toothbrush or toothette for mouth care.
   f. Use water-soluble lubricants, as needed, during sexual activity.
3. Advise the patient to avoid exposure to potential bone marrow toxins: solvents, sprays, paints, and pesticides.
4. Teach the patient to take only prescribed medications; avoid aspirin and nonsteroidal anti-inflammatory drugs (NSAIDs),

which may interfere with platelet function. As some vitamins and herbs may also affect platelet function, instruct the patient to check with physician before using any supplements.
5. Resources for the patient and family include the Aplastic Anemia & MDS International Foundation (*www.aamds.org*).

Evaluation: Expected Outcomes

- Remains afebrile with no signs or symptoms of infection.
- Episodes of bleeding rapidly controlled.

MYELOPROLIFERATIVE DISORDERS

 See additional online content: Patient Education Guidelines 26-1, 26-2 and Nursing Care Plan 26-1

Myeloproliferative disorders are disorders of the bone marrow that result from abnormal proliferation of cells from the myeloid line of the hematopoietic system. They include polycythemia vera, acute lymphocytic and AML, and chronic myelogenous leukemia (CML).

Polycythemia Vera

Polycythemia vera is a chronic myeloproliferative disorder that involves all bone marrow elements, resulting in an increase in RBC mass and hemoglobin.

Pathophysiology and Etiology

1. Hyperplasia of all bone marrow elements results in the following:
   a. Overproduction of all three blood cell lines, most prominently RBCs.
   b. Increased red cell mass.
   c. Increased blood volume and viscosity.
   d. Decreased marrow iron reserve.
   e. Splenomegaly.
2. Increased mass of blood cells increases viscosity and leads to engorgement of blood vessels and possible thrombosis.
3. Underlying cause is unknown.
4. Usually occurs in middle and later years.

Clinical Manifestations

Result from increased blood volume and viscosity.
1. Reddish purple skin and mucosa, pruritus (especially after bathing).
2. Splenomegaly, hepatomegaly.
3. Epigastric discomfort, abdominal discomfort.
4. Painful fingers and toes from arterial and venous insufficiency, paresthesia.
5. Headache, fullness in head, dizziness, visual abnormalities, altered mentation from disturbed cerebral circulation.
6. Weakness, fatigue, night sweats, bleeding tendency.
7. Hyperuricemia from increased formation and destruction of erythrocytes and leukocytes and increased metabolism of nucleic acids.
8. Itching related to histamine release from basophils.

Diagnostic Evaluation

1. CBC—elevated RBC and hemoglobin and hematocrit (greater than 60%); elevated platelets.
2. Bone marrow aspirate and biopsy—hyperplasia.
3. Elevated uric acid.

Management

1. Of hyperviscosity: phlebotomy (withdrawal of blood) at intervals determined by CBC results to reduce RBC mass; generally, 250 to 500 mL removed at a time to maintain hematocrit less than 45%. The British Committee for Standards in Hematology recommendations also include aspirin at 75 mg/day unless contraindicated.
2. Of marrow hyperplasia: chronic myelosuppressive therapy, generally using hydroxycarbamide (formerly known as hydroxyurea) or IV radioactive phosphorus; biologic response modifier (ie, alpha interferon). Aggressive chemotherapy is not recommended because of increased risk of secondary leukemia.
3. Of hyperuricemia: allopurinol.
4. Of pruritus: antihistamines (cimetidine or cyproheptadine); low-dose aspirin; certain antidepressants (doxepin, paroxetine); phototherapy; cholestyramine; alpha interferon.

 EVIDENCE BASE Tefferi, A., & Barbui, T. (2017). Polycythemia vera and essential thrombocythemia: 2017 update on diagnosis, risk-stratification, and management. *American Journal of Hematology, 92*(1), 94–108.

Complications

1. Thromboembolic events caused by hyperviscosity, including deep vein thrombophlebitis, myocardial and cerebral infarction, transient ischemic attacks, pulmonary embolism, retinal vein thrombosis, and thrombotic occlusion of the splenic, hepatic, portal, and mesenteric veins.
2. Spontaneous hemorrhage caused by venous and capillary distention and abnormal platelet function.
3. Gout caused by hyperuricemia.
4. Heart failure caused by increased blood volume and hypertension.
5. Myelofibrosis or acute myeloid leukemia may be terminal complications.

Nursing Assessment

1. Obtain history of symptoms, including changes in skin, epigastric discomfort, bleeding tendencies, circulatory problems, or painful, swollen joints.
2. Monitor for signs of bleeding or thromboembolism.
3. Monitor for hypertension and signs and symptoms of heart failure, including shortness of breath, distended neck veins.

Nursing Diagnosis

• Ineffective Tissue Perfusion (multiple organs) related to hyperviscosity of blood.

Nursing Interventions

Preventing Thromboembolic Complications

1. Encourage or assist with ambulation. Employ thromboembolism precautions during periods of immobility.
2. Assess for early signs of thromboembolic complications—swelling of limb, increased warmth, pain, shortness of breath, and chest pain. Report immediately.
3. Monitor CBC and assist with phlebotomy, as ordered.

Patient Education and Health Maintenance

1. Educate the patient about risk of thrombosis; encourage the patient to maintain normal activity patterns and avoid long periods of bed rest.
2. Advise the patient to avoid taking hot showers or baths because rapid skin cooling worsens pruritus; use skin emollients; take antihistamines, as prescribed; may find starch baths helpful.
3. Instruct the patient to take only prescribed medications.
4. Encourage the patient to report at prescribed intervals for follow-up blood (hematocrit) studies and phlebotomies.
5. Instruct the patient in technique of subcutaneous injection for alpha interferon.

Evaluation: Expected Outcomes

• Hematocrit less than 45%; no signs or symptoms of thromboembolism, heart failure, or bleeding.

Acute Lymphocytic and Acute Myelogenous Leukemia

Leukemias are malignant disorders of the blood and bone marrow that result in an accumulation of dysfunctional, immature cells that are caused by loss of regulation of cell division. They are classified as acute or chronic based on the development rate of symptoms and further classified by the predominant cell type. Acute leukemias affect immature cells and are characterized by rapid progression of symptoms. When lymphocytes (B or T cell) are the predominant malignant cell, the disorder is *acute lymphocytic leukemia (ALL)*; when monocytes or granulocytes are predominant, it is *acute myelogenous leukemia (AML)*.

Pathophysiology and Etiology

1. The development of leukemia has been associated with the following:
   a. Exposure to ionizing radiation.
   b. Exposure to certain chemicals and toxins (eg, benzene, alkylating agents).
   c. Human T-cell leukemia—lymphoma virus (HTLV-1 and HTLV-2) in certain areas of the world, including the Caribbean and southern Japan.
   d. Familial susceptibility.
   e. Genetic disorders (eg, Down syndrome, Fanconi anemia).
   f. Childhood leukemia is often not associated with a specific cause.
2. Approximately one half of new leukemias are acute. Approximately 85% of acute leukemias in adults are AML. ALL is most common in children, with peak incidence between ages 2 and 9.
3. Childhood ALL is usually cured with chemotherapy alone (greater than 75%), whereas only 30% to 40% of adults with ALL are cured.
4. AML is a disease of older people, with a median age at diagnosis of 67. However, it does also occur in children, though much less common than ALL. Even in the younger adults (patients who are younger than age 60), AML is difficult to treat, with a median survival of 5 to 6 months, despite intensive therapy.

Clinical Manifestations

1. Common symptoms include pallor, fatigue, weakness, fever, weight loss, abnormal bleeding and bruising, lymphadenopathy (in ALL), and recurrent infections.
2. Other presenting symptoms may include bone and joint pain, headache, splenomegaly, hepatomegaly, and neurologic dysfunction.

Diagnostic Evaluation

1. CBC and blood smear—peripheral WBC count varies widely from 1,000 to 100,000/mm³ and may include significant numbers of abnormal immature (blast) cells; anemia may be profound; platelet count may be abnormal and coagulopathies may exist.
2. Bone marrow aspiration and biopsy—cells also studied for chromosomal abnormalities (cytogenetics) and immunologic markers to classify type of leukemia further.
3. Lumbar puncture and examination of cerebrospinal fluid for leukemic cells (especially in ALL).

Management

1. National Comprehensive Cancer Network (NCCN; *www.nccn.org*) guidelines provide recommendations for workup, management, and supportive care of patients with various subtypes of AML. Evidence-based treatment guidelines for management of ALL are published by the National Cancer Institute (*www.cancer.gov/cancertopics/pdq/treatment/adultALL/HealthProfessional*).
2. Management of AML and ALL is designed to eradicate leukemic cells and allow restoration of normal hematopoiesis.
   a. High-dose chemotherapy given as an induction course to obtain remission (disappearance of abnormal cells in bone marrow and blood) and then in cycles as consolidation or maintenance therapy to prevent recurrence of disease (see Table 26-4).
   b. Leukapheresis (or exchange transfusion in infants) may be used when abnormally high numbers of white cells are present to reduce the risk of leukostasis and tumor burden before chemotherapy.
   c. Radiation, particularly of central nervous system (CNS) in ALL.
   d. Targeted therapies are being developed to stop cancer cell growth by targeting specific genes or proteins; may be used in conjunction with other chemotherapy.
   e. Autologous or allogeneic bone marrow or stem cell transplantation.

Complications

1. Leukostasis: in setting of high numbers (greater than 50,000/mm³) of circulating leukemic cells (blasts), blood vessel walls are infiltrated and weakened, with high risk of rupture and bleeding, including intracranial hemorrhage.

Table 26-4 Common Chemotherapeutic Drugs Used in Acute Leukemias

DRUG	MAJOR ADVERSE EFFECTS	CLASSIFICATION	PRIMARY USE
All-trans retinoic acid	Dry skin and mucous membranes, headaches, eyesight changes, bone pain, flulike symptoms, bone marrow suppression, and retinoic acid syndrome (includes weight gain, peripheral edema, dyspnea, and fever)	Retinoid	Therapy for AML subtype M3 (APL)
Cyclophosphamide	Bone marrow suppression, alopecia, nausea and vomiting, diarrhea, hemorrhagic cystitis, and cardiomyopathy	Alkylating agent	Induction and consolidation therapy for ALL
Cytarabine	Bone marrow suppression, nausea and vomiting, pulmonary toxicity, mucositis, lethargy, cerebellar toxicity, dermatitis, and keratoconjunctivitis	Antimetabolite	Induction and consolidation therapy for AML
Daunorubicin	Bone marrow suppression, nausea and vomiting, alopecia, cardiotoxicity, and vesicant	Antibiotic	Induction and consolidation therapy for AML
Doxorubicin	Leukopenia, nausea and vomiting, alopecia, cardiotoxicity, photosensitivity, and vesicant	Antibiotic	Induction and consolidation therapy for AML
Imatinib mesylate	Edema, nausea and vomiting, musculoskeletal pain, and rash	Tyrosine kinase inhibitor	Induction and consolidation therapy for Philadelphia chromosome–positive adult ALL
L-Asparaginase	Liver dysfunction, nausea and vomiting, hypersensitivity reaction, depression, and lethargy	Miscellaneous: enzyme	Induction therapy for ALL
6-Mercaptopurine	Mild bone marrow suppression, GI disturbances, and hepatotoxicity	Antimetabolite	Maintenance therapy for ALL
Methotrexate	Bone marrow suppression, stomatitis, nausea, diarrhea, hepatotoxicity, and neurotoxicity with intrathecal doses	Antimetabolite	Intrathecal central nervous system treatment and prophylaxis for ALL; maintenance therapy for ALL
Prednisone	Appetite stimulation, mood alteration, Cushing syndrome, hypertension, diabetes, and peptic ulcer	Corticosteroid	Induction therapy for ALL
Vincristine	Neurotoxicity, alopecia, and vesicant	Plant alkaloid	Induction therapy for ALL

ALL, acute lymphocytic leukemia; AML, acute myelogenous leukemia; APL, acute promyelocytic leukemia.

2. Disseminated intravascular coagulation (DIC).
3. Tumor lysis syndrome: rapid destruction of large numbers of malignant cells leads to alterations in electrolytes (hyperuricemia, hyperkalemia, hyperphosphatemia, and hypocalcemia), renal failure, and other complications.
4. Infection, bleeding, organ damage.

 DRUG ALERT Allopurinol and/or rasburicase are commonly used as part of a regimen to prevent tumor lysis syndrome. In rare cases, they may cause severe, even lethal, skin reactions (toxic epidermolysis syndrome). Allopurinol should be discontinued for any patient who develops a new skin rash.

Nursing Assessment

1. Take nursing history, focusing on weight loss, fever, frequency of infections, progressively increasing fatigability, shortness of breath, palpitations, and visual changes (retinal bleeding).
2. Ask about difficulty in swallowing, coughing, and rectal pain.
3. Examine the patient for enlarged lymph nodes, hepatosplenomegaly, evidence of bleeding, abnormal breath sounds, and skin lesions.
4. Look for evidence of infection: mouth, tongue, and throat for reddened areas or white patches. Examine skin for breakdown, which is a potential source of infection.

Nursing Diagnoses

- Risk for Infection related to granulocytopenia of disease and treatment.
- Risk for Bleeding secondary to bone marrow failure and thrombocytopenia.

Nursing Interventions

Preventing Infection

1. Especially monitor for pneumonia, pharyngitis, esophagitis, perianal cellulitis, urinary tract infection, and cellulitis, which are common in leukemia and which carry significant morbidity and mortality.
2. Monitor for fever, flushed appearance, chills, and tachycardia; appearance of white patches in mouth; redness, swelling, heat, or pain of eyes, ears, throat, skin, joints, abdomen, and rectal and perineal areas; cough, changes in sputum; skin rash.
3. Check results of granulocyte counts. Concentrations less than 500/mm³ put the patient at serious risk for infection. Administer granulocyte-stimulating and erythropoiesis-stimulating agents, as ordered (eg, epoetin alfa or darbepoetin alfa).
4. Avoid invasive procedures and trauma to skin or mucous membrane to prevent entry of microorganisms.
5. Use the following rectal precautions to prevent infection:
   a. Avoid diarrhea and constipation, which can irritate the rectal mucosa.
   b. Avoid use of rectal thermometers.
   c. Keep the perianal area clean.
6. Care for the patient in private room with strict hand washing practice. Patients with prolonged neutropenia may benefit from high-efficiency particulate air filtration.
7. Encourage and assist the patient with personal hygiene, bathing, and oral care.
8. Obtain cultures and administer antimicrobials promptly, as directed. Prophylactic antimicrobials, antifungals, and

antivirals serve to protect the patient from life-threatening infections.

Preventing and Managing Bleeding

1. Watch for signs of minor bleeding, such as petechiae, ecchymosis, conjunctival hemorrhage, epistaxis, bleeding gums, bleeding at puncture sites, vaginal spotting, and heavy menses.
2. Be alert for signs of serious bleeding, such as headache with change in responsiveness, blurred vision, hemoptysis, hematemesis, melena, hypotension, tachycardia, and dizziness.
3. Monitor urine, stools, and emesis for gross and occult blood.
4. Monitor platelet counts daily.
5. Administer blood components, as directed.
6. Keep the patient on bed rest during bleeding episodes.

Patient Education and Health Maintenance

1. Teach infection precautions (see page 761).
2. Teach signs and symptoms of infection and advise whom to notify.
3. Encourage adequate nutrition to prevent emaciation from chemotherapy.
4. Teach avoidance of constipation with increased fluid and fiber and good perianal care.
5. Teach bleeding precautions (see page 761).
6. Encourage regular dental visits to detect and treat dental infections and disease.
7. Provide the patient and family with information about resources in the community, see Box 26-1.

Evaluation: Expected Outcomes

- Afebrile, without signs of infection.
- No signs of bleeding.

Chronic Myelogenous Leukemia

Chronic myelogenous leukemia (CML) (ie, involving more mature cells than acute leukemia) is characterized by proliferation of myeloid cell lines, including granulocytes, monocytes, platelets, and, occasionally, RBCs.

Pathophysiology and Etiology

1. Specific etiology unknown, associated with exposure to ionizing radiation and family history of leukemia. Results from malignant transformation of pluripotent hematopoietic stem cell.
2. First cancer associated with chromosomal abnormality (the Philadelphia [Ph] chromosome), present in more than 90% of patients.
3. Accounts for 25% of adult leukemias and less than 5% of childhood leukemias. Generally presents between ages 25 and 60 with peak incidence in the mid-40s.
4. May progress to an accelerated phase or blast crisis, resembling an acute leukemia.

Clinical Manifestations

1. Insidious onset; may be discovered during routine physical examination.
2. About 70% of patients have symptoms at diagnosis such as fatigue, pallor, activity intolerance, fever, weight loss, night sweats, and abdominal fullness (splenomegaly).

Diagnostic Evaluation

1. CBC and blood smear: large numbers of granulocytes (usually more than 100,000/mm³), platelets may be decreased.

2. Bone marrow aspiration and biopsy: hypercellular, usually demonstrates Philadelphia (Ph[1]) chromosome.

Management

Treatment guidelines for the management of CML are provided by NCCN (*www.nccn.org*).

Chronic Phase

1. Tyrosine kinase inhibitors are oral agents used as primary treatment for most patients with CML. They include imatinib mesylate, dasatinib, and nilotinib.
   a. These agents work by inhibiting proliferation of abnormal cells and inducing cell death (apoptosis) in abnormal cells.
   b. Adverse effects vary based on the agent used but include edema, diarrhea, headache, muscle cramps, muscle and bone pain, rash, and, rarely, hepatotoxicity, pleural or pericardial effusion, and myelosuppression.
2. For patients who do not respond to tyrosine kinase inhibitors, allogeneic (related or unrelated) BMT may be an option.

Accelerated Phase or Blast Crisis

1. High-dose tyrosine kinase inhibitors or chemotherapy (ALL or AML regimens) may be used to attempt to regain chronic phase.
2. Supportive care and palliative care may be appropriate because this phase is usually terminal.

Complications

1. Leukostasis.
2. Infection, bleeding, and organ damage.
3. If untreated, CML is a terminal disease with unpredictable survival, on average 3 years.

Nursing Assessment

1. Obtain health history, focusing on fatigue, weight loss, night sweats, and activity intolerance.
2. Assess for signs of bleeding and infection.
3. Evaluate for splenomegaly and hepatomegaly.
4. Assess for weight gain and edema in patients taking tyrosine kinase inhibitors.

Nursing Diagnosis

• Fear related to disease progression and death.

Nursing Interventions

Also see nursing interventions for acute leukemia, page 762.

Allaying Fear

1. Encourage appropriate verbalization of feelings and concerns.
2. Provide comprehensive patient teaching about disease, using methods and content appropriate to the patient's needs.
3. Assist the patient in identifying resources and support (eg, family and friends, spiritual support, community or national organizations, support groups).
4. Facilitate use of effective coping mechanisms.

Patient Education and Health Maintenance

1. Teach the patient to take medications, as prescribed, and monitor for adverse effects.
2. Teach the patient method of subcutaneous injection for self-administration of alpha interferon and teach strategies for managing such adverse effects as fatigue and fever.
3. Provide the patient and family with information about resources in the community (see Box 26-1).

BOX 26-1 Resources for Patients with Hematologic Malignancies

AMERICAN CANCER SOCIETY
250 Williams Street NW
Atlanta, GA 30303
(404) 320-3333 or (800) 227-2345
www.cancer.org
Patient education materials, Can Surmount and I Can Cope educational and support programs, and durable medical equipment loans

CORPORATE ANGEL NETWORK, INC.
Westchester County Airport, 1 Loop Road
White Plains, NY 10604
(914) 328-1313 or (866) 328-1313
www.corpangelnetwork.org
Use of corporate aircraft to provide free travel to cancer patients going to checkups, treatments, or consultations

LEUKEMIA AND LYMPHOMA SOCIETY
1311 Mamaroneck Avenue
Suite 310
White Plains, NY 10605
(914) 949-5213 or (800) 955-4572
Patient education materials, support groups, financial assistance (patient aid) program for patients with leukemia, Hodgkin and non-Hodgkin lymphoma, and multiple myeloma

NATIONAL COALITION FOR CANCER SURVIVORSHIP
1010 Wayne Ave., Suite 707
Silver Spring, MD 20910

(301) 650-9127
www.canceradvocacy.org
Network related to survivorship issues, sponsors National Cancer Survivors' Day, publishes Cancer Survivors Almanac of Resources

NATIONAL MARROW DONOR PROGRAM
3001 Broadway Street NE, Suite 100
Minneapolis, MN 55413
(800) 507-5427
www.bethematch.org
Information for patients and volunteer donors regarding unrelated bone marrow transplant

NATIONAL CANCER INSTITUTE
National Institutes of Health
Bethesda, MD 20892
(800) 4-CANCER
www.cancer.gov
National telephone hotline for information, patient education materials, and research reports

BLOOD & MARROW TRANSPLANT INFORMATION NETWORK
2900 Skokie Valley Road, Suite B
Highland Park, IL 60035
(888) 597-7674
www.bmtinfonet.org
Resources, support, and educational materials for patients and families

Evaluation: Expected Outcomes

• Demonstrates effective coping skills.

LYMPHOPROLIFERATIVE DISORDERS

Lymphoproliferative disorders result from proliferation of cells from the lymphoid line of the hematopoietic system. They include chronic lymphocytic leukemia, Hodgkin lymphoma, non-Hodgkin lymphoma, and multiple myeloma.

Chronic Lymphocytic Leukemia

Chronic lymphocytic leukemia (CLL) (ie, involving more mature cells than acute leukemia) is characterized by proliferation of morphologically normal but functionally inert B lymphocytes. In CLL, the abnormal lymphocytes are found in the bone marrow and blood, whereas in *small lymphocytic lymphoma (SLL)*, the same abnormal lymphocytes are found predominantly in lymph nodes. The differential diagnosis includes *hairy cell leukemia* and *Waldenström macroglobulinemia*.

Pathophysiology and Etiology

1. Specific etiology unknown. Tends to cluster in families, much more common in Western hemisphere. Male hormones may play role.
2. Most common adult leukemia in the United States and Europe. Disease of later years (90% over age 50); 1.5 times more common in men than in women.
3. Lymphocytes are immunoincompetent and respond poorly to antigenic stimulation.
4. In late stages, organ damage may occur from direct lymphocytic infiltration of tissue.
5. Variable course: may be indolent for years, with gradual transformation to more malignant or aggressive disease with 1- to 2-year course.

Clinical Manifestations

1. Insidious onset; may be discovered during routine physical examination.
2. Early symptoms may include painless lymph node swelling, commonly in cervical area, history of frequent skin or respiratory infections, mild splenomegaly and hepatomegaly, and fatigue.
3. Symptoms of more advanced disease include fever, night sweats, weight loss, pallor, activity intolerance, easy bruising, skin lesions, bone tenderness, and abdominal discomfort.

Diagnostic Evaluation

1. CBC and blood smear: large numbers of lymphocytes (10,000 to 150,000/mm^3); may also be anemia, thrombocytopenia, and hypogammaglobulinemia.
2. Bone marrow aspirate and biopsy: lymphocytic infiltration of bone marrow.
3. Lymph node biopsy to detect spread.

Management

Symptom Control and Treatments

1. The patient with newly diagnosed and indolent CLL is generally observed and followed closely until symptoms develop. Treatment is individualized; NCCN guidelines suggest clinical trial or various chemotherapy and monoclonal antibody combinations (*www.nccn.org*).
2. Lymphocyte proliferation can be suppressed with chlorambucil, cyclophosphamide, and prednisone.
3. The purine analogue fludarabine has significant activity in CLL alone or in combination with rituximab and/or cyclophosphamide.
4. Monoclonal antibodies, such as alemtuzumab and rituximab, may be used.
5. Hairy cell leukemia, a distinctive type of B-cell leukemia with hairlike projections of cytoplasm from lymphocytes, may be successfully treated with cladribine, pentostatin, or alpha interferon.
6. Splenic irradiation or splenectomy for painful splenomegaly or platelet sequestration, hemolytic anemia.
7. Irradiation of painful enlarged lymph nodes.
8. Allogeneic bone marrow transplant is also used to treat CLL.

Supportive Care

1. Transfusion therapy to replace platelets and RBCs.
2. Antibiotics, antivirals, and antifungals, as needed, to control infections.
3. IV immunoglobulins or gamma globulin to treat hypogammaglobulinemia.

Complications

1. Thrombophlebitis from venous or lymphatic obstruction caused by enlarged lymph nodes.
2. Infection, bleeding.
3. Median survival depends on severity of disease; varies from 2 to 7 years.

Nursing Assessment

1. Obtain health history, focusing on history of infections, fatigue, bruising and bleeding, and swollen lymph nodes.
2. Assess for signs of anemia, bleeding, or infection.
3. Evaluate for splenomegaly, hepatomegaly, and lymphadenopathy.

Nursing Diagnoses

• Acute Pain related to tumor growth, infection, or adverse effects of chemotherapy.
• Activity Intolerance related to anemia and adverse effects of chemotherapy.

Nursing Interventions

Reducing Pain

1. Assess the patient frequently for pain and administer or teach the patient to administer analgesics on regular schedule, as prescribed; monitor for adverse effects.
2. Teach the patient the use of nonpharmacologic methods, such as music, relaxation breathing, progressive muscle relaxation, distraction, and imagery to help manage pain.

Improving Activity Tolerance

1. Encourage frequent rest periods alternating with ambulation and light activity, as tolerated.
2. Assist the patient with hygiene and physical care, as necessary.
3. Encourage balanced diet or nutritional supplements, as tolerated.
4. Teach the patient to use energy conservation techniques while performing activities of daily living, such as sitting while bathing, minimizing trips up and down stairs, using shoulder bag or push cart to carry articles.

Patient Education and Health Maintenance

1. Teach the patient to minimize risk of infection (see page 761).
2. Teach the patient use of medications, as ordered, and possible adverse effects and their management; also teach the patient to avoid aspirin and NSAIDs, which may interfere with platelet function.
3. Provide the patient and family with information about resources in the community (see page 765).

Evaluation: Expected Outcomes

- States pain relief.
- Performs activities without complaints of fatigue.

Hodgkin Lymphoma

Lymphomas are malignant disorders of the reticuloendothelial system that result in an accumulation of dysfunctional, immature lymphoid-derived cells. They are classified according to the predominant cell type and by the degree of malignant cell maturity (eg, well differentiated, poorly differentiated, or undifferentiated). Hodgkin lymphoma originates in the lymphoid system and involves predominantly lymph nodes. It accounts for about 12% of all lymphomas.

Pathophysiology and Etiology

1. Etiology is unknown.
2. Characterized by appearance of "Reed-Sternberg" multinucleated giant cell in tumor.
3. Generally spreads via lymphatic channels, involving lymph nodes, spleen, and ultimately extralymphatic sites. May also spread via bloodstream to such sites as GI tract, bone marrow, skin, upper air passages, and other organs.
4. Incidence demonstrates two peaks, between ages 20 and 30 and after age 55. Risk is increased in males, for patients with HIV, in individuals with previous Epstein-Barr viral infection, and in individuals with first-degree relative with Hodgkin lymphoma.

Clinical Manifestations

1. Common symptoms include painless enlargement of lymph nodes (generally unilateral cervical or supraclavicular), splenomegaly, fever, chills, night sweats, weight loss, and pruritus.
2. Various symptoms may occur with pulmonary involvement, superior vena cava obstruction, and hepatic or bone involvement.

Diagnostic Evaluation

Tests are used to determine extent of disease involvement before treatment and followed at regular intervals to assess response to treatment.

1. CBC—determines abnormal cells.
2. Lymph node biopsy—determines type of lymphoma.
3. Bilateral bone marrow aspirate and biopsy—determine whether bone marrow is involved.
4. Radiographic tests (eg, x-rays, positron emission tomography [PET] scan, computed tomography [CT] scan, magnetic resonance imaging [MRI])—detect deep nodal involvement.
5. Gallium-67 scan—detects areas of active disease and may be used to determine aggressiveness of disease.
6. Liver function tests—determine hepatic involvement; liver biopsy may be indicated if results abnormal.
7. Lymphangiogram—detects size and location of deep nodes involved, including abdominal nodes, which may not be readily seen via CT scan.
8. Surgical staging (laparotomy with splenectomy, liver biopsy, and multiple lymph node biopsies)—in selected patients.

Management

Choice of treatment depends on extent of disease, histopathologic findings, and prognostic indicators. Hodgkin lymphoma is more readily cured than other lymphomas, with a 5-year survival rate of 80%. The NCCN guidelines for Hodgkin lymphoma (*www.nccn.org*) provide recommendations for diagnosis and treatment with chemotherapy, chemotherapy and radiation, and/or hematopoietic stem cell transplant for select patients. Hodgkin lymphoma arising in presence of HIV requires specialized treatment.

1. Radiation therapy.
   a. Treatment of choice for localized disease.
   b. Areas of body where lymph node chains are located can generally tolerate high radiation doses.
   c. Vital organs are protected with lead shielding during radiation treatments.
2. Chemotherapy.
   a. Initial treatment commonly consists of ABVD regimen of doxorubicin (Adriamycin), bleomycin, vinblastine (Velban), and dacarbazine; or MOPP regimen of nitrogen mustard (Mustargen), vincristine (Oncovin), procarbazine, and prednisone.
   b. Three or four drugs may be given in intermittent or cyclical courses with periods off treatment to allow recovery from toxicities.
   c. Brentuximab vedotin is an antibody drug conjugate that targets CD30 positive cells and has shown to be effective in treating Hodgkin lymphoma, both as part of upfront therapy and therapy for relapsed disease.
3. Autologous or allogeneic bone marrow or stem cell transplantation.

Complications

1. Adverse effects of radiation or chemotherapy (see page 763).
2. Dependent on location and extent of malignancy, but may include splenomegaly, hepatomegaly, thromboembolic complications, and spinal cord compression.

Nursing Assessment

1. Obtain health history, focusing on fatigue, fever, chills, night sweats, and swollen lymph nodes.
2. Evaluate splenomegaly, hepatomegaly, and lymphadenopathy.

Nursing Diagnoses

- Impaired Tissue Integrity related to high-dose radiation therapy.
- Impaired Oral Mucous Membrane related to high-dose radiation therapy.

Nursing Interventions

Maintaining Tissue Integrity

1. Avoid rubbing, powders, deodorants, lotions, or ointments (unless prescribed) or application of heat and cold to treated area.
2. Encourage the patient to keep the treated area clean and dry, bathing area gently with tepid water and mild soap.
3. Encourage wearing loose-fitting clothes.
4. Advise the patient to protect skin from exposure to sun, chlorine, and temperature extremes.

Preserving Oral and GI Tract Mucous Membranes

1. Encourage frequent small meals, using bland and soft diet at mild temperatures.
2. Teach the patient to avoid irritants, such as alcohol, tobacco, spices, and extreme food temperatures.
3. Administer or teach self-administration of pain medication or antiemetic before eating or drinking, if needed.
4. Encourage mouth care at least twice per day and after meals using gentle flossing, soft toothbrush or toothette, and mild mouth rinse.
5. Assess for ulcers, plaques, or discharge that may be indicative of superimposed infection.
6. For diarrhea, switch to low-residue diet and administer antidiarrheals, as ordered.

Patient Education and Health Maintenance

1. Teach the patient about risk of infection (see page 761).
2. Teach the patient how to take medications, as ordered, and instruct about possible adverse effects and management.
3. Explain to the patient that radiation therapy may cause sterility; men should be given opportunity for sperm banking before treatment; women may develop ovarian failure and require hormone replacement therapy.
4. Reassure the patient that fatigue will decrease after treatment is completed; encourage frequent naps and rest periods.
5. Provide the patient and family with information about resources in the community (see page 765).

Evaluation: Expected Outcomes

- Skin intact without erythema or swelling.
- Oral mucosa intact, patient eating.

Non-Hodgkin Lymphomas

Non-Hodgkin lymphomas are a group of malignancies of lymphoid tissue arising from T or B lymphocytes or their precursors; it includes both indolent and aggressive forms. In the United States, B-cell lymphomas represent about 80% of all cases. Types of non-Hodgkin lymphomas include chronic lymphocytic leukemia or small lymphocytic lymphoma (CLL/SLL; see page 766), follicular lymphoma, diffuse large B-cell lymphoma, and primary cutaneous B-cell lymphoma.

Pathophysiology and Etiology

1. Association with defective or altered immune system; higher incidence in patients receiving immunosuppression for organ transplant, in HIV-positive people, and in people with some viruses (eg, HTLV-1 and Epstein-Barr). Other risk factors include family history, male gender, white ethnicity, autoimmune diseases such as rheumatoid arthritis, history of *Helicobacter* gastritis (for gastric B-cell lymphoma), history of Hodgkin lymphoma, history of radiation therapy, diet high in meats and fat, and exposure to certain pesticides.
2. Arise from malignant transformation of lymphocyte at some stage during development; level of differentiation and type of lymphocyte influences course of illness and prognosis.
3. Incidence rises steadily from age 40.

Clinical Manifestations

1. Common symptoms include painless enlargement of lymph nodes (generally unilateral); fever; chills; night sweats; weight loss; unexplained pain in chest, abdomen, or bones. Unlike Hodgkin lymphoma, is more likely to be advanced disease at presentation.
2. Various symptoms may occur with pulmonary involvement, superior vena cava obstruction, and hepatic or bone involvement.

Diagnostic Evaluation

1. Incisional or excisional lymph node biopsy to detect type.
2. CBC, bone marrow aspirate, and biopsy to detect bone marrow involvement.
3. CT scan of the chest, abdomen, and pelvis with oral and intravenous contrast or PET with CT scan to detect deep nodal involvement.
4. Liver function tests, liver scan to detect liver involvement. Hepatitis B testing is recommended because of risk of reactivation.
5. Lumbar puncture to detect CNS involvement (for some lymphoma types).
6. Surgical staging (laparotomy with splenectomy, liver biopsy, multiple lymph node biopsies).

Management

1. The NCCN guidelines for non-Hodgkin lymphomas (*www.nccn.org*) describe a variety of regimens, using radiation therapy, chemotherapy, monoclonal antibodies, radioimmune therapy, and hematopoietic stem cell transplant. Precise diagnosis and staging is needed to ensure appropriate treatment.
2. Radiation therapy is generally palliative, not curative.
3. Chemotherapy: various regimens available, including CHOP regimen of cyclophosphamide, doxorubicin (Adriamycin), vincristine (Oncovin), and prednisone; or BACOP regimen of bleomycin, doxorubicin (Adriamycin), cyclophosphamide, vincristine (Oncovin), and prednisone.
4. Monoclonal antibody therapy: rituximab may be given alone or with chemotherapy to patients with CD20 positive lymphomas. Hepatitis B-positive patients receiving rituximab are at high risk for reactivation and need antiviral prophylaxis and close monitoring.
5. Radioimmune therapies, such as yttrium-90–labeled ibritumomab tiuxetan and ^{131}I tositumomab, have been effective

for patients with certain lymphomas who do not respond to rituximab.

6. There are also many new therapies currently being studied as a more targeted approach to the treatment of specific gene mutations found in non-Hodgkin lymphoma.

7. Autologous or allogeneic bone marrow or stem cell transplantation.

Complications

1. Of radiation therapy and chemotherapy (see page 763).
2. Of disease: depends on location and extent of malignancy, but may include splenomegaly, hepatomegaly, thromboembolic complications, and spinal cord compression.

Nursing Assessment

1. Obtain health history, focusing on fatigue, fever, chills, night sweats, swollen lymph nodes, and history of illness or therapy causing immunosuppression.
2. Evaluate splenomegaly, hepatomegaly, and lymphadenopathy.

Nursing Diagnosis

- Risk for Infection related to altered immune response because of lymphoma and leukopenia caused by chemotherapy or radiation therapy.

Nursing Interventions

Minimizing Risk of Infection

1. Care for patient in protected environment with strict hand washing observed.
2. Avoid invasive procedures, such as urinary catheterization, if possible.
3. Assess temperature and vital signs, breath sounds, LOC, and skin and mucous membranes frequently for signs of infection.
4. Notify the health care provider of fever greater than 101°F (38.3°C) or change in condition.
5. Obtain cultures of suspected infected sites or body fluids.

Patient Education and Health Maintenance

1. Teach the patient infection precautions (see page 761).
2. Encourage frequent follow-up visits for monitoring of CBC and condition.
3. Provide the patient and family with information about resources in the community (see page 765).

Evaluation: Expected Outcomes

- Remains afebrile with no signs or symptoms of infection.

Multiple Myeloma

Multiple myeloma is a malignant disorder of plasma cells accounting for approximately 13% of all hematologic malignancies.

 EVIDENCE BASE Terpos, E., International Myeloma Society. (2017). Multiple myeloma: Clinical updates from the American Society of Hematology Annual Meeting 2016. *Clinical Lymphoma, Myeloma and Leukemia,* 17(6), 329–339.

Pathophysiology and Etiology

1. Etiology unknown; genetic and environmental factors, such as chronic exposure to low levels of ionizing radiation and agricultural exposures to herbicides, may play a part.
2. Characterized by proliferation of neoplastic plasma cells derived from one B lymphocyte (clone) and producing a homogeneous immunoglobulin (M protein or Bence Jones protein) without any apparent antigenic stimulation.
3. Plasma cells produce osteoclast-activating factor leading to extensive bone loss, severe pain, and pathologic fractures.
4. Abnormal immunoglobulin affects renal function, platelet function, resistance to infection, and may cause hyperviscosity of blood.
5. Generally affects older people (median age at diagnosis is 68) and is twice as common among African Americans as among Caucasians.

Clinical Manifestations

1. Constant, usually severe bone pain caused by bone lesions and pathologic fractures; sites commonly affected include thoracic and lumbar vertebrae, ribs, skull, pelvis, and proximal long bones.
2. Fatigue and weakness related to anemia caused by crowding of marrow by plasma cells.
3. Proteinuria and renal insufficiency.
4. Electrolyte disturbances, including hypercalcemia (bone destruction) and hyperuricemia (cell death, renal insufficiency).

Diagnostic Evaluation

1. Bone marrow aspiration and biopsy—demonstrate increased number and abnormal form of plasma cells.
2. CBC and blood smear—changes reflect anemia.
3. Urine and serum analysis for presence and quantity of abnormal immunoglobulin.
4. Skeletal x-rays—osteolytic bone lesions.

Management

1. Patients with "smoldering" multiple myeloma do not require treatment.
2. The NCCN guidelines for symptomatic multiple myeloma (*www.nccn.org*) and other clinical guidelines currently recommend two treatment approaches: either melphalan plus thalidomide or melphalan plus bortezomib as initial treatment.
   a. Melphalan is a chemotherapy agent.
   b. Thalidomide is an antiangiogenesis agent and bortezomib is a proteasome inhibitor.
   c. Another option is low-dose dexamethasone plus lenalidomide, a structural analogue of thalidomide.
3. Autologous bone marrow or peripheral blood stem cell transplant in selected cases (usually younger than age 65 with no renal failure, few bone lesions, and good organ function).
4. Supportive care options:
   a. Plasmapheresis to treat hyperviscosity or bleeding.
   b. Radiation therapy for bone lesions.
   c. Bisphosphonates (eg, pamidronate), potent inhibitors of bone resorption, to treat hypercalcemia and alleviate bone pain.
   d. Allopurinol and fluids to treat hyperuricemia.
   e. Hemodialysis to manage renal failure.
   f. Surgical stabilization and fixation of fractures.

DRUG ALERT Pamidronate and other bisphosphonates may cause transient temperature elevations, hypophosphatemia, hypomagnesemia, hypocalcemia, and local reactions at the site of IV administration, such as thrombophlebitis, pain, and erythema. Bisphosphonates are administered as IV infusions, generally during 4 or more hours; rapid IV administration may cause renal failure. Long-term bisphosphonate use has been associated with jaw osteonecrosis—patients should be monitored closely and advised to maintain good oral health and avoid invasive dental procedures.

Complications

1. Pathologic fractures, spinal cord compression.
2. Recurrent infections, particularly bacterial.
3. Electrolyte abnormalities (hypercalcemia, hypophosphatemia).
4. Renal failure, pyelonephritis.
5. Bleeding.
6. Thromboembolic complications caused by hyperviscosity.
7. Patients with multiple myeloma treated by chemotherapy have a median survival of 2 to 3 years; the impact of newer treatment options on survival is still unknown.

Nursing Assessment

1. Obtain health history, focusing on pain, fatigue.
2. Evaluate for evidence of bone deformities and bone tenderness or pain.
3. Assess the patient's support system and personal coping skills.

Nursing Diagnoses

- Acute Pain related to destruction of bone and possible pathologic fractures.
- Impaired Physical Mobility related to pain and possible fracture.
- Fear related to poor prognosis.
- Risk for Injury related to complications of disease process.

Nursing Interventions

Controlling Pain

1. Assess for presence, location, intensity, and characteristics of pain.
2. Administer pharmacologic agents, as ordered, to control pain. Use adequate doses of regularly scheduled, around-the-clock analgesics.
3. Teach the use of nonpharmacologic methods, such as music, relaxation breathing, progressive muscle relaxation, distraction, and imagery, to help manage pain.
4. Assess effectiveness of analgesics and adjust dosage or drug used, as necessary, to control pain.

Promoting Mobility

1. Encourage the patient to wear a back brace for lumbar lesion.
2. Recommend physical and occupational therapy consultation.
3. Discourage bed rest to prevent hypercalcemia but ensure safety of environment to prevent fractures.
4. Assist the patient with measures to prevent injury and decrease risk of fractures. Advise avoidance of lifting and straining; use walker and other assistive devices, as appropriate.

Relieving Fear

1. Develop trusting, supportive relationship with the patient and his or her significant others.
2. Encourage the patient to discuss medical condition and prognosis with the health care provider when the patient is ready.
3. Assure the patient that you are available for support, to provide comfort measures, and to answer questions.
4. Encourage use of the patient's own support network, religious and community services, and national agencies.

Monitoring for Complications

1. Report sudden, severe pain, especially of back, which could indicate pathologic fracture.
2. Provide assistance, safety precautions, and supervision to prevent injury.
3. Watch for nausea, drowsiness, confusion, polyuria, which could indicate hypercalcemia caused by bony destruction or immobilization. Monitor serum calcium levels.
4. Check results of blood urea nitrogen (BUN) and creatinine and urine protein tests to detect renal insufficiency, caused by nephrotoxicity of abnormal proteins in multiple myeloma.
5. Increase fluid intake, monitor intake and output, and weigh the patient daily.

Community and Home Care Considerations

1. Make sure that the patient has appropriate housing and equipment to support decreased mobility and risk of pathologic fractures (eg, stair handrails, cane or walker, commode chair).
2. Inspect home environment for throw rugs, cluttered furnishings, dark hallways, or difficult stairs that may cause a fall and possible fracture.

Patient Education and Health Maintenance

1. Teach the patient about risk of infection caused by impaired antibody production and chemotherapy (see page 761).
2. Teach the patient to take medications, as prescribed, and monitor for possible adverse effects; avoid aspirin and NSAIDs unless prescribed by health care provider because these drugs may interfere with platelet function.
3. Teach the patient to minimize risk of fractures. Use proper body mechanics and assistive devices, as appropriate; avoid bed rest, remain ambulatory.
4. Advise the patient to report new onset of pain, new location, or sudden increase in pain intensity immediately. Report new onset or worsening of neurologic symptoms (eg, changes in sensation) immediately.
5. Encourage the patient to maintain high fluid intake (2 to 3 L/day) to avoid dehydration and prevent renal insufficiency; also not to fast before diagnostic tests.
6. Provide the patient and family with information about resources in the community (see page 765).

Evaluation: Expected Outcomes

- States decreased pain.
- Ambulates without injury.
- Asks questions about disease; contacts support group.
- No development of complications.

BLEEDING DISORDERS

Bleeding disorders may be congenital or acquired and may be caused by dysfunction in any phase of hemostasis (clot formation and dissolution). Bleeding disorders seen in adults include thrombocytopenia, idiopathic thrombocytopenic purpura (ITP), DIC, and von Willebrand disease.

Thrombocytopenia

Thrombocytopenia is characterized by a decreased platelet count (less than 150,000/mm³), the most common cause of bleeding disorders.

Pathophysiology and Etiology

Classification by Etiology

1. Decreased platelet production—infiltrative diseases of bone marrow, leukemia, aplastic anemia, myelofibrosis, myelosuppressive therapy, and radiation therapy; may include inherited disorders, such as Fanconi anemia and Wiskott-Aldrich syndrome.
2. Increased platelet destruction—infection (eg, HIV or hepatitis C), drug-induced (eg, heparin or quinidine), ITP, and DIC.
3. Abnormal distribution or sequestration in spleen.
4. Dilutional thrombocytopenia—after hemorrhage, RBC transfusions.

Clinical Manifestations

1. Usually asymptomatic.
2. When platelet count drops below 20,000/mm³:
   a. Petechiae occur spontaneously.
   b. Ecchymoses occur at sites of minor trauma (venipuncture, pressure).
   c. Bleeding may occur from mucosal surfaces, nose, GI and GU tracts, respiratory system, and within CNS.
   d. Menorrhagia is common.
3. Excessive bleeding may occur after procedures (dental extractions, minor surgery, biopsies).
4. Thrombotic complications (arterial and venous) and areas of skin necrosis are associated with heparin-induced thrombocytopenia.

Diagnostic Evaluation

1. CBC with platelet count—decreased hemoglobin, hematocrit, platelets.
2. Bleeding time, prothrombin time (PT), partial thromboplastin time (PTT)—prolonged.
3. Platelet aggregation test for heparin-dependent platelet antibodies—positive.

Management

1. Treat underlying cause.
2. Platelet transfusions.
3. Steroids or IV immunoglobulins may be helpful in selected patients.
4. Heparin-induced thrombocytopenia: discontinue heparin, use alternate anticoagulant therapy because of high risk of venous and arterial thromboses in these patients (direct thrombin inhibitors, such as lepirudin or argatroban hirudin), and avoid platelet transfusions. Although incidence varies dependent upon patient population and heparin preparation, any exposure to heparin can precipitate this serious autoimmune syndrome.

Complications

Severe blood loss or bleeding into vital organs may be life threatening.

Nursing Assessment

1. Obtain health history, focusing on prior illnesses and episodes of bleeding, past surgical experiences, exposure to toxins or ionizing radiation, and family history of bleeding.
2. Obtain list of current and recent medications (including OTC preparations, herbal and dietary supplements).
3. Perform complete physical examination for signs of bleeding.

Nursing Diagnosis

• Risk for Bleeding related to thrombocytopenia.

Nursing Interventions

Minimizing Bleeding

1. Institute bleeding precautions.
   a. Avoid use of plain razor, hard toothbrush or floss, IM injections, tourniquets, rectal procedures, and suppositories.
   b. Administer stool softeners, as necessary, to prevent constipation.
   c. Restrict activity and exercise when platelet count is less than 20,000/mm³ or when active bleeding occurs.
2. Monitor pad count and amount of saturation during menses; administer or teach self-administration of hormones to suppress menstruation, as prescribed.
3. Administer blood products, as ordered. Monitor for signs and symptoms of allergic reactions, anaphylaxis, and volume overload.
4. Evaluate urine, stools, and emesis for gross and occult blood.

Patient Education and Health Maintenance

1. Teach the patient bleeding precautions (see page 761).
2. Demonstrate the use of direct, steady pressure at bleeding site if bleeding develops.
3. Encourage routine follow-up for platelet counts.

Evaluation: Expected Outcomes

• Episodes of bleeding rapidly controlled; platelet count maintained at goal (usually 20,000/mm³).

Idiopathic Thrombocytopenic Purpura

Idiopathic thrombocytopenic purpura (ITP), is an acute or chronic bleeding disorder that results from immune destruction of platelets by antiplatelet antibodies.

Pathophysiology and Etiology

1. Proteins on the platelet cell membrane stimulate production of autoantibodies that bind to circulating platelets, leading to destruction of platelets in spleen and liver.
2. Acute disorder more common in childhood, typically following viral illness; has good prognosis, with 80% to 90% recovering uneventfully within 6 months.
3. Chronic disorder (more than 6-month course) most common between ages 20 and 50, three times more common in women, may last for years or even indefinitely. May be associated with pregnancy or with development of systemic lupus erythematosus, thyroid disease, and infections (eg, *Helicobater pylori*, cytomegalovirus, varicella zoster, hepatitis C, and HIV) or malignancy (eg, CLL).

Clinical Manifestations

May have no signs and symptoms with mild disease (platelet counts 30,000 to 100,000/mm³). Platelet counts less than 30,000/mm³: bruising, petechiae, bleeding from nares and gums, and menorrhagia.

Diagnostic Evaluation

1. CBC demonstrates platelet count less than 100,000/mm³; may also be lymphocytosis and eosinophilia.
2. Testing for hepatitis C, HIV, *Helicobacter pylori*, and Epstein-Barr virus, which have been found to be associated with ITP.
3. Bone marrow aspirate (not necessary for most patients with typical features of ITP) shows increased numbers of young megakaryocytes, sometimes increased numbers of eosinophils.
4. Assay for platelet autoantibodies sometimes helpful.
5. Bleeding times are typically normal.

Management

1. Supportive care: judicious use of platelet transfusions, control of bleeding.
2. High-dose corticosteroids, IV immunoglobulins, and parenteral anti-D (for Rhesus-positive patients with spleens). Thrombopoietin receptor agonists may be used to treat patients at risk for bleeding with chronic or relapsed ITP.
3. Splenectomy (see page 756) removes potential site for sequestration and destruction of platelets and is used to treat chronic refractory ITP in adults.

Complications

Severe blood loss or bleeding into vital organs may be life threatening.

Nursing Assessment

1. Obtain history of bleeding episodes, including bruising and petechiae, bleeding of gums, and heavy menses.
2. Perform physical examination for signs of bleeding.

Nursing Diagnosis

• Risk for Bleeding related to thrombocytopenia.

Nursing Interventions

Minimizing Bleeding

1. Institute bleeding precautions.
2. Monitor pad count and amount of saturation during menses; administer or teach self-administration of hormones to suppress menstruation, as prescribed.
3. Administer blood products, as ordered. Monitor for signs and symptoms of allergic reactions, anaphylaxis, and volume overload.
4. Evaluate all urine and stools for gross and occult blood.

Patient Education and Health Maintenance

1. Teach the patient bleeding precautions (see page 761).
2. Demonstrate the use of direct, steady pressure at bleeding site if bleeding does develop.
3. Encourage routine follow-up for platelet counts.

Evaluation: Expected Outcomes

• Episodes of bleeding rapidly controlled.

Disseminated Intravascular Coagulation

Disseminated intravascular coagulation (DIC) is an acquired thrombotic and hemorrhagic syndrome characterized by abnormal activation of the clotting cascade and accelerated fibrinolysis. This results in widespread clotting in small vessels with consumption of clotting factors and platelets, so that bleeding and thrombosis occur simultaneously.

Pathophysiology and Etiology

1. A syndrome arising secondary to an underlying disorder or event.
   a. Overwhelming infections, particularly bacterial sepsis.
   b. Obstetric complications: abruptio placentae, eclampsia, amniotic fluid embolism, retention of dead fetus.
   c. Massive tissue injury: burns, trauma, fractures, major surgery, fat embolism, organ destruction (eg, severe pancreatitis, hepatic failure).
   d. Malignancy: particularly lung, colon, stomach, and pancreas.
   e. Vascular and circulatory collapse, shock.
   f. Severe toxic or immunologic reactions: hemolytic transfusion reaction, snake bites, recreational drugs.

Clinical Manifestations

1. Signs of abnormal clotting:
   a. Coolness and mottling of extremities.
   b. Acrocyanosis (cold, mottled extremities with clear demarcation from normal tissue).
   c. Dyspnea, adventitious breath sounds.
   d. Altered mental status.
   e. Acute renal failure.
   f. Pain (eg, related to bowel infarction).
2. Signs of abnormal bleeding:
   a. Oozing, bleeding from sites of procedures, IV catheter insertion sites, suture lines, mucous membranes, and orifices.
   b. Internal bleeding leading to changes in vital organ function, altered vital signs.

Diagnostic Evaluation

1. Platelet count—diminished.
2. PT, PTT, and thrombin time—prolonged.
3. Fibrinogen—decreased level.
4. Fibrin split (degradation) products—increased level.
5. D-dimer fibrin degradation product—increased level.
6. Antithrombin III—decreased level.
7. Protein C—decreased level.

Management

1. Treat underlying disorder.
2. Replacement therapy for serious hemorrhagic manifestations:
   a. Fresh frozen plasma replaces clotting factors.
   b. Platelet transfusions.
   c. Cryoprecipitate replaces clotting factors and fibrinogen.
3. Supportive measures including fluid replacement, oxygenation, maintenance of BP, and renal perfusion.
4. Heparin or other anticoagulant therapy (controversial) inhibits clotting component of DIC.

Complications

1. Thromboembolic: pulmonary embolism; cerebral, myocardial, splenic, or bowel infarction; acute renal failure; tissue necrosis or gangrene.
2. Hemorrhagic: cerebral hemorrhage is the most common cause of death in DIC.

Nursing Assessment

1. Be aware that seriously ill patients are at risk; monitor condition closely.
2. Assess for signs of bleeding and thrombosis, including chest pain, shortness of breath, hematuria, abdominal pain, headache, and numbness and coolness of an extremity.

Nursing Diagnoses

- Risk for Bleeding related to thrombocytopenia.
- Ineffective Tissue Perfusion (all tissues) related to ischemia due to microthrombi formation.

Nursing Interventions

Minimizing Bleeding

1. Institute bleeding precautions.
2. Monitor pad count and amount of saturation during menses; administer or teach self-administration of hormones to suppress menstruation, as prescribed.
3. Administer blood products, as ordered. Monitor for signs and symptoms of allergic reactions, anaphylaxis, and volume overload.
4. Avoid dislodging clots. Apply pressure to sites of bleeding for at least 20 minutes, use topical hemostatic agents. Use tape cautiously.
5. Maintain bed rest during bleeding episode.
6. If internal bleeding is suspected, assess bowel sounds and abdominal girth.
7. Evaluate fluid status and bleeding by frequent measurement of vital signs, central venous pressure, intake, and output.

Promoting Tissue Perfusion

1. Keep the patient warm.
2. Avoid vasoconstrictive agents (systemic or topical).
3. Change the patient's position frequently and perform range-of-motion exercises.
4. Monitor electrocardiogram and laboratory tests for dysfunction of vital organs caused by ischemia—arrhythmias, abnormal arterial blood gas levels, and increased BUN and creatinine levels.
5. Monitor for signs of vascular occlusion and report immediately.
   a. Brain—decreased LOC, sensory and motor deficits, seizures, and coma.
   b. Eyes—visual deficits.
   c. Bone—bone pain.
   d. Pulmonary vasculature—chest pain, shortness of breath, tachycardia.
   e. Extremities—cold, mottling, numbness.
   f. Coronary arteries—chest pain, arrhythmias.
   g. Bowel—pain, tenderness, decreased bowel sounds.

Patient Education and Health Maintenance

Explain the syndrome and its management to the patient and family members as part of reassurance and support during this critical illness.

Evaluation: Expected Outcomes

- Episodes of bleeding rapidly controlled.
- Alert, vital signs stable, urine output adequate, and no complaints of chest pain or shortness of breath.

von Willebrand Disease

von Willebrand disease is an inherited (autosomal dominant) or acquired bleeding disorder characterized by decreased level of von Willebrand factor and prolonged bleeding time.

Pathophysiology and Etiology

1. von Willebrand factor synthesized in vascular endothelium, megakaryocytes, and platelets; enhances platelet adhesion as first step in clot formation, also acts as carrier of factor VIII in blood.
2. von Willebrand is most common inherited bleeding disorder, with estimated incidence as high as 1 in 90 people; includes multiple subtypes with varying severity; affects males and females.
3. Acquired form is rare, generally appears late in life, typically in association with lymphoma, leukemia, multiple myeloma, or autoimmune disorder.

Clinical Manifestations

1. Mucosal and cutaneous bleeding (eg, bruising, gingival bleeding, epistaxis, menorrhagia).
2. Prolonged bleeding from cuts or after dental and surgical procedures.

Diagnostic Evaluation

1. Bleeding time—prolonged.
2. Ristocetin cofactor—abnormal.
3. von Willebrand factor—decreased.
4. von Willebrand factor multimers—demonstrate defective von Willebrand factor in some types.
5. Factor VIII—generally decreased.

Management

1. Replacement of von Willebrand factor and factor VIII using clotting factor concentrates.
2. Antifibrinolytic medications (aminocaproic acid, tranexamic acid) to stabilize clot formation before dental procedures and before minor surgery.
3. Desmopressin acetate, a synthetic analogue of vasopressin, may be used to manage mild to moderate bleeding.
4. Estrogen and progesterone stimulate production of von Willebrand factor and factor VIII and may be particularly helpful in control of menorrhagia.

Complications

Severe blood loss or bleeding into vital organs may be life threatening.

Nursing Assessment

1. Obtain history of bleeding episodes such as menstrual flow. Ask quantitative questions (eg, how many nosebleeds do you have each year?) as the patient may not realize his or her experience is abnormal.
2. Perform physical examination for signs of bleeding.

Nursing Diagnosis

- Risk for Bleeding related to decreased level of von Willebrand factor and factor VIII.

Nursing Interventions

Minimizing Bleeding

1. Institute bleeding precautions:
   a. Avoid use of plain razor, hard toothbrush, or floss.
   b. Avoid IM injections, tourniquets, rectal procedures, or suppositories.
   c. Administer stool softeners, as necessary, to prevent constipation.
   d. Restrict activity and exercise when platelet count less than 20,000/mm^3 or when active bleeding occurs.
2. Monitor pad count and amount of saturation during menses; administer or teach self-administration of hormones to suppress menstruation, as prescribed.
3. Administer blood products, as ordered. Monitor for signs and symptoms of allergic reactions, anaphylaxis, and volume overload.
4. Use topical hemostatic agents, such as absorbable gelatin, oxidized cellulose, topical adrenaline, or phenylephrine, if pressure and use of ice does not stop bleeding.

Patient Education and Health Maintenance

1. Teach the patient bleeding precautions (see page 761).
2. Demonstrate the use of direct, steady pressure at bleeding site if bleeding develops.

Evaluation: Expected Outcomes

- Episodes of bleeding rapidly controlled.

SELECTED REFERENCES

Alaqzam, T.S., Stanley, A.C., Simpson, P. M., et al. (2018). Treatment modalities in adolescents who present with heavy menstrual bleeding. *Journal of Pediatric & Adolescent Gynecology*. Advanced online publication. doi: 10.1016/j.jpag.2018.02.130.

Blaisdel, F. W. (2012). Causes, prevention, and treatment of intravascular coagulation and disseminated intravascular coagulation. *Journal of Trauma and Acute Care Surgery, 72*(6), 1719–1722.

Boddu, P. C., & Kadia, T. M. (2017). Updates on the pathophysiology and treatment of aplastic anemia: A comprehensive review. *Expert Review of Hematology, 10*(5), 433–448.

Castaman, G., & Linari, S. (2017). Diagnosis and treatment of von Willebrand disease and rare bleeding disorders. *Journal of Clinical Medicine, 6*(4), 45.

Cao, J., Wang, G., Cheng, H., et al. (2018). Potent anti-luxemica activities of humanized CD19-targeted CAR-T cells in patients with relapsed/refractory acute lymphoblastic leukemia. *American Journal of Hematology*. Advanced online publication. doi: 10.1002/ajh.25108.

Cornell, R. F., & Palmer, J. (2012). Adult acute leukemia. *Disease-A-Month, 58*, 219–238.

Dragomir, M., Petrescu, D. G. E., Manga, G. E., Călin, G. A., & Vasilescu, C. (2016). Patients after splenectomy: Old risks and new perspectives. *Chirurgia, 111*(5), 393–399.

Grimaldi-Bensouda, L., Nordon, C., Leblanc, T., et al. (2017). Childhood immune thrombocytopenia: A nationwide cohort study on condition management and outcomes. *Pediatric Blood and Cancer, 64*(7).

Hartmann, J., & Croteau, S. E. (2016). Clinical trials update: Innovations in hemophilia therapy. *American Journal of Hematology, 91*(12), 1252–1260.

Lambert, M. P., & Gernsheimer, T. B. (2017). Clinical updates in adult immune thrombocytopenia. *Blood, 129*(21), 2829–2835.

Larsen, M.A., Larsen, J.B., & Hvas, A. M. (2018). Platelet function in disseminated intravascular coagulation: a systemic review. *Platelets*. Advanced online publication. doi: 10.1080/09537104.2018.1442567.

Meenaghan, T., Dowling, M., & Kelly, M. (2012). Acute leukaemia: Making sense of a complex blood cancer. *British Journal of Nursing, 21*(2), 76–83.

Peslak, S.A., Olson, T., & Babushok, D.V. (2017). Diagnosis and treatment of aplastic anemia. *Current Treatment Options in Oncology, 18*(12), 70.

Rodeghiero, F. (2018). A critical appraisal of the evidence for the role of splenectomy in adults and children with ITP. *British Journal of Haematology*. Advance online publication. doi: 10.1111/bjh.15090.

Tefferi, A., & Barbui, T. (2017). Polycythemia vera and essential thrombocythemia: 2017 update on diagnosis, risk-stratification, and management. *American Journal of Hematology, 92*(1), 94–108.

Terpos, E.; International Myeloma Society. (2017). Multiple myeloma: Clinical updates from the American Society of Hematology Annual Meeting 2016. *Clinical Lymphoma, Myeloma and Leukemia, 17*(6), 329–339.

Weiss, J. A. (2012). Just heavy menses or something more? Raising awareness of von Willebrand disease. *American Journal of Nursing, 112*(6), 38–44.

27

Transfusion Therapy and Blood and Marrow Stem Cell Transplantation

TRANSFUSION THERAPY

 See additional online content: Procedure Guidelines 27-1

Principles of Transfusion Therapy

Because of the potentially life-threatening consequences of blood type ABO incompatibility and disease transmission through blood products, transfusion therapy is limited to occasions when it is absolutely necessary, and stringent screening techniques are required before transfusion begins. Alternatives to transfusion therapy should also be considered, as appropriate, such as erythropoietin-stimulating agents, iron supplementation, blood loss prevention during surgery, and volume replacement with other solutions. Blood product procurement, storage, preparation, and testing are regulated by the Food and Drug Administration (FDA), the American Association of Blood Banks, and the Joint Commission.

Blood Compatibility

Antigens

1. The surface membrane of the red blood cell (RBC) is characterized by glycoproteins known as antigens.
2. More than 400 different antigens have been identified on the RBC membrane.
3. There are fewer than a dozen clinically significant antigens, and of these, only two antigenic systems (ABO and Rh) require routine prospective matching before the transfusion.
4. The ABO blood group system is clinically the most significant because A and B antigens elicit the strongest immune response.
5. The presence or absence of A and B antigens on the RBC membrane determines the person's ABO group (see Table 27-1). The ability to make A or B antigens is inherited.

6. Antibody formation without specific exposure to the antigen is unique to the ABO system. Antibody directed against the missing antigens is produced in neonates by 3 months of age.

Antibodies

1. Antibodies (or immunoglobulins) are proteins produced by B lymphocytes; they consist of two light and two heavy chains that form a Y shape.
2. Antibodies generally have a high degree of specificity and interact only with the antigen that stimulated their production.
3. The five classes of immunoglobulins are determined by differences in their heavy chains: immunoglobulins (Ig) G, IgA, IgM, IgD, and IgE.
4. The interaction of antibodies and antigens triggers the humoral immune response.
5. Antibodies against the A and B antigens are large IgM molecules. When they interact with and coat the A and B antigens on the RBC surface, the antibody/RBC complexes clump together (agglutinate).
6. Antibody/RBC complexes also activate the complement cascade, resulting in the release of numerous active substances and RBC lysis. The large antibody/RBC complexes also become trapped in capillaries, where they may cause thrombotic complications to vital organs, and in the reticuloendothelial system, where they are removed from circulation by the spleen.
7. The extent of the humoral response elicited by anti-A and anti-B interaction with A and B antigens depends on the quantity of antibody and antigen.

Other Red Blood Cell Antigens

1. Non-ABO RBC antigen–antibody reactions usually do not produce powerful immediate hemolytic reactions but several have clinical significance.
2. After A and B, D is the most immunogenic antigen. It is part of the rhesus system, which includes C, D, and E antigens.

Table 27-1	Blood Group Antigens and Antibodies of ABO System		
BLOOD GROUP	**ANTIGEN ON RBC**	**ANTIBODY IN PLASMA**	**APPROXIMATE FREQUENCY OF OCCURRENCE IN POPULATION**
A	A	Anti-B	45%
B	B	Anti-A	8%
AB	A and B	None	3%
O	None	Anti-A and anti-B	44%

a. D (Rh)–negative people do not develop anti-D without specific exposure, but have a high incidence of antibody development (alloimmunization) after exposure to D.

b. Two common methods of sensitization to these RBC antigens are by transfusion or fetomaternal hemorrhage during pregnancy and delivery.

c. Anti-D can complicate future transfusions and pregnancies. For the D (Rh)–negative person, exposure to D should be avoided by the use of Rh-negative blood products. In the case of Rh-negative mother and Rh-positive fetus, prophylaxis for exposure to D uses Rh immunoglobulin (RhoGAM), which will prevent anti-D formation.

d. Exposure to RBC antigens from other antigenic systems (such as Lewis, Kidd, or Duffy) may also cause alloimmunization, which becomes clinically significant in people who receive multiple blood products for extended periods of time.

Blood Transfusion Options

Autologous Transfusion

1. Before elective procedures, the patient may donate blood to be set aside for later transfusion. Patients may donate up to 3 days prior to surgery provided hemoglobin is greater than 11 g/dL.

2. Autologous RBCs can also be salvaged during some surgical procedures or after trauma-induced hemorrhage by use of automated cell-saver devices or by manual suction equipment.

3. Autologous blood products must be clearly labeled and identified.

4. Autologous transfusion eliminates the risks of alloimmunization, immune-mediated transfusion reactions, and transmission of disease, making it the safest transfusion choice.

 NURSING ALERT Patients who do not meet standard criteria for blood donation may still be eligible to donate autologous blood before elective surgeries. The nurse should encourage suitable candidates to consider this underused option.

Homologous Transfusion

1. With this most common option, volunteer donors' blood products are assigned to patients randomly.

2. Before donation, volunteer donors receive information about the process, potential adverse effects, tests that will be performed on donated blood, postdonation instructions, and education regarding risk of human immunodeficiency virus (HIV) infection and signs and symptoms.

3. Donors are screened against eligibility criteria designed to protect donor and recipient (see Table 27-2).

Table 27-2	General Blood Donor Eligibility Criteria
Age	≥17 years *or* 16 years with parental consent if state law allows
Weight	Minimum 110 lb (49.9 kg) (additional rules apply for donors ≤18 years)
Vital signs	Afebrile, normotensive, pulse 50–100, blood pressure < 180/100 mm Hg
Hemoglobin	≥12.5 g/dL
History	Travel, exposures, and past illnesses or events may defer or disallow blood donation. *Examples*: travel to malarial areas, living in areas exposed to bovine spongiform encephalopathy, blood transfusion or tattoo within 12 months, recent surgery or pregnancy, corneal transplant, history of hepatitis or unexplained jaundice, history of blood cancer or recent cancer, history of behaviors at high risk for human immunodeficiency virus.
Immunizations	Recent attenuated and live vaccines generally result in deferral.
Illnesses	A variety of current illnesses may defer or disallow blood donation. *Examples*: clotting disorders, sickle cell disease, systemic lupus erythematosus, multiple sclerosis, Lyme disease, tuberculosis, chronic fatigue syndrome.
Medications	Blood thinners, such as heparin and warfarin, disallow donation. Some other medications may result in deferral.

 EVIDENCE BASE American Red Cross. (2017). *Donate blood: Eligibility requirements.* Available: *www.redcrossblood.org/donating-blood/eligibility-requirements.*

Directed Transfusion

1. In directed transfusion, blood products are donated by a person for transfusion to a specified recipient.

2. This option may be used in certain circumstances (eg, a parent who provides sole transfusion support for a child), but in general, no evidence exists that directed donation reduces transfusion risks.

Blood Product Screening

Serologic Testing

1. Routine laboratory testing is performed to assess the compatibility of a particular blood product with the recipient before release of the blood product from the blood bank (see Table 27-3).

   a. ABO group and Rh type: determines the presence of A, B, and D antigens on the surface of the patient's RBCs.

   b. Direct Coombs test: determines the antibody attached to the patient's RBCs.

   c. Crossmatch (compatibility test): detects agglutination of donor RBCs caused by antibodies in the patient's serum.

   d. Indirect Coombs test: identifies lower molecular weight antibodies (IgG) directed against blood group antigens.

Table 27-3   ABO and Rh Compatibility Chart

This chart identifies ABO and Rh compatibility when transfusing whole blood, red blood cells, and plasma. Components suspended in plasma, such as platelets and cryoprecipitate, usually follow plasma compatibility rules if the total volume exceeds 120 mL for an adult patient.

WHOLE BLOOD

	Donor					
Recipient	A	B	O	AB	Rh positive	Rh negative
A	✓					
B		✓				
O			✓			
AB				✓		
Rh positive					✓	✓
Rh negative						✓

RED BLOOD CELLS

	Donor					
Recipient	A	B	O	AB	Rh positive	Rh negative
A	✓		✓			
B		✓	✓			
O			✓	✓		
AB	✓	✓	✓			
Rh positive					✓	✓
Rh negative						✓

PLASMA

	Donor					
Recipient	A	B	O	AB	Rh positive	Rh negative
A	✓			✓		
B		✓		✓		
O	✓	✓	✓	✓		
AB				✓		
Rh positive					✓	✓
Rh negative					✓	✓

Screening for Infectious Diseases

1. Routine laboratory testing is performed to identify antigens or antibodies in donor blood that may indicate prior exposure to specific blood-borne diseases.
2. Such testing supplements other principles of donation designed to decrease the risk of disease transmission via blood products, including the use of volunteer donors, the exclusion of high-risk populations, and the screening of donors via health and social history.
3. Through the use of donor screening and blood testing, the risk of infections transmitted with donated blood is less than 1% and continues to decline.
4. Specific conditions screened for include:
   a. Hepatitis: Per FDA recommendations, each unit of blood is tested for the presence of hepatitis B core antibody, surface antigen, and more recently hepatitis B viral DNA through nucleic acid testing (NAT). Hepatitis C antibody and viral DNA tests (NAT) are also completed.
   b. HIV-1 and HIV-2: tests for prior exposure to the virus.
      i. All blood products in the United States have been screened since the test first became available in 1985. Current tests include testing for antibodies with enzyme-linked immunosorbent assay or enzyme immunoassay or antigen with the P24 test. NAT is becoming more widely used and provides a mechanism to look for the presence of HIV-1 and HIV-2 before antibody formation.
      ii. Because antibody to the virus is not produced until at least 6 weeks after exposure, diligent donor screening and exclusion of high-risk groups (eg, homosexual men, intravenous [IV] drug abusers, prostitutes, and sexual partners of high-risk people) remain important parts of preventing transmission of HIV via blood products.
      iii. A low risk of HIV transmission (estimated to be less than 1/2,000,000 units of blood) remains.
   c. Cytomegalovirus (CMV): tests for the antibody against CMV.
      i. Approximately 50% to 75% of blood donors have been exposed to CMV, and 10% to 20% carry CMV virus in their white blood cells (WBCs).
      ii. Patients with impaired immune function (eg, bone marrow and organ transplant recipients, premature babies) are at risk for CMV infection from transfused blood. It is recommended that these patients receive CMV-seronegative blood or leukoreduced products.
   d. Syphilis: tests for the presence of antibody against the spirochete.
   e. Bacteria: contamination of blood products with bacteria may occur during and after collection of blood. This risk is managed by adherence to sterile technique during phlebotomy and blood-processing procedures, correct storage techniques, visual inspection of blood products, and limitations on shelf life.
   f. Other infections that may be transmitted via blood transfusions include West Nile virus, human T-cell lymphoma virus (HTLV) 1 and 2, human herpesvirus 8 (implicated as the causative agent of Kaposi sarcoma), malaria, babesiosis, Chagas disease, and *Yersinia*. Variant Creutzfeldt-Jakob disease has also been transmitted via blood transfusions, which has led to restrictions on donation by individuals who have lived in areas with bovine spongiform encephalopathy or "mad cow" disease.

Administration of Whole Blood and Blood Components

Whole blood and blood components are administered to increase the amount of oxygen being delivered to the tissues and organs, to prevent or stop bleeding because of platelet defects or because of deficiencies or coagulation abnormalities, and to combat infection caused by decreased or defective WBCs or antibodies. See Standard of Care Guidelines 27-1, page 778.

General Considerations

1. A unit of whole blood is usually separated into its various components shortly after collection.
2. The use of blood components conserves the limited supply of blood, provides optimal therapeutic benefit, and reduces the risk of circulatory overload. Less than 3% of the blood collected nationwide is transfused as whole blood.

STANDARDS OF CARE GUIDELINES 27-1
Blood Transfusion

When administering whole blood or blood components, ensure the following:

- Follow up on results of complete blood count (CBC) and report to health care provider so appropriate blood product can be ordered based on patient's condition.
- Verify informed consent.
- Contact the blood bank with health care provider's order and ensure timely delivery of blood product.
- Establish a patent IV line with compatible IV fluid.
- Use appropriate administration setup, filter, warmer, etc.
- Obtain baseline vital signs.
- Ensure proper blood product is given to the right patient by verifying at least two identifiers (eg, full name and date of birth) with patient, blood product, and original order.
- Transfuse at prescribed rate during prescribed time, as tolerated by patient.
- Observe for acute reactions—allergic, febrile, septic, hemolytic, air embolism, and circulatory overload—by assessing vital signs, breath sounds, edema, flushing, urticaria, vomiting, headache, and back pain.
- Stop transfusion and notify patient's health care provider or available house officer if signs of reaction or other abnormalities occur.
- Be aware of delayed reactions and educate patient on risk and what to look for: hemolytic, iron overload, graft versus host disease, hepatitis, and other infectious diseases.

This information should serve as a general guideline only. Each patient situation presents a unique set of clinical factors and requires nursing judgment to guide care, which may include additional or alternative measures and approaches.

3. Because of the risks, blood components should be administered only with informed consent, meticulous identification procedures, careful protocol, and close monitoring.

 DRUG ALERT Crystalloid solutions other than 0.9% saline and all medications are incompatible with blood products. They may cause agglutination or hemolysis.

 KEY DECISION POINT Observe the patient closely and check vital signs at least hourly until 1 hour after transfusion. Observe for fever, chills, flushing, urticaria, difficulty breathing, anxiety, and change in vital signs. Stop transfusion and report signs of adverse effect to health care provider immediately if acute reaction is suspected.

Whole Blood

Description

1. Consists of RBCs, plasma, plasma proteins, and approximately 60-mL anticoagulant/preservative solution in a total volume of approximately 500 mL.

2. Indications include acute, massive blood loss of greater than 1,000 mL, requiring the oxygen-carrying properties of RBCs and the volume expansion provided by plasma. In general, even acute loss of as much as one third of a patient's total blood volume (1,000 to 1,200 mL) can be safely and rapidly replaced with crystalline or colloidal solutions.

Nursing and Patient Care Considerations

1. For rapid infusions of large volumes of whole blood, additional steps may be taken to deliver product rapidly and safely.
   a. A small-pore (20 to 40 mm) filter may be used to remove microaggregates (platelets, WBCs) that have been identified in the lungs of massively transfused patients.
   b. An approved blood warmer may be indicated to prevent hypothermia and cardiac arrhythmias associated with the rapid infusion of refrigerated solutions.
   c. Electromechanical infusion devices to deliver blood at high flow rates can hemolyze RBCs and should be used with caution.
2. Observe closely for the most common acute complication associated with whole blood transfusion—circulatory overload (rise in venous pressure, distended neck veins, dyspnea, cough, crackles at bases of lungs).

Packed RBCs

Description

1. Consist primarily of RBCs, a small amount of plasma, and approximately 100-mL anticoagulant/preservative solution in a total volume of approximately 250 to 300 mL/unit.
2. Packed RBCs may be contaminated with WBCs that may increase the risk of minor transfusion reactions and alloimmunization. For patients who receive multiple blood products during a specific period (eg, patients with leukemia or aplastic anemia), packed RBCs may be further manipulated to remove WBCs (leukoreduced) by washing or freezing the product in the blood bank or by the use of small-pore (20 to 40 mm) leukoreduction filters during administration.
3. Indications include restoration or maintenance of adequate organ oxygenation with minimal expansion of blood volume.
4. Dosage: average adult dose administered is 2 units; pediatric doses are generally calculated as 5 to 15 mL/kg.

Nursing and Patient Care Considerations

1. Infuse at the prescribed rate. Generally, a unit can be given to an adult in 90 to 120 minutes. Pediatric patients are usually transfused at a rate of 2 to 5 mL/kg/hour.
2. To reduce the risk of bacterial contamination and sepsis, RBCs must be transfused within 4 hours of leaving the blood bank.
3. Observe closely (particularly during first 15 to 30 minutes) for the most common acute complications associated with packed RBCs, allergic and febrile transfusion reactions. Signs and symptoms of the more serious, but rare, hemolytic transfusion reactions are usually manifested during infusion of the first 50 mL.

Platelet Concentrates

Description

1. Consist of platelets suspended in plasma. Products vary according to the number of units (each unit is a minimum of 5.5×10^{10} platelets) and the volume of plasma (50 to 400 mL).

2. Platelets may be obtained by centrifuging multiple units of whole blood and expressing off the platelet-rich plasma (multiple-donor platelets) or from a single volunteer platelet donor using automated cell separation techniques (apheresis). The use of single-donor products decreases the number of donor exposures, thus decreasing the risk of alloimmunization and transfusion-transmitted disease.

3. Patients may become alloimmunized to human leukocyte antigens (HLAs) through exposure to multiple platelet products. When this occurs, apheresis products from HLA-matched platelet donors may be necessary. However, HLA-matched transfusions are commonly difficult to obtain because of the vast number of possible HLA combinations among the human population.

4. Indications include prevention or resolution of hemorrhage in patients with thrombocytopenia or platelet dysfunction.

5. Platelet transfusions are generally contraindicated in heparin-induced thrombocytopenia, where they may precipitate arterial thrombosis, and in immune (idiopathic) thrombocytopenia, where they may worsen this autoimmune destruction of platelets.

6. Dosage: average dose is generally 1 unit of platelets for each 10 kg of body weight; however, patients who are actively bleeding or undergoing surgical procedures may require more.

Nursing and Patient Care Considerations

1. Infuse at the rate prescribed. Generally, the infusion can be completed within 20 to 60 minutes, depending on total volume.

2. Observe closely for the most common acute complications associated with platelet transfusions, allergic and febrile transfusion reactions.

3. Platelets are stored at 68°F to 75°F (20°C to 24°C), a warmer environment than other blood products and more conducive to bacterial growth. This increases the risk of bacterial contamination of a platelet product, which occurs in 4 to 10 per 10,000 units, limiting their shelf life.

Plasma (Fresh or Fresh Frozen)

Description

1. Consists of water (91%), plasma proteins including essential clotting factors (7%), and carbohydrates (2%). Each unit is the volume removed from a unit of whole blood (200 to 250 mL).

2. May be stored in a liquid state or frozen within 6 hours of collection.

3. Indications include treatment of blood loss or blood-clotting disorders related to liver disease and failure, disseminated intravascular coagulation (DIC), overanticoagulation with warfarin, all congenital or acquired clotting factor deficiencies, and dilutional coagulopathy resulting from massive blood replacement. Storage in liquid state results in the loss of labile clotting factors V and VIII, so that only plasma that has been fresh-frozen can be used to treat factor V and VIII deficiencies.

4. Dosage: depends on the clinical situation and assessment of prothrombin time, partial thromboplastin time, or specific factor assays.

Nursing and Patient Care Considerations

1. Infuse at the rate prescribed. Generally, the infusion can be completed within 15 to 30 minutes, depending on total volume.

2. Observe closely for the most common acute complication associated with plasma infusion, volume overload.

Cryoprecipitate

Description

1. Consists of certain clotting factors suspended in 10 to 20 mL plasma. Each unit contains approximately 80 to 120 units of factor VIII (antihemophilic and von Willebrand factors), 250 mg fibrinogen, and 20% to 30% of the factor XIII present in a unit of whole blood.

2. Indications include correction of deficiencies of factor VIII (ie, hemophilia A and von Willebrand disease), factor XIII, and fibrinogen (ie, DIC).

3. Dosage: adult dosage is generally 10 units, which may be repeated every 8 to 12 hours until the deficiency is corrected or until hemostasis is achieved.

Nursing and Patient Care Considerations

Infuse at the rate prescribed. Generally, the infusion can be completed within 3 to 15 minutes.

Fractionated Plasma Products

Description

1. Various highly concentrated plasma protein products are commercially prepared by pooling thousands of single plasma units and by extracting the desired protein. Most techniques involve heat or chemical treatments, which eliminate the risk of transmitting blood-borne viruses, such as hepatitis B and HIV.

2. Colloid solutions provide volume expansion in situations where crystalloid solutions are not adequate, such as therapeutic plasma exchange, shock, and massive hemorrhage. They may also be used in the treatment of acute liver failure, burns, and hemolytic disease of the neonate.
   a. Albumin is available as a 5% solution, which is oncotically equivalent to plasma, and as a concentrated 25% solution.
   b. Plasma protein fraction (PPF) is available as a 5% solution. Rapid infusion of PPF has been associated with hypotension.
   c. Albumin and PPF are pasteurized and carry no risk of viral disease. They do not contain preservatives and should be used immediately after opening.

3. Immune serum globulins (ISGs) are concentrated aqueous solutions of gamma globulin that contain high titers of antibody.
   a. Must be administered by deep intramuscular (IM) injection.
   b. Nonspecific ISG is prepared from random donor plasma and is used to increase gamma globulin levels and to enhance general immune response in mild inherited or acquired immune disorders such as hypogammaglobulinemia.
   c. Specific ISG is prepared from donors who have high antibody titers to known antigens and is used to treat specific disorders or conditions. Hepatitis B immunoglobulin, varicella-zoster immunoglobulin, and Rh immunoglobulin are examples of specific ISGs.
   d. ISGs carry no risk of hepatitis B, HIV, or other blood-borne infections.
   e. Problems associated with use include pain at the injection site, limitations on volume administered, loss of IgG into extravascular tissue, or by degradation at the injection site.

4. IV immunoglobulins (IVIGs) are aqueous solutions of immunoglobulins at a higher concentration and are given in larger volumes than ISGs.

a. Like ISGs, they may be nonspecific or specific.

b. Indications include chronic replacement therapy in patients with congenital or acquired immunodeficiency syndromes, acute autoimmune disorders such as immune (idiopathic) thrombocytopenia, and the treatment of chronic lymphocytic leukemia. Also, there are numerous investigational uses, such as Guillain-Barré syndrome, myasthenia gravis, rheumatoid arthritis, multiple sclerosis, lupus, and viral infections such as CMV, adenovirus, and influenza. IVIGs may also be used to treat platelet alloimmunization.

c. IVIGs do not appear to transmit HIV, but have been reported to transmit hepatitis C.

d. Administration of IVIG should be closely monitored because of the possibility of anaphylactic reactions. Dosage and rate of infusion depend on the manufacturer's formulation.

5. Factor VIII concentrate is a lyophilized concentrate used to treat moderate to severe hemophilia A and severe von Willebrand disease.

6. Factor IX concentrate is a lyophilized concentrate used to treat factor IX deficiency (Christmas disease).

Nursing and Patient Care Considerations

1. These products are often distributed by a pharmacy rather than by a blood bank.

2. Check order and product insert to ensure proper dosage and administration route.

Granulocyte Concentrates

Description

1. Consist of a minimum of 1×10^{10} granulocytes, variable amounts of lymphocytes (usually less than 10% of the total number of WBCs), 6 to 10 units of platelets, 30 to 50 mL RBCs, and 200 to 400 mL plasma.

2. Obtained via apheresis, generally of multiple donors.

3. Indications include treatment of life-threatening bacterial or fungal infection unresponsive to other therapy in a patient with severe neutropenia.

4. Dosage: generally 1 unit daily for approximately 5 to 10 days, discontinuing if no therapeutic response.

Nursing and Patient Care Considerations

1. Product must be ABO compatible and, if possible, Rh compatible because of the high erythrocyte content. Granulocytes are irradiated prior to transfusion to prevent the risk of graft-versus-host disease.

2. Transfuse granulocytes as soon as they are available. WBCs have a short survival time and therapeutic benefit is directly related to dose and viability.

3. Premedicate per order to prevent adverse effects, generally with antihistamine and acetaminophen. Steroids may also be required.

4. Begin the transfusion slowly and increase to the rate prescribed and as tolerated. The recommended length of infusion is 1 to 2 hours.

5. Observe the patient closely throughout the transfusion for signs and symptoms of febrile, allergic, and anaphylactic reactions, which may be severe. Have emergency medications and equipment readily available.

6. Agitate the bag approximately every 15 minutes to prevent granulocytes from clumping at the bottom of the bag.

7. Do not administer amphotericin products immediately before or after granulocyte transfusion because pulmonary insufficiency has been reported with concurrent administration of amphotericin and granulocytes. Many institutions recommend a 4-hour gap to avoid this risk.

Modified Blood Products

Purpose

1. To reduce the risk of specific transfusion-related complications, blood products may receive further processing or treatment.

   a. Leukocytes are removed from blood products through filtration, washing, and freezing to reduce the risk of febrile, nonhemolytic transfusion reactions and alloimmunization to HLA.

   b. Function and proliferation of donor lymphocytes are inhibited by irradiation, to decrease the risk of posttransfusion graft-versus-host disease (GVHD) in immunocompromised patients including oncology patients, lung or heart transplant patients, and pediatric patients under age 6.

Methods

1. Filtration.

   a. Standard filters (170 μm) effectively remove gross fibrin clots.

   b. Microaggregate filters (approximately 40 μm) remove microscopic aggregates of fibrin, platelets, and leukocytes that accumulate in RBC products during storage. Their use is recommended during rapid, massive transfusion of whole blood or packed RBCs to prevent pulmonary complications. They reduce the risk of CMV transmission and may also decrease the incidence of febrile transfusion reactions by removing many of the leukocytes present.

   c. Special leukocyte-depletion filters have been developed for use with platelet products that remove 80% to 95% of leukocytes and that retain 80% of the platelets. These filters also reduce the risk of CMV transmission.

   d. A product may be filtered before release from the blood bank, but more commonly is released with the appropriate filter that must be attached to the standard infusion set at the bedside per manufacturer's or blood bank's instructions.

2. Washing.

   a. Washing RBCs or platelets with a normal saline solution removes 80% to 95% of the WBCs and virtually all of the plasma to reduce the incidence of febrile, nonhemolytic transfusion reactions.

   b. Washing requires an additional hour of processing time, and the shelf life of the product is reduced to 24 hours after this additional manipulation.

3. Freezing.

   a. RBCs can be frozen within 7 days of blood collection and then remain viable for 7 to 10 years.

   b. Removal of the hypertonic freezing preservative (glycerol) before transfusion eliminates all of the plasma and 99% of WBCs.

   c. Thawing and deglycerolization of RBCs require an additional 90 minutes of preparation time and reduce shelf life to 24 hours after this additional manipulation.

   d. Freezing is also an effective method of storing rare blood types and autologous RBCs.

4. Irradiation.
   a. Exposure of blood products to a measured amount of gamma irradiation inhibits lymphocyte function and proliferation without damaging RBCs, platelets, or granulocytes. This eliminates the ability of transfused lymphocytes to engraft in the immunocompromised transfusion recipient and the accompanying risk of posttransfusion GVHD.
   b. Patients at risk for posttransfusion GVHD include bone marrow and peripheral stem cell transplant recipients, lung or heart transplant patients, premature neonates, and patients with congenital immunodeficiency disorders, Hodgkin and non-Hodgkin lymphomas, and HIV.

Transfusion Reactions

Every transfusion of blood components can result in an adverse effect. Reactions can be placed into two general categories: acute and delayed.

Acute Reactions

1. Acute reactions may occur during the infusion or within minutes to hours after the blood product has been infused.
2. Acute reactions include allergic, febrile, septic, and hemolytic reactions, air embolism, and circulatory overload. Patients who also receive multiple blood products within a short time frame may also be at risk for hyperkalemia, hypocalcemia, and hypothermia.
3. Because reactions may exhibit similar clinical manifestations, every symptom should be considered potentially serious and the transfusion should be discontinued until the cause is determined.
4. When a reaction is suspected, the health care provider should be notified immediately, and blood bags with tubing from all products recently transfused should be returned to the blood bank for evaluation.

5. The following samples should also be obtained if an acute reaction is suspected.
   a. A clotted blood specimen to examine serum for hemoglobin and confirm RBC group and type.
   b. An anticoagulated blood sample for a direct Coombs test to determine the presence of antibody on the RBCs.
   c. The first-voided urine specimen to test for hemoglobinuria (this does not need to be a clean-catch specimen).
6. Precautions must be taken to avoid the hemolysis of RBCs during venipuncture and sample collection because this could lead to invalid test results. Whenever possible, blood samples should be drawn from a fresh venipuncture and not from existing needles or catheters.
7. If the only symptoms are those resulting from a mild allergic reaction (eg, urticaria), extensive evaluation may not be necessary. In the event of a severe reaction (eg, hypotension, tachypnea), more tests may be required to determine the cause of the reaction.
8. Causes, clinical manifestations, management, and prevention of acute reactions are summarized in Table 27-4.

Delayed Reactions

1. Delayed reactions occur days to years after the transfusion.
2. Delayed reactions include delayed hemolytic reactions, iron overload (hemosiderosis), GVHD, and infectious diseases (eg, hepatitis B, hepatitis C, CMV, Epstein-Barr virus, malaria, HIV, HTLV).
3. Symptoms of a delayed reaction can vary from mild to severe. Diagnosis may be complicated by the long incubation period between transfusion and reaction and the complexity of diagnostic tests.
4. Causes, clinical manifestations, management, and prevention of delayed reactions are summarized in Table 27-5, pages 783 and 784.

Table 27-4 Acute Reactions to Blood Transfusion				
ACUTE REACTION	**CAUSE**	**CLINICAL MANIFESTATIONS**	**MANAGEMENT**	**PREVENTION**
Allergic	Sensitivity to plasma protein or donor antibody, which reacts with recipient antigen	• Flushing • Itching, rash • Urticaria, hives • Asthmatic wheezing • Laryngeal edema • Anaphylaxis	• Stop transfusion immediately. Keep vein open (KVO) with normal saline. Notify health care provider and blood bank. • Give antihistamine, as directed (diphenhydramine). • Observe for anaphylaxis—prepare epinephrine if respiratory distress is severe. • If hives are the only clinical manifestation, the transfusion can sometimes continue at a slower rate. • Send blood samples and blood bags to blood bank. Collect urine specimens for testing.	• Before transfusion, ask patient about past reactions. If patient has history of anaphylaxis, alert health care provider, have emergency drugs available, and remain at bedside for the first 30 minutes.

(continued)

Table 27-4 Acute Reactions to Blood Transfusion (*Continued*)

ACUTE REACTION	CAUSE	CLINICAL MANIFESTATIONS	MANAGEMENT	PREVENTION
Febrile, nonhemolytic	Hypersensitivity to donor white blood cells, platelets, or plasma proteins	• Sudden chills and fever • Headache • Flushing • Anxiety	• Stop transfusion immediately and KVO with normal saline. Notify health care provider and blood bank. • Send blood samples and blood bags to blood bank. Collect urine specimens for testing. • Check temperature 30 minutes after chill and as indicated thereafter. • Give antipyretics, as prescribed—treat symptomatically.	• Give antipyretic (acetaminophen or aspirin) before transfusion as directed. • Leukocyte-poor blood products may be recommended for future transfusions.
Septic reactions	Transfusion of blood or components contaminated with bacteria	• Rapid onset of chills • High fever • Vomiting, diarrhea • Marked hypotension	• Stop transfusion immediately and KVO with normal saline. Notify health care provider and blood bank. • Obtain cultures of patient's blood and return blood bags with administration set to blood bank for culture. • Treat septicemia, as directed—antibiotics, IV fluids, vasopressors, and steroids.	• Do not permit blood to stand at room temperature longer than necessary. Warm temperatures promote bacterial growth. • Inspect blood for gas bubbles, clotting, or abnormal color before transfusion. • Complete infusions within 4 hours. Change administration set after 4 hours of use.
Circulatory overload	Fluid administered at a rate or volume greater than the circulatory system can accommodate. Increased blood in pulmonary vessels and decreased lung compliance	• Rise in venous pressure • Distended neck veins • Dyspnea • Cough • Crackles at base of lungs	• Stop transfusion and KVO with normal saline. Notify health care provider. • Place patient upright with feet in dependent position. • Administer prescribed diuretics, oxygen, morphine, and aminophylline.	• Concentrated blood products should be given whenever positive. • Transfuse at a rate within the circulatory reserve of the patient. • Monitor central venous pressure of patient with heart disease.
Hemolytic reaction	Infusion of incompatible blood products: • Antibodies in recipient's plasma attach to transfused red blood cells (RBCs), hemolyzing the cells either in circulation or in the reticuloendothelial system. • Antibodies in donor plasma attach to recipient RBCs, causing hemolysis (may result from infusion of incompatible plasma—less severe than incompatible RBCs).	• Chills; fever • Lower back pain • Feeling of head fullness; flushing • Oppressive feeling • Tachycardia, tachypnea • Hypotension, vascular collapse • Hemoglobinuria, hemoglobinemia • Bleeding • Acute renal failure	• Stop transfusion immediately—KVO with 0.9% saline. Notify health care provider and blood bank. • Treat shock, if present. • Draw testing samples; collect urine specimen. • Maintain blood pressure with IV colloid solutions. • Give diuretics, as prescribed, to maintain urine flow, glomerular filtration, and renal blood flow. • Insert indwelling catheter to monitor hourly urine output. Patient may require dialysis if renal failure occurs.	• Meticulously verify patient identification—from sample collection to product infusion. • Begin infusion slowly and observe closely for 30 minutes—consequences are in proportion to the amount of incompatible blood transfused.

Table 27-5   Delayed Reactions to Transfusion Therapy

DELAYED REACTION	CAUSE	CLINICAL MANIFESTATIONS	MANAGEMENT	PREVENTION
Delayed hemolytic reaction	The destruction of transfused red blood cells by antibody not detectable during crossmatch, but formed rapidly after transfusion. Rapid production may occur because of antigen exposure during previous transfusions or pregnancy.	• Fever • Mild jaundice • Decreased hematocrit	• Generally, no acute treatment is required, but hemolysis may be severe enough to cause shock and renal failure. If this occurs, manage as outlined under acute hemolytic reactions.	• The crossmatch blood sample should be drawn within 3 days of blood transfusion. Antibody formation may occur within 90 days of transfusion or pregnancy.
Iron overload (hemosiderosis)	Deposition of iron in the heart, endocrine organs, liver, spleen, skin, and other major organs as a result of multiple, long-term transfusions (aplastic anemia, thalassemia).	• Diabetes • Decreased thyroid function • Arrhythmias • Heart failure and other symptoms related to major organ failure	• Treat symptomatically. • Deferoxamine, which chelates and removes accumulated iron through the kidneys; administered via IV line, IM, or SubQ	—
Graft-versus-host disease	Engraftment of lymphocytes in the bone marrow of immunosuppressed patients, setting up an immune response of the graft against the host	• Erythematous skin rash • Liver function test abnormalities • Profuse, watery diarrhea	• Immunosuppression with corticosteroids, cyclosporine A • Symptomatic management of pruritus, pain • Fluid and electrolyte replacement for diarrhea	• Transfuse with irradiated blood products.
Hepatitis B	Hepatitis B virus transmitted from blood donor to recipient via infected blood products	• Elevated liver enzymes (ALT/AST) • Anorexia, malaise • Nausea and vomiting • Fever • Dark urine • Jaundice	• Usually resolves spontaneously within 4–6 wk. Can result in permanent liver damage. Treat symptomatically.	• Screen blood donors, temporarily rejecting those who may have had contact with the virus. Those with a history of hepatitis after age 11 are permanently deferred; pretest all blood products (EIA).
Hepatitis C (formerly non-A, non-B hepatitis)	Hepatitis C virus transmitted from blood donor to recipient via infected blood products	• Similar to serum B hepatitis, but symptoms are usually less severe. • Chronic liver disease and cirrhosis may develop.	• Symptoms usually mild. Interferon and ribavirin may be used to treat chronic liver disease.	• Pretest all blood donors (ALT, anti-HBc antibody, anti-hepatitis C antibody).
Epstein-Barr virus, cytomegalovirus, malaria	Transmitted through infected blood products	• Fever • Fatigue • Hepatomegaly • Splenomegaly	• Rest and supportive management	• Question prospective blood donors regarding colds, flu, and foreign travel.
Acquired immunodeficiency syndrome (AIDS)	Human immunodeficiency virus (HIV) transmitted from blood donor to recipient via infected blood products	• Night sweats • Unexplained weight loss • Lymphadenopathy • Pneumocystis pneumonia • Kaposi sarcoma • Diarrhea	• Combination antiretroviral therapy	• Test each donor for HIV antibody. • Reject prospective high-risk donors: males who have had sex with another male since 1977; users of self-injected IV drugs; male or female partners of prostitutes; hemophiliacs or their sexual partners; partners of those with AIDS or high risk for AIDS; immigrants from Haiti or sub-Saharan Africa.

(continued)

Table 27-5 Delayed Reactions to Transfusion Therapy (*Continued*)

DELAYED REACTION	CAUSE	CLINICAL MANIFESTATIONS	MANAGEMENT	PREVENTION
Human T-lymphotropic virus type 1 (HTLV-1) associated myelopathy and tropical spastic paraparesis (HAM/TSP) Adult T-cell leukemia	HTLV-1 transmitted from blood donor to recipient via blood products	• Signs of neuromuscular disease • Signs of T-cell leukemia	• HTLV-1–infected individuals have a low risk of developing disease (3%–5%). Incubation period 10–20 yr. • Should disease occur, treat symptomatically.	• Screen all prospective blood donors for anti–HTLV-1 antibody.
Syphilis	Spirochetemia caused by *Treponema pallidum*. Incubation 4–18 wk.	• Presence of chancre • Regional lymphadenopathy • Generalized rash	• Penicillin therapy	• Test blood before transfusion (rapid plasma reagin). Organism will not remain viable in blood stored 24–48 hr at 39.2°F (4°C).

TRANSITIONAL CARE ALERT Nurses must educate patients about the potential for a delayed blood transfusion reaction at the time of discharge, including signs and symptoms to be on the lookout for and notify their health care provider for timely diagnosis and outpatient treatment.

BLOOD AND MARROW STEM CELL TRANSPLANTATION

Blood and marrow stem cell transplantation is a potentially lifesaving treatment with application in many malignant and nonmalignant disorders. Decades of research have advanced this technology from an experimental treatment of last resort to the preferred method of intervention for selected diseases. Although the basic procedures are now well established, this field continues to grow rapidly through ongoing research in areas such as nonmyeloablative ("mini") allogeneic transplants, the application of biologic response modifiers to modulate the immune response, and the use of donor lymphocyte infusions to prevent or treat posttransplant relapse.

Principles of Blood and Marrow Stem Cell Transplantation

Types of Stem Cell Transplant

The type of transplant selected is contingent on a variety of factors, such as the underlying disorder, the availability of a histocompatible (HLA-matched) donor, and the clinical condition of the patient. Stem cells may come from the patient (autologous), an identical twin (syngeneic), or another donor (allogeneic). Stem cells are found in bone marrow, in peripheral blood (especially if the donor is treated to increase the numbers of circulating stem cells), and in umbilical cord blood.

Autologous Bone Marrow Transplantation

1. Bone marrow is removed from the patient during an operative harvesting procedure, frozen, and reinfused after the patient has undergone high-dose chemotherapy and possibly radiotherapy.

2. Advantages: readily available and usually lower morbidity and mortality than allogeneic bone marrow transplantation (BMT).
3. Disadvantages: operative procedure; marrow must be disease-free; sufficient quantity of cellular marrow must be aspirable; in most cases has higher rate of relapse than allogeneic BMT.

Syngeneic Bone Marrow Transplantation

1. Bone marrow is removed from an identical twin during an operative harvesting procedure and infused into the recipient, who has undergone high-dose chemotherapy and possibly radiotherapy.
2. Advantages: recipient's marrow does not need to be harvestable (as in hypocellular or tumor-contaminated bone marrow), generally lower morbidity and mortality than allogeneic BMT.
3. Disadvantages: higher disease relapse rate than in allogeneic BMT.

Allogeneic Bone Marrow Transplantation

1. Bone marrow is removed from a donor who is most commonly a sibling or other close relative (related) but may be a volunteer donor (unrelated).
   a. Identical or mismatched HLA phenotypes may be used, though identical phenotypes are often preferred. HLA mismatches require additional immunosuppression and GVHD prophylaxis and can be associated with higher morbidity and mortality.
   b. Bone marrow is removed from the donor during an operative harvesting procedure and infused into the recipient, who has undergone high-dose chemotherapy and possibly radiotherapy.
   c. Allogeneic bone marrow may be treated in various ways before infusion, including removing RBCs if ABO incompatible and removing T lymphocytes to reduce the risk of GVHD.
2. Advantages: recipient's marrow does not need to be harvestable (as in hypocellular or tumor-contaminated bone marrow) and lowest rate of relapse.
3. Disadvantages: risk for GVHD and generally higher morbidity and mortality than other types of BMT. Unrelated and HLA-mismatched transplants have higher risk of GVHD and infectious complications and some risk of graft rejection or failure.

Autologous, Syngeneic, or Allogeneic Peripheral Blood Stem Cell Transplantation

1. Although hematopoietic stem cells are primarily found in the bone marrow, they can also be found in the peripheral circulation in smaller numbers.
2. Peripheral blood stem cells are collected using one or more apheresis procedures after the patient or donor has been treated to increase the number of circulating stem cells. This is done by methods such as timed administration of chemotherapy (patient only) and stem cell growth factors. After the collection, the cells are frozen and stored for reinfusion into the patient after high-dose chemotherapy and possibly radiotherapy.
3. Advantages: patient's marrow does not need to be harvestable (as in hypocellular or tumor-contaminated bone marrow); there is no operative risk to the patient or donor.
4. Disadvantages: for allogeneic donors, the long-term risks of boosting healthy bone marrow production with growth factors, and in some cases chemotherapy, are not yet known. Research has shown that allogeneic peripheral blood stem cell transplant may be associated with a higher incidence of chronic GVHD than allogeneic bone marrow transplant.

Umbilical Cord Blood Stem Cell Transplantation

1. Umbilical cord blood is rich in stem cells and may be stored at birth for later autologous use, related allogeneic use, or unrelated allogeneic use. Cord blood transplantation requires less stringent HLA matching because mismatched cord blood stem cells are less likely to cause GVHD than mature stem cells from other sources.
2. Advantages: may provide lifesaving allogeneic stem cells from new sibling to older child at no risk to the donor. Cord blood banks provide options for unrelated donor transplantation when there is an urgent need.
3. Disadvantages: may have higher risk of graft failure than other types of transplants; number of stem cells may be insufficient for older patients.

Nonmyeloablative or "Mini" Transplants

1. Conventional conditioning for blood and marrow stem cell transplants requires high doses of chemotherapy and radiotherapy (myeloablative) to destroy existing bone marrow cells. This results in significant morbidity and mortality, particularly in certain patient populations (eg, older patients, those with poor organ function).
2. Research has demonstrated that under certain conditions, individuals can exist with bone marrow stem cells from two sources (self and allogeneic donor), a state known as *mixed chimerism*. These changes in the immune system appear to enhance the antitumor immune response, creating a desired graft-versus-tumor effect.
3. The goals of nonmyeloablative conditioning regimens are to prevent graft rejection and promote mixed chimerism. The nonmyeloablative preparative regimen uses combinations of agents such as cyclophosphamide, fludarabine, antithymocyte globulin, and low-dose total body irradiation. Alemtuzumab is often considered as well. After the completion of the reduced intensity regimen, the allogeneic bone marrow or peripheral blood stem cells are then infused.
4. Donor lymphocytes may also be given at specific intervals following transplant to enhance the immune antitumor effect further.
5. Advantages: patients otherwise ineligible for allogeneic transplant because of age, comorbid conditions, or organ function are more likely to tolerate the less-toxic preparative regimen. Patients do not usually experience significant neutropenia, thrombocytopenia, anemia, and other complications that typically accompany myeloablative therapy. Patients generally have shorter episodes of neutropenia and a reduced need for RBC and platelet transfusions, allowing an opportunity for outpatient transplants to be performed.
6. Disadvantages: Increased risk of graft failure.

The Human Leukocyte Antigen System and Transplantation

1. The human leukocyte antigen (HLA) system is part of the major histocompatibility complex.
2. The immune-mediated recognition of the differences in each individual's HLA system is the first step in the rejection of a transplanted organ or graft or in GVHD.
3. The HLA antigens are complex proteins expressed on the surface of all nucleated cells (A, B, C antigens—class I) or cells of the immune system (D antigens—class II).
   a. More than 100 different antigens have been identified.
   b. Antigens are classified according to their location on chromosome 6, which encodes them.
   c. A person's genetically inherited mixture of antigens expressed on cell surfaces is their individual phenotype or tissue type.
4. Determination of an individual's HLA type is completed by complex DNA phenotyping or gene sequencing.
   a. The gold standard for HLA typing in bone marrow transplantation is to complete the above testing at high resolution (allelic level), identifying both the class I (A, B, C) and class II (D) groups.
   b. A phenotypically identical donor is considered to be one who matches at all 10 antigens at their associated allelic level—A, B, C, DR, and DQ.
5. Siblings have a 1-in-4 chance of having identical sets of HLA antigens. With a decreasing national birthrate, however, only 35% of people in the United States can anticipate having an HLA-identical sibling.
6. Because of the complexity of the HLA system, unrelated people have less than a 1-in-5,000 chance of being HLA identical.
7. The National Bone Marrow Donor Program (BeTheMatch Registry), established in 1987, maintains a computerized list of potential HLA-matched peripheral blood stem cell and bone marrow donors, providing assistance to patients who seek an unrelated donor. Information on becoming a volunteer bone marrow donor or on initiating a computerized search for a donor can be obtained by calling the National Marrow Donor Program ((800) 507-5427 or www.marrow.org), for additional resources for patients undergoing blood and marrow stem cell transplantation.

Indications

1. If an HLA-matched related donor is available, allogeneic bone marrow or stem cell transplantation is generally considered the treatment of choice in certain disorders, including:
   a. Severe aplastic anemia.
   b. Inherited immunodeficiency disorders, such as severe combined immunodeficiency disease and Wiskott-Aldrich syndrome.
   c. Allogeneic bone marrow and peripheral blood stem cell transplantation has also been used with varying success in the treatment of other genetic disorders (eg, thalassemia, sickle cell disease).
2. Allogeneic, syngeneic, and autologous bone marrow and peripheral blood stem cell transplantation is also widely

BOX 27-1	Indications for Blood and Marrow Stem Cell Transplantation

ALLOGENEIC

Nonmalignant
- Aplastic anemia.
- Myelofibrosis.
- Wiskott-Aldrich syndrome.
- Thalassemia.
- Severe combined immunodeficiency diseases.
- Mucopolysaccharidoses.
- Sickle cell disease.

Malignant
- Acute myeloid leukemia.
- Acute lymphocytic leukemia.
- Hodgkin lymphoma.
- Non-Hodgkin lymphoma.
- Myelofibrosis.
- Multiple myeloma.
- Selected solid tumors.

AUTOLOGOUS
- Hodgkin lymphoma.
- Non-Hodgkin lymphoma.
- Multiple myeloma.
- Selected solid tumors.

applied in the treatment of malignancies, where success rates depend largely on factors such as the age of the patient, disease status at time of transplant, the extent of prior treatment, and existing comorbidities.

3. Autologous peripheral blood stem cell transplantation is used in the treatment of certain lymphomas, multiple myeloma, and solid tumors such as Ewing sarcoma and neuroblastoma. Allogeneic bone marrow and peripheral blood stem cell transplantation is generally used in the treatment of leukemias as well as certain lymphomas.

4. Diseases and disorders treated with this technology are summarized in Box 27-1.

Harvesting of Bone Marrow and Peripheral Blood Stem Cells

Evaluation of Recipient

1. Eligibility criteria include age (generally younger than age 65 for allogeneic myeloablative transplants and autologous and syngeneic transplants and younger than age 75 for allogeneic nonmyeloablative transplants) and availability of suitable donor and stem cell source.

2. Before undergoing transplantation, an extensive workup is completed to ensure that the patient's disease is treatable with the selected type of transplant and that the patient has no limitations that will increase the risk of mortality.

3. Specific criteria may vary among transplant centers and treatment protocols, but generally include:
   a. Disease-specific evaluation of severity and extent of current disease manifestations.
   b. Adequate cardiac function: generally left ventricular ejection fraction greater than 45%.
   c. Adequate pulmonary function: generally, forced expiratory capacity and forced vital capacity greater than 50%.
   d. Adequate renal function: generally, creatinine less than 2 mg/dL.

e. Adequate hepatic function: generally, bilirubin less than 2 mg/dL.
   f. No active infections (including HIV).
   g. No coexisting severe or uncontrolled medical conditions.

Evaluation of Blood and Marrow Donors

1. Because bone marrow donation for allogeneic or syngeneic BMT is an elective procedure with no benefit to the donor, great care is taken to ensure that the potential donor is fit for surgery and understands the potential risks. Autologous bone marrow donors must generally meet the same criteria. Evaluation includes:
   a. Thorough medical history and physical examination.
   b. Chest x-ray.
   c. Electrocardiogram.
   d. Laboratory evaluation (CBC; chemistry profile; testing for CMV, hepatitis B and C, HIV, HTLV, and syphilis; ABO and Rh determination; coagulation studies).

2. Informed consent including potential donor complications must be obtained.

3. Relatively common complications include:
   a. Bruising.
   b. Pain at aspiration sites.
   c. Mild bleeding.

4. Rare complications include:
   a. Adverse effects of anesthesia (general, spinal, or epidural).
   b. Infection of aspiration sites.
   c. Persistent pain.
   d. Transient neuropathies.

5. Because of the significant loss of blood volume and RBCs during the harvest procedure, donors are advised to give one or two units of autologous blood 1 to 3 weeks before surgery, which may be reinfused during marrow collection, if needed.

6. Evaluation of donors for peripheral blood stem cell transplantation is similar, but less stringent as there is generally no anesthesia required. The apheresis procedure is similar to donating platelets.

Stem Cell Collection Procedure

Bone Marrow Harvest (Autologous, Syngeneic, or Allogeneic)

1. Performed under epidural, spinal, or general anesthesia under sterile conditions in operating room.

2. An aspiration needle is used to puncture the skin and puncture the iliac crest multiple times without exiting the skin, removing marrow in 2- to 5-mL aliquots (samples).

3. Marrow is drawn up into heparinized syringes and filtered to remove fibrin clots and other debris.

4. Marrow may be infused immediately, treated and infused, or frozen in a preservative solution containing dimethyl sulfoxide (DMSO) until needed.

5. Bone marrow donation is a relatively safe operative procedure with few serious complications.

Postharvest Care of the Bone Marrow Donor

1. Procedure is generally done as same-day care, with discharge after recovery from anesthesia.

2. Observe for potential complications (bleeding, hypotension caused by fluid loss).

3. Instruct patient to resume normal activities gradually during the week after donation.

4. Instruct patient to keep aspiration sites clean and dry and observe for signs of infection (redness, swelling, warmth or discharge at sites, fever, malaise).

5. Provide adequate analgesia and instruct patient about pain management.

Harvesting of Peripheral Blood Stem Cells

1. Involves donor preparation by "priming" hematopoietic system with timed chemotherapy (autologous stem cell collection only) and sequential growth factor administration to increase the number of circulating stem cells.
2. A large-bore central catheter suitable for apheresis procedures is inserted.
3. One to ten apheresis procedures may be needed to collect sufficient numbers of suitable cells.
4. Cells are frozen in a preservative solution that contains DMSO until needed.
5. Acute complications of apheresis include citrate toxicity, which may be managed by increasing dietary calcium intake 2 to 3 days before procedure and by using calcium-based antacids during the procedure. Blood calcium levels are carefully monitored throughout the procedure and IV calcium is given, as needed.

TRANSITIONAL CARE ALERT After donation of bone marrow and peripheral blood stem cells, attention to follow-up should be given to the donor to ensure there are no signs of complications from the donation procedure. It is also important that adequate pain management medications be prescribed and that the donor and caregiver are instructed on concerns that warrant medical attention such as fever, numbness or tingling, or severe pain not relieved by medications.

Preparation and Performance of the Transplant

Preparation of Recipient

1. A long-term central catheter is inserted for multiple IV treatments, including blood products, total parenteral nutrition, and blood drawing.

2. High-dose chemotherapy or radiotherapy is administered to:
   a. Destroy residual tumor cells.
   b. Suppress immune response against new stem cells.
   c. Create space within recipient's marrow for the new stem cells.
3. Symptoms immediately associated with high-dose chemotherapy or radiotherapy regimens used in blood and marrow stem cell transplantation may include:
   a. Severe nausea and vomiting (with most regimens).
   b. Cardiomyopathy and hemorrhagic cystitis (with cyclophosphamide).
   c. Seizures (with busulfan).
   d. Fever, generalized erythema, and parotitis (with total body irradiation).

Infusion of Bone Marrow or Peripheral Blood Stem Cells

See Table 27-6.

 NURSING ALERT Unlike all other blood products administered to transplant recipients, stem cells should never be irradiated. In addition, infusion pumps and filters should be avoided because they may remove or damage stem cells.

Posttransplant Care

General Considerations

1. Significant complications that require specialized medical and nursing care may occur during the first few weeks and months after blood and marrow stem cell transplantation.
   a. Risk is highest in mismatched unrelated allogeneic BMT.
   b. Followed by matched unrelated and mismatched related allogeneic BMT.
   c. Followed by matched related allogeneic BMT.

TYPE OF STEM CELLS	PROCESSING PRIOR TO INFUSION	VOLUME	POTENTIAL ADVERSE EFFECTS	NURSING CONSIDERATIONS
ABO-compatible untreated allogeneic bone marrow	Filtered to remove large particles	500–2,000 mL	Volume overload, allergic reactions, pulmonary compromise (fat emboli, cell aggregates)	Emergency medications available, close monitoring
ABO-incompatible bone marrow	Removal of red blood cells and plasma	200–600 mL	Allergic reactions, intravascular hemolysis (rare)	Prehydrate to ensure adequate renal perfusion and alkaline urine, emergency medications available, close monitoring
Autologous bone marrow	Filtered and frozen with DMSO as preservative, thawed in warm water bath immediately prior to infusion	100–500 mL	Related to DMSO: histamine release reaction (flushing, chest tightness, abdominal cramping, nausea), cardiac arrhythmias, anaphylaxis	Emergency medications available, close monitoring, cardiac monitoring recommended
Peripheral blood stem cells	Frozen with DMSO as preservative, thawed in warm water bath immediately prior to infusion	100–1,000 mL	Related to DMSO: histamine release reaction (flushing, chest tightness, abdominal cramping, nausea), cardiac arrhythmias, anaphylaxis	Administer as tolerated (may be high volume and DMSO content), premedicate with antihistamine and antiemetic, emergency medications available, close monitoring, cardiac monitoring recommended

Table 27-6 Infusion Guidelines for Bone Marrow or Peripheral Blood Stem Cells

DMSO, dimethyl sulfoxide.

    d. Followed by syngeneic BMT.

    e. Followed by autologous BMT.

    f. Followed by autologous peripheral blood stem cell transplantation (lowest risk).

2. Nursing care is aimed at early identification and treatment of problems and includes:

    a. Comprehensive physical and psychosocial assessment.

    b. Immediate notification of health care provider of any abnormal assessment parameters found.

    c. Early recognition and intervention for life-threatening complications, such as sepsis, respiratory failure, gastrointestinal (GI) bleeding, renal and hepatic failure, and veno-occlusive disease (VOD).

    d. Prevention of infection.

    e. Prevention of bleeding.

    f. Expert symptom management of problems that may occur after blood and marrow stem cell transplantation, such as nausea, vomiting, diarrhea, pain, fatigue, anxiety, and delirium.

Hematopoietic Complications

1. Blood and marrow stem cell transplant patients, particularly allogeneic recipients, are at risk for life-threatening bacterial, viral, and fungal infections because of their profound neutropenia and prolonged immunosuppression.

    a. Transplant recipients are usually cared for in a protective environment, most commonly single HEPA-filtered rooms.

    b. In an ambulatory or home setting, the patient and family must pay strict attention to methods of preventing infection, including wearing high-filtration masks, handwashing, safe food handling, and avoidance of crowded areas and exposure to illnesses.

    c. Blood and marrow stem cell recipients are at high risk for nosocomial bloodstream infections related to long-term central venous catheters, neutropenia, and immunosuppression. Strict adherence to an evidence-based procedure for insertion and management of central venous catheters is essential in this population.

    d. Colony-stimulating factors such as GCSF and GM-CSF have been shown to reduce the duration of neutropenia, though the optimal timing for administration has not been determined.

    e. Additional preventive interventions vary widely and include elaborate disinfection procedures, modified or sterile diets, prophylactic antibiotics, antivirals, and antifungals, and surveillance cultures.

2. The megakaryocyte is generally the last cell produced by new stem cells, and platelet counts may take months to return to normal.

    a. Blood and marrow stem cell transplant patients require frequent assessment for signs and symptoms of overt or covert bleeding, protection from injury, and support with platelet products.

3. Anemia is a common complication caused by loss of RBCs through aging, destruction, bleeding, and routine phlebotomy. Blood and marrow stem cell transplant patients require frequent RBC transfusions. Erythropoietin alfa and darbepoetin alfa may also be used to stimulate RBC production. Delayed erythropoiesis and immune hemolytic anemia are complications of ABO-incompatible allogeneic stem cell transplants.

Gastrointestinal Complications

1. Mucositis may develop because of high-dose chemotherapy and radiation therapy that destroy rapidly dividing cells, including cells lining the mouth, esophagus, and GI tract. Management includes meticulous oral hygiene, local and systemic analgesia, and antimicrobial therapy.

2. Nausea and vomiting may arise from multiple causes, including high-dose chemotherapy, infection, GI bleeding, acute GVHD, and medications. Management includes pharmacologic and nonpharmacologic interventions, adequate replacement of fluids and electrolytes, and support of nutritional requirements.

3. Diarrhea may have multiple causes, including high-dose chemotherapy, infection, GI bleeding, GVHD, and medications. Management includes cautious use of antidiarrheals, adequate replacement of fluids and electrolytes, support of nutritional requirements, and protection of perirectal skin from excoriation.

Renal and Genitourinary Complications

1. Renal failure may arise from multiple factors, including drug toxicity, infection, and ischemia. Management includes maintenance of fluid and electrolyte balance, monitoring of drug levels, and hemodialysis or continuous venovenous hemodialysis.

2. Hemorrhagic cystitis may occur as a result of high-dose cyclophosphamide or with certain viral infections, such as adenovirus and BK virus (a polyoma virus, named for the first patient). Management includes hydration, blood product support, continuous bladder irrigation, and rare invasive procedures, such as instillation of alum or formalin, or surgery.

Hepatic Complications

Sinusoidal obstruction syndrome or VOD may occur as a result of damage to the liver from high-dose chemotherapy and radiation therapy; incidence is approximately 30%.

1. Signs and symptoms include hepatomegaly (generally painful), hyperbilirubinemia, and weight gain.

2. May progress to hepatic encephalopathy, coagulopathies, coma, and death in up to 50% of patients with VOD.

3. Management is generally aimed at preventing further damage and at treating symptoms. The antithrombotic and thrombolytic agent defibrotide may be administered for severe VOD; however, the risk of bleeding is high with the administration of this agent; other agents being studied include heparin, recombinant tissue plasminogen activator, and ursodeoxycholic acid.

Pulmonary Complications

1. Life-threatening pulmonary infections in stem cell recipients include bacterial pneumonias, fungal infections including aspergillosis, viral infections such as CMV (especially in allogeneic recipients), respiratory syncytial virus, parainfluenza, and, less commonly, *Pneumocystis carinii* pneumonia (PCP), Legionnaires' disease, toxoplasmosis, and tuberculosis.

    a. Preventive measures include hand hygiene, encouragement of exercise, deep breathing, and coughing; routine CMV polymerase chain reaction monitoring if recipient or donor is CMV IgG positive at the time of transplant; administration of CMV-screened and/or leukoreduced blood products, high-dose acyclovir or ganciclovir, and IVIG for allogeneic BMT patients at high risk for CMV; and prophylactic co-trimoxazole for patients at risk for PCP.

    b. Staff, patient, and family education regarding risk factors and transmission of these infectious agents may help prevent primary and nosocomial infections.

    c. Supportive care if symptomatic includes pulmonary hygiene, oxygen therapy, and mechanical ventilation.

2. Noninfectious pulmonary disease includes idiopathic pneumonitis, diffuse alveolar hemorrhage, pulmonary fibrosis, and bronchiolitis obliterans.

Graft-Versus-Host Disease

1. Acute GVHD occurs in 40% to 60% of allogeneic recipients even with HLA matching, generally within first 3 months after transplant as a manifestation of the immune system's response to activated donor T lymphocytes against the recipient's cells and organs.
   a. Primarily affects the skin, liver, and GI tract; may also affect conjunctivae and lungs.
   b. Severity ranges from mild and self-limited erythematous rash to widespread blistering of the skin, profuse watery diarrhea, and liver failure.
   c. Prophylaxis generally includes immunosuppression with such medications as cyclosporine, tacrolimus, and methotrexate; may also include T-cell depletion of bone marrow.
   d. Recently, research has demonstrated that administration of high-dose cyclophosphamide a few days after the stem cell transplant decreases the rate of acute GVHD.
   e. Treatment generally includes increased doses of routine immunosuppressive drugs and additional drugs, such as corticosteroids, antithymocyte globulin, and monoclonal antibodies.

2. Chronic GVHD occurs in approximately 20% of long-term survivors; usually appears within first year after allogeneic blood and marrow stem cell transplant.
   a. It has many similarities to autoimmune disorders such as scleroderma.
   b. It affects the skin, mouth, salivary glands, eyes, musculoskeletal system, liver, esophagus, GI tract, and vagina.
   c. Treatment generally consists of corticosteroids and other immunosuppressive drugs, such as mycophenolate and thalidomide.
   d. Immune system frequently suppressed beyond the effects of medications; patient is at risk for infections, particularly from encapsulated bacteria, and should receive prophylaxis with suitable antibiotic such as penicillin.

Long-Term Sequelae and Survivorship Issues

1. Long-term, disease-free survival varies from 5% to 20% for patients with resistant, aggressive leukemias or lymphomas to 75% to 80% for aplastic anemia.

2. Long-term complications of blood and marrow stem cell transplantation include:
   a. Relapse of original disease.
   b. Secondary malignancy, including skin, oral mucosa, brain, thyroid, bone, and acute leukemia.
   c. Sterility.
   d. Endocrine dysfunction, including reduced levels of human growth hormone, estrogens, and testosterone.
   e. Cataracts (risk increased with radiation therapy, corticosteroids).
   f. Chronic GVHD (allogeneic).
   g. Aseptic necrosis and osteoporosis (risk increased with corticosteroids).
   h. Encephalopathy (risk increased with cranial irradiation and intrathecal chemotherapy).

3. Survivorship issues after this intensive and potentially life-threatening treatment include:
   a. Feelings of isolation, guilt, and loss.
   b. Altered family dynamics.
   c. Delayed puberty, decreased libido, early menopause, and other physical problems that have an impact on sexual relationships.
   d. Readjustment to school or work setting.
   e. Financial burden of blood and marrow stem cell transplantation.
   f. Chronic health problems and fatigue.
   g. Difficulty obtaining adequate health insurance.

4. Despite the complex issues blood and marrow stem cell transplant survivors face, several quality-of-life studies have demonstrated that the majority rate their quality of life highly and would choose to undergo transplant again.

SELECTED REFERENCES

Bertaina, A., & Andreani, M. (2018). Major histocompatibility complex and hematopoietic stem cell transplantation: beyond the classical HLA polymorphisim. *International Journal of Molecular Science, 19*(2), 621–635.

Broxton, S., Medeiros, R., Abuzeid, A., et al. Implementation of a massive transfusion protocol: Evaluation of Its use and efficacy. *Journal of Trauma Nursing, 25*(2), 92–97.

DeLisel, J. (2018). Is this a blood transfusion reaction? Don't hesitate; check it out. *Journal of Infusion Nursing. 41*(1), 43–51.

DeSimone, R.A., Nowak, M.D., Lo, D.T., et al. (2018). *https://www.ncbi.nlm.nih.gov/pubmed/29624677*. Logistical and safety implications of temperature-based acceptance of returned red blood cell units. *Transfusion*. Advanced online publication. doi: 10.1111/trf.14615.

Dierckx de Casterlé, I., Billiau, A.D., & Sprangers, B. (2018). *https://www.ncbi.nlm.nih.gov/pubmed/29678553*. Recipient and donor cells in the graft-versus-solid tumor effect: It takes two to tango. *Blood Reviews*. Advanced online publication. doi: 10.1016/j.blre.2018.04.002.

Gallo, A.M., Patil, C., Adeniyi, T., et al. (2018). Health related quality of life and personal life goals of adults with Sickle cell disease after hematopoietic stem cell transplantation. *Western Journal of Nursing Research*. Advanced online publication. doi: 10.1177/0193945918768277.

Gordon, L. I. (2017). Strategies for management of relapsed or refractory Hodgkin lymphoma. *Journal of the National Comprehensive Cancer Network, 15*(5S), 716–718.

Jones, A. (2018). Safe transfusion of blood components. *Nursing Standard, 32*(25), 50–61.

Khetan, D., Katharia, R., Pandey, H. C., et al. (2018). *https://www.ncbi.nlm.nih.gov/pubmed/29563672*. Assessment of bedside transfusion practices at a tertiary care center: A step closer to controlling the chaos. Asian Journal of Transfusion Science, 12(1),27–33.

Li, Y., Duan, F., Xiao, H., et al. (2018). *https://www.ncbi.nlm.nih.gov/pubmed/29677078*. Therapeutic outcomes of haploidentical allogeneic hematopoietic stem cell transplantation in patients with severe aplastic anemia: a multicenter study. *Transplantation. Advanced online publication.* doi: 10.1097/TP.0000000000002200.

Liu, L., Zhang, X., & Feng, S. (2018). Epstein-barr virus-related post-transplantation lymphoproliferative disorders after allogeneic hematopoietic stem cell transplantation. *Biology of Blood and Marrow Transplant*. Advanced online publication. doi: 10.1016/j.bbmt.2018.02.026.

Moalic-Allain, V. (2018). *https://www.ncbi.nlm.nih.gov/pubmed/29555414*. Medical and ethical considerations on hematopoietic stem cells mobilization for healthy donors. *Transfusion Clinical Biology*. Advanced online publication. doi: 10.1016/j.tracli.2018.02.004.

Ní Chonghaile, M., & Wolownik, K. (2018). Identification and management: sinusoidal obstruction syndrome/veno-occlusive disease related to hematopoietic stem cell transplantation. *Clinical Journal of Oncology Nursing, 22*(1), E7–E17.

Passwater, M. (2018). Antibody formation in transfusion therapy. *Journal of Infusion Nursing, 41*(2), 87–95.

Revol, B., Bickert, L., Sarrot-Reynauld, F., & Allenet, B. (2017). *https://www.ncbi.nlm.nih.gov/pubmed/28941580*. Immunoglobulins: Benefits and risks from the patient's point of view. *Therapie, 72*(6),683–684.

Santoro, N., Labopin, M., Giannotti, F., et al. (2018). *https://www.ncbi.nlm.nih.gov/pubmed/29661208*. Unmanipulated haploidentical in comparison with matched unrelated donor stem cell transplantation in patients 60 years and older with acute myeloid leukemia: a comparative study on behalf of the ALWP of the EBMT. *Journal of Hematology Oncology, 11*(1), 55.

28
Asthma and Allergy

OVERVIEW AND ASSESSMENT

See additional online content: Procedure Guidelines 28-1–28-2.

The Allergic Reaction

An allergic reaction results from antigen–antibody reaction on sensitized mast cells or basophils, causing the release of chemical mediators. The reaction may be characterized by inflammation, increased secretions, and bronchoconstriction.

Definitions

1. Antigen (Ag)—a protein that is found on the surface of a pathogen and stimulates an immune reaction, causing the production of antibodies.
2. Antibody (Ab)—immunoglobulin (Ig)(protein) secreted by B cells as a defense mechanism against foreign material such as antigen.
3. Atopy—ability to produce immunoglobulin E antibodies to common allergens. The genetic tendency to develop classic allergic disease or hypersensitivity reaction.
4. Immunity:
   a. Humoral—process by which B lymphocytes produce and secrete circulating antibodies to act against antigens.
   b. Cell-mediated—part of the immune system comprised of T lymphocytes responsible for antigen-specific cell-mediated immunity (CMI) by activating cytotoxic T cells that identify infectious pathogens such as virus, bacteria, fungi, and protozoan cells. Cell-mediated response also fights cancers.

5. Mast cell—type of WBC tissue cell similar to peripheral blood basophil, which contains granules with chemical mediators. Known for its role in allergic and anaphylactic reactions
6. Basophil—leukocyte with large granules that contain the vasodilator histamine and the anticoagulant heparin.
7. Hypersensitivity—reaction to an antigen after reexposure; there are four types.
   a. Type I (immediate, IgE)—allergic reactions such as atopy, anaphylaxis, asthma
   b. Type IV (delayed)—occurs 48 to 72 hours after exposure, as in contact dermatitis, tuberculin reaction, and transplant rejection (also considered allergic reaction).
   c. Type 2 (IgM, IgG antibody dependent)—autoimmune hemolytic anemia.
   d. Type 3 (IgG)—immune complex disease as in rheumatoid arthritis.

Immunoglobulins

Antibodies that are formed by lymphocytes and plasma cells in response to an immunogenic stimulus comprise a group of serum proteins called *immunoglobulins*.

1. The abbreviation for immunoglobulin is Ig.
2. Antibodies combine with antigens in lock-and-key style.
3. There are five major classes of immunoglobulins.
   a. IgM—produced by B cells constitutes 10% of immunoglobulin pool; found mostly in intravascular fluid and primarily engaged in initial defense; levels elevated with recent infection or exposure to antigen.
   b. IgG—major immunoglobulin that accounts for 70% to 75% of secondary immune responses and combats tissue infection.

c. IgA—15% to 20% of immunoglobulins; predominantly found in seromucous secretions (such as saliva, tears, sweat, and secretions from the gastrointestinal tract, genitourinary tract, prostate, and respiratory epithelium). It provides a primary defense mechanism.

d. IgD—less than 1% of immunoglobulin pool; found on circulating B lymphocytes, and signals B cells to become activated.

e. IgE—only a trace found in serum; attaches to surface membrane of basophils and mast cells; responsible for immediate types of allergic reactions (Type 1 hypersensitivity).

Immunologic Reactions

Immediate Hypersensitivity (Type I)

1. Characterized by:
   a. IgE-mediated allergic reaction Mast cells and/or basophils (see Figure 28-1).
   b. Occurs immediately after contact with the antigen.
   c. Causes release and neo-synthesis of preformed chemical mediators.
   d. Can occur 2nd to medications.
2. Examples—anaphylaxis, allergic rhinitis, urticaria.

Products of Immediate Hypersensitivity (Chemical Mediators)

1. Histamine—bioactive amine stored in granules of mast cells and basophils.
2. Leukotrienes—newly synthesized potent bronchoconstrictors; cause increased venous permeability.
3. Prostaglandins—potent vasodilators and potent bronchoconstrictors.
4. Platelet-activating factor—has many properties; causes the aggregation of platelets.
5. Cytokines—control and regulate immunologic functions (eg, interleukins, tumor necrosis factor).
6. Proteases—enzymes, such as tryptase and chymase, increase vascular permeability.
7. Eosinophil chemotactic factor of anaphylaxis—causes an influx of eosinophils into the area of allergic inflammation (fevers, stomatitis, sepsis).

8. Examples—drug-induced hemolytic anemia, drug-induced thrombocytopenia, drug-induced neutropenia.

Effects of Chemical Mediators and Their Manifestations

1. Generalized vasodilation (histamine, nitric oxide, prostaglandin) hypotension, flushing.
2. Increased permeability (histamine, bradykinin, leukotrienes, among others)
   a. Capillaries of the skin—edema.
   b. Mucous membranes—edema.
3. Smooth muscle contraction.
   a. Bronchioles—bronchospasm.
   b. Intestines—abdominal cramps, diarrhea.
4. Increased secretions.
   a. Nasal mucous glands—rhinorrhea.
   b. Bronchioles—increased mucus in airways.
   c. GI—increased gastric secretions.
   d. Lacrimal—tearing.
   e. Salivary—salivation.
5. Pruritus (itching).
   a. Skin.
   b. Mucous membrane.

Delayed Hypersensitivity (Type IV)

1. Characterized by a cell-mediated reaction between antigens and antigen-responsive T lymphocytes (IgG, IgM).
2. Maximal intensity occurs between 24 and 48 hours.
3. Usually consists of erythema and induration.
4. Examples—tuberculin skin test, contact dermatitis such as poison ivy, Hashimoto thyroiditis

Allergy Assessment

Subjective and Objective Data

1. Evaluate for symptoms related to hay fever, asthma, skin reactions, insect allergy, and food allergy.
2. Determine exacerbating factors such as contact with pets, outdoor exposure, a certain season, contact with mold, exposure to dust.

REACTION TO ALLERGEN EXPOSURE

Figure 28-1. Type I immediate hypersensitivity. During the initial exposure, T cells recognize foreign allergens and release chemicals to instruct B cells to produce immunoglobulin (Ig) E. These antibodies attach themselves to mast cells. Upon reexposure, the allergen comes in contact with the IgE antibodies attached to mast cells, causing degranulation and release of chemical mediators. (Stewart, J.G. [2017]. Anatomical Chart Company Atlas of Pathophysiology [4th ed.]. Philadelphia: Lippincott Williams & Wilkins.)

3. Obtain complete medical history for past illnesses, medication allergies, family history, medications that have been tried, exercise, smoking, and work environment.
4. Perform physical examination based on patient presentation and specific allergy condition, usually skin, head, chest, eye, ear, nose, and throat examination.

Skin Testing

The purpose of skin testing is to identify antigens responsible for immediate hypersensitivity. The types of skin tests used in clinical allergy are epicutaneous (prick, puncture, or scratch) and intradermal methods. The skin test remains unequaled as a sensitive, specific, and effective test for the diagnosis of allergies.

Epicutaneous (Prick) Method
1. Advantages:
   a. Efficient—results within 15 minutes.
   b. Little discomfort to the patient/relatively safe.
   c. Only rare instances of anaphylaxis because of minimal systemic absorption.
2. Disadvantages:
   a. Old or thick, leathery skin decreases reactivity.
   b. Lack of standardization and quantification.
   c. Drops have a tendency to run together, which would affect the accuracy of the test.

Intradermal Method
1. Advantages:
   a. Useful to confirm equivocal epicutaneous results with some antigens.
   b. Moderate sensitivity and reproducibility.
2. Disadvantages:
   a. Less specific than prick testing/subjective interpretation.
   b. Increased possibility for anaphylactic reactions.
   c. Requires more time and skill to perform.
   d. Increased discomfort to the patient/variation in wheal size and erythema.

In Vitro Testing

Description
1. *In vitro*—using blood samples—tests for IgE antibodies to specific allergens. Instead of looking for a reaction *in vivo* (with the patient's body—as in skin testing), *in vitro* testing measures the IgE response to specific antigens added to blood samples.
2. Advantages over skin testing include the following:
   a. Can be done without special knowledge of skin testing or availability of allergen extract.
   b. Patient does not need to stop antihistamine before testing.
   c. Can be done even with severe eczema or other skin-related diseases.
   d. There is no risk of systemic anaphylactic reaction.
3. An immunofluorescent process is preferred for specific IgE testing because of high degree of sensitivity and specificity.
4. Some labs may offer a radioallergosorbent test (RAST); measures the allergen-specific IgE antibodies in serum samples after panel of allergens have been added to samples.

Nursing and Patient Care Considerations
1. Tell the patient that it is allergy testing without the risk of causing severe allergic reaction.
2. Obtain adequate venous blood for each allergen panel to be tested.
3. A positive result depends on the standards for that particular laboratory. The test does not indicate clinical significance of symptoms and must be interpreted with patient's history.

4. Arrange for a follow-up visit for the patient with the health care provider to discuss test results.

GENERAL PROCEDURES AND TREATMENT MODALITIES

 See additional online content: Procedure Guidelines 28-3.

Immunotherapy

Immunotherapy is the modulation of the immune system to develop tolerance to a known allergen that causes IgE, type I (immediate) hypersensitivity. Given in appropriate doses, it can significantly decrease patient symptoms in most patients. It is indicated for significant symptoms of allergic rhinitis, allergic conjunctivitis, allergic asthma, and stinging insect allergy that cannot be controlled by avoidance of the allergen. Considerable compliance and time commitment are essential for successful therapy.

Features of Immunotherapy
1. Specific allergens are identified by skin or blood testing.
2. Serial injections are begun that contain extracts from identified allergens (allergy vaccine).
3. Initially, a small amount of dilute allergy vaccine is given, usually at weekly intervals.
4. Amount and concentration are slowly increased to maximum tolerable dose.
5. The maintenance dose is injected every 2 to 4 weeks for a period of several years to achieve maximal benefit.
6. Several allergens are now standardized (dust mite, cat, grass and ragweed pollens, Hymenoptera venoms [yellow jacket, yellow and white-faced hornet, honey bee, wasp]).

Precautions and Considerations
1. Anaphylaxis rarely occurs after injection but risk remains.
   a. Usually given in health care facility with epinephrine, trained personnel, and emergency equipment available. See Standards of Care Guidelines 28-1, page 793.
   b. Patient should remain in office for 30 minutes after injection, after which the risk of anaphylaxis is greatly reduced.
   c. If large, local reaction (erythema, induration) occurs after an injection, the next dose should not be increased without checking with prescribing health care provider because a systemic reaction may occur.
2. If several weeks are missed, dosage may need to be decreased to prevent a reaction.
3. Medication, such as antihistamines and decongestants, should be continued until significant symptom relief occurs (may take 12 to 24 months).
4. Environmental controls should be maintained to enhance effectiveness of therapy.

 NURSING ALERT With immunotherapy (allergy shots), the risk of systemic reaction is always present, occurring in 0.02% of injections. Skin testing can also result in systemic reactions. Have epinephrine 1:1,000 available during these procedures (with syringe and tourniquet) and have patient remain in office or clinic for at least 30 minutes after administration.

To perform immunotherapy or allergy testing, have Epinephrine 1:1,000 available with a 1-mL syringe and a 1-inch (2.5 cm) needle.

- Make sure that the patient remains under observation for at least 30 minutes after injection and assess for local reaction and respiratory distress before the patient leaves.
- If a significant reaction occurred after the last injection or if the patient is late for his or her dosage, follow written protocol for those cases or call the patient's health care provider for instructions.
- Be prepared to inject 0.3 to 0.5 mL (or 0.01 mL/kg for children less than 30 kg) of epinephrine IM as directed by health care provider present or facility protocol if signs of anaphylaxis develop. Call for immediate help and transfer to an acute care facility.

This information should serve as a general guideline only. Each patient situation presents a unique set of clinical factors and requires nursing judgment to guide care, which may include additional or alternative measures and approaches. IM, intramuscular.

ALLERGIC DISORDERS
Anaphylaxis

Anaphylaxis is an immediate, life-threatening systemic reaction that can occur on exposure to a particular substance. It can occur within an hour or longer. It is a result of a type I hypersensitivity reaction in which chemical mediators released from mast cells and basophils affect many types of tissue and organ systems. It can be an IgE-mediated allergen such as immunotherapy or a non–IgE-mediated allergen as in contrast media.

 EVIDENCE BASE Lieberman, P., Nicklas, R. A., Randolph, C., et al. (2015). Anaphylaxis—a practice parameter update 2015. *Annals of Allergy, Asthma and Immunology, 115*, 341–384.

Pathophysiology and Etiology

1. May be caused by:
   a. Immunotherapy.
   b. Stinging insects such as honeybee, Australian native ants, wasps
   c. Skin testing.
   d. Medications, most commonly antibiotics and nonsteroidal anti-inflammatory drugs (NSAIDs).
   e. Contrast media infusion.
   f. Foods such as peanuts, seeds, cow's milk, sea food, dairy products, eggs.
   g. Exercise and exposure to cold.
   h. Latex.
2. Mast cell activation causes release of chemical mediators (histamine, leukotrienes, tumor necrosis factor, cytokines), which results in massive vasodilation, increased capillary permeability, smooth muscle contraction, and increased mucosal secretions, which results in bronchoconstriction and decreased peristalsis.

Clinical Manifestations

1. Respiratory—laryngeal edema, bronchospasm, cough, wheezing, dyspnea, feeling of lump in throat.
2. Cardiovascular—hypotension, tachycardia (as a compensatory response to the hypotension), palpitations, syncope, bradycardia with cardiovascular collapse can occur before cutaneous changes occur.
3. Cutaneous—urticaria (hives), angioedema, pruritus, erythema (flushing).
4. GI—nausea, vomiting, diarrhea, abdominal pain, bloating.

 DRUG ALERT Before administering any drug, ask if the patient has ever had a reaction to it. Do not rely on the medical record alone.

Management

Prompt identification of signs and symptoms and immediate intervention are essential; a reaction that occurs quickly tends to be more severe.

Immediate Treatment
www.aaaai.org/conditions-and-treatments/allergies/anaphylaxis
1. Place patient supine and check vital signs.
2. Immediately administer epinephrine 1:1,000—adolescents and adults, 0.3 to 0.5 mL; children, 0.01 mL/kg via intramuscular (IM) route into vastus lateralis muscle. This may be repeated every 5 to 10 minutes if necessary—causes vasoconstriction, decreases capillary permeability, relaxes airway smooth muscle, and inhibits mast cell mediator release.
3. Monitor vital signs continuously.
4. Administer oxygen, if needed.
5. A tourniquet is applied above site of antigen injection (allergy injection, insect sting, etc.) or skin test site to slow the absorption of antigen into the system.

Subsequent Adjunct Treatment
1. An adequate airway is established, and bronchodialtor (albuterol or salbutamol) is administered by nebulization (using face mask or handheld mouthpiece), as needed.
2. Hypotension and shock are treated with IV fluids (normal saline) and vasopressors.
3. Additional bronchodilators are given to relax bronchial smooth muscle.
4. Histamine-1 (H_1) antihistamines, such as diphenhydramine, and, possibly, H_2 antihistamines, such as ranitidine, are given to block the effects of histamine by relieving itching and urticaria.
5. Corticosteroids such as methylprednisolone are given to decrease vascular permeability and diminish the migration of inflammatory cells; may be helpful in preventing late-phase responses.

Complications
1. Cardiovascular collapse.
2. Respiratory failure.

Nursing Assessment
1. Promptly assess airway, breathing, and circulation (ABCs) with severe presentation and intervene with cardiopulmonary resuscitation, as appropriate.
2. When ABCs are stable, assess vital signs, degree of respiratory distress, and angioedema.
3. Obtain a history of onset of symptoms and of exposure to allergen.

Nursing Diagnoses

- Ineffective Breathing Pattern related to bronchospasm and laryngeal edema.
- Decreased Cardiac Output related to vasodilation.
- Anxiety related to respiratory distress and life-threatening situation.

Nursing Interventions

Restoring Effective Breathing

1. Establish and maintain an adequate airway.
   a. If epinephrine has not stabilized bronchospasm, assist with endotracheal intubation, emergency tracheostomy, or cricothyroidotomy, as indicated.
   b. Continually monitor respiratory rate, depth, and breath sounds for decreased work of breathing and effective ventilation.
2. Administer nebulized albuterol or other bronchodilators, as ordered. Monitor heart rate (increased with bronchodilators).
3. Provide oxygen via nasal cannula at 2 to 5 L/minute or by alternative means, as ordered.
4. Administer intravenous (IV) corticosteroids, as ordered.

Increasing Cardiac Output

1. Monitor blood pressure (BP) by continuous automatic cuff, if available.
2. Administer rapid infusion of IV fluids to fill vasodilated circulatory system and raise BP.
3. Monitor central venous pressure (CVP) to ensure adequate fluid volume and to prevent fluid overload.
4. Insert indwelling catheter and monitor urine output hourly to ensure kidney perfusion.
5. Initiate and titrate vasopressor, as ordered, based on BP response.

Reducing Anxiety

1. Provide care in a prompt, calm, and confident manner.
2. Remain responsive to the patient, who may remain alert but not completely coherent because of hypotension, hypoxemia, and effects of medication.
3. Keep family or significant others informed of patient's condition and the treatment being given.
4. When patient is stable and alert, give a simple, honest explanation of anaphylaxis and the treatment that was given.

Community and Home Care Considerations

1. Make sure that patient who has experienced anaphylaxis or severe local reactions obtains a prescription for self-injectable epinephrine to have available at all times.
2. Even if treatment is given successfully at home, encourage the patient to follow-up with the health care provider immediately.
3. Make sure that the patient with history of anaphylaxis has access to emergency medical system and does not spend time alone if risk of reaction is present.

Patient Education and Health Maintenance

1. Teach the patient at risk for anaphylaxis about the potential seriousness of these reactions, avoiding allergens, and identifying early signs and symptoms of anaphylaxis.
2. Instruct the patient and family members on the injection technique upon exposure to known antigen or at the first signs of a systemic reaction.
   a. Provide patient with information on epinephrine, including dose, drug action, possible adverse effects, and the importance of prompt administration at the first sign of a systemic reaction.
   b. Encourage the patient to check expiration date regularly and obtain replacement of outdated epinephrine.
   c. Ensure day care providers, coworkers, and school personnel are aware of patient's potential for anaphylaxis and have access to and are able to administer epinephrine.
3. People allergic to venom stings should avoid wearing brightly colored or black clothes, perfumes, and hair spray. Shoes should be worn at all times.
4. For exercise-induced anaphylaxis, patient should exercise in moderation, preferably with another person, and in a controlled setting, where assistance is readily available.
5. Instruct patient to wear a medical alert tag at all times.
6. For potential drug allergies, teach the patient to:
   a. Read labels and be familiar with the generic name of the drug thought to cause a reaction.
   b. Discard all unused drugs. Make sure any drug kept in the medicine cabinet is clearly labeled.
   c. Become familiar with drugs that may cross-react with a drug to which patient is allergic.
   d. Always know the name of every drug taken.
   e. Clear all herbals and nutraceuticals with health care provider.
7. Advise patient with a known sensitivity to a food product to be extremely careful about everything he or she eats—allergen compounds may be hidden in a preparation (such as caseinate, lactalbumin).
8. Advise that if food is associated with exercise-induced anaphylaxis, wait at least 2 hours after eating to exercise.

Evaluation: Expected Outcomes

- Respirations unlabored with clear lung fields, minimal wheezing.
- BP and CVP within normal range; urine output adequate.
- Responsive and cooperative.

Allergic Rhinitis

Allergic rhinitis is an inflammation of the nasal mucosa caused by an allergen that affects 10% to 30% of the population and up to 40% of children.

Pathophysiology and Etiology

1. Type I hypersensitivity causes local vasodilation and increased capillary permeability.
2. Caused by airborne allergens.
3. IgE-mediated inflammatory process is now believed to be the same disease process for asthma and allergic rhinitis. IgE antibodies bind to IgE receptors on mast cells in respiratory mucosa. When patient is exposed to the same allergen, then mast cells activates chemical mediators resulting in allergic rhinitis.
4. Allergic rhinitis was formerly classified as seasonal or perennial; current classifications are intermittent or persistent.
   a. Intermittent—symptoms present less than 4 days per week and less than 4 weeks per year.
   b. Persistent—symptoms present more than 4 days per week and more than 4 weeks per year.
5. Severity is classified as mild (no interference with daily activities or troublesome symptoms) or moderate-severe (presence of at least one: impaired sleep, daily activity, work, or school; troublesome symptoms).

Clinical Manifestations

1. Nasal—mucous membrane congestion, edema, itching, rhinorrhea with clear secretions, sneezing, nasal obstruction, or nasal drip.
2. Eyes—edema, itching, burning, tearing, redness, dark circles under eyes (allergic shiners).
3. Ears—itching, fullness.
4. Other—postnasal drainage, palatal itching, throat itching, nonproductive cough.

Diagnostic Evaluation

1. Skin testing—confirms a hypersensitivity to certain allergens. Quick and cost-effective.
2. Nasal smear—increased number of eosinophils suggests allergic disease.
3. ImmunoCAP or other *in vitro* IgE-specific antigen testing—positive test result for offending allergens.
4. Rhinoscopy—allows better visualization of the nasopharynx; helps rule out physical obstruction (septal deviation, nasal polyps).
5. Evaluation for asthma.

Management

Avoidance

1. Patient should minimize contact with offending allergens, regardless of other treatment.
2. Patient may be instructed to reduce dust mite exposure by encasing bed pillows and mattress in allergen-proof covering; however, studies have not shown that this alone improves symptoms. Use of allergen-proof bedding should be carried out in conjunction with broad environmental controls (see Patient Education Guidelines 28-1).

Medications: Antihistamines

H_1 antihistamines—block the effects of histamine on smooth muscle and blood vessels by blocking histamine receptor sites, thereby preventing the symptoms of allergic rhinitis.

1. Loratadine, fexofenadine, and cetirizine are long-acting antihistamines sold over-the-counter (OTC) and are considered nonsedating (cetirizine is considered less sedating).
2. Long-acting, nonsedating antihistamines available by prescription include desloratadine and levocetirizine.
3. Topical antihistamine nasal spray available by prescription (azelastine or olopatadine).
4. Older, sedating antihistamines (diphenhydramine, chlorpheniramine) are inexpensive, available OTC, short-acting, and effective if tolerated by the patient. Older antihistamines are sedating. They also have an anticholinergic effect—inhibit mucous secretions, act as drying agents.

Medications: Controllers

1. Intranasal corticosteroids: beclomethasone, flunisolide, budesonide, mometasone
   a. Reduce inflammation of nasal mucosa.
   b. Prevent mediator release.
   c. Can be used safely every day.
   d. May be given systemically for a short course during a disabling attack.
2. Mast cell stabilizers—such as intranasal cromolyn sodium or ophthalmic cromolyn and lodoxamide hinder the release of chemical mediators. These medications are used before and during allergen season.
3. Leukotriene receptor antagonists, including montelukast and zafirlukast, are systemic agents used for asthma; montelukast also has an indication in allergic rhinitis and reduces the inflammation, edema, and mucous secretion of allergic rhinitis.

Medications: Symptom Relief

1. Oral corticosteroids may be given systematically for a short course during a disabling attack.
2. Decongestants—shrink nasal mucous membrane by vasoconstriction; oral and topical, many available OTC and in combination with antihistamines, pain relievers, and anticholinergics.
3. Topical eye preparations—sold OTC and by prescription; reduce inflammation and relieve itching and burning.

Immunotherapy

1. Regimen consists of administering subcutaneous injections of increasing amounts of an allergen to which the patient is sensitive to decrease sensitivity and reduce the severity of symptoms (see page 792).

PATIENT EDUCATION GUIDELINES 28-1

Environmental Control for Allergic Rhinitis

The following environmental modifications may help reduce symptoms of allergic rhinitis (hay fever):

- Encase pillows and mattress in allergen-proof covers.
- Wash all bed linens (mattress pad, sheets, blanket, comforter, and bedspread) in hot water weekly.
- Keep clothing in a closet with door shut or in dresser drawers that are kept closed.
- Use easily cleaned shades, blinds, and curtains.
- Avoid stuffed animals and other items that collect dust.
- Vacuum and damp-dust weekly; wear a mask while doing it.
- If you have severe symptoms of dust allergy, leave the house during cleaning. Allergic reaction is possible for about 30 minutes after vacuuming because dust mite feces and other allergens become airborne. Fine-filtering face masks may provide some protection.
- Eliminate upholstered furniture, carpets, and draperies.
- Use air conditioning and keep windows closed during high pollen and mold seasons to reduce antigen load indoors.
- Change furnace and air conditioner filters frequently.
- Using a high-efficiency air filtering system may help.
- Avoid smoking and smoke-filled areas.
- Avoid rapid changes in temperature.
- If you are allergic to animal dander, you should not have household pets. If pets are present in your household, keep them out of the bedroom and run a high-efficiency particulate air filter (place on table).
- Avoid mold growth by dehumidification (less than 45% ambient humidity) and use of a fungicide in bathrooms, damp basements, food storage areas, and garbage containers.
- Avoid outdoor activities when pollen or other pollutants are in the air.

2. Immunotherapy produces the following immunologic changes:
   a. Production of IgG-blocking antibody that combines with antigen before it reacts with IgE antibodies.
   b. Decreases IgE antibodies against specific antigens.
   c. Modulation from T helper (Th) 2 to Th1 T lymphocytes (Th2 associated with allergy).
3. Possible adverse effects of immunotherapy.
   a. Systemic reactions—anaphylaxis is rare, but potentially fatal.
   b. Local reactions—consist of erythema and induration at the site of injection.

 NURSING ALERT Immunotherapy should be administered with caution to patients taking beta-adrenergic blockers and should not be given to patients whose asthma is not controlled.

Complications

1. Allergic asthma.
2. Chronic otitis media, hearing loss.
3. Chronic nasal obstruction, nasal polyps, sinusitis.
4. Orthodontic malocclusion in children.

Nursing Assessment

1. Obtain history of severity and seasonality of symptoms.
2. Inspect for characteristic tearing, conjunctival erythema, pale nasal mucous membranes with clear discharge, allergic shiners, and mouth breathing.
3. Auscultate lungs for wheezing or prolonged expiration characteristic of asthma.

Nursing Diagnosis

- Ineffective Breathing Pattern related to nasal obstruction.

Nursing Interventions

Facilitating Normal Breathing Pattern

1. Reassure patient that suffocation will not occur because of nasal obstruction; mouth breathing will occur.
2. Use intranasal saline to soothe irritated mucous membranes and increase oral fluid intake to prevent drying of mucous membranes and increased insensible loss through mouth breathing.
3. Administer and teach self-administration of antihistamines, decongestants, intranasal corticosteroids and antihistamine, and other medications, as directed.
   a. Instruct patients on proper use of nasal sprays—clear mucus from nose first, exhale, flex neck to point nose downward, direct spray away from the nasal septum (toward the eye), activate the spray, and gently sniff while releasing medication. Report any nasal irritation or nose bleeds to provider.
   b. Warn patient to avoid driving or other situations that require alertness if sedating antihistamines, such as diphenhydramine or chlorpheniramine, are being used.
   c. Do not use OTC nasal decongestants for more than 4 to 5 days because their effect is short term and a rebound effect, which causes nasal mucosal edema, commonly occurs.

 DRUG ALERT Long-term use of nasal corticosteroids may cause nasal septum rupture. Teach patients to direct spray or aerosol away from septum.

Patient Education and Health Maintenance

1. Provide information on purpose, administration method, time frame of expected results, and possible risks involved (local reactions, anaphylaxis) with immunotherapy.
2. Inform the patient that close observation for 30 minutes is essential after each injection.
3. Alert patient to the possibility of a delayed reaction during immunotherapy that should be reported to the nurse or health care provider.
4. Teach lifestyle and environmental changes to reduce exposure to allergens.
5. For additional information and support, refer to American Academy of Allergy, Asthma, and Immunology (*www.aaaai.org*), American College of Allergy, Asthma & Immunology (*www.acaai.org*), and National Institute of Allergy and Infectious Diseases Office of Communications (*www.niaid.nih.gov*).

Evaluation: Expected Outcomes

- Decreased nasal congestion, no mouth breathing, and no complaints of dry mouth.

Urticaria and Angioedema

Urticaria, or hives, may affect 25% of the population at any given time. Lesion is intensely pruritic erythematous. *Angioedema* is a similar lesion but involves deep dermis and subcutaneous tissues. Urticaria and angioedema can occur individually or in combination.

Pathophysiology and Etiology

1. Acute urticaria:
   a. Hives that last less than 6 weeks.
   b. A detectable cause is often determined.
2. Chronic urticaria:
   a. Hives that last 6 weeks or longer.
   b. Up to 50% of cases may be autoimmune chronic urticaria with autoantibodies against high-affinity IgE receptor or IgE.
   c. At least 50% are idiopathic.
3. Cause may be undetermined or may include:
   a. Ingested substances—food, food additives, latex, drugs (such as penicillins, cephalosporins).
   b. Infections—viral, bacterial, parasitic.
   c. Physical factors—heat, sunlight, cold, pressure, vibration.
   d. Emotional stress.
   e. Insect stings (bees, wasps, hornets, fire ants).

Clinical Manifestations

1. Raised, red, edematous wheals.
2. Intense pruritus.
3. May affect any body region.
4. Diffuse swelling with angioedema, especially of the lips, eyelids, cheeks, hands, and feet.
5. Symptoms may develop within seconds or over 1 to 2 hours and may last up to 24 to 36 hours.

Diagnostic Evaluation

1. Laboratory—serum tryptase is elevated in the acute phase, complement study results can be abnormal, total serum IgE elevated.
2. Challenge testing to determine physical cause.
   a. Dermographism (most common).
   b. Exercise challenge.
   c. Ice cube challenge.
   d. Heat challenge.
   e. Pressure challenge.

Management

Acute Urticaria

1. Identification and elimination of causative factors.
2. Medications.
   a. H_1 antihistamines, such as diphenhydramine and cetirizine.
   b. Corticosteroids—limited to severe cases; unresponsive to antihistamines.
   c. Epinephrine 1:1,000 (0.3 to 0.5 mL IM) for severe angio-edema or urticaria.

Chronic Urticaria

1. Avoid causative factors.
2. Medications.
   a. H_1 antihistamines.
   b. H_2 antihistamines, such as ranitidine, may be of some value.
   c. Tricyclic antidepressants, such as doxepin, given for anti-histaminic effect.
   d. Topical agents to relieve itching (moisturizer or oatmeal baths).
3. Severe, unremitting urticarial treatment may include low-dose cyclosporine, tacrolimus, or omalizumab therapy.

Complications

1. Neurovascular impairment because of swelling.
2. Rarely, edema of the larynx or bronchi.

Nursing Assessment

1. Assess for time frame during which lesions appear and disappear.
2. Assess for triggering factors.
3. Assess for family history of angioedema; may indicate heredi-tary angioedema rather than allergic reaction.

Nursing Diagnosis

- Impaired comfort related to pruritus.

Nursing Interventions

Relieving Pruritus

1. Administer or teach self-administration of antihistamines, corticosteroids, and additional medications, as prescribed.
2. Encourage the proper use of topical and OTC agents, as directed.
3. Advise patient to avoid exposure to heat, exercise, sunburn, and alcohol and to promptly control fever and anxiety—factors that may aggravate reactions caused by vasodilation.
4. Warn patient to avoid identified triggers.
5. Teach relaxation techniques and methods of distraction to enhance coping.
6. Assess effectiveness of therapy.

Patient Education and Health Maintenance

1. Warn the patient to monitor for symptoms of laryngeal edema and to seek medical intervention immediately if respiratory distress occurs.
2. Instruct patients with laryngeal edema how to self-administer epinephrine.

Evaluation: Expected Outcomes

- Reports relief of pruritus with antihistamines and distraction methods.

Food Allergies

Food allergies result when the body's immune system overreacts to certain, otherwise harmless, substances. Food allergies occur in 8% of children and in 2% of adults, although the perceived prevalence is much higher because other existing adverse food reactions cause similar symptoms.

Pathophysiology and Etiology

1. Food hypersensitivity—a true food allergy is an IgE-mediated response to a food allergen (protein).
2. Food intolerance—an abnormal physical response to a food or additive; may be immunologic but not IgE-mediated.
   a. Toxicity (poisoning)—caused by toxins contained in foods, microorganisms, or parasites.
   b. Pharmacologic (chemical)—such as caffeine.
   c. Idiosyncratic—etiology unknown.
3. Common food allergens include cow's milk, eggs, shellfish, peanuts, tree nuts, soybean, and wheat.

Clinical Manifestations

1. Respiratory—rhinoconjunctivitis, sneezing, laryngeal edema, wheezing.
2. Cutaneous—urticaria, angioedema, atopic dermatitis.
3. Gastroenteritis—lip swelling, palatal itching, nausea, abdomi-nal cramping, diarrhea, vomiting.
4. Neurologic—migraine headache in some patients.

Diagnostic Evaluation

1. Skin testing.
   a. Limited to those foods suspected of provoking symptoms based on history.
   b. Only epicutaneous testing is recommended.
   c. Intradermal testing has not been demonstrated to have a high degree of clinical correlation.
2. ImmunoCAP, RAST, or other IgE-specific antigen *in vitro* testing—positive result.
3. Oral challenge—the suspected food is given to the patient to identify the allergen by reproducing the symptoms caused by the initial reaction.
   a. Open—may be used if the suspected food skin test result is negative; suspected food is openly administered and the patient is monitored for a reaction.
   b. Single-blind—suspected food is disguised in capsules, liquids, or other foods and administered to the patient in increasing doses at intervals determined by history and may be interspersed with placebo. Some bias exists, however.
   c. Double-blind placebo-controlled—the "gold standard" and most definitive technique to confirm or refute food allergy. The suspected food is administered in capsules or via some other vehicle that masks its identity; it is interspersed with pla-cebo so neither the health care provider nor the patient knows whether the suspected food or placebo is being ingested.
4. Elimination diet.
   a. To determine if the patient's symptoms will stop when cer-tain foods are avoided.
   b. Restrict one or two foods at a time if certain foods are suspected.
   c. If no particular food is suspected, a highly restricted diet for 14 days is preferable.

Management

1. Avoidance of specific foods is the only way of effectively preventing food allergy reactions.
2. Medications:
   a. Antihistamines—may modify IgE-mediated symptoms but will not eliminate them.
   b. Corticosteroids—only used in the treatment of food allergy if associated with eosinophilic gastroenteritis or gastroenteropathy.
   c. Epinephrine—if history of anaphylaxis, patient should carry subcutaneous self-injection at all times.
3. Oral desensitization may be considered under careful observation.

Complications

Anaphylaxis.

Nursing Assessment

1. Assist with assessment for offending foods; encourage the patient to keep a food and symptom diary.
2. Auscultate lungs and document any wheezing.
3. Assess adherence with prescribed diet and relief of symptoms.

Nursing Diagnosis

- Imbalanced Nutrition: Less Than Body Requirements related to restrictive diet.

Nursing Interventions

Promoting Adequate Nutrition

1. Consult with dietitian to ensure a balanced diet that excludes identified allergens and incorporates patient's food preferences.
2. Administer dietary supplements, as needed.
3. Discuss alternative food preparation techniques and methods of substitution (such as using extra baking powder in place of eggs).
4. Administer and teach self-administration of medications, if necessary, to reduce abdominal cramping and diarrhea, which may deter food intake.
5. Monitor weight.

Patient Education and Health Maintenance

1. Instruct the patient with history of anaphylactic reaction about self-injection technique for the administration of epinephrine.
2. Caution highly allergic patient about restaurant food; when eating out, avoid buffets and patient should request ingredient information; brochures listing ingredients of various dishes are now available in many restaurants, including fast food establishments.
3. Explain hidden sources of foods to decrease the risk of unexpected exposure to an offending allergen. Some foods may contain allergens not as primary ingredients but as fillers or additives. Likewise, a food that has been prepared or stored in the same container or cooled on the same surface as an allergen-containing food may become contaminated with a sufficient quantity of the allergen to cause a reaction. Encourage label reading.
4. Advise patient that most young children and about one third of older children and adults lose their food sensitivity after several years of avoidance. Compliance with elimination is the key. Sensitivity to shellfish and nuts is rarely lost, however.
5. Provide resource for patient to obtain more information: The Food Allergy & Anaphylaxis Network (*www.foodallergy.org*).

Evaluation: Expected Outcomes

- Decreased frequency and severity of food allergy reactions by log; verbalizes acceptance of diet; weight stable.

Latex Sensitivity

Latex sensitivity is becoming a major health concern for health care workers, patients, and others at risk by occupation. Allergic reaction may be immediate or delayed. Latex is present in approximately 40,000 medical and other products, including household products and toys. The prevalence of latex sensitivity is estimated to be 1% in the general population, 20% in nurses, and more than 60% in children with spina bifida.

Pathophysiology and Etiology

1. Natural rubber latex, manufactured from the sap of rubber trees, is highly irritating and allergenic in some people.
2. Increased use of latex, in the form of sterile and unsterile gloves, has made latex sensitivity a problem for many health care workers since the inception of Universal Precautions in the 1980s.
3. Three types of reactions to latex may occur:
   a. Irritant dermatitis—not an allergic reaction.
   b. Type IV (cell-mediated, delayed) hypersensitivity—a localized contact allergic reaction.
   c. Type I (IgE-mediated, immediate)—a systemic allergic reaction.
4. No predictable pattern exists for the progression of reactions; anaphylaxis may occur at any time. More severe reaction occurs with latex contact with mucous membrane than with intact skin.
5. Those at risk include children with spina bifida, health care workers, people with atopic allergies, people with a history of multiple surgeries, and workers in factories that produce latex products.

Clinical Manifestations

1. Irritant dermatitis—may be caused by powder or chemical residue on gloves; erythema and pruritus localized to area of contact; occurs immediately.
2. Type IV (delayed) hypersensitivity—contact allergic reaction; erythema, pruritus, urticaria; possible flushing, localized edema, rhinitis, coughing, and conjunctivitis. Symptoms occur 1 to 48 hours after contact with product.
3. Type I (immediate) hypersensitivity—urticaria, angioedema, conjunctivitis, dyspnea, pharyngeal edema, arrhythmias, and anaphylaxis. Symptoms are immediate and may be moderate to life-threatening in intensity.

Diagnostic Evaluation

1. History of symptoms gives presumptive diagnosis, but confirmation is difficult because standardized tests are not yet widely available.
2. A crude skin prick test uses a fragment of latex glove soaked in saline for 15 minutes as the solution. This is not standardized, but a positive test result is considered proof of latex sensitivity.
3. A challenge test can be done by having the patient wear a latex glove or fingertip of a glove for 15 minutes; look for a reaction. Latex-free gloves can be used as a control. Severe reactions may occur with this test.
4. Standardized skin testing will become more available pending Food and Drug Administration approval of standardized latex solution, but the threat of anaphylaxis will still exist.
5. RAST or other IgE *in vitro* blood testing is safe but expensive and is limited due to both false-positive and false-negative results.

Management

1. Avoidance is the key. See Box 28-1 for safety and prevention techniques in the health care workplace.
2. For irritant reactions, changing brands of gloves or changing to a powder-free glove may be sufficient.
3. Decreasing length of exposure time or wearing cotton liners in gloves may help, but may not solve the problem.
4. Use of latex-free gloves and products is usually necessary. Although more hospitals and medical offices are making latex-free products available, a job change may be necessary for some people.
5. A latex-free environment is necessary for treatment.
6. Topical corticosteroid creams may be used for local reactions.
7. Oral antihistamines may be used for mild to moderate reactions.
8. Epinephrine, oral or parenteral corticosteroids, and IM antihistamines are given for severe reactions.
9. IV fluids, oxygen, and intubation may be needed for cardiovascular and pulmonary support with severe reactions.

Complications

Unpredictable anaphylaxis and death.

Nursing Assessment

1. Assess patient for history of risk factors and pattern of suspected reactions.
2. Assess skin for erythema, swelling, vesicles, and other lesions.
3. Assess mucous membranes for conjunctivitis, rhinitis, and other lesions.
4. For suspected systemic reactions, assess vital signs for hypotension, tachycardia, arrhythmia, and respiratory distress.
5. Assess respiratory status for stridor caused by laryngeal edema and breath sounds for wheezing.
6. Assess for signs of internal edema with systemic reaction, such as nausea, vomiting, and diarrhea.

Nursing Diagnosis

- Deficient Knowledge related to sources of latex and how to avoid latex.

BOX 28-1	Latex Safety for Patients and Health Care Workers

- Use latex-free gloves of synthetic rubber, vinyl, nitrile, neoprene, or other material.
- Be aware that removing latex gloves with power may cause latex particles to become aerosolized for up to 5 hours and be carried to other areas on clothing and equipment.
- Do not enter OR with latex gloves or without having scrubbed after removing latex gloves in another area and remove possibly latex-laden clothing.
- Schedule latex-sensitive patients early in the day or as first surgical case.
- Post signs indicating Latex Allergy or Latex Alert.
- Encourage latex-sensitive individuals to wear identification bracelets.
- Evaluate all equipment for latex prior to use.
- A latex-free cart should accompany a latex-sensitive patient throughout the facility.
- Each facility should form a latex allergy task force with representatives from all departments.

Nursing Interventions and Patient Education

Increasing Knowledge about Latex Avoidance

1. Educate patients about the widespread use of latex; latex-free alternatives are usually available (see Table 28-1).
2. Ensure that patients with history of type I reaction have self-injectable epinephrine and antihistamines on hand at all times to use at first sign of a reaction.
3. Encourage patients who have had immediate hypersensitivity reactions to wear a medical alert tag.
4. Encourage patients to notify all their health care providers, labs, and clinics before they make a visit, to facilitate the use of latex-free products. These patients should be given the first appointment of the day and all supplies that contain latex should be removed from the room or covered with a cotton cloth. Only latex-free products should be used, and staff members should be careful to avoid wearing or removing latex gloves in the hall while the patient is in the office.
5. Support the patient who has had a severe reaction in the workplace. Remind the patient that the Americans with Disabilities Act guarantees workers reasonable modifications to the workplace to accommodate a disability. However, the area of latex sensitivity as a disability is controversial.
6. For further information, contact the American Latex Allergy Association (*www.latexallergyresources.org*) and the National Institute for Occupational Safety and Health (*www.cdc.gov/NIOSH/homepage.html*).

Evaluation: Expected Outcomes

- Verbalizes signs of reaction and appropriate treatment.

Table 28-1	Sources of Latex in Health Care Facilities and at Home
HEALTH CARE FACILITY	**HOME AND COMMUNITY**
Syringes	Mattresses and foam in furniture
Medication vial stoppers	Undergarments and clothing
Intravenous catheters, tubing	Bathmats and rugs
Stopcocks	Pacifiers and diapers
Tourniquet	Toys such as balls and dolls
Tape, dressings, drains	Pet toys
Elastic wraps	Bicycle helmets
Waterproof pads	Cosmetics
Blood pressure cuff	Food storage bags
Stethoscope	Drain stoppers
Reflex hammer	Spatulas
Electrocardiograph electrodes	Earphones
Oximetry sensor	Garden hose
Manual resuscitation bag	Rubber-handled tools
Oxygen canula, mask, tubing	Weather stripping
Airways, endotracheal tube	Plants—rubber, poinsettia, ficus
Urinary catheters	Scratch-off tickets and advertisements
Suction catheters	Raincoats and waterproof boots
Casting materials	Glue, envelopes, stamps

Bronchial Asthma

 EVIDENCE BASE National Heart, Lung and Blood Institute, National Asthma Education and Prevention Program Expert Panel Report 3. (2007). Guidelines for the diagnosis and management of asthma. *Summary Report 2007, NIH Publication No. 08–5846.* Bethesda, MD: National Institutes of Health. Available: *www.nhlbi.nih.gov/guidelines/asthma/asthsumm.pdf.*
Global Initiative for Asthma. (2016). Global strategy for asthma management and prevention. Available: *www.gin-asthma.org*

Asthma is a chronic inflammatory disease of the airways, characterized by airflow obstruction, which is at least partially reversible; bronchial hyperreactivity; and mucus production. The course of asthma is highly variable. In 2007, the National Asthma Education and Prevention Program Expert Panel Report 3 and in 2010, the Global Initiative for Asthma guidelines were updated. These updates are evidence-based and continue to recommend treatment that is stepwise and based on severity; however, the updates emphasize assessment of control, impairment of daily function, and risk for exacerbation at subsequent patient visits. Although severity is best established prior to the use of asthma medications, it may be determined based on the medications necessary to gain control and directs initial therapy.

Asthma therapy is characterized by periodic follow-up visits and continual reassessment. One such factor that is always assessed includes control, which can be measured at home by the patient and family and evaluated and discussed at subsequent visits. The level of control guides adjustment of medications. Nurses can use control assessment to identify patients and families who need more asthma education to gain better control of asthma.

Pharmacotherapy for asthma is now based on three age groups: ages 0 to 4 years, ages 5 to 11 (see Chapter 44), and ages 12 and older. It is comprised of six steps and has expanded to include more medications for asthma; however, inhaled corticosteroids continue as the preferred long-term control therapy for all ages.

Pathophysiology and Etiology

The basic defect appears to be an abnormality in the host, which intermittently leads to an increased constriction of smooth muscle, hypersecretion of mucus in the bronchial tree, and mucosal edema.

Neuromechanisms (Autonomic Nervous System)

1. Stimulation of the vagus nerve (which is responsible for bronchomotor tone) by viral respiratory infections, air pollutants, and other stimuli causes bronchoconstriction, increased secretion of mucus, and dilation of the pulmonary vessels.
2. Beta-adrenergic receptor cells that line the airways are also responsible for bronchomotor tone. Abnormal functioning of these cells predisposes patients to bronchoconstriction.

Antigen–Antibody Reaction

1. Susceptible individuals form abnormally large amounts of IgE when exposed to certain allergens. Most children and more than half of adults with asthma are sensitized to at least one common inhaled allergen.
2. Antigen-specific IgE fixes itself to the mast cells of the bronchial mucosa.
3. When the person is exposed to certain allergens, the resulting antigen combines with the cell-bound IgE molecules, causing the mast cell and basophil to degranulate and release chemical mediators.

4. These chemical mediators act on bronchial smooth muscle to cause bronchoconstriction, on dilated epithelium to reduce mucociliary clearance, on bronchial glands to cause mucus secretion, on blood vessels to cause vasodilation and increased permeability, and on leukocytes to cause cellular infiltration and inflammation.
5. Late-phase reactions (these occur 4 to 8 hours after the initial response) include the influx of eosinophils, neutrophils, lymphocytes, and monocytes.

Bronchial Inflammation

1. Occurs in both the immediate- and late-phase reactions caused by antigen–antibody response.
2. Factors other than allergens (such as noxious environmental stimuli) cause bronchial inflammation and hyperreactivity by mast cell activation.

Classification

Extrinsic Asthma

1. Hypersensitivity reaction to inhalant allergens (dust mites, animal allergens, cockroaches, pollen, and mold are the major ones).
2. Mediated by immunoglobulin E (IgE mediated).

Intrinsic Asthma

1. No inciting allergen.
2. Infection, typically viral.
3. Environmental stimuli (such as air pollution).

Mixed Asthma

Immediate type I reactivity appears to be combined with intrinsic factors.

Aspirin-Induced Asthma

1. Induced by ingestion of aspirin and related compounds.
2. "Samter Triad" has been described as a combination of aspirin-induced asthma, nasal polyps, and sinusitis.

Exercise-Induced Bronchoconstriction

Symptoms vary from slight chest tightness and cough to severe wheezing and cough and shortness of breath that usually occurs after 5 to 20 minutes of sustained exercise.

Occupational Asthma

Caused by inhalation of industrial fumes, dust, allergens, and gases.

Classification by Severity

1. Asthma severity for purposes of treatment is classified as intermittent, mild persistent, moderate persistent, and severe persistent based on level of impairment and risk for exacerbation.
2. Level of impairment parameters include degree of symptoms, nighttime awakenings, need to use short-acting beta$_2$-agonist for symptom control, interference with normal activity, and lung function by spirometry.
3. Risk level is based on the number of exacerbations that required oral corticosteroids within the past year and how severe they were.
4. See details of classifying asthma severity at *www.nhlbi.nih.gov/guidelines/asthma/asthgdln.pdf.*

Clinical Manifestations

1. Episodes of coughing.
2. Wheezing.
3. Dyspnea.
4. Feeling of chest tightness.

NURSING ALERT Do not be fooled by lack of wheezing on auscultation when the patient reports severe shortness of breath. Airflow may be so restricted that wheezing ceases.

Diagnostic Evaluation

1. Pulmonary function testing (spirometry)—more than 12% increase over baseline in forced expiratory volume in first second of exhalation (FEV_1) following inhalation of bronchodilator. Peak flow more than 20% variability between A.M. and P.M. measurements.
2. Bronchial challenge with airborne agent resulting in airway hyperreactivity; a positive challenge is determined by decrease in FEV_1 from baseline.
   a. Methacholine bronchial challenge (nebulized)—20% decrease in FEV_1.
   b. Mannitol (dry powder inhalation)—15% decrease in FEV_1.
3. Skin testing to identify causative allergens.
4. Chest x-ray to exclude other lung diseases in new-onset asthma in adult.

Management

The goal is to allow the person with asthma to live a normal life. The treatment plan should be as simple as possible and individualized to the patient's lifestyle. See Figure 28-2 for stepwise therapy for those ages 12 and older; see pages 1183 and 1184 for stepwise therapy for children younger than age 12. See Table 28-2, pages 802 and 803, and Table 28-3, page 803, for medication information. For additional information on treatment and specific dosages, see "Expert Panel Report 3: Guidelines for the Diagnosis and Management of Asthma" (National Heart, Lung and Blood Institute, 2007), pages 346–352 (*www.nhlbi.nih.gov/guidelines/asthma/asthgdln.pdf*).

Long-Term Controllers

1. Inhaled corticosteroids (ICSs), such as beclomethasone, budesonide, ciclesonide, flunisolide, fluticasone, mometasone.
2. Long-acting inhaled beta-agonists (LABA) include salmeterol, formoterol. *Note:* arformoterol is a LABA that is indicated for long-term control of chronic obstructive pulmonary disease, not asthma.
3. Combination inhalers, such as fluticasone and salmeterol, budesonide and formoterol, mometasone and formoterol.
4. Leukotriene modifiers, such as montelukast and zafirlukast.
5. Inhaled mast cell stabilizer: cromolyn sodium.

Intermittent Asthma	Persistent Asthma: Daily Medication Consult with asthma specialist if step 4 care or higher is required. Consider consultation at step 3.

Step 1

Preferred:

SABA PRN

Step 2

Preferred:

Low-dose ICS

Alternative:

Cromolyn, LTRA, Nedocromil, or Theophylline

Step 3

Preferred:

Low-dose ICS + LABA OR Medium-dose ICS

Alternative:

Low-dose ICS + either LTRA, Theophylline, or Zileuton

Step 4

Preferred:

Medium-dose ICS + LABA

Alternative:

Medium-dose ICS + either LTRA, Theophylline, or Zileuton

Step 5

Preferred:

High-dose ICS + LABA

AND

Consider Omalizumab for patients who have allergies

Step 6

Preferred:

High-dose ICS + LABA + oral corticosteroid

AND

Consider Omalizumab for patients who have allergies

Step up if needed

(first, check adherence, environmental control, and comorbid conditions)

Assess control

Step down if possible

(and asthma is well controlled at least 3 months)

Each step: Patient education, environmental control, and management of comorbidities.

Steps 2–4:   Consider subcutaneous allergen immunotherapy for patients who have allergic asthma.

Quick-Relief Medication for All Patients

- SABA as needed for symptoms. Intensity of treatment depends on severity of symptoms: up to 3 treatments at 20-minute intervals as needed. Short course of oral systemic corticosteroids may be needed.
- Use of SABA >2 days a week for symptom relief (not prevention of EIB) generally indicates in adequate control and the need to step up treatment.

Key: **Alphabetical order is used when more than one treatment option is listed within either preferred or alternative therapy.** EIB, exercise-induced bronchospasm; ICS, inhaled corticosteroid; LABA, long-acting inhaled beta–agonist; LTRA, leukotriene receptor antagonist; SABA, inhaled short-acting beta$_2$–agonist

Figure 28-2. Stepwise approach for managing asthma in youths age 12 or older and adults.

Table 28-2 Long-Term Control Medications

DRUG/INDICATION	MECHANISM	POTENTIAL ADVERSE EFFECTS
Inhaled Corticosteroids		
Beclomethasone, budesonide, flunisolide, ciclesonide, fluticasone, mometasone *Indications:* Long-term suppression of symptoms of asthma; suppression, control, and reversal of airway inflammation; reduced need for oral corticosteroids.	*Anti-inflammatory:* Block late reaction to allergen and reduce airway hyperresponsiveness; inhibit cytokine production, adhesion protein activation, and inflammatory cell migration and activation. Reverse beta$_2$-receptor down-regulation. Inhibit microvascular leakage.	Cough, dysphonia, oral candidiasis. In high doses, systemic effects may occur (adrenal suppression, osteoporosis, skin thinning, easy bruising), although studies are not conclusive, and clinical significance has not been established. In low to medium doses, suppression of growth velocity has been observed in children, but this effect may be transient and the clinical significance has not been established.
Systemic Corticosteroids		
Methylprednisolone, prednisolone, prednisone *Indications:* Short-term burst therapy to gain control of inadequately controlled asthma; long-term prevention of symptoms in severe persistent asthma.	*Anti-inflammatory:* Block late reaction to allergen and reduce airway hyperresponsiveness; inhibit cytokine production, adhesion protein activation, and inflammatory cell migration and activation. Reverse beta$_2$-receptor down-regulation. Inhibit microvascular leakage.	Short-term use: reversible abnormalities in glucose metabolism, increased appetite, fluid retention, weight gain, mood alteration, hypertension, peptic ulcer, and, rarely, aseptic necrosis. Long-term use: adrenal axis suppression, growth suppression, dermal thinning, hypertension, diabetes, Cushing syndrome, cataracts, muscle weakness, and, rarely, impaired immune function. Consideration should be given to coexisting conditions that could be worsened by systemic corticosteroids, such as herpes virus infections, varicella, tuberculosis, hypertension, peptic ulcer, diabetes mellitus, osteoporosis, and *Strongyloides.*
Mast Cell Stabilizers		
Cromolyn sodium (nebulizer solution only) *Indications:* Long-term prevention of symptoms in mild persistent asthma; may modify inflammation; preventive treatment prior to exposure to exercise or known allergen.	*Anti-inflammatory:* Block early and late reaction to allergen; interfere with chloride channel function. Stabilize mast cell membranes and inhibit activation and release of mediators from eosinophils and epithelial cells. Inhibit acute response to exercise, cold dry air, and SO$_2$.	Cough and irritation.
Immunomodulators		
Omalizumab *Indications:* Long-term control and prevention of symptoms in patients (≥age 12) who have moderate or severe persistent allergic asthma inadequately controlled with ICS.	Binds to circulating IgE, preventing it from binding to high-affinity receptors on basophils and mast cells. Decreases mast cell mediator release from allergen exposure and the number of high-affinity receptors in basophils and submucosal cells.	Pain and bruising at injection sites has been reported in 45% of patients. Anaphylaxis has been reported in 0.2% of treated patients. Malignant neoplasms have been reported in 0.5% of patients compared to 0.2% of patients receiving placebo; however, relationship to drug is unlikely.
Leukotriene Modifiers		
Montelukast, zafirlukast, zileuton *Indications:* Long-term control and prevention of symptoms in mild persistent asthma; may be used in combination with ICS in moderate persistent asthma. Montelukast is indicated in patients >age 1; zafirlukast, >age 7; zileuton, >age 12.	*Leukotriene receptor antagonist* (montelukast and zafirlukast): Selective competitive inhibitors of CysLT1 receptor. *5-Lipoxygenase inhibitor* (zileuton): Inhibits the production of leukotrienes—LTB$_4$ and cysteinyl leukotrienes—from arachidonic acid.	With zafirlukast, rare cases of Churg-Strauss have occurred, but the association is unclear; postmarketing surveillance has reported cases of reversible hepatitis and, rarely, irreversible hepatic failure resulting in liver transplantation and death. Elevation of liver enzymes has been reported with zileuton. There have been limited case reports of reversible hepatitis and hyperbilirubinemia.
Long-Acting Beta$_2$-Agonists		
Formoterol, salmeterol, oral sustained-release albuterol *Indications:* Long-term prevention of symptoms, added to ICS; prevention of exercise-induced bronchospasm. *Note:* Not to be used to treat acute exacerbations; only used in combination with inhaled corticosteroid.	*Bronchodilation:* Smooth muscle relaxation following adenylate cyclase activation and increase in cyclic AMP, producing functional antagonism of bronchoconstriction. Compared to SABA, salmeterol (but not formoterol) has slower onset of action (15 to 30 min). Both salmeterol and formoterol have longer duration (>12 hr) compared to SABA.	Tachycardia, skeletal muscle tremor, hypokalemia, prolongation of QTc interval in overdose. A diminished bronchoprotective effect may occur within 1 wk of chronic therapy (clinical significance has not been established). Potential risk of severe, life-threatening, or fatal exacerbation.

Table 28-2 Long-Term Control Medications (*Continued*)

DRUG/INDICATION	MECHANISM	POTENTIAL ADVERSE EFFECTS
Methylxanthines		
Theophylline sustained release *Indications:* Long-term control and prevention of symptoms in mild persistent asthma or as an adjunct to ICS in moderate or persistent asthma.	*Bronchodilation:* Smooth muscle relaxation from phosphodiesterase inhibition and possibly adenosine antagonism. May affect eosinophilic infiltration into bronchial mucosa as well as decreases T-lymphocyte numbers in epithelium. Increases diaphragm contractility and mucociliary clearance.	Dose-related acute toxicities include tachycardia, nausea and vomiting, tachyarrhythmias (supraventricular tachycardia), central nervous system stimulation, headache, seizures, hematemesis, hyperglycemia, and hypokalemia. Adverse effects at usual therapeutic doses include insomnia, gastric upset, aggravation of ulcer or reflux, increase in hyperactivity in some children, difficult urination in older males who have prostatism.

ICS, inhaled corticosteroid; SABA, short-acting beta-agonist.
Modified from Heart, Lung and Blood Institute, National Asthma Education and Prevention Program. (2007). Expert Panel Report 3: Guidelines for the diagnosis and management of asthma. Full Report 2007 (pp. 245–246). Available: www.nhlbi.nih.gov/guidelines/asthma/asthgdln.pdf.

Table 28-3 Quick Relief Medications

DRUG/INDICATION	MECHANISM	POTENTIAL ADVERSE EFFECTS
Short-Acting Beta$_2$-Agonists		
Albuterol, levalbuterol, pirbuterol *Indications:* Relief of acute symptoms; preventive treatment for exercise-induced bronchospasm prior to exercise.	*Bronchodilation:* Bind to the beta$_2$-adrenergic receptor, producing smooth muscle relaxation following adenylate cyclase activation and increase in cyclic AMP, producing functional antagonism of bronchoconstriction.	Tachycardia, skeletal muscle tremor, hypokalemia, increased lactic acid, headache, hyperglycemia. Inhaled route, in general, causes few systemic adverse effects. Patients with preexisting cardiovascular disease, especially older adults, may have adverse cardiovascular reactions with inhaled therapy.
Anticholinergic		
Ipratropium *Indications:* Acute bronchospasm; reverses only cholinergically mediated bronchospasm; does not modify reaction to antigen; does not block exercise-induced bronchospasm. Multiple doses of ipratropium in the emergency department provide additive effects to SABA. May be alternative for patients who do not tolerate SABA. Treatment of choice for bronchospasm because of beta-blocker medication.	*Bronchodilation:* Competitive inhibition of muscarinic cholinergic receptors. Reduces intrinsic vagal tone of the airways. May block reflex bronchoconstriction secondary to irritants or to reflux esophagitis. May decrease mucous gland secretion.	Drying of mouth and respiratory secretions, increased wheezing in some individuals, blurred vision if sprayed in eyes. If used in the emergency department, produces less cardiac stimulation than SABAs.
Systemic Corticosteroids		
Methylprednisolone, prednisolone, prednisone *Indications:* For moderate or severe exacerbations to prevent progression of exacerbation, reverse inflammation, speed recovery, and reduce rate of relapse.	*Anti-inflammatory:* Block late reaction to allergen and reduce airway hyperresponsiveness; inhibit cytokine production, adhesion protein activation, and inflammatory cell migration and activation. Reverse beta$_2$-receptor down-regulation. Inhibit microvascular leakage.	Short-term use: reversible abnormalities in glucose metabolism, increased appetite, fluid retention, weight gain, facial flushing, mood alteration, hypertension, peptic ulcer, and, rarely, aseptic necrosis. Consideration should be given to coexisting conditions that could be worsened by systemic corticosteroids, such as herpes virus infections, varicella, tuberculosis, hypertension, peptic ulcer, diabetes mellitus, osteoporosis, and *Strongyloides*.

SABA, short-acting beta agonist.
Modified from Heart, Lung and Blood Institute, National Asthma Education and Prevention Program. (2007). Expert Panel Report 3: Guidelines for the diagnosis and management of asthma. Full Report 2007 (pp. 247–248). Available: www.nhlbi.nih.gov/guidelines/asthma/asthgdln.pdf.

6. Long-acting oral beta-agonists, such as albuterol extended-release tablets.
7. Oral corticosteroids (maintenance dose).
8. Methylxanthines such as theophylline.
9. Muscarinic agents, namely tiotropium, as adjunct therapy.
10. An IgE blocker (omalizumab) can be added to standard maintenance therapy to reduce exacerbations in moderate to severe allergic asthma.
    a. It is given by subcutaneous injection every 2 to 4 weeks.
    b. The most common adverse reactions are injection site reactions and viral infection.

 NURSING ALERT The most convenient and inexpensive method of aerosol delivery to patients is the metered-dose or dry powder inhaler; however, nebulization offers alternative delivery for those with unreliable inhaler technique.

 DRUG ALERT Beta-adrenergic blockers, such as propranolol, have the potential to cause bronchoconstriction and should not be given to patients with asthma. Cardiac selective beta-blockers can be used such as carvedilol.

Quick-Relief Medications

1. Short-acting bronchodilators by inhalation.
   a. Short-acting beta-agonists (SABAs), such as albuterol, pirbuterol, and levalbuterol.
   b. Anticholinergic agent, such as ipratropium bromide.
2. Systemic corticosteroids (short course)—prednisone, prednisolone, and methylprednisolone.

 DRUG ALERT Patients should be encouraged to use SABAs appropriately when needed and not to wait for severe symptoms.

Other Measures

1. Environmental control (see page 795).
2. Immunotherapy (see page 792).
3. Avoidance of foods that contain tartrazine (yellow dye number 5) in aspirin-sensitive patients.
4. Regular aerobic exercise should be encouraged.
5. Use of an inhaled beta-adrenergic agonist or cromolyn taken 5 to 10 minutes before exercise will decrease exercise-induced bronchoconstriction.
6. Antibiotics are prescribed only during acute exacerbations if signs and symptoms of bacterial infection are present.
7. Alternative and complementary therapies that include acupuncture, herbal preparations, yoga, and chiropractic treatment have been suggested for acute and chronic asthma control; however, none is a substitute for usual medical treatment. In fact, glucosamine and chondroitin have been suspected of causing asthma exacerbation in some patients.

Nursing Assessment

1. Review patient's record: ask about coughing, dyspnea, chest tightness, wheezing, exertional changes, nighttime awakenings with asthma, use of SABA, and recent unscheduled or ER visits. Use an assessment tool such as the Asthma Control Test, Asthma Control Questionnaire, and Asthma Therapy Assessment Questionnaire. These tools quantify symptoms, quick-relief medication usage, effect of asthma on quality of life, and patient/family perception of control. They can be found at *www.nhlbi.nih.gov/guidelines/asthma/asthgdln.pdf.*
2. Observe the patient and assess the rate, depth, and character of respirations, especially on expiration; observe for hyperinflation. Assess peak flow.
3. Auscultate the chest for breath sounds or wheezing.
4. Assess for triggers of asthma that include the following:
   a. Allergens.
   b. Respiratory infections.
   c. Inhalation of irritating substances (dust, fumes, and gases).
   d. Environmental factors (weather, air pollution, and humidity).
   e. Exercise, particularly in cold weather.
   f. Aspirin and its derivatives.
   g. Sulfite-containing agents used as food preservatives.
   h. Emotional factors.
5. After acute episode subsides, attempt to determine patient's degree of adherence with medications and management regimen.
6. Observe and correct inhalation technique and discuss care of inhaler (eg, cleaning, priming).

Nursing Diagnoses

- Ineffective Breathing Pattern related to bronchospasm.
- Anxiety related to fear of suffocating, difficulty in breathing, death.
- Readiness for Enhanced Knowledge related to drug treatment and potential adverse effects.

Nursing Interventions

Attaining Relief of Dyspneic Breathing

1. Monitor vital signs, skin color, retraction, oxygen saturation, and degree of restlessness, which may indicate hypoxia.
2. Provide medication and oxygen therapy, as prescribed.
3. Monitor airway functioning through peak flow meter or spirometry (FEV_1, FEV_1/FVC) to assess effectiveness of treatment.
4. Encourage intake of fluids to liquefy secretions.
5. Instruct patient on positioning to facilitate breathing—sitting upright (leaning forward on a table).
6. Encourage patient to use adaptive breathing techniques (eg, pursued-lip breathing) to decrease the work of breathing.

Relieving Anxiety

1. Explain rationale for interventions to gain patient's cooperation. Provide care in prompt, confident manner.
2. Help patient clarify sources of anxiety; suggest measures to reduce anxiety and to control breathing.
3. Encourage active participation and support efforts to adhere to management plan.

Preventing Adverse Effects of Drugs

1. Teach patient to rinse mouth and spit out after using ICS to prevent growth of fungi and be alert for sore throat or mouth caused by oropharyngeal candidiasis.
2. Suggest a spacer if patient is prone to candidiasis and ensure proper dosing and inhalation technique. Blood glucose testing may also be indicated to rule out hyperglycemia.

3. Monitor liver function enzymes, as directed, for patients taking zileuton and zafirlukast, and advise patient to report signs of liver dysfunction: abdominal pain, nausea, itching, and jaundice.
4. Make sure patient is aware that LABAs are not used for acute symptoms or as anti-inflammatory therapy or monotherapy for asthma. Duration of protection against exercised-induced bronchospasm may decrease with regular use.
5. Monitor serum theophylline concentration periodically and maintain steady-state serum concentrations between 5 and 15 mcg/mL. Routine serum concentration monitoring is essential because of significant toxicities, narrow therapeutic range, and individual differences in metabolism. Absorption variation can produce significant changes in steady-state serum theophylline concentrations.
6. Warn patients that regular use (greater than 2 days/week) of SABA for symptom control (not prevention of exercise-induced bronchospasm), increasing use, or lack of expected effect indicates inadequate asthma control. For patients frequently using SABA, anti-inflammatory medication should be initiated or intensified.

Community and Home Care Considerations

1. Initiate peak flow monitoring, if indicated. This may be done twice daily by the patient with persistent asthma. Provide written and verbal instruction and have the patient demonstrate the procedure.
2. The patient can buy a peak flow meter from a pharmacy or from a medical supply company.
3. Once optimal asthma control is obtained, daily peak flow measurements in the early morning and early afternoon should be used during a 2- to 3-week period to determine the patient's personal best. The personal best peak flow measurement will be used to monitor control and to guide self-therapy in an individualized action plan.
4. Teach the patient how to obtain peak flow measurement.
   a. Place the indicator at the base of the numbered scale.
   b. Stand (preferably) or sit upright.
   c. Take a deep breath.
   d. Place the meter in mouth and close lips around mouthpiece, with tongue under the mouthpiece.
   e. Blow out as hard and as fast as possible. Coughing or spitting will result in a falsely elevated level.
   f. Note the measurement that the indicator is pointing to on the number scale.
   g. Repeat previous steps twice more and record the highest number.
5. Provide written and verbal instruction on an action plan for self-management of asthma exacerbation as outlined by the health care provider. National Asthma Education and Prevention Program Guidelines suggest the following:
   a. For symptomatic worsening of asthma or asymptomatic decrease in peak flow measurement, use initial inhalation of a short-acting beta-adrenergic agonist by metered-dose inhaler (MDI), two to four puffs for up to three treatments at 20-minute intervals, or a single nebulization treatment.
   b. After initial treatment, recheck peak flow; if it is more than 80% of personal best and no wheezing or shortness of breath, continue beta-adrenergic agonist every 3 to 4 hours for 24 to 48 hours. The patient should contact the health care provider for further instructions.
   c. If peak flow is 40% to 80% of personal best, or if the patient has persistent wheezing and shortness of breath, an oral corticosteroid should be initiated and beta-adrenergic agonist should be continued. The patient should contact the health care provider the same day for further instructions.
   d. If peak flow is less than 40% of personal best or if the patient has significant wheezing and shortness of breath, an oral corticosteroid should be started, beta-adrenergic agonist should be repeated immediately, and the patient should proceed to the emergency department.

Patient Education and Health Maintenance

1. Provide information on the nature of asthma and methods of treatment.
2. Provide information regarding medications, including the difference between long-term controllers and quick-relief medications and the proper use of inhalers and spacer devices; stress avoiding overuse of inhalers and nebulizers. Ensure that patient understands that long-acting bronchodilating inhalers, such as salmeterol, are not effective for asthma exacerbations.
3. Demonstrate the use of MDIs (see Patient Education Guidelines 28-2) and nebulization equipment.
   a. Inhalers vary widely with hydrofluoroalkane (HFA) propellant and breath-actuated devices currently on the market; familiarize yourself with the manufacturer's instructions to help the patient.
   b. Teach patients how to clean inhalers according to manufacturer's instructions.
   c. Advise patients to count number of inhalations if the inhaler does not have an automatic counter.
4. Help the patient to identify what triggers asthma, warning signs of an impending attack, and strategies for preventing and treating an attack.
5. Teach adaptive breathing techniques and breathing exercises such as pursed lip breathing.
6. Discuss environmental control.
   a. Avoid people with respiratory infections. Get an annual flu shot.
   b. Avoid substances and situations known to precipitate bronchospasm, such as allergens, irritants, strong odors, gases, fumes, and smoke.
   c. Wear a mask if cold weather precipitates bronchospasm.
   d. Stay inside when air pollution is high.
   e. Also see Patient Education Guidelines 28-1, page 795.
7. Promote optimal health practices, including nutrition, rest, and exercise.
   a. Encourage regular exercise to improve cardiorespiratory and musculoskeletal conditioning.
   b. Drink liberal amounts of fluids to keep secretions thin.
   c. Try to avoid upsetting situations.
   d. Use relaxation techniques, biofeedback management.
   e. Use community resources for smoking-cessation classes, stress management, exercises for relaxation, asthma support groups, etc.
8. Make sure that patient knows with whom to follow-up and the frequency of follow-up. Discuss with patient how to overcome any barriers to follow-up, such as transportation, limited office or clinic hours, childcare, and work requirements.
9. For additional information and support, refer to American Academy of Allergy, Asthma and Immunology (www.aaaai.org).

PATIENT EDUCATION GUIDELINES 28-2

How to Use an Inhaler and Spacer

Using an Inhaler

1. Make sure that the medication canister is attached to the plastic inhaler and shake well or, if using a dry powder inhaler system (DPI), load the medication according to the manufacturer's instructions.
2. If recommended, attach a spacer to your metered-dose inhaler (MDI) (see Using a Spacer, below).
3. If using the closed-mouth method (recommended for DPI and HFA systems):
   a. Exhale fully and place the mouthpiece of the inhaler in your mouth and close lips tightly around it.
   b. While starting to inhale, use your index finger to press down firmly on the top of the canister.
   c. Continue to inhale for 3 to 5 seconds to obtain a full breath, then hold your breath for 5 to 10 seconds.
   d. Remove the inhaler from your mouth before you exhale and breathe normally.
4. If more than one inhalation of a beta$_2$-agonist is prescribed, wait 30 seconds before taking another inhalation, then repeat steps 1 to 5.
5. Replace the mouthpiece cap after each use.
6. Clean the inhaler according to the manufacturer's instructions.
7. Discard the canister after you have used the labeled number of inhalations. You should not use it beyond this indicated number because the correct dose amount can no longer be guaranteed.
8. For dry powdered inhalers, use a forceful, rapid inhalation with closed-mouth technique. See the instructions provided by the manufacturer of the device you use.

Using a Spacer

Unless you use your inhaler correctly, much of the medicine can end up on your tongue, on the back of your throat, or in the air. If you experience this problem, your health care provider may recommend using a spacer. Also called a valved holding chamber, a spacer is a device that attaches to a MDI. It holds the medicine in its chamber long enough for you to inhale it in one or two slow, deep breaths, thereby enabling you to get your full dose of medicine. It also prevents you from coughing and may prevent a yeast infection in your mouth if you use a steroid inhaler. Several types of spacers are available; these devices may be purchased through your pharmacist.

1. Attach the inhaler to the spacer or holding chamber as shown in the product instructions.
2. Shake well.
3. Press the canister on the inhaler, which will put one puff of medicine into the holding chamber.
4. Place the mouthpiece of the spacer into your mouth and inhale slowly.
5. Hold your breath a few seconds, then exhale.

 EVIDENCE BASE Center for Disease Control and Prevention. (2018). Know how to use your asthma inhaler. [multimedia] Available: https://www.cdc.gov/asthma/inhaler_video/default.htm

 DRUG ALERT Never submerge an inhalation canister in water to determine if any medication remains. Moisture in the tip will ruin the canister.

Evaluation: Expected Outcomes

- Symptoms (wheezing, coughing, dyspnea, chest tightness) reduced; peak flow improved.
- Verbalizes relief of anxiety.
- No adverse reactions to drug therapy reported.

Status Asthmaticus

Status asthmaticus is a severe form of asthma in which the airway obstruction is unresponsive to usual drug therapy.

Contributing Factors

1. Infection.
2. Inhalation of air pollutants and allergens to which sensitized.
3. Noncompliance in taking medications, including overuse of bronchodilators.
4. Ingestion of aspirin or related drugs in aspirin-sensitive patient.
5. Aspiration of gastric acid.

Clinical Manifestations

1. Tachypnea, labored respirations, with increased effort on exhalation.
2. Suprasternal retractions, use of accessory muscles of respiration.
3. Diminished breath sounds, decreased ability to speak in phrases or sentences.
4. Anxiety, irritability, fatigue, headache, impaired mental functioning.
5. Muscle twitching, somnolence, diaphoresis—from continued carbon dioxide retention.
6. Tachycardia, elevated BP.
7. Heart failure and death from suffocation.

Management and Nursing Interventions

1. Monitor respiratory rate and oxygen saturation continuously; frequently monitor arterial blood gas levels, BP, electrocardiogram.

2. Administer repeated aerosol treatments with beta$_2$-agonist bronchodilators, such as albuterol or levalbuterol; add anticholinergic ipratropium, as prescribed—administer with caution until the metabolic and respiratory acidosis and hypoxemia have been corrected.

3. Monitor IV therapy.

    a. Corticosteroids are given to treat inflammation of airways; because these act slowly, their beneficial effects may not be apparent for several hours.

    b. Fluids are given to treat dehydration and loosen secretions.

4. Provide continuous humidified oxygen via nasal cannula, as prescribed. (Patients with associated chronic obstructive pulmonary disease or emphysema are at risk for depressed hypoxemic ventilatory drive, thus compounding respiratory insufficiency, so use oxygen cautiously.)

5. Initiate mechanical ventilation, if necessary.

6. Assist with mobilization of obstructing bronchial mucus.

    a. Perform chest physiotherapy (chest wall percussion and vibration).

    b. Administer expectorant and mucolytic drugs, as prescribed.

    c. Remove secretions by suctioning or prepare for bronchoscopy, if needed.

7. Provide adequate hydration.

8. Obtain portable chest x-ray and administer antibiotic, as prescribed, to treat any underlying respiratory infection.

9. Alleviate the patient's anxiety and fear by acting calmly and by reassuring the patient during an attack. Stay with the patient until the attack subsides.

NURSING ALERT In status asthmaticus, the return to normal or increasing partial pressure of carbon dioxide does not necessarily mean that the patient with asthma is improving—it may indicate a fatigue state that develops just before the patient slips into respiratory failure.

SELECTED REFERENCES

Bernstein, J. A., Lang, D. M., Kuhn, D. A., et al. (2014). The diagnosis and management of acute and chronic urticaria: 2014 update. *Journal of Allergy and Clinical Immunology, 135*(5), 1270–1277.

Bernstein, I. L., Li, J. T., Bernstein, D. I., et al. (2008). Allergy diagnostic testing: An updated practice parameter. *Annals of Allergy and Asthma Immunology, 100*(3 Suppl 3), S1–S148.

Bernstein, J. A., & Moellman, J. (2012). Emerging concepts in the diagnosis and treatment of patients with undifferentiated angioedema. *Internal Journal of Emergency Medicine, 5*, 39.

Bonilla, F. (2017). The adaptive cellular immune response. *UpToDate.* New York: Wolters Kluwer.

Center for Disease Control and Prevention. (2018). Know how to use your asthma inhaler. [multimedia] Available: *https://www.cdc.gov/asthma/inhaler_video/default.htm*

Chowdhury, B. A., & Dal Pan, G. (2010). The FDA and safe use of long-acting beta-agonists in the treatment of asthma. *New England Journal of Medicine, 362*, 1169–1171.

Cox, L. S., Nelson, H. A., Lockey, R., et al. (2011). Allergen immunotherapy: A practice parameter third update. *Journal of Allergy and Clinical Immunology, 127*(1 Suppl), S1–S55.

Dao, A. & Bernstein, D.I. (2018). Occupational exposure and asthma. *Annals of Allergy, Asthma & Immunology, 120*(5), 468–475.

Dinakar, C., Fineman, S.M., Chipps, B.E. et al. (2018). Recent advances in our understanding of the environment's role in allergy. *Annals of Allergy, Asthma & Immunology, 120*(5), 465–467.

Global Initiative for Asthma. (2016). *Global strategy for asthma management and prevention.* Available: *www.ginasthma.org*

Golden, D. B., Demain, J., Freeman, T., et al. (2017). Stinging insect hypersensitivity: A practice parameter update 2016. *Annals of Allergy, Asthma and Immunology, 118*, 28–54.

Hayden, M. L., Stoloff, S. W., Colice, G. L., et al. (2012). Exercise-induced bronchospasm: A case study in a nonasthmatic patient. *Journal of the American Academy of Nurse Practitioners, 24*, 19–23.

Hellings, P. W., Fokkens, W. J., Akdis, C., et al. (2013). Uncontrolled allergic rhinitis and chronic rhinosinusitis: Where do we stand today? *Allergy, 68*(1), 1–7.

Jones, S. M., & Burks, A. W. (2013). The changing CARE of patients with food allergy. *Journal of Allergy and Clinical Immunology, 131*(1), 3–11.

Kelley, K. J. (2012). *Latex allergy 101: Allergy fact sheet.* Slinger, Wisconsin: American Latex Allergy Association. Available: *www.latexallergyresources.org/allergy-fact-sheet*

Lieberman, J.A., Greenhaut, M., Nowak-Wegrzyn, A. (2018). The environment and food allergy. *Annals of Allergy, Asthma & Immunology, 120*(5), 455–457.

Lieberman, P., Nicklas, R. A., Randolph, C., et al. (2015). Anaphylaxis—a practice parameter update 2015. *Annals of Allergy, Asthma and Immunology, 115*, 341–384.

National Heart, Lung and Blood Institute, National Asthma Education and Prevention Program. (2007). Guidelines for the diagnosis and management of asthma. *Full report 2007, NIH Publication No. 08–4051.* Bethesda, MD: National Institutes of Health. Available: *www.nhlbi.nih.gov/guidelines/asthma/asthsumm.pdf*

National Heart, Lung and Blood Institute, National Asthma Education and Prevention Program Expert Panel Report 3. (2007). Guidelines for the diagnosis and management of asthma. *Summary Report 2007, NIH Publication No. 08–5846.* Bethesda, MD: National Institutes of Health. Available: *www.nhlbi.nih.gov/guidelines/asthma/asthsumm.pdf*

Nurmatov, U., Van Schayck, C. P., Hurwitz, B., et al. (2012). House dust avoidance measure for perennial allergic rhinitis: An update. *Allergy, 67*, 158–165.

Portnoy, J., Miller, J. D., Williams, B., et al. (2013). Environmental assessment and exposure of dust mites: A practice parameter. *Annals of Allergy, Asthma and Immunology, 111*, 465–507.

Sadatsafavi, M., Tavakoli, H., Lynd, L., FitzGerald, J. M. (2017). Has asthma medication use caught up with the evidence?: a 12-year population-based study of trends. *Chest, 151*, 612–618.

Sampson, H. A., Aceves, S., Bock, A., et al. (2014). Food allergy: A practice parameter update-2014. *Journal of Allergy, Asthma, and Clinical Immunology, 134*(5), 1016–1025.

Schitt, N., & Ueno, H. (2015). Regulation of human helper T-cell subset differentiation by cytokines. *Current Opinion in Immunology, 34*, 130–136.

Solensky, R., Khan, D. A., Berstein, I. L., et al. (2010). Drug allergy: An updated practice parameter. *Annals of Allergy and Asthma Immunology, 105*(4), 259–273.

Steiner, M., Huber, S., & Harrer, A. H. (2016). The evolution of human basophil biology from neglect towards understanding of their immune functions. *BioMed Research International, 2016*, Article ID 8232830, 16. Available: *www.hindawi.com/journals/bmri/2016/8232830/*

Tavakoli, H., FitzGerald, J. M., Lynd, L. D., Sadatsafvi, M. (2018). Predictors of innapropriate and excessive use of reliever medications in asthma: A 16-year population-based study. *BMC Pulmonary Medicine 2018, 18*(33). Available: *https://doi.org/10.1186/s12890-018-0598-4.*

van den Berge, M., ten Hacken, N. H., van der Wiel, E., et al. (2013). Treatment of the bronchial tree from beginning to end: Targeting small airway inflammation in asthma. *Allergy, 68*(1), 16–26.

Wallace, D. V., Dykewicz, M. S., Bernstein, D. I., et al. (2008). The diagnosis and management of rhinitis: An updated practice parameter. *Journal of Allergy and Clinical Immunology, 122*, S1–S84.

Weiler, J. M., Brennan, J. D., Randolph, C., et al. (2016). Exercise-induced bronchoconstriction update-2016. *Journal of Allergy and Clinical Immunology, 138*, 1292–1295.e36.Epub.

29

HIV Infection and AIDS

OVERVIEW

Human immunodeficiency virus (HIV) is an RNA retroviral infection that is transmitted from person to person most often through sexual and blood-to-blood contact. Over time, HIV interferes with the immune system's ability to coordinate an effective response against infection. This loss of immune function takes years to occur, eventually leading to the stage of disease called *acquired immune deficiency syndrome (AIDS)*, which is marked by vulnerability to opportunistic infections. Without antiretroviral treatment, HIV infection is almost universally fatal.

Since the immune deficiency syndrome associated with HIV was first described in 1981, great strides have been made in care and treatment of persons living with HIV. Medication regimens have been simplified into fixed dose combination tablets with once daily dosing. The cost of medication has decreased globally, clearing the way for more widespread access to treatment. There is international will to test and treat more people and prevent new infection among those who are at risk for acquiring HIV. Life expectancy on antiretroviral therapy (ART) has increased significantly across all income settings of the world. The Joint United Nations Programme on HIV/AIDS (UNAIDS) is rolling out effective treatment across the globe with the aim of an AIDS-free generation by 2030. This program sets ambitious 90-90-90 goals: 90% of people with HIV diagnosed, 90% of them on ART, and 90% being virally suppressed by 2020. In support of this momentum toward an AIDS-free generation, the US President's Emergency Plan for AIDS Relief (PEPFAR) has committed to interventions that target persons at high risk in areas of the world with the highest HIV incidence. Scientists are actively modeling a cure strategy.

Nevertheless, HIV has claimed more than 35 million lives in the past 35 years, and approximately 37 million persons were living with HIV in 2016 globally. As of 2015, the Centers for Disease Control (CDC) estimates that more than 1.1 million persons are living with HIV in the United States. The Patient Protection and Affordable Care Act (ACA) has provided expanded opportunity to millions who had been uninsured or underinsured; however, only 40% of HIV-infected persons in the United States are in care, 35% are receiving treatment, and 30% have a very low or undetectable viral load (see Figure 29-1). A goal of the National HIV/AIDS Strategy is to achieve 80% viral suppression by 2020. There is work to do. Nurses are present at each point in the HIV care continuum: testing, treatment, retention to care, and preventing new infections. Endless possibility exists for nursing's contribution toward achieving national and international goals.

EVIDENCE BASE Center for Disease Control and Prevention. (2017) HIV Surveillance Report. Atlanta, GA: Author. Available: *https://www.cdc.gov/hiv/statistics/overview/index.html.*

Mignano, J. L. (2016). 80% viral suppression by 2020? Understanding the concept of engagement in HIV care and a call to action for nursing. *Journal of the Association of Nurses in AIDS Care, 27*(5), 550–562.

UNAIDS. (2014). *90-90-90 An ambitious treatment target to help end the AIDS epidemic.* Geneva: Author. Available: *www.unaids.org/sites/default/files/media_asset/90-90-90_en_0.pdf*

World Health Organization. (2018). *WHO HIV/AIDS fact sheet (No. 360).* Geneva: WHO. Available: *http://www.who.int/en/news-room/fact-sheets/detail/hiv-aids.*

Transmission and Natural History

Epidemiology and Pathophysiology

1. Today, most new HIV infections are found among men who have sex with men (MSM) (67% of new infections in 2015). Among MSM, adult racial minorities and adolescent/young adult Black and Hispanic men aged 13 to 24 are disproportionately affected. Heterosexual transmission accounted for 24% of new HIV infections in 2015. The trend in new infections from injection drug use has declined to approximately 6%.

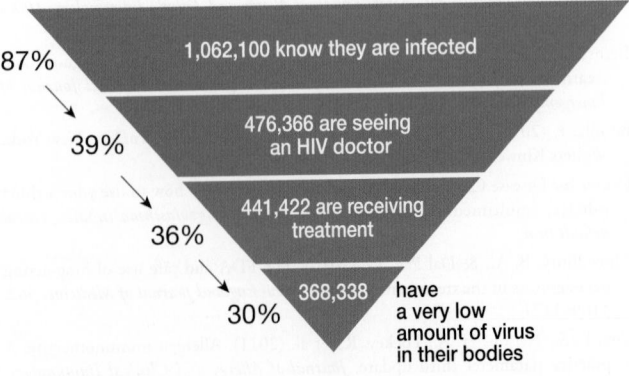

Figure 29-1. The Continuum of HIV Care in the United States. (From Centers for Disease Control and Prevention. [2016]. *CDC fact sheet: Today's HIV/AIDS epidemic.* Atlanta, GA: Author. www.cdc.gov/nchhstp/newsroom/docs/factsheets/todaysepidemic-508.pdf.)

Geographic distribution of new infections is uneven across the United States. The South represented the highest burden of incident infections (16.8), the Northeast (11.6), the West (9.8), and the Midwest (7.6). The availability of HIV prevention and treatment programs across all regions will be important to decreasing the rate of new infections.

2. HIV enters the body through condomless sexual contact or blood-to-blood transmission and then targets T helper immune cells that carry CD4+ receptors. Once inside the host cell, HIV uses the cell's components as a factory to reproduce. Replicating HIV within the host cell ruptures the cell membrane, releasing more HIV virions into the plasma that bind to and disable other CD4+ cells.

3. Antiretroviral drugs interfere with viral replication at specific points in the viral life cycle.

4. HIV infection can be viewed as a chronic condition in patients who strictly adhere to antiretroviral treatment and care. Some patients have difficulty managing highly structured medication and appointment regimens. They need encouragement or special interventions to support their treatment plan. Nursing is important for working with patients to tailor a plan that optimizes their opportunity for successful and enduring treatment.

 NURSING ALERT Globally, approximately 1.8 million persons became infected in 2016. Despite prevention efforts, there have been a persistent 40,000 new infections in the United States each year, pointing to the inadequacy of efforts to reach everyone who is at risk.

Natural History of HIV Infection

1. Approximately 50% to 90% of patients who become infected experience some symptom of primary HIV infection at around 2 to 4 weeks after exposure to HIV. Typical symptoms of acute HIV seroconversion include fever, lymphadenopathy, sore throat, rash, myalgia/arthralgia, diarrhea, weight loss, and headache. Many new HIV infections evade diagnosis because symptoms of acute HIV infection mimic other common infections. Seroconversion is marked by a sudden decrease in T4 helper cells and a sharp increase in HIV viral load for a brief period before establishing a steady viral set point.

2. The time to detection of s depends upon the test being used. A fourth-generation antigen/antibody combination HIV-1/2 immunoassay can capture early infection, because the assay detects HIV p24 antigen prior to antibody formation. If positive, a confirmatory antigen/antibody combination HIV-1/2 immunoassay is performed. If a patient is suspect of being in the window period before antibody formation, a plasma HIV RNA level can be drawn.

3. The CDC provides a case definition for staging HIV infection and defining progression to AIDS (see Table 29-1). A normal CD4+ count is approximately 1,000/mm³. HIV replication destroys CD4+ T cells, causing the number of CD4 cells to diminish slowly over time.

4. Waning immunity in persons who have untreated infection or are on a failing antiretroviral regimen leads to frequent infections, severe opportunistic infections, and malignancies. See Figure 29-2.

 NURSING ALERT The period around acute seroconversion is a time when the patient is highly infectious to others. High HIV viral load is linked to a high rate of transmission. Counsel patients to use effective measures to prevent transmission through sexual contact and/or needle sharing. Encourage and refer newly diagnosed persons into care and treatment. Ask patients to talk with their partner(s) about preexposure prophylaxis (PrEP) or refer them to a PrEP center for advice.

Diagnostic Evaluation

EVIDENCE BASE Dumitru, G., Irwin, K., & Tailor, A. (2017). Updated federal recommendations for HIV prevention with adults and adolescents with HIV in the United States: The pivotal role of nurses. *Journal of the Association of Nurses in AIDS Care, 28*(1), 8–18.

Simeone, C. A., Seal, S. M., & Savage, C. (2017). Implementing HIV testing in substance use treatment programs: A systematic review. *Journal of the Association of Nurses in AIDS Care, 28*(2), 199–215.

Table 29-1	AIDS Surveillance Case Definition for Adolescents and Adults		
	CLINICAL CATEGORIES*		
	A	**B**	**C**
CD4+ CELL CATEGORIES	**ASYMPTOMATIC OR PGL OR ACUTE HIV INFECTION**	**SYMPTOMATIC†** (NOT A OR C)	**AIDS INDICATOR CONDITION (1987)**
1 ≥500/mm³ (≥29%)	A1	B1	C1
2 200–499 mm³ (14%–8%)	A2	B2	C2
3 200/mm³ (<14%)	A3	B3	C3

* All patients in categories A3, B3, and C1–3 are reported as acquired immunodeficiency syndrome (AIDS), based on the AIDS indicator conditions and a CD4 cell count less than 200/mm³. AIDS indicator conditions include three new entries: recurrent bacterial pneumonia, invasive cervical cancer, and pulmonary tuberculosis.
†Symptomatic conditions not included in category C that are (a) attributed to human immunodeficiency virus (HIV) infection or indicative of a defect in cell-mediated immunity or (b) considered to have a clinical course or management that is complicated by HIV infection. Examples of B conditions include, but are not limited to, bacillary angiomatosis; thrush; vulvovaginal candidiasis that is persistent, frequent, or poorly responsive to therapy; cervical dysplasia (moderate or severe); cervical carcinoma in situ; constitutional symptoms, such as fever (101.3°F [38.5°C]) or diarrhea for 1 month; oral hairy leukoplakia; herpes zoster involving two episodes or more than one dermatome; idiopathic thrombocytopenic purpura; listeriosis; pelvic inflammatory infection (especially if complicated by a tubo-ovarian abscess); and peripheral neuropathy.
PGL, persistent generalized lymphadenopathy.
Centers for Infection Control and Prevention. (1993). AIDS surveillance case definition for adolescents and adults. Morbidity and Mortality Weekly Report, 41(RR-17), 2.

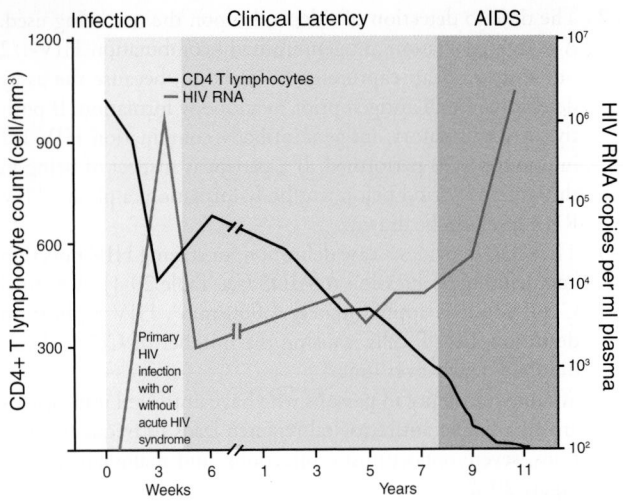

Figure 29-2. Natural history of untreated HIV Infection.

HIV Testing

Description

1. Enzyme-linked immunoassay (ELISA) is a method of serologic testing.
    a. First- and second-generation tests detect HIV IgG antibody. Their approximate time to positivity is 25 to 45 days after exposure.
    b. Third-generation tests detect HIV IgM and IgG antibody within approximately 20 to 30 days from exposure.
    c. Fourth-generation tests detect HIV IgM and IgG antibody and p24 antigen within approximately 15 to 20 days from exposure.
2. Western blot is considered a confirmatory test and detects HIV IgM and IgG antibody within approximately 45 to 60 days from exposure. Indeterminate results may occur prior to this interval.
3. HIV viral load assays detect HIV RNA.
    a. Assays that are sensitive to less than 50 copies/mL can measure viral load within 10 to 15 days of exposure.
    b. Ultrasensitive assays that are sensitive to less than 5 copies/mL can measure viral load within 5 days of exposure.

Nursing and Patient Care Considerations

1. Occasionally, a positive ELISA screen may yield an indeterminate result by Western blot.
    a. The cause of an indeterminate result may be early HIV seroconversion, HIV vaccine, infection with O strain or HIV-2, or a false-positive in a low-risk individual.
    b. The test should be repeated at 1, 2, and 6 months until Western blot becomes positive or there is no longer suspicion of HIV infection. If a conclusive test is needed quickly, HIV RNA viral load testing can be done.
2. The CDC recommends opt-out HIV testing for patients age 13 to 64 informing them that screening is routine, but allowing that they may decline. Written consent and pretest and posttest counseling are no longer recommended, but consult state law to be in local compliance.

Other Laboratory Tests

1. Lymphocyte panel may show decreased CD4+ count. In early infection or in long-term nonprogressors and elite controllers, CD4+ count may be nearly normal.

2. A complete blood count (CBC) may show anemia, leukopenia, and/or thrombocytopenia.
3. HIV viral load testing is a measure of the amount of HIV in the blood. The lower the better, with an undetectable level being the goal. High viral loads (greater than 750,000) tend to be found in acute seroconversion and late untreated infection.
4. Resistance testing is done to determine if the patient is infected with or has acquired a drug-resistant virus. The test uses genotypic assays that amplify HIV virus for mutations in the viral genotype, which block or impair the efficacy of specific antiretrivirals (ARVs).

 NURSING ALERT An undetectable HIV viral load result does not indicate that the patient is free of HIV. Latent reservoirs exist in lymphoid tissue and resting memory CD4+ T cells indefinitely. These reservoirs are not reached by antiretroviral agents. Therefore, counsel patients that they must still maintain strict adherence to ART.

MANAGEMENT
Pharmacologic Treatment

 EVIDENCE BASE U.S. Department of Health and Human Services, Panel on Antiretroviral Guidelines for Adults and Adolescents. (2018). Guidelines for the use of antiretroviral agents in adults an adolescents living with HIV. Rockville, MD: Author. Available: *https://aidsinfo. nih.gov/contentfiles/lvguidelines/AdultandAdolescentGL. pdf.*
Turner, L., Roepke, A., Wardell, E., & Teitelman, A. (2017). Do you PrEP? A review of primary care provider knowledge of PrEP and attitudes on prescribing PrEP. *Journal of the Association of Nurses in AIDS Care, 29*(1), 83–92.

Treatment Overview

1. ART serves a four-part purpose: (1) to decrease HIV viral burden and increase immune function, (2) to reduce morbidity and mortality, (3) to increase quality of life and life expectancy, and (4) to prevent HIV transmission. Successful treatment requires strict adherence to medication, which means taking about 95% of doses.
    a. Before initiating antiretrovirals, patients should be assessed for readiness to start, as treatment is lifelong. However, some trepidation is expected and is not a complete barrier to initiating treatment.
    b. An emerging treatment strategy encourages real-time testing and treatment if positive, or, testing and prevention using PrEP, if negative and at high risk for acquiring HIV infection. See Table 29-2.
2. New guidelines recommend universal treatment for all HIV-positive patients regardless of CD4 count. The purpose of earlier treatment is to prevent patients from experiencing a decline in CD4 count that places them at risk for consequences of ongoing inflammatory response and for acquiring opportunistic infections.

Table 29-2 Summary of Guidance for Preexposure Prophylaxis for the Prevention of HIV

	MEN WHO HAVE SEX WITH MEN	HETEROSEXUAL WOMEN AND MEN	INJECTION DRUG USERS
Detecting substantial risk of acquiring HIV infection	HIV-positive sexual partner Recent bacterial STI High number of sex partners History of inconsistent or no condom use Commercial sex work	HIV-positive sexual partner Recent bacterial STI High number of sex partners History of inconsistent or no condom use Commercial sex work In high-prevalence area or network	HIV-positive injecting partner Sharing injection equipment Recent drug treatment (but currently injecting)
Clinically eligible	Documented negative HIV test result before prescribing PrEP No signs/symptoms of acute HIV infection Normal renal function; no contraindicated medications Documented hepatitis B virus infection and vaccination status		
PRESCRIPTION	DAILY, CONTINUING, ORAL DOSES OF TDF/FTC (TRUVADA), ≤90-DAY SUPPLY		
Other services	Follow-up visits at least every 3 months to provide the following: HIV test, medication adherence counseling, behavioral risk reduction support, side effect assessment, STI symptom assessment At 3 months and every 6 months thereafter, assess renal function Every 6 months, test for bacterial STIs		
	Do oral rectal STI testing	Assess pregnancy intent Pregnancy test every 3 mo	Access to clean needles/syringes and drug treatment services

STI, sexually transmitted infection.
From Centers for Disease Control and Prevention. (2017). US Public Health Service preexposure prophylaxis for the prevention of HIV infection in the United States—2017 Update: A clinical practice guideline. Atlanta, GA: Author. Available: https://www.cdc.gov/hiv/pdf/risk/prep/cdc-hiv-prep-guidelines-2017.pdf.

3. When a patient's CD4 counts falls below 200 cells/mm³, some opportunistic infections can be prevented by prophylactic medication. This is known as primary prophylaxis. See Table 29-3.
   a. All persons with CD4 less than 200 cells/mm³ must receive prophylaxis against PCP.
   b. Those who have CD4 less than 100 cells/mm³ and are *Toxoplasma gondii* serum IgG+ must receive prophylaxis against toxoplasmosis.
   c. Those who have CD4 less than 50 cells/mm³ must receive prophylaxis against *Mycobacterium avium* complex, after initial culture for *M. avium intracellulare* is negative.
4. Care and treatment of HIV infection and AIDS can require consultation with the expertise of many specialties including infectious diseases, nephrology, pulmonology, gastroenterology, neurology, obstetrics and gynecology, dentistry, dermatology, cardiology, oncology, surgery, psychiatry, rheumatology, nursing, nutrition, and social work.
5. Many patients are coinfected with hepatitis C, which is now curable with 8 to 12 weeks of treatment. Referral to specialty hepatitis C care can significantly reduce morbidity and mortality that is associated with chronic liver disease.

Initiating Antiretroviral Therapy in Treatment-Naive Patients

1. Universal treatment is recommended for all HIV-infected persons, regardless of CD4 count. ART medications belong to six drug classifications that interfere with HIV replication at six different points in the viral life cycle. To simplify medication taking and reduce pill burden, there is a growing arsenal of multiclass combination products.
2. The standard of care for ART is to use a minimum of three different drugs from at least two different drug classifications.

Treatment guidelines make specific drug choice recommendations and are updated frequently.

3. Classes of antiretroviral drugs:
   a. Nucleoside/nucleotide reverse transcriptase inhibitors (NRTI).
   b. Nonnucleoside reverse transcriptase inhibitors (NNRTIs).
   c. Protease inhibitors (PIs).
   d. Entry/fusion inhibitor.
   e. Entry inhibitor/CCR5 antagonist.
   f. Integrase inhibitor (INSTI).
   g. Multiclass combination products.

Adverse Effects of Antiretroviral Medications

 EVIDENCE BASE Panel on Antiretroviral Guidelines for Adults and Adolescents. Guidelines for the Use of Antiretroviral Agents in Adults and Adolescents Living with HIV. (2018) Department of Health and Human Services. Available at *http://aidsinfo.nih.gov/contentfiles/lvguidelines/AdultandAdolescentGL.pdf.*

1. New medications have simplified medication dosing and reduced side effects significantly.
2. Bone density reduction is especially associated with tenofovir disoproxil fumarate (TDF). Effect can be reduced by switching to the newer formulation tenofovir alafenamide (TAF).
3. Cardiac disease and/or cardiac effects are associated with NRTIs, some NNRTIs, and PIs.
4. Diabetes mellitus and insulin resistance are associated with NRTIs and some PIs.
5. Dyslipidemia is associated with NRTIs, NNRTIs, PIs, and INSTI.
6. Gastrointestinal effects such as nausea, vomiting, and diarrhea are associated with NRTIs and some PI-containing regimens.

Table 29-3 Opportunistic Infections and Drug Therapies

NAME	CLINICAL MANIFESTATIONS	DIAGNOSTIC TESTS	MEDICATIONS
Pneumocystis jirovecii pneumonia (PCP)	• Low-grade fever • Shortness of breath • Cough: dry or scant white sputum production	• Chest x-ray • Induced sputum specimen • Bronchoscopy • Microscopy • PCR	• Co-trimoxazole (+/− steroids) • Clindamycin with primaquine +/− steroids • Atovaquone
Oral *Candida* and *Candida* esophagitis	• White coating in mouth • White coating down throat • Sensation of food getting caught in throat while swallowing	• Gross observation • Microscopy for hyphae • Endoscopy	• Nystatin • Clotrimazole • Itraconazole • Fluconazole • Liposomal amphotericin B
Mycobacterium avium complex (MAC)	• Fever • Weakness • Weight loss • Diarrhea • Bone marrow suppression	• Blood culture for acid-fast bacilli • Bone marrow biopsy	• Rifabutin • Ethambutol • Azithromycin • Clarithromycin
Kaposi sarcoma	• Pink, purple, or brown spots or nodules • +/− Pain, edema of affected area	• Gross observation • Biopsy	• ART (improved immune function) • Chemotherapy
Toxoplasmosis	• Fever • Headache • Change in mental status • Confusion • Lethargy • Psychosis	• CT • MRI • Serum *Toxoplasma* IgG antibodies	• Pyrimethamine • Sulfadiazine • Folinic acid
Tuberculosis	• Fever • Cough: none, dry or scant frothy white or pink sputum, hemoptysis • Shortness of breath • Weight loss • Lymphadenopathy	• Chest x-ray • Sputum for acid-fast bacilli (AFB) smear, microscopy, Gene Xpert, and culture • Positive purified protein derivative (PPD) (≥5 mm induration) • Interferon-gamma release assays (IGRAs) • * Note that PPD and IGRAs detect evidence of past exposure and are not conclusive for TB disease)	• Rifampin • Isoniazid • Pyrazinamide • Ethambutol • Pyridoxine
Cryptosporidium	• Severe watery diarrhea • Severe abdominal cramping	• Stool microscopy for Cryptosporidium	• ART (improved immune function) • Nitazoxanide +aggressive ART
Cryptococcal meningitis	• Headache • Confusion, memory loss • Nausea • Seizures • Change in mental status • Fever • Photophobia	• Serum and CSF cryptococcal antigen • CSF fungal culture	• Liposomal amphotericin B • Flucytosine • Fluconazole
Cytomegalovirus (CMV)	• Visual changes; floaters, flashes or blind spots, and blindness • Difficulty swallowing • Nausea, vomiting • Abdominal cramping • Altered mental status • Adrenal insufficiency	• Ophthalmologic examination • Blood, urine, tissue culture for CMV • PCR • Immunohistochemistry • Histopathology (visualization of characteristic owl's eyes inclusion bodies)	• Valganciclovir • Ganciclovir • Foscarnet • Cidofovir • Intraocular ganciclovir release device
Herpes simplex virus 1 and 2	• Blisters or ulcerations: mouth, lips, genitalia, perianal area	• PCR • Viral culture • Clinical observation	• Acyclovir • Famciclovir • Valacyclovir
Herpes zoster	• Painful vesicular rash on one or more dermatome(s)	• PCR • Viral culture • Clinical observation	• Famciclovir • Valacyclovir • Acyclovir

ART, antiretroviral therapy; CMV, cytomegalovirus; CSF, cerebrospinal fluid; CT, computed tomography; IV, intravenous; MRI, magnetic resonance imaging.

7. Hepatotoxicities can occur with most NRTIs, some NNRTIs, and all PIs. Check hepatitis B status before discontinuing the NRTIs TAF, TDF, lamivudine, or emtricitabine, as discontinuation can cause severe HBV flares. The PI combination TPV/r is contraindicated in patients with hepatic disease that is characterized as Child-Pugh B or C.

8. Hypersensitivity reaction (HSR) is associated with the NRTI abacavir (ABC), the NNRTI nevirapine (NVP), and the INSTI raltegravir (RAL) and can present with any combination of the following symptoms: fever, rash, malaise, nausea, headache, myalgia, chills, diarrhea, vomiting, abdominal pain, dyspnea, fatigue, blisters, oral lesions, facial swelling, eosinophilia, granulocytopenia, arthralgia, lymphadenopathy, and respiratory symptoms.

9. Lactic acidosis/steatohepatitis occurs with some NRTI medications; presents with nausea, vomiting, fatigue, and abdominal pain. May progress rapidly to a life-threatening condition.

10. Myopathy and elevated creatinine phosphokinase (CPK) are associated with the NRTI ZDV and the INSTI RAL.

11. Central nervous system and psychiatric effects are associated with the NRTI d4T, the NNRTI efavirenz (EFV), and all INSTI.

12. Rash is associated with nearly all ARVs.

13. Renal effects such as elevated serum creatinine and kidney stones are associated with the NRTI TDF (elevated creatinine) and some PIs (elevated creatinine and stone/crystal formation).

14. Stevens-Johnson syndrome and toxic epidermal necrosis have been reported among NRTIs, NNRTIs, PIs, and INSTI.

15. Treatment fatigue is an emotional reaction to medication dosing and adverse effects. It can be managed effectively by switching to a simplified regimen, if possible, and by offering supportive care. Drug "holidays" are not recommended, since HIV replication recurs almost immediately.

 DRUG ALERT If a patient decides to stop taking antiretroviral therapy, then all ARV medications should be stopped at the same time. Taking only some of the ARVs creates resistance to HIV, which could lead to loss of effective treatment options for this patient in the future. Resistance can develop within a few days to a few weeks of inadequate dosing. Special rules exist for stopping a regimen that contains drugs with a different half-life. Consult the literature before a planned treatment interruption or discontinuation and counsel patients to contact their provider for advice before stopping a regimen on their own.

Health Maintenance

EVIDENCE BASE U.S. Department of Health and Human Services, Panel on Opportunistic Infections in HIV-Infected Adults and Adolescents. (2018). Guidelines for the prevention and treatment of opportunistic infections in HIV-infected adults and adolescents: recommendations from the Centers for Disease Control and Prevention, the National Institutes of Health, and the HIV Medicine Association of the Infectious Diseases Society of America. Rockville, MD: Author. Available: *http://aidsinfo.nih.gov/contentfiles/lvguidelines/adult_oi.pdf.*

Patient Education and Health Maintenance

1. Emphasize importance of ART to improve health, to promote longevity, and to prevent transmission to others.

2. Encourage patient to disclose HIV status to sex partner(s) and/or needle-sharing partner(s).

3. Discuss risk of acquiring and/or transmitting other sexually transmitted infections and assist patient in developing a prevention strategy.

4. Discuss advances in hepatitis C treatment that now make cure possible in 8 to 12 weeks.

5. Discuss family planning with all patients, if relevant. Some ARVs should not be taken by women who could become pregnant.

6. Encourage routine health maintenance such as dental care, immunizations, eye exams, annual cervical Pap smear for women and consider anal Pap smear for MSM, lipid screening, glucose and A1C monitoring, and routine screening for the ageing patient.

7. Teach patient to recognize and report a new symptom or complaint.

8. Discuss smoking cessation.

9. Ask patient if he or she uses complementary or alternative therapies, such as vitamins, herbs, and teas.

10. Refer patient to resources such as:
    a. Patient-oriented site with many resources including a list of hotlines for persons at risk for acquiring HIV and HIV-infected consumers, *www.thebody.com.*
    b. Consumer-oriented magazine, which is available online and by mail, *www.poz.com.*
    c. *100 Question and Answers about HIV and AIDS*, by Joel Gallant, Third Edition (2016) (paperback available online and at bookstores). Excellent resource for patients in easy to understand language.
    d. 100 Questions and Answers about HIV/AIDS, (updated 2014) by the New York State Health Department, *www. health.ny.gov/publications/0213.pdf.*
    e. Information about hepatitis C testing, treatment and support at The American Liver Foundation *http://hepc.liverfoundation.org/.*
    f. Information about clinical trials that are open to enrollment at ClinicalTrials.gov, *https://clinicaltrials.gov/.*
    g. Preexposure prophylaxis. *www.cdc.gov/hiv/risk/prep/index.html.*

11. Resources for health care professionals:
    a. U.S. Department of Health and Human Services, *https://aidsinfo.nih.gov.* Comprehensive website with links to a variety of information sources, including a list of resources for consumers.
    b. Centers for Disease Control and Prevention, *https://cdc.gov/hiv.* General HIV/AIDS information, publications, resources, and statistics.
    c. Johns Hopkins University AIDS Service, *www.hopkinsguides.com/hopkins/ub.* Look up testing, treating infections, complications, pathogens, management, and resistance.
    d. International resources, *www.unaids.org/en/.* Provides statistics and guidance about the international HIV/AIDS epidemic with links to other international resources.

 DRUG ALERT Oral contraceptives interact with many protease inhibitors and NNRTI medications. Encourage patient to discuss this with her women's health provider because she may need alternative contraception.

DRUG ALERT PI levels can be affected by St. John's wort and grapefruit products. Discourage patients who are on PIs from using this over-the-counter herbal remedy and taking grapefruit products.

Preventing Opportunistic Infections

1. *Pneumocystis jirovecii* pneumonia (PCP) prophylaxis is started when the CD4⁺ count is ≤200/mm³. The most effective medication is trimethoprim/sulfamethoxazole (TMP/SMZ); others are dapsone, atovaquone, and aerosolized pentamidine. To reduce pill burden and prevent unnecessary antibiotic exposure, primary PCP prophylaxis should be discontinued when the CD4 count has increased to ≥200 cells/mm³ for greater than 3 months.
2. Toxoplasmosis prophylaxis is appropriate in patients who are *Toxoplasma* IgG ab+ when the CD4⁺ count is ≤100/mm³. TMP/SMZ is the preferred agent, which is an added benefit when the patient is on concomitant PCP prophylaxis using TMP/SMZ. Alternative drug combinations are available for patients who cannot tolerate sulfa drugs, and these combinations are also effective prophylaxis against PCP. The recommendation for discontinuation of primary prophylaxis follows the model for primary PCP prophylaxis above.
3. *Mycobacterium avium* complex (MAC) prophylaxis is started when the CD4⁺ count is ≤50/mm³ and blood cultures for *M. avium* are negative; medications include azithromycin or clarithromycin. Alternative therapy is available for patients who cannot tolerate a macrolide antibiotic.
4. CMV end-organ prophylaxis, including for CMV retinitis, is no longer recommended, owing to high cost and toxicities. The best prevention is effective ART that maintains the CD4 count above 100/mm³. Clinician monitoring for symptoms of disseminated disease and patient education about the hallmark symptoms of CMV retinitis (decreased visual acuity/floaters/flashes) are the current recommendations for preventing severe CMV progression.

Immunizations

1. Pneumococcal pneumonia—all patients should receive both types of pneumococcal vaccine (PPV13 and PPV23) and immunization should be repeated when a patient attains a CD4⁺ count of ≥200/mm³.
2. Influenza—all patients should receive the inactivated flu vaccine each Fall.
3. Tetanus booster—all patients should receive routine booster every 10 years, or in the case of a wound, after 5 years.
4. Hepatitis A—recommended if at risk and baseline total antibody test is negative.
   a. Risk factors include MSM, IDU, travel to endemic areas, and hemophiliacs.
   b. Persons who are coinfected with viral hepatitis or chronic liver disease should be vaccinated to prevent morbidity and mortality associated with acute hepatitis A infection.
5. Hepatitis B—recommended if baseline antibody test is negative.
6. Human papilloma virus—Gardasil is recommended for women and men aged 9 to 26.
7. Meningococcal—recommended if a risk exists (college freshman living in dormitory, military recruits, asplenia, complement component deficiency, travel to or residence in area with outbreaks, occupational exposure).

8. Measles, Mumps, Rubella (MMR)— recommended for all nonimmune patients with CD4 ≥ 200/mm³ (live virus is contraindicated in patients with CD4 ≤ 200/mm³).

Nursing Management of HIV Infection and AIDS

See Standards of Care Guidelines 29-1.

STANDARDS OF CARE GUIDELINES 29-1
HIV/AIDS

When caring for patients with HIV infection
- Practice standard precautions.
- Protect confidentiality.
- Educate the patient about methods that prevent HIV transmission to others.
- Perform a psychosocial assessment and identify mental health needs.
- Develop adherence strategies for patients taking antiretroviral therapy.
- Provide education and interventions for HIV symptom management.
- Assist with tobacco, alcohol, and substance abuse cessation.

Nursing Assessment

1. Obtain history of date of HIV diagnosis, CD4⁺ count at time of diagnosis, risk factors for infection, constitutional signs and symptoms, recent infections, positive test result for HIV, most recent CD4⁺ count, and HIV RNA viral load.
2. Review patient's present complaints, if any.
3. Assess patient's knowledge about HIV/AIDS, including causes, signs and symptoms, modes of transmission, methods for preventing transmission to others, disease progression, and importance of CD4⁺ count and HIV RNA viral load monitoring.
4. Assess the patient's adherence to medications by reviewing all prescribed drugs, dosing, and frequency. Ask the patient how many times over the last day or week he or she missed a dose. Encourage honest reporting by acknowledging that missed doses occur.

TRANSITIONAL CARE ALERT Medication reconciliation should occur periodically, especially after hospitalizations or specialty consultations, to check for possible interactions and ensure that the patient is taking all medications appropriately. Some antiretrovirals may have drug–drug interactions with new medications. Encourage patient to use the same pharmacy for all prescription drugs, so the pharmacist can detect possible interactions.

5. Evaluate nutritional and general health status by assessing weight, body mass index, anemia, lipid profile, fasting glucose, hemoglobin A1C, and other pertinent labs and anthropometric measures.

6. Assess respiratory rate and depth and auscultate lungs for breath sounds; assess skin color and temperature, palpate lymph nodes, and ask about fever and night sweats.
7. Inspect mouth for lesions and dentition.
8. Examine skin for temperature, condition, and presence of rash, sores, and other changes.
9. Ask about bowel movement patterns, changes in habits, constipation, abdominal cramping, number and volume of stools, and presence of perianal pain and ulceration.
10. Assess patient's orientation to time, place, and person. Note patient's affect. Ask about any problem with memory and concentration, headaches, seizures, visual changes.
11. Find out as much as possible about patient's lifestyle (assessing for ongoing risk behavior), experience and skills, social support system.

Clinical Manifestations of HIV/AIDS with Advancing Infection

1. Pulmonary manifestations.
   a. Persistent or acute cough, with or without sputum production, shortness of breath, chest pain, fever, hemoptysis.
   b. Possible causes: *Pneumocystis jiroveci* pneumonia (PCP), bacterial pneumonia (community-acquired pneumonia), *Mycobacterium* tuberculosis, disseminated *Mycobacterium avium* complex, *Aspergillus*, *Pseudomonas*, cytomegalovirus (CMV), *Histoplasma*, Kaposi sarcoma, lung cancer, lymphoma, *Cryptococcus*, *Legionella*, or other pathogens and malignancies.
2. GI manifestations.
   a. Diarrhea, weight loss, anorexia, abdominal cramping, feeling of fullness, rectal urgency (tenesmus).
   b. Possible causes: enteric pathogens or malignancies including *Salmonella*, *Shigella*, *Campylobacter*, *Entamoeba histolytica*, *C. difficile*, CMV, *M. avium* complex, herpes simplex, *Strongyloides*, *Giardia*, *Cryptosporidium*, *Isospora belli*, *Chlamydia*, lymphoma, Kaposi's sarcoma, and others.
   c. Difficulty swallowing or substernal pain upon swallowing (feeling of food being stuck), usually caused by *Candida* esophagitis. Also, consider an esophageal ulcer caused by herpes simplex, CMV, or aphthous stomatitis, malignancy.
3. Oral manifestations.
   a. Appearance of oral lesions, white plaques on oral mucosa, particularly in the posterior pharynx, and angular cheilitis from *Candida albicans* of mouth.
   b. Vesicles with ulceration from herpes simplex virus.
   c. White, thickened lesions on lateral margins of tongue from oral hairy leukoplakia.
   d. Oral warts because of human papillomavirus.
   e. Periodontitis progressing to gingival necrosis.
   f. Painful, solitary lesions with raised margins may be aphthous ulcers of unclear etiology.
   g. Appearance of flat or nodular purple lesions on the hard or soft palate, buccal mucosa, posterior pharynx from Kaposi sarcoma.
4. CNS manifestations.
   a. Cognitive, motor, and behavioral symptoms may be caused by HIV encephalopathy, AIDS dementia, acute infection, toxicity from alcohol or drugs, adverse reaction to medication, psychiatric condition, and other infectious and malignant causes.
   b. Acute symptoms of infection with fever, malaise, headache, and/or mental status change, seizure, hemiparesis, abnormal gait or speech may be caused by toxoplasmosis, cryptococcal meningitis, herpes virus infections, CMV encephalitis, progressive multifocal leukoencephalopathy, CNS lymphoma, neurosyphilis, or other pathogens and malignancies.
   c. May also have sensory symptoms that present as numbness, tingling, and neuropathic pain of the feet or hands.
5. Ocular manifestations.
   a. Seeing floaters in the visual field, flashes of light, or sudden loss of a visual field in persons with less than 100 CD4/mm^3 because of CMV retinitis with or without retinal detachment, a sight-threatening infection that requires urgent evaluation by an ophthalmologist.
   b. Blurry vision, dry eyes, double vision, or swelling of the eyelid or conjunctiva, caused by bacterial or viral conjunctival infection, adverse reaction to medication, syphilis, Kaposi's sarcoma, or other pathogens and malignancies.
6. Malignancies—may be AIDS-defining cancer (ADC) or non-ADC.
   a. Kaposi's sarcoma (ADC).
   b. Non-Hodgkin's lymphoma (ADC) and other lymphomas (non-ADC).
   c. Cervical cancer (ADC).
   d. Liver cancer (non-ADC).
   e. Lung cancer (non-ADC).
   f. Anal cancer (non-ADC).
7. Skin manifestations.
   a. Pruritic rash with raised, erythematous papules, located on surfaces that contain hair follicles known as HIV folliculitis. Check for eosinophilia.
   b. Abscess caused by methicillin-sensitive and methicillin-resistant *S. aureus* infections, Streptococcus, or other common skin pathogens.
   c. Pruritic nodular rash located on any skin surface, known as prurigo nodularis.
   d. Purple, flat, or nodular lesions located on any skin surface including soles of feet, palms of hands, oral mucosa including hard palate is likely to be Kaposi's sarcoma and should be biopsied.

Nursing Diagnoses

- Ineffective Therapeutic Regimen Management related to complicated regimen of medications, treatment plans, clinical appointments, lack of social support, impaired cognitive functioning, substance use, or psychiatric illness.
- Fear of infection progression, treatment effects, isolation, and death related to having HIV/AIDS.
- Risk for infection related to immunodeficiency.
- Imbalanced Nutrition: Less Than Body Requirements related to infection or medication side effects, More than Body Requirements related to diet choices and exercise deficit.
- Impaired Oral Mucous Membranes related to infection or adverse effects of medication.
- Diarrhea related to infection or adverse effects of medication.
- Confusion related to infection or adverse effects of medicine.
- Hyperthermia related to opportunistic infection or malignancy.
- Ineffective Breathing Pattern related to infection or malignancy.
- Other nursing diagnoses may include:
  - Fatigue related to underlying HIV infection or depression.
  - Disturbed Body Image related to body changes from disease process or adverse effects of medication.
  - Hopelessness related to chronic illness, sense of loss of control, depression, or vulnerability associated with HIV/AIDS.

- Acute and Chronic Pain related to infection, peripheral neuropathy, avascular necrosis, or other condition.
- Anticipatory Grieving related to awareness of implications of HIV/AIDS, changes in lifestyle, possible death.
- Disabled Family Coping related to crisis created by HIV/AIDS, guilt, fear, overwhelming caretaking responsibilities.

Nursing Interventions

Managing ART

1. Assess patient's adherence to medications and clinical appointments; work together to problem solve a plan to improve adherence.
2. Provide education about prescribed medications before ART is started and periodically thereafter; provide educational materials that the patient can take home.
3. Develop a medication schedule for the patient that incorporates his or her usual day-to-day activities; place pills in a medication box per the schedule.
4. Encourage the involvement of a household member in the education and administration of the patient's medications.
5. Continue to monitor for medication adherence after patient has achieved an undetectable viral load.
6. Routinely ask about adverse effects. Encourage patient to call if these become a problem and teach management of common symptoms.
7. Encourage patient to keep his or her insurance and prescription drug coverage active and up to date, to prevent lapses in refills and periods without insurance.

 DRUG ALERT Successful ART requires about 95% adherence to medication dose and frequency. Stress this before starting ART and at every visit. Problem-solve barriers to adherence. Develop strategies that anticipate going off course, such as late or missed doses, change in daily routine, vacation, spending the night away from home, and other life events.

Promoting Dignity and Reducing Fear

1. Maintain nonjudgmental approach.
2. Anticipate that the patient may pass through a series of stages: initial crisis, transitional stage, acceptance state, and possibly preparation for death if treatment options have been exhausted.
3. Allow patient to use some degree of denial as a protective mechanism, which gives some control over when and how patient will confront the diagnosis and his or her prognosis.
   a. Expect some displaced anger; avoid being personally affronted by patient's anger.
   b. Allow patient to acknowledge reality of the situation without giving false assurance.
4. Acknowledge that symptoms of anxiety and depression are common initially but generally improve with time and support. Refer patient to counseling or psychiatric care, if needed.
5. Anticipate that patients who have active substance use may exhibit antisocial behaviors and feelings of alienation and isolation. Refer for counseling and treatment.
6. Provide careful discussion and clarification of treatment options.
7. Help patient set realistic goals and expectations.
8. Obtain social work consult for available insurance-related, prescription drug and other social resources, and community-based case management.

9. Help patient identify and strengthen personal resources, such as positive coping skills, relaxation techniques, support network, and optimistic outlook.
10. Encourage patient to join a support group.
11. Observe for emerging psychiatric problems, especially in patients who are socially isolated, those who have guilt or shame about sexuality and lifestyle, and those with a history of psychiatric illness.
12. Discuss the importance of advance directives and legal guardianship for minor children. Cognitive deterioration may make it impossible for patient to act on his or her own behalf in the future.
13. The population of HIV-infected patients is ageing, with approximately half of patients being over age 50. Consider the needs of an ageing population with regard to health maintenance, socialization, adaptive equipment, and home safety considerations. Consultation with a geriatrician may be helpful.

 NURSING ALERT Never assume that the patient's family or friends know the patient's HIV status. Always ask the patient who knows of his or her status. Encourage the patient to share his or her diagnosis to decrease isolation. Offer to be with the patient when the diagnosis is shared with family or friend(s); role-playing before disclosing status can be helpful.

Preventing Infection

1. Assess for overt and subtle signs of infection at every visit.
2. Follow standard precautions with all patients.
3. Discuss food safety regarding storage and preparation.
4. Promote proper skin care to prevent breaks in the skin.
5. Teach wound care and management; monitor wound for signs of worsening or infection, if applicable.
6. Discuss preventing STIs at every visit, if relevant.
7. Teach patient to take all antibiotics as directed.
8. Teach patient to maintain a clean living environment.
9. Use aseptic techniques when performing invasive procedures.
10. Counsel the patient to have someone else clean a cat box or bird cage. If no one else is available, then use rubber gloves, wear a mask, change clothes, and wash hands afterward.
11. Ensure that the patient is up to date with immunizations.

Improving Nutritional Status

1. Monitor nutritional status by weighing patient, calculating BMI, and reviewing dietary choices
2. Include patient in decision making regarding nutritional care. Consult with dietitian to develop strategies for optimizing patient's nutritional status.
3. Review ART dosing in relation to meal times to optimize ART absorption; some medications should be taken with food and others should be taken on an empty stomach.
4. Administer or teach patient to take prescribed antiemetic 30 minutes before meals or medication, if nausea is a problem. Use antidiarrheal medication if advised after consultation with provider.
5. For patient with oral or esophageal pain from *Candida* esophagitis or another cause:
   a. Administer prescribed antifungal and/or antiviral therapy.
   b. Avoid highly seasoned or acidic foods.
   c. Offer fluids and pureed or soft foods to minimize chewing and ease swallowing. Offer liquid nutritional supplements.

6. Discourage alcohol use because it has immunosuppressive effect and is contraindicated in patients with chronic hepatitis.
7. Make appropriate community referral if patient is unable to grocery shop or prepare meals. Inform patient of local online grocery shopping options and services that deliver prepared meals.

Relieving Oral Discomfort
1. Ask about tooth pain, sore throat, dysphagia, and heartburn.
2. Examine mouth for oral candida and other lesions and teach patient to do the same.
3. Administer antifungal treatment as indicated.
4. Refer to dental care in the community for poor dentition and/or gum disease.

Minimizing the Effects of Diarrhea
1. Diarrhea is common and can have many causes.
2. Review medication list for causative agents.
3. Send new diarrheal stool for ova and parasite studies, microscopy, and culture.
4. Counsel patient to monitor stools, and report frequency, consistency, and presence of blood.
5. Monitor intake and output; assess skin and mucous membranes for poor turgor and dryness, indicating dehydration.
6. Monitor electrolytes. Administer fluids and electrolytes as prescribed.
7. Follow contact precautions and practice strict handwashing.
8. Plan skin care regimen that includes bathing and drying by blotting. Apply ointment or skin barrier cream to the area.
9. Advise patient to eliminate caffeine, alcohol, dairy products, high fat foods, and acidic juices.
10. Drink liquids at room temperature.
11. Advise patient to avoid foods that increase motility and distention such as gas-forming fruits and vegetables.

Managing Altered Mental Status
1. HIV has an affinity for the brain and is a target organ for opportunistic infections in advanced HIV infection.
2. Take measures to keep the patient safe. Refer altered outpatients to an acute care appointment or to the emergency department.
3. In inpatients, promote patient safety: bed alarm on, call signal available, articles within patient's reach. Anticipate a plan for toileting the patient. Make frequent checks.
4. Assess for depressive or suicidal symptoms.
5. Provide daily assessment of mental status; monitor for changes in behavior, memory, concentration ability, and motor dysfunction.
6. Check labs for abnormalities, diagnostic test results, and medication side effect profiles for possible cause.
7. Maintain a low stimulus environment such as dim lighting, low noise, promote sleep/wake cycle, quiet activities such as coloring or doing puzzles, light socialization, light exercise, and listening to quiet music.
8. Reorient patient frequently: use calendar, clock, family and friends' pictures, lists, and structured care plan.
9. Provide reassurance.
10. Anticipate need for advance directives or guardianship, durable power of attorney for health care and financial matters, and managing the process of informed consent if patient has impaired cognition.

Reducing Fever
1. Assess for chills, fever, tachycardia, and tachypnea.
2. Aggressively treat the underlying cause.
3. Encourage high fluid intake to replace insensible water losses incurred by fever or diaphoresis.
4. Administer or teach patient to administer antipyretics as prescribed.

Improving Breathing Pattern
1. Provide supplemental oxygen as ordered. Monitor for increased oxygen demand.
2. Position patient to optimize effective breathing, elevate head of bed, support head and neck to maintain patent airway.
3. Monitor for change in respiratory status.
4. Administer or teach patient to take cough medication.
5. Encourage smoking cessation.
6. Answer questions and provide support if patient has made decision for or against resuscitation and mechanical ventilation.

Community and Home Care Considerations for the Patient with End-Stage AIDS
1. Assist patient, family, or significant other to locate care and support services in the community.
2. If patient is homebound, contact an agency that offers help specifically for HIV-infected patients and provides home visits for services such as light housekeeping and food delivery.
3. Assess the home for safety and function; provide durable medical goods that can enhance safety and comfort, and improve function.
4. Provide latex gloves to the family for handling body fluids of the HIV-positive household member.
5. Reinforce that routine household cleaning of the bathroom, dishes, and laundry is sufficient to prevent household transmission of HIV.

 TRANSITIONAL CARE ALERT If the patient is inpatient and transitioning to home for care by the family or friends, invite the caretakers to learn basic care from the hospital nurses. Invite caretakers to spend the night to learn the treatments and care that occur around the clock. This can help caretakers to identify gaps in services in the home and decide their readiness to take responsibility prior to the patient's discharge.

For family members/friends who are taking care of a patient at home over a long period, provide information about day care services that the patient can attend or about respite care so that caregivers can receive a break from the caretaking role.

Evaluation: Expected Outcomes
- Takes prescribed ART at least 95% of the time; maintains an undetectable viral load.
- Speaks openly about HIV infection with health care providers and significant others; manages life stressors effectively.
- No signs of opportunistic infections; practices safe sex.
- Eating balanced meals.
- Oral mucosa moist and without lesions.
- Having formed stools and no perianal skin breakdown.
- Oriented to time, person, and place.
- Afebrile.
- Respirations unlabored, no cough or sputum production.

SELECTED REFERENCES

Bartlett, J. G. (2016). The natural history and clinical features of HIV infection in adults and adolescents. *UpToDate*. New York: Wolters Kluwer. Available: *www. uptodate.com/contents/the-natural-history-and-clinical-features-of-hiv-infection-in-adults-and-adolescents*

Centers for Disease Control and Prevention. (1993). AIDS surveillance case definition for adolescents and adults. *Morbidity and Mortality Weekly Report, 4*(RR-17), 2.

Center for Disease Control and Prevention. (2017). HIV Surveillance Report. Atlanta, GA: Author. Available: *https://www.cdc.gov/hiv/statistics/overview/index.html*.

Center for Disease Control and Prevention. (2014). *US Public Health Service preexposure prophylaxis for the prevention of HIV infection in the United States 2014: A clinical practice Guideline*. Atlanta, GA: Author. Available: *www.cdc.gov/hiv/pdf/prepguidelines2014.pdf*

Dumitru, G., Irwin, K., & Tailor, A. (2017). Updated federal recommendations for HIV prevention with adults and adolescents with HIV in the United States: The pivotal role of nurses. *Journal of the Association of Nurses in AIDS Care, 28*(1), 8–18.

Gallant, J. E. (2016). *100 questions and answers about HIV and AIDS*. Sudbury, MA: Jones & Bartlett.

HRSA HIV/AIDS Bureau. (2014). *Guide for HIV/AIDS clinical care: Health care maintenance and disease prevention*. Washington, DC: USDHHS. Available: *www.careacttarget. org/library/guide-hivaids-clinical-care-health-care-maintenance-and-disease-prevention*

Marcus, J. L., Chao, C. R., & Leyden, W. A. (2016). Narrowing the gap in life expectancy between HIV-infected and HIV-uninfected individuals with access to care. *Journal of Acquired Immune Deficiency Syndromes, 73*(1), 39–46.

Mignano, J. L. (2016). 80% viral suppression by 2020? Understanding the concept of engagement in HIV care and a call to action for nursing. *Journal of the Association of Nurses in AIDS Care, 27*(5), 550–562.

Sax, P. E. (2017). Acute and early HIV infection: Clinical manifestations and diagnosis. *UpToDate*. New York: Wolters Kluwer. Available: *www.uptodate.com/contents/acute-and-early-hiv-infection-clinical-manifestations-and-diagnosis?source=see_link &sectionName=DIAGNOSIS&anchor=H18410709#H18410709*

Sexton, D. J., & Pien, B. C. (2014). Immune reconstitution inflammatory syndrome. *UpToDate*. New York: Wolters Kluwer. Available: *www.uptodate.com/contents/immune-reconstitution-inflammatory-syndrome*

Siliciano, J. D., & Siliciano, R. F. (2016). Recent developments in the effort to cure of HIV infection: going beyond N = 1. *Journal of Clinical Investigation, 126*(2), 409–414.

Simeone, C. A., Seal, S. M., & Savage, C. (2017). Implementing HIV testing in substance use treatment programs: A systematic review. *Journal of the Association of Nurses in AIDS Care, 28*(2), 199–215.

Singh, H. K., Del Carmen, T., Freeman, R., et al. (2017). From one syndrome to many: Incorporating geriatric consultation into HIV care. *Clinical Infectious Diseases, 65*, 501–506. doi:*10.1093/cid/cix311*.

Swanson, B (Ed.). (2010). *ANAC's core curriculum for HIV/AIDS nursing* (3rd ed.). Sudbury, MA: Jones & Bartlett.

Turner, L., Roepke, A., Wardell, E., & Teitelman, A. (2017). Do you PrEP? A review of primary care provider knowledge of PrEP and attitudes on P prescribing PrEP. *Journal of the Association of Nurses in AIDS Care, 29*(1), 83–92.

UNAIDS. (2014). *90-90-90 An ambitious treatment target to help end the AIDS epidemic*. Geneva: Author. Available: *www.unaids.org/sites/default/files/media_asset/90-90-90_en_0.pdf*

U.S. Department of Health and Human Services, Panel on Antiretriviral Guidelines for Adults and Adolescents. (2018). Guidelines for the use of antiretroviral agents in adults an adolescents living with HIV. Rockville, MD: Author. Available: *https://aidsinfo.nih.gov/contentfiles/lvguidelines/AdultandAdolescentGL. pdf*.

U.S. Department of Health and Human Services, Panel on Opportunistic Infections in HIV-Infected Adults and Adolescents. (2018). Guidelines for the prevention and treatment of opportunistic infections in HIV-infected adults and adolescents: Recommendations from the Centers for Disease Control and Prevention, the National Institutes of Health, and the HIV Medicine Association of the Infectious Diseases Society of America. Rockville, MD: Author. Available at *http://aidsinfo. nih.gov/contentfiles/lvguidelines/adult_oi.pdf*.

Wells, J. S., Holstad, M. M., Thomas, T., & Bruner, D. W. (2014). An integrative review of guidelines for anal cancer screening in HIV-infected persons. *AIDS Patient Care & STDs, 28*(7), 350–357.

World Health Organization. (2018). *WHO HIV/AIDS fact sheet (No. 360)*. Geneva: WHO. Available: *http://www.who.int/en/news-room/fact-sheets/detail/hiv-aids*

30
Connective Tissue Disorders

OVERVIEW AND ASSESSMENT

Connective tissue is a fibrous tissue that supports and connects internal organs, forms bones and the walls of blood vessels, attaches muscles and bones to bones (tendons and ligaments), and replaces tissue following injury (scar tissue). The long fibers of connective tissue contain a protein called *collagen*.

Connective tissue disorders are also known as *rheumatologic disorders*. They affect the integrity of the musculoskeletal system and may also affect blood vessels, the skin, and a variety of organs. They are chronic and may lead to disability; however, they can usually be controlled with medication.

Musculoskeletal and Related Assessment

Assessment for connective tissue disorders not only focuses on the musculoskeletal system but also involves remote body systems. Clues to connective tissue disorders may be found in the skin, eyes, lungs, and neurologic system. Functional assessment is also important; many questionnaires and scales have been developed to assess patient function or disability related to connective tissue disorders, such as the Health Assessment Questionnaire first published in 1980, available: *www.chcr.brown.edu/pcoc/ehaqdescrscoringhaq372.pdf.*

Subjective Data

Obtain history of presenting symptoms, including duration and intensity, course of the illness, and impact of symptoms on the patient's life.
1. Musculoskeletal pain—characteristics.
   a. Joint swelling.
   b. Morning stiffness.
2. Constitutional symptoms.
   a. Fever.
   b. Weight loss and anorexia.
   c. Fatigue.
3. Involvement of other body symptoms.
   a. Skin.
   b. Ocular.
   c. Pulmonary.
   d. Neurologic.
   e. Mucous membranes.
   f. Gastrointestinal (GI).
4. Depression or psychosis.
5. Self-care activities and functional ability.
6. Social activities and roles.
7. Family history of rheumatic or autoimmune disorders.

Objective Data

1. Musculoskeletal examination:
   a. Pain on palpation or range of motion (ROM).
   b. Joint swelling, warmth, or erythema.
   c. Joint motion restriction.
   d. Pain, swelling, or warmth of soft tissues surrounding joints.
   e. Deformities.
2. Skin:
   a. Skin rash or other abnormalities such as thickening.
   b. Alopecia.
3. Oral mucosa:
   a. Ulcerations.
   b. Dryness.
4. Ocular:
   a. Conjunctival inflammation.
   b. Dryness.
5. Pulmonary:
   a. Adventitious sounds.
   b. Friction rub.
6. Neurologic:
   a. Foot drop.
   b. Muscle weakness.
   c. Neurologic deficits.

Laboratory Studies

Anti–Double-Stranded DNA

Anti–double-stranded DNA (anti-dsDNA) is a highly specific marker for diagnosing systemic lupus erythematosus (SLE). This antibody is also useful for monitoring disease progression because anti-dsDNA levels fluctuate with disease activity.

Nursing and Patient Care Considerations

1. High anti-dsDNA levels are associated with the development of lupus nephritis.
2. There is a low false-positive rate (about 5%) in patients with other connective tissue disorders; in patients taking medications such as minocycline, etanercept, infliximab, and penicillamine; in first-degree relatives of patients with lupus; and in some laboratory workers.
3. There is no special preparation for this blood test.

Anticyclic Citrullinated Peptide

Anticyclic citrullinated peptide (anti-CCP) is a marker that helps diagnose rheumatoid arthritis (RA). These autoantibodies are produced in the joint as a result of the synovial immune response of patients with RA.

Nursing and Patient Care Considerations

1. Anti-CCP is about as sensitive, but more specific (95% to 98%), than the rheumatoid factor (RF) test. Found in approximately 50% to 55% of patients with RA.
2. It may be valuable in cases of early arthritis when symptoms are mild and nonspecific and aggressive treatment is being contemplated. Anti-CCP antibody is now used with the RF as the gold standard in making the diagnosis of RA.
3. No specific preparation is needed for this blood test, but the specimen may need to be sent out for processing, as not all labs perform this test.

Antinuclear Antibody

Antinuclear antibody (ANA) is a test for antibodies to nucleoprotein (autoantibodies or a heterogeneous group of gamma globulins); it is highly sensitive for detecting SLE but is nonspecific (high false-positive rate).

Nursing and Patient Care Considerations

1. Be alert for drugs that may cause false-positive results.
2. Results will be reported in a staining pattern (speckled, homogeneous, peripheral, nucleolar) if positive, which correlates to various types of connective tissue disorders and various subsets of SLE (see Table 30-1).
3. Titer will also be reported with positive ANA but does not reflect disease activity or prognosis.

Complement

1. *Complement* is a complex cascade system that activates proteins as part of the body's defense against infection.
2. Specific components include CH50 (total complement), C3, and C4; measurement helps determine immune complex formation or agammaglobulinemia.
3. Complement levels are decreased in certain autoimmune diseases, particularly SLE, because of complement consumption and because of activation of proteolytic enzymes and tissue damage. C3 and C4 are often monitored to evaluate activity in SLE.

Table 30-1	ANA Staining Patterns and Connective Tissue Disorders
ANA PATTERN	**CONNECTIVE TISSUE DISORDER**
Peripheral (rim, ring, membranous)	Active SLE, usually with renal disease
Homogenous (diffuse)	SLE, RA
Speckled	SLE, RA, scleroderma, Sjögren syndrome, mixed connective tissue disorder
Nucleolar	Scleroderma

ANA, antinuclear antibody; RA, rheumatoid arthritis; SLE, systemic lupus erythematosus.

Nursing and Patient Care Considerations

1. Obtain venous blood sample and refrigerate; send to laboratory promptly because complement deteriorates at room temperature.
2. Serial measurements may be helpful in monitoring the activity of some rheumatic diseases; decreased levels indicate increased disease activity.

C-Reactive Protein

C-reactive protein (CRP) is produced by the liver and is a nonspecific marker for infection and inflammation. It can be used to support the diagnosis for immune-mediated inflammatory diseases such as psoriatic arthritis, RA, and Crohn disease.

Nursing and Patient Care Considerations

1. CRP reacts quicker to inflammatory changes than erythrocyte sedimentation rate (ESR); it rises within a few hours of an infection or inflammatory condition and then decreases quickly when inflammation resolves.
2. CRP can be used to differentiate inflammatory from noninflammatory conditions and to monitor effectiveness of treatment.
3. Normal CRP is usually below 10 mg/L; a level over 100 mg/L usually indicates infection or inflammation; however, some inflammatory conditions can raise CRP a thousandfold.

Erythrocyte Sedimentation Rate

1. *Erythrocyte sedimentation rate (ESR)* determines the rate at which red blood cells (RBCs) fall out of unclotted blood in 1 hour.
2. The test is based on the premise that inflammatory and other disease processes create changes in blood proteins, thus causing aggregation of RBCs that makes them heavier.

Nursing and Patient Care Considerations

1. ESR is generally elevated in most rheumatic illnesses.
2. The test is sensitive for inflammatory condition, but not specific to connective tissue disorders.
   a. Result may be elevated by pregnancy, menstruation, medications (such as heparin and oral contraceptives), infection, malignancy, anemia, and advanced age.
   b. Result may be reduced by elevated blood glucose or albumin, high phospholipids, or drugs, such as corticosteroids or high-dose aspirin.
3. Most beneficial in monitoring inflammatory disease activity.

Table 30-2   Synovial Fluid Analysis

	NORMAL COLOR	WHITE BLOOD CELL COUNT	VISCOSITY	CRYSTALS
Normal	Clear, yellow	200/μm³	Normal	None
Osteoarthritis	Clear, slightly turbid	200–600/μm³	Low	None
Gout	Turbid	2,000–75,000/μm³	Low	Monosodium urate
Inflammatory Arthritis	Turbid, yellow	2,000–75,000/μm³	Low	None
(Rheumatoid arthritis, systemic lupus erythematosus, Sjögren syndrome, psoriatic)				
Septic Arthritis	Pus, very turbid	Generally 80,000/μm³	Low	None

Rheumatoid Factor

Rheumatoid factor (RF) is a test for macroglobulin found in the blood of patients with RA and other disorders. RF has properties of an antibody and may be directed against immunoglobulin.

Nursing and Patient Care Considerations

1. It is not a highly sensitive or specific test.
2. May be positive in 50% to 75% of patients with RA, SLE, and Sjögren syndrome. May be false-positive with endocarditis, tuberculosis, syphilis, sarcoidosis, cancer, viral infections, hepatitis C, patients with skin or renal allographs, and in some liver, lung, or kidney diseases.
3. Negative RF does not exclude the diagnosis of RA.
4. Certain disease manifestations, such as severe joint involvement and extra-articular manifestations, may be more frequent in those with high-titer RF.

Other Tests

Synovial Fluid Analysis

1. A sample of synovial (joint) fluid is analyzed for several components.
   a. Color.
   b. Clarity/turbidity.
   c. Viscosity.
   d. White blood cell (WBC) count with differential.
   e. Crystals and their identification.
2. Arthrocentesis, a sterile procedure, requires antiseptic cleaning agent, local anesthetic, a 20-G needle (an 18-G needle if infected fluid is suspected), and a 10- to 20-mL syringe.

Nursing and Patient Care Considerations

1. Patients are generally apprehensive about having a needle inserted into a joint. They require reassurance and explanation of the importance of information derived from test results.
2. Assist the health care provider with the test by collecting supplies, maintaining a sterile field, sending joint fluid samples for testing, and monitoring for bleeding following the procedure.
3. Results help to differentiate infection, inflammation, and crystal deposition in a painful joint (see Table 30-2).

GENERAL PROCEDURES AND TREATMENT MODALITIES
Pharmacologic Agents

EVIDENCE BASE American College of Rheumatology. (2012). *Update of the 2008 American College of Rheumatology recommendations for the use of* disease-modifying antirheumatic drugs and biologic agents in the treatment of rheumatoid arthritis. Atlanta, GA: Author. Available: www.rheumatology.org/Practice-Quality/Clinical-Support/Clinical-Practice-Guidelines.

Connective tissue disorders may be treated with various drugs to relieve pain and to halt or minimize the disease process. Types of agents include nonsteroidal anti-inflammatory drugs (NSAIDs), corticosteroids, immunosuppressive agents, and a group of unrelated drugs known as disease-modifying antirheumatic drugs (DMARDs). Drug therapy may be long term and may require frequent evaluation for adverse effects (see Table 30-3). Patient education information about pharmacologic agents used to treat various disorders can be obtained from the National Institute of Arthritis and Musculoskeletal and Skin Disease (*www.niams.nih.gov/Health_Info/default.asp*) or from the American College of Rheumatology (ACR; *www.rheumatology.org*).

Physical and Occupational Therapy

Physical and occupational therapy provides a multimodal program to help reduce pain and to improve joint function. Many other measures can be taught to patients for home practice. Components of the program may include:

- Joint conservation.
- Energy conservation.
- Splinting (in rare instances).
- ROM exercises.
- Application of heat and cold.
- Endurance or aerobic conditioning.
- Modification of home and work environment.

Joint Conservation

Teach or reinforce the following practices:
1. Perform activities using good body mechanics.
2. Avoid overuse of joints. Pace task and include rest in long or repetitive activities.
3. Use large joints to perform activities—spread the load over as many joints as possible.
4. Perform activities in smooth movements to avoid trauma induced by abrupt movements.

Energy Conservation

Teach or reinforce the following practices:
1. Organize materials, utensils, and tools.
2. Perform lengthy activities in a seated position.
3. Work at an even pace—avoid rushing.
4. Delegate work to others when possible.

Table 30-3 Drug Therapy for Connective Tissue Disorders

DRUG	ACTION	ADVERSE EFFECTS
Anti-Inflammatory Agents		
Salicylates		
• Aspirin (may be buffered or enteric coated)	• Anti-inflammatory, antipyretic, and analgesic effects	• Tinnitus, gastric intolerance or GI bleeding, and purpuric tendencies
Nonsteroidal Anti-Inflammatory Drugs (NSAIDs)		
• Ibuprofen • Fenoprofen • Naproxen • Tolmetin • Sulindac • Meclofenamate • Ketoprofen • Salsalate • Diclofenac • Nabumetone • Ketorolac • Oxaprozin • Flurbiprofen • Diflunisal • Piroxicam • Etodolac • Indomethacin • Trisalicylate	• Anti-inflammatory and analgesic effects • Mechanism of action may be related to inhibition of prostaglandin synthesis (prostaglandins have a role in inflammatory process, pain, and fever). • Nonsteroidal anti-inflammatory agents for adjunctive treatment of rheumatoid arthritis • Sometimes remarkably effective in the control of articular symptoms	• GI irritation: nausea, vomiting, epigastric distress, precipitation and reactivation of peptic ulcer, hepatitis • Hematologic: bone marrow depression, anemia, leukopenia, thrombocytopenia purpura • Decrease in renal function can precipitate renal failure. • Central nervous system: headache, dizziness, drowsiness, aseptic meningitis • Cardiovascular: edema, dyspnea palpitations
COX-2 Inhibitors		
• Celecoxib • Meloxicam	• Selective prostaglandin inhibition so that the inflammatory process is reduced without reducing protective prostaglandin effects on gastric mucosa	• Same adverse effects as other NSAIDs, with less risk for GI bleeding
Disease-Modifying Agents		
Antimalarial Agents		
• Hydroxychloroquine sulfate • Chloroquine phosphate	• Remission-induction agents for inflammatory arthritis usually in combination with other DMARDs • Used frequently for lupus	• Ocular toxicity (retinopathy that can result in permanent loss of vision; blurred vision, night blindness, scotoma)
Sulfonamides		
• Sulfasalazine	• Salicylate, sulfonamide	• Anorexia, rash, hemolytic anemia
Immunomodulators		
• Etanercept • Adalimumab • Golimumab • Certolizumab pegol	• Tumor necrosis factor blocker (subcutaneous)	• Infection, injection site reaction (SQ), dyspepsia, aplastic anemia, demyelinating disorders, activation of latent TB infection, reactivation of hepatitis B
• Infliximab • Golimumab	• IV tumor necrosis factor blocker	• Infusion reaction (IV), headache, optic neuritis, lupuslike syndrome, risk of severe infection
• Abatacept	• Selective costimulation modulator; available as IV or SC	• Risk of serious infection • Worsening of COPD
• Tocilizumab	• Interleukin 6-receptor blocker available as IV or SC	• Risk of severe infection, hypersensitivity reaction, gastrointestinal perforation, demyelinating disorder, malignancy, injection site reaction (SQ), infusion reaction (IV)
Immunosuppressives		
• Methotrexate	• Exert anti-inflammatory effect by inhibition of cellular replication	• Bone marrow suppression, hepatic and pulmonary toxicity, reduced resistance to infection, teratogenic
• Azathioprine	• Suppresses cell-mediated hypersensitivities and alters antibody production	• Bone marrow depression, GI and hepatic toxicity, carcinogenesis
• Cyclophosphamide	• Alkylating agent that interferes with the growth of rapidly dividing cells	• Possibility of a malignancy occurring many years later after initiating therapy can cause sterility, urinary bladder, fibrosis, cystitis

Table 30-3 Drug Therapy for Connective Tissue Disorders (Continued)

DRUG	ACTION	ADVERSE EFFECTS
• Cyclosporine	• Inhibition of immunocompetent lymphocytes also inhibits lymphokine production and release.	• Renal dysfunction, tremor, hypertension, gum hyperplasia
• Leflunomide	• Pyrimidine synthesis inhibitor	• Diarrhea, liver function test abnormalities, alopecia, rash, upper respiratory infection, hypertension
• Mycophenolate mofetil	• Inhibits T lymphocyte activation	• Bone marrow suppression, hepatic, reactivation of hepatitis B or C, reduced resistance to infection, teratogenic
Corticosteroids		
• Prednisone • Prednisolone • Triamcinolone • Betamethasone • Hydrocortisone • Dexamethasone • Methylprednisolone	• Alter immune response by binding to intracellular corticosteroid receptors • Potent anti-inflammatory action • Usually used for short-term management of patients with severe limitations	• Osteoporosis, fractures, avascular necrosis • Gastric ulcers, infection susceptibility • Hirsutism, acne, moon facies, abnormal fat deposition, edema, emotional disorders, menstrual disorders • Hyperglycemia, hypokalemia • Hypertension, cataracts

IV, intravenous; SC, subcutaneous.

Splinting

1. May be used for wrists and hands.
2. Ensure proper application.
3. Periodically inspect for skin irritation, neurovascular compromise, or improper fit.
4. Usually worn during acute stage of inflammation to protect joint.

Exercise

Instruct and reinforce correct method of exercise:

1. Avoid exercising inflamed joints—putting these joints through ROM exercises one to two times per day when inflamed is sufficient.
2. Perform exercises daily, as prescribed.
3. Aerobic conditioning exercises may be indicated when disease activity permits.
4. Walking, biking, swimming, and water walking for 30 minutes, three times per week. Regular exercise three times per week for at least 20 minutes for 6 months has been shown to reduce fatigue and disability in patients with RA compared to those who didn't exercise.

Other Measures

1. Reinforce correct use and application of heat and cold.
2. Obtain and teach correct use of assistive devices.
3. Reinforce use of behavior-modification and relaxation techniques as adjuncts to therapy.
4. Suggest discussion with health care provider about complementary and alternative therapies. A wide variety of herbal and nutraceutical products have been used and studied, but data remain inconclusive about efficacy (see Table 30-4).
   a. Many herbal and supplemental products are marketed for pain, inflammation, repair of cartilage, and boosting the immune system; however, scientific evidence for clear-cut treatment benefit is lacking. There is preliminary evidence for fish oil, gamma linolenic acid, and the herb thunder god vine.
   b. Reflexology, tai chi, and acupressure or acupuncture have benefited some patients with arthritis and connective tissue disorders. Assist the patient in finding certified providers in these disciplines, if desired.
   c. Use of magnets to relieve pain has not shown effectiveness in numerous studies since the concept was introduced.
   d. For more information, refer patients to the National Center for Complimentary and Alternative Medicine at *https://nccam.nih.gov/health/RA/getthefacts.htm.*
5. Advise patient to modify home and work environments, as needed, to install safety devices, and to maintain a safe environment.
6. Advise patient to seek counseling regarding sexuality if joint pain and inflammation are barriers to performance.
7. Reinforce the chronic waxing-and-waning nature of the illness to lessen susceptibility to quackery.

 EVIDENCE BASE National Center for Complementary and Alternative Medicine. (2013). *Rheumatoid arthritis and complementary and alternative medicine.* Bethesda, MD: Author. Available: *https://nccam.nih.gov/health/RA/getthefacts.htm.*

Cameron, M., Gangier, J. J., & Chrubasik, S. (2011). Herbal therapy for treating rheumatoid arthritis. *The Cochrane Database of Systematic Reviews,* (2), CD002948.

DISORDERS

Rheumatoid Arthritis

Rheumatoid arthritis (RA) is a chronic inflammatory disease that affects joints and other organ systems. RA affects 0.5% to 1% of the population worldwide. The 2010 criteria include synovitis in any joint where no alternative diagnosis can explain the synovitis, and a score of 6/10 in four domains: number and site of involved joints, serologic abnormality, elevated acute phase response (markers of inflammation), and symptom duration. Joint erosions as seen on imaging confirm diagnosis regardless of score.

Table 30-4   Complementary and Alternative Drug Therapy for Arthritis

DRUG	EFFECT	COMMENTS
Fish oil (omega-3 fatty acid)	May reduce tenderness and stiffness; may reduce the need for NSAIDs	May interact with blood thinners, antihypertensives. Avoid high-dose fish liver oil, which may cause vitamin A and D toxicity.
Gamma-linoleic acid (GLA) (omega-6 fatty acid, evening primrose oil, borage, black currant)	Converted into substances that reduce inflammation to relieve joint pain, stiffness, tenderness, and possibly NSAID use	Appears to be safe but some borage oil preparations contain hepatotoxic chemicals. More research on dose and duration is needed.
Thunder god vine (*Tripterygium wilfordii*)	May fight inflammation and suppress the immune system; may relieve rheumatoid arthritis symptoms	May cause serious side effects—diarrhea, stomach upset, hair loss, headache, skin rash, menstrual changes, male infertility; long-term use may reduce bone mineral density.
Boswellia	Anti-inflammatory and analgesic effects	Generally safe. Lab and animal studies have been done; need clinical studies.
Ginger	Anti-inflammatory and analgesic effects	Large doses may cause GI adverse effects; may cause bleeding if given with anticoagulant. Lab studies have been done; need clinical studies.
Green tea	Substances might be useful in rheumatoid arthritis and osteoarthritis.	More information is needed.
Turmeric (curcumin)	Animal studies show protection of joints from inflammation and damage.	Generally safe, no adverse effects; however, may cause stomach ulcers in high doses with prolonged use. Animal studies have been done; need clinical studies.
Cayenne pepper (capsicum)	Thought to deplete substance P, reducing pain transmission. Applied topically to the skin over joints in concentrations of 0.025%–0.25%	Takes several days to obtain pain relief; do not use with heat application.
Glucosamine and chondroitin	Cartilage repair, pain relief Glucosamine: 1,000–2,000 mg daily chondroitin: 800–1,600 mg daily, based on weight	Bleeding risk if ASA taken with chondroitin; may be effective either alone or as combination; must be taken for several months to achieve noticeable effect. Studies showed conflicting results.

GLA, gamma-linoleic acid.

EVIDENCE BASE American College of Rheumatology. (2015). *2015 American College of Rheumatology guideline for the treatment of rheumatoid arthritis.* Atlanta, GA: Author. Available: *https://www.rheumatology. org/Portals/0/Files/ACR%202015%20RA%20Guideline.pdf.*

Pathophysiology and Etiology

1. Immunologic processes result in inflammation of synovium, producing antigens and inflammatory by-products that lead to destruction of articular cartilage and bone, synovitis, and production of a granular tissue called *pannus* (see Figure 30-1).
2. Granulation tissue forms adhesions that lead to decreased joint mobility.
3. Similar adhesions can occur in supporting structures, such as ligaments and tendons, and cause contractures and ruptures that further affect joint structure and mobility.
4. The etiology is unknown but is probably a combined effect of environmental, epidemiologic, infectious, and genetic factors. Smoking is known to worsen the symptoms of RA.
5. Women are affected more frequently than men.
6. Differential diagnosis includes reactive arthritis, psoriatic arthritis, and other inflammatory arthritides.

Clinical Manifestations

1. Arthritis—2010 criteria include synovitis in any joint, rather than symmetrical joints in the 1987 ACR criteria (see Figure 30-2, page 825).
2. Skin manifestations.
   a. Rheumatoid nodules—elbows, occiput, and sacrum.

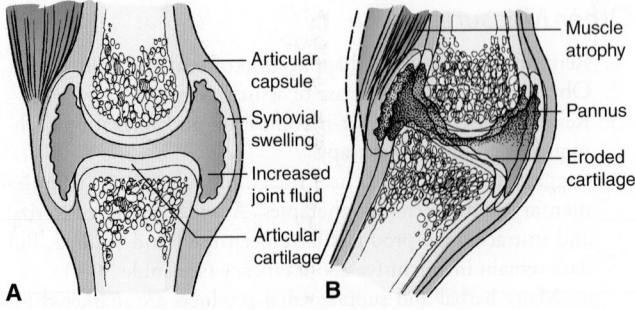

Figure 30-1. Pathophysiology of rheumatoid arthritis. **(A)** Joint structure with synovial swelling and fluid accumulation in the joint. **(B)** Pannus, eroded articular cartilage with joint space narrowing, muscle atrophy, and ankylosis.

Figure 30-2. Rheumatoid arthritis characteristically involves the joints of the hands, wrist, feet, ankles, knees, and elbows, the glenohumeral and acromioclavicular joints, and the hips. The articulations of the cervical spine are also affected.

   b. Vasculitic changes—brown, splinter-like lesions in fingers or nail folds.
3. Cardiac manifestations.
   a. Acute pericarditis.
   b. Conduction defects.
   c. Valvular insufficiency.
   d. Coronary arteritis.
   e. Cardiac tamponade—rare.
   f. Myocardial infarction and sudden death—rare.
4. Pulmonary manifestations.
   a. Asymptomatic pulmonary disease.
   b. Pleural effusion and pleurisy.
   c. Interstitial fibrosis.
   d. Laryngeal obstruction caused by involvement of the cricoarytenoid joint—rare.
   e. Pulmonary nodules.
5. Neurologic manifestations.
   a. Mononeuritis multiplex—wrist drop and foot drop.
   b. Carpal tunnel syndrome.
   c. Compression of spinal nerve roots (cervical spine only).
   d. Distal sensory neuropathy.
6. Other manifestations.
   a. Fever.
   b. Fatigue.
   c. Weight loss.
   d. Episcleritis.

Diagnostic Evaluation

1. Complete blood count (CBC)—normochromic, normocytic anemia of chronic disease; may also have iron deficiency anemia (hypochromic, microcytic); platelets may be elevated with inflammation.
2. RF—positive in up to 70% to 80% of patients with RA; CCP is more specific for RA than RF testing.

3. ESR and CRP—often elevated due to active inflammation.
4. Synovial fluid analysis may be done in acute swollen large joint—see page 821.
5. X-rays—changes develop within 2 years.
   a. Hands/wrists—marginal erosions of the proximal interphalangeal (PIP), metacarpophalangeal, and carpal joints; generalized osteopenia.
   b. Cervical spine—erosions that produce atlantoaxial subluxation (generally after many years).
6. Magnetic resonance imaging (MRI)—detects spinal cord compression that results from C1 to C2 subluxation and compression of surrounding vascular structures. Also detects erosions earlier than x-ray.
7. Ultrasound—detects synovitis and erosion (very user dependent).

Management

 EVIDENCE BASE Singh, J. A., Furst, D. E., Bharat, A., et al. (2012). 2012 update of the 2008 American College of Rheumatology Recommendations for the use of disease-modifying antirheumatic drugs and biologic agents in the treatment of rheumatoid arthritis. *Arthritis Care Research, 64,* 625–639.

1. NSAIDs to relieve pain and inflammation.
2. DMARDs to reduce disease activity.
   a. Monotherapy or combination of older agent, such as methotrexate or hydroxychloroquine, with newer agents immunomodulatory referred to as biologics.
   b. TNF inhibitor and methotrexate have shown greater benefit in improving signs and symptoms, preventing radiologic deterioration of the joint, and improving physical function in comparison with monotherapy.
   c. The goal is to have long-term impact on the joints and to prevent disability.
3. Corticosteroids (by mouth or intra-articular administration) to reduce inflammatory process. Generally used for short periods, because of multiple side effects.
4. Local comfort measures:
   a. Application of heat and cold did not show benefit in a meta-analysis, but treatment can be individualized.
   b. Use of splints to support painful, swollen joints.
   c. Paraffin wax baths with exercise may be of some benefit.
5. Nonpharmacologic modalities:
   a. Behavior modification.
   b. Relaxation techniques.
6. Surgery:
   a. Synovectomy.
   b. Arthrodesis—joint fusion.
   c. Total joint replacement.

 DRUG ALERT Do not give biologic DMARDs (immunomodulators) within 2 to 3 weeks of any live vaccine. Oral DMARDs, such as methotrexate, leflunomide, hydroxychloroquine, and sulfasalazine, may be used. Watch for signs of infection, including reactivation of viral infection, while patients are receiving these medications.

Complications

1. Loss of joint function because of bony adhesions, erosions, and damage of supporting structures—7% of patients become disabled within 5 years of onset; 32% cannot work after 10 years.

2. Anemia of chronic disease.
3. Felty syndrome—neutropenia, splenomegaly, frequent infections, and leg ulcers; occurs in 1% of patients.

Nursing Assessment

1. Perform joint examination, if indicated, noting which joints affected; ROM of each joint; presence of heat, redness, synovial swelling; and possible joint effusion.
2. Note presence of deformities (see Figure 30-3):
   a. Swan neck—PIP joints hyperextend.
   b. Boutonniere—PIP joints flex.
   c. Ulnar deviation—fingers point toward the ulna.
3. Assess pain using a pain measurement scale such as the visual analog scale (10-cm straight line scored 0 to 100; patient makes a mark indicating intensity of pain).
4. Assess functional status using the ACR revised criteria for classification for global functional status.
   a. Class I—Completely able to perform usual activities of daily living (ADLs).
   b. Class II—able to perform usual self-care and vocational activities, but limited in avocational activities.
   c. Class III—able to perform usual self-care activities, but limited in vocational and avocational activities.
   d. Class IV—limited ability to perform usual self-care, vocational, and avocational activities.
5. Assess for adherence to treatment plan, any complementary methods used, and any adverse reactions to medications.

Nursing Diagnoses

- Chronic Pain related to disease process.
- Impaired Physical Mobility related to pain and limited joint motion.
- Risk for Infection related to side effects/toxicities of DMARD therapy.
- Dressing or Grooming Self-Care Deficit related to limitations secondary to disease process.
- Ineffective Coping related to pain, physical limitations, and chronicity of RA.

Nursing Interventions

Controlling Pain

1. Apply local heat or cold to affected joints for 15 to 20 minutes, three to four times per day. Avoid temperatures likely to cause skin or tissue damage by checking temperature of warm soaks or by covering cold packs with a towel.
2. Administer or teach self-administration of pharmacologic agents.
   a. Advise patient when to expect pain relief, based on mechanism of action of the drug.
3. Encourage use of adjunctive pain control measures.
   a. Progressive muscle relaxation.
   b. Biofeedback.
   c. Meditation.
   d. Acupuncture or similar therapies.
4. Note frequency, location, and degree of pain. Tracking and trending "flares" of disease important in setting plan of care and change in medication regime.

Optimizing Mobility

1. Encourage warm bath or shower in the morning to decrease morning stiffness.
2. Encourage measures to protect affected joints.
   a. Perform gentle ROM exercises.
   b. Use splints, if necessary.
   c. Assist with ADLs, if necessary.
3. Encourage exercise consistent with degree of disease activity.
4. Refer to physical therapy and occupational therapy.

Preventing Infection and Adverse Reactions to Drug Therapy

1. Review drug information before administration to ensure that baseline blood work, such as CBC and liver function tests, has been done; there are no drug interactions; and you understand reconstitution and administration information.
2. Ensure that a tuberculin test has been done prior to starting biologics. If positive, treatment for latent tuberculosis (TB) and biologic may be started simultaneously.
   a. In immunocompromised individuals, including those with autoimmune diseases, greater than 5-mm reaction to tuberculin skin test is considered positive.
   b. Interferon-gamma release assays for tuberculosis screening are preferred method of detecting mycobacterial exposure.
3. Make sure that no live vaccines have been administered in the past 2 to 3 weeks before initiating biologic therapy because infection with vaccine agent could result. Oral DMARDs may be used safely.
4. Ensure that the patient has no active or untreated infections. Be aware that suppressed viral infections, such as hepatitis, herpes, and varicella, can result from immune therapy.

Figure 30-3. Swan neck (**A**) and boutonniere (**B**) deformities.

5. Administer or teach patient to administer medication subcutaneously by rotating sites of the abdomen, thigh, and upper arm, as directed.
   a. Many biologics, such as etanercept, adalimumab, certolizumab, golimumab, and abatacept, ustekinumab, and secukinumab are available in prefilled syringe or pen form. Etanercept and certolizumab are also available in powder form for reconstitution.
   b. Give IV drugs (abatacept, rituximab, infliximab, golimumab, belimumab, and tocilizumab) by recommended time as identified in the prescribing information, monitoring for fever and chills and cutaneous reaction (as per infusion protocol).

 TRANSITIONAL CARE ALERT Teach patients taking biologics the early signs and symptoms of infection and the appropriate action to take (call provider or proceed to emergency department) to reduce the risk of overwhelming infection and readmission. Also, teach patients that biologics are generally held when an antibiotic is prescribed.

Promoting Self-Care

1. Provide pain relief before self-care activities.
2. Provide privacy and an environment conducive to performance of daily activities.
3. Schedule adequate rest periods during flare.
4. Discuss importance of promoting the patient's self-care at an appropriate level with patient and family.
5. Help patient attain appropriate assistive devices, such as raised toilet seats, special eating utensils, and zipper pulls. Contact occupational therapist, social worker, or Arthritis Foundation for information.

Strengthening Coping Skills

1. Be aware of potential job, childcare, home maintenance, and social and family functioning problems that may result from RA.
2. Encourage patient to vocalize problems and feelings.
3. Assist with problem-solving approach to explore options and to gain control of problem areas, such as cost of drugs and medical care and limited resources at home.
   a. Patient assistance programs are available for drug therapy through the manufacturer or Partnership for Prescription Assistance (*www.pparx.org*). There are also several foundations that may be able to assist with copays and other costs.
   b. Obtain order for home care nursing or physical or occupational therapy for treatment and monitoring, as needed.
   c. Consult social worker, the Arthritis Foundation, or other community resources for additional services, as needed.
4. Reinforce effective coping mechanisms.
5. Refer to social worker or mental health counselor, as needed.

Patient Education and Health Maintenance

1. Instruct patient and family in the nature of disease.
   a. Chronic nature of RA with characteristic exacerbations and remissions with time.
   b. Disease can have systemic effects that result in constitutional symptoms and involvement of other organ systems.
   c. Severity of RA is variable, but most patients are *not* confined to bed or wheelchair.
   d. RA has no cure; avoid "miracle cures."

2. Educate patient about pharmacologic agents.
   a. Medication must be taken consistently to achieve maximum benefit.
   b. Most medications used in the treatment of RA require periodic laboratory testing, such as CBC and liver functions, to monitor for potential adverse effects.
   c. Advise patient of possible adverse effects of medications and need to report adverse effects to health care provider, including fever, chills, lethargy, rash, difficulty breathing, swelling, worsening of arthritis, and severe diarrhea.
   d. Advise patients to discuss the use of any complementary or alternative therapies with their health care provider.
   e. Reinforce to patient the need for lifelong treatment.
3. During periods of remission, encourage patient to exercise regularly, choosing an activity that is inexpensive, convenient, enjoyable, and not dependent on the weather. Suggest dancing, mall walking, use of stationary bicycle in the home, or contacting the local YMCA about special programs for arthritis.
4. For additional information and support, refer to the Arthritis Foundation (*www.arthritis.org*) or the American College of Rheumatology (*www.rheumatology.org/public/factsheets/index.asp*).

Evaluation: Expected Outcomes

- Reports reduction in pain and fatigue.
- Protects joints from overuse. No signs of infection and no adverse reactions to drug therapy.
- Maintains independent toiletry, bathing, and feeding.
- Verbalizes concerns about cleaning and cooking; meets with occupational therapist.

Systemic Lupus Erythematosus

Systemic lupus erythematosus (SLE) is a chronic, multisystem autoimmune disease. Discoid lupus may also occur with predominant skin lesions.

Diagnostic criteria for SLE include the presence of at least 4/17 findings, as outlined in the Systemic Lupus International Collaborating Clinics classification criteria, updating the SLICC/ACR Damage Index for SLE. Criteria include clinical manifestations and laboratory criteria.

 EVIDENCE BASE Petri, M., Orbai, A. M., Alarcon, G. S., et al. (2012). Derivation and validation of the Systemic Lupus International Collaborating Clinics classification criteria for systemic lupus erythematosus. *Arthritis and Rheumatism*, 64(8), 2677–2686.

Pathophysiology and Etiology

1. The T-lymphocyte system is affected for unknown reasons, and the failure of its regulatory system may result in an inability to slow or to halt the production of inappropriate autoantibodies.
2. B-lymphocyte–stimulating factors are produced and this too may lead to production of autoantibodies.
3. Autoantibodies may combine with other elements of the immune system to activate immune complexes. These immune complexes and other immune system constituents combine to form complement, which is deposited in organs, causing inflammation and tissue necrosis.
4. More women, particularly in child-bearing years, are affected than men.

Clinical Manifestations

1. Skin:
   a. Butterfly-shaped rash of the malar region of the face, characterized by erythema and edema.
   b. Discoid lesions are scarring, ring-shaped, involving the shoulders, arms, and upper back.
   c. Discoid lesions may also result in erythematous, scaly plaques on the face, scalp, external ear, and neck, resulting in alopecia.
2. Arthritis:
   a. Generally bilateral and symmetric, involving the hands, wrists, and other joints.
   b. Can resemble RA and may be mistaken for it, especially early in the course of the disease.
   c. Unlike RA, the arthritis is primarily nonerosive; may (occasionally) be erosive, representing some overlap with RA.
   d. Tendon involvement is common and may lead to deformities or tendon rupture.
3. Cardiac:
   a. Pericarditis.
   b. Pleural effusion.
   c. Myocarditis.
   d. Endocarditis.
   e. Coronary artery disease.
4. Pulmonary:
   a. Pleuritis.
   b. Pleural effusion.
   c. Lupus pneumonitis.
   d. Pulmonary hemorrhage.
   e. Pulmonary embolism.
5. GI:
   a. Oral ulcers.
   b. Acute or subacute abdominal pain.
   c. Pancreatitis.
   d. Spontaneous bacterial peritonitis.
   e. Bowel infarction.
6. Renal: occurs in 50% of patients, with as many as 15% of patients developing renal failure. Renal thrombosis is rare. Lupus nephritis is more common.
   a. Mesangial nephritis—mild form, can be reversible, best prognosis.
   b. Focal segmental glomerulonephritis—active necrotic or sclerosing lesions.
   c. Proliferative—may be focal or diffuse; diffuse carries good prognosis.
   d. Membranous nephritis—may persist for years without serious renal function decline; may present as nephrotic syndrome.
   e. Sclerosing nephritis—increase in the amount of matrix material in the glomeruli.
7. Central nervous system:
   a. Neuropsychiatric disorders—depression and psychosis.
   b. Transient ischemic attacks and stroke.
   c. Seizures.
   d. Migraine headache.
   e. Myelopathy.
   f. Guillain-Barré syndrome.
   g. Chorea and other movement disorders.
   h. Poor concentration and "lupus fog."
8. Hematologic:
   a. Hemolytic anemia.
   b. Leukopenia.
   c. Thrombocytopenia.

Figure 30-4. Characteristic pallor because of vasospasm in Raynaud phenomenon.

9. Vascular:
   a. Hypertension.
   b. Raynaud phenomenon (see Figure 30-4).
10. Constitutional:
    a. Fever.
    b. Weight loss.
    c. Fatigue.

Diagnostic Evaluation

1. CBC—leukopenia, anemia (may be hemolytic), and thrombocytopenia.
2. ANA—positive in more than 90% of patients with SLE; predominant pattern is homogeneous.
3. Anti-dsDNA—97% specific for lupus.
4. ESR—generally elevated.
5. Complement levels—generally decreased when disease is active.
6. Urinalysis—hematuria, proteinuria, and active sediment (RBC casts).
7. Twenty-four–hour urine for protein and creatinine clearance.
8. Chest x-ray may show changes.
9. X-ray of hands and wrists—nondestructive arthritis.
10. Computed tomography (CT) or MRI may be clinically indicated.
    a. Brain—to define any neurologic manifestations.
    b. Abdomen—to rule out other abdominal processes in a patient with abdominal pain.
    c. Cerebral arteriogram—to look for evidence of cerebral vasculitis.
    d. Magnetic resonance angiography.

Management

Pharmacologic

1. NSAIDs to reduce pain and inflammation.
2. Antimalarials to decrease disease activity.
3. Corticosteroids to reduce inflammatory process.
4. Immunosuppressives to suppress immune process and to act as steroid-sparing agents.
   a. Research is ongoing to develop lymphocyte-specific immunosuppressants and biologic modifiers to stop autoantibody production.
   b. Belimumab is a human monoclonal antibody that neutralizes the B-cell survival factor and B-lymphocyte stimulator (BLyS). Belimumab is available in SQ or IV delivery systems.

5. Antihypertensives and diuretics to treat hypertension and fluid overload, if present due to renal disease.
6. Calcium channel blockers, angiotensin receptor blockers, or sildenafil for Raynaud phenomenon.

 EVIDENCE BASE Stohl, W., & Hilbert, D. M. (2012). The discovery and development of belimumab: The anti BLyS–lupus connection. *Nature Biotechnology, 30*(1), 69–77.

Nonpharmacologic
1. Avoid direct exposure to sunlight to reduce the chance of exacerbation. Protective clothing and sunblock with an SPF of 50 should also be used.
2. Behavior modification to prevent exacerbations and to reduce symptoms.
3. Joint protection and energy conservation.

Other Management
1. Close follow-up for evaluation of cardiac, neurologic, renal, and other body systems.
2. Referral to specialists for systemic manifestations.

Complications
1. Renal failure.
2. Permanent neurologic impairment.
3. Infection.
4. Death caused by disease process.

Nursing Assessment
1. Obtain clinical history, review systems, and perform physical examination for characteristic findings.
2. Assess for signs and symptoms of infection and other adverse effects to medications.
3. Assess patient's and family's ability to cope with impact of prolonged disease.

Nursing Diagnoses
- Chronic Pain related to inflammation of joints and juxta-articular structures.
- Powerlessness related to unpredictable course of disease.
- Risk for Impaired Skin and Oral Mucous Membrane Integrity related to skin/oral lesions.
- Fatigue related to chronic inflammatory process.
- Impaired Urinary Elimination related to renal involvement.

Nursing Interventions

Reducing Pain
1. Administer and teach self-administration of medications to reduce disease activity and of additional analgesics as ordered.
2. Suggest the use of hot or cold applications, relaxation techniques, and nonstrenuous exercise to enhance pain relief.
3. Monitor for adverse reactions to corticosteroids (see page 823).

Increasing Control over Disease Process
1. Instruct patient to avoid factors that may exacerbate disease.
   a. Avoid exposure to sunlight and ultraviolet light.
      i. Use sunscreen with sun protection factor of 30 or greater. Avoid prolonged sun exposure.
      ii. Wear protective, lightweight clothing with long sleeves and wide-brimmed hats.
      iii. Avoid use of tanning beds.
   b. Avoid exposure to drugs and chemicals.
      i. Avoid exposure to hairspray.
      ii. Avoid exposure to hair-coloring agents.
      iii. Medications—obtain provider advice before taking any medications or supplements.
2. Teach self-administration of pharmacologic agents to reduce disease activity. Reinforce importance of adhering to antimalarial therapy (hydroxychloroquine).
3. Encourage good nutrition, sleep habits, exercise, rest, and relaxation to improve general health and to help prevent infection.
4. Encourage expression of feelings, counseling, or referrals to social work and occupational therapy, as needed.

Maintaining Skin and Mucous Membrane Integrity
1. Apply topical corticosteroids to skin lesions, as ordered.
2. Suggest alternative hairstyles, scarves, and wigs to cover significant areas of alopecia.
3. Encourage good oral hygiene and inspect mouth for oral ulcers.
   a. Avoid hot or spicy foods that may irritate oral ulcers.
   b. Apply topical agents or analgesics to reduce pain and to promote eating.

Reducing Fatigue
1. Advise patient that fatigue level will fluctuate with disease activity.
2. Encourage patient to modify schedule to include several rest periods during the day; pace activity and exercise according to body's tolerance; use energy conservation techniques in daily activities.
3. Teach relaxation techniques, such as deep breathing, progressive muscle relaxation, and imagery, to reduce emotional stress that causes fatigue.

Preserving Urinary Elimination
1. Assist with monitoring of urinary status as indicated by degree of renal involvement.
   a. Monitor intake and output and urine specific gravity.
   b. Measure urine protein and microalbumin, or obtain 24-hour creatinine clearance, as ordered.
   c. Check test results of serum blood urea nitrogen and creatinine.
2. See page 595 for care of patients on dialysis.

Patient Education and Health Maintenance
1. Stress that close follow-up is essential, even in times of remission, to detect early progression of organ involvement and to alter drug therapy.
2. Advise on the use of special cosmetics to cover skin lesions.
3. Advise about reproduction.
   a. Avoid pregnancy during the time of severe disease activity. Should have stable disease for 1 year before planning pregnancy.
   b. Immunomodulators may have teratogenic effects.
   c. Use of some drugs for treatment of SLE can result in sterility.
   d. Hydroxychloroquine is proven safe during pregnancy.
4. Stress that any complementary or alternative therapies should be discussed with the health care provider.
5. For additional information and support, refer to agencies such as the Lupus Foundation (*www.lupus.org*) or the American Occupational Therapy Association (*www.aota.org*).

Evaluation: Expected Outcomes
- Reports pain reduction.
- Verbalizes appropriate use of medications, avoidance of sun and chemicals, and need for nutrition and sleep to minimize disease process.

- Reports oral ulcers healing without interference with appetite.
- Reports resting three times per day, with adequate energy to carry out activities.
- Urine output adequate; specific gravity stable.

Systemic Sclerosis

Systemic sclerosis is a generalized disorder of connective tissue, characterized by hardening and thickening of the skin (scleroderma), blood vessels, synovium, skeletal muscles, and internal organs. Fibrotic, degenerative, and inflammatory changes result in changes in joints and several organ systems. New diagnostic criteria being evaluated and validated by the ACR and EULAR include 23 items.

 EVIDENCE BASE Johnson, S. R., Fransensen, J., Khanna, D., et al. (2012). Validation of potential classification criteria for systemic sclerosis. *Arthritis Care Research, 64*(3), 358–367.

Pathophysiology and Etiology

1. The changes seen in the skin and internal organs in systemic sclerosis are most likely caused by overproduction of collagen by fibroblasts.
2. The etiology of systemic sclerosis is unknown.
3. Systemic sclerosis affects three to four times as many women as men.
4. Major subtypes include:
   a. Diffuse scleroderma—rapidly progressive, generalized skin thickening of the proximal and distal extremities and trunk and tendency toward early internal organ involvement.
   b. Limited scleroderma—skin thickening is limited to the distal extremities and face.
   c. Localized forms of scleroderma—do not include visceral involvement.
   d. Overlap with other connective tissue disorders.

Clinical Manifestations

Skin

1. Bilateral symmetric swelling of the hands and, sometimes, the feet.
2. After the edematous phase, the skin becomes hard and thick.
3. Digits, dorsum of the hand, neck, face, and trunk are involved.
4. Normal landmarks in the skin are absent—no skin folds.
5. Increased or decreased skin pigmentation (salt and pepper skin).
6. Skin changes may regress after several years.
7. Telangiectasia—on/under the tongue, face, fingers, and lips.
8. Areas of calcinosis—late in the course of disease.
9. Raynaud phenomenon.
10. Decreased oral aperture.

GI

1. Esophageal dysmotility—resulting in reflux and dysphagia.
2. Distal esophageal dilation and esophagitis.
3. Barrett metaplasia—may predispose to adenocarcinoma of the esophagus.
4. Duodenal atrophy dilation—may cause postprandial abdominal pain, malabsorption, diarrhea, and abdominal distention.
5. Colonic hypomotility—results in constipation.

Musculoskeletal

1. Joint pain.
2. Polyarthritis—large and small joints affected.

3. Carpal tunnel syndrome.
4. Flexion contractures.
5. Inflammatory muscle atrophy.

Cardiac

1. Left ventricular dysfunction.
2. Myocardial involvement—heart failure and atrial and ventricular arrhythmias.
3. Right ventricular involvement—secondary to pulmonary disease.

Pulmonary

1. Interstitial fibrosis.
2. Restrictive lung disease.
3. Pulmonary hypertension.

Renal

Scleroderma renal crisis—rapid malignant hypertension with encephalopathy.

Localized Scleroderma

1. CREST—calcinosis (calcium deposits of the subcutaneous tissue and periarticular tissue), *R*aynaud phenomenon, *e*sophageal dysmotility, *s*clerodactyly (shiny, tight, atrophic appearance of the skin of the fingers or toes), *and telangiectasia.*
2. Morphea—scattered patches may be several centimeters and may have a purple border.
3. Linear—lesions appear as streaks or bands.
4. Generally, no visceral involvement exists in localized scleroderma.

Diagnostic Evaluation

1. CBC and ESR—generally normal.
2. RF—positive in approximately 30% of patients.
3. ANA—generally positive with speckled or nucleolar patterns.
   a. Antiscleroderma antibody (Scl-70)—positive in diffuse cutaneous disease.
   b. Anticentromere antibody—highly specific for limited cutaneous disease.
4. Additional antibodies that have been identified include anti-RNA polymerase III antibody and antitopoisomerase I antibody.
5. X-ray of hands and wrists—muscle atrophy, osteopenia, and osteolysis.
6. Barium swallow—esophageal dysmotility.
7. Pulmonary function test—decreased diffusion capacity and vital capacity; CT of the chest to evaluate for pulmonary fibrosis.
8. Multiple-gated acquisition scan—to determine left ventricular function; echocardiogram to evaluate for pulmonary hypertension.
9. Endoscopy—to biopsy for Barrett metaplasia.
10. Esophageal manometry—to determine contractile capacity of esophageal muscles.

Management

Pharmacologic

1. Calcium channel blockers; losartan or other angiotensin receptor blockers or sildenafil for more severe cases of Raynaud phenomenon. Nitroglycerin ointment is sometimes used. Prazosin, an alpha-adrenergic agent, has a modest effect but may cause dizziness, headache, and lack of energy.
2. NSAIDs and/or other analgesics for arthralgias, polyarthritis, and painful calcinosis.
3. Proton pump inhibitors for reflux.
4. Antibiotics for malabsorption because of bacterial overgrowth or secondarily infected skin ulcerations.

5. Antihypertensive agents, particularly a high-dose angiotensin-converting enzyme inhibitor such as enalapril.
6. Bronchodilators for pulmonary involvement; oxygen and cyclophosphamide may also be used in severe cases.
7. For Raynaud phenomenon, topical L-arginine has been used on the hands to stimulate formation of nitric oxide, a vasodilator. Sildenafil may be helpful with symptoms. Severe symptoms may also respond to injections of Botox.

 DRUG ALERT L-Arginine should not be used with nitrates and antihypertensives; vasodilating effect may cause excessive drop in blood pressure.

Nonpharmacologic

1. Skin lubricants and care for ulcerations to promote healing.
2. Lifestyle modification for control of Raynaud phenomenon:
   a. Increased environmental temperature.
   b. Appropriate dress with gloves and heavy socks.
   c. Avoidance of handling cold and frozen items without gloves.
   d. Avoidance of wind and exposure to cold weather.
   e. Use of hand and foot warmers.
   f. Smoking cessation.
3. Raynaud attack can possibly be aborted by placing the hand or foot in tepid water.
4. Biofeedback to abort or prevent Raynaud attack.
5. Smoking cessation and immunization against pneumococcal pneumonia and influenza for pulmonary involvement.
6. Dietary modifications for GI involvement:
   a. Avoidance of caffeinated beverages.
   b. Eating smaller meals.
   c. Remaining upright after meals for at least 3 hours.
   d. Avoidance of alcohol.
   e. Elevating the head of the bed.
7. Physical therapy to help prevent contractures.

Complications

1. Skin ulcers.
2. Malabsorption.
3. Esophageal adenocarcinoma.
4. Pulmonary hypertension.
5. Renal failure.
6. Heart failure.
7. Death caused by disease process.

Nursing Assessment

1. Focus physical assessment on:
   a. Skin ulcers, thickening, subcutaneous deposits, and secondary infection.
   b. Joint examination—flexion contractures.
   c. Pulmonary examination—for shortness of breath and wheezing.
   d. Blood pressure and renal status.
2. Determine nutritional intake.
3. Assess mood, support system, and coping ability.

Nursing Diagnoses

- Ineffective Peripheral Tissue Perfusion related to Raynaud phenomenon.
- Risk for Impaired Skin Integrity related to effects of disease process.
- Imbalanced Nutrition: Less Than Body Requirements related to impaired swallowing and GI involvement.
- Disturbed Body Image related to effects of disease.

Nursing Interventions

Maintaining Tissue Perfusion

1. Teach patient to identify Raynaud phenomenon.
   a. Characteristic color change of the fingers—white, blue, and red.
   b. Coldness, pallor, numbness, and pain.
2. Teach patient to reduce factors associated with precipitation or exacerbation of Raynaud phenomenon.
   a. Dress warmly—cover head and extremities; keep trunk warm.
   b. Discontinue tobacco usage.
   c. Avoid prolonged exposure to cold.
      i. Weather.
      ii. Artificially controlled environments (eg, air conditioning).
      iii. Limit contact with cold food items, such as frozen foods and ice cube trays—use gloves or tongs.
3. Protect ulcerated digits and report signs of infection.

Preserving Skin Integrity

1. Use moisturizers on the skin daily.
2. Advise patient to avoid use of drying soaps and detergents.
3. Use protective padding (eg, elbow pads) to protect the skin from friction or trauma.
4. Inspect the skin daily for cracking, ulceration, and signs of infection.
5. Soak ulcerations, apply topical antibiotic, and use occlusive dressings, as directed.

Achieving Optimal Nutritional Status

1. Make sure patient is in proper position for meals to avoid aspiration (ie, in chair if possible).
2. Provide smaller, more frequent feedings of a well-balanced diet.
3. Encourage patient to remain upright after meals for 45 to 60 minutes and raise head of bed during sleep to avoid reflux.
4. Administer or teach self-administration of medications to prevent nausea and reflux, as ordered.
5. Encourage good oral hygiene and frequent dental visits.
6. Advise the use of lubricating agents, if necessary, to treat dry mouth and to teach stretching exercises of the mouth to maintain aperture.
7. Weigh weekly and ask patient to keep food diary.

Strengthening Body Image

1. Encourage patient to take an active role in treatment plan to feel in control of body changes.
2. Explain that changes may be gradual and slow; although not noticeable, internal organ involvement is even more important than external changes.
3. Suggest continuance of activities that patient enjoys and foster strong support network.
4. Refer for counseling, as needed.

Patient Education and Health Maintenance

1. Explain diagnostic tests and their purpose in detecting GI, pulmonary, or renal involvement.
2. Teach about drug treatment and adverse effects.

3. Advise on modifying activity and using bronchodilators and oxygen to prevent dyspnea caused by restrictive lung disease.
4. Encourage regular follow-up visits and prompt attention to worsening symptoms.
5. Refer to agencies such as United Scleroderma Foundation (*www.scleroderma.org*).

Evaluation: Expected Outcomes

- Relates factors that precipitate Raynaud phenomenon.
- Reports no skin cracking or ulceration.
- Reports no weight loss.
- Reports participating in community and church activities and groups.

Gout

Gout is a disorder of purine metabolism, characterized by elevated uric acid levels and deposition of urate (usually in the form of crystals) in joints and other tissues. More common in men, but may affect postmenopausal women, especially those taking diuretics.

Pathophysiology and Etiology

Gout results from an overabundant accumulation and subsequent deposition of monosodium urate crystals in joints and other connective tissue. This can occur in one of two ways.

Overproduction of Uric Acid (10% of Cases)
1. Inherited enzyme defects.
2. Certain conditions:
   a. Myeloproliferative disorders.
   b. Lymphoproliferative disorders.
   c. Cancer chemotherapy.
   d. Hemolytic anemias.
   e. Psoriasis.

Underexcretion of Uric Acid (90% of Cases)
1. Renal disease.
2. Endocrine disorders.
3. Medications and chemicals:
   a. Diuretics, beta-blockers, and angiotensin-converting enzyme inhibitors.
   b. Ethanol (alcohol).
   c. Low-dose aspirin.
   d. Pyrazinamide—antituberculosis agent.
   e. Lead.
4. Volume depletion states—nephrogenic diabetes insipidus.

Clinical Manifestations

Acute Gouty Arthritis
1. Generally affects one joint—commonly the first metatarsophalangeal joint (called podagra); however, in women is often polyarticular.
2. Other joints can be affected, such as the ankle, tarsals, and knee; upper extremities are less commonly involved.
3. Pain, warmth, erythema, and swelling of tissue surrounding the affected joint.
4. Fever may occur.
5. Onset of symptoms is sudden; intensity is severe.
6. Duration of symptoms is self-limiting; lasts approximately 3 to 10 days without treatment.

Chronic Tophaceous Gout
1. Occurs if acute gout is inadequately treated or if it goes untreated.
2. Characterized by development of tophi or deposits of uric acid in and around joints, cartilage, and soft tissues.
3. Arthritis is more prolonged in nature with discrete attacks less common.
4. Arthritis can produce bone erosions and subsequent bony deformities that can resemble RA.

Hyperuricemia
1. Produces no symptoms but is characterized by persistent elevation of uric acid in the blood.
2. Renal calculi composed of uric acid may develop.
3. Deposition of uric acid in kidney tissue causing nephropathy.

Diagnostic Evaluation
1. Synovial fluid analysis.
   a. Identification of monosodium urate crystals under polarized microscopy.
   b. Synovial WBC count can range from 2,000 to 100,000/mm^3.
   c. Culture of synovial fluid to rule out infection.
2. Twenty-four–hour urine for uric acid to determine overproduction of uric acid versus underexcretion.
3. ESR—elevated.
4. X-rays of affected joints may show changes consistent with diagnosis of gout.

Management

Acute Management
1. NSAIDs for acute attacks to relieve pain and swelling; considered first-line therapy.
2. Colchicine for acute treatment and prevention of attacks; considered second-line therapy.
   a. May be given orally at onset of an attack, taken bid to tid as tolerated (may cause nausea, cramping, diarrhea).
   b. Taken once daily on continuous basis to prevent attack, usually while transitioning to urate-lowering medications. May be used every other day for patients with chronic kidney disease.
3. Corticosteroids.
   a. Intra-articular if attack confined to one or two joints.
   b. Oral—in short-tapering course if other treatments are contraindicated or if attack involves many joints.
4. Increase fluids (orally because usually treated as outpatient) and rest joint for 48 hours.

Chronic Management
1. Urate-lowering agents (antihyperurecemic agents) are taken to prevent progressive articular damage in cases of asymptomatic hyperuricemia and chronic tophaceous gout.
   a. Allopurinol—interferes with conversion of hypoxanthine and xanthine to uric acid. May also be given to prevent renal calculi and kidney disease.
   b. Febuxostat—a xanthine oxidase inhibitor, lowers uric acid and is associated with fewer drug interactions than allopurinol.
   c. Uricosuric drugs, such as probenecid—interfere with tubular reabsorption of uric acid.
   d. Lesinurad, a URAT1 inhibitor indicated in combination with a xanthine oxidase inhibitor (XOI) for the treatment of hyperuricemia associated with gout in patients who have not achieved target serum uric acid levels with an XOI alone.
   e. Pegloticase is a pegylated uric acid–specific enzyme indicated for the treatment of chronic gout in adult patients refractory to conventional therapy.
2. Adverse reactions for these drugs include headache, anorexia, nausea and vomiting, allergic reaction, hemolytic anemia and other blood dyscrasias, and worsening of gout. Urinary frequency and uric acid kidney stones may occur with probenecid.

3. Rapid increase or decrease of uric acid may precipitate a gout flare, so medication usually started at a low dose and titrated up.
4. Uric acid levels and renal function are monitored during chronic therapy. A small percentage of patients develop elevated liver functions with urate-lowering treatment.

 DRUG ALERT Exfoliative dermatitis (sometimes fatal) and liver and biliary dysfunction may occur with use of allopurinol and febuxostat.

Lifestyle Modification
1. Avoidance of obesity and fluctuations in weight.
2. Avoidance of alcohol—can precipitate gout attacks through overproduction and decreased excretion of urate.
3. Low-purine diet gives only a minor decrease in serum uric acid levels.
4. Moderate coffee consumption has been linked to decreased uric acid levels.

Complications
1. Uric acid renal calculus.
2. Urate nephropathy.
3. Erosive, deforming arthritis/contractures.

Nursing Assessment
1. Obtain history for factors predisposing to gout, such as malignancy, alcoholism, and renal insufficiency.
2. Perform physical examination.
   a. Inspect the involved joint for pain, swelling, redness, warmth, and effusion.
   b. Observe for tophi over the pinna of the ear, olecranon bursa, Achilles tendon, and fingertips.
3. Assess pain and pain relief pattern if attack is acute.

Nursing Diagnoses
- Acute Pain related to acute arthritis.
- Impaired Physical Mobility related to arthritis.

Nursing Interventions
Relieving Pain
1. Administer and teach self-administration of pain-relieving medications, as prescribed.
2. Encourage adequate fluid intake to assist with excretion of uric acid and to decrease likelihood of stone formation.
3. Instruct patient to take prescribed medications consistently because interruptions in therapy can precipitate acute attacks.
4. Encourage patient to follow-up as directed, usually in 48 hours and then 4 to 8 weeks after acute attack to evaluate for chronic therapy.

Facilitating Mobility
1. Elevate and protect affected joint during acute attack.
2. Assist with ADLs.
3. Encourage exercise and maintenance of routine activity in chronic gout, except during acute attacks.
4. Protect draining tophi by covering and applying antibiotic ointment, as needed.

Patient Education and Health Maintenance
1. Instruct patient and family in the nature of disease.
   a. Generally, acute attacks are followed by periods of remission.
   b. Once need for chronic treatment has been determined, it will generally be lifelong.
2. Encourage avoidance of alcohol.
3. Avoid rapid weight loss by fasting or crash diets because rapid weight loss results in production of chemicals that compete with uric acid for excretion from the body, resulting in increased uric acid levels.
4. Avoid medications known to increase uric acid levels, such as aspirin, diuretics, and cyclosporine.
5. Advise prompt treatment of acute attack to reduce joint damage associated with repeated attacks.
6. Instruct about signs and symptoms of allopurinol hypersensitivity syndrome and need to report promptly.
7. Advise patients to avoid foods containing purines (ie, sardines, anchovies, shellfish, organ meats) and, in general, to consume meat, seafood, and high-calorie food in moderation.

Evaluation: Expected Outcomes
- Reports relief from pain.
- Performs ADLs with minimal assistance.

Sjögren Syndrome

Sjögren syndrome is a chronic inflammatory autoimmune process that affects the lacrimal and salivary glands. The disease can be primary or secondary. Secondary Sjögren syndrome is seen most commonly in RA but can be seen in SLE and some other connective tissue diseases. Diagnostic criteria involve at least two of three items (presence of antibodies, ocular staining score, lymphocytic sialadenitis).

 EVIDENCE BASE Shiboski, S. C., Shiboski, C. H., Criswell, L., et al. (2012). American College of Rheumatology classification criteria for Sjögren's syndrome: A data-driven, expert consensus approach in the Sjögren's International Collaborative Clinical Alliance cohort. *Arthritis Care and Research, 64*(4), 475–487.

Pathophysiology and Etiology
1. The etiology of the syndrome is unknown, but is thought to include several factors: genetic predisposition, immunologic, infectious, and hormonal.
2. It is thought that antibodies directed at exocrine glands are produced, leading to disturbed function of the involved tissue.
3. Lymphocytes are found infiltrating affected tissues.
4. Sjögren syndrome occurs primarily in middle-aged women.

Clinical Manifestations
1. Ocular—xerophthalmia (dry eyes) because of decreased tear formation that leads to keratoconjunctivitis and photophobia, greater than 3 months. Positive Schirmer or positive vital dying test.
2. Oral—xerostomia (dry mouth) caused by diminished production of saliva, mucosal ulcers, and stomatitis, greater than 3 months. Need for fluids to swallow food.
3. Recurrent or persistent salivary gland enlargement—unilateral or bilateral.
4. Dryness of the skin, vagina, and other tissues may also occur.
5. Extraglandular features include rash, dysphagia, Raynaud phenomenon, arthralgias/arthritis, and myalgias.
6. Less commonly, major organ dysfunction, such as interstitial pneumonitis, glomerulonephritis, vasculitis, thyroid disease, and central and peripheral neuropathy may occur.

Diagnostic Evaluation

1. CBC—mild anemia and leukopenia present in 30% of patients.
2. ESR—elevated in 90% of patients.
3. RF—positive in 75% to 90% of patients.
4. ANA—positive in 70% of patients; speckled and nucleolar patterns are most common; titer more than 1:320.
5. Antibodies to SSA/SSB—detects antibodies to specific nuclear proteins.
   a. SSA (Ro antibody)—positive in patients with Sjögren syndrome and SLE.
   b. SSB (La antibody)—positive in patients with Sjögren syndrome; also in patients with SLE.
6. Organ-specific antibodies—antibodies directed against specific organ tissues have been found (eg, antithyroid antibodies).
7. Salivary scintigraphy—salivary gland function is measured by determining excretion of radioisotope dye.
8. X-rays of affected joints to rule out erosive arthritis.
9. Salivary gland biopsy—to determine lymphocytic infiltration of tissue and confirm diagnosis; usually done on one of the minor salivary glands and in the lower lip.

Management

Systemic Drugs

1. NSAIDs and hydroxychloroquine may be used to try to control symptoms.
2. Corticosteroids and immunosuppressants may be used in severe cases.
3. Antifungal agents—used for oral candidiasis.
4. Pilocarpine or cevimeline, systemic parasympathomimetic agents—used to improve salivation when there is some salivary gland function.

Topical Agents

1. Cyclosporine emulsion eye drops to reduce ocular inflammation and increase tear production.
2. Over-the-counter products that contain salivary stimulants or substitutes.
   a. A meta-analysis of 36 randomized controlled trials showed slight benefit with oxygenated glycerol triester sprays over enzyme sprays as saliva substitutes.
   b. Integrated mouth care systems (toothpaste, gel, mouthwash) and oral reservoir devices show promising results, but more research is needed.
   c. Chewing gum is effective for people with residual salivary capacity.
3. Symptomatic relief of dryness.
   a. Artificial tears and lubricant inserts.
   b. Frequent use of sugar-free liquids, gums, and candies.
   c. Vaginal lubricants.
4. Dental care.
   a. Frequent brushing and flossing.
   b. Topical fluoride treatments.
   c. Avoidance of high-sucrose foods.
5. Avoidance of drying.
   a. Avoid windy, low-humidity environments and cigarette smoke.
   b. Avoid anticholinergic medications, such as antihistamines.
   c. Use of occlusive goggles at bedtime to prevent drying.

Complications

1. Ocular complications, such as corneal ulceration, corneal opacification, vascularization of the cornea, infection, glaucoma, and cataract formation.

2. Dental caries and tooth loss.
3. Lymphoma.

Nursing Assessment

1. Obtain history of signs and symptoms, emphasizing dryness.
2. Perform complete physical examination, focusing on the oral cavity, eyes, skin, lungs, GI, and neurologic systems.
3. Assess nutritional status because decreased saliva may make eating difficult.

Nursing Diagnoses

- Impaired Oral Mucous Membrane related to disease process.
- Risk for Impaired Skin Integrity related to dryness.
- Imbalanced Nutrition: Less Than Body Requirements related to disturbances in saliva production, taste, and difficulty swallowing.
- Sexual Dysfunction related to discomfort of decreased vaginal secretions.

Nursing Interventions

Maintaining Mucous Membranes

 EVIDENCE BASE Furness, S., Worthington, H. V., Bryan, G., et al. (2011). Interventions for the management of dry mouth: Topical therapies. *The Cochrane Database of Systematic Reviews*, (12), CD008934.

1. Inspect oral mucosa for oral *Candida*, ulcers, saliva pools, and dental hygiene.
2. Instruct and assist patient in proper oral hygiene.
   a. At least twice-daily brushing.
   b. Frequent rinsing with antiseptic mouthwash.
3. Encourage frequent intake of noncaffeinated, nonsugared liquids. Keep pitcher filled with cool water.
4. Promptly report any ulcers or signs of infections.

Protecting Skin Integrity

1. Instruct and assist patient with daily inspection of the skin for areas of trauma or for potential breakdown.
2. Apply lubricants to the skin daily.
3. Avoid shearing forces and encourage or perform frequent position changes.

Promoting Adequate Nutritional Intake

1. Increase liquid intake with meals.
2. Assist and instruct patient to avoid choosing spicy or dry foods from menu choices.
3. Suggest small, more frequent meals.
4. Weigh weekly and review diet history for deficiency in basic nutrients.

Promoting Optimal Sexual Functioning

1. Encourage patient to discuss sexual difficulty and to explain its relation to disease process.
2. Advise on proper use of water-soluble vaginal lubrication.
3. Suggest alternative positioning and practices to prevent discomfort.
4. Teach patient to report symptoms of vaginitis—discharge, irritation, and itching—because infection may result from altered mucosal barrier.

Patient Education and Health Maintenance

1. Advise patient of commercially available artificial saliva preparations, artificial tears, moisturizing nasal sprays, and artificial vaginal moisturizers.

2. Encourage frequent dental visits. Dental cavities are more frequent in Sjögren syndrome.
3. Advise patient to check with health care provider before using any medications because many, such as diuretics, tricyclic antidepressants, and antihistamines, have the adverse effect of mouth dryness.
4. Advise patient to wear protective eyewear while outdoors.
5. Encourage support through Sjögren's Syndrome Foundation (*www.sjogrens.org*) or the American College of Rheumatology (*www.rheumatology.org/public/factsheets/index.asp*).

Evaluation: Expected Outcomes

- Demonstrates proper oral hygiene.
- Reports skin without cracking, scaling, or other lesions.
- Maintains weight.
- Describes correct use of water-soluble lubricants.

Fibromyalgia

Fibromyalgia is a syndrome characterized by fatigue, diffuse muscle pain and stiffness, sleep disturbance, and tender points on physical examination. The American College of Rheumatology has stated that fibromyalgia is not a rheumatic disease.

Pathophysiology and Etiology

1. Etiology is unknown.
2. It affects 3 to 6 million Americans, usually women between ages 29 and 37.
3. Fibromyalgia most likely represents a complex pain syndrome in which there is abnormality in central sensory processing, dysregulation of peripheral pain receptors, and psychoneuroendocrine dysfunction.
4. Clinical features include:
   a. Reduction in pain threshold.
   b. Increased response to painful stimuli.
   c. Mild muscle contraction or tension results in postexertion muscle pain.
   d. Decreased muscle strength and endurance, resulting in deconditioning.

Clinical Manifestations

EVIDENCE BASE Wolfe, F., Clauw, D. J., Fitzcharles, M., et al. (2010). The American College of Rheumatology preliminary diagnostic criteria for fibromyalgia and measurement of symptom severity. *Arthritis Care and Research, 62*(5), 600–610.

1. Widespread pain and tenderness on physical exam. Diagnostic criteria proposed in 2010 include a widespread pain index, fatigue, and awakening unrefreshed.
2. Additional symptoms include:
   a. Chronic fatigue and easy fatigability.
   b. Sleep is poor or nonrestorative.
   c. Possible joint pain and stiffness.
   d. Additional somatic complaints such as headache, nausea, and abdominal pain.
3. Exacerbation of symptoms occurs due to cold weather, stress, poor sleep, infection, and exertion.

Diagnostic Evaluation

1. To rule out other disorders—test results generally normal in fibromyalgia.

2. Complete history and physical examination.
3. Sleep study may be done to rule out organic sleep disorder causing fatigue.

Management

EVIDENCE BASE Macfarlane, G., Kronisch, C., Dean, L. (2016). EULAR revised recommendations for the management of fibromyalgia. *Annuls of Rheumatic Disease, 76*(2), 318–328.

Treatment is aimed at symptom management and should be individualized, comprehensive, and goal-oriented.

Pharmacologic

1. Nonopioid analgesics are used to relieve pain.
   a. NSAIDs and acetaminophen are rarely effective alone.
   b. Tramadol may be effective if taken regularly at 50 to 100 mg every 4 to 6 hours.
   c. Naltrexone has been shown to relieve symptoms.
2. Low-dose tricyclic antidepressants improve sleep quality and help control chronic pain and depression. Other antidepressants may also be used for concomitant depression.
3. Sleep medication may be used occasionally or on a regular basis in some cases.
4. Periodic limb movements and restless leg syndrome that interfere with sleep can be treated with such medication as ropinirole or clonazepam.
5. Gabapentin and pregabalin, antiepileptics, may be tried for chronic pain control. Dosage is titrated and effects are seen over time for some patients.
6. Duloxetine and milnacipran, serotonin and norepinephrine reuptake inhibitors, are approved by the FDA for symptom relief in fibromyalgia.

DRUG ALERT There are risks for birth defects for women and men of child-bearing years while taking pregabalin.

Nonpharmacologic

1. Exercise is important and should be initiated at a level below the level expected for the patient and gradually increased.
   a. Overtraining is to be avoided to prevent muscle microtrauma, which increases pain.
   b. Stretching, strength training, and aerobic exercise should be included in every patient's exercise plan.
   c. Walking; water aerobics; daily activities, such as gardening; and use of exercise equipment, such as a bike or treadmill, can be part of the patient's exercise routine.
2. Relaxation training through visualization, electromyogram biofeedback, and other techniques.
3. Cognitive–behavioral therapy for feelings of depression, confusion, and irritability.
   a. Patient may learn to think nonnegatively by visualizing a stop sign when negative thoughts enter the mind.
   b. Patient can be taught to control anxiety by learning to stop, become aware of his body, and take deep breaths.
4. Meditation, prayer, and other spiritual practices.

Complications

1. Deconditioning.
2. Work disability.

3. Inability to fulfill social role.
4. Unnecessary diagnostic and therapeutic maneuvers.

Nursing Assessment

1. Assess pain level because it varies during the day/week.
2. Assess functional ability.
3. Assess mood, support system, and coping mechanisms.
4. Assess lifestyle factors that may be impairing well-being—smoking, lack of exercise, and poor posture.

Nursing Diagnoses

- Chronic Pain related to disease process.
- Disturbed Sleep Pattern related to disease process.
- Ineffective Role Performance related to disabling disease process.

Nursing Interventions

Controlling Pain

1. Encourage regular use of analgesics and antidepressants, as directed.
2. Encourage regular exercise routine, including stretching, aerobic activity, and muscle-strengthening exercises.
3. Suggest referrals to physical therapist or pain specialist for additional pain-control modalities, as needed.
4. Suggest referral to psychiatrist or therapist for anxiety, depression, and cognitive or behavioral impairments. Up to 80% of fibromyalgia patients have these symptoms, but only 10% are referred.

Improving Sleep

1. Suggest regular nighttime ritual to promote sleep. Advise avoidance of reading, watching television, or using a computer while in bed.
2. Discourage staying up late and other erratic sleep habits.
3. Encourage relaxation periods or short naps during the day, as needed, for fatigue.
4. Advise limiting caffeine intake during the day, especially after 4:00 P.M.
5. Discourage alcohol as a sleep aid; instead, advise patient to discuss sleep problems with health care provider.

Strengthening Roles

1. Encourage patient to look at fibromyalgia as a chronic condition that can be controlled.
2. Suggest a fibromyalgia support group.
3. Tell the patient that fibromyalgia is not a progressive debilitating disease and that most people gain control of their symptoms.
4. Help patient plan schedule and pace activities to accomplish routine activities.

Patient Education and Health Maintenance

1. Educate patient and family that fibromyalgia is a real disorder that causes pain and fatigue despite normal test results and lack of ill appearance.
2. Explain proper use of analgesics and potential adverse effects.
3. Encourage regular activity as much as possible and avoid physical and emotional stress.
4. Advise patient to discuss all types of alternative and complementary therapy with health care provider.
5. Encourage regular follow-up visits with primary care provider, rheumatologist, and physical therapist, as indicated.
6. Suggest further help and information from Fibromyalgia Network (*www.fmnetnews.com*) or the Arthritis Foundation (*www.arthritis.org*). Many local support groups are also available through community hospitals.

Evaluation: Expected Outcomes

- States pain at 0 to 2 level.
- Sleeping 8 hours per night with 0 to 1 short awakenings.
- Goes to work; takes care of children.

Other Rheumatologic Disorders

A number of other conditions affect the joints and periarticular tissue. Nursing care for patients with these disorders is similar to that for RA (see page 826).

Seronegative Spondyloarthropathies

Seronegative spondyloarthropathies are inflammatory conditions with negative RF or other autoantibodies, but are associated with HLA-B27 antigen. NSAIDs are generally used for treatment, but DMARDs and biologic agents may also be used. Seronegative spondyloarthropathies include the following:

1. Ankylosing spondylitis (AS)—characterized by lower back stiffness (sacroiliac involvement), uveitis, cardiac, and decreased chest expansion. Untreated AS may result in fusion of affected joints.
2. Reiter disease—characterized by the triad of urethritis, arthritis, and conjunctivitis.
3. Arthritis-associated inflammatory bowel disease—overlap of ulcerative colitis and arthritis of the large and small joints, with synovitis.
4. Psoriatic arthritis—characterized by arthritis with synovitis, enthesitis, and the skin lesions of psoriasis.

Additional Common Rheumatic Diseases

1. Polymyositis (dermatomyositis if rash around the eyes is present)—an inflammatory disease of striated muscles that most commonly affects the proximal limb girdle, neck, pharynx, proximal third of the esophagus, and occasionally the heart. Corticosteroids and methotrexate are used for treatment, but response is slow.
2. Calcium pyrophosphate dihydrate crystal deposition disease, also known as pseudogout—results in crystal deposition in the joint cartilage and menisci, bursae, and periarticular tissue and can present similar to gout. Treatment is similar, although urate-lowering therapies have no place in treatment.
3. Polymyalgia rheumatica—an inflammatory disease with elevated ESR that affects mostly women older than age 50 and presents with profound stiffness, usually in the shoulder girdle and hips. It responds well to low-dose corticosteroids.
4. Sarcoidosis—a chronic, granulomatous multisystem disorder that most notably affects the lungs but can mimic rheumatic disease by causing fever, arthritis, uveitis, myositis, and rash. May also be treated with steroid-sparing DMARDs and biologic agents, such as infliximab or adalimumab.

SELECTED REFERENCES

Aletaha, D., Neogi, T., Silman, A. J., et al. (2010). 2010 rheumatoid arthritis classification criteria: An American College of Rheumatology/European League Against Rheumatism Collaborative Initiative. *Annals of Rheumatic Disease*, 69(9), 1580–1588.

American College of Rheumatology. (2016). *Position statement: Complementary and alternative medicine for rheumatic diseases*. Atlanta, GA: Author. Available: https://www.rheumatology.org/Portals/0/Files/Complementary-and-Alternative-Medicine-for-Rheumatic-Diseases-Position-Statement.pdf.

American College of Rheumatology. (2012). *Update of the 2008 American College of Rheumatology recommendations for the use of disease-modifying antirheumatic drugs and biologic agents in the treatment of rheumatoid arthritis.* Atlanta, GA: Author. Available: *www.rheumatology.org/Practice-Quality/Clinical-Support/Clinical-Practice-Guidelines*

American Nurses Association and Rheumatology Nurses Society. (2013). *Rheumatology nursing: Scope and standards of practice.* Silver Spring, MD: Author.

American College of Rheumatology. (2015). *2015 American College of Rheumatology guideline for the treatment of rheumatoid arthritis.* Atlanta, GA: Author. Available: *https://www.rheumatology.org/Portals/0/Files/ACR%202015%20RA%20Guideline.pdf.*

Anderson, J., Liron, C., Jinoos, Y., et al. (2012). Rheumatoid arthritis disease activity measures: American College of Rheumatology recommendations for use in clinical practice. *Arthritis Care and Research, 64*(5), 640–647.

Bryant, P., & Baddley, J. (2017). Opportunistic infections in biological therapy, risk and prevention. *Rheumatic Disease Clinics of North America, 43*(1), 27–42.

Cameron, M., Gangier, J. J., & Chrubasik, S. (2011). Herbal therapy for treating rheumatoid arthritis. *The Cochrane Database of Systematic Reviews,* (2), CD002948.

Chakravarty, S. D., & Markenson, J. A. (2013). Rheumatic manifestations of endocrine disease. *Current Opinion in Rheumatology, 25*(1), 37–43.

Dejaco, C., Singh, Y., Perel, P., et al. (2015). 2015 recommendation for the management of polymyalgia rheumatica: A European League Against Rheumatism/American College of Rheumatology collaborative initiative. *Arthritis and Rheumatism, 67*(10), 2569–2580.

Dougados, M., Khanna, D., King, C. M., et al. (2012). Multinational evidence-based recommendations for pain management by pharmacotherapy in inflammatory arthritis: Integrating systematic literature research and expert opinion of a broad panel of rheumatologists in the 3e Initiative. *Arthritis Care and Research, 64*(5), 625–639.

Dures, E., & Hewlett, S. (2012). Cognitive-behavioral approaches to self-management in rheumatic disease. *Nature Reviews Rheumatology, 8*, 553–559.

Fink, L., Lewis, D. (2017). Exercise as a treatment for fibromyalgia: A scoping review. *Journal for Nurse Practitioners, 13*(8), 546–551.

Furness, S., Worthington, H. V., Bryan, G., et al. (2011). Interventions for the management of dry mouth: Topical therapies. *The Cochrane Database of Systematic Reviews,* (12), CD008934.

Johnson, S. R., Fransensen, J., Khanna, D., et al. (2012). Validation of potential classification criteria for systemic sclerosis. *Arthritis Care Research, 64*(3), 358–367.

Koutsianas, C., Konstantinos, T., Vassilopoulos, D. (2017). Hepatitis B reactivation in rheumatic diseases: Screening and prevention. *Rheumatic Disease Clinics of North America, 43*(1), 133–150.

Lam N., Ghetu M., & Bieniek M. (2016). Systemic lupus erythematosus: Primary care approach to diagnosis and management. *American Family Physician, 94*(4), 284–294.

Macfarlane, G., Kronisch, C., Dean, L., et al. (2016). EULAR revised recommendations for the management of fibromyalgia. *Annals of the Rheumatic Disease, 76*(2), 318–328.

Moore, R. A., Straube, S., Wiffen, P. J., et al. (2010). Pregabalin for acute and chronic pain in adults. *The Cochrane Database of Systematic Reviews,* (3), CD007676.

Moore, R. A., Wiffen, P. J., Derry, H., et al. (2011). Gabapentin for chronic neuropathic pain and fibromyalgia in adults. *The Cochrane Database of Systematic Reviews,* (3), CD007938.

National Center for Complementary and Integrative Health. (2013). *Rheumatoid arthritis and integrative health.* Bethesda, MD: Author. Available: *https://nccih.nih.gov/health/RA/getthefacts.htm*

Petri, M., Orbai, A. M., Alarcon, G. S., et al. (2012). Derivation and validation of the systemic lupus international collaborating clinics classification criteria for systemic lupus erythematosus. *Arthritis and Rheumatism, 64*(8), 2677–2686.

Pruitt, R., Lemanski, A., Carroll, A. (2018). Herbal supplements: Research and safety. *Nurse Practitioner, 43*(5), 32–37.

Shiboski, S. C., Shiboski, C. H., Criswell, L. A., et al. (2012). American College of Rheumatology classification criteria for Sjögren's syndrome: A data-driven, expert consensus approach in the Sjögren's international collaborative clinical alliance cohort. *Arthritis Care and Research, 64*(4), 475–487.

Singh, J. A., Christensen, R., Wells, G. A., et al. (2009). Biologics for rheumatoid arthritis: An overview of Cochrane reviews. *The Cochrane Database of Systematic Reviews,* (4), CD007848.

Singh, J. A., Furst, D. E., Bharat, A., et al. (2012). 2012 Update of the 2008 American College of Rheumatology recommendations for the use of disease-modifying antirheumatic drugs and biologic agents in the treatment of rheumatoid arthritis. *Arthritis Care Research, 64*, 625–639.

Stohl, W., & Hilbert, D. M. (2012). The discovery and development of belimumab: The anti BLyS-lupus connection. *Nature Biotechnology, 30*(1), 69–77.

Straube, S., Derry, S., Straube, C., & Moore, R. A. (2015). Vitamin D for the treatment of chronic painful conditions in adults. *The Cochrane Database of Systematic Reviews,* (5), CD007771.

Tort, S., Urrutia, G., Nishishinya, M. B., et al. (2012). Monoamine oxidase inhibitors (MAOIs) for fibromyalgia syndrome. *The Cochrane Database of Systematic Reviews,* (4), CD009807.

Villeneuve, E., Nam, J. L., Bell, M. J., et al. (2013). A systematic literature review of strategies promoting early referral and reducing delays in the diagnosis and management of inflammatory arthritis. *Annals of the Rheumatic Diseases, 72*(1), 13–22.

Winthrop, K. L., Baxter, R., Liu, L., et al. (2013). Mycobacterial diseases and antitumour necrosis factor therapy in USA. *Annals of the Rheumatic Diseases, 72*(1), 37–42.

Yachoui, R., & Kolasinski, S. L. (2012). Complementary and alternative medicine for rheumatic diseases. *Aging Health, 8*(4), 403–412.

Younger, J., Noor, N., McCue, R., et al. (2013). Low-dose naltrexone for the treatment of fibromyalgia: Findings of a small, randomized, double-blind, placebo-controlled, counterbalanced, crossover trial assessing daily pain levels. *Arthritis and Rheumatism 65*(2), 529–538.

31

Infectious Diseases

OVERVIEW AND ASSESSMENT

An infection results when a microorganism or pathogen colonizes a host organism, using its resources to live and replicate. A disease results when there is a change or impairment of normal tissue function because of the pathogen. An infectious disease differs from other types of disease, in that it is transmissible from the host to other individuals.

Public health experts agree and literature supports that infection prevention can positively impact patient outcomes. Being a primary advocate of patient safety, nurses have a significant responsibility to learn about and ensure that infection prevention strategies are part of practice and being upheld at the bedside as well as in the community settings.

The Infectious Disease Process

The chain of infection includes six components that must be in succession for any infectious disease to evolve. If one link is eliminated from the chain, then transmission of the pathogen will not occur. Infection control strategies are based on breaking the chain of infection. The six components of the chain of infection include the pathogenic microorganism, reservoir, portal of exit from reservoir, mode of transmission, portal of entry into host, and susceptible host (Figure 31-1).

Pathogenic Microorganism

Must be able to enter the body and invade or colonize host tissue by attaching to specific host cells then cause damage to those cells

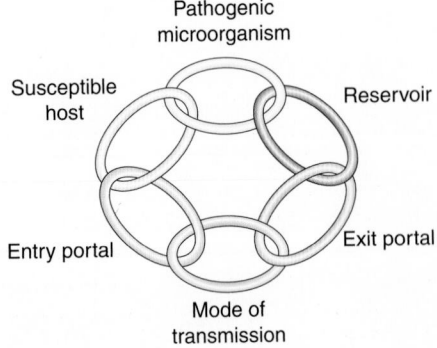

Figure 31-1. Chain of infection.

by production of toxins or destructive enzymes. The pathogen may enter the body through a body orifice or broken skin.

Types

There are six types of infectious agents: bacteria (including mycobacteria), viruses, fungi, protozoa, helminths, and prions.

Characteristics

1. Pathogenicity—ability to produce disease.
2. Virulence—disease severity.
3. Infectious dose—number of organisms needed to initiate infection.
4. Toxigenicity—capacity to produce injurious substances that damage the host.
5. Adaptability—ability to adjust to changing conditions, that is, resistance to antimicrobial agents (see Table 31-1).

Reservoir

The environment in which a pathogenic microorganism lives and survives naturally, can be human, animal, or environmental. Examples of each type include:

1. Human—*Mycobacterium tuberculosis* in human lungs.
2. Animal—Zika virus via *Aedes aegypti* and/or *Aedes albopictus* mosquitoes.
3. Environment—Legionnaires disease (*Legionella pneumophila*) through water.
4. Fomite—Methicillin (oxacillin)-resistant *Staphylococcus aureus* bacteria on a bedside table.

Portal of Exit from Reservoir

The portal of exit are routes in which infectious agents leave their reservoir and include:

1. Droplets from the respiratory tract.
2. Vomitus and feces.
3. Body fluids (except for sweat).

Mode of Transmission

How the pathogenic microorganism is spread to a host by an infectious source. Horizontal transmission is the spread of a pathogen from one individual to another individual. Vertical transmission is from mother to offspring via transplacental transmission, contact through the birth canal, or through breastfeeding or close contact after birth.

There are two main types of transmission: direct and indirect.

Table 31-1　Multidrug-Resistant Organisms (MDROs)

ORGANISM	OVERVIEW AND TRANSMISSION	PREVENTION (ALL)
Methicillin-resistant *Staphylococcus aureus* (MRSA)	Found in various body sites but especially in nares and on skin. Can produce toxins and invade body tissues. Transmitted via direct and indirect contact. Drug of choice: vancomycin.	• Hand hygiene with soap or alcohol-based hand sanitizer. • Use of gloves and gowns for patient contact. • Isolate patient in private room or cohort patients with the same organisms on contact isolation. • Use disposable equipment or disinfect reusable items after removal from room. • Utilize a system for prompt identification and isolation of patients upon readmission and for discharge planning. • Health care worker, patient and family education.
Vancomycin-resistant enterococci (VRE)	Found in GI tract and female GU tract. Not highly pathogenic but can cause serious illness in immunocompromised persons. If infection occurs, treatment options are limited. Transmitted via direct and indirect contact.	
Vancomycin-intermediate or -resistant *Staphylococcus aureus* (VISA/VRSA)	Transmitted via direct and indirect contact. Must be reported to the Centers for Disease Control and Prevention (CDC) and the local health department. Strictly follow contact precautions and dedicate staff for one-to-one care. Treatment options are limited.	
Multidrug-resistant gram-negative rods such as *Escherichia coli, Klebsiella pneumoniae, Acinetobacter* species, and *Pseudomonas aeruginosa*.	Found in various body sites, especially sputum. Spread via direct and indirect contact.	
Emerging MDROs • Extended-spectrum metallo-beta lactamase (ESBLs) producers • Carbapenem-resistant enterobacteriaceae (CRE) • New Delhi metallo-beta lactamase	Produced by some gram-negative bacteria, making them resistant to multiple antibiotics. Spread via direct and indirect contact. Limited treatment options because of resistance. There is worldwide concern for growing pan-resistance creating "super-bugs".	

Direct Transmission

1. Direct contact—by touching the reservoir (eg, touching a wound infection with MRSA) or sexual contact (eg, human papillomavirus).
2. Droplet transmission.
   a. Droplets of large particles more than 5 microns in size usually from respiratory secretions.
   b. Transmitted through coughing, sneezing, or talking to an infected person (eg, human metapneumovirus spread through coughing).
   c. Transmitted through aerosolizing procedures (eg, sprays of infectious agents during a nebulization treatment or a sputum induction).
3. Airborne transmission.
   a. Droplet nuclei—less than 5 microns that remains suspended in air (eg, Tuberculosis and Varicella [Primary Chickenpox]).
   b. Dust particles in the air containing the infectious agent (eg, *Aspergillus* fungi through dust).

Indirect Transmission

Touching an inanimate object or fomite that has had direct contact with the reservoir (eg, touching a tissue of a child with Influenza virus or touching a bedside table contaminated with *Clostridium difficile*).

1. Common vehicle route (through contaminated items).
   a. Food (eg, *Salmonella* and *Campylobacter*).
   b. Water (eg, *Vibrio cholera* and *Legionella* species).
   c. Medications (eg, bloodborne pathogens including Hepatitis B, Hepatitis C, and HIV from contaminated multidose vials).

2. Vector-borne transmission.
   a. A living creature acts as an intermediary acquiring a pathogen from one living host and transmits the disease agent to another living organism, often an arthropod (fly, mosquito, tick).
   b. Can be mechanical or biological vectors. Mechanical transmission occurs when the vector transports the pathogen on its feet or body surfaces to the host. Biological transmission occurs when the vector takes the pathogen into its body where it develops, produces copies, and then is put in the host by bite or sting, such as the plague transmitted by infected fleas from rats to humans.

Portal of Entry

Defined as how an infectious agent enters a new host. Entry sites include:

1. Respiratory tract
2. Gastrointestinal/genitourinary
3. Mucous membranes
4. Nonintact skin
5. Blood

Susceptible Host

Host susceptibility is determined by a complex interrelationship between host and an infectious agent, by factors that influence infection or disease, such as:

1. Pathogenicity—the ability to produce disease in a host. The organism invades a host, enters tissue, colonizes then spreads from host to host while not necessarily causing death to the host.
2. Virulence—the wide range of damage that can occur to the host because of the toxic capabilities of the pathogen. Given that the host–pathogen relationship is fluid, the outcome can be dictated by:

a. Number of pathogens to which the host is exposed; route and duration of exposure.

b. Invasiveness of the pathogen and its ability to produce toxins.

c. Ability to bypass or overcome host defense mechanisms (immunologic response).

3. Host factors—susceptibility of the new host to infection including age, nutritional status, immune status (eg, vaccination), genetic constitution, and general physical, mental, and emotional health and nutritional status of host.

Collection of Specimens for Infectious Disease Identification

 EVIDENCE BASE Leber, A. L. et al. (Ed.-in-Chief). (2016). *Clinical microbiology procedures handbook* (4th ed.). Washington, DC: American Society for Microbiology Press.

Proper collection and transport of laboratory specimens is important to maximize the outcome of tests for the diagnosis of infectious diseases. A variety of laboratory tests can be performed to make a presumptive or definitive diagnosis so that therapy can begin.

Principles

1. Review local laboratory guidelines for the specimen collection recommendations for each test. These guidelines should be readily available and include information on the appropriate specimen containers, sample size, and transport requirements (temperature, time, etc.).

2. It is imperative that specimens be collected and handling carefully by following standard precautions (see Standards of Care Guidelines 31-1).

3. Specimen collection should occur before the initiation of antibiotic therapy whenever possible.

4. To prevent contamination, specimens should be collected using aseptic technique.

5. Obtain an adequate amount of the specimen necessary for all tests.

6. Label the container properly according to local laboratory protocol with at least two patient identifiers (eg, patient's name, date of birth, medical record number) and include on a requisition the source of the specimen, date and time collected, test to be performed, and any special instructions.

7. Seal specimen containers tightly and place in a biohazard bag to transport the specimen to the laboratory as soon as possible according to laboratory guidelines.

8. Be familiar with hospital policy recommending the transport of specified pathogens by staff personnel to the laboratory instead of via a pneumatic tube system.

Types of Specimen Collection

Blood Culture

1. Normally a sterile body fluid.

2. Specimens obtained by peripheral venipuncture are preferred over sampling from vascular catheters because of contamination of the catheter. Culturing hardware to determine a central line infection is not recommended in the literature.

3. Aseptic technique is essential to avoid contaminating the specimen with organisms colonizing the skin or the collector's hands.

STANDARDS OF CARE GUIDELINES 31-1
Universal Precautions (Referenced OSHA 1910.1030)

These infection control precautions are mandated by the Occupational Safety and Health Administration (OSHA) and recommend that all blood and certain body fluids are treated as potentially infectious for human immunodeficiency virus (HIV), hepatitis B virus (HBV), hepatitis C virus (HCV), and other bloodborne pathogens:

- Employers are required to provide appropriate personal protective equipment (PPE) and other engineering/work practice controls to eliminate or minimize employee exposure to bloodborne pathogens as mandated in OSHA regulation 1910.

- Gloves are to be worn when there is anticipation of contact with blood, other potentially infectious materials, mucous membranes, and nonintact skin.

- Gowns, aprons, or other protective body clothing are to be worn when contamination of clothing with blood or other potentially infectious materials is anticipated.

- Masks in combination with protective eyewear are to be worn when performing procedures likely to generate sprays or splashes of blood or other potentially infectious materials into the eyes, nose, or mouth.

- Hands and other skin surfaces are to be washed immediately if contaminated with blood or other potentially infectious materials.

- Utilize safety devices for needles and other sharps and do not manipulate by hand (eg, recapping, purposely bending or breaking, or removing from syringes, etc.).

- Needles and other sharps are to be placed in puncture-resistant containers for disposal.

- All specimens and items with blood or other potentially infectious materials are to be transported in containers that prevent leakage.

- Blood and body fluid spills are to be cleaned up promptly with an appropriate germicide, such as a bleach solution or phenolic.

---

4. Cleanse the venipuncture site with 70% alcohol followed by povidone iodine or chlorhexidine gluconate and allow to fully dry.

5. The diaphragm tops of the culture bottles are not sterile and must be cleaned with alcohol before injection of blood.

Urine Culture

1. Normally a sterile body fluid.

2. A clean-catch, midstream urine collection provides the best method for obtaining a specimen to detect a urinary tract infection.

3. Patients who are catheterized should have the specimen withdrawn using a sterile syringe from the catheter sampling port.

4. Urine specimens must be transported to the laboratory promptly. If not cultured within 30 minutes of collection, urine must be refrigerated and cultured within 24 hours.

5. Other types of urine specimens may be collected, such as a straight in-and-out catheter specimen or suprapubic bladder drainage.

Stool Culture

1. Obtained to culture organisms that are not part of the normal bowel flora (eg, *Salmonella* species, *Shigella* species).
2. Patient should defecate into a sterilized container or bedpan. Stool specimens should not contain urine or water from the toilet bowl.
3. Stool specimens can also be obtained directly from the rectum using a sterile swab.

Sputum Culture

1. Specimen needs to be from the lower respiratory tract, not oropharyngeal secretions. The laboratory will perform a Gram stain on all sputum specimens to determine if they are representative of pulmonary secretions and appropriately collected. A specimen containing a majority of cells from squamous epithelium may be rejected.
2. The most common method of collection is expectoration from a cooperative patient with a productive cough. Early morning is the optimal time to collect sputum specimens.
3. A sputum specimen can be collected in a sputum trap from patients who have artificial airways and require suctioning.
4. If a patient cannot produce sputum, sputum induction using an aerosol nebulizer may assist with loosening thickened secretions.
5. Bronchoscopy may be required to obtain sputum if induction fails.

Wound Culture

1. Specimens are usually cultured for aerobic and anaerobic organisms.
2. Specimens may be collected by multiple techniques, depending on the depth of the wound, including tissue samples, needle aspiration, and swabbing the surface.
3. Surface cultures are not as valuable as can often be heavily contaminated and hard to distinguish the causative infectious agent.
4. To collect a wound culture using a sterile swab, cleanse the surface with 70% alcohol and collect as much exudate as possible from the advancing margin of the lesion. Avoid swabbing surrounding skin.
5. Place the swab immediately in appropriate transport culture tube and send to the laboratory.
6. Label with the specific anatomic site.

Throat Culture

1. Use a tongue depressor to hold the tongue down.
2. Carefully yet firmly rub swab over areas of exudate or over the tonsils and posterior pharynx, avoiding the cheeks, teeth, and gums.
3. Insert swab into packet and follow directions for handling the transport medium.

Laboratory Tests

Microbiologic Evaluation

Microscopy

1. Microscopic examination distinguishes tissue cells from microorganisms.
2. Various stains are used to highlight the structural characteristics of microorganisms (eg, Gram stain to identify groups of bacteria, acid-fast stains to isolate mycobacteria).

3. Classification is conducted according to physical appearance such as shape, size, or tendency to form chains or clusters and stain reactions such as gram-positive versus gram-negative.
4. Results of microscopy are usually available within minutes, which permits early initiation of treatment based on a presumptive diagnosis.

Culture

1. Culture was the gold standard for positive identification of many microorganisms, although technological advances have transitioned to molecular and other innovative testing for several microbes.
2. Different culture media are used for suspected pathogens and can be selective (allow growth of only certain microorganisms) and/or differential (distinguish between different bacteria based on different characteristics).
   a. A liquid medium is used for blood specimens because lower numbers of microorganisms are detectable.
   b. A solid medium is used to isolate mixtures of organisms and grow pure cultures of each type of organism found.
3. Recovery of pathogens from culture varies depending on the microorganism type, test selected, and stage of illness.
   a. Most common pathogens, such as staphylococci, streptococci, and enterococci, are often identifiable to genus and species within 48 hours.
   b. Fungal organisms may take 10 to 14 days to grow in culture medium.
   c. Viruses may take 2 to 3 weeks to grow in culture medium.
   d. Mycobacteria may take up to 6 weeks to grow in culture medium.

Mass Spectrometry

1. Biomolecules absorb energy from a short laser pulse to become ionized which are then accelerated in an electrical field and collide with a detector. They are then separated based upon their mass to charge ratio and leads to molecular detections into mass spectrum.
2. Based upon databases of mass spectrum profiles, identifies a microorganism, including bacteria and fungus, to the genus and species level within minutes versus several hours to days with traditional cultures.

Antibiotic Susceptibility Testing

1. Used to determine minimal concentration of antibiotics that will inhibit growth of an organism.
   a. Minimum inhibitory concentration (MIC) is the lowest concentration of an antimicrobial drug that will inhibit organism growth and is measured by the size of the zone around the antimicrobial disk in which growth is inhibited.
   b. Based on Clinical and Laboratory Standards Institute (CLSI) guidelines for each organism, the size of the inhibitory zone diffusion tests are interpreted as resistant (R), sensitive (S), and intermediate (I).

Molecular Testing

1. There are several technologies to detect specific genetic portions of pathogenic organisms or to identify the specific host's response to the presence of the pathogen. Examples include DNA probe testing and polymerase chain reaction (PCR).
2. These tests may be more sensitive for lower amounts of organism and often yield a more rapid result than culture.

3. Some tests including multiplex PCRs, detect the presence of multiple organisms at once such as respiratory viruses or gastrointestinal infectious agents.

White Blood Cell Count

1. An increase in white blood cell count or "leukocytosis" may indicate infection, inflammatory response, tissue necrosis, or bone marrow failure.
2. The total number of circulating leukocytes and the differential (given as a percent of the total white blood cell [WBC] count) may change during a bacterial or viral infection.
3. During an acute bacterial infection, the WBC count often increases (greater than $11,000/mm^3$), accompanied by increased neutrophils and increased bands (immature neutrophils) in the differential. The shift (to the left) in differential reflects phagocytic activity.

Immunologic Tests

1. Pathogens that are antigenic stimulate antibodies that can be detected in the serum of patients.
2. Detection of antibodies is not necessarily diagnostic of current infection.
3. Antigen–antibody reactions must be evaluated over a period of time.
4. Immunoglobulin M (IgM) antibody production peaks during active infection and decreases during convalescence.
5. IgG antibodies peak during convalescence and persist.

6. A fourfold rise in antibody titer between the acute and convalescence samples indicates recent infection.

GENERAL PROCEDURES AND TREATMENT MODALITIES

Immunity

The human body is equipped with defense mechanisms to protect against disease. These include anatomical barriers, such as the skin, and physiological barriers, such as enzymes in saliva. The normal flora of microorganisms on and in the body also helps to prevent invasion of pathogens. If these nonspecific defense mechanisms fail, the body's specific immune response usually provides protection. Specific immunity to a particular organism implies that an individual has either generated the appropriate antibody in his or her own body or received ready-made antibodies from another source. Immunity may be natural or acquired or passive or active.

Natural active immunity occurs when antibodies are acquired following an infection. Antibodies are also acquired through natural passive immunity, such as from mother to fetus through the placenta or to infant via breast milk.

Passive artificial immunity is achieved through administration of immune globulin or antitoxin. *Active artificial immunity* occurs when antibodies are produced in response to a vaccine or toxoid (see Table 31-2).

There has been debate over the possibility of a link between childhood vaccines and subsequent development of autism.

Table 31-2	Recommended Immunization Schedule for Adults Aged 19 Years or Older, United States, 2018				
Vaccine	19–21 years	22–26 years	27–49 years	50–64 years	≥65 years
Influenza	1 dose annually				
Tdap or Td	1 dose Tdap, then Td booster every 10 yrs				
MMR	1 or 2 doses depending on indication (if born in 1957 or later)				
VAR	2 doses				
RZV (preferred) or ZVL					2 doses RZV (preferred) or 1 dose ZVL
HPV–Female	2 or 3 doses depending on age at series initiation				
HPV–Male	2 or 3 doses depending on age at series initiation				
PCV13					1 dose
PPSV23		1 or 2 doses depending on indication			1 dose
HepA	2 or 3 doses depending on vaccine				
HepB	3 doses				
MenACWY	1 or 2 doses depending on indication, then booster every 5 yrs if risk remains				
MenB	2 or 3 doses depending on vaccine				
Hib	1 or 3 doses depending on indication				

Recommended for adults who meet the age requirement, lack documentation of vaccination, or lack evidence of past infection

Recommended for adults with other indications

No recommendation

Public fear and refusal to obtain childhood vaccines for preventable diseases has shown an increase of these diseases in the community. There have been multiple studies in the scientific community to refute these fears (see *cdc.gov/vaccinesafety/research/index.html*).

Vaccines are the best protection against infections that may cause serious complications and possible poor outcomes in children and adults.

For further updated recommendations see *www.cdc.gov/vaccines/schedules/hcp/imz/adult.html* and *www.cdc.gov/vaccines/schedules/hcp/imz/child-adolescent.html*.

Infection Prevention

Health care–associated infections (HAIs) occur when a patient comes to a health care facility and acquires a new infection during their care. HAIs affect 722,000 patients a year (2011) and 75,000 of those people die annually as a result. Approximately 1 in 25 hospital patients has a HAI. The majority of these infections, however, are potentially preventable by following infection prevention practices.

Infection prevention efforts include surveillance and reporting, monitoring transmission of multidrug-resistant organisms (MDROs), hospital-wide hand hygiene compliance, antimicrobial stewardship, and cleaning and disinfection. In addition, occupational health measures include vaccine compliance, staff education, and performance improvement initiatives to reduce HAIs. Infection prevention strategies are aimed at breaking the chain of infection.

HAI Surveillance

1. The four most common HAIs for which hospitals perform surveillance are:
   a. Surgical site infection (SSI).
   b. Central line–associated bloodstream infection (CLABSI).
   c. Ventilator-associated events (VAE).
   d. Catheter-associated urinary tract infection (CAUTI).
2. HAI rates are increasingly being used as indicators of quality and patient safety in health care facilities.
3. Hospitals are reporting infection rates to the National Health Safety Network, part of the Centers for Disease Control and Prevention (CDC), and the data is being published and made available to the public via state/local health department Web sites and Centers for Medicare and Medicaid's Hospital Compare site.
4. Each year, the bottom quartile of performers in hospital quality metrics including HAI rates receive a penalty of reduced CMS reimbursement of expenses.

Fundamentals of Standard Precautions

Standard precautions were issued by the CDC as an isolation guideline for hospitals but have become common practice for the care of all patients in any setting, every time. They apply to (1) blood; (2) all body fluids, secretions, and excretions, regardless of whether or not they contain visible blood; (3) nonintact skin; and (4) mucous membranes. If there is a chance of coming into contact with a potentially infectious material, a barrier is recommended to be placed between the patient and the care provider. The barrier may be a gown, glove, mask, or goggles, depending on the reason and area of contact.

Hand Hygiene

1. Hand hygiene is the single most recommended measure to reduce the risks of transmitting microorganisms.
2. Hand hygiene should be performed between patient contacts; after contact with blood, body fluids, secretions, excretions, and contaminated equipment or articles; before donning and after removing gloves is vital for infection control. It may be necessary to clean hands between tasks on the same patient to prevent cross-contamination of different body sites.
3. To perform hand hygiene, clean hands with soap and water, applying friction for 15 seconds upon all surfaces of the hands, or applying alcohol-based waterless hand sanitizer covering all surfaces of both hands until completely dry.
4. Waterless hand cleaners are recommended unless there is visible soil on the hands, before eating, after using the restroom, and when there is significant buildup of waterless hand cleaners.
5. If caring for a patient with a spore-producing pathogen such as *C. difficile*-associated disease (CDAD), then use hand hygiene with soap and water applying friction for 15 seconds, as the spores this organism forms are resistant to alcohol hand gel.
6. Similarly, for other pathogens known or suspected to be resistant to alcohol waterless hand gels—such as *Norovirus*—hand hygiene with soap and water while applying friction for 15 seconds.

Respiratory Hygiene/Cough Etiquette

1. When coughing or sneezing, cover the mouth and nose with a tissue or the fabric of your sleeve.
2. Use the nearest waste receptacle to dispose of the tissue after use.
3. Perform hand hygiene immediately.
4. Apply a mask when coughing or sneezing to contain secretions.
5. Sit at least 3 feet from others.

Transmission-Based Precautions

In addition to standard precautions, the CDC recommends instituting transmission-based precautions when there is a suspicion for, or a laboratory confirmed case involving, an epidemiologically significant pathogen. There are three types of transmission-based precautions recommended by the CDC: contact, droplet, and airborne. Each type of isolation takes into account the pathogen and its mode of transmission. Always refer to each health care facility's infection control policies as hospitals may be more restrictive than the CDC recommendations influenced by endemic or newly emerging pathogens in that region. Care should be taken when donning and doffing personal protective equipment (PPE) to avoid contamination. See Figure 31-2.

 NURSING ALERT Standard precautions are recommended for the care of each patient in all circumstances even if already on another type of isolation. When possible, dedicate the use of noncritical patient care equipment to a single patient. Thoroughly clean and disinfect reusable equipment before use on another patient.

Contact Precautions

1. Used for patients known or suspected to be infected or colonized with epidemiologically significant microorganisms, which can be transmitted by direct contact with the patient

SEQUENCE FOR PUTTING ON PERSONAL PROTECTIVE EQUIPMENT (PPE)

The type of PPE used will vary based on the level of precautions required, such as standard and contact, droplet or airborne infection isolation precautions. The procedure for putting on and removing PPE should be tailored to the specific type of PPE.

1. GOWN

- Fully cover torso from neck to knees, arms to end of wrists, and wrap around the back
- Fasten in back of neck and

2. MASK OR RESPIRATOR

- Secure ties or elastic bands at middle of head and neck
- Fit flexible band to nose bridge
- Fit snug to face and below chin
- Fit-check respirator

3. GOGGLES OR FACE SHIELD

- Place over face and eyes and adjust to fit

4. GLOVES

- Extend to cover wrist of isolation gown

USE SAFE WORK PRACTICES TO PROTECT YOURSELF AND LIMIT THE SPREAD OF CONTAMINATION

- Keep hands away from face
- Limit surfaces touched
- Change gloves when torn or heavily contaminated
- Perform hand hygiene

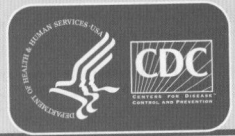

Figure 31-2. CDC guide to donning and doffing PPE (*https://www.cdc.gov/hai/pdfs/ppe/ppe-sequence.pdf*).

HOW TO SAFELY REMOVE PERSONAL PROTECTIVE EQUIPMENT (PPE) EXAMPLE 1

There are a variety of ways to safely remove PPE without contaminating your clothing, skin, or mucous membranes with potentially infectious materials. Here is one example. **Remove all PPE before exiting the patient room** except a respirator, if worn. Remove the respirator **after** leaving the patient room and closing the door. Remove PPE in the following sequence:

1. GLOVES

- Outside of gloves are contaminated!
- If your hands get contaminated during glove removal, immediately wash your hands or use an alcohol-based hand sanitizer
- Using a gloved hand, grasp the palm area of the other gloved hand and peel off first glove
- Hold removed glove in gloved hand
- Slide fingers of ungloved hand under remaining glove at wrist and peel off second glove over first glove
- Discard gloves in a waste container

2. GOGGLES OR FACE SHIELD

- Outside of goggles or face shield is contaminated!
- If your hands get contaminated during goggle or face shield removal, immediately wash your hands or use an alcohol-based hand sanitizer
- Remove goggles or face shield from the back by lifting head band or ear pieces
- If the item is reusable, place in designated receptacle for reprocessing. Otherwise, discard in a waste container

3. GOWN

- Gown front and sleeves are contaminated!
- If your hands get contaminated during gown removal, immediately wash your hands or use an alcohol-based hand sanitizer
- Unfasten gown ties, taking care that sleeves don't contact your body when reaching for ties
- Pull gown away from neck and shoulders, touching inside of gown only
- Turn gown inside out
- Fold or roll into a bundle and discard in a waste container

4. MASK OR RESPIRATOR

- Front of mask/respirator is contaminated — DO NOT TOUCH!
- If your hands get contaminated during mask/respirator removal, immediately wash your hands or use an alcohol-based hand sanitizer
- Grasp bottom ties or elastics of the mask/respirator, then the ones at the top, and remove without touching the front
- Discard in a waste container

5. WASH HANDS OR USE AN ALCOHOL-BASED HAND SANITIZER IMMEDIATELY AFTER REMOVING ALL PPE

PERFORM HAND HYGIENE BETWEEN STEPS IF HANDS BECOME CONTAMINATED AND IMMEDIATELY AFTER REMOVING ALL PPE

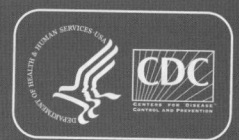

Figure 31-2. (*Continued*)

HOW TO SAFELY REMOVE PERSONAL PROTECTIVE EQUIPMENT (PPE) EXAMPLE 2

Here is another way to safely remove PPE without contaminating your clothing, skin, or mucous membranes with potentially infectious materials. **Remove all PPE before exiting the patient room** except a respirator, if worn. Remove the respirator **after** leaving the patient room and closing the door. Remove PPE in the following sequence:

1. GOWN AND GLOVES

- Gown front and sleeves and the outside of gloves are contaminated!
- If your hands get contaminated during gown or glove removal, immediately wash your hands or use an alcohol-based hand sanitizer
- Grasp the gown in the front and pull away from your body so that the ties break, touching outside of gown only with gloved hands
- While removing the gown, fold or roll the gown inside-out into a bundle
- As you are removing the gown, peel off your gloves at the same time, only touching the inside of the gloves and gown with your bare hands. Place the gown and gloves into a waste container

2. GOGGLES OR FACE SHIELD

- Outside of goggles or face shield is contaminated!
- If your hands get contaminated during goggle or face shield removal, immediately wash your hands or use an alcohol-based hand sanitizer
- Remove goggles or face shield from the back by lifting head band and without touching the front of the goggles or face shield
- If the item is reusable, place in designated receptacle for reprocessing. Otherwise, discard in a waste container

3. MASK OR RESPIRATOR

- Front of mask/respirator is contaminated — DO NOT TOUCH!
- If your hands get contaminated during mask/respirator removal, immediately wash your hands or use an alcohol-based hand sanitizer
- Grasp bottom ties or elastics of the mask/respirator, then the ones at the top, and remove without touching the front
- Discard in a waste container

4. WASH HANDS OR USE AN ALCOHOL-BASED HAND SANITIZER IMMEDIATELY AFTER REMOVING ALL PPE

PERFORM HAND HYGIENE BETWEEN STEPS IF HANDS BECOME CONTAMINATED AND IMMEDIATELY AFTER REMOVING ALL PPE

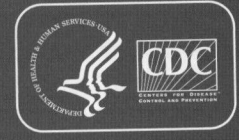

Figure 31-2. (Continued)

or indirect contact with environmental surfaces (fomites) or patient care items in the patient's environment.

2. Examples of microorganisms requiring contact precautions:
   a. Methicillin (oxacillin)-resistant *Staphylococcus aureus* (MRSA).
   b. Vancomycin-resistant *Enterococcus*.
   c. Vancomycin-intermediate or vancomycin-resistant *S. aureus*.
   d. CDAD.
3. Place the patient in a private room or in a room with a patient who has the same microorganism (cohorting).
4. Wear PPE when entering a room marked as contact isolation, including gloves and a gown (see Box 31-1). Many hospitals encourage visitors to follow the same precautions.
5. All equipment, including intravenous poles, handles on carts, and other devices, should be cleaned, disinfected, and identified as clean prior to transport in halls, elevators, or before provided to a new patient—doing so protects the environment, staff, visitors, and patients from contamination with potentially infectious germs.

BOX 31-1 Personal Protective Equipment

GLOVES

Gloves are worn to provide a protective barrier and prevent gross contamination of the hands of health care workers; if used properly, they reduce the transmission of microorganisms and help prevent cross-contamination within a patient. Wearing gloves does not replace the need for hand hygiene because gloves may have small defects or may be torn during use, and during the removal of gloves, hands may become contaminated.

- Perform hand hygiene before putting on gloves.
- Change gloves after contact with infective material, such as feces and wound drainage.
- Remove gloves before leaving the patient's environment and perform appropriate hand hygiene immediately with soap and water or alcohol-based waterless antiseptic agent.
- Gloves also must be changed between procedures on the same patient, such as central line dressing change and wound care or catheter drainage bag manipulation.
- As a general practice, examination gloves are not to be worn outside a patient's room.

GOWNS

Gowns are to be worn during the care of patients infected with epidemiologically significant pathogens to reduce contamination of the health care worker's clothing. Contaminated clothing can transmit pathogens to patients.

- The gown must be tied at the neck and sides, covering the nurse completely.
- If the gown is too small, two gowns can be used to cover any exposed areas of the nurse.
- Water-impermeable gowns, leg coverings, boots, or shoe covers provide greater protection to the skin when large splashes of blood or body fluid are possible such as in the OR.
- Gowns must be removed and discarded prior to leaving the patient's environment, and appropriate hand hygiene must be performed.

Droplet Precautions

1. Designed for care of patients known or suspected to be infected with microorganisms transmitted by large-particle droplets generated by the patient when coughing, sneezing, talking, or during the performance of certain procedures, such as sputum induction or nebulization.
2. These large-particle droplets fall out of the air 3 to 6 feet from the patient's mouth so use of surgical mask, eye protection, gown, and gloves is mandatory.
3. Examples of illnesses requiring droplet precautions: *Neisseria meningitidis*, pneumonic plague, scarlet fever, pertussis, adenoviruses, parainfluenza viruses, influenza, respiratory syncytial virus, human metapneumovirus, rhinovirus, mumps, parvovirus B12, rubella.
4. Place the patient in a private room.
   a. When a private room is not available, place patients with the same microorganism together (cohorting).
   b. If neither of these is possible, maintain spatial separation of at least 3 feet between the infected patient and other patients and visitors.
5. Special air handling and ventilation are not necessary and the door may remain open.
6. PPE includes surgical masks; gowns and gloves may also be required based on the disease, refer to the disease-specific hospital policy.
   a. Wear a mask when working within 3 feet (0.9 m) of the patient.
   b. To protect the mucous membranes of the eyes, nose, and mouth, masks and goggles or face shields are worn by health care workers during patient care to protect against splashes or sprays of blood, body fluids, or secretions.
7. Limit transport of the patient from the room for essential purposes only. If transport is necessary, minimize dispersal of droplets by masking the patient immediately prior to and during transport. See below for additional measures.

Airborne Precautions

1. Designed to reduce the risk of airborne transmission of infectious agents through dissemination of small-droplet nuclei less than 5 microns in size, which remain suspended in the air for long periods of time.
2. Microorganisms can be dispersed widely by air currents and may become inhaled by or deposited on a susceptible host within the same room or over a longer distance from the source patient. Therefore, special air handling, filtration, and ventilation are required.
3. Examples of illnesses requiring airborne precautions: measles, varicella (including disseminated zoster), and tuberculosis.
4. PPE—respirators are required (N95 respirator, a high-efficiency particulate air [HEPA] filter respirator, or a powered air-purifying respirator [PAPR]); gowns and gloves may also be required based on the disease, refer to the disease-specific hospital policy.
   a. Staff members are required to be trained in the use of protective respirators and/or PAPRs annually in a program of respiratory protection that includes a "fit test." This test ensures that the respirator seals to the face of the staff member, teaches the staff member how to use the respirator, and optimizes the protection for the staff member.
   b. Persons immune to rubeola or varicella need not wear a mask but must wear gown and gloves when having exposure to lesions, to prevent carrying contaminant to a non-immune patient outside of the room.

5. Place the patient in a private room that has:
    a. Monitored negative air pressure in relation to the surrounding areas.
    b. At least 6 but preferably 12 air changes per hour.
    c. Appropriate discharge of air outdoors or monitored high-efficiency filtration of room air before recirculation.
    d. Door that is closed at all times with the patient in the room.
6. Limit the transport of the patient from the room to essential purposes only. If transport is necessary, minimize patient dispersal of droplet nuclei by placing a surgical or procedural mask on the patient. See below for additional measures.

Other Considerations

Limiting the Movement of Patients
1. Limiting the movement of patients with epidemiologically significant microorganisms reduces transmission. Every effort should be made to limit the movement of patients on airborne precautions.
2. When transport is necessary for a contact, droplet, or airborne patient:
    a. Patient should be in a clean hospital gown with clean linens.
    b. Appropriate barriers (such as masks and impervious dressings) are to be worn by the patient.
    c. Personnel in the area to which the patient is taken need notification with time to collect PPE, prepare a room that will meet specifications for the identified isolation, and communicate with cleaning staff and ensure the patient will not sit in a waiting area with other patients, visitors, and staff.
    d. Unless transporting staff are giving care during the transport, there is no need to wear PPE. If the patient may require care in the hallway, consider having two transporters: one to remain without PPE to open doors, touch elevator buttons and push the patient, whereas the other person with PPE will only touch the patient.
3. When appropriate, patients are taught how they can assist in preventing transmission.

Attention to Equipment, Linens, and Supplies
1. Medical equipment should be cleaned in-between each patient according to the equipment manufacturer's instructions for use (IFUs) according to the Spaulding classification of medical equipment.
    a. Noncritical equipment are devices such as a stethoscope and blood pressure cuff used on intact skin. Routine cleaning and low-level to intermediate-level disinfection are required.
    b. Semicritical equipment are devices such as a vaginal speculum or fiberoptic endoscope, used on mucous membranes or nonintact skin. High-level disinfection is required.
    c. Critical equipment are devices used in sterile areas of the body such as the blood stream and for surgical procedures. Sterilization is required.
2. Soiled linen should be handled, transported, and laundered in a manner that avoids transfer of microorganisms to patients, personnel, and environments in consistent with best practice guidelines. With some organisms, such as smallpox or anthrax, care must be taken to not expel the air from plastic linen bags outside of airborne patient rooms.
3. There is currently no evidence indicating a need for special precautions for dishes, glasses, cups, or eating utensils because the combination of hot water and detergents used in hospital dishwashers is sufficient for decontamination for most infectious diseases. However, appropriate hand hygiene is required when removing food trays from some isolated rooms.

4. Patient-care equipment that is soiled with blood, body fluids, secretions, and excretions must be handled in a manner that prevents skin and mucous membrane exposures, contamination of clothing, and transfer of microorganisms to other patients and environments.
    a. There must be a procedural mechanism in place labeling or otherwise identifying used equipment as not to be used on another patient.
    b. Clean and dirty equipment should be stored in separate physical locations.
    c. Reusable equipment must be transported in a manner to prevent contamination of the staff, the environment, and visitors until it reaches the area where it will be cleaned, disinfected, and reprocessed appropriately before use for another patient.
    d. Single-use items must be discarded properly.
5. Care must be taken to prevent injuries from needles, scalpels, and other sharp objects. Used needles must never be recapped using both hands, removed from syringes, bent, broken, or otherwise manipulated. Used needles and sharps must have the engineered sharps injury protection activated and be disposed of immediately into an OSHA-approved puncture-resistant container. These containers should be mounted per the National Institute of Occupational Safety and Health guidelines and be located as close as is practical to the area of use.
6. Protective mouthpieces, resuscitation bags, or other ventilation devices are used instead of mouth-to-mouth resuscitation methods.

Infection Prevention Bundles
In addition to standard and isolation precautions, hand hygiene, and appropriate equipment/supply handling, there are inclusive, grouped steps called bundles, which are evidence-based practices shown to prevent specific HAIs when all steps are followed. Bundled practices exist for the prevention of CLABSI, CAUTI, VAE, CDAD, and VAE. Bundles prevent infection through aseptic/sterile technique at the time of device insertion as well as properly maintaining devices. An essential component is daily review of necessity for indwelling devices and prompt early removal of devices and to avoid infection.

TRANSITIONAL CARE ALERT Provide education on basic infection prevention practices for all patients who will be discharged with devices and caring for them while at home. For example, for central lines, the patient should be taught to wash hands before and after touching the lines; when and how to change dressings; how to shower or bathe with the dressing (depending on the type of supplies used); ongoing monitoring for early signs and symptoms of infection; and to communicate to the health care provider immediately. Proper care of devices in the home setting will reduce the risk for infections and other complications and potential readmission to the hospital.

SELECTED INFECTIOUS DISEASES

Infectious disorders are covered throughout the book in a variety of body system chapters. See Table 31-3 for selected infectious disorders. Be aware that new data on infectious diseases are emerging daily. For the latest information on infectious diseases, contact your state public health department or the CDC at *www.cdc.gov*.

Table 31-3 Selected Infectious Diseases

DISEASE, INFECTIOUS AGENT, AND TRANSMISSION	PRESENTATION	NURSING CONSIDERATIONS
Rocky Mountain Spotted Fever		
Rickettsia rickettsii • Transmission usually occurs via an infected tick bite with a minimum of 4–6 hr of attachment for infection to occur. May also be transmitted via contamination of breaks in the skin or mucous membranes with crushed tissues or feces of the tick. • Reservoir includes the American dog tick in the east and south, the Rocky Mountain wood tick in the northwest, and the brown dog tick. • Coinfection with other tickborne pathogens should be considered.	• Incubation period is 2–14 d. • Sudden high fever, malaise, headache, chills, and conjunctival injection (red eyes). • Maculopapular rash may begin on day 2–5 on the extremities, which progresses to the soles, palms, and body trunk (in 35%–60%) into petechia and purpura on or after the 6th day. • Mortality ranges depending on the region but occurs in 3%–5% of cases after treatment.	• Not communicable person to person. • Instruct patient to report reoccurrence of symptoms immediately; may be relapse. • Stress prevention through avoidance of tick-infested areas, wearing protective clothing and tick repellent, inspecting body and clothes for ticks every 3–4 hr. • Remove ticks with tweezers or forceps to avoid leaving mouth parts of the skin. Avoid folklore remedies of painting tick with nail polish or petroleum jelly or using heat to make tick detach from the skin. Remove tick from skin as soon as it is found.
Lyme Disease		
Borrelia burgdorferi • Endemic in the Northern Hemisphere temperate regions but found worldwide. • Ixodid ticks reservoir (affecting primarily small mammals and deer). • Coinfection with other tickborne pathogens should always be considered.	• Incubation period is 3–32 d. • Erythema migrans rash occurs in 70%–80% of infected patients after a delay of 3–30 d. Appears at the site of the tick bite and gradually expands over a period of days. May be anywhere on the body. Feels warm but is rarely itchy or painful. May have a bull's-eye appearance. • Flulike symptoms—malaise, fever, headache, stiff neck, myalgia, migratory arthralgias, lymphadenopathy. • Weeks to months—limb weakness, pain and swelling in the large joints, facial palsy, aseptic meningitis. • Months to years—arthritis with severe joint pain and swelling, chronic neurologic symptoms.	• Not communicable person to person. • Preventive measures include: (a) avoiding tick-infested areas; (b) wearing protective clothing; (c) using insect repellent; (d) inspecting the body and clothing daily while working or playing in tick-infested areas. • Ticks should be removed from the skin with tweezers or forceps, using gentle, steady traction to avoid leaving mouth parts in the skin. Protect hands with gloves, cloth, or tissue when removing ticks. • Condition of most patients improves after initial antibiotic treatment. The literature doesn't show a benefit for long-term treatment so is not recommended.
Influenza		
• Acute viral disease of the respiratory tract. • Spread from person to person by large-particle respiratory droplet transmission or by contact with articles recently contaminated with respiratory secretions. • Animal influenza viruses may also be spread via direct contact with infected animals.	• Incubation is 1–4 d. • Usually self-limited febrile illness associated with upper and lower respiratory infection. • Characterized by sudden onset of fever, chills or rigors, headache, malaise, myalgia, and nonproductive cough, typically followed by sore throat, nasal congestion, and rhinorrhea. • Among children—otitis media, abdominal pain, and vomiting are commonly reported. • Cough may last 2 wk or more but other symptoms generally resolve within 5–7 d.	• Highly infectious via aerosolization or droplets from the respiratory tract of infected persons. • Implement droplet precautions for patients for the duration of symptoms. • Best means of prevention—annual influenza vaccination for individuals 6 mo and older, particularly for high-risk groups and HCWs. • Maintain bed rest for at least 48 hr after fever subsides. Encourage fluids. Report symptoms of secondary infection (purulent nasal drainage or sputum, ear pain, increase in fever) to health care provider. • Stay home. • At onset of symptoms contact medical provider for antiviral treatment (including children, pregnant women and those at high risk for severe flu complications). • Bacterial coinfection with Flu can cause severe complications such as with MRSA. • Continue antibiotics prescribed for bacterial complications for defined time period (usually 7–10 d). • Educate on the misuse of antibiotics to treat viral illness.

(continued)

Table 31-3 Selected Infectious Diseases (*Continued*)

DISEASE, INFECTIOUS AGENT, AND TRANSMISSION	PRESENTATION	NURSING CONSIDERATIONS
Mononucleosis Most common cause: Epstein-Barr virus (EBV) Spread via bodily fluids, especially saliva but also through blood, semen, and transplant.	• Incubation period is 4–6 wk. • Fever, sore throat (exudative pharyngo-tonsillitis), fatigue, splenomegaly, and lymphadenopathy.	• Person-to-person spread via saliva is prolonged—can be months to a year or more after infection. • Convalescence may be as long as several months. • Patients with splenomegaly should avoid activity that may increase the risk of injury to the spleen, such as contact sports and heavy lifting. • Report any excess bruising or bleeding, jaundice, or abnormal CNS functioning.
Cytomegalovirus (CMV) Spread by intimate contact with mucous membranes, secretions, and excretions and by blood transfusion and organ transplant. A fetus may be infected in utero or at delivery.	• Incubation period is 3–8 wk following transplant or transfusion; 3–12 wk delivery. • Ordinarily asymptomatic, especially in children. • Can be a cause of mononucleosis. • More extensive organ involvement in the immunosuppressed host: colitis, pneumonitis, and retinitis may occur. • GI tract disorders. • Congenital infections are serious and lead to irreversible CNS and liver damage.	• Patients with splenomegaly should avoid activity that may increase the risk of injury to the spleen, such as contact sports and heavy lifting. • Report any excess bruising or bleeding, jaundice, or abnormal CNS functioning. • Pregnant personnel should be counseled about potential risks and urged to practice. • Good hygiene (especially hand hygiene) and to follow standard precautions. • Most healthy nonpregnant people do not require treatment.
Rabies Rabies virus Spread by direct contact of virus-laden saliva of a rabid animal into a bite or scratch; may also be transmitted via transplanted corneas and, possibly, other organs removed from patients dying of undiagnosed rabies.	• Incubation is highly variable, usually 3–8 wk; if the bite occurs on the head rather than on an extremity, incubation is shorter. • Initial symptoms apprehension, malaise, fatigue, headache, and fever; possible pain or paresthesia at the site of exposure. • Usually lasts 2–6 d. • Progresses to paresis or paralysis, hydrophobia, eventually to delirium and convulsions. • Respiratory arrest usually occurs, followed by death.	• Avoid contact with respiratory secretions, especially saliva, for duration of illness. • Preexposure prophylaxis should be offered to persons at high risk for exposure to rabies, such as veterinarians, veterinary students, wildlife personnel, park rangers, staff of kennels, and laboratory workers working with rabies. • Bites from animals, particularly dogs and cats, should be thoroughly flushed and cleaned with soap and water immediately. Wounds should not be sutured unless unavoidable. • Domestic dogs and cats should be quarantined for 10 d. • Wild animal carriers include skunks, bats, foxes, coyotes, raccoons, bobcats, wolves, jackals, and other carnivores. • Contact local health department and provider for treatment.
Malaria *Plasmodium vivax, P. falciparum, P. malariae,* and *P. ovale* Malaria is vector-borne through the bite of a female *Anopheles* mosquito; may be congenital or transmitted by transfusions or dirty needles.	• Incubation is 7 d to 10 mo, depending on the strain. • Malarial paroxysm characterized by variations of high fever, chills, sweats, headache, rigor, cough, diarrhea, respiratory distress, nausea, vomiting, and arthralgia. • As infection becomes synchronized, fever and paroxysms are generally cyclic. • Moderate splenomegaly and tender hepatomegaly.	• Maintain standard precautions. • Obtain a travel history. • Fever and recent travel to malaria endemic area should be evaluated using diagnostics. • Symptoms may recur; instruct patient to report recurrence immediately. • Travelers to malaria endemic countries should follow preventive measures: 1. Proper use of mosquito netting at night. 2. Clothing that minimizes contact with mosquitoes. 3. Use of insect repellents. 4. Chemoprophylaxis with suppressive drugs, based on local endemicity and resistance.

Table 31-3 Selected Infectious Diseases (*Continued*)

DISEASE, INFECTIOUS AGENT, AND TRANSMISSION	PRESENTATION	NURSING CONSIDERATIONS
Amebiasis		
Entamoeba histolytica Transmitted by ingestion of fecally contaminated food or water, or sexually by oral–anal contact. Amebic dysentery is a severe form.	• Incubation usually 2–4 wk but range is 3 d to as long as months or even years. • Only 10%–20% of infected people become sick. • Intestinal disease: may be asymptomatic or mild symptoms such as abdominal distention, flatulence, constipation, and, occasionally, loose stools. • Nondysenteric colitis: recurring episodes of loose stools; vague abdominal pain; hemorrhoids with occasional rectal bleeding. • Dysenteric colitis: abdominal cramps and diarrhea containing blood and mucus, alternating with periods of constipation or remission.	• Maintain standard precautions. • Instruct patient to wash hands thoroughly after defecating to prevent transmission to others. • Household and sexual contacts should seek medical examination and treatment. • Instruct patient on safer sex practices. • Travelers to areas where the water supply is not chemically treated or protected from sewage should boil all water used for drinking and cooking.
Giardiasis		
Giardia lamblia Transmitted by ingestion of fecally contaminated water or food, or sexually.	• Incubation is 1–3 wk. • Acute: explosive, watery diarrheal stool; abdominal cramping and flatulence; nausea. • Lasts 2–6 wk. • Chronic: intermittent foul-smelling diarrheal stools; increased flatulence and distention; anorexia.	• Maintain standard precautions. • Instruct patient to wash hands thoroughly after defecating to prevent transmission to others. • Household and sexual contacts should seek medical examination and treatment. • Instruct patient on safer sex practices. • Travelers to areas where the water supply is not chemically treated or protected from sewage should boil all water used for drinking and cooking. • Can be tolerant to chlorine disinfection. • Spread mostly in drinking water and recreational water not properly disinfected.
Hookworm		
Ancylostoma duodenale, Necator americanus Transmitted by entry into the skin of soil contaminated with feces from humans, or animals.	• Incubation is a few weeks to many months, depending on intensity of infection. • Chronic, debilitating disease leading to iron deficiency and hypochromic, microcytic anemia because of intestinal blood loss to the hookworm.	• Follow-up examination of the stool 2 wk after therapy is necessary. Repeat therapy if heavy worm burden persists. • Nutrition counseling and taking iron supplements are recommended until deficiencies are corrected. • Family members and close contacts should be examined and treated for parasites. • Educate public about dangers of soil contamination and importance of wearing shoes.
Trichinosis, Trichinellosis		
Trichinella spiralis Transmitted by ingestion of raw or insufficiently cooked meat, chiefly pork and pork products infected with the larvae. Other meats are wild carnivores and omnivores—bear, cougar, fox, dog, wolf, horse, seal, walrus, wild boar.	• Incubation is 1–2 d for abdominal symptoms; further symptoms start 2–8 wk after eating contaminated meat. • Clinical disease is highly variable, from inapparent infection to a fulminating fatal disease. • During first week: abdominal discomfort, nausea, vomiting, and, possibly, diarrhea. • Early signs: sudden appearance of muscle soreness and pain accompanied by edema of upper eyelids, pain, and photophobia; ocular signs may progress to subconjunctival, subungual, and retinal hemorrhages. • Remittent fever is usual, sometimes as high as 104°F (40°C).	• Instruct patient to thoroughly wash hands after defecation. • Do not eat raw or uncooked meats; curing, smoking, or microwaving meat doesn't consistently kill infected worms; homemade jerky and sausage cause many cases. • Proper cooking of meats: pork to 160°F (71°C) is necessary. • Family members and close contacts of patients should be examined and treated for parasites.

(continued)

Table 31-3 Selected Infectious Diseases (*Continued*)

DISEASE, INFECTIOUS AGENT, AND TRANSMISSION	PRESENTATION	NURSING CONSIDERATIONS

Histoplasmosis
 	
Histoplasma capsulatum
Transmitted by inhalation of airborne particles from soil or dust that harbor chicken or other bird droppings or bat droppings.
	• Incubation is variable, 3–17 d after exposure.
	• May be asymptomatic with only hypersensitivity to histoplasmin.
	• Four other clinical forms of disease:
	  1. Acute benign respiratory—mild respiratory illness to temporary flulike illness.
	  2. Acute disseminated—debilitating fever, GI symptoms, bone marrow suppression, hepatosplenomegaly, and lymphadenopathy; usually fatal in infants and immunocompromised unless treated.
	  3. Chronic disseminated—intermittent fever, weight loss, weakness, hepatosplenomegaly, hematologic abnormalities, and focal disease, such as endocarditis, meningitis, and mucosal ulcers; usually fatal unless treated.
	  4. Chronic pulmonary disease—resembles pulmonary tuberculosis with cavitation; occurs most commonly with underlying emphysema.
		• Investigation for the common source of infection should be done in outbreaks.
		• Educate public to minimize exposure to dust in chicken coops, attics, and caves—use protective masks, gloves, and disposable clothing.

Typhoid Fever *Salmonella typhi* Typhoid Fever Transmitted by ingestion of food and water contaminated by feces, sewage, or by direct contact with excrement.	• Incubation usually 8–14 d; may range 3–30 d. • Systemic—insidious onset of fever, severe headache, malaise, anorexia, bradycardia, and splenomegaly. • Ulceration of the distal ileum; can progress to hemorrhage or perforation.	• Instruct patient to wash hands thoroughly after defecation and before preparing food. • Educate public—control flies, avoid raw shellfish, thoroughly rinse raw fruits and vegetables. • Family and close contacts should be examined and treated.
Botulism *Clostridium botulinum* Transmitted by ingestion of contaminated food or by contact with a contaminated wound.	• Incubation usually 18–36 hr or up to 10 d after eating contaminated food; 4–14 d when transmitted through a wound. • Severe intoxication characterized by visual difficulty, dysphagia, and dry mouth, followed by descending symmetrical flaccid paralysis. • Vomiting and constipation or diarrhea may be present initially.	• All patient contacts known to have eaten the same food should have gastric lavage, high enemas, and cathartics and be kept under close medical supervision. • Instruct patient/patient contacts to wash hands thoroughly after defecation and before handling food. • No questionable canned food should ever be tasted.
Tetanus *Clostridium tetani* Transmitted by direct contact of soil contaminated with animal or human feces into a wound (primarily puncture wounds), burn, or laceration.	• Usually 3–21 d (average is 10 d); may range from 1 d to several months. • Painful muscular contractions, primarily of the masseter and neck muscles. • Abdominal rigidity. • Generalized spasms frequently induced by sensory stimuli—opisthotonos (arching of the trunk) and risus sardonicus (distorted grin).	• Refer persons with skin injuries for tetanus prophylaxis. • Remind adults to receive a tetanus booster every 10 yr. • For major wounds, booster dose of vaccine should be given if none received in past 5 yr.

Table 31-3 Selected Infectious Diseases (Continued)

DISEASE, INFECTIOUS AGENT, AND TRANSMISSION	PRESENTATION	NURSING CONSIDERATIONS
Staphylococcal Infections		
Staphylococcus aureus, S. epidermidis, S. haemolyticus, coagulase-negative *staphylococci* Transmitted by direct contact with draining lesions or by autoinfection from colonized nares; hands are the most common vehicle of transmission.	• Incubation usually 4–10 d. • Skin and soft tissue infections—furuncles (boils), impetigo, carbuncles, cellulitis, abscesses, and infected lacerations. • Seeding of the bloodstream may lead to pneumonia, lung abscess, osteomyelitis, septicemia, endocarditis, bacteremia, pyarthrosis, meningitis, and brain abscess.	• Monitor patient's response to prescribed therapy. • Emphasize meticulous hand hygiene among patients and visitors. • Contain purulent drainage with a dressing. • Place soiled dressings in a paper bag before disposal.
Group A Streptococcal Infections		
Streptococcus pyogenes, group A, with ~ 80 serologically distinct types Transmitted by large respiratory droplets or direct contact with secretions, or by ingestion of contaminated food and milk.	• Incubation usually 2–5 d. • Streptococcal pharyngitis (most common). • Wound and skin infections—impetigo, cellulitis, and erysipelas. • Scarlet fever—streptococcal sore throat with a rash that occurs if infectious agent produces erythrogenic toxin to which patient is not immune.	• Repeated attacks of sore throat or other streptococcal disease because of different types of streptococci are relatively frequent. • Make sure the patient understands the importance of completing the course of antimicrobial therapy. • Emphasize the relationship of streptococcal infections to heart disease and glomerulonephritis. • Children should not return to school and HCWs should not return to work until afebrile and at least 24 hr after appropriate antimicrobial therapy has begun.
Syphilis		
Treponema pallidum, a spirochete Transmitted sexually or by direct contact with infectious exudates; transplacental infection of fetus can occur.	• Incubation usually 3 wk or up to 3 mo; signs of secondary syphilis develop 6 wk to 6 mo after primary syphilis. • Congenital: can result in spontaneous abortion or stillbirth, hydrops fetalis, prematurity, and multisystem abnormalities, including deafness. • Primary: indurated, painless, clean ulcer (chancre) with serous exudates. May not see it. Will heal without treatment. • Secondary: generalized macular-papular rash including palms and soles; fever; generalized lymphadenopathy, condylomata, malaise, headache, and splenomegaly. • Tertiary: aortitis, neurosyphilis; ocular syphilis gummatous changes of skin, bone, viscera, and mucosal surfaces.	• Ensure that sexual activity is not resumed until treatment is complete for patient and partner. • Consider testing for HIV and other sexually transmitted diseases. • Encourage follow-up at 3 mo for repeat serologic testing. • All women should be screened serologically for syphilis early in pregnancy. • All individuals, including HCWs, who have had close, unprotected contact with patient with early congenital syphilis before or during the first 24 hr of therapy should be examined for lesions in 3 wk and again in 3 mo.
Prion Disease		
Creutzfeldt-Jakob disease (CJD) and variant CJD (vCJD) Prion proteinaceous infectious particles. Transmission unknown in most cases; transmission of vCJD probably occurs through consumption of beef infected with BSE. Potential infectious organs and body fluids include the brain, spinal cord, eye, and CSF.	• Incubation is 15 mo to more than 30 yr. • Insidious onset with confusion, progressive defects in memory and personality, ataxia, rigidity, and myoclonus. • vCJD is distinguished by onset at early age, absence of EEG changes, and prolonged duration.	• Prion is extremely hardy and resistant to many disinfectants and to normal sterilization practices. • Use disposables as much as possible. • Health care facilities should have protocols in place for identification of cases and for instrument reprocessing at a higher temperature and for longer periods than typical. • Tissue from infected patients must not be used for transplants.

Hot Topics in Communicable Diseases

Ebola Virus

The Ebola virus disease epidemic of 2013 to 2016 in Guinea, Liberia, and Sierra Leone was the largest ever reported. Likely originating in Guinea in 2013 as an epizootic case in a remote village, it spread person to person quickly, moving across borders and to more populated areas. As of June 2016, there were 28,616 cases and 11,310 deaths. The World Health Organization (WHO) in August 2014, declared Ebola in West Africa to be a public health emergency of international concern. Vaccine trials are underway with efforts in several countries. Marburg virus is another filovirus with similar symptoms.

1. Filoviruses cause severe hemorrhagic fevers, commonly accompanied by hepatic and renal damage.
2. Wildlife reservoir host exposure and human-to-human transmission.
3. Central nervous system (CNS) involvement and shock with multiorgan failure can occur.
4. Case mortality rate—Ebola virus, 50% to 90%; Marburg virus, 23% to 90%.

Symptoms

1. Sudden onset of fever, myalgia, and headache; followed by vomiting, diarrhea, and maculopapular rash.
2. Commonly leads to hepatic damage, renal failure, CNS involvement, and terminal shock with multiorgan dysfunction.

Transmission

1. Person to person by direct contact to infected blood and body fluids (included but not limited to feces, saliva, sweat, urine, vomit, breast milk and semen).
2. Direct contact with objects that have been contaminated with infectious blood or body fluids (e.g., equipment and supplies, bathroom surfaces).
3. Risk is highest during later stages when patient is vomiting, experiencing diarrhea, and hemorrhaging.
4. Enters the body through broken skin or mucous membranes.

Implications for Nursing

1. When caring for someone with suspected, probable or confirmed cases of illness, follow strict adherence to use of PPE that fully covers skin and clothing preventing exposure to the eyes, nose, and mouth.
2. HAI have occurred frequently; virtually all Ebola cases in outbreaks that were acquired from contaminated syringes and needles have been fatal.
3. To decrease the likelihood of exposure, there are recommendations for facilities to maintain safety for all workers including clinical and nonclinical staff and visitors who may come in contact with infected patients, equipment or the environment.
   a. Administrative oversight is recommended to ensure strict adherence to infection control policies, such as having a "buddy" not helping with the equipment but to directly observe staff donning and doffing PPE.
   b. The CDC recommends a combination of measures targeted at prevention of virus transmission and infection in hospitals.

Zika Virus

Since its discovery in Uganda in the mid-1900s, outbreaks of Zika virus have occurred in Africa, Southeast Asia, South America, and the Pacific Islands. Zika has made international headlines after the discovered link between the virus and infant microcephaly and other birth defects in 2016. There is no treatment beyond supportive therapy.

Symptoms

1. Often asymptomatic, or signs and symptoms may last up to a week and death is extremely rare.
2. Fever, rash.
3. Joint and muscle pain, headache.
4. Complications include Guillain-Barré syndrome and birth complications including microcephaly, miscarriage, and stillbirth.

Transmission

1. Mosquito bites.
2. Transplacental from mother to baby.
3. Vaginal, oral, and anal sex.
4. Potentially via blood transfusions (not confirmed in the United States, however).

Implications for Nursing

1. Conduct a thorough travel history assessment of the patient.
2. Educate patients who are traveling to areas with known Zika transmission on safe sex practices and mosquito bite prevention including long-sleeves and insect repellent.
3. Educate patients who are trying to conceive on safe conception after travel to areas with Zika transmission and after Zika infection to reduce risk of complications.
4. Follow standard precautions and routine cleaning/disinfection practices when caring for patients suspected or known to have Zika virus.
5. Zika virus is a reportable condition so participate in reporting to the local/state health department in accordance with state/local laws.

Avian Flu

 EVIDENCE BASE Centers for Disease Control and Prevention. (2017). Avian influenza A virus infections of humans. Atlanta, GA: Author. Available: *www.cdc.gov/flu/avian/gen-info/facts.htm*.

Avian flu refers to novel influenza A viruses found in wild and domestic birds, and rare cases of human-to-human transmission have occurred. Asian lineage H7N9 and H5N1 viruses have been of most concern for causing serious illness or death. Because there is a potential for the virus to change becoming more virulent and potentially more easily transmissible from person to person, monitoring human infection is important for public health safety.

Symptoms

1. Conjunctivitis.
2. Fever, cough, sore throat, muscle aches.
3. Pneumonia, acute respiratory distress.
4. Nausea, vomiting.
5. Neurologic changes.

Transmission

1. Reports of human-to-human transmission have been limited; however, because the virus has the potential to change, transmission is being monitored.
2. Direct contact or inhaling particles associated with sick or dead, infected birds or poultry.

Implications for Nursing

1. Conduct a thorough travel history assessment of the patient.
2. Teach patients that for those at risk because of contact with birds or poultry, good hand hygiene and use of PPE are recommended (mask, gloves).

3. Do not rub your eyes, nose, or mouth when around infected poultry or the environment where they live. Infection can occur without touching poultry because of contaminated dust and scratching, flapping, or head-shaking bird behavior.

4. Avoid contact with birds that appear sick and avoid contact with surfaces contaminated with feces from wild or domestic birds.

5. Report the presence of dead birds to the public health agency in your area.

6. For suspected contact with an infected bird, the patient should be monitored for symptoms throughout the week following exposure.

7. The CDC and World Health Organization recommend oseltamivir, peramivir, and zanamivir (as with other types of influenza A) for treatment of infection and as prophylaxis for exposure to infection.

Clostridium difficile-*Associated Disease*

Clostridium difficile is the most common HAI in US hospitals and is usually associated with previous antibiotic use. This organism is a spore-forming bacteria, shed in feces and spread by touching surfaces contaminated by stool then subsequently ingest or contact mucous membranes without proper hand washing. The bacterium causes inflammation of the colon, known as colitis.

1. The use of antibiotics disrupts the indigenous gut microbiota allowing the *C. difficile* to overgrow causing anything from mild to severe diarrhea. The disease is associated with the use of almost every class of antibiotics, but the use of fluoroquinolones has become the leading class of antibiotics associated with this disease.

2. This bacterial spore producer is highly resistant to most cleaning supplies and alcohol-based hand sanitizers routinely used in hospital settings.

3. An especially toxic strain, NAP-1, has emerged as the leading cause of outbreaks in hospitals across the world.

Symptoms

1. Although incubation rates have not been clearly established, they can range from less than 7 days to 6 months depending on the clinical picture of the patient.

2. The patient may be an asymptomatic carrier or may present with abdominal cramps, diarrhea, colitis, pseudomembranous colitis, fulminant colitis, and toxic megacolon.

3. The most common presentation is nonbloody, watery diarrhea (at least three bowel movements per day for two or more days), cramps, fever, and loss of appetite.

4. Recurrence of the disease is common.

Transmission

1. Contaminated environment and the contaminated hands of those who touch surfaces in that environment leads to transmission.

2. The use of alcohol hand gels is not recommended following care of a patient with CDAD. Staff and visitors should wash their hand with soap, warm water, and friction for 15 seconds to perform adequate hand hygiene.

3. The use of sodium hypochlorite at 5,000-ppm, bleach diluted 1:10, buffered commercially prepared bleach solutions, or FDA-approved sporicidal disinfectant is recommended for cleaning the patient's environment and equipment.

Implications for Nursing

1. Collect stool samples for testing for *C. difficile* or its toxins only on diarrheal (unformed) stool, unless ileus because of *C. difficile* is suspected.

2. Follow contact precautions strictly and use diligent hand hygiene with soap and water, for all who enter the environment.

3. Dedicate patient equipment and disposable items as much as possible.

4. Closely monitor antimicrobial use and advocacy judiciously for discontinuation of antibiotics when appropriate.

5. Consider using a bleach-based disinfectant (or other FDA-approved sporicidal) and a highly trained environmental staff.

6. Studies show that patients continue to shed following cessation of diarrhea so consider isolation practices for several days beyond resolution of symptoms or for the rest of the hospitalization.

7. Advocate for an antimicrobial stewardship program if not one in your facility, see Box 31-2.

Transmissible Spongiform Encephalopathy/ Prion Disease

Transmissible spongiform encephalopathies (TSEs) are rare and a family of progressive neurodegenerative disorders that affect both animals and humans. The causative agent is called a "prion." This pathogen is not well understood but thought to be transmissible and induce abnormal folding of normal proteins called prion proteins found mostly in the brain. This group of diseases has long incubation periods, associated with neuronal loss and a failure to induce inflammatory response. Once the symptoms begin, it progresses rapidly and is always fatal. Prion diseases in humans include— Creutzfeldt-Jakob disease (CJD), Variant Creutzfeldt-Jakob disease

BOX 31-2	Antimicrobial Resistance and Antimicrobial Stewardship

Antimicrobial resistance (AMR) occurs when microorganisms (such as bacteria, fungi, viruses, and parasites) evolve or mutate after exposure to antimicrobial drugs (such as antibiotics, antifungals, antivirals, antimalarials, and antihelmintics). Resistance occurs naturally overtime, however, has accelerated due to overuse and misuse of antibiotics without oversight. Examples for types of misuse is prescribing antibiotics for viruses such as the common cold or Influenza or giving them to animals such as fish or livestock as growth promoters. AMR is an increasing global concern and has been recognized as a major public health threat. Antimicrobial stewardship in institutions is the coordinated effort by infectious disease and pathology leaders to educate providers, develop treatment strategies, and enact treatment standards to drive the appropriate use of antibiotics based on the established evidence. The concern for overuse and misuse of antibiotics and subsequent antibiotic resistance has prompted national discussion and convergence of the Antibacterial Resistance Leadership Group (ARLG). This group's focus is to prioritize and promotion research trials for an ongoing acquisition of knowledge while collaborating with international partners to combat and reduce the threat of resistance.

(vCJD), Gerstmann-Sträussler-Scheinker syndrome, fatal familial insomnia, and Kuru. Transmission has been reported in 250 cases worldwide and linked to human growth hormone, dura mater and corneal grafts, or neurosurgical equipment. Special considerations are taken with treatments, procedures or surgeries involving contact with high infectivity tissues (brain, spinal cord, and eyes) of patients thought to have TSEs. The CDC and WHO have developed infection control guidelines for individuals caring for CJD patients. For more information, see (*www.cdc.gov/prions/index.html*).

SELECTED REFERENCES

AHRQ's Healthcare-Associated Infections Program. Content last reviewed April 2018. *Agency for Healthcare Research and Quality*, Rockville, MD. Available: *http://www.ahrq.gov/professionals/quality-patient-safety/hais/index.html*.

Alfaraj, S.H., Al-Tawfig, J. A., Altuwaijri, T. A. et al. (2018). Middle East Respiratory Syndrome Coronavirus transmission among healthcare workers: implication for infection control. *American Journal of Infection Control*, 46(2), 165–168.

Baron, E. J., Miller, J. M., Weinstein, M. P., et al. (2013). A guide to utilization of the microbiology laboratory for diagnosis of infectious diseases: 2013 recommendations by the Infectious Disease Society of America (IDSA) and the American Society for Microbiology (ASM). *Clinical Infectious Diseases*, 57(4), e22–e121.

Berende, A., ter Hofstede, H., Vos, F., et al. (2016). Randomized trial of longer-term therapy for symptoms attributed to Lyme disease. *New England Journal of Medicine*, 374, 1209–1220.

Britton, R. A., & Young, V. B. (2014). Role of the intestinal microbiota in resistance to colonization by *Clostridium difficile*. *Gastroenterology*, 146, 1547–1553.

Brown, E. D., & Wright G. D. (2016). Antibacterial drug discovery in the resistance era. *Nature*, 529, 336–343.

Carter, E., Greendyke, W. G., Furuya, E. Y., et al. (2018). Exploring the nurses' role in antibiotic stewardship: a multisite qualitative study of nurses and infection preventionists. *American Journal of Infection Control*, 46, 492–497.

Cauley, L., & Vella, A. (2015). Why is co-infection with Influenza virus and bacteria so difficult to control? *Discovery Medicine*, 19(102), 33–40.

Centers for Disease Control and Prevention. (2002). Guideline for hand hygiene in health-care settings: Recommendations of the Healthcare Infection Control Practices Advisory Committee and the HICPAC/SHEA/APIC/IDSA Hand Hygiene Task Force. *Morbidity and Mortality Weekly Report*, 51, RR-16.

Centers for Disease Control and Prevention. (2017). *Avian influenza A virus infections of humans*. Atlanta, GA: Author. Available: *www.cdc.gov/flu/avian/gen-info/facts.htm*

Centers for Disease Control and Prevention. (2012). *CRE toolkit—guidance for control of carbapenem-resistant enterobacteriaceae (CRE)*. Atlanta, GA: Author. Available: *www.cdc.gov/hai/organisms/cre/cre-toolkit/index.html*

Centers for Disease Control and Prevention. (2012). *Healthcare associated infections*. Atlanta, GA: Author. Available: *www.cdc.gov/ncidod/dhqp/pdf/isolation2007.pdf*.

Centers for Disease Control and Prevention. (2012). *Frequently asked questions about Clostridium difficile for healthcare providers*. Atlanta, GA: Author. Available: *www.cdc.gov/hai/organisms/cdiff/cdiff_faqs_hcp.html*

Centers for Disease Control and Prevention. (2017). Recommended adult immunization schedule. *Morbidity and Mortality Weekly Report*, 61(4). Available: *www.cdc.gov/vaccines/schedules/hcp/imz/adult.html, www.cdc.gov/vaccines/schedules/hcp/imz/child-adolescent.html*

Centers for Disease Control and Prevention. (2017). *Healthcare exposure to Zika and infection control*. Atlanta, GA: Author. Available: *www.cdc.gov/zika/hc-providers/infection-control.html*

Centers for Disease Control and Prevention. (2017). *Zika virus overview*. Atlanta, GA: Author. Available: *www.cdc.gov/zika/about/overview.html*

Centers for Disease Control and Prevention. (2016). *HAI data and statistics*. Atlanta, GA: Author. Available: *www.cdc.gov/hai/surveillance/index.html*

Center for Disease Control and Prevention. (2015). *Facility guidance for control of carbapenem-resistant enterobacteriaceae (CRE)-November 2015 Update CRE toolkit, 1–24 pp*. Atlanta, GA: Author. Available: *www.cdc.gov/hai/pdfs/cre/CRE-guidance-508.pdf*

Centers for Disease Control and Prevention. (2015). *Prion diseases*. Atlanta, GA. *https://www.cdc.gov/prions/*.

Chambers, H., & Fowler, V. *Antibacterial Resistance Leadership Group (ARLG)*. January 2016 Stockholm, Sweden. Available: *Jpiamr.eu/wp-content/uploads/2016/03/Vance-Fowler.pdf*

Cohen, S. H., Gerding, D. N., Johnson, S., et al. (2010). Clinical practice guidelines for *Clostridium difficile* infection in adults: 2010 update by the Society for Healthcare Epidemiology of America (SHEA) and the Infectious Diseases Society of America (IDSA). *Infection Control and Hospital Epidemiology*, 31(5), 431–455. (Update in progress: Projected publication, Fall 2017.)

Dahl, B. A., Kinzer, M. H., Raghunathan, P. L., et al. (2016). CDC's response to the 2014–2016 *Ebola* epidemic-Guinea, Liberia, and Sierra Leone. *MMWR*, 65(Suppl-3), 12–20.

Ibeneme, S., Maduako, V., Ibeneme, G. C., et al. (2017). Hygiene practices and microbial investigation of hand contact swab among physiotherapists in an Ebola endemic region: Implications for public health. *BioMed Research International*, Volume 2017, Article ID 5841805, 13 pages. *http://doi.org/10.1155/2017/5841805*

Louh, I. K., Greendyke, W. G., Hermann, E. A., et al. (2017). *Clostridium difficile* infection in acute care hospitals: Systematic review and best practices for prevention. *Infection Control & Hospital Epidemiology*, 38(4), 476–482.

Magill, S. S., Edwards, J. R., Bamberg, W., et al. (2014). Multistate point-prevalence survey of health care-associated infections. *The New England Journal of Medicine*, 370, 1198–1208.

McAlearney, A. S., Hefner, J. L., Sieck, C. J., et al. (2017). Searching for management approaches to reduce HAI transmission (SMART): A study protocol. *Implementation Science*, 12, 82.

Melia, M., & Auwaerter, P. (2016). Time for a different approach to Lyme disease and long-term symptoms. *New England Journal of Medicine*, 374, 1277–1278.

Occupational Safety & Health Administration. (1992). *Standard number 1910.1030 Bloodborne Pathogens*. Washington, DC: U.S. Department of Labor, OSHA. Available: *www.osha.gov/pls/oshaweb/owadisp.show_document?p_table=standards&p_id=10051*

O'Grady, N. P., Alexander, M., Burns, L. A., et al. (2011). *Guidelines for the prevention of intravascular catheter-related infections*. Atlanta, GA: Centers for Disease Control and Prevention. Available: *www.cdc.gov/hicpac/pdf/guidelines/bsi-guidelines-2011.pdf*

Rosenberg, K. (2018). Improved patient hand hygiene reduces C. difficile infections in hospitals. *American Journal of Nursing*, 118(1), 156.

Rutala, W. A., Weber, D. J., & the Healthcare Infection Control Practices Advisory Committee (HICPAC). (2008). *Guideline for disinfection and sterilization in healthcare facilities, 2008*. Atlanta, GA: Center for Disease Control and Prevention. Available: *www.cdc.gov/hicpac/pdf/guidelines/disinfection_nov_2008.pdf*

Sickbert-Bennett, E. E., DiBiase, L. M., Schade Willis, T. M., et al. (2016). Reduction of healthcare associated infections by exceeding high compliance with hand hygiene practices. *Emerging Infectious Diseases*, 22(9), 1628–1630.

Siegel, J. D., Rhinehart, E., Jackson, M., et al. (2006). *Management of multidrug-resistant organisms in healthcare settings, 2006*. Atlanta, GA: Centers for Disease Control and Prevention. Available: *www.cdc.gov/hicpac/pdf/guidelines/MDROGuideline2006.pdf*

Siegel, J. D., Rhinehart, E., Jackson, M., et al. (2007). *2007 guideline for isolation precautions: Preventing transmission of infectious agents in healthcare settings*. Atlanta, GA: Centers for Disease Control and Prevention. Available: *www.cdc.gov/hicpac/pdf/isolation/Isolation2007.pdf*

Sun, K., & Metzger, D. W. (2014). Influenza infection suppresses NADPH oxidase-dependent phagocytic bacterial clearance and enhances susceptibility to secondary methicillin-resistant staphylococcus aureus infection. *The Journal of Immunology*, 192(7), 3301–3307.

Surawicz, C. M., Brandt, L. J., Binion, D. G., et al. (2013). Guidelines for diagnosis, treatment, and prevention of *Clostridium difficile* infections. *The American Journal of Gastroenterology*, 108, 474–498.

Taylor, L. E., Swerdfeger, A. L., & Eslick, G. D. (2014). Vaccines are not associated with autism: An evidence-based meta-analysis of case-control and cohort studies. *Vaccine*, 32(29), 3623–3629.

University of Geneva. (2017). *Measuring the safety, efficacy of a vaccine against Ebola virus disease. Science Daily April 18, 2017*. Available: *www.sciencedaily.com/releases/2017/04/170418114348.htm*

Van Belkum, A., Welker, M., Erhard, M., & Chatellier, S. (2012). Biomedical mass spectrometry in today's and tomorrow's clinical microbiology laboratories. *Journal of Clinical Microbiology*, 50(5), 1513–1517.

Vong, S., Reuben, S., Philip, G., et al. (2016). Assessment of *Ebola* virus disease preparedness in the WHO South-East Asia region. *Bulletin of the World Health Organization*, 94, 913–924.

World Health Organization. (2018). *Antimicrobial resistance key facts*. Available: *http://www.who.int/en/news-room/fact-sheets/detail/antimicrobial-resistance*.

Yoldas, O., Altindis, M., Cafali, D., et al. (2016). A diagnostic algorithm for the detection of *Clostridium difficile*-associated diarrhea. *Journal of Balkan Medicine*, 33(1), 80–86.

32
Musculoskeletal Disorders

OVERVIEW AND ASSESSMENT
Subjective Data

Much can be learned about musculoskeletal disorders from subjective data. History of injury, description of symptoms, and associated personal health and family history can give clues to the underlying problem and appropriate care for that problem.

Common Manifestations of Musculoskeletal Problems

Pain
1. Where is the pain located?
   a. Joints, as in osteoarthritis (OA).
   b. Muscles or soft tissue, as in contusions, sprains, or strains.
   c. Bone, as in fractures or tumors.
2. Is it sharp, as in a fracture or sprain, or dull, as in a bone tumor?
3. Does the pain radiate?
   a. To buttocks or legs, as in lower back pain.
   b. To thigh or knee, as in hip fracture, or arm, as in shoulder injury.
4. What makes the pain increase? What makes it better?
5. When was the onset of pain?

Limited Range of Motion
1. Is stiffness present? How long does it last?
   a. Present in the morning for less than 30 minutes or after sitting for long period when due to OA.

   b. May persist and is associated with acute pain when due to spasm of lower back strain.
2. Is swelling present and limiting mobility?
   a. May be due to fracture.
   b. May be soft tissue injury, such as sprain, strain, or contusion.
3. How does limited mobility affect activities of daily living (ADLs)?

Associated Symptoms
1. Any sensory or motor deficits, such as numbness, paresthesias, or weakness, indicating neurovascular compromise?
2. Any weight loss, fever, or malaise, as in bone tumors?
3. Any bony nodules or deformity, as in rheumatoid arthritis?

History

Mechanism of Injury
1. How did the injury occur? Essential for all trauma, including fractures, contusions, sprains, and strains, to help identify the extent of injury.
2. What was the progression of symptoms?
3. If not an acute injury, was there any repetitive movement or strain that may have contributed to problem, as in tendinitis?

Medical History
1. What medications are you taking (include name, dosage schedule, and last time taken—include prescription medications, vitamins, over-the-counter [OTC] medications, and herbal products)?

857

2. Any history of corticosteroid use that predisposes to osteoporosis?
3. Is the woman postmenopausal? On estrogen replacement? If estrogen deficient, may predispose to osteoporosis.
4. Any history of prostate, breast, or lung cancer, which may metastasize to the bone?
5. What are other conditions that may affect immobility imposed by casting, traction, or surgery?
6. Any chronic illnesses such as diabetes that may affect healing?

Social History

1. What is the patient's occupation and specific job activities, which may contribute to lower back strain or OA?
2. Does the patient exercise? What type of exercise is performed, how frequently, and what is the duration of exercise? When was the last time this was performed?
3. What activities or sports does the patient participate in, such as running or tennis, which may cause repetitive injury?
4. Are there risk factors for osteoporosis, such as smoking, inactivity, low calcium intake, or lack of exposure to the sun?
5. Is there a family history of osteoporosis or arthritis?
6. What cultural issues/religious beliefs contribute to this history?
7. Does the patient drink alcohol? If yes, what is the daily alcohol consumption?

Objective Data

Data on current condition and functional abilities are secured through inspection, palpation, and measurement. Always compare with contralateral side (one side of the body to the other).

Musculoskeletal System

Skeletal Component

1. Note deviation from normal structure—bony deformities, length discrepancies, alignment, symmetry, amputations.
2. Identify abnormal motion and crepitus (grating sensation), as found with fractures.

Joint Component

1. Identify swelling that may be due to inflammation or effusion.
2. Note deformity associated with contractures or dislocations.
3. Evaluate stability, which may be altered.
4. Estimate active and passive range of motion (ROM).

Muscle Component

1. Inspect for size and contour of muscles.
2. Assess coordination of movement.
3. Palpate for muscle tone.
4. Estimate strength through resistance testing using scaled criteria (ie, 0 = no palpable contraction; 5 = normal ROM against gravity with full resistance).
5. Measure girth to note increases due to swelling or bleeding into muscle or decreases due to atrophy (difference of more than 1 cm is significant).
6. Identify abnormal clonus (rhythmic contraction and relaxation) or fasciculation (contraction of isolated muscle fibers).

Additional Assessment

Neurovascular Component

1. Assess circulatory status of involved extremities by noting skin color and temperature, peripheral pulses, capillary refill response, pain, and edema.
2. Assess neurologic status of involved extremities by the patient's ability to move distal muscles and description of sensation (eg, paresthesia).

3. Test reflexes of extremities.
4. Compare all to uninjured/unaffected extremity.

Skin Component

1. Inspect traumatic injuries (eg, cuts, bruises).
2. Assess chronic conditions (eg, dermatitis, stasis ulcers, scars overlying joints).
3. Note hair distribution and nail condition.
4. Inspect for Heberden or Bouchard nodes.
5. Assess for warmth or coolness of skin.

 NURSING ALERT The subjective and objective data will help to differentiate acute from chronic processes. Signs and symptoms of infection, neurovascular compromise, and fracture require immediate diagnostic testing.

Radiologic and Imaging Studies

Many radiologic and imaging studies are helpful in evaluating musculoskeletal problems to rule out fracture or skeletal changes and to differentiate soft tissue injury.

 DRUG ALERT Many radiologic studies include injection or oral contrast. Check the patient's allergies and make sure a recent creatinine level has been obtained. To prevent contrast-induced nephropathy, make sure that elevated creatinine or reduced estimated glomerular filtration (eGFR) is reported to the radiology department. Ensure that nephrotoxic drugs and metformin are held according to facility protocol (usually if eGFR is less than 30 mL/minute, for 48 hours before the procedure and for 48 hours following). The patient should be well hydrated before and after the procedure.

X-rays

1. Of bone—to determine bone density, texture, integrity, erosion, changes in bone relationships.
2. Of cortex—to detect any widening, narrowing, irregularity.
3. Of medullary cavity—to detect any alteration in density.
4. Of involved joint—to show fluid, irregularity, spur formation, narrowing, changes in joint contour.
5. Tomogram—special x-ray technique for detailed view of special plane of bone.

Nursing and Patient Care Considerations

1. Tell the patient that proper positioning is important to obtain a good x-ray, so cooperation is essential.
2. Advise the patient to remove all jewelry, clothing with zippers or snaps, change from pockets, or other items that may interfere with x-ray.
3. Medicate the patient for pain prior to x-ray, as needed.

Bone Scan

A *bone scan* consists of parenteral injection of bone-seeking radiopharmaceutical (such as gallium); concentration of isotope uptake revealed in primary skeletal disease (osteosarcoma), metastatic bone disease, inflammatory skeletal disease (osteomyelitis); fracture.

Nursing and Patient Care Considerations

1. There is usually no special preparation prior to the scan.
2. Injectable radionuclide is given several hours before the scan.

3. Reassure the patient that the procedure will not cause pain and that the scan will take 1 to 2 hours.
4. Analgesics or sedatives may be ordered for patients for whom lying immobile for any length of time is difficult.
5. Breast-feeding should be discontinued for at least 4 weeks after test to prevent radionuclide exposure to infant.
6. Inform the patient that the exposure to radioactive substances is small (dose of radiation is less than a chest x-ray), and substances are excreted quickly by the body.

Bone Densitometry

Bone densitometry is a noninvasive study that yields an actual measurement of bone density and is diagnostic for osteoporosis (see page 152). It is most often performed on the lower spine and hips; however, simple portable screening tests that analyze the wrist or heel are also available.

Nursing and Patient Care Considerations
1. Calcium supplements should be avoided 24 hours prior to exam.
2. DXA scan should be avoided for 10 to 14 days if the patient recently had a barium examination or has been injected with a contrast material for a computed tomography (CT) scan or radioisotope scan.
3. Have the patient remove clothing and all jewelry or other metal objects.
4. Advise the patient to lie still with hips flexed for 10 to 30 minutes; during test; technician will remain in the room.
5. Reassure the patient that radiation exposure is minimal.

Magnetic Resonance Imaging

Magnetic resonance imaging (MRI) uses magnetic fields to demonstrate differences in hydrogen density of various tissues. Demonstrates tumors and soft tissue (muscle, ligament, tendon) abnormalities. Although it is more costly than CT scans, the cost is typically validated through the diagnostic accuracy. MRI not only clearly defines internal organs but also is able to detect nerve damage and changes, such as edema or bruises, of bone. Bone bruises (osseous contusions) with traumatic injuries have some predictive value for future development of posttraumatic arthritis.

Nursing and Patient Care Considerations
1. Prepare the patient for the need to lie still for about 1 hour; repetitive clanging noise of machine will be heard; patients may feel closed in.
2. Practice relaxation techniques, such as relaxation breathing and imagery, ahead of time.
3. Some patients may need sedation; claustrophobic patients may be unable to undergo procedure or may need open MRI.
4. May be contraindicated for patients with some types of metal implants and devices. Notify the technologist or radiologist of any surgical implants, medical devices, or hardware for evaluation prior to MRI.
   a. In general, metal objects used in orthopedic surgery pose no risk during MRI. However, a recently placed artificial joint may require the use of another imaging procedure. If there is any question of their presence, an x-ray may be taken to detect the presence of and identify any metal objects.
   b. Patients who might have metal objects in certain parts of their bodies may also require an x-ray prior to an MRI. Notify the technologist or radiologist of any shrapnel, bullets, or other pieces of metal that may be present because of accidents.
   c. Dyes used in tattoos may contain iron and could heat up during MRI, but this is rarely a problem.

d. Tooth fillings and braces usually are not affected by the magnetic field but they may distort images of the facial area or brain, so the radiologist should be aware of them.
e. Parents who accompany children into the scanning room also need to remove metal objects and notify the technologist of any medical or electronic devices they may have.

 NURSING ALERT In most cases, an MRI exam is safe for patients with metal implants, except for a few types. People with the following implants cannot be scanned and should not enter the MRI scanning area unless cleared by a radiologist:

- Internal (implanted) defibrillator or pacemaker
- Cochlear (ear) implant
- Some types of clips used on brain aneurysms
- Some types of metal coils placed within blood vessels

Other Tests
1. CT scan—narrow beam of x-ray that scans the area in successive layers to evaluate disease, bone structure, joint abnormalities, and trauma (fractures).
2. Arthrogram—injection of radiopaque substance or air into joint cavity to outline soft tissue structures (eg, meniscus) and contour of joint.
3. Myelogram—injection of contrast medium into subarachnoid space at lumbar spine to determine level of disk herniation or site of tumor.
4. Diskogram—injection of small amount of contrast medium into lumbar disk abnormalities.
5. Arthrocentesis—insertion of needle into joint and aspiration of synovial fluid for purposes of examination or injection of therapeutic medications.
6. Arthroscopy—endoscopic procedure that allows direct visualization of joint structures (synovium, articular surfaces, menisci, ligaments) through a small needle incision. May be combined with arthrography.
7. Nerve studies—to differentiate nerve root compression, muscle disease (eg, dystrophy, myositis), peripheral neuropathies, central nervous system–anterior horn cell neuropathies, neuromuscular junction problems.
   a. Electromyography (EMG)—measures electrical potential generated by the muscle during relaxation and contraction.
   b. Nerve conduction velocities—measure the rate of potential generation along specific nerves (speed of impulse conduction).

GENERAL PROCEDURES AND TREATMENT MODALITIES

 See additional online content: Procedure Guidelines 32-1–32-3

Crutch Walking

Crutches are artificial supports that assist patients who need aid in walking because of disease, injury, or a birth defect.

Preparation for Crutch Walking

The goals are to develop power in the shoulder girdle and upper extremities that bear the patient's weight in crutch walking and strengthen and condition the patient.

Strengthening the Muscles Needed for Ambulation

Instruct the patient as follows:

1. For quadriceps setting:
   a. Contract the quadriceps muscle while attempting to push the popliteal area against the mattress and raise the heel.
   b. Maintain the muscle contraction for a count of 5.
   c. Relax for the count of 5.
   d. Repeat this exercise 10 to 15 times hourly.
2. For gluteal setting:
   a. Contract or pinch the buttocks together for a count of 5.
   b. Relax for the count of 5.
   c. Repeat 10 to 15 times hourly.

Strengthening the Muscles of the Upper Extremities and Shoulder Girdle

Instruct the patient as follows:

1. Flex and extend arms slowly while holding traction weights; gradually increase poundage of weight and number of repetitions to increase strength and endurance.
2. Do push-ups while lying in a prone position.
3. Squeeze rubber ball—increases grasping strength.
4. Raise the head and shoulders from the bed; stretch the hands forward as far as possible.
5. Sit up on bed or chair.
   a. Raise the body from the chair by pushing hands against chair seat (or mattress).
   b. Raise the body out of the seat. Hold. Relax.

Measuring for Crutches

1. When the patient is lying down (an approximate measurement):
   a. Measure from the anterior fold of the axilla to the sole. Then add 2 inches (5 cm).
   b. Alternatively, subtract 16 inches (40 cm) from the patient's height.
2. When the patient is standing erect:
   a. Stand the patient against the wall with feet slightly apart and away from the wall.
   b. The crutches should be fitted with large rubber suction tips.
   c. The elbow is flexed 30 degrees with the hand resting on the grip.
   d. There should be a two-finger-width insertion between the axillary fold and the underarm piece grip. A foam rubber pad on the underarm piece will relieve pressure on the upper arm and thoracic cage.
   e. The tip of the crutch is placed 6 to 8 inches (15 to 20 cm) lateral to the forefoot.

Teaching the Crutch Stance

1. Have the patient wear well-fitting shoes with firm soles.
2. Before using the crutches, have the patient stand by a chair on the unaffected leg to achieve balance.
3. Position the patient against a wall with head in a neutral position.
4. Tripod position—basic crutch stance for balance and support.
   a. Crutches rest approximately 8 to 10 inches (20 to 25 cm) in front of and to the side of the patient's toes (see Figure 32-1).
   b. A taller patient requires a wider base, whereas a shorter patient needs a narrower base.
5. Teach the patient to support weight on hands; weight borne on the axillae can damage the brachial plexus nerves and produce "crutch paralysis."

Figure 32-1. The tripod position is the basic crutch stance for balance and support. (From Smeltzer, S., & Bare, B. [2000]. *Brunner and Suddarth's textbook of medical-surgical nursing* [9th ed.]. Philadelphia, PA: Lippincott Williams & Wilkins. Photo by Barbara Proud.)

Teaching the Crutch Gait

1. Crutch walking requires balance, coordination, and a high expenditure of energy; these can be acquired with diligent and regular practice.
2. Practice balancing with crutches while leaning against the wall.
3. Practice shifting body weight in different positions while standing with crutches.
4. The selection of the crutch gait depends on the type and severity of the disability, weight-bearing status, and the patient's physical condition, arm and trunk strength, and body balance.
5. Teach the patient at least two gaits—a faster gait to be used for swiftness and a slower one to be used in crowded places.
6. Instruct the patient to change from one gait to another—relieves fatigue because a different combination of muscles is used.

Crutch Gaits

See Figure 32-2 and Patient Education Guidelines 32-1.

Four-Point Gait (Four-Point Alternate Crutch Gait)

1. Four-point gait is a slow but stable gait; the patient's weight is constantly being shifted.
2. Four-point gait can be used only by patients who can move each leg separately and bear a considerable amount of weight on each of them.
3. Crutch-foot sequence:
   a. Right crutch.
   b. Left foot.
   c. Left crutch.
   d. Right foot.

4 POINT GAIT	3 POINT GAIT	2 POINT GAIT
• Partial weight bearing both feet • Maximal support provided • Requires constant shift of weight	• Non-weight bearing • Requires good balance • Requires arm strength • Faster gait • Can use with walker	• Partial weight bearing both feet • Provides less support • Faster than a 4 point gait
4. Advance right foot	4. Advance right foot	4. Advance right foot and left crutch
3. Advance left crutch	3. Advance left foot and both crutches	3. Advance left foot and right crutch
2. Advance left foot	2. Advance right foot	2. Advance right foot and left crutch
1. Advance right crutch	1. Advance left foot and both crutches	1. Advance left foot and right crutch
Beginning stance	Beginning stance	Beginning stance

Figure 32-2. Crutch gaits. Shaded areas are weight bearing. *Arrow indicates advance of foot or crutch.* (From Smeltzer, S., & Bare, B. [2000]. *Brunner and Suddarth's textbook of medical-surgical nursing* [9th ed.]. Philadelphia, PA: Lippincott Williams & Wilkins.)

Three-Point Gait

1. Three-point gait is used when one leg is affected.
2. Both crutches and the affected lower leg are moved forward simultaneously.
3. Then the stronger lower extremity is moved forward while most of the body weight is put on the crutches.

Two-Point Gait

1. Two-point gait is a progression from the four-point gait that allows faster ambulation.
2. Weight is borne on both lower extremities and both crutches.
3. Advance left foot and right crutch together.
4. Then advance right foot and left crutch together.

Ambulation with a Walker

A walker provides more support than crutches or a cane for the patient who has poor balance and cannot use crutches.

Technique for Using a Walker

1. Be aware that a walker gives stability but does not permit a natural reciprocal walking pattern.
2. Rolling walkers may assist the patient who has painful joints in the lower extremities, decreased balance, or decreased cardiopulmonary function.
3. Teach the following sequence for a patient using a stationary (nonrolling) walker:
   a. Lift the walker, placing it in front of you while leaning your body slightly forward.
   b. Take a step or two into the walker.
   c. Lift the walker and place it in front of you again.
4. Teach the following sequence for a patient using a rolling walker:
   a. Roll the walker and move it forward about 12 inches.
   b. If the patient has an injured leg, a new joint, or a weaker side, step forward with that foot first. Instruct the patient to use the walker to help keep the balance as the patient takes the step.
   c. Bring the other foot forward to the center of the walker.
   d. Repeat the sequence.

Ambulation with a Cane

A cane is used for balance and support. Canes come in a variety of shapes, but the majority have a curved handle and a rubber tip. Quad canes may offer greater support.

PATIENT EDUCATION GUIDELINES 32-1

Crutch-Maneuvering Techniques

STANDING UP
1. Move forward to the edge of the chair with the strong leg slightly under the seat.
2. Place both crutches in the hand on the side of the affected extremity.
3. Push down on the hand pieces while raising the body to a standing position.

SITTING IN A CHAIR
Grasp the crutches at the hand pieces for control and bend forward slightly while assuming a sitting position.

GOING UP STAIRS
1. Advance the stronger leg first up to the next step.
2. Advance the crutches and the weaker extremity.

GOING DOWN STAIRS
1. Place the feet forward as far as possible on the step.
2. Advance the crutches to the lower step. The weaker leg is advanced first and then the stronger one—the stronger extremity shares the work of raising and lowering the body weight with the patient's arms.

Note: Strong leg goes up stairs first and down stairs last.

Purposes

1. To assist the patient to walk with greater balance and support and less fatigue.
2. To compensate for deficiencies of function normally performed by the neuromuscular skeletal system.
3. To relieve pressure on weight-bearing joints.
4. To provide forces to push or pull the body forward or to restrain the forward motion of the patient while walking.

Principles of Cane Use

1. An adjustable aluminum cane fitted with a 1½-inch (3.8-cm) rubber suction tip to provide traction while walking gives optimal stability to the patient.
2. With bilateral disease, using two canes gives better balance and weight relief.
3. To fit for a cane:
   a. Have the patient flex elbow at a 30-degree angle and hold the cane 6 inches (15 cm) lateral to the base of fifth toe.
   b. Adjust the cane so that the handle is approximately level with the greater trochanter.
4. Alternatively, while the patient is standing with arms at side, the handle of the cane should line up with the crease in wrist.

Technique for Walking with a Cane

1. Hold the cane in the hand opposite to the affected extremity (ie, the cane should be used on the good side)—allows partial weight-bearing relief because the cane is in contact with the floor at the same time as the affected extremity.
2. Advance the cane at the same time the affected leg is moved forward.
3. Keep the cane fairly close to the body to prevent leaning.
4. If the patient cannot use the cane in the opposite hand, the cane may be carried on the same side and advanced when the affected leg is advanced.
5. To go up and down stairs:
   a. Step up on the unaffected extremity.
   b. Then place the cane and affected extremity on the step.
   c. Reverse this procedure for the descending steps.
   d. The strong leg goes up first and comes down last.
6. When using a quad cane, ensure that all four tips are touching the ground.

Casts

A *cast* is an immobilizing device made up of layers of plaster or fiberglass (water-activated polyurethane resin) bandages molded to the body part that it encases.

Purposes

1. To immobilize and hold bone fragments in reduction.
2. To apply uniform compression of soft tissues.
3. To permit early mobilization.
4. To correct and prevent deformities.
5. To support and stabilize weak joints.

Types of Casts

1. Short arm cast—extends from below the elbow to the proximal palmar crease.
2. Gauntlet cast—extends from below the elbow to the proximal palmar crease, including the thumb (thumb spica).
3. Long arm cast—extends from upper level of axillary fold to proximal palmar crease; elbow usually immobilized at right angle.
4. Short leg cast—extends from below knee to base of toes.
5. Long leg cast—extends from upper thigh to the base of toes; foot is at right angle in a neutral position.
6. Body cast—encircles the trunk stabilizing the spine.
7. Spica cast—incorporates the trunk and extremity.
   a. Shoulder spica cast—a body jacket that encloses trunk, shoulder, and elbow.
   b. Hip spica cast—encloses trunk and a lower extremity.
      i. Single hip spica—extends from nipple line to include pelvis and extends to include pelvis and one thigh.
      ii. Double hip spica—extends from nipple line or upper abdomen to include pelvis and extends to include both thighs and lower legs.
      iii. One-and-a-half hip spica—extends from upper abdomen, includes one entire leg and extends to the knee of the other.
8. Cast brace—external support about a fracture that is constructed with hinges to permit early motion of joints, early mobilization, and independence.
   a. Cast bracing is based on the concept that some weight bearing is physiologic and will promote the formation of bone and contain fluid within a tight compartment that compresses soft tissues, providing a distribution of forces across the fracture site.
   b. Cast brace is applied after initial edema and pain have subsided and there is evidence of fracture stability.
9. Cylinder cast—can be used for upper or lower extremity. Used for fracture or dislocation of knee (lower extremity) or elbow dislocation (upper extremity).

Complications Associated with Casts

1. Pressure of cast on neurovascular and bony structures causes necrosis, pressure sores, and nerve palsies.
2. Compartment syndrome is a condition resulting from increased progressive pressure within a confined space, thus compromising the circulation and the function of tissues within that space. This is a medical emergency and can be limb threatening. A tight cast, trauma, fracture, prolonged compression of an extremity, bleeding, and edema put patients at risk for compartment syndrome.
3. Immobility and confinement in a cast, particularly a body cast, can result in multisystem problems.
   a. Nausea, vomiting, and abdominal distention associated with cast syndrome (superior mesenteric artery syndrome, resulting in diminished blood flow to the bowel), adynamic ileus, and possible intestinal obstruction.
   b. Acute anxiety reaction symptoms (ie, behavioral changes and autonomic responses—increased respiratory and heart rate, elevated blood pressure [BP], diaphoresis) associated with confinement in a space.
   c. Thrombophlebitis and possible pulmonary emboli associated with immobility and ineffective circulation (eg, venous stasis).
   d. Respiratory atelectasis and pneumonia associated with ineffective respiratory effort.
   e. Urinary tract infection—renal and bladder calculi associated with urinary stasis, low fluid intake, and calcium excretion associated with immobility.
   f. Anorexia and constipation associated with decreased activity.
   g. Psychological reaction (eg, depression) associated with immobility, dependence, and loss of control.

Nursing Assessment

1. Assess neurovascular status of the extremity with a cast for signs of compromise.
   a. Pain (pain out of proportion to injury is an indication for compartment syndrome).
   b. Swelling.

c. Discoloration—pale or blue.
d. Cool skin distal to injury.
e. Tingling or numbness (paresthesia).
f. Pain on passive extension (muscle stretch).
g. Slow capillary refill; diminished or absent pulse.
h. Paralysis.
2. Assess skin integrity of casted extremity. Be alert for the following:
   a. Severe initial pain over bony prominences; this is a warning symptom of an impending pressure ulcer. Pain increases when ulceration occurs.
   b. Odor.
   c. Drainage on the cast.
3. Carefully assess for positioning and potential pressure sites of the casted extremity (see Figure 32-3).
   a. Lower extremity—heel, malleoli, dorsum of foot, head of fibula, anterior surface of patella.
   b. Upper extremity—medial epicondyle of humerus, ulnar styloid.
   c. Plaster jackets or body spica casts—sacrum, anterior and superior iliac spines, vertebral borders of scapulae.
4. Assess cardiovascular, respiratory, and GI systems for possible complications of immobility.
5. Assess psychological reaction to illness, cast, and immobility.

NURSING ALERT Signs and symptoms of compartment syndrome include pain, paresthesia, pallor, pulselessness, poikilothermia, and paralysis. Pain is the first sign and is usually described as deep, constant, poorly localized, and out of proportion to the injury. The pain is not relieved by analgesia and worsens with stretching of the muscle group. The other signs occur late in the course of compartment syndrome. Unrelenting pain and other signs of compartment syndrome should be reported immediately. The cast may have to be split and removed.

Figure 32-3. Pressure areas in different types of casts.

Nursing Diagnoses
- Risk for Neurovascular Injury related to swelling and constrictive bandage or cast.
- Impaired Physical Mobility related to condition and casting.
- Risk for Impaired Gastrointestinal Motility related to cast syndrome.

Nursing Interventions
Maintaining Adequate Tissue Perfusion
1. Elevate the extremity on a cloth-covered pillow above the level of the heart. Keep the heel off the mattress.
2. Avoid resting the cast on hard surfaces or sharp edges that can cause denting or flattening of the cast and consequent pressure sores.
3. Handle moist cast with palms of hands.
4. Turn the patient every 2 hours while cast dries and feel cast for abnormal warm areas when dry.
5. Instruct the patient not to place objects into the cast. Advise the patient of alternative methods of managing itching such as blowing cool air under the cast.
6. Assess neurovascular status hourly during the first 24 hours and then less frequently as condition warrants and swelling resolves.
7. If symptoms of neurovascular compromise occur:
   a. Notify the health care provider immediately.
   b. Bivalve the cast—split cast on each side over its full length into two halves.
   c. Cut the underlying padding—blood-soaked padding may shrink and cause constriction of circulation.
   d. Spread cast sufficiently to relieve constriction.
8. If symptoms of pressure area occur, cast may be "windowed" (hole cut in it) so the skin at the pain point can be examined and treated. The window must be replaced so the tissue does not swell and cause additional pressure problems at window edge.

Minimizing the Effects of Immobility
1. Encourage the patient to move about as normally as possible.
2. Encourage compliance with prescribed exercises to avoid muscle atrophy and loss of strength.
   a. Active ROM for every joint that is not immobilized at regular and frequent intervals.
   b. Isometric exercises for the muscles of the casted extremity. Instruct the patient to alternately contract and relax muscles without moving affected part.
3. Reposition and turn the patient frequently.
4. Avoid pressure behind knees, which reduces venous return and predisposes to thromboembolism.
5. Use antiembolism stockings and sequential compression devices (SCDs), on unaffected limb, as indicated.
6. Administer prophylactic anticoagulants, as prescribed.
7. Encourage deep-breathing exercises and coughing at regular intervals to prevent atelectasis and pneumonia.
8. Encourage the patient to drink liberal quantities of fluid to avoid urinary infection and calculi secondary to immobility.
9. Facilitate patient participation in care planning and activities. Encourage verbalization of feelings and concerns regarding restriction of activities.
10. Provide and encourage diversional activities.
11. Pay special attention to positioning and turning for patients in spica or body cast (see Box 32-1).

BOX 32-1 Specific Care for the Patient in Spica or Body Cast

POSITIONING

1. Place a bed board under the mattress for uniform support of the body.
2. Support the curves of the cast with cloth-covered flexible pillows—prevents cracking and flat spots while cast is drying.
   a. Place three pillows crosswise on bed for body cast.
   b. Place one pillow crosswise at the waist and two pillows lengthwise for affected leg for spica cast. If both legs are involved, use two additional pillows.
3. Encourage the patient to maintain physiologic position by the following:
   a. Using the overhead trapeze.
   b. Placing good foot flat on bed and pushing down while lifting self up on the trapeze.
   c. Avoiding twisting motions.
   d. Avoiding positions that produce pressure on groin, back, chest, and abdomen.

TURNING

1. Move the patient to the side of the bed using a steady, even pulling motion.
2. Place pillows along the other side of the bed—one for the chest and two (lengthwise) for the legs.
3. Instruct the patient to place the arms at the side or above the head.
4. Turn the patient as a unit. Avoid twisting the patient in the cast.
5. Turn the patient toward the leg not encased in plaster or toward the unoperated side if both legs are in plaster.
   a. One nurse stands at other side of bed to receive the patient's shoulders.
   b. Second nurse supports leg in plaster while the third nurse supports the patient's back as he or she is turned.
   c. Turn the patient in body cast to a prone position twice daily—provides postural drainage of bronchial tree; relieves pressure on back.
6. Keep the cast level by elevating the lumbar sacral area with a small pillow when the head of the bed is elevated.

 NURSING ALERT Do not grasp crossbar of spica cast to move the patient. The purpose of the bar is to maintain the integrity of the cast.

OTHER CARE

1. Protect cast from soiling.
   a. Cover perineum with a towel. Tuck 4-inch (10-cm) strips of thin polyethylene sheeting under perineal area of cast and tape to cast exterior. Replace when soiling occurs.
   b. Clean outside of soiled cast with a mild powdered cleanser and a *slightly* dampened or dry, clean cloth and pat dry completely, only when necessary.
2. Roll the patient onto fracture bedpan; use small pillow in lumbosacral area for support.
3. Inspect skin for signs of irritation around cast edge, under cast using a flashlight for illumination.
4. Reach up under the cast and massage accessible skin.
5. Protect the toes from the pressure of the bedding.

NURSING ALERT People at high risk for pulmonary emboli include older adults and persons with previous thromboembolism, obesity, heart failure, or multiple trauma. These patients require prophylaxis against thromboembolism.

Preventing Gastrointestinal Impairment

1. Encourage balanced nutritional intake.
   a. Assess the patient's food preferences. Serve small meals.
   b. Provide natural bowel stimulants (eg, fiber) and good fluid intake.
   c. Monitor bowel movements, bowel sounds, and use a bowel program, if necessary.
2. Observe for symptoms of cast syndrome—nausea, vomiting, abdominal distention, abdominal pain, and decreased bowel sounds.
3. If symptoms of cast syndrome develop, report immediately to the health care provider.
   a. Place the patient in a prone position, if tolerated, to relieve pressure symptoms.
   b. Use nasogastric suction as prescribed.
   c. Maintain electrolyte balance by intravenous (IV) replacement of fluids, as prescribed.
   d. Prepare the patient for removal of the cast or surgical relief of duodenal obstruction, if necessary.

NURSING ALERT Cast syndrome (superior mesenteric artery syndrome) is a rare sequela of body cast application, yet it is a potentially fatal complication. It is important to teach patients about this syndrome because this can develop as late as several weeks after cast application.

Patient Education and Health Maintenance

Neurovascular Status

1. Instruct the patient to check neurovascular status and to control swelling.
   a. Watch for signs and symptoms of circulatory disturbance, including blueness or paleness of fingernails or toenails accompanied by pain and tightness, numbness, cold or tingling sensation.
   b. Elevate the affected extremity and wiggle fingers or toes.
   c. Apply ice bags, as prescribed (one third to one half full), to each side of the cast, making sure they do not make indentations in plaster.
   d. Call the health care provider promptly if excessive swelling, paresthesia, persistent pain, pain on passive stretch, or paralysis occurs.
2. Instruct the patient to alternate ambulation with periods of elevation to the cast when seated. Encourage the patient to lie down several times daily with cast elevated.

Skin Irritation

Advise the patient to prevent skin irritation at the cast edge by padding the edges of the cast with moleskin or "petaling" cast edges with strips of tape.

Exercise

1. Instruct the patient to actively exercise every joint that is not immobilized and to perform isometric exercises (contract muscles without moving joint) of those immobilized to maintain muscle strength and to prevent atrophy.

2. Tell the patient to perform hourly when awake:
    a. Leg cast—push down on the popliteal space, hold it, relax, repeat. Move toes back and forth; bend toes down, then pull them back.
    b. Arm cast—make a fist, hold it, relax, repeat. Move shoulders.
3. Encourage ambulation with weight-bearing restrictions.

Cast Care
1. Advise to avoid getting cast wet, especially padding under cast—causes skin breakdown as plaster cast becomes soft.
2. Warn against covering a leg cast with plastic or rubber boots because this causes condensation and wetting of the cast.
3. Instruct to avoid weight bearing or stress on plaster cast for 24 hours.
4. Instruct to report to the health care provider if the cast cracks or breaks; instruct the patient not to try to fix it.
5. Teach how to clean the cast:
    a. Remove surface soil with slightly damp cloth.
    b. Rub soiled areas with mild powder cleanser and slightly dampened cloth, and then pat dry completely.
    c. Wipe off residual moisture.

Teaching Safety Measures
To prevent falls, avoid walking on wet floors or sidewalks. To prevent pressure and injury to the skin, do not place objects inside the cast.

After Cast Removal
1. Instruct to clean skin with mild soap and water, blot dry, and apply emollient lotion to dry skin.
2. Warn against scratching the skin.
3. Advise to continue prescribed exercises. Gradually resume activities and elevate extremity to control swelling.

Evaluation: Expected Outcomes
- No pain, discoloration, or sensory or motor impairment of affected extremity; warm, with good capillary refill.
- Ambulates with assistance; performing active ROM and isometric exercises every 1 to 2 hours.
- No signs of cast syndrome.

Traction

Traction is the force applied in a specific direction. To apply the force needed to overcome the natural force or pull of muscle groups, a system of ropes, pulleys, and weights is used.

Purposes of Traction
1. To reduce and immobilize fracture.
2. To regain normal length and alignment of an injured extremity.
3. To lessen or eliminate muscle spasm.
4. To prevent deformity.
5. To give the patient freedom for "in-bed" activities.
6. To reduce pain.

Types of Traction
Running Traction
1. A form of traction in which the pull is exerted in one plane.
2. May use either skin or skeletal traction.
3. Buck extension traction (see Figure 32-4) is an example of running skin traction.

Balanced Suspension Traction
1. Uses additional weights to counterbalance the traction force and floats the extremity in the traction apparatus.
2. The line of pull on the extremity remains fairly constant despite changes in the patient's position.

Application of Traction
Traction may be applied to the skin or to the skeletal system.

Skin Traction
1. Accomplished by applying a light force that pulls on tape, sponge rubber, or special device (boot, cervical halter, pelvic belt) that is in contact with the skin.
2. The pulling force is transmitted to the musculoskeletal structures.
3. Skin traction is used as a temporary measure in adults to control muscle spasm and pain.
4. It is used before surgery in the treatment of hip fracture (Buck extension) and femoral shaft fractures (Russell traction).
5. It may be used definitively to treat fractures in children.

Skeletal Traction
See Figure 32-5.
1. Traction applied by the orthopedic surgeon under aseptic conditions using wires, pins, or tongs placed through bones and provides a strong, steady, continuous pull.
2. Skeletal traction is used most frequently in treating fractures of the femur, humerus (supracondylar fractures), tibia, and cervical spine.

Figure 32-4. Buck extension traction. **(A)** Skin traction is accomplished through a boot device in contact with the skin. **(B)** Weight is applied to exert running traction in one plane, while the body acts as a counterweight. (Courtesy Position Health, *www.positionhealth.com*.)

Figure 32-5. Balanced skeletal traction using **(A)** Thomas leg splint and Pearson attachment and **(B)** slings for support and suspension. **(A,** From Smeltzer, S., & Bare, B. [2000]. *Brunner and Suddarth's textbook of medical-surgical nursing* [9th ed.]. Philadelphia, PA: Lippincott Williams & Wilkins. **B,** Hinkle, J.L., and Cheever, K.H. [2017]. *Brunner and Suddarth's textbook of medical-surgical nursing* [14th ed.]. Philadelphia, PA: Lippincott Williams & Wilkins.)

Complications

1. Infection of pin tracts in skeletal traction.
2. Skin breakdown and dermatitis under skin traction.
3. Neurovascular compromise resulting in increased pain, muscle spasms, numbness, tingling, and loss of sensation.
4. Inadequate fracture alignment resulting in posttreatment arthritis.
5. Complications of immobility include the following:
   a. Stasis pneumonia.
   b. Thrombophlebitis.
   c. Pressure ulcers.
   d. Urinary infection and calculi.
   e. Constipation.

Nursing Assessment

1. Assess for pain, deformity, swelling, motor and sensory function, and circulatory status of the affected extremity.
2. Assess skin condition of the affected extremity, under skin traction and around skeletal traction, as well as over bony prominences throughout the body.
3. Assess for alignment of the affected body part.
4. Assess for signs and symptoms of complications.
5. Assess traction equipment for safety and effectiveness.
   a. The patient is placed on a firm mattress.
   b. The ropes and the pulleys should be in alignment.
   c. The pull should be in line with the long axis of the bone.
   d. Any factor that might reduce the pull or alter its direction must be eliminated.
      i. Weights should hang freely.
      ii. Ropes should be unobstructed and not in contact with the bed or equipment.
      iii. The patient's bed should have an overhead trapeze set up to assist the patient to pull self up in bed at frequent intervals.
   e. The amount of weight applied in skin traction must not exceed the tolerance of the skin. The condition of the skin must be inspected frequently.
   f. Cover exposed sharp ends of skeletal pins with cork or other pin covering to protect the patient and caregivers from injury.
6. Assess emotional reaction to condition and traction.
7. Assess understanding of the treatment plan.

 NURSING ALERT Traction is *not* accomplished if the knot in the rope or the footplate is touching the pulley or the foot of the bed or if the weights are resting on the floor. Never remove the weights when repositioning the patient who is in skeletal traction because this will interrupt the line of pull and cause the patient considerable pain.

Nursing Diagnoses

• Impaired Physical Mobility related to traction therapy and underlying pathology.
• Risk for Impaired Skin Integrity related to pressure on soft tissues.
• Risk for Infection related to bacterial invasion at skeletal traction site.
• Risk for Peripheral Neurovascular Dysfunction related to injury or traction therapy.

Nursing Interventions

Minimizing the Effects of Immobility

1. Encourage active exercise of uninvolved muscles and joints to maintain strength and function. Dorsiflex feet hourly to avoid development of footdrop and aid in venous return.
2. Encourage deep breathing hourly to facilitate expansion of lungs and movement of respiratory secretions.
3. Auscultate lung fields at least twice per day.
4. Encourage fluid intake of 2,000 to 2,500 mL daily.
5. Provide balanced high-fiber diet rich in protein; avoid excessive calcium intake.
6. Establish bowel routine through the use of diet and stool softeners, laxatives, and enemas, as prescribed.
7. Prevent pressure on the calf and evaluate twice daily for the development of thrombophlebitis.
8. Check traction apparatus at repeated intervals—the traction must be continuous to be effective, unless prescribed as intermittent, as with pelvic traction.
   a. With *running traction*, the patient may not be turned without disrupting the line of pull.
   b. With *balanced suspension traction*, the patient may be elevated, turned slightly, and moved as desired.
9. Use SCDs and compression stockings, as indicated.
10. Administer prophylactic anticoagulants, as prescribed.

 NURSING ALERT Every complaint of the patient in traction should be investigated immediately to prevent injury.

Maintaining Skin Integrity

1. Examine bony prominences frequently for evidence of pressure or friction irritation.
2. Observe for skin irritation around the traction bandage.
3. Observe for pressure at traction–skin contact points.
4. Report complaint of burning sensation under traction.
5. Relieve pressure without disrupting traction effectiveness.
   a. Make sure that linens and clothing are wrinkle free.

b. Use lambs' wool pads, heel and elbow protectors, and special mattresses, as needed.
6. Special care must be given to the back every 2 hours because the patient maintains a supine position.
   a. Have the patient use trapeze to pull self up and relieve back pressure.
   b. Provide backrubs.

Avoiding Infection at Pin Site

1. Monitor vital signs for fever or tachycardia.
2. Watch for signs of infection, especially around the pin tract.
   a. The pin should be immobile in the bone, and the skin surrounding the wound should be dry. Small amount of serous oozing from pin site may occur.
   b. If infection is suspected, percuss gently over the tibia; this may elicit pain if infection is developing.
   c. Assess for other signs of infection: heat, redness, fever.
3. If directed, clean the pin tract with sterile applicators and prescribed solution or ointment (ie, normal saline, sterile water, chlorhexidine)—to clear drainage at the entrance of tract and around the pin because plugging at this site can predispose to bacterial invasion of the tract and bone.

Preventing Neurovascular Injury

1. Assess motor and sensory function of specific nerves that might be compromised.
   a. Peroneal nerve—have the patient point the great toe toward the nose; check sensation on the dorsum of the foot; presence of footdrop.
   b. Radial nerve—have the patient extend the thumb; check sensation in the web between the thumb and index finger.
   c. Median nerve—thumb–middle finger apposition; check sensation of index finger.
2. Determine adequacy of circulation (eg, color, temperature, motion, capillary refill of peripheral fingers or toes).
   a. With Buck traction, inspect the foot for circulatory difficulties within a few minutes and then periodically after the elastic bandage has been applied.
3. Report promptly if change in neurovascular status is identified.

Patient Education and Health Maintenance

1. Teach the patient the purpose of traction therapy.
2. Delineate limitations of activity necessary to maintain effective traction.
3. Teach the use of patient aids (eg, trapeze).
4. Instruct the patient not to adjust or modify traction apparatus.
5. Instruct the patient in activities designed to minimize effects of immobility on body systems.
6. Teach the patient necessity for reporting changes in sensations, pain, movement.

Evaluation: Expected Outcomes

- Exercises as instructed; deep breaths hourly; fluid intake 2,000 to 2,500 mL/24 hours.
- No signs of skin breakdown under traction bandage or over bony prominences.
- No drainage, redness, or odor at pin site.
- No motor or sensory impairment; good capillary refill, color, and warmth of extremity.

External Fixation

External fixation is a technique of fracture immobilization in which a series of transfixing pins is inserted through bone and attached to a rigid

Figure 32-6. External fixation device used for reduction and immobilization of open fracture, allowing treatment of soft tissue wounds. (From Smeltzer, S., & Bare, B. [2000]. *Brunner and Suddarth's textbook of medical-surgical nursing* [9th ed.]. Philadelphia, PA: Lippincott Williams & Wilkins.)

external metal frame (see Figure 32-6). The method is used mainly in the management of open fractures with severe soft tissue damage.

Advantages

1. Permits rigid support of severely comminuted open fractures, infected nonunions, and infected unstable joints.
2. Facilitates wound care (frequent debridements, irrigations, dressing changes) and soft tissue reconstruction (delayed wound closure, muscle flaps, skin grafts).
3. Allows early function of muscles and joints.
4. Allows early patient comfort.

Circular Fixators

Purpose

May be used for limb lengthening, correction of angulation and rotation defects, and in treatment of nonunion.

Components

1. This fixator apparatus consists of through-the-bone tension wires placed above and below the treatment site.
2. The wires are attached to fixator rings surrounding the limb.
3. The rings are connected to one another by telescoping rods.

Management

1. Adjustments are made daily at about 1 mm/day, stimulating callus and bone formation.
2. Patient compliance is essential.
3. Weight bearing is encouraged.
4. When the desired length or correction is achieved, the fixator is left in place without further adjustment until bone healing occurs.

Application of External Fixator

1. Under general anesthesia, the skin is cleaned and transfixing pins are inserted into the bone through small incisions above and below the fracture.
2. After reduction of the fracture, the appliance is stabilized by adjusting and tightening the bars connecting the sets of pins.
3. The sharp pinheads are covered with plastic, cork, or rubber covers to protect the other extremity and caregivers.

Nursing Assessment

1. Determine the patient's understanding of procedure and fixation device.
2. Evaluate neurovascular status of involved body part.
3. Inspect each pin site for redness, drainage, tenderness, pain, and loosening of the pin.
4. Inspect open wounds for healing, infection, or devitalized tissue.
5. Assess functioning of other body systems affected by injury or immobilization.

Nursing Diagnoses

- Anxiety related to appearance of external fixation device and wound.
- Risk for Peripheral Neurovascular Dysfunction related to swelling, fixator, and underlying condition.
- Risk for Infection related to open injury and skeletal pin insertion.
- Impaired Physical Mobility related to presence of fixator and condition.

Nursing Interventions

Relieving Anxiety

1. If possible, before placement of the device, reassure the patient that, although the fixator appears clumsy and cumbersome, it should not hurt once it is in place.
2. Emphasize the positive aspects of this device in treating complex musculoskeletal problems.
3. Encourage the patient to verbalize reaction to the device.
4. Inform the patient that greater mobility can be achieved with an external fixation device, thereby minimizing the development of other system problems.
5. Involve the patient in care and in the management of external fixator.

Maintaining Intact Neurovascular Status

1. Assess neurovascular status frequently—every 15 minutes to 1 hour while swelling is significant and later, every 2 to 8 hours.
2. Establish baseline of functioning for comparative monitoring. Complex musculoskeletal injuries frequently result in disruption of soft tissue functioning.
3. Elevate extremity to reduce swelling.
4. Report any change in neurovascular status.

 NURSING ALERT Assess neurovascular status frequently and record findings. Report abnormal findings or change in status.

Preventing Infection

1. Provide site and fixator care.
   a. Clean pin sites and remove crusts with sterile cotton applicator, using solution as prescribed, or established standard of care.
      i. Crusts formed by serous drainage can prevent fluid from draining and can cause infection.
      ii. A small amount of serous drainage from the pin sites is normal.
   b. Note and report inflammation, swelling, tenderness, and purulent drainage at pin site.
   c. Note skin tension at pin site—tension can cause discomfort.
   d. Report loosened pins.
   e. Clean fixator with clean cloth and water, as needed.
2. Provide wound care.
   a. The open wounds at the fracture site are usually treated by daily dressing changes.
   b. Use sterile technique.
   c. Note wound appearance. Monitor healing. Report signs of infection.
3. Monitor for local and systemic indicators of infection.

Encouraging Mobility

1. Encourage the patient to participate in care activities.
2. Assure the patient that pain associated with injury will diminish as tissue reactions to injury and manipulation resolve and healing progresses.
3. Inform the patient that the external fixator maintains the fracture in a stable position and that the extremity can be moved. Adjustment of the fixator is done by the health care provider. (The patient is taught how to adjust the circular fixator.)
4. To move the extremity, do not grasp the frame, rather support the entire extremity and assist the patient to move. Reassure the patient that the fixator can withstand normal movement.
5. Teach quadriceps exercises and ROM exercises for joints; usually started on first postoperative day.
6. Teach crutch walking when soft tissue swelling has diminished; encourage weight bearing, as prescribed.

Patient Education and Health Maintenance

1. Instruct the patient to inspect around each pin site daily for signs of infection and loosening of pins. Watch for pain, soft tissue swelling, and drainage.
2. Teach the patient how to clean around each pin daily, using aseptic technique. Do not touch the wound with hands.
3. Advise the patient to clean the fixator regularly—to keep it free of dust and contamination.
4. Warn against tampering with clamps or nuts—can alter compression and misalign fracture.
5. Review weight bearing and other restrictions associated with injury and treatment regimen.
6. Encourage the patient to follow rehabilitation regimen.

Evaluation: Expected Outcomes

- Verbalizes understanding of and comfort with fixator device.
- Swelling relieved; neurovascular status intact.
- No drainage or signs of infection at pin sites; pin tracts remain intact, no loosening of pins.
- Ambulating with ambulatory device, as directed.

Orthopedic Surgery

 EVIDENCE BASE National Association for Orthopaedic Nursing. (2017). *Orthopaedic Surgery Manual*, (3rd ed.). Chicago, IL: Author.

Types of Surgery

1. Open reduction—reduction and alignment of the fracture through surgical incision.
2. Closed reduction—manipulation of bone fragments or joint dislocation without surgical incision.
3. Internal fixation—stabilization of the reduced fracture with the use of metal screw, plates, nails, or pins.
4. Bone graft—placement of autologous or homologous bone tissue to replace, promote healing of, or stabilize diseased bone.
5. Arthroplasty—repair of a joint through realignment or reconstruction; may be done through arthroscope (arthroscopy) or open joint repair.
6. Joint replacement—type of arthroplasty that involves replacement of joint surfaces with metal or plastic materials.
7. Total joint replacement—replacement of both articular surfaces within a joint.
8. Meniscectomy—excision of damaged meniscus (fibrocartilage) of the knee.
9. Tendon transfer—movement of tendon insertion point to improve function.
10. Fasciotomy—cutting muscle fascia to relieve constriction or contracture.
11. Amputation—removal of a body part.

Note: Joint replacement and amputation will be covered separately.

Preoperative Management

1. Hydration, protein, and caloric intake are assessed. The goal is to maximize healing and reduce risk of complications by providing IV fluids, vitamins, and nutritional supplements, as indicated.
2. Medications, including prescribed, OTC, and herbals, are reviewed, and the patient is instructed on which medications should be held prior to surgery and for how long.
   a. Aspirin, anti-inflammatories, anticoagulants, and anti-platelet agents that may affect clotting may be held for up to a week prior to surgery.
   b. If the patient has had previous corticosteroid therapy, it could contribute to current orthopedic condition (aseptic necrosis of the femoral head, osteoporosis) as well as affect the patient's response to anesthesia and the stress of surgery. History of corticosteroid therapy must be documented.
   c. Metformin is usually held for 48 hours prior to surgery to prevent lactic acidosis due to fasting, a rare complication.
   d. Antidepressants, particularly monoamine oxidase inhibitors, and herbals should be explored for interaction with anesthetics.
3. Signs of infection (respiratory, dental, skin, urinary), which could contribute to development of osteomyelitis after surgery, are ruled out.
4. Coughing and deep breathing, frequent vital sign and wound checks, repositioning are described to prepare the patient.
5. Prepare the patient for voiding in bedpan or urinal in recumbent position before surgery, if indicated. This helps reduce the need for postoperative catheterization.
6. The patient is acquainted with traction apparatus and the need for splint or cast, as indicated by type of surgery.
7. Type and cross-match is ordered if there is a potential need for the patient to receive blood products. Autologous blood donation may be done several weeks before surgery.
8. Discharge planning is begun prior to surgery with plan for rehabilitation options postoperatively.

 GERONTOLOGIC ALERT Many older patients are at risk for poor healing due to poor nutritional status. Suggest obtaining albumin, prealbumin, and transferrin evaluation and nutrition consult in advance of surgery.

Postoperative Management

1. Neurovascular status is monitored, and swelling caused by edema and bleeding into tissues (causing a hematoma) should be assessed and controlled.
2. The affected area is immobilized and activity limited to protect the operative site and stabilize musculoskeletal structures.
3. Hemorrhage is watched for to prevent hypovolemic shock, which may result from significant blood loss.
4. Complications of immobility are prevented through aggressive and vigilant postoperative care. Deconditioning is limited through isometric and isotonic exercises.

Complications

1. Compartment syndrome.
2. Blood loss, shock, anemia.
3. Atelectasis and pneumonia.
4. Osteomyelitis, wound infections.
5. Venous thromboembolic events.
6. Fat embolus.

Nursing Diagnoses

- Risk for Deficient Fluid Volume related to hemorrhage.
- Ineffective Breathing Pattern related to effects of anesthesia, analgesics, and immobility.
- Risk for Peripheral Neurovascular Dysfunction related to swelling.
- Acute Pain related to surgical intervention.
- Risk for Infection related to surgical intervention.
- Impaired Physical Mobility related to immobilization therapy and pain.
- Imbalanced Nutrition: Less Than Body Requirements related to blood loss and the demands of healing and immobility.

Nursing Interventions

Monitoring for Shock and Hemorrhage

1. Evaluate BP and pulse rates frequently—rising pulse rate, widening pulse pressure, or slowly falling BP indicate persistent bleeding or development of a state of shock.
2. Monitor for hemorrhage—orthopedic wounds have a tendency to ooze more than do other surgical wounds.
   a. Measure suction drainage, if used.
   b. Anticipate up to 500 mL of drainage in the first 24 hours, decreasing to less than 30 mL/8 hours within 48 hours, depending on surgical procedure.
   c. Report increased wound drainage or steady increase in pain of the operative area.
3. Administer IV fluids and blood products, as ordered.

Promoting Effective Breathing Pattern

1. Give respiratory depressant drugs cautiously. Monitor respiration depth and rate frequently. Opioid analgesic effects may be cumulative.
2. Change position every 2 hours—mobilizes secretions and helps prevent bronchial obstruction.
3. Encourage the use of incentive spirometer and coughing and deep-breathing exercises every 2 hours.
4. Auscultate the lungs for atelectasis and retention of secretions.

Monitoring Peripheral Neurovascular Status

1. Monitor circulation distal to the part where cast, bandage, or splint has been applied.
2. Prevent constriction leading to interference with blood or nerve supply.
3. Elevate affected extremity and apply covered ice packs, as directed, to reduce swelling and bleeding into tissues.
4. Observe toes and fingers for healthy color and good capillary refill.
5. Check pulses of affected extremity; compare with unaffected extremity.
6. Note skin temperature and sensation.
7. Document observations.

 NURSING ALERT If neurovascular problems are identified, loosen cast or dressing at once and notify surgeon.

Relieving Pain

1. Institute comfort measures, as prescribed, as well as nursing measures, as indicated: backrubs; soft light; soft, tranquil music.
2. Be aware that muscle spasms may contribute to discomfort.
3. Use patient-controlled analgesia according to standards of care.
4. Facilitate progression from IV medications to by mouth when tolerated.
5. Prevent constipation due to opioids by obtaining order for bowel regimen and instituting diet regimen.

Preventing Infection

1. Monitor vital signs for fever, tachycardia, or increased respiratory rate, which may indicate infection.
2. Examine incision for redness, increased temperature, swelling, and induration. Document findings.
3. Note and document character of drainage.
4. Evaluate complaints of recurrent or increasing discomfort.
5. Administer antibiotic therapy, as prescribed.
6. Maintain aseptic technique for dressing changes and wound care.

Minimizing the Effects of Immobility

1. Encourage the patient to exercise by self with a planned program of exercise as soon as possible after surgery.
2. Have the patient exercise the unaffected extremity (unless instructed by physical therapist to exercise affected extremity as well): flex knee, extend the knee with hip still flexed, and then lower the extremity to the bed. Passive motion devices may be used to maintain ROM.
3. Encourage the patient to move fingers and toes hourly.
4. Advise the patient to move joints that are not fixed by traction or appliance through their ROM as fully as possible.
5. Suggest muscle-setting exercises (quadriceps setting) if active motion is contraindicated.
6. Apply antiembolism stockings, foot pumps, or SCDs as prescribed by the surgeon.
7. Give prophylactic anticoagulants as directed (eg, heparin, warfarin, aspirin, a low molecular weight heparin).
8. Encourage early resumption of activity.

Providing Adequate Nutrition

1. Provide a balanced diet and increase fluids and fiber to promote healing and reduce incidence of constipation associated with immobility.
2. Encourage a high-iron diet and administer blood products and iron supplements to counteract significant blood loss, as directed.
3. Monitor hemoglobin and hematocrit levels. Report below-normal results to the health care provider.

4. Watch for signs and symptoms of anemia, especially after fracture of long bones:
   a. Fatigue.
   b. Shortness of breath.
   c. Pallor.
   d. Tachycardia.
5. Maintain good fluid intake and urinary output to prevent infection and calculi. Watch for urinary retention—especially in older men with some degree of prostatism who may have difficulty voiding.

Patient Education and Health Maintenance

1. Teach the patient activities that will minimize the development of complications (eg, turning, ankle pumps, antiembolism stockings, SCDs, coughing, and deep breathing, early mobilization as able).
2. Instruct the patient in dietary considerations to facilitate healing and minimize development of constipation and renal calculi.
3. Inform the patient of techniques that facilitate moving while minimizing associated discomforts (eg, supporting injured area and practicing smooth, gentle position changes).
4. Encourage long-term follow-up and physical therapy (PT) exercises, as prescribed, to regain maximum functional potential.

 TRANSITIONAL CARE ALERT When working with musculoskeletal patients, the main focus is the return of function to one's previous physical condition. Upon discharge from the hospital, equipment will be necessary for assistance at home, as well as the help of a caregiver to provide support and safety. Help prepare the patient and caregiver by teaching safe body mechanics and use of mobility aids. Facilitate referrals for durable medical equipment, home health nursing and therapy services, and ongoing caregiver education and support through community resources to help prevent complications and reduce the risk of readmission.

Evaluation: Expected Outcomes

- BP stable; drainage from wound less than 30 mL.
- Respirations, deep; performing effective deep breathing and coughing every 2 hours.
- Extremity beyond operative site neurovascularly intact.
- Verbalizes decreased pain.
- Afebrile; incision without drainage.
- Ambulating as directed.
- Eats a balanced diet high in iron; hemoglobin within normal range.

Arthroplasty and Total Joint Replacement

Arthroplasty is reconstructive surgery to restore joint motion and function and to relieve pain. It generally involves replacement of bony joint structure by a prosthesis. *Total joint arthroplasty* is the replacement of both articular surfaces with metal or plastic components. The most common types of joint replacement (see Figure 32-7) include the following:

Total hip arthroplasty—replacement of a severely damaged hip with an artificial joint. A large number of implants are available, often with a metal femoral component topped by a spherical ball fitted into a plastic acetabular socket. Surgical approach is anterior (muslce sparing) or posterior (involves cutting and reattachment of muscles and longer healing time).

Acetabular
(pelvic) component

Femoral (distal)
component

Femoral
(proximal)
component

Tibial component

Figure 32-7. Hip and knee replacement. (From Smeltzer, S., & Bare, B. [2000]. *Brunner and Suddarth's textbook of medical-surgical nursing* [9th ed.]. Philadelphia, PA: Lippincott Williams & Wilkins.)

Total knee arthroplasty—implant procedure in which tibial, femoral, and patellar joint surfaces are replaced because of destroyed knee joint.

Total shoulder arthroplasty—replacement of the humeral head and the glenoid surface with prostheses.

Clinical Indications

1. For patients with unremitting pain and irreversibly damaged joints:
   a. Primary OA.
   b. Rheumatoid arthritis (RA).
2. Selected fractures (eg, femoral neck fracture).
3. Failure of previous reconstructive surgery (osteotomy, cup arthroplasty, femoral neck fracture complications—nonunion, avascular necrosis).
4. Congenital hip disease.
5. Pathologic fractures from metastatic cancer.
6. Joint instability.

Considerations

1. The prostheses are of various designs and may be fixed to the remaining bone by cement, press fit, or bone ingrowth.
2. Selection of the prosthesis and fixation technique depends on the patient's bone structure, joint stability, and other individual characteristics, including age, weight, and activity level.
3. Arthroplasty is an exacting and meticulous procedure. To reduce the risk of an infected prosthesis, special precautions are carried out in the operating room (impermeable operating room attire, clean air system) to reduce particulate matter and bacterial count of the air.

Preoperative Management

1. Infections (urinary, dental, skin, respiratory) are ruled out or treated because they are potential foci of infection for seeding prosthesis infection.
2. Preoperative patient teaching is provided.
   a. Postoperative regimen (eg, extended exercise program) that will be carried out after surgery is explained; atrophied muscles must be reeducated and strengthened.
   b. Isometric exercises (muscle setting) of quadriceps and gluteal muscles are taught.
   c. Bed-to-wheelchair transfer without going beyond the hip flexion limits (usually 60 to 90 degrees) is taught.
   d. Non–weight- and partial weight-bearing walking with ambulatory aid (walker, crutches) is taught to facilitate postoperative ambulation.
   e. Abduction splint, knee immobilizer, or continuous passive motion is demonstrated if equipment will be used postoperatively.
3. Antiembolism stockings are applied to minimize development of thrombophlebitis.
4. Skin preparation includes antimicrobial solution to reduce skin microorganisms, a potential source of infection.
5. Antibiotics are administered timely, as prescribed, to ensure therapeutic blood level during and immediately after surgery. Antimicrobials usually are given immediately preoperatively, intraoperatively, and postoperatively to reduce incidence of infection.
6. Cardiovascular, respiratory, renal, and hepatic function are assessed, and measures are taken to maximize general health condition.
7. Discharge planning is begun, including rehabilitation options postoperatively.

Postoperative Management

Use of Appropriate Positioning

To prevent dislocation of prosthesis and facilitate healing, numerous modifications are required in positioning these patients postoperatively.

1. After hip arthroplasty (posterior approach):
   a. The patient is usually positioned supine in bed.
   b. The affected extremity is held in slight abduction by either an abduction splint or pillow or Buck extension traction to prevent dislocation of the prosthesis.
   c. Two nurses turn the patient on the unoperated side while supporting the operated hip securely in an abducted position; the entire length of leg is supported by pillows.
      i. Use pillows to keep the leg abducted; place pillow at back for comfort.
      ii. If the bed is equipped, use overhead trapeze to assist with position changes.
   d. The bed is usually not elevated more than 45 to 60 degrees; placing the patient in an upright sitting position puts a strain on the hip joint and may cause dislocation.
   e. A fracture bedpan is used. Instruct the patient to flex the unoperated hip and knee and pull up on the trapeze to lift buttocks onto pan. Instruct the patient *not* to bear down on the operated hip in flexion when getting off the pan.
2. Following anterior hip arthroplasty, the patient can flex the hip and bear weight often within hours. Restrictive positioning is not necessary to prevent dislocation.
3. After knee arthroplasty:
   a. The knee may be immobilized in extension with a firm compression dressing and an adjustable soft extension splint or long-leg plaster cast.

b. Leg is elevated to control swelling being mindful to assure that there is nothing causing the knee to remain bent if it is not in an immobilizer.

c. Alternatively, continuous passive motion may be started to facilitate joint healing and restoration of joint ROM.

 NURSING ALERT The patient must not adduct the hip or flex it beyond recommended degree, as indicated by the surgeon, as this may lead to subluxation or dislocation of the hip. Signs of joint dislocation include shortened extremity, increasing discomfort, inability to move joints.

Deterring Complications

1. Aggressive care and frequent assessment can reduce the complication rate.
2. Prevent thromboembolism by continuous use of elastic hose and SCD while the patient is in bed. Discontinue SCD when the patient is ambulatory.
3. C-reactive protein and erythrocyte sedimentation rate (ESR) can be used to quantify the risk of periprosthetic joint infection. High serum levels indicate a high risk of infection and require further diagnostic testing or biopsy.

Promoting Early Ambulation

1. Ambulation may begin on the day of surgery or the first postoperative day.
2. Transfers to the chair or ambulation with aids, such as walkers, are encouraged as tolerated and based on the patient's condition and type of prosthesis.
3. Caution is taken in moving the patient to upright position, and the patient is monitored for orthostatic hypotension.

Nursing Diagnoses

Also see "Orthopedic Surgery," page 869.

• Impaired Physical Mobility related to prosthetic joint.

Nursing Interventions

Also see page 869.

Promoting Mobility

After posterior hip arthroplasty:
1. Use an abduction splint or pillows while assisting the patient out of bed.
   a. Keep the hip at maximum extension.
   b. Instruct the patient to pivot on unoperated extremity.
   c. Assess the patient for orthostatic hypotension.
2. When ready to ambulate, teach the patient to advance the walker and then advance the operated extremity to the walker, permitting weight bearing, as prescribed.
3. With increased stability, assist the patient to use crutches or cane, as prescribed.
4. Encourage practice of PT exercises to strengthen muscles and prevent contractures.
5. Encourage bed mobility by providing an overhead frame/trapeze.

After knee arthroplasty:
1. Assist the patient with transfer out of bed into wheelchair with extension splint in place, if applicable.
2. Encourage weight bearing, as directed by the surgeon.
3. Apply continuous passive motion equipment or carry out passive ROM exercises, as prescribed.

Community and Home Care Considerations

1. Encourage the patient to continue to wear compression stockings after discharge until full activities are resumed.
2. Ensure that the patient avoids excessive hip adduction, flexion, and rotation for 6 weeks after hip arthroplasty (posterior hip precautions).
   a. Avoid sitting in a low chair or toilet seat to avoid flexing the hip more than 90 degrees.
   b. Keep the knees apart; do not cross the legs.
   c. Limit sitting to 30 minutes at a time—to minimize hip flexion and the risk of prosthetic dislocation and to prevent hip stiffness and flexion contracture.
   d. Avoid internal rotation of the hip.
   e. Follow weight-bearing restrictions from the surgeon.
3. Encourage quadriceps setting and ROM exercises, as directed.
   a. Have a daily program of stretching, exercise, and rest throughout lifetime.
   b. Do not participate in any activity placing undue or sudden stress on joint (jogging, jumping, lifting heavy loads, gaining weight, excessive bending and twisting).
   c. Use a cane when taking fairly long walks.
4. Suggest self-help and energy-saving devices.
   a. Handrails by toilet.
   b. Raised toilet seat if there is some residual hip flexion problem.
   c. Bar-type stool for kitchen work.
   d. Occupational therapy (OT) devices for dressing, reaching.
   e. Adequate home lighting to prevent falls.
   f. Removal of scatter rugs.
5. Advise the patient to sleep with two pillows between legs to prevent turning over in sleep. The patient should get out of bed with nonoperative leg.
6. Tell the patient to lie prone when able twice daily for 30 minutes to promote full extension of hip.
7. Monitor for late complications—deep infection, increased pain or decreased function associated with loosening of prosthetic components, implant wear, dislocation, fracture of components, avascular necrosis or dead bone caused by loss of blood supply; heterotrophic ossification (formation of bone in periprosthetic space).
8. Assess home for safety to prevent falls—long phone cords, scatter rugs, pets that run underfoot, slippery floors.

Patient Education and Health Maintenance

1. Teach the patient use of supportive equipment, such as walkers and raised toilet seat, as prescribed.
2. Advise the patient to notify all health care providers about prosthetic joint because prophylactic antibiotic (to prevent implant infection) will be needed prior to other surgical procedures or any procedure known to cause bacteremia (tooth extraction, manipulation of genitourinary tract). Patients with inflammatory arthropathies, immunosuppressive therapies, and immunocompromising conditions are especially at risk.

 EVIDENCE BASE American Association of Orthopaedic Surgeons and American Dental Association. (2012). *Prevention of orthopaedic implant infection in patients undergoing dental procedures: Evidence-based guideline and evidence report.* Rosemont, IL: Author.

3. Avoid MRI studies because of implanted metal component.
4. Advise the patient that metal component in hip or knee may set off metal detectors (airports, some buildings). The patient should carry a medical identification card.

5. New hip or knee is designed for low-impact exercise, such as walking, golf, dancing. High-impact exercises, such as jogging, may cause the prosthesis to loosen.

Evaluation: Expected Outcomes

- Maintains proper positioning without evidence of complications.

Amputation

Amputation is the total or partial surgical removal of digits, foot, lower leg, or forearm. Amputation is considered a surgical reconstructive procedure.

Indications

1. Inadequate tissue perfusion caused by peripheral vascular diseases.
2. Severe trauma.
3. Malignant tumor.
4. Congenital deformity.
5. Osteomyelitis/infection.

Types of Amputation

Open (Guillotine)

1. Used with infection and for patients who are poor surgical risks.
2. Wound heals by granulation over time or secondary closure 1 week later.

Closed (Myoplastic or Flap)

1. Residual limb is covered by a flap of skin.
2. Flap of skin is sutured posteriorly.
3. Most common technique used for vascular disease.

Surgical Considerations

1. The surgeon considers possible limb-salvage techniques.
   a. Revascularization (research is focusing on angiogenesis and stem cell therapy).
   b. Hyperbaric oxygenation.
   c. Tumor resection with bone grafting.
2. Determines level for amputation based on level of maximal viable tissue for wound healing.
3. Develops a functional, nontender, pressure-tolerant residual limb.

Types of Dressings

Soft Dressing

1. Secured with elastic bandage.
2. Permits wound inspection.
3. Used with patients who should avoid early weight bearing (eg, those with peripheral vascular disease).

Closed, Rigid Plaster Dressing

1. Applied immediately after surgery (ie, immediate postoperative prosthesis).
2. Controls edema.
3. Supports circulation, promoting healing.
4. Minimizes pain on movement.
5. Shapes residual limb.
6. Permits attachment of prosthetic extension (pylon) and early ambulation.

Preoperative Management

1. Hemodynamic evaluation is performed through testing, such as angiography, arterial blood flow, and xenon 133 scan, to determine optimal amputation level.

2. Culture and sensitivity tests of draining wounds are done to assist in control of infection preoperatively.
3. Evaluation of contralateral extremity is performed to determine functional potential postoperatively.
4. Evaluation of cardiovascular, respiratory, renal, and other body systems is necessary to determine preoperative condition of the patient and reduce the risks of surgery by optimizing function.
5. Nutritional status is evaluated and optimized with adequate protein to enhance wound healing.
6. Exercises are taught to strengthen muscles for the use of ambulatory aids (lower-limb amputee).
   a. Flex and extend arms while holding traction weights.
   b. Do push-ups from a prone position, if feasible.
   c. Do sit-ups from a seated position, if feasible.
7. Use of ambulatory aids taught to maintain mobility, prepare for postoperative status, and instill confidence in ability.
8. Phantom sensation is explained—the patient will continue to "feel" the amputated body part for some time.
9. Emotional support is given.
   a. Support concept of amputation as a surgical reconstructive procedure.
   b. Explore the patient's perception of procedure and effect on lifestyle.
   c. Avoid unrealistic and misleading reassurance—management of prosthesis can be slow and painful.

 GERONTOLOGIC ALERT Amputation of the lower extremity can be a life-threatening procedure, especially in patients older than age 60 with peripheral vascular disease. Significant morbidity accompanies above-knee amputations because of associated poor health and disease as well as the complications of sepsis and malnutrition and the physiologic insult of amputation.

Postoperative Management

1. The extremity should be in full extension and may be elevated, if possible. An extension splint/immobilizer may be indicated.
2. Complications are monitored—hemorrhage, infection, unrelieved phantom pain, nonhealing wound.
3. Rehabilitation is initiated through PT and prosthetic fitting, if indicated.
4. Optimal treatment is provided for diabetes mellitus, heart disease, infection, stroke, chronic obstructive pulmonary disease, peripheral vascular disease, and age-related deterioration, which are factors limiting rehabilitation.
5. If wound breakdown, infection, or delay in healing of residual limb occurs, therapy is provided to prevent delay in rehabilitation.
6. Acceptance of body image change is promoted.

Nursing Diagnoses

- **Risk for Deficient Fluid Volume** related to hemorrhage from disrupted surgical homeostasis.
- **Ineffective Tissue Perfusion** related to edema and tissue responses to surgery and prosthesis.
- **Ineffective Coping** related to change in body image.
- **Acute Pain** related to surgical procedure.
- **Impaired Physical Mobility** related to amputation, muscle weakness, alteration in body weight distribution.

Nursing Interventions

 NURSING ALERT Prevention of complications associated with a major operation and facilitation of early rehabilitation are essential to prevent prolonged disability. Frequent monitoring of the patient's physiologic responses to anesthesia, surgery, and immobility is required.

Monitoring Fluid Balance

1. Monitor the patient for systemic symptoms of excessive blood loss—hypotension, widening pulse pressure, tachycardia, diaphoresis, decreased level of consciousness.
2. Watch for excessive wound drainage.
   a. Keep tourniquet (in view) attached to end of bed to apply to residual limb (stump) if excessive bleeding occurs.
   b. Reinforce dressing, as required, using aseptic technique.
   c. Measure suction drainage.
   d. Maintain accurate record of bloody drainage on dressing and in drainage system.
3. Monitor intake and output for fluid balance.

Maintaining Adequate Tissue Perfusion

1. Control edema.
   a. Elevate residual limb to promote venous return.
   b. Use air splint, if prescribed.
2. Maintain pressure dressing.
   a. Reapply, if necessary, using sterile dressing secured with elastic bandage.
   b. Notify the surgeon if rigid cast dressing comes off.

Supporting Effective Coping

1. Accept patient responses to the loss of body part (ie, depression, withdrawal, denial, frustration).
2. Encourage expression of fears and concerns.
3. Recognize that modification of body image takes time.
4. Encourage participation in rehabilitation planning and self-care.
5. Assist the patient to adapt to changes in self-care activities.
   a. Upper-extremity amputation—encourage independence in one-handed self-care activities using one-handed aids (eg, one-handed knife), as needed.
   b. Lower-extremity amputation—encourage mobility using transfer assistance and ambulatory aids, as needed.

Controlling Pain

1. Surgical pain.
   a. Assess the patient's pain experience.
   b. Administer prescribed medications, as needed, to control postoperative pain.
   c. Use nonpharmaceutical pain-management techniques, such as progressive muscle relaxation and imagery.
   d. Recognize that increasing discomfort may indicate presence of hematoma, infection, or necrosis.
2. Phantom sensations (pain).
   a. Anticipate complaint of pain and sensation located in the missing limb ("phantom pain").
   b. The use of adjunctive pain medications may be prescribed, such as gabapentin.
   c. Use physical modalities (eg, wrapping, temperature changes) and transcutaneous electrical nerve stimulation (TENS), if prescribed, in relieving discomfort.
   d. Encourage patient activity to decrease awareness of phantom limb pain.
   e. Reassure the patient that phantom limb pain will diminish over time.
   f. Patients may benefit from cognitive behavioral therapy to assist in pain management. Virtual reality–based interventions may also be effective.

Promoting Physical Activity

1. Encourage frequent repositioning in bed.
2. Teach the patient to avoid long periods in one position.
   a. Avoids dependent edema.
   b. Avoids flexion deformity.
   c. Avoids skin pressure areas.
3. Prevent deformities.
   a. Lower-extremity amputations—hip flexion contracture (avoid placing residual limb on pillow; encourage prone position twice per day) and abduction deformity (use trochanter roll; avoid pillow between legs).
   b. Upper-extremity amputations—postural abnormalities (encourage good posture).
4. Encourage active ROM and muscle-strengthening exercises when prescribed to
   a. Minimize muscle atrophy.
   b. Increase muscle strength.
   c. Prepare residual limb for prosthesis.
5. Promote reestablishment of balance (amputation alters distribution of body weight).
   a. Transfer to chair within 48 hours after surgery.
   b. Instruct and guard lower-limb amputee during balance exercises (ie, arise from chair; stand on toes holding on to chair; bend knee holding on to chair; balance on one leg without support; hop on one foot while holding on to chair).
6. Supervise ambulation, use of wheelchair, and self-care activities.

Patient Education and Health Maintenance

1. Teach the patient and family how to wrap residual limb with elastic bandage to control edema and to form a firm conical shape for prosthesis fitting (see Figures 32-8 and 32-9).
   a. Wrapping generally begins 1 to 3 days after surgery or after hard plaster dressing is removed.
   b. Use diagonal figure-of-8 bandaging technique.
   c. Wrap distal to proximal to maintain pressure gradient and to control edema.

Figure 32-8. Wrapping above-elbow residual limb. Elastic bandaging reduces edema and shapes the residual limb for the prosthesis. Bandage may need to be secured by wrapping across back and shoulders. (From Smeltzer, S., & Bare, B. [2000]. *Brunner and Suddarth's textbook of medical-surgical nursing* [9th ed.]. Philadelphia, PA: Lippincott Williams & Wilkins.)

Figure 32-9. Wrapping above-knee residual limb. Elastic bandaging reduces edema and shapes the residual limb in a firm conical form for the prosthesis. (From Smeltzer, S., & Bare, B. [2000]. *Brunner and Suddarth's textbook of medical-surgical nursing* [9th ed.]. Philadelphia, PA: Lippincott Williams & Wilkins.)

    d. Begin wrapping with minimal tension and increase as wound heals and sutures are removed.
    e. Flatten skin at ends of incision to ensure conical stump shape.
    f. Rewrap residual limb a couple of times per day and as necessary to achieve a smooth, graded tension dressing.
    g. Rewrap if the patient complains of more pain—dressing is probably too tight.
    h. Keep residual limb wrapped at all times except when bathing (when the patient is cleared for bathing by physician).
2. Teach the patient residual limb conditioning.
    a. Push the residual limb against a soft pillow.
    b. Gradually push residual limb against harder surfaces.
    c. Massage healed residual limb to soften scar, decrease tenderness, and improve vascularity.
3. Fitting of prosthesis.
    a. Note residual limb contour.
    b. Assess for residual limb contraction.
    c. When maximum shrinkage occurs, the prosthetist measures and fits the prosthesis.
    d. Adjustments are made by the prosthetist to minimize skin problems.
4. Continuing care of residual limb and prosthesis.
    a. Instruct the patient to wash and dry the limb thoroughly at least twice per day, removing all soap residue, to prevent skin irritation and infection.
    b. Avoid soaking residual limb because it results in edema.
    c. Inspect residual limb and skin under prosthesis harness daily for pressure, irritation, and actual skin breakdown.
    d. Wear residual limb sock or cotton underwear—to absorb perspiration and to avoid direct contact between the prosthetic socket or harness and skin.
    e. Avoid wrinkles in residual limb sock—potential pressure areas.

    f. Wipe the socket of the prosthesis with a damp cloth when the prosthesis is removed for the evening.
    g. Have the prosthesis checked periodically.
5. Teach the patient to protect the remaining extremity from injury and to secure prompt treatment of problems.

Evaluation: Expected Outcomes

- Vital signs stable; dressing reinforced once in 4 hours.
- Pressure dressing intact; stump elevated without edema.
- Participates in care plan; expresses concerns about independence.
- Verbalizes relief of incisional pain; dull phantom sensation tolerable.
- Performs ROM actively; transfers to wheelchair with assistance; participates in PT and OT activities.

MUSCULOSKELETAL TRAUMA

See Standards of Care Guidelines 32-1.

Contusions, Strains, and Sprains

A *contusion* is an injury to the soft tissue produced by a blunt force (blow, kick, or fall). A *strain* is a microscopic tearing of the muscle caused by excessive force, stretching, or overuse. A *sprain* is an injury to ligamentous structures surrounding a joint; it is usually caused by a overstretching, sudden twisting, or hyperextension of the joint, resulting in a decrease in joint stability.

> **STANDARDS OF CARE GUIDELINES 32-1**
> Caring for a Patient with Musculoskeletal Trauma, Surgery, Casting, or Immobilization
>
> When caring for a patient with musculoskeletal trauma, surgery, casting, or immobilization, provide the following care, as indicated:
> - Check neurovascular status of involved extremities.
> - Palpate for intact and equal pulses bilaterally.
> - Palpate for proper warmth of the skin.
> - Check for brisk capillary refill.
> - Test sensation to light touch and pain.
> - Observe for unusual or increased swelling.
> - Ensure that the patient can move affected parts.
> - Ensure proper positioning for comfort and alignment.
> - Determine pressure points and take precautions to prevent pressure sores.
> - Medicate to control pain, particularly before movement, procedures, and physical therapy.
> - Provide diversional activities and emotional support during long immobilizations.
> - Always document assessments and interventions meticulously, realizing that the patient may be involved in workers' compensation claim or litigation due to accident and that records will be essential to the patient's future well-being.
>
> This information should serve as a general guideline only. Each patient situation presents a unique set of clinical factors and requires nursing judgment to guide care, which may include additional or alterative measures and approaches.

Clinical Manifestations

Contusion

1. Hemorrhage into injured part (ecchymosis)—from rupture of small blood vessels; also associated with fractures.
2. Pain, swelling, and ecchymosis.
3. Hyperkalemia may be present with extensive contusions, resulting in destruction of body tissue and loss of blood.

Strain

1. Hemorrhage into the muscle.
2. Swelling.
3. Tenderness.
4. Pain with isometric contraction.
5. May be associated spasm.

Sprain

1. Rapid swelling—due to extravasation of blood within tissues.
2. Pain on passive movement of joint.
3. Increasing pain during first few hours due to continued swelling.

Management

1. X-ray may be done to rule out fracture.
2. Immobilize in splint, elastic wrap, or compression dressing to support painful structures and control swelling.
3. Apply ice while swelling is present.
4. Analgesics usually include nonsteroidal anti-inflammatory drugs (NSAIDs).
5. Severe sprains may require surgical repair or cast immobilization.
6. The acronym PRICE-M is often used to guide treatment at home for minor injuries: Protection—of the affected part from injury; Rest—to promote healing; Ice—to control swelling (do not use heat until acute swelling is relieved); Compression—with an elastic wrap or splint to control swelling and prevent stiffness, can be removed at night; Elevation—above the level of the heart to reduce swelling; Medication—analgesic and antiinflammatories, often over the counter.

Nursing Interventions and Patient Education

1. Elevate the affected part to reduce swelling. Maintain splint or immobilization, as prescribed.
2. Apply cold compresses for the first several days (15 to 20 minutes at a time every few hours)—to produce vasoconstriction, decrease edema, and reduce discomfort (do not apply ice directly to skin). Ice may be needed for up to a week to control acute swelling.
3. Assess neurovascular status of contused extremity every 1 to 4 hours as the patient's condition indicates.
4. Instruct the patient on the use of pain medication, as prescribed.
5. Ensure the correct use of crutches or other mobility aid with or without weight bearing, as prescribed.
6. Educate on the need to rest injured part for about a month to allow for healing.
7. Teach the patient to resume activities gradually.
8. Teach the patient to avoid excessive exercise of injured part.
9. Teach the patient to avoid reinjury by "warming up" before exercise and stretching tendons and muscles before and after exercise.
10. Complementary methods, such as acupuncture, biofeedback, and imagery, may contribute to healing by reducing anxiety and pain.

Tendinitis

Tendinitis is an inflammation of a tendon caused by a lack of sufficient lubrication of the tendon sheath. May be caused by acute stress on tendon structure or by chronic overuse.

Clinical Manifestations

1. Onset of pain may occur immediately after activity or delayed up to a day later. ROM and resistance testing is painful.
2. Mild swelling occurs and the tendon sheath is tender to the touch.
3. Sudden onset of sharp pain in extremity and hearing or feeling a "snap" are associated with tendon rupture, as in Achilles tendinitis due to running injuries or stop–start activities such as basketball. Also occurs in gastrocnemius and biceps.

Management

1. X-rays are not usually diagnostic.
2. Thompson test helps with diagnosis of Achilles rupture. The patient kneels on a chair or lies prone. Examiner squeezes the calf of the affected leg. Normal response: foot flexes, denoting intact tendon. If the foot does not move, tendon is assumed to be ruptured.
3. Initial treatment includes protection, rest, ice, compression, elevation (PRICE).
4. Splinting or casting for up to 6 weeks in functional position is usually necessary.
5. Surgical intervention may be necessary if rupture is complete.
6. PT to regain strength and function.
7. Corticosteroid injection.
8. NSAIDs for pain and inflammation.

Nursing Interventions and Patient Education

1. Ensure understanding of the need for proper immobilization for full time period even though fracture is not present.
2. Encourage the use of warm compresses after 24 hours to relieve pain and inflammation.
3. Advise the patient not to return to full activity until strength is equal to unaffected extremity.
4. Teach proper warm-up before exercise and sports activities (stretching of all major tendons).

Bursitis

Bursitis is a painful inflammation of the bursae, fluid-filled sacs lined with synovium similar to the lining of the joint spaces. Bursae reduce friction between tendons and bones or tendons and ligaments. They are found over joints with bony prominences, such as the trochanter, patella, and olecranon. Friction between skin and musculoskeletal tissues may result in bursitis.

Clinical Manifestations

1. Pain around a joint—commonly the knee, elbow, shoulder, and hip.
2. Varying degrees of redness, warmth, and swelling may be visible.
3. There is point tenderness and limited ROM on examination.

Management and Nursing Interventions

1. Rest and immobilization of affected joint.
2. Ice for the first 48 hours; moist heat every 4 hours thereafter.
3. Nonopioid analgesics such as NSAIDs.
4. ROM exercises.
5. Corticosteroid injection into the area.
6. Surgery indicated when calcified deposits or adhesions have diminished function.

Plantar Fasciitis

Plantar fasciitis is inflammation of the fascia that runs along the bottom of the foot from heel to toes. As the fascia is stretched, microscopic tears develop at the point where fascia attaches to the calcaneus.

Clinical Manifestations

1. Pain along the sole of the foot, usually unilateral but may be bilateral.
2. Worse upon arising, long period of standing, and walking.
3. Tenderness of heel area.

Management and Nursing Interventions

1. Rest—decrease walking, running, exercise, standing.
2. NSAIDs for pain and inflammation.
3. Good supportive footwear.
4. Orthotic devices may be beneficial.
   a. Heel cup to cushion the heel (OTC).
   b. Arch support orthotics for pes planus (flat foot).
   c. Cushioning of arches for pes cavus (high arch).
5. Stretching exercises several times per day.
6. Massage of the bottom of the foot.
7. Steroid injection into the painful area.
8. Low-intensity extracorporeal shock wave therapy, also known as orthotripsy, may be tried when conservative management has failed.
   a. Using a handheld device, shock waves are focused directly at the painful area, causing microtraumas to the tissue causing the plantar fasciitis.
   b. An inflammatory response occurs, causing increased blood supply to the painful area, as well as breaking down injured tissue and calcifications, allowing a natural healing process.
   c. One or more 15-minute treatments take place in the office setting without anesthesia or any special preparation.
9. Surgery for the release of fascia as last resort.

Traumatic Joint Dislocation

Dislocation of a joint occurs when the surfaces of the bones forming the joint are no longer in anatomic contact. This is a medical emergency because of associated disruption of surrounding blood and nerve supplies. Shoulder, fingers, and elbow are the most commonly dislocated joints. Mechanism of injury can be anterior, posterior (most common), lateral, or medial force.

Clinical Manifestations

1. Pain.
2. Deformity.
3. Change in the length of the extremity.
4. Loss of normal movement.
5. X-ray confirmation of dislocation without associated fracture.

Management

1. Immobilize the part while the patient is transported to emergency department, x-ray department, or clinical unit.
2. Secure reduction of dislocation (bring displaced parts into normal position) as soon as possible to prevent circulatory or nerve impairments; usually performed under anesthesia.
3. Stabilize reduction until joint structures are healed to prevent permanently unstable joint or aseptic necrosis of bone.

Nursing Interventions and Patient Education

1. Assess neurovascular status of extremity before and after reduction of dislocation.
2. Administer or teach self-administration of pain medications such as NSAIDs.

3. Ensure proper use of immobilization device after reduction.
4. Review instructions for activity restrictions and need for PT and follow-up.

Knee Injuries

The knee ligaments provide stability to the knee joint. These ligaments promote rotational stability (*anterior cruciate ligament [ACL]* and *posterior cruciate ligament*) and prevent varus and valgus instability (*medial and lateral collateral ligaments*). Pieces of cartilage that stabilize the knee internally are known as the medial and lateral menisci. *ACL injuries* and *medial meniscus tears* are common because of sports injuries.

Clinical Manifestations

1. Severe stresses are applied to the knee during many sports activities (eg, soccer, skiing, running).
2. Injury to knee structures occurs during rapid position changes involving flexing and twisting of the joint.
3. Torn cartilage (meniscus) causes pain, tenderness, joint effusion, clicking sensations, and decreased ROM.
4. Knee ligaments may be torn, resulting in pain on ambulation, swelling, and joint instability. The patellar tendon may rupture.

Management

1. Special assessment techniques are done to detect ACL injury (see Table 32-1).
2. MRI shows injury to soft tissue involved.
3. Some injuries may be immobilized (splint, brace, or cast) and treated with PT.

Table 32-1 Assessment Techniques for Anterior Cruciate Ligament Injury

TEST	DESCRIPTION	POSITIVE FINDING
Anterior drawer test	Place the patient supine with knee in 90 degrees of flexion with foot flat on table. Proximal tibia is pulled forward by examiner using two hands.	Tibia subluxes (dislocates) forward on femur.
Lachman test	Place the patient supine with knee in 15 to 20 degrees of flexion. Distal femur is grasped by examiner with one hand while the other hand grasps the proximal tibia and applies forward pressure.	Tibia subluxes forward on femur.
Pivot shift test (evaluates anterolateral rotational stability)	Place the patient supine with knee slightly flexed. The examiner grasps the patient's ankle in one hand and places the palm of the other hand over the lateral aspect of the knee distal to the joint. Lower leg is extended and internally rotated, applying a valgus (lateral) stress to knee.	Tibia subluxes and reduces itself ("pivots and shifts").

4. ACL reconstruction frequently indicated.
   a. Arthroscopic surgery preferred; synthetic ligaments selected where ligaments failed. Graft rejection is a complication.
   b. Postoperative continuous passive motion used.
   c. Postoperative ACL rehabilitation program includes progressive ROM, bracing (not done with synthetic ligaments).
   d. Long-term bracing during sports controversial.
5. Meniscal injury—damaged cartilage removed.
   a. Arthroscopic or open meniscectomy.
   b. Rehabilitation includes progressive ROM and quadriceps strengthening.

Nursing Interventions and Patient Education

1. After arthroscopic surgery, ensure proper use of crutches, as indicated, and encourage pain control through medications, as prescribed, and RICE.
2. For open joint surgery, see care of the patient undergoing orthopedic surgery, page 868.
3. Teach the patient strengthening exercises for affected extremity.
4. Teach the patient to prevent fatigue through rest periods, conservation of energy.
5. Advise on prevention of injuries using proper equipment and footwear for sports.

Fractures

A *fracture* is a break in the continuity of bone. A fracture occurs when the stress placed on a bone is greater than the bone can absorb. Muscles, blood vessels, nerves, tendons, joints, and other organs may be injured when fracture occurs.

Types of Fractures

1. Complete—involves the entire cross section of the bone, usually displaced (abnormal position).
2. Incomplete—involves a portion of the cross section of the bone or may be longitudinal.
3. Closed (simple)—skin not broken.
4. Open (compound)—skin broken, leading directly to fracture.
   a. Grade I—minimal soft tissue injury.
   b. Grade II—laceration greater than 1 cm without extensive soft tissue flaps.
   c. Grade III—extensive soft tissue injury, including skin, muscle, neurovascular structure, with crushing.
5. Pathologic—through an area of diseased bone (osteoporosis, bone cyst, bone tumor, bony metastasis).

Patterns of Fracture

See Figure 32-10.
1. Greenstick—one side of the bone is broken and the other side is bent.
2. Transverse—straight across the bone.
3. Oblique—at an angle across the bone.
4. Spiral—twists around the shaft of the bone.
5. Comminuted—bone splintered into more than three fragments.
6. Depressed—fragments are driven inward (seen in fractures of the skull and facial bones).
7. Compression—bone collapses in on itself (seen in vertebral fractures).
8. Avulsion—fragment of bone pulled off by ligament or tendon attachment.
9. Impacted—fragment of bone wedged into other bone fragment.

Figure 32-10. Patterns of fractures. (From Smeltzer, S., & Bare, B. [2000]. *Brunner and Suddarth's textbook of medical-surgical nursing* [9th ed.]. Philadelphia, PA: Lippincott Williams & Wilkins.)

10. Fracture dislocation—fracture complicated by the bone being out of the joint.
11. Other—described according to anatomic location: epiphyseal (end of large bones containing growth plate), supracondylar (above the articular prominence of a bone), midshaft, intra-articular.

 GERONTOLOGIC ALERT Osteoporosis is a major risk for fractures, particularly hip and vertebral compression fractures.

Clinical Manifestations
Physical Findings
1. Pain at the site of injury.
2. Swelling.
3. Tenderness.
4. False motion and crepitus (grating sensation).
5. Deformity.
6. Loss of function.
7. Ecchymosis.
8. Paresthesia.

Altered Neurovascular Status
1. Injured muscle, blood vessels, nerves.
2. Compression of structures resulting in ischemia.
3. Findings:
   a. Progressive uncontrollable pain.
   b. Pain on passive movement.
   c. Altered sensations (paresthesia).
   d. Loss of active motion.
   e. Diminished capillary refill response, diminished distal pulse.
   f. Pallor.

Shock
1. Bone is very vascular.
2. Overt hemorrhage through open wound.
3. Covert hemorrhage into soft tissues (especially with femoral fracture) or body cavity, as with pelvic fracture.
4. May be fatal if not detected.

Diagnostic Evaluation
1. X-ray and other imaging studies to determine integrity of bone.
2. Blood studies (complete blood count [CBC], electrolytes) with blood loss and extensive muscle damage—may show decreased hemoglobin level and hematocrit.
3. Arthroscopy to detect joint involvement.
4. Angiography if associated with blood vessel injury.
5. Nerve conduction and electromyogram studies to detect nerve injury.

Management
For emergency management, see page 947.
Principles of Management
1. Factors influencing choice of management include the following:
   a. Type, location, and severity of fracture.
   b. Soft tissue damage.
   c. Age and health status of the patient, including type and extent of other injuries.
2. Goals include the following:
   a. To regain and maintain correct position and alignment.
   b. To regain the function of the involved part.

Figure 32-11. Method for immobilizing a clavicular fracture with a clavicular strap. (From Smeltzer, S., & Bare, B. [2000]. *Brunner and Suddarth's textbook of medical-surgical nursing* [9th ed.]. Philadelphia, PA: Lippincott Williams & Wilkins.)

   c. To return the patient to usual activities in the shortest time and at the least expense.
3. The management process is a three-step process:
   a. Reduction—setting the bone; refers to restoration of the fracture fragments into anatomic position and alignment.
   b. Immobilization—maintains reduction until bone healing occurs (see Figures 32-11 and 32-12).
   c. Rehabilitation—regaining normal function of the affected part.

Approaches to Management
Vary by specific site of fracture (see Table 32-2, pages 880 to 882).
1. Closed reduction.
   a. Bony fragments are brought into apposition (ends in contact) by manipulation and manual traction restoring alignment.
   b. May be done under anesthesia for pain relief and muscle relaxation.
   c. Cast or splint applied to immobilize extremity and maintain reduction (see "Casts," page 862).

Figure 32-12. Immobilization of fracture of upper humerus can be achieved with conventional sling and swathe. (From Smeltzer, S., & Bare, B. [2000]. *Brunner and Suddarth's textbook of medical-surgical nursing* [9th ed.]. Philadelphia, PA: Lippincott Williams & Wilkins.)

Table 32-2   Fractures of Specific Sites

SITE AND MECHANISM	MANAGEMENT	NURSING CONSIDERATIONS
Clavicle Fall on shoulder	• Closed reduction and immobilization with clavicular strap (see Figure 32-11) figure-of-8 bandage or sling. • ORIF for marked displacement, severely comminuted fracture, and extensive soft tissue injury.	• Pad the axilla to prevent nerve damage from pressure of immobilizer. • Assess neurovascular status of arm. • Teach exercises of elbow, wrist, and fingers. • Teach shoulder exercises through full ROM, as prescribed.
Proximal Humerus Fall on outstretched arm; osteoporosis is predisposing factor	• Many remain in alignment and are supported by a sling and swathe or Velpeau bandage for comfort (see Figure 32-12). • If displaced, treated with reduction under x-ray control, open reduction, or replacement of humeral head with prosthesis.	• Place a soft pad under the axilla to prevent skin maceration. • Encourage shoulder ROM exercises after specified period of immobilization to prevent frozen shoulder. • Instruct the patient to lean forward and allow affected arm to abduct and rotate.

Shaft of Humerus
Direct fall, blow to arm, or auto injury; damage to radial nerve may occur
	• Immobilize with sling and swathe, splint, or hanging cast.
	• A hanging cast is applied for its weight to correct displaced fractures with shortening of the humeral shaft.
	• ORIF for associated vascular injury or pathologic fracture, followed by support in sling.
		• Hanging cast must remain unsupported to maintain traction.
		  • Teach the patient to avoid supporting elbow in lap or arm on pillow.
		  • The patient should sleep in upright position to maintain 24-hour traction.
		• Encourage exercise of fingers immediately after application of cast.
		• Teach pendulum exercises of arm, as prescribed, to prevent frozen shoulder.

Elbow and Forearm Fall on elbow, outstretched hand, or direct blow (side-swipe injury)	• Treatment depends on specific characteristics of fracture—ORIF, arthroplasty, external fixation, casting. • Closed drainage system may be used to decrease hematoma formation and swelling.	• Assess neurovascular status of forearm and hand. • If radial pulse weakens or disappears, report immediately to prevent irreversible ischemia. • Elevate arm to control edema. • Encourage finger and shoulder exercises.

Wrist
Colles fracture is common (½–1 inch [1.2–2.5 cm] above the wrist with dorsal displacement of lower fragment); caused by fall on out-stretched palm; commonly associated with osteoporosis
	• Closed reduction with splint or cast support.
	• Percutaneous pins and external fixator or plaster cast.
		• Elevate arm above level of heart for 48 hours after reduction to promote venous and lymphatic return and reduce swelling.
		• Watch for swelling of fingers and check for constricting bandages or cast.
		• Teach finger exercises to reduce swelling and stiffness.
		  • Hold the hand above the level of the heart.
		  • Move fingers from full extension to flexion.
		  • Hold and release.
		  • Repeat at least 10 times every half hour when awake for as long as swelling occurs.
		• Encourage daily-prescribed exercises to restore full extension and supination.

Hand Caused by numerous injuries	• Splinting for undisplaced fractures of fingers. • Debridement, irrigation, and Kirchner wire fixation for open fractures. • Reconstructive surgery may be necessary for complex injuries.	• Provide aggressive care and encouragement with rehabilitation plan to regain maximal function of hand.

Table 32-2 Fractures of Specific Sites (Continued)

SITE AND MECHANISM	MANAGEMENT	NURSING CONSIDERATIONS

Hip (Proximal Femur)
Occur frequently in older adults, women with osteoporosis, and with fall types:
• Intracapsular—femoral neck within joint capsule
• Extracapsular—femoral neck between greater and lesser trochanter (intertrochanteric) or of femoral shaft
• Subtrochanteric—of femur just below level of lesser trochanter
	• Hip fracture identified by shortening and external rotation of affected leg; pain in hip or knee; inability to move leg.
	• Immobilization with Buck extension traction until surgery.
	• Surgery as soon as medically stable; choice depends on location, character, and patient factors.
	  • Internal fixation with nail, nail–plate combination, multiple pins, screw, or sliding nails.
	  • Femoral prosthetic replacement.
	  • Total hip arthroplasty.
		• Provide constant monitoring and nursing care to reduce the risk of complications, such as pneumonia, thrombophlebitis, fat emboli, dislocation of prosthesis, infection, and pressure sores.
		• Administer aspirin, warfarin, subcutaneous heparin, or low molecular weight heparin, as ordered.
		• Use sequential compression devices, as ordered.
		• Provide meticulous skin care to prevent breakdown.
		  • Use trapeze for the patient to assist with position changes.
		  • Use a special bed or mattress, as indicated.
		  • Inspect heels daily and use heel protection measures.
		• Prevent UTI by increasing fluids, limiting use of indwelling catheter, and encouraging frequent voiding.
		• Keep affected leg in abduction and neutral rotation.
		• Teach quadriceps setting exercise to prevent muscle atrophy of affected leg.

Femoral Shaft	• Closed reduction and stabilization with skeletal traction—Thomas leg splint with Pearson attachment; followed by use of orthosis (cast brace) to allow weight bearing. • Open reduction with hardware or with bone grafting may be necessary. • External fixator may be used.	• Marked concealed blood loss may occur; watch for signs of shock initially and anemia later. • Examine skin under the ring of the Thomas splint for signs of pressure.
Knee Direct blow to knee area; involve distal shaft of femur (supracondylar), articular surfaces, or patella	• Closed reduction and immobilization through casting, traction, braces, splints. • ORIF. • Goal is to preserve knee mobility.	• Elevate extremity by raising foot gatch of bed. • Evaluate for effusion—report and loosen pressure dressing if pain is severe; prepare for joint aspiration. • Teach quadriceps setting exercises and limited weight bearing, as prescribed.
Tibia and Fibula/Ankle Distal tibia or fibula, malleoli, or talus fractures generally result from forceful twisting of ankle and commonly associated with ligament disruption; also high incidence of open fractures of tibial shaft because tibia lies superficially beneath the skin	• Closed reduction and toe-to-groin cast for closed fractures, later replaced by short leg cast or orthosis. • ORIF may be necessary for some closed fractures. • External fixator for open fracture.	• Elevate lower leg to control edema. • Avoid dependent position of extremity for prolonged periods. • Prepare the patient for long immobilization period, as union is slow (12–16 weeks, longer for open and comminuted fractures). • Prepare the patient for stiff ankle joint following immobilization.
Foot Metatarsal fracture due to crush injuries of the foot	• Immobilization with cast, splint, or strapping.	• Encourage partial weight bearing, as allowed. • Elevate the foot to control edema.
Thoracic and Lumbar Spine Trauma from falls, contact sports, or auto accidents, or excessive loading may cause fracture of vertebral body, lamina, spinous and transverse processes; usually stable compression fractures	• Suspected with pain that is worsened by movement and coughing and radiates to extremities, abdomen, or intercostal muscles and presence of sensory and motor deficits. • Bed rest on firm mattress and pain relief followed by progressive ambulation and back strengthening to treat stable fractures; takes about 6 weeks to heal. • ORIF with Harrington rod, body cast, or laminectomy with spinal fusion may be necessary for unstable or displaced fractures.	• Use log roll technique to change positions. • Monitor bowel and bladder dysfunction, as paralytic ileus and bladder distention may occur with nerve root injury. • Assist the patient to ambulate when pain subsides, no neurologic deficit exists, and x-rays reveal no displacement. • Teach proper body mechanics and back preservation techniques. • Encourage weight reduction. • Teach the patient with osteoporosis the importance of safety measures to avoid falls.

(continued)

Table 32-2 Fractures of Specific Sites (*Continued*)

SITE AND MECHANISM	MANAGEMENT	NURSING CONSIDERATIONS
Pelvis		

Sacrum, ilium, pubic, ischium, and coccyx fractures may occur from auto accidents, crush injuries, and falls; most are stable fractures that do not involve the pelvic ring and have minimal displacement	• Emergency management to treat multiple trauma, shock from intra-peritoneal hemorrhage, and injury to internal organs is necessary (see pages 948 to 952).
	• Bed rest for several days followed by progressive weight bearing for stable fracture.
	• Prolonged bed rest, external fixation, ORIF, skeletal traction, and pelvic sling are options for unstable fracture.
		• Monitor and support vital functions, as indicated.
		• Observe urine output for blood indicating genitourinary injury.
		• Do not attempt to insert urethral catheter until patency of urethra is known; incidence of urethral injury in males is high with anterior fractures.
		• Assist the patient being treated in pelvic sling.
		  • Fold sling back over buttocks to enable the patient to use bedpan.
		  • Reach under the sling to give skin care; line the sling with sheepskin.
		  • Loosen sling only as directed.

ORIF, open reduction with internal function; ROM, range of motion; UTI, urinary tract infection.

2. Traction.
   a. Pulling force applied to accomplish and maintain reduction and alignment (see "Traction," page 865).
   b. Used for fractures of long bones.
   c. Techniques.
      i. Skin traction—force applied to the skin using foam rubber, tape.
      ii. Skeletal traction—force applied to the bony skeleton directly, using wires, pins, or tongs placed into or through the bone.
3. Open reduction with internal fixation.
   a. Operative intervention to achieve reduction, alignment, and stabilization.
      i. Bone fragments are directly visualized.
      ii. Internal fixation devices (metal pins, wires, screws, plates, nails, rods) used to hold bone fragments in position until solid bone healing occurs (may be removed when bone is healed).
      iii. After closure of the wound, splints or casts may be used for additional stabilization and support.
4. Endoprosthetic replacement.
   a. Replacement of a fracture fragment with an implanted metal device.
   b. Used when fracture disrupts nutrition of the bone or treatment of choice is bony replacement.
5. External fixation device.
   a. Stabilization of complex and open fracture with the use of a metal frame and pin system.
   b. Permits active treatment of injured soft tissue.
      i. Wound may be left open (delayed primary wound closure).
      ii. Repair of damage to blood vessels, soft tissue, muscles, nerves, and tendons, as indicated.
      iii. Reconstructive surgery may be necessary (see "External Fixation," page 867).

Complications

Complications Associated with Immobility
1. Muscle atrophy, loss of muscle strength, and endurance.
2. Loss of ROM due to joint contracture.
3. Pressure sores at bony prominences from immobilizing device pressing on skin.

4. Diminished respiratory, cardiovascular, GI function, resulting in possible pooling of respiratory secretions, orthostatic hypotension, ileus, anorexia, and constipation.
5. Psychosocial compromise resulting in feelings of isolation and depression.

Other Acute Complications
1. Venous stasis and thromboembolism—particularly with fractures of the hip and lower extremities.
2. Neurovascular compromise.
3. Infection, especially with open fractures.
4. Shock due to significant hemorrhage related to trauma or as a postoperative complication.
5. Pulmonary emboli.

Fat Emboli Syndrome
1. Associated with embolization of marrow or tissue fat or platelets and free fatty acids to the pulmonary capillaries, producing rapid onset of symptoms.
2. Clinical manifestations.
   a. Respiratory distress—tachypnea, hypoxemia, crackles, wheezes, acute pulmonary edema, interstitial pneumonitis.
   b. Mental disturbances—irritability, restlessness, confusion, disorientation, stupor, coma due to systemic embolization, and severe hypoxia.
   c. Fever.
   d. Petechiae in buccal membranes, hard palate, conjunctival sacs, chest, anterior axillary folds, due to occlusion of capillaries.

NURSING ALERT Restlessness, confusion, irritability, and disorientation may be the first signs of fat embolism syndrome. Confirm hypoxia with arterial blood gas (ABG) analysis. Young adults (age 20 to 30) and older adults (age 60 to 70) with multiple fractures or fractures of long bones or pelvis are particularly susceptible to development of fat emboli.

Bone Union Problems
1. Delayed union (takes longer to heal than average for type of fracture).
2. Nonunion (fractured bone fails to unite).
3. Malunion (union occurs but is faulty—misaligned).

Nursing Assessment

1. Ask the patient how the fracture occurred—mechanism of injury important in determining possible associated injuries.
2. Ask the patient to describe location, character, and intensity of pain to help determine possible source of discomfort.
3. Ask the patient to describe sensations in injured extremity to aid in evaluation of neurovascular status.
4. Observe the patient's ability to change position to assess functional mobility.
5. Note the patient's emotional status and behavior—indicators of ability to cope with stress of injury.
6. Assess the patient's support system; identify current and potential sources of support, assistance, and caregiving.
7. Review findings on past and present health status to aid in formulating care plan.
8. Conduct physical examination.
   a. Examine skin for lacerations, abrasions, ecchymosis, edema, and temperature.
   b. Auscultate lungs to establish baseline assessment of respiratory function.
   c. Assess pulses and BP; assess peripheral tissue perfusion, especially in injured extremity, to establish circulatory status baseline.
   d. Determine neurologic status (sensations and movement) of extremity distal to injury.
   e. Note length, alignment, and immobilization of injured extremity.
   f. Evaluate behavior and cognitive functioning of the patient to determine ability to participate in care planning and patient education activities.

 NURSING ALERT Change in behavior or cerebral functioning may be an early indicator of cerebral anoxia from shock or pulmonary or fat emboli.

 GERONTOLOGIC ALERT Assessment of the patient's health and functional abilities before a fracture along with available support systems facilitates development of realistic rehabilitation and discharge goals.

Nursing Diagnoses

- Risk for Deficient Fluid Volume related to hemorrhage and shock.
- Impaired Gas Exchange related to immobility and potential pulmonary emboli or fat emboli.
- Risk for Peripheral Neurovascular Dysfunction.
- Risk for Vascular Trauma related to thromboembolism.
- Acute Pain related to injury.
- Risk for Infection related to open fracture or surgical intervention.
- Bathing or Hygiene Self-Care Deficit related to immobility.
- Impaired Physical Mobility related to injury/treatment modality.
- Risk for Disuse Syndrome related to injury and immobilization.
- Risk for Posttrauma Syndrome related to cause of injury.

Nursing Interventions

Evaluating for Hemorrhage and Shock

1. Monitor vital signs as frequently as clinical condition indicates, observing for hypotension, elevated pulse, widening pulse pressure, cold clammy skin, restlessness, pallor.
2. Watch for evidence of hemorrhage on dressings or in drainage containers.
3. Review laboratory data; report abnormal values.
4. Administer prescribed fluids/blood to maintain circulating volume.
5. Monitor intake and output. Goal is to maintain at least 30 mL/hour and establish individual's normal voiding pattern.

 NURSING ALERT Patients with hip and long bone fractures are at high risk for hemorrhage. Frequent checks for hemodynamics, neurovascular status, and drainage should be performed, particularly in patients with other comorbidities who may not tolerate changes in hematocrit and hemoglobin levels.

Monitoring for Impaired Gas Exchange

1. Evaluate changes in mental status and restlessness that may indicate hypoxia.
2. Review diagnostic evaluation data—especially ABG values and chest x-ray.
3. Position to enhance respiratory effort. Report any sudden or progressive changes in respiratory status.
4. Encourage coughing and deep breathing to promote lung expansion and diminish pooling of pulmonary secretions.
5. Monitor pulse oximetry; administer oxygen, as prescribed.
6. Maintain cervical spine precautions if spinal injury is suspected.

Preventing Neurovascular Compromise

1. Monitor neurovascular status for compression of nerve, diminished circulation, development of compartment syndrome.
   a. Pain—progressive, localized, deep throbbing, persistent, unrelieved by immobilization and medications.
   b. Pain on passive stretch.
   c. Weakness progressing to paralysis.
   d. Altered sensation, hypoesthesia, paresthesia.
   e. Poor capillary refill (greater than 3 seconds).
   f. Skin color—pale, cyanotic.
   g. Elevated compartment pressure—palpable tightness of muscle compartment, elevated measured tissue pressure.
   h. Pulselessness—a late sign.
2. Reduce swelling.
   a. Elevate injured extremity (unless compartment syndrome is suspected—may contribute to vascular compromise).
   b. Apply cold to injury, if prescribed.
3. Relieve pressure caused by immobilizing device, as prescribed (such as bivalving cast, rewrapping elastic bandage, or splinting device).
4. Relieve pressure on skin to prevent development of pressure sore.
   a. Frequent repositioning.
   b. Skin care—do not massage bony prominences.
   c. Special mattresses.

 NURSING ALERT Monitoring the neurovascular integrity of the injured extremity is essential. Development of compartment syndrome (increased tissue pressure causing hypoxemia) leads to permanent loss of function in 6 to 8 hours. This situation must be identified and managed promptly.

Preventing Development of Thromboembolism

1. Encourage active and passive ankle exercises.
2. Use elastic stockings, foot pumps, or SCDs, as prescribed.
3. Elevate legs to prevent stasis, avoiding pressure on blood vessels.
4. Encourage mobility; change position frequently; encourage ambulation.
5. Administer anticoagulants, as prescribed.
6. Monitor for development of thrombophlebitis.
   a. Note complaint of pain and tenderness in calf.
   b. Report calf pain.
   c. Report increased size and temperature of calf.
   d. Homans sign has not been proved to be an effective screen for deep vein thrombosis (DVT); therefore, it is no longer an acceptable measure for assessing DVT.

GERONTOLOGIC ALERT Older adults with fractures, trauma, immobility, obesity, or history of thrombophlebitis are at high risk for developing thromboembolism.

Relieving Pain

1. Perform a comprehensive pain assessment.
   a. Have the patient describe the pain, location, characteristics (dull, sharp, continuous, throbbing, bony, radiating, aching).
   b. Ask the patient what causes the pain, makes the pain worse, relieves the pain. Evaluate the patient for proper body alignment, pressure from equipment (casts, traction, splints, appliances).
2. Initiate activities to prevent or modify pain.
   a. Assist the patient with pain-reduction techniques—cutaneous stimulation, distraction, guided imagery, TENS, biofeedback.
   b. Immobilize injured part.
   c. Position the patient in correct alignment.
   d. Support splinted fracture above and below fracture when repositioning or moving the patient.
   e. Reposition the patient with slow and steady motion; use additional personnel, as needed.
   f. Elevate painful extremity to diminish venous congestion.
   g. Apply heat or cold modalities, as prescribed. Heat versus cold is controversial. One randomly controlled trial found significantly less edema with cold packs versus heat 3 to 5 days postinjury.
   h. Modify environment to facilitate rest and relaxation.
3. Administer prescribed medications, as indicated. Encourage the use of less potent drugs as severity of discomfort decreases.
4. Establish a supportive relationship to assist the patient to deal with discomfort.
5. Encourage the patient to become an active participant in rehabilitative plans.

DRUG ALERT Meperidine may cause toxicity as it breaks down into the metabolite normeperidine, which has a 15- to 20-hour half-life, especially in patients with impaired renal function or older patients.

Monitoring for Development of Infection

1. Clean, debride, and irrigate open fracture wound, as prescribed, as soon as possible to minimize risk of infection.
   a. All open fractures are contaminated.
   b. Begin prescribed antibiotic therapy promptly after wound culture obtained.
2. Use sterile technique during dressing changes to minimize infection of wound, soft tissues, and bone.
3. Evaluate the patient for elevation of temperature every 4 hours as indicated by facility or provider order.
4. Note and report elevated white blood cell (WBC) counts.
5. Report areas of inflammation and swelling around incision or open wound.
6. Report purulent odiferous drainage.
7. Obtain specimens for culture and sensitivity to determine causative organism.

Promoting Adequate Hygiene

1. Encourage participation in care.
2. Arrange the patient area and personal items for patient convenience and to promote independence.
3. Modify activities to facilitate maximum independence within prescribed limits.
4. Allow time for the patient to accomplish the task.
5. Teach safe use of mobility and necessary aids.
6. Assist with ADLs, as needed.
7. Teach family how to assist the patient while promoting independence in self-care.

Promoting Physical Mobility

1. Perform active and passive exercises to all nonimmobilized joints.
2. Encourage patient participation in frequent position changes, maintaining support to fracture during position changes.
3. Minimize prolonged periods of physical inactivity, encouraging ambulation when prescribed.
4. Administer prescribed analgesics judiciously to decrease pain associated with movement.

Preventing Disuse Syndrome

1. Teach and encourage isometric exercises to diminish muscle atrophy.
2. Encourage the use of immobilized extremity within prescribed limits.

Minimizing the Psychological Effects of Trauma

1. Monitor the patient for symptoms of posttraumatic stress disorder.
   a. Memory of event; anger, helplessness, vulnerability, mood swings, depression, cognitive impairment, sleep disturbance, increased dependency, and social withdrawal.
2. Assist the patient to move through phases of posttraumatic stress (outcry, denial, intrusiveness, working through, completion).
3. Establish trusting therapeutic relationship with the patient.
4. Encourage the patient to express thoughts and feelings about traumatic event.
5. Encourage the patient to participate in decision-making to reestablish control and overcome feelings of helplessness.
6. Teach relaxation techniques to decrease anxiety.
7. Encourage development of adaptive responses and participation in support groups.
8. Refer the patient to psychiatric liaison nurse or refer for psychotherapy, as needed.

Community and Home Care Considerations

1. Assist the patient to actively exercise joints above and below the immobilized fracture at frequent intervals.
   a. Isometric exercises of muscles covered by cast—start exercise as soon as possible after cast application.
   b. Increase isometric exercises as fracture stabilizes.
2. After removal of immobilizing device (eg, cast, splint), have the patient start isotonic exercises and continue with isometric exercises.
3. Assess the home for any fall hazards when the patient ambulates.
4. Obtain PT/OT consultation for assistance with ADLs, transferring technique, gait strengthening, and conditioning after lengthy immobilization, as needed.
5. Assess orthostatic BP when the patient begins to ambulate to prevent falls.

Patient Education and Health Maintenance

1. Explain the basis for fracture treatment and need for patient participation in therapeutic regimen.
2. Promote adjustment of usual lifestyle and responsibilities to accommodate limitations imposed by fracture.
3. Instruct the patient on exercises to strengthen upper-extremity muscles if crutch walking is planned.
4. Instruct the patient in methods of safe ambulation—walker, crutches, cane.
5. Emphasize instructions concerning amount of weight bearing that will be permitted on fractured extremity.
6. Discuss prevention of recurrent fractures—safety considerations, avoidance of fatigue, proper footwear.
7. Encourage follow-up medical supervision to monitor for union problems.
8. Teach symptoms needing attention, such as numbness, decreased function, increased pain, elevated temperature.
9. Encourage adequate balanced diet to promote bone and soft tissue healing.

Evaluation: Expected Outcomes

- Vital signs within normal parameters; urine output at least 30 mL/hour.
- Respirations unlabored; alert and oriented.
- No signs of neurovascular compromise (ie, circulation, motor, sensory intact).
- No calf pain reported.
- Reports decreased pain with elevation, ice, and analgesic.
- Afebrile; no wound drainage.
- Performing hygiene and dressing practices with minimal assistance.
- Performing active ROM correctly.
- Using affected extremity for light activity, as allowed.
- Denies acute symptoms of stress; reports working through feelings about trauma.

OTHER MUSCULOSKELETAL DISORDERS

Lower Back Pain

 EVIDENCE BASE Qaseem, A., Wilt, T. J., McLean, R. M., Forciea, M. A.; for the Clinical Guidelines Committee of the American College of Physicians. (2017). Noninvasive treatments for acute, subacute, and chronic low back pain: A clinical practice guideline from the American College of Physicians. *Annals of Internal Medicine, 166*(7), 514–530.

Lower back pain is characterized by an uncomfortable or acute pain in the lumbosacral area associated with severe spasm of the paraspinal muscles, usually with pain radiating to the lower extremities.

Pathophysiology and Etiology

Acute low back pain lasts up to 4 week, subacute low back pain lasts 4 to 12 weeks, and chronic low back pain lasts longer than 12 weeks. There are multiple causes:
1. Mechanical (joint, muscular, or ligamentous sprain).
2. Degenerative disk disease; acute herniation of disks.
3. Lack of physical activity and exercise; weakness of musculature of back.
4. Arthritic conditions.
5. Diseases of bone (osteoporosis, vertebral fracture, Paget disease, metastatic carcinoma).
6. Congenital disorders.
7. Systemic diseases.
8. Infections of disk spaces or vertebrae.
9. Spinal cord tumors.
10. Referred pain from other areas.

Clinical Manifestations

1. Pain localized or radiating to buttocks or to one or both legs.
2. Paresthesias, numbness, and weakness of lower extremities.
3. Spasm in acute phase.
4. Bowel or bladder dysfunction in cauda equina syndrome.

Diagnostic Evaluation

1. X-rays of lumbar spine are usually negative.
2. CT of spine—to detect arthritic changes, degenerative disk disease, tumor, and other abnormalities.
3. Myelography—to confirm and localize disk herniation.
4. MRI—to detect pathology, disk herniation, soft tissue injury, stenosis, nerve impingement.
5. EMG of lower extremities—to detect nerve changes related to back pathology.
6. Diskogram—to evaluate herniated disk.

Management

For management of herniated disk, see page 428. For management of spinal cord tumors, see page 417. Guidelines call for conservative, nonpharmacologic management as first-line treatment. Most people with acute and subacute low back pain improve over time.
1. Avoid activities that may strain the back until healed, but bed rest is to be avoided as well because it may significantly decrease the rate of recovery, increase pain and disability, and lengthen time spent absent from work.
2. Exercise, PT, and tai chi may be helpful for chronic pain.
3. Heat or ice is used to relax muscle spasm and relieve discomfort. Follow heat with massage.
4. Medications.
    a. Oral analgesic and anti-inflammatory agent—usually NSAID is first-line agent, unless contraindicated because of history or high risk of GI bleeding, renal insufficiency, or allergy. If there is a high risk of GI bleeding, COX-2 inhibitors may be used unless the patient has a sulfa or aspirin allergy or is in the third trimester of pregnancy.
    b. Painful trigger points may be injected with hydrocortisone/xylocaine for pain relief.
    c. Opioids may be sedating.
    d. Muscle relaxant to relieve spasm and tense muscles. Muscle relaxants may be sedating.
    e. Adjunct medications to reduce chronic neuropathic pain include duloxetine.
5. Lumbosacral support may be used—provides abdominal compression and decreases load on lumbar intervertebral disks.
6. Acupuncture is helpful for acute and chronic pain; TENS may be helpful in relieving chronic pain.
7. Behavioral intervention such as mindfulness-based stress reduction techniques is helpful for chronic pain.
    a. Psychotropic medication may be used for treatment of depression and anxiety, which potentiate pain.
    b. Focus on getting back to functional state after long disability.

NURSING ALERT Risk factors of chronic low back pain include high severity of pain, depression, lack of positive coping skills, beliefs that the patient cannot control his or her pain, and high rate of missing work because of low back pain. Cognitive behavioral strategies can be used to help the patient with pain management and strengthen positive coping skills. Screening tools are available to help identify risk factors and guide treatment decisions.

Complications

1. Spinal instability, infection, sensory and motor deficits.
2. Chronic pain.
3. Malingering and other psychosocial reactions.

Nursing Assessment

1. Obtain history to determine when, where, and how the pain occurs, aggravating or relieving factors, relationship of pain to specific activities, presence of numbness or paresthesia.
2. Perform physical examination of neurologic system—spots localized weakness of extremities and reflex and sensory loss.
3. Perform musculoskeletal examination for changes in strength, tone, and ROM.
4. If condition is chronic, assess coping ability of the patient and family or significant others.
5. Assess effect of illness on daily living—work, school.

Nursing Diagnoses

- Acute Pain related to injury.
- Chronic Pain related to injury.
- Impaired Physical Mobility related to pain.

Nursing Interventions

Relieving Pain

1. Advise the patient to stay active and avoid bed rest, in most cases.
2. Keep pillow between flexed knees while in side-lying position—minimizes strain on back muscles.
3. Apply heat or ice, as prescribed.
4. Administer or teach self-administration of pain medications and muscle relaxants, as prescribed.
   a. Give NSAIDs with meals to prevent GI upset and bleeding.
   b. Muscle relaxants and opioids may cause drowsiness.

Coping with Chronic Pain

1. Administer adjunct pain medications, as directed. Explain that medications may not completely relieve pain but will reduce level of discomfort so that the patient can increase daily activities. Encourage adherence to therapy.
2. Teach relaxation techniques such as progressive muscle relaxation and imagery (see page 25).
3. Encourage balanced diet, exercise program, and avoidance of smoking.
4. Suggest consultation with physical/occupational therapist, psychologist, or pain management clinician, as needed.

Promoting Mobility

1. Encourage ROM of all uninvolved muscle groups.
2. Suggest gradual increase of activities and alternating activities with rest in semi-Fowler position.
3. Avoid prolonged periods of sitting, standing, or lying down.
4. Encourage the patient to discuss problems that may be contributing to backache.

5. Encourage the patient to do prescribed back exercises. Exercise keeps postural muscles strong, helps recondition the back and abdominal musculature, and serves as an outlet for emotional tension.

Patient Education and Health Maintenance

Instruct the patient to avoid recurrences as follows:

1. Standing, sitting, lying, and lifting properly are necessary for a healthy back.
2. Alternate periods of activity with periods of rest.
   a. Avoid prolonged sitting (intradiskal pressure in lumbar spine is higher during sitting), standing, and driving.
   b. Change positions and rest at frequent intervals.
   c. Avoid assuming tense, cramped positions.
   d. Sit in a straight-back chair with the knees slightly higher than the hips. Use a footstool, if necessary.
   e. Flatten the hollow of the back by sitting with the buttocks "tucked under." Pelvic tilt (small of back is pressed against a flat surface) decreases lordosis.
   f. Avoid knee and hip extension. When driving a car, have the seat pushed forward as necessary for comfort. Place a cushion in the small of the back for support.
3. When standing for any length of time, rest one foot on a small stool or platform to relieve lumbar lordosis.
4. Avoid fatigue that contributes to spasm of back muscles.
5. Use good body mechanics when lifting or moving about.
6. Daily exercise is important in the prevention of back problems (see Patient Education Guidelines 32-2).
   a. Do prescribed back exercises twice daily—strengthens back, leg, and abdominal muscles.
   b. Walking outdoors (progressively increasing distance and pace) is recommended.
   c. Reduce weight, if necessary—decreases strain on back muscles.

Evaluation: Expected Outcomes

- Verbalizes relief of pain with rest and medication.
- Able to participate in ADLs with sedation or pain greater than 3/10.
- Performs back exercises correctly.

Osteoarthritis

 EVIDENCE BASE National Institute for Health and Clinical Excellence. (2014). *Osteoarthritis: Care and management.* London: Author.
   American Association of Orthopaedic Surgeons. (2017). *Management of osteoarthritis of the hip evidence-based clinical practice guideline.* Rosemont, IL: Author.
   American Association of Orthopaedic Surgeons. (2013). *Treatment of osteoarthritis of the knee: Evidence-based guideline* (2nd ed.). Rosemont, IL: Author.

Osteoarthritis, or degenerative joint disease, is a chronic, noninflammatory, slowly progressing disorder that causes deterioration of articular cartilage. It affects weight-bearing joints (hips and knees) as well as joints of the distal interphalangeal and proximal interphalangeal joints of the fingers.

Pathophysiology and Etiology

1. Changes in articular cartilage occur first; later, secondary soft tissue changes may occur.

PATIENT EDUCATION GUIDELINES 32-2

Taking Care of Your Lower Back

Almost everyone has lower back pain at some time. Chronic pain will develop in some, and a few will become disabled because of it. Risk factors for chronic lower back pain include being overweight, being deconditioned (out of shape), having poor posture, and having poor abdominal muscle tone. You can relieve pain and avoid disability by adhering to the following instructions.

DO BACK EXERCISES EVERY DAY

- Lie on your back on the floor or a firm mattress. Bend one knee and bring that leg up toward your chest. Hold it against your chest a few seconds. Then repeat with the other leg. Alternate legs several times.
- Lie on your back with your knees bent and feet flat on the floor. Tighten your abdomen and buttocks, and push your lower back to the floor. Hold for a few seconds, and then relax. Repeat several times.
- Lie on your back with knees bent and feet flat on the floor. Do a partial sit-up by crossing your arms on your chest or behind your head and lifting your shoulders off the floor 6 to 12 inches (15 to 30.5 cm). Repeat several times.

BE CAREFUL HOW YOU LIFT

- Move your body close to an object before picking it up.
- Bend at the knees, not the back, to pick up an object that is low.
- Hold the object close to your abdomen and chest.
- Bend at the knees again to put down an object.
- Avoid reaching, twisting, or turning your back as you lift or carry an object.

PROTECT YOUR BACK WHILE SITTING AND STANDING

- Avoid sitting in soft, cushioned chairs too long.
- If you sit for long periods at work, make sure your knees are level with your hips. Use a step stool, if necessary.
- If you stand for long periods, try to put one foot up on a stool and then the other. Walk around and change position periodically.

Back exercises to strengthen abdominal and postural muscles, to stretch contracted back muscles, and to maintain flexibility.

- Adjust your car seat so there is a bend in your knees. Do not stretch.
- Put a firm pillow behind your lower back if it does not feel supported while you are sitting.

STAY ACTIVE AND IN GOOD HEALTH

- Take a walk every day wearing comfortable, low-heeled shoes.
- Eat a balanced, low-fat diet with plenty of fruits and vegetables to avoid constipation.
- Get plenty of sleep on a firm mattress.
- See your health care provider promptly for worsening pain or new injury.

---

2. Progressive wear and tear on cartilage leads to thinning of joint surface and ulceration into bone.
3. Leads to inflammation of the joint and increased blood flow and hypertrophy of subchondral bone.
4. New cartilage and bone formation at joint margins result in osteophytosis (bone spurs), altering the size and shape of bone.
5. Generally affects adults age 50 to 90; equal in males and females.
6. Cause is unknown, but aging and obesity are contributing factors. Previous trauma may cause secondary OA.

Clinical Manifestations

1. Pain in one or more joints, may be long-standing pain that increases with weight bearing or use of joint; may have been a gradual, insidious onset, or may have been some history of trauma to the joint in the past.
2. Less than 30 minutes of morning stiffness.
3. Bony deformity (osteophyte) or enlargement of the joint.
4. Possible crepitation, effusion.

Diagnostic Evaluation

1. No specific laboratory examination or imaging is necessary to make the diagnosis if person is 45 years or older with activity-related joint pain and less than 30 minutes of morning stiffness.
2. X-rays of affected joints show joint space narrowing, osteophytes, and sclerosis.
3. Radionuclide imaging (bone scan) shows increased uptake in affected bones.
4. Analysis of synovial fluid differentiates OA from RA.

Management

Conservative Management

1. Exercise for muscle strengthening and general fitness, including low-impact aerobic self-management programs; may involve PT and OT to maintain function while preserving the joints. Manipulation and stretching may be added with hip arthritis.

2. Weight loss if overweight or obese to reduce stress on joints.
3. Pain management using nonopioid analgesics, particularly NSAIDs which have proven more effective in many studies than acetaminophen, but side effects must be considered; tramadol may need to be added and opioids should be avoided unless benefits outweigh risks.
4. Hyaluronate and hylan G-F 20, agents known as viscosupplements, have been approved by the Food and Drug Administration. These drugs are administered over time through intra-articular injections into the knee. However, current guidelines no longer recommend their use because of lack of sufficient improvement for a majority of patients.
5. TENS as adjunct to pain management.
6. Proper nutrition, sleep, and stress reduction to improve well-being.
7. OTC supplements glucosamine and chondroitin sulfate are commonly used but have not proven to be more effective than placebo.

NURSING ALERT The patient's body mass index can be used to determine the need for weight loss, a major factor in preventing chronic pain due to osteoarthritis. Long-term management with a primary care provider or weight-loss specialist may assist the patient in successful weight reduction.

Surgical Intervention
Surgical intervention is considered when the pain becomes intolerable to the patient and mobility is severely compromised. Options include osteotomy, debridement, joint fusion, arthroscopy, and arthroplasty.

Complications
1. Limited mobility.
2. Neurologic deficits associated with spinal involvement.

Nursing Assessment
1. Obtain history of pain and its characteristics, including specific joints involved.
2. Evaluate ROM and strength.
3. Assess effect on ADLs and emotional status.

Nursing Diagnoses
- Acute or Chronic Pain related to joint degeneration and muscle spasm.
- Impaired Physical Mobility related to pain and limited joint motion.
- Bathing, Hygiene, Feeding, and Toileting Self-Care Deficits related to pain and limited joint movement.

Nursing Interventions
Relieving Pain
1. Advise the patient to take prescribed NSAIDs or OTC analgesics as directed to relieve inflammation and pain. If tramadol or opioids are prescribed, ensure that the patient is taking them as directed.
2. Provide rest for involved joints—excessive use aggravates the symptoms and accelerates degeneration.
   a. Use splints, braces, cervical collars, traction, and lumbosacral corsets, as ordered by health care provider.
   b. Have prescribed rest periods in recumbent position.
3. Advise the patient to avoid activities that precipitate pain.
4. Apply heat, as prescribed—relieves muscle spasm and stiffness; avoid prolonged application of heat—may cause increased swelling and flare symptoms.
5. Teach correct posture and body mechanics—postural alterations lead to chronic muscle tension and pain.
6. Advise sleeping with a rolled terry cloth towel under the neck—for relief of cervical OA.
7. Provide crutches, braces, walker, or cane when indicated—to reduce weight-bearing stress on hips and knees. Teach proper use of assistive devices, see page 859.
8. Advise wearing corrective shoes and metatarsal supports for foot disorders—also helps in the treatment of arthritis of the knee.
9. Encourage weight loss to decrease stress on weight-bearing joints.
10. Support the patient undergoing orthopedic surgery for unremitting pain and disabling arthritis of joints (see page 868).

 GERONTOLOGIC ALERT Older patients are at greater risk for GI bleeding and renal failure associated with NSAID use. Encourage administration with meals and monitor stool for occult blood. Celecoxib and meloxicam are associated with less risk of GI bleeding but may cause an increased risk of cardiovascular embolic events and deleterious effects on the kidneys.

Increasing Physical Mobility
1. Encourage activity as much as possible without causing pain.
2. Teach ROM exercises to maintain joint mobility and muscle tone for joint support, to prevent capsular and tendon tightening, and to prevent deformities. Avoid flexion and adduction deformities.
3. Teach isometric exercises and graded exercises to improve muscle strength around the involved joint.
4. Advise putting joints through ROM after periods of inactivity (eg, automobile ride).

Promoting Self-Care
1. Suggest performing important activities in morning, after stiffness has been abated and before fatigue and pain become a problem.
2. Advise on modifications, such as wearing looser clothing without buttons, placing bench in tub or shower for bathing, sitting at table or counter in kitchen to prepare meals.
3. Help with obtaining assistive devices, such as padded handles for utensils and grooming aids, to promote independence.
4. Refer to OT for additional assistance.

Patient Education and Health Maintenance
1. Suggest swimming or water aerobics (offered by the YMCA) as a form of nonstressful exercise to preserve mobility.
2. Encourage adequate diet and sleep to enhance general health.
3. Advise the patient to discuss the use of complementary therapies, such as glucosamine and chondroitin sulfate, with health care provider.
4. For additional information and support, refer to the Arthritis Foundation (*www.arthritis.org*).

Evaluation: Expected Outcomes
- Reports reduction in pain while ambulatory.
- Performs ROM exercises.
- Dresses, bathes self, and grooms with assistive devices.

Neoplasms of the Musculoskeletal System

Musculoskeletal neoplasms include primary *sarcomas, metastatic bone disease*, and benign tumors (*osteoma, chondroma, osteoclastoma*) of the bone. More than 60% of bone neoplasms are metastatic from other sites of cancer.

Pathophysiology and Etiology

Benign Bone Tumors

Osteoid osteoma, chondroma, and osteoclastoma (benign giant cell tumor) are examples of benign bone tumors. Malignant transformation occurs with some.

Malignant Bone Tumors

1. Chondrosarcoma and osteosarcoma are examples of primary malignant bone tumors.
   a. Tumors develop in areas of rapid growth.
   b. Risk factors include Paget disease, previous radiation therapy to the bone, and other bone diseases.
   c. Hematogenous spread to the lung occurs.
2. Multiple myeloma is a malignant neoplasm arising from the bone marrow.

Metastatic Bone Tumors

1. Metastatic bone tumors are most frequently associated with cancers of the breast, prostate, and lung (primary malignancy site).
2. Bone metastasis most frequently occurs in the vertebrae and results in pathologic fracture.

Clinical Manifestations

1. Pain in the involved bone—from effects of tumor (destruction, erosion, and expansion of tumor).
   a. Generally mild to constant pain, which may be worse at night or with activity.
   b. Pain will be acute with fracture.
   c. Neurologic symptoms may present with nerve root compression.
2. Swelling and limitation of motion and joint effusion.
3. Physical findings.
   a. Palpable, tender, fixed bony mass.
   b. Increase in skin temperature over mass.
   c. Superficial veins dilated and prominent.

Diagnostic Evaluation

1. X-ray will usually reveal bone tumor; may show increased or decreased bone density. Tomograms may be helpful for some benign osseous lesions.
2. CT and MRI demonstrate soft tissue involvement and location of tumors.
3. Bone scan—helpful in detecting initial extent of malignancy, planning therapy, defining level of amputation, and following course of radiation or chemotherapy.
4. Ultrasound may help with identification of the lesion.
5. Serum alkaline phosphatase—usually increased.
6. Bence Jones protein in urine with multiple myeloma.
7. Biopsy of bone—to confirm suspected diagnosis.
8. Chest x-ray and lung scan—to determine if metastasis is present.
9. Arteriography—to assess soft tissue involvement.

Management

A multidisciplinary approach in a cancer center is usually preferred. The basic objective is to halt the progression of the tumor by destroying or removing the lesion. Treatment depends on the type of tumor. Combinations of chemotherapy, surgery, and radiation may be indicated as most appropriate for specific type of tumor.

Surgery

1. Tumor curettage or resection with bone grafting may be used.
2. Limb-salvaging procedures involve resection of affected bone and surrounding normal muscle tissue and reconstruction using metallic prostheses or allografts for bone or joint replacement and skin grafting, as needed.
3. Amputation is necessary in some cases.

Chemotherapy

May be used as preoperative, adjunctive, and palliative treatment.
1. Chemotherapy may be administered before (to shrink the tumor) and after (to destroy metastasis) surgery.
2. Chemotherapy used in combination to achieve a greater patient response at a lower toxicity rate and to minimize potential problems of drug resistance and may be given in varying courses separated by rest periods.

Radiotherapy

1. Tumor irradiation may be used.
2. Prophylactic lung irradiation may be performed—to suppress metastasis.

Other Therapies

1. Immunotherapy—interferon.
2. Hormone therapy may be used with metastatic tumors of the breast and prostate.
3. If pathologic fracture occurs, the fracture is managed with open reduction and internal fixation or other fracture treatment method.

Complications

1. Lack of tumor control and metastases.
2. Pathologic fracture.
3. Hypercalcemia from bone destruction.

Nursing Assessment

1. Obtain history of progression of disease; presence of pain, fever, weight loss, malaise.
2. Examine for painless mass.
3. Review records for evidence of pathologic fracture.
4. Assess knowledge of cancer, experiences with family or others, and present coping.

Nursing Diagnoses

- Acute Pain related to effects of tumor.
- Risk for Injury related to altered bone structure.
- Ineffective Coping related to diagnosis and treatment options.

Nursing Interventions

See also "Orthopedic Surgery," page 868, and "Amputation," page 873.

Relieving Pain

1. Use multiple approaches to reduce discomfort (see page 1508).
2. Administer pain medications 30 minutes before ambulation or other uncomfortable movement.
3. Support painful extremities on pillows.

Preventing Pathologic Fractures

1. Assist the patient in movement with gentleness and patience.
2. Avoid jarring the patient or bed.
3. Support joints when repositioning the patient.
4. Guard the patient to avoid falls.
5. Create a hazard-free environment.
6. Provide patient education on safety.

Strengthening Coping Ability

1. Create a supportive environment.
2. Use psychological support services, as needed.
3. Answer questions and clear up misconceptions about treatment options.

Patient Education and Health Maintenance

1. Teach about particular treatment selected. See page 112 for information on chemotherapy and page 122 for radiation therapy information.
2. Encourage appropriate follow-up and diagnostic testing for recurrence.
3. Refer for additional information and support to the American Cancer Society (*www.cancer.org*).

Evaluation: Expected Outcomes

- Reports decreased pain with ambulation.
- No signs or symptoms of fractures.
- Verbalizes understanding of treatment options and strength to make decisions.

Osteomyelitis

Osteomyelitis is a severe pyogenic infection of the bone and surrounding tissues, which requires immediate treatment.

Pathophysiology and Etiology

1. Generally, bacteria gain entry to the bone via three routes:
   a. Bloodstream (hematogenous spread).
   b. Adjacent soft tissue infection (contiguous focus).
   c. Direct introduction of microorganisms into the bone.
2. Bacteria lodge and multiply in bone.
3. Pressure increases as pus collects in confined rigid bone, contributing to ischemia and vascular occlusion and leading to bone necrosis.
4. *Staphylococcus aureus* is the most common infecting microorganism, although others are prevalent: *Escherichia coli*, *Pseudomonas*, *Klebsiella*, *Salmonella*, and *Proteus*.

Clinical Manifestations

1. Infection of long bones with acute pain and signs of sepsis.
2. Localized pain and drainage.
3. Symptoms vary in adults and children according to the site of involvement.

Diagnostic Evaluation

1. Acute osteomyelitis diagnosis made on initial clinical signs (history, physical examination, CBC, ESR).
2. Aerobic and anaerobic cultures of bone and deep tissue to identify the organism. Wound cultures are not reliable.
3. ESR elevated, WBC and hemoglobin decreased.
4. Radiographic evidence of osteomyelitis lags behind symptoms by up to 14 days.
5. Radionuclide bone scans used to diagnose early acute osteomyelitis.
6. MRI used increasingly—distinguishes between soft tissue and bone marrow.

Management

1. Acute: full recovery possible with minimal loss of function.
2. Chronic: develops with inadequate or ineffective course of antibiotics or delayed treatment.

Surgical Intervention

1. Needle aspiration or needle biopsy done initially.
2. Surgical intervention may be needed to obtain culture and sensitivity of specimen.
3. Surgical decompression considered when the patient does not improve after 36 to 48 hours of antimicrobial therapy.
4. Debridement may be done, or antibiotic-impregnated beads used in wound (removed after 2 to 4 weeks and replaced with bone graft).
5. Hyperbaric oxygen therapy may be used as an adjunctive therapy.

Pharmacologic Intervention

1. Employ quickly after presentation of symptoms to avoid chronicity.
2. Parental antimicrobial therapy based on blood/wound cultures.
3. Medications depend on organism but include the following:
   a. Penicillins (penicillin G, penicillin V).
   b. Semisynthetic penicillins (nafcillin, oxacillin, methicillin).
   c. Extended-spectrum penicillins (ampicillin, carbenicillin, amoxicillin).
   d. Beta-lactam agents (imipenem).
   e. Tetracyclines.
   f. Cephalosporins.
   g. Aminoglycosides.
4. Requires 6 to 8 weeks of IV antibiotic therapy, requiring a peripherally inserted central catheter line or other long-term access device and coordination of home care services.

Complications

1. Nonhealing wound.
2. Sepsis.
3. Immobility.
4. Amputation.

Nursing Assessment

1. Obtain detailed history of injury.
2. Assess pain and functional deficits.
3. Be aware that systemic symptoms are acute in children but vary in intensity with adults.
4. Perform general systemic assessment because adults with long bone involvement generally have more systemic septic symptoms.

Nursing Diagnoses

- Acute Pain related to inflammatory process.
- Deficient Knowledge related to disease and medications.
- Impaired Physical Mobility related to rest of affected part.

Nursing Interventions

Relieving Pain

1. Administer opioids for acute pain; nonopioids for chronic pain.
2. Administer medications around the clock versus as necessary to establish a consistent blood level.
3. Report any increase in pain that may indicate worsening infection.

Increasing Knowledge

1. Describe the infectious process and rationale for prolonged treatment with osteomyelitis.
2. Explain IV antibiotic therapy, potential adverse effects, and reactions.
3. Explain strict adherence to infection control practices (sterile technique, hand washing, selection of roommate) to prevent spread of infection in some cases.

4. Initiate home care nursing and infusion service referrals before discharge.

Promoting Rest without Complications

1. Support the affected extremity (splint, traction) to minimize pain.
2. If the patient is on bed rest, prevent hazards of immobility (passive ROM, position changes, coughing, and deep breathing).
3. Encourage distraction activities.

Patient Education and Health Maintenance

1. Advise the patient to adhere to infection control principles—proper hand washing, disposal of wound drainage, dressings to prevent reinfection or transmission of infection at home.
2. Stress adherence to medication regimen, which may be prolonged, with frequent follow-up visits.
3. Teach care of indwelling device for medication delivery.
4. Educate the patient on signs and symptoms of infection to monitor for and when to notify physician.

Evaluation: Expected Outcomes

- Pain managed with nonopioid analgesics.
- Infectious process minimized.
- Functional status of affected joint intact.

Paget Disease (Osteitis Deformans)

Paget disease of the bone is a skeletal disorder resulting from excessive osteoclastic activity, affecting the long bones, pelvis, lumbar vertebrae, and the skull predominantly.

Pathophysiology and Etiology

1. The cause of this disease is unknown, although there is evidence of familial tendency (25% to 40% have at least one affected relative).
2. More common in men than in women.
3. Rare before age 40 and increases as age does—12% after age 80.
4. May be caused by infection from blood-borne viruses. After acute viremia, osteoclasts become chronically infected, stimulating osteoclastic proliferation. See Figure 32-13.

Clinical Manifestations

1. Generally asymptomatic.

2. Most common symptoms are pain and predisposition to fracture.
3. Pagetic lesions can lead to OA, joint destruction, spinal deformity.
4. Decrease in hearing, tinnitus, and vertigo as a result of skull abnormality.
5. Waddling gait due to abnormality of pelvis.
6. Radiculopathy and nerve palsies due to effects from the vertebral column.
7. Rarely, heart failure and other cardiovascular effects from increased blood supply over abnormal bone.
8. Malignant bone tumors occur in 5% to 10%.

Diagnostic Evaluation

1. Elevated serum alkaline phosphatase and urine hydroxyproline.
2. Serum calcium, phosphorus, and albumin levels usually normal.
3. Generally confirmed with radiologic examinations showing characteristic abnormalities.
4. Bone scans can evaluate rapid bone turnover.
5. Bone biopsy to differentiate from osteomyelitis or bone tumor.

Management

1. No treatment for asymptomatic Paget.
2. Pain management—NSAIDs, aspirin.
3. Medications—calcitonin is the main medication used to suppress bone turnover, reduce pain, and prevent progression.
4. Other medications used to block bone resorption—the bisphosphonates etidronate disodium, alendronate, pamidronate, risedronate; an antineoplastic agent, plicamycin.
5. Tibial osteotomy done to realign knees and relieve pain.

Nursing Assessment

1. Assess pain and functional ability.
2. Observe for bowing (legs) or complaint that hats feel tight.
3. Assess for cardiovascular complications.
4. Assess for auditory symptoms—tinnitus, vertigo, and hearing loss.

Nursing Diagnoses

- Chronic Pain related to pathophysiologic process.
- Risk for Injury related to falls.

Figure 32-13. Pathophysiology of Paget disease.

Nursing Interventions

Reducing Pain
1. Administer and teach self-administration of analgesics.
2. Avoid sedation due to opioids, which may increase risk of falls.

Preventing Injury
1. Establish exercise protocols through a PT consult to maintain physical abilities and prevent falls.
2. Teach safe transferring and make sure that the patient can alert nurses if he or she needs help.
3. Assist the patient with activities, as necessary.
4. Provide function and mobility aids such as heel lifts, walking aids, as needed, through an OT consult.

Patient Education and Health Maintenance

1. Teach safety measures in the home—removal of loose rugs and obstacles to prevent falls, good lighting.
2. Provide education about the disease process and medication treatment.
3. Make sure that the patient knows how to use mobility aids.
4. Initiate home care referral, as indicated.
5. Advise the patient that laboratory testing to monitor serum calcium, phosphorous, vitamin D, and kidney function may be ordered.
6. Provide information about The Paget Foundation (*www. paget.org*).
7. Encourage follow-up for periodic hearing tests and blood work.

Evaluation: Expected Outcomes

- The patient reports reduced pain scale score
- No falls

Hallux Valgus

Also called *bunion*, *hallux valgus* is a deformity of the foot involving the first metatarsal and great toe. Occurs in females more frequently than in males and incidence increases with age; may have a genetic predisposition. Commonly occurs with other deformities of the feet, such as hammertoe, mallet toe, and claw toe.

Clinical Manifestations

1. Pain.
2. Possible callus of skin overlying bunion and accompanying toe deformities.
3. Diminished ROM.
4. Generally associated with tight footwear.

Management and Nursing Interventions

Conservative Management
1. Wearing footwear made of soft material with a wider toe box, rounded rather than pointed, and with low heel.
2. Special orthoses can be ordered.
3. Steroid injections to relieve pain.

Surgical Management
Surgical alignment of the great toe by osteotomy of metatarsal or proximal phalanx of the great toe or fusion of the metatarsal–metatarsophalangeal joint.

Postoperative Care
1. Elevation of the foot to reduce pain.

2. Initial non–weight-bearing activity, with very gradual progress in activity.
3. Crutch walking initially, followed by wooden shoe immobilizer for several weeks.
4. NSAIDs and opioid analgesics for pain.
5. Bandages changed by the surgeon initially.

SELECTED REFERENCES

A'Court, J., Lees, D., Harrison, W., Ankers, T., & Reed, M. (2017). Pain and analgesia requirements with hip fracture surgery. *Orthopaedic Nursing, 36*(3), 224–228.

American Academy of Orthopaedic Surgeons. (2013). *Treatment of osteoarthritis of the knee: Evidence-based guideline* (2nd ed.). Rosemont, IL: Author.

American Academy of Orthopaedic Surgeons. (2014). *Management of anterior cruciate ligament injuries: Evidence-based clinical practice guideline.* Rosemont, IL: Author.

American Association of Orthopaedic Surgeons. (2014). *Management of hip fractures in the elderly: Evidence-based clinical practice guideline.* Rosemont, IL: Author.

American Academy of Orthopaedic Surgeons. (2017). *Management of osteoarthritis of the hip evidence-based clinical practice guideline.* Rosemont, IL: Author.

American Association of Orthopaedic Surgeons and American Dental Association. (2012). *Prevention of orthopaedic implant infection in patients undergoing dental procedures: Evidence-based guideline and evidence report.* Rosemont, IL: Author.

Georgiades, D. (2018). Systematic integrative review of pin site crusts. *Orthopaedic Nursing, 37*(1), 36–42.

Graham, P. (2017). Calcific tendinitis of the shoulder. *Orthopaedic Nursing, 36*(6), 439–441.

Gwynne-Jones, D., Martin, G., & Crane, C. (2017). Enhanced recovery after surgery for hip and knee replacements. *Orthopaedic Nursing, 36*(3), 203–210.

Liebert, R. (2016). Establishment and evaluation of an anterior cruciate ligament injury prevention program. *Orthopaedic Nursing, 35*(3), 161–171.

Mori, C., Hageman, D., & Zimmerly, K. (2017). Nursing care of the patient undergoing an anterior approach to total hip arthroplasty. *Orthopaedic Nursing, 36*(2), 124–130.

National Association of Orthopaedic Nurses. (2018). *An Introduction to Orthopaedic Nursing,* 5th Edition. Chicago: Author.

National Association of Orthopedic Nurses. (2015). *Clinical Practice Guideline for Thromboembolic Disease Prevention.* Chicago: Author.

National Association of Orthopaedic Nurses. (2013). *Clinical Practice Guideline for Surgical Site Infection Prevention.* Chicago: Author.

National Association of Orthopaedic Nurses. (2013). *Acute Pain Management Algorithms for the Adult Orthopaedic Patient.* Chicago: Author.

National Association of Orthopaedic Nurses. (2017). *Orthopaedic Surgery Manual,* 3rd Edition. Chicago: Author.

National Association of Orthopaedic Nurses. (2016). *Safe Patient Handling and Mobility Algorithms for the Adult Orthopaedic Patient.* Chicago: Author.

National Institute for Health and Clinical Excellence. (2014). *Osteoarthritis: Care and management.* London: Author.

Oliveira, M., Campos, M., Padilha, J., et al. (2011). Exploring the family caregiving phenomenon in nursing documentation. *Online Journal of Nursing Informatics, 15*(1).

Powell-Cope, G., Thomason, S., Bulat, T. (2018). Preventing falls and related injuries at home. *American Journal of Nursing, 118*(1), 58–61.

Prah, A., Richards, E., Griggs, R., Simpson, V. (2017). Enhancing osteoporosis efforts through lifestyle modifications and goal-setting techniques. *Journal for Nurse Practitioners, 13*(8), 552–561.

Qaseem, A., Wilt, T. J., McLean, R. M., Forciea, M. A.; for the Clinical Guidelines Committee of the American College of Physicians. (2017). Noninvasive treatments for acute, subacute, and chronic low back pain: A clinical practice guideline from the American College of Physicians. *Annals of Internal Medicine, 166*(7), 514–530.

Salt, E., Gokun, Y., Rankin Kerr, A., & Talbert, J. (2016). A description and comparison of treatments for low back pain in the United States. *Orthopaedic Nursing, 35*(4), 214–221.

Slaughter, A., Reynolds, K. A., Jambhekar, K., et al. (2014). Clinical orthopedic examination findings in the lower extremity: Correlation with imaging studies and diagnostic efficacy. *RadioGraphics, 34*(2), e41–e55.

Whitehead, P.B. (2018). The effects of yoga on chronic nonspecific backpain. *American Journal of Nursing, 118*(2), 64.

33
Dermatologic Disorders

OVERVIEW AND ASSESSMENT
Description of Skin Lesions

The description of dermatologic conditions always includes the morphology of the lesions that appear on the skin (ie, their size, shape, color, pattern, and distribution; see Figure 33-1).

Primary Lesions

1. Macule—flat, circumscribed discoloration of the skin; may have any size or shape.
2. Papule—solid, elevated lesion less than 1 cm wide.
3. Nodule—raised, solid lesion larger than 1 cm wide.
4. Vesicle—circumscribed elevated lesion less than 0.5 cm, containing fluid.
5. Bulla—a vesicle or blister larger than 0.5 cm wide.
6. Pustule—circumscribed raised lesion that contains pus; may form as a result of purulent changes in a vesicle.
7. Wheal—elevation of the skin that lasts less than 24 hours, caused by edema of the dermis; may be surrounded by erythema or blanching.
8. Plaque—solid, elevated lesion on the skin or mucous membrane, larger than 1 cm in diameter; psoriasis is commonly manifested as plaques on the skin; leukoplakia is an example of plaques on mucous membranes.
9. Cyst—soft or firm mass in the skin, filled with semisolid or with liquid material contained in a sac.

Secondary Lesions

Secondary lesions involve changes that take place in primary lesions that modify them.
1. Scale—heaped-up, horny layer of dead epidermis; may develop as a result of inflammatory changes.
2. Crust—covering formed by the drying of serum, blood, or pus on the skin (scab).
3. Excoriation—linear scratch marks or traumatized areas of the skin.
4. Fissure—linear cracks in the skin, usually from marked drying and long-standing inflammation.
5. Ulcer—lesion formed by local destruction of the epidermis and by part or all of the underlying dermis.
6. Lichenification—thickening of the skin accompanied by accentuation of skin markings.
7. Scar/keloid—abnormal new formation of connective tissue that replaces the loss of substance in the dermis as a result of injury or disease. A keloid is a hypertrophic scar that is larger than the original lesion or injury.
8. Atrophy—diminution in size or in loss of skin cells that causes thinning of the skin.

Other Lesions

1. Petechiae—circumscribed deposits of blood or blood pigment 1 to 2 mm wide.
2. Purpura—circumscribed deposits of blood or blood pigment greater than 0.5 cm wide.

Primary lesions

Figure 33-1. Types of skin lesions. (From Smeltzer, S., & Bare, B. [2000]. *Brunner and Suddarth's textbook of medical-surgical nursing* [9th ed.]. Philadelphia, PA: Lippincott Williams & Wilkins.)

3. Comedones—hair follicle obstructed by a sebum and keratin plug; blackheads and whiteheads.
4. Telangiectasia—small, irregular blood vessels visible in the epidermis.
5. Burrow—linear, irregular, elevated tunnel produced by parasites in the skin.

Shape and Configuration

After the type of lesion is identified, the shape, configuration or arrangement (in relation to each other), and pattern of distribution are noted (see Figure 33-2). The following are descriptions commonly used:

1. Annular—ring shaped.
2. Circinate—circular.
3. Confluent—lesions run together or join.

4. Discoid—disk shaped.
5. Discrete—lesions remain separate.
6. Generalized—widespread eruption.
7. Grouped—clustering of lesions.
8. Guttate—droplike.
9. Herpetiform—grouped vesicles.
10. Iris—ring or a series of concentric circles (bull's eye).
11. Linear—in lines.
12. Nummular—coin shaped.
13. Polymorphous—occurring in several or many forms.
14. Reticulated—lacelike network.
15. Serpiginous—snakelike or creeping eruption.
16. Telangiectatic—a tiny red thread or line.
17. Zosteriform or dermatomal—bandlike distribution, limited to one or more dermatomes of the skin.

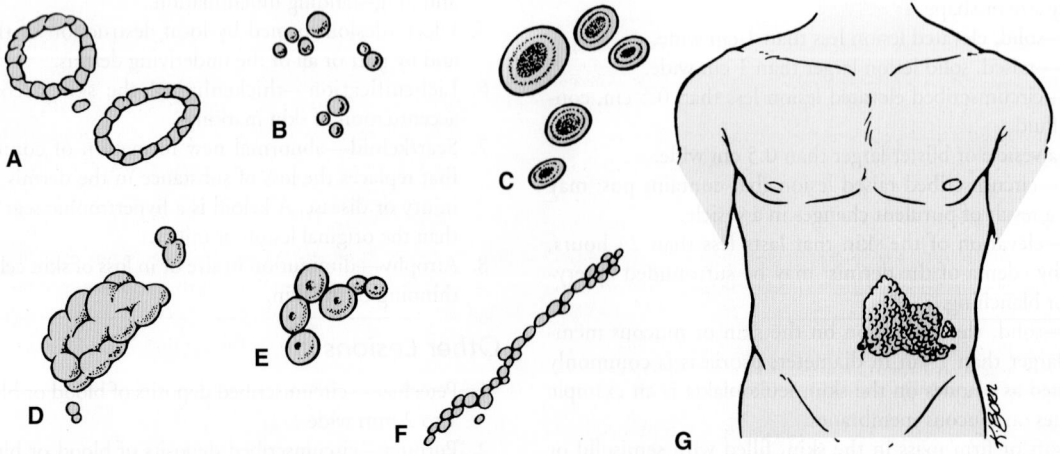

Figure 33-2. Shape and arrangement of skin lesions: **(A)** annular, **(B)** grouped, **(C)** iris, **(D)** confluent, **(E)** herpetiform, **(F)** linear, **(G)** zosteriform or dermatomal.

History

Obtaining a thorough history is the key to diagnosing and developing a plan of care for dermatologic conditions, as well as understanding the characteristics of the problem and its effect on the patient.

Characteristics of Rash

1. When did the rash first occur? Was the onset sudden or gradual?
2. What site was first affected? Describe the spread and its severity.
3. What was the initial color and configuration of the rash? Has it changed?
4. Is there associated itching, burning, tingling, pain, or numbness?
5. Has it been constant or intermittent?

Associated Factors

1. What makes the rash worse or better? Is it seasonal? Is it affected by stress?
2. What medications are being taken? What topical products have been used? What effect did they have?
3. What skin products are used? What chemicals have come into contact with the skin: such as laundry detergent, cleaning products, insecticides, or nickel?
4. Has there been pet contact?
5. What is the patient's occupation? Any hobbies, such as gardening or hiking, that may have contributed? Are latex gloves worn routinely? Is frequent handwashing required?
6. What is the sexual history and chance of sexually transmitted disease exposure (if relevant)?
7. Any international travel?

Medical History

1. Is there a history of hay fever, asthma, hives, eczema, or allergies?
2. Has the patient had this particular rash or other skin disorders in the past?
3. What is the family history of skin disorders?
4. Are there any long-standing medical problems? Immunosuppressive therapy?

Physical Examination

1. Focus your examination on the skin, hair, and nails. Some dermatologic conditions affect other body systems (eg, hair loss may be associated with thyroid disease or anemia); perform a general physical exam, as indicated.
2. Ask the patient to show you the area of concern and examine the skin surface under good lighting. Patients should be undressed, in a gown, and the skin of the total body should be examined, not just the area affected.
3. Note the distribution and configuration of skin lesions. Compare right and left sides of the body.
4. Note the shape, border, texture, and surface of the lesions.
5. Palpate the lesions for texture, warmth, and tenderness.
6. Use a metric ruler to determine size of lesions to serve as a baseline for comparison with subsequent measurements.
7. Examine the scalp, nails, and oral mucosa.
8. Perform diascopy—gently press a glass slide or Lucite rule over a skin lesion to detect blanching (caused by dilated blood vessels).
9. Use a Wood light to inspect for fluorescent changes with some fungal infections. Clean the skin prior to examination because some ointments, soaps, or deodorant may fluoresce.
10. For dark-skinned patients, look for black, purple, or gray lesions; palpate carefully to determine if rash is present.

Laboratory Tests

Some dermatologic conditions can be evaluated by laboratory tests such as microscopy and culture.

Microscopy

Description

1. Sample taken by scraping, swabbing, or aspirating a lesion is transferred to a glass slide for microscopic examination or staining.
   a. Direct visualization of scrapings mixed with mineral oil to detect scabies, mites, or lice nits that cling to the hair.
   b. A Tzanck smear is obtained from vesicular fluid or a moist ulcer and stained to detect characteristics of herpes simplex virus, herpes zoster, and varicella. This is rarely done in the office, but properly obtained specimen could be sent to the lab.
   c. Potassium hydroxide may be added to skin scrapings on a glass slide and heated to dissolve skin cells to detect hyphae and spores in fungal infections.
   d. Gram stain may be performed by the lab or dermatopathologist to tentatively identify bacteria or fungi in certain skin infections.

Nursing and Patient Care Considerations

1. To obtain the specimen for microscopy, use the side of a glass slide or a scalpel held at a 45-degree angle to gently scrape the active border of a dry lesion or of an inflamed area; only mild discomfort and pinpoint bleeding should occur.
2. For moist or semimoist ulcerations or crusted lesions, roll saline-soaked cotton or Dacron-tipped swab over the lesion; for weeping lesions, use a dry swab.
3. For intact vesicles, aspirate fluid from the edge with a 25-G sterile needle; if vesicle is partially broken, gently unroof with forceps and obtain fluid on a swab.

Culture

Description

1. Drainage from lesions may be cultured on specific media to detect causative organism and sensitivity to antimicrobial therapy; also, portions of the skin, hair, and nails may be submitted for fungal culture.
2. Usually takes 24 to 48 hours for results; fungal cultures may take 4 to 5 weeks.

Nursing and Patient Care Considerations

1. Obtain specimen with cotton- or Dacron-tipped swab, and send to laboratory in bacterial culture container clearly labeled with the patient's name, the date, and the site where the specimen was obtained or in a viral culture container also clearly labeled. Refrigerate viral culture if laboratory pickup is delayed.
2. To obtain specimen for fungal culture, scrape or clip the affected skin, hair, or nails; then, place into a dry, sterile container for transport or onto a dermatophyte test medium.

Other Tests

Patch Testing

Description

1. *Patch testing* is an office procedure done to determine if patients are sensitive to contact materials.

2. Materials are applied in patches to the skin and checked for reaction 48 hours after application and possibly again in 1 week.
3. Erythema, itching, swelling, papules, and vesicles indicate an allergic contact dermatitis rather than an irritant contact dermatitis or no reaction.

Nursing and Patient Care Considerations

1. Confirm that patient has been off oral corticosteroids at the time of the test; topical corticosteroids should be discontinued 1 to 2 weeks before testing to prevent a weak reaction or false-negative results. Make sure the patient has followed the health care provider's instructions.
2. When patient returns in 48 hours for the first reading, mark the outline of the patch strip on the patient's back; then, remove the strip. A skin marker or an ultraviolet skin pen marker may be used.
3. Wait 30 minutes; then, do the first reading. Document based on the outcome as follows or take a picture for the patient's record:
   a. 1+ Weak reaction. Nonvesicular, but with erythema, induration, and possible papules.
   b. 2+ Strong reaction. Edematous and vesicular, with erythema, edema, papules, and vesicles.
   c. 3+ Extreme reaction. Spreading, bullous, ulcerative IR (irritant reaction).
   d. Negative reaction.

GENERAL PROCEDURES AND TREATMENT MODALITIES
Baths and Wet Dressings

A therapeutic bath is used to apply medication to the entire skin surface and is useful in treating widespread eruptions and general pruritus. Baths soothe, soften, and reduce inflammation and relieve itching and dryness. See Table 33-1 for types and desired effects. Wet dressings and soaks are damp compresses that contain water,

Table 33-1 Therapeutic Baths

BATH SOLUTION AND MEDICATION	DESIRED EFFECT
Water	• Removes crusts and relieves inflammation
Saline	• Used for widely disseminated lesions
Colloidal Oatmeal	• Antipruritic and demulcent
Sodium Bicarbonate	• Cooling
Starch	• Soothing
Tar Baths (follow package directions)	• Used for psoriasis and chronic eczematous conditions
Bath Oils	• Used for antipruritic and emollient soothing properties • Used for acute and subacute eczematous eruptions
Bleach Baths	• Reduces colonization of harmful bacteria that contribute to acute and chronic eczema

normal saline solution, aluminum acetate (Burow) solution, or magnesium sulfate solution. They may be sterile or clean, or warm or cool, depending on the skin condition and the area to which they are applied.

Therapeutic Baths
Indications
1. Vesicular disorders, eczema, atopic dermatitis.
2. Acute inflammatory conditions.
3. Erosions and exudative, crusted surfaces.

Nursing and Patient Care Considerations
1. Prepare the bath or teach patient to prepare a lukewarm bath at 90°F to 100°F (32.2°C to 37.8°C); with the tub half-full, add the prescribed quantity of medication and mix thoroughly to prevent sensitivity reaction. Add oatmeal products or oils to emulsifying baths.
   a. Bleach baths may be used for acute and chronic atopic dermatitis.
   b. Add ½ cup of bleach to full tub or ¼ cup to half tub of warm water, and soak limbs and torso for 5 to 10 minutes (do not submerge head), no more than twice a week.
2. Do not rub the skin. Soaking for at least 5 to 10 minutes will promote removal of loosened scales.
3. Keep the room and water at comfortable temperatures and limit bathing to 20 to 30 minutes; the bath area should be well ventilated if tars are used because they are volatile.
4. Tell patient to use a bath mat inside the tub and to use a rug outside the tub when bathing at home because medication may make the tub and other wet surfaces slippery.
5. Blot skin dry with a towel and apply emollient or topical medication to moist skin. While the skin is wet, apply steroid to inflamed areas, if prescribed.

Open Wet Dressings
Indications
1. Bacterial infections that require drainage.
2. Inflammatory and pruritic conditions.
3. Oozing and crusting conditions.

Nursing and Patient Care Considerations
1. Apply dressing to affected area or teach patient to apply. Moisten to the point of slight dripping; remoisten as necessary.
2. Use warm tap water if warming is desired.
3. Application may be from 5 to 15 minutes three to four times per day, unless otherwise indicated.
4. Keep patient warm and do not treat more than one third of the body at a time because open wet dressings can cause chilling and hypothermia.
5. Teach patients to prevent burns by measuring temperature of solution with a bath thermometer or by testing tap water on the wrist before applying compress. Advise them not to use microwave ovens to warm dressings because uneven heating can occur.

Other Dressings
Occlusive Dressing

An *occlusive dressing* is formed by an airtight plastic or vinyl film applied over medicated areas of the skin (usually with corticosteroids) to enhance absorption of medication and to promote moisture retention.

Indications

Skin conditions with thick scaling, such as psoriasis, eczema, and lichen simplex chronicus.

Nursing and Patient Care Considerations

1. Wash area and pat dry.
2. Apply medication while the skin is still moist.
3. Cover with plastic wrap, vinyl gloves, or plastic bag.
4. Seal with paper tape at edges or cover with other self-adhesive dressing to hold in place.
5. Do not apply to ulcerated or abraded skin; removal is recommended within 12 to 24 hours. High-potency steroids are for short-term use only.

 DRUG ALERT Excessive use of occlusive dressings that contain corticosteroids may cause skin atrophy, striae, telangiectasia, folliculitis, nonhealing ulceration, erythema, and systemic absorption of corticosteroids.

Nonocclusive Dressings

Other dressing materials may be used as dry dressings to protect the skin, keep affected areas clean, absorb drainage, or cover medication or hold occlusive dressings in place.

Nursing and Patient Care Considerations

1. Apply dry gauze dressing using clean technique (unless sterile technique is indicated by open wounds).
2. Wrap extremities with elastic or cotton-rolled bandages or apply tape. Avoid constricting circulation.
3. Alternative dressing materials can be used for home care, such as disposable or white cotton gloves for the hands, cotton socks for the feet, sheets or towels for large areas, disposable diapers or towels folded in diaper fashion for the groin, washcloths for the axilla, cotton T-shirt or cotton pajamas for the trunk, turban or plastic shower cap for the scalp, or mask made from gauze for the face, with holes cut for the eyes, mouth, and nose.

Skin Biopsy

Removal of a piece of the skin by shave, punch, or excision technique to detect malignancy or other characteristics of skin disorders.

Types of Biopsy

1. Shave biopsy—scalpel used to remove raised lesions, leaving lower layers of the dermis intact.
2. Punch biopsy—special instrument used to remove round core of lesion, containing all layers of the skin. Biopsy site is usually closed with sutures.
3. Excisional biopsy—scalpel and scissors used to remove the entire lesion, usually with prescribed margins; suturing required.

Nursing and Patient Care Considerations

1. Position patient comfortably with the site exposed; explain that a local anesthetic will be given.
2. Check if patient has any known allergies to local anesthetics.
3. Ask patient what current medication he or she is taking. Aspirin, some herbal supplements, or anticoagulants may cause increased postoperative bleeding.

4. Explain the procedure.
5. Obtain written consent.
6. After the biopsy, apply hemostatic agent and pressure to the site to stop bleeding, along with an appropriate dressing. Pressure dressing may be required for larger wounds or wounds that are bleeding.
7. Place the biopsy specimen in a clearly labeled container with 10% formaldehyde, and transport it to the dermatopathology lab for hematoxylin and eosin staining. It is essential that skin biopsies be sent to a specialized dermatopathology lab for examination by a dermatopathologist to get the best analysis and most complete information on the histology of the skin disease or lesion.

Patient Education

1. Keep the bandage on surgery site for 24 to 48 hours. During this time, keep site clean and dry.
2. After this time, remove the bandage and do the following daily:
   a. Wash the incision with soap and water.
   b. Dry the incision well.
   c. Apply petroleum- or mineral oil–based ointment, such as Vaseline or Aquaphor, one to four times per day, keeping the incision moist at all times.
3. After a few days, the dressing is no longer needed but continue to apply ointment one to four times per day to keep the site moist and help reduce scarring.
4. Do not apply makeup directly to the stitches.
5. Repeat wound care for 2 or 3 days after stitches have been removed, unless otherwise instructed.
6. Use caution when shaving around stitches on the face.

 DRUG ALERT Many patients are allergic to neomycin, a component of triple antibiotic ointment. Petrolatum- or mineral oil–based ointments pose less risk of allergic dermatitis.

Wound Coverage: Grafts and Flaps

Wound coverage, using grafts and flaps, is a type of reconstructive (plastic) surgery performed to improve the skin's appearance and function. These are sometimes used following Mohs micrographic surgery to remove skin cancers, especially on the face, head, and neck.

Skin Graft

1. A section of skin tissue is separated from its blood supply and transferred as free tissue to a distant (recipient) site; it must obtain nourishment from capillaries at the recipient site.
2. In dermatology, skin grafting is used to repair defects that result from excision of skin tumors and to cover areas of denuded skin.
3. Definitions.
   a. Autografts—grafts done with tissue transplanted from the patient's own skin.
   b. Allografts—involve the transplant of tissue from one individual of the same species; these grafts are also called allogenic or homografts.
   c. Xenograft or heterograft—involves the transfer of tissue from another species.
4. Classification by thickness.

a. Split thickness (thin, intermediate, or thick)—graft that is cut at varying thicknesses and is used to cover large wounds because its total potential donor area is virtually unlimited.

b. Full thickness—graft consists of epidermis and all of the dermis without the underlying fat; used to cover wounds that are too large to close primarily. They are used frequently to cover facial defects because they provide a better contour match and less postoperative contracture.

Skin Flaps

1. A flap is a segment of tissue that has been left attached at one end (called a base or pedicle); the other end has been moved to a recipient area. It is dependent for its survival on functioning arterial and venous blood supplies and on lymphatic drainage in its pedicle or base.
   a. Free flap or free-tissue transfer—one that is completely severed from the body and is transferred to another site; receives early vascular supply from microvascular anastomosis with vessels at recipient site.
2. Flaps may consist of the skin, mucosa, muscle, adipose tissue, and omentum.
3. Used for wound coverage and to provide bulk, especially when bone, tendon, blood vessels, or nerve tissue are exposed.
4. Flaps offer the best aesthetic solution because a flap retains the color, texture, and thickness match of the donor area.
5. Flaps are classified according to the method of movement, composition, location, or function.

Procedure for Skin Grafts

1. Split-thickness skin graft is obtained by razor blade, skin-grafting knife, or electric or air-powered dermatome or drum dermatome. Most commonly obtained from the inner aspect of the upper arm or outer thigh.
2. A full-thickness skin graft is primarily excised, defatted, and tailored to fit accurately over the defect area.
3. Skin is taken from the donor or host site and applied to the wound or defect site, called the recipient site or graft bed.
4. A bolster (pressure) dressing is applied to the graft to enhance the survival of the skin graft by providing stable approximation of the graft to the recipient bed.
5. The bolster dressing is left in place for 1 week. The process of revascularization and reattachment of the skin graft to the recipient bed is referred to as a take.
6. The donor site is maintained clean and dry.
   a. If Scarlet Red (a single-layer dressing impregnated with epithelial growth promoter) is used on the donor site for split-thickness grafts, it is left in place for 2 to 3 weeks to allow the wound to heal.
   b. Occlusive dressings, such as Omniderm or Allevyn, may also be used to decrease pain, alleviate frequent wound care, and speed healing.
   c. Daily wound care and dressing change with an antimicrobial ointment and nonstick dressing may also be used.

 NURSING ALERT Patients usually find the donor site more painful than the graft site.

Preoperative Management and Nursing Care

1. Aspirin and nonsteroidal anti-inflammatory drugs (NSAIDs) and vitamin E are discontinued 14 days before the procedure.

Coumadin should be held for several days before the procedure, and prothrombin time and international normalized ratio should be measured before the procedure, as ordered. Herbal supplements, such as ginkgo, ginseng, green tea, and vitamin E, can inhibit coagulation.
2. Efforts should be made to enhance wound healing several months to several weeks before the procedure, such as smoking cessation, alcohol avoidance, and proper nutrition.
3. Medical history and examination should be evaluated, particularly for latex sensitivity, cardiovascular problems requiring endocarditis antibiotic prophylaxis, bleeding problems, and high blood pressure (BP).
4. The procedure is usually done under local anesthetic, so no meals are withheld.
5. The operative site should be free from makeup.
6. The patient should have someone available to drive him or her home after surgery unless otherwise notified.

Postoperative Management and Nursing Care

Educate the patient with a skin graft on the following care:
1. Initial pressure dressing will be left in place for 24 to 48 hours.
2. If wound begins to ooze, apply firm pressure for 10 to 15 minutes (without peeking). If bleeding persists, contact surgeon.
3. Do not take aspirin or aspirin-containing medication for pain. May take one to two acetaminophen tablets every 4 to 6 hours, as needed.
4. Most skin grafts are held in place by a bolster dressing (cotton ball or foam). Do not remove the bolster dressing during the next week.
5. May clean site and apply ointment to the surrounding area of the bolster dressing.
6. Do not get the bolster dressing wet.
7. When the bolster dressing is removed, may shower, but *do not* let the water hit the graft directly.
8. Keep the graft edges moist with ointment.
9. Protect the graft from the sun. The sun will cause pigmentation changes in the graft. A sunscreen may be used in 2 to 3 weeks.
10. Skin grafts to the lower leg must be kept elevated because the new capillary connections are fragile and excess venous pressure may cause rupture. Keep leg elevated as much as possible during the next week.
11. Inspect the dressing daily. Report unusual drainage or signs of an inflammatory reaction.
12. After 2 to 3 weeks, any water-based moisturizer may be applied to the skin donor site for split-thickness skin grafts.
13. Expect some loss of sensation in the grafted area for a time.
14. Avoid strenuous exercise (jogging, lifting heavy objects). Anything that causes face flushing will raise BP, cause bleeding, and impair healing.

Aesthetic Procedures

Aesthetic procedures (cosmetic surgery) consist of reconstructive (plastic) surgery or the use of injected substances, which may be performed to reconstruct or to alter congenital or acquired defects or to restore or improve the body's appearance. Noninvasive procedures alter the skin surface through the use of light sources or chemical applications.

Types of Procedures

Rhytidectomy

1. Done through various techniques and incisions to alleviate skin folds and wrinkles to improve the appearance of the aging face (face-lift).
2. The correction can last as long as 10 years, but results vary with each individual. The skin relaxes with time and the muscles may also relax, but seldom does the face revert to its preoperative condition.
3. Surgical procedures include:
   a. Operative: Standard incisions that are either temporal (hidden in hairline) or submental.
   b. Laser: Several laser modalities are now used in facial plastic surgery, including radiofrequency tissue tightening, which causes collagen shrinkage and reduction of deep wrinkles and lines.

Blepharoplasty

1. Removes loose skin, muscle, and excess fat from upper or lower eyelids. It will not remove lines at the lateral corners of the eyes ("crow's feet").
2. The procedure is generally done by either scalpel under local or general anesthetic or by carbon dioxide laser.

Dermabrasion, Chemical Peel, Laser Resurfacing, and Fillers

1. Patients with weathered skin, fine wrinkles (especially at the corners of the eyes and along the vermilion border), or acne pitting and scarring may benefit from these procedures.
2. The use of laser technology allows for a more predictable result and eliminates the porcelain appearance resulting from such chemicals as trichloroacetic acid. There is less risk of hypopigmentation than with dermabrasion.
3. Chemical peels using tretinoin cream and alpha hydroxy acids result in the destruction of portions of the epidermis and dermis, with subsequent regeneration of new tissues.
4. New nonablative laser resurfacing is used for fine wrinkles, smoker lines, sun-damaged skin, and shallow acne scarring with minimal downtime.
5. Contraindications of laser resurfacing include:
   a. History of isotretinoin therapy 6 to 12 months prior to treatment.
   b. Status of postradiation or scleroderma.
   c. History of herpes simplex—requires perioperative treatment.
6. Hyperpigmentation can occur in persons with dark skin.
7. Purified botulinum toxin and fillers (collagen, hyaluronic acid, autologous fat) are used to correct deep wrinkles and facial hollows. Results may last 3 to 12 months.

Liposuction

1. Also called body contouring, liposuction reduces localized deposits of fat not amenable to weight loss with a cannula aided by suction or fitted to a syringe.
2. May be done on the face, neck, breasts, abdomen, flanks, hips, buttocks, and extremities.

Preoperative Management and Nursing Care

1. Local or general anesthetic will be administered. For local anesthetic, patient may eat and drink before surgery. For general anesthetic:
   a. Preoperative assessment may be necessary, depending on health status and patient's age.
   b. No eating or drinking for several hours before surgery.
   c. Patient should have escort and must be reminded not to drive home alone after surgery.
2. Review patient's allergies and medication before surgery.
3. Instruct patient to cleanse the skin with antiseptic agent the night before surgery, if prescribed.
4. Make sure patient thoroughly understands the procedure and has discussed the risks and benefits with the health care provider before surgery.
5. Make sure a consent form is signed before any procedure.
6. Make sure aspirin, warfarin, and NSAIDs have been discontinued for 2 weeks before surgery, unless otherwise indicated. Herbal supplements, such as ginkgo, ginseng, green tea, and vitamin E, can inhibit coagulation.
7. If applicable, instruct the patient to stop smoking for the 2 weeks leading up to rhytidectomy and to continue cessation for 2 weeks postprocedure and permanently, if possible.
8. Be aware of signs of topical lidocaine toxicity (if used)—drowsiness, tingling of lips, and metallic taste—which may lead to seizures.

Postoperative Management and Nursing Care

Rhytidectomy

1. Mild exercise can be resumed in 3 days postoperatively.
2. No strenuous exercise (that will increase the BP) for 1 month.
3. Dressings are usually removed on the first postoperative day. Elastic facial support garment is recommended for 1 to 3 weeks.
4. Eyelid sutures are removed in 3 to 5 days; facial sutures in 7 days.
5. Showering and gentle hair washing may begin on day 2 or 3.
6. The patient is to apply ointment (petroleum or a similar ointment) to all suture lines.
7. Stress to the patient not to remove crusts by "picking" at them along suture lines or scarring may result.
8. Elevate the head at night for 2 weeks after the procedure. Avoid bending and lifting, which may increase edema and provoke bleeding.
9. Expect the face or affected part to be swollen, bruised, and numb for several days to weeks.
10. Be aware that complications include bleeding and hematoma, sloughing of the skin, and possible facial nerve damage. Notify surgeon if the areas become increasingly red or swollen or if they become more tender or painful.

Blepharoplasty

1. Apply iced gauze compresses to eyes for 10 minutes four to six times per day to reduce edema after surgery.
2. Head of bed should be elevated to reduce internal pressure that might cause bleeding.
3. Avoid strenuous exercise for 1 week.
4. Bruising and swelling generally resolve in 2 weeks.
5. Watch for such complications as eyelid hematomas, ocular mobility dysfunction, and postsurgical ectropion (eversion of the edge of the eyelid).

Dermabrasion and Chemical Peel

1. Instruct patients to not pick at crusts because new epithelium will be injured; soak face several times per day and apply emollient, as directed. Crusts form in 2 to 3 days and start to separate by 7 to 10 weeks. Total separation can take up to 3 weeks.
2. Keep treated areas clean and moist.

3. Avoid sun on treated areas. Apply sunscreen with sun protection factor (SPF) of 15 to 30 when outdoors.
4. Manage bruising and swelling from injectables with ice packs.

Laser Resurfacing

1. Dressings, such as hydrogel dressings (see page 152), may be applied to the affected areas immediately and left in place for 24 to 48 hours.
2. Alternately, the open technique involves using petroleum gel and daily face washes with tepid water.

Liposuction

1. After liposuction, increased fluids are required.
2. Aspirin and NSAIDs should be avoided for at least 1 week to prevent bleeding.
3. Wear compression garment, as instructed.
4. Notify the surgeon if increased swelling develops; could indicate development of a seroma.
5. Expect blood-tinged fluids from cannula injection sites for 2 to 3 days.
6. Keep sutured areas moist with ointment, as instructed.
7. Avoid jarring exercise.
8. Complications include development of seromas, lumpiness in treated areas, excessive bruising.

 NURSING ALERT Advise all postoperative patients to notify health care provider if sudden pain, swelling, or bruising develops; these suggest hematoma or abscess. Do not take aspirin for postoperative discomfort; follow surgeon's orders.

DERMATOLOGIC DISORDERS
Cellulitis

Cellulitis is a diffuse inflammation of the deep dermal and subcutaneous tissue that results from an infectious process.

Pathophysiology and Etiology

1. Caused by infection with group A beta-hemolytic streptococci, *Staphylococcus aureus*, *Haemophilus influenzae*, or other organisms.
2. Usually results from break in the skin that may be as simple as athlete's foot.
3. Infection can spread rapidly through lymphatic system.

 NURSING ALERT Methicillin-resistant *S. aureus* (MRSA) is a significant problem outside of the hospital as well as within. It is resistant to previously effective antistaphylococcal antibiotics and may be fatal.

Clinical Manifestations

1. Tender, warm, erythematous, and swollen area that is poorly demarcated.
2. Tender, warm, erythematous streak that extends proximally from the area, indicating lymph vessel involvement.
3. Possible fluctuant abscesses or purulent drainage.
4. Possible fever, chills, headache, malaise.

Diagnostic Evaluation

1. Gram stain and culture of drainage.
2. Blood cultures.

Management

1. Oral antibiotics (penicillinase-resistant penicillins, cephalosporins, quinolones, or sulfa-based) may be adequate to treat small, localized areas of cellulitis of legs or the trunk.
2. Parenteral antibiotics may be needed for cellulitis of the hands, face, or lymphatic or widespread involvement.
3. Surgical drainage and debridement for suppurative areas recommended for MRSA infections.

Complications

1. Tissue necrosis.
2. Septicemia.

Nursing Assessment

1. Obtain history of trauma to the skin, needlestick, insect bite, or wound.
2. Observe for expanding borders and lymphatic streaking; palpate for fluctuance of abscess formation.
3. Watch for signs of antibiotic sensitivity—shortness of breath, urticaria, angioedema, maculopapular rash, or severe skin reaction, such as erythema multiforme or toxic epidermal necrolysis.
4. Assess for patient and caretaker ability to provide care at home, keep affected area clean, and adhere to medication prescribed.

Nursing Diagnoses

- Impaired Skin Integrity related to infectious process.
- Acute Pain related to inflammation of subcutaneous tissue.

Nursing Interventions

Protecting Skin Integrity

1. Administer or teach patient to administer antibiotics, as prescribed; teach dosage schedule and adverse effects. Assess ability to swallow pills. Recommend crushing or taking with food to avoid stomach irritation, if applicable.
2. Maintain intravenous (IV) infusion or venous access to administer IV antibiotics, if indicated.
3. Elevate affected extremity to promote drainage from area and reduce swelling.
4. Prepare patient for surgical drainage and debridement, if necessary.

Relieving Pain

1. Encourage comfortable position and immobilization of affected area.
2. Administer or teach patient to administer analgesics, as prescribed; monitor for adverse effects.
3. Use bed cradle to relieve pressure from bed covers.

Patient Education and Health Maintenance

1. Make sure that patient understands dosage schedule of antibiotics and the importance of complying with therapy to prevent complications.
2. Advise patient to notify health care provider immediately if condition worsens; hospitalization may be necessary.
3. Outpatient-treated cellulitis should be observed within 24 to 48 hours of starting antibiotics to determine efficacy.
4. Teach patient with impaired circulation or impaired sensation how to perform proper skin care and how to inspect skin for trauma.

Evaluation: Expected Outcomes

- Skin is normal color and temperature, nontender, nonswollen, and intact.
- Actively moves extremity; verbalizes no pain.

Necrotizing Fasciitis

Necrotizing fasciitis is a type of necrotizing infection of the soft tissue that spreads quickly along fascia. It rapidly progresses toward death if not treated quickly.

Pathophysiology and Etiology

1. Usually caused by group A *Streptococcus*, known as flesh-eating bacteria, but may also be a clostridia or polymicrobial infection. It is emerging as a complication of MRSA infection.
2. May result postoperatively or from local injury with superficial or deep infection.
3. More common in patients with diabetes, those that abuse drugs, and other immunocompromised populations.
4. Spreads along fascia, causing extensive necrosis of the skin and subcutaneous tissue.

Clinical Manifestations

1. Increasing pain or pain out of proportion to local infection or injury; increasing redness, edema, and warmth.
2. Fever, rapid pulse.
3. Tissue appears darkened under the skin.
4. Possible bullae or petechiae or appears hemorrhagic.
5. May be foul odor and drainage (delayed).

Diagnostic Evaluation

1. Surgical excision and debridement are diagnostic to determine extent as well as therapeutic.
2. Gram stain and culture from deep tissue to determine exact etiology.
3. Blood cultures to rule out septicemia.

Management

1. Immediate hospitalization with intensive care support.
2. Prompt and repeated surgical debridement.
3. IV antibiotic regimen using multiple agents, including clindamycin, penicillin G, erythromycin, ceftriaxone, and others.

Complications

1. Muscle gangrene—requires amputation.
2. Loss of tissue and function.
3. Death.

Nursing Assessment

1. After trauma, surgery, or with cellulitis, frequently assess for increasing pain, fever, and changes in skin appearance, which may indicate necrotizing fasciitis.
2. Be aware of underlying conditions that may cause immunocompromise, such as diabetes, alcoholism, malnutrition, IV drug use, cancer and cancer treatment, and HIV/AIDS, which increases the risk and worsens the course of necrotizing fasciitis.
3. Monitor vital signs frequently for any change (rise or fall in BP, temperature, pulse, and respirations) that may indicate worsening condition.

4. Monitor wound dressings after debridement for amount, color, and odor of drainage. Wounds will usually be left open to heal by secondary intention.

 NURSING ALERT Inform the health care provider immediately if pain is out of proportion to injury or if progressive skin changes occur. The patient should be assessed for necrotizing fasciitis.

Nursing Diagnoses

- Hyperthermia related to infectious process.
- Acute Pain related to necrosis.

Nursing Interventions

Normalizing Body Temperature
1. Administer antipyretics, as directed.
2. Encourage oral fluids and administer IV fluids, as directed.
3. Monitor intake and output to ensure adequate hydration because of fluid loss through fever and insensible loss.
4. Provide cool compresses, sponge baths, and clothing and linen changes as comfort measures.

Relieving Pain
1. Administer analgesics, as directed and based on pain assessment; however, be alert for sedation that may mask signs of worsening condition.
2. Assist patient to position of comfort that will not place pressure on affected area.
3. Administer analgesic 30 to 60 minutes before wound care and dressing changes.

Education and Health Maintenance

1. Make sure that patient can complete wound care at home and will follow-up as directed.
2. Make home care nursing referral, as necessary.
3. Teach patient signs of infection and to notify health care provider immediately if experiencing increasing pain, fever, redness, swelling, warmth, or increased and odorous drainage.
4. Advise patient to eat a balanced diet rich in protein, vitamin C, iron, and zinc for wound healing.

Evaluation: Expected Outcomes

- Core temperature 97.6°F to 98.8°F (36.4°C to 37.1°C).
- Patient turning in bed, verbalizing minimal pain.

Toxic Epidermal Necrolysis

Toxic epidermal necrolysis is a severe, potentially fatal skin disease associated with erythema, blistering, and epidermal sloughing. A less severe form is known as *Stevens-Johnson syndrome*.

Pathophysiology and Etiology

1. Exact mechanism is unknown, but can be induced by various drugs, including sulfonamides, anticonvulsants, NSAIDs, allopurinol.
2. Resembles second-degree burns, with sloughing of the skin at epidermal or dermal junction.
3. Mortality ranges from 3.2% to 90%, based on an illness severity score with factors such as age, presence of malignancy, heart rate, and percentage of epidermal detachment.

Clinical Manifestations

1. Malaise, fatigue, vomiting, cough, fever, and diarrhea may be prodromal symptoms.
2. Sudden onset of urticaria and large dark red areas; within 5 to 8 days, large, flaccid bullae appear.
3. Within hours, coma may develop.
4. Bullae become confluent and slough in large sheets, leaving moist, erythematous surface.
5. Positive Nikolsky sign (desquamation of the skin on light pressure).
6. Erosions of mucosal sites, including lips, oral pharynx, or urinary tract.

Diagnostic Evaluation

1. Skin biopsy to determine level of separation.
2. Possible cultures of blood and body fluids to differentiate infection.

Management

1. Treatment in intensive care unit or regional burn center because toxic epidermal necrolysis has similar pathophysiologic characteristics to those of extensive burns (see page 924).
2. Treatment of affected skin.
   a. Wounds are cleaned in operating room under anesthesia; loose skin and blisters are removed, and necrotic areas are debrided to prevent infection.
   b. Temporary biologic dressings (porcine cutaneous xenografts, amnion, collagen-based skin substitute, or plastic semipermeable dressings) applied to prevent secondary skin infection while awaiting reepithelialization.
3. All nonessential drugs are stopped immediately.
4. Fluid replacement therapy, as necessary, and possible enteral nutrition if oral involvement.
5. Topical antimicrobial dressings to enhance reepithelialization.
6. Ophthalmologic examination and removal of corneal adhesions, as necessary.
7. Use of systemic corticosteroids is not recommended and use of human IV immunoglobulin is controversial.

Complications

1. Sepsis.
2. Pneumonia.
3. Blindness.

Nursing Assessment

1. Obtain medication and immunization history.
2. Monitor vital signs and level of consciousness closely because the condition is rapidly progressive.
3. Monitor fluid and nutritional status through daily weight, vital signs, and laboratory test results (electrolytes, especially glucose, bicarbonate, blood urea nitrogen, creatinine, albumin, and total protein).

Nursing Diagnoses

- Impaired Skin Integrity related to sloughing.
- Risk for Deficient Fluid Volume related to transudation of fluid into bullae.
- Acute Pain related to exposed dermal nerve endings.
- Impaired Oral Mucous Membranes related to oral lesions.

Nursing Interventions

Restoring Skin Integrity

1. Place patient on warmed air-fluidized bed to distribute weight with minimal shearing forces.
2. Use extreme care in handling patient because the skin is very fragile; obtain assistance to move patient.
3. Gently apply warm, wet compresses of prescribed antiseptic solution to reduce bacterial population of wound surface.
4. Inspect xenograft several times daily for dislodgment or purulence; these will require new xenograft.
5. Watch for new areas of toxic epidermal necrolysis; note and record progression of skin slough and chart progress.
6. Patient should be in private room on reverse isolation to prevent infection.
7. Provide nutritional supplements through enteral feeding to ensure healing.

Maintaining Fluid Balance

1. Monitor vital signs for falling BP or for rising pulse that indicates hypovolemia; use an indwelling arterial catheter to provide continuous measurement while avoiding cuff pressure on the skin.
2. Measure hourly urine output.
3. Weigh patient daily.
4. Give IV fluids, as prescribed.
5. Assess bowel sounds and give oral or enteral fluids, as tolerated.

Reducing Pain

1. If patient cannot verbalize, watch for facial expressions, for guarding, or for increased pulse and respirations to indicate pain.
2. Administer analgesics, as prescribed and as required, possibly around the clock; monitor for adverse effects and document effectiveness.
3. Provide distraction through music or other measures to promote relaxation.
4. Provide emotional support and encouragement. Emotional/psychological support to patient and family is crucial.

Protecting Mucous Membranes

1. Use meticulous oral hygiene.
   a. Inspect oral cavity daily; note any changes.
   b. Rinse mouth with normal saline, diluted hydrogen peroxide, or other solution to remove debris and to cleanse ulcerations.
   c. Apply petroleum jelly or other lubricant/protectant to cracked, swollen lips.
2. Assess urethral, vaginal, and anal regions for ulcerations or bleeding.
3. Inspect eyes and remove crusts from eyelid margins using damp compresses or saline-soaked swabs; apply eyedrops as prescribed.

Patient Education and Health Maintenance

1. Encourage follow-up appointments with plastic surgeon and other health care providers as indicated.
2. Encourage compliance with physical therapy, as indicated, to restore function.
3. Advise patient to use sunscreen of at least SPF 15, avoid direct sunlight during the healing phase, and continue to use sunscreen.
4. Advise patient to avoid suspected medication in the future.

Evaluation: Expected Outcomes

- New epithelium noted without scarring.
- Output equals input; weight and vital signs remain stable.
- Patient verbalizes reduced pain.
- Oral mucosa intact.

Herpes Zoster

Herpes zoster (varicella–zoster, shingles) is an inflammatory condition in which reactivation of the chickenpox virus produces a vesicular eruption along the distribution of the nerves from one or more dorsal root ganglia (dermatome). The prevalence increases with age. A varicella–zoster vaccine is available for people older than age 50 to prevent reactivation.

Pathophysiology and Etiology

1. Caused by a varicella–zoster virus, which is a member of a group of deoxyribonucleic acid viruses.
2. Virus is identical to the causative agent of varicella (chickenpox). After the primary infection, the varicella–zoster virus may persist in a dormant state in the dorsal nerve root ganglia. The virus may emerge from this site in later years, either spontaneously or in association with immunosuppression, to cause herpes zoster.

Clinical Manifestations

1. Eruption may be accompanied or preceded by fever, malaise, headache, and pain; pain may be burning, lancinating, stabbing, or aching.
2. Inflammation is usually unilateral, involving the cranial, cervical, thoracic, lumbar, or sacral dermatome in a bandlike configuration.
3. Vesicles appear in 3 to 4 days.
   a. Characteristic patches of grouped vesicles appear on erythematous, edematous skin.
   b. Early vesicles contain serum; they later rupture and form crusts; scarring usually does not occur unless the vesicles are deep and they involve the dermis.
   c. If ophthalmic branch of the facial nerve is involved, patient may have a painful eye. (This can be a medical emergency.) Vesicles on the tip of the nose suggest eye involvement.
   d. In healthy host, lesions resolve in 2 to 3 weeks.
4. A susceptible person can acquire chickenpox if there is contact with the infective vesicular fluid of a zoster patient. A person with a history of chickenpox or who has received the immunization is immune and thus is not at risk from infection after exposure to zoster patients.

 NURSING ALERT Varicella–zoster virus may be a life-threatening condition to the patient who is immunosuppressed, who is receiving cytotoxic chemotherapy, or who is a bone marrow transplant recipient.

Diagnostic Evaluation

1. Usually diagnosed by clinical presentation.
2. Culture of varicella–zoster virus from lesions or detection by fluorescent antibody techniques, including viral detection that uses monoclonal antibodies or by electron microscopy, to confirm diagnosis.

Management

1. Antiviral drugs, such as acyclovir, famciclovir, and valacyclovir, interfere with viral replication; may be used in all cases, but especially for treatment of immunosuppressed or debilitated patients. Must be started within 72 hours of onset.
2. Corticosteroids early in illness (controversial)—given for severe herpes zoster if symptomatic measures fail; given for anti-inflammatory effect and for relief of pain.
3. Pain management—aspirin, acetaminophen, NSAIDs, opioids—useful during the acute stage, but not generally effective for postherpetic neuralgia. If treated early (48 to 72 hours), may decrease risk of postherpetic neuralgia.
4. Postherpetic neuralgia may be treated with anticonvulsant agents, such as gabapentin or pregabalin, and 5% lidocaine patch.

Complications

1. Approximately 20% of patients will experience chronic pain syndrome (postherpetic neuralgia), characterized by constant aching and burning pain or by intermittent lancinating pain or hyperesthesia of affected skin after it has healed.
2. Ophthalmic complications with involvement of ophthalmic branch of trigeminal nerve with keratitis, uveitis, corneal ulceration, and possibly blindness.
3. Facial and auditory nerve involvement, resulting in hearing deficits, vertigo, and facial weakness (Ramsay Hunt syndrome).
4. Visceral dissemination—pneumonitis, esophagitis, enterocolitis, myocarditis, pancreatitis.

Nursing Diagnoses

- Acute Pain related to inflammation of cutaneous nerve endings.
- Impaired Skin Integrity related to rupture of vesicles.

Nursing Interventions

Controlling Pain

1. Assess patient's level of discomfort and medicate, as prescribed; monitor for adverse effects of pain medications.
2. Teach patient to apply wet dressings, such as aluminum acetate (Burow) solution, for soothing effect.
3. Encourage distraction techniques such as music therapy.
4. Teach relaxation techniques, such as deep breathing, progressive muscle relaxation, and imagery, to help control pain.

Improving Skin Integrity

1. Apply wet dressings to cool and dry inflamed areas by means of evaporation.
2. Administer antiviral medication in dosage prescribed (usually high dose); warn the patient of adverse effects such as nausea.

Patient Education and Health Maintenance

1. Teach patient to use proper handwashing technique to avoid spreading herpes zoster virus.
2. Advise patient not to open the blisters to avoid secondary infection and scarring.
3. Reassure patient that shingles is a viral infection of the nerve endings; nervousness does not cause shingles.
4. A caregiver may be required to assist with dressings and meals. In older patients, the pain is more pronounced and incapacitating. Dysesthesia and skin hypersensitivity are distressing.

Evaluation: Expected Outcomes

- Verbalizes decreased pain.
- Reepithelialization of the skin without scarring.

Pemphigus

Pemphigus is a serious autoimmune disease of the skin and of the mucous membranes, characterized by the appearance of flaccid blisters (bullae and vesicles) of various sizes on apparently normal skin and mucous membranes (mouth, esophagus, conjunctiva, or vagina) (see Figure 33-3). Familial benign chronic pemphigus (Hailey-Hailey disease) is a familial type of pemphigus that appears in adults, particularly affecting the axillae and groin.

Pathophysiology and Etiology

1. The exact cause is unknown.
2. Certain drugs, other autoimmune diseases, and genetics may play a role in its development.
3. Many variants of pemphigus exist.

Clinical Manifestations

1. Initial lesions may appear in the oral cavity; flaccid blisters (bullae) may arise on normal or erythematous skin.
   a. The bullae enlarge and rupture, forming painful, raw, and denuded areas that eventually become crusted. These areas can become secondarily infected.
   b. The eroded skin heals slowly; eventually, widespread areas of the body may become involved.
   c. In the mouth, the blisters are usually multiple, of varying size and irregular shape, painful, and persistent. Oral lesions may appear initially, with lesions of the mucous membranes of the pharynx and esophagus; the conjunctivae, larynx, urethra, cervix, and rectum may become affected as well.
2. An offensive odor may emanate from the bullae because of infection.
3. Positive Nikolsky sign—separation of the epidermis when minimal pressure is applied to the skin; downward pressure on a bulla will cause it to expand laterally.

Diagnostic Evaluation

1. Skin biopsies of blisters and surrounding skin—demonstrate acantholysis (separation of epidermal cells from each other).

Figure 33-3. Pemphigus vulgaris blisters on the forearm. (From Smeltzer, S., & Bare, B. [2000]. *Brunner and Suddarth's textbook of medical-surgical nursing* [9th ed.]. Philadelphia, PA: Lippincott Williams & Wilkins.)

2. Immunofluorescence of skin cells shows antibodies that bind to the epidermis in a lacy pattern network (pemphigus antibodies).

Management

1. Corticosteroids in large doses to control the disease and keep skin free from blisters.
2. Immunosuppressive agents, such as cyclophosphamide and azathioprine, are used alone or in combination with steroids, for immunosuppressive and steroid-sparing effect.
3. Plasmapheresis—reinfusion of specially treated plasma cells; temporarily decreases serum level of antibodies.
4. Treatment of denuded skin.

Complications

1. Infections (skin, pneumonia, septicemia).
2. Adverse effects from acute and chronic corticosteroids: GI bleeding, secondary infection, psychosis, hyperglycemia, and others.

Nursing Assessment

1. Assess for odor or drainage from lesions, which may indicate infection.
2. Assess for fever and signs of systemic infection.
3. Assess for adverse effects of corticosteroids, such as abdominal pain, white patches in the mouth that indicate *Candida* infection, and emotional changes.

Nursing Diagnoses

- Impaired Oral Mucous Membrane related to ruptured bullae.
- Impaired Skin Integrity related to ruptured bullae.
- Risk for Deficient Fluid Volume related to transudation of fluid into bullae.
- Disturbed Body Image related to widespread or chronic skin lesions.

Nursing Interventions

Restoring Oral Mucous Membrane Integrity

1. Inspect oral cavity daily; note and report any changes—oral lesions heal slowly.
2. Keep oral mucosa clean and allow regeneration of epithelium.
3. Give topical oral therapy, as directed.
4. Offer prescribed mouthwashes through a straw to rinse the mouth of debris and to soothe ulcerative areas.
5. Teach patient to apply petrolatum to lips frequently.
6. Use cool mist therapy to humidify environmental air.

Restoring Skin Integrity

1. Keep skin clean and eliminate debris and dead skin—the bullae will clear if epithelium at the base is clean and not infected.
2. Obtain swab of bullous fluid for cultures—most common organism is *S. aureus*.
3. Administer cool, wet dressings or baths or teach patient to administer to soothe and cleanse the skin. Large areas of blistering have a characteristic odor that is lessened when secondary infection is under control.
   a. After the bath, dry and cover with talcum powder, as directed; this enables the patient to move more freely in bed. Large amounts are necessary to keep clothes and sheets from sticking.

4. The nursing management of patients with blistering or with bullous skin conditions is similar to that of the patient with a burn (see page 930).

Restoring Fluid Balance

1. Evaluate for fluid and electrolyte imbalance—extensive denudation of the skin leads to fluid and electrolyte imbalance.
   a. Monitor serum albumin and protein levels.
   b. Monitor vital signs for hypotension or tachycardia.
   c. Weigh patient daily.
   d. Monitor intake and output.
2. Administer IV saline solutions, as directed.
3. Encourage the patient to maintain hydration; suggest cool, nonirritating fluids.
   a. Suggest soft, high-protein, high-calorie diet or liquid supplements that will not be irritating to oral mucosa but will replace lost protein.

Promoting Positive Body Image

1. Develop a trusting relationship with the patient.
2. Educate patient and family about the disease and its treatment; this reduces uncertainty and clears up misconceptions.
3. Encourage expression of anxieties, embarrassment, and discouragement.
4. Encourage patient to maintain social contacts and activities among support network.

Patient Education and Health Maintenance

Instruct the patient as follows:
1. The disease may be characterized by relapses that require continuing therapy to maintain control.
2. Long-term administration of immunosuppressive drugs is associated with numerous adverse effects and risks—hyperglycemia, osteoporosis, psychosis, adrenal suppression, and increased risk of cancer. Report for health care follow-up visits regularly.
3. Monitor the skin and mouth for recurrence of pemphigus activity.

Evaluation: Expected Outcomes

- Oral mucous membranes pink with healing lesions and no signs of infection.
- Skin with intact bullae, healing lesions, and no signs of infection.
- Vital signs stable; urine output adequate.
- Patient expresses concerns and plans activities.

Psoriasis

Psoriasis (see Figure 33-4) is a chronic T-cell–mediated inflammatory disorder causing secondary epidermal turnover, which occurs at a rate six to nine times faster than normal.

Pathophysiology and Etiology

1. Affects 2% to 3% of people.
2. Classified as mild if less than 2% of body surface area affected; moderate, if 2% to 10% affected; and severe, if more than 10%.
3. Types of psoriasis include:
   a. Plaque—most common type (about 80% of cases); occurs on the knees, elbows, scalp, and other areas.
   b. Guttate—droplike pattern occurs on the trunk, arms, or legs; often starts in childhood or young adulthood; comes on suddenly, often triggered by streptococcal infection.

Figure 33-4. The lesions of psoriasis appear as red, raised patches of the skin covered with silvery scales that in time coalesce, forming irregularly shaped patches.

   c. Inverse—affects flexural areas, such as the axilla and groin.
   d. Erythrodermic—scalded appearance that affects most of the body; can lead to protein and fluid loss.
   e. Pustular—primarily seen in adults; exacerbated by the sun; blisters contain purulent material on palms and soles or on widespread area.
   f. Psoriatic arthritis—joint involvement, pain, and other abnormalities accompany skin involvement.
4. Formerly considered idiopathic, now thought to be genetically linked and immune system modulated.
   a. May be caused by some antigenic stimuli that activate cytokines and T cells, thus causing an extreme dermal response.
   b. Genes are being identified that may predispose a person to developing psoriasis.
5. Condition tends to last a person's life span, with flares and remissions. May be exacerbated by infection (particularly beta-hemolytic streptococcal infection), stress, injury, hormonal changes, and drugs, such as lithium, beta-adrenergic blockers, angiotensin-converting enzyme inhibitors, antimalarial drugs, and indomethacin.
6. Recent research may indicate that the inflammatory nature of disease may be associated with increased coronary artery calcification. Appropriate medical follow-up should be recommended.

Clinical Manifestations

1. Characteristic rash.
   a. Plaque type—erythematous plaques with silvery scales, symmetric involvement, may be pruritic and painful; often appears at areas of epidermal injury (Koebner reaction).
   b. Guttate—small red individual spots, not as thick as plaque psoriasis.
   c. Inverse—bright red patches that are smooth and shiny, involving skin folds.
   d. Pustular—white blisters and noninfectious pus surrounded by red skin.
   e. Erythrodermic—redness of most of the body, shedding of the skin, severe itching, and signs of systemic illness.

2. Characteristic pitting of nails in 50% of patients.
3. Arthritis in approximately 30% of patients; most frequently occurs between age 30 and 50.

Management

1. Diagnosed by clinical features; rarely, a biopsy may be needed.
2. Coal tar and anthralin preparations inhibit excessive skin turnover.
   a. Applied topically, with no systemic adverse effects.
   b. Application may be messy, odorous, and may stain clothing.
3. Topical corticosteroids are the mainstay topical treatment. Adverse effects may include striae, thinning of the skin, adrenal suppression (rare). Tachyphylaxis may result if used for extended periods.
4. Topical calcipotriene, a vitamin D derivative, used for mild to moderate psoriasis, generally produces no adverse effects.
5. Another topical preparation is tazarotene, a receptor selective retinoid, which is potentially teratogenic (pregnancy category X).
6. Phototherapy—20 to 30 short treatments. Narrowband ultraviolet B (UVB) light is safer than ultraviolet A (UVA), which carries the risk of sunburn and skin cancer.
   a. Photochemotherapy—ingestion of an oral photosensitizer (psoralen) followed by exposure to UVA light therapy (PUVA).
   b. Cataracts, nausea, and malaise are possible adverse effects of systemic PUVA.
7. Oral methotrexate, the retinoid acitretin, and cyclosporine also are used.
   a. Hepatotoxicity may occur with methotrexate.
   b. Hypertension and renal failure may occur with cyclosporine.
   c. Acitretin is a potent teratogen and should not be used if any risk of pregnancy up to 3 years posttreatment in women of childbearing age.
8. Biologic agents, such as etanercept, infliximab, ustekinumab, alefacept, and adalimumab, have demonstrated efficacy in the control of moderate to severe symptoms as well as psoriatic arthritis.

 DRUG ALERT Cyclosporine is contraindicated in patients with renal disease, uncontrolled hypertension, active infection, internal malignancy, immune deficiency, gout, hepatic disease, and concomitant use of nephrotoxic drugs. Serum creatinine must be followed closely throughout the treatment.

Nursing Interventions and Patient Education

1. Assist patient, as needed, with daily tub bath to soften scales and plaques.
2. Apply topical preparations after bath and gentle debridement of scale removal.
3. Warn patient that coal tar and anthralin preparations may stain clothing; let it dry before dressing.
4. Advise patient to wear goggles for phototherapy to prevent cataracts and to follow-up with periodic eye exams.
5. Encourage patient to follow-up closely with primary care provider or with dermatologist and to report for blood work to check renal function and liver function tests as indicated.

6. Reinforce to women of childbearing age that retinoids and methotrexate are teratogenic; must be using birth control.
7. Encourage patients to try to identify triggers that may cause flare-ups and to practice avoidance techniques, such as relaxation therapy, to avoid stress.
8. Teach patients to avoid direct sun exposure by wearing protective clothing and sunscreen, especially on the day of phototherapy.
9. Advise patients to use good lubricants to prevent drying and cracking of the skin, which can lead to hyperkeratinization.
10. Encourage verbalization of frustration of condition, treatment, and impact on social network.
11. For more information, contact the National Psoriasis Foundation (*www.psoriasis.org*).

Benign Tumors

Benign tumors are common skin growths. Most do not require any treatment but are important to recognize to differentiate from malignant lesions.

Characteristics and Management

Seborrheic Keratoses
1. Lesions are benign and wartlike of varying size and color, ranging from light tan to black that may appear to be stuck on; they are the most common skin tumors in middle-aged and older people.
2. Treatment is usually unnecessary, but lesions can be removed by liquid nitrogen cryotherapy or curettage.

Verrucae (Warts)
1. Common, benign skin tumors caused by human papillomavirus.
2. Often disappear spontaneously without scarring and may not need treatment.
3. Many topical treatment options are available for office and self-treatment, but some may cause scarring.
   a. Cryotherapy with liquid nitrogen—destroys wart and spares rest of the skin.
   b. Area may be treated surgically with curettage or electrodesiccation.
   c. Application of salicylic acid, topical fluorouracil, imiquimod, topical vitamin A acid, cantharidin, or other irritants may be helpful, especially for flat warts, except on the face.
   d. Occlusion with duct tape is controversial. Modest clinical effectiveness has been shown in studies, but not statistically significant.
   e. Apple cider vinegar soak. Apply petroleum ointment on the surrounding skin to protect it. Apply small piece of cotton soaked in vinegar and tape it to the wart overnight and repeat until the wart is gone.
   f. Suggestive therapy (placebo) often works with children through age 10.

 NURSING ALERT Several studies have not revealed sufficient evidence in favor of treatment other than salicylic acid and aggressive cryotherapy.

 EVIDENCE BASE Habif, T. P. (2016). *Clinical dermatology: A color guide to diagnosis and therapy* (6th ed.). St. Louis, MO: Mosby.

Hemangiomas

1. Hemangiomas are benign tumor of the capillaries, which present shortly after birth.
2. They grow rapidly for 6 to 18 months, followed by stabilization and subsequent regression. Most hemangiomas resolve by age 9.
3. Surgery is reserved for complicated hemangiomas that may be obstructing the airway.
4. Hemangiomas blocking the visual axis or compressing against the eye are treated with high doses of corticosteroids or interferon.
5. For hemangiomas that do not threaten vision or life, no intervention is preferred.
6. Lasers can be used for ulcerated hemangiomas.

Pigmented Nevi (Moles)

1. Common skin tumors of various sizes and shapes, ranging from yellowish to brown to black; may be flat, macular lesions, elevated papules, or nodules that occasionally contain hair.
2. Most pigmented nevi are harmless; however, in rare cases, malignant changes supervene and a melanoma develops at the site of the nevus.
3. Nevi at sites subject to repeated irritation from clothing or jewelry can be removed for comfort.
4. Nevi that show change in size, shape, or color, become symptomatic (itch or bleed), or develop notched borders should be removed to determine if malignant changes have occurred. This is especially true for nevi with irregular borders or variations of red, blue, and blue-black.
5. Use "ABCDE" to recall criteria for evaluation of nevi: A = asymmetry, B = border (irregular), C = color (lack of uniform), D = diameter (greater than 6 mm), and E = evolving or changing.

Keloids

1. Benign overgrowths of connective tissue expanding beyond the site of scar or trauma in predisposed individuals.
2. More prevalent among dark-skinned individuals.
3. Usually asymptomatic—may cause disfigurement and cosmetic concern.
4. Management—intralesional corticosteroid therapy, surgical removal, radiation, or silicone gel sheeting.

Premalignant Lesions: Actinic (Solar) Keratoses

1. Premalignant skin lesions appearing as rough, scaly patches with underlying erythema, which develop as a consequence of prolonged exposure to ultraviolet rays.
2. Develop in areas of the body that experience prolonged sun exposure such as the scalp, face, dorsal hands, and arms; may gradually transform into squamous cell carcinoma.
3. Many topical treatments are available, including the antineoplastic fluorouracil, the immune response modifier imiquimod, liquid nitrogen cryosurgery, and curettage.
4. Photodynamic therapy with application of aminolevulinic acid and exposure to blue light that destroys abnormal cells.

Cancer of the Skin

Skin cancer is the most common malignancy, accounting for about half of all cancers. Nonmelanoma skin cancers are categorized as basal cell carcinoma (BCC) (80%) or squamous cell carcinoma (SCC) (20%). BCCs are more easily curable because of early diagnosis and slow progression. These cancers are locally invasive and tend not to metastasize. SCCs have an increased potential for metastasis. Conversely, malignant melanomas are least common and have a higher risk of metastasis.

 EVIDENCE BASE Wernli, K., Henrikson, N., Morrison, C., et al. (2016). Screening for skin cancer in adults: Updated evidence report and systematic review for the US Preventive Services Task Force. *Journal of the American Medical Association, 316*(4), 436–447.

Pathophysiology and Etiology

1. Most BCCs and SCCs are located on sun-exposed areas and are directly related to ultraviolet radiation. Sun damage is cumulative.
2. Risk factors for skin cancer include:
   a. Fair complexion, blue eyes, and blond or red hair; Fitzpatrick skin—type I or II (see page 909).
   b. Working outdoors.
   c. Older people with sun-damaged skin.
   d. History of radiation treatment of skin conditions.
   e. Exposure to certain chemical agents (arsenicals, nitrates, tar and pitch, oils, and paraffins).
   f. Burn scars, damaged skin in areas of chronic osteomyelitis, fistulae openings.
   g. Long-term immunosuppressive therapy, including organ transplants.
   h. Genetic susceptibility.
   i. Multiple dysplastic nevi—moles that are larger, irregular, more numerous, or variable colors — or family history of dysplastic nevi.
   j. Congenital nevi that are large (more than 20 cm in size).
   k. Presence of human papillomavirus.
3. Types of skin cancer:
   a. Basal cell carcinoma—arises from basal layers of the epidermis or hair follicle; most common type but rarely metastasizes; can be locally invasive.
   b. Squamous cell carcinoma—arises from the epidermis; metastasis occurs more commonly than with basal cell carcinoma.
   c. Malignant melanoma—a malignancy of melanocytes; can metastasize.

 NURSING ALERT Although only 3% of skin cancers are melanoma, this form of skin cancer causes the majority of skin cancer deaths. Melanoma incidence is increasing at about 3% per year.

Clinical Manifestations

Basal Cell Carcinoma

1. Lesions typically begin as small nodules with a rolled, pearly, translucent border with telangiectasia, crusting, and occasionally ulceration (see Figure 33-5A).
2. Appear most frequently on sun-exposed skin, frequently on the face between the hairline and upper lip or back.
3. If neglected, may cause local destruction, hemorrhage, and infection of adjacent tissues, producing severe functional and cosmetic disabilities.

Figure 33-5. (A) Basal cell carcinoma, (B) squamous cell carcinoma. (From Smeltzer, S., & Bare, B. [2000]. *Brunner and Suddarth's textbook of medical-surgical nursing* [9th ed.]. Philadelphia, PA: Lippincott Williams & Wilkins.)

Squamous Cell Carcinoma

1. Appears as reddish, rough, thickened, scaly lesion with bleeding and soreness—may be asymptomatic; border may be wider, more indurated, and more inflammatory than BCC (see Figure 33-5B).
2. May be preceded by leukoplakia (premalignant lesion of mucous membrane) of the mouth or tongue, actinic keratoses, scarred or ulcerated lesions.
3. Seen most commonly on the lower lip, rims of ears, head, neck, and backs of the hands.

Malignant Melanoma

See Figure 33-6.

1. Melanoma in situ; earliest phase, difficult to recognize because clinical changes are minimal.
2. Superficial spreading melanoma (most common).
   a. Circular, with irregular outer portions; the margins may be flat or elevated and palpable.
   b. Has combination of colors—hues of tan, brown, and black mixed with gray, bluish black, or white.
   c. May be dull pink-rose color in a small area within the lesion.
   d. Occurs anywhere on the body; usually affects middle-aged people.

Figure 33-6. (A) Superficial spreading melanoma; note irregular border. (B) Nodular melanoma. (C) Lentigo maligna melanoma; note irregular pigment pattern. (A, B: From Smeltzer, S., & Bare, B. [2000]. *Brunner and Suddarth's textbook of medical-surgical nursing* [9th ed.]. Philadelphia, PA: Lippincott Williams & Wilkins; C: Hall J.C., Hall B.J. [2017]. *Sauer's Manual of Skin Diseases* [11th ed.] Philadelphia, PA: Lippincott Williams & Wilkins.)

3. Nodular melanoma.
   a. Spherical blueberry-like nodule with relatively smooth surface and uniform blue-black, blue-gray, or reddish-blue color.
   b. May be polypoidal and elevated, with smooth surface of rose-gray or black color.
   c. Occurs commonly on the torso and extremities.
   d. Invades directly into the subjacent dermis (vertical growth) and hence has a poorer prognosis.
4. Lentigo malignant melanoma.
   a. First appears as tan, flat macule—malignant degeneration is manifested by changes in color, size, and topography.
   b. Evolves slowly; occurs on sun-exposed skin surfaces of people in their 40s or 50s.
5. Acrolentiginous melanoma (uncommon).
   a. Irregular pigmented macules, which develop nodules; may become invasive early.
   b. Occurs on palms, soles, nail beds, and rarely on mucous membranes.
   c. Most common type of melanoma in Blacks and Asians.

Diagnostic Evaluation

Excisional biopsy (for histopathologic diagnosis) and microstaging determination of thickness and level of invasion; helps determine treatment and prognosis. Shave biopsy is usually performed for suspected BCC or SCC lesions.

Management

Basal Cell Carcinoma and Squamous Cell Carcinoma

Method of treatment depends on tumor location, cell type (location and depth), history of previous treatment, whether it is invasive, or if metastasis has occurred.

1. Curettage followed by electrodesiccation—usually done on small tumors of basal or squamous cell type (less than 1 to 2 cm).
2. Surgical excision by Mohs surgery for larger lesions or for those in areas more likely to recur or located in cosmetically sensitive areas (around the nose, eyes, ears, lips); may be followed by simple closure, flap, or graft.
   a. Microscopically controlled excision, with immediate examination of frozen or chemically fixed sections for evidence of cancer cells.
   b. Layers are removed until a reasonable cancer-free margin is achieved.
3. Radiation therapy—should be reserved for older adults, may be used for extensive malignancies where goal is palliation or when other medical conditions contraindicate other forms of therapy.
4. Other therapeutic regimens—topical fluorouracil, the immune response modifier imiquimod, photodynamic therapy.

Malignant Melanoma

1. Complete excision of lesion. If depth is between 1 and 4 mm or there is ulceration present, sentinel lymph node biopsy may be done at the time of reexcision. Margins of 1 to 2 cm are required on reexcision. Close subsequent follow-up is necessary.
2. Systemic chemotherapy—generally used for recurrence of metastasis or palliation; may be combined with autologous bone marrow transplantation or several agents used in combination.

3. Early detection has a 5-year survival rate approaching 95% for thin (less than 1 mm) lesions in primary melanoma. The 10-year survival rate for lesions of 1.01 to 2 mm in thickness is 89% but drops off to 32% for lesions at greater than 4 mm.

Complications

1. BCC arising around the eyes, nasolabial folds, ear canal, or posterior sulcus may invade deeply and cause extensive destruction into muscle, bone, and dura mater. Hemorrhage may result from eroded vessels.
2. SCC may metastasize in 3% to 4% of cases.
3. If left untreated, melanoma will metastasize over months to years.

Nursing Assessment

1. Have a high index of suspicion for people at risk. Fitzpatrick skin type can be used to assess risk for sun damage to the skin.
   a. Type I: very white skin, always burns.
   b. Type II: white, burns easily, tans with difficulty.
   c. Type III: white to olive, tans after initial burn.
   d. Type IV: light brown, tans easily.
   e. Type V: brown, tans easily.
   f. Type VI: black, does not burn.
2. Ask about sunbathing habits and sunburn history. Question patient about pruritus, tenderness, pain, or bleeding, which are not features of a benign nevus (mole).
3. Ask about changes in preexisting moles or about development of a newly pigmented lesion.
4. Use a magnifying lens or dermatoscope in a brightly lit room to look for variegated color and irregular border and surface in the nevus. Use side lighting to assess subtle elevation.
5. Examine entire skin surface, including the scalp, genital area, gluteal folds, and soles of feet.
6. Examine diameter of mole; melanomas are usually larger than 6 mm; look for lesions situated near the mole.

 NURSING ALERT Any skin lesion that changes in size or color, bleeds, ulcerates, or becomes infected may be skin cancer.

Nursing Diagnoses

- Deficient Knowledge related to risk factors for skin cancer.
- Anxiety related to diagnosis of cancer.

Nursing Interventions

Increasing Knowledge and Awareness

1. Encourage follow-up skin examinations and instruct the patient to examine the skin monthly as follows:
   a. Use a full-length mirror and a small hand mirror to aid in examination.
   b. Learn where moles and birthmarks are located.
   c. Inspect all moles and other pigmented lesions; report any change in color, size, elevation, thickness, or development of itching or bleeding.
2. Teach the patient to use a sunscreen with at least SPF 30 routinely and to avoid becoming sunburned. Reapply sunscreen at least every 2 hours.
   a. Sunlight permanently damages DNA in the skin and the cumulative effects of the sun may result in skin cancers.

b. Avoid tanning, especially if the skin burns easily, never tans, or tans poorly.
c. Avoid unnecessary exposure to the sun, especially during times when ultraviolet radiation is most intense (10:00 A.M. to 3:00 P.M.).
d. Wear protective clothing (long sleeves, broad-brimmed hat, high collar, long pants). However, clothing does not provide complete protection of UVA rays.
e. Do not use sunlamps for indoor tanning; avoid commercial tanning salons.

 NURSING ALERT Indoor tanning beds are not safe. All sources of ultraviolet light have been determined to be carcinogenic by the World Health Organization.

Reducing Anxiety

1. Provide dressing changes and wound care while teaching patient to take control, as directed, after surgical intervention.
2. Administer chemotherapy with attention to possible adverse effects, as directed.
3. Allow patient to express feelings about the seriousness of diagnosis.
4. Answer questions, clarify information, and correct misconceptions.
5. Emphasize use of positive coping skills and support system.

Patient Education and Health Maintenance

1. Encourage lifelong follow-up appointments with dermatologist or primary care provider with examinations every 6 months.
2. Encourage all individuals to have moles removed that are accessible to repeated friction and irritation, congenital, or suspicious in any way.
3. Teach all individuals the importance of sun avoidance measures; teach proper use of sunscreen:
   a. Sunscreens with SPF 15 or greater offer good protection. Sunscreen should provide UVA and UVB protection.
   b. Sunscreens should be used from 6 months through old age.
   c. Sunscreens should be applied before going outdoors to all areas that may be exposed, preferably before dressing. They should be applied liberally to achieve the stated SPF.
   d. Newly developed sunscreens are more resistant to removal by water, clothing, sweating; however, periodic reapplication is necessary when spending prolonged periods outdoors, especially when swimming.
   e. Protect lips with a lip balm that contains a sunscreen with the highest SPF.
4. For more information, refer patients to agencies such as the Skin Cancer Foundation (*www.skincancer.org*).

Evaluation: Expected Outcomes

- Uses high-SPF sunscreen, wears protective clothing, and performs monthly skin examinations.
- Verbalizes decreased anxiety.

Other Dermatologic Disorders

See Table 33-2.

Table 33-2	Other Dermatologic Disorders

NAME AND DESCRIPTION	CLINICAL MANIFESTATIONS
Bacterial Infections	
Folliculitis Inflammation of the hair follicle	• Single or multiple papules or pustules. • Commonly seen in the beard area of men and on women's legs from shaving.
Furunculosis Perifollicular abscess (boil) caused by *Staphylococcus aureus*; carbuncles are two or more confluent furuncles	• Tender, circumscribed, erythematous area whose center may become fluctuant and suppurate. • Commonly occur on the back of the neck, axillae, or buttocks. • Common organism is methicillin-resistant *Staphylococcal aureus* (MRSA).
Paronychia Inflammation of skin folds surrounding the fingernail; may be bacterial or fungal or both	• Tender, purulent, erythematous swelling of nail border. • Chronic and recurrent paronychia causes horizontal ridges at the base of the nail.
Erysipelas Streptococcal infection involving the superficial dermal lymphatics of the head or extremities, may be *S. aureus* of the face	• Prodromal—malaise, fever, chills, headache, vomiting, and joint pain. • Local—redness, warmth, swelling, and characteristic raised indurated border. • Leukocytosis. • Advancing edge of the patch with extension. • May vesiculate.
Intertrigo Superficial inflammation and secondary infection where two skin surfaces are in apposition; may be bacterial or fungal or both	• Erythematous and macerated rash under breasts, in abdominal skin fold, or in the groin. • Rash may exhibit erosions, fissures, and drainage. • Burning and itching.
Mycotic (Fungal) Infections	
Tinea Pedis Ringworm of the footTinea corporis—ringworm of the bodyTinea cruris—ringworm of the groinTinea capitis—ringworm of the scalp	• Caused by the dermatophytes *Trichophyton*, *Epidermophyton*, or *Microsporum* • Erythematous, inflamed, and vesicular lesions of feet. • Scaling erythematous patches of the body or head with central clearing. • Dull red or brownish rash of upper inner thighs and groin with scaling borders. • Itching and irritation.

 DRUG ALERT Oral antifungal agents are associated with significant drug interactions with such agents as warfarin, simvastatin, lovastatin, triazolam, cisapride, digoxin, cyclosporine, phenytoin, cimetidine, and rifampin. Baseline and periodic liver function test monitoring is recommended. More frequent monitoring of INR or blood levels may be required.

NAME AND DESCRIPTION	CLINICAL MANIFESTATIONS
Tinea Versicolor Superficial fungal infection by *Malassezia furfur*	• Patchy macular or mildly scaly rash of the upper trunk and upper arms; yellowish or brownish in light-skinned people, hypopigmented in those with dark skin. • Mild itching and scaling.

MANAGEMENT	NURSING CONSIDERATIONS
• Twice daily cleansing with moisturizing soap and/or BPO. • Topical antibiotic treatment, as prescribed by health care provider. • Systemic antibiotics for recurrent or recalcitrant cases.	• Suggest warm compresses to relieve inflammation and promote drainage.
• Warm compresses to reduce inflammation and promote drainage. • When area becomes fluctuant, incision and drainage can be performed, followed by packing. • Furuncles of the ear canal, nares, upper lip, and nose may require systemic antibiotic treatment because these areas drain directly into cranial venous sinuses.	• Suggest warm compresses. • Warn patient not to squeeze or incise the lesion. • Suggest mild analgesics, if needed. • If severe or recurrent, look for underlying immunosuppression by disorders, such as diabetes, AIDS, alcoholism, or malnutrition.
• Incision and drainage for acutely inflamed paronychia. • Fungicidal or bactericidal ointment for chronic paronychia. • Systemic antibiotic treatment usually is not necessary. • Prevention of trauma and maceration.	• Encourage soaking in warm water for 10 to 15 minutes three to four times per day while acutely inflamed to relieve pain and promote drainage. • Identify persons with work-related chronic paronychia (such as bartenders, dishwashers, and housekeepers) and recommend use of rubber gloves over thin cotton gloves when working around moisture.
• Oral, IM, or IV antibiotics, usually penicillinase-resistant penicillin derivatives; cephalosporin or macrolide antibiotic may be used.	• Ice or cold compresses may be soothing. • Prompt treatment required in patient with diabetes to prevent extensive spread and necrotizing fasciitis.
• Topical antibacterial and antifungal agents, as prescribed by health care provider.	• Teach patient to prevent skin maceration by separating opposing skin surfaces with gauze or cotton material. • Skin surfaces should be dried thoroughly after bathing with a hair dryer on low setting. • Absorbent powder can be applied lightly to the area after drying as long as no redness or irritation is present. • Loose, air-permeable clothing should be worn.
• Examination of rash under Wood light differentiates erythrasma, which will fluoresce; most tinea patches will not. • Skin scraping from leading edge shows characteristic spores and hyphae with KOH preparation under microscope. • Treat with topical antifungals or systemic antifungals for severe cases. • Reduction of moisture in the groin, between toes.	• Advise washing one to two times per day with water and mild soap and then applying talcum powder or cornstarch to well-dried area. • Use hair dryer set on low temperature to dry tender areas. • Encourage wearing cotton socks and underwear and light, air-permeable clothing to promote evaporation. • Warn about contamination from feet to the groin or other areas of the body by hands or clothing. • In tinea pedis, encourage use of open shoes or canvas sneakers and avoidance of tight shoes or plastic or rubber-soled shoes or boots. • Wash contaminated clothing in hot water.
• On Wood light examination, may fluoresce and will show hypopigmented patches. • Microscopic examination with KOH preparation of skin scraping shows characteristic "spaghetti and meatball" appearance of hyphae and spores. • Treat with selenium sulfide shampoo (leave on for 40 minutes before showering) daily for 1 week. • Topical or systemic antifungal treatment may be used as prescribed by health care provider.	• Common in high-temperature, high-humidity environments. • Advise patient that discoloration may persist after fungus has been eradicated; lost pigmentation will resolve with sun exposure. • Tell patient that recurrence is common after 2 to 12 weeks if prophylactic treatment is not given periodically.

(continued)

Table 33-2	Other Dermatologic Disorders (*Continued*)
NAME AND DESCRIPTION	**CLINICAL MANIFESTATIONS**
Onychomycosis (Tinea Unguium)	
Fungal infection of the nail	• Discoloration (white, yellow, or darkened) of the nail. • Nail becomes brittle, cracked, irregular, and loosened. • May be some inflammation and pain.
Parasitic and Other Infestations	
Pediculosis	
Pediculosis capitis—head lice Pediculosis corporis—body lice Pediculosis pubis—crab louse infestation of the genital region **DRUG ALERT** Caution pregnant patients who have pediculosis capitis not to use antiparasitic preparations.	• Itching is primary complaint. • Lice and nits may be seen in seams of clothing (body lice) or clinging to hairs (pubic lice). • Skin excoriation in affected area. • Erythematous macules or wheals may appear at puncture sites. • Gray-blue macules may appear on the trunk or inner thighs with pediculosis pubis.
Scabies	
Superficial infestation by itch mite; transmitted by close personal contact **GERONTOLOGIC ALERT** Infestation with scabies may be a problem in nursing homes, particularly among debilitated patients who require extensive hands-on care.	• Itching, more intense at night. • Small erythematous papules and short, wavy burrows are seen on skin surface. • Frequently seen between fingers or in groin area. • Spares head and scalp except in children under age 1. • Atypical scabies may be found in immunocompromised people and may be resistant to standard treatment.
Bedbugs	
Small, nocturnal, blood-sucking insects requiring weekly meals to advance in their life cycle; however can survive up to a year without a meal. Bedbugs hide during the day in seams, crevices, and cracks in mattresses, box springs, walls, and floors.	• Pruritic papules often assume a linear configuration of 3 to 4 lesions ("breakfast, lunch, and dinner"). • Found on exposed areas. • Affected individuals often awake in the early morning because of pruritus as this is the time bedbugs are most active. • May be variance in reaction to bedbugs in household members (not all individuals react to bedbug bites to the same degree).

MANAGEMENT	NURSING CONSIDERATIONS
• Identification of offending fungus by microscopic examination of shavings with KOH or by culture. • Treatment with appropriate systemic antifungal for prolonged period—usually at least 6 weeks for fingernails and at least 12 weeks for toenails. • Surgical removal of the nail may be necessary.	• Encourage patient to comply with lengthy treatment, as fungal infections of the nail are difficult to treat. • Examine patient for other areas of tinea infection (feet, groin), encourage treatment, and teach patient that infection may be spread from fingernails by scratching. • After nail removal, advise patient to keep hand or foot elevated for several hours and change dressing daily by applying gauze and antibiotic ointment or other prescribed medication until nail bed is free of exudate or blood.

• Treatment for pediculosis corporis involves washing with soap and water and washing all infested clothing and linens with hot water. Alternatively, clothes may be dry-cleaned or ironed, paying close attention to the seams.
• Pediculosis capitis and pubis are treated with a topical antiparasitic preparation, such as lindane or permethrin.
• Manual removal of nits (eggs) may be performed; retreatment with topical antiparasitic in 3 to 7 days is recommended.
• Petroleum may be applied to eyelashes and then lice and nits removed with swab or tweezers, or pilocarpine drops can be used to paralyze the lice.
• Items that cannot be washed or dry-cleaned can be stored for 30 days without use.
	• Advise patient that pediculosis pubis is considered a sexually transmitted disease; partners must be examined and treated.
	• Teach patient the proper use of medication:
	  • Apply lotion or cream after bathing to affected hairy and adjacent areas; wash off after 8 to 12 hours.
	  • Alternatively, apply shampoo to affected hairy areas and lather for 4 to 5 minutes, rinse, and let hair dry.
	  • Use fine-tooth comb to remove nits.
	• Urge patient to wash all clothing, towels, linens, combs, and hair items by soaking in hot water for 10 minutes.
	• Advise patient not to use antiparasitic preparations more frequently than recommended.

• Parasite identified by microscopic examination of skin scraping.
• Treated with antiparasitic, such as permethrin or crotamiton, and oral treatment with ivermectin 0.2 mg/kg × 1 dose, if indicated.
• Machine wash and dry clothing and linens on hot cycle.
• Topical or systemic steroids may be needed to treat symptoms of allergic reaction to mites.
	• Teach proper use of medication:
	  • Apply thin layer from the neck downward, with particular attention to hands, feet, and intertriginous areas; every inch of the skin must be treated because mites are migratory. Apply to dry skin. (Wet skin allows more penetration and the possibility of toxicity.)
	  • Leave medication on for 8 to 12 hours—but no longer, as doing so will irritate the skin. Wash thoroughly.
	• Advise patient to avoid close contact for 24 hours after treatment to prevent transmission.
	• Encourage treatment of sexual and close contacts simultaneously.
	• Tell patient that itching may persist for days to weeks following treatment because of an allergic reaction to mites; retreatment is not necessary.

• Bedbug bite lesions will resolve on their own in 1 to 2 weeks. • Treatment aimed at controlling symptoms: oral antihistamines and topical corticosteroids per health care provider.	• Advise close examination of mattress seams for brown spots (excrement of bedbugs), especially when traveling and staying in hotels (to prevent transporting of bedbugs home on luggage) • Advise professional extermination to eradicate infestation • Explain to patient that scratching will make itching worse and may lead to secondary skin infection such as impetigo • Reassure patient that bedbugs do not carry disease and are not associated with uncleanliness.

(continued)

Table 33-2 Other Dermatologic Disorders (*Continued*)

NAME AND DESCRIPTION	CLINICAL MANIFESTATIONS
Viral Infections	
Herpes Simplex	
Acute vesicular eruption caused by herpes simplex virus type 1 or 2	• Prodromal pain, burning, or tingling, possible fever and malaise. • Tiny vesicles appear on erythematous, swollen base; they rupture, forming painful ulcers and crusting; healing occurs but outbreaks are recurrent. • Can occur anywhere, especially near mucocutaneous junctions. • Viral shedding may occur between symptomatic periods, leading to transmission of the infection.
Other Conditions	
Contact Dermatitis	
Inflammatory condition caused by exposure to irritating or allergenic substances, such as plants, cosmetics, cleaning products, soaps and detergents, hair dyes, metals, and rubber	• Itching, burning, erythema, and vesiculation at point of contact. • Progresses to weeping, crusting, drying, fissuring, and peeling. • Lichenification (thickening of the skin) and pigmentation changes may occur with chronicity.
Exfoliative Dermatitis	
Chronic extensive scaling and inflammation of the skin; may be idiopathic or related to preexisting skin conditions, drug reactions, or underlying malignancy	• Starts as patchy erythema, with possible fever, chills, and malaise. • Rapid spread until whole integument is involved. • Skin color changes to scarlet, desquamates, and may ooze serous fluid. • Pruritus, hair loss, and secondary infection.
Alopecia	
Hair loss, may be idiopathic (alopecia areata), male-pattern, physiologic, or because of hair pulling (trichotillomania); also because of scarring from other skin or systemic disorders	• Patterned, patchy, or diffuse hair loss. • Inflammation and scarring with some types. • Physiologic alopecia may be associated with hormonal changes, such as childbirth, nutritional factors, or toxin exposure.
Seborrheic Dermatitis	
Chronic, superficial inflammatory skin disorder	• Crusted pinkish or yellow patches. • Loose scales that may be dry, moist, or greasy. • Mild itching. • Affects the scalp, eyebrows, eyelids, nasolabial creases, lips, ears, chest, axillae, umbilicus, and groin.

MANAGEMENT	NURSING CONSIDERATIONS
• Tzanck smear from scraping of ulcer or fluid from vesicle shows characteristic giant cells with intranuclear inclusions; also diagnosed by fluorescent antibody detection or viral culture. • Antiviral treatment with acyclovir, famciclovir, or valacyclovir for acute infection or continuous suppressive therapy to prevent or lessen recurrence. • Analgesics may be needed for widespread and genital eruptions.	• Teach patient that herpes simplex can be transmitted by close and sexual contact; good personal and hand hygiene is required for facial cases; sexual abstinence or condom use is required for genital cases. • Recurrence may be brought on by fever, illness, emotional stress, menses, pregnancy, sunlight, and other factors. • Advise patients with active herpes simplex infection to avoid contact with immunosuppressed individuals, such as those with diabetes, HIV disease, cancer (including those undergoing cancer treatment), alcoholism, and malnutrition, because herpes simplex infection can be severe in these individuals. • Tell patients that lesions usually resolve in 1 to 2 weeks without scarring.
• Topical or oral steroids, depending on severity. Oral steroids usually given in tapered dose—start with high dose and gradually decrease to provide greatest anti-inflammatory effect without adrenal suppression. • Removal or avoidance of causative agent. • Antipruritics—systemic or topical antihistamines or topical calamine preparations. • Desensitization to poison ivy and other substances may be accomplished for those who have severe reactions and cannot avoid contact.	• Take thorough history to determine causative agent or contributing factors; have patient keep log of activities and symptoms if unsure of irritant. • Teach patient to use allergen-free products, wear gloves and protective clothing, wash and rinse skin thoroughly, and wash clothing after contact with potential irritants. • Advise patient that rash—even oozing lesion of poison ivy—is not contagious; however, contaminated clothing may cause spread of poison ivy in those who are sensitive. • Advise patient to perform patch test by applying substance behind the ear or on inside of the wrist before trying new cosmetics, soaps, or hair products.
• Discontinuation of offending drug or treatment of underlying condition. • Systemic corticosteroids should control most cases. • Supportive treatment—bed rest, warm environment, and fluid and electrolyte replacement. • Soothing baths and topical emollients for symptomatic relief • Possible use of immunosuppressants—azathioprine, methotrexate, and cyclophosphamide.	• Monitor fluid balance and electrolyte values. • Watch for signs of secondary infection and report; antimicrobial therapy may be necessary. • Watch for signs of heart failure caused by chronically increased cutaneous blood flow. • Teach patient how to relieve itching with oatmeal baths and emollient creams. • Tell patient to avoid environments with temperature fluctuations to avoid chilling. • Advise patient to avoid all irritants.
• Treatment of underlying causes. • Minoxidil may cause fine hair regrowth in male-pattern baldness and alopecia areata. Finasteride, an oral agent, can be used by men only, with good results. • Other methods of hair replacement—surgical grafting of hair follicles, hair weaving, or hairpieces.	• Explain that alopecia areata and physiologic hair loss are usually temporary and self-limiting. • Encourage female patient to change hairstyle or wear hairpieces or turbans until hair grows back after childbirth. • Counsel male patient on the slow, limited effects of minoxidil treatment and stress that effects reverse when treatment is stopped.
• Apply selenium sulfide, tar, zinc, or resorcinol shampoo to the scalp several times per week. • Corticosteroid lotions or creams. • For eyelid margin involvement (blepharitis), daily debridement with cotton-tipped applicator and baby shampoo and application of ophthalmic steroid ointment or lotion. • Zinc soap or selenium lotion for washing once controlled. • For external ear canal involvement, corticosteroid cream.	• Advise patient of chronic nature of seborrhea and that condition may be exacerbated by perspiration, neuroleptic drugs, and emotional stress; also seen more frequently in persons with Parkinson disease, HIV disease, diabetes mellitus, malabsorption syndromes, and epilepsy. • Teach patient to apply topical preparations, as prescribed. • Advise using only baby shampoo and gently rubbing with swab near the eyes to prevent irritation of conjunctiva in seborrheic blepharitis.

(continued)

Table 33-2 Other Dermatologic Disorders (Continued)

NAME AND DESCRIPTION	CLINICAL MANIFESTATIONS
Hidradenitis Suppurativa Chronic follicular plugging and secondary infection of the apocrine glands of the groin and axilla	• Development of tender red nodules that enlarge, rupture, and suppurate. • Sinus tracts develop with recurrent lesions, leading to continuous inflammation and drainage.
Bullous Pemphigoid Chronic bullous disease of autoimmune etiology; occurs in older adults	• Tense vesicles and bullae arise on normal or erythematous skin, rupture, and heal without scarring. • Occurs on flexor aspects of the body, axilla, inguinal areas, abdomen, and, occasionally, on mucous membranes.
Acne Vulgaris Obstruction and inflammation of sebaceous glands and follicles	• Closed comedones (whiteheads). • Open comedones (blackheads). • Papules, pustules, nodules, cysts, or abscesses may develop. • Primary sites are the face, chest, upper back, and shoulder.
Rosacea Erythematous, pustular eruption of the malar cheeks, forehead, nose or around the eyes; most common in adults ages 40 to 60; unknown cause; may affect the eyes in 20% to 50% of cases	• Diffuse redness, papules, and pustules develop over malar cheeks, forehead, nose, or around the eyes. • Later, dilated blood vessels and flushing are seen. • Rhinophyma (hypertrophic, bulbous nose) may develop. More common in men, rare in women.

AIDS, acquired immunodeficiency syndrome; HDL, high-density lipoprotein; HIV, human immunodeficiency virus; IM, intramuscular; INR, international normalized ratio; IV, intravenous; KOH, potassium hydroxide.

MANAGEMENT	NURSING CONSIDERATIONS
• Initially, prolonged (2 months or more) administration of an antibiotic, such as tetracycline, clindamycin, or erythromycin, as well as systemic or intralesional corticosteroids; however, progression of the condition is likely. • Surgical treatment necessary when chronic suppuration and fistulas develop. • Incision and drainage or laser stripping. • Cauterization of sinus tracts. • Exteriorization with curettage and electrodesiccation. • Excision with possible skin grafting. • Isotretinoin, antiandrogens, and intralesional or systematic steroid therapy may relieve exacerbations.	• Advise patient to use moisturizing soap and keep axilla and groin dry to reduce bacterial colonization of the skin. • Teach patient the signs of bacterial infection—purulent drainage, odor, pain—that call for notification of health care provider and treatment with antibiotics. • Encourage use of warm compresses to relieve inflammation. • Obesity and cigarette smoking contribute to the disease. Encourage weight loss and smoking cessation, if applicable.
• Systemic corticosteroid treatment in widespread involvement. Topical corticosteroids if limited lesions. Immunosuppressant for resistant cases. • Condition may remit within 2 to 4 years even without treatment.	• Keep skin clean and dry to reduce chances of secondary infection. • If patient is immobilized, encourage positioning to prevent undue pressure on lesions to avoid risk of premature rupture and secondary infection. • Make sure to differentiate from early pressure sore development and treat pressure sores appropriately. • Advise patient that lesions usually heal without scarring.
• Topical benzoyl peroxide—antibacterial and comedolytic. • Topical retinoic acid, a comedolytic, or adapalene, a more potent synthetic retinoid. • Topical antibiotics—suppress growth of *Propionibacterium* acnes and decrease comedones, papules, and pustules without systemic adverse effects. • Azelaic acid, a topical agent with multiple antiacne effects. • Systemic antibiotics—long-term, low-dose therapy for more inflammatory and extensive causes. • Retinoid therapy—inhibits sebum production and secretion; for severe, disfiguring cystic acne. • Estrogen therapy—antiandrogenic effect decreases sebum production in women taking oral contraceptives. Spironolactone may be added, if needed, to increase antiandrogenic effect. • Intralesional steroid injection—for inflamed lesions. • Dermabrasion—surgical planning or chemical peels to smooth surface configuration of old scars. Should not be done within 6 to 12 months of Accutane use.	• Advise patient to wash face gently with mild soap and water one to two times per day. • Teach proper application of topical preparation—use sparingly and decrease frequency if irritation and redness develop. • Inform patient about adverse effects of systemic antibiotics. • Ensure that women of childbearing potential are using contraceptives and that a negative pregnancy test has been obtained before starting isotretinoin therapy. Female patients must be on two forms of birth control. All patients must be enrolled in the iPLEDGE system. • Encourage follow-up and monitoring of laboratory tests during treatment with isotretinoin for elevated liver enzymes, cholesterol, and triglycerides and for decreased HDL. • Advise patient taking isotretinoin to notify health care provider of persistent headache—could signal pseudotumor cerebri. • Tell patient that initiation of therapy may worsen symptoms for several weeks, but to continue treatment. • Advise patient not to squeeze pimples and avoid friction around the face. • Suggest use of water-based and hypoallergenic cosmetics. • Encourage stress management, balanced diet, and avoidance of foods believed to aggravate acne.
• Topical metronidazole gel applied bid. • Oral doxycycline. • Treatment necessary for 4 to 6 weeks and repeated if recurrence. May need long-term suppression with oral antibiotics. • Avoid exercise, stress, hot beverages, and spicy foods.	• Teach patient to avoid flushing by reducing stress, replacing strenuous exercise with low-intensity workouts, staying cool, and avoiding the sun. • Suggest contacting the National Rosacea Society (*www.rosacea.org*).

SELECTED REFERENCES

Aldridge, A. (2015). Dealing with common skin lesions in older people. *Journal of Community Nursing*, *29*(6), 53–61.

Armstrong, K. (2014). Common skin problems in the community and primary care. *British Journal of Community Nursing*, *19*(10), 482–488.

Bale, T. (2017). Dermatology across healthcare settings. *British Journal of Nursing*, *26*(5), 263.

Bibbins-Domingo, K., Grossman, D., Curry, S., et al. (2016). Screening for skin cancer: US Preventive Services Task Force recommendation statement. *Journal of the American Medical Association*, *316*(4), 429–435.

Cantrell, W. (2017). Psoriasis and psoriatic therapies. *The Nurse Practitioner*, *42*(7), 35–39.

Casey, G., & Kai, T. (2016). Disorders of the skin. *Nursing New Zealand*, *22*(3), 20–24.

Centers for Disease Control and Prevention (2018). *Shingles (Herpes Zoster) Vaccination*. Available at *https://www.cdc.gov/vaccines/vpd/shingles/index.html*.

Driscoll, D., & Darcy, J. (2015). Indoor tanning legislation: Shaping policy and nursing practice. *Pediatric Nursing*, *41*(2), 59–88.

Edwards, J. (2016). Scars: An overview of current management and nursing care. *Dermatological Nursing*, *15*(2), 18–23.

Habif, T. P. (2016). *Clinical dermatology: A color guide to diagnosis and therapy* (6th ed.). St. Louis, MO: Mosby.

Hall, J. C. (2017). *Sauer's manual of skin diseases* (11th ed.). Philadelphia, PA: Lippincott Williams & Wilkins.

Haras, M. (2017). All things bed bugs: A primer for nephrology nurses. *Nephrology Nursing Journal*, *44*(2), 181–185.

Hilton, R. (2016). Impact of psoriasis affecting high impact sites. *Dermatological Nursing*, *15*(4), 23–27.

Jackson, K. (2016). Assessing and treating the patient with psoriasis. *Dermatological Nursing*, *15*(3), s10–s13.

Jackson, K., & Brown, D. (2017). Nursing management of Stevens-Johnson Syndrome and toxic epidermal necrolysis: What the new BAD guidelines recommend. *Dermatological Nursing*, *16*(2), 46–50.

James, W. D., Berger, T. G., & Elston, D. M. (2015). *Andrews' diseases of the skin clinical dermatology* (12th ed.). Philadelphia, PA: Elsevier.

Kathrotiya, H. (2015). The treatment and demographics of warts: An analysis of national trends. *The Foot and Ankle Quarterly*, *26*(2), 111–113.

Kaylor, M., Wenning, P., & Eddy, C. (2015). Prevalence, knowledge, and concern about bed bugs. *Journal of Environmental Health*, *78*(1), 20–24.

Kirkland-Kyhn, H., Zaratkiewicz, S., Teleten, O. (2018). Caring for aging skin. *American Journal of Nursing*, *118*(2), 60–63.

Langa, Y., & Van der Merwe, E. (2016). Atopic dermatitis: Tacrolimus vs topical corticosteroid use. *Professional Nursing Today*, *20*(3), 50–56.

Lawton, S. (2016). Identifying, diagnosing, and managing skin allergies. *Primary Health Care*, *26*(4), 34–40.

Moyal, D., & Seité, S. (2016). Towards a broader sun protection. *Dermatological Nursing*, *15*(2), s5–s9.

Osier, E., Matiz, C., Ghali, F., & Eichenfield, L. (2015). Staphylococcus aureus infections in atopic dermatitis. *Contemporary Pediatrics*, *32*(10), 34–37.

Renton, C. (2018). Late-onset psoriasis: Diagnosis, assessment and management. *British Journal of Community Nursing*, *23*(2), 58–63.

Shostak, K., & Conceicao, V. (2015). Understanding the development and management of shingles. *Journal of Community Nursing*, *29*(2), 74–78.

US Preventive Services Task Force. (2016). Screening for skin cancer: Recommendation statement. *American Family Physician*, *94*(6), 479–481.

Van Onselen, J. (2018). Dermatology prescribing update: Skin infestations. *Nurse Prescribing*, *16*(4), 162–166.

Van Onselen, J. (2018). Dermatology prescribing update: Skin infections. *Nurse Prescribing*, *16*(1), 19–24.

Watkins, J. (2015). An itch to scratch: Skin diseases in the older person. *Nursing and Residential Care*, *17*(5), 262–265.

Weidinger, S., & Novak, N. (2016). Atopic dermatitis. *Lancet*, *367*, 1109–1122.

Wernli, K., Henrikson, N., Morrison, C., et al. (2016). Screening for skin cancer in adults: Updated evidence report and systematic review for the US Preventive Services Task Force. *Journal of the American Medical Association*, *316*(4), 436–447.

Wheatley, B. (2018). Improving dermatologic screening in primary care. *Nurse Practitioner*, *43*(4), 19–24.

Zaenglein, A.L., Pathy, A.L., Schlosser, B.J. et al. (2016). Guidelines of care for the management of acne vulgaris. *Journal of the Academy of Dermatology*, *74*(5), 945–973.

34
Burns

OVERVIEW AND ASSESSMENT

Burns are a form of traumatic injury caused by thermal, electrical, chemical, or radioactive agents.

Inhalation injury and associated pulmonary complications are a significant factor in mortality and morbidity from burn injury.

Etiology and Pathophysiology

 EVIDENCE BASE American Burn Association. (2016). *Resources: Burn incidence and treatment in the United States fact sheet.* Chicago, IL: Author. Available: *www.ameriburn.org/resources_factsheet.php.*

Incidence

1. In the United States, an estimated 436,000 patients seek medical treatment for burn injuries in emergency departments each year, with about 40,000 requiring hospitalization. Seventy-five percent of those patients are admitted to burn centers.
2. With an estimated 3,275 fire-related deaths per year, one civilian fire death occurs every 2 hours and 41 minutes. More than 83% of these deaths are from residential fires and 9% are from vehicle collision fires. Fire deaths decreased by more than 11% from 2005 to 2014.
3. Burns less than 10% total body surface area (TBSA) account for 75% of admissions to burn centers, with a mortality rate of 0.6%. Mortality increases with burn size. Patients with a TBSA of 80% or greater have a mortality rate of 80%. Overall national mortality rate for all admissions to a burn center is 3.3%.
4. Males (68%) are more commonly injured by burns than are females.
5. Flame injury (41%) is the leading cause of burn injuries. Other etiologies include scald (33%), contact with a hot object (9%), electrical injuries (3%), and chemical injuries (3%). Scald burns are more prevalent in children under 5.
6. Most burn injuries occur in the home (73%). Other places of occurrence include industrial environments, streets or highways, and places of recreation and sport.
7. An estimated 7% of patients admitted to burn centers have an inhalation injury, with a mortality rate of 19%. Patients without inhalation injuries have a mortality rate of less than 2%.

Burn Injury

1. A burn injury usually results from energy transfer from a heat source to the body. The type of burn injury may be flame/flash, contact, scald (water, grease), chemical, electrical, inhalation, or any thermal source. Many factors alter the response of body tissues to these sources of heat.
   a. Local tissue conductivity—bone is most resistant to the heat source accumulation. Lesser resistance is seen in nerves, blood vessels, and muscle tissue.
   b. Adequacy of peripheral circulation.
   c. Skin thickness, insulating material of clothing, or dampness of the skin.
2. Physiologic reaction to a burn is dependent on burn size and depth. Smaller burns produce a local response of pain, erythema, and edema at the site of injury. Severe burns, generally described as 20% TBSA or more, may produce a systemic response with widespread hemodynamic and cardiovascular changes.
3. Systemic response to burn injury is a unique combination of distributive and hypovolemic shock. The release of mediators such as tumor necrosis factor-α produce a profound effect on the circulatory system. In burns greater than 20% TBSA, there is an intravascular depletion, low pulmonary artery occlusion pressures, elevated systemic vascular resistance, and depressed cardiac output.
   a. Systemic microcirculation loses its vessel wall integrity, and proteins are lost into the interstitium.
   b. Protein loss causes intravascular colloid osmotic pressure to drop and allows fluid to leak from the vessels.
   c. There is an increase of fluid leaking into the interstitium, caused by decreased interstitial pressure and increased capillary permeability to protein.
   d. Over 24 hours, there is a loss of intravascular fluids, electrolytes, and proteins into the interstitium.
   e. The resultant changes are reflected in massive edema formation, loss of circulating plasma volume, hemoconcentration, decreased urine output, and depressed cardiac function.
4. Burns may be superficial thickness (first-degree), partial-thickness (second-degree), or full-thickness (third-degree) (see Figure 34-1).
   a. Superficial thickness burns are commonly termed first-degree burns. Only the epidermis is involved, remaining intact with no blistering. Local redness and blanching occur similar to a sunburn. Epidermal-only injuries heal within 5 to 7 days.

919

Figure 34-1. Cross-section of the skin depicting blood supply, depth of burn, and relative thickness of skin grafts.

b. Partial-thickness burn injuries, commonly known as second-degree burns, involve the epidermis and upper portions of the dermis. Sweat glands, hair follicles, and nerves remain intact. The wound is moist and very painful. Partial-thickness injuries can be categorized as superficial or deep depending on how far into the dermis the damage extends. In superficial partial-thickness burns, some of the dermal appendages remain, from which the wound can spontaneously reepithelialize and heal on its own. A deep partial-thickness burn injury can convert to a full-thickness burn injury if patient is underresuscitated or develops an infection. Healing time is 5 to 35 days.

c. Full-thickness injuries, commonly known as third-degree burns, involve all layers of the skin, and sometimes, underlying tissues are destroyed. The burn wound is dry, white, brown, or leathery in appearance. Patients typically do not have pain with full-thickness injuries because of the destruction of the nerve endings. At the core is the burn injury. There is then a zone of coagulation surrounded by a zone of stasis, surrounded by hyperemia (erythema) very similar to a bull's-eye pattern, the burn being in the center (see Figure 34-2). Grafting is usually required to close the wound.

5. Burn depth is directly related to the temperature of the burning agent and the duration of contact with body tissue.
   a. Below 112°F (44.4°C), no local damage occurs unless exposure is for a protracted period.
   b. At 120°F (48.9°C), it takes 5 minutes' exposure to create a full-thickness burn.
   c. At 125°F (51.7°C), the time requirement is 2 minutes, and at 140°F (60°C), only 6 seconds is required.
   d. At 159°F (70.6°C), it takes 1 second to create a full-thickness burn in a healthy adult—less time or temperature in children or older adults.

Inhalation Injury

EVIDENCE BASE Herndon, D. N. (2018). *Total Burn Care*, 5th Edition. New York: Elsevier.

1. Inhalation injury is broadly defined as damage to the airway and pulmonary tissue by heat or chemical irritants. Patients with larger flame burns and those who were trapped in a burning, enclosed space are at the highest risk for inhalation injury. Inhalation injuries combined with extensive cutaneous injury greatly increase risk of mortality.

2. Most inhalation injuries that result in death are a result of hypoxia and inhalation of the toxic by-products of combustion.

3. A patient's smoke exposure will contain a variety of poisonous gases such as cyanide, aldehydes, benzenes, and hydrogen chloride as a result of the synthetic and natural materials that burned near them.

4. Breathing toxic smoke creates a lower airway injury characterized by bronchial casts and constriction, increased pulmonary capillary permeability, and the leakage of protein-filled fluid into the alveolar space.

5. Impaired gas exchange from inhalation injury can be considered a type of acute lung injury (ALI) and may progress to acute respiratory distress syndrome (ARDS).

6. Carbon monoxide toxicity is a complication of inhalation injury and exposure to smoke. Carbon monoxide is a colorless, odorless, tasteless, nonirritating gas produced from incomplete combustion of carbon-containing materials.

7. Carbon monoxide's affinity for hemoglobin is 200 times greater than for oxygen.

8. Toxicity depends on concentration of carbon monoxide in inspired air and the length of time of exposure.

9. Although oxygen content of the blood is diminished, the amount of dissolved oxygen in the plasma (PaO_2) is unaffected by carbon monoxide poisoning; therefore, the arterial blood gas (ABG) will appear normal.

A

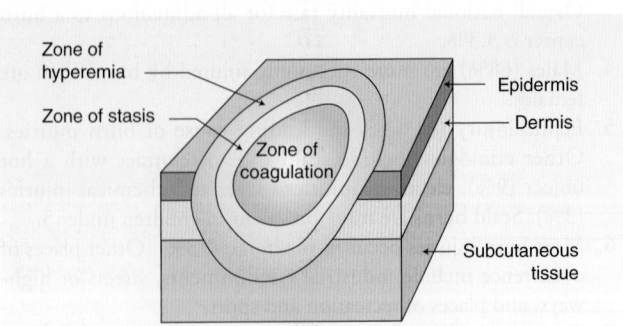

B

Figure 34-2. **(A)** Cross-section. **(B)** Surface view and depth.

10. Pulse oximetry only detects saturated hemoglobin and does not measure carbon monoxide; therefore, the pulse oximetry will appear normal.

11. A serum carboxyhemoglobin level must be measured in any patient with possible exposure to carbon monoxide in a fire.
    a. A carboxyhemoglobin level of less than 10% is not a cause for alarm. Normal carboxyhemoglobin in nonsmokers is less than 5%, and smokers can have carboxyhemoglobin levels as high as 10%.
    b. From 10% to 20%, severe headache, flushing, and dilation of skin vessels occur.
    c. Levels of 30% to 50% can produce disorientation, nausea, irritability, dizziness, vomiting, prostration, tachypnea, and tachycardia.
    d. Levels above 50% result in coma, seizures, convulsions, and Cheyne-Stokes respirations, and death is possible.

Systemic Changes in Major Burns

 EVIDENCE BASE Rowan, M. P., et al. (2015). Burn wound healing and treatment: Review and advancements. *Critical Care, 19*(1), 243.

 NURSING ALERT Smaller burn injuries (TBSA less than 20%) are typically characterized by a local response of pain, erythema, and edema at the site of injury. Major burns involving more than 20% TBSA are at risk for exhibiting systemic cardiovascular and hemodynamic changes resulting in burn shock.

Fluid Shifts

1. The water vapor barrier for the body is the outermost layer of the epidermis. When it is rendered nonfunctioning, severe systemic reactions from fluid losses can occur.
2. Fluid volume deficit is directly proportional to the extent and depth of burn injury.
3. Capillary permeability increases, permitting fluid and protein to move from vascular to interstitial spaces (edema results) for the first 24 to 36 hours, peaking at 12 hours postburn. Protein-rich fluid is lost in blebs of the burned tissues as well as by weeping of second-degree wounds and surface of full-thickness wounds. With reduced vascular volume, the patient will go into shock if untreated.
4. Capillary permeability starts to change in about 48 hours, but protein lost in interstitial spaces may remain there for 5 days to 2 weeks before returning to the vascular system.
    a. When fluid mobilizes (moves from interstitial spaces back to vascular compartment), patients with good cardiac and renal function will diurese.
    b. Patients with impaired cardiac or renal function are in danger of fluid overload and pulmonary edema at this time.
5. Red blood cell (RBC) mass is also diminished because of thrombosis, sludging, and RBC death from thermal injury; as fluid escapes from capillary walls, however, blood concentrates and the hematocrit rises, causing sluggish flow (see Figure 34-3).
6. Capillary stasis may cause ischemia and even necrosis.
7. The body attempts to compensate for losses of plasma volume.
    a. Constriction of vessels.
    b. Withdrawal of fluid from undamaged extracellular space.
    c. Patient thirst.

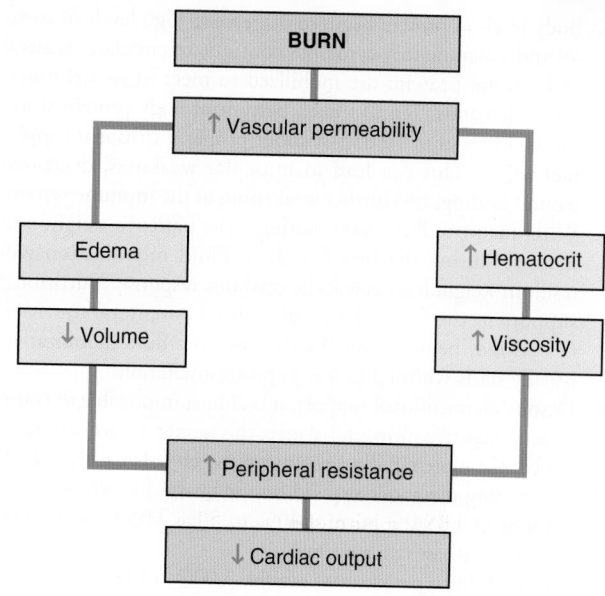

Figure 34-3. Hemodynamic changes in burn injury.

Hemodynamic Changes

1. Decreased circulating blood and plasma volume results in decreased cardiac output initially and increased pulse rate as a result of hypovolemia.
2. Afterload is increased due to a marked increase in systemic vascular resistance resulting from vasoactive mediators such as catecholamines.
3. A decrease in cardiac contractility is a predominant feature of full-thickness injuries covering more than 40% TBSA.
4. This results in inadequate tissue perfusion, which may in turn cause metabolic acidosis, renal failure, and irreversible burn shock.
5. Electrolyte imbalance may also occur.
    a. Hyponatremia usually occurs during the 3rd to 10th day because of fluid shift.
    b. The burn injury also causes hyperkalemia initially because of cell destruction, followed by hypokalemia as fluid shifts occur if potassium is not replaced.

Metabolic Demands

1. The initial metabolic response is thought to be activated by proinflammatory cytokines. The release of catecholamines, cortisol, glucagon, renin–angiotensin, antidiuretic hormone, and aldosterone is also increased. The major fuel source is stored glycogen. Major hypermetabolism and catabolism occur immediately postburn. The degree of the response is directly proportionate to the size of the burn injury.
2. Tachycardia, ranging from 100 to 120 beats/minute, is common and results from persistent elevation of catecholamine levels.
3. "Burn fever" (usually seen during the first week) is common and is dependent on depth of burn and percentage of TBSA involved. An increase of 1°F to 2°F makes it difficult to assess for infection.
4. Total body glucose stores are limited and stored liver and muscle glycogen is exhausted within the first few days postburn, hepatic glucose synthesis (gluconeogenesis) increases, and patients with glucose intolerance (obese patients and older adults) usually develop hyperglycemia.
5. Increased catabolism leads to increased urea production, especially in nutritionally depleted patients.

6. Body levels of protein begin to decrease as high levels of cortisol and inflammatory cytokines continue to circulate. Skeletal and visceral proteins are mobilized to meet increased nutritional demands. Ten to fifteen percent of body protein stores can be lost within 10 days without proper nutritional supplementation. This can lead to muscular weakness, decreased wound healing, and further weakening of the immune system.
7. With adequate fluid resuscitations, the patient's weight will increase during the first few days. Fluid mobilization will result in weight loss, as will the catabolic response. Nutritional support in the form of enteral or total parenteral nutrition (TPN) may be necessary. Weight loss from fluid mobilization usually starts within 3 to 4 days postresuscitation.
8. Despite all nutritional support, it is almost impossible to counteract a negative nitrogen balance; the sooner a burn wound is closed, the more rapidly a positive nitrogen balance is reached.
9. The resting metabolic expenditure increases linearly with the amount of TBSA; a burn of 40% to 50% TBSA has a metabolic rate almost twice normal.
10. The adult burn patient may require 3,000 to 5,000 calories or more per day.
    a. A burn of less than 10% usually requires minimal supplementation.
    b. A high-protein, high-calorie diet is necessary for a 10% to 20% burn.
    c. For burns 20% and greater, beginning enteral nutrition within 24 hours of the injury is recommended.

Renal Needs
1. Glomerular filtration may be decreased in extensive injury.
2. Without resuscitation or with delay, decreased renal blood flow may lead to high output or oliguric renal failure and decreased creatinine clearance.
3. Hemoglobin and myoglobin, present in the urine of patients with deep muscle damage commonly associated with electrical injury, may cause acute tubular necrosis and call for a greater amount of initial fluid therapy and osmotic diuresis.

Pulmonary Changes
1. Hyperventilation and increased oxygen consumption are associated with major burns.
2. The majority of deaths from fire are due to smoke inhalation.
3. Overzealous fluid resuscitation and the effects of burn shock on cell membrane potential may cause pulmonary edema, contributing to decreased alveolar exchange. Therefore, with an inhalation injury, it may be necessary to keep the patient slightly less hydrated.
4. Initial respiratory alkalosis resulting from hyperventilation may change to respiratory acidosis associated with pulmonary insufficiency as a result of major burn trauma.

Hematologic Changes
1. Thrombocytopenia, abnormal platelet function, depressed fibrinogen levels, inhibition of fibrinolysis, and a deficit in several plasma clotting factors occur postburn.
2. Anemia results from the direct effect of destruction of RBCs because of burn injury, reduced life span of surviving RBCs, and blood loss during diagnostic and therapeutic procedures.

Immunologic Activity
1. The loss of the skin barrier and presence of eschar favor bacterial growth. Methicillin-resistant *Staphylococcus aureus* (MRSA) is now being seen in the immunocompromised burn patient.
2. Polymorphonuclear chemotactic activity is suppressed, which results in decreased oxygen consumption and impaired bactericidal activity.

3. Abnormal inflammatory response after burn injury causes a decreased delivery of antibiotics, white blood cells, and oxygen to the injured area.
4. Hypoxia, acidosis, and thrombosis of vessels in the wound area impair host resistance to pathogenic bacteria.
5. Sera IgA, IgM, and IgG are depressed, reflecting depressed B-cell function.
6. Depressed cellular immunity is reflected by lymphocytopenia, delayed skin sensitivity, decreased allograft rejection potential, depletion of thymus-dependent lymphoid tissue, and increased susceptibility to fungi, viruses, and gram-negative organisms.
7. Burn wound sepsis.
   a. After colonization of the burn wound surface by bacteria, subeschar and intrafollicular colonization develops. Intraeschar and subeschar colonization may progress to invasion of subadjacent, nonburned, previously viable tissue.
   b. A bacterial count of 10^5 per gram of tissue as determined by burn wound biopsy (quantitative culture) indicates burn wound sepsis. Usually, only a swab culture is done of the wound surface.
   c. The wound is fully colonized in 3 to 5 days.
8. Seeding of bacteria from the wound may give rise to systemic septicemia.

GI Impact
1. As a result of sympathetic nervous system response to trauma, peristalsis decreases and gastric distention, nausea, vomiting, and paralytic ileus may occur.
2. Ischemia of the gastric mucosa and other etiologic factors put the burn patient at risk for duodenal and gastric ulcers. Curling ulcers, a gastric ulcer associated with severe burn injuries and well-known for causing life-threatening bleeding, have been noticeably declining in the literature. Although definitive data are lacking, researchers believe Curling ulcers have nearly been eradicated due to the early enteral feeding and gastrointestinal ulcer prophylaxis now routinely given to patients with severe burns.

Immediate Assessment

Immediate assessment of the burned patient is imperative, particularly burn size and depth, as fluid resuscitation is hallmark for initial management of severe burns. As with all trauma patients, it is important to start with the primary and secondary trauma survey. Do not become distracted by the visual appearance of the burn injury. Consider the mechanism of injury and assess for concomitant traumatic injuries.

Severity of Burns
Severity of burns is determined by:
1. Depth—first-, second- (partial-thickness), and third-degree (full-thickness). Patients with deeper burns may experience a greater systemic response. Full-thickness injuries require surgical excision and grafting.
2. Extent—percentage of TBSA. The higher the TBSA, the higher the risk of a systemic response and burn shock.
3. Age—mortality rate increases with age.
4. Area of the body burned—face, hand, feet, perineum, and circumferential burns require special care.
5. Medical history and concomitant injuries and illness. Preexisting conditions such as diabetes, renal failure, and congestive heart failure can complicate the management of even a small burn injury.
6. Inhalation injury.

Table 34-1	Signs and Symptoms of Toxicity from Carbon Monoxide
CO BLOOD LEVEL	**MANIFESTATIONS**
0%–10%	• None. • Smokers may have 10% carbon monoxide level or greater.
10%–20%	• Headache, vision disturbance, angina in patients with cardiovascular disease, and slowed mental function.
20%–40%	• Tight feeling in the head, rapid fatigue from muscular effort, decreased muscular coordination, confusion, irritability, ataxia, nausea, vomiting, increased pulse rate, decreased blood pressure, and dysrhythmias.
40%–60%	• Pulmonary and cardiac dysfunction, collapse, coma, and convulsions.
>60%	• Commonly fatal.

Assessment for Inhalation Injury

1. If victim was burned in a closed area, there should be a high index of suspicion that smoke inhalation has occurred.
2. Evaluate all patients in closed-space fires for symptoms of carbon monoxide poisoning—headache, visual changes, confusion, irritability, decreased judgment, nausea, ataxia, and collapse (see Table 34-1).

3. Observe for upper body burn erythema or blistering of lips, buccal mucosa, or pharynx; singed nasal hair; soot in the oropharynx; and dark gray or black sputum (see Figure 34-4).
4. Listen for hoarseness and crackles. Increasing hoarseness, stridor, and drooling are indicators of increasing need for intubation.
5. Obtain ABGs, carboxyhemoglobin levels, and spirometry.
6. Direct visualization of the vocal cords may be necessary. Further visualization may be accomplished through bronchoscopy, if necessary.
7. A chest x-ray should be obtained as a baseline.

Extent of Body Surface Burned

1. Anatomic location—burns affecting hands, feet, face, and perineum require specialized care. Circumferential burns also require special attention, possibly escharotomy.
2. Determination is based on the use of tables for this purpose, such as the "rule of nines" (see Figure 34-5), the Lund and Browder chart (see page 1436), or the rule of the palm. The patient's palm (including the fingers) is approximately 1% of the TBSA burned. The Lund and Browder chart is the most accurate. Calculation of the percentage of TBSA burned serves as a guide for fluid therapy. Full fluid resuscitation is necessary for partial- or full-thickness burns of 20% TBSA or greater.
3. Repeat assessment may be performed on the 2nd or 3rd day to verify demarcation of burned areas.

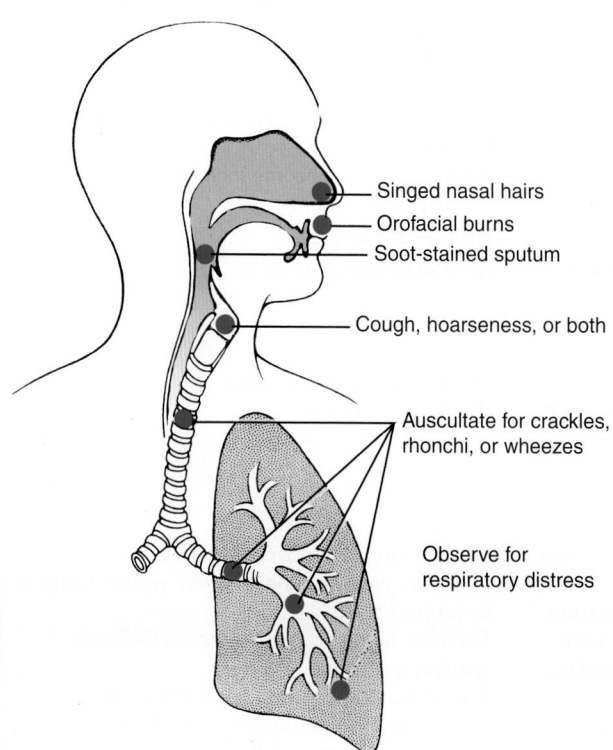

Figure 34-4. Respiratory system signs of inhalation injury.

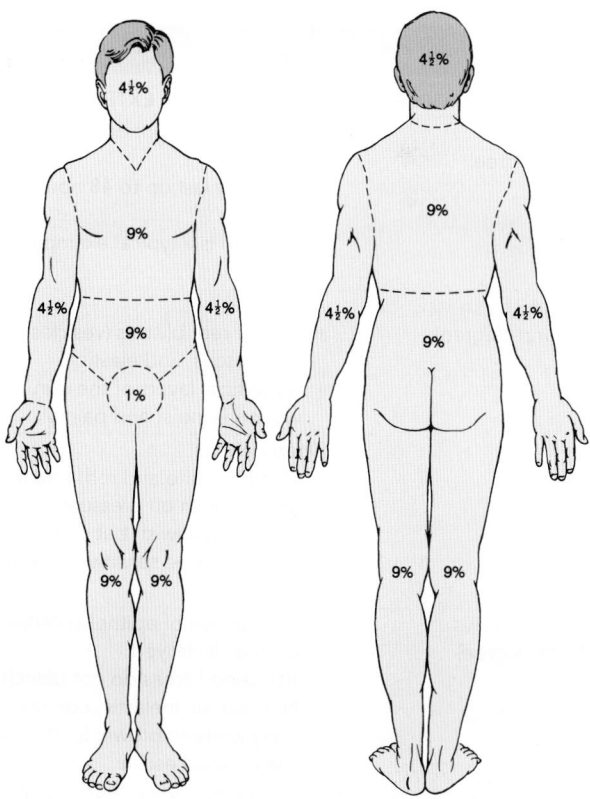

Figure 34-5. Rule of nines for calculating total burn surface area (TBSA).

Depth of Burn and Triage Criteria

1. It may be difficult to differentiate between second- and third-degree wounds initially.
   a. If the areas appear wet and pink and are particularly sensate, then a second-degree (partial-thickness) injury is likely. Blistering is another classic sign of a second-degree (partial-thickness) injury.
   b. If the area is dry, leathery, and firm to the touch, then it is most likely a third-degree (full-thickness) burn. Third-degree (full-thickness) burns can be a variety of colors such as white, mottled, or charred and may also have decreased sensation to light touch (see Table 34-2).
2. Reassess daily for the first few days because a partial-thickness burn can convert or progress to a full-thickness burn injury.
3. Deep partial-thickness burns of certain extent, full-thickness burns, chemical burns, electrical burns, burns of certain areas of the body, and any airway or inhalation injury should be transferred to a regional burn center (see Box 34-1).

MANAGEMENT

Management of the acute burn injury includes hemodynamic stabilization, metabolic support, wound debridement, use of topical antibacterial therapy, biologic dressings, and wound closure. Prevention and treatment of complications, including infection and pulmonary damage, and rehabilitation are also of major importance. The patient will also require physical and occupational therapy and psychiatric and nutritional support.

| BOX 34-1 | Burn Center Referral Criteria |

- Partial-thickness burns of greater than 10% TBSA.
- Involvement of the face, hands, feet, and genitalia.
- Third-degree burns.
- Electrical burns.
- Chemical burns.
- Inhalation injury.
- Preexisting medical conditions that could complicate management.
- Concomitant trauma where burn injury poses greatest risk.
- Burned children where facilities lack qualified staff and equipment.
- Patients who require special social, emotional, or rehabilitative intervention.

Hemodynamic Stabilization

IV Fluid Therapy

 EVIDENCE BASE American Burn Association. (2016). *Advanced Burn Life Support Provider Manual.* Chicago: Author.

1. The goal of fluid resuscitation is to maintain tissue perfusion and organ function. Careful and continuous fluid

---

| Table 34-2 | Assessment of Burn Injury |

EXTENT OR DEGREE	ASSESSMENT OF EXTENT	REPARATIVE PROCESS
Superficial (First-degree)	• Pink to red; slight edema, which subsides quickly. • Pain may last up to 48 hours; relieved by cooling. • Sunburn is a typical example.	• In about 5 days, epidermis peels and heals spontaneously. • Itching and pink skin persist for about 1 week. • No scarring. • If burn does not become infected, heals spontaneously within 10–14 days.
Partial-Thickness (Second-degree)	Superficial: • Pink or red; blisters (vesicles) form; weeping, edematous, and elastic. • Superficial layers of the skin are destroyed; wound is moist and painful.	• Heals in 2–3 weeks. • Little to no scarring.
	Deep dermal: • Mottled white and red; edematous reddened areas blanch on pressure. • May be yellowish but soft and elastic—may or may not be sensitive to touch; sensitive to cold air.	• Takes several weeks to heal. • Scarring may occur.
Full-Thickness (Third-degree)	• Destruction of epithelial cells—epidermis and dermis destroyed. • Reddened areas do not blanch with pressure. • Not painful; inelastic; coloration varies from waxy white to brown; leathery devitalized tissue is called eschar. • Destruction of epithelium, fat, muscles, and bone.	• Eschar must be removed. Granulation tissue forms to nearest epithelium from wound margins or support graft. • For areas larger than 1¼–2 inches (3–5 cm), grafting is required. • Expect scarring and loss of skin function. • Area requires debridement, formation of granulation tissue, and grafting.

management is critical to minimize complications associated with overresuscitation and underresuscitation.

a. Overzealous fluid resuscitation has been associated with acute coronary syndrome, compartment syndrome of the extremities, ARDS, airway obstruction, and pulmonary edema.

b. Underresuscitation may lead to inadequate organ and cellular perfusion, stress ulcer development, acute tubular necrosis, and conversion of deep partial-thickness burns to full-thickness burns.

2. The American Burn Association recommends fluid resuscitation for partial-thickness and full-thickness burns exceeding 20% TBSA.

a. Immediate intravenous (IV) fluid resuscitation is indicated for patients with electrical injury, older patients, or those with cardiac or pulmonary disease.

b. These patients require meticulous monitoring and may require a modification of fluid requirements.

3. Two large-bore peripheral IV catheters are established for fluid resuscitation and pain management, preferably through non-burned skin. If unable to obtain peripheral IV access, intraosseous or central line catheters may be used.

4. Generally, a crystalloid (Ringer lactate) solution is used for fluid resuscitation. One of several formulas may be used to determine the amount of fluid to be given in the first 48 hours.

a. Any formula that is utilized is only a guide and a starting point. Some patients will require more or less fluid depending on their response.

b. The consensus formula (formerly known as the Parkland formula) is most commonly used.

c. Some burn centers utilized albumin as a rescue therapy for patients requiring excessive amounts of fluids during resuscitation. Albumin may also be used postresuscitation on the 2nd day.

5. The consensus formula:

a. First 24 hours: 2 to 4 mL of Ringer lactate × weight in kg × % TBSA.

b. One-half amount of fluid is given in the first 8 hours, calculated from the time of injury. If the starting of fluids is delayed, then the same amount of fluid is given over the remaining time. Remember to deduct any fluids given in the prehospital setting.

c. The remaining half of the fluid is given over the next 16 hours.

d. Example:
Patient's weight: 70 kg; % TBSA: 80%.
4 mL × 70 kg × 80% TBSA = 22,400 mL of Ringer lactate.
First 8 hours: 11,200 mL or 1,400 mL/hour.
Second 16 hours: 11,200 mL or 700 mL/hour.

 NURSING ALERT Several regional burn centers have developed protocols for fluid resuscitation, such as the Michigan State Burn Coordinating Center, and a number of computer-driven algorithms have been developed, utilizing technology to more precisely guide fluid management.

Wound Care

Diligent wound care is essential to getting the burn wound healed as soon as possible. Treatment of the partial-thickness burn wounds includes daily or twice-daily wound cleansing with debridement or hydrotherapy (tubbing/showering) and dressing changes. Treatment of deep partial-thickness and full-thickness burns requires early surgical excision of eschar, skin grafting, and postoperative wound care.

Cleansing and Debridement

1. Burn wounds must be cleansed initially and usually daily with a mild antibacterial cleansing agent and saline solution or water.
a. May be done in the hydrotherapy tub, in the bathtub or shower, or at the bedside.
b. See "Hydrotherapy," below.

2. Nonviable tissue (eschar) may be removed through natural, enzymatic, mechanical, and/or surgical debridement.

3. Burn eschar will begin to separate from the underlying viable tissue by a natural process of bacterial growth, which causes a lysis of protein at the viable–nonviable tissue interface.

4. Loose eschar, dried blood, and exudate can be debrided at the time of wound cleansing.

Hydrotherapy Principles

1. Hydrotherapy ("tubbing," "tanking," or "showering") is bathing of the burn patient in a tub of water or with a water shower to facilitate cleansing and debridement of the burned area. Even ventilator-dependent patients can be safely bathed when a shower table is used.

2. Advantages
a. Topical medications, adherent dressings, and eschar are more easily removed.
b. Provides an opportunity for the patient to practice range-of-motion (ROM) exercises.
c. Total assessment of the burn area is facilitated; total body cleansing can be achieved.

3. Disadvantages
a. Loss of body heat; loss of sodium.
b. Uncomfortable and at times painful for the patient.
c. Maintenance of IV lines and ventilator care may be difficult during bathing and showering.

NURSING ALERT Adequately premedicating the patient with an opioid and anxiolytic allows the patient to participate in and tolerate the bathing and dressing change process.

Hydrotherapy Process

1. Describe the procedure to the patient who is experiencing hydrotherapy for the first time.

2. Select the time for future hydrotherapy sessions in collaboration with the patient; administer a pain control medication, as prescribed, before the treatment so that maximum benefit is realized. Use nursing activities to assist patient with the pain experience.

3. If the patient has an indwelling catheter, drain and plug it or maintain a closed system to avoid contamination.

4. Sterile technique is adhered to as closely as possible in preparing the patient for hydrotherapy, during hydrotherapy, and in redressing the patient's wounds after therapy.

5. During hydrotherapy, after cleansing of the wounds, debride wound, shave adjacent areas at health care provider's direction, shampoo hair, and gently wash normal skin.

6. Limit hydrotherapy to as brief a time as possible to decrease the loss of body temperature and subsequent chilling.

7. Never leave the patient unattended in the tub.
8. Respect the patient's feelings and expressions of stress, pain, cold, and fatigue.
9. After treatment, the patient may be weighed before being carefully dressed and returned to the unit.
10. Document significant data, including status of the wound.

Topical Antimicrobials

1. Topical medications are used to cover burn areas and to reduce the number of organisms. See Table 34-3. Identifying the most effective topical antimicrobial and dressing medium is an essential aspect in promoting wound closure.
2. Factors such as location of burn, burn depth, ease of application and removal, pain, frequency of dressing changes, and cost need to be considered.
3. They are applied directly to the burn area as ointments, creams, or solutions, or they may be incorporated in single-layer dressings that do not stick to the wound but permit drainage.
4. Dressings may take the form of commercial multilayered pads, standard 4 × 4-gauze pads, or several layers of stretch bandage (Kerlix type).
5. If gauze or pads are used, they may be held in place by stretch gauze or net tube dressings.
6. When wet dressings are used, that is, after a surgical procedure, then the same dressings are maintained. They are remoistened every 4 to 6 hours, as ordered. Heat loss may be prevented by limiting evaporative loss with a dry blanket and by warming the bed and room. When wet dressings are used, 20-ply gauze will help retain solution at the proper concentration if rewet every 4 hours. A dry top layer of stockinette or a cotton bath blanket prevents evaporative heat loss.
7. Desired characteristics in a topical antimicrobial:
   a. Demonstrates action against a broad spectrum of bacteria.
   b. Has the ability to diffuse through the wound and penetrate the eschar.
   c. Nontoxic and noninjurious to body tissue.
   d. Is inexpensive, is pleasant to use, is odorless or has pleasant odor; will not stain the skin or clothing.
   e. Will not cause resistant strains of pathogenic organisms to develop.
8. Generally, all of the previously applied topical cream should be removed and the wound gently cleansed before applying new cream with each dressing change. Extremity dressings should be wrapped distally to proximally, taking care to avoid circulatory compromise when edema occurs or dressing is too tight.
9. Some silver-based dressings can be left in place on second-degree (partial-thickness) wounds or donor sites for several days. Most require an outer wrap to secure the dressing in place and this can be changed as needed.
10. Identifying the best evidence on dressings for superficial and partial-thickness burn injuries has produced limited results. A Cochrane Database systematic review of 30 randomized controlled trials showed some evidence that biosynthetic dressings, silver-based dressings, and silicon nylon decrease healing time over silver sulfadiazine. However, methodological shortcomings of the individual studies limit usefulness of the review.

 EVIDENCE BASE Wasiak, J., Cleland, H., Campbell, F., et al. (2013). Dressings for superficial and partial thickness burns. *Cochrane Database of Systematic Reviews*, (4), CD0002106.

Surgical Management

Early excision and skin grafting are the goal to early wound closure for deep partial-thickness and full-thickness burn injuries. For types of burn wound coverings, see Table 34-4, page 928.

General Considerations

1. Early surgical intervention reduces the potential for wound infection and potentially reduces the length of stay.
2. Operative excision is very stressful metabolically and incurs heavy blood loss; therefore, more conservative measures may be indicated for some patients.
3. As a general consideration, up to 190 mL of blood may be lost per 1% of burn excised in the adult patient.
4. With tangential excision, a special blade is used to remove thin layers of damaged skin until live tissue is evidenced by capillary bleeding. It is commonly used with deep partial-thickness burns and full-thickness burns and followed with immediate coverage with a biosynthetic or biologic dressing or an autograft.
5. With fascial (primary) excision, the skin, lymphatics, and subcutaneous tissue are removed down to fascia, with either immediate autografting or temporary coverage with biologic or biosynthetic dressings. This is repeated until all deep burn areas are removed.

Biologic Dressings

1. Biologic dressings are used to temporarily cover large surfaces of the body. Usually, they are split-thickness grafts harvested either from human cadavers or from other mammalian donors such as pigs.
   a. An allograft is a graft of the skin taken from a person other than the burn patient and applied to a burn wound (most common type of biologic dressing). A cadaver is the most common source. Other sources may be live donors having a panniculectomy or other surgery.
   b. A xenograft or heterograft is a segment of the skin taken from an animal such as a pig.
2. Allograft can provide temporary wound closure for large surface area burns when there is not enough healthy skin available for autografting. They typically adhere for 2 to 3 weeks before sloughing off.
   a. Skin color is unimportant because it is only a temporary graft.
   b. Donor should be an adult, free from infection. All donated skin must be tested and free from contagious diseases before it can be used for donation.

Purpose and Benefits

1. Decreases heat, fluid, and protein losses.
2. Reduces bacterial proliferation.
3. Closes wound temporarily; enhances production and protection of granulation tissue.
4. Protects exposed neurovascular and muscle tissue as well as tendons.
5. Reduces pain and facilitates patient comfort.
6. Acts as a test graft to determine when granulating wounds will accept autograft successfully.
7. Provides an effective donor site dressing.

Clinical Procedures

1. Devitalized tissue is first removed surgically or enzymatically.
2. Allograft is applied directly (shiny side down) to the denuded area. Before applying, it may be dipped in saline solution. It may be trimmed to fit the wound.

Table 34-3	Topical Antimicrobial Agents for Burns		
TOPICAL AGENT	**DESCRIPTION AND INDICATIONS**	**DISADVANTAGES**	**NURSING CONSIDERATIONS**
Silver Sulfadiazine 1%			
	• White, crystalline, highly insoluble compound in an opaque, odorless, water-miscible cream. • Exerts antimicrobial effect against gram-negative and gram-positive bacteria and yeasts at level of cell membrane and cell wall. • Penetration of silver sulfadiazine into wound is intermediate between silver nitrate and mafenide. • Systemic toxicity is rare. • Most widely used agent and least common incidence of adverse effects.	• May cause transient leukopenia that disappears after 2–3 days of treatment. • May increase possibility of kernicterus; should not be used in pregnant women in the last trimester, premature neonates, or infants younger than age 2 months. • Impairment of hepatic and renal function that results in decreased excretion of drug constituents may preclude therapeutic benefits of continued silver sulfadiazine administration. • Exposure to sunlight produces gray discoloration. • Crystalluria and methemoglobinemia are rare toxic effects. • Protracted use may be associated with emergence of sulfadiazine resistance.	• Use with open treatment or with light or occlusive dressings. • Apply with sterile gloved hand directly to the wound or to gauze dressing 1/16 inch (0.2 cm) thick, once or twice per day after a thorough wound cleansing. • Silver sulfadiazine will be discontinued if white blood cell (WBC) count is <1,500 in an adult or <2,000 in a child; WBC count usually returns to normal in 2–4 days, after which application may be resumed.
Mafenide Acetate 10% cream or 5% solution	• Usually supplied in water-miscible, hydroscopic cream base. • Active against most gram-positive organisms, particularly *Clostridia* spp. • Active against common gram-negative burn wound pathogens but has little antifungal activity. • Not significantly bound by protein and wound exudate. • Good penetrating power and useful for control of established invasive burn wound infection.	• Painful during and for a short period following application. • A potent carbonic anhydrase inhibitor resulting in metabolic acidosis, therefore not used if total body surface area is >20%. • Brisk alkaline diuresis and inappropriate polyuria may result when used on patients with a large burn surface area. • Compensatory hyperventilation and pulmonary failure may ensue if mafenide is not discontinued. • Hemolytic anemia is a rare complication.	• Cream is applied without dressing, if possible and must be reapplied every 12 hours to maintain therapeutic effectiveness. • Therapeutic solution concentration is maintained with bulky wet dressings; rewet every 2–4 hours. • Application is associated with significant pain. • Hypersensitivity evidenced by maculopapular rash; is treated with antihistamines or by discontinuing use. • Requires careful monitoring of pulmonary status and acid–base and fluid balance.
Silver Nitrate (0.5% solution)	• Clear solution with low toxicity and significant antimicrobial effect against common burn wound pathogens. • Absorption is minimal because of the insolubility of its chloride and other salts. • Nonallergenic and not usually painful on application. • Best use is prophylaxis against infection.	• Can cause electrolyte abnormalities by depleting serum sodium, chloride, potassium, and magnesium. • Methemoglobinemia is a rare complication. • Stains everything (including normal skin) brown or black.	• Monitor electrolyte balance carefully; supplementation with sodium and potassium salts is routinely needed for patients with extensive burns. • Use bulky dressings; rewet every 2–4 hours to maintain therapeutic concentration. • Maintain patient warmth and minimize transcutaneous evaporative water loss with dry top layer, such as stockinette or bath blanket.
Silver Sheeting	• Silver impregnated on a neutral backing.	• Cannot be moistened until time of application. • Moisten with sterile water only; saline deactivates the silver. • Need to keep moist with sterile water every 8 hours.	• Dressing change required only every 4–7 days, reducing pain. • Can be used on an outpatient basis.
Mupirocin	• Ointment. • Active against methicillin-resistant *Staphylococcus aureus* (MRSA).	• Allergy is a major contraindication. • Prolonged use may result in super-infection. • Apply bid to tid.	• May be ordered based on culture or prophylactically.

Table 34-4   Burn Wound Coverings

COVERING AND DESCRIPTION	INDICATIONS	SOURCE OR FORM	NURSING CONSIDERATIONS
Allograft/Homograft • Human cadaver skin, about 0.015 inch thick • Preferred biologic dressing	• To debride untidy wounds. • To protect granulation tissue after escharotomy. • To cover excised wound immediately. • To serve as test graft before autograft.	Fresh, cryopreserved homografts available from tissue banks throughout the United States.	• Remember: Length of time dressing is left in place varies greatly. • Observe for exudate; also, watch for local and systemic signs of infection and rejection.
Xenograft Heterograft • Pigskin similar to human skin, harvested after slaughter, then cryopreserved, or lyophilized for long-term storage	• Same as for homograft. • To cover meshed autografts. • To protect exposed tendons. • To cover partial-thickness burns that are eschar-free and clean or only slightly contaminated.	Available in fresh, frozen, or lyophilized form, in rolls or sheets; also available meshed and impregnated with silver sulfadiazine.	• Change every 2–5 days; wound may be dressed or left open. • Observe for signs of infection.
Biobrane • Nylon fabric bonded to silicon rubber membrane, containing collagenous porcine peptides • Elastic and durable; adheres to wound surface until removed or sloughed by spontaneous re-epithelialization	• To cover donor graft sites. • To protect clean, superficial, partial-thickness burns and excised wounds awaiting autografts. • To cover meshed autografts.	Individually packaged sterile sheets of various sizes; also in glove-shaped form for hand burns.	• Useful for wounds awaiting autograft because it can be left in place 3–14 days and is permeable to antimicrobials, which can be applied over it.
DuoDERM • Hydroactive dressing that interacts with moisture on the skin, creating bond that makes it adhere • Interacts with wound exudate to produce soft, moist gel, facilitating removal	• To cover small partial-thickness burns. • To prevent bacterial contamination.	Individual, peelable, "blister" packages containing sheets of various sizes (from 3 × 3 inches to 8 × 12 inches).	• Use size that allows dressing to extend beyond wound onto healthy skin. • Be careful to distinguish pus from liquefied material that normally remains in the wound. • Used until it falls off, usually 7–10 days.
Integra Artificial Skin • Permanent bilayer membrane composed of a dermal portion consisting of a porous lattice of fibers of cross-linked bovine collagen and glycosaminoglycan composite and an epidermal layer of synthetic polysiloxane polymer	• To create a template for dermal regeneration by formation of a "neodermis." Provides an immediate postexcisional physiologic wound closure. Allows use of a thinner autograft.	Sterile individual sheets.	• Dermal regeneration layer is very soft and fragile. No hydrotherapy immersion should occur while the silicone layer is still in place. • Change outer dressing every 4–5 days. • Removal of the silicon layer is usually done in 14–21 days.
Acticoat • Temporary covering of a nanocrystalline film of pure ionic silver	• To provide a temporary layer with optimal antimicrobial protection. May be used for immediate wound coverage as well as for postgraft site coverage. May also be used as donor site coverage.	Sterile individual sheets.	• Must be moistened immediately before application. It must also be moistened with sterile water every 4–6 hours. Do not apply any topical antimicrobial over or onto the silver sheeting.
Aquacel AG	• To provide wound coverage for superficial to middepth partial-thickness wounds. It dries and remains on the wound until healed, at which time it will loosen and can be peeled from the wound.	Individual sterile rolls.	• Do not try to wet or remove before the wound has healed.

3. Grafts are usually secured with adhesive strips or with staples or sutures. The graft is covered with wet nonadherent gauze (antibiotic solution or saline) and covered with stretch gauze; this is again wet down with the appropriate solution.

4. The wound remains unchanged initially for 3 to 5 days, during which time it is wet down every 4 to 6 hours. Sheet grafts do not require the wet-down procedure.

5. After the initial takedown (typically known as the first postoperative dressing removal), dressings are changed daily.

6. If allograft or xenograft is used, the wound bed may be prepared for permanent autografting.

Biosynthetic Dressings

1. Temporary biosynthetic dressings help prevent bacterial contamination.

2. Used when permanent autograft is unavailable or unnecessary (as when partial-thickness wounds will heal spontaneously over time).

3. Biobrane (Woodruff Laboratories) consists of a custom-knit nylon fabric mechanically bonded to an ultrathin silicone rubber membrane, to which collagenous peptides of porcine skin are covalently bonded.
   a. Has a longer shelf life and lower cost than biologic dressings such as pigskin.
   b. Is widely used for coverage of shallow wounds awaiting epithelialization, excised wounds awaiting autografts, widely meshed autografts until closure of interstices, and donor sites awaiting healing.

Artificial Dermis

1. Method being studied in selected burn centers to improve survival of patients with massive burns and little donor skin available.

2. Composed of a porous collagen–chondroitin 6-sulfate fibrillar mat covered with a thin Silastic sheet.

3. Used with an epidermal graft to provide a permanent cover that is at least as satisfactory as other available grafting techniques.

4. Used with donor sites that are thinner and that heal faster; seems to result in less hypertrophic scarring than the usual grafting methods.

Wound Closure

1. Skin grafting is usually required or preferred with full-thickness burns greater than 1¼ to 2 inches (3 to 5 cm) in diameter or in deep partial-thickness wounds or in areas of function.

2. After gradual eschar removal and development of a base of granulating tissue or in the presence of viable tissue after excision, grafts of the patient's own skin (autografts) are applied.

3. Sheet grafts or meshed grafts, providing wider expansion from donor sites, may be used.

4. Blood flow is established by the 3rd or 4th day, and postgrafting, vascular continuity, and wound closure have been established by the 7th to 10th day.

5. Definitive wound closure in patients with extensive full-thickness injuries may require multiple operations over many weeks or even months. To hasten healing, cultured epithelial autografts (cultured skin) may be used for patients with large burns and little available donor skin.

   a. Biopsies of unburned skin are cultured in a specialized laboratory to yield confluent sheets of epithelial cells suitable for grafting in about 3 weeks.
   b. Available donor sites can be used for coverage of the most functional or posterior surfaces, and the more delicate cultured epithelial autografts can be used to cover other large areas.
   c. The sheets of epithelial cells are at higher risk of shearing because they lack a dermis and seem to be less resistant to infection. Some burn centers have improved graft take by using an allograft dermis underneath.
   d. Additional experience is needed to determine the long-term durability of cultured epithelial autografts, which may be lifesaving treatment for the severely burned.

6. Many partial-thickness burn wounds will heal spontaneously within a few weeks, provided they are protected from infection.

7. The donor site requires meticulous care and may be covered with a synthetic dressing, scarlet red, silver sheeting, or an antimicrobial cream such as silver sulfadiazine 1%.

Other Interventions

Pain Management

1. Pain relief should be considered in the primary assessment of all initial burn injuries. A burn injury is one of the most feared painful injuries; all burn injuries are painful.

2. All pain medication should be given via IV line. Pain medication that is given intramuscularly may not be metabolized properly through burned tissue. Acceptable IV pain medications are morphine, hydromorphone, and fentanyl.

3. Careful administration of opioids for pediatrics, older adults, and patients with higher pain tolerances to avoid respiratory suppression or overdose.

Nutrition Support

1. Initially, institute nothing-by-mouth (NPO) status until bowel sounds return (1 to 2 days). However, small amounts (5 to 10 mL/hour) of isotonic enteral tube feedings are typically started within 24 hours to help maintain a functioning GI tract. Small amounts of erythromycin may be used to encourage GI motility.

2. Reduce metabolic stress by allaying pain, fear, and anxiety and maintaining a warm environment.

3. Nutritional management must be aggressive to combat acute nutritional deficiency and weight loss; a positive nitrogen balance should be the goal throughout postburn care.

4. When bowel sounds return, administer oral fluids and advance diet, as tolerated.

5. Offer more solid food after 2 to 3 days postburn as tolerance to food improves.
   a. Build up daily caloric intake to match daily caloric expenditure.
   b. Provide 3-g protein/kg body weight: 20% of needed calories in the form of fats; remainder in carbohydrates.

6. Oral anabolic steroids (oxandrolone) have shown good results in helping to maintain lean muscle mass.

7. When caloric requirements cannot be met by enteral feedings, it may be necessary to initiate TPN (amino acids, carbohydrates, and fat emulsions).

8. Provide potassium and vitamin and mineral supplements (zinc, iron, and vitamin C).

Prevention and Treatment of Complications

Primary causes of morbidity and mortality in burn patients are those related to infection and pulmonary problems.

1. Topical antibacterial agents help to retard the proliferation of pathogenic organisms until wound closure occurs spontaneously or through surgical intervention.
2. Broad-spectrum antibiotics may be necessary to treat systemic gram-positive and gram-negative infections and sometimes fungal infection.
3. Critical diagnostic parameters include observing for signs of burn wound sepsis, obtaining quantitative and qualitative wound biopsy, checking for signs of systemic septicemia, and taking blood for cultures.
4. Meticulous pulmonary care is essential because pneumonia (especially if patient remains intubated) is common.
5. Severe inhalation injury, including ARDS, can contribute significantly to mortality, even though the burn wound size may be small.

Nursing Management of the Burn Patient

See Box 34-2.

Nursing Assessment

1. Obtain a thorough history, including:
   a. Causative agent—hot water, chemical, gasoline, flame, tar, radiation PUVA light, etc.
   b. Duration of exposure.
   c. Circumstances of injury, including whether in closed or open space, accidental or intentional, or self-inflicted.
   d. Initial treatment, including first aid, prefacility emergency care (including fluids, intubation, etc.), or care rendered in another facility (emergency department, etc.).
   e. Patient's age and preexisting medical problems, such as heart disease, human immunodeficiency virus, drug abuse, diabetes, ulcers, alcoholism, chronic obstructive pulmonary disease (COPD), epilepsy, psychosis, or hepatitis.
   f. Current medications—include both prescription and over the counter.
   g. Concomitant injuries (eg, from fall, explosions, assaults).
   h. Evidence of inhalation injury.
   i. Medication and food allergies and tetanus immunization status.
   j. Height and weight.
2. Perform ongoing assessment of hemodynamic and respiratory status, condition of wounds, and signs of infection.
3. Perform pain assessment using simple pain scale and observing for signs of pain.

Nursing Diagnoses

- Impaired Gas Exchange related to inhalation injury.
- Ineffective Breathing Pattern related to circumferential chest burn, upper airway obstruction, or ARDS.
- Decreased Cardiac Output related to fluid shifts and hypovolemic shock.
- Ineffective Tissue Perfusion: Peripheral related to edema and circumferential burns.

BOX 34-2   **Innovation in Patient Care**

Over a century ago, Parkland Hospital in Dallas, Texas, opened to fulfill a mission created by inherent goodwill. None envisioned the fledgling haven for medical treatment to the poor would become the institution it is today. Parkland is a renowned burn care facility and noted for a number of other firsts including the first high-risk maternity unit and the first pediatric trauma unit in the United States. In 1962, Parkland opened one of the largest civilian burn units in the United States and advanced burn care through the fluid resuscitation formula used in more than 80% of the burn units throughout the country.

The new Parkland hospital, opened in 2015, promotes excellence in clinical care, teaching, and research in a technologically advanced and easily accessible environment. The new hospital was designed and built in a thoughtful, deliberate manner using evidence-based healing concepts and involved nursing at every step. The entire hospital is designed with the patient in mind. The patient-centered approach creates a healing environment with single-patient rooms, windows, and natural light as well as more space for family and visitors. An onstage/offstage model provides comfort for patients as well as efficiency for staff. Vendors and staff utilize separate hallways and elevators from those of patients and visitors. The facility is adaptable to future needs.

- Risk for Imbalanced Fluid Volume related to fluid resuscitation and subsequent mobilization 3 to 5 days postburn.
- Impaired Skin Integrity related to burn injury and surgical interventions (donor sites).
- Impaired Urinary Elimination related to indwelling catheter.
- Ineffective Thermoregulation related to loss of skin microcirculatory regulation and hypothalamic response.
- Risk for Infection related to loss of skin barrier and altered immune response.
- Impaired Physical Mobility related to edema, pain, and skin and joint contractures.
- Imbalanced Nutrition: Less Than Body Requirements related to hypermetabolic response to burn injury.
- Risk for Bleeding related to stress response.
- Acute Pain related to burn injury.
- Ineffective Coping related to fear and anxiety.
- Disturbed Body Image related to cosmetic and functional sequelae of burn wound.
- Disturbed Sleep Pattern related to unfamiliar surroundings and pain.

Nursing Interventions

Achieving Adequate Oxygenation and Respiratory Function

1. Provide humidified 100% oxygen until carbon monoxide level is known. (*Caution:* Adjust oxygen flow rate for patient with COPD, as prescribed.) If the patient is stable, try to get the initial ABG on room air.
2. Assess for signs of hypoxemia (anxiousness, tachypnea, tachycardia) and differentiate this from pain.
3. Suspect respiratory injury if burn occurred in an enclosed space.
4. Observe for and report erythema or blistering of the buccal mucosa; singed nasal hairs; burns of lips, face, or neck; and increasing hoarseness.
5. Monitor respiratory rate, depth, rhythm, and cough.
6. Auscultate chest and note breath sounds.
7. Note character and amount of respiratory secretions; report carbonaceous sputum.
8. Observe for signs of inadequate ventilation and begin serial monitoring of ABG levels and oxygen saturation.
9. Provide mechanical ventilation, continuous positive airway pressure, or positive end-expiratory pressure, if requested.
10. Keep intubation equipment nearby and be alert for signs of respiratory obstruction.
11. In mild inhalation injury:
    a. Provide humidification of inspired air.
    b. Encourage coughing and deep breathing.
    c. Promote clearance of secretions through chest physical therapy (see page 187) or intrapulmonary percussive ventilation.
12. In moderate to severe inhalation injury:
    a. Initiate more frequent bronchial suctioning.
    b. Closely monitor vital signs, urine output, and ABG levels.
    c. Administer bronchodilator treatments, as ordered.
    d. For additional respiratory problems, it may be necessary to have patient intubated and placed on mechanical ventilation.

 NURSING ALERT Be prepared to assist with early intubation if inhalation injury is suspected. Progressive airway edema is expected in the first 24 hours following a patient with an inhalation injury.

Maintaining Adequate Tidal Volume and Unrestricted Chest Movement

1. Observe rate and quality of breathing; report if progressively more rapid and shallow.
2. Assess tidal volume; report decreasing volume to health care provider.
3. Encourage deep breathing and incentive spirometry (may use sigh control on ventilator, as needed).
4. Place patient in semi-Fowler position to permit maximal chest excursions if there are no contraindications, such as hypotension or trauma.
5. Make sure that chest dressings are not constricting.
6. Prepare the patient for escharotomy and assist, as indicated.

Supporting Cardiac Output

1. Position the patient to increase venous return.
2. Give fluids, as prescribed.
3. Monitor vital signs, including apical pulse, respirations, central venous pressure, pulmonary artery pressures, and urine output at least hourly.
4. Determine cardiac output, as requested.
5. Monitor sensorium.
6. Document all observations and particularly note trends in vital sign changes.

Promoting Peripheral Circulation

1. Remove all jewelry and clothing.
2. Elevate extremities.
3. Monitor peripheral pulses hourly; use Doppler, as necessary.
4. Prepare the patient for escharotomy if circulation is impaired.
5. Avoid tight, constrictive dressings.

Facilitating Fluid Balance

1. Titrate fluid intake, as tolerated. The initial resuscitation formula is only a base.
2. Maintain accurate intake and output records.
3. Weigh the patient daily.
4. Monitor results of serum potassium and other electrolytes.
5. Be alert to signs of fluid overload and heart failure, especially during initial fluid resuscitation and immediately afterward, when fluid mobilization is occurring.
6. Administer diuretics, as ordered.

 GERONTOLOGIC ALERT Older patients and those with impaired renal function, cardiovascular disease, and pulmonary disease are more likely to develop fluid overload. Proceed with caution.

Protecting and Reestablishing Skin Integrity

1. Cleanse wounds and change dressings one to two times per day. Use an antimicrobial solution or mild soap and water. Dry gently. This may be done in the hydrotherapy tank, bathtub, shower, or bedside.
2. Perform debridement of dead tissue at this time. May use gauze, scissors, or forceps as appropriate. Try to limit time to 20 to 30 minutes depending on the patient's tolerance. Additional analgesia may be necessary.
3. Apply topical bacteriostatic agents, as directed. Cream or ointment is applied 1/8 inch (3 mm) thick.
4. Dress wounds, as appropriate, using conventional burn pads, gauze rolls, or any combination. Dressings may be held in place, as necessary, with gauze rolls or netting.
5. For grafted areas, use extreme caution in removing dressings; observe for and report serous or sanguineous blebs or purulent drainage. Redress grafted areas according to facility protocol.
6. Observe all wounds daily and document wound status on the patient's record. Report any odor, drainage, cellulitis, bleeding, or signs of infection.
7. Promote healing of donor sites by:
    a. Preventing contamination of donor sites that are clean wounds.
    b. Opening to air for drying postoperatively if gauze or impregnated gauze dressing is used.
    c. Following health care provider's or manufacturer's instructions for care of sites dressed with synthetic materials.
    d. Allowing dressing to peel off spontaneously.
    e. Cleansing healing donor site with mild soap and water when dressings are removed; lubricating site twice daily and as needed.

Preventing Urinary Infection

1. Maintain closed urinary drainage system and ensure patency. Use a catheter impregnated with an antimicrobial agent whenever possible.
2. Frequently observe color, clarity, and amount of urine.
3. Empty drainage bag per facility protocol.
4. Provide catheter care per facility protocol.
5. Encourage removal of catheter and use of urinal, bed pan, or commode as soon as frequent urine output determinations are not required.

Promoting Stable Body Temperature

1. Be efficient in care; do not expose wounds unnecessarily.
2. Maintain warm ambient temperatures.
3. Use radiant warmers, warming blankets, or adjustment of the bed temperature to keep the patient warm.
4. Obtain urine, sputum, and blood cultures for temperatures above 102°F (38.9°C) rectal or core temperature or if chills are present.
5. Provide a dry top layer for wet dressings to reduce evaporative heat loss.
6. Warm wound cleansing and dressing solutions to body temperature.
7. Use blankets in transporting patient to other areas of the hospital.
8. Administer antipyretics, as prescribed.

Avoiding Wound and Systemic Infection

1. Wash hands with antibacterial cleansing agent before and after all patient contact.
2. Use barrier garments—isolation gown or plastic apron—for all care requiring contact with the patient or the patient's bed.
3. Cover hair and wear mask when wounds are exposed or when performing a sterile procedure.
4. Use sterile examination gloves for all dressing changes and all care involving patient contact.
5. Maintain proper concentration of topical antibacterial agents used in wound care.
6. Be alert for reservoirs of infection and sources of cross-contamination in equipment and assignment of personnel.
7. Check history of tetanus immunization and provide passive or active tetanus prophylaxis as prescribed.
8. Change IV tubing and central line catheters according to Centers for Disease Control and Prevention recommendations.
9. Administer antibiotics, as prescribed, and be alert for toxic effects and incompatibilities.
10. Assess wounds daily for local signs of infection—swelling and redness around wound edges, purulent drainage, discoloration, and loss of grafts.
11. Be alert for early signs of septicemia, including changes in mentation, tachypnea, and decreased peristalsis as well as later signs, such as increased pulse, decreased blood pressure (BP), increased or decreased urine output, facial flushing, increased and later decreased temperatures, increasing hyperglycemia, and malaise. Report to health care provider promptly.
12. Promote optimal personal hygiene for the patient, including daily cleansing of unburned areas, meticulous care of teeth and mouth, shampooing of hair every other day, shaving of hair in or near burned areas, and meticulous care of IV and urinary catheter sites.
13. Inspect the skin carefully for signs of pressure and breakdown.
14. Observe for and report signs of thrombophlebitis or catheter-induced infections.
15. Prevent atelectasis and pneumonia through chest physical therapy, postural drainage, meticulous pulmonary technique, and, if indicated, tracheostomy care.

 DRUG ALERT Although pseudomonas has been and continues to be a danger to the burn patient, hospital-acquired MRSA is now another serious threat. Staple antibiotics, such as vancomycin and gentamicin, are not effective. Now, linezolid, clindamycin, sulfamethoxazole–trimethoprim, and even mupirocin ointment are being used to combat MSRA—not only in the hospital setting, but in most burn clinics as well.

Promoting Mobility and Ability to Perform Activities of Daily Living (ADLs)

1. Ensure consultation with physical and occupational therapists, who will exercise the patient at least once or twice daily, as necessary.
2. Encourage the patient to be as active as possible and to perform active ROM exercises throughout the day.
3. Maintain splints in proper position as prescribed by occupational therapist; remove splints on regular schedule and observe for signs of skin irritation before reapplying.
4. Position the patient to decrease edema and avoid flexion of burned joints.
5. Coordinate pain management and other care to allow optimal effort during periods of physical exercise.
6. Initiate passive and active ROM and breathing exercises during early postburn period.
7. Plan with therapists for a conditioning regimen that gradually increases energy expenditure and tolerance for activity.
8. Act as advocate for the patient's need for rest by coordinating the patient's therapeutic and social activities and prioritizing interventions and visits.
9. Help the patient achieve adequate relaxation and sleep through medication and environmental measures.

Ensuring Adequate Nutrition

1. Weigh the patient daily with dressings removed.
2. Obtain consultation from dietitian for calculation of nutritional needs based on age, weight, height, and burn size. Two of the more popular formulas used to estimate nutritional needs are the Harris-Benedict and Curreri formulas.
3. Administer vitamins and mineral supplements, as prescribed. Deficiencies in zinc, copper, and selenium can occur after a burn.
4. Minimize metabolic stress by allaying fears, pain, and anxiety and by maintaining a warm environmental temperature.
5. Generally, for burns less than 10% TBSA, a well-balanced diet with emphasis on protein intake is necessary. For 10% to 20% TBSA, a high-protein, high-calorie diet is ordered. For 20% TBSA and greater, early enteral nutrition believed to decrease the metabolic response and improve outcomes. When the patient is ready for oral fluids, observe tolerance. If there are no problems, advance the diet, as tolerated.
6. Provide nasogastric (NG) tube feedings, as prescribed.
7. Administer IV hyperalimentation and fat emulsions prescribed with usual nursing precautions.
8. Keep record of caloric intake.
9. Encourage the patient to feed self.

10. Supplement meals with between-meal high-protein, high-calorie snacks, such as milkshakes or foods brought from home according to patient's preference.

Preventing Paralytic Ileus and Stress Ulcer

1. Keep on NPO status until bowel sounds resume.
2. Assess bowel sounds every 2 to 4 hours while acutely ill. (Decreased peristalsis may be an early sign of septicemia.)
3. Recent practice now encourages beginning tube feeds within 24 hours of the initial injury to help preserve the function of the gut and prevent paralytic ileus or stress ulcer.
4. Administer histamine-2 blockers and antacids, as prescribed. This will help prevent or diminish the occurrence of stress (Curling's) ulcers.
5. Heed complaints of nausea while intubated by checking for abdominal distention, tube placement, and residual aspirate.
6. Provide mouth care every 2 hours while intubated.

 EVIDENCE BASE Mandell, S. P., & Gibran, N. S. (2014). Early enteral nutrition for burn injury. *Advances in Wound Care, 3*(1), 64–70.

Reducing Pain

1. Assess for pain periodically; do not wait for complaints of pain to intervene. Common opioids used include morphine, fentanyl, hydromorphone, and propofol administered via IV line or by patient-controlled analgesia. Oral agents such as oxycodone, hydrocodone, and long-acting continuous-release agents are appropriate once the patient is tolerating PO food and fluids.
2. Determine previous experience with pain, the patient's response, and coping mechanisms.
3. Offer analgesics before wound care or before particularly painful treatments. Analgesia given orally should be administered 30 to 45 minutes before the procedure. Ketamine IV is now more commonly used than before. It is also becoming more popular to use conscious sedation for dressing changes.
4. Change the patient's position when possible, supporting extremities with pillows.
5. Reduce anxiety by such approaches as sensory-oriented explanations of procedures.
6. Teach relaxation techniques, such as imagery, breathing exercises, and progressive muscle relaxation, to help the patient cope with pain.
7. Allow the patient to make choices regarding care whenever possible, thus allowing some measure of input and control in care.
8. Greater emphasis is now focusing on pain management both from an inpatient and an outpatient perspective. Midrange analgesics are often used rather than just morphine. Medication dosages are being increased if patient is on a ventilator. It is not always possible to make a conscious patient completely pain-free, but increased comfort is the goal.

NURSING ALERT Check with your state board of nursing and facility policy to determine requirements for administering conscious sedation. Requirements may dictate that an anesthesiologist be in attendance or that the nurse be trained in intubation and airway management.

Enhancing Coping

1. Assess the patient's coping mechanisms from past history and current behavior.

2. Provide opportunities for the patient to express thoughts, feelings, fears, and anxieties regarding injury.
3. Explore with the patient alternative mechanisms for coping with the burn injury and its consequences.
4. Assure the patient of the normality of responses and the effect that time and healing will likely have on current concerns.
5. Interpret patient behavior to concerned family members and significant others.
6. Respect current coping mechanisms and discourage them only when an appropriate alternative can be provided.
7. Support family and friends' communications and visits if this is noted to help the patient.
8. Assess need for mental health consultation.
9. Offer antianxiety medications, as prescribed.

Preserving Positive Body Image

1. Gather data on the patient's preburn self-image and lifestyle.
2. When ready, encourage the patient to express concerns regarding changes in self-image or lifestyle that may result from burn injury.
3. Be honest, but positive, in responding to the patient and family.
4. Positively reinforce appropriate, effective coping mechanisms.
5. Arrange for the patient to see face (if burned) with appropriate supportive personnel before being placed/transferred to a room with access to a mirror.
6. Arrange for the patient to talk with other patients who have had a similar injury and are progressing satisfactorily.
7. Encourage participation in a burn survivor's group such as the Phoenix Society or other local support group.
8. Use and emphasize the concept of being a burn survivor. Survivors continue onward. Avoid the use of the term "burn victim" because it enhances the sick role.
9. Refer to psychological services, as needed. Consider other areas of the patient's traumatic experience that may require intervention as well.

Promoting Sleep

1. Assess patient's pain level at hour of sleep and administer pain medications, as needed.
2. Ensure comfort with room temperature and splints.
3. Administer sleep medications, as needed.
4. Schedule dressing changes accordingly to accommodate patient's sleep–wake cycle.

Community and Home Care Considerations

1. Demonstrate and explain wound care procedures to be continued after discharge:
   a. Wash hands.
   b. Clean small open wounds with mild soap in tub or shower.
   c. Rinse well with tap water.
   d. Pat dry with clean towel.
   e. Apply prescribed topical agent and dressing.
2. Assess for and teach patient to observe for local signs of wound infection:
   a. Increased redness of normal skin around burn area.
   b. Increased or purulent drainage.
   c. Increased pain and foul odor in burn area.
   d. Elevated body temperature.
3. Coordinate physical therapy consultation, and encourage patient to develop a schedule to incorporate exercise regimen as prescribed by physical therapist.
   a. Suggest scheduling exercises immediately after wound cleansing and application of topical agent because the skin may be more pliable and less sensitive to stretching then.

4. Instruct the patient in use and care of splints and pressure garments.
   a. Cleanse with mild soap and rinse well daily.
   b. Keep away from heat; dry garment by laying it flat on towels.
   c. Wear garment, as prescribed. This is usually 23 out of 24 hours/day. The garment is usually worn for 1 to 1½ years.
   d. Small open wounds should be covered with a light dressing under splints or pressure garments.
   e. Observe for signs of skin breakdown. Reassure the patient that small blister formation is normal and generally lessens after the first year.
   f. Wear/bring splints and pressure garments to follow-up visits to be checked for proper fit.

 TRANSITIONAL CARE ALERT Ensure the patient or family member is able to demonstrate how they will perform a dressing change from start to finish prior to going home. Confidence with wound care upon discharge may decrease the risk of the patient returning with an infection because of fear of changing the dressings on their own.

Patient Education and Health Maintenance

Health education is closely related to rehabilitation as the burn patient prepares to return to a productive place in society. Functional and cosmetic reconstruction is accomplished and the patient attempts to integrate a new self-concept into social realities. Broadly viewed, health education focuses on biologic, psychological, and social parameters.

1. Assist the patient in transition from dependence on the health team to independence by assisting the patient to communicate needs and functional abilities to others.
2. Guide the patient in thinking positively about self. Promote ability to redirect others' attention from the scarred body to the self within.
3. Instruct the patient in measures to lubricate and enhance comfort of healing skin:
   a. After cleaning, use moisturizers such as cocoa butter or other nonperfumed hand lotion at least twice per day or more frequently, as needed.
   b. Wear clean white underwear and clothing free from irritating dyes until wounds are well healed.
   c. Take antipruritics, as prescribed.
   d. Stay in a cool environment if itching occurs.
   e. Protect the skin from further trauma; use a sunscreen with a sun protection factor of 24 or higher.
   f. Discuss summer precautions, which should include a hat with a full, wide brim if there were facial or neck burns. Also, limit exposure to sun because the affected areas will sunburn more easily and tan more deeply.
   g. Advise the patient that if wearing a pressure vest with or without sleeves, or tights, the Occupational Safety and Health Administration standards for work in a hot environment should be used. The patient should also be aware of the need for oral fluid replacement.
4. Review with the patient and family common emotional responses during convalescence (depression, withdrawal, grieving, dreaming, anxiety, guilt, excessive sensitivity, emotional lability, insomnia, and fear of future), and discuss usual temporary nature of these as well as effective coping mechanisms.
   a. There may be some psychological sequelae that will require long-term intervention, such as image adjustment disorders or posttraumatic stress issues. If not already in place, psychological referral is appropriate as an outpatient.
   b. Make sure that the patient has a phone number or referral to the counselor to make follow-up appointments, if desired.
5. Make sure that information has been given about follow-up evaluations and home health care services, as needed, in the interim.
6. Offer to connect the patient with a peer support program for burn survivors if available.
7. For additional information and support, contact agencies such as the American Burn Association (*www.ameriburn.org*) or the Phoenix Society for Burn Survivors (*www.phoenix-society.org*). The Phoenix Society is a national foundation with local chapters whose primary function is support of other burn survivors. It has a toll-free number that burn survivors may use: (800) 888-BURN (2876).

Evaluation: Expected Outcomes

- Carboxyhemoglobin level below 10%, ABG levels within normal limits, and respiratory rate 12 to 28 breaths/minute.
- Tidal volume within normal limits.
- Pulse 110 to 120 mm Hg or below and BP stable.
- Peripheral pulses strong.
- Weight stable, no edema, and lungs clear.
- Wounds clean and granulating.
- Catheter patent, urine clear, and quantity sufficient.
- Temperature normal to low-grade fever; no chills.
- No signs of infection.
- Normal ROM achieved and performing ADLs independently.
- Less than 5% weight loss from baseline.
- No gastric distention and aspirate and stool Hemoccult negative.
- Reports minimal pain after analgesic administration.
- Uses appropriate coping mechanisms.
- Verbalizes fears and concerns after viewing self in mirror.
- Sleeping 2- to 4-hour intervals; falls back to sleep easily.

SELECTED REFERENCES

Abboud, E. C., Legare, T. B., Settle, J. C., Boubekri, A. M., Barillo, D. J., & Marcet, J. E. (2014). Do silver-based wound dressings reduce pain? A prospective study and review of the literature. *Burns, 40*(Suppl 1), S40–S47. doi:10.1016/j.burns.2014.09.012.

Abdullahi, A., & Jeschke, M. G. (2014). Nutrition and anabolic pharmacotherapies in the care of burn patients. *Nutrition in Clinical Practice, 29*(5), 621–630. doi:10.1177/0884533614533129.

American Burn Association. (2016). *Advanced burn life support provider manual.* Chicago, IL: Author.

American Burn Association. (2016). *Resources: Burn incidence and treatment in the United States fact sheet.* Chicago, IL: Author. Available: *www.ameriburn.org/resources_factsheet.php*

American Burn Association. (2016). *2016 National burn repository report of data from 2006–2015.* Chicago, IL: Author.

Cancio, L. C. (2014). Initial assessment and fluid resuscitation of burn patients. *The Surgical Clinics of North America, 94*(4), 741–754.

Ching, J. A., Ching, Y. H., Shivers, S. C., et al. (2016). An analysis of inhalation injury diagnostic methods and patient outcomes. *Journal of Burn Care & Research*, *37*(1), e27–e32.

Culleiton, A. L., & Simko, L. M. (2013). Caring for patients with burn injuries. *Nursing*, *43*(8), 26–34.

Greenlaugh, D. G. (2016). *Burn care for general surgeons and general practitioners.* New York, NY: Springer.

Grieve, B., Shapiro, G. D., Wibbenmeyer, L., et al. (2017). Long-term social reintegration outcomes for burn survivors with and without peer support attendance: A Life Impact Burn Recovery Evaluation (LIBRE) Study. *Archives of physical medicine and rehabilitation.* 2017 Oct 31. pii: S0003-9993(17)31328-X. [Epub ahead of print]

Herndon, D. N. (2018). *Total Burn Care*, 5th Edition. New York: Elsevier.

Jacobson, K., Fletchall, S., Dodd, H., & Starnes, C. (2017). Current concepts burn rehabilitation, part I: care during hospitalization. *Clinics in Plastic Surgery*, *44*(4), 703–712.

Jeschke, M. G., Pinto, R., Costford, S. R., & Amini-Nik, S. (2016). Threshold age and burn size associated with poor outcomes in the elderly after burn injury. *Burns*, *42*(2), 276–281.

Kanchan, T., Geriani, D., & Savithry, K. S. B. (2015). Curling's ulcer: Have these stress ulcers gone extinct? *Burns*, *41*(1), 198–199.

Liu, H. F., Zhang, F., & Lineaweaver, W. C. (2017). History and advancement of burn treatments. *Annals of Plastic surgery*, *78*(2), S2–S8.

Mandell, S. P., & Gibran, N. S. (2014). Early enteral nutrition for burn injury. *Advances in Wound Care*, *3*(1), 64–70.

Nielson, C. B., Duethman, N. C., Howard, J. M., et al. (2017). Burns: Pathophysiology of systemic complications and current management. *Journal of Burn Care & Research*, *38*(1), e469–e481.

Rowan, M. P., Cancio, L. C., Elster, E. A., et al. (2015). Burn wound healing and treatment: Review and advancements. *Critical Care*, *19*(1), 243.

Veeravagu, A., Yoon, B. C., Jiang, B., et al. (2015). National trends in burn and inhalation injury in burn patients: Results of analysis of the nationwide inpatient sample database. *Journal of Burn Care & Research*, *36*(2), 258–265.

Wasiak, J., Cleland, H., Campbell, F., & Spinks, A. (2013). Dressings for superficial and partial thickness burns. *The Cochrane Database of Systematic Reviews*, (3), CD002106.

Wiechman, S. A., McMullen, K., Carrougher, G. J., et al. (2017). Reasons for distress among burn survivors at 6, 12 and 24 months post-discharge: A Burn Injury Model System investigation. *Archives of Physical Medicine and Rehabilitation.* 2017, Dec 16. pii: S0003-9993(17)31402-8. [Epub ahead of print]

35

Emergent Conditions

OVERVIEW AND ASSESSMENT

Emergency medicine is the care, diagnosis, and treatment of unforeseen illness or injury. It is provided to patients with conditions ranging from minor to serious or life-threatening. The philosophy of emergency care includes the concept that an emergency is whatever the patient or family considers it to be. Emergency nursing is a dynamic and evolving practice that deals with unstable, undiagnosed patients usually presenting unexpectedly. See Standards of Care Guidelines 35-1, page 937.

Emergency Assessment

When first making contact with an emergency patient, it is essential that a systematic approach is used to ensure all factors are identified. The primary and secondary surveys provide the emergency nurse with a methodical approach to help identify and prioritize patient needs.

Primary Survey

The initial, rapid ABCD (**a**irway, **b**reathing, **c**irculation, and neurologic **d**isability) assessment of the patient is meant to identify life-threatening problems. If conditions are identified that present an immediate threat to life, you must stop and take corrective action prior to moving on to the next steps.

ABCD–AVPU

1. **A**—Airway: Does the patient have an open airway? Is the patient able to speak, swallow, or cry? Check for airway obstructions such as loose teeth, foreign objects, bleeding, vomitus, or other secretions. Immediately treat anything that compromises the airway. Never do a blind finger sweep of an airway.

2. **B**—Breathing: Is the patient breathing adequately? Assess for equal rise and fall of the chest (check for bilateral breath sounds), respiratory rate and pattern, skin color, use of accessory muscles, adventitious breath sounds, integrity of the chest wall, and position of the trachea. All major trauma patients require supplemental oxygen via a nonrebreather mask at 12 to 15 L/minute. Dress any penetrating chest injuries with occlusive dressings.

3. **C**—Circulation: Is circulation adequate? Can you palpate central and peripheral pulses? What are the quality of the pulses (strong, weak, slow, rapid)? Is the skin warm and dry? Is the skin color normal? What is the capillary refill? Obtain a blood pressure (BP; in both arms if chest trauma or dissecting aortic aneurysm is suspected). Is there any major bleeding?

STANDARDS OF CARE GUIDELINES 35-1
Emergency Assessment and Intervention

When a patient presents with a potentially life-threatening condition, proceed swiftly with the following:

- Call for help.
- Ensure the area is safe for you to enter, with no live electric current, hazardous materials, dangerous persons, or other threats.
- Remove the patient from potential source of danger, such as live electric current, water, or fire. If hazardous materials are present, consult protocols from the Occupational Safety and Health Association (OSHA) for decontamination procedures.
- Determine whether patient is conscious.
- Assess for adequate airway, breathing, and circulation in systematic manner. If any of these are absent, or inadequate, begin basic life support.
- Assess pupillary reaction and level of responsiveness to voice or touch, as indicated.
- If the patient is unconscious or has sustained a significant head injury, assume there is a spinal cord injury and maintain C-spine stabilization.
- Remove clothing to assess for wounds and skin lesions as indicated. Control any hemorrhage, as needed.
- When help arrives, assist with further assessment and transport, as needed.

This information should serve as a general guideline only. Each patient situation presents a unique set of clinical factors and requires nursing judgment to guide care, which may include additional or alternative measures and approaches.

4. **D**—Disability: Assess level of consciousness and pupils (a more thorough neurologic survey will be completed in the secondary survey). Assess level of consciousness using the AVPU scale:
   a. **A**—Is the patient alert? Are they looking at you and responding?
   b. **V**—Does the patient respond to voice? Do they open their eyes or respond when you call them?
   c. **P**—Does the patient respond to painful stimulus? Do they respond to sternal rub or nail bed pressure?
   d. **U**—The patient is unresponsive even to painful stimulus.

Secondary Assessment

The secondary assessment is a brief, but thorough, systematic assessment designed to identify all injuries. The steps include *Expose/environmental* control, *Full* set of vital signs, *Five* interventions, *Facilitate* family presence, and *Give* comfort measures. If your emergency department (ED) has enough staff, these interventions may be assigned to multiple staff members and performed simultaneously.

1. Expose/environmental control: It is necessary to remove all of the patient's clothing to identify all injuries. You must then prevent heat loss by using warm blankets, overhead warmers, and warmed intravenous (IV) fluids unless induced hypothermia is indicated. If your facility has a dedicated trauma or resuscitation room, keep the ambient temperature elevated to prevent heat loss.

2. Full set of vital signs:
   a. Obtain a full set of vital signs including BP, heart rate, respiratory rate, temperature, and oxygen saturation.
   b. As stated previously, obtain BP in both arms if chest trauma or dissecting aortic aneurysm is suspected.
   c. Institute continuous cardiac monitoring.
   d. Assess Glasgow Coma Scale (GCS) (see page 354) and pain scores.

3. Five potential interventions:
   a. Vascular access with two large-bore IV catheters, if possible.
   b. Pulse oximetry to measure the oxygen saturation; consider capnography to measure end-tidal carbon dioxide ($EtCO_2$), noninvasive ultrasonic cardiac output monitor, and 12-lead electrocardiogram (ECG).
   c. Indwelling urinary catheter (do not insert if you note blood at the meatus, blood in the scrotum, or if you suspect a pelvic fracture).
   d. Gastric tube (if there is evidence of facial fractures, insert the tube orally rather than nasally).
   e. Laboratory studies may include type and cross-matching, complete blood count (CBC), urine drug screen, blood alcohol, electrolytes, prothrombin time and partial thromboplastin time, arterial blood gas (ABG), venous blood gases (VBG), lactate, lipase, amylase, and pregnancy test, if applicable.

4. Facilitate family presence: Family presence is important during unexpected, potentially life-threatening events. They often have information that is critical in formulating the correct treatment plan. It is important to assess and respect the family's needs and wishes. Resuscitation rooms are often loud and appear chaotic. Assigning a staff member to any family wishing to be present can do much to alleviate their anxiety and assure them that everything is being done to help their loved one. If a family member does not wish to be present, providing them with a quiet area to wait and assigning a staff member as a contact person or liaison can be helpful.

5. Give comfort measures including pain management and verbal reassurance: Do not forget to give comfort measures to the family as well as the patient during the resuscitation process.

History

1. Obtain prehospital information from emergency personnel, patient, family, or bystanders using the mnemonic MIVT.
   M—Mechanism of injury: It is helpful to understand the mechanism of injury to anticipate probable injuries. It is particularly helpful in motor vehicle accidents to know such information as external and internal damage to the car (or at least if the car was drivable after the accident), if the patient was ejected, if they were wearing a seat belt, if airbags were deployed, and the period of time elapsed before the patient received medical attention.
   I—Injuries sustained or suspected: Ask prehospital personnel to list any injuries that they have identified. Most prehospital providers will have completed a rapid trauma survey, including looking for DCAP/BTLS (deformities, contusions, abrasions, punctures/burns, tenderness, lacerations, and swelling).
   V—Vital signs: What were the prehospital vital signs?
   T—Treatment: What treatment did the patient receive before arriving at the hospital and what was the patient's response to those interventions?

2. If the patient is conscious, it is essential to ask what happened. How did the accident occur? Why did it happen? A fall, for example, may not be a simple fall—perhaps, the patient blacked out and then fell. If the patient is conscious and time permits, explore the chief complaint through the OPQRST mnemonic.

   O—Onset: When did they first notice symptoms? Was today the first time? Has it been ongoing? Is it getting progressively worse?

   P—Provokes, Palliates, and Precipitates: What makes the symptoms better or worse?

   Q—Quality: How would they describe the discomfort? Burning, throbbing, aching, and like an electric shock are all commonly used to describe the quality of pain.

   R—Region and Radiates: Can the patient point to the pain with one finger? Does it move or shoot anywhere?

   S—Severity and Associated Symptoms: How do they rate their symptom? Is it accompanied by anything else such as numbness, tingling, or nausea?

   T—Timing: Have the symptoms been constant or do they come and go? How often?

3. Obtain past medical history from the patient or a family member or friend; it may be helpful to utilize the mnemonic SAMPLE to assist in organizing history information:

   S—Signs and symptoms, including chief complaint and OPQRST.

   A—Allergies to foods and medications.

   M—Medications, including herbal supplements and over-the-counters.

   P—Past medical and surgical history.

   L—Last oral intake.

   E—Events leading up to the incident.

4. Plus any history of alcohol or illicit drug use.

 NURSING ALERT To obtain a good descriptive history, use open-ended questioning.

Head-to-Toe Assessment

The head-to-toe assessment begins with assessment of the patient's general appearance, including body position or any guarding or posturing. Work from the head down, systematically assessing the patient one body area at a time.

1. Head and face.
   a. Inspect for any lacerations, abrasions, contusions, avulsions, puncture wounds, impaled objects, ecchymosis, or edema. The hair can hide injuries, so take time to do a complete inspection. Scalp lacerations also tend to bleed profusely, further obscuring the area from quick inspections.
   b. Gently palpate for crepitus, crackling, or bony deformities.
   c. Inspect ears and nares for any bleeding or drainage; if present, check for halo sign.

2. Neck (ensure proper C-spine stabilization is maintained).
   a. Inspect for any punctures, lacerations, contusions, swelling, tracheal deviation, JVD, or subcutaneous emphysema.
   b. Check for stomas or MedicAlert tags.
   c. Gently palpate for midline cervical tenderness.

3. Chest.
   a. Inspect for breathing effectiveness, paradoxical (uneven) chest wall movement, and disruptions in chest wall integrity (lacerations, punctures, subcutaneous emphysema).

   b. Auscultate for bilateral breath sounds and adventitious breath sounds.
   c. Auscultate heart tones (muffled).
   d. Gently palpate for bony crepitus or deformities.

4. Abdomen/flanks.
   a. Inspect for lacerations, abrasions, contusions, avulsions, puncture wounds, impaled objects, ecchymosis, edema, scars, eviscerations, or distention.
   b. Auscultate for the presence of bowel sounds.
   c. Gently palpate for rigidity, guarding, masses, or areas of tenderness.

5. Pelvis/perineum.
   a. Inspect for lacerations, abrasions, contusions, avulsions, puncture wounds, impaled objects, ecchymosis, edema, or scars. Look for blood at the urinary meatus and vagina in females. Look for priapism in males (which could indicate spinal cord injury).
   b. Gently palpate for pelvic instability or tenderness (do not rock the pelvis).

6. Neurologic/spinal (maintaining proper stabilization).
   a. Reassess mental status.
   b. Gently palpate for midline bony spinal tenderness.
   c. Check for paresthesias and determine sensory level.
   d. Check motor function and sphincter tone.

7. Extremities.
   a. Inspect skin color and temperature. Look for signs of injury and bleeding. Does the patient have movement in all four extremities? Touch the patient on a distal extremity and ask them to identify the part you are touching.
   b. Gently palpate peripheral pulses, any bony crepitus, or areas of tenderness.
   c. Check capillary refill.
   d. Gently palpate extremities for compartment firmness or signs of compartment syndrome.

 NURSING ALERT Any penetrating chest wound has the potential to rapidly cause a life-threatening tension pneumothorax and must be treated immediately.

 NURSING ALERT Pregnant trauma patients present a unique set of challenges. While performing assessments and interventions, a towel or roll should be placed under the right side of the backboard, tipping the patient slightly to the left and preventing fetal compression of the inferior vena cava and decreased blood return to the heart.

Focused Assessment

Any injuries that were identified during the primary and secondary surveys require a detailed assessment, which will typically include a team approach and radiographic studies.

Emergency Triage

Triage is a French verb meaning "to sort." Emergency triage is a subspecialty of emergency nursing, which requires specific, comprehensive educational preparation. The goal of an efficient triage system is to rapidly connect a patient with the proper level of care and the correct resources in the shortest amount of time. Upon entering an ED, patients are greeted by a triage nurse, who will perform a rapid assessment, to include a general impression, chief complaint, immediate or potential life threats, and pertinent history, and then make a decision about the patient's acuity and the resources needed. These decisions can often be difficult if the patient has an altered mental status, is intoxicated, or is otherwise impaired. Thus, the primary role of the triage nurse is to make acuity and disposition decisions and set priorities while maintaining awareness for potentially violent or communicable disease situations. Secondary triage decisions involve the initiation of triage-extended practices, such as the ordering of standardized labs or radiology studies. With the waiting times in EDs because of overcrowding becoming an increasing problem, the accuracy of the triage nurse in assigning acuity level is of critical importance. With extended wait times, triage is an ongoing process, with the triage nurse frequently reevaluating those who are waiting for changes in condition and updating their status, as needed.

Priorities of Care and Triage Categories

Standardized 5-level triage systems, such as the Australasian Triage Scale, the Canadian Triage and Acuity Scale, and the Emergency Severity Index, have been developed and proven through research to possess utility, validity, reliability, and safety. All three systems utilize similar time frames and are evidence based (the Manchester Triage System is a consensus-based algorithm approach, which utilizes longer time frames).

Triage Level 1: Immediately Life-Threatening or Resuscitation

1. Conditions requiring immediate clinician assessment. Any delay in treatment is potentially life- or limb-threatening. These are the patients that are in active danger of dying if there is no immediate intervention.
2. Includes conditions such as:
   a. Airway or severe respiratory compromise.
   b. Cardiac arrest.
   c. Severe shock.
   d. Symptomatic cervical spine injury.
   e. Multisystem trauma.
   f. Altered level of consciousness (LOC) (GCS less than 10).
   g. Eclampsia.
   h. Acute mental status changes or unresponsiveness.

Triage Level 2: Imminently Life-Threatening or Emergent

1. These are conditions that are not in immediate danger, but have the potential to deteriorate rapidly if not treated.
2. Conditions include:
   a. Head injuries.
   b. Trauma.
   c. Conscious overdose.
   d. Severe allergic reaction without airway compromise.
   e. Chemical exposure to the eyes.
   f. Chest pain without hemodynamic instability.
   g. Back pain.
   h. GI bleed with unstable vital signs.
   i. Stroke with deficit.
   j. Severe asthma without airway compromise.
   k. Abdominal pain in patients older than age 50.
   l. Vomiting and diarrhea with dehydration.
   m. Fever in infants younger than age 3 months.
   n. Acute psychotic episode.
   o. Severe headache.

p. Any pain greater than 7 on a scale of 1 to 10.
q. Any sexual assault.
r. Any neonate age 7 days or younger.

Triage Level 3: Potentially Life-Threatening/Time Critical or Urgent

1. Conditions requiring urgent care-level activities with stable vital signs, but have the potential to deteriorate and utilize multiple resources.
2. Conditions include:
   a. Alert head injury with vomiting.
   b. Mild to moderate asthma.
   c. Moderate trauma.
   d. Abuse or neglect.
   e. GI bleed with stable vital signs.
   f. History of seizure and alert on arrival.

Triage Level 4: Potentially Life-Serious/Situational Urgency or Semiurgent

1. Stable conditions that use few resources.
2. Conditions include:
   a. Alert head injury without vomiting.
   b. Minor trauma.
   c. Vomiting and diarrhea in patient older than age 2 without evidence of dehydration.
   d. Earache.
   e. Minor allergic reaction.
   f. Corneal foreign body.
   g. Chronic back pain.

Triage Level 5: Less/Nonurgent

1. Stable conditions that utilize little to no resources.
2. Conditions include:
   a. Minor trauma, such as minor cuts, abrasions, bruises, etc.
   b. Minor symptoms such as rhinorrhea, sneezing, conjunctivitis, etc.

 NURSING ALERT When working with pediatric patients in a triage setting, it is important to remember that they can deteriorate rapidly. Pediatric patients should be triaged by those experienced in identifying the subtle clues that often precede this rapid deterioration.

Psychological Considerations

Serious illness or trauma is an insult to physiologic and psychological homeostasis; it requires physiologic and psychological healing. Both patients and families experience high levels of anxiety when being treated in the emergency department. It is important for the emergency nurse to recognize, understand, and alleviate these anxieties whenever possible.

Approach to the Patient

1. Understand and accept the basic anxieties of the acutely ill or traumatized patient. Be aware of the patient's fear of death, disablement, and isolation.
   a. Personalize the situation as much as possible. Speak, react, and respond in a warm manner; give reassurance.
   b. Give explanations on a level that the patient can grasp. An informed patient can cope with psychological/physiologic stress in a more positive manner.
   c. Accept the rights of the patient and family to have and display their own feelings.

d. Maintain a calm and reassuring manner—helps the emotionally distressed patient or family to mobilize their psychological resources.

e. Include the patient's family or significant others if the patient wishes.

f. Encourage the patient or family to reach out to their support system. Often friends, other family members, or clergy can be of great comfort.

2. Understand and support the patient's feelings concerning loss of control (emotional, physical, and intellectual). Whenever possible, give the patient options and choices. This can help alleviate some of their feelings of helplessness.

3. Speak to the unconscious patient. Touch, call by name, and explain every procedure that is done. Avoid making negative comments about the patient's condition.

a. Orient the patient to person, time, and place as soon as he or she is conscious; reinforce by repeating this information.

b. Bring the patient back to reality in a calm and reassuring way.

c. Encourage the family, when possible, to touch the patient and aid in orienting the patient to reality.

4. Be prepared to handle all aspects of acute illness and trauma; know what to expect and what to do. When in doubt, stop, take a deep breath, and refocus. This will help alleviate the nurse's anxiety and increase the patient's confidence.

Approach to the Family

1. Inform the family where the patient is and give as much information as possible about the treatment he or she is receiving.

2. Consider allowing a family member to be present during the resuscitation. Assign a staff person to the family member to explain procedures and offer comfort.

3. Recognize the anxiety of the family and allow them to talk about their feelings. Acknowledge expressions of remorse, anger, guilt, and criticism.

4. Allow the family to relive the events, actions, and feelings preceding admission to the ED.

5. Deal with reality as gently and quickly as possible; avoid encouraging and supporting denial.

6. Assist the family to cope with sudden and unexpected death. Some helpful measures include the following:

a. Take the family to a private place.

b. Talk to all of the family together so they can mourn together.

c. Assure the family that everything possible was done; inform them of the treatment rendered.

d. Avoid using euphemisms such as "passed on." Show the family that you care by touching, offering coffee.

e. Allow family to talk about the deceased—permits ventilation of feelings of loss. Encourage family to talk about events preceding admission to the ED.

f. Encourage family to support each other and to express emotions freely—grief, loss, anger, helplessness, tears, and disbelief.

g. Avoid volunteering unnecessary information (eg, patient was drinking).

h. Avoid giving sedation to family members—may mask or delay the grieving process, which is necessary to achieve emotional equilibrium and prevent prolonged depression.

i. Be cognizant of cultural and religious beliefs and needs.

j. Encourage family members to view the body if they wish—to do so helps to integrate the loss (cover mutilated areas).

   i. Prepare the family for visual images and explain any legal requirements.

   ii. Go with family to see the body.

   iii. Show acceptance of the body by touching to give family permission to touch and talk to the body.

   iv. Spend a few minutes with the family, listening to them.

   v. Allow the family some private time with the body, if appropriate.

7. Encourage the ED staff to discuss among themselves their reaction to the event to share intense feelings for review and for group support. Organize a formal debriefing session for staff if warranted by circumstances of the event.

Pain Management

Pain is an unpleasant sensory and emotional experience associated with actual or potential tissue damage and is also associated with significant morbidity. Pain inhibits immune function and has detrimental effects on cardiovascular, respiratory, GI, and other body systems. Over 60% of patients report pain on arrival at ED, making pain the most common patient complaint. It is imperative to adequately assess, monitor, and relieve pain in the ED. Despite this, significant evidence–practice gaps continue to be identified with underestimation and undertreatment of pain, as well as gaps in pain documentation, despite available clinical practice guidelines. In general, geriatric and pediatric patients tend to have their pain underestimated and undertreated more frequently than adults do. Pain may be somatic or visceral, acute or chronic, or centrally or peripherally generated.

Primary Assessment

1. ABCD.

2. Evaluate pain using the OPQRST mnemonic.

3. Assess pain score using a pain rating tool, such as the numeric rating scale, visual analogue scale, Wong-Baker FACES pain scale (see page 1151), FLACC (faces, legs, activity, cry, and consolability) behavioral scale, verbal rating scale, or Abbey pain scale.

Primary Interventions

1. Pain is always subjective. Never doubt that a patient has pain based on how they look.

2. Establish a supportive relationship with the patient.

3. Respect the patient's response to pain and its management.

4. Educate the patient regarding methods of pain relief, preventive measures, and expectations.

5. Establish a baseline pain level, as well as a pain level the patient would consider tolerable.

6. Administer pharmaceutical and nonpharmaceutical pain control.

7. Monitor the patient's response to and effectiveness of treatment.

8. If initial interventions do not bring pain down to the tolerable level, explore other options.

9. Always reassure your patient and let them know you take their pain seriously.

 NURSING ALERT Pain relief is a moral, humane, and physiologic imperative.

CARDIOPULMONARY RESUSCITATION AND AIRWAY MANAGEMENT

See additional online content: Procedure Guidelines 35-1–35-4

EVIDENCE BASE American Heart Association. (2015). American Heart Association 2015 guidelines for CRP and ECC. *Circulation, 122*(Suppl. 3).
  Mathiesen, C., McPherson, D., Ordway, C., & Smith, M. (2015). Caring for patients treated with therapeutic hypothermia. *Critical Care Nurse, 35*(5), e1–e12.

Cardiopulmonary Resuscitation

Cardiopulmonary resuscitation (CPR) is a technique of basic life support for the purpose of oxygenating the brain and heart until appropriate, definitive medical treatment can restore normal heart and ventilatory action. Management of foreign body airway obstruction or cricothyroidotomy may be necessary to open the airway while CPR is performed.

Over the years, many changes have been made to the CPR guidelines. The emphasis is now on performing good, high-quality chest compressions, with a minimum of interruptions, in an effort to not only preserve life but prevent anoxic brain injuries as well. The traditional "look–listen and feel" for breathing has been eliminated, as well as the A–B–C order for assessing the unresponsive patient. For the lay public, the focus has changed to a compressions-only resuscitation model, with no interruptions to deliver breaths. For the professional provider, airway, breathing, and circulation are all still important parts of the resuscitation effort; however, A–B–C has become C–A–B, or circulation, airway, and then breathing. All efforts begin with good, high-quality chest compressions.

Indications

1. Cardiac arrest.
   a. Ventricular fibrillation.
   b. Ventricular tachycardia.
   c. Asystole.
   d. Pulseless electrical activity.
2. Respiratory arrest.
   a. Drowning.
   b. Stroke.
   c. Foreign-body airway obstruction.
   d. Smoke inhalation.
   e. Drug overdose.
   f. Electrocution/injury by lightning.
   g. Suffocation.
   h. Accident/injury.
   i. Coma.
   j. Epiglottitis.

Assessment

1. Immediate loss of consciousness.
2. Absence of palpable carotid or femoral pulse; pulselessness in large arteries.
3. Absence of breath sounds or air movement through the nose or mouth.

Interventions

1. Kneel as close to the side of the patient's chest as possible, placing the heel of one hand on the lower half of the sternum, taking care to avoid the xiphoid process. Fingers may be interlaced or extended, but care must be taken to keep them off the chest.
2. Keep your arms straight and your elbows locked. Ensure your shoulders are directly over your hands, and quickly and forcefully depress the patient's sternum straight down to a depth of at least 2 inches.
3. Deliver 30 compressions at a rate of at least 100 compressions a minute. Always allow for complete chest recoil after each compression without taking your hands off of the chest between compressions.
4. Taking no more than 10 seconds, open the airway and deliver 2 breaths.
5. Continue resuscitation at a rate of 30:2 with one or two rescuers.
6. Utilize the automatic external defibrillator according to audio instructions (see page 251).

Complications

1. Postresuscitation distress syndrome (secondary derangements in multiple organs).
2. Neurologic impairment and brain damage.

NURSING ALERT The patient who has been resuscitated is at risk for another episode of cardiac arrest.

Induced Hypothermia Post Cardiac Arrest

In adults with persistent coma (post cardiac arrest), initiating induced hypothermia to a temperature of 89°F to 93°F (32°C to 34°C) for 12 to 24 hours results in neuroprotection, improving neurologic function, and decreasing mortality. It is also associated with beneficial hemodynamic, renal, and acid–base effects. Hypothermia should be initiated within 6 hours of collapse.

Indications

1. Persistent coma in the adult patient following cardiac arrest and return of spontaneous circulation (ROSC).
2. Traumatically induced cerebral anoxia with or without cardiac arrest.
3. Time frame from cardiac arrest to ROSC is less than 60 minutes.
4. SBP greater than 90 mm Hg with a mean arterial pressure (MAP) greater than 60 mm Hg with or without pressors.

NURSING ALERT The patient who responds to verbal stimuli after cardiac arrest should not be treated with induced hypothermia.

Assessment

1. Institute continuous cardiac monitoring. Monitor for bradycardia caused by cooling or other dysrhythmias.
2. Institute continuous temperature monitoring, preferably core temperature.

3. Frequently monitor blood pressure to avoid hypotension, particularly during rewarming.
4. Monitor CBC for signs of infection, because temperature will not be an accurate sign. Monitor electrolyte panel for hypokalemia caused by hypothermia. ABGs should be analyzed at patient's actual body temperature.
5. Assess the skin every 2 hours for pressure and cold injury.
6. Monitor pupils every hour and consider continuous EEG monitoring.

Interventions

1. Apply ice packs to the groin, axillae, sides of the chest, and neck, or apply cooling device according to manufacturer's instructions. A number of commercially available cooling devices are currently available, including cooling blankets, cooling gel pads applied to the skin, and centrally inserted heat exchange catheters.
2. Instill 30 mL/kg of refrigerated lactated Ringer solution over 30 minutes through a femoral line (if patient is not in acute pulmonary edema).
3. Remove ice packs once temperature is less than 91°F (33°C). Target temperature is 91.4°F (32°C).
4. Replace ice packs and consider further ice-cold lactated Ringer solution if temperature remains above 92.3°F (33.5°C).
5. Use nondepolarizing neuromuscular blockade to prevent shivering. Provide sedation according to standard ICU protocol.
6. Maintain patient at target temperature for a period of 12 to 24 hours once temperature is reached.
7. After the targeted time has elapsed, allow passive rewarming slowly over 8 to 12 hours.

Complications

1. Shivering—patient will require sedation and neuromuscular blockade to relieve shivering, which will interfere with hypothermia.
2. Seizures—continuous neuromuscular blockade may mask postcardiac arrest seizure activity.
3. Ileus because of slowing of metabolic processes.
4. Hypotension because of vasodilation.

Foreign-Body Airway Obstruction

Foreign-body obstruction of the airway may be either partial or complete. Abdominal thrusts (the Heimlich maneuver) are recommended for relieving foreign-body airway obstruction in the conscious adult. Back blows and chest thrusts are used in the conscious infant or toddler.

Assessment

1. Weak, ineffective cough.
2. High-pitched noises on inspiration.
3. Respiratory distress.
4. Inability to speak or breathe.
5. Cyanosis.
6. Hands at the throat (universal choking sign).

Interventions

1. If the patient is conscious, stand behind the patient; wrap your arms around patient's waist, and proceed as follows:
   a. Make a fist with one hand, placing the thumb side of the fist against the patient's abdomen in the midline, slightly

above the navel and well below the xiphoid process. Grasp the fist with your other hand.
   b. Press your fist into the patient's abdomen with a quick upward thrust. Each new thrust should be a separate and distinct maneuver.
   c. Continue until the obstruction is cleared, help arrives, or the patient becomes unresponsive.
   d. Should the patient become unresponsive, immediately begin CPR, checking the airway after each set of compressions and prior to attempting ventilations.
2. If the patient is obese or pregnant, making abdominal compressions ineffective, follow these steps:
   a. Stand behind the patient with your arms under the axillae to encircle his or her chest.
   b. Place the thumb side of your fist on the middle of the patient's sternum, taking care to avoid the xiphoid process and rib cage margins.
   c. Grasp your fist with your other hand and perform backward thrusts until the foreign body is expelled. If the patient becomes unconscious, stop and begin CPR.

Cricothyroidotomy

Cricothyroidotomy is the puncture or incision of the cricothyroid membrane to establish an emergency airway in certain emergency situations when placement of an endotracheal tube or laryngeal mask airway is not possible or is contraindicated and when adequate oxygenation cannot be maintained utilizing a bag-valve-mask device with 100% oxygen.

Indications

1. Compromised airway and inability to intubate or perform tracheostomy:
   a. Complete foreign-body airway obstruction.
   b. Trauma to the head and neck.
2. Allergic reaction causing laryngeal edema.

Contraindications

1. Laryngeal fracture.
2. Tracheal rupture.
3. Tracheal transection with distal tracheal retraction into the mediastinum.

Interventions

Assist the physician or emergency health care provider as follows:

1. Preoxygenate the patient, if possible.
2. Extend the patient's neck. Place a towel roll beneath the shoulders.
3. Attach a 10-mL syringe containing 5 mL of saline to the insertion catheter.
4. Identify the prominent thyroid cartilage (Adam's apple), and allow your finger to descend in the midline to the depression between the lower border of the thyroid cartilage and the upper border of the cricoid cartilage (see accompanying figure).
5. Scrub insertion site and maintain sterility throughout procedure.
6. Provide skin tension and hold the trachea in place with the nondominant hand, using the index finger to palpate the cricothyroid membrane.
7. Place the catheter at the inferior margin of the cricothyroid membrane, in the midline of the neck, and direct it caudally at a 30- to 45-degree angle.

8. While maintaining negative pressure on the syringe, advance the catheter through the skin and tissue until air bubbles are seen in the syringe.

9. Thread the catheter off of the needle until the hub rests on the skin surface and withdraw the needle.

10. Listen for air passing back and forth through the needle synchronously with the patient's respirations.

11. Secure the needle with adhesive tape or sutures.

12. Ventilate with bag-valve-mask device, allowing for a prolonged exhalation time.

Complications

1. Bleeding.
2. Aspiration.
3. Subcutaneous emphysema.

INJURIES TO THE HEAD, SPINE, AND FACE

Head Injuries

Head injuries can include fractures to the skull and face, direct injuries to the brain (as from a bullet), and indirect injuries to the brain (such as a concussion, contusion, or intracranial hemorrhage). Head injuries commonly occur from motor vehicle accidents, assaults, or falls.

Concussion—a mild diffuse axonal injury resulting in a transient disturbance of neurological function that may or may not include a loss of consciousness.

Contusion—a focal injury resulting in bruising of the brain tissue. Actual small amounts of bleeding into the brain tissue associated with edema formation and possible tissue necrosis and infarction.

Intracranial hemorrhage—significant bleeding into a space or a potential space between the skull and the brain. This is a serious complication of a head injury with a high mortality because of rising intracranial pressure (ICP) and the potential for brain herniation. Intracranial hemorrhages can be classified as *epidural hematomas*, *subdural hematomas*, or *subarachnoid hemorrhages*, depending on the site of bleeding.

 NURSING ALERT Always assume a cervical spine fracture for any patient with a significant head injury until proven otherwise.

Primary Assessment

1. Airway: assess for vomitus, bleeding, and foreign objects. Ensure cervical spine immobilization.
2. Breathing: assess for abnormally slow or shallow respirations. An elevated carbon dioxide partial pressure can worsen cerebral edema.
3. Circulation: assess pulse and bleeding.
4. Disability: assess the patient's neurologic status.

Primary Interventions

1. Open the airway using the jaw-thrust technique without head tilt. Oral suction equipment (to handle heavy vomitus) should be at hand. Make sure that you do not stimulate the gag reflex as this can cause increases in ICP.
2. Administer high-flow oxygen.
3. Assist inadequate respirations with a bag-valve-mask, as necessary. Prophylactic hyperventilation is contraindicated.

4. Control bleeding—do not apply pressure to the injury site. Apply a bulky, loose dressing.
5. Initiate two IV lines. The administration of fluid and rate of flow should be determined by the patient's hemodynamic status.

Subsequent Assessment

1. History.
   a. Mechanism of injury.
   b. Presence and duration of loss of consciousness.
   c. Amnesia of the event.
   d. Position found.
2. LOC.
   a. Change in mental status is the most sensitive indicator of a change in the patient's condition.
   b. GCS (see page 354).
3. Vital signs.
   a. Hypertension and bradycardia are late signs of increasing ICP.
   b. Patients with a head injury may have associated cardiac dysrhythmias, noted by an irregular or rapid pulse.
   c. Changing patterns of respiration or apnea may indicate a head injury.
   d. Elevated temperature—high temperatures may be associated with head injury.
4. Unequal or unresponsive pupils.
5. Confusion or personality changes.
6. Impaired vision.
7. One or both eyes appear sunken.
8. Seizure activity.
9. Periauricular ecchymosis—"Battle sign," a bluish discoloration behind the ears (indicates a possible basal skull fracture).
10. Rhinorrhea or otorrhea (indicative of leakage of CSF).
11. Periorbital ecchymosis (indicates anterior basilar fracture).

 NURSING ALERT If basilar skull fracture or severe midface fractures are suspected, a nasogastric (NG) tube is contraindicated. An orogastric tube may be considered for insertion.

General Interventions

1. Keep the neck in a neutral position with the cervical spine immobilized.
2. Establish an IV line of normal saline or lactated Ringer solution—fluid volume should be based on the patient's hemodynamic status.
3. Be prepared to manage seizures—if seizures occur, they should be controlled immediately.
4. Maintain normothermia.
5. Pharmacologic interventions may include:
   a. Anticonvulsants—to control seizures.
   b. Mannitol or hypertonic saline—to reduce cerebral edema and decrease ICP.
   c. Antibiotics.
   d. Antipyretics to control hyperthermia.

Cervical Spine Injuries

Injuries to the cervical spine are serious because the crushing, stretching, and rotational shear forces exerted on the cord at the time of trauma can produce severe neurologic deficits. Edema and cord swelling contribute further to the loss of spinal cord function.

Any person with a head, neck, or back injury or fractures to the upper leg bones or to the pelvis should be suspected of having a potential spinal cord injury until proven otherwise.

Primary Assessment

1. Provide immediate immobilization of the spine and maintain immobilization throughout assessment.
2. Airway—determine patency.
3. Breathing.
   a. Intercostal paralysis with diaphragmatic breathing indicates cervical spinal cord injury.
   b. In conscious patient, observe for increased respiratory rate and difficulty in speaking because of shortness of breath.
4. Circulation—heart rate, blood pressure, presence and quality of pulses, and capillary refill.
5. Disability—assess neurologic status.

Primary Interventions

1. Immobilize the cervical spine.
2. Open the airway using the jaw-thrust technique without head tilt.
3. If the patient needs to be intubated, consider nasal intubation.
4. If respirations are shallow, assist with a bag-valve-mask.
5. Administer high-flow oxygen to minimize potential hypoxic spinal cord damage.

Subsequent Assessment

1. Assess the position of the patient when found; this may indicate the type of injury incurred.
2. Hypotension and bradycardia accompanied by warm, dry skin—suggests spinal shock.
3. Neck and back pain/extremity pain or burning sensation to the skin.
4. History of unconsciousness.
5. Total sensory loss and motor paralysis below level of injury.
6. Loss of bowel and bladder control; usually urinary retention and bladder distention.
7. Loss of sweating and vasomotor tone below level of cord lesion.
8. Priapism—persistent erection of the penis.
9. Hypothermia—because of the inability to constrict peripheral blood vessels and conserve body heat.
10. Loss of rectal tone.

General Interventions

 NURSING ALERT A spinal cord injury can be made worse during the acute phase of injury, resulting in permanent neurologic damage. Proper positioning and movement of the patient is an immediate priority.

1. Ensure adequacy of airway, breathing, and circulation. Frequently monitor vital signs.
2. Insert an NG/OG tube.
3. Keep the patient warm.
4. Initiate IV access.
5. Insert an indwelling urinary catheter to avoid bladder distention.
6. Continue with repeated neurologic examinations to determine if there is deterioration of the spinal cord injury.

7. Be prepared to manage seizures if head injury is also suspected.
8. Pharmacologic interventions: possible steroids or antiepileptics.

 NURSING ALERT Patients with spinal cord injuries can experience autonomic dysreflexia, an exaggerated sympathetic response to noxious stimuli. It has the potential to be life-threatening if signs are not immediately recognized and treated, along with the removal of the offending stimuli.

Maxillofacial Trauma

Injuries to the head frequently result in facial lacerations and fractures to the facial bones (ie, nasal fractures, orbital fractures, maxillary fractures, and mandibular fractures).

Primary Assessment

1. Maintain immobilization of the spine while performing assessment.
2. Airway—obstruction can occur due to tongue swelling, bleeding, or broken or missing teeth.
3. Breathing—have suction ready to prevent aspiration of blood or broken teeth.
4. Circulation—control bleeding; monitor vital signs for signs of instability.
5. Disability—neuro assessment.

Primary Interventions

1. Establish and maintain an airway. Apply high-flow oxygen and assist with intubation. Oral and nasopharyngeal airways should be used with caution. Do not use a nasopharyngeal airway if there is evidence of nasal fractures or CSF leakage from the nose.
2. Control bleeding—do not apply pressure to the injury site. Apply a bulky, loose dressing.

Subsequent Assessment

1. Examine the mouth for broken or missing teeth.
2. Assess for a potential eye injury, vision loss, double vision, or pain in the eye.
3. Examine the eye for disconjugate gaze—uncoordinated eye movements.
4. Paralysis of the upward gaze is indicative of an inferior orbit fracture (blow-out fracture).
5. Crepitus or a crackling feeling on palpation around the nose usually indicates a nasal fracture.
6. Malocclusion of the teeth is indicative of a maxilla or mandible fracture.
7. A palpable flattening of the cheek and a loss of sensation below the orbit may indicate a zygoma (cheek bone) fracture.
8. Spasms of the jaw (trismus) and mobility of the jaw indicate a maxilla fracture.
9. Rhinorrhea or otorrhea (indicative of leakage of CSF).

General Interventions

1. Gently apply ice to areas of swelling or ecchymosis. This may reduce further swelling and pain. However, if you suspect an injury to the eye itself, do not apply ice.
2. If other injuries permit, elevate the head of the bed.
3. Possible pharmacologic interventions:
   a. Pain management.
   b. Sedation.

4. With the potential for a CSF leak, the patient should be instructed not to blow the nose because of the potential for transmitting infection to the brain or eyes.

INJURIES TO SOFT TISSUE, BONES, AND JOINTS

Soft Tissue Injuries

Soft tissue injuries involve the skin and underlying subcutaneous tissue and muscles. They can be classified as closed or open injuries. A *closed wound* is an injury to the soft tissue but without an associated break in the skin. Closed wounds include:

1. Contusion—bleeding beneath the skin into the subcutaneous tissue. Discoloration, swelling, and pain may be present.
2. Hematoma—well-defined pocket of blood and fluid beneath the skin resulting from a disruption of the deeper veins and arteries. Hematomas present as an appreciable soft mass on palpation.

An *open wound* is an injury to soft tissue with an associated break in the skin. Generally, they are more serious than closed injuries because of the potential for blood loss and infection. Open wounds include:

1. Abrasion—superficial loss of the skin resulting from rubbing or scraping the skin over a rough or uneven surface.
2. Laceration—a tear or cut in the skin. They can be a partial- or full-thickness cut, incisional or jagged.
3. Puncture—occurs when the skin is penetrated by a pointed object. Can be penetrating (entrance wound only) or perforating (entrance and exit wound). Generally, puncture wounds do not cause serious external bleeding, but there may be significant internal bleeding and damage to vital organs, as well as significant risk of infection.
4. Avulsion—involves a tearing off or loss of a full-thickness flap of the skin.
5. Amputation—traumatic cutting or tearing off of an appendage (eg, finger, toe, arm, or leg).
6. Burn—tissue injury that results from thermal, chemical, electrical, or radiation energy.

Primary Assessment

1. Always ensure the adequacy of airway, breathing, and circulation.
2. If the bleeding from the injury has been significant, be aware of the clinical signs and symptoms of shock.
   a. Restlessness, confusion, and anxiety.
   b. Skin pale, mottled, cold, and diaphoretic.
   c. Tachycardia (rapid pulse).
   d. Tachypnea (rapid, shallow breathing).
   e. Hypotension (falling BP is a late sign of shock).
3. Assess for arterial or venous bleeding. Arterial bleeding is bright red and usually spurts from the wound. Venous bleeding is darker red and will flow steadily from a wound.

Primary Interventions

The primary goal and nursing intervention are to control severe bleeding.

 NURSING ALERT Wounds that result in severe arterial bleeding should be considered life-threatening, and treatment is second only to CPR.

Direct Pressure

1. Most external bleeding can be controlled with firm direct pressure.
2. Cover the injury with sterile dressings.
3. While maintaining pressure, assess for distal pulses.
4. Pressure should be maintained until the bleeding stops, a pressure dressing is applied, or definitive treatment is undertaken.
5. If the dressing becomes saturated, reinforce the dressing; do not remove the dressing.
6. After bleeding has stopped, apply a pressure dressing.
   a. A pressure bandage is made by securing several gauze pads over the injury with a rolled gauze bandage.
   b. A pressure dressing allows the nurse freedom to continue assessing the patient or attend to other injuries.
   c. After applying a pressure dressing, always ensure that the patient has a pulse distal to the dressing. If no pulse is present, the dressing may be too tight.

Elevation

1. Elevating the injured area while applying direct pressure helps to control bleeding. This measure uses gravity to slow the blood flow.
2. If possible, the injured area should be elevated above the level of the heart.
3. Do not raise a limb if a fracture is suspected or if elevation causes the patient pain or discomfort.

Pressure Points

1. Pressure points are used when direct pressure and elevation cannot control bleeding alone or when direct pressure cannot be applied to a bleeding site because of a protruding bone or an embedded object.
2. Pressure points are located between the site of injury and the heart where a main artery passes over a bone or underlying muscle mass (see Figure 35-1).
3. Locate the pressure point and apply firm, steady pressure with the heel of the hand.
4. If heavy bleeding is still not controlled, the patient may exsanguinate and a tourniquet should be used or a vascular clamp can be applied to the artery.

Subsequent Assessment

1. Expose the wound; cut away clothing, if necessary. Secure any impaled objects in place.
2. Assess for the presence of concomitant injuries. The obvious wound is not necessarily the most life-threatening.
3. Assess vascular status distal to the injury and compare it to the uninjured extremity.
   a. Color of the injured extremity—pallor suggests poor arterial perfusion and cyanosis suggests venous congestion.
   b. Test capillary refill time by depressing the nail bed until it blanches and seeing how long until the nail bed returns to pink. A capillary refill time greater than 2 to 3 seconds suggests decreased capillary perfusion.
   c. Test pulses distal to the injury—generally, they should be full and strong.
4. Perform a neurologic assessment of the injured extremity to determine peripheral nerve insult, possibly caused by direct injury, compression, or edema.
   a. Sensory function—while the patient's eyes are closed, lightly touch the area distal to the injury and ask them to identify the area being touched. Have them discriminate between sharp and dull touch.
   b. Motor function—have patient move extremity distal to the injury.
5. Determine tetanus immunization status.

A. Temporal

B. Facial

C. Carotid

D. Subclavian

E. Brachial

F. Radial and Ulnar

G. Femoral

Figure 35-1. Pressure points for control of hemorrhage. (Smeltzer, S. & Bare, B. [2000]. *Brunner and Suddarth's textbook of medical–surgical nursing* [9th ed.]. Philadelphia, PA: Lippincott Williams & Wilkins.)

6. History of the injury, including when and how the wound occurred. Any wound that is more than 6 hours old is considered at high risk for infection, and primary closure by suturing may not be an option.
7. Allergies to local anesthesia, epinephrine, and antibiotics.

General Interventions

Wound Preparation
1. Shaving is not recommended; instead, clip only the required area. Eyebrows are never clipped.
2. Irrigate gently and copiously with isotonic sterile saline solution to remove dirt and debris. All wounds must be thoroughly explored for retained foreign objects before closure. If the wound is grossly contaminated, it may need to be cleansed with a surgical scrub sponge and then irrigated. If the patient is in pain, anesthetize the wound prior to cleansing and irrigating.
3. Topical anesthetic may be applied to the wound (prior to infiltration with local anesthetic) intradermally through the wound margins or by regional nerve block.
4. Devitalized tissue and foreign matter are removed—devitalized tissue inhibits wound healing and enhances chance of bacterial infection.

Wound Closure
1. Closure by primary intent.
   a. Wound is repaired without delay after the injury; yields the fastest healing.

   b. Primary closure may be with sutures, skin tapes, staples, or tissue adhesives. Location and size of the wound are key factors in determining closure material used.
2. Closure by secondary intent.
   a. Wound is allowed to granulate on its own without surgical closure.
   b. Wound is cleaned and covered with a sterile dressing.
3. Closure by secondary intent with delayed closure.
   a. Wound is cleaned and dressed.
   b. Patient returns in 3 to 4 days for definitive closure.

Wound Dressing
1. Dressing should be applied in three layers.
   a. The first layer is the contact layer. This should consist of a nonabsorbent hydrophilic dressing that will allow exudate to pass through to the second layer without wetting the contact layer. Examples of contact layer dressings are Adaptic, petroleum gauze, and Xeroform gauze.
   b. The second layer is the absorbent layer and is usually constructed of surgical dressing pads or 4 × 4-gauze dressings.
   c. The third layer is the outer wrap that holds the dressing in place. The outer wrap may consist of rolled gauze and tape.
2. There are many different proprietary dressings available for application.

Pharmacologic Interventions
1. Give antimicrobial treatment, as directed, depending on how the injury occurred, age of wound, presence of soil, and infection potential.

2. Give tetanus prophylaxis, as indicated, based on patient's immunization status and wound.
3. Rabies prophylaxis, as indicated. For more information on four-dose postexposure rabies prophylaxis, go to *www.cdc.gov/vaccines/pubs/ACIP-list.htm#rabies*.

Patient Education

1. Inform the patient that pain should subside over the course of the next 24 to 48 hours.
2. Acetaminophen, ibuprofen, or prescribed analgesic to be taken for the first 24 hours after a simple laceration.
3. If pain reappears, a wound infection may be suspected.
4. Recommend that the wound be monitored for signs of infection.
5. Advise that health care provider be contacted if there is sudden or persistent onset of pain, fever/chills, bleeding, rapid swelling, foul odor, purulent fluid, or redness surrounding the wound.

Injuries to Bones and Joints

Injuries to bones and joints are common. *Fractures* may be caused by direct trauma (eg, projectiles, crush injuries) or by indirect trauma (ie, bones being pulled apart or rotational forces). In addition, bones may be fractured due to pathologic reasons. A pathologic fracture is due to a weakness in the bone secondary to a disease process such as metastatic cancer. For the classification of fractures, see page 878.

Other injuries include:

1. Dislocation—complete displacement or separation of a bone from its normal place of articulation. It may be associated with a tearing of the ligaments. The shoulder, elbow, fingers, hips, and ankles are the joints most frequently affected.
2. Subluxation—partial disruption of the articulating surfaces.
3. Sprains—injuries in which ligaments are partially torn or stretched. These types of injuries are usually caused by a twisting of a joint beyond its normal range of motion. The severity can range from mild to severe. The more seriously injured ligaments may resemble a fracture.
4. Strains—stretching or tearing of muscle and tendon fibers. Usually caused by overexertion or overextension.

Primary Assessment

1. Always ensure the adequacy of airway, breathing, and circulation before initiating treatment.
2. Occult blood loss into a closed space from the fracture may be significant enough to produce hypovolemic shock. Death by exsanguination can occur from pelvic and femoral fractures. Estimated blood loss in an adult from closed fractures in liters:
   a. Tibia—1.5 L.
   b. Femur—2 L.
   c. Pelvis—6 L.
   d. Humerus—2 L.
3. A fractured cervical spine, pelvic fracture, or fractured femur may produce life-threatening injuries. Posterior dislocations of the hip are life- and limb-threatening emergencies because of the potential for blood loss and the disruption in blood supply to the head of the femur. Unless this dislocation is promptly reduced, the patient may develop avascular necrosis of the femoral head and subsequently may require a hip replacement.

Primary Interventions

1. Support airway, breathing, and circulation, if compromised.
2. Initiate IV line and treat for shock, if evident.
3. Assess circulation distal to the site of injury. Loss of distal pulses requires immediate intervention.
4. Protect injured part from movement or further trauma. Splinting in the position the patient was found may be helpful if circulation is not compromised.
5. Pain management is essential.

Subsequent Assessment

1. Seek information on the mechanism of injury.
   a. How did the injury occur and when did the injury occur?
   b. In what position was the limb after the injury?
   c. If the mechanism of injury was a fall, how many feet did the person fall? What type of surface did they land on?
   d. If the mechanism was a motor vehicle crash, where was the patient? What was the direction and amount of force? Certain musculoskeletal injuries commonly occur together.
2. Assess for the presence of concomitant injuries.
   a. A fractured calcaneus as the result of a fall from a great height may also include a compression fracture of the spine.
   b. A person with a fractured patella from a motor vehicle accident may also have a fractured or dislocated femur.
   c. A fractured pelvis may occur with lumbosacral spine fractures and bladder injuries.
3. Perform a neurovascular assessment to include the area above and below the injury.
   a. Assess for ischemia to the extremity.
   b. Pallor suggests poor arterial perfusion, whereas cyanosis suggests venous congestion.
      i. A capillary refill time greater than 2 seconds suggests decreased arterial capillary perfusion.
   c. Assess neurologic supply of the injured extremity to determine peripheral nerve insult. Damage to a peripheral nerve can be the result of a direct injury, compression, stretching, or edema.
      i. Test sensory function—with the patient's eyes closed, lightly touch the area distal to the injury. Ask the patient to identify the area being touched.
      ii. Test motor function—have patient move extremity distal to the injury.
      iii. Numbness or paralysis indicates pressure on the nerves and may require immediate medical intervention.
4. Examine the bones and joints adjacent to the injury. If there was enough force to produce one injury, there may be other injuries.
5. Signs and symptoms of fractures:
   a. Pain and tenderness over the fracture site, called "point tenderness."
   b. A grating or crepitus over the fracture site.
   c. Swelling, because of internal bleeding and edema.
   d. Deformity, unnatural position, or movement where there is no joint.
   e. Loss of use or guarding.
   f. Discoloration because of bleeding into the surrounding tissue.
   g. Shortening of an extremity or rotation of the extremity.
6. Signs and symptoms of dislocations:
   a. Loss of joint motion—the joint may appear "frozen."
   b. Obvious deformity—lump, ridge, or excavation.
   c. Pain.

7. Signs and symptoms of sprains:
   a. Pain in the joint area.
   b. Swelling.
   c. Limited use or movement.
   d. Ecchymosis.
8. Signs and symptoms of strains:
   a. Pain located in a muscle or its tendon, not a bone or a joint.
   b. Swelling is usually minimal.
9. Closely monitor vital signs.

General Interventions

Interventions for the Severely Injured Patient

1. Ensure adequacy of airway, breathing, and circulation. Closely monitor vital signs.
2. Initiate two IV lines and start volume replacement with lactated Ringer solution or normal saline.
3. Immobilize the injury—this will prevent further damage and will help to relieve the pain.
4. Prepare the patient for the possibility of needing to go to the OR (operating room)—keep the patient NPO (nothing by mouth).
5. Antibiotics may be started if warranted.

Other Interventions

1. Elevate to prevent or limit swelling.
2. Apply ice packs or cold compresses; ice should not be placed directly on the skin.
3. Cover open fractures with a sterile dressing. If bone is protruding, do not attempt to tuck the ends under the skin. Cover with a sterile dressing.
4. Splint the extremity in as good alignment as possible until definitive care is complete. Immobilize the joint above and below the fracture.
5. Handle the injured part gently and as little as possible.
6. Pain management may include ice packs, simple or opioid analgesics, nonsteroidal anti-inflammatory drugs, or regional nerve blocks.
7. High-flow oxygen should be administered to patients with pelvic or femoral fractures, compartment syndrome, or signs of shock.

Assess for Compartment Syndrome

1. Increased pressure within an extremity resulting from bleeding and swelling into a closed space, causing pressure on vital structures.
2. The six Ps (signs and symptoms) of compartment syndrome are:
   a. Pain—development of a different type of pain, the return of pain after treatment/splinting had caused pain relief, or pain out of proportion to the severity of the injury.
   b. Pallor—deterioration in skin color and an increase in the capillary refill time.
   c. Pulselessness.
   d. Paresthesias.
   e. Paralysis—late sign.
   f. Puffiness—late sign.

 NURSING ALERT Compartment syndrome is a limb-threatening event; therefore, if suspected, do not elevate limb above the level of the heart. This may decrease perfusion to the compromised extremity. Emergent fasciotomy is often required.

 NURSING ALERT Patients with long bone or pelvic fractures are at risk for developing fat emboli and should be monitored closely.

SHOCK AND INTERNAL INJURIES
Shock

Shock is the common denominator in a wide variety of disease processes that present as an immediate threat to life. Simply defined, *shock* is inadequate tissue perfusion. This inadequate tissue perfusion is the result of failure of one or more of the following: (1) the heart–pump failure, (2) blood volume, (3) arterial resistance vessels, and (4) the capacity of the venous beds. Any condition that significantly affects any of the above may precipitate a shock state. Shock can be classified as compensated (hemodynamically stable) or uncompensated (hemodynamically unstable).

Types of shock are:

1. Hypovolemic shock—occurs when a significant amount of fluid is lost from the intravascular space. May result from hemorrhage, burns, GI losses, or fluid shifts.
2. Cardiogenic shock—occurs when the heart fails as a pump. Primary causes of this failure are myocardial infarction (MI), serious cardiac dysrhythmias, and myocardial depression from diseases such as myocarditis, endocarditis, and pericarditis. Secondary causes include mechanical restriction of cardiac function or venous obstruction, such as occurs with cardiac tamponade, vena cava obstruction, or tension pneumothorax.
3. Distributive—occurs as the result of a loss of vascular tone. It may be anaphylactic, septic, neurogenic, or because of an acute adrenal insufficiency. Septic shock may occur with or without an infection. Sepsis is characterized by a systemic inflammatory response in the presence of suspected or confirmed infection. Systemic inflammatory response syndrome (SIRS) is the body's systemic clinical response to an insult with an acute inflammatory reaction. See Table 35-1 for defining characteristics of SIRS and sepsis.

Table 35-1	Defining Characteristics of Sepsis
SEPTIC CONDITION	**CHARACTERISTIC**
SIRS, two or more of:	Temperature >100.4°F (38°C) or <96.8°F (36°C)
	HR > 90, RR > 20, arterial CO_2 < 32 mm Hg or need for mechanical ventilation
	WBC > 12,000/mm³ or <4,000/mm³ or more than 10% immature band forms
Sepsis	SIRS criteria
	Suspected or confirmed infection
Severe sepsis	Serum lactate level >2 mmol/L
	Hypovolemia responsive to fluid resuscitation
	Signs of tissue hypoperfusion
Septic shock	Profound hypovolemia, hypoxia, and hypoperfusion
	Hypovolemia unresponsive to fluid resuscitation
	Multiple organ failure

bpm, beats per minute; HR, heart rate; RR, respiratory rate; SIRS, systemic inflammatory response syndrome; WBC, white blood cell.

Primary Assessment and Interventions

1. Rapid recognition and prompt intervention are essential to increase the chance of survival because a downward spiral of physiologic responses culminating in multiorgan dysfunction syndrome and eventual death will occur if shock is not treated.
2. The initial priorities in the assessment are the same for all types of shock.
   a. Is the airway open?
   b. Is the patient breathing?
   c. Is there a circulation problem?
3. Initiate immediate interventions, as indicated.
   a. Resuscitate as necessary. Fluid replacement with isotonic fluids and eventually blood products is essential.
   b. Administer oxygen.
   c. Start cardiac monitoring.
   d. Control hemorrhage or other fluid loss, if present.
4. Pain management is essential.

Subsequent Assessment

1. Assess level of consciousness—important indicator of shock because it reflects cerebral perfusion. Changes may include:
   a. Confusion.
   b. Irritability.
   c. Anxiety.
   d. Agitation.
   e. Inability to concentrate.
2. Watch for increasing lethargy progressing to obtundation and coma, indicating progression of shock.
3. Monitor arterial BP.
   a. If the patient can compensate for the shock state, the BP may initially rise approximately 20%. A significant decrease in BP may not occur until late in the shock state.
   b. Narrowing pulse pressure—early in shock, the diastolic pressure may rise due to an initial vasoconstriction produced by release of catecholamines from the sympathetic nervous system.
   c. Fall in the systolic pressure—there is no absolute value in BP that indicates a shock state. It is the deviation from normal that is important. However, it is generally accepted that a systolic pressure below 80 mm Hg or a mean arterial pressure below 60 mm Hg is indicative of shock.
4. Assess pulse quality and rate change.
   a. The rate is usually increased.
   b. Weak, thready pulse because of decreased cardiac output and increased peripheral vascular resistance.
5. Assess urine output.
   a. A decrease in renal blood flow or pressure will result in decreased urine output.
   b. Ideally in an adult, the urine output should be 50 mL/hour. An output of less than 25 mL/hour may indicate shock in a patient without renal dysfunction.
6. Assess capillary perfusion.
   a. Pale, ashen, mottled, cold, and sweaty skin indicates potent vasoconstriction.
   b. Capillary refill greater than 2 seconds indicates vasoconstriction.
7. Also assess for:
   a. Subjective feeling of impending doom.
   b. Metabolic acidosis because of anaerobic metabolism within the cells.
   c. Excessive thirst.

NURSING ALERT Rapid identification and treatment of SIRS or sepsis are essential in the treatment of septic shock. Although a source of infection may not be identified, signs include fever, tachypnea, tachycardia, and leukocytosis.

General Interventions

1. Administer 100% O_2 by nonrebreather face mask to maintain the partial pressure of arterial oxygen at 90% to 100%.
2. Assist with intubation if the patient is unable to maintain airway.
3. Fluid resuscitation.
   a. Two large-bore IV lines should be established.
   b. Administer IV fluids—lactated Ringer or normal saline. Rate of infusion depends on severity of blood loss and clinical evidence of hypovolemia.
   c. Packed red blood cells or whole blood are infused when there is hypovolemic shock because of blood loss.
   d. Additional platelets and coagulation factors are given when large amounts of blood are needed because replacement blood is deficient in clotting factors.
   e. Warm the blood and fluids using a commercial fluid warmer—massive blood replacement has a cooling effect that can cause cardiac dysrhythmias, paradoxical hypotension, decreased oxyhemoglobin dissociation, or cardiac arrest.
4. Insert an indwelling urinary catheter.
   a. Record urine output every 15 to 30 minutes.
   b. Urinary volume reveals adequacy of kidney and visceral perfusion.
5. Maintain patient in supine position with the legs slightly elevated. (This position is contraindicated in patients with head injuries.)
6. ECG monitoring—dysrhythmias may contribute to shock.
7. Maintain ongoing nursing surveillance of total patient—BP, heart rate, respiratory rate, temperature, color, central venous pressure (CVP), ABG levels, urine output, ECG, hematocrit, hemoglobin, coagulation profiles, and electrolytes—to assess patient response to treatment.
8. Immobilize fractures to minimize blood loss.
9. Maintain normothermia.
   a. Too much heat produces vasodilatation, which counteracts the body's compensatory mechanism of vasoconstriction and also increases fluid loss through perspiration.
   b. A patient who is in septic shock should be kept cool because high fever will increase the cellular metabolic effects of shock.
10. Provide pharmacologic interventions:
    a. Vasopressors may be indicated but should not be used in place of volume replacement except as dictated by cardiogenic or neurogenic shock states.
    b. Antibiotics—broad spectrum for septic shock.

NURSING ALERT Trendelenburg position is no longer recommended because of the potential for respiratory compromise caused by pressure from abdominal organs.

Abdominal Injuries

Abdominal injuries account for a large percentage of trauma-related injuries and deaths. The visceral organs contained within the abdomen can be classified as either hollow or solid.

Damage to a hollow organ can result in acute peritonitis, leading to shock within a few hours, and damage to a solid organ can result in lethal hemorrhage. Abdominal injuries may be classified as either penetrating or blunt.

Penetrating abdominal injury—usually the result of gunshot wounds or stab wounds. The mechanism that caused the penetrating abdominal trauma may cross the diaphragm and enter the chest. The opposite can also occur.

Blunt abdominal injury—usually caused by motor vehicle accidents or falls. Trauma to the abdomen is commonly associated with extra-abdominal injuries (ie, chest, head, and extremity injuries) and severe concomitant trauma to multiple intraperitoneal organs. Blunt abdominal injury is often associated with delayed complications, especially if there is injury to the liver, spleen, or blood vessels, which can lead to substantial blood loss into the peritoneal cavity.

Primary Assessment and Interventions

1. Assess airway, breathing, and circulation.
2. Initiate resuscitation, as indicated.
3. Control bleeding and prepare to treat shock.
4. If there is an impaled object in the abdomen, leave it there. Stabilize the object in place with bulky dressings along the sides of the object.

Subsequent Assessment

1. Obtain a history of the mechanism of the injury, type of weapon, and estimated amount of blood loss.
   a. If the patient was stabbed, how long was the blade?
   b. Was the person who stabbed the patient a man or a woman?
      i. Men usually hold a knife underhand and stab/thrust upward.
      ii. Women usually will stab/thrust downward with an overhand motion.
   c. If the patient sustained a gunshot wound, attempt to ascertain the type of gun and range at which shot.
   d. Time of onset of symptoms.
   e. Passenger location (driver frequently sustains spleen/liver rupture). Were seat belts worn? Did the airbag deploy? Were there other injured parties or fatalities involved in the same accident?
2. Inspect the abdomen for obvious signs of injury (penetrating injury, bruises).
3. Evaluate for signs and symptoms of hemorrhage—usually accompanies abdominal injury, especially if the liver and spleen have been traumatized.
4. Note tenderness, rebound tenderness, guarding, rigidity, and spasm.
   a. Firmly press, with the whole hand, the area of maximal tenderness (let the patient point to the area).
   b. Remove the fingers quickly to check for rebound tenderness; pain at suspected point indicates peritoneal irritation.
5. Ask about referred pain: Kehr sign—pain radiating to the left shoulder may be a sign of blood beneath the left diaphragm; pain in the right shoulder can result from laceration of the liver. The patient must be lying flat for this type of shoulder pain to occur.
6. Look for increasing abdominal distention. Measure abdominal girth at umbilical level early in your assessment—serves as a baseline from which changes can be determined. Making a mark where you measured can also assist in assuring the same place is measured each time.

7. Auscultate—a silent abdomen accompanies peritoneal irritation or ileus. The presence of bowel sounds in the chest indicates a ruptured diaphragm. Bruits over the aorta or other large arteries may indicate disrupted arterial blood flow.
8. Percuss—tympani over solid organs (liver, spleen)—indicates presence of free air; dullness over regions normally containing gas may indicate presence of blood or other fluids.
9. Look for chest injuries, which frequently accompany intra-abdominal injuries.
10. Cullen sign, a slight bluish discoloration around the navel, is a sign of blood in the abdominal wall. Grey Turner sign, or flank ecchymosis, is indicative of renal injuries or retroperitoneal bleeding.
11. Pain is a poor indicator of the extent of an abdominal injury. Rebound tenderness and boardlike rigidity are indicative of a significant intra-abdominal injury.
12. A rectal examination and examination of the perineum should be done on all patients. The presence of blood may be indicative of trauma.
13. Continually assess vital signs, urine output, CVP readings, hematocrit values, and neurologic status. Tachypnea, tachycardia, and hypotension may be clues to intra-abdominal bleeding.

General Interventions

1. Assess adequacy of airway, breathing, and circulation. Begin frequent monitoring.
2. Goals are to control bleeding, maintain blood volume, and prevent infection.
3. Keep the patient quiet and on the stretcher because movement may fragment or dislodge a clot in a large vessel and produce massive hemorrhage.
4. Cut the clothing away from the wound. Do not cut through bullet holes or stab marks. These will be needed by law enforcement authorities as forensic evidence.
5. Count the number of wounds.
6. Look for entrance and exit wounds.
7. If the patient is comatose, immobilize the cervical spine until after cervical films are taken and cleared.
8. Apply compression to external bleeding.
9. Insert two large-bore IV lines and infuse fluid as dictated by the patient's hemodynamic status.
10. Be prepared to insert an NG tube to decompress the abdomen. This will serve to empty the stomach, relieve gastric distention, and facilitate abdominal assessment. In addition, if blood is found, it may indicate stomach injury or esophageal injury.
11. Cover protruding abdominal viscera; do not attempt to replace the protruding organs into the abdomen. Use sterile saline dressings to protect viscera from drying.
12. Cover open wounds with dry dressings.
13. Withhold oral fluids to prevent increased peristalsis and vomiting.
14. Insert an indwelling urethral catheter to ascertain the presence of hematuria and to monitor urine output. If a fracture of the pelvis is suspected, a catheter should not be placed until the integrity of the urethra is ensured.
15. Pharmacologic interventions.
    a. Analgesics.
    b. Tetanus prophylaxis.
    c. Broad-spectrum antibiotics because bacterial contamination is a frequent complication (depending on history and nature of wound).

16. Prepare for focused ultrasound when there is uncertainty about intraperitoneal bleeding. Focused assessment with sonography in trauma (FAST) is a standard for rapid bedside assessment with ultrasound performed by providers to identify free fluid in the abdomen, pericardium, or peritoneum.

17. Prepare for surgery if the patient shows evidence of unexplained shock, unstable vital signs, peritoneal irritation, bowel protrusion or evisceration, significant penetrating injury, significant GI bleeding, or peritoneal air.

18. Prepare the patient for diagnostic procedures.
    a. Catheterization and urinalysis—as a guide to possible urinary tract injury and to monitor urine output.
    b. Type and crossmatch and serial hemoglobin and hematocrit levels—their trend reflects presence or absence of bleeding.
    c. Complete blood count (CBC)—white blood cell count is generally elevated with trauma.
    d. Serum amylase elevation usually indicates pancreatic injury or perforations of GI tract.
    e. Computed tomography (CT) scans permit detailed evaluation of abdominal and retroperitoneal injuries.
    f. Abdominal and chest x-rays may reveal free air beneath the diaphragm, indicating ruptured hollow viscus.

Multiple Injuries

The patient with multiple injuries requires rapid and definitive interventions during the first hour after the trauma to increase chance of survival; this first hour has been called the "golden hour." During this time, multiple assessments and interventions may be performed simultaneously by the health care team.

Primary Assessment and Interventions

Airway

1. Assume a cervical spine injury and open the airway using the jaw-thrust technique without head tilt.
2. Apply suction to clear the trachea and bronchial tree. Remove debris from the mouth (ie, broken teeth, mucus).
3. Insert an oropharyngeal airway—to prevent occlusion by the tongue. Oropharyngeal airways are used in unconscious patients only to prevent stimulation of the gag reflex.
4. Prepare for endotracheal intubation if adequate airway cannot be maintained.
5. If upper airway trauma or edema exists, a cricothyroidotomy may be indicated.

Breathing

1. Note the character and symmetry of chest wall motion and pattern of breathing. Assess for open wounds, deformity, and flail segments.
2. Auscultate the lungs and assess for tracheal deviation. If a tension pneumothorax is present, the trachea will shift away from the injury. Tracheal deviation is a late sign.
3. Ask the conscious patient if experiencing difficulty in breathing or chest pain with breathing.
4. Administer oxygen by 100% nonrebreather mask or assist the patient's ventilations by bag-valve-mask.
5. Suspect serious intrathoracic injuries if respiratory distress continues after adequate airway has been established.
6. Assess the overall effectiveness of ventilations.

Circulation

1. Assess cardiac function and treat cardiac arrest (hypoxia, metabolic acidosis, and chest trauma may precipitate cardiac arrest).
2. For cardiac arrest, start CPR.

3. Control hemorrhage.
   a. Apply direct pressure over bleeding points, if able.
   b. Expect significant blood loss in patients with fractures to the shaft of the femur, multiple fractures, or pelvic trauma.
   c. Use tourniquet(s) for massive arterial bleeding from extremities that cannot be halted with pressure.
   d. Prepare for immediate surgical intervention if patient is bleeding internally.

4. Palpate the carotid pulse and note its rate and quality. Palpate both central and peripheral pulses and compare their quality. Patients will lose their peripheral pulses before losing their central pulse. In addition, assess the femoral and radial pulses to determine an approximate systolic pressure.
   a. If the carotid pulse is present, the systolic pressure is at least 60 mm Hg.
   b. If the femoral pulse is present, the systolic pressure is at least 70 mm Hg.
   c. If the radial pulse is present, the systolic pressure is at least 80 mm Hg.

5. Prevent and treat hypovolemic shock.
   a. Insert at least two IV lines.
   b. If indicated, place a central venous catheter to monitor the patient's response to fluid infusion—to prevent fluid overload and as a route for fluid infusion.
   c. Fluid resuscitation—lactated Ringer solution or normal saline is given for volume replacement until blood is available.
   d. Administer blood—massive transfusions have a cooling effect that can cause cardiac irritability and arrest; blood should be warmed.

6. Note presence or absence of pulses in fractured extremities.

Neurologic

1. Assess level of responsiveness, pupil size and reactivity, strength, and reflexes.
2. Determine a Glasgow Coma Score as a baseline (see page 354).
3. If signs of increased ICP exist, ICP monitoring may be instituted.
4. Agitation or other mental status changes are often the first sign of impending problems.

Subsequent Assessment and Interventions

1. The goals are rapid determination of the extent of the injuries and treatment prioritization.
2. Monitor ECG—to detect life-threatening dysrhythmias.
3. Insert indwelling urethral catheter and monitor urine output to aid in diagnosis of shock as well as monitor effectiveness of therapy. Do not force the catheter—the patient may have a ruptured urethra.
4. Perform an ongoing clinical evaluation to observe for improvement or deterioration, such as changes in vital signs, improvement in level of responsiveness, skin warmth, and speed of capillary filling.
5. Prepare for immediate surgical intervention if the patient does not respond to fluids or blood. Inability to restore BP and circulatory volume in the patient usually indicates major internal bleeding.
6. Splint fractures to prevent further trauma to soft tissues and blood vessels and to relieve pain.
7. Examine the patient for abdominal pain, rigidity, tenderness, rebound tenderness, diminished bowel sounds, hypotension, and shock.
8. Prepare for FAST exam or CT scan to assess for intraperitoneal bleeding.

9. Draw blood for laboratory studies (type and cross-matching, hemoglobin, hematocrit, baseline CBC, electrolytes, blood urea nitrogen [BUN], glucose, coagulation studies).
10. Insert an NG tube to prevent vomiting and aspiration.
11. Prepare for laparotomy if the patient shows continuing signs of hemorrhage and deterioration.
12. Continue to monitor urine output every 30 minutes—reflects cardiac output and state of perfusion of vital organs.
13. Assess for hematuria and oliguria.
14. Evaluate the patient for other injuries and institute appropriate treatment, including tetanus immunization.
15. Perform a more thorough physical examination after resuscitation and management of the aforementioned priorities.

ENVIRONMENTAL EMERGENCIES

Heat Exhaustion

Heat exhaustion is the inadequacy or the collapse of peripheral circulation because of volume and electrolyte depletion. Heat exhaustion is one condition in the spectrum of heat-related illnesses, including heat rash, heat edema, heat cramps, and heat syncope. Untreated heat exhaustion may progress to heatstroke.

Primary Assessment and Interventions

1. Expect the patient to be alert without significant cardiorespiratory or neurologic compromise.
2. If vital functions are significantly impaired, suspect secondary condition, such as MI or stroke.

Subsequent Assessment

1. Ask patient about headache, fatigue, dizziness, muscle cramping, and nausea.
2. Inspect the skin—usually pale, ashen, and moist.
3. The temperature may be normal, slightly elevated, or as high as 104°F (40°C).
4. Measure vital signs for hypotension, orthostatic changes, tachycardia, and tachypnea.
5. The patient will be awake but may give a history of syncope or confusion.
6. Laboratory analysis will show hemoconcentration and hyponatremia (if sodium depletion is the primary problem) or hypernatremia (if water depletion is the primary problem).
7. The ECG may show dysrhythmias without evidence of infarction.

General Interventions

1. Move the patient to a cool environment and remove all clothing.
2. Position the patient supine with feet slightly elevated.
3. If the patient complains of nausea or vomiting, do not give fluids by mouth.
4. Start an IV line with normal saline until electrolyte results are confirmed.
5. Monitor the patient for changes in the cardiac rhythm and vital signs. Vital signs should be taken at least every 15 minutes until the patient is stable.
6. Provide fans and cool sponge baths as cooling methods.
7. Provide patient education.
   a. Advise the patient to avoid immediate reexposure to high temperatures; the patient may remain hypersensitive to high temperatures for a considerable length of time.

b. Emphasize the importance of maintaining an adequate fluid intake, wearing loose clothing, and reducing activity in hot weather.
c. Athletes should monitor fluid losses, replace fluids, and use a gradual approach to physical conditioning, allowing sufficient time for acclimatization.

 NURSING ALERT Identify those at increased risk for heat exhaustion and heatstroke so preventive measures can be taken. Risk factors include such underlying conditions as cardiovascular disease, alcohol abuse, malnutrition, diabetes, skin diseases, and major burn scarring; very young or very old age; drugs such as anticholinergics, phenothiazines, diuretics, antihistamines, antidepressants, and beta-adrenergic blockers; and such behaviors as working outdoors, wearing inappropriate clothing, inadequate fluid intake, and living in poor environmental conditions.

Heatstroke

Heatstroke is a medical emergency that can result in significant morbidity and mortality. It is defined as the combination of hyperpyrexia greater than 104°F (40°C) and neurologic symptoms. It is caused by a shutdown or failure of the heat-regulating mechanisms of the body. It can be classified as exertional or nonexertional.

Primary Assessment and Interventions

1. Assess airway, breathing, and circulation.
2. LOC may be altered.
3. Expect to intervene immediately if cardiovascular collapse occurs.

Subsequent Assessment

1. Obtain a history from accompanying person about environmental conditions, activity, underlying health, and medications that may have contributed to heatstroke.
2. Perform a neurologic assessment.
   a. Initially, the patient may exhibit bizarre behavior or irritability. This may progress to confusion, combativeness, deliriousness, and coma.
   b. Other central nervous system (CNS) disturbances include tremors, seizures, fixed and dilated pupils, and decerebrate or decorticate posturing.
3. Assess vital signs.
   a. Temperature greater than 104°F (40°C).
   b. Hypotension.
   c. Rapid pulse; may be bounding or weak.
   d. Rapid respirations.
4. The skin may appear flushed and hot; in early heatstroke, the skin may be moist, but, as the heatstroke progresses, the skin will become dry as the body loses its ability to sweat.
5. ABGs show metabolic acidosis.

General Interventions

 NURSING ALERT When the diagnosis of heatstroke is made or suspected, it is imperative to reduce the patient's temperature.

1. Protect the airway in patients with deteriorating mental status or absent gag reflex.
2. Provide cooling measures.
   a. Reduce the core (internal) temperature to 102°F (38.9°C) as rapidly as possible.
   b. Evaporative cooling is the most efficient. Spray tepid water on the skin while electric fans are used to blow continuously over the patient to augment heat dissipation.
   c. Apply ice packs to the neck, groin, axillae, and scalp (areas of maximal heat transfer).
   d. Soak sheets/towels in ice water and place on patient, using fans to accelerate evaporation/cooling rate.
   e. Immersion in cold or ice water is contraindicated.
   f. If the temperature fails to decrease, initiate core cooling: iced saline gastric lavage, cool fluid peritoneal dialysis, cool fluid bladder irrigation, or cool fluid chest irrigation.
   g. Cooling blankets may be used after temperature is stabilized.
   h. Discontinue active cooling when the temperature reaches 102°F (38.9°C). In most cases, this will reduce the chance of overcooling because the body temperature will continue to fall after cessation of cooling.
3. Oxygenate patient to supply tissue needs that are exaggerated by the hypermetabolic condition: 100% nonrebreather mask or intubate the patient, if necessary, to support a failing cardiorespiratory system.
4. Monitor condition.
   a. Monitor and record the core temperature continually during cooling process to avoid hypothermia; also, hyperthermia may recur spontaneously within 3 to 4 hours.
   b. Monitor the vital signs continuously, including ECG, CVP, BP, pulse, and respiratory rate.
   c. Perform frequent (every 30 minutes) neurologic assessments.
   d. Monitor lab values for signs of coagulopathy and liver or renal damage.
5. Replace fluids.
   a. Start IV infusion using normal saline solution to replace fluid losses, maintain adequate circulation, and facilitate cooling.
   b. If possible, a central line should be established.
   c. Fluid replacement is based on the patient's response and laboratory results.
6. Other potential measures:
   a. Dialysis for renal failure.
   b. Diuretics, such as mannitol, to promote diuresis.
   c. Anticonvulsant agents to control seizures.
   d. Potassium for hypokalemia and sodium bicarbonate to correct metabolic acidosis, depending on laboratory results.
   e. Antipyretics are not useful in treating heatstroke. They may contribute to the complications of coagulopathy and hepatic damage.
   f. Intense shivering may be controlled by diazepam. Shivering will generate heat and increase the metabolic rate.
   g. Patients with depleted clotting factors may be treated with platelets or fresh frozen plasma.
7. Monitor urine output, likely with an indwelling catheter—acute tubular necrosis is a complication of heatstroke.
8. Perform continuous ECG monitoring and frequent cardiovascular assessments for possible ischemia, infarction, and dysrhythmias.
9. Perform serial laboratory testing (coagulation studies, electrolytes, glucose, and serum enzymes).
10. The patient should be admitted to an intensive care unit (ICU); complications can occur, including heart failure, cardiovascular collapse, hepatic failure, renal failure, disseminated intravascular coagulation, and rhabdomyolysis.
11. Monitor the patient for the development of seizures and provide for a safe environment in case of seizures.

 GERONTOLOGIC ALERT Vigorous fluid replacement in older adults or those with underlying cardiovascular disease may cause pulmonary edema.

Frostbite

Frostbite is trauma because of exposure to freezing temperatures that cause freezing of the tissue fluids in the cell and intracellular spaces, resulting in vascular damage. The areas of the body most likely to develop frostbite are the ear lobes, cheeks, nose, fingers, and toes. Frostbite may be classified as frostnip (initial response to cold, reversible), superficial frostbite, and deep frostbite.

Primary Assessment and Interventions

1. Assess airway, breathing, and circulation.
2. Deficits may indicate coexisting hypothermia or underlying condition.
3. Protect frostbitten tissue while performing other interventions.

Subsequent Assessment

Frostnip
1. History of gradual onset.
2. The skin appears pale.
3. Complaints of numbness or tingling.

Superficial Frostbite
1. Damage is limited to the skin and subcutaneous tissue.
2. The skin will appear white and waxy.
3. On palpation, the skin will feel stiff, but the underlying tissue will be pliable and soft and have its normal "bounce."
4. Sensation is absent.

Deep Frostbite
1. The skin will appear white, yellow–white, or mottled blue–white.
2. On palpation, the surface will feel frozen and the underlying tissue will feel frozen and hard.
3. The affected part is completely insensitive to touch.

General Interventions

1. Frostnip may be treated by placing a warm hand over the chilled area.
2. Leave the frostbitten area alone until definitive rewarming is undertaken. Pad the extremity to prevent damage from trauma.
3. Handle the part gently to avoid further mechanical injury.
4. Remove all constricting clothing that can impair circulation, including watchbands and rings.
5. Rewarming:
   a. Rewarm the extremity by controlled and rapid rewarming. Rewarm with a temperature of 98.6°F to 104°F (37°C to 40°C) in a fairly large, tepid water bath where the part can be fully immersed without touching the side or bottom. If clothing, socks, or gloves are frozen to the extremity, they should be left on and removed after rewarming.

b. More warm water may be added to the container by removing some cooled water and adding warm water.

c. Slow rewarming is less effective and may increase tissue damage.

d. Dry heat is not recommended for rewarming.

e. The rewarming procedure may take 20 to 30 minutes.

f. Rewarming is complete when the area is warm to the touch and pink or flushed.

g. Do not rub or massage a frostbitten extremity. The ice crystals in the tissue will lacerate delicate tissue.

6. Pharmacologic interventions:

a. Opioids or nonsteroidals for pain control.

b. Antibiotics if there is an open wound.

c. Tetanus prophylaxis.

 NURSING ALERT When definitive rewarming of a frostbitten extremity has started, it must not be stopped. Refreezing of a partially thawed extremity may increase tissue damage and loss.

Postrewarming Care

1. Protect the thawed part from infection. Large blisters may develop in 1 hour to a few days after rewarming; these blisters should not be broken. If necessary, fluid may be aspirated from the blister with a sterile needle.

2. Place sterile gauze or cotton between affected fingers/toes to absorb moisture.

3. Use strict sterile technique during dressing changes.

4. Elevate the part to help control swelling. Make sure dressings are applied loosely.

5. Use a foot cradle to prevent contact with bedding if the feet are involved—prevent further tissue injury.

6. Perform a physical assessment to look for concomitant injury (soft tissue injury, dehydration, alcohol coma, fat embolism because of fracture, immobility).

7. Restore electrolyte balance; dehydration and hypovolemia are common in frostbite victims.

8. Whirlpool bath for the affected extremity—to aid circulation, debride dead tissue, and help prevent infection.

9. Potential escharotomy (incision through the eschar)—to prevent further tissue damage, allow for normal circulation, and permit joint motion.

10. Potential fasciotomy (incision in fascia to release pressure on the muscles, nerves, blood vessels)—to treat compartment syndrome.

11. Encourage hourly active motion of the affected digits to promote maximum restoration of function and to prevent contractures.

12. Advise patient not to use tobacco because of the vasoconstrictive effects of nicotine, which further reduce the already deficient blood supply to injured tissues.

13. Perform serial laboratory testing (urinalysis, electrolytes, and serum enzymes) to monitor for the complications of rhabdomyolysis and subsequent renal failure.

Hypothermia

Hypothermia is a condition in which the core (internal) temperature of the body is less than 95°F (35°C) as a result of exposure to cold or a loss of thermoregulation. In response to a decreased core temperature, the body will attempt to produce or conserve more heat by (1) shivering, which produces heat through muscular activity; (2) peripheral vasoconstriction, to decrease heat loss; and (3) raising the basal metabolic rate. Hypothermia may be classified as mild, moderate, or severe.

 GERONTOLOGIC ALERT Older patients are at greater risk for hypothermia because of altered compensatory mechanisms.

Primary Assessment and Interventions

 NURSING ALERT Extreme caution should be used in moving or transporting hypothermia patients because of the increased risk of cardiac arrhythmias.

1. Assess airway and breathing.

a. Spontaneous respirations may be extremely slow and imperceptible.

b. Assist breathing and oxygenation with supplemental oxygen at 100% or a bag-valve-mask device.

c. If intubation is necessary, extreme caution should be used because ventricular fibrillation may be precipitated.

2. Assess circulation.

a. If the body temperature falls below 86°F (30°C), the heart sounds may not be audible even if the heart is still beating. Tissues conduct sound poorly at low temperatures.

b. BP readings may be extremely difficult to hear because cold tissue conducts sound waves poorly.

c. Pupil reflexes may be blocked by a decrease in cerebral blood flow, so the pupils may appear fixed and dilated.

d. A patient with severe hypothermia may present like a patient in cardiac arrest with fixed dilated pupils, no pulse or perfusing rhythm, and no BP. If there is any doubt about whether a pulse is present, begin CPR.

Subsequent Assessment

1. There is progressive deterioration marked by apathy, poor judgment, ataxia, dysarthria, drowsiness and, eventually, coma.

2. Speech is slow and may be slurred.

3. Shivering may be suppressed below a temperature of 90°F (32.2°C).

4. Cardiac dysrhythmias—cold disrupts the conduction system of the heart and a variety of dysrhythmias may be seen. A hypothermic heart is extremely susceptible to conduction delays. Ventricular fibrillation may occur if the temperature falls below 81°F (25°C). Patients with core temperatures below 86°F (30°C) do not respond to drugs or defibrillation.

5. The heartbeat and the BP may be so weak that the peripheral pulsations become undetectable. Always check a central pulse.

6. Urine output may increase in response to peripheral vasoconstriction—cold diuresis.

7. Initial tachypnea is usually followed by slow and shallow respirations, possibly two or three per minute in severe hypothermia.

General Interventions

The goal is to rewarm without precipitating cardiac dysrhythmias.

Supportive Measures

1. Handle the patient carefully and gently—to avoid triggering arrhythmias.

2. Continuously monitor core temperatures with a low-reading rectal thermometer.

3. Continuously monitor ECG and central pulses. Loss of a central pulse indicates a nonperfusing rhythm and the need for immediate CPR and ACLS interventions.
4. Monitor the patient's condition through vital signs, CVP, urine output, ABG values, and blood chemistry determinations.
5. Maintain an arterial line for recording BP and to facilitate blood sampling—allows rapid detection of acid–base disturbances and assessment of adequacy of ventilation and oxygenation.
6. Start IV therapy with warmed normal saline. Lactated Ringer solution is not recommended because the cold liver may not be able to metabolize the lactate.

Rewarming Techniques

The type of rewarming depends on the degree of hypothermia. Rewarming should continue until the core temperature is 93.2°F (34°C). Death in hypothermia is defined as a failure to revive after rewarming.

1. Passive external rewarming (mild hypothermia).
   a. Remove all the wet or cold clothing and replace with warm clothing.
   b. Provide insulation by wrapping the patient in several blankets.
   c. Provide warmed fluids to drink.
   d. Disadvantage: slow process.
2. Active external rewarming (moderate to severe hypothermia or hemodynamic instability).
   a. Provide external heat for the patient—warm hot water bottles to the armpits, neck, or groin. (Do not apply hot water bottles directly to the skin.)
   b. Warm water immersion.
   c. Disadvantages:
      i. Causes peripheral vasodilation, returning cool blood to the core, causing an initial lowering of the core temperature.
      ii. Acidosis because of the "washing out" of lactic acid from the peripheral tissues.
      iii. An increase in the metabolic demands before the heart is warmed to meet these needs.
      iv. A combination of active external rewarming and active core rewarming can be used to minimize rewarming shock.
3. Active core rewarming (severe hypothermia less than 82.4°F [less than 28°C]).
   a. Inhalation of warmed, humidified oxygen by mask or ventilator.
   b. Warmed IV fluids.
   c. Peritoneal dialysis with warmed standard dialysis solution.
   d. Mediastinal irrigation through open thoracotomy has been used successfully but has serious complications.
   e. Cardiopulmonary bypass.
   f. Disadvantage: invasiveness of the procedures.

TOXICOLOGIC EMERGENCIES

Toxicology is the study of the harmful effect of various substances on the body. Toxins are substances that are harmful to the body no matter how much or in what manner they enter the body. Drugs become toxic when they are taken in excess quantities or manners that are not therapeutic. Alcohol is considered a drug. The treatment goals of toxicological emergencies are, first, to support; second, to prevent or minimize absorption; and third, to provide an antidote.

Ingested Poisons

Ingested poisons can produce immediate or delayed effects. Immediate injury is caused when the poison is caustic to the body tissues (ie, a strong acid or a strong alkali). Other ingested poisons must be absorbed into the bloodstream before they become harmful. Ingested poisoning may be accidental or intentional.

Primary Assessment and Interventions

1. Maintain an open airway—some ingested substances may cause soft tissue swelling of the airway.
2. Attain control of the airway, ventilation, and oxygenation; in the absence of cerebral or renal damage, the patient's prognosis depends largely on successful management and support of vital functions.

Subsequent Assessment

1. Identify the poison.
   a. Try to determine the product taken: where, when, why, how much, who witnessed the event, and time since ingestion. Histories obtained from the patient are often inaccurate and should be confirmed if at all possible.
   b. Always contact the local poison control center for assistance in identifying the toxin, if unknown, treatment recommendations, and antidote information. In the United States, local poison control centers can all be reached by calling (800) 222-1222.
2. Continue the focused assessment, observing any significant deviations from normal. Different poisons will affect the body in different ways.
3. Obtain blood and urine tests for toxicology screening. Gastric contents may also be sent for toxicology screening in serious ingestions.
4. Monitor neurologic status, including mentation; monitor the course of vital signs and neurologic status over time.
5. Monitor for fluid and electrolyte imbalance.

General Interventions

Supportive Care

1. Assess and protect the patient's airway, as needed.
2. Administer oxygen and assist ventilations, as needed.
3. Monitor and treat shock.
4. Insert two large-bore IV lines.
5. Give supportive care to maintain vital organ systems.
6. Insert an indwelling urinary catheter to monitor renal function.
7. Support the patient having seizures; many poisons excite the CNS or the patient may convulse from oxygen deprivation.
8. Monitor and treat for complications: hypotension, coma, cardiac dysrhythmias, and seizures.
9. Psychiatric evaluations should be done after the patient is stabilized.

Minimizing Absorption

1. The primary method for preventing or minimizing absorption is to administer activated charcoal. Newer superactivated charcoals can reduce absorption of a toxic substance by as much as 50%. Administering activated charcoal alone is recommended. Insertion of a large-bore orogastric tube and gastric lavage are no longer recommended. The routine use of a cathartic in combination with activated charcoal is also no longer recommended.

a. Administration of premixed oral-activated charcoal adsorbs the poison on the surface of its particles and allows it to pass with the stool. Multiple doses may be administered.

b. A routine NG tube may be inserted to facilitate emptying of stomach contents (without lavage) within 30 minutes of ingestion or to instill charcoal if the patient is unable to drink the mixture.

 NURSING ALERT Contact your local poison control center for recommendations on giving charcoal. Do not give charcoal if the patient may not be able to maintain airway unless you have an artificial airway established.

2. Gastric lavage is contraindicated due to poor outcomes and complications.

3. Procedures to enhance the removal of the ingested substance if the patient is deteriorating.
   a. Forced diuresis with urine pH alteration—to enhance renal clearance.
   b. Hemoperfusion (process of passing blood through an extracorporeal circuit and a cartridge containing an adsorbent, such as charcoal, after which the detoxified blood is returned to patient).
   c. Hemodialysis—used in selected patients to purify blood and accelerate the elimination of circulating toxins.
   d. Repeated doses of charcoal—for binding nonabsorbed drugs/toxins.

NURSING ALERT Do not induce emesis after ingestion of caustic substances, hydrocarbons, iodides, silver nitrates, strychnine, or petroleum distillates, to a patient having seizures, or to pregnant patients.

Providing an Antidote

1. An antidote is a chemical or physiologic antagonist that will neutralize the poison.
2. Administer the specific antidote as early as possible to reverse or diminish effects of the toxin.
3. Repeated antidote doses may be necessary.
4. Follow the recommendations of your poison control center.

Carbon Monoxide Poisoning

Carbon monoxide poisoning is an example of an inhaled poison and is the result of the inhalation of the products of incomplete hydrocarbon combustion. It may occur as an industrial or household accident or as an attempted suicide. Carbon monoxide exerts its toxic effect by binding to circulating hemoglobin to reduce the oxygen-carrying capacity of the blood. The affinity between carbon monoxide and hemoglobin is 200 to 250 times more than between oxygen and hemoglobin. (Carbon monoxide combines with hemoglobin to form carboxyhemoglobin.) As a result, tissue anoxia occurs.

Primary Assessment

1. Assess airway and breathing. Assist with ventilations, as needed.
   a. Respiratory depression may be present.
   b. If the carbon monoxide poisoning is due to smoke inhalation, stridor (indicative of laryngeal edema because of thermal injury) may be present. Check for soot on the back of the hard palate or pharynx if smoke inhalation is suspected.

Primary Interventions

1. Provide 100% oxygen by tight-fitting mask. (The elimination half-life of carboxyhemoglobin, in serum, for a person breathing room air is 5 hours and 20 minutes. If the patient breathes 100% oxygen, the half-life is reduced to 80 minutes; 100% oxygen in a hyperbaric chamber will reduce the half-life to 23 minutes [treatment of choice].)
2. Intubate, if necessary, to protect the airway.

Subsequent Assessment

1. A thorough history is important: determine the type and length of exposure as well as possible other fumes inhaled. An underlying anemia, cardiac disease, or pulmonary disease may place a person at higher risk.
2. Determine LOC—the patient may appear intoxicated from cerebral hypoxia; confusion may progress rapidly to coma.
3. Assess complaints of headache, muscular weakness, palpitation, and dizziness.
4. Inspect the skin: may be pink, cherry red, or cyanotic and pale—skin color is not a reliable sign.
5. Monitor vital signs: increased respiratory and pulse rates are generally present. Be alert for altered breathing patterns and respiratory failure.
6. Listen for rales or wheezes in the lungs (with smoke inhalation, indicates acute respiratory distress syndrome).
7. Obtain arterial or venous blood samples for carboxyhemoglobin levels.
   a. Normal levels for a nonsmoking patient are less than 3%. For a patient who smokes one to two packs per day, 4% to 5%, and two or more packs per day, 8% to 10%.
   b. Toxic concentrations are considered to be greater than 20%.

General Interventions

1. History of exposure to carbon monoxide justifies immediate treatment.
2. Goals are to reverse cerebral and myocardial hypoxia and hasten carbon monoxide elimination.
3. Give 100% oxygen at atmospheric or hyperbaric pressures to reverse hypoxia and accelerate elimination of carbon monoxide. Patients should receive hyperbaric oxygen for CNS or cardiovascular system dysfunction.
4. Use continuous ECG monitoring, treat dysrhythmias, and correct acid–base and electrolyte abnormalities.
5. Observe the patient constantly—psychoses, spastic paralysis, vision disturbances, and deterioration of personality may persist after resuscitation and may be symptoms of permanent CNS damage.

Insect Stings

Insect stings or bites are injected poisons that can produce either local or systemic reactions. Local reactions are characterized by pain, erythema, and edema at the site of injury. Systemic reactions usually begin within minutes and produce mild to severe and life-threatening reactions.

Primary Assessment and Interventions

1. Assess airway, breathing, and circulation.
2. Anaphylactic reactions may produce unconsciousness, laryngeal edema, and cardiovascular collapse.

3. Epinephrine is the drug of choice—the amount and route depend on the severity of the reaction.
4. Administer a bronchodilator to help relieve the bronchospasm.
5. Initiate an IV line with lactated Ringer solution.
6. Prepare for CPR.

Subsequent Assessment

1. Obtain history of insect sting, previous exposure, and allergies.
2. Inspect the skin for local reaction—erythema, edema, and pain at site of injury—as well as generalized pruritus, urticaria, and angioedema.
3. Continue to monitor BP and respiratory status for dyspnea, wheezing, and stridor.

General Interventions

1. Apply ice packs to site to relieve pain.
2. Elevate extremity with large edematous local reaction.
3. Administer oral antihistamine for local reactions.
4. Clean the wound thoroughly with soap and water or an antiseptic solution.
5. Administer tetanus prophylaxis if not up to date.
6. Provide patient education.
   a. Always have epinephrine on hand.
   b. Wear medical emergency bracelets indicating hypersensitivity.
   c. Instructions when sting occurs:
      i. Take epinephrine immediately if stung.
      ii. Remove stinger with one quick scrape of fingernail.
      iii. Do not squeeze venom sac because this may cause additional venom to be injected.
      iv. Report to the nearest health care facility for observation.
   d. Avoid exposure and become desensitized.
      i. Avoid locales with stinging insects (camp and picnic sites).
      ii. Stay away from insect-feeding areas—flower beds, ripe fruit orchards, garbage, and fields of clover.
      iii. Avoid going barefoot outdoors—yellow jackets may nest on ground.
      iv. Avoid perfumes, scented soaps, and bright colors, which attract bees.
      v. Keep car windows closed.
      vi. Spray garbage cans with rapid-acting insecticide and keep areas meticulously clean.

Snakebites

The majority of snakes in the United States are not poisonous. The poisonous varieties are pit vipers (rattlesnakes and copperheads) and coral snakes. Bites by these snakes may result in envenomation, an injected poisoning. Other parts of the world have many snakes capable of lethal bites. Snakebites can cause neurotoxic muscle paralysis, coagulopathy, and hemolysis. Therefore, knowledge of snakes indigenous to your area is important for swift and appropriate treatment.

Primary Assessment and Interventions

1. Assess airway, breathing, and circulation.
2. Severe envenomation may lead to neurotoxicity with respiratory paralysis, shock, coma, and death.
3. Be prepared to resuscitate and provide advanced life support.

Subsequent Assessment

1. Get a description of the snake, the time of the snakebite, and the location of the bite. Bites to the head and trunk may progress more rapidly and be more severe.
   a. Pit vipers have triangular heads, vertical pupils, indentations between the eyes and nostrils, and long fangs.
   b. Coral snakes are small and brightly colored, with short fangs and teeth behind them and a series of bands of yellow, red, yellow, and black (in that order).
   c. Venom detection kits are available in some areas of the world such as Australia where venomous snakes are not uncommon. Specific antivenom may be available.
2. Assess for local reactions—burning, pain, swelling, and numbness at the site. Local reactions to coral snakebites may be delayed by several hours and may be very mild.
3. A few hours after the bite, hemorrhagic blisters may occur at the site and the entire extremity may become edematous.
4. Watch for signs of systemic reactions, including nausea, sweating, weakness, light-headedness, initial euphoria followed by drowsiness, difficulty in swallowing, paralysis of various muscle groups, signs of shock, seizures, and coma.
5. Monitor vital signs closely because tachycardia or bradycardia may develop.

 NURSING ALERT Patients will, on occasion, bring the snake that bit them into the emergency department for identification. Even dead, a snake can reflexively bite for several hours. Caution should be used to avoid becoming a second victim.

General Interventions

1. Keep the patient calm and at rest in a recumbent position with the affected extremity immobilized. Remove jewelry or other constricting items, as the area may become edematous.
2. Administer oxygen.
3. Start an IV line with normal saline or lactated Ringer solution.
4. Administer antivenin and be alert to allergic reaction.
5. Administer vasopressors in the treatment of shock.
6. Monitor for bleeding and administer blood products for coagulopathy.

Drug Intoxication

Substance abuse includes the use of specific substances that are intended to alter mood or behavior.

Drug abuse is the use of drugs for other than legitimate medical purposes. There is a growing tendency among drug users to take a variety of drugs simultaneously (polypharmacy abuse), including alcohol, sedatives, hypnotics, and marijuana, which may have addictive effects. The clinical manifestations may vary with the drug used (see Table 35-2), but the underlying principles of management are essentially the same.

Overdose refers to the toxic effects that occur when a drug is taken in a larger-than-normal dose.

Primary Assessment and Interventions

1. Assess airway, breathing, and circulation.
2. Attain control of the airway, ventilation, and oxygenation.
3. Intubate and provide assisted ventilation in patients with severe respiratory depression or in patients lacking gag or

Table 35-2   Specific Drug Overdose Presentations and Interventions

TYPE OF DRUG	PRESENTATION	INTERVENTIONS
CNS Stimulants		
• Amphetamines • Designer drugs (MDMA, ecstasy, ice, Eve, bath salts) • Cocaine (can be smoked in freebase or crack form, snorted, or injected)	Palpitations, feeling of impending doom, tachycardia, hypertension, dysrhythmia, myocardial ischemia or infarction, euphoria, agitation, combativeness, confusion, hallucinations, paranoia, aggressive or violent behavior, suicide attempts, hyperpyrexia, and seizures. When the drug wears off, depression, exhaustion, irritability, and sleeplessness.	• Secure airway, breathing, and circulation. • Monitor ECG and provide oxygen for ischemia. • Sedate, as necessary. • Administer antiarrhythmics for ventricular dysrhythmia. • Administer diazepam for seizures. • Closely monitor hemodynamic status and provide IV fluids, as indicated.
Hallucinogens		
• Lysergic acid diethylamide (LSD) • Phencyclidine HCl (PCP) • Mescaline • Psilocybin mushrooms • Jimson weed seeds • Salvia	Marked anxiety bordering on panic, confusion, incoherence, hyperactivity, hallucinations, hazardous behavior, convulsions, coma, circulatory collapse, and death. Flashbacks may occur months to years after initial drug use.	• Reduce sensory stimuli, encourage patient to keep eyes open, and stay with patient. • Monitor for hypertensive crisis and evidence of trauma. • Sedate if hyperactivity cannot be controlled and place patient in a protected environment.
Opioids		
• Heroin (may be cut with other ingredients in 20:1–200:1 ratios) • Morphine and its derivatives • Codeine and its derivatives	Hypotension, respiratory depression leading to apnea, miosis, and drowsiness progressing to stupor and coma.	• Administer naloxone 0.4–2 mg via IV line or by endotracheal tube (effective in 1–2 min). • Maintain an open airway but defer intubation until naloxone is given, if possible. • Monitor for reappearance of symptoms and readminister naloxone. • Protect the patient from harm (may be combative on awakening).
Sedatives		
• Barbiturates, such as amobarbital and secobarbital • Benzodiazepines, such as diazepam and flurazepam • Other sedative/hypnotics, such as chloral hydrate and glutethimide	Incoordination, ataxia, impaired thinking and speech, lethargy to coma, early miosis; later, fixed and dilated pupils, hypoventilation, hypotension, hypothermia, and decreased reflexes.	• Administer flumazenil to reverse or diminish effects of benzodiazepines. • Administer activated charcoal. • Protect the airway. • For hypotension, infuse with lactated Ringer solution and give vasopressors.
Alcohol		
Intoxication generally occurs with blood levels >100 mg/dL. Levels more than 400 mg/dL are due to rapid consumption of alcohol and represent a medical emergency.	Slurred speech, incoordination, ataxia, belligerent behavior progressing to stupor and coma, odor of alcohol on breath and clothing, and respiratory depression.	• Protect the airway. • Closely monitor for CNS and respiratory depression. • Draw blood for ethanol concentration, electrolytes, glucose, and drug screen, using nonalcohol skin cleanser. • Assess for head injury and other trauma, as well as organic disease. • Administer IV fluids, magnesium sulfate (to reduce risk of seizures), thiamine (to prevent Wernicke-Korsakoff syndrome), and glucose (to treat hypoglycemia).

CNS, central nervous system; ECG, electrocardiogram.

cough reflexes. If possible, intubation should be held off until a trial dose of naloxone is given.

4. Begin CPR in the absence of pulse.

Subsequent Assessment

1. Do a thorough physical examination to rule out insulin shock, meningitis, head injury, stroke, or trauma.
2. If the patient is unconscious, consider all possible causes of loss of consciousness.

3. Monitor LOC continuously.
4. Monitor vital signs frequently—some drugs will cause depressed vital signs; others will elevate the vital signs.
5. Monitor the pupils: extreme miosis (pinpoint pupils) may indicate opioid overdose.
6. Look for needle marks and external evidence of trauma.
7. Perform a rapid neurologic survey: level of responsiveness, pupil size and reactivity, reflexes, and focal neurologic findings; these can all give clues for identifying the drug taken.

8. Keep in mind that many drug abusers take multiple drugs simultaneously.
9. Be aware that there is a high incidence of human immunodeficiency virus (HIV), tuberculosis, and infectious hepatitis among drug users.
10. Examine the patient's breath for characteristic odor of alcohol, acetone, and so forth.
11. Try to obtain a history of drug experiences (from the person accompanying the patient or from the patient).

General Interventions

1. Goals:
   a. Support the respiratory and cardiovascular functions.
   b. Give definitive treatment for drug overdose, such as naloxone.
   c. Prevent further absorption, enhance drug elimination, and reduce its toxicity.
2. Measure ABGs for hypoxia because of hypoventilation or for acid–base derangements.
3. Continuously monitor ECG.
4. Draw blood samples for testing glucose, electrolytes, BUN, creatinine, and appropriate toxicology screen.
5. Initiate IV fluids.
6. Administer oxygen.
7. Pharmacologic interventions:
   a. Give specific drug antagonist if drug is known.
   b. Naloxone for CNS depression because of opioids.
   c. Dextrose 50% IV to rule out hypoglycemic coma.
8. If the drug was taken by mouth, the primary method for preventing or minimizing absorption is to administer activated charcoal. Multiple doses may be administered. A routine NG tube may be inserted to facilitate emptying of stomach contents (without lavage) within 30 minutes of ingestion, or charcoal may be instilled if the patient is unable to drink.
9. In unconscious or semiconscious patients who are or may be lacking gag or cough reflexes, use an NG tube only after intubation with cuffed endotracheal tube to prevent aspiration of charcoal stomach contents.
10. Take rectal temperature—extremes of thermoregulation (hyperthermia/hypothermia) must be recognized and treated.
11. Treat seizures with diazepam.
12. Assist with hemodialysis/peritoneal dialysis for potentially lethal poisoning.
13. Catheterize the patient because the drug or its metabolites are excreted in urine.
14. Do not leave the patient alone; there is a potential for the patient to harm self or ED staff.
15. Anticipate complications—sudden death from cerebral hypoxia, dysrhythmias, seizures, respiratory arrest, and MI.
16. Always suspect mixtures of medications and alcohol.

 DRUG ALERT Antidotes generally have a shorter half-life than the drugs they are used to treat. Repeated dosing is often necessary.

 NURSING ALERT Many drugs will not or cannot be detected in a standard toxicology screen. A negative drug screen does not mean an overdose is not the cause of the emergency.

Alcohol Withdrawal Delirium

Alcohol withdrawal delirium (*delirium tremens* or *alcoholic hallucinosis*) is an acute toxic state that follows a prolonged bout of steady drinking or sudden withdrawal from prolonged intake of alcohol. It may be precipitated by acute injury or infection. Symptoms can begin as early as 4 hours after a reduction of alcohol intake and usually peak at 24 to 48 hours, but may last up to 2 weeks.

 NURSING ALERT Alcohol withdrawal delirium is a serious complication of inadequate withdrawal management and is life-threatening.

Primary Assessment and Interventions

1. Patient may present alert, unless experiencing a seizure.
2. Ensure adequacy of airway, breathing, and circulation.

Subsequent Assessment

1. Assess for major symptoms—may occur independently or in combination.
   a. Nausea.
   b. Tremors.
   c. Paroxysmal sweating.
   d. Anxiety.
   e. Agitation.
   f. Headache.
   g. Mental status.
   h. Hallucinations (may be tactile, visual, or auditory).
2. Utilizing a standard Clinical Institute Withdrawal Assessment for Alcohol scale may assist in identifying those at risk for withdrawal problems and guide treatment. See Box 35-1.
   a. Each category is given a score and the total added. The cumulative score provides a basis for treatment. Generally, a score of 8 to 10 or greater is the threshold for treatment to alleviate symptoms and prevent seizures.
   b. Reassess frequently during the first 48 hours and discontinue treatment and assessments when three subsequent determinations have been below the threshold.
3. Obtain drinking history, including the severity of past withdrawal episodes and any recent drug intake. Be aware that people tend to underestimate drinking habits.
4. Perform a thorough examination for signs of autonomic hyperreactivity—tachycardia, diaphoresis, elevated temperature, and dilated but reactive pupils—as well as any coexisting illnesses or injuries (head injury, pneumonia, metabolic disturbances).
5. Observe behavior for talkativeness, restlessness, agitation, or preoccupation.

General Interventions

1. Protect the patient from injury. Not all patients have hallucinations; however, if they do, the hallucinations may be visual, tactile, or auditory and are frequently frightening. Seizures may also occur.
2. Using a nonalcoholic skin preparation, draw blood for measurement of ethanol concentration, toxicology screen for other drugs of abuse, and other tests, as directed.

BOX 35-1   Clinical Institute of Withdrawal from Alcohol Scale Revised (Ciwa-Ar)*

NAUSEA AND VOMITING
Ask: "Do you feel sick to your stomach? Have you vomited?"
0 = No nausea, no vomiting
1 = Mild nausea with no retching or vomiting
4 = Intermittent nausea with dry heaves
7 = Constant nausea, frequent dry heaves, and/or vomiting

TACTILE DISTURBANCES
Ask, "Have you any itching, pins-and-needles sensation, burning or numbness, or do you feel bugs crawling on or under your skin?"
0 = None
1 = Very mild
2 = Mild
3 = Moderate
4 = Moderately severe hallucinations
5 = Severe hallucinations
6 = Extremely severe hallucinations
7 = Continuous hallucinations

TREMOR
Arms extended and fingers spread apart.
0 = No tremor
1 = Not visible, but can be felt fingertip to fingertip
4 = Moderate with patients arm extended
7 = Severe, even with arms not extended

AUDITORY DISTURBANCES
Ask, "Are you more aware of the sounds around you? Are they harsh? Do they frighten you? Are you hearing anything disturbing? Are you hearing things you know are not there?"
0 = Not present hallucinations
1 = Very mild
2 = Mild
3 = Moderate
4 = Moderately severe
5 = severe hallucinations
6 = Extremely severe hallucinations
7 = Continuous hallucinations

SWEATING
0 = No sweat visible
1 = Barely perceptible sweating, palms moist
4 = Beads of sweat obvious on the forehead
7 = Drenching sweat over the face and chest

VISUAL DISTURBANCES
Ask, "Does the light appear to be too bright? Is its color different? Does it hurt your eyes? Are you seeing anything disturbing to you? Are you seeing things you know are not there?"
0 = Not present
1 = Very mild
2 = Mild
3 = Moderate
4 = Moderately severe
5 = Severe hallucinations
6 = Extremely severe hallucinations
7 = Continuous hallucinations

ANXIETY
Ask, "Do you feel nervous?"
0 = No anxiety, at ease
1 = Mildly anxious
4 = Moderately anxious or guarded, so anxiety is inferred
7 = Equivalent to acute panic states, as seen in severe delirium or acute schizophrenic reaction

HEADACHE, FULLNESS IN HEAD
Ask, "Does your head feel different? Does it feel like there is a band around your head?" Do not rate dizziness or lightheadedness. Otherwise, rate severity.
0 = Not present
1 = Very mild
2 = Mild
3 = Moderate
4 = Moderately severe
5 = Severe
6 = Very severe
7 = Extremely severe

AGITATION
0 = Normal activity
1 = Somewhat more than normal activity (may move legs up and down, shift position occasionally)
4 = Moderately fidgety and restless, shifting position frequently
7 = Paces back and forth or constantly thrashes about

ORIENTATION AND CLOUDING OF SENSORIUM
Ask, "What day is this? Where are you? Who am I?"
0 = Oriented and can do serial additions
1 = Cannot do serial additions or is uncertain about date
2 = Disoriented for date by no more than 2 calendar days
3 = Disoriented for date by more than 2 calendar days
4 = Disoriented for place and/or person

*Assessment is made in each category and cumulative score is used to determine treatment (institutional protocols vary).
From Sullivan, J. T., Sykora, K., Schneiderman, J., et al. (1989). Assessment of alcohol withdrawal: The revised Clinical Institute Withdrawal Assessment for Alcohol scale (CIWA-Ar). British Journal of Addiction, 84(11), 1373–1357.

3. Pharmacologic interventions:
   a. Diazepam or chlordiazepoxide for sedation. Sedate the patient with sufficient dosage of medication to produce adequate relaxation and to reduce agitation, prevent exhaustion, and promote sleep without compromising airway.
   b. Diazepam or phenytoin for seizure control.
4. Monitor vital signs every 30 minutes.
5. Maintain close observation.
6. Maintain electrolyte balance and hydration through oral or IV route—fluid losses may be extreme because of profuse perspiration, vomiting, and agitation.
7. Assess respiratory, hepatic, and cardiovascular status of patient—pneumonia, liver disease, and cardiac failure are complications.
8. Observe for hypoglycemia and treat appropriately. Hypoglycemia may accompany alcoholic withdrawal because alcohol depletes liver glycogen stores and impairs gluconeogenesis; many patients also suffer from malnutrition.
   a. Administration of thiamine is common.

BEHAVIORAL EMERGENCIES

A *behavioral emergency* is an urgent, serious disturbance of behavior, affect, or thought that makes the patient unable to cope with his or her life situation and interpersonal relationships. A patient presenting with a psychiatric emergency may be overactive or violent, depressed, or suicidal.

Violent Patients

Violent and aggressive behavior is usually episodic and is a means of expressing feelings of anger, fear, or hopelessness about a situation.

Assessment

1. Assess for overactivity, aggression, or anger out of proportion to the circumstances.
2. Determine risk factors for violence, including:
   a. Intoxicated with drugs/alcohol.
   b. Going through drug or alcohol withdrawal.
   c. Acute paranoid schizophrenic states, acute organic brain syndrome, acute psychosis, paranoia, or borderline personality.
3. Obtain psychiatric assessment.

General Interventions

1. Goals are to bring violence under control and protect patient and staff from harm.
2. Establish control.
   a. Keep room door open, and be in clear view of the staff. Always leave a clear exit pathway. Never allow the patient to be between you and safety.
   b. Help the patient bring violence under control.
      i. Give patient space; do not make sudden moves.
      ii. Avoid touching agitated patients or standing close.
      iii. Ask if the patient has a weapon; request that it be placed in a neutral area.
      iv. If the patient will not surrender weapon, leave the room and allow security personnel/police to handle the situation.
   c. Try not to leave the patient alone unless your safety is in jeopardy; this may be interpreted as rejection or the patient may try to harm self.

   d. Adopt a calm nonconfrontational approach and remain in control of the situation. External calm and structure may help the patient gain control.
   e. Give the patient choices and options about treatments or timing of events if at all possible.
3. Provide emotional support.
   a. Talk and listen to the patient.
   b. Crisis intervention is best done with an attitude of interest in the patient's well-being and with an attempt to "tune in" to the patient while remaining firm.
   c. Acknowledge the patient's state of agitation (eg, "I want to work with you to relieve your distress").
   d. Give the patient the opportunity to ventilate anger verbally; avoid challenging the delusional state.
   e. Try to hear what the patient is saying.
   f. Convey the expectation of appropriate behavior and make the patient aware that help is available for him or her to gain control.
   g. Administer prescribed medications to reduce anxiety and hyperactivity, if verbal management techniques fail to attenuate the patient's tension.
4. Secure assistance.
   a. Allow security personnel/police to intervene if patient does not become calm.
   b. Use of a dedicated safe room is encouraged. The room should be free of cords, cables, or any object capable of being used as a weapon and be easily seen by staff. Shatterproof windows and/or cameras are encouraged. Use restraints when absolutely necessary and per the facility's policy.
   c. Have a specific plan and enough well-trained personnel available when applying restraints; if patient is intoxicated, restrain in a left lateral position and monitor closely for aspiration.
   d. Talk reassuringly while applying restraints; use empathic and supportive verbal interactions.
   e. Monitor patient continuously after restraints are applied; check circulation of restrained extremities.

Depression

Depression may be seen as the presenting condition at the health care facility or may be masked by the presentation of anxiety and somatic complaints.

Assessment

1. Observe for sadness, apathy, feelings of worthlessness, self-blame, suicidal thoughts, desire to escape, worsening of mood in morning, anorexia, weight loss, sleeplessness, lessening interest in sex, reduction of activity, or ceaseless activity.
2. The agitated, depressed person may exhibit motor restlessness and severe anxiety.

General Interventions

1. Listen to the patient in a calm, unhurried manner.
2. The patient will benefit from ventilation of feelings.
3. Give the patient an opportunity to talk about problems.
4. Anticipate that the patient may be suicidal.
5. Attempt to find out if the patient has thought about or attempted suicide and the lethality of the suicide plan.
   a. "Have you ever thought about taking your own life?"
   b. The patient is generally relieved because of the opportunity to discuss feelings.
6. Find out if there is an illness, perceived or real.

7. Assess whether there has been sudden worsening of depression.
8. Notify relatives about a seriously depressed patient. Do not leave the patient alone because suicide is usually an act committed in solitude.
9. Give antidepressant and antianxiety agents, as prescribed.
10. Point out to the patient that depression is treatable.
11. Be aware of crisis and supportive services in the community: telephone counseling and referral, suicide prevention centers, group therapy, marital and family counseling, drug/alcohol counseling, adolescent counseling, or befriending programs.
12. Refer for psychiatric consultation or to psychiatric unit.

Suicide Ideation

According to the Centers for Disease Control and Prevention (CDC), suicide is the 11th leading cause of death in the United States and the third most common cause of death in young people.

Assessment

1. Assess for risk factors:
   a. Associated psychiatric illness (affective disorders and substance abuse in adults; conduct disorders and depression in young people).
   b. Personality traits, such as aggression, impulsivity, depression, hopelessness, borderline personality disorder, or antisocial personality.
   c. Persons who have experienced early loss, decreased social support, chronic illness, or recent divorce.
   d. Genetic and familial factors: family history of suicide, certain psychiatric disorders or alcoholism, alcohol and substance abuse.
2. Determine whether patient has communicated suicidal intent, such as preoccupation with death or talking about someone else's suicide.
3. Determine whether patient has ever attempted suicide—the risk is much greater in these people.
4. Determine whether there is a specific plan for suicide and a means to carry out the plan.

General Interventions

1. Treat the consequences of the suicide attempt, if one has been made.
2. After the patient has been stabilized, or if there was no active attempt made, use crisis intervention (a form of brief psychotherapy) to determine suicide potential, discover areas of depression and conflict, find out about the patient's support system, and determine whether hospitalization, psychiatric referral, and so forth are warranted.
3. Prevent further self-injury—a patient who has made a suicide gesture may do so again.
4. Admit to ICU (if condition warrants), arrange follow-up care, or admit to psychiatric unit, depending on assessment of suicide potential.

SEXUAL ASSAULT
Rape

Rape is defined as any kind of penetration of another person, without her or his consent. This definition includes men and women, as well as the use of objects, rather than just body parts. Lack of consent is the key. *Lack of consent* can imply either force or the incapacity or inability to consent. Children, mentally handicapped

individuals, and persons who are intoxicated or drugged are all considered unable to consent to sexual acts.

 NURSING ALERT The management of the sexual assault is important, but immediate physical health should be ensured first. A complete primary and focused assessment should take place, being alert for signs of internal hemorrhage, shock, or respiratory distress. If the victim has suffered trauma in the form of physical assault (eg, head or abdominal trauma), the trauma should be managed in the order of established priorities.

Assessment
Initiating a Supportive Relationship

1. The manner in which the patient is received and treated in the ED is important to her or his future psychological well-being. Many areas have sexual assault nurse examiners. These nurses have specialized education and clinical experience to prepare them for forensic examination of sexual assault victims. Some areas of the country have a designated center for treatment of sexual assault victims. If this is true in your area, the patient should have any life-threatening injuries stabilized and then be transferred to the dedicated facility for examination.
   a. Call a rape crisis intervention counselor (if available), who will meet the patient/family in the ED.
   b. Do not leave patient alone. Accept the emotional reactions of the patient (hysteria, stoicism, overwhelmed feeling, etc.).
2. Emotional trauma may be present for weeks, months, or years. Patients may experience complex posttraumatic stress disorder or rape trauma syndrome. Patients may go through phases of psychological reactions:
   a. Acute phase (disorganization)—shock, disbelief, fear, anxiety, guilt, humiliation, and suppression of feelings—may be for a few days to several weeks.
   b. Outward adjustment phase—victim resumes what appears to be a normal life but internally faces continued turmoil, manifested as fear, flashbacks, sleep disturbances, hyperalertness, and psychosomatic reactions.
   c. Resolution phase—the rape is no longer the central focus of the victim's life and she or he is able to move on from the incident.

Interviewing the Patient

1. Consent should be obtained for the examination, the collecting of cultures/evidence, and for release of information to law enforcement agencies.
2. Record history of event in the patient's own words.
3. Ask if the patient has bathed, douched, gargled or brushed teeth, changed clothes, or urinated or defecated since attack—may alter interpretation of subsequent findings.
4. Record time of admission, time of examination, date and time of sexual assault, and the general appearance of the patient.
   a. Document any evidence of trauma—discoloration, bruises, lacerations, secretions, and torn and bloody clothing.
   b. Record emotional state.

 NURSING ALERT Most EDs have commercially prepared rape evidence collection kits as well as written protocols for treatment of injuries, legal documentation, prevention of sexually transmitted infection (STI), HIV testing and postexposure prophylaxis, and pregnancy prevention. Remember that the evidence collection kit is meant to preserve forensic evidence.

Interventions

Preparing for Physical Examination

1. Assist the patient to undress over a sheet/large piece of paper to obtain debris.
2. Place each item of clothing in a separate paper bag (plastic bags promote moisture retention, which may lead to formation of mold and mildew, which can destroy evidence).
3. Label bags appropriately; give to appropriate law enforcement authority.
4. Advise the patient of the nature and necessity of each procedure; give the rationale for each question asked.

Physical Examination

1. Examine the patient (from head to toe) for injuries, especially to the head, neck, breasts, thighs, back, and buttocks.
2. Assess for external evidence of trauma (bruises, contusions, lacerations, stab wounds).
3. Assess for dried semen stains (appearing as crusted, flaking areas) on the patient's body.
4. Inspect fingers for broken nails and tissue and foreign materials under nails. Obtain scrapings or clippings of fingernails.
   a. Conduct an oral examination looking for any contusions and petechiae, and obtain swabs for DNA testing.
5. Document evidence of trauma with body diagrams and photographs if available.

Pelvic and Rectal Examinations

1. Examine the perineum and thighs with an ultraviolet light (Wood lamp) if available. Areas that are found to fluoresce may indicate semen stains. Urine and other stains may also fluoresce.
2. Note color and consistency of any discharge present.
3. Examine external vaginal area and rectum for any bleeding, contusion, ecchymosis, erythema, lacerations, scars, or any other injuries or abnormalities.
4. Use water-moistened vaginal speculum for examination; do not use lubricant (contains chemicals that may interfere with later forensic testing of specimens and acid phosphatase determinations).

Obtaining Laboratory Specimens

1. Obtain separate swabs from the oral, labial, vaginal, and anal areas.
2. Obtain swabs of body orifices for gonorrhea and chlamydia testing, or send a urine sample to test for gonorrhea, chlamydia, and trichomonas if the facility has that testing capability.
3. Comb and trim areas of pubic hair suspected of containing semen; obtain several pubic hairs with follicles; place in separate containers and identify these as patient's pubic hairs.
4. Obtain blood sample for syphilis and hepatities B and C, and offer the patient HIV testing.
5. Collect foreign material or debris (leaves, grass, dirt, loose hair, string) and place in appropriate container.
6. Conduct a pregnancy test on all females of child-bearing capability.
7. Label all specimens with name of patient, date, time of collection, body area from which specimen was obtained, and names of personnel collecting specimens to preserve chain of evidence; give to designated person (eg, crime laboratory), and document who you gave the collected evidence to in the medical record.
8. Photographs, if taken, should be preserved according to facility policy.

Other Interventions

1. Treat physical trauma as with any patient.
2. Offer the patient treatment for STIs, pregnancy prevention, and HIV postexposure prophylaxis. CDC recommendations for prophylactic treatment following a sexual assault are: Ceftriaxone 250 mg IM in a single dose.
   plus
   Metronidazole 2 g by mouth (PO) in a single dose.
   plus
   Azithromycin 1 g PO in a single dose *or* doxycycline 100 mg PO twice per day for 7 days.
3. Protect patient against pregnancy.
   a. It is important to determine whether pregnancy existed before the attack.
   b. Negative pregnancy test should be obtained before administering postcoital therapy.
   c. Hormonal treatment to prevent pregnancy—morning-after pill, as indicated, with patient's consent.
4. Provide the patient with cleansing facilities, including a cleansing douche, shower, and mouthwash after forensic exam is completed.

Providing for Follow-Up Services

1. Ensure the patient has follow-up for results of her STI cultures, HIV test, and any other lab testing that was done.
2. Ensure the patient has follow-up with counseling services. This is imperative to prevent long-term psychological effects of the assault. Families of the victim may need counseling services as well. Stress to the patient the importance of postassault counseling to return to her previous level of functioning.
3. Provide support to the patient in her decision to involve law enforcement.
4. Ensure a safety plan for the patient prior to discharge. The patient should be accompanied by a family member or friend when leaving the health care facility.

BIOLOGICAL WEAPONS AND PREPAREDNESS

Following the September 11, 2001, terrorist attacks on the United States, bioterrorism has become a real possibility. As frontline responders, emergency nurses must be aware of possible acts of bioterrorism and be familiar with their facilities' policies regarding such emergencies.

Biological Agents

Terrorism may consist of the intentional release of a chemical, biological, radiological, nuclear, or explosive device intended to cause widespread illness or death. Explosive devices tend to announce themselves rather quickly and definitively. Bioterrorism, however, can have a slow, insidious onset, leaving the population with little idea they have been the victim of an attack. The emergency nurse should be on the alert for possible signs of terrorism:

1. Large numbers of people with similar disease.
2. Cases of unexplained illness or death.
3. More severe illness than would normally be expected for a specific pathogen.
4. An illness that is resistant to usual treatment.
5. Unusual routes of exposure for a specific pathogen.
6. Disease that is unusual for an area.
7. A single case of unusual disease (smallpox, hemorrhagic fever).
8. Disease unusual for an age group.

Table 35-3   Potential Biological Weapons

AGENT AND METHOD OF TRANSMISSION	CLINICAL MANIFESTATIONS	MANAGEMENT
Smallpox		
Transmitted by inhalation or direct contact with the variola virus; has a 2-week incubation period.	High fever, fatigue, muscle aches, and rash that progresses to blisters after 3 days. The rash first develops on the face and around the wrists and then spreads to the trunk. Smallpox lesions progress at the same rate, unlike lesions of chickenpox, which may be seen in various stages of progression.	The patient should be isolated (preferably at home) until all of the scabs have fallen off. Management includes IV hydration. Health care providers should use masks, gowns, and gloves when caring for these patients and should receive smallpox vaccination within 2–3 days of exposure. Persons who have had contact with the patient should be isolated for 17 days.
Anthrax		
Transmitted through consumption of contaminated animal products, ingestion of raw meat, or inhalation of airborne spores of *Bacillus anthracis*, a gram-positive, spore-forming bacterium. The incubation period is 1–6 days.	Fever, fatigue, cough, chest discomfort, widened mediastinum on chest x-ray, and respiratory distress	Ensure that standard precautions are observed and that all surfaces are disinfected. Persons who have had contact with the patient should be started on the vaccine schedule and treated with ciprofloxacin or doxycycline.
Pneumonic Plague		
Transmitted by inhalation of *Yersinia pestis*. The incubation period is 2–6 days.	Fever, headache, weakness, and upper respiratory symptoms often including hemoptysis.	Treatment must begin within 24 hours and should include gentamicin or streptomycin drug. Isolate the patient for 48 hours after antibiotics are started. Postexposure prophylaxis consists of tetracycline or doxycycline for 7 days.
Botulism		
Transmitted primarily by ingestion of food contaminated with a preformed toxin produced by *Clostridium botulinum*. An inhalation form has been developed specifically as a biological agent.	Blurred or double vision, slurred speech, nausea, vomiting, diarrhea, and descending muscle weakness.	An antitoxin is effective if used early in the disease. Standard precautions are satisfactory; botulism is not contagious.

See Table 35-3 for specific agents of bioterrorism, such as smallpox, anthrax, plague, and botulism.

For additional information regarding bioterrorism, consult the following web site:

- Center for Disease Control and Prevention, Emergency Preparedness and Response *https://emergency.cdc.gov/bioterrorism/prep.asp*.

SELECTED REFERENCES

American Heart Association. (2015). *ACLS provider manual 2015*. Dallas, TX: Author.

Arrich, J., Holzer, M., Havel, C., et al. (2012). Hypothermia for neuroprotection in adults after cardiopulmonary resuscitation (Review). *The Cochrane Library*, CD004128.pub3.

Carleo, S. & Vallejos, B. S. (2016). Sepsis: The medicine, claims and defenses. *The Journal of Legal Nurse Consulting, 27*(3), 22–30.

Chernyak, V., Patlas, M., Menias, C., et al. (2015). Traumatic and non-traumatic adrenal emergencies. *Emergency Radiology, 22*(6), 697–704.

Emergency Nurses Association. (2017). *Emergency nursing core curriculum* (7th ed.). Philadelphia, PA: W.B. Saunders.

Emergency Nurses Association. (2014). *Trauma nursing core course* (7th ed.). Des Plaines, IL: Author.

Guidelines 2015/CPR and ECC. (2015). *Channing Bete Company, South Deerfield, MA.*

Makic, M.B., Bridges, E. (2018). Managing sepsis and septic shock current guidelines and definitions. *American Journal of Nursing, 118*(2), 34–39.

Mathiesen, C., McPherson, D., Ordway, C., & Smith, M. (2015). Caring for patients treated with therapeutic hypothermia. *Critical Care Nurse, 35*(5), e1–e12.

Mitchell, C. (2016). Tissue oxygenation monitoring as a guide for trauma resuscitation. *Critical Care Nurse, 36*(3), 12–19.

Sullivan, J. T., Sykora, K., Schneiderman, J., et al. (1989). Assessment of alcohol withdrawal: The revised Clinical Institute Withdrawal Assessment for Alcohol scale (CIWA-Ar). *British Journal of Addiction, 84*(11), 1373–1357.

Zhan, L., Yang, L., Huang, Y. et al. (2017). Continuous chest cmpressions vs. interrupted chest compressions for cardiopulmonary resuscitation of non-asphyxial out of hospital cardiac arrest. *Cochrane Database of Systematic Reviews* 2017; 3: CD010134.

Maternal and Fetal Health

PART THREE

MATERNITY AND NEONATAL NURSING

36

Maternal and Fetal Health

INTRODUCTION TO MATERNITY NURSING

According to the World Health Organization (WHO), social determinants of health (SDH) directly impact maternal-fetal outcomes. The nurse today faces many evolving challenges to achieve positive birth outcomes. In addition to health concerns during pregnancy, pregnancies with existing health conditions including diabetes and hypertension, lifestyle factors such as substance abuse, late or no prenatal care, and those occurring at extreme ages of reproductive life face unique complications. Furthermore, advances in assisted reproductive technologies (ART) have afforded people opportunities once thought impossible; however, they may experience additional inherent risks. Today's child-bearing families have many options. Childbirth may take place in the traditional hospital setting, a birthing center, or at home. Primary care provider includes physicians, certified registered nurse midwives, or lay midwives. Birth-related choices commonly include the use of labor, delivery, and recovery rooms or labor, delivery, recovery, and postpartum rooms; various birthing positions and analgesic methods; alternative pain-relief strategies such as hydrotherapy; and the decision to allow children and others to be present during labor and delivery. Regionalization of obstetric services has provided child-bearing families with access to the technologic advances and skilled personnel capable of managing pregnancy or neonatal complications. The combination of advancing technology, pregnancy risk factors, and changing economics because of the rising cost of health care challenges the nurse to be proficient in areas of neonatal resuscitation, external fetal monitoring, assessment, and interprofessional communication.

 EVIDENCE BASE National Institutes of Health. (2017). What are the factors that put a pregnancy at risk? Bethesda, MD: Author.
World Health Organization. (2017). Social determinants of health. Geneva, Switzerland: Author.

Terminology Used in Maternity Nursing

1. Gestation—pregnancy or maternal condition of having a developing fetus in the body.
2. Embryo—human conceptus up to the 10th week of gestation (8th week postconception).
3. Fetus—human conceptus from 10th week of gestation (8th week postconception) until delivery.

4. Periviability—alternately termed the limit of viability; is considered the stage of fetal maturity needed for extrauterine survival between 20 0/7 and 25 6/7 weeks gestation.

 EVIDENCE BASE American College of Obstetricians and Gynecologists and Society for Fetal Medicine. (2016). *Periviable birth: Obstetric care consensus.* Washington, DC: ACOG.

5. Gravida (G)—woman who is or has been pregnant, regardless of pregnancy outcome.
6. Nulligravida—woman who is not now and never has been pregnant.
7. Primigravida—woman pregnant for the first time.
8. Multigravida—woman who has been pregnant more than once.
9. Para (P)—refers to past pregnancies that have reached viability.
10. Nullipara—woman who has never completed a pregnancy to the period of viability. The woman may or may not have experienced an abortion.
11. Primipara—woman who has completed one pregnancy to the period of viability regardless of the number of infants delivered and regardless of the infant being live or stillborn.
12. Multipara—woman who has completed two or more pregnancies to the stage of viability.
13. Living children—refers to the number of children a woman has delivered who are living.

A woman who is pregnant for the first time is a primigravida and described as gravida 1 para 0 (or G1P0). A woman who delivered one fetus carried to the period of viability and who is pregnant again is described as gravida 2, para 1. A woman with two pregnancies ending in abortions and no viable children is gravida 2, para 0.

Obstetric History

TPAL

In some obstetric services, a woman's obstetric history is summarized by a series of four digits, such as 5-0-2-5. These digits correspond with the abbreviation TPAL.

1. **T**—represents full-term deliveries, 37 completed weeks or more.
2. **P**—represents preterm deliveries, 20 to less than 37 completed weeks.

3. **A**—represents abortions, elective or spontaneous loss (miscarriage) of a pregnancy before the period of viability.
4. **L**—represents the number of children living. If a child has died, further explanation is needed for clarification.
5. If, for example, a particular woman's history is summarized as G7, P5-0-2-5, then she has been pregnant seven times and had five term deliveries, zero preterm deliveries, two abortions, and five living children.

GTPALM

In some institutions, a woman's obstetric history can also be summarized as GTPALM, especially when multiple gestations or births are involved.
1. **G**—represents gravida.
2. **T**—represents full-term deliveries, 37 completed weeks or more.
3. **P**—represents preterm deliveries, 20 to less than 37 completed weeks.
4. **A**—represents abortions, elective or spontaneous loss of a pregnancy before the period of viability.
5. **L**—represents the number of children living. If a child has died, further explanation is needed for clarification.
6. **M**—represents the number of multiple gestations and births (not the number of neonates delivered).

If, for example, a particular woman's history is summarized as G5, P5-0-0-6-1, then she has been pregnant five times and had five term deliveries, zero preterm deliveries, zero abortions, six living children, and one multiple gestation/birth.

THE EXPECTANT MOTHER

 EVIDENCE BASE Records, K., & Tanaka, L. (2016). Physiology of pregnancy. In S. Mattson & J. E. Smith (Eds.), *Core curriculum for maternal–newborn nursing* (5th ed., pp. 83–107). St. Louis, MO: Saunders Elsevier.
Blackburn, S. T. (2014). Physiologic changes of pregnancy. In K. R. Simpson & P. A. Creehan (Eds.), *AWHONN's perinatal nursing* (4th ed., pp. 71–88). Philadelphia PA: Wolters, Kluwer|Lippincott.

Manifestations of Pregnancy

Pregnancy may be determined by the cessation of menses, enlargement of the uterus, ultrasound, and/or a positive human chorionic gonadotropin (hCG) test. These and the many other manifestations of pregnancy are classified into three groups: presumptive, probable, and positive.

Presumptive Signs and Symptoms

Physical signs and symptoms that suggest, but do not prove, pregnancy.
1. Abrupt cessation of menses—pregnancy is suspected if more than 10 days have elapsed since the time of the expected onset in a healthy woman who previously had predictable menstrual periods.
2. Breast changes:
   a. Breasts enlarge and become tender. Veins in breasts become increasingly visible.
   b. Nipples become larger and more pigmented. Nipple tingling may also be present.
   c. Colostrum—a thin, milky fluid—may be expressed in the second half of pregnancy.
   d. Montgomery glands—small elevations on the areolae—may appear.
3. Skin pigmentation changes:
   a. Chloasma or melasma gravidarum (the mask of pregnancy)—brownish pigmentation appearing on the face in a butterfly pattern in 50% to 70% of women that is progressive throughout the pregnancy; usually symmetric and distributed on the forehead, cheeks, and nose; more common in dark-haired, brown-eyed women.
   b. Linea nigra—dark vertical line on the abdomen between the sternum and the symphysis pubis.
   c. Striae gravidarum (stretch marks)—reddish or purplish linear markings sometimes appearing on the breasts, abdomen, and buttocks, because of the stretching, rupture, and atrophy of the deep connective tissue of the skin.
4. Nausea (morning sickness)—with or without vomiting occurs mainly in the morning but may occur at any time of the day, lasting a few hours. Begins between 2 and 6 weeks after conception and usually disappears spontaneously near the end of the first trimester (12 weeks).
5. Urinary frequency:
   a. Caused by pressure of the expanding uterus on the bladder.
   b. Decreases when the uterus rises out of the pelvis (around 12 weeks).
   c. Reappears when the fetal head engages in the pelvis at the end of pregnancy.
6. Constipation—because of the decreased absorption of fluid by the gut.
7. Fatigue—characteristic of early pregnancy in response to increased hormonal levels.

Probable Signs and Symptoms

Objective findings detected by 12 to 16 weeks of gestation.
1. Enlargement of abdomen—at about 12 weeks gestation, the uterus can be felt through the abdominal wall, just above the symphysis pubis.
2. Uterine changes:
   a. Uterus enlarges, elongates, and decreases in thickness as pregnancy progresses. The uterus changes from a pear shape to a globe shape.
   b. Hegar sign—lower uterine segment softens 6 to 8 weeks after the onset of the last menstrual period.
3. Cervical changes:
   a. Chadwick sign—bluish or purplish discoloration of cervix and vaginal wall.
   b. Goodell sign—softening of the cervix; may occur as early as 4 weeks.
   c. With inflammation and carcinoma during pregnancy, the cervix may remain firm.
4. Braxton-Hicks contractions—intermittent contractions of the uterus generally painless, palpable contractions occurring at irregular intervals, more frequently felt after 28 weeks. They usually disappear with walking or exercise.
5. Ballottement—sinking and rebounding of the fetus in its surrounding amniotic fluid in response to a sudden tap on the uterus (occurs near midpregnancy).
6. Leukorrhea—increase in vaginal discharge.

7. Quickening—the sensations of fetal movement in the abdomen occurring between the 16th and 20th week after the onset of the last menses.
8. Positive hCG—laboratory (urine or serum) test for pregnancy.

Positive Signs and Symptoms

Diagnostic of Pregnancy
1. Fetal heart tones (FHTs)—usually heard between 16th and 20th week of gestation with a fetoscope or the 10th and 12th week of gestation with a Doppler stethoscope.
2. Fetal movements felt by the examiner (after about 20 weeks gestation).
3. Outlining of the fetal body through the maternal abdomen in the second half of pregnancy with Leopold maneuvers.
4. Sonographic evidence (after 4 weeks gestation) using vaginal ultrasound. Fetal cardiac motion can be detected by 6 weeks gestation.

Maternal Physiology During Pregnancy

Duration of Pregnancy
1. Averages 280 days or 40 weeks (10 lunar months, 9 calendar months) from the first day of the last normal menses.
2. Duration may also be divided into three equal parts, or trimesters, of slightly more than 13 weeks or 3 calendar months each.
3. Estimated date of confinement (EDC), more commonly referred to now as estimated date of delivery (EDD), is calculated by adding 7 days to the date of the first day of the last menses and counting back 3 months (Nägele rule). Additionally, most antenatal clinics have obstetric wheels where the outer wheel has markings for the calendar and an inner, sliding wheel with weeks and days of gestation. These wheels facilitate the estimation of gestational age (GA) and the calculation of the EDD. The accuracy of these wheels may vary.
   a. For example, if a woman's last menstrual period (LMP) began on September 10, 2018, her EDC would be June 17, 2019. The calculation would start with September 10, 2018, plus 7 days (September 17, 2018), minus 3 months (June 17, 2018). If the date of the woman's LMP begins after March 31, an additional year must be added to give a correct EDD.
   b. Another method of calculating the EDD is McDonald rule: after 24 weeks gestation, the fundal height measurement will correspond to the week of gestation plus 2 to 4 weeks.
   c. EDD can also be calculated using ultrasound technology, which is the most accurate assessment—preferably in the first trimester. Gestational age in the first trimester is usually calculated from the fetal crown–rump length (CRL). This is the longest demonstrable length of the embryo or fetus, excluding the limbs and the yolk sac. The correlation between CRL and GA is excellent until about 12 weeks gestation, and the estimate has a 95% confidence interval of plus or minus 6 days.

Reproductive Tract Changes

Uterus
1. Enlargement during pregnancy involves stretching and marked hypertrophy of existing muscle cells secondary to increased estrogen and progesterone levels.
2. In addition to an increase in the size of the uterine muscle cells, there is an increase in fibrous tissue and elastic tissue. The size and number of blood vessels and lymphatics increase.
3. Enlargement and thickening of the uterine wall are most marked in the fundus.
4. By the end of the 3rd month (12 weeks), the uterus is too large to be contained wholly within the pelvic cavity—it can now be palpated suprapubically.
5. As the uterus rises out of the pelvis, it rotates somewhat to the right because of the presence of the rectosigmoid colon on the left side of the pelvis.
6. By 20 weeks gestation, the fundus has reached the level of the umbilicus.
7. By 36 weeks, the fundus has reached the xiphoid process.
8. By the end of the 5th month, the myometrium hypertrophy ends and the walls of the uterus become thinner, allowing palpation of the fetus.
9. During the last 3 weeks, the uterus descends slightly because of fetal descent into the pelvis.
10. Changes in contractility occur from the first trimester with irregular painless contractions beginning later in the second trimester.
11. There is a progressive increase in uteroplacental blood flow during pregnancy.

Cervix
1. Pronounced softening and cyanosis—because of increased vascularity, edema, hypertrophy, and hyperplasia of the cervical glands.
2. Endocervical glands secrete thick mucus that forms a cervical plug and obstructs the cervical canal. This plug prevents bacteria and other substances from entering and ascending into the uterus.
3. Erosions of the cervix, common during pregnancy, represent an extension of proliferating endocervical glands and columnar endocervical epithelium.
4. Evidence of Chadwick sign, the bluish, purplish coloring of the cervix. This sign is due to the increased vascularity and hyperemia caused by increased estrogen levels.

Ovaries
1. Ovulation ceases during pregnancy, and maturation of new follicles is suspended.
2. The corpus luteum functions during early pregnancy (first 10 to 12 weeks), producing progesterone. However, small levels of estrogen and relaxin are also produced by the corpus luteum.
3. After 8 weeks gestation, the corpus luteum remains the source for the hormone relaxin. However, relaxin is not required for a successful pregnancy outcome and normal delivery.

Vagina and Outlet
1. Increased vascularity, hyperemia, and softening of connective tissue occurs in skin and muscles of the perineum and vulva.
2. Vaginal walls prepare for labor as mucosa increases in thickness, connective tissue loosens, and small muscle cells hypertrophy. Secretions are thick, white, and acidic in nature and play a major role in the prevention of infections.
3. Vaginal secretions increase; pH is 3.5 to 6—because of increased production of lactic acid from glycogen in the vaginal epithelium by *Lactobacillus acidophilus*. (Acid pH probably aids in keeping vagina relatively free of pathogenic bacteria.)
4. Hypertrophy of the structures, along with fat deposits, causes the labia majora to close and cover the vaginal introitus (vaginal opening).

Abdominal Changes

1. Striae gravidarum (stretch marks) may develop on the skin of abdomen, breast, and thighs (become glistening silvery lines after pregnancy).
2. Linea nigra may form characterized by a line of dark pigment extending from the umbilicus down the midline to the symphysis. Commonly seen in the first pregnancy, the linea nigra occurs at the height of the uterus. During subsequent pregnancies, the entire line may be present early in gestation.
3. Diastasis recti may occur as muscles (rectus) separate. If severe, a part of the anterior uterine wall may be covered by only a layer of skin, fascia, and peritoneum.

Breast Changes

1. Tenderness and tingling occur in early weeks of pregnancy.
2. Increase in size by 2nd month because of the hypertrophy of mammary alveoli. Veins become more prominent and striae may develop as the breasts enlarge.
3. Nipples become larger, more deeply pigmented, and more erectile early in pregnancy.
4. Colostrum, a yellow secretion rich in antibodies, may be expressed by second trimester.
5. Areolae become broader and more deeply pigmented. The depth of pigmentation varies with the woman's pigmentation.
6. Glands of Montgomery are hypertrophic sebaceous glands scattered through the areola surrounding the nipple.

Metabolic Changes

Numerous and concentrated changes occur in response to rapidly growing fetus and placenta.

Weight Gain Average
Twenty-five to thirty-five pounds (11.5 to 16 kg) (see Table 36-1).

Water Metabolism
1. Total body water increases to 6 to 8 L during the pregnancy because of hormonal influence with approximately 4 to 6 L of fluid moving to the extracellular spaces (ECF) resulting in an increase in blood volume.
2. Many pregnant women experience a normal accumulation of fluid in their legs and ankles at the end of the day. This is most common in the third trimester and is referred to as physiologic edema.
3. Additional sodium is required during pregnancy to meet the need for increased intravascular and extracellular fluid volumes and to maintain a normal isotonic state. The limitation of sodium is discouraged in pregnancy because it can result in decreased kidney function, resulting in decreased urine output and a potential adverse outcome.

4. Sodium excretion in the pregnant woman is similar to that of the nonpregnant woman.
5. Sodium retention is usually directly proportional to the amount of water accumulated during the pregnancy. However, pregnancy lends itself toward sodium depletion, making sodium regulation more difficult.

Protein Metabolism
1. The fetus, uterus, and maternal blood are rich in protein rather than in fat or carbohydrates.
2. At term, the fetus and placenta contain approximately 500 g of protein or approximately half of the total protein increase of pregnancy.
3. Approximately 500 g more of protein is added to the uterus, breasts, and maternal blood in the form of hemoglobin and plasma proteins.

Carbohydrate Metabolism
1. Carbohydrate metabolism during pregnancy is controlled by glucose levels in the plasma and the metabolism of glucose in the cells.
2. The liver controls the plasma glucose level. Not only does it store glucose as glycogen, but also it converts it into glucose when the woman's blood glucose levels are low.
3. Early in pregnancy, the effects of estrogen and progesterone can induce a state of hyperinsulinemia. As pregnancy advances, there is increased tissue resistance partnered with increased hyperinsulinemia.
4. Approximately 2% to 3% of all women will develop gestational diabetes mellitus during pregnancy regardless if they have a history of carbohydrate intolerance.
5. Pregnant women with preexisting diabetes mellitus (type 1 or 2) may experience a worsening of the disease attributed to hormonal changes occurring with pregnancy.
6. During pregnancy, there is a "sparing" of glucose used by maternal tissues and a shunting of glucose to the placenta for use by the fetus.
7. Human placental lactogen (hPL) promoting lipolysis, increasing plasma-free fatty acids, and thereby providing alternative fuel sources for the mother.
8. Human placental lactogen, estrogen, progesterone, and cortisol oppose the action of insulin during pregnancy and promote maternal lipolysis as well.

Fat Metabolism
1. Lipid metabolism during pregnancy causes an accumulation of fat stores, mostly cholesterol, phospholipids, and triglycerides.
2. This accumulation of fat stores has no negligible effect on the fetus.
3. Fat storage occurs before the 30th week of gestation. After 30 weeks gestation, fat mobilization occurs correlating with increased utilization of glucose and amino acids by the fetus.

Nutrient Requirements

Caloric Requirements
1. Additional calories are usually not required during the first trimester because of the limited metabolic demands.
2. During the second trimester, pregnant women should take in 340 additional calories per day, and in the third trimester, caloric intake should increase to 452 calories daily. However, because of the variety of women and their individualized

Table 36-1	Components of Weight Gain	
AREA	KG	POUND
Fetus	3.2–3.4	7–7.5
Placenta	0.5–0.7	1–1.5
Amniotic fluid	0.9	2
Uterus	1.1	2.5
Breast tissue	0.7–1.4	1.5–3
Blood volume	1.6–2.3	3.5–5
Maternal stores	1.8–4.3	4–9.5

needs, the exact caloric requirements need to be established on an individual basis.

3. Caloric expenditure varies throughout pregnancy. There is a slight increase in early pregnancy and a sharp increase near the end of the first trimester, continuing throughout pregnancy.

Protein Requirements

1. Protein is required for adequate amino acids to accommodate the normal development of the fetus, blood volume expansion, and growth of maternal breast and uterine tissue. Pregnant women should take in 60 to 80 g of protein daily.
2. The ratio of low-density proteins to high-density proteins is increased during pregnancy.

Carbohydrate and Fat Requirements

1. As in the nonpregnant woman, carbohydrates should supply 55% to 60% of calories in the diet and should be in the form of complex carbohydrates, such as whole-grain cereal products, starchy vegetables, and legumes.
2. Fat intake should not exceed 30% of the diet. Saturated fats should not exceed 10% of the total calories.

Iron Requirements

1. Total circulating red blood cells (RBCs) increase about 20% to 30% (250 to 450 mL) during pregnancy; therefore, iron requirements are increased to 500 mg of iron needed: 270 mg by fetus; 90 mg by the placenta. This equates to 0.8 g/day in early pregnancy and 7.5 mg/day by term. This usually exceeds dietary intake.
2. Supplemental iron is valuable and necessary during pregnancy and for several weeks after pregnancy or lactation.
3. During the last half of pregnancy, iron is transferred to the fetus and stored in the fetal liver. These store lasts 3 to 6 months.

Other Nutritional Requirements

1. If a woman has not increased folic acid intake in preparation for conception, a pregnant woman should increase folic acid intake from 400 to 800 mcg per day.
2. Vitamin D deficiency is the most common nutritional deficit globally. Additionally, vitamin D deficiency has been associated with increased rates of preeclampsia and cesarean births; therefore, pregnant women should take 400 IU (10 mcg) daily. Many manufactured prenatal vitamins increase vitamin D levels.

TRANSITIONAL CARE ALERT Because of the increasing rates of obesity, diabetes, and hypertension in women of reproductive age, it is essential for nurses to focus on maternal and fetal well-being to include nutritional education and appropriate weight gain during pregnancy. The promotion of healthy behaviors may decrease risk for hospitalization and improve maternal and fetal outcomes.

Cardiovascular System Changes

Heart

1. The diaphragm progressively elevates during pregnancy causing displacement of the heart to the left and upward with the apex moved laterally.
2. Heart sounds are exaggerated, splitting of the first heart sound with a loud, easily heard third sound.
3. Heart murmurs—systolic murmurs are common and usually disappear after delivery.

Blood Volume Changes

1. Cardiac output increases by 30% to 50% (1,450 to 1,750 mL), beginning as early as 6 weeks and peaking by 28 to 34 weeks' gestation causing slight hypertrophy of the heart and increased cardiac output. Women with multiple gestation can have higher cardiac outputs, especially after 20 weeks gestation.
2. Cardiac output peaks in the second trimester and plateaus until term, reaching a volume of 6 to 7 L/minute by term.
3. Position greatly influences cardiac output, especially in the third trimester.
   a. In the supine position, the large uterus compresses the venous return from the lower half of the body to the heart. This may cause arterial hypotension, referred to as *supine hypotensive syndrome*.
   b. When the woman turns from her back to lateral position (either left or right side), cardiac output increases by 25% to 30%, with an increase in uterine and renal blood flow.
4. Femoral venous pressure increases due to the slowing of blood flow from lower extremities as a result of pressure of enlarged uterus on pelvic veins and inferior vena cava.
5. Increased cutaneous blood flow dissipates excess heat caused by increased metabolism of pregnancy.
6. Plasma volume increases 40% to 60% (1,200 to 1,600 mL) by term, resulting in hemodilution, more commonly referred to as *physiologic anemia of pregnancy* or *physiologic dilutional anemia*. This "anemic" state is not a true pathologic state and decreases the risk of thrombosis. It is due to the rapid increase in plasma volume and the later increase in RBC volume.

Blood Pressure Changes

1. Blood pressure (BP)—during the first half of pregnancy, there is a slight (5 to 10 mm Hg) decrease in systolic BP (SBP) and diastolic BP (DBP), with the lowest point occurring in the second trimester. By the third trimester, the BP gradually returns to prepregnancy levels.
2. Maternal position influences BP: the highest reading is obtained in the sitting position, the lowest reading is obtained in the left lateral position, and an intermediate reading is obtained in the supine position. Sitting or standing positions show minimal change in SBP readings; however, they can decrease the DBP by about 10 to 15 mm Hg.
3. Maternal BP will also rise with uterine contractions and returns to the baseline level after the uterine contraction is over.
4. Hypertensive disease affects up to 22% of pregnancies and is associated with maternal and fetal death. According to the National Institutes of Health, women with hypertension in pregnancy should be referred to as having hypertensive disorders of pregnancy. Additionally, the term "gestational hypertension" replaces the term "pregnancy-induced hypertension" to describe cases in which elevated BP without proteinuria occurs in a woman beyond 20 weeks of gestation who previously had a normal BP. Essentially, gestational hypertension is an elevated BP past 20 weeks of gestation without proteinuria.

Hematologic Changes

1. Total volume of circulating RBCs increases 17% to 33%; hemoglobin concentration at term averages 12 to 16 g/dL; hematocrit concentration at term averages 37% to 47%.
2. Average leukocyte (white blood cell [WBC]) count in the third trimester is 5 to 12,000/mm³. WBC count can be elevated as high as 30,000 or more during labor—cause unknown; probably represents the reappearance in the circulation of leukocytes previously shunted from of active circulation.

3. Pregnancy is a hypercoagulable state because of the increased levels of essential coagulation factors including factor I (fibrinogen by 50%), factor V (proaccelerin or labile factor), factor VII (proconvertin or serum prothrombin conversion accelerator), factor VIII (antihemophilic factor or antihemophilic globulin), factor IX (plasma thromboplastin component or Christmas factor), factor X (Stuart or Prower factor), factor XII (Hageman or glass or contact factor), and vWF (von Willebrand factor antigen). Factor II (prothrombin) increases slightly, whereas factors XI (plasma thromboplastin antecedent) and XIII (fibrin-stabilizing factor) decrease during pregnancy.

4. There is no significant change in the number, appearance, or function of platelets. Average platelet count is 150,000 to 400,000/mm³, which increases the risk to the pregnant woman for venous thrombosis.

Respiratory Tract Changes

1. Nasal stuffiness and epistaxis (nosebleeds) are also common during pregnancy, secondary to vascular congestion caused from the increased estrogen levels.

2. Approximately 60% to 70% of pregnant women experience shortness of breath.

3. Diaphragm is elevated (about 4 cm) during pregnancy—chiefly by the enlarging uterus that decreases the length of the lungs. Breathing is more diaphragmatic rather than costal.

4. Thoracic cage expands its anteroposterior diameter (by 2 cm). The increased pressure from the uterus also widens the substernal angle by about 50%, causing slight flaring of the ribs—result of increased mobility of rib attachments.

5. Oxygen consumption increases 15% to 20% and as much as 300% in labor. This increase leads to increased maternal alveolar and arterial oxygen partial pressure levels.

6. Hyperventilation—an increase in respiratory rate, tidal volume (amount of air inspired and expired with normal breath) increases by 30% to 40%, and minute ventilation (amount of air inspired in 1 minute) increases by 40%.

7. Total lung volume (amount of air in lungs at maximum inspiration) decreases by about 5%. Residual volume (amount of air in lungs after maximum expiration), respiratory reserve volume (maximum amount of air expired during rest), and functional residual capacity (amount of air remaining in lungs at rest and allowing for gas exchange) drop by about 18% to 20%.

8. Increased total volume lowers partial pressure of arterial carbon dioxide ($PaCO_2$), causing mild respiratory alkalosis that is compensated for by lowering of the bicarbonate concentration.

9. Partial pressure of arterial oxygen (PaO_2) elevates to 106 to 108 mm Hg in first trimester and 101 to 104 mm Hg at term. $PaCO_2$ is decreased to 27 to 32 mm Hg. Bicarbonate decreases to 18 to 21 mEq/L. Normal pH during pregnancy is 7.40 to 7.45. These changes allow for removal of fetal carbon dioxide via passive diffusion in the placenta.

Renal System Changes

1. Ureters dilate and elongate during pregnancy because of mechanical pressure and perhaps because of the effects of progesterone. When the uterus rises out of the uterine cavity, it rests on the ureters, compressing them at the pelvic brim. Dilation is greater on the right side—the left side is cushioned by the sigmoid colon.

2. Renal plasma flow (RPF) increases by 60% to 80% by the end of the first trimester because of the increases in blood volume and cardiac output as well as a decrease in systemic vascular resistance due to the effects of progesterone. RPF increases early in pregnancy and decreases to nonpregnant levels in the third trimester. These changes may be due to placental lactogen hormone (hPL).

3. Glomerular filtration rate (GFR) increases 40% to 50% by the second trimester and persists almost to term. Glucosuria may be a result from an increase in GFR without an increase in tubular resorptive capacity for filtered glucose.

4. Protein excretion is also increased to a rate not always handled by the kidneys' tubular resorptive capability. Therefore, protein can spill into the urine. However, protein in the urine should not be considered an abnormal finding until 24-hour urine values exceed 300 mg/dL.

5. Toward the end of pregnancy, pressure of the presenting part impedes drainage of blood and lymph from the bladder base, typically leaving the area edematous, easily traumatized, and more susceptible to infection.

6. Because of the increased RPF and GFR, the amount of glucose the kidneys filter increases 10- to 100-fold. The kidneys cannot always keep up with this increase; therefore, whatever glucose that is not filtered is lost in the urine, contributing to glycosuria.

7. Protein excretion is also increased to a rate not always handled by the kidneys' tubular resorptive capability. Therefore, protein can spill into the urine. However, protein in the urine should not be considered an abnormal finding until 24-hour urine values exceed 300 mg/dL.

Gastrointestinal Tract Changes

1. Gums may become hyperemic and soft; bleeding easily.

2. *Epulis of pregnancy*—a localized vascular swelling of the gums may appear.

3. Stomach and intestines are displaced upward and laterally by the enlarging uterus. Heartburn (pyrosis) is commonly caused by reflux of acid secretions in the lower esophagus.

4. Peptic ulcer formation or exacerbation is uncommon during pregnancy because of decreased hydrochloric acid (caused by increased estrogen levels).

5. Tone and motility of GI tract decrease leading to prolonged gastric emptying because of the large amount of progesterone produced by the placenta. Decreased motility, mechanical obstruction by the fetus, and decreased water absorption from the colon leads to constipation.

6. Hemorrhoids are common because of elevated pressure in veins below the level of the large uterus and constipation.

7. Distention and hypotonia of the gallbladder are common, causing stasis of bile. Additionally, there is a decrease in emptying time and the thickening of bile, resulting in hypercholesterolemia and gallstone formation.

8. Liver function tests are altered. With pregnancy, bilirubin, aspartate aminotransferase, and alanine aminotransferase values are unchanged; prothrombin time may show a slight increase or be unchanged. Liver size and morphology are unchanged.

9. The appendix is pushed superiorly.

Endocrine Changes

1. Anterior pituitary gland enlarges in both weight (30% increase) and volume (twofold increase). Its shape also changes from convex to dome shaped; posterior pituitary gland remains unchanged.

2. Thyroid is moderately enlarged because of hyperplasia of glandular tissue and increased vascularity.
   a. Basal metabolic rate increases progressively during normal pregnancy (as much as 25%) because of metabolic activity of fetus.
   b. Level of protein-bound iodine and thyroxine rises sharply and is maintained until after delivery because of increased circulatory estrogen and hCG.
   c. Hyperthyroidism during pregnancy is rare. Although levels of thyroxine (T_4) and triiodothyronine (T_3) are elevated by as much as 40% to 100% by term, this is a result of estrogen, hCG, and increased urinary iodide secretion, resulting in "euthyroid hyperthyroxinemia."
3. Parathyroid gland size is known to increase, but there is a decrease in the parathyroid hormone (PTH) during pregnancy. This decrease is balanced by the increased production of PTH by the fetus and placenta.
4. Adrenal secretions considerably increased—amounts of aldosterone increase as early as the 15th week to accommodate for the increased sodium excretion.
5. Pancreas—because of the fetal glucose needs for fetal growth, there are alterations in maternal insulin production and usage.
   a. Estrogen, progesterone, cortisol, and human placental lactogen (hPL) decrease the maternal utilization of glucose.
   b. Cortisol also increases maternal insulin production.
   c. Insulinase, an enzyme produced by the placenta, deactivates maternal insulin.
   d. These changes cause an increased demand for insulin triggering the islets of Langerhans to increase production of insulin.

Integumentary Changes

1. Pigment changes occur because of melanocyte-stimulating hormone as a result of increased estrogen and progesterone and is elevated from the 2nd month of pregnancy until term.
2. Striae gravidarum appear in later months of pregnancy as reddish, slightly depressed streaks in the skin of the abdomen and occasionally over the breasts and thighs and occur in as much at 50% of all pregnant women.
3. Linea nigra—a brownish-black line of pigment is usually formed in the midline of the abdominal skin.
4. Chloasma or melasma (mask of pregnancy)—brownish patches of pigment may form on the face. Chloasma usually disappears after pregnancy but can reappear with excessive exposure to the sun or with oral contraceptive treatment.
5. Angiomas (vascular spider nevus)—minute red elevations commonly on the skin of the face, neck, upper chest, legs, and arms may develop.
6. Palmar erythema—reddening of the palms may also occur.
7. Increased warmth to the skin and variation in hair and nail growth occur.

Musculoskeletal Changes

1. The increasing mobility of sacroiliac, sacrococcygeal, and pelvic joints during pregnancy is a result of hormonal changes, specifically the hormone relaxin.
2. The center of gravity shifts secondary to increased weight gain, fluid retention, lordosis, and mobile ligaments. This mobility and the change in the center of gravity contribute to alteration of maternal posture and to back pain.
3. Late in pregnancy, aching, numbness, and weakness in the upper extremities may occur because of lordosis and paresthesia, which ultimately produces traction on the ulnar and median nerves.
4. Separation of the rectus muscles because of the pressure of the growing uterus creates what is called a diastasis recti. If this is severe, a portion of the anterior uterine wall is covered by only a layer of skin, fascia, and peritoneum.

Neurologic Changes

1. Usually no system changes.
2. Mild frontal headaches are common in the first and second trimester and are usually related to tension or hormonal changes.
3. Dizziness is common and related to vasomotor instability, postural hypotension, or hypoglycemia following long periods of standing or sitting.
4. Tingling sensations in the hands are common and are due to excessive hyperventilation, which decreases maternal $PaCo_2$ levels.

Hormonal Changes

Steroid Hormones

1. Estrogen:
   a. Secreted by the ovaries in early pregnancy, with over half of the estrogen secreted by the placenta by 7 weeks gestation.
   b. The three classic estrogens during pregnancy are estrone, estradiol, and estriol. More than 90% of the estrogen secreted during pregnancy is estriol.
   c. Estrogens also ensure uterine growth and development, maintenance of uterine elasticity and contractility, maintenance of breast growth and its ductal structures, and enlargement of the external genitalia.
2. Progesterone:
   a. Is initially secreted by the corpus luteum and later by the placenta playing a critical role in the maintenance of the pregnancy by suppressing the maternal immunologic response to the fetus and the rejection of the trophoblasts.
   b. Progesterone helps maintain the endometrium, inhibits uterine contractility, helps in the development of breast lobules for lactation, stimulates the maternal respiratory center, and relaxes smooth muscle.

Placental Protein Hormones

1. Human chorionic gonadotropin (hCG):
   a. Secreted by the syncytiotrophoblasts and stimulates the production by the corpus luteum of progesterone and estrogen until the fully developed placenta takes over.
   b. In multiple gestations, hCG can be twice as high as in a single pregnancy.
   c. hCG levels peak around 10 weeks gestation (50,000 to 100,000 mIU/mL), then decrease to 10,000 to 20,000 mIU/mL by 20 weeks gestation.
2. Human chorionic somatomammotropin (hCS) also called human placental lactogen (hPL) is produced by the syncytiotrophoblasts of the placenta; detected in maternal serum as early as 6 weeks gestation.
   a. Serum hCS levels rise concomitantly with placental growth.
   b. hCS is an antagonist of insulin. It increases the amount of free fatty acids available to the fetus for metabolic needs and decreases the maternal metabolism of glucose allowing for protein synthesis. This action allows the fetus to have the needed nutrients when the woman is not eating.

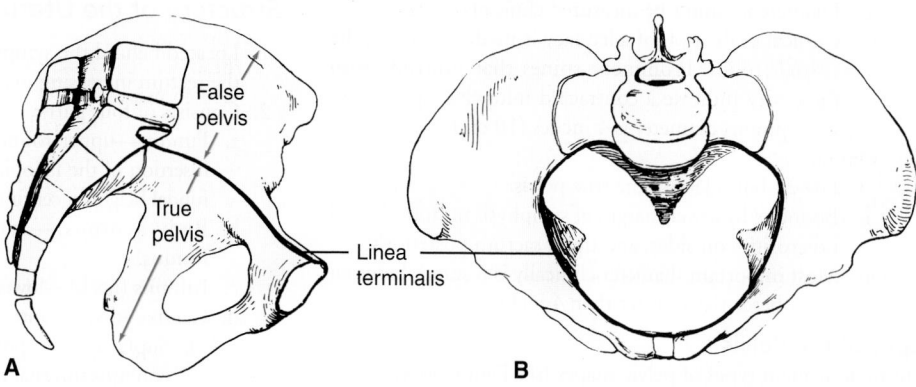

Figure 36-1. **(A)** Side view of the true and false pelvis. **(B)** Front view showing linea terminalis (pelvic brim).

Other Hormones

1. Prostaglandins:
   a. Exact function is still unknown but is essential for the cardiovascular adaptation to pregnancy, cervical ripening, and initiation of labor.
   b. Affect smooth muscle contractility with increased levels leading to vasodilation.
2. Relaxin:
   a. Secreted primarily by the corpus luteum and be secreted in small amounts by the decidua and the placenta.
   b. Inhibits uterine activity and decreases the strength of uterine contractions and cervical ripening.
3. Prolactin:
   a. Released from the anterior pituitary gland and responsible for sustaining milk protein, casein, fatty acids, lactose, and the volume of milk secretion during lactation.

Structure of the Pelvis

Bones of the Pelvis

1. The pelvis is composed of four bones:
   a. Two innominate bones (hip bones) form the sides and front.
   b. Sacrum and coccyx form the back.
2. Pelvic bones are held together by fibrocartilage of the symphysis pubis and several ligaments.

Divisions of the Pelvis

1. False pelvis—lies above an imaginary line called the *linea terminalis* or *pelvic brim* (see Figure 36-1). Function of the false pelvis is to support the enlarged uterus.

2. True pelvis lies below the pelvic brim or linea terminalis; it is the bony canal through which the fetus must pass. It is divided into three planes: the inlet, the midpelvis, and the outlet.
   a. Inlet:
      i. Upper boundary of the true pelvis—Bound by the upper margin of symphysis pubis in front, linea terminalis on the sides, and sacral promontory (first sacral vertebra) in the back.
      ii. Largest diameter of inlet is transverse (see Figure 36-2).
      iii. Smallest diameter of inlet is anteroposterior.
      iv. Anteroposterior diameter is most important diameter of inlet: measured clinically by diagonal conjugate—distance from lower margin of symphysis to the sacral promontory (usually 5½ inches [14 cm]) (see Figure 36-3).
      v. Obstetric (true) conjugate—distance between inner surface of symphysis and sacral promontory measured by subtracting ½ to ¾ inch (1.5 to 2 cm) (thickness of symphysis) from the diagonal conjugate. Adequate diameter is usually 4½ inches (11.5 cm). This is the shortest anteroposterior diameter through which the fetus must pass.
   b. Midpelvis:
      i. Bounded by inlet above and outlet below—true bony cavity. Midpelvis contains the narrowest portion of the pelvis.

Figure 36-2. Inlet of normal female pelvis showing transverse and anteroposterior diameters.

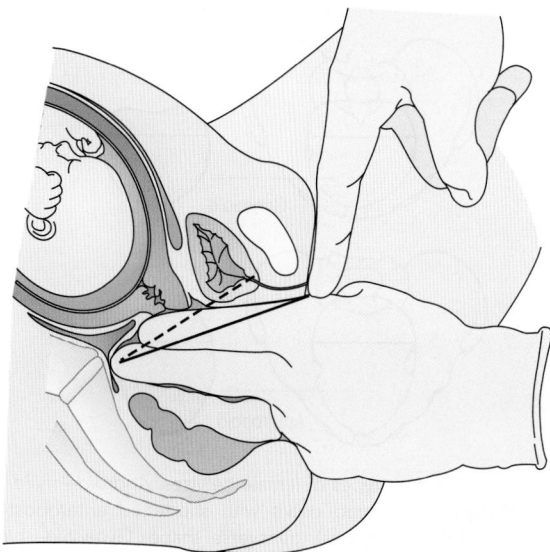

Figure 36-3. Measurement of diagonal conjugate diameter. *Straight line* shows diagonal conjugate; *dotted line* shows true conjugate.

ii. Diameters cannot be measured clinically.

iii. Clinical evaluation of adequacy is made by noting the ischial spines. Prominent spines that protrude into the cavity indicate a contracted midpelvic space. The interspinous diameter is 4 inches (10 cm).

c. Outlet:

i. Lowest boundary of the true pelvis.

ii. Bounded by lower margin of symphysis in front, ischial tuberosities on sides, and tip of sacrum posteriorly.

iii. Most important diameter clinically is distance between the tuberosities (greater than 4 inches).

Shapes of the Pelvis

There are four main types of pelvic shapes (see Figure 36-4).

1. Gynecoid (normal female pelvis); optimal diameters in all three planes; 50% of all women.

2. Android (normal male pelvis); posterior segments are decreased in all three planes; deep transverse arrest of descent of the fetus and failure of rotation of the fetus are common; 20% of all women.

3. Anthropoid (apelike pelvis with long anteroposterior diameter); may allow for easy delivery of an occiput-posterior presentation of the fetus; 25% of all women.

4. Platypelloid (flat female pelvis with wide transverse diameter); arrest of fetal descent at the pelvic inlet is common; labor progress can be poor in 5% of all women.

Figure 36-4. The four types of female pelvises. *Android*—male-type pelvis. *Platypelloid*—broad pelvis with shortened anteroposterior diameter and flattened, oval, transverse shape. *Gynecoid*—typical female pelvis in which inlet is round instead of oval. *Anthropoid*—pelvis in which anteroposterior diameter is equal to or greater than the transverse diameter.

Structure of the Uterus

1. Located behind the symphysis pubis between the bladder and the rectum increasing in size after childbirth.

2. Consists of four parts:

a. Fundus—upper rounded segment that extends above the insertion of the fallopian tubes; fetal growth is measured by fundal height in centimeters correlating with weeks gestation.

b. Body (corpus)—main portion between cervix and fundus.

c. Isthmus (neck)—lower uterine segment.

d. Cervix—divided into two sections:

i. Supravaginal—portion that extends inside the uterus; contains internal os that opens into the uterine cavity.

ii. Vaginal—portion that extends outside the uterus into the vagina; contains the external os that is the visible opening of the cervix; portion that is felt during vaginal examination in assessing cervical dilation.

3. Consists of three layers:

a. Parietal peritoneum—serous coat; covers most of uterus except cervix and anterior portion of body.

b. Myometrium—three layers:

i. Outer layer—provides power to expel the fetus.

ii. Middle layer—provides contractions after childbirth to control blood loss.

iii. Inner layer—provides sphincter action to help keep cervix closed during pregnancy.

c. Endometrium—highly vascular mucous membrane; responds to hormonal stimulation with hypertrophy and secretion; sloughs if pregnancy does not occur.

Prenatal Assessment

 EVIDENCE BASE Association of Women's Health, Obstetric, Neonatal Nurses. (2015). *Fetal heart monitoring: Principles and practices* (5th ed.). Dubuque, IA: Kendall Hunt Publishing Company.

Health History

Age

Babies born to women at the extremes of reproductive life defined as women younger than 19 years and older than 35 years have an increased risk of prematurity, congenital anomalies, as well as other risks of pregnancy.

1. Adolescent mothers have an increased incidence of anemia, gestational hypertension, preterm labor (PTL), small-for-gestational age (SGA) infants, intrauterine growth–restricted infants, cephalopelvic disproportion, and dystocia.

2. Women of advanced maternal age (AMA) have an increased incidence of hypertension with pregnancies complicated by underlying medical problems such as diabetes, multiple gestation, and infants with genetic abnormalities.

Family History

Includes maternal and paternal history for conditions such as congenital disorders, hereditary diseases, multiple pregnancies, diabetes, heart disease, hypertension, mental retardation, renal disease, and any recent global travel destinations.

Maternal Medical History

1. Childhood diseases and immunization records especially rubella, measles, and chickenpox.

2. Major illnesses, surgery (especially of the reproductive tract, spinal surgery, or appendectomy), blood transfusions.
3. Existing medical conditions, such as epilepsy, cardiac disease, endocrine disorders (eg, diabetes, thyroid disease), asthma, and hypertension.
4. Drug, food, and environmental allergies.
5. Urinary tract infections (UTIs) and sexually transmitted infections (STIs).
6. Menstrual history (onset of menarche, length, amount, regularity, and dysmenorrhea). Also, assess for bleeding between menses.
7. Gynecologic history (reproductive history, contraceptive use, and sexual history).
8. Use of medications (prescription, herbal, and over the counter [OTC]), recreational drugs, alcohol, nicotine, tobacco, and caffeine.
9. History of tuberculosis, hepatitis, group B beta-hemolytic streptococcus (GBS), or human immunodeficiency virus (HIV).

Maternal Nutritional History

1. Adherence to special dietary practices (religious, social, or cultural preferences).
2. History of eating disorders (obesity, bulimia, anorexia nervosa), gastric bypass, absorption problems (eg, phenylketonuria [PKU] and celiac disease), and food allergies.
3. Eating patterns (times and frequency of eating daily), number of servings of food from the five food groups, calories, protein, vitamins, and minerals consumed daily.
4. Additional factors to be considered include where the food was eaten, quantity of food eaten, how food was prepared (ie, fried, baked), and which foods are limited and why.
5. The U.S. Department of Agriculture provides an online interactive diet program, Daily Food Plan for Moms, specifically tailored to pregnant and breastfeeding women. This program gives a personalized plan for nutrition for pregnancy including multiples and lactating women.
6. Weight gain of less than 10 pounds (4.5 kg) or loss of more than 5 pounds (2.3 kg).

 EVIDENCE BASE United States Department of Agriculture. (2017). Nutritional needs during pregnancy. Washington, DC: Author. Available: www.choosemyplate.gov/nutritional-needs-during-pregnancy.

Woman's Past Obstetric History

1. Infertility issues, dates of previous pregnancies and deliveries, infant weights, length of labors, types of deliveries, anesthesia use, multiple births, abortions, stillbirths, and maternal, fetal, and neonatal complications. Include history of infertility to include treatments, medications, and conceived or lost pregnancies.
2. Last delivery less than 1 year before present conception.
3. Woman's perception of past pregnancy, labor, and delivery experience for herself and effect on her family.

Woman's Current Obstetric Experience

1. Gravidity, parity.
2. Date of last menses.
3. Estimated date of birth—EDC (estimated date of confinement)/EDD (estimated date of delivery).
4. Signs and symptoms of pregnancy—amenorrhea, breast changes, nausea and vomiting, fetal movement, fatigue, urinary frequency, and skin pigment changes.

5. Expectations for her present pregnancy, labor, and delivery.
6. Expectations for her health care providers and her perception of her relationship between herself and her nurse.
7. Rest and sleep patterns—length, quality, and regularity of rest and sleep.
8. Activity and employment—exercise patterns, type and hours of employment, exposure to hazardous material (occupational hazards), and plans for continued employment.
9. Sexual activity and contraceptive practices.
10. Inadequate prenatal care, intrauterine growth problems, Rh sensitization, or preterm labor.

Psychosocial History

1. Psychiatric and mental status history: history of mood or anxiety disorders; mental illness; medications or treatments for psychiatric or mental problems. Past history of depression, with or without an association with pregnancy.
2. Self-concept or self-esteem issues.
3. Support systems available, including ones she has made contact with.
4. Stressors: personal and occupational stressors that may affect her pregnancy and the fetus; include coping strategies she may use or lack of coping skills.
5. Emotional changes and adjustment to pregnancy.
6. The Psychosocial Screening Tool can be used to determine factors that impact a woman's physical and mental health and may interfere with her following through with prenatal care. Any positive response to the following questions deserves further investigation and intervention.
   a. Do you have any problems (job, transportation, etc.) that prevent you from keeping your health care appointments?
   b. Do you feel unsafe where you live?
   c. In the past 2 months, have you used any form of tobacco?
   d. In the past 2 months, have you used drugs or alcohol (including beer, wine, or mixed drinks)?
   e. On a scale of 1 to 5, how do you rate your current stress level?
   f. How many times have you moved in the past 12 months?
   g. If you could change the timing of this pregnancy, would you want it earlier, later, not at all, no change?

 EVIDENCE BASE American College of Obstetricians and Gynecologists. (2016). Screening for perinatal depression (2010/Reaffirmed 2016). (Committee Opinion No. 630). Washington, DC: Author.

7. In addition to the Perinatal Screening Tool, the pregnant woman can be asked about intimate partner violence. Examples of questions for this interview are:
   a. Has your current partner ever threatened you or made you feel afraid? Threatened to hurt you or your children if you did or did not do something?
   b. Has current partner ever hit, choked, or physically hurt you? (Includes being slapped, kicked, bitten, pushed, or shoved.)
   c. Has current partner ever forced you to do something sexually that you did not want to do or refused your request to use condoms?
   d. Has current partner ever tampered with your birth control or tried to get you pregnant when you did not want to be pregnant?
   e. Has current partner prevented you from using a wheelchair, cane, respirator, or other assistive devices?

EVIDENCE BASE American College of Obstetricians and Gynecologists. (2012). Intimate partner violence (Committee Opinion No. 518). Washington, DC: Author.

Laboratory Data

Urinalysis

1. Urine is tested for glucose, ketones, and protein. Urine is usually collected by a clean-catch, midstream technique.
2. Glucose (glucosuria) may be present in small amounts because the glomerular filtration rate is increased without the same increase in kidney tubular reabsorption. Glucosuria should be investigated to rule out diabetes.
3. Protein in the urine that exceeds 300 mg/dL/24-hour urine collection should be reported because it may be a sign of pre-eclampsia, renal problems, or UTI.
4. Ketones in the urine should be reported because ketonuria may be a sign of excessive weight loss, dehydration, or electrolyte imbalance. Ketonuria is commonly secondary to nausea and vomiting of pregnancy.
5. If the urine is cloudy and bacteria or leukocytes are present (more than four leukocytes per high-powered field), a urine culture is performed.
6. The presence of bilirubin is indicative of liver or gallbladder disease or breakdown of RBCs.
7. The presence of blood in the urine (hematuria) is suggestive of UTI, kidney disease, or vaginal contamination.

Complete Blood Count

1. Determination of hematocrit and hemoglobin levels and description of the morphology of the RBCs are done to find evidence of anemias, such as sickle cell or thalassemia.
2. Hemoglobin levels average 12 to 16 g/dL.

Blood Type and Screening

1. Blood type, Rh factor, and antibody screen—if the woman is found to be Rh negative or to have a positive antibody screen, her partner is screened and a maternal antibody titer is drawn, as indicated.
    a. Coombs test—retested at 28 weeks in the Rh-negative woman for detection of antibodies.
    b. Rh_o (D) immune globulin (RhoGAM) given at 28 weeks, as indicated. Also administered following chorionic villus sampling (CVS), percutaneous umbilical sampling, amniocentesis, trauma, or placental separation (abruptio placentae or placenta previa).
    c. Given within 72 hours of birth to a Rh_o (D) mom or Du– and without antibodies if the newborn is Rh positive.
2. Glucose testing—diabetic screening for women who are at average risk conducted at 24 to 28 weeks using a 1-hour 50-g glucose load test. According to the American Diabetes Association, average risk includes age 25 or older, obese women of any age, family history of diabetes mellitus in a first-degree relative, previous delivery resulting in a macrosomic infant, member of an ethnic group with a high prevalence of diabetes (Hispanic, Black, Pacific Islander, Native American, Asian American), history of abnormal glucose tolerance, and history of poor obstetric outcome.
3. Maternal serum alpha-fetoprotein (MS-AFP)—may be done at 15 to 18 weeks. High maternal levels may indicate an open neural tube defect in the fetus; low levels have been associated with Down syndrome. Inaccurate pregnancy dating is the most common cause for an abnormal MS-AFP.

Infection

1. Rapid plasma reagin (RPR), Venereal Disease research lab (VDRL) or fluorescent treponemal antibody absorption test for syphilis is done on the initial visit; repeat testing at 32 weeks, as indicated.
2. Gonorrhea—cervical cultures are usually done at the initial visit and when symptoms are present.
3. HSV—all visible lesions are cultured, and the cervix is cultured weekly beginning 4 to 8 weeks before delivery.
4. Chlamydia—done at the initial visit and when symptoms are present.
5. Rubella titer—immunity is 10 IU/mL or greater.
6. Hepatitis B surface antigen.
7. HIV—screening is recommended for all pregnant women.

Other Tests

1. Toxoplasmosis—done as indicated for women at risk.
2. Tuberculin skin tests—done as indicated.
3. Papanicolaou (Pap) smear—done unless recent results available.
4. Sickle cell screen—done to detect presence of sickle hemoglobin in at-risk women.
5. Group B beta streptococcus (rectovaginal swab)—done to detect carriers or active GBS.
6. Drug screen—done to decrease possible neonatal abstinence syndrome.

Physical Assessment

General Examination

1. The woman is asked to empty her bladder before the examination to enhance her comfort and to facilitate palpation of her uterus and pelvic organs during the vaginal examination.
2. Evaluation of the woman's weight and BP.
3. Examination of the eyes, ears, and nose—nasal congestion during pregnancy may occur as a result of peripheral vasodilation.
4. Examination of the mouth, teeth, throat, and thyroid—the gums may be hyperemic and softened because of increased progesterone.
5. Inspection of breasts and nipples—the breasts may be enlarged and tender; nipple and areolar pigment may be darkened.
6. Auscultation of the heart.
7. Auscultation and percussion of the lungs.

Abdominal Examination

1. Examination for scars or striations, diastasis recti (separation of the rectus muscle), or umbilical hernia.
2. Palpation of the abdomen for fundal height (palpable after 13 weeks of pregnancy); measurement recorded and used as guideline for subsequent calculations.
3. Palpation of the abdomen for fetal outline and position (Leopold maneuvers)—third trimester.
4. Check of FHTs—FHTs are audible with a Doppler after 10 to 12 weeks and at 18 to 20 weeks with a fetoscope.
5. Record fetal position, presentation, and FHTs.

Figure 36-5. Vaginal speculum examination. **(A)** Blades held obliquely on entering the introitus. **(B)** Blades rotated to horizontal position and pushed toward the cervix. **(C)** Blades separated to encircle the cervix. **(D)** Blades removed with gentle pulling.

Pelvic Examination

1. The woman is placed in lithotomy position.
2. Inspection of external genitalia.
3. Vaginal examination—done to rule out abnormalities of the birth canal and to obtain cytologic smear (Pap and, if indicated, smears for gonorrhea, vaginal trichomoniasis, candidiasis, herpes, group B beta streptococcus, and chlamydia) (see Figure 36-5).
4. Examination of the cervix for position, size, mobility, and consistency. Cervix is softened and bluish (increased vascularity) during pregnancy.
5. Identification of the ovaries (size, shape, and position).
6. Rectovaginal exploration to identify hemorrhoids, fissures, herniation, or masses.
7. Evaluation of pelvic inlet—anteroposterior diameter by measuring the diagonal conjugate.
8. Evaluation of midpelvis—prominence of the ischial spines.
9. Evaluation of pelvic outlet—distance between ischial tuberosities and mobility of coccyx.

Subsequent Prenatal Assessments

1. Uterine growth and estimated fetal growth (see Figure 36-6).
   a. Fundus at symphysis pubis indicates 12 weeks gestation.
   b. Fundus at umbilicus indicates 20 weeks gestation.
   c. Fundal height corresponds with gestational age between 22 and 34 weeks.
   d. Fundus at lower border of rib cage indicates 36 weeks gestation.
   e. Uterus becomes globular and drop indicates 40 weeks gestation.
2. A greater fundal height suggests:
   a. Multiple pregnancy.
   b. Miscalculated due date.
   c. Polyhydramnios (excessive amniotic fluid).
   d. Gestational throphoblastic disease (degeneration of villi into grapelike clusters; fetus does not usually develop).
   e. Uterine fibroids.
3. A lesser fundal height suggests:
   a. Intrauterine fetal growth restriction.
   b. Error in estimating gestation.
   c. Fetal or amniotic fluid abnormalities.
   d. Intrauterine fetal death.
   e. SGA.
4. FHTs—palpate abdomen for fetal position.
   a. Normal—110 to 160 beats/minute (bpm).
5. Weight—major increase in weight occurs during second half of pregnancy; usually between 0.5 pound (0.2 kg)/week and 1 pound (0.5 kg)/week. Greater weight gain may indicate fluid retention and hypertensive disorder.
6. BP—should remain near woman's prepregnant baseline.
7. Complete blood count at 28 and 32 weeks gestation; VDRL—rechecked at 36 to 40 weeks gestation.
8. Antibody serology screen if Rh negative at 36 weeks gestation.

Figure 36-6. Height of fundus. (Pillitteri, A. [2013]. *Maternal and child health nursing: Care of the childbearing and childrearing family* [7th ed.]. Philadelphia, PA: Lippincott Williams & Wilkins.)

9. Culture smears for gonorrhea, chlamydia, group B beta-hemolytic streptococcus, and herpes, as indicated; usually at 36 and 40 weeks gestation.
10. Urinalysis—for protein, glucose, blood, and nitrates.
11. AFP—done at 15 to 20 weeks.
12. Diabetic screening—done, as indicated, at 24 to 28 weeks.
13. Administer RhoGAM, as indicated, at 28 weeks.
14. Edema—check the lower legs, face, and hands.

15. Evaluate discomforts of pregnancy—fatigue, heartburn, hemorrhoids, constipation, and backache.
16. Evaluate eating and sleeping patterns, general adjustment and coping with the pregnancy.
17. Evaluate concerns of the woman and her family.
18. Evaluate preparation for labor, delivery, and parenting. See Patient Education Guidelines 36-1.

Nursing Interventions and Patient Education

Nursing Diagnoses

- Acute Pain (backache, leg cramps, breast tenderness) related to physiologic changes of pregnancy.
- Imbalanced Nutrition: Less Than Body Requirements related to morning sickness, heartburn, lack of knowledge of requirements in pregnancy and growing fetus.
- Impaired Urinary Elimination (frequency) related to increased pressure from the uterus.
- Constipation related to physiologic changes of pregnancy and pressure from the uterus.
- Impaired Tissue Integrity related to pressure from the uterus and increased blood volume.
- Anxiety or Fear related to the birth process and infant care.
- Ineffective Role Performance related to the demands of pregnancy.
- Activity Intolerance related to physiologic changes of pregnancy and enlarging uterus.

Nursing Interventions

Minimizing Pain
1. Teach the woman to use good body mechanics—wear comfortable, low-heeled shoes with good arch support; try the use of a maternity girdle.
2. Instruct the woman in the technique for pelvic-rocking exercises.
3. Encourage the woman to take rest periods with her legs elevated.

PATIENT EDUCATION GUIDELINES 36-1

Prenatal Care

- It is important to keep scheduled prenatal care appointments:
  - Weeks 1 to 28: Every month.
  - Weeks 28 to 36: Every 2 weeks.
  - Weeks 36 to delivery: Every week.
- Expect the following discomforts of pregnancy, and speak with your nurse or health care provider about strategies for relief:
  - Back pain, leg cramps, breast tenderness.
  - Morning sickness, heartburn.
  - Frequent urination.
  - Constipation.
  - Swelling of legs, varicose veins.
  - Fatigue.
- Follow a healthy, balanced diet with three meals per day and take prenatal vitamins as directed by your health care provider.

- Get regular exercise and use proper body mechanics to avoid injury.
- Be aware of danger symptoms of pregnancy; these must be reported to your health care provider promptly:
  - Vision disturbances—blurring, spots, or double vision.
  - Vaginal bleeding, new or old blood.
  - Edema of the face, fingers, and sacrum.
  - Headaches—frequent, severe, or continuous.
  - Fluid discharge from vagina; unusual or severe abdominal pain.
  - Chills, fever, or burning on urination.
  - Epigastric pain (severe stomachache).
  - Muscular irritability or convulsions.
  - Inability to tolerate food or liquids, leading to severe nausea and hyperemesis.

4. Inform the woman that adequate calcium intake may decrease leg cramps.

5. Instruct the woman to dorsiflex the foot while applying pressure to the knee to straighten the leg for immediate relief of leg cramps.

6. Instruct the woman to wear a fitted, supportive bra.

7. Instruct the woman to wash her breasts and nipples with water only.

8. Instruct the woman to apply vitamin E or lanolin cream to the breast and nipple area. Lanolin is contraindicated for women with allergies to lamb's wool.

Minimizing Morning Sickness and Heartburn and Maintaining Adequate Nutrition

1. Encourage the woman to eat a few bites of a soda cracker or dry toast before getting out of bed in the morning.

2. Instruct the woman to rise from bed slowly.

3. Encourage the woman to eat low-fat protein foods and dry carbohydrates, such as toast and crackers.

4. Encourage the woman to eat small, frequent meals.

5. Advise the woman to eat slowly.

6. Teach the woman the importance of good nutrition for herself and her fetus. Review the basic food groups with appropriate daily servings for essential vitamins and nutrients.
   a. Seven servings of protein-rich foods, including one serving of a vegetable protein.
   b. Three servings of dairy products or other calcium-rich foods.
   c. Seven servings of grain products.
   d. Two or more servings of vitamin C–rich vegetable or fruit.
   e. Three servings of other fruits and vegetables.
   f. Three servings of unsaturated fats.
   g. Two or more servings of other fruits and vegetables.

7. Encourage the woman to drink soups and liquids between meals to avoid stomach distention and dehydration.

8. Instruct the woman in the use of antacids; caution against the use of sodium bicarbonate because it results in the absorption of excess sodium and fluid retention.

9. Instruct the woman to avoid brushing her teeth soon after eating.

10. Instruct the woman to avoid offensive foods or cooking odors that may trigger nausea.

11. Recommended dietary reference intakes for pregnant women can be obtained from *www.choosemyplate.gov/nutritional-needs-during-pregnancy*. If the woman is a vegetarian, inform her of appropriate intake. Assess type of vegetarian and food intake.
    a. Two broad groups of vegetarians:
       i. Traditional—cultural or religious affiliation prescribes their diet.
       ii. New—adopted vegetarian dietary patterns as a personal or philosophical choice.
    b. Subgroups exist within the above two groups:
       i. Vegan—eat foods from a plant origin; eat no animal foods or anything derived from an animal (ie, eggs, milk, cream, etc.).
       ii. Lacto—eat milk/dairy products, but eat no meat, poultry, fish, seafood, or eggs.
       iii. Lacto-ovo—eat milk/dairy products and eggs, but eat no meat, poultry, fish, or seafood.
       iv. Pesce—eat foods from a plant origin and fish or cheese, but no meat, poultry, or eggs.

c. Partial vegetarians may exclude a specific type of animal food, usually meat, but may consume fish and poultry.
    d. Recommend iron and folic acid supplements.

12. Inform the woman that average weight gain in pregnancy is 25 to 35 pounds (11 to 16 kg). About 2 to 5 pounds (0.9 to 2.3 kg) are gained in the first trimester and about 1 pound (0.5 kg) per week for the remainder of the gestation.
    a. Average weight gain for obese women is 15 pounds (6.8 kg).
    b. Adolescent weight gain should be about 5 pounds more than for adult women if within 2 years of starting menses.
    c. Women with a multiple pregnancy should gain between 35 and 45 pounds (16 and 20 kg).
    d. Average weight gain for underweight women is 28 to 40 pounds (13 to 18 kg).
    e. Assess for any cultural or religious times of fasting (eg, Lent or Ramadan).

13. Advise the woman to limit the use of caffeine.

14. Inform the woman that alcohol should be eliminated during pregnancy as no safe level of intake has been established.

15. Inform the woman that smoking should be eliminated or severely reduced during pregnancy related to the increased risk of spontaneous abortion, fetal death, low birth weight, and neonatal death.

16. Inform the woman that ingesting any drug during pregnancy may affect fetal growth and should be discussed with her health care provider.

Minimizing Urinary Frequency and Promoting Elimination

1. Instruct the woman to limit fluid intake in the evening and to void before going to bed.

2. Encourage the woman to void after meals, with the urge to void, and after sexual intercourse.

3. Encourage the woman to wear loose-fitting cotton underwear.

4. Cranberry or blueberry juice may be recommended to help prevent UTIs.

5. Caffeine should be avoided.

Avoiding Constipation

1. Instruct the woman to increase fluid intake to at least eight glasses of water per day. One to 2 quarts of fluid per day is desirable.

2. Encourage daily intake of foods high in fiber.

3. Encourage the woman to establish regular patterns of elimination.

4. Encourage daily exercise such as walking.

5. Inform the woman that OTC laxatives should be avoided. Providers may recommend stool softeners or bulk-forming agents as indicated.

Maintaining Tissue Integrity

1. Encourage the woman to take frequent rest periods with her legs elevated.

2. Instruct the woman to wear support stockings and wear loose-fitting clothing for leg varicosities.

3. Instruct the woman to avoid constipation, apply cold compresses, take sitz baths, and use topical anesthetics, such as Tucks, for the relief of anal varicosities (hemorrhoids).

Reducing Anxiety and Fear and Promoting Preparation for Labor, Delivery, and Parenthood

The nurse should facilitate education to the woman and her partner related to the following:

1. Current, knowledge, perceptions, cultural values, and expectations of the labor and delivery process and parenting.

2. Availability of childbirth preparation classes that include infant care, breastfeeding, and parenting and encourage attendance.
3. Availability of sibling and grandparent preparation, as indicated.
4. A tour of the birth facility.
5. Common procedures that may be performed during labor and birth.
6. Creating a personalized birth plan to include coping and relaxation techniques and pain management options both nonpharmacologic and pharmacologic, for labor and birth.
7. General guidelines for coming to the birth facility.
8. Preparations for the infant, such as a sleeping space, clothing, feeding, changing, and bathing equipment.

> **NURSING ALERT** Women who attended childbirth preparation have reported an increased satisfaction with their birth experience. Additional benefits to childbirth preparation include improved breastfeeding rates and decreased use of pharmacologic pain management.

Enhancing Role Changes

1. Encourage discussion of feelings and concerns regarding the new role of mother and father.
2. Provide emotional support to the woman/partner regarding the altered family roles.
3. Discuss physiologic causes for changes in sexual relationships, such as fatigue, loss of interest, and discomfort from advancing pregnancy. Some women experience heightened sexual activity during the second trimester.
4. Teach the woman/partner that there are no contraindications to intercourse or masturbation to orgasm provided the woman's membranes are intact, there is no vaginal bleeding, and she has no current problems or history of premature labor.
5. Teach the woman or partner that female superior or sidelying positions are usually more comfortable in the latter half of pregnancy.

Minimizing Fatigue

1. Teach the woman reasons for fatigue and have her plan a schedule for adequate rest.
   a. Fatigue in the first trimester is due to increased progesterone and its effects on the sleep center.
   b. Fatigue in the third trimester is due mainly to carrying increased weight of the pregnancy.
   c. About 8 hours of rest are recommended with frequent 15- to 30-minute rest periods to avoid overfatigue.
   d. Whenever possible, the woman should work while sitting with her legs elevated.
   e. The woman should avoid standing for prolonged periods, especially during the third trimester.
   f. To promote placental perfusion, the woman should not lie flat on her back—left lateral position provides the best placental perfusion; however, either side is acceptable. In the third trimester of pregnancy, sleeping with a small pillow under the abdomen may enhance comfort.
2. Help the woman plan for adequate exercise (if not contraindicated).
   a. In general, exercise during pregnancy should be in keeping with the woman's prepregnancy exercise pattern and type.
   b. Activities or sports that have a risk of bodily harm (skiing, snowmobiling, ice skating, inline skating, horseback riding) should be avoided.
   c. During pregnancy, endurance during exercise may be decreased.
   d. Exercise classes for pregnant women that concentrate on toning and stretching have resulted in enhanced physical condition, increased self-esteem, and greater social support as a result of being in the exercise group.
   e. Contraindications to aerobic exercise during pregnancy include hemodynamically significant heart disease, restrictive lung disease, incompetent cervix, cerclage, multiple gestations at risk for PTL, persistent second- or third-trimester bleeding, placenta previa after 26 weeks gestation, ruptured membranes, PTL in current pregnancy, and preeclampsia.
   f. Exercise that increases the risk of injury or a woman diagnosed with a pregnancy complication should avoid any strenuous exercise.

> **NURSING ALERT** Exercise in pregnancy benefits both the mother and fetus by enhancing overall health and fitness by promoting adequate weight gain, strengthened muscle tone, and reduced blood sugar. Outcomes demonstrate a decrease in operative delivery, gestational diabetes, and hypertension.

> **EVIDENCE BASE** American College of Obstetricians and Gynecologists. (2016). Exercise during pregnancy FAQs. Washington, DC: Author. *www.acog.org/patients/FAQS/exercise-during-pregnancy*.

Community and Home Care Instructions

1. Community and home care is prevention oriented.
2. Case management coordinates health care management collaboratively.
3. Search out and register for prepared childbirth classes. Preferable to attend those associated with the family's intended delivery facility.
4. Social support available from Women, Infants, and Children's Special Supplemental Feeding Program, breastfeeding groups (La Leche League), and father/partner support groups.
5. Prenatal education should focus on nutrition, sexuality, stress reduction, lifestyle behaviors, and hazards at home or work.
6. Consider cultural practices as they have implications for the provision of nursing care.

Alternative Therapies

General Measures

1. Alternative therapies range from nutrition and lifestyle changes to mind and body programs.
2. Encourage the woman to discuss options with her health care provider and consult a credentialed naturopath, acupuncturist, or other complementary practitioner.
3. Physical activities—maintaining an active lifestyle and healthy diet. Some use macrobiotic diets and isometric exercise.
4. Attitudinal activities—maintaining a positive attitude and self-image; have fun and laugh.
5. Relational activities—maintaining social relationships—friends, pets, and family.
6. Spiritual activities—having faith, hope, prayer, and music and meditating as an active part of daily life.

7. Self-caring activities—taking care of self, balancing life, personal integrity, knowing and trusting self, and own time management.
8. Help-seeking activities—seeking assistance in health care ranging from prescribed treatments to biomedicine (self-healing touch). Help-seeking activities include ethnomedicine (Chinese herbal medicine and acupuncture), structure/energy therapies (therapeutic touch and osteopathy), pharmacologic/biologic treatments (antioxidants), biofeedback, guided imagery, music therapy, meditation, and prayer.

Alternative Therapies Specific to the Prenatal Period

1. It is essential that the woman and her family discuss the use of herbs with her obstetric provider before use, become familiar with manufacturers, and ask questions. Although herbs are natural, they can be harmful if misused. Herbs should be used with the same respect as medications.
2. Many herbs are available to be used during pregnancy including the labor and delivery process. Herbs come in different forms—capsules, tablets, extracts, tinctures, powders, dried and prepared as teas or juices, in combinations, and as external preparations.
3. Herbal therapies that are Food and Drug Administration–approved include:
   a. Aloe, cascara (sacred bark, bitter bark), psyllium (plantago seed), senna as a laxative.
   b. Capsicum or cayenne pepper (chili pepper, red pepper) as a topical analgesic; marketed as a cream and used topically.
   c. Slippery elm (red elm) as an oral demulcent; marketed as throat lozenges.
4. Other herbal preparations including Catnip, fennel, lobelia, papaya, spearmint, and wild yams decrease colic stomach cramps, gas, and heartburn and improve the appetite.
5. Cranberry or blueberry juice for UTI prevention.
6. Nausea is sometimes attributed to vitamin B deficiencies but does not always improve with simple vitamin supplements. Red raspberry, peppermint, spearmint, or chamomile tea and ginger root or ginger ale may be used to alleviate the nausea. To increase the effectiveness of red raspberry tea, alfalfa may be added to the tea.
7. Certain acupressure or acupuncture points may assist with the relief of nausea.
8. Other therapies include therapeutic touch and yoga.

 EVIDENCE BASE Louik, C., Gardiner, P., Kelley, K., & Mitchell, A. A. (2010). Use of herbal treatments in pregnancy. *American Journal of Obstetrics and Gynecology, 202*(5), 439.e1–439.e10.

Evaluation: Expected Outcomes

- Verbalizes understanding of proper body mechanics and wears low-heeled shoes.
- Identifies the basic food groups and describes meals to include needed servings for pregnancy.
- Reports limited fluid intake in the evening.
- Describes foods high in fiber.
- Wears support stockings and loose-fitting clothing.
- Discusses expectations for labor, delivery, and parenthood and attends educational classes.
- Verbalizes an understanding of the physiologic causes that may change the sexual relationship.
- Reports engaging in regular exercise.

Psychosocial Adaptation of Pregnancy

 EVIDENCE BASE Link, D. G. (2016). Psychology of pregnancy. In S. Mattson & J. E. Smith (Eds.), *Core curriculum for maternal–newborn nursing* (5th ed., pp. 108–122). St. Louis, MO: Saunders Elsevier.

Rubin's Framework for Maternal Role Assumption

1. Attainment of motherhood role occurs with each pregnancy.
2. Involves a series of cognitive operations:
   a. Mimicry—woman begins observing and modeling her behavior after other pregnant women.
   b. Role-play—woman begins acting out behaviors of a mother (eg, rocking a baby to sleep).
   c. Searching for a role "fit"—woman has perceptions of how the motherhood role will be. She observes others' behaviors to determine how well they fit with her expectations of the motherhood role.
   d. Grief work—woman experiences a sense of loss of her "old" self as she prepares to begin her new role as a mother.
3. Maternal tasks—commonly divided by trimesters.
   a. First trimester:
      i. Acceptance of pregnancy—moves from a state of conflict and ambivalence to one of acceptance of the pregnancy, the child, and the motherhood role.
      ii. Realignment of roles—expectant parents begin to realign their roles and responsibilities as they relate to the child.
      iii. Safe passage—although the mother seeks to ensure a safe passage for her fetus and self throughout her pregnancy, the main focus during this trimester is on self-safety.
   b. Second trimester
      i. Safe passage—in this trimester, the mother's main focus is on appropriate nutrition and exercise.
      ii. Acceptance by others—acceptance of the child by each family member.
      iii. Binding-in to the child—maternal perception of the child as a real person.
   c. Third trimester
      i. Safe passage—during this trimester, the main focus is on the safety of the fetus and is inseparable from self-safety.
      ii. Giving of oneself—the most complex task, in which the mother is learning to give to the unborn child and placing the unborn child's need in relation to her own needs.
      iii. Critical to this trimester is the preparation of the nursery because it solidifies the acceptance of the unborn child.

Rubin's Framework for Paternal Role Assumption

1. The fatherhood role can also be attained with the pregnancy.
2. Paternal tasks can also be divided by trimesters.
   a. First trimester
      i. Announcement and realization of the pregnancy—father will exhibit excitement over the announcement of the pregnancy and is more interested in maternal changes. Usually, he will insist on accompanying the mother to each prenatal appointment.

ii. Some fathers will even begin to experience the same signs and symptoms of pregnancy experienced by the mother. This is more commonly referred to as *couvade syndrome.*

b. Second trimester
   i. Anticipation—father anticipates and adapts to the role of fatherhood.
   ii. Fantasy and exploration—along with the mother, the father begins to imagine what his child will look like and may also begin to explore the talents and attributes of the unborn child.
   iii. Adjustment of sexual expression to accommodate the pregnancy.

c. Third trimester
   i. Preparation—now, serious preparation for the forthcoming child includes preparation of the nursery and childbirth education courses to prepare for labor and delivery.
   ii. Reassurance—provided by the father to ease the anxious mother's fears regarding labor and delivery.

THE FETUS

 EVIDENCE BASE Callahan, L. (2016). Fetal and placental development and functioning. In S. Mattson & J. E. Smith (Eds.), *Core curriculum for maternal–newborn nursing* (5th ed., pp. 37–62). St. Louis, MO: Saunders Elsevier.

Fetal Growth and Development

Advances in knowledge and technology have provided newer methods for assessing fetal well-being and maturity. Improved methods for assessment and diagnosis enable early intervention for improved outcome. See Figure 36-7 for critical periods of fetal growth.

Stages of Growth and Development

The growth and development of the fetus is typically divided into three stages.

Preembryonic Stage: Fertilization to 2 to 3 Weeks
1. Rapid cell division and differentiation.
2. Develop embryonic membranes and germ layers.

Embryonic Stage: 4 to 8 Weeks Gestation
1. Most critical stage of physical development.
2. Organogenesis.

Fetal Stage: 9 Weeks to Birth
1. Every organ system and external structure present.
2. Refinement of fetus and organ function occurs.

Development by Month

First Lunar Month
1. Fertilization to 2 weeks of embryonic growth.
2. Implantation is complete.
3. Primary chorionic villi forming.
4. Embryo develops into two cell layers (trophoblast and blastocyst).
5. Amniotic cavity appears.

Second Lunar Month
1. Three to six weeks of embryonic growth.
2. At the end of 6 weeks of growth, the embryo is approximately ½ inch (1.3 cm) long.
3. Arm and leg buds are visible; arm buds are more developed with finger ridges beginning to appear.
4. Rudiments of the eyes, ears, and nose appear.
5. Lung buds are developing.
6. Primitive intestinal tract is developing.
7. Primitive cardiovascular system is functioning.
8. Neural tube, which forms the brain and spinal cord, closes by the 4th week.

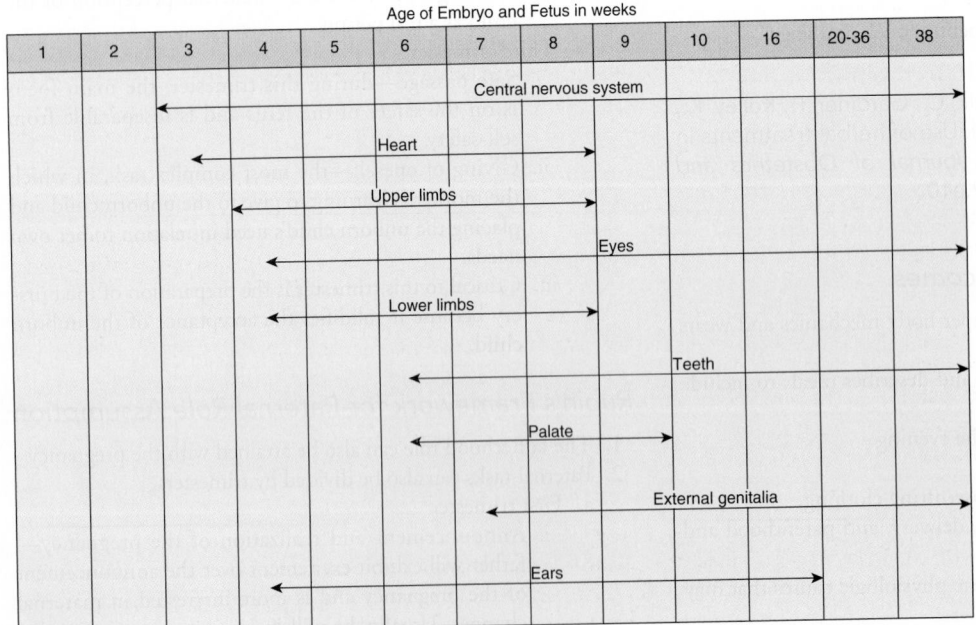

Figure 36-7. Critical periods of fetal growth. (Pillitteri, A. [2013]. *Maternal and child health nursing* [7th ed.]. Philadelphia, PA: Lippincott Williams & Wilkins.)

Third Lunar Month

1. Seven to ten weeks of growth.
2. The middle of this period (9 weeks) marks the end of the embryonic period and the beginning of the fetal period.
3. At the end of 10 weeks of growth, the fetus is approximately 2½ inches (6.3 cm) from crown to rump and weighs ½ oz (14 g).
4. Appearance of external genitalia.
5. By the middle of this month, all major organ systems have formed.
6. The membrane over the anus has broken down.
7. The heart has formed four chambers (by 7th week).
8. The fetus assumes a human appearance.
9. Bone ossification begins.
10. Rudimentary kidney begins to secrete urine.

Fourth Lunar Month

1. Eleven- to fourteen-week-old fetus.
2. At the end of 14 weeks of growth, the fetus is approximately 4¾ inches (12 cm) crown–rump length and 3¾ oz (110 g).
3. Head erect; lower extremities well developed.
4. Hard palate and nasal septum have fused.
5. External genitalia of male and female can now be differentiated.
6. Eyelids are sealed.

Fifth Lunar Month

1. Fifteen- to eighteen-week-old fetus.
2. At the end of 18 weeks of growth, the fetus is approximately 6¼ inches (16 cm) crown–rump length and 11¼ oz (320 g).
3. Ossification of fetal skeleton can be seen on x-ray.
4. Ears stand out from head.
5. Meconium is present in the intestinal tract.
6. Fetus makes sucking motions and swallows amniotic fluid.
7. Fetal movements may be felt by the mother (end of month).

Sixth Lunar Month

1. Nineteen- to twenty-two-week-old fetus.
2. At the end of 22 weeks of growth, the fetus is approximately 8¼ inches (21 cm) crown–rump length and 1 pound, 6¼ oz (630 g).
3. Vernix caseosa covers the skin.
4. Head and body (lanugo) hair visible.
5. Skin is wrinkled and red.
6. Brown fat, an important site of heat production, is present in neck and sternal area.
7. Nipples are apparent on the breasts.

Seventh Lunar Month

1. Twenty-three- to twenty-six-week-old fetus.
2. At the end of 26 weeks of growth, the fetus is approximately 10 inches (25 cm) crown–rump length and 2 pounds, 3¼ oz (1,000 g).
3. Fingernails present.
4. Lean body.
5. Eyes partially open; eyelashes present.
6. Bronchioles are present; primitive alveoli are forming.
7. Skin begins to thicken on hands and feet.
8. Startle reflex present; grasp reflex is strong.

Eighth Lunar Month

1. Twenty-seven- to 30-week-old fetus.
2. At the end of 30 weeks of growth, the fetus is approximately 11 inches (28 cm) crown–rump length and 3 pounds, 12 oz (1,700 g).
3. Eyes open.
4. Ample hair on head; lanugo begins to fade.
5. Skin slightly wrinkled.
6. Toenails present.
7. Testes in inguinal canal, begin descent to scrotal sac.
8. Surfactant coats much of the alveolar epithelium.

Ninth Lunar Month

1. Thirty-one- to 34-week-old fetus.
2. At the end of 34 weeks of growth, the fetus is approximately 12½ inches (32 cm) crown–rump length and 5 pounds, 8 oz (2,500 g).
3. Fingernails reach fingertips.
4. Skin pink and smooth.
5. Testes in scrotal sac.

Tenth Lunar Month

1. Thirty-five- to 38-week-old fetus; end of this month is also 40 weeks from onset of last menses.
2. At the end of 38 weeks of growth, fetus is approximately 14½ inches (37 cm) crown–rump length and 7 pounds, 8 oz (3,400 g).
3. Ample subcutaneous fat.
4. Lanugo almost absent.
5. Toenails reach toe tips.
6. Testes in scrotum.
7. Vernix caseosa mainly on the back.
8. Breasts are firm.

Fetal Circulation

See Figure 36-8.

Assessment of Fetal Maturity and Well-Being

 EVIDENCE BASE American College of Obstetricians and Gynecologists. (2015). Diagnostic tests for birth defects FAQ's 164. Washington, DC: Author. American College of Obstetricians and Gynecologists. (2014, July) (1999/Reaffirmed 2016). Antepartum fetal surveillance (Practice Bulletin #145). Washington, DC: Author.
Association of Women's Health, Obstetric, Neonatal Nurses. (2015). *Fetal heart monitoring: Principles and practices* (5th ed.). Dubuque, IA: Kendall Hunt Publishing Company.

Maternal History and Examination

1. Comprehensive family medical history, personal medical history, and reproductive health history including previous pregnancy experience/outcomes and STIs.
2. Comprehensive physical examination, history of current pregnancy, and identified risk factors.
3. Routine prenatal labs.
4. Fetal assessment after first trimester and individualized fetal surveillance, as indicated.

Fetal Heart Tones

Description

Fetal heart tones (FHTs) are representative of the fetal heart rate (FHR) and are an indicator of oxygen perfusion to the fetal brain, heart, and adrenals. The evaluation of FHTs is indicated in routine assessment of fetal well-being, in determining gestational age, and

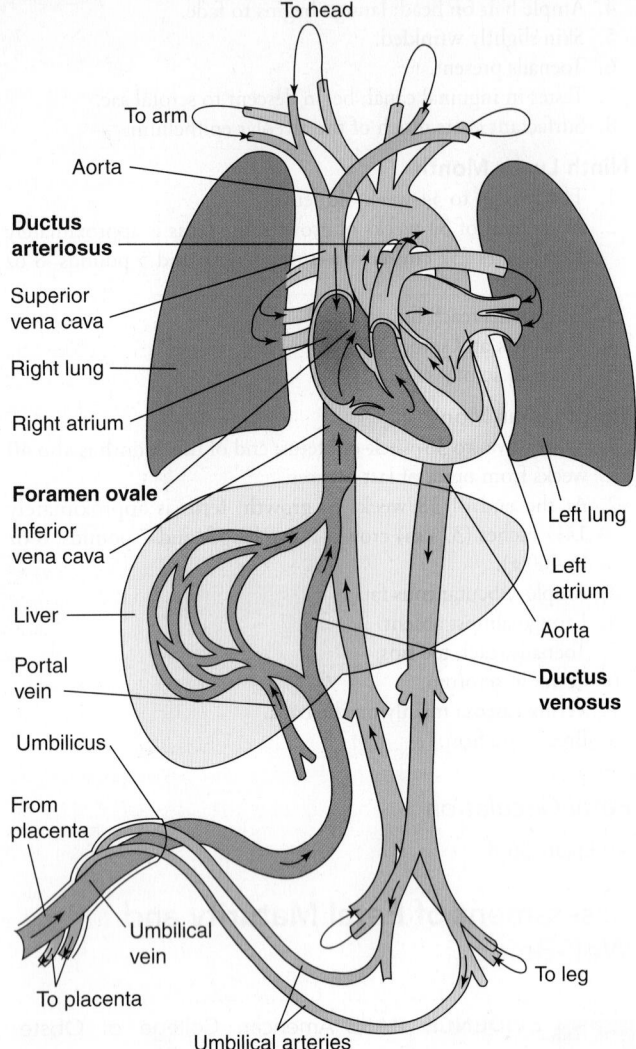

To head
To arm
Aorta
Ductus arteriosus
Superior vena cava
Right lung
Right atrium
Foramen ovale
Inferior vena cava
Liver
Portal vein
Umbilicus
From placenta
Umbilical vein
To placenta
Umbilical arteries
Left lung
Left atrium
Aorta
Ductus venosus
To leg

Figure 36-8. Diagram of the fetal circulation shortly before birth. *Arrows* indicate course of blood. (Pillitteri, A. [2013]. *Maternal and child health nursing: Care of the childbearing and childrearing family* [7th ed.]. Philadelphia, PA: Lippincott Williams & Wilkins.)

in cases of threatened abortion or other abnormalities. FHTs can be heard using techniques that amplify sound.

1. Doppler at approximately 10 to 12 weeks fetal gestation.
2. Fetoscope (fetal stethoscope) at approximately 18 to 20 weeks fetal gestation.
3. Electronic fetal monitoring testing is usually done when the fetus is considered viable, around 24 weeks gestation.
4. Rate—between 110 and 160 bpm.
5. In latter months of pregnancy, fetal heart sounds found:
   a. Near the woman's midline in fetal occipitoanterior positions.
   b. Lateral to midline in fetal occipitotransverse positions.
   c. In the woman's flank in fetal occipitoposterior positions.
   d. Below the woman's umbilicus in cephalic presentations.
   e. At or above the woman's umbilicus in breech presentations.
   f. Position may affect the ability to clearly hear the heart tones.
6. Failure to hear FHTs at the expected time may be due to maternal obesity, polyhydramnios, error in date calculation, or fetal death.

Nursing and Patient Care Considerations

1. Explain equipment, purpose, and procedure to patient.
2. Assist patient to a sidelying or semi-Fowler position. Perform Leopold maneuvers.
3. Document findings on patient's chart and monitor strip along with date, time, activity level, medications, and other information per your health care facility's guidelines.
4. Discontinue electronic fetal monitoring, as indicated, according to facility guidelines.
5. Document and communicate appropriate information in the patient record to the patient and provider.
6. Monitor tracings become part of the neonate's and mother's chart and are legal documents that may be used in litigation.

Assessment of Fetal Movement

Description

Fetal movement or "kick counts" may be evaluated daily by the pregnant woman to provide reassurance of fetal well-being. Several methods are used in practice but study comparisons do not provide sufficient evidence to influence practice related to the ideal number of kicks or the ideal interval for movement counting. Methods are facility specific, and policy should be standardized for consistently. Testing can be as short as 5 minutes or as long as 2 hours.

Nursing and Patient Care Considerations

1. Instruct patient to lie on her side in a quiet place with no distractions. Have her place her hands on the largest part of her abdomen and concentrate on fetal movement.
2. Instruct patient to use a clock and record the movements felt. Once the tenth movement is felt, the testing is stopped. If fewer than 10 movements are felt in 2 hours or if the time it takes to get the 10 movements takes longer to achieve than earlier testing, she should contact her primary care provider.
3. Instruct patient that fetal movements are best assessed after meals, after or with light abdominal massage, or after short walks, and if she has not smoked for the last 2 hours.
4. Instruct patient that the fetus can sleep for up to 40 minutes.
5. Request patient to explain the procedure so her understanding is ensured.

Alpha-Fetoprotein

Description

Alpha-fetoprotein is produced by the fetus' liver and present in amniotic fluid. Small amounts cross the placenta into the maternal circulation.

1. MS-AFP levels are analyzed at 15 to 20 weeks gestation to identify neural tube defects and Down syndrome (trisomy 21) and may be tested alone or with a triple or quad screening. This testing is not diagnostic, and further diagnostic testing may be indicated for conclusive results.
   a. Elevated MS-AFP levels may be associated with birth defects and chromosomal abnormalities, such as open neural tube defects, open abdominal defects, and congenital nephrosis. Also associated with Rh isoimmunization, multiple gestation, maternal diabetes mellitus, and fetoplacental dysfunction.
   b. Decreased levels have been associated with Down syndrome and other chromosome anomalies (eg, gestational trophoblastic disease) but are not diagnostic.
   c. Follow-up for abnormal high or low levels includes ultrasound examination and amniocentesis.

2. Triple marker screening (TMS) can also be used for the evaluation of trisomy 18 and 21 and neural tube defects. This test is costly when compared to MS-AFP; thus, it is limited in its use. The TMS evaluates unconjugated estriol and hCG: Down syndrome shows increased hCG and decreased estriol levels; trisomy 18 shows decreased hCG and decreased estriol levels.

3. The quadruple screen, which includes a measurement of the substance dimeric inhibin A, provides a more sensitive and accurate detection of trisomy 21.

Nursing and Patient Care Considerations

1. Obtain health and pregnancy history, including the date of patient's last menses and risk factors. Accurate dating of the pregnancy is crucial to interpret the results of the serum levels.

2. Explain the purpose and procedure for the test.

3. Explain that the testing is for screening purposes only and not diagnostic. If an abnormal result is detected, further testing may be recommended.

4. Discuss patient's concerns.

Ultrasound and Doppler Studies

Description

Ultrasonography is a noninvasive, safe technique that uses reflected sound waves as they travel in tissue to produce a picture. In the abdominal approach, a clear gel is applied to the woman's abdomen or to the transducer, and the transducer is moved along the abdomen by the examiner. Images are produced onto a screen. During the early weeks of gestation, when the uterus remains a pelvic organ, a full bladder may be necessary to facilitate visualization. In the transvaginal approach, a lubricated transducer probe is inserted (either by the woman or by the examiner) into the vagina. No full bladder is necessary, and this technique is especially useful during the early weeks of pregnancy or when cervical evaluation is important (ie, for assessment of preterm labor). Three-dimensional ultrasonography is a newer technology that is believed to offer improved assessment of fetal growth and weight parameters.

1. Indications for a first trimester (prior to 13 6/7 weeks gestation) ultrasonography:
   a. Early confirmation of intrauterine pregnancy.
   b. To confirm cardiac activity.
   c. Estimated date of confinement.
   d. Estimate gestational age.
   e. To evaluate for an ectopic pregnancy or gestational trophoblastic disease.
   f. Detection of an intrauterine device.
   g. Evaluation of placental location.
   h. Diagnosis of a multiple gestation.
   i. Guidance for chorionic villous sampling (CVS) between 10 and 13 weeks requiring a small sample of placental tissue for prenatal diagnosis of certain chromosomal abnormalities when early diagnosis is preferred.
   j. Nuchal translucency at 11 to 14 weeks to screen for fetal aneuploidy.

2. Indications for second- and third-trimester ultrasonography that may be standard, limited, or specialized as necessary:
   a. Fetal survey for anatomy, growth, weight, gestational age, and anomalies.
   b. Evaluation of the placenta position and attachment.
   c. Evaluation of fetal presentation and position.
   d. Evaluation of fetal viability and cardiac activity.
   e. Biophysical profile (BPP).
   f. Evaluation of amniotic fluid volume.
   g. Guidance for amniocentesis or fetal blood sampling.

3. Doppler flow study, also known as Doppler velocimetry, is a noninvasive way to analyze uteroplacental blood flow within the umbilical, uterine, and cerebral arteries. The use of this technology primarily focuses on placental analysis to identify patients at risk for increased perinatal mortality. Systolic and diastolic ratios are measured within the arteries. If the ratios rise above normal, it means that blood flow to the placenta is decreased.

4. Three- and four-dimensional (3-D and 4-D) ultrasonography evaluates major and superficial vessels of the placenta, including the cord, fetal physiologic development, and fetal behavior. There are a number of advantages to 3-D and 4-D ultrasonography over Doppler velocimetry, such as decreased time of fetal exposure to ultrasound beam (2 to 5 minutes for 3-D vs. 15 to 30 minutes for velocimetry), off-line image processing, and identification of placental anastomoses, to mention a few.

Nursing and Patient Care Considerations

1. Explain the purpose and procedure to patient, emphasizing the need to remain still.

2. Inform patient of the need for a full bladder, if indicated, before the procedure.

3. When indicated, instruct patient to drink three to four glasses of water if the bladder is not full.

4. Instruct patient not to void until the procedure is over.

5. Remove the lubricant from patient's abdomen after the procedure or provide perineal cleaning products, as needed.

Note: Nurse can perform ultrasound if credentialed in limited ultrasound.

Amniocentesis

Description

Amniocentesis is a diagnostic procedure requiring informed consent, in which amniotic fluid is removed from the uterine cavity by insertion of a needle through the abdominal and uterine walls and into the amniotic sac. The procedure, when performed between 15 and 20 weeks gestation, is used genetic evaluation. In later pregnancy, amniocentesis is performed for the assessment of fetal lung maturity and to treat polyhydramnios. Risks are associated with the procedure such as miscarriage (1:300 to 500 procedures), chorioamnionitis, and preterm premature rupture of membranes. In determination of genetic or metabolic diseases, the procedure is performed between 16 and 18 weeks gestation. It is useful for women age 35 or older, for those with a family history of metabolic disease, a previous child with a chromosomal abnormality, a family history of chromosomal abnormality, a patient or husband with a chromosomal abnormality, or a possible female carrier of an X-linked disease.

1. In determination of lung maturity, the lecithin/sphingomyelin (L/S) ratio of the amniotic fluid is analyzed.
   a. When the L/S ratio is 2:1 or greater, the fetal lung is considered mature and the incidence of respiratory distress syndrome in the neonate is low.
   b. Results may be less reliable with maternal diabetes or if the fluid is contaminated with blood or meconium.

2. The presence of phosphatidylglycerol (PG), one of the last lung surfactants to develop, is the most reliable indicator of fetal lung maturity. PG is not present until 36 weeks gestation and is measured as being present or absent. Unlike the L/S ratio, PG is not affected by hypoglycemia, hypoxia, or hypothermia.

3. In the treatment of polyhydramnios also called hydramnios (2,000 mL amniotic fluid or greater than 25 cm amniotic fluid index [AFI]), amniocentesis may be performed to drain excess fluid and relieve pressure. Polyhydramnios can be associated with specific fetal abnormalities, such as trisomy 18, anencephaly, spina bifida, and esophageal atresia or tracheo-esophageal fistula.

Nursing and Patient Care Considerations

1. Reduce anxiety related to the procedure.
   a. Reduce the parents' anxiety by determining their understanding of the procedure and the meaning it holds for them.
   b. Reexplain the procedure before it begins and answer any questions they have. Ensure informed consent is signed.
   c. Provide explanations during the procedure, correct misinformation they may have, and make sure they know when the results will be available and how they may obtain the results as soon as possible.
2. Reduce pain and discomfort related to the procedure.
   a. Reduce discomfort by having patient lie comfortably on her back with her hands and a pillow under her head. Relaxation and controlled breathing may help.
   b. Ensure adequate time between infiltration of local anesthetic and introduction of needle into the amniotic sac.
   c. IV access in accordance with facility policy. Tocolytics such as terbutaline may be administered per facility policy.
3. Reduce potential for traumatic injury to fetus, placenta, or maternal structures.
   a. Have patient empty her bladder if the fetus is more than 20 weeks gestation to avoid injury to patient's bladder. If the fetus is less than 20 weeks gestation, patient's full bladder will hold the uterus steady and out of the pelvis. The placenta is localized with the use of ultrasound.
   b. Obtain maternal vital signs and a 20-minute FHR tracing to serve as a baseline to evaluate possible complications.
   c. Monitor patient during and after the procedure for signs of premature labor or bleeding.
   d. Tell patient to report signs of bleeding, unusual fetal activity or abdominal pain, cramping, or fever while at home after the procedure.
   e. If woman in Rh negative, may need to administer RhoGAM.

Chorionic Villus Sampling

Description

Chorionic villus sampling (CVS) involves obtaining samples of chorionic villus (placental tissue [fetal origin]) to test for chromosomal (via deoxyribonucleic acid [DNA]) and enzymatic disorders of the fetus. CVS is ideally performed between 10 and 14 weeks gestation.

1. Using ultrasound, a catheter is passed vaginally into the uterus, where a specimen of chorionic villus tissue is removed.
2. Results from CVS are available in 4 days.
3. Complications include rupture of membranes, intrauterine infection, spontaneous abortion, hematoma, fetal trauma, or maternal tissue contamination.
4. Incidence of fetal loss is about 2% to 5%.

Nursing and Patient Care Considerations

1. Obtain maternal vital signs.
2. Instruct patient to void.
3. Offer reassurance and compassionate presence during the procedure.

4. If woman in Rh negative, may need to administer RhoGAM.
5. Inform patient that a small amount of spotting is normal, but heavy bleeding or passing clots or tissue should be reported to provider immediately.
6. Instruct patient to rest at home for a few hours after the procedure.

Percutaneous Umbilical Blood Sampling

Description

Percutaneous umbilical blood sampling (PUBS), or *cordocentesis*, involves a puncture of the umbilical cord (vein) for aspiration of fetal blood under ultrasound guidance.

1. It is used in the diagnosis of fetal blood disorders, infections, Rh isoimmunization, metabolic disorders, and karyotyping.
2. Transfusion to the fetus may be conducted with this procedure.
3. Using ultrasound picture, the provider inserts a needle (guided by ultrasound) into one of the umbilical vessels. A small amount of blood is withdrawn.
4. Can also be used for fetal therapies, such as RBC and platelet transfusion.

Nursing and Patient Care Considerations

1. Explain the procedure to patient.
2. Provide support to patient during the procedure.
3. Monitor patient after the procedure for uterine contractions and the FHR for distress.
4. If woman in Rh negative, may need to administer RhoGAM.

Biochemical Markers

Description

1. *Fetal fibronectin (fFN)* is a protein that is secreted by the trophoblast of the implanted egg. The exact function is unknown; however, this protein is thought to play a key role in placental–uterine attachment. It is considered to be a better marker of women who will *not* go into PTL than those who *will* go into PTL.
   a. Normally present in cervical or vaginal fluid before 20 weeks gestation.
   b. After 20 weeks' gestation, the presence of fFN can indicate a detachment of the fetal membranes and should be evaluated as an early marker for preterm birth.
   c. Specimen is collected no earlier than 24 weeks and no later than 34 weeks and 6 days.
   d. A positive finding for fetal fibronectin alone is not predictive of PTL.

Nursing and Patient Care Considerations

1. Explain the procedure to patient.
2. Collect specimen with a Dacron swab placed in the posterior fornix of the vagina and rotated for 10 seconds. Sexual activity within 24 hours of sample collection, recent cervical examination, and vaginal bleeding may result in a false-positive test.
3. Provide support to patient during the procedure.

 EVIDENCE BASE DeFranco, E. A., Lewis, D. F., & Odibo, A. O. (2013). Improving the screening accuracy for preterm labor: Is the combination of fetal fibronectin and cervical length in symptomatic patients a useful predictor of preterm birth? A systematic review. *American Journal of Obstetrics and Gynecology, 208*(3), 233. e1–233.e6.

Nonstress Test

Description

The *nonstress test (NST)* is used to evaluate FHR accelerations that normally occur in response to fetal activity as a measure of utero-placental function. Accelerations are indicative of an intact central and autonomic nervous system and are a sign of fetal well-being. Absence of FHR accelerations in response to fetal movements may be associated with hypoxia, acidosis, drugs (analgesics, barbiturates), fetal sleep pattern, and some fetal anomalies.

1. Maternal indications include postdates, Rh sensitization, maternal age 35 or older, chronic renal disease, hypertension, collagen disease, sickle cell disease, diabetes, premature rupture of membranes, history of stillbirth, trauma, and vaginal bleeding in the second and third trimesters.
2. There are no contraindications or known adverse effects associated with the NST.
3. Fetal indications include decreased fetal movement, intrauterine growth restriction, fetal evaluation after an amniocentesis, external cephalic version, oligohydramnios, or polyhydramnios.
   a. Criteria for a reactive NST for a fetus greater than 32 weeks gestation include two accelerations within 20 minutes, each lasting at least 15 seconds with an FHR increased by 15 bpm above baseline in response to fetal activity. The quality of the tracing is an important factor in the test interpretation.
   b. Criteria for a reactive NST in a preterm fetus (less than 32 completed weeks gestation) include two accelerations within 20 minutes, each lasting at least 10 seconds with an FHR increased by 10 bpm above baseline in response to fetal activity.
   c. Testing time for the term NST can be as long as 40 minutes. Testing time for the preterm NST can be as long as 60 to 90 minutes.
   d. In a nonreactive NST, the above criteria are not met.
4. Significance/management
   a. Reactive NST—is reassuring and suggests a less than 1% chance of fetal death within 1 week of the NST. However, nonpreventable fetal death for abruptio placentae, sepsis, and cord accidents are excluded.
   b. Nonreactive NST—suggests a fetus that may be compromised and there needs to be further follow-up with a BPP, modified BPP, contraction stress test (CST), or oxytocin challenge test (OCT).

Nursing and Patient Care Considerations

1. Explain the procedure and equipment to the patient. Make sure the patient has had adequate nutrition and fluid intake and, if a smoker, has not been smoking within the past 2 hours.
2. Instruct the patient to void prior to NST for comfort.
3. Assist patient to a semi-Fowler position in bed. Perform Leopold maneuvers, and apply the external fetal and uterine monitors.
4. Event markers do not need to be used unless the fetal movement is not observed on the fetal monitor. If fetal movement not observed, instruct patient to make a mark on the monitor strip each time fetal movement is felt. The nurse will do this if patient cannot.
5. Evaluate the response of the FHR immediately after fetal activity.
6. Monitor patient's BP and uterine activity during the procedure.

Fetal Acoustic Stimulation Test and Vibroacoustic Stimulation Test

Description

Acoustic (sound) and vibroacoustic stimulation (VAS) are sound plus vibration involving the use of handheld battery-operated devices (usually a laryngeal stimulator) placed over the mother's abdomen near the fetal head. This technique produces a low-frequency vibration and a buzzing tone intended to induce fetal movement along with associated FHR accelerations. The sound stimulus should last for up to 3 seconds. The *fetal acoustic stimulation test (FAST)* and *vibroacoustic stimulation test (VST)* are used as an adjunct following a nonreactive NST; these tests may also be used with fetuses that exhibit a nonreassuring FHR cardiotocographic (CTG) tracing during labor. If no FHR accelerations occur in response to the stimulus, it is repeated at 1-minute intervals up to three times (total of 6 seconds). If the FHR tracing remains nonreactive, further evaluation with BPP or CST is indicated. In the light of advanced ultrasound technology, this test is being used less frequently. However, there are still facilities that do not have the ultrasound capabilities; therefore, this testing is appropriate.

1. It is not known whether the fetus responds more to the sound or to the vibration.
2. Both methods of testing are noninvasive, easy to perform, and yield rapid results.
3. No adverse neurologic or auditory effects noted in the fetus after testing.

Nursing and Patient Care Considerations

1. Explain procedure, equipment, and purpose to patient.
2. Instruct the patient to void prior to NST for comfort.
3. Assist patient to a semi-Fowler position in bed.
4. Apply external fetal monitors to patient.
5. Demonstrate how the stimulus may feel on patient's forearm or leg.
6. Observe for reactivity.

Contraction Stress Test (Oxytocin Contraction Test)

Description

Contraction stress test (CST) or OCT is used to evaluate the ability of the fetus to withstand the stress of uterine contractions as would occur during labor.

1. The test is generally used when a woman has a nonreactive NST or FAST/VST, although in many areas, the CST has been replaced by the BPP.
2. The test is contraindicated in women with third-trimester bleeding, multiple gestation, incompetent cervix, placenta previa, previous classic uterine incision, hydramnios, history of PTL, or premature rupture of membranes.
3. Contractions may occur spontaneously (unusual), or they may be induced endogenously producing oxytocin with nipple or breast stimulation.
4. The OCT utilizes exogenous oxytocin, which is administered by titrated IV infusion with continuous fetal monitoring.

Nursing and Patient Care Considerations

1. Obtain maternal vital signs, especially BP.
2. Instruct patient to void for comfort.
3. Assist patient to a semi-Fowler or sidelying position in bed.
4. Obtain a 20-minute strip of the FHR and uterine activity for baseline data.

5. For CST:
   a. Apply warm packs to the breasts for 10 minutes before the CST.
   b. Instruct patient on nipple stimulation. Instruct patient to brush or roll the nipple, using the palmar surface of the index finger and thumb. The patient can do this through her clothes or skin-to-skin. If using skin-to-skin, provide the patient with some lubricant to use on her fingers to ease stimulation. Stimulation occurs in 4 cycles of 2 minutes *on* and 2 to 5 minutes off (*for ease of memory: 1 cycle = 2 minutes on and 2 minutes off*). The nipple is stimulated until contractions begin *or* 2 minutes have passed.
   c. If contractions occur during stimulation, instruct the patient to stop the stimulation; she can begin the stimulation again when the contraction is over. If no contractions after four cycles, two different methods can be used:
      i. Let the patient rest for 5 to 10 minutes, then begin bilateral continuous stimulation for 5 to 10 minutes, stopping when contractions begin (have the patient resume stimulation when contraction ends).
      ii. Let the patient rest for 5 to 10 minutes, then begin stimulation again, alternating nipples, stopping when contractions begin (have the patient resume stimulation when contraction ends).
   d. Stop the stimulation if:
      i. Three or more contractions occur within 10 minutes that last more than or equal to 40 seconds.
      ii. Hyperstimulation or tachysystole occurs.
      iii. Unsuccessful nipple stimulation (two rounds of four cycles without contractions). Notify health care provider and prepare for OCT, BPP, or modified BPP.
6. For OCT: Follow steps 1 through 4 above. In addition:
   a. Administer low-dose oxytocin infusion using a pump, as indicated, until three contractions occur within 10 minutes and last ≥40 seconds. Maintain mainline IV fluids in accordance with facility policy.
   b. Discontinue the infusion when:
      i. Criteria are met.
      ii. Maximum dose of 16 milliunits per minute has been achieved.
      iii. Hyperstimulation or tachysystole occurs. Prolonged deceleration, bradycardia, or late decelerations are observed.

Interpretation of CST/OCT

1. Negative (normal/reassuring)—absence of late or variable decelerations.
2. Positive (abnormal/nonreassuring)—late decelerations with more than 50% of uterine contractions even if frequency is less than three contractions in 10 minutes; usually associated with absent or minimal variability.
3. Equivocal—intermittent late decelerations (less than 50% of uterine contractions) or significant variables.
4. Unsatisfactory—quality of tracing inadequate to assess or less than three contractions in 10 minutes or contractions less than 40 seconds in duration.
5. Equivocal and unsatisfactory results can be repeated in 24 hours or sooner unless indication for delivery is present.
6. Regardless of the result, if variable decelerations are present, further testing should be done to evaluate for oligohydramnios.

Biophysical Profile

Description

The *biophysical profile (BPP)* uses ultrasonography and NST to assess five biophysical variables in determining fetal well-being. A BPP is performed during a 30-minute time frame by someone credentialed in ultrasonography.

1. For each variable, if the criteria are met, a score of 2 is given. For an abnormal observation, a score of 0 is given.
2. A score of 8 to 10 is reassuring, 6 is equivocal and requires further evaluation, and 4 or less is nonreassuring and requires further evaluation and delivery may be considered.
   a. NST—assessing for FHR acceleration (fetal reactivity) in relation to fetal movements.
   b. AFI volume—assessing for one or more pockets of amniotic fluid measuring at least (2 cm) or more in two perpendicular planes.
   c. Fetal breathing movements—one or more episodes lasting at least 30 seconds within 30 minutes.
   d. Gross fetal body movements—three or more body or limb movements, in 30 minutes.
   e. Fetal muscle tone—one or more episodes of active extension with return to flexion of spine, hand, or limbs within 30 minutes.

Nursing and Patient Care Considerations

1. Explain the purpose and procedure to the patient; provide emotional support.
2. Instruct patient to empty her bladder for comfort.
3. Assist patient onto the examination table and help her to assume a position of comfort.
4. Remove the lubricant from patient's abdomen after the procedure.
5. Assist patient in rising from the examination table.

Modified BPP

Description

The modified BPP is more common today than the BPP. It consists of an NST and an assessment of AFI. The modified BPP performed twice per week provides the same predictive results as the weekly CST.

1. Normal interpretation is a reactive NST with an AFI greater than 5 cm. A normal AFI is 9 to 25 cm with a borderline "normal" being 5 to 8 cm.
2. An abnormal AFI of less than 5 cm of amniotic fluid (oligohydramnios) requires a full ultrasound evaluation, and the fetus is evaluated for functioning renal tissue.

Nursing and Patient Care Considerations

1. Explain NST and AFI check in accordance with previously stated guidelines, as noted in this chapter.
2. Document findings in patient's prenatal record.

SELECTED REFERENCES

American Academy of Pediatrics & American College of Obstetricians and Gynecologists. (2012). *Guidelines for perinatal care* (7th ed.). Washington, DC: Author.

American College of Obstetricians and Gynecologists. (2016). *Management of preterm labor. Practice Bulletin # 171*. Washington, DC: Author.

American College of Obstetricians and Gynecologists. (2015). *Diagnostic tests for birth defects FAQ's*. Washington, DC: Author. Available: www.acog.org/Patients/FAQs/Diagnostic-Tests-for-Birth-Defects.

American College of Obstetricians and Gynecologists. (2016). *Exercise during pregnancy FAQs*. Washington, DC: Author. www.acog.org/patients/FAQS/exercise-during-pregnancy.

American College of Obstetricians and Gynecologists. (2010/Reaffirmed 2016). *Screening for perinatal depression (Committee Opinion No. 630)*. Washington, DC: Author.

American College of Obstetricians and Gynecologists. (2014) (1999/Reaffirmed 2016). *Antepartum fetal surveillance. Practice Bulletin #145*. Washington, DC: Author.

American College of Obstetricians and Gynecologists. (2013). *Screening and diagnosis of gestational diabetes mellitus. Practice Bulletin # 137*. Washington, DC: Author.

American College of Obstetricians and Gynecologists. (2012). *Intimate partner violence (Committee Opinion No. 518)*. Washington, DC: Author.

American College of Obstetricians and Gynecologists and Society for Fetal Medicine. (2016). *Periviable birth: Obstetric care consensus*. Washington, DC: ACOG. Available: *www.acog.org/Resources-And-Publications/Obstetric-Care-Consensus-Series/Periviable-Birth*.

Association of Women's Health, Obstetric, Neonatal Nurses. (2015). *Fetal heart monitoring: Principles and practices* (5th ed.). Dubuque, IA: Kendall Hunt Publishing Company.

Barron, M. L. (2014). Antenatal care. In K. R. Simpson & P. A. Creehan (Eds.), *Perinatal nursing* (4th ed., pp. 89–121). Philadelphia, PA: Wolters, Kluwer.

Blackburn, S. T. (2014). Physiologic changes of pregnancy. In K. R. Simpson & P. A. Creehan (Eds.), *Perinatal nursing* (4th ed., pp. 71–88). Philadelphia, PA: Wolters, Kluwer.

Callahan, L. (2016). Fetal and placental development and functioning. In S. Mattson & J. E. Smith (Eds.), *Core curriculum for maternal–newborn nursing* (5th ed., pp. 37–62). St. Louis, MO: Saunders Elsevier.

Cypher, L. (2016). Antepartum fetal surveillance and prenatal diagnosis. In S. Mattson & J. E. Smith (Eds.), *Core curriculum for maternal–newborn nursing* (5th ed., pp. 135–156). St. Louis, MO: Saunders Elsevier.

Jain, V., Chari, R., Maslovitz, S., & Farine, D. (2015). Guidelines for the management of a pregnant trauma patient. *Journal of Obstetrics and Gynaecology Canada, 37*(6), 553–571.

Kaimal, A. J. (2014). Assessment of fetal health. In M. F. Greene, R. K. Creasy, J. D. Resnick, J. D. Iams, C. J. Lockwood, & T. Moore (Eds.). (2014). *Maternal–fetal medicine: Principles and practice* (7th ed., pp. 473–506). Philadelphia, PA: Elsevier Saunders.

Kennedy, D. A., Lupattelli, A., Koren, G., & Nordeng, H. (2016). Safety classification of herbal medicines used in pregnancy in a multinational study. *BMC Complementary and Alternative Medicine, 16*(102), 1–9.

Ladwig, G. B., Ackley, B. J., & Flynn-Makic, M. B. (2017). *Mosby's guide to nursing diagnosis* (5th ed.). St. Louis, MO: Elsevier.

Link, D. G. (2016). Psychology of pregnancy. In S. Mattson & J. E. Smith (Eds.), *Corecurriculum for maternal–newborn nursing* (5th ed., pp. 108–122). St. Louis, MO: Saunders Elsevier.

Link, D. G. (2016). Reproductive anatomy, physiology, and the menstrual cycle. In S. Mattson & J. E. Smith (Eds.), *Core curriculum for maternal–newborn nursing* (5th ed., pp. 4–5). St. Louis, MO: Saunders Elsevier.

Manqesi, L. Hofmeyr, G. J., Smith, V., & Smyth R. M. (2015). Fetal movement counting for assessment of fetal wellbeing. *Cochrane Database System Reviews* (10), CD004909.

Mattson, S., & Smith, J. (2016). *Core curriculum for maternal-newborn nursing* (5th ed.) St. Louis, MO: Saunders Elsevier.

Monga, M. & Mastrobattista, J. M. (2014). Maternal cardiovascular, respiratory, and renal adaptation to pregnancy. In M. F. Greene R. K. Creasy, & J. D. Resnick, J. D. Iams C. J. Lockwood & T. Moore (Eds.), *Maternal–fetal medicine: Principles and practice* (7th ed., pp. 93–99). Philadelphia, PA: Elsevier Saunders.

National Institutes of Health. (2017). *What are the factors that put a pregnancy at risk?* Bethesda, MD: Author. Available: *www.nichd.nih.gov/health/topics/high-risk/conditioninfo/pages/factors.aspx*.

Records, K. (2015). Obesity and women's health. *Journal of Obstetric, Gynecologic & Neonatal Nursing, 44*(6), 758–759.

Records, K., & Tanaka, L. (2016). Physiology of pregnancy. In S. Mattson & J. E. Smith (Eds.), *Core curriculum for maternal–newborn nursing* (5th ed., pp. 83–107). St. Louis, MO: Saunders Elsevier.

Ricci, S. S. (2017). *Essentials of maternity, newborn, and women's health nursing* (4th ed.). Philadelphia, PA: Wolters, Kluwer.

Son, M., & Miller, E.S. (2017). Predicting preterm birth: Cervical length and fetal fibronectin. *Seminars in Perinatology, 41*(8), 445–451.

Stotland, N. E., Bodnar, L. M., & Abrams, B. (2014). Maternal nutrition. In M. F. Greene R. K. Creasy, & J. D. Resnick, J. D. Iams C. J. Lockwood & T. Moore (Eds.), *Maternal–fetal medicine: Principles and practice* (7th ed., pp. 131–138). Philadelphia, PA: Elsevier Saunders.

United States Department of Agriculture. (2017). *Nutritional needs during pregnancy*. Available: *www.choosemyplate.gov/nutritional-needs-during-pregnancy*.

World Health Organization. (2017). *Social determinants of health*. Geneva, Switzerland: Author. Available: *www.who.int/social_determinants/en*.

37

Nursing Management During Labor and Delivery

THE LABOR PROCESS

The phases of pregnancy, labor, and birth are normal physiologic processes. A pregnant woman typically approaches the birth process with possible concerns of personal well-being, that of her unborn child, and fear of labor pain. Addressing these concerns, minimizing her discomfort, and optimizing patient safety should be of paramount importance to all participants involved in the care of the mother and her fetus during the intrapartum period.

General Considerations

 EVIDENCE BASE Lowdermilk, D., Perry, S., Cashion, C., & Alden, K. R. (2016). *Maternity and women's health care* (11th ed.). St. Louis, MO: Elsevier.
  Mattson, S., & Smith, J. E. (2016). *Core curriculum for maternal–newborn nursing* (5th ed.). St. Louis, MO: Elsevier.

Prepared Childbirth

Historically, the term *natural childbirth* has evolved to mean (1) delivery outside in nature, (2) home birth, (3) nonhospital birth (birthing center), (4) facility birth—no medical intervention (eg, no intravenous [IV] medications)—and, most recently, (5) facility birth without analgesia or anesthesia. Preparation through education and training prior to labor gives the pregnant woman a method of coping with the discomforts of labor and delivery. This method is known as *prepared childbirth* and incorporates analgesia and anesthesia into the process. The latter method dominates current culture in the United States. Variances in prepared childbirth are outlined.

Psychoprophylactic or Lamaze Method
1. Psychoprophylactic childbirth has a rationale based on Pavlov concept of pain perception and his theory of conditioned reflexes (the substitution of favorable conditioned reflexes for unfavorable ones). The Lamaze method is an example of this technique.
2. The woman learns to replace responses of restlessness, fear, and loss of control with more controlled measures, which can excite the cerebral cortex efficiently to inhibit other stimuli such as pain in labor.
3. The mother learns exercises that strengthen the abdominal muscles and relax the perineum.
4. The mother/partner/support person learns various breathing techniques to help maintain focus and a sense of control during the labor process.

The mother learns to respond with respiratory measures and disassociation or relaxation of the uninvolved muscles while controlling her perception of the stimuli associated with labor.

The Bradley Method of Delivery
1. Commonly referred to as "partner-coached childbirth." A coach may be *any* significant other designated by the mother.
2. Involves the concepts of leading, guiding, supporting, caring, and fostering specific skills and confidence.
3. Coaches attend classes and learn to help the woman prior to labor.
4. The coach serves as a conditioned stimulus using the sound of his or her voice, use of particular words, and repetition of practice.
5. Relaxation is the core component and medications are not encouraged for pain relief. Increased tolerance to pain is accomplished by decreased mental anxiety and fear, which ultimately decreases the awareness of the pain stimulus. This occurs through cognitive and physical rehearsal.

The Dick-Read Method
1. Dr. Grantly Dick-Read wrote the landmark book, Childbirth without Fear in 1944.
2. Fear is the primary factor that creates tension and therefore increases pain perception.
3. Classes include a detailed explanation of the normal labor process to enhance understanding of the normal physiological changes associated with labor.
4. Women learn strategies such as abdominal breathing to break the fear–tension–pain cycle.

Planned Home Birth

1. Motivations for home delivery:
   a. Increases patient choices and flexibility during the birth process while decreasing patient separation and fear of medical intervention.
   b. Desire to avoid medical intervention such as anesthesia and operative procedures.
2. Contraindications:
   a. High-risk pregnancy such as placental abnormalities, multiple gestation, preeclampsia, and gestational diabetes.
   b. History of premature or postdate delivery in previous or current pregnancy or previous cesarean delivery.
   c. Diagnosed fetal abnormalities.
3. Alternatives to home delivery:
   a. Family-centered hospital setting.
   b. Birthing centers with adequate facilities for emergency care for low-risk women.

 NURSING ALERT Women interested in a planned home birth should weigh the risks and benefits for this method of delivery. Current evidence supports that the risk of perinatal death in home births is double that of facility births (however, still low at 1 to 2 per 1,000 births). Additionally, the risk of neonatal seizures or neurologic dysfunction is three times more likely to occur (0.4 to 0.6 per 1,000 births). Nurses working with the maternal–child population should provide women with educational resources that foster informed decision-making.

 EVIDENCE BASE American College of Obstetricians and Gynecologists. (2017). *Planned home birth* (Committee Opinion #697). Washington, DC: Author.

Initiation of Labor

 EVIDENCE BASE Cunningham, F. G., Leveno, K., Bloom, S., et al. (2014). *Williams obstetrics* (24th ed.). New York: McGraw-Hill.

Parturition is a multifactorial physiologic process and the exact mechanism initiating labor is unknown. The inhibition of labor during pregnancy is maintained by a constant release of progesterone and other uterotonic inhibitors (eg, PgI$_2$, relaxin, nitric oxide, and parathyroid hormone). Progesterone is the primary hormone of pregnancy, which prevents uterine contractility during the pregnancy. As the pregnancy approaches term, progesterone levels begin to decrease and estrogen levels increase reciprocally stimulating uterine contractility. Labor onset involves both maternal and fetal influences as outlined:
1. Maternal factors:
2. In preparation for labor, prostaglandin (PG) is released as the uterus stretches to accommodate the fetus.
3. The posterior pituitary releases oxytocin because of pressure on the cervix.
4. Oxytocin and PG jointly aid in the inhibition of calcium binding in muscle cells, thus increasing the calcium levels intracellularly causing uterine contractions.
5. Placental and fetal factors:
   a. Placental maturation triggers the onset of contractions.
   b. The concentration of fetal cortisol increases in response to the increase in maternal oxytocin.

Factors Affecting Labor Process

The five Ps: the success of labor and delivery depends on five factors: *passageway (birth canal)*, *passenger (fetus)*, *powers (contractions)*, *position (maternal)*, and *psychological response*.

 EVIDENCE BASE Ricci, S. S. (2017). *Essentials of maternity, newborn and women's health nursing* (4th ed.). Philadelphia, PA: Wolters Kluwer Health/ Lippincott Williams & Wilkins.

Passageway: Pelvic Dimensions
1. Pelvic inlet (anteroposterior diameter): The obstetric conjugate anteroposterior measurement is typically more than 10 cm. Over 50% of women have a gynecoid-shaped pelvis to accommodate proper descent.
2. Midpelvis (ischial spines): Intraspinous diameter is typically more than 10 cm; protrusion of the spines into the birthing canal may complicate descent.
3. Pelvic outlet (intertuberous diameter + suprapubic arch): Dimensions are estimated as the anteroposterior diameter from the coccyx to the symphysis pubis. This is typically 13 cm in length, but again one must subtract 1.5 to 2 cm from the calculation because of the thickness of the symphysis. A prominent coccyx may impede descent.

Passenger: Fetal Dimensions
1. Size—assessed via palpation using Leopold maneuvers or ultrasound. Excessive size may lead to inadequate or asynclitic descent, labor dystocia, shoulder dystocia, or postpartum hemorrhage.
2. Attitude—typically, the fetal head and extremities are flexed while the back is rounded. Flexion of the head allows for the smallest diameter (occiput) to present and pass through the birth canal with ease (see Figure 37-1). Nonflexed presentations may increase risk of asynclitic conditions.
3. Lie—constitutes the comparison of the fetal long axis to the long axis of the mother. Variances include transverse, longitudinal, or oblique; 99% of fetuses present as a longitudinal lie parallel to the mother's spine. This improves ease of access into the birth canal.
4. Presentation—the fetal body part presenting into the birth canal first and is felt on vaginal exam (see Figure 37-2).
   a. Cephalic (head)—occiput, sinciput, brow, face, or chin (mentum).
   b. Breech (feet)—frank, complete, or footling (single or double).
   c. Shoulder (transverse).
   d. Compound—two or more parts presenting at the same time.
5. Position—specific landmark of fetal presenting part (occiput, mentum, sacrum, scapula) in comparison to the anterior, posterior, or transverse portion of the woman's pelvis and the maternal left or right side; designated by a three-letter abbreviation.
   a. The first letter L or R represents the side (right or left) in the maternal pelvis the presenting part is facing.
   b. The second letter represents the landmark that is presenting: O for occiput, M for mentum (chin), S for sacrum, and Sc for scapula or shoulder.
   c. The third letter represents the direction (anterior [A], posterior [P], or transverse [T]) the presenting part is facing in the pelvis.

Figure 37-1. **(A)** Complete flexion allows smallest diameter of the head to enter the pelvis. **(B)** Moderate extension causes larger diameter to enter the pelvis. **(C)** Marked extension forces largest diameter against pelvic brim, but the head is too large to enter the pelvis.

d. For example, the fetus with the head presenting and facing toward the maternal right anterior pelvis is right–occiput–anterior (ROA).

 EVIDENCE BASE American College of Obstetricians and Gynecologists. (2009/Reaffirmed 2016). *Induction of labor* (Practice Bulletin # 107). Washington, DC: Author.

Passenger: Fetal Head (Vertex)

In approximately 95% of all births, the fetal head (vertex) presents first. Sutures and fontanelles provide important landmarks for determining fetal position during a vaginal examination (see Figure 37-3).

1. Bones of the fetal skull:
   a. One occipital bone posteriorly.
   b. Two parietal bones bilaterally.
   c. Two temporal bones bilaterally.
   d. Two frontal bones anteriorly.
2. Sutures of the fetal skull—membranous spaces between the bones of the fetal skull:
   a. Frontal—between the two frontal bones.
   b. Sagittal—between the two parietal bones.
   c. Coronal—between the frontal and parietal bones.
   d. Lambdoidal—between the back of the parietal bones and the margin of the occipital bone.
3. Fontanelles of the fetal skull—irregular spaces formed where two or more sutures meet. Sutures and fontanelles allow fetal skull bones to overlap to pass through the maternal pelvis.
   a. Anterior—largest fontanelle; junction of the sagittal, frontal, and coronal sutures; closes by age 18 to 24 months; "diamond" shaped.

Figure 37-2. Fetal presentations. **(A)** Cephalic; **(B)** breech; **(C)** face; **(D)** transverse.

b. Posterior—located where the sagittal suture meets the lambdoidal suture (smaller than anterior); closes by 1 year; "triangle" shaped.

Powers: Uterine Contractions

Successful labor depends on regular uterine contractions of adequate intensity that lead to cervical advancement and facilitate fetal descent. The following are characteristics of labor contractions:
   a. Uterine contractions typically increase in intensity, frequency, and duration as labor progresses.
   b. Uterine contractions may cause vasoconstriction of the umbilical cord leading to potential alterations in the fetal heart rate (eg, variable decelerations).
   c. The active upper portion of the uterus (fundus) stimulates activation of contractions during labor (referred to as fundal dominance).

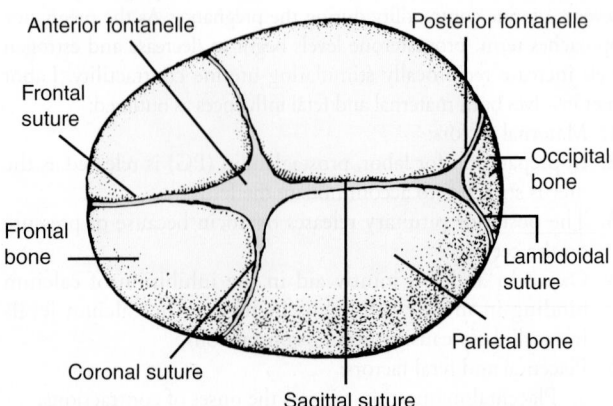

Figure 37-3. Fetal head.

d. At the completion of a contraction, the upper uterine segment retains its shortened, thickened cell size and, with each succeeding contraction, becomes thicker and shorter. As a result, the upper uterine segment never totally relaxes during labor. Cells of the lower uterine segment become thinner and longer with each contraction. This mechanism is greatly responsible for the progress of the fetus through the birth canal.

e. The differentiation point between the upper and lower uterine segment is known as the "physiologic retraction ring."

f. Intrabdominal pressure increases with voluntary maternal pushing efforts during the second stage of labor.

Position (Maternal)

1. The maternal position may influence pelvic size and contour and fetal position and assist fetal rotation.
2. The upright position may facilitate a shortened first and second stage.
3. Allows for the use of gravity for fetal decent.

Psychological Responses

1. A woman's psyche is essential to the labor process in the following ways:
   a. To maintain a sense of well-being and control.
   b. Assists the woman in facing the challenge of labor and sense of accomplishment.

Events Leading to Labor

1. Lightening is the settling of the fetus in the lower uterine segment occurring 2 to 3 weeks before term in the primigravida and typically during labor in the multigravida.
   a. Breathing becomes easier as the fetus falls away from the diaphragm.
   b. Lordosis of the spine is increased as the fetus enters the pelvis and moves more anteriorly. Walking may become more difficult as leg cramping may increase.
   c. Urinary frequency occurs due to pressure on the adjacent bladder.
2. Vaginal secretions may increase due to hormonal changes.
3. Mucus plug may be discharged from the cervix along with a small amount of blood from surrounding capillaries—referred to as "bloody show."
4. The cervix softens and effaces (shortens and thins) and gradually moves from a posterior to an anterior position.
5. Membranes may rupture spontaneously.
6. False labor contractions (Braxton Hicks) may occur (see Table 37-1) in preparation for true labor.
7. Backaches may occur due to fetal size and lightening.
8. Gastrointestinal alterations (eg, diarrhea) and weight loss of 1 to 3 pounds (0.5 to 1.5 kg) may occur with advanced pregnancy.
9. Energy may increase (referred to as "nesting") or decrease in the last few weeks.

Stages of Labor

First Stage of Labor (Labor Onset to Full Cervical Dilation and Effacement)

1. Begins with regular and rhythmic true labor contractions and ends with complete effacement (100%) and dilation of the cervix (10 cm).
2. The length of the first stage varies and is almost double in a primiparous patient; this stage of labor consists of three phases:

Table 37-1	True and False Labor Contractions
TRUE LABOR CONTRACTIONS	**FALSE LABOR CONTRACTIONS**
Result in progressive cervical dilation and effacement	Do not result in progressive cervical dilation and effacement
Occur at regular intervals	Occur at irregular intervals
Interval between contractions decreases	Interval between contractions remains the same or increases
Frequency, duration, and intensity increase	Intensity decreases or remains the same
Located mainly in the back and abdomen	Located mainly in the lower abdomen and groin
Generally intensified by walking	Generally unaffected by walking
Not easily disrupted by medications	Generally relieved by mild sedation

a. Latent phase (early):
   i. Dilation from 0 to 3 cm; effacement tends to precede dilation in the primiparous patient.
   ii. At the end of the phase, contractions typically occur regularly every 5 minutes on average and are mild via palpation.
b. Active phase:
   i. Dilation from 4 to 7 cm; completion of effacement evolves over this period in multiparous patients.
   ii. Contractions are more frequent at every 2 to 5 minutes, lasting 40 to 60 seconds and of moderate to strong intensity by palpation or 60 to 80 mm Hg when an internal uterine pressure catheter (IUPC) is in use. Dilation averages 1.2 cm/hour in the nullipara and 1.5 cm/hour in the multipara.
c. Transition phase: Dilation from 8 to 10 cm with contractions occurring every 2 to 3 minutes, lasting 60 to 90 seconds with strong intensity (nonindentable by palpation or 70 to 90 mm Hg with an IUPC).

Second Stage of Labor (Fetal Expulsion)

1. Begins with complete effacement and dilation ending with delivery of the fetus.
2. The second stage may last from 1 to 4 hours in the nullipara and typically less than 1 hour in the multipara. Variance in time depends on maternal pushing efforts, contraction pattern, anesthesia, and fetal descent and position.

Third Stage of Labor (Placental Expulsion)

1. Begins with delivery of the fetus and ends with delivery of the placenta.
2. The third stage may last from a few minutes to 30 minutes typically. Prolonged periods may be attributable to abnormal placentation (ie, placenta accreta) and may require further evaluation and intervention related to the increased risk of hemorrhage.

Fourth Stage (Immediate Postpartum)

This period lasts from delivery of the placenta until the postpartum condition of the woman has become stabilized. With the increase for improved outcomes related to hemorrhage, the fourth stage of labor lasts at least the first 2 hours and may require further assessment and evaluation based on maternal status.

Engagement, Descent, Flexion

Internal Rotation

External Rotation (Restitution)

Extension Beginning (rotation complete)

External Rotation (Shoulder rotation)

Extension Complete

Expulsion

Figure 37-4. Seven fetal cardinal movements of labor (vertex presentation). (Pillitteri, A. [2013]. *Maternal and child health nursing: Care of the childbearing and childrearing family* [7th ed.]. Philadelphia, PA: Lippincott Williams & Wilkins.)

Seven Cardinal Fetal Movements of Labor

When the biparietal diameter (BPD) of the fetal head has passed through the pelvic inlet, engagement occurs. Once the fetus enters the pelvis, seven "cardinal movements" occur to facilitate passage through the maternal pelvis during labor and birth (see Figure 37-4).

Descent

1. The downward movement of the fetus through the birth canal is accomplished by the force of uterine contractions and pressure of the amniotic fluid; during second stage of labor, "maternal bearing-down" efforts increase intra-abdominal pressure, thus augmenting effects of uterine contractions.
2. *Station* refers to the relationship of the presenting part to the ischial spines. Subsequently, station has a direct correlation to the degree of descent, as described below (see Figure 37-5):
   a. Floating—fetal presenting part is not engaged in pelvic inlet; may be ballotable via cervical exam.
   b. Engagement—fetal presenting part enters the pelvis as the BPD passes through the inlet.
   c. The pelvis is divided into sections measured in centimeters; a 5-cm scale is used (see Figure 37-6).

Flexion

Resistance to descent causes the fetal head to flex down, leading to convergence onto the chest.

1. Flexion results in the smallest head diameter, the suboccipito-bregmatic, to present through the canal.
2. This position relocates the posterior fontanelle to the center of the cervix, easily palpable on vaginal examination.
3. Flexion begins at the pelvic inlet and continues until the fetal head (or presenting part) reaches the pelvic floor.

Figure 37-5. Engagement, floating, and dipping.

-4 (floating)
-3
-2
-1
0 (engaged)
+1
+2
+3
+4 (at outlet)

Figure 37-6. Stations of presenting part. The location of the presenting part in relation to the level of the ischial spines is designated station and indicates the degree of advancement of the presenting part through the pelvis. Stations are expressed in centimeters above (minus) or below (plus) the level of the ischial spines (zero). (Pillitteri, A. [2013]. *Maternal and child health nursing: Care of the childbearing and childrearing family* [7th ed.]. Philadelphia, PA: Lippincott Williams & Wilkins.)

Internal Rotation

To accommodate the birth canal, the fetal occiput rotates 45 or 90 degrees from its original position toward the symphysis.

1. The rotation is usually anteriorly, but if the pelvis cannot accommodate the occiput anteriorly because of a narrow fore-pelvis, it will rotate posteriorly, resulting in an occipitoposterior (OP) position of the fetus.
2. This movement results from the shape of the fetal head and maternal pelvis, as well as the contour of the perineal muscles.
3. The ischial spines project into the midpelvis, causing the fetal head to rotate anteriorly to accommodate the available space.

Extension

1. As the fetal head meets the pelvic floor, it meets resistance from the perineal muscles and is forced to extend up and outward.
2. The fetal head becomes visible at the vulvovaginal ring; its largest diameter is encircled (crowning) and later emerges from the vagina.

External Rotation

1. Initial phase is called *restitution*. Once the fetal head realigns with the shoulders, restitution is complete.
2. The second phase of external rotation occurs as the body rotates so that the shoulders are in the anteroposterior diameter of the pelvis.

Expulsion

1. After delivery of the fetal head and internal rotation of the shoulders, the anterior shoulder resets beneath the symphysis pubis.
2. The posterior shoulder is expelled, followed by the anterior shoulder, leading to total body expulsion.

NURSING ASSESSMENT AND INTERVENTIONS
Initiation of Labor

Nursing responsibilities begin with an initial assessment once a patient presents in labor.

Collection of History and Baseline Data

EVIDENCE BASE Lowdermilk, D., Perry, S., Cashion, C., & Alden, K. R. (2016). *Maternity and women's health care* (11th ed.). St. Louis, MO: Elsevier.

American College of Obstetricians and Gynecologists. (2017). *Emergent therapy for acute-onset, severe hypertension during pregnancy, and the postpartum period* (Committee Opinion #692). Washington, DC: Author.

1. Introduce yourself; maintain eye contact as culturally appropriate; ask for name of woman's health care provider; inquire if the provider has been notified that the woman was coming to the facility or birth center; ask about presenting complaints/concerns; orient woman and partner to surroundings and explain the plan of care.
   a. Establish baseline obstetric, medical, and surgical information. Inquire and validate patient information with the prenatal care record, if available. Complete brief review of past medical (including allergies), surgical, and obstetric history.
   b. Obtain a history of the current pregnancy: gravidity, parity, expected date of delivery or confinement, complications, fetal growth, antepartal testing results, sexually transmitted infections, recent travel abroad, and group β streptococcus status if tested.
   c. Inquire about current labor status and validate uterine contraction data with palpation: when did contractions begin, frequency, intensity, and duration; fetal movement; bloody show; have the membranes ruptured, time of rupture, color, consistency, amount of fluid, and any odor?
   d. Assess patient's comfort level.
   e. Inquire about a birth plan, participation in childbirth preparation classes, and pain management plans.
   f. Last oral intake of solids and liquids.
   g. Medications taken—prescription, over the counter, illicit drugs, herbals, or supplements?
   h. Inquire about the woman's support system.
2. Obtain baseline maternal and fetal vital signs.
   a. Temperature—elevation more than 100.0°F (37.8°C) suggests a possible infection or dehydration.
   b. Pulse—elevated over the resting rate during contractions; may be elevated between contractions because of medications, bleeding, or drug use; goal: 60 to 100 bpm.
   c. Respirations—increase as labor progresses; goal: 12 to 24 breaths/minute.
   d. Blood pressure (BP)—slight elevation over baseline may be attributed to anxiety and pain.
      i. BP more than 140 diastolic or 90 systolic (mm Hg) may be suggestive of hypertensive disorder of pregnancy and requires further evaluation and notification to primary care provider.
      ii. BP of more than 160/110 requires immediate attention and notification of the primary health care provider because of potential for stroke or seizure (see page 1048).
      iii. Goal: Systolic more than 90 and less than 140 mm Hg; diastolic more than 60 and less than 90 mm Hg; mean arterial pressure (MAP) less than 100.

e. Complete fetal heart rate assessment; if a fetal monitor is to be used, run a 20-to 30-minute strip for baseline data and assessment of fetal well-being.

f. Physical assessment—complete review of systems on admission to include heart and lung sounds and deep tendon reflexes as indicated based on assessment.

3. Obtain a urine specimen—if indicated for symptoms of urinary tract infection or in cases of hypertension to check protein.

Methods for Determining Fetal Presentation

Leopold Maneuvers

The manual manipulation of the maternal abdomen to determine fetal placement in relation to maternal structures (see Figure 37-7).

1. First maneuver (fundal grip) (see Figure 37-7A)—determines fetal parts (fetal head or breech) located in the uterine fundus.

   a. While facing the woman, place both hands laterally on each side of the fundus and palpate; note the size, shape, and consistency.

   b. A head feels smooth, hard/firm, and round, mobile, and ballotable; breech position feels irregular, rounded, soft, and not independently mobile.

2. Second maneuver (lateral grip) (see Figure 37-7B)—identifies the relationship of the fetal back and the small parts to the front, back, or sides of the maternal abdomen (fetal lie).

   a. In the same position, lower hands bilaterally along the lateral borders of the maternal abdomen.

   b. Select one hand to stabilize one side of the uterus while the opposite hand palpates downward over the opposite side. Repeat on the opposing side.

   c. Determine fetal anatomy by palpated contents: firm, smooth, and a hard continuous structure = fetal back; if small, knobby, irregular, protruding, and moving = fetal extremities.

3. Third maneuver (1st pelvic grip) (see Figure 37-7C)—determines the portion of the fetus that is presenting into the pelvic inlet (fetal presentation). This maneuver is also known as Pallach's maneuver or grip.

   a. Grasp the part of the fetal presenting part situated in the lower uterine segment between the thumb and middle finger of one hand.

   b. Assess contents as described in the first maneuver; findings should be opposite of information found in the fundus.

4. Fourth maneuver (2nd pelvic grip) (see Figure 37-7D)—determines flexion or attitude of the fetal vertex or the greatest prominence of the fetal head over the pelvic brim.

   a. Face woman's feet and place hands on each side of the uterus, below the umbilicus and pointing toward the symphysis pubis.

   b. Press deeply with the fingertips toward the symphysis pubis, locating the cephalic prominence.

      i. If the cephalic prominence is felt on the same side as the small parts, sinciput (fetus' forehead), fetal vertex is flexed.

      ii. If the cephalic prominence is felt on the same side as the back, occiput (or crown), fetal vertex is flexed.

      iii. If the cephalic prominence is felt equally on both sides, military position (common in posterior position), fetal vertex is nonflexed.

   c. As hands move toward the pelvic brim, assess for the following: if the hands converge (come together) around the presenting part, it is floating; if the hands diverge (move apart), the presenting part is either dipping or engaged in the pelvis.

Ultrasonography

See page 985.

Vaginal Examination

See Figure 37-8.

1. Explain the procedure to the woman and assist her to a lithotomy position.

2. Keep patient covered as much as possible to maintain privacy.

3. Conduct examination gently using a sterile glove.

4. Perineum—visually assess the perineum for lesions, ulcerations, bruising, discharge, odor, rupture of membranes, or bleeding. If infection is suspected (ie, syphilis or genital herpes) or active bleeding exists, stop the examination and notify the health care provider for further evaluation.

5. Perform manual examination with dominant hand (may use nondominant hand over fundus to stabilize fetal presenting part against the cervix):

   a. Cervical assessment.

      i. Location: Posterior, mid, or anterior (facing the introitus and aligned parallel to the vagina).

      ii. Hard or soft: The cervix softens during latent phase of labor.

      iii. Long or short? As effacement occurs, the cervix shortens and thins. Measured in percentages from 0% to 100%.

      iv. Open or closed: Measure degree of dilation in centimeters from 1 to 10 cm (complete).

   b. Presentation.

      i. Breech, cephalic/vertex face, shoulder, transverse, or compound.

      ii. Caput succedaneum (edema occurring in and under fetal scalp) present (mild, moderate, severe) or absent.

      iii. Station identified: signifies descent in relation to maternal pelvis (−5 to +5).

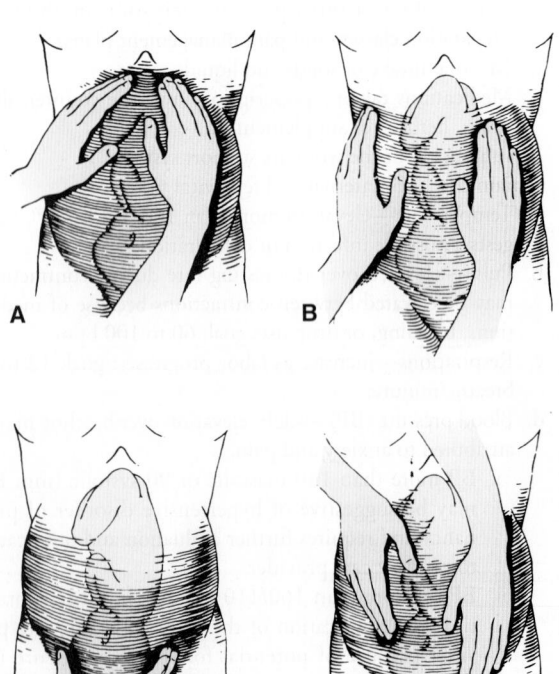

A   B   C   D

Figure 37-7. Leopold maneuvers.

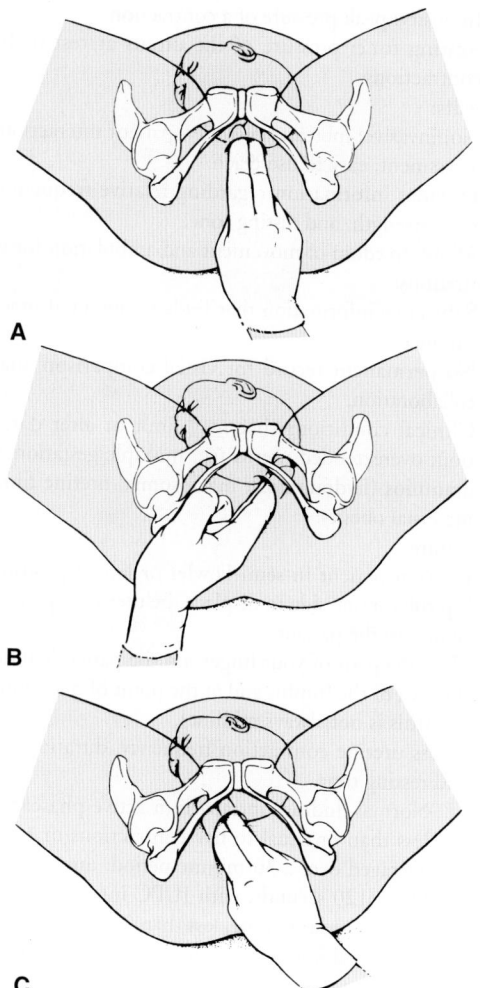

7. Explain each step of the procedure to decrease anticipatory anxiety of the patient.
8. With the nondominant hand separating the labia, place two fingers just inside the introitus, and gently press down on the base of the vagina. Next, insert the closed speculum past the fingers at a 45-degree downward angle such that the handle is perpendicular to the introitus.
9. Once the speculum enters the vagina, remove your fingers and turn the blades of the speculum into a horizontal position with the handle now parallel to the introitus; maintain a moderate and constant downward pressure (alleviates pain to the urethra).
10. As the speculum enters the posterior fornix, gently open the blades to visualize the cervix. If you still cannot visualize, close the blades, withdraw the speculum slightly, and move the blades toward the back of the vagina and try again. Once the cervix is in view, tighten the thumbscrew to maintain the blades in an open position. Complete a visual cervical assessment and obtain any samples necessary.
11. When the examination is complete, release the thumbscrew and withdraw in reverse order of placement.
12. Wipe any moisture or discharge from the perineal area and tell the patient the procedure is over; offer her assistance to a comfortable position.

Fetal Heart Assessment

 EVIDENCE BASE Association of Women's Health, Obstetric and Neonatal Nurses. (Ed.). (2015). *Fetal heart monitoring principles and practices* (5th ed.). Dubuque, IA: Kendall-Hunt Publishing Co.

Fetal heart rate (FHR) assessment was established in Europe during the 17th century and utilized in the United States by Dr. Edward Hon. As FHR analysis evolved, so too has its purpose.

Providers caring for patients during labor and delivery must be skilled in utilizing correct instrumentation for the current clinical scenario, interpreting FHR characteristics and patterns, applying appropriate interventions, and communicating both routine and critical data to the perinatal team as the patient's (mother, fetus, or both) condition warrants.

Maternal Risk Factors, Fetal/Neonatal Risks, and Fetal Heart Rate Implications

One cannot sufficiently interpret FHR variances without considering the impact of maternal physiology and pathophysiology during gestation. Maternal conditions that may negatively impact oxygenation and perfusion of the mother may lead to oxygen deprivation and hypoxemia in the fetus. The large majority of maternal and fetal couplets tolerate physiologic challenges of pregnancy, labor, and birth without consequence. Under extreme conditions (ie, asthma attack, seizure, hemorrhage), the maternal patient diverts blood and oxygen away from the nonvital uterus to vital organs at the expense of the fetus. Several maternal conditions outlined below explain risk factors to the fetus and subsequent FHR changes possibly witnessed during the intrapartum period.

1. Cardiovascular—acquired or congenital cardiac disease, anemias (sickle cell), or hypertensive disorders.
   a. *Fetal/neonatal secondary risks*: small for gestational age (SGA), intrauterine growth restriction (IUGR), hydrops fetalis, hypoxemia, decreased amniotic fluid volume (AFV), preterm labor (PTL)/birth, and placental abruption.

Figure 37-8. Vaginal examination. **(A)** Determining the station and palpating the sagittal suture. **(B)** Identifying the posterior fontanelle. **(C)** Identifying the anterior fontanelle.

   c. Position.
      i. Cephalic presentation (in relation to maternal pelvis anterior, posterior, transverse).
      ii. Location of fontanelles.
   d. Membranes—intact or ruptured.
      i. Amount, color, and any odor of fluid.
      ii. Passage of meconium and consistency.

Sterile Speculum Examination

In some situations (eg, premature rupture of membranes, or positive group β streptococcus), a vaginal examination may be deferred and a sterile speculum examination may be required or preferred.

1. Explain the procedure to the woman, ask her to empty her bladder and remove all clothing from the waist down, and give her a sheet to cover herself.
2. Assist the patient into a lithotomy position (place hip roll under one hip to displace the uterus).
3. Drape her legs and abdomen and adjust lighting at the perineum.
4. After selecting a sterile speculum, utilizing sterile technique, open the package.
5. Put on sterile gloves using proper technique.
6. Ask the woman to relax her legs for proper visualization.

b. *Potential FHR alterations*: tachycardia, bradycardia, minimal or absent variability, absent accelerations, late decelerations, variable decelerations, prolonged decelerations, or sinusoidal patterns.

2. Respiratory—*chronic disease*: asthma and smoking; *acute disease*: status asthmaticus, acute respiratory distress syndrome, pulmonary embolus, sickle cell crisis, amniotic fluid embolus, or infections.
   a. *Fetal/neonatal secondary risks*: SGA, IUGR, hypoxemia, PTL/birth, and presence of meconium.
   b. *Potential FHR alterations*: tachycardia, bradycardia, minimal or absent variability, absent accelerations, late decelerations, or prolonged decelerations.

3. Neurologic—*chronic disease*: epilepsy and underlying; *acute disease*: stroke and eclampsia.
   a. *Fetal/neonatal secondary risks*: hypoxemia and PTL/birth.
   b. *Potential FHR alterations*: bradycardia, minimal or absent variability, absent accelerations, late decelerations, or prolonged decelerations.

4. Renal—*chronic disease*: dialysis and transplant; *acute disease*: acute tubular necrosis, acute renal failure, development of calculi, fluid/electrolyte imbalance, and infection.
   a. *Fetal/neonatal secondary risks*: SGA, IUGR, hypoxemia, decreased AFV, decreased/reversed umbilical blood flow, and PTL/birth. (*Note*: Altered electrolytes may adversely affect the fetus if prolonged.)
   b. *Potential FHR alterations*: tachycardia, bradycardia, minimal or absent variability, absent accelerations, variable decelerations, late decelerations, or prolonged decelerations.

5. Psychosocial and other risk factors—lack of prenatal care, medications, malnutrition/inadequate weight gain, excessive stress, domestic violence, and substance abuse (eg, alcohol, illicit drug use).
   a. *Fetal/neonatal secondary risks*: SGA, IUGR, congenital anomalies, placental anomalies, hypoxemia, decreased AFV, or PTL/birth.
   b. *Potential FHR alterations*: tachycardia, bradycardia, minimal or absent or marked variability, absent accelerations, variable decelerations, late decelerations, or prolonged decelerations.

Fetal Heart Monitoring Instrumentation: External Options

Uterine Contraction Assessment by Palpation

1. Uterine palpation is performed periodically throughout labor to validate labor adequacy and progression; if applicable, palpation is also utilized to validate information received from internal equipment (eg, intrauterine pressure catheter).

2. Intensity may be described as follows (this may be taught to patient and labor coach):
   a. The uterus easily indented: feels like the tip of the nose (mild intensity).
   b. Able to slightly indent the uterus: feels like the chin (moderate intensity).
   c. Unable to indent the uterus: feels like the forehead (strong intensity).

3. Uterine contraction data include:
   a. Frequency: beginning of one contraction to the beginning of the next.
   b. Duration: beginning of one contraction to the end of the same contraction.

c. Intensity: peak pressure of a contraction.
d. Resting tone: pressure of the uterus at rest or between contractions.

4. Benefits:
   a. Noninvasive; increases provider–patient interaction; direct assessment; easy to use/teach.
   b. Provides information regarding relative frequency, duration, strength, and resting tone.
   c. Allows freedom of movement and ambulation for woman.

5. Limitations:
   a. Subjective information that leads to potential practitioner variance.
   b. No permanent record for visual comparison analysis or collaboration.
   c. Clinical conditions that may limit or alter data collection: overextended uterus (eg, multiple gestation, polyhydramnios (hydramnios), macrosomia, uterine fibroids) or maternal obesity.

6. Procedure:
   a. Position patient in semi-Fowler or lateral position; place hip roll on one side to displace the uterus; explain the procedure to the patient.
   b. Place the pads of your fingers on the patient's abdomen in the area of the fundus and at the point of maximum intensity (this is not always midline).
   c. Assess uterine contraction frequency, duration, intensity, and resting tone.
      i. Normal findings/intrapartum active phase: frequency, less than or equal to five contractions in 10 minutes, averaged over a 30-minute period; duration, less than 90 to 120 seconds; with IUPC intensity, less than 80 mm Hg; resting tone, less than 20 to 25 mm Hg.
      ii. Abnormal findings—tachysystole, more than five contractions in 10 minutes; hypertonus, intensity. With IUPC intensity, greater than 80 mm Hg; resting tone greater than 20 to 25 mm Hg or Montevideo units (MVUs) greater than 400.

Uterine Contraction Assessment by Tocodynamometer

1. A *tocodynamometer* (TOCO, tocotransducer) detects changes in tension or muscular tone over the fundus on the outside layer of the maternal abdomen. The electronic data are then converted into a number and printed on the lower half of the electronic fetal monitor (EFM) paper. However, proper placement is key for accuracy:
   a. If patient is at term—place over the point of maximum intensity in the fundal region of the maternal abdomen.
   b. If patient is preterm—place over the lower uterine segment below the umbilicus, typically beside the ultrasound device if the fetus is vertex.

2. Benefits:
   a. Noninvasive and easy to use.
   b. Detects relative uterine resting tone, frequency, intensity, and duration of uterine contraction.
   c. Does not require ruptured amniotic membranes.
   d. Generates a tracing for future assessment and permanent record keeping.

3. Limitations:
   a. Nonspecific data are gathered, particularly intensity and resting tone. External uterine monitoring identifies contraction frequency and duration. Contraction intensity is subjectively identified by patient and manual palpation.

b. Difficult to obtain data in patients with the following conditions: obesity, polyhydramnios, macrosomia, PTL, maternal vomiting, and maternal bearing-down efforts/pushing during second stage or during procedures.

c. Location sensitive; placement may result in false or inadequate information.

d. Sensitive to maternal and fetal movement—may be superimposed on contraction waveform.

e. May limit maternal movement and ambulation during labor.

4. Procedure:

a. Position patient in a semi-Fowler or lateral position; place hip roll on one side to displace the uterus; explain the procedure to the patient and support persons.

b. Palpate the point of maximum intensity over the fundus and secure belt.

c. Press the uterine activity (UA) reference button on the EFM between contractions to set the resting tone between 5 and 15 mm Hg.

d. Palpate the fundus and compare printed data.

e. Reposition the device periodically, as needed, for patient comfort and during labor as the fetus descends.

f. Interpret data and document and communicate findings.

Fetal Heart Rate Assessment by Auscultation

1. *Auscultation* is a FHR counting technique accompanied by a listening device (ie, fetoscope or Doppler). The examiner counts the FHR over a specified time frame (see Table 37-2).

2. Interpretation of data includes FHR baseline rate, rhythm, variability, and accelerations and decelerations in the FHR.

3. Devices for interpretation may include Doptone/Doppler, fetoscope, or Leffscope or Pinard stethoscope.

4. Capabilities of a fetoscope—detects:

a. Differentiation of fetal and maternal heart rates—eliminates error because of fetal demise and EFM with nonelectrical device (ie, fetoscope).

b. Verification of FHR dysrhythmias visualized on EFM tracing.

c. Clarification of halving or doubling (may occur due to dysrhythmia) on the EFM tracing.

5. Benefits:

a. Neonatal outcomes comparable to the use of EFM, in low-risk populations and with 1:1 nurse–patient ratios.

b. Noninvasive, easy to use, and most methods require no electricity.

c. Patient has increased freedom of movement and ambulation.

d. Patient can be monitored if submerged in water (eg, water/Jacuzzi births).

6. Limitations:

a. Subjective data collection; variances between practitioners may exist.

b. Conditions may limit the practitioner's ability to assess the FHR (obesity, increased fetal movement, or amniotic fluid).

c. Cannot assess FHR variability or periodic/episodic decelerations or accelerations.

d. Lack of continuous recording from monitor for visual comparative analysis.

e. Requires education, practice, and skill in auditory assessment.

f. Requires a 1:1 nurse–patient ratio during intrapartum; therefore, may create need to increase or realign labor and delivery staff.

7. Procedure:

a. Position patient in a semi-Fowler or lateral position; place hip roll on one side to displace the uterus; explain the procedure to the patient and her support persons.

b. Palpate the maternal abdomen to locate the fetal back by using Leopold maneuvers (see page 996). Figure 37-9 outlines FHR locations and corresponding fetal positions.

c. When using Doppler device, apply conduction gel to underside of device.

d. Position the bell of the fetoscope or Doppler on the area of the abdomen where maximum fetal heart sounds can be heard, usually over the back or chest of fetus. If using a fetoscope, use firm pressure. If using Doppler device, avoid friction noises caused by fingers on the abdominal surface area.

e. Assess and compare maternal heart rate (radial pulse) against the FHR; confirm differentiation.

f. Palpate uterine contractions simultaneously and compare with FHR data.

g. Differentiate between fetal heart rate/tone and other abdominal sounds.

Table 37-2 Frequency of Auscultation: Recommended Assessment and Documentation

ORGANIZATION	LATENT PHASE	ACTIVE PHASE	SECOND STAGE
ACOG			
Low risk	—	q30min	q15min
High risk	—	q15min	q5min
AWHONN			
Low risk	—	q30min	q15min
High risk		q15min	q5min
SOGC	Regularly after rupture of membranes or clinically significant change	q15min	q5min when pushing is initiated

Assess fetal heart rate (FHR) before initiation of labor-enhancing procedures, ambulation, administration of medications, administration or initiation of analgesia or anesthesia, and transfer or discharge of patient.

Assess FHR after admission of patient, artificial or spontaneous rupture of membranes, ambulation, recognition of abnormal uterine activity patterns, and administration of medications.

ACOG, American College of Obstetrics and Gynecologists; AWHONN, Association of Women's Health, Obstetric and Neonatal Nurses; SOGC, Society of Obstetrics and Gynecology of Canada.

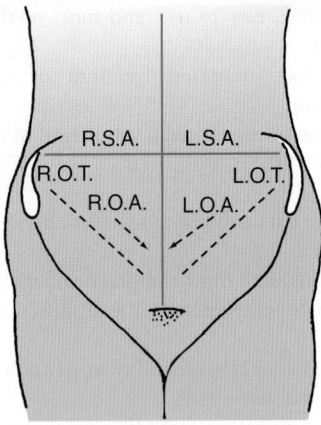

Figure 37-9. Fetal heart tone locations on the abdominal wall indicating possible corresponding fetal positions and the effects of the internal rotation of the fetus.

    i. FHR—a rapid crisp ticking or galloping sound.

    ii. Uterine bruit—a soft murmur, caused by the passage of blood through dilated uterine vessels; synchronous with maternal pulse.

    iii. Funic souffle (uterine souffle)—a hissing sound produced by passage of blood through the umbilical arteries; synchronous with the FHR.

h. Count the FHR between contractions for at least 30 to 60 seconds (60 seconds per Society of Obstetricians and Gynaecologists of Canada).

i. Interpret findings to include FHR baseline rate, rhythm, and increases or decreases; further evaluation via EFM is indicated if:

    i. Baseline FHR less than 110 or more than 160, irregular rhythm, and abrupt or gradual decreases in FHR during, immediately after, or 30 seconds after a contraction.

j. Document and communicate findings with woman and her support persons.

k. Communicate abnormal findings to primary practitioner immediately.

8. Troubleshooting interventions:

a. Verify placement; utilize Leopold maneuvers to verify fetal position.

b. Assess all four quadrants of the maternal abdomen slowly; fetal malpresentation or demise may exist.

c. Repositioning the patient may reposition the fetus.

d. Reaffirm and compare data to the maternal pulse.

e. Use alternative equipment options (ie, EFM) if unable to assess.

f. Consult with other members of the perinatal team (patient care team) and notify the practitioner as warranted.

g. Multiple gestations require a keen sense of auscultation; each FHR should be documented by location. For example, baby A/#1 = left lower quadrant, 150 beats/minute; baby B/#2 = right upper quadrant, 120 beats/minute. Ultrasound may be warranted to discern two separate FHRs.

Fetal Heart Rate Assessment by Ultrasound Transducer

Monitoring the FHR via ultrasound transducer allows detection of the FHR baseline rate, variability, accelerations, and decelerations.

1. Benefits:

a. Noninvasive.

b. Rupture of membranes not required.

c. Provides permanent record for review and collaboration.

2. Limitations:

a. Signal transmission may be influenced by maternal obesity, polyhydramnios, or anterior placental placement providing a weak, absent, or false signal.

b. Restricts maternal mobility.

c. Episodic maternal and fetal movement may interfere with continuous recording.

d. Half or double counting of FHR may occur, especially with fetal tachycardia or bradycardia.

e. May document maternal pulse with undiagnosed intrauterine fetal demise; always validate and compare data to maternal pulse.

3. Procedure:

a. Gather equipment, explain procedure to patient, and perform Leopold maneuvers to locate the fetal back or chest (point of maximum intensity [PMI]).

b. Lubricate the face of the transducer with a thin layer of ultrasonic gel to aid in the transmission of sounds. Place the transducer over the PMI.

c. Readjust the device periodically to maximize signal quality. Maintain a constant strip of FHR data as diligently as possible during course of labor.

Fetal Heart Monitoring Instrumentation: Internal Options

Uterine Contraction Assessment by Intrauterine Pressure Catheter

An *intrauterine pressure catheter* (IUPC) is the most objective technique to evaluate all uterine contraction characteristics and patterns. The device may be utilized for amniotic fluid testing and to perform an intrapartum amnioinfusion. IUPCs are either fluid-filled or solid-tipped catheters. Currently, there is no absolute indication for use of the IUPC in labor. Although not required, many practitioners utilize this device during labor of a woman with a previous uterine scar (eg, vaginal birth after cesarean). IUPCs are typically placed by the health care provider.

1. Benefits (fluid-filled and solid-tipped catheters):

a. Utilized to calculate MVUs. Uterine activity (frequency, duration, intensity, and resting tone) can be calculated and documented using mm Hg and MVUs. MVUs are derived by subtracting the resting tone of the uterus from the peak pressure of the contraction (in mm Hg) for each contraction occurring in a 10-minute period. These numbers are then added together for the total number of MVUs during that 10-minute period. IUPC data should also be periodically checked against manual palpation until delivery.

b. Assists in the interpretation of the FHR (ie, comparison of a variable vs. late deceleration).

c. Tracing generated as a permanent part of the medical record.

d. Offers a portal for amniotic fluid sampling and amnioinfusion.

e. Solid-tipped—easy, quick setup with decreased pressure artifact.

f. Fluid-filled—least expensive; most accurate readings if correctly installed.

2. Limitations (fluid-filled and solid-tipped catheters):

a. Rupture of membranes (ROM) and adequate cervical dilation are required for insertion.

b. Invasive procedure.

c. Increased risk of uterine infection.

d. Improper insertion can lead to maternal or fetal trauma (ie, uterine perforation, uterine cord prolapse, extraovular placement).

e. Limits maternal ambulation during labor.

f. May be contraindicated in presence of vaginal bleeding and infection where ROM is discouraged to prevent maternal–fetal transmissions (eg, human immunodeficiency virus [HIV], herpes, group B strep).

g. Differences may occur in readings between fluid-filled and sensor-tipped catheters.

h. Solid-tipped—pressure readings higher than fluid-filled catheters.

i. Fluid-filled—lengthy setup; may be difficult to maintain with maternal repositioning; may become compressed between the uterine wall and fetus, distorting the waveform.

3. Contraindications: placenta previa, active vaginal or cervical herpes, active hepatitis, or HIV infection, and active vaginal bleeding.

Fetal Heart Assessment by Fetal Spiral Electrode

The use of the *fetal spiral electrode* (FSE) to monitor the FHR allows for detection of FHR baseline rate, variability, accelerations, decelerations, and FHR dysrhythmias. Indications for use during labor include FHR not detected or abnormal findings via an external device.

1. Contraindications:
   a. Face, shoulder, compound, or footling breech presentations.
   b. Unable to identify presenting part.
   c. Presence of placenta previa; active vaginal or cervical herpes; active hepatitis, or HIV infection; active vaginal bleeding; or category III FHR pattern.

2. Benefits:
   a. Ability to detect FHR characteristics to include dysrhythmias and direct FHR variability.
   b. Maternal position change does not alter quality of tracing.
   c. Continuous detection of FHR; permanent recording in health record.
   d. Enhanced maternal comfort with removal of abdominal belt from external device.

3. Limitations:
   a. Invasive procedure; requires ROM, cervical dilation, and accessible/appropriate fetal presenting part.
   b. Potentially small risk of fetal hemorrhage, injury, or infection.
   c. May record maternal heart rate in the presence of fetal demise.
   d. Fetal arrhythmias may be missed (not detected) if EFM logic or electrocardiogram activation switch is turned on.
   e. A moist environment is necessary for FHR detection.
   f. Electronic interference and artifact may occur (ie, may become twisted in fetal hair).

4. Procedure:
   a. Gather equipment and explain procedure to patient.
   b. Perform EFM test if turning on EFM for the first time.
   c. Open FSE package utilizing sterile technique and place sterile glove on dominant hand.
   d. Following completion of a cervical exam, secure hand inside the cervix with second and third fingers pressed against presenting part, avoiding the face, genitalia, and fontanelles.
   e. Press catheter against presenting part and turn clockwise one full turn, pinch locking device at end, remove introducer, and attach to the EFM while securing to maternal abdomen or inner thigh.
   f. Interpret and document data.

Interpretation of Fetal Heart Rate

 EVIDENCE BASE Association of Women's Health, Obstetric and Neonatal Nurses. (Ed.). (2015). *Fetal heart monitoring principles and practices* (5th ed.). Dubuque, IA: Kendall-Hunt Publishing Co.

American College of Obstetricians and Gynecologists. (2010/Reaffirmed 2017). *Management of intrapartum fetal heart rate tracings* (Practice Bulletin #116). Washington, DC: Author.

American College of Obstetricians and Gynecologists. (2009/Reaffirmed 2017). *Intrapartum fetal heart rate monitoring: Nomenclature, interpretation, and general management principles* (Practice Bulletin #106). Washington, DC: Author.

The following FHR interpretation criteria meet the current National Institute of Child Health and Human Development (NICHD) terminology and update and guidelines adopted by American College of Obstetricians and Gynecologists and Association of Women's Health, Obstetric and Neonatal Nurses in 2005, as well as management updates by ACOG in 2009 and 2010 and reaffirmed by ACOG 2017.

Fetal Heart Rate Baseline

1. *Fetal heart rate baseline* (FHRB) is the approximate mean FHR rounded to increments of 5 beats/minute during a 10-minute segment and excluding periodic/episodic changes, periods of marked FHR variability, and segments of the baseline that differ by more than 25 beats/minute; interpretation between contractions is recommended but not required.

2. Documented as a single number.

3. Normal FHRB, 110 to 160 beats/minute; tachycardia, more than 160 beats/minute for 10 minutes or greater; bradycardia, less than 110 beats/minute for 10 minutes or greater.

4. In any 10-minute window, the minimum baseline duration must be at least 2 minutes or the baseline for that period is indeterminate. In this case, one may need to refer to the previous 10-minute segment for determination of the baseline. Two consecutive minutes are recommended but not required.

5. FHRB is calculated by determining the range of FHRV first and then calculating the mean in increments of 5 (if FHRV equals 10 [ie, 140 to 150], mean FHRB = 145; if FHRV equals 15 [ie, 120 to 135], mean = 7.5, round up to FHRB of 130).

6. Variations from the normal baseline rate are tachycardia, bradycardia, and sinusoidal patterns.

Tachycardia

1. Etiology—maternal causes:
   a. Maternal fever.
   b. Maternal infection.
   c. Dehydration.
   d. Hyperthyroidism.
   e. Endogenous adrenaline or anxiety.
   f. Medications.
      i. Sympathomimetics (eg, terbutaline, albuterol, epinephrine, ephedrine).
      ii. Parasympathomimetics (eg, atropine, hydralazine, phenothiazines, hydroxyzine).
      iii. Selected positive inotropic agents (dobutamine and positive chronotropic drugs).
      iv. OTC medications (decongestants, appetite suppressants, and caffeine).

     v. Illicit drugs (cocaine, methamphetamines, and heroin).

    vi. Nicotine, if inhaled (if inhaled, nicotine may increase FHR; if absorbed through a nicotine patch, it may decrease FHR).

   vii. Labor enhancement agents (ie, oxytocin, misoprostol), leading to persistent abnormal uterine contraction patterns.

2. Etiology—fetal causes:

  a. Infection.

  b. Fetal activity or stimulation.

  c. Compensatory response to early/acute hypoxemia.

  d. Fetal hyperthyroidism.

  e. Fetal tachyarrhythmias (supraventricular tachycardia).

  f. Prematurity.

  g. Congenital anomalies—cardiac abnormalities or heart failure.

  h. Anemia.

3. Interventions:

  a. Monitor vital signs: maternal temperature and pulse; compare to FHR data.

  b. Assess maternal hydration (initiate or increase IV fluids, as needed).

  c. Decrease maternal temperature, if elevated, via an antipyretic, as ordered.

  d. Decrease maternal anxiety, give explanations for treatment measures, provide comfort measures, and assist with breathing/relaxation techniques.

  e. Assess additional FHR characteristics: if decelerations exist, consider the need to:

    i. Change patient to a lateral position.

    ii. Administer oxygen via face mask (8 to 10 L/minute); prolonged use discouraged.

   iii. Assess medication history and use.

   iv. Assess for tachydysrhythmia.

    v. If auscultating, apply EFM, as needed.

   vi. Notify the primary health care provider and perinatal team.

Bradycardia

Bradycardia in the fetus may result from maternal or fetal conditions and defined as less than 110 bpm for 10 minutes or greater. Severe bradycardia is defined as FHR less than 60 beats/minute. Sudden and sustained bradycardia accompanied by absent FHR variability (FHRV) has the highest risk of fetal and neonatal morbidity or mortality.

1. Etiology—maternal causes:

  a. β-Blocking agents (propranolol).

  b. Connective tissue disease (systemic lupus erythema).

  c. Prolonged maternal hypoglycemia.

  d. Maternal hypotension (r/t supine positioning, hypovolemia).

  e. Hypothermia.

  f. Anesthetics (epidural, spinal, pudendal, or paracervical).

  g. Conditions that may cause acute maternal cardiopulmonary compromise (amniotic fluid embolus, pulmonary embolus, cerebral vascular ischemia, hemorrhage, uterine rupture, trauma).

2. Etiology—fetal causes:

  a. Congenital heart block.

  b. Mature parasympathetic nervous system (post gestation).

  c. Acute hypoxemia.

  d. Cardiac structural defects.

  e. Impaired fetal oxygenation: (eg, umbilical cord occlusion, cord prolapse, uterine rupture, abruptio placentae).

  f. Maternal or fetal sentinel event precipitating hypoxia.

3. Hypoxic causes: umbilical cord prolapse or compression, uterine rupture, maternal hemorrhage, prolonged maternal hypoglycemia, placental abruption, maternal trauma, and persistent abnormal uterine contraction patterns (ie, tachysystole). A FHR category III pattern of lengthy and severe bradycardia accompanied by absent FHR variability may lead to permanent central nervous system (CNS) injury or death in the fetus or neonate.

4. Interventions:

  a. Validate maternal heart rate versus FHR with pulse oximetry if available; validate if fetus has complete heart block.

  b. Perform vaginal examination to assess for umbilical cord prolapse.

  c. Assess maternal vital signs to rule out hypotension; increase fluids.

  d. Assess FHR variability and other FHR characteristics—consider:

    i. Maternal lateral position change.

    ii. Discontinue oxytocin administration or augmentation agents.

   iii. Modify maternal pushing techniques or stop pushing during second stage of labor until FHR resolves.

   iv. Administer oxygen via face mask (8 to 10 L/minute) as necessary; prolonged use discouraged.

  e. If auscultating, apply EFM to assess FHR variability.

  f. Notify the primary health care provider and perinatal team.

Sinusoidal

1. This pattern differs from variability in that it has a smooth, sine wavelike pattern (equal deflections above and below the FHRB) of regular frequency and amplitude and is excluded in the definition of variability; described as *sinusoidal* or *pseudosinusoidal (medication induced)*.

2. Etiology:

  a. Severe fetal anemia: Rh isoimmunization.

  b. Fetal–maternal hemorrhage.

  c. Severe fetal hypoxia or asphyxia.

  d. Maternal opioid administration; may lead to pseudosinusoidal pattern.

3. Interventions:

  a. Lateral positioning.

  b. Administer IV hydration.

  c. Administer oxygen via face mask (8 to 10 L/minute); prolonged use discouraged.

  d. Assess patient for hemorrhage and treat accordingly.

  e. Notify the primary health care provider and perinatal team.

  f. If etiology necessitates, consider:

    i. Kleihauer-Betke test to assess for fetal red cells in maternal blood because of hemorrhage.

    ii. Expeditious delivery.

Fetal Heart Rate Variability

1. *Fetal heart rate variability* (FHRV) is the result of electrical impulses received by the cardiac muscle from the brain stem's medulla oblongata. The medulla oblongata receives information from both the parasympathetic (slow) and the sympathetic (fast) nervous systems; the combined effect leads to a cyclic push and pull of the heart rate over time (heart rates are never static unless permanent CNS damage has occurred). Oxygenation must remain constant for communication to occur between the CNS and cardiac muscle.

2. At the time of observation, variability indicates adequate oxygenation of the fetal CNS.

3. FHRV is defined as fluctuations in the baseline FHR. These fluctuations are irregular in amplitude and frequency and are visually quantified as the *amplitude of the peak-to-trough range* in beats per minute as follows:
   a. Absent FHRV—undetectable.
   b. Minimal FHRV—more than undetectable but less than or equal to 5 beats/minute.
   c. Moderate FHRV—6 to 25 beats/minute.
   d. Marked FHRV—more than 25 beats/minute.
4. Calculation of FHRV range is determined by the mean peak-to-trough range rounded to increments 5 beats/minute (ie, 120 to 135, 115 to 130, 150 to 155); the mean is reported as the FHRB.
5. Absent or minimal variability may be due to preterm gestation (less than 28 to 32 weeks), alteration in nervous system function, medications, abnormal uterine contraction patterns, or inadequate oxygenation.
6. Normal sleep and wake states, medications, alcohol, and illicit drugs that cause fetal neurologic damage; morphine; methadone; anomalies; and previous insults that have damaged the fetal brain can affect the baseline variability.
7. Moderate FHRV, even in the presence of decelerations, is strongly associated (98%) with an umbilical pH more than 7.15 (nonacidemic) or newborn vigor (Apgar score ≥ 7 at 5 minutes).
8. Abnormal findings: prolonged periods of absent, minimal, or marked FHRV; if absent FHRV is accompanied by recurrent decelerations (late, variable, or prolonged), fetal or neonatal morbidity or mortality may result.
9. Interventions for category III pattern: recurrent late, variable, or prolonged decelerations accompanied by absent FHRV (caused by CNS dysfunction, hypoxia, asphyxia):
   a. Notification to primary practitioner and perinatal team for expeditious delivery.
   b. Prepare for expeditious and immediate delivery; route dependent on clinical conditions.
   c. Discontinue oxytocin administration, if applicable.
   d. Assess maternal vital signs (initiate/increase intravenous infusion [IVF], as needed).
   e. Administer oxygen via face mask (8 to 10 L/minute); prolonged use discouraged.
   f. Change maternal lateral position.
10. Interventions for minimal FHRV (caused by sleep state, medications, hypoxia, CNS dysfunction, dysrhythmias):
   a. Rule out nonhypoxic causes: sleep state and medications.
   b. If minimal FHRV is accompanied by recurrent late, variable, or prolonged decelerations, extended time to complete all interventions outlined in 9a to f (previous paragraph) is afforded.
   c. If pattern does not resolve within 60 to 90 minutes, delivery via the most expeditious route is recommended.
11. Interventions for marked FHRV (possibly caused by cord entanglement, excessive release of fetal catecholamines, asphyxia): same as for minimal FHRV.

Periodic/Episodic Fetal Heart Rate Patterns

Periodic or episodic changes are visually apparent increases or decreases in the FHRB in the form of an acceleration or deceleration. Their duration is greater than 15 seconds and less than 2 minutes. After 2 minutes, they are considered prolonged. If duration exceeds 10 minutes, a baseline rate change has occurred.

Periodic patterns occur simultaneously with contractions and *episodic* patterns occur in the absence of contractions. Periodic and episodic patterns are distinguished on the basis of waveforms, currently accepted as "abrupt" (onset to peak or nadir [lowest point] is less than 30 seconds) or "gradual" (onset to nadir is equal to or greater than 30 seconds). Decelerations are defined as recurrent if they appear with 50% or greater of uterine contractions in any 20-minute period, or intermittent, if they occur with less than 50% of uterine contractions, in any 20-minute period.

1. Acceleration: visually apparent, abrupt increase in the FHR above the baseline rate; calculated from the most recently determined FHRB.
   a. The following criteria reflect gestational age implications:
      i. Term (greater than or equal to 32 weeks): peak of acceleration is 15 or more beats/minute (bpm) above the FHR baseline and 15 seconds or more in duration but less than 2 minutes.
      ii. Preterm (less than 32 weeks): peak of acceleration is at least 10 bpm above the FHR baseline and at least 10 seconds in duration but less than 2 minutes.
      iii. Prolonged: duration 2 minutes or longer but less than 10 minutes.
   b. Etiology: fetal movement, uterine contraction, partial umbilical cord occlusion, breech presentation, occipitoposterior position of the fetal vertex, vaginal examination, fetal scalp stimulation, following application of vibroacoustic stimulator, and application of FSE.
   c. Accelerations are associated with a nonhypoxic fetus and normal fetal pH at the time of observation.
   d. Interventions—none required.
2. Early deceleration—visually apparent usually symmetrical gradual decrease and return of the FHR associated with a uterine contraction; calculated from the most recently determined portion of the FHR baseline. It is coincident in timing, with the nadir of the deceleration occurring with the peak of a contraction. In most cases, the onset, nadir, and recovery of the deceleration occur with the beginning, peak, and end of the contraction, respectively.
   a. Physiology—head compression causing a vagal response. It is a benign pattern and not associated with fetal hypoxemia; may evolve into variable decelerations.
   b. Interventions—none required.
3. Late decelerations—visually apparent, usually symmetrical gradual decrease and return of the FHR associated with a uterine contraction. The decrease in FHR is calculated from the onset to the nadir of the deceleration. The deceleration is delayed in timing, with the nadir of the deceleration occurring after the peak of the contraction. In most cases, the onset, nadir, and recovery of the deceleration occur after the beginning, peak, and ending of the contraction, respectively.
   a. Physiology.
      i. Reflex—chemoreceptor stimulation leading to the transient decrease in FHR accompanied by normal FHRB and moderate variability. Prolonged supine positioning may precipitate reflex late decelerations; repositioning patient laterally often resolves pattern.
      ii. Myocardial depression—decreased oxygen transfer at the placental interface may lead to uteroplacental insufficiency (UPI). Prolonged periods of UPI may lead to progressive fetal hypoxia and metabolic acidosis. Metabolic acidosis can directly influence electrical

conduction and performance of the fetal heart, causing direct myocardial depression. These late decelerations are "myocardial mediated" and may be accompanied by a change in the fetal heart baseline (tachycardia or bradycardia), absent or minimal variability, and the absence of accelerations, usually indicative of a fetus in metabolic acidemia. A category III FHR pattern of recurrent late decelerations accompanied by absent FHRV requires immediate delivery via the most expeditious route.

 b. Maternal factors that may promote UPI:

  i. Hypotension (may also be associated with reflex late decelerations).

  ii. Severe hypertension.

  iii. Placental changes that may affect uteroplacental gas exchange (ie, postmaturity, premature placental aging, calcification, placental abruption, placenta previa, or placental malformations).

  iv. Physiologic conditions that may be associated with decreased maternal oxygen saturation or hemoglobin levels (ie, asthma attack, cardiopulmonary disease, or trauma).

  v. Persistent abnormal uterine contraction patterns (ie, tachysystole, tetany, or hypertonus).

 c. Interventions—aimed at increasing uteroplacental perfusion by correcting cause.

  i. Alter maternal position: lateral position (right or left) or knee–chest.

  ii. Correct maternal hypotension with hydration and/or medication.

  iii. Discontinue labor stimulation or cervical ripening agents.

  iv. Administer oxygen by face mask at 8 to 10 L/minute via a nonrebreather mask; prolonged use discouraged.

  v. If category III FHR pattern of recurrent late decelerations accompanied by absent FHRV, immediate delivery is warranted by the most expeditious route. Notification of the primary practitioner and perinatal team is indicated. Preparations for emergent delivery are warranted.

4. Variable deceleration—visually apparent abrupt decrease in FHR from the onset of the deceleration to the beginning of the FHR nadir is less than 30 seconds. When variable decelerations are associated with uterine contractions, their onset, depth, and duration commonly vary with successive uterine contractions. It is important to note that variable decelerations vary in shape, timing, and return to baseline. Severe variable decelerations last more than 60 seconds yet less than 2 minutes and fall more than 70 beats below the FHRB. Therefore, deceleration depth correlates with the degree of academia.

 a. Physiology—decreased umbilical cord perfusion, resulting from compression or stretch. Compression may result from maternal positioning, prolapsed cord, cord entanglement, second-stage labor, short cord, and a true knot in the cord.

 b. Interventions.

  i. Change maternal position, which may dislodge an occluded cord.

  ii. Perform a vaginal examination to assess for cord prolapse or imminent delivery.

  iii. If prolapse, elevate presenting part off the cord while palpating for an umbilical pulse and FHR.

  iv. Amnioinfusion, if appropriate.

  v. Decrease or discontinue oxytocin, if appropriate.

  vi. Provide oxygen by face mask at 8 to 10 L/minute; prolonged use discouraged.

  vii. Discontinue or alter second-stage pushing technique if repetitive, severe variables occur in second stage.

  viii. If category III FHR pattern of recurrent variable decelerations accompanied by absent FHRV, immediate delivery is warranted by the most expeditious route. Notification of the primary practitioner and perinatal team is indicated. Preparations for emergent delivery are warranted.

5. Prolonged deceleration—visually apparent decrease of FHR of at least 15 beats/minute or more below the baseline and lasting more than 2 minutes but less than 10.

 a. Physiology—causes may reflect similar pathophysiology of late or variable deceleration.

 b. Interventions—if more than 4 to 5 minutes and causes unknown or unresolved, perinatal team should prepare for an emergent delivery.

6. Document all findings and classify patterns as normal (category I FHR), indeterminate (category II FHR), or abnormal (category III FHR) per NICHD guidelines (see Table 37-3).

Table 37-3	Three-Tier Fetal Heart Rate Interpretation System
CATEGORY	**FHR PATTERNS**
Category I: normal patterns	Baseline rate: 110 to 160 beats/minute Baseline FHR variability: moderate Late or variable decelerations: absent Early decelerations: present or absent Accelerations: present or absent
Category II: indeterminate patterns (includes all tracings not categorized in categories I or III)	Bradycardia not accompanied by absent baseline variability Tachycardia Minimal variability Absent variability not accompanied by recurrent decelerations Marked variability Absence of induced accelerations after fetal stimulation Recurrent variable decelerations accompanied by minimal or moderate variability Prolonged decelerations Recurrent late decelerations with moderate variability Variable decelerations with other characteristics, such as slow return to baseline, overshoots, or "shoulders"
Category III: abnormal patterns	Absent variability plus any of the following: Recurrent late or variable decelerations Bradycardia Sinusoidal pattern

EVIDENCE BASE AWHONN. (2014). *Women's health and perinatal nursing care quality refined draft specifications.* Washington, DC: Author.

 TRANSITIONAL CARE ALERT Obstetric units should have comprehensive policies and procedures in place detailing evidence-based labor and delivery supportive practices based on AWHONN and ACOG guidelines. Research supports that maternal–fetal outcomes, hospital readmission rates, and patient satisfaction with the birth experience are improved with continuous nursing support.

First Stage of Labor: Latent Phase (0 to 3 cm)

Nursing Diagnoses

- Deficient Fluid Volume related to decreased oral intake, dietary restrictions, and energy requirement of labor.
- Anxiety related to concern for self and fetus.
- Acute Pain related to uterine contractions, position of fetus, and advancement of labor.
- Knowledge Deficit related to safe and effective use of alternative interventions.

Nursing Interventions

Maintaining Nutrition and Hydration

1. Provide clear liquids and ice chips, as allowed.
2. Initiate IV access and infuse fluids, if ordered.
3. Assess intake and output, and evaluate urine for ketones and glucose, per facility policy.

Relieving Anxiety

1. Establish a relationship with the woman/partner/support persons.
2. Inform the woman/partner/support persons of maternal status, fetal status, and labor progress periodically during the labor process. Ensure appropriate permission for information sharing.
3. Explain all procedures and equipment used during labor; answer questions and offer support.
4. Review birth plan and explain rationales for necessary revisions, if applicable.

Promote partner/support persons' participation in the labor experience.

5. Monitor maternal vital signs as the patient's condition warrants.
   a. Temperature every 2 to 4 hours, unless elevated or membranes ruptured, and then every 1 to 2 hours per facility policy.
   b. Pulse and respirations, as indicated by facility policy, medical condition, or medication administration (eg, oxytocin or magnesium sulfate infusions).
   c. BP is obtained typically every hour unless hypertension or hypotension exists or woman has received pain medication or anesthesia; then, evaluate more frequently based on findings or as indicated.
6. Monitor FHR periodically per facility policy (refer to Table 37-2, page 999).

Promoting Comfort

1. Encourage ambulation and frequent repositioning, as tolerated.
2. Encourage diversional activities, such as reading, talking, watching TV, playing cards, and listening to music.

3. Review, evaluate, and teach proper breathing techniques:
   a. Slow chest breathing (slow paced/)—relax, take one deep cleansing breath, and exhale slowly and completely. Breathe deeply, slowly, rhythmically throughout the contraction. Average 10 to 12 breaths/minute. Breathe slowly and deeply in through the nose and out through the nose or slightly pursed lips.
   b. Modified-paced breathing—used when slow chest breathing no longer effective, typically as labor progresses. Take one deep breath and exhale slowly and completely. As contractions intensify, breathe with more frequent shallow breaths during a contraction. At conclusion of contraction, take a deep breath and exhale slowly. Maintain a pace not to exceed twice the woman's average respiratory rate or less than 24 breaths/minute. Encourage HOOT–HOUT breathing with emphasis on a "crisp T" for exhalation.
   c. Patterned-paced breathing (pant–blow breathing)—utilized in later stages of labor as contractions intensify and deep long breaths are not obtainable. Concentrate on breathing in a controlled manner. Take a deep breath and exhale slowly and completely. Then, take four shallow breaths through the mouth, making a "hee" or "heh" sound; maintain steady rhythm. Finish with a deep cleansing breath at the end of contraction. This breathing pattern is most commonly used during transition prior to active pushing.
4. Teach effleurage—light touch and massage over maternal skin, typically the abdomen, with fingertips; can be used with slow chest and modified-paced breathing. Start at the pubic bone and move hands slowly up sides of the abdomen in wide circular sweep; during exhalation, move fingertips down the center of the abdomen. Usually performed by laboring mother, but can be done with one hand if sidelying or coach assisted (see Figure 37-10).

Figure 37-10. Effleurage. **(A)** During uterine contractions, a woman creates the pattern on her bare abdomen with her fingers. **(B)** If electronic fetal monitoring is being used, effleurage may be performed on the thigh. (Pillitteri, A. [2013]. *Maternal and child health nursing: Care of the childbearing and childrearing family* [7th ed.]. Philadelphia, PA: Lippincott Williams & Wilkins.)

5. Encourage a warm shower or whirlpool, if approved by primary practitioner.
6. Provide comfort measures.
   a. Give back or foot rubs.
   b. Assist the woman to change position. Walking, rocking chairs, squatting, semisitting, hands-and-knees, kneeling, standing, sidelying, or sitting on the toilet assist fetal descent and alleviate pain. Sidelying position or hands-and-knees position will assist to rotate a persistent OP position to an anterior position.

Educate for Safe and Effective Use of Alternative Therapies

Provide information and clear up misconceptions about alternative therapies if patient is interested.
1. Birthing Balls—sturdy inflatable vinyl balls approximately 2½ feet (0.8 m) in diameter. The laboring woman can sit on the ball and sway from side to side, or she may kneel and lean forward resting on the birthing ball to assist in fetal descent.
2. Self-hypnosis—women are trained to rehearse the birth mentally and to control physical reactions to labor, such as BP, pulse, or pain. The American Psychotherapy and Medical Hypnosis Association (*www.apmha.com*) can provide referrals.
3. Acupuncture—although there are no current US studies on acupuncture, this practice is active, and past research findings indicate relief of as much as 90% of the pain in early labor and 60% of the pain during transition. Referrals can be made to the American Academy of Medical Acupuncture (*www.medicalacupuncture.org*).
4. Herbal therapies—although many of the herbs used are not approved by the Food and Drug Administration, they have been researched and found to be effective in laboring women and are documented in myriad medical and nursing references.
   a. Evening primrose oil—rubbed on the abdomen in prelabor to stimulate uterine activity.
   b. Corn silk—stimulates sluggish labor.
   c. Nutmeg—enhances uterine contractions; if added, cayenne and bayberry help to reduce bleeding after delivery.
   d. Nutmeg with yarrow, mistletoe, and corn silk—utilized as a treatment for postpartum hemorrhage.

 EVIDENCE BASE Kennedy, D. A., Lupattelli, A., Koren, G., & Nordeng, H. (2016). Safety classification of herbal medicines used in pregnancy in a multinational study. *BMC Complementary and Alternative Medicine, 16*(102), 1–9.

Evaluation: Expected Outcomes

- Tolerates fluids well and urine negative for ketones and glucose.
- Verbalizes positive statements about self and fetus.
- Reports pain decreased from comfort strategies.
- Use of birthing ball and evening primrose oil with provider consent and partner assistance.

First Stage of Labor: Active and Transition Phase (4 to 10 cm)

 EVIDENCE BASE Davidson, M. W., London, M. L., & Ladewig, P. W. (2016). *Olds' maternal–newborn nursing and women's health across the lifespan* (10th ed.). Upper Saddle River, NJ: Prentice Hall.

Nursing Diagnoses

- Anxiety related to concern for self and fetus.
- Acute Pain related to uterine contractions, nausea, and vomiting.
- Impaired Urinary Elimination related to epidural anesthesia or from pressure of the fetus.
- Ineffective Coping related to discomfort.
- Risk for Infection related to rupture of the membranes and prolonged labor.
- Impaired Physical Mobility related to medical interventions and discomfort.
- Ineffective Breathing Pattern related to pain and fatigue.

Nursing Interventions

Relieving Anxiety

1. Monitor maternal vital signs every hour if low-risk pregnancy or every 30 minutes if high-risk pregnancy; assess FHR as outlined in Table 37-2, page 999. Reassure mother of her progress and of the well-being of her baby.
2. Provide encouragement and continuous labor support, and involve the patient/partner/support persons in the maternal–fetal plan of care.

Minimizing Pain

1. Encourage frequent position changes for comfort.
2. Assist the woman with breathing and relaxation techniques, as needed.
3. Provide back, leg, and shoulder massage, as needed.
4. Evaluate cervical status as needed to monitor progression. Cervical checks should be kept to a minimum with ROM and positive β-streptococcus status.
5. Assist with preparation for analgesia and anesthesia following patient request (see Table 37-4).
6. Intervene for analgesia as follows:
   a. Confirm known allergies.
   b. Assess and document baseline temperature, BP, pulse, and respiratory rate.
   c. Monitor FHR before and after intramuscular (IM) or IV administration of analgesic medication.
   d. Assess efficacy of analgesics.
   e. Monitor FHR, continuous or intermittent, per facility policy and patient status.
7. Intervene for regional anesthesia as follows:
   a. Communicate maternal health information, laboratory results, labor status, and current obstetric complications with members of the health care team.
   b. Administer IV fluid bolus of lactated Ringer solution (500 to 1,000 mL) as directed, if not contraindicated (ie, severe preeclampsia, pulmonary edema).
   c. Assist anesthesia care provider by helping to position and hold patient for catheter insertion (lateral decubitus or sitting with feet supported, head flexed forward, elbows resting on knees with feet supported on a stool).
   d. Monitor maternal BP, pulse, and respiratory rate after initiation or rebolus of regional anesthesia per facility protocol; typically every 5 minutes for the first 15 minutes.
8. Support patient to comfortable position as labor progresses—lateral or semi-Fowler position, side of bed with legs dangling, or Taylor sitting position with uterine displacement.
9. Intervene for maternal hypotension by assisting to lateral positioning; infusing additional IV fluids, as directed; and administering ephedrine per facility protocol.

Table 37-4 Obstetric Analgesia and Anesthesia

DRUG	COMMENTS
Analgesics/Parenteral Opioids	
Meperidine Butorphanol Nalbuphine Fentanyl Morphine sulfate	Decreases fear and anxiety, promotes physical relaxation and rest between contractions; may cause nausea and vomiting; respiratory depression is the main adverse effect and is seen primarily in the neonate. Most commonly given via IV line or IM every 3 to 4 hours.
Tranquilizers	
Promethazine Hydroxyzine	May be used in combination with opioids; potentiates opioids; may be used as an antiemetic. Used in latent and first stage of labor to relieve anxiety, increase sedation and rest, and decrease nausea and vomiting.
Sedatives	
Sodium pentobarbital Sodium secobarbital Zolpidem tartrate	Produces sedation and hypnosis. Used for latent stage of labor to decrease anxiety, inhibit uterine contractions, and allow for rest. Does not relieve pain. Given orally or IM.
Regional Anesthesia/Analgesia	
Epidural opioids	Used with a local anesthetic to provide pain relief with a decreased motor block in labor. Used postoperatively to promote long-acting analgesia.
Epidural block	Used for labor to provide a sensory block up to the T10 to T12 level. Medication is given through the epidural catheter. Used for cesarean delivery and postpartum tubal ligation by increasing the level of anesthesia up to T4 to T6.
Subarachnoid block (spinal/intrathecal)	Used for such surgical procedures as a cesarean delivery and postpartum tubal ligation. The procedure is quicker and easier to perform. There is no catheter left in place for the procedure. Medication lasts for a finite period.
Local anesthesia	Used for pain control of the perineal area for an episiotomy or repair during a vaginal delivery.
Pudendal block	Used during the second stage of labor just before delivery to numb the lower vaginal canal, vulva, and the perineum for delivery. May also be used to provide pain relief for a forceps delivery if the woman does not have an epidural and for perineal repair.
General anesthesia	Used for emergency delivery involving cesarean delivery; if the woman refuses regional anesthesia; if regional anesthesia cannot be performed.

10. Monitor for adverse reactions from IV injection of local anesthetic: maternal tachycardia or bradycardia, hypertension, dizziness, tinnitus, metallic taste in the mouth, loss of consciousness, or cardiopulmonary collapse.
11. Monitor for adverse effects of opioids or anesthetics:
    a. Pruritus (itching on the chest, face, and arms), especially during the first hour after medication administration (usually begins within 30 to 60 minutes and decreases during the next hour).
    b. Nausea/emesis—can occur in up to 50% of women; administer medications to help with nausea/emesis, as directed by provider.
    c. Headache (pain in the frontal/occipital regions or radiating to the neck, stiff neck); increases in upright position and may decrease in horizontal position; relieved by abdominal compression; and may be accompanied by nausea/vomiting, ocular symptoms (photophobia, diplopia, difficulty in accommodation), and auditory symptoms (hearing loss, hyperacusis, tinnitus).
    d. Urine retention—observe for bladder distention; may utilize straight or indwelling catheter to empty the bladder if patient loses ability to sense fullness.
12. Assess dermatomes following procedure and periodically as indicated.
13. Periodically evaluate and document maternal pain level on a continuum using pain assessment tools in accordance with facility policy.
14. Evaluate labor progress; anesthetics may slow labor progression; realize that augmentation agents may be necessary.
15. Following delivery, assess neonate for effects of analgesia or anesthesia (neurobehavioral change, such as decreased motor tone and decreased respiratory rate). Initiate neonatal resuscitation, as indicated.

Encouraging Bladder Emptying
1. Encourage the woman to void every 2 hours at least 100 mL, if possible.
2. Palpate the lower abdomen; evaluate for a distended bladder periodically throughout labor.
3. Provide privacy to the patient to complete task. Running water or providing a perineal bottle of warm water for the woman to squirt against her perineum may assist success.
4. Catheterize patient if unable to void voluntarily.
5. Monitor intake and output per facility policy, particularly for certain medical conditions or following medication administration of IV oxytocin or magnesium sulfate.

Strengthening Coping with Active Labor and Transition
1. Assist the woman with breathing and relaxation techniques.
2. Encourage partner/support persons to assist with coping strategies.
3. Provide comfort measures, which may include:
    a. Effleurage, back rubs, and leg stroking.
    b. Cool cloth to the face, neck, abdomen, or back.
    c. Ice chips to moisten the mouth.

d. Peri care and change pads and linens, as needed.
e. Quiet, calm environment.
f. Repositioning frequently for comfort with pillow and blanket.
4. Assist patient to pace herself and to encourage her to deal with one contraction at a time.
5. Provide information on the contraction's ascent, peak, and descent; encourage resting between contractions. Anticipatory guidance helps to assist with the patient's ability to tolerate labor.
6. Encourage the woman not to push with feelings of rectal pressure until complete cervical dilation has occurred. Short panting breaths may assist to divert bearing-down sensation.

Preventing Intrauterine Infection
1. Assess temperature every 2 hours if membranes are not ruptured. If ruptured, assess temperature every hour.
2. Periodically change pads and linens when wet or soiled.
3. Provide perineal care after voiding and as needed.
4. Discourage the use of perineal pads or folded towels against the perineum because they create a warm, moist environment for bacteria.
5. Minimize vaginal examinations.
6. Observe for fetal tachycardia and warmth of maternal skin as signs of infection.
7. Assess complete blood count, as indicated and available.

Maintaining Mobility
1. Provide information regarding limitations and opportunities for movement with EFM.
2. Encourage ambulation or sitting in a chair while being monitored, if appropriate.
3. Encourage frequent upright or lateral position changes.

Encouraging Effective Breathing Techniques
1. Assist the woman to alter her breathing and utilize relaxation techniques, as needed, to maintain pain control.
2. Inform the woman that the urge to push is common during transition and occurs as the fetal presenting part meets the perineal floor muscles. Pushing with feelings of rectal pressure before complete cervical dilation should be avoided due to risks of increasing cervical edema and lacerations.
3. Assist the woman to avoid pushing prematurely by:
   a. Maintaining close eye contact during breathing and keeping patient focused.
   b. Breathing with the woman, having her blow out strong, short breaths (pant–blow).

Evaluation: Expected Outcomes
- Verbalizes positive statements about self and fetus.
- Reports pain decreased from comfort strategies and medical interventions.
- The bladder remains nondistended.
- Directs strategies for decreasing discomfort.
- Absence of fever and signs of infection.
- Changes position during labor.
- Utilizes patterned breathing techniques during contractions.

Second Stage of Labor
The second stage of labor is typically the most challenging for both the mother and fetus. As contractions become more frequent and increase in intensity, perineal pressure is heightened as the fetus completes the last few cardinal movements through the birth canal. Breathing techniques and positioning may either help or hinder descent and oxygenation. It is important for each practitioner to assist the maternal–fetal couplet with strategies to optimize oxygenation, encouragement, descent, and patient safety.

Positioning
It is most beneficial for practitioners who offer labor support to encourage the patient to utilize upright positions to facilitate fetal descent. Research supports that the most successful position is the squat; additional options exist (ie, standing, upright kneeling, leaning against a wall). Advanced imaging techniques have verified an increase in the pelvic outlet during squat positioning of approximately 1 to 2 cm. Subsequent findings also conclude that a squat position is accompanied by a shorter second stage, higher Apgar scores, reduced pain, decreased perineal trauma, and decreased need for neonatal resuscitation intervention. With advancements in anesthesia preparations and dosing, patients have increased mobility during anesthetic infusions. Therefore, encouraging and assisting the epidural-induced patient into a squat position is achievable. Additional positions are available to encourage fetal rotation and descent: sidelying, knee–chest, hands-and-knees, and forward lean accompanied by a pelvic tilt or pelvic rocking. Supine positioning is inappropriate during labor—at all stages—as it promotes maternal aortocaval compression syndrome with subsequent deoxygenation and perfusion of the mother and fetus.

Pushing Techniques
For optimum success, pushing techniques should be initiated once the cervix is fully dilated, fetal presenting part is on the pelvic floor (+1, +2, or greater than station), and the patient has a sense to push/bear down (Ferguson reflex). Because of the expanded use and effects of anesthetics during labor and birth, some women lose sensitivity to perineal pressure, requiring guidance and instruction with pushing efforts. Two methods of pushing exist: passive pushing or laboring down and active pushing.
1. Passive pushing ("laboring down"/"rest and descend")—this technique offers no active participation by the patient or practitioner to facilitate descent; strength of second-stage labor contractions moves the fetus down the birth canal. Reasons that may necessitate the need for this method include the following:
   a. Because of epidural anesthesia/analgesia, the woman does not feel the urge to push.
   b. Maternal clinical conditions such as cardiac disease, respiratory distress, or trauma.
   c. Fetal clinical conditions such as category III FHR or persistent abnormal UA data.
   d. Maternal exhaustion; need for periods of rest during prolonged second stage.
   e. Lack of nursing personnel to provide 1:1 support.
   f. Absence or unavailability of primary practitioner to assist with delivery.
2. Active pushing—this technique involves active participation (breathing techniques and positioning) by the patient and practitioner to assist in fetal descent. It is essential facilitate pushing efforts through spontaneous pushing and supporting the woman's preferred pushing choice. Closed-glottis (ie, breath holding) is no longer recommended during second stage as it limits oxygenation and encourages CO_2 retention. If prolonged, this technique may negatively impact the fetus and potentially lead to abnormal FHR patterns. Strategies that promote oxygen exchange in the mother include:
   a. Open-glottis pushing—this technique allows the woman to maintain a patent airway for gas exchange while enhancing bearing-down efforts with several short, quick breaths over the duration of a contraction (60 to 90 seconds). The

method includes several short, quick breaths of 4 to 6 seconds accompanied by bearing-down efforts that utilize muscles in the upper abdomen; improves maternal–fetal oxygenation.

b. Tug-of-war—utilization of a gown or short sheet tied in a knot at both ends. When the mother has the urge to push, she grabs one end of the gown or sheet and pulls as much as she can while the coach or nurse provides resistance by holding the other end (alternative way is to tie knot in one end and tie the other end to squat bar of labor bed); relaxes the perineum and has been found to decrease the second stage of labor by as much as 20 minutes.

c. Birthing aids—birthing balls, squat bars, birthing stools, and cushions may also be utilized to support the woman and her fetus.

Nursing Diagnoses

- Fear or Anxiety related to impending delivery.
- Acute Pain related to descent of the fetus.
- Knowledge Deficit related to the delivery process.

Nursing Interventions

Minimizing Fear and Anxiety
1. Monitor maternal vital signs per facility policy.
2. Assess FHR and contraction every 5 to 15 minutes per facility policy and patient status.
3. Explain procedures, breathing technique, and equipment during the delivery process.
4. Keep the mother informed of her progress and alterations in care plan.
5. Provide frequent, positive encouragement and utilize a mirror to assist the woman to see her progress.
6. Assist with positioning and pushing, as outlined above.

Promoting Comfort
1. Change positions frequently to increase comfort and promote fetal descent.
2. Evaluate bladder fullness and encourage voiding or catheterize, as needed.
3. Evaluate effectiveness of analgesia or anesthesia, as indicated; notify if alterations in dosing are needed to facilitate progression while maintaining pain control.

Facilitating an Uncomplicated Delivery Process
1. Explain delivery process and equipment to patient/partner/support persons.
2. Prepare the delivery equipment maintaining sterile technique, and prepare the delivery area to maximize work area and accessibility of equipment.
3. Prepare the infant resuscitation equipment and preheat radiant warmer; notify pediatric personnel, per facility policy as appropriate; if category III pattern, have two practitioners available to administer neonatal resuscitation, as indicated.
4. Notify necessary obstetric personnel and primary practitioner to prepare for delivery.
5. If delivery room is to be used, safely transfer the patient to the delivery bed before the birth is imminent.
6. If delivering in a birthing room, prepare labor bed for delivery.
7. Position the woman for vaginal birth in a semi-Fowler position (C-position) supported by pillows for her head, back, and shoulders. Positioning may vary by patient preference, practitioner, and facility.
   a. If used, gently place legs in padded stirrups or footrests symmetrically to avoid ligament strain, backache, or injury.

b. Under buttock drapes are recommended to evaluate blood loss during birth process. Accurate blood loss should be assessed and documented at every birth.

c. Follow facility protocol or provider preference for cleansing the perineal area.

8. Support and guide the woman step by step during the delivery process. When the birth is imminent, encourage the woman to breath and maintain focus. Controlled pushing may decrease the risk of lacerations, tears, and episiotomy. Evidence-based criteria do not support routine use of episiotomy to facilitate the second stage of labor; however, clinical judgment is the best guide based on individualized patient and fetal status.

a. An episiotomy may be performed when the fetal head is encircled by the vulvovaginal ring.

b. Once the head is delivered, the mother is instructed to stop pushing. Mucus is wiped from the infant's face and the mouth and nose. A bulb syringe may be used. Neonatal resuscitation guidelines no longer recommend suctioning of any kind on the perineum for the presence of meconium.

c. Nuchal cord intervention—loops of umbilical cord found around the neonate's neck are loosened and slipped over the head, whenever possible. If the cord cannot be slipped over the head, it is clamped with two clamps and cut between the two clamps.

d. Next, the woman is instructed to give a gentle push to assist with delivery of the neonate's body and placed skin-to-skin on the maternal abdomen as the neonatal condition allows.

e. Cord clamping—depending on the newborn's condition, some providers may delay clamping until the umbilical cord stops pulsating. This is done primarily to increase neonatal weight and hemoglobin and iron stores. The cord is clamped with two cord clamps and cut between the two clamps. It is common for the mother's partner or support person to cut the cord with assistance from the provider.

f. If color and tone are adequate and accompanied by a vigorous cry, basic neonatal care can be delayed to support skin-to-skin contact and family bonding. If additional resuscitative support is indicated, the baby is passed to the neonatal team for immediate care.

9. Practice standard precautions during labor and delivery.

 TRANSITIONAL CARE ALERT Evidence clearly supports the routine implementation of uninterrupted skin-to-skin between the mother and her healthy newborn. Studies demonstrate improved neonatal outcomes with respect to stabilized cardiorespiratory status and blood glucose levels. Maternal benefits include improved breastfeeding, pain management, and reduced anxiety. Nurses should make this a routine process after delivery as the neonate's condition allows. Discharge teaching should include the importance of skin-to-skin contact to facilitate infant comfort, temperature and glucose stability, and bonding.

Evaluation: Expected Outcomes

- Verbalizes positive statements about delivery outcome.
- Reports decreased pain from proper positioning.
- Infant is delivered without complications.

Third Stage of Labor: Delivery of the Placenta

Nursing Diagnoses

- Impaired Tissue Integrity related to placental separation.

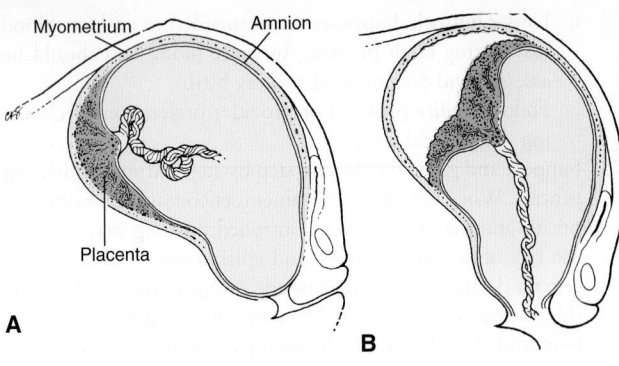

Figure 37-11. Placental separation. (LifeART image.) **(A)** Placenta attached to uterine wall. **(B)** Placenta separated from uterine wall.

Nursing Interventions

Promoting Tissue Integrity

1. Observe for signs of placental separation (see Figure 37-11):
   a. The uterus becomes globular in shape and rises upward in the abdomen.
   b. Umbilical cord lengthens.
   c. Small amount (gush) of blood appears.
2. Once signs of placental separation are observed, instruct the woman to assist delivery of the placenta with gentle bearing-down efforts. Be aware that delivery of the placenta typically occurs within the first 5 to 10 minutes, but may persist past 30 minutes, particularly in preterm gestations.
3. Administer and titrate oxytocin as directed to maintain uterine tone. Once the neonate has been delivered, oxytocin 10 units IM or 10 to 40 units IV per 1,000 mL is often utilized as the first line of treatment to prevent obstetric hemorrhage because of uterine atony.

 NURSING ALERT When oxytocin has been in use for prolonged periods, it may be ineffective in the fourth stage of labor to control hemorrhage. Additionally, high doses of oxytocin can lead to hypotension. Oxytocin is never administered IV push as it can cause cardiac dysrhythmia and death.

1. Inspect the placenta for size, shape, insertion site of cord, and intact cotyledons. The presence of even one cotyledon remaining intact within the uterus may lead to a postpartum hemorrhage. Umbilical cord should be inspected for true/false knots, clots, length, and a three-vessel cord. Abnormalities in the placenta, cord, or foul odor should be documented in the labor record and may necessitate the provider to request the placenta be sent for pathology.

Fourth Stage of Labor: Immediate Postpartum

 EVIDENCE BASE American College of Obstetricians and Gynecologists. (2006/Reaffirmed 2011). *Postpartum hemorrhage* (Practice Bulletin #76). Washington, DC: Author.

Nursing Diagnoses

• Risk for Bleeding related to uterine atony and hemorrhage.

• Deficient Fluid Volume related to decreased oral intake, bleeding, and diaphoresis.
• Acute Pain related to tissue trauma and birth process, intensified by fatigue.
• Impaired Urinary Elimination related to epidural or spinal anesthesia and tissue trauma.
• Risk for Injury related to disturbed sensation of lower extremities after regional anesthesia.
• Risk for Impaired Parenting related to inexperience or birth trauma.

Promoting Normal Involution and Controlled Bleeding

Also, see postpartum hemorrhage, page 1073.

1. Monitor BP, pulse, respirations, and oxygen saturation every 15 minutes for 1 to 2 hours and then every half to 1 hour until stable or transferred to the postpartum unit. Vital signs are assessed as the patient's condition warrants; increased frequency during periods of instability is necessary. Take temperature during the first hour postpartum and every 4 hours unless elevated or additional signs of infection present.

 NURSING ALERT Hypotension is a late sign of hypovolemia; increased pulse rate is the first indicator.

2. Immediately after delivery of the placenta, assess uterine fundal tone, height, and position every 15 minutes for 1 to 2 hours. Place a hand over the lower uterine segment above the symphysis pubis to inhibit uterine inversion, and gently massage the fundus with the other hand. Visual inspection of the perineum should occur simultaneously to assess lochia.
3. Note that the uterus is firm at or around the level of the umbilicus and midline. If deviated to the side (usually the right side), it is indicative of a full bladder. Assist the mother to void spontaneously or utilize a straight catheter to empty her bladder if anesthesia effects remain.
4. Gently massage uterine fundus at least every 15 minutes for the 1 to 2 hours to promote firmness and expression of clots to decrease the risk of hemorrhage. Also, teach the woman how to massage the uterus. Uterine massage may be performed with a bimanual technique when indicated by a provider.
5. Utilize an under-buttock drape after the placenta is delivered to improve accuracy of blood loss calculation and identify obstetrical hemorrhage.
6. Assess vaginal bleeding (lochia):
   a. Scant—blood only on tissue when wiped or less than 1-inch (2.5-cm) stain on perineal pad.
   b. Small/light—less than 4-inch (10.2-cm) stain on perineal pad.
   c. Moderate—less than 6-inch (15.2-cm) stain on perineal pad.
   d. Heavy—saturated perineal pad.
   e. Clots—note size and frequency; weigh for ABL.
7. Assess the perineum for pain, edema, discoloration, bleeding, odor, or hematoma formation, if excessive perineal pain.
8. Assess episiotomy/lacerations for approximation, drainage, bleeding, or infection.
9. Report and document all assessments.
   a. The woman is stable if the fundus remains firm or firms quickly with massage and moderate amount of lochia for 1 hour and then reduce to small or trace moderate amounts over 2 to 4 hours postpartum.

b. The woman is unstable if mean arterial pressure (MAP) is less than 60, a systolic blood pressure less than 90, or a 15% drop from normal baseline blood pressure (clinical indicators of obstetrical hemorrhage).

c. Severe tachycardia (≥120) and severe tachypnea (greater than 30/minute) are signs of impending compromise and require immediate evaluation and intervention by a provider.

Maintaining Fluid Volume

1. Maintain IV fluids as clinical condition warrants. Administer oxytocin as above if not given in the third stage.
2. Maintain accurate measurement of intake and output during the immediate postpartum.
3. Provide oral fluids and a snack or meal, as tolerated, if vital signs are stable and bleeding is controlled.

Relieving Discomfort and Fatigue

1. Apply a covered ice pack to the perineum immediately after delivery and periodically during the first 24 hours for an episiotomy, perineal laceration, or edema.
2. Administer analgesics, as indicated. Excessive perineal pain unrelieved by medications suggests hematoma formation and mandates careful examination of the vulva, vagina, and rectum.
3. Ensure that epidural catheter has been removed by anesthesia provider, if appropriate.
4. Assist the woman in finding comfortable positions.
5. Assist the woman with a partial bath and perineal care. Periodically change linens and pads, as necessary.
6. Allow for privacy and promote rest periods between postpartum checks.
7. Provide warm blankets and reassure the woman that tremors are common during this period because of intravascular fluid shifts.

Encouraging Bladder Emptying

1. Evaluate the bladder for distention.
2. Encourage the woman to void periodically.
   a. Provide adequate time and privacy.
   b. The sound of running water may stimulate voiding.
   c. Gently squirting tepid water on the perineum may facilitate voiding.
3. Catheterize the woman if the bladder is full and she is unable to void.
   a. Birth trauma, anesthesia, and pain from lacerations and episiotomy may reduce or alter the voiding reflex.
   b. Bladder distention may displace the uterus upward and to the right side, impairing tone.

Preventing Injury Pending Return of Sensation

1. Evaluate mobility and sensation of the lower extremities.
2. Evaluate vital signs.
3. Remain with the woman and assist her out of bed for the first time. Evaluate her ability to support her weight and ambulate safely.

Promoting Parenting

1. Once stable, bring neonate to the mother and support person immediately after birth.
2. Encourage the parents to hold infant as soon as possible.
3. Assist and teach parents to hold the neonate close to their faces, about 8 to 12 inches (20.5 to 30.5 cm) to engage neonate.
4. Assist parents to inspect the infant's body to familiarize themselves with their child.

5. Assist with breastfeeding as soon as possible once both mother and newborn are stable. This is typically a period of quiet alert time for the neonate often optimizing successful breastfeeding.
6. Document appropriate and inappropriate bonding; notify primary practitioner and social services if suspect lack of or inappropriate response in mother, father, or any other potential caregiver.

Evaluation: Expected Outcomes

- Vital signs remain stable, vaginal bleeding remains light to moderate, and the uterus remains firm at the midline below the umbilicus.
- Tolerates fluids and food well after delivery.
- Verbalizes decreased perineal pain and feels rested.
- Voids within 2 hours of delivery.
- Ambulates without assistance.
- Interacts with the neonate.

Precipitous Delivery or Delivery in the Absence of Health Care Provider (Nurse-Assisted)

A precipitous delivery is an emergent event. During this event, consider the woman and infant as a unit. Coordination to prevent maternal and fetal infection, injury, and hemorrhage is key.

Interventions

1. Provide reassurance and instruct the woman in a calm, controlled manner. Sustain eye contact and assist the mother to utilize pant–blow breathing until told to push. Do not break down the birthing bed. The lower half of the bed will be utilized as a table and promotes fetal safety.
2. Position patient for comfort and enhance visualization of the perineum.
3. Wash hands, put on gloves, and clean the perineum as time permits.
4. Exert gentle pressure against the head of the fetus, using pads of the thumb, index finger, and middle fingers or cupped palm of the hand, to control progress and prevent precipitous delivery; this prevents undue stretching of the perineum and sudden expulsion through the vulva with subsequent infant and maternal complications.
5. Encourage the woman to pant at this time to prevent bearing down.
6. If membranes are intact at the time of delivery, rupture can be achieved by applying pressure to the membranes
7. Wipe the infant's face and mouth with a clean towel. Suction the mouth and nose with a bulb syringe, if available.
8. Check for nuchal cord and reduce, if possible. If the cord is too tight to permit slipping over the infant's head, it must be clamped in two places and cut between the clamps before the rest of the body is delivered.
9. Allow head to restitute. Place one hand over each ear bilaterally to support the infant's head; gently exert downward pressure toward the floor, thus slipping the anterior shoulder under the symphysis pubis.
10. As soon as the anterior shoulder is delivered, provide upward, outward traction to the head to deliver the posterior shoulder.
11. Support the infant's body and head in the lower hand. As the body is delivered, place skin-to-skin on maternal abdomen.

12. Gentle rubbing of the back may stimulate breathing with warm blankets
13. Cover mother and infant with warm blankets.
14. Watch for signs of placental separation (gush of dark blood from introitus, lengthening of umbilical cord, change in uterine contour). Avoid pulling on the cord, which might break and cause hemorrhage.
15. Clamp and cut cord as outline above.
16. Assess fundal tone and massage the uterus as outlined above. Putting the baby to breast may assist uterine contraction to promote oxytocin release.
17. Place identification bands on both the mother and infant.
18. Offer the patient fluids (IV or by mouth).
19. Teach the woman to massage her fundus.
20. Record the time and date of birth, as well as:
    a. Notifications and preparations for the birth.
    b. Fetal presentation and position.
    c. Presence of nuchal or body cord.
    d. Rupture of membranes: character, color, odor, and amount of amniotic fluid.
    e. Time of placental expulsion.
    f. Placental appearance.
    g. Maternal condition.
    h. Unusual occurrences during birth (ie, shoulder dystocia).
21. Assist and transport as necessary.

Immediate Care of the Neonate

 EVIDENCE BASE Ricci, S. S. (2017). *Essentials of maternity, newborn, and women's health nursing* (4th ed.). Philadelphia, PA: Wolters Kluwer Health/Lippincott Williams & Wilkins.
American Academy of Pediatrics & American Heart Association. (2015). *Textbook of neonatal resuscitation* (7th ed.). Elk Grove Village, IL: American Academy of Pediatrics.

Nursing Diagnoses

- Ineffective Airway Clearance related to nasal and oral secretions from delivery.
- Ineffective Thermoregulation related to environment and immature ability for adaptation.
- Risk for Infection related to immature defenses of the neonate.

Nursing Interventions

Promoting Airway Clearance and Transitioning of the Neonate

1. Over 90% of newborns complete intrauterine to extrauterine transition without compromise or assistance. Close observation of all neonates is recommended for a minimum of 4 to 6 hours after birth.
2. Clean mucus from the face, mouth, and nose. Aspirate with a bulb syringe, as necessary.
    a. Neonatal resuscitation protocols no longer require suctioning on the perineum if meconium is present in the amniotic fluid.
    b. A vigorous newborn demonstrating strong respiratory effort, good muscle tone and a heart rate greater than 100 may only require bulb suctioning of the mouth an nose if needed.
    c. In the presence of meconium-stained amniotic fluid and a non-vigorous infant, deep suctioning of the mouth and trachea may be necessary to prevent aspiration.

Table 37-5	Apgar Scoring Chart		
SIGN	**0**	**1**	**2**
Heart rate	Absent	Slow (<100)	>100
Respiratory effort	Absent	Slow, irregular	Good, crying
Muscle tone	Flaccid	Some flexion of extremities	Active motion
Reflex irritability	No response	Cry	Vigorous cry
Color	Blue, pale	Body pink, extremities blue	Completely pink

3. Assess neonate's transition using the Apgar scoring system (see Table 37-5) at 1 and 5 minutes after birth. When the 5-minute score is less than 7, scoring continues every 5 minutes up to 20 minutes after delivery. An Apgar score of 0 to 3 at 20 minutes is associated with increased neonatal morbidity. Wear gloves at all times when handling an unbathed newborn and maintain standard precautions.

Promoting Thermoregulation

1. Dry the neonate immediately after delivery, remove wet towels, and place skin-to-skin on mother's abdomen if vigorous and cover with a blanket and hat to prevent heat loss. If newborn is nonvigorous, place under a prewarmed radiant warmer for further evaluation. A neonate can lose up to 200 cal/kg/minute through evaporation, convection, conduction, and radiation.
2. Double wrap the neonate in warm blankets, with hat, and return to mother after stabilization.
3. Provide a warm, draft-free environment for the neonate.
4. Assess neonate's axillary temperature—a normal temperature is between 97.7°F and 99.3°F (36.5°C and 37.4°C).

Preventing Infection and Other Complications

1. Prophylactic eye care: Administer a 1-cm ribbon of erythromycin 0.5% or tetracycline 1% ophthalmic ointment to the lower conjunctival sac to prevent ophthalmia neonatorum (gonorrheal or chlamydial). This can be delayed up to 1 hour after birth to facilitate breastfeeding and parental bonding. Ointment may be gently wiped away after 1 minute with a sterile cotton ball.
    a. If the mother has a positive gonococcal or chlamydial culture, the neonate will require further treatment.
    b. Treatment is mandatory in all states.
2. Vitamin K: Administer a single prophylactic dose of vitamin K_1 (phytonadione) 0.5 to 1 mg IM to the vastus lateralis and document site.
    a. Given to prevent a vitamin K–dependent hemorrhagic disease of the newborn.
    b. If the parents decline vitamin K administration, inform the parents that if they desire a circumcision, it may not be performed related to the increased risk of bleeding.
    c. Additionally, inform parents that vitamin K levels will reach their peak (without neonatal injection) at 8 days after birth.
3. Security and Identification: place identical identification bracelets on the mother and the neonate per facility policy. An additional electronic security device may also be secured at this time to prevent infant abduction.

a. Information on bands may include mother's name, hospital/admission number, neonate's sex, race, primary practitioner, and date and time of birth and other information specified in the facility's policy.

b. The father, partner, or other designated person may also wear an identical bracelet matching the mother's and infant's band.

c. Foot printing and fingerprinting the neonate are not adequate methods of patient identification and may or may not be performed based on facility policy.

d. Complete all identification procedures before the infant leaves the delivery room.

4. Measurements: Weigh and measure the infant shortly after birth.
   a. Average neonate weight is 5 to 8 pounds (2,500 to 4,000 g).
   b. Average neonate length is 18 to 22 inches (46 to 56 cm).
   c. Head, chest, and abdominal circumferences are also measured (facility dependent).

5. After birth, nursery/mother–baby personnel should evaluate the neonate's status and assess risks of birth trauma or injury.

6. Administer hepatitis B vaccine according to your facility's policy.
   a. Vaccination of all infants born in the United States is recommended regardless of mother's hepatitis status. If the mother's hepatitis B surface antigen (HBsAg) status is negative, the vaccine is given within 12 hours of birth to age 2 months and then again at 1 to 2 months after the initial dose with the final vaccine (#3) given at 6 to 18 months. The vaccine is given for the prevention of acute and chronic hepatitis B infection.
   b. If the mother is hepatitis B positive, the infant will receive hepatitis B immunoglobulin (HBIG) and the HBV vaccine at birth to within 12 hours. Additionally, infants of hepatitis-positive mothers will receive HBV at ages 1 to 2 months and age 6 months.
   c. Neonates born to nonscreened mothers will receive the HBV at birth within 12 hours of birth. If the mother later proves to be hepatitis B positive, the neonate will also receive HBIG (0.5 mL) IM as soon as possible, but no later than 1 week after birth. The infant will also receive HBV at 1 to 2 months and another injection at 6 to 18 months.

Community and Home Care Considerations

1. Issues regarding promoting airway clearance, transitioning, and thermoregulation promotion are essentially unchanged for home births; Apgar scores are not always given at home deliveries.

2. Eye prophylaxis is required using an antimicrobial ointment (ie, erythromycin) to prevent ophthalmia neonatorum.

3. Vitamin K administration is not a requirement for home deliveries. Vitamin K levels naturally increase at 8 days of life. If infant is a boy and parents desire circumcision, the procedure is withheld until after day 8.

4. Make sure attendants are familiar with neonatal resuscitation and that emergency numbers and procedures are readily available.

5. Identification procedures are not required for home births, although required state paperwork must be completed by the health care provider.

Evaluation: Expected Outcomes

- Neonate transitions appropriately, as evidenced by Apgar score between 7 and 10.
- Temperature remains between 97.5°F and 99°F (36.4°C and 37.2°C).
- Eye prophylaxis and other procedures completed before leaving delivery room.

SPECIAL CONSIDERATIONS
Neonatal Resuscitation

 EVIDENCE BASE American Academy of Pediatrics & American Heart Association. (2015). *Textbook of neonatal resuscitation* (7th ed.). Elk Grove, IL: American Academy of Pediatrics.

Neonatal resuscitation is most effective with an organized and efficient team. At every delivery, there should be at least one person whose primary responsibility is the neonate and who is capable of initiating neonatal resuscitation. Any high-risk delivery (requiring more advanced neonatal resuscitation) requires at least two people to be present to manage the resuscitation—one with complete resuscitation skills (intubation and umbilical catheter placement) and one to assist.

Causes

Perinatal asphyxia is the main cause for neonatal resuscitation. When the infant is deprived of oxygen, an initial period of rapid respirations occurs followed by apnea, decreased heart rate, and decreased neuromuscular tone. This is a period of primary apnea.

Primary Apnea

1. Intrauterine asphyxia may result in passage of meconium, fetal tachycardia, absent variability, recurrent late or variable decelerations, or prolonged bradycardia.
2. Infants born with primary apnea will need sensory stimuli (tactile or positive-pressure ventilation) to initiate respirations.
3. May occur in utero or after birth.

Secondary Apnea

1. Secondary apnea occurs when primary apnea is unresolved. The heart rate continues to drop lower (begins to drop about the same time the infant enters into primary apnea), the BP drops, the infant becomes flaccid, and spontaneous gasps occur.
2. May occur in utero or after birth.
3. At birth, these infants are pale, flaccid, and bradycardia.
4. Anticipation and preparation of neonatal resuscitation should occur at every birth.
5. When the infant is apneic at birth, it is difficult to distinguish between primary and secondary apnea; therefore, one must assume secondary apnea and resuscitation must begin immediately.

Initial Steps in Neonatal Resuscitation

1. A: Airway
2. B: Breathing
3. C: Circulation

How to Achieve Initial Steps

Performing the initial steps should take no more than 30 seconds.

1. Call for assistance, if needed.
2. Place infant on a warm, dry radiant warmer.
3. Dry infant thoroughly with warmed towels, dispose of wet towels, and stimulate infant by rubbing back or slapping soles of feet, if necessary.
4. Assess respirations (rise and fall of the chest, air moving in the lungs) and pulse (heart rate more than 100 bpm).
5. If apnea or the heart rate is less than 100 bpm, begin positive-pressure ventilation (PPV; bag and mask ventilation) and SpO$_2$ monitoring. Breaths are administered at a rate of 40 to 60 per minute. Resuscitation starts with room air (21%) and increases are made to the concentration of oxygen demonstrated by an uncompromised term neonate.
   a. Observe chest movement and auscultate for air movement in all lung fields.
   b. To prevent air filling, the stomach during PPV, an orogastric tube can be inserted orally.
6. If heart rate is less than 60 bpm, start chest compressions. New recommendations are to intubate infant prior to beginning chest compressions to improve circulation of oxygenated blood. One cycle of events consists of three compressions plus one ventilation, resulting in 120 "events" per 60 seconds or 90 compressions plus 30 breaths.
   a. If the heart rate increases to above 60 bpm, cease chest compressions and maintain ventilation at a rate of 40 to 60 breaths/minute.
   b. Once the heart rate exceeds 100 and spontaneous breathing resumes, gradually decrease rate of PPV.
7. Assist with endotracheal intubation, if needed.
8. Assist with insertion of an umbilical catheter for administration of medications and fluids, if needed. If heart rate remains below 60 bpm for over 60 seconds of PPV and chest compressions, medications (eg, epinephrine) should be considered and administered intravenously via an umbilical catheter or endotracheally.
9. Continue to assess neonate periodically once stabilization is reestablished and transport accordingly.

SELECTED REFERENCES

Adams, J., Frawley, J., Steel, A., et al. (2015). Use of pharmacological and nonpharmacological labor pain management techniques and their relationship to maternal and infant birth outcome: Examination of a nationally representative sample of 1835 pregnant women. *Midwifery, 31*(4), 458–463.

American Academy of Pediatrics & American College of Obstetricians and Gynecologists. (2012). *Guidelines for perinatal care* (7th ed.). Washington, DC: Author.

American Academy of Pediatrics & American College of Obstetricians and Gynecologists. (2015). *The Apgar score* (Committee Opinion). Washington, DC: Author.

American Academy of Pediatrics & American Heart Association. (2015). *Textbook of neonatal resuscitation* (7th ed.). Elk Grove Village, IL: American Academy of Pediatrics.

American College of Obstetricians and Gynecologists. (2006/Reaffirmed 2015). *Postpartum hemorrhage* (Practice Bulletin #76). Washington, DC: Author.

American College of Obstetricians and Gynecologists. (2009/Reaffirmed 2016). *Induction of labor* (Practice Bulletin # 107). Washington, DC: Author.

American College of Obstetricians and Gynecologists. (2009/Reaffirmed 2017). *Intrapartum fetal heart rate monitoring: Nomenclature, interpretation, and general management principles* (Practice Bulletin #106). Washington, DC: Author.

American College of Obstetricians and Gynecologists. (2010/Reaffirmed 2017). *Management of intrapartum fetal heart rate tracings* (Practice Bulletin #116). Washington, DC: Author.

American College of Obstetricians and Gynecologists. (2012). *Optimizing protocols in obstetrics: Management of hemorrhage.* Series 2. Washington, DC: Author.

American College of Obstetricians and Gynecologists. (2017). *Delayed umbilical cord clamping after birth* (Committee Opinion # 684). Washington, DC: Author.

American College of Obstetricians and Gynecologists. (2017). *Emergent therapy for acute-onset, severe hypertension during pregnancy, and the postpartum period* (Committee Opinion #692). Washington, DC: Author.

American College of Obstetricians and Gynecologists. (2017). *Episiotomy: Procedures and repair techniques.* Washington, DC: Author.

American College of Obstetricians and Gynecologists. (2017). *Planned home birth* (Committee Opinion #697). Washington, DC: Author.

Association of Women's Health, Obstetric and Neonatal Nurses. (Ed.). (2015). *Fetal heart monitoring principles and practices* (5th ed.). Dubuque, IA: Kendall-Hunt Publishing Co.

Association of Women's Health, Obstetric and Neonatal Nurses. (2015). Quantification of blood loss: AWHONN practice brief number 1. *Journal of Obstetric, Gynecologic, and Neonatal Nursing, 44,* 158–160.

Cheng, Y.W., & Caughey, A. B. (2015). Second stage of labor. *Clinical Obstetrics and Gynecology, 58*(2), 227–240.

Crenshaw, J. (2014). Healthy birth practice #6: Keep mother and baby together—It's best for mother, baby, and breastfeeding. *Journal of Perinatal Education, 23*(4), 211–217.

Cunningham, F. G., Leveno, K., Bloom, S., et al. (2014). *Williams obstetrics* (24th ed.). New York: McGraw-Hill.

Davidson, M. W., London, M. L., & Ladeweig, P. W. (2016). *Olds' maternal–newborn nursing and women's health across the lifespan* (10th ed.). Upper Saddle River, NJ: Pearson Education.

Diaz, V., Abalos, E., & Carroli, G. (2014). Methods for blood loss estimation after vaginal birth (Protocol). *Cochrane Database of Systematic Reviews* (2), CD010980.

Gizzo, S., Di Gangi, S., Noventa, M., et al. (2014). Women's choice of positions during labor: Return to the past of modern way of giving birth? A Cohort Study in Italy. *BioMed Research International, 2014*(2014), 7. Article ID 638093.

Handcock, A., Weeks, A. D., & Lavender, T. D. (2015). Is accurate and reliable blood loss estimation the 'crucial step' in early detection of postpartum haemorrhage: An integrative review of the literature. *BMC Pregnancy and Childbirth, 15,* 1–9.

Hanson, L., & VandeVusse, L. (2014). Supporting labor progress toward physiologic birth. *J Perinatal Neonatal Nursing, 28*(2), 101–107.

Kennedy, D. A., Lupattelli, A., Koren, G., & Nordeng, H. (2016). Safety classification of herbal medicines used in pregnancy in a multinational study. *BMC Complementary and Alternative Medicine, 16*(102), 1–9.

Kolkman, D. G., Verhoeven, C. J., Brinkhorst, S. J., et al. (2013). The Bishop score as a predictor of labor induction success: A systematic review. *American Journal of Perinatology, 30*(8), 625–630.

Lertbunnaphong, T., Lapthanapat, N., Leetheeragul, J., et al. (2016). Postpartum blood loss: Visual estimation versus objective quantification with a novel birthing drape. *Singapore Medical Journal, 57*(6), 325–328.

Lothian, J. (2016). Does childbirth education make a difference?. *Journal of Perinatal Education, 25*(3), 139–141.

Lowdermilk, D., Perry, S., Cashion, C., & Alden, K. R. (2016). *Maternity and women's health care* (11th ed.). St. Louis, MO: Mosby.

Macones, G. A., Hankins, G. D., Spong, C. Y., et al. (2008). The 2008 National Institute of Child Health and Human Development workshop report on electronic fetal monitoring: Update on definitions, interpretation, and research guidelines. *Obstetrics and Gynecology, 112,* 661–666.

Mattson, S, & Smith, J. (2016). *Core curriculum for maternal–newborn nursing* (5th ed.). St. Louis, MO: Saunders Elsevier.

Mhyre, J. M., D'Oria, R., Hameed, A. B., et al. (2014). The maternal early warning criteria: a proposal from the national partnership for maternal safety. *Journal of Obstetric, Gynecologic, and Neonatal Nursing, 43*(6), 771–779.

Moore, E. R., Bregman, N., Anderson, G. C., & Medley, N. (2016). Early skin-to-skin contact for mothers and their healthy newborn infants. *Cochrane Database of Systematic Reviews,* CD003519.

Ricci, S. S. (2017). *Essentials of maternity, newborn, and women's health nursing* (4th ed.). Philadelphia, PA: Wolters, Kluwer Health/Lippincott Williams & Wilkins.

Simpson, K. R., & Creehan, P. A. (2014). *Perinatal nursing* (4th ed.). Philadelphia, PA: Wolters, Kluwer, Lippincott.

World Health Organization, UNICEF, United Nations Fund for Population Activities, et al. (2014). *Trends in maternal mortality, 1990 to 2013: Estimates by WHO, UNICEF, UNFPA, The World Bank Estimates, and the United Nations Population Division.* Geneva, Switzerland: Author.

38

Care of Mother and Neonate During the Postpartum Period

NURSING CARE OF THE MOTHER

The Puerperium

The *puerperium* is the period beginning after delivery and ending when the woman's body has returned as closely as possible to its prepregnant state. The period lasts approximately 6 weeks. (See Standards of Care Guidelines 38-1, page 1016.)

Physiologic Changes of the Puerperium

 EVIDENCE BASE Cunningham, F. G., Leveno, K. J., Bloom, S. L., et al. (2014). *Williams obstetrics* (24th ed.). New York: McGraw-Hill.
Mattson, S., & Smith, J. E. (Eds.). (2016). *Core curriculum for maternal-newborn nursing* (5th ed.). St. Louis, MO: Saunders Elsevier.

1. Uterine and cervical changes.
   a. Uterine involution begins immediately after delivery where the fundus is palpable halfway between the umbilicus and symphysis pubis. At 1 hour postpartum, the fundus is usually level with or slightly below the level of the umbilicus. The fundus is usually midline. Within 12 hours of delivery, the fundus may be ½ inch (1.3 cm) above the umbilicus and, by 24 hours, ¼ inch (1 cm) below the umbilicus. After this, the level of the fundus descends approximately 1 fingerbreadth (or ½ inch) each day; until by the 10th to 14th day, it has descended into the pelvic cavity and can no longer be palpated (see Figure 38-1). At approximately 6 weeks postpartum, uterine involution is complete.
   b. After delivery, *lochia*—a vaginal discharge that consists of fatty epithelial cells, shreds of membrane, decidua, and blood—is red or dark brown with clots (lochia rubra) for approximately 2 to 3 days. It then progresses to a paler pink or more brown-tinged color of serosanguineous consistency (lochia serosa) for 4 to 10 days, followed by a whitish or yellowish color (lochia alba) in the 10th to 14th day. Lochia usually ceases by 2 to 4 weeks, and the placental site is completely healed by the 6th week.
   c. Lochial flow can be scant (less than 2.5 cm stain [1 inch]/hour), light (less than 10 cm stain [4 inches]/hour), moderate (less than 15.2 cm stain [6 inches]/hour), or heavy (one pad saturated within 1 hour). Lochial flow is considered to be "excessive" if the perineal pad becomes saturated in less than 15 minutes (see Figure 38-2).
2. Immediately after delivery of the placenta, the cervix has little tone or resemblance to the prepregnant state.
   a. In approximately 2 to 3 days, the cervix appears more like the prepregnant state and is dilated to 2 to 3 cm. By the end of the first postpartum week, it is approximately 1 cm in diameter.
   b. The cervical opening is more slitlike than the prepregnant dimple and remains that way. (If the cervix has never been dilated, it will remain more prepregnant dimple-like.)
   c. The vaginal walls, uterine ligaments, and muscles of the pelvic floor and abdominal wall regain most of their tone during the puerperium.
   d. Immediately after delivery, the vaginal walls are smooth and swollen because the vaginal rugae are absent. Rugae reappear approximately 3 weeks postpartum.
   e. Postpartum diuresis begins within 12 hours after birth and continues for 2 to 5 days postpartum, as extracellular water accumulated during pregnancy is excreted.
   f. Diuresis may also occur shortly after delivery if urine output was obstructed because of the pressure of the presenting part or if IV fluids were given during labor.

Postpartum Care

- Perform focused assessment regularly using the BUBBLE-HE acronym—breasts, uterus (size and consistency), bladder (distention), bowel elimination, lochia, episiotomy (lacerations), Homans sign, and emotional status/bonding.
- Notify health care provider immediately if abnormalities are present:
  - Increased respiration and pulse, decreased blood pressure, and orthostatic changes may indicate hemorrhage.
  - Excessive vaginal bleeding (saturation of peripad within 1 hour for 2 or more hours), expulsion of large clots, or steady increase in vaginal bleeding, which indicates hemorrhage.
  - Boggy uterine fundus that does not become firm and remain firm with massage, indicating atony.
  - Inability to void and bladder distention, which may displace uterus, leading to uterine atony.
  - Decreased urine output, which may indicate hemorrhage.
  - Elevated temperature, increased pain, swelling, and redness from incisions, indicating infection.
  - Calf tenderness, swelling, redness, or warmth, which may indicate a blood clot.
  - Excessive irritability, crying, moodiness, withdrawal, insomnia, and loss of interest in activities, which may indicate postpartum depression (PPD).
- Encourage rest, nutrition, and bonding with the infant.
- Provide education on feeding, bathing, changing, safety measures, signs of illness, and when to call infants pediatric care provider with questions.

This information should serve as a general guideline only. Each patient situation and facility policy present a unique set of clinical factors and requires nursing judgment to guide care, which may include additional or alternative measures and approaches.

3. Breasts—with loss of the placenta, circulating levels of estrogen and progesterone decrease and levels of prolactin increase, initiating lactogenesis.
   a. *Colostrum*—a thick, yellowish fluid that contains more minerals and protein but less sugar and fat than mature breast milk and has a laxative effect on the infant—is secreted for the first 2 days postpartum.
   b. Mature milk secretion is usually present by the third postpartum day but may be present earlier if a woman breastfeeds immediately after delivery. Usually by the end of the 2nd postpartum week, mature breast milk is present.
   c. Breast engorgement with milk and venous and lymphatic stasis with swollen, tense, and tender breast tissue may occur between days 3 and 5 postpartum.
4. Endocrine/metabolic function.
   a. Human chorionic gonadotropin declines rapidly and is nonexistent by the end of the first postpartum week.
   b. Thyroid levels are normal by 4 to 6 weeks postpartum.
   c. Glucose levels are low secondary to decreased human placental lactogen, decreased cortisol, decreased estrogen, and decreased growth hormone.
   d. Blood glucose levels of women with gestational diabetes mellitus (GDM) may return to normal limits shortly after birth. However, ACOG and the CDC recommend all women with GDM should glucose tested 6 to 12 weeks postpartum and screened for diabetes every 1 to 3 years for early identification of type 2 diabetes mellitus.
5. Ovarian function.
   a. Estrogen and progesterone levels decrease rapidly after delivery of the placenta and are usually their lowest by the 7th postpartum day.
   b. Estrogen reaches the follicular phase by 3 weeks after birth, as long as the woman is not lactating.
   c. Ovulation may occur as early as 27 days after delivery. The average time is 70 to 75 days postdelivery and 190 days postdelivery if breast-feeding.
   d. The start of menses after delivery is individualized. Usually, the first menses occurs approximately 7 to 9 weeks after delivery in nonnursing mothers, although breast-feeding women may not start their first menses until as late as 18 months.

A   B   C

Figure 38-1. Changes in uterine size and shape following delivery. **(A)** Uterus after delivery. **(B)** Uterus at 6th day. **(C)** Nongravid uterus. (Reeder, S., Martin, L., & Koniak-Griffin, D. [1997]. *Maternity nursing: Family newborn, and women's health care* [18th ed.]. Philadelphia, PA: Lippincott-Raven Publishers.)

Scant amount
Blood only on tissue
when wiped or less
than 1-inch (2.5 cm)
stain on peripad.

Light amount
Less than 4-inch
(10-cm) stain on
peripad.

Moderate amount
Less than 6-inch
(15.2-cm) stain on
peripad.

Heavy amount
Saturated peripad
within 1 hour.

Figure 38-2. Assessing the volume of lochia by peri-pad saturation.

6. Urinary function.
   a. Mild proteinuria (+1 on urine dipstick) is common for 1 to 2 days after delivery in 40% to 50% of postpartum women.
   b. Spontaneous voiding should return by 6 to 8 hours postpartum. Bladder tone returns between 5 and 7 days postpartum.
   c. The catabolic process of involution can cause an increase in blood urea nitrogen levels during the postpartum period.
   d. Stress incontinence is common during the first 6 weeks postpartum, and Kegel exercises should be encouraged.
   e. Hematuria immediately after normal spontaneous vaginal birth can be indicative of bladder trauma. If hematuria occurs after the first 24 hours, it may be indicative of urinary tract infection.
7. Neurologic function.
   a. Discomfort and fatigue are common.
   b. Afterpains because of the involution process and discomfort from the delivery, lacerations, episiotomy, and muscle aches are common for the first 2 to 3 days postdelivery.
   c. Frontal and bilateral headaches are common and are caused by fluid shifts in the first week postpartum.
   d. Non–rapid eye movement (REM) sleep is absent after birth and increases during the next 2 weeks. REM sleep decreases as non-REM sleep increases.
   e. Carpal tunnel syndrome (resulting from physiologic edema causing pressure on the median nerve) is usually relieved by postpartum diuresis.
   f. Postpartum eclamptic seizures can begin more than 48 hours and less than 4 weeks postdelivery. They are commonly preceded by severe headache or vision disturbances (spots before the eyes, double vision, etc.). Extra care is taken to observe for these symptoms, especially in women with prenatal diagnosis of preeclampsia or hypertension.
8. Cardiovascular function.
   a. Most dramatic changes occur in this system and can take between 6 and 12 weeks to return to the prepregnant state.
   b. Cardiac output decreases to prelabor values within a one hour postpartum and may be dependent on multiple factors including anesthesia use and method of delivery. However, it can remain elevated for as much as 48 hours postpartum. Cardiac output values return to normal by 6 to 12 weeks postpartum.
   c. Blood volume decreases immediately after birth. Average blood loss in a vaginal birth is between 200 to 500 mL and 600 to 800 mL in caesarean deliveries.

   d. Hematocrit increases and increased red blood cell (RBC) production stops.
   e. Leukocytosis (increased white blood cells [WBCs]) is common during the first postpartum week.
   f. A positive Homans sign may indicate thrombophlebitis and should be reported to the primary care provider. The woman should be instructed not to massage her legs.
9. Respiratory function.
   a. Returns to normal by approximately 6 to 8 weeks postpartum.
   b. Basal metabolic rate increases for 7 to 14 days postpartum, secondary to mild anemia, lactation, and psychological changes.
   c. Partial pressure of arterial oxygen (PaO_2), partial pressure of carbon dioxide ($PaCO_2$), and pH usually return to normal by 3 weeks postpartum.
10. GI/hepatic function.
    a. GI tone and motility decrease in the early postpartum period, commonly causing gaseous distention of the abdomen and constipation.
    b. Normal bowel function, including normal bowel movements, returns at about 2 to 3 days postpartum.
    c. Liver function returns to normal approximately 10 to 14 days postpartum.
    d. Gallbladder contractility increases to normal, allowing for expulsion of small gallstones.
    e. GI function can be inhibited by surgical intervention, analgesia, anesthesia, and decreased muscle tone.
11. Musculoskeletal function.
    a. Generalized fatigue and weakness are common.
    b. Decreased abdominal tone is common.
    c. Diastasis recti heals and resolves by the 4th to 6th week postpartum. Until healing is complete, usually 1 to 2 weeks postpartum, abdominal exercises are contraindicated.
    d. Joint instability returns to normal between 6 and 8 weeks postpartum.
12. Integumentary function.
    a. Striae gravidarum lighten, and melasma is usually gone by 6 weeks postpartum.
    b. Hair loss can increase for the first 4 to 20 weeks postpartum and then regrowth will occur, although the hair may not be as thick as it was before pregnancy.
13. A good method to remember how to check the postpartum changes is the use of the acronym **BUBBLE-HE**:
    a. **B**—Breast.
    b. **U**—Uterus.
    c. **B**—Bladder.
    d. **B**—Bowels.
    e. **L**—Lochia.
    f. **E**—Episiotomy/lacerations.
    g. **H**—Homans sign/extremities.
    h. **E**—Emotional status/bonding.

Emotional and Behavioral (Psychosocial) Status

EVIDENCE BASE American College of Obstetricians and Gynecologists. (2008/Reaffirmed 2016). *Use of psychiatric medications during pregnancy and lactation* (Practice Bulletin #92). Washington, DC: Author.
   Bigelow, A., Power, M., MacLellan-Peters, J., et al. (2012). Effect of mother/infant skin-to-skin contact on postpartum depressive symptoms and maternal physiological stress. *Journal of Obstetric, Gynecologic, & Neonatal Nursing, 41*(3), 369–382.

1. Reva Rubin, the noted nursing theorist, developed the developmental tasks of pregnancy documenting maternal changes and role attainment. After delivery, the woman may progress through Rubin's stages of taking in, taking hold, and letting go.
   a. Taking in (extends over first 24 hours postpartum):
      i. May begin with a refreshing sleep after delivery. Restorative sleep should occur within first 24 hours postdelivery.
      ii. Woman exhibits passive, dependent behavior.
      iii. Woman is concerned with sleep and the intake of food, mainly for herself.
   b. Taking hold (if not in the first 24 hours postpartum, then between days 2 and 4 postpartum):
      i. Woman begins to initiate action and to function more independently. The first sign mother is in this phase is alert interest in her infant.
      ii. Woman may require more explanation and reassurance that she is functioning well, especially in caring for her infant.
      iii. Openness to teaching on care of self and neonate.
      iv. Today, with early hospital discharge, this phase may occur earlier, or it may occur after discharge.
   c. Letting go:
      i. May begin near the end of the first week; no specific end time noted.
      ii. Is influenced by cultural beliefs.
      iii. Reestablishment of couple relationship.
      iv. As the woman meets success in caring for the neonate, her concern extends to other family members and to their activities.
2. Some women may experience euphoria in the first few days after delivery and set unrealistic goals for activities after discharge.
3. Many women may experience temporary mood swings during this period because of the discomfort, fatigue, and exhaustion following labor and delivery and because of hormonal changes after delivery.
4. Up to 60% to 80% of women may experience a transient period of depression termed postpartum blues. They can last for a few days to 1 to 2 weeks and usually peak at approximately the 5th postpartum day. Women may exhibit irritability, poor appetite, insomnia, tearfulness, or crying. This is a normal reaction to the physiologic shifts that occur postdelivery and temporary.
5. Postpartum depression is a more serious problem affecting as many as 20% of postpartum women. Cultural and ethnic influences may impact the postpartum period; therefore, cultural awareness of pregnancy practices is important to consider when working with postpartum women. A prenatal diagnosis of depression is considered a significant risk factor for PPD. Women may experience an increase in the manifestations listed above as well inability to adequately care for themselves and the baby. These women are at increased risk of suicide and in need of further evaluation (see Chapter 39 Postpartum Depression).
6. Nursing research findings indicate that new mothers commonly identify postpartum needs such as coping with:
   a. The physical changes and discomforts of the puerperium, including a need to regain their prepregnancy figure.
   b. Changing family relationships and meeting the needs of family members, including the infant.
   c. Fatigue, emotional stress, feelings of isolation, and being tied down.
   d. A lack of time for personal needs and interests.

Nursing Assessment

 EVIDENCE BASE Lowdermilk, D., Perry, S., Cashion, C., & Alden, K. R. (2016). *Maternity and women's health care* (11th ed.). St. Louis, MO: Mosby.

Immediate Postpartum Assessment

The first hour after delivery of the placenta (fourth stage of labor) is a critical period; postpartum hemorrhage is most likely to occur at this time (see page 1073).

Subsequent Postpartum Assessment

1. Check the fundus at regular intervals for tone and location. Perform fundal massage if the uterus is boggy (not firm) (see Figure 38-3).
2. Teach patient self-fundal massage and warning signs to report
   a. Inspect the perineum regularly for bleeding. Note color, amount, clots, and odor of the lochia.
3. Count and/or weigh the number of perineal pads that are saturated as necessary. Assess mother's ability to perform self-care. Provide support and education as needed.
4. Assess vital signs at least twice daily and more frequently, if indicated.
5. Assess bowel and bladder elimination.

Figure 38-3. Fundal massage. With hands correctly positioned, gentle fundal massage stimulates the uterine muscles to contract, helping to restore normal tone and control bleeding. (Reeder, S., Martin, L., & Koniak-Griffin, D. [1997]. *Maternity nursing: Family newborn, and women's health care* [18th ed.]. Philadelphia, PA: Lippincott-Raven Publishers.)

6. Evaluate interaction and the new family's ability to provide care to the newborn. Provide support and education as needed.
7. Assess breasts for colostrum, milk production, engorgement, and condition of the nipples if breast-feeding.
8. Assess Homans sign for possible thrombophlebitis.
9. Assess incisions for signs of infection and healing.
10. Assess the perineum using the REEDA acronym. REEDA is based on a 3-point scale. A score of 3 indicates an assessment of very poor wound healing. On the first postpartum day, the REEDA score may range from 0 to 3; by the second postpartum week, the score should be 0 to 1.
    a. **R**—Redness.
    b. **E**—Edema.
    c. **E**—Ecchymosis (purplish patch of blood flow).
    d. **D**—Discharge.
    e. **A**—Approximation or the closeness of the skin edges.
11. If the patient is Rh negative, evaluate her need for Rho(D) immune globulin (RhoGAM). If the newborn is Rh positive, administer the RhoGAM within 72 hours of delivery.
12. If the woman is rubella and/or varicella nonimmune, these vaccinations may be administered at discharge. During the flu season, the influenza vaccine should also be offered if the mother has not been previously immunized during the pregnancy. Note: If the rubella vaccine is administered at discharge, educate the mother to avoid pregnancy for at least 3 months to minimize fetal risks of congenital defects.

Nursing Management

 EVIDENCE BASE Mattson, S., & Smith, J. E. (Eds.). (2016). *Core curriculum for maternal-newborn nursing* (5th ed.). St. Louis, MO: Saunders Elsevier.

Nursing Diagnoses

- Risk for Deficient Fluid Volume related to blood loss and effects from anesthesia.
- Impaired Urinary Elimination related to birth trauma.
- Constipation related to physiologic changes from birth.
- Risk for Infection related to birth process.
- Fatigue related to labor.
- Acute Pain related to perineal discomfort from birth trauma, hemorrhoids, and physiologic changes from birth.
- Readiness for enhanced self-health management pertaining to postpartum care.
- Breast-feeding: Ineffective related to lack of knowledge and inexperience.

Nursing Interventions

Monitoring for Obstetrical Hemorrhage

1. Monitor vital signs every 4 hours during the first 24 hours and then every 8 to 12 hours or as delineated by facility policy. Observe for the following:
   a. Increased respiratory rate greater than 24 breaths/minute may be caused by increased blood loss, pulmonary edema, or a pulmonary embolus.
   b. Increased pulse rate greater than 100 beats/minute (bpm) may in response to increased blood loss, fever, or pain.
   c. Decrease in blood pressure (BP) 15 to 20 mm Hg below baseline pressures may indicate decreased fluid volume or increased blood loss.
2. Assess the woman for light-headedness and dizziness when sitting upright or before walking.
   a. Assist patient out of bed until stable.
   b. Emphasize to the patient the need for assistance out of bed.
   c. Encourage patient to sit at the bedside prior to ambulating.
3. Evaluate lower extremity sensory function and motor function before ambulation if the woman had regional anesthesia.
   a. Assess regional anesthesia site (epidural/spinal) if applicable.
   b. Evaluate orthostatic BP if symptoms persist.
   c. Have the woman maintain bed rest if symptoms persist.
4. Assess lochia for amount and presence of clots.
5. Maintain IV access and infusion, as ordered.
6. Monitor postpartum hemoglobin levels and hematocrit if ordered.
7. Encourage oral fluids, as tolerated.

Promoting Urinary Elimination

1. Assess for voiding within 6 to 8 hours after delivery.
2. Palpate the abdomen for bladder distention if the woman cannot void or if she complains of fullness after voiding.
   a. Uterine displacement from the midline suggests bladder distention.
   b. Frequent voiding of small amounts of urine suggests urine retention with overflow.
   c. Bladder distention may lead to uterine atony.
3. Utilize a bladder scanner if available to document urine volume.
4. Catheterize the woman with a straight catheter if indicated.
5. Instruct the woman to void every several hours and after meals to keep her bladder empty.

Promoting Bowel Function

1. Teach the woman that bowel activity is sluggish because of decreased abdominal muscle tone, anesthetic effects, effects of progesterone, decreased solid food intake during labor, and opioid use.
2. Inform the woman that pain from hemorrhoids, lacerations, and episiotomies may cause her to delay her first bowel movement.
3. Review the woman's dietary intake with her, and encourage adequate intake of fiber through fresh fruit, vegetables, and at least eight glasses of water daily.
4. Encourage frequent ambulation.
5. Administer stool softeners, as indicated.

Preventing Infection

1. Encourage patient to change peri-pads frequently and use cleansing bottle with warm water.
2. Observe for elevated temperature above 100.4°F (38°C) exclusive of the first 24 hours.
3. Evaluate episiotomy/perineum for REEDA.
4. Assess for pain, burning, and frequency on urination.
5. Assess epidural/spinal site.
6. Administer antibiotics as directed.

Reducing Fatigue

1. Provide a quiet and minimally disturbed environment.
2. Organize nursing care to keep interruptions to a minimum.
3. Encourage the woman to minimize visitors and phone use.
4. Encourage the woman to sleep while the baby is sleeping and specifically to lie down at least 30 minutes/day.

Adequate Pain Management

1. Instruct the woman to apply ice packs to her perineal area for the first 24 hours for perineal trauma or edema and then to apply heat to the area.
   a. Commercial or handmade packs may be used.
   b. Ensure a barrier between the skin and ice.
2. Initiate the use of a warm water sitz baths for 15 to 20 minutes for perineal discomfort after the first 24 hours as needed.
3. Instruct the woman to contract her buttocks before sitting to reduce perineal discomfort.
4. Assist the woman in the use of positioning cushions and pillows while sitting or lying.
5. Encourage frequent perineal cleansing.
6. Provide witch hazel pads or topical creams or ointments for hemorrhoids, as indicated.
7. Administer analgesics as indicated.
   a. Assess for decreased respiratory rate below 12 breaths/minute after receiving opioid analgesics.
8. Assess breasts for signs of engorgement (swollen, tender, tense, shiny breast tissue).
   a. Engorgement in breast-feeding mothers:
      i. Nurse infant on both breasts to ensure adequate emptying of breasts.
      ii. Apply cold packs to breasts after feeding.
      iii. Encourage a warm-to-hot shower water to flow over the breasts to improve comfort, or warm compresses on the breasts may improve comfort.
      iv. Express some milk manually or by breast pump to improve comfort and to make the nipple more available for infant feeding.
      v. OTC analgesics may be used to enhance comfort.
   b. Engorgement in non–breast-feeding mothers:
      i. Instruct the mother to wear a snug and supportive bra at all times and avoid handing her breasts.
      ii. Teach the mother to avoid any stimulation to her breasts including the avoidance of letting warm water fall on her breasts during showers because the heat stimulates milk production.
      iii. Suggest the application of ice or cabbage leaves to the breasts to provide comfort.
      iv. OTC analgesics may be needed to provide comfort.

Promoting Postpartum Health Maintenance

1. **Perineal care:**
   a. Teach the woman to perform perineal care using warm water over the perineum after each voiding and/or bowel movement to promote comfort, cleanliness, and healing.
   b. Promote sitz baths for the same purpose.
   c. Teach the woman to apply perineal pads by touching the outside only keeping the side that will touch her perineum clean.
2. **Breasts:**
   a. Assess the condition of the woman's breasts and nipples inspecting nipples for intactness, reddening, ecchymosis, fissures, and pain.
   b. Encourage the mother to ensure an adequate latch and utilize different breast-feeding positions to decrease the risk of sore nipples.
   c. Advise that reddened areas may be improved by expressing colostrum and air-drying nipples.
   d. Commercially prepared lanolin-based creams and ointments may also enhance comfort.
   e. Instruct mother to read labels carefully to determine if ointment needs to be removed before breast-feeding her infant.
   f. Teach the woman to wash her breasts using warm water *without* soap to maintain the protective skin oils and avoid dryness.
   g. Encourage wearing a support bra without underwires for comfort.
3. **Nutrition:**
   a. Instruct mother to eat foods from all food groups with three to four servings of protein, four to six servings of dairy, and four servings each of fruits, grains, and vegetables. Occasional use of caffeine is allowable.
   b. Encourage the woman to continue her prenatal vitamins until her 6-week follow-up appointment.
   c. Increase fluid intake to keep urine pale in color.
   d. Breast-feeding mothers should add 300 to 500 additional calories daily for milk production.
4. **Activity:**
   a. Anatomical and physiologic changes during pregnancy are necessary to consider before beginning an exercise program. Women with uncomplicated pregnancies may resume activity as tolerated to maintain a healthy lifestyle. Women with medical and surgical complications should consult with their provider before doing beginning any exercise program.
   b. Common exercises for all postpartum women may include Kegel exercises, short walks that gradually increase in duration, stationary cycling low-impact aerobics, and modified yoga.

Promoting Breast-Feeding

1. Assist the woman and infant in the breast-feeding process.
   a. Have the mother wash her hands before feeding to help prevent infection.
   b. Encourage the mother to assume a comfortable position, such as sitting upright in the bed or in a chair or side lying.
   c. Have the woman hold the baby so that they are facing each other. Common positions for holding the baby are the cradle hold, with the baby's head and body supported against the mother's arm, with buttocks resting in her hand; the football hold, in which the baby's body and legs are supported under the mother's arm and the head is at the breast, resting in the mother's hand; and side lying with mother and baby facing each other.
   d. Teach the woman to hold the baby close for control and to prevent back, shoulder, and arm strain.
   e. Have the woman cup the breast in her hand in a C-position, with bottom of the breast in the palm of her hand and the thumb on top, or the U position, with the fingers and the thumb to the sides of the breast and the breast resting in the palm of the hand.
   f. Have the woman place her nipple against the side of the baby's mouth, and when the mouth opens, guide the nipple and the areola into the mouth. The baby should latch on so that as much of the areola as possible is in his or her mouth. If the baby has latched on to the nipple only, break the latch by putting the tip of the mother's finger in the corner of the baby's mouth to break the suction, and then reposition on the breast to prevent nipple pain and trauma.

g. Encourage the woman to alternate the breast with which she begins feeding at each feeding to ensure emptying of both breasts and stimulation for maintaining milk supply.

h. Advise the mother to use each breast at each feeding. Begin with at least 10 minutes at each breast and then increase the time at each breast, allowing the infant to suck until he or she stops sucking actively.

i. Have the mother breast-feed frequently (8 to 12 times/24 hours) to maintain the milk supply. Although there is no time limit on each breast-feeding session, it is recommended to last at least 10 to 15 minutes on each breast.

j. Have the mother express colostrum/milk and apply to nipples; then, air-dry for approximately 15 to 20 minutes after feeding to help prevent nipple trauma.

2. Encourage burping between breasts and at the end of the feeding. Alert the mother that uterine cramping (afterpains) may occur, because of the release of oxytocin needed for milk ejection during feeding. Multiparous women may experience increased discomfort related to decreased uterine tone.

3. Teach the mother to provide for adequate rest periods and nutrition. She should also avoid stress, which can inhibit the let-down reflex and make breast milk less available at feeding.

4. Advise the woman to consult her provider prior to taking any OTC and prescription medications as many substances pass into the breast milk and may also affect milk production or the infant.

Evaluation: Expected Outcomes

- Vital signs within normal limits; decreasing color and amount of lochia.
- Voids freely and without discomfort.
- Lack of constipation; eats high-fiber foods and uses stool softeners.
- Afebrile, no abnormal redness of the perineum, no purulent discharge or foul odor of lochia.
- Verbalizes feeling rested.
- Verbalizes decreased pain.
- Incorporates postpartum care into activities of daily living.
- Demonstrates successful breast-feeding; breasts and nipples intact and without redness or cracks.

Postpartum Patient Education

1. Advise the woman that healing occurs within 2 to 4 weeks; however, evaluation by the health care provider during the follow-up visit is necessary.

2. Inform the woman that intercourse may be resumed when perineal and uterine wounds have healed and when vaginal bleeding has stopped. Inform the woman that normal vaginal secretions may not occur for up to 6 months and use of vaginal lubricants may be helpful. Also, inform the mother that for the first 3 months following delivery, her sexual arousal and desire may be diminished due to infant needs and fatigue. Review methods of contraception. Sexual arousal may cause milk to leak from her breasts; encourage breast-feeding her infant prior to sexual activity. Breast-feeding is not a reliable method of contraception.

3. Inform the woman that menstruation usually returns within 4 to 8 weeks if bottle-feeding; if breast-feeding, menstruation usually returns within 4 months, but may return between 2 and 18 months postpartum. Nursing mothers may ovulate even if they are experiencing amenorrhea. Thus, a form of contraception should be used if pregnancy is to be avoided.

4. Encourage mother to sleep when the baby sleeps and rest when possible. Encourage resuming activities as tolerated and medically indicated (see Activity section). Driving restrictions may be indicated.

5. Counsel the woman to provide quiet times for herself at home and to help her establish realistic goals for resuming her own interests and activities.

6. Encourage the couple to provide times to reestablish their own relationship and to renew their social interests and relationships apart from the infant.

7. Encourage the couple to discuss child care arrangements and return to work plans if appropriate.

NURSING CARE OF THE NEONATE

 EVIDENCE BASE American Academy of Pediatrics & American College of Obstetricians and Gynecologists. (2012). *Guidelines for perinatal care* (7th ed.). Washington, DC: Author.

Lowdermilk, D., Perry, S., Cashion, C., & Alden, K. R. (2016). *Maternity and women's health care* (11th ed.). St. Louis, MO: Mosby.

Verklan, M. T., & Walden, M. (Eds.). (2015). *Core curriculum for neonatal intensive care nursing* (5th ed.). St. Louis, MO: Saunders Elsevier.

Physiology of the Neonate

The first 24 hours of life constitutes a highly vulnerable time where the infant must make major physiologic adjustments to extrauterine life. Most neonates transition without difficulty within the first 6 to 10 hours of life.

Transitional Stages

During the period of postnatal transition, six overlapping stages have been identified:

- Stage 1. Receives stimulation (during labor) from the pressure of the uterine contractions and from changes in pressure when the membranes rupture.
- Stage 2. Encounters various foreign stimuli—light, cold, gravity, and sound.
- Stage 3. Initiates breathing.
- Stage 4. Changes from fetal circulation to neonatal circulation.
- Stage 5. Undergoes alteration in metabolic processes, with activation of the liver and GI tract for passage of meconium.
- Stage 6. Achieves a steady level of equilibrium in metabolic processes (production of enzymes, increased blood oxygen saturation, decrease in acidosis associated with birth, and recovery of the neurologic tissues from the trauma of labor and delivery).

Respiratory Changes

Factors Initiating Respiration

1. Mechanical—pressure changes (eg, compression of the fetal chest with delivery) from intrauterine life to extrauterine life produce stimulation to initiate respirations.

2. Chemical—changes in the blood, as a result of transitory asphyxia, include:

   a. Cessation of placental blood flow.

   b. Lowered oxygen level.

c. Increased carbon dioxide level.

d. Lowered pH—if asphyxia is prolonged, depression of the respiratory center (rather than stimulation) occurs and resuscitation is necessary.

3. Sensory—light (visual), sound (auditory), olfactory, and tactile stimulation, beginning in utero with uterine contraction and when the infant is touched and dried, contribute to the initiation of respiration by stimulating the neonate's respiratory center in the brain.

4. Thermal—a drop in environmental temperature produced by sudden chilling of the moist infant stimulates the respiratory center in the brain.

5. First breath—maximum effort is required to expand the lungs and to fill the collapsed alveoli.

   a. Surface tension in the respiratory tract and resistance in lung tissue, thorax, diaphragm, and respiratory muscles must be overcome.

   b. First active inspiration comes from a strong contraction of the diaphragm, which creates a high negative intrathoracic pressure, causing a marked retraction of the ribs and distention of the alveolar space. (Any remaining fluid is reabsorbed rapidly if the pulmonary capillary blood flow is adequate because the fluid is hypotonic and passes easily into the capillaries.)

6. Contributing factors, such as pulmonary blood flow, surfactant production, and respiratory musculature, also increase the respiratory effort of the neonate.

Character of Normal Respirations

1. First period of reactivity occurs immediately after birth. Vigorous, diffuse, purposeless movements alternate with periods of relative immobility/inactivity.

2. Respirations are rapid, as frequent as 80 breaths/minute, accompanied by tachycardia, 160 to 180 breaths/minute.

3. Relaxation occurs and the infant usually sleeps; he or she then awakes to a second period of activity. Oral mucus may be a major problem during this period.

4. Respirations are reduced to 30 to 60 breaths/minute and become quiet and shallow; respiration is carried out by the diaphragm and abdominal muscles.

5. Period of dyspnea and cyanosis may occur suddenly in an infant who is breathing normally; this may indicate an anomaly or a pathologic condition.

6. Pauses in respirations of less than 20 seconds are normal in the neonatal period.

Circulatory Changes

1. Cord clamping causes increased systemic vascular resistance (SVR), an increase in blood pressure, and increased pressures in the left side of the heart.

2. Functional closure of the ductus venosus shunt and anatomic closure the first week of life (see page 984).

3. With the neonate's first breath, the foramen ovale shunt functionally closes. Permanent closure occurs by 3 months of age.

4. Increased SVR, falling pulmonary vascular resistance (PVR), and increased sensitivity to rising arterial oxygen concentrations in the blood = closure of ductus arteriosus shunt. The shunt is completely closed in all infants by 96 hours of age with permanent closure within 3 weeks to 3 months of age.

5. Blood volume can be as high as 300 mL/kg immediately after birth and then decrease to 80 to 85 mL/kg shortly after birth. Factors that influence blood volume:

   a. Maternal blood volume (affected by maternal diseases and iron intake).

   b. Placental function.

   c. Uterine contractions during labor.

   d. Amount of blood loss associated with delivery.

   e. Placental transfusion at birth with delayed cord clamping—increase in blood volume of 60% if cord is clamped and cut after pulsation ceases.

6. Acrocyanosis (cyanosis in hands and feet) is a normal finding related to sluggish peripheral circulation in the first 24 hours after birth.

7. Normal apical pulse rate 110 to 160 bpm; may rise to 180 bpm when the infant is crying or drop to 80 to 110 bpm during deep sleep.

8. Blood pressure in the term newborn ranges from 60 to 80 mm Hg systolic and 30 to 60 mm Hg diastolic at birth and varies with gestational age, weight, activity, and appropriate cuff size (slightly higher in legs).

   a. A systolic BP in the upper extremities that is 20 mm Hg greater than in the lower extremities strongly suggests coarctation of the aorta.

   b. BP measurement is best accomplished with an automated noninvasive blood pressure (NIBP) device while the infant is at rest.

9. Coagulability is temporarily diminished due to a vitamin K deficiency because a sterile gastrointestinal tract. Vitamin K synthesis begins after 5 hours of bacterial colonization in the intestinal tract.

   a. Coagulation time is 5 to 8 minutes (in a glass tubes), 5 to 15 minutes (room temperature), or 30 minutes (silicone tube).

   b. Bleeding time is 2 to 4 minutes.

   c. Prothrombin 50%, decreasing to 20% to 30% (approximately 13 to 18 seconds).

10. Values for blood components in the neonate:

    a. Hemoglobin, 14.5 to 22 g/dL.

    b. Hematocrit, 14% to 72%.

    c. Reticulocytes, 4% to 6%.

    d. Leukocytes, 9,000 to 34,000/mm³.

Temperature Regulation

1. Temperature instability in the term newborn can be the result of anatomical and physiological factors such as a thin subcutaneous adipose tissue, blood vessels closer to the skin, and larger body surface to body weight ratio.

2. Heat loss in term newborns may occur at birth by radiation, convection, evaporation, and conduction.

   a. Radiation—transfer of heat from neonate to cooler object not in direct contact with the infant.

   b. Convection—transfer of heat when flow of cool air passes over infant's skin.

   c. Evaporation—loss of heat when water on infant's skin is converted to vapor.

   d. Conduction—transfer of heat when neonate comes into direct contact with cooler surface/object.

3. Infants respond readily to environmental heat and cold stimuli and develop mechanisms to counterbalance heat loss.

   a. Vasoconstriction—blood directed away from skin surfaces.

   b. Insulation—from subcutaneous adipose tissue.

   c. Heat production—by nonshivering thermogenesis (brown fat metabolism) elicited by the sympathetic nervous system's response to decreased temperatures; activated by adrenaline.

   d. Fetal position—by assuming a flexed position.

Basal Metabolism

1. Surface area of infant, especially the head, is large in comparison to weight.
2. Basal metabolism per kilogram of body weight is higher than that of an adult.
3. Calorie requirements are high—110 to 130 calories/kg of body weight per day.

Renal Function

Neonatal kidneys have functional deficiency in concentrating urine and coping with fluid and electrolyte fluctuations. Low arterial BP and increased renal vascular resistance lead to the following effects:

1. Decreased ability to concentrate urine because of low tubular resorption rate and low levels of antidiuretic hormone.
2. Limited ability to maintain water balance by excretion of excess water or retention of needed water.
3. Decreased ability to maintain acid–base mechanism; slower excretion of electrolytes, especially sodium and hydrogen ions, results in accumulation of these substances, which predisposes the infant to dehydration, acidosis, and hyperkalemia.
4. Excretion of large amount of uric acid during neonatal period—appears as brick dust stain on diaper.

Hepatic Function

Function limited because of lack of GI tract activity, deficiency in forming plasma proteins, and limited blood supply; consequences include the following:

1. Decreased ability to conjugate bilirubin (rationale for physiologic jaundice).
2. Decreased ability to regulate blood glucose concentration (less glycogen stores) (rationale for neonatal hypoglycemia).
3. Deficient production of prothrombin and other coagulation factors that depend on vitamin K for synthesis (rationale for neonate's predisposition to hemorrhage).

Endocrine Function

Endocrine glands are better organized than other systems: disturbances are most commonly related to maternally provided hormones. This can cause the following:

1. Vaginal discharge (or bleeding [pseudomenstruation]) in female infants.
2. Enlargement of mammary glands (breast engorgement) in both sexes—related to increased estrogen, luteal, and prolactin activity. Milky secretions may be present (witch's milk).
3. Disturbances related to maternal endocrine pathology (eg, mother with diabetes or mother with inadequate iodine intake).

GI Changes

The neonate's intestinal tract is proportionately longer than the adult's; however, elastic tissue and musculature are not fully developed and neurologic control is variable and inadequate.

1. Most digestive enzymes are present, with the exception of pancreatic amylase and lipase. Protein and carbohydrates are easily absorbed, but fat absorption is poor.
2. Limitations relate primarily to anatomic structures and neutrality of the gastric contents.
3. Limited production of pancreatic amylase leads to inadequate utilization of complex carbohydrates.
4. Immaturity of the cardiac and pharyngoesophageal sphincters and neurological control causes mild regurgitation or slight vomiting.
5. Irregularities in peristaltic motility slow stomach emptying.
6. Peristalsis increases in the lower ileum, resulting in stool frequency—one to six stools per day. No stools within 48 hours after birth may be indicative of intestinal obstruction such as imperforate anus.

Neurologic Changes

Neurologic mechanisms are immature; they are not fully developed anatomically or physiologically. As a result, uncoordinated movements, labile temperature regulation, and poor control over musculature are characteristic of the infant. Reflexes are important indicators of infant neural development (see page 1027).

Nursing Assessment

Delivery of effective neonatal care is enhanced by effective communication of information about the mother and her infant with the interprofessional team.

Pertinent Maternal History

1. Mother's age, socioeconomic status, ethnic or cultural group, educational level, and marital status.
2. Mother's/family's past medical history.
3. Mother's past obstetric history.
4. Mother's prenatal history with current pregnancy includes rubella status, hepatitis B testing, mental health history, domestic violence, or history of previous child abuse or neglect and also includes other maternal test results relevant to neonatal care (ie, human immunodeficiency virus test results and colonization with group B hemolytic streptococci, STIs).
5. Labor and delivery (includes intrapartum maternal antibiotic therapy, along with type and dosage of antibiotics).

Physical Assessment Findings and Physiologic Functioning

Posture

1. Full-term neonate assumes symmetric posture; face turns to side with full mobility; flexed extremities; hands tightly fisted with thumb covered by fingers.
2. Asymmetric posture may be caused by fractures of the clavicle and humerus or nerve injuries (commonly of the brachial plexus).
3. Infants born in the breech position may keep knees and legs straightened or in frog position, depending on the type of breech birth.

Length

Newborn (full-term) length ranges from 18 to 22 inches (46 to 56 cm) with an average of 20 inches (51 cm).

Weight

The weight of a full-term infant ranges from 2,500 to 4,000 g (5 pounds 8 ounces to 8 pounds 13 ounces).

Skin

Infants should be examined under natural light and observed for the following:

1. Hair distribution—term infant will have some lanugo over back; most of the lanugo will have disappeared on extremities and other areas of the body.
2. Turgor—term infant should have good skin turgor (ie, after gently pinching small portion of the skin and releasing it, the skin should return to its original position).
3. Color.
   a. Peripheral cyanosis (acrocyanosis) is bluish discoloration of the hands and feet related to vasoconstriction and sluggish peripheral circulation. It is a normal finding and may be exacerbated by cold temperatures.
   b. Central cyanosis is an indication of reduced arterial oxygen saturation. Persistent central cyanosis requires immediate intervention.
   c. Pallor—may indicate cold, stress, anemia, or cardiac failure.
   d. Plethora—reddish (ruddy) coloration may be caused by a high level of RBCs to total blood volume from intrauterine intravascular transfusion (twins), cardiac disease, or diabetes in the mother.
   e. Jaundice—physiologic jaundice caused by immaturity of the liver is common beginning on day 2, peaking at 1 week, and disappearing by the 2nd week. It first appears in the skin over the face or upper body and then progresses over a larger area; it can also be seen in conjunctivae of the eyes.
   f. Meconium staining of the skin, fingernails, and umbilical cord indicates passage of meconium in utero (possibly caused by fetal hypoxia in utero).
4. Dryness/peeling—marked scaling and desquamation are signs of postmaturity.
5. Vernix—in full-term infants, it may be found in skin folds under the arms and in the groin under the scrotum (in males) and in the labia (in females). Increased amounts of vernix may indicate prematurity.
6. Nails—should reach end of fingertips and be well developed in the full-term infant. There should be no evidence of pits, ridges, aplasia, or hypertrophy.
7. Edema—some edema may occur over buttocks, back, and occiput if the infant has been supine; pitting edema may be caused by erythroblastosis, heart failure, and electrolyte imbalance.
8. Ecchymosis—may appear over the presenting part in a precipitous or prolonged delivery; may also indicate infection or a bleeding problem.
9. Petechiae—pinpoint hemorrhages on the skin caused by increased intravascular pressure, infection, or thrombocytopenia; usually resolves within 48 hours.
10. Erythema toxicum (newborn rash)—small white, yellow, or pink to red papular rash that appears on the trunk, face, and extremities.
11. Hemangiomas—vascular lesions present at birth; some may fade, but others may be permanent.
    a. Strawberry (nevus vasculosus)—bright red, raised, lobulated tumor that occurs on the head, neck, trunk, or extremities; soft, palpable, with sharp demarcated margins; increases in size for approximately 6 months and then regresses after several years.
    b. Cavernous—larger, more mature vascular elements; involves dermis and subcutaneous tissues; soft, palpable, with poorly defined margins; increases in size the first 6 to 12 months and then involutes spontaneously.
12. Telangiectatic nevi (stork bites)—flat red or purple lesions most commonly found on the back of the neck, lower occiput, upper eyelid, and bridge of the nose; regress by age 2, although the ones on the neck may persist through adulthood.
13. Milia—enlarged sebaceous glands found on the nose, chin, cheeks, brow, and forehead; regress in several days to a few weeks. They appear as multiple yellow or pearly white papules, approximately 1 mm in diameter. When found in the mouth, they are referred to as Epstein pearls.
14. Mongolian spots—blue-green or gray pigmentation on the lower back, sacrum, and buttocks; common in Blacks (90%), Asians, and infants of southern European heritage; regress by age 4. May be mistaken for signs of child abuse.
15. Café au lait spots—tan or light brown macules or patches. When less than 1¼ inches (3 cm) in length and less than 6 in number, there is no pathologic significance; if greater than 1¼ inches or more than 6 in number, it may indicate cutaneous neurofibromatosis.
16. Harlequin color change—when on side, dependent half turns red and upper half pale; caused by gravity and vasomotor instability.
17. Abrasions or lacerations can result from internal monitoring and instruments used at birth.
18. Cutis marmorata—bluish mottling or marbling of the skin in response to chilling, stress, or overstimulation.
19. Port-wine nevus (nevus flammeus)—flat pink or reddish-purple lesion consisting of dilated, congested capillaries directly beneath the epidermis; does not blanch.

Head

1. Examine the head and face for symmetry, paralysis, shape, swelling, movement.
   a. Caput succedaneum—swelling of soft tissues of the scalp because of pressure; swelling crosses suture lines. May be associated with vacuum-assisted birth or prolonged second stage of labor (pushing).
   b. Cephalohematoma—subperiosteal hemorrhage with collection of blood between the periosteum and bone; swelling does not cross suture lines. May result from vacuum-assisted birth or prolonged second stage of labor.
   c. Molding—overlapping of skull bones, caused by compression during labor and delivery (disappears in a few days).
   d. Examine symmetry of facial movements.
   e. Forceps marks—U-shaped bruising usually on the cheeks following forceps delivery.
2. Measure head circumference—13 to 14 inches (33 to 35.5 cm), approximately ¾ inch (2 cm) larger than the chest. Measure just above the eyebrows and over the occiput.
3. Fontanelles—area where more than two skull bones meet; covered with strong band of connective tissue; also called the soft spot.
   a. Enlarged or bulging—may indicate increased intracranial pressure (ICP).
   b. Sunken—commonly indicates dehydration.
   c. Size—posterior may be obliterated because of molding; generally closes in 2 to 3 months. Anterior is palpable; generally closes in 12 to 18 months.
4. Sutures—junctions of adjoining skull bones.
   a. Overriding—caused by molding during labor and delivery.
   b. Separation—extensive separation may be found in malnourished infants and with increased ICP.

Face

1. Eyes—examine the following:
    a. Color—the sclera in most full-term infants is white; subconjunctival hemorrhages are common from the birth process; blue sclera is indicative of osteogenesis imperfecta. Eye color is usually slate gray, brown, or dark blue; final eye color is evident by 6 to 12 months.
    b. Hemorrhagic areas—subconjunctival hemorrhages may appear as a red band from pressure during delivery; regress within 2 weeks.
    c. Edema—edema of the eyelids may be caused by pressure on the head and face during labor and delivery.
    d. Conjunctivitis or discharge—may be caused by instillation eye prophylaxis or infections from organisms, such as staphylococcus, chlamydia trachomatis, or gonococcus. Tear formation does not usually begin until age 2 to 3 months.
    e. Jaundice—may be seen in the sclera because of physiologic or pathological jaundice.
    f. Pupils—equal in size and should constrict equally in bright light.
    g. Infant can see and discriminate patterns; limited by imperfect oculomotor coordination and inability to accommodate for varying distances.
    h. Red reflex—red-orange color seen when light from an ophthalmoscope is reflected from the retina. No red reflex indicates cataracts.
    i. Brushfield spots—white or yellow pinpoint areas on the iris that may indicate trisomy 21 or even a normal variant.
    j. Abnormal placement of eyes or small eye openings can signify a syndrome or chromosomal anomaly.
    k. Strabismus—cross-eyed appearance that is common; nystagmus (constant, rapid, involuntary movement of the eye) is also common and disappears by age 4 months.
2. Nose—examine the following:
    a. Patency—necessary because infants are obligate nose breathers.
    b. Nasal flaring—abnormal and may indicate respiratory distress. Check for appropriate size and shape of the nose; should be placed vertically midline in the face.
    c. Discharge—stuffiness is normal unless chronic nasal discharge is present; may be caused by possible infection.
    d. Sense of smell—infants will turn toward familiar odors and away from noxious odors.
    e. Septum should be midline; low nasal bridge with broad base may be associated with Down syndrome.
    f. Periodic sneezing is common to clear nasal passages. Excessive sneezing may be an indication of neonatal abstinence syndrome.
3. Ears—Formation: large, flabby ears that slant forward may indicate abnormalities of the kidney or other parts of the urinary tract.
    a. Position in relation to the eye—helix (top of the ear) on the same plane as the eye; low-set ears may indicate chromosomal or renal abnormalities.
    b. Cartilage—full-term infant has sufficient cartilage to make the ear feel firm.
    c. Hearing—auditory canals may be congested for a day or 2 after birth; the infant should hear well in a few days. Hearing screening may be performed prior to discharge.
    d. Observe for skin tags; preauricular sinus located in front of the ear may be normal or may be associated with genetic disorders.
4. Mouth—examine the following:
    a. Size—small mouth found in trisomy 18 and 21; corners of the mouth turn down (fish mouth) in fetal alcohol syndrome. Mucous membranes should be pink.
    b. Palate—examine hard and soft palate for closure.
    c. Size of the tongue in relation to the mouth—normally does not extend much past the margin of gums. Excessively large tongue seen in congenital anomalies, such as cretinism and trisomy 21.
    d. Teeth—predeciduous teeth are found on rare occasions; if they interfere with feeding or pose an aspiration risk, they may be removed.
    e. Epstein pearls—small white nodules found on sides of hard palate (commonly mistaken for teeth); regress in a few weeks.
    f. Ankyloglossia—thin or thick ridge of tissue running from base of the tongue along undersurface to the tip of the tongue. Most require no intervention, but depending on the extent of ankyloglossia, breast-feeding and speech may be impacted and require further evaluation.
    g. Sucking blisters (labial tuberales)—thickened areas on midline of the upper lip that may be filled with fluid or callous; no treatment necessary.
    h. Infections—thrush, caused by *Candida albicans*, may appear as white patches on the tongue and/or insides of cheeks that do not wash away with fluids; treated with nystatin suspension.

Neck

1. Mobility—can the infant move the head from side to side; palpate for lymph nodes; palpate the clavicle for fractures, especially after a difficult delivery.
2. Torticollis—observe for spasmodic, one-sided contraction of neck muscles; generally from a shortened sternocleidomastoid muscle; physical therapy may be indicated.
3. Excessive skin folds may be associated with congenital abnormalities such as trisomy 21.
4. Stiffness and hyperextension may be caused by trauma or infection.
5. Clavicle—assess for intactness, fractures, and masses such as cystic hygroma, soft and usually seen laterally or over the clavicle.

Chest

1. Circumference and symmetry—average circumference is 12 to 13 inches (30.5 to 33 cm), approximately ¾ inch (2 cm) smaller than head circumference.
2. Breast.
    a. Engorgement—may occur at day 3 because of maternal hormones, especially estrogen; no treatment required. Regresses in 2 weeks.
    b. Nipples and areolae—less formed and pronounced in preterm infants.

Respiratory System

1. Rate—normally between 30 and 60 breaths/minute; influenced by sleep–wake status, hunger, medication, and temperature.
2. Rhythm—respirations may be shallow with irregular rhythm.
    a. Respiratory movements are symmetric and mainly diaphragmatic because of weak thoracic muscles. For example, the lower thorax pulls in and the abdomen bulges with each respiration.
    b. Periodic breathing—resumption of respiration after 5- to 15-second period without respiration; decreases with time;

more common in preterm infants. Substernal retractions, if accompanied by gasps or stridor, are indicative of upper airway obstruction.

    c. Observe for abnormal respiratory signs.

3. Breath sounds—determined by auscultation.

    a. Bronchial sounds are heard over most of the chest.

    b. Crackles may be heard immediately after birth.

    c. Expiratory grunting may be indicative of respiratory distress.

Cardiovascular System

1. Rate—normal between 110 and 160 bpm (80 to 110 normal with deep sleep); influenced by behavioral state, environmental temperature, and medication; take apical count for 1 minute.

2. Rhythm—common to find periods of deceleration followed by periods of acceleration.

3. Heart sounds—second sound higher in pitch and sharper than first; third and fourth sounds rarely heard; murmurs common; majority are transitory and benign.

4. Pulses—examine equality and strength of brachial, radial, pedal, and femoral pulses; lack of femoral pulses indicative of inadequate aortic blood flow (coarctation).

5. Cyanosis—examine for central cyanosis. Record location of any cyanosis and color changes with time and when crying.

6. Blood pressure—blood pressure in the term newborn ranges from 60 to 80 mm Hg systolic and 30 to 60 mm Hg diastolic at birth and varies with gestational age, weight, activity, and appropriate cuff size. BP is usually higher in the lower extremities than in the upper extremities. BP assessment may not be conducted routinely on healthy neonates. Measurement of BP is essential for infants who show signs of distress, are premature, or are suspected of having a cardiac anomaly.

Abdomen

1. Shape—cylindrical, protrudes slightly, moves synchronously with chest in respiration. Diastasis recti is a common occurrence in the newborn and characterized by a separation of the right and left sides of the rectus abdominis muscle.

2. Distention may be caused by bowel obstruction, organ enlargement, or infection.

3. Palpate the abdomen for masses; palpate the liver and spleen.

    a. The liver has decreased ability to conjugate bilirubin (rationale for physiologic jaundice).

    b. The liver has decreased production of prothrombin and factors that depend on vitamin K for synthesis (rationale for neonate's predisposition to hemorrhage).

4. Auscultate abdomen in all four quadrants for bowel sounds; usually bowel sounds occur 1 hour after delivery.

5. Kidneys—palpate kidneys for size and shape.

    a. Infant has decreased ability of the kidney to concentrate urine, excrete a solute load, and maintain water and electrolyte balance.

    b. Urine may contain uric acid crystals, which appear on diaper as reddish blotches; uric acid crystals may yield false-positive result when the infant's urine is tested for protein.

6. Umbilical cord.

    a. Normally contains two arteries, one vein; single artery sometimes associated with renal and other congenital abnormalities.

    b. Signs of infection (omphalitis) around insertion into abdominal wall—redness, discharge.

    c. Meconium staining—associated with intrauterine compromise or postmaturity.

    d. By 24 hours, becomes yellowish brown; dries and falls off in approximately 10 to 14 days.

    e. Umbilical hernia—defect in abdominal wall.

7. Genitalia.

    a. Female:

        i. Labia majora cover labia minora and clitoris in full-term female infants.

        ii. Hymenal tag (tissue) may protrude from the vagina—regresses within several weeks.

        iii. Vaginal discharge—white mucus discharge common; pink-tinged mucus discharge (pseudomenstruation) may be present because of the drop in maternal hormones; no treatment necessary.

    b. Male:

        i. Full-term—testes in scrotal sac; scrotal sac appears markedly wrinkled because of rugae.

        ii. Edema may be present in scrotal sac if the infant was born in breech presentation; a collection of fluid in the scrotal sac is a hydrocele—regresses in approximately a month.

        iii. Examine glans penis for urethral opening—normally central; opening ventral (hypospadias); opening dorsally (epispadias); abnormally adherent foreskin (phimosis).

    c. Check for patent anus—infant should stool within 24 hours after delivery.

Back

1. Examine spinal column for normal curvature, closure, and pilonidal dimple or sinus; also for fluid-filled sac, exposed nerves, or other skin abnormality seen with spinal bifida.

2. Examine anal area for position, anal opening, response of anal sphincter (anal wink reflex), and fissures.

Musculoskeletal System

1. Examine extremities for fractures, paralysis, range of motion, and irregular position.

2. Examine fingers and toes for number and separation: extra digits (polydactyly) and fused digits (syndactyly).

3. Examine hips for dislocation—with the infant in supine position, flex knees and abduct hips to side and down to table surface; clicking sound (Ortolani sign) and clunking sound (Barlow sign) indicate dislocation or subluxation. Asymmetrical gluteal folds may also indicate congenital hip dislocation.

4. Examine feet for structural and positional deformities, that is, club foot (talipes equinovarus) or metatarsus adductus (inward turning of the foot).

Neurologic System

1. Neurologic mechanisms are immature anatomically and physiologically; as a result, uncoordinated movements, temperature instability, and lack of control over musculature are characteristic of the infant.

2. Examine muscle tone, head control, and reflexes.

3. Two types of reflexes are present in the neonate:

    a. Protective in nature (blink, cough, sneeze, gag)—remain throughout life.

    b. Primitive in nature (rooting/sucking, Moro, startle, tonic neck, stepping, and palmar/plantar grasp)—either disappear within months or become highly developed and voluntary (sucking and grasping) (see Figure 38-4, page 1027).

Figure 38-4. Newborn reflexes. **(A)** Rooting. **(B)** Grasp. **(C)** Moro. **(D)** Startle. **(E)** Tonic neck. **(F)** Stepping. (Reeder, S., Martin, L., & Koniak-Griffin, D. [1997]. *Maternity nursing: Family newborn, and women's health care* [18th ed.]. Philadelphia, PA: Lippincott-Raven Publishers.)

Behavioral Assessment

Response to Stimulation

1. Neonates exhibit predictable, directed responses in social interactions with nurturing adults or in response to attractive auditory or visual stimuli.
2. Neonate responses are influenced by states of consciousness, such as:
   a. Quiet, deep sleep (sleep state)—no spontaneous activity, eyes closed, and respirations regular, with delayed response to external stimuli.
   b. Light, active sleep (sleep state)—random startles, eyes closed, REMs, and frequent change of state with response to stimulation.
   c. Drowsy awake (transitional state)—eyes open or closed, appearing dull and heavy lidded, eyelids flutter, variable activity level, mild startles periodically, and delayed response to stimulation.
   d. Quiet alert (awake state)—eyes open, little motor activity, focuses on source of stimulation. Interacts most with environment; respirations regular.
   e. Alert active (awake state)—eyes open, less bright and attentive, much motor activity, and increase in startles in response to stimulation.
   f. Crying (awake state)—intense crying that is difficult to interrupt with stimulation; increased motor activity and color changes.

Sleeping Pattern

1. Length of sleep cycles (REM, active and quiet sleep) changes with maturation of the central nervous system (CNS).
2. Quiet sleep should increase with time in relation to REM sleep.
3. Neonates usually sleep 20 hours/day.
4. Safe sleep positions should be discussed with families.
5. Prone positioning has been shown to increase the risk of sudden infant death syndrome. The AAP recommends that all healthy infants be positioned supine for sleep.

Feeding Pattern

1. Most breast-fed neonates eat 10 to 12 times per day with 2 to 4 hours between feedings; establish fairly regular feeding patterns in approximately 2 weeks. Formula-fed babies eat every 3 to 4 hours.
2. Caloric requirements are high—110 to 130 calories/kg of body weight daily.
3. Most digestive enzymes are present at birth.
4. Immaturity of the cardiac and pharyngoesophageal sphincters and neurological control causes mild regurgitation or slight vomiting.

Pattern of Elimination

1. Stools.
   a. Meconium is usually passed in 24 to 48 hours.
   b. Passage of meconium (tarry green-black stools) continues for about 72 hours, followed by transitional stools (greenish brown to yellowish brown; thin; may contain milk curds). Milk stools (for breast-fed, yellow to golden; pasty; odor like sour milk; for formula-fed, pale yellow to light brown; firmer; more offensive odor) are passed by day 4 to 5.
   c. Neonate has up to six stools per day in the first weeks after birth.
2. Voiding.
   a. Neonate voids within first 24 hours.
   b. After first few days, infant voids from at least six to eight times per day.

Temperature Regulation

1. Infant's body responds readily to changes in environmental temperature.
2. Heat loss at birth may occur through evaporation, convection, conduction, and radiation.
3. Physiologic mechanisms to avoid heat loss include:
   a. Vasoconstriction.
   b. Nonshivering thermogenesis elicited by sympathetic nervous system in response to decreased temperature.
   c. Adipose tissue and brown fat—the latter contains many small blood vessels, fat vacuoles, and mitochondria and is a site of heat production. Brown fat is found between scapulae, around the neck and thorax, behind the sternum, and around kidneys and adrenals.
   d. Flexed position of full-term neonate.

Universal Newborn Screening

EVIDENCE BASE American Academy of Pediatrics. (2015). Hospital stay for healthy term newborn infants. *Pediatrics, 135*(5), 949–953.

Public health law requires newborn screening for disorders caused by inborn errors of metabolism, hemoglobinopathies, infectious diseases, and specific genetic and endocrine disorders. The United States requires testing for 31 core disorders and 26 secondary disorders. In addition, infants are screened for hearing loss, hyperbilirubinemia, and cardiac defects.

1. Blood spot testing—obtain blood by heel stick for the following conditions.
   a. Phenylketonuria—inability of the infant to metabolize phenylalanine; scheduled after 24 hours of protein feedings.
   b. Galactosemia—inborn error of carbohydrate metabolism, in which galactose and lactose cannot be converted to glucose.
   c. Hypothyroidism—thyroid hormone deficiency.
   d. Maple syrup urine disease—inability to metabolize leucine, isoleucine, and valine.
   e. Homocystinuria—inborn error of sulfur amino acid metabolism.
   f. Sickle cell anemia—abnormally shaped RBCs with lower oxygen solubility.
   g. Cystic fibrosis—autosomal recessive genetic disorder affecting the respiratory, endocrine, and gastrointestinal systems.
   h. Human immunodeficiency virus (HIV)—weakens the immune system by reducing CD4 cells (T cells) and increasing the risk for opportunistic infection and acquired immunodeficiency syndrome (AIDS).
2. Hearing screening—screen newborn before discharge using an automated auditory brainstem hearing device or an otoacoustic emission device.
   a. If the infant passes the screening, no further action is needed.
   b. If the infant fails the screening, the testing should be repeated before discharge or on an outpatient basis.
   c. With repeated failed screening, the infant should be evaluated by a pediatric audiologist.
3. Hyperbilirubinemia screening—complete a systematic risk screening for hyperbilirubinemia prior to discharge. Use the serum bilirubin result from the blood spot metabolic screen and plot it on the Hour-Specific Nomogram (*www.bilitool.org*).
   a. A treatment plan should be identified for infants at risk.
   b. Parents should be provided with information on feeding, symptoms of increasing jaundice, and follow-up care.
4. Critical congenital heart disease (CCHD) screening—obtain oxygen saturation by pulse oximetry, according to recommendation by the U.S. Department of Health and Human Services (HHS). Screen after 24 hours of age using pre and post ductal oxygen saturation values taken for 60 seconds.

Discharge Readiness

EVIDENCE BASE American Academy of Pediatrics & American College of Obstetricians and Gynecologists. (2012). *Guidelines for perinatal care* (7th ed.). Washington, DC: Author.

1. The American Academy of Pediatrics (AAP established guidelines with suggested criteria for newborn discharge where readiness for discharge is determined in consultation with the maternal and newborn providers and the mother. The following criteria apply to the term newborn (37 0/7 to 41 6/7 weeks' gestation):
   a. Family, environmental, and social risk factors have been assessed for safety.
   b. Physical assessment and clinical course were unremarkable for abnormalities.

c. The newborn is stable with documented vital signs within normal ranges for 12 hours prior to discharge; temperature 36.5°C to 37.4°C (97.7°F to 99.3°F); respirations below 60 bpm; no signs of respiratory distress; heart rate 100 to 190 while awake.

d. Pertinent laboratory data have been reviewed and within normal limits for mother and neonate. Cord or infant blood type and direct Coombs results (if required) have been reviewed.

e. Neonate has spontaneously passed at least one stool spontaneously and urinated.

f. Neonate stable, maintaining thermal homeostasis in an open crib, and feeding well with at least two successful feedings with coordinated sucking, swallowing, and breathing. If breast-feeding, the infant latch has been assessed by a qualified caregiver.

g. If circumcised, no excessive bleeding from circumcision site for 2 hours post procedure.

h. All necessary vaccines have been administered to the newborn (eg, hepatitis B) according to current AAP immunization schedules.

i. Maternal immunizations such as Tdap, varicella, rubella, and influenza are administered if not previously immunized. Additionally, any adolescent or adults with close contact to infant should be immunized for Tdap and influenza.

j. Risk assessment for jaundice has been determined with appropriate home management and follow-up according to AAP guidelines.

k. Adequate evaluation for sepsis has been completed according to AAP guidelines.

l. Hearing screening, congenital hip dysplasia screening, newborn metabolic screening, and pulse oximetry for critical congenital heart disease (CCHD) have been completed per facility protocol.

m. The mother's ability to provide appropriate care to her newborn is documented with teaching related to feeding, elimination, infant care, temperature assessment, signs and symptoms of illness, common newborn problems, and infant safety (nicotine-free environment, safe sleep, car seat, and sibling safety).

n. An appropriate car seat for infant's maturity and medical condition is available at discharge.

o. Family members and support persons are available for support.

p. Mother aware of possible complications for self and neonate.

q. Facility has in place mechanisms to address patient questions after discharge.

r. Plan for follow-up medical care is in place. For infants discharged before 48 hours of birth, follow-up should occur within the next 48 hours.

s. Provide mother with lactation support resources.

2. Assess the parents ability to provide daily care of the infant.

a. Advise the parents to attend or view parenting and baby care classes offered during their stay at the birth facility.

b. Assess the parents' ability to bathe and diaper the infant, perform circumcision care, and initiate either breast- or bottle-feeding.

c. Assess bonding and encourage skin-to-skin contact, infant eye contact, and talking to and touching the infant.

3. Assess parents' knowledge of signs of illness and when to notify health care provider.

a. Fever above 100.4°F (37.8°C).

b. Loss of appetite for two consecutive feedings.

c. Inability to awaken the baby to his or her usual activity state.

d. Vomiting all or part of two feedings.

e. Diarrhea—three watery stools.

f. Extreme irritability or inconsolable crying.

4. Assess the parents' technique to properly use an infant car seat in the back seat, facing back.

5. Provide positive reinforcement and reassurance to the parents.

6. Further assess any knowledge gaps and provide written instructions and educational material on discharge.

 TRANSITIONAL CARE ALERT Newborn readmission to the hospital increases with primiparity, maternal morbidity, prematurity, operative vaginal delivery, and small for gestational age infants. Discharge readiness should be assessed by the interprofessional team. Discharge instructions should include a thorough discussion of the infant's sleeping, eating, activity, and response patterns for the first month of life. Parents should be alert for signs and symptoms of illness including when to call the provider.

Nursing Management

In caring for the neonate, the nurse establishes an ongoing care plan for the infant and the family until discharge. The nurse's assessment of the neonate includes observing and recording vital signs, daily weight gain or loss, bowel and bladder function, activity and sleep patterns, and thermoregulation. Observation for potential problems in the neonate, ensuring safety, and the prevention of infection are the main goals of nursing care.

Another main component of caring for the neonate is to assist with establishing a healthy family unit. Because so much of the baby's time is spent with parents, the nurse has the opportunity to assist them with promoting health maintenance by teaching feeding methods and by demonstrating baby care techniques, such as diapering, bathing, and circumcision care. The nurse provides health counseling and education and answers questions to enable the parents to gain confidence, control, and satisfaction in caring for their child at home.

PROBLEMS OF THE NEWBORN

 See additional online content: Procedure Guidelines 38-1

Premature Infant

 EVIDENCE BASE American College of Obstetricians and Gynecologists. (2013/Reaffirmed 2015). *Medically indicated late-preterm and early-term deliveries.* (Committee Opinion #560). Washington, DC: Author.
Verklan, M. T., & Walden, M. (Eds.). (2016). *Core curriculum for neonatal intensive care nursing.* St. Louis, MO: Saunders Elsevier.

The *premature neonate* is a neonate born before the completion of 37 weeks' gestation. Other classifications include moderately preterm (32 to 36 weeks), late preterm (34 0/7 to 36 6/7 weeks), early term (37 0/7 to 38 6/7 weeks), and very preterm birth (less than 32 weeks).

A low-birth-weight (weight at birth) neonate is one whose birth weight is less than 2,500 g (5 pounds, 8 ounces), regardless of gestational age.

A very-low-birth-weight neonate is one whose birth weight is below 1,500 (3 pounds, 5 ounces), regardless of gestational age.

An extremely-low-birth-weight neonate is one whose birth weight is below 1,000 g (2 pounds, 2 ounces), regardless of gestational age.

Pathophysiology and Etiology

1. A wide range of maternal factors is associated with prematurity.
2. Possible risk factors associated with prematurity include, but are not limited to:
   a. Chronic health problems, such as hypertension, obesity, or diabetes.
   b. Behavioral and environmental risks, such as late or no prenatal care, smoking, substance abuse, domestic violence, stress, or lack of social support.
   c. Demographic risks, such as non-Hispanic black race, younger than age 17, older than age 35, or low socioeconomic status.
   d. Genetic endowment.
   e. Assisted reproductive technologies (ART).
   f. Medical risks in current pregnancy, such as preeclampsia or gestational hypertension, bleeding, placenta previa or abruptio placentae, uterine or cervical anomalies (incompetent cervix), premature rupture of membranes, preterm premature rupture of membranes, polyhydramnios or oligohydramnios, infection, or periodontal disease.
   g. Changes in delivery practices, concern about postmaturity complications, or risk of stillbirth (late preterm).
3. Fetal factors associated with prematurity include:
   a. Chromosomal abnormalities.
   b. Anatomic abnormalities, such as tracheoesophageal atresia or fistula and intestinal obstruction.
   c. Fetoplacental unit dysfunction.
4. The premature infant has altered physiology because of immature and typically poorly developed systems. The severity of any problem that occurs depends on the gestational age of the infant. Systems and situations that are most likely to cause problems in the premature infant include:
   a. Respiratory system.
   b. Digestive system.
   c. Thermoregulation.
   d. Immune system.
   e. Neurologic system.

Nursing Assessment and Interventions

1. Notice physical characteristics of the premature neonate:
   a. Hair—lanugo, fluffy.
   b. Poor ear cartilage.
   c. Skin—thin; capillaries are visible (may be red and wrinkled).
   d. Lack of subcutaneous fat.
   e. Sole of the foot is smooth.
      i. 36 weeks' gestation—anterior one third of the foot is creased.
      ii. 38 weeks' gestation—two third of the foot is creased.
   f. Breast buds 5 mm.
      i. 36 weeks' gestation—none.
      ii. 38 weeks' gestation—1¼ inches (3 cm).
   g. Testes—undescended.
   h. Labia majora—undeveloped.
   i. Rugae of scrotum—fine.
   j. Fingernails—soft.
   k. Abdomen—relatively large.
   l. Thorax—relatively small.
   m. Head—appears disproportionately large.
   n. Muscle tone poor and possibly weak reflexes.
2. Obtain accurate body measurements.
   a. Head circumference—frontal–occipital circumference one finger above eyebrows, using parallel lines of tape around the head.
   b. Abdominal girth—one finger above umbilicus, mark location.
   c. Heel to crown.
   d. Shoulder to umbilicus—used to calculate proper length of catheter for umbilical catheter placement.
   e. Weight in grams.
3. Assess gestational age (see Figure 38-5) using a tool such as the New Ballard scoring system (recommended by the Committee of Fetus and Newborn of AAP):
   a. Observation of physical and neurologic characteristics that change predictably with growth and maturation. Ideally done in the first 12 to 24 hours of life.

	0	1	2	3	4	5
SKIN	gelatinous red, transparent	smooth pink, visible veins	superficial peeling &/or rash, few veins	cracking pale area, rare veins	parchment, deep cracking, no vessels	leathery, cracked, wrinkled
LANUGO	none	abundant	thinning	bald areas	mostly bald	
PLANTAR CREASES	no crease	faint red marks	anterior transverse crease only	creases ant. 2/3	creases cover entire sole	
BREAST	barely percept.	flat areola, no bud	stippled areola, 1–2 mm bud	raised areola, 3–4 mm bud	full areola, 5–10 mm bud	
EAR	pinna flat, stays folded	sl. curved pinna, soft with slow recoil	well-curv. pinna, soft but ready recoil	formed & firm with instant recoil	thick cartilage, ear stiff	
GENITALS Male	scrotum empty, no rugae		testes descending, few rugae	testes down, good rugae	testes pendulous, deep rugae	
GENITALS Female	prominent clitoris & labia minora		majora & minora equally prominent	majora large, minora small	clitoris & minora completely covered	

	0	1	2	3	4	5
Posture						
Square Window (Wrist)	90°	60°	45°	30°	0°	
Arm Recoil	180°		100°-180°	90°-100°	<90°	
Popliteal Angle	180°	160°	130°	110°	90°	<90°
Scarf Sign						
Heel to Ear						

Score	Wks
5	26
10	28
15	30
20	32
25	34
30	36
35	38
40	40
45	42
50	44

Figure 38-5. Ballard assessment of gestational age criteria. (Reprinted from *Journal of Pediatrics*, 119/3, Ballard J. L., Khoury J. C., Wedig K., et al., New Ballard score, expanded to include extremely premature infants, 417–423, Copyright 1991, with permission from Elsevier.)

b. Later, adjusted, or corrected age will be determined once the neonate reaches term (40 weeks after conception). Chronological age is adjusted for prematurity by taking gestational age − 40 + chronologic age = developmental or corrected age. This is the age the neonate would have been if he or she had been born at 40 weeks' gestation.

4. Assist with laboratory testing, as indicated, for blood gases, blood glucose, complete blood count or hemoglobin and hematocrit, electrolytes, calcium, and bilirubin.

5. Monitor closely for respiratory or cardiac complications.
   a. Respirations above 60 per minute and an oxygen saturation below 92% may indicate respiratory difficulty. Expiratory grunting, retractions, chest lag, or nasal flaring should be reported immediately. Respiratory distress syndrome (RDS) is a common complication of prematurity where the etiologic cause is the decreased level of surfactant production.
   b. Watch for cyanosis (other than acrocyanosis—coldness and cyanosis of hands and feet) and other signs of respiratory distress.
   c. Increased (greater than 180 bpm) or irregular heart rate may indicate cardiac or circulatory difficulties.
   d. Muscle tone and activity should be evaluated.
   e. Hypotension, indicated by BP measurement, may be caused by hypovolemia.
   f. Hypoglycemia may result from inadequate glycogen stores, respiratory distress, and cold stress.

6. Institute cardiac monitoring and care for infant in isolette or radiant heater. Defer bathing until infant's temperature has stabilized. Temperature instability is a risk factor for hypoglycemia.

7. Observe for early signs of jaundice and check maternal history for any blood incompatibilities. Also, be aware of maternal factors that can lead to additional complications, such as drug use, diabetes, and infection.

8. Once the infant is admitted to the nursery, be aware that the first 24 to 48 hours after birth is a critical time, requiring constant observation and intensive care management. Assess for the following:
   a. Umbilicus—if umbilical lines are in use, observe for bleeding—apply pressure and notify provider.
   b. Urinary output—first void within 24 hours and monitor every 2 to 4 hours. Stools—abdominal distention and lack of stools may indicate intestinal obstruction or other intestinal tract anomalies. Measure abdominal girth at regular intervals.
   c. Activity and behavior—look for sucking movement and hand-to-mouth maneuver, which can help to determine oral feeding initiation depending on gestational age.
   d. Observe for a tense and bulging fontanelle; palpate suture lines, noting separation or overriding—may indicate intracranial hemorrhage. Be alert to twitching and seizures.
   e. Color—cyanosis, jaundice, rashes, paleness, and ruddiness.
   f. Carefully monitor, document, and report vital signs to the interprofessional team as necessary.

9. Have resuscitative equipment, oxygen, and suction available.
   a. A bulb syringe is used for clearing the mouth and nose.
   b. Frequent suctioning of the pharynx may not be necessary and should be used judiciously.

c. May need to assist with intubation for administration of exogenous surfactant depending on the infant's gestational age and clinical presentation.

10. Position to optimize ventilation, with careful attention to maintaining body alignment nesting extremities with blankets.
    a. Elevate head and trunk to decrease pressure on the diaphragm from abdominal organs.
    b. Change position from side to side.

 NURSING ALERT Prone positioning offers some advantage for oxygenation in preterm neonate with respiratory compromise. During the initial phase of illness, these infants are cared for with cardiorespiratory monitoring and may be placed prone according to your facility's policy.

Before discharge, these neonates should be placed supine for sleep with alternating head position. Positioning should be reinforced with the parents.

11. Provide humidified oxygen therapy in percentages necessary to maintain appropriate oxygen saturation and/or blood gas values.
    a. Continuous oxygen saturation monitoring is recommended when oxygen is in use and until infant is stable.
    b. Continuous cardiac monitoring is recommended to assess for apnea and bradycardia episodes.

12. Monitor for apnea (pauses more than 20 seconds) versus periodic breathing (regular repetition of breathing pauses of less than 15 seconds, alternating with breaths of regularly increasing then decreasing amplitude for 10 to 15 seconds). Medications (ie, theophylline and caffeine) may be given to reduce apneic episodes.

13. Protect the infant from infection by maintaining standard and aseptic practices at all times. Follow facility policies related to visitation by family members.

14. Provide meticulous skin care avoiding adhesives and providing adequate hydration.

15. Avoid deformational plagiocephaly (misshapen head) by frequent repositioning and facility-approved devices such as the "cranial cup" or gel pads.

16. Protect the neonate's eyes from bright lights.

17. Continue to provide IV and oral feedings according to neonate's needs. Assist the mother with breast pumping, as needed, and encourage parents to hold and feed infant based on infant status.

18. Continue to monitor for complications, such as hypo/hyperglycemia, respiratory distress syndrome (see page 1186), apnea, pneumothorax, infection, hypocalcemia, cardiac abnormalities, necrotizing enterocolitis (NEC), intracranial hemorrhage, and hyperbilirubinemia. Long-term complications may include retinopathy of prematurity, chronic lung disease, hearing loss, and learning disabilities.

19. Make every effort to include parents in their infant's care and update them frequently on the infant's condition.

The Postterm Infant

The postterm newborn infant is one whose gestation is 42 weeks or longer and who may show signs of weight loss with placental insufficiency.

EVIDENCE BASE American Academy of Pediatrics & American Heart Association. (2016). *American Academy of Pediatrics & American Heart Association, Textbook of neonatal resuscitation* (7th ed.). Chicago, IL: American Academy of Pediatrics.

Mattson, S., & Smith, J. E. (Eds.). (2014). *Core curriculum for maternal-newborn nursing* (5th ed.). St. Louis, MO: Saunders Elsevier.

Pathophysiology and Etiology

1. Cause is not known in many cases. Maternal factors associated with postmaturity include nulliparity, a prior postterm pregnancy, carrying a male fetus, and maternal obesity.
2. Anencephaly and placental sulfatase deficiency are disorders associated with postterm delivery.
3. Maternal risks include:
   a. Trauma to the perineum related to possible fetal macrosomia.
   b. Increased risk of infection, hemorrhage, operative vaginal delivery (forceps, vacuum), and cesarean delivery.
   c. Psychological stress and anxiety.
4. Fetal risks include:
   a. Increased risk of mortality and morbidity.
   b. Increased risk of hypoxia related to an aging placenta and decreased amount of amniotic fluid.
   c. Increased risk of meconium aspiration syndrome (MAS).
   d. Increased risk of trauma related to macrosomia and shoulder dystocia.
   e. Increased risk of seizures.
   f. Increased risk of an Apgar score of less than 4 at 5 minutes of life.

Nursing Assessment and Interventions

1. Be alert for the physical appearance of a postterm neonate. The following characteristics are most commonly seen in postterm neonate:
   a. Reduced subcutaneous tissue—loose skin, especially of buttocks and thighs.
   b. Long, curved fingernails and toenails.
   c. Minimal amount of vernix caseosa.
   d. Abundant scalp hair.
   e. Wrinkled, macerated skin; possibly pale, peeling skin.
   f. Having the alert appearance of a 2- to 3-week-old neonate after delivery.
   g. Greenish-yellow staining of the skin, fingernails, or cord may indicate fetal stress in utero.
2. Determine gestational age by physical examination and New Ballard Scale. Measure weight, length, and head circumference.
3. Monitor blood glucose per facility policy; below 40 mg/100 mL indicates hypoglycemia.
4. Assess for asphyxia neonatorum by Apgar score and blood gas analysis.
5. Assess for meconium aspiration; signs include:
   a. Thick meconium in amniotic fluid at delivery.
   b. Tachypnea, increasing signs of cyanosis; difficulty breathing, with need for ventilation.
   c. Tachycardia.
   d. Inspiratory nasal flaring and retraction of the chest.
   e. Expiratory grunting.
   f. Increased anteroposterior diameter of the chest.
   g. Crackles and rhonchi on chest auscultation.
   h. Concomitant cerebral irritation—jitteriness, hypotonia, and seizures.

   i. X-ray—classic coarse, patchy, streaky areas with irregular pulmonary infiltrates ranging in severity.
   j. Additional signs: metabolic acidosis, hypotension, hypoglycemia, and hypocalcemia.
6. Provide supportive care for the prevention of meconium aspiration syndrome (MAS). The consistency of the meconium in the amniotic fluid (thin vs. thick) is no longer used to determine the need for tracheal suctioning.
   a. The indication for *selective* intubation and tracheal suctioning of an infant exposed to meconium in utero includes any infant who is nonvigorous. The neonatal resuscitation program (NRP) defines a nonvigorous infant as an infant who meets one or more of the following conditions: depressed respirations, depressed muscle tone, or heart rate below 100 beats/minute.
   b. A contraindication to *selective* intubation and tracheal suctioning is apparent vigor. The NRP defines a vigorous infant as one with all of the following: strong respiratory effort, good muscle tone, or heart rate above 100 beats/minute.
7. Supportive care measures include:
   a. Warmth—maintain a thermoregulated environment to reduce oxygen and calorie consumption and preserve glycogen stores.
   b. Adequate humidified oxygenation to maintain oxygen saturation of 90% to 95%.
   c. Respiratory support with a ventilator may be necessary.
   d. Adequate administration of calories and fluid.
   e. Accurate monitoring of vital signs and intake and output—to assess possible alteration in kidney function caused by hypoxia.
   f. Administration of antibiotics prophylactically.
8. Provide oral feeding or IV glucose soon after birth to treat or prevent hypoglycemia. If oral feedings are not contraindicated, they can begin 1 to 2 hours after birth. Monitor blood sugar until condition stabilizes per facility policy.
9. Be alert for persistent pulmonary hypertension of the newborn (PPHN)—physiologic disorder characterized by severe, labile cyanosis arising from persistent or return to suprasystemic pulmonary vascular resistance and pressure normally found in the fetus.
   a. Cyanosis, pronounced respiratory distress, murmur, and heart failure.
   b. Treatment is aggressive respiratory support in a tertiary care nursery.
10. Provide psychological support to the parents and encourage participation.

Infant of a Diabetic Mother

A mother may have a diabetes diagnosis prior to pregnancy, overt (unrecognized, preexisting) diabetes or gestational diabetes (GDM). The severity of neonatal problems will depend on the maternal diabetic control of blood glucose prenatally and perinatally. A neonate may be termed infant of diabetic mother (IDM).

Pathophysiology and Etiology

Hyperinsulinemia in utero, secondary to elevated maternal glucose levels, results in the following in the neonate:
1. Macrosomia/large for gestational age (LGA)—increased amount of body fat, not edema.
   a. Total body water is somewhat reduced at birth.
   b. High urine output during the first 2 days of life, probably from freeing of intracellular water.
   c. Large trunk and chest increasing risk of shoulder dystocia.

2. Hypoglycemia (defined as serum glucose less than 40 mg/dL).
   a. In utero, the fetus produces insulin to metabolize glucose independently of maternal endocrine function. With the cessation of maternal glucose transfer at birth, fetal hyperinsulinemia may result in hypoglycemia.
   b. Occurs within first ½ to 12 hours of life; may occur within minutes after birth.
   c. The neonate's response to glucose is excessive (ie, insulin blood level has a slight elevation, will drop, and then peak within 1 hour). This response is probably caused by maternal hyperglycemia.
   d. Neonate may be asymptomatic; therefore, care assessment for hypoglycemia is essential to improve outcomes.
   e. When hypoglycemia is present, symptoms may include the following: lethargy, jitteriness, poor feeding, vomiting, pallor, apnea, irregular respirations, hypotonia, tremors, seizure activity, and high-pitched cry.
3. Hypocalcemia (less than 7 mg/dL).
   a. Associated with prematurity, difficult labor and delivery, asphyxia at birth, and decreased functioning of parathyroid glands.
   b. Generally occurs during the first 24 to 72 hours of life.
   c. Tremors are characteristic and may be secondary to prematurity or stress during pregnancy, labor, and birth.
   d. The infant may also have hypomagnesemia (less than 1.4 mg/dL) resulting from functional hypoparathyroidism because of maternal magnesium loss.
4. Polycythemia and hyperbilirubinemia.
   a. Most likely to occur within 48 to 72 hours after birth.
   b. Immature liver results in inability to conjugate bilirubin.
   c. Hematocrit is higher on the third day after birth and extracellular volume is decreased.
   d. Because of large size, birth trauma may increase risk of cephalohematoma.
   e. May be premature or small for gestational age when associated with placental insufficiency in some cases.
   f. Respiratory function is similar to that of other premature neonates. Thus, neonate is prone to RDS.
5. Polycythemia.
   a. Venous hematocrit greater than 65% or venous hemoglobin 22 g/100 mL.
   b. Polycythemia increases the risks of occurrence of jaundice, renal vein thrombosis, respiratory distress, hypoglycemia, and hypocalcemia.
6. Congenital anomalies.
   a. Increased incidence of congenital anomalies may be caused by:
      i. Divergent gene pattern.
      ii. High glucose concentrations early in pregnancy.
      iii. Episodes of ketoacidosis in early pregnancy.
   b. Common anomalies are renal, CNS, caudal regression syndrome, small colon syndrome, facial clefts, and cardiac defects such as patent ductus arteriosus, transposition of the great vessels, and ventricular septal defect.
7. Infection.
   a. Prematurity and lowered passive immunity.
   b. Possible maternal UTI and chorioamnionitis.

Nursing Assessment and Interventions

1. Assess for typical appearance of IDM—macrosomia, large chest and shoulders, cardiomegaly, hepatomegaly, large umbilical cord and placenta, plethora, full-face, tendency to be large for gestational age (some may be normal weight or small for gestational age), abundant fat, abundant hair, liberally coated with vernix caseosa, and hypertrichosis pinnae (excessive hair growth on the external ear).
2. Assist with diagnostic evaluation of the infant.
   a. Maternal history of diabetes.
   b. Physical assessment of neonate and determination of gestational age.
   c. Laboratory tests—serum glucose, calcium, phosphorus, magnesium, electrolytes, bilirubin, arterial blood gas analysis, blood hemoglobin, and hematocrit as ordered.
3. Monitor for hypoglycemia.
   a. Monitor serum glucose levels every 30 to 60 minutes beginning immediately after birth for 24 hours and then every 4 to 8 hours until stabilized per facility policy.
   b. May be asymptomatic or may show signs of jitteriness, tremors, convulsions, sweating, cyanosis, weak or high-pitched cry, uncoordinated and/or diminished suck/swallow reflex, hypotonia, apnea, and temperature instability.
4. Hypoglycemia may be prevented or treated by early breast or formula feeding. Persistent hypoglycemia may require an IV infusion of 10% dextrose to maintain serum glucose concentrations above 40 mg/dL. Facility protocols should be followed.
5. Monitor neonate closely for changes in acid–base status, respiratory distress, temperature instability, hypocalcemia, and sepsis.
6. Observe for hyperbilirubinemia.
   a. IDM infants have a higher incidence of hyperbilirubinemia.
   b. Levels will be elevated 48 to 72 hours after birth.
7. Be aware that the neonate may require phototherapy. An exchange transfusion may also be necessary to prevent kernicterus. Monitor intake and output, ensure adequate fluid intake, and assess for dehydration.
8. Observe for possible cardiac anomalies and secondary heart failure.
9. Observe for other complications, including RDS, renal vein thrombosis, infection, hypermagnesemia or hypomagnesemia, birth injuries (encephalohematomas, facial nerve paralysis, fractured clavicles, brachial nerve plexus injuries), prematurity, asphyxia neonatorum, and organomegaly.
10. Provide supportive care to the family and encouraging full participation in care.

Jaundice in the Newborn (Hyperbilirubinemia)

 EVIDENCE BASE American Academy of Pediatrics & American College of Obstetricians and Gynecologists. (2012). *Guidelines for perinatal care* (7th ed.). Washington, DC: Author.

Hyperbilirubinemia (jaundice) in the neonate is an accumulation of serum bilirubin above normal levels. Onset of clinical jaundice is seen when serum bilirubin levels are 5 to 7 mg/100 dL. Jaundice appears first on the face and progresses and serum bilirubin levels increase. Bilirubin levels above 20 mg/100 dL cross the blood–brain barrier.

Kernicterus is the yellow discoloration of specific areas of brain tissue by unconjugated bilirubin and can be confirmed only by death and autopsy. Bilirubin encephalopathy best describes the occurrence of the syndrome and the accompanying neurologic sequela in neonates.

Pathophysiology and Etiology

Causes

1. Increased bilirubin load.
   a. Hemolytic disease—Rh and ABO incompatibility.
   b. Morphologic abnormalities of RBCs.
   c. RBC enzyme defects.
   d. Physiologic jaundice.
   e. Sepsis.
2. Extravascular blood.
   a. Cephalohematoma.
   b. Pulmonary or cerebral hemorrhage.
   c. Any enclosed occult blood.
3. Decrease or inhibition of bilirubin conjugation.
   a. Inherited bilirubin conjugation defect: Crigler-Najjar syndrome (deficiency of glucuronyl transferase needed to conjugate bilirubin).
   b. Acquired bilirubin conjugation defect: breast milk jaundice, Lucey-Driscoll syndrome, IDM, asphyxiated infant with respiratory distress.
4. Increased extrahepatic circulation.
   a. Intestinal obstruction.
   b. Ileus.
5. Polycythemia.
   a. Twin–twin transfusion.
   b. Maternal–fetal transfusion.
   c. IDM.
   d. Infant small for gestational age.
6. Hypothyroidism.
7. Familial, transient—associated with inhibiting factor in plasma.
8. Obstructive disorders (ie, biliary atresia).
9. Intrauterine infection.
10. Postterm infants.

Physiologic Jaundice

1. Increased bilirubin load for conjugation on immature liver cells.
   a. Increased bilirubin production related to rapid hemolysis because of higher level of circulating RBCs per kg of body weight and a shorter RBC life span.
   b. Enterohepatic circulation—reabsorption of unconjugated bilirubin.
2. Decreased clearance of bilirubin from plasma.
   a. Predominant bilirubin-binding protein in liver cells may be deficient in the first days of life.
   b. Glucuronyl transferase enzyme activity may be decreased, resulting in impaired conjugation of bilirubin.
   c. The liver may show decreased ability to excrete large amounts of conjugated bilirubin.
   d. Poor portal blood supply may decrease the liver's capacity to act effectively.
3. Physiologic jaundice occurs 2 to 5 days after birth.
   a. Increase in unconjugated bilirubin levels; levels should not exceed 5 mg/100 dL/day with physiological jaundice.
   b. Full-term infant peak levels are reached 48 to 72 hours after birth; clinical jaundice generally declines in 1 week.
   c. Premature infant peak levels are reached by 5 to 6 days of age; clinical jaundice declines in 2 weeks.
   d. Jaundice progresses in head-to-toe fashion. A yellow hue can be seen on the face and on the abdomen with levels of 10 to 15 mg/dL and on the soles of the feet with levels of more than or equal to 20 mg/dL.

4. Pathologic unconjugated hyperbilirubinemia.
   a. Jaundice usually appears in the first 24 hours of life.
   b. Total serum bilirubin usually increases greater than 5 mg/dL/day; total serum bilirubin greater than 12.9 mg/dL in term infant or 15 mg/dL in preterm infant.
   c. Direct serum bilirubin usually exceeds 1 to 2 mg/dL.

Erythrocyte Destruction

1. Erythroblastosis fetalis (isoimmunization caused by Rh factor or ABO incompatibility).
   a. Immune hemolysis or Rh/ABO blood group incompatibility; the mother's and fetus's blood are different. Rh factor; different ABO blood groups (see Coombs test, page 976).
   b. Fetal cells frequently cross the placenta and may cause the mother to produce antibodies against the antigen of the fetus's blood.
   c. Antibodies of the mother's blood are in the infant's blood at birth, causing hemolysis of the neonate's RBCs, leading to a rising level of indirect bilirubin.
2. Glucose-6-phosphate dehydrogenase deficiency—nonimmune hemolytic disease (erythrocyte biochemical factor).
   a. Deficiency results in reduced stability to oxidative destruction from substances that act as oxidizing agents (ie, vitamin K, naphthalene, salicylates).
   b. X-linked recessive disease that affects primarily Black and Mediterranean Asian groups.
   c. Screen maternal blood for carrier state and screen neonatal blood in high-risk groups.
3. Other conditions associated with increased erythrocyte destruction:
   a. Infection—bacterial, viral, or protozoan.
   b. Structural abnormal erythrocyte.
   c. Sequestered blood (ie, cephalohematoma, ecchymoses).

Nursing Assessment and Interventions

1. Assess for signs and symptoms of jaundice:
   a. Sclerae appear yellow before the skin appears yellow.
   b. The skin appears light to bright yellow or orange.
   c. Lethargy.
   d. Dark amber, concentrated urine.
   e. Poor feeding.
   f. Meconium stools.
2. Make observations in daylight, sunlight, or white fluorescent light.
   a. Blanch the skin during the observation to clear away capillary coloration: forehead, cheeks, and clavicle sites allow for clear view.
   b. Be alert to the neonate's age in connection with the appearance of jaundice.
   c. With dark-skinned neonates, observing the color of the sclera and buccal mucosa is useful.
   d. If available, utilize the transcutaneous bilirubin (TCB) monitor to trend bilirubin levels.
3. Monitor serum bilirubin levels as ordered.
   a. Utilize the Hour-specific Nomogram for Risk Stratification on the BiliTool Web site (www.bilitool.org) to evaluate treatment needs.
4. Assist with treatment.
   a. Fluids—ensure adequate hydration and increase elimination. Encourage frequent feeding of newborn to facilitate excretion of bilirubin. Breast-feeding infants may require supplementation with formula.

b. Phototherapy—uses blue light to convert bilirubin molecules into water-soluble isomers for excretion. Therapy will depend on infant's age in hours, serum bilirubin level, and risk zone (see *www.bilitool.org*).

c. Exchange transfusion—mechanically remove bilirubin.

d. Enzyme induction agent—used in rare cases (Crigler-Najjar syndrome type 1) to reduce bilirubin levels by inducing hepatic enzyme system involved in bilirubin clearance (ie, phenobarbital).

5. Provide nursing care related to phototherapy.

a. Photoisomerization of tissue bilirubin occurs when the neonate is exposed to blue light-emitting diodes. The number of lights used will depend on the clinical presentation of the infant.

b. Check light intensity for therapeutic range daily with a phototherapy radiometer to ensure adequate light intensity.

c. Undress infant to expose maximum skin surface to light. A small diaper may be used to cover genitalia.

d. Keep the neonate's eyes covered with a size-appropriate mask, to protect from constant exposure to high-intensity light, which may cause retinal injury.

e. Develop a systematic schedule of turning neonate so all body surfaces are exposed (ie, every 2 hours).

f. Maintain thermoregulation of infant to prevent cold stress—lights affect the ambient temperature.

g. Obtain bilirubin levels, as ordered. The diminishing icterus (ie, the lowering of unconjugated bilirubin from cutaneous tissue) does not reflect the serum bilirubin concentration. Lights should be turned off when blood is being collected to eliminate false-low bilirubin levels.

h. During feedings, remove the neonate from under the lights, remove eye covers, and encourage parent participation.

i. A fiberoptic blanket (biliblanket), which delivers continuous phototherapy by wrapping light around the neonate's torso, may be used. This method allows the neonate to remain in the mother's room in an open crib. Encourage the mother to remove the infant from the biliblanket and hold for feedings. An eye mask is not required when using the biliblanket.

Septicemia Neonatorum

Septicemia neonatorum (sepsis of the neonate) is a generalized infection that is characterized by the proliferation of bacteria in the bloodstream and commonly involves the meninges (as distinguished from simple bacteremia, congenital infection, septicemia after major diseases or surgery, or major congenital anomalies). Mortality is high.

Pathophysiology and Etiology

1. The distribution of etiologic agents varies from year to year and from facility to facility.

a. Gram-negative organisms include *Escherichia coli*, *Klebsiella* (Enterobacteriaceae), *Pseudomonas*, *Proteus*, *Salmonella*, and *Haemophilus influenzae*.

b. Gram-positive organisms include group B beta-hemolytic *Streptococcus*, *Listeria monocytogenes*, *Staphylococcus aureus* (coagulase-negative and coagulase-positive), *Staphylococcus epidermidis*, *Streptococcus pneumoniae*, and *Streptococcus faecalis*.

2. Preterm infants are at increased risk of fungal infections from the organism *Candida albicans* because of immature immune system and diminished integumentary integrity.

3. Predisposing factors include a wide range of maternal perinatal complications; iatrogenic factors, such as use of catheters, oxygen, and resuscitative equipment; and infant complications, such as prematurity, congenital anomalies, RDS, skin infections, and asphyxia.

4. Infection occurs because of a temporary breakdown or depression of the neonate's defense mechanism for an unknown reason.

5. Risk factors for bacterial infection: prematurity, prolonged rupture of membranes (≥18 hours), foul-smelling amniotic fluid, maternal temperature, urinary tract infection with group B *Streptococci*, chorioamnionitis, low socioeconomic status, no or limited prenatal care, or antenatal or intrapartum asphyxia.

Nursing Assessment and Interventions

1. Assess for early signs of sepsis, which are vague and subtle.
   a. Poor feeding; gastric retention; weak sucking.
   b. Lethargy, limpness; weak crying, irritability.
   c. Temperature alteration—generally hypothermia, but infant may have hyperthermia or temperature instability.
   d. Hypoglycemia or hyperglycemia.
   e. Tachycardia (because of inability to change contractility of the heart).
   f. Decreased perfusion and pulses.
2. Assist with diagnostic testing.
   a. Cultures from the blood, urine, cerebral spinal fluid (CSF), skin lesions, nose, throat, rectum, and gastric fluid may be obtained.
   b. WBC and differential, hemoglobin, and hematocrit. Be alert for neutrophils less than 5,000 cells/mm³ or greater than 25,000 cells/mm³; absolute neutrophil count less than 1,800 cells mm³; immature/total neutrophils greater than 0.2; platelets less than 150,000.
   c. Blood chemistries—glucose, calcium, pH, electrolytes.
   d. C-reactive protein (CRP) and erythrocyte sedimentation rate (ESR).
   e. Acid–base studies (acidosis).
   f. Bilirubin.
   g. TORCH (toxoplasmosis–rubella–cytomegalic inclusion virus–herpes–other) detects antibodies against common intrauterine-infective agents.
   h. Arterial blood gases.
   i. Chest x-ray—may demonstrate pulmonary infection.
   j. Urinalysis.
   k. CSF: look for protein 150 to 200 mg/L term and 300 mg/L preterm; glucose, 50% to 60% or more of blood glucose level.
3. Assist with treatment.
   a. Before the specific organism is identified and after cultures have been obtained, the antibacterial therapy is based on the more common causative agents and their anticipated susceptibilities.
   b. Supportive therapy includes observation, standard precautions, hydration, nutrition, oxygen, regulation of thermal environment, blood transfusion to correct anemia and shock, and protection from further infection.
4. Observe for complications, such as meningitis, shock, adrenal hemorrhage, disseminated intravascular coagulation, PPHN, seizures, pneumonia, UTI, and heart failure.

Neonatal Abstinence Syndrome

Maternal abuse of such substances as drugs, alcohol, and tobacco may have an impact on the growth, development, and well-being of her fetus or neonate. According to the National Institute on Drug Abuse, there has been a fivefold increase in opioid use during pregnancy since 2000. Working mechanisms include direct toxic effects on fetal circulation and CNS (heroin/cocaine), indirect toxic and vasoconstrictive effects impacting placental circulation (alcohol and marijuana), and both direct and indirect toxic effects (polydrug use).

Pathophysiology and Etiology

1. Drugs and alcohol cross the placental barrier and enter the fetal circulation. The supply to the neonate is abruptly terminated at delivery, causing withdrawal symptoms.
2. Alcohol is a CNS depressant, and fetal alcohol spectrum disorders (FASD) are caused by direct ethanol toxicity to the developing fetus. Additional effects on the fetus come from maternal malnutrition, maternal hypoglycemia, smoking, and alcohol-induced illness.
3. Cocaine is a CNS stimulant which produces increased norepinephrine levels resulting in vasoconstriction, tachycardia, hypertension, and uterine contractions, which may lead to cerebral hemorrhage. This can result in fetal complications such as decreased uterine blood flow, increased fetal mean arterial pressure, increased FHR, decreased fetal oxygen, and damage to fetal brain transmitters.
4. Opioids are morphine derivatives with three sources of dependence: pain management (misuse of prescribed opioids), an untreated opioid use disorder (heroin addiction), and pharmacologically supported dependence with methadone and buprenorphine. The long-term biologic effects on the neonate of a drug-dependent mother are not fully known.
5. These children will be at risk for:
   a. Abnormal psychomotor development associated with intrauterine growth restriction because of the decreased perfusion/blood flow.
   b. Behavioral disturbances, such as hyperactivity, brief attention spans, temper tantrums, and seizures, because of exposure to large doses of the drug.
   c. Fetal anoxia (because of decreased perfusion) and meconium aspiration, prematurity (because of uterine hypertension and hyperirritability), and a wide variety of complications to include but not limited to limb reduction defects, uterine tract anomalies such as urethral obstruction malformation, prune belly syndrome, or hydronephrosis.
   d. Neurodevelopmental abnormalities because of damage to the fetal brain neurotransmitters; this may be permanent.
6. Infants and children with FASD may develop intellectual impairment, poor fine motor control, difficulty feeding, hyperactivity, delay of gross motor skills, and brain dysfunction.
7. Complications of cocaine abuse include spontaneous abortion, premature labor, abruptio placentae, uterine rupture, meconium staining, congenital anomalies, and neonatal death.

Nursing Assessment and Interventions

Treatment of a newborn with NAS requires a multidisciplinary approach to care and will depend upon the infant's gestational age, clinical presentation, length of exposure, and type of drug abused. Hallmark signs of neonatal withdrawal include excessive high-pitched cry, reduced quality and length of sleep following a feeding, hypertonia, tremors, and convulsions. Autonomic dysregulation may be present with sweating, frequent yawning and sneezing, and increased respirations. Gastrointestinal manifestations with excessive sucking, poor feeding, regurgitation or vomiting, and loose or watery stools may also present.

1. Obtain maternal history of drug, dosage, time of last dose, and length of use. Be alert and assess for onset of symptoms of withdrawal.
   a. Heroin—several hours after birth to 3 to 4 days of life.
   b. Methadone—7 to 10 days after birth to several weeks of life.
   c. Alcohol—3 to 12 hours after birth.
   d. Barbiturates—1 to 14 days after birth with a mean of 4 to 7 days.
   e. Sedative hypnotics—withdrawal can begin as late as 12 days (diazepam) to 21 days (chlordiazepoxide).
2. Assess infant for NAS using the Neonatal Abstinence Scoring System (see Figure 38-6).
   a. Assessment and scoring of the neonate utilizing the NASS tool should be every 2 hours for the first 2 days following birth and then deceased to every 8 hours as long as withdrawal symptoms continue.
   b. A score is awarded based upon observations of the neonates' psychomotor behavior. The use of a scoring tool provides a more objective approach when determining a plan of care.
   c. When a neonate receives a score greater than 8 on three consecutive screenings, and nursing interventions implemented have not assisted in decreasing the neonates' withdrawal behaviors, initiation of medications should be considered.
3. Assess for symptoms of FASD.
   a. Difficulty establishing respirations.
   b. Metabolic problems.
   c. Irritability.
   d. Increased muscle tone, tremulousness.
   e. Lethargy.
   f. Opisthotonos.
   g. Poor sucking reflex.
   h. Abdominal distention.
   i. Seizure activity.
   j. Facial abnormalities.
4. Assess the neonate born to mother of cocaine abuse—does not appear to experience classic neonatal abstinence syndrome because cocaine metabolites are stored in the fetal liver compartment. Symptoms may not occur for several days and the infant may exhibit:
   a. Mild tremulousness.
   b. Increased irritability and startle response.
   c. Muscular rigidity.
   d. Difficulty in being consoled.
   e. Pronounced state of lability.
   f. Tachycardia and tachypnea.
   g. Poor tolerance for oral feedings, diarrhea.
   h. Disturbed sleep pattern.
5. Collect urine and/or meconium for toxicology screen within 24 hours after birth. Obtain blood gases, blood glucose, and other laboratory tests.
6. Administer medications, as directed.
   a. Opioid antagonist such as naloxone for opioid-induced respiratory depression at birth.

SYSTEM	SIGNS AND SYMPTOMS	SCORE	A^M				P^M				COMMENTS
	NEONATAL ABSTINENCE SCORING SYSTEM										
CENTRAL NERVOUS SYSTEM DISTURBANCES	Excessive High Pitched (Or other) Cry	2									Daily Weight
	Continuous High Pitched (Or other) Cry	3									
	Sleeps < 1 Hour After Feeding	3									
	Sleeps < 2 Hours After Feeding	2									
	Sleeps < 3 Hours After Feeding	1									
	Hyperactive Moro Reflex	2									
	Markedly Hyperactive Moro Reflex	3									
	Mild Tremors Disturbed	1									
	Moderate-Severe Tremors Disturbed	2									
	Mild Tremors Undisturbed	3									
	Moderate-Severe Tremors Undisturbed	4									
	Increased Muscle Tone	2									
	Excoriation (Specific Area)	1									
	Myoclonic Jerks	3									
	Generalized Convulsions	5									
METABOLIC/VVASOMOTOR/RESPIRATORY DISTURBANCES	Seating	1									
	Fever<101 (99-100.8 F./37.2-38.2C.)	1									
	Fever>101 (38.4C. and Higher)	2									
	Frequent Yawning (> 3-4 Times/Interval)	1									
	Mottling	1									
	Nasal Stuffiness	1									
	Sneezing (> 3-4 Times/Interval)	1									
	Nasal Flaring	2									
	Respiratory Rate > 60/min	1									
	Respiratory Rate > 60/min with Retractions	2									
GASTRO-INTESTINAL DISTURBANCES	Excessive Sucking	1									
	Poor Feeding	2									
	Regurgitation	2									
	Projectile Vomiting	3									
	Loose Stools	2									
	Watery Stools	3									
TOTAL SCORE											
INITIALS OF SCORES											

Figure 38-6. Neonatal abstinence scoring system. (Finnegan, L. P. [1986]. Neonatal abstinence syndrome: assessment and pharmacolotherapy. In Rubaltelli, F. F. and Granati, B. (Eds.), Neonatal therapy: An update. New York, NY: Excerpta Medica; 122–146.)

b. Drug therapy for alleviation of signs of withdrawal. Duration of therapy using decreasing dosages will depend on clinical presentation.
    i.   Morphine.
    ii. Tincture of opium.
    iii. Phenobarbital.
    iv. Chlorpromazine.
    v.   Diazepam.
    vi. Methadone.
    vii. Lorazepam.

7. Provide nursing care to support infant and to relieve symptoms.
    a. Irritability and restlessness, high-pitched crying.
        i.   Swaddle infant with legs flexed.
        ii. Minimize handling.
        iii. Gentle rocking.
        iv. Decrease environmental stimuli (ie, light, noise).
        v.   Skin to skin with snug blanket.
        vi. Organize care to allow for periods of uninterrupted sleep.

vii. Supervised prone positioning may help the infant organize motor movements.

viii. Give medications with feedings.

b. Tremors—protect the skin from irritation and abrasions.

   i. Change position frequently.

   ii. Give frequent skin care—keep the neonate clean and dry.

c. Frantic sucking—use pacifier between feedings; protect the neonate's hands and chin from excoriation.

d. Poor feeding—give small, frequent feedings; maintain caloric and fluid intake requirement for the neonate's desired weight. Higher-calorie formulas may be used.

e. Vomiting/diarrhea—position the neonate to prevent aspiration; provide good skin care to areas exposed to vomitus or stools.

f. Muscle rigidity, hypertonicity.

   i. Change position frequently to minimize development of pressure areas.

g. Increased salivation and nasal stuffiness.

   i. Aspirate nasopharynx as needed; avoid overuse.

   ii. Provide frequent nose and mouth care.

   iii. Note respiration rate and characteristics and infant's color.

h. Tachypnea.

   i. Note onset and severity of accompanying signs of respiratory distress; place the infant on respiratory monitor.

   ii. Position the infant for easier ventilation—semi-Fowler position; tilt head back slightly.

   iii. Minimize handling.

   iv. Have resuscitative equipment available.

i. Tachycardia and hypertension—monitor vital signs closely; cardiopulmonary monitor may be indicated.

8. Provide supportive care to parents to promote bonding and nonjudgmental therapeutic communication is essential. Teaching should include infant care, bathing, and feeding.

SELECTED REFERENCES

Abraham, K., & Wilk, N. (2014). Living with gestational diabetes in a rural community. *MCN: The American Journal of Maternal Child Nursing, 39*(4), 239–245.

American Academy of Pediatrics. (2012). Male circumcision. *Pediatrics, 130*(3), e756–e785.

American Academy of Pediatrics. (2015). Hospital stay for healthy term newborn infants. *Pediatrics, 135*(5), 949–953.

American Academy of Pediatrics. (2016). Umbilical cord care in the newborn infant. *Pediatrics, 138*(3), e20162149.

American Academy of Pediatrics & American College of Obstetricians and Gynecologists. (2012). *Guidelines for perinatal care* (7th ed.). Washington, DC: Author.

American Academy of Pediatrics & American College of Obstetricians and Gynecologists. (2015). *The Apgar score.* (Committee Opinion). Washington, DC: Author.

American Academy of Pediatrics & American Heart Association. (2016). *American Academy of Pediatrics & American Heart Association, Textbook of neonatal resuscitation* (7th ed.). Chicago, IL: American Academy of Pediatrics.

American Academy of Pediatrics, Newborn Screening Task Force. (2000). Newborn screening: A blueprint for the future. *Pediatrics, 106*(2), 389–427.

American Academy of Pediatrics, Task Force on Sudden Infant Death Syndrome and Other Sleep-Related Infant Deaths. (2011). Expansion of recommendations for a safe infant sleeping environment. *Pediatrics, 128*(5), 1341–1367.

American College of Obstetricians and Gynecologists. (2006/Reaffirmed 2015). *Postpartum hemorrhage* (Practice Bulletin #76). Washington, DC: Author.

American College of Obstetricians and Gynecologists. (2008/Reaffirmed 2016). *Use of psychiatric medications during pregnancy and lactation* (Practice Bulletin #92). Washington, DC: Author.

American College of Obstetricians and Gynecologists. (2011/Reaffirmed 2016). *Prevention of early-onset group B streptococcal disease in newborns.* (Committee Opinion #485). Washington, DC: Author.

American College of Obstetricians and Gynecologists. (2012/Reaffirmed 2016). *Opioid abuse, dependence, and addiction in pregnancy.* (Committee Opinion #524). Washington, DC: Author.

American College of Obstetricians and Gynecologists. (2014). *Postpartum depression.* Washington, DC: Author.

American College of Obstetricians and Gynecologists. (2014/Reaffirmed 2016). *Management of late-term and postterm pregnancies* (Practice Bulletin #146). Washington, DC: Author.

American College of Obstetricians and Gynecologists. (2017). *Episiotomy: Procedures and repair techniques.* Washington, DC: Author.

American College of Obstetricians and Gynecologists. (2017). *Delayed umbilical cord clamping after birth.* (Committee Opinion # 684). Washington, DC: Author.

Association of Women's Health, Obstetric, Neonatal Nurses. (2014). Quantification of blood loss: AWHONN practice brief number 1. *Journal of Obstetric, Gynecologic, and Neonatal Nursing, 44,* 158–160.

Association of Women's Health, Obstetric, Neonatal Nurses. (2016). Newborn screening: Position statement. *Journal of Obstetric, Gynecologic, and Neonatal Nursing, 45*(1), 135–136.

Ballard, J. L., Khoury, J. C., Wedig, K., et al. (1991). New Ballard score, expanded to include extremely premature infants. *Journal of Pediatrics, 119,* 417–423.

Charafeddine, L., Tamim, H., Hassouna, H., Akel, R., & Nabulsi, M. (2014). Axillary and rectal thermometry in the newborn: Do they agree? *BMC Research Notes, 7,* 584–590.

Clapp, J. C. (2015). Multidisciplinary team approach to management of postpartum hemorrhage. *Journal of Obstetric, Gynecologic, and Neonatal Nursing, 44,* S22.

Creasy, R. K., Resnick, R., Iams, J. D., et al. (2014). *Maternal–fetal medicine* (7th ed.). Philadelphia, PA: Saunders.

Cunningham, F. G., Leveno, K. J., Bloom, S. L., et al. (2014). *Williams obstetrics* (24th ed.). New York: McGraw-Hill.

Finnegan, L. P. (1990). Neonatal abstinence syndrome: Assessment and pharmacotherapy. In N. Nelson (Ed.), *Current therapy in neonatal–perinatal medicine* (2nd ed.). St. Louis, MO: Mosby.

Geissler, C., & Powers, H. (Eds.). (2017). *Human nutrition* (13th ed.). United Kingdom: Oxford University Press.

George, S., Phillips, K., Mallory, S., et al. (2015). A pragmatic descriptive study of rewarming the newborn after the first bath. *Journal of Obstetric, Gynecologic & Neonatal Nursing, 44,* 203–209.

Jegatheesan, P., Song, D., Angell, C., et al. (2013). Oxygen saturation nomogram in newborns screened for critical congenital heart disease. *Pediatrics, 131*(6), e1803–e1810.

Knorr, A., Gauvreau, K., Porter, C. L., et al. (2016). Use of the cranial cup to correct positional head shape deformities in hospitalized premature infants. *Journal of Obstetric, Gynecologic & Neonatal Nursing, 45*(4), 542–552.

Lisenko, S. A., & Kugeiko, M. M. (2014). Method for estimation bilirubin isomerization efficiency in phototherapy to treat neonatal jaundice. *Journal of Applied Spectroscopy, 81*(5), 834–842.

Lowdermilk, D., Perry, S., Cashion, C., & Alden, K. R. (2016). *Maternity and women's health care* (11th ed.). St. Louis, MO: Mosby.

Mattson, S., & Smith, J. E. (Eds.). (2016). *Core curriculum for maternal–newborn nursing* (5th ed.). St. Louis, MO: Saunders Elsevier.

Moore, E. R., Bregman, N., Anderson, G. C., & Medley, N. (2016). Early skin-to-skin contact for mothers and their healthy newborn infants. *Cochrane Database of Systematic Reviews,* CD003519.

Patrick, S. W., Davis, M. M., Lehmann, C. U., & Cooper, W. O. (2015). Increasing incidence and geographic distribution of neonatal abstinence syndrome: United States 2009 to 2012. *Journal of Perinatology, 35,* 650–655.

Purnell, L. D. (2014). *Guide to culturally competent healthcare* (3rd ed.). Philadelphia, PA: FA Davis.

Rubin, R. (1984). *Maternal identity and the maternal experience.* New York: Springer.

Seabra, G., Saunders, C., de Carvalho Padilha, P., et al. (2015). Association between maternal glucose levels during pregnancy and gestational diabetes mellitus: An analytical cross-sectional study. *Diabetology & Metabolic Syndrome, 7,* 17.

Simpson, K. R., & Creehan, P. A. (2014). *Perinatal nursing* (4th ed.). Philadelphia, PA: Wolters Kluwer/Lippincott.

Verklan, M. T., & Walden, M. (Eds.). (2015). *Core curriculum for neonatal intensive care nursing* (5th ed.). St. Louis, MO: Saunders Elsevier.

Zuppa, A., Riccardi, R., Catenazzi, P., et al. (2015). Clinical examination and pulse oximetry as screening for congenital heart disease in low-risk newborn. *Journal of Maternal-Fetal & Neonatal Medicine, 28*(1), 7–11.

39

Complications of the Childbearing Experience

ANTEPARTUM/OBSTETRIC COMPLICATIONS

 NURSING ALERT Many obstetric complications involve the possibility of hemorrhage, requiring blood replacement. Determine the patient's feelings and cultural beliefs regarding the possibility of transfusions, and notify health care providers if transfusion is refused.

Ectopic Pregnancy

Ectopic pregnancy is a gestation that implants outside the uterine cavity. Locations typically include the fallopian tube (96%), ovary, cervix, or abdominal cavity (Figure 39-1). Most tubal pregnancies occur in the distal (ampullary) two thirds of the tube. Some are located in the proximal portion of the extrauterine part of the tube (isthmic).

Pathophysiology and Etiology

1. Clinical or structural factors that prevent or delay the passage of the fertilized ovum:
   a. Pelvic inflammatory disease.
   b. History of ectopic pregnancy.
   c. Prior tubal surgery and/or ligation.
   d. Diethylstilbestrol (DES) exposure.
   e. Endometriosis.
   f. Increased maternal age.
   g. Sexually transmitted infections.
2. Assisted reproduction technologies (ART) especially with multiple embryo transfer.
3. The growing ectopic pregnancy may result in inflammation, rupture, hemorrhage, peritonitis, or death.

Clinical Manifestations

1. Abdominal or pelvic pain (typically unilateral). Pain may become severe if the fallopian tube ruptures; clinical presentation will evolve into shock.
2. Irregular vaginal bleeding—usually scanty and dark (most common).
3. Amenorrhea—75% of the cases.
4. Uterine enlargement: size equates to normally implanted pregnancy.
5. Abdominal tenderness on palpation.
6. Radiating shoulder pain (because of bleeding aggravating nerves in the peritoneal cavity).
7. Increased pulse and anxiety.
8. Nausea, vomiting, faintness, vertigo, or syncope.
9. Pelvic examination may reveal a pelvic mass, posterior or lateral to the uterus, adnexal tenderness, and cervical pain with movement of the cervix.

Diagnostic Evaluation

1. Serial quantitative levels of the beta subunit of human chorionic gonadotropin (β-hCG) can be used in combination with ultrasound in most cases to confirm diagnosis.
   a. Serum β-hCG (produced by trophoblastic cells)—serial evaluations will not show characteristic rise as in intrauterine pregnancy and assists in determining management of care when an ectopic pregnancy is identified through use of ultrasound.
   b. Transvaginal ultrasound—identifies absence of gestational sac within the uterus and is most accurate and rapid method of diagnosis.
2. Serum progesterone—reflects production of progesterone by the corpus luteum stimulated by a viable pregnancy; 97.5%

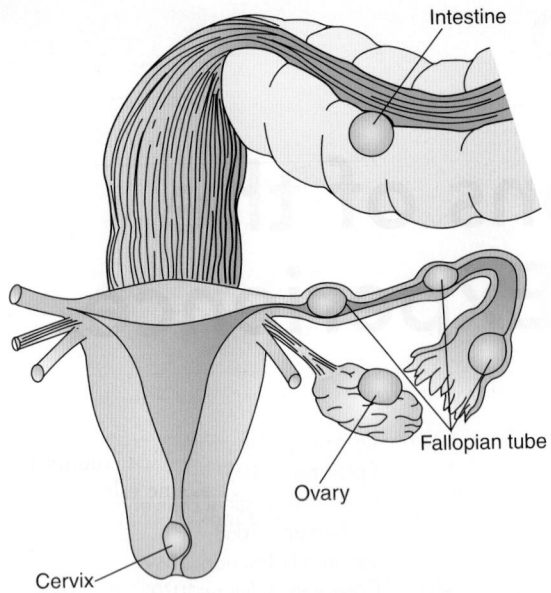

Figure 39-1. Sites of ectopic pregnancy. (From Pillitteri, A. [2013]. *Maternal and child health nursing: Care of the childbearing and childrearing family* [7th ed.]. Philadelphia, PA: Lippincott Williams & Wilkins.)

sensitivity if serum progesterone levels are greater than or equal to 25 ng/mL (greater than or equal to 79.5 nmol/L), signifying further testing is warranted; is not a good predictor for diagnosis of an ectopic pregnancy.

3. Culdocentesis—bloody aspirate from the cul-de-sac of Douglas, the posterior fornix of the vagina, indicates intraperitoneal bleeding from tubal rupture.
4. Laparoscopy—abdominal visualization of tubal.
5. Laparotomy—indication for surgery if there is any question about the diagnosis.

Management

Conservative Therapy

1. Conservative therapy is chosen should the patient desire future childbearing and clinical condition is stable.
2. Methotrexate is considered first-line treatment, if applicable.
   a. Hemodynamically stable without active bleeding or signs of hemoperitoneum.
   b. General anesthesia poses a risk.
   c. Patient is unable to return for follow-up care.
3. Contraindications to methotrexate include breastfeeding, immunodeficiency, alcoholism, liver disease, pulmonary disease, peptic ulcer disease, renal dysfunction, or blood dyscrasias.
4. May be single or multiple dosing.
   a. Weight-based, single-dose methotrexate (50 mg/m²)—may need to be divided into 2 syringes related to volume required for safe intramuscular administration
   b. Multiple dose may be necessary if hCG levels remain elevated and patient is hemodynamically stable.
5. Goal of treatment is to resolve the ectopic pregnancy and preserve tubal patency and reproductive function. Following treatment, absorption of the pregnancy will take approximately 4 to 6 weeks.

Surgical Treatment

1. If methotrexate is not an option based on clinical presentation, surgical intervention is recommended. The surgical procedure depends on the extent of tubal involvement and if rupture has occurred.
   a. The surgery of choice used to preserve future fertility is a salpingostomy (removes conceptus leaving tube intact but may cause adhesions).
   b. Should a woman not desire future fertility, the surgery of choice is salpingectomy (removal of portion of fallopian tube with conceptus).
   c. Other surgeries range from removal of ectopic pregnancy with tubal resection, salpingostomy, and possibly salpingo-oophorectomy (removal of tube and ovary on affected side).
2. Treat shock and hemorrhage accordingly as clinical condition warrants.
3. Administer Rho(D)Immune Globulin (RhIG) if woman is Rh negative.

Complications

1. Infertility.
2. Hemorrhage and death.

Nursing Assessment

Evaluate the following to determine pregnancy status and to monitor for clinical changes in patient, such as ectopic rupture or hemorrhage:

1. Maternal vital signs.
2. Presence and amount of vaginal bleeding.
3. Amount, type, and evolving intensity of pain.
4. Presence of abdominal tenderness on palpation accompanied by radiating shoulder pain.
5. Date of last menses.
6. Presence of positive pregnancy test.
7. Rh type.

Nursing Diagnoses

- Deficient Fluid Volume relative to blood loss from ruptured fallopian tube.
- Acute Pain related to ectopic pregnancy or rupture and bleeding into the peritoneal cavity.
- Grieving related to loss of pregnancy.

Nursing Interventions

Maintaining Fluid Volume

1. Establish an intravenous (IV) line with a large-bore catheter (16G to 18G) and infuse fluids; blood component therapy may be prescribed.
2. Obtain blood samples for complete blood count (CBC) and type and screen, as directed.
3. Monitor vital signs and urine output as the patient's condition warrants.

Promoting Comfort

1. Administer analgesics, as needed and prescribed.
2. Encourage the use of relaxation techniques.

Providing Support through the Grieving Process

1. Be available to patient and provide emotional support; listen to concerns of patient and significant others.
2. Be aware that patient/family may be experiencing denial or other stages of grief; compassionate presence and empathy are essential.
3. Offer bereavement resources.

Patient Education and Health Maintenance

1. Teach signs and symptoms of ectopic pregnancy to women at risk: increased vaginal bleeding, moderate to severe abdominal pain (typically unilateral and low), shoulder pain, nausea, and vomiting.
2. Instruct woman to report relative signs and symptoms to primary practitioner or emergency department immediately.
3. Encourage grief counseling and supportive care at home.
4. Discuss contraception.
5. If methotrexate is used reinforce that women should not become pregnant for 3 months.

Evaluation: Expected Outcomes

- Vital signs stable.
- Verbalizes pain relief.
- Patient and support person express appropriate grief response.

Gestational Trophoblastic Disease

Gestational trophoblastic disease (GTD) ("molar pregnancy") comprises a myriad of interrelated conditions, originating from anomalous development of the placenta that can be uterine or extrauterine (rare). It is characterized by the conversion of the chorionic villi into a mass of clear vesicles (moles). GTD is observed in 1 in 1,500 pregnancies and 1 in 600 therapeutic abortions. Molar pregnancies are usually diagnosed during the first trimester of pregnancy and may be classified as incomplete (partial) or complete. In a complete GTD pregnancy, the fetus, placenta, and amniotic membranes or fluid are absent. Incomplete molar pregnancies may contain embryonic or fetal parts and an amniotic sac. The majority of women experiencing a molar pregnancy will have nonmetastatic invasive moles; however, 20% will develop a malignancy. The use of chemotherapy will be dependent on presentation and pathology.

Pathophysiology and Etiology

1. GTD occurs due an excess of paternal chromosomes.
   a. Complete homozygous moles are generally the result of abnormal fertilization of an ovum devoid of genetic material (empty egg without DNA) with a single sperm containing a haploid set (single set of unpaired chromosomes) of 23X chromosomes (80%) that duplicates to 46XX.
   b. A heterozygous mole (20% of complete moles) occurs when 2 sperm fertilize an empty egg (46XX/46XY).
   c. Partial moles are triploid and occur due to paternal dispermic fertilization. The mole has a karyotype of 69XXX, 69XXY, or 69XYY.
2. Malignancy results from one of the following: invasive hydatidiform mole (most common), choriocarcinoma, placental trophoblastic tumor, or an epithelioid trophoblastic tumor.
3. Complete moles account for approximately 50% of all choriocarcinomas with the heterozygous mole presenting the greater risk of developing a malignancy.

Clinical Manifestations

1. First-trimester vaginal bleeding.
2. Absence of fetal heart tones and fetal structures.
3. Uterine enlargement greater than dates (size may double if complete mole exists).
4. β-hCG titers greater than expected for gestational age.
5. Expulsion of the vesicles.

6. Hyperemesis gravidarum (severe nausea and vomiting).
7. Early onset of preeclampsia; first half of pregnancy.

Diagnostic Evaluation

1. β-hCG levels—excessive elevations.
2. Ultrasound—diffuse mixed echogenic pattern replacing the placenta. May be described as villous cavitation—clear "grape-like" structures fill the uterine cavity accompanied by an absent fetus or partial development.

Management

1. Suction curettage is the method of choice for immediate evacuation of the mole with possibility of laparotomy; hysterectomy may be an option but rare.
2. Serial quantitative β-hCG determinations should be performed to confirm resolution to baseline values (less than 5 mIU/mL). Persistent elevations indicate malignant postmolar GTD.
3. Hormonal contraception during β-hCG monitoring.
4. Chemotherapy for patients with a malignant invasive GTD.
5. Administer RhIG per your facility's policy if woman is Rh negative.

Complications

1. Significant blood loss.
2. Malignancy (10% to 20%).
3. Infertility.

Nursing Assessment

1. Monitor vital signs; note symptoms of early-onset preeclampsia (see page 1048).
2. Assess the amount and type of vaginal bleeding; note the presence of other vaginal discharge.
3. Assess for proteinuria (elevated levels of protein in urine).
4. Determine date of last menstrual period (LMP) and date of positive pregnancy test.
5. Measure fundal height, via tape or palpation, and compare to LMP.
6. Evaluate CBC results and Rh type.

Nursing Diagnoses

- Risk for deficient Fluid Volume related to maternal hemorrhage.
- Anxiety related to loss of pregnancy and medical interventions.

Nursing Interventions

Maintaining Fluid Volume

1. Obtain blood samples for type and screen; blood component therapy may be indicated, prepare accordingly.
2. Establish and maintain peripheral IV line; start with a large gauge needle (16G to 18G) to accommodate anticipatory need for transfusion and/or large quantities of fluid.
3. Assess maternal vital signs and evaluate bleeding as patient's condition warrants.
4. Monitor laboratory results to evaluate patient's status.

Decreasing Anxiety

1. Prepare the patient for surgery. Explain preoperative and postoperative care along with intraoperative procedures.
2. Educate patient and family on the disease process—acute and chronic aspects.
3. Allow the family to grieve over the loss of pregnancy and possible infertility.

Patient Education and Health Maintenance

1. Advise the woman on the importance of continuous follow-up care, including weekly evaluation of β-hCG level until levels return to normal and remain normal for 3 weeks, and then monitor once a month for 6 months.
2. Provide reinforcement of follow-up procedures; typically lasts at least 1-year postdiagnosis.
3. Encourage ongoing discussion of care and fertility options with health care provider.

Evaluation: Expected Outcomes

- Vital signs stable; laboratory work within normal limits.
- Verbalizes concerns about self and related procedures; describes follow-up care and its importance.

Spontaneous Abortion

 EVIDENCE BASE American College of Obstetricians and Gynecologists. (2005/Reaffirmed 2016). *Medical management of abortion* (Practice Bulletin #143). Washington, DC: Author.

Spontaneous abortion occurs as a natural termination of pregnancy prior to 20 weeks. Variations are outlined in Table 39-1. Medical termination of a pregnancy is known as a *therapeutic* (maternal or fetal indications) accomplished through medication administration or surgical intervention.

Pathophysiology and Etiology

1. Natural causes commonly unknown, yet up to 50% are due to chromosomal anomalies.
2. Exposure or contact with teratogenic agents.
3. Poor maternal nutritional status.
4. Maternal illness with virus, such as rubella, cytomegalovirus, varicella, active herpes, and toxoplasmosis, or specific bacterial microorganisms that put the pregnancy at risk.
5. Endocrine imbalance: Luteal phase defect, insulin-dependent diabetes mellitus, thyroid disease.
6. Systemic lupus erythematosus and other immunologic factors: antiphospholipid antibodies.
7. Smoking, substance abuse, and high caffeine intake.
8. Genetic factors.
9. Morbid obesity.
10. Abnormal uterine development or structural defect in the maternal reproductive system (ie, incompetent cervix, uterine fibroids, bicornuate uterus).
11. Presence of intrauterine device.
12. Environmental factors such as chemicals, radiation, or trauma.
13. Bleeding during first trimester.

Clinical Manifestations

1. Uterine cramping, lower back pain.
2. Vaginal bleeding usually begins as dark spotting and then progresses to frank bleeding.
3. hCG levels may be elevated for as long as 2 weeks after loss of embryo.

Table 39-1	Types of Spontaneous Abortions	
CLASSIFICATION	**CLINICAL MANIFESTATIONS**	**MANAGEMENT**
Threatened	• Vaginal bleeding or spotting • Mild cramps • Tenderness over uterus, simulates mild labor or persistent lower backache with feeling of pelvic pressure • Cervix closed or slightly dilated • Symptoms subside or develop into inevitable abortion	• Vaginal examination • Bed rest (some clinicians will not limit activity in belief that the embryo will be aborted anyway) • Pad count
Inevitable	• Bleeding more profuse • Cervix dilated • Membranes rupture • Painful uterine contractions	• Embryo delivered, followed by dilatation and evacuation (D&E)
Habitual	• Spontaneous abortion occurs in successive pregnancies (three or more)	• D&E • Treatment of possible causes: hormonal imbalance, tumors, thyroid dysfunction, abnormal uterus, incompetent cervix; with treatment, 70% to 80% carry a pregnancy successfully • Hysterogram to rule out uterine abnormalities, infections • Surgical suturing of the cervix if incompetent cervix is a causative factor
Incomplete	• Fetus usually expelled • Placenta and membranes retained	• D&E
Missed	• Fetus dies in utero and is retained • Maceration • No symptoms of abortion, but symptoms of pregnancy regress (uterine size, breast changes)	• Real-time ultrasound, and if second trimester, fetal monitoring to determine if fetus has died • D&E if early pregnancy • If fetus is not passed after diagnosis, oxytocin induction may be used; retained dead fetus may lead to development of DIC or infection • Fibrinogen concentrations should be measured weekly

Diagnostic Evaluation

1. Ultrasonic evaluation of the gestational sac or embryo.
2. Visualization of the cervix; presence of dilation or tissue expulsion.

Complications

1. Hemorrhage.
2. Uterine infection.
3. Septicemia may occur due to missed/undiagnosed abortion.
4. Disseminated intravascular coagulation (DIC) is rare but may occur with a missed abortion.

Nursing Assessment

1. Determine date of LMP and date of positive pregnancy test.
2. Monitor maternal vital signs: assess for hemorrhage or infection.
3. Evaluate blood loss: initiation, duration, estimated total amount, precipitating factors.
4. Evaluate any blood or clot tissue for the presence of amniotic membranes, placenta, or fetus.

Nursing Diagnoses

- Risk for Deficient Fluid Volume related to maternal bleeding.
- Anticipatory Grieving related to loss of pregnancy, cause of the abortion, future childbearing.
- Risk for Infection related to dilated cervix and open uterine vessels.
- Acute Pain related to uterine cramping.

Nursing Interventions

Maintaining Fluid Volume

1. Draw blood for CBC as well as type and screen, as directed, to assess blood loss and prepare for possible transfusion.
2. Assess and report to the perinatal team signs of hemorrhage: tachycardia, hypotension, hyperventilation, altered level of consciousness (LOC), diaphoresis, or pallor.
3. Establish and maintain an IV access with large gauge catheter (16G to 18G) for possible transfusion and large quantities of fluid replacement; two IV lines may be warranted.
4. Inspect all expelled tissue and assess for completeness; retained products of conception may lead to further bleedin and, possibly, hemorrhage if not completely expelled.
5. Administer RhIG per your facility's policy if woman is Rh negative.

Providing Support through the Grieving Process

1. Evaluate need for grievance counseling; offer emotional support to mother, partner, and family.
2. Do not minimize the loss by focusing on future childbearing; rather, acknowledge the loss and allow grieving. Every pregnancy, irrelevant to the length of gestation, deserves recognition and respect of acknowledgment.
3. Provide time alone for the couple/family to discuss their feelings and to grieve.
4. Discuss the prognosis of future pregnancies with the patient and support persons.
5. Provide an opportunity for viewing the fetus per patient request.
6. Screen for signs and symptoms of depression.

7. Offer spiritual support and case management opportunities as indicated.

Preventing Infection

1. Evaluate temperature and pulse for signs of infection periodically.
2. Assess vaginal drainage for increased amount and odor; may indicate infection.
3. Educate and encourage perineal care after each urination and defecation to prevent contamination.

Promoting Comfort

1. Instruct patient on the cause of pain to decrease anxiety.
2. Instruct and encourage the use of relaxation techniques to augment analgesics.
3. Administer pain medications, as needed and prescribed.

Community and Home Care Considerations

1. Review symptoms of hemorrhage if a threatened abortion is suspected.
2. Discuss an emergency access care plan with patient and support personnel.
3. Instruct the patient to collect any expelled specimen and to bring to facility for evaluation.

Patient Education and Health Maintenance

1. Provide the names of local bereavement support groups; Resolve Through Sharing (*www.gundersenhealth.org/resolve-through-sharing/*) groups may be available.
2. Discuss with the patient desired method of contraception to be used.
3. Explain the need to wait 2 to 4 months before attempting another pregnancy.
4. Teach the woman to observe for signs of infection (fever, pelvic pain, change in character and amount of vaginal discharge) and advise to report to provider immediately.
5. Provide information regarding genetic testing of the products of conception, if indicated; send the specimen according to facility policy.

Evaluation: Expected Outcomes

- Vital signs remain normal; minimal blood loss.
- Expresses feelings regarding the loss of the pregnancy by demonstrating normal signs of grief and coping.
- No signs of infection, temperature normal, performs perineal care.
- Verbalizes relief of pain and discomfort.

Hyperemesis Gravidarum

 EVIDENCE BASE American College of Obstetricians and Gynecologists. (2015 # 153). *Nausea and vomiting in pregnancy* (Practice Bulletin #52). Washington, DC: Author.

Hyperemesis gravidarum is exaggerated and persistent nausea and vomiting that occurs during pregnancy. It is a clinical diagnosis of exclusion based on a typical presentation in the absence of other diseases that could explain the findings, such as GI conditions, metabolic disease, neurologic disorders, drug use, or acute fatty liver or preeclampsia during pregnancy. Early identification and treatment at onset of nausea and vomiting may decrease the incidence of developing hyperemesis gravidarum.

Pathophysiology and Etiology

1. Typically occurs during the first 16 weeks' gestation but may last into the third trimester in severe cases.
2. Etiology is unknown, but two theories prevail: psychosomatic or hormonal stimulus (high levels of β-hCG or estrogen).
3. Accompanied by appetite disturbances that are intractable in nature.
4. Psychological factors, including neurosis or altered self-concept, may be contributory.
5. Seen in molar pregnancies, multiple gestation, and history of hyperemesis in previous pregnancies.
6. Decreased gastric motility often accompanies the condition.
7. Persistent vomiting may result in fluid and electrolyte imbalances, dehydration, jaundice, and elevation of serum transaminase.

Clinical Manifestations

1. Persistent vomiting; inability to tolerate anything by mouth.
2. Dehydration—fever, dry skin, decreased urine output, large ketonuria.
3. Weight loss (up to 5% to 10% of body weight).
4. Severity of symptoms commonly increases as the condition progresses.

Diagnostic Evaluation

1. Tests may be done to rule out other conditions causing vomiting (cholecystitis, appendicitis, pancreatitis, thyroid disease, or hepatitis) or to confirm hyperemesis gravidarum diagnosis.
2. Liver enzymes LDH, AST, and ALT elevated.
3. Serum bilirubin elevated (less than 4 mg/dL).
4. Complete blood count may indicate anemia.
5. Blood urea nitrogen (BUN) and creatinine—may be slightly elevated.
6. Serum electrolytes—may result in hypokalemia, hyponatremia, or hypernatremia; loss of hydrogen and chloride.
7. Urine may show ketones and elevated specific gravity.
8. Ultrasound may be considered to identify multiple gestation or molar pregnancy.

Management

1. Try withholding food and fluid for 24 to 48 hours or until vomiting stops and appetite returns; then restart small meals.
2. Control of vomiting may require pharmacological treatment with antiemetics and prokinetic agents (benefits to therapy may outweigh the risks of drugs), such as:
   a. Pyridoxine (vitamin B₆) with or without doxylamine—first line of treatment for nausea and vomiting of pregnancy.
   b. Ondansetron (Zofran)—most commonly prescribed parenterally and orally.
   c. Meclizine.
   d. Dimenhydrinate.
   e. Metoclopramide—do not give in combination with phenothiazines.
   f. Methylprednisolone (recently found to be more helpful than promethazine; 16 mg three times per day for 3 days then tapered over 2 weeks).
   g. Over the counter remedies may include ginger capsules of 250 mg taken four times a day.
   h. Aromatherapy, acupressure, and acupuncture have been used.
3. Treat dehydration with IV fluids—typically 1 to 3 L of dextrose solution with electrolytes and vitamins, as needed.
4. Most women respond quickly to restricting oral intake and giving IV fluids, but repeated episodes may occur.
5. Total parenteral nutrition rarely needed.

Complications

1. Hypovolemia and renal insufficiency.
2. Electrolyte imbalance.
3. Malnutrition.
4. Hepatic or renal failure with coma could result from disease progression but rare.

Nursing Assessment

1. Evaluate weight loss pattern; compare to prepregnant weight.
2. Evaluate 24- or 48-hour dietary recall.
3. Evaluate environmental factors that may affect the woman's appetite. Determine if woman is ingesting nonfood substances (pica), such as starch, clay, or toothpaste.
4. Monitor vital signs for tachycardia, hypotension, and fever because of dehydration.
5. Assess skin turgor, mucous membranes, and urine for signs of dehydration.

Nursing Diagnoses

- Risk for Deficient Fluid Volume related to prolonged vomiting.
- Imbalanced Nutrition: Less Than Body Requirements related to prolonged vomiting.
- Anxiety related to threat to self and fetus/infant.
- Fear related to concerns for fetal well-being.

Nursing Interventions

Maintaining Fluid Volume

1. Establish an IV line and administer IV fluids, as prescribed.
2. Monitor serum electrolytes and report abnormalities.
3. Medicate with antiemetics, as prescribed.
4. Maintain nothing-by-mouth status until vomiting has stopped; introduce ice chips slowly and add clear fluids once tolerated; solid food in small amounts introduced later as tolerated.
5. Assess intake and output, urine-specific gravity and ketones, vital signs, skin turgor, and fetal heart rate (FHR), as indicated by condition.

Encouraging Adequate Nutrition

1. Advise the woman that oral intake can be restarted as tolerated.
2. Begin small bland meals (ie, rice and chicken). Avoid greasy, gassy, and spicy foods.
3. Suggest or provide an environment conducive to eating.
4. Administer parenteral calorie replacement if multiple antiemetic treatments and enteral tube feeding have been unsuccessful.
5. Consult with a dietitian, as indicated.

Strengthening Coping Mechanisms

1. Therapeutic communication and compassionate presence allowing patient to verbalize feelings regarding this pregnancy and associated stressors.
2. Refer the patient to social service and counseling services, as needed.

Allaying Fears

1. Explain the effects of all medications and procedures on maternal as well as fetal well-being.
2. Once confirmed, accentuate the positive signs o fetal well-being.
3. Praise and support patient for attempts at following nutritious diet and healthy lifestyle.

Patient Education and Health Maintenance

1. Educate the woman about proper diet, nutrition, and healthy weight gain.
2. Educate the woman on the need to take antiemetics continuously during the nausea phase to alleviate vomiting episodes.
3. Recommend to take prenatal vitamins 3 months prior to pregnancy as may decrease nausea and vomiting in subsequent pregnancy.

Evaluation: Expected Outcomes

- Demonstrates signs of normal hydration with no ketosis; urine output adequate; urine-specific gravity within normal limits; blood pressure (BP) stable.
- Tolerates clear liquids then small, bland diet without vomiting.
- Verbalizes concerns and stresses related to pregnancy.
- Expresses confidence in fetal well-being.

Placenta Previa

Placenta previa is the abnormal implantation of the placenta in the lower uterine segment, partially or completely covering the internal cervical os (Figure 39-2). Classification may change over the course of the pregnancy or during labor as the cervix dilates. Placenta previa occurs in 1 in 200 live births and is associated with intrauterine growth restriction (IUGR) and increased risk for hemorrhage. The improvement in ultrasound technology has increased the accuracy of assessing the placental location and cervical os.

Pathophysiology and Etiology

1. *Classifications* of placenta previa:
   a. Complete: placenta covers the cervical os completely.
   b. Partial: placenta partially covers the cervical os.
   c. Marginal: placenta lies at the margin of the internal os, but does not cover it.
   d. Low-lying placenta: placental implantation in the lower uterine segment next to the cervical os; the placenta may migrate and be pulled upward as the uterus stretches and grows during the course of the pregnancy.

Figure 39-2. Degrees of placenta previa. **(A)** Low implantation. **(B)** Partial placenta previa. **(C)** Total placenta previa. (From Pillitteri, A. [2013]. *Maternal and child health nursing: Care of the childbearing and childrearing family* [7th ed.]. Philadelphia, PA: Lippincott Williams & Wilkins.)

2. *Causation* is unknown, but risk factors include:
   a. Previous myomectomy.
   b. Endometritis.
   c. Scarred uterus to include vaginal birth after cesarean delivery (VBAC).
   d. Induced or spontaneous abortions involving suction curettage.
   e. Advanced maternal age, multiparity, cigarette smoking.
   f. Fetal hydrops fetalis.
   g. Previous placenta previa.

Clinical Manifestations

1. Cardinal sign is sudden onset of painless bright red vaginal bleeding during the second or third trimester; some women may not exhibit bleeding until labor starts.
2. Initial episode of bleeding is rarely life-threatening and usually stops spontaneously. Bleeding can be intermittent or continuous.
3. With a complete placenta previa, bleeding typically occurs earlier in the pregnancy.

Diagnostic Evaluation

1. Ultrasound (transabdominal, transvaginal, or translabial) is the method of choice to identify location of placental implantation.

Management

1. Conservative management is usually possible with immature fetus and maternal stability.
2. Avoid vaginal examinations in patients with active vaginal bleeding as this may aggravate the condition.
3. Once viable and fetal lung maturity is established, delivery may be attempted based on maternal–fetal status.
4. If repeated episodes or heavy bleeding, IV access should be established immediately, along with CBC, blood type, screen, and crossmatch, as indicated.
5. Typically, in the medical facility setting, continuous maternal and fetal monitoring may be necessary.
6. Cesarean delivery is usually indicated if maternal–fetal status unstable or complete previa.
7. Vaginal delivery may be attempted in a marginal or low-lying placenta without active bleeding. Operating room and neonatal teams should be available.

Complications

1. Placenta accreta (abnormally adherent placenta difficult to expel); increased incidence if placenta previa exists with maternal history of uterine surgery.
2. Placenta increta (placenta attaches very deeply into muscle layer of uterus) and placenta percreta (placenta grows through the uterus possibly to surrounding organs).
3. Immediate hemorrhage, possible shock, and maternal death.
4. Postpartum hemorrhage.
5. Uterine rupture.
6. Fetal malpresentation.
7. Prematurity.

Nursing Assessment

1. Estimate current episode of blood loss; review history of bleeding throughout current pregnancy.

2. Assess pain in association with the bleeding.
3. Assess maternal and fetal vital signs through electronic fetal monitoring (EFM).
4. Assess for symptoms of labor: preterm or term.
5. Evaluate laboratory data to assess signs of hemorrhage: hemoglobin and hematocrit.

Nursing Diagnoses

- Risk for Ineffective Peripheral Tissue Perfusion: Placental related to excessive bleeding causing fetal compromise.
- Risk for Deficient Fluid Volume related to excessive bleeding.
- Anxiety related to excessive bleeding, procedures, and possible maternal–fetal complications.

Nursing Interventions

Promoting Tissue Perfusion

1. Monitor both the mother and fetus frequently; pulse, respirations, and BP should be taken as the patient's condition warrants; continuous EFM if fetus viable.
2. Administer IV fluids, as prescribed.
3. Prepare for emergency delivery and neonatal resuscitation, as needed.
4. Administer antenatal corticosteroids (betamethasone) if gestational age is between 24 and 34 weeks to enhance fetal lung maturity.

Maintaining Fluid Volume

1. Establish and maintain IV access as indicated; obtain CBC, type and screen/cross for blood replacement, platelets, PT/PTT, and fibrinogen. Repeat periodically as patient's condition warrants.
2. Assess bleeding frequently to note changes in frequency and volume.
3. Activity may be restricted while hospitalized based on mother and fetal condition.
4. If bleeding is profuse and delivery cannot be delayed, prepare for a cesarean delivery.
5. Administer blood transfusion, as necessary.

Decreasing Anxiety

1. Explain all treatments and procedures; answer related questions to patient satisfaction.
2. Offer compassionate presence and emotional support.

Community and Home Care Considerations

1. Home care for patients with placenta previa and other antenatal bleeding disorders can occur if the following criteria are met:
   a. No active bleeding.
   b. No signs and symptoms of preterm labor (PTL).
   c. Follow up plan with health care team in place. Emergency support readily available.
2. Teach the woman signs and symptoms of hemorrhage; patient report to labor and delivery immediately if bleeding occurs.
3. Monitor vaginal discharge and bleeding after each urination and bowel movement.
4. Instruct the woman on home uterine activity monitoring, if ordered; use of palpation and electronic telemetry units included.
5. Instruct the woman on performing daily fetal movement counts (kick counts).
6. Antepartum testing may be increased, as indicated periodically; biophysical profile (BPP), nonstress test (NST), and amniotic fluid index (AFI) may be ordered to be conducted weekly.
7. Instruct the woman to have support persons readily available.
8. Instruct patient of the need for vaginal and sexual abstinence; discuss options.

Patient Education and Health Maintenance

1. Educate the woman and her family about the diagnosis, etiology, and treatment of placenta previa.
2. Educate the woman who is discharged from the hospital with placenta previa to avoid intercourse or inserting anything into her vagina, limit physical activity, have an accessible person in the event of an emergency, and report to the hospital immediately if repeat bleeding, more than six uterine contractions per hour, or decreased fetal movement.

Evaluation: Expected Outcomes

- Fetal condition stable.
- Absence of shock, stable vital signs, absence of bleeding.
- Verbalizes concerns and understanding of procedures and treatments.

Abruptio Placentae

Abruptio placentae results from the premature separation of a normally implanted placenta before the birth of the fetus; typically occurs after 20 weeks' gestation. Classifications include partial, complete, or marginal (Figure 39-3). Hemorrhage can be concealed (occult/hidden) or revealed (exposed). During an occult hemorrhage, the placenta detaches from the center, leaving the edges attached; this offers a concealed area for blood to pool behind the placenta. Even though bleeding is not evident at the perineum, concealed hemorrhage is accompanied by constant cramping or general abdominal pain. Prompt intervention is warranted.

Pathophysiology and Etiology

1. Typically, the etiology is unknown, but risks include:
   a. History of abdominal trauma, prior cesarean birth, uterine anomalies (fibroids, septum).
   b. Maternal hypertension: 50% of placental abruptions are associated with some form of hypertension.
   c. Cigarette smoking, cocaine, or amphetamine abuse.
   d. Thrombophilias, such as Factor V Leiden or antiphospholipid antibody.
   e. Previous history of abruptio placentae or partial abruption in current pregnancy.
   f. Rapid decompression of the uterus (reduction of fluid with polyhydramnios).
   g. Preterm premature rupture of membranes: less than 34 weeks.
2. Hemorrhage occurs into the decidua basalis behind the placenta and forms a hematoma. This hematoma will expand as bleeding increases; enlargement further detaches the placenta from the uterine wall.

Partial Separation (Concealed Hemorrhage) Partial Separation (Apparent Hemorrhage) Complete Separation (Concealed Hemorrhage)

Figure 39-3. Abruptio placentae—premature separation of the placenta. (From Pillitteri, A. [2013]. *Maternal and child health nursing: Care of the childbearing and childrearing family* [7th ed.]. Philadelphia, PA: Lippincott Williams & Wilkins.)

Clinical Manifestations

1. Sudden-onset, intense, constant, generalized abdominal pain/tenderness with (revealed) or without (concealed) vaginal bleeding; approximately 10% of women present with concealed hemorrhage.
2. Uterine contractions are typically low amplitude and high frequency. Uterine baseline resting tone may be elevated over course of evolving abruption.
3. Changes in the FHR may commonly be the first sign of maternal hemodynamic imbalance. Category II or III patterns may present to include tachycardia or bradycardia, recurrent late decelerations with minimal or absent variability. Fetal response depends on amount of blood loss and extent of uteroplacental insufficiency present.
4. Patient may exhibit signs and symptoms of rapid labor progress and delivery.

Diagnostic Evaluation

1. Based on woman's history, physical examination, laboratory studies, EFM data, and signs and symptoms to include vaginal bleeding, abdominal pain, uterine contractions, uterine tenderness, and/or maternal–fetal distress. Presentations vary per patient.
2. Ultrasound is performed to exclude placenta previa, but may not be sensitive enough to diagnose or rule out abruptio placentae; EFM is frequently more accurate.
3. Kleihauer-Betke lab test may be ordered to determine maternal–fetal hemorrhage by assessing maternal blood for the presence of fetal RBCs.

Management

1. Management depends on maternal and fetal status and degree of bleeding. Any viable fetus and patient with suspected abruptio placentae should be admitted immediately and continuous EFM applied.
2. In fetal compromise, severe hemorrhage, coagulopathy, or increasing uterine activity dysfunction, emergent cesarean delivery is highly recommended.
3. If the mother is hemodynamically stable and the fetus is stable (normal FHR/Uterine Activity data) or has an intrauterine fetal demise, vaginal delivery may be recommended.
4. If mother is hemodynamically unstable, she may need stabilization with IV/blood/blood products replacement to maintain urine output and appropriate hematocrit levels. With rapid infusion of fluids, monitor woman for signs/symptoms of pulmonary edema.
5. A neonatal specialty team is necessary at delivery because of prematurity and neonatal complications.

Complications

1. Maternal shock, DIC.
2. Anaphylactoid syndrome of pregnancy (formerly amniotic fluid embolism).
3. Postpartum hemorrhage.
4. Acute respiratory distress syndrome.
5. Sheehan syndrome (postpartum pituitary necrosis).
6. Renal tubular necrosis.
7. Precipitous labor and delivery.
8. Prematurity.
9. Maternal or fetal death.

Nursing Assessment

See Table 39-2.

1. Determine the amount and type of bleeding along with the presence or absence of pain; labor pain is episodic, whereas placental abruption pain is constant.
2. Monitor maternal and fetal vital signs, especially maternal BP, pulse, FHR, FHR characteristics, and uterine activity data.
3. Palpate the abdomen.
   a. Note presence of contractions and note relaxation between each subsequent contraction.
   b. If contractions are not present, assess abdominal firmness (relaxed or tight).
4. Measure and record fundal height periodically to evaluate accumulation of concealed bleeding.
5. Prepare for possible delivery.

Nursing Diagnoses

Ineffective Peripheral Tissue Perfusion: Placental related to excessive bleeding

- Deficient Fluid Volume related to excessive bleeding.
- Fear related to excessive bleeding, procedures, and unknown outcome.

Table 39-2	Characteristics of Abruptio Placentae and Placenta Previa	
CHARACTERISTIC	**ABRUPTIO PLACENTAE**	**PLACENTA PREVIA**
Onset	Third trimester	Third trimester (commonly at 32–36 weeks)
Bleeding	May be concealed, external dark hemorrhage, or bloody amniotic fluid	Mostly external, small to profuse in amount, bright red
Pain and uterine tenderness	Usually present; irritable uterus, progresses to boardlike consistency	Usually absent; uterus soft
Fetal heart tone	May be irregular or absent	Usually normal
Presenting part	May be engaged	Usually not engaged
Shock	Moderate to severe depending on extent of concealed and external hemorrhage	Usually not present unless bleeding is excessive
Delivery	Immediate delivery, usually cesarean delivery	Delivery may be delayed, depending on size of fetus and amount of bleeding

Nursing Interventions

Maintaining Tissue Perfusion

1. Evaluate amount of bleeding by weight of pads (actual blood loss) and direct visualization, rather than estimated blood loss, particularly if moderate to severe. Monitor CBC results and vital signs.
2. Position in the left lateral position, with head elevated.
3. Administer oxygen via face mask at 8 to 10 L/minute. Maintain oxygen saturation level above 90% to 95%. Limit prolonged use, particularly if delivery is imminent.
4. Evaluate fetal status with continuous external fetal monitoring.
5. Encourage relaxation techniques.
6. Prepare for possible cesarean delivery if maternal or fetal compromise is evident.

Maintaining Fluid Volume

1. Establish and maintain IV access for fluids and blood component therapy, as prescribed.
2. Evaluate coagulation studies and intake and output totals.
3. Monitor maternal vital signs and uterine activity.
4. Monitor vaginal bleeding and evaluate fundal height to detect an increase in bleeding.

Decreasing Fear

1. Inform the woman and her family about maternal–fetal status frequently.
2. Explain all procedures in advance when possible or as they are performed.
3. Answer questions in a calm manner, using simple terms.
4. Encourage the presence of a support person.

Patient Education and Health Maintenance

1. Provide information regarding etiology and treatment for abruptio placentae.
2. Encourage involvement from the neonatal team regarding education related to fetal/neonatal outcome.
3. Teach high-risk women the signs and symptoms of placental abruption.
4. Instruct woman to report to labor and delivery immediately should excessive bleeding or constant pain occur at home.
5. Instruct woman to have emergency plan in place for transport to medical facility. It is important to have support persons aware of procedures as well.

Evaluation: Expected Outcomes

- FHR remains as category I or II with minimal fetal deterioration noted.
- Absence of shock, demonstrated by stable maternal vital signs after initiation of treatment.
- Verbalizes concerns; asks questions.

Hypertensive Disorders of Pregnancy

EVIDENCE BASE American College of Obstetricians and Gynecologists. (2017). *Emergent therapy for acute-onset, severe hypertension during pregnancy, and the postpartum period* (Committee Opinion #692). Washington, DC: Author.

Simpson, K. R., & Creehan, P. A. (2014). *Perinatal nursing* (4th ed.). Philadelphia, PA: Wolters Kluwer/Lippincott.

Hypertensive disorders of pregnancy are considered the most common medical complications of pregnancy, affecting 10% of all pregnancies globally and of the leading cause of maternal deaths in the United States. Classification varies from prepregnancy disease and beyond 12 weeks postpartum.

Classification

Chronic Hypertension

Hypertension is defined as mild, systolic BP ≥ 140 mm Hg *or* diastolic BP ≥ 90 mm Hg, or severe, systolic BP ≥ 160 mm Hg *or* diastolic BP ≥ 110 mm Hg. The condition may be observable before pregnancy, diagnosed before the 20th week of gestation, or persisting beyond 12 weeks postpartum. Condition increases risk of placental abruption.

Gestational Hypertension

1. New onset of hypertension (systolic BP ≥ 140 mm Hg *or* diastolic BP ≥ 90 mm Hg), generally after 20 weeks' gestation in the absence of gestational proteinuria; replaces the term *pregnancy-induced hypertension*.
2. BP typically normalizes to prepregnancy values by 12 weeks postpartum; if it remains elevated past 12 weeks, then a diagnosis of chronic hypertension is confirmed.

Preeclampsia and Eclampsia

1. Preeclampsia—elevated BP after 20 weeks' gestation accompanied by proteinuria.
   a. Gestational proteinuria greater than 300 mg on random specimen or greater than 1+ on dipstick.
   b. Urinary excretion ≥0.3 g protein in a 24-hour specimen (24-hour specimens are recommended for diagnosis).
   c. Both must be present for a diagnosis.
2. Severe preeclampsia: diagnosis considered if preeclampsia evident and at least one of the following is also present: systolic BP ≥ 160 mm Hg; diastolic BP ≥ 110 mm Hg; proteinuria 5 g or greater than 24-hour specimen or 3+ on two or more random urine specimens; oliguria of less than 500 mL/24 hours, cerebral or visual disturbances, pulmonary edema or cyanosis, epigastric or right upper quadrant pain, impaired liver function (elevated AST/SGOT, ALT/SGPT, or LDH), thrombocytopenia (less than 150,000/mm^3 platelets), or fetal growth restriction.
3. HELLP syndrome—acronym stands for **H**emolysis: microangiopathic hemolytic anemia, **E**levated **L**iver enzymes, and **L**ow **P**latelets; form of severe preeclampsia (refer to Box 39-1).
4. Eclampsia—new onset of seizure activity or coma in a preeclamptic patient that cannot be attributed to any underlying neurologic condition or preexisting disease.

Preeclampsia/Eclampsia Superimposed on Chronic Hypertension

1. Diagnosis based on presence of one or more of the following in woman with hypertension and proteinuria prior to 20 weeks' gestation:
   a. New onset of proteinuria.
   b. Sudden increase in proteinuria.
   c. Sudden increase in hypertension.
   d. Development of HELLP syndrome.

Pathophysiology and Etiology

1. The etiology of preeclampsia is unknown; however, inadequate placentation related to inadequate trophoblastic invasion of uterine spiral arteries is characteristic. Additional

HELLP Syndrome

HELLP syndrome—consisting of Hemolysis of RBCs, Elevated Liver enzymes, and Low Platelets (<100,000 mm³)—is a severe complication with or without preeclampsia.

- These findings are commonly associated with DIC and, in fact, may be diagnosed as DIC.
- The hemolysis of erythrocytes is seen in the abnormal morphology of the cells.
- The elevated liver enzyme measurement is associated with decreased blood flow to the liver as a result of fibrin thrombi.
- The low platelet count is related to vasospasm and platelet adhesions.
- Treatment is similar to treatment for preeclampsia with close monitoring of liver function and bleeding.
- These women are at increased risk for postpartum hemorrhage.
- Complaints range from malaise, epigastric pain, and nausea and vomiting to nonspecific viral syndrome-like symptoms.

theories include immunologic, genetic, and endocrine factors. These factors lead to endothelial dysfunction, systemic inflammatory response, and subsequent increased capillary permeability resulting in multisystem organ dysfunction.
2. The disease is more commonly seen in primigravidas.
3. Risk factors—history of preeclampsia, African descent, first pregnancy with a new partner, chronic hypertension, hydatidiform mole, multiple gestation, polyhydramnios, preexisting vascular disease, obesity, and diabetes mellitus. Adolescents (younger than age 19) and women older than age 40 are at higher risk.

Diagnostic Evaluation

1. Evaluate BP with appropriate cuff size and placement.
2. A 24-hour urine for protein-creatinine ratio is recommended to confirm diagnosis of preeclampsia.
3. Serum BUN, serum creatinine, and serum uric acid levels evaluate renal function and glomerular filtration capability, signaling advanced disease.
4. Liver function tests (AST, ALT, LDH); elevations indicative of organ dysfunction and disease.
5. CBC with platelets.
6. Ultrasound assesses fetal growth, amniotic fluid volume, and placental implantation and function.
7. Periodic antepartum testing may be required to assess advanced or evolving disease and maternal–fetal tolerance: nonstress test (NST), oxytocin challenge test (OCT), biophysical profile (BPP).
8. Deep tendon reflexes (DTRs) and clonus evaluation assesses evolving disease and level of medications administered to treat disease.

Management

Treatment for hypertensive disorders of pregnancy focus on stabilization of the mother and pregnancy prolongation while observing for fetal intolerance. Delivery may be necessary for maternal indications, fetal indications, or both.

Expectant Management

Expectant management can be considered if the following maternal and fetal factors are present:
1. Maternal factors:
   a. Controlled hypertension.
   b. Urinary protein not severe; organ function adequate.
   c. Oliguria (less than 0.5 mL/kg/hour) that resolves with hydration.
   d. Liver enzymes not excessive, organ function adequate.
2. Fetal factors:
   a. BPP greater than 6.
   b. Amniotic fluid index (AFI) greater than 2 cm.
   c. Ultrasound fetal weight greater than 5th percentile.

Delivery

Delivery may be considered if any of the following occur:
1. Maternal factors:
   a. Uncontrolled hypertension: persistent greater than 160 systolic or 110 diastolic.
   b. Eclampsia unresolved or controlled.
   c. Thrombocytopenia: platelet count less than 100,000/mm³.
   d. Compromised liver function.
   e. Pulmonary edema.
   f. Compromised renal function.
   g. Abruptio placentae.
   h. Persistent and unresolved severe headache or visual changes.
   i. Evidence of hemorrhagic stroke or coma.
2. Fetal factors:
   a. Evolving category II patterns or category III FHR patterns (see page 1004).
   b. BPP less than 4 on two occasions, 4 hours apart.
   c. AFI less than 2 cm.
   d. Ultrasound fetal weight less than 5th percentile.
   e. Reverse umbilical artery diastolic flow.
   f. Evidence of acute placental abruption.

Antihypertensive Drug Therapy

Acute and persistent (greater than 15 minutes) onset of severe preeclampsia, systolic greater than 160 or diastolic greater than 110, is considered a hypertensive emergency warranting prompt medical management. A clinical relationship between severe systolic hypertension and risk of hemorrhagic stroke has been observed in pregnant and nonpregnant adults. Therefore, a systolic BP of 160 mm Hg or greater is widely adopted as the definition of severe hypertension in pregnant or postpartum women. The goal of antihypertensive therapy is not to achieve normotension but to reduce risk of stroke and coma. BP is maintained with a margin of safety (less than 100 mm Hg) without compromising adequate uterine perfusion.

1. Hydralazine—relaxes vascular arterioles and stimulates cardiac output via direct peripheral vasodilation.
   a. Use with caution in women with coronary artery disease.
   b. Dosage: 5 to 10 mg IV push over 2 minutes every 15 to 20 minutes to a maximum dose of 20 mg; dose cautiously and avoid hypotension. Cardiac monitoring is required for IV administration. Oral dosing will depend on clinical presentation.
   c. Onset of action can occur in 10 to 20 minutes, with peak action in 20 minutes; duration of the drug can last 3 to 8 hours.
   d. Monitor BP and pulse closely. If desired response is not obtained after 20 mg, change agents or consider hemodynamic monitoring.

e. Adverse effects: flushing, headache, maternal and fetal tachycardia, palpitations, uteroplacental insufficiency with subsequent fetal tachycardia, late decelerations, and worsening hypertension (if due to elevated cardiac output). Rebound hypotension is possible if drug is given too rapidly.

2. Labetalol—alpha/beta-adrenergic blocker that decreases systemic vascular resistance without reflex tachycardia; it slows the maternal heart rate.
   a. Contraindicated in women with asthma, heart failure, and/or second- or third-degree heart block.
   b. Administered as 20 mg IV bolus dose, followed by 40 mg if no effect is seen in 10 minutes, then 80 mg every 10 minutes to a maximum dose of 220 mg. Cardiac monitoring is required for IV administration. Oral dosing will depend on clinical presentation.
   c. Onset of action is 1 to 2 minutes, with peak of action at 10 minutes; duration of drug effect lasts 6 to 16 hours.
   d. Adverse effects: transient fetal and neonatal hypotension, bradycardia, and hypoglycemia. Small doses excreted in breast milk.

3. Nifedipine—a calcium channel blocker that inhibit calcium reuptake and smooth muscle cell contractility.
   a. Administer 10 mg orally.
   b. Onset of action is 20 minutes, may repeat ×1 after 30 minutes if necessary.
   c. Sublingual route is contraindicated related excessive hypotension and acute myocardial ischemia and death.

Anticonvulsant Therapy

1. Magnesium sulfate is the primary medication for prophylactic treatment of seizure activity precipitated by hypertension; may be given either via IV line or IM, yet IV route is preferred; IM administration is reserved for eclamptic patients without IV access.
   a. A 4-g loading dose of 50% magnesium sulfate is usually given via IV line over 15 to 30 minutes followed by a maintenance dose (secondary infusion) of 1 to 2 g/hour.
   b. The therapeutic level for magnesium sulfate is a serum level of 4 to 7 mEq/dL. Periodic laboratory analysis of serum levels is required.
   c. Actions: decreases neuromuscular irritability and blocks release of acetylcholine at the neuromuscular junction; depresses vasomotor center; depresses central nervous system (CNS) irritability.
   d. Signs of magnesium sulfate toxicity (magnesium sulfate levels greater than 8 mEq/dL): loss of DTRs, including patellar reflex, respiratory depression, oliguria, respiratory arrest, and cardiac arrest.
   e. Calcium gluconate is maintained bedside (but must remain secure) as a reversal agent for magnesium toxicity; dosage is 1 g (10 mL of 10% solution) by slow IV push.

2. Phenytoin, although proposed for eclampsia prophylaxis, is considered second-line therapy in the United States; preferred for patients with kidney dysfunction.

Complications

Complications of preeclampsia affect many organ systems to include cardiovascular, renal, hematologic, neurologic, hepatic, and uteroplacental.

1. Abruptio placentae.
2. DIC.
3. HELLP syndrome.
4. Maternal or fetal death.
5. Hypertensive crisis, hemorrhagic stroke, or coma.
6. Pulmonary edema; cerebral edema.
7. Oliguria; acute renal dysfunction or failure.
8. Thrombocytopenia; acute liver dysfunction or failure.
9. Postpartum hemorrhage.
10. Blindness; retinal detachment.
11. Fetal intolerance of labor; evolving category II or category III patterns.
12. Hypoglycemia.
13. Hepatocellular dysfunction; hepatic rupture.
14. Prematurity.
15. Growth restriction and placental dysfunction.

 DRUG ALERT To improve maternal–fetal outcomes, severe headaches that occur after 20 weeks' gestation, accompanied by visual changes, elevated BP (systolic > 140 mm Hg or diastolic > 90 mm Hg), and proteinuria should be evaluated immediately by the health care provider to decrease associated risk to mother and fetus during pregnancy and prevent hospitalization.

Nursing Assessment

1. Evaluate BP with appropriate cuff size and placement.
2. Assess urine protein and creatinine as ordered.
3. Assess DTRs and clonus on admission and per facility policy.
4. Evaluate fetal status with NST, fetal movement (kick) counts, BPP, contraction stress test (CST) via nipple stimulation or OCT, and continuous EFM, as directed.
5. Evaluate uterine activity for high-frequency, low-intensity uterine contractions; possible signs and symptoms of PTL or placental abruption.
6. Periodically observe for signs and symptoms of advancing disease.
7. Monitor for signs of magnesium sulfate toxicity—absent knee-jerk reflex, respiratory depression, oliguria, absent FHR variability; if evident, discontinue magnesium sulfate and notify health care provider immediately.
8. Monitor serum magnesium serum level based on patient's clinical status and per facility's policy.

Nursing Diagnoses

- Risk for Imbalanced Fluid Volume related to pathophysiologic aspects of disease leading to fluid overload.
- Risk for Decreased Cardiac Tissue Perfusion (Placental) related to altered vascular perfusion caused by vasospasm and thrombosis formation.
- Risk for Injury related to seizures, prolonged bed rest, or other therapeutic regimens.
- Anxiety related to diagnosis and concern for self and fetus.
- Decreased Cardiac Output related to antihypertensive therapy.

Nursing Interventions

Maintaining Fluid Balance

1. Strict intake and output—control IV fluid intake using an infusion pump. Foley catheter with urometer for strict assessment of output may be ordered. Notify health care provider if urine output is less than 25 mL/hour.
2. Monitor vital signs per facility protocol and as the patient's condition warrants.

3. Auscultate breath sounds at admission and periodically; report signs of pulmonary edema (ie, wheezing, crackles, shortness of breath, increased pulse rate, increased respiratory rate, or reduced SpO$_2$ saturation).

Promoting Adequate Tissue Perfusion
1. Maintain bed rest and position laterally to optimize maternal and placental perfusion.
2. Evaluate NST and continuous EFM, if applicable, to determine fetal status.

Preventing Injury
1. Instruct patient on importance of reporting signs of advancing disease: headaches, visual changes, dizziness, respiratory distress, and/or epigastric pain.
2. Keep the environment quiet and calm as possible, minimizing visitors.
3. Implement seizure precautions with padded side rails and maintain safe environment
4. Hospitalized patients should have oxygen, suction, and emergency medications immediately available for seizure management.
5. Assess DTRs and clonus facility protocol; increase frequency as patient's condition warrants.

Decreasing Anxiety and Increasing Knowledge
1. Explain disease process and care plan including signs and symptoms of evolving disease.
2. Discuss the effects of all medications on mother and fetus.
3. Allow time to ask questions and discuss feelings regarding the diagnosis and treatment plan.

Maintaining Cardiac Output
1. Maintain strict intake and output monitoring.
2. Monitor maternal vital signs and pulse oximetry. Report abnormalities to provider.
3. Assess formation of edema: peripheral and pulmonary. Report pitting edema of +2 or less or evidence of pulmonary edema to primary care provider immediately.

Community and Home Care Considerations
1. Mild preeclampsia, if stable, may be considered for home care at the discretion of the primary practitioner.
2. Ensure patient has access to primary care provider.
3. Periodic home visits by nursing personnel may be warranted.
4. Teach woman signs and symptoms of evolving disease. Home BP and urine output monitoring is recommended.
5. Teach woman to assess daily fetal movement (kick) counts; arrange for weekly NST, if indicated.

Patient Education and Health Maintenance
1. Teach the woman the importance of bed rest, medication use, and lateral positioning.
2. Encourage support of family and friends; suggest diversional activities on bed rest.
3. Include support of the neonatal team for discussion of fetal prognosis with the woman and her family.

Evaluation: Expected Outcomes
- BP and other vital parameters stable.
- Absence of evolving category II or category III FHR patterns.
- No seizure activity.
- Expresses concern for self and fetus.
- No evidence of pulmonary edema; urine output adequate.

Hydramnios

Hydramnios also called poly*hydramnios* is excess amniotic fluid and occurs in 1% to 5% of pregnancies; volume typically exceeds 2 L between 32 and 36 weeks' gestation. Although about 50% of cases result in normal outcomes, hydramnios often leads to preterm delivery, fetal malpresentation, and umbilical cord prolapse.

Pathophysiology and Etiology
1. Amniotic fluid is 98% to 99% water, with the remainder consisting of proteins, carbohydrates, fats, electrolytes, enzymes, hormones, urinary by-products, fetal cells, lanugo, and vernix.
   a. Amniotic fluid volume is influenced by fetal urination and fetal lung liquid production.
   b. Volume facilitates normal lung and neuromuscular maturity.
   c. A fetus near term will produce 500 to 1,200 mL of urine and swallow 210 to 760 mL of amniotic fluid daily.
   d. At 36 weeks' gestation, approximately 1 L of fluid is present with subsequent decreases over the duration of gestation.
2. Polyhydramnios is idiopathic in 60% of women but is associated with multiple gestation, immune and nonimmune hydrops fetalis, chromosomal anomalies such as Down syndrome, and fetal GI–cardiac–neural tube abnormalities.

Clinical Manifestations
1. Excessive weight gain, dyspnea.
2. Abdomen may be tense and shiny.
3. Edema of the vulva, legs, and lower extremities may be evident.
4. Increased uterine size for gestational age; usually accompanied by difficulty in palpating fetal parts or auscultation of the FHR.
5. Possible evolving category II or category III FHR patterns.

Diagnostic Evaluation
1. Ultrasound evaluation: AFI greater than 20 cm or single deepest pocket depth greater than 8 cm or total volume greater than 2 L.
2. Difficult to palpate fetus or auscultate FHR.
3. Fundal height (FH) greater than age of gestation.

Management
1. Treatment is based on severity and underlying conditions; may include direct fetal therapy, amnioreduction, or administration of prostaglandin inhibitors such as indomethacin.
2. Indomethacin decreases fetal urine output through the constriction of the renal arteries. Used cautiously after 30 weeks' gestation to prevent premature closure of the patent ductus arteriosus.
3. Amnioreduction:
   a. Accomplished with amniocentesis where fluid is slowly removed under ultrasound-guided needle aspiration; rapid removal can result in a premature separation of the placenta.
   b. Usually 500 to 1,000 mL of fluid is removed during one procedure. Fluid should be removed slowly, no faster than 1,000 mL over 20 minutes.

Complications

1. Potential for dysfunctional labor with increased risk for cesarean delivery.
2. Postpartum hemorrhage because of uterine atony from prolonged gross distention of the uterus.
3. Acute fetal hypoxia secondary to prolapsed cord or trauma.
4. Potential for preterm delivery.

Nursing Assessment

1. Evaluate maternal respiratory status; dyspnea may be present as hydramnios increases.
2. Evaluate EFM, to assess fetal status.
3. Inspect abdomen and evaluate uterine height and compare with previous findings.
4. Evaluate for abdominal pain, edema, varicosities of lower extremities, and vulva.

Nursing Diagnoses

- Ineffective Breathing Pattern related to pressure on the diaphragm.
- Impaired Physical Mobility related to edema and discomfort from the enlarged uterus.
- Anxiety related to fetal outcome.
- Risk for Bleeding at delivery and postpartum related to prolonged overdistention of the uterus.

Nursing Interventions

Promoting Effective Breathing
1. Position to alleviate dyspnea.
2. Limit activities and plan for frequent rest periods.
3. Maintain adequate intake and output.

Promoting Mobility
1. Assist the woman with position changes and ambulation, as needed.
2. Advise on alternating activity with rest periods to promote circulation.
3. Instruct the woman to wear loose-fitting clothing and low-heeled shoes with good support.

Decreasing Anxiety
1. Explain probable causes of polyhydramnios, if known.
2. Encourage the patient and family to ask questions and express feelings regarding any treatment or procedure.
3. Prepare patient for mode of delivery that is anticipated and for the expected findings at the time of delivery.
4. Encourage presence and participation of support person in plan of care.

Preventing Hemorrhage During Labor and Postpartum
1. Notify primary care provider of inadequate or abnormal labor curve.
2. Maintain IV access and administer parenteral fluids as ordered (LR).
3. Administer medications (ie, oxytocin, misoprostol) to decrease postpartum bleeding, as necessary.
4. Observe for alterations in vital signs indicating excessive blood loss.

Patient Education and Health Maintenance

1. Instruct the woman to notify her health care provider if she experiences respiratory distress.
2. Teach the woman signs of PTL and hemorrhage and to report them to health care provider.

Evaluation: Expected Outcomes

- Respirations: rate of 18 to 22 and unlabored.
- Verbalizes improved comfort; moves freely.
- Discusses pregnancy outcome realistically; asks questions regarding treatment for self and fetus.
- Labor progresses and involution occurs without hemorrhage.

Oligohydramnios

Oligohydramnios is the marked decrease of amniotic fluid of less than 500 mL in the amniotic sac. It is rarer than hydramnios and is associated with a 43% perinatal mortality risk.

Pathophysiology and Etiology

1. Commonly related to amnion abnormalities, placental insufficiency, severe preeclampsia, premature rupture of membranes, and fetal problems, such as obstruction in the urinary tract, renal agenesis, pulmonary hypoplasia (Potter syndrome), and IUGR (any condition that prevents the formation of urine or the entry of urine into the amniotic sac usually results in oligohydramnios).
2. Commonly seen in postdate pregnancies.

Clinical Manifestations

1. Prominent fetal parts on palpation of the abdomen.
2. Small-for-date uterine size.
3. FHR variable decelerations or repetitive late decelerations may present on EFM tracing.

Diagnostic Evaluation

1. Ultrasound evaluation of the AFI—decrease of amniotic fluid in all four vertical plane quadrants of the uterus of less than 500 mL, single deep pocket depth less than 2 cm, or AFI less than 5 cm at term.

Management

1. Frequent evaluation of fetal status through NST, BPP, CST, or OCT, as indicated.
2. Periodic ultrasound evaluations performed to evaluate fetal renal dysfunction and abnormal fetal growth.
3. Amnioinfusion (the installation of fluid into the amniotic cavity to replace depleted volumes of amniotic fluid) during labor is optional to decrease occurrence and severity of FHR variable decelerations.
4. Delivery may be indicated for such conditions as IUGR or fetal compromise.

Complications

1. Preterm labor.
2. Umbilical cord compression.
3. Passage of meconium.
4. Fetal/neonatal death.
5. Neonatal respiratory distress because of pulmonary hypoplasia related to fetal compression and growth restriction.

Nursing Interventions and Patient Education

1. Evaluate fetal status with EFM.
2. Evaluate maternal vital signs per facility protocol; note signs of infection, especially if oligohydramnios is secondary to PROM.

3. Assist with an amnioinfusion, as indicated.

4. Inform health care provider of fetal intolerance to labor and treat, as indicated.

Multiple Gestation

Multiple gestation or *multifetal pregnancy* results when two or more fetuses are present in the uterus at the same time. Since 1980, there has been a 76% increase in the frequency of twins and a 400% rise in triplet and high-order multiples because of advanced maternal age and assisted reproductive technology (ART). Multiple gestation is not a complication of pregnancy; rather, it is a condition that presents an increased risk of morbidity and mortality for mother and neonates.

 EVIDENCE BASE American College of Obstetricians and Gynecologists. (2014/Reaffirmed 2016). *Multiple gestation: Complicated twin, triplet, and high-order multifetal pregnancy* (Practice Bulletin #169). Washington, DC: Author.

Pathophysiology and Etiology

1. Types of twinning (Figure 39-4): The degree to which structures are shared (amnion, chorion, placenta) is related to the time of zygotic division after conception (within 72 hours).
   a. Monozygotic (identical)—one ovum fertilizes with one sperm, later dividing early in gestation resulting in two embryos. Each embryo has identical genetic makeup and gender identity but may vary in size because of unequal splitting of the cytoplasm; etiology unclear; rarest type of twinning with increased risk of twin-to-twin transfusion syndrome.
   b. Dizygotic, trizygotic (fraternal, nonidentical)—two or more ova are fertilized by two or more separate sperm. The twins do not always share same genetic makeup or gender identity.

2. Artificially induced ovulation, as well as in vitro fertilization with multiple embryos transferred into the uterus, increases risk of multiple gestation.

3. Increasing maternal age and parity increase odds of twinning.

4. Other terminology:
   a. Monochorionic—one chorionic membrane.
   b. Monoamniotic—one amniotic sac.
   c. Dichorionic—two chorionic membranes.
   d. Diamniotic—two amniotic sacs.

Clinical Manifestations

1. Uterine size is large for gestational age. Fundal height is typically 2 cm larger than normal.

2. Auscultation of two or more distinct and separate fetal hearts may occur with a Doppler late in the first trimester or with a fetoscope after 20 weeks' gestation.

3. Ultrasound is the primary diagnostic tool; used for 95% to 100% of cases. Gestation sacs identified as early as 6 to 8 weeks.

4. High initial quantitative β-hCG is one of the earliest indicators. However, because of the possibility of false-positive results, ultrasound should be used to confirm the diagnosis in the presence of elevated β-hCG levels.

Complications

1. Cardiopulmonary.
   a. Pulmonary edema.
   b. Complications from tocolysis.
   c. Hypertension or preeclampsia.
   d. Aortocaval compression syndrome
   e. Peripartum and postpartum cardiomyopathy.

2. GI.
   a. Acute fatty liver of pregnancy.
   b. Cholestasis of pregnancy.

3. Hematologic—anemia.

4. Obstetric.
   a. PTL or preterm birth.
   b. Incompetent cervix.
   c. Increased incidence of cesarean delivery.

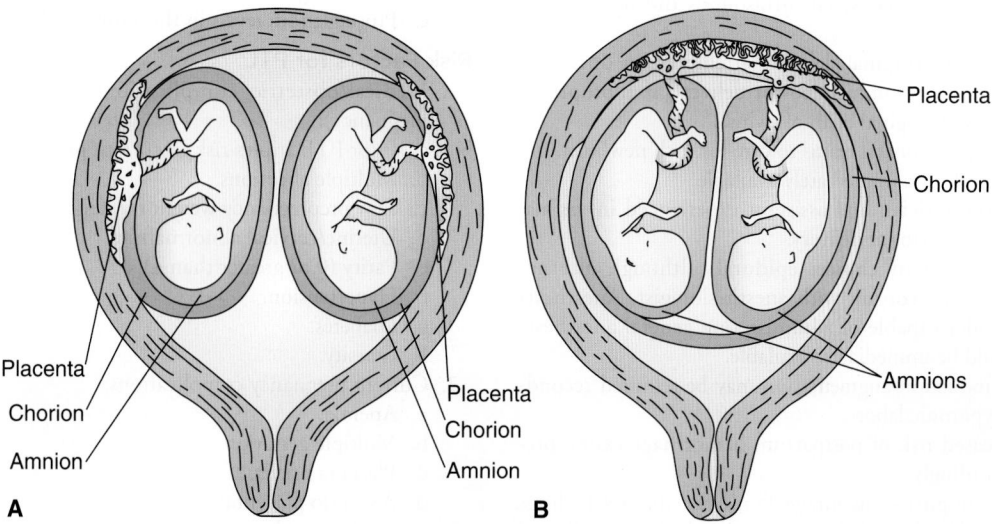

Figure 39-4. Multiple gestations. **(A)** Dizygotic twins showing two placentas, two chorions, and two amnions. **(B)** Monozygotic twins with one placenta, one chorion, and two amnions. (From Pillitteri, A. [2013]. *Maternal and child health nursing: Care of the childbearing and childrearing family* [7th ed.]. Philadelphia, PA: Lippincott Williams & Wilkins.)

d. Increased use of tocolysis.

e. Antepartum and postpartum hemorrhage.

f. Abruptio placentae.

g. Uterine rupture.

h. Gestational diabetes.

i. Polyhydramnios; oligohydramnios common with twins.

j. Spontaneous abortion.

k. IUGR.

l. Umbilical cord problems, such as entanglement, cord prolapse, or vasa previa.

5. Fetal risks—structural abnormalities, such as congenital heart defects, intestinal tract anomalies, neural tube defects, hydrocephaly, craniofacial defects, skeletal defects, anencephaly, and encephalocele.

6. Conjoined twins.

7. Twin-to-twin transfusion syndrome leads to anastomoses of placental vessels; increased risk with one placenta.

Management and Nursing Interventions

1. Nutrition counseling—increased caloric and protein intake as well as vitamin supplements are needed to meet demands of multiple fetuses.

2. Fetal evaluation—serial sonograms during the pregnancy evaluate growth and development to growth inconsistencies. NST, BPP, and amniocentesis are utilized for detection of fetal lung maturity and fetal tolerance. Percutaneous umbilical cord sampling may be used to establish fetal well-being if twin-to-twin transfusion is suspected.

3. PTL prevention—hospitalization may be necessary for signs and symptoms of PTL.

a. Encourage bed rest and hydration.

b. Institute fetal monitoring and assist with tocolytic therapy, if ordered.

4. Mode of delivery—dependent on the presentation of the twins, maternal and fetal status, and gestational age. Cesarean delivery is commonly used for multiples other than twins.

5. Intrapartum management.

a. Establish IV access.

b. Provide for EFM for each fetus; triplets and high-order multiples may need serial ultrasounds during labor or preoperatively.

c. Double setup (vaginal delivery attempted in operating room suite) is recommended for delivery, if appropriate. Guidelines for vaginal birth of twins:

i. Multiple neonatal teams to care for each newborn.

ii. Surgical suite immediately available.

iii. An obstetrician and assistant experienced in vaginal births of twins at delivery.

iv. Anesthesia of choice: epidural, although alternatives exist; consult with anesthesiologist. Anesthesia provider capable of administering general anesthesia should be immediately available.

d. Pitocin induction/augmentation may be required secondary to hypotonic labor.

e. An increased risk of postpartum hemorrhage exists; prepare accordingly.

6. Emotional support—encourage family to discuss feelings about multiple births and identify ways in which they will need assistance. Refer to resources such as National Organization of Mothers of Twins Clubs (*www.nomotc.org*).

Community and Home Care Considerations

1. Discuss the warning signs of PTL.

2. Home care may include nursing visits and fetal assessments.

3. Ensure provider contact information is available.

INTRAPARTUM COMPLICATIONS OF LABOR

Preterm Labor

Preterm labor (PTL) is defined as regular contractions associated with cervical change between 20 and 37 completed weeks of gestation. PTL is second, only to birth defects, as a leading cause of infant mortality. The preterm birth rate in the United States was 9.6% for 2016. However, neonatal intensive care and technology has advanced to meet the various needs of extrauterine transition of the preterm fetus.

It is important to differentiate PTL from other sequelae to avoid misdiagnosis. For example, uterine irritability without cervical change is not PTL. Likewise, preterm birth (PTB) and low birth weight (LBW) are not synonymous; preterm birth is any birth that occurs before 37 completed weeks of pregnancy, whereas LBW refers to birth weight alone (less than 2,500 g [5½ lb]), regardless of gestational age.

Pathophysiology and Etiology

1. The exact etiology for PTL remains unknown, but may include:

a. Decidual hemorrhage (placental abruption).

b. Mechanical factors such as uterine overdistention or cervical incompetence.

c. Hormonal dysfunction.

d. Anatomical and structural abnormalities.

e. Infectious etiology (eg, bacterial vaginosis, group B beta strep).

2. Physiologic alterations occur with onset of spontaneous labor.

a. Cervical changes occur: softening, shortening, and location.

b. Oxytocin receptors present in the myometrium respond to circulating levels.

c. Prostaglandin levels in the amniotic fluid rise.

Risk Factors for PTL

1. Medical/obstetric complications (predating the current pregnancy):

a. Prior PTB triples risk in current pregnancy.

b. Multiple abortions.

c. Low prepregnancy weight for height.

d. Uterine/cervical abnormalities.

e. Parity (0 or greater than 4).

f. Hypertension.

g. Diabetes.

h. Obesity.

2. Current pregnancy complications:

a. Anemia.

b. Multiple gestation.

c. Placenta previa.

d. Abruptio placentae.

e. Fetal anomaly.

f. Hydramnios (polyhydramnios, oligohydramnios).

g. Abdominal surgery.

h. Infection.
i. Bleeding in first trimester.
j. Short interpregnancy interval.
k. PROM.
l. Cervical incompetence.
m. UTIs/pyelonephritis.

3. Demographic data:
   a. Maternal age younger than 17 or older than 35.
   b. African American (doubles the risk).
   c. Low socioeconomic status.

4. Behavioral and environmental:
   a. DES exposure.
   b. Smoking (especially if more than 11 cigarettes/day).
   c. Poor nutrition or excessive stress.
   d. Substance abuse.
   e. Late or no prenatal care.
   f. Intimate partner violence.

Clinical Manifestations

1. Uterine cramping (menstrual-like, intermittent, or constant).
2. Uterine contractions occurring at intervals of 10 minutes or less.
3. Low abdominal pain or pressure (pelvic pressure).
4. Dull low backache (intermittent or constant).
5. Increase or change in vaginal discharge.
6. Feeling that baby is "pushing down" or that "something" is in the vagina.

Diagnostic Evaluation

1. Transvaginal cervical ultrasound can predict cervical length and direct internal changes.
2. Fetal fibronectin (fFN): protein produced by fetal membranes and functions as an adhesive to hold membranes against the uterine myometrium. It is normally absent in cervical secretions after 16 to 20 weeks and reappears after 34 weeks. Therefore, a mid-trimester assay with positive fFN is an indicator of risk for PTL/PTB and possible infection. (See Chapter 36.)

Management

Management of PTL is focused on early education, prevention, and limiting neonatal morbidity.

Preconception Care

1. Baseline assessment of health and risks; advise patient to decrease risks attributable to PTL/PTB.
2. Pregnancy planning and identification of barriers to care.
3. Periodontal care.
4. Adjustment of prescribed and over-the-counter medications that may pose a threat to the developing fetus.
5. Nutritional counseling, as needed.
6. Genetic counseling, as indicated.

Antepartum Treatment

1. Educate mother regarding signs/symptoms of PTL.
2. Instruct mother and provide resources for lifestyle modifications:
   a. If applicable, encourage smoking-cessation classes.
   b. Discuss aspects of a healthy diet and adequate maternal weight gain during pregnancy.
3. Early therapy options include bed rest, hydration, and abstention from intercourse and orgasm; effectiveness of each method is uncertain.

Tocolytic Therapy

If antepartum therapy is not successful, tocolytic therapy may be instituted, with no one medication recognized to stop PTL. These drugs should be used only when the potential benefit to the fetus outweighs the potential risk. If tocolytic drugs are used, the choice of drug should be individualized and based on maternal condition, potential drug side effects, and gestational age.

1. Betamimetic—terbutaline: acts on β_2 receptor cells located in smooth muscle, inhibiting uterine contractions. Injectable (subcutaneous) terbutaline should not be used in pregnant women for prevention or prolonged treatment (beyond 48 to 72 hours) of PTL in either the hospital or outpatient setting because of the potential for serious maternal heart problems and death. In addition, oral terbutaline should not be used for prevention or any treatment of PTL because it has not been shown to be effective and has similar safety concerns.
   a. Withhold medication for a maternal pulse greater than 120.
   b. Contraindications: cardiac arrhythmias.
   c. Potential maternal adverse effects: tachycardia, cardiac arrhythmias, pulmonary edema, myocardial ischemia, hypotension, and death.
   d. Potential fetal adverse effects: tachycardia, hyperinsulinemia, hyperglycemia, myocardial or septal hypertrophy, myocardial ischemia.

2. Magnesium sulfate—interferes with smooth-muscle contractility, although its exact mechanism of action is unknown.
   a. Dosage: 4 to 6 g IV piggyback bolus over 15 to 30 minutes and then 1 to 2 g maintenance dose via continuous IV drip.
   b. Contraindications: myasthenia gravis and renal disease.
   c. Potential maternal adverse effects: flushing, lethargy, headache, muscle weakness, diminished DTR, diplopia, dry mouth, pulmonary edema, and cardiac arrest.
   d. Potential fetal adverse effects: lethargy, hypotonia, respiratory depression, and demineralization with prolonged use.
   e. Monitor serum magnesium levels.
   f. Antidote for magnesium toxicity: calcium gluconate.

3. Prostaglandin inhibitors—Indomethacin: inhibits prostaglandin stimulation of contractions; however, after 34 weeks' gestation, indomethacin may cause premature closure of the fetal ductus arteriosus.
   a. Dosage: loading dose of 50 mg orally and then 25 mg orally every 6 hours for 48 hours maximum.
   b. Contraindications: significant renal or hepatic impairment.
   c. Potential maternal adverse effects: nausea, heartburn, postpartum hemorrhage.
   d. Potential fetal adverse effects: constriction of the ductus arteriosus, pulmonary hypertension, reversible decreased renal function with oligohydramnios, intraventricular hemorrhage, hyperbilirubinemia, necrotizing enterocolitis (NEC).

4. Calcium channel blocker—nifedipine: relaxes smooth muscle by inhibiting the transport of calcium negating contraction formation.
   a. Dosage: 10 to 40 mg oral loading dose and then 30 to 60 mg every 8 to 12 hours for 48 hours maximum.
   b. Contraindications: cardiac disease, use caution with renal disease, maternal hypotension (less than 90/50 mm Hg), avoid concomitant use with magnesium sulfate.
   c. Potential maternal adverse effects: flushing, dizziness, headache, nausea, transient hypotension.
   d. Potential fetal adverse effects: none currently known.

5. Antibiotic therapy: several regimens exist for intrapartum antimicrobial prophylaxis for perinatal group B streptococcal (GBS) disease prevention. Treatment should be started as presumptive positive for GBS.

General Contraindications to Tocolytic Therapy
1. Category III FHR patterns.
2. Intra-amniotic infection.
3. Eclampsia or severe preeclampsia.
4. Fetal demise.
5. Fetal maturity.
6. Maternal hemodynamic instability.
7. Severe bleeding of any cause.
8. Fetal anomaly incompatible with life.
9. Severe IUGR.
10. Cervix dilated more than 5 cm.

Acceleration of Fetal Lung Maturity
1. Corticosteroid administration—betamethasone or dexamethasone.
   a. Given to potential PTL patients between 24 and 34 weeks' gestation.
   b. Betamethasone is given IM in two doses of 12 mg each, 24 hours apart.
   c. Dexamethasone is given IM in four doses of 6 mg each, every 12 hours.
      i. Decreases intraventricular hemorrhage (IVH), NEC, and respiratory distress syndrome (RDS), mortality that may be a result of prematurity.
   d. Timely administration is essential; given before delivery to mother; postponing delivery for administration is an option.
   e. Serial administration of the agents is no longer recommended.
   f. Administered to woman at risk for PTB within the next 7 days.

Complications
1. Prematurity and associated neonatal complications include:
   a. Intraventricular hemorrhage (IVH), necrotizing enterocolitis (NEC).
   b. Respiratory distress syndrome (RDS) because of lung immaturity related to lack of surfactant production.
   c. Patent ductus arteriosus (PDA).
   d. Necrotizing enterocolitis (NEC).

Nursing Assessment
During tocolytic therapy, assess the following:
1. Fetal status and uterine activity (UA) data by EFM.
2. Respiratory status (pulmonary edema is an adverse effect).
3. Muscular tremors.
4. Palpitations.
5. Dizziness/light-headedness.
6. Urine output.
7. Patient education to signs and symptoms of PTL.
8. Patient education to signs and symptoms of infection.

Nursing Diagnoses
- Anxiety related to use of tocolytic drugs and change in role function.
- Risk for Injury to fetus secondary to prematurity.
- Potential Complications of Drug Therapy related to tocolytic therapy.
- Ineffective Coping related to situational crisis.

Nursing Interventions
Decreasing Anxiety
1. Know the contraindications and potential complications of tocolytic therapy.
2. Explain the purpose and common adverse effects of tocolytic therapy.
3. Provide accurate information on the status of the fetus and progressive labor.
4. Allow the woman and her support person to verbalize their feelings.
5. Encourage relationship with other patients who are also experiencing PTL.

Minimizing Injury to Fetus
1. Encourage the woman to assume lateral positions that will enhance placental perfusion.
2. Monitor fetal status and labor progress.
3. Assist with delivery of infant, as needed.
4. Notify the interprofessional team of progressing labor.

Minimizing Risk of Drug-Related Complications
1. Maintain accurate intake and output at least per facility protocol based on tocolytic agent and dosing.
2. Assess maternal vital signs in accordance with facility policy. Notify the primary health care provider if maternal pulse greater than 120 beats/minute.
3. Assess for signs and symptoms of pulmonary edema.
4. Assess DTRs per facility policy noting hyporeflexia because of magnesium sulfate infusion; excessive dosage or poor renal clearance may lead to magnesium toxicity.
5. Discontinue infusion if adverse effects occur; notify health care provider.
6. Educate the woman and partner on tocolytic therapy, explaining the purpose and common adverse effects.

Promoting Maternal–Family Coping
1. Provide support and direction, but also encourage private time for woman and partner.
2. Encourage asking questions and verbalization of feelings.
3. Facilitate social worker referral as needed.

Community and Home Care Considerations
1. Ensure that woman meets the following criteria for home management of PTL:
   a. No evidence of active PTL.
   b. No evidence of infection.
   c. Cervical dilatation less than 3 cm.

Patient Education and Health Maintenance
1. Educate the patient about the importance of continuing the pregnancy until term related to improved outcomes with enhanced fetal lung maturity.
2. Encourage compliance with a decreased activity level or bed rest, pelvic rest, adequate nutrition, and hydration.
3. Teach the woman signs and symptoms of infection and to report them immediately.

Evaluation: Expected Outcomes
- Demonstrates concern about treatment and pregnancy outcome.
- No fetal compromise or complications; term delivery.
- Vital signs stable.
- Family focused on maternal–fetal well-being.

Premature Rupture of Membranes

Premature rupture of membranes (PROM) is defined as rupture of the membranes before the onset of labor. PROM is independent of gestational age; when it occurs prior to term it is referred to as preterm PROM. This condition occurs in approximately one third of preterm births and 8% of term pregnancies. PROM increases the risk of variable decelerations in the FHR tracing related to decreased amniotic fluid volume.

Pathophysiology and Etiology

1. Rupture of membranes occurs during the normal course of labor. The exact etiology of PROM is not clearly understood, although nonpathologic causes, such as the combination of stretching of the membranes and biochemical changes, are suspected to contribute; infection has commonly been found to be a primary cause.
2. PROM is manifested by a gush of amniotic fluid or leaking of fluid through the vagina, which usually persists; flow may decrease in the sitting or supine position.

Diagnostic Evaluation

1. Patient history and physical exam.
2. Sterile speculum examination for identification of "pooling" of fluid in the vagina, cervicitis, umbilical or fetal prolapse, and cervical advancement. Collect cultures as appropriate.
3. Nitrazine test—amniotic fluid changes pH paper from yellow–green to blue. False-positives may result when blood, semen, alkaline antiseptics, and bacterial vaginosis are present.
4. Fern test—swab of the posterior vaginal fornix is taken to obtain amniotic fluid. Positive test will reveal arborization or "ferning" (visually appears as a fern leaf) on a slide viewed under a microscope.
5. Ultrasound to assess amniotic fluid volume.

Management (>34 Weeks)

1. When PROM is confirmed, the gestational age, fetal presentation, and well-being will determine if hospitalization is warranted.
2. At any gestational age, a patient with evident intrauterine infection, placental abruption, or evidence of category III FHR pattern is best cared for by expeditious delivery.
3. If immediate delivery is not indicated, cultures of the cervix should be obtained to identify best antibiotic management (chlamydia, gonorrhea, and group B beta-hemolytic *Streptococcus*, if appropriate).
4. Expectant management: offer adequate time for the latent phase of labor to progress (may be as long as hours to days or at the discretion of the primary practitioner) and EFM.
   a. Vaginal examinations are kept to a minimum to prevent infection.
   b. Once the decision to deliver is made, GBS prophylaxis should be initiated based on prior culture results or risk factors.
5. Active management:
   a. Oxytocin induction/augmentation may be initiated at the time of presentation to reduce:
      i. Risk of chorioamnionitis.
      ii. Postpartum febrile morbidity.
      iii. Neonatal antibiotic treatments.

Complications

1. Maternal infection—intrapartum (chorioamnionitis) and postpartum (endometritis).
2. Potential increased rates of cesarean delivery.
3. Fetal or neonatal infection or compromise.

Nursing Assessment

1. Evaluate maternal BP, respirations, pulse, and temperature per facility policy. Temperatures should be done every 2 hours. If temperature or pulse is elevated, continue monitoring more frequently.
2. Monitor the amount and type of amniotic fluid that is leaking. Observe for purulent, foul-smelling discharge that may indicate chorioamnionitis and report immediately.
3. Assess patient periodically for diffuse abdominal pain or pain on palpation, signs of increased infection.
4. Evaluate periodic CBC with differentials results; any shift to the left (ie, increase of immature forms of neutrophils/WBCs) signals infection.
5. Communicate any findings related to signs of infection to the primary practitioner and perinatal team.
6. Evaluate fetal status per facility policy depending on stages of labor; maternal infection is the primary cause of fetal tachycardia.
7. Allow patient activity as clinical status warrants.

Nursing Diagnosis

- Risk for Infection related to ascending bacteria, rupture of amniotic sac.

Nursing Interventions

Preventing Infection

1. Evaluate amount and odor of amniotic fluid leakage.
2. Use sterile gloves with vaginal exams that should be kept to a minimum.
3. Place patient on disposable pads to collect leaking fluid and change pads every 1 to 2 hours or more frequently, as needed.
4. Review the need for good hand-washing technique and hygiene after urination and defecation.
5. Monitor FHR and fetal activity per facility policy, as indicated.
6. Monitor maternal temperature, pulse respirations, BP, and uterine tenderness frequently, as indicated.
7. Administer GBS therapy or antibiotics, as indicated.

Evaluation: Expected Outcomes

- No signs of infection.

Preterm Premature Rupture of Membranes

Preterm premature rupture of membranes (PPROM) is defined as rupture of membranes before 37 completed weeks' gestation without the onset of spontaneous labor. Regardless of management or clinical presentation, delivery within 1 week is the most likely outcome. However, approximately 3% to 13% of patients can anticipate cessation of fluid leakage and possible restoration of normal amniotic fluid volume over remaining course of gestation.

PPROM patients are at high risk for infection during the intrapartum and postpartum phases. Secondary complications include fetal malpresentation, placental abruption, and prematurity. Neonatal complications are respiratory distress syndrome, infection, and death.

Pathophysiology and Etiology

1. Although the exact cause is unknown, PPROM is likely to be either a pathologic intrinsic weakness or related to an extrinsic factor that causes the membranes to rupture prematurely.
2. The primary cause of PPROM is infection, particularly in earlier gestations (amnionitis; group B beta-hemolytic *Streptococcus*).
3. Other causes:
   a. History of PROM/PTB.
   b. Low body mass index (less than 19.8).
   c. Nutritional deficiencies.
   d. Connective tissue disorders.
   e. Maternal smoking.
   f. Cervical conization or cerclage.
   g. Pulmonary disease.
   h. Uterine overdistention.
   i. Amniocentesis.

See PROM, page 1057, and Preterm Labor, page 1054, for management and nursing interventions.

Induction and Augmentation of Labor

 EVIDENCE BASE Troiano, N., Harvey, C., & Chez, B. (Eds.). (2013). *High-risk and critical care obstetrics* (3rd ed.). Philadelphia, PA: Lippincott Williams & Wilkins.

Association of Women's Health, Obstetric, Neonatal Nurses. (2011). AWHONN Position statement: Non-medically indicated induction and augmentation of labor. *Journal of Obstetric, Gynecologic, and Neonatal Nursing, 40,* 665–666.

Induction of labor (IOL) refers to utilization of exogenous labor enhancement agents or procedures resulting in rhythmic contractions and spontaneous onset of labor. Cervical ripening utilizes medications and procedures to effect the physical properties (softening and dilation) of the cervix in preparation for labor and delivery. Benefits of induction must outweigh the risks to the maternal–fetal unit. Inductions may be medically indicated or elective. Elective procedures prior to 39 completed weeks of gestation are contraindicated.

Augmentation refers to the administration of uterine stimulants once labor dystocia (dysfunction) ensues. Dysfunctional labor may result for several reasons (outlined in the next section) and remains the number one cause for primary cesarean deliveries. Similar medications are utilized for induction, augmentation, and sometimes cervical ripening.

Indications for Induction

Medically Indicated

1. Abruptio placentae.
2. Chorioamnionitis (intra-amniotic infection).
3. Fetal demise.
4. Hypertensive disorders: chronic, gestational, preeclampsia, or eclampsia.
5. Premature rupture of membranes.
6. Postterm pregnancy.
7. Maternal medical conditions: diabetes mellitus, renal disease, chronic pulmonary disease, or underlying cardiac disease.
8. Fetal conditions: severe fetal growth restriction, anomalies, isoimmunization, evolving category II FHR pattern, or category III FHR pattern, oligohydramnios.

Elective

1. Patient or provider preference.
2. Logistic reasons: risk of rapid labor, distance from hospital.
3. Psychosocial indications.
4. In addition to the other reasons for elective induction, there must also be fetal lung maturity or 39 or more weeks' gestational age determined by one of the following criteria:
   a. Fetal heart tones documented from 20 weeks onward by nonelectronic fetoscope or for at least 30 weeks by Doppler.
   b. Thirty-six weeks or more since a positive serum or urine hCG pregnancy test from a reliable laboratory.
   c. An ultrasound measurement of the crown to rump length obtained at 6 to 12 weeks, which supports a gestational age of at least 39 weeks.
   d. An ultrasound examination between 13 and 20 weeks, confirming at least 39 weeks' gestation as determined by clinical history and physical exam.

Contraindications for Induction

1. Vaginal bleeding, known placenta previa or vasa previa.
2. Abnormal presentation: transverse or funic (cord).
3. Previous transfundal ("classic") uterine incision or extensive myomectomy.
4. Pelvic structural deformities.
5. Active or culture-proven genital herpes infection.
6. Invasive cervical carcinoma.
7. Umbilical cord prolapse.
8. Fetal presenting part above pelvic inlet.
9. Category III FHR pattern.

Indications for Augmentation

1. Uterine hypocontractility.
2. Dystocia (slow, abnormal progression of labor).
3. Augmentation should be considered in the absence of cervical change if the frequency of contractions is less than 3 over 10 minutes or the intensity of contractions is less than 25 mm Hg above baseline with intrauterine pressure catheter or both.

Contraindications for Augmentation

1. Same as induction.

Management

Bishop score refers to a scoring system that documents cervical favorability, giving a score of 0 to 3 for each of five parameters: dilation, position of cervix, effacement, station, and cervical consistency. With a Bishop score of 8 or greater, the likelihood of a vaginal delivery is similar to spontaneous labor. A Bishop score should be documented along with fetal presentation prior to induction.

Cervical Ripening

Cervical ripening is performed if induction is indicated and the cervix is unfavorable. Typically, the cervix is evaluated according to the Bishop pelvic scoring system; if the score is 8 or more, the probability of vaginal delivery after labor induction is similar to that of spontaneous labor.

1. Mechanical methods:
   a. Laminaria digitata—a seaweed preparation that is inserted directly into and dilates the cervix by absorption of water.
   b. Transcervical balloon catheter is inserted through the cervix, balloon is inflated, and gentle traction is applied to dilate the cervix.

2. Prostaglandin E₂ (PGE₂): Dinoprostone is a solid, time-released 10 mg insert placed into the vagina and can be removed.
   a. Requires continuous fetal monitoring as evidenced by manufacturer and research guidelines.
   b. Keep frozen until immediately before use; unstable at room temperature; stable up to 3 years when frozen.
   c. Patient is to remain supine for 2 hours after insertion; may ambulate after 2 hours if EFM telemetry is available for continuous monitoring.
   d. Removal may be required if evidence of uterine tachysystole response or fetal intolerance (evolving FHR category II or category III pattern).
   e. Removal after 12 hours or at onset of labor; oxytocin should be delayed at least 30 to 60 minutes after removal.
   f. Should be administered at or near labor and delivery/birthing suite with continuous EFM to monitor fetal and uterine status and for at least 15 minutes after removal.
3. PGE₂ gel is given via catheter or diaphragm (pessary) in doses ranging from 0.5 to 5 mg.
   a. Unstable at room temperature; store in refrigerator; bring to room temperature just before administration (do not use microwave; warm water, or any other heating method to speed the warming process as the gel is sensitive to heat and may be inactivated).
   b. Patient should stay recumbent for at least 30 minutes. If no response, additional doses may be administered every 6 hours.
   c. Uterine tachysystole is a complication with increased risk of uterine rupture.
   d. Removal may be required if evidence of uterine tachysystole response or fetal intolerance (evolving FHR category II or category III pattern).
   e. Oxytocin should be delayed for 6 to 12 hours after last dose of gel.
   f. Should be administered at or near labor and delivery/birthing suite (to monitor fetal and uterine status—continue monitoring for 30 minutes to 2 hours after administration).

Stripping/Swiping of Membranes
1. Mechanical method of induction.
2. Following a cervical exam, the procedure entails separating the membranes from the lower uterine segment, without rupturing the membranes, to induce labor.
3. Complications include maternal–fetal infection, PPROM, umbilical cord prolapse, precipitous labor and birth, and maternal discomfort.

Amniotomy
1. Mechanical method of induction through artificial rupture of membranes (AROM).
2. Insert amnihook through cervix and perform a slight twisting motion to catch a small area of the membranes. Fluid should be clear or cloudy without odor.
3. Data show when amniotomy is used alone it has unpredictable results with often long intervals before the onset of labor; increasing risk of infection.
4. Utilized with oxytocin at onset, induction to delivery is shorter than with amniotomy alone.
5. Monitor UA and FHR data at periodic intervals.
6. Complications include umbilical cord prolapse or compression and possible maternal or fetal infection.

Pharmacologic Methods of Induction
1. Prostaglandin E₁–misoprostol is not FDA-approved but has off-label use for cervical ripening or labor induction.

   a. Various dosing regimens are available; however, lower doses are associated with less uterine tachysystole; 25 to 50 mcg administered orally or intravaginally—every 4 hours.
   b. Adverse effects include shivering, backache, vomiting, diarrhea, shortness of breath, uterine hypertonus, or uterine rupture.
   c. Redosing is withheld if more than five contractions occur in 10 minutes, adequate cervical ripening is achieved (cervix 80% effaced and 3 cm dilated), the patient is in active labor, or FHR category III pattern.
   d. Patient should be observed for up to 2 hours after spontaneous rupture of membranes. If the cervix remains unfavorable, the uterine activity is minimal, there is absence of category III FHR pattern, and the last dose was given at least 3 hours, redosing is acceptable.
   e. Oxytocin can be initiated 4 hours after the last dose.
   f. Misoprostol should be administered at or near the labor and delivery/birthing suite to allow continuous monitoring of fetal and uterine status.

 DRUG ALERT Misoprostol is not recommended for women with a history of prior cesarean delivery or other uterine scarring (myomectomy).

2. Oxytocin is naturally produced peptide hormone by hypothalamus and released by the posterior pituitary. Synthetic oxytocin is one of the most common drugs utilized in the United States. Based on pharmacokinetic studies, uterine response begins within 3 to 5 minutes of infusion and reaches a steady state in 40 minutes; however, patient sensitivity varies. Cervical dilation, parity, and gestational age predict the dose response of oxytocin.
   a. Oxytocin infusion is administered as a secondary infusion connected to the lowest port of the primary IV. Solution concentrations vary and may be mixed by pharmacy or on labor and delivery by a staff registered nurse per facility policy. Oxytocin is only given via infusion pump accompanied by constant monitoring of maternal and fetal status with EFM in the inpatient setting.
   b. Due to the antidiuretic property of oxytocin, water intoxication may occur, which can lead to heart failure. Symptoms of water intoxification include headache, nausea and vomiting, mental confusion, decreased urine output, hypotension, tachycardia, and cardiac arrhythmia.
   c. Dosing requirements adequate for labor vary as low-and high-dose options. Typical starting doses vary from 0.5 to 2 milliunits (mU) and increasing 1 to 2 mU every 30 to 60 minutes until an adequate contraction pattern is achieved.
   d. The goal is to establish regular uterine contractions leading to cervical change and fetal descent. Cervical dilation of 0.5 to 1 cm/hour in the active phase of labor—contractions occurring every 2 to 3 minutes lasting 60 to 90 seconds and an intensity of 50 to 70 mm Hg (moderate) or greater than 180 Montevideo units but less than 400. Montevideo units are measures using an intrauterine pressure catheter.

 NURSING ALERT Be aware that cervical dilation, effacement, and subsequent fetal descent are the true indicators of adequate labor progression, not uterine activity.

e. If oxytocin is discontinued for 20 to 30 minutes, it may be restarted at least below the prior rate of infusion, once reassuring UA and FHR data are established. However, if the oxytocin has been discontinued for over 30 to 40 minutes, it must be restarted at the initial dose.

3. Complications of oxytocin include:
   a. Uterine tachysystole (more than 5 contractions in 10 minutes).
   b. Uterine hypertonus (resting tone greater than 20 to 25 mm Hg, depending on the type of intrauterine pressure catheter; intensity greater than 80 mm Hg).
   c. Contractions longer than 2 minutes in duration.
   d. Increased incidence of cesarean delivery.
   e. Hypotension with rapid infusion.
   f. Uterine tachysystole accompanied by fetal bradycardia may be treated with tocolytics prior to emergent delivery, if indicated.

Nursing Assessment

Prior to Induction of Labor
1. Obtain an NST to assess fetal well-being.
2. Evaluate maternal vital signs, especially BP.
3. Place an IV and evaluate patency prior to initiation.
4. Follow facility policy. Fetal presentation, Bishop score, fetal assessment, and vaginal exam should be documented prior to IOL.

Following Administration of Oxytocin
1. Monitor FHR and uterine activity every 30 minutes and as indicated.
2. Assess maternal vital signs in accordance with facility policy; BP and pulse should be assessed at each dose interval.
3. Limit vaginal examinations, especially after the membranes have ruptured.
4. Maintain intake and output records and watch for signs of water intoxication—dizziness, headache, confusion, nausea and vomiting, hypotension, tachycardia, and decreased urine output.

Nursing Diagnoses

- Anxiety related to medical interventions and maternal fetal outcomes.
- Risk for Impaired Tissue Perfusion: Placental, related to hyperstimulatory uterine response.
- Acute Pain related to uterine activity and evolution of labor and birth process.

Nursing Interventions

Decreasing Anxiety
1. On admission, review hospital policies and protocols for induction with patient and partner.
2. Solicit feedback related to birth plan and cultural preferences.
3. Teach or review the use of relaxation and distraction techniques.
4. Answer questions and offer emotional support.

Enhancing Uteroplacental Oxygenation
1. Assess fetal status and uterine contractions periodically. Assess for signs of uteroplacental insufficiency (minimal-absent variability, abnormal baseline FHR, recurrent or repetitive late or variable decelerations).
2. Place patient in lateral position and assess vital signs; increase IV fluids if hypotension occurs.

3. Administer prescribed oxygen (8 to 10 L/minute by nonrebreather face mask) if nonreassuring FHR characteristics develop (evolving category II or category III FHR pattern) and notify provider.
4. If any persistent hyperstimulatory uterine response (eg, tachysystole or hypertonus) develops, discontinue the augmentation or induction agent, if possible; induce intrauterine resuscitation techniques; and notify health care provider immediately. Administer tocolytics, as ordered, and prepare for emergent cesarean delivery.

Pain Control
1. Encourage use of breathing/relaxation techniques, distraction, positioning, and nonpharmacologic comfort measures.
2. Encourage active partner participation.
3. Administer analgesia/anesthesia as requested and prescribed.
4. Support mother and partner through the process with presence and empathy.

Evaluation: Expected Outcomes

- Verbalizes understanding of the induction process.
- No evidence of hyperstimulatory uterine response or category III FHR pattern.
- Labor progressing and pain controlled.

Dystocia

Dystocia is characterized by slow, abnormal labor progression typically resulting from abnormal uterine activity patterns or maternal expulsive forces. Dystocia is the leading indication for augmentation and primary cesarean delivery. Causes include power (contractions), passageway (pelvis), or passenger (fetus) abnormalities. (Refer to Chapter 37.)

Pathophysiology and Etiology

Power Abnormalities
1. Inadequate contractions result in poor labor progression and slow fetal descent. Common causes include increased uterine tone, abnormal contraction pressure, hypotonic labor (prolonged latent phase, protracted or arrested active phase, or prolonged second stage of labor), and abnormal contraction pressure.
2. Problems with the force of labor result in ineffective contractions or bearing-down efforts (pushing) during the second stage of labor.
3. Etiology of abnormalities in the force of labor includes:
   a. Early or excessive use of analgesia.
   b. Overdistention of the uterus (hydramnios, macrosomia, multiple gestation).
   c. Excessive cervical rigidity.
   d. Grand multiparity (greater than 6).

Passageway Abnormalities
1. Abnormalities in the passageway may be the result of pelvic or soft tissue anomalies.
2. Pelvic abnormalities that interfere with the engagement, descent, and expulsion of the fetus include:
   a. Size and shape of the pelvis.
   b. Obstruction that may result from soft tissue problems, such as a uterine or ovarian fibromyoma, and obesity.
3. Contractions of the inlet are noted when the anteroposterior diameter is less than 10 cm or the greatest transverse diameter is less than 12 cm. Contracted inlets may be of genetic origin or a result of rickets.

4. Cephalopelvic disproportion (CPD) is a disparity between the size of the maternal pelvis and fetal head that prevents or precludes fetal descent and subsequent vaginal birth; cesarean birth is indicated if unresolved.

Passenger Abnormalities

1. Breech presentations occur in approximately 3% of all deliveries.
   a. This presentation is more common in multiple gestations, increased parity, hydramnios, congenital dislocated hip, placenta previa, and preterm neonates.
   b. Usually, the method of choice for delivery is a cesarean delivery.
2. Shoulder presentation (transverse lie) occurs when the infant lies perpendicular to the maternal spine and cervical os. The infant is delivered by cesarean delivery if external cephalic version (ECV) is unsuccessful.
3. A large fetus increases the risk of trauma, both maternal and fetal; CPD may result.

Diagnostic Evaluation

1. Inadequate progress of cervical effacement, dilation, or descent of the presenting part as determined by vaginal examination.
2. Comparison of serial evaluations of labor progress using Friedman curve criteria, if available.
   a. A prolonged latent phase in the primigravida is greater than 20 hours and greater than 14 hours in the multigravida.
   b. During the active phase, the cervix of a primigravida will normally dilate at a rate of 1.2 cm/hour and a multigravida 1.5 cm/hour. In addition, the fetus should descend at a typical rate of 1 cm/hour in a primigravida and 2 cm/hour for a multigravida.

Management

1. Treatment for contraction abnormalities involves stimulation of labor through the use of labor enhancement medications such as oxytocin (see page 1059); an intrauterine pressure catheter may be utilized for direct assessment of uterine contraction data.
2. Management for maternal passageway or fetal passenger problems involves delivery in the safest manner for the mother and fetus.
   a. If the problem is related to the inlet or midpelvis, a cesarean delivery is indicated.
   b. If the problem is related to the pelvic outlet, an operative vaginal delivery with forceps or vacuum extraction may be performed.

Complications

1. Maternal exhaustion.
2. Infection.
3. Postpartum hemorrhage.
4. Fetal intolerance: evolving category II or category III FHR patterns.
5. Fetal or maternal trauma from operative vaginal delivery.

Nursing Assessment

1. Perform Leopold maneuvers and evaluate fetal presentation, position, and size.
2. Using Friedman labor curve, periodically evaluate progress of labor.

3. Monitor FHR and contraction status periodically per facility policy.

Nursing Diagnoses

- Acute Pain related to physical and psychological factors of difficult labor.
- Anxiety related to threat of possible operative delivery.

Nursing Interventions

Promoting Comfort

1. Review relaxation techniques.
2. Encourage use of breathing techniques learned in prenatal classes.
3. Encourage frequent change of position, especially the use of the upright posture to facilitate descent.
4. Encourage voiding at regular intervals to decompress the bladder.
5. Provide back rubs and sacral pressure, as needed.
6. Offer ice chips and clear fluids as permitted.
7. Provide frequent encouragement to the woman and her support person.
8. Administer pain medication as ordered.
9. Assist with the administration of anesthesia, as requested and indicated.

Decreasing Anxiety

1. Provide anticipatory guidance regarding labor process and progress, the use of medication, equipment, and procedures.
2. Educate the woman regarding augmentation agents: oxytocin.
3. Prepare the family for cesarean delivery, if necessary.

Evaluation: Expected Outcomes

- Verbalizes increased comfort.
- Verbalizes understanding of procedures.

Shoulder Dystocia

Shoulder dystocia is the dysfunctional descent and expulsion of the fetal shoulders, resulting in impaction of the anterior shoulder behind the maternal pubis symphysis or posterior shoulder on the sacral promontory during the second stage of labor. This condition is often relieved with gentle manipulation but may turn into an obstetric emergency within minutes. Approximately 50% of shoulder dystocia incidents have no risk factors.

Pathophysiology and Etiology

1. Antepartum risk factors:
   a. Fetal macrosomia.
   b. Maternal diabetes.
   c. Fetal macrosomia more than 5,000 g or more than 4,500 g with maternal diabetes (women with 2 or more risk factors have highest rate of shoulder dystocia).
   d. Postterm gestation.
   e. Previous history of shoulder dystocia, macrosomia, or postterm pregnancy.
2. Intrapartum factors:
   a. Labor induction.
   b. Epidural anesthesia.
   c. Protraction or arrest of labor.
   d. Prolonged second stage.
   e. Operative vaginal delivery.
3. None of the risk factors noted above individually, or collectively, can predict shoulder dystocia. Facilities should develop

interprofessional protocols to effectively manage and anticipate shoulder dystocia at every delivery. Simulation exercises are recommended to enhance team communication and function during this emergency.

Management

1. Compare labor progression to a labor progression model such as the Friedman labor graph per facility policy, and communicate dysfunctional patterns early and prepare accordingly.
2. Prevention is the key because shoulder dystocia is difficult to predict.
   a. Early identification and treatment of gestational diabetes mellitus.
   b. Antepartum glucose control of insulin-dependent diabetes mellitus.
   c. Periodic estimated fetal weight measurements; third-trimester ultrasound measurements are significantly inaccurate.
   d. Avoid postterm deliveries.
   e. Prevent abnormal progression of labor or treat early.
   f. Promote adequate maternal weight gain.
3. Once shoulder dystocia is identified, the following interventions may be indicated based on individual clinical conditions:
   a. Document the time shoulder dystocia is called.
   b. Perform appropriate nursing maneuvers and assist with appropriate medical maneuvers, if applicable (see below). Fundal pressure is contraindicated. Performing fundal pressure may further impact the shoulder; utilize other maneuvers to dislodge shoulder.
   c. Call for assistance to support maneuvers and to treat immediate postpartum complications.
   d. Notify neonatal team.
   e. Document delivery time and calculate total time frame from the delivery of the fetal head to the delivery of the infant. List all maneuvers performed during incident, time of application, and individual(s) who performed the intervention(s). Record Apgar scores and neonatal resuscitative interventions, if applicable. Lastly, manage and document any postpartum complications.
   f. Perform critical assessment of neonate after delivery, particularly face and upper limbs.
4. Nursing maneuvers; begin with least invasive; no particular order is recommended:
   a. McRoberts maneuver—exaggerated flexion of the mother's legs, simulating a supine squat position. The squat position increases pelvic diameter by 1 to 3 cm.
   b. Suprapubic pressure—place the heel or palm of one hand over the suprapubic area and press down and to the left or right, as directed by the primary practitioner, to assist in dislodging the anterior shoulder under the maternal pubic bone. Have a step stool available to assist position of staff.
   c. Gaskin maneuver—Hands-and-knees position; assist the patient onto her hands and knees in an "all-fours" position; it is suspected the anterior shoulder drops posteriorly in this position, releasing the dystocia and resulting in delivery. This may be difficult but obtainable in the patient with epidural anesthesia.
5. Medical maneuvers:
   a. Episiotomy is no longer routinely recommended and is performed based on clinical presentation.
   b. Rotation of the anterior shoulder to oblique position.
   c. Barnum maneuver-delivery of posterior arm across fetal chest.
   d. Rubin maneuver—displacement of the posterior shoulder anteriorly, with respect to fetus.
   e. Wood screw maneuver—rotation of the shoulders to an oblique position.
   f. Zavanelli maneuver—replacement of the head by reverse cardinal movements into the vagina and delivery by cesarean.

Complications

Fetal

1. Fetal hypoxia and asphyxia; neonatal hypoxic ischemic encephalopathy.
2. Brachial plexus injury.
3. Fractured clavicle or humerus.
4. Facial nerve paralysis.
5. Neuropsychiatric dysfunction or death.

Maternal

1. Postpartum hemorrhage.
2. Vaginal lacerations.
3. Cervical lacerations.

Nursing Assessment

1. Continuously evaluate labor curve for signs of dystocia.
2. Maintain EFM until delivery is successful.
3. Notify all perinatal team members of delivery time frame.

Nursing Diagnoses

- Fear and Anxiety related to inability of fetus to deliver.
- Acute Pain associated with operative and instrumented procedures or uterine manipulation.
- Risk for Injury to fetus or mother secondary to instrumented delivery or manual maneuvers.

Nursing Interventions

Reducing Fear and Anxiety

1. Inform patient of complication and offer support.
2. Limit family members in the delivery room should shoulder dystocia occur, as additional health care personnel may be required.
3. Keep voice calm and controlled during delivery process.
4. Keep patient focused on pushing efforts and positioning.

Decreasing Pain

1. Maintain appropriate anesthesia/analgesia for pain relief during maneuvers.
2. Offer additional anesthesia/analgesia after delivery, as needed or indicated.

Reducing Risk of Injury

See Nursing maneuvers above.

Evaluation: Expected Outcomes

- Verbalizes understanding of situation and is cooperative with plan.
- Verbalizes control of pain.
- No maternal or neonatal injury.

Uterine Rupture

 EVIDENCE BASE American College of Obstetricians and Gynecologists. (2010/Reaffirmed 2017). *Vaginal birth after cesarean* (Practice Bulletin #115). Washington, DC: Author.

Uterine rupture is a spontaneous or traumatic tear in the uterus exposing the internal uterine compartment to the peritoneal cavity; extrusion of the umbilical cord, fetus, or fetal parts may occur. *Uterine dehiscence* occurs due to partial separation of an old scar prior to full rupture. Uterine rupture is a rare, catastrophic event with significant risk of maternal, fetal, and neonatal morbidity and mortality.

Pathophysiology and Etiology

Risk factors:
1. Number of prior cesarean births and scar type (vertical uterine incision).
2. Interpregnancy interval (time frame of the end of one gestation to the beginning of the subsequent gestation).
3. Trial of labor after cesarean (TOLAC).
4. Uterine closure technique: single-layer closure has higher risk over double-layer closure.
5. Trauma.
6. Obstetric maneuvers.
7. Uterine abnormalities.

Clinical Manifestations

Clinical manifestations depend on location, size, and duration of rupture. Clinical conditions may evolve acutely (within minutes) or chronically (hours) during the intrapartum period. Signs and symptoms may be absent or present individually or collectively.
1. Constant abdominal pain and tenderness (may be dulled by anesthesia or analgesia).
2. Uterine contractions will usually continue but may diminish in intensity and tone.
3. Vaginal or abdominal bleeding into the peritoneal cavity.
4. Nausea/vomiting.
5. Syncope.
6. Vital sign instability: early (tachycardia, tachypnea, hypertension); late (signs of shock: rapid, weak pulse); hypotension; cold, clammy skin; pale color.
7. Uteroplacental insufficiency as evidenced by evolving category II or category III FHR patterns.
8. Clinical signs of placental abruption or cord prolapse (sudden onset of FHR variable decelerations).

Management

1. Immediate stabilization of maternal hemodynamics followed by emergent cesarean delivery. Anticipatory preparations may require intraoperative blood component therapy.
2. Fetus is delivered expeditiously and neonatal resuscitation is performed, as indicated. The uterus is repaired, if possible; otherwise, a hysterectomy may be indicated.
3. Adequate fluid replacement is maintained.
4. Antibiotic therapy.

Complications

Maternal
1. Urologic injury.
2. Hysterectomy.
3. Concurrent complete or partial abruptio placentae; hemorrhage.
4. Hypovolemic shock.
5. Severe blood loss or anemia, with possibility of transfusion.
6. Bowel laceration, with possibility of peritonitis.
7. Infection.
8. Death.

Fetal
1. Hypoxia leading to fetal acidosis and perinatal asphyxia (occurs 39% to 91%).
2. Hypoxic–ischemic encephalopathy; neonatal brain injury.
3. Death.

Nursing Assessment

1. Continuously evaluate maternal vital signs for clinical triggers of decompensation.
2. Observe for signs and symptoms of impending rupture periodically during labor progression, particularly during VBAC delivery or a history of uterine surgery (see Box 39-2).
3. Assess fetal status by continuous monitoring.
4. Communicate with family and debrief them on event following stabilization of mother and newborn as HIPAA allows.

Nursing Diagnoses

- Deficient Fluid Volume related to active fluid loss secondary to hemorrhage.
- Risk for Decreased Cardiac Tissue Perfusion: Maternal and Fetal, related to hypovolemia.
- Fear related to outcome for fetus and mother.

Nursing Interventions

Maintaining Fluid Volume
1. Maintain primary IV line and start a secondary line, as indicated by the patient's condition; if patient is unstable with lactated Ringer solution with rapid infusion.
2. Monitor vital signs frequently to observe for maternal decompensation.

BOX 39-2 Vaginal Birth After Cesarean

- Selection criteria to identify women eligible for vaginal birth after cesarean (VBAC):
  - One or two low-transverse cesarean births.
  - Clinically adequate pelvis.
  - No other uterine scars or previous rupture.
  - Physician (capable of monitoring labor and performing an emergent cesarean delivery) is immediately available throughout active labor.
  - Anesthesia and surgical team available for emergent cesarean delivery.
- Contraindications for VBAC (because of high risk of uterine rupture):
  - Prior classic or T-shaped incision or other transfundal uterine surgery.
  - Contracted pelvis.
  - Medical or obstetric complication that prevents/precludes vaginal delivery.
  - Inability to perform emergency cesarean delivery because of unavailability of surgeon, anesthesia provider, sufficient personnel, physician capable of performing cesarean delivery, or sufficient facility.

3. Assist with and maintain central venous pressure and arterial lines, as indicated, for hemodynamic monitoring.
4. Maintain bed rest to decrease metabolic demands.
5. Place indwelling urinary catheter and monitor urine output hourly or as indicated.
6. Obtain and administer blood component therapy, per obstetric hemorrhage (OH) guidelines.
7. Monitor for signs of DIC—spontaneous bleeding from IV sites, oral mucous membranes, and vagina; bruising.

Maintaining Maternal Vital Organ and Fetal Tissue Perfusion

1. Administer oxygen using a face mask at 8 to 10 L/minute or as indicated; prolonged use prior to delivery is not recommended unless clinical conditions dictate.
2. Apply pulse oximeter and monitor oxygen saturation, as indicated. Pulse oximeter is unreliable during episodes of severe hemorrhage; therefore, monitor patient closely.
3. Monitor arterial blood gas levels and serum electrolyte levels, as indicated, to assess respiratory status, observing for hypoxemia and electrolyte imbalance.
4. Continually monitor maternal vital signs and FHR and UA data on EFM for clinical triggers of decompensation; rapid deterioration may indicate shock and report any abnormalities to the health care team.
5. Evaluate actual blood loss as determined by weight.

Reducing Fear

1. Offer explanation and answer questions of events and procedures to the patient and her support person.
2. Maintain a quiet and calm atmosphere to enhance relaxation.
3. Remain with the patient during anesthesia administration; offer support, as needed.
4. Update family members on the current situation, while the woman is in surgery, and then again postoperatively. Debrief family with the family about the emergency situation and discuss expected outcomes of mother and newborn.

Patient Education and Health Maintenance

1. Provide information and support regarding the possibility for future pregnancies.
2. Encourage the support of family and friends.
3. Offer dietary options high in iron to improve secondary anemia.
4. Inform patient of the postoperative care to reduce risk for thrombophlebitis, pneumonia, infection, and inadequate pain management.

Evaluation: Expected Outcomes

- Vital signs stable; no evidence of shock.
- Hemoglobin and hematocrit stable.
- Verbalizes concerns about self and her fetus.

Amniotic Fluid Embolism

Amniotic fluid embolism (AFE), also known as *anaphylactic syndrome of pregnancy*, is an unpredictable and unpreventable catastrophic even occurring once amniotic fluid containing fetal cells and debris enters the maternal circulation. Deposits of fluid or debris into the pulmonary arterioles result in rapid onset of respiratory distress, shock, and possible development of DIC. The incidence is 1 in 10,000 to 1 in 80,000 pregnancies with a mortality rate of 60% to 90%.

Pathophysiology and Etiology

1. The exact mechanism or portal of entry is uncertain, yet many researchers have postulated the following theories:
   a. Fluid and debris may enter through small endocervical tears, vessels of the lower uterine segment, or cervical veins.
   b. Diffusion across amniotic membranes.
   c. Once fluid and debris enter the maternal vasculature, the maternal system may stimulate an immunologic (allergic) response to the foreign entity similar to rejection of a transplanted organ or infusion of the wrong blood type; this often stimulates the coagulation system, resulting in DIC (see Figure 39-5).
   d. Debris may be large enough to block the perfusion through the pulmonary artery, leading to pulmonary hypertension and right-sided heart failure; over a short time, subsequent left-sided heart failure ensues, accompanied by hypoxia and acidosis.
2. If prolonged, DIC, shock, and cardiopulmonary collapse may occur.
3. It can occur in the intrapartum or postpartum period.
4. Although AFE is unpredictable, the following conditions have a potentially higher association to AFE.
   a. Intrapartum period.
   b. Multiparous.
   c. Abruptio placentae.
   d. Multiple gestations.
   e. Genetic influences.
   f. Previous cesarean delivery.
   g. Chorioamnionitis.
   h. Hydramnios.

Clinical Manifestations

1. Sudden dyspnea and chest pain.
2. Cyanosis, tachycardia.
3. Pulmonary edema.
4. Seizures.
5. Increasing restlessness and anxiety.
6. Feeling of impending doom.
7. DIC.
8. Cardiac dysrhythmias.
9. Cardiopulmonary collapse.

Diagnostic Evaluation

1. Clinical picture of sudden onset of respiratory collapse, shock, and cardiopulmonary arrest.
2. DIC confirmed by coagulation studies (prolonged thrombin time, PT, and PPT; decreased factor V, VIII, X; decreased platelets; increased fibrin split products).
3. Pulmonary aspirate evaluation for fetal cells.
4. Autopsy evaluation to confirm fetal cells and debris intravascularly.

Management

Also see Disseminated Intravascular Coagulation, page 772.

1. Respiratory support with oxygen therapy and intubation, as necessary.
2. Administration of IV crystalloid fluids in the treatment of shock.

Figure 39-5. Pathogenesis of disseminated intravascular coagulation from amniotic fluid embolism.

3. Administration of blood component therapy to combat hemorrhage, shock, and DIC.
4. Establishment of a pulmonary artery catheter, if appropriate.
5. Cardiopulmonary resuscitation in a wedge position or abdominal displacement if undelivered.
6. Perimortem cesarean delivery within 5 minutes of cardiopulmonary collapse.

Nursing Assessment and Interventions

See page 773 for additional nursing care.
1. Be alert and suspicious to signs and symptoms of potential AFE and patients at risk (see above risk factors).
2. Monitor maternal vital signs to assess for signs of shock.
3. Monitor FHR if undelivered.
4. Administer oxygen to assist respiratory status.
5. Alert the interprofessional team immediately and assist with emergency procedures, such as delivery and cardiopulmonary resuscitation, as needed.
6. Provide information and comfort to the family or support persons as the situation allows.

Umbilical Cord Prolapse

If the umbilical cord precedes the presenting part of the fetus or lies adjacent to the primary presenting part, prolapse has occurred. Types of cord prolapse include:

Complete—the cord completely and significantly precedes the primary fetal presenting part; may be in the vagina or visible outside the introitus.
Occult—the cord is beside or just in front of the presenting part of the fetus (hidden).
Funic—the cord can be felt on vaginal examination through intact membranes preceding the fetal presenting part.

Pathophysiology and Etiology

Predisposing factors include:
1. Rupture of membranes before the presenting part is engaged in the pelvis.
2. More common in abnormal fetal positions, such as shoulder and foot presentations.
3. Prematurity.
4. Polyhydramnios (hydramnios).
5. Multifetal gestation.
6. Cephalopelvic disproportion.
7. Abnormally long umbilical cord.
8. Result of interventions or maneuvers (ie, external cephalic version or amniotomy).
9. Low-lying placenta.

Clinical Manifestations

1. Cord may be seen protruding from vagina or palpated in the vagina or through the cervix.
2. Compression of the cord may cause variable decelerations; prolonged decelerations or bradycardia may develop over time.

 NURSING ALERT Prolapsed cord should be suspected with FHR prolonged deceleration or bradycardia resulting immediately after spontaneous or artificial rupture of membranes.

Management

1. Deliver fetus as soon as possible via the most expeditious route.
2. When prolapsed cord is identified, relieve pressure off the umbilical cord by positioning the cord between your two examination fingers and elevating the fetal presenting part up and off the cord.

3. Change maternal positions to potentially alleviate compression (typically knee–chest position or side-lying is adequate).
4. Prepare for emergent delivery.

Complications

Maternal
1. Infection.
2. Risk of increased perineal trauma from emergency operative delivery.

Fetal
1. Prematurity.
2. Hypoxia and perinatal asphyxia.
3. Meconium aspiration.
4. Fetal death if delayed or undiagnosed.

Nursing Assessment and Interventions

1. Observe for variable or prolonged FHR deceleration following spontaneous or artificial rupture of membranes.
2. Perform vaginal exam with sterile gloves; if cord is palpated, call for assistance and prepare for emergent delivery. Keep pressure off the cord as described above. Do not remove hand from vagina (see Figure 39-6). Extreme conditions may include lack of additional staff to assist; if so, remove hand and place patient in a reverse Trendelenburg position or up on all four extremities so that she is supported by knees and elbows to alleviate pressure on the cord while preparing for emergent delivery.
3. A cord exposed to room air may exhibit a reflex constriction of the umbilical blood vessels. These conditions may further restrict oxygen and blood flow to the fetus. Do not pinch or squeeze the umbilical cord as this may cause the cord to spasm, decreasing umbilical blood flow and oxygen to the fetus.
4. Explain procedures as much as possible to the woman during this emergent situation.
5. Administer oxygen at 8 to 10 L/minute via nonrebreather mask.

Uterine Inversion

Uterine inversion is a potentially life-threatening complication in which the uterus turns inside out during the third stage of delivery. Uterine inversions may be classified as:

Complete—fundus inverts and passes through the cervical os into the vagina and may prolapse through the introitus.

Incomplete—fundus of uterus partially inverts but not beyond the cervical os.

Pathophysiology and Etiology

1. Excessive traction on the cord while the placenta is still attached.
2. Aggressive fundal pressure.
3. Lax or thin uterine wall.
4. Spontaneous inversion.
5. Abnormally short umbilical cord.
6. Prolonged labor.
7. Uterine atony.
8. Uterine anomalies.
9. Fundal placentation.
10. Abnormally adherent placental tissue (placenta accreta or increta).
11. Fetal macrosomia.

Clinical Manifestations

1. Sudden onset of maternal hemorrhage, shock, and instability accompanied severe pelvic pain (anesthesia may dull pain sensation).
2. Inability to palpate fundus in association with clinical manifestations.
3. Confirmed with bimanual examination.

Management

1. Prevention is the most effective therapy. Proper management of the third stage of labor may prevent most uterine inversions. Immediate identification and interventions essential.
2. Goal is to manually restore the uterus to its normal position.
3. Typically, anesthesia is necessary to complete manual manipulation and to alleviate associated pain.
4. If manipulation is difficult or lengthy. Administer tocolytic therapy (terbutaline or magnesium sulfate) as ordered.
5. Monitor maternal vital signs for signs for deterioration and shock.
6. After the uterus has been restored, oxytocin is administered to alleviate uterine atony.
7. Abdominal or vaginal surgery may be necessary if manual replacement fails.
8. Administer a broad-spectrum antibiotic if ordered.

Figure 39-6. Prolapsed cord. Reduction of cord compression using gloved examiner's hand in vagina to elevate presenting part. **(A)** Vertex. **(B)** Breech. (From Reeder, S., Martin, L., & Koniak-Griffin, D. [1997]. *Maternity nursing: Family newborn, and women's health care* [18th ed.]. Philadelphia, PA: Lippincott-Raven Publishers.)

A   B

Complications

1. Infection.
2. Anemia.
3. Hysterectomy.
4. Hemorrhagic shock.
5. Death.

Nursing Assessment and Interventions

Also see page 949 for additional nursing care.

Before Correction of the Inversion

1. Check maternal vital signs and evaluate blood loss.
2. Assist practitioner, as needed, for manual replacement.
3. Administer oxygen, as warranted.
4. Maintain primary IV line and establish a second line with a 16G or 18G catheter for administration of fluids, blood products, and/or medications.
5. Apply a pulse oximeter to determine oxygen saturation.
6. If replacement of the uterus is unsuccessful, prepare the woman and her support persons for surgery.

After Correction of the Inversion

1. Check maternal vital signs, and monitor CBC for signs of bleeding and infection.
2. Administer oxytocin and other uterotonic agents, as ordered.
3. Measure and record accurate intake and output.
4. Evaluate uterine fundus carefully for position and firmness and avoid vigorous massage.
5. Evaluate lochia for amount of blood loss.
6. Evaluate for transfusion reactions (ie, itching, wheezing, anaphylaxis).
7. Administer antibiotics, as ordered, to minimize risk of infection.
8. Provide support to the woman and encourage her to express her feelings.

OPERATIVE OBSTETRICS

See additional online content: Procedure Guidelines 39-1

Episiotomy

 EVIDENCE BASE American College of Obstetricians and Gynecologists. (2016). *Prevention and management of obstetric lacerations at vaginal delivery* (Practice Bulletin 165). Washington, DC: Author.

An *episiotomy* is a surgical incision of the perineum to increase the vaginal opening for delivery of the fetus during the second stage of labor. In the United States, the rates have episiotomies performed have decreased to about 12% of vaginal births. The common type of episiotomy in the United States is the midline (median) and the mediolateral episiotomy is more prevalent in Europe. Routine episiotomies are not recommended in current practice. Episiotomies are only recommended for such maternal or fetal indications as avoiding severe maternal lacerations or facilitating or expediting difficult deliveries.

Types of Episiotomies

See Figure 39-7.

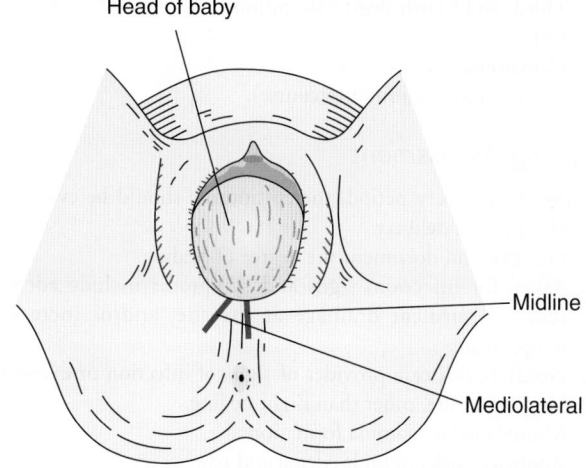

Figure 39-7. Position of episiotomy incision in a woman during second stage of labor. Baby's head is presenting to vaginal outlet (crowning). (From Pillitteri, A. [2013]. *Maternal and child health nursing: Care of the childbearing and childrearing family* [7th ed.]. Philadelphia, PA: Lippincott Williams & Wilkins.)

Median (Midline)

1. Incision is made midline down the perineum directed toward the rectum.
2. This method is believed to heal with few complications, is more comfortable for the woman during healing, is easy to repair, and is associated with minimal blood loss.
3. Increases risk of third- and fourth-degree lacerations.
4. Decreased postpartum dyspareunia.
5. Most commonly performed in the United States.

Mediolateral

1. Incision 45 degrees or more from the midline.
2. This method avoids the anal sphincter if an extension is needed.
3. Women find it extremely uncomfortable during healing.
4. Difficult to repair.
5. Associated with increased blood loss.
6. Necessitates longer wound healing time.

Management

1. The application of warm compresses to the perineum during the second stage of labor has demonstrated a reduction in third- and fourth-degree lacerations.
2. Pain relief.
   a. The stretching of the perineum and pressure from the fetal head may provide a natural numbing effect.
   b. Local perineal infiltration with lidocaine provides anesthesia for performing and repairing the episiotomy.
   c. A pudendal block provides anesthesia to the lower two thirds of the perineum and vagina using lidocaine injection into the vaginal walls.
   d. Epidural anesthesia provides anesthesia from the level of the umbilicus to the midthigh area.
3. The episiotomy is performed once the fetal head is 3 to 4 cm visible with a contraction.
4. The repair of the episiotomy usually begins after the delivery of the placenta.

Complications

1. Infection.
2. Bleeding.

3. Third- and fourth-degree lacerations.
4. Pain.
5. Hematoma.
6. Dyspareunia (painful intercourse).

Nursing Assessment

During the recovery period, the episiotomy should be evaluated periodically after delivery.
1. Describe and document the degree of healing.
2. Assess for infection; signs and symptoms include edema, redness, purulent drainage at the site, and/or increased temperature.
3. Notify health care provider of signs of infection or excessive bleeding at site, other than slight oozing.
4. Monitor for hematoma formation.
5. Apply ice packs to limit edema and pain.

Nursing Diagnoses

• Risk for Infection related to traumatized tissue.
• Acute Pain related to tissue trauma.

Nursing Interventions

Preventing Infection
1. Instruct the woman to clean the perineum from front to back.
2. Provide instructions on perineal care.
   a. Provide a peri bottle; teach patient to squirt the water gently on her perineum after voiding.
3. Instruct patient to change the perineal pad each time after urination and defecation; dispose of in proper biohazard receptacle.
4. Explain the importance of proper handwashing before and after perineal care.
5. Explain that perineal care should be performed after urination and defecation.
6. Encourage a diet that is high in protein and vitamin C and encourage hydration.

Promoting Comfort
1. Apply covered ice packs to the perineal area for the first 24 hours after delivery. The ice packs should not remain in place longer than 20 minutes at a time to get the maximum benefit from the treatment.
2. Encourage sitz baths with either warm or cool water.

3. Administer pain medication and topical anesthetics, as ordered.
4. Instruct the woman to tighten her buttocks and perineal muscles before sitting in a chair and to release the muscles once seated.
5. Abstain from sexual intercourse until healing is complete, typically 4 to 6 weeks.

Evaluation: Expected Outcomes

• No evidence of infection; afebrile.
• Demonstrates increase in comfort.

Operative Vaginal Delivery: Forceps

Obstetric forceps (see Table 39-3) are used to facilitate delivery of the fetal head during the second stage and expedite a safe vaginal delivery when indicated for maternal and fetal health. Most forceps are placed on each side of the fetal vertex and others are utilized for special considerations (pipers: vaginal breech birth). Forceps consist of two pieces: a right blade, which is slipped into the right side of the mother's pelvis, and a left blade, which is slipped into the left side. Unfortunately, forceps increase the diameter of the presenting part, which may hinder delivery. Special training and skill are required.

Types of Forceps Deliveries

American College of Obstetricians and Gynecologists definitions for obstetric forceps:

Outlet Forceps
1. Scalp is visible at the introitus without separating labia.
2. Fetal skull has reached pelvic floor.
3. Sagittal suture in anteroposterior diameter or right or left occiput anterior or posterior position.
4. Fetal head is at or on perineum.
5. Rotation does not exceed 45 degrees.

Low Forceps
1. Leading point of fetal skull is at station +2 cm or above and not on the pelvic floor.
   a. Rotation is less than 45 degrees (left or right occiput anterior to occiput anterior or left or right occiput posterior to occiput posterior).
   b. Rotation is greater than 45 degrees.

Table 39-3	Representative Types of Forceps*
MAJOR CLASSIFICATIONS	**USE**
Simpson—separated shanks (eg, DeLee forceps)	Extract fetus with elongated, molded head; commonly used with nulliparas who have long labors
Elliot—overlapping shanks (eg, Tucker-McLean)	Extract fetus with unmolded, rounder heads; commonly used with multiparas who have briefer labors
Specialized Types Piper	Deliver aftercoming head in a breech presentation
Kielland	Rotate head from transverse or posterior position to an anterior position; used with women with anthropoid pelves
Barton	Rotate head from transverse to an anterior position; designed for use in women with flat pelves

*There are more than 600 types of forceps.

Indications for Forceps Delivery

1. No absolute indication exists. The fetal head must be engaged and the cervix fully dilated.
2. Suspicion of immediate or potential fetal compromise.
3. Shortening of the second stage of labor for maternal benefit.
4. Prolonged second-stage labor.
   a. Nulliparous women: lack of continuing progress for 3 hours with regional anesthesia or 2 hours without regional anesthesia.
   b. Multiparous women: lack of continuing progress for 2 hours with regional anesthesia or 1 hour without regional anesthesia.
5. Category III FHR pattern.
6. Cardiac or neurologic disease.

Contraindications

1. Malpresentations: face or brow presentation.
2. Incomplete dilation of the cervix.
3. Unengaged fetal head.
4. Gestational age less than 34 weeks.
5. Live fetus with bone demineralization.
6. Fetal coagulopathies.
7. Inexperience of practitioner or unavailable operative personnel.

Management

1. The woman is placed in lithotomy position.
2. The bladder should be emptied, and may be done by catheterization.
3. Regional anesthesia may be used.
4. The neonatal staff is in attendance at delivery.
5. An episiotomy should not be routinely performed for an operative delivery.
6. Each blade is placed bilaterally over the fetal ear, avoiding the face.
7. Gentle traction is administered in a downward motion.

Complications

Maternal

1. Perineal trauma: lacerations of the vulva, cervix, vagina, and rectum; coccyx fracture.
2. Extensions of an episiotomy into the rectum: fourth-degree laceration.
3. Bladder trauma, uterine rupture.
4. Postpartum infection, postpartum hemorrhage secondary to uterine atony.
5. Anemia secondary to uterine atony/hemorrhage.
6. Urinary or fecal incontinence; fistula formation.

Fetal

1. Bruising.
2. Cephalohematoma.
3. Nerve injuries.
4. Facial lacerations and facial nerve palsy.
5. Skull fracture.
6. Ocular trauma.
7. Intracranial hemorrhage.

Nursing Assessment

1. After application of forceps, the FHR should be evaluated frequently per facility policy until delivery.

2. Evaluate bladder fullness—bladder should be empty before the application of the forceps.
3. Ensure sterile technique is maintained.

Nursing Diagnoses

- Anxiety related to fetal outcome.
- Acute Pain related to procedures.

Nursing Interventions

Decreasing Anxiety

1. Provide education and support for the woman and her partner when use of a vaginal assisted birth is expected.
2. Explain that a sensation of pressure will be felt.
3. Stay with the woman and provide guidance during the delivery process.

Promoting Comfort

1. Encourage use of breathing and relaxation techniques.
2. Make sure bladder is completely empty.
3. Encourage relaxation between contractions and use of abdominal muscles and pushing with the contractions.
4. Use blankets and pillows for support when positioning the woman for delivery.

Evaluation: Expected Outcomes

- Verbalizes concerns regarding forceps; responds to instructions.
- Demonstrates increased level of comfort.

Vacuum Extraction

Vacuum extraction applies suction to the fetal vertex, which is slowly increased to assist in delivery. Advantages include ease of application with a decrease in intensity to the fetal vertex. It is also associated with less maternal trauma, decreased injuries to fetus, and less need for general or regional anesthesia.

Indications

1. Same as forceps.

Contraindications

1. Same as forceps.

Management

1. Fetus is in vertex presentation.
2. Fetus should not be below 34 weeks' gestation.
3. The woman is in the lithotomy position.
4. The bladder is emptied by catheterization.
5. Pressure is applied during contractions and released between contractions. Fetal descent should occur with each contraction.
6. Anesthesia may be indicated.
7. Unsuccessful extraction is followed by a cesarean delivery.
8. Neonatal staff is in attendance at delivery.

Complications

Complications are usually less frequent and less severe with vacuum extraction than with forceps.

Maternal

1. Lacerations of the cervix or vagina.
2. Pain.

3. Infection.
4. Bladder trauma.
5. Hemorrhage.

Fetal

1. Cephalohematoma.
2. Caput succedaneum (swelling of the scalp) from the vacuum.
3. Intracranial hemorrhage.
4. Retinal hemorrhage.
5. Abrasions and lacerations to scalp.
6. Subgaleal hemorrhage.

Nursing Assessment

1. After application of the vacuum extractor, the FHR should be assessed frequently per facility policy until delivery.
2. Evaluate maternal sensation.
3. Evaluate bladder fullness—bladder should be empty before the application of the vacuum extractor.
4. Make sure sterile technique is maintained.
5. Monitor the vacuum pressure of the equipment according to your facility's protocol and document maternal–fetal response during procedure.
6. Monitor "pop-offs" (vacuum extractor cup pops off the fetal head); if three pop-offs have occurred or greater than 20 minutes have passed, other options should be considered.

Nursing Interventions

Same as for forceps delivery, page 1069.

Cesarean Delivery

Cesarean delivery is the surgical removal of the infant from the uterus through an abdominal and uterine incision. Cesarean births after increasing for more than a decade have begun to decrease from 32.9% to 32%. A decision to perform a cesarean section is for maternal and fetal well-being. It is recommended that prior to performing an elective cesarean section (based upon maternal request) that fetal gestational age of 39 weeks be confirmed.

Types of Cesarean Delivery

Uterine Incisions

Incision choice is based on the clinical scenario and future fertility.

1. Low transverse—transverse incision made across the lower uterine segment.
   a. Incision is made across the thickest section and away from uterine activity (fundus); minimizes blood loss and improves the integrity of the scar, decreasing risk of future dehiscence or rupture.
   b. Incidence of postoperative adhesions and danger of intestinal obstruction are reduced.
   c. First-line choice of incision in most clinical scenarios.
2. Classic or Vertical incision from the fundus down the body of the uterus to the lower uterine segment; may be utilized for emergent or preterm deliveries.
   a. Useful when bladder and lower segment are involved in extensive adhesions.
   b. Surgery of choice with a diagnosed anterior placenta previa, which inhibits the use of the low transverse incision.
   c. Increased blood loss versus low transverse.
   d. Increased risk of uterine rupture in subsequent deliveries.

Indications for Cesarean Delivery

1. Maternal medical complications, such as asthma, chronic hypertension, diabetes, cardiac disease, and active herpes infection.
2. Labor complications: dystocia, malpresentation, CPD, category III FHR pattern, prolonged or arrest of first or second stage of labor, early labor induction prior to cervical ripening.
3. Obstetric complications: placenta previa, breech, elective induction of nulliparous (50% higher risk than spontaneous labor).
4. Possible indications for cesarean hysterectomy:
   a. Ruptured uterus.
   b. Intrauterine infection.
   c. Postpartum hemorrhage: unresponsive to conservative management options.
   d. Laceration of major uterine vessel.
   e. Severe dysplasia or carcinoma in situ of the cervix.
   f. Placenta accreta.
   g. Gross multiple fibromyomas.
   h. Uterine inversion unresponsive to manual replacement.

Management

Preoperative

1. Assess patient's last intake of food; surgery should be delayed for 8 hours following last meal; consult anesthesia.
2. A blood sample should be typed, screened with Rh status, and available to be cross matched, if needed; a CBC is obtained including platelets.
3. Anesthesia, regional or general, depends on indication for surgery.
4. Informed consents signed and witnessed.
5. A large gauge IV is established with Lactated Ringers (LR).
6. Insert indwelling urinary catheter; may wait until after anesthesia placement to minimize discomfort.
7. Administer an antacid; reduces gastric acidity, limiting complications should aspiration occur.
8. Shaving of pubic hair with a razor just prior to the incision is discouraged related to increased risk of SSI. Clipping pubic hair is preferred. Refer to facility guidelines.
9. Cleanse incision area with antimicrobial wash per facility protocol.
10. Antibiotics may be given prophylactically, as directed.

Intraoperative

1. Patient is moved to the operating suite.
2. Application of pneumatic compression devices is recommended.
3. Grounding pad applied per manufacturer's instructions.
4. Assist in application of monitors (cardiorespiratory).
5. Ensure facility verification process is completed prior to beginning of procedure, including "Time Out" Per facility policy.
6. Cleanse lower abdominal area (incision site) with FDA-approved antiseptic agent based on provider preference and facility policy.
7. Perform instrument, needle/knife, and lap pad counts periodically: before, during, and after surgery.
8. Verify that neonatal resuscitation equipment is readily accessible and radiant warmer is preheated.
9. Receive newborn and perform neonatal assessment; maintain asepsis.
10. Provide hand-off communication per facility policy.

Postoperative

In addition to routine postoperative recovery room care (see page 94), fundal checks must be performed as with the fourth stage of labor (page 1010).

Complications

1. Hemorrhage.
2. Endometritis.
3. Paralytic ileus (intestinal obstruction).
4. Pulmonary embolism.
5. Thrombophlebitis.
6. Anesthesia complications.
7. Bowel or bladder injury.
8. Respiratory depression of the infant from anesthetic drugs.
9. Possible delay in mother–infant bonding.

Nursing Assessment

Before Delivery

1. Assess knowledge of procedure.
2. Perform admission assessment.
3. Obtain 20- to 30-minute fetal tracing strip to assess fetal and uterine status.
4. Obtain maternal vital signs.
5. Identify drug allergies; identify other allergies (eg, latex, iodine, tape).

After Delivery (Also See Chapter 37)

1. Assess maternal vital signs every 15 minutes the first 1 to 2 hours or more frequently as the patient's condition warrants.
   a. Respiratory status: airway patency, oxygen needs, rate/quality/depth of respirations, auscultation of breath sounds, oxygen saturation readings.
   b. Circulation: BP, pulse, electrocardiogram monitoring for assessing dysrhythmias, color; assess dressing for drainage.
   c. LOC: orientation and response to verbal/tactile/painful stimulation.
2. Assess mobility and sensation of extremities if regional anesthesia is used.
3. Assess postpartum status (same intervals for assessment): fundal position and contractions, condition of incision and abdominal dressing, maternal–neonatal attachment, lochia (color, amount), neonate condition (if applicable), feeding preferences.
4. Assess hourly intake and output and reestablishment of bowel sounds.
5. Perform pain assessment: evaluate level of anesthesia, medications given (amount/time/results).
6. Assess knowledge and performance of breastfeeding.

Nursing Diagnoses

- Anxiety related to change in childbirth plan.
- Acute Pain related to surgical procedure.
- Risk for Infection related to open abdominal cavity.
- Interrupted family process related to unmet expectations for childbirth experience.

Nursing Interventions

Relieving Anxiety

1. Explain the purpose of all interventions and answer questions.
2. Allow the support person to attend the birth, if appropriate.

Promoting Comfort

1. Encourage use of relaxation techniques after medication has been given for pain.

2. Monitor for respiratory depression up to 24 hours after epidural opioid administration.
3. Monitor and instruct patient on use of patient-controlled anesthesia pump, as applicable.
4. Use a back rub and a quiet environment to promote the effectiveness of the medication.
5. Support and splint the abdominal incision when moving or coughing and deep breathing.
6. Encourage frequent rest periods.
7. To reduce pain caused by gas, encourage ambulation or use of rocking chair.
8. Administer pain medications as ordered. Do not administer parenteral opioids if patient is receiving epidural opioids unless ordered by anesthesia provider.

Preventing Infection

1. Establish protocol to decrease surgical site infections (SSI) per national guidelines.
2. Maintain sterile technique during surgery and use sterile technique when changing dressings postoperatively.
3. Be aware that the most effective method of infection prevention is handwashing.
4. Provide perineal care along with vital signs every 4 hours or as needed.
5. Provide routine postoperative care measures to prevent urinary or pulmonary infection.
6. Utilize incentive spirometer every hour while awake.

Promoting Effective Family Unit

1. Encourage infant bonding as soon as possible.
2. Emphasize the positive outcomes of operative delivery—avoidance of maternal–fetal complications and healthy baby.
3. Provide parent education and family time as tolerated by the mother.
4. Emphasize that adjustments to parenting under any circumstances are necessary and normal.

Patient Education and Health Maintenance

1. Teach and assist the woman with the "football hold" for breastfeeding; alleviates pressure on the abdominal incision.
2. Teach incisional care per facility policy and instruct to observe for signs of infection (foul-smelling lochia, elevated temperature, increased pain, redness and edema at the incision site) and to report them immediately through 12 weeks' postpartum.
3. Assist the woman in planning for the assistance of friends and family during the period immediately after discharge.

Evaluation: Expected Outcomes

- Verbalizes an understanding of the cesarean delivery procedure and postdelivery care.
- Reports relief of pain.
- Absence of infection.
- Able to care of self and infant by discharge.

POSTPARTUM COMPLICATIONS
Postpartum Infection

Postpartum (puerperal) infection should be suspected if the patient's temperature exceeds 100°F (37.8°C) on two occasions at least 6 hours apart during the first 10 days postpartum exclusive of the first 24 hours postpartum. The infection may remain localized or extend to various parts of the body such as connective tissue by lymphatic dissemination (parametritis). The broad ligament is the main pathway for systemic infection.

Pathophysiology and Etiology

The most common cause is polymicrobial ascent to the uterus from the lower genital tract. Hematogenous bacterial spread may also occur.

1. Types of infection include:
   a. Endometritis: inflammation of the endometrium.
   b. Endomyometritis: inflammation of the endometrium and myometrium.
   c. Parametritis: inflammation of the endometrium and parametrial tissue.
2. Other infections include:
   a. Wound or UTIs.
   b. Pneumonia.
   c. Mastitis.
   d. Pelvic thrombophlebitis.
   e. Necrotizing fasciitis.
3. Risk factors:
   a. Operative birth.
   b. Prolonged labor or rupture of membranes.
   c. Use of invasive procedures (ie, internal monitoring, amnioinfusion, fetal scalp sampling).
   d. Multiple pelvic examinations.
   e. Excessive blood loss.
   f. Pyelonephritis or diabetes.
   g. Socioeconomic and nutritional factors compromising host defense mechanisms.
   h. Anemia and systemic illness.
   i. Smoking.
   j. Mastitis-specific risk factors: infrequent breastfeeding, incomplete breast emptying, plugged milk duct, cracked or bleeding nipples (may be secondary to improper latch-on and removal).

Clinical Manifestations

Endometritis Postpartum
1. Fever occurring around third day postpartum is the most important finding.
2. Uterus usually larger than expected for postdelivery day and tender.
3. Lochia may be profuse, bloody, and foul-smelling.
4. Chills, malaise, and fever occur if lochial discharge is obstructed by clots.
5. WBC greater than 20,000/mm³ with increased neutrophils.
6. Infection may spread to myometrium (endomyometritis), parametrium, fallopian tubes, peritoneum, and blood.

Parametritis (Pelvic Cellulitis)
1. Chills, fever (38.9°C to 40°C [102°F to 104°F]), tachycardia.
2. Severe unilateral or bilateral pain in lower abdomen.
3. Enlarged and tender uterus.
4. Uterine position may become fixed as it is displaced by the exudate along the broad ligament.
5. Commonly, the result of an infected wound in the cervix, vagina, perineum, or lower uterine segment.

Diagnostic Evaluation and Management

1. Obtain urinalysis and urine culture to rule out UTI.
2. Obtain blood sample for CBC and report results; assess for leukocytosis more than 20,000/mm³.

3. Antibiotic therapy: obtain cultures to identify causative agent prior to administration of broad-spectrum antibiotics including penicillins, cephalosporins (cefoxitin, cefazolin), clindamycin, and aminoglycosides (gentamicin, tobramycin). Antibiotics are given until the woman is afebrile for 48 hours (maternal response usually occurs within 48 to 72 hours) and may include home therapy.
4. Increase daily fluid intake.
5. Encourage increased intake of 300 to 500 calories if lactating; diet should include a variety of foods, usually high in protein and vitamin C (promotes wound healing).
6. Ensure adequate urine output (30 mL/hour).
7. Supportive therapy is used to control pain and to maintain hydration and nutritional status.
8. Drainage is indicated for abscess development.

Complications

1. Thrombophlebitis may result from postpartum infection spread along the veins or immobility.
   a. Femoral thrombophlebitis—appears 10 to 20 days after delivery as pain in calf, fever, edema; affected leg circumference is 2 cm greater than unaffected leg.
   b. Pelvic thrombophlebitis—infection of the veins of uterine wall and broad ligament usually caused by anaerobic streptococci; presents 14 days after delivery with severe chills and wide range of temperature changes.
   c. Treatment may include bed rest, compression stockings anticoagulants, and antibiotics.
2. Pulmonary embolus may occur—respiratory distress and chest pain.
3. Peritonitis—spread of infection through lymphatic channels.

Nursing Assessment

1. Perform postpartum assessment: note uterine tenderness on palpation and the color, amount, and odor of lochia; assess for proper breastfeeding techniques.
2. Monitor vital signs for signs of infection per facility policy.
3. Assess patient hygienic practices, and encourage frequent handwashing.

Nursing Diagnoses

- Hyperthermia related to infection.
- Risk for impaired attachment because of management of infection.

Nursing Interventions

Restoring Normothermia
Teach proper technique and assist, if necessary.
1. Provide for adequate rest periods.
2. Increase fluid intake to make up for insensible loss.
3. Position in high-Fowler position to promote drainage.
4. Administer antibiotics and analgesics, as ordered.
5. Explain the benefit of perineal washing or sitz baths; assist, as needed.
6. Explain importance of good handwashing technique; proper cleaning (front to back) during voiding or defecation.
7. Assist with perineal pads and medications; encourage changing pads with each voiding, bowel movement, and periodically throughout the day.
8. Observe for signs of septic shock: severe tachycardia, hypotension, tachypnea, changes in sensorium, and decreased urine output. Report to interprofessional team.

Promoting Infant Attachment

1. Encourage minimal separation from the infant and continuation of breastfeeding, as able.
2. Promote good handwashing technique for the mother before contact with the infant.
3. Encourage father/family participation in care of mother/baby unit.

Evaluation

- Afebrile, tolerating antibiotics well, using good hand hygiene.
- Infant bonding time uninterrupted.

Postpartum Hemorrhage

Postpartum hemorrhage, also known as obstetric hemorrhage (OH), reflects a blood loss in excess of 500 mL for a vaginal delivery or greater than 1,000 mL in a cesarean delivery. Early postpartum hemorrhage occurs in the first 24 hours and may be considered late after 24 hours up until 12 weeks after birth. The greatest risk is during the first hour following delivery. Hemorrhage may also be defined as a decrease in hematocrit of at least 10%, but determinations of hemoglobin and hematocrit concentrations may not reflect current hematologic status. The World Health Organization (WHO) found 25% of pregnancy-related deaths in the world were attributed to OH, and it is the single greatest cause of maternal deaths. In the United States, the mortality rate is 13% and on the rise. Worldwide, a woman dies of OH every 4 minutes.

 EVIDENCE BASE American College of Obstetricians and Gynecologists. (2006/Reaffirmed 2015). *Postpartum hemorrhage* (Practice Bulletin #76). Washington, DC: Author.

Pathophysiology and Etiology

Excessive bleeding from a point between the uterus and perineum (see Figure 39-8).

Early Postpartum Hemorrhage (the First 24 Hours After Birth)

1. Main cause: uterine atony (80%)—relaxation of the uterus secondary to:
   a. Overdistention of uterus secondary to multiple pregnancy, polyhydramnios, or macrosomia.
   b. High parity (more than six pregnancies).
   c. Prolonged labor.
   d. Medications—oxytocin, magnesium sulfate, tocolytics, anesthetics.
   e. Fibroids—prevents uterus from contracting.
   f. Retained placental fragments—result from manual removal of placenta, succenturiate (additional) lobe, abnormally adherent placenta (placenta accreta), or spontaneous Duncan placenta delivery (periphery detaches first instead of central detachment).
2. Uterine inversion.
3. Bleeding disorders such as DIC.
4. Trauma, laceration, or hematomas of the vagina, cervix, or perineum secondary to:
   a. Forceps delivery, especially rotation forceps.
   b. Large infant.
   c. Multiple gestation.
5. Difficult third stage of labor (aggressive fundal manipulation or cord traction).
6. Sepsis.

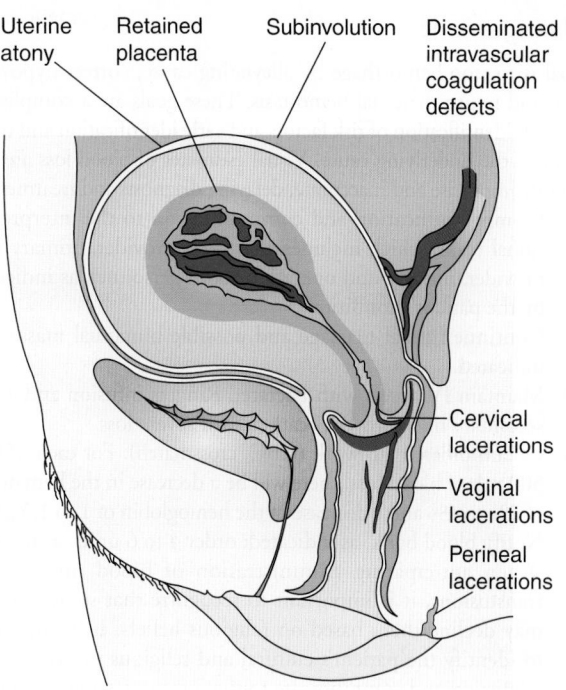

Figure 39-8. Common causes of postpartum hemorrhage. (From Pillitteri, A. [2013]. *Maternal and child health nursing: Care of the childbearing and childrearing family* [7th ed.]. Philadelphia, PA: Lippincott Williams & Wilkins.)

7. Uterine rupture; uterine inversion.
8. Other risk factors include augmented or induced labor, rapid labor, history of postpartum hemorrhage, preeclampsia, or Asian or Hispanic ethnicity.

Late Postpartum Hemorrhage (24 Hours to 6 Weeks Postpartum)

1. Main cause is retained placental fragments.
2. Infection.
3. Subinvolution (delayed healing) of placental site.

Clinical Manifestations

Early Postpartum Hemorrhage

1. With uterine atony, uterus is soft or boggy, usually difficult to palpate, and will not remain contracted; excessive vaginal bleeding occurs.
2. Lacerations of the vagina, cervix, or perineum cause bright red, continuous bleeding even when the fundus is firm.
3. Tachycardia, hypotension, dizziness, pallor, and decreased urine output occur after loss of 10% total blood volume.

Late Postpartum Hemorrhage

1. Uterus is soft or boggy.
2. Slow, reddish oozing or heavy bleeding (first 6 weeks postdelivery).
3. Low persistent backache.
4. Abdominal pain or tenderness.
5. Fatigue.
6. Loss of appetite.

 NURSING ALERT Over 50% of deaths because of OH were preventable and the result of ineffective medical management. Early assessment, identification, and intervention in the event of an OH is essential to improving obstetric outcomes.

Management

Goal is to stop hemorrhage by alleviating cause, correct hypovolemia, and return maternal hemostasis. These goals are accomplished through identification of risk factors and early identification and treatment of the underlying cause. Visual estimates of blood loss are frequently imprecise and inaccurate, delaying diagnosis and treatment.

1. Prompt notification and communication to the interprofessional team, which includes anesthesia provider, primary care provider, nursing and operating room personnel, as indicated by the patient's condition.
2. Continue fundal massage and possible bimanual massage if indicated.
3. Maintain IV access with Lactated Ringers infusion and add a secondary line with 16G catheter for severe loss.
4. Obtain ordered lab work (CBC, crossmatch). For each 450 to 500 mL of blood loss, there will be a decrease in the hematocrit of 2% to 4% and a decrease in the hemoglobin of 1 to 1.5 g/dL.
5. Notify blood bank, as indicated; order 4 to 6 units, as needed. When anticipating administration of blood products or transfusions, it is important to recognize that some patients may decline them based on religious beliefs. It is important to identify the patient's cultural and religious practices upon admission and communicate to the interprofessional team.
6. Administer medications, as ordered: for uterine atony—
   a. IV administration of oxytocin, IV or IM (see Chapter 37 stage 4 of labor).
   b. When oxytocin is ineffective to control bleeding, anticipate the need for additional medications to treat postpartum hemorrhage:
   c. Methylergonovine 0.2 mg IM every 2 to 4 hours. (Contraindicated in women with hypertension, Raynaud syndrome, scleroderma).
   d. Misoprostol 800 to 1,000 mcg per rectum (single dose) (may cause fever and tachycardia).
   e. Carboprost tromethamine 0.25 mg IM every 15 to 90 minutes (8 dose maximum)—contraindicated in women with asthma, active cardiac, hepatic, or renal disease; may cause fever, chills, nausea, vomiting, diarrhea).
7. In the presence of continuous bleeding and a firm uterus, notify the provider for evaluation and possible intervention.
   a. Repair of lacerations, transfusion of blood products, dilation and curettage, B-lynch suture, uterine tamponade, and selective arterial embolization.
   b. Intrauterine balloon tamponade using, for example, the Bakri SOS (surgical obstetric silicone) to control bleeding (see Figure 39-9).
      i. 250 to 500 mL of saline is introduced into the balloon to maintain pressure against the uterine walls. Pooled blood above the balloon is removed through the drainage port of the catheter.
      ii. Vaginal packing is also placed to increase the tamponade effect on the lower uterine segment, and a urinary catheter is placed for bladder drainage.
8. Opioid analgesics may be needed to counter the pain of uterine contractions.
9. Emergency hysterectomy may be necessary.

Complications

1. Hypovolemic shock.
2. Hysterectomy.
3. Death.

Figure 39-9. The Bakri SOS provides balloon tamponade to stop postpartum hemorrhage.

Nursing Assessment

1. Assess maternal history for risk factors; plan accordingly and communicate to the perinatal team.
2. Perform ongoing cumulative assessment of blood loss during the entire postpartum period. As the patient changes hands between practitioners and departments, blood loss is commonly estimated only by what one practitioner visualizes over his or her own shift, not taking into consideration what has transpired over the course of the entire postpartum period. Therefore, documentation and communication should reflect a cumulative total and any acute changes relative to the changes in the patient's immediate status. See Box 39-3 for blood loss estimates.
3. Evaluate for presence of clots expelled or passed during voiding; note number of pads saturated in 1 hour or shorter time frame, if applicable. Weigh pads, as necessary, to determine loss.
4. Assess vital signs, pulse pressure, and oxygen saturation per facility policy and increase assessments if the patient shows signs of instability—tachycardia, hypotension, pallor, diaphoresis, altered LOC, tachypnea, nausea and vomiting, feelings of impending doom—all of which may indicate hypovolemic shock.

BOX 39-3   Estimation of Blood Loss

Accurate evaluation of blood loss is critical to maternal outcomes. Studies validate the inaccuracy of blood loss estimation with visual inspection. The use of under buttock drapes to collect blood loss during delivery has been valuable in improving the ability to measure blood loss during childbirth. Estimation by weight using a scale is desirable. Follow these steps:

- Obtain the dry weight (in grams) of commonly used items such as disposable underpad, perineal pad, 4 × 4.
- Weigh the saturated items and subtract the dry weight of the items to determine blood loss.
- 1 gram weight = 1 mL of blood. In the absence of a scale, the following estimations may be utilized:
- Saturated 12-ply surgical sponge (4 × 4 in.) = 5 mL.
- Standard perineal pad 50% saturated = 25 mL.
- Saturated 18 × 18 inch surgical laparotomy pad = 100 mL.
- Clot the size of a golf ball = 50 mL.
- Clot the size of a tennis ball = 140 mL.

a. Normal vital signs are not an indication that the woman is *not* in shock. Traditional signs of hypovolemic shock are not evident until approximately 15% to 20% of total maternal blood volume is lost.

b. Continuous BP monitor readings may falsely lower diastolic and raise systolic readings. Assessments more frequent than 2 minutes apart may not allow for vessels within the extremity to reperfuse between assessments.

5. Assess intake and output (maintain greater than 25 mL/hour); make sure intake includes a cumulative total to include all labor and delivery infusions as well as any fluids administered during surgery, such as with cesarean delivery. Foley catheter may be used for bladder decompression.

6. Assess location and firmness of uterine fundus.

7. Percuss and palpate for bladder distention, which may interfere with contracting of the uterus.

8. Inspect for intactness of any perineal repair.

9. Because of rapid infusion of fluid during fluid resuscitation, assess breath sounds for signs of pulmonary edema.

Nursing Diagnoses

- Anxiety related to unexpected blood loss and uncertainty of outcome.
- Deficient Fluid Volume related to uterine atony.
- Risk for Infection related to blood loss and vaginal examinations.

Nursing Interventions

Decreasing Anxiety

1. Maintain a quiet and calm atmosphere; provide emotional support.
2. Provide information about the current clinical situation; answer questions.
3. Encourage the presence of a support person.
4. Explain changes to care plan.

Maintaining Fluid Volume

1. Maintain primary IV access and place a second large gauge 16G catheter infusing crystalloids and blood products, as indicated.
2. Monitor and maintain accurate intake and output; use of indwelling urinary catheter provides accurate output measurements.
3. Make sure that cross-matched blood is available; administer per facility protocol when necessary.
4. Provide supplemental oxygen by face mask; monitor oxygen saturation with pulse oximetry.
5. Administer medications, as ordered.
6. Change patient positions to facilitate perfusion to vital organs: elevate legs 20 to 30 degrees.
7. Monitor CBC and additional ordered lab work.

Preventing Infection

1. Maintain standard precautions and asepsis.
2. Evaluate for symptoms of infection: chills, elevated temperature, increased WBCs, uterine tenderness, and odor of lochia.
3. Administer antibiotics, as prescribed.
4. Maintain adequate rest and proper nutrition.

Patient Education and Health Maintenance

1. Educate the woman about the cause of hemorrhage.
2. Teach the woman the importance of eating a balanced diet high in iron-rich options and taking vitamin supplements.

3. Advise the woman she may feel tired and fatigued and to schedule daily rest periods.
4. Teach woman and family signs and symptoms of hemorrhage for home care.
5. Advise the woman to notify her health care provider of increased bleeding or other changes in her status.

Evaluation: Expected Outcomes

- Verbalizes concerns about her well-being.
- Vital signs stable, urine output adequate, hematocrit stable.
- Remains afebrile, WBC count within normal limits.

Postpartum Hematomas

Postpartum hematomas are localized collections of blood in loose connective tissue beneath the skin of external genitalia, beneath the vaginal mucosa, or in the broad ligaments. Usually occurs without laceration of the overlying tissue. Excessive perineal pain unrelieved by medications suggests hematoma formation and mandates careful examination of vulva, vagina, and rectum.

Pathophysiology and Etiology

1. Trauma during spontaneous labor or operative vaginal delivery.
2. Inadequate suturing of an episiotomy.
3. Delayed homeostasis or difficult or prolonged second stage of labor or both.

Clinical Manifestations

1. Complaints of pressure and pain; pain may be verbalized as excruciating.
2. Discolored skin that is tight, full feeling, and painful to the touch.
3. Possible decrease in BP, tachycardia.
4. Decrease or absence of lochia flow if the vagina is impeded.

Management

1. Small hematomas (less than 3 cm) are left to resolve on their own—ice packs may be applied. Sitz baths may also increase comfort.
2. Large hematomas (greater than 3 cm) may require evacuation of the blood and ligation of the bleeding vessel.
3. Analgesics and broad-spectrum antibiotics may be ordered (because of increased chance of infection).

Complications

1. Hypovolemia and shock from extreme blood loss.
2. Anemia, infection.
3. Increased length of postpartum recovery period.
4. Sepsis.
5. Calcification and scar tissue.
6. Dyspareunia (painful intercourse).

Nursing Interventions and Patient Education

1. Inspect perineal and vulvar area for signs of a hematoma periodically postpartum.
2. Inspect vaginal area for signs of a hematoma if woman is unable to void.
3. Monitor vital signs and evaluate for signs of shock.

4. Relieve pain of a hematoma by applying an ice bag to perineal area, medicating with mild analgesics, and positioning for comfort to decrease pressure on the affected area.
5. Help relieve voiding problems by assisting to bathroom if able to ambulate. If patient is unable to ambulate, then assist her on to a bedpan with legs hanging over side of bed. Provide privacy and run water while the woman is attempting to void.
6. Catheterize patient if unable to void.
7. Teach the woman the importance of eating a balanced diet and to include food high in iron.
8. Encourage the woman to take vitamin supplements and to take medications, as ordered.
9. Instruct the woman in the use of a sitz bath to provide perineal comfort after the first 24 hours and at home.

Postpartum Depression

 EVIDENCE BASE American College of Obstetricians and Gynecologists. (2015). *Screening for depression during and after pregnancy* (Committee Opinion #630). Washington, DC: Author.

There is no consensus regarding the classification of postpartum depression. Is it estimated to complicate 13% to 19% of pregnancies. Severity and presenting symptoms vary.

Pathophysiology and Etiology

Social, cultural, physiologic, and psychological factors may contribute to postpartum depression. Predisposing factors include:
1. Stressful life events during pregnancy or the postpartum period.
   a. Loss of loved one (fetus, neonate, partner, or other child).
   b. Illness of loved one.
   c. Financial difficulties.
   d. Loss of job.
   e. Move to new area, home, or job.
   f. Previous mental health history.
2. Poor interpersonal relationships.
3. Inadequate support.
4. History of sexual abuse or domestic violence.
5. High levels of anxiety, neurotic behavior, and depression or emotional distress.
6. Personal or family history of psychopathology, especially depression.

Common Presentations
1. Maternity blues; postpartum blues; baby blues; mother's blues; or 3rd-, 4th-, or 10th-day blues.
2. Postpartum or postnatal depression.
3. Postpartum or puerperal psychosis.
4. Postpartum panic disorder.
5. Postpartum obsessive–compulsive disorder.

Clinical Manifestations
1. Confusion.
2. Exaggerated and prolonged periods of irritability, moodiness, hostility, and fatigue.
3. Ineffective coping.
4. Withdrawal and inappropriate response to the infant or family.
5. Loss of interest in activities.
6. Insomnia or sleep disturbances.
7. Headache.
8. Constipation or other gastrointestinal symptoms.
9. Hair loss.
10. Dysmenorrhea.
11. Difficulties with lactation.
12. Decreased sexual responsiveness.

Evaluation and Management
1. Signs and symptoms may be overlooked, making the diagnosis of depression difficult. Several assessment tools, designed to screen for women who may need further evaluation for postpartum depression, are available. The psychosocial screening tool recommended by the American College of Obstetricians and Gynecologists can be used by the nurse or health care provider as a means of communication. Questions should be worded empathically and nonjudgmentally to stimulate an honest response from the mother.
2. Counseling with a mental health professional, medication, and continuous support from family and friends may be helpful in managing the depressed patient. If untreated, the woman may possibly harm the infant, herself, or others.
3. The use of psychotropic medications during breastfeeding remains a controversial issue. All of the major classes of psychotropic drugs are expressed in breast milk. Use will depend on the risk versus benefits of treatment. Consultation with the interprofessional team including lactation consultant is recommended.
4. Any indication of suicide or harm to infant requires immediate intervention to relieve the danger and referral to mental health professional.

Nursing Interventions and Patient Education
1. Actively listen to the woman regarding her adjustment to role of mother and observe for any clinical manifestations suggesting depression.
2. Teaching related to signs and symptoms should include the mother and her partner.
3. Provide multimedia resources if available.
4. Ask the woman about the infant's behavior. Negative statements about the infant may suggest that the woman is having difficulty coping. Notify the woman's obstetric or primary care provider.
5. Consult or refer woman to health care provider and other resources skilled in postpartum depression, as indicated. Refer patients to Postpartum Support International (*www.postpartum.net*).
6. Provide support and encourage family and friends to support and assist with the infant and mother. Physical support as well as emotional support may be indicated.
7. Educate the woman that treatment may help alleviate her symptoms and allow her to better care for herself and her infant.
8. Encourage the woman to engage in activities that enhance attachment: rooming-in, breastfeeding, and becoming involved in the medical examination of the neonate.
9. Realize that effective attachment behaviors differ from culture to culture and do not necessarily indicate maladaptive parenting behaviors.

SELECTED REFERENCES

American College of Obstetricians and Gynecologists. (2004/Reaffirmed 2016). *Diagnosis and treatment of gestational trophoblastic disease* (Practice Bulletin #53). Washington, DC: Author.

American College of Obstetricians and Gynecologists. (2006/Reaffirmed 2015). *Postpartum hemorrhage* (Practice Bulletin #76). Washington, DC: Author.

American College of Obstetricians and Gynecologists. (2008/Reaffirmed 2016). *Use of psychiatric medications during pregnancy and lactation* (Practice Bulletin #92). Washington, DC: Author.

American College of Obstetricians and Gynecologists. (2009/Reaffirmed 2017). *Intrapartum fetal heart rate monitoring: Nomenclature, interpretation, and general management principles* (Practice Bulletin #106). Washington, DC: Author.

American College of Obstetricians and Gynecologists. (2009/Reaffirmed 2016). *Induction of labor* (Practice Bulletin #107). Washington, DC: Author.

American College of Obstetricians and Gynecologists. (2010/Reaffirmed 2016). *Screening for perinatal depression* (Committee Opinion No. 630). Washington, DC: Author.

American College of Obstetricians and Gynecologists. (2010/Reaffirmed 2017). *Vaginal birth after cesarean* (Practice Bulletin #115). Washington, DC: Author.

American College of Obstetricians and Gynecologists. (2011/Reaffirmed 2016). *Prevention of early-onset group B streptococcal disease in newborns* (Committee Opinion #485). Washington, DC: Author.

American College of Obstetricians and Gynecologists. (2012/Reaffirmed 2016). *Opioid abuse, dependence, and addiction in pregnancy* (Committee Opinion #524). Washington, DC: Author.

American College of Obstetricians and Gynecologists. (2014/Reaffirmed 2016). *Management of late-term and postterm pregnancies* (Practice Bulletin #146). Washington, DC: Author.

American College of Obstetricians and Gynecologists. (2014). *Medical management of first trimester abortion* (Practice Bulletin #143). Washington, DC: Author.

American College of Obstetricians and Gynecologists. (2014). *Postpartum depression.* Washington, DC: Author.

American College of Obstetricians and Gynecologists. (2015). *Nausea and vomiting of pregnancy* (Practice Bulletin #153). Washington, DC: Author.

American College of Obstetricians and Gynecologists. (2015). *Operative vaginal delivery* (Practice Bulletin #154). Washington, DC: Author.

American College of Obstetricians and Gynecologists. (2016). *Magnesium sulfate use in obstetrics* (Committee Opinion #652 #171). Washington, DC: Author.

American College of Obstetricians and Gynecologists. (2016). *Prevention and management of obstetric lacerations at vaginal delivery* (Practice Bulletin #165). Washington, DC: Author.

American College of Obstetricians and Gynecologists. (2016). *Multifetal gestations: Twin, triplet, and higher-order multifetal pregnancies* (Practice Bulletin #169). Washington, DC: Author.

American College of Obstetricians and Gynecologists. (2016). *Premature rupture of membranes* (Practice Bulletin #171). Washington, DC: Author.

American College of Obstetricians and Gynecologists. (2017). *Shoulder dystocia* (Practice Bulletin #178). Washington, DC: Author.

American College of Obstetricians and Gynecologists. (2017). *Emergent therapy for acute-onset, severe hypertension during pregnancy, and the postpartum period* (Committee Opinion #692). Washington, DC: Author.

American College of Obstetricians and Gynecologists. (2017). *Episiotomy: Procedures and repair techniques.* Washington, DC: Author.

Association of Women's Health, Obstetric, Neonatal Nurses. (2014). Quantification of blood loss: AWHONN practice brief number 1. *Journal of Obstetric, Gynecologic, and Neonatal Nursing*, 1–3.

Association of Women's Health, Obstetric, Neonatal Nurses. (2015). Mood and anxiety disorders in pregnant and postpartum women. Position Statement. *Journal of Obstetric, Gynecologic, and Neonatal Nursing*, 44(5), 687–689.

Association of Women's Health, Obstetric and Neonatal Nurses (Ed.). (2015). *Fetal heart monitoring principles and practices* (5th ed.). Dubuque, IA: Kendall-Hunt Publishing Co.

Bakri, Y. N., Amri, A., & Abdul, J. F. (2001). Tamponade-balloon for obstetrical bleeding. *International Journal of Gynaecology and Obstetrics*, 74(2), 139–142.

Beck, C. T. (1993). Teetering on the edge: A substantive theory of postpartum depression. *Nursing Research*, 44, 293–304.

Bishop, E. H. (1964). Pelvic scoring for elective induction. *Obstetrics and Gynecology*, 24, 266–268.

Clapp, J. C. (2015). Multidisciplinary team approach to management of postpartum hemorrhage. *Journal of Obstetric, Gynecologic, and Neonatal Nursing*, 44, S22.

Cunningham, F. G., Leveno, K. J., Bloom, S. L., et al. (2014). *Williams obstetrics* (24th ed.). New York, NY: McGraw-Hill.

Davidson, M. W., London, M. L., & Ladewig, P. W. (2016). *Olds' maternal-newborn nursing and women's health across the lifespan* (10th ed.). Upper Saddle River, NJ: Pearson Education.

Deussen, A. R., Ashwood, P., & Martis, R. (2011). Pain relief for after pains (uterine cramping/involution) after the baby's birth. *Cochrane Database of Systematic Reviews: Plain Language Summaries*. doi:10.1002/14651858.CD004908.pub2.

Diaz, V., Abalos, E., & Carroli, G. (2014). Methods for blood loss estimation after vaginal birth (Protocol). *Cochrane Database of Systematic Reviews*, 2.

Dildy, G. A., Paine, A. R., George, N. C., & Velasco, C. (2004). Estimating blood loss: Can teaching significantly improve visual estimation? *Obstetrics and Gynecology*, 104(3), 601–606.

Friedman, E. A. (1978). *Labor: Clinical evaluation and management* (2nd ed.). New York, NY: Appleton.

Gibbins, K. J., Weber, T., Holmgren, C. M., et al. (2015). Fetal morbidity associated with uterine rupture of the unscarred uterus. *American Journal of Obstetrics and Gynecology*, 213(3), 382.e1–382.e6.

Handcock, A., Weeks, A. D., & Lavender, T. D. (2015). "Is accurate and reliable blood loss estimation the crucial step" in early detection of postpartum haemorrhage: An integrative review of the literature. *BMC Pregnancy and Childbirth*, 15, 1–9.

Heller, D. S. (2015). *OB-GYN pathology for the clinician*. New York, NY: Springer.

Jacquemyn, Y., Zecic, A., Van Laere, D., & Roelens, K. (2015). The use of intravenous magnesium in non-preeclamptic pregnant women: Fetal/neonatal neuroprotection. *Archives of Gynecology and Obstetrics*, 291(5), 969–975.

Ko, J. Y., Rockhill, K. M., Tong, V. T., et al. (2017). Trends in postpartum depressive symptoms—27 States, 2004, 2008, and 2012. *MMWR. Morbidity and Mortality Weekly Report*, 66, 153–158.

Kolkman, D. G., Verhoeven, C. J., Brinkhorst, S. J., et al. (2013). The Bishop score as a predictor of labor induction success: A systematic review. *American Journal of Perinatology*, 30(8), 625–630.

Liu, A., Lv, J., Hu, Y., Ma, L., & Chen, W. (2014). Efficacy and safety of intravaginal misoprostol versus intracervical dinoprostone for labor induction at term: A systematic review and meta-analysis. *Journal of Obstetrics and Gynaecology Research*, 40, 897–906.

Lowdermilk, D., Perry, S., Cashion, C., & Alden, K. R. (2016). *Maternity and women's health care* (11th ed.). St. Louis, MO: Mosby.

Mattson, S., & Smith, J. E. (Eds.). (2016). *Core curriculum for maternal-newborn nursing* (5th ed.). St. Louis, MO: Saunders Elsevier.

Moroz, L. A., Simpson, L. L., & Rochelson, B. (2016). Management of severe hypertension in pregnancy. *Seminars in Perinatology*, 40, 112–118.

Pawluski, J. L., Lonstein, J. S., & Fleming A. S. (2017). The neurobiology of postpartum anxiety and depression. *Trends in Neurosciences*, 40(2), 106–120.

Perkins, K. M., Boulet, S. L., Kissin, D. M., et al.; the National ART Surveillance (NASS) Group. (2015). Risk of ectopic pregnancy associated with assisted reproductive technology in the United States, 2001–2011. *Obstetrics and Gynecology*, 125(1), 70–78.

Queenan, J. T., Spong, C. Y., & Lockwood, C. J. (Eds.). (2015). *Protocols in high risk pregnancies: An evidence-based approach* (6th ed.). UK: Wiley Blackwell.

Ricci, S. S. (2017). *Essentials of maternity, newborn, and women's health nursing* (4th ed.). Philadelphia, PA: Wolters Kluwer Health/Lippincott Williams & Wilkins.

Royal College of Obstetricians and Gynaecologists. (2016). *The management of nausea and vomiting of pregnancy and hyperemesis gravidarum.* Green-top Guideline No. 69. London, UK: Author.

Rubin, R. (1984). *Maternal identity and the maternal experience.* New York, NY: Springer.

Seabra, G., Saunders, C., de Carvalho Padilha, P., et al. (2015). Association between maternal glucose levels during pregnancy and gestational diabetes mellitus: An analytical cross-sectional study. *Diabetology and Metabolic Syndrome*, 7, 17.

Sekharan, P. K. (2016). Gestational trophoblastic disease. In A. Gandhi, N. Malhotra, J. Malhotra, N. Gupta, & N. Malhotra Bora (Eds.), *Principles of critical care in obstetrics: Volume 2* (pp. 197–212). New York, NY: Springer.

Simpson, K. R., & Creehan, P. A. (2014). Chapter 14: Labor and birth. In *Perinatal nursing* (4th ed.). Philadelphia, PA: Wolters Kluwer/Lippincott Williams & Wilkins.

Smith, R. (2017). *Netter's obstetrics and gynecology* (3rd ed.). Philadelphia, PA: Elsevier.

Smith, D. Stringer, E., Vladutiu, C. J., Hickman Zink, A., & Strauss, R. (2015). Risk of uterine rupture among women attempting vaginal birth after cesarean with an unknown uterine scar. *American Journal of Obstetrics and Gynecology,* *213*(1), 80–85. doi.org/10.1016/j.ajog.2015.01.056

Son, M., & Miller, E. S. (2017). Predicting preterm birth: Cervical length and fetal fibronectin. *Seminars in Perinatology, 41*(8), 445–451.

Thomas, J., Fairclaough, A., Kavanaugh, J., & Kelly, A. J. (2014). Vaginal prostaglandin (PGE2 and PGF2a) for induction of labour at term. *Cochrane Database of Systematic Reviews,* (6). doi:10.1002/14651858.CD003101.pub3.

Troiano, N., Harvey, C., & Chez, B. (Eds.). (2013). *High-risk and critical care obstetrics* (3rd ed.). Philadelphia, PA: Lippincott Williams & Wilkins.

Verklan, M. T., & Walden, M. (Eds.) (2015). *Core curriculum for neonatal intensive care nursing* (5th ed.). St. Louis, MO: Saunders Elsevier.

Ward, S. L., Hilsey, S. M., & Mitchell-Kennedy, A. (2016). *Maternal-child nursing care: Optimizing outcomes for mothers, children, & families.* Philadelphia, PA: F.A. Davis.

PART FOUR

PEDIATRIC NURSING

40

Pediatric Growth and Development

GROWTH AND DEVELOPMENT

Infant to Adolescent Growth and Development

Growth and development begin with birth. As infants and children grow and mature, they pass through predictable stages of development. Knowledge and assessment of growth and development help the nurse provide screening for physical and emotional problems, offer anticipatory guidance to parents and caregivers, develop a rapport with the child to enhance the provision of health care, and provide education to the family to build a healthy lifestyle for the future. For assessment of the neonate, see Chapter 38, page 1023. This chapter covers the beginning of infancy (age 1 month) to adolescence (ages 12 to 14). See Table 40-1.

Developmental Screening

Assessment tools have been created to determine the overall developmental age of a child or to detect specific areas of development that are lacking. The most widely used developmental screening tool is the Denver II Developmental Screening Test (Denver II). This tool provides for a quick overview of development in children from birth to age 6 years and identifies areas of strength and weakness relative to age norms. Denver II test forms, and an instruction manual can be obtained from *www.denverii.com.* This test has been criticized for a lack of sensitivity in detecting children with more subtle developmental delays. The American Academy of Pediatrics recommends that developmental surveillance be conducted at all well-child exams and screening tests administered at the 9-, 18-, and 30-month visits; however, they do not recommend a specific test.

Another method for developmental screening involves interviewing the parent or caregiver about attainment of developmental milestones. Persistent deficits or deficits in multiple areas indicate a more serious problem than deficits in a single area (Table 40-2, pages 1092 and 1093).

Table 40-1 Infant to Adolescent Growth and Development

AGE AND PHYSICAL CHARACTERISTICS	BEHAVIOR PATTERNS	NURSING CONSIDERATIONS
Birth to 4 Weeks (1 Month) • Significant neurologic disorganization. • Strong Moro reflex. • Sleep cycle disorganized. • GI system too immature for solid foods.	**Motor development** • Momentary visual fixation on objects and human face. • Eyes follow bright moving objects. • Lies awake on back. • Immediately drops objects placed in hands. • Responds to sounds of a bell and other similar noises. • Keeps hands fisted. **Socialization and vocalization** • Mews and makes throaty noises. • Shows interest in human face. **Cognitive and emotional development** • Reflexive. • External stimuli are meaningless. • Responses are generally limited to tension states or discomfort. • Gains satisfaction from feeding and being held, rocked, fondled, and cuddled. • Has an intense need for sucking pleasure. • Quiets when picked up.	**Play stimulation** • Use human face—smile and talk. • Dangle bright moving object (eg, mobile) in field of vision. • Hold, touch, caress, fondle, and kiss. • Rock, pat, and change position. • Play soft music or have infant listen to ticking clock or sing. • Talk to infant; call by name. **Parental guidance** • Begin to expose infant to different household sounds. • Change crib location in the room. • Use brightly colored clothing and linens. • Put infant to sleep on back until old enough to roll. • Keep infant nearby. • Play with infant when awake. • Hold during feeding. **NURSING ALERT** Educate parents about infant sleep stages and putting infant to sleep on back.
4 to 8 Weeks (2 Months) • Crossed extensor reflex disappears. • Tonic neck reflex begins to fade.	**Motor development** • Reflexive behavior is slowly being replaced by voluntary movements. • Turns from side to back. • Begins to lift head momentarily from prone position. • Shows improved eye coordination. • If a bell is sounded nearby, infant will stop activity and listen. • Eyes more accurately follow vertical and horizontal alignment. Focuses well. **Socialization and vocalization** • Begins vocalization—coos, especially to a voice. • Crying becomes differentiated. • Visually looks for sounds. • May squeal with delight when stimulated by touching, talking, or singing. • Begins to smile socially. • Eyes follow person or object more intently. **Cognitive and emotional development** • Recognizes familiar face. • Becomes more aware and interested in environment. • Anticipates being fed when in feeding position. • Enjoys sucking—puts hand in the mouth.	**Play stimulation** • Securely arrange mobile over crib. • Hang wind chimes near infant. • Hang brightly colored pictures on the wall. • Use cradle gym and infant seat. • Use rattles. • Hold infant and walk around the room. • Allow freedom of kicking with clothes off. **Parental guidance** • Talk to infant and smile; get excited when infant coos. • Place infant seat on a secure surface (eg, floor, center of a table—never near the edge of the table) near mother's activities. • Put infant in prone position in bed or on floor for supervised periods. • Expose infant to different textures. • Exercise infant's arms and legs. • Sing to infant. • Provide tactile experience during bathing, diapering, and feeding.
8 to 12 Weeks (2 to 3 Months) • Landau reflex appears at 3 to 4 months. • Positive support reflex disappears.	**Motor development** • When prone, will rest on forearms and keep head in midline—makes crawling movements with legs, arches back, and holds head high; may get chest off surface.	**Play stimulation** • Encourage socialization, smiling, and laughing. • Place on mat on the floor. • Continue to introduce new sounds.

(continued)

Table 40-1 Infant to Adolescent Growth and Development (*Continued*)

AGE AND PHYSICAL CHARACTERISTICS	BEHAVIOR PATTERNS	NURSING CONSIDERATIONS
8 to 12 Weeks (2 to 3 Months) (*Continued*) • Posterior fontanelle closes. • Increase in body fluids—real tears appear, drooling and GI juices increase.	**Motor development (Continued)** • Indicates preference for prone or supine. • Discovers hands—bats objects with hands. • Holds objects in the hands and brings to the mouth. • Has fairly good head control. **Socialization and vocalization** • Smiles more readily, babbles, and coos. • Stops crying when parent enters the room or when caressed. • Enjoys playing during feeding. • Stays awake longer without crying. • Turns head to follow familiar person. **Cognitive and emotional development** • Shows active interest in environment. • Recognizes familiar faces and objects. • Focuses and follows objects. • Shows repetitiveness in play activity. • Is aware of strange situations. • Derives pleasure from sucking—purposefully gets hand to the mouth. • Begins to establish routine preceding sleep.	**Parental guidance** • Take outdoors with proper clothing (similar warmth as that of adults), hat, and PABA-free sunscreen. • Bounce on bed. • Play with infant during feeding. • Rattles can be used effectively for visual following and for hand play. • Encourage older siblings to "make faces," sing, and talk to infant. **NURSING ALERT** Children of all ages should avoid intense sun exposure, particularly during the middle of the day. PABA-free broad spectrum sunscreen with a sun protection factor of at least 15 (SPF 15) should be used on children of all ages, particularly if sun exposure is longer than 30 minutes with frequent reapplication.
12 to 16 Weeks (3 to 4 Months) • Moro reflex fades. • Stepping reflex disappears. • Rooting reflex disappears. • By 4 to 5 months, infant's weight approximately doubles birth weight. • Average weekly weight gain, 4 to 7 ounces (113.5 to 198.5 g). • Average monthly height gain, 1 inch (2.5 cm). • Pulse rate slows to 100 to 140 beats/minute. • Respirations, 20 to 40 breaths/minute. • Grasp becomes voluntary. • Sucking becomes voluntary.	**Motor development** • Eyes focus on small objects; may pick a dangling ring. • Holds head up (when being pulled to sitting position). • Becomes more interested in environment. • Hand comes to meet rattle. • Listens—turns head to familiar sound. • Sits with minimal support. • Intentional rolling over, back to side. • Reaches for offered objects. • Grasps objects with both hands and everything goes into the mouth. **Socialization and vocalization** • Laughs and chuckles socially. • Demands social attention by fussing. • Recognizes mother. • Begins to respond to "No, no." • Enjoys being propped in sitting position. **Cognitive and emotional development** • Actively interested in environment. • Enjoys attention; becomes bored when alone for long periods. • Recognizes bottle. • More interested in mother. • Indicates increasing trust and security. • Sleeps through the night; has defined nap time.	**Play stimulation** • Encourage mirror play. • Provide soft squeeze toys in vivid colors of varying textures. • Allow infant to splash in bath. • Infant still enjoys holding and playing with rattles. • Enjoys old-fashioned clothespins and playing pat-a-cake and peekaboo. **Parental guidance** • Be certain button eyes on toys and other small objects cannot be pulled off. • Hold rattle and let infant reach and grasp it. • Secure infant in high chair or infant seat. • Move mobile out of reach—infant may grab it and cause injury. • Repeat child's sounds. • Talk in varying degrees of loudness. • Begin looking at and naming pictures in book. • Begin physically active play by both parents. • Give space in playpen or on sheet on the floor to practice rolling over. • Place on the abdomen for part of playtime.
16 to 26 Weeks (4 to 7 Months) • By 5 to 6 months, tonic neck reflex disappears. • By 6 to 7 months, palmar grasp disappears.	**Motor development** • Shows momentary sitting with hand support. • Bounces and bears some weight when held in standing position. • Transfers and mouths objects in one hand.	**Play stimulation** • Enjoys social games, hide-and-seek with adult, toys, and large blocks. • Likes to bang objects. • Plays in bounce chair and walker.

Table 40-1 Infant to Adolescent Growth and Development (*Continued*)

AGE AND PHYSICAL CHARACTERISTICS	BEHAVIOR PATTERNS	NURSING CONSIDERATIONS
16 to 26 Weeks (4 to 7 Months) (*Continued*) • Two central lower incisors erupt. • Spine "C-shaped"—lacks lordotic and lumbar curves • Eustachian tube short and horizontal, which may be a factor in ear infections • GI system mature enough for solid foods	***Motor development*** (*Continued*) • Discovers feet. • Bangs objects together. • Rolls over well. • May begin some form of mobility. ***Socialization and vocalization*** • Discriminates between strangers and familiar people. • Crows and squeals. • Starts to say "Ma," and "Da." • Play is self-contained. • Laughs out loud. • Makes "talking" sounds in response to others' talking. ***Cognitive and emotional development*** • Secures objects by pulling on string. • Searches for lost objects that are out of sight. • Inspects objects; localizes sounds. • Likes to sit in high chair. • Drops and picks up objects. • Displays exploratory behavior with food. • Exhibits beginning fear of strangers. • Becomes fretful when mother leaves. • Shows much mouthing and biting.	***Play stimulation*** (*Continued*) • Enjoys large nesting toys (round rather than square). • Likes to drop and retrieve things. • Likes metal cups, wooden spoons, and things to bang with. • Loves crumpled paper. • Enjoys squeeze toys in bath. • Likes peekaboo, bye-bye, and pat-a-cake. ***Parental guidance*** • Will play as long as you can. • Let play with extra spoon at feeding. • Give soft finger foods in small amounts. • Because infant puts everything in the mouth, use safety precautions. • Keep small items away from infant, which could choke on them. • Show excitement at achievements. • Supply safe kitchen items for toys.
26 to 40 Weeks (7 to 10 Months) • By 7 to 9 months, develops eye-to-eye contact while talking; engages in social games. • Four upper incisors erupt around 7 to 9 months. • By 9 to 12 months, plantar reflex disappears. • By 9 to 12 months, neck righting reflex disappears. **6 to 12 months** • Average weekly weight gain, 3 to 5 ounces (85 to 141.7 g). • Average monthly height gain, ½ inch (1.25 cm).	***Motor development*** • Sits without support. • Recovers balance. • Manipulates objects with hands. • Unwraps objects. • Creeps. • Pulls self upright at crib rails. • Uses index finger and thumb to hold objects. • Rings a bell. • Can feed self a cracker and can hold a bottle. Chewing reflex develops. • Can control lips around cup. • Does not like supine position. • Can hold index finger and thumb in opposition. ***Socialization and vocalization*** • Claps hands on request. • Responds to own name. • Is very aware of social environment. • Imitates gestures, facial expressions, and sounds. • Smiles at image in the mirror. • Offers toy to adult, but does not release it. • Begins to test parental reaction during feeding and at bedtime. • Will entertain self for long periods. • Begins fear of strangers, 8½ to 10 months. ***Cognitive and emotional development*** • Begins to imitate. • Shows more interest in picture books. • Enjoys achievements. • Has strong urge toward independence—locomotion, feeding, and dressing.	***Play stimulation*** • Encourage use of motion toys—rocking horse and stroller. • Supervised water play. • Imitate animal sounds. • Allow exploration outdoors. • Provide for learning by imitation. • Offer new objects (blocks). • Child likes freedom of creeping and walking, but closeness of family is important. • Good toys: plastic milk carton; beanbag for tossing; fabric books; things to move around, fill up, and empty out; pileup and knockdown toys. ***Parental guidance*** • Protect from dangerous objects—cover electrical outlets, block stairs, and remove breakable objects from tables. • Have child with family at mealtime. • Offer cup. • Talk and sing to infant.

(continued)

Table 40-1   Infant to Adolescent Growth and Development (*Continued*)

AGE AND PHYSICAL CHARACTERISTICS	BEHAVIOR PATTERNS	NURSING CONSIDERATIONS

10 to 12 Months (1 Year)
 	
 • Develops lordotic and lumbar curves to make walking possible.
 • Weight should approximately triple birth weight.
 • Two lower lateral incisors appear.
 • Four first molars appear by 14 months.
 	
 Child development theories
 • Freudian: Behavior
   • Birth to 1 year—Oral Stage
 • Eriksonian: Emotion/ Personality
   • Birth to 1 year—Sense of Trust vs. Mistrust
 • Piagetian: Intellectual Activity (Thought Process)
   • Birth to 2 years— Sensorimotor Period
	Motor development
	 • Cruises around furniture.
	 • Beginning to stand alone and toddle.
	 • Turns pages in book.
	 • Tries tossing object.
	 • Shows hand dominance.
	 • Navigates stairs; climbs on chairs.
	 • Builds a tower of two blocks.
	 • Puts balls in the box.
	 • May use spoon.
	 • Can release objects at will.
	 • Has regular bowel movements.
	
	 Socialization and vocalization
	 • Uses jargon.
	 • Points to indicate wants.
	 • Loves give-and-take game.
	 • Responds to music.
	 • Enjoys being center of attention and will repeat laughed-at activities.
	
	 Cognitive and emotional development
	 • Shows fear, anger, affection, jealousy, anxiety, and sympathy.
	 • Experiments to reach new goals.
	 • Displays intense determination to remove barriers to action.
	 • Begins to develop concepts of space, time, and causality.
	 • Has increased attention span.
		Play stimulation
		 • Ball play.
		 • Cloth doll.
		 • Motion objects and toys.
		 • Transporting objects.
		 • Name and point to body parts.
		 • "Put in" and "take out" toys.
		 • Sandbox with spoons and other simple objects.
		 • Blocks.
		 • Music.
		
		 Parental guidance
		 • Allow self-directed play rather than adult-directed play.
		 • Continue to expose to foods of different texture, taste, smell, and substance.
		 • Offer cup.
		 • Show affection and encourage child to return affection.
		 • Safety teaching: Child gets into everything within reach. Place medications in safe, locked place. Create a safe environment for child. Use stair guards, faucet protectors, and drawer locks. Have poison control center phone number readily available.

12 to 18 Months • *Note:* Between ages 1 and 3 years, the child is called a "toddler." • By 12 to 24 months, Landau reflex disappears. • Anterior fontanelle closes. • The abdomen protrudes; arms and legs lengthen. • Large muscles become well developed. • Four cuspids appear by 18 months. • Fine muscle coordination begins to develop. • Average yearly weight gain, 4½ to 6½ pounds (2 to 3 kg). • Average height gain during second year, 4¾ inch (12 cm).	***Motor development*** • Walks up stairs with help and creeps downstairs. • Walks without support and with balance. • Falls less frequently. • Throws ball. • Stoops to pick up toys and looks at bug. • Turns pages of book. • Holds and lifts cup. • Builds three-block tower. • Picks up and places small beads in a container. • Begins to use spoon. ***Cognitive and emotional development*** • Has vocabulary of 10 words that have meanings. • Uses phrases and imitates words. • Points to objects named by adult. • Follows directions and requests. • Imitates adult behavior. • Retrieves toy from several hiding places. ***Psychosocial development*** • Develops new awareness of strangers. • Wants to explore everything in reach. • Plays alone, but near others. • Is dependent on parents, but begins to reach out for autonomy. • Finds security in a blanket, toy, or thumb-sucking.	***Play stimulation*** • Allow unrestricted motor activity (within safety limits). • Offer push–pull toys. • Child selects favorite toy. • Child likes blocks, pyramid toys, teddy bears, dolls, pots and pans, cloth picture books with large colorful pictures, telephone, musical top, and nested blocks. ***Parental guidance*** • Begin to teach toothbrushing to establish good dental habits; however, continue to brush child's teeth with specially formulated pediatric toothpaste. • Establish limits to give toddler sense of security, but encourage exploration. • Reinforce safety teaching.

Table 40-1 Infant to Adolescent Growth and Development (*Continued*)

AGE AND PHYSICAL CHARACTERISTICS	BEHAVIOR PATTERNS	NURSING CONSIDERATIONS
1½ to 2 Years • Protruding abdomen less noticeable. • During first 2 years, 14 inches (35 cm) is added to height. • Slight bowing of legs with a wide-based walk. • Hand preference may become apparent.	**Motor development** • Walks up and down stairs. • Opens doors; turns knobs. • Has steady gait. • Holds drinking cup well with one hand. • Uses spoon without spilling food (may prefer fingers). • Kicks a ball in front of him or her without support. • Builds a tower of four to six blocks. • Scribbles. • Rides tricycle or kiddie car (without pedals). **Cognitive development** • Has 200 to 300 words in vocabulary. • Begins to use short sentences. • Refers to self by pronoun. • Obeys simple commands. • Does not know right from wrong. • Begins to learn about time sequences. **Psychosocial development** • Uses word "mine" constantly. • Is possessive with toys. • Displays negativism—uses "no" as assertion of self. • Routine and rituals are important. • May begin cooperation in toilet training. • Resists restrictions on freedom. • Has fear of parents leaving. • Shows parallel play. • Dawdles. • Resists bedtime—uses transitional objects (blanket, toy). • Vacillates between dependence and independence.	**Play stimulation** • Shows parallel play, although enjoys having other children around. • Has very short attention span. • Enjoys same toys as child of 18 months. • Likes doll play and balls. • Imitates parents in domestic activities. • Likes swing, hammering, paper, and large crayons. **Parental guidance** • Has need for peer companionship (parallel play) although displays immaturity by inability to share and take turns. • A decrease in appetite normally occurs at this stage. • Toilet training readiness should be assessed and started if appropriate (each child follows own pattern). • Begin to have child eat meals with family if not already doing so. • Begin to read to child; child likes storybooks with large pictures.

2 to 3 Years
• Height approximates one-half adult height.
• Legs are about 34% of body length.
• Begins 5 pounds (2.3 kg) or more weight gain per year until age 5 years.
• At 2½ years, has full set (20) of baby teeth.
• Four second molars appear by 2½ years.
• Height gain, 2⅜ to 3¼ inches (6 to 8 cm).
• Lordosis and protuberant abdomen of toddler disappear.
 	
Child development theories
• Freudian:
  • 1 to 3 years—Anal Stage
• Eriksonian:
  • 1 to 3 years—Sense of Autonomy versus Shame and Doubt
	Motor development
	• Throws objects overhead.
	• Pedals tricycle.
	• Walks backward.
	• Washes and dries hands.
	• Begins to use scissors.
	• Can string large beads.
	• Can undress him- or herself.
	• Feeds himself well.
	• Tries to dance.
	• Jumps in place.
	• Builds tower of eight blocks.
	• Balances on one foot.
	• Swings and climbs.
	• Can eat an ice cream cone.
	• Drinks from a straw.
	• Chews gum without swallowing it.
	
	Cognitive development
	• Shows increased attention span.
	• Gives first and last name.
	• Begins to ask "why."
	• Is egocentric in thought and behavior.
	• Beginning ability to reflect on own behavior.
	• Talks in short sentences.
		Play stimulation
		• Plays simple games with other children.
		• Enjoys storytelling and dress-up play.
		• Plays "house."
		• Colors.
		• Uses scissors and paper.
		• Rides tricycle.
		• Reads simple books to child.
		• Will assist in developing memory skills, visual discrimination skills, and language.
		
		Parental guidance
		• From 2 to 3 years, the child develops a seeming maturity; do not expect more than child is able to do.
		• Arrange first visit to the dentist to have teeth checked if not done prior.
		• Be aware that negativistic and ritualistic behavior is normal.
		• Be consistent in discipline.
		• Control temper tantrums.
		• Begin to teach stranger, animal and traffic safety.
		• Supervise outdoor play.

(continued)

Table 40-1 Infant to Adolescent Growth and Development (*Continued*)

AGE AND PHYSICAL CHARACTERISTICS	BEHAVIOR PATTERNS	NURSING CONSIDERATIONS
2 to 3 Years (*Continued*) • Piagetian: • 2 to 7 years—Preoperational Period; shows egocentrism and centering	***Cognitive development*** (**Continued**) • Uses plurals. • May attempt to sing simple songs. • Has vocabulary of 900 words. • Begins fantasy. • Begins to understand what it means to take turns. • Can repeat three numbers. • Shows interest in colors. ***Psychosocial development*** • Negativism grows out of child's sense of developing independence—says "no" to every command. • Ritualism is important to toddler for security (follows certain pattern, especially at bedtime). • Temper tantrums may result from toddler's frustration in wanting to do everything for self. • Shows parallel play as well as beginning interaction with others. • Engages in associative play. • Fears become pronounced. • Continues to react to separation from parents but shows increasing ability to handle short periods of separation. • Has daytime bladder control and is beginning to develop nighttime bladder control. • Becomes more independent. • Begins to identify sex (gender) roles. • Explores environment outside the home. • Can create different ways of getting desired outcome.	
3 to 4 Years *Note:* Between ages 3 and 5 years, the child is called a "preschooler." May appear "knock-kneed."	***Motor development*** • Drawings have form and meaning, not detail. • Copies a circle and a cross. • Buttons front and side of clothes. • Laces shoes. • Bathes self, but needs direction. • Brushes teeth. • Shows continuous movement going up and down stairs. • Climbs and jumps well. • Attempts to print letters. ***Cognitive development*** • Awareness of body is more stable; child becomes more aware of own vulnerability. • Is less negativistic. • Learns some number concepts. • Begins naming colors. • Can identify longer of two lines. • Has vocabulary of 1,500 words. • Uses mild profanities and name-calling. • Uses language aggressively. • Asks many questions. • May not be abstract enough to understand body parts that cannot be seen or felt. • Can be given simple explanation as to cause and effect. • Thinks very concretely; demonstrates irreversibility of thought.	***Play stimulation*** • Plays and interacts with other children. • Shows creativity. • Likes ring-around-the-rosy. • "Helps" adults. • Likes costumes and enjoys dramatic play. • Toys and games: record player, nursery rhymes, housekeeping toys, transportation toys (tricycle, trucks, cars, wagon), blocks, hammer and peg bench, floor trains, blackboard and chalk, easel and brushes, clay, crayon and finger paints, outside toys (sandbox, swing, small slide), books (short stories, action stories), drum, and scrapbook. ***Parental guidance*** • Base your expectations within child's limitations. • Provide limited frustrations from environment to assist in coping. • Give small tasks to do around the house (putting silverware on table, drying an unbreakable dish). • Expand child's world with trips to the zoo, to the supermarket, to restaurant, etc. • Prevent accidents.

Table 40-1 Infant to Adolescent Growth and Development (*Continued*)

AGE AND PHYSICAL CHARACTERISTICS	BEHAVIOR PATTERNS	NURSING CONSIDERATIONS
3 to 4 Years (*Continued*)	**Cognitive development (Continued)** • Immature concept of death—believes it is reversible. • Has beginning understanding of past and future. • Is egocentric in thought. **Psychosocial development** • Is more active with peers and engages in cooperative play. • Performs simple tasks. • Frequently has imaginary companion. • Dramatizes experiences. • Is proud of accomplishments. • Exaggerates, boasts, and tattles on others. • Can tolerate separation from mother longer without feeling anxiety. • Is keen observer. • Has good sense of "mine" and "yours." • Behavior still frequently ritualistic. • Becomes curious about life and sex. Often masurbates.	**Parental guidance (Continued)** • Provide for brief nonthreatening separation from parents and home. • Reinforce correct use of language. • Use opportunities for simple sexual education as child's needs arise. • Accept masturbation as a normal phenomenon to be discouraged in public. • Provide consistent discipline, motivated by love rather than anger. • Consider nursery school/preschool opportunities.

4 to 5 Years
• By 2 to 5 years, adds 9½ inches (25 cm) to height
• At age 4, legs comprise about 44% of body length.
 	
Child development theories
• Freudian:
  • 3 to 6 years—Phallic Stage
• Eriksonian:
  • 3 to 6 years—Sense of Initiative versus Guilt
• Piagetian:
  • 2 to 7 years—Preoperational Period; shows egocentrism and centering
	Motor development
	• Hops two or more times.
	• Dresses without supervision.
	• Has good motor control—climbs and jumps well.
	• Walks up stairs without grasping handrail.
	• Walks backward.
	• Washes self without wetting clothes.
	• Prints first name and other words.
	• Adds three or more details in drawings.
	• Draws a square.
	
	Cognitive development
	• Has 2,100-word vocabulary.
	• Talks constantly.
	• Uses adult speech forms.
	• Participates in conversations.
	• Asks for definitions.
	• Knows age and residence.
	• Identifies heavier of two objects.
	• Knows weeks as time units.
	• Names days of week.
	• Begins to understand kinship.
	• Knows primary colors.
	• Can count to 10.
	• Can copy a triangle.
	• Has a high degree of imagination.
	• Questioning is at a peak.
	• Begins to develop power of reasoning.
	
	Psychosocial development
	• May have an imaginary companion.
	• Has a sense of order (likes to finish what was started).
	• Is obedient and reliable.
	• Is protective toward younger children.
	• Begins to develop an elementary conscience with some influence in governing behavior.
	• Has increased self-confidence.
		Play stimulation
		• Demonstrates gross motor activity—likes to jump rope, skip, climb on jungle gym, etc.
		• Prefers group play and cooperates in projects.
		• Plays simple letter, number, form, and picture games.
		• Plays with cars and trucks.
		• Still likes being read to.
		• Continues to enjoy fantasy play.
		
		Parental guidance
		• Child may no longer require an afternoon nap
		• Prepare child for kindergarten.
		• Tell him or her stories.
		• Provide opportunities and reassurance for group play; have his or her friends visit for lunch and an afternoon of playing.
		• Prevent accidents.
		• Encourage child's participation in household activities.

(*continued*)

Table 40-1   Infant to Adolescent Growth and Development (*Continued*)

AGE AND PHYSICAL CHARACTERISTICS	BEHAVIOR PATTERNS	NURSING CONSIDERATIONS
4 to 5 Years (*Continued*)	**Psychosocial development (*Continued*)** • Accepts responsibility for acts. • Is less rebellious. • Has dreams and nightmares. • Is cooperative and sympathetic. • Shows generosity with toys. • Begins to question parents' thinking. • Identifies strongly with parent of same sex.	

Middle Childhood (5 to 9 Years)
• Growth rate is slow and steady.
• Gains an average of 7 pounds (3.2 kg) per year. Height increases approximately 2½ inch (6.3 cm) per year.
• Among children, there is considerable variation in height and weight.
• Appears taller and slimmer.
• Early lordosis disappears.
• Begins to lose baby teeth; permanent teeth appear at a rate of about 4 teeth per year from 7 to 14 years.
• Neuromuscular and skeletal development allows improved coordination.
• Eyes become fully developed; vision approaches 20/20.
• Handedness should be well developed.
 	
Child development theories
• Freudian:
  • 5 to 9 years—Beginning of Latency Period
• Eriksonian:
  • 5 to 9 years—Industry versus Inferiority
• Piagetian:
  • 5 to 9 years—Enters Stage of Concrete Operations
	Motor development
	6 years
	• Is active and impulsive.
	• Balance improves.
	• Uses hands as manipulative tools in cutting, pasting, and hammering.
	• Can draw large letters or figures.
	
	7 years
	• Has lower activity level.
	• Capable of fine hand movements; can print sentences.
	• Nervous habits, such as nail biting, are common.
	• Muscular skills, such as ball throwing, have improved.
	
	8 years
	• Moves with less restlessness.
	• Has developed grace and balance, even in active sports.
	• Has developed coordination of fine muscles, allowing child to write in script.
	
	9 years
	• Uses both hands independently.
	• Has become skillful in manual activities because of improved eye–hand coordination.
	
	Cognitive development
	6 years
	• Begins to learn to read. Defines objects in terms of use. Time sense is as much in past as present.
	• Is interested in relationship between home and neighborhood; knows some streets.
	• Uses sentences well; uses language to share others' experiences; may swear or use slang.
	• Distinguishes morning from afternoon.
	
	7 years
	• More reflective and has deeper understanding of meanings.
	• Interested in conclusions and logical endings. Begins to have scientific interests in cause and effect.
	• More responsible in relation to time, more punctual. Sense of space is more realistic; child wants some space of own.
	• Knows value of coins.
	• Concept of death maturing—includes idea of irreversibility.
	
	8 years
	• Thinking is less animistic. Is aware of impersonal forces of nature. Begins to understand logical reasoning, conclusions, and implications.
		Parental guidance
		• Family atmosphere continues to have an impact on the child's emotional development and future response within the family.
		• The child needs ongoing guidance in an open, inviting atmosphere. Limits should be set with conviction. Deal with only one incident at a time. When punishment is necessary, the child should not be humiliated. Child should know that it was the act that the adult found undesirable, not the child.
		• Needs assistance in adjusting to new experiences and demands of school. Should be able to share experiences with family. Parents need to have communication with the teacher to work together for the health of the child.
		• Convey love and caring in communication. The child understands language directed at feelings better than at intellect. Get down to eye level with the child.
		• Focus attention on child's abilities and accomplishments rather than shortcomings and limitations.
		• The child is sex-conscious and should be able to discuss questions at home rather than with friends. Requires simple, honest answers to questions.
		• Common problems include teasing, quarreling, nail biting, enuresis, whining, poor manners, swearing, lying, cheating, and stealing. These are usually fleeting phases and should not be handled negatively. The causes for such behavior should be investigated and dealt with constructively.
		• The child needs order and consistency to help in coping with doubts, fears, unacceptable impulses, and unfamiliar experiences.
		• Encourage peer activities as well as home responsibilities and give recognition to child's accomplishments and unique talents.
		• Television may stimulate learning in several spheres, but should be monitored.
		• Accidents are a major cause of disability and death. Safety practices should be continued. (Refer to section on safety, page 1127.)

Table 40-1 Infant to Adolescent Growth and Development (*Continued*)

AGE AND PHYSICAL CHARACTERISTICS	BEHAVIOR PATTERNS	NURSING CONSIDERATIONS
Middle Childhood (5 to 9 Years) (*Continued*)	***Cognitive development (Continued)*** • Less self-centered in thinking. Personal space is expanding; goes places on own. Aware of time; plans events of the day. Understands right from left. *9 years* • Intellectually energetic and curious. Realistic; reasonable in thinking. Able to plan in advance. Breaks complex activities into steps. • Focuses on detail. • Sense of space includes the entire earth. • Participates in family discussions. • Likes to have secrets. ***Psychosocial development*** *5 to 9 years* • Still requires parental support, but pulls away from overt signs of affection. • Peer groups provide companionship in widening circle of persons outside the home. Child learns more about self as he or she learns about others. • "Chum" stage occurs at about age 9 or 10. Child chooses a special friend of same sex and age in whom to confide. This is usually child's first love relationship outside of home, when someone becomes as important to him or her as oneself. • Play teaches the child new ideas and independence. Child progressively uses tools of competition, compromise, cooperation, and beginning collaboration. • Body image and self-concept are fluid because of rapid physical, emotional, and social changes. • Latency-stage sexual drive is controlled and repressed. Emphasis is on the development of skills and talent. ***Patterns of play*** *6 to 7 years* • Child acts out ideas of family and occupational groups with which he or she has contact. • Painting, pasting, reading, simple games, watching television, digging, running games, skating, riding bicycle, and swimming are all enjoyed activities. *8 years* • Child enjoys collections; loosely formed, short-lived clubs, table games, card games, books, television, and music.	***Parental guidance (Continued)*** • Exercise is essential to promote motor and psychosocial development. The child should have a safe place to play and simple pieces of equipment. • A school health program should be available and concerned with the child's physical, emotional, mental, and social health. This should be augmented by information and example at home. • Medical supervision should continue with yearly examination to detect developmental delay and disease. Appropriate immunizations should be administered. • The child frequently has "quiet days"—periods of shyness, which should be tolerated as part of growing up and deciding who he or she is. • The child may be subject to nightmares, a situation that requires reassurance and understanding. • Parents, teachers, and health professionals should be available and able to provide information and answer questions about the physical changes that occur.
Late Childhood (9 to 12 Years) • Vital signs approach adult values. • Loses childish appearance of face and takes on features that will characterize individual as an adult.	***Motor development*** • Energetic, restless, active movements such as finger drumming or foot tapping appear. • Has skillful manipulative movements nearly equal to those of adults. • Works hard to perfect physical skills.	***Parental guidance*** • Continue appropriate interventions related to early childhood. • Continue sex education and preparation for adolescent body changes. • Understanding is important.

(continued)

Table 40-1 Infant to Adolescent Growth and Development (*Continued*)

AGE AND PHYSICAL CHARACTERISTICS	BEHAVIOR PATTERNS	NURSING CONSIDERATIONS

Late Childhood (9 to 12 Years) (*Continued*)
 	
• Growth spurt occurs and some secondary sex characteristics appear: in girls, between ages 10 and 12 years, and in boys, between ages 12 and 14 years.
 	
Physical changes of puberty
• Increased height and weight, increased perspiration and activity of sebaceous glands; vasomotor instability; increased fat deposition.
 	
Physical changes in girls
• The pelvis increases in transverse diameter; hips broaden; tenderness in developing breast tissue; enlargement of areola diameter; appearance of pubic hair.
 	
Physical changes in boys
• Size of testes increases; scrotum color changes; breasts enlarge, temporarily; height and shoulder breadth increase.
• Appearance of lightly pigmented hair at the base of the penis.
• Increase in length and width of the penis.
 	
Child development theories
• Freudian:
  • 9 to 12 years—Latency Period continues.
• Eriksonian:
  • 9 to 12 years—Industry versus. Inferiority continues.
• Piagetian:
  • 9 to 12 years—Stage of Concrete Operations continues.
	Cognitive development
	
	10 years
	• Likes to reason and enjoys learning.
	• Thinking is concrete and matter of fact.
	• Wants to measure up to challenge.
	• Likes to memorize and identify facts.
	• Attention span may be short. Space is rather specific (ie, where things are).
	• Can write for relatively long time with speed.
	• Likes action in learning.
	• Concentrates well when working competitively.
	• Can understand relational terms, such as weight and size.
	• Perceives space as nothingness that goes on forever.
	• Can discuss problems.
	• Can conceptualize symbolically enough to understand body parts.
	• Can describe some abstract terms.
	
	12 years
	• Enjoys learning.
	• Considers all aspects of a situation.
	• Motivated more by inner drive than by competition.
	• Able to classify, arrange, and generalize.
	• Likes to discuss and debate.
	• Begins conceptual thinking.
	• Verbal, formal reasoning now possible.
	• Can recognize moral of a story.
	• Defines time as duration; likes to plan ahead.
	• Understands that space is abstract.
	• Can be critical of own work.
	
	Psychosocial development
	• Gang becomes important and gang code takes precedence over nearly everything. Gang codes are typically characterized by collective action against the mores of the adult world. Here, children begin to work out their own social patterns without adult interference. Early gangs may include both sexes; later gangs are separated by sex.
	• May strive for unreasonable independence from adult control.
	• Usually interested in religion and morality.
	• Has increased interest in sexuality.
	• May reach puberty; resurgence of sexual drives causes recapitulation of Oedipal struggle.
	
	Patterns of play
	• Continues to enjoy reading, TV, and table games.
	• More interested in active sports as a means to improve skills.
	• Creative talents may appear; may enjoy drawing and modeling clay. By age 10, gender differences in preferred play activities may be more pronounced.
	• Occasional privacy is important.
	• Begins to have vocational aspirations, may be seemingly unrealistic and frequently changing.
		Parental guidance (*Continued*)
		• Encourage participation in organized clubs and youth groups.
		• Democratic guidance is essential as child works through a conflict between dependence (on parents) and independence. The child needs realistic limits set.
		• Needs help channeling energy in proper direction—work and sports
		• Requires adequate explanation of body changes prior to changes appearing. Special understanding is required for the child who lags in physical development compared to peers or to those who develop significantly earlier than peers.
		• Continue consistent disciplinary style.

Table 40-1	Infant to Adolescent Growth and Development (*Continued*)

AGE AND PHYSICAL CHARACTERISTICS	BEHAVIOR PATTERNS	NURSING CONSIDERATIONS

Early Adolescence (12 to 14 Years)
 	
• Phase of development begins when reproductive organs become functionally operative; the phase ends when physical growth is completed.
• Skeletal system grows faster than supporting muscles.
• Hands and feet grow proportionately faster than the rest of the body.
• Large muscles develop more quickly than small muscles.
 	
Girls
• Physical changes include beginning of menarche, growth of axillary and perineal hair, deepened voice, ovulation, and further development of breasts.
• Nutritional need for iron and calcium increases dramatically.
 	
Boys
• Physical changes include growth of axillary, perineal, facial, chest hair, deepening of voice, production of spermatozoa, and nocturnal emissions.
 	
Child development theories
• Freudian:
  • 12 to 14 years—Begins Stage of Sexuality
• Eriksonian:
  • 12 to 14 years—Identity versus Role Diffusion.
• Piagetian:
  • 12 to 14 years—Begins Stage of Formal Operations
	Motor development
	• Usually uncoordinated; has poor posture.
	• Tires easily.
	
	Cognitive development
	• Mind has great ability to acquire and use knowledge.
	• Abstract thinking is sufficient to learn multivariable ideas such as the influence of hormones on emotions.
	• Categorizes thoughts into usable forms.
	• May project thinking into the future.
	• Is capable of highly imaginative thinking.
	
	Psychosocial development
	• Interest in opposite sex increases.
	• Often revolts from adult authority to conform to peer–group standards.
	• Continues to rework feelings for parent of opposite sex and unravel the ambivalence toward parent of same sex.
	• Affection may turn temporarily to an adult outside of the family (eg, crush on family friend, neighbor, or teacher).
	• Uses peer–group dialect—highly informal language or specially coined terminology.
	• Peer groups are especially important and help adolescent to define own identity, to adapt to changing body image, to establish more mature relationships with others, and to deal with heightened sexual feelings. Cliques may develop.
	• Dating generally progresses from groups of couples to double dates and finally single couples.
	• Teenage "hangouts" become important centers of activity.
	• Begins questioning existing moral values
		Parental guidance
		• Stresses frequently result from conflicting value systems between generations. The parents may need help to see that the adolescent is a product of the times and that actions reflect what is happening around the adolescent.
		• The parents' limits and rules should be realistic and consistent. They should convey the parent's love and concern and should be a source of comfort and reassurance, protecting the child from activities for which he or she is not ready.
		• The home should be an accepting, emotionally stable environment.
		• Continue sex education, including discussion of ovulation, fertilization, menstruation, pregnancy, contraception, masturbation, nocturnal emissions, and hygiene.
		• Adolescents have an increased need for rest and sleep because they are expending large amounts of energy and are functioning with an inadequate oxygen supply.
		• Recreational interests should be fostered. Favorite activities include sports, dating, dancing, reading, hobbies, and social media. Socializing via telephone or computer and listening to music are favorite pastimes.
		• Adolescent health problems that require preventive education are accidents, obesity, acne, pregnancy, sexually transmitted disease, and drug abuse.
		• Allow the adolescent to handle his or her own affairs as much as possible, but be aware of physical and psychosocial problems that may require help. Encourage independence but allow child to seek support and guidance from parents or trusted adults when frightened or unable to attain goals.
		• Adolescents with special problems should have access to specialists, such as adolescent clinics and psychologists.
		• Requires reassurance and help in accepting a changing body image. Parents should make the most of the child's positive qualities.
		• Give gentle encouragement and guidance regarding dating. Avoid strong pressures in either direction.
		• Understand conflicts as the child attempts to deal with social, moral, and intellectual issues.

Table 40-2 Developmental Milestones

AGE	GROSS MOTOR	VISUAL–MOTOR/ PROBLEM SOLVING	LANGUAGE	SOCIAL/ADAPTIVE
1 month	Raises head slightly from prone, makes crawling movements	*Birth*: visually fixes *1 month*: has tight grasp, follows to midline	Alerts to sound	Regards face
2 months	Holds head in midline, lifts chest off table	No longer clenches fist tightly, follows object past midline	Smiles socially (after being stroked or talked to)	Recognizes parent
3 months	Supports on forearms in prone, holds head up steadily	Holds hands open at rest, follows in circular fashion, responds to visual threat	Coos (produces long vowel sounds in musical fashion)	Reaches for familiar people or objects, anticipates feeding
4 months	Rolls front to back, supports on wrists, and shifts weight	Reaches with arms in unison, brings hands to midline	Laughs, orients to voice	Enjoys looking around environment
5 months	Rolls back to front, sits supported	Transfers objects	Says "ah-goo," blows raspberries, orients to bell (localizes laterally)	—
6 months	Sits unsupported, puts feet in the mouth in supine position	Unilateral reach, uses raking grasp	Babbles	Recognizes strangers
7 months	Creeps	—	Orients to bell (localized indirectly)	—
8 months	Comes to sit, crawls	Inspects objects	"Dada" indiscriminately	Finger-feeds
9 months	Pivots when sitting, pulls to stand, cruises	Uses pincer grasp, probes with forefinger, holds bottle, throws objects	"Mama" indiscriminately, gestures, waves bye-bye, inhibits to "no"	Starts to explore environment; plays gesture games (eg, pat-a-cake)
10 months	Walks when led with both hands held	—	"Dada/mama" discriminately; orients to bell (directly)	—
11 months	Walks when led with one hand held	—	One word other than "dada/mama," follows one-step command with gesture	—
12 months	Walks alone	Uses mature pincer grasp, releases voluntarily, marks paper with pencil	Uses two words other than "dada/mama," immature jargoning (runs several unintelligible syllables together)	Imitates actions, comes when called, cooperates with dressing
13 months	—	—	Uses three words	—
14 months	—	—	Follows one-step command without gesture	—
15 months	Creeps up stairs, walks backward	Scribbles in imitation, builds tower of two blocks in imitation	Uses four to six words	*15 to 18 months:* uses spoon, uses cup independently
17 months	—	—	Uses 7 to 20 words, points to five body parts, uses mature jargoning (includes intelligible words in jargoning)	—

Table 40-2 Developmental Milestones (Continued)

AGE	GROSS MOTOR	VISUAL–MOTOR/ PROBLEM SOLVING	LANGUAGE	SOCIAL/ADAPTIVE
18 months	Runs, throws objects from standing without falling	Scribbles spontaneously, builds tower of three blocks, turns two to three pages at a time	Uses two-word combinations	Copies parent in tasks (sweeping, dusting), plays in company of other children
19 months	—	—	Knows 8 body parts	—
21 months	Squats in play, goes up steps	Builds tower of five blocks	Uses 50 words, two-word sentences	Asks to have food and to go to toilet
24 months	Walks up and down steps without help	Imitates stroke with pencil, builds tower of seven blocks, turns pages one at a time, removes shoes, pants, etc.	Uses pronouns (*I, you, me*) inappropriately, follows two-step commands	Parallel play
30 months	Jumps with both feet off the floor, throws ball overhand	Holds pencil in adult fashion, performs horizontal and vertical strokes, unbuttons	Uses pronouns appropriately, understands concept of "1," repeats two digits forward	Tells first and last names when asked; gets self drink without help
3 years	Can alternate feet when going up steps, pedals tricycle	Copies a circle, undresses completely, dresses partially, dries hands if reminded	Uses minimum 250 words, three-word sentences; uses plurals, past tense; knows all pronouns; understands concept of "2"	Group play, shares toys, takes turns, plays well with others, knows full name, age, sex
4 years	Hops, skips, alternates feet going down steps	Copies a square, buttons clothing, dresses self completely, catches ball	Knows colors, says song or poem from memory, asks questions	Tells "tall tales," plays cooperatively with a group of children
5 years	Skips alternating feet, jumps over low obstacles	Copies triangle, ties shoes, spreads with knife	Prints first name, asks what a word means	Plays competitive games, abides by rules, likes to help in household tasks

SELECTED REFERENCES

Abo, E., Tawfik, M., Abo, E., et al. (2017). Screening for developmental delay in preschool-aged children using parent-completed Ages and Stages Questionnaires: Additional insights into child development. *Postgraduate Medical Journal, 93*, 597–602.

American Academy of Pediatrics. (2018). Developmental Surveillance and Screening in Preventative Health Care Visits. *https://www.aap.org/en-us/about-the-aap/Committees-Councils-Sections/Council-on-Children-with-Disabilities/Pages/Description-and-Policy.aspx*

Augustyn, M., Zuckerman, B., & Caronna, E. (2010). *The Zuckerman Parker handbook of developmental and behavioral pediatrics: A handbook for primary care* (3rd ed.). Philadelphia, PA: Lippincott Williams & Wilkins.

Brown, A., & Elder, J. (2014). Communication in Autism Spectrum disorder: A guide for pediatric nurses. *Pediatric Nursing, 40*(5), 219–225.

Burns, C., Dunn, A., Brady, M., et al. (2016). *Pediatric primary care* (6th ed.). Philadelphia, PA: Saunders.

Dixon, S., & Stein, M. (2005). *Encounters with children: Pediatric behavior and development* (4th ed.). St. Louis, MO: Mosby.

Johns Hopkins Hospital; Hughes, H., Kahn, L. (Eds.). (2017). *The Harriet Lane handbook* (21st ed.). Philadelphia, PA: Elsevier Mosby.

Kyle, T. (Ed.). (2016). *Essentials of pediatric nursing* (3rd ed.). Philadelphia, PA: Wolters Kluwer Health.

MacLaughlin, S., Gillespie, L., & Parlakia, R. (2017). Using Pediatric Visits to Support Children and Families. *Zero to Three, 37*(4), 46–52.

National Institute of Child Health and Human Development. (2012). SIDS: Back to sleep public education campaign. Available: *www.nichd.nih.gov/sids/*

Nelson, K., & McKinney, E. (2017). *Maternal-child nursing* (5th ed.). St. Louis, MO: Saunders.

Pillitteri, A. (2013). *Maternal and child health nursing: Care of the childbearing and childrearing family* (7th ed.). Philadelphia, PA: Lippincott Williams & Wilkins.

Reading, R. (2015). How best to teach developmental assessment? A single-blinded randomized study. *Child: Care, Health and Development, 41*(2), 334.

Sheldrick, R.C., & GArfinkel, D. (2017). Is a Positive Develpomental-Behavioral Screening Score Sufficient to Justify Referral? A Review of Evidence and Theory. *Pediatrics, 17*(5), 464–170.

Vehkavuori, S., & Stolt, S. (2018). Screening language skills. *Infant Behavior & Development, 50*, 174–197.

41

Pediatric Physical Assessment

HISTORY

Obtaining a History

A history of the child is obtained to establish a relationship with the child and family, to assess family understanding about the child's health, to formulate an individual care plan, and to correct misinformation the family may have.

Focus on specific topics in the history, depending on the child's age, including:

- Infant—prenatal and postnatal history, nutrition, development.
- Toddler—home environment, safety issues, development, parent's response.
- School age—school, friends, reaction to previous hospitalizations.
- Adolescent—alcohol, drugs, friends, sexual history, relationships with parents, identity.

Identifying Information

Type of Information Needed

1. Date and time.
2. Health care provider's name and telephone number, if known.
3. Insurance data.
4. Patient's name, address, telephone number, birth date.
5. Referring health care source (eg, school, other health care provider, clinic).

Note: Permission from the legal guardian must be obtained to treat a child unless it is an emergency.

Method of Collecting Data

1. Identify the care person in charge of the patient by name and relationship to the patient; obtain a relative's or caregiver's address and home, cell and work telephone numbers, if different from those of the parent.
2. To make the informant feel more at ease, the questions should begin in a friendly, nonthreatening manner. Questions addressed to the parent should be phrased appropriately.
3. Casual, friendly responses or remarks on the part of the interviewer may also help break the ice, such as:
   a. "Whoever takes care of this baby certainly does a good job."
   b. "That is a lovely outfit the baby is wearing." (Remember that families will usually put good clothes on a baby for a visit to a health care agency.)

4. Sometimes, repeat the information to verify data. This will give you a better judgment of the care person's cooperation and reliability.
5. If age appropriate, get some data directly from the child.

Chief Complaint

Method of Recording

1. Record who arrived with child and write an exact description of the complaint.
2. Use quotation marks to clearly indicate that the informant's words are being used. It is helpful to explain:
   a. "I will write it down so there will be no mistake."
   b. "Let me read this back to you to make sure it is correct."
3. Quotation of the care person's exact words may give an indication of how he feels about the symptoms; it may reflect fear, guilt, and defensiveness.

Method of Collecting Information

1. Begin with a helpful, open-ended question. That is the first overture made to this patient:
   a. "How have things been going?"
   b. "Please tell me the reason for your coming here today."
   c. "Do you have any particular worries or concerns about the baby?"
2. Then, proceed to more specific questions.

Duration of Complaint

1. The information obtained may indicate the natural history of the disease, if one is present, and its gradual evolution. Pursue the information with a series of probing questions.
   a. "How long has the baby (child) had this problem?"
   b. If the informant cannot remember, try another route: "When did the child last act well? Before summer vacation? Last Christmas? Did the baby have the trouble then?"
2. Write down the responses; try to assess, as more questions are asked, how accurate the informant's answers may be. Remember, a child that is a reliable historian, may be the most accurate source of information regarding their health history, treatments, and other health needs.

History of Present Illness

Type of Information Needed

For an infant, a preverbal, or nonverbal child, information will consist mainly of what the informant has been able to observe. Having established what the chief complaint is, identify further problems, if any. Obtain the following information for each problem:

1. Body location—of pain, itching, weakness.
2. Quality and quantity of complaint—both type (a burning pain) and severity (knifelike, comes and goes).
3. Degree of symptom—(eg, pain, how severe; cough, day and night; eye drainage, amount).
4. Chronology—indicate time sequence and whether the problem is episodic (lasts for a while and then clears up completely).
5. Environment or setting—where and when the symptoms occur.
6. Aggravating and alleviating factors—what makes the pain worse or better.
7. Associated manifestations or symptoms—accompanied by vomiting, blurred vision.

Importance of Detail

1. Typically, a carefully written description of a symptom will be the source of a future diagnosis and will serve all who are involved in helping the patient.
2. Do not worry about how many notes you have to take at first.
3. You will be able to recheck this information when you do the review of systems.

Family History

1. Family members—parents' age and state of health, siblings-who is at home with you?
2. Family health history:
   a. Eyes, ears, nose, throat—nosebleeds, sinus problems, glaucoma, cataracts, myopia, strabismus, other problems of eyes, ears, nose, throat.
   b. Cardiorespiratory—tuberculosis, asthma, hay fever, hypertension, heart murmurs, heart attacks, strokes, rheumatic fever, pneumonia, emphysema, other problems.
   c. Gastrointestinal—ulcers, colitis, vomiting, diarrhea, other problems.
   d. Genitourinary—kidney infections, bladder problems, congenital abnormalities.
   e. Musculoskeletal—congenital hip or foot problems, muscular dystrophy, arthritis, other problems.
   f. Neurologic—seizures, epilepsy, nervous disorder, mental retardation, emotional problems, comas, headaches, others.
   g. Chronic disease—diabetes, liver disease, cancer, tumors, anemia, thyroid problems, congenital disorder.
   h. Special senses—anyone deaf or blind.
   i. Miscellaneous—other medical problem not mentioned.
3. Family social history:
   a. Residence—apartment or house and size. Yard, stairs, proximity to transportation, shopping, playground, school, safe neighborhood? City or well water?
   b. Financial situation—who works, where employed, occupation, welfare, food stamps.
   c. Primary care person—babysitters, day care center.
   d. Family interrelationships—happy, cooperative, antagonistic, chaotic, multiproblem, violent.

Past History

Prenatal

1. Pregnancy—planned or not; source of care; approximate date of seeking care; birth order of this pregnancy, including miscarriages. This area of the history may be one of great sensitivity. Try to make the questions gentle and supportive:
   a. "Did you plan a baby around this time?"
   b. "When was your first checkup for the pregnancy?"
   c. "Were there any unusual problems related to your pregnancy or delivery?"
2. Maternal health—includes illnesses and dates, abnormal symptoms (eg, fever, rash, vaginal bleeding, edema, hypertension, urine abnormalities, sexually transmitted disease). Avoid technical words, if possible.
   a. "Were the doctors or nurses worried about your health?"
   b. "Were your rings or shoes tight?"
   c. "Do you know if your blood pressure went up?"
   d. "Did you have trouble with your urine?"
3. Weight gain—validate by trying to get a figure for nonpregnant weight and weight at delivery.
4. Medications taken—for example, vitamins, iron, calcium, aspirin, cold preparations, tranquilizers ("nerve medicine"), antibiotics; use of ointments, hormones, injections during pregnancy; special or unusual diet; radiation exposure; sonography; and amniocentesis.
5. Quality of the fetal movements—when felt?
6. Use of alcohol, tobacco, or drugs during pregnancy.

Natal

1. Expected date of delivery and approximate duration of pregnancy.
2. Place of delivery and name of person who conducted the delivery.
3. Labor—spontaneous or induced, duration, and intensity.
4. Analgesia or anesthesia.
5. Type of delivery—vaginal (breech or vertex presentation); cesarean delivery; forceps delivery.
6. Complications (eg, need for blood transfusion or delay in delivery).

Neonatal

1. Condition of infant.
2. Color (if seen) at delivery.
3. Activity of infant.
4. Type of crying heard.
5. Breathing abnormality.
6. Birth weight and length.
7. Problems that occurred immediately at birth.

Postnatal

1. Duration of hospitalization of the mother and infant.
2. Problems with baby's breathing or feeding.
3. Need of supportive care (eg, oxygen, incubator, special care nursery, isolation, medications).
4. Weight changes, weight at discharge, if known.
5. Color—cyanosis or jaundice.
6. Bowel movements—when.
7. Problems—seizures, deformities identified, consultation required.
8. Hearing—was a hearing screen conducted in the nursery? The United States Preventative Services Task Force recommends universal screening for all newborns using otoacoustic emissions and/or auditory brain stem response testing. The guideline is available online at *www.guideline.gov/summaries/summary/47317/preventive-services-for-children-and-adolescents?q=newborns+otoacoustic*.
9. Mother's contact with the baby and her first impression:
   a. "What was it like when you first saw your baby?"
   b. "What did the baby do when you were first together?"

Nutrition

1. Breast- or bottle-fed? What formula? How prepared?
2. Amounts offered and consumed.
3. Frequency of feeding—weight gain.
4. Addition of juice or solid foods.

5. Food preferences or allergies.
6. Feeding problems—variations in appetite.
7. Age of weaning.
8. Vitamins—type, amount, regularity.
9. Pattern of weight gain.
10. Current diet—frequency and content of meals.

Growth and Development

1. Past weights and lengths, if available.
2. Milestones—sat alone unsupported; walked alone; used words, then sentences.
3. Teeth—eruption, difficulty, cavities, brushing, flossing.
4. Toilet training.
5. Current motor, social, and language skills.
6. Sexual development.
   a. Infant—swollen breast tissue, vaginal discharge, hypertrophy of the labia.
   b. Toddler or school-age child—early development of breasts or pubic hair.
   c. Prepubertal or pubertal child—in girls, time of development of breasts and pubic hair and onset of menstruation. In boys, time of enlargement of testes and penis, development of pubic and facial hair, and voice changes.

Health Maintenance

1. Immunizations—rubella, rubeola, mumps, polio, diphtheria, pertussis, tetanus toxoid, varicella, pneumococcal, bacille Calmette-Guérin, influenza, *Haemophilus influenzae* type b, hepatitis A and B, meningococcal conjugate, human papillomavirus, and rotavirus. Indicate number and dates. Recommended immunization schedules are available online at *www.cdc.gov/vaccines/recs/schedules/*.
2. Screening procedures—hematocrit or hemoglobin level, urinalysis, tuberculin testing, visual and auditory acuity, color vision, lead testing, cholesterol screening, syphilis testing, HIV testing, gonorrhea and Chlamydia screening.
3. Dental care—source and frequency of care, dental hygienist visits, fillings, extractions, last checkup.

Acute Infectious Diseases

Rubella, rubeola, mumps, chickenpox, group A beta-hemolytic pharyngitis, parvovirus B19 (fifth disease), hepatitis, infectious mononucleosis, sexually transmitted disease, tuberculosis, influenza. Recent exposure to a communicable disease.

Hospitalizations and Surgeries

1. Dates, hospital, health care provider.
2. Indications, diagnosis, procedures.
3. Complications.
4. Reactions to previous hospitalizations.

Injuries

1. Emergency department or urgent care visits-frequency and diagnosis.
2. Fractures, injuries, burns—location and treatment.
3. Ingestions.
4. Ask the parents about provision of a safe environment; for example, cleaning supplies out of reach, electrical outlets with appropriate covers, guns in the house unloaded and kept in a locked room or cabinet, water safety education (bathtub and pools). Ask about use of safety equipment, such as seat belts, bike helmets, childproof safety caps on medications, smoke and carbon monoxide detectors in home.

Medications

1. For general use, such as vitamins, antihistamines, laxatives.
2. Special or fad diets.

3. Recent antibiotics.
4. Herbal or complementary remedies.
5. Routine use of aspirin.
6. Hormonal contraceptives—types, dose, duration.
7. Drugs, opioids, marijuana, hallucinogens, mood elevators, tranquilizers, alcohol.
8. Determine when last dose of medication was taken; is the medication with the patient? How does the child take the medication?
9. Allergy or adverse reaction to medication?

School History

Type of Information Needed

1. Present and past schooling, attendance, grade, and performance.
2. Favored and least-favored subjects.
3. School-related behavior—anxious to go, anxious to stay home.
4. General attitude toward school and career plans.
5. General attitude toward peer groups, attempt to avoid or be included.

Method of Collecting Data

1. Straightforward questions to a child (eg, "What grade are you in?" "Who are your friends?").
2. Three wishes offered to the child:
   a. "If your birthday were here, what would you ask for?"
   b. "If you could be anyone, who would it be?"
   c. "What would be the best thing that could happen to you?"
3. "Do you have friends?," "Who is your best friend?"
4. Questions to parents: "Do you know the friends your child identified?
5. Adolescents—Interviews with older children and teens may start with the parents present, but the child should also be provided with some private time away from the parents to discuss concerns. The parents should also be allowed a brief time away from their child to voice any concerns.
6. Emphasize the positive (eg, "What is your best subject?").

Social History

Type of Information Needed

1. Environment—rural, urban.
2. Housing—type, location, heating, sewage, water supply, family pets, other animal exposure.
3. Parents' occupations (employment) and marital status.
4. Number of individuals living in home, sleeping arrangements.
5. Religious affiliations.
6. Previous utilization of social agencies.
7. Health insurance and usual source of care.
8. After assuring older children of the confidentiality of their answers, inquire about risk-taking behaviors, such as cigarette smoking, alcohol and drug use, drinking and driving, and sexual history.

Method of Collecting Data

Parents are proud, so use tact and diplomacy when asking some questions. Ask permission.
1. "Can you tell me a little bit about your home?"
2. "I need to know more about how you live to help you with your child's problem."

Personal History

Type of Information Needed

1. Hygiene.
2. Exercise.

3. Sleep habits.
4. Elimination habits.
5. Activities, hobbies, special talents.
6. Friends, teacher relationships.
7. Sibling and parent relationships.
8. Expression of emotions.
   a. Blows up easily.
   b. Quiet.
9. Idiosyncratic behavior and habits (eg, thumb-sucking, nail-biting, temper tantrums, head banging, pica, breath-holding, rituals, tics).
10. Emotional issues, such as school avoidance, somatic complaints.

Review of Systems

Type of Information Needed

1. General—activity, appetite, affect, sleep patterns, weight changes, edema, fever, behavior.
2. Allergy—eczema, hay fever, asthma, hives, food or drug allergy, sinus disorders.
3. Skin—rash or eruption, nodules, pigmentation or texture change, sweating or dryness, infection, hair growth, itching.
4. Head—headache, head trauma, dizziness.
5. Eyes—visual acuity, corrective lenses, strabismus, lacrimation, discharge, itching, redness, photophobia.
6. Ears—auditory acuity, earaches (frequency, ages, response to specific medications), infection, drainage.
7. Nose—colds and runny nose (frequency), infection, drainage.
8. Teeth—hygiene practices, frequency of brushing, general condition, cavities, malocclusions.
9. Throat—sore throat, tonsillitis, difficulty swallowing.
10. Speech—peculiarity of or change in voice, hoarseness, clarity, enunciation, stuttering, development of articulation, vocabulary, use of sentences.
11. Respiratory—difficulty breathing, shortness of breath, chest pain, cough, wheezing, croup, pneumonia, tuberculosis or exposure.
12. Cardiovascular—cyanosis, fainting, exercise intolerance, palpitations, murmurs.
13. Hematologic—pallor, anemia, tendency to bruise or bleed.
14. Gastrointestinal—appetite (amount, frequency, cravings), nausea, vomiting, abdominal pain, abnormal size, bowel habits and nature of stools, parasites, encopresis (incontinence of feces), colic.
15. Genitourinary—age of toilet training, frequency of urination, straining, dysuria, hematuria (or unusual color or odor of infant's soiled diaper), previous urinary tract infection, enuresis (age of onset; day or nighttime), urethral or vaginal discharge. Girls and young women: age at menarche, last menses, cramps, changes in interval and duration.
16. Musculoskeletal—deformities, fractures, sprains, joint pains or swelling, limited motion, abnormality of nails.
17. Neurologic—weakness or clumsiness, coordination, balance, gait, dominance, fatigability, tone, tremor, seizures or paroxysmal behavior, personality changes.

PHYSICAL EXAMINATION
General Principles

1. Establish the order of all data collection according to the needs of the patient. For example:
   a. An exhausted parent with a screaming baby will not give a careful, comprehensive history.
   b. Alternative care may not be available for preschoolers when the neonate comes in for his or her first checkup.
2. If the parent has come in with more than one child, try to organize some supervision of the other children so that you can have a little time alone with the parent.
3. Remember that the safest place for a young child is on the parent's lap. Privacy may not be possible when other children are present.
4. Attempt to develop rapport with the young patient from the moment you first see or meet him or her.
5. Explain to the school-age child or teenager what you are looking for as you proceed with the examination and provide feedback.

APPROACH TO THE PATIENT

1. Offer the young child a choice of being examined on the parent's lap or on your "special table."
2. Start with examination of the lungs and heart. You will need to listen to at least 10 heartbeats. Consider the use of a pacifier for a screaming infant.
3. The part to be examined should be completely exposed, but if an apprehensive child objects to having clothes removed, slip your stethoscope under the shirt.
4. After listening to the heart, begin with parts of the body that are already exposed.
5. Start with either the head or the toes and work thoroughly and systematically toward the other end.
6. Gradually remove the child's clothes (may best be done by usual caregiver); look for asymmetry very carefully in the bodies of all children.
7. Develop a pattern appropriate to the patient's age.
   a. With infants, it may be wise to leave the diaper area until last.
   b. Adolescents and school-age children are usually embarrassed at the genital examination—you may want to leave this until last, covering areas already examined.
8. Using a cold stethoscope may result in a frightened and screaming child, so warm and clean the stethoscope before bringing it into contact with the child.
9. Some children are less frightened if allowed to hold the examination equipment first.
10. Show the child the procedure by demonstrating on the parent first.
11. Many young children enjoy listening to their own hearts.
12. Toddlers and preschoolers enjoy blowing your otoscope light out.

Pediatric Physical Assessment

Technique	Findings

VITAL SIGNS

1. Obtain temperature, pulse rate, respiratory rate, and blood pressure as often as necessary, based on the child's condition.

2. Measure core temperature, whenever possible, via rectal or ear route. A mercury thermometer must remain in place 3 to 5 minutes. Alternately, use an electronic thermometer. Avoid taking temperature via oral route following fluid or food intake.

3. Obtain apical pulse rate on an infant or small child; radial, temporal, or carotid pulse may be measured on an older child. Pulse may be counted for 30 seconds and multiplied by 2.

4. Count respirations on an infant for 1 full minute; observe the chest as well as the abdomen. Respirations may be counted for 30 seconds and multiplied by 2 in an older child.

5. Obtain blood pressure by auscultatory method, rather than palpation method, whenever possible. Make sure the cuff covers no less than ½ and no more than 2/3 the length of the upper arm or leg.

Temperature

Oral	Rectal	Axillary
97.6°F–99.3°F	97°F–100°F	96.6°F–98°F
(36.4°C–37.4°C)	(36.1°C–37.8°C)	(35.9°C–36.7°C)

Pulse and respiratory rates

Age	Pulse	Respirations
Neonate	70–170	30–50
11 months	80–160	26–40
2 years	80–130	20–30
4 years	80–120	20–30
6 years	75–115	20–26
8 years	70–110	18–24
10 years	70–110	18–24
Adolescent	60–110	12–20

Blood pressure

Varies with age, height, and weight of child.

STANDING HEIGHT, HEAD CIRCUMFERENCE, AND CHEST CIRCUMFERENCE

1. Use a tape measure to obtain accurate head circumference. Measure the widest part of head.

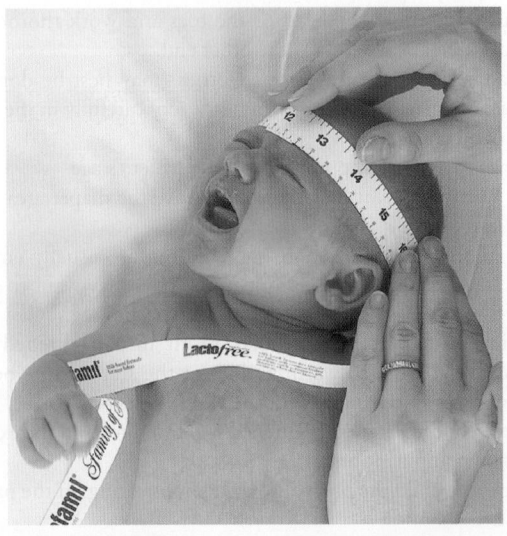

2. Measure the chest at the level of the nipples.

3. Record height and weight at each visit. Plot on growth chart.

4. Calculate body mass index (BMI) and plot on appropriate chart.

3. A variety of clinical growth charts on which to record length, head, circumference, BMI, and weight can be downloaded from *https://www.cdc.gov/growthcharts/index.htm*. Trends in growth are as important as the basic measurements.

4. BMI is calculated by following the formula on page 566, or for online pediatric BMI calculator, *https://nccd.cdc.gov/dnpabmi/calculator.aspx*.

Pediatric Physical Assessment (*Continued*)

Technique	Findings

GENERAL APPEARANCE

1. Begin your observations with the first contact with the patient, taking into account that there are at least two people to observe (child and parent).

2. The patient's interaction with the caretaker, whether it be the mother, father, a babysitter, an older sibling, or a friend of the family, is vital in the assessment of the child. As you observe for race, sex, general physical development, nutritional state, mental alertness, evidence of pain, restlessness, body position, clothes, apparent age, hygiene, and grooming, remember that many of these things are a measure of the parent's caretaking.

1. If the child is easily distracted or sleepy, it may be nap time.

2. Careful observation of the general state of the child will provide many clues about the child's relationship with the family and its response to the child.

SKIN AND LYMPHATICS

Examine as you move through each body region (include hair and skin).

Inspection

Inspection of the skin is the same as for the adult.

1. Observe for skin color, pigmentation, lesions, jaundice, cyanosis, scars, superficial vascularity, moisture, edema, color of mucous membranes, hair distribution.

2. Describe any variation in color, particularly in children with increased pigmentation. No pigment, or vitiligo, in darker children can be noted.

3. Birthmarks of any type are recorded. (May change as child grows older.)

4. Bruises or unusual marks, wounds or insect bites, scratch marks, or scars may have particular significance.

5. Draw a picture of anything unusual such as a scar and measure the dimensions of the lesion when recording the findings.

6. To ascertain suspected jaundice, take the child to the window to get a true picture of the color of the skin. (A room with yellow walls and artificial lighting may create a wrong impression when jaundice is suspected.)

7. The skin of neonates will still be covered with vernix caseosa, the oily material that covers the fetus's body while in utero.

8. Postmature infants may have scaliness or peeling that persists for several weeks after birth, particularly around the feet. The color of the skin may change as the child gets a little older.

9. Note striae.

10. Dark-skinned children may have Mongolian spots at the base of spine or elsewhere.

1. In young infants, the skin is soft, smooth, and velvety in texture.

2. Pigmentations vary in children, depending on race, and will change as the child gets older.

3. A suntan, freckles, and small, light-brown patches or café au lait spots may occur.

4. Bruises are particularly important because of the possibility of reoccurring injury and/or child abuse.

5. If you have difficulty describing something, use ordinary words rather than inaccurate technical terms.

6. Carotenemia, which causes the nose and palms to have a yellowish tinge, may lead the parents to suspect jaundice; however, carotenemia is caused by eating a large amount of yellow vegetables (sweet potatoes, squash, carrots). In carotenemia, the sclerae are clear; this is not the case in jaundice.

7. Swollen sebaceous glands over the nose and chin are commonly seen immediately after birth and are called *milia*.

8. The blotchy, pink patches over the eyelid, bridge of the nose, and the back of the neck may persist until the child is almost 2 years of age.

9. May indicate rapid weight gain or loss.

10. Important to distinguish from child abuse.

continued on following page

Pediatric Physical Assessment (*Continued*)

Technique	Findings

SKIN AND LYMPHATICS (*Continued*)

Palpation

1. Use the tips of your fingers to palpate—fingertips are more sensitive.

2. Check the tension of the skin by pinching up a fold of skin—normal skin quickly falls back, but dehydrated skin remains in pinched position.

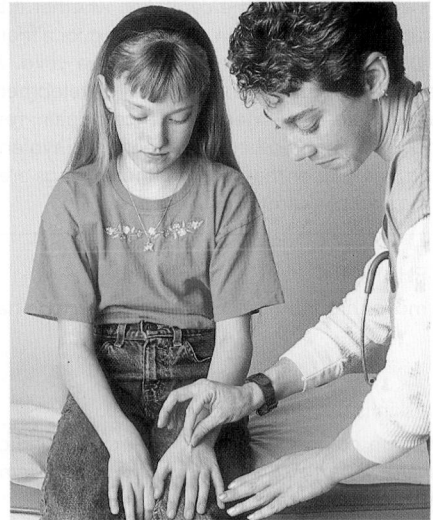

3. Feel the skin for texture, moisture, temperature, turgor, elasticity, masses, tenderness.

3. Skin that is rough and dry in texture may actually have a discrete rash that can be felt but not seen.

Lymph

1. Observe and palpate for lymph node enlargement in lymph chain areas.
   a. Neck.
   b. Axilla.
   c. Inguinal.
   d. Epitrochlear.
2. Note tenderness, size, and consistency.

1. May be large or readily palpable, but should be non-tender, mobile, and slightly spongy.

Nails

1. Observe for color, shape, irregularities in surface, and general nail care; cleanliness, evidence of biting.
2. Palpate the skin around the fingernails for firmness. Palpate any part that appears inflamed.

1. Nail beds should be pink, nails convex.

2. General care of the child is frequently reflected in good care of nails.

Hair

1. Observe for color and distribution.
   a. Note according to the age of the child and race.
   b. Be aware that tufts of hair over the spine or sacral area may mark an underlying abnormality.

2. Note changes in pigmentation.
3. Palpate the hair for texture and thickness.
4. Examine to see if there are patches on the head where hair is missing.

5. Separate thick hair on the head to get a good view of the scalp. Check for dandruff or scaliness in older children.
6. Check scalp for signs of lice infestation.

7. Inspect in the axillae and over the pubis and the extremities for hair and its quantity, to gauge the development and level of puberty.

1. *Neonate:* Normally varies from no hair to a thick bush. Infant: lanugo, a soft, downy covering commonly seen over the shoulders, back, arms, face, and sacral area, especially in dark-skinned children; lanugo is present for the first 1 to 2 months, after which it disappears.
2. Remember, children may experiment with hair dye or rinse.
3. Texture may be thick or thin, coarse or fine, straight or curly.
4. May denote underlying skin infection; however, some children pull their hair out; sometimes, the hair is braided so tightly that it falls out. Infants who sleep consistently on their backs may have thinning or absent hair in the occiput.
5. Look carefully for broken hairs, for scaliness on the scalp, or cradle cap in infants.
6. Nits (louse eggs) appear on the hair as little white dots. Lice may be seen on the scalp; they move quickly and may jump.
7. The child does not need to be totally undressed at one time, a prepubertal child will usually be embarrassed if all clothes are removed.

Pediatric Physical Assessment (*Continued*)

Technique	Findings

HEAD AND NECK

1. Unless specifically requested, examine the eyes and ears last, especially in the younger child.
2. Also, examine the throat toward the end of the examination, unless the child exhibits concern about the "throat stick." It is then best to examine the throat right away to "get it over with." If a child cries or can open mouth widely with encouragement, you may be able to avoid using a tongue blade.
3. To avoid frightening the child when palpating the head, make a game out of it—ask, "Where is your nose?" "Where are your eyes?"

Inspection

1. Observe the face and skull for asymmetry, deformity, and abnormal or limited movements.

2. Closely observe facial expressions and blinking, if the child is not crying. This may be one of your few moments to see the child when he or she is not crying. If you are examining a crying infant, watch particularly for asymmetry of the face.
3. Observe the movement of the head on the neck as the infant looks around. When turning an infant over, observe the head for control, position, and movement.
4. Because an infant's neck is typically short and there are usually several folds of skin under the chin, it is necessary to lift the chin a little to observe the skin completely—to see that it is clear and free from perspiration rash or irritation.

1. An infant's head may be asymmetrical because of pressure during pregnancy and delivery. The rounded head of an infant born by breech delivery contrasts with the long, pointed head of an infant who is a firstborn and whose head was molded during a prolonged labor.
2. In an infant born by forceps delivery, there may be signs of weakness of the facial nerve caused by pressure of the forceps over the front of the ear where the facial nerve emerges. When the infant cries, the involved side will show weakness and downturning of the mouth.
3. There should be very little head lag after age 3 months.

4. In the back, the neck should be free of webbing or extra folds of skin extending from just beneath the ear toward the shoulder.

Palpation

1. Palpate the skull for the suture lines. Feel the face for masses, noting size, consistency, surface, temperature, and tenderness.

1. The suture lines of the skull may be felt to override as a result of the pressure applied when contractions occurred during labor. This is usually most marked between the frontal and the parietal bone, where the coronal suture is located.

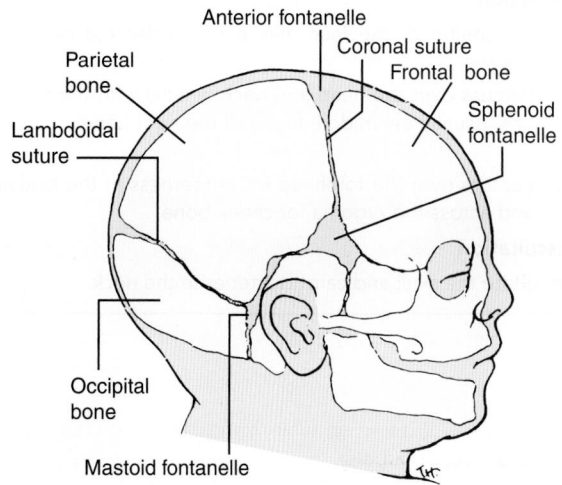

continued on following page

Pediatric Physical Assessment (*Continued*)

Technique	Findings
HEAD AND NECK (*Continued*)	
Palpation (*Continued*)	

2. Palpate the anterior and posterior fontanelles.

2. The fontanelles are soft and flat when the child is quiet. Tense or bulging fontanelles may indicate hydrocephalus. Depressed fontanelles are often a sign of dehydration. The posterior fontanelle usually closes by 1 to 2 months; anterior fontanelle by 18 months.

3. Palpate along the lambdoidal suture at the back of the head between the parietal bones and the occipital bone.
4. Palpate the neck for swollen lymph nodes, noting tenderness, mobility, location, and consistency.

4. Palpation of the lymph nodes may reveal slightly enlarged nodes in the anterior cervical chain secondary to sore throat.

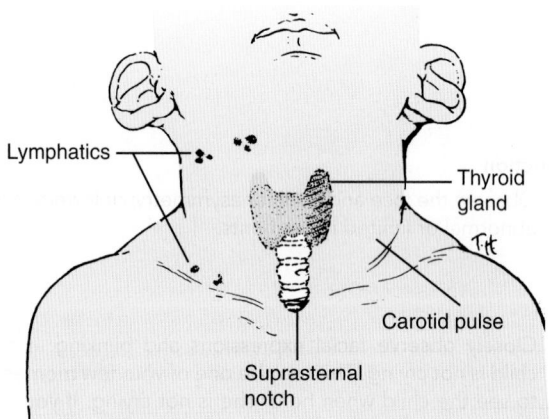

5. Note that there are other nodes, which are normally not palpable.

5. These include the preauricular and postauricular, the posterior cervical (behind the sternomastoid), the submental and submandibular (under the jaw), the supraclavicular, and the occipital nodes (along the prominence of the occiput).

6. Feel the pulses in the neck for location, strength, and equality.
7. Check the thyroid for enlargement, position, texture, and tenderness.
8. Locate the trachea in the suprasternal notch for position in the center of the neck.
9. Palpate the sternocleidomastoids, making sure they are equal in size.

Percussion

1. Percussion of the face may elicit tenderness over the sinuses.

1. Tenderness may be caused by a tooth cavity or by a sinus infection.

2. Percuss over the head and neck directly with the fingertips, usually the middle finger of the right hand.

2. Gentle tapping over the skull elicits a typical sound when the sutures are open and elicits a different sound when the sutures are closed.

3. Percuss over the forehead for tenderness in the sinuses and across the zygoma, or cheek bone.

3. Determines underlying tenderness in the frontal or maxillary sinus.

Auscultation

Auscultate the skull and carotid arteries in the neck.

To determine bruits.

Pediatric Physical Assessment (*Continued*)

Technique	Findings

EYES AND VISION

Inspection

Similar to adult examination; see pages 45 to 46.

1. Pay particular attention to the lacrimal duct and excessive tearing.

2. Note the distance between the eyes and the distribution of the eyebrows.

3. Test the eyes for light perception.

4. Do cover–uncover test.

5. Beginning at about age 3 years, a visual acuity screen using an age-appropriate chart should be attempted at every well-child checkup.

Palpation

If the child is old enough, have him or her squeeze the eyes tightly (not possible in younger children) while you try to open them.

Funduscopic examination

1. Check to see that the child's eyes move in conjugate fashion. Ask the mother if she has noticed signs of squinting, especially when the child is tired.

2. This is a difficult examination to conduct because children tend to watch the light and stare directly at you, which constricts their pupils. If the child cannot cooperate, it may be necessary to dilate the pupil to see the fundus and this is only infrequently necessary.

3. Start your examination at about 1 foot (0.3 m) from the patient. Look for the red reflex, which should be readily observable.

4. Look for opacities and then slowly approach the patient, turning the ophthalmoscope dial to the smaller plus (+) numbers. Start originally at +8 to +10.

5. To help guide your gaze, put your hand on top of the child's head or at the side, with your thumb at the corner of the eye at the outer edge. If you lose the fundus, you can return to your thumb and get your bearings by directing your gaze medial to the tip of your thumbnail.

---

1. Discharge from the eyes along the lower lid or from the lacrimal duct can occur as a result of infection or reaction to silver nitrate administered to the neonate.

2. Hypertelorism denotes a wider than normal area between the eyes. Excessively long and full eyebrows that meet in the midline and extra-long eyelashes may signify a developmental abnormality from a genetic disorder.

3. It is difficult to prevent children from blinking their eyes or closing them when testing light response.

4. To discover strabismus.

Weakness of the muscles around the eyes is difficult to demonstrate in the young child. Muscle strength or weakness can be evaluated when the child cries.

1. Loss of vision can occur if the eyes are not working together properly. Squinting can indicate vision problems.

2. A picture can be pinned to the wall opposite the child, who is then instructed to look at the picture during the examination. If the child is examined while lying down, a picture can be placed on the ceiling.

3. The corneal light reflex and red reflex should be symmetrical.

4. The red reflex is diminished if there is something obstructing your view. A cataract or opacity in the retina can cause this, as would a tumor filling the posterior chamber. If there is any paleness in the red reflex or difficulty in identifying it, a consultation should be sought immediately.

continued on following page

Pediatric Physical Assessment (*Continued*)

Technique	Findings

EARS AND HEARING

Equipment
- Otoscope with insufflator (pneumatic bulb and tubing)
- Varying sizes of ear speculum
- Fresh batteries to ensure a bright light

Inspection

1. When examining the external ear, the auricle, or the pinna, be sure to note the position of the ear.

2. If you cannot get the child to cooperate by offering an explanation or by playing a game, the child will need to be restrained. Many children will enjoy watching the light on their legs or seeing the red glow of their fingers with the light shining through or blowing the light out. If restraint is needed:

   a. The child can be seated on the parent's knee, facing the parent, with arms and legs wrapped around the parent. The parent can then use one hand to hold the child's head firmly against the parent's chest and the other hand to hold the child's back.

   b. An older child may be held in a supine position, with the parent controlling the head by holding the child's arms above his head.

Inspection with otoscope

1. Attach the insufflator, a small bulb and tube device, to the otoscope. Hold the otoscope gently with the handle between the thumb and forefinger. This will enable you to control the head of the otoscope while keeping your hand steady on the child's head.

2. With your free hand, pull the pinna back and slightly upward to straighten the canal. Examine the canal.

3. Use the insufflator to inspect the eardrum and test for mobility. Do not use an insufflator if there is any suspicion of a perforated eardrum.

Palpation
Palpate behind the ear over the mastoid process.

Special testing

1. Most children will be able to respond to a test of gross hearing.

2. More specific tests using an electric screening device are used before school age.

Findings

1. The top of the ear should cross an imaginary line drawn between the edge of the eye and the back of the occiput. If the ear is positioned more obliquely or is low set, some underlying abnormality, particularly of the genitourinary system, may be present.

2. If the child is in a supine position, be sure to remove the child's shoes because some children will kick when frightened.

   a. This allows a good secure hold and provides the child with the security of a "hug."

1. Small children will jerk about, so be careful not to push the speculum into the eardrum. The insufflator allows assessment of mobility of the tympanic membrane.

2. Cerumen or wax may interfere with your view of the eardrum. You may need to remove the wax with an ear curette or hydrogen peroxide instillation.

3. The normal eardrum moves slightly when air is introduced into the ear canal.

Tenderness behind the ear may denote infection. Sometimes, a lymph node can be felt in this area.

1. A small bell, such as that found in the Denver kit, can be used to determine hearing ability by noting if the child stops moving when the bell is rung and turns his or her head toward the sound.

Pediatric Physical Assessment (*Continued*)

Technique	Findings

NOSE AND SINUSES

Equipment

- Nasoscope
- Small speculum

Inspection

1. Observe for general deformity.
2. With a nasoscope, examine the nasal septum, mucous membranes, and turbinates and observe for discharge and nasal obstruction (see "Adult Physical Examination," page 48).
3. Check for the presence of a foreign body. Always remember that a foul odor may indicate a foreign body in the nose, ear, or any other body orifice including the anus or the vagina.
4. Observe for nasal flaring.

2. Dry mucous membranes may bleed and cause clots of blood to form in the nares. Scratches may also occur if the child picks at his or her nose or scratches when itching occurs.
3. A foreign body in the nose will cause a foul odor, purulent discharge, and possibly cause bleeding.

4. Indicates respiratory distress.

Palpation

Palpate the sinuses, remembering the order of development.

Sinuses develop in a set order; the ethmoid and maxillary sinuses are present at birth. The frontal sinuses begin to develop at about 7 years and are fully formed by adolescence. The sphenoid sinuses develop after puberty.

MOUTH AND THROAT

Equipment

- Penlight
- Tongue blade

Inspection

Note: The child may gag when the tongue blade is placed on the tongue. The use of the tongue blade may be avoided by encouraging the child to open widely, or perform oral inspection if a young child is crying during ear exam (lying in supine position on exam table).

A child may also be allowed to place the tongue blade directly on own tongue while you guide with your hand.

1. Observe the lips, noting the color. (Remember that cyanosis is difficult to detect in a black child.)

2. Count the teeth (see page 1106) and note any extra or missing teeth and any evidence of caries, staining, tartar, and malocclusion.
3. Check the gums for swelling and signs of easy bleeding. Also note mouth odor.
4. Check the tongue for movement, color, and taste buds on the surface. Check to see that the frenulum under the tongue is the proper length.

5. As the gag reflex is elicited, note how the palate moves upward and the uvula springs into view.
6. Examine the roof of the mouth.

7. Inspect the height of the arch of the palate.

1. *Infants:* There may be a protuberance on the upper lip, the so-called sucking blister.
   Children: May have dry lips and redness around the lips caused by allergy.

4. If the frenulum is too short, the child may be tongue-tied (meaning that he or she cannot advance the tip of the tongue beyond the lips), which may interfere with sucking or speech.
5. It should be midline and single, although occasionally, it will be divided or bifurcated.
6. Whitish lesions, called Epstein pearls, may be noted on the roof of the mouth at the junction of the hard and soft palate and persist through infancy.
7. With experience, an unusually high arch is easily recognizable.

continued on following page

Pediatric Physical Assessment (*Continued*)

Technique	Findings

MOUTH AND THROAT (*Continued*)

Inspection (*Continued*)

8. Note the tonsils on each side of the uvula and immediately posterior to it for position, surface, size, equality, and color.

9. As the child cries, note the odor of the breath and any hoarseness of the voice; note difficulty on inspiration, as in croup, or wheezing on expiration.

8. Any coating with pus or ulcers or a pocket or cryptic appearance should be recorded.

9. These signs may indicate throat and chest disturbances.

Palpation

1. Palpate the lips and cheeks manually using a finger cot or glove.

2. Note evidence of swelling.

3. Palpate for submucous cleft.

1. By comparing one side with the other, differences caused by abnormality can be detected.

3. Submucous cleft may indicate a genetic disposition toward cleft palate.

PRIMARY

	(Upper)	(Lower)
1 Central incisor	8 to 12 months	5 to 9 months
2 Lateral incisor	8 to 12 months	12 to 18 months
3 Cuspid	18 to 24 months	18 to 24 months
4 First molar	12 to 18 months	12 to 18 months
5 Second molar	24 to 30 months	24 to 30 months

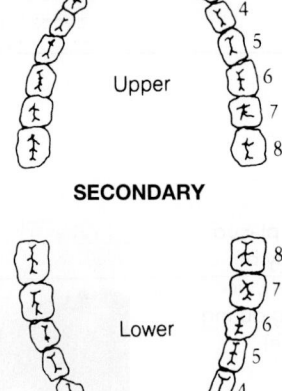

SECONDARY

	(Upper)	(Lower)
1 Central incisor	6 to 7 years	7 to 8 years
2 Lateral incisor	7 to 8 years	8 to 9 years
3 Cuspid	9 to 10 years	11 to 12 years
4 First bicuspid	10 to 11 years	10 to 11 years
5 Second bicuspid	11 to 12 years	10 to 12 years
6 First molar	6 to 7 years	6 to 7 years
7 Second molar	11 to 13 years	12 to 13 years
8 Third molar	17 years	17 to 18 years

BREAST

1. Realize that a child may be resistant to examination because of not wanting to remove clothes.

2. The following approaches may help overcome this problem:
   a. Distract the child by having him or her listen to a few heartbeats.
   b. Have the parent (while the child is sitting on parent's knee) remove the underclothing while you stand by.
   c. For an older child entering puberty, provide an examination sheet or gown.

1. Resistance may be due to modesty or fear of being exposed.

Inspection

1. Check to see if there are any small extra nipples present.

2. In the neonate, the nipples appear a little darker than normal and breast tissue underneath may form a small knot with occasional leakage of fluid.

3. In the child, a lump may be found under or near one or both nipples in either males or females, causing parents to worry about cancer.

4. Occasionally, the breasts begin to develop earlier than normal, at about age 5 or 6 years.

1. These would appear along a line extending from the anterior axillary line through the normal nipple down toward the symphysis pubis.

2. This leakage is a secondary effect of the hormone level in the mother; instruct the mother not to try to express the fluid because of the danger of infection.

3. Such lumps are almost always secondary to hormone stimulation and occur toward puberty or during the neonatal period.

4. This may indicate the need for referral to an endocrinologist.

Pediatric Physical Assessment (*Continued*)

Technique	Findings

THORAX

Inspection

1. Observe the entire thorax as the child breathes; note symmetry and equal expansion of both sides as the lungs inflate.

2. Confirm the respiratory rate as you observe the child with shirt off.

3. Observe for substernal, suprasternal, and intercostal retractions.

1. Diaphragm excursion is more marked than intercostal expansion in infants (especially an infant lying on the parent's knee) and young children. Thus, the abdomen goes up and down more than the chest expands.

3. Indicates respiratory distress.

Percussion

Percussion of the child's chest is difficult. Because the underlying structures are crowded, little information is gathered. The heart edge is difficult to outline.

Light percussion is necessary; a hyperresonant note may be elicited over air, particularly of a stomach bubble that projects up into the left side of the chest.

Palpation

1. Use warmed hands as you palpate the shape and angle of the sternum. Note if there is depression of the sternum.

2. Palpate the costochondral junctions for tenderness and enlargement.

3. As you palpate, vibration may be felt through your hands as the child cries.

4. Vocal fremitus is difficult to elicit in the smaller child since it is difficult to have him or her make repetitive sounds on command.

1. The shape of the sternum may vary, although a large depression of the sternum (funnel sternum) may cause subsequent trouble because of pressure on underlying structures.

2. May suggest an underlying inflammatory response.

3. Normal inspiration and expiration do not give a sensation under the fingers, except for the expansion of the chest.

4. In the older child, it is worth trying to obtain transmission of sound through the lung tissue (see page 55).

Auscultation

1. Try to examine the child before crying begins.

2. Warm the stethoscope before using by rubbing it between your hands.

3. Be aware that breathing is louder in younger children with slightly increased length of inspiration, almost to the point of bronchovesicular breathing in the adult.

4. Crackles (discontinuous; interrupted, explosive sounds) may be heard more easily in children.

5. Wheezes.

1. Note, however, that crying increases lung expansion.

2. A cold stethoscope will startle the child.

3. Bronchial breathing with equal inspiration and expiration is very loud and easy to hear in children with respiratory tract infections.

4. Added coarse-quality sounds in the chest are commonly associated with mucus in the trachea or in the back of the nose and usually clear with cough.

5. Recurrent wheeze is an important finding in children.

HEART

Inspection

In thin children, the apical beat or the point of maximal impulse can easily be seen, particularly if you look obliquely across the chest wall.

Measurement and documentation of the distance from the midline and the exact rib space are worth noting.

Palpation

The apical beat may be felt in the 6th intercostal space about 2 inches (5 cm) from the midline in the school-age child. It is more difficult to feel in the infant, particularly a plump child, and would not be so far out toward the anterior axillary line.

The apical beat will be deviated to the left with cardiac enlargement or a collapsed lung on that side. The apical pulse could be pushed toward the right by a tumor or a collapsed lung on the right. Pneumothorax under tension will push the heart away from the side of the increased pressure.

continued on following page

Pediatric Physical Assessment (*Continued*)

Technique | **Findings**

HEART (*Continued*)

Auscultation

1. Identify the first heart sound (S₁) (occurs during systole).

   a. Locate the apical beat (closing of the mitral valve) by placing the stethoscope over the maximum impulse area, concentrating on the first heart sound. (As the ventricle on the left contracts, pushing the blood up into the aorta, the sound of the mitral valve closing is heard.)

   b. That sound can be identified by placing the thumb on the carotid pulse of the neck, which will coincide very closely with the heart sounds.

2. Identify the second heart sound (S₂).

   a. Move the stethoscope up toward the sternum and to the left.

   b. At the base of the heart, both over the aortic and pulmonic areas, S₂ is louder than S₁.

3. Move the stethoscope in small jumps from the apical area medially toward the sternum. Go up to the left side of the sternum, listening at each interspace next to the sternum.

4. Move next to the child's right second intercostal space—again next to the sternum.

5. Listen to only one sound; concentrate on that to the exclusion of all others. Can you identify this sound? Is it clear? Compare it with your own heart sound or that of the parent.

6. If there is question of a heart murmur or added sounds, refer to the health care provider.

7. As you listen to the heart sounds, you are also listening to the rhythm to confirm your findings on pulse.

   a. If the child breathes in and out deeply, a sinus arrhythmia may be detected.

   b. If the child holds his or her breath, the sinus arrhythmia will disappear.

8. Be sure to note a rapid heart rate that is present even when the child is at rest and quiet.

9. In the infant, heart sounds are just a series of taps; they occur so fast that it may be very difficult to determine which sound is S₁.

---

1. Consists of the "lub" portion of the "lub–dub" heart sound.

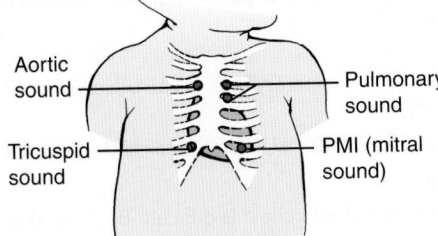

Aortic sound — Pulmonary sound

Tricuspid sound — PMI (mitral sound)

2. Represents the "dub" portion of the "lub–dub" heart sound.

   b. In a child, S₂ can be heard as two heart sounds because the two valves in the aorta and pulmonary vessels do not close at the same time. This split will increase with inspiration and decrease with expiration.

3. Represents the area of maximum intensity of sound of the pulmonary vessels.

4. It is at this area that you will hear the aortic sound best.

5. The child will enjoy this comparison if allowed to listen.

7. The typical rhythm of a child is called *sinus arrhythmia*. As the heart speeds up, the child is breathing in; the heart slows down on expiration.

8. This may be indicative of a tachycardia that requires further investigation.

9. In the infant, the S₁ and S₂ are equal in intensity.

ABDOMEN

1. For examination of the abdomen, the child should be lying down, relaxed, and not crying. Placing a small child, particularly those between ages 1 and 3, on a high table on cold paper can be frightening; as a result, his or her abdomen will not be relaxed.

2. Infants up to age 1 do not seem to be perturbed and will usually lie down and play nicely as long as they can see the parent, who should be stationed at the head of the child while you examine the abdomen.

3. Having the child lie across the parent's knees with the legs dangling on one side and the head cradled in his or her arms will enable you to feel the abdomen quite well.

   a. You may find that with the infant's head in the parent's left arm, you can use your left hand to examine the infant's abdomen on the right, feeling up under the right costal margin and into the right hypochondrium.

   b. You may need to turn the infant around and use your right hand to examine the left side of the infant's abdomen.

---

1. The abdomen needs to be relaxed to palpate abnormal masses or enlarged liver or spleen as well as to auscultate for abnormal sounds.

Pediatric Physical Assessment (*Continued*)

Technique	Findings

ABDOMEN (*Continued*)

Inspection

1. Observe the abdomen for contour and any markings while the child is standing and when lying down. As you inspect, you may see some abdominal movement with respiration. (Remember that the diaphragm, as it goes up and down, will move the contents of the abdomen.)

2. Check for early signs of puberty as evidenced by pubic hair over the symphysis pubis.

3. Carefully inspect the umbilicus for cleanliness and the presence of scar tissue.

1. Sometimes superficial veins are seen on the abdomen, particularly in a very blond infant. Striae are commonly noticed on the flank following rapid loss or gain of weight.

2. Early pubic hair in younger children (ages 8 to 10 years) may appear long and silky. This will ultimately become curly toward the onset of puberty.

3. A deep umbilicus may be difficult to keep clean. Immediately after the cord has dropped off, a granuloma may occur.

Auscultation

1. Because percussion and palpation will stimulate the small bowel and increase bowel sounds, auscultation should precede these two techniques.

2. To obtain the child's cooperation, you can conduct a running commentary as you listen, saying such things as, "I can hear the Cheerios in there."

1. Bowel sounds are heard as tinkling, irregular sounds that indicate that fluid is moving from one section of the bowel to the next.

2. In a quiet infant who has just eaten, not many bowel sounds will be heard. In a hungry child, noisy bowel sounds can be heard, even without a stethoscope.

Percussion

1. On the right side, percuss for the liver. Confirm on palpation.
2. Percuss over the left upper quadrant (LUQ).

3. Percuss the lower abdomen, particularly above the symphysis pubis.

1. Liver dullness can frequently be outlined to determine size of the liver.
2. Percussion over a gas-filled bowel or stomach results in a high-pitched, hollow sound.

3. Above the symphysis pubis, a filled bladder can produce a duller sound, as does a pregnant uterus. (A mass in the abdomen of a female over age 10 years may be a fetus.)
   a. The liver is frequently felt about $^3/_8$ inch (1 cm) below the right costal margin and in some instances as low as ¾ inch (2 cm). This is a common finding in the neonate and through the early school-age years.

Palpation

1. Divide the abdomen into imaginary quadrants, palpating each with the fingertips.
2. In the right upper quadrant, palpate for the liver edge.
   a. Although the liver is easily palpable in many children, you may have to press quite firmly.

3. In the LUQ, palpate for the spleen. Less resistance is encountered as you feel up under the left costal margin.

3. Typically, only the tip of the spleen can be felt in the outer LUQ in the early months of life and in very thin children of preschool age.

continued on following page

Pediatric Physical Assessment (*Continued*)

Technique	Findings

ABDOMEN (*Continued*)
Palpation (*Continued*)

4. In the upper quadrants, also try to palpate for the kidneys. Deep palpation for both kidneys should routinely be a part of the examination to make sure there is no enlargement of the kidney. Normally, the kidney is not palpable.

5. In the iliac fossa or the left lower quadrant, palpate for the descending bowel.

6. Palpate on the right lower quadrant (RLQ) where the appendix is located.

7. If the child has pain in any area or has pointed to the umbilicus when asked to show where the pain is, avoid the area demonstrated and leave it until last. Note whether the pain is with pressure or rebound.

8. Palpate around the umbilicus for any masses that may indicate a hernia, especially in preterm and black children. As you press over the protruding hernia, you can feel the sensation of gurgling under your fingers as the bowel returns to the abdomen.

4. Kidney palpation is difficult, but during the neonatal period, the lower pole of the right kidney may be felt and sometimes the left as well. (This applies to the period immediately after delivery, when the neonate's abdomen is relaxed and the bowel is not distended.)

5. The descending colon can be felt, particularly if it's filled with firm stool and the child is quiet. It may be slightly tender, but it should not cause severe pain on gentle palpation.

6. In the RLQ, usually, the only sensation is that of gas-filled bowel. Tenderness in this area could be related to an inflamed appendix.

7. If the painful area is palpated first, the child may tense up when the other areas of the abdomen are examined.

8. Most of these hernias heal naturally by age 6 years. A hernia above the umbilicus can be revealed by asking the child to lift his or her head from the table. (Widening of the muscles above the umbilicus is called *diastasis recti*.)

RECTUM AND ANUS

1. Rectal examinations are rarely necessary in infants and young children.

2. If the child will be examined by another health care provider, it is not necessary to duplicate this part of the examination.

3. Rectal examinations are embarrassing and uncomfortable for most children. Explain the procedure before performing the examination.

4. Positioning for a rectal examination:
   a. Infants can be placed on their abdomens, sides, or backs with their legs raised to their chests.
   b. Young children and teenagers can be positioned on their sides.

Inspection

1. When examining an infant or toddler, place the child on a flat surface so that the weight is evenly distributed on the front of the pelvis. As the infant moves about on the abdomen, observe the entire back, the lower back, the upper thigh, and the tightening of the buttocks.

2. Check particularly the lower part of the back for hairiness or a mass.

3. As the child moves away, part the buttocks and look at the cleft between them.

4. Pay careful attention to the outer appearance of the anus and the perineum, the underside of the scrotum in the male, and the labia majora in the female.

1. If one buttock is larger than the other, you will see that side projected above the other. Weakness of one side will be obvious as the infant moves around, although a child in the early stages of crawling will tend to use one knee as a predominant leader, dragging the other.

2. This may indicate an underlying abnormality of the vertebrae in spina bifida.

3. A pilonidal dimple or sinus may be seen over the lower back. This is a common finding, but parents should be told about it for cleaning purposes. Make sure there is no drainage.

4. The anus is inspected for blood, fissures, or splitting in the external tissue, redness, swelling, or pads of extra flesh. On occasion, small white pinworms may be seen adhering to the anal skin.

Pediatric Physical Assessment (*Continued*)

Technique	Findings

RECTUM AND ANUS (*Continued*)
Palpation

1. Consider the child's age and feelings; ask the mother to assist, if necessary. This part of the examination is not always needed.

2. Start by parting the buttocks with the left hand and introducing a well-lubricated finger (with finger cot) into the anus.

3. Gently apply pressure on the anal sphincter to allow the muscles to relax and the fingertip to slide into the rectum.

4. Gently palpate the inner ring, feeling for areas of thickening and tenderness and simultaneously judging the sphincter tone.

5. If the rectum is full of stool, it will be impossible to feel any other mass.

6. Palpate the walls of the rectum.

7. In the adolescent male, gently turn your finger through 180 degrees and feel the posterior surface of the prostate. Note size, consistency, tenderness, and contour.

8. In the female, perform a bimanual examination and palpate the cervix.

2. When an infant is being examined, the small finger should be used.

3. Apply pressure with pulp of the finger rather than jab at the anus with the fingertip.

4. As the perianal area is pressed on from the inside, tenderness will be elicited if a deep fissure exists or if an infection has occurred around a fissure.

5. In a young child, particularly an infant, dilation provided by the finger may result in a bowel movement. In an older child, a suppository or even an enema may be required.

6. The mucosal walls should be smooth, and deep palpation should elicit mild tenderness and no acute pain.

EXAMINING MALE GENITALIA

1. This part of the examination requires a direct, matter-of-fact approach. Acknowledge that it is normal to feel embarrassed during an examination of the genitals. Explain what you are looking for as you proceed through the examination with a teenager.

2. Reassure the child after the examination that his genitals are normal. This decreases anxiety.

3. When examining the testes in a young boy, you may need to block the canals to prevent them from retracting into the abdomen.

Scrotum and Testes
Inspection

1. Before touching the child, determine by observation of the testes whether they are in the scrotum.

2. Observe the skin over the scrotum for color and surface appearance, noting the presence of wrinkles, or rugae.

1. Retraction of the testes into the abdomen occurs frequently in young children; the development of the scrotum depends on the presence of the testes.

2. The skin over the scrotum varies in color, being a darker brown to black in the more pigmented races and reddish in children with light complexions. The wrinkles, or rugae, are more developed as the child grows older.

Palpation

1. Check the scrotum wall for swelling or sensitivity. Gently feel the testes, palpating across the upper pole and feeling for the epididymis. (Remember the scrotum is extremely sensitive to pressure.)

2. Estimate the size of the testes and identify the spermatic cord, tracing it from the testis up toward the groin.

3. Make a special effort to locate the testis in a young child whose testes may be retracted into the abdomen via a hyperactive cremasteric reflex. You may need to have the child in a sitting or standing position. Occasionally, you may need to ask a parent to check at home with the child sitting in a warm bathtub.

(Findings column:)

1. The epididymis is a ridge of soft, bumpy tissue extending from the superior pole and running down and behind the testis.

2. The spermatic cord, with the vas deferens, feels firm and is accompanied by softer nerves, arteries, veins, and a few muscle fibers.

3. Ascertaining the presence of the testes in the scrotum is vital in older infant or toddler. Nondescent of the testes requires further evaluation.

continued on following page

Pediatric Physical Assessment (*Continued*)

Technique	Findings

EXAMINING MALE GENITALIA (*Continued*)
Scrotum and Testes (*Continued*)
Palpation (*Continued*)

a. If the testes cannot be felt in the scrotum, gently run the skin of the upper scrotum between your fingers, moving superiorly and approaching the external inguinal ring.

b. Try to milk the testis down toward the scrotum from above with your hand.

c. If this fails, have the child sit cross-legged to abolish the reflex of the cremaster muscle.

4. When examining a boy in the early stages of puberty, it is important to note the size of the testis as well as the greater number of rugae on the scrotum and the appearance of pubic hair around the penis. If appropriate, discuss importance of self testicular exam.

a. During this period, the testis is about ½ to ¾ inch (1.5 to 2 cm) in length. In the quiescent period before puberty, the male genitalia remain fairly infantile.

4. In early puberty, the testes start to grow. Onset of puberty varies, occurring between the ages of 10 and 14 years. In most teenagers, the findings are similar to those in adults.

Penis

1. Evaluate the penis on all sides by lifting up the shaft.

2. If the child is not circumcised, partially retract the foreskin to observe the glans and meatus.

3. Observe the position of the meatus and evert the lips of the meatus to reveal an adequate orifice.

4. In the older child, inspect the penis for ulcers, sores, or discharge from the meatus.

1. The shaft of the penis contains the urethra on the under, or ventral, surface and is easily palpable.

2. The foreskin may adhere to the glans for the first few years of life. It is not necessary for the parent to "stretch" the foreskin by retraction.

3. The meatus may be positioned off center. If the meatus is located on the dorsal or ventral surface of the shaft, the child should be evaluated by a pediatric urologist.
    Whitish discharge around the glans under the foreskin is normal and not a sign of infection. The foreskin should completely encircle the glans.

4. Consider sexually transmitted infections in children of all ages; the possibility of sexual abuse must be considered.

Inguinal Area
Palpation

1. Palpate for a hernia over the external inguinal ring. Have the child cough to enhance your observation.

1. Having the child stand with the parent either holding him or placing him against the parent's knee will help you in locating a hernia in the inguinal area.

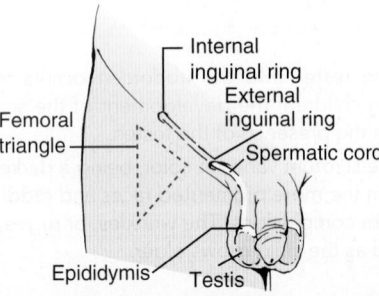

2. An increased cough reflex or swelling in the area should be checked by carefully placing a finger on the scrotal skin and invaginating the skin over your fingers toward the external ring. You are trying to follow the course of a hernia that would descend into the scrotum while you feel the external ring from below. A hernia in the inguinal region presents as a bulge that can be either seen or felt from below by placing the finger in the scrotum pointing up toward the external inguinal ring.

3. Also palpate for the inguinal lymph nodes.

3. The inguinal lymph nodes in an infant are palpable as small and "shotty." Anything more than this should alert you to possible infection because the perianal area drains into the superficial inguinal lymph nodes. For example, diaper rash may explain enlargement of the lymph nodes, which should be noted and reported.

Pediatric Physical Assessment (*Continued*)

Technique	Findings

EXAMINING MALE GENITALIA (*Continued*)
Femoral Area

Palpation

Palpate the femoral triangle carefully for a hernia and for lymph nodes.

In the femoral area, a swelling that can be reduced with a gurgling sound is an unusual finding.

Auscultation

If you are trying to reduce a mass, listen over the scrotum to determine if there is a gurgling sound.

This will locate the bowel and confirm a hernia.

Transillumination

1. To locate the testis, darken the room and shine a bright light from behind the scrotum. In a normal child, the testis will stand out as a darker area.
2. Transilluminate any suspicious mass to help locate a hernia.

1. A scrotal sac that is swollen by fluid (hydrocele) will transilluminate. Fluid around the testes or cord must be differentiated from a hernia.
2. Any mass in this area must be reported to a health care provider immediately.

EXAMINING FEMALE GENITALIA

1. If the child will be examined by a health care provider, it is not necessary to duplicate this part of the examination.
2. Place the infant or toddler on the table or on her parent's knee while the parent holds the child's knees in an abducted and flexed position.
3. A preschool child can be allowed to lean over her parent's knee. However, remember that the structures are being visualized upside down.
4. The older child or teenager should be draped as an adult would and should be placed in a lithotomy position with the aid of stirrups.

Equipment

- Disposable gloves
- Speculum
- Light source

1. Carefully inspect the perineal area for cleanliness, inflammation, and abnormality.

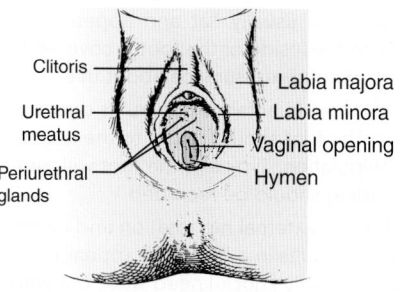

1. This includes the mons pubis, clitoris, labia, urethra, and perineum. The labia minora are seen as two slender folds of tissue inside the labia majora. In some instances, adhesions of the labia minora occur because of the lack of natural hormones.

2. If the mother of a neonate has noted a bloody discharge from the infant's vagina during the first few days of life, reassure her that this is not an uncommon occurrence; the discharge will disappear, as will swelling of the labia majora and clitoris and enlargement of the infant's breasts.

2. Hormone stimulation from the mother's body accounts for this occurrence. The discharge usually stops after the hormones are excreted. The bloody appearance on the diaper may be confused with the presence of urates, which are also orange-red and appear normally in urine.

3. Note the vaginal opening, which may vary in size because of the presence of a thin membrane, the hymen. The hymen varies in appearance according to the child's age.

3. The lack of an opening into the vagina may result in the retention of menstrual fluid when the child reaches puberty. In the sexually active adolescent, vestigial remains on the hymen may appear as small particles (caruncles) at the fringe of the vagina.

   The possibility of sexual abuse should always be considered and, if necessary, the child referred to a specialist in sexual abuse.

4. In the young child, it is usually unnecessary to examine inside the vagina. If a young child requires an extensive vaginal exam, it is frequently done under sedation.

4. A foreign body or sexually transmitted infection may be suspected if there is a vaginal discharge, bleeding, or odor.

continued on following page

Pediatric Physical Assessment (*Continued*)

Technique	Findings

MUSCULOSKELETAL SYSTEM

1. Evaluation of the musculoskeletal system can be done both in an informal manner, while watching the child at rest and at play, and in a formal manner as specific findings are methodically checked.

2. In the neonate, observe the position of the extremities during sleep and the quality of movement when the child is awake.

3. Various aspects of size, shape, and movement are evaluated as the child is observed pushing up on his or her arms and turning his or her head toward the mother.

4. A child in the early stages of walking offers many opportunities for evaluation of muscle strength and movement.

5. At the same time, rapport with the mother can be reinforced by your admiring the child's ability and by inquiring if she is concerned about the manner in which the child is walking.

6. A more mobile child can be evaluated as you watch him or her play and explore the room.

7. Having the older child reach for crayons, run after a ball, or walk around the room enables you to evaluate the musculoskeletal system and the child's sense of balance.

Upper Extremities

1. In the infant, evaluate the status of the clavicles when examining the skull and neck.

    1. During a difficult delivery, the clavicle that has been exposed to traction may snap. A lump can be felt on the bone at about age 3 weeks.

2. Carefully examine the hands to note the shape of the hand, shape and length of the fingers, changes in the nails, and creases on the palms.

    2. Variation in the hands or unusual length of the fingers should be noted. An incurved little finger or low-set thumb with the single simian crease may reflect Down syndrome.

Lower Extremities

1. Examine the appearance of the infant's foot, noting arch formation.

    1. The foot of an infant is usually flat and appears broad because the arch on the inside of the foot is covered by a fat pad. Parents may need reassurance about this.

2. Inspect the angle of the foot and lower leg and then manipulate the ankle to evaluate the range of motion.

    2. Full flexibility of the foot (plantar flexion) rules out underlying abnormality. The foot should return to the neutral position after manipulation. Typically, the foot will turn in, or adduct. Such a finding should be recorded.

3. Place the legs together and see how far the ankles and knees are separated.

    3. Toddlers typically have external hip rotation and internal knee rotation, which results in a "bowed" appearance. The preschooler has a normally knock-kneed walk, but with knees touching, ankles should be no more than two finger-breadths apart.

4. Evaluate the child's ability to walk, noting the appearance of his or her legs and foot placement. Remember to look at the child's shoes and see which side of the sole is worn down.

    4. Infants commonly appear to be bowlegged when they first start to walk because the feet are kept wide apart and turn slightly in. The ankles appear curved when viewed from behind.

Hip

When examining children under age 1, check for signs of hip dislocation. See page 1424.

Pediatric Physical Assessment (*Continued*)

Technique	Findings

MUSCULOSKELETAL SYSTEM (*Continued*)
Spine

1. Check the spine for signs of abnormal curvature.

2. Observe the child from the side and back in the standing position to see forward curving of the shoulders.

3. Have the child bend forward with the arms hanging down. A unilateral rib prominence will be seen in children with scoliosis.

1. The normal young child has a curve inward at the lumbar region (lordosis), but this should not be exaggerated. It is normally more exaggerated in black children.

2. These appear most commonly during school-age years and adolescence.

Kyphosis   Scoliosis

Kyphosis: Forward curvature of the shoulders.

Scoliosis: Side-to-side curvature of the spine.

NEUROLOGIC EXAMINATION

1. The neurologic system at birth is different from that in an infant age 3 months. There is an even greater contrast between the infant and children and adults.

2. The central nervous system at birth is underdeveloped and the functions tested are below the level of the cortex.

Equipment

- Flashlight
- Noisemaker
- Ophthalmoscope
- Tongue depressor
- Tuning fork

Procedure for the neonate and young infant

1. Observe the neonate for general appearance, positioning, activity, crying, and alertness. Take note of the posture—including head, neck, and extremities.

2. Note the pitch, volume, and character of his or her cry.

3. Observe the infant's facial expression and the symmetry of his or her face when crying or sucking.

4. Most of the cranial nerves are difficult to check at this early age.

1. Stiffness of the neck or marked extension of the head will cause a position of opisthotonos and necessitates referral.

2. The high-pitched cry of the infant who has intracranial irritation is distinctive.

3. Poor sucking, with dribbling, is abnormal. Transient weakness of the mouth caused by cranial nerve VII paralysis is commonly seen as a result of a forceps delivery in which the forceps is pressed on the facial nerve where it emerges from the ear.

continued on following page

Pediatric Physical Assessment (Continued)

Technique	Findings

NEUROLOGIC EXAMINATION (*Continued*)
Procedure for the neonate and young infant (*Continued*)
Automatic Reflexes

1. *Blinking reflex because of loud noise*
   Clap your hands or produce a loud clicking noise. Be careful not to clap near the infant to prevent a wave of air from causing a blinking of the eyes.

2. *Blinking reflex because of bright light*
   Shine a bright light into the infant's eyes to elicit the blinking reflex.

3. Cranial nerve X can be checked by using a tongue blade to gag the infant.

4. *Palmar grasp reflex*
   Place your fingers across the infant's palm from the ulnar side. The infant needs to be in a relaxed position with head in a central position. Reinforcement may be offered by having the infant suck on a bottle at the same time.

5. *Rooting reflex*
   Touch the edge of the infant's mouth.

6. *Incurving of the trunk (Galant reflex)*
   Hold the infant horizontally and prone in one arm while using the other hand to stimulate one side of the infant's back from the shoulders to the buttocks. The trunk curves toward the stimulated side as the shoulders and pelvis move toward the stroking hand (persists until the infant is about age 2 months).

7. *Vertical suspension position*
   Place your hands under the infant's axillae with thumbs supporting the back of the head and hold the infant upright.

8. *Stepping response*
   Hold the infant under its axillae with thumbs supporting the back of the head. Allow the infant's foot to touch a firm surface.

A   B

---

1. Lack of a blink in response to a loud noise may indicate deafness.

2. Failure to blink may indicate blindness.

3. Palate moves upward.

4. Both hands will flex and can be compared for strength. Weakness on one side may be indicated by a failure to grasp when the palm is stimulated.

5. The infant's mouth will open and the head will turn toward the side stimulated. This reflex is marked during the early weeks of life.

7. The legs flex at the hips and knees (persists for about 4 months).

8. Normally, the infant responds by lifting one knee and hip into a flexed position and moving the opposite leg forward—making a series of stepping movements (see 8A).
   a. Difficulty with the stepping reflex and stiffness or spasticity connected with crossing of the feet and scissoring (see 8B) is indicative of spastic paraplegia or diplegia.
   b. It should be noted that the stepping response may be affected by breech delivery. (It may also be affected by weakness.)
   c. The stepping response is evident toward the end of the first week after birth and persists for a variable time.

Pediatric Physical Assessment (Continued)

Technique	Findings

NEUROLOGIC EXAMINATION (Continued)
Procedure for the neonate and young infant (Continued)
Automatic Reflexes (Continued)

9. Tonic neck reflex
    Hold the infant in a supine position with the head turned to one side and the jaw held in place over the shoulder.

9.
a. The arm and leg on the side to which the head is turned will extend, whereas those on the other side will flex (the so-called fencing reflex).
b. This reflex persists for about 5 to 6 months; it may be present at birth or delayed until the infant is age 6 or 8 weeks.
c. Persistence beyond 6 months suggests major cerebral damage.

10. *Mass reflexes* (Moro or startle reflex)
    Hold the infant along your arm with the other hand below the lower legs. Lower the feet and body in a sudden motion.

10. The arms will spring up and out, abducting and extending; the fingers are also extended. The arms then return forward over the body with a clasping motion. At the same time, the legs flex slightly and the hips abduct.

    a. The Moro reflex is present at birth and disappears at approximately the end of the third month. Persistence beyond 6 months is significant.
    b. Asymmetrical response may be caused by paralysis of the arm after difficult delivery, tension and injury to the brachial plexus, or a fracture of the clavicle or humerus. A dislocated hip would produce an asymmetrical response in the lower extremities.

11. *Perez reflex*
    Hold the infant in a prone position along your arm; place the thumb of the other hand on the sacrum and move it firmly toward the head, along the entire length of the spine.

11. The head and spine will extend and the knees will flex upward.

Summary
1. Some of the jerking and shaking movements seen in neonates are normal, but they should be rechecked frequently during the first few weeks of life.
2. Variants in the findings caused by the infant's sleepiness or hunger should be taken into account and reevaluations should be carried out under different conditions.
3. Severe neurologic damage may be completely asymptomatic and impossible to detect during the first few weeks of life.

continued on following page

Pediatric Physical Assessment (*Continued*)

Technique	Findings
NEUROLOGIC EXAMINATION (*Continued*) **Procedure for the toddler and early school-age child** 1. The neurologic examination for the toddler and the early school-age child is similar to that for the adult (see page 66). 2. The Draw-A-Person Test and the Denver Developmental Assessment are both well-accepted methods for testing areas in the development of the child. 3. Beyond the neonatal period, specific gross and fine motor coordination testing, accompanied by appropriate evaluation of the Denver test, will assist in assessing the child's level of development. 4. 4. These tests also assess social and language development and are important screening devices. 5. Interview techniques can also be useful in assessing development in the preschool child.	2. See *www.denverii.com* for instructions and findings of the Denver Development Assessment.

SELECTED REFERENCES

American Academy of Pediatrics. (2008). *Bright futures: Guidelines for health supervision of infants, children, and adolescents* (3rd ed.). Elk Grove Village, IL: Author.

American Academy of Pediatrics. (2011). *Bright futures: Nutrition* (3rd ed.). Elk Grove Village, IL: Author.

Bickley, L. (2016). *Bates' guide to physical examination and history taking* (12th ed.). Philadelphia, PA: Lippincott Williams & Wilkins.

Burns, C., Dunn, A., Brady, M., et al. (2016). *Pediatric primary care* (6th ed.). Philadelphia, PA: Saunders.

Centers for Disease Control and Prevention. (2010). *Growth charts.* Atlanta, GA: Author. Available: *www.cdc.gov/growthcharts/*

Duderstadt, K. G. (2013). *Pediatric physical examination: An illustrated handbook* (2nd ed.). St. Louis, MO: Mosby Elsevier.

Guerrerp, N., Small, A., Schwei, R. & Jacobs, E. (2018). Informing physician strategies to overcome language barriers in encounters with pediatric patients. *Patient Education & Counseling, 101*(4), 653–658.

Johns Hopkins Hospital; Hughes, H., & Kohl, L. (Eds.). (2017). *The Harriet Lane handbook* (21st ed.). Philadelphia, PA: Elsevier Mosby.

McDonald, K., & Eckhardt, A. (2017). Evidence-based practice in action: Ensuring quality of pediatric assessment frequency. *Journal of Pediatric Nursing, 35,* 134–138.

Nelson, K., & McKinney, E. (2017). *Maternal-child nursing* (5th ed.). St. Louis, MO: Saunders.

Pillitteri, A. (2013). *Maternal and child health nursing: Care of the childbearing and childrearing family* (7th ed.). Philadelphia, PA: Lippincott Williams & Wilkins.

42

Pediatric Primary Care

HEALTH MAINTENANCE

 See additional online content: Patient Education Guidelines 42-1 and Procedure Guidelines 42-1

Pediatric primary care includes health promotion and disease prevention interventions that will positively affect the well-being of children and their families. The goal of pediatric primary care is to achieve physical, emotional, and developmental health for all children. Primary prevention—through immunizations, proper nutrition, and safety counseling—is an essential component of pediatric health care.

Immunizations

Disease prevention through immunizations has significantly reduced childhood morbidity and mortality from infectious diseases. However, despite effective immunization availability, vaccine-preventable diseases are still present in the United States and continue to pose significant public health problems. The rate of immunization in the United States exceeds 90% for children aged 19 to 35 months for poliovirus vaccine; measles, mumps, rubella (MMR); hepatitis B, and varicella vaccine. However, rates vary by state and decrease after this age. Rates of immunization for routine vaccines for adolescents aged 13 to 17 have risen over the past 10 years from 26.7% to 41.7% (human papillomavirus vaccine) and 84.7% to 86.7% (Tdap vaccine).

Nurses are in a vital position to promote child health by assessing, recommending, and administering immunizations. Also, nurses are frequently asked to provide documentation (to parents or caregivers) of the immunizations that have been administered to facilitate children's enrollment in day care, school programs, and summer camp participation. A review of immunizations and administration of needed vaccines should be done at every health care visit.

 EVIDENCE BASE Centers for Control Disease and Prevention. (2016). National and state vaccination coverage among children aged 19–35 months—United States, 2015. *Morbidity and Mortality Weekly Report,* 65(39), 1065–1071.

Barriers to Vaccination

 EVIDENCE BASE Carpiano, R., & Fritz, N. (2017). Public attitudes toward child undervaccination: A randomized experiment on evaluations, stigmatizing orientations, and support for policies. *Social Science & Medicine, 185,* 127–136.

Rutten, L., St. Sauver, J., Beebe, T., et al. (2017). Clinician knowledge, clinician barriers and perceived parental barriers regarding human papillomavirus vaccination: Association with initiation and completion rates. *Vaccine, 35*(1), 164–169.

There are many reasons that parents or caregivers may give to refuse vaccinations for their children.

1. Safety concerns, such as concerns that the child may develop learning disabilities. Information about vaccine safety can be obtained from the Centers for Disease Control and Prevention (CDC) at *www.cdc.gov/vaccinesafety/Concerns/Index.html.*
2. Concern for the pain inflicted on the child.
3. Because of success of vaccine programs for many years, many parents have no memory or knowledge of the serious vaccine-preventable illnesses that have been near eradicated.
4. Unfortunately, many parents may be influenced by high-impact negative media information regarding vaccinations despite the fact that most is not supported by evidence.

 NURSING ALERT Nurses can be instrumental in assisting caregivers in discerning factual information from myths and erroneous information that may be presented in the media.

General Considerations

Requirements of National Childhood Vaccine Injury Act (Effective 1988)
1. This act mandated providers to notify all patients and parents about the risks and benefits associated with vaccines.
2. The patient, parent, or legal guardian should be informed about the benefits and risks of immunizations. Before

administration of the vaccine, they must be provided with the current Vaccine Information Statement (VIS), developed by the CDC. Health care providers must record the name of the VIS publication (eg, polio), date of VIS publication, and the date the VIS was given to the patient or his or her family on the child's medical record.

3. Federal law mandates that all health care providers must record the following information in the patient's permanent medical record: month, day, and year of administration; vaccine or other biologic administered; manufacturer, lot number, and expiration date; and name, address, and title of the health care provider administering the vaccine.

4. In addition, the site and route of administration should be documented in the patient's record.

5. Health care providers are required to report selected events occurring after vaccination to the Vaccine Adverse Events Reporting System, part of the CDC Immunization Safety Office, which monitors and investigates possible vaccine adverse effects.

Routine Vaccinations for Children in the United States

The Advisory Committee on Immunization Practices (ACIP) annually develops written recommendations for the CDC regarding the routine administration of vaccines, along with schedules detailing the appropriate timing, dosage, and contraindications for children and adults in the civilian population in the United States. The most recent recommendations are reviewed below, but complete immunization schedules can be found at *www.cdc.gov/vaccines*.

Childhood-recommended vaccines (ages 0 to 6 years) include diphtheria, tetanus toxoid, acellular pertussis (DTaP); inactivated poliovirus vaccine (IPV); MMR; *Haemophilus influenzae* type b (Hib) vaccine; hepatitis B vaccine (HBV); *Varicella*; pneumococcal conjugate vaccine (PCV7 and PCV13); rotavirus (Rota); hepatitis A (HepA); and meningococcal vaccine (MCV4). An influenza vaccine is recommended to be given annually for healthy children aged 6 months to 19 years old. In many areas of the United States, influenza vaccine is a requirement for day-care attendance.

The recommended immunization schedule for persons ages 7 to 18 years includes tetanus toxoid, diphtheria, and acellular pertussis (Tdap); human papillomavirus vaccine (HPV); MCV4; pneumococcal polysaccharide vaccine (PPV)—to certain groups at high risk; annual influenza vaccine (trivalent inactivated influenza vaccine [TIV]); HepA—for certain groups of children; HBV; MMR; *Varicella*; and IPV, if necessary, to equal a total of four doses. While not required by schools, the HPV is recommended to start by age 9 years, but can be given until age 26 years. If the child receives the vaccine before age 14 years, he or she only needs a two-dose vaccine series; after age 14 years, three doses of the vaccine are required.

Immunization Schedules

1. Routine immunizations are started in infancy. However, if a child is not immunized in infancy, immunizations may be started at any age and a slightly different schedule may be followed, depending on the child's age and the prevalence of specific diseases at that time.

2. Usually, an interrupted primary series of immunizations does not need to be restarted; rather, the original series should be resumed regardless of the length of time that has elapsed.

3. In special circumstances involving some cancer treatments and severe immunologic disorders, immunization schedules will require adjustment.

4. The immunoresponse is limited in a significant proportion of infants, and the recommended booster doses are designed to ensure and maintain immunity.

5. Current recommended immunization schedules can be found at *www.cdc.gov/vaccines/*.

6. When using a combination vaccine, if there is a contraindication to any of the components, do not vaccinate.

Contraindications and Precautions

It is important to read the manufacturer's insert for each vaccine before administration.

1. Contraindications to all vaccines:
   a. Anaphylactic reaction to a vaccine or a vaccine constituent.
   b. Moderate or severe illnesses with or without a fever. Children with moderate or severe illnesses, with or without fever, can be vaccinated as soon as they are recovering and no longer acutely ill.

2. All live virus vaccines (live oral poliovirus vaccine [OPV], MMR, *Varicella*) are contraindicated in pregnancy, immunosuppression or immunodeficiency, and household or close contact with those who are immunosuppressed or immunodeficient.
   a. MMR vaccine should be considered for all symptomatic human immunodeficiency virus (HIV)–infected persons who do not have evidence of severe immunosuppression or evidence of measles immunity.
   b. *Varicella* vaccine should be considered for asymptomatic or mildly symptomatic HIV-infected children.

3. Diphtheria, tetanus, and pertussis (DTP)/DTaP—encephalopathy within 7 days of administration of previous dose of DTP/DTaP.
   a. Infants and children with stable neurologic conditions, including well-controlled seizures, may be vaccinated; however, such vaccination should be decided on an individual basis.

4. IPV—anaphylactic reaction to neomycin, streptomycin, or polymyxin B.

5. MMR and *Varicella*—anaphylactic reactions to neomycin or gelatin.

6. Influenza—anaphylactic reaction to eggs or egg protein. Persons with asthma, reactive airway disease, or other chronic pulmonary or cardiovascular disorders should not receive LAIV.

7. HBV—anaphylactic reaction to baker's yeast.

8. Meningococcal vaccines—can be given to pregnant women; should not be administered with other vaccines for children with sickle cell disease or those without a functioning spleen.

Misconceptions Concerning Vaccine Contraindications

1. Some health care providers and parents inappropriately consider certain conditions or circumstances to be contraindications to vaccination. Conditions most commonly regarded as such include the following:
   a. Mild acute illness with low-grade fever or mild diarrheal illness in an otherwise well child.
   b. Current antimicrobial therapy or the convalescent phase of illness.
   c. Reaction to a previous DTaP dose that involved only soreness, redness, swelling in the immediate vicinity of the vaccination site, or temperature of less than 105°F (40.5°C).

d. Prematurity.

e. Person using aerosolized steroids, short course of oral steroids (less than 14 days), or topical steroids.

f. Pregnancy of mother or other household contact.

g. Recent exposure to an infectious disease.

h. Breast-feeding.

i. History of nonspecific allergies or relatives with allergies.

j. Allergies to penicillin or other antibiotic, except anaphylactic reactions to neomycin or streptomycin.

k. Allergies to duck meat or duck feathers.

l. Family history of seizures in people considered for pertussis or measles vaccination.

m. Family history of sudden infant death syndrome in children considered for DTaP vaccination.

n. Family history of an adverse event, unrelated to immunosuppression, after vaccination.

o. Malnutrition.

2. In most cases, children with the above conditions can still be immunized.

Vaccine Administration Considerations

1. Strict adherence to the manufacturer's storage and handling recommendation is vital. Failure to observe these precautions and recommendations may reduce the potency and effectiveness of vaccines.

2. Health care personnel administering vaccines should be immunized against MMR, hepatitis B, influenza, tetanus, pertussis, and diphtheria. *Varicella* vaccine is recommended for health care providers with no serologic proof of immunity, prior vaccination, or previous disease. Gloves should be worn when administering vaccines. Good hand-washing technique is mandatory before and after vaccine administration.

3. Sterile, disposable needles and syringes should be discarded promptly in appropriate biohazard containers. Do not recap needles.

4. Parenteral vaccines should be administered in the anterolateral aspect of the upper thigh in infants and in the deltoid area of the upper arm in older children and adolescents. Recommended routes of administration are included in the package inserts of vaccines.

5. Before administering a subsequent dose of any vaccine, question patients and parents about adverse effects and possible reactions from previous doses.

6. Routine vaccines can be safely and effectively administered simultaneously in most healthy children.

Specific Immunizations

DTaP

1. Administered IM.

2. A time lapse of 8 weeks is recommended between the first three DTaP injections for desirable maximum effects.

3. Administration of acetaminophen at the time of immunization and at 4 and 8 hours after immunization decreases the incidence of febrile and local reactions.

4. Tdap is recommended for children over age 7 years. As of 2006, vaccination guidelines recommend that Tdap be routinely used in adolescents 11 to 18 years of age and single doses for adults 19 to 64 years of age in attempts to control recent pertussis outbreaks.

5. For contaminated wounds, a booster dose of tetanus should be given if more than 5 years have elapsed since the last dose.

6. For infant pertussis protection, ACIP has recommended that Tdap be given during each pregnancy between 27 and 36 weeks of gestation to maximize the maternal antibody response and passive antibody transfer to the infant.

Tuberculin Skin Test

1. It is recommended that, if indicated, the tuberculin test be given before or at the time of the MMR vaccine. The measles vaccine may temporarily suppress tuberculin reactivity for 4 to 6 weeks, so result may not be accurate during that time frame.

2. The frequency of repeated tuberculin testing depends on the following:

a. Risk of tuberculosis exposure to the child.

b. Prevalence of tuberculosis in the population group.

c. Presence of underlying host factors in the child (immunosuppressive conditions or HIV infection).

3. Children who have immigrated or been adopted from another country may have received an immunization for tuberculosis (BCG vaccine). It is not recommended in the United States because of low effectiveness.

a. BCG may cause a false-positive tuberculosis (TB) skin test; however, screening for tuberculosis should still occur.

b. Interferon-gamma release assays (IGRAs) are the preferred method of testing for tuberculosis in those immunized with BCG. An IGRA measures how strong a person's immune system reacts to TB bacteria by testing the person's blood in a laboratory.

c. Chest x-ray confirms pulmonary disease.

 EVIDENCE BASE Fry, S., Barnabas, S., & Cotton, M. (2018). Update on trends in childhood tuberculosis. *Current Opinion in Pediatrics, 30*(1), 152–160.

Measles Vaccine

1. Usually given between ages 12 and 15 months, but should be given at 12 months in high-risk areas. Second dose is recommended between ages 4 and 6 years.

2. Administered subcutaneously.

3. During an outbreak, infants as young as age 6 months can be immunized. A second dose should be given between ages 12 and 15 months and again at school entry.

4. Mild postimmunization symptoms include transient skin rashes and fever up to 2 weeks after vaccination.

5. Immunoglobulin preparations will interfere with the serologic response to measles vaccine; therefore, wait the specified time after administration for vaccination.

Meningococcal Vaccine

1. Usually given between the ages of 11 and 12 years, with a booster dose at age 16 years for healthy children. Is administered earlier (minimum age of 9 months) for some children with underlying conditions or children who are resident or travel to countries with epidemic disease.

2. Administer the MPSV4 vaccine subcutaneously into the fat of the arm. The MCV4 vaccines are given IM.

3. Mild postimmunization symptoms such as local discomfort may occur. A small percentage of those who receive the vaccine may develop a fever. Severe reactions (such as an allergic reaction) are very rare.

Mumps Vaccine

1. Usually administered in combination with measles and rubella vaccine between ages 12 and 15 months.

2. Second dose administered as MMR is important because a substantial number of cases have occurred in people with previous immunizations.
3. Important to immunize susceptible children approaching puberty, adolescents, and adults.

Rubella Vaccine

1. Two doses of rubella vaccine are recommended to avoid consequences such as congenital rubella syndrome; usually administered in combination with mumps and measles.
2. Important to immunize postpubertal individuals, especially college students and military recruits.
3. Women should avoid pregnancy within 3 months of vaccine because of the theoretical risk to the fetus.

Polio Vaccine

1. Two types of trivalent vaccine have been developed—OPV and IPV (given IM or subcutaneously). Both are effective in preventing poliomyelitis; however, as of 2000, both the ACIP and CDC recommend exclusive use of IPV for infants and children in the United States, to reduce the risk of vaccine-induced polio from OPV.
2. Because live OPV is excreted in the stool for up to 1 month after vaccination, vaccine-induced polio is a risk to both the nonimmune child and any immunosuppressed contact.

Haemophilus Influenzae Type B Vaccine

1. Incidence of invasive disease caused by Hib has declined dramatically since the introduction of the conjugate vaccine.
2. Several different types of Hib vaccines are available. Different vaccines have different schedules.
3. Minimal adverse reactions (pain, redness, or swelling at immunization site for less than 24 hours).

Hepatitis B Vaccine

1. There are two schedules for this vaccine. Infants born to hepatitis B surface antigen (HBsAg)–negative mothers should receive the routine schedule. Infants born to HBsAg-positive mothers should be on an accelerated vaccination schedule.
2. Recommended for all infants born to HBsAg-negative mothers. Three-dose schedule is initiated in neonatal period or by age 2 months; the second dose is given 1 to 2 months later; the third dose, 6 to 18 months later.
3. All infants born to HBsAg-positive mothers, including premature neonates, should receive hepatitis B immunoglobulin and HBV within 12 hours after birth. The second dose is given between ages 1 and 2 months; the third dose is given at age 6 months.
4. Preterm neonates weighing less than 2,000 g may have lower seroconversion rates. Initiation of HBV should be delayed until just before hospital discharge if the infant weighs 2,000 g or more or until about age 2 months when other routine immunizations are given.
5. All children and adolescents who have not had HBV should be immunized.
6. Administered IM.

Pneumococcal Vaccines

1. There are two types of pneumococcal vaccines:
   a. PCV7/Prevnar (must be administered IM).
   b. 23-valent PPV/Pneumovax (may be given IM or subcutaneously).
2. Since 2000, the pneumococcal has been included in the recommended childhood vaccines for all children ages 2 to 23 months and for certain children ages 2 to 5 years.
3. Efficacy for the vaccine is 97%, and the adverse effects are mild (fever and localized tenderness and redness at the injection site).

4. PPV is recommended for children ages 2 to 5 years in certain high-risk groups (sickle cell disease, functional or anatomic asplenia, nephrotic syndrome, chronic renal failure, immunosuppressive disorders, HIV infection, and cerebrospinal fluid leak).

Influenza Vaccine

1. The influenza vaccine known as TIV or LAIV contains three virus strains and is changed yearly, based on predictions of predominate strains expected to circulate in the upcoming influenza season. LAIV was approved for use in those ages 2 through 49 years in the United States in 2003 and is administered intranasally. TIV is available in both pediatric and adult formulations and is administered IM.
2. The influenza vaccine should be given annually to children ages 6 months through 18 years. The "Recommended Immunization Schedule" provides more specifics.
3. This vaccine is given annually, before flu season, usually in October, November, or December.
4. In children ages 8 years and younger, the first time influenza vaccine is administered, two doses should be given 1 month apart. In subsequent years, only one dose is needed.
5. TIV should be used for children with asthma, children 2 to 4 years who had wheezing in the past 12 months, or children who have any other underlying medical contraindications to the LAIV.
6. In recent years, LAIV has been less effective than the TIV, and therefore, many providers have chosen not to offer it to patients.

Rotavirus Vaccine

1. In 2006, a live, oral vaccine—RotaTeq—was licensed. In the United States, routine vaccination of infants—with three doses of rotavirus vaccine administered at 2, 4, and 6 months—is recommended.

Varicella Virus Vaccine

1. Varicella virus vaccine contains live, attenuated virus; approved for children 12 months and older and for adults.
2. Administered subcutaneously at 12 to 15 months; second dose at 4 to 6 years (or at least 3 months after first dose).
3. May be given to older children and adults who do not have immunity. In those older than age 13, the second dose may be delayed only 4 weeks following first dose.

 NURSING ALERT Millions of children travel overseas every year, risking exposure to infectious diseases not covered by routine immunizations. Refer families to their local public health department or retail travel clinic for special immunizations and malaria prophylaxis.

Nutrition in Children

The nutritional status of the child is an important aspect of health maintenance. A balanced diet influences child growth and psychosocial development. Feeding provides emotional and psychological benefits in addition to nutritional needs. In the United States, obesity in childhood has become a major problem, and in developing countries, undernutrition—due to scarcity of nutrient-rich foods—leads to malnutrition and illness. In addition, anorexia, bulimia, and other dietary restrictions may place children and adolescents at risk for serious health consequences. Good eating habits, nutrient-rich foods, and physical activity introduced early in life can help foster good nutrition practices into adulthood. Nurses can be instrumental in providing factual information to both parents and children on typical nutritional needs and those required for specific sport participation. Table 42-1 presents nutritional guidelines based on age and developmental maturation.

text continues on page 1127

Table 42-1 Nutrition in Children

AGE AND DEVELOPMENTAL INFLUENCE ON NUTRITIONAL REQUIREMENTS AND FEEDING PATTERNS	FEEDING PATTERN AND DIET	NURSING CONSIDERATIONS AND PARENTAL GUIDANCE
Neonate		

Birth–4 weeks
 • Neonate's rapid growth makes infant especially vulnerable to dietary inadequacies, dehydration, and iron deficiency anemia.
 • Feeding process is basis for infant's first human relationship, formation of trust.
 • Neonates require more fluid relative to their size than do adults.
 • Sucking ability is influenced by individual neuromuscular maturity.
	• Breast milk or formula is generally given in 6–8 feedings per day, spaced 2–4 hours apart.
	 • Feeding schedules should be individualized according to infant's needs.
	 • Breast-fed infants should receive 400 IU of supplemental vitamin D daily, beginning in the first few days of life. Supplementation should continue until baby is weaned to at least 1 qt (1 L) of whole milk per day. Whole milk should not be used until after 12 months of age.
	 • Human milk contains little iron, so infants who are exclusively breast-fed are at increased risk of iron deficiency after 4 months of age. It is recommended that infants be given 1 mg/kg/day of a liquid iron supplement until iron-containing solid foods are introduced at about 6 months of age.
	 • Infant formula should be iron fortified to prevent anemia.
	 • All formulas sold in the United States have at least 400 IU/L of vitamin D; if baby is drinking at least 32 ounces of formula, vitamin D supplementation is not needed.
		• Provide information to help parents make decision concerning breast- or bottle-feeding.
		 • Support parents in their decision.
		 Breast-fed infant:
		 • Help mother assume comfortable and satisfying position for self and baby.
		 • Help mother to determine schedule, timing, and when infant is satisfied.
		 • Provide specific information about:
		   • Feeding technique: position, "bubbling/burping"
		   • Care of breasts
		   • Manual expression of milk from breast
		   • Maternal diet
		 Bottle-fed infant:
		 • Provide specific information about:
		   • Type of formula
		   • Preparation of formula: measuring and sterilization
		   • Equipment—types of bottles and nipples
		   • Sterilization of equipment
		   • Technique of feeding: position, "bubbling/burping"
		 • Help mother to determine when infant is satisfied; develop schedule for feeding.
		 • Provide information about normal characteristics of stools, signs of dehydration, constipation, colic, milk allergy.
		 • Discuss need for prescribed supplements and how to administer (by dropper).
		 • Discuss need for additional fluids during periods of hot weather and with fever, diarrhea, and vomiting.
		 • Observe for evidence of common problems and intervene accordingly:
		   • Overfeeding
		   • Underfeeding
		   • Difficulty digesting formula because of its composition
		   • Improper feeding technique; holes in nipples too large or too small; formula too hot or too cold; uncomfortable feeding position; failure to "bubble/burp"; improper sterilization; bottle propping
		   • Bottles should never be given to infants to take to bed.

Infant		
1–3 months • Infants consume more formula or breast milk with each feeding and sleep for longer periods. • Infants have increased interaction during feeding because of cooing and development of a social milestone. • Bowel movements become less frequent. Breast-fed infants may not have a bowel movement after each feeding.		
Infant		
3 months–1 year overview • Increased neuromuscular development allows infant to make transition from a totally liquid diet to a diet of milk and solid foods as well as to more active participation in the feeding process. **3–6 months** • Sucking reflex becomes voluntary and chewing action begins; infant can approximate lips to rim and cup and may begin drinking from cup at 6 months.	• Number of feedings per day decreases through the first year. • By ages 4–6 months, generally ready to begin strained foods. The usual sequence of foods is cereal followed by vegetables and fruits. Meats may be started between 8 and 9 months. Sequence may vary according to preferences of the family and health care provider.	• The person feeding should be calm, gentle, relaxed, and patient in approach. • When first offered puréed foods with a spoon, the child expects and wants to suck. The protrusion of the tongue, which is needed in sucking, makes it appear as if the child is pushing the food out of the mouth. This response should not be interpreted as dislike for the food; it is a result of immature muscle coordination and surprise at the taste and feel of the new food. • The baby foods selected should be high in nutrients without providing excessive calories. Personal and cultural preferences should be considered. Iron-fortified formulas and cereals are needed to prevent physiologic anemia. • New foods should be offered one at a time and early in the feeding while the infant is still hungry. Allow 3–5 days between new foods to assess for any allergic reaction.

(continued)

Table 42-1 Nutrition in Children (Continued)

AGE AND DEVELOPMENTAL INFLUENCE ON NUTRITIONAL REQUIREMENTS AND FEEDING PATTERNS	FEEDING PATTERN AND DIET	NURSING CONSIDERATIONS AND PARENTAL GUIDANCE
Infant (Continued)		
6–12 months • Loses maternal iron stores at 6 months; first tooth erupts between ages 6 and 9 months; eyes and hands can work together; infant can sit without support and has developed grasp; can feed self a biscuit; bangs objects on table; able to hold own bottle between ages 9 and 12 months; can "pincer" grasp food; able to be weaned from bottle as child becomes developmentally able to take sufficient fluids from the cup. • Food provides the infant with a variety of learning experiences; motor control and coordination in self-feeding; recognition of shape, texture, and color; stimulation of speech movement through use of mouth muscles. • Mealtime allows the infant to continue development of trust in a consistent, loving atmosphere. The infant is forming lifetime eating habits; it is therefore important to make mealtime a positive experience.	• Mashed table foods or junior foods are generally started between ages 6 and 8 months, when infant begins chewing action. • Infant begins to enjoy finger foods between ages 10 and 12 months. • The transition from iron-fortified formula or breast milk to cow's milk is usually advised at about age 12 months. • By age 1 year, most infants are satisfied with three meals and additional fluids throughout the day.	• Infants should be observed for allergic reactions when new foods are added. Common allergies are to citrus juices, egg whites, and cow's milk. These foods should be avoided until age 12 months. New research has shown early introduction of peanuts into the diet of infants at high risk of peanut allergy can play a role in the prevention of peanut allergies. Health care providers may recommend introducing peanut containing products into the diets of infants between ages 4 and 11 months. • Honey should be avoided until age 12 months because of the risk of infantile botulism. • Finger foods should be selected for their nutritional value. Good choices include teething biscuits, cooked vegetables, bananas, cheese sticks, and enriched cereals. Avoid nuts, raisins, and raw vegetables, which can cause choking. • Parents can be taught to prepare their own strained or junior foods using a commercial baby food grinder or blender. • Weaning is a gradual process. • Assist parents to recognize indications of readiness. • Do not expect the infant to completely drop old pattern of behavior while learning a new one; allow overlap of old and new techniques. • Evening feedings are usually the most difficult to eliminate because the infant is tired and in need of sucking comfort. • During illness or household disorganization, the infant may regress and return to sucking to relieve his or her discomfort and frustration.

 NURSING ALERT Obtain a thorough nursing history for the hospitalized infant that includes feeding pattern and schedule; types of foods that have been introduced; likes and dislikes; breast- or bottle-fed; type of bottle; and temperature at which infant prefers foods and fluids.

AGE AND DEVELOPMENTAL INFLUENCE ON NUTRITIONAL REQUIREMENTS AND FEEDING PATTERNS	FEEDING PATTERN AND DIET	NURSING CONSIDERATIONS AND PARENTAL GUIDANCE
Toddler		
1–3 years • Growth slows at the end of the first year. The slower growth rate is reflected in a decreased appetite. • The toddler has a total of 14–16 teeth, making him or her more able to chew foods. • Increased self-awareness causes the toddler to want to do more for self. Refusal of food or refusal of assistance in feedings are common ways in which the toddler asserts self. • Because body tissues, especially muscles, continue to grow quite rapidly, protein needs are high.	• Transition from a bottle to a cup before, or at the age of 1 is recommended to prevent tooth decay. • Appetite is sporadic; specific foods may be favored exclusively or refused from time to time. • Child may be ritualistic concerning food preferences, schedule, and manner of eating. • Diet should include a full range of foods: milk, meat, fruits, vegetables, breads, and cereals. Iron-fortified dry cereals (rice, barley) are an excellent source of iron during the second year of life.	• Provide foods with a variety of colors, textures, and flavors. Toddlers need to experience the feel of foods. • Offer small portions. It is fun for the child to ask for more. It is more effective to give small helpings than to insist that he or she eat a specific amount. • Maintain a regular mealtime schedule. • Provide appropriate mealtime equipment: • Silverware scaled to size • Dishes—colorful, unbreakable; shallow, round bowls are preferable to flat plates • Plastic bibs, placemats, and floor coverings permit a relaxed attitude toward child's self-feeding attempts • Comfortable seating at good height and distance from table • Adults who help toddlers at mealtime should be calm and relaxed. Avoid bribes or force-feeding because this reinforces negative behavior and may lead to a dislike for mealtime. Encourage independence, but provide assistance when necessary. Do not be concerned about table manners.

Table 42-1 Nutrition in Children (Continued)

AGE AND DEVELOPMENTAL INFLUENCE ON NUTRITIONAL REQUIREMENTS AND FEEDING PATTERNS	FEEDING PATTERN AND DIET	NURSING CONSIDERATIONS AND PARENTAL GUIDANCE
Toddler (Continued)	• Older toddler can be expected to consume about one half the amount of food than an adult consumes. • Whole milk is recommended up to age 2 years.	• Avoid the use of soda or "sweets" as rewards or between-meal snacks. Instead, substitute fruit or cereal. • Toddlers who show little interest in eggs, meat, or vegetables should not be permitted to appease their appetite with carbohydrates or milk because this may lead to iron deficiency anemia. Milk should be limited to ~16 ounces a day and should be offered after solid foods. **NURSING ALERT** Nursing history for the hospitalized toddler should include feeding pattern and schedule; food likes and dislikes; food allergies; special eating equipment and utensils; whether child is weaned; and what child is fed when ill.

Preschooler
 	
3–5 years
• Increased manual dexterity enables child to have complete independence at mealtime.
• Psychosocially, this is a period of increased imitation. The preschooler identifies with parents at the table and will enjoy what parents enjoy.
• Additional nutritional habits are developed that become part of the child's lifetime practices.
• Slower growth rate and increased interest in exploring his or her environment may decrease the preschooler's interest in eating.
• Eating assumes increasing social significance. Mealtime promotes socialization and provides the preschooler with opportunities to learn appropriate mealtime behavior, language skills, and understanding of family rituals.
 	
 NURSING ALERT Consider cultural differences. Allow parents to bring in favorite foods or eating utensils from home for the hospitalized preschooler. Encourage family members to be present at mealtime.
	• Appetite tends to be sporadic.
	• Child requires the same basic four food groups as the adult, but in smaller quantities.
	• Generally likes to eat one food from plate at a time.
	• Likes vegetables that are crisp, raw, and cut into finger-sized pieces. Often dislikes strong-tasting foods.
		• Emphasis should be placed on the quality rather than the amount of food ingested.
		• Foods should be attractively served, mildly flavored, plain, as well as separated and distinctly identifiable in flavor and appearance.
		• Nutritional foods (eg, crackers and cheese, yogurt, fruit) should be offered as snacks.
		• Desserts should be nutritious and a natural part of the meal, not used as a reward for finishing the meal or omitted as punishment.
		• Unless they persist, periods of overeating or not wanting to eat certain foods should not cause concern. The overall eating pattern from month to month is more pertinent to assess.
		• Frequent causes of insufficient eating:
		  • Unhappy atmosphere at mealtime
		  • Overeating between meals
		  • Parental example
		  • Attention-seeking.
		  • Excessive parental expectations
		  • Inadequate variety or quantity of foods
		  • Tooth decay
		  • Physical illness
		  • Fatigue
		  • Emotional disturbance
		• Measures to increase food intake:
		  • Allow child to help with preparations, planning menu, setting table, and other simple chores.
		  • Maintain calm environment with no distractions.
		  • Avoid between-meal snacks.
		  • Provide rest period before meal.
		  • Avoid coaxing, bribing, threatening.
		• Place children in small groups, preferably at tables during mealtime. Use nursing history to determine likes and provide simple foods in small portions. Peanut butter and jelly sandwiches are often favorites. Allow and encourage children to feed themselves. Do not punish children who refuse to eat. Offer alternative foods.

(continued)

Table 42-1 Nutrition in Children (*Continued*)

AGE AND DEVELOPMENTAL INFLUENCE ON NUTRITIONAL REQUIREMENTS AND FEEDING PATTERNS	FEEDING PATTERN AND DIET	NURSING CONSIDERATIONS AND PARENTAL GUIDANCE
School-Age Child • Slowed growth rate during middle childhood results in gradual decline in food requirements per unit of body weight. • The preadolescent growth spurt occurs about age 10 in girls and about age 12 in boys. At this time, energy needs increase and approach those of the adult. Intake is particularly important because reserves are laid down for the demands of adolescence. • The child becomes dependent on peers for approval and makes food choices accordingly. • The child experiences increased socialization and independence through opportunities to eat away from home (eg, at school and homes of peers).	• By this time, food practices are generally well established, a product of the eating experiences of the toddler and preschool period. • Many children are too busy with other affairs to take time out to eat. Play readily takes priority unless a firm understanding is reached and mealtime is relaxed and enjoyable.	• Nutrition education should help the child to select foods wisely and to begin to plan and prepare meals. • Parental attitudes continue to be important as the child copies parental behavior (eg, skipping breakfast, not eating certain foods, consuming fast foods frequently). • Most children require a nutritious breakfast to avoid lassitude in late morning. • Mealtime should continue to be relaxed and enjoyable. Diversions, such as television, should be avoided. • Calcium and vitamin D intake warrant special consideration. They must be adequate to support the rapid enlargement of bones. • Parents and health care professionals should be alert to signs of developing obesity. Intake should be altered accordingly. • Table manners should not be overemphasized. The young child typically stuffs mouth, spills food, and chatters incessantly while eating. Time and experience will improve habits. • Provide some companionship and conversation at the child's level during meals. Peers should be invited occasionally for meals. **NURSING ALERT** Nursing history of the hospitalized child should include food preferences; mealtime patterns and snacks; food allergies; and food preferences when ill. Provide opportunities for children to eat in small groups at tables. Consider cultural differences. Allow parents to bring in favorite foods from home. Allow child to order his or her own meal.
Adolescent **11–17 years** • Dietary requirements vary according to stage of sexual maturation, rate of physical growth, and extent of athletic and social activity. • When rapid growth of puberty appears, there is a corresponding increase in energy requirements and appetite. • Menstruating teen is particularly susceptible to iron deficiency anemia.	• Previously learned dietary patterns are difficult to change. • Food choices and eating habits may be quite unusual and are related to the adolescent's psychological and social milieu. • Generally, a significant percentage of the daily caloric intake of the adolescent comes from snacking.	• Continue nutrition education, with emphasis on: • Selecting nutritious foods high in iron • Nutritional needs related to growth • Preparing favorite "adolescent foods" • Foods and physical fitness • Informal sessions are generally more effective than lectures on nutrition. • Special problems requiring intervention: • Obesity • Excessive dieting • Extreme fads—eccentric and grossly restricted diets • Anorexia nervosa and bulimia • Adolescent pregnancy • Iron deficiency anemia • Provide nutritious foods relevant to the adolescent's lifestyle. • Discourage cigarette smoking, which may contribute to poor nutritional status by decreasing appetite and increasing the body's metabolic rate. **NURSING ALERT** Allow hospitalized adolescent to choose own foods, especially if on a special diet. Provide a refrigerator in the recreation room for snacks or utilize a snack cart. Serve foods that appeal to adolescents. Use a nursing history similar to that for the school-age child.

EVIDENCE BASE Lewis, E., Richard, C., Larsen, B., & Field, C. (2017). The importance of human milk for immunity in preterm infants. *Clinics in Perinatology,* 44(1), 23–47.

Breast-Feeding

1. Breast-feeding is the natural and ideal nourishment that will supply an infant with adequate nutrition as well as immunologic and anti-infection properties. With breast milk being at the proper temperature, it may prevent other GI disturbances as well. The development of allergies is reduced in breast-fed babies.
2. Breast-feeding is recommended solely for infants up to 6 months of age. As the infant grows and develops, the breast milk properties change in respect to amounts of fat, carbohydrates, and protein as well as physical properties such as pH needed for the respective age of the infant.
3. Breast-feeding provides psychological and emotional satisfaction for the infant and mother and can promote bonding. The physical closeness may also provide comfort after a frightening or painful procedure.
4. Breast-feeding can be continued through most illnesses and hospitalizations of the infant. In times of stress, the infant may cope with breast-feeding better than bottle-feeding. Because breast milk is more easily and quickly digested, shorter periods without food preoperatively and postoperatively may be necessary. Attempts should be made to maintain the breast-feeding bond and routines of the child and mother.
   a. Supplemental artificial formula can be given to the infant if the mother is not available.
   b. The mother can pump her breasts so that milk can be given to the infant by way of bottle when she is not available.
   c. Breast milk can be frozen for up to 6 months (check the facility's specific policy).
   d. Thaw frozen breast milk for use in tepid water. Do not use a microwave, which may destroy vitamins and nutritional properties as well as result in extreme overheating of portions of the breast milk.
5. Stress of new motherhood or illness in the infant or mother may decrease the mother's milk supply and inhibit her "let-down" reflex, as well as increase or decrease the infant's desire to suckle. Pumping may be initiated to help stimulate the mother's milk supply. An electronic pump may be necessary if prolonged pumping is expected or if manual pumping is not successful.
6. Education and encouragement should be offered to all new mothers and those having difficulty or concerns about breast-feeding.

Bottle-Feeding

1. Bottle-feeding is a method of supplying nutrition to the infant by oral feedings, using a bottle and nipple setup.
2. Bottle-feeding can supplement breast-feeding with formula or water or can be the sole means of nutritional intake for the infant.
3. Bottle-feeding can also provide intermittent feedings of expressed breast milk when the mother cannot be present at the time of the feeding.
4. Bottle-feeding can be a time of bonding between the mother and infant. The father or other capable members of the family should be taught bottle-feeding technique as well.

5. Some mothers may have chosen bottle-feeding for a variety of reasons, ranging from poor milk production, discomfort (psychological or physical) with breast-feeding, or drug treatment not compatible with breast-feeding. It is important that health care providers offer mothers information on all methods of feeding, but not be judgmental when the mother chooses one method over another.

Safety

Safety is an important aspect of child health and well-being. Injuries are the leading cause of death for children in the United States. Additionally, injury is a significant cause of childhood morbidity. Although childhood deaths from other causes have decreased, deaths from injuries remain constant.

Role of the Nurse

1. Identify environmental hazards and act to reduce or eliminate them.
2. Identify behavioral characteristics of individual children that may be related to accidental liability and caution parents accordingly. Pay particular attention to children who show the following:
   a. Characteristics that increase exposure to hazards, such as excessive curiosity, inability to delay gratification, hyperactivity, and daringness.
   b. Characteristics that reduce the child's ability to cope with hazards, such as aggressiveness, stubbornness, poor concentration, low frustration threshold, poor impulse control, and lack of self-control.
3. Provide anticipatory guidance about child development as it relates to accidents. Direct preventive teaching toward the intended audience, be it individuals or groups, children or adults.
4. Participate in policy setting for accident prevention, with great emphasis on effective public health measures.

Principles of Safety

1. The type of accident likely to occur is influenced by the child's age and developmental level. Parents who have knowledge of their own child's typical behavior patterns may foresee potential accident situations.
2. Children are naturally curious, impulsive, and impatient. The young child needs to touch, feel, and investigate. Consistent adult supervision will enable children to learn in a safe environment.
3. Children copy the behavior of their parents and absorb parental attitudes. Parents and other adults should be a role model for using proper and safe methods.
4. Children become less careful and less willing to listen to warnings and to observe routine safety precautions when they are tired or hungry.
5. An estimated 90% of all accidents are preventable.

General Areas of Adult Responsibility for Child Safety

Motor Vehicle

EVIDENCE BASE Evidence Base American Academy of Pediatrics. (2017). Car seats: Information for families. Available: *https://healthychildren.org/ English/safety-prevention/on-the-go/Pages/Car-Safety-Seats-Information-for-Families.aspx.*

1. Automobiles should be in good mechanical condition.
2. Use properly fitted and installed car seats and seat belts. Be aware of the guidelines for restraints based on the child's age, weight, and height.
   a. Rear-facing car seat until age 2, or if child has outgrown the manufacturer's recommendation for maximum height and weight.
   b. Front-facing car seat from age 2 until the child has outgrown the manufacturer's recommendation for maximum height and weight.
   c. Belt-positioning booster seat until the vehicle seat belt fits properly, typically when the child has reached 4 feet, 9 inches in height, between 8 and 12 years of age.
3. All children younger than 13 years should be restrained in the rear seats of vehicles (when the vehicle has a rear seat with lap and shoulder belts) for optimal protection. The center rear seat is the safest seat for a child.
4. The driver should look carefully in front and back of the car before getting into the car.
5. Lock all car doors.
6. Never leave young children in a car alone.
7. Do not place heavy or sharp objects on the same seat with a child.

Sports and Recreation
1. Keep equipment in good condition and proper working order.
2. Ensure that children are aware of the correct use of sports equipment.
3. Encourage the routine use of bike helmets (see Figure 42-1).
4. Wear appropriate clothing and safety equipment for the activity (see Figure 42-2).
5. Do not attempt activities beyond one's physical endurance.
6. Keep firearms and ammunition locked in different locations.

Electrical and Mechanical Equipment
1. Only underwriter-approved devices should be installed; they should be inspected periodically.
2. Dry hands before touching appliances. Keep radios, transportable heaters, and hair dryers out of the bathroom.
3. Disconnect appliances after each use and before attempting minor repairs.

Figure 42-1. Use of bike helmets by all children for safety.

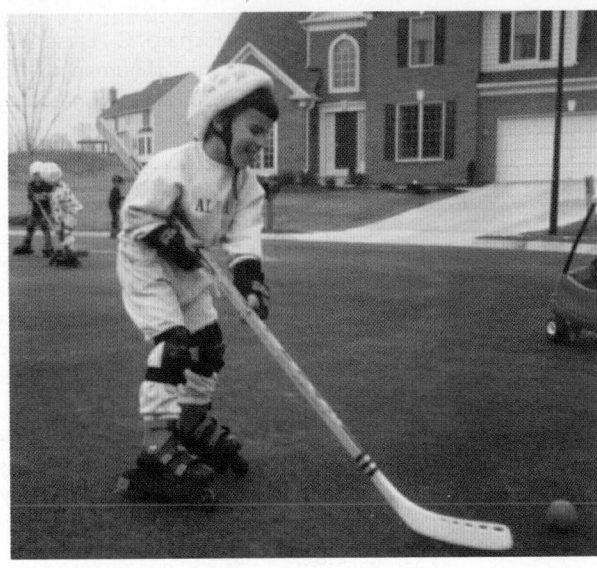

Figure 42-2. Use of appropriate pads and helmets for safety.

4. Keep garden equipment and machinery in a restricted area. Teach proper use of the equipment as soon as the child is old enough.
5. Avoid overloading electrical circuits.
6. Discourage children from playing with or being in area where appliances or power tools (eg, washing machine, clothes dryer, saw, lawn mower) are in operation.

Prevention of Falls
1. Keep stairs well lit and free from clutter.
2. Use gates at tops and bottoms of stairways where toddlers have access.
3. Provide sturdy railings.
4. Anchor small rugs securely.
5. Use rubber mats in the bathtub and shower.
6. Use only sturdy ladders for climbing.
7. The American Academy of Pediatrics and the National Association of Children's Hospitals and Related Institutions have recommended that baby walkers be banned as most injuries using these walkers will occur even when adults are present (rolling down stairs, burns, drowning, reaching unsafe objects because of greater stability provided by walkers).

Poisonings and Ingestions
1. Do not mix bleaches with ammonia, vinegar, and other household cleaners.
2. See section on ingested poisons and pediatric poisoning (see page 1133).
3. Label poisonous household materials, and keep them out of child's reach.
4. Become familiar with the telephone number for poison control centers where available. Post local poison control phone number in easily accessible location (eg, refrigerator door).

Fire
1. Maintain an adequate fire escape plan and routinely conduct home fire drills. Teach children escape routes as soon as they are old enough.
2. Keep a pressure-type, handheld fire extinguisher on each floor. Regularly check expiration or necessary inspection dates.

Consider additional units in areas where there are higher risk of fires (kitchen, laundry room, garage). Instruct all family members who are old enough in its use.

3. Fit fireplaces with snug fireplace screens.
4. Store gasoline and other flammable fluids in tightly covered containers that are clearly labeled, away from heat and sparks, and out of reach.
5. Dispose of paint- and oil-soaked cloths promptly.
6. Use flame-retardant sleepwear.
7. Mark children's rooms so they are obvious to firefighters.
8. Teach children about the danger of smoke inhalation.
9. Teach children to stop, drop, and roll if their clothing catches fire.
10. Maintain smoke and carbon monoxide detectors in working order.
11. Keep lighters and matches out of the reach of children.
12. Keep children away from heated oven, stovetop, and outdoor grill.

Swimming Pools

1. Completely enclose pool with a fence that complies with local regulations. The gate should be self-closing and have a lock.
2. Indicate water depth with numbers on the edge of the pool. Place a safety float line where the bottom of the slope begins to deepen.
3. Install at least one ladder at each end of the pool. Ladders should have handrails on both sides, and the diameter of the rails should be small enough for a child to grasp.
4. Use nonslip materials on ladders, deck, and diving boards.
5. If the pool is used at night, install underwater lighting as well as outdoor lights.
6. Install a ground fault circuit interrupter on the pool circuit to cut off electrical power and thus prevent electrocutions should electrical fault occur.
7. Instruct children about safety rules, such as not swimming alone, need for adult supervision, not running around the pool, and not pushing others. Avoid using radios or other electrical appliances around the pool.
8. Warn children not to attempt to walk on any remaining pool water after the season—frozen water or pool-covering equipment.
9. Keep essential rescue devices and first-aid equipment close to the pool.

Emergency Precautions

1. Record emergency telephone numbers in an obvious and easily accessible place.
2. Keep a well-stocked first-aid kit immediately available for emergencies. It is helpful to also carry a small first-aid kit in family vehicles.
3. Give instruction in principles of first aid to all family members who are old enough.
   a. Responsible adults should enroll in first-aid courses offered by the American Red Cross and adult education programs.
   b. Be aware of first-aid procedure for the following conditions: burns, electric shock, poisoning, bites and stings, wounds, near drowning, fractures, cardiopulmonary arrest.
   c. Teach children safety precautions concerning bicycles, answering the telephone or door, strangers outside the home, and street safety.
4. Know the location of gas, water, and electrical switches and how to turn them off in an emergency.
5. Teach children their addresses and telephone numbers and how to dial 911 in case of emergency.

Miscellaneous

1. Take advantage of preventive health care.
   a. Obtain recommended immunizations.
   b. Have regular physical and dental examinations.
2. Seek immediate treatment of all diseases and health problems.
3. Balance periods of work, rest, and exercise in daily living.

PEDIATRIC CARE TECHNIQUES
Nursing Management of the Child with Fever

 EVIDENCE BASE Peetoom, K., Sits, J., & Ploum, L. (2017). Does well-child care education improve consultations and medication management for childhood fever and common infections: A systematic review. *Archives of Disease in Childhood, 102*, 261–267.

Fever is an abnormal elevation of body temperature. Prolonged elevation of temperature above 104°F (40°C) may produce dehydration and harmful effects on the central nervous system (CNS).

General Considerations

1. Consider basic principles related to temperature regulation in pediatric patients.
   a. Usually, an infant's temperature does not stabilize before age 1 week. A neonate's temperature varies with the temperature of the environment.
   b. The degree of fever does not always reflect the severity of the disease. A child may have a serious illness with a normal or subnormal temperature.
   c. Febrile seizures may occur in some children when the temperature rises rapidly.
   d. The range for normal temperature varies widely in children. A common explanation for "fever" is misinterpretation of a normal temperature reading.
   e. A child's temperature is influenced by activity and by the time of day; temperatures are highest in late afternoon.
2. Temperature interpretation depends on accurate temperature measurement in a child. The mode should be appropriate for the child's age and condition, and the thermometer should be left in place for the required time period. Parents or caregivers should be taught the appropriate assessment of temperature as the child grows.

Causes of Fever in Children

1. Infection.
2. Inflammatory disease.
3. Dehydration.
4. Tumors.
5. Disturbance of temperature-regulating center.
6. Extravasation of blood into the tissues.
7. Drugs or toxins.

Nursing Assessment

1. Assess history of present illness for source of fever.
   a. Age of the child.
   b. Pattern of the fever.
   c. Length of the illness.
   d. Change in normal patterns of eating, elimination, and recreation.

e. Other symptoms—poor feeding, cough, earache, diarrhea, vomiting, and rash.
f. Exposure to any illness.
g. Recent immunizations or drugs.
h. Treatment of fever and effectiveness of treatment, including appropriate dosing of antipyretic medications.
i. Previous experiences with fever and its control.
2. Assess the general appearance of the child.
3. Perform a systematic physical assessment.
  a. Inspection of the skin for rashes, sores, or flushed appearance.
  b. Inspection of eyes, ears, nose, and throat for redness and drainage.
  c. Auscultation of the lungs for abnormal sounds.
  d. Neurologic observation for changes in state of consciousness, pupillary reaction, strength of grip, abnormal muscle movement, or lack of movement.
  e. Inspection of external genitals for redness and drainage.
  f. Presence of abdominal or flank tenderness.
4. Assist with laboratory tests, as indicated. Initial tests typically include complete blood count; urinalysis; cultures of the throat, nasopharynx, urine, blood, and spinal fluid; and chest x-ray.
5. Attempt to identify the pattern of the fever. Take the child's temperature by the same method every hour until stable, then every 2 hours until normal, then every 4 hours for 24 hours.

Nursing Measures to Reduce Fever

Fever does not necessarily require treatment. The presence of fever should not be obscured by the indiscriminate use of antipyretic measures. However, if the child is uncomfortable or appears toxic because of fever, an attempt should be made to reduce it by any of the following nursing measures or by a combination of these measures:

1. Increase the child's fluid intake to prevent dehydration.
2. Expose the skin to the air by leaving the child lightly dressed in absorbent material. Avoid warm, binding clothing and blankets.
3. Administer antipyretic drugs, as prescribed. Avoid aspirin/acetyl salicylic acid as its use is known to result in Reye syndrome (encephalopathy, fatty degeneration of the liver with associated hypoglycemia) in some children. Children ages 4 to 12 years with a viral illness are at greatest risk for Reye syndrome.
4. Use a tepid tub or sponge bath or a hypothermia blanket. Do not allow the child to shiver, as that may increase the body temperature.

Administering Medications to Children

Administration of medication can be traumatic for children. The proper approach to administration can facilitate the process and enhance the child's understanding of the importance of taking medications.

Important Considerations

1. The manner of approach should indicate that the nurse firmly expects the child to take the medication. This manner usually convinces the child of the necessity of the procedure.

2. Establishing a positive relationship with the child will allow expression of feelings, concerns, and misconceptions regarding medications.
3. Explanation about medication should be directed to the child's level of understanding (ie, through play or comparison to something familiar).
4. The nurse must mask her or his own feelings regarding the medication.
5. Always be truthful when the child asks, "Does it taste bad?" or "Will it hurt?" Respond by saying, "The medication does not taste good, but I will give you some juice as soon as you swallow it," or "It will hurt for just a minute."
6. It is typically necessary to mix distasteful medications or crushed pills with a small amount of carbonated drink, cherry syrup, ice cream, or applesauce. After mixing, monitor to ensure that the child finishes the preparation.
7. Never threaten a child with an injection when refusing oral medication.
8. Do not mix medications with large quantities of food or with any food that is taken regularly (eg, milk).
9. Avoid giving medications to a child at mealtime unless specifically prescribed.
10. For each medication administered, the nurse should know the common use, safe dosage based on the child's weight, contraindications, adverse effects, and toxic effects.
11. The child must be accurately identified before medication is given.
12. When preparing IM injections, draw 0.2 cc of air into the syringe, in addition to the correct amount of medication. This clears the medication from the needle on injection and prevents backflow and the depositing of medication in subcutaneous fat when the needle is withdrawn.
13. Physical intervention (through swaddling, side or stomach position, shushing, swinging, sucking) and oral sucrose administration have been shown through research to reduce pain reactions in infants ages 2 and 4 months during vaccine injections.

 EVIDENCE BASE Saleh, E., Swamy, G., Moody, A. & Walter, E. (2017). Parental Approach to the Prevention and Management of Fever and Pain Following Childhood Immunizations. *Clinical Pediatrics*, 56(5), 435–442.

Calculating the Pediatric Dosage

General Principles
1. The nurse is responsible for knowing the safe dosage range for the medication she administers.
2. Factors determining the amount of drug prescribed include the following:
  a. Action, absorption, detoxification, and excretion of the drug are related to the maturity and metabolic rate of the child.
  b. Neonates and premature neonates require a reduced dosage because of:
    i. Deficient or absent detoxifying enzymes.
    ii. Decreased effective renal function.
    iii. Altered blood–brain barrier and protein-binding capacity.
  c. Dosage recommendations based on age groups are not satisfactory because a child may be much smaller or larger than the average child in the age group.
  d. Dosages based on child's weight are more accurate; however, these calculations have limitations.

3. Consult drug references for recommended dosage and other information, and be alert for prescription that would be inappropriate for a child.

4. Advise parents not to save unused medications that are unneeded or outdated, and do not give one child's prescription to another child.

Calculating by Body Surface Area

The following formulas are used to estimate the pediatric dosage based on the child's body surface area (BSA). BSA calculations are generally preferred because many physiologic processes in the child (eg, blood volume, glomerular filtration) are related to BSA.

1. Surface area in square meters × dose per square meter = approximate child dose.
2. Surface area of child/surface area of adult × dose of adult = approximate child dose.
3. Surface area of child in square meters/1.75 × adult dose = child dose.

Calculating by Clark Rule

Clark rule may be used as an estimate of the pediatric dosage based on the child's weight in respect to the adult dose of the drug:

Child's weight in pounds/150 × Adult dose = Approximate dose for child

 NURSING ALERT Ensure proper identification of all patients via the identification bracelet before administration of medication.

Oral Medications

Infants

1. Draw up medication in a plastic dropper or disposable syringe.
2. Elevate the infant's head and shoulders; depress chin with thumb to open mouth.
3. Place dropper or syringe on the middle of the tongue and slowly drop the medication on the tongue.
4. Release thumb and allow the child to swallow.
5. When the correct amount of medication has been measured, it can be placed in a nipple and the infant can suck the medication through the nipple.
6. If the nurse feels comfortable managing the infant in her or his lap, it is acceptable to hold the infant for medication administration.

Toddlers

1. Draw up liquid medications in a syringe or measure into medicine cup. Medications may be placed in a medicine cup or spoon after being measured accurately in a syringe.
2. Elevate the child's head and shoulders.
3. Squeeze the cup and put it to the child's lips or place the syringe (without needle) in the child's mouth, positioning the syringe tip in the space between the cheek mucosa and gum, and slowly expel the medicine. Child may prefer using a familiar teaspoon.
4. Allow the child time to swallow.
5. Allow the child to hold the medicine cup if able and to drink it at his or her own pace. (This may be a more agreeable method.) Offer a favorite drink as a "chaser," if not contraindicated.
6. The small, safe medicine cups can be given to the child for play.

School-Age Children

1. When a child is old enough to take medicine in pill or capsule form, teach the child to place the pill near the back of the tongue and immediately swallow fluid such as water or fruit juice. If swallowing of the fluid is emphasized, the child will no longer think about the pill.
2. Always give praise after a child takes medication.
3. If the child finds it particularly difficult to take oral medications, express understanding and offer help.

Subcutaneous and Intramuscular Medications

General Considerations

1. After the medication to be given IM is drawn from the vial, draw up an additional 0.2 to 0.3 cc of air into the syringe, thus clearing the needle of medication and preventing medication seepage from the injection site.
2. When injecting less than 1 mL of medication, use a tuberculin syringe for accuracy.
3. Clean site thoroughly, using friction with an antiseptic solution; let site dry.
4. Establish anatomic landmarks and prepare to position the needle at a 45-degree angle for subcutaneous (SC) injection and a 90-degree angle for IM injection (see Figure 42-3). Alternate injection sites and keep record at bedside or on medication card.
5. With IM injections, after penetrating site, aspirate to check for blood vessel puncture. If this occurs, withdraw the needle, discard the medicine, and start again.
6. After injection, massage site (unless contraindicated). When multiple injections are being administered, such complications as fibrosis and contracture of the muscle can be diminished by massage, warm soaks, and range-of-motion exercises to disrupt and stretch immature scar tissue.

Infants

1. Acceptable sites for IM injections include the rectus femoris (anterior thigh, middle third), vastus lateralis (lateral thigh, middle third), or ventrogluteal, as these sites are relatively free from major nerves and blood vessels. The gluteus maximus and deltoid muscles are underdeveloped in the infant and use of these sites can result in nerve damage.

2. Rectus femoris injection.
   a. Place the child in a secure position to prevent movement of the extremity.
   b. Do not use a needle longer than 1 inch.
   c. Bunch the muscle between your thumb and forefinger.
   d. Insert needle at 90-degree angle or slightly toward the knee.

3. Vastus lateralis injection.
   a. Place the child in a prone or supine position.
   b. Area is a narrow strip of muscle extending along a line from the greater trochanter to lateral femoral condyle below.
   c. Insert needle at 90-degree angle, ¾ to 1½ inches (2 to 4 cm) deep.

4. Ventrogluteal injection.
   a. This site provides a dense muscle mass that is relatively free from the danger of injuring the nervous and vascular systems.
   b. The disadvantage is that the injection site is visible to the child.
   c. Administration.
      i. Position the child supine.
      ii. Place the index finger on the anterosuperior spine.
      iii. With the middle finger moving dorsally, locate the iliac crest; drop finger below the crest. The triangle formed

Figure 42-3. IM and subcutaneous injections in children. Sites for IM injections: **(A)** rectus femoris, **(B)** deltoid, **(C)** ventrogluteal, **(D)** subcutaneous, and **(E)** IM. (From Pillitteri, A. [2013]. *Maternal and child health nursing: Care of the childbearing and childrearing family* [7th ed.]. Philadelphia, PA: Lippincott Williams & Wilkins.)

by the iliac crest, index finger, and middle finger is the injection site.
  iv. Inject needle perpendicular to the surface on which the child is lying.
5. After administration of medication, hold and cuddle the infant.
6. Administer subcutaneous injection in the fatty tissue over the anterolateral thigh.

Toddlers and School-Age Children

1. Posterogluteal injection—upper outer quadrant for IM injection.
   a. Gluteal muscles do not develop until a child begins to walk; they should be used only when the child has been walking for 1 year or more. Complications include sciatic nerve injury or subcutaneous injury (because of medication being injected) and poor absorption.
   b. Upper outer quadrant of the young child's buttock is smaller in diameter than that of an adult; thus, accuracy in determining the area constituting the upper outer quadrant is essential.
   c. Administration.
      i. Do not use a needle longer than 1 inch.
      ii. Position the child in a prone position.
      iii. Place thumb on the trochanter.
      iv. Place middle finger on the iliac crest.
      v. Let index finger drop at a point midway between the thumb and middle finger to the upper outer quadrant of the buttock. This is the injection site.
      vi. Insert needle perpendicular to the surface on which the child is lying, not to the skin.

2. Ventrogluteal injection for IM injection.
   a. May be used for the older child who is difficult to restrain.
   b. See description given above.
3. Deltoid injection for IM injection.
   a. May be used for older, larger children.
   b. Inaccurate site injection can result in damage to the radial nerve or brachial artery.
   c. Determine injection site by palpating the acromion process of the shoulder and placing two fingers down from the acromion process.
   d. Inject needle at 90-degree angle or slightly toward the shoulder.
4. Lateral and anterior aspect of the thigh for IM injection.
   a. Do not use a needle longer than 1 inch.
   b. Use the upper outer quadrant of the thigh.
   c. Insert needle at 45-degree angle in a downward direction, toward the knee.
5. Administer subcutaneous injection in the fatty tissue over the anterolateral thigh or outer aspect of upper arm.
6. Nursing support of toddlers and older children.
   a. Prepare all equipment before approaching the child.
   b. Explain to the child where you are going to give the injection (site) and why you are giving it.
   c. Allow the child to express fears.
   d. Carry out the procedure quickly and gently. Have needle and syringe completely prepared and ready before contact with the child.
   e. Numb the site of injection by rubbing the skin firmly with cleaning swab or with ice (older children may assist with this).

Minimize pain of an IM injection by injecting the needle into the muscle with a quick, darting motion.

f. Always secure the assistance of a second nurse or a family member to help immobilize the child and divert his or her attention as well as to offer support and comfort.

g. Praise the child for behavior after the injection. Allowing the child to assist with applying an elastic bandage will give some feeling of comfort.

h. Also encourage activity that will use the muscle site of the injection, this promotes dispersal of medication and decreases soreness. This can also be done by firmly massaging the muscle after injection, unless contraindicated.

i. Accurately record the injection site to ensure proper site rotation.

Intravenous Medications

1. Intravenous (IV) administration of medications may be done through a variety of techniques, including piggyback or through a heparin lock, volume control set, or implantable port. See pages 71 to 74 for information on these techniques.
2. Prepare mixtures aseptically (laminar flow hood) and use sterile technique when accessing the IV line. (Sepsis is a constant threat when a child is receiving IV medications.)
3. Be aware that an exaggerated pharmacologic effect may exist with IV medications. As with any medication, know the use, adverse effects, and toxic effects of the drug as well as the pharmacologic effect on the body.
4. Dilute IV medications and inject slowly—never less than 1 minute (this allows peripheral blood flow through the entire circulating system to dilute the medication and prevent high concentrations of the drug from reaching the brain and heart).
5. Be knowledgeable about compatibilities of drugs, electrolytes in IV solutions, and the fluid itself.
6. Observe the IV site frequently. Restrain the child, as needed, to prevent infiltration. Infiltration of fluids containing medications can cause rapid and severe tissue necrosis.

SPECIAL CONSIDERATIONS IN PEDIATRIC PRIMARY CARE

Acute Poisoning

Exposure to poisons can occur by ingestion, inhalation, or skin or mucous membrane contact. This section focuses on the most common poisoning, toxic ingestions. Poisoning by ingestion refers to the oral intake of a harmful substance that, even in a small amount, can damage tissues, disturb body functions, and, possibly, cause death. The substances may include such medications as acetaminophen and iron, household products, and plants.

Children are at risk for acute poisoning. Every day, over 300 Children in the United States ages 0 to 19 years of age are treated in an emergency department and two will die as a result of being poisoned. The most common agents ingested by children younger than age 6 include cosmetics and personal care products; however, cleaning products, analgesics, plants, pesticides, vitamins, and cough and cold medications also pose risk.

Pathophysiology and Etiology

1. Improper or dangerous storage of potentially toxic substances.
2. Poor lighting—causes errors in reading.

3. Human factors:
   a. Failure to read label properly.
   b. Failure to return poisons to their proper place.
   c. Failure to recognize the material as poisonous.
   d. Lack of supervision of the child.
   e. Purposeful use of poison.
4. Toxin is ingested and may have limited local effects or continue to a stage of absorption and interference with metabolic processes and organ function.
5. Typically occurs in children younger than age 6, with a peak incidence between 12 and 24 months.
6. Acute poisoning may result in arrhythmias or permanent multiorgan damage due to initial loss of airway, breathing, and circulation (ABCs) and specific organ toxicity.

Poisoning with Acetaminophen

Acetaminophen is a common drug poisoning agent in children because of its replacement of salicylates and the pleasant taste of the preparations developed to facilitate administration. Ingestion by adolescents is frequently intentional. Acetaminophen is toxic to the liver, resulting in cell necrosis and, possibly, cell death.

Clinical Manifestations
Phase I (first 24 hours after ingestion):
1. May be asymptomatic.
2. Anorexia.
3. Nausea and vomiting.
4. Diaphoresis.
5. Malaise.
6. Pallor.

Phase II (24 to 48 hours after ingestion):
1. Symptoms of phase I diminish or disappear.
2. Right upper quadrant pain due to liver damage.
3. Liver enlargement with elevated bilirubin and hepatic enzymes and prolonged prothrombin time.
4. Oliguria.

Phase III (days 3 to 5 after ingestion):
1. Signs of hepatic failure, such as jaundice, hypoglycemia, coagulopathy, and encephalopathy.
2. Peak liver function abnormalities.
3. Anorexia, nausea, vomiting, and malaise may reappear.
4. Renal failure and cardiomyopathy may occur.

Phase IV:
1. Associated with recovery or progression to complete liver failure and death.

Diagnostic Evaluation
1. Serum acetaminophen level 4 hours after ingestion.
2. Serial liver function tests.
3. Urine and serum chemistry studies for renal function.

Management
1. Activated charcoal should be given if treatment is instituted within 6 to 8 hours after ingestion; if treatment is begun after this time frame, activated charcoal is not used unless another toxic substance was ingested.
2. *N*-Acetylcysteine as an antidote given orally or via IV line. This is the most extensively studied regimen for acetaminophen overdose.
3. As with all poisons, ABCs and treatment of shock are always the priority in management.

Iron Poisoning

Iron poisoning occurs frequently in childhood because of the prevalence of iron-containing preparations. The severity of iron poisoning is related to the amount of elemental iron absorbed. The range of potential toxicity is between 50 and 60 mg/kg.

Clinical Manifestations

1. Thirty minutes to 2 hours after ingestion:
   a. Local necrosis and hemorrhage of GI tract.
   b. Nausea and vomiting, including hematemesis.
   c. Abdominal pain.
   d. Diarrhea, usually bloody.
   e. Severe hypotension.
   f. Symptoms subside after 6 to 12 hours.
2. Six to twenty-four hours—period of apparent recovery.
3. Twenty-four to forty hours:
   a. Systemic toxicity with cardiovascular collapse, shock, hepatic and renal failure, seizures, coma, and, possibly, death.
   b. Metabolic acidosis.
4. Two to 4 weeks after ingestion:
   a. Pyloric and duodenal stenosis.
   b. Hepatic cirrhosis.

Diagnostic Evaluation

1. Measurement of serum-free iron.
   a. Total serum iron.
   b. Total serum iron-binding capacity.
2. Abdominal x-ray to visualize iron tablets; limited use for visualizing liquid toxins.

Management

1. Gastric lavage may be of some benefit because iron is not absorbed by activated charcoal; however, wide lumen must be used, which may not be possible in small children.
2. Whole-bowel irrigation reduces the absorption of iron and sustained-release drugs.
3. Administration of deferoxamine for severe cases—iron-chelating agent that binds with iron and is excreted in urine (urine will be bright red).

Primary Assessment in Acute Poisoning

1. Initial assessment should include evaluation of ABCs, level of consciousness, vital signs, and neurologic assessment.
2. Assess for symptomatic effects of poisoning by systems.
   a. GI—common in metallic acid, alkali, and bacterial poisoning. These may include nausea and vomiting, diarrhea, abdominal pain or cramping, and anorexia.
   b. CNS—may include seizures (especially with CNS depressants, such as alcohol, chloral hydrate, barbiturates) and behavioral changes. Dilated or pinpoint pupils may be noted.
   c. Skin—rashes; burns to the mouth, esophagus, and stomach; eye inflammation; skin irritations; stains around the mouth; lesions of the mucous membranes. Cyanosis may be visible, especially with cyanide and strychnine.
   d. Cardiopulmonary—dyspnea (especially with aspiration of hydrocarbons) and cardiopulmonary depression or arrest.
   e. Other—odor around the mouth.
3. Identify the poison when possible.
   a. Determine the nature of the ingested substance from the child's history or by reading the label on the container. Nursing intervention may need to be implemented immediately after this assessment.

b. Call the nearest poison control center or toxicology section of the medical examiner's office to identify the toxic ingredient and obtain recommendations for emergency treatment. The United States toll-free number is (800) 222-1222.
c. Save vomitus, stool, and urine for analysis when the child reaches the hospital.

 NURSING ALERT It may be necessary to initiate emergency respiratory and circulatory support at this time. If needed, obtain venous access, maintain safety during seizure activity, and treat shock. Otherwise, continue with assessment.

Primary Interventions

Assisting the Family by Telephone Management

1. Calmly obtain and record the following information:
   a. Name, address, and telephone number of caller.
   b. Evaluation of the severity of the ingestion.
   c. Age, weight, and signs and symptoms of the child, including neurologic status.
   d. Route of exposure.
   e. Name of the ingested product, approximate amount ingested, and time of ingestion.
   f. Brief past medical history.
   g. Caller's relationship to victim.
2. Instruct the caller about appropriate emergency actions or refer to (800) 222-1222.
3. Direct the patient to the nearest emergency department. Dispatch an ambulance, if necessary.
4. Instruct the caller to clear the child's mouth of any unswallowed poison.
5. Identify what treatments have already been initiated.
6. Instruct the parents to save vomitus, unswallowed liquid or pills, and the container and to bring them to the hospital as aids in identifying the poison.
7. Identify whether other children were involved in the poisoning to initiate treatment for them also.

 DRUG ALERT Do not administer household neutralizing foods or products (unless recommended by poison control specialist) because the heat generated by the chemical reaction could result in a burn (or exacerbation of an existing burn).

Intervention Related to the Patient's Condition

Support ABCs, as needed.

Removing the Poison from the Body

1. If the poison is nonpharmaceutical, have the child drink 100 to 200 mL of water if told to do so by Poison Control. If a medication was ingested, do not dilute with water, as this may speed absorption.
2. For skin or eye contact, remove contaminated clothing and flush with water for 15 to 20 minutes.
3. For inhalation poisons, remove from the exposed site.
4. Administer gastric lavage if the toxin is not bound by charcoal (most effective within 50 minutes after ingestion).
5. Follow lavage with a cathartic and activated charcoal to hasten removal of the poison from the GI tract. Use cautiously with young children.

6. Be aware of the dangers associated with lavage.
   a. Esophageal perforation—may occur in corrosive poisoning.
   b. Gastric hemorrhage.
   c. Impaired pulmonary function resulting from aspiration.
   d. Cardiac arrest.
   e. Seizures—may result from stimulation in strychnine ingestion.
7. Follow lavage (if performed) with activated charcoal (preferably within 1 hour after ingestion) to hasten removal of the poison from the GI tract.
   a. Charcoal poorly absorbs most electrolytes, iron, lithium, mineral acids and bases, alcohols, cyanide, most solvents, and hydrocarbons.
   b. Administer 30 to 50 g for an adolescent, in 6 to 8 ounces (180 to 240 mL) of water with sweetener.
   c. It is sometimes easier to administer in an opaque beverage container as some children are hesitant to drink the charcoal because of its unusual dark color.

EVIDENCE BASE Mowry, J., Spyker, D., Brooks, D., et al. (2016). 2015 Annual Report of the American Association of Poison Control Centers' National Poison Data System (NPDS): 33rd Annual Report. *Clinical Toxicology, 54*(10), 924–1109.

Reducing the Effect of the Poison by Administering an Antidote

1. An antidote may either react with the poison to prevent its absorption or counteract the effects of the poison after its absorption.
2. Not all poisons have specific antidotes.
3. Information about appropriate antidotes for specific poisons is available through all poison control centers. Antidotes for the most common poisons should be listed in the emergency department of the hospital.
4. Effectiveness of the antidote usually depends on the amount of time that elapses between ingestion of the poison and administration of the antidote.

Eliminating the Absorbed Poison

1. Force dieresis.
   a. Administer large quantities of fluid either orally or via IV line.
   b. Carefully monitor intake and output.
2. Assist with kidney dialysis, which may be necessary if the child's kidneys are not functioning effectively.
3. Assist with exchange transfusion if this method is indicated for removing the poison.

Providing Emotional Support

1. Remain calm and efficient while working rapidly.
2. Reassure the child and his or her family that therapeutic measures are being taken immediately.
3. Discourage anxious parents from holding, caressing, and over-stimulating the child.

Subsequent Nursing Assessment and Interventions

Observing the Child for Progression of Symptoms

1. CNS involvement.
   a. Observe for restlessness, confusion, delirium, seizures, lethargy, stupor, or coma.
   b. Administer sedation with caution—to avoid CNS depression and masking of symptoms.
   c. Avoid excessive manipulation of the child.
   d. See nursing care of the child with seizures, page 1252.
   e. See nursing care of the unconscious patient, Chapter 15.
2. Respiratory involvement.
   a. Observe for respiratory depression, obstruction, pulmonary edema, pneumonia, or tachypnea.
   b. Have artificial airway and tracheostomy set available.
   c. Be prepared to administer oxygen and provide artificial respiration.
   d. Other nursing concerns:
      i. Nursing care for mechanical ventilation, see page 1166.
      ii. Procedures for administration of oxygen, see page 181.
      iii. Procedure for cardiopulmonary resuscitation, see page 1162.
3. Cardiovascular involvement.
   a. Observe for peripheral circulatory collapse, disturbances of heart rate and rhythm, or heart failure.
   b. Maintain IV therapy, as directed, to prevent shock. Assess for complications of overhydration.
   c. Be prepared for cardiac arrest.
4. GI involvement.
   a. Observe for nausea, pain, abdominal distention, and difficulty swallowing.
   b. Maintain IV therapy to replace water and electrolyte losses.
   c. Offer a diet that is easily swallowed and digested.
      i. Begin with clear liquids.
      ii. Progress to full liquids, soft foods, and then a regular diet as the child's condition improves.
5. Kidney involvement.
   a. Observe the child for decreased urine output. Record oral and IV intake and urine output exactly.
   b. Observe for hypertension.
   c. Insert indwelling catheter, if necessary, for urinary retention.
   d. Administer appropriate amounts of fluids and electrolytes.
   e. See nursing care of child with renal failure, page 1329.
   f. Correct and monitor acid–base balance.

Providing Supportive Care

1. Maintain adequate caloric, fluid, and vitamin intake. Oral fluids are preferable if they can be retained.
2. Avoid hypothermia or hyperthermia. (Control of body temperature is impaired in many types of poisoning.) Monitor the child's temperature frequently.
3. Observe closely for inflammation and tissue irritation.
   a. This is especially important in ingestion of kerosene or other hydrocarbons, which cause chemical pneumonitis.
   b. Isolate the patient from other children, especially those with respiratory infections.
   c. Administer antibiotics, as prescribed by the physician.
4. Counsel parents who typically feel guilty about the accident.
   a. Encourage parents to talk about the poisoning.
   b. Emphasize how their quick action in getting treatment for the child has helped.
   c. Discuss ways that they can be supportive to their child during the hospitalization.
   d. Do not allow prolonged periods of self-incrimination to continue. Refer parents to a psychologist for assistance in resolving these feelings, if necessary.

5. Involve the young child in therapeutic play to determine how he or she views the situation.
   a. The child commonly sees nursing measures as punishments for misdeed involving the poisoning.
   b. Explain treatment and correct misinterpretations in a manner appropriate for child's age.
6. Initiate a community health nursing referral for any childhood poisoning incident. A home assessment should be made to identify any potential or actual problems and provide proper poisoning prevention interventions and education.

Family Education and Health Maintenance

Stressing Prevention

1. Information concerning poison prevention should be available on every hospital pediatric unit and during every child health care visit.
   a. Many free booklets and home safety checklists are available from such sources as insurance companies and drug companies.
   b. Teaching may be done with any parent regardless of the reason for the child's hospitalization or office visit.
2. Teach the following precautions:
   a. Keep medicines and poisons out of the reach of children.
   b. Provide locked storage for highly toxic substances; select cabinet that is higher than child can reach or climb.
   c. Do not store poisons in the same areas as foods.
   d. Make sure all containers are properly marked and labeled. Keep medicines, drugs, and household chemicals in their original containers.
   e. Do not discard poisonous substances in receptacles where children can reach them; however, do discard used containers of poisonous substances.
   f. Teach children not to taste or eat unfamiliar substances.
   g. Clean out medicine cabinets periodically.
   h. Keep medications in childproof containers that are securely closed.
   i. Read all labels carefully before each use.
   j. Do not give medicines prescribed for one child to another.
   k. Never refer to drugs as candy or bribe children with such inducements.
   l. Never give or take medications in the dark.
   m. Encourage parents not to take medication in front of young children because children role-play adult behavior.
   n. Suggest that mothers avoid keeping medications in their purses or on the kitchen table.
   o. Keep baby creams and ointments away from young children.
   p. Never puncture or heat aerosol containers.
   q. Store lawn and garden pesticides in a separate place under lock and key outside of the house; do not store large quantities of cleaning products or pesticides.
3. Advise parents to dispose of syrup of ipecac if they keep it in the household. According to the American Academy of Pediatrics, there is no evidence supporting improved outcomes of poisonings with the use of ipecac. In addition, there is potential for abuse of ipecac with bulimic or anorexic teenagers; therefore, the recommendation for keeping ipecac on hand to induce vomiting has been rescinded.
4. Tell family to keep a list of emergency telephone numbers including the poison control center, health care provider's number, nearest hospital, and ambulance service.
5. Reinforce the need for vigilance and consistent supervision of infants and young children because of their increased mobility, increased curiosity, and increased dexterity.

Teaching Emergency Actions

1. Suspect poisoning with the occurrence of sudden, bizarre symptoms or peculiar behavior in toddlers and preschoolers.
2. Read label on the ingested product or call the health care provider, hospital, or poison control center for instructions about treatment for the poisoning. Give all relevant information about the child, condition, and substance ingested.
3. Maintain an adequate airway in a child who is convulsing or who is not fully conscious.
4. Dilute the poison with 100 to 200 mL of water, if advised by Poison Control or other medical provider.
5. Transport the child promptly to the nearest medical facility.
   a. Wrap the child in a blanket to prevent chilling.
   b. Bring the container and any vomitus or urine to the hospital with the child.
6. Avoid excessive manipulation of the child.
7. Act promptly but calmly.
8. Do not assume the child is safe simply because the emesis shows no trace of the poison or because the child appears well. The poison may have produced a delayed reaction or may have reached the small intestine where it is still being absorbed.

Lead Poisoning

There are approximately half a million children with elevated blood lead levels (greater than 5 mcg/dL) in the United States. Lead poisoning, referred to as *plumbism*, results from some form of lead consumption. Blood lead levels even lower than the prior accepted level of 10 mcg/dL can affect intellectual functioning in children. This has resulted in the acceptable lead level being lowered to 5 from 10 mcg/dL as of 2017.

Millions of children live in housing built before 1950, which contains the highest surface soil level and internal household dust contaminated with lead. Normal hand-to-mouth activities of children may introduce leaded household dust, soil, and nonfood items into their GI tract. Pica (eating nonfood substances, particularly leaded paint chips) is generally associated with more severe degrees of lead poisoning.

Pathophysiology and Etiology

Etiologic Factors

1. Multiple episodes of chewing on, sucking, or ingestion of nonfood substances.
   a. Toys, furniture, windowsills, household fixtures, and plaster painted with lead-containing paint.
   b. Cigarette butts and ashes.
   c. Acidic juices or foods served in lead-based earthenware pottery made with lead glazes.
   d. Colored paints used in newspapers, magazines, children's books, matches, playing cards, and food wrappers.
   e. Water from lead pipes.
   f. Fruit treated with insecticides.
   g. Dirt containing lead fallout from automobile exhaust.
   h. Antique pewter, especially when used to serve acidic juices or foods.
   i. Lead weights (curtain weights, fishing sinkers).
   j. Continuous proximity to lead-processing center.
   k. Occupations or hobbies that use lead.
   l. Imported folk remedies, cosmetics, food, or cookware that contains lead.
2. Inhalation of fumes containing lead (less common cause in children).
   a. Leaded gasoline.

b. Burning storage batteries.

c. Dust containing lead salts.

d. Dust in the air at shooting galleries and in enclosed firing ranges with poor ventilation.

e. Cigarette smoke.

3. Highest incidence in children between ages 1 and 6 years, especially those between ages 1 and 3 years.

a. High incidence in individuals living in old homes or deteriorated housing conditions.

b. No significant difference in incidence by sex.

c. High incidence among siblings.

4. Symptomatic lead poisoning occurs most frequently in summer months.

> **! NURSING ALERT** Legislation stipulates that toys, children's furniture, and the interior of homes be painted with lead-free paint; however, the problem arises when deeper layers of paint and plaster on older products are contaminated with lead. One paint chip contains much more lead than is considered safe.

Systemic Effects

1. Lead absorption from GI tract is affected by age, diet, and nutritional deficiency. Young children absorb 40% to 50% and retain 20% to 25% of dietary lead.

2. It takes the body twice as long to excrete lead as it does to absorb lead.

3. Lead is stored in two places in the body:

a. Bone.

b. Soft tissue.

4. Principal toxic effects occur in nervous system, bone marrow, and kidneys.

5. Nervous system.

a. Brain—increased capillary permeability results in edema, increased intracranial pressure, and vascular damage; destruction of brain cells causes seizures, mental retardation, paralysis, blindness, and learning disabilities.

b. Neurologic damage cannot be reversed.

c. CNS of young children and fetuses is most sensitive to lead.

6. Bone marrow.

a. Lead attaches to red blood cells (RBCs).

b. Inhibition of a number of steps in the biosynthesis of heme, thus reducing the number of RBCs, increasing fragility, and reducing half-life.

c. The decreased production of hemoglobin results in anemia and respiratory distress.

7. Kidneys—injury to the cells of the proximal tubules, causing increased excretion of amino acids, protein, glucose, and phosphate.

8. Recurrence rate is high, especially if the lead is not removed from the home environment.

Clinical Manifestations

Symptoms in young children may develop insidiously and may abate spontaneously.

1. GI—anorexia, sporadic vomiting, intermittent abdominal pain (colic), constipation.

2. CNS—hyperirritability; decreased activity; personality changes; loss of recently acquired developmental skills; falling, clumsiness, loss of coordination (ataxia); local paralysis; peripheral nerve palsies.

3. Hematologic—anemia, pallor.

4. Cardiovascular—hypertension, bradycardia.

Diagnostic Evaluation

1. Detailed history with emphasis on the presence or absence of clinical symptoms; evidence of pica; family history of lead poisoning; possible source of exposure to lead; recent change in behavior, developmental delay, or behavior problems; recent change of address; or recent renovations in the home.

2. Assess serum lead level and repeat confirmatory, preferably by way of venipuncture. Recent changes in screening recommendations have been made to include targeted screening of all Medicaid-enrolled and Medicaid-eligible children. Additionally, all children born outside the United States should be screened.

a. For levels greater than 5 µg/dL, a more extensive environmental history should be reviewed.

b. For levels between 10 and 14 µg/dL, level should be confirmed and repeated in 3 months. Education on decreasing exposure and limiting absorption of lead should be done on all levels greater than 10 µg/dL.

c. Levels between 15 and 19 µg/dL should be repeated within 2 months, while an environmental history additionally is reviewed.

d. Levels between 20 and 44 µg/dL should be repeated within 2 days and referred to local health department plus a thorough medical history and physical examination added to education as noted above.

e. Levels between 45 and 69 µg/dL should be confirmed immediately, referred to the local health department, and should be considered for chelation therapy in consultation with an expert.

f. Immediate hospitalization is required for levels greater than 70 µg/dL.

3. Hematologic evaluation for iron deficiency anemia.

4. Flat plate of abdomen—may reveal radiopaque material if lead has been ingested during the preceding 24 to 36 hours.

5. Erythrocyte protoporphyrin level—not sensitive enough for identifying lead levels below 25 mg/dL. Can be used to follow levels after medical and environmental interventions for poisoned children have occurred. A progressive decline in erythrocyte protoporphyrin levels indicates that management is successful.

6. 24-Hour urine—more accurate than a single voided specimen in determining elevated urinary components that correspond with elevated blood lead levels.

7. Radiologic examination of long bones—unreliable for diagnosis of acute lead poisoning; may provide some indication of past lead poisoning or length of time poisoning has occurred.

8. Edetate calcium disodium provocation chelation test—used only in selected medical centers treating large numbers of lead-poisoned children; demonstrates increased lead levels in urine over an 8-hour period after injection of edetate disodium.

> **! NURSING ALERT** Venous sampling is the best method for assessing the level of lead in the blood as it limits cutaneous contamination. If a fingerstick sample is being used, careful collection should include a free flowing specimen.

EVIDENCE BASE American Academy of Pediatrics. (2016). Prevention of childhood lead toxicity. *Pediatrics*, *138*(1). Available: www.pediatrics.aappublications. org/content/pediatrics/early/2016/06/16/peds.-1493.

Management

Removal of Lead from the Environment
1. Remove leaded paint and paint chips or objects containing lead from the child's environment.
2. Remove child from environment during lead abatement process.

Nutritional Considerations
1. Consume adequate amounts of iron. Iron supplementation may be indicated to correct anemia.
2. Reduced-fat diet and small, frequent meals will reduce the GI absorption of lead.
3. Encourage foods high in vitamin C (such as fruits and juices) and calcium (such as milk, yogurt, and ice cream).

Chelation Therapy
According to the CDC, although chelation therapy is considered a mainstay in the medical management of children with blood lead levels greater than 45 mg/dL, it should be used with caution. An expert in the management of lead chemotherapy should be consulted prior to using chelation agents. State lead poisoning programs, local poison control centers, or the Lead Poisoning Prevention Branch at the CDC can be used as resources to identify accessible experts.

EVIDENCE BASE Barber, C., Huebner, J., Marquez, E., et al. (2018). Effective Recruitment Strategies for Lead Hazard Control and Healthy Homes Programs. *Journal of Environmental Health, 80*(7), 20–26.

Complications
1. Severe and usually permanent mental, emotional, and physical impairment.
2. Neurologic deficits.
   a. Learning disabilities.
   b. Mental retardation.
   c. Seizures.
   d. Encephalopathy.

Nursing Assessment
1. Partake in primary prevention through screening for lead poisoning—should target high-risk groups. This includes children:
   a. Who live in homes built before 1950.
   b. With iron deficiency anemia.
   c. Who are exposed to contaminated dust or soil.
   d. Who have developmental delays.
   e. Who are victims of abuse or neglect.
   f. Whose parents are exposed to lead through occupational hazards or hobbies.
   g. Who live in low-income families.
2. Screening should also be targeted at children who live in communities with more than 27% of houses built before 1950

or in populations where 12% or more of the children have elevated lead levels.
3. Assess all children for signs of lead toxicity, including hyperactivity, developmental delay, constipation, anorexia, colicky abdominal pain, clumsiness, and pallor.
4. Inquire about presence of pica behavior in children younger than age 6 years.
5. Assess the child's level of development. The Denver Developmental Screening Test II or other standardized developmental assessment tools may be useful for this purpose and will help detect delays possibly caused by lead poisoning.

Nursing Diagnoses
- Risk for Injury related to seizures and encephalopathy.
- Acute Pain related to chelation therapy injections.
- Delayed Growth and Development related to the effects of chronic lead exposure.
- Compromised Family Coping related to guilt and concern for child.

Nursing Interventions

Protecting the Child with Seizures and Encephalopathy
1. Maintain seizure precautions.
   a. Crib or bed rails elevated and padded.
   b. Tongue blade (if indicated per institutional guidelines) and suction equipment at bedside.
2. Be aware that encephalopathy may occur 4 to 6 weeks after first symptoms:
   a. Sudden onset of persistent vomiting.
   b. Severe ataxia.
   c. Altered state of consciousness.
   d. Coma.
   e. Seizures.
   f. Massive cerebral edema in younger children.
3. Observe for signs of increased intracranial pressure (ICP) in the child with encephalopathy:
   a. Rising blood pressure.
   b. Papilledema.
   c. Slow pulse.
   d. Seizures.
   e. Unconsciousness.
4. Provide supportive care to maintain vital functions.

Reducing Pain Associated with Chelation Therapy
1. Plan appropriate play activities to prepare the child for the injections and as an outlet for the pain and anger the child feels.
2. Implement measures to decrease pain at injection site.
   a. Rotate injection sites.
   b. Apply warm packs to the site to decrease pain.
   c. Move painful areas slowly.
3. Provide diversion activities, fluids, and meals between injections.
4. Monitor intake and output and blood studies, such as electrolytes and liver and renal function tests, as directed.

Promoting Growth and Development
1. Provide and encourage activities that will help the child to learn and progress from his or her present developmental state to meet the next appropriate milestone.

2. Initiate appropriate referrals in cases of obvious developmental delays or learning difficulties. The referrals may be to such professionals as psychologists, psychiatrists, and specialists in early child education.
3. Share the results of developmental testing with the parents and discuss ways to provide stimulation for the child at home.

Strengthening Family Coping

1. Use sensitivity in interviewing and teaching to avoid causing or increasing guilt feelings about the poisoning and to establish a positive, trusting relationship between the family and the health care facility.
2. Explain the treatment and its purpose because parents are commonly faced with putting an asymptomatic child through painful treatments.
3. Encourage frequent visits by parents and siblings and facilitate family involvement.

Community and Home Care Considerations

1. Carry out lead screening in the community. It is recommended that all high-risk children be screened for high lead levels between ages 9 and 12 months and, if feasible, again at 24 months. Screening policies, universal or targeted, are determined by local departments of health, based on the prevalence of risk factors in the community.
2. Coordinate community care efforts to return the child to a safe home. Communicate with community outreach workers so that environmental case management is conducted. Lead abatement must be conducted by experts, not untrained parents, property owners, or contractors.
3. Suggest periodic, focused household cleaning to remove the lead dust; use a wet mop.
4. Encourage hand washing before meals and at bedtime to eliminate lead consumption from normal hand-to-mouth activity.
5. Observe the child and other children in the home for pica.
   a. Observe and record the child's eating habits and food preferences.
   b. Report any attempted eating of nonfood substances.
   c. Encourage caregivers to provide regular meals and make mealtime a pleasurable time for the child.
   d. Teach caregivers to discourage oral activity and to substitute activity that contributes to play, social skills, and ego development.
   e. Refer the family for additional social or psychiatric casework, if indicated, to reduce economic and other factors that result in pica in the child.
6. Screen siblings and playmates of known cases immediately.
7. Make sure that the family is able to provide close supervision of the child or assist them to make arrangements to ensure that the child is adequately supervised at home.

Family Education and Health Maintenance

Ensuring Long-Term Follow-Up

1. Teach the parents why long-term follow-up is important. Tell them that residual lead is liberated gradually after treatment and:
   a. May result in the renewal of symptoms.
   b. May increase serum lead to a dangerous level.
   c. May cause additional damage to the CNS, which may not become apparent for several months.

2. Stress that acute infections must be recognized and treated promptly because these may reactivate the disease.
3. Teach that iron supplementation may be continued to treat anemia. Advise the parents about medication administration and adverse effects and periodic complete blood count monitoring.

Preventing Re-Exposure of the Child to Lead

1. Advise the parents that the single most important factor in managing childhood lead poisoning is reducing the child's re-exposure to lead.
2. Instruct the parents about the seriousness of repeated lead exposure.
3. Initiate referrals to home health nursing and community agencies, as indicated.

 NURSING ALERT Children should not return home until their home environment is lead free.

Providing Community Education

1. Initiate and support educational campaigns through schools, day care centers, and news media to alert parents and children to hazards and symptoms of lead poisoning.
2. Provide literature in clinics, waiting rooms, and other appropriate settings that stresses the hazards of lead, sources of lead, and signs of lead intoxication.
3. Support legislation to study the nature and extent of the lead poisoning problem and to eliminate the causes of lead poisoning.
4. Include the topic of pica and lead poisoning in nutritional teaching.
5. For additional information, contact the state or local health department or CDC (*www.cdc.gov*).

Evaluation: Expected Outcomes

- Seizure precautions maintained; no signs of increased ICP.
- Tolerates chelation therapy injections; expresses anger through doll play.
- Parents provide appropriate play and stimulation for development.
- Family involved in care; provides support to the child.

Communicable Diseases

With the dramatic success of immunizations, many childhood diseases have decreased in frequency. However, a number of communicable diseases still cause significant morbidity in children (see Table 42-2). Many other infections that occur in childhood are covered elsewhere in the book such as Chapter 31, Infectious diseases, or the chapters of each body system.

Child Abuse and Neglect

 EVIDENCE BASE Thomas, R. (2018). School Nurses and Child Sexual Exploitation: Keep on looking and listening. *British Journal of School Nursing, 13*(3), 150–151.

Child abuse is any type of maltreatment of children or adolescents by their parents, guardians, or caretakers. It is considered a major problem worldwide, with most countries tracking the problem and allocating some resources toward services to prevent and treat

Table 42-2 Communicable Diseases

DISEASE, AGENT, MODE OF TRANSMISSION, AGE WHEN MOST COMMON	INCUBATION AND COMMUNICABILITY PERIODS	SYMPTOMS
Chickenpox **Varicella-zoster virus** • Highly communicable; acquired in direct contact, droplet spread, and airborne transmission • 2–9 years; January to May *Diagnostic tests:* Tzanck smear shows multinucleated giant cells; a culture may be done for confirmation.	*Incubation (I):* 11–21 days after exposure. *Communicability (C):* onset of fever (1–2 days before first lesion) until last vesicle is dried (5–7 days)	• General malaise, low-grade fever, and anorexia for 24 hours • Rash—macules to papules and vesicles to crusts within several hours • Pruritus of lesions may be severe and scratching may cause scarring • *Rash characteristics:* rash appears first on the head and mucous membranes and then becomes concentrated on body and sparse on extremities, papulovesicular eruption.
Rubella (German 3-Day Measles) **Rubella virus; RNA toga virus** • Oral droplet or transplacentally • School age, young adults; spring, winter *Diagnostic tests:* tissue culture of throat, blood, or urine; latex agglutination, enzyme immunoassay, passive hemagglutination, fluorescent immunoassay tests *Passive immunity:* birth to age 6 months from maternal antibodies	*I:* 14–21 days after exposure. *C:* virus can be passed from 7 days before to 5 days after rash appears.	• Enlarged lymph nodes in postauricular, auricular, suboccipital, and cervical areas 24 hours before rash develops • Enanthem: discrete rose spots on soft palate • Exanthem: variable; begins on face, spreads quickly over entire body; usually maculopapular; clears by third day
Roseola Infantum (Exanthem subitum) **Human herpesvirus 6** • Direct contact or droplet • 6–24 months; late fall to early spring	*I:* 5–15 days. *C:* not known—believed not to be highly contagious	• Fever of 103°F–106°F (39.4°C–41.1°C), either intermittent or sustained 3–4 days with no clinical findings • Fever suddenly drops and macular or maculopapular rash develops on trunk, spreading to arms and neck; mild involvement of face and legs; rash fades quickly.
Rubeola (Hard, Red, 7-Day Measles) **Measles virus, RNA-containing paramyxovirus** • Direct contact with droplets from infected persons, respiratory route • *Diagnostic tests:* serologic procedures not routinely done • *Passive immunity:* birth to between ages 4 and 6 months if mother is immune before pregnancy • 5–10 years, adolescents; spring	*I:* 10–12 days. *C:* fifth day of incubation to fourth day of rash	• Fever, lethargy, cough, coryza, and conjunctivitis • 2–3 days later; Koplik spots on buccal pharyngeal mucosa (grayish white spots with reddish areolae), which disappear within 12–18 hours • 2 days later: maculopapular rash appears at hairline and spreads to feet in 1 day; rash begins to clear after 3–4 days
Mumps **Mumps virus, paramyxovirus** • Direct contact, through families, airborne droplets, saliva, and possibly urine • School age; all seasons but slightly more frequent in late winter and early spring *Diagnostic tests:* serologic testing and viral culture from throat swab *Passive immunity:* birth to age 6 months if mother is immune before pregnancy	*I:* 16–18 days. *C:* 3 days before to 9 days after swelling appears; virus in saliva greatest just before and after parotitis onset	• Headache, anorexia, generalized malaise; fever 1 day before glandular swelling; fever lasts 1–6 days • Glandular swelling usually of parotid—one side or bilaterally • Enlargement and reddening of Wharton duct and Stensen duct • Subclinical infection may occur

TREATMENT	COMPLICATIONS	NURSING CONSIDERATIONS
• Symptomatic: shorten fingernails to prevent scratching • Daily antiseptic baths • Oral antihistamines to decrease pruritus • Treatment of itching: baking soda (sodium bicarbonate) or oatmeal baths, calamine lotion to lesions • Isolation until all lesions have crusted • Acyclovir by mouth (PO) within first 24 hours • Avoid salicylates.	• Complications are rare in otherwise healthy children • Secondary bacterial infection of lesions • Hemorrhagic varicella, pneumonia, encephalitis, and thrombocytopenia are not common but they can occur. • Reye syndrome	• Severe in neonate and pregnant women • Varicella-zoster immune globulin is available for high-risk susceptible children who have been exposed to varicella zoster. • Prevention through immunization is the best practice.
• Symptomatic—isolation	• In adolescent females: arthritis; arthralgias • Encephalitis • Thrombocytopenia	• Exposure of nonimmune pregnant women in the first trimester results in a high percentage of affected fetuses and infants born with various birth defects: cataracts, deafness, growth retardation, congenital heart disease, mental retardation • Prevention is the best practice.
• Symptomatic—antipyretic	• Seizures due to high fever • Encephalitis (rare)	• Reassure family that this is a self-limiting illness.

• Symptomatic:
  • Sedatives
  • Antipyretic
  • Bed rest in humid, comfortably warm room
  • Dark room for photophobia
  • Adequate fluids
	• Otitis media
	• Pneumonia, laryngitis
	• Mastoiditis, encephalitis
	• Appendicitis
		• Provide symptomatic care and respiratory isolation.
		• Prevention through immunization is the best practice.

• Isolation until swelling has subsided
• Symptomatic:
  • Analgesics
  • Hydration
  • Alimentation
  • Antipyretics
  • Rest
	• Meningoencephalitis
	• Orchitis, epididymitis
	• Auditory nerve involvement, resulting in unilateral deafness
		• Provide symptomatic care.
		• Prevention through immunization is the best practice.

(continued)

Table 42-2 Communicable Diseases (*Continued*)

DISEASE, AGENT, MODE OF TRANSMISSION, AGE WHEN MOST COMMON	INCUBATION AND COMMUNICABILITY PERIODS	SYMPTOMS
Diphtheria		
Corynebacterium diphtheriae • Acquired through secretions of carrier or infected individual by direct contact with contaminated articles and environment • Unimmunized children under 15 years old; incidence increased in autumn and winter *Diagnostic tests:* cultures of nose and throat	*I:* 2–4 days. *C:* 2–4 weeks untreated; 1–2 days with antibiotic treatment	**Nasal diphtheria** • Coryza with increasing viscosity, possibly epistaxis, low-grade fever • Whitish gray membrane may appear over nasal septum **Pharyngeal and tonsillar diphtheria** • General malaise, low-grade fever, anorexia • 1–2 days later, whitish gray membranous patch on tonsils, soft palate, and uvula • Lymph node swelling, fever, rapid pulse, "bull neck" **Laryngeal diphtheria** • Usually spread from pharynx to larynx • Fever, harsh voice, stridor, barking cough; respiratory difficulty with inspiratory retraction **Nonrespiratory diphtheria** • Affects eye, ear, genitals, or, rarely, skin
Pertussis (Whooping Cough)		
Bordetella pertussis • Direct contact or respiratory droplet spread • Infants and young children; females more than males *Diagnostic tests:* culture of nasopharyngeal mucus	*I:* 3–12 days; mean of 7 days. *C:* 7 days after exposure (greatest just before catarrhal stage) to 3 weeks after onset of paroxysms or until cough has ceased	**Stage I (catarrhal stage)** • Lasts 1–2 weeks • Rhinorrhea, conjunctival injection, lacrimation, mild cough, and low-grade fever **Stage II (paroxysmal stage)** • Lasts 2–4 weeks or longer • Frequent severe, violent coughing attacks occurring in clusters, leading to vomiting, cyanosis, and exhaustion **Stage III (convalescent stage)** • Lasts 2 weeks to several months • Coughing attacks decrease, but may return with each respiratory infection • Duration: 9 months to 2 years
Staphylococcal Scalded Skin Syndrome (Ritter Disease)		

Group II phage-type *Staphylococcus aureus*
• Disseminated from a primary infection site (usually nose or around eyes)
• Infants and children under 10 years old
Diagnostic tests: cultures of skin, conjunctiva, nasopharynx, stools, and blood. Biopsy of exfoliated epidermis
	I: few days. *C:* onset of rash until after antibiotics initiated	• Malaise, fever, irritability, or asymptomatic
		• Rash develops in three phases:
		  • Erythematous—macular involving face, neck, axilla, and groin
		  • Exfoliative—upper layer of epidermis becomes wrinkled and can be removed by light stroking (Nikolsky sign); crusting around eyes, mouth, and nose produces characteristic "sunburst," radial pattern; irritable because of extreme tenderness of skin
		  • Desquamative—epidermis peels away, leaving moist areas that dry quickly and heal in 10–14 days

Erythema Infectiosum (Fifth Disease or Slapped Cheek)		

Parvovirus B19
• Respiratory route
• School-age children
Diagnostic tests: not widely available; IgM antibody test, polymerase chain reaction detection test
	I: 6–14 days. *C:* until rash develops	• Mild fever, chills, fatigue, or nonpruritic rash develops in three stages:
		  • Sudden appearance of bright erythema on cheeks
		  • Erythematous, maculopapular rash on trunk and extremities
		  • Rash on body fades with central clearing, giving a lacy or reticulated appearance
		• Rash lasts 2–39 days; frequently pruritic without desquamation
		• Occasional joint arthropathy

TREATMENT	COMPLICATIONS	NURSING CONSIDERATIONS

• Diphtheria antitoxin via IV line or IM
• Antibiotic therapy (penicillin, erythromycin)
• Supportive treatment:
  • Respiratory support and cardiac monitoring
  • Isolation until three cultures are negative after antibiotic therapy is completed
  • Bed rest for 2–3 weeks
  • Hydration
  • Immunization with diphtheria toxoid after recovery
	• Myocarditis
	• Neuritis
	• Paralysis
	• Toxic neurosis and hyaline degeneration of heart, liver, adrenal glands, and kidneys
	• Gastritis, hepatitis
	• Nephritis
		• Identify close contacts and monitor for illness; culture nose, throat, and cutaneous lesions and administer prophylactic antimicrobial therapy.
		• Prevention through immunization is the best practice.

• Specific:
  • Erythromycin estolate
  • Azithromycin
  • Clarithromycin
• Supportive:
  • Antipyretics
  • Bed rest
  • Quiet environment to reduce coughing
  • Gentle suctioning
  • Increase fluid intake
  • Oxygen
	• Respiratory: pneumonia, atelectasis, emphysema, aspiration pneumonia, pneumothorax
	• CNS: convulsions, encephalopathy, coma
	• Death may occur among the unvaccinated
		• Erythromycin should be given to all close and household contacts for 14 days.
		• Neither immunization nor natural disease confers complete or lifelong immunity.

• Specific:
  • Therapy with penicillinase-resistant penicillin PO, IM, or via IV line
• Symptomatic:
  • Gentle cleaning of skin with compresses
	• Excessive fluid loss, electrolyte imbalance, pneumonia, septicemia, cellulitis	• Provide symptomatic care.

• Symptomatic treatment • Immunoglobulin for immunocompromised patients	• Complications are rare among otherwise healthy children. • Children with abnormal RBCs (sickle cell disease, hereditary spherocytosis, and thalassemia) can develop transient aplastic anemia and may require multiple transfusions. • Immunocompromised patients may develop severe, chronic anemia.	• Avoid contact of child with pregnant female (<5% of exposed unborn children will have severe anemia; rare chance of miscarriage).

(continued)

Table 42-2 Communicable Diseases (Continued)

DISEASE, AGENT, MODE OF TRANSMISSION, AGE WHEN MOST COMMON	INCUBATION AND COMMUNICABILITY PERIODS	SYMPTOMS
Rotavirus **Reoviridae group A** • Most common agent responsible for infantile diarrhea • Fecal–oral route • Ages 6 months to 2 years; most common in winter in temperate climates *Diagnostic tests:* enzyme-linked immunosorbent assay	*I:* 1–3 days. *C:* until 2–5 days after diarrhea	• Fever • Vomiting • Profuse, watery, non–foul-smelling diarrhea
Hand, Foot, Mouth Disease **Coxsackie virus A16 or other enteroviruses** • Moderately contagious by direct contact with nose and throat secretions, fluid from blisters, and stool • Most common in children under age 10 during summer and fall *Diagnostic tests:* throat swab or stool culture for virus; rarely indicated	*I:* 3–7 days. *C:* first week of illness	• Mild fever, poor appetite, malaise, and sore throat • Painful sores develop in the mouth 1–2 days after fever begins (usually on the tongue, gums, and buccal mucosa). A nonpruritic rash follows on the palms and soles, occasionally on the buttocks.

child abuse. Child abuse includes physical or emotional abuse, injury, trauma, neglect, or sexual abuse of a child that is intentional and nonaccidental. Abuse includes the following:

• Battering—physical injury.
• Drug abuse—intentional administration of harmful drugs, especially during pregnancy.
• Sexual abuse.
• Sexual assault or molestation (non–family member).
• Incest (family offender).
• Emotional abuse—scapegoating, belittling, humiliating, lack of mothering.

Neglect is the omission of certain appropriate behaviors, with such omission having detrimental physical or psychological effects on development. Neglect includes:

• Child abandonment.
• Lack of provision of the basic needs of survival, including shelter, clothing, stimulation, medical care, food, love, supervision, education, attention, emotional nurturing, and safety.

Etiology and Incidence

 EVIDENCE BASE U.S. Department of Health and Human Services, Administration for Children and Families. (2017). *Child maltreatment 2015.* Washington, DC: Author.

The cause of child abuse and maltreatment is multidimensional. The abuse may be related to the combined presence of three factors: special kind of child, special kind of parent or caretaker, special circumstances of crisis. Abuse occurs in all ethnic, geographic, religious, educational, occupational, and socioeconomic groups.

1. In 2015, there were 683,000 reported victims of child abuse and neglect in the United States. Furthermore, 1,670 reported fatalities occurred. Maltreatment occurred approximately 91.6% of the time at the hands of one or both parents.
2. The most common type of abuse is neglect (75.3% of cases), followed by physical abuse (17.2%), sexual abuse (8.4%), and the remainder of reported cases (6.9%) suffered from other types of abuse, which include emotional maltreatment and medical neglect.

Contributing Factors

1. Incidents of child abuse may develop as a result of disciplinary action taken by the abuser who responds in uncontrolled anger to real or perceived misconduct of the child. The parents may confuse punishment with discipline. "Good parenting" may be equated with physical contact to eradicate child behavior. The abuser may be a stern, authoritarian disciplinarian.
2. Incidents of child abuse may develop out of a disagreement between caretakers. The child may come to the aid of one parent and may be entered into the midst of the quarrel; marital discord is common.
3. The abuser may be under a great deal of stress because of life circumstances (debt, poverty, illness) and may thus resort to child abuse. Crisis and stress may be ongoing. The abuser may have a low frustration tolerance level and may not have a well-developed means of coping with stress in general.
4. The abuser may be intoxicated with alcohol or drugs at the time of the abuse; only 10% of abusers have a history of mental illness.
5. Child abuse may occur by a surrogate caregiver, such as a babysitter or boyfriend.
6. Lack of effective parenting, inappropriate parent–child bonding, and punitive treatment as a child may contribute to the parent becoming an abuser.

TREATMENT	COMPLICATIONS	NURSING CONSIDERATIONS
• Oral fluid and electrohydrate solution	• Isotonic dehydration with acidosis • Malnourished infants may develop malabsorption dehydration and die.	• Excellent hygiene (hand washing) is necessary to avoid spreading disease. • Current vaccine will prevent 74% of all cases and 98% of severe cases.
• Symptomatic for fever, aches, and mouth lesions	• Rare, asymptomatic meningitis	• Provide pain relief and monitor fluid intake to prevent dehydration from not eating.

7. Specific characteristics evident in many abusing parents include:
   a. Low self-esteem—a sense of incompetence in role, unworthiness, unimportance, or have difficulty controlling aggressive impulses; commonly live in social isolation.
   b. Unrealistic attitudes and expectations of the child, little regard for the child's own needs and age-appropriate abilities, lack of knowledge related to parenting skills.
   c. Fear of rejection—a deep need to feel wanted and loved, but a feeling of rejection when love is not obvious; a crying infant may elicit a feeling of rejection.
   d. Inability to accept help—isolation from the community, loneliness.
   e. Unhappiness due to unsatisfactory relationships; may look to child for satisfaction of own emotional needs.
   f. Child abusers are commonly the children of abuse or victims of spousal abuse.
8. Incidents of child abuse may develop from a general attitude or resentment or rejection on the part of the abuser toward the child.
9. Atypical child behavior (eg, hyperactivity or a technology-dependent child who needs additional care) may unintentionally provoke the abuser.
10. The degree of the family crisis is not usually in proportion to the degree of abuse.

Clinical Manifestations

Characteristics of the Child that Should Raise Suspicion
1. The child is usually younger than age 3 years. School-age children and adolescents are also subject to abuse. The average age of a sexually abused child is 9 years.
2. General health of the child indicates neglect (diaper rash, poor hygiene, malnutrition, unattended physical problem).
3. Characteristic distribution of fractures (scattered over many parts of body).
4. Disproportionate amount of soft tissue injury.
5. Evidence that injuries occurred at different times (healed and new fractures, resolving and fresh bruises).
6. Cause of recent trauma in question.
7. History of similar episodes in the past.
8. No new lesions during the child's stay in the hospital.
9. May show a wide range of reactions—may be either very withdrawn or overactive. The child may be anxious, tense, or nervous or show regressive behavior.
10. The child may show unusual affection for strangers or may be overly fearful of adults and avoid any physical contact with them.
11. For sexual abuse: the child may fear no one will believe him or her; may experience self-blame; most know their abusers.
12. Children may not "tell" about abuse from parents, fearing a loss of security; "a bad parent is better than no parent at all."
13. Behavior problems, depression, acting-out behaviors, and aggression toward younger children may result.
14. For abuse that occurs in school or daycare, the child may exhibit fear of the teacher, have nightmares, decrease school attendance, or develop psychosomatic illnesses.

Injuries or Types of Abuse that May Occur
1. Bruises, welts (linear or looplike).
2. Abrasions, contusions, lacerations (most common).
3. Wounds, cuts, punctures.
4. Burns (cigarette, radiator), scalding—stocking or glove distribution.
5. Bone fractures.
6. Sprains, dislocations.
7. Subdural hemorrhage or hematoma; "shaken baby syndrome."
8. Brain damage.
9. Internal injuries.

10. Drug intoxication.
11. Malnutrition (deliberately inflicted).
12. Freezing, exposure.
13. Whiplash-type injury.
14. Eye injuries, periorbital injuries, ear bruises.
15. Dirty, infected wounds or rashes.
16. Unexplained coma in infant.
17. Failure to thrive—developmental delay, malnutrition with decreased muscle mass, decreased interaction with environment and with others, dental caries, listlessness, behavior problems.
18. Sexually transmitted diseases—genital trauma, recurrent urinary tract infection, pregnancy.

> **NURSING ALERT** Munchausen syndrome by proxy is a condition in which symptoms are induced in a child by the actions of a parent or caregiver. A wide range of methods have been noted as the basis for the fabricated illness, with most falling into one of four general categories: poisoning, bleeding, infections, and injuries. Many of the conditions cannot be observed by a health care provider nor can diagnosis be confirmed by further evaluation. Munchausen syndrome by proxy is a serious form of child abuse and is associated with a high rate of morbidity and mortality. It is important for nurses to obtain thorough histories of any illness or injury and be observant in any unusual cases.

Management

1. The goal of treatment is to ensure the physical and emotional safety of the child. Therefore, treatment is inclusive of other family members and caretakers and is often focused on the parents. A team approach is employed to determine the most effective use of community resources to protect the child and help the parents.
2. It is estimated that 80% to 90% of abusing parents can be rehabilitated. The ideal approach is to return the child to the biological parents after treatment concludes.
3. Counseling is offered to help parents do the following:
   a. Understand and redirect their anger.
   b. Develop an adequate parent–child relationship.
   c. See their child as an individual with his or her own needs and differences.
   d. Understand child development and normal behaviors of developing children.
   e. Learn about effective discipline techniques.
   f. Enjoy the child.
   g. Develop realistic expectations of their child.
   h. Decrease their use of criticism.
   i. Increase parents' self-esteem and confidence.
   j. Establish supportive relationships with others.
   k. Improve their economic situation (if appropriate).
   l. Show progress toward the physical, emotional, and intellectual development of their child.

Nursing Assessment

1. Identify family or child at risk.
   a. Alcohol or drug abuser.
   b. Adolescent parent.
   c. Low-income, single-parent family.
   d. Multiple births.
   e. Unwanted child.
   f. Sickly and more demanding child.
   g. Premature child with long separation from mother at birth.
2. Inspect for evidence of possible abuse.
   a. Describe completely on the medical record all bruises, lacerations, and similar lesions as to location and state of healing. Look carefully at areas generally covered with clothing (ie, buttocks, underarms, behind knees, bottom of feet).
   b. Ask how injuries occurred and record descriptions of the injury, including the date, time, and place of the event.
3. Collect necessary specimens for identification of organisms, sperm, or semen.
4. Take color photographs, as indicated.
5. Assess developmental level of the child.
6. Observe for behaviors common in abusing or neglecting parents. Be aware that not all abusing parents exhibit these behaviors but be alert for the parent who:
   a. Anxiously volunteers information or withholds information related to an injury.
   b. Gives explanation of the injury that does not fit the condition or gets story confused concerning the injury.
   c. Shows inappropriate reaction or concern to severity of injury.
   d. Becomes irritable about questions being asked.
   e. Seldom touches or speaks to the child; does not respond to child. May be critical or indicate unreal expectations of child (or may be over solicitous to the child).
   f. Delays seeking medical help; refuses to sign permit for diagnostic studies; frequently changes hospitals or health care providers.
   g. Shows no involvement in the care of the hospitalized child; does not inquire about the child.
   h. Obtains little or no prenatal care and shows inappropriate response to the neonate; acts disinterested or unhappy with the child.
7. Assess the parent–child relationship in the areas of appropriate involvement in care, show of affection, reaction to arrival and leaving, expectations, role portrayal.
8. Assess for signs of sexual abuse. Sexual abuse should be suspected when the young, prepubertal child presents with:
   a. Genital trauma not readily explained.
   b. Gonorrhea, syphilis, or other sexually transmitted organisms.
   c. Blood in urine or stool.
   d. Painful urination or defecation.
   e. Penile or vaginal infection or itch.
   f. Penile or vaginal discharge.
   g. Report of increased, excessive masturbation.
   h. Report of increased, unusual fears.
   i. Trauma to genitalia, inner thigh, breast.
9. Establish a relationship with the child based on mutual respect, empathy, and sensitivity to facilitate further investigation.
   a. Consideration of the child's emotions in conjunction with a good relationship may encourage the child to express feelings either verbally or through drawings or play.
   b. Prepare the child physically and psychologically for the necessary physical and pelvic examination.
   c. Talk with the child without the presence of the parents, especially when incest is possible.

10. Report suspicion of child abuse based on your assessment. All states (as well as the District of Columbia) have mandatory reporting laws. All states provide statutory immunity for those who report real or suspected child abuse. There is no immunity from civil or criminal liability for failure to report such. Notify the appropriate officials.

 NURSING ALERT If the alleged sexual abuse occurred within 72 hours of the health care visit, or if trauma or bleeding is present, an immediate physical examination should be done. Assessment and evidence collection is very important and every attempt should be made to enlist the assistance of a health care provider experienced in this task. Many emergency departments have SANE-Ps (Sexual Abuse Nurse Examiners–Pediatric) who have had extensive training in the acute management of sexual abuse and also in managing the long-term needs of the abused child. If more than 72 hours have passed since the alleged sexual abuse, the physical examination might be delayed. After child abuse has been reported, additional children in the family may be examined as well.

 NURSING ALERT Every nurse is morally and legally responsible to report and provide protective services for the abused child. Become familiar with laws, procedures, and protective services in your community and state.

Nursing Diagnoses

- Fear related to experiences with abuse.
- Impaired Parenting related to abusive treatment of a child.

Nursing Interventions

Relieving Fear and Fostering Trust

1. Be aware that some of these children have never learned how to trust an adult; they are fearful of giving affection for fear of rejection.
2. Assign one nurse to care for the child over a period of time so that a therapeutic relationship can be established.
3. Make no threatening moves toward the child. The child will indicate readiness and awareness of the environment by verbal or facial expressions.
4. Touch the child gently.
5. Provide nonthreatening physical contact (hold and frequently cuddle the child). Pick up and carry child around; encourage any exploration of your face and hair.
6. Provide appropriate opportunities for play.
7. Set limits for the child.
8. Provide therapeutic play to allow the child to express fears and anger in a nonverbal manner; be nonjudgmental and supportive with expression of feelings; correct misconceptions.
9. Provide additional help in these areas:
   a. Having ambivalent feelings toward the parents or any adult caretaker.
   b. Overcoming low self-image and the fear that something is wrong with him or her.
   c. Fearing future abuse upon his or her return home or for misbehavior in the hospital.

Providing Support in Parenting

1. Assume a nonjudgmental attitude that is neither punitive nor threatening. Convey a desire to help the parents through the healing process.
2. Refrain from questioning them about the incident of abuse. The health care provider, social worker, and investigative authority will interview the suspected abuser.
3. Include the parents in the hospital experience (ie, orient them to the unit and to any procedure to be done to the child). Serve as a role model in the management of the child's behavior as well as their own. Try to give the parents as much information as possible about the care of their child. Listen to what they are saying.
4. Refrain from challenging all the information they may give.
5. Express appropriate concern and kindness. Remain objective, yet empathic. This will help foster the parents' self-respect and improve their self-image and dignity.
6. Discuss the reporting to the authorities with them because of the widespread nature of the problem and the need for education and assistance.
7. Support the parents who may have feelings of guilt, anger, and helplessness. Explain to them the extent of trauma and educate them. Allow them to express their feelings. Support their parental role in handling the child (eg, allow the child to talk about or play out the incident, but do not force it).
8. Build a relationship by working with the parents' strengths rather than their weaknesses. Use compliments as positive reinforcement.
9. Assist the parents to learn safe and appropriate parenting skills.
   a. Remember that many of these parents were abused as children and have no role models or personal experience with nurturing behaviors.
   b. Foster attachment between child and parents, not between child and nurse, when the parents are present; the latter would increase their feelings of incompetence in the parenting role.
   c. Correct erroneous expectations as to what is appropriate behavior for a particular age group.
   d. Encourage the parents to take time out from caring for their children to meet their own needs; assist them in identifying safe and appropriate resources for their child's care.
10. Provide the parents with psychological support and reinforcement for appropriate parenting behaviors.
11. Work with the parents in planning for the child's future care.
12. Determine the areas in which the parents need help. Does the infant cry often? How does this make the parents feel? How do the parents comfort the child? Is there someone the parents can call for help?

 NURSING ALERT A critical part of working in this area is learning to recognize, examine, and work with your own feelings of anger, disgust, and contempt toward the parents. It may help to do the following:

1. Realize that most abusive parents do love their children and want the best for them despite their ambivalent feelings toward their children.
2. Understand the dynamics of child abuse and neglect. This crisis is due to stress, with which the parents are unable to cope, and to deprivations they have themselves suffered in the past.

Community and Home Care Considerations

Nurses typically provide home care visits as part of a multidisciplinary team engaging in extensive community follow-up. Education and continued assessment are the focus.

1. Teach the parents about normal growth and development (see Chapter 40).
   a. Give specific information about and examples of the types of behavior to expect at the various stages of development. Point out in a nonthreatening way normal behavior exhibited by their child.
   b. Provide specific strategies for dealing with whatever behavior the child exhibits.
   c. Serve as a role model and teacher; minimize intensity when the parents become threatened.
2. Teach the parents how to use discipline without resorting to physical force.
   a. Discipline must be consistent. Offer suggestions for alternative ways of handling undesirable behavior (eg, time-out).
   b. Suggest using a reward system for acceptable behavior (eg, a trip to the zoo, staying up later than usual for a special television show, a special treat).
   c. Instruct the parents to withhold rewards for unacceptable behavior.
3. Teach children how to avoid being the victims of abuse.
   a. Teach them about "good touch" and "bad touch."
   b. Emphasize that they can say no to anyone who wants to touch their body.
   c. Provide names or places where they can go if they feel they are being abused.
   d. Assist them in dealing with their fears that their parents will be sent to jail or that they will be removed from the home.
4. Be alert for signs of abuse in the school. If a teacher is suspected of being the abuser, the child may:
   a. Display increased fear of the teacher.
   b. Decrease school attendance.
   c. Develop psychosomatic symptoms during school days.
   d. Develop nightmares.
   e. Worry excessively over school performance

Bullying

Bullying is a form of abuse, frequently initiated among children. It is defined by the CDC as unwanted aggressive behaviors against a youth, initiated by another youth or groups of youths. Bullying can take many forms and can include physical, verbal, or social aggression. These behaviors can be direct with actual violence with verbal and/or physical results or indirect involving social media (spreading rumors). Bullying can cause physical and/or psychological symptoms in the victims of this abuse. Nurses should be aware of the possibility of bullying and refer to a primary health care provider, mental health counselor, or social worker for further care.

Family Education and Health Maintenance

1. Teach the parents and child (if age is appropriate) any specific instructions relative to injury and follow-up care.
2. Ensure that the family knows where and when to follow-up.
3. Review schedule for well-child visits and immunizations so the family can keep up with routine care.

4. Make known to the parents your continued concern and your availability as a source of help. Help them to use resources in the community, including the home health nurse, social worker, and therapists.
5. Refer those interested in learning more about abuse to the following agencies: Prevent Child Abuse America (*www.preventchildabuse.org*, 1-800-CHILDREN) and Child Welfare Information Gateway (*www.childwelfare.gov*).

Evaluation: Expected Outcomes

- Exhibits appropriate developmental behavior.
- Both parents participate in feeding and playing with child.

SELECTED REFERENCES

Akehurst, R. (2015). Child neglect identification: The health visitor's role. *Community Practitioner, 88*(11), 38–42.

American Academy of Pediatrics. (2016). Prevention of Childhood Lead Toxicity. *Pediatrics, 138*(1). Available: *http://pediatrics.aappublications.org/content/pediatrics/early/2016/06/16/peds*

American Academy of Pediatrics. (2017). Car seats: Information for families. Available: *https://healthychildren.org/English/safety-prevention/on-the-go/Pages/Car-Safety-Seats-Information-for-Families.aspx*

Barber, C., Huebner, J., Marquez, E., et al. (2018). Effective Recruitment Strategies for Lead Hazard Control and Healthy Homes Programs. *Journal of Environmental Health, 80*(7), 20–26.

Blosser, C., O'Keefe, C., & Sanderson, S. (2017) Infectious diseases and immunizations. In C. Burns, A. Dunn, M. Brady, et al. (Eds.), *Pediatric primary care* (pp. 474–493). Philadelphia, PA: Elsevier.

Braham M. (2017). Caregiver-Fabricated Illness in a Child. *Journal of Forensic Nursing, 13*, 39–42.

Carpiano, R., & Fritz, N. (2017). Public attitudes toward child undervaccination: A randomized experiment on evaluations, stigmatizing orientations, and support for policies. *Social Science & Medicine, 185*, 127–136.

Carter, J., & Wilson, F. (2015). Cyberbullying: A 21st century health care phenomenon. *Pediatric Nursing, 41*(3), 115–125.

Centers for Disease Control and Prevention. (2017). Childhood lead poisoning prevention. Available: *www.cdc.gov/nceh/lead/about/program.htm*

Centers for Disease Control and Prevention. (2016). Child Safety and Injury Prevention. Available: *https://www.cdc.gov/safechild/poisoning.index.html*.

Centers for Disease Control and Prevention. (2016). Tuberculosis: Testing and diagnosis. Atlanta, GA: Author. Available: *www.cdc.gov/tb/topic/testing/default.htm#bcg*

Centers for Disease Control and Prevention. (2017). Recommended immunization schedules for persons aged 0 through 18 years. Available: *www.cdc.gov/vaccines/schedules/downloads/child/0-18yrs-combined schedule*

Davidson, M. (2017). Vaccination as a cause of autism—myths and controversies. *Dialogues in Clinical Neuroscience, 19*(4), 403–407.

Feldman-Winter, L. (2013). Evidence-based interventions to support breastfeeding. *Pediatric Clinics of North America, 60*(1), 169–187.

Flaherty, E., & MacMillian, H. (2013). Caregiver-fabricated illness in a child: A manifestation of child maltreatment. *Pediatrics, 132*(3), 590–597.

Fry, S., Barnabas, S., & Cotton, M. (2018). Update on trends in childhood tuberculosis. *Current Opinion in Pediatrics, 30*(1), 152–160.

Guix-Comellas, E., Rozas-Quesada, L., Force-Sanmartin, E., et al. (2015). Influence of nursing interventions on adherence to treatment with antituberculosis drugs in children and young people: research protocol. *Journal of Advanced Nursing, 71*(9), 2189–2199.

Hensley, V. (2017). Childhood bullying: Assessment practices and predictive factors associated with assessing for bullying by health care providers. *Kentucky Nurse, 65*(2), 17–18.

Holmes, A. (2017). Breastfeeding considerations for mothers of infants with neonatal abstinence syndrome. *Pharmacotherapy, 37*(7), 861–869.

Hughes, H., & Kahl, L. (Eds.) (2017). *The Harriet Lane handbook* (21st ed.). Philadelphia, PA: Elsevier.

Hunt, S. (2015). New clinical protocols on breastfeeding and substance abuse. *Nursing for Women's Health, 19*(4), 371–373.

Infant Nutrition Council. (2013). Safe preparation, storage and handling of powdered infant formulas. Available: *http://infantnutritioncouncil.com/safe-prep-and-handling/*

Jin, J. (2016). Interventions to support breastfeeding. *JAMA, 316*(16), 1688–1693.

Kimberlin, D. W., Brady, M., Jackson, M., et al. (Eds.). (2015). *Red book: 2015 reports of the Committee on Infectious Diseases* (30th ed.). Elk Grove Village, IL: American Academy of Pediatrics.

Mahan, J., Betz, C., Okumura, M., et al. (2017). Self-management and transition to adult health care in adolescents and young adults: A team process. *Pediatrics in Review, 38*(7), 305–319.

Meissner, H. (2016). 2016 immunization schedule including several updates. *AAP News.* Available: *http://aappublications.org/news/2016/02/01/immunizations*

Mowry, J., Spyker, D., Brooks, D., McMillan, N., & Schauben, J. (2015). 2014 Annual Report of the American Association of Poison Control Centers' National Poison Data System (NPDS): 32nd Annual Report. *Clinical Toxicology, 53*(10), 962–1147.

Mowry, J., Spyker, D., Brooks, D., et al. (2016). 2015 Annual Report of the American Association of Poison Control Centers' National Poison Data System (NPDS): 33rd Annual Report. *Clinical Toxicology, 54*(10), 924–1109.

Paterson, P., Meurice, F., Stanberry, L., et al. (2016). Vaccine hesitancy and health-care providers. *Vaccine, 33*(4), 6700–6706.

Peetoom, K., Sits, J., & Ploum, L. (2017). Does well-child care education improve consultations and medication management for childhood fever and common infections: A systematic review. *Archives of Disease in Childhood, 102*, 261–267.

Raffaeli, G., Orenti, A., Gambino, M., et al. (2016). Fever and pain management in childhood healthcare providers and parents adherence to current recommendations. *International Journal of Environmental Research and Public Health, 13*(5), 499–515.

Reagan-Steiner, S., Yankey, D., Jeyarajah, J., et al. (2014). National, regional, and selected local area vaccination coverage among adolescents aged 13–17 year—United States, 2014. *Morbidity and Mortality Weekly Report, 64*(29), 784–792.

Rutten, L., St. Sauver, J., Beebe, T., et al. (2017). Clinician knowledge, clinician barriers and perceived parental barriers regarding human papillomavirus vaccination: Association with initiation and completion rates. *Vaccine, 35*(1), 164–169.

Saleh, E., Swamy, G., Moody, A. & Walter, E. (2017). Parental approach to the prevention and management of fever and pain following childhood immunizations. *Clinical Pediatrics, 56*(5), 435–442.

Shaikhkhalil A., Groleau, V., & Wendel, D. (2016). Feeding healthy infants, children, and adolescents. In R. Kliegman, B. Stanton, J. St Geme, III, N. Schor (Eds.), *Nelson's textbook of pediatrics* (20th ed., pp. 286–295). Philadelphia, PA: Elsevier.

Skoff, T., & Martin, S. (2016). Impact of tetanus toxoid, reduced diphtheria toxoid, and acellular pertussis vaccinations on reported pertussis cases among those 11 to 18 years of age in an era of waning pertussis immunity: A follow-up analysis. *JAMA Pediatrics, 170*(5), 453–458.

Taylor, L., Swerdfeger, A., & Eslick, G. (2014). Vaccines are not associated with autism: An evidence-based meta-analysis of case-control and cohort studies. *Vaccine, 32*(29), 3623–3629.

Thomas, R. (2018). School nurses and child sexual exploitation: Keep on looking and listening. *British Journal of School Nursing, 13*(3), 150-151.

U.S. Department of Health and Human Services, Administration for Children and Families. (2017). *Child maltreatment 2015.* Washington, DC: Author.

Willis, E., Sabnis, S., Hamiliton, L., Xionf, F., Coleman, K., et al. (2016). Improving immunization rates through community-based participatory research: Community health improvement for Milwaukee's Children Program. *Progress in Community Health Partnership—Research, Education and Action, 10*(1), 19–30.

Zhai, Y., Santibanez, T., Kahn, K., & Srivastav, A. (2017). Parental-Reported Full Influenza Vaccination Coverage of Children in the U.S. *American Journal of Preventive Medicine, 52*(4), e103–e113.

43

Care of the Sick or Hospitalized Child

GENERAL PRINCIPLES

Hospitalization of a child brings about a range of emotions in the child and his or her family. To care for the hospitalized child, one must take into consideration the child's development and family coping skills. Being hospitalized versus receiving care at home affects the child's response to his or her illness. In addition, family presence is often an integral part of pediatric patient care. Facilitating family-centered care allows the family to fully support the child during his or her hospitalization. Knowledge of these aspects will assist the registered nurse in providing appropriate pediatric patient care.

Pain Management

 EVIDENCE BASE Sng, Q., He, H., Wang, W. (2017). A Meta-Synthesis of Children's Experiences of Postoperative Pain Management. *Worldviews on Evidence-Based Nursing, 14*(1), 46–54.

Accurate assessment and timely management of pain in children is an important and challenging nursing responsibility because infants and young children cannot express their pain, as adults can.

General Considerations

1. Pain experienced by infants and children often is not effectively identified or managed by health care providers.
2. There are still misunderstandings about the ways pain is experienced and expressed by infants and children. Studies have shown that long-term effects can occur from inadequately treated pain.
3. Behavioral and physiologic cues are used to assess pain in infants. Special rating tools are available to involve children in assessing the intensity of their pain, including the Pain Experience Inventory, CRIES Neonatal Postoperative Pain Measurement Scale, Oucher Pain Rating Scale, numerical or visual analog scale, FLACC Behavioral Pain Assessment Scale, and the Wong-Baker FACES Pain Rating Scale (see Figure 43-1).
4. Pain caused by a condition is not always proportional to the seriousness of the illness or injury. For example, a relatively minor illness, such as an earache, is a very painful experience, whereas an enlarging tumor may not cause pain in early stages.
5. It is important to consider pain when a child is noncommunicative, has decreased consciousness, is intubated, or whose chosen language is not understood by the health caregivers. Changes in vital signs (such as heart rate, respiratory rate, and blood pressure) may indicate pain.
6. It is equally important to consider pain when a child requires an injection, blood test, or noninvasive or invasive diagnostic test.
7. Consider parents when assessing and managing the pain of their child. It is well documented that parents are important influences on their children.
   a. Consider the way in which the parents view the situation experienced by the child and work with them to intervene effectively.
   b. Presence of the parents during a procedure can be very positive, especially when the family has been prepared.
   c. At other times, it is recommended that the parents mutually agree to wait in a nearby area.
   d. Arbitrary rules against parental presence are often designed to meet the needs of staff, not the needs of the child and his or her parents.

Nursing Interventions

1. Anticipate pain and intervene early.
2. Use a rating scale that the child can understand and use it consistently with that child for initial pain assessment and to determine the effectiveness of interventions. Attempt to introduce the pain rating scale to the child prior to the surgery or procedure.
3. Use self as therapeutic presence to help ease pain.
4. Teach self-regulation and self-control techniques.
5. Utilize distraction by sounds, music, audio images, and movies.
6. Allow self-soothing maneuvers (thumb-sucking, clinging to blanket, rocking).
7. Reposition patient, as needed.
8. Decrease environmental light and noise when possible.
9. Consider referral for self-hypnosis and conscious relaxation techniques.

Figure 43-1. Wong-Baker FACES Pain Rating Scale. (© 1983 Wong-Baker FACES Foundation. *www.WongBakerFACES.org*. Used with permission. Originally published in Whaley & Wong's Nursing Care of Infants and Children. © Elsevier Inc.)

| 0 No Hurt | 1 Hurts Little Bit | 2 Hurts Little More | 3 Hurts Even More | 4 Hurts Whole Lot | 5 Hurts Worst |

10. Utilize medication delivered by way of noninvasive routes where possible.

11. Administer premedication—anesthetizing, antianxiety, and antiemetic medications—as indicated.

12. Assist with conscious sedation when indicated, following standards of practice related to assessment, staffing, care, and documentation.

13. Reassess the patient's response to the intervention and document appropriately. This is important to evaluate effectiveness and identify possible new pain issues.

The Child Undergoing Surgery

EVIDENCE BASE Al-Sagarat, A. Y., Al-Oran, H. M., Obeidat, H., et al. (2017). Preparing the family and children for surgery. *Critical Care Nursing Quarterly, 40*(2), 99–107.

Physical and emotional preparation for surgery will minimize stress and will help the child and family cope effectively with surgery. Also, see Chapter 7, Perioperative Nursing.

Psychological Preparation and Support

1. Potential threats for the hospitalized child anticipating surgery are as follows:
   a. Physical harm—bodily injury, pain, mutilation, death.
   b. Separation from parents; peers for the older child or adolescent.
   c. The strange and unknown—possibility of surprise.
   d. Confusion and uncertainty about limits and expected behavior.
   e. Relative loss of control of their world, loss of autonomy.
   f. Fear of anesthesia.
   g. Fear of the surgical procedure itself.
   h. Misinterpretation of medical jargon (eg, *dye/die*).

2. The attitudes of the parents toward hospitalization and surgery largely determine the attitudes of their child.
   a. The experience may be emotionally distressing.
   b. Parents may have feelings of fear or guilt.
   c. The preparation and support should be integrated for parent, child, and family unit.
   d. Give individual attention to parents; explore and clarify their feelings and thoughts; provide accurate information and appropriate reassurance.
   e. Stress parents' importance to the child. Help parents understand how they can care for their child.

Preoperative Teaching

1. All preparation and support must be based on the child's age, developmental stage, and level, personality, past history and experience with health professionals and hospitals, and background including religion, socioeconomic circumstances, culture, and family attitudes and dynamics. Anxiety level and coping skills should be taken into consideration.

2. Inquire as to what information the child has already received.

3. Determine what the child knows or expects; identify family myths and possible misunderstandings.

4. Additional guidelines in preparation include the following:
   a. Use illustration or model of a child's body, concrete examples, and simple terms (not medical jargon).
   b. Identify changes that may occur as a result of the procedure, in both body and daily routine.
   c. Give explanations slowly and clearly, saving anxiety-producing aspects until the end. Repeat as needed.
   d. Make use of the child's creative ability and logical thinking powers to aid in preparation for procedures.
   e. Involve parents, as indicated, depending on the situation.
   f. Allow and encourage the child to participate as able.
   g. Suggest ways for the child to cope—crying is okay.
   h. Offer constant reassurance; speak in a calm manner.
   i. Evaluate the child's understanding of your teaching. Repeat and correct information, as necessary.

5. Orient the patient and family to the unit, room, location of playroom, operating room, and recovery room (if applicable) and introduce them to appropriate personnel. Make arrangements for the child to meet the anesthesiologist as well as the operating room nurse and recovery room nurse.

6. Allow and encourage questions. Give honest answers.
   a. Such questions will give the nurse a better understanding of the child's fears and perceptions of what is happening.
   b. Infants and young children need to form a trusting relationship with those who care for them.
   c. The older the child, the more reassuring information can be.

7. Provide opportunity for the child and parents to work out concerns and feelings (play, talk). Such supportive care should result in less upset behavior and more cooperation.

8. Prepare the child for what to expect postoperatively (ie, equipment to be used or attached to child, where the child will wake up, how the child will feel, what the child will be expected to do, diet, any physical restrictions). Be honest about what pain they may experience.

9. Educate parents regarding the option to be with their child, if available at the facility, during induction of anesthesia to reduce separation anxiety and fear.

Physical Preparation

1. Assist with necessary laboratory studies. Explain to the child what is going to happen before the procedure and how he or she may respond. Give continual support during the procedure.

2. See that the patient has nothing by mouth (NPO). Explain to the child and his or her parents what NPO means and the importance of it. Place signs on the patient's hospital door

indicating the NPO status to ensure that nonfamily members and nonstaff members do not give the patient food.

3. Assist with fever reduction.
   a. Fever can result from some surgical problems (eg, intestinal obstruction).
   b. Fever increases risk of anesthesia and need for fluids and calories.

4. Administer appropriate medications, as prescribed. Sedatives and drugs to dry the secretions are often given on the unit preoperatively.

5. Establish good hydration. Parental therapy may be necessary to hydrate the child, especially if the child is NPO, vomiting, or febrile.

6. With the parents in attendance, assist the surgeon with marking the patient's intended surgical site, as recommended by the Joint Commission as part of the National Safety Goals.

7. Allow the child to carry a toy or other comfort item to the preoperative area.

Immediate Postoperative Care

1. Maintain a patent airway and prevent aspiration.
   a. Position the child as ordered depending on his or her surgical procedure; position as needed to allow secretions to drain and to prevent the tongue from obstructing the pharynx.
   b. Suction any secretions present. Avoid causing a gag reflex or spasm during suctioning.

2. Make frequent observations of general condition and vital signs. Postoperative protocols may vary per procedure and facility.
   a. Take vital signs every 15 minutes until the child is awake and his or her condition is stable.
   b. Note temperature, respiratory rate and quality, pulse rate and quality, blood pressure, and skin color.
   c. Watch for signs of shock.
      i. Children in shock may have signs of pallor, coldness, increased pulse, and irregular respiration.
      ii. Older children have decreased blood pressure and respiration.
   d. Change in vital signs may indicate airway obstruction or compromise, hemorrhage, atelectasis, and altered hemodynamics.
   e. Restlessness may indicate pain or hypoxia. Medication for pain is not usually given until anesthesia has worn off. Give analgesics and sedatives per the pain management team orders.
   f. Check dressings for drainage, constriction, and pressure. Perform dressing changes per protocol.

3. See that all drainage tubes are connected and functioning properly. Gastric decompression relieves abdominal distention and decreases the possibility of respiratory compromise. Chest tubes evacuate pleural air and fluid. Ensure all tubes are secure to prevent accidental removal.

4. Monitor parenteral fluids, as prescribed.

5. Be physically near as the child awakens to offer soothing words and a gentle touch. Reunite the parents and child as soon as possible after the child recovers from anesthesia. If a language barrier exists, the parents should be with the child during recovery from anesthesia and an interpreter should be present when medical explanations are being given to the parents or child.

After Recovery from Anesthesia

After undergoing simple surgery and receiving a small amount of anesthesia, the child may be ready to play and eat in a few hours. More complicated and extensive surgery debilitates the child for a longer period of time.

1. Continue to make frequent and astute observations in regard to behavior, comfort level and pain control, vital signs, dressings or operative site, and special apparatus (intravenous [IV] lines, chest tubes, oxygen, nasogastric tubes).
   a. Note signs of dehydration—dry skin and membranes, sunken eyes, poor skin turgor, sunken fontanelle in an infant, poor urine output.
   b. Record any passage of flatus or stool and bowel sounds. Observe for intestinal ileus. Gastric distention may be caused by swallowed air in the crying child.
   c. Record vomiting including time, amount, and characteristics.

2. Assess behavior for signs of pain and medicate appropriately.

3. Record intake and output accurately.
   a. Parenteral fluids and oral intake.
   b. Drainage from gastric tubes or chest tubes, colostomy, wound, and urinary output.
   c. Parenteral fluid is evaluated and prescribed by considering output and intake. It is usually maintained until the child is taking adequate oral fluids.

4. Advance diet as tolerated, according to the child's age and the health care provider's directions.
   a. First feedings are usually clear fluids; if tolerated, advance slowly to full diet for age. Note any vomiting or abdominal distention.
   b. Because anorexia may occur, offer what the child likes in small amounts and in an attractive manner.

5. Prevent infection.
   a. Keep the child away from other children or personnel with respiratory or other infections.
   b. Change the child's position every 2 to 4 hours; support infant with a blanket roll.
   c. Encourage the child to cough and breathe deeply; let the infant cry for short periods of time, unless contraindicated. Offer older children incentive spirometry every hour while awake.
   d. Keep operative site clean—change dressing, as ordered; in infant, keep the diaper away from the wound.
   e. Enforce diligent handwashing by family members and staff before any contact with the patient.
   f. Do not cohort surgical patients with patients with a proven or presumptive infection.
   g. Administer prophylactic antibiotics, as ordered.

6. Provide good general hygiene and opportunities for exercise and diversional activity; encourage sleep and rest.

7. Provide emotional support and psychological security. Reassure the child that things are going well; if there are complications, offer honest information based on the patient's health and developmental level and the parents' willingness to share this information with their child. Talk about going home, if appropriate.

 TRANSITIONAL CARE ALERT Hospitalization can be anxiety provoking for both the child and caregivers. Identify caregivers early, and try to coordinate nursing care and education with their visits. This includes teaching special procedures, providing written instructions, and arranging for home nursing and/or supplies.

The Dying Child

The nursing role is to assist the child and family to cope with the experience in such a way that it will promote growth rather than destroy family integrity and emotional well-being.

> **EVIDENCE BASE** Kubler-Ross, E. (1997). *On death and dying.* New York: Scribner.
> Schonfield, D. J., Demaria, T., & AAP Committee on Psychosocial Aspects of Child and Family Health, Disaster Preparedness Advisory Council. (2016). Supporting the grieving child and family. *Pediatrics, 138*(3), e20162147.

Recognize the Stages of Dying

See Table 43-1.
1. Be aware that the patient, his or her family, and the health care providers all progress through these stages; however, not necessarily at the same time.
2. Children experience the stages with much variation. They tend to pass more quickly through the stages and may merge some of these stages.
3. The nursing goal is to accept the child and his or her family at whatever stage they are experiencing, not to push them through the stages.
4. Understand the meaning of illness and death at various stages of growth and development (see Table 43-2).
5. Be aware of other factors that influence a child's personal concept of death. Of particular importance are the following:
   a. The amount and type of direct exposure a child has had to death.
   b. Cultural values, beliefs, and patterns of bereavement.
   c. Religious beliefs about death and an afterlife.
6. Meet with the parents separately from the child and discuss their wishes regarding dissemination of information to their child.

Communicate with the Child about Death

Research indicates that children generally can cope with more than adults will allow and that children appreciate the opportunity to know and understand what is happening to them. It is important that the child's questions be answered simply but truthfully. The answers should be based on the child's particular level of understanding. The following responses have been suggested by Easson in *The Dying Child: The Management of the Child or Adolescent Who Is Dying* and may be useful as a guide:

Preschool-Age Child

1. When the child at this age is comfortable enough to ask questions about illness, questions should be answered. When death is anticipated at some future time and the child asks, "Am I going to die?," a response might be, "We will all die someday, but you are not going to die today or tomorrow."
2. When death is imminent and the child asks, "Am I going to die?," the response might be, "Yes, you are going to die, but we will take care of you and stay with you."
3. When the child asks, "Will it hurt?," the response should be truthful and factual.
4. Death should never be described as a form of sleep. Some children may fear sleep as the result of this type of explanation. Anesthesia is sometimes called a "special sleep" so it is not currently recommended to refer to death as "sleep."
5. Parents can express to the child the fact that they do not want the child to go and that they will miss the child very much; they feel sad, too, that they are going to be separated.

School-Age Child

1. Responses to the school-age child's questions about death should be answered truthfully. The child looks for support from those he or she trusts.
2. The school-age child should be given a simple explanation of his or her diagnosis and its meaning; the child should also receive an explanation of all treatments and procedures.
3. The child should be given no specific time in terms of days or months because each individual and each illness is different.
4. When the school-age child asks, "Am I going to die?" and death is inevitable, the child should be told the truth. The school-age child has the emotional ability to look to parents and those he or she trusts for comfort and support.
5. The school-age child believes in his or her parents. The child should be allowed to die in the comfort and security of his or her family.

Table 43-1	Stages of Dying as Identified by Dr. Elizabeth Kübler-Ross
STAGE	**NURSING CONSIDERATIONS**
I. Denial, shock, disbelief	• Accept denial, but function within a reality sphere. Do not tear down the child's (or family's) defenses. • Be aware that denial usually breaks down in the early morning when it may be dark and lonely. • Be certain that it is the child or family who is using denial, not the staff.
II. Anger, rage, hostility	• Accept anger and help the child express it through positive channels. • Be aware that anger may be expressed toward other family members, nursing staff, physicians, and other persons involved. • Help families recognize that it is normal for children to express anger for what they are losing.
III. Bargaining (from "No, not me," to "Yes, me, but …")	• Recognize this period as a time for the child and family to regain strength. • Encourage the family to finish any unfinished business with the child. This is the time to do things such as take a promised trip or buy a promised toy.
IV. Depression (the child and/or family experiences silent grief and mourns past and future losses)	• Recognize this as a normal reaction and expression of strength. • Help families to accept the child who does not want to talk and excludes help. This is the usual pattern of behavior. • Reassure the child that you can understand his or her feelings.
V. Acceptance	• Assist families to provide significant loving human contact with their child and one another.

Table 43-2   Stages in the Development of a Child's Concept of Death

AGE OF CHILD	STAGE OF DEVELOPMENT
Child up to age 3	• At this stage, the child cannot comprehend the relationship of life to death because the child has not developed the concept of infinite time. • The child fears separation from protecting and comforting adults. • The child perceives death as a reversible act.
Preschool child	• At this age, the child has no real understanding of the meaning of death; the child feels safe and secure with parents. • The child may view death as something that happens to others. • The child may interpret the separation that occurs with hospitalization as punishment; the painful tests and procedures that the child is subjected to support this idea. • The child may become depressed because of not being able to correct these wrongdoings and regain the grace of adults. • The concept may be connected with magical thoughts of mystery.
School-age child	• The child at this age sees death as the cessation of life; child understands that he or she is alive and can become "not alive"; child fears dying. • The child differentiates death from sleep. Unlike sleep, the horror of death is in pain, progressive mutilation, and mystery. • The child is vulnerable to guilt feelings related to death because of difficulty in differentiating death wishes and the actual event. • The child believes death may be caused by angry feelings or bad thoughts. • The child learns the meaning of death from own personal experiences, such as the death of pets, family members, and public figures. • Television and movies have contributed to the concept of death and understanding of the meaning of illness. There may be more knowledge in the meaning of the diagnosis and an awareness that death may occur violently.
Adolescent	• The adolescent comprehends the permanence of death as the adult does, although the adolescent may not comprehend death as an event occurring to persons close to self. • The adolescent wants to live—sees death as thwarting pursuit of goals: independence, success, achievement, physical improvement, and self-image. • The adolescent fears death before fulfillment. • The adolescent may become depressed and resentful because of bodily changes that may occur, dependency, and the loss of social environment. • The adolescent may feel isolated and rejected because adolescent friends may withdraw when faced with impending death of a friend. • The adolescent may express rage, bitterness, and resentment; especially resents the fact that fate is to die.

6. The school-age child knows death means final separation and knows what will be missed. The child must be allowed to mourn this loss. The dying child may be sad and bitter and demonstrate aggressive behavior. The child must be allowed the opportunity to verbalize this if able to do so.

Adolescent

1. The adolescent should be given an explanation of his or her illness and all necessary treatments and procedures.
2. The adolescent feels deprived and reasonably resentful regarding his or her illness because he or she wants to live and reach fulfillment.
3. As death approaches, the adolescent becomes emotionally closer to his family.
4. The adolescent should be allowed to maintain emotional defenses—including absolute denial. The adolescent will indicate by questions what types of answers are desired.
5. If the adolescent states, "I am not going to die," he or she is pleading for support. Be truthful and state, "No, you are not going to die right now."
6. The adolescent may ask, "How long do I have to live?" Adolescents are able to face reality more directly and can tolerate more direct answers. No absolute time should be given because that blocks all hope. If an adolescent has what is felt to be a prognosis of approximately 3 months, the response might be, "People with an illness like yours may die in 3 to 6 months, but some may live much longer."

Support Parents' Adaptation to Child's Death

1. Develop a care plan that includes this approach:
   a. The primary responsibility for communicating with the parents should be designated to one nurse.
   b. Information regarding the parents' concerns should be communicated to all staff members and should be included in the patient's care plan.
2. Accept parental feelings about the child's anticipated death and help parents deal with these feelings.
   a. It is not unusual for parents to reach the point of wishing the child dead and to experience guilt and self-blame because of this thought.
   b. The parents may withdraw emotional attachments to the child if the process of dying is lengthy. This occurs because the parents complete most of the mourning process before the child reaches biologic death. They may relate to the child as if he or she were already dead.
3. Provide anticipatory guidance regarding the child's actual death and immediate decisions and responsibilities afterward.

a. Describe what the death will probably be like and how to know when it is imminent. This is necessary to dispel the horrifying fantasies that many parents have. Reassure the parents that all measures will be taken to keep the child comfortable at the time of death. (*Note:* Certain diseases, despite appropriate medical interventions, may cause an uncomfortable or painful death. Parents should be promised complete comfort for their child only if this expectation is realistic.)

b. Clarify the parents' wishes about being present at the child's death and respect their desires. See if they want to hold the child—before, during, or after the death.

c. If appropriate, allow the parents to discuss their feelings about issues such as autopsy and organ donation in order that they may make appropriate decisions. Do not make them feel guilty if they do not consent.

d. If necessary, assist the parents to think about funeral arrangements.

4. Be aware of factors that affect the family's capacity to cope with fatal illness, especially social and cultural features of the family system, previous experiences with death, present stage of family development, and resources available to them.

5. Contact the appropriate clergy if the family desires. Contact other extended family members for support if they wish.

6. During final hours, do not leave the family alone, unless they request it.

7. Encourage parents and siblings to share their thoughts with the dying child.

8. Provide information on bereavement support groups, usually available through hospital or church.

PEDIATRIC PROCEDURES

 See additional online content: Procedure Guidelines 43-1–43-7

Restraints

 EVIDENCE BASE Longo, M. A., & Miller-Hoover, S. (2016). Effective decision making in the use of pediatric restraints. *Journal of Pediatric Nursing, 31,* 217–221.

Protective measures to limit movement may be necessary for restraining children in the health care setting (see Figure 43-2). They can be a short-term restraint to facilitate examination and minimize the child's discomfort during special tests, procedures, and specimen collections. Restraints can also be used for a longer period of time to maintain the child's safety, protection from injury, and/or protection of medically necessary devices.

General Considerations

1. Protective devices should be used only when necessary and after all other considerations are exhausted, never as a substitute for careful observation of the child.

Figure 43-2. Types of restraints.

A Mummy device

B Belt device

C Jacket device

D

Papoose board

2. Protective devices cannot be used on a continuous basis without an order. Continuous use requires justification and full documentation of the type of restraint used, reason for use, and the effectiveness of the restraint used. Ongoing monitoring, documentation, and renewal of the order, with the length of time the restraint will be in place, are required.

3. The reason for using the protective device should be explained to the child and parents to prevent misinterpretation and to ensure their cooperation with the procedure. Children often interpret restraints as punishment.

4. Teach the child and family about specific devices they may be using in the hospital (ie, side rails) and after discharge (ie, mitts, elbow restraints).

5. Any protective device should be checked frequently to make sure it is effective and is not causing any ill side effects. It should be removed periodically to prevent skin irritation or circulation impairment. Provide range of motion and skin care routinely.

6. Do not cover an IV site with a restraint when possible.

7. Protective devices should always be applied in a manner that maintains proper body alignment and ensures the child's comfort.

8. Any protective device that requires attachment to the child's bed should be secured to the bed springs or frame, never the mattress or side rails. This allows the side rails to be adjusted without removing the restraint or injuring the child's extremity.

9. Any required knots should be tied in a manner that permits their quick release. This is a safety precaution.

10. When a child must be immobilized, an attempt should be made to replace the lost activity with another form of motion. For example, although restrained, a child can be moved in a stroller, in a wheelchair, or in bed. When arms are restrained, the child may be allowed to play kicking games. Water play, mirrors, body games, and blowing bubbles are helpful replacements.

11. Restraints should be removed as soon as the child is no longer considered a danger to self or others or when medical devices are no longer in place.

> **! NURSING ALERT** An order from a health care provider is needed to initiate continuous restraints. Proper documentation is required when restraints are in use. Do not secure restraints to bed rails or mattresses. Hourly assessment of the restrained extremity is needed to ensure there has been no impairment of circulation and constriction or respiratory compromise with chest restraints.

Mummy Device

The *mummy device* involves securing a sheet or blanket around the child's body in such a way that the arms are held to the sides and leg movements are restricted (see Figure 43-2). This short-term type of restraint is used on infants and small children during treatments and examinations involving the head and neck.

Equipment
Small sheet or blanket.

Nursing Action

1. Place the blanket or sheet flat on the bed.
2. Fold over one corner of the blanket.
3. Place the child on the blanket with shoulder at the edge of the fold.

4. Pull the right side of the blanket firmly over the child's right shoulder.
5. Tuck the remainder of the right side of the blanket under the left side of the child's body.
6. Repeat the procedure with the left side of the blanket.
7. Separate the corners of the bottom portion of the sheet and fold it up toward the child's neck.
8. Tuck both sides of the sheet under the child's body.
9. Secure by crossing one side over the other in the back and tucking in the excess or by pinning or taping the blanket in place.

Special Precautions
Make certain the child's extremities are in a comfortable position during this procedure. Make sure that the restraint is not obstructing the child's airway.

Jacket Device

The *jacket device* is a piece of material that fits the child like a jacket or halter. Long tapes are attached to the sides of the jacket (see Figure 43-2). Jacket device restraints are used to keep the child in a wheelchair, high chair, or crib.

Nursing Action

1. Put the jacket on the child so the opening is in the back.
2. Tie the strings securely with a knot that can be easily released, if necessary.
3. Position the child in a wheelchair, high chair, or crib.
4. Secure the long tapes appropriately:
   a. Under the arm supports of a chair.
   b. Around the back of the wheelchair or high chair.
   c. To the springs or frame of a crib.

Special Precautions
Children in cribs must be observed frequently to make certain they do not become entangled in the long tapes of the jacket device. Release, reposition, and perform range-of-motion exercises as per hospital policy.

Belt Device

The *belt device* is exactly like the jacket method of restraining, except that the material fits the child like a wide belt and buckles in the back (see Figure 43-2).

Elbow Device

The *elbow device* is a plastic device that fits around the arm at the elbow bend and is secured with a Velcro strap. This type of restraint prevents flexion of the elbow. It is especially useful for pediatric patients receiving IV therapy, those with eczema or other skin rashes, and those following a cleft lip repair, eye surgery, or any other type of procedure or surgery in which touching the upper extremities, head, or neck should be prevented.

Equipment
1. Elbow device.
2. Skin protective material for under the device (long-sleeved shirt or gauze).

Nursing Action

1. Cover the elbow with a long-sleeved shirt or gauze if irritation or sweating is expected.
2. Place the child's arm in the center of the appropriately sized elbow restraint.
3. Wrap the restraint around the child's arm.
4. Secure with Velcro.

Special Precautions

1. The child's fingers should be observed frequently for coldness or discoloration and the skin under the device should be checked for signs of irritation.
2. The device should be removed periodically according to facility policy or standards of care to provide skin care and range of motion.

Devices to Limit Movement of the Extremities

Many different kinds of devices are available to limit motion of one or more extremities. One commercial variety consists of a piece of material with tapes on both ends to be secured to the frame of the bed. The material also has two small flaps sewn to it for securing the child's ankles or wrists. Similar devices are available that use sheepskin flaps. These should be used when the device will be necessary over a prolonged period or for children with sensitive skin. This restraining device may be used to restrain infants and young children for procedures, such as IV therapies and urine collection.

Equipment

1. Extremity restraint of appropriate size for the child (small, medium, or large).

Nursing Action

1. Secure the device to the crib or bed frame.
2. Velcro the small flaps securely around the child's ankles or wrists.

Special Precautions

1. The child's fingers or toes should be observed frequently for coldness or discoloration and the skin under the device should be checked for signs of irritation.
2. The device should be removed periodically according to policy or standards of care to provide skin care and range-of-motion exercises and documentation should be completed.

Abdominal Device

The *abdominal device* is used for restraining a small child in a crib. It operates exactly like the method described for limiting the movements of extremities. However, the strip of material is wider and has only one wide flap sewn in the center for fastening around the child's abdomen.

Mitts

Mitts are used to prevent a child from injuring self with his or her hands and from removing tubes or IV lines. They are especially useful for children with dermatologic conditions such as eczema or burns and for those with nasogastric or nasojejunal feeding tubes. Mitts can be purchased commercially or made by wrapping the child's hands in Kling gauze or by covering the child's hands with a pair of clean socks and securing them to the wrist with tape.

 NURSING ALERT Mitts should be removed at least every 4 hours to permit skin care and to allow the child to exercise fingers.

Crib Top Device

A *crib top device* is used to prevent an infant or small child from climbing over the crib sides. Several types of commercial devices are available, including nets, plastic tops, and domes. A crib top device should be applied to the crib of a child capable of climbing over the crib sides (usually between ages 1 and 4).

 NURSING ALERT In all instances, it is essential to be certain that the crib sides are kept all of the way up and latched securely.

Papoose Board

A papoose board is a restraint device to be used for procedures of the head, chest, and abdomen. Straps restrain the child or infant at the forehead, lower arms, and thighs (see Figure 43-2, page 1155).

Specimen Collection

Evaluation of specimens such as blood, urine, and stool is important in determining the status of the child. The nurse should be adept in the techniques for obtaining specimens, as well as meticulous in labeling and recording them.

 KEY DECISION POINT Anticipate bleeding if venipuncture was difficult. Hold pressure over the area until oozing has stopped (longer if the child is being treated with aspirin or an anticoagulant). Assess frequently and reapply pressure, if needed; report continued oozing or hematoma formation.

 EVIDENCE BASE Bowden, V. R., & Greenberg, C. S. (2015). *Pediatric nursing procedures* (4th ed.). Philadelphia, PA: Lippincott Williams & Wilkins.

For catheterization of the urinary bladder, refer to Chapter 21. For infants and children, the catheter size is 6 to 10 F, depending on the size of the child.

 EVIDENCE BASE Patel, V., Romano, M., Corkins, M., et al. American Society for Parenteral and Enteral Nutrition. (2014). Nutrition screening and assessment in hospitalized patients: A survey of current practice in the United States. *Nutrition in Clinical Practice*, 29(4), 483–490.

Feeding and Nutrition

Nutritional requirements may increase while infant or child is ill, but the ability to feed naturally may be impaired by illness or the child's response to illness. If existing feeding patterns cannot be maintained, alternate methods may be necessary. The ability to feed enterally is preferred over parenteral nutrition because of decreased risk of complications as well as improved physiological response.

Gavage Feeding

 KEY DECISION POINT If improper placement occurs and the catheter enters the trachea, the patient may cough, fight, and become cyanotic. Remove the catheter immediately and allow the patient to rest before attempting to insert the tube again.

KEY DECISION POINT If bradycardia occurs, remove tube and allow the patient to relax. If the child appears to be in distress, follow basic life support protocols and contact the health care provider. When the patient's vital signs normalize, attempt tube replacement.

 EVIDENCE BASE Clifford, P., Heimall, L., Brittingham, L., et al. (2015). Following the evidence: Enteral tube placement and verification in neonates and young children. *The Journal of Perinatal & Neonatal Nursing, 29*(2), 149–161.

1. *Gavage feeding* is a means of providing food by way of a catheter passed through the nares or mouth, past the pharynx, down the esophagus, and into the stomach, slightly beyond the cardiac sphincter. Feedings may be continuous or intermittent.
2. Gavage feedings can provide a method of feeding or administering medications that require minimal patient effort when the child is unable to suck or swallow adequately.
3. Gavage feedings can be used to administer supplemental calories to a patient who is unable to meet their caloric needs by mouth. They also can be used to provide full calories to those unable to tolerate oral intake.
4. Gavage feedings can prevent fatigue or cyanosis that can occur from bottle-feeding in susceptible infants. They can provide supplements for an infant who is a poor bottle-feeder.
5. Gavage feedings can provide a safe method of feeding patients with hypotonia, patients experiencing respiratory distress, patients with uncoordinated suck and swallow, patients that are intubated, patients with a debilitation, and patients with anomalies of the digestive tract.

Gastrostomy Feeding

1. Gastrostomy feeding is a means of providing nourishment and fluids by way of a tube that is surgically inserted through an incision made through the abdominal wall into the stomach. A gastrostomy tube may also be placed surgically or by endoscopy using interventional radiology. Gastrostomy placement is the method of choice for those requiring tube feedings for an extended period of time (usually longer than 4 to 6 months).

 KEY DECISION POINT If the gastrostomy tube becomes dislodged and if it is newly placed (less than 6 weeks), replace tube (if allowed in scope of practice) with gastrostomy tube or Foley catheter and secure tube. Frequently, a smaller size must be used if the stoma is closing. Notify health care provider before using the tube, as oftentimes imaging will be needed to confirm correct tube placement, and accurately record events.

If gastrostomy tube is established (more than 6 weeks) and dislodged, replace with a Foley catheter or comparable-sized gastrostomy tube and aspirate the tube for gastric contents. If gastric contents are obtained, feeds may be resumed. If there is difficulty verifying placement, notify the health care provider.

2. Gastrostomy feedings provide a safe method of feeding a hypotonic or debilitated patient or one who cannot tolerate alternative methods. Prolonged feeding problems occur frequently in those with physical disabilities, prematurity, and chronic disease. Gastrostomy feedings may provide a route that allows adequate calorie or fluid intake in a child with chronic lung disease or in one who does not have continuity of the GI tract, such as in esophageal atresia, chronic reflux, or aspiration processes.
3. Gastrostomy tubes can also allow better decompression of the stomach because of larger tube size.

Community and Home Care Considerations

 TRANSITIONAL CARE ALERT If gastrostomy feedings are likely to be ordered upon discharge, involve caregivers in early education. Ensure that home health team is ready to support patient and family immediately upon discharge.

1. Teach the child (if age appropriate) and caregivers about the gastrostomy tube and feeding regimen.
   a. Anatomy of tube placement.
   b. Type of gastrostomy tube (button or tube).
   c. Amount and timing of feedings.
   d. Signs and symptoms of problems—tube obstruction or displacement, distended stomach, infection.
   e. Appropriate actions to be taken if problems occur—call home care nurse or health care provider.
2. Teach use of equipment: syringes, feeding bag, feeding tubing.
3. Teach the use of feeding pump (for continuous feedings or slow boluses).
4. Teach care of the gastrostomy tube—how to clamp, observe for leakage, determine amount of water in the balloon, and how to change a gastrostomy tube at home, if the site is mature and family is willing to learn.
5. Teach stoma care—clean area with soap and water, observe for breakdown, and apply skin barrier cream or powder, as appropriate.
6. Instruct about formula—proper mixing if not reconstituted; need to refrigerate if opened; discard any unused and nonrefrigerated formula after 4 hours.
7. Teach measures to take in an emergency.
   a. Procedure to follow if the tube falls out—replace tube (gastrostomy or Foley catheter), secure and cover site with gauze dressing, and call health care provider or proceed to emergency room if the tube has been in place less than 6 weeks. If tube has been in place for longer than 6 weeks, the tube may be replaced by the family or home care nurse.
   b. Troubleshooting for nonfunctioning equipment—ensure that the pump is plugged in and turned on; tubing is unclamped, not kinked; and abdomen is not distended.
   c. Proper phone numbers available to have as a resource or to obtain assistance.
8. Perform regular home visits as prescribed to assess nutritional and hydration status of the child, check tube placement and stoma site, and modify the care plan, as needed.

Nasojejunal and Nasoduodenal Feedings

 KEY DECISION POINT If abdominal pain, distention, diarrhea, or vomiting occurs, stop feeds and check emesis and stools for gross blood and report to health care provider immediately—this may be a sign of necrotizing enterocolitis.

1. Nasojejunal (NJ) or nasoduodenal (ND) feedings are means of providing full enteral feedings by way of a catheter passed through the nares, past the pharynx, down the esophagus, through the stomach, through the pylorus into the duodenum or jejunum.
2. Duodenal or jejunal feedings may decrease the risk of aspiration and can minimize regurgitation and gastric distention because the feeding bypasses the stomach and pylorus.
3. ND and NJ feedings provide a route that allows for adequate calorie or fluid intake (a full enteral feeding) by way of continuous drip.
4. ND or NJ feedings may also provide a route for administration of enteral medications.
5. ND or NJ feedings can provide a method of feeding that requires minimal patient effort when the child or infant is unable to tolerate alternative feeding methods (low birth weight, increased respiratory effort, and intubated patient).
6. ND or NJ feeding tubes may be placed under fluoroscopy, endoscopically, or at the bedside.

Fluid and Electrolyte Balance

 EVIDENCE BASE Parker, S., Benzies, K., Hayden, K., et al. (2017). A systematic review: effectiveness of pediatric peripheral intravenous catheterization strategies. *Journal of Advanced Nursing, 73*(7), 1570–1582.

Basic Principles

1. Infants and small children have different proportions of body water (see Table 43-3) and body fat than adults.
   a. The body water of a neonate is approximately 75% of body weight compared with that of an average adult man, which is approximately 60%.
   b. The normal neonate demonstrates a rapid physiologic decline in the ratio of body weight to body water during the immediate postpartum period.
   c. Proportion of body water declines more slowly throughout infancy and reaches the characteristic value for adults by about age 2 years.
2. Compared with adults, a greater percentage of the body water of infants and small children is contained in the extracellular compartment.
   a. Infants—approximately one half of the body water is extracellular.
   b. Adults—approximately one third of the body water is extracellular.

3. Compared with adults, the water turnover rate per unit of body weight is three or more times greater in infants and small children.
   a. The child has more body surface in relation to weight.
   b. The immaturity of kidney function in infants may impair their ability to conserve water.
4. Electrolyte balance depends on fluid balance and cardiovascular, renal, adrenal, pituitary, parathyroid, and pulmonary regulatory mechanisms (see Table 43-4).
5. Infants and children are more vulnerable to dehydration than adults.
   a. The basic principles relating to fluid balance in children make the magnitude of fluid losses considerably greater in children than in adults.
   b. Children are prone to severe disturbances of the GI tract that result in diarrhea and vomiting.
   c. Young children cannot independently respond to increased losses by increased intake. They depend on others to provide them with adequate fluid.

Common Fluid and Electrolyte Therapy

1. Repair of preexisting deficits that may occur with prolonged or severe diarrhea or vomiting.
   a. Deficits are estimated and corrected as soon and as safely as possible.
   b. Initial therapy is aimed at restoring intravascular and intracellular fluid volume to relieve or prevent shock and restore renal function.
   c. Intracellular deficits are replaced slowly over an 8- to 12-hour period after the circulatory status is improved.
2. Provision of maintenance requirements.
   a. Maintenance requirements occur as a result of normal expenditures of water and electrolytes because of metabolism.
   b. Maintenance requirements bear a close relationship to metabolic rate and are ideally formulated in terms of caloric expenditure.
3. Correction of concurrent losses that may occur by way of the GI tract as a result of vomiting, diarrhea, or drainage of secretions.
4. Replacement should be similar in type and amount to the fluid being lost.
5. Replacement is usually formulated as milliliters of fluid and milliequivalents of electrolytes lost.

Intravenous Fluid Therapy

IV therapy refers to the infusion of fluids directly into the venous system. This may be accomplished through the use of a needle or by venous cut down and insertion of a small catheter directly into the vein (see Figure 43-3). IV therapy is used to restore and maintain the child's fluid and electrolyte balance and body homeostasis when oral intake is inadequate to serve this purpose

1. Infusion pumps are often used in pediatrics to provide a controlled, constant rate of infusion.
2. Because infants and children are vulnerable to fluid shifts, the rates need to be monitored carefully.
3. During an IV infusion, every hour, check the following:
   a. Rate of infusion.
   b. Volume delivered.
   c. IV site for infiltration, because many pumps will continue to infuse solution even if infiltration has occurred.

See Standards of Care Guidelines 43-1.

Table 43-3	Body Fluids Expressed as Percentage of Body Weight		
FLUID	**ADULT**		
	MALE (%)	**FEMALE (%)**	**INFANT (%)**
Total body fluids	60	54	75
Intracellular	40	36	35
Extracellular	20	18	40

Table 43-4 Common Abnormalities of Fluid and Electrolyte Metabolism

SUBSTANCE AND MAJOR FUNCTION	ABNORMALITY	CAUSE	CLINICAL MANIFESTATION	LABORATORY DATA
Water Medium of body fluids, chemical changes, body temperature, lubricant	Volume deficit	• Primary—inadequate water intake • Secondary—loss following vomiting, diarrhea, and GI obstruction	Oliguria, weight loss, signs of dehydration including dry skin and mucous membranes, lassitude, sunken fontanelles, lack of tear formation, increased pulse rate, decreased blood pressure	Concentrated urine; azotemia; elevated hematocrit, hemoglobin level, erythrocyte count, and sodium level
	Volume excess	• Failure to excrete water in the presence of normal intake, such as in cardiac disease or failure or renal disease • Water intake in excess of output	Weight gain, peripheral edema, signs of pulmonary congestion	Variable urine volume, low specific gravity of urine, decreased hematocrit
Potassium Intracellular fluid balance, regular heart rhythm, muscle and nerve irritability	Potassium deficit	• Excessive loss of potassium because of vomiting, diarrhea, prolonged cortisone, corticotropin or diuretic therapy, diabetic acidosis • Shift of potassium into the cells, such as occurs with the healing phase of burns, recovery from diabetic acidosis	Signs and symptoms variable, including weakness, lethargy, irritability, abdominal distention, and, eventually, cardiac arrhythmias	Low plasma potassium level (<3.5 mEq/L) may be normal in some situations; hypochloremic alkalosis; ECG changes
	Potassium excess	• Excessive administration of potassium-containing solutions, excessive release of potassium because of burns, severe kidney disease, adrenal insufficiency • Beta-blocker therapy	Variable, including listlessness, confusion, heaviness of the legs, nausea, diarrhea, abdominal cramping, ECG changes, and, ultimately, paralysis and cardiac arrest	Elevated potassium plasma level; decreased arterial pH; ECG abnormalities
Sodium Osmotic pressure, muscle and nerve irritability	Sodium deficit	• Water intake in excess of excretory capacity, replacement of fluid loss without sufficient sodium; excessive sodium losses	Headache, nausea, abdominal cramps, confusion alternating with stupor, diarrhea, lacrimation, salivation, later hypotension; early polyuria, later oliguria	Sodium plasma level may be normal or low (<135 mEq/L).
	Sodium excess	• Inadequate water intake especially in the presence of fever or sweating; increased intake without increased output; decreased output	Thirst, oliguria, weakness, muscular pain, excitement, dry mucous membranes, hypotension, tachycardia, fever, agitation	Elevated sodium plasma level (>148 mEq/L), high plasma volume
Bicarbonate Acid–base balance	Primary bicarbonate deficit	• Diarrhea (especially in infants), diabetes mellitus, starvation, infectious disease, shock or cardiac failure producing tissue anoxia and renal failure	Progressively increasing rate and depth of respiration—ultimately becoming Kussmaul respiration; flushed, warm skin; weakness; disorientation progressive to coma	• Urine pH usually <6.0 • Plasma bicarbonate < 20 mEq/L • Plasma pH < 7.35
	Primary bicarbonate excess	• Loss of chloride through vomiting, gastric suction, or the use of excessive diuretics; excessive ingestion of alkali	Depressed respiration, muscle hypertonicity, hyperactive reflexes, tingling of fingers and toes, tetany, and, sometimes, convulsions	Urine pH usually >7, plasma bicarbonate > 26 mEq/L (30 mEq/L in adults), plasma pH > 7.45

ECG, electrocardiographic.

Venipuncture of scalp vein

Paper cup taped over venipuncture site for protection. A clear plastic cup may also be used.

Restraint of arm when hand is site of infusion

Infant's leg taped to sandbag for immobilization (IV site should be visible)

Figure 43-3. IV fluid therapy.

STANDARDS OF CARE GUIDELINES 43-1
Pediatric IV Therapy

When caring for a child undergoing IV therapy:
- Check IV site hourly, noting skin color and evidence of swelling. Compare to the opposite extremity or look for asymmetry. Feel area for sponginess. Observe for leakage.
- Check the IV tubing and equipment hourly. Stop the infusion if any cracks are noted in the tubing or there is discoloration of the IV fluid.
- Record the reading on the container or reservoir, amount of fluid absorbed in the hour, flow rate.
- Check for blood return in the tube by stopping IV fluid flow. It may be normal not to see blood return due to small catheter size.
- Check function of pump rate set versus amount infused.
- Maintain accurate intake and output record and 24-hour totals.
- Describe consistency and approximate volume of all stools and vomitus.
- Weigh child at regular intervals, using the same scale each time. An increase or decrease of 5% body weight in a relatively brief time period is usually significant.
- Monitor electrolytes (see Table 43-4, page 1160).
- Report evidence of electrolyte imbalances: decreased skin turgor, marked increase or decrease in urination, fever, sunken or bulging fontanelles, sudden change in vital signs, diarrhea, weakness, lethargy, apathy, pyrogenic reactions, and arrhythmias.
- If the child is experiencing severe reactions, the IV should be discontinued and the solution saved for possible analysis.
- Change the IV container and tubing every 24 hours or as per facility policy.
- If infiltration occurs, remove the IV, raise the affected extremity, apply heat to the site, and restart the IV at an alternative site. Notify the health care provider if irritation develops or toxic medication has infiltrated.

This information should serve as a general guideline only. Each patient situation presents a unique set of clinical factors and requires nursing judgment to guide care, which may include additional or alternative measures and approaches.

Cardiac and Respiratory Monitoring

Cardiac and respiratory monitoring refers to electrical surveillance of heart and respiratory rates and patterns. It is indicated for patients whose conditions are unstable, patients with cardiac or respiratory disorders, and patients receiving anesthesia or conscious sedation.

Nursing Management

1. Select a monitor that is appropriate for the child's needs. This will depend on the child's age and ability to cooperate, purpose for monitoring, information desired, and equipment available.
2. Stabilize the device to reduce the amount of mechanical noise and for safety considerations. Ensure the equipment is functioning well and there are no frayed cords. Plug into an emergency power outlet.
3. Reduce the child's anxiety:
   a. Provide age-appropriate explanations of the equipment.
   b. When possible, involve the child in care, including change of electrodes.
4. Select lead placement sites according to equipment specifications:
   a. Cardiac monitors frequently use three leads located at:
      i. Right upper chest wall below the clavicle.
      ii. Left lower chest wall in the anterior axillary line.
      iii. Left upper chest wall below the clavicle.
   b. Respiratory monitors frequently use three electrodes located:
      i. On either side of the chest (anterior axillary line in fourth or fifth intercostal space).
      ii. A reference electrode placed on the manubrium or other suitable distal point.
5. Apply electrodes by:
   a. Cleaning the appropriate areas on the chest with soap and water.
   b. Placing pregelled, disposable electrodes to dry skin.
6. Plug the leads into the lead cable at appropriate insertion points.
7. Make sure that the monitor alarms are in the "on" position. High- and low-alarm limits should be set according to the child's age and condition so that apnea, tachypnea, bradycardia, and tachycardia can be readily detected.
8. Avoid skin breakdown by changing lead placement sites, as needed. Clean and dry old sites and expose them to air.

9. Check integrity of the entire system at least once per shift.
   a. Carefully inspect lead wires and cable for breaks and proper attachment.
   b. If malfunction is suspected, change equipment and notify the engineering department or manufacturer immediately.
10. Continue to count respiratory and apical rates at least once per shift.
    a. Compare with monitor rates to verify accuracy of equipment.
    b. It must be remembered that monitors cannot substitute for close observation and nursing assessments of the child.

 EVIDENCE BASE American Heart Association. (2015). *BLS for the healthcare provider: Student manual.* Dallas, TX: Author.

Cardiopulmonary Resuscitation

Cardiopulmonary resuscitation (CPR) involves measures instituted to provide effective ventilation and circulation when the patient's heart and lungs have ceased to function. In children, the most common initial cause is respiratory distress.

Underlying Considerations

Cardiac Arrest
1. Signs—absence of heartbeat and absence of carotid and femoral pulses.
2. Causes—asystole, ventricular fibrillation, cardiovascular collapse, shock, or progression of respiratory failure.

Respiratory Arrest
1. Signs—apnea and cyanosis.
2. Causes—obstructed airway, depression of the central nervous system, neuromuscular paralysis.

Emergency Preparation
1. Every hospital should have a well-defined and organized plan to be carried out in the event of cardiac or respiratory arrest.
2. Emergency carts should be placed in strategic locations in the hospital and checked daily to ensure that all equipment is available.
3. Personnel should be trained in up-to-date CPR maneuvers and be certified in basic life support at least every 2 years.

Equipment

1. Emergency cart—assembled and ready for use.
2. Positive pressure breathing bag with nonrebreathing valve and universal 15-mm adapter.
3. Mask (premature neonate, child, adult sizes).
4. Oropharyngeal airway tubes, sizes 0 to 4.
5. Laryngoscope with blades of various sizes.
6. Extra batteries and light bulbs for laryngoscope.
7. Endotracheal tubes with connectors (complete sterile set, 2.5- to 8-mm inner diameter).
8. Portable suction equipment and sterile catheters of various sizes.
9. Bulb syringe, DeLee trap.
10. Oxygen source—portable supply, gauge, and tubing.
11. Cardiac board (30 × 50 cm).
12. Emergency drugs:
    a. Sodium bicarbonate.
    b. Epinephrine.
    c. Isoproterenol.
    d. Normal saline solution (for dilution).
    e. Diphenhydramine.
    f. Diazepam.
    g. Hydrocortisone sodium succinate.
    h. Digoxin.
    i. Naloxone.
    j. Calcium gluconate.
    k. Calcium chloride 10%.
    l. Dextrose 50%.
    m. Lidocaine.
    n. Atropine.
    o. Phenytoin.
    p. Insulin.
    q. Procainamide.
    r. Propranolol.
    s. Dopamine.
    t. Bretylium tosylate.
    u. Volume expanders (lactated Ringer solution, normal saline solution).
    v. Vasopressin.
    w. Amiodarone.
    x. Magnesium sulfate.
    y. Vecuronium.
13. Intracardiac needles, 20G and 22G, 2 to 3 inches long.
14. IV equipment, including infusion set, IV fluids.
15. Tourniquet, armboards, and tape.
16. Scalp vein needles of various sizes.
17. Gloves, mask, gown, other protective barriers.
18. Nasogastric tubes of various sizes.
19. Syringes and syringe needles of various sizes.
20. Intraosseous needles.
21. Long dwell catheters of various sizes.
22. Three-way stopcock.
23. Cutdown set.
24. Alcohol wipes.
25. Tongue blades.
26. Sterile 4″ × 4″ gauze pads.
27. Sterile hemostat.
28. Sterile scissors.
29. Blood specimen tubes.
30. Electrocardiograph (ECG) monitor, lead wires.
31. Defibrillator and paddles (pediatric and adult), lubricating jelly.
32. Arrest documentation record and patient-specific labels.

Artificial Ventilation

Mouth-to-Mouth Technique
1. Infants:
   a. Slightly extend neck by gently pulling chin up and forward and the head back by pressing forehead into a neutral position (known as head tilt–chin lift; use jaw thrust if cervical trauma is suspected). Place a rolled towel or diaper under the infant's shoulder or use one hand to support the neck in an extended position. Do not hyperextend the neck because this narrows the airway.
   b. Check the mouth and throat, and clear mucus or vomitus with finger or suction, if visible.
   c. Take a breath.
   d. Make a tight seal with your mouth over the infant's mouth and nose.
   e. Gently blow air from the cheeks and observe for chest rise. Give a total of two slow breaths.

f. Remove your mouth from infant's mouth and nose and allow the infant to exhale.

g. If spontaneous respiration does not return, continue breathing at a rate and volume appropriate for the size of the infant (usually 12 to 20 times/minute or 1 breath every 3 to 5 seconds).

2. Children older than age 1 year:

a. Clear mouth of mucus or vomitus with fingers or suction.

b. Extend neck with one hand or a rolled towel (head tilt, chin lift, or jaw thrust, if cervical trauma is suspected).

c. Clamp the nostrils with the fingers of one hand, which also continues to exert pressure on the forehead to maintain the neck extension.

d. Take a deep breath.

e. Make a tight seal with your mouth over the child's mouth.

f. Force air into the lungs until the chest expansion is observed.

g. Release your mouth from the child's mouth and release nostrils to allow the child to exhale passively. Give a total of two slow breaths.

h. Repeat approximately 10 to 12 times/minute or 1 breath every 5 to 6 seconds if spontaneous breathing does not occur.

Hand-Operated Ventilation Devices

1. Remove secretions from mouth and throat and move chin forward.

2. Appropriately extend the neck with one hand or place a diaper roll behind the neck.

3. Select an appropriate-sized mask to obtain an adequate seal and connect mask to bag.

4. Hold the mask snugly over the mouth and nose, holding the chin forward and the neck in extension.

5. Squeeze the bag, noting inflation of the lungs by chest expansion. If there is no chest expansion, realign the patient's head and adjust the mask; retry.

6. Release the bag, which will expand spontaneously. The child will exhale and the chest will fall.

7. Repeat 12 to 20 times/minute (depending on the size of the child).

8. Because this technique is commonly difficult to master, it should be practiced in advance, under supervision.

Indications of Effective Technique

1. Victim's chest rises and falls.

2. Rescuer can feel in his or her own airway the resistance and compliance of the victim's lungs as they expand.

3. Rescuer can hear and feel the air escape during exhalation.

4. Victim's color improves.

Management of Complications

1. Gastric distention (occurs frequently if excessive pressure is used for inflation).

a. Turn victim's head and shoulders to one side.

b. Exert moderate pressure over the epigastrium between the umbilicus and the rib cage.

c. A nasogastric tube may be used to decompress the stomach.

2. Vomiting.

a. Turn patient on side for drainage.

b. Clear the airway with finger or suction.

c. Resume ventilations after the airway is clear and patent.

Artificial Circulation

General Principles Related to Artificial Circulation

See Table 43-5, page 1164. See also Figure 43-4, page 1164.

1. A backward tilt of the head lifts the back in infants and small children. A firm support beneath the back is therefore essential if external cardiac compression is to be effective.

2. A supine position on a firm surface is mandatory. Only in this position can chest compression squeeze the heart against the immobile spine enough to force blood into the systemic circulation.

   Because most infant/child cardiac arrests are the result of respiratory failure or shock, there is a decrease in the oxygen levels in the blood prior to the arrest. Thus, chest compressions alone are not an effective method for delivering oxygen to the heart and brain.

3. This is different from cardiac arrest in an adult, in which the blood usually has a high level of oxygen and compressions alone are an effective way to deliver oxygen to the heart and brain.

4. Compressions must be regular, smooth, and uninterrupted. Avoid sudden or jerking movements. Push hard and push fast. Compressions should be done at a rate of at least 100 compressions/minute.

5. The chest must recoil (return to normal position) fully after each compression.

6. Between compressions, the fingers or heel of the hand must completely release their pressure but should remain in constant contact with the chest. This allows for complete recoil of the chest while minimizing interruptions to the compressions.

7. Fingers should not rest on the patient's ribs during compression. Pressure with fingers on the ribs or lateral pressure increases the possibility of fractured ribs and costochondral separation.

8. Never compress the xiphoid process at the tip of the sternum. Pressure on it may cause laceration of the liver.

9. Indications of effective technique include the following:

a. A palpable femoral or carotid pulse.

b. Decrease in size of pupils.

c. Improvement in the patient's color.

Nursing Management

1. Recognize cardiac and respiratory arrest.

2. Send for assistance and note time.

3. Initiate CPR:

a. Check for responsiveness and breathing; if the patient is unresponsive and not breathing, palpate a pulse. Checking for a pulse should not take more than 10 seconds.

b. If no pulse is felt, institute artificial circulation using appropriate technique.

c. For an infant or child, each cycle contains a ratio of 30 compressions to two breaths, starting with compressions.

d. Continue repeating this cycle until help arrives.

e. If alone, perform CPR as previously described for five cycles or 2 minutes of CPR, then call for help. After call, resume CPR until help arrives.

4. When help arrives:

a. One rescuer performs mouth-to-mouth resuscitation or institutes bag breathing.

b. Another rescuer performs cardiac compressions.

c. A ratio of 15 compressions to two breaths is maintained for both infants and children.

d. Cardiac compression should not be stopped for respiration. Breaths should be interposed on the upstroke of each fifth cardiac compression.

5. Anticipate and assist with emergency procedures.

Table 43-5 Technique of Artificial Circulation

SIZE OF CHILD	PREPARATORY PHASE	ACTION PHASE	COMPRESSION	RATE
Neonate, premature, or otherwise small infant	1. Place in supine position. 2. Encircle the chest with the hands, with thumbs over the midsternum. *or* Use method for a larger infant.	1. Compress midsternum with both thumbs, gently but firmly.	1/3 the depth of the chest (~1½ inches)	At least 100/min
Larger infant	1. Place on a firm, flat surface. 2. Support the back with one hand or use a small blanket under the shoulders. 3. Place the tips of the index and middle fingers of one hand over the midsternum, just below the nipple line.	1. Compress the midsternum with the tips of the index and middle fingers.	1/3 the depth of the chest (~1½ to 2 inches)	At least 100/min
Small child	1. Place on a firm, flat surface. 2. Support the back by slipping one hand beneath it, or use a small blanket. 3. Place the heel of one hand over the midsternum, parallel with the long axis of the body (at the nipple line).	1. Apply a rapid downward thrust to the midsternum, keeping the elbow straight. 2. Instantly and completely release the pressure so the chest wall can recoil. 3. Do not remove the heel of the hand from the chest.	1/3 the depth of the chest (~2 inches)	At least 100/min
Larger child, adolescent	1. Place on a flat, firm surface, or place a board under the thorax. 2. Place the heel of one hand on the lower half of the sternum, about 1 to 1½ inches (2.5 to 3.8 cm) from the tip of the xiphoid process and parallel with the long axis of the body. 3. Place the other hand on top of the first one (may interlock fingers). 4. Place shoulders directly over child's sternum, to use own weight in application of pressure.	1. Exert pressure vertically downward to depress lower sternum, keeping elbows straight. 2. Instantly and completely release the pressure so the chest wall can recoil. 3. Do not remove the hands from the chest.	2 inches (5 cm)	At least 100/min

Premature infant

Infant

Young child

Older child/adolescent

Figure 43-4. Cardiopulmonary resuscitation in children. In the young child, the heel of the hand is placed over the lower sternum at the nipple line. In older children and adolescents, both hands are used.

a. Assist with intubation, monitoring, placement of intravascular access, administration of IV fluids, defibrillation, and other definitive measures.

b. Prepare and administer emergency medications, as prescribed. Record dose and time.

c. Notify family of current management and CPR.

6. After resuscitation:

a. Care for the child, as required.

b. Determine if family members have been notified and are being cared for.

c. Record all events.

d. Restock emergency cart.

 TRANSITIONAL CARE ALERT After the stress of having a hospitalized child, families will need support in the transition to home or another aftercare location. It is crucial that they have complete and understandable care instructions on home care, medications, and follow-up appointments. If arrangements have been made for nursing care in the home, families should be aware of the agency providing services and when they can expect communication regarding care arrangements. Families should have thorough written (and if necessary to assist understanding, pictorial) instructions on signs and symptoms to monitor that could suggest worsening of status.

SELECTED REFERENCES

Al-Sagarat, A. Y., Al-Oran, H. M., Obeidat, H., et al. (2017). Preparing the family and children for surgery. *Critical Care Nursing Quarterly, 40*(2), 99–107.

American Heart Association. (2015). *BLS for the healthcare provider: Student manual.* Dallas, TX: Author.

Bennett, R., & Proudfoot, J. (2016). What does the staff think? Factors associated with clinical staff perceptions of what constitutes high-quality dying and death at a tertiary pediatric hospital. *Journal of Hospice & Palliative Nursing, 18*(5), 470–476.

Bowden, V. R., & Greenberg, C. S. (2015). *Pediatric nursing procedures* (4th ed.). Philadelphia, PA: Lippincott Williams & Wilkins.

Clifford, P., Heimall, L., Brittingham, L., et al. (2015). Following the evidence: Enteral tube placement and verification in neonates and young children. *The Journal of Perinatal & Neonatal Nursing, 29*(2), 149–161.

Curran, J. A., Bishop, A., Plint, A., et al. (2017). Understanding discharge communication behaviours in a pediatric emergency care context: A mixed methods observation study protocol. *BMC Health Services Research, 17,* 276. doi 10.1186/s12913-017-2204-5.

Davidson, F., Snow, S., Hayden, J. A., et al. (2016). Psychological interventions in managing postoperative pain in children: A systematic review. *Pain, 157*(9), 1872–1886.

Easson, W. (1981). *The dying child: The management of the child or adolescent who is dying* (2nd ed.). Springfield, IL: Charles C. Thomas Publishing.

Forster, E., & Hafiz, A. (2015). Paediatric death and dying: Exploring coping strategies or health professionals and perceptions of support provision. *International Journal of Palliative Nursing, 21*(6), 294–301.

Hughes, H. K., Kahl, H. K. (Eds.). 2017). *The Harriet Lane handbook* (21st ed.). Philadelphia, PA: Elsevier.

Irving, A. Y., Lyman, B., Northington, L., et al. (2014). Nasogastric tube placement and verification in children: Review of the current literature. *Critical Care Nurse, 34*(3), 67–78.

Jain, A. (2015). Body fluid composition. *Pediatrics in Review, 36*(4), 141–152.

Kirwan, L., & Coyne, I. (2017). Use of restraint with hospitalized children: A survey of nurses' perceptions of practices. *Journal of Child Health Care, 21*(1), 46–54.

Kuo, H., Pan, H., Creedy, D. K., et al. (2016). Distraction-based interventions for children undergoing venipuncture procedures: A randomized controlled study. *Clinical Nursing Research,* 1–16. doi: 10.1177/1054773816686262.

Longo, M. A., & Miller-Hoover, S. (2016). Effective decision making in the use of pediatric restraints. *Journal of Pediatric Nursing, 31,* 217–221.

Manworren, R., & Stinson, J. (2016). Pediatric pain measurement, assessment, and evaluation. *Seminars of Pediatric Neurology, 23,* 189–200.

Margonari, H., & Hannon, M. (2017). Quality Improvement Initiative on Pain Knowledge, Assessment, and Documentation Skills of Pediatric Nurses. *Pediatric Nursing, 43*(2), 65–70.

McNab, S. (2016). Intravenous maintenance fluid therapy in children. *Journal of Paediatrics and Child Health, 52,* 137–140.

O'Meara, M., & Trethewie, S. (2016). Managing paediatric death in the emergency department. *Journal of Paediatrics and Child Health, 52,* 164–167.

Oh, G., & Sutherland, S. (2016). Perioperative fluid management and postoperative hyponatremia in children. *Pediatric Nephrology, 31,* 53–60.

Parker, S., Benzies, K., Hayden, K., et al. (2017). A systematic review: effectiveness of pediatric peripheral intravenous catheterization strategies. *Journal of Advanced Nursing, 73*(7), 1570–1582.

Patel, V., Romano, M., Corkins, M., et al. American Society for Parenteral and Enteral Nutrition. (2014). Nutrition screening and assessment in hospitalized patients: A survey of current practice in the United States. *Nutrition in Clinical Practice, 29*(4), 483–490.

Ramira, M. L., Instone, S., & Clark, M. (2016). Pediatric pain management: An evidence-based approach. *Pediatric Nursing, 42*(1), 39–49.

Schonfield, D. J., Demaria, T., & AAP Committee on Psychosocial Aspects of Child and Family Health, Disaster Preparedness Advisory Council. (2016). Supporting the grieving child and family. *Pediatrics, 138*(3), e20162147.

Sean Quadros, D., Kamenwa, R., Akech, S., et al. (2018). Hospital-acquired malnutrition in children at a tertiary care hospital. *South African Journal of Clinical Nutrition, 31*(1), 8–13.

Sng, Q., He, H., & Wang, W. (2017). A meta-synthesis of children's experiences of postoperative pain management. *Worldviews on Evidence-Based Nursing, 14*(1), 46–54.

Svendsen, E., Pedersen, R., Moen, A., et al. (2017). Exploring perspective on restraint during medical procedures in paediatric care: a qualitative interview study with nurses and physicians. *International Journal of Qualitative Studies on Health & Well-being, 12*(1).

Thornton, S. (2017). Supporting the siblings of terminally ill children. *British Journal of School Nursing, 13*(9), 459–461.

Thrane, S., Wanless, S., Cohen, S., et al. (2016). The assessment and non-pharmacologic treatment of procedural pain from infancy to school age through a developmental lens: A synthesis of evidence with recommendations. *Journal of Pediatric Nursing, 31*(1), e23–e32.

White, M., Lawson, K., Ramsey, R., et al. (2016). Simple nutrition screening tool for pediatric inpatients. *Journal of Parenteral and Enteral Nutrition, 40*(3), 392–398.

44

Pediatric Respiratory Disorders

PEDIATRIC RESPIRATORY PROCEDURES

> *See additional online content: Procedure Guidelines 44-1*

Oxygen Therapy

Children with respiratory problems may receive oxygen therapy via nasal cannula, mask, face tent, endotracheal (ET) tube, or tracheostomy device (see pages 179 to 181). An Isolette or oxygen hood may also be used for infants and young children.

Mechanical Ventilation

Infants and children requiring mechanical ventilation need specialized care. These patients are typically treated in facilities that focus on providing a safe environment for technology-dependent children, with care provided by highly skilled nurses, respiratory therapists, and pediatricians. Specific nursing procedures and interventions and management of technology-dependent infants and children are beyond the scope of this text. General considerations are as follows:

Maintenance of a Patent Airway

1. Artificial airway options include nasotracheal, orotracheal, and tracheostomy. ET and tracheostomy tubes are available in several sizes, cuffed and uncuffed, for the pediatric population.
   a. Several methods are available to determine the appropriate size, such as ET tube size = age in years + 16 divided by 4 (consult facility policy).

2. The patient should be closely monitored for hypoxia and bradycardia during intubation.
   a. Only experienced and highly trained and skilled practitioners should perform intubation.
   b. Resuscitation and reintubation equipment and access to oxygen and suction equipment must always be readily available.
   c. An appropriately sized self-inflating bag with reservoir for oxygenation and mask should remain with the patient.

3. Action should be taken to prevent dislodgement of the artificial airway (especially during movement of the child) and obstruction of the airway.
   a. Pediatric ET tubes have small diameters and are easily obstructed by thick secretions.
   b. Adequate humidification will loosen secretions, and suctioning will prevent airway obstruction.
   c. Frequent vital signs and respiratory assessments are necessary. Cardiorespiratory monitors, pulse oximeter, end-tidal carbon dioxide, or transcutaneous carbon dioxide monitors are also necessary.

4. Nursing care should address issues of hydration, nutrition, sedation, skin integrity, tissue perfusion, infection control, communication, safety, and parental support and education.

5. Available ventilators for pediatric use have a wide range of capabilities, versatility, and clinical application. Some are more suitable for use with infants; others with older children.
   a. Nurses must be well acquainted with the characteristics of the particular machine being used and the meaning of the settings and alarms on each of the various machines.

Nursing Management

See Chapter 10, page 183. In addition the nurse who is caring for a pediatric patient should remember the following.

Setting Controls

In setting controls, inspiratory flow rate will be less and the respiratory rate will be greater than in the adult patient. These parameters depend on the patient's size and condition and are determined by the health care provider or respiratory therapist.

Humidification

During ventilation of an infant in an incubator, the amount of ventilator tubing outside the incubator should be kept to a minimum. The warm temperature inside the incubator helps decrease the amount of condensation in the tubing and thus provides higher water content in the inspired gas.

Oxygen Concentration

1. In infants, inspired concentrations of oxygen should always be kept as low as possible (while still providing for physiologic requirements) to prevent the development of retinopathy of prematurity or pulmonary oxygen toxicity.
2. The oxygen concentration should be checked periodically with an analyzer.

Blood Gases

1. Blood gas analysis, via arteriopuncture or umbilical or arterial lines, is necessary to monitor oxygenation.
2. The arterialized capillary sample method is inaccurate for infants in respiratory distress because the constricted peripheral circulation may not reflect the ABG (arterial blood gases) levels accurately.

Sterile Precautions

The neonate has only those antibodies transferred across the placenta from the mother. Therefore, sterile precautions are essential.

1. Ventilator tubing should be changed every 24 hours.
2. Routine cultures should be taken after intubation: may include frequent Gram staining of secretions.
3. Suctioning requires aseptic technique.

Tubing Support

1. Special frames are available to support ventilator tubing; this helps to prevent accidental decannulation in infants and small children.
2. Infants may require support or padding on either side and at the top of their heads to decrease mobility and take up space between the head and the frame.

Monitoring the Ventilator

1. Pressure gauges should be checked at frequent intervals as this gives an indication of changing compliance or increased airway resistance.
2. Volume measurements are difficult to obtain in infants because most spirometers incorporated into ventilators and meters do not read accurately at low volumes and flows. However, they are helpful with older children.
3. Measure respiratory rates of the machine and the patient at least every hour and record.

DISORDERS

 See additional online content: Procedure Guidelines 44-2

Common Pediatric Respiratory Infections

Respiratory tract infection is a frequent cause of acute illness in infants and children. Many pediatric respiratory infections are seasonal. The child's response to the infection will vary based on the age of the child, causative organism, general health of the child, and existence of chronic medical conditions. Information about specific respiratory infections, including bacterial pneumonia, viral pneumonia, *Pneumocystis* pneumonia, *Mycoplasma* pneumonia, bronchiolitis, croup, and epiglottitis, may be found in Figure 44-1 and Table 44-1, pages 1168 to 1177.

Nursing Assessment

Determine the severity of the respiratory distress that the child is experiencing. Make an initial nursing assessment.

1. Observe the respiratory rate and pattern. Count the respirations for 1 full minute, document, and note level of activity, such as awake or asleep. Determine if the rate is appropriate for the child's age (see page 1098).
2. Observe respiratory rhythm and depth. Rhythm is described as regular, irregular, or periodic. Depth is normal, hypopnea or too shallow, and hyperpnea or too deep.
3. Auscultate breath sounds for a full cycle of inspiration and expiration over all lung fields. Note airflow and presence of adventitious sounds such as crackles, wheeze, or stridor.
4. Observe degree of respiratory effort—normal, difficult, or labored. Normal breathing is effortless and easy.
5. Document character of dyspnea or labored breathing; continuous, intermittent, worsening, or sudden onset. Note relation to activity, such as rest, exertion, crying, feeding, and association with pain, positioning, or orthopnea.

Figure 44-1. Characteristic posture of a child with acute epiglottitis: leaning forward on hands, in the "tripod" position; mouth open, tongue out, head forward, and tilted up in a sniffing position in an effort to relieve the acute airway obstruction secondary to swollen epiglottis.

text continues on page 1176

Table 44-1   Common Pediatric Respiratory Infections

CONDITION AND CAUSATIVE AGENT	AGE AND INCIDENCE	CLINICAL MANIFESTATIONS

Bacterial Pneumonia

Bacterial infection of the lung parenchyma.

General considerations: In the normal child, bacterial pneumonias are not common. A viral respiratory infection commonly occurs before bacterial pneumonia. The initial viral infection alters the lungs' defense mechanisms.

CONDITION AND CAUSATIVE AGENT	AGE AND INCIDENCE	CLINICAL MANIFESTATIONS
Pneumococcal pneumonia The most common causative agent is *Streptococcus pneumoniae*.	• Responsible for the majority of bacterial pneumonias in ages 1 month through 6 years. However, it is seen in all age groups. • The incidence has declined because of the use of the vaccine. • Most common in winter and spring.	• *Infants:* Mild URI of several days' duration, poor feeding, decreased appetite. • Abrupt onset of fever 102.2°F (39°C) or higher; restlessness, respiratory distress, air hunger, pallor, cyanosis (common), nasal flaring, retractions, grunting, tachypnea, tachycardia, irritability; may see abdominal distention due to swallowed air or ileus. • *Older child:* Mild URI, followed by fever up to 104.9°F (40.5°C), shaking chills, headache, decreased appetite, abdominal pain, vomiting, drowsiness, restlessness, irritability, lethargy, rhonchi, fine crackles, dry hacking cough, increased respirations, anxiety, occasionally circumoral cyanosis, pleuritic pain, diminished breath sounds, may develop a pleural effusion, empyema.

> **! NURSING ALERT** Pneumococcal polysaccharide vaccine provides protection from 23 types of *S. pneumoniae*. It is recommended for children age 2 years and older with sickle cell disease, functional or anatomic asplenia, nephrotic syndrome, human immunodeficiency virus (HIV) infection, and Hodgkin disease before beginning cytoreduction therapy.

CONDITION AND CAUSATIVE AGENT	AGE AND INCIDENCE	CLINICAL MANIFESTATIONS
Streptococcal pneumonia • Beta-hemolytic Streptococcus group A	• Ages 3–5 years. Uncommon, serious. • An endemic influenza predisposes to streptococcal pneumonia and tracheobronchitis.	• Sudden onset, high fever, chills, worsening cough, pleuritic pain, respiratory distress, grunting, retractions, altered mental status, signs of shock, decreased capillary refill, tachycardia. • May be insidious, mildly ill, low-grade fever. • Severe infections—toxic shock syndrome with erythematous rash, desquamation, hypotension, hepatic dysfunction, renal involvement, vomiting and diarrhea, hematologic abnormalities, acute respiratory distress syndrome.
Staphylococcal pneumonia • *Staphylococcus aureus*, Gram-positive	• Most common in children ages 6 months to 1 year. October–May (rare).	• Predisposing factors: cystic fibrosis, maternal infection, immunodeficiency. • Usually preceded by a viral URI. Changes abruptly to high fever, cough, respiratory distress, tachypnea, grunting, nasal flaring, cyanosis, retractions. • Anxiety, lethargic, occasionally vomiting, diarrhea, anorexia, abdominal distention, toxic appearance.

DIAGNOSTIC EVALUATION	TREATMENT	NURSING CONSIDERATIONS	COMPLICATIONS
• Chest x-ray: Commonly does not correspond to clinical findings. • *Infants:* Patchy, diffuse areas follow a bronchial distribution, many limited areas of consolidation around smaller airways. • *Young and older child:* Lobar or segmental consolidation; pleural fluid may be present. • WBC count elevated, ABG analysis indicates hypoxemia. • *Cultures:* Sputum, nasopharyngeal secretions, pleural fluid, blood.	• Oxygen. • Penicillin G; penicillin allergy: erythromycin, trimethoprim–sulfamethoxazole, alternately amoxicillin, ampicillin, cefuroxime, cefotaxime, ceftriaxone, clindamycin, chloramphenicol. • Because of the increased incidence of penicillinase-resistant pneumococci, all pneumococcal isolates should be tested for resistance. Vancomycin has been recommended for penicillin-resistant strains. • Bronchodilators.	• Bed rest, monitor fluids, intake and output. Give oral fluids cautiously to avoid aspiration. Do not give oral fluids to a child in respiratory distress. • Administer oxygen with humidification. Perform frequent, thorough respiratory assessment. • Administer antipyretics as prescribed. • Change position frequently. Isolation procedures, as ordered or per facility policy.	• Rare, but include bacteremia, empyema, pleural effusion, otitis media, sinusitis, meningitis, hemolytic uremic syndrome, lung abscess, necrotizing pneumonia.
• Initial chest x-ray may be normal or slightly abnormal. Within 24 hours, chest x-ray worsens. • Unilateral lobar disease, bilateral diffuse infiltrates with severe disease. • Blood cultures, nasopharyngeal secretions cultured, throat swab, culture pleural fluid and lung aspirate. • Leukocytosis, sedimentation rate increased, elevated serum ASO titer.	• Penicillin G.	• Administer antipyretics. • Provide humidified oxygen, as needed. Rest. Monitor intake and output.	• Empyema, toxic shock syndrome, severe respiratory compromise, pneumatoceles. Can be life threatening.
• *Older infant/child:* Elevated WBC count, especially polymorphonuclear cells. • *Young infant:* WBC count may be normal, mild to moderate anemia. • Cultures—pleural fluid, lung aspirate, sputum, gastric aspirate, blood. • If pulmonary fluid is purulent and of a large amount, closed chest drainage may be utilized. • Chest x-ray: Patchy infiltrate, may involve entire lobe or hemithorax. Right lung involvement common; bilateral involvement is also seen. Pleural effusion, empyema, pyopneumothorax, pneumatoceles, pneumothorax, lung abscesses.	• Thoracentesis. • Nafcillin, oxacillin, methicillin, cefazolin, clindamycin, vancomycin. MRSA exists, especially in long-term care facilities or in patients with a prolonged hospital stay.	• Isolation per policy, check for MRSA, prevent nosocomial infection. • Rapid treatment is important. Administer antibiotics as soon as possible. Monitor for signs of tension pneumothorax. Monitor fluid status closely. • Strict hand washing. • Staphylococcal pneumonia is rare and must be treated aggressively because of rapid onset and deterioration.	• Empyema, tension pneumothorax, abscess, fibrothorax, bronchiectasis, osteomyelitis, staphylococcal pericarditis. Consider screening infants for cystic fibrosis and immunodeficiency.

(continued)

Table 44-1   Common Pediatric Respiratory Infections (*Continued*)

CONDITION AND CAUSATIVE AGENT	AGE AND INCIDENCE	CLINICAL MANIFESTATIONS
Bacterial Pneumonia (*Continued*)		
***Haemophilus influenzae*, type B**	• Majority of children younger than age 4 years. • Infants and children who are not immunized. • Winter and spring.	• Usually preceded by URI. Associated with otitis media, epiglottitis, and meningitis; appears toxic. • Insidious onset; cough, febrile, tachypneic, nasal flaring, retractions.
Viral Pneumonia		
• Respiratory syncytial virus (RSV); parainfluenza virus types 1, 2, 3; adenovirus types 1, 2, 5, 6 and types 3, 7, 11, 21; influenza A and B.	• Peak age for bronchiolitis is within the first year of life. Peak age for viral pneumonia is age 2.3 years. • Typically seen in the winter months.	• Usually preceded by URI with symptoms of cough, rhinitis, and mild fever. Progressing to tachypnea, poor feeding in infants and retractions (suprasternal, intercostal, subcostal, and substernal), leading to nasal flaring. Along with use of accessory muscles, wheezing, severe cough, cyanosis, and respiratory fatigue. • Viral pneumonia may present concurrently with bacterial pneumonia. Adenovirus types 3, 7, 11, and 21 may cause severe necrotizing pneumonia in infants.
• RSV subgroup A (more virulent, associated with more severe disease); RSV subgroup B.	• In infants, RSV is the most common cause of pneumonia, bronchiolitis, and hospitalizations. • Severity of RSV infection decreases with age and subsequent infections. • Peak age is 2–7 months, October–April.	• Typically begins with URI, rhinorrhea, fever usually <102°F (38.9°C), otitis media, and conjunctivitis. • Progressing to coughing, wheezing, tachypnea (>70 breaths/minute), intercostal and subcostal retractions, poor air exchange, hypoxia, decreased breath sounds, cyanosis, lethargy, listless apneic episodes, and irritability. Infants will present with poor feeding, inability to suck and breathe.

DIAGNOSTIC EVALUATION	TREATMENT	NURSING CONSIDERATIONS	COMPLICATIONS

• Chest x-ray: Usually lobar infiltrates; however, segmental, single, or multiple lobe infiltrates are also seen. Pleural effusion, pneumatocele. CBC: elevated WBC, lymphopenia.
• Cultures: blood, pleural fluid, lung aspirates, and nasal secretions. In the absence of a positive culture, a positive urine latex agglutination can confirm diagnosis.
• If atelectasis is present, bronchoscopy to rule out foreign body.
	• Patients may present receiving antibiotics for otitis media.
	• Ceftriaxone and other cephalosporins, ampicillin, chloramphenicol, azithromycin.
		• Administer antibiotics on time.
		• Ensure adequate hydration. Monitor for signs of upper respiratory impairment, drooling, stridor, and dusky color.
		• Respiratory isolation until 24 hours after appropriate antibiotic therapy is initiated.
		• Rifampin prophylaxis should be considered for close household contacts if there are:
		  • Incomplete or unvaccinated members younger than age 2 years.
		  • Immunocompromised child.
		  • Day care setting with two or more cases of invasive disease within 2 months and incompletely vaccinated children in attendance.
		• Not recommended for pregnant women.
			• Frequently in young infants, bacteremia, pericarditis, cellulitis, empyema, meningitis, pyarthrosis.

• Chest x-ray shows patchy infiltrates, transient lobular infiltration, and hyperinflation. • CBC: slightly elevated WBC count. • Cultures: blood and nasopharyngeal secretions. • Viral antigens for rapid diagnosis.	• If bacterial pneumonia is suspected, administer antibiotics. • Supportive measures: IV fluids, antipyretics, humidified oxygen, assisted ventilation. • Avoid aspirin because of risk of Reye syndrome. • Oseltamivir or zanamivir for influenza infection.	• Monitor closely for signs of respiratory fatigue or distress. • Monitor oxygen saturation levels and response to oxygen therapy if hypoxic. • Close cardiac monitoring may be indicated. • Monitor for adequate hydration and nutritional status. Elevate infants up to an angle of 10–30 degrees to ease breathing. Infants and children who require mechanical ventilation require close supervision and frequent monitoring. Institute contact precautions with strict hand washing. • Prevention: influenza vaccine.	• Influenza: severe fulminant pneumonia with hemorrhagic exudate. Death may result. Severe disease may be seen in children with cardiopulmonary disease, cystic fibrosis, bronchopulmonary dysplasia, and neurovascular disease. • Type B—myositis.
• Nasopharyngeal secretions for rapid antibody or assay for RSV antigen detection. • Chest x-ray: chest hyperexpanded, air trapping, multiple lobe infiltrates, atelectasis. • ABG analysis. • Pulse oximetry.	• Supportive measures, such as oxygen, respiratory support, hydration. • Bronchodilators should not be used routinely. • Racemic epinephrine can be effective in bronchiolitis. • Glucocorticoids and ribavirin are not supported in the literature. • Antibiotics only if a secondary bacterial infection is suspected.	• Prevent nosocomial spread. Institute contact isolation. Strict hand washing. • RSV-positive patients should not be in contact with other high-risk patients, such as those with chronic cardiac or respiratory illness or immunocompromised patients. • Assess frequently for signs of respiratory failure. • Use noninvasive oxygen monitoring.	• RSV can be fatal, especially in children with chronic cardiac and respiratory diseases, premature infants, and those with underlying neuromuscular or immunologic diseases. • Respiratory failure, intubation, and mechanical ventilation. • In older children with asthma, RSV can cause an acute asthmatic episode.

(continued)

Table 44-1	Common Pediatric Respiratory Infections (Continued)	
CONDITION AND CAUSATIVE AGENT	**AGE AND INCIDENCE**	**CLINICAL MANIFESTATIONS**

Viral Pneumonia (Continued)

Respiratory syncytial virus (continued)

Pneumocystis carinii Pneumonia

• *P. carinii*, also known as *P. jiroveci*, is a fungus with similarities to protozoa. The organism exists in three forms in the tissues: trophozoite, sporozoite, and cyst.	• Most healthy humans are infected before age 4 years and are asymptomatic. • Life-threatening pneumonia is seen in the immunosuppressed host. PCP in severely immunocompromised children with acquired or congenital immunodeficiency disorders, malignancies, organ transplant recipients, and debilitated, malnourished, and premature infants. In HIV-infected children, it most commonly occurs between ages 3 and 6 months. PCP can occur during remission or relapse in patients with leukemia or lymphoma.	• Slow onset, tachypnea, retractions, and nasal flaring cyanosis. • Sporadic form in immunocompromised patients. Signs may vary; onset may be acute or fulminant. • Fever, tachypnea, dyspnea, cough, nasal flaring, cyanosis, subacute, diffuse pneumonitis with dyspnea at rest, tachypnea and decreasing oxygen saturation. Extrapulmonary sites rarely occur and usually produce no symptoms.

Mycoplasma Pneumonia

• *Mycoplasma pneumoniae*, microorganisms with properties between bacteria and viruses.	• Fall and winter. • Crowded living conditions. Seen frequently in school age children and adolescents.	• Slow onset; 2- to 3-week incubation period. Coryza, malaise, headache, anorexia, normal temp or low-grade fever, sore throat, muscle pain, vomiting, subacute tracheobronchitis, shortness of breath, dry cough that progresses to mucopurulent cough, mild chest pain, wheezing. May present with maculopapular rash.

Bronchiolitis

• Inflammation of the bronchioles. Causative agents: RSV, adenovirus, parainfluenza type 1 or 3, influenza virus, and *M. pneumoniae*.	• Winter and spring. • Most common in infants younger than 6 months old, may occur up to age 2 years. • Greater incidence in males than in females. • Increased in day care centers.	• Gradual onset after exposure to an individual with URI. Coryza, tachypnea, respiratory rate >50 bpm, retractions, wheezing, paroxysmal cough, fever, cyanosis, dehydration, poor feeding, vomiting, tachycardia, irritability, dyspnea. • Apnea may be first sign in infants with RSV. Decreased breath sounds with prolonged expiratory phase. Hypoxemia may persist for 4–6 weeks.

DIAGNOSTIC EVALUATION	TREATMENT	NURSING CONSIDERATIONS	COMPLICATIONS
	• Early detection is important in hospitalized patients. Institute contact precautions with strict hand washing. RSV immune globulin (RSV-IGIV) and palivizumab may be given to prevent infection in select patient populations. Consult AAP Guidelines for specific information.	• In tachypneic patients and those in respiratory distress, oral fluids are contraindicated because of risk of aspiration.	
• Chest x-ray: Bilateral, diffuse, alveolar disease with a granular pattern, initially perihilar densities, which progress to peripheral and apical areas. • Organism cannot be cultured from routine specimens. • Open lung biopsy is the most reliable method. • Bronchoalveolar lavage is also utilized to obtain samples. Needle aspiration of the lung. IgM-ELISA: elevated. CBC: mild leukocytosis, moderate eosinophilia.	• PCP mortality is 5%–40% in immunocompromised patients; if untreated, 100%. • Trimethoprim–sulfamethoxazole; rate of adverse reactions is high in HIV-infected patients. • Pentamidine, parenterally or aerosolized. IV form associated with increased risk of adverse reactions. Aerosolized for children ages 5 and older. • Corticosteroids recommended for children older than age 13, may be used in younger children.	• Close monitoring of respiratory status, hydration, and nutrition. • Monitor for adverse reactions to therapy: vomiting, nausea, rash. • Respiratory isolation should be instituted for 48 hours after initiation of therapy. • PCP prophylaxis (see page 1392). **NURSING ALERT** Pentamidine is associated with a high incidence of adverse reactions: pancreatitis, renal dysfunction, hypoglycemia, hyperglycemia, hypotension, fever, and neutropenia. Pentamidine should not be used with didanosine, which also causes pancreatitis, and in patients with hepatic dysfunction.	—
• Chest x-ray: bronchopneumonic, diffuse bilateral infiltrates. • Complement fixation test: increased. Cold agglutinins: increased. Immunofluorescent and enzyme immunoassay tests. • Positive sputum culture.	• Erythromycin, azithromycin, clarithromycin, tetracycline, and doxycycline may be used in children ages 8 and older. Rule out pregnancy in female patients prior to use.	• Children should be on secretion precautions. • Monitor fever. • Assess need for cough suppressants.	• May be fatal if infection becomes systemic or if the child has a preexisting chronic lung disease, sickle cell anemia, immunodeficiencies, or cardiac disease. Those with Down syndrome can develop severe pneumonia. • Pleural effusions.
• Chest x-ray: patchy or peribronchial infiltrates, hyperinflation of lungs with flattening of diaphragms. Some will present with a normal chest x-ray. • Nasopharyngeal viral cultures. • Serologic studies for specific organisms. ABG analysis for children with respiratory distress.	• Humidified oxygen, ventilatory assistance as needed. (Note treatment for RSV above regarding bronchodilators, glucocorticoids, antibiotics.) • Antipyretics for fever. • Continuous cardiac monitoring for apnea or bradycardia. • Pulse oximetry.	• Avoid high-density humidity; may cause bronchospasm. • Monitor fluid and electrolyte balance closely. Place infant on apnea monitor. • Keep nasal passages free of secretions; infants are obligate nose breathers. • Position patient upright to facilitate breathing. Monitor closely for signs of impending respiratory failure. • There is a high risk of cross-contamination to noninfected children. Institute contact precautions and respiratory isolation. • Monitor oxygenation levels with noninvasive monitoring.	• Increasing respiratory distress resulting in the need for mechanical ventilation. • Secondary bacterial infection. • Pneumothorax and pneumomediastinum. Apneic episodes, may be life-threatening in children with chronic respiratory or cardiac disease. • Some infants demonstrate abnormal lung functions months after infection.

(continued)

Table 44-1 Common Pediatric Respiratory Infections (Continued)

CONDITION AND CAUSATIVE AGENT	AGE AND INCIDENCE	CLINICAL MANIFESTATIONS
Croup Syndromes		
Croup syndromes refer to infections of the supraglottis, glottis, subglottis, and trachea.		
Acute laryngotracheobronchitis (subglottic croup) • Parainfluenza types 1, 2, 3; RSV; influenza A and B; adenovirus; measles.	• Ages 3 months to 5 years. Peak ages 1–2 years. • Greater incidence in males than in females. • Late autumn, early winter.	• Usually a preceding URI is seen. Initially, a mild brassy or barking cough, hoarse, intermittent stridor, progresses to continuous stridor. • Nasal flaring, suprasternal, infrasternal, intercostals, retractions. • Breathing labored, prolonged expiratory phase. Temperature slightly elevated. • Crying and agitation aggravate signs. • Child prefers to be held upright or sit up in bed. Symptoms are worse at night. • Severe croup: restlessness, air hunger, decreased breath sounds, hypoxemia, hypercapnia, anxiety, cyanosis, tachycardia, and cessation of breathing.

 NURSING ALERT If ABG analysis is done, a normal partial pressure of arterial carbon dioxide may not indicate decreased severity. By the time hypercapnia is seen, intubation will be required. Children decompensate very quickly.

CONDITION AND CAUSATIVE AGENT	AGE AND INCIDENCE	CLINICAL MANIFESTATIONS
Spasmodic croup and acute spasmodic laryngitis • No infectious agents seen. Thought to be related to spasm of laryngeal muscle. • Cause may be viral in a few cases, allergic or psychological.	• Ages 1–6 years. • Peak incidence 7–36 months.	• Similar to acute laryngotracheobronchitis. Symptoms are sudden, in the evening. • Afebrile, barking, brassy cough, hoarse, stridor. Child may be anxious and frightened. • Breathing is noisy on inspiration, slow, and labored; respiratory distresses. • Tachycardia. Skin cool, moist. Dyspnea is worse with excitement. • Cyanosis is rare; severity decreases over time. Patient appears well in the morning, may cough or sound hoarse. The symptoms may recur for subsequent nights; however, they will be less severe.
Bacterial tracheitis (pseudomembranous croup) • Tracheal inflammation in the subglottic region. • *S. aureus, H. influenzae,* streptococci groups A and B, *Escherichia coli, Klebsiella, Moraxella catarrhalis, Pseudomonas, Chlamydia trachomatis,* and *Corynebacterium diphtheriae* should be considered in the nonvaccinated patient.	• No season variation. • Age is variable, 1 month to 6 years; however, most are younger than age 3 years.	• Usually follows a viral illness. Slow or sudden deterioration, child appears toxic. • High fever, stridor, hoarse, respiratory distress. Thick, purulent, copious airway secretions. • Mucosal necrosis, brassy or barking cough. Epiglottitis may coexist. May cause life-threatening airway obstruction.
Acute epiglottitis • Supraglottitis, inflammation of the epiglottis and edema of the arytenoepiglottic folds. • *H. influenzae* type B, most common. *S. pneumoniae, S. aureus,* group A. Beta-hemolytic streptococcus, *Streptococcus pyogenes, Moraxella catarrhalis,* and *Candida albicans* (in the immunocompromised).	• Range ages 2–7 years; peak ages 3–5 years. • Autumn and winter. • Incidence significantly decreased because of the routine use of the *H. influenzae* vaccine.	• Sudden fulminating course, high fever, toxic appearance, sore throat, drooling, dysphagia, aphonia, retractions, air hunger, anxiety, tachycardia, hoarseness, irritability, restlessness, rapid progression to respiratory distress. • Sitting forward, neck hyperextended, mouth open, tongue protruding. Older child will sit in tripod position. Drooling, agitation, and absence of spontaneous cough are predictive of epiglottitis. • Absence of croupy cough.

DIAGNOSTIC EVALUATION	TREATMENT	NURSING CONSIDERATIONS	COMPLICATIONS
• Diagnosis is made by clinical evaluation and careful history. A croup score may be assigned to grade severity. Lateral neck x-ray: subglottic edema, narrowing with normal supraglottic structures. Anterior/posterior neck film: steeple sign. • Lower airway involvement.	• Racemic epinephrine nebulized with oxygen. Monitor pulse and cardiac rhythm. • Severe airway edema may require intubation. • Corticosteroid therapy. • Antibiotic therapy.	• Maintain a calm environment, avoid agitating the child, and disturb as little as possible. Monitor oxygenation with noninvasive pulse oximeter. Monitor respiratory status closely and frequently. Closely observe response to racemic epinephrine. Have intubation equipment at bedside and available during transport. Increasing tachypnea may be first sign of hypoxia. If severe distress does not respond to initial treatment, ABG analysis should be obtained. In a hypoxic, pale, cyanotic, or obtunded patient, do not manipulate larynx and do not examine with a tongue blade; it may lead to sudden cardiopulmonary arrest.	• Dehydration, intubation, airway obstruction, death.
• CBC is normal, x-ray: subglottic narrowing. • Endoscopic exam: inflammation of the arytenoids cartilage, epithelium intact, pale mucosa.	• Corticosteroid therapy. • Racemic epinephrine, nebulized.	• Same as for acute laryngotracheobronchitis (above). • Allow the parent to hold the child, remain in upright position. • Use racemic epinephrine with caution and provide cardiac monitoring, because of possible tachycardia.	
• Neck x-ray: subglottic narrowing, large epiglottis, thick arytenoepiglottic folds, pseudomembrane in trachea. • Tracheal culture. Laryngoscopy, CBC, leukocytosis, bandemia.	• Humidified oxygen as required, mist, antibiotic therapy, cephalosporin, antipyretics. • Admit to the intensive care unit (ICU), intubation, and frequent suctioning. • Racemic epinephrine ineffective.	• Monitor closely for airway obstruction.	• Airway obstruction, death, tracheostomy, pneumothorax, toxic shock syndrome.
• Clinical evaluation and history, determining the onset of symptoms. • Monitor oxygen saturation level. • Lateral neck films: while sitting in parent's lap with portable radiology, swollen epiglottis.	• Medical emergency. • Establish a stable artificial airway first. Approach child in a calm manner; emotional upset and agitation may result in complete airway obstruction.	• Allow the parents to remain with and hold the child. Before transport to the operating room, observe closely for signs of airway obstruction. Allow the child to maintain a position of comfort (not supine).	• Airway obstruction, death, tracheostomy, pneumothorax, toxic shock syndrome. **NURSING ALERT** Do not attempt to visualize the epiglottis with a tongue blade or take a throat culture. May cause laryngospasm and airway obstruction. Have intubation equipment ready.

(continued)

Table 44-1   Common Pediatric Respiratory Infections (*Continued*)

CONDITION AND CAUSATIVE AGENT	AGE AND INCIDENCE	CLINICAL MANIFESTATIONS
Croup Syndromes (*Continued*) **Acute epiglottitis (*Continued*)**		• Complete fatal airway obstruction and death may occur within hours if not treated. In group A beta-hemolytic streptococcus and *H. influenzae*, patient will present with acute respiratory distress. • Stridor and breath sounds decrease as child begins to tire. • A brief episode of air hunger with restlessness and agitation may rapidly progress into increasing cyanosis, coma, and death.

ABG, arterial blood gas; ASO, antistreptolysin; CBC, complete blood count; HIV, human immunodeficiency virus; ICU, intensive care unit; MRSA, methicillin-resistant *S. aureus*; PCP, *Pneumocystis carinii* pneumonia; RSV, respiratory syncytial virus; URI, upper respiratory infection.

6. Note presence of additional signs of respiratory distress: nasal flaring, grunting, and retractions. Note location of retractions (see Figure 44-2) and character (mild, moderate, or severe).

7. Observe for head bobbing, usually noted in a sleeping or exhausted infant. The infant should be held by the caregiver with head supported on the caregiver's arm at the suboccipital area. The head bobs forward with each inspiration.

8. Observe the child's color. Note the presence and location of cyanosis—peripheral, perioral, facial, and trunk. Note degree of color changes, duration, and association with activity such as crying, feeding, and sleeping.

9. Observe the presence of cough, noting type and duration, such as dry, barking, paroxysmal, or productive. Note any pattern, such as time of day or night, association with activity, physical exertion, or feeding. Severity of croup may be determined by cough and signs of respiratory effort.
   a. Mild croup—occasional barking cough, no audible stridor at rest, and either mild or no suprasternal or intercostal retractions.
   b. Moderate croup—frequent barking cough, easily audible stridor at rest, and suprasternal and sternal retractions at rest, but little or no agitation.
   c. Severe croup—frequent barking cough, prominent inspiratory and occasional expiratory stridor, marked sternal retractions, and agitation and distress.

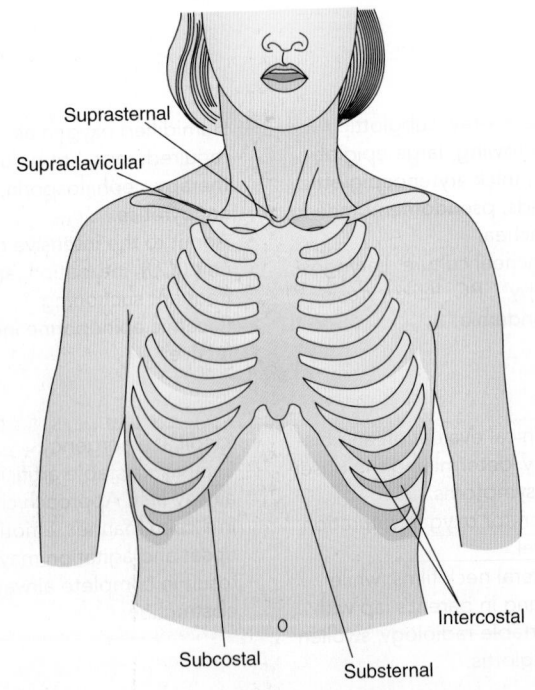

Figure 44-2. Sites of respiratory retractions. (Pillitteri A. [2013]. Maternal and child health nursing: Care of the childbearing and childrearing family [7th ed.]. Philadelphia: Lippincott Williams & Wilkins.)

DIAGNOSTIC EVALUATION	TREATMENT	NURSING CONSIDERATIONS	COMPLICATIONS
• Direct exam or laryngoscopy: large, swollen cherry-red epiglottis, edema of arytenoepiglottic folds. CBC, cultures, IV catheters must be done after intubation.	• Proceed to the operating room or ICU with personnel skilled and equipped to intubate or perform a percutaneous tracheostomy. • Lateral neck films should be done in the operating room or ICU after airway is established. • Antibiotics: intravenous cefotaxime, ceftriaxone, ampicillin with sulbactam. • Supplemental humidified oxygen; mechanical ventilation, if necessary. • If epiglottitis is strongly suspected, examination of the throat is contraindicated; because of reflex laryngospasm, acute airway obstruction, aspiration, and cardiopulmonary arrest during or immediately after examination of the pharynx with a tongue blade. Do not attempt throat culture.	• Equipment for intubation and tracheostomy must remain with the patient at all times. A practitioner skilled in intubation and tracheostomy procedures must accompany the child to the operating room or ICU. After intubation, the child should remain in the ICU with frequent assessment of oxygenation levels and need for mechanical ventilation. Prevent self-extubation; use arm boards or restraints to prevent arm movements, extubation, and death. After intubation, administer sedation, as needed. When the decision is made to extubate the child, emergency tracheostomy and intubation equipment must be at bedside.	

d. Impending respiratory failure—barking cough (often not prominent), audible stridor at rest (may be hard to hear), sternal retractions (may be marked), lethargy or decreased level of consciousness, and often dusky appearance in the absence of supplemental oxygen.

10. Note the presence of sputum, including color, amount, consistency, and frequency.
11. Observe the child's fingernails and toenails for cyanosis and the presence and degree of clubbing, which indicate underlying chronic respiratory disease.
12. Evaluate the child's degree of restlessness, apprehension, level of responsiveness, and muscle tone.
13. Note the presence or complaint of chest pain and its location, whether it is local or generalized, dull or sharp, and associated with respiration or grunting.
14. Assess for signs of infection, such as elevated temperature; enlarged cervical lymph glands; purulent discharge from nose or ears; sputum; or inflamed mucous membranes.

 EVIDENCE BASE Grundfast, K., Insalaco, L., & Levi, J. (2017). The 10 commandments of management of acute upper airway obstruction in infants and children. *JAMA Otoloaryngology, Head and Neck Surgery, 143*(6), 539–540.

Nursing Diagnoses
- Ineffective Airway Clearance related to inflammation, obstruction, secretions, or pain.
- Ineffective Breathing Pattern related to inflammatory process or pain.
- Deficient Fluid Volume related to fever, decreased appetite, and vomiting.
- Fatigue related to increased work of breathing.
- Anxiety related to respiratory distress and hospitalization.
- Parental Role Conflict related to hospitalization of the child.

Nursing Interventions
Promoting Effective Airway Clearance
1. Provide a humidified environment enriched with oxygen to combat hypoxia and to liquefy secretions.
2. Advise the parents to use a jet or ultrasonic nebulizer at home if prescribed and to encourage fluids, as tolerated.
3. Keep nasal passages free of secretions. Infants are obligate nose breathers. Use a bulb syringe to clear nares and oropharynx.

Improving Breathing Pattern
1. Place the child in a comfortable position to promote easier ventilation.
   a. Maintain semi-Fowler position—use infant seat or elevate head of bed.

b. Do not place the infant in prone position. Occasional side or abdominal position will aid drainage of liquefied secretions.

c. Do not position the child in severe respiratory distress in a supine position. Allow the child to assume a position of comfort.

2. Provide measures to improve ventilation of the affected portion of the lung.

   a. Change position frequently.

   b. Provide postural drainage, if prescribed.

   c. Relieve nasal obstruction that contributes to breathing difficulty. Instill normal saline solution or prescribed nose drops and apply nasal suctioning.

   d. Quiet prolonged crying, which can irritate the airway, by soothing the child; however, crying may be an effective way to inflate the lungs.

   e. Realize that coughing is a normal tracheobronchial cleansing procedure, but temporarily relieve coughing by allowing the child to sip water; use extreme caution to prevent aspiration.

   f. Insert a nasogastric tube, as ordered, to relieve abdominal distention, which can limit diaphragmatic excursion.

3. Ensure that the child's oxygen input is not compromised.

   a. Monitor oxygen saturations, as indicated; pulse oximetry should be performed if hypoxia is suspected.

   b. If compressed air or oxygen is to be administered to a small infant, use a method that is best tolerated, monitoring excess carbon dioxide concentrations and increased respiratory rate.

4. Administer appropriate antibiotic or antiviral therapy.

   a. Observe for drug sensitivity.

   b. Observe the child's response to therapy.

5. Administer specific treatment for respiratory syncytial virus (RSV), if ordered.

   a. There is presently no evidence that supports the use of ribavirin or inhaled corticosteroids in acute bronchiolitis; however, some health care providers do consider these options in the management of RSV, especially in high-risk populations such as children who have undergone a stem cell transplant.

6. If the decision is made to initiate ribavirin therapy, appropriate precautions should be implemented to protect personnel and caregivers.

   a. Information about the potential but unknown risk of exposure to ribavirin.

   b. Pregnant women should not provide direct care to patients who are receiving ribavirin therapy. Pregnant women should not enter the patient's room while ribavirin is being administered.

   c. Methods to reduce environmental exposure to ribavirin should be employed:

      i. Stop aerosol administration before opening hood or tent.

      ii. Use room with adequate ventilation of at least six air exchanges per hour. Place the patient in a negative pressure room if indicated by organizational policy.

      iii. Consider the use of scavenger devices to help decrease the escape of ribavirin into the air.

      iv. Gowns and N95 face masks should be used for the duration of the time the nebulizer is in use.

7. For cases of severe respiratory distress, assist with intubation or tracheostomy and mechanical ventilation.

a. Tracheostomy and ET tubes are generally not cuffed for infants and small children because the tube itself is big enough relative to the size of the trachea to act as its own sealer.

b. Position the infant with a tracheostomy with the neck extended by placing a small roll under the shoulders to prevent occlusion of the tube by the chin. Support his or her head and neck carefully when moving the infant to prevent dislodgement of the tube.

c. When feeding, cover the tracheostomy with a moist piece of gauze, or use a bib for older infants or young children.

d. See page 1166 in this chapter as well as Chapter 10 for care of the patient on mechanical ventilation.

EVIDENCE BASE Pascoal, L., Lopes, M., da Silva, V., et al. (2016). Clinical differentiation of respiratory nursing diagnoses among children with acute respiratory infection. *Journal of Pediatric Nursing, 31*(1), 85–91.

Fisk, A.C. (2018). The effects of endotracheal suctioning in the pediatric population: An integrative review. *Dimens Crit Care Nurs*, Jan/Feb, 37(1), 44–56.

NURSING ALERT Infants with a history of very low birth weight and bronchopulmonary dysplasia have chronic, compensated carbon dioxide retention. Careful attention must be given to oxygen administration to avoid respiratory depression by suppressing their hypoxic drive.

Promoting Adequate Hydration

1. Administer fluids via intravenous (IV) route at the prescribed rate.

2. To prevent aspiration, withhold oral food and fluids if the child is in severe respiratory distress.

3. Offer the child small sips of clear fluid when respiratory status improves.

   a. Note any vomiting or abdominal distention after the oral fluid is given.

   b. As the child begins to take more fluid by mouth, notify the health care provider and modify the IV fluid rate to prevent fluid overload.

   c. Do not force the child to take fluids orally as this may cause increased distress and possibly vomiting. Anorexia will subside as the condition improves.

4. Assist in the control of fever to reduce respiratory rate and fluid loss.

   a. Give antipyretics, as prescribed.

5. Record the child's intake and output and monitor urine-specific gravity.

6. Provide mouth care or offer mouth rinse if child is able to perform this safely.

Promoting Adequate Rest

1. Disturb the child as little as possible by organizing nursing care, and protect the child from unnecessary interruptions.

2. Be aware of the age of the child and be familiar with the level of growth and development as it applies to hospitalization.

3. Encourage the parents to stay with the child as much as possible to provide comfort and security.

4. Provide opportunities for quiet play as the child's condition improves.

Reducing Anxiety

1. Explain procedures and hospital routine to the child as appropriate for age.
2. Provide a quiet, stress-free environment.
3. Observe the child's response to the oxygen therapy environment such as a mist tent or head box and provide reassurance.
   a. The child may experience fear of confinement or suffocation.
   b. Vision is distorted through the plastic.
   c. The environment is noisy and damp.
   d. Physical and diversional activities are restricted.
   e. Parental contact is decreased.
   f. The environment is often uncomfortable.
4. Avoid the use of sedatives and opiates, which may obscure restlessness. Restlessness may be a sign of increasing respiratory distress or obstruction.
5. Allow the child to assume a position of comfort.

Strengthening the Parents' Role

1. Help the parents understand the purpose of the oxygen therapy/humidifier and how to work with it.
2. Discuss their fears and concerns about the child's therapy.
3. Include the parents in planning for the child's care. Promote their participation in caring for the child.
4. Recognize that the parents will need rest periods. Encourage them to take breaks and eat on a regular basis.

Family Education and Health Maintenance

1. Teach the importance of good hygiene. Include information on hand washing and appropriate ways to handle respiratory secretions at home.
2. Teach the family when it is appropriate to keep the child home from school (any fever, coughing up secretions, and significant runny nose in toddler or younger child).
3. Teach methods to keep the ill child well hydrated.
   a. Provide small amounts of fluids frequently.
   b. Offer clear liquids and prepared electrolyte preparations.
   c. Offer frozen juice pops.
   d. Avoid juices with a high sugar content.
4. Teach ways to assess the child's hydration status at home.
   a. Decreased number of wet diapers or number of times the child urinates per day.
   b. Decreased activity level.
   c. Dry lips and mucous membranes.
   d. No tears when the child cries.
5. Teach the parents when to contact their health care provider—signs of respiratory distress, recurrent fever, decreased appetite and activity, and signs of dehydration.
6. Teach about medications and follow-up.
7. If a tracheostomy was required, teach care of the tracheostomy, use of equipment, safety, and referral for home nursing care before discharge.

Evaluation: Expected Outcomes

- Breath sounds clear and equal.
- Easy, regular, unlabored respirations on room air (or back to baseline if the child is on oxygen).
- Mucous membranes moist; urine output adequate.
- Bathing and feeding tolerated well.
- Child calm and interacts appropriately with family and staff.
- Parents participate in the child's care.

Disorders Requiring Surgery of the Tonsils and Adenoids

 EVIDENCE BASE Kenney, K., & Gropman, R. (2013). What immediate post-operative nursing care contributes to a better patient outcome after a child has had a day surgery tonsillectomy and adenoidectomy (T and A)? *Journal of Perianesthesia Nursing, 28*(3), e44.

Tonsillectomy and *adenoidectomy* are the surgical removal of the adenoidal and tonsillar structures, part of the lymphoid tissue that encircles the pharynx. These are one of the most frequently performed surgical procedures in the child. The most common disease processes that require tonsillectomy and adenoidectomy are obstructive sleep apnea; chronic, persistent tonsillitis or adenoiditis; and chronic persistent otitis media.

Pathophysiology and Etiology

Function of Tonsils and Adenoids

1. They are a first line of defense against respiratory infections.
2. Because the growth of the tonsils and adenoids in the first 10 years of life exceeds general somatic growth, these structures are proportionally larger in the child.
3. The natural process of involution of tonsillar and adenoidal lymphoid tissue in the prepubertal years is associated with decreased frequency of throat and ear infections.

Obstructive Sleep Apnea

1. Adenotonsillar hypertrophy causes airway obstruction, leading to persistent hypoventilation during sleep.
2. Peak incidence in children is between ages 3 and 6 years.
3. Incidence is increased in children with Down syndrome.

Tonsillitis and Adenoiditis

1. In tonsillitis and adenoiditis, structures that are already large become inflamed because of an infectious agent and cause airway obstruction, decreased appetite, and pain.
2. Infection may be caused by bacterial or viral organisms, with viral organisms most commonly implicated.
3. Group A beta-hemolytic *Streptococcus* is the most common bacterial cause.
4. Enlarged adenoids may block nasal passages, resulting in persistent mouth breathing.
5. Chronic adenoiditis without tonsillitis is typically seen in children younger than in age 4 years.

Otitis Media

1. Bacterial infection caused most commonly by *Streptococcus pneumoniae* or *Haemophilus influenzae*.
2. Chronic infection may be associated with enlarged adenoids that block drainage from the eustachian tubes.

Clinical Manifestations

Obstructive Sleep Apnea

1. Loud snoring or noisy breathing in sleep.
2. Excessive daytime sleepiness.
3. Mouth breathing.

Chronic Infection of Tonsils and Adenoids

1. Mouth breathing or difficulty breathing.
2. Frequent sore throat.
3. Anorexia, decreased growth velocity.
4. Fever.

5. Obstruction to swallowing or breathing.
6. Nasal, muffled voice.
7. Night cough.
8. Offensive breath.

Chronic Otitis Media
1. Ear pain or general irritability in young children.
2. Alterations in hearing.
3. Fever.
4. Enlarged lymph nodes.
5. Anorexia.

Diagnostic Evaluation
1. Thorough ear, nose, and throat examination and appropriate cultures to determine presence and source of infection.
2. Preoperative blood studies to determine risk of bleeding—clotting time, smear for platelets, prothrombin time, and partial thromboplastin time.

Management
Appropriate antibiotics are given, and the decision is made to perform surgery. Tonsillectomy and adenoidectomy may be performed together or separately. Debate continues over indications for and benefits of surgery.

Indications for Tonsillectomy
1. Conservative.
   a. Recurrent or persistent tonsillitis. The widely accepted criteria for surgery are seven episodes of tonsillitis in the previous 12 months or five episodes in each of the preceding 2 years.
   b. Marked hypertrophy of tonsils, which distorts speech, causes swallowing difficulties, and causes subsequent weight loss.
   c. Tonsillar malignancy.
   d. Diphtheria carrier.
   e. Cor pulmonale due to obstruction.
2. Controversial.
   a. Peritonsillar abscess or retrotonsillar abscess.
   b. Suppurative cervical adenitis with tonsillar focus.
   c. Persistent hyperemia of anterior pillars.
   d. Enlarged cervical lymph nodes.

Indications for Adenoidectomy
1. Conservative.
   a. Adenoid hypertrophy resulting in obstruction of airway, leading to hypoxia, pulmonary hypertension, and cor pulmonale.
   b. Hypertrophy with nasal obstruction accompanied by breathing difficulty and severe speech distortion.
   c. Hypertrophy associated with chronic suppurative or serous otitis media and sensorineural or conductive hearing loss, chronic mastoiditis, or cholesteatoma.
   d. Mouth breathing due to hypertrophied adenoids.
2. Controversial.
   a. Enlarged adenoids.
   b. Chronic otitis media and no evidence of complications.
   c. Child younger than age 4 years, unless life-threatening situation.

Contraindications to Surgery
1. Bleeding or coagulation disorders.
2. Uncontrolled systemic disorders (eg, diabetes, rheumatic fever, cardiac or renal disease).

3. Presence of upper respiratory infection in the child or immediate family.
4. Specific for adenoidectomy—certain palate abnormalities (ie, cleft palate or submucous cleft palate).

Complications
1. If untreated, obstructive sleep apnea in the child may result in pulmonary hypertension, cor pulmonale, failure to thrive, respiratory failure, attention-deficit disorders, and cardiac arrhythmias.
2. Untreated chronic tonsillitis may result in failure to thrive, peritonsillar or retropharyngeal abscess, difficulty swallowing, and poor eating.
3. Untreated chronic otitis media may result in hearing loss, scarring of the eardrum (tympanosclerosis), mastoiditis, and meningitis.
4. Complications of surgery include hemorrhage, reactions to anesthesia, otitis media, and bacteremia.

Nursing Assessment

Preoperative Assessment
1. Assess the child's developmental level.
2. Assess the parents' and child's understanding of the surgical procedure.
3. Assess psychological preparation of the child for hospitalization and surgery.
   a. Does the child understand what will happen?
   b. Do the parents know the importance of telling the child the truth, and do they have a good understanding of the procedure?
   c. Does the child have preconceived ideas that may pose a threat?
4. Obtain thorough nursing history from the child and parents to gather any pertinent information that would impact the child's care.
   a. Has the child had a recent infection? It is desirable for the child to be free of respiratory infection for at least 2 weeks.
   b. Has the child recently been exposed to any communicable diseases?
   c. Does the child have any loose teeth that may pose the threat of aspiration?
   d. Are there any bleeding tendencies in the child or family?
   e. Are there any family members with a history of adverse reactions to anesthesia?
5. Obtain the child's baseline vital signs along with his or her height and weight.
6. Assess the child's hydration status.

 NURSING ALERT The preschool child is especially vulnerable to psychological trauma as a result of surgical procedures or hospitalization.

Postoperative Assessment
1. Assess respiratory status and pain often.
2. Assess frequently for signs of postoperative bleeding; monitor vital signs, as warranted.
3. Assess oral intake.
4. Assess for indications of negative psychological sequelae related to the surgery and hospitalization.

Nursing Diagnoses

- Fear related to painful procedure, unfamiliar environment.
- Anxiety of the parents related to concept of surgery.
- Risk for Deficient Fluid Volume related to reduced intake post-operatively and blood loss.
- Ineffective Airway Clearance related to pain and effects of anesthesia.
- Acute Pain related to surgical incision.

Nursing Interventions

Reducing Fear

1. Prepare the child and parents by encouraging participation in hospital tours and preadmission programs specifically for children.
2. Share information with the child, commensurate with their development stage and cognitive ability, as well as the family.
3. Prepare the child specifically for what to expect postoperatively, using techniques appropriate to the child's developmental level (books, dolls, drawings). Include the following:
   a. Where the child will wake up.
   b. Temporary sore throat, emesis of blood, position, and foul taste and smell in mouth.
   c. Medications.
   d. Fluid regimen and possible IV infusion.
4. Talk to the child about the new things to be seen in the operating room and clear up any misconceptions. Whenever possible, allow the child to see, touch, and examine equipment, such as thermometers, beds, tubings, and suction equipment.
5. Where available, involve the play specialist in the preparation.

Relieving Parental Anxiety

1. Help the parents prepare the child by talking at first in general terms about surgery and progressing to more specific information.
2. Reassure the parents that complication rates are low and that recovery is usually swift.
3. Encourage the parents to stay with the child and help provide care.

Maintaining Adequate Fluid Volume

1. Assess the child frequently for postoperative bleeding. Check all secretions and emesis for the presence of fresh blood. These are indications of hemorrhage:
   a. Increased pulse.
   b. Frequent swallowing while awake and asleep.
   c. Pallor.
   d. Restlessness.
   e. Clearing of throat and vomiting of blood.
   f. Continuous slight oozing of blood over a number of hours.
   g. Oozing of blood in back of throat.
2. Have suction equipment, oxygen, and packing material readily available in case of emergency.
3. Provide adequate fluid intake.
   a. Give ice cubes 1 to 2 hours after awakening from anesthesia.
   b. When vomiting has ceased, cautiously advance to clear liquids.
   c. Offer cool fruit juices without pulp at first because they are best tolerated, avoid fluids that are red or purple in color; then offer ice pops and cool water for the first 12 to 24 hours. Avoid red and brown fluids.
   d. There is some debate regarding the intake of milk and ice cream the evening of surgery. It can be soothing and can reduce swelling; however, it coats the mouth and throat,

causing the child to clear the throat more often, which may initiate bleeding.

 NURSING ALERT Notify the surgeon immediately if bleeding is suspected.

Promoting Effective Airway Clearance

1. Assist the child in maintaining a patent airway by draining secretions and preventing aspiration of vomitus.
2. Assess the child for signs and symptoms of airway obstruction and respiratory distress (stridor, drooling, restlessness, agitation, tachypnea, and cyanosis), which may result from edema or the accumulation of secretions.
   a. Place the child prone or semiprone with his or her head turned to side while still under the effects of anesthesia.
   b. Allow the child to assume a position of comfort when alert. (The parent may hold the child.)
   c. The child may vomit old blood initially. If suctioning is necessary, avoid trauma to the oropharynx.
   d. Remind the child not to cough, clear throat, or blow nose.

Improving Comfort

1. Give analgesics, as ordered, parenteral or rectally.
2. Rinse the child's mouth with cool water or alkaline solution.
3. Keep the child and environment free from blood-tinged drainage to help decrease anxiety.
4. Encourage the parents to be with the child when the child awakens.
5. When the parents must leave, reassure the child that they will return.

Family Education and Health Maintenance

1. Explain and write instructions concerning the care of the child at home after discharge.
   a. Diet should still consist of large amounts of fluids and soft, cool, nonirritating foods. (Supply a list of suggestions for the family.)
   b. Eating helps promote healing because it increases the blood supply to the tissues.
   c. Bed rest should be maintained for 1 to 2 days and then daily rest periods for about 1 week. Resume normal eating and activities within 2 weeks after surgery.
   d. Avoid contact with people with infections.
   e. Discourage the child from blowing nose and frequent coughing and clearing of his or her throat.
   f. Avoid gargling. Mouth odor may be present for a few days after surgery; only mouth rinsing is acceptable.
   g. Discourage use of red dye–enhanced foods or analgesics if possible—can be difficult to differentiate from bleeding.
2. Advise the parents to call the health care provider if the following occur. (Ensure that the parents have the phone numbers of the health care provider and hospital emergency department.)
   a. Earache accompanied by fever.
   b. Any bleeding, often indicated only by frequent swallowing; most common between the 5th and 10th postoperative days when membrane sloughs from surgical site.
3. Teach about medications prescribed or suggested for pain relief.
4. Discuss with the parents what results they can expect from the surgery.
   a. Decreased number of sore throats.
   b. Lessened evidence of obstructive symptoms.

c. Decreased incidence of cervical lymphadenitis.
d. Improvement in nutritional status.
e. No improvement in nasal allergies.
f. No improvement in secretory otitis media.

5. Guide the parents in helping the child think of the experience as a positive one after the surgery is over, to make subsequent health care experiences easier.
   a. Talk about what happened and the positive outcomes.
   b. Let the child play out his or her feelings.

Evaluation: Expected Outcomes

- Acts out surgery with dolls, asks questions.
- Parents interact with the child, ask appropriate questions.
- Takes fluids well; no signs of bleeding.
- No vomiting; breathing without difficulty.
- Verbalizes reduced pain.

Asthma

Asthma is a chronic, inflammatory disease of the airways, characterized by airflow obstruction, bronchial hyperreactivity, and increased mucus production. The course of asthma is highly variable. Many cells and mediators play a role, including mast cells, eosinophils, neutrophils, and epithelial cells. Classic signs and symptoms include cough, wheezing, shortness of breath/dyspnea, and chest tightness. Children may also report stomach pain when they are experiencing an asthma exacerbation. The Global Initiative for Asthma (GINA) guidelines (2017), published by the World Health Organization, and the National Asthma Education and Prevention Program of the National Institutes of Health provide evidence-based categorization, treatment, and ongoing control information.

Assessment of Asthma Control

1. Although severity is best evaluated prior to the use of asthma medications, it can be established based on the medications necessary to gain control and direct initial therapy.
2. Two domains of asthma control are assessed at each encounter: risk and impairment.
   a. Risk is measured by exacerbations.
   b. Impairment is determined both on initial diagnosis and ongoing assessment.
3. Factors that affect impairment include the following:
   a. Day and nighttime asthma symptoms.
   b. Use of quick-relief medication.
   c. Pulmonary function tests/peak flow measurements if the child is capable.
   d. Limitations of daily activities.
   e. Adverse effects of medications.
   f. Progression of lung disease.
4. Several validated tools are available for patients aged 12 years and older to complete, including the Asthma Control Test, Asthma Control Questionnaire, and Asthma Therapy Assessment Questionnaire.
   a. These tools quantify symptoms, quick-relief medication usage, effect of asthma on quality of life, and patient/family perception of control.
   b. To assist in the diagnosis of asthma, particularly in very small children who cannot perform lung function tests, an asthma predictive index can help identify children likely to have asthma.

 NURSING ALERT Level of control guides adjustment of medications, and nurses can use this assessment to identify patients/families who need more asthma education for better gain control of asthma.

 EVIDENCE BASE Johnson, D. P., Arnold, D. H., Gay, J. C., et al. (2018). Implementation and improvement of pediatric asthma guideline improves hospital-based care. *Pediatrics, 141*(2), 1–9.

Variations of Asthma

Cough Variant Asthma
Cough variant asthma is typically seen in children, where cough (especially at night) is the principal symptom. The child may never wheeze. Although the symptoms are chronic and commonly mild in many children, severe exacerbations (attacks) may arise, even resulting in respiratory failure and death.

Exercise-Induced Bronchospasm
Exercise-induced bronchospasm refers to symptoms of cough, shortness of breath, chest pain, tightness, wheezing, and endurance problems during or after vigorous activity. Typically, symptoms begin during exercise and peak 5 to 10 minutes after stopping; they may resolve spontaneously within 20 to 30 minutes. Diagnosis is confirmed by documenting a decrease in peak expiratory flow (PEF) or forced expiratory volume in 1 second (FEV_1), before and after exercise and at 5-minute intervals for 20 to 30 minutes. This condition may occur without chronic asthma and has a different pathophysiology from asthma that is triggered by exercise. The preferred treatment consists of short-acting beta-2 agonists, taken 15 minutes prior to exercise. Cromolyn sodium, available only for a nebulizer, is an alternative, although less effective.

Factors that Increase Risk of Asthma Death

 EVIDENCE BASE Kim, C. K., Callawayc Z., & Gern, J. E. (2018). Viral infections and associated factors that promote acute exacerbations of asthma. *Allergy Asthma Immunol Res, 10*(1),12–17.

Global Initiative for Asthma. (2017). Pocket guide for asthma management and prevention. Available: www.ginasthma.org.

1. Previous severe exacerbation (intubation or intensive care admission).
2. Hospitalization two or more times within the year, three or more emergency department (ED) visits in the last year.
3. Use of more than two canisters per month of short-acting beta-adrenergic (SABA).
4. Difficulty perceiving airway obstruction or the severity of worsening asthma.
5. Low socioeconomic status or inner-city residence.
6. Illicit drug use.
7. Major psychological problems or psychiatric disease.
8. Comorbidity, such as cardiovascular disease or other chronic lung disease.
9. Other factors, lack of asthma action plan, sensitivity to *Alternaria*.

Management

The Stepwise Approach to Managing Asthma, developed by the EPR 3, identifies classifications of asthma according to symptoms and suggests pharmacologic options for the control of asthma. Medications may be "stepped up or down" depending on the patient's response to therapy. See Table 44-2 and Table 44-3, page 1184, for the recommended management of asthma for infants and children age 0 to 4 and 5 to 12 years. See page 801 for the management of older children with asthma.

For additional information on treatment and specific dosages, see Expert Panel Report 3: Guidelines for the Diagnosis and Management of Asthma, National Heart, Lung and Blood Institute, National Asthma Education and Prevention

Table 44-2 Stepwise Approach for Managing Asthma in Children 0–4 Years of Age

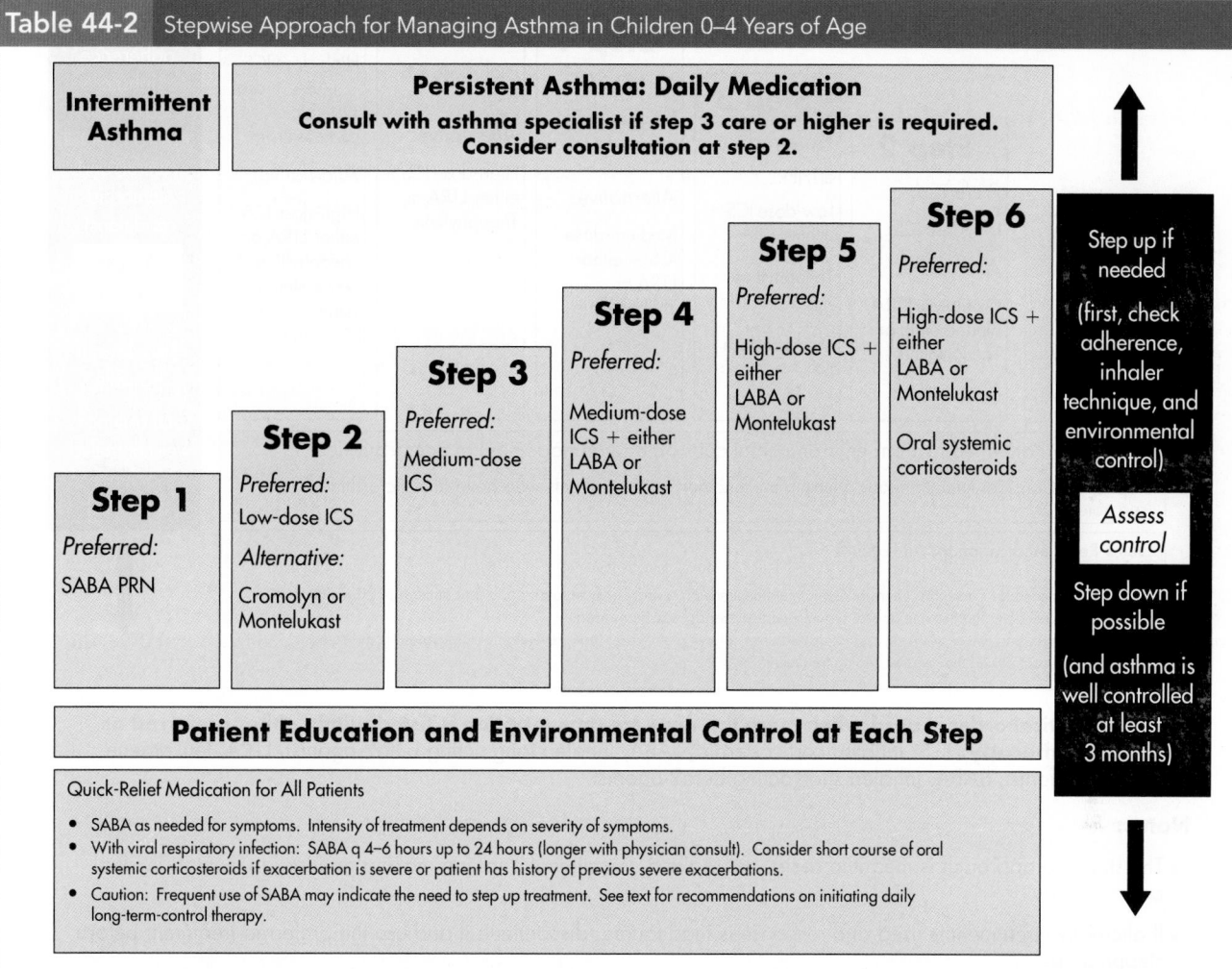

Key: **Alphabetical order is used when more than one treatment option is listed within either preferred or alternative therapy.** ICS, inhaled corticosteroid; LABA, inhaled long-acting beta2-agonist; SABA, inhaled short-acting beta2-agonist.

Notes:

■ The stepwise approach is meant to assist, not replace, the clinical decisionmaking required to meet individual patient needs.

■ If alternative treatment is used and response is inadequate, discontinue it and use the preferred treatment before stepping up.

■ If clear benefit is not observed within 4–6 weeks and patient/family medication technique and adherence are satisfactory, consider adjusting therapy or alternative diagnosis.

■ Studies on children 0–4 years of age are limited. Step 2 preferred therapy is based on Evidence A. All other recommendations are based on expert opinion and extrapolation from studies in older children.

From National Heart, Lung and Blood Institute, National Asthma Education and Prevention Program. (2007). Expert panel report 3: Guidelines for the diagnosis and management of asthma (p. 305). Available: *www.nhlbi.nih.gov/guidelines/asthma/asthgdln.pdf.*

Table 44-3 Stepwise Approach for Managing Asthma in Children 5–11 Years of Age

Intermittent Asthma	Persistent Asthma: Daily Medication Consult with asthma specialist if step 4 care or higher is required. Consider consultation at step 3.

Step 1

Preferred:

SABA PRN

Step 2

Preferred:

Low-dose ICS

Alternative:

Cromolyn, LTRA, Nedocromil, or Theophylline

Step 3

Preferred:

EITHER:

Low-dose ICS + either LABA, LTRA, or Theophylline

OR

Medium-dose ICS

Step 4

Preferred:

Medium-dose ICS + LABA

Alternative:

Medium-dose ICS + either LTRA or Theophylline

Step 5

Preferred:

High-dose ICS + LABA

Alternative:

High-dose ICS + either LTRA or Theophylline

Step 6

Preferred:

High-dose ICS + LABA + oral systemic corticosteroid

Alternative:

High-dose ICS + either LTRA or Theophylline+ oral systemic corticosteroid

Step up if needed

(first, check adherence, inhaler technique, environmental control, and comorbid conditions)

Assess control

Step down if possible

(and asthma is well controlled at least 3 months)

Each step: Patient education, environmental control, and management of comorbidities.

Steps 2–4: Consider subcutaneous allergen immunotherapy for patients who have allergic asthma (see notes).

Quick-Relief Medication for All Patients

- SABA as needed for symptoms. Intensity of treatment depends on severity of symptoms: up to 3 treatments at 20-minute intervals as needed. Short course of oral systemic corticosteroids may be needed.
- Caution: Increasing use of SABA or use >2 days a week for symptom relief (not prevention of EIB) generally indicates inadequate control and the need to step up treatment.

Key: Alphabetical order is used when more than one treatment option is listed within either preferred or alternative therapy. ICS, inhaled corticosteroid; LABA, inhaled long-acting beta2-agonist, LTRA, leukotriene receptor antagonist; SABA, inhaled short-acting beta2-agonist.

Notes:

- The stepwise approach is meant to assist, not replace, the clinical decision making required to meet individual patient needs.

- If alternative treatment is used and response is inadequate, discontinue it and use the preferred treatment before stepping up.

- Theophylline is a less desirable alternative due to the need to monitor serum concentration levels.

- Step 1 and step 2 medications are based on Evidence A. Step 3 ICS + adjunctive therapy and ICS are based on Evidence B for efficacy of each treatment and extrapolation from comparator trials in older children and adults—comparator trials are not available for this age group; steps 4–6 are based on expert opinion and extrapolation from studies in older children and adults.

- Immunotherapy for steps 2–4 is based on Evidence B for house-dust mites, animal danders, and pollens; evidence is weak or lacking for molds and cockroaches. Evidence is strongest for immunotherapy with single allergens. The role of allergy in asthma is greater in children than in adults. Clinicians who administer immunotherapy should be prepared and equipped to identify and treat anaphylaxis that may occur.

Program, Full Report, NIH Publication No. 08-4051, 2007. Available: *www.nhlbi.nih.gov/guidelines/asthma/asthgdln.pdf.*

Acute Exacerbation

1. Be alert for severe asthma exacerbation. Exacerbations may be associated with viral respiratory infections.
2. In a severe exacerbation, the child is short of breath, may be audibly wheezing with a prolonged expiratory phase, restless, apprehensive, anxious, diaphoretic, and tachycardic; color may be pale or flushed and lips may be dark red or cyanotic.
   a. There are signs of respiratory distress, such as nasal flaring, use of accessory muscles, retractions, one- to two-word dyspnea (speaking in short phrases), tachypnea, hypoxemia, and respiratory alkalosis progressing to respiratory acidosis.
   b. Breath sounds may be decreased and there may be decreased level of consciousness.
   c. A young child will assume tripod position; an older child will sit upright with shoulders hunched.
3. Signs of respiratory distress in infants include use of accessory muscles, inspiratory and expiratory wheezing, paradoxical breathing, cyanosis, respiratory rate greater than 60, and oxygen saturation less than 90%. These infants are at greater risk of respiratory failure.
4. The goals of emergency management are to quickly reverse airflow obstruction, to correct hypoxemia, and to reduce the likelihood of recurrence.
5. Assess PEF rate or FEV_1 upon arrival; assess degree of respiratory distress or fatigue.
6. Obtain an oxygen saturation level by pulse oximetry.
7. Obtain arterial or capillary blood gas levels in infants with an oxygen saturation of 90% or less and in a child with moderate to severe respiratory distress.
8. Deliver humidified oxygen via nasal cannula, hood, or face mask at lowest level necessary to maintain adequate oxygenation. Obtain a brief history and physical and focus on prior treatment and possible triggers of the episode, such as respiratory infection or lack of medication.
9. Administer emergency treatment, as indicated.
   a. SABA with ipratropium, either by nebulization or by MDI with spacer (with face mask in young child).
   b. Systemic corticosteroids should be administered early in treatment.
   c. Adjunctive treatments include IV leukotriene modifiers, heliox, and magnesium sulfate.
   d. Antibiotics are generally not used unless there is evidence of bacterial infection.
10. Hospitalized patients will need frequent assessment, repeat or continuous SABA treatments, corticosteroids, and treatment of any comorbid condition, such as sinusitis.
11. Discharge planning for patients with exacerbations should include an action plan for medications, recognition and treatment of acute asthma, and plans for follow-up.
12. Children in severe status asthmaticus unresponsive to the above therapy may require the following:
    a. Intubation and mechanical ventilation with 100% oxygen for impending or actual respiratory distress, decreased mental alertness, increased fatigue, or partial pressure of arterial carbon dioxide ($Paco_2$) greater than or equal to 42 mm Hg.
    b. Nebulized beta-2 agonist, hourly or continuously.
    c. Anticholinergic such as ipratropium, although generally limited to the emergency department.
    d. IV corticosteroid therapy.
    e. Admission to ICU.

f. Pharmacologic paralysis to ventilate effectively.
g. Cardiopulmonary monitoring of the child's response to treatment.
h. Placement of an arterial line for blood monitoring.

13. Therapies not recommended for treating an exacerbation, based on the 2007 National Heart, Lung, and Blood Institute Expert Panel Report:
    a. Subcutaneous beta-2 agonist provides no advantage over inhaled medication.
    b. Theophylline or aminophylline therapy is not recommended in the ED. It does not provide additional benefit to short-acting beta-2 agonists; it may produce adverse effects.
    c. Chest physiotherapy (CPT) and mucolytics.
    d. Antibiotics are not recommended for asthma treatment. However, antibiotics may be needed in patients with fever, purulent sputum, and evidence of bacterial pneumonia.
    e. Anxiolytic and hypnotic drugs are contraindicated.
    f. Aggressive hydration is not recommended in older children. Assess fluid status; make corrections, as needed, for infants and young children to decrease risk of dehydration.

 NURSING ALERT Cyanosis of the lips and nail beds is an ominous sign.

 NURSING ALERT Absence of wheezing with decreased breath sounds and inability to blow a PEF indicates minimal air exchange. This situation requires immediate, swift attention to prevent respiratory failure. Respiratory failure tends to progress quickly and is difficult to reverse.

 TRANSITIONAL CARE ALERT To prevent readmission for acute asthma exacerbation in the transitional period from hospitalization to outpatient/community care, strategies prior to discharge should target medication adherence and parental knowledge of asthma. Compliance with treatment plan has been cited as the most important factor in preventing readmission.

 EVIDENCE BASE Hewner, S., Sullivan. S. & Yu, G. (2018). Reducing Emergency Room Visits and Inpatient Hospitalizations by Implementing Best Practice for Transitional Care Using Innovative Technology and Big Data. *Worldviews Evidence Based Nursing,* 23, [epub ahead of print].

Long-Term Management

1. As the child becomes stabilized, begin to develop a home and school management plan. Components of the plan should include the following:
   a. The use of quick-relief medications (SABA); expected effect and side effects.
   b. The use of long-term controllers, which include corticosteroids, leukotriene modifiers, mast cell stabilizers, and long-acting beta agonists (LABA). See page 802 for mechanism and adverse reactions. Note: LABA should only be prescribed if poor control with other medications due to increased risk of asthma-related deaths.

Figure 44-3. Multidose inhaler use with spacers.

Figure 44-4. Peak flow monitoring.

c. Inhalation technique with nebulizer or multidose inhaler with spacer (see Figure 44-3).
d. Peak flow and symptom monitoring.
e. Use of PEF zone system, if indicated (see below).
f. Identification of triggers (eg, exercise, weather change, infection, allergen exposure [pollen, mold, dust mite, animal dander, cockroach or mouse exposure]).
g. Environmental control by removal of suspected stimuli.
h. Hydration, nutrition, rest, and exercise regimens.
i. Emergency action plans.

2. Plan a team conference involving the child, parents, school nurse, and teacher, if possible. Ideally, the plan should be clear and easy for the child and family to follow, adapted to their lifestyle, and using the least amount of medications necessary to control and prevent the child's asthma symptoms. A written action plan should be submitted to the school, including information on medications (possible self-medication by the adolescent), identified triggers, steps in an emergency plan, and emergency contact information. Emergency action plans may need to include multiple family caregivers, and residences. An example of this form can be found at *https://www.nhlbi.nih.gov/files/docs/public/lung/asthma_actplan.pdf*. Stress that, without exception, no smoking should be permitted in the home or car of a child with asthma. Even if the child is out of the home, the residual odor will cause symptoms. Opening windows or using sprays and air cleaners are not acceptable alternatives.

3. Encourage the parents to pay particular attention to environmental control in the child's bedroom, including elimination of dust, not allowing any pets, and avoidance of any strong smells or sprays. If using wood stoves in the home, find out if there is an alternative source of heat.

4. Obtain more information from the National Asthma Education Program (*https://www.nhlbi.nih.gov/science/national-asthma-education-and-prevention-program-naepp*) the American Academy of Allergy, Asthma and Immunology (*www.aaaai.org*), or the American Lung Association (*http://lung.org/*).

Peak Expiratory Flow Monitoring and the Zone System

1. Teach the family and child about PEF monitoring at home as well as other important indicators, as directed (see Figure 44-4).
   a. PEF monitoring is not emphasized as much in current guidelines as in the past.
   b. Other indicators of severity include symptom assessment, need for medication, and measures of control such as the asthma control questionnaire.

2. A PEF meter measures the PEF rate that can be produced during a forced expiration. It measures airflow through the large airways; the result is effort dependent. PEF measurements can be initiated in children as young as age 5. Given time and practice, consistent readings will be produced. (See page 805 for directions on use of PEF meter.)

3. A table of predicted PEF values should be included in the packaging of the home PEF meter. These values are based on age and height. A few patients may find their readings above or below the published values. Therefore, each child should establish a personal best PEF value. Ideally, this should be implemented during a time when the child is symptom free. If PEF readings are consistently below predicted values, the health care provider should be contacted and additional medications may be necessary.

4. Use of the PEF zone system along with a home asthma management plan can assist families in the proper use of medications, and assists in decision making regarding the degree of airflow obstruction. After the personal best PEF value is identified, teach the patient that subsequent PEF measurements can be classified into three zones that will dictate a home management plan.
   a. Green Zone = 80% to 100% of personal best. No asthma symptoms are present. Continue usual medications.
   b. Yellow Zone = 50% to less than 79% of personal best. Signals caution. May be experiencing an asthma episode or day-to-day control is suboptimal. Need to use short-acting inhaled beta-2 agonist, follow emergency plan, and contact health care provider for further instructions.
   c. Red Zone = less than 50% of personal best value. This zone signals danger. Must take a short-acting inhaled beta-2 agonist immediately and, if PEF does not return to yellow or green zone, contact health care provider or proceed to the ED immediately.

Respiratory Distress Syndrome (Hyaline Membrane Disease)

Respiratory distress syndrome (RDS), formerly known as hyaline membrane disease, is a syndrome of premature neonates that is characterized by progressive and usually fatal respiratory failure resulting from atelectasis and immaturity of the lungs. RDS occurs most commonly in premature neonates (primarily weighing between 1,000 and 1,500 g) and between 28 and 37 weeks' gestation. In neonates 26 to 28 weeks' gestation, the incidence is 50% to 70% and increases with degree of prematurity. RDS can be fatal; those who survive are at risk for chronic respiratory and neurologic complications.

Pathophysiology and Etiology

1. Adequate pulmonary function at birth depends on the following:
   a. An adequate amount of surfactant (a lipoprotein mixture) lining the alveolar cells, which allows for alveolar stability and prevents alveolar collapse at the end of expiration.
   b. An adequate surface area in air spaces to allow for gas exchange (ie, sufficient pulmonary capillary bed in contact with this alveolar surface area).
2. RDS is ultimately the result of decreased pulmonary surfactant, incomplete structural development of lung, and a highly compliant chest wall.
3. Contributing factors are any factor that decreases surfactant, such as the following:
   a. Prematurity and immature alveolar lining cells.
   b. Acidosis.
   c. Hypothermia.
   d. Hypoxia.
   e. Hypovolemia.
   f. Diabetes.
   g. Elective cesarean delivery.
   h. Fetal or intrapartum stress that compromises blood supply to fetal lungs: vaginal bleeding, maternal hypertension, difficult resuscitation associated with birth asphyxia. (Some situations, such as steroid therapy or a heroin-addicted mother, result in the acceleration of surfactant.)
   i. RDS due to nonpulmonary factors such as cardiac defects, sepsis, airway obstruction, intraventricular hemorrhage, hypoglycemia, and acute blood loss.
4. Surfactant production is deficient by type II alveolar cells. (Although some surfactant may be present at birth, it may not be regenerated at an adequate rate.) Surfactant production may be reduced because of the following:
   a. Extreme immaturity of alveolar lining cells.
   b. Diminished or impaired production rate resulting from fetal or early neonatal stress.
   c. Impairment of release mechanism for phospholipid from type II alveolar cells.
   d. Death of many of these cells responsible for decreased surfactant production.
5. Intra-alveolar surface tension is increased, and alveoli are unstable and collapse at the end of expiration. Functional reserve capacity—the amount of air left in the lungs after expiration—is decreased; thus, the next breath requires almost as much effort as the first breath after birth.
6. More oxygen and energy are required to expand the alveoli with each breath, causing fatigue.
7. The number of alveoli that expand progressively decreases, leading to alveolar instability and atelectasis.
8. Pulmonary vascular resistance increases, causing hypoperfusion of lung.
9. Persistence of fetal circulation right-to-left shunt results, leading to hypoxemia and hypercapnia, which lead to respiratory and metabolic acidosis.

10. Hypoxemia and pulmonary vascular pressure cause ischemia in the alveoli, leading to transudate in the alveoli and formation of a membranous layer (see Figure 44-5).
11. Gas exchange becomes inhibited. Lungs become stiff (decreased compliance), requiring more pressure to expand them.
12. Airway obstruction leads to increased hypoxia and vasoconstriction, and the cycle continues.
13. RDS is usually a self-limiting disease and symptoms peak in about 3 to 4 days, at which time surfactant synthesis begins to accelerate and pulmonary function and clinical appearance begin to improve.
    a. Moderately ill infants or those who do not require assisted ventilation usually show slow improvement by about 48 hours and rapid recovery over 3 to 4 days with few complications.
    b. Severely ill and very immature infants who require some ventilatory assistance usually demonstrate rapid deterioration, such as decreased cardiac inflow, decreased arterial pressure, apneic episodes, cyanosis, pallor, and flaccid, unresponsive shocklike state. Ventilatory assistance may be required for several days, and chronic lung disease and other complications are common.

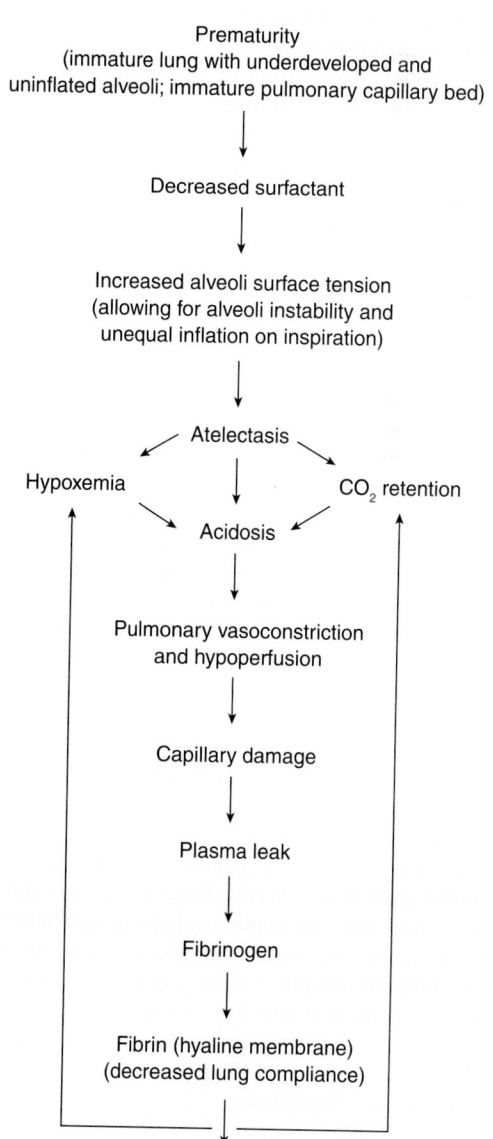

Figure 44-5. Schematic outline of respiratory distress syndrome.

Clinical Manifestations

Symptoms are usually observed soon after birth and may include those listed here and increase in severity over the first 2 days of life.

Primary Signs and Symptoms

1. Expiratory grunting.
2. Sternal, suprasternal, substernal, and intercostal retractions progressing to paradoxical seesaw respirations.
3. Inspiratory nasal flaring.
4. Tachypnea less than 60 breaths/minute.
5. Hypothermia.
6. Cyanosis when child is in room air (infants with severe disease may be cyanotic even when given oxygen), increasing need for oxygen.
7. Decreased breath sounds and dry "sandpaper" breath sounds.
8. Pulmonary edema.
9. As the disease progresses:
   a. Seesaw retractions become marked with marked abdominal protrusion on expiration.
   b. Peripheral edema increases.
   c. Muscle tone decreases.
   d. Cyanosis increases.
   e. Body temperature drops.
   f. Short periods of apnea occur.
   g. Bradycardia may occur.
   h. Changes in distribution of blood throughout the body result in pale gray skin color.
   i. Diminished breath sounds.

Secondary Signs and Symptoms

1. Hypotension.
2. Edema of the hands and feet.
3. Absent bowel sounds early in the illness.
4. Decreased urine output.

Diagnostic Evaluation

1. Prenatal diagnosis: evaluation of amniotic fluids to assess fetal lung maturity.
   a. Lecithin/sphingomyelin ratio—tests of surfactant phospholipids in amniotic fluid.
   b. Phosphatidylcholine and phosphatidylglycerol (PG)—phospholipids that stabilize surfactant.
   c. Fetal maturity assay—determines PG levels in amniotic fluid or neonatal tracheal aspirates.
   d. Lamellar bodies test—measures a storage form of surfactant in amniotic fluids.
2. Laboratory tests:
   a. $PaCO_2$—elevated.
   b. Partial pressure of arterial oxygen (PaO_2)—low.
   c. Blood pH—low because of metabolic acidosis.
   d. Calcium—low.
   e. Serum glucose—low.
3. Chest x-ray—diffuse, fine granularity; "whiteout," very heavy, uniform granularity reflecting fluid-filled alveoli and atelectasis of some alveoli, surrounded by hyperdistended bronchioles; "ground glass" appearance with prominent air bronchogram extending into periphery of lung fields. Pulmonary interstitial emphysema is observed in premature neonates with RDS because of overdistension of distal airways.
4. Pulmonary function studies—stiff lung with a reduced effective pulmonary blood flow.

Management

EVIDENCE BASE Liu, J., Wang, W., Liu, F., & Li, Z. (2018). Pediatric acute respiratory distress syndrome - current views. *Exp Ther Med, 5*(2), 1775–1780.
Pacheco, G.S., Mendelson, J., & Gaspers, M. (2018). Pediatric ventilator management in the emergency department. *Emerg Med Clin North Am., 36*(2), 401–413.

Early recognition is imperative so that treatment may be initiated to halt the progression of RDS. In fact, treatment should begin prior to birth if the mother is at risk for delivering the baby preterm. Transportation to a facility providing specialized care is desirable, when possible.

Supportive

1. Maintenance of oxygenation—PaO_2 at 60 to 80 mm Hg to prevent hypoxia; frequent arterial pH and blood gas measurements and use of a pulse oximeter.
2. Maintenance of respiration with ventilatory support, if necessary.
   a. Intermittent mandatory ventilations delivered via ET tube. Allows the infant to breathe spontaneously at his or her own rate while the ventilator provides a preset cycle of respirations and pressure.
   b. Positive end-expiratory pressure (PEEP) via ET tube. The ventilator is pressure or volume limited. Provides increased PEEP during expiration to prevent alveolar collapse; residual airway pressure is maintained.
   c. Continuous positive airway pressure (CPAP) delivered via mask or nasal prongs. Used in spontaneous respiration to improve oxygenation by preventing collapse of the alveoli and increasing diffusion time.
   d. Synchronized intermittent mandatory ventilation allows the infant to breathe spontaneously between mechanical breaths. In assist or control mode, mechanical breaths are delivered at a regular rate if spontaneous breaths are not detected.
3. Maintenance of normal body temperature.
4. Maintenance of fluid, electrolyte, and acid–base balance—metabolic acidosis buffered with sodium bicarbonate.
5. Maintenance of nutrition—IV fluids, as prescribed.
6. Antibiotics, as needed, to treat infection.
7. Constant observation for complications—pneumothorax, disseminated intravascular coagulation (DIC), patent ductus arteriosus (PDA) with heart failure, chronic lung disease.
8. Care appropriate for a small, premature neonate.
9. Prevent hypotension.
10. Maintain a hematocrit of 40% to 45%.

Aggressive (Offered in Tertiary Care Centers)

1. Administration of exogenous surfactant into lungs early in the disease.
   a. Especially beneficial in the very low birth weight (VLBW) infant.
   b. May be given preventively to VLBW infants at birth.
   c. Available preparations are natural (derived from animal lungs) and synthetic (protein free): bovine and synthetic surfactant.
   d. Administered into the ET tube.

2. Surfactant replacement therapy.
   a. Prophylactic surfactant therapy: infants at increased risk for RDS, infants of less than 27 weeks' gestational age, and infants with a birth weight of less than 1,250 g.
   b. Treatment initiated after infant is stabilized in the delivery room or within 15 minutes of life.
   c. Rescue surfactant therapy: infants with moderate to severe RDS, requiring ventilatory assistance, with an oxygen requirement greater than 40%.
   d. Benefits of surfactant: decreases oxygen requirement and mean airway pressure; decreases pulmonary leaks.
   e. Complications observed in surfactant administration: pulmonary hemorrhage, PDA, mucus plugging.
   f. Nursing assessment with surfactant administration: suctioning delayed for 1 hour or as indicated by protocol. Assist with delivery of surfactant, collection and monitoring of ABG studies, meticulous monitoring of oxygenation status with pulse oximeter or transcutaneous monitor ($Tcpco_2$).
   g. Assess the infant's tolerance of the procedure: increase in respiratory compliance, which will require adjustments of the ventilator.
3. High-frequency ventilation—mechanical ventilation that uses rapid rates (can be greater than 900 breaths/minute) and tidal volumes near and, commonly, less than anatomical dead spaces.
   a. Jet ventilator delivers short burst of gases at high flow.
      i. Exhalation is passive.
      ii. Necrotizing tracheitis is a significant complication, along with hypotension and pneumopericardium.
   b. Oscillator ventilator delivers gases by vibrating columns of air.
      i. Exhalation is active.
      ii. The child appears to shake on the bed, which may be frightening for the parents.
4. Extracorporeal membrane oxygenation (ECMO)—indicated in infants with reversible cardiac or respiratory failure. ECMO is a modified heart–lung bypass machine used to allow gas exchange outside the body.
   a. Blood is removed from the venous system by a catheter placed in the internal jugular vein or right atrium.
   b. Oxygen is added and carbon dioxide is removed with a membrane oxygenator.
   c. Oxygenated blood is returned by way of the right common carotid (in venoarterial ECMO) or the femoral vein (in venovenous ECMO).
   d. The infant must be heparinized for the procedure, increasing the risk of intraventricular hemorrhage. For this reason, VLBW infants or infants of decreased gestational age are usually not candidates for the procedure.
   e. One nurse and one ECMO specialist must be present at the bedside at all times to monitor the patient and equipment. The patient will receive paralytic agents as well as analgesia and sedation; therefore, diligent continuous monitoring is required.
   f. Cannula dislodgement or tubing separation will result in immediate hemorrhage. Tubing and cannula must be secured and visible.
   g. Administration of vasoactive medications may be required to support alteration in cardiac output and blood pressure.
   h. Blood transfusions may be indicated because of blood loss from frequent sampling or anemia of prematurity.
5. Ventilatory support modalities for RDS currently under study: nitric oxide, liquid ventilation (tidal or partial), and perfluorocarbon-assisted gas exchange.

Complications

1. Complications related to respiratory therapy are as follows:
   a. Air leak: pneumothorax, pneumomediastinum, pneumopericardium, and pneumoperitoneum.
   b. Pneumonia, especially Gram-negative organisms.
   c. Pulmonary interstitial emphysema.
2. PDA or heart failure.
3. Hypotension.
4. Intraventricular hemorrhage—typically seen in infants weighing less than 1,500 g.
5. DIC.
6. Chronic problems associated with long-term use of oxygen:
   a. Bronchopulmonary dysplasia (BPD)—cystic-appearing lungs with hyperinfiltration, obstructive bronchiolitis, dysplastic changes, and pulmonary fibrosis.
   b. Chronic respiratory infections.
7. Necrotizing enterocolitis.
8. Tracheal stenosis.
9. Retinopathy of prematurity (retrolental fibroplasia).
10. Other complications related to prematurity.
11. Renal failure requiring use of dialysis.

Nursing Assessment

1. Review the birth history.
   a. Apgar scores 1 and 5 minutes after birth.
   b. Type of resuscitation required.
   c. Treatments or medications administered.
   d. Medications or anesthesia administered to the mother during labor.
   e. Estimated gestational age.
   f. Maternal history—contributing factors or complications.
2. Carefully assess the infant's respiratory status to determine the degree of respiratory distress.
   a. Determine the degree and severity of retractions.
   b. Count the respiratory rate for 1 full minute, note level of activity, and determine if they are regular or irregular.
   c. Identify periods of apnea, length, and type of stimulation necessary.
   d. Listen for expiratory grunting or whining sounds from the infant when quiet. This indicates an attempt to maintain PEEP and prevent alveoli from collapse.
   e. Note nasal flaring.
   f. Note cyanosis—location, improvement with oxygen.
   g. Auscultate chest for diminished breath sounds and presence of crackles.
3. Determine the infant's cardiac rate and rhythm.
   a. Count the apical pulse for 1 full minute.
   b. Note irregularities in the rate or bounding pulses.
4. Observe the infant's general activity.
   a. Lethargic or listless.
   b. Active and responds to stimuli.
   c. Infant's cry.
5. Assess the skin for cyanosis, jaundice, mottling, paleness or grayness, and edema.

Nursing Diagnoses

- Impaired Gas Exchange related to disease process.
- Imbalanced Nutrition: Less than Body Requirements related to prematurity and increased energy expenditure on breathing.
- Ineffective Thermoregulation related to immaturity.
- Impaired Parenting related to separation from the neonate due to hospitalization.

Nursing Interventions

Promoting Adequate Gas Exchange

1. Have emergency equipment readily available for use in the event of cardiac or respiratory arrest.
2. Institute cardiorespiratory monitoring to continuously monitor heart and respiratory rates.
3. Administer supplemental oxygen.
   a. Incubator with oxygen at prescribed concentration.
   b. Plastic hood with oxygen at prescribed concentration when using radiant warmer.
   c. CPAP, if indicated, using nasal prongs or ET tube.
4. Assist with ET intubation and maintain mechanical ventilation, as indicated.
5. Measure oxygen concentration every hour and record.
6. Monitor ABG levels, as appropriate. Obtain sample of blood through indwelling umbilical line, arterial puncture, or capillary puncture. (Capillary gas analysis for monitoring $Paco_2$ and pH but not Pao_2.)
7. Institute pulse oximetry, if available, for continuous monitoring of the blood's arterial oxygen saturation (SaO_2).
   a. Avoid using adhesive to secure the sensor when the infant is active. Wrap it snugly enough to reduce sensitivity to movement but not tight enough to constrict blood flow.
   b. If transcutaneous Pao_2 monitor is used, reposition the probe every 3 to 4 hours to avoid burns caused by heating the probe to achieve sufficient arterialization.
8. Observe the infant's response to oxygen.
   a. Observe for improvement in color, respiratory rate and pattern, and nasal flaring.
   b. Note response by improvement in arterial or capillary blood gas levels.
   c. Observe closely for apnea.
9. Stimulate the infant if apnea occurs. If unable to produce spontaneous respiration with stimulation within 15 to 30 seconds, initiate resuscitation.
10. Position the infant to allow for maximal lung expansion.
    a. Prone position provides for a larger lung volume because of the position of the diaphragm, decreases energy expenditure, and increases the time spent in quiet sleep; however, it may be contraindicated because of placement of the umbilical catheter. The risk for sudden infant death syndrome (SIDS) is increased, but the infant is continuously monitored.
    b. Change position frequently.
11. Suction, as needed, because the gag reflex is weak and cough is ineffective.
12. Try to minimize time spent on procedures and interventions and monitor effects on respiratory status. (Infants undergoing multiple procedures lasting 45 minutes to 1 hour have shown a moderate decrease in Pao_2.)
13. The decision to suction should be based on assessment of the infant, such as auscultation of chest, decrease in oxygenation, excessive moisture in the ET tube, and irritability.
    a. Nasopharyngeal, tracheal, or ET tube suctioning should be done gently, quickly, 5 seconds or less, with intermittent suction applied as the catheter is withdrawn.
    b. To prevent hypoxemia, observe oximeter before, during, and after the procedure.
    c. Suctioning of the ET tube is done to maintain a patent airway. The practice of inducing a catheter into the tube until resistance is met and then withdrawn has been shown to cause trauma to the tracheal wall. Instead, the suction catheter should be premeasured according to the size of the infant's ET tube length and documented. When suctioning, do not insert the catheter beyond this predetermined length. This will prevent damage to the mucosa.
14. Observe for complications of suctioning: bronchospasm, vagal nerve stimulation, bradycardia, hypoxia, increased intracranial pressure, trauma to airway, infection, and pneumothoraces.
15. VLBW and extremely low birth weight neonates cannot tolerate percussion and vibration. Trendelenburg position is contraindicated in premature neonates and may result in increased intracranial pressure.
16. Record all nursing observations.

 NURSING ALERT Prone position may present several problems: Turning head to side can compromise upper airway and increase airflow resistance; observation of chest is obstructed, making retractions difficult to detect; and abdominal distention is more difficult to recognize.

Promoting Adequate Nutrition and Hydration

1. Administer IV fluids or enteral feeding, as ordered, and observe infusion rate closely to prevent fluid overload.
2. Observe IV sites for infiltration or infection; use meticulous technique to prevent sepsis.
3. If umbilical artery catheter is in place, observe for bleeding.
4. Provide adequate caloric intake (80 to 120 kcal/kg/24 hours) through the following:
   a. Nasojejunal tube (best tolerated by VLBW neonates).
   b. Nasogastric tube.
   c. Parenteral nutrition—$D_{10}W$ or hyperalimentation fluid usually required, especially in the acute phase of illness.
5. Monitor for hypoglycemia, which is especially common during stress. Maintain serum glucose greater than 45 mg/dL.
6. Monitor intake and output closely.
   a. Include amount of blood drawn (small infants can become anemic because of frequent blood sampling).
   b. Apply urine collection bag to obtain sample of urine and measure specific gravity periodically.
7. Weigh the infant daily and record.

Maintaining Thermoregulation

1. Provide a neutral thermal environment to maintain the infant's abdominal skin temperature between 97°F and 98°F (36.1°C and 36.7°C) to prevent hypothermia, which may result in vasoconstriction and acidosis.
2. Adjust incubator or radiant warmer to obtain desired skin temperature. For the infant weighing less than 1,250 g, the radiant warmer should be used with caution because of increased water loss and potential for hypoglycemia.
3. Prevent frequent opening of incubator.
4. Ensure that oxygen is warmed to a temperature between 87.6°F and 93.2°F (30.9°C and 34°C) with 60% to 80% humidity.

Encouraging Parental Attachment

1. Identify factors that may prohibit the parents' visitation and communication: geographic distance, lack of transportation, care of siblings, employment restrictions, economic issues, lack of telephone in the home, and fear. Refer to social services for assistance and intervention, if required.

2. If the neonate was transported to a tertiary care center immediately after birth, send the mother a photograph of the neonate.

3. Call the parents daily to update them on the infant's condition until they are able to visit the child. Emphasize positive aspects of the infant's status.

4. Refer to the child by his or her first name when speaking with the parents.

5. Prepare the parents for the neonatal intensive care unit (NICU) environment and how their child will appear before their first visit.

6. Assist the parents to participate in the child's care, as appropriate.

7. Demonstrate for the parents how they can touch and speak to the child while the child is in an Isolette/incubator.

8. Allow the parents to hold the infant as soon as possible.

9. If the mother plans to breast-feed, assist her with expressing her milk and use the breast milk to feed the infant when enteral feedings are initiated.

10. If the infant has siblings, provide the parents with information on how to discuss the infant's illness with them.

11. If unit policies allow and the situation is appropriate, encourage sibling visitation with adequate preparation.

12. Provide the parents with information concerning the disease process, expected outcomes, and usual course of the NICU stay. Encourage the parents to ask questions and participate in the care plan.

13. Help parents work through their distress at the birth of a premature child.

14. Assess parents' support mechanisms (eg, grandparents, friends).

Family Education and Health Management

1. Prepare the family for long-term follow-up, as appropriate. Infants with BPD may eventually go home on oxygen therapy.

2. Stress the importance of regular health care, periodic eye examinations, and developmental follow-up with the parents.

3. Ensure that the family receives information on routine well-baby care.

4. Before discharge, parents should feel comfortable in their abilities to care for the infant. Referrals for home nursing visits should be completed and a physician identified for follow-up care.

Evaluation: Expected Outcomes

- Respiratory rate within normal range for age; pattern regular and unlabored.
- Tolerates enteral feedings well; weight gain noted.
- Maintains temperature within normal limits.
- Parents interact with infant, participate in care, and ask appropriate questions.

Cystic Fibrosis

EVIDENCE BASE Schmid-Mohler, G. (2018). Patient-reported outcome measures for symptom perception during a cystic fibrosis exacerbation. *Respiratory Care*, 63(3), 353–366.

Cystic fibrosis (CF) is an autosomal recessive disorder affecting the exocrine glands, causing abnormal viscosity of secretions. It primarily affects the pulmonary and GI systems. Approximately 4% to 5% of Caucasians are symptomless carriers of the CF gene. Slightly more males than females are affected. Incidence is estimated at approximately 1 in 3,500 live Caucasian births. CF is found in all racial groups. There are approximately 30,000 people living with CF in the United States, 45% of who are aged 18 or older. Presently, the predicted survival age extends to the late 40s, compared with a life expectancy of less than 1 year in the 1950s.

Pathophysiology and Etiology

1. CF is caused by a genetic defect in a single gene located on the long arm of chromosome 7 that encodes the cystic fibrosis transmembrane conductance regulator (CFTR).

2. The variations in the onset of the disease, symptomatology, and clinical presentation within the CF population are attributed to the over 1,000 mutations of the CF gene. CFTR is responsible for the fluid balance across epithelial cells.

3. The malfunction of CFTR results in the following:
   a. Decreased chloride secretion into the airway lumen.
   b. Increased sodium reabsorption, which leads to decreased airway surface liquid volume.
   c. Thickened mucus, impaired mucociliary clearance, chronic infection, plugged bronchi.
   d. Chronic inflammation, airway damage, atelectasis, and hyperinflation of lungs.
   e. Progressive bronchiectasis, irreversible fibrotic changes in lungs.

4. GI and pancreatic involvement includes the following:
   a. Acini and ducts of pancreas become filled with thick mucus and are obstructed.
   b. Trypsin, chymotrypsin, lipase, and amylase do not reach the small intestine.
   c. Digestion is impaired. Interruption of the enterohepatic circulation of bile acids probably results in interference with normal pancreatic lipolysis and fat absorption through the intestinal wall.
   d. Stools are abnormal and indicate malabsorption syndrome.
   e. Meconium ileus often occurs in infants, indicating that bowel is obstructed by thick intestinal secretions.
   f. Biliary cirrhosis occurs because the intrahepatic biliary tract is obstructed by thick secretions.
   g. In 30% of CF patients, the gallbladder is small, with suboptimal function. Gallstones develop in up to 10% of patients.

5. Sweat gland involvement includes the following:
   a. Secretions contain excessive amount of sodium and chloride, leading to excessive loss, especially with hot weather, fever, or exertion.
   b. Saliva also contains an excess of sodium and chloride.

Clinical Manifestations

Presentation usually occurs younger than age 6 months but may occur at any age. Signs and symptoms and severity of the disease vary and change over time as the disease progresses.

Respiratory Manifestations

1. Recurrent pulmonary infections—*H. influenzae*, *S. aureus*, *P. aeruginosa*.

2. Cough, dry to productive. Chronic clearing of throat may indicate increased mucus production.

3. Wheezing, crackles on auscultation are indicative of respiratory exacerbation.
4. Dyspnea.
5. Barrel-shaped chest (increased anteroposterior chest diameter).
6. Cyanosis.
7. Clubbing of fingers and toes.
8. Nasal polyps and pansinusitis.
9. Progressive chronic obstructive pulmonary disease (COPD). A 10% drop in FEV_1 is a sign of an acute exacerbation or worsening lung disease.
   a. Mild form of CF—slightly decreased FEV_1 (70% to 90%).
   b. Moderate CF—FEV_1 of 40% to 69%.
   c. Severe forms of CF—life-threatening pulmonary disease with FEV_1 of less than 40%.

GI Manifestations

1. Meconium ileus found in neonates.
2. Failure to thrive and failure to gain weight in the presence of a good appetite.
3. Abdominal distention.
4. Vomiting, dehydration, and electrolyte imbalance.
5. Maldigestion, steatorrhea (fatty stools, loss of fat-soluble vitamins).
6. Rectal prolapse.
7. Distal intestinal obstructive syndrome.
8. Biliary cirrhosis, obstructive jaundice.
9. Pancreatitis.

Other Manifestations

1. Thin extremities, sallow skin, wasted buttocks.
2. Hyperglycemia, glucosuria, polyuria, weight loss.
3. Salty taste when parents kiss skin.
4. Sterility in males.
5. Hypoproteinemia and anemia.
6. Bleeding diathesis.
7. Hyponatremia and heat prostration.
8. Kyphosis.

Diagnostic Evaluation

1. Quantitative sweat chloride test; pilocarpine iontophoresis, performed at a CF Foundation accredited center by skilled personnel. Measures sodium and chloride content in sweat.
   a. Chloride level greater than 60 mEq/L is virtually diagnostic.
   b. Chloride of 40 to 60 mEq/L is borderline and should be repeated, followed by genotype for the most frequent CFTR mutations.
   c. Sodium level greater than 60 mEq/L is diagnostic.
2. Measurement of trypsin concentration in duodenal secretions; absence of normal concentration virtually diagnostic.
3. Analysis of digestive enzymes (trypsin and chymotrypsin) in stool—reduced, used for initial screening for CF.
4. Chest x-ray—may be normal initially; later shows areas of infection, overinflation, bronchial thickening and plugging, atelectasis, fibrosis, and emphysema.
5. Sinus radiograph or computed tomography shows mucus plugging.
6. Analysis of stool for steatorrhea.
7. Meconium strip test for stool includes lactose and protein content; used for screening.
8. Sputum or throat cultures to rule out infection.
9. Pulmonary function studies (after age 4 years).
   a. Decreased vital capacity and flow rates.
   b. Increased residual volume or increased total lung capacity.

10. Diagnosis made when a positive sweat test is seen in conjunction with one or more of the following:
    a. Positive family history for CF.
    b. Typical COPD.
    c. Documented exocrine pancreatic insufficiency.
    d. Failure to thrive.
    e. History of frequent respiratory infections.
11. Prenatal diagnostic tests—prenatal genetic screening for families affected with CF:
    a. Chorionic villus sampling at approximately 12 weeks' gestation.
    b. Deoxyribonucleic acid (DNA) probes.
    c. Microvillar enzymes.
12. Neonatal screening: immunoreactive trypsinogen; if elevated, DNA assay for single and multiple CFTR mutations.

Management

Goals of treatment are to prevent and minimize pulmonary complications, ensure adequate nutrition for growth, and assist the family and child to adapt to chronic disease.

Pulmonary Interventions

1. Antimicrobial therapy, as indicated, for pulmonary infection.
   a. Oral antibiotics may be given prophylactically or when symptomatic.
   b. IV antibiotics are given when the child fails to respond to oral antibiotics; this may be inpatient or at-home therapy.
   c. Inhaled antibiotics such as tobramycin. Colistin may be used for severe lung disease or colonization of organisms. Recently, some practitioners advocate using nebulized antibiotics earlier in therapy.
   d. Patients with CF metabolize antibiotics rapidly; if drug dosage is higher than normal, monitor for signs of toxicity.
2. Bronchodilators to increase the airway size and assist with mucociliary clearance. Many CF patients also have airway hyperreactivity.
   a. Long-term clinical improvement with inhaled bronchodilators has not been well supported in the literature. Salmeterol, a long-acting bronchodilator, has demonstrated improvements in pulmonary function and is effective in decreasing nocturnal hypoxia.
   b. Inhaled steroids for treatment of airway hyperreactivity.
3. Aerosols, expectorants, and mucolytic agents to decrease viscosity of secretions.
   a. Recombinate human DNase administered via nebulizer improves pulmonary function and decreases sputum viscosity and pulmonary exacerbations.
   b. Hypertonic saline solution 3% to 7%.
   c. Improves airway clearance and lung function, although it is not as effective as recombinant human DNase.
   d. Acetylcysteine solution is not recommended because of irritant effect on airways.
4. CPT for bronchial drainage, especially during acute exacerbations.
   a. Postural drainage (see Figure 44-6, page 1193).
   b. Some patients use a vibrating vest that utilizes a shaking motion rather than manual postural drainage.
   c. Coughing and deep-breathing exercises; huffing helps move secretions from smaller airways.
   d. Increase physical activity—aerobic activity.

Figure 44-6. Positions for postural drainage.

e. Active cycle of breathing, a new technique, improves lung function without decreasing oxygenation. Consists of breathing control, thoracic expansion, forced expiratory technique, and huffing. An assistant is not required.

f. Autogenic drainage—breathing at various lung volumes to move and evacuate mucus. Oxygenation should not be affected during procedure.

g. Positive expiratory pressure (PEP) and flutter. PEP airway technique is utilized by those with severe disease. It reduces airway collapse due to bronchiectasis. Available as low-pressure PEP, high-pressure PEP, and oscillating PEP with a flutter or acapella device.

h. High-frequency chest compressions—externally applied device provides oscillation to the chest, resulting in release of mucus from the airway wall.

5. Bronchopulmonary lavage—treatment of atelectasis and mucoid impaction using large volumes of saline (used in some institutions in the United States).

6. Lobectomy—resection of symptomatic lobar bronchiectasis to retard progression of lesion to total lung involvement.

 EVIDENCE BASE Mikesell, C., Kempainen, B., Laguna, T., et al. (2017). Objective measurement of adherence to out-patient airway clearance therapy by high-frequency chest wall compression in cystic fibrosis. *Respiratory Care, 62*(7), 920–927.

GI Interventions

1. Pancreatic enzyme supplementation is provided with each feeding.
   a. Favored preparation is pancrelipase.
   b. Antacids are occasionally helpful to improve tolerance of enzymes.
   c. Favorable response to enzymes is evidenced by tolerance of fatty foods, decreased stool frequency, absence of steatorrhea, improved appetite, and lack of abdominal pain.

2. Provide a high-energy diet by increasing carbohydrates, protein, and fat (possibly as high as 40%). Increases in dietary intake should consider growth and repair, infection, the work of breathing and energy expenditure for coughing, malabsorption, and physical activity.

3. Provide zinc and iron supplements and water-soluble and fat-soluble vitamins.

4. Ensure adequate fluid and salt intake.

Controversial and Experimental Treatments

1. Heart–lung, double-lung, or single-lung transplantation for end-stage lung disease.
   a. This treatment is limited by availability of donor organs.
   b. Long-term survival at 5 years is approximately 50%.
   c. Bilateral lobar transplantation using a new method, called bipartitioning of a single-donor lung, is under study. This method could result in increased availability of donor organs.

2. Liver transplant.

3. Gene therapy.
   a. This treatment is at present only being undertaken by a small number of centers because of its complexity.
   b. Therapy is based on somatic gene correction; an attempt to correct the defect in the cells of the individual is made by adding the correct gene sequence to the cells.
   c. One trial method will use a virus carrying DNA with the appropriate gene sequence, which will be introduced into the affected lung cells by nebulization.
   d. A second method being investigated is the introduction into the lungs of DNA by nebulization with the appropriate gene sequence suspended in liposomes.
   e. It is thought that the treatment will need to be repeated at regular intervals.

4. *Pseudomonas aeruginosa* genome is complete, which should lead to the development of new medications to combat this common lung infection in CF.

Complications

1. Pulmonary infections:
   a. Most frequently caused by *P. aeruginosa*, *S. aureus*, *H. influenzae*, and *Burkholderia cepacia*. *Pseudomonas* is the most difficult organism to treat.
   b. Bronchiectasis and bronchiolitis.

2. Other pulmonary complications—emphysema, atelectasis, pneumothorax, hemoptysis (primarily seen in adolescents), and pulmonary hypertension.

3. Biliary cirrhosis, leading to portal hypertension, esophageal varices, and splenomegaly.

4. Pancreatic fibrosis with islets of Langerhans involvement, resulting in glucose intolerance and CF-related diabetes.

5. Cor pulmonale.

6. Chronic sinusitis.

7. Rectal polyps (3 months to 3 years).

8. Rectal prolapse.

9. Intussusception (younger than 2 years).

10. Pancreatitis.

11. Hypertrophic pulmonary osteoarthropathy—arthritis, clubbing, periosteitis; the long tubular bones are most commonly involved.

12. Bone thinning and demineralization.

13. Depression.

14. Heat prostration.

15. Fibrosis of epididymis and vas deferens in male; aspermia.

16. Growth retardation.

17. Gastroesophageal reflux.

18. Allergic bronchopulmonary aspergillosis.

19. Respiratory failure and death.

 NURSING ALERT *B. cepacia* affects approximately 5% of CF patients, is associated with a rapid decline in pulmonary function, and is multiple antibiotic-resistant. Twenty percent of colonized patients develop fulminant septicemia and necrotizing pneumonia, leading to death.

Nursing Assessment

1. Check for family history of CF, failure to thrive, and unexplained infant death; check the child's history and physical condition. Carefully listen for subtle information that may suggest CF.

2. Assess respiratory status—respiratory rate, presence of tachypnea, wheeze, cough, character of sputum, and oxygen saturation level.
   a. Increased work of breathing.
   b. Quality of breath sounds by auscultation.
   c. Child's perception of respiratory status.
   d. Ability to participate in activities of daily living, exercise tolerance, quality of sleep.
   e. Assess for oxygen desaturation with sleep.

3. Assess nutritional status and characteristics of stool.

Nursing Diagnoses

- Ineffective Airway Clearance related to thick pulmonary secretions.
- Risk for Infection related to thick, tenacious secretions.
- Imbalanced Nutrition: Less than Body Requirements related to decreased appetite or inadequate absorption.

- Disturbed Body Image related to chronic disease process.
- Interrupted Family Processes related to the child with a chronic disease.

Nursing Interventions

Promoting Airway Clearance
1. Use intermittent nebulizer therapy three to four times per day when child is symptomatic.
   a. Use pretreatment postural drainage.
   b. Administer bronchodilators and other medications, diluted in normal saline, in aerosol form to penetrate respiratory tract. Proper technique is necessary to deliver the correct dose of medication. If using a face mask, it should fit snugly; movement of the mask by ¾ inch (2 cm) could decrease the delivery of medication by 85%.
2. Perform CPT three to four times per day after nebulizer therapy; perform more frequently if infection is present.
   a. Perform prior to meals or 1 hour after eating to prevent vomiting or discomfort.
   b. Place the child in a position that gives the greatest access to the affected lobes of the lung and facilitates gravity drainage of mucus from specific lung areas.
   c. Children with gastroesophageal reflux should not use the head-down position during CPT.
3. Help the child to relax to cough more easily after postural drainage.
4. Suction the infant or young child when necessary if he or she is unable to cough.
5. Teach child breathing exercises using pursed lips to increase duration of exhalation.
6. Monitor child's oxygen saturation levels during procedures.
7. Maintain cautious oxygen therapy because of chronic carbon dioxide retention.
8. Monitor for signs and symptoms of pneumothorax, such as tachypnea, tachycardia, pallor, dyspnea, and cyanosis.
9. Monitor for hemoptysis, which requires immediate treatment and may be life threatening.
10. Provide treatment of hemoptysis: bed rest, cough suppressants, and antibiotics.
    a. Bronchoscopy is used to locate the site, cauterize, or embolize.
    b. Administer vitamin K, as directed.

NURSING ALERT Mist therapy is no longer recommended because water droplets may cause bronchospasm in some patients, and the equipment required to deliver the therapy is frequently contaminated with opportunistic organisms.

Preventing Infection
Adherence to infection control procedures must be enforced to prevent the spread of nosocomial infections.
1. Provide frequent mouth care to reduce the chance of infection because mucus is present.
2. Restrict contact with people with respiratory infections.
3. Administer antibiotics, as prescribed, to treat specific organisms when the child is symptomatic.
4. Most institutions change nebulizers after each use for CF patients.
5. Monitor closely for deteriorating respiratory status.

6. Provide good skin care and position changes to prevent skin breakdown of malnourished child.
7. Change diapers promptly to prevent diaper rash and superimposed infection.

 NURSING ALERT To decrease the risk of transmission of *B. cepacia* within the hospital setting, children who test positive for the pathogen are placed on room isolation.

Promoting Adequate Nutrition
1. Refer to dietitian for dietary assessment.
2. Encourage diet composed of foods high in calories and protein and moderate to high in fat because absorption of food is incomplete. Provide 120% to 150% of recommended dietary allowances because only 80% to 85% of intake is absorbed.
3. Administer fat-soluble vitamins in water-miscible solution in two to three times the normal dose, as prescribed, to counteract malabsorption.
   a. Give vitamins A, D, and E on a daily basis.
   b. Give vitamin K when the child has an infection or is being treated with antibiotics.
4. Administer pancreatic enzymes with each meal and snack. Dose is based on the child's weight, weight gain, growth, food intake, and number and character of bowel movements.
   a. Mix capsule, granules, or powder with small portion of food for infant or small child; do not mix with formula, which may not be finished.
   b. Offer the older child capsules or tablets.
   c. Withhold enzymes, as ordered, if the child is taking only clear liquid diet or enteral feedings.
   d. Beads should not be chewed or crushed.
   e. The CF Foundation discourages the use of generic enzymes.
5. Increase salt intake during hot weather, fever, or excessive exercise to prevent sodium depletion and cardiovascular compromise.
6. To prevent vomiting, allow ample time for feeding, especially if irritable because of not feeling well and coughing.
7. Check weights at least weekly to assess nutritional interventions. Document and plot height and weight every 3 months.
8. Infants who are breast-fed will need enzyme supplementation. If supplementation with formula is necessary, choose a high-calorie preparation.
9. Administer supplemental parenteral or enteral feedings, as required.
10. Constipation, due to malabsorption, decreased gastric motility; viscous intestinal secretions may be treated with laxatives, stool softeners, or rectal administration of x-ray contrast material.

Enhancing Self-Esteem and Body Image
1. Explain each procedure, medication, and treatment to the child as appropriate for age.
2. Allow the child to show frustrations, fears, and feelings by talking, complaining, or crying.
3. Support and comfort the child by talking to and holding him or her.
4. Provide diversional activities related to the child's interests and praise the child for his or her accomplishments.
5. Encourage the older child to take an active role in his or her self-management and be involved in the care plan.

6. Help the child to identify strengths and limitations and to feel good about self.
7. Help to redirect feelings of anger, fear, or frustration, to increase compliance with CPT.
8. Encourage regular exercise and activity to foster a sense of accomplishment and independence and improve pulmonary function. Consent from health care provider is necessary prior to the initiation of an exercise program. Oxygenation status during exercise should be assessed.

Enhancing Family Processes

1. Provide opportunities for the parents to learn all aspects of care for the child.
2. Provide education and support during hospitalization to make home care easier.
3. Encourage maintenance of family activities and involvement with other children.
4. Initiate social work referral, as needed.
5. Encourage information sharing about CF with friends, teachers, and relatives. Explain that one of the most important things people can do to help a child with CF is to treat him or her just as they would any other child.
6. Help family share and interpret feelings about CF and its impact on all of their lives.
7. Encourage families to foster the older child's independence when the time comes.

Family Education and Health Maintenance

1. Teach parents to have a thorough understanding of the dietary regimen and special need for calories, fat, and vitamins. Consultation with a registered dietitian is recommended.
2. Discuss the child's need for salt replacement and free access to salt as well as the increased need for salt during hot weather or in the presence of fever, vomiting, or diarrhea.
3. Help the parents to become skilled at CPT and other pulmonary treatments. Demonstrate and explain procedures and evaluate their return demonstration.
4. Help the family to schedule care for the child within the framework of family life.
   a. CPT should be done at least 1 hour after meals.
   b. Nebulizer treatments should be done before CPT.
   c. Mild exercise and activity are beneficial to the child.
   d. Vacations and major family outings can be planned for remissions of the child's symptoms.
5. Help the parents to provide emotional support to their child. The child needs love, understanding, and security, not overprotection.
6. Stress the importance of regular medical care.
   a. Routine immunizations.
   b. Prompt attention to infection.
   c. Continued evaluation and supervision in home management.
   d. Attention to developments through research that may change therapy.
   e. Prevention or early detection of complications.
7. Stress the importance of following up with regular health care provider for routine follow-up according to Cystic Fibrosis Foundation.
   a. Outpatient visits, four per year.
   b. Pulmonary function tests, two or more per year.
   c. Respiratory cultures, at least one per year.
   d. Creatinine level, every year.
   e. Glucose level, every year if older than age 13.
   f. Liver enzymes, every year.

8. Discuss with parents the limitations and expectations for the child.
   a. With proper care, the child will most likely live to adulthood but may be smaller and shorter than peers.
   b. Play and school participation depends on severity of illness.
   c. Involve teachers and school nurses in planning of the child's day.
9. Suggest parents and child meet other CF families. Investigate location and participation in summer camps for children with CF.
10. Investigate home care options for families, especially respite services for caregivers.
11. After the diagnosis is confirmed, refer the parents to genetic counseling. It is important for the parents to realize that the affected child inherits the defective gene from both parents. Each pregnancy will result in a 25% chance that the infant will have CF, a 50% chance that it will be a carrier of the CF gene and *not* have CF, and a 25% chance that the infant will neither be a carrier of the CF gene nor have CF.
12. Refer families for additional information and support to agencies such as Cystic Fibrosis Foundation (*www.cff.org*). Most areas have local chapters of the organization.
13. The pediatric health care team should discuss with the patient and parents the concept of eventual transitioning of care from a pediatric CF center to an adult CF center as early as possible—an important issue that should not be left until adolescence. Facilitate a planned, efficient, and smooth transition by
   a. Encouraging the child to gradually assume responsibility for health care.
   b. Encouraging the parents to foster the adolescent's independence.
   c. Providing patient and family time to adjust and educate themselves about the transitioning process.
   d. Identifying and introducing the child and his or her family to members of the adult care team.
   e. Advocating for the patient in regard to any restrictions superimposed by the patient's health insurance plan.
14. Sadly, at some point, it will become apparent to the health care team that the time has arrived to discuss end-of-life issues. Use a family-centered approach to provide care for the child and family facing a life-threatening illness or death. Discuss hospice care and other available services with the family (see page 1153).

 EVIDENCE BASE Butler, A., Hall, H., & Copnell, B. (2018). The changing nature of relationships between parents and healthcare providers when a child dies in the paediatric intensive care unit. *Journal of Advanced Nursing, 74*(1), 89–99.

Lynch, J., III, Savah, D., Belperio, J., & Weigt, S. S. (2015). Lung transplantation for cystic fibrosis: Results, indicators, complications, and controversies. *Seminars in Respiratory Critical Care Medicine, 36*(2), 299–320.

Evaluation: Expected Outcomes

- Tolerates CPT four times per day for 30 minutes with stable oxygen saturation.
- No signs of respiratory infection.
- Eats well with no vomiting; weight stable.
- Plays, interacts appropriately.
- Parents ask questions; meet, as necessary, with a social worker; and take part in care of their child.

Apnea of Infancy and Brief Resolved Unexplained Events in Infants

Apnea of infancy (AOI) is defined as an unexplained episode of cessation of breathing for 20 seconds or longer or a shorter respiratory pause associated with bradycardia, cyanosis, pallor, and marked hypotonia in an infant of 37 weeks' gestation or more at the onset of apnea.

Apnea of prematurity (AOP) is defined as sudden cessation of breathing that lasts for 20 seconds and may or may not be accompanied by bradycardia and cyanosis in an infant younger than 37 weeks' gestation.

Brief Resolved Unexplained Event in Infants are defined as an episode that is frightening to the observer and is characterized by some combination of apnea (central or obstructive), color change, cyanosis, pallor or plethora, marked change in muscle tone, extreme limpness, choking, or gagging.

Pathophysiology and Etiology

1. Cause is often unknown—may result from many different pathologic processes; may be idiopathic.
2. Apnea may be related to organic disorders, such as seizure disorders, sepsis, severe infection, hypoglycemia, and impaired regulation of breathing while sleeping or feeding, gastroesophageal reflux, upper airway abnormalities, metabolic disorders, or abuse.
3. Abnormal properties of surfactant have been reported in some children with recurrent ALTE.
4. A diagnosis of AOI is made when no identifiable cause of ALTE is found.
5. AOP is related to immature neurologic and respiratory control mechanisms.

Clinical Manifestations

1. The infant may be found by parents or caretaker to be limp, cyanotic, and pale with no respiration. Skin is cool to the touch.
2. Some form of resuscitation may be required.
3. The infant usually exhibits symptoms when asleep, although the syndrome may occur during waking hours.
4. Types of AOP are as follows:
   a. Central or diaphragmatic—chest movement ceases, absence of airflow.
   b. Obstructive—chest and diaphragm move, but there is no air exchange.
   c. Mixed—cessation of airflow and chest movement, followed by respiratory effort without airflow.

Diagnostic Evaluation

Complete history, physical examination, and diagnostic tests are aimed at ruling out other medical problems that could result in respiratory failure as a secondary cause.

1. Complete blood count with differential, serum glucose, electrolytes, calcium, phosphate, magnesium, and ABG levels, as indicated.
2. Chest x-ray.
3. Electrocardiogram.
4. Electroencephalogram (may not be routine) and neurologic examination.
5. Respiratory studies—a 12- to 24-hour pneumogram recording of small changes in electrical resistance with each breath or respiratory pattern; multichannel sleep test with continuous printout, monitoring heart rate, chest impedance, nasal airflow, and oxygen saturation.
6. Continuous cardiac and apnea monitoring for recurrence of event, prolonged apnea, or bradycardia.
7. Barium swallow for GER.
8. Because of hypoxemia that may have occurred, the child should be assessed for learning difficulties, discrete neurologic impairments, impaired hearing or vision, and personality disorders.
9. Polysomnograph—records brain waves, eye movements, esophageal manometry, and end-tidal carbon dioxide.

Management

1. BRUE may require hospitalization and cardiorespiratory monitoring.
2. Specific treatment of the underlying cause, if identified.
3. Theophylline may be used to decrease apneic episodes (therapeutic levels of 6 to 13 mcg/mL). Caffeine, which also acts as a central nervous system stimulant for breathing, may be given to maintain a trough level of 5 to 20 mcg/mL.
4. Long-term follow-up for physiologic and neurologic behavioral functions.
5. Prevention of SIDS: the most effective method of prevention is public education to avoid prone sleeping. More education is needed, with an emphasis on poor, underserved areas (see Box 44-1).

 NURSING ALERT Infants who have experienced apnea may be at risk for recurrent apnea, hypoxia, and sudden death and should be monitored closely. Research has shown that SIDS is more likely in infants sleeping prone. It is now recommended that all infants be put to sleep on their backs or sides.

Nursing Assessment

1. Obtain a nursing history, including the parents' description of the events that preceded the hospitalization, and their understanding of prolonged apnea.
   a. This information may provide clues for factors to observe during hospitalization and provides data for the development of a teaching plan.
   b. It allows for the correction of misinformation and misconceptions.
2. Have the parents describe sleep patterns, feeding habits, prior health problems, immunizations, and medications; this may provide data regarding possible influencing factors or causes of the condition.
3. Have the parents describe a typical day in the life of the infant and the family unit. This provides important data on how home monitoring may affect family life and contributes to the effective development of home management and family teaching plans; it also provides a basis for continuity of care for the infant.

Nursing Diagnoses

- Ineffective Breathing Pattern related to periods of apnea.
- Anxiety of the parents related to life-threatening event.
- Deficient Knowledge regarding home monitoring.

BOX 44-1   Sudden Infant Death Syndrome

EVIDENCE BASE Goldber, N., Rodriguez-Prado, Y., Tillery, R., et al. (2018). Sudden Infant Death Syndrome: A Review. *Pediatric Annals,* 47(3), e118–e123.

Stiffler, D., Ayers, B., Fauvergue, C., et al. (2018). Sudden infant death and sleep practices in the Black community. *Journal of Specialists in Pediatric Nursing, 23*(2), e1.

Sudden infant death syndrome (SIDS) is sudden death of an infant under the age of 1 year, which remains unexplained after a thorough case investigation, including performance of a complete autopsy, examination of the death scene, and review of clinical history.

The peak incidence occurs between 2 and 3 months of age. In addition, it has been found that there is a higher rate of incidence, two to three times the national average, in children who are black or American Indian or of Alaskan origin. Additional infant risk factors include male gender, prematurity, preterm birth or low birth weight, low Apgar scores, prone sleeping position, overheating, sleeping on soft surfaces, and twin victim of SIDS. Maternal risk factors include young maternal age, late or no prenatal care, smoking or exposure to smoking during pregnancy, history of sexually transmitted disease or urinary tract infection, anemia, and poverty.

There has generally been a reduction in death rate, with 1.2 deaths per 1,000 live births reported in 1992 and 0.5% deaths per 1,000 live births in 2002. However, since 2001, there has been a slightly higher proportion of deaths occurring in the neonatal period and after 6 months of age, possibly due to classification.

Current theories on the cause of SIDS focus on abnormalities of the brain stem and its network. Recent autopsy results from victims of SIDS have indicated deficits in serotonin receptors in this network, which are responsible for breathing, body temperature, blood pressure, and arousal.

The American Academy of Pediatric's Task Force on Sudden Infant Death Syndrome introduced a policy statement in November 2005 that put forth a number of recommendations that were developed to reduce the risk of SIDS. The recommendations are as follows:

- Infants should be placed in the supine position for sleep.
- A firm sleep surface should be used. For example, soft items, such as quilts or pillows, should not be placed under the infant.
- Soft objects and loose bedding should not be part of the infant's sleeping environment.
- Smoking and exposure to passive smoke during pregnancy should be avoided.
- Infants should not share the same bed as adults.
- Overheating should be avoided.
- Using a pacifier, when placing the infant down to sleep, should be considered.
- Home monitors should not be used as a strategy to reduce the risk of SIDS as there is no evidence that proves their effectiveness for this purpose. This is only suggested for infants who have had an apparent life-threatening event.

Nursing Interventions

Maintaining Breathing Pattern

1. Be prepared for the infant's admission and have all equipment, including apnea monitor, ready for use. Continuous cardiac monitoring is also recommended.
   a. Select a room that is clearly visible from the nursing station; the room should be quiet to reduce sensory stimulation, which may reduce the likelihood of a recurring episode.
   b. Be aware that the family has just experienced the extreme stress of feeling that their infant has almost died. Reassure them with empathy and efficiency at the time of admission.
2. Continuously monitor respirations. Document apnea along with state of consciousness; sleep state; color; position of infant; muscle tone; respiratory effort before, during, and after event; relationship to activity (eg, feeding); and intervention necessary (nothing, gentle stimulation, vigorous stimulation, resuscitation).
3. Administer theophylline, if prescribed. Observe for signs of toxicity: apical rate above 200, vomiting, and agitation. Concentration of theophylline for apnea is lower than the concentration for bronchospasm.
4. Continue the infant's normal activities whenever possible (eg, holding him or her for feedings, playing with him or her, disconnecting from monitor for bathing); allow for continuation of usual eating or sleeping patterns. Simulating the home environment as much as possible will encourage deep sleep patterns, which may stimulate apnea and provide valuable diagnostic information.

Minimizing Anxiety

1. Encourage the parents to continue involvement in infant care during hospitalization.
2. Clarify any misconceptions about apnea and SIDS.
3. Allow ventilation of feelings and concerns.
4. Assess family dynamics for any conflicts or maladapted responses; intervene or refer, as appropriate.
5. Use anticipatory guidance in preparing the parents for emotional responses to home monitoring.
   a. Increased anxiety or tension.
   b. Constant worry about the alarm even when it does not go off.
   c. Fatigue.
   d. Financial and emotional burdens encountered by the family.
   e. Perceived loss of "normal, healthy child"; parents may grieve when given the diagnosis.

Increasing Confidence in Home Monitoring

1. Demonstrate operation and maintenance of the monitor. Reinforce teaching by equipment supplier. Provide information on contacting a monitor technician. Teach parents proper electrode and belt placement and skin care.
   a. Do not adjust monitor to eliminate false alarms.
   b. Maintain an unobstructed view of the monitor. Plug power cord directly into outlet—do not use extension cords. Check battery and charger. Place monitor on firm surface.
   c. Monitored infant should not share his or her bed.
2. Identify the presence of a telephone in the home and, if not, devise an alternative plan in the event of an emergency situation.

3. Describe how to record apnea in relation to activity and position and when to report apnea to health care provider.
4. Teach methods of responding to alarms; what to observe and document in diary (eg, color, presence or absence of breathing) and how to respond (gentle vs. vigorous stimulation, cardiopulmonary resuscitation [CPR]). Never vigorously shake the child.
5. Discuss the necessary adjustments in daily living and anticipated changes.
   a. Emphasize that responsibility must be shared by family members.
   b. Discuss the possible impact on siblings.
   c. Advise the parents to eliminate noises that would interfere with their ability to hear the alarm (eg, showering, vacuuming). Someone must always be available to hear and respond to the alarm. Be aware of electrical interference from appliances or cellular phones and in public places such as airports.
   d. Avoid traveling long distances alone with the infant.
   e. Encourage the parents to enlist the assistance of a third person who is willing to learn CPR and to help care for the infant and provide the parents with an opportunity for respite time.
6. Emphasize the healthy aspects of the infant. Encourage the parents to continue as many usual routines as possible. Provide specific things parents can do to encourage normal development and a healthy parent–child relationship.
7. Encourage the parents to provide total care for their infant 24 hours before discharge so they regain confidence in caring for their child.

Family Education and Health Maintenance

1. Advise the family to keep emergency numbers near the telephone or set on speed dial.
2. Educate about feeding precautions: frequent burping, no bottle in bed, upright position after feeding, positioning the infant on his or her back or side, not abdomen. Avoid soft, moldable sleeping surfaces and pillows; toys and stuffed animals should be removed from the crib.
3. Have parents contact local emergency service to inform them about their infant and to be certain that they have infant resuscitation equipment. Arrange for notification of the utility company to plan for the event of a power outage.
4. Instruct the parents in the administration of any new medications.
5. Teach CPR to all those involved in providing care for the infant.
6. Refer the family to a home care agency for home nursing visits, additional teaching, and support.

Evaluation: Expected Outcomes

- Monitoring maintained; respirations regular without apnea.
- Parents verbalize concern over infant's well-being.
- Parents demonstrate correct operation of respiratory monitor and response to alarms.

 TRANSITIONAL CARE ALERT Respiratory disorders are among the most common conditions in the pediatric population due to their developing airways and their potential for rapid decompensation. Children being discharged with respiratory disorders may require oxygen therapy, suction procedures, and a multitude of medications delivered in many routes (oral, nebulizer, etc.). If arrangements have been made for nursing care in the home, families should be aware of the agency providing services and when they can expect communication regarding care arrangements. Families should have thorough written (and if necessary to assist understanding, pictorial) instructions on signs and symptoms to monitor for worsening of status. Nurses responsible for discharging children should ensure that families understand (and can demonstrate if possible) proper use of necessary treatments.

> **EVIDENCE BASE** Tieder, J., Bonkowsky, J., Etzel, R., et al. (2016). Brief resolved unexplained events (formerly apparent life-threatening events) and evaluation of lower risk infants. *Pediatrics, 137*(5), e1–e32.
> Rabasco, J., Vigo, A., Vitelli, O., et al. (2016). Apparent life-threatening events could be a wake-up call for sleep disordered breathing. *Pediatric Pulmonology, 51*(12), 1403–1408.

SELECTED REFERENCES

Askew, K., Bamford, J., Hudson, N., et al. (2017). Current characteristics, challenges and coping strategies of young people with cystic fibrosis as they transition to adulthood. *Clinical Medicine, 17*(2), 121–125.

Auger, K., Kahn, R., Davis, M., & Simmons, J. M. (2015). Pediatric asthma readmission: Asthma knowledge is not enough. *Journal of Pediatrics, 166*(1), 101–108.

Barreira, E., Munoz, G., Cavalheiro, P., et al.; Pediatric Acute Respiratory Distress Syndrome Study Group. (2015). Epidemiology and outcomes of acute respiratory distress syndrome in children according to the Berlin definition: A multicenter prospective study. *Critical Care Medicine, 43*(5), 947–953.

Berlinger, N., Barfield, R., & Fleischman, A. (2013). Facing persistent challenges in pediatric decision-making: New Hastings Center guidelines. *Pediatrics, 132*(5), 789–791. doi: 10.1542/peds.2013-1378.

Blake, K., & Hengameh, R. (2018). Asthma Guidelines from the National Asthma Education and Prevention Program: Where Are We Know? *Pediatric Allergy, Immunology, and Pulmonology, 31*(1), eupdate.

Boroughs, D., & Dougherty, J. (2015). Pediatric tracheostomy care. *American Nurse Today, 10*(3), 8–10.

Bruce, C., Hoare, C., Mukherjee, A., & Paul, S. P. (2016). Managing acute respiratory tract infections in children. *British Journal of Nursing, 26*(11), 602–609.

Caffrey, O., & Clarke, J. (2016). 2016 NICE clinical guideline: Bronchiolitis in children. *Archives of Disease in Childhood—Education and Practice, 101*(1), 46–48.

Dalton, H. J., Macrae, D. J.; Pediatric Acute Lung Injury Consensus Conference Group. (2015). Extracorporeal support in children with pediatric acute respiratory distress syndrome: Proceedings from the Pediatric Acute Lung Injury Consensus Conference. *Pediatric Critical Care Medicine, 16*(5 Suppl 1), S111–S117.

Debiasi, L. (2018). Older adolescent with cystic fibrosis: Transitioning to adult care. *Pediatric Nursing, 44*(2), 95–97.

Deschildre, A., Pin, I., El Abd, K., et al. (2014). Asthma control assessment in a pediatric population: Comparison between GINA/NAEPP guidelines, Childhood Asthma Control Test (C-ACT), and physician's rating. *Allergy, 69*(6), 784–790.

Ekim, A., & Ocaki, A. (2016). Efficacy of a transition theory-based discharge planning program for childhood asthma management. *International Journal of Nursing Knowledge, 27*(2), 70–78.

Goldber, N., Rodriguez-Prado, Y., Tillery, R., et al. (2018). Sudden infant death syndrome: A review. *Pediatric Annals, 47*(3), e118–e123.

Grundfast, K., Insalaco, L., & Levi, J. (2017). The 10 commandments of management of acute upper airway obstruction in infants and children. *JAMA Otolaryngology—Head and Neck Surgery, 143*(6), 539–540.

Hewner S, Sullivan SS, Yu G. (2018). Reducing Emergency Room Visits and In-Hospitalizations by Implementing Best Practice for Transitional Care Using Innovative Technology and Big Data. Worldviews Evid Based Nurs. Mar 23

Hill, C. (2016). Nurse-led implementation of a ventilator-associated pneumonia care bundle in a children's critical care unit. *Nursing Children and Young People, 28*(4), 23–27.

Huang, M., Parker, A., Bienvenu, O., et al.; National Institutes of Health, National Heart, Lung, and Blood Institute Acute Respiratory Distress Syndrome Network. (2016). Psychiatric symptoms in acute respiratory distress syndrome survivors: A 1-year national multicenter study. *Critical Care Medicine, 44*(5), 954–965. doi: 10.1097/CCM.0000000000001621.

Johnson, D., Arnold, D., Gay, J., et al. (2018). Implementation and Improvement of Pediatric Asthma Guideline Improves Hospital-Based Care. *Pediatrics, 141*(2), 1–9.

Jones, B., Fleming, G., Otillio, J., et al. (2016). Pediatric acute asthma exacerbations: Evaluation and management from emergency department to intensive care unit. *Journal of Asthma, 53*(6), 607–617.

Karlekar, M., Doherty, K., Guyer, D., & Slovis, B. (2015). Integration of palliative care into the routine care of cystic fibrosis patients. *Palliative Medicine, 29*(3), 282–283.

Kenney, K., & Gropman, R. (2013). What immediate post-operative nursing care contributes to a better patient outcome after a child has had a day surgery tonsillectomy and adenoidectomy (T and A)? *Journal of Perianesthesia Nursing, 28*(3), e44.

Kyle, U., Lucas, L., Mackey, G., et al. (2016). Implementation of nutrition support guidelines may affect energy and protein intake in the pediatric intensive care unit. *Journal of the Academy of Nutrition and Dietetics, 116*(5), 844–885.

Lahiri, T., Hempstead, S., Brady, C., et al. (2016). Clinical practice guidelines from the cystic fibrosis foundation for preschoolers with cystic fibrosis. *Pediatrics, 137*(4).

Lee, G. Y., Yamada, J., Kyololo, O., et al. (2014). Pediatric clinical practice guidelines for acute procedural pain: A systematic review. *Pediatrics, 133*(3), 500–515.

Leyenaar, J. K., Rizzo, P. A., Khodyakov, D., et al. (2018). Importance and feasibility of transitional care for children with medical complexity: Results of a multistakeholder delphi process. *Acad Pediatr, 18*(1), 94–101

Liu, J., Wang, W., Liu, F., Li, Z. (2018). Pediatric acute respiratory distress syndrome - current views. *Exp Ther Med, 5*(2), 1775–1780.

Lynch, J., III, Savah, D., Belperio, J., & Weigt, S. S. (2015). Lung transplantation for cystic fibrosis: Results, indicators, complications, and controversies. *Seminars in Respiratory and Critical Care Medicine, 36*(2), 299–320.

Meissner, H. (2016). Viral bronchiolitis among children. *NEJM, 347*(1), 62–72.

Mikesell, C., Kempainen, B., Laguna, T., et al. (2017). Objective measurement of adherence to out-patient airway clearance therapy by high-frequency chest wall compression in cystic fibrosis. *Respiratory Care, 62*(7), 920–927.

Moheet, A., Moran, A. (2018). Pharmacological management of cystic fibrosis related diabetes. *Expert Rev Clin Pharmacol, 11*(2), 185–191.

Nierengarten, M., & Lahiri, T. (2017). Cystic fibrosis guidelines for preschool children. *Contemporary Pediatrics, 34*(3), 26–28.

Nikolopoulos, T. (2014). To give or not to give antibiotics in non-severe acute otitis media? The American Academy of Pediatrics guidelines that do not guide. *International Journal of Pediatric Otorhinolaryngology, 78*(7), 983–984.

Okumura, M., & Kleinhenz, M. (2016). Cystic fibrosis transitions of care: Lessons learned and future directions for cystic fibrosis. *Clinics in Chest Medicine, 37*(1), 119–126; 607–617.

Ozen, M., Kocabas Sandal, G., & Dinleyici, E. C. (2014). Probiotics for the prevention of pediatric upper respiratory tract infections: A systematic review. *Expert Opinion on Biological Therapy, 15*(1), 9–20.

Pacheco, G.S., Mendelson, J., Gaspers, M. (2018). Pediatric ventilator management in the emergency department. *Emerg Med Clin North Am., 36*(2), 401–413.

Pakhale, S., Armstrong, M., Holly, C., et al. (2014). Assessment of stigma in patients with cystic fibrosis. *BMC Pulmonary Medicine, 14*, 76.

Pascoal, L., Lopes, M., da Silva, V., et al. (2016). Clinical differentiation of respiratory nursing diagnoses among children with acute respiratory infection. *Journal of Pediatric Nursing, 31*(1), 85–91.

Pedraza-Bernal, A., Rodriguez-Martinez, C., & Acuna-Cordero, R. (2016). Predictors of severe disease in a hospitalized population of children with acute viral lower respiratory tract infections. *Journal of Medical Virology, 88*(5), 754–759.

Pomicino L, Maccacari E, Buchini S.(2018). Levels of anxiety in parents in the 24 hr before and after their child's surgery: A descriptive study. *J Clin Nurs., 27*(1-2), 278–287.

Porter, S., Holly, C., & Echevarria, M. (2016). Infant delirium: Keys to management and assessment. *Pediatric Nursing, 42*(5), 223–229.

Rabasco, J., Vigo, A., Vitelli, O., et al. (2016). Apparent life-threatening events could be a wake-up call for sleep disordered breathing. *Pediatric Pulmonology, 51*(12), 1403–1408.

Sanders, R., Nett, S., Davis, K., et al. (2016). Family presence during pediatric intubations. *JAMA Pediatrics, 170*(3), 1–8.

Schmid-Mohler, G. (2018). Patient-Reported Outcome Measures for Symptom Perception During a Cystic Fibrosis Exacerbation. *Respiratory Care, 63*(3), 353–366.

Soyer, T., Yalcin, S., & Arslan, S. (2017). Pediatric Eating Assessment Tool-10 as an indicator to predict aspiration in children with esophageal atresia. *Journal of Pediatric Surgery, 52*(10), 1576–1579.

Stiffler, D., Ayers, B., Fauvergue, C., et al. (2018). Sudden infant death and sleep practices in the Black community. *Journal of Specialists in Pediatric Nursing, 23*(2), e1.

Strychowsky, J. E., Albert, D., Chan, K., et al. (2016). International Pediatric Otolaryngology Group (IPOG) consensus recommendations: Routine peri-operative pediatric tracheotomy care. *International Journal of Pediatric Otorhinolaryngology, 86*, 250–255.

Styne, D., Arslanian, S., Connor, E., et al. (2017). Pediatric obesity-assessment, treatment, and prevention: An Endocrine Society Clinical Practice Guideline. *Journal of Clinical Endocrinology and Metabolism, 102*(3), 709–757.

Sullivan, J. E., Gillam, L. H., Monagle, P. T. (2018). The enactment stage of end-of-life decision-making for children. *Palliat Support Care*, Jan 11, 1–7.

Terry, K., Disabato, J., & Krajicek, M. (2015). Snoring, Trouble Breathing, Un-Refreshed (STBUR) Screening Questionnaire to reduce perioperative respiratory adverse events in pediatric surgical patients: A quality improvement project. *AANA Journal, 83*(4), 256–262.

Tieder, J., Bonkowsky, J., Etzel, R., et al. (2016). Brief resolved unexplained events (formerly apparent life-threatening events) and evaluation of lower risk infants. *Pediatrics, 137*(5), e1–e32.

Torretta, S., Rosazza, C., Pace,M., et al. (2017). Impact of adenotonsillectomy on pediatric quality of life: review of the literature. *Italian Journal of Pediatrics, 42*, 1–8.

Volsko, M. (2013). Airway clearance therapy: Finding the evidence. *Respiratory Care, 58*(10), 1669–1678.

Walls, T., Hughes, N., Mullan, P., et al. (2017). Improving Pediatric Asthma Outcomes in a Community Emergency Department. *Pediatrics, 139*(1), 55–55.

Zimlich, R., (2018). Children still prescribed postop codeine despite warnings: A new study reveals that too many children are still given codeine or codeine-containing medications after surgery. *Contemporary Pediatrics, 35*(2), 25–26.

45

Pediatric Cardiovascular Disorders

CARDIAC PROCEDURES

Cardiac Catheterization

Cardiac catheterization is an invasive procedure used to identify cardiac anatomy; measure intracardiac pressures, shunts, and oxygen saturations; and calculate systemic and pulmonary vascular resistance.

Procedure

1. Catheter insertion sites include femoral vein or artery, umbilical vein or artery, brachial vein, or internal jugular vein.
2. Under fluoroscopy, catheters are guided through the heart, collecting pressure measurements and oxygen saturations.
3. Contrast dye is injected through the catheters to visualize blood flow patterns and structural abnormalities.
4. Cardiac catheterization is usually an outpatient procedure for children who undergo an elective procedure. After interventional procedures, some children are observed in the hospital for 12 to 24 hours.

Indications

1. To confirm or establish the diagnosis.
2. To measure cardiac output.
3. To measure pressures and oxygen saturations.
4. To calculate intracardiac shunting and pulmonary and systemic vascular resistance.
5. To visualize coronary arteries.
6. To assess for myocarditis or rejection following heart transplantation.
7. To intervene in congenital heart disease (see Box 45-1 for definitions of abbreviations):
   a. Balloon atrial septostomy (Rashkind) for restrictive atrial septum.
   b. Balloon valvuloplasty (arterial stenosis [AS], pulmonary stenosis [PS]) and angioplasty (recurrent coarctation of the aorta [CoA]).
   c. Endomyocardial biopsy.

d. To occlude vessels (coil embolization) or defects (atrial septal defect [ASD], ventricular septal defect [VSD], or patent ductus arteriosus [PDA] closure devices).
   e. To stent vessels open (branch pulmonary artery [PA] stenosis, recurrent CoA).
   f. To dilate stenotic valves (mitral, pulmonary, tricuspid).
   g. To dilate conduits used to repair defect.

Complications

1. Arrhythmias (usually catheter induced).
2. Infection.
3. Bleeding at catheter insertion site; large hematoma.
4. Allergic reaction to contrast material.
5. Loss of pulse in the extremity used for cannulation.
6. Perforation of heart or vessels.
7. Stroke.
8. Dislodgment of coils, closure devices, or stents.
9. Death.

Nursing Diagnoses

Preoperative
- Fear related to surgical procedure.
- Deficient Knowledge regarding surgical procedure and associated nursing care.

Postoperative
- Risk for Injury related to complications of cardiac catheterization.

Nursing Interventions

Reducing Fear in Child and Parents
1. Provide specific instructions in nonthreatening manner:
   a. Day and time of the procedure.
   b. Nothing-by-mouth (NPO) guidelines.
   c. Sedation versus general anesthesia.
   d. Site of the planned arterial and venous puncture.
   e. Routine postprocedure care.

BOX 45-1	Abbreviations Used for Congenital Heart Disease
ASD	Atrial septal defect
AV	Atrioventricular
CoA	Coarctation of the aorta
HLHS	Hypoplastic left heart syndrome
IAA	Interrupted aortic arch
IVC	Inferior vena cava
LVOTO	Left ventricular outflow tract obstruction
PA	Pulmonary artery
PAPVR	Partial anomalous pulmonary venous return
PDA	Patent ductus arteriosus
PFO	Patent foramen ovale
PS	Pulmonary stenosis
PVR	Pulmonary vascular resistance
SVC	Superior vena cava
TA	Tricuspid atresia
TAPVR	Total anomalous pulmonary venous return
TGA	Transposition of great arteries
TOF	Tetralogy of Fallot
VSD	Ventricular septal defect

2. Provide appropriate teaching geared toward the child's age and level of cognitive development. Use diagrams and models, as appropriate.
3. Provide parents an opportunity, without the child present, to discuss the procedure, risks, benefits, and alternative choices.
4. Give the child an opportunity to express fears and ask questions.
5. Provide tour of the cardiac catheterization laboratory, if appropriate.
6. Use of child life specialist, if available, to prepare for procedure, aid in insertion of IV.

Explaining and Providing Nursing Care
1. Obtain baseline set of vital signs: heart rate, BP, respiratory rate, and oxygen saturation.
2. Measure and record the child's height and weight.
3. Note the time of last oral intake: solids and liquids.
4. Identify known allergies.
5. List current medications and note time last taken.
6. Help the child change into a hospital gown.
7. Start peripheral IV, as needed.
8. Administer sedation, as prescribed.
9. Assess and mark the location of pulses (dorsalis pedis, posterior tibial).

Observe for and Prevent Complications
1. Monitor and record routine vital signs (q 15 min × 4, q 30 min × 2, then q 1 hr); extremity temperature, color, and pulse check with vital signs.
2. Notify health care provider for:
   a. Heart rate, respiratory rate, or BP outside normal parameters for age.
   b. Bleeding or increasing hematoma at puncture site.
   c. Change in oxygen saturations.
   d. Fever.
   e. Cool, pulseless extremity.

3. Observe puncture site for redness, pain, swelling, or induration.
4. Maintain the child in a reclining position for 4 to 6 hours after the procedure, with no ambulation.
5. Offer fluids as soon as the child is ready.

Family Education and Health Maintenance
1. Provide discharge information:
   a. Care of incision or puncture site (keep dry for 48 hours).
   b. Activity restrictions (usually for 48 hours, but may be up to 2 weeks following placement of closure devices).
   c. Observe for and report late complications: redness, swelling, drainage from puncture site.
   d. Follow-up medical care.
   e. Reinforce infective endocarditis precautions.
2. If cardiac catheterization was a preoperative procedure, use the recovery time to teach the child and family about upcoming hospital stay.

Evaluation: Expected Outcomes
• Child describes procedure in own words; parents and child discuss procedure and ask appropriate questions.
• Child cooperative with preoperative nursing care.
• Insertion site intact without drainage, redness, or hematoma.

Cardiac Surgery

The ultimate goal of treatment of cardiovascular disease in children is to restore normal heart structure and function. Most types of CHDs can be palliated or definitively repaired.

Procedures

Closed-Heart Surgery
1. Surgical approach: lateral thoracotomy or mediastinal incision.
2. Indications:
   a. PDA ligation.
   b. PA banding.
   c. CoA repair.
   d. Vascular ring repair.
   e. Blalock-Taussig shunt (BT shunt) placement.
   f. Occasionally, Glenn and Fontan procedures.

Open-Heart Surgery
1. Surgery is done through a mediastinal incision.
2. With the use of cardiopulmonary bypass, the surgeon can stop the heart and operate inside to repair the defects.
3. Deep hypothermia with circulatory arrest, and/or aortic cross clamping, allows the surgeon to safely stop cardiopulmonary bypass and remove arterial or venous cannulas to better visualize and repair the defects.
4. Indications:
   a. Anomalous coronary arterial anatomy.
   b. ASD, VSD, atrioventricular (AV) canal defect.
   c. Aortic stenosis, pulmonary stenosis.
   d. Tetralogy of Fallot (TOF).
   e. Transposition of great arteries (TGA).
   f. Tricuspid atresia.
   g. Total anomalous pulmonary venous return (TAPVR) or partial APVR.
   h. Truncus arteriosus.
   i. Hypoplastic left heart syndrome (HLHS).
   j. Complex single ventricle.

Potential Complications of Specific Surgeries

1. PDA ligation: laryngeal nerve damage, phrenic nerve damage, diaphragm paralysis, thoracic duct injury.
2. CoA: rebound hypertension, mesenteric arteritis (abdominal pain), coarctation restenosis.
3. Aorta-pulmonary shunt (modified BT shunt): shunt occlusion, PA distortion, pulmonary overcirculation.
4. ASD: atrial arrhythmias, sinoatrial node dysfunction.
5. VSD: transient or permanent heart block, residual VSD, ventricular dysfunction.
6. TOF: low cardiac output, residual right ventricular outflow tract obstruction (RVOTO) or VSD, ectopic junctional tachycardia or arrhythmias, thoracic duct injury.
7. TGA: arterial switch operation—coronary artery injury, ventricular dysfunction, suprapulmonary stenosis.
8. TGA: atrial switch operation—baffle obstruction, RV failure, atrial arrhythmias.
9. Valvotomy (for valve stenosis): valve insufficiency.
10. Bidirectional Glenn shunt: superior vena cava (SVC) syndrome, low cardiac output, hypoxia, pleural effusions.
11. Fontan completion: low cardiac output, pleural effusions, ventricular dysfunction, thrombus formation, arrhythmias, hepatic dysfunction, lymphatic dysfunction.

Cardiac Transplant Surgery

Cardiac transplantation is a treatment option for children with progressive congestive heart failure (CHF) or certain cardiac diseases not amenable to conventional medical–surgical therapy. Children who cannot grow and meet developmental milestones or who have unacceptable quality-of-life issues may benefit from cardiac transplant surgery. However, approximately one in four children dies while waiting for an organ donor. Those children who receive a donor heart can develop significant complications and must take lifelong immunosuppression medications to prevent organ rejection.

Indications for Cardiac Transplantation

1. End-stage cardiomyopathy.
2. Untreatable complex CHD.
3. Malignant arrhythmia.
4. Retransplant for cardiac graft failure.

Immunosuppressive Medications

 EVIDENCE BASE Rossano, J. W., Cherikh, W. S., Chambers, D., et al. (2017). The registry of the International Society for Heart and Lung Transplantation: Twentieth pediatric heart transplantation report - 2017; Focus theme: Allograft ischemic time. *The Journal of Heart and Lung Transplantation, 36*(10), 1060–1069.

Immunosuppressive therapy is divided into two phases, induction and maintenance. Induction therapies reduce early rejection and may help to reduce the child's overall exposure to corticosteroids. Combination therapy is usually used in the maintenance phase to ensure ongoing protection against rejection.

1. Phase I: Induction.
   a. Polyclonal antibodies.
      i. Antibodies harvested from equine (Atgam) or rabbit (thymoglobulin).
      ii. Interlukin-2 receptor antibodies.
         1) Daclizumab.
         2) Basiliximab.

2. Phase II: Maintenance therapies.
   a. Calcineurin inhibitors.
      i. Cyclosporine.
      ii. Tacrolimus.
   b. Antiproliferative agent.
      i. Azathioprine.
      ii. Mycophenolate mofetil.
   c. Mammalian target of rapamycin inhibitors.
      i. Sirolimus.
      ii. Everolimus.
      iii. Less nephrotoxic than calcineurin inhibitors.
   d. Corticosteroids.
   e. Oral prednisone and prednisolone most common.
      i. Used in higher doses early post-transplant, gradually tapering over time.
      ii. Short burst IV doses of methylprednisolone can be used in acute rejection.

Complications

1. Organ rejection: routine surveillance endomyocardial biopsies are performed to assess for rejection.
   a. With mild to moderate rejection, children may initially be asymptomatic.
   b. With severe rejection, children are usually symptomatic with hemodynamic instability.
2. Infection.
3. Adverse effects of immunosuppressive agents.
   a. Polyclonal antibodies—fever, chills, urticaria, headaches, severe hypotension, abdominal pain, leukopenia, and thrombocytopenia
   b. Reactions can be minimized by premedicating with corticosteroids, acetaminophen, diphenhydramine
   c. Calcineurin inhibitors.
      i. Ciclosporin—nephrotoxicity, hypertension, diabetes mellitus, hirsutism, gingival hyperplasia, tremor.
      ii. Tacrolimus—nephrotoxicity, diabetes mellitus, hypertension, hyperkalemia, hypomagnesemia, tremor.
   d. Antiproliferative agent.
      i. Azathioprine—leukopenia, thrombocytopenia, nausea, hepatic dysfunction, pancreatitis.
      ii. Mycophenolate mofetil—leukopenia, nausea, vomiting, diarrhea, anorexia.
   e. Mammalian target of rapamycin inhibitors—hyperlipidemia, thrombocytopenia, anemia, leukopenia, interference with wound healing, oral lesions.
   f. Prednisone—hypertension, Cushing syndrome, growth retardation.
4. Graft dysfunction/failure.
   a. Leading cause of death posttransplant.
   b. The most severe cases become apparent in the immediate post-operative period.
   c. Treat with inotropic drugs, short-term mechanical circulatory support with extracorporeal membrane oxygenation (ECMO) or ventricular assist device (VAD), eventual retransplantation.
5. Cardiac allograft vasculopathy (CAV).
   a. Occurs late after transplant.
   b. Unique and progressive atherosclerosis affecting only transplanted hearts.
   c. Treat with mechanical circulatory support, discontinuation of all immunosuppressive agents.
6. Posttransplant lymphoproliferative disease.

Routine Follow-Up

1. Routine well-child care visits to primary care provider.
    a. Transplant children should not receive any live virus immunizations (oral polio, measles–mumps–rubella, varicella). Monitor for adverse effects of chronic steroids and immunosuppressive medications.
2. Routine cardiology clinic visits.
    a. Laboratory studies: chemistry, hematology, therapeutic drug levels.
    b. Vital signs.
    c. Electrocardiogram (ECG).
    d. Echocardiography.
3. Serial cardiac catheterizations and endomyocardial biopsies.
4. Yearly coronary angiography.

Nursing Assessment

Baseline Assessment on Day of Surgery

1. Measure and record height and weight.
2. Document vital signs: heart rate, respiratory rate, BP, and oxygen saturation.
3. Assess for preoperative infection: fever, signs of upper respiratory infection (cough, runny nose, crackles), vomiting, or diarrhea might necessitate delaying surgery.
4. Document last oral intake.
5. Void on call to the operating room.

Nursing Diagnoses

Preoperative

- Fear related to surgical procedure.

Postoperative

- Delayed Surgical Recovery related to complications.
- Impaired Adjustment related to postsurgery care.

Nursing Interventions

Preparing the Child and Family and Reducing Fear

1. Be honest and use nonthreatening language the child can understand.
2. The following are frequently asked questions from parents. Address them with the parents:
    a. What to tell the child.
    b. When to tell the child.
    c. What to bring to the hospital.
    d. Anticipated hospital course: how long in the operating room; how many days in the intensive care unit (ICU); how many days on the general care unit; visiting policy, rooming-in accommodations.
3. Review preoperative instructions.
    a. NPO guidelines.
    b. Where to report on the day of the surgery.
    c. Time to arrive at the hospital; time of surgery.
    d. Preoperative medications (injection, liquid, inhalation).
    e. What the operating room looks like; what the people wear in the operating room (hats, gowns, and masks).
4. Explain the preoperative period.
    a. Change into a hospital gown.
    b. Parents stay with the child.
    c. Transportation to the operating room (walking, wheelchair, or stretcher).
5. Explain the operative period.
    a. Operating room waiting room.
    b. Updates during the surgery will come from the surgical scrub nurses.
    c. Surgeon will meet the family after surgery to review the surgical findings and to describe the operation.
6. Explain the postoperative period. Use models and diagrams.
    a. Pediatric ICU routines and procedures.
    b. Monitoring lines and equipment.
    c. Ventilators, oxygen therapy.
    d. Protective restraints.
7. Offer medical equipment to handle and play with (ECG leads, face mask, BP cuff), age-appropriate books about surgery and hospital stays, and tour of ICU and surgical area, as available.
8. Prehospital tour of the pediatric ICU and general pediatric care unit.
9. Allow an opportunity for the child and family to ask questions, express their concern, or ask for more detail.

Observing for and Preventing Complications

1. Assess respiratory status and maintain respiratory support.
    a. Maintain ventilatory support, as needed.
    b. Maintain patent airway with routine endotracheal suctioning.
    c. Auscultate breath sounds frequently. Decreased breath sounds may indicate pleural effusions, atelectasis, pneumothorax, or hemothorax.
    d. Report results of routine chest x-ray.
    e. Perform frequent position changes: side-back-side.
    f. Monitor arterial blood gas levels and oxygen saturations.
    g. Assess chest or mediastinal tube drainage; examine characteristics and quantify hourly in the initial postoperative period.
    h. Identify those patients at risk for pulmonary hypertension in the postoperative period.
    i. Treatment includes oxygen, analgesia and sedation, prevention of acidosis, chemical paralysis, and inhaled nitric oxide.
    j. Extubate when hemodynamically stable and when patient meets extubation criteria.
    k. Administer oxygen therapy, as needed, after extubation.
2. Assess cardiac status.
    a. Monitor vital signs and oxygen saturations.
    b. Auscultate heart sounds immediately upon admission, noting quality and presence of any residual murmurs.
    c. If patient has had a BT shunt placed, frequently assess shunt murmur presence and volume. Sudden or progressive muting of this could indicate shunt occlusion and is an emergency.
    d. Maintain continuous ECG monitoring.
        i. Daily 12-lead ECG to assess rhythm.
        ii. Temporary epicardial pacemaker wires available for atrial and/or ventricular pacing, as needed.
        iii. In presence of these, keep pacer located at the bedside.
    e. Continuous BP monitoring (arterial line).
    f. Monitor intracardiac pressures (central venous pressure [CVP], left atrial [LA], PA).
    g. Monitor peripheral perfusion, capillary refill, toe temperature.
    h. Titrate vasopressors (dopamine, dobutamine, epinephrine, milrinone), as prescribed.

3. Assess fluid status.
   a. Record hourly intake (IV fluids, blood products, fluid boluses).
   b. Record hourly output (urine, chest/mediastinal tube drainage, nasogastric drainage).
   c. Concerning if chest/mediastinal tube output exceeds 5 to 10 cc/kg/hour.
   d. Take note if chest/mediastinal tube drainage suddenly decreases, concern for obstruction in tube with resultant pericardial or pleural effusion.
   e. Perform daily weights.
   f. Administer diuretics, as prescribed, noting response.
4. Assess neurologic status.
   a. Monitor level of responsiveness, response to verbal commands, and response to pain.
   b. Check pupil size and reactivity to light.
   c. Document movement of all extremities.
   d. Monitor all invasive lines for air bubbles and potential air embolism.
   e. Observe for signs of neurologic injury related to hypoperfusion or embolism.
5. Monitor for potential specific complications related to particular surgery for CHD.
6. Assess for postoperative pain.
   a. Monitor level of responsiveness, agitation.
   b. Implement pediatric pain scale rating to assist the child in identifying the severity of pain.
   c. Administer pain and anxiolytic medication, as prescribed: continuous IV infusion and IV boluses, as necessary to control pain and hypertension related to pain and anxiety.
   d. Utilize patient-controlled analgesia continuous pump, as appropriate.
7. Assess serum electrolyte balance. Obtain blood tests and report results. Treat deficits with supplements, paying particular attention to potassium, calcium, and magnesium levels.
8. Assess packed cell volume, platelet count, and coagulation studies.
   a. Low hematocrit (less than 30): consider directed donor transfusion or blood bank transfusion.
   b. Low platelet count: continue to monitor; if bleeding persists, transfuse platelets.
   c. Prolonged coagulation studies: continue to monitor; if bleeding or oozing persists, give fresh frozen plasma, protamine.

Enhancing Adjustment Postoperatively

1. Provide continuity of care (primary nursing and consistent medical team).
2. Explain all procedures and routines to the child and parents to minimize fear.
3. Explain to the parents a child's typical reactions to stressful events.
   a. Regression—temporary loss of developmental milestones.
   b. Fear of any medical personnel (white coat anxiety).
   c. Sibling jealousy that one child is receiving a lot of attention.
   d. Withdrawal—related to stimulation overload and lack of undisturbed sleep.
   e. Nightmares.
   f. Increased dependency; clinging behavior.
4. Suggest parent and patient support groups, Child Life Therapy, community resources, and counseling, as needed.

Family Education and Health Maintenance

1. Provide the child and family with oral and written discharge instructions and recommendations.
   a. Medications.
   b. Activity restrictions.
   c. Sternal precautions
      i. No strenuous activity or contact sports for 6 to 8 weeks after surgery.
      ii. Most children are ready to return to school at least part time about 2 weeks after surgery.
      iii. If child needs prolonged recovery time at home, may need to consider home tutoring.
      iv. No gym class until full recovery.
   d. Care of the incision.
   e. Dietary recommendations.
   f. Bathing or showering guidelines.
2. Provide the child and family with a list of potential signs of complications and instructions to notify the health care provider.
   a. Fever greater than or equal to 101.5°F (38.6°C).
   b. Any redness, swelling, or drainage from chest incision.
   c. Partial opening of the chest incision.
   d. Poor appetite, nausea, vomiting.
   e. Breathing difficulties, shortness of breath.
   f. Lethargy, sustained.
   g. For neonates and infants, increased fussiness or sudden inconsolability.
3. Provide the family with the names and phone numbers of people to call for questions and emergencies.
4. Make follow-up appointments for the child to be seen by his or her primary care provider 2 to 3 days after discharge from the hospital and 10 to 14 days to be seen by their pediatric cardiologist.
5. Review American Heart Association's recommendations for infective endocarditis prophylaxis. In children with CHD, prophylaxis is indicated only for patients who:
   a. Have cyanotic heart disease that has not been fully repaired.
   b. Have prosthetic material or device for the first 6 months postoperatively.
   c. Have residual cardiac lesions even after repair, such as abnormal flow or regurgitation at patches or valves.

Community and Home Care Considerations

1. Arrange skilled home nursing visits, as needed, to:
   a. Review medications.
   b. Assess wound healing.
   c. Monitor vital signs and oxygen saturations.
   d. Monitor growth for single ventricle infants post-operatively, during the interstage period, optimize nutrition.
   e. Assess oral intake; nutritional status.
   f. Resource for family.
2. Make referral to community agencies, as needed (infant and toddler program).
3. Arrange for home medical equipment (oxygen, feeding pump, and supplies), as needed.
4. Review safety precautions in the home:
   a. Childproof medication bottles.
   b. Poison control phone number for accidental medication overdose.
   c. Infant and child CPR techniques.

d. Bleeding precautions for children on anticoagulation therapy. No aspirin or ibuprofen products. Be sure to read the labels on over-the-counter cold and cough syrups. Avoid activities with high risk of injury. All head injuries need to be evaluated by a physician. Signs of bleeding:
  i. Blood in the urine.
  ii. Black tarry stools.
  iii. Prolonged nosebleeds.
  iv. Bleeding gums.
  v. Bruising for no known trauma.
  vi. Spitting or coughing up blood.
  vii. Any unusual swelling or pain.
  e. MedicAlert bracelet or tags.
5. Discuss developmental issues with the family.
  a. A child on diuretics may have difficulty with toilet training.
  b. Disciplining, establishing behavioral expectations, and setting limits in a child with CHD should be similar to those for a child without CHD.
6. Discuss the need for home schooling or tutoring during recovery time. Return to the classroom as soon as the child is ready.
7. Discuss infants with CHD in daycare situations—address each case individually. Daycare programs usually have increased risk of URIs and other communicable diseases.
8. Encourage routine dental visits to prevent dental caries (dental caries predispose to bacteremia and endocarditis).
9. Encourage heart-healthy eating and exercise routines.
10. Encourage age-appropriate activities. A few children will need exercise restrictions. Children with CHD should be allowed to participate in activities with rest periods, as needed. Children with pacemakers and children on anticoagulation therapy should refrain from contact sports.
11. Maintain standard childhood immunization schedule. Delay vaccines around the perioperative time until fully recovered from surgery (no immunizations for 6 weeks postoperatively).
12. Encourage yearly influenza vaccine for children with unrepaired or complex CHD.
13. Encourage respiratory syncytial virus (RSV) immunization for children younger than age 2 with complex CHD and those at risk of CHF or pulmonary hypertension.

Evaluation: Expected Outcomes

- Child describes procedure without fear; parents and child discuss procedure and ask appropriate questions.
- Vital signs stable, no signs of infection.
- Parents offer support to child.

CONGENITAL HEART DISEASE
Overview

 EVIDENCE BASE Bouma, B. J., & Mulder, B. J. M. (2017). Changing landscape of congenital heart disease. *Circulation Research, 120*, 908–922.

Congenital heart disease (or *defects*) *(CHD)* is one of the most common forms of congenital anomalies. It involves the chambers, valves, and vessels arising from the heart (see Figure 45-1, page 1207). In most cases, the cause of CHD is not known. Some infants and children with CHD may appear perfectly healthy, whereas others may present as critically ill. Most infants and children with CHD can be successfully managed with medications and surgeries.

Etiology and Incidence

1. CHD affects 8 of every 1,000 live births (range from 3 to 10).
2. Exact cause of CHD is unknown in approximately 85% of cases.
3. The heart begins as a single cell and develops into a four-chambered pumping system during the 3rd to 8th weeks of gestation.
4. Associated factors for CHD include:
  a. Fetal or maternal infection during the first trimester (rubella).
  b. Chromosomal abnormalities (trisomy 21, 18, 13).
  c. Maternal insulin-dependent diabetes.
  d. Phenylketonuria
  e. Systemic lupus erythematosus.
  f. Teratogenic effects of drugs and alcohol.
    i. Lithium—Ebstein anomaly.
    ii. Phenytoin—aortic and pulmonic stenosis.
    iii. Alcohol—ASD and VSD.
5. Syndromes that include CHD:
  a. Marfan syndrome—mitral valve prolapse (MVP), dilated aortic root.
  b. Turner syndrome—aortic valve stenosis (AVS), CoA.
  c. Noonan syndrome—dysplastic pulmonary valve.
  d. William syndrome—supravalvular PS.
  e. DiGeorge syndrome—interrupted aortic arch (IAA), truncus arteriosus, TGA, and TOF.
  f. Down syndrome (trisomy 21)—endocardial cushion can develop abnormally, commonly AV canal defect, VSD. About 50% of children with Down syndrome have a CHD.

 DRUG ALERT Teratogenic drugs also include amphetamines, estrogen, progesterone, retinoic acid, selective serotonin reuptake inhibitors, trimethadione, and valproic acid.

Common Congenital Heart Malformations

Congenital heart defects can be classified into three categories: obstruction to blood flow, increased pulmonary blood flow (acyanotic lesions), and decreased pulmonary blood flow (cyanotic lesions).
1. Obstructive lesions:
  a. AS—valvular, subvalvular, or supravalvular.
  b. CoA.
  c. PS—valvular, subvalvular, or supravalvular.
  d. IAA.
2. Increased pulmonary blood flow (acyanotic):
  a. PDA.
  b. ASD.
  c. VSD.
  d. AV canal (balanced or unbalanced).
  e. PAPVR.
3. Decreased pulmonary blood flow (cyanotic):
  a. TOF.
  b. TA.
  c. TAPVR.
  d. TGA.
  e. Truncus arteriosus.
  f. HLHS.
  g. DORV.

Patent Ductus Arteriosus

Patent ductus arteriosus (PDA) is a vascular connection that, during fetal life, shunts blood from the pulmonary artery to the aorta. Functional closure of the ductus normally occurs soon after birth. If the ductus remains patent after birth, the direction of blood flow in the ductus is reversed from aorta to pulmonary circuit by the higher pressure in the aorta.

Ventricular Septal Defect

Ventricular septal defect (VSD) is an abnormal opening between the right and left ventricle. VSDs vary in size and may occur in either the membranous or muscular portion of the ventricular septum. Due to the higher pressure in the left ventricle, a shunting of blood from the left to right ventricle occurs during systole. If pulmonary hypertension or obstruction to pulmonary flow exists, the shunt of blood is then reversed from the right to the left ventricle, with cyanosis resulting.

Pulmonary Stenosis

Pulmonary stenosis refers to any lesion that obstructs the blood flow from the right ventricle to the pulmonary artery. This obstruction may cause right ventricular hypertrophy and eventual right-sided heart failure.

Aortic Stenosis

Aortic stenosis may be at the subvalvular, valvular (with thickening or fusion of the cusps), or supravalvular level. Subaortic stenosis is caused by a fibrous ring below the aortic valve in the outflow tract of the left ventricle. At times, valvular and subaortic stenosis exist in combination. The obstruction presents an increased workload for the normal output of the left ventricular blood and results in left ventricular enlargement.

Coarctation of the Aorta

Coarctation of the aorta is characterized by a narrowed aortic lumen. It normally occurs in the juxtaductal position. Coarctations exist with great variation in anatomic features. The lesion produces an obstruction to the flow of blood through the aorta, causing increased left ventricular pressure and workload.

Tetralogy of Fallot

Tetralogy of Fallot is characterized by the combination of four defects: (1) pulmonary stenosis, (2) ventricular septal defects, (3) overriding aorta, (4) hypertrophy of right ventricle. It is the most common defect causing cyanosis in patients surviving past age 2. The severity of symptoms depends on the degree of pulmonary stenosis, the size of the VSD, and the degree to which the aorta overrides the ventricular septal defect.

Complete Transposition of Great Vessels

The aorta originates from the right ventricle and the pulmonary artery from the left ventricle. An abnormal communication between the two circulations (atrial septal defect [ASD] or VSD) must be present to sustain life.

Atrial Septal Defect

An atrial septal defect (ASD) is an abnormal opening between the right and left atria. Basically, three types of abnormalities result from incorrect development of the atrial septum: (1) sinus venosus at the top of the atrial septum, (2) ostium secundum at the middle of the atrial septum, (3) ostium primum at the bottom of the atrial septum. In general, left-to-right shunting of blood occurs in all ASDs.

Tricuspid Atresia

Tricuspid valvular atresia is characterized by absence of the tricuspid valve, a small right ventricle, and usually diminished pulmonary circulation. Cyanosis is present because blood from the right atrium passes through an ASD into the left atrium, mixes with oxygenated blood returning from the lungs, flows into the left ventricle, and is propelled into the systemic circulation. The lungs may receive blood through one of three routes: (1) VSD, (2) PDA, and (3) collateral aortopulmonary vessels.

Hypoplastic Left Heart Syndrome

A collection of complex congenital heat lesions results in the abnormal development of the left side of the heart. These lesions include: (1) mitral stenosis/atresia, (2) aortic stenosis or atresia, (3) aortic arch hypoplasia, and (4) hypoplastic left ventricle. The right ventricle pumps blood through the pulmonary and systemic circulations. A patent foramen ovale allows a left-to-right shunt and blood is shunted from left atrium back to right atrium. A PDA is often the sole supply of blood to the systemic circulation.

Figure 45-1. Congenital heart abnormalities.

Aortic Stenosis

 EVIDENCE BASE Friedland-Little, J. M., Zampi, J. D., & Gajarski, R. J. (2016). Aortic stenosis. In H. D. Allen, R. E. Shaddy, D. J. Penny, T. F. Feltes, & F. Cetta (Eds.), *Moss and Adams' heart disease in infants, children, and adolescents* (9th ed., pp. 1085–1101). Philadelphia, PA: Lippincott Williams & Wilkins.

Congenital *aortic stenosis (AS)* is a left ventricular outflow tract obstructive lesion. It may be caused by a bicuspid aortic valve with fused commissures that does not open completely, by a hypoplastic aortic valve annulus, or by stenosis above or below the aortic valve (subvalvular or supravalvular stenosis). The result is turbulent blood flow across the aortic valve and into the ascending aorta. Patients with AS must be evaluated for additional left heart lesions that include coarctation of the aorta, mitral valve stenosis, hypertrophic cardiomyopathy, and hypoplastic left heart. AS is the most common form of left ventricular outflow tract obstruction (LVOTO). It accounts for 3% to 6% of CHDs. AS may occur at any age, and it occurs more commonly in boys than in girls.

Pathophysiology and Etiology

1. Blood flows at an increased velocity across the obstructive valve or stenotic area and into the aorta.
2. During systole, left ventricular pressure rises dramatically to overcome the increased resistance at the aortic valve.
3. Myocardial ischemia may occur because of an imbalance between the increased oxygen requirements related to the hypertrophied left ventricle (LV) and the amount of oxygen that can be supplied.
4. A consistent increased pressure load on the LV causes pathologic ventricular remodeling. Progression to left-sided heart failure and eventual cellular changes is reflected in clinical signs of failure.

Clinical Manifestations

Neonate
Onset of symptoms occurs quickly with critical AS, upon the closure of the ductus arteriosus.
1. Severe CHF.
2. Metabolic acidosis.
3. Tachypnea.
4. Faint peripheral pulses, poor perfusion, poor capillary refill, cool skin.
5. Poor feeding and feeding intolerance.

Child and Adolescent
Symptoms may be slower to progress and develop over time.
1. Chest pain on exertion, decreased exercise tolerance.
2. Dyspnea, fatigue, shortness of breath.
3. Syncope, light-headedness.
4. Palpitations.
5. Sudden death.

Diagnostic Evaluation

1. Auscultation.
   a. Systolic ejection murmur heard best at right upper sternal border, radiates to neck.
   b. Ejection click. May be absent with severe stenosis.
   c. S_2 splits normally or narrowly.
2. Four-limb blood pressure.
   a. Systolic blood pressure normally 5 to 10 mm higher in lower extremities.
   b. For patients with supravalvar aortic stenosis, right arm may have a 15 to 20 mm Hg increase in systolic pressure as compared to left arm.
3. Palpation.
   a. Thrill may be palpable over suprasternal notch with mild valvar aortic stenosis, right upper sternal border in moderate or worse stenosis.
4. Auscultation.
   a. May hear harsh crescendo–decrescendo systolic ejection murmur, at the right upper sternal border for valvar and supravalvar stenosis, at the left mid-sternal border for subvalvar stenosis.
5. ECG: left ventricular hypertrophy (LVH) with a strain pattern may be seen in severe cases.
6. Chest x-ray: increased cardiac silhouette, increased pulmonary vascular markings. A prominent aortic knob may be seen occasionally from poststenotic dilatation with valvular AS.
7. Echocardiogram: two-dimensional echocardiogram with Doppler study and color flow mapping to visualize the anatomy and to estimate the gradient across the valve and through the aorta.

Management

Neonate
1. Stabilize with prostaglandin E_1 (PGE_1) infusion to maintain cardiac output through the PDA.
2. Inotropic support, as needed.
3. Intubation and ventilation, as needed.
4. Cardiac catheterization after initial stabilization: aortic balloon valvuloplasty or aortic balloon angioplasty.
5. Surgical valvotomy, commissurotomy, or myectomy/myotomy.

Child and Adolescent
1. Medical management with close follow-up to monitor increasing gradient across the aortic valve or through the aorta.
2. Continued hypertension can significantly dilate the aortic root over time.
3. Exercise testing to determine recommended level of activity. Those who have more abnormal results and/or EKG changes should stay away from sports with a high aerobic component.
4. Aortic balloon valvuloplasty or aortic balloon angioplasty.
5. Surgical intervention.
   a. Surgical valvotomy, commissurotomy, or myectomy/myotomy.
   b. In neonates with critical aortic stenosis, success of a biventricular repair has to be determined, gauging the strength of the LV and its associated structures. If damage is too great, then a single ventricle staged repair approach may be used.
   c. Aortic valve replacement.
      i. Mechanical prosthesis (St. Jude valve).
      ii. Ross procedure (pulmonary autograft, placement of right ventricle to pulmonary artery conduit).

Complications

1. CHF and pulmonary edema.
2. Dizziness, light-headedness, and syncope.
3. Palpitations, arrhythmias.
4. Infective endocarditis.
5. Sudden death.

Coarctation of the Aorta

EVIDENCE BASE Kaya, U., Colak, A., Becil, N., et al. (2018). Surgical management of aortic coarctation from infant to adult. *Eurasian Journal of Medicine, 50*(1), 14–18.

Coarctation of the aorta (CoA) is a discrete narrowing or a long segment hypoplasia of the aortic arch, usually in the juxtaductal position. It accounts for 6% to 8% of CHDs and is two to five times more common in males. Thirty percent of infants with Turner syndrome have CoA. Commonly associated defects include VSD, mitral valve stenosis, and bicuspid aortic valve.

Pathophysiology and Etiology

1. The discrete narrowing or hypoplastic segment of the aorta increases the workload of the left ventricle (increased LV systolic pressure).
2. In a neonate with critical CoA, lower body blood flow occurs through the PDA (right-to-left shunting).
3. In the older child, collateral vessels grow and bypass the coarctation to perfuse the lower body.

Clinical Manifestations

1. The neonate with critical CoA (ductal dependent lesion):
   a. Asymptomatic until the PDA begins to close, rapid decompensation at 8 to 10 days of life.
   b. After PDA closure: severe CHF, poor lower body perfusion, tachypnea, acidosis, progressive circulatory shock, absent femoral and pedal pulses.
2. The child or adolescent with CoA:
   a. Usually asymptomatic—normal growth and development.
   b. Hypertension in the upper extremities, with absent or weak femoral pulses.
   c. Murmur present.
   d. Nosebleeds, headaches, leg cramps with exercise.

Diagnostic Evaluation

1. Auscultation—varies; nonspecific systolic ejection murmur. Murmur may be heard over the base or posteriorly in the left scapular region. Single S_2 loud S_3 gallop is usually present.
2. Four-limb blood pressure.
   a. Systolic blood pressure elevated in upper extremities, proximal to coarctation, as compared to lower extremities. A significant gradient exists between the two.
3. Chest x-ray—cardiomegaly and pulmonary edema or pulmonary venous congestion.
4. ECG—varies; normal or right ventricular hypertrophy (RVH) in infants and LVH in older children.
5. Two-dimensional echocardiography with Doppler and color flow mapping identifies area of aortic arch narrowing and associated lesions (bicuspid aortic valve, VSD, PDA).
6. Invasive studies (cardiac catheterization) usually not needed to make the initial diagnosis; may need aortic angiography to identify collateral vessels before surgery.
7. Cardiac magnetic resonance imaging may be done to noninvasively assess the location and degree of narrowing and identify collateral vessels.

Management

Critical Coarctation in the Neonate

1. Medical management:
   a. Resuscitation and stabilization with PGE_1 infusion: monitor for complications related to PGE_1 therapy (fever, apnea).
   b. Intubation and ventilation, as needed.
   c. Anticongestive therapy (digoxin and Lasix) and inotropic support, as needed.
   d. Assessment of renal, hepatic, and neurologic function.
2. Balloon angioplasty may be indicated for infants who are at high surgical risk.
3. Surgical intervention: usually performed as soon as the diagnosis is made.
   a. Subclavian flap repair (Waldhausen procedure).
   b. End-to-end anastomosis.
   c. Dacron patch repair.
   d. Stent implantation.

Coarctation in the Child or Adolescent

1. Surgical intervention.
   a. End-to-end anastomosis.
   b. Dacron patch.
   c. Stent implantation.
2. Medical management for hypertension (beta-adrenergic blockers).

Recurrent Coarctation in the Neonate or Child

More common in the patient who underwent repair in infancy.

1. Balloon angioplasty in the cardiac catheterization laboratory.
2. Redo surgical intervention.

Complications

1. Systemic hypertension.
2. CHF—occurs in 20% to 30% of all infants with CoA by age 3 months.
3. Intracranial hemorrhage.
4. Left ventricular failure.
5. Aortic aneurysm.

Pulmonary Stenosis

EVIDENCE BASE Nielsen, E., & Vibeke, E. (2016). Surgically treated pulmonary stenosis: over 50 years of follow up. *Cardiology of the Young, 26*(5), 860–866.

The pulmonary valve opens during systole to let blood flow from the right ventricle into the main PA. Obstruction to flow can occur at three levels: subvalvular, valvular, or supravalvular. The most common cause of RV outflow tract obstruction is pulmonary valve stenosis (PS). PS accounts for 8% to 10% of CHDs.

Pathophysiology and Etiology

1. Critical PS in the neonate: blood flows into the right atrium, across a patent foramen ovale (PFO) into the left side of heart; pulmonary blood flow comes from a left-to-right shunt through a PDA.
2. Right ventricular pressure increases to pump blood across the obstructive pulmonary valve.

3. Right ventricular hypertrophy develops in response to the increased pressure gradient across the pulmonary valve.
4. Signs of right-sided heart failure include hepatic congestion, neck vein distention, and elevated CVP.

Clinical Manifestations

Critical PS in the Neonate
1. Hypoxia.
2. Tachypnea.
3. RV failure.

Mild to Moderate PS in the Child and Adolescent
1. Asymptomatic.
2. Decreased exercise tolerance, fatigue, exertional dyspnea.
3. Chest pain.

Diagnostic Evaluation

1. Auscultation: systolic ejection murmur heard best at the left upper sternal border; ejection click.
2. ECG: varies; normal in mild cases and RVH in moderate to severe cases.
3. Chest x-ray: varies; may show right ventricular enlargement; poststenotic dilatation of PA.
4. Two-dimensional echocardiography with Doppler study and color flow mapping to visualize the sites of obstruction, observe the degree of RVH, and estimate the pressure gradient across the valve.
5. Cardiac catheterization is usually not needed for the initial diagnosis.

Management

Neonate with Critical PS
1. Medical management:
   a. Stabilize and improve oxygen saturations with PGE_1 infusion.
   b. Intubation and ventilation, as needed.
   c. Inotropic support, as needed.
2. Balloon pulmonary valvuloplasty.
3. Blalock-Taussig shunt (Gore-Tex graft between the subclavian artery and the PA to supply pulmonary blood flow), as initial intervention.

Child and Adolescent with PS
1. Medical management:
   a. Close follow-up to monitor and record RV to PA gradient and assess RV function.
   b. Restrict strenuous exercise.
   c. Refer for intervention when RV pressure is greater than two thirds of the systemic pressure.
2. Balloon pulmonary valvuloplasty in the cardiac catheterization laboratory.
3. Surgical intervention:
   a. Valvotomy or valvectomy for dysplastic pulmonary valve.
   b. Patch repair of the right ventricular outflow tract.
   c. Placement of an RV-to-PA conduit.

Complications

1. Cyanosis (critical PS in the neonate as a result of suprasystemic pulmonary pressures through anatomic shunt).
2. Arrhythmia; sudden death.
3. Infective endocarditis.
4. Right ventricular failure.

Patent Ductus Arteriosus

 EVIDENCE BASE Taggart, N. W. & Qureshi, M. Y. (2016). In H. D. Allen, R. E. Shaddy, D. J. Penny, T. F. Feltes, & F. Cetta (Eds.), *Moss and Adams' heart disease in infants, children, and adolescents* (9th ed., pp. 803–813). Philadelphia, PA: Lippincott Williams & Wilkins.

The *ductus arteriosus* is a normal fetal connection between the left PA and the descending aorta. During fetal life, blood flow is shunted away from the lungs through the ductus arteriosus and directly into the systemic circulation. PDAs occur in up to 60% of premature neonates who weigh less than 1,000 g. In term infants, PDAs account for 5% to 10% of CHDs; the male to female ratio is 1:2.

Pathophysiology and Etiology

1. During fetal life, the ductus arteriosus allows blood to bypass the pulmonary circulation (fetus receives oxygen from the placenta) and flow directly into the systemic circulation.
2. After birth, the ductus arteriosus is no longer needed. Functional closure usually occurs within 24 to 72 hours after birth. Anatomic closure is completed by age 2 to 3 weeks.
3. When the ductus arteriosus fails to close, blood from the aorta (high pressure) flows into the low-pressure PA, resulting in pulmonary overcirculation.
4. Increased pulmonary blood flow leads to a volume-loaded LV.

Clinical Presentation

Small- to Moderate-Sized PDA
Usually asymptomatic.

Large PDA
1. CHF, tachypnea, frequent respiratory tract infections.
2. Poor weight gain, failure to thrive.
3. Feeding difficulties.
4. Decreased exercise tolerance.
5. Infective endocarditis.

Diagnostic Evaluation

1. Auscultation: continuous murmur heard best at left upper sternal border. Hyperactive precordium with large PDAs.
2. Wide pulse pressure; bounding pulses.
3. Chest x-ray: varies; normal or cardiomegaly with increased pulmonary vascular markings.
4. ECG: varies; normal, LVH, or RVH.
5. Two-dimensional echocardiogram with Doppler study and color flow mapping to visualize the PDA with left-to-right blood flow.
6. Elevated levels of N-terminal pro-B-type natriuretic peptide and cardiac troponin T.
7. Cardiac catheterization is not needed for the initial diagnosis.

Management

1. In the symptomatic premature neonate—NSAIDs (indomethacin and ibuprofen) are given via IV line. These drugs are not effective in term infants.

2. Medical management:
   a. Monitor growth and development.
   b. Reassess for spontaneous PDA closure.
   c. Diuretics (furosemide, chlorothiazide) for pulmonary congestion.
   d. Increase caloric intake as needed for normal weight gain.
   e. Infective endocarditis prophylaxis for 6 months after surgery or coil occlusion.
3. Cardiac catheterization:
   a. For small PDAs, coil occlusion.
   b. For larger PDAs, a closure device may be used.
4. Surgical management through PDA ligation.

Complications

1. CHF, pulmonary edema.
2. Infective endocarditis.
3. Pulmonary hypertension/pulmonary vascular occlusive disease.
4. Recurrent pneumonia.

Atrial Septal Defect

 EVIDENCE BASE Sachdeva, R. (2016). Atrial septal defect. In H. D. Allen, R. E. Shaddy, D. J. Penny, T. F. Feltes, & F. Cetta (Eds.), *Moss and Adams' heart disease in infants, children, and adolescents* (9th ed., pp. 743–753). Philadelphia, PA: Lippincott Williams & Wilkins.

Atrial septal defect (ASD) is an abnormal communication between the left and right atria. ASDs account for 8% to 10% of CHDs. There are four types:
1. Ostium secundum ASD: most common type of ASD (accounts for 50% to 70%); abnormal opening in the middle of the atrial septum.
2. Ostium primum ASD (accounts for 30%): abnormal opening at the bottom of the atrial septum; increased association with cleft mitral valve and atrioventricular defects.
3. Sinus venosus ASD (accounts for 10%): abnormal opening at the top of the atrial septum; increased association with partial anomalous pulmonary venous return.
4. Coronary sinus defect (rare): abnormal opening between coronary sinus and left atrium.

Pathophysiology and Etiology

1. Blood flows from the higher pressure left atrium across the ASD into the lower pressure right atrium (left-to-right shunt).
2. Increased blood return to the right side of the heart leads to right ventricular volume overload and right ventricular dilation.
3. Increased pulmonary blood flow leads to elevated pulmonary artery pressures.

Clinical Manifestations

1. Usually asymptomatic.
2. Clinical symptoms vary depending on type of associated defects and degree of shunting:
   a. CHF (usually not until the third or fourth decade of life).
   b. Frequent upper respiratory infections (URIs).
   c. Poor weight gain.
   d. Decreased exercise tolerance.
   e. Dyspnea and fatigue.

Diagnostic Evaluation

1. Auscultation: soft systolic ejection murmur heard best at the left upper sternal border; widely split, fixed second heart sound.
2. Prominent systolic impulse.
3. Chest x-ray: varies; normal to right atrial and ventricular dilation, increased pulmonary markings.
4. ECG: varies; right axis deviation and mild RVH or right bundle-branch block. Alterations are present only when the shunt is large and the pulmonary resistance to systemic resistance ratio is greater than 1.5:1 (Qp:Qs > 1.5:1).
5. Two-dimensional echocardiogram with Doppler study and color flow mapping to identify the site of the ASD and associated lesions and document left-to-right flow across the atrial septum.
6. Cardiac catheterization is usually not needed for initial diagnosis; performed if defect can be closed using an atrial occlusion device (device can be used only in ostium secundum defects).

Management

1. Medical management:
   a. Monitor and reassess (spontaneous closure rate is small but may occur up to age 2).
   b. Treatment with diuretics may be necessary if signs of CHF are present (usually not until third to fourth decade of life if ASD unrepaired).
   c. Infective endocarditis prophylaxis for 6 months after surgery or atrial occlusion device is used.
2. Cardiac catheterization for placement of an atrial occlusion device for ostium secundum defects.
3. Surgical intervention:
   a. Primary repair: suture closure of the ASD.
   b. Patch repair of the ASD.

Complications

1. CHF (rare).
2. Infective endocarditis.
3. Embolic stroke.
4. Pulmonary hypertension.
5. Atrial arrhythmias.

Ventricular Septal Defect

 EVIDENCE BASE Cohen, M. S., & Lopez, L. (2016). Ventricular septal defects. In H. D. Allen, R. E. Shaddy, D. J. Penny, T. F. Feltes, & F. Cetta (Eds.), *Moss and Adams' heart disease in infants, children, and adolescents* (9th ed., pp. 783–800). Philadelphia, PA: Lippincott Williams & Wilkins.

A *ventricular septal defect (VSD)* is an abnormal communication between the right and left ventricles. It is the most common type of CHD, accounting for up to 40% of CHDs. VSD is slightly more common in females and is the most common lesion found in chromosomal syndromes (Trisomy 13, 18, 21). VSDs vary in size (small and restrictive to large and nonrestrictive), number (single vs. multiple), and type (perimembranous or muscular).

Pathophysiology and Etiology

1. Blood flows from the high-pressure left ventricle across the VSD into the low-pressure right ventricle and into the PA, resulting in pulmonary overcirculation. The size of the defect determines the physiologic effect on the infant.
2. A left-to-right shunt because of a VSD results in increased right ventricular pressure and increased PA pressure.
3. The increased pulmonary venous return to the left side of the heart results in left atrial dilation.
4. Long-standing pulmonary overcirculation causes a change in the pulmonary arterial bed, leading to increased pulmonary vascular resistance. High pulmonary vascular resistance (PVR) can reverse the blood flow pattern that leads to a right-to-left shunt across the VSD (Eisenmenger syndrome), resulting in cyanosis. Once this develops, the child is no longer a candidate for surgical repair.

Clinical Manifestations

1. Small VSDs—usually asymptomatic; high spontaneous closure rate during the first year of life. Ongoing risk of endocarditis.
2. Moderate VSDs—present with similar symptoms as the larger VSDs, but in milder form that is not quite as pronounced or significant.
3. Large VSDs—typical presentation at 4 to 8 weeks of age.
   a. CHF: tachypnea, tachycardia, excessive sweating associated with feeding, hepatomegaly.
   b. Frequent URIs.
   c. Poor weight gain, failure to thrive presenting at age 2 to 3 months.
   d. Feeding difficulties.
   e. Fatigue.

Diagnostic Evaluation

1. Auscultation: harsh systolic regurgitant murmur heard best at the lower left sternal border (LLSB); systolic thrill felt at LLSB, narrowly split S_2. The murmur may radiate toward the head along the left parasternal border or to the right of the sternum.
2. Chest x-ray: varies; normal or cardiomegaly and increased pulmonary vascular markings. Pulmonary vascular markings are directly proportionate to the amount of left-to-right shunting.
3. ECG: varies; normal to biventricular hypertrophy.
4. Two-dimensional echocardiogram with Doppler study and color flow mapping to identify the size, number, and sites of the defects; estimate pulmonary artery pressure; and identify associated lesions.
5. Cardiac catheterization usually not needed for initial diagnosis; may be needed to calculate the size of the shunt or to assess PVR. May be performed if defect can be closed using a ventricular occlusion device (device can be used only in muscular defects).

Management

Small VSD

1. Medical management:
   a. Usually no anticongestive therapy is needed.
   b. Infective endocarditis prophylaxis for 6 months after surgical implantation of a ventricular occlusion device.

2. Cardiac catheterization for placement of a ventricular occlusion device for muscular defects (for Qp:Qs > 1.5:1).
3. Surgical intervention is usually not necessary.

Moderate to Large VSD

1. Medical management:
   a. CHF management: digoxin, ACE inhibitors, and diuretics.
   b. Avoid oxygen; oxygen is a potent pulmonary vasodilator and will increase blood flow into the PA.
   c. Maximize nutrition: increase caloric intake by fortifying formula or breast milk to make 24 to 30 cal/ounce; supplemental nasogastric feeds, as needed.
   d. Infective endocarditis prophylaxis for 6 months after surgery/ventricular device occluder.
2. Cardiac catheterization for placement of a ventricular occlusion device for muscular defects (for Qp:Qs > 1.5:1).
3. Refer for surgical intervention.
   a. Usually repaired before age 2.
   b. Patch closure of VSD.

Long-Term Follow-Up

1. Monitor ventricular function.
2. Monitor for subaortic membrane and double-chamber RV.
3. Monitor for formation of residual VSD following patch closure.

Complications

1. CHF.
2. Frequent URIs.
3. Failure to thrive; poor weight gain.
4. Infective endocarditis.
5. Arrhythmias (right bundle branch block, transient complete heart block in postop period).
6. Eisenmenger syndrome.
7. Pulmonary hypertension.
8. Aortic insufficiency.

Tetralogy of Fallot

 EVIDENCE BASE Roche, S. L., Greenway, S., & Redington, A. (2016). Tetralogy of Fallot with pulmonary stenosis, pulmonary atresia, and absent pulmonary valve. In H. D. Allen, R. E. Shaddy, D. J. Penny, T. F. Feltes, & F. Cetta (Eds.), *Moss and Adams' heart disease in infants, children, and adolescents* (9th ed., pp. 1029–1047). Philadelphia, PA: Lippincott Williams & Wilkins.

Tetralogy of Fallot (TOF) is the most common complex CHD. The four abnormalities of TOF include:

1. A large, nonrestrictive VSD.
2. Overriding aorta.
3. Pulmonary stenosis (right ventricular outflow tract obstruction).
4. Right ventricular hypertrophy.

Pathophysiology and Etiology

1. Degree of cyanosis depends on the size of the VSD and the degree of RVOTO.
2. Obstruction of blood flow from the right ventricle to the PA results in deoxygenated blood being shunted across the VSD and into the aorta (right-to-left shunt causes cyanosis).

3. RVOTO can occur at any or all of three levels: pulmonary valve stenosis, infundibular stenosis, or supravalvular stenosis.
4. The right ventricle becomes hypertrophied as a result of the increased gradient across the RVOT.
5. Minimal RVOTO results in a pink TOF variant, with the physiology behaving more like a large, nonrestrictive VSD. As pulmonary vascular resistance decreases, signs/symptoms may become more apparent as a result of increased shunting.

Clinical Manifestations

1. Clinical manifestations are variable and depend on the size of the VSD and the degree of RVOTO.
2. Cyanosis.
   a. Neonate may have normal oxygen saturations; as the infant grows, the RVOTO increases and the oxygen saturation falls.
   b. Neonate with unacceptably low oxygen saturation needs PGE_1 infusion to maintain ductal patency and adequate oxygen saturation (necessary for the TOF with pulmonary atresia).
   c. Cyanosis may initially be observed only with crying and with exertion (increasing PVR and right to left shunting).
3. Loud second heart sound with a harsh systolic ejection murmur.
4. Polycythemia.
5. Decreased exercise tolerance.
6. A common clinical manifestation years ago was squatting, a posture characteristically assumed by older children to increase systemic vascular resistance and to encourage increased pulmonary blood flow. Squatting is rarely seen currently, however, because TOF is now surgically repaired during the first year of life.
7. Hypercyanotic spells (formerly known as Tet spells): life-threatening hypoxic event with a dramatic decrease in oxygen saturations; mechanism is usually infundibular spasm, which further obstructs pulmonary blood flow and increases right-to-left flow across the VSD.
   a. Typical hypoxic spells occur in the morning soon after awakening; during or after a crying episode; during or after a feeding; during painful procedures such as blood draws.
   b. Typical scenario includes tachypnea, irritability, and increasing cyanosis, followed by flaccidity and loss of consciousness.
   c. Home treatment for the caregiver: soothe the infant and place him or her in a knee–chest position; notify the health care provider immediately.
   d. Hospital treatment includes knee–chest position, sedation (morphine), oxygen, beta-adrenergic blockers (propranolol) to relax the infundibulum, and administration of medications to increase systemic vascular resistance (phenylephrine, norepinephrine).
   e. Intubation and ventilation as needed to reduce work of breathing and oxygen consumption.
   f. Hypercyanotic spells usually prompt the cardiologist to refer for surgical intervention.

Diagnostic Evaluation

1. Auscultation: harsh systolic ejection murmur heard best at the upper left sternal border (RVOT murmur); single loud second heart sound; aortic ejection click. Murmur is caused by pulmonary stenosis—in mild stenosis, the murmur is louder and longer than when stenosis is more severe; during a hypercyanotic spell, the murmur disappears.
2. Palpation: systolic thrill palpable along left lower and left middle sternal border (50% of cases). RV tap at left sternal border.
3. Chest x-ray: varies; normal or decreased pulmonary vascular markings. The heart may appear "boot shaped" because of a concave main PA with an upturned apex resulting from RVH.
4. ECG: varies; normal or RVH.
5. Two-dimensional echocardiogram with Doppler study and color flow mapping to identify the structural abnormalities, estimate the degree of RVOTO, and assess the coronary artery pattern.
6. Cardiac catheterization is usually not needed for the initial diagnosis. May be performed before surgical intervention to identify the location and number of VSDs, the PVR, the degree of RVOTO, and the presence of any coronary abnormalities.

Management

1. Medical management:
   a. Monitor oxygen saturation level.
   b. Monitor growth and development.
   c. Monitor for hypercyanotic spells (many spells go unnoticed by parents).
   d. Infective endocarditis prophylaxis (lifelong).
   e. Restrict strenuous activity and participation in competitive sports.
2. Balloon pulmonary angioplasty (rarely).
3. Infants with severe pulmonary stenosis may require PGE_1 to maintain ductal patency.
4. Surgical intervention: palliative versus definitive repair.
   a. Many centers prefer definitive, one-stage repair.
   b. Potential obstacles for one-stage repair: abnormal coronary artery distribution (left anterior descending arises from right coronary artery and crosses RVOT); multiple VSDs; hypoplastic branch pulmonary arteries; small infant weighing less than 5.5 pound (2.5 kg).
   c. Palliative surgery: modified BT shunt-tube Gore-Tex graft between the left subclavian artery and the PA; increased pulmonary blood flow results in higher oxygen saturations.
   d. Reparative surgery: patch closure of VSD, relief of right ventricular outflow tract obstruction; with or without transannular patch across the pulmonary valve.
   e. For patients with pulmonary atresia, a RV to PA conduit is placed, bypassing the atretic RVOT. As the patient grows, this conduit will need to be upsized, up to several times throughout childhood.
5. Long-Term Follow-Up
   a. Assess RV outflow tract, monitor degree of pulmonary insufficiency.
   b. Monitor RV function and exercise tolerance.
   c. Monitor for arrhythmias.
   d. Continue monitoring for incompletely understood sequelae of long-term effects of repaired physiology, extending to adulthood.

Complications

1. Hypoxia.
2. Hypercyanotic spells.
3. Polycythemia.
4. CHF: rare; associated with pink TOF.
5. Right ventricular dysfunction.
6. Ventricular arrhythmias.
7. Infective endocarditis.

Transposition of the Great Arteries

 EVIDENCE BASE Qureshi, A. M., Justino, H., & Heinle, J. S. (2016). Transposition of the great arteries. In H. D. Allen, R. E. Shaddy, D. J. Penny, T. F. Feltes, & F. Cetta (Eds.), *Moss and Adams' heart disease in infants, children, and adolescents* (9th ed., pp. 1164–1183). Philadelphia, PA: Lippincott Williams & Wilkins.

Transposition of the great arteries (TGA) occurs when the PA arises off the left ventricle and the aorta arises off the right ventricle. It accounts for 5% of CHDs and is more common in males. The most commonly associated additional lesion is a ventricular septal defect. Ten percent of infants with TGA also have noncardiac malformations.

Pathophysiology and Etiology

1. This defect results in two parallel circulations:
   a. The right atrium receives deoxygenated blood from the inferior vena cava (IVC) and SVC; blood flow continues through the tricuspid valve into the right ventricle and is pumped back to the aorta.
   b. The left atrium receives richly oxygenated blood from the pulmonary veins; blood flow continues through the mitral valve into the left ventricle and is pumped back into the PA.
2. To sustain life, there must be an accompanying defect that allows mixing of deoxygenated blood and oxygenated blood between the two circuits, such as PDA, ASD, PFO, or VSD.
3. Neonates born with TGA with an intact ventricular system are usually more cyanotic and sicker than neonates born with TGA with a VSD.

Clinical Manifestations

Symptoms evident soon after birth; clinical scenario and varying degrees of clinical manifestations are influenced by the extent of intercirculatory mixing (presence or absence of intact ventricular septum).
1. Cyanosis.
2. Tachypnea.
3. Metabolic acidosis.
4. CHF.
5. Feeding difficulties.

Diagnostic Evaluation

1. Auscultation: varies; no murmur or a murmur related to an associated defect, single loud S₂.
2. Chest x-ray: varies; neonate chest x-ray usually normal; cardiomegaly with a narrow mediastinum (egg-shaped cardiac silhouette) and increased pulmonary markings; or decreased pulmonary markings with pulmonary stenosis.
3. ECG: right atrial enlargement, RVH, or biventricular hypertrophy.
4. Two-dimensional echocardiogram with Doppler study and color flow mapping identifies the structural abnormalities: transposed vessels, coronary artery pattern, and degree of mixing across the atrial septum plus associated lesions.

Management

Medical Management
1. Stabilize with PGE₁ infusion.
2. Correct metabolic acidosis.
3. Supplemental oxygen to decrease PVR.
4. Treat pulmonary overcirculation with digoxin and diuretics, as needed.
5. Intubate and ventilate, as needed.
6. Inotropic support, as needed.
7. Infective endocarditis prophylaxis (lifelong).

Cardiac Catheterization
1. Balloon atrial septostomy (Rashkind) is indicated for severe hypoxia to create or improve atrial level mixing, for those patients who have an intact ventricular septum.

Surgical Management
1. Arterial switch operation (Jatene)—procedure of choice:
   a. Ideally performed during the first 1 to 2 weeks of life—center-specific timing.
   b. The aorta and PA are switched back to their anatomically correct ventricle above the level of the valve.
   c. Coronary arteries are transferred to the new aorta.
   d. Associated lesions are also repaired at this time.
2. Rastelli operation—performed for TGA, VSD, and PS.
   a. Repaired during the first year of life.
   b. VSD patch repaired to include LV to aortic outflow continuity with pulmonary blood flow provided via an RV to PA homograft.
3. Atrial switch operation—Mustard or Senning procedure:
   a. Rerouting of atrial blood flow: RA → mitral valve → LV → PA and LA → tricuspid valve → RV → Ao.
   b. Restores oxygenated blood into the systemic system and deoxygenated blood guided to the pulmonary system.
   c. Disadvantages:
      i. RV is left as the systemic ventricle—will develop RV dysfunction.
      ii. Increased incidence of atrial dysrhythmias and baffle obstruction.

Complications

1. Severe hypoxia.
2. Multiorgan ischemia.
3. Arrhythmias.
4. RV dysfunction.
5. Coronary artery obstruction leading to myocardial ischemia or death.
6. Long-term follow up is necessary for pediatric and adult patients, regardless of surgical repair technique.

Tricuspid Atresia

 EVIDENCE BASE Cetta, F., Dearani, J. A., O'Leary, P. W., & Driscoll, D. J. (2016). Tricuspid valve disorders: Atresia, dysplasia, and Ebstein anomaly. In H. D. Allen, R. E. Shaddy, D. J. Penny, T. F. Feltes, & F. Cetta (Eds.), *Moss and Adams' heart disease in infants, children, and adolescents* (9th ed., pp. 950–958). Philadelphia, PA: Lippincott Williams & Wilkins.

Tricuspid atresia involves the absence of the tricuspid valve and hypoplasia of the right ventricle. Such associated defects as ASD, VSD, or PDA are necessary for survival. Tricuspid atresia accounts for about 3% of CHDs.

Pathophysiology and Etiology

1. With tricuspid atresia, systemic venous return enters the right atrium and cannot continue into the RV; blood flows across an atrial septal opening into the left atrium.
2. Pulmonary blood flow occurs through a PDA or VSD.

Clinical Manifestations

1. Cyanosis.
2. Tachypnea.
3. Feeding difficulties.
4. Additional signs of failure.

Diagnostic Evaluation

1. Auscultation: murmurs vary depending on the associated lesions; single S_2.
2. Palpation: if a restrictive VSD is present, a thrill may be palpated.
3. Chest x-ray: pulmonary vascular markings related to the amount of pulmonary blood flow (usually decreased); normal to slightly increased cardiac silhouette.
4. ECG: superior axis; right and left atrial hypertrophy; LVH. First-degree AV block can be common.
5. Two-dimensional echocardiogram identifies the atretic tricuspid valve and hypoplastic RV; Doppler study and color flow mapping documents the right-to-left atrial shunt and the size of the PDA or VSD.
6. Cardiac catheterization may be necessary to delineate anatomy.

Management

Medical Management

1. Stabilize with PGE_1 infusion.
2. Maintain oxygen saturation at greater than 75%.
3. Intubate and ventilate, as needed.
4. Inotropic support, as needed.

Surgical Management

1. First surgery—neonate:
   a. BT shunt—indicated if pulmonary blood flow is insufficient.
   b. Pulmonary artery band—indicated if pulmonary blood flow is excessive.
   c. No treatment is required if pulmonary blood flow is balanced.
   d. If the great arteries are transposed, Damus-Kaye-Stansel (DKS) may be performed—placement of a modified BT shunt as well as joining of the aorta and main pulmonary artery.
2. Second surgery—ages 6 to 9 months:
   a. Bidirectional Glenn shunt: end-to-side anastomosis of the SVC to the right PA.
3. Third surgery—ages approximately 3 to 4 years
   a. Fontan completion: IVC to PA connection (extracardiac conduit with or without fenestration or intracardiac baffle).

Complications

1. CHF.
2. Persistent pleural effusion (especially after stage II and stage III repairs).
3. Thrombus formation in the systemic venous system.
4. Infective endocarditis.
5. Rarely, heart block.
6. Eventual Fontan circulation can result in lifelong multisystem complications, to varying degrees, in childhood, as well as adulthood.

Hypoplastic Left Heart Syndrome

 EVIDENCE BASE Spillane, N. T., Kashyap, S., Bateman, D., Weindler, M., & Krishnamurthy, G. (2016). Comparison of feeding strategies for infants with hypoplastic left heart syndrome. *World Journal for Pediatric and Congenital Heart Surgery, 7*(4), 446–453.

Tweddell, J. S., et al. (2016). Hypoplastic left heart syndrome. In H. D. Allen, R. E. Shaddy, D. J. Penny, T. F. Feltes, & F. Cetta (Eds.), *Moss and Adams' heart disease in infants, children, and adolescents* (9th ed., pp. 1085–1101). Philadelphia, PA: Lippincott Williams & Wilkins.

Hypoplasic left heart syndrome (HLHS) is a constellation of left-sided heart abnormalities that include:

1. Critical mitral stenosis or atresia.
2. Hypoplastic LV.
3. Critical aortic stenosis or atresia.
4. Hypoplastic ascending aorta with severe coarctation of the aorta.
5. Associated anomalies include CoA (75%), ASD (15%), and VSD (10%).

HLHS accounts for 1.4% to 3.8% of all CHDs. It is the most common cause of death from cardiac defects in the first month of life.

Pathophysiology and Etiology

1. The left side of the heart is underdeveloped and essentially nonfunctional.
2. The right ventricle supports the pulmonary and systemic circulations.
3. An ASD allows blood to flow from the left atrium into the right heart.
4. Blood flows right to left across the PDA and into the descending aorta to deliver oxygen and nutrients to the body.

Clinical Manifestations

1. Neonate may appear completely well initially but becomes critically ill when the PDA closes.
2. Once the PDA begins to close:
   a. Tachypnea due to CHF.
   b. Decreased urine output.
   c. Poor feeding and feeding intolerance.
   d. Lethargic; change in level of alertness.
   e. Pallor; gray.
   f. Weak peripheral pulses.
   g. Cyanosis.
   h. Metabolic acidosis.

Diagnostic Evaluation

1. Auscultation: single S_2; usually no heart murmur is present, but occasionally, a soft systolic ejection murmur may be heard. As CHF develops, gallop rhythm may be heard.
2. Chest x-ray: cardiac silhouette varies (normal to increased size); increased pulmonary markings and pulmonary edema.
3. ECG: RV hypertrophy; decreased electrical forces in V_5 and V_6.

4. Two-dimensional echocardiogram with Doppler study and color flow mapping identifies the structural abnormalities and the altered blood flow patterns.
5. A cardiac catheterization is usually not needed for initial diagnosis. It may be performed if a balloon atrial septostomy is needed to improve oxygenation.

Management

Medical Management

1. Resuscitation and stabilization with PGE_1 infusion.
2. Inotropic support, as needed (dopamine, dobutamine).
3. Intubate and ventilate, as needed.
4. Correct metabolic acidosis.
5. Assess hepatic, renal, and neurologic function.
6. Infective endocarditis prophylaxis (lifelong).
7. Refer for surgical intervention.

Cardiac Catheterization

1. May need balloon atrial septostomy to allow unrestrictive LA to RA blood flow.
2. Hybrid approach to first stage palliation, combining both catheterization and surgery; often consists of stenting the PDA and placement of bilateral PA bands.

Surgical Management

1. Palliative, staged repair:
   a. Stage I Norwood (neonate): reconstruction of the hypoplastic aorta using the PA and an aortic or pulmonary allograft, an atrial septectomy, repair of the coarctation, and placement of a BT shunt or RV-PA conduit (Sano modification).
   b. Postoperatively, desire to have a balanced systemic and pulmonary circulation, maintaining oxygen saturations at approximately 75% to 85%.
   c. Stage II bidirectional Glenn shunt (ages 6 to 9 months): transect the SVC off the right atrium and directly suture end to side to right PA; ligate BT shunt.
   d. Expect goal oxygen saturations postoperatively to be approximately 75% to 85%.
   e. Stage III Fontan (ages 18 months to 4 years): IVC to PA connection (extracardiac conduit with or without fenestration or intracardiac baffle).
   f. Expect goal oxygen saturations postoperatively to be greater than 85%, increasing to near normal postdischarge.
2. Cardiac transplantation.

Complications

1. Cyanosis.
2. Metabolic acidosis.
3. Persistent pleural effusion (especially after stage II or III repair).
4. Thrombus formation in the systemic venous system.
5. Infective endocarditis.
6. Cardiovasclar collapse, multisystem failure, possible death.
7. Interstage period, between stage I and II of surgical repair, has been identified as a vulnerable period for neonates, the second highest risk for mortality. As a result, most programs have adopted interstage monitoring, consisting of oxygen saturation and weight checks, designed to be completed in the home. This may identify top risk factors that can be recognized early and treated during this time.

Nursing Care of the Child with Congenital Heart Disease

EVIDENCE BASE Cao, J. Y., Lee, S. Y., Phan, et al. (2018). Early outcomes of hypoplastic left heart syndrome infants: Meta-analysis of studies comparing the Hybrid and Norwood procedures. *World Journal for Pediatric and Congenital Heart Surgery, 9*(2), 224–233.

Peterson, J. K., & Evangelista, L. S. (2017). Developmentally supportive care in congenital heart disease: A concept analysis. *Journal of Pediatric Nursing, 36*, 241–247.

Nursing Assessment

1. Obtain a thorough nursing history.
2. Discuss the care plan with the health care team (cardiologist, cardiac surgeon, nursing case manager, social worker, and nutritionist). Discuss the care plan with the patient, parents, and other caregivers.
3. Measure and record height and weight and plot on a growth chart.
4. Record vital signs and oxygen saturations.
   a. Measure vital signs at a time when the infant/child is quiet.
   b. Choose appropriate-size blood pressure (BP) cuff.
   c. Check four extremity BP × 1.
5. Assess and record:
   a. Skin color: pink, cyanotic, mottled.
   b. Mucous membranes: moist, dry, cyanotic.
   c. Extremities: check peripheral pulses for quality and symmetry; dependent edema; capillary refill; color and temperature.
6. Assess for clubbing (cyanotic heart disease).
7. Assess chest wall for deformities; prominent precordial activity.
8. Assess respiratory pattern.
   a. Before disturbing the child, stand back and count the respiratory rate.
   b. Loosen or remove clothing to directly observe chest movement.
   c. Assess for signs of respiratory distress: increased respiratory rate, grunting, retractions, and nasal flaring.
   d. Auscultate for crackles, wheezing, congestion, and stridor.
9. Assess heart sounds.
   a. Determine rate (bradycardia, tachycardia, or normal for age) and rhythm (regular or irregular).
   b. Identify murmur (type, location, and grade).
10. Assess fluid status.
    a. Daily weights.
    b. Strict intake and output (number of wet diapers; urine output).
11. Assess and record the child's level of activity.
    a. Observe the infant while feeding. Does the infant need frequent breaks or does he or she fall asleep during feeding? Assess for sweating, color change, or respiratory distress while feeding.
    b. Observe the child at play. Is play interrupted to rest? Ask the parent if the child keeps up with peers while at play.
    c. Assess and record findings relevant to the child's developmental level: age-appropriate behavior, cognitive skills, gross and fine motor skills.

Nursing Diagnoses

- Impaired Gas Exchange related to altered pulmonary blood flow or pulmonary congestion.
- Decreased Cardiac Output related to decreased myocardial function.
- Activity Intolerance related to hypoxia or decreased myocardial function.
- Imbalanced Nutrition: Less Than Body Requirements related to excessive energy demands required by increased cardiac workload.
- Risk for Infection related to chronic illness.
- Fear and Anxiety related to life-threatening illness.

Nursing Interventions

Relieving Respiratory Distress

1. Position the child in a reclining, semi-upright position.
2. Suction oral and nasal secretions, as needed.
3. Identify target oxygen saturations and administer oxygen, as prescribed.
4. Administer prescribed medications and document response to medications (improved, no change, or worsening respiratory status).
   a. Diuretics.
   b. Bronchodilators.
5. May need to change oral feedings to nasogastric feedings because of increased risk of aspiration with respiratory distress.

Improving Cardiac Output

See Table 45-1.

1. Organize nursing care and medication schedule to provide periods of uninterrupted rest.
2. Provide play or educational activities that can be done in bed with minimal exertion.
3. Maintain normothermia.
4. Administer diuretics (furosemide, spironolactone), as prescribed.
   a. Give the medication at the same time each day. For older children, do not give a dose right before bedtime.
   b. Monitor the effectiveness of the dose: measure and record urine output.
   c. Monitor serum electrolytes. Can experience hypokalemia, hypocalcemia with diuretic use.
5. Administer digoxin, as prescribed.
   a. Check heart rate for 1 minute. Withhold the dose and notify the physician for bradycardia (heart rate less than 90 beats/minute).
   b. Lead II rhythm strip may be ordered for PR interval monitoring. Prolonged PR interval indicates first-degree heart block (dose of digoxin may be withheld).
   c. Give medication at the same time each day. For infants and children, digoxin is usually divided and given twice per day.
   d. Monitor serum electrolytes. Increased incidence of digoxin toxicity associated with hypokalemia.
6. Administer afterload-reducing medications (captopril, enalapril), as prescribed.
   a. When initiating medication for the first time: check BP immediately before and 1 hour after dose.
   b. Monitor for signs of hypotension: syncope, light-headedness, and faint pulses.
   c. Withhold medication and notify the physician according to ordered parameters.

Improving Oxygenation and Activity Tolerance

1. Place pulse oximeter probe (continuous monitoring or measure with vital signs) on finger, earlobe, or toe. Preductal and postductal saturation monitoring provides the most comprehensive information about oxygenation.
2. Administer oxygen, as needed.
3. Titrate amount of oxygen to reach target oxygen saturations.
4. Assess response to oxygen therapy: increase in baseline oxygen saturations, improved work of breathing, and change in patient comfort.
5. Explain to the child how oxygen will help. If possible, give the child the choice for face mask oxygen or nasal cannula oxygen.

Table 45-1 Common Cardiac Drugs

DRUG CLASSIFICATION	MECHANISM OF ACTION	EXAMPLES
Beta-adrenergic blockers	Antagonize epinephrine receptors resulting in decreased cardiac contractility and decreased heart rate	Propranolol, esmolol, atenolol
Angiotensin-converting enzyme (ACE) inhibitor	Lowers blood pressure by decreasing blood vessel tone (reduces afterload)	Captopril, enalapril
Angiotensin II receptor blockers	Decrease blood pressure by causing dilation of blood vessels	Losartan, valsartan
Calcium-channel blockers	Decrease intracellular calcium leading to reduced cardiac and vascular smooth muscle contraction and lower blood pressure	Amlodipine, diltiazem, felodipine, isradipine, intravenous nicardipine, nifedipine, and verapamil
Vasopressors	Increase cardiac contractility and vascular muscle tone resulting in increased blood pressure	Dopamine, dobutamine, milrinone, epinephrine
Diuretics	Reduce blood volume by increasing urinary output. Used to treat high blood pressure and congestive heart failure	Furosemide, spironolactone
Antiarrhythmics	Various classifications used to treat cardiac dysrhythmias	Lidocaine, amiodarone, disopyramide adenosine
Cardiac glycosides	Strengthens cardiac contractility and decreases heart rate. Used to treat congestive heart failure	Digoxin

Providing Adequate Nutrition

1. For the infant:
   a. Small, frequent feedings.
   b. Fortified formula or breast milk (up to 30 cal/ounce).
   c. Limit oral feeding time to 15 to 20 minutes.
   d. Supplement oral feeds with nasogastric feedings, as needed, to provide weight gain (ie, continuous nasogastric feedings at night with ad-lib by-mouth feeds during the day).
2. For the child:
   a. Small, frequent meals.
   b. High-calorie, nutritional supplements.
   c. Determine child's likes and dislikes and plan meals accordingly.
   d. Allow the parents to bring the child's favorite foods to the hospital.
3. Report feeding intolerance: nausea, vomiting, and diarrhea.
4. Document daily weight (same time of day, same scale, same clothing).
5. Record accurate intake and output; assess for fluid retention.
6. Fluid restriction not usually needed for children; manage excess fluid with diuretics.

Preventing Infection

1. Maintain routine childhood immunization schedule. With the exception of RSV and influenza, immunizations should not be given for 6 weeks after cardiovascular surgery.
2. Administer yearly influenza vaccine.
3. Administer RSV immunization for children younger than age 2 with complex CHD and those at risk for CHF or pulmonary hypertension.
4. Prevent exposure to communicable diseases.
5. Good handwashing.
6. Report fevers.
7. Report signs of URI: runny nose, cough, and increase in nasal secretions.
8. Report signs of GI illness: diarrhea, abdominal pain, and irritability.

Reducing Fear and Anxiety

1. Educate the patient and family.
2. Provide the family with contact phone numbers: how to schedule a follow-up visit; how to reach a cardiologist during the work week, evenings, weekends, and holidays.

Family Education and Health Maintenance

1. Instruct the family in necessary measures to maintain the child's health:
   a. Complete immunization.
   b. Adequate diet and rest.
   c. Prevention and control of infections.
   d. Regular medical and dental checkups. The child should be protected against infective endocarditis when undergoing certain dental procedures.
   e. Regular cardiac checkups.
2. Teach the family about the defect and its treatment.
   a. Provide patients and families with written and verbal information regarding the CHD. Offer appropriate Internet resources for information about CHD and medical and surgical treatment options.
   b. Provide individualized resources for parents and patient if applicable. Visual aid of current physiology as well as repair, medication list, emergency action cards, upon discharge.
   c. Signs and symptoms of CHF (see page 1219).

d. Signs of hypercyanotic spells associated with cyanotic defects and need to place child in knee–chest position.
e. Need to prevent dehydration, which increases risk of thrombotic complications.
f. Emergency precautions related to hypercyanotic spells, pulmonary edema, cardiac arrest (if appropriate).
g. Special home care equipment, monitors, oxygen.

3. Encourage the parents and other people (teachers, peers) to treat the child in as normal a manner as possible.
   a. Avoid overprotection and overindulgence.
   b. Avoid rejection.
   c. Promote growth and development with modifications. Facilitate performance of the usual developmental tasks within the limits of the child's physiologic state.
   d. Prevent adults from projecting their fears and anxieties onto the child.
   e. Help family deal with anger, guilt, and concerns related to the disabled child.
4. Initiate a community health nursing referral, if indicated.
5. Stress the need for follow-up care.
6. Encourage attendance in support groups for patients and families.

Evaluation: Expected Outcomes

- Improved oxygenation evidenced by easy, comfortable respirations.
- Improved cardiac output demonstrated by stable vital signs, adequate peripheral perfusion, and adequate urine output.
- Increased activity level.
- Maximal nutritional status demonstrated by weight gain and increase in growth curve percentile.
- No signs or symptoms of infection.
- Parents discuss diagnosis and treatment together and with child.

Congestive Heart Failure

 EVIDENCE BASE Benhase, C. (2018). Nursing aspects of heart failure. In Benhase, C., Faulkner, T.J., Hendricks, K., Sublett, J. (Eds.), *Heart Failure in the Child and Young Adult: From Bench to Bedside*, (p. 481–492). Cambridge, MA: Academic Press.
Jayaprasad, N. (2016). Heart failure in children. *Heart Views*, 17(3), 92–99.
Kirk, R., Dipchand, A. I., & Rosenthal, D. N. (2014). *International Society for Heart and Lung Transplantation guidelines for the management of pediatric heart failure.* Volume 8. Birmingham, AL, UAB Printing.

Congestive heart failure (CHF) occurs when cardiac output cannot meet the metabolic demands of the body.

Pathophysiology and Etiology

1. May result from:
   a. CHDs with a volume or pressure overload (moderate to large left-to-right shunt [PDA, VSD], AV valve insufficiency, or outflow obstruction [HLHS, CoA]).
   b. Acquired heart disease: myocarditis, cardiomyopathy, acute rheumatic fever.
   c. Chronic pulmonary disease: cor pulmonale, bronchopulmonary dysplasia.
   d. Arrhythmias: prolonged SVT, complete heart block.
   e. Anemia.
   f. Iatrogenic fluid overload.

2. In an attempt to meet the metabolic needs of the body, the heart rate increases to increase cardiac output.
   a. Cardiac output = heart rate × stroke volume.
   b. Stroke volume is the amount of blood (mL) ejected from the heart with each heartbeat; it depends on preload and vascular resistance.
3. Preload (CVP) increases as the failing heart contracts poorly.
4. With decreased cardiac output, the systemic vascular resistance increases to maintain BP. This increase in afterload limits cardiac output.
5. With decreased blood flow to the kidneys, the glomerular filtration rate decreases as tubular reabsorption increases sodium and water retention, resulting in decreased urine output.
6. Long term, these compensatory mechanisms are detrimental to the failing myocardium. The chronic increase in preload and afterload contributes to chamber dilation and myocardial hypertrophy, leading to progressive CHF.

Clinical Manifestations

1. Impaired myocardial function.
   a. Tachycardia, S_3 gallop.
   b. Poor peripheral perfusion: weak peripheral pulses, cool extremities, delayed capillary refill.
   c. Pallor.
   d. Exercise or activity intolerance.
2. Pulmonary congestion.
   a. Tachypnea.
   b. Cyanosis.
   c. Retractions, nasal flaring, grunting.
   d. Cough.
3. Systemic venous congestion.
   a. Hepatomegaly.
   b. Peripheral edema: scrotal and orbital.
   c. Water weight gain.
   d. Decreased urine output.

Diagnostic Evaluation

1. Characteristic physical examination findings.
2. Chest x-ray shows cardiomegaly and pulmonary congestion.
3. B-type natriuretic peptide (BNP) as a biomarker for diagnostic, prognostic, and therapeutic monitoring use for pediatric patients with congenital heart disease, cardiomyopathy.

Management

1. Diuretics to reduce intravascular volume (furosemide, spironolactone).
2. Digoxin to increase myocardial contractility for symptomatic patients with low ejection fraction. Not necessary for those asymptomatic patients with left ventricular dysfunction.
3. Afterload reduction to decrease the workload of the ailing myocardium (angiotensin-converting enzyme inhibitors—captopril, enalapril, lisinopril).
4. Beta-adrenergic blockers to counteract increased sympathetic activity and reduce systemic vascular resistance (metoprolol, carvedilol).
5. Angiotensin II receptor blockers (ARBs) for patients who are intolerant of ACE inhibitors, but who can benefit from RAAS blockade.
6. Inotropic support, as needed.

Complications

1. Pulmonary edema.
2. Metabolic acidosis.
3. Failure to thrive.
4. URIs.
5. Arrhythmia.
6. Death.

Nursing Assessment

1. Assess response to medical treatment plan.
2. Document vital signs and oxygen saturations.
3. Observe infant or child during feeding or activity. Assess for diaphoresis, need for frequent rest periods, and inability to keep up with peers.
4. Follow growth curve.

Nursing Diagnoses

- Decreased Cardiac Output related to myocardial dysfunction.
- Excess Fluid Volume related to decreased cardiac contractility and decreased excretion from the kidney.
- Impaired Gas Exchange related to pulmonary venous congestion.
- Activity Intolerance related to myocardial dysfunction and pulmonary congestion.
- Risk for Infection related to pulmonary congestion.
- Imbalanced Nutrition: Less Than Body Requirements related to increased metabolic demands with decreased caloric intake.
- Anxiety related to diagnosis and prognosis.

Nursing Interventions

Improving Myocardial Efficiency

1. Administer digoxin, as prescribed.
   a. Measure heart rate. Hold medication and notify health care provider for heart rate less than 90 beats/minute.
   b. Check most recent potassium level. Hold medication and notify health care provider for potassium less than 3.5 mEg/L.
   c. Run lead II ECG, if ordered, to monitor PR interval. If first-degree AV block occurs, notify health care provider and hold medication, as directed.
   d. Report signs of possible digoxin toxicity: vomiting, nausea, visual changes, and bradycardia.
   e. Double-check dose of digoxin with another nurse before administering the dose. Make sure the digoxin order has two signatures.
2. Administer afterload reduction medications, as prescribed.
   a. Measure BP before and after giving the patient the medication. Hold the medication and notify the health care provider for low BP (greater than a 15-mm Hg drop from baseline).
   b. Observe for other signs of hypotension: dizziness, lightheadedness, and syncope.

Maintaining Fluid and Electrolyte Balance

1. Administer diuretics, as prescribed.
   a. Obtain daily weights.
   b. Keep strict intake and output record.
   c. Monitor serum electrolytes. Provide potassium supplements, as needed.

2. Sodium restriction: not usually needed in children; provide dietary assistance, as needed.
3. Fluid restriction: not usually needed in children.

Relieving Respiratory Distress

1. Administer oxygen therapy, as prescribed.
2. Elevate head of bed; infants may be more comfortable in an upright infant seat.

Promoting Activity Tolerance

1. Organize nursing care to provide periods of uninterrupted sleep/rest.
2. Avoid unnecessary activities.
3. Respond efficiently to a crying infant. Provide comfort and treat the source of distress: wet or dirty diaper, hunger.
4. Provide diversional activities that require limited expenditure of energy.
5. Provide small, frequent feedings.

Decreasing Risk of Infection

1. Ensure good handwashing by everyone.
2. Avoid exposure to ill children or caretakers.
3. Monitor signs of infection: fever, cough, runny nose, diarrhea, and vomiting.

Providing Adequate Nutrition

1. For the older child: provide nutritious foods that the child likes, along with supplemental high-calorie snacks (milkshake, pudding).
2. For the infant:
   a. High-calorie formula (24 to 30 cal/ounce).
   b. Supplement oral intake with nasogastric feedings. Allow ad-lib oral intake through the day with continuous nasogastric feedings at night.

Reducing Anxiety and Fear

1. Communicate the care plan to the child and family.
2. Educate the family about CHF and provide home care nursing referral to reinforce teaching after discharge.
3. Encourage questions; answer questions as able or refer to another member of the health care team.

Family Education and Health Maintenance

1. Teach the signs and symptoms of CHF.
2. Teach medications: brand name and generic name, expected effects, adverse effects, and dose.
3. Demonstrate medication administration.
4. With the family, design a medication administration time schedule.
5. Provide guidelines for when to seek medical help.
6. Teach infant and child cardiopulmonary resuscitation (CPR), as needed.
7. Reinforce dietary guidelines; provide a recipe to the parent on how to make high-calorie formula.
8. Reinforce ways to prevent infection.
9. Make sure that follow-up visit with health care providers is scheduled, prior to discharge.
10. Educate the patient and family on infective endocarditis guidelines and provide them with written materials. Standard general prophylaxis for children at risk: amoxicillin 50 mg/kg (maximum dose = 2 g) given orally 1 hour before the procedure.

Evaluation: Expected Outcomes

- Heart rate within normal range for age; adequate urine output.
- No unexpected weight gain.
- Clear lungs; normal respiratory rate and effort.
- Participates in quiet diversional activities.
- No signs or symptoms of infection.
- Adequate intake of small, frequent feedings.
- Parents express understanding of disease process and treatment.

ACQUIRED HEART DISEASE

Note: Kawasaki disease is discussed in Chapter 53.

Acute Rheumatic Fever

 EVIDENCE BASE Tani, L. (2016). Rheumatic fever and rheumatic heart disease. In H. D. Allen, R. E. Shaddy, D. J. Penny, T. F. Feltes, & F. Cetta (Eds.), *Moss and Adams' heart disease in infants, children, and adolescents* (9th ed., pp. 1799–1801). Philadelphia, PA: Lippincott Williams & Wilkins.

Acute rheumatic fever (ARF) is an acute autoimmune disease that occurs as a sequela of group A beta-hemolytic streptococcal infection. It is characterized by inflammatory lesions of connective tissue and endothelial tissue, primarily affecting the joints and heart.

Pathophysiology and Etiology

1. Most initial attacks of ARF occur 1 to 5 weeks (average 3 weeks) after a streptococcal infection of the throat or of the upper respiratory tract.
2. Peak incidence occurs in children ages 5 to 15 years. Incidence after a mild streptococcal pharyngeal infection is 0.3%; after a severe streptococcal infection, 1% to 3%.
3. Family history of rheumatic fever is usually positive.
4. Streptococcal infection abates with or without treatment; however, autoantibodies attack the myocardium, pericardium, and cardiac valves.
   a. Aschoff bodies (fibrin deposits) develop on the valves, possibly leading to permanent valve dysfunction, especially of the mitral and aortic valves.
   b. Severe myocarditis may cause dilation of the heart and CHF.
5. Inflammation of the large joints causes painful arthritis that may last 6 to 8 weeks.
6. Involvement of the nervous system causes chorea (sudden involuntary movements).

Clinical Manifestations

Documented or undocumented group A beta-hemolytic streptococcal infection is usually followed (within several weeks) by fever, malaise, and anorexia. Major symptoms of ARF may appear several weeks to several months after initial infection.

Major Manifestations (Jones criteria)

1. Carditis—manifested by sinus tachycardia, a soft blowing pansystolic murmur, prolonged PR and QT intervals on ECG, and possibly by signs of CHF (see page 1219).

2. Polyarthritis—pain and limited movement of two or more joints; joints are swollen, red, warm, and tender.
3. Chorea—purposeless, involuntary, rapid movements commonly associated with muscle weakness, involuntary facial grimaces, speech disturbance, and emotional lability.
4. Erythema marginatum—nonpruritic pink, macular rash mostly of the trunk with pale central areas; migratory.
5. Subcutaneous nodules—firm, painless nodules over the scalp, extensor surface of joints, such as wrists, elbows, knees, and vertebral column.

Minor Manifestations

1. History of previous rheumatic fever or evidence of preexisting rheumatic heart disease.
2. Arthralgia—pain in one or more joints without evidence of inflammation, tenderness, or limited movement.
3. Fever—temperature greater than 100.4°F (38°C).
4. Laboratory abnormalities—elevated erythrocyte sedimentation rate, positive C-reactive protein, elevated white blood cell count.
5. ECG changes—prolonged PR interval.

Diagnostic Evaluation

1. Diagnosed clinically through use of the Jones criteria from the American Heart Association—presence of two major manifestations or one major and two minor manifestations (as listed above), with supporting evidence of a recent streptococcal infection.
2. ECG to evaluate PR interval and other changes.
3. Laboratory tests listed above. In addition, group A streptococcal culture and/or antistreptolysin-O titer to detect streptococcal antibodies from recent infection.
4. Chest x-ray for cardiomegaly, pulmonary congestion, or edema.

Management

1. Course of antibiotic therapy to completely eradicate streptococcal infection (may be given despite previous treatment).
   a. Usually benzathine penicillin is given IM in a single dose or a 10-day course of oral penicillin V.
   b. Oral erythromycin may be used for children who are allergic to penicillin.
2. Nonsteroidal anti-inflammatory drugs (naproxen sodium) usually used to control pain and inflammation of arthritis. Aspirin for acute carditis.
3. Corticosteroids may be used in severe cases to try to control cardiac inflammation; however, there is limited evidence to support their use.
4. Phenobarbital, diazepam, or other neurologic agent to control chorea.
5. Bed rest during the acute phase to rest the heart. Gradual return to activities is recommended once acute symptoms resolve.
6. Mitral valve replacement may be necessary in some cases.
7. Secondary prevention of recurrent ARF:
   a. Risk of recurrence greatest within first 5 years, with multiple episodes of ARF, and with rheumatic heart disease. Prophylactic antibiotic treatment may be lifelong.
   b. For those at low risk for recurrence, antibiotic prophylaxis may be continued for 5 years or longer.

   c. Antibiotic regimens may include:
      i. Benzathine penicillin IM once.
      ii. Penicillin V 250 mg orally twice per day for children less than 27 kg, 500 mg orally twice per day for patients greater than 27 kg.
      iii. Patients with penicillin allergies may be prescribed cephalosporin, clindamycin, azithromycin, or clarithromycin.

Complications

1. CHF.
2. Pericarditis, pericardial effusion.
3. Permanent damage to the aortic or mitral valve, possibly requiring valve replacement.

Nursing Assessment

1. Assess for signs of cardiac involvement by auscultation of the heart for murmur and cardiac monitoring for prolonged PR interval.
2. Monitor pulse for 1 full minute to determine heart rate.
3. Assess temperature for elevation.
4. Observe for involuntary movements: stick out tongue or smile; garbled or hesitant speech when asked to recite numbers or the ABCs; hyperextension of the wrists and fingers when trying to extend arms.
5. Assess child's ability to feed self, dress, and do other activities if chorea or arthritis present.
6. Assess pain level using scale appropriate for child's age.
7. Assess parents' ability to cope with illness and care for child.
8. Assess need for home schooling while the patient is on bed rest.

Nursing Diagnoses

- Decreased Cardiac Output related to carditis.
- Acute and Chronic Pain related to arthritis.
- Risk for Injury related to chorea.

Nursing Interventions

Improving Cardiac Output

1. Explain to the child and family the need for bed rest during the acute phase and as long as CHF is present. In milder cases, light indoor activity is allowed.
2. In severe cases, organize care to minimize exertion and provide uninterrupted rest.
3. Maintain cardiac monitoring, if indicated.
4. Administer course of antibiotics, as directed. Be alert to adverse effects, such as nausea, vomiting, and GI distress.
5. Administer medications for CHF, as directed. Monitor BP, intake and output, and heart rate.

Relieving Pain

1. Administer anti-inflammatory medication, analgesics, and antipyretics, as directed.
   a. Monitor for side effects of corticosteroid use—GI distress, acne, weight gain, and emotional disturbances—or long-term effects, such as rounded face, ulcer formation, and decreased resistance to infection.
   b. Administer all anti-inflammatory medications with food to reduce GI injury.
   c. Be aware that anti-inflammatories may not alter the course of myocardial injury.
2. Teach family the importance of maintaining dosage schedule, continuing medication until all signs and symptoms of the

ARF have gone, and tapering the dose, as directed by health care provider.

3. Assist child with positioning for comfort and protecting inflamed joints.

4. Suggest diversional activities that do not require use of painful joints.

Protecting the Child with Chorea

1. Use padded side rails if chorea is severe.
2. Assist with feeding and other fine-motor activities, as needed.
3. Assist with ambulation if weak.
4. Avoid the use of straws and sharp utensils if chorea involves the face.
5. Make sure that child consumes nutritious diet with recommended vitamins, protein, and calories.
6. Be patient if speech is affected and offer emotional support.
7. Protect the child from stress.
8. Administer phenobarbital or other medication for chorea, as directed. Observe for drowsiness.

Family Education and Health Maintenance

1. Teach the appropriate administration of all medications, including prophylactic antibiotic.
2. Encourage all family and household members to be screened for streptococcus and receive the appropriate treatment.
3. Instruct on additional prophylaxis for endocarditis with dental procedures and surgery, as indicated.
4. Encourage following activity restrictions, resuming activity gradually, and resting whenever tired.
5. Encourage keeping appointments for follow-up evaluation by cardiologist and other health care providers.
6. Advise the parents that child cannot return to school until health care provider assesses that all disease activity is gone. Parents may need to discuss with teachers how the child can catch up with schoolwork.
7. Instruct on follow-up with usual health care provider for immunizations, well-child evaluations, hearing and vision screening, and other health maintenance needs.

Provide general health education about early identification and treatment seeking for any possible streptococcal infection (fever, sore throat). Compliance with 10 to 14 days of antibiotics can greatly reduce the risk of ARF and other poststreptococcal sequelae.

Evaluation: Expected Outcomes

- Heart rate and PR interval within normal range for age; no signs of CHF.
- Compliant with anti-inflammatory therapy; reports pain as 1 to 2 on scale of 1 to 10.
- Feeds self, washes face and hands, and ambulates to bathroom without injury.

Cardiomyopathy

EVIDENCE BASE Yuan, S. M. (2018). Cardiomyopathy in the pediatric patients. *Pediatrics and Neonatology*, 59(2), 120–128.

Glotzbach, K., May, L., & Wray, J. (2018). Health related quality of life and functional outcomes in pediatric cardiomyopathy. *Progress in Pediatric Cardiology*, 48, 26–35.

According to the type of myocardial changes, *cardiomyopathy* can be classified into three categories: dilated, hypertrophic, and restrictive. The most common type in children is dilated cardiomyopathy. Hypertrophic cardiomyopathy is a leading cause of death in young athletes.

Pathophysiology and Etiology

1. Familial (family history, genetic predisposition) tendency.
2. Idiopathic in most cases.
3. May be related to:
   a. Nutritional deficiency (carnitine or selenium).
   b. Viral infection (myocarditis), human immunodeficiency virus.
   c. Collagen vascular disease (systemic lupus erythematosus).
   d. Cardiotoxic drugs (doxorubicin).
   e. Cocaine abuse.
   f. Infants of diabetic mothers.
   g. Ion channelopathies.
   h. Catecholamine surge; hyperthyroidism.
4. Dilated cardiomyopathy involves dilatation of one or both ventricles associated with normal septal and LV free wall thickness.
5. Decreased systolic function (contractility) results in CHF.
6. Increasing end-systolic dimension results in AV valve insufficiency, further worsening CHF.

Clinical Manifestations

1. Signs of CHF—tachycardia, tachypnea, dyspnea, crackles, hepatosplenomegaly.
2. Decreased exercise tolerance, fatigue, sweating.
3. Poor weight gain, nausea, abdominal tenderness.
4. Ventricular arrhythmia.
5. Chest pain.
6. Syncope.

Diagnostic Evaluation

1. Auscultation: systolic regurgitant murmur (if mitral or tricuspid insufficiency is present), S_2 is normal or narrowly split, prominent S_3 gallop.
2. ECG: tachycardia, abnormal ST segments, arrhythmia, ectopic atrial tachycardia, deep Q waves, LVH.
3. Chest x-ray: cardiomegaly, pulmonary congestion.
4. Two-dimensional echocardiogram: increased wall thickness, poor ventricular systolic function, dilated heart chambers; AV valve insufficiency.
5. Cardiac MRI will provide useful information on cardiac function and may demonstrate ventricular hypertrophy or fibrosis.
6. Cardiac catheterization: not needed for initial diagnosis; endomyocardial biopsy (to rule out myocarditis); assess PVR.

Management

General Measures

1. Identify and treat the underlying cause.
2. Maximize caloric intake: fortify formula; supplemental nasogastric feedings.
3. Supplemental oxygen, as needed.
4. Activity restriction (usually self-imposed by the younger child and infant). Restrict participation in strenuous and competitive sports.

Treatment of Systolic Dysfunction with Dilated Cardiomyopathy

1. Diuretics: furosemide, spironolactone.
2. Inotropes for patients with poor perfusion: milrinone, dopamine, epinephrine.
3. Afterload reduction: captopril, enalapril, lisinopril.
4. Anticoagulation: warfarin, low-molecular-weight heparin (enoxaparin).
5. Antiarrhythmics.
6. Placement of an automatic implantable cardioverter defibrillator.
7. Biventricular pacing.
8. Cardiac transplant.

Treatment of Diastolic Dysfunction with Hypertrophic Cardiomyopathy

1. Beta-adrenergic blockers: propranolol.
2. Calcium channel blockers: verapamil.
3. AV sequential pacing.
4. Myomectomy or myotomy.

Treatment of Diastolic Dysfunction with Restrictive Cardiomyopathy

1. Diuretics.
2. Anticoagulation.
3. Permanent pacemaker for advanced heart block.

Complications

1. Severe CHF.
2. Increased pulmonary vascular resistance.
3. Intracardiac thrombus.
4. Embolus.
5. Malignant arrhythmias.
6. Sudden death.

Nursing Assessment

Perform a thorough nursing assessment as for CHD (see page 1216).

Nursing Diagnoses

- Decreased Cardiac Output related to impaired systolic or diastolic ventricular function.
- Imbalanced Nutrition: Less Than Body Requirements related to increased metabolic demands and poor feeding from dyspnea, fatigue, and poor appetite.
- Ineffective Family Coping related to chronic illness.

Nursing Interventions

Maximizing Cardiac Output

1. Monitor vital signs; notify physician for hypotension, tachycardia, arrhythmia; increasing tachypnea.
2. Administer oxygen therapy, as prescribed.
3. Administer medications, as prescribed.
   a. Maintain bleeding precautions for anticoagulated patients.
   b. Document response to diuretics; monitor intake and output.
4. Monitor electrolytes.
5. Restrict level of activity.

Providing Maximal Nutritional Support

1. Encourage frequent, small meals. Provide foods the child likes.
2. Provide high-calorie supplements (milkshakes, pudding).
3. Administer supplemental tube feedings if nutritional needs are not being met.

4. Administer parenteral hyperalimentation and intralipids, as directed (rarely needed).

Promoting Effective Coping and Control within the Family

1. Organize a family meeting with various members of the health care team to review the child's medical condition and to explain the treatment plan.
2. Allow the child and family to express their questions, fears, and concerns.
3. Identify support systems and services for the child and family: extended family members, clergy, support groups, community resources.

Family Education and Health Maintenance

1. Teach child and family medication administration: purpose of the drug, drug dosage, drug schedule, and adverse effects.
2. Help family design a realistic medication schedule.
   a. Identify usual wake-up time and bedtime. Schedule medications accordingly.
   b. Do not give a diuretic right before bedtime or nap time.
   c. If possible, avoid having to give medications at school.
3. Teach bleeding precautions if the child is on anticoagulation agents (coumadin).
   a. Monitor prothrombin International Normalized Ratio regularly.
   b. Observe for signs of bleeding.
   c. Counsel regarding menses and pregnancy.
   d. Instruct on foods and medications that interfere with coumadin.
4. Give guidelines for notifying the physician.
   a. Worsening shortness of breath.
   b. Irregular pulse; palpitations.
   c. Syncope, dizziness, or light-headedness.
   d. Increasing fatigue, exercise intolerance.
5. Teach infant and child CPR to family members and other caregivers.

Evaluation: Expected Outcomes

- Stable vital signs.
- Maximal nutritional status, as evidenced by weight gain and growth.
- Compliance with the treatment plan and follow-up visits.

 TRANSITIONAL CARE ALERT Many children discharged from the hospital diagnosed with a complex cardiac condition will have extensive discharge needs. Families will need support in the transition to home or another aftercare location. It is crucial that they have complete and understandable care instructions on home care, medications, and follow-up appointments. If arrangements have been made for nursing care in the home, families should be aware of the agency providing services and when they can expect communication regarding care arrangements. Families should have thorough written (and if necessary to assist understanding, pictorial) instructions on signs and symptoms to monitor, for that could suggest worsening of status. Instructions should include clear understanding of acceptable discharge expectations as many children may be in different phases if a surgical repair is necessary. Parents should be aware of when and where they should seek further emergency care if the child's condition deteriorates.

SELECTED REFERENCES

American Heart Association. (2016). Infective endocarditis. In *The impact of congenital heart defects*. Dallas, TX: American Heart Association.

Anton, K. (2016). Challenges caring for adults with congenital heart disease in pediatric settings: How nurses can aid in the transition. *Critical Care Nursing, 36*(4), e1–e8.

Beekman, R. H. (2016). Coarctation of the aorta. In H. D. Allen, R. E. Shaddy, D. J. Penny, T. F. Feltes, & F. Cetta (Eds.), *Moss and Adams' heart disease in infants, children, and adolescents* (9th ed., pp. 1085–1101). Philadelphia, PA: Lippincott Williams & Wilkins.

Bouma, B. J., & Mulder, B. J. M. (2017). Changing landscape of congenital heart disease. *Circulation Research, 120*, 908–922.

Campbell, J. (2015). Education and simulation training of pediatric intensive care unit nurses to care for open heart surgery. *Critical Care Nurse, 35*(3), 76–81.

Cohen, M. S., & Lopez, L. (2016). Ventricular septal defects. In H. D. Allen, R. E. Shaddy, D. J. Penny, T. F. Feltes, & F. Cetta (Eds.), *Moss and Adams' heart disease in infants, children, and adolescents* (9th ed., pp. 783–800). Philadelphia, PA: Lippincott Williams & Wilkins.

Dijkema, E. J., Leiner, T., & Grotenhuis, H. B. (2017). Diagnosis, imaging and clinical management of aortic coarctation. *Heart, 103*, 1148–1155.

Friedland-Little, J. M., Zampi, J. D., & Gajarski, R. J. (2016). Aortic stenosis. In H. D. Allen, R. E. Shaddy, D. J. Penny, T. F. Feltes, & F. Cetta (Eds.), *Moss and Adams' heart disease in infants, children, and adolescents* (9th ed., pp. 1085–1101). Philadelphia, PA: Lippincott Williams & Wilkins.

Glotzbach, K., May, L., & Wray, J. (2018). Health related quality of life and functional outcomes in pediatric cardiomyopathy. *Progress in Pediatric Cardiology, 48*, 26–35.

Huang, H., Chen, C., Chen, C., Yang, H., et al. (2018). A positive perspective of knowledge, attitude, and practices for health -promoting behaviors of adolescents with congenital heart disease. *European Journal of Cardiovascular Nursing, 17*, 217–225.

Jenkins, E. (2015). Feeding protocols for neonates with hypoplastic left heart syndrome: A review. *AACN Advances in Critical Care Nursing, 26*(3), 576–580.

Kaya, U., Colak, A., Becil, N., et al. (2018). Surgical management of aortic coarctation from infant to adult. *Eurasian Journal of Medicine, 501*, 14–18.

Kevat, P., Reeves, B., Ruben, A., et al. (2017). Adherence to secondary prophylaxis for acute rheumatic fever and rheumatic heart disease: A systematic review. *Current Cardiology Previews, 13*(2), 155–166.

Kirk, R., Dipchand, A. I., & Rosenthal, D. N. (2014). *International Society for Heart and Lung Transplantation guidelines for the management of pediatric heart failure*. Volume 8. Birmingham, Alabama: UAB Printing.

Lawrence, K., Stilley, C. S., Pollock, S. A., et al. (2011). A family-centered educational program to promote independence in pediatric heart transplant recipients. *Progress in Transplantation, 21*(1), 61–66.

Lopez, R., Frangini, P., Ramirez, M., Valenzuela, P. M., et al. (2016). Well-being and agency in parents of children with congenital heart disease: A survey in Chile. *World Journal for Pediatric and Congenital Heart Surgery, 7*(2), 139–145.

March, S. (2017). Parents' perceptions during the transition to home for their child with a congenital heart defect: How can we support families of children with hypoplastic left heart syndrome? *Journal for Specialists in Pediatric Nursing, 22*(3), 11.

Masarone, D., Valente, F., Rubino, M., et al. (2017). Pediatric heart failure: A practical guide to diagnosis and management. *Pediatric Neonatalogy, 58*(4), 303–312.

Nielsen, E., & Vibeke, E. (2016). Surgically treated pulmonary stenosis: over 50 years of follow up. *Cardiology of the Young, 26*(5), 860–866.

Nieves, J., Uzark, K., Rudd, N., et al. (2017). Interstage home monitoring after newborn first-stage palliation for hypoplastic left heart syndrome: Family education strategies. *Critical Care Nurse, 37*(2), 72–88.

Niwa, K. (2015). Adults with congenital heart disease transition. *Current Opinion in Pediatrics, 27*(5), 576–580.

Park, M. (2014). *Pediatric cardiology for practitioners* (6th ed.). St. Louis, MO: Mosby.

Prieto, L. R., & Latson, L. A. (2016). Pulmonary stenosis. In H. D. Allen, R. E. Shaddy, D. J. Penny, T. F. Feltes, & F. Cetta (Eds.), *Moss and Adams' heart disease in infants, children, and adolescents* (9th ed., pp. 1085–1101). Philadelphia, PA: Lippincott Williams & Wilkins.

Roche, S. L., Greenway, S., & Redington, A. (2016). Tetralogy of Fallot with pulmonary stenosis, pulmonary atresia, and absent pulmonary valve. In H. D. Allen, R. E. Shaddy, D. J. Penny, T. F. Feltes, & F. Cetta (Eds.), *Moss and Adams' heart disease in infants, children, and adolescents* (9th ed., pp. 1029–1047). Philadelphia, PA: Lippincott Williams & Wilkins.

Rossano, J. W., Cabrera A. G., & Shaddy, R. E. (2016). Heart transplantation—The pediatric cardiac critical care perspective. *Pediatric Critical Care Medicine, 17*(8S), 171–177.

Rossano, J. W., Cherikh, W. S., Chambers, D., et al. (2017). The registry of the International Society for Heart and Lung Transplantation: Twentieth pediatric heart transplantation report - 2017; Focus theme: Allograft ischemic time. *The Journal of Heart and Lung Transplantation, 36*(10), 1060–1069.

Sachdeva, R. (2016). Atrial septal defect. In H. D. Allen, R. E. Shaddy, D. J. Penny, T. F. Feltes, & F. Cetta (Eds.), *Moss and Adams' heart disease in infants, children, and adolescents* (9th ed., pp. 743–753). Philadelphia, PA: Lippincott Williams & Wilkins.

Samuel, B., Stuive, A., & Eding, D. (2016). Nursing assessment, education, and care of extremely premature neonates with patent ductus arteriosus. *Current Pediatric Reviews, 12*(2), 106–109.

Schermehil, C., Malhotra, D., & Patel, D. (2017). Cardiac screening to prevent sudden death in young athletes. *Translational Pediatrics, 6*(3), 199–206.

Spillane, N. T., Kashyap, S., Bateman, D., et al. (2016). Comparison of feeding strategies for infants with hypoplastic left heart syndrome. *World Journal for Pediatric and Congenital Heart Surgery, 7*(4), 446–453.

Taggart, N. W., & Qureshi, M. Y. (2016). In H. D. Allen, R. E. Shaddy, D. J. Penny, T. F. Feltes, & F. Cetta (Eds.), *Moss and Adams' heart disease in infants, children, and adolescents* (9th ed., pp. 803–813). Philadelphia, PA: Lippincott Williams & Wilkins.

Tani, L. (2016). Rheumatic fever and rheumatic heart disease. In H. D. Allen, R. E. Shaddy, D. J. Penny, T. F. Feltes, & F. Cetta (Eds.), *Moss and Adams' heart disease in infants, children, and adolescents* (9th ed., pp. 1799–1801). Philadelphia, PA: Lippincott Williams & Wilkins.

Tweddell, J. S., et al. (2016). Hypoplastic left heart syndrome. In H. D. Allen, R. E. Shaddy, D. J. Penny, T. F. Feltes, & F. Cetta (Eds.), *Moss and Adams' heart disease in infants, children, and adolescents* (9th ed., pp. 1085–1101). Philadelphia, PA: Lippincott Williams & Wilkins.

Ware, S. (2017). Genetics of pediatric cardiomyopathies. *Current Opinion in Pediatrics, 29*(5), 534–540.

Wehman, B., Stafford, K. A., Bittle, G. J., et al. (2016). Modern outcomes of mechanical circulatory support as a bridge to pediatric heart transplantation. *Annals of Thoracic Surgery, 101*, 2321–2328.

Yuan, S. M. (2018). Cardiomyopathy in the pediatric patients. *Pediatrics and Neonatology, 59*(2), 120–128.

46

Pediatric Neurologic Disorders

NEUROLOGIC AND NEUROSURGICAL DISORDERS

It is essential to have strong knowledge of growth and development and use physical assessment skills while caring for a child with a neurological or neurosurgical condition. Children are not little adults. They have their own unique physiology, which is important to consider when assessing and understanding the manifestation of neurological conditions in children. Young children often cannot either speak or express how they feel; therefore, a complete ongoing physical assessment is essential. Parents and caregivers are an invaluable source of information and know their child the best and should always be included in all aspects of care delivery.

Cerebral Palsy

Cerebral palsy (CP) is a nonprogressive disorder of posture, muscle tone, and movement. There are a number of causes, but CP is a result of abnormalities of the developing brain. The prevalence of CP is 2 per 1,000 live births with a higher prevalence in preterm than term infants. Preterm infants account for less than half of all cases of CP.

Pathophysiology and Etiology

1. Prematurity.
2. Perinatal hypoxic–ischemic injury.
3. Congenital abnormalities.
4. Genetic susceptibility.
5. Multiple births.
6. Stroke.
7. Intracranial hemorrhage.
8. Intrauterine postnatal causes.

Classification of Cerebral Palsy

Spastic Subtypes
1. Spastic Diplegia
   a. 13% to 25% of CP cases.
   b. Most commonly associated with periventricular leukomalacia.
   c. Lower limbs more affected than upper limbs.

   d. Presence of flexion, adduction, and internal rotation of the hips with contractures of hip flexors and hamstring muscles.
   e. Variable degrees of flexion at elbows and knees.
   f. Reduced limb length and muscle bulk in lower extremities.
2. Spastic Hemiplegia
   a. 21% to 40%
   b. One side of the body affected.
   c. The arm typically more affected than the leg.
   d. The arm adducted at the shoulder and flexed at the elbow with forearm pronated with the wrist and fingers flexed with hand closed.
   e. The hip partially flexed and adducted, the knee and ankle are flexed, and the foot may be in equinovarus or calcaneo-valgus position.
   f. Sensory deficits present in most children.
   g. Postural abnormalities more apparent during walking or running in mildly affected children; walking occurs at appropriate developmental stage unless in the presence of intellectual disability.
3. Spastic Quadriplegia
   a. 20% to 43%.
   b. All limbs affected.
   c. Upper limbs may be equally or more involved than lower limbs.
   d. Children often severely affected.
   e. Feeding difficulties, chronic respiratory insufficiency, and seizure disorders are common.

Dyskinetic Subtypes
1. 12% to 14%.
2. Involuntary movements.
3. Contractures not common but may evolve later in life.
4. Variable degree of dysarthria and intellectual disability.
5. Choreoathetotic CP
   a. Rapid, irregular, unpredictable contractions of individual muscles or small muscle groups that involve the face, bulbar muscles, proximal extremities, fingers, and toes.
   b. Athetosis—slow, smooth, writhing movements involving the distal muscles.
      i. Movements may be induced or may be heightened by emotions or change in posture.
      ii. Very obvious during reaching.

iii. Chorea may be aggravated by fever, stress, or excitement.

iv. Persistent primitive reflexes.

v. Commonly seen are oropharyngeal difficulties.

6. Dystonic CP
   a. Slow or rapid repetitive, patterned, twisting, and sustained movements of the trunk and limbs.
   b. May have pyramidal signs and anarthria.
   c. Sudden involuntary increase (tension) in tone may affect flexor and extensor muscles during attempted movement or with emotion.
   d. It may be difficult to elicit tendon reflexes or they may be normal.
   e. Absence of clonus and extensor plantar responses.

7. Ataxic CP
   a. 4% to 13%.
   b. Ataxic movements.
   c. Widespread disorder of motor function.
   d. Over time, ataxia will usually improve.
   e. Speech is slow, jerky, and explosive.

Clinical Manifestations

Common associated findings include:

1. Pain (50% to 75%).
2. Intellectual disability (50%).
3. Speech–language disorders (40%).
4. Epilepsy (25% to 40%).
5. Visual impairment (30%).
6. Hip displacement (30%).
7. Behavior disorder (25%).
8. Bladder control problems (30% to 60%).
9. Sleep disorder (20%).
10. Drooling (20%).
11. Hearing impairment (10% to 20%).
12. Gastrostomy tube dependence (7%).

Diagnostic Evaluation

Diagnosis is based on clinical examination and history. Various diagnostic tests also help determine the cause and evaluate for associated problems.

History and Physical Examination

1. Review of prenatal and birth history.
2. Review of newborn screening results.
3. Review of family history
   a. Intellectual disability/developmental disabilities.
   b. Seizures.
   c. CP.
   d. Neuromotor/movement disorders.
   e. Neurobehavioral disorders.
   f. Joint contractures/stiffness.
   g. Thromboses/vascular accidents.
   h. Congenital anomalies.
   i. Infertility.
   j. Recurrent miscarriages/stillborn.
   k. Adult-onset neurodegenerative conditions.

Diagnostic Tests

Although CP is diagnosed based on clinical findings, diagnostic evaluation should be completed to identify underlying causes of CP and to rule out other conditions.

1. Magnetic resonance imaging (MRI) of the brain

a. Should be obtained in all children with CP of undetermined etiology.
b. MRI is preferred to computed tomography (CT) because of its higher diagnostic yield and it can help determine etiology and timing of insult.
c. Abnormalities on MRI seen in patients with CP include hypoxic–ischemic lesions (periventricular leukomalacia or PVL), cortical malformations, and lesions in the basal ganglia.

2. Electroencephalography (EEG) should be obtained in children who are suspected of having seizure activity.
   a. 45% of children with CP have seizures.

3. Lumbar puncture (LP) should be obtained in children with drug-resistant seizures or movement disorders such as ataxic–spastic gait or dyskinesias.
   a. Screening is done for pediatric neurotransmitter disorders, to evaluate low cerebrospinal fluid (CSF) glucose concentration, which may be caused by glucose transporter deficiency (GLUT1).

4. Metabolic and genetic testing should be done if:
   a. Testing should be done if the history reveals features that are atypical for CP but suggestive of a genetic or metabolic etiology (eg, history of progressive encephalopathy, metabolic decompensation, family history of childhood neurologic disorder associated with CP, and history of consanguinity).
   b. If there is a developmental brain malformation on brain imaging (eg, lissencephaly, schizencephaly, pachygyria) or frontal/temporal atrophy.
   c. When no etiology has been identified on history and physical examination and on neuroimaging.
   d. If there are atypical symptoms or a brain malformation on MRI.

5. Thrombophilia screening should be done in children with hemiplegic CP or MRI evidence of a cerebral infarction.
   a. 50% to 60% of patients with hemiplegic CP have at least one prothrombotic coagulation abnormality.
   b. Test for factor V Leiden mutation, prothrombin 202210 mutation, antithrombin deficiency, protein C deficiency, protein S deficiency, hyperhomocysteinemia, antiphospholipid antibodies, and elevated factor VIII.

Management

Management of CP requires a multidisciplinary team that will look at medical, psychological, educational, social, and therapeutic needs. Management of CP includes the following:

Functional Evaluation

1. Important in planning treatment as functional evaluation is based on the limitations of the patient with respect to body structure and function.
2. Treatment is guided by standardized measurement of functional status such as the Gross Motor Function Classification System (GMFCS), Modified Ashworth Scale, Manual Ability Classification System (MACS), and Communication Function Classification System (CFCS).

Management of Spasticity

1. Botulinum toxin injections of botulinum type A (BTXA) into affected muscles
   a. Most commonly used in calf muscles in patients with diplegia or hemiplegia.
   b. To maintain efficacy, injections are repeated every three to eight months.

c. Used to treat children who have increased muscle tone that negatively affects function, which, over time with growth, will likely result in formation of contractures.

2. Antispastic Drugs
    a. Although less effective than Botox, oral antispastic drugs such as baclofen, benzodiazepines (eg, diazepam), and dantrolene are sometimes used to treat spasticity in CP.

Intrathecal Baclofen

1. Administered via the intrathecal route to achieve higher cerebrospinal fluid (CSF) drug levels as opposed to oral administration, which results in lower CSF drug levels.
2. Reduces spasticity in severely affected children.
3. Has significant complications and is therefore reserved for children with severe spasticity that is unresponsive to other treatment modalities.

Surgical Treatment

1. Selective dorsal rhizotomy (SDR) is the primary surgical intervention used in the treatment of spasticity.
2. Deep brain stimulation (DBS) is an emerging therapy that has been used in the treatment of severe primary dystonia in adults who have failed to respond to pharmacotherapy such as Botox; however, further studies are needed to establish efficacy in treating dyskinetic CP.

Orthopedic Interventions

1. Gait analysis is utilized in identifying muscles that may benefit from surgical lengthening and is used postoperatively to evaluate surgical outcomes on function.
    a. Gait analysis is typically used in children aged 6 to 10 years who have a mature gait.
    b. Ankle–foot orthoses are often used to try to stabilize or improve range of motion or gait.
2. Casting
    a. Serial casting is often used to stretch and shorten muscles in lower limbs as well as improve range of motion.
3. Muscle–Tendon Surgery
    a. To reduce restrictions in joint motion or malalignment, surgical intervention to release or recess limb muscles and tendons is performed when function is affected by fixed contractures.
4. Surgical Treatment of Hip Disorders
    a. Children with spastic CP commonly have hip disorders including subluxation, dislocation, and dislocation with degeneration and pain.
    b. Soft tissue lengthening is done to correct hip subluxation, whereas reconstructive hip surgery is done in children younger than four years old who are more severely affected but who have not developed degenerative changes of the femoral head.

Physical Therapy

1. Physical therapy is a vital component of treatment programs for the management of CP and includes establishing methods to promote posture, mobility, and transfer and to allow for effective methods of promoting activities of daily living.
2. Bimanual training for hemiplegic CP.
    a. The child is trained to use two hands together through repetitive tasks.
    b. Constraint-induced movement therapy (CIMT)—used in children who have hemiplegic CP to promote limb function through the use of intermittent restraint of the unaffected limb during therapeutic tasks and often involves casting of the unaffected limb.

c. Context-focused therapy—the task or environment is changed to promote successful task performance rather than changing the child's approach.
    d. Goal-directed/functional training—promotes the focus of activities that are based on goals set by the child using a motor learning approach.
3. Occupational therapy for the upper limbs—involves physical therapy approaches and can be done concurrently with botulinum toxin treatment.

Feeding and Nutrition

Children with CP often have oromotor difficulties and feeding problems. Infants should be assessed for their ability to suck and for swallowing difficulties. School-aged children should be assessed for their height and weight status, as well as for any difficulty feeding, need for assistance with feeding, duration of feeding time, choking, and/or frequent vomiting and their nutritional status to ensure they receive adequate intake. Gastrostomy feeding should be considered in children with failure to thrive or who have chronic aspiration.

Management of Drooling

1. Children with CP who have oromotor dysfunction often drool. Management of drooling includes medication, behavior therapy, and surgery. Noninvasive methods such as behavior therapy and medications are often tried before surgical intervention.
2. Medications to manage drooling include anticholinergic agents such as benzhexol hydrochloride, scopolamine, or glycopyrrolate.
3. Botox injections into the salivary glands to decrease the flow of saliva are often used.
4. Surgical treatment of drooling targets the reduction of salivary production.
5. Behavior management includes behavior management techniques and biofeedback techniques.

Management of Osteopenia

1. For children with CP who have severe reductions in bone mineral density and/or pathological extremity fractures or vertebral compression, treatment with bisphosphonates is employed.

Urinary Incontinence

1. Anticholinergic medication is often used to treat urinary incontinence.
2. Children with CP who have a neurogenic bladder are managed with anticholinergic medication, modification of the toileting schedule or environment, and/or intermittent catheterization, which is contingent upon features of a neurogenic bladder.

EVIDENCE BASE Linsell, L., Malouf, F., Morris, J., et al. (2016). Prognostic factors for cerebral palsy and motor impairment in children born very preterm or very low birthweight: A systematic review. *Developmental Medicine and Child Neurology, 58*(6), 554–569.

DRUG ALERT Intrathecal baclofen lowers the seizure threshold. Children may develop severe withdrawal syndrome characterized by fever, hypertension, tachycardia, agitation, and hallucinations, which may occur in situations of pump malfunction, catheter breakage, or improper filling of pump.

EVIDENCE BASE Ozel, S., Switzer, L., Macintosh, A., et al. (2016). Informing evidence-based clinical practice guidelines for children with cerebral palsy at risk of osteoporosis: An update. *Developmental Medicine and Child Neurology, 58*(9), 918–923.

Complications

1. Contractures.
2. Hip subluxation/dislocation.
3. Malnutrition.
4. Scoliosis.
5. Osteopenia/fractures.
6. Gastroesophageal reflux.
7. Constipation.
8. Seizures.
9. Spasticity.
10. Pain.

Nursing Assessment

1. Perform a functional assessment; determine ability to perform activities of daily living (ADL).
2. Perform a developmental assessment; use Denver II developmental or other screening tools.
3. Evaluate ability to protect airway—gag reflex and swallowing.
4. Assess nutritional status—growth (height, weight, head circumference, ideal body weight), signs of nutritional deficiency, risk of aspiration, length of time it takes to feed, food diary to determine quantify of food and fluid consumed, and hydration.
5. Assess neuromuscular function and mobility—range of motion (ROM), spasticity, coordination, and scoliosis.
6. Assess speech, hearing, and vision.
7. Evaluate parent–child interaction.
8. Determine parents' understanding of and compliance with treatment plan.
9. Assess the skin for pressure sores, especially in areas of friction (splints).
10. Assess for the presence of pain (chronic or acute because of hip subluxation, dislocation).

Nursing Diagnoses

- Impaired Physical Mobility related to altered neuromuscular functioning.
- Delayed Growth and Development related to the nature and extent of the disorder.
- Interrupted Family Processes related to nature of disorder, role disturbances, and uncertain future.
- Risk for Injury related to deficit in motor activity and coordination.

Nursing Interventions

Increasing Mobility and Minimizing Deformity

1. Teach the parents to carry out appropriate exercises under the direction of the physical therapist and occupational therapist, and encourage them to incorporate this into their child's daily routine. Ensure they understand the rationale/importance of completing the exercises.
2. Use splints and braces to facilitate muscle control and improve body functioning.
   a. Apply, as directed.
   b. Remove for recommended time.
   c. Inspect the underlying skin for redness, irritation, skin breakdown, and signs of improper application or fit of splints or orthoses.
   d. Regularly inspect orthoses for cracks, loose screws, or broken Velcro straps.
   e. Use splint as directed for constraint-induced therapy in children with unilateral CP.
3. Use assistive devices, such as adapted grooming tools, writing implements, and utensils, to enhance independence. Handles for toothbrushes, spoons, and forks can be built up with sponges or specially curved to make holding easier.
4. Encourage self-dressing with easy pull-on pants, large sweat-shirts, Velcro closures, and other loose clothing.
5. Use play, such as board games, ball games, pegboards, puzzles, computers, and tablets, to improve coordination.
6. Maintain good body alignment to prevent contractures.
7. Provide adequate rest periods.
   a. Employ good sleep hygiene practices.
   b. Administer or teach parents about side effects of medications and how to administer medications safely, as prescribed.

Maximizing Growth and Development

1. Evaluate the child's developmental level and then assist with age-appropriate tasks.
2. Provide for continuity of care at home, daycare, therapy centers, and the hospital.
   a. Obtain a thorough history from the parents regarding the child's usual home routines, weaknesses and strengths, and likes and dislikes.
   b. Communicate with representatives from all disciplines involved in the child's care to ensure that the specific needs of the child are identified.
   c. Formulate a consistent care plan that incorporates the goals of all related disciplines and aligns with the goals of the child and family. Include in the care plan guidelines for the following:
      i. Feeding.
      ii. Sleeping.
      iii. Physical therapy/occupational therapy.
      iv. Play.
      v. Other ways to foster growth and development.
      vi. Medications.
      vii. Psychosocial needs.
      viii. Family needs.
      ix. Pain assessment/management.
3. During feeding, maintain a pleasant, distraction-free environment.
   a. Provide a comfortable chair.
   b. Serve the child alone, initially. After the child begins to master the task of eating, encourage the child to eat with other children.
   c. Do not attempt feedings if the child is very fatigued.
   d. Find the eating position in which the child can be most self-sufficient.
   e. Allow the child to hold the spoon even if self-feeding is minimal.
   f. Stand behind and reach over the child's shoulder to guide the spoon from the plate to the child's mouth.
   g. Serve foods that stick to the spoon, such as thick applesauce or mashed potatoes.

h. Encourage finger foods that the child can handle to self-feed.

i. Provide appropriate assistive devices for independent feeding, such as a spoon and fork with special handles, plate and glass holders, and special feeding chair.

j. Disregard "messy" eating; use a large plastic bib, smock, or towel to protect the child's clothes.

4. If the child requires assistance with feeding, do so slowly and carefully. Be aware of difficulty sucking and swallowing caused by poor muscle control. Cut large pieces of food into small pieces or serve pureed foods.

5. Be alert for associated sensory deficits that delay development and could be corrected.

a. Hearing, speech, and vision.

b. Squinting, failure to follow objects, or bringing objects very close to the face.

Strengthening Family Processes

1. Assess parental coping and provide anticipatory guidance, emotional support, access to peer support, and contact with social worker, as needed.

2. Help the parents to recognize immediate needs and identify short-term goals that can be integrated into the long-term plan.

3. Assess for caregiver burden because of the numerous challenges of daily care, and link with appropriate resources (eg, home care, respite, funding) and provide access to social work for assistance in obtaining such support.

4. Provide positive feedback for effective parenting skills and positive approaches to caring for the child.

5. Assist the parents to deal with siblings' responses to the disabled child.

a. Encourage parents to find time to spend with each sibling separately.

b. Encourage family to maintain contact with friends and community and engage in outside activities as much as possible.

c. Suggest family counseling.

6. Assist parents to find local resources to help in the child's care.

a. Contact hospital social worker or discharge planner for information about local CP organizations, chapters, funding sources, community supports, or charities.

b. Help to navigate through the national and regional programs that may have local chapters.

Protecting the Child from Injury

1. Evaluate the child's need for specific safety equipment, such as a suction machine, helmet, and walker, and modify the environment as appropriate to ensure the child's safety.

2. Provide for frequent position changes and adequate fit on orthotics, wheelchairs, and walking or standing devices to prevent skin breakdown. Assess skin integrity regularly.

Community and Home Care Considerations

1. Assess the home environment for safety. Stairs should be gated and paths should be cleared for walking with assistive devices or for adequate passage of wheelchairs, walkers, etc.

2. Assist parents in arranging for equipment that may be required in the home (eg, wheelchair, pump for intermittent G-tube feedings, walkers, home suction machine).

3. Check all adaptive equipment, braces, and walkers for correct fit. Arrange for replacement, as needed.

Family Education and Health Maintenance

1. Instruct the parents in all areas of the child's physical care.

2. Encourage regular medical and dental evaluations.

3. Advise parents that the child needs discipline to feel secure.

4. Refer parents to such agencies as the United Cerebral Palsy Association of America (*www.ucp.org*).

5. Connect families with other families who have a child with CP so that they may provide a supportive network.

6. Encourage maintenance of good nutritional status.

7. Help the child engage in regular exercise to maintain health.

Evaluation: Expected Outcomes

- Dresses and feeds self as independently as possible; minimal contractures noted.

- Consistent growth curve maintained; sequential developmental milestones consistent with condition achieved.

- Family participates in usual school and community activities; uses respite care when available.

- Safety equipment used; no injury reported.

Hydrocephalus

Hydrocephalus is characterized by an increased volume of cerebrospinal fluid (CSF) that accumulates in the ventricles and/or subarachnoid spaces and is associated with progressive ventricular dilatation. There are two main categories of hydrocephalus: communicating and noncommunicating. Hydrocephalus occurs with such conditions as tumors, infections, congenital malformations, and hemorrhage. The incidence of hydrocephalus is 0.5 to 4 per 1,000 live births.

Pathophysiology and Etiology

1. Noncommunicating hydrocephalus—obstruction of CSF flow within the ventricular system or blockage of CSF flow from the ventricular system to the subarachnoid space.

a. May be partial, intermittent, or complete.

b. More common than communicating type.

c. Congenital causes.

i. Aqueductal stenosis.

ii. Congenital lesions (vein of Galen malformation, congenital tumors).

iii. Arachnoid cyst.

iv. Chiari malformations (with or without myelomeningocele).

v. X-linked hydrocephalus.

vi. Dandy-Walker malformation.

d. Acquired causes.

i. Aqueductal gliosis (posthemorrhagic or postinfectious).

ii. Space-occupying lesions (tumors or cysts).

iii. Head injuries.

2. Communicating hydrocephalus—CSF circulates through the ventricular system into the subarachnoid space with no obstruction.

a. Congenital causes.

i. Achondroplasia.

ii. Arachnoid cyst.

iii. Craniofacial syndromes.

b. Acquired causes.

i. Posthemorrhagic (intraventricular or subarachnoid).

ii. Choroid plexus papilloma or choroid plexus carcinoma.

iii. Venous obstruction (eg, superior vena cava syndrome).

iv. Postinfectious.

Clinical Manifestations

May be rapid, slow and steadily advancing, or intermittent. Clinical signs depend on the age of the child, whether the anterior fontanelle has closed, whether the cranial sutures have fused, and the type and duration of hydrocephalus.

Infants

1. Excessive head growth (may be seen up to age 3 years).
2. Delayed closure of the anterior fontanelle.
3. Fontanelle tense and elevated above the surface of the skull.
4. Signs of increased intracranial pressure (ICP) (see Box 46-1).
5. Alteration of muscle tone of the extremities, including clonus or spasticity.
6. Later physical signs:
   a. Forehead becomes prominent ("bossing").
   b. Scalp appears shiny with prominent scalp veins.
   c. Eyebrows and eyelids may be drawn upward, exposing the sclera above the iris.
   d. Infant cannot gaze upward, causing "sunset eyes."
   e. Strabismus, nystagmus, and optic atrophy may occur.
   f. Infant has difficulty holding head up.
   g. Child may experience physical or mental developmental lag.
7. Pseudobulbar palsy (difficulty sucking, feeding, and phonation, which leads to regurgitation, drooling, and aspiration).

 NURSING ALERT It is important to measure head circumference because the infant's skull is highly elastic and can accommodate an increase in ventricular size. Ventriculomegaly may progress without obvious signs of increased ICP.

Older Children

Older children have closed sutures and present with signs of increased ICP.

BOX 46-1	Signs and Symptoms of Increased Intracranial Pressure in Infants and Children

- Vomiting.
- Restlessness and irritability.
- High-pitched, shrill cry (infants).
- Rapid increase in head circumference (infants).
- Tense, bulging fontanelle (infants).
- Changes in vital signs:
  - Increased systolic blood pressure.
  - Decreased pulse.
  - Decreased and irregular respirations.
  - Increased temperature.
- Pupillary changes.
- Papilledema.
- Possible seizures.
- Lethargy, stupor, and coma.
- Older children may also experience:
  - Headache, especially on awakening.
  - Lethargy, fatigue, and apathy.
  - Personality changes.
  - Separation of cranial sutures (may be seen in children up to age 10).
  - Visual changes such as double vision.

Diagnostic Evaluation

1. Percussion of the infant's skull may produce a typical "cracked pot" sound (Macewen sign).
2. Ophthalmoscopy may reveal papilledema.
3. MRI is the diagnostic tool of choice.
4. CT is also used for diagnosis in cases where sedation poses added risk because of need for general anesthetic or in situations in which MRI is not available.
5. Ultrasonography is also used.

Management

Hydrocephalus can be treated through a variety of surgical procedures, including direct operation on the lesion causing the obstruction, such as a tumor; intracranial shunts for selected cases of noncommunicating hydrocephalus to divert fluid from the obstructed segment of the ventricular system to the subarachnoid space; and extracranial shunts (most common) to divert fluid from the ventricular system to an extracranial compartment, frequently the peritoneum or right atrium. CSF production may also be reduced by medication or surgical intervention.

Extracranial Shunt Procedures

1. Ventriculoperitoneal (VP) shunt (see Figure 46-1):
   a. Diverts CSF from a lateral ventricle or the spinal subarachnoid space to the peritoneal cavity.
   b. A tube is passed from the lateral ventricle through an occipital burr hole subcutaneously through the posterior aspect of the neck and paraspinal region to the peritoneal cavity through a small incision in the right lower quadrant.
   c. A ventricular access device is an implanted reservoir and catheter used for premature neonates <2,000 g in lieu of a shunt. The catheter drains fluid from the ventricles into the reservoir, which can then be emptied using aseptic technique. When infant weight exceeds 2,000 g, a shunt can be placed.
2. Ventriculoatrial (VA) shunt:
   a. A tube is passed from the dilated lateral ventricle through a burr hole in the parietal region of the skull.

Figure 46-1. A ventriculoperitoneal shunt removes excessive cerebrospinal fluid from the ventricles and shunts it to the peritoneum. A one-way valve is present in the tubing behind the ear. (From Pillitteri, A. [2013]. *Maternal and child health nursing: Care of the childbearing and childrearing family* [7th ed.]. Philadelphia, PA: Lippincott Williams & Wilkins.)

b. It then is passed under the skin behind the ear and into a vein down to a point where it discharges into the right atrium or superior vena cava.

c. A one-way pressure-sensitive valve will close to prevent reflux of blood into the ventricle and open as ventricular pressure rises, allowing fluid to pass from the ventricle into the bloodstream.

3. Ventriculopleural shunt:
   a. Diverts CSF to the pleural cavity.
   b. Indicated when the VP or VA route cannot be used.

4. Ventricle–gall bladder shunt:
   a. Diverts CSF to the common bile duct.
   b. Used when all other routes are unavailable.

5. Most shunts have the following components:
   a. Ventricular tubing.
   b. A one-way or unidirectional pressure-sensitive flow valve.
   c. A pumping chamber.
   d. Distal tubing.

6. Programmable shunts are available. These can be programmed to a certain flow pressure and pressure settings can be readjusted based on patient response. A magnetic device is used to adjust the pressure setting of the shunt valve. The use of a programmable shunt eliminates the need for multiple surgeries or hospital visits to adjust shunt pressure.

Shunt Complications

1. Need for shunt revision frequently occurs because of occlusion, infection, or malfunction, especially in the first year of life.

2. Shunt revision may be necessary because of growth of the child. Newer models, however, include coiled tubing to allow the shunt to grow with the child.

3. Shunt dependency frequently occurs. The child rapidly manifests symptoms of increased ICP if the shunt does not function optimally. Onset may be sudden or insidious.

4. Children with VA shunts may experience endocardial contusions and clotting, leading to bacterial endocarditis, bacteremia, and ventriculitis or thromboembolism and cor pulmonale.

5. Children with VA shunts require biannual or annual chest x-ray to check length of tubing. Chest x-ray is also done during growth spurts, especially during puberty. When tubing is short or close to being out of the right atrium, shunt replacement needs to be scheduled.

Prognosis

1. Prognosis depends on early diagnosis and prompt therapy and the underlying etiology.

2. With improved diagnostic and management techniques, the prognosis is becoming considerably better.
   a. Many children experience normal motor and intellectual development.
   b. The severity of neurologic deficits is directly proportional to the interval between onset of hydrocephalus and the time of diagnosis.

3. Approximately two thirds of patients will die at an early age if they do not receive surgical treatment.

4. Surgery reduces mortality and decreases morbidity, with a survival rate of >90%.

Complications

1. Seizures and headaches.
2. Herniation of the brain.
3. Spontaneous arrest because of natural compensatory mechanisms, persistent increased ICP, and brain herniation.

4. Developmental delays.
5. Depression in adolescents is common.
6. Shunt malfunctions.

Nursing Assessment

Infants

1. Assess head circumference.
   a. Measure at the occipitofrontal circumference—point of largest measurement.
   b. Measure the head at approximately the same time each day.
   c. Use a centimeter measure for greatest accuracy.

2. Palpate fontanelle for firmness and bulging.
3. Assess pupillary response.
4. Assess level of consciousness (LOC).
5. Evaluate breathing patterns and effectiveness.
6. Assess feeding patterns and patterns of emesis.
7. Assess motor function.
8. Assess developmental milestones.

Older Children

1. Measure vital signs for signs of increased ICP.
2. Assess patterns of headache and emesis.
3. Determine pupillary response.
4. Evaluate LOC using the Glasgow Coma Scale.
5. Assess motor function.
6. Evaluate attainment of milestones and school performance.
7. Assess for behavioral changes.

Nursing Diagnoses

- Ineffective Cerebral Tissue Perfusion related to increased ICP before surgery.
- Imbalanced Nutrition: Less Than Body Requirements related to reduced oral intake and vomiting.
- Risk for Impaired Skin Integrity related to alterations in LOC and enlarged head.
- Anxiety of parents related to child undergoing surgery.
- Risk for Injury related to malfunctioning shunt.
- Risk for Deficient Fluid Volume related to CSF drainage and decreased intake postoperatively.
- Risk for Infection related to bacterial infiltration of the shunt.
- Ineffective Family Coping related to diagnosis and surgery.

Nursing Interventions

Maintaining Cerebral Perfusion

1. Observe for evidence of increased ICP and report immediately.
2. Assist with diagnostic procedures to determine cause of hydrocephalus and indication for surgical intervention.
   a. Explain the procedure to the child and parents at their levels of comprehension.
   b. Administer prescribed sedatives 30 minutes before the procedure to ensure their effectiveness.
   c. Organize activities so that the child is permitted to rest after administration of the sedative.
   d. Observe closely after ventriculography for the following:
      i. Leaking CSF from the sites of subdural or ventricular taps. These tap holes should be covered with a small piece of gauze or other dressing per institutional policy.
      ii. Reactions to the sedative, especially respiratory depression.
      iii. Changes in vital signs indicative of shock.
      iv. Signs of increased ICP, which may occur if air has been injected into the ventricles.

NURSING ALERT Brain stem herniation can occur with increased ICP and is manifested by opisthotonic positioning (flexion of the head and feet backward). This is a grave sign and may be followed by respiratory arrest. Prepare for emergency resuscitation and corrective measures, as directed.

DRUG ALERT Sedatives are contraindicated in many cases because increased ICP predisposes the child to hypoventilation or respiratory arrest. If they are administered, the child should be observed very closely for evidence of respiratory depression.

Providing Adequate Nutrition

1. Be aware that feeding is frequently difficult because the child may be listless, have a diminished appetite, and be prone to vomiting.
2. Complete nursing care and treatments before feeding so that the child will not be disturbed during feeding.
3. Hold the infant in a semireclined position with head well supported during feeding. Allow ample time for bubbling.
4. Offer small, frequent feedings.
5. Place the child on side with head elevated after feeding to prevent aspiration.

Maintaining Skin Integrity

1. Prevent pressure sores (pressure sores of the head are a frequent problem) by placing the child on a sponge rubber or lamb's wool pad or an alternating-pressure or eggcrate mattress to keep weight evenly distributed. Be mindful of latex allergies and the type of padding used.
2. Keep the scalp clean and dry.
3. Turn the child's head frequently; change position at least every 2 hours.
   a. When turning the child, rotate head and body together to prevent strain on the neck.
   b. A firm pillow may be placed under the child's head and shoulders for further support when lifting the child.
   c. Keep weight off incision during immediate postoperative period.
4. Provide meticulous skin care to all parts of the body and observe the skin for signs of breakdown or pressure.
5. Give passive ROM exercises to the extremities, especially the legs.
6. Keep the eyes moistened with artificial tears if the child is unable to close the eyelids normally. This prevents corneal ulcerations and infections.

Reducing Anxiety

1. Prepare the parents for their child's surgery by answering questions, describing what nursing care will take place postoperatively, and explaining how the shunt will work.
2. Encourage the parents to discuss all the risks and benefits with the surgeon. Help them to understand the prognosis and what to expect of the child's neurologic and cognitive development.
3. Prepare the child for surgery by using dolls or other forms of play to describe what interventions will occur or solicit the help of a child life specialist to prepare the child for surgery through play.

Improving Cerebral Tissue Perfusion Postoperatively

1. Monitor the child's temperature, pulse, respiration, blood pressure (BP), and pupillary size and reaction every 15 minutes until stable; then, monitor every 1 to 2 hours or as indicated by child's condition and institutional policy.
2. Maintain normothermia.
   a. Provide appropriate blankets or covers, an Isolette or infant warmer, or hypothermia blanket.
   b. Administer a tepid sponge bath or antipyretic medication for temperature elevation.
3. Aspirate mucus from the nose and throat, as necessary, to prevent respiratory difficulty.
4. Turn the child frequently.
5. Promote optimal drainage of CSF through the shunt by pumping the shunt and positioning the child, as directed.
   a. If pumping is prescribed, carefully compress the valve at specified number of times at regularly scheduled intervals.
   b. Report any difficulties in pumping the shunt.
   c. Gradually elevate the head of child's bed to 30 to 45 degrees, as ordered. Initially, the child will be positioned flat to prevent excessive CSF drainage.
6. Assess for excessive drainage of CSF.
   a. Sunken fontanelle, agitation, and restlessness (infant).
   b. Decreased LOC (older child).
7. Assess closely for increased ICP, indicating shunt malfunction.
   a. Note especially change in LOC, change in vital signs (increased systolic BP, decreased pulse rate, decreased or irregular respirations), vomiting, and pupillary changes.
   b. Report these changes immediately to prevent cerebral hypoxia and possible brain herniation.
8. Prevent excessive pressure on the skin overlying shunt by placing cotton behind and over the ears under the head dressing and avoiding positioning the child on the area of the valve or the incision until the wound is healed.

Maintaining Fluid Balance

1. Accurately measure and record total fluid intake and output.
2. Administer intravenous (IV) fluids, as prescribed; carefully monitor infusion rate to prevent fluid overload.
3. Use a nasogastric tube, if necessary, for abdominal distention. This is most frequently used when a VP shunt has been performed.
   a. Measure the drainage and record the amount and color.
   b. Monitor for return of bowel sounds after nasogastric suction has been disconnected for at least 30 minutes.
4. Give frequent mouth care while the child is to have nothing by mouth.
5. Begin oral feedings when the child is fully recovered from the anesthetic and displays interest.
   a. Begin with small amounts of dextrose 5% in water.
   b. Gradually introduce formula.
   c. Introduce solid foods suitable to the child's age and tolerance.
   d. Encourage a high-protein diet.
   e. Observe for and report any decrease in urine output, increased urine specific gravity, diminished skin turgor, dryness of mucous membranes, or lethargy, indicating dehydration.

Preventing Infection

1. Assess for fever (temperature normally fluctuates during the first 24 hours after surgery), purulent drainage from the incision, or swelling, redness, and tenderness along the shunt tract.
2. Administer prescribed prophylactic antibiotics.

NURSING ALERT All children who have had surgery require assessments for pain. Although pain management is institution specific, acetaminophen is often the medication of choice. Also, use alternative modes of pain management, such as distraction and relaxation techniques, and ensure a quiet environment.

Strengthening Family Coping

1. Begin discharge planning early, including specific techniques for care of the shunt and suggested methods for providing daily care.
   a. Turning, holding, and positioning.
   b. Skin care over the shunt.
   c. Exercises to strengthen muscles—incorporated with play.
   d. Feeding techniques and schedule.
   e. Pumping the shunt.
2. Accompany all instructions with reassurance necessary to prevent the parents from becoming anxious or fearful about assuming the care of the child.
3. Offer opportunities for care by parent during hospitalization so that parents may become familiar and capable of care delivery in the home setting through practice.
4. Help the parents to assist siblings to understand hydrocephalus and the child's special needs. Encourage parents to spend individual time with siblings. Suggest family counseling and social work support, if needed.
5. Assist parents in locating additional resources.
   a. Social worker, discharge planner, or department of social services.
   b. Visiting or home health nurses or aides.
   c. Parent groups.
   d. Community agencies.
   e. Special programs at school.

Community and Home Care Considerations

1. Follow the community and home care considerations listed under "Cerebral Palsy" on page 1229. Check shunt functioning regularly, and reinforce parental performance of shunt checks and assessment for shunt malfunction and increased ICP.
2. Perform total physical assessment regularly, looking for signs of trauma or skin breakdown.
3. Patient should wear a medical alert bracelet when he or she starts to attend school or daycare.
4. Ensure parents or caregivers are certified in cardiopulmonary resuscitation (CPR).

Family Education and Health Maintenance

1. Stress the importance of recognizing symptoms of increased ICP and reporting them immediately.
2. Advise parents to report shunt malfunction or infection immediately to prevent increased ICP.
3. Teach parents that illnesses that cause vomiting and diarrhea or illnesses that prevent an adequate fluid intake are a great threat to the child who has had a shunt procedure. Advise parents to consult with the child's health care provider about immediate treatment of fever, control of vomiting and diarrhea, and replacement of fluids.
4. Tell the parents that few restrictions are required for children with shunts and to consult with the health care provider about specific concerns.
5. Alert parents that additional information and support are available from the Hydrocephalus Association (*www.hydroassoc.org*).

Evaluation: Expected Outcomes

- No changes in vital signs, LOC, or head size; no vomiting; pupils equal and responsive.
- Feeds every 4 hours without vomiting; no significant weight loss.
- No erythema, blanching, or skin breakdown; wound healing evident.
- Parents have an understanding of operative procedure, risks, and benefits.
- Shunt pumping without resistance; stable LOC and vital signs.
- Urine output equal to intake; skin turgor normal; electrolytes within normal limits.
- Afebrile; no drainage from shunt site.
- Parents actively seeking resources.

Spina Bifida

Spina bifida, also called *spinal dysraphia*, is a malformation of the spine in which the posterior portion of the laminae of the vertebrae fails to close. It occurs in approximately 1 per 1,000 live births in the United States and is the most common developmental defect of the central nervous system (CNS). It is more common in Caucasians than in other races. The incidence of spina bifida defects has been declining in the United States and United Kingdom because of antenatal screening and changes in environmental factors such as the consumption of folic acid in early pregnancy.

Several types of spina bifida are recognized, of which the following three are most common (see Figure 46-2, page 1234).

Spina Bifida Occulta

Spina bifida occulta is seen in 10% of the US population. It is a result of the posterior vertebral arches failing to fuse. A fat pad, dermal sinus, hairy tuft, or dimple in the lower back/lumbosacral region is often seen.

Meningocele

Meningocele is a herniation of the meninges through the defective posterior arches. The sac does not contain neural elements.

Myelomeningocele (or Meningomyelocele)

The spinal nerve roots and cord membranes protrude through the defect in the laminae of the vertebral column. Myelomeningoceles are covered by a thin membrane.

Pathophysiology and Etiology

1. Unknown etiology, but generally thought to result from genetic predisposition triggered by something in the environment.
   a. Certain drugs, including valproic acid, have been known to cause neural tube defects if administered during pregnancy.
   b. Women who have spina bifida and parents who have one affected child have an increased risk of producing children with neural tube defects.
2. Involves an arrest in the orderly formation of the vertebral arches and spinal cord that occurs between the 4th and 6th weeks of embryogenesis.
3. Theories of causation include:
   a. Incomplete closure of the neural tube during the 4th week of embryonic life.
   b. The neural tube forms adequately and then ruptures.
4. In spina bifida occulta, the bony defect may range from a very thin slit separating one lamina from the spinous process to a complete absence of the spine and laminae.
   a. A thin, fibrous membrane sometimes covers the defect.
   b. The spinal cord and its meninges may be connected with a fistulous tract extending to and opening onto the surface of the skin.
5. In meningocele, the defect may occur anywhere on the cord. Higher defects (from the thorax and upward) are usually meningoceles.

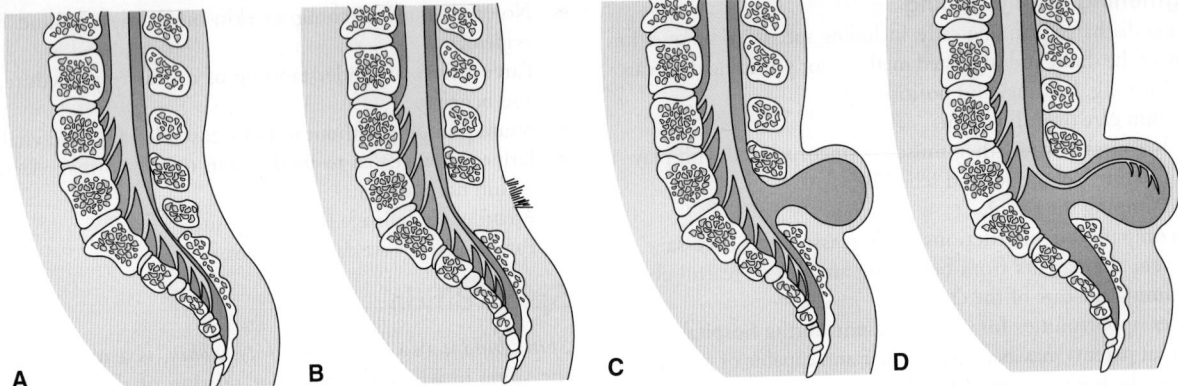

Figure 46-2. Spina bifida. **(A)** Normal spine. **(B)** Spina bifida occulta. **(C)** Spina bifida with meningocele. **(D)** Spina bifida with myelomeningocele. (From Pillitteri, A. [2013]. *Maternal and child health nursing: Care of the childbearing and childrearing family* [7th ed.]. Philadelphia, PA: Lippincott Williams & Wilkins.)

    a. Surgical correction is necessary to prevent rupture of the sac and subsequent infection.

    b. Prognosis is good with surgical correction.

6. In myelomeningocele (meningomyelocele), the lesion contains both the spinal cord and cord membranes.

    a. A bluish area may be evident on the top because of exposed neural tissue.

    b. The sac may leak in utero or may rupture after birth, allowing free drainage of CSF. This renders the child highly susceptible to meningitis.

    c. Of all defects known as spina bifida cystica, 95% are myelomeningoceles and 5% are meningoceles.

 DRUG ALERT Maternal periconceptional use of folic acid supplementation reduces by 50% or more the incidence of neural tube defects in pregnancies at risk.

Clinical Manifestations

Spina Bifida Occulta

1. Most patients have no symptoms.

    a. They may have a dimple in the skin or a growth of hair over the malformed vertebra.

    b. There is no externally visible sac.

2. With growth, the child may develop foot weakness or bowel and bladder sphincter disturbances.

3. This condition is occasionally associated with more significant developmental abnormalities of the spinal cord, including syringomyelia and tethered cord.

Meningocele

1. An external cystic defect can be seen in the spinal cord, usually in the midline.

    a. The sac is composed only of meninges and is filled with CSF.

    b. The cord and nerve roots are usually normal.

2. There is seldom evidence of weakness of the legs or lack of sphincter control.

Myelomeningocele

1. A round, raised, and poorly epithelialized area may be noted at any level of the spinal column. However, the highest incidence of the lesion occurs in the lumbosacral area.

2. Hydrocephalus occurs in approximately 90% of children with myelomeningocele because of associated Arnold-Chiari malformation, which causes a block in the flow of CSF through the ventricles.

3. Loss of motor control and sensation below the level of the lesion can occur. These conditions are highly variable and depend on the size of the lesion and its position on the cord.

    a. A low thoracic lesion may cause total flaccid paralysis below the waist.

    b. A small sacral lesion may cause only patchy spots of decreased sensation in the feet.

4. Contractures may occur in the ankles, knees, or hips. Hips may become dislocated.

    a. Nature and degree of involvement depend on size and location of the lesion.

    b. This occurs because some fibers of innervation get through. One side of a hip, knee, or ankle may be innervated, whereas the opposing side may not be. The unopposed side then becomes pulled out of position.

5. Clubfeet are a common accompanying anomaly; thought to be related to the position of paraplegic feet in the uterus.

6. Bladder dysfunction occurs because of how the sacral nerves that innervate the bladder are affected. The bladder fails to respond to normal messages that it is time to void and simply fills and overflows, causing incontinence and susceptibility to urinary tract infections (UTIs) because of incomplete emptying.

7. Fecal incontinence and constipation are caused by poor innervation of the anal sphincter and bowel musculature.

8. Most children have average intellectual ability despite hydrocephalus. Developmental disabilities include the following:

    a. Gross motor development—children will need assistance in gaining and maintaining mobility.

    b. Most children are able to learn in a "mainstream" school environment, provided they are able to overcome other barriers (architectural and attitudinal).

Diagnostic Evaluation

1. Prenatal detection is done through prenatal ultrasound and fetal MRI. This testing should be offered to all women at risk (women who are affected or who have had other affected children).

2. Diagnosis is primarily based on clinical manifestations.

3. CT scan and MRI may be performed to further evaluate the brain and spinal cord.

Management

Surgical Intervention

1. Procedure: laminectomy and closure of the open lesion or removal of the sac usually can be done soon after birth.
2. Purpose:
   a. To prevent further deterioration of neural function.
   b. To minimize the danger of rupture and infection, especially meningitis.
   c. To improve cosmetic effect.
   d. To facilitate handling of the infant.

Multidisciplinary Follow-Up for Associated Problems

1. A coordinated team approach will help maximize the physical and intellectual potential of each affected child.
2. The team may include a neurologist, neurosurgeon, orthopedic surgeon, urologist, primary care provider, social worker, physical therapist, occupational therapist, nurse practitioners, and a variety of community-based and hospital staff nurses, and the child and family.
3. Numerous neurosurgical, orthopedic, and urologic procedures may be necessary to help the child achieve maximum function.

Prognosis

1. Influenced by the site of the lesion and the presence and degree of associated hydrocephalus. Generally, the higher the defect, the greater the extent of neurologic deficit and the greater the likelihood of hydrocephalus.
2. In the absence of treatment, most infants with meningomyelocele die early in infancy.
3. Surgical intervention is most effective if it is done early in the neonatal period, preferably within the first few days of life.
4. Even with surgical intervention, infants can be expected to manifest associated neurosurgical, orthopedic, or urologic problems.
5. New techniques of treatment, intensive research, and improved services have increased life expectancy and have greatly enhanced the quality of life for most children who receive treatment.

Complications

1. Hydrocephalus associated with meningocele; may be aggravated by surgical repair.
2. Scoliosis, contractures, and joint dislocation.
3. Skin breakdown in sensory denervated areas and under braces.

Nursing Assessment

1. Assess sensory and motor response of lower extremities.
2. Assess ability to void spontaneously, retention of urine, and symptoms of UTI.
3. Assess usual stooling patterns and need for medications to facilitate elimination.
4. Assess mobility and use of orthoses, casts, and other special equipment.

Nursing Diagnoses

Neonates (Preoperative)

- Risk for Impaired Skin Integrity related to impaired motor and sensory function.
- Risk for Infection related to contamination of the myelomeningocele site.
- Impaired Urinary Elimination related to neurologic deficits.
- Ineffective Tissue Perfusion: Cerebral related to potential hydrocephalus.
- Fear (parents) related to neonate with neurologic disorder and to surgery.

Infants and Children (Postoperative)

- Ineffective Thermoregulation following surgery.
- Impaired Urinary Elimination related to sacral denervation.
- Bowel Incontinence or Constipation related to impaired innervation of anal sphincter and bowel musculature.
- Disturbed Body Image related to the child's appearance, difficulties with locomotion, and lack of control over excretory functions.

Nursing Interventions

Protecting Skin Integrity

1. Avoid positioning on the infant's back to prevent pressure on the sac. Check position at least once every hour.
2. Do not place a diaper or other covering directly over the sac.
3. Observe the sac frequently for evidence of irritation or leakage of CSF.
4. Use prone positioning and prevent hip flexion to decrease tension on the sac.
5. Place a foam rubber pad covered with a soft cloth between the infant's legs to maintain the hips in abduction and to prevent or counteract subluxation. A diaper roll or small pillow may be used in place of the foam rubber pad.
6. Allow the infant's feet to hang freely over the pads or mattress edge to prevent aggravation of foot deformities.
7. Provide meticulous skin care to all areas of the body, especially ankles, knees, tip of the nose, cheeks, and chin.
8. Provide passive ROM exercises for muscles and joints that the infant does not use spontaneously. Avoid hip exercises because of common hip dislocation, unless otherwise recommended.
9. Use a foam or fleece pad to reduce pressure of the mattress against the infant's skin.
10. Avoid pressure on the infant's back during feeding by holding the infant with your elbow rotated to avoid touching the sac or feeding while infant is lying on side or prone on your lap. Encourage the parents to use these positions to provide infant stimulation and bonding.

Preventing Infection

1. Be aware that infection of the sac is most commonly caused by contamination by urine and feces.
2. Keep the infant's buttocks and genitalia scrupulously clean.
   a. Do not diaper the infant if the defect is in the lower portion of the spine.
   b. Use a small plastic drape taped between the defect and the anus to help prevent contamination.
3. Apply a sterile gauze pad or towel or a sterile, moistened dressing over the sac, as directed.
   a. When the sterile covering is used, it should be changed frequently to keep the area free from exudate and to maintain sterility.
   b. Care must be taken to prevent the covering from adhering to and damaging the sac.
4. Monitor and report immediately any signs of infection.
   a. Oozing of fluid or pus from the sac.
   b. Fever.
   c. Irritability or listlessness.
   d. Seizure.

Promoting Urinary Elimination

1. Use Crede method for emptying the bladder (unless contraindicated by vesicoureteral reflux) and teach parents the technique.
   a. Apply firm, gentle pressure to the abdomen, beginning in the umbilical area and progressing toward the symphysis pubis.
   b. Continue the procedure as long as urine can be manually expressed.
2. Ensure fluid intake to dilute the urine.
3. Administer prescribed prophylactic antibiotics.
4. Monitor and report concentrated or foul-smelling urine.

Maintaining Cerebral Tissue Perfusion

1. Monitor for signs of hydrocephalus and report immediately.
   a. Irritability.
   b. Feeding difficulty, vomiting, and decreased appetite.
   c. Temperature fluctuation.
   d. Decreased alertness.
   e. Tense fontanelle.
   f. Increased head circumference.

Reducing Fear

1. Encourage parents to express feelings of guilt, fear, lack of control, or helplessness.
2. Provide accurate information about spina bifida and what to expect postoperatively.
3. Include the parents in all of infant's care and encourage private bonding time.

Maintaining Thermoregulation and Preventing Complications

1. Frequently monitor temperature, pulse, respirations, color, and level of responsiveness postoperatively, based on the infant's stability.
2. Use an Isolette or infant warmer to prevent temperature fluctuation.
3. Prevent respiratory complications.
   a. Periodically reposition the infant to promote lung expansion.
   b. Watch for abdominal distention, which could interfere with breathing.
   c. Have oxygen available.
4. Maintain hydration and nutritional intake.
   a. Administer IV fluids, as ordered; keep accurate intake and output log.
   b. Administer gavage feedings, as ordered.
   c. Begin bottle-feeding when infant is responsive and tolerating feedings. Give small, frequent feedings slowly so air can be expelled naturally without bubbling.
5. Keep the surgical dressing clean and dry and observe for drainage. Avoid pressure to the area and diapers that cover the incision until healed.
6. Monitor for and teach parents to recognize signs of hydrocephalus. Report immediately.
7. Limit or prevent direct contact of the child to products routinely used that contain latex, because of risk of latex allergy and severe reaction. Latex products include BP cuffs, tourniquets, tape, indwelling catheters, gloves, and IV tubing injection ports. Develop protocols specifying modification of care for children at risk for latex allergy.

> **! NURSING ALERT** Be aware that children with spina bifida have a far greater risk of latex allergy than the general population. It is estimated that up to 20% of spina bifida patients have a latex allergy. Symptoms include hives, itching, wheezing, and anaphylaxis. Incidence increases with time and may be related to repeated exposure to products containing latex.

Achieving Continence

1. Teach parents that continence can usually be achieved with clean, intermittent self-catheterization.
   a. Children can generally be taught to catheterize themselves by age 6 or 7.
   b. Parents can catheterize younger children.
2. Teach the following procedure:
   a. Gather equipment: catheter, water-soluble lubricant, soap and water, and urine collection container.
   b. Wash hands.
   c. Position patient.
   d. Clean the area around the urethral meatus.
   e. Lubricate the catheter tip.
   f. Insert the catheter until urine starts to flow. Have urine collection container or diaper available.
   g. Remove catheter when urine is drained from the bladder.
   h. Clean any lubricant off the child.
   i. Dispose of urine.
   j. Wash hands.
3. Teach about the action of medications, such as imipramine and ephedrine, if prescribed, which are used to help children retain urine rather than dribbling. When used with self-catheterization, many children can stay dry for 3 to 4 hours at a time.
4. Teach the signs of UTI (concentrated, foul-smelling urine; irritability; pain or burning; and fever) and the proper administration of antibiotics either prophylactically or when prescribed for infection.
5. For children who cannot achieve urinary continence through intermittent catheterization, provide information about options, such as surgically implanted mechanical urinary sphincters and bladder pacemakers, indwelling catheters, external collecting devices, and urinary diversion (may be necessary in some cases).

Achieving Regular Bowel Elimination

1. Assist with bowel training program to compensate for decreased sacral sensation.
   a. Children are placed on a toileting schedule and are taught to push.
   b. Medications, such as stool softeners, suppositories, or enemas, may be used initially to help determine scheduling.
2. To prevent constipation and enhance bowel control, encourage intake of high-fiber, high-fluid diet. Such medications as psyllium may be used to increase bulk or soften stool.

Fostering Positive Body Image

1. Emphasize rehabilitation that makes use of the child's strengths and minimizes disabilities.
2. Continually reassess functional abilities and offer suggestions to increase independence. Periodically consult with physical or occupational therapists to help maximize function.
3. Encourage the use of braces and specialized equipment to enhance ambulation while minimizing the appearance of the equipment. For example, wear pants instead of dresses or shorts to cover leg braces; choose a compact wheelchair that can be decorated or personalized for the child.
4. Encourage participation with peer group and in activities that build on strengths, such as cognitive abilities and interest in music or art.
5. Periodically reassess bowel and bladder programs. The ability to stay dry for reasonable time intervals is one of the greatest factors in enhancing self-esteem and positive body image.

Community and Home Care Considerations

1. Follow the community and home care considerations listed under "Cerebral Palsy" on page 1229.
2. Survey the home environment for latex and substitute products obtained, if possible. Toys and equipment for children, such as nipples, pacifiers, and elastic on the legs of disposable diapers, also contain latex. Teach the parents how to recognize latex allergy and to notify the child's health care provider.
3. Teach the family how to clean and reuse urinary catheters. The catheter should be washed in warm, soapy water and rinsed well in warm water. The catheter should be air-dried and, when completely dried, placed in a clean jar or plastic bag. A catheter should be replaced when it becomes dry, cracked, and stiff or if the child develops a UTI.
4. Instruct the parents to notify the health care provider for signs of associated problems, such as hydrocephalus, meningitis, UTI, and latex sensitivity.

 NURSING ALERT Ensure there is an emergency epinephrine injection available in case of inadvertent latex exposure.

Family Education and Health Maintenance

1. Prepare the parents to feed, hold, and stimulate their infant as naturally as possible.
2. Teach the parents the special techniques that may be required for holding and positioning, feeding, caring for the incision, emptying the bladder, and exercising muscles.
3. Alert the parents to safety needs of the child with decreased sensation, such as protection from prolonged pressure, the risk of burns because of bathwater that is too warm, and avoidance of trauma from contact with sharp objects.
4. Urge continued follow-up and health maintenance, including immunizations and evaluation of growth and development.
5. Advise parents that children with paralysis are at risk for becoming overweight because of inactivity, so they should provide a low-fat, balanced diet; control snacking; and encourage as much activity as possible.
6. For additional resources, refer families to agencies such as the Spina Bifida Association of America *www.spinabifidaassociation.org*.

Evaluation: Expected Outcomes

- No signs of meningeal sac or skin breakdown.
- Afebrile, alert, and active.
- Clear urine without odor; adequate elimination; no infection.
- Fontanelle soft; head circumference stable.
- Parents asking questions about surgery, showing affection for infant.
- Vital signs stable; incisional dressing dry and intact.
- Parents or child demonstrates proper catheterization technique.
- Passes stool once per day; adequate elimination; no constipation.
- Verbalizes participation in school and other social activities.

Muscular Dystrophy

Muscular dystrophy (MD) refers to a group of genetically determined, progressive, degenerative myopathies affecting a variety of muscle groups—most patients are children. The most common pediatric muscular dystrophies include Duchenne MD (DMD) and Becker MD (BMD). A 2015 US report estimated the prevalence of DMD and BMD at approximately 2 per 10,000. Most with Duchenne MD rarely survive beyond ages 20 to 25.

Pathophysiology and Etiology

1. Inherited; may be X-linked, autosomal dominant, or recessive.
2. Genetic coding defect causes abnormal muscle development and function—mutations of the dystrophin gene in DMD and BMD are termed dystrophinopathies.
3. Degeneration and loss of skeletal muscle fibers, but no associated structural abnormalities in peripheral nerves or spinal cord.
4. Marked reduction of dystrophin, a protein vital to muscle function. The amount of dystrophin levels varies with the type of MD.

Clinical Manifestations

1. Progressive muscular weakness, calf enlargement, and leg pain (see Table 46-1).
2. Gower sign is a hallmark feature of Duchenne MD, characterized by a child's difficulty rising from the floor. The child must take the following steps to assume a standing position:
   a. Roll onto hands and knees.
   b. Bear weight with legs by creating a wide base of support, while using hands on the floor to support some weight.
   c. Use arms to climb up legs.
   d. Push torso to an upright stance with legs remaining wide apart.
3. Heart muscle weakens and tachycardia develops.
4. Respiratory muscles weaken, causing ineffective cough and frequent infections.
5. May have mild cognitive impairment in Duchenne MD.

Diagnostic Evaluation

1. Nerve conduction test and electromyography show abnormalities.
2. Serum creatinine kinase—elevated.
3. Deoxyribonucleic acid (DNA) analysis of blood.
4. Muscle biopsy may provide definitive diagnosis.
5. Electrocardiogram and echocardiogram to determine degree of cardiomyopathy.

Management

1. Goals of treatment are directed toward maintaining mobility, quality of life, and prevention of complications.
2. Medications to control symptoms, such as antiarrhythmics and bronchodilators.
3. Promotion of ambulation with appropriate aid after loss of ability to walk.
4. Provision of spinal orthotic supports.
5. Surgical tendon releasing to treat contractures.
6. Physical therapy, such as passive stretching, to preserve function.
7. Vigorous respiratory therapy, such as chest percussion, inspirometry, and assisted cough.
8. Pulmonary function monitoring.
9. Carrier detection and genetic counseling to explain implications of MD to parents and detect sibling carriers.
10. Glucocorticoids for DMD patients 4 years of age and older to delay the progression of muscle weakness.

Table 46-1　Clinical Manifestations of Muscular Dystrophies

TYPE	ONSET	CLINICAL MANIFESTATIONS	OTHER INFORMATION
Duchenne	Age 2 to 6 years	Muscle atrophy and weakness over time affecting the pelvis, thighs, upper arms, and eventually all voluntary muscles; waddling gait, need for wheelchair by age 12; pulmonary and cardiac abnormalities; survival beyond age 20 is rare	Affects only males Most common type of MD in children
Becker	Age 2 to 16 years	Similar to Duchenne, but less severe, very mild in some cases; slower progression. Survival into middle age	Affects only males
Limb–girdle	Late teen to adult	Progressive weakness of the pelvic and shoulder girdles and then arms and legs. Walking becomes difficult over a 20-year period. Survival may be to late adulthood	Affects males and females Most common type overall
Facioscapulohumeral	Teen to early adult	Weakness of fascial muscles, wasting of shoulders and upper arms; slow progression with short periods of rapid deterioration. Causes problems with chewing, swallowing, speaking; characteristic "Popeye" arms and scapular winging. Survival well into adulthood	Affects males and females Severity varies widely
Congenital	At birth	General muscle weakness; possible joint deformities because of contractures; slow progression. Seizures and other brain abnormalities with Fukuyama type. Shortened life span	Affects males and females Several types have been identified
Emery-Dreifuss	Childhood to early teen	Slowly progressive weakness and atrophy of the shoulder, upper arm, and lower leg muscles; joint deformities; possible cardiac problems causing sudden death. Cardiac problems may affect carriers (including women)	Affects males only Rare form

11. May require early surgical intervention to correct scoliosis.
12. Nutritional management to prevent obesity is necessary as this may affect quality of life, life expectancy, and burden of care.
13. Frequent surveillance of cardiac function.

Complications

1. Infections (pulmonary, urinary, systemic).
2. Cardiac dysrhythmias.
3. Respiratory insufficiency and failure secondary to weakness of the diaphragm and chest muscles.
4. Aspiration pneumonia because of oropharyngeal dysfunction.
5. Depression.
6. Orthopedic deformities—contractures, lordosis, and scoliosis.
7. Learning and behavioral disorders.
8. Malignant hyperthermia—may develop in small number of children with mild or nonapparent muscle disease.
9. Osteopenia related to immobility.

Nursing Assessment

1. Assess muscle strength, atrophy, gait, age-related motor development, and progressive loss of function.
2. Evaluate respiratory and cardiac status—breath sounds, heart sounds, pulse rate and rhythm, BP, and peripheral perfusion.
3. Evaluate ADLs.
4. Assess degree of pain.
5. Identify psychosocial issues, such as altered self-concept, decreased socialization, and family discord.

Nursing Diagnoses

- Ineffective Breathing Pattern related to muscle weakness.
- Impaired Physical Mobility related to disease process.
- Acute pain related to neurologic effects from the disease process.
- Decreased Cardiac Output related to cardiac muscle involvement.
- Impaired Swallowing related to muscle weakness.
- Deficient Diversional Activity related to weakness.

Nursing Interventions

Maintaining Breathing Pattern

1. Encourage upright positioning to provide for maximum chest excursion.
2. Encourage energy conservation techniques and avoidance of exertion.
3. Teach deep breathing exercises to strengthen respiratory muscles.
4. Assess rate, depth, and pattern of respirations; listen to breath sounds; and report any change in condition.
5. Note results of arterial blood gas levels, sputum cultures, and chest x-rays.
6. Encourage coughing and deep breathing or perform chest physiotherapy, as indicated.

Preserving Optimal Motor Function

1. Refer to physical therapy for stretching and strengthening exercises to optimize remaining motor function.
2. Perform ROM exercises to preserve mobility and prevent atrophy.

3. Schedule activity with consideration to energy highs throughout the day.
4. Consult with occupational therapist for assistive devices to maintain independence.
5. Apply braces and splints to prevent contractures.
6. Ensure adequate pain management.

Improving Cardiac Output

1. Monitor vital signs, cardiac rhythm, and signs of heart failure, such as edema, adventitious breath sounds, and weight gain.
2. Monitor intake and output and maintain IV or oral fluid intake, as ordered.

Monitoring Swallowing Function

1. Assess cranial nerve function for swallowing (gag reflex) and chewing.
2. Provide a diet that the patient can handle; a pureed diet may be necessary.
3. Diet should be high protein and controlled calories to provide optimal nutritional value.
4. Encourage eating in upright position without talking and encourage consumption of smaller, frequent meals.
5. Administer alternative enteral feeding if gag reflex is diminished.

Encouraging Diversional Activities

1. Encourage diversional activities that prevent overexertion and frustration, but discourage long periods of bed rest and inactivity such as TV watching.
2. If upper extremities are mostly affected, suggest walking or riding a stationary bike; if lower extremities are mostly affected, encourage use of a wheelchair to promote mobility and performing simple crafts.
3. Discuss patient's interests and assist with preferred activities.
4. Investigate with the patient various methods of stress management to deal with frustration.
5. Administer analgesics and antidepressants, as ordered, to facilitate participation in activities.

Community and Home Care Considerations

1. Follow the community and home care considerations listed under "Cerebral Palsy" on page 1229.
2. Obtain services and devices that will promote maximal functioning, such as wheelchair ramp, wheelchair van for transportation, and assistive devices.
3. Explore physical and recreational activities with family such as Special Olympics.
4. Assess child's educational progress and ability to attend school versus home schooling.
5. Collaborate with patient and family to establish daily plan of activities that incorporates patient's interests, ability, and need for rest periods.

Family Education and Health Maintenance

1. Offer genetic counseling, if indicated, to determine options of family planning.
2. Instruct the patient and family in ROM exercises, pulmonary care, and methods of transfer and locomotion.
3. Refer to community respite and counseling services.
4. Stress the importance of fluids to decrease risk of urinary/pulmonary infection and minimize constipation.
5. Advise patient or family to report signs of respiratory infection immediately to obtain treatment and prevent heart failure.

6. Refer patient and family to agencies such as the Muscular Dystrophy Association (*www.mdausa.org*).

Evaluation: Expected Outcomes

- Deep, unlabored respirations with clear breath sounds.
- Ambulates unassisted; no contractures noted.
- Vital signs stable; no edema.
- Tolerates small pureed feeds without aspiration.
- Out of bed most of day; engages in diversional and social activities.

Bacterial Meningitis

Bacterial meningitis is an inflammation of the meninges that follows the invasion of the spinal fluid by a bacterial agent. Inflammation occurs in the leptomeninges and tissues surrounding the brain and spinal cord. Since the introduction of the *Haemophilus influenzae* type B (1990) and pneumococcal conjugate (2000) vaccines to the pediatric immunization schedule, the incidence of bacterial meningitis has decreased in all age groups except in children under 2 months old. In 2006 to 2007, the US population–based surveillance found the peak incidence occurred under age 2 months (80.69 per 100,000) with the 2- to 23-month age group significantly less (6.91 per 100,000), dropping even further in the 2- to 10-year age group (0.56 per 100,000).

Pathophysiology and Etiology

1. The proportion of cases because of a specific organism varies from year to year; there is also considerable geographic difference. The organisms most commonly causing bacterial meningitis in different age groups include:
   a. ≥1 month and <3 months: *Escherichia coli*, *Streptococcus* group B, *Listeria monocytogenes*, *Pseudomonas aeruginosa*, *Staphylococcus* species, *Streptococcus pneumoniae*, *Neisseria meningitidis*, and gram-negative bacilli.
   b. ≥3 months to <3 years: *Streptococcus pneumoniae*, *Neisseria meningitidis* (meningococcal meningitis), and group B *Streptococcus*.
   c. ≥3 years to <10 years: *S. pneumoniae* and *N. meningitidis*.
   d. ≥10 years and <19 years: *N. Meningitidis*.
2. Bacterial meningitis is frequently preceded by an upper respiratory infection, which is complicated by bacteremia. Bacteria in the circulating blood then invade the CSF.
   a. Less commonly, bacterial meningitis may occur as an extension of a local bacterial infection, such as otitis media, mastoiditis, or sinusitis.
   b. Bacteria may also gain direct entry through a penetrating wound, spinal tap, surgery, or anatomic abnormality.
3. The infective process results in inflammation, exudation, and varying degrees of tissue damage in the brain.

Clinical Manifestations

1. Signs and symptoms are variable, depending on the patient's age, the etiologic agent, and the duration of the illness when diagnosed. Onset may be insidious or fulminant.
2. Infants younger than age 2 months usually display irritability, lethargy, vomiting, lack of appetite, temperature instability (fever or hypothermia), respiratory distress, poor tone, tremors, seizures, high-pitched cry, and full (possibly bulging) fontanelle.

3. Infants up to age 2 manifest symptoms similar to those of the young infant and may have a rash, altered sleep patterns, fever, tenseness of the fontanelle, nuchal rigidity, and positive Kernig or Brudzinski signs (see page 380).
4. Children older than age 2 initially have vomiting, headache, fever, mental confusion, lethargy, irritability, and photophobia. Later symptoms include nuchal rigidity within 12 to 24 hours after onset, positive Kernig or Brudzinski sign, seizures, and progressive decline in responsiveness.
5. Petechiae or purpura may develop.
   a. Characteristic skin lesions are most commonly observed in cases of meningococcal or *Pseudomonas* infection.
   b. Hemorrhagic rashes may occur in any child with overwhelming bacterial sepsis because of disseminated intravascular coagulation (DIC).
6. Septic arthritis suggests either meningococcal or *H. influenzae* infection.

Diagnostic Evaluation

1. Diagnosis is usually established through lumbar puncture and examination of CSF.
   a. Cloudy or turbid appearance.
   b. Elevated CSF pressure.
   c. High cell count with mostly polymorphonuclear cells.
   d. Low glucose level.
   e. Elevated protein level (also may be normal).
   f. Positive Gram stain and cultures (identifies the causative organism).
2. Additional laboratory studies include:
   a. Complete blood count (CBC)—total white blood cell count usually increased, with a preponderance of young neutrophils in the differential blood count (known as "shift to the left").
   b. Blood, urine, and nasopharyngeal cultures to look for source of infection.
   c. Platelet count, serum electrolytes, glucose, blood urea nitrogen and creatinine, and urinalysis usually done to monitor critically ill patient as well as clotting function if petechiae or purpuric lesions are noted.

Management

1. IV administration of the appropriate antimicrobial agents to promote rapid destruction of the bacteria and to suppress the emergence of resistant strains. The first dose of antibiotics should be administered as soon as possible (cultures should be taken before an antibiotic is given).
2. Recognition and treatment of hyponatremia caused by syndrome of inappropriate antidiuretic hormone (SIADH).
3. Supportive management of the comatose child or the child with seizures including neuroprotective measures.
4. Appropriate prophylactic treatment provided for contacts when indicated.

Complications

1. Acute—seizures, cerebral edema and increased ICP, shock, ischemia, infected subdural effusion, disseminated illness (septic arthritis, pericarditis), and SIADH.
2. Long term—sensorineural hearing loss, hydrocephalus, blindness, learning disabilities, or developmental delays.
3. Disseminated intravascular coagulation (DIC).

Nursing Assessment

1. Obtain a history from the parents about recent upper respiratory or other infection.
2. Assess LOC and neurologic status.
   a. Evaluate for *Kernig sign*—with the child in the supine position and knees flexed, flex the leg at the hip so the thigh is brought to a position perpendicular to the trunk. Attempt to extend the knee. If meningeal irritation is present, this cannot be done, and attempts to extend the knee result in pain.
   b. Evaluate for *Brudzinski sign*—flex the patient's neck. Spontaneous flexion of the lower extremities indicates meningeal irritation.
3. Monitor breathing pattern and circulatory status.

Nursing Diagnoses

- Ineffective Tissue Perfusion: Cerebral related to endotoxin release into the CSF.
- Hyperthermia related to infectious process.
- Acute Pain related to neurologic effects from the disease process.
- Anxiety related to infection transmission precautions.
- Ineffective Tissue Perfusion: Cerebral related to complications of infectious process.
- Anxiety of parents related to severity of illness and hospitalization.

Nursing Interventions

See Standards of Care Guidelines 46-1, page 1241.

Maintaining Cerebral Tissue Perfusion

1. Administer antimicrobial agents at specified time intervals to obtain optimal serum levels. Obtain blood studies for peak and trough levels, as ordered.
2. Maintain patent IV line for medication administration; observe for signs of infiltration and phlebitis.
3. Monitor closely for signs of complications affecting cerebral perfusion.
   a. Monitor vital signs, LOC, and neurologic status at frequent intervals.
   b. Monitor intake and output, weight, and head circumference daily to assess for hydrocephalus.
   c. Be especially alert for lethargy or subtle changes in condition, which may indicate cerebral edema.
   d. Accurately chart child's behavior and clinical signs.

Reducing Fever

1. Administer antipyretics, tepid sponge baths, and hypothermia blanket, as ordered, to reduce fever. Fever increases metabolic rate and energy requirements by the brain; this may lead to hypoxemia and brain damage in the child with cerebral vascular compromise.
2. Monitor for seizures and use seizure precautions in the febrile child.
   a. There is an increased potential for seizures in the febrile child.
   b. Ensure safety by using padded bed or crib rails and having airway and suction equipment on hand.

Relieving Pain and Irritability

1. Reduce the general noise level around the child and prevent sudden loud noises.
2. Organize nursing care to provide for periods of uninterrupted rest.
3. Keep general handling of the child at a minimum. When necessary, approach the child slowly and gently.

6. Maintain sterile technique for procedures, when indicated.
7. Identify close contacts of the child with meningitis caused by *H. influenzae* or *N. meningitidis* who might benefit from prophylactic treatment.

Avoiding Complications

1. Monitor for and report any of the following:
   a. Decreased respirations, decreased pulse rate, increased systolic BP, pupillary changes, or decreased responsiveness, which may indicate increased ICP.
   b. Decreased urine volume and increased body weight, which may indicate SIADH.
   c. Sudden appearance of a skin rash and bleeding from other sites, which may indicate DIC.
   d. Persistent or recurring fever, bulging fontanelle, signs of increased ICP, focal neurologic signs, seizures, or increased head circumference, which may indicate subdural effusion.
   e. Hearing disturbances and apparent deafness, indicating cranial nerve involvement.
2. Observe for episodes of apnea and initiate measures to stimulate respiration.
   a. Institute respiratory monitoring.
   b. Stimulate the infant when apnea does occur.
      i. Pinch feet and provide more vigorous stimulation, if necessary.
      ii. When spontaneous respiration does not occur within 15 to 20 seconds, provide bag or mask ventilation.
   c. Report any periods of apnea.
   d. Record length of apneic episode and response to stimulation.

Allaying Parental Anxiety

1. Encourage the parents to engage in quiet activities with their child, such as reading or listening to soft music.
2. Provide the parents with an opportunity to express their concerns and answer questions they may have regarding the child's progress and care.
3. Engage the parents in the supportive care of the child so they may feel some control over the situation.

Family Education and Health Maintenance

1. Provide parents with appropriate information if they and other family members are to receive antibiotic prophylaxis.
2. Discuss symptoms for which the parents should watch as signs of possible latent complications, especially hydrocephalus.
3. Give specific instructions about medications to be administered at home.
4. Encourage regular health maintenance visits to chart growth and development and assess for any delays.
5. Parents can obtain more information about meningitis at *http://kidshealth.org/en/parents/meningitis.html*.

Evaluation: Expected Outcomes

- Alert without signs of increased ICP.
- Fever below 101°F (38.3°C); no subsequent infection.
- Resting comfortably; verbalizing reduced pain.
- Child expresses understanding of infection precautions.
- Vital signs stable; breathing pattern regular without apnea.
- Parents participate in child's care and ask questions.

STANDARDS OF CARE GUIDELINES 46-1
Caring for a Child with Neurologic Dysfunction

- Monitor vital signs, level of consciousness, pupillary reaction, and behavior, as indicated, and observe for signs of increased intracranial pressure; report significant changes immediately.
- Make sure that the patient receives all seizure medications and antibiotics, as directed, and that any deviation from dosage schedule or change in therapeutic serum drug levels is reported immediately.
- Assess for adequate elimination: ability for the child to urinate, or caregiver or child to do catheterization. Report deviation from normal pattern and take measures to prevent constipation and stool impaction.
- Assess for signs of secondary infection: postoperative incision infection; shunt malfunction and infection; pneumonia; skin breakdown. Report abnormality in timely fashion.
- Monitor for seizures and maintain safety. Document and report all seizures, including type, time of onset, duration, and behavior afterward. Administer medications, as needed, and as directed.
- Make sure that any assistive devices fit adequately to avoid tissue breakdown. Check more frequently if child is restless.
- Observe and assist with ambulation for safety.
- Train all caregivers in standards of home safety, including cardiopulmonary resuscitation, seizure control, and accident prevention.
- Make sure that the patient and family are aware of all community resources, including respite and support groups, educational assistance, and social services.
- Teach caregivers to do range of motion exercises to prevent contractures. Utilize physical and occupational therapy, as needed.
- Encourage regular health maintenance visits to monitor growth, development, and general health.

This information should serve as a general guideline only. Each patient situation presents a unique set of clinical factors and requires nursing judgment to guide care, which may include additional or alternative measures and approaches.

---

4. Maintain subdued lighting as much as possible.
5. Speak in a low, well-modulated tone of voice.
6. Medicate for pain, as ordered, avoiding opioids that cause CNS and respiratory depression.

Preventing Transmission of Infection without Anxiety

1. Use infection control precautions at all times to prevent transmission of infection.
2. Practice careful hand-washing technique.
3. Explain the use of all protective equipment and procedures to child and family to allay anxiety.
4. Make sure that personnel with colds or other infections avoid contact with infants with meningitis and wear a mask when it is necessary to enter the nursery.
5. Teach parents and other visitors proper hand-washing and gown techniques.

Seizures and Epilepsy

Neonates, infants, and children with epilepsy differ from adults in many ways because of their immature brains: variances are noted in the etiology of seizures, clinical manifestations, responses to antiepileptic medications, and electroencephalogram (EEG) patterns. Although the immature brain is more prone to seizures, as the child grows and develops, some seizures may change and even disappear. In a nationally representative sample of US children, the estimated lifetime prevalence of epilepsy/seizure disorder was 10.2/1,000 (1%) and of current reported epilepsy/seizure disorder was 6.3/1,000. It is estimated that 1% of US children and teens will have at least one afebrile seizure by age 14 years.

Obtaining a thorough history and physical examination is crucial because the diagnosis of epilepsy is primarily based on clinical features.

The terms seizures and epilepsy are often used interchangably. A seizure is a physical minifestation of abnormal, excessive, synchronous neuronal discharges generated primarily from the cerebral cortex. The discharges are intermittent in nature and often self-limited and may last for several seconds to minutes.

Epilepsy is diagnosed when any one of the following exists:

- At least two unprovoked (or reflex) seizures that occur more than 24 hours apart.
- One unprovoked (or reflex) seizure with the likelihood of further seizures with a similar recurrence risk after two unprovoked seizures, occurring over the next 10 years (eg, in cases of remote structural lesions related to CNS infection, stroke, or certain types of traumatic brain injury).

Classification of Epilepsy Syndrome

1. A recent update to the International League Against Epilepsy (ILAE) Classification of the Epilepsies was published in March 2017 along with the revised ILAE 2017 Classification of Seizure Types.
2. This new classification of the epilepsies has three levels of diagnosis: seizure type, epilepsy type, and epilepsy syndrome.
3. The ILAE is aware neonatal seizures may have motor manifestations, and minimal or no behavioral manifestations. A Neonatal Seizure Task Force is currently developing a separate classification of neonatal seizures.

Seizure Type

1. The first step is to rule out another type of paroxysmal event and provide a definitive diagnosis of an epileptic seizure type based on the initial manifestation of the seizure.
2. There are three seizure types:
   a. Focal.
   b. Generalized.
   c. Unknown.

Epilepsy Based on Seizure Type

1. The second level of diagnosis for patients with epilepsy includes four categoires, two are new categories.
   a. Focal.
   b. Generalized.
   c. Combined generalized and focal.
   d. Unknown.

Epilepsy Syndromes

1. An epilepsy syndrome refers to a group of findings that occur together and define a clinically recognizable seizure disorder.
2. This cluster of findings includes certain seizure types, imaging and EEG features along with particular ages of onset, triggers, comorbidities, and prognoses, which may have specific treatment recommendations.
3. A new ILAE educational website EpilepsyDiagnosis.org provides diagnostic guidelines, videos of seizure types, and more relevant information on epilepsy syndromes.
4. Epilepsy syndromes recognized in the neonatal period include:
   a. Benign neonatal seizures.
   b. Benign familial neonatal epilepsy.
   c. Early myoclonic encephalopathy.
   d. Ohtahara syndrome.
5. Epilepsy syndromes of infancy (onset under 2 years) include:
   a. West syndrome.
   b. Dravet syndrome.
   c. Epilepsy of infancy with migrating focal seizures.
   d. Benign infantile epilepsy.
   e. Benign familial infantile epilepsy.
   f. Febrile seizures plus.
6. Epilepsy syndromes of childhood include:
   a. Lennox-Gastaut syndrome.
   b. Landau-Kleffner syndrome.
   c. Epileptic encephalopathy with continuous spike and wave during sleep (CSWS).
   d. Febrile seizures plus (may start in infancy).
   e. Childhood absence epilepsy.
   f. Epilepsy with myoclonic absences.
   g. Late-onset childhood occipital epilepsy (Gastaut type).
   h. Panayiotopoulos syndrome (early childhood onset occipital epilepsy).
   i. Epilepsy with myoclonic atonic (previously astatic) seizures.
   j. Benign epilepsy with centrotemporal spikes.
7. Epilepsy syndromes of adolescence to adulthood include:
   a. Juvenile absence epilepsy (JAE).
   b. Juvenile myoclonic epilepsy (JME).

Infantile Spasms

1. These seizures occur in infants; they are second in incidence only to generalized seizures in this age group.
2. Children with infantile spasms (IS) typically develop epileptic spasms with an associated EEG pattern known as hypsarrhythmia.
3. The triad of spasms, hypsarrhythmia, and developmental regression is known as West syndrome.
4. Peak incidence is in children between ages 3 and 7 months; onset after age 2 years is rare.
5. Clinical signs include the following:
   a. Sudden, forceful, myoclonic contractions involving the musculature of the trunk, neck, and extremities.
      i. Flexor type—infant adducts and flexes the extremities, drops the head, and doubles on him- or herself.
      ii. Extensor type—infant extends neck, spreads out arms, and bends body backward in a position described as "spread eagle."
      iii. Mixed—combination of the above two types, occurring in clusters or volleys of each.
   b. A cry or grunt may accompany severe attacks.
   c. The infant may grimace, laugh, or appear fearful during or after the attack.
6. Duration is momentary (usually <1 minute).
7. Frequency varies from a few attacks per day to hundreds per day.
8. Almost always associated with cerebral abnormalities. Mental retardation usually accompanies this disorder in 95% of cases.

9. Usually, this type of seizure disappears spontaneously by the time the child reaches age 4 years. Subsequent generalized or other types of seizures usually develop.

 NURSING ALERT Occurrence of infantile spasms is a pediatric emergency. Delay in treatment could lead to permanent cognitive impairment and developmental delay.

Pathophysiology and Etiology

Etiologic Factors

1. *Structural etiology* refers to abnormalities seen on structural neuroimaging where the imaging along with the electroclinical findings indicates the abnormality is the probable cause of the seizures, such as hippocampal sclerosis. Structural abnormalities can be congenital such as tuberous sclerosis and cortical dysplasia or acquired by hypoxic–ischemic encephalopathy, infection, stroke, trauma, tumors, neurosurgery, and genetic cortical malformations.
2. *Genetic etiology* refers to a pathogenic genetic variant (mutation) of significant effect that causes epilepsy. A large number of epilepsy gene mutations have been identified in both severe and mild epilepsies, many being de novo mutations. Examples of genetic etiologies in children include SCN1A mutations associated with Dravet syndrome and genetic/generalized epilepsy with febrile seizures plus (GEFS+) and mutations in the potassium channel genes KCNQ2 and KCNQ3 (benign familial neonatal epilepsy).
3. *Infectious etiology* refers to epilepsy resulting from a known infection including tuberculosis, cerebral malaria, HIV, neurocysticercosis, congenital infections (Zika virus, cytomegalovirus), cerebral toxoplasmosis, and subacute sclerosing panencephalitis (SSPE). Epilepsy, which develops after an acute infectious illness, may also fall in this category.
4. *Metabolic etiology* refers to epilepsy, which directly results from a presumed or known metabolic disorder, in which seizures are a main symptom. Often, metabolic disorders and epilepsies will be related to a genetic mutation, but some might be acquired. An example in children is pyridoxine deficiency.
5. *Immune etiology* refers to epilepsy, which directly results from a presumed or known immune disorder, in which seizures are a main symptom and where autoimmune-mediated central nervous system inflammation is noted. An example of this is anti-NMDA receptor encephalitis.
6. *Unknown etiology* refers to epilepsy in which the cause is not yet determined.

Altered Physiology

1. The basic mechanism for all seizures appears to be prolonged depolarization and other chemical changes, causing neurons to discharge in an uncontrolled manner.
2. This paroxysmal burst of electrical energy spreads to adjacent areas of the brain or may jump to distant areas of the CNS, resulting in a seizure.
3. Some seizures appear to occur under the influence of a triggering factor.
   a. Hormonal factors, such as those related to the menstrual period, menarche, and menopause.

b. Nonsensory factors, such as hyperthermia; hyperventilation; metabolic disorders such as hypoglycemia, hyponatremia, and hypocalcemia; sleep deprivation; emotional disturbances; and physical stress.
c. Sensory factors, such as those related to vision, hearing, touch, the startle reaction, and those that are self-induced.

Clinical Manifestation Based on the ILAE 2017 Classification of Seizure Types

Focal Onset Seizures

1. Focal onset seizures originate in networks limited to one hemisphere and include focal aware and focal impaired awareness seizures.
   a. Focal aware seizures were formerly known as simple partial seizures.
      i. No impairment of consciousness; retains awareness of self and environment even if immobile.
      ii. Caused by abnormal activation of a limited number of neurons that allow for localization of the epileptic focus.
   b. Focal impaired awareness seizures
      i. Includes all seizures with impaired consciousness during any portion of the event.
      ii. Formerly known as complex partial seizures.
2. Focal seizures are also subgrouped into those with motor or nonmotor signs and symptoms at the onset and can be further classified by the earliest prominent motor-onset or non–motor-onset characteristic:
   a. Motor Onset seizures
      i. Automatisms—mouth movements (ie, chewing, lip smacking), hand movements (ie, picking at clothing, "pill rolling," grasping at objects), rubbing genitalia, eye blinking, head turning, and raising of arms.
      ii. Atonic—loss of tone (degree of awareness usually not specified).
      iii. Clonic—jerking of limbs, often asymmetric and irregular.
      iv. Epileptic spasms—spasms of muscles of the neck, trunk, and extremities (degree of awareness usually not specified).
      v. Hyperkinetic.
      vi. Myoclonic—brief synchronous jerks of one or more muscle groups.
      vii. Tonic—sustained muscle contraction with no clonic phase.
   b. Nonmotor Onset
      i. Autonomic—changes in skin color, BP, heart rate, pupil size, piloerection, drooling, rising epigastric sensation, retching, and vomiting.
      ii. Behavioral arrest.
      iii. Emotional—fear, depression, anger, and irritability.
      iv. Sensory—tingling or numbness, simple visual phenomenon, hallucinations (visual, auditory, gustatory, olfactory), illusions of perception (size [macro- or micropsia], shape, weight, distance, sound), dysphasia, or aphasia.
3. Focal to Bilateral Tonic–Clonic Seizure:
   a. Formerly known as partial-onset seizure with secondary generalization.
   b. A special seizure type, which indicates a propagation pattern of a seizure.

Generalized Onset Seizures

1. Generalized onset seizures are characterized by global synchronized activation of neurons resulting in impaired consciousness, bilateral motor changes, and EEG abnormalities.
    a. Motor
        i. Tonic–clonic—consists of tonic phase (10 to 30 seconds), clonic phase (30 to 60 seconds), and postictal phase (2 to 30 minutes); postictal phase consists of confusion and fatigue.
        ii. Clonic—jerking that is often asymmetric and irregular; occurs more frequently in neonates, infants, and young children.
        iii. Tonic—sustained muscle contractions with no clonic phase, can occur at any age, frequently seen in children with diffuse cerebral damage and Lennox-Gastaut syndrome.
        iv. Myoclonic—brief involuntary muscle contractions of one or several muscle groups; may be triggered by action, noise, percussion, being startled, or photic stimulation; may occur alone or in clusters.
        v. Myoclonic–tonic–clonic—combination of three seizure manifestations.
        vi. Myoclonic–atonic—brief involuntary muscle contractions of one or several muscle groups and then sudden loss of tone.
        vii. Atonic—sudden loss of tone.
        viii. Epileptic spasms—involve spasms of muscles of the neck, trunk, and extremities.
    b. Nonmotor (Absence)
        i. Typical—abrupt onset of activity arrest, brief loss of consciousness, may have eye flickering, lasts 10 seconds, easily provoked by hyperventilation or photic stimulation, no postictal phase with resumption of normal activity, may occur in clusters.
        ii. Atypical—frequently associated with symptomatic epilepsies and mixed seizure disorders, may have aura or automatisms; partial impairment of consciousness, may last several minutes; postictal headache, confusion, and emotional disturbances are common.
        iii. Myoclonic—brief involuntary muscle contractions of one or several muscle groups; may be triggered by action, noise, percussion, being startled, or photic stimulation.
        iv. Eyelid myoclonia.

Unknown Onset and Unclassified Seizures

1. Unknown onset seizures are those in which there is an absence of knowledge of the seizure's onset, but it can be provisionally classified based on key characteristics.
    a. Motor
        i. Tonic–clonic—consists of tonic phase (10 to 30 seconds), clonic phase (30 to 60 seconds), and postictal phase (2 to 30 minutes); postictal phase consists of confusion and fatigue.
        ii. Epileptic spasms—involve spasms of muscles of the neck, trunk, and extremities.
    b. Nonmotor
        i. Behavioral arrest—abrupt onset of activity arrest.
2. Unclassified—this category is for seizures for which there is a lack of or inadequate information or if the seizure cannot be placed in other categories because of its unusual presentation.

Status Epilepticus

1. A prolonged seizure or repeated seizures lasting longer than 30 minutes with no interictal recovery.

2. Most common pediatric neurologic emergency, possibly resulting in permanent neurologic sequelae.
3. May be overt seizure activity (convulsive) or subclinical (nonconvulsive).
4. Generalized tonic–clonic status epilepticus is life-threatening.
5. Causes include new acute illness, progressive neurologic disease, loss of seizure control in an epileptic, or a febrile seizure in a child who is otherwise in good health.
6. Recurrence occurs more often in children who have other neurologic abnormalities; recurrence is rare in children who experience febrile seizures.
7. Absence and complex partial status epilepticus are often difficult to identify, and children often appear to be in a mildly confused state.

Psychogenic Nonepileptic Seizures

1. Previously known as "hysterical" or "pseudoseizures" and are usually a method of seeking attention and secondary gain.
2. Occur most frequently in adolescents and more often in girls than boys (3:1).
3. History of sexual abuse is common in women with nonepileptic seizures.
4. May occur in people with true seizures that have come under control.
5. Difficult to distinguish by observation alone.
6. Most episodes of psychogenic nonepileptic seizures (PNES) occur in front of witnesses and tend not to occur during sleep.
7. Forced eye closure suggests PNES as eyes are usually open during the ictus of an epileptic seizure.
8. Often include three broad patterns:
    a. Unilateral or bilateral motor activity that may include tonic posturing or tremulousness—movements are thrashing or jerking, rather than tonic–clonic, and often different movements occur simultaneously.
    b. Behavioral or emotional changes—distress or discomfort, followed by semipurposeless—but not stereotyped—behaviors and may include walking or fumbling with objects.
    c. Periods of unresponsiveness with precipitation or cessation of the attack occurring after suggestion—no self-harm occurs, with no associated incontinence during these episodes.

Diagnostic Evaluation

Electroencephalogram

1. Used to confirm the clinical diagnosis, classify type of epilepsy, localize the area of epileptic focus, and determine when it is safe to discontinue treatment.
2. A normal EEG does not preclude the diagnosis of epilepsy. Indeed, about 10% to 20% of children who have epilepsy have a normal EEG.

Brain Imaging

1. CT scan and MRI—provide an anatomic picture of the brain; essential in ruling out the presence of a lesion. MRI is the gold standard in evaluation of epilepsy, although CT scan is used when MRI is not available.
2. Single-photon emission computed tomography (CT), positron emission tomography (PET), and functional MRI (fMRI)—brain imaging techniques that measure local vascular or metabolic changes associated with neuronal activity; they can also map cortical function when resective surgery is being planned.
3. Magnetoencephalography (MEG)—noninvasive technology that helps map the sensory and language cortex when resective surgery is being planned.

Neuropsychological Evaluation

1. Used to evaluate the specific learning needs of children with epilepsy because many have learning difficulties.
2. Part of the presurgical workup is to determine cognitive deficits and predict long-term consequences of epilepsy, particularly when surgery is performed in an eloquent area.
3. WADA testing (named after its inventor, Juhn Wada) evaluates hemisphere dominance for language and memory when resective surgery is being planned.
   a. Involves the intracarotid administration of amobarbital to anesthetize each hemisphere of the brain separately.
   b. The patient is then shown objects to name and recall over a short period of time.
   c. Some facilities now use alternative anesthetic agents such as etomidate as amobarbital has not been readily available (ie, "eSAM"—etomidate speech and memory test).

Laboratory Studies

1. Serum electrolytes, magnesium, calcium, and fasting blood sugar to rule out metabolic causes.
2. Toxicology screen—drug overdoses may cause seizures.
3. Blood cultures—fever and CNS infections may cause seizures.
4. Lumbar puncture may be done if fever is present.
5. Serum levels of seizure medications should follow therapy.
6. Metabolic workup in infants or children with developmental delay.
7. Genetic testing to determine underlying epilepsy syndrome.

Management

Pharmacologic Management

1. Selection of the most effective drug depends on correct identification of the clinical seizure type (see Table 46-2).
2. A desirable drug level is one that will prevent seizures without producing undesirable adverse effects.

Table 46-2 Drugs Used to Treat Seizures in Children

DRUGS AND DOSAGE	ADVANTAGES	ADVERSE EFFECTS	NURSING CONSIDERATIONS
Phenobarbital			
Maintenance dosage: 3 to 5 mg/kg given qid or bid *Status epilepticus:* 10 to 20 mg/kg, may repeat to maximum 40 mg/kg	Relatively safe and inexpensive	Excitement, hyperactivity, rash, GI distress, dizziness, ataxia, worsening of psychomotor seizures, drowsiness; toxicity causing respiratory depression, circulatory collapse, and renal impairment	• Contraindicated in hepatic or renal dysfunction, hypersensitivity • IM or IV loading dose can be given • IV rate should not exceed 1 mg/kg/min
Phenytoin			
Loading dose: 20 mg/kg *Maintenance:* 3 to 9 mg/kg given qid or bid	Safest drug for psychomotor seizures; does not cause drowsiness	Hypertrophy of gums, hirsutism, rickets, nystagmus, ataxia, rash; may accentuate absence seizures; toxicity may cause blood dyscrasias and liver damage	• May interact with a wide variety of drugs because of extensive protein binding • Daily gum massage may prevent gum disease • Avoid IM administration • If given IV, do not exceed rate of 0.5 mg/kg/min • Dilute with normal saline to prevent formation of precipitant
Ethosuximide			
Maintenance: 20 to 40 mg/kg given qid by oral route only	Used for absence seizures	Drowsiness, GI distress, lethargy, euphoria; may aggravate generalized seizures; toxicity causes blood dyscrasias and psychiatric symptoms	• This is contraindicated in hepatic or renal disease • Dosage should not be increased more frequently than every 4 to 7 days
Primidone			
Children younger than age 8 years: 10 to 25 mg/kg given tid *Children older than age 8 years:* 750 to 1,500 mg tid or qid by oral route only	May control generalized seizures not responsive to treatment by other drugs	Ataxia, vertigo, GI symptoms; megaloblastic anemia is a rare idiosyncratic reaction; drowsiness in breastfed infants of treated mothers; Stevens-Johnson syndrome, gum hypertrophy, night terrors	• Contraindicated in those hypersensitive to phenobarbital and those with porphyria • Commonly used with other drugs for mixed seizure • Dosage increases are usually done weekly until effect is seen
Diazepam			
IV dosage: 0.04 to 0.2 mg/kg to maximum of 10 mg if age 5 years or older; maximum of 5 mg if younger than age 5 years *Rectal dosage:* 0.5 mg/kg	Given IV, IM, or rectally for status epilepticus or as adjunct therapy	Ataxia, drowsiness, fatigue, venous thrombosis or phlebitis at injection site, confusion, depression, headache; tonic status epilepticus when given IV for absence seizures; toxicity may cause somnolence, confusion, diminished reflexes, hypotension, coma, apnea, cardiac arrest	• If administered IV, give no faster than 1 mg/min. Drug used cautiously in children with limited pulmonary reserve • Monitor respiratory status closely

(continued)

Table 46-2   Drugs Used to Treat Seizures in Children (*Continued*)

DRUGS AND DOSAGE	ADVANTAGES	ADVERSE EFFECTS	NURSING CONSIDERATIONS
Carbamazepine 20 to 30 mg/kg tid or qid *Maximum dose:* 1,000 mg/day if older than age 12 years; 100 mg bid if ages 6 to 12 years; 20 mg/kg/day if younger than age 6 years	Especially useful for major motor and psychomotor seizures	Most likely to occur during initiation of therapy: dizziness, drowsiness, nausea, and vomiting; toxicity may cause bone marrow depression (fever, sore throat, oral ulcers, easy bruising)	• Administration with phenytoin reduces half-life of phenytoin; higher dose of phenytoin may be needed • Contraindicated in previous bone marrow depression and is used cautiously in patients with cardiac, hepatic, or renal problems • Erythromycin increases plasma levels • Give with food
Lorazepam 0.05 to 0.1 mg/kg q 10 to 15 minutes *Maximum dose:* 4 mg	Given IV or rectally for status epilepticus; longer acting; may cause less respiratory depression	Sedation, dizziness, respiratory depression, hypotension, ataxia, weakness	• Use with caution in patients with hepatic or renal dysfunction • Monitor respiratory status closely
Valproic Acid *Loading dose:* 10 mg/kg/day *Maximum dose:* 30 to 60 mg/kg tid or qid	Adjunct for poor seizure control; some success with behavioral problems	Nausea, vomiting, anorexia, amenorrhea, sedation tremor, weight gain, alopecia, hepatotoxicity	• Use caution with hepatic dysfunction. Increases serum levels of phenytoin, phenobarbital, and primidone
Gabapentin *Loading dose:* 10 to 15 mg/kg/day in three divided doses *Maximum dose:* 25 to 40 mg/kg/day in three divided doses	Recommended for add-on therapy in children over age 3 with refractory partial seizures	May interfere with the action of other drugs, including cimetidine; nausea/dizziness	• Must exercise caution in patients with renal impairment
Topiramate *Loading dose:* 25 mg/day at bedtime for the first week *Maximum dose:* 200 to 400 mg/day in two divided doses	Recommended for patients aged 2 to 16 with partial-onset seizures and those seizures related to Lennox-Gastaut syndrome	Most commonly associated with fatigue, dizziness, sleepiness	• Must exercise caution in patients with renal impairment • Interacts with other anticonvulsants, altering drug concentrations; may interfere with effectiveness of hormonal contraceptives
Oxcarbazepine *Loading dose:* 8 to 10 mg/kg/day in two divided doses *Maximum dose:* children 2 to <4 years—60 mg/kg/day; children 4 to 16 years—900 to 1,800 mg/day based on weight	Adjunctive therapy in children aged 4 to 16 years for partial seizures	Fatigue, abnormal gait, sedation, difficulty in concentration, and memory impairment	• Need to monitor serum sodium • May interfere with other anticonvulsants by increasing serum concentration; decreases the effectiveness of hormonal contraceptives
Zonisamide *Loading dose:* 2 to 4 mg/kg/day *Maximum dose:* 12 mg/kg/day in two to three divided doses	Adjunctive therapy in children older than age 16; especially effective in refractive seizures, such as absence, Lennox-Gastaut syndrome, or infantile spasms	Drowsiness, ataxia, loss of appetite, GI upset, and slowing of mental activity, psychiatric symptoms (ie, depression, psychosis)	• Must exercise caution in patients with renal and/or hepatic impairment, and patients with sensitivity to sulfonamides • Pediatric patients may be at increased risk and may have more severe metabolic acidosis

Table 46-2 Drugs Used to Treat Seizures in Children (*Continued*)

DRUGS AND DOSAGE	ADVANTAGES	ADVERSE EFFECTS	NURSING CONSIDERATIONS
Lacosamide *Adolescents ≥17 years*, monotherapy initial dose 100 mg bid, adjunctive therapy initial dose: 50 mg bid; maintenance dose: 200 to 400 mg/day *Children and adolescents under <17 years*: 1 to 2 mg/kg/day divided bid, may titrate to 1 mg/kg/day weekly to effect	Adjunctive therapy in the treatment of partial-onset seizures and severe refractory seizures in children <17 years	Dizziness, ataxia, light-headedness, excessive drowsiness, headaches, nausea, vomiting, tremors, change in vision or multiorgan sensitivity reactions Report signs of suicide ideation or depression	• Carbamazepine, fosphenytoin, phenobarbital, and phenytoin may decrease lacosamide serum concentration • May prolong PR interval (patients with conduction problems or severe cardiac disease should have ECG tracing prior to/during treatment)
Clobazam Lennox-Gastaut (adjunctive), US labeling: *Children ≥2 years*: refer to adult dosing Epilepsy (monotherapy or adjunctive), oral: *children <2 years, initial dose*: 0.5 to 1 mg/kg/day; *Children 2 to 16 years, initial dose*: 5 mg/day; *maximum*: 40 mg/day	Adjunctive treatment of seizures associated with Lennox-Gastaut syndrome (FDA-approved in ages ≥2 years and adults); has also been used as monotherapy and adjunctive treatment for other forms of epilepsy	Somnolence, fever, lethargy, upper respiratory tract infection, GI issues, muscle weakness, paradoxical reactions including hyperactive or aggressive behavior, anterograde amnesia, suicidal ideation **US Boxed Warning: Risks from concomitant use of benzodiazepines and opioids**	• May be administered with or without food • Tablets can be crushed and mixed in applesauce • Tolerance and loss of seizure control have been reported with chronic administration • Rebound or withdrawal symptoms may occur following abrupt discontinuation or large decreases in dose • Use caution, adjust dose in patients with hepatic impairment, respiratory disease, and pre-existing muscle weakness (Canadian labeling contraindicates use in myasthenia gravis)
Rufinamide, Oral Lennox-Gastaut syndrome: *Children ≥4 years, initial dose*: 10 mg/kg/day in two equally divided doses; *target dose*: 45 mg/kg/day; *maximum dose*: 3,200 mg/day)	Adjunctive therapy of seizures associated with Lennox-Gastaut syndrome (FDA-approved in ages ≥4 years and adults)	Cardiovascular: QT shortening (46% to 65%; may be dose-related), headache, somnolence, dizziness, fatigue, aggression, anxiety, ataxia/gait disturbance, vertigo, tremor, attention disturbance, back pain, hyperactivity, seizures, status epilepticus, suicidal thinking, pruritus, rash, frequent urination, anemia, leucopenia; visual, respiratory or GI disturbances	• Contraindicated in patients with familial short QT syndrome • Administer with food • Monitor for signs and symptoms of anxiety, depression, unusual mood or behavior changes, suicide ideation
Vigabatrin FDA approved in ages ≥ 10 years and adults: *Children, oral, initial dose*: 40 mg/kg/day in two divided doses, maintenance dosages based on patient weight Infantile spasms: *FDA approved in children 1 month to 2 years, initial dose*: 50 mg/kg/day in two divided doses; *maximum dose*: 150 mg/kg/day	Treatment of infantile spasms; adjunct therapy for refractory complex partial seizures in patients with inadequate response to several alternative treatments and for whom the potential benefits outweigh the potential risk of vision loss	Anemia, somnolence, headache, fatigue, irritability, sedation, nystagmus, tremor, insomnia, GI issues, weight gain, edema, peripheral neuropathy, neurotoxicity, suicidal ideation, vision loss, abnormal MRI changes have been reported in some infants **US Boxed Warning: Permanent Vision Loss** Only available in the United States under the Sabril REMS Program	• May be administered without regard to meals • Assess vision prior to initiating therapy or within 4 weeks from start, at least every 3 months during therapy and at 3 to 6 months after therapy has been discontinued • Assess for CNS depression, changes in behavior, and suicidal tendencies

(continued)

Table 46-2   Drugs Used to Treat Seizures in Children (Continued)

DRUGS AND DOSAGE	ADVANTAGES	ADVERSE EFFECTS	NURSING CONSIDERATIONS
Levetiracetam Partial-onset seizures: *Children 1 to <6 months, initial dose: 7 mg/kg bid; maximum dose: 21 mg/kg bid* *Children 6 months to <4 years, initial dose: 10 mg/kg bid; maximum dose: 25 mg/kg bid* *Children 4 to <16 years, initial dose: 10 mg/kg/day bid; maximum dose: 30 mg/kg/day bid (maximum daily dose: 3,000 mg/day)* Tonic–clonic seizures: *Children 6 to <16 years, initial dose: 10 mg/kg bid; recommended dose: 30 mg/kg twice daily.*	Adjunctive therapy in the treatment of partial-onset, myoclonic, and/or primary generalized tonic–clonic seizures	Behavioral/psychiatric symptoms, agitation, amnesia, anxiety, somnolence, fatigue, anorexia and other GI symptoms, ataxia and coordination problems, hypertension	• Be aware of neuropsychiatric adverse events as incidence of behavioral abnormalities and psychiatric symptoms may be increased in children • Use with caution and decrease dose in patients with renal dysfunction • May be administered without regard to meals
Stiripentol *Children ≥3 years and adults,* in conjunction with clobazam and valproic acid: *increased over 3 days to a final dose of 50 mg/kg/day in 2 to 3 divided doses with food*	Treatment of refractory generalized tonic–clonic seizures in conjunction with clobazam and valproic acid in patients with severe myoclonic epilepsy in infancy (Dravet syndrome) whose seizures are not adequately controlled with clobazam and valproic acid alone	Clobazam concentrations have increased 2- to 3-fold when given with stiripentol; a clobazam dosage reduction of 25% per week may be required in the presence of clobazam toxicity (drowsiness, hypotonia, and irritability)	• Product available in various countries; not currently available in the United States • Should be given with food, excluding fruit juice, dairy, or caffeinated or carbonated products
Perampanel *Children ≥ 12 years and adolescents—with no enzyme inducing AED's:* initial dose 2 mg HS, increase by 2 mg/week to recommended dose 8 to 12 mg; *with enzyme-inducing AEDs:* initial dose 4 mg HS, increase by 2 mg/week to 8 to 12 mg HS	Adjunctive therapy in treatment of partial-onset seizures with or without secondarily generalized seizures	Headache, nausea, vomiting, abdominal pain, fatigue, loss of strength and energy, back pain or weight gain, dizziness, passing out, change in balance or abnormal gait **US Boxed Warning: Serious psychiatric and behavioral reactions** such as depression, suicidal ideation, illogical thinking, aggression, anger, hostility, homicidal ideation	• Not recommended (not studied) in cases of severe renal and hepatic impairment; with mild to moderate renal and hepatic impairment, use caution and lower doses with slower titration • To be administered once daily at HS
Midazolam *Infants 1 to 5 months:* 0.2 mg/kg single dose; *infants ≥ 6 months, children and adolescents:* 0.2 to 0.3 mg/kg, maximum single dose 10 mg (intranasal dosing parameters)	For acute treatment of prolonged seizures	Antegrade amnesia, potential respiratory depression, and respiratory arrest if used with other CNS depressants; hypotension, CNS depression, paradoxical reactions such as agitation hyperactive or aggressive behavior **US Boxed Warning: Respiratory depression; IV dosing; neonates (injection); risk from concomitant use with opioids**	• Use a MAD nasal drug delivery device to administer intranasal • Maximum 1 mL per nostril (0.5 mL for infants < 1 year old) • Vial can be stored in cool, dry area at room temperature; an open vial can be stored up to 28 days and then must be discarded • Use with caution in children with cardiac, lung, hepatic, or renal impairment

bid, twice a day; CNS, central nervous system; ECG, electrocardiogram; FDA, Food and Drug Administration; GI, gastrointestinal; IM, intramuscular; IV, intravenous; qid, four times a day; tid, three times a day.

3. Dosages are adjusted according to blood level, clinical signs, and the child's weight.
4. Accurate timing is essential to prevent seizures. This is especially true when the child tends to have seizures at a certain time each day.
5. Enteric-coated tablets, which have a delayed effect, should be used for children who are prone to attacks during sleep.
6. Most anticonvulsants are available in liquid form and in capsules or tablets. Some drugs are less well absorbed in liquid form.
7. It may take several months to find the best combination of medications and the best dosages of each to control the child's seizures. Monotherapy is attempted initially. If this is not successful, a second drug may be tried or added on.
8. Symptoms may not be controlled 100% in every patient.
9. Dosage adjustments may be required from time to time because of the child's growth and clinical progress.
10. Blood counts, urinalysis, therapeutic drug levels, and liver function studies are done at regular intervals in children receiving certain anticonvulsants.
11. Medication is commonly not discontinued until 2 to 3 years after the last seizure and if the EEG is normal.
12. Weaning from medication should always be gradual, with stepwise reduction of dosage and withdrawal of one drug at a time.
13. There is some evidence to suggest that long-term use of some antiepileptic agents may cause intellectual impairment in children with epilepsy.
14. Monitor bone health and provide calcium supplementation if inadequate calcium intake.

Surgical Management
1. If a cerebral lesion, such as a tumor, is found, surgical removal is the treatment of choice.
2. Surgical treatment, such as hemispherectomy, resection of localized seizure focus/epileptogenic zone, or corpus callosotomy, may be performed in children with severe, medically intractable seizure disorders.

Ketogenic Diet Therapy
1. The ketogenic diet is a high-fat, adequate protein, and low-carbohydrate diet is used for control of seizures refractory to medications. The diet consists of precisely calculated portions of protein, fat, and carbohydrates. The diet causes the child to become ketotic because fats are used for fuel rather than carbohydrates. It is thought that ketones may inhibit seizures, although the mechanism of action is not known.
2. There are several ketogenic diet types: classic, medium-chain triglyceride, modified Atkins, and the low glycemic index diet.
3. Children on this diet should not be given IV fluids with dextrose.
4. All medications should be in sugar-free and carbohydrate-free suspensions, tablets, or capsules.
5. The child will be on strict fluid restriction.
6. This diet must be carefully monitored by a dietitian. Ongoing surveillance monitors the child's growth and nutritional status as well as other parameters including kidney functions and lipid and micronutrient levels.
7. There is some evidence that this diet may put the child at increased risk for developing kidney stones. The risk may be increased when the child receives concomitant therapy with topiramate. Renal and abdominal ultrasounds are done periodically to monitor for stones.
8. Periodic electrocardiograms are performed to monitor for heart rhythm abnormalities.
9. Another form of the ketogenic diet is the medium-chain triglyceride (MCT) diet. The MCT diet allows for consumption of more carbohydrates than the classic ketogenic diet, reducing the side effects of vomiting and lack of energy.
10. Valproic acid must be weaned off prior to commencing treatment with the MCT ketogenic diet to prevent hepatic toxicity.

 EVIDENCE BASE Cai, Q., Zhou, Z., Luo, R., et al. (2017). Safety and tolerability of the ketogenic diet used for the treatment of refractory childhood epilepsy: A systematic review of published prospective studies. *World Journal of Pediatrics, 13*(6), 528–536.

Modified Atkins Diet
1. Emerging as another form of diet therapy for seizure control.
2. Carbohydrates are restricted to 10 to 20 g per day, with no restriction of protein, fluid, or calories.
3. Hospital admission is not required to initiate the diet. The diet is often self-administered.

Vagal Nerve Stimulation
The vagal nerve stimulator is a pacemaker-like device that is surgically implanted into the chest and attached to coiled electrodes, which are tunneled to the left cervical vagus nerve. The generator emits a programmed stimulus to stop seizures of long duration (usually 1 minute or longer), and children/families may activate the generator to allow for additional stimulus at times of seizure activity. Vagal nerve stimulation is an adjunctive treatment for intractable epilepsy—although the mechanism of action is unknown, studies have shown that VNS therapy reduces seizure frequency and is well tolerated.

 EVIDENCE BASE Vaiman, M., Heyman, E., & Lotan, G. (2017). Neurological results of the modified treatment of epilepsy by stimulation of the vagus nerve. *Child's Nervous System, 33*(11), 2017–2022.

Behavioral Management
1. Psychiatric disorders, especially attention deficit hyperactivity disorder, depression, and anxiety, are common in children and adolescents who have epilepsy. They are more prevalent in this population than in children and adolescents in the general population or children who have other chronic conditions. Psychosis occurs infrequently.
2. It is important to monitor children with epilepsy for these disorders to ensure early recognition and treatment to minimize lifelong negative sequelae.
3. Further studies are needed to identify the most effective treatments.

General Prognosis
1. General prognosis depends on type and severity of seizure disorder, coexisting mental retardation, organic disorders, and the type of medical management.
2. Medically treated seizures—spontaneous cessation of seizures may occur. Drugs may be gradually discontinued when the child has been free from seizures for an extensive period and the EEG pattern has reverted to normal.
3. Untreated epilepsy—seizures tend to become more numerous.

Complications

1. Apnea/hypoventilation.
2. Hypoglycemia in status epilepticus.
3. Injuries sustained during a seizure.
4. Sudden unexpected death in epilepsy (SUDEP).
5. Osteopenia—because of restrictions in physical activity as a result of seizures or other conditions, such as CP, or treatment with antiepileptic medications, such as valproic acid and carbamazepine.

Nursing Assessment

1. During a seizure, assess the following:
   a. Indications of difficulties with airway or breathing.
   b. Significant preseizure events, such as noise, excitement, and lethargy.
   c. Behavior before the seizure, aura.
   d. Types of movements observed.
   e. Time seizure began and ended.
   f. Site where twitching or contraction began.
   g. Areas of the body involved.
   h. Movements of the eyes and changes in pupil size.
   i. Incontinence.
   j. Color change—pallor, cyanosis, and flushing.
   k. Mouth—teeth clenched, abnormal movements, and tongue bitten.
   l. Degree of consciousness during the seizure.
2. After a seizure, assess the following:
   a. Degree of memory for recent events.
   b. Types of speech.
   c. Coordination, paralysis, or weakness.
   d. Length of time the child is postictal.
   e. Pupillary reaction.

NURSING ALERT A devastating phenomenon of epilepsy is sudden unexpected death in epilepsy (SUDEP). The American Academy of Neurology and the American Epilepsy Society have created a practice guideline that directs clinicians to incorporate the following in their discussions:

- The incidence in children is 1 in 4,500 annually.
- For those children who have active generalized tonic–clonic seizures, they are strongly encouraged to pursue therapies to manage their epilepsy while incorporating individual treatment preferences in the context of a risk/benefit approach.
- Inform patients and families that freedom from generalized tonic–clonic seizures greatly decreases the risk of SUDEP.

Nursing Diagnoses

- Risk for Injury related to seizure activity.
- Ineffective Breathing Pattern related to spasms of respiratory musculature.
- Social Isolation related to the child's feelings about seizures or public fears and misconceptions.
- Chronic Low Self-Esteem related to lack of control over seizures.

Nursing Interventions

Ensuring Safety during a Seizure

1. Remove hard toys from the bed.
2. Pad the sides of the crib or side rails of the bed.

3. Assess level of consciousness.
4. Make sure the child can be readily observed.
5. During a seizure, monitor vital signs and assess neurologic status frequently.
6. After a seizure, check the child frequently and report the following:
   a. Behavior changes.
   b. Irritability.
   c. Restlessness.
   d. Listlessness.
   e. Neurologic signs.

Preventing Respiratory Arrest and Aspiration

1. During a seizure, take the following emergency actions:
   a. Clear the area around the child.
   b. Do not restrain the child.
   c. Loosen the clothing around the neck.
   d. Turn the child on side so saliva can flow out of the mouth.
   e. Place a small, folded blanket under the head to prevent trauma if the seizure occurs when the child is on the floor.
2. Do not give anything by mouth or attempt to place anything in the mouth.
3. After the seizure, place the child in a side-lying position.

Promoting Socialization

1. Advise the parents that the child should be in an environment that is as normal as possible.
2. Encourage regular attendance at school after the school nurse and teachers have been notified and emergency treatment of seizures is understood.
3. Encourage the child to participate in organizations and outside activities with limited restrictions.
   a. Each child must be treated individually; the kind of activity depends on the degree of seizure control.
   b. Generally, children with seizure disorders should not be allowed to climb in high places or to swim alone.
   c. Responsible adults should be made aware of the child's disorder.
   d. Children with seizures should wear a MedicAlert bracelet at all times.

Strengthening Self-Esteem

1. Offer reassurance and praise to the parents and child for coping effectively with seizures.
2. Observe parent–child interactions for evidence of rejection or overprotection.
   a. Tell the parents that the child should not be made to feel that he or she can never be left alone.
   b. Advise the parents that the child needs to be disciplined as any other child and should not gain attention directly or indirectly by having seizures.
3. Help the child gain more control by providing education about seizure disorders.
   a. Include the child in treatment planning.
   b. Allow the opportunity to ask questions and answer them honestly.
   c. Make sure the child is aware of restrictions and can deal with them.
   d. Encourage parents gradually to give the child responsibility for taking medications.
4. Help the older child or adolescent to achieve independence.
   a. Encourage the parents to give the older child the opportunity for privacy to discuss concerns with the physician.

b. Encourage parents to allow the older child to use his or her own judgment in making decisions.

c. Help the older child to develop realistic educational and career goals.

5. Help parents deal with a noncompliant child. Refusal to take medications requires prompt intervention. Children need to be reassured that they are not abnormal, but that they do require medication to control seizures. Children need to be taught that they are normal and can have normal lives. This is most commonly seen during adolescence. Family counseling may be necessary.

6. Teach the parents and child seizure safety.

Community and Home Care Considerations

1. Follow community and home care considerations listed under "Cerebral Palsy" on page 1229.

2. Make sure that the home environment is safe, especially where the child sleeps and plays. Remove toys with sharp edges or parts or small pieces the child could choke on if they are put in the mouth, and cover very hard surfaces, such as the floor, against which the child could fall.

3. Reinforce parents' knowledge and ability to dispense seizure medications.

4. Help the family acquire a medical alert tag that the child should wear at all times, especially when attending daycare or school.

5. Make sure that parents and caregivers know the seizure type, name of all medications, when to call the health care provider, and when to call 911.

a. The health care provider should be notified of an increased frequency of seizures or new onset of symptoms.

b. Emergency response should be activated when the child has been seizing for longer than 5 minutes or is unresponsive after a seizure.

6. Make sure that parents and caregivers are trained in CPR and seizure management.

Family Education and Health Maintenance

1. Describe completely any examinations, evaluations, and treatments that the child is receiving.

2. Provide information regarding the disorder itself.

a. Epilepsy is not contagious, is seldom dangerous, and does not indicate insanity or mental retardation.

b. Most children with epilepsy have infrequent seizures and with medications can completely control their convulsions.

c. The child may have normal intelligence and can live a useful and productive life.

3. Prepare the parents for the fact that it may take several months of regulating drug dosages before adequate control is obtained.

4. Encourage parents and older children to obtain genetic counseling.

a. As genetic research progresses, an increasing number of mutations have been found in patients with both sporadic and inherited epilepsy syndromes. There is a genetic predisposition with certain types of seizures, such as absence, febrile, and juvenile myoclonic seizures.

b. It is impossible to predict accurately the possibility of the seizure disorder appearing in siblings or offspring of the affected child.

5. Teach the parents and child factors that may precipitate a seizure.

a. The child should be kept in optimal physical condition with routine immunizations, medical care, dental care, and eye care and should receive prompt evaluation and treatment of infections.

b. Excessive fatigue, dehydration, and sleep deprivation should be avoided.

c. Irregular, fluctuating schedules are detrimental. Advise the parents to maintain a daily routine.

d. Fever or illness of any kind can trigger seizures in children diagnosed with epilepsy even though their seizures may otherwise be under control.

6. For additional resources, refer families to *www.aboutkid-shealth.ca/En/ResourceCentres/Epilepsy/Pages/default.aspx*.

Evaluation: Expected Outcomes

- Padded bed rails in place.
- Breathing unlabored after seizure, with lungs clear.
- Parents and child verbalize understanding of child's ability to participate in activities.
- Child participates in treatment plan and takes medications as ordered without reminders; serum drug levels are therapeutic.

Febrile Seizures

Febrile seizures occur in childhood after 1 month of age and are associated with a febrile illness that is not caused by an infection of the central nervous system. There is no history of a previous neonatal seizure or a previous unprovoked seizure and the child does not have an acute symptomatic seizure. Most febrile seizures occur between 6 and 36 months of age, with the peak incidence at 12 to 18 months. In North America, 2% to 4% of all children will have at least one febrile seizure before age 5 years.

Febrile seizures may be simple or complex:

- Simple febrile seizures—brief, last <10 minutes; tonic–clonic convulsion occurs once in 24 hours; absence of focal features; resolve spontaneously; 70% to 75% of febrile seizures are simple.
- Complex febrile seizures—prolonged, last more than 10 to 15 minutes; focal in nature; may recur within the same febrile illness over 24 hours; approximately 20% of febrile seizures are complex in most series.

Pathophysiology and Etiology

1. Febrile seizures are associated with first- or second-degree relatives with a history of febrile seizure, daycare attendance, developmental delay, influenza A viral infection, herpes virus-6 infection, metapneumovirus, and iron-deficiency anemia.

2. Seizures often accompany intercurrent infections, especially viral illness, tonsillitis, pharyngitis, and otitis.

3. They appear to occur in a familial pattern, although exact pattern of inheritance is not completely understood. Children with a positive family history of febrile seizures have a greater risk of recurrent febrile seizures.

4. Clinical studies have now demonstrated that it is the actual maximum temperature attained rather than the rate of rise, which is the determinant of risk in febrile seizures. One key

variable that alters fever effect is seizure threshold, which is lower in infants.

5. Most febrile seizures consist of generalized tonic–clonic seizures and the majority occur on the first day of illness (see above).

Clinical Manifestations

1. Fever is usually more than 101.8° F (38.8° C) rectally.
2. Seizures usually occur near the onset of fever rather than after prolonged fever.

Diagnostic Evaluation

Measures are directed toward delineating the cause of any seizure as precisely as possible so its implications and prognosis may be discussed with the parents. Diagnostic methods may include the following:

1. Careful history taking and physical examination.
2. CSF examination to detect CNS infection—strongly recommended in children experiencing their first febrile seizure, especially in children age < 12 months, those who have had a prolonged seizure including febrile status epilepticus, if there are any meningeal signs, if the child is on antibiotics (could mask meningitis signs and symptoms) and for seizures that occur after the second day of febrile illness.
3. CBC and urinalysis to detect signs of infection.
4. Cultures of nasopharynx, blood, or urine, as appropriate, to determine cause of fever.
5. Blood glucose, calcium, and electrolyte levels to detect abnormalities that may cause seizures.
6. EEG (for atypical seizures or for a child at risk for epilepsy).
   a. Demonstrates mild, postictal slowing soon after the attack.
   b. Pattern is generally normal after a few days.

Management

The goals of treatment are to control seizures and decrease temperature.

1. Administration of antipyretics and other cooling measures.
2. Prevention of febrile seizures with anticonvulsants is not common practice. Prompt control of fevers is the desired course of action.
3. Rectal diazepam gel is the preferred method of acute seizure management for prolonged seizures >5 minutes or for someone who is at risk for status epilepticus. It is used only in extreme cases.
   a. Intermittent therapy with phenobarbital during febrile episodes is apparently of no value because of the length of time required to achieve therapeutic serum levels of the drug.
4. Airway management, as required.
5. Prognosis—likelihood of recurrence is about 33% in those who have had two febrile seizures. The younger the child is at the time of the first seizure, the greater the risk for additional febrile seizures.
6. The risk of development of nonfebrile seizures is relatively low (about 5%). At risk are children who demonstrate the following characteristics:
   a. Prolonged or complex febrile seizures.
   b. Abnormal or suspected abnormal development before the first seizure.
   c. Family history of nonfebrile seizures.
   d. Persistent EEG abnormalities.

Complications

Injury may occur during seizure.

Nursing Assessment and Interventions

Nursing assessment and interventions are the same as for seizure disorders, page 1250.

Family Education and Health Maintenance

1. Reinforce realistic, reassuring information, such as the following:
   a. A seizure does not necessarily imply that the underlying disease is serious.
   b. Febrile seizures are relatively common in children.
   c. The prognosis depends on the cause of the seizure.
      i. A single febrile seizure does not indicate later chronic epilepsy.
      ii. Children usually outgrow the tendency to develop febrile seizures by age 4 or 5.
      iii. Occasional or brief seizures are thought to not have any effect on the child's overall development, although this is controversial.
2. Discuss and demonstrate emergency management of seizures.
   a. The child should be positioned on the side, on a flat surface from which he or she cannot fall.
   b. The surface should be padded, if possible, to prevent injury.
   c. An adult should stay with the child to monitor the airway and breathing until the seizure is complete.
   d. If the child vomits, immediately clear the mouth of all foreign material.
3. Stress that medical evaluation is indicated as soon as the child develops a fever.
   a. Review technique of temperature measurement.
   b. Prompt administration of antipyretic measures is necessary when the child is febrile but may not prevent a febrile seizure.
4. Review administration schedule, adverse reactions, and appropriate follow-up regarding anticonvulsant therapy.
5. Let the family know that when a child is diagnosed with febrile seizures, future events can be adequately managed at home and do not require emergency transport if <5 minutes in duration. However, parents should notify pediatrician of febrile illness and seizure occurrence.

Subdural Hematoma

Subdural hematoma refers to an accumulation of fluid, blood, and its degradation products within the potential space between the dura and arachnoid membranes (subdural space). Subdural hematomas are classified as acute or chronic, depending on the time between injury and the onset of symptoms.

Also, see for care of unconscious patient, ICP monitoring, and other neurologic care.

Pathophysiology and Etiology

Causes

1. Direct or indirect trauma to the head:
   a. Birth trauma.
   b. Accidental causes.
   c. Purposeful violence, as in cases of child abuse.
2. Meningitis.

Classification

1. Acute syndrome—presents as an acute problem, closely related to the time of presumed injury.
2. Chronic:
   a. Signs and symptoms are nonlocalizing and subacute.
   b. This is the most common type of subdural hematoma in children.
   c. It is usually difficult to delineate the exact time and type of injury because the precipitating episode may appear relatively insignificant.

Altered Physiology

1. Trauma to the head causes tearing of the delicate subdural veins, resulting in small hemorrhages into the subdural space. (Bleeding may be of arterial origin in cases of acute subdural hematoma.)
2. As the blood breaks down, there is an increased capillary permeability and effusion of blood cells and protein into the subdural space.
3. The breakdown products of blood stimulate the growth of connective tissue and capillaries largely from the dura.
4. A membrane is formed that usually extends frontally and laterally over the hemispheres, surrounding the clot.
5. Fluid accumulates within the membrane and increases the width of the subdural space.
6. Further hemorrhages occur.
7. The lesion enlarges, compressing the brain and expanding the skull, and, if unrelieved, ultimately causes cerebral atrophy or death from compression and herniation.
8. The lesion may arrest spontaneously at any point.
9. Further bleeding may occur into an already existing sac and may increase symptoms.
10. In long-standing subdural hematoma, the fluid may disappear, leaving a constricting membrane that prevents normal brain growth.

Clinical Manifestations

Acute

1. Typically present with continuous unconsciousness from the time of injury, but child may present with a lucid interval.

2. Ensuing manifestations include deterioration of LOC, progressive hemiplegia, focal seizures, and signs of brain stem involvement and herniation (pupillary enlargement, changes in vital signs, decerebrate posturing, and respiratory failure; see Figure 46-3).

Chronic

This has a slow, gradual onset; symptoms are variable and are related to the age of the child.

1. Infants—early signs:
   a. Anorexia, difficulty feeding, and vomiting.
   b. Irritability.
   c. Low-grade fever.
   d. Retinal hemorrhages.
   e. Failure to gain weight.
2. Infants—later signs:
   a. Enlargement of the head.
   b. Bulging and pulsation of the anterior fontanelle.
   c. Tight, glossy scalp with dilated scalp veins.
   d. Strabismus, pupillary inequality, and ocular palsies (rare).
   e. Hyperactive reflexes.
   f. Seizures.
   g. Retarded motor development.
3. Older children—early signs:
   a. Lethargy and anorexia.
   b. Symptoms of increased ICP (vomiting, irritability, headache).
4. Older children—later signs (may also occur immediately if bleeding takes place rapidly):
   a. Seizures.
   b. Coma.

Diagnostic Evaluation

1. Clinical features.
   a. In infants who are irritable, have failed to gain weight, and have developed an enlarged and tense fontanelle, chronic subdural hematoma should be suspected.
   b. Biparietal bulge of the head.
2. Imaging.
   a. Diagnosis and size of hematoma are confirmed by CT and, if necessary, by MRI.

Figure 46-3. Primitive posturing in unconscious states because of loss of motor control. **(A)** Decorticate posturing occurs when cortical loss is present. **(B)** Decerebrate posturing occurs when the midbrain is involved. (From Pillitteri, A. [2013]. *Maternal and child health nursing: Care of the childbearing and childrearing family* [7th ed.]. Philadelphia, PA: Lippincott Williams & Wilkins.)

Management

Acute Subdural Hematoma

This requires evacuation of the clot through a burr hole or craniotomy.

Chronic Subdural Hematoma

1. Repeated subdural taps are done to remove the collecting fluid.
   a. In infants, the needle can be inserted through the fontanelle or suture line.
   b. In older children, burr holes into the skull are necessary before the needle can be inserted.
   c. Subdural taps may be the only treatment required if the fluid disappears entirely and symptoms do not recur.
   d. Concurrently, treatment is instituted to correct anemia, electrolyte imbalance, and malnutrition.
2. Shunting procedure may be indicated if repeated taps fail to significantly reduce the volume or protein content of the subdural collections. Shunting is usually to the peritoneal cavity.

Prognosis

1. Treatment is usually successful when the diagnosis is made before cerebral atrophy and a fixed neurologic deficit have occurred. In such cases, subsequent development is normal.
2. Prognosis depends on the effect of the initial trauma on the brain and the effect of continued fluid collection.
3. Mortality in massive, acute subdural bleeding is very high, even if promptly diagnosed.

Complications

1. Mental retardation.
2. Ocular abnormalities.
3. Seizures.
4. Spasticity and paralysis.
5. Brain stem herniation and death.
6. Neurologic impairment (cognitive or physical).

Nursing Assessment

Assess the child's neurologic status to evaluate the effectiveness of treatment or to identify disease progress.

1. Observe general behavior, especially irritability, lethargy, and evidence of personality changes. It is important to obtain a thorough history from the parents regarding normal behavior and level of functioning so abnormalities can be more easily recognized.
2. Evaluate appetite and feeding difficulties, including vomiting.
3. Assess vital signs for signs of increased ICP—be alert for the following:
   a. Increased systolic BP.
   b. Widened pulse pressure.
   c. Decreased pulse or irregularities.
   d. Changes in respiratory rate or difficulty breathing.
4. Assess LOC; describe response explicitly, including what type of stimulus was required to elicit a response.
5. Assess pupillary and visual changes, especially dilated pupil, double vision, lack of response to light, alterations in visual acuity, and nonsymmetric or abnormal eye movements.
6. Monitor for seizures.
7. Evaluate motor function, including ability to move all extremities. The ability to grasp should be checked and compared bilaterally.
8. Inspect for drainage of CSF from the nose or ears, indicating fractured skull with CSF leak.

Nursing Diagnoses

- Ineffective Tissue Perfusion: Cerebral related to disease process.
- Impaired Physical Mobility related to decreased LOC.
- Imbalanced Nutrition: Less Than Body Requirements related to decreased LOC.
- Ineffective Family Coping: Compromised related to hospitalization of child.

Nursing Interventions

Maintaining Cerebral Tissue Perfusion

1. Avoid additional increase in ICP.
   a. Maintain a quiet environment.
   b. Avoid sudden changes in position.
   c. Organize nursing activities to allow for long periods of uninterrupted rest.
   d. Carefully regulate fluid administration to avoid danger of fluid overload.
   e. Measure urine output and record specific gravity.
   f. Administer laxatives or suppositories to prevent straining during a bowel movement.
2. Assist with subdural taps.
   a. Protect and restrain the child, as needed (see page 1222).
   b. Hold the child securely to avoid injury caused by sudden movement.
   c. Apply firm pressure over the puncture site for a few minutes after the tap has been completed to prevent fluid leakage along the needle tract.
   d. Observe the child frequently after the procedure for shock or drainage from the site of the tap.
   e. Note whether there is serous drainage or frank blood.
   f. Reinforce the dressing, as needed, to prevent contamination of the wound.
   g. Monitor temperature frequently and monitor for signs of developing infection.
   h. Report purulent drainage from the site of the subdural tap.
3. Avoid discussing the child's condition near the bed. Even though comatose, the child may be able to hear.
4. Have emergency equipment available for resuscitation.

Preventing Complications of Immobility

1. Change the child's position frequently and provide meticulous skin care to prevent hypostatic pneumonia and decubitus ulcers.
2. Prevent contractures.
   a. Apply passive ROM exercises to all extremities.
   b. Place pillows appropriately to support the child's body in good alignment.
   c. Use splints designed by physical therapy, as instructed.
3. Suction the child as necessary to remove secretions in the mouth and nasopharynx.
4. Observe for signs of respiratory or urinary infection related to stasis.
5. Keep the child's eyes well lubricated to prevent corneal damage.

Maintaining Nutritional Status

1. Provide nutrition and fluids through nasogastric feedings, as ordered. Observe for gastric distention.
2. Monitor urine output and specific gravity daily.
3. Monitor electrolyte and protein levels on laboratory work.
4. Do not neglect mouth care, even if child is not eating.

Strengthening Family Coping

1. Encourage the parents to hold and cuddle their child as much as possible.

2. Encourage the parents to bring diversional activities from home.
   a. Infants—mobiles or musical toys.
   b. Older children—quiet games, books, and dolls.
3. Provide emotional support to the parents.
   a. Encourage as much parental participation in the child's care as possible.
   b. Support parents and suggest pastoral counseling, as indicated.
4. Be nonjudgmental in cases caused by intentional or accidental trauma.
5. Make sure that cases of suspected child abuse have been reported to the appropriate agency and that parents have been referred for counseling.
6. Encourage visitation by siblings.

Community and Home Care Considerations

1. Follow community and home care considerations listed under "Cerebral Palsy" on page 1229.
2. Perform periodic developmental assessments and reinforce the need to report any signs of developmental delay to the health care provider.
3. Discuss return-to-activity/play as the child progresses, as directed by health care provider.

Family Education and Health

1. Reinforce explanations in the following areas:
   a. Condition.
   b. Causes of the child's specific symptoms.
   c. Need and rationale for treatment.
   d. Postoperative and recovery expectations.
2. Encourage parents to keep all follow-up appointments for medical evaluation and physical and occupational therapy.
3. Teach parents safety measures to prevent injuries in the future.
4. Assist parents in seeking additional support and resources through social work department, church groups, community agencies, or private counseling.

Evaluation: Expected Outcomes

- Drowsy but responsive to verbal stimuli; pupils equal and reactive to light; vital signs stable; ventricular tap site without drainage.
- Skin without signs of erythema or breakdown; full ROM of all joints; functional position maintained.
- Tolerates nasogastric feedings without distention; urine output sufficient.
- Parents participate in child's care, hold, and read to child; parents receive counseling.

 TRANSITIONAL CARE ALERT The proper transition of pediatric patients to adult care has always been important to health care providers but has received more attention over the past several years as an increased number of children with serious and complex medical conditions are surviving into adulthood. Because of the need for proper transition of this population, many organizations have studied the myriad of transition issues and developed programs to ensure a smooth transition of children and their families to adult care.

The goal of transition is to help teens with chronic medical conditions (and their families) develop the knowledge and skills required to successfully manage their health care in the adult system while they are still within the pediatric system. With proper guidance, children and youth can acquire the skills to advocate for themselves (or through others), attain self-management of care when possible, and learn to successfully navigate and access adult health care services.

Many issues must be considered for a successful transition such as different levels of patient complexity, comorbid conditions, the need for multidisciplinary services, and the required links with appropriate community agencies. When these needs are all met, teens and their families will have a more positive experience with the transition process.

SELECTED REFERENCES

Aaberg, K. M., Bakken, I. J., Losius, M. I., et al. (2018). Short-term seizure outcomes in childhood epilepsy. *Pediatrics, 2018 May 22.* [epub ahead of print]

Aschenbrenner, D. (2017). New treatment for Duchenne muscular dystrophy. *American Journal of Nursing*, 117(6), 22–23.

Ashwal, S., Russman B. S., Blasco, P. A., et al. (2004). Practice parameter: diagnostic assessment of the child with cerebral palsy: report of the Quality Standards Subcommittee of the American Academy of Neurology and the Practice Committee of the Child Neurology Society. *Neurology*, 62(6), 851–863.

Barty, E., Caynes, K., & Johnston, M. (2016). Development and reliability of the Functional Communication Classification System for children with cerebral palsy. *Developmental Medicine and Child Neurology*, 58(10), 1036–41.

Benson, A., Lambert, V., Gallagher, P., Shahwan, A., & Austin, J. K. (2017). Parent perspectives of the challenging aspects of disclosing a child's epilepsy diagnosis to others: Why don't they tell? *Chronic Illness*, 13(1), 28–48.

Benson, A., O'Toole, S., Lambert, V., et al. (2016). The stigma experiences and perceptions of families living with epilepsy: implications for epilepsy-related communication within and external to the family unit. *Patient Education and Counseling*, 99(9), 1473–1481.

Bloemen, M., Van Wely, L., Mollema, J., et al. (2017). Evidence for increasing physical activity in children with physical disabilities: A systematic review. *Developmental Medicine and Child Neurology*, 59(10), 1004–1010. doi: 10.1111/dmcn.13422.

Borlot, F., Tellez-Zenteno, J. F., Allen, A., et al. (2014). Epilepsy transition: Challenges of caring for adults with childhood-onset seizures. *Epilepsia*, 55(10), 1659–1666.

Buxton, K., Morgan, A., & Rogers, J. (2017). Nurse Practitioner Lead Pediatric Baclofen Pump Program: Impact on safety and quality of care. *Journal of Neuroscience Nursing*, 49(5), 324–329.

Cai, Q., Zhou, Z., Luo, R., et al. (2017). Safety and tolerability of the ketogenic diet used for the treatment of refractory childhood epilepsy: A systematic review of published prospective studies. *World Journal of Pediatrics*, 13(6), 528–536.

Caplan, E., Dey, I., Scammell, A., et al. (2016). Recognition and management of seizure in children in emergency departments. *Emergency Nurse*, 24(5), 30–38.

Decker, K. A., Miller W. R., & Bluelow, J. M. (2016). Parent perceptions of family social supports in families with children with epilepsy. *Journal of Neuroscience Nursing*, 48(6), 336–341.

Demarest, S. T., Shellbass, R. A., Gaillard, W. D., et al. and the Pediatric Epilepsy Research Consortium. (2017). The impact of hypsarrhythmia on infantile spasms treatment response: observational cohort study from the national Infantile Spasms Consortium. *Epilepsia*, 58(12), 2098–2103.

Fisher, R. S., Cross, J. H., French, J. A., et al. (2017). Operational classification of seizure types by the International League Against Epilepsy: Position paper of the ILAE Commission for Classification and Terminology. *Epilepsia*, 58(4), 522–530.

Gloss, D., Moxley, R. T. III, Ashwal, S., et al. (2016). Practice guideline update summary: Corticosteroid treatment of Duchenne muscular dystrophy: Report of the Guideline Development Subcommittee of the American Academy of Neurology. *Neurology*, 86, 465.

Good 2 Go Transition Program, SickKids. Accessed April 22, 2017. Available at: *www.sickkids.ca/good2go/*

Greenwood, J., & Valdes, J. (2016). Perampanel (Fycompa): A review of clinical efficacy and safety in epilepsy. *P & T*, 41(11), 683–698.

Guilfoyle, S.M., Follansbee-Junger, K., Smith, A.W. et al. (2018). Antiepileptic drug behavioral side effects and baseline hyperactivity in children and adolescents with new onset epilepsy. *Epilepsia*, 59(1), 146–154.

Guiraud, S., & Davies, K. (2017). Pharmacological advances for treatment in Duchenne muscular dystrophy. *Current Opinion in Pharmacology, 6*, 36–48.

Hanak, B., Bonow, R., Harris, C., et al. (2017) Cerebrospinal fluid shunting complications in children. *Pediatric Neurosurgery, 52*(6), 381–400.

Harden, C., Tomson, T., & Grloss, D. (2017). Practice guideline summary: Sudden unexpected death in epilepsy incidence rates and risk factors: report of the Guideline development, dissemination, and implementation subcommittee of the American Academy of Neurology and the American Epilepsy Society. *Neurology, 88*(17), 1674–1680.

Hénaff, F., Levy, C., Cohen, R., et al. (2017). Risk factors in children older than 5 years with pneumococcal meningitis: Data from a national network. *Pediatric Infectious Disease Journal, 36*(5), 457–461.

Hill, E., Glass, H. C., Kelley, K., et al. (2017). Seizures and antiseizure medications are important to parents of newborns with seizures. *Pediatric Neurology, 67*, 40–44.

Hirvonon, M., Ojata, R., Korhonen, P., et al. (2014). Cerebral palsy among children born moderately and late preterm. *Pediatrics, 134*(6), e1584–e1593.

Innes, R. F. (2015). Understanding the pathophysiology behind febrile convulsions. *Nursing Children and Young People, 27*(2), 20–23.

Kellermann, T. S., Wagner, J. L., Smith, G., et al. (2016). Surgical management of pediatric epilepsy: Decision-making and outcomes. *Pediatric Neurology, 64*, 21–31.

Lager, C., & Kroksmark, A. K. (2015). Pain in adolescents with spinal muscular atrophy and Duchenne and Becker muscular dystrophy. *European Journal of Paediatric Neurology, 19*(5), 537–546.

Lambert, V., Gallagher, P., O'Toole, S., et al. (2014). Stigmatising feelings and disclosure apprehension among children with epilepsy. *Nursing of Children and Young People, 26*(6), 22–26.

Lindsay, S., Proulx, M., Maxwell, J., et al. (2016). Gender and transition from pediatric to adult health care among youth with acquired brain injury: Experiences in a transition model. *Archives of Physical Medicine and Rehabilitation, 97*(2 Suppl 1), S33–S39.

Linsell, L., Malouf, F., Morris, J., et al. (2016). Prognostic factors for cerebral palsy and motor impairment in children born very preterm or very low birthweight: A systematic review. *Developmental Medicine and Child Neurology, 58*(6), 554–569.

Lundbo, L. F., & Benfield, T. (2017). Risk factors for community-acquired bacterial meningitis. *Infectious Diseases, 49*(6), 433–444.

Mendes, T. P., Crespo, C. A., & Austin, J. K. (2017). Family cohesion, stigma, and quality of life in dyads of children with epilepsy and their parents. *Journal of Pediatric Psychology, 42*(6), 689–699. doi: 10.1093/jpepsy/jsw105.

Miller, W. R. (2017). Self-management behaviors of children with spina bifida. *Pediatric Nursing, 49*(1), 22.

Nabbout, R, Andrade, D. M., Bahi-Buisson, N., et al. (2017). Outcome of childhood-onset epilepsy from adolescence to adulthood: Transition issues. *Epilepsy and Behavior, 69*, 161–169.

Offringa, M., Newton, R., Cozinsen, M. A., et al. (2017). Prophylactic drug management for febrile seizures in children. *Cochrane Database of Systematic Reviews.* doi: 10.1002/14651858.CD003031.pub3.

O'Toole, S., Lambert, V., & Gallagher, P. (2016). "I don't like talking about it because that's not who I am": Challenges children face during epilepsy-related family communication. *Chronic Illness, 12*(3), 216–226.

Ozel, S., Switzer, L., Macintosh, A., et al. (2016). Informing evidence-based clinical practice guidelines for children with cerebral palsy at risk of osteoporosis: An update. *Developmental Medicine and Child Neurology, 58*(9), 918–923.

Panebianco M., Prabhakar H., Marson A. G. (2018). Rufinamide add-on therapy for refractory epilepsy. *Cochrane Database of Systematic Reviews,* 2018, Issue 4. Art. No.: CD011772.

Patel, N., Kerr-Liddell, R., Challis, L., et al. (2017). Nursing management of reflex anoxic seizures in children. *Emergency Nurse, 25*(1), 22–26.

Paul, S. P., Kirkham, E. N., & Shirt, B. (2015). Recognition and management of febrile convulsion in children. *Nursing Standard, 29*(52), 36–43.

Paul, S. P., Rogers, E., & Wilkinson, R. (2015). Management of febrile convulsion in children. *Emergency Nurse, 23*(2), 18–25.

Pidcock, F. S. (2017). Pediatric constraint induced movement therapy: Harnessing adaptive neuroplasticity, *Journal of Pediatric Medicine, 10*(1), 1–89. doi: 10.3233PRM-170413.

Polfuss, M., Simpson, P., Neff Greenley, R., et al. (2017). Parental feeding behaviors and weight-related concerns in children with special needs, *Western Journal of Nursing Research, 39*(8), 1070–1093. doi: 10.1177/0193945916687994.

Romitti, P. A., Zhu, Y,, Puzhankara, S., et al. (2015). Prevalence of Duchenne and Becker muscular dystrophies in the United States. *Pediatrics, 135*(3), 513–521.

Sands, T. T., & Choi, H. (2017). Genetic testing in pediatric epilepsy. *Current Neurology and Neuroscience Reports, 17*(5), 45.

Scheffer, I. E., Berkovic, S., Capovilla, G., et al. (2017). ILAE classification of the epilepsies: Position paper of the ILAE Commission for Classification and Terminology. *Epilepsia, 58*(4), 512–521.

Smith, J. (2015). Parent-professional collaboration when a child presents with potential shunt malfunction. *Nursing Children and Young People, 27*(1), 22–27.

Takasaki, K., Diaz Stransky, A., & Miller, G. (2016). Psychogenic nonepileptic seizures: Diagnosis, management, and bioethics. *Pediatric Neurology, 62*, 3–8.

Vaiman, M., Heyman, E., & Lotan, G. (2017). Neurological results of the modified treatment of epilepsy by stimulation of the vagus nerve. *Child's Nervous System, 33*(11), 2017–2022.

Wagner, J. L., Ferguson, P. L., Kellermann, T., et al. (2016). Behavioral health referrals in pediatric epilepsy. *Epilepsy Research, 127*, 72–77.

Wein, N., Alfano, L., & Flanigan, K. M. (2015). Genetics and emerging treatments for Duchenne and Becker muscular dystrophy. *Pediatric Clinics of North America, 62*(3), 723–742.

Woll, C., Neuman, M. I., Pritt, C. M., et al. and the Febrile Young Infant Research Collaborative. (2018) *Epidemiology and Etiology of Invasive Bacterial Infection in Infants ≤ 60 Days Old Treated in Emergency Departments. Journal of Pediatrics, May 18.* [epub ahead of print]

47

Pediatric Eye and Ear Problems

CONDITIONS OF THE EYE

Also see Chapter 16 for additional information on eye problems.

Infectious Processes

Infectious processes of the eye include conjunctivitis, periocular cellulitis, hordeolum (stye), or chalazion. They are characterized by inflammation, infectious exudate, and tissue damage caused by microbes, such as bacteria or viruses. Conjunctivitis is a common problem, affecting almost all children at some time or another.

Pathophysiology and Etiology

1. Microbes are usually introduced into the eye or surrounding tissues including eyelids, eyebrow, and cheeks by direct contact with infected objects. Orbital infections occur secondary to microbial spread from an adjacent sinus, direct inoculation from trauma, surrounding skin infection, or hematogenous spread from sepsis or dental infection.
2. An inflammatory response develops with engorgement and dilation of conjunctival blood vessels with or without discharge and chemosis or edema of the conjunctiva.
3. Common bacterial agents include nontypeable *Haemophilus influenzae*, *Streptococcus pneumoniae*, and *Staphylococcus aureus*. Pathogens in neonates and adolescents can include *Neisseria gonorrhoeae* and *Chlamydia trachomatis*. Viral infections are common and are usually caused by adenoviruses. Less commonly, coxsackievirus, enterovirus, Zika, and herpesvirus may occur.
4. The infecting agents are contagious and easily spread via hand to eye contact from infected objects (fomites). Outbreaks in which multiple children in the same family, classroom, or community are infected may occur.
5. Environmental allergens such as pollen are major contributors to conjunctivitis.

Clinical Manifestations

Redness of the eye is a common ophthalmic symptom comprising 1% of primary care office visits. The cause of this redness can arise from within or outside the globe. Causes range from minor eye dryness to life-threatening systemic illness. Such diverse causes of redness must be differentiated from the red eye of noninfectious processes (see Table 47-1).

Conjunctivitis
1. Acute onset of inflammation of palpebral and bulbar conjunctival layer leads to dilation of the blood vessels. Usually starts initially in one eye followed by the second a few days later.
2. Eyelid and conjunctiva edema.
3. Excessive tearing or exudate.
4. Gritty or burning feeling in the eye and itching.
5. Photophobia with fluctuating blurring and cloudy vision.
6. Accompanied by preauricular lymphadenopathy.

Preseptal Cellulitis
1. Unilateral swelling and redness of the eyelid and surrounding tissues that does not involve eyeball or internal structures.
2. No significant fever.
3. No pain with or limitation of eye movement.
4. No impaired vision.
5. Age less than 5 years.

Postseptal Cellulitis
1. Marked redness and swelling of eyelid and soft tissues surrounding the eye.
2. Pain and tenderness of the eye area.
3. Proptosis (forward displacement of the eye).
4. Purulent discharge from the eye.
5. Fever.
6. Limited mobility of the eye with reduced visual acuity.
7. Age over 5 years.

Hordeolum (Stye)
1. Acute inflammation of lubricating glands of eyelids and eyelashes.
2. Unilateral pustule of eyelash follicle accompanied by tenderness.
3. Does not respond to antibiotics.

Chalazion
1. Chronic, localized eyelid swelling and erythema.
2. "Lump under the eyelid."
3. Does not respond to antibiotics.

Table 47-1 Common Causes of Eye Redness in Children

CAUSE	ASSOCIATED SYMPTOMS	MANAGEMENT
Conjunctivitis		
Viral	Commonly associated with other symptoms of generalized viral illnessCommonly known as "pink eye," itchy, burning eye	Hygiene (see page 1261), rest, cool compresses, artificial tears
Bacterial	Yellow, green, or white discharge, photophobia, tender eye	Antibiotic eyedrops or ointment, hygiene
Chlamydial	Cough, history of maternal infection	Systemic antibiotic
Herpetic	Pain, photophobia, skin lesions	Evaluation by specialist, antiviral agents
Allergic	Marked itching, bilateral, watery discharge, seasonal onset, other allergic symptoms (rhinorrhea, allergic shiners), cobblestoning of inner eyelids	Topical mast cell stabilizer/antihistamine eyedrops, oral antihistamines, avoidance of allergens
Chemical	Watery discharge, onset of symptoms when exposed to cigarettes or other irritants	Avoidance of irritating substances
Trauma	Pain, photophobia, increased tear production	May require eye protection, referral to specialist
Congenital glaucoma	Increased tear production, cloudiness of the cornea	Referral to specialist

Diagnostic Evaluation

1. Because of the cost of and the delay in results, laboratory testing is limited to cases that fail to respond to treatment. Appropriate laboratory media must be used to transport a swab of eye exudate for bacterial culture, viral culture, and antigen testing. Swabs should be obtained immediately but treatment not delayed, especially in the cases of suspected *N. gonorrhea* or *C. trachomatis*.
2. Screening vision exam should be done.
3. A dendritic ulcer caused by herpesvirus can be visualized by instilling fluorescein dye and examining the cornea with a cobalt-filtered blue light, looking for the dendrite lesion.
4. Clinical evaluation and computed tomography scan are the best methods to distinguish preseptal from postseptal cellulitis.

NURSING ALERT A child who has a painful red eye should be referred immediately for medical evaluation because this could indicate an infectious process, exposure to a chemical or foreign body, or other traumatic etiology.

Management

1. Allergic conjunctivitis may respond to removal of the underlying allergen and avoidance of eye rubbing. Treatment includes systemic or topical agents such as antihistamines, mast cell stabilizers, and/or corticosteroids.
2. Antibiotic eyedrops or ointment—such as erythromycin, trimethoprim sulfate and polymyxin B, sulfacetamide, ciprofloxacin, tobramycin, azithromycin, or doxycycline—will shorten the course of bacterial conjunctivitis and make the child more comfortable.
3. Hordeolum and chalazion resolve without antibiotic treatment. Warm compresses applied four times daily are recommended. Lid washes of diluted baby shampoo in water aid with drainage. Incision and drainage may be necessary to promote healing of long-standing chalazion.

4. Systemic antibiotic treatment is indicated for postseptal cellulitis. These children require close follow-up as hospitalization and IV antibiotics may be necessary. A multidisciplinary approach, including an ophthalmologist, pediatrician, otolaryngologist, and, possibly, a neurosurgeon, may be indicated.

 DRUG ALERT Topical corticosteroids should only be prescribed by an ophthalmologist because they may aggravate a herpetic infection.

Complications

1. Permanent scarring of the cornea and visual impairment with herpetic infection, *N. gonorrhoeae*, and *C. trachomatis*.
2. Spread of postseptal cellulitis to the central nervous system, with optic nerve damage, vision loss, ptosis, and strabismus.
3. Eyelid deformity.
4. Septicemia.

Nursing Assessment

1. Assess nature and extent of symptoms and their effect on child's activities.
2. Assess visual acuity.
3. Determine resources available to family for treatment and rehabilitation.

Nursing Diagnoses

- Risk for Infection (spread, secondary, transmission to others) related to hand-to-hand or hand-to-object contact.
- Acute Pain and Discomfort related to tissue swelling, inflammation, and light sensitivity.

Nursing Interventions

Preventing Spread of Infection

1. Perform or teach proper cleansing of drainage.
   a. Use warm water or saline and a disposable applicator, such as cotton balls or gauze.
   b. Use a separate applicator for each eye.

c. Wipe from inner to outer canthus to avoid contamination of the other eye.

2. Teach self-care measures to prevent spread to others.
   a. Observe good handwashing practices.
   b. Wipe eyes and nose with tissues and dispose promptly. Do not wipe the nose and then eyes with same tissue.
   c. Avoid rubbing eyes to prevent spread.

3. Administer and teach proper instillation of eyedrops or ointment (see page 436).

4. Administer oral or IV antibiotics, as prescribed.

5. Advise parents to only use eyedrops prescribed or recommended by a health care provider and dispose of leftover medication at end of treatment period.

Minimizing Pain

1. Apply warm compresses to affected area.
2. Suggest darkened room and sunglasses for patients with photophobia.
3. Administer an analgesic, as prescribed.
4. Administer lubricating eyedrops and ointment, as needed.
5. Minimize environmental stimulation.

Family Education and Health Maintenance

1. Advise of ways to prevent transmission to others.
   a. Handwashing is the most important factor in infection control.
   b. Do not share washcloths or towels or handkerchiefs.
   c. Change pillowcases frequently.
   d. Avoid swimming until infection is resolved.
   e. Return child to school only after having received antibiotic treatment for 24 hours.
   f. Dispose of contaminated items in proper receptacles.
   g. Discontinue use of contact lenses until infection is cleared.
2. Advise parents of indications for reevaluation by health care provider.
   a. Lack of response to antibiotic treatment.
   b. Increased swelling and tenderness; any eye pain.
   c. Worsening of visual acuity.
   d. Identification of dry eye.
   e. Development of additional symptoms such as fever.
3. Encourage routine follow-up visits and vision evaluation.
4. Advise about proper detection and early treatment of sinus, dental, and other infection.
5. Recommend updated immunization, including the *Haemophilus influenzae* type B vaccine in children.

Evaluation: Expected Outcomes

- Parents perform treatment correctly; hygiene procedures followed.
- Patient verbalizes less pain; tolerates bright light.

Congenital Problems

Congenital problems of the eye include structural defects present at birth or developing soon thereafter. These are usually genetically transmitted and include cataract, dacryostenosis, glaucoma, ptosis, and strabismus. See Table 47-2 for pathophysiology, clinical manifestations, and management of each.

Nursing Assessment

1. Assess for red light reflex, especially in neonates and infants. Absence or asymmetry of the red light reflex may indicate congenital cataract or an intraocular tumor or other eye disease.
2. Inspect the eyes for redness of conjunctiva, cloudiness of the cornea, excessive tearing, drooping eyelids that partially occlude the pupil, or obvious misalignment, which provide clues to congenital eye problems.
3. Assess visual acuity routinely in infants and children. Changes in acuity may be the first manifestation of a problem or indication of effectiveness of treatment. Prompt referral to a specialist is necessary.
4. Perform pupillary light reflex test using a penlight or "muscle light" or use a distant light source to help detect strabismus.
   a. Hirschberg test for symmetry of the pupillary light reflexes—normally, the light reflexes are in the same position in each pupil when a light is shone on the bridge of the nose, but asymmetrical reflection will occur with strabismus (positive Hirschberg test).
5. Perform the cover–uncover test to detect latent strabismus caused by weak eye muscles. When the patient is fixated on an object approximately 12 inches (30.5 cm) away, cover one eye. The eye with weak muscles will drift when covered and will snap back when uncovered. An eye with normal muscles will remain straight.

Nursing Diagnoses

- Disturbed Sensory Perception (Visual) related to reduction in visual acuity or no visual stimulation.
- Disturbed Body Image related to the need for patch or glasses.
- Risk for Injury related to reduced visual acuity and modified depth perception.
- Delayed Growth and Development related to altered visual stimulation and possible overprotective behavior of parents.

Nursing Interventions

Minimizing Effects of Vision Loss

1. Participate in visual acuity problem identification and encourage prompt treatment to minimize functional impairment. Accurate assessment of (corrected) monocular visual acuity is the single most important element in an examination.
   a. Effective newborn screening in the nursery helps to detect congenital eye problems.
   b. All children should be screened for visual acuity and strabismus. In young children, this is accomplished by physical examination and assessment of developmental milestones (ie, looks at parent's face, smiles responsively, reaches for objects). Instrument-based photoscreening can assess preverbal children. Special assessment tools are available to assess preverbal children. By age 3 to 5 years, most children can cooperate for performance of accurate visual acuity screening tests.
2. Encourage and assist parents in obtaining corrective lenses for the child.
3. Advise and encourage parents to adhere to the postoperative treatment plan, such as occlusion therapy following cataract surgery or proper use of eyedrops after glaucoma surgery.
4. Encourage and assist parents in providing normal experiences for child to achieve maximum potential:
   a. Assist parents in locating and accessing resources, such as financial assistance, special education in Braille, or parent support groups.
   b. Remind parents of their child's right to an education.

Minimizing Body Image Disturbance

1. Encourage parents to focus on normalization rather than on overprotection. Place expectations on the child's abilities rather than on disabilities, provide opportunities for interaction with peers, and make the child's life as normal as possible.
2. Encourage acceptance of appearance and emphasize the positive aspects of treatment.

Table 47-2   Congenital Eye Problems

CONDITION AND DESCRIPTION	CLINICAL MANIFESTATIONS	MANAGEMENT
Congenital Cataract Opacity of the lens. Possible causes include abnormal embryonic development, intrauterine infection, metabolic disorders, retinopathy of prematurity. Incidence is 1 in 250 neonates.	• Absence of red reflex • Visible clouding of lens • Varying impairment of vision, depending on size, location, and density of cataract • May result in amblyopia	• Surgical removal within first 3 months to promote visual stimulation. • Postoperative care: sedation for first 24 hours to prevent crying, vomiting, and increased IOP; dilating eyedrops; antibiotic and steroid ointments to prevent infection; eye patch and shield for several days. • Aggressive optical therapy and patching of nonoperative eye; monitoring for IOP.
Dacryostenosis Relatively common obstruction of the nasolacrimal duct caused by incomplete duct development and persistence of membrane at lower end of duct. Tears cannot exit via the duct into the nasal cavity and continuously spill over onto the cheek. May be unilateral or bilateral.	• Excessive tearing and spilling onto cheek • Crusted eyelashes and lids • Excoriated cheek • Normal-appearing eye structures and vision • Possible episodes of secondary conjunctivitis and lacrimal duct infection • Increased risk of dacryocystitis	• Resolves spontaneously in 90% of infants in first year of life. • Gentle massage of lacrimal duct four times daily. • Topical antibiotics for secondary infection. • Surgical probing of duct if persists beyond age 12 months; more complex surgery if probing unsuccessful.
Glaucoma Rare, congenital, or acquired abnormality in which the balance between aqueous fluid production and outflow is disrupted. Increased pressure of fluid in anterior chamber causes damage to the retina, cornea, and other structures.	• Corneal enlargement • Haziness of the cornea • Photophobia and intolerance to ordinary light • Excessive tearing • Decreased visual acuity (symptoms present in 35% at birth) • Amblyopia and permanent loss may result without treatment	• Early diagnosis is essential. • Monitoring of IOP by tonometry and central corneal thickness by pachymetry and fundoscopy. • Medical therapy. • Surgical intervention is first-line treatment. • Postoperatively, a patch and shield may be worn for several days to protect sutures. • Lifetime follow-up.
Ptosis Drooping of the upper eyelid caused by weakness of levator palpebrae or, less frequently, Möller muscle. May be congenital or acquired. Affects either the muscle or the nerve that innervates it. Particularly challenging to treat if amblyopia is also present.	• Drooping is visible on inspection • Vision may be impaired if eyelid covers the pupil • May be unilateral or bilateral • If unilateral, amblyopia may result without treatment	• Surgical correction to raise the eyelid and increase visual field. • Patching not necessary postoperatively. • Nonsurgical modalities, such as the use of "crutch" glasses to support the eyelid.
Strabismus Malalignment of the eyes caused by muscle imbalance or by paralysis, which prevents both eyes from focusing correctly on the same image. Affects 2% to 5% of the preschool population. Can cause visual and psychological disability.	• Asymmetric pupillary light reflexes • Asymmetric extraocular movements • Diplopia, impaired depth • Tendency to close one eye or tilt head during vision testing • Amblyopia may result without treatment	• Early and rigorous amblyopic occlusion therapy (patching of the stronger eye for a prescribed period each day may correct latent strabismus by exercising the muscles of the weaker eye). • Correction of refractive error. • Surgical repositioning of the extraocular muscles for severe or fixed cases. • Postoperatively: antibiotic ointment, no eye patch.

IOP, intraocular pressure.

Preventing Injury

1. Encourage the family to be aware of safety in the home, school, and community.
   a. Suggest the use of impact-resistant polycarbonate eyeglasses and devices to keep eyeglasses in place.
   b. Advise the family to maintain a consistent and uncluttered furniture arrangement; notify child of planned changes.
   c. Instruct child in the use of a cane or other assistive device, if warranted.
   d. Teach traffic safety and personal security measures.
2. Orient visually impaired children to their immediate environment.
   a. Orient child to food placement on meal trays.
   b. Assist child with ambulation, and use side rails on bed or crib to prevent falls.

Promoting Normal Growth and Development

1. Encourage parents to provide many sensory opportunities, such as manipulating objects, hearing various sounds, noting the smells in the environment, and tasting an assortment of substances.
2. Allow child to perform activities of daily living (ADLs) as independently as possible.

Family Education and Health Maintenance

Postoperative Teaching

1. In the interest of hygiene and safety, the patient (if older) and parent should be taught correct handwashing technique before and after instilling eye medication, particularly eyedrops. This must be reinforced before discharge.
2. Teach about instillation of medications and use of eye shield to prevent injury to the operative eye after surgery.
3. Teach about activity restrictions after glaucoma surgery.
   a. Bed rest may be required immediately postoperatively.
   b. Older children should not engage in strenuous activity or contact sports for 2 weeks.
4. Advise that activity is not usually restricted after repair of ptosis.
5. Following strabismus repair, strenuous activity, contact sports, and swimming are restricted for 2 to 4 weeks.
6. After cataract surgery because of inflammatory reaction, encourage behaviors to reduce the risk of damage to sutures from increased intraocular pressure (IOP):
   a. Prevent vomiting.
   b. Minimize crying.
   c. Encourage intense occlusion therapy and use of optical correction with glasses or contact lenses as advised.
7. Encourage parents to remove eye discharge or crusts on lashes regularly by wiping the eyes with warm water. Separate washcloths should be used for each eye and each child. Moistened cotton balls may be used.
8. Advise and encourage about the importance of keeping postoperative follow-up appointments.
9. Advise of indications that would require reevaluation by health care provider:
   a. Worsening of visual acuity.
   b. Evidence of inflammation and infection, such as pain, redness, swelling, drainage, and increased temperature.
10. Refer family to Prevent Blindness America (*www.prevent-blindness.org*) for information on eye disease and safety measures. For cataract and glaucoma patients, refer to the Pediatric Glaucoma and Cataract Family Association (*www.pgcfa.org*). Lighthouse International (*www.lighthouse.org*) aids with rehabilitation of visual impairment.

Evaluation: Expected Outcomes

- Child wears glasses or contact lens, as prescribed; good visual outcome with adequate optical rehabilitation.
- Parents and child report involvement in activities, satisfactory school performance, and positive peer interactions.
- No injuries reported.
- Achieves age-appropriate developmental milestones.

Eye Trauma

 EVIDENCE BASE Bagheri, N., Wajdi, B. N. (2017). *The Wills Eye manual: Office and emergency room diagnosis and treatment of eye disease* (7th ed.). Philadelphia, PA: Wolters Kluwer.

Eye trauma causes structural damage to the eye and is produced by mechanical force or contact with a corrosive chemical. Some common types of eye trauma are corneal abrasions, blunt trauma, perforating injuries, and chemical injuries. Eye injuries are common among children and are usually related to their involvement in vigorous play activities.

Pathophysiology and Etiology

Corneal Abrasion

1. Injury to corneal epithelium.
2. This may happen when a foreign object becomes lodged in the eye (eg, flying dust particle; contact lens rubbing against the eye because of inadequate tear production; injury from a fingernail, tree branch, or other sharp object entering the eye, and scraping the cornea).
3. May occur from the effects of general anesthetic, which cause decreased tear production, decreased eyelid reflexes, decreased perception of pain, and failure of the eye to close properly.
4. May result from corneal exposure with such conditions as ptosis or pressure on the globe, especially in the presence of dry eyes.
5. May result from contact with household or industrial chemicals.

Blunt Trauma

1. Occurs when the eye or surrounding tissues are struck by a blunt object such as a ball, a hockey puck, a bat, or a stick. May occur with airbag deployment in a motor vehicle accident.
2. The resulting injury depends on the size, hardness, and velocity of the blunt object and the force imparted. Injury may include tissue swelling and seepage of blood into the surrounding tissues.
3. The bony structures surrounding the eye may be fractured.
4. Subconjunctival hemorrhage, lens dislocation, hyphema (blood in the anterior chamber of the eye), and a retinal detachment may occur.

 TRANSITIONAL CARE ALERT Care should be made to ensure that patients can safely transition from inpatient management (surgery, medical management, outpatient surgery, or emergency management) to home. Patients should be discharged with full instructions on medication administration including type and frequency of application as well as instructions for administration procedures. Patients with hyphema should have a rigid shield placed over the involved eye. However, this should not be a patch as any change in vision noted by the patient may indicate rebleeding into the orbit.

Perforating Injury

1. When an object penetrates the eyeball, there may be loss of vitreous material and/or damage to the internal structures of the eye—vitreous hemorrhage, choroidal rupture, retinal tears, retinal detachment, and ruptured globe.
2. Bacteria may also be introduced into the interior of the eye causing infection.

Chemical Injury

1. Corrosive chemicals burn the delicate tissues of the cornea and may penetrate into deeper layers of the eye.
2. Healing may occur with scarring.

 NURSING ALERT A chemical injury is a medical emergency.

Clinical Manifestations

1. Pain or sensation of a foreign body in the affected eye—because of the high concentration of nerve endings in the cornea from the ciliary body.
2. Increased tear production—one of the eye's defenses against injury or irritation.
3. Injection of the blood vessels of the cornea—increase of blood flow to the cornea is another protective mechanism; most likely seen with foreign bodies, abrasions, or chemical burns that affect the cornea.
4. Impaired visual acuity caused by:
   a. Swelling of the cornea, reducing its clarity.
   b. Swelling of the soft tissues surrounding the eye, causing the eye to partially or completely close.
   c. Excessive tear production, impairing vision.
   d. Damage to internal structures of the eye, altering or obstructing visual pathways.
5. Visible signs of injury—bruising, swelling, or a foreign object visible in the eye.

 NURSING ALERT At times, pain may be useful in distinguishing a serious eye problem from a self-limiting condition.

Diagnostic Evaluation

1. Thorough inspection of the eye, including eversion of the upper lid to inspect for a foreign object.
2. A slit-lamp examination to determine the extent of the corneal abrasion.
3. Fundoscopic examination may detect abnormalities, such as a dislodged lens, retinal hemorrhage, retinal detachment, or papilledema with increased IOP.
4. Staining with fluorescein dye reveals lesions of the cornea such as abrasions.
5. Assessment of eye function, including near and far acuity, extraocular movements, and visual field testing.
6. CT scan of orbit(s) and brain if concern for fracture or brain hemorrhage.

Management

Most childhood injuries will resolve spontaneously with no adverse long-term consequences. Early detection and prompt intervention may help reduce the incidence of ocular morbidity.

Corneal Abrasion

1. Removal of the offending foreign body, such as contact lens.
2. Antibiotic drops or ointment for superficial abrasion.
3. For infected or inflamed abrasion, antibiotic eyedrops or ointment to prevent infection and anti-inflammatory drops to decrease inflammation.
4. Follow up for any recurrent symptoms because recurrent corneal erosion can occur months or years following injury because of spontaneous disruption of corneal epithelium that occurs near the site of the corneal abrasion.

 NURSING ALERT Avoid topical anesthetic after the initial examination because this will slow down the healing process. Avoid the use of contact lens until the abrasion has healed. Patching is no longer recommended because it reduces the removal of pathogens by the tear film.

Blunt Trauma

1. The head should be elevated 45 degrees to facilitate settling of hyphema, if present.
2. Hospitalization may be necessary for noncompliant patients, patients with blood disorders such as sickle cell trait or disease, or if suspicion for child abuse.
3. Surgery may be required because of damage to underlying bones or eye structures.

Perforating Injury

1. Surgery is usually necessary to remove the object and reconstruct damaged tissues.
2. The head should be elevated 30 degrees. Avoid sneezing, nose blowing, and any activity.
3. The child should be kept on nothing-by-mouth status in preparation for surgery. Avoid topical medications. Tetanus toxoid should be given if greater than 7 years since last dose or unknown immunization status.

 NURSING ALERT Never remove a penetrating object from the eye. It should be stabilized, and the eye should be shielded with a Fox shield, with no pressure applied. In an emergency, use a foam cup with part of the bottom cut off, if necessary, to support the object. Patch the unaffected eye during transport to the hospital.

Chemical Injury

1. Continuous, gentle flushing of the affected eye(s) with any available water until able to change to normal saline solution or Ringer lactate solution for at least 30 minutes (see page 436) to help remove the offending chemical. Evert the eyelids and flush from the inner aspect of the eye outward to prevent contaminated water from flowing into the other eye. Wash the patient's face and hands.
2. Further management depends on the nature and extent of the injury.

 NURSING ALERT Acid chemicals coagulate the conjunctival protein, leaving the blood vessels undamaged. Alkaline chemicals rapidly permeate the eye's structure, thus causing more damage.

Complications

1. Infection.
2. Bleeding.

3. Refractive problems because of corneal scar, cataract, glaucoma, shrinkage of the affected eye, and inflammation of the unaffected eye may result in vision impairment or loss of vision.
4. Disfigurement may result from severe or extensive tissue damage.

Nursing Assessment

1. Obtain history of injury, including the child's account of how the injury occurred, and a description of symptoms experienced.
2. Inspect for location and extent of swelling and bruising, asymmetry, or abnormality in appearance of any part of the eye.
3. Obtain visual history preinjury. Assess visual acuity. This should include near and far acuity in each eye. If the patient cannot see well enough to read a Snellen chart, assess ability to count fingers or perceive light. Compare findings with preinjury visual history.

Nursing Diagnoses

- Acute Pain related to inflammation, photophobia, or trauma to eye tissue.
- Risk for Injury related to impaired vision and adverse effects of pain medications.
- Feeding, Dressing, and Grooming Self-Care Deficit related to impaired vision and adverse effects of pain medications.

Nursing Interventions

Minimizing Pain

1. Apply cold compresses to the affected area to help reduce swelling and discomfort.
2. Keep the child's room as dark as possible to help reduce pain for photophobic patients.
3. Administer analgesics, as prescribed.
4. Encourage quiet activities to act as a distraction to pain.

Preventing Injury

1. Enforce safety measures:
   a. Use of bed side rails.
   b. Assistance with ambulation.
   c. Close observation.

Maintaining ADLs

1. Provide assistance with eating, bathing, toileting, and other ADLs, as needed.
2. Teach child location of self-care items and positioning of food on tray to promote independence.
3. Encourage child to attempt self-care and offer praise even if unsuccessful.

Family Education and Health Maintenance

1. Teach indications for reevaluation by health care provider.
   a. Increase in swelling, tenderness, discoloration, or pain.
   b. Worsening of visual acuity.
   c. Development of additional symptoms, such as fever, alteration in sensorium, or other indications of neurologic injury.
2. Provide safety education to all families to prevent common causes of injury. Encourage families to use protective eyewear when participating in sports or other activities; proper use of infant car seat, booster seat, and seat belt; proper storage of household chemicals.
3. Provide families with information and support as they cope with having a visually impaired child in the home. The American Council of the Blind has multiple resources for families at its Web site (*https://acb.org*).

Evaluation: Expected Outcomes

- Demonstrates decreased pain.
- No injuries reported.
- Dressing and feeding self with minimal assistance.

Functional Problems

Functional problems of the eye involve vision impairment because of refractive errors or disuse of visual pathways. Such problems frequently result in amblyopia—impaired vision in one or both eyes because of poor visual stimulation rather than an structural problem. Abnormal vision screening with referral occurs in 1.2% of 5-year-old patients and increases to 9.1% by the time the child reaches age 13. Amblyopia affects 1% to 3% of the population and 2% to 4% of children in North America.

Pathophysiology and Etiology

1. Refractive errors are usually caused by a genetic predisposition to shortened or elongated eyeballs or by individual variations in growth.
   a. In an elongated or shortened eyeball, the visual image is focused either in front of or behind the retina, resulting in unclear images.
   b. The nearsighted (myopic) child can see near objects, such as print in schoolbooks, but cannot focus clearly on far objects, such as words on the blackboard.
   c. The farsighted (hyperopic) child can see far objects clearly but has difficulty seeing near objects.
   d. The problem may be unilateral or bilateral.
2. Amblyopia may result from any condition that causes the two retinas to receive different images. Etiology may include:
   a. Diplopia caused by strabismus.
   b. Significant difference in acuity of the two eyes.
   c. Cataract.
   d. Unilateral severe ptosis.
3. When a discrepancy exists between images received on the two retinas, the more unclear image is suppressed.
   a. Over time, a young child will become permanently unable to use the visual pathways of the suppressed eye.
   b. Although the visual pathways are structurally normal, the child is visually impaired in that eye because of poor visual stimulation.

Clinical Manifestations

Children usually do not complain that they cannot see well but may exhibit other signs of vision problems, including:
1. Poor academic performance or behavioral problems in school.
2. Dislike for reading.
3. Head tilting.
4. Squinting.
5. Sitting close to the television or holding reading materials close to the face.
6. Refusal or resistance to covering one eye during vision screening.

Diagnostic Evaluation

1. Standardized vision screening tests using optotype symbols such as HOTV or LEA may be used for acuity screening.
   a. Tests can be administered to children as young as age 3 years.
   b. Each eye should be tested separately making sure the nontested eye is occluded.
   c. A 2-line difference between eyes requires referral to an ophthalmologist.

Management

1. Most visual acuity problems can be treated by the use of corrective lenses or refractive surgery.
2. Amblyopia management focuses on prevention through early identification and treatment of conditions that caused it.
   a. Strabismus is treated with patching the stronger eye to strengthen the weaker eye. Glasses may also be prescribed to improve the vision. In some cases, however, surgery may be required.
   b. Topical miotic drops may be used if the child is not able to tolerate the daily patching required to correct amblyopia.
   c. Surgery may also be required to correct ptosis.
   d. Acuity problems because of refractive error are usually managed with the use of corrective lenses.
3. Optimal outcome is accomplished when treatment is begun early in life, whereas visual pathways are still developing. However, some visual function may be recovered even if the problem is treated in adolescence or adulthood. Ideally, the problem can be prevented by early identification and treatment of factors that may cause it.

 EVIDENCE BASE DeSantis, D. (2014). Amblyopia. *Pediatric Clinics of North America, 61*(3), 505–518. Donahue, S. P., Baker, C. N.; Committee on Practice and Ambulatory Medicine, Section on Ophthalmology, American Association of Certified Orthoptists, American Association for Pediatric Ophthalmology and Strabismus & American Academy of Ophthalmology. (2016). Procedures for the evaluation of the visual system by pediatricians. *Pediatrics, 137*(1), 1–9.

Complications

Injuries caused by visual impairment.

Nursing Assessment

1. Begin visual acuity screening early, in the preschool years and whenever a child displays behaviors suggestive of acuity problems.
2. Assess Hirschberg test for symmetry of the pupillary light reflexes routinely, beginning at birth.
3. Perform the cover–uncover test as part of routine eye assessment.
4. Assess the effect of the functional deficit on the child's overall function, including academic progress, self-esteem, and safety.

Nursing Diagnoses

- Disturbed Sensory Perception (Visual) related to reduced acuity or inability to use one eye.
- Risk for Injury related to impaired visual acuity or lack of depth perception.
- Chronic Low Self-Esteem related to lowered performance caused by poor vision.

Nursing Interventions

Minimizing Effects of Sensory Deficits

1. Encourage the consistent use of corrective lenses, as prescribed.
2. Teach the parents ways to help develop the child's skills in interpreting information through the senses of hearing, smell, and touch.
   a. Familiarize the child with common sounds and smells in the environment. Also, orient the child to traffic sounds and sounds associated with danger, such as animals and speeding vehicles, and instruct the child how to respond.
   b. Use voice or touch, rather than facial expressions or gestures, to express emotion.
   c. Speak to the child before touching to reduce startling.
   d. Allow the child to touch and handle unfamiliar objects to learn about them.
   e. Have the child practice such things as retelling stories and giving the home telephone number and address.
   f. Explain unfamiliar sounds and smells to the hospitalized child.

Preventing Injury

1. Recommend the use of shatterproof eyeglasses with flexible frames.
2. Recommend the use of eye protection on a routine basis because eye trauma can occur unexpectedly. This is especially important for children who rely on only one eye.
3. Suggest extra protection, such as shatterproof goggles or shields, when participating in contact or ball sports and activities.
4. Maintain a stable arrangement of furniture in the home, adequate lighting, and an uncluttered environment to minimize falls.
5. Orient hospitalized children to the hospital room and offer assistance when walking.

Promoting a Positive Sense of Self-Esteem

1. Provide opportunities for mastery of developmentally appropriate activities such as tablet computer applications.
2. Encourage interactions with sighted children to decrease feelings of isolation. Also, suggest interactions with children with similar alterations in vision.
3. Encourage the child to discuss feelings and strategies for coping with negative peer reactions such as teasing.
4. Encourage independence in self-care activities to promote autonomy, such as dressing, cooking, feeding, and use of bathroom.
5. Assist the patient and family with effective coping mechanisms to promote family stability.

Community and Home Care Considerations

1. Perform a safety inspection of the home environment and make changes as necessary to help prevent falls and other injuries.
2. Assist family access to financial and social resources, as needed.
3. Make sure that the child is receiving early intervention services and individualized educational resources.

Family Education and Health Maintenance

1. Teach the importance of patching for amblyopia and the wearing of corrective lenses, as prescribed, and their proper care.
2. Refer families of blind children to community resources that can help their child learn special skills, such as reading Braille, using a cane, or developing self-care skills. Information can be obtained from agencies such as the American Foundation for the Blind (*www.afb.org*).

Evaluation: Expected Outcomes

- Identifies common sounds.
- No injury reported; wears protective eyeglasses.
- Reports good school performance and participation in extracurricular activities; can eat and dress independently.

CONDITIONS OF THE EAR

Also see Chapter 17 for additional information on ear, nose, and throat problems.

Eustachian Tube Dysfunction

Eustachian tube dysfunction (ETD) is an umbrella term describing disorders that arise from closure of the eustachian tube, which ventilates the middle ear to equalize pressure on both sides of the tympanic membrane. ETD may be associated with otitis media with effusion (OME), also known as serous otitis; acute otitis media (AOM); and recurrent otitis media. Approximately 90% of children experience one or more episodes of middle ear effusion by age 2.

Pathophysiology and Etiology

1. Inflammation of the eustachian tube lining is caused by an acute upper respiratory infection, an allergic response, trauma, or inflammation of middle ear mucosa.
   a. Infected secretions may pass through the tube from the nasal area into the middle ear.
   b. When inflammation and swelling causes the eustachian tube to close, the passage of air into and out of the middle ear is prevented.
   c. The air in the middle ear is absorbed into the middle ear lining and a vacuum is created.
   d. The vacuum is filled by serous fluid that seeps out of the middle ear lining.
   e. The warm, moist environment of the middle ear and nutrients in the serous fluid are conducive to the growth of viruses or bacteria that may be present in the middle ear cavity.
2. Children between ages 6 and 24 months are predisposed to the development of AOM because their short, floppy, relatively straight eustachian tubes more easily allow the passage of infected nasal secretions into the middle ear cavity. See Box 47-1 for additional risk factors.
3. Viruses account for 15% to 20% of AOM cases. In 30% of AOM cases, there is no identifiable bacterial pathogen. The most common bacterial agents include:
   a. *S. pneumoniae.*
   b. Nontypeable *H. influenzae.*
   c. *Moraxella catarrhalis.*

BOX 47-1	Risk Factors for Eustachian Tube Dysfunction

- Frequent episodes of upper respiratory infections in younger children.
- Nasal allergies.
- Genetic predisposition to floppy eustachian tube.
- Native American or Eskimo heritage.
- Craniofacial abnormalities such as cleft lip and palate and Down syndrome.
- Enlarged adenoids.
- Lower socioeconomic status.
- Exposure to tobacco smoke.
- Bottle-feeding.
- Male gender.
- Day care attendance with greater than six attendees.
- Parental or sibling history of OM.
- Immune deficiencies such as cystic fibrosis.

---

4. Barotrauma, caused by rapid changes in atmospheric pressure, may also lead to closure of the eustachian tube and to the development of serous otitis. This is less likely to involve introduction of microorganisms through infected nasal secretions; development of AOM is less common.

 EVIDENCE BASE Chonmaitree, T., Trujillo, R., Jennings, K., et al. (2016). Acute otitis media and other complications or viral respiratory infection. *Pediatrics, 137*(4), 1–10.

Clinical Manifestations

1. OME—decreased hearing, sensation of fullness in the affected ear(s) without pain or fever.
2. AOM—ear pain (otalgia) and signs of infection fever, fussiness, or decreased appetite.
3. ETD—popping sensations in the affected ear(s).

Diagnostic Evaluation

1. Otoscopic examination.
   a. OME—nonpurulent mucoid or serous effusion, prominent bony landmarks, a diffuse light reflex, and decreased mobility of tympanic membrane.
   b. AOM—inflamed tympanic membrane with purulent effusion and decreased or absent mobility; bulging of the tympanic membrane may obscure the bony landmarks and light reflex.
2. Tympanometry—quick and simple way to assess tympanic membrane mobility in children over 7 months of age
   a. A probe occludes the ear canal while pressure is varied and a test sound is emitted. The test produces a graphic display that shows the mobility of the tympanic membrane at various air pressures. A normal reading has a distinct peak in the middle of the graph.
   b. A flat tympanogram (no peak) indicates lack of mobility of the tympanic membrane, usually caused by serous otitis or AOM.
   c. A peak to the left of the center indicates negative pressure in the middle ear.

Management

 EVIDENCE BASE Rosenfeld, R. M., Shin, J. J., Schwartz, S. R., et al. (2016). Clinical practice guideline: Otitis media with effusion (update). *Otolaryngology-Head and Neck, 154*(1 suppl), S1–S41.

American Academy of Family Physicians, American Academy of Otolaryngology- Head and Neck Surgery, American Academy of Pediatrics Subcommittee on Otitis Media With Effusion. (2004). Otitis media with effusion. *Pediatrics, 113*(5), 1412–1429.

Otitis Media with Effusion

1. Usually resolves spontaneously, but 30% to 40% of patients have repeated episodes, and approximately 25% have persistent effusion after 3 months.
2. OME is the leading cause of hearing loss, so interval visits for reexamination and hearing testing should be done. Hearing levels (HLs) of ≥40 dB requires an immediate, complete audi-

ologic evaluation and may indicate pressure equalization tubes (PETs). Persistent effusions of greater than 3 months and any concern for speech and language delay indicate need for referral to an otolaryngologist.

3. Patients less than 4 years of age with persistent OME should have PETs placed, and patients 4 years of age and older should have PETs placed with or without adenoidectomy.
4. Pharmacology treatment such as antihistamines, decongestants, antimicrobials, and corticosteroids is not indicated.
5. Tonsillectomy is not recommended.

 EVIDENCE BASE Lieberthal, A. S., Carroll, A. E., Chonmaitree, T., et al. (2013). The diagnosis and management of acute otitis media. *Pediatrics, 131*(3), e964–e999.

Acute Otitis Media

1. All infants and children should be assessed for pain and inflammation of the inner ear.
2. All infants under age 6 months with presumed or certain AOM should be treated with antibiotics and analgesics.
3. Children ages 6 to 24 months with certain AOM accompanied by acute onset, moderate or severe otalgia, or temperature 39°C (102.2°F) or higher should be treated. Infants with unilateral AOM but no severe symptoms may be monitored. Those with bilateral AOM or severe symptoms should receive antibiotic therapy.
4. For children over age 2 years, observation may be considered for those with certain AOM but who do not have severe illness.
5. If not treating, the clinician should ensure that an adult caregiver is able to observe the child, recognize signs of serious illness, and be able to provide prompt access to medical care if improvement does not occur. If there is worsening of illness or no improvement in 48 to 72 hours, antibacterial therapy should be considered.
6. First-line treatment includes amoxicillin (80 to 90 mg/kg divided in 2 divided doses) or, for the penicillin allergic, cefdinir (14 mg/kg in 1 or 2 doses), cefuroxime (30 mg/kg in 2 divided doses), or cefpodoxime (10 mg/kg in 2 divided doses) for 10 days.
7. Children who have received amoxicillin in the past 30 days, have concurrent purulent conjunctivitis, or have a history of recurrent AOM unresponsive to amoxicillin should receive high-dose amoxicillin–clavulanate (90 mg/kg/day of amoxicillin with 6.4 mg/kg/day of clavulanate in 2 divided doses).
8. Alternative antibiotics for treatment failures include ceftriaxone (50 mg/kg/day IM or IV for 3 days) or clindamycin (30 to 40 mg/kg/day in 3 divided doses), with or without a second- or third-generation cephalosporin.

Recurrent Otitis Media

1. Placement of ventilating tubes by myringotomy (incision into the tympanic membrane) may be considered for children who experience three or more episodes in 6 months or four or more episodes per year (see Figure 47-1).
2. Antibiotic prophylaxis is no longer recommended because it may contribute to the problem of antibiotic-resistant bacteria.

Complications

1. Perforations of the tympanic membrane, scarring because of healed perforations, or damage to the ossicles of the middle ear may occur; permanent hearing loss is a rare complication.
2. Delayed speech and language development.

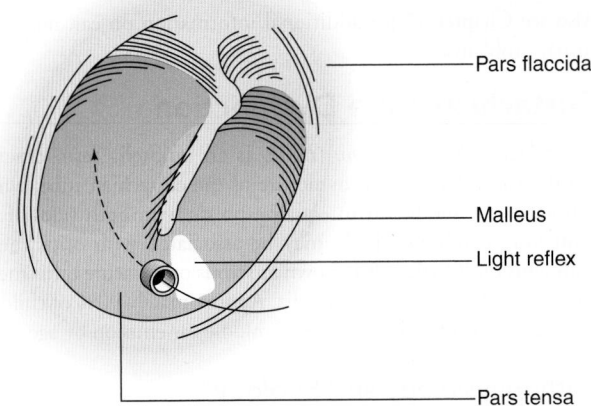

Figure 47-1. A ventilating (myringotomy) tube provides air to the middle ear to prevent otitis media. (From Pillitteri, A. [2013]. *Maternal and child health nursing: Care of the childbearing and childrearing family* [7th ed.]. Philadelphia, PA: Lippincott Williams & Wilkins.)

3. Mastoiditis, meningitis, lateral sinus thrombosis, or intracranial abscess; spread of bacterial infection may occur, although all are uncommon.

Nursing Assessment

1. Assess for etiologic factors that contribute to ETD.
2. Assess for symptoms of serous otitis and AOM to identify and to document the nature and severity of the illness.
3. Assess hearing after the middle ear effusion is resolved. Promptly identify any hearing loss that may have social and educational consequences.
4. Assess speech and language development in children who experience recurrent or prolonged infections to determine deficits.
5. Assess for effects of illness on family, such as sleep deprivation of parents caused by staying up with child at night or decreased attendance at work caused by keeping child out of school.

 NURSING ALERT Prompt identification of speech and language delays is important in young children because speech and language development is quite rapid at this time. Young children may demonstrate either rapid regression or failure of progression of speech and language skills.

Nursing Diagnoses

• Acute Pain related to increased pressure in the middle ear.
• Impaired Verbal Communication caused by conductive hearing loss.

Nursing Interventions

Minimizing Discomfort

1. Administer and teach parents to administer antibiotics. Provide instruction in:
   a. Measurement of correct dosage.
   b. Time of doses.
   c. Importance of administering all doses.
   d. Proper storage and disposal of unused medication.
   e. Adverse effects.
2. Administer acetaminophen or ibuprofen, as directed, for pain or fever.
3. Apply warm compresses to the external ear.

4. Advise elevation of head to facilitate drainage of fluid from the middle ear into the pharynx.
5. Teach older children to stimulate opening of their eustachian tubes by yawning or performing Valsalva maneuver.

Facilitating Verbal Communication

1. Assess hearing, speech, and language development regularly.
2. Alert parents to report signs of hearing difficulty or delayed speech immediately to ensure early intervention.
3. Refer to a specialist for evaluation and treatment, if necessary.

Family Education and Health Maintenance

1. Teach parents that episodes of otitis may be minimized by:
   a. Breast-feeding.
   b. Placing older, bottle-fed infants in a sitting position during feeding.
   c. Identifying and eliminating allergens, such as particular foods, molds, and dust.
   d. Not exposing the child to cigarette smoke.
   e. Immunization with pneumococcal and influenza vaccines.
2. Teach the importance of taking antibiotics at prescribed times for the indicated length of therapy to prevent partial treatment and the development of resistance.
3. Teach all parents the difference between viral and bacterial infections, emphasizing that overuse of antibiotics for viral infections contributes to the development of resistant bacteria.
4. If ventilating tubes are placed, instruct parents to do the following.
   a. Prevent water or other fluids from entering the ear canal. Encourage use of earplugs when the child is bathing or swimming.
   b. Discourage instillation of eardrops or other medications in the external ear unless they have been prescribed by the health care provider.
   c. Tubes will fall out of the ear spontaneously, usually in 6 to 12 months.

 EVIDENCE BASE Pettigrew, M. M., Alderson, M. R., Bakaletz, L. O., et al. (2017). Research conference report from the 18th international conference on recent advances in otitis media—Panel 6: Vaccines. *Otolaryngology-Head and Neck Surgery, 156*(4 suppl), S76–S87.

Evaluation: Expected Outcomes

- Demonstrates improved comfort; family states proper treatment regimen.
- Speech and language development appropriate for age; reports regular assessment; receives therapy from specialist, if indicated.

External Otitis

Acute *otitis externa* is inflammation in the external ear canal. It is frequently unilateral but may be bilateral. Commonly known as "swimmer's ear."

Pathophysiology and Etiology

1. Caused by bacteria or fungi. Common pathogens include:
   a. *Pseudomonas aeruginosa.*
   b. *Staphylococcus aureus.*
   c. *Proteus mirabilis.*
   d. *Streptococcus pyogenes.*
   e. Fungi *(Candida, Aspergillus).*
2. Risk factors include:
   a. Frequent swimming.
   b. Insertion of objects, such as cotton swabs, into the ear canals.
   c. AOM with perforation of the tympanic membrane.
   d. Ventilation tubes with drainage.
   e. Poorly fitting ear plugs.
3. When water remains in the external ear canal, a warm, moist environment is created.
4. Skin lining the canal is irritated, causing breakdown of its protective barrier.
5. Bacteria or fungi overgrow in the conducive environment and cause symptoms of inflammation and infection in 1 to 2 days.
6. Breakdown of protective barrier and introduction and proliferation of infectious organisms can also occur through trauma to the ear canal, such as cleaning the ear with an inappropriate object or using an improper technique.

Clinical Manifestations

1. Intense ear pain, itching, and white, yellow, or greenish drainage.
2. Inflammation of the external ear canal and structures.
3. Pain when the ear pinna is manipulated.

Diagnostic Evaluation

1. Otoscopic examination may be difficult because of severe pain and swelling; redness, swelling, and drainage in external canal are noted while tympanic membrane appears normal.
2. Ear pain may be severe.
3. Cellulitis of the surrounding structures can result in displacement of the external ear out and away from the head.
4. Cultures are usually not necessary.

Management

1. Ear pain may be severe, and appropriate analgesia should be provided.
2. Effective topical treatments include acetic and boric acid solutions, which dry and modify the pH of the ear canal.
3. Topical antibiotic solution, possibly combined with a steroid to reduce significant discomfort and swelling.
4. Ear canal may be gently cleansed with curette, cotton swab, mild suctioning, or irrigation to remove drainage.
5. An ear wick may be used to aid in medication getting to the lining of the deeper ear canal.
6. Oral antibiotics may be used in addition to topical medications in severe cases or if cellulitis extends beyond the external canal.

Nursing Assessment

1. Assess severity of symptoms and need for pain relief.
2. Assess ear hygiene and the need for earplugs.

Nursing Diagnosis

- Acute Pain related to inflammation and irritation of drainage.

Nursing Interventions

Relieving Pain

1. Administer eardrops or teach parents administration, as prescribed.
   a. Have child lie on side with affected ear upward.
   b. Instill drops, using caution not to contaminate dropper, and press gently on tragus.
   c. Have child maintain position for 5 minutes to facilitate penetration of medication into ear canal.
   d. Repeat on other side, if ordered.
2. Administer analgesics, such as acetaminophen or ibuprofen, as directed.
3. Suggest application of warm or cold compresses to outer ear to relieve discomfort.
4. Frequently clean drainage from area surrounding opening of ear canal to relieve irritation.

Family Education and Health Maintenance

1. Teach proper ear hygiene.
   a. Insert nothing into ear canal for cleaning or scratching.
   b. Clean the outer area with a washcloth only.
   c. Drain water promptly from ear by leaning the child over and pulling auricle slightly downward and outward.
2. Instruct in the use of well-fitting earplugs, if necessary.
3. Instruct in the use of routine acetic acid solution instillation after water activity, if prescribed.

Evaluation: Expected Outcomes

- Reports pain relieved; uses compresses and analgesics, if necessary.

Functional Hearing Disorders

Functional hearing disorders arise from problems in the function of the ear. In a quiet environment, the healthy child can hear tones between 0 and 25 dB. Categories of hearing impairment include slight, 15 to 25 dB; mild, 25 to 40 dB; moderate, 40 to 65 dB; severe, 65 to 95 dB; and profound, 95 or more dB. In the United States, moderate to profound bilateral sensorineural hearing loss occurs in 0.5 to 1.0 per 1,000 live births each year. Factors that place an infant at high risk for hearing loss include low birth weight, craniofacial anomalies, family history of hereditary childhood hearing loss, and certain infections, such as rubella or bacterial meningitis.

Pathophysiology and Etiology

1. Hearing loss may be conductive, sensorineural, or mixed.
2. Conductive loss may uncommonly result from a congenital ear deformity. More commonly, conductive loss is acquired and occurs when sound transmission through the outer and/or middle ear is impaired, caused by impaction of cerumen in the external ear canal, fluid in the middle ear cavity, or scarring of the tympanic membrane.
   a. A mechanical obstruction, such as cerumen or a foreign object blocking the external ear canal, may block the passage of sound waves to the tympanic membrane.
   b. With otitis media or OME, fluid in the middle ear cavity does not transmit sound as well as air.
   c. A scarred or perforated tympanic membrane has lost its normal mobility and does not transmit sound as well as a normal one.

d. Most cases of conductive hearing loss in children are reversible and produce no permanent effect.
3. Sensorineural hearing loss results from damage to the cochlea or auditory nerve and congenital defects of the cochlea. Examples include damage caused by ototoxic drugs, damage resulting from prenatal infections, and damage caused by prolonged exposure to loud noise.
   a. Damage to the auditory nerve prevents transmission of sound impulses to the brain for interpretation.
   b. Damage to hair cells of the cochlea may be caused by prolonged exposure to loud noise, resulting in hearing loss, especially pronounced for high-pitched sounds.
   c. Sensorineural problems are usually irreversible.

Clinical Manifestations

1. Infants may be noted to be unresponsive to sound. Response to sound, however, is not sufficiently reliable as a screening method, especially for high-risk infants.
2. Children usually do not complain that they cannot hear well. They may exhibit other signs of hearing problems, including:
   a. Poor academic performance or behavior problems in school.
   b. Lack of response to sounds.
   c. Delayed language development.
   d. Listening to the television or radio at a loud volume.
   e. Speaking loudly.

Diagnostic Evaluation

 EVIDENCE BASE Harlor, A. D, Jr., Bower, C.; Committee on Practice and Ambulatory Medicine. (2009). Hearing assessment in infants and children: Recommendation beyond neonatal screening. *Pediatrics, 124,* 1252–1263.
Bass, P. F. (2016). *Hearing loss & the pediatrician.* Available: www.ContemporaryPediatrics.com, 14–17.

1. Universal newborn hearing screening using a two-stage process is advocated by the American Academy of Pediatrics and the Agency for Healthcare Research and Quality and is widely accepted as the standard of care for infants in the United States. This is accomplished by an initial automated transient evoked otoacoustic emission (OAE) before discharge from the hospital newborn nursery. If indicated, an automated auditory brain response test is used to confirm a positive OAE screen.
2. Infants who fail their initial screening need a follow-up evaluation at 1 month of age. Any infants with a second abnormal result should be evaluated by an audiologist as soon as possible. Infants with risk factors such as sepsis at birth requiring antibiotics require a repeat hearing evaluation at 3 months of age.
3. Infants with documented hearing loss need referral to specialists (otolaryngology and ophthalmology) by 3 months of age. Referral to other subspecialists (genetics, nephrology, neurology, etc.) may be necessary. The infant should be enrolled in Early Intervention Services (Part C) through the local school system in the United States no later than 6 months of age, which will supply physical therapy, occupational therapy, speech therapy, and visual intervention, as indicated.

4. Infants whose initial hearing screen is normal should be routinely assessed for their response to sound and achievement of developmental speech language milestones.
5. Routine audiometric screening should be done beginning as soon as the child can cooperate and follow instructions (between ages 3 and 5 years). It is important that the child be screened and hearing deficits addressed before entry into school.

Management

1. Treatment of the underlying problem, such as impacted cerumen or otitis media.
2. Hearing aids may be helpful for both conductive and sensorineural hearing loss.
3. Cochlear implants help some children with sensorineural hearing loss.
   a. Consists of an external microphone and speech processor, which sends radio signals to an internal electrode array implanted in the cochlea.
   b. Most effective in the young child who has had shorter hearing deprivation but requires a long period of rehabilitation.
4. If the problem cannot be corrected, the focus of treatment is on development of adaptive skills through special education, sign language or other communication alternatives, and/or technical devices for the hearing impaired.

Complications

1. Speech and language delays.
2. Inadequate social development.
3. Academic failure.

Nursing Assessment

1. Periodically assess hearing in the child with an identified hearing impairment to follow up promptly on changes in ability to hear.
2. Assess speech and language development frequently so that children may obtain special assistance, as indicated.
3. Assess social development and academic progress periodically so that counseling and intervention can be instituted.

Nursing Diagnoses

- Disturbed Sensory Perception (Auditory) related to limited ability to hear.
- Impaired Verbal Communication related to inability to hear and imitate speech sounds.
- Risk for Injury related to inability to hear warning sounds of impending danger.
- Chronic Low Self-Esteem related to social and academic difficulties.

Nursing Interventions

Minimizing Effects of Hearing Loss

1. Face the child, use appropriate facial expressions, and make sure the child can see your face clearly when communicating.
2. Approach the child so that you can be seen; touch the deaf child on the shoulder to get attention.
3. Assist the child in utilizing hearing aid, as prescribed, or assistive technology.

Promoting Effective Communication

1. Determine usual method of communication: ability to write, using verbal cues, or reading lips. Do not depend on gestures to communicate with child or with a third party who does not know sign language.
2. Obtain an interpreter, when necessary, for children who communicate using sign language. Adequate communication is especially important when providing health education or when treating children who may have been abused.
3. Help the parents of a young child to stimulate and communicate with him or her using visual language.
   a. Teach them to use gestures, mime, and nonverbal communication.
   b. Teach them to help the infant to develop watching behavior by giving rewards of pleasure and praise.
   c. Teach them to talk to the child while looking directly into his or her eyes and using appropriate facial expressions.

Preventing Injury

1. Advise parents that home safety devices, such as smoke detectors, may require visual or tactile alarms (flashing lights or vibration) rather than auditory alarms.
2. Encourage the use of other senses to compensate for inability to hear. For example, the child should be especially careful to look in all directions when crossing the street.
3. Do not leave the child alone in an unfamiliar environment without means of communication.
4. Provide close surveillance and frequent visual contact for the hospitalized child.

Increasing Self-Esteem

1. Inform families of the child's right to a public education in the least restrictive setting and promote use of augmented communication devices.
2. Encourage interaction with hearing and nonhearing children to promote integration.
3. Encourage mastery of developmental milestones and skills through self-care activities and play.
4. Help parents understand that the child may not be able to express anxiety or frustration and may act out instead.
5. Teach them to be consistent in their use of discipline and to provide alternative ways for the child to gain attention or to relieve stress.
6. Praise the child for accomplishments and attempts at social interaction.

Family Education and Health Maintenance

1. Encourage families to learn sign language and alternative methods of communication with the child.
2. Advise on proper hearing aid cleaning and maintenance.
3. Encourage attention to health maintenance needs, such as immunizations and well-child visits.
4. For additional support and information, refer to groups such as the American Society for Deaf Children (*deafchildren.org*).

Evaluation: Expected Outcomes

- Responds appropriately to environmental stimuli.
- Communicates effectively through sign language, interpreter, and visual cues.
- Reports no injuries.
- Reports adequate progress in school and participation in extracurricular activities.

1270 Chapter 47 • PEDIATRIC EYE AND EAR PROBLEMS

TRANSITIONAL CARE ALERT Patients discharged with ear conditions and disorders may require complex care at home. Family caregivers may not be experienced in administering otic medications and will require detailed instructions. Education may also be required if a child is discharged without an intact tympanic membrane (conditions that resulted in a perforation or surgical intervention for tympanostomy tubes) for injury and infection prevention. Children discharged to home with acute or chronic ear conditions may not have full hearing ability, and safety measures should be reviewed.

SELECTED REFERENCES

American Academy of Family Physicians, American Academy of Otolaryngology-Head and Neck Surgery, & American Academy of Pediatrics Subcommittee on Otitis Media with Effusion. (2004). Otitis media with effusion. *Pediatrics, 113*(5), 1412–1429.

Bagheri, N., & Wajda, N. B. (2017). *The Wills eye manual: Office and emergency room diagnosis and treatment of eye disease* (7th ed.). Philadelphia, PA: Wolters Kluwer.

Bass, P. F. (2016). *Hearing loss & the pediatrician.* Available: *www.ContemporaryPediatrics. com.* 14–17.

Beal, C., & Giordano, B. (2016). Clinical evaluation of red eyes in pediatric patients. *Journal of Pediatric Health Care, 30*(5), 506–514.

Beal, C. R., & Rosenblum, L. P. (2018). Evaluation of the effectiveness of a tablet computer application (App) in helping students with visual impairments solve mathematics problems. *Journal of Visual Impairment & Blindness,* 5–19.

Chonmaitree, T., Trujillo, R., Jennings, K., et al. (2016). Acute otitis media and other complications or viral respiratory infection. *Pediatrics, 137*(4), 1–10.

DeSantis, D. (2014). Amblyopia. *Pediatric Clinics of North America, 61*(3), 505–518.

Donahue, S. P., Baker, C. N.; Committee on Practice and Ambulatory Medicine, Section on Ophthalmology, American Association of Certified Orthoptists, American Association for Pediatric Ophthalmology and Strabismus & American Academy of Ophthalmology. (2016). Procedures for the evaluation of the visual system by pediatricians. *Pediatrics, 137*(1), 1–9.

Harlor, A. D., Jr., Bower, C.; Committee on Practice and Ambulatory Medicine, The Section on Otolaryngology-Head and Neck Surgery. (2009). Hearing assessment in infants and children: Recommendation beyond neonatal screening. *Pediatrics, 124*(4), 1252–1263.

Hoberman, A., Paradise, J. L., Rockette, H. E., et al. (2016). Shortened antimicrobial treatment for acute otitis media in young children. *New England Journal of Medicine, 375*(25), 2446–2456.

Kohli, M. A., Farkouh, R. A., Maschio, M. J., et al. (2015). Despite high cost, improved pneumococcal vaccine expected to return 10-year net savings of $12 billion. *Health Affairs, 34*(7), 1234–1240.

Lieberthal, A. S., Carroll, A. E., Chonmaitree, T., et al. (2013). The diagnosis and management of acute otitis media. *Pediatrics, 131*(3), e964–e999.

Linsenbigler, K., Petersen, S., & Lieberman, L. (2018). Barriers to physical activity for children with visuals impairments: How far have we come and where do we still need to go? *PALAESTRA, 32*(1), 26–31.

McCulloch, J. (2015). Ocular emergencies and trauma. In K. Curtis & C. Ramsden (Eds.), *Emergency and trauma care for nurses and paramedics* (2nd ed., pp. 793–820). Australia: Elsevier.

Miraldi Utz, V., & Kaufman, A. R. (2014). Allergic eye disease. *Pediatric Clinics of North America, 61*(3), 607–620.

Nierengarten, M. B. (2016). *Early hearing detection and intervention.* Available: *www.ContemporaryPediatrics.com,* 22–25.

Nye, C. (2014). A child's vision. *Pediatric Clinics of North America, 61*(3), 495–503.

Pettigrew, M. M., Alderson, M. R., Bakaletz, L. O., et al. (2017). Research conference report from the 18th international conference on recent advances in otitis media—Panel 6: Vaccines. *Otolaryngology-Head and Neck Surgery, 156*(4 suppl), S76–S87.

Puodziuviene, E., Jokubauskiene, G., Vieversyte, M., et al. (2018). A five-year retrospective study of the epidemiological characteristics and visual outcomes of pediatric ocular trauma. *BMC Ophthalmology, 18,* 1–9.

Rosenfeld, R. M., Shin, J. J., Schwartz, S. R., et al. (2016). Clinical practice guideline: Otitis media with effusion (update). *Otolaryngology-Head and Neck Surgery, 154*(1 suppl), S1–S41.

Scanga, H. L., & Nischal, K. K. (2014). Genetics and ocular disorders. *Pediatric Clinics of North America, 61*(3), 555–565.

Schilder, A. G., Marom, T., Bhutta, M. F., et al. (2017). Research conference report from the 18th international conference on recent advances in otitis media—Panel 7: Otitis media: Treatment and complications. *Otolaryngology-Head and Neck Surgery, 154*(1 suppl), S88–S105.

Ting, C., & McPherson, B. (2017). Hearing loss in children with otitis media with effusion: a systematic review. *International Journal of Audiology, 56*(2), 65–76.

Wong, M. M., & Anninger, W. (2014). The pediatric red eye. *Pediatric Clinics of North America, 61*(3), 591–606.

Yang, C. O., Reilly, B. K., & Preciado, D. A. (2018). Barriers to pediatric cochlear implantation: A parental survey. *International Journal of Pediatric Otorhinolaryngology, 104,* 224–227.

48

Pediatric Gastrointestinal and Nutritional Disorders

COMMON PEDIATRIC GASTROINTESTINAL DISORDERS

Cleft Lip and Palate

Cleft lip and palate are congenital anomalies, known as *orofacial clefts*, resulting in structural facial malformation. These defects are usually present in early fetal development, are one of the most common birth defects in the United States, and are associated with any of more than 400 syndromes. The lip, or the lip and palate, fails to close in approximately 1 in every 1,000 neonates. This equals approximately 7,000 infants born each year in the United States. Infants born with cleft lip with or without cleft palate number 4,440 per year.

Cleft lip and palate are most prevalent among Native Americans. Cleft lip (with or without cleft palate) occurs more frequently in males, and isolated cleft palate is more frequent in females. The chance of having a child with an orofacial cleft increases if one or both parents have a defect and if there is a sibling born with a defect.

EVIDENCE BASE National Institute of Dental and Craniofacial Research, National Institutes of Health. *https://nidcr.nih.gov/DataStatistics/FindDataByTopic/CraniofacialBirthDefects/PrevalenceCleft%20LipCleftPalate.htm.* Accessed 20 March, 2017.

Pathophysiology and Etiology

EVIDENCE BASE Saal, H. (2016). Genetic evaluation for craniofacial conditions. *Facial Plastic Surgery Clinics, 24*(4), 405–425.

1. A failure of fusion of lip/palate tissue between 5 and 7 weeks of gestation, resulting in defect in morphogenesis. It involves patterns of DNA signaling, gene and biochemical organizers, nuclear and cellular differentiation, proliferation, and migration. A major impact is at the level of the neural crest cell.

2. Although the syndrome is not well understood, genetic/hereditary factors may play a role; a fetus with an affected parent or sibling has a 3% to 5% risk of being affected.

3. In 2004, a gene variant was identified as being a major contributor to orofacial clefts. This gene variant may triple the risk of developing the defect in signaling and transcription proteins that are involved in development and differentiation. There is a 50% risk in monozygotic twins.

4. Environmental factors may include the following:
   a. Vitamin B and folic acid deficiency. Some studies have shown that consumption of multivitamins with folic acid prior to conception and during the first trimester may lower the incidence of cleft lip and palate. A study by the National Institute of Environmental Health Sciences in 2007 suggests taking a multivitamin containing 400 mcg of folic acid. New data suggests a correlation between Vitamins A and D and cleft palate phenotypes.
   b. Medications taken during pregnancy, including antiseizure drugs and corticosteroids.
   c. Maternal alcohol and smoking.
   d. Infections.
   e. Diabetes.

EVIDENCE BASE Sarwer, D., Kazak, A., Clarke, A., et al. (2017). Body Image and Quality of Life in Adolescents with Craniofacial Conditions. *Cleft Palate-Craniofacial Journal, 54*(1), 2–12.

Types of Defects

1. Cleft lip—prealveolar cleft (see Figure 48-1):
   a. Varies from a notch in the lip to complete separation of the lip into the nose.
   b. May be unilateral or bilateral.
   c. Failure of maxillary process to fuse with nasal elevations on frontal prominence; normally occurs during 5th and 6th weeks of gestation.
   d. Merging of upper lip at midline complete between 7th and 8th weeks of gestation.

Figure 48-1. Cleft lip. (Nath, J. [2016]. *Stedman's Medical Terminology* [2nd ed.]. Philadelphia: Lippincott Williams & Wilkins.)

2. Isolated cleft palate—postalveolar cleft:
   a. Cleft of uvula.
   b. Cleft of soft palate.
   c. Cleft of both soft and hard palate through roof of mouth.
   d. Unilateral or bilateral.
   e. Failure of mesodermal masses of lateral palatine process to meet and fuse; normally occurs between 7th and 12th weeks of gestation.
3. Submucous cleft:
   a. Muscles of soft palate not joined.
   b. Not recognized until child talks; cannot be seen at birth.
4. Pierre Robin syndrome—cleft palate, glossoptosis (tongue lays back on pharynx), and micrognathia (underdeveloped mandible):
   a. This causes feeding difficulties, potential airway obstruction by tongue, slow weight gain, and ear infections.
   b. By age 3 to 4 months, the mandible has grown enough to accommodate the tongue, and respiratory difficulty is greatly diminished.

Clinical Manifestations

1. Physical appearance of cleft lip or palate:
   a. Incompletely formed lip—varies from slight notch in vermilion to complete separation of lip.
   b. Opening in roof of mouth felt with examiner's finger on palate.
2. Eating difficulty:
   a. Suction cannot be created for effective sucking.
   b. Food returns through the nose.
3. Nasal speech.
4. Increased incidence of otitis media, which may lead to mild to moderate hearing loss.
5. Speech delay secondary to lip defect as well as related to chronic otitis media.
6. Dental problems.

Diagnostic Evaluation

 EVIDENCE BASE Woo, A. (2017). Evidence-based medicine: Cleft palate. *Plastic & Reconstructive Surgery, 139*(1), 191e–203e.

1. Prenatal ultrasonography to detect cleft lips and some cleft palates *in utero*.
2. Magnetic resonance imaging (MRI) and three-dimensional computed tomography to evaluate extent of abnormality before treatment.
3. Photography to document the abnormality.
4. Serial x-rays before and after treatment.
5. Dental impressions for expansion prosthesis.
6. Genetic evaluation to determine recurrence risk.

Management

 EVIDENCE BASE Burg, M., Chait, Y., Yao, C., et al. (2016). Epidemiology, Etiology, and Treatment of Isolated Cleft Palate. *Frontiers in Physiology, 7*(67), epages.

Interdisciplinary approach begins early and continues into late adolescence. Craniofacial team consists of a plastic surgeon, otolaryngologist, pediatric dentist, prosthodontist, orthodontist, feeding specialist, speech pathologist, audiologist, geneticist, psychologist, and community health nurse. Each team member has a role at some point in the child's care.

1. General management is focused on proper growth and nutrition, closure of the clefts, prevention of complications, oral–motor rehabilitation, and facilitation of normal growth and development of the child.
2. Patients with isolated cleft lips have a greater chance of overcoming feeding difficulties than do those with combined defects.
3. The cleft lip is repaired before the palate defect, generally around age 3 months.
   a. Techniques performed include the Millard repair, which results in a zigzag scar on the lip, or placement of sutures where the line of the columella would have been.
   b. The surgical goals are adherence and the most cosmetically pleasing and naturally appearing lip.
4. Cleft palate repair may be done any time between ages 6 and 18 months. Surgery and timing are based on degree of deformity, width of oropharynx, neuromuscular function of palate and pharynx, and surgeon's preference. Some children may require more than one reconstructive surgery.
   a. Palatoplasty is the reconstruction of the palatal musculature.
   b. The surgical goal is adherence, development of normal speech pattern, and safe/appropriate eating skills. Additionally, it should decrease the incidence of otitis media.
   c. Surgery may be performed by craniofacial or plastic surgeon in conjunction with other specialists, including oral surgeon and dentist.

Complications

1. Respiratory distress.
2. Infection.

3. Palatal fistulas.
4. Dehydration and electrolyte imbalance.
5. Bleeding.

Nursing Assessment

1. If the newborn has a cleft lip, assess for cleft palate by direct visualization and palpation with finger.
2. Obtain family history of cleft lip or palate.
3. Evaluate feeding abilities.
   a. Effectiveness of suck and swallow.
   b. Amount taken.
   c. Vomiting, regurgitation, or formula coming from nose.
4. Observe for other syndromic features, such as small jaw, abnormal facies, micro/macrocephaly, heart murmur, anal–rectal defects.

Nursing Diagnoses

- Ineffective Infant Feeding Pattern related to defect.
- Risk for Infection related to open wound created by malformation, ear infections.
- Risk for Impaired Attachment related to malformation and special care needs of the infant.
- Risk for Aspiration related to tongue and palate deformities in Pierre Robin syndrome.
- Deficient Knowledge related to home management of infant with cleft malformation.
- Fear related to surgery.
- Deficient Knowledge related to postoperative care.

Nursing Interventions

 EVIDENCE BASE Baylis, A. L., Pearson, G. D., Hall, C., et al. (2018). A quality improvement initiative to improve feeding and growth of infants with cleft lip and/or palate. *The Cleft Palate Craniofacial Journal*, Jan 01, 1545–1569.

Maintaining Adequate Nutrition

1. Facilitate nutrition and speech therapy for all infants.
2. Encourage the mother to begin feeding the infant as soon as possible to enhance bonding and to strengthen the oral structures needed for mastication and speech production.
3. If sucking is permitted:
   a. Encourage breast-feeding.
   b. Encourage and demonstrate breast pump.
   c. Use a soft nipple with crosscut to facilitate feeding.
4. If sucking is ineffective because of inability to create a vacuum, try alternate oral feeding methods.
   a. Feeding devices include preemie nipple, crosscut nipple, NUK nipple, Ross Cleft Palate Nurser, Mead Johnson Cleft Palate Nurser, Pidgeon nipple bottle system, Haberman Feeder, or palatal obturator.
   b. Avoid enlarging nipple holes because of infant's inability to control flow of milk, which will result in choking. Crosscut nipples allow milk to flow only when infant squeezes the crosscut open.
   c. Using a squeezable bottle (eg, Mead Johnson Cleft Palate Nurser) or plastic liner can be helpful by applying rhythmic pressure along with the infant's normal sucking and swallowing.
   d. Rubber-tipped Asepto syringe or dropper; the rubber extension should be long enough to extend back into the mouth to prevent regurgitation through the nose. Direct tip to side of mouth and feed slowly.
5. Feed infant in an upright, sitting position or the upright side-lying position if airway support is needed. This decreases possibility of fluid being aspirated or returned through the nose or back to the auditory canal.
   a. Feeding is usually easier if the nipple is angled to the side of the mouth away from the cleft so that the infant's tongue can press the nipple against the upper gum or dental arch.
   b. Feed slowly over approximately 18 to 30 minutes. Feedings longer than 45 minutes expend too many calories and tire the infant.
   c. Smaller but more frequent feedings may be necessary if the infant tires or requires extended time to eat.
   d. Burp frequently during feeding to decrease amount of air swallowed.
   e. If micrognathia exists, use of the pinky finger under the chin for support aids in improved sucking ability.
   f. Feed the infant before he or she becomes too hungry. If the infant is too agitated, feeding becomes a problem.
6. Administer enteral tube feedings if nipple feeding is to be delayed.
7. Advance diet as appropriate for age and needs of infant. Eating usually improves when solids are introduced because they are easier for the infant to manipulate.
8. Assess and calculate adequate nutritional intake.

Preventing Infection

1. Protect the child from infection so that surgery will not be delayed.
   a. Use and teach good hand-washing practice.
   b. Avoid patient contact with anyone who has an infection.
   c. Provide frequent assessment for otitis media.
2. Clean the cleft after each feeding with water and a cotton-tipped applicator.
3. Observe for fever, irritability, redness, or drainage around cleft and report promptly.
4. Monitor vital signs; report temperature greater than 101°F (38.3°C).

Promoting Acceptance and Adjustment

1. Show acceptance of the infant; maintain composure and do not show negative emotion when handling the infant. The manner in which the nurse handles the infant can make a lasting impression on the parents.
2. Support parents when showing a neonate for the first time. Demonstrate acceptance of the infant's and the parents' feelings. Parents may be grieving about the infant's cosmetic imperfections and may harbor ambivalent feelings.
3. Offer information and answer any questions in a simple, matter-of-fact manner. The better informed the family, the easier it will be for them to see the infant as a normal child with a physical difference that will require surgery, dental work, and possibly speech therapy.
4. Be aware that the normal sequence of parental responses may include shock, disbelief, worry, grief, and anger and then proceed to a state of equilibrium and reorganization.
5. Encourage parental involvement in infant's care: frequent holding, cuddling, and playing.

Preventing Aspiration and Airway Obstruction

1. Prevent respiratory obstruction by the tongue, especially on inspiration and when the infant is quiet.
   a. Positioning: elevated and side-lying.

b. Tilt head back as tolerated by the infant, and elevate upper trunk slightly.

c. Tongue/lip suture may be placed by otolaryngologist to prevent the tongue from interfering with airway. Assess for slippage, infection, pain, interference with eating.

d. Suction nasopharynx, as needed.

2. Infants with Pierre Robin syndrome are at greater risk for airway compromise, especially when feeding.

a. Feeding can be done with a nursing bottle (feeding techniques similar to those used for cleft palate).

b. Generally use orthopneic position—vertical and slightly forward; this allows the infant to push the jaw forward to suck and allows the feeder a clear view of the infant.

c. Use gentle finger pressure at mandibular attachment to bring the jaw forward.

Preparing for Home Management

1. Prepare family for home feedings by providing several days to practice feeding and to become familiar with the infant's feeding pattern.

2. Alert the caregiver to difficulties with feeding and how to manage them.

a. Nasal regurgitation: feed in more upright position or stop feeding and allow the infant to cough and clear the airway; then continue with smaller feedings.

b. Respiratory distress: feed slowly, give smaller feedings. Observe for signs of aspiration, such as coughing, color changes, increased respiration, fever, and/or formula coming from nose.

c. Prolonged feeding: if oral feedings take longer than 20 to 30 minutes, energy expenditure increases. Smaller, more frequent feedings are indicated, or enteral tube feeding supplements may be warranted.

3. Suggest that about 1 week before scheduled admission for surgery, the mother begin using feeding techniques preferred by multidisciplinary team. Infants who feed well prior to surgery may do better postoperatively than poor feeders.

4. Encourage the parents to prepare siblings at home for the arrival of the infant. Suggest they show a picture of the new infant.

5. Offer parents available resources regarding children with cleft lip and palate.

6. Encourage parental involvement with local self-help groups that provide information and parent-to-parent contact.

7. Initiate referrals, as indicated, for additional support and financial assistance and early intervention programs.

8. Describe and reinforce surgical treatment plans to the parents to promote communication and hope.

9. Stress compliance with follow-up care with the pediatrician, plastic surgeon, dentist, orthodontist, psychologist, and speech therapist to prevent chronic otitis media, hearing loss, speech impairment, and emotional problems.

10. Initiate a community nurse referral to continue emotional support and teaching progress at home.

Providing Preoperative Care and Allaying Fear in the Child Undergoing Surgery

1. Prepare the infant or toddler for the postoperative experience to decrease fear and increase cooperation.

a. Practice the feeding measure that will be used postoperatively—cup, side of spoon, or syringe.

b. Use elbow immobilizers for short periods; allow the child to play with them and the caregiver to use them. Check your facility's policy regarding the use of immobilizers because this is considered a form of restraint but may be deemed medically necessary.

c. Demonstrate and practice mouth irrigation because it will be done postoperatively for cleft palate repair; allow the child to assist if age appropriate.

2. Prepare the parents emotionally for the postoperative appearance of the child.

a. Explain the use of the Logan bow (a curved metal wire that prevents stress on the suture line for cleft lip repair) and restraints.

b. Encourage a parent to be with the child, especially when awakening from anesthesia, to offer security and comfort.

3. Address and explain pain management, collaborating with the parents as to what comforts their child.

Providing Postoperative Care

1. Protect surgical site:

a. Apply elbow immobilizers to prevent hands from reaching the mouth while still allowing some freedom of movement; follow your institution's policy regarding medical restraints.

i. Assess the patient's skin and/or intravenous (IV) line every 2 hours while the immobilizer is in place.

ii. Remove the immobilizer to exercise the arms.

iii. Do not allow anything in the child's mouth, such as straw, eating utensils, or fingers.

2. Maintain adherence device: check that Logan bow or other device is intact and maintaining adherence of lip repair.

a. Prevent wetting tape or it will loosen.

b. Observe for and report bleeding or dislodgement of Logan bow.

3. Prevent the child from stressing the suture site—not crying, blowing, sucking, talking, or laughing.

4. Assess and manage pain.

a. Consult institution's pain management team, if necessary.

b. Use pain medications appropriate for age, weight, and condition.

c. Use pain assessment tools appropriate for age (see page 1150).

d. Recognize signs of pain, such as crying, agitation, poor feeding, increased vital signs.

e. Discourage pacifiers until cleared by surgeon.

f. Encourage the mother to hold the infant, swaddle, and use security/comfort items from home.

5. Positioning—elevated head of bed and side-lying.

a. An infant seat may be useful for variation of position, comfort, and entertainment and to prevent interference with suture line.

b. Provide for appropriate diversional activity, hanging toys, and mobiles.

c. If only cleft palate was repaired, child may lie on abdomen.

6. Monitor respiratory effort after cleft palate repair.

a. Be aware that breathing with a closed palate is different from the child's customary way of breathing; the child must also contend with increased mucus production.

b. Provide humidified air, if needed, to provide moisture to mucous membranes that may become dry from mouth breathing.

7. Prevent infection.

a. Clean suture line after every feeding.

b. Gently wipe lip incision with cotton-tipped applicator and solution of choice, such as water, saline, or diluted hydrogen peroxide. Gently pat dry and apply antibiotic ointment or petroleum jelly, if ordered.

c. Rinse the mouth with water or offer a drink of water after each feeding.

d. Irrigate the mouth with normal saline solution or water after cleft palate repair. Technique may vary based on preference of surgeon. You can direct a gentle stream over the suture line using an ear bulb syringe with the child in a sitting position with head forward.

8. Avoid tension on the suture line during feeding for several days after lip repair.

a. Use dropper or syringe with a rubber tip and insert from the side to avoid suture line or to avoid stimulating sucking.

b. Use side of spoon. Never put spoon into the mouth.

c. Perform enteral tube feedings, if prescribed; usually this is the last treatment of choice.

d. Advance slowly to nipple feeding, as directed. The infant should be able to suck more efficiently after the lip is repaired.

e. After palate repair, feed the child in the manner used preoperatively (cup, side of spoon, or rubber-tipped syringe). Never use straw, nipple, or plain syringe.

f. Consult with speech/occupational therapy if feeding/swallowing continues to be difficult.

9. Facilitate adequate nutrition.

a. Obtain nutrition consult, if indicated.

b. Diet progresses from clear liquids to full liquids to soft foods.

c. Soft foods are usually continued for about 1 month after surgery, at which time a regular diet is started, but excludes hard food.

d. Ensure that the child is receiving adequate calories.

e. Weigh daily and plot on growth charts (*www.cdc.gov/growthcharts/*).

f. Early feeding intervention relates to appropriate growth.

10. Administer an antibiotic, if prescribed, to prevent infection, as the mouth and skin contain bacteria.

Community and Home Care Considerations

1. As the patient's advocate, alert members of the craniofacial team when a family is overwhelmed by too many appointments and interventions. Act as liaison to case manager, social worker, and home care agency.

2. Continue to assess weight gain, feeding behavior, overall development, parent–child bonding and interactions.

3. Advise the parents to discuss the child's problem with teachers and other responsible adults in close contact with the child.

a. Aesthetic touch-up and bone graft surgery performed later may interfere with schooling.

b. Speech differences require early identification and intervention.

c. Monitor for reading and learning problems related to speech and language delays.

d. Hypernasality may develop at ages 10 to 14 years because of normal shrinkage of adenoid tissue occurring at this time.

4. Assess the child's self-perception and coping skills. Assess the family's support systems and coping mechanisms.

5. Help school-age children deal with teasing (as a result of being "different" from their peers) by allowing them to express their feelings and guiding their response: ignoring the remark, responding with a joke or good-natured tease, or educating the teaser.

6. The school nurse can also help by performing frequent hearing evaluations, communicating with staff, and educating the school community on the child's condition and individual needs.

 EVIDENCE BASE Sischo, L., Clouston, S., & Phillips, C. (2016). Caregiver responses to early cleft palate care: A mixed method approach. *Health Psychology, 35*(4), 474–482.

Family Education and Health Maintenance

1. Instruct on continued protection of the mouth after surgery. Child cannot put anything in mouth, including lollipops.

2. Demonstrate how to rinse mouth after eating.

3. Advise parents on the introduction of solid foods; semi-upright position or upright position; avoid spicy or acidic foods, which may irritate the oral and nasal cavities; avoid hard, sharp-edged foods, such as raw carrots or potato chips.

4. Advise on increased risk of ear infections and need to seek medical attention for colds, ear pain, fever, or other signs and symptoms. Frequent hearing screens and tympanometry should be done to monitor the effects of middle ear pathology. *Note:* Hearing should be monitored at least every 6 months during the 1st year of life and then annually to prevent hearing impairment.

5. Encourage modeling "good speech" by providing a stimulating language environment, and encourage spontaneous imitations of sounds at home.

6. Stress the importance of speech therapy and practicing exercises as directed by the speech therapist.

7. Encourage thorough brushing of teeth, regular dental examinations, and fluoride treatment as indicated because of risk of tooth decay related to defective enamel and abnormally positioned teeth with clefts.

8. Advise the parents on current therapies available: bone grafting providing permanent teeth support, dental implants to replace missing teeth, and speech prosthesis for incomplete velopharyngeal closure.

9. Help the parents realize that, although rehabilitation is extensive, their child can live a normal life.

10. For additional information and support, refer patients and family to the American Cleft Palate-Craniofacial Association (*www.acpa-cpf.org*).

11. Refer families to companies that manufacture bottles for cleft palate: Enfamil (Mead Johnson) Cleft Palate Nurser, 1-800-222-9123; Medela Haberman Feeder, 1-800-435-8316; Pigeon Bottle (Children's Medical Ventures), 1-888-766-8443.

Evaluation: Expected Outcomes

• Infant feeds with appropriate feeding device in small amounts every 2 to 3 hours.

• No signs of infection.

• Parents involved with care; demonstrate contact with infant as seen by holding and talking to infant.

• Proper positioning maintained, no signs of aspiration.

• Parents demonstrate proper feeding technique as evidenced by adequate nutrition and weight gain.

• Parents and child prepared for surgery.

• Parents express understanding of postoperative home care procedures and identify supportive resources.

Esophageal Atresia with Tracheoesophageal Fistula

EVIDENCE BASE Krishnan, U., Mousa, H., Dall'Oglio, L., et al. (2016). ESPGHAN-NASPGHAN guidelines for the evaluation and treatment of gastrointestinal and nutritional complications in children with esophageal atresia-tracheoesophageal fistula. *Journal of Pediatric Gastroenterology and Nutrition, 63*(5), 550–570.

Okata, Y., Maeda, K., & Bitoh, Y. (2016). Evaluation of the intraoperative risk factors for esophageal anastomotic complications after primary repair of esophageal atresia with tracheoesophageal fistula. *Pediatric Surgery International, 32*(9), 869–873.

Esophageal atresia (EA) is failure of the esophagus to form a continuous passage from the pharynx to the stomach during embryonic development. EA can occur with *tracheoesophageal fistula (TEF)*, which is an abnormal connection between the trachea and esophagus. EA/TEF occurs in approximately 1 in 3,500 births.

Clinically, EA/TEF is divided equally into isolated EA and syndromic EA. Additional defects vary in severity, with cardiac anomalies as the most common (14.7% to 28%) and life threatening. Currently, an overall survival of 85% to 90% has been reported from developed countries. In developing countries, however, several factors contribute to higher mortality rates. Such factors include prematurity, delay in diagnosis with an increased incidence of aspiration pneumonia, and a shortage of qualified nurses.

Pathophysiology and Etiology

1. Cause is unknown in most cases and likely multifactorial. Possible influences include:
   a. Low evidence for inheritable genetic factor.
   b. Six to ten percent due to chromosomal (structural) abnormalities, including trisomies (12, 18, 21), and partial deletions such as 13q13-qter, 22q11.2.
   c. Teratogenic stimuli, such as the anticancer drug adriamycin and diethylstilbestrol (DES).
2. Failure of proper separation of the embryonic channel into the esophagus and trachea occurring during the 4th and 5th weeks of gestation.
3. Esophageal atresia can be classified as (see Figure 48-2):
   a. *Type I* (Type A): proximal and distal segments of esophagus are blind; there is no connection to trachea; accounts for approximately 7% of cases; second most common.
   b. *Type II* (Type B): proximal segment of esophagus opens into trachea by a fistula; distal segment is blind; rare, 0.8% of cases.
   c. *Type III* (Type C): proximal segment of esophagus has blind end; distal segment of esophagus connects into trachea by a fistula; most common, with 86% of cases. (Discussion is limited to this type.)
   d. *Type IV* (Type D): esophageal atresia with fistula between proximal and distal ends of trachea and esophagus (rare, 0.7% of cases).
   e. *Type V* (Type E): proximal and distal segments of esophagus open into trachea by a fistula; no esophageal atresia but sometimes referred to as an H-type fistula; occurs in 4.2% of cases; not usually diagnosed at birth.

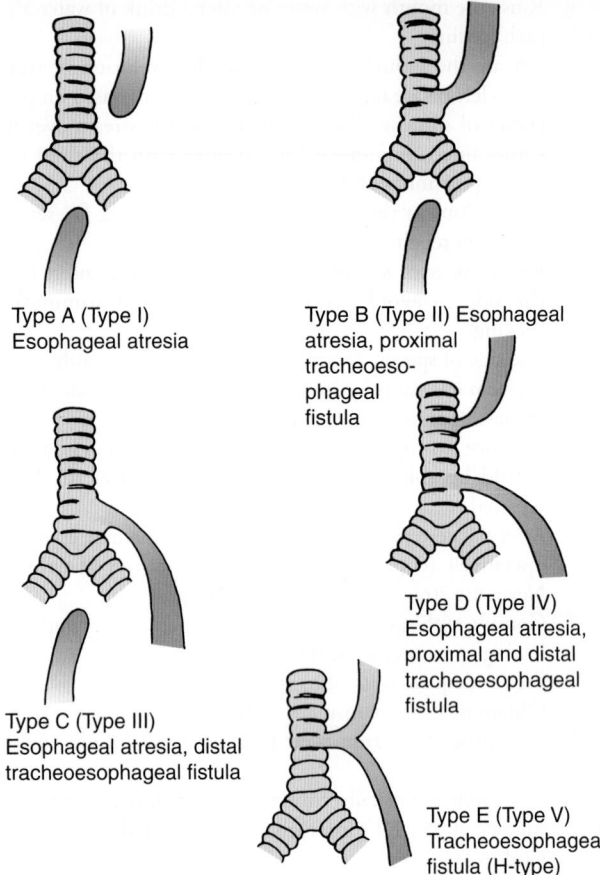

Type A (Type I) Esophageal atresia

Type B (Type II) Esophageal atresia, proximal tracheoesophageal fistula

Type C (Type III) Esophageal atresia, distal tracheoesophageal fistula

Type D (Type IV) Esophageal atresia, proximal and distal tracheoesophageal fistula

Type E (Type V) Tracheoesophageal fistula (H-type)

Figure 48-2. Types of esophageal atresia: esophageal atresia and tracheoesophageal fistula.

4. Associations:
   a. Down syndrome.
   b. VACTERL syndrome (vertebral defects, anal atresia, cardiac anomaly, TEF fistula with EA, renal defects, and radial limb dysplasia).
   c. Feingold syndrome.

 EVIDENCE BASE Svoboda, E., Fruithof, J., Widenmann-Grolig, A., et al. (2018). A patient led, international study of long term outcomes of esophageal stresia: EAT 1. *Journal of Pediatric Surgery, 53*(4), 610–615.

Clinical Manifestations

These appear soon after birth.
1. Excessive secretions.
   a. Constant drooling.
   b. Large amount of secretions from nose.
   c. Saliva or formula accumulates in upper esophageal pouch and is aspirated into airway.
2. Intermittent, unexplained cyanosis and laryngospasm.
   a. Caused by aspiration of accumulated saliva in blind pouch.
   b. Gastric acid is regurgitated through distal fistula.
3. Abdominal distention.
   a. Occurs as a result of air entering the lower esophagus through the fistula and passing into the stomach, especially when the child is crying.

4. Violent response after first or second swallow of feeding.
   a. Infant coughs and chokes.
   b. Fluid returns through nose and mouth.
   c. Cyanosis occurs.
   d. Infant struggles.
5. Poor feeding.
6. Inability to pass catheter through nose or mouth into stomach; tip of catheter stops at blind pouch, or atresia. *Note:* Be aware of coiling of catheter; coiling may make catheter appear to be descending into stomach.
7. Infant can be premature and pregnancy complicated by polyhydramnios. Look for other birth anomalies.

Diagnostic Evaluation

1. Ultrasound scanning techniques enable TEF to be identified *in utero* for some infants.
2. Failure to pass a 10F catheter (smaller catheters may coil) into the stomach through nose or mouth. Catheter is left *in situ* while an x-ray confirms the diagnosis.
3. pH of tracheal secretions is acidic.
4. Flat-plate x-ray of abdomen and chest may reveal presence of gas in stomach and catheter coiled in the blind pouch. Barium x-ray may be used in some cases.
5. Electrocardiogram and echocardiogram are performed because there is a high association with cardiac anomalies.

Management

Immediate Treatment

1. Propping infant at 30-degree angle, supine or side-lying, to prevent reflux of gastric contents.
2. Nasogastric (NG) tube remains in the esophagus and is aspirated frequently to prevent aspiration until continuous low suction is applied.
3. Pouch is washed out with normal saline to prevent thick mucus from blocking the tube.
4. Gastrostomy to decompress stomach and prevent aspiration; later used for feedings.
5. Nothing by mouth (NPO); IV fluids.
6. Comorbidities, such as pneumonitis and heart failure, are treated.
7. Supportive therapy includes meeting nutritional requirements, IV fluids, antibiotics, respiratory support, and maintaining thermally neutral environment.

Surgery

1. Prompt primary repair: fistula found by bronchoscopy is divided, followed by esophageal anastomosis of proximal and distal segments if infant weight permits and is without pneumonia.
2. Short-term delay: subsequent primary repair is used to stabilize infant and prevent deterioration when the patient's condition contraindicates immediate surgery.
3. Staging: initially, fistula division and gastrostomy are performed with later secondary esophageal anastomosis or colonic transposition performed approximately 1 year later to effect total repair. Approach may be used with a very small, premature infant or a very sick neonate or when severe congenital anomalies exist.
4. Circular esophagomyotomy may be performed on proximal pouch to gain length and allow for primary anastomosis at initial surgery.
5. Cervical esophagostomy: when ends of esophagus are too widely separated, esophageal replacement with segment

of intestine (colonic transposition) is done at ages 18 to 24 months.
6. Fiber-optic tracheoscopy-assisted repair of TEF can expedite and facilitate surgery on ventilated patients.
7. Staged repair resulted in least amount of GI dysmotility postoperatively.

 EVIDENCE BASE Lal, D., Gadepalli, S., Downard, C., et al. (2017). Perioperative management and outcomes of esophageal atresia and tracheoesophageal fistula. *Journal of Pediatric Surgery, 52*(8), 1245–1251.

Complications

Note: Higher rates of complications occur in patients with cardiac anomalies and low birth weight.
1. Death from asphyxia.
2. Pneumonitis/pneumonia secondary to salivary aspiration and/or gastric acid reflux.
3. Leak at anastomosis site: most common and dangerous complication (15% to 20%).
4. Recurrent fistulas.
5. Esophageal strictures (30% to 40%).
6. Abnormal function of distal esophagus sphincter (gastroesophageal reflux (GER) can be found in approximately 50% of these infants).
7. Esophagitis.
8. Tracheomalacia (10% to 20% of these patients).
9. Gastroesophageal Reflux Disease (GERD) (40% to 65%).
10. Feeding problems with older children due to esophageal dysmotility (95%).

Nursing Assessment

Assessment begins immediately after birth.
1. Be alert for risk factors of polyhydramnios and prematurity.
2. Suspect in infant with the following:
   a. Excessive amount of mucus.
   b. Difficulty with secretions.
   c. Cyanotic episodes (unexplained).
3. Report suspicion to health care provider immediately.

Nursing Diagnoses

Preoperative

- Risk for Aspiration related to structural abnormality.
- Risk for Deficient Fluid Volume related to inability to take oral fluids.
- Anxiety of parents related to critical situation of neonate.

Postoperative

- Ineffective Airway Clearance related to surgical intervention.
- Ineffective Infant Feeding Pattern related to defect.
- Acute Pain related to surgical procedure.
- Impaired Tissue Integrity related to postoperative drainage.
- Risk for Injury related to complex surgery.
- Risk for Impaired Attachment related to prolonged hospitalization.

Nursing Interventions

Preventing Aspiration

1. Position the infant supine with head and chest elevated 20 to 30 degrees to prevent or decrease reflux of gastric juices into the tracheobronchial tree.

a. This position may also ease respiratory effort by dropping the distended intestines away from the diaphragm.

b. Side-lying position can be used if the risk of aspiration from being supine is greater than the risk of sudden infant death syndrome (SIDS); supine positioning is preferred to reduce the risk of SIDS.

c. Turn frequently to prevent atelectasis and pneumonia.

2. Perform intermittent nasopharyngeal suctioning or maintain indwelling Sump tube with constant suction to remove secretions from esophageal blind pouch.

a. Tip of tube is placed in the blind pouch.

b. Sump tube allows air to be drawn in through a second lumen and prevents tube obstruction by mucous membrane of pouch.

c. Maintain indwelling tube patency by irrigating with 1 mL normal saline solution frequently.

3. Place the infant in an Isolette or under a radiant warmer with high humidity to aid in liquefying secretions and thick mucus. Maintain the infant's temperature in thermoneutral zone and ensure environmental isolation to prevent infection by using Isolette.

4. Administer oxygen, as needed.

5. Suction mouth to keep it clear of secretions and prevent aspiration. Provide mouth care.

6. Be alert for indications of respiratory distress.

a. Retractions.

b. Circumoral cyanosis.

c. Restlessness.

d. Nasal flaring.

e. Increased respiration and heart rate.

7. Maintain NPO status.

8. Administer antibiotics, as ordered, to prevent or treat associated pneumonitis.

9. Observe infant carefully for any change in condition; report changes immediately.

a. Check vital signs, color and amount of secretions, abdominal distention, and respiratory distress.

b. Evaluate for complications that can occur in any neonate or premature infant.

10. Be available and recognize need for emergency care or resuscitation.

a. Have resuscitation equipment on hand.

b. Accompany the infant to other departments and the operating room in Isolette with portable oxygen and suction equipment.

11. Monitor for signs or symptoms that may indicate additional congenital anomalies or complications.

12. Gastrostomy tube (GT) may be placed before definitive surgery to aid in gastric decompression, prevention of reflux, or nutrition.

Preventing Dehydration

1. Administer parenteral fluids and electrolytes as prescribed.

2. Monitor vital signs frequently for changes in blood pressure (BP) and pulse, which may indicate dehydration or fluid volume overload.

3. Record intake and output, including gastric drainage (if GT for decompression is present) and weight of diapers.

Reducing Parental Anxiety

1. Explain procedures and necessary events to parents as soon as possible.

2. Orient parents to hospital and intensive care nursery environment.

3. Allow family to hold and assist in caring for infant.

4. Offer reassurance and encouragement to family frequently. Provide for additional support by social worker, clergy, and counselor, as needed.

Maintaining Patent Airway

1. Keep endotracheal (ET) tube patent by frequent lavage and suction. *Note:* Reintubation could damage the anastomosis.

2. Suction frequently; every 5 to 10 minutes may be necessary, but at least every 1 to 2 hours.

3. Observe for signs of obstructed airway. Ventilatory support is continued until clinically stable (usually 24 to 48 hours).

4. Request that the surgeon mark a suction catheter, indicating how far the catheter can be safely inserted without disturbing the anastomosis (usually 2 to 3 cm).

5. Administer chest physiotherapy, as prescribed.

a. Change the infant's position by turning; stimulate crying to promote full expansion of lungs.

b. Elevate head and shoulders 20 to 30 degrees.

c. Use mechanical vibrator 2 to 3 days postoperatively (to minimize trauma to anastomosis), followed by more vigorous physical therapy after the 3rd day.

6. Continue use of Isolette or radiant warmer with humidity.

7. Be prepared for an emergency: have emergency equipment available, including suction machine, catheter, oxygen, laryngoscope, ET tubes in varying sizes.

 NURSING ALERT Care should be taken not to hyperextend the neck, causing stress to the operative site.

Providing Adequate Nutrition

Feedings may be given by mouth, by gastrostomy, or (rarely) by a feeding tube into the esophagus, depending on the type of operation performed and the infant's condition.

1. The gastrostomy is generally attached to gravity drainage postoperatively, then elevated and left open to allow for air to escape and gastric secretions to pass into the duodenum before feedings are begun.

2. Practice patterns differ regarding when to start feedings but generally minimal enteral nutrition is beneficial in promoting gut motility, decreasing bacterial overgrowth, and decreasing the stress on the liver; these "trickle" feedings are given at a rate of 5 to 20 mL/kg per day.

3. Give the infant a pacifier to suck during feedings, unless contraindicated.

4. Use care to prevent air from entering the stomach, thereby causing gastric distention and possible reflux.

5. Continue gastrostomy feedings until the infant can tolerate full feedings orally.

Providing Comfort Measures

1. Position comfortably.

2. Avoid restraints when possible.

3. Administer mouth care frequently.

4. Offer pacifier frequently.

5. Assess for pain and administer analgesics, as ordered (see page 1150).

6. Caress and speak or sing to the infant frequently. Handling should be kept to a gentle minimum.

Maintaining Chest Drainage

1. Assess type of chest drainage present (determined by surgical approach). Report saliva or hemorrhage.

a. Retropleural—small tube in posterior mediastinum; may be left open for drainage.

b. Transthoracic—chest tube placed in pleural space and connected to suction.

2. Keep tubing patent: free from clots, unkinked, and without tension.

3. If a break occurs in the closed drainage system, immediately clamp tubing close to the infant to prevent pneumothorax.

Observing for Complications

1. Inspect for leak at the anastomosis, causing mediastinitis, pneumothorax, and saliva in chest tube: hypothermia or hyperthermia, severe respiratory distress, cyanosis, restlessness, and weak pulses.

2. Continue to monitor for complications during the recovery process.

a. Stricture at the anastomosis: difficulty in swallowing, vomiting, or spitting-up of ingested fluid; refusing to eat; fever secondary to aspiration and pneumonia.

b. Recurrent fistula: coughing, choking, and cyanosis associated with feeding; excessive salivation; difficulty in swallowing associated with abnormal distention; repeated episodes of pneumonitis; general poor physical condition (no weight gain).

c. Atelectasis or pneumonitis: aspiration, respiratory distress.

3. Provide meticulous care for cervical esophagostomy—artificial opening in the neck that allows for drainage of the upper esophagus.

a. Keep the area clean of saliva.

b. Wash with clear water.

c. Place an absorbent pad over the area.

4. As soon as possible, allow the infant to suck a few milliliters of milk at the same time gastrostomy feeding is being done. Advance the infant to solid foods, as appropriate, if esophagostomy is maintained for a few months.

a. Encourage sucking and swallowing.

b. Familiarize the infant with food so that when able to eat orally, infant will be used to it.

5. Begin oral feedings 10 to 14 days postoperatively after anastomosis, as directed.

a. Feed slowly to allow the infant time to swallow.

b. Use upright sitting position to avoid risk of regurgitation.

c. Burp frequently or vent GT.

d. Do not allow the infant to become overtired at feeding time. Note heart rate.

e. Try to make each feeding a pleasant experience for the infant. Use a consistent approach and patience. Encourage parental involvement.

Stimulating Parent–Infant Attachment

1. Gently hold and cuddle the infant for feedings and after feedings.

2. Encourage parents to cuddle and talk to the infant.

3. Provide for visual, auditory, and tactile stimulation, as appropriate, for the infant's physical condition and age.

4. Provide opportunities for the parents to learn all aspects of care of their infant.

5. Encourage the parents to talk about their feelings, fears, and concerns.

6. Help to develop a healthy parent–child relationship through flexible visiting, frequent phone calls, and encouraging physical contact between child and parents.

Community and Home Care Considerations

 EVIDENCE BASE Holscher, A., Laschat, M., Choinitzki, V., et al. (2017). Quality of life after surgical treatment for esophageal atresia: Long-term outcomes of 154 patients. *European Journal of Pediatric Surgery*, 27(5), 443–448.

1. Teach carefully and thoroughly all procedures to be done at home. Show the parents how to do them and then watch return demonstration of the following procedures:

a. Gastrostomy feedings and care.

b. Esophagostomy care with feeding technique.

c. Suctioning.

d. Identifying signs of respiratory distress.

2. Advise parents that esophageal motility will be affected for many years, because of the narrowed abnormal esophagus emptying slowly and tension on the stomach from the anastomosis.

3. Reflux may increase after surgery and thus should be maximally treated because of the risk of developing esophageal strictures.

4. Monitor weight gain and developmental progress.

5. Observe parental feeding technique.

6. Encourage parents to discuss child's condition with day care workers, teachers, school nurse, or other responsible adults in close contact with the child so that they will be able to recognize possible problems and reinforce good eating habits.

7. To compensate for altered motility, encourage cutting food into small pieces, chewing food well, swallowing food with fluid, and sitting upright while eating.

8. Observe parent–child interaction to assess for overprotection and appropriate coping skills.

Family Education and Health Maintenance

 EVIDENCE BASE Menzies, J., Hughes, J., Leach, S., et al. (2017). Prevalence of malnutrition and feeding difficulties in children with esophageal atresia. *Journal of Pediatric Gastroenterology & Nutrition*, 64(4), 100–105.

Singh, A., Middlesworth, W., & Khlevner, J. (2017). Surveillance in patients with esophageal atresia/tracheoesophageal fistula. *Current Gastroenterology Reports*, 19(1), 4.

1. Help the parents understand the psychological needs of the infant for sucking, warmth, comfort, stimulation, and affection. Suggest that activity be appropriate for age.

2. Encourage the parents to continue close medical follow-up, and help them learn to recognize possible problems.

a. Eating problems may occur, especially when solids are introduced.

b. Repeated respiratory tract infection should be reported.

c. Occurrence of stricture at site of anastomosis weeks to months later may be recognized by difficulty in swallowing, spitting of ingested fluid, and fever. Continue all reflux medications until advised otherwise. Medications should be adjusted by weight as infant grows.

d. Dilatation of esophagus may be necessary to treat stricture at the site of the anastomosis.

e. Signs of fistula leakage are dusky color or choking with feeding.

3. Help the parents understand the need for good nutrition and the need to follow the diet regimen suggested by the health care provider.
4. Reassure parents that an infant's raspy cough is normal and will gradually diminish as the infant's trachea becomes stronger over 6 to 24 months (most infants have some tracheomalacia).
5. Teach parents to guard against the child swallowing foreign objects.
6. Help and support can be given by introducing the parents to other parents of children with TEF.
7. For additional information and support, refer parents to EA/TEF Family Support Connection (*www.eatef.org*), TEF Vater (*www.tefvater.org*), Birth Defect Research for Children (*www.birthdefects.org*), International Foundation for Functional Gastrointestinal Disorders (*www.aboutkidsgi.org*), Boston Children's Hospital (*www.childrenshospital.org*), or the March of Dimes Foundation (*www.marchofdimes.org*).

Evaluation: Expected Outcomes

- No cyanosis or respiratory distress.
- Hydrated; urine output adequate.
- Parents hold and talk to infant; express concerns.
- Postoperatively, tolerates gastrostomy feedings without distention or regurgitation.
- Infant thrives, with adequate weight gain.
- Infant sleeps and rests without irritability or pain.
- Chest tube in place with minimal drainage.
- Feeds without regurgitation 12 days postoperatively.
- Parents caring for infant postoperatively and assisting with feedings.

Gastroesophageal Reflux and Gastroesophageal Reflux Disease

 EVIDENCE BASE Rosen, R., Vandenplas, Y., Singendonk, M., et al. (2018). Pediatric gastroesophageal reflux clinical practice guidelines: Joint recommendations of the North American Society for Pediatric Gastroenteroloyg, Hepatology, and Nutrition and the European Society for Pediatric Gastroenterology, Hepatology, and Nutrition. *JPGN, 66*(3), 516–544.

GER is the passage of gastric contents into the esophagus. The barrier between the stomach and esophagus is controlled primarily by pressure at the lower esophageal sphincter (LES). GER is a normal physiologic process and occurs in all healthy infants and children, usually several times a day, without symptoms or sequelae. Of all infants with GER, 50% will be symptomatic (vomiting or regurgitation) during the first 3 months of life; 67% of infants ages 4 to 9 months will have symptoms; and 5% of ages 10 to 12 months will have symptoms. Symptomatic GER often self-resolves by 12 to 14 months of age.

GERD is defined as the symptom complex that results as a complication of GER. GERD is used to describe a condition when this reflux process causes bothersome symptoms and complications, such as significant discomfort and altered feeding and sleeping patterns. Clinical manifestations include vomiting, dysphagia, food refusal, poor weight gain, failure to thrive (FTT), esophagitis, irritability/excessive crying, abdominal pain, substernal pain, respiratory disorders, asthma, and apparent life-threatening events (ALTE) or apnea.

The North American Society for Pediatric Gastroenterology, Hepatology, and Nutrition has formulated guidelines for the diagnosis and management of GER and GERD in infants and children; however, these guidelines are not intended for the management of neonates less than 72 hours old, premature neonates, or infants/children with neurologic or anatomic abnormalities of the upper GI tract. The American Academy of Pediatrics has also endorsed these guidelines.

Supportive care by nurses and other health care staff regarding feeding techniques and nutrition is often sufficient for patients with GER. GERD may require additional interventions such as changes to feeding regimen or medication therapy.

Pathophysiology and Etiology

Gastroesophageal Reflux
1. The LES is a physiologic, rather than an anatomic, segment that forms an antireflux barrier.
   a. 2 to 5 cm in length.
   b. Characterized by a pressure greater than that found proximally in the esophagus or distally in the stomach.
   c. Constitutes an effective barrier to protect the esophageal mucosa and airway passages from damage by gastric contents (acid, pepsin, bile salts, food).
   d. Neuromuscular connection is weak in infants, and GER peaks at age 6 months and usually resolves by 12 months.

Gastroesophageal Reflux Disease
1. Episodes of GERD with aspiration of refluxed material are more likely to occur during the nocturnal period—when the esophagus and stomach are leveled and the swallowing response to reflux and airway protection mechanisms are blunted by sleep.
2. Cause is undetermined in most patients; however, possible causes include:
   a. Delayed neuromuscular development.
   b. Cerebral defects.
   c. Obstruction at or just below the pylorus (eg, pyloric stenosis, malrotation).
   d. Physiologic immaturity.
   e. Increased abdominal pressure.
   f. Obesity.
   g. Cystic fibrosis.
   h. Congenital esophageal disease.
3. Associated conditions that contribute to reflux include:
   a. Chronic lung disease—there is a higher incidence of reflux in infants with this condition. It appears to be related to the duration of the episode and how proximal the reflux occurs, possibly contributing to poor clearance.
   b. Trauma/mechanical causes that affect the LES.
      i. Indwelling orogastric/NG enteric feeding tube.
      ii. Surgery on the esophagus or stomach.
      iii. Mechanical ventilation.
      iv. Extreme changes in position; lying completely flat; seating devices for infants greater than a 30% incline (increases intra-abdominal pressure).
      v. Hiatal hernia.
   c. Studies show a reduced incidence of reflux in the prone position versus the supine position; however, the American Academy of Pediatrics' "Back to Sleep" program discourages prone positioning because of increased incidence of SIDS.
   d. Protein allergy: increased inflammation in the mucosa of the esophagus and stomach, altering motility.
   e. Medications/drugs that affect LES and increase gastric acidity, such as bronchodilators, antihypertensives,

diazepam, meperidine, morphine, prostaglandins, calcium channel blockers, nitrate heart medications, anticholinergics, adrenergic drugs, caffeine, alcohol, and nicotine.
f. Cystic fibrosis, cardiac disease, and other chronic illnesses.

Clinical Manifestations of GERD

Infants
1. Vomiting or regurgitation of formula or breast milk.
2. Irritability, excessive crying with or without association with vomiting.
3. Sleep disturbances.
4. Arching, stiffening.
5. It is recommended that the infant be referred to a pediatric gastroenterologist if the following manifestations occur:
   a. Refusal to eat.
   b. Weight loss or failure to gain weight.
   c. Dehydration.
   d. Recurrent respiratory symptoms, such as cough, wheezing, stridor, pneumonia, otitis media, bronchitis.
   e. BRUE (brief, resolved, unexplained event): blue spell, decreased responsiveness, limp, apnea, bradycardia. (*Note:* The exact relationship between GER and BRUE is not clear despite continued investigation. Indeed, both apnea and reflux are common in premature neonates.)
   f. Eructation (belching).
   g. Sandifer syndrome (rare)—dystonic posturing caused by reflux.
   h. Anemia (from chronic esophagitis).
   i. Hematemesis (vomitus with blood).
   j. Occult blood in stool.
   k. Hypoproteinemia: low albumin due to severe inflammation and protein losses in the GI tract; can be seen with or without malnutrition and FTT.

Older Children
1. Intermittent vomiting.
2. Chronic heartburn or regurgitation.
3. Upper abdominal discomfort; pressure or "squeezing" feeling.
4. Chronic respiratory/airway symptoms, such as cough, stridor, otitis media, bronchitis, asthma.
5. Food refusal.
6. Dysphagia: difficulty swallowing.
7. Odynophagia: painful swallowing.
8. Anemia (from chronic esophagitis).
9. Hematemesis.
10. Hypoproteinemia.
11. Occult blood in stool.

Diagnostic Evaluation

1. History and physical exam can diagnose most cases.
2. Multiple intraluminal impedance and esophageal pH monitoring can be performed on all ages; no sedation necessary.
   a. Performed over 24 hours but does not indicate whether aspiration is occurring.
   b. Used as an index of esophageal acid exposure; however, esophageal impedance studies have been found to be more accurate, especially in the neurologically impaired child.
   c. The child must be off acid-suppressing medications for 48 to 72 hours so that acid pH can be detected.

d. Gastric motility medications may or may not be held depending on the reason for performing the study.
e. Most centers allow the patient to go home and return 24 hours later. Exceptions include the fragile child, premature infant, infant with active respiratory symptoms, or the child with significant symptoms who requires close observation because reflux may exacerbate while off reflux medications.
f. Not indicated in the infant/child who is vomiting, unable to tolerate bolus feedings, or acutely ill. Because the probe is inserted in nares, infant/children with oxygen requirements may not tolerate the study.
3. Endoscopy and biopsy allow for visualization of esophageal, gastric, and duodenal mucosa.
   a. Indicated for severe GERD or failure of medical management.
   b. Biopsy can determine cause: allergy (eosinophilic), inflammation, chemical injury, or Barrett esophagus.
   c. Mechanical problems such as strictures, webs, and duplication/cysts will be visualized.
   d. For this procedure, sedation and anesthesia are necessary.
   e. Reflux medications do not have to be discontinued for the study.
   f. Can be done on the child who is not tolerating feedings. However, severity of illness may prevent study from being performed because of risk associated with procedure, such as with anesthesia, infection, bleeding, and cardiac.
4. Technetium scintigraphy (milk/emptying scan) to assess gastric emptying and associated aspiration. This is not a reliable test for determining GERD.
   a. Sedation is not necessary, and the study can be performed on children of all ages.
   b. Involves drinking/eating food with radionuclide, followed by dynamic sequenced imaging.
   c. Not indicated in the infant/child who is vomiting, unable to tolerate bolus feedings, or acutely ill.
   d. Acid suppression medications do not interfere with the study.
5. Modified barium swallow—also called *videofluoroscopy*.
   a. Assesses oral pharyngeal function and potential for aspiration from oral intake using several consistencies of feedings. This is not a reliable test for determining GERD.
   b. Sedation is not necessary for this procedure but does require cooperation with eating.
   c. Should not be performed on the infant/child with acute respiratory symptoms or one identified by speech therapy or occupational therapy as being at risk for aspiration.
   d. Reflux medications do not have to be discontinued for the study.
   e. Speech therapist can be present for the exam to offer detailed assessment of oral–motor skills and swallowing.
6. Esophageal manometry to measure pressure inside the LES.
   a. It is a cooperative, nonsedated procedure and can only be used on an older child.
   b. Reflux medications generally do not have to be discontinued for the study.
7. Intraluminal esophageal impedance to detect the flow of liquids and gas through the esophagus may be used in combination with manometry.
8. Polysomnography may be used for evaluation of infant apnea and sleep apnea.

Complications

Complications result from frequent and sustained reflux of gastric contents into lower esophagus.
1. Recurrent pulmonary disease.
2. Chronic esophagitis.
3. FTT.
4. Anemia.
5. ALTE, although evidence is not strong.
6. Esophageal stricture from scarring.
7. Barrett esophagus: the replacement of distal esophageal mucosa with a potentially malignant metaplastic epithelium caused by chronic exposure to acid.
8. Chronic sinusitis/otitis media.
9. There is an unclear relationship between GERD and dental erosion/caries.

Management

Goal of treatment is to alleviate and relieve symptoms and prevent complications. May be treated medically through careful positioning, feeding techniques, and medication or surgically.

Positioning for GER
1. Esophageal monitoring has demonstrated that infants have significantly fewer episodes of GER when prone. Several studies support less incidence of reflux episodes in the prone and left-side sleeping position; however, the North American Society for Pediatric Gastroenterology, Hepatology and Nutrition, along with the American Academy of Pediatrics, endorses the following recommendations:
   a. Place infant with head elevation or left lateral position after feeding when awake, not for sleep.
   b. Handle the infant gently, with minimal movement during and after feeding.

Feeding for GER
1. Small, frequent feedings followed by upright positioning with infant held over the shoulder.
2. Thickened feedings with dry rice cereal (1 tbsp per ounce of formula) or commercial thickening agent may be used. Thickening does not decrease episodes of reflux but does decrease episodes of vomiting. Commercial formulas thickened with rice starch are now available, but no studies regarding their efficacy have been published. Thickening of breast milk may be necessary in infants with poor weight gain.
3. Continuance of breast-feeding with the mother eliminating milk and soy products is encouraged, as allergen sensitivity can contribute to GER. No studies support the need for dietary restriction in mothers who breast-feed, but in anecdotal reports, infants appear to improve when dairy products are reduced. Two to four week trial of partially hydrolyzed formula is useful for refractory symptoms or for those infants/children with signs of allergy, anemia, constipation, occult positive stools, and vomiting. Hypoallergenic (elemental) formula may be used if symptoms persist.
4. Pectin liquid partially decreases GER, as measured by esophageal pH monitoring, and might improve vomiting and respiratory symptoms in children with cerebral palsy.
5. Concentrating formula is a method of increasing calories for the volume-sensitive infant.
6. Avoid constant feeding (grazing), which reduces appetite and, ultimately, caloric intake.
7. Comfort the infant to reduce crying before and after meals, which increases intra-abdominal pressure and swallowing of air, increasing the likelihood of reflux.
8. Use a pacifier for nonnutritive sucking after eating to avoid overeating.

Feeding for GERD
1. Transgastric (transpyloric) enteric feeding tube used for infants when reflux medical management fails and symptoms persist; can reduce number of reflux episodes, but has not been shown to significantly reduce episodes of apnea.
   a. There are concerns regarding using these feeding tubes in neonates; however, the rate of complications does not appear to be statistically significant in recent reports.
   b. The procedure should be performed by a skilled pediatric radiologist or neonatal intensive care nurse, using a small-caliber soft polyurethane nonweighted feeding tube.
   c. Considered a temporary feeding method (to help infant/child gain weight and improve respiratory symptoms) until further options can be explored, such as surgery—Nissen fundoplication or jejunostomy.
   d. To prevent clogging, tubes should be flushed at least four to six times per day and before and after medication administration. If the tube clogs or dislodges, the family must return to a qualified center for reinsertion.
   e. If feeding difficulty persists, consult dietitian and speech and/or occupational therapist.
2. Older child:
   a. Nothing to eat 2 hours before bedtime.
   b. Avoid spicy and acidic foods (onions, citrus products, apple juice, tomatoes), esophageal irritants (chocolate, caffeinated beverages, peppermint, and secondhand smoke), and carbonated beverages.
   c. Chew gum (stimulates parotid secretions, which augment esophageal clearance and provide a buffering effect).

Other Lifestyle Changes for GERD
1. Prevent obesity.
2. Avoid tight or constrictive clothing.
3. Avoid nonsteroidal anti-inflammatory drugs, especially at bedtime.

Drug Therapy for GERD
1. Often used in combination with lifestyle changes. Prescribed for a 4 to 8 week trial and can be tapered and discontinued if symptoms resolve.
2. Antacids—buffer existing acids and also increase serum gastrin levels, leading to increase in LES pressure (symptomatic relief). Chronic antacid therapy is generally not recommended unless ordered by a gastroenterologist.
3. Histamine-2 (H_2) receptor antagonists—act by reducing hydrochloric acid and pepsinogen secretion by blocking histamine receptors on the parietal cells.
   a. Cimetidine, ranitidine, famotidine, nizatidine.
   b. Oral dosing of tid versus bid has demonstrated improved duration of acid suppression in one study of infants (44% vs. 90%).
   c. Tolerance to IV dosing within 6 weeks of usage has been observed.
4. Proton-pump inhibitors (PPIs)—block all gastric acid secretion by binding and deactivating the H^+/K^+ ATPase enzyme pumps. To be activated, PPIs require acid in the parietal cell

canaliculus; therefore, they are most effective when the parietal cells are stimulated by a meal following a fast.

a. Omeprazole, lansoprazole, pantoprazole, esomeprazole, rabeprazole.

b. Generally given 15 to 30 minutes before a meal, one to two times per day.

c. Generally not recommended in combination with H_2-antagonists because of interference with absorption (H_2 reduces the acid necessary for PPI to work).

d. Reserved for infants and children resistant to H_2-antagonist therapy. Gastroenterology specialist should be involved. Data on the pharmacology in infants and children are limited.

e. Dominant regurgitation in neonates and infants responds poorly to PPIs.

5. Prokinetic agents—enhances esophageal peristalsis and accelerates gastric emptying. However there is insufficient evidence of efficacy in GERD.

a. Metoclopramide—an antidopaminergic agent whose efficacy is not well observed in clinical trials. Adverse effects include parkinsonian reactions, tardive dyskinesia, irritability, sleeplessness, and lowered seizure threshold.

b. Erythromycin at low dose: motility receptor agonist. Can be associated with dysrhythmia and increased incidence of hypertrophic pyloric stenosis. Contraindicated in some patients with preexisting cardiac conditions.

6. A surface agent sucralfate may be used—an aluminum complex that acts by adhering to mucosal lesions, reducing symptoms, and promoting healing.

a. May be used as an adjunct to an H_2 blocker or PPI, and usually for a period of several weeks or less.

b. If used for esophagitis, should be made into a liquid preparation.

c. If used for ulcer or gastritis, it is inhibited by H_2 blockers and PPIs because of the need for an acidic environment.

 DRUG ALERT All acid-altering medications may affect the efficacy of pH-dependent medications. Additionally, PPIs are metabolized to varying degrees by the hepatic cytochrome P450 enzymatic system and may alter drug metabolism by induction or inhibition of the cytochrome P enzymes.

 DRUG ALERT The potential adverse effects of aluminum in infants and children should be considered before administering sucralfate; data on its efficacy and safety in children are inadequate.

Surgical Management for GERD

 EVIDENCE BASE Jancelewicz, T., Lopez, M., Downward, C., et al. (2016). Surgical management of gastroesophageal reflux disease (GERD) in children: A systematic review. *Journal of Pediatric Surgery, 52*(8), 1228–1238.

1. Nissen fundoplication is the most commonly used surgical method to treat moderate to severe GERD that is unresponsive to medication therapy. Decisions concerning appropriate long-term feeding access must be individualized.

a. Involves wrapping of the fundus around the LES (see Figure 48-3).

View of stomach after the surgery

Figure 48-3. Nissan fundoplication for gastroesophageal reflux disease.

b. Overall complication rate ranges from 2.2% to 45%.

c. Other surgical approaches include ventral (Thal) or dorsal (Toupet) semifundoplication.

d. In some studies, recurrence of reflux in the neurodisabled child is as high as 46%.

e. Simultaneous gastrostomy is usually performed for feeding purposes or as a temporary measure to decompress the stomach.

f. The most commonly reported complications of surgery include breakdown of the wrap, small bowel obstruction, gas bloat syndrome, infection, perforation, leaking at the anastomosis site, persistent esophageal stricture, esophageal obstruction, dumping syndrome, incisional hernia, and gastroparesis.

g. Reoperation rates range from 3% to 18%.

h. The greater the complexity of the infant or child's health status, the greater the chance of complications.

2. Jejunostomy feeding tubes can be placed but are usually restricted to severe cases of recurrent GERD and/or failed Nissen procedure.

a. Most surgeons use either a standard GT or a low-profile tube (button).

b. Complications include intestinal obstruction and leaking.

Other Treatments under Investigation

Investigation is underway to identify pathways and mechanisms that interfere or control the transient relaxation of the LES. Future understanding of this mechanism will aid in the development of lifestyle changes and medical management, which will assist in inhibiting transient relaxations. Reduction of gastric mechanoreceptor signaling to the brain has emerged as one of the likely sites of action for new reflux inhibitor drugs. The most promising among these appear to be the $GABA_B$ receptor agonists and metabotropic glutamate receptor 5 (mGluR5).

Nursing Assessment

1. Obtain history of infant's or child's eating habits, including formula history, food allergies, volume tolerated at each meal.

2. Obtain history of complications from GER (ie, recurrent respiratory infections, asthma, poor weight gain).

3. Observe infant's or child's feeding behaviors. (Does child eat with a bottle, spoon, fingers? Can child feed self?)

4. Assess general appearance, skin integrity, and growth and development.

Nursing Diagnoses

- Risk for Aspiration related to reflux of gastric contents.
- Imbalanced Nutrition: Less Than Body Requirements related to decreased oral intake.
- Risk for Deficient Fluid Volume related to frequent vomiting.
- Fear of eating related to distress.

Nursing Interventions

Preventing Aspiration

1. Administer medications via IV line until tolerating enteral feedings.
   a. Administer prokinetics (motility agents) and acid suppressants 30 minutes before meals when bolus feeding schedule is instituted. Monitor for adverse effects.
   b. Unless abnormal gastric dysmotility prior to surgery, most prokinetics are discontinued after Nissen fundoplication.
2. Maintain positioning, as stated above.
3. Use cardiac and apnea monitors for infants and children with severe reflux.
   a. Observe for apneic periods of more than 20 seconds or accompanied by cyanosis, pallor, or bradycardia.
   b. Document apnea episodes, associated symptoms, and recovery efforts.
4. Provide chest physiotherapy before rather than after meals, if ordered.

 NURSING ALERT Avoid slouching position because this may change angle of esophagus in relation to stomach, increase intra-abdominal pressure, and facilitate reflux of stomach contents.

Maintaining Adequate Nutrition

See also section on feeding, page 1282.
1. Provide concentrated formula if volume cannot be tolerated.
2. Seek nutrition consult if patient continues to have difficulty feeding.
3. Monitor for fatigue during feeding; increased effort to suck requires higher energy expenditures. If noted, referral to occupational/speech therapy and possible modified barium swallow study are advised.
4. Monitor weight on the same scale.
5. Accurately record activity of infant.
   a. Amount of feeding taken; whether retained.
   b. Any change in behavior as a result of feeding technique.
6. Explain to the breast-feeding mother that feeding modifications may need to be made, especially in infants with poor weight gain. Assist her to express milk, quantitate volume, thicken with cereal, and fortify breast milk with formula, as needed.
7. Follow postoperative instructions on initiation of feedings.
8. If the child has a GT:
   a. Usually elevated and vented until return of bowel function.
   b. Monitor drainage, avoid kinking, and follow orders for positioning for straight drainage, elevation, or clamping.

Maintaining Fluid and Electrolyte Balance

1. Monitor vital signs and assess skin turgor for signs of dehydration.
2. Observe and record accurately urine output.
   a. Weigh diapers.
   b. Measure amount, frequency, color, and concentration of voided urine.
   c. Check specific gravity, if possible.
3. Monitor IV therapy, if ordered.
4. Monitor serum electrolytes, magnesium, phosphorus, and calcium. Replace, as ordered. Particular close monitoring is warranted if infant/child has draining gastrostomy.
5. Promote good skin care to prevent lesions of dry and delicate tissues.
   a. Change position frequently.
   b. Change soiled diapers promptly.
   c. Apply lotion and gently massage any reddened areas.

 NURSING ALERT If patient is malnourished, monitor for refeeding syndrome until laboratory studies are stable. Refeeding syndrome can cause intracellular shifting of electrolytes including calcium, magnesium, and phosphorus, resulting in death. Laboratory studies should be monitored daily or more frequently if abnormal.

Reducing Fear of Eating

1. Provide thickened feedings to increase satisfaction for the infant.
2. Identify and attempt to reduce stress, especially around mealtime.
3. Feed the child in a quiet, calm environment.
4. Children like routines; feed at routine intervals by the person with whom the child is familiar and comfortable.
5. For the older child, encourage participation in family dinnertime so the child observes eating as a pleasurable experience.
6. Advise parents that clinical specialists in feeding disorders are available.

Community and Home Care Considerations

1. Recognize that home health care referral is appropriate for the following situations:
   a. FTT: medication teaching and monitoring, teaching of formula preparation, positioning, weight.
   b. Respiratory complications/ALTE: medication teaching and monitoring, assessment of respiratory status, teaching of monitor/cardiopulmonary resuscitation (CPR), use of nebulizer.
   c. Nissen fundoplication (with GT): medication teaching and monitoring; wound assessment; monitoring of bloating; dumping syndrome; formula intolerance; GT teaching, including pump teaching, venting, medication administration, tube changing.
2. Recommend careful feeding and behavioral diary to monitor symptoms and improvements.
3. Recognize that school and community activities may affect compliance for older children; work with the family to devise individualized management strategies.
4. Assist parents to discuss medication and lunchtime behaviors with teacher and school nurse so consistency can be maintained.
5. Assess need for community services, such as respite care, especially for single parent.

Family Education and Health Maintenance

 EVIDENCE BASE Baird, D., Harker, D., & Karmes, A. (2015). Diagnosis and treatment of gastroesophageal reflux in infants and children. *American Family Physician, 92*(8), 705–714.

1. Plan a program of intensive parental teaching on how to handle and care for the infant. Explain rationale to parents. Make sure that they have proper equipment for propping the infant. Help the parents understand that it is not necessary to keep infant in infant seat or propped up at all times.
   a. Bathe or play with the infant before feeding.
   b. Change position about 1 hour after feeding.
   c. During the night after feeding, the infant can sleep in a semi-reclining (30 degrees) position.
   d. Expect occasional small amounts of vomiting.
2. Offer clear, concise instructions. Focus on parental fears. Discuss techniques to promote development of infants while facilitating bonding and normal parental behavior.
3. If infant or child is not demonstrating complication of GER (ie, GERD), assist parents in understanding that GER is self-limited; symptoms usually disappear within 12 months.
4. If complications exist (GERD), referral to pediatric gastroenterology and nutrition specialists is recommended.
5. If Nissen fundoplication has been performed:
   a. Teach gastrostomy care, if applicable (see page 1158). Make sure that the parents know how to use, clear, vent, assess, and replace the tube. Help them to understand the purpose of GT placement (feedings, venting, medications) and the need for surgical or gastroenterology follow-up care.
   b. Explain about potential complications and when to call the health care provider. Such complications include gagging, retching, bloating, abdominal distention, fever, vomiting, diaphoresis, lethargy, diarrhea, and weight loss. Generally, the family should contact the surgeon within the first 6 weeks postoperatively, whereas eventual follow-up is with the gastroenterologist.
   c. It usually takes 12 weeks to heal; if the GT becomes dislodged in this period, the patient should be taken to the emergency department immediately.
   d. Complications of a dislodged GT in the early postoperative period include peritonitis and bacteremia.
6. Help the parents understand the importance of follow-up for assessment of weight gain and development.
7. Assist with community resource planning (eg, education, advocacy, and financial assistance). Identify support groups.
8. Instruct parents and caregivers in CPR training before discharge of infant, if indicated.
9. Provide written and verbal instructions for medications and adverse effects.
10. Advise parents on when to call their health care provider in regard to their child's symptoms. Danger signs of dehydration include a decrease in wet diapers, listlessness, lethargy, reduced appetite, sunken fontanelle; those for aspiration include respiratory distress and cyanotic spells, fever.
11. Encourage family to contact their health care provider immediately with treatment concerns or problems.
12. For additional information and support, contact the North American Society of Pediatric Gastroenterology, Hepatology and Nutrition (*www.naspghan.org*), the United Ostomy Association *www.ostomy.org*, or the Pediatric/Adolescent Gastroesophageal Reflux Association (*www.reflux.org*).

Evaluation: Expected Outcomes

- Mild regurgitation immediately after feeding; no apnea or cyanosis noted.
- Takes regular feedings without significant symptoms; weight gain noted.
- Urine output adequate.
- Exhibits pleasure in eating.

Failure to Thrive/Malnutrition

 EVIDENCE BASE Becker, P., Carney, L., Corkins, L., et al. (2014). Consensus statement of the Academy of Nutrition and Dietetics/American Society for Parenteral and Enteral Nutrition: Indicators recommended for the identification and documentation of pediatric malnutrition (undernutrition). *Journal of the Academy of Nutrition and Dietetics, 114*(12), 1988–2000.

FTT, or *malnutrition*, is the inadequate physical development of an infant or child manifested as a deceleration in weight gain, a low weight/height ratio, or a low weight/height/head circumference ratio. The exact prevalence is unknown, although research suggests FTT accounts for 3% to 5% of pediatric hospital admissions. Children with FTT are at risk for adverse outcomes, such as short stature, behavior problems, and developmental delay. The Agency for Healthcare Research and Quality has an evidence-based practice program on which clinical guidelines can be developed. The primary causative factors of FTT are insufficient nutrition availability, inadequate absorption and/or utilization of nutrients, and added metabolic requirements.

Previously practitioners diagnosed FTT when a child's weight for age falls below the fifth percentile of the standard National Center for Health Statistics growth chart or if it crosses two major percentile lines. Recent research has validated using z scores, or standard deviations from the mean, of weight for height or body mass index to classify malnutrition:

Mild malnutrition: z score –1 to –1.9
Moderate malnutrition: z score –2 to –2.9
Severe malnutrition: z score –3 or greater

About 25% of normal infants will shift to a lower growth percentile in the first 2 years of life and then follow that percentile; this should not be diagnosed as FTT (see Standards of Care Guidelines 48-1, page 1286).

Pathophysiology and Etiology

1. FTT is a nutritional disorder having organic and nonorganic components.
   a. Organic FTT implies a major illness or organ system dysfunction as the etiology of the growth failure. It occurs equally in all populations and accounts for approximately 25% of FTT cases.
   b. Nonorganic FTT is the result of multiple psychosocial factors, including disturbances in parent–child interaction. This type accounts for 50% of cases of FTT and is most common among the psychosocially and economically deprived.
   c. The remaining 25% of cases represent mixed etiology.

STANDARDS OF CARE GUIDELINES 48-1
Care of a Child with a GI or Nutritional Disorder

When caring for a child with a GI or nutritional disorder:
- Monitor weight.
- Monitor urinary and bowel elimination.
- Monitor intake and output.
- Assess developmental milestone attainment.
- Provide and teach appropriate feeding products and techniques.
- Use most efficient position for feeding.
- Facilitate a calm, pleasant environment for feeding.
- Avoid foods that may inhibit absorption of nutrients or cause such symptoms as gas.
- Encourage and support parental involvement in care and feeding of the child.
- Encourage and support normal play and other activities for the child as condition allows.
- Identify and respond to signs and symptoms that may indicate lack of adequate nutrition or sign of complications.

This information should serve as a general guideline only. Each patient situation presents a unique set of clinical factors and requires nursing judgment to guide care, which may include additional or alternative measures and approaches.

---

2. Organic FTT has a pathophysiologic cause that reduces the availability of nutrients for maintenance and growth and is best divided into three categories:
   a. Insufficient nutrition because of the child's inability to feed properly, which may be a result of severe neurologic dysfunction, GER, or cleft palate/lip.
   b. Nutrition is adequate but poorly absorbed and/or utilized (malabsorption syndromes), which may result from chronic ileocecal intussusception, GER, milk protein allergy, malrotation of the colon, hypoplastic stomach, short bowel syndrome (anatomic and functional), pancreatic insufficiency (including cystic fibrosis), pyloric stenosis, inflammatory bowel disease, and acquired immunodeficiency syndrome.
   c. Associated disorders include asthma, cardiac failure, thyroiditis, congenital heart disease, neurologic lesions, hydronephrosis, adrenal hyperplasia, diabetes insipidus, cystic fibrosis, chronic or recurrent urinary tract infection (UTI), hypothyroidism, autoimmune disorders, and immunodeficiency.
3. Nonorganic FTT occurs in the absence of GI, endocrine, congenital, or chronic diseases. It is usually associated with psychological deprivation but can also be related to behavioral or economic problems. Multiple features of the parents, child, and environment interact over time, resulting in parent–child interaction that ultimately leads to under nutrition and under nurturance of the child.

Clinical Manifestations
Organic FTT
1. Retarded growth accompanied by manifestations of the underlying disease.

2. Weight loss in early stages. If poor intake continues, linear growth slows down or ceases. In latent stage, head circumference growth is retarded, indicating compromised brain development.
3. Developmental delays.
4. Infant stress—irritability, fussiness, jitteriness.
5. Feeding disorders—ineffective sucking, difficulty chewing, difficulty swallowing.
6. Clinical symptoms can include vomiting, hypothermia, lethargy, muscle wasting, decreased subcutaneous tissue, hypoalbuminemia, eczema, hair loss, and diarrhea.

Nonorganic FTT
1. Retarded growth.
2. Infant stress—irritability, fussiness, jitteriness.
3. Feeding disorders—ineffective sucking, difficulty chewing, difficulty swallowing.
4. Reduced energy level.
5. Difficult temperament.
6. Fitful sleep.
7. Reduced responsiveness and interaction with the environment.
8. Social isolation, lack of vocalization.
9. Spasticity or rigidity when touched.
10. Inability to make eye contact or smile.
11. Refusal to eat; rejection of foods.
12. Spits up, gags, coughs with feeding, rumination.

Parental Characteristics
1. Characteristics associated with parents of nonorganic FTT include lack of social and financial support, maladaptive relationships, alcohol or drug abuse, history of anxiety or depression, lack of parenting skills, family stress and crisis, absent father.
2. Postnatal depression corresponds to a higher association of FTT, but on its own, depression does not contribute to a higher incidence of FTT.

Diagnostic Evaluation
Comprehensive Assessment
1. FTT suggested if a child is falling off a previously established growth curve or falls below the 5th percentile. If FTT is of recent onset, weight but not height will fall below accepted standards. Depression of weight and height indicates chronic malnutrition.
2. Technique for evaluating growth—look at growth percentage of the median for that age. Divide the actual value of height or weight by median value for that age. For example, 12-month-old female weighs 15 pounds (6.8 kg); the median for age is 21 1/2 pounds (9.8 kg). Child is 70% of median for age.
3. Complete health and dietary history—feeding, eating patterns, 3-day calorie count.
4. Physical examination for evidence of organic causes, with particular attention to ears, facial structure, mouth, heart, lungs, abdomen, and neurologic system.
5. Assessment of prenatal, perinatal, and postnatal infections.
6. Developmental assessment.
7. Family assessment—family short stature syndrome, family dynamics.
   a. With the assistance of endocrinologist and dietitian, calculate the midparental height:
   {(Father's height in cm + mother's height in cm) + 13 cm} divided by 2

Note: Subtract 13 cm for girls and add 13 cm for boys. For example, if the father is 180 cm and the mother is 167 cm, the daughter's equation would be {(180 + 167) – 13} ÷ 2.

 NURSING ALERT Children whose weight is less than 60% of the median value for age or less than 70% for height are in acute danger of severe morbidity and malnutrition.

Tests to Rule Out Organic Conditions

1. Complete blood count (CBC) with differential and indices, sedimentation rate to rule out anemia or hematologic or inflammatory cause.
2. Blood cultures if fever present.
3. Urinalysis and urine culture as baseline for bladder and renal function.
4. Thyroid-stimulating hormone and free thyroxine to rule out hypothyroidism.
5. Blood chemistry: provide data on electrolyte balance, renal function, and skeletal disorders.
6. Neonate screening tests, TORCH studies.
7. Stool screening tests to be ordered if diarrhea/abnormal stools are present:
   a. Infection: culture, ova and parasite, *Clostridium difficile*, white blood cell (WBC) count (may have false-negative results if recently on antibiotics).
   b. Protein malabsorption: alpha-one antitrypsin (may have false-negative results if not fed during collection).
   c. Carbohydrate malabsorption: pH, reducing substances (time sensitive, need to be fresh stool; may have false-negative results if not fed during collection).
   d. Fat malabsorption: random qualitative fecal fat (one-time sample); if needed, a 72-hour quantitative fecal fat should be collected. Results are more accurate when sample is collected while patient is receiving adequate nutrition.
   e. Pancreatic sufficiency: stool pancreatic elastase, stool chymotrypsin, and serum trypsin to detect primary or secondary pancreatic insufficiency.
8. Radiologic studies including upper GI series, barium swallow, reflux workup, upper endoscopy, and sweat test.

 NURSING ALERT One of the best tests to distinguish organic from nonorganic FTT is through observed feedings or enteral tube feedings to assess weight gain and caloric intake.

Management

1. Immediate treatment is directed at reversing malnutrition.
2. All children with FTT need additional calories for catch-up growth (typically 150% of the caloric requirement for their expected, not actual, weight).
3. Nutritional treatment is aimed at providing sufficient calories to support "catch-up" growth to restore deficits in weight and height. Protein and energy requirements for normal and FTT children are outlined in Table 48-1.
   a. This may require NG tube feedings for safe refeeding.
   b. If fat malabsorption present, may need formula with high level of medium-chain triglycerides for direct absorption of fat.
4. Multivitamin supplementation containing zinc and iron is usually recommended, fat-soluble vitamins (A, D, E, K) if fat malabsorption is present.

Table 48-1	Protein and Energy Requirements			
	NORMAL CHILDREN		**FTT CHILDREN**	
AGE (YEARS)	**PROTEIN (G/KG)**	**ENERGY (KCAL/KG)**	**PROTEIN (G/KG)**	**ENERGY (KCAL/KG)**
0–0.5	2.2	0.08	3.2	150–250
0.5–1	1.6	98	3.2	150–250
1–3	1.2	102	2.5	150–250
4–6	1.1	90	2.5	150–250
7–10	1.0	70	2.5	150–250

5. If cause is organic, the underlying disease entity is treated or managed.
6. In nonorganic FTT, hospitalization is avoided (unless the child is in imminent danger) because it further disrupts the parent–child relationship. Therefore, frequent home or clinic visits are necessary. Referral to feeding disorder clinic or rehabilitation center may be necessary.
7. Developmental interventions through occupational and physical therapy are instituted, if necessary, to prevent further delay.
8. Support, education, and financial assistance are offered to the family.
9. Nutrition, occupational therapy, and physical therapy consults are indicated.

Complications

Studies are inconsistent regarding the long-term complications of FTT.

1. Anemia, fatigue, hypothermia.
2. Vulnerability to infection.
3. Delayed healing.
4. Behavior problems, poor academic performance.
5. Developmental, speech, and language delays.
6. Perceptual difficulties.

Nursing Assessment

1. Obtain accurate anthropometric measurements.
   a. Weight of children younger than age 3 should be done unclothed in a supine position using a calibrated beam scale. Children older than age 3 should be done standing on a standard scale wearing same clothing each time. Effort should be made to use the same scale each time.
   b. Height should be recumbent up to age 2. All children should be measured without shoes.
   c. Head circumference is measured each visit until age 2 with a nonstretchable tape placed firmly from maximal occipital prominence to just above the eyebrow.
   d. All measurements need to be corrected for prematurity up to the second birthday by subtracting the number of weeks premature from the chronological age.
   e. Measurements should be plotted on growth chart using a straight edge or plot grid. Birth measurements should be obtained and entered for comparison.
2. Obtain nutritional history regarding eating patterns; nutritional beliefs for food allocation; 24-hour recall; who normally feeds the child; the type, amount, and frequency of feedings; the amount of time and effort required for meals; the child's reactions (physiologic and psychological) to feedings; food likes and dislikes; and environmental factors.

3. Observe parent–child interactions, such as sensitivity to child's needs, eye-to-eye contact, if and how the infant is held, and how the parent speaks to the child.
4. If possible, observe the parent feeding the child. Assess child's overall tone, sucking pattern, oral sensitivity (gag reflex), lip and tongue function, and swallowing ability. A videotape of the child eating in the home can be reviewed later to reduce the chance of observer distraction.
5. Assess neurologic and cardiovascular status for alertness, attentiveness, developmental delays, cardiac arrhythmias, or murmurs.
6. Assess skin, hair, and musculoskeletal system.
7. Assess developmental status using a Denver II developmental tool, as indicated.

Nursing Diagnoses

- Imbalanced Nutrition: Less Than Body Requirements related to FTT process.
- Delayed Growth and Development related to malnutrition.
- Impaired Parenting related to inability to meet the needs of the FTT child.

Nursing Interventions

Promoting Adequate Nutrition

1. Facilitate nutritional consultation.
2. If hospitalized, provide a primary core of staff to feed the child. Ask the parents to do so when present in a nonthreatening manner.
3. Develop individualized teaching plan to instruct parents of child's dietary needs. Specify type of diet, essential nutrients, serving sizes, and method of preparation.
4. Provide a quiet, nonstimulating environment for eating.
5. Demonstrate proper feeding techniques including details on how to hold and how long to feed the child.
6. Administer multivitamin supplements, as prescribed.
7. Encourage nutritious, high-calorie, and fortified fluids to increase nutrient density. For infants, use 24 to 30 cal/ounce rather than 20 cal/ounce. For older children, suggest fruit smoothies using whole milk and ice cream.
8. Refeed the malnourished child with caution, monitoring electrolytes, calcium, magnesium, and phosphorus daily or more frequently, if abnormal.
   a. Gradually increase nutrients and use small, frequent feedings with adequate fluids to ensure hydration.
   b. Monitor intake and output.
9. Maintain high-nutrient diet until weight is appropriate for height (usually age 4 to 9 months).
10. Advise family that some nutritional intervention will be continued until appropriate height for age is reached.

 NURSING ALERT If patient is malnourished, monitor for refeeding syndrome until laboratory studies are stable. Refeeding syndrome can cause intracellular shifting of electrolytes, calcium, magnesium, and phosphorus, resulting in death. Laboratory studies should be monitored daily or more frequently, if abnormal.

 NURSING ALERT Be alert for signs of dehydration due to sudden change to a high-calorie, high-protein diet. A dramatic increase in protein can increase renal solute load to the point that a child is at risk for dehydration.

Promoting Adequate Growth and Development

1. Obtain accurate weight at every visit or every day, if hospitalized.
2. Assess child's growth by using age- and gender-appropriate growth charts. Extremely low-birth-weight infants born with major anomalies have nearly twice the risk of neurodevelopmental impairment and increased risk of poor growth.
3. Assess child's development by interviewing the parent or caregiver or using developmental screening tests, such as the Denver II (Denver Developmental Materials, Inc., *http://denverii.com/denverii/*).
4. Observe interactions between parents and child and among family members, including eye contact, communication patterns, and coping ability.
5. Provide the infant with visual and auditory stimulation by exposing to bright colors, shapes, and music. Provide the older child with age-appropriate stimulation, such as books, games, and toys. Place the infant prone, while awake, on the floor to encourage trunk control.
6. Encourage periods of scheduled rest and sleep.

 EVIDENCE BASE Stobaugh, H., Rogers, B., Rosenberg, I., et al. (2018). Children with poor linear growth are at risk for repeated relapse to wasting after recovery from moderate acute malnutrition. *Journal of Nutrition*, May 3. Epub ahead of print.

Promoting Effective Parenting

1. Teach the parents (especially the mother) normal parenting skills by demonstrating proper holding, stroking, feeding, and communication using age-appropriate words and gestures.
2. If hospitalized, encourage and facilitate the parents to spend as much time as possible with the child.
3. Educate the parents to recognize and respond to the child's distress and hunger calls.
4. Help the parents to develop organizational skills—write down daily schedule with mealtimes, time for shopping, and so forth.
5. Refer for counseling, if necessary, to help parents overcome feelings of mistrust or neglect resulting from adverse personal childhood experiences.
6. Refer to social services to help resolve any social and financial difficulties that might interfere with providing a nurturing environment.
7. Monitor parents' progress and provide positive reinforcement.

Community and Home Care Considerations

Early intervention home visiting has been shown to reduce the long-term complications associated with FTT. This may be due to promotion of maternal sensitivity and helping children build strong work habits that enables them to flourish at school.

1. Make regular home visits to:
   a. Observe for continued parent–child interaction.
   b. Encourage continued developmentally appropriate play.
   c. Monitor feeding status and assess intake amount.
   d. Determine frequency of voiding and stooling.
   e. Assess child's weight, height, and head circumference.
   f. Monitor vital signs and watch for signs of dehydration.
   g. Auscultate bowel sounds.
   h. Assess muscle tone and vigor of activity.
   i. Assess family dynamics and use of support systems.
2. Inform parents of community resources, such as Women in Crisis program, food banks, parenting groups.

3. Make sure that day care providers can meet child's special needs in terms of diet, feeding, and developmentally appropriate play. Day care may be beneficial in the presence of family dysfunction by providing structure.
4. Make referrals to social work and occupational or physical therapy, as needed.

Family Education and Health Maintenance

1. Reinforce the need for a quiet, nonthreatening, nurturing environment.
2. Encourage the parents to be consistent with feedings. Although forced feeding is avoided, strict adherence to appropriate feeding is essential for growth.
3. Advise the parents to introduce new foods slowly and follow the child's rhythm of feeding.
4. Review the importance of providing a routine rest schedule in an environment that is conducive to sleep.
5. Review development, stressing need for visual, auditory, and tactile stimulation and age-appropriate toys for continued development.
6. Reinforce the need for follow-up care, well-child visits, and immunizations.

Evaluation: Expected Outcomes

- Increases weight steadily.
- Attains developmental milestones at appropriate age.
- Parents participating in child's care, using appropriate feeding technique.

Hypertrophic Pyloric Stenosis

 EVIDENCE BASE Gezer, H., Oguzkurt, P., Temiz, A., et al. (2015). Hypertrophic pyloric stenosis in twins; genetic or environmental factors. *Clinical Genetics*, *87*(4), 388–391.

Hypertrophic pyloric stenosis is an acquired condition in which the circumferential muscle of the pyloric sphincter becomes thickened, causing a high-grade gastric outlet obstruction that results in dilation, hypertrophy, and hyperperistalsis of the stomach. It is the second most common condition (after inguinal hernia) requiring surgery, which rarely occurs before age 2 weeks or later than age 5 months. Incidence is 1 in 250 live births and is predominant in males (5:1) and more common in first-born males. Incidence peaks in spring and fall. It is more likely to affect a full-term infant than a premature infant.

Pathophysiology and Etiology

1. Unknown cause, although new research has identified several genetic markers associated with the condition. Multiple theories of etiology exist, including immature or degenerated pyloric neural elements, variations in infant feeding regimens, excessive production of gastrin (maternal or infant), dyscoordination between gastric peristalsis and pyloric relaxation, deficiency of nitric acid, abnormalities in enteric nervous system, and abnormalities in neurotransmitters.
2. Current studies of combined imaging (pressure recordings, MRI, ultrasound, and fluid-mechanical analysis) have offered new understanding of the role of the pylorus in gastric emptying and digestion. Other studies have shown that persistent duodenal hyperacidity can lead to increased incidence of pyloric stenosis. This is associated with repeated contractions of the pylorus.
3. The use of erythromycin to treat reflux and gastric dysmotility has led to research regarding the association with pyloric stenosis. The published evidence has concluded that young infants exposed to erythromycin in the first few weeks of life are at greater risk for developing hypertrophic pyloric stenosis. The highest risk seems to be in the first 2 weeks of life in term or near-term infants, with a course of more than 14 days.
4. Increase in size of the circular musculature of the pylorus with thickening (size and shape of an olive). The pylorus muscle becomes elongated and thickened and is enlarged to about twice the usual size. On clinical exam, palpation of an "olive" is diagnostic.
5. Hypertrophy of the pylorus musculature occurs with narrowing of the pyloric lumen.
6. Constriction of the lumen of the pyloric canal (at the distal end of the stomach) causes the stomach to become dilated.
7. Gastric emptying is delayed.

 EVIDENCE BASE Zhu, J., Zhu, T., Lin, Z., et al. (2017). Perinatal risk factors for infantile hypertrophic pyloric stenosis: A meta-analysis. *Journal of Pediatric Surgery, 52*(9), 1389–1397.
Murchison, L., De Coppi, P., & Eaton, S. (2016). Postnatal erythromycin exposure and risk of infantile hypertrophic pyloric stenosis: A systematic review and meta-analysis. *Pediatric Surgery International, 32*(12), 1147–1152.

 DRUG ALERT Erythromycin should only be used in young infants (less than 4 weeks) when the therapeutic benefits outweigh the risks and no alternative agent is available.

Clinical Manifestations

Onset usually occurs between ages 3 and 12 weeks.
1. Cardinal sign is projectile, nonbilious vomiting.
   a. Initially, occasional regurgitation (similar to GER) may be present, but eventually vomiting increases in frequency and intensity.
   b. Vomitus contains milk and gastric juices; however, it may be blood-streaked or have a "coffee ground" appearance.
   c. Emesis occurs just after or near the end of a feeding.
2. Constipation or decreased quantity of stools.
3. Loss of weight or failure to gain weight.
4. Epigastric distention.
5. Visible gastric peristaltic waves, left to right, seen just after infant vomits.
6. Excessive hunger—willingness to eat immediately after vomiting.
7. Dehydration—electrolyte disturbance with alkalosis, hypoglycemia, hypochloremia.
8. Decreased urine output.
9. Palpable pyloric mass in upper right quadrant of abdomen, to the right of the umbilicus and best felt during feeding or immediately after vomiting.
10. Jaundice.

Diagnostic Evaluation

1. Palpation of pyloric mass ("olive") in conjunction with persistent, projectile vomiting is pathognomonic.
2. Ultrasound evaluation—broadly used, noninvasive method to evaluate the length and diameter of the pyloric muscle.
   a. Criteria for a positive diagnosis: pyloric muscle thickness (PMT) ≥ 3 mm and pyloric muscle length (PML) ≥ 17 mm.
   b. Sensitivity and specificity of PMT, 91% and 85%, respectively; for PML, 76% and 85%, respectively.
   c. No significant correlation among age, weight, or prematurity and a sonographic diagnosis of infantile hypertrophic pyloric stenosis; therefore, the same ultrasound criteria should apply irrespective of prematurity, age, or weight. Borderline PMT and PML measurements necessitate repeat ultrasound or alternative imaging.
3. Barium upper GI series—indicated if ultrasound is inconclusive.
4. Flat film of abdomen—dilated, air-filled stomach; nondilated pyloric canal.
5. Tests for metabolic alkalosis (seen in less than 10% because of more prompt diagnosis over the past 20 years).
6. Urinalysis—urine alkaline and concentrated.
7. Blood hemoglobin and hematocrit—elevated due to hemoconcentration.

 EVIDENCE BASE Ayaz, U., Dogen, M., Dilli, A., et al. (2015). The use of ultrasonography in infantile hypertrophic pyloric stenosis: does the patient's age and weight affect pyloric size and pyloric ratio? *Medical Ultrasonography, 17*(1), 28–33.

Management

 EVIDENCE BASE Sathya, C., Wayne, C., Gotsch, A., et al. (2017). Laparoscopic versus open pyloromyotomy in infants: A systematic review and meta-analysis. *Pediatric Surgery International, 33*(3), 325–333.

1. Considered a medical emergency because of dehydration and electrolyte imbalance, with initial treatment to rehydrate to correct electrolytes and alkalosis.
2. Surgical treatment is corrective and takes place when electrolytes are stable—Rammstedt pyloromyotomy is procedure of choice, performed through a short transverse incision in the right upper quadrant over the rectus muscle at or above the liver edge. Laparoscopic pyloromyotomy may also be done but the open procedure continues to be the most performed technique.
   a. Hypertrophy of the pyloric muscle regresses to normal size about 12 weeks postoperatively.
   b. Some postoperative vomiting is expected but should decrease over 48 hours. If persistent vomiting continues, a contrast study should be completed to rule out gastric leak, fluid collection obstructing the gastric outlet, or other causes of obstruction. If these are ruled out, incomplete pyloromyotomy should be considered.
   c. Postoperative complications include duodenal perforation, gastric leak, wound infection, small bowel obstruction, and postoperative vomiting.

3. Good outcomes following surgery appear to be strongly related to the qualifications of the pediatric surgeon, the use of pediatric certified anesthesiologists, qualified pediatric nurses, adequate correction of fluids and electrolytes preoperatively.

Complications

1. Starvation.
2. Dehydration.
3. Severe electrolyte imbalance.
4. Hematemesis.

Nursing Assessment

1. Obtain a thorough history of infant's feeding behaviors and history of vomiting.
2. Assess hydration status and for signs and symptoms of electrolyte imbalance.
3. Assess and chart growth and development parameters.

Nursing Diagnoses

Preoperative

- Deficient Fluid Volume related to frequent vomiting.
- Imbalanced Nutrition: Less Than Body Requirements related to vomiting.
- Acute Pain related to gastric distention.
- Anxiety of parents related to illness, hospitalization, and impending surgery of child.

Postoperative

- Risk for Injury related to postoperative complications.
- Risk for Deficient Fluid Volume after surgery.
- Impaired Tissue Integrity related to surgical incision.

Nursing Interventions

Maintaining Fluid and Electrolyte Balance

1. Administer IV therapy, as ordered, to treat dehydration, metabolic alkalosis, and electrolyte deficiency.
2. Carefully monitor output, including amount and characteristics of urine (check specific gravity), vomiting, and stools.
3. Accurately measure daily weight as a guide for calculating need for parenteral fluid.
4. Monitor laboratory data for serum electrolytes.
5. Position infants to prevent interference with fluid therapy.
6. Provide pacifier for infants who are NPO.
7. Monitor vital signs, as indicated by condition. Watch for tachycardia, hypotension, change in respirations.

 NURSING ALERT Irregular respiratory rate with apnea is a sign of severe alkalosis.

Maintaining Nutrition

 EVIDENCE BASE Sullivan, K., Chan, E., & Vincent, J. (2016). Feeding post-pyloromyotomy: A meta-analysis. *Pediatrics, 137*(1), epub.

1. Emphasize rehydration, electrolyte balance, and replacement of body fat and protein stores. This depends on severity of depletion and may require total parenteral nutrition for several days or weeks before surgery to reduce surgical risk.

Figure 48-4. Pyloric stenosis. **(A)** Normal passage through pyloric sphincter. **(B)** Stoppage of flow due to stenotic sphincter. **(C)** Postoperative treatment: child propped upright, slightly on right side, aids in gastric emptying.

2. Maintain NPO status with indwelling NG tube (inserted to remove any residual barium and retained formula), as ordered. Ensure placement, position, and patency. Record drainage type, color, and amount.
3. If oral feedings are to be continued, do the following:
   a. Provide small, frequent feedings, given slowly.
   b. Burp frequently before, during, and after feeding.
   c. Allow breast-feeding, as tolerated.
4. Prop the patient in 30-degree upright position (see Figure 48-4).
5. Handle gently and minimally after feeding.

Providing Comfort
1. Provide mouth care and wet lips frequently if NPO.
2. Let the infant suck on a pacifier.
3. Provide for physical contact or nearness without excessive stimulation.
4. Provide for audio and visual stimulation that may be soothing.
5. Do not palpate pyloric "olive" to decrease risk of postoperative wound infection from bruising abdominal wall and excoriating tissue in operative site.
6. Administer analgesics, as ordered.

Alleviating Parental Anxiety
1. Assess understanding of diagnosis and care plan.
2. Help minimize guilt feelings by providing adequate, specific information and clarifying any misconceptions.
3. Prepare the parents for the surgery of their child.
   a. Be honest with them.
   b. Prepare them for the expected postoperative appearance of the infant.
   c. Show them where the operating room and recovery room are located and where to wait during surgery.

4. Allow them to hold the infant to maintain bonding.
5. Encourage them to rest to care better for the infant postoperatively.
6. Accept and explore negative displays of emotion, which may be due to fatigue and frustration because of the extensive care given to the child before hospitalization.
7. Reassure them that surgery is considered curative and normal feeding should resume shortly afterward.

Preventing Complications
1. Assess vital signs to evaluate for fluid and electrolyte imbalances.
2. Assess skin and mucous membranes for hydration status.
3. Weigh daily to assess gain or loss.
4. Elevate head slightly.
5. If placed intraoperatively, maintain patent NG tube to prevent gastric distention. Record losses.
6. Monitor blood glucose levels to prevent hypoglycemia.

Maintaining Hydration
1. Administer IV fluids until adequate intake has been established.
2. Resume oral feeding 2 to 8 hours (standard is 6 hours) after surgery when infant is alert or as ordered.
3. After surgery, infants may progress to ad-lib feedings within 12 to 16 hours provided they did not have a prolonged preoperative course.
4. Start with small, frequent feedings of glucose water and slowly advance to full-strength (FS) formula and regular diet, as tolerated. An example of a postoperative feeding schedule includes:
   a. NPO for 6 hours.
   b. Sugar water solution orally 30 mL every 2 hours for two feedings.
   c. Then half-strength formula 30 mL every 2 hours for two feedings.
   d. Then FS formula 45 mL every 2 hours for two feedings.
   e. Then FS formula 60 mL every 3 hours for two feedings.
   f. Then formula ad lib every 4 hours.
5. Report any vomiting—amount and characteristics. Feeding schedule may be withheld 2 hours and then reinitiated.
6. Feed slowly and burp frequently.
7. Note how feeding is taken and if it is retained.
8. Increase the amount of feeding as the time interval between feedings is lengthened.
9. Allow breast-feeding to resume, as tolerated, if permitted by the operating surgeon, beginning with limited nursing of 5 to 8 minutes and gradually increase.
10. Continue to elevate the infant's head and shoulders after feeding for 45 to 60 minutes for several feedings after surgery. Place on right side to aid gastric emptying.
11. Expect that regurgitation may continue for a short period after surgery.

Promoting Healing
1. Provide analgesia and comfort measures, such as a pacifier, rocking, and other soothing stimulation to keep infant quiet and prevent tension on incision.
2. Involve parents in care of infant postoperatively to prepare them for care of wound after discharge.
3. Observe for drainage or signs of inflammation at incision site and provide care to incision, as ordered.
4. Note that poor nutritional status may delay wound healing.

Community and Home Care Considerations

1. Teach proper care of the operative site.
   a. Check for signs and symptoms of inflammation.
   b. Observe for drainage.
   c. Provide specific care of site, as ordered by provider.
2. Monitor weight and feeding behavior. Encourage close follow-up for growth and development.
3. Observe for signs of delayed gastric emptying or GER.
4. Assess parent–infant interaction and parental coping.

Family Education and Health Maintenance

1. Teach feeding technique to be continued at home; length of feeding technique varies depending on wound healing, nutritional status, and growth.
2. Provide written and verbal instructions as to infant's care and follow-up schedule.
3. Review with family when medical attention is needed and appropriate resources:
   a. Signs of infection.
   b. Frequent vomiting, vomiting longer than 5 days, or poor feeding with signs of dehydration.
   c. Abdominal distention.

Evaluation: Expected Outcomes

- Vital signs stable; urine output adequate.
- Tolerates 1- to 2-ounce feedings in upright position without vomiting.
- Rests quietly with pacifier.
- Parents verbalize understanding of surgery and postoperative care.
- Vital signs stable; blood glucose within normal limits.
- No signs of dehydration.
- Incision healing without signs of infection.

Celiac Disease

EVIDENCE BASE Hill, I., Fasano, A., Guandalini, S., et al. (2016). NASPGHAN clinical report on the diagnosis and treatment of gluten-related disorders. *Journal of Pediatric Gastroenterology & Nutrition, 63*(1), 156–165.

Paul, S. P., Sandhu, B. K., Spray, C. H., et al. (2018). Evidence supporting serology-based pathway for diagnosing celiac disease in asymptomatic children from high-risk groups. *Journal of Pediatric Gastroenterology & Nutrition, 66*(4), 641–644.

Celiac disease (CD), or *gluten-sensitive enteropathy*, is a complex autoimmune genetic disorder with multiple contributing genes. CD affects the small intestine and is characterized by a permanent inability to tolerate dietary gluten; however, it can have systemic manifestations as well. Gluten is a protein found in wheat, rye, and barley (see Figure 48-5). The disease process is reversible with strict adherence to a gluten-free diet.

CD occurs more frequently in Caucasians; however, it is found in all ethnic groups. In the United States and Europe, the prevalence of CD in the pediatric population is between 1 in 300 and 1 in 80, respectively. It is thought to be grossly underdiagnosed.

Pathophysiology and Etiology

1. CD is an immune-mediated disease. The two necessary components of the disease are exposure to gluten and a genetic predisposition resulting in immune activation to gluten. Linkage studies have identified several genomic regions that probably contain CD-susceptibility genes.

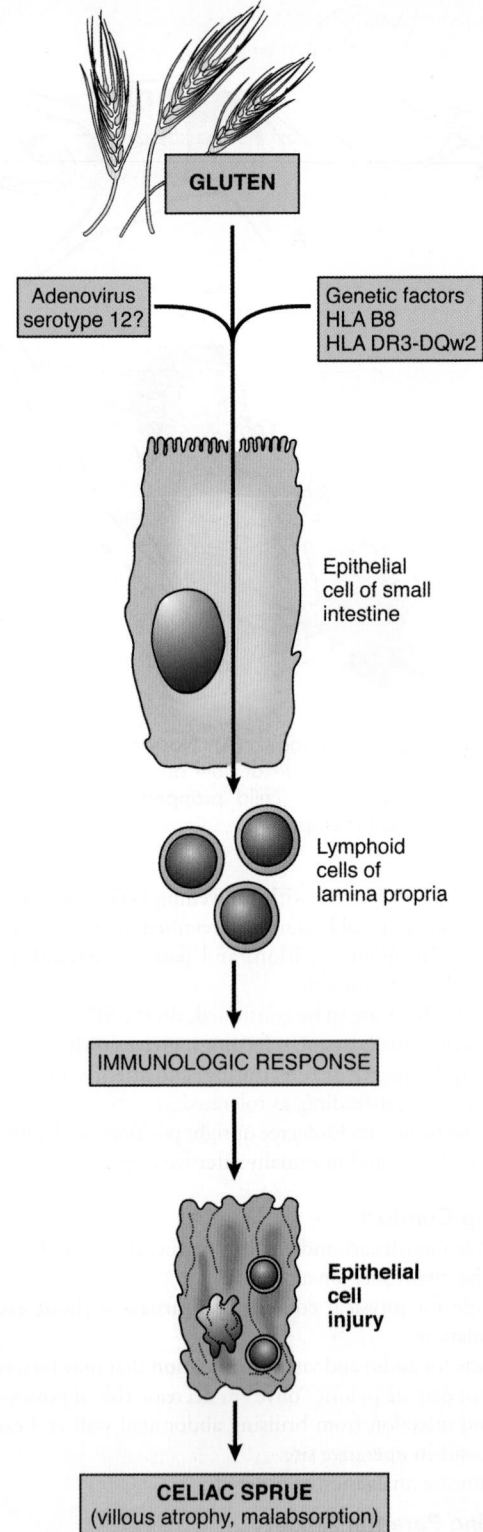

Figure 48-5. Mechanisms in the pathogenesis of celiac disease. (Rubin, R., & Strayer, D. S. [2011]. *Rubin's Pathology: Clinicopathologic Foundations of Medicine* [6th ed.]. Philadelphia: Lippincott Williams & Wilkins.)

a. The genes implicated in celiac disease are HLA-DQ2 and HLA DQ8. However, these genes can be found in 30% of the normal population as well.
b. A familial connection is found in 5% to 15% of celiac patients, with an 83% to 86% concordance rate among monozygotic twins.

2. The disease results in inflammation in the mucosa of the small bowel, especially the duodenum and jejunum. This results in damage to the villi, which can be shortened or totally lost.
3. The mucosal damage results in deficiency of enzymes on the mucosal surface, such as disaccharidase and peptidase. This, along with a reduced surface area, leads to malabsorption.
4. The body may be unable to absorb fats, fat-soluble vitamins (A, D, E, and K), minerals, and some protein and carbohydrates.
5. The severity of symptoms depends on the extent of affected intestine. If involvement is focal and limited to the proximal bowel, GI symptoms may be absent.
6. A number of conditions may be associated with celiac disease, including:
    a. Type 1 diabetes mellitus.
    b. Mucocutaneous manifestations, dermatitis herpetiformis.
    c. Cystic fibrosis, seizures, peripheral neuropathy.
    d. Autoimmune thyroiditis, adrenal insufficiency.
    e. Systemic lupus erythematosus, rheumatoid arthritis, and other connective tissue disorders.
    f. Sclerosing cholangitis.
    g. Trisomy 21.
    h. Unexplained folate or iron deficiency, refractory to treatment.
    i. Alopecia areata.
    j. Dental enamel hypoplasia.
    k. Risk of thromboembolism.

Clinical Manifestations

The age and mode of presenting signs and symptoms are extremely variable. Diagnosis may be made by ages 6 to 24 months when infants are introduced to cereal; however, more subtle gastrointestinal and extraintestinal symptoms often lead to diagnosis much later in life.

Ages 6 to 18 months
Presentation may include the following:
1. Impaired growth.
    a. Normal growth during early months of life.
    b. Slackening of weight followed by weight loss.
2. Diarrhea—more frequent, pale, soft, bulky, greasy (steatorrhea) with offensive odor.
3. Recalcitrant constipation (occasionally).
4. Abdominal distention.
5. Anorexia.
6. Muscle wasting—most obvious in buttocks and proximal parts of extremities.
7. Vomiting.
8. Seizures.
9. Loss of tooth enamel.
10. Painful/pruritic skin rash called "dermatitis herpetiformis."

Older Children
1. Complications of malabsorption:
    a. Anemia, vitamin deficiency.
    b. Hypoproteinemia (hypoalbuminemia) with edema.
    c. Hypocalcemia, hypokalemia, hypomagnesemia.
    d. Hypoprothrombinemia resulting from impaired vitamin K absorption.
    e. Disaccharide intolerance—with acid sugar-containing stools (secondary to the altered small-bowel mucosa).
    f. Low bone density, osteoporosis secondary to decreased calcium absorption.
2. Diarrhea or constipation.
3. Overweight status.

4. Linear growth delay.
5. Abdominal pain.
6. Fatigue.

 EVIDENCE BASE Jericho, H., Assiri, A., & Guandalini, S. (2017). Celiac disease and wheat intolerance syndrome: A critical update and reappraisal. *Journal of Pediatric Gastroenterology & Nutrition, 64*(1), 15–19.

Diagnostic Evaluation

 EVIDENCE BASE Allen, P. (2015). Gluten-related disorders: Celiac disease, gluten allergy, non-celiac gluten sensitivity. *Pediatric Nursing, 41*(3), 146–150.

1. Thorough history, including family history of autoimmune disorders, diabetes, dietary history, growth history, and general status of the child.
2. Serologic testing is done to screen the individual at risk. It has been recommended that all short-stature children be screened irrespective of GI symptoms. Assays detect immunoglobulin (Ig) A antibody to endomysium or tissue transglutaminase. These antibodies have a very high sensitivity and specificity for CD; however, they may be falsely low in a child with IgA deficiency. Therefore, the total IgA level must also be checked. Maintain usual diet during testing.
3. An upper endoscopy is the gold-standard test to confirm the diagnosis and must be done in all individuals whose serologic screening is positive. It might show infiltration of the mucosa with lymphocytes and variable degrees of flattened villi.
4. Videocapsule endoscopy shows good sensitivity and excellent specificity for the detection of villous atrophy in patients with suspected CD but is not often practical in the pediatric population; the gold standard of diagnosis remains the small intestinal biopsy.

 NURSING ALERT Age 3 to 6 months is too early to be able to detect celiac disease with testing because of the length of time of gluten exposure.

Management

 EVIDENCE BASE Isaac, D., Wu, J., Mager, D., et al. (2016). Managing the pediatric patient with celiac disease: A multidisciplinary approach, *Journal of Multidisciplinary Healthcare, 9*, 529–536.

1. Lifelong gluten-free diet.
    a. Avoid all foods containing wheat, rye, and barley and their derivatives because even a small amount, such as a trace contaminant, may cause a pathologic response. Oats are naturally gluten-free; however, they are often cross-contaminated during the manufacturing process, so their exclusion may be recommended.
    b. The small intestinal mucosa will always respond abnormally to dietary gluten, although clinical signs may not be immediately evident.
    c. Biopsy and serologic screening revert to normal with appropriate diet.
    d. Clinical signs of improvement are often seen days to weeks after proper diet is initiated but can take up to 1 year in the case of more insidious symptoms such as delayed linear growth.

2. Adequate caloric and nutrient intake.
3. Supplemental vitamins and minerals may be used when clinically indicated. Folic acid may be used if low level is suspected or detected.
   a. Vitamins A and D.
   b. Iron supplements until anemia resolves.
   c. Vitamin K if evidence of hypoprothrombinemia and bleeding.
   d. Calcium if milk is restricted.
4. Temporary restriction of lactose and sucrose (disaccharidases) from diet for 6 to 8 weeks may be indicated in some cases, if these products are shown to worsen symptoms.
5. Enzyme therapy that protects the mucosal lining from gluten exposure is being investigated in clinical trials.

Complications

1. Nutritional deficiencies (most important short-term risks, which can lead to anemia, osteoporosis, and growth failure).
2. Long-term risks of untreated CD include increased risk of lymphoma and adenocarcinoma of small intestine.
3. Refractory CD.
4. Seizures related to inadequate absorption of folic acid and buildup of calcium deposits on the brain.

Nursing Assessment

1. Obtain family dietary history as it relates to onset of symptoms.
2. Assess child's nutritional status.
3. Check for signs of infection.
4. Assess growth and developmental parameters.

Nursing Diagnoses

- Imbalanced Nutrition: Less Than Body Requirements related to malabsorption of nutrients, diarrhea, and vomiting.
- Impaired Parenting related to inability to control behavioral problems.

Nursing Interventions

Provide Adequate Nutrition and Dietary Restrictions

1. Provide gluten-free diet, being careful to avoid accidental exposure via cross-contamination while food is prepared and/ or cooked.
2. An initial diet high in protein, relatively low in fat, low in lactose, and free from gluten may be necessary if the newly diagnosed child exhibits severe malabsorption.
   a. Initiate a referral with a dietitian for precise diet recommendations.
   b. Soy milk or lactaid drops may be indicated if the patient is exhibiting signs of lactose intolerance.
   c. Watch for fat intolerance in infants and young children.
3. Maintain NPO status during the initial treatment of celiac crisis or during diagnostic testing. Take special precautions to ensure proper restriction if the child is ambulatory.
4. Encourage small, frequent, appetizing meals, but do not force eating if the child has anorexia.
5. Note the child's reaction to food. Close observation of the child's responses to food may reveal other intolerances. Note and record
   a. Foods taken and refused.
   b. Appetite.
   c. Change in behavior after eating.
   d. Characteristics and frequency of stools.

e. General disposition—behavior improvement commonly seen within 2 to 3 days after diet control is initiated.
6. Be prepared to temporarily eliminate new food introduced if symptoms increase.
7. A gluten-challenged diet is not routinely indicated.
8. Provide the family with assistance to obtain a variety of gluten-free foods. Studies demonstrate that poor availability and expense of gluten-free foods lead to dietary noncompliance.

 EVIDENCE BASE Barnes, C. (2016). An introduction to the management of paediatric patients with celiac disease. *Gastrointestinal Nursing, 14*(9), 39–45.

Promoting Effective Parenting

1. Teach the parents to develop an awareness of the child's behavior; recognize changes and care for child accordingly.
2. Explain that diet and eating have a direct effect on behavior and that behavior may indicate how the child is feeling.
3. Help the parents recognize and understand mood swings, from having temper tantrums to being very timid, nervous, or unstable.
4. Advise the parents to allow the child to express feelings freely through safe and age-appropriate media.
5. Encourage parents to define limits of behavior for the child and convey them to all family members.
6. Encourage patience, routines, and consistency.
7. Advise parents to record changes in behavior, especially in relation to eating and diet, to document effectiveness of therapy.
8. Help the parents to maintain a balance between the child with celiac disease, the other family members, and additional roles and responsibilities.
9. If the child is withdrawn, advise providing opportunity for play with other children, especially when the child begins to feel better.
10. Explain that the toddler may cling to infantile habits for security. Allow this behavior; it may disappear as physical condition improves.
11. Suggest offering the child other sensory stimulation to compensate for lack of eating pleasure.
12. Help the parents to understand that, after initial rapid weight gain, further improvement may be slow.
13. Provide emotional support for the child and parents.
14. Refer for counseling, if indicated.

Family Education and Health Maintenance

 EVIDENCE BASE Haas, K., Martin, A., & Park, K. T. (2017). Text message intervention (TEACH) improves quality of life and patient activation in celiac disease: A randomized clinical trial. *Journal of Pediatrics, 185,* 62–67.

1. Teach parents about celiac disease and how it is controlled by diet. Help them to understand that severe, long-term damage to the intestinal lining has occurred and must be controlled to allow for normal growth and development.
2. Long-term follow-up with a qualified dietitian has been shown to improve compliance based on symptoms and follow-up serological testing.
3. Provide a specific list of restricted and acceptable foods to get the family started; because there is much variation among

brands of packaged foods, it is best for the family to check with the manufacturers.

4. Teach the parents how to read labels on foods to identify those containing wheat, rye, and barley glutens, thus avoiding them.
   a. Advise that any ingredient of unknown or unspecified grain origin should be assumed to contain gluten, unless the manufacturer confirms that it is gluten-free.
   b. Advise that medications should also be checked; filler and excipients, such as alcohol in cough medication, may be wheat based.
   c. Advise parents that gluten is found in many manufactured products as a filler or thickener, such as gravy powder.
5. Provide information on substitutes for wheat, rye, and barley such as corn, rice, potato, soybean flour, and gluten-free starch.
6. Help the parents become comfortable in situation problem solving (eg, supplying gluten-free cupcakes for birthday party to which child has been invited).
7. Initiate referral to dietitian to ensure that nutrient and energy requirements are being met. There is no standardized vitamin regimen.
8. Discuss the importance of continued adherence to gluten-free diet, even though the child is feeling well, eating well, and has normal stools. Encourage child to become involved in diet.
9. Adolescent compliance may be variable. Encourage support and understanding.
10. Alteration in diet may have significant cultural, ethnic, and religious implications. Help parents identify how adjustments can be made.
11. Advise parents on eating out—check ahead of time with fast-food chains and restaurant chefs or management to determine if they can ensure gluten-free items. (Be aware that even a gluten-free hamburger cooked on a grill with a breaded chicken breast cannot be considered gluten free.)
    a. Many gluten-free menus at chain restaurants can be found on the Internet by searching keyword "gluten-free."
    b. Inform friends before visiting and bring gluten-free products, if necessary.
    c. If necessary, consider implementation of formalized plan of necessary dietary restrictions for appropriate accommodations in school settings.
12. Advise parents to investigate support groups, Internet companies, natural food stores, and major food brands that offer information and sell gluten-free products.
13. Tell parents that common problems with long-term gluten-free diet are constipation due to low dietary fiber intake and weight gain due to now normal absorption; therefore, encourage regular physical activity and avoidance of high-calorie foods.
14. Impress on the parents the importance of regular medical follow-up.
15. Encourage the parents to practice good hygiene to prevent infection because the child may be especially prone to infection if malnutrition and/or anemia are present.
16. Advise the family that patients with CD have a predisposition to nonresponse of the hepatitis B vaccine; therefore, titers should be considered.
17. Help the parents to understand that the emotional climate in the home and around the child is vitally important in maintaining the child's medical and physical stability. Stress the importance of not making the child feel abnormal or a nuisance to the family. Family support is invaluable in facilitating acceptance of the diet.
18. Stress that the disorder is lifelong; however, changes in the mucosal lining of the intestine and the general clinical condition of the child are reversible when dietary gluten is avoided.
19. Advise screening for all first-degree relatives, because of hereditary nature of the disease.
20. For additional information and support, refer to Celiac Sprue Association (*www.csaceliacs.org*), Canadian Celiac Association (*www.celiac.ca*), or Celiac Disease Foundation (*www.celiac.org*).

Evaluation: Expected Outcomes

- Tolerates gluten-free diet well. Poor growth is not the symptom for every child; therefore gaining weight is not an appropriate expected outcome for each child.
- Parents setting limits with child and documenting behavior in relation to meals.

Diarrhea

Diarrhea is the rapid movement of fecal matter through the intestine, resulting in an excessive loss of water and electrolytes and producing more frequent loose, unformed, or watery stools. It is a symptom of many conditions and may be caused by many diseases (see Table 48-2). Commonly, the cause is difficult to determine; occasionally, it is unknown. Worldwide, approximately 1.8 million children die from diarrhea annually. Studies show that approximately 40% of cases of diarrhea have no direct cause, although some viruses have yet to be identified.

Pathophysiology and Etiology

 EVIDENCE BASE Lo Vecchio, A., Dias, J., Berkley, J. et al. (2016). Comparison of recommendations in clinical practice guidelines for acute gastroenteritis in children. *Journal of Pediatric Gastroenterology & Nutrition, 63*(2), 226–235.
Lo Vecchio, A., Vandenplas, Y., Benninga, M., et al. (2016). An International Consensus Report on a new algorithm for the management of infant diarrhea. *Acta Paediatrica, 105*(8), 384–389.

Mechanisms of Diarrhea
1. Secretory—decreased absorption, increased secretion.
2. Osmotic—maldigestion, transport defects, ingestion of unabsorbable solute.
3. Intestinal dysmotility—intact absorption with decreased intestinal transit time.
4. Inflammatory—malabsorption; can be caused by infectious or noninfectious agents.

Physiologic Effects of Diarrhea
1. Dehydration (extracellular fluid [ECF] loss).
   a. Large loss of fluid and electrolytes in watery stools.
   b. May be compounded by vomiting, decreased fluid intake, and increased insensible loss due to fever and rapid respirations.
2. Electrolyte imbalance.
   a. Potassium—may be hyper or hypokalemic.
   b. Sodium and chloride are directly related and may be increased or decreased.
      i. Hypernatremic hyperchloremic (hypertonic) dehydration occurs with acute diarrhea.
      ii. Hyponatremic hypochloremic (hypotonic) hypervolemia occurs with too rapid fluid replacement.

Table 48-2 Differential Diagnosis of Diarrhea

	INFANT	CHILD	ADOLESCENT
Acute			
Common	• Gastroenteritis • Systemic infection • Antibiotic associated • Overfeeding	• Gastroenteritis • Food poisoning • Systemic infection • Antibiotic associated	• Gastroenteritis • Food poisoning • Antibiotic associated
Rare	• Primary disaccharidase deficiency • Hirschsprung toxic colitis • Adrenogenital syndrome	• Toxic ingestion	• Hyperthyroidism
Chronic			
Common	• Postinfectious secondary lactase deficiency • Cow's milk or soy protein intolerance • Chronic nonspecific diarrhea of infancy • Celiac disease • Cystic fibrosis • AIDS enteropathy	• Postinfectious secondary lactase deficiency • Irritable bowel syndrome • Celiac disease • Lactose intolerance • Giardiasis • Inflammatory bowel disease • AIDS enteropathy	• Irritable bowel syndrome • Inflammatory bowel disease • Lactose intolerance • Giardiasis • Laxative abuse (anorexia nervosa)
Rare	• Primary immune defects • Familial villous atrophy • Secretory tumors • Acrodermatitis enteropathica • Lymphangiectasia • Abetalipoproteinemia • Eosinophilic gastroenteritis • Short-bowel syndrome • Intractable diarrhea syndrome • Autoimmune enteropathy	• Acquired immune defects • Secretory tumors • Pseudo-obstruction	• Secretory tumor • Primary bowel tumor • Anal intercourse (inflammation confined to the rectum) • Kaposi sarcoma–associated diarrhea

AIDS, acquired immunodeficiency syndrome.

3. Acid–base imbalance—metabolic acidosis.
   a. From large losses of potassium, sodium, and bicarbonate in stools.
   b. From impaired renal function.
4. Monosaccharide intolerance and protein hypersensitivity.

Pathogenic Etiology
1. Bacteria—*Escherichia coli* O157:H7, *Salmonella*, *Shigella*, *Yersinia enterocolitica*, *Campylobacter jejuni*, *Clostridium difficile*, dysentery, cholera.
2. Antibiotic-associated diarrhea, such as *C. difficile* diarrhea, is a leading cause of nosocomial outbreaks.
3. Viral—rotavirus (most common; peaks during winter months), enteroviruses (echovirus), adenoviruses, human Reovirus-like agent, Norwalk virus.
4. Fungal—*Candida enteritis*.
5. Parasitic—*Giardia lamblia, Cryptosporidium parvum*.
6. Protozoal.

Noninfectious Etiologic Factors
1. Malabsorption—lactase deficiency, cow's milk protein allergy, food protein-induced enteropathy, celiac disease, cystic fibrosis, microvillus inclusion disease.
2. Inflammatory bowel disease—ulcerative colitis, Crohn disease, rare in infants.
3. Immune deficiency—severe combined immunodeficiency, IgA deficiency.
4. Infant exposed to overeating.

5. Direct irritation of GI tract by foods, medications, chemicals, radiation.
6. Inappropriate use of laxatives and purgatives.
7. Mechanical disorders—malrotation, incomplete small-bowel obstruction, intermittent volvulus.
8. Congenital anomalies (eg, Hirschsprung disease–related enterocolitis).
9. Drug consumption—increases the risk of colitis, especially in predisposed persons; some agents may just exacerbate underlying colitis.
10. Functional—diagnosis of exclusion, although etiology may be a virus that has not been identified. For example, child exposed to excessive stress, emotional excitement, and fatigue.

Acute Diarrhea
1. Sudden increase in frequency of stools.
2. Usually self-limited but can result in dehydration.

Chronic or Persistent Diarrhea
1. Defined as three loose or liquid bowel movements a day for at least 2 to 4 weeks and a stool weight greater than 200 g/day.
2. Associated with disorders of malabsorption, anatomic defects, abnormal bowel motility, hypersensitivity reaction, or a long-term inflammatory response.
3. May be due to behaviors that continue to expose children to pathogens as well as increased resistance of bacteria to commonly used antibacterial agents.

COMMON PEDIATRIC GASTROINTESTINAL DISORDERS

 NURSING ALERT Infants and young children in day care centers may be at increased risk for diarrhea due to *Shigella*, *Salmonella*, rotavirus, endopathogenic *E. coli*, and giardiasis. Hand washing is the major preventive measure. These infections are usually reportable to the health department. Bloody diarrhea should be immediately referred for medical evaluation.

Risk Factors for Diarrhea

 EVIDENCE BASE Adams, D., Eberly, M., Rajnik, M., et al. (2017). Risk factors for community-associated *Clostridium difficile* infection in children. *Journal of Pediatrics, 186*, 105–109.

1. Age—the younger the child, the greater the susceptibility and severity.
   a. ECF volume is proportionately larger in the infant and young child.
   b. Nutritional reserves are relatively smaller in the young child.
2. Impaired health—susceptibility is increased in the malnourished or debilitated child.
3. Climate—susceptibility is increased in warm weather.
4. Environment—frequency is increased where there is overcrowding, poor sanitation, inadequate refrigeration of food, and inadequate health care and education.
5. Virulence of a potential pathogen affects severity.
6. Internationally adopted child.

Clinical Manifestations

Symptoms vary with severity, specific cause, and type of onset (insidious vs. acute).
1. Low-grade fever to 100°F (37.8°C).
2. Anorexia.
3. Vomiting (can precede diarrhea by several days); mild and intermittent to severe.
4. Stools—appearance of diarrhea from a few hours to 3 days.
   a. Loose and fluid consistency.
   b. Greenish or yellow-green, although can be any color.
   c. May contain mucus, pus, or blood.
   d. Frequency varies from 3 to 20 per day.
   e. Expelled with force; may be preceded by pain.
5. Behavioral changes.
   a. Irritability and restlessness.
   b. Weakness.
   c. Extreme prostration.
   d. Stupor and convulsions.
   e. Flaccidity.
6. Physical changes.
   a. Little to extreme loss of subcutaneous fat.
   b. Up to 50% total body weight loss.
   c. Poor skin turgor; capillary refill longer than 2 seconds.
   d. Dry mucous membranes and dry, cracked lips.
   e. Pallor.
   f. Sunken fontanelles and eyes.
   g. Petechiae may be seen with bacterial infections.
   h. Excoriated buttocks and perineum.
   i. Urine with blood.
7. Vital sign and urine output changes (signal imminent cardiovascular collapse).
   a. Low BP.
   b. High pulse rate.
   c. Respirations rapid and hyperpneic.
   d. Decreased or absent urine output.

Diagnostic Evaluation

Studies to Evaluate Condition
1. Thorough history and physical examination to determine hydration status.
2. Electrolyte and kidney function tests—serum sodium, chloride, potassium, and blood urea nitrogen variable.
3. Acid–base balance—serum carbon dioxide; arterial pH and carbon dioxide possibly abnormal.
4. CBC to determine plasma volume by hematocrit; infection by WBC count and differential.
5. Sedimentation rate—elevated in infection and inflammation.

 NURSING ALERT A postural change in heart rate and blood pressure is a useful clue in assessing the fluid state of a toddler (or any child). An increase greater than 20 beats/minute when moving from lying to standing is an indicator of hypovolemia. A decrease of at least 20 mm Hg in systolic BP or a decrease of at least 10 mm Hg in diastolic BP when moving from lying to standing is considered orthostatic and likely indicates hypovolemia.

Studies to Determine Cause
1. Thorough history to determine recent contact or exposure, contact with potentially contaminated water (swimming in lakes and ponds, well water), travel to at-risk countries, antibiotic therapy, and possible immunosuppression.
2. Enzyme immunoassay tests such as Rotazyme to test stool for rotavirus.
3. Multiple stool and rectal swab for bacterial cultures, ova and parasites, and *C. difficile*. Some labs require the sample specify for *Giardia* profile, *Cryptosporidium*, and *E. coli* O157:H7 serotyping. If immunosuppressed, add *Microsporidian*, *Cryptosporidium*, and *G. lamblia* antigen 65.
4. Stool for WBC count, calprotectin or lactoferrin, to screen for colitis that may be of a bacterial or inflammatory nature.
5. Stool pH, reducing substances—decreased pH may indicate various noninfectious causes; acid stool containing sugar is characteristic of disaccharide intolerance, abnormality of bile salt reabsorption.
6. Blood cultures can rule out septicemia.
7. Serologic studies can detect viral pathogens.
8. Breath hydrogen test can determine carbohydrate malabsorption and bacterial overgrowth.
9. Urinalysis can exclude UTI as cause of nonspecific diarrhea and screen for blood, which may be part of hemolytic uremic syndrome associated with *E. coli* O157:H7 infection.

Management

 EVIDENCE BASE Carson, R., Mudd, S., & Jamil, P. (2017). Evaluation of a nurse-initiated acute gastroenteritis pathway in the Pediatric Emergency Department. *Journal of Emergency Nursing, 43*(5), 406–412.
Hendrickson, M., Zaremba, J., Wey, A., et al. (2017). The use of a triage-based protocol for oral rehydration in a Pediatric Emergency Department. *Pediatric Emergency Care, 34*(4), 227–232.

Table 48-3 Assessment for Dehydration in Children

CLINICAL SIGNS	DEGREE OF DEHYDRATION		
	MILD	MODERATE	SEVERE
General			
Infant's behavior	Thirsty, alert, restless	Restless or lethargic; irritable to touch	Limp, drowsy; cyanotic extremities
Child's behavior	Thirsty, alert, restless	Thirsty, alert; postural hypotension	Usually conscious; cyanotic extremities
Respirations	Slightly increased	Increased	Deep and rapid
Pulse	Slightly increased	Increased	Rapid
Blood pressure	Normal	Decreased	May be unrecordable
Capillary refill	2 sec	2–3 sec	≥3 sec
Skin turgor	Normal	Slightly reduced	Reduced
Skin color	Pale	Gray	Mottled
Weight loss	Up to 5%	Up to 10%	Up to 15%
Mucous membrane	Tacky	Tacky/dry	Parched
Anterior fontanelle	Flat	Slightly depressed	Sunken
Urine volume	Small	Oliguria	Oliguria/anuria
Specific gravity	1.020	1.030	1.035

Treatment is based on the degree of dehydration; mild (loss of less than 5% of body weight), moderate (5% to 10% loss), and severe (greater than 10% loss) (see Table 48-3).

1. Goal is to prevent spread of disease; communicable disease is suspected until proved otherwise; enteric precautions are followed.
2. Bowel rest may be required based on degree of diarrhea and vomiting, if blood present, or electrolyte abnormalities.
3. For mild to moderate dehydration, oral rehydration solution is given to maintain fluid and electrolyte balance (WHO solution, Pedialyte, Infalyte). BRAT (banana, rice, apple, tea) diet is no longer recommended, as it is nutritionally suboptimal.
   a. For oral rehydration, 100 mL/kg over 4 hours, with additional fluids after each liquid bowel movement.
   b. Candidates for oral rehydration include mild to moderate dehydration, older than age 4 months, no persistent vomiting, and probable gastroenteritis.
4. For moderate to severe dehydration, IV fluid and electrolyte replacement is given slowly, as ordered (usually 20 mL/kg), usually over 2 days to prevent hypotonic hypervolemia (water intoxication). Administration of larger amounts of IV dextrose is associated with reduced return visits in children with gastroenteritis and dehydration.
5. Supportive care is given: monitoring oral and IV fluid intake, output from all sources, and patient's response to treatment.
6. Specific antimicrobial therapy may be given in some cases such as immunosuppression, bacteremia, documented *C. difficile*, and traveler's diarrhea.
   a. Metronidazole 30 mg/kg/day in divided doses orally or via IV line may be used to treat *C. difficile* infection, although IV dosing may be less efficacious.
   b. Vancomycin PO for resistant *C. difficile*. Fidaxomicin PO is another antimicrobial FDA approved treatment for *C. difficile*–associated diarrhea in adults, but its use is not yet approved in children.
   c. Rifampin has been shown to be effective in traveler's diarrhea without associated side effects.
7. Probiotics (*Saccharomyces boulardii*, *Lactobacillus rhamnosus* GG, and probiotic mixtures) significantly reduced the development of antibiotic-associated diarrhea. *S. boulardii* was effective for *C. difficile* infection.
8. The World Health Organization and the American Academy of Pediatrics discourage the use of antidiarrheal agents in children. In children who are younger than age 3 years, malnourished, moderately or severely dehydrated, systemically ill, or who have bloody diarrhea, adverse events outweigh benefits. In children who are older than age 3 years, with no/minimal dehydration, loperamide may be a useful adjunct to oral rehydration and early refeeding.

 EVIDENCE BASE Johnston, B., Goldenberg, J., & Parkin, P. (2016). Probiotics and the prevention of antibiotic-associated diarrhea in infants & children. *Journal of the American Medical Association*, 316(14), 1484–1485.

Complications

1. Severe dehydration and acid–base derangements with acidosis.
2. Shock.

Nursing Assessment

1. Obtain accurate history of signs and symptoms: nature and frequency of stools, type of onset, length of illness, and associated symptoms.
2. Assess degree of dehydration (see Table 48-3).
3. Monitor intake and output including oral and IV fluids, fluid loss from diarrhea, urine output, and vomitus; monitor weight.
4. Note color and consistency of stool and vomitus.
5. Successful rehydration (at 4 hours) is defined as resolution of moderate dehydration, production of urine, weight gain, and the absence of severe emesis (≥5 mL/kg).

 NURSING ALERT Assess child's behavior to determine comfort level. Crying or legs drawn up to abdomen usually indicates pain.

Nursing Diagnoses

- Deficient Fluid Volume related to diarrhea and ECF loss.
- Risk for Infection and transmission to others related to infectious diarrhea.

- Risk for Impaired Skin Integrity related to irritation by frequent stools.
- Imbalanced Nutrition: Less Than Body Requirements related to malabsorption.
- Anxiety and Fear related to hospitalization and illness.

Nursing Interventions

Restoring Fluid Balance
1. Monitor amount and rate of IV fluid therapy, which have been calculated by the health care provider. Fluid needs are based on fluid deficit, ongoing losses, and body weight.
2. Prevent overload of circulatory system.
   a. Check flow rate and amount absorbed hourly and totally.
   b. Adhere to prescribed volume carefully when oral feedings are given in conjunction with IV fluid.
   c. Never administer IV fluids to pediatric patient without safeguard of a volume-control infusion device or pump.
   d. Observe for signs of fluid overload: edema, increased BP, bounding pulse, labored respirations, and crackles in lung fields.
3. Check IV site for infiltration or improper flow, so site can be changed as necessary.
4. Use appropriate protective devices to prevent the child from injuring involved extremity or causing IV to malfunction.
5. Weigh the patient daily as a guide for fluid needs and patient status.
6. Monitor urine output and keep accurate intake and output record, including vomitus and liquid stools.
7. If NPO, provide frequent mouth care and nonnutritive sucking with a pacifier. Continue to burp infant to expel air swallowed while crying or sucking.
8. If oral rehydration solution is used, reassess hydration status every 2 to 4 hours; once rehydrated, continue for 8 to 12 hours, then resume breast-feeding with increased frequency of feedings or formula at full strength or increased frequency if half strength.

Note: Unless vomiting is severe, do not deprive the patient of nutrition for longer than 1 or 2 days. If adequate nutrition cannot be provided, parenteral nutrition should be instituted.

 NURSING ALERT Diluted fruit juices and soft drinks are not recommended. High disaccharide content aggravates diarrhea by osmotic effect.

Preventing Spread of Infection
1. Ensure adherence to good hand washing and gown technique protocols for all people having contact with infant or child.
2. Follow your facility's policy on care of diapers.
3. Handle specimens collected using universal precautions and transport to laboratories in appropriate containers per policy. Collect stool sample for culture before instituting antibiotic therapy.
4. Teach good hygiene measures to older children.

Preventing Skin Impairment
1. Protect infant's diaper area from becoming excoriated by making frequent diaper changes.
2. Expose to air and light as much as possible.
3. Avoid commercial baby wipes, which contain alcohol and may sting inflamed or excoriated diaper area. Use mild soap and water, place infant in tub of water or baking soda bath (soothing and neutralizing) for cleaning.
4. Prevent scratching or rubbing of the irritated area. Holding the infant on the parent's protected lap may provide comfort and stimulation for the parent and infant.

5. Use protective barrier creams, such as zinc oxide; if excoriated, soak off cream and pat dry—do not rub. Not all cream barrier has to be removed because this can denude skin.
6. Leave diaper area open to air until thoroughly dried.

Resuming Adequate Nutritional Intake
1. After rehydration, advance slowly from clear liquids to half-strength formula, to regular diet.
   a. If chronic diarrhea, bloody diarrhea, or secretory diarrhea, limit milk products containing lactose.
   b. In older infants and children, offer nonlactose, bland, carbohydrate-rich foods shortly after successful rehydration.
2. As diet is advanced, note any vomiting or increase in stools and report it immediately. Oral feedings should not be resumed too early or advanced too rapidly because diarrhea may recur.

Reducing Fear and Anxiety
1. Acknowledge that hospitalization is frightening, especially when it is sudden, as with diarrhea.
2. Many treatments and procedures may be painful. Give reassurance to the child before, during, and after treatment.
   a. Explain treatment in age-appropriate language.
   b. Include family in care and treatments when possible.
3. Explain to family that intermittent abdominal cramps may be painful and provide support.
4. Provide some means of pleasant stimulation, entertainment, or diversion, especially while child remains in bed.
   a. Infant—mobile, musical toy.
   b. Young child—books, tapes.
   c. Older child—television, videos.
5. Provide physical closeness to provide comfort, if child displays interest.
   a. Petting, stroking.
   b. Holding, rocking.

Community and Home Care Considerations
1. Infants and young children in day care centers may be at increased risk for diarrhea due to *Shigella, Salmonella,* rotavirus, *E. coli, Cryptosporidium, Campylobacter, C. difficile,* and *Giardia.* Good hand washing is the major preventive measure. This is especially important with rotavirus because it can be excreted for as long as 57 days in some cases.
2. If infectious agent is identified, it should be reported because other children may be at risk.
   a. Encourage parents to contact the child day care center and report.
   b. A child with diarrhea containing blood or mucus should be excluded from day care and medically evaluated. Exclusion from day care should occur until the diarrhea resolves.
   c. Stool cultures positive for *E. coli* O157:H7 or *Shigella* are reportable to the county health department, and the child should be excluded until the diarrhea resolves and two cultures, from two different stools, are negative for these organisms.
3. Assess sanitation and hygiene practices in the home or day care center for overcrowding, number of working toilets in the home for number of people, availability of working sinks with soap and towels in the bathrooms and their proximity to food preparation areas, disposal of diapers, and hand washing practices of caregivers and children.
4. Because most treatment for diarrhea is done on an outpatient basis, nurses in the community need to be available to answer questions.

Family Education and Health Maintenance

1. After the cause of the diarrhea is determined, it may be necessary to teach proper hygiene, formula or food preparation, handling, and storage.
   a. Use hand washing before bottle and food preparation.
   b. Use disposable bottles or sterilize or use dishwasher for reusable bottles.
   c. Refrigerate reconstituted formula and all other fluids between uses. Milk may become contaminated within 1 hour if left out at room temperature; juice becomes contaminated within several hours.
   d. Discard small amounts of food or fluid from containers already used.
2. Explain the fecal–oral mode of transmission of infectious diarrheal illnesses.
3. Explain the early symptoms of a diarrheal illness and of dehydration, which requires notification of the health care provider.
4. Discourage the use of antiemetics and antidiarrheal medications for infants and children with gastroenteritis; they have little effect on infantile diarrhea, may cause toxicity, and can mask signs and symptoms of more serious illness.
5. Advise parents when traveling internationally with their children to eat and drink only boiled, bottled, or carbonated water, be aware of drinks with ice cubes, food rinsed with water, and make sure all food is well cooked.
6. Help parents understand the importance of medical care and general good hygiene.
7. For additional information and support, refer to National Institute of Diabetes and Digestive and Kidney Diseases (*www.niddk.nih.gov*).

 DRUG ALERT Bismuth subsalicylate, an over-the-counter drug that is readily available, has shown only modest beneficial effects in children and may increase the risk of Reye syndrome due to salicylate absorption.

Evaluation: Expected Outcomes

- Vital signs stable; urine output adequate.
- Family, staff members hand washing properly and frequently.
- No redness or excoriation of diaper area.
- Tolerates small feedings of clear liquids without diarrhea or vomiting.
- No signs or symptoms of pain or discomfort.

Hirschsprung Disease

 EVIDENCE BASE Moore, S. (2016). Genetic impact on the treatment and management of Hirschsprung disease. *Journal of Pediatric Surgery, 52,* 218–222.
Westfal, M., & Goldstein, A. (2017). Pediatric enteric neuropathies: Diagnosis and current management. *Current Opinion in Pediatrics, 29*(3), 347–353.

Hirschsprung disease (congenital aganglionic megacolon) is a form of chronic intestinal obstruction affecting primarily full-term infants.

It occurs because of the congenital absence of the parasympathetic ganglion nerve cells from within the muscle wall of the intestinal tract, usually at the distal end of the colon. Ganglion cells are located throughout the intestinal tract from the mouth down to the rectum. It occurs in 1 in 5,000 (ranges 1:4,400 to 1:7,000) live births with no racial predilection.

The male:female ratio is reported as 2:1, except in long segment disease, in which it is closer to 1:1, possibly favoring females. Strong evidence supports a genetic component and the association of other congenital anomalies such as Down syndrome, small/large intestinal atresias, trisomy 18, and other rare disorders.

Pathophysiology and Etiology

1. An arrest in embryologic development affecting the migration of parasympathetic nerve innervation of the intestine.
   a. Normally, the nerve cells migrate to the upper end of the alimentary tract and then proceed in the caudal direction, with migration to the distal colon complete by 12 weeks.
   b. Migration occurs first in the intermuscular layer, called *Auerbach plexus*, and then moves into the submucosal plexus, moving along the GI tract in a descending manner.
2. The process of aganglionosis is almost always continuous within the affected segment, ending in proximal segment with ganglion cells. Intermittent ganglion cells in the colon have been reported, but this is extremely unusual.
   a. Most commonly affected site is the rectosigmoid colon (referred to as short-segment disease) (80%).
   b. Long-segment disease extends to the upper descending colon and transverse colon (10%) and occasionally throughout the entire colon, involving the small bowel (5%).
   c. Total angiogliosis of the bowel, involving the entire small and large bowel, is rare.
3. No peristalsis occurs in the affected portion of intestine (ie, spastic and contracted). This section is usually narrow; therefore, no fecal material passes through it.
4. Proximal to the narrow affected section, the colon is dilated (see Figure 48-6).
   a. Filled with fecal material and gas.
   b. Hypertrophy of muscular coating.
   c. Ulceration of mucosa may be seen in neonate.
5. The internal rectal sphincter fails to relax and evacuation of fecal material and gas is prevented. Abdominal distention and constipation result.

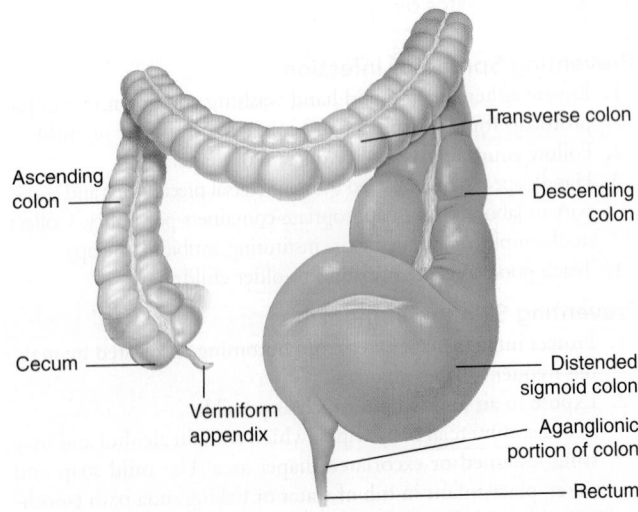

Figure 48-6. Bowel dilation in Hirschsprung disease. (Anatomical Chart Company.)

Clinical Manifestations

Clinical manifestations vary depending on degree of involved bowel.

1. Neonate—symptoms appearing at birth or within first weeks of life.
   a. No meconium passed in the first 48 hours of life.
   b. Vomiting—bile-stained or fecal.
   c. Abdominal distention.
   d. Constipation—occurs in 100% of patients.
   e. Overflow-type diarrhea.
   f. Dehydration; FTT.
   g. Temporary relief of symptoms with enema.
   h. Bowel perforation—uncommon presentation.
2. Older child—symptoms not prominent at birth. Short-segment disease commonly presents later.
   a. History of obstipation at birth.
   b. Progressive abdominal distention.
   c. Peristaltic activity observable over abdomen.
   d. Absence of retentive posturing (ability to contract the internal and external sphincter to purposefully avoid defecation).
   e. Constipation—unresponsive to conventional remedies.
   f. Presence of encopresis.
   g. Ribbon-like, fluidlike, or pellet stools.
   h. Failure to grow—loss of subcutaneous fat; appears malnourished, stunted growth.
   i. Presentation insidious or catastrophic as with enterocolitis.
3. Enterocolitis—consists of severe toxemia and a proliferation of bacteria in the colonic lumen.
   a. Abdominal distention.
   b. Explosive diarrhea.
   c. Vomiting.
   d. Fever.
   e. Lethargy.
   f. Rectal bleeding.
   g. Shock.

Diagnostic Evaluation

1. Supportive findings on history and physical examination indicate Hirschsprung disease.
2. Digital rectal examination—reveals a tight anal sphincter and a rectum that is narrow and empty of stool (in long-segment disease). In short-segment disease, rectal impaction may be present; removal of finger may be associated with a rush of stool as the obstruction is relieved.
3. Plain films—show severe gaseous distention of the bowel, with absence of air in the rectum.
4. Barium enema—used to demonstrate a transition zone between the proximal dilated, normal innervated colon and the distal, narrow, aganglionic colon.
   a. May be nondiagnostic in young infants who have not had sufficient time to develop a transition zone.
   b. Delayed passage of barium is suggestive but not definitive for Hirschsprung disease.
   c. Must be an unprepped study, as results may be falsely negative if laxatives or rectal stimulation have been used to facilitate defecation.
5. Anorectal manometry—demonstrates failure of the intestinal sphincter to relax in response to transient rectal distention. Requires cooperation of the child.
6. Full thickness or suction rectal biopsy—absence or reduced number of ganglion nerve cells; definitive diagnosis.
7. Radiopaque markers, ingested, measure intestinal transit time. Use of these markers is not part of the standard diagnostic workup for Hirschsprung disease; however, children with short-segment disease retain the markers in the rectum for long periods.

Management

Definitive treatment is removal of the aganglionic, nonfunctioning, dilated segment of the bowel, followed by anastomosis and improved functioning of internal rectal sphincter.

1. Initially, a colostomy or ileostomy is performed to decompress intestine, divert fecal stream, and rest the normal bowel.
2. Definitive surgery includes the following reconstructive procedures:
   a. Swenson—abdominoperineal pull-through leaving the smallest amount of aganglionic bowel remaining.
   b. Duhamel—retrorectal transanal pull-through creating a neorectum with aganglionic anterior wall and ganglionic posterior wall.
   c. Soave—endorectal pull-through in which the ganglionic segment is pulled through the aganglionic muscular cuff, preserving the internal sphincter; may be done laparoscopically. May be delayed until infant is age 9 to 12 months or until weight reaches 15 to 20 pounds (6.5 to 9 kg).
3. Many surgeons are now performing the endorectal pull-through without colostomy in neonates. This depends on the degree of defect, degree of dilatation of the colon, and the clinical status of the infant.
4. In older child whose symptoms are chronic but not severe, treatment may consist of isotonic enemas, stool softeners, and low-residue diet until surgery is performed.
5. Treatment of enterocolitis.
   a. Broad-spectrum IV antibiotics.
   b. Colonic irrigation and decompression with saline solution is initial emergency treatment. Hypertonic phosphate enemas are contraindicated because they may be retained, leading to electrolyte abnormalities.
   c. Surgical decompression colostomy.
   d. At least 1 month after, abdominal perineal pull-through.

 NURSING ALERT Enterocolitis is a potentially life-threatening event. Notify health care provider immediately if change in abdominal distention occurs in an infant or child with Hirschsprung disease (whether preoperatively or postoperatively), especially if accompanied by fever, diarrhea, vomiting, or lethargy.

Complications

 EVIDENCE BASE Gosain, A., Frykman, P., Cowles, R., et al. (2017). Guidelines for the diagnosis and management of Hirschsprung-associated enterocolitis. *Pediatric Surgery International, 33*(5), 517–521.

Langer, J., Rollins, M., Levitt, M., et al. (2017). Guidelines for the management of postoperative obstructive symptoms in children with Hirschsprung disease. *Pediatric Surgery International, 33*(5), 523–526.

1. Preoperative.
   a. Enterocolitis—a major cause of death.
   b. Hydroureter or hydronephrosis.

    c. Water intoxication from tap water enemas.

    d. Bowel perforation.

2. Postoperative.

    a. Enterocolitis: remains the major cause of morbidity and mortality (mortality 6% to 30%).

    b. Diarrhea (69%).

    c. Vomiting (51%).

    d. Fever (34%).

    e. Lethargy (27%).

    f. Leaking of anastomosis and pelvic abscess.

    g. Stenosis, sudden inability to evacuate colon.

    h. Intestinal obstruction from adhesions, volvulus, or intus-susception can develop late.

    i. Fecal incontinence is common but can improve with a proper bowel regimen.

    j. Adverse reaction to foods.

    k. Enuresis.

Nursing Assessment

1. Observe neonate for constipation.

2. Obtain parents' history, especially on infant's bowel and feeding habits.

    a. Onset of constipation.

    b. Character of stools (ribbon-like or fluid filled).

    c. Frequency of bowel movements.

    d. Enemas needed.

    e. Suppositories or laxatives needed.

3. Observe for irritability, feeding difficulty, distended abdomen, and signs of malnutrition (pallor, muscle weakness, thin extremities, fatigue).

 NURSING ALERT Diagnosis of Hirschsprung disease should be suspected in any infant who fails to pass meconium within the first 24 hours and requires repeated rectal stimulation to induce bowel movements.

Nursing Diagnoses

Preoperative

- Ineffective Breathing Pattern related to abdominal distention.
- Acute Pain related to intestinal obstruction.
- Imbalanced Nutrition: Less Than Body Requirements related to poor intake.
- Constipation due to pathophysiologic process.

Postoperative

- Impaired tissue integrity related to postoperative intervention.
- Risk for Infection of surgical incision.
- Risk for Dysfunctional Gastrointestinal Motility related to decreased peristalsis postoperatively.
- Ineffective Family Coping related to care of child with colostomy.

Nursing Interventions

Improving Breathing Pattern

1. Monitor for respiratory compromise that may result from abdominal distention; watch for rapid, shallow respirations; cyanosis; sternal retractions.

2. Elevate infant's head and chest by tilting the mattress to facilitate an open airway

3. Administer oxygen, as ordered, to support respiratory status.

Relieving Pain

1. Note degree of abdominal tenderness.

    a. Infant's legs drawn up.

    b. Chest breathing.

2. Note color of abdomen and presence of gastric waves; take sequential measurements of abdominal girth for evidence of changes.

3. Assist in emptying the bowel by giving repeated colonic irrigations.

    a. Procedure for irrigation in an infant is similar to that in an older child, except that less fluid and pressure are used.

    b. Physiologic saline solution (warmed) should be used for irrigations. Tap water may result in large quantities of water being absorbed and in water intoxication.

4. Administer medications (antibiotics), as ordered, to reduce the bacterial flora of the bowel.

5. Note any change in degree of distention before and after irrigation. Record if location of distention changes (ie, upper or lower abdomen).

6. Record all intake and output of irrigant and drainage. Report marked discrepancies in retention or loss of fluid.

7. Insert rectal tube for escape of accumulated fluid and gas, as ordered.

8. If abdominal distention is not relieved by irrigation and decompression and discomfort is significant, insert an NG tube, as ordered.

    a. Note drainage from NG tube and chart characteristics.

    b. Check for patency; saline irrigations may be requested. Carefully record intake and output.

    c. Perform frequent mouth care.

    d. Alternate nares when changing NG tube, and use minimal amount of tape to prevent skin irritation.

9. Offer pacifier for nonnutritive sucking if NPO, on parenteral fluids.

10. Encourage parents to hold and rock infant.

11. Maintain position of comfort with head elevated. Offer soothing stimulation (eg, music, touch, play therapy).

Providing Adequate Nutrition

1. Obtain a dietary history regarding food and eating habits.

    a. Discuss history with dietitian to facilitate potential dietary alterations.

    b. Explain to parents that eating problems are common with Hirschsprung disease.

2. Monitor IV fluids appropriately; measure all output.

3. Offer small, frequent feedings.

    a. Feed child slowly.

    b. Provide as comfortable a position as possible for child during feedings.

4. Inform parents that defect can be corrected, but it may take some time for the child's physical status and feeding habits to improve.

    a. Feeding may cause additional discomfort because of distention and nausea.

    b. Parenteral nutrition may be necessary.

Controlling Constipation in the Older Child

1. Note and record frequency and characteristics of stools (constipation is likely to occur).

2. Provide demonstration and written and verbal instructions to family for saline enema administration and use of stool softeners.

3. Obtain dietary consultation for teaching of dietary alterations.

Preventing Complications Related to Colostomy

1. Monitor vital signs and respiratory status closely.
2. Monitor for proper functioning of colostomy, if present.
   a. Note drainage from colostomy: characteristics, frequency, fecal material, or liquid drainage.
   b. Record stoma color, size, and return of function.
   c. Note abdominal distention.
   d. Measure fluid loss from colostomy because the amount will affect fluid replacement.
3. Report signs of obstruction from peritonitis, paralytic ileus, handling bowel during surgery, or swelling.
   a. No output from colostomy.
   b. Increased abdominal tenderness.
   c. Irritability.
   d. Vomiting.
   e. Increased temperature.
   f. Firm abdomen.
4. Place child in a lateral position on a flat or only slightly elevated bed. When head of bed is elevated, the residual carbon dioxide in the child's abdominal cavity may cause referred pain in neck and shoulder.
5. Differentiate type and cause of pain to determine appropriate pain management interventions. Proper positioning, patent catheters and tubes, and timely administration of analgesics are key to ensuring patient comfort.
6. "Nothing per rectum" sign should be placed at head of bed so that no rectal temperatures, rectal medications, or digital rectal examinations are done.

 NURSING ALERT Prevent injury to rectal mucosa by taking axillary or external ear temperature.

 NURSING ALERT Any rectal examination or procedure has the potential to cause serious harm to the patient and surgical site.

Preventing Postoperative Infections

1. Change wound dressing using sterile technique. If done laparoscopically, wound is minimal.
2. Prevent contamination from diaper.
   a. Apply diaper below dressing.
   b. Change diaper frequently.
3. Be aware that 7 to 10 stools per day may be passed postoperatively via ostomy bag. When cleared by surgery, prevent perianal and anal excoriation by thorough cleansing sitz baths and application of zinc oxide paste after soiling.
4. If skin is denuded and moist, apply a skin barrier, and provide specific instruction to the family to prevent further damage to skin with aggressive removal.
5. Use careful hand-washing technique.
6. Report wound redness, swelling or drainage, evisceration, or dehiscence immediately.
7. Suction secretions frequently to prevent infection of the tracheobronchial tree and lungs.
8. Encourage frequent coughing and deep breathing to maintain respiratory status.
9. Allow the infant to cry for short periods to prevent atelectasis.
10. Change the infant's position frequently to increase circulation and allow for aeration of all lung areas.

Preventing Abdominal Distention

1. Maintain patency of NG tube immediately postoperatively.
   a. NG suction, as ordered, for 24 to 48 hours or until adequate bowel sounds, gas from rectum or gas from ostomy.
   b. Watch for increasing abdominal distention; measure abdominal girth.
   c. Measure fluid loss because amount will affect fluid replacement.
2. Maintain NPO status until bowel sounds return, and the bowel is ready for feedings as determined by provider.
3. Administer fluids to maintain hydration and replace lost electrolytes.
4. Maintain Foley catheter for 24 to 48 hours, as ordered.
5. Provide frequent oral hygiene while NPO.
6. Begin oral feedings, as ordered.
   a. Avoid overfeeding.
   b. Burp frequently during feeding.
   c. Turn head to side or elevate after feeding to prevent aspiration.

Supporting the Parents

1. Acknowledge that even a temporary colostomy can be a difficult procedure to accept and learn to manage.
   a. Initiate ostomy referral.
   b. Support the parents when teaching them to care for the colostomy.
   c. Include the parents in dressing changes and any other appropriate activities soon after surgery.
   d. Assist and encourage the parents to treat the infant or child as normally as possible.
   e. Reassure parents that colostomy will not cause delay in the child's normal development.
2. Encourage the parents to talk about their fears and anxieties. Anticipating future surgery for resection may be confusing and frightening.
3. Initiate community-nurse referral to help the parents care for the child at home away from the comforting situation of the hospital and obtain necessary equipment.
4. Initiate a genetic counseling referral, especially if the parents plan to have more children.

Ostomy Care in Children

 EVIDENCE BASE Colwell, J., McNichol, L., & Boarini, J. (2017). North America wound, ostomy, and continence and enterostomal therapy nurses current ostomy care practice related to peristomal skin issues. *Journal of Wound Ostomy Continence Nursing, 44*(3), 257–261.

Care of the colostomy and ileostomy in the infant and young child is based on the same principles and is essentially the same as that for an adult (see Chapter 18), with the following exceptions:

1. Colostomy irrigation is not part of management in small children. Irrigation is primarily for the purpose of regulating the colostomy to empty at regular intervals. Because children have bowel movements at more frequent intervals, this type of control is not feasible. Irrigation may be done only in preparation for tests or surgery and occasionally for the treatment of constipation.
2. Dehydration occurs quickly in the infant or small child; therefore, it is particularly important to observe drainage for amount and characteristics. Drainage should be measured

to provide an accurate basis for computation of fluid replacement.

3. Prevention and treatment of skin excoriation around the stoma are of primary concern. With the advent of better skin shields and equipment designed especially for the pediatric patient, keeping an ostomy appliance in place is now less difficult. Through careful application and trying different types of pouches until a proper fit is obtained, most children can be kept clean and dry for at least 24 hours between changes. This is a significant factor in preventing skin breakdown and subsequent infections in the peristomal area. Remember, however, that infant dressings must be checked frequently.
   a. Check ostomy bag for leakage every 2 hours and change bag as soon as leakage is suspected.
   b. Teach the parents the importance of emptying the bag, when it is one quarter to one- third full.
   c. Skin breakdown is more frequent. Reinforce to parents to treat breakdown with method and products recommended by ostomy nurse.
   d. Be aware that infant elimination is more frequent than in the older child.
4. For older children with ostomies:
   a. "Potty training" may be achieved for colostomy pouch emptying. This will not be possible for a child with an ileostomy.
   b. Pouching optimizes socialization and developmental activities.
   c. Encourage a matter-of-fact and accepting attitude to help build child's self-confidence.
   d. Encourage the child to participate in ostomy care.
   e. Encourage child to join age-appropriate ostomy support group.
5. Additional information and support can be obtained from the United Ostomy Associations of America (*www.ostomy.org*).

Community and Home Care Considerations

1. Begin early teaching about the colostomy (preoperatively, before discharge, and at home), including how it works and how to care for it and the child. Explanations should be thorough and in accordance with family readiness. Encourage care of the ostomy as part of normal activities of daily living.
2. Arrange frequent home visits to carry out comprehensive teaching plan. Consult with ostomy nurse, as needed, for any skin breakdown or other ostomy problems.
3. Involve the entire family in teaching colostomy care to enhance acceptance of body change of the child. An older child should become totally responsible for own colostomy care.
4. Assess family's self-care of the ostomy, including such procedures as preparation of skin, application of collecting appliance, care of appliance, and control of odor.
5. Observe for and teach family about signs of stomal complications, including ribbon-like stool, diarrhea, failure of evacuation of stool or flatus, and bleeding.
6. Assess hydration status and teach increased fluid intake because colon absorption is decreased or may be absent if an ileostomy is present.
7. Review GT feeding techniques, if ordered.
8. Assist family to discuss the child's needs with day care workers, teachers, and school nurse, as applicable. Review care of ostomy with child's care providers.

9. Assist with preoperative preparation for colostomy closure when the time comes.

Family Education and Health Maintenance

1. Instruct the parents to serve small, frequent meals to the child and be alert for and eliminate foods that cause gas and diarrhea, such as cabbage, spicy foods, beans, brussels sprouts, fruits, and fruit juices.
2. Advise parents that colds or viruses may cause loose stools, which increases risk of dehydration, especially in long-segment disease, so to increase fluids in these situations.
3. Alert parents of common postoperative problems, including bacterial overgrowth, colitis or enterocolitis, and lactose intolerance. Advise parents to contact their health care provider if persistent diarrhea, abdominal distention, abdominal pain, fever, vomiting, or constipation occur.
4. Encourage parents to practice all procedures long before the infant is to be discharged.
5. Emphasize the importance of treating the child as normally as possible to prevent behavior problems later.
6. Teach the basics of good nutrition and diet. Involve the dietitian, as necessary.
7. Encourage close medical follow-up and general good health and hygiene.
   a. Safety.
   b. General growth and development.
   c. Immunizations.
8. Advise older children without colostomies that fecal staining may occur, but this will improve with time.

Evaluation: Expected Outcomes

- Respirations unlabored; no cyanosis.
- Abdominal girth decreased; resting comfortably.
- Tolerates 1- to 2-ounce feedings every hour, depending on the age of the child.
- Passes stool at least every 2 days spontaneously or after enema.
- Vital signs within normal limits, afebrile, no abdominal distention.
- Stoma pink without drainage, redness, warmth, and tenderness.
- Bowel sounds present, NG tube discontinued.
- Parents listen, ask questions about care of child, and demonstrate adequate care/technique for device care/maintenance.

Intussusception

 EVIDENCE BASE Savoie, K., Thomas, F., Nouer, S., et al. (2017). Age at presentation and management of pediatric intussusception: A Pediatric Health Information System database study. *Surgery, 161*(4), 995–1003.

Intussusception is the invagination or telescoping of a portion of the intestine into an adjacent, more distal section of the intestine, which creates a mechanical obstruction. Intussusception is one of the most common causes of intestinal obstruction in infancy. It can occur at any time in life but most commonly occurs in children younger than age 3, with the greatest incidence between ages 5 and 10 months. It is twice as common in male infants as in female infants. Incidence in the United States is 1.5 to 4 cases per 1,000 births. Intussusception should be high on the differential list when a child younger than age 1 presents with sudden onset of abdominal pain.

Pathophysiology and Etiology

1. The cause can fall into one of three categories: idiopathic, lead point, or postoperative.
    a. Idiopathic: this is the most common type, with no identifiable cause. It is not unusual, however, to obtain a history of a recent upper respiratory or GI virus. It is hypothesized that hypertrophy of Peyer patches creates a thickened segment. It is most common in infants.
    b. Lead point: an identifiable change in the intestinal mucosa can be discovered, usually during surgical treatment, and is most common in children ages 2 to 3. Malformations include polyps, cysts, tumors, Meckel diverticulum, and hematomas (seen in Henoch-Schönlein purpura). Children with cystic fibrosis are at risk for lead point intussusception due to mucus and thick stool.
    c. Postoperative: uncommon but can occur after surgery of the abdomen and even the chest. It may be due to interrupted motility from anesthesia or direct handling of the intestine. It can also occur from placing long tubes into the bowel.
2. Invagination results in complete intestinal obstruction.
    a. Mesentery/lymphatics/blood vessels pulled into intestine when invagination occurs.
    b. Intestine becomes curved, sausage-like; blood supply is cut off.
    c. Bowel begins to swell; hemorrhage may occur.
    d. Necrosis of involved segment occurs.
    e. If not recognized and treated, bowel death occurs, possibly resulting in significant loss of intestine, shock, and death.
3. Classification of location:
    a. Ileocecal (most common): when ileum and the attached mesentery, lymphatic tissue, and blood vessels invaginate into the cecum (see Figure 48-7).
    b. Ileocolic: ileum invaginates into colon.
    c. Colocolic: colon invaginates into colon.
    d. Ileo–ileo (enteroenteric): small bowel invaginates into small bowel.
4. An increase in cases of intussusception was noted after the introduction of the first rotavirus vaccine (RotaShield), so this vaccine was taken off the market. The second generation of rotavirus vaccines (RotaTeq and Rotarix) carries a much lower (though not zero) risk of intussusception. It is felt that the small risk is outweighed by the benefit of the vaccine.

 EVIDENCE BASE Haber, P., Parashar, U., Haber, M., et al. (2015). Intussusception after monovalent rotavirus vaccine—United States, Vaccine Adverse Event Reporting (VAERS), 2008–2014. *Vaccine, 33*(38), 4873–4877.

Clinical Manifestations

1. Classic four signs of intussusception—vomiting, abdominal pain, bloody/red currant jelly–like stool, and abdominal mass—only occur in about 45% of children.
2. Pain is usually paroxysmal.
    a. "Attacks of pain" that awaken child from sleep; inconsolable, drawing up legs, colicky.
    b. Cyclic repetition of symptoms at approximately 5- to 30-minute intervals.
    c. Between episodes, child may act normal.
3. Stool may be like currant jelly—sloughed mucosa of dark red color with a mucoid consistency.
4. Vomiting may begin with decreased appetite and progress to bilious vomiting.
5. Bowel sounds vary:
    a. During a crisis of pain, bowel sounds may be hyperperistaltic rushes (borborygmi).
    b. Ileus/peritonitis: bowel sounds are diminished or absent.
6. Decreasing frequency of bowel movements.
7. Increasing abdominal distention and tenderness.
8. Sausage-like mass palpable in abdomen. This is pathognomonic and is known as *Dance sign*—elongated mass in the right upper quadrant of the abdomen with absence of bowel sounds in the right lower quadrant.
9. Unusual-looking anus; may look like rectal prolapse.
10. Dehydration, fever, lethargy; shocklike state with rapid pulse, pallor, marked sweating.
11. Hematochezia (maroon-colored stools)—not always present.
    a. Rectal examination is significant if bloody mucus on examiner's finger.
    b. Occult or gross blood on rectal exam in 60% to 90% of patients.
12. The groin should be inspected for incarcerated hernia or torsion of testicle or ovary as differential diagnosis.

 NURSING ALERT Currant jelly–like stool indicates damage to the intestine and can be a late sign. *Any* gross blood in the stool should raise suspicion of intussusception, especially when associated with abdominal pain; one should not wait for currant jelly–like stool to report.

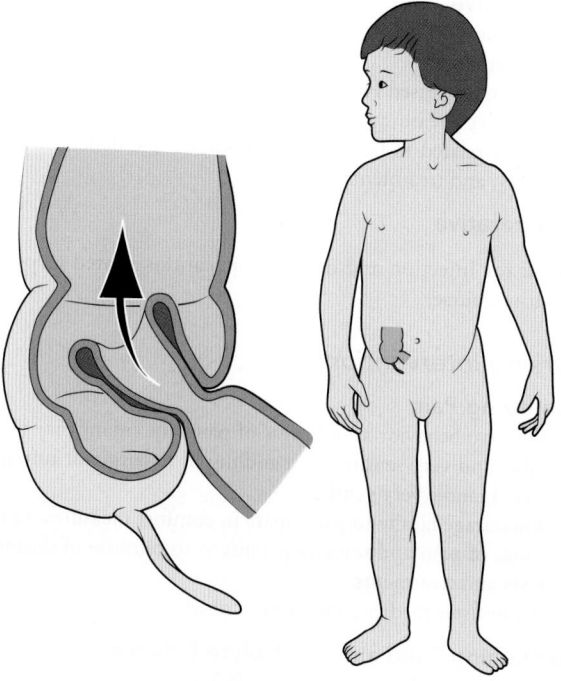

Figure 48-7. Intussusception. A portion of the ileum has been pushed into the lumen of the adjoining cecum. (LifeArt image.)

Diagnostic Evaluation

 EVIDENCE BASE Territo, H., Wrotniak, B., Qiao, H., et al. (2014). Clinical signs and symptoms associated with intussusception in young children undergoing ultrasound in the emergency room. *Pediatric Emergency Care, 30*(10), 718–722.

1. X-ray examination.
   a. Supine and upright abdomen film. Early course may be normal, but as it progresses absence of gas in the colon is found. Can also have finding of right upper quadrant mass and/or the meniscus/crescent sign.
   b. If no intraperitoneal air found on abdominal film, an air or barium enema is attempted.
   c. Commonly, a concave filling defect is seen in the transverse colon that can be reduced to the cecum.
2. Ultrasonogram to locate area of telescoped bowel and color Doppler sonography used to determine whether reducible or not. Absence of blood flow (color) indicates ischemia, and therefore, enema reduction should be avoided. Ultrasound will usually be obtained prior to contrast enema because of the low risk and excellent accuracy.

 NURSING ALERT Enemas are contraindicated in cases involving clinical findings of peritonitis, shock, or signs of perforation on abdominal x-ray.

Management

 EVIDENCE BASE Kim, J., Lee, J., Ryu, J., et al. (2018). Risk factors for recurrent intussusception after fluoroscopy-guided air enema. *Pediatric Emergency Care, 34*(7), 484–487.

1. Air or barium enema—both for diagnosis and treatment (hydrostatic reduction) in reducing intussusception.
   a. A surgeon should be present during the barium enema because of risk of perforation.
   b. A noninflatable tube is passed into rectum; contrast enters by gravity under fluoroscopic guidance. If air is used, it is delivered under constant pressure.
   c. As the intussusception is reduced, the contrast or air should reflux freely into the small intestine; this radiographic evidence is needed to confirm a successful reduction.
   d. Success ranges from 70% to 90%. Recurrence is the most common complication, but perforation can also occur.
   e. Nonoperative reduction using air enema or other hydrostatic reduction methods has been the standard treatment in most cases. The success rate can be as high as 84%. However, if nonoperative method is not indicated or fails, open surgery is still necessary.
2. Surgical reduction of intussusception may be necessary when radiologic reduction is unsuccessful, a pathologic lead point or peritonitis is suspected or with multiple recurrences. Factors associated with increased risk of intestinal resection include abdominal distension (32%), bowel obstruction on abdominal x-ray (27%), and hypovolemic shock (40%).
3. Surgery involves a laparotomy—manual milking-out of the intussuscepted segment from the distal to proximal end, followed by resection of the nonviable bowel and, commonly, an incidental appendectomy. Up to 86% successful in reduction.
4. Recurrence is 5% to 7% regardless of the type of treatment undertaken.

 EVIDENCE BASE Wong, C., Jin, S., Tam, P., et al. (2016). Predictors for bowel resection and the presence of a pathological lead point for operated childhood intussusception: A multi-center study. *Journal of Pediatric Surgery, 51*, 1998–2000.

Complications

1. Perforation.
2. Peritonitis.
3. Shock.
4. Loss of bowel resulting in short bowel syndrome.

Nursing Assessment

1. Obtain careful history of infant's or child's physical and behavioral symptoms, including any recent or chronic illness.
2. Perform physical examination, which may reveal a well-developed, well-nourished, afebrile infant with abdominal tenderness and distention.
3. Observe for dehydration; may be mild or severe. Poor capillary refill, decreased mental status, and decreased urine output are reliable indicators of shock in children.

 NURSING ALERT Report of episodic, severe, colicky abdominal pain combined with vomiting suggests intussusception.

Nursing Diagnoses

Preoperative
- Acute Pain related to paroxysmal abdominal pain, fever, and treatments.
- Risk for Decreased Fluid Volume related to vomiting.
- Ineffective Breathing Pattern related to abdominal distention.
- Anxiety related to hospitalization, knowledge deficit of illness, surgery, and treatments.

Postoperative
- Risk for Infection and other complications related to postoperative course.

Nursing Interventions

Minimizing Pain
1. Observe behavior as indicator of pain; the infant may be irritable and very sensitive to handling or lethargic or unresponsive. Handle very gently.
2. Encourage family to participate in comfort measures. Explain cause of pain and reassure parents as to purpose of diagnostic tests and treatments.
3. Administer medications, as prescribed.

Maintaining Fluid and Electrolyte Balance
1. Monitor fluids and maintain NPO status.
2. Restrain infant, as necessary, for IV therapy.
3. Monitor intake and output.

Promoting Effective Breathing

1. Be alert for respiratory distress because of abdominal distention. Watch for grunting or shallow and rapid respirations if in shocklike state.
2. Insert NG tube, if ordered, to decompress stomach.
   a. Irrigate, as ordered
   b. Note drainage and return from irrigation.
3. Maintain NPO status, as ordered.
   a. Wet lips and perform mouth care.
   b. Give infant pacifier to suck.
4. Continually reassess condition because disordered breathing or respiratory distress may indicate progression of disease process.

 NURSING ALERT Passage of one normal brown stool may occur, clearing the colon distal to the intussusception. Passage of more than one normal brown stool may indicate that the intussusception has reduced itself. Report any stools immediately to the physician.

Preparing for Surgery

1. Offer support to the parents during time of crisis and fear.
2. Offer specific teaching to parents.
   a. Compare intussusception to a collapsible telescope or antenna or by drawing a picture.
   b. Visual aids, such as a rubber glove with one finger into itself, may be helpful. Reduction can be demonstrated by filling glove with water until inverted finger resumes its normal position.
3. Children need brief, simple explanations in age-appropriate language.

Preventing Infection and Other Postoperative Complications

1. Monitor vital signs and general condition and notify health care provider of any change or unexpected trend.
2. Assess temperature and administer antipyretics and other cooling measures. Fever may be present from the translocation of bacteria into the bloodstream through the damaged intestinal wall.
3. Assess for abdominal tenderness, bowel sounds, and distention of abdomen. Maintain NG suction, as ordered.
4. Assess pain and level of consciousness.
5. When able to take fluids, assess tolerance carefully, and advance intake slowly.

Family Education and Health Maintenance

1. Explain that recurrences may occur and usually occur within 24 to 48 hours after reduction. Review signs and symptoms with parents.
2. Review activity restrictions with parents (eg, positioning on back or side, quiet play, and avoidance of water sports until wound heals).
3. Encourage follow-up care.
4. Provide anticipatory guidance for developmental age of child.
5. Encourage awareness of symptoms that require prompt medical attention among day care centers and other childcare providers (eg, paroxysmal abdominal pain, blood or mucus in stool).

Evaluation: Expected Outcomes

- Decreased irritability/pain.
- Urine output adequate.
- Respirations unlabored; abdominal distention relieved.
- Parents verbalize understanding of condition and surgery.
- Postoperative vital signs stable; audible bowel sounds; passes stool postoperatively.

Anorectal Malformations

 EVIDENCE BASE Van der Steeg, J., Schmiedeke, E., Bagolan, P., et al. (2015). European consensus meeting of ARM-Net members concerning diagnosis and early management of newborns with anorectal malformations. *Techniques in Coloproctology, 19*(3), 181–185.

The term *anorectal malformation* encompasses multiple congenital anomalies of the rectum, urinary tract, and reproductive system. Incidence is 1 in 2,500 to 1 in 4,000 live births, with a slight male predominance. Complexity varies from isolated imperforate anus to the extremely rare cloacal exstrophy (occurs in males and females 1 in every 250,000 births).

Pathophysiology and Etiology

 EVIDENCE BASE Kovacic, K., Matta, S., Kovacic, K., et al. (2018). Healthcare utilization and comorbidities associated with anorectal malformations in the United States. *Journal of Pediatrics, 194*, 142–146.

1. An arrest in embryologic development of the anus, lower rectum, and urogenital tract at the 6th week of embryonic life; however, cause is unknown.
2. Approximately 40% of infants with anorectal malformations have associated major anomalies, including:
   a. Down syndrome.
   b. VACTERL syndrome (vertebral defects, anal atresia, cardiac anomaly, TEF with EA, renal defects, and radial limb dysplasia).
   c. Congenital heart disease.
   d. Renal abnormalities.
   e. Cryptorchidism.
   f. Esophageal atresia.
   g. Malformation of the spine.
   h. Variant of infantile hemangioma occurring in the extremity.
3. Abnormal development of the terminal hindgut ranges from mild anal stenosis, corrected by simple dilatation, to complex deformities, such as rectal atresia and fistula, with varying degrees of fecal and urinary incontinence.
4. BMP4 and Hox genes may play a role.

Types

See Figure 48-8.

1. Imperforate anal membrane—infant fails to pass meconium; greenish, bulging membrane is seen; bowel and sphincter return to normal after excision.
2. Rectoperineal fistula—rectum opens into the perineum; excellent function.
3. Anal atresia and stenosis—complete obstruction (atresia) or stenosis (decrease in caliber) is present approximately 2 cm above the anal opening.
4. Imperforate anus without fistula (anal agenesis)—rectum is completely blind, ending 2 cm from perineum; intestinal obstruction occurs if no associated fistula.

Figure 48-8. Anorectal malformations. **(A)** Anal stenosis. **(B)** Imperforate anal membrane. **(C)** Anal agenesis. **(D)** Rectal agenesis. **(E)** Rectoperineal fistula. **(F)** Small orifice located in the perineum. (Adapted with permission from Wong, D. L. [1995]. *Whaley and Wong's nursing care of infants and children* [5th ed.]. St. Louis, MO: Mosby.)

5. Anorectal malformation with rectourinary fistula in males (present in 80% of males with anorectal malformations).
   a. Rectourethral bulbar fistula.
   b. Rectourethral prostatic fistula.
   c. Rectobladder neck fistula.
6. Anorectal malformation with fistula and cloaca in females.
   a. Vestibular fistula—rectum opens through an abnormal narrow orifice located in the vestibule of the genitalia outside the hymen; most common defect in females.
   b. Vagina fistula—rectum opens via fistula into vagina; exceptionally rare malformation.
   c. Persistent cloaca—complex defect in which the rectum, vagina, and urinary tract are fused together into one common channel ending in a single perineal orifice at the site of the urethra; requires colostomy, urinary diversion, or vaginal diversion.
7. Cloacal exstrophy—complex anorectal anomaly that includes omphalocele, two exstrophied hemibladders with cecum between them, imperforate anus, and abnormalities of sexual structures; rare; occurs in males and females.
8. Ectopic anus—mild displacement of the anus, which causes constipation. It is not a true anorectal malformation but may require dilatations or surgery. The anal position can be measured using the anal position index, which is the ratio of anus–fourchette distance in girls and anus–scrotum distance in boys to the distance between coccyx and fourchette/scrotum.

Degree of Incontinence

1. It may be difficult to absolutely predict what pediatric patients will obtain bowel and bladder continence for those with congenital GI/GU abnormalities or those who have suffered an injury to the area.

2. Bowel and bladder incontinence can be caused by damage to the nerves that control the sphincter muscles that control the outflow or damage to the muscle wall itself.
3. Complications may also occur from extensive surgical repairs required for surgery of the gastrointestinal or urologic system.
4. Gender and the type of abnormality will impact the likelihood of continence.
5. Some disorders; such as perineal fistula, rectal atresia, and rectal stenosis frequently result in 100% of patients having neither bowel nor bladder control.
6. Disorders such as rectobladder neck fistulas usually cause incontinence of urine but allow for bowel control.

Clinical Manifestations

1. Absence of anal opening; stimulation of perineum leads to puckering.
2. Displaced anal opening.
3. Anal opening near vaginal opening in female.
4. Thermometer, small finger, or rectal tube cannot be inserted into the rectum.
5. Meconium stool is absent or delayed.
6. Stool passed by way of the vagina or urethra may appear as green-tinged urine.
7. Progressive abdominal distention.
8. Fistula is likely to be present.
9. Vomiting if infant is fed.

Diagnostic Evaluation

1. Urine examination for presence of meconium and epithelial debris indicates presence of fistula.

2. Cross-table lateral abdominal x-ray—infant in prone position with pelvis elevated.
   a. Gas in blind rectum gives a radiolucent image.
   b. Measurement from the skin (radiopaque marker) and the blind rectum allow estimate of the height of the defect.
3. Abdominal ultrasound to detect urinary obstruction and locate rectal pouch.
4. Voiding cystourethrogram to detect commonly associated urinary tract anomalies such as vesicoureteral reflux.
5. MRI.

Management

 EVIDENCE BASE Youssef, F., Arbash, G., Puligandla, P., et al. (2017). Loop versus divided colostomy for the management of anorectal malformations: A systematic review and meta-analysis. *Journal of Pediatric Surgery, 52*(5), 783–790.

Rigueros Springfield, L., Connor, M., Jones, K., et al. (2016). Prevalence of active long-term problems in patients with anorectal malformations: A systematic review. *Diseases of the Colon and Rectum, 59*(6), 570–580.

Imperforate Anal Membrane
1. Internal and external sphincters are intact, so usually requires only a membrane excision from the anal opening.
2. Repaired at birth; no colostomy required.

Anal Stenosis
1. Internal and external sphincters are intact, so usually treated with anal dilation.
2. Occasionally requires myotomy (cutting of anal muscle).
3. Treated at birth; no colostomy required.

Imperforate Anus (Anal Agenesis)
1. Low lesion.
   a. Can usually be repaired with perineal anoplasty, which creates an anal opening for passage of stool.
   b. Usually accompanied by fistulas that need to be closed at the same time.
   c. Repaired at birth; colostomy usually not needed unless a fistula is present or more time for healing is needed.
2. High lesion.
   a. Requires more extensive surgery because of missing innervation.
   b. Usually requires a two-stage procedure, occasionally three-stage if complex defect is present.
   c. First step is a colostomy.
   d. Second step is anal repair, colon/rectum anastomosis, possible colostomy closure.
      i. Posterior sagittal anorectoplasty, also known as the *Pena procedure* (after the surgeon who developed it). The rectum is "pulled down" and sewn into a newly made anal opening in the perineum.
      ii. Most surgeons wait 4 to 6 months to complete it to allow for growth.
   e. Third step is colostomy closure if defect is complex and more healing time is needed.

Complex Fistulas and Cloaca
1. Complex rectal, urologic, and vaginal reconstruction are necessary.
2. Urinary diversion is performed in the neonate if a urologic emergency is apparent.

Note: Rectal dilation may be needed for any condition after the final surgery.

Complications
1. Infection.
2. Intestinal obstruction.
3. Loss of bladder or urinary sphincter control.

 NURSING ALERT Condition is usually discovered immediately after birth or within several hours. A delay in diagnosis is not uncommon and can significantly increase the risk of serious early complications and death.

Nursing Assessment
1. Perform physical assessment of neonate for abnormalities.
   a. Presence of perineal fistula.
   b. Meconium from vagina or presence of meconium-stained urine.
   c. No anal opening or inability to pass thermometer into rectum.
2. Perform thorough examination for other congenital anomalies.
3. Assess parents' level of understanding of condition and ability to cope with infant's surgery.

 NURSING ALERT A neonate who does not pass a stool in the first 24 hours after birth requires further assessment.

Nursing Diagnoses
Preoperative
- Risk for Activity Intolerance related to instability before surgery.

Postoperative
- Risk for Infection related to surgical incision of anoplasty.
- Risk for Impaired Skin Integrity related to ostomy and anoplasty.
- Risk for Decreased Fluid Volume related to restricted intake.
- Readiness for Enhanced Family Processes related to increased needs of infant.
- Delayed Surgical Recovery related to definitive repair surgery.

Nursing Interventions
Maintaining Stability Before Surgery
1. Maintain NPO status. Note any vomiting: color and amount.
2. Minimize energy expenditure due to altered nutritional status.
3. Maintain NG tube passed to decompress the stomach, as ordered. Measure abdominal girth.
4. Observe the patient carefully for any signs of distress and report. Check vital signs frequently.
5. Use an Isolette or radiant warmer to maintain temperature stability.
6. Minimal handling; cluster procedures together to encourage rest and sleep.
7. Keep fistula area clean to prevent UTI.
8. Administer good oral care.

Preventing Infection of Suture Line

1. Following anoplasty, do not put anything in the rectum.
   a. Position the infant for easy access to perineum for cleansing and minimal irritation to site (ie, place the infant on his or her abdomen, possibly with hips elevated, to prevent pressure on perineal surfaces; turn side-to-side).
   b. Expose the perineum to air.
   c. Observe incision site for redness, drainage, poor healing.
   d. Apply antibiotic ointment to perineum, as directed.
2. Following colostomy, observe wound and stoma for redness, drainage, poor healing.
3. Administer IV antibiotics, as directed (usually 2 to 3 days).

Preventing Skin Breakdown

See "Ostomy Care in Children," page 1303.

Maintaining Fluid and Electrolyte Balance

1. Monitor for return of peristalsis; NG tube may be discontinued by the health care provider when bowel sounds present.
2. Start oral feedings, as ordered.
   a. Anoplasty: usually within hours.
   b. Colostomy: when bowel sounds present and colostomy has output.
3. Monitor parenteral fluids and discontinue when oral intake is sustained.
4. Report vomiting.
5. Describe stool frequency, consistency, and character. Report blood in stool or lack of stool output.
6. Monitor urine output, particularly important with urethral defects (including cloaca).

Strengthening Coping

1. Assure the parents that colostomy is temporary (unless complex surgery performed).
2. Encourage the parents to participate in care of the child and to provide emotional security for the child.
3. Provide thorough teaching program for special care needed at home.
   a. Colostomy care.
   b. Anal dilatation to prevent a stricture at site of anastomosis from scar tissue (after instructions by health care provider).
4. Initiate referral to community nurse, especially if the parents are particularly anxious about caring for the child at home.
5. Encourage the parents to talk about their concerns.
6. Enlist help of enterostomal nurse specialist before the child leaves the hospital and for continued home care needs.
7. Assist breast-feeding mother to maintain milk supply through frequent pumping.

Maximizing Recovery Following Definitive Pull-Through Surgery

1. Maintain GT or NG tube decompression until peristalsis returns.
2. If a bladder catheter is used, provide care, as directed, and measure urine output accurately.
3. Observe carefully for abdominal distention, bleeding from perineum, and respiratory compromise. Report immediately.
4. Carry out perineal care.

Family Education and Health Maintenance

1. Review special care and procedures to be continued at home. Involve parents and other caregivers in teaching. Advise parents to make day care providers, teachers, and school nurse aware of child's needs.

2. It is important that the family understands the rationale and technique for anal dilation as indicated by the surgeon. Provide written instructions and assess their understanding of the procedure.
3. Help the parents to understand situations that may be encountered as a result of anorectal malformation repair as the infant gets older.
   a. Fecal impaction due to lack of sensation to defecate.
   b. Future surgery if primary repair was not done or defect complicated.
   c. Toilet training—may be delayed, especially after a pull-through procedure.
   d. Inability to control fecal seepage from rectum.
4. Offer practical guidelines to help parents cope.
   a. Fecal control may not be achieved until age 10; however, about 85% of children achieve normal or socially acceptable continence if defect limited to imperforate anus.
   b. If incontinence occurs, anorectal manometric evaluation in postoperative period can give more realistic information about future incontinence.
   c. Encourage bowel habit training or patterning of defecation (eg, after breakfast).
   d. Promote diet modifications; teach foods that produce laxative effect (plums, prunes, chocolate, nuts, corn) and foods that have binding effect (peanut butter, hot cereal, cheese).
   e. Stool softeners or antidiarrheal medication as ordered by the health care provider.
   f. Rectal inertia may cause fecal impaction in rectosigmoid colon with soiling from fluid overflow. Bisacodyl suppository or cleansing enema provides assistance in management.
5. Antegrade continence enema procedures may allow for continence in children without anal sphincter function.
6. Encourage mutual support from other families who have a child with an anorectal malformation.
7. For additional information and support, refer the parents to the National Organization for Rare Disorders (*www.rarediseases.org*) or the United Ostomy Associations of America (*www.ostomy.org*).

 DRUG ALERT Antidiarrheal medications should be used with caution in children.

Evaluation: Expected Outcomes

- Vital signs stable, abdominal girth stable.
- No signs of infection of suture line.
- Skin intact surrounding ostomy.
- Bowel sounds present; oral feeding tolerated without vomiting; NG tube discontinued.
- Family discusses plans for home care with enterostomal therapist.

 TRANSITIONAL CARE ALERT Children discharged to home with a gastrointestinal disorder may require a complex level of care by family caregivers. Ensure that the caregivers understand procedures and outcomes for nutritional support. It is crucial that nurses discharging these patients ensure that the families have the financial means and access to secure necessary nutritional requirements as well as the ability to store items (if refrigeration is required). Gastrointestinal disorders frequently cause alteration in means of elimination, or incontinence. Ensure that all necessary equipment is available to maintain optimal hygiene and infection disease containment. This is also crucial for the child (who has successfully toilet trained) to maintain social interactions without embarrassment. If long term management is expected for nutrition and elimination in the school-age child, the nurse may be called on to assist in training and education of school personnel to assist in the care.

SELECTED REFERENCES

Adams, D., Eberly, M., Rajnik, M., et al. (2017). Risk factors for community-associated *Clostridium difficile* infection in children. *Journal of Pediatrics, 186,* 105–109.

Allen, P. (2015). Gluten-related disorders: Celiac disease, gluten allergy, non-celiac gluten sensitivity. *Pediatric Nursing, 41*(3), 146–150.

Baird, D., Harker, D., & Karmes, A., (2015). Diagnosis and Treatment of Gastroesophageal Reflux in Infants and Children. *American Family Physician, 92*(8), 705–714.

Barnes, C. (2016). An introduction to the management of paediatric patients with celiac disease. *Gastrointestinal Nursing, 14*(9), 39–45.

Baylis, A. L., Pearson, G. D., Hall, C., et al. (2018). A Quality improvement initiative to improve feeding and growth of infants with cleft lip and/or palate. *The Cleft Palate Craniofacial Journal.* Jan 01, 1545–1569.

Becker, P., Carney, L., Corkins, L., et al. (2014). Consensus statement of the Academy of Nutrition and Dietetics/American Society for Parenteral and Enteral Nutrition: Indicators recommended for the identification and documentation of pediatric malnutrition (undernutrition). *Journal of the Academy of Nutrition and Dietetics, 114*(12), 1988–2000.

Burg, M., Chait, Y., & Yao, C., et al. (2016). Epidemiology, etiology, and treatment of isolated cleft palate. *Frontiers in Physiology, 7*(67), epages.

Carson, R., Mudd, S., & Jamil, P. (2017). Evaluation of a nurse-initiated acute gastroenteritis pathway in the Pediatric Emergency Department. *Journal of Emergency Nursing, 43*(5), 406–412.

Colwell, J., McNichol, L., & Boarini, J. (2017). North America wound, ostomy, and continence and enterostomal therapy nurses current ostomy care practice related to peristomal skin issues. *Journal of Wound Ostomy & Continence Nursing, 44*(3), 257–261.

Costanzo, C., Vinocur, C., & Berman, L. (2018). Postoperative outcomes of open versus laparoscopic pyloromyotomy for hypertrophic pyloric stenosis. *Journal of Surgical Residency,* Apr, 240–244. Epub.

Dahl, R., Curns, A., Tate, J., et al.(2018). Effect of Rotavirus Vaccination on Acute Diarrheal Hospitalizations Among Low and Very Low Birth Weight US Infants, 2001–2015. *Pediatric Infectious Disease Journal,* Feb 3, Epub ahead of print.

Feragen, K., & Stock, N. (2017). Psychological adjustment to craniofacial conditions (excluding oral clefts): A review of the literature. *Psychology & Health, 32*(3), 253–288.

Gezer, H., Oguzkurt, P., Temiz, A., et al. (2015). Hypertrophic pyloric stenosis in twins; genetic or environmental factors. *Clinical Genetics, 87*(4), 388–391.

Gosain, A., Frykman, P., Cowles, R., et al. (2017). Guidelines for the diagnosis and management of Hirschsprung-associated enterocolitis. *Pediatric Surgery International, 33*(5), 517–521.

Haaland, Ø. A., Lie, R. T., Romanowska, J., et al. (2018). A genome-wide search for gene-environment effects in isolated cleft lip with or without cleft palate triads points to an interaction between maternal periconceptional vitamin use and variants in *ESRRG. Frontiers in Genetics, 9,* 60. *http://doi.org/10.3389/fgene.2018.00060.*

Haas, K., Martin, A., & Park, K. T. (2017). Text message intervention (TEACH) improves quality of life and patient activation in celiac disease: A randomized clinical trial. *Journal of Pediatrics, 185,* 62–67.

Haber, P., Parashar, U., Haber, M., et al. (2015). Intussusception after monovalent rotavirus vaccine—United States, Vaccine Adverse Event Reporting (VAERS), 2008–2014. *Vaccine, 33*(38), 4873–4877.

Hendrickson, M., Zaremba, J., Wey, A., et al. (2017). The use of a triage-based protocol for oral rehydration in a Pediatric Emergency Department. *Pediatric Emergency Care, 34*(4), 227–232.

Hill, I., Fasano, A., Guandalini, S., et al. (2016). NASPGHAN clinical report on the diagnosis and treatment of gluten-related disorders. *Journal of Pediatric Gastroenterology and Nutrition, 63*(1), 156–165.

Holscher, A., Laschat, M., Choinitzki, V., et al. (2017). Quality of life after surgical treatment for esophageal atresia: Long-term outcomes of 154 patients. *European Journal of Pediatric Surgery, 27*(5), 443–448.

Isaac, D., Wu, J., Mager, D., et al. (2016). Managing the pediatric patient with celiac disease: A multidisciplinary approach. *Journal of Multidisciplinary Healthcare, 9,* 529–536.

Jancelewicz, T., Lopez, M., Downward, C., et al. (2016). Surgical management of gastroesophageal reflux disease (GERD) in children: A systematic review. *Journal of Pediatric Surgery, 52*(8), 1228–1238.

Jericho, H., Assiri, A., & Guandalini, S. (2017). Celiac disease and wheat intolerance syndrome: A critical update and reappraisal. *Journal of Pediatric Gastroenterology and Nutrition, 64*(1), 15–19.

Johnston, B., Goldenberg, J., & Parkin, P. (2016). Probiotics and the prevention of antibiotic-associated diarrhea in infants & children. *Journal of the American Medical Association, 316*(14), 1484–1485.

Kaye, A., Thaete, K., Snell, A., et al. (2017). Initial nutritional assessment of infants with cleft lip and/or palate: interventions and return to birth weight. *Cleft Palate Craniofac J, 54*(2), 127–136.

Kim, J., Lee, J., Ryu, J., et al. (2017). Risk factors for recurrent intussusception after fluoroscopy-guided air enema. *Pediatric Emergency Care.* [Epub ahead of print].

Kovacic, K., Matta, S., Kovacic, K., et al. (2018). Healthcare utilization and comorbidities associated with anorectal malformations in the United States. *Journal of Pediatrics, 194,* 142–146.

Krishnan, U., Mousa, H., Dall'Oglio, L., et al. (2016). ESPGHAN-NASPGHAN guidelines for the evaluation and treatment of gastrointestinal and nutritional complications in children with esophageal atresia-tracheoesophageal fistula. *Journal of Pediatric Gastroenterology and Nutrition, 63*(5), 550–570.

Kuijpers, M., Chiu, Y., Nada, R., et al. (2014). Three-dimensional imaging methods for quantitative analysis of facial tissues and skeletal morphology in patients with orofacial clefts: A systematic review. *PLoS ONE, 9*(4), e93442.

Lal, D., Gadepalli, S., Downard, C., et al. (2017). Perioperative management and outcomes of esophageal atresia and tracheoesophageal fistula. *Journal of Pediatric Surgery, 52*(8), 1245–1251.

Langer, J., Rollins, M., Levitt, M., et al. (2017). Guidelines for the management of postoperative obstructive symptoms in children with Hirschsprung disease. *Pediatric Surgery International, 33*(5), 523–526.

Lo Vecchio, A., Dias, J., Berkley, J., et al. (2016). Comparison of recommendations in clinical practice guidelines for acute gastroenteritis in children. *Journal of Pediatric Gastroenterology and Nutrition, 63*(2), 226–235.

Lo Vecchio, A., Vandenplas, Y., Benninga, M., et al. (2016). An international consensus report on a new algorithm for the management of infant diarrhea. *Acta Paediatrica, 105*(8), 384–389.

Mcguire, E. (2017). Cleft lip and palates and breastfeeding. *Breastfeeding Review, 25*(1), 17–23.

Menzies, J., Hughes, J., Leach, S., et al. (2017). Prevalence of malnutrition and feeding difficulties in children with esophageal atresia. *Journal of Pediatric Gastroenterology and Nutrition, 64*(4), 100–105.

Moore, S. (2016). Genetic impact on the treatment and management of Hirschsprung disease. *Journal of Pediatric Surgery, 52,* 218–222.

Morini F, Conforti A, Bagolan P. (2018). Perioperative complications of esophageal atresia. *Eur J Pediatr Surg, 28*(2), 133–140. *https://www.ncbi.nlm.nih.gov/pubmed/29534254.*

Murchison, L., De Coppi, P., & Eaton, S. (2016). Post-natal erythromycin exposure and risk of infantile hypertrophic pylori stenosis: A systematic review and meta-analysis. *Pediatric Surgery International, 32*(12), 1147–1152.

National Institute of Dental and Craniofacial Research, National Institutes of Health. *https://nidcr.nih.gov/DataStatistics/FindDataByTopic/CraniofacialBirthDefects/PrevalenceCleft%20LipCleftPalate.htm.* Accessed: 9 May 2018

Okata, Y., Maeda, K., & Bitoh, Y. (2016). Evaluation of the intraoperative risk factors for esophageal anastomotic complications after primary repair of esophageal atresia with tracheoesophageal fistula. *Pediatric Surgery International, 32*(9), 869–873.

Paul, S. P., Sandhu, B. K., Spray, C. H., et al. (2018). Evidence supporting serology-based pathway for diagnosing celiac disease in asymptomatic children from high-risk groups. *Journal of Pediatric Gastroenterology & Nutrition, 66*(4), 641–644.

Rao, A., Ahmed, M., Taub, P., et al. (2016). The correlation between maternal exposure to air pollution and the risk of orofacial clefts in infants: A systematic review and meta-analysis. *Journal of Oral & Maxillofacial Research, 7*(1), e2.

Rigueros Springfield, L., Connor, M., Jones, K., et al. (2016). Prevalence of active long-term problems in patients with anorectal malformations: A systematic review. *Diseases of the Colon and Rectum, 59*(6), 570–580.

Rosen, R., Vandenplas, Y., Singendonk, M., et al. (2018). Pediatric Gastroesophageal Reflux Clinical Practice Guidelines: Joint Recommendations of the North American Society for Pediatric Gastroenteroloyg, Hepatology, and Nutrition and the European Society for Pediatric Gastroenterology, Hepatology, and Nutrition. *JPGN, 66*(3), 516–544

Saal, H. (2016). Genetic evaluation for craniofacial conditions. *Facial Plastic Surgery Clinics of North America, 24*(4), 405–425.

Sarwer, D., Kazak, A., Clarke, A., et al. (2017) Body image and quality of life in adolescents with craniofacial conditions. *Cleft Palate-Craniofacial Journal, 54*(1), 2–12.

Sathya, C., Wayne, C., Gotsch, A., et al. (2017). Laparoscopic versus open pyloromyotomy in infants: A systematic review and meta-analysis. *Pediatric Surgery International, 33*(3), 325–333.

Savoie, K., Thomas, F., Nouer, S., et al. (2017). Age at presentation and management of pediatric intussusception: A pediatric health information system database study. *Surgery, 161* (4), 995–1003.

Singh, A., Middlesworth, W., & Khlevner, J. (2017). Surveillance in patients with esophageal atresia/tracheoesophageal fistula. *Current Gastroenterology Reports, 19*(1), 4.

Sischo, L., Clouston, S., & Phillips, C. (2016). Caregiver responses to early cleft palate care: A mixed method approach. *Health Psychology, 35*(4), 474–482.

Stobaugh, H., Rogers, B., Rosenberg, I., et al. (2018). Children with poor linear growth are at risk for repeated relapse to wasting after recovery from moderate acute malnutrition. *Journal of Nutrition*, May 3. Epub ahead of print.

Sullivan, K., Chan, E., & Vincent, J. (2016). Feeding post-pyloromyotomy: A meta-analysis. *Pediatrics, 137*(1), epub.

Svoboda, E., Fruithof, J., Widenmann-Grolig, A., et al. (2018). A patient led, international study of long term outcomes of esophageal stresia: EAT 1. *Journal of Pediatric Surgery, 53*(4), 610–615.

Territo, H., Wrotniak, B., Qiao, H., et al. (2014). Clinical signs and symptoms associated with intussusception in young children undergoing ultrasound in the emergency room. *Pediatric Emergency Care, 30*(10), 718–722.

Van der Steeg, J., Schmiedeke, E., Bagolan, P., et al. (2015). European consensus meeting of ARM-Net members concerning diagnosis and early management of newborns with anorectal malformations. *Techniques in Coloproctology, 19*(3), 181–185.

Vandenplas, Y., & Hauser, B. (2015). An updated review on gastro-esophageal reflux in pediatrics. *Expert Review of Gastroenterology and Hepatology, 9*(12), 1511–1521.

Westfal, M., & Goldstein, A. (2017). Pediatric enteric neuropathies: diagnosis and current management. *Current Opinion in Pediatrics, 29*(3), 347–353.

Wong, C., Jin, S., Tam, P., et al. (2016). Predictors for bowel resection and the presence of a pathological lead point for operated childhood intussusception: A multi-center study. *Journal of Pediatric Surgery, 51*, 1998–2000.

Woo, A. (2017). Evidence-based medicine: Cleft palate. *Plastic & Reconstructive Surgery, 139*(1), 191e–203e.

Youssef, F., Arbash, G., Puligandla, P., et al. (2017). Loop versus divided colostomy for the management of anorectal malformations: A systematic review and meta-analysis. *Journal of Pediatric Surgery, 52*(5), 783–790.

Zhu, J., Zhu, T., Lin, Z., et al. (2017). Perinatal risk factors for infantile hypertrophic pyloric stenosis: A meta-analysis. *Journal of Pediatric Surgery, 52*(9), 1389–1397.

49

Pediatric Renal and Genitourinary Disorders

ACUTE DISORDERS

Acute Glomerulonephritis

Acute glomerulonephritis is a broad term used to describe several disease processes that result in glomerular injury. The glomerular injury is the result of antigen–antibody deposits within the glomeruli. It occurs most frequently in school-age children, is rare in children younger than age 2, and occurs more frequently in males than in females (2:1).

Pathophysiology and Etiology

1. Presumed cause—antigen–antibody reaction secondary to an infection elsewhere in the body (see Figure 49-1).
2. The initial infection is usually either an upper respiratory infection (URI) or a skin infection.
3. Most frequent causative agent—nephritogenic strains of group A beta-hemolytic streptococcus.
4. It is speculated that the streptococcal infection is followed by the release of a membrane-like material from the organism into the circulation.
5. Antibodies produced to fight the invading organism also react against the glomerular tissue, thus forming immune complexes.
6. The immune complexes become trapped in the glomerular loop and cause an inflammatory reaction in the affected glomeruli.
7. Changes in the glomerular capillaries reduce the amount of the glomerular filtrate, allow passage of blood cells and protein into the filtrate, and reduce the amount of sodium and water that is passed to the tubules for reabsorption.
8. General vascular disturbances, including loss of capillary integrity and spasm of arterioles, are secondary.

Clinical Manifestations

Onset

1. Usually 7 to 15 days after acute pharyngitis. In streptococcal skin infections, the latency period may be as long as 4 to 6 weeks.

2. May be abrupt and severe or mild and detected only by laboratory measures.

Signs and Symptoms

1. Urinary symptoms:
   a. Decreased urine output.
   b. Bloody or brown-colored urine.
2. Edema.
   a. Present in most patients.
   b. Usually mild.
   c. Commonly manifested by periorbital edema in the morning.
   d. May appear only as rapid weight gain.
   e. May be generalized and influenced by posture.
3. Hypertension.
   a. Present in up to 70% of those hospitalized with glomerulonephritis.
   b. Usually mild.
   c. Rise in blood pressure (BP) may be sudden.
   d. Usually appears during the first 4 to 5 days of the illness.
4. Pallor.
5. Malaise, lethargy.
6. Low-grade fever.
7. Mild headache.
8. GI disturbances, especially anorexia and vomiting.

Diagnostic Evaluation

1. Urinalysis:
   a. Decreased output (oliguria)—may approach anuria.
   b. Microscopic or gross hematuria (noted in 30% to 70% of all cases).
   c. Specific gravity—moderately elevated.
   d. Proteinuria may be mild to severe.
   e. Microscopic—red blood cells, leukocytes, epithelial cells, and casts.
   f. Low urinary sodium may be noted.
2. Blood urea nitrogen (BUN) and creatinine—usually mildly to moderately elevated; however, normal in 50% of cases.

Figure 49-1. Sequence of events in acute glomerulonephritis. (Smeltzer, S., & Bare, B. [2000]. *Brunner and Suddarth's textbook of medical-surgical nursing* [9th ed.]. Philadelphia: Lippincott Williams & Wilkins.)

3. Antistreptolysin-O titer—elevated initially.
4. Anti-DNase B titer—elevated.
5. Erythrocyte sedimentation rate—elevated.
6. Complement C3 and complement C4—depressed.
7. If chest x-ray indicated—may show pulmonary congestion, cardiac enlargement during the edematous phase.

Management

1. Antibiotic therapy may be initiated if there is any concern that streptococci or other organisms are still present.
2. Other management is mostly symptomatic; in most patients, spontaneous recovery is expected. Hospitalization is usually not necessary.
3. Salt and fluid intake should be restricted during the acute phase of the disease.
4. Diuretics should be administered if significant edema or hypertension develops.
5. A renal biopsy may be indicated if the child does not recover from apparent acute poststreptococcal glomerulonephritis.

Complications

The following complications occur infrequently.

1. Circulatory congestion—if severe can lead to pulmonary edema.

2. Hypertensive encephalopathy.
3. Acute renal failure.
4. Anemia.

Nursing Assessment

1. Obtain history regarding recent streptococcal infection.
2. Obtain appropriate cultures and assess for current infection.
3. Measure urine output and degree of hematuria and proteinuria.
4. Weigh the child and document areas and extent of edema.
5. Obtain baseline BP reading to assess for hypertension.

Nursing Diagnoses

• Impaired Urinary Elimination related to glomerular dysfunction.
• Excess Fluid Volume related to impaired renal function.
• Deficient Diversional Activity related to prolonged illness and restrictions.
• Deficient Knowledge regarding acute glomerulonephritis and its management.

Nursing Interventions

Promoting Normal Urine Output

1. Monitor daily intake and output.
2. Test and record urine for hematuria and proteinuria, as directed. Note color of urine.
3. Monitor daily weight.

Reducing Excess Fluid Volume

1. Provide a no-salt-added diet during the acute phase of the illness. Other restrictions may be indicated if renal function is impaired. Protein intake is not usually restricted because of the possible risk of malnutrition.
2. Restrict fluids in children with hypertension, edema, heart failure, or renal failure.
3. Place a sign that indicates dietary restrictions on the child's bed so that staff and visitors will be aware of special needs.
4. With fluid restrictions, offer small amounts of fluids spaced at regular intervals throughout the day and evening. Use an appropriate-size cup for the amount of fluid being offered.
5. Check BP, as ordered or needed, and observe for signs of hypertension (eg, headache, blurry vision, fussy, fatigue). Administer antihypertensive and diuretic drugs, as ordered by health care provider.

Promoting Diversional Activity

1. Explain fluid restriction at an age-appropriate level and direct the child's focus away from restrictions.
2. Provide the child with diversional activity and play therapy.
3. Encourage activity, as tolerated.

Providing Information

1. Explain all aspects of the diagnostic tests and treatment in terms the family can understand.
2. Explain the purpose of all medications and the restricted diet, including a review of high-sodium foods to avoid and sample menus.
3. Encourage family participation in the child's care.
4. Help the family plan for adaptation of the child's nursing care to the home environment.
5. Arrange for appointments for continued medical supervision and initiate referrals when appropriate.

Family Education and Health Maintenance

1. Reinforce medical explanation of the disease process.
   a. Alert the family to signs and symptoms of disease recurrence.
   b. Be aware that microscopic hematuria may persist for several months.
2. Reinforce activity recommendation; usually not restricted.
3. Advise that tonsillectomy or other oral surgery is not recommended for several months after the acute phase of glomerulonephritis.
   a. If this type of surgery is necessary, penicillin may be recommended before and after the procedure to prevent bacterial infection.
   b. Obtain information regarding drug allergies before administering penicillin.

Evaluation: Expected Outcomes

- Output remains adequate.
- Weight returns to baseline.
- Child does age-appropriate activities, as tolerated, and does not complain of thirst.
- Parents and child can state rationale for treatment.

Nephrotic Syndrome

Nephrotic syndrome is characterized by heavy proteinuria, hypoalbuminemia, and edema. The syndrome can be subdivided into congenital, primary, and secondary types. Primary nephrotic syndrome includes idiopathic, minimal change and childhood types. Approximately 85% to 95% of primary cases in preadolescents are classified as minimal-change nephrotic syndrome (MCNS) and are associated with minimal histologic change in the glomeruli. Nephrotic syndrome afflicts approximately 16 per 100,000 children younger than age 16 in the United States annually; in young children, it is slightly more common in males than in females, but it disappears in teenagers and adults. The most common age for presentation is 2 years, and 70% to 80% of cases occur in children younger than age 6 years.

Pathophysiology and Etiology

1. Underlying defect is thought to be caused by the loss of charge selectivity of the glomerular basement membrane, which permits negatively charged proteins, primarily albumin, to pass easily through the capillary walls into the urine.
2. Excessive urinary loss of protein and catabolization by the kidney of circulating albumin leads to a decrease in serum protein (hypoalbuminemia).
3. The colloidal osmotic pressure that holds water in the vascular compartments is reduced because of the decrease in the amount of serum albumin. This allows fluid to flow from the capillaries into the interstitial spaces, thus producing edema.
4. The shift of fluid from the plasma to the interstitial spaces reduces the vascular fluid volume (hypovolemia), which in turn stimulates the renin–angiotensin system and the secretion of antidiuretic hormone and aldosterone.
5. Tubular reabsorption of sodium and water is increased for intravascular volume.
6. The loss of proteins, particularly immunoglobulins, predisposes the child to infection.

Clinical Manifestations

1. Onset is insidious—thought to be caused by immune system disturbances because it commonly occurs after a mild URI.
2. Edema is typically the presenting symptom.
   a. Edema may be minimal or massive.
   b. Edema is usually first apparent around the eyes.
   c. Dependent edema occurs in areas of the body such as the hands, ankles, feet, and genitalia.
   d. Fluid that accumulates in the body spaces may give rise to ascites and pleural effusions.
   e. Striae may appear on the skin from overstretching.
3. Profound weight gain caused by edema; the child may actually double normal weight.
4. Decreased urine output during the edematous phase—urine appears concentrated and frothy.
5. Pallor, irritability, lethargy, and fatigue.
6. GI disturbances, including vomiting, diarrhea, abdominal pain, and anorexia caused by edema of intestinal mucosa.

Diagnostic Evaluation

1. Urinalysis:
   a. Proteinuria (tests for albumin)—2+ (greater than 1.0 g/L) on urine dipstick; should be sent for urine protein to creatinine ratio (first voided or random spot urine) to confirm. Considered nephrotic range if greater than 200 to 250 mg/mmol.
   b. Blood—gross hematuria is not present but microscopic hematuria may be found in about 20% of patients.
2. Twenty-four-hour urine collection is the gold standard for quantification of urine protein—nephrotic range greater than 40 mg/m^2/hour.
3. Blood tests.
   a. Total protein—reduced.
   b. Albumin—less than 2.5 g/dL.
   c. Complete blood count may show decreased hematocrit due to hemodilution.
   d. BUN may be elevated, indicating general renal function.
   e. Creatinine—usually normal but may be increased if intravascularly depleted.
   f. Electrolytes—may have sodium, potassium, CO_2, and calcium imbalances.
   g. Increased serum cholesterol and triglycerides—due to reactive protein synthesis by the liver in response to hypoproteinemia.
4. Renal biopsy is indicated to look for other cause of renal dysfunction if the patient has persistent proteinuria after 4 to 8 weeks of steroid therapy (median time to remission is 10 days—negative or trace proteinuria for 3 consecutive days). Biopsy also indicated if atypical presentation such as persistent renal failure, age less than 1 year or greater than 10 years, use of nephrotoxic drugs, or persistent hematuria.

Management

Steroid Therapy

1. Corticosteroid therapy—prednisone or prednisolone are drugs of choice because of lower cost and are less likely to induce salt retention and potassium loss.
2. No standard program of therapy exists; however, the 2012 Kidney Disease: Improving Global Outcomes guidelines recommend the following:

a. Corticosteroid therapy be given for at least 12 weeks.

b. Oral prednisone be administered as a single daily dose starting at 60 mg/m²/day or 2 mg/kg/day to a maximum 60 mg/day.

c. Daily oral prednisone be given for 4 to 6 weeks followed by alternate-day medication as a single daily dose starting at 40 mg/m² or 1.5 mg/kg (maximum 40 mg on alternate days) and continued for 2 to 5 months with tapering of the dose.

3. Corticosteroid therapy should be discontinued slowly to avoid complications of steroid withdrawal, particularly benign intracranial hypertension.

4. Children with nephrotic syndrome may respond to steroid therapy in several ways:

a. Steroid sensitive: achieving remission within 28 days of the start of corticosteroid therapy.

b. Steroid dependent: relapses on alternate-day dosing or relapses within 14 days of corticosteroid discontinuation.

c. Steroid resistant: persistent proteinuria after 8 weeks of corticosteroid therapy.

5. Children with steroid-responsive MCNS have a favorable long-term prognosis.

 EVIDENCE BASE Kidney Disease: Improving Global Outcomes (KDIGO) Work Group. (2012). Clinical practice guideline for glomerulonephritis. *Kidney International, 2*(2), 139–274.

Copeman, H. (2014). Renal care in the paediatric setting: an overview of common conditions. *Journal of Renal Nursing, 6*(6), 280–283.

Intravenous (IV) Albumin 25%

1. To shift fluid from interstitial space into the vascular system.

2. Only a temporary treatment to relieve edema but may be used in severe cases of edema that cause respiratory distress or severe discomfort.

3. Diuretic therapy is used in combination with IV albumin to help relieve edema. In cases of hypovolemia, diuretics may not be indicated.

Alternative Drug Therapies

1. Should be considered when children relapse frequently (greater than four relapses in 1 year or two relapses in 6 months), become steroid resistant or steroid dependent, or demonstrate unacceptable adverse effects of steroid therapy (steroid toxicity). The decision to use alternative therapy in conjunction with steroids should be made by an experienced pediatric nephrologist.

2. Immunosuppressants.
   a. Cyclophosphamide.
   b. Cyclosporin A.
   c. Tacrolimus.
   d. Mycophenolate mofetil.
   e. Rituximab.

Complications

1. Infections:
   a. Peritonitis, most commonly caused by *Streptococcus pneumoniae* but may also be caused by *Escherichia coli* and *Haemophilus influenzae*.
   b. Gram-negative septicemia.
   c. Staphylococcal cellulitis.

2. Thromboembolic events.

3. Hypertension.

4. Hyperlipidemia.

5. Pulmonary edema.

6. Bone disease secondary to corticosteroid therapy.

7. Acute renal failure.

Nursing Assessment

1. Obtain history of onset of illness and symptoms.
   a. Precipitating events.
   b. Recent immunizations.
   c. Recent URIs.
   d. Flulike symptoms.
   e. Time of onset and location of edema.
   f. Urinary pattern changes.

2. Perform physical examination focusing on vital signs; auscultation of breath sounds to determine adventitious sounds; areas and extent of edema, especially periorbital region, extremities, genitalia, abdomen; and peripheral perfusion, including pulses, color, and warmth of extremities.

Nursing Diagnoses

- Excess Fluid Volume related to fluid accumulation in tissues.
- Risk for Infection related to urinary loss of proteins and chronic steroid use.
- Imbalanced Nutrition: Less Than Body Requirements related to loss of proteins through urine and anorexia.
- Interrupted Family Processes related to childhood illness.

Nursing Interventions

Relieving Excess Fluid

1. Administer corticosteroids, as directed.
   a. Observe for adverse effects and complications of therapy, such as Cushing syndrome—increased body hair (hirsutism), rounding of the face ("moon face"), abdominal distention, striae, increased appetite with weight gain, cataracts, and aggravation of adolescent acne.
   b. Stress that these physical changes are not harmful or permanent and that they will disappear after the steroid treatment is stopped.
   c. Observe for serious adverse effects and uncommon complications of corticosteroids (see pages 702 to 704).

2. Administer immunosuppressive drugs, as prescribed.
   a. Make sure that the patient and parents understand the desired and adverse effects of therapy.
   b. Observe for complications of therapy, such as decreased white blood cell (WBC) count, increased susceptibility to infection, hair loss or increased hair growth (hirsutism), gingival hyperplasia, and hemorrhagic cystitis.

3. Administer diuretics, as prescribed.
   a. Be aware of those diuretics that may cause potassium depletion.
   b. Offer foods high in potassium, such as orange juice, bananas, and dried fruits (eg, raisins, apricots).
   c. Administer supplemental potassium chloride, as ordered, and if the urine output is adequate.

4. Encourage activity, as tolerated.

5. Restrict fluids as ordered (usually only during the extreme edematous phases).
   a. Restriction is carefully calculated at frequent intervals, based on the urine output of the previous day plus estimated insensible losses.
   b. Offer small amounts of fluids spaced at regular intervals throughout the day and evening. Use a cup of appropriate size for the amount of fluid being offered.

c. Measure fluids accurately in graduated containers. Do not estimate fluid intake or output.

d. Place a sign on the child's bed to make sure that no urine is accidentally discarded and that all intake is recorded.

e. Determine total intake and output every 8 hours. In children who are not toilet trained, a fairly accurate record of output can be obtained by weighing diapers before and after voiding.

f. Record other causes of fluid loss, such as the number of stools per day, perspiration.

6. In refractory or extreme cases, assist with abdominal paracentesis; this may be required because of marked ascites. During the procedure, fluid is withdrawn from the peritoneal cavity to relieve pressure symptoms and respiratory distress.

7. Restrict sodium, as ordered (usually done while the child is on corticosteroid therapy). A starting point is 1.5 to 2 g/day.

a. Use a low-sodium menu when ordering meals from the hospital.

b. Assist family in making food choices that are low in sodium.

c. Foods that should be limited include cured, salted, canned, or smoked meats; processed cheese; regular canned or frozen soups and bouillon cubes; and salted crackers and other snack foods.

 NURSING ALERT No live vaccinations or immunizations should be given during active episodes of nephrosis or while the child receives immunosuppressive therapy.

 DRUG ALERT Administer cyclophosphamide in the morning, with large volumes of fluid, to prevent concentration of the drug in the urine and increased susceptibility to cystitis.

Preventing Infection

1. Monitor complete blood count for decreased WBC count and neutropenia.

2. Closely observe the child who takes corticosteroids for signs of infection. Be aware that fever and other symptoms may be masked.

3. Provide meticulous skin care to edematous areas of the body.

a. Bathe the child frequently and apply powder. Areas of concern are moist parts of the body and edematous male genitalia. Support the scrotum with a cotton pad held in place by a T-binder, if necessary, for the child's comfort.

b. Position the child so that edematous skin surfaces are not in contact. Place a pillow between the child's legs when lying on side.

c. Elevate the child's head to reduce edema.

4. If possible, avoid invasive procedures, such as femoral venipunctures and IM injections, to decrease the chance of introducing pathogens. Venipuncture of the lower extremities may also predispose the child to thromboembolism because of hypovolemia, stasis, and increased plasma concentration of clotting factors.

5. Educate the parents regarding signs and symptoms of possible infections.

Enhancing Nutritional Status

1. Assess nutritional intake, growth, and development as appropriate for age.

2. Provide a diet low in sodium, fat, and sugar. Place a sign on the child's bed that indicates dietary restrictions so that everyone will be aware of special needs.

3. Provide food choices that appeal to the child and that are easy to eat according to stage of development.

4. Provide nutritional supplements, as needed.

Providing Emotional Support

1. Encourage frequent visiting and allow as much parental participation in the child's care as possible. Hospitalization, if necessary, is usually brief.

2. Allow the child as much activity as tolerated.

a. Balance periods of rest, recreation, and quiet activities during the convalescent phase.

b. Allow the child to eat meals with family or other children.

3. Encourage the child and family to verbalize fears, frustrations, and questions.

a. Be aware that young children frequently fear abandonment by their parents.

b. Allow parents to express frustrations regarding the uncertainties associated with the cause of the disease, the clinical course, and the prognosis.

c. Explain the difference between nephritis and nephrosis if parents have questions.

4. Help the child adjust to changes in body image, such as cushingoid appearance, by explaining changes ahead of time.

5. Discuss the problems of discipline with the parents. Encourage them to set consistent limits and reasonable expectations of their child's behavior.

6. Suggest parents get involved with a support group for families of children with chronic illnesses, as needed.

Family Education and Health Maintenance

1. Prepare the family for home management of the child's care plan.

a. Have the dietitian discuss special diets with the parents.

b. Teach the parents about the child's medication—the desired effects and the potential adverse effects.

c. Demonstrate urine testing for protein.

d. Initiate a community health nursing referral, if necessary, for reassessment and reinforcement of teaching.

2. Encourage continued medical follow-up visits.

3. Emphasize the necessity of taking medication according to the prescribed schedule and for an extended time. Discuss complications encountered with steroid therapy.

4. Teach prevention and recognition of signs and symptoms of infection.

5. Advise family on necessary activity restrictions.

6. Teach signs and symptoms of relapse (proteinuria on urine dipstick at home, increased edema, and decreased urine output) and whom and when to call with questions.

7. Teach signs and symptoms of fluid imbalances (excess or dehydration).

Evaluation: Expected Outcomes

- Decreased edema and ascites; adequate urine output.
- Exhibits no signs of infection.
- Family verbalizes and follows dietary restrictions as demonstrated by appropriate weight gain/loss.
- Family verbalizes concerns regarding child's illness as demonstrated by open communication with staff and other family members.

Urinary Tract Infection

 EVIDENCE BASE American Academy of Pediatrics. (2016). Urinary tract infection: Clinical practice guidelines for the diagnosis and management of the initial UTI in febrile infants and children 2 to 24 months. Subcommittee on Urinary Tract Infection. Steering Committee on Quality Improvement and Management. *Pediatrics, 138*(6), e20163026.

The RIVUR Trial Investigators. (2014). Antimicrobial prophylaxis for children with vesicoureteral reflux. *New England Journal of Medicine, 371*(11), 1071–1072.

American Urological Association. (Published 2010, Reviewed and Validity Confirmed 2017). Management and Screening of Primary Vesicoureteral Reflux in Children.

Urinary tract infection (UTI) is defined as bacteria that exist anywhere between the renal cortex and the urethral meatus. Because it is usually difficult to determine the exact location of the infection, the term UTI is used to explain microorganisms anywhere within the urinary tract. UTIs are categorized as cystitis or urethritis (located in the bladder or urethra), upper tract (located in the ureters or collecting system), and pyelonephritis (renal parenchyma). The greatest incidence of UTI in males occurs in the first year of life (most common in uncircumcized males), after which it rapidly declines, remaining low through childhood and adolescence. Incidence in females is also highest in the first year of life and steadily declines through adolescence but remains higher than the incidence for males at a rate of 10:1.

Pathophysiology and Etiology

1. Causative organisms—*E. coli* (80%), *Klebsiella* species, *Proteus* species, *Staphlyococcus saprophyticus* (female adolescents and sexually active females), *Enterococcus species, Streptococcus* group B (neonates), *Pseudomonas aeruginosa*.
2. Route of entry:
   a. Ascent from the urethra (most common).
   b. Circulating blood (rare).
3. Contributing causes:
   a. Female specific.
      i. Perineal location of urethral orifice and shorter urethra.
      ii. Sexual intercourse (mechanics of vaginal penetration).
      iii. Vaginal voiding—reflux of urine into the vagina while voiding, with subsequent dribbling of urine.
   b. Male specific—foreskin (prepuce can be a reservoir for bacteria).
   c. Abnormal bladder or voiding with or without incontinence.
      i. High pressures in the bladder.
      ii. Incomplete bladder emptying, infrequent voiding.
      iii. Difficulty relaxing pelvic floor.
   d. Constipation and bowel/bladder dysfunction.
   e. Congenital urinary tract anomalies—vesicoureteral reflux, posterior urethral valves, prune belly syndrome, hydronephrosis, bladder exstrophy.
   f. Neurogenic bladder (spina bifida, spinal injury).
   g. Catheterization, urinary drains/tubes.
   h. Bacterial colonization.
   i. Alteration in periurethral flora by antibiotic therapy
4. Pathophysiology—colonization of uropathogens in periurethral area that ascend into bladder via urethra affecting portions of urinary tract, spreading from bladder to kidneys through the ureter (pyelonephritis) and possibly to bloodstream (bacteremia)
   a. Clumps of bacteria may be present.
   b. Inflammation results in urine retention and stasis of urine in the bladder.
   c. Backflow of urine into the kidneys may occur through the ureters; this is called *vesicoureteral reflux* (VUR).
   d. Inflammatory changes in the renal pelvis, and throughout the kidney, occur when the kidney is involved.
   e. Scarring of the kidney parenchyma occurs in chronic infection and interferes with kidney function, particularly with the ability to concentrate urine.
   f. If pyelonephritis is left untreated, the kidney tissue may be destroyed, and renal function could fail.

Clinical Manifestations

1. Onset may be abrupt or gradual; may be asymptomatic.
2. Failure to thrive in infancy.
3. Young children: may be nonspecific (vomiting, irritability, poor feeding, diarrhea); fever is often the only presenting complaint.
4. Older children and adolescents: urinary frequency, urgency or voiding hesitancy, dysuria, suprapubic tenderness, dribbling, and nocturnal enuresis (more common in lower UTI).
5. Hematuria: often occurs with viral cystitis.
6. Fever.
   a. May be moderate or severe.
   b. May fluctuate rapidly.
   c. May be accompanied by chills or convulsions.
7. Anorexia and general malaise.
8. Foul odor or change in the appearance of urine.
9. Abdominal or suprapubic pain (more common in upper tract disease).
10. Tenderness over one or both kidneys.
11. Systemic symptoms: flank pain, fever, chills, nausea, and vomiting may occur with pyelonephritis.

Diagnostic Evaluation

1. Urinalysis:
   a. Leukocytes, nitrites suggestive but not indicative.
   b. Casts, especially WBC casts, may be present and are indicative of intrarenal infection.
   c. Hematuria—occurs occasionally.
   d. Decreased specific gravity due to decreased renal concentrating ability.
2. Urine culture:
   a. Urinalysis for proteinuria and bacteriuria should be obtained as part of the general medical evaluation. If the urinalysis indicates an infection, both urine culture and sensitivity are recommended.
   b. Documentation of a single pathogenic organism in the urine is the only means of definitive diagnosis. Multiple organisms found in the culture are suspicious of perineal flora contamination and warrant repeat culture.
   c. A urine culture demonstrating more than 100,000 bacteria per mL indicates significant bacteriuria.
   d. A catheterized urine specimen, with growth greater than 50,000 colonies of bacteria per mL, is considered significant and required in the non–toilet trained child to prevent contamination from perineal flora.
   e. To avoid contamination, discard first few milliliters of urine (if quantity is sufficient). A new catheter should be used for each subsequent attempt if unsuccessful.

3. Urologic and radiologic studies to identify anatomic abnormalities or renal changes that stem from recurrent infections—renal bladder ultrasound (ensure child is well hydrated with distended bladder), voiding cystourethrogram (VCUG).
   a. Dimercaptosuccinic acid scan—evaluates renal function and scarring.

Management

See Table 49-1.

1. Treatment depends on child's age, severity of infection, and antimicrobial resistance rates in the community.
2. Oral antibiotic therapy for uncomplicated UTI. Usually 10- to 14-day antibiotic therapy for febrile UTIs.
3. IV antibiotics for complicated UTI—infections that do not respond to oral therapy or that develop into pyelonephritis or those that appear septic or dehydrated.
4. Repeat culture following therapy if still symptomatic, has chronic renal disease, or has known colonization of bacteria.

Complications

1. A tendency for recurrent infection exists.
2. Children with obstructive lesions of the urinary tract and those with severe VUR are at highest risk for kidney damage. These patients may need prophylactic oral antibacterial therapy.

Nursing Assessment

1. Obtain history to determine if UTI is initial or recurrent and to determine if there may be other disease processes contributing to this infection.
2. Focus assessment on identifying clinical manifestations and determining location of infection, such as presence and appearance of urethral discharge, high-grade fever (more common with upper UTI), or low-grade fever (more common with lower UTI).
3. Determine urinary pattern (ie, amount and frequency) and associated discomfort.
4. Determine bowel pattern and possibility of constipation.

Nursing Diagnoses

- Impaired Urinary Elimination related to infection.
- Acute Pain related to inflammatory changes and fever.
- Anxiety related to exposure and manipulation of the genitourinary tract.

Nursing Interventions

Promoting Urinary Elimination

1. Obtain a clean urine specimen for urinalysis or culture (see pages 588 and 591).
   a. Obtain freshly voided early morning specimen, if possible (most accurate). This urine is usually acidic and concentrated, which tends to preserve the formed elements.
   b. Provide fluids to help the child void.
   c. Perform catheterization, if necessary, to obtain a sterile specimen; however, this procedure may cause emotional trauma and the accidental introduction of additional bacteria. In girls, pulling the labia majora out versus splaying them will help identify the meatus and prevent catheter insertion into the vagina. In the event that there is inadvertent catheterization of the vagina, leaving the catheter in situ and using a new sterile catheter should prevent recatheterization of the vagina. In boys, pulling back the foreskin is required to identify the location of the meatal opening.
   d. Send urine to the laboratory immediately or refrigerate to avoid a falsely high bacterial count.
2. Administer antibiotics, as ordered by the health care provider (after specimen has been obtained for culture).
   a. Antibiotic therapy is generally determined by the results of the urine cultures and sensitivities and by the child's response to therapy; however, empirical therapy may be started before culture results are back.
   b. Become familiar with toxic effects of antimicrobial agents and assess the child regularly for any signs and symptoms.

Maintaining Comfort and Providing Symptomatic Relief

1. Administer analgesics and antipyretics, as ordered.
2. Maintain the child on bed rest while febrile.

Table 49-1	Antimicrobial Agents Commonly Used in the Management of Childhood Urinary Tract Infection	
DRUG	**ADVERSE EFFECTS**	**NURSING CONSIDERATIONS**
Amoxicillin	• Occasional nausea, vomiting, diarrhea • Hypersensitivity reactions of skin	• Readily absorbed. • May be taken with food.
Ampicillin	• Diarrhea, urticaria • Anaphylactic reaction	• Contraindicated in penicillin-sensitive children. Package insert should be consulted regarding reconstitution, administration, and storage of IM and IV preparation Absorption of oral preparations may be decreased with food. Dose must be repeated q6h to ensure therapeutic blood level.
Cephalexin	• Diarrhea, nausea, vomiting	• May be taken with food. Dose should be reduced if renal function is impaired.
Gentamicin	• Renal and auditory toxicity; respiratory paralysis	• Toxic effects can be minimized by slow IV infusion (over 1 hour).
Nitrofurantoin	• Fever, nausea, vomiting, peripheral neuropathy	• Recommended for prolonged use. Give with food or milk to decrease GI adverse effect May cause urine to be amber or brown in color. Contraindicated in renal failure and in infants younger than 3 months old.
Co-trimoxazole	• Nausea, vomiting, fever, rash, photosensitivity	• Commonly used if bacterial resistance is anticipated or the child fails to respond to initial therapy.

3. Encourage fluids to reduce the fever and dilute the concentration of the urine. (Water is the best clear fluid.)
4. Administer IV fluids, if necessary.

Promoting Self-Esteem

1. Reinforce medical explanations of the disease and its therapy.
2. Explain all diagnostic tests and procedures to the child, allowing time for questions and answers.
3. Encourage verbalizing. Correct any misconceptions and particularly address concerns about the functioning of the urinary tract and sexual function. Reassure the child that he or she did not cause the problem.
4. Maintain privacy for the child as much as possible.
5. Provide an environment that is as close to normal as possible during hospitalization. Include opportunities for the child to play.
6. Prepare the child and family for discharge and begin discussions of rest, fluids, and medications.

Family Education and Health Maintenance

1. Review long-term antibiotic therapy, if prescribed, to prevent recurrence of UTI. Schedules for prolonged therapy vary from several months to continuous prophylaxis.
2. Encourage scheduled follow-up visits because of the possibility of disease recurrence.
   a. Emphasize that even though this disease may have few symptoms, it can lead to serious, permanent disability.
   b. Advise family that subsequent suspected UTIs should be assessed and followed by health care provider.
3. Teach measures of prevention:
   a. Minimize spread of bacteria from the anal and vaginal areas to the urethra in female children by cleansing the perianal area from the urethra back toward the anus.
   b. Encourage adequate fluid intake, especially water.
   c. Avoid carbonated and caffeinated beverages because of their irritative effect on bladder mucosa.
   d. Encourage the child to void frequently and to empty the bladder completely with each voiding (double voiding).
   e. Encourage a high-fiber diet to avoid constipation.

Evaluation: Expected Outcomes

- Voids regularly in adequate amounts.
- No complaints of pain during or after voiding; afebrile.
- Shows less anxiety about hospitalization; appears more relaxed about appearance, body image, tests.

ABNORMALITIES OF THE GENITOURINARY TRACT THAT REQUIRE SURGERY

See Figure 49-2 for congenital abnormalities of the urinary tract, extrophy of the bladder and hypospadias.

Exstrophy of the Bladder

Bladder exstrophy is an abnormality present at birth in which the bladder and associated structures are improperly formed. Rather than being its normal round shape, the bladder is flattened. The skin, muscle, and pelvic bones joining the lower part of the abdomen did not form properly, so the inside of the bladder is exposed outside the abdomen. There are also associated deficiencies of the abdominal muscles and pelvic bones. These occur at a rate of 1:10,000 to 50,000 live births. It is more common in males. Recent published evidence suggests that the risk of bladder extrophy in children born as a result of assisted fertility techniques is seven times greater than in children conceived naturally without assistance. Evidence exists genetic predisposition in likelihood of exstophy parent with a 1 in 70 chance of having a child with bladder exstrophy and reoccurrence probability of 1 in 100.

Pathophysiology and Etiology

1. Results from failure of the abdominal wall and its underlying structures to fuse in utero during the 3rd to 4th week of gestation. Presumed cause is persistence of cloacal membrane during fetal development that ruptures to produce extrophy.
2. In classic exstrophy (about 60% of bladder anomalies), the posterior bladder wall is externalized and lies open on the lower part of the abdomen with an epispadial urethra, allowing constant passage of urine to the outside.

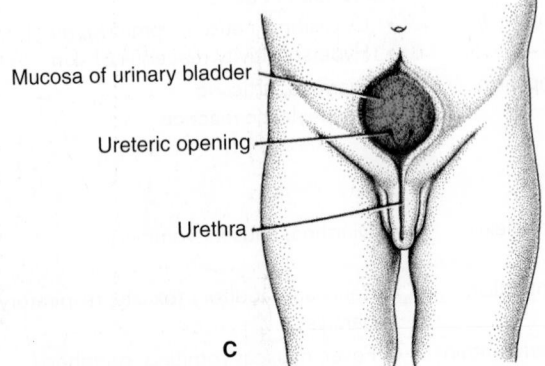

Abnormal urethral orifices

Hypospadias

Mucosa of urinary bladder

Ureteric opening

Urethra

A   B   C

Figure 49-2. (A) Hypospadias showing the various locations of abnormal urethral orifice. **(B)** Patient with hypospadias. The urethra is open on the ventral surface of the penis. **(C)** Epispadias combined with exstrophy of the bladder. Bladder mucosa is exposed. (**A** and **C** courtesy of Dr. R. J. Gorlin, Department of Oral Pathology and Genetics, University of Minnesota; **B,** Dudek, R. W. [2013]. *High-Yield Embryology* [5th ed.]. Philadelphia: Lippincott Williams & Wilkins.)

3. Epispadias may occur without exstrophy (about 30% of bladder anomalies); the bladder remains an internal organ, but the urethra is laid open, possibly with a split glans penis and the meatus located proximally.
4. Cloacal anomalies (about 10% of bladder anomalies) involve externalization of the bladder and portions of the GI tract.

Clinical Manifestations

1. Urine dribbles constantly.
2. Infection and ulceration of the bladder mucosa may occur.
3. Genitalia may be ambiguous.
4. Affected children may walk with a waddling or an unsteady gait due to diastasis (separation) of pelvic bones.

Diagnostic Evaluation

1. May be diagnosed prenatally by ultrasound.
2. Newborn inspection is the most important tool in evaluation. The obvious anomaly may involve multiple systems.
3. Diagnostic procedures, such as radiography, ultrasound, magnetic resonance imaging, and urodynamic testing, determine extent of the anomaly.
4. Spinal ultrasound for infant with sacral dimples to rule out spinal cord tethering.

Management

1. Surgical closure of bladder within first 24 to 48 hours of life by means of primary complete bladder closure and epispadias repair. This approach allows for maximal continence postrepair.
2. Urinary diversion should be rare.

Complications

1. Skin excoriation, infection.
2. Trauma to bladder mucosa.

Nursing Assessment

1. Assess for growth and development milestones during reconstruction.
2. Assess the family for coping ability.

Nursing Diagnoses

- Impaired Urinary Elimination related to anatomical defect.
- Risk for Infection as a complication of surgery.

Nursing Interventions

Facilitating Urine Output Preoperatively

1. Protect the bladder area from trauma and infection.
   a. Apply smooth common kitchen plastic wrap
   b. Warm sterile saline can be squirted over bladder to keep tissue moist.
   c. Position on back or side.
   d. Ensure umbilical cord is sutured and not clamped.
2. Observe the infant closely for signs of infection.
3. Involve other members of the health care team for parental support because of the psychosocial implications of a child who has special needs.
4. Assist the parents in dealing with their emotional reactions regarding the child's defect.
5. Prepare child and parents for the proposed surgery (see page 1151).
6. While previously repaired at birth, recent trend includes delayed closure to 3 months for better care outcomes including physiologic testosterone surge for penile growth in male patients.

Providing Postoperative Care to Prevent Infection

1. Goal of reconstruction is to preserve renal function, urinary continence and volitional voiding, functional and cosmetically acceptable external genitalia.
2. Provide care for the ureteral and urethral catheters. Observe and record the amount of urinary drainage, catheter positions, and bladder spasms.
3. Care for dressings, castings, stents and/or skin traction as necessary.
4. Provide care and instruction for an ileal conduit, as necessary (see page 597).
5. Antibiotic prophylaxis and pain control as ordered.
6. Observe for complications.
   a. Urinary or incisional infections.
   b. Fistulae in the suprapubic or penile incisions.
7. Recommend long-term support for children and families to help them deal with concerns about appearance of genitalia, sexual function, reproduction, and rejection by peers.

Family Education and Health Maintenance

1. Specific teaching and preparation depending on type of closure (primary or staged). Staged closures will likely require additional surgery at 4 to 5 years of age.
2. Provide community nursing referral, as needed, to support family and make sure that family understands the importance of follow-up with the various specialists.
3. Act as a liaison, as necessary, to coordinate care.
4. For more information and support, refer families to the following resources:
   a. Association for the Bladder Exstrophy Community (ABC) (*www.bladderexstrophy.com*).
   b. Book—*Living with Bladder Exstrophy: A Book for Families* (Murrey and Schremmer, 1996). Available through ABC.

Evaluation: Expected Outcomes

- No skin breakdown or infection.
- Incision healing well without infection or fistula; eventually, voiding without difficulty.

Vesicoureteral Reflux

 EVIDENCE BASE Cara-Fuentes, G., Gupta, N., & Garin, E. H. (2015). The RIVUR study: A review of its findings. *Pediatric Nephrology, 30*(5), 703.
American Urological Association. (Published 2010, Reviewed and Validity Confirmed 2017). Management and Screening of Primary Vesicoureteral Reflux in Children.

Vesicoureteral reflux (VUR) is the abnormal retrograde flow of urine from the bladder into the upper urinary tract. In the absence of bacterial infection, VUR is not considered to be critical. In the presence of bacteria, however, VUR is a risk factor for the development of UTIs and pyelonephritis, which can lead to renal damage and scarring. With linear growth, spontaneous resolution of VUR occurs in most children.

Pathophysiology and Etiology

VUR occurs as a result of congenital deficiency in the formation of the ureterovesical junction, resulting in a laterally displaced ureteral orifice. Secondary VUR is acquired as a result of increased bladder pressure.

Clinical Manifestations

1. Febrile UTI-culture confirmed, catheterized specimen for non–toilet trained child.
2. Unexplained febrile illnesses.
3. Associated urogenital anomalies (bladder exstrophy, posterior urethral valves, neurogenic bladder).
4. Prenatal diagnosis (hydronephrosis detected on prenatal screening ultrasounds).

Diagnostic Evaluation

1. VCUG—to establish diagnosis of VUR but should not be performed routinely after first febrile UTI, indicated after ultrasound reveals hydronephrosis, scarring or findings of high grade VUR or obstructive uropathy, recurrent UTI or atypical complex clinical circumstances.
2. Renal ultrasound—to assess for renal damage, associated hydronephrosis.
3. DMSA—recommended when renal ultrasound is abnormal w/greater concern for scarring (breakthrough UTI, grade 3 to 4 VUR, elevated creatinine)

Management

1. The goals of medical and/or surgical management are to prevent pyelonephritis, recurrent UTIs, and formation of renal cortical scarring.
2. Continuous prophylactic antibiotic recommended for some children based on age, history of febrile UTI and degree of VUR.
3. Surgical intervention is indicated when medical therapy is unsuccessful.
   a. Circumcision offered for infant males with VUR-protective for babies before the age of 1 year
   b. Endoscopic polymer injection into the ureter(s)—83% success rate
   c. Ureter reimplantation—98.1% success rate
4. Yearly ultasounds to monitor renal growth and kidney parenchymal scarring.

Complications

1. Recurrent UTI can lead to renal damage and failure.
2. Recurrence of VUR following surgical intervention-postoperative UTI in children close to or toilet trained age is strongly associated with incidence of preoperative UTI and presence of BBD (bladder bowel dysfunction).
3. Postoperative renal obstruction rate of 0.4%.

Family Education and Health Maintenance

1. Association of bowel/bladder dysfunction
2. General routine evaluation for patients with renal scarring prior to VUR resolution or recurrent urinary tract infection after resolution of VUR—BP, height, weight, and urinalysis for protein screening for patients with abnormal ultrasound/DMSA
3. Communication of long-term concerns of hypertension (especially in pregnancy), renal function loss, recurrent urinary tract infection, and familial VUR in siblings and offspring to be discussed when child at an appropriate age
4. Evidence-based study conducted (RIVUR) concluding that prophylaxis reduces risk of recurrent urinary tract infection but not renal scarring

For nursing assessment, diagnoses, and interventions, see "Care of the Child Who Undergoes Urologic Surgery," page 1324.

Obstructive Lesions of the Lower Urinary Tract

Obstruction of the lower urinary tract may be caused by structural lesions, such as posterior or anterior urethral valves, bladder neck obstruction, meatal stricture, and urolithiasis (stones), or by functional lesions, such as neuromuscular dysfunction. The effect of obstruction on ureteral and renal function depends on the degree and duration of obstruction, on the rate of urine formation, and whether infection exists.

Pathophysiology and Etiology

Types of Obstruction

1. Urethral valves—filamentous valves that obstruct urine flow.
2. Congenital narrowing of the urethra.
3. Bladder neck obstruction—most common site of lower urinary tract obstruction.
4. Meatal stricture.
5. Neuromuscular dysfunction.
6. Severe phimosis (rare).
7. Inflammatory processes.
8. Neoplasia.
9. Urolithiasis.
10. Trauma.

Effects of Obstruction

1. Urinary tract becomes distended, proximal to the point of obstruction.
2. The bladder dilates and hypertrophies.
3. Stasis of urine occurs.
4. The ureters become elongated, dilated, and tortuous.
5. Hydronephrosis and destruction of kidney tissue inevitably result if left untreated.

Clinical Manifestations

1. Abnormal urination.
   a. Dysuria, frequency.
   b. Enuresis, dribbling.
   c. Reduced force of urine stream.
   d. Difficulty starting urine stream.
   e. Straining during urination.
   f. Abrupt cessation during urination.
2. Signs of infection—fever, pain, irritability, and, occasionally, hematuria.
3. Lower obstruction: suprapubic pain, prolapse via urethra in females (ureterocele) presenting as bulging vulvar mass in females.

Diagnostic Evaluation

1. Physical examination may reveal abdominal mass.
2. Laboratory findings depend on the degree that renal function is compromised.
3. Renal ultrasound may show hydronephrosis.
4. Radionuclide scanning.
5. Endoscopic examination.
6. Ureteroscopy.
7. Urodynamic examination.

Management

1. Prevention or eradication of infection with antibiotics.
2. Dilation of urethral stenosis or stricture.
3. Urinary diversion may be necessary.
4. Surgical relief of the obstruction.

Complications

1. Urinary stasis and recurrent UTI could lead to renal failure.
2. Severe and recurrent UTI.
3. Recurrence of the obstruction.

For nursing assessment, diagnoses, and interventions, see "Care of the Child Who Undergoes Urologic Surgery," page 1324.

Obstructive Lesions of the Upper Urinary Tract

Obstructive lesions of the upper urinary tract include ureteropelvic junction obstruction, ureterovesical junction obstruction, ureteral stricture, congenital absence or duplication of a ureter, and urolithiasis. These obstructive lesions are primarily congenital.

Pathophysiology and Etiology

1. Congenital anomalies develop in the upper urinary tract.
   a. Ureteropelvic junction obstruction.
   b. Ureterovesical junction obstruction.
   c. Stricture of a ureter.
   d. Congenital absence of one ureter.
   e. Duplication of the ureter of one kidney.
2. Urolithiasis (renal calculi) is rare in children but may be associated with metabolic disease, such as cystinosis or oxalosis.

Clinical Manifestations

1. Hydronephrosis may present as an abdominal mass.
2. Commonly asymptomatic (seldom any problem with voiding).
3. Vague signs, such as failure to thrive, may be present.
4. UTIs may be frequent.
5. Hypertension may occur.

Diagnostic Evaluation

1. Laboratory tests to determine renal function.
2. Renal ultrasound, radionuclide imaging, and ureteroscopy to determine the extent of the lesion.

Management

1. Prevention or eradication of infection.
2. Surgical correction of the obstruction.

Complications

Renal failure.
For nursing assessment, diagnoses, and interventions, see "Care of the Child Who Undergoes Urologic Surgery," page 1324.

Hypospadias

 EVIDENCE BASE Baskin, L. S. (2019). Hypospadias. In L. Baskin & B. Kogan (eds.), *Handbook of pediatric urology* (Chapter 2). Philadelphia, PA: Lippincott Williams & Wilkins.
Pfeil, M., Parr, J., & Milind, M., (2012). Hypospadias repair: the nursing contribution. *International Journal of Urological Nursing*, 6(3), 152–158.

Hypospadias is a congenital defect of the penis, resulting in the incomplete development of the anterior urethra, corpora cavernosa, and prepuce (foreskin). Hypospadias is also associated with penile ventral curvature (chordee) which depending on the severity of the defect may result in infertility secondary to difficulty in semen delivery. Hypospadias is a common birth defect, occurring in one out of every 150 to 300 boys. The goal of treatment is to achieve cosmetic and functional repair. See Figure 49-2 on page 1320.

Pathophysiology and Etiology

1. At 1 month gestation, the male and female genitalia are indistinguishable. However, under the influence of testosterone, the male genitalia become masculinized. By the end of the first trimester, the penile urethra and foreskin are completely formed. Abnormalities in this development, such as subsequent, decreased testosterone production, can lead to hypospadias.
2. Classification is determined by the location of the urethral meatus.
3. Majority of cases have no known etiology but may show genetic inheritability—14% incidence in siblings; 8% incidence in offspring.
4. Undescended testicle, hydrocele, or inguinal hernia may be associated.

Clinical Manifestations

1. Inability to void with penis in normal elevated position.
2. Spraying of urine when voiding.
3. 70% urethral meatus located distal on penile shaft
4. 30% proximal location and often more complex
5. In case of concomitant unilateral or bilateral undescended testis, endocrine evaluation advised to exclude disorders of sexual differentiation

Diagnostic Evaluation

1. Usually not difficult to diagnose because of visual anomaly. Assess glans penis for possible hypospadias before circumcision.
2. Severe cases require genotypic/phenotypic sex determination, chromosomal, and hormonal studies.

Management

Surgical reconstruction between ages 6 and 18 months, if possible (to minimize psychological issues surrounding toileting and genital awareness), and before circumcision because foreskin is essential for most complex repairs. Phalloplasty is also considered as a surgical option for removal of dorsal hooded foreskin in mild hypospadias.
   Postop temporary stent in situ for complex hypospadias repair that is typically removed/falls out in 7 to 10 days to allow newly created urethra and opening to heal.
   Dressings are typically removed within the first few days at home and bathing is encouraged to keep incision site clean and prevent bacteria from developing.

Complications

1. Urethrocutaneous fistula,
2. Meatal stenosis.
3. Urethral diverticulum.
4. Residual penile curvature
5. Wound dehiscence or infection.
6. Urinary tract symptoms
7. Esthetic result

Family Education and Health Maintenance

Follow-up post reconstruction typically is few months after reconstruction, 1 year after the repair, after toilet training, and after puberty to ensure satisfaction and understanding of congenital anomaly. Complications are seen as needed.

For nursing assessment, diagnoses, and interventions, see "Care of the Child Who Undergoes Urologic Surgery."

Cryptorchidism

 EVIDENCE BASE Kolon, T., Herndon, A., Baker, L., et al. (2014). Evaluation and Treatment of Cryptorchidism: AUA guideline. *Journal of Urology, 192*, 337–345.

American Urological Association. (Published 2010, Reviewed and Validity Confirmed 2017). Management and Screening of Primary Vesicoureteral Reflux in Children.

Cryptorchidism refers to the failure of one or both testes to descend through the inguinal canal to the normal position in the scrotum. A testis is considered undescended if on examination, the testicle is palpable elsewhere and cannot be brought down into the scrotum. It is more common in premature infants and is the most common surgical problem in pediatric urology.

Pathophysiology and Etiology

1. Possibly caused by delayed descent, prevention of descent by mechanical lesion, or endocrine disorder (rare).
2. Testicular and ductal development are abnormal. It is unclear whether this is because of congenital dysplasia or because of underdevelopment.
3. Degeneration of the sperm-forming cells occurs after puberty because of the higher temperatures of the abdomen, compared with normal location in the scrotum.

Clinical Manifestations

Testicle nonpalpable within the scrotum.

Spontaneous descent of the testes may occur in the first corrected 6 months of life

Diagnostic Evaluation

1. Imaging for cryptorchidism is not recommended prior to referral. Ultrasonography may reveal undescended testicle but is not as reliable as physical examination.
2. Serum testosterone measurements may be decreased.

Management

Complications for cryptorchidism can include testicular malignancy later in life, potential impairment in fertility, testicular torsion, trauma to testicle, and associate hernias.

1. Specialist referral should ensure surgical evaluation by 6 months of age because of low probability of descent and probable damage should the testes remain in a nonscrotal location.
2. Bilateral nonpalpable testicles require immediate urology consultation to evaluate for possible disorder of sex development (DSD)
3. Surgical laparoscopic exploration must be performed after exam under anesthesia confirms that testicles are not palpable on all nonpalpable unilateral and bilateral cryptorchid patients. Open approach is used for palpable testicles.

4. Orchiopexy surgery to achieve permanent fixation of the testis in the scrotum. Surgery should be perform between ages 6 and 15 months to prevent damage to the tissues and to lessen emotional concerns related to body image.
5. Surgical placement of testicular prosthesis, if testicle(s) absent.
6. Lack of evidence in long-term success of testicular descent in administration of human chorionic gonadotropin and has noted low response rates

Family Education and Health

1. Primary care provider should palpate testes with every well-child visit for quality and position.
2. Retractile testes are at increased risk for secondary testicular ascent due to hyperactive cremasteric reflex, short patent processus vaginalis, or entrapping adhesions.
3. Previously cryptorchid boy should be assessed with each well-child visit for quality and position postoperatively and eventually taught how to perform monthly testicular self-examination after puberty to facilitate early cancer detection.
4. Former bilateral cryptorchid men have a greatly reduced fertility compared to men with history of unilateral cryptorchidism and general male population.

For nursing assessment, diagnoses, and interventions, see "Care of the Child Who Undergoes Urologic Surgery."

Care of the Child Who Undergoes Urologic Surgery

Also see Chapter 21, pages 596 and 597, for a discussion of kidney surgery and urinary diversion.

Nursing Assessment

1. Obtain history from prenatal and birth record, family, and child.
2. Assess feeding and crying patterns, indicating potential obstruction or abdominal pain.
3. Assess urinary elimination pattern to determine degree of disorder.
4. Assess for associated congenital defects.
5. Assess for failure to thrive.
6. Determine family's response to body image changes. Expect anxieties regarding sterility and gender identity and perceptions of the child as defective or inadequate.
7. Measure and record vital signs, height, weight, abdominal girth, and compare with previous measurements, if available. Renal insufficiency may alter growth. Fever may be indicative of infection.
8. Visually and manually inspect genitalia and record abnormalities (eg, if bladder mucosa is visible, describe signs of irritation).
9. Palpate abdomen; note masses.
10. Obtain urine for culture and sensitivity. Note color, amount, odor, and degree of cloudiness.
11. Review results of all laboratory and diagnostic procedures.

Nursing Diagnoses

- Deficient Knowledge related to surgery.
- Impaired Urinary Elimination related to surgical intervention.
- Disturbed Body Image related to appearance of genitalia.

- Risk for Infection related to surgical incision and drainage tubes.
- Risk for Deficient Fluid Volume related to surgical losses.
- Acute Pain related to surgical incision and drainage tubes.

Nursing Interventions

Promoting Understanding of Surgical Treatment
1. Determine the child's expectation regarding illness and hospitalization through discussion and play therapy.
2. Explain the anatomy and physiology of the urinary system in terms the child can understand.
   a. Use a body outline appropriate for the age of the child.
   b. Explain how the child differs from the normal. Relate defect to symptoms whenever possible.
3. Explain all diagnostic tests before their occurrence. These may include urinalysis, 24-hour urine collections, IV, retrograde pyelography, ultrasound, and/or VCUG. Descriptions should include such information as:
   a. Preparation required—fasting, enemas, catheterization.
   b. Location of the test—operating room, radiology department.
   c. Appearance and attire of personnel.
   d. Positioning.
   e. Anesthesia.
   f. Pain or discomfort.
   g. Expectations after the procedure—diet, rest, urine collections.
4. Determine the child's understanding of the procedure.
   a. Ask simple, direct questions.
   b. Allow the child to perform the procedure on a doll or to demonstrate it on a diagram.
5. Explain the surgical procedure, including the following:
   a. Preparation required—fasting, enemas.
   b. Description of the operating room, including the appearance of the personnel.
   c. Anesthesia.
   d. Postoperative appearance—urinary drainage tubing and collection devices, appearance of urine, sutures, bandages, IV infusion.
6. Reassess the child's understanding of the surgery and reinforce teaching when necessary.
7. Emphasize additional points:
   a. The child is in no way to blame for illness.
   b. No other part of the body will be operated on.

Promoting Normal Urine Output
1. Monitor daily intake and output.
2. Encourage adequate fluids and monitor daily weight.
3. Care for all catheters and urinary tubes according to facility policy. Maintain appropriate position of tubes.
4. Observe and record amount and appearance of urinary drainage, occurrence of bladder spasms, and symptoms of urinary or incisional infection.

Providing Emotional Support Regarding Body Image
1. Continue reassurance about appearance of genitalia.
2. Maintain discussions regarding reactions. This may need to be done with patient and family alone as well as the family unit.
3. If additional surgical intervention is required, discuss plans for interim period from initial surgery until secondary or reconstructive procedures can be performed.
4. Initiate independence of care.
5. Focus on activities the child can perform and accomplish.

Preventing Infection
1. Administer antibiotics and IV fluids, as ordered.
2. Maintain patency of catheters. Provide catheter care, as directed.
3. Administer wound care using aseptic technique. Inspect incision for drainage or signs of infection.

Maintaining Fluid Volume
1. Administer fluids, as ordered.
2. Monitor vital signs for hypotension or tachycardia.
3. Assess patient's skin turgor and mucous membranes for signs of dehydration.
4. Measure and record accurate intake and output.

Promoting Comfort
1. Administer analgesics, as ordered and according to assessment of complaints of pain, restlessness, crying, or withdrawal.
2. Administer antispasmodics, as ordered, for bladder spasm.
3. Provide distraction and comfort measures.

Family Education and Health Maintenance
1. Advise the family about follow-up appointments, additional surgeries, or procedures.
2. Teach care of incision, signs of infection.
3. Advise on avoidance of straddle toys for 6 weeks to promote healing.
4. Encourage good nutrition to promote healing and to prevent infection.
5. Provide contact names and phone numbers for families to call to update on status with complications, urgent concerns, and where to go in the case of an emergency.

Evaluation: Expected Outcomes
- Child and family verbalize understanding of surgery.
- Clear urine draining via catheter.
- Child and family verbalize relief that defects can be surgically repaired and reconstructed.
- Incision without drainage or signs of infection.
- Vital signs stable; urine output adequate.
- Decreased crying and increased restful periods and sleep noted.

RENAL FAILURE AND DIALYSIS
Acute Renal Failure

Acute renal failure is a sudden, usually reversible deterioration in normal renal function. This results in fluid and electrolyte imbalance and accumulation of metabolic toxins. Nursing care of children with acute renal failure is generally the same as that of adults (see pages 602 to 604), although there are special considerations for pediatric patients.

Pathophysiology and Etiology
1. Causes are divided into *prerenal* (problem occurs in blood supply to the kidneys), *intrarenal* (problem is within the kidney or kidneys), and *postrenal* (problem occurs in urinary system after the kidneys).
   a. Prerenal causes: conditions causing hypovolemia (dehydration, shock, trauma, or burns) cause decreased blood flow to the kidneys. The nephrons, however, are structurally and functionally intact.
   b. Intrarenal causes: conditions causing a reduction in glomerular filtration rate (GFR), renal ischemia, and tubular

damage. May be due to vascular diseases (hemolytic uremic syndrome, thrombosis), tubular nephropathies (myoglobinuria, hemoglobinuria, toxins), or interstitial nephritis (penicillins, allergies). These are the largest group to require extended medical management.

    c. Postrenal causes: conditions causing obstruction to urine flow. Uncommon, except for obstructive uropathies in the first year of life. Renal function is restored with relief of the obstruction.

2. The exact pathophysiology of acute renal failure is not always known. Three phases of acute renal failure are recognized in children:

    a. Initiating phase: begins when kidney is injured and lasts from hours to days. Signs and symptoms of renal impairment are present.

    b. Oliguric phase: usually lasts 5 to 15 days but can persist for weeks; shorter in infants and young children (3 to 5 days) and longer in older children and adolescents (10 to 14 days). Not all patients have an oliguric phase.

    c. Diuretic phase: highly variable, from mild and lasting only a few days to profound.

3. Trauma, burns, and nephrotoxic agents may cause acute tubular necrosis and temporary cessation of renal function. Myoglobin (a protein released from muscle when injury occurs) and hemoglobin are released, causing renal toxicity, ischemia, or both.

4. Severe transfusion reactions may result in hemoglobin that filters through the kidney glomeruli. This becomes concentrated in the kidney tubules. Resulting precipitation interferes with the excretion of urine.

5. Nonsteroidal anti-inflammatory drugs (NSAIDs) interfere with prostaglandins that normally protect renal blood flow, decreasing GFR.

 DRUG ALERT Nephrotoxic agents include aminoglycosides, penicillins, cephalosporins, sulfonamides, calcineurin inhibitor immunosuppressives, NSAIDs and certain antineoplastic drugs. Large doses of vitamin A, chemicals that contain arsenic, and mercury are also nephrotoxic.

Clinical Manifestations

1. Nausea and vomiting.
2. Diarrhea.
3. Decreased tissue turgor.
4. Dry mucous membranes.
5. Lethargy.
6. Difficulty in voiding; changes in urine flow; decreased urine output.
7. Steady rise in serum creatinine.
8. Fever.
9. Edema—periorbital, pitting lower leg edema, ascites.
10. Changes in mental status or mood.
11. Headaches and blurry vision due to hypertension.
12. Seizures.

Diagnostic Evaluation

1. Serum creatinine level—the most reliable measure of the GFR, found to be rising.
2. Radionuclide studies—evaluate GFR and renal blood flow and distribution.

3. Urinalysis—reveals proteinuria, hematuria, casts.
4. Ultrasonography—determines anatomic abnormalities.

Management

1. Seventy-five percent of children with acute renal failure attain complete recovery.
2. Treatment is directed toward the underlying cause.
3. Correction of any reversible cause of acute renal failure (ie, surgical relief of obstruction).
4. Correction and control of fluid and electrolyte imbalances.
5. Restoration and maintenance of stable vital signs.
6. Maintenance of nutrition with low-sodium, low-potassium, low-phosphate, and low-protein diet.
7. Initiation of dialysis (hemodialysis, peritoneal dialysis, or continuous venovenous hemofiltration) for patients with life-threatening complications.

Complications

1. Fluid and electrolyte imbalance, especially hyperkalemia—when GFR is reduced, patient cannot excrete potassium.
2. Metabolic acidosis, caused by decreased acid excretion and reduced bicarbonate reabsorption (see Box 49-1).
3. Insufficient nutritional intake because of metabolic abnormalities and symptoms, such as nausea and vomiting.

Nursing Assessment

1. Obtain history of all medications, recent and past illnesses or injuries, allergies, and potential exposure to toxic substances.

BOX 49-1	Clinical Manifestations of Metabolic Acidosis

GI
- Anorexia.
- Nausea and vomiting.
- Abdominal pain.

NEUROLOGIC
- Lethargy.
- Stupor.
- Coma.

CARDIOVASCULAR
- Decreased heart rate.
- Cardiac dysrhythmias.
- Peripheral vasodilation.

OTHER MANIFESTATIONS
- Warm and flushed skin.
- Weakness and malaise.
- Bone resorption (with chronic acidosis).
- Increased rate and depth of respirations (Kussmaul breathing due to compensation).

LABORATORY FINDINGS
- Decreased pH.
- Decreased HCO_3^- (initially).
- Decreased PCO_2 (compensatory).
- Hyperkalemia.
- Acidic urine (compensatory).

2. Measure intake and output. Insert indwelling urinary catheter, as indicated.
3. Monitor vital signs, especially BP. Institute cardiac monitoring, as indicated.
4. Assess for edema and fluid overload (cardiac and respiratory assessment).
5. Monitor urine-specific gravity, as directed. Fixed specific gravity of 1.010 indicates the kidneys' inability to concentrate or dilute urine.

Nursing Diagnoses

- Risk for Imbalanced Fluid Volume related to inability of the kidneys to maintain fluid balance.
- Risk for electrolyte imbalance: hyperkalemia.

Nursing Interventions

Maintaining Fluid Volume
1. Administer IV fluids slowly to prevent heart failure.
2. Maintain fluid restriction, as ordered.
3. Keep strict intake and output records.
4. Weigh child daily.
5. Promptly report signs of heart failure—edema, bounding pulse, third heart sound, shortness of breath, and adventitious breath sounds.

Preventing Severe Electrolyte Disturbance
1. Monitor blood test results (creatinine, BUN, electrolytes, calcium) and notify health care provider promptly of abnormal levels.
2. Watch for signs of hyperkalemia—weak, irregular pulse, abdominal cramps, and muscle weakness.
3. Do not administer IV fluids with potassium while renal function is impaired.
4. Maintain low-protein, low-potassium, low-sodium, and high-carbohydrate diet.
5. Administer treatments for hyperkalemia, as ordered, such as IV sodium bicarbonate and IV glucose and insulin (requires careful glucose monitoring), both of which drive potassium into cells and temporarily out of the bloodstream.
6. Administer cation exchange medications to reduce potassium, as ordered.
7. Watch for signs of hypocalcemia—muscle twitching and tetany.

Family Education and Health Maintenance

1. Explain all steps of the diagnostic and treatment process to the family.
2. Teach about dialysis if this becomes necessary.
3. Explain that as kidney function resumes, diuresis may occur to eliminate excess fluid the body was storing.
4. Educate about prompt medical attention for illnesses that may cause dehydration to prevent renal injury in the future.
5. Avoid nephrotoxins, including NSAIDs during recovery period

Evaluation: Expected Outcomes

- No signs of heart failure.
- Potassium remains within upper range of normal; kidney function returns to baseline.

Chronic Renal Failure

Chronic renal failure (CRF) is irreversible destruction of nephrons so that they are no longer capable of maintaining normal fluid and electrolyte balance. *Chronic kidney disease (CKD)* refers to kidney damage with a decreased GFR of less than 60 mL/min/1.73 m² for 3 months or greater. Nursing care of children with CRF is similar to that of adults (see page 606). The following considerations are important for pediatric patients.

Pathophysiology and Etiology

1. Congenital renal and urinary tract abnormalities are the most common causes in children younger than age 5 (eg, polycystic kidney disease, congenital nephrotic syndrome, hyperoxaluria).
2. Most common causes in ages 5 to 15 years:
   a. Glomerular disease (eg, glomerulonephritis).
   b. Urologic abnormalities.
   c. Cystic kidney disease.
3. Similar progression regardless of cause.
   a. Nephron damage that results in hypertrophy and hyperplasia of remaining nephrons.
   b. Overload results in decreased ability for nephrons to excrete effectively.
   c. Results in azotemia and clinical uremia.
   d. Inability of kidney to excrete phosphate causes hypocalcemia, which results in osteodystrophy.
   e. Kidneys cannot synthesize vitamin D, thus impairing calcium absorption. Bones may become so calcium depleted that growth halts and bones become brittle (renal rickets).
   f. Kidneys cannot synthesize erythropoietin, thus resulting in anemia.
   g. Excretion of nitrogenous waste through sweat causes pruritus.
   h. Overload of fluid results in edema and hypertension.
4. Severity of CRF is indicated by GFR. The lower the GFR, the greater the loss of renal function.

Clinical Manifestations

Variable and not chronological.
1. Nausea and vomiting, decreased appetite, and energy level.
2. Initial polyuria caused by kidneys' inability to concentrate urine; later oliguria and anuria.
3. Bone or joint pain.
4. Dryness and itching of skin.
5. Poor growth.
6. Fatigue, lethargy due to anemia.

Diagnostic Evaluation

1. Serum studies:
   a. Anemia and iron studies: decreased hemoglobin, hematocrit, iron levels
   b. Decreased Na+, Ca++, and CO_2 (metabolic acidosis); increased K+ and phosphorus.
   c. As renal function declines, BUN, uric acid, and creatinine values continue to climb.
   d. Elevated PTH.
2. Urine studies:
   a. Specific gravity—increased or decreased.

b. Twenty-four-hour urine for creatinine clearance is decreased (increased creatinine in urine), thus reflecting decreased GFR.
c. Changes in total output (may initially be polyuric because of difficulty concentrating urine, then oliguric).
d. Proteinuria.
3. Many other tests may be ordered to evaluate other systems and extent of disease (eg, chest x-ray, echocardiogram, bone age).

Management

1. Correction of calcium-phosphorus imbalance. Initiate low-phosphorus diet. Administer activated vitamin D to increase calcium absorption and phosphate binders with meals to bind phosphate in the GI tract.
2. Correction of acidosis with buffers, such as sodium bicarbonate tablets.
3. Correction of hyperkalemia through low-potassium diet or administration of potassium-lowering agents such as sodium polystyrene.
4. Diets should meet caloric needs of the child and contain adequate protein for development (0.9 to 1.5 g/kg/day).
5. Correction of anemia through the use of oral iron and erythropoietin administered subcutaneously at home.
6. BP should be managed with appropriate antihypertensive medications (angiotensin-converting enzyme inhibitors, angiotensin receptor blockers, calcium channel blockers, or diuretics).
7. Growth retardation should be evaluated for possible use of growth hormone. Consult dietitian to ensure optimal nutrition for use of growth hormone.
8. Renal replacement options for end-stage renal disease include hemodialysis, peritoneal dialysis, transplantation, or no treatment, typically initiated when GFR < 15 mL/min/1.73 m².
9. Dialysis, while renal transplant workup is in progress.

Complications

1. Growth retardation.
2. Delayed or absent sexual maturation.
3. Severe anemia—kidneys cannot stimulate erythropoietin; uremic toxins deplete erythrocytes; nutritional deficiencies.
4. Hypertension—renal ischemia stimulates renin–angiotensin system.
5. Cardiovascular disease (left ventricular hypertrophy, heart failure).
6. Renal osteodystrophy due to vitamin D deficiency and secondary hyperparathyroidism.
7. Azotemia/uremia—nitrogen waste products accumulate in blood. Toxic levels manifest themselves in many ways, such as coma, headache, GI disturbances, and neuromuscular disturbances.
8. Neurodevelopmental delay due to uremic effects.
9. Metabolic acidosis, which may cause poor growth, confusion, dull headache, and lethargy.
10. Electrolyte imbalance—hypocalcemia, hyperkalemia.

Nursing Assessment

1. Perform a comprehensive, multisystem assessment to help in planning care.
2. Assess nutrition, growth, and developmental status.
3. Assess coping, support systems, and other resources.

Nursing Diagnoses

Children with CRF are in multisystem physiologic crises. The nursing diagnoses throughout the chapter are applicable, but focus may be:

- Risk for Electrolyte Imbalance: hypocalcemia, hyperkalemia.
- Risk for Imbalanced Fluid Volume related to renal failure and dialysis.
- Imbalanced Nutrition: Less Than Body Requirements related to GI disturbances, diet restrictions, and protein loss.
- Activity Intolerance related to fatigue and anemia.
- Ineffective Coping related to changes in lifestyle and body image on dialysis.

Nursing Interventions

Ensuring Safety

1. Protect the child from the effects of decreased level of consciousness and involuntary movements by maintaining crib or bed side rails up and padded, as necessary.
2. Monitor for seizure activity and have airway or tongue blade and suction equipment on hand.
3. Monitor BUN, creatinine, electrolyte, and calcium levels and report abnormalities promptly.

Promoting Fluid Balance

See "Acute renal failure," page 1325.

Ensuring Adequate Nutrition

1. Ensure adequate protein in diet. Obtain consultation from a registered dietitian.
2. Encourage appropriate fluid intake between meals.
3. Consult with dietitian regarding appropriate milk intake and alternatives because of high phosphate, sodium, and potassium content. Instead, administer feedings high in calories and low in wastes, as directed.

Increasing Activity Tolerance

1. Plan activities when child is rested.
2. Encourage activity as tolerated
3. Administer blood transfusions or IV iron therapy, as ordered (if patient is resistant to erythropoietin therapy and unable to tolerate oral iron supplementation).

Enhancing Coping

Because numerous issues may interfere with the child's psychological and social development and education, help the child and family to cope with:

1. Uncertainty regarding the course of the disease and ultimate prognosis.
2. Abnormal lifestyle necessitated by dialysis (including interference with school).
3. Burden of dialysis and continuous administration of medications.
4. Problems of adjustment related to growth failure.
5. Fear of death, present in most children, adolescents, and family members.
6. Possible kidney transplantation, involving major surgery and prolonged hospitalization, followed by altered body image that is caused by high-dose steroids and potential for rejection, which may threaten survival.

Family Education and Health Maintenance

1. Teach child to avoid high-sodium foods, such as chips, pretzels, and popcorn; luncheon meats; canned foods; and fast foods, if sodium is restricted.
2. Encourage follow-up as advised by kidney specialist and primary health care provider.
3. Encourage family to keep up with regular dental care, immunizations, and health assessments to help prevent infections, problems with growth, and more severe childhood diseases.
4. Teach about medications and support child who may be taking multiple medications—calcium, phosphate binder, acid neutralizer, recombinant erythropoietin, antihypertensives, and others.
5. Teach about maintaining good hygiene and peritoneal dialysis catheter care.
6. Advise the family about support services and media resources available—for example, *Children & Teens with Kidney Disease*, by the National Kidney Foundation (*www.kidney.org*).

Evaluation: Expected Outcomes

- Side rails up with airway and suction at bedside.
- Fluid restriction maintained, weight stable, no signs of heart failure.
- Taking 100% of renal diet.
- Engaging in play without shortness of breath.
- Parents asking questions and discussing treatment with child.

The Child Who Undergoes Dialysis

Dialysis is the passage of a solute through a semipermeable membrane. The purpose of dialysis is to preserve life by replacing some of the normal kidney functions. See pages 593 to 594 for a complete description of different types of dialysis.

General Considerations

The following principles should be considered by the nurse who works with pediatric patients:

1. Peritoneal dialysis:
   a. This mode of dialysis continues to be the favored mode in young children.
   b. Because of the child's small size, the volume of dialysate is 1,100 to 1,400 mL/m².
   c. The child can be expected to participate at a developmentally appropriate level with his or her own care.
   d. Peritoneal dialysis is a continual treatment and therefore can constantly dialyze metabolic waste and fluids off.
2. Hemodialysis:
   a. When possible, subcutaneous or IM injections are avoided because the child is anticoagulated with heparin.
   b. BP cuff and tourniquets should not be applied to a limb with a fistula and peripheral IVs should not be placed in a limb with a graft or fistula.
3. Specific care for the child during dialysis is generally provided by specially trained personnel in a dialysis unit. However, the following considerations should be noted:
   a. Choice for vascular access depends on patient size and availability of peripheral blood vessels of suitable size (see Figure 49-3). A central venous catheter may also be used.

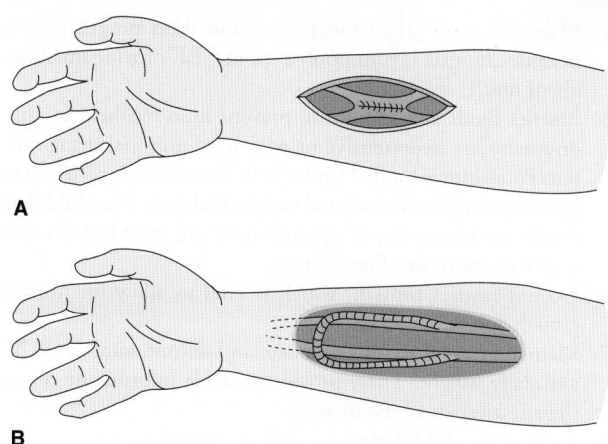

Figure 49-3. Vascular access devices for hemodialysis. **(A)** An internal arteriovenous fistula. **(B)** An internal arteriovenous graft. (Pillitteri, A. [2013]. *Maternal and child healthnursing: Care of the childbearing and childrearing family* [7th ed.]. Philadelphia: Lippincott Williams & Wilkins.)

   b. Extracorporeal blood volume (blood outside of the body at any given time) should be as small as possible. It should not exceed 8% to 10% of the child's total blood volume.
   c. Efficiency or adequacy of the dialyzer, relative to the child's weight, should be noted and blood pump speed adjusted accordingly.
   d. External catheter should be secured to make sure catheter is not traumatized.

Nursing Care of the Child Who Undergoes Dialysis

1. Prepare the child for the procedure. Dialysis is threatening to most children and may evoke fears of pain, mutilation, immobilization, helplessness, and dependency. Many children have fears of losing all of their blood during hemodialysis. A child who is well prepared will be less frightened and better able to cooperate during the procedure.
   a. Explain the procedure in terms that the child can understand.
   b. Allow the child to handle equipment similar to that which will be used during dialysis.
   c. Encourage the child to express fears so that misinterpretations can be corrected.
   d. Provide simple pictures and diagrams, if appropriate.
   e. Allow the child to talk with peers who have undergone dialysis.
2. Explain the procedure to family members and answer questions so that they will be in the best position to support the child.
3. Protect the child from infection.
   a. Keep the dressings and area around the catheter (if used) clean and dry.
   b. Use aseptic technique throughout the dialysis procedure.
   c. Provide supplemental vitamins because diet may be low in vitamins.
   d. Provide meticulous daily hygiene.

4. Maintain appropriate nutritional and fluid modifications. Because anorexia is commonly seen in CRF, provide small frequent meals.

5. Restrict fluids and sodium to prevent fluid overload in children who are hypertensive or who have minimal urine output. Potassium is limited (more so in hemodialysis patients) to prevent complications related to hyperkalemia. The child may see dietary restrictions as a punishment and must be helped to realize the purpose of restrictions.

6. Do not restrict protein, which is vital to allow for normal growth and development.

7. Maintain careful records of intake and output, vital signs, BP, and daily weight. These provide valuable information about the effectiveness of the therapy.

8. Support the child during the dialysis procedure.
   a. Provide symptomatic relief of nausea, vomiting, malaise, muscle cramping, or headache. Notify the health care provider if these symptoms are severe.
   b. Involve the child in diversional activities, such as play therapy, crafts, television, and books.
   c. Encourage the family to bring in articles that will make the child's room appear more homelike (eg, pictures, posters).
   d. Encourage the child to be as independent as possible in daily care.

9. Help the child to keep up with schoolwork by initiating a referral to a tutor and providing study times.

Community and Home Care Considerations

1. Be aware that although life is preserved, it is by no means normal during the time on dialysis or between dialysis treatments. These measures may increase the child's feeling of self-esteem and diminish regression and social isolation. By serving as role models, health professionals may encourage parents to recognize and foster the normal, healthy aspects of the child's daily life.

2. Offer appropriate support to the family.
   a. Provide opportunity for family members to discuss their feelings, fears, and frustrations and to ask questions.
   b. Allow family members to become involved in the child's care.
   c. Provide for continuity of personnel.
   d. Initiate appropriate referrals and provide resources. These may include referrals to a social worker, psychiatrist, dietitian, community health agency, or other families who are coping with dialysis.

3. Be aware that families usually need extensive support from many health professionals to cope with the physical, psychological, financial, and logistical aspects of renal failure and dialysis. Attention must be focused on siblings and parents because sibling relationships are usually strained and difficult.

4. Teach the child and family about all of the important aspects of renal failure and dialysis, including the following:
   a. Protection from infection.
   b. Dietary restrictions and recommendations; ways of incorporating the special diet into the family meal plan.
   c. Dialysis schedule.
   d. Medications.
   e. Emergency procedures.
   f. Reintegration into the community and school.

5. Empower the family to care for the child at home. Learning about the child's care also helps restore some sense of control in a frightening situation.

Renal Transplantation

Renal (kidney) transplantation is the optimal therapeutic modality for end-stage renal disease in the pediatric age group. With successful transplantation, there is a greater likelihood of optimum rehabilitation than with any other form of dialytic therapy. The potential for normal growth and pubertal development is significantly increased after transplantation. However, it should be noted that post transplant growth is affected by many variables: age of onset of chronic renal disease, caloric intake, corticosteroid dosage, bone age at transplantation, transplant function, and rejection episodes. Requirements of preoperative management and nursing care of children or teens for renal transplantation are similar to that of adults (see page 596). However, they are also more exhaustive because the recipient as well as the parents must be included. The emotional, psychological, and financial needs of the recipient and the family must be evaluated. An appropriate care plan must then be designed to address identified needs; this care plan must be appropriate for the developmental age of the recipient.

Evaluation of Recipient

The major issues that must be evaluated when considering renal transplantation in children are:

1. Patient age and size.
2. Primary renal disease.
3. Psychological status.
4. Live versus deceased donor allograft.
5. Optimal immunosuppressive regimen.
6. Maximization of growth and pubertal development.

Donor Selection (by Priority)

A tissue-compatible transplantation from a relative is 90% successful.

1. Identical twin sibling.
2. Siblings cannot be used as donors until they are of legal age to give consent for removal of a kidney.
3. Parent.
4. Other relative.
5. Unrelated live donor such as a family friend.
6. Deceased donor.

Operative Procedure

A child who weighs more than 22 pounds (10 kg) usually receives the kidney of an adult. In a very small child, the kidney transplant is placed within the abdomen, with vessel anastomosis to the aorta and superior vena cava.

Potential Emotional Concerns of Children with Transplants

1. The concept of a foreign body, especially a cadaver kidney, inside one's own body may be disturbing.
2. Fear that the kidney may wear out sooner if it is from an older person.
3. Altered body image because of growth failure and the effects of steroid therapy.
4. Guilt feelings if a live donor transplant fails, especially that of a family donor.

Nursing Interventions

Also see "After kidney transplantation," page 597.

1. Support the child and family through the preoperative phase, including diagnostic testing and blood transfusions.
2. After surgery, maintain strict infection precautions.
3. Administer immunosuppressants and other medications, as directed.
4. Continue support through dialysis, if necessary.
5. Monitor urine output, bloodwork results, and urine-specific gravity.
6. Watch for signs of rejection—fever, oliguria, proteinuria, weight gain, hypertension, and tenderness over transplanted kidney. Acute rejection usually occurs in the first 3 months after transplant. Chronic rejection may develop at any time. It occurs slowly over months to years and leads to progressive loss of renal function.
7. Watch for signs of infection: fever, leukopenia, neutropenia.
8. Infection can be bacterial (most common are pneumonia and UTIs) or viral (cytomegalovirus and Epstein-Barr virus are the most common infections).

Community and Home Care Considerations

The practice of discharging patients from an in-hospital setting as quickly as possible is also true for the pediatric transplant recipient. Community and home care nurses must have:

1. The knowledge to care for a child who receives IV and immunosuppressive medications.
2. The ability to access and heparinize central venous lines and peripheral IV catheters.
3. The ability to aid in reinforcing discharge teaching, aid in BP monitoring, and assess medication adherence.

Family Education and Health Maintenance

1. Teach families about the signs of rejection and infection.
2. Encourage close follow-up for proper dosing of immunosuppressants.
3. Education, communication, and employ strategies to promote medication adherence.
4. Advise family that close medical surveillance will always be necessary because the incidence of malignant disease is six times more likely in transplant recipients than in the general population.
5. Teach parents not to overprotect the child. When the child has healed from surgery, regular activity can be resumed. This includes returning to school; however, the school needs to be aware of the patient's immunosuppressive status.
6. Teach families and patients the importance of good hand washing.
7. Encourage patient to wear a MedicAlert bracelet or necklace, and inform the community emergency services of transplant status.
8. Advise parents that no live vaccine should be given to the child who is immunosuppressed.
9. Advise the family about resources available.

 TRANSITIONAL CARE ALERT After the stress of having a hospitalized child, families will need support in the transition to home or another aftercare location. It is crucial that they have complete and understandable care instructions on home care, medications, and follow-up appointments. If arrangements have been made for nursing care in the home, families should be aware of the agency providing services and when they can expect communication regarding care arrangements. Families should have thorough written (and if necessary to assist understanding, pictorial) instructions on signs and symptoms to monitor for that could suggest worsening of status. Children with renal and genitourinary disorders require careful monitoring of intake and output to prevent electrolyte unbalance. Family caregivers will need additional instructions on signs and symptoms that would indicate hydration alterations.

SELECTED REFERENCES

American Academy of Pediatrics. (2011). Urinary tract infection: Clinical practice guideline for the diagnosis and management of the initial UTI in febrile infants and children 2 to 24 months. Subcommittee on Urinary Tract Infection. Steering Committee on Quality Improvement and Management. *Pediatrics, 128,* 595–610.

American Urological Association. (Published 2010, Reviewed and Validity Confirmed 2017). Management and Screening of Primary Vesicoureteral Reflux in Children.

Cara-Fuentes, G., Gupta, N., & Garin, E. H. (2015). The RIVUR study: A review of its findings. *Pediatric Nephrology, 30*(5), 703.

Copeman, H. (2014). Renal care in the paediatric setting: An overview of common conditions. *Journal of Renal Nursing, 6*(6), 280–283.

Doyle, S., Carter, B., Bray, L., et al. (2016). Bladder augmentation in children and young adults: A review of the published literature. *International Journal of Urological Nursing, 10*(2), 97–106.

Fantasia, J., Aidlen, J., Lathrop, W., et al. (2015). Undescended testes: A clinical and surgical review. *Urologic Nursing, 35*(3), 117–126.

Kidney Disease: Improving Global Outcomes (KDIGO) Work Group. (2012). Clinical practice guideline for glomerulonephritis. *Kidney International, 2*(2), 139–274.

Kim, S., & Choi, H. (2016). Experiences of Korean adolescent renal transplant recipients. *Journal for Specialists in Pediatric Nursing, 21*(3), 158–165.

Kolon, T., Herndon, A., Baker, L., et al. (2014). Evaluation and treatment of cryptorchidism: AUA guideline. *Journal of Urology, 192,* 337–345.

Merguerian, P., & Rowe, C. (2018). Developmental abnormalities of the genitourinary system. In *Avery's Diseases of the Newborn* (10th ed.) (pp.1260–1273). Elsevier: Philadelphia.

Merkel, S., Danaher, J., & Williams, J. (2015). Pain management in the postoperative pediatric urologic patient. *Urologic Nursing, 35*(2), 75–100.

Micklos, L. (2014). Transition and interprofessional collaboration in moving from pediatric to adult renal care. *Nephrology Nursing, 41*(3), 311–317.

Pfeil, M., Parr, J., & Milind, M. (2012). Hypospadias repair: The nursing contribution. *International Journal of Urological Nursing, 6*(3), 152–158.

Sanders, C., & Bray, L. (2013). Young People's evaluation of a nurse-led bladder training service: Working towards developing a patient reported experience and outcome measure. *International Journal of Urological Nursing, 7*(1), 25–32.

Stermer, K. (2012). MR urogram in the pediatric population. *Journal of Radiology Nursing, 31*(2), 73.

The RIVUR Trial Investigators. (2014). Antimicrobial prophylaxis for children with vesicoureteral reflux. *New England Journal of Medicine, 371*(11), 1071–1072.

Wang, P., Djahanirian, O., & Wehbi, E. (2018). Urinary tract infections and VUR. In *Avery's Diseases of the Newborn* (10th ed.) (pp.1308–1313). Elsevier: Philadelphia.

Wiliams, L. (2016). Zeroing in on safety: A pediatric approach to preventing catheter-associated urinary tract infections. *AACN Advanced Critical Care, 27*(4), 372–378.

50

Pediatric Metabolic and Endocrine Disorders

OVERVIEW AND ASSESSMENT

Common Nursing Assessment for Growth and Development

Endocrine dysfunction in children frequently leads to altered growth and development. Accurate nursing assessment can help detect variations in growth and developmental patterns, identify such factors as diet and medications that may have an impact on growth and development, and obtain information about compliance and understanding of treatment.

Evaluation of Growth Patterns

1. Perform frequent and accurate measurements of height and weight.
2. Accurately plot measurements on growth curve for absolute chronologic age.
3. Assess growth pattern for any deviation from the child's percentile or from the parallel of the growth curve for age (includes both an upward as well as a downward deviation).
4. Calculate growth velocity—take the difference of current height from previous height and divide by the time period. Growth rate for a prepubertal child should be 2 to 3 inches (5 to 7 cm) on an annual basis.
5. Report any child whose pattern deviates from the expected pattern for age to health care provider.

General Health History

1. Dietary history—what is the child's meal frequency, volume, and food preferences? Be vigilant while obtaining the history of a child when anorexia may be possible—growth velocity will usually be low, in addition to poor weight gain.
2. History of major illnesses or surgeries that have altered the child's growth and development.
3. Family history—is there a family history of growth or developmental issues? Is there a family history of delayed puberty?

Are family members unusually short or tall in stature, or is there obvious dysmorphology?
4. Clothing—outgrowing clothing and shoes?
5. Social history relative to friendships.
6. Academic and school performance—recent changes?
7. Activity—activities the child participates in? Intensity and type of exercise?

Medication History and Compliance

1. Is the child on any steroid medications (such as prednisone) that would suppress growth? Inquire about over-the-counter medications or herbal supplementation.
2. When pubertal signs are present on physical examination, does the child have access to any gonadal steroids (ie, birth control pills, anabolic steroids)?
3. Do the child and family understand treatment medication indication and usage instructions?
4. Are the child and family compliant with medications according to dose, frequency, and route? Is medication stored properly?
5. If the child is taking oral medication, is it being taken with food, if indicated? If pills are being chewed, are teeth being brushed soon after, which could be rinsing out the medications?
6. If injectable, are injection sites being rotated appropriately? Review technique.

Physical Examination Relative to Development

1. Dental development—eruption of teeth and presence of permanent teeth (see page 1106).
2. Pubertal development—Tanner staging of pubic hair and gonadal development (see Table 50-1).
3. Presence of genetic dysmorphology—such as short-limbed dwarfism and various atypical stigmata.

Table 50-1 Tanner Staging of Puberty

BOYS' GENITAL DEVELOPMENT	GIRLS' BREAST DEVELOPMENT	BOTH SEXES: PUBIC HAIR
Stage I		
Preadolescent. Testes, scrotum, and penis are of about the same size and proportion as in early childhood.	Preadolescent. Elevation of papilla only.	Preadolescent. The vellus over the pubis is not further developed than that over the abdominal wall (ie, no pubic hair).
Stage II		
Enlargement of scrotum and testes. Skin of scrotum reddens and changes in texture. Little or no enlargement of penis at this time.	Breast bud stage. Elevation of breast and papilla as small mound. Enlargement of areola diameter.	Sparse growth of long, slightly pigmented downy hair. Straight or slightly curled at base of penis or along labia.
Stage III		
Enlargement of penis that occurs at first mainly in length. Further growth of testes and scrotum.	Further enlargement and elevation of breast and areola with no separation of their contours.	Considerably darker, coarser, and more curled. The hair spreads sparsely over the symphysis pubis.
Stage IV		
Increased size of penis with growth in breadth and development of glans. Testes and scrotum larger; scrotal skin darkened.	Projection of areola and papilla to form a secondary mound above level of the breast.	Hair now adult in type, but area covered is still considerably smaller than in adult. No spread to medial surface of thighs.
Stage V		
Genitalia adult in size and shape.	Mature stage: projection of papilla only, due to recession of the areola to the general contour of the breast.	Adult in quantity and type; distribution of the horizontal (or classically "feminine") pattern. Spread to medial surface of thighs or above base of the inverse triangle occurs late (stage VI).

Adapted from Tanner, J. M. (1975). Growth and endocrinology of the adolescent. In: Gardner, L. (Ed.), Endocrine and genetic diseases of childhood and adolescence (2nd ed.). Philadelphia, PA: W.B. Saunders.

Causes of Disorders of Growth and Stature

It is important to realize that growth and stature problems are caused by a wide variety of factors. Thorough history, physical examination, and diagnostic testing can help reveal the underlying cause. Many of the disorders are associated with other anomalies, such as mental retardation, cardiac problems, metabolic issues, and secondary sex characteristic abnormalities. The cause may be treatable to resolve the growth problem, may be amenable to growth hormone supplementation, or may be untreatable because of genetic cause.

Short Stature and Growth Failure

Genetic Causes

1. Familial short stature—short target height relative to U.S. standards; however, growth rate is normal.
2. Constitutional delay—short stature with retarded linear growth beginning in the first 3 years of life followed by short stature relative to peers; however, final height normal upon completion of pubertal development. Puberty is usually delayed.
3. Genetic disorders:
   a. Dwarfism—multiple types and causes relative to chondrodysplasias.
   b. Turner syndrome—occurs in about 1 in 2,500 female births worldwide. Characterized by short stature, ovarian dysgenesis (underdeveloped, degenerate ovaries), and, in some cases, unusual physical appearance (see page 1461).
   c. Russell-Silver syndrome—characterized by unilateral poor growth, short stature, characteristic facies, and mental delays. Whenever unilateral change in growth is present, abdominal tumor needs to be ruled out.
   d. Prader-Willi syndrome—rare syndrome characterized by below-normal intelligence, small stature, hypogonadism (see page 31, failure to thrive in infancy followed by obesity and insatiable appetite, binge-type eating behaviors.
   e. Down syndrome—occurs in 1 in 700 live births; characterized by growth retardation and developmental delays (see page 1458).
   f. Cystic fibrosis—occurs in 1 in 2,500 live births. In addition to respiratory and GI symptoms, growth retardation occurs (see page 1191).

Endocrine Disorders

1. Hypothyroidism.
2. Growth hormone (GH) deficiency.
3. Glucocorticoid excess—Cushing syndrome.

Nonendocrine Disorders

1. Glucocorticoid (prednisone) therapy for asthma, prevention of transplant rejection, adjunct medication in cancer chemotherapy, and severe dermatological disorders.
2. Nutritional deficiency.
3. Psychosocial issues.
4. Chronic diseases—cardiovascular, renal, hematologic, pulmonary, malabsorptive disorders, and inborn errors of metabolism.
5. Medical interventions—surgical tumor resection and radiation for brain tumors.

Tall Stature and Excessive Growth

Genetic Causes

1. Familial tall stature—tall stature relative to U.S. standards; however, normal for family. Growth rate is usually normal.
2. Genetic disorders:
   a. Marfan syndrome—tall, long extremities, long fingers and toes; cardiac and other anomalies.
   b. Klinefelter syndrome—tall, slim, underweight, gynecomastia, small testicles, infertile.

Endocrine Disorders

1. Congenital adrenal hyperplasia.
2. Precocious puberty (see page 1344).
3. Hyperthyroidism (see page 1340).
4. Acromegaly—overproduction of GH usually related to pituitary tumors; very rare in children.

Nonendocrine Disorders

1. Exogenous use of androgens (ie, testosterone injections):
   a. Although stature and growth will initially be above the normal expected for age, ultimate height will be decreased because of undue advance of bone maturation at growth plate.
   b. The child will ultimately end up shorter than genetically determined.
2. Sotos syndrome (cerebral gigantism)—usually large at birth with rapid growth in first year of life, intellectual impairment. Hypothesized to be a hypothalamic defect; normal endocrine function.

DISORDERS OF THE ANTERIOR PITUITARY

The anterior pituitary is under the control of the hypothalamus and secretes six specific hormones: GH, thyroid-stimulating hormone (TSH), adrenocorticotropic hormone (ACTH), luteinizing hormone (LH), follicle-stimulating hormone (FSH), and prolactin. GH is the only hormone that does not have a target gland to induce further hormonal secretion. Hypopituitarism is a deficiency of one, some, or all of the hormones secreted by the pituitary gland. With the exception of GH, decreased secretion results in hypofunction of the consequential target gland.

TSH deficiency, ACTH deficiency, and LH/FSH deficiency are discussed under disorders of the thyroid gland, disorders of the adrenal glands, and disorders of gonadal function, respectively.

Growth Hormone Deficiency

 EVIDENCE BASE Collin, J., Whitehead, A., & Walker, J. (2016). Educating children and families about growth hormone deficiency and its management: Part 1. *Nursing Children and Young People, 28*(1), 32–37.
Collin, J., Whitehead, A., & Walker, J. (2016). Educating children and families about growth hormone deficiency and its management: Part 2. *Nursing Children and Young People, 28*(2), 30–36.

Insufficient secretion of GH is caused by lack of pituitary production or hypothalamic stimulation on the pituitary. Incidence is approximately 1 in 3800 for classic GH insufficiency and is unknown for varying degrees of insufficiency.

Pathophysiology and Etiology

1. The lack of GH impairs the body's ability to perform the following functions:
   a. Protein metabolism—growth through increased protein synthesis; nitrogen, phosphorus, and potassium storage.
   b. Fat metabolism—increases lipolysis and oxidation of fat.
   c. Carbohydrate metabolism—decreases conversion of glucose to fat in adipose tissue.
2. Organic etiology:
   a. Intracranial cyst.
   b. Central nervous system (CNS) tumor (hypothalamic–pituitary structural lesions).
   c. CNS irradiation.
   d. Exogenous (head trauma from various causes such as birth injury, infection, pituitary infarction, or aneurysm).
   e. Histiocytosis X.
   f. Septo-optic dysplasia (abnormal forebrain development).

3. Idiopathic causes:
   a. Isolated GH deficiency; aplasia.
   b. Traumatic birth or breech delivery.
   c. Genetic (GH gene deletion).
   d. Nutritional deprivation; psychosocial issues.
4. Genetic cause—Turner syndrome:
   a. The pituitary and hypothalamus are not abnormal in Turner syndrome and GH secretion measurement is usually normal; however, GH is bioinactive because of binding problems.
   b. Hypothyroidism is common with Turner syndrome and Down syndrome.
   c. Growth rate usually declines within the first year of life.
   d. Treatment with GH is a commonly accepted therapy to restore growth.

Clinical Manifestations

1. Hypoglycemia, prolonged jaundice, microphallus (small penis); usually in the neonate.
2. Growth velocity usually less than the 5th percentile for chronologic age.
3. Delayed skeletal maturation—bone age at least 1 year delayed from chronologic age.
4. "Pudgy" when the weight age (50% for weight) exceeds the height age (50% for height).
5. Frequently delayed eruption of primary and secondary teeth (not as severe as in hypothyroidism).
6. Delayed or lack of sexual development.
7. In young adulthood after epiphyseal fusion, the following symptoms may develop, requiring evaluation from an adult endocrinologist:
   a. Altered body composition (increased fat mass, decreased lean body mass).
   b. Reduced aerobic exercise capacity or performance.
   c. Decreased muscle strength.
   d. Abnormal blood lipid (fat and cholesterol) concentrations.
   e. Decreased bone mineral density or content.
   f. Impaired cardiac function.
   g. Impaired health-related quality of life (low energy level, decreased physical mobility, difficulties with concentration and memory, increased emotional lability, irritability, difficulty relating to others, or increased social isolation).

Diagnostic Evaluation

1. Rule out organic, nonendocrine causes of short stature (ie, chronic illness, nutritional deficiencies, genetic disorders, psychosocial factors).
2. Calculate growth velocity. (Does growth pattern parallel or deviate from the growth curve?)
3. Bone age assessment—(usually left wrist and hand), ascertain age of physical development; usually delayed.
4. General physical examination—physical development that of a younger-appearing child, microphallus in the neonate.
5. Chromosome testing of females (rule out Turner syndrome).
6. Thyroid function tests to rule out hypothyroidism.
7. GH secretion laboratory indicators: IGF-1 (insulin-like growth factor 1), IGF-binding protein 3 are decreased. (Malnutrition can cause low IGF-1.)
8. Subnormal secretion of GH in response to two provocative stimuli:
   a. Insulin-induced hypoglycemia.

b. Abnormal stimulatory response to arginine infusion, L-dopa, clonidine, or glucagon—all of which have specific actions resulting in GH secretion from pituitary. Pharmacologic agent is given, followed by blood sampling for GH response; GH levels less than 10 ng/mL are abnormal.
9. In the neonate with hypoglycemia, GH release is reduced at time of documented hypoglycemia (concomitant GH level relative to documented hypoglycemia is abnormally low).
10. GH has been associated with reduction in serum levels of free T4. Patients starting on GH should have their thyroid function monitored in the first 6 months of treatment.
11. Magnetic resonance imaging (MRI) of head to rule out tumor (MRI is gold standard).

 NURSING ALERT In the neonate with hypoglycemia, always draw blood for cortisol and GH *before* initiating corrective action for the hypoglycemia. Early detection and diagnosis will protect the child from future episodes if related to hypopituitarism.

Management

1. Goal of treatment is to restore normal growth and development, as well as to maximize growth potential and prevent hypoglycemia.
2. Replacement of deficiency uses recombinant deoxyribonucleic acid–derived GH given as subcutaneous injection.
3. Typical dose is 0.2 to 0.3 mg/kg per week divided in six or seven doses weekly until final height is achieved. In treatment of Turner syndrome, dose is generally 0.375 mg/kg per week divided in doses as above. *Note*: Administration three times per week is not as effective as six to seven times per week.
4. Therapy is being recommended for adult replacement. Depending on the degree of insufficiency, continued treatment into adulthood may be useful. Dosing recommendations range from less than 0.006 mg/kg/day to as high as 0.0125 mg/kg/day after epiphyseal fusion has occurred.

 EVIDENCE BASE Collin, J., Whitehead, A., & Walker, J. (2016). Educating children and families about growth hormone deficiency and its management: Part 1. *Nursing Children & Young People, 28*(1), 32–37.

Complications

1. Altered carbohydrate, protein, and fat metabolism.
2. Hypoglycemia—seizures/death in neonates.
3. Adverse effects of therapy.
   a. Leukemia.
   b. Recurrence of CNS tumors.
   c. Pseudotumor cerebri.
   d. Slipped capital femoral epiphysis.
   e. Glucose intolerance/diabetes.

Nursing Assessment

1. See "Common nursing assessment for growth and development," page 1332.
2. Obtain family history related to parental heights and ages of pubertal maturation.

Nursing Diagnoses

- Delayed Growth and Development related to lack of GH.
- Impaired Social Interaction related to short stature and peer acceptance.
- Chronic Low Self-Esteem related to discordant expectations by peers and adults.

Nursing Interventions

Providing Education and Evaluation

1. Teach method of injecting GH through written and verbal instructions. Give demonstration and encourage return demonstration.
2. Encourage rotation of sites in the subcutaneous tissue of the upper arms or thighs to prevent skin irritation and hypertrophy.
3. Document growth every 3 to 6 months while on therapy.
4. If poor growth response, evaluate for appropriate dose, compliance, and injection technique. There may be initial "catch-up" growth that will be exhibited by a growth velocity above normal.
5. Instruct patient and family to report adverse effects: severe headache, hip and knee pain, limp, and increased thirst and urination.

Encouraging Social Interaction

1. Encourage the child to verbalize feelings regarding short stature.
2. Have the child describe what he or she likes about certain people to help the child understand that friendships and social value are based on personality traits rather than absolute height.
3. Suggest involvement in activities that do not use height as an advantage, such as music, art, and gymnastics.
4. Ask the child to identify behaviors that may deter socialization (may or may not be related to short stature) and find ways to change behavior.

Strengthening Self-Esteem

1. Help the child and parents to identify age-appropriate behaviors and develop a plan for maintaining consistent behaviors in the home and socially.
2. Make sure the parents have realistic expectations of the child.
3. Encourage the use of positive feedback rather than punishment.

Community and Home Care Considerations

1. Become familiar with the GH preparation being used and develop a teaching plan for home injection (mixing and injection technique). Provide periodic evaluation and ongoing support.
2. If home injections are difficult relative to family learning or parental availability, attempt to include school nurse in administering daily injections.
3. Review storage and stability of GH product relative to manufacturer's specifications for the home, as well as use in travel.

Family Education and Health Maintenance

1. Tell the child and family that short stature is not a "disease."
   a. Growth often catches up with peers usually when peers have stopped growing.
   b. After initial startup of treatment, growth rate should be 4 to 5 inches (10 to 12 cm)/year in year 1 and 2¾ to 3½ inches (7 to 9 cm)/year over the next 2 years. Growth will slow after that.
   c. Treatment is not to make the child tall; rather, its purpose is to optimize final height potential.
2. Review medication dosage and injection technique periodically.
3. Tell family to think of GH as a replacement that is essential rather than a medication; therefore, it should always be given regardless of illness or other medication therapies.
4. Encourage regular follow-up for growth evaluation and maintenance of therapy.
5. Discuss potential lifelong therapy, which may be necessary depending on the degree of deficiency. Many hypopituitary patients require lifelong replacement therapy.
6. Recommend counseling about probable infertility for female with Turner syndrome. This should be done with a genetic counselor, if available.

Evaluation: Expected Outcomes

- Growth rate in initial 2 years of therapy should be two to four times pretreatment growth velocity with final gain of one to two standard deviations in height.
- The child reports interest in school activities and playing with friends.
- Parents report more positive behavior relative to self-esteem.

DISORDERS OF THE POSTERIOR PITUITARY

The posterior pituitary is under the control of the hypothalamus and secretes two hormones, vasopressin (antidiuretic hormone [ADH]) and oxytocin. Abnormality of ADH function is the most common disorder seen in children. The function of ADH is to conserve water at the distal tubules and collecting ducts of the kidney and to act on smooth muscle to increase blood pressure (BP).

Diabetes Insipidus

EVIDENCE BASE Hunter, F., & Calikoglu, A. (2016). Etiological and clinical characteristics of central diabetes insipidus in children: a single center experience. *International Journal of Pediatric Endocrinology*, 2/11/2016, 1–5.

Diabetes insipidus (DI) is failure of the body to conserve water due to a deficiency of ADH, decreased renal sensitivity to ADH, or suppression of ADH secondary to excessive ingestion of fluids (primary polydipsia).

Pathophysiology and Etiology

1. The function of water metabolism in the body is to maintain a constant plasma osmolality near the mean level of 287 mOsm/kg.
2. Intake and output of water are governed by the centers in the hypothalamus to control thirst and synthesis of ADH.
3. Thirst ensures adequate intake of water, and ADH prevents water loss through the kidney.
4. Patients with DI are unable to produce appropriate levels or action of ADH, leading to polyuria, increased plasma osmolality, and increased thirst (see Figure 50-1).

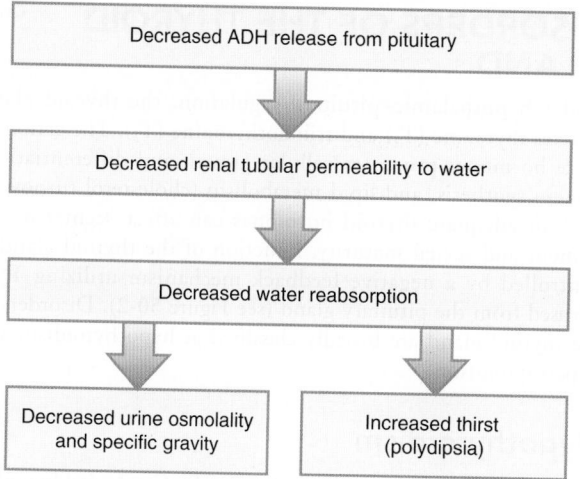

Figure 50-1. Mechanism of antidiuretic hormone (ADH) deficiency in diabetes insipidus.

5. Classified as central or nephrogenic DI:
  a. Central DI—low levels of ADH; may be congenital or acquired.
    i. Congenital causes—CNS defects, hereditary.
    ii. Acquired causes—CNS tumors, head trauma (orbital trauma), infections, vascular disorders, idiopathic.
  b. Nephrogenic DI—renal unresponsiveness to vasopressin; usually caused by chronic renal disease.
  c. Acquired causes—dietary abnormalities such as primary polydipsia, decreased sodium chloride intake, severe protein restriction or depletion, sickle cell disease, drugs (alcohol, lithium, diuretics, medications such as tetracycline).

Clinical Manifestations

1. Sudden onset of excessive thirst and polyuria.
2. In infants:
  a. Excessive crying—quieted with water more than milk feeding.
  b. Rapid weight loss—caloric loss due to water preference over feedings.
  c. Constipation.
  d. Growth failure—weight loss, failure to thrive.
  e. Dehydration—sunken fontanelle, rapid heart rate, headache, fever, low blood pressure.
3. In children:
  a. More abrupt onset, excessive thirst and drinking, preference for ice water.
  b. Polyuria (usually more than 2 L/day) with nocturia and enuresis.
  c. Pale, dry skin with reduced sweating.
  d. Lethargy.

Diagnostic Evaluation

Tests document inability to produce ADH in the face of hyperosmolality of plasma.
1. Urine-specific gravity, sodium, and osmolality are decreased.
2. Serum osmolality and sodium are elevated.
3. Serum measurement of ADH is low in conjunction with high plasma osmolality.
4. Water deprivation test (potentially dangerous):
  a. Fluids are restricted, and the urinary volumes and concentrations are monitored hourly along with the child's weight.

  b. Test is terminated if the child loses more than 3% to 5% of body weight. Serum sodium and osmolality are measured at completion of test and are high; urine osmolality remains lower.
  c. Test is completed by giving the child a dose of ADH, which should stop the abnormal diuresis. If it does not, child may have nephrogenic DI.
5. Assess for underlying cause:
  a. MRI of hypothalamic–pituitary region.
  b. High incidence of associated anterior pituitary disorders.

Management

1. Daily replacement of ADH using desmopressin (DDAVP), a synthetic analogue.
2. Available as a metered nasal spray, measured insufflation (nasal) tube, or tablets. In children with cleft lip and palate, sublingual administration has been shown to be effective.
3. Thiazide diuretics in nephrogenic DI.

Complications

1. Dehydration.
2. Hypernatremia.
3. Adverse reactions to DDAVP therapy—hyponatremia and hypertension.

Nursing Assessment

1. Assess children with complaints or behaviors of polyuria and polydipsia for dehydration.
2. Obtain a thorough history of symptoms and behaviors—specific attention to changes in sleep patterns (may be caused by enuresis) and choices of fluids, including sources of water (eg, does child drink from toilet bowls or dog dishes?).
3. Evaluate height and weight—assess for weight loss related to possible decrease in calories due to excessive drinking, which decreases appetite.
4. For the child on treatment, assess for hydration status. Obtain history of fluid intake and output from the parents to assess appropriate dosage, frequency, and administration of medication.

Nursing Diagnoses

- Deficient Fluid Volume related to disease process.
- Imbalanced Nutrition: Less Than Body Requirements due to fluid preference over food.
- Disturbed Sleep Pattern related to nocturia and enuresis.

Nursing Interventions

Regaining Fluid Balance

1. Assess for and teach parents assessment of dehydration—dry mucous membranes, weight loss, increased pulse, listlessness or irritability, sunken fontanelle in infants, fever, and poor skin turgor.
2. Administer fluid via intravenous (IV) route, as ordered, if acutely dehydrated.
3. Monitor intake and output and teach parents to maintain record of fluid intake and output in child. Reduced output may require restriction of fluids to prevent hyponatremia if overdosage of DDAVP is suspected.
4. Keep record of daily weight.
5. Family education of DDAVP administration includes nurse demonstration and family administration. Proper management should eliminate symptoms.

6. Teach parents to provide free access to fluid (water) sources at all times. However, caution parents that child is unprotected from water excess.
7. Calculate general estimated total daily (24 hours) fluid requirements based on body size to assess fluid replacement versus excess: 100 mL/kg for first 10 kg of body weight, 50 mL/kg for second 10 kg of body weight, and 20 mL/kg for each additional kilogram.

 NURSING ALERT Watch for and report signs of water intoxication due to excess free water and hyponatremia—drowsiness, listlessness, headache, confusion, anuria, and weight gain. Hold DDAVP to prevent seizures, coma, and death.

Maintaining Adequate Nutrition
1. Make sure that adequate formula is ingested between plain water bottles.
2. For older child, provide liquid nutritional supplements.
3. Stress to parents or caregivers the importance of providing nutritional requirements with fluids to ensure meeting caloric demands for growth.
4. Consult with dietitian about need for vitamin or other supplements.
5. Monitor length and weight and developmental milestones at regular intervals.

Normalizing Sleep Pattern
1. Ensure adequate evening administration of DDAVP to prevent nighttime water craving and enuresis.
2. Suggest the use of diapers at night and plastic padding on bed to make controlling bedwetting easier until optimum management of condition is attained.
3. Encourage easy access to fluids and toilet or commode for older child during night.

Family Education and Health Maintenance
1. Teach family insufflation method (for infants and young children):
   a. Correct dose is measured and drawn up into catheter.
   b. Catheter is inserted into patient's nostril.
   c. Parent or patient inserts other end of catheter into mouth and gently blows.
   d. Older children may be able to inhale the solution.
2. Advise that nostrils should be as clear as possible before administration of dose.
3. Advise that, if dose is thought to be swallowed, do not readminister because of potential overdosage. Split the dose into both nares if swallowing is occurring.
4. Tell family to store drug away from heat and direct light and moisture (not in bathroom).
5. Advise parents that children should wear MedicAlert bracelet for DI.
6. Tell parents that school or daycare personnel should be aware of condition and symptoms needing attention (water intoxication).
7. Advise routine follow-up; treatment may be temporary or lifelong, depending on cause.

Evaluation: Expected Outcomes
- No signs of dehydration; intake equals output.
- No weight loss, growth curve maintained.
- Child sleeping through night.

DISORDERS OF THE THYROID GLAND

Under hypothalamic–pituitary regulation, the thyroid gland secretes thyroxine (T_4) and triiodothyronine (T_3). The action of these hormones promotes cellular growth and differentiation, protein synthesis, and lipid metabolism (cholesterol turnover). Lack of adequate thyroid hormones can affect mental development and sexual maturity. Function of the thyroid gland is controlled by a negative feedback mechanism utilizing TSH released from the pituitary gland (see Figure 50-2). Disorders of the thyroid gland are broadly classified as hypothyroidism and hyperthyroidism.

Hypothyroidism

Hypothyroidism is low circulating level of T_4. Congenital hypothyroidism occurs in 1 in 4,000 live births with females more commonly affected.

Pathophysiology and Etiology

1. Circulating levels of T_4 are dependent on hypothalamic–pituitary stimulation (TRH [thyrotropin-releasing hormone]/TSH) of the thyroid gland.
2. Low levels of T_4 cause an increase in TSH level.
3. Absent or decreased levels of T_4 result in abnormal development of the CNS of the neonate.
4. In older children, hypothyroidism results in a decrease in metabolism, growth, and physical maturation.
5. Congenital causes:
   a. Thyroid agenesis or dysgenesis.
   b. Hormone synthesis defect.
   c. Maternal thyroid antibodies crossing placenta.
   d. Iodine deficiency.

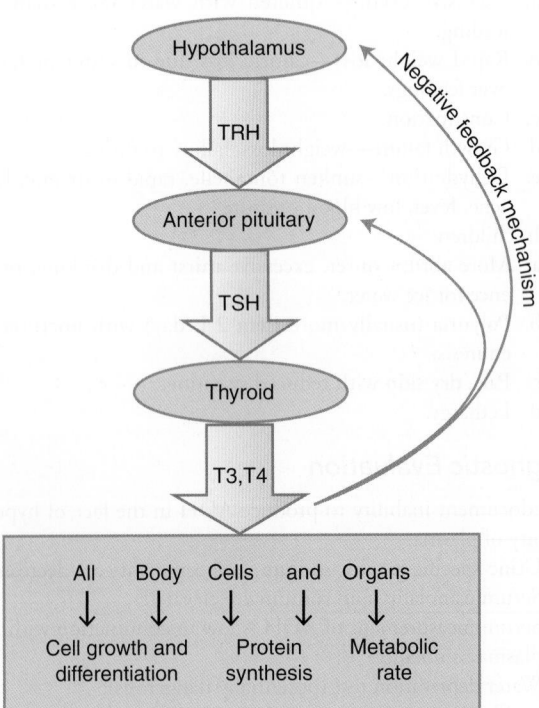

Figure 50-2. Normal thyroid hormone function.

e. Drug-induced destruction (thioamides for treatment of hyperthyroidism, iodide excess).

f. Peripheral T_4 resistance.

6. Acquired (postnatal) causes:

a. Autoimmune thyroiditis (Hashimoto disease or chronic lymphocytic thyroiditis).

b. Cranial/spinal radiation.

c. Surgical ablation (thyroidectomy).

d. Antithyroid drugs.

e. Iodine deficiency.

f. Central hypothyroidism (TRH/TSH deficiency).

Clinical Manifestations

Neonates

1. Very subtle physical signs, if any.
2. Markedly open posterior fontanelle.
3. Prolonged physiologic jaundice.
4. Feeding difficulties.
5. Skin cool to touch, mottled.
6. Poor muscle tone—hypotonia, umbilical hernia.

After Age 6 Months

1. Growth failure.
2. Large, protruding tongue.
3. Coarse facial features.
4. Poor feeding and constipation.

Acquired Cases

1. Growth retardation—slow growth rate, increased weight gain.
2. Lethargy—obedient, nonaggressive, somnolent.
3. Cold intolerance.
4. Possible poor school performance.
5. Constipation.

Diagnostic Evaluation

1. Neonatal screening of TSH with backup T_4; elevation of TSH or a low T_4 may indicate congenital hypothyroidism.

a. Testing is ideally done at 2 to 4 days of life or immediately before the neonate is discharged from the hospital. TSH levels in the first 24 to 28 hours of life may be falsely elevated.

b. Abnormal screening test should be confirmed and treatment begun within 2 weeks after birth.

2. Thyroid nuclear scan—reduced uptake.
3. Abnormal growth rate.
4. Bone age x-ray; delayed.
5. Blood studies:

a. Free T_4 decreased; TSH elevated.

b. Thyroid antibodies—elevated in autoimmune thyroiditis.

 EVIDENCE BASE Nierengarten, M. (2016). Hypothyroidism in children. *Contemporary Pediatrics, 33*(5), 29–33.

Management

1. Replacement of thyroid hormone: levothyroxine.
2. Treatment must not be delayed.
3. Therapy goal is to maintain normalcy of thyroid function tests (free T_4, T_4, and T_3 concentrations) in the upper half of normal range.

Complications

1. Developmental delays in neonate who is undiagnosed or untreated.
2. Short stature, growth failure, and delayed physical maturation and development in the older child.

Nursing Assessment

1. Assess the neonate for clinical manifestations listed above.
2. Perform behavioral assessment to include sleeping, eating, bowel patterns, level of alertness, and school performance.
3. Assess growth patterns: growth velocity (rate of growth over time), weight gain, and head circumference.

Nursing Diagnoses

- Delayed Growth and Development related to effects of hypothyroidism.
- Deficient Knowledge regarding hypothyroidism and its treatment.

Nursing Interventions

 EVIDENCE BASE Erlichman, I., Mimouni, F., Erlichman, M., et al. (2016). Thyroxine-based screening for congenital hypothyroidism in neonates with Down syndrome. *Journal of Pediatrics, 173*, 165–168.

Promoting Growth and Development

1. Administer or teach parents to administer thyroid hormone replacement daily.
2. Discourage mixing thyroid medication with liquid in bottle that may not be completely finished during a feeding; instead, mix with small amount of fluid and give with dropper or syringe or crush tablet and place in teaspoon of infant food. Do not mix with soy formula.
3. If thyroid pill is being chewed rather than swallowed, have the patient avoid brushing the teeth immediately after to protect against rinsing away dose.
4. Monitor growth and developmental milestones at regular intervals.

Increasing Knowledge

1. Encourage the parents to verbalize feelings about the child and the condition.
2. Educate the parents as to the importance of the therapy so the child will grow and develop normally.
3. Stress that with replacement therapy, the child can participate in all usual activities.

Family Education and Health Maintenance

1. Encourage follow-up by a primary care provider or pediatric endocrinologist for blood studies to assess and monitor thyroid levels and evaluation of neurologic development to ensure adequate treatment and optimal cognitive development.
2. Make sure the family understands that therapy is usually lifelong. May do a 6-week trial off medication after age 3 years under health care provider's supervision.
3. Support the parents and refer child for special testing and therapy if mental retardation is suspected.
4. Teach family the importance of avoiding overdosage of levothyroxine and of being alert for signs of overdosage (weight loss, restlessness, heat intolerance, fatigue, muscle weakness, tachycardia).

Evaluation: Expected Outcomes

- Growth curve and developmental milestones appropriate for age.
- Parents verbalize understanding and acceptance of therapy.

Hyperthyroidism

Hyperthyroidism is a disorder of the thyroid gland in which a high circulating level of T_4 results in abnormally increased body metabolism (thyrotoxicosis).

Pathophysiology and Etiology

1. May be caused by autoimmune process—thyrotropin receptor antibodies of a stimulating nature are produced.
   a. Graves disease—most common cause of hyperthyroidism in children, affecting 1% to 2% of school-age children.
   b. Chronic thyroiditis—Hashimoto disease; usually short-term hyperthyroidism (6 to 18 months duration) before developing hypothyroidism.
2. Autoantibodies stimulate thyroid gland to produce and secrete T_4.
3. Elevated circulating thyroid hormone increases the body's metabolic rate, causing an increase in excitability of the neuromuscular, cardiovascular, and sympathetic nervous systems.
4. May also be caused by ingestion or overdosage of thyroid medication (iatrogenic) or pituitary adenoma (TSH initiated).

Clinical Manifestations

1. Thyromegaly—enlargement of the thyroid, possibly with a bruit.
2. Polyphagia with weight loss.
3. Exophthalmos, proptosis, lid retraction.
4. Hyperactivity—restlessness, nervousness, hand tremors, perspiration, sleeping disturbances, emotional lability; inability to concentrate, decreased school performance.
5. Heat intolerance, excessive diaphoresis.
6. Fatigue (proximal), muscle weakness.
7. Tachycardia, palpitations, wide pulse pressure.
8. Tall stature, underweight for height.

Diagnostic Evaluation

1. Serum thyroid function tests—elevated T_4, T_3 resin uptake with a suppressed TSH.
2. Microsomal antibodies—positive.
3. Thyroid radionuclide scan of goiter—rules out cold nodules that could indicate thyroid carcinoma.

Management

1. Propranolol, a beta-adrenergic blocking agent, for cardiac effects, antipyretics, and anxiolytics.
2. Inorganic iodide preparation, such as propylthiouracil or methimazole, to block release of thyroid hormone. Adverse effects include headache, nausea, diarrhea, skin rash, itching, liver disease, jaundice, arthralgia, and, rarely, agranulocytosis (severe leukopenia).
3. Radioactive ablation of thyroid gland using radioiodine—preferred over thyroidectomy. This is chosen when medical management is ineffective and results in permanent hypothyroidism that requires treatment.

Complications

1. Development of a goiter (glandular enlargement due to overstimulation).
2. Cardiac problems of tachycardia and hypertension.
3. Exophthalmos—abnormal protrusion of the eyeball.

Nursing Assessment

1. Perform physical assessment to include temperature, heart rate, BP, height, and weight.
2. Obtain history of symptoms specific to onset and subsequent development of symptoms.
3. Elicit history of any changes in behavior, school performance, emotions, or sleep patterns.
4. Assess for presence of goiter—pain with swallowing or talking, palpation of thyroid.

Nursing Diagnoses

- Activity Intolerance related to effects of excessive metabolic activity.
- Imbalanced Nutrition: Less Than Body Requirements due to increased metabolic demand.
- Disturbed Sleep Pattern related to high metabolic rate.
- Fear related to radioiodine ablation of gland if therapy choice.

Nursing Interventions

Improving Activity Tolerance

1. Administer and teach parents to administer medications and comply with treatment to gradually lower the metabolic rate and improve activity tolerance.
2. Assess activity tolerance periodically. Ascertain if fatigue is present at rest, with activities of daily living, or with exercise. Promote relaxation and rest between activities.
3. Avoid overactivity.

Ensuring Adequate Diet

1. Encourage high-calorie, nutritious diet until thyroid hormone levels are stabilized to try to maintain weight.
2. Advise the parents that effective treatment will lower metabolic rate and facilitate appropriate weight gain.
3. Periodically assess growth and development parameters.

Normalizing Sleep Pattern

1. Assess sleep pattern, including naps and sleeping through the night.
2. Adjust schedule to allow maximum amount of rest until sleeping through the night.
3. Allow short naps, as needed.

Reducing Fear

1. Encourage the parents and child to verbalize fears related to the thyroid ablation.
2. Teach them about the procedure and clear up misconceptions.
   a. Ablation is accomplished through radioactive destruction of thyroid tissue by administration of a radioactive iodine pill.
   b. The thyroid gland is the only tissue in the body that absorbs iodine; therefore, the radiation only destroys thyroid tissue.
   c. Radiation will be eliminated through the child's urine and feces; precautions for disposal must be followed according to nuclear medicine department policies.
3. Tell them that the resultant effect will most likely be hypothyroidism, which can be managed with lifelong treatment of T_4 replacement.

Family Education and Health Maintenance

1. Review prescribed medications and their functions. Stress the importance of compliance.
2. Advise about periodic blood testing and monitoring for adverse effects of antithyroid medication.
3. Educate family about possibility of oversuppression, from which hypothyroidism could develop.
4. If midday dose of medication is necessary, have family contact school nurse to coordinate dosing.
5. If gland is radioactively ablated, be certain family and other caregivers are appropriately instructed on storage and disposal of human waste after ablative therapy.
6. Encourage follow-up to monitor treatment through blood tests, growth and development evaluation, and size of thyroid gland.

 DRUG ALERT Antihyperthyroid medications may cause agranulocytosis (severe leukopenia), thrombocytopenia, and aplastic anemia. Periodic blood testing is necessary to monitor blood counts. Agranulocytosis may present with sore throat and fever. Drug should be discontinued immediately and health care provider notified.

Evaluation: Expected Outcomes

- The child can play normally without early fatigue.
- No weight loss noted.
- The child displays normal sleep patterns through the night as well as during naps.
- Parents and child verbalize understanding of radiation procedure agnd its rationale.

DISORDERS OF THE ADRENAL GLANDS

The adrenal glands are responsible for the life-sustaining production of mineralocorticoids (aldosterone) for sodium retention, glucocorticoids (cortisol) for blood glucose regulation, and androgens (Dehydroepiandrosterone [DHEA], androstenedione) for phallic and secondary sex characteristic development (adrenarche).

Adrenocortical insufficiency is the inability of the adrenal gland to produce aldosterone and cortisol due to adrenal failure or lack of adrenal stimulation. With the exception of congenital adrenal hyperplasia (discussed below), pediatric adrenocortical insufficiency is similar in adults (see page 720).

Hyperadrenalism, although rare in children, does occur, causing tissue to be exposed to excessive glucocorticoids (cortisol). This is commonly called *Cushing syndrome*. Additionally, hyperfunction of the adrenal medulla, in which epinephrine, norepinephrine, and other catecholamines are secreted, is commonly seen in the disorder of pheochromocytoma. See pages 718 and 721 for a discussion of these conditions.

Congenital Adrenal Hyperplasia

Congenital adrenal hyperplasia (CAH) is the most common type of adrenocortical insufficiency in children. Adrenal dysfunction is a result of an enzyme deficiency in the steroid pathway converting cholesterol to cortisol, resulting in overproduction of androgens (sex hormones). The most common form of the condition is life threatening and requires diagnosis and treatment soon after birth.

Pathophysiology and Etiology

1. Production of adrenal mineralocorticoids and glucocorticoids is blocked by an enzyme deficiency in the steroid pathway. "Blocks" may be severe or partial.
   a. Deficiency of 21-hydroxylase (90% to 95% of CAH cases)—insufficiency in cortisol and usually aldosterone production.
   b. Deficiency of 11-β-hydroxylase (5% to 8%)—insufficiency of cortisol and aldosterone; however, precursor block to aldosterone is a potent mineralocorticoid.
   c. Deficiency of 3-β-hydroxysteroid dehydrogenase (5%)—insufficiency in cortisol, aldosterone, and androgen production.
2. Because of lack of feedback suppression, ACTH and renin are secreted to stimulate adrenal gland production, causing hyperplasia of the gland.
3. Aldosterone insufficiency results in fluid and electrolyte imbalance.
   a. Loss of sodium at the kidney results in loss of fluid and an increase in serum potassium (cation exchange).
   b. Depletion of extracellular fluid leads to decreased BP.
   c. Low BP stimulates renin in the kidney to activate the adrenal aldosterone pathway.
4. Cortisol insufficiency results in diminished hepatic gluconeogenesis and tissue glucose uptake.
   a. Diminished production/secretion results in low blood sugar levels—more pronounced in times of stress.
   b. Low blood sugar, stress, or low cortisol stimulates feedback to hypothalamic–pituitary axis to release ACTH to stimulate adrenal activity, which also stimulates the release of melanocyte-stimulating hormone (MSH).
   c. Constant ACTH stimulation of gland causes overproduction and "backup" of blocked steroid pathways, resulting in "spillover" production of adrenal androgens.
5. Depending on etiology, overproduction of androgens will virilize female external genitalia or underproduction of androgens will block virilization of male external genitalia.

Clinical Manifestations

1. Ambiguous female genitalia—varying degrees of virilization due to exposure of androgens during development in utero:
   a. Clitoromegaly (may be penile shaped).
   b. Labial fusion (partial or complete).
   c. Rugated labia-appearing scrotal.
   d. Vagina may be incomplete, ending in a blind pouch.
2. Ambiguous male genitalia (3-β-dehydrogenase)—incomplete virilization development of external genitalia:
   a. Small phallic development.
   b. Incomplete scrotal fusion.
3. Hyperpigmentation (due to MSH secretion).
4. Dehydration.
5. Vomiting/poor feeding.
6. Shock.
7. Latent signs—basal cortisol levels are normal because of compensated chronic ACTH stimulation:
   a. Weakness, fatigue.
   b. Anorexia, nausea, diarrhea.
   c. Weight loss (failure to thrive).

   d. Hyperpigmentation.

   e. Hypotension/postural dizziness.

   f. Rapid growth rate—adrenal androgen effect.

   g. Premature adrenarche—pubic hair, axillary hair, acne, body odor.

Diagnostic Evaluation

Neonates

1. Pelvic ultrasound for identification of uterus, ovaries, or testes to determine true sex (internal development of gender-specific organs depends on presence or absence of Y chromosomal activity; external genital development depends on the presence or absence of androgens).
2. Karyotyping.
3. Serum electrolytes—sodium depletion.
4. Serum glucose levels—hypoglycemia.
5. Serum 17-hydroxyprogesterone (most common precursor to 21-hydroxylase)—elevated.

Latent Diagnosis

1. Rapid growth velocity, premature adrenarche.
2. Advanced bone age x-ray for chronologic age.
3. Elevated serum 17-hydroxyprogesterone.
4. Elevated plasma renin activity—compensated prevention of salt loss.

Management

1. Glucocorticoid replacement—physiologic production of cortisol is 15 to 20 mg/m²/day. Doses are individually dependent. Replacement is with hydrocortisone twice or three times per day or prednisone once per day when final growth has been achieved.
2. Mineralocorticoid replacement—aldosterone is replaced with fludrocortisone tablets at 0.05 to 0.20 mg daily.
3. Added salt to the diet of neonates if salt loss is severe.
4. Surgical correction of ambiguous genitalia—can require multiple corrections over time.

 DRUG ALERT Overdosage of chronic corticosteroid use will result in growth failure. If child fails to grow and exhibits excessive hunger, corticosteroid dosing should be reviewed.

Complications

1. Aldosterone insufficiency:
   a. Hyponatremia, hyperkalemia.
   b. Hypotension.
   c. Shock.
   d. Hypertension in 11-β-hydroxylase insufficiency in which aldosterone precursor is potent mineralocorticoid.
2. Cortisol insufficiency—hypoglycemia.

Nursing Assessment

Neonates

 NURSING ALERT In male-appearing genitals, at least one testis must be palpated; if not, assumption must be that child is female with severe virilization. Notify health care provider so diagnostic evaluation can be initiated.

BOX 50-1	Manifestations of Hyponatremia and Hyperkalemia

HYPONATREMIA

- Caused by dilution of sodium (Na^+) when water intake exceeds output. Signs and symptoms occur when Na^+ level falls below 120 mEq/L.
- Gradual fall: anorexia, apathy, mild nausea, and vomiting
- Rapid fall: headache, mental confusion, muscular irritability, delirium, convulsions

HYPERKALEMIA

- Caused by a shift of potassium out of cells to compensate for decreased Na^+ caused by an oliguric state. Usually asymptomatic, except for electrocardiogram (ECG) changes.
- ECG characteristics: (progressive) shortened QT interval; tall, peaked T waves; ventricular arrhythmias; degeneration of QRS complex; ventricular asystole or fibrillation.

1. Assess genitalia for ambiguity.
2. Assess for signs of hypoglycemia, hyponatremia, and hyperkalemia (see Box 50-1).
3. Assess feeding pattern of the neonate.
4. Look for hyperpigmentation—may be subjective.

Latent Diagnosis of Child on Treatment

1. Assess growth and development.
2. Monitor vital signs; include sitting and recumbent BP for orthostatic changes.
3. Assess skin for hyperpigmentation.
4. Obtain history to include level of activity/fatigue, dietary history, salt craving, behavior, and school performance.

Nursing Diagnoses

- Fatigue related to hypoglycemia and electrolytic imbalances.
- Risk for Deficient Fluid Volume related to aldosterone deficiency.
- Deficient Knowledge related to risk of acute insufficiency.
- Anxiety of parents related to gender, sexual ambiguity, and chronic illness.

Nursing Interventions

Minimizing Fatigue

1. Administer glucocorticoids and emphasize compliance to increase energy level.
2. Encourage frequent rest periods and prevent overactivity.
3. Assess activity tolerance to determine adequacy of replacement therapy.
4. Tell the family that the child's activity level as well as growth rate should be normalized on therapy.
   a. If growth rate is too high, review corticosteroid dose and compliance with family.
   b. If growth rate is too low, overdosage of corticosteroid should be suspected.
   c. Review dosing with family.

Maintaining Fluid Balance

1. Assess fluid status and review history of fluid intake and output for appropriate volumes. Assess the hydration status of the child.

2. If the child is vomiting and unable to take oral fluids and mineralocorticoids, administer IV fluids. Start with 5% dextrose in normal saline and monitor serum sodium level.
3. Emphasize compliance with mineralocorticoid replacement.

 NURSING ALERT No less than 0.5% normal saline should be infused in the child who is aldosterone deficient, because of the inability to retain mineralocorticoid replacement.

Preventing Acute Adrenocortical Insufficiency

1. Identify times of stress, such as acute infections, surgical procedures, or extreme emotional stress, which require increased corticosteroid replacement.
2. Teach the parents how to use and give intramuscular (IM) injections of hydrocortisone for stress management, when oral supplementation is not possible because of vomiting.
3. Make sure that the child is evaluated by the primary care provider and treated for the cause of stress.

Reducing Anxiety

1. Encourage the parents to verbalize feelings regarding diagnosis, gender decisions or changes, and treatment plans.
2. Explain to the parents that the ambiguity is a result of the development process not being completed, rather than being a "mistake."

Family Education and Health Maintenance

1. Stress and reinforce the function of and need for constant replacement of adrenal steroid therapy to maintain normal daily activities.
2. Encourage the parents to obtain a MedicAlert bracelet, which indicates steroid dependency, for the child.
3. Facilitate instructions to the school nurse to notify the parents and health care provider of signs of illness and for emergency injection of hydrocortisone should it become necessary.
4. Explain to the parents and child why pubic hair may be developing and encourage discussion with teachers and school officials to prevent embarrassment of child in the locker room and other situations.

Evaluation: Expected Outcomes

- Parents report the child is more active.
- No signs of dehydration.
- Parents verbalize understanding when to call health care provider or when to use emergency hydrocortisone injection; parents also demonstrate correct technique for hydrocortisone injection.
- Parents verbalize understanding of disorder and need for reconstructive surgery.

DISORDERS OF GONADAL FUNCTION

Proper gonadal function is necessary for developing sexual maturation (puberty). The process involves the hypothalamic release of gonadotropin-releasing hormone (GnRH), which in turn stimulates the pituitary to release LH and FSH. In turn, these stimulate the gonads to produce and release the gonadal steroid testosterone from the testes in males or estrogen from the ovaries in females. The actions of these steroids lead to the development of secondary sexual characteristics and maturation.

Delayed Sexual Development

 EVIDENCE BASE Palmert, M., & Dunkel, L. (2012). Delayed puberty. *New England Journal of Medicine,* 355(5), 443–453.

Delayed sexual development is the lack of pubertal development or progression.

Pathophysiology and Etiology

1. Lack of production or secretion of gonadal steroids from the testes (testosterone) or ovaries (estrogen), due either to the lack of pituitary stimulation (secondary delayed sexual development) or to gonad dysfunction (primary delayed sexual development).
2. Primary delayed sexual development—absence or dysfunction of the gonads.
   a. 45 XO Turner syndrome (chromosomal variants).
   b. Sporadic gonadal dysgenesis.
   c. Bilateral gonadal failure due to radiation, chemotherapy, infection, defect in gonadal steroid synthesis, trauma.
3. Secondary delayed sexual development—lack of hypothalamic–pituitary stimulation to gonads.
   a. Hypothalamic lesions due to infections, trauma, irradiation, or isolated deficiency of GnRH (Kallmann syndrome).
   b. Pituitary lesions due to infection, trauma, or irradiation; also hypopituitarism or isolated LH and FSH deficiencies.
4. Failure of end organs to respond to circulating gonadal steroid—androgen insensitivity.
5. Other causes include chronic illness, anorexia nervosa, and autoimmune atrophy.
6. Resultant effect is failure to achieve sexual maturity.

Clinical Manifestations

1. Females—lack of breast development by age 13 years or failure to progress through puberty.
2. Males—lack of testicular enlargement by age 14 years or failure to progress through puberty.
3. Emotional lability.

Diagnostic Evaluation

1. Bone age x-ray to determine physical age—pubertal delay is not consistent with bone age.
2. Laboratory measurement of sex steroids (testosterone and estrogen) and gonadotropins (LH, FSH).
   a. Gonadal failure will show elevated LH and FSH with low estrogen.
   b. No good test is available to distinguish isolated gonadotropin deficiency (LH or FSH).
3. End organ insensitivity (lack of gonadal steroid receptor)—sex steroid and gonadotropins will be elevated. Hypothalamic receptors for feedback inhibition are the same as the end organ receptors; therefore, there is no hypothalamic "shutoff."
4. Abdominal ultrasound to view internal organ structure and development.

Management

1. Replacement of gonadal steroid—should be as close to the physiologic level as possible; however, maximal adult height may be compromised because of potential adverse effect of acceleration of skeletal maturation.
   a. Males—testosterone supplement; 50 to 100 mg monthly by injection until final height is achieved, then 200 mg monthly.
   b. Females—conjugated estrogen 0.3 to 0.625 mg daily by oral tablet. When appropriate, a progestational agent is added to the therapy for normal periods to occur. An alternative is the use of birth control pills that have the combination of estrogen and progesterone.
2. There is no pituitary or hypothalamic agent for use in secondary gonadal failure.

Complications

1. Sterility.
2. Ambiguity—in androgen insensitivity, male genital development does not respond to circulating level of testosterone from testes; may result in mistaken gender assignment.
3. Potential for dysfunctional dormant gonad to become malignant.

Nursing Assessment

1. Assess growth and development, particularly height.
2. Assess sexual development at regular intervals.

Nursing Diagnoses

1. Delayed Growth and Development related to lack of sexual development.
2. Disturbed Body Image related to delayed sexual maturation.
3. Chronic Low Self-Esteem related to delayed sexual maturation.

Nursing Interventions

Promoting Sexual Development

1. Administer or teach self-administration of medication, as prescribed.
2. Teach technique for IM injections of testosterone enanthate. Watch return demonstration.
3. Stress compliance with prescribed dose and not to exceed recommended dose. Excessive use of testosterone will stunt potential statural growth.

Improving Body Image

1. Discuss strategies for assisting the child to become more comfortable with appearance and ways that may minimize appearance of physical delay in sex characteristics.
2. Stress the importance of cautious therapy to prevent loss of potential height, therefore making sexual development a slow process.

Improving Self-Esteem

1. Encourage the child to discuss self-concept; list positive and negative characteristics.
2. Explore ways to strengthen and add to positive characteristics.
3. Encourage participation in age-appropriate activities and social functions.

Family Education and Health Maintenance

1. Teach the patient about adverse effects of testosterone replacement—possible behavioral changes (aggressiveness, moodiness) and an increase in acne.
   a. Suggest over-the-counter acne products or referral to dermatologist if indicated.
   b. Alert the family to report behavioral changes to the health care provider.
2. Teach the patient taking estrogen replacement the importance of daily compliance. Missed doses could result in breakthrough bleeding or spotting due to drop in circulatory estrogen levels. Alert patient to notify health care provider if spotting does occur with estrogen replacement.
3. In both treatments, stress to child not to exceed prescribed dose to prevent loss of final adult height.

Evaluation: Expected Outcomes

- At follow-up visit, there is an increase in height and progression of sexual development.
- Child verbalizes improved feelings of body image.
- Child lists more positive concepts of self.

Advanced Sexual Development and Precocious Puberty

Advanced sexual development is secondary sexual development earlier than the normal timing for a child's maturation. There is abnormal early production and secretion of the gonadal steroids or adrenal androgens. Normal pubertal development occurs abnormally early. Skeletal maturation is also advanced under presence of sex steroids and adrenal androgens.

Pathophysiology and Etiology

Central Precocious Puberty

1. Central precocious puberty (CPP)—early activation of the hypothalamic–pituitary gonadotropin axis.
2. May be idiopathic or caused by:
   a. Tumors of hypothalamus/pituitary.
   b. Cranial irradiation.
   c. Trauma.
   d. Infection—meningitis.
   e. Hydrocephalus.
3. Most common form of precocious puberty.

Peripheral Precocious Puberty

1. Peripheral precocious puberty (PPP)—sex hormone production at the glandular level independent of central stimulation.
2. Ovarian PPP caused by estrogen-producing tumors or cysts.
3. Testicular PPP caused by androgen- and estrogen-producing tumors or autonomous production of testosterone.
4. Adrenal PPP caused by enzyme defects (CAH) or androgen- and estrogen-producing tumors.

Other Causes

1. Hypothyroidism.
2. Exogenous estrogen or androgen exposure.

Clinical Manifestations

1. Males:
   a. Testicular enlargement (4 mL): younger than age 9½ years.
   b. Tanner stage II pubic hair: younger than age 9 years.
   c. Tanner stage III pubic hair: younger than age 10 years.
2. Females:
   a. Breast bud (stage II): younger than age 8 years.
   b. Tanner stage III pubic hair: younger than age 8½ years.
   c. Menarche: younger than age 9½ years.
3. In both sexes, rapid growth (increased growth velocity) evident.

Diagnostic Evaluation

1. Physical assessment—Tanner staging:
   a. If adrenarche is present without thelarche (breast development) or testicular enlargement, adrenal cause is likely.
   b. In females, if only thelarche is present, ovarian or exogenous estrogen involvement is likely.
   c. If adrenarche and pubarche (gonadal signs) are present, central cause is likely.
2. Skeletal x-ray for bone age—usually advanced. Pubertal stage development is usually commensurate with bone age maturation.
3. Laboratory analysis:
   a. Gonadal steroid levels—may be elevated; however, secretion is diurnal early in development.
   b. Elevated gonadotropins to GnRH stimulation if CPP. Basal levels are frequently unreliable. Lack of elevation of gonadotropins may indicate peripheral source.
   c. Thyroid function to rule out hypothyroidism.
4. MRI of head to rule out central etiology.
5. Ultrasound of abdomen, pelvis, testes for presence of cysts or tumors.

Management

For CPP, most common form of advanced sexual development in children.

1. Goal is to inhibit puberty to preserve psychosocial well-being and to delay epiphyseal closure to maximize adult height.
2. GnRH agonist—down-regulates GnRH receptors of the pituitary against endogenous GnRH.
   a. Nafarelin—intranasal spray, twice daily.
   b. Leuprolide—daily subcutaneous injection.
   c. Depot-leuprolide—monthly IM injection.
   d. Histrelin—subcutaneous daily injection.
3. Progestins.
   a. Medroxyprogesterone injections—biweekly IM injections.
   b. Medroxyprogesterone tablets—oral daily dosing.

 DRUG ALERT IM injections of leuprolide have, rarely, been linked to sterile abscesses. The site should not be reused, and the health care provider should be notified immediately if abscess occurs.

Complications

1. Complications of underlying tumor.
2. Behavioral problems.
3. Short stature for final height due to early epiphyseal closure.

Nursing Assessment

1. Assess sexual development using Tanner scale.
2. Obtain history of when signs and symptoms began with specific attention to chronology of events.
3. Perform psychosocial assessment relative to peer relations.
4. While the child is on treatment, perform ongoing assessment of height and sexual characteristics.

Nursing Diagnoses

- Disturbed Body Image related to early presence of secondary sexual characteristics.
- Deficient Knowledge regarding maturing body and sexuality.

- Disturbed Personal Identity due to societal height expectations versus appropriate age-related expectations.

Nursing Interventions

Fostering Positive Body Image

1. Encourage the child to verbalize concerns regarding body development changes.
2. Stress to child that the changes are normal events that peers will go through; however, they are occurring early.
3. Teach the child that therapy will halt the process and soon peers will catch up.

Teaching about the Effects of Treatment

1. Assist and encourage parents to teach the child about sexual development to reduce fear of the unknown.
2. Encourage proper hygiene practices for body odor, hair growth, and menses.
3. Teach administration techniques for medication treatment, including intranasal, IM, or subcutaneous administration, as indicated.
4. In GnRH-agonist treatment in females, instruct child and parents that it takes 10 to 12 days to fully down-regulate the pituitary receptors. The suppression results in a fall of estrogen and may cause breakthrough bleeding or even a period to occur. This will happen only once if child remains suppressed on therapy.

Promoting Sense of Identity

1. Encourage the child and parents to discuss normal age-related behaviors and identify inappropriate behaviors that are associated with society's expectations of advanced height and development.
2. Encourage the child to wear age-appropriate clothing, participate in age-appropriate activities, and socialize with peers.
3. Suggest counseling, as needed.

Family Education and Health Maintenance

1. Encourage follow-up at regular intervals while on treatment and, if condition is not treated, to monitor progress and address behavioral issues.
2. Discuss with parents that child may act out relative to advancing pubertal development. (This may include masturbation.) This behavior needs to be dealt in an understanding way, not necessarily through punishment.
3. Encourage parents to meet with school personnel regarding potential embarrassment in a locker room situation; alternatives to changing clothes in front of peers may be necessary.
4. Prepare family for the start of menstruation if puberty is advanced. The school nurse may need to assist with feminine hygiene during the cycle. Parents may need to meet with the nurse to plan for assistance during school days.
5. Teach family to inspect injection sites and notify health care provider immediately upon noticing a hard, painful, reddened area, which may be a sterile abscess from Lupron injections and require treatment.
6. Teach family to maintain strict adherence to hormonal therapy. Failure to maintain suppression of gonadotropins can result in relative rise in estrogen. Subsequent suppression may cause breakthrough bleeding.

Evaluation: Expected Outcomes

- Child accepts body changes through verbalization at follow-up visits.

- Parents or child give adequate return demonstration of IM injection; verbalizes understanding of sexual development.
- Child participates in school activities and socializes with peers of same age.

DISORDERS OF THE PANCREAS

The pancreas manufactures powerful enzymes for digestion as well as the hormones insulin and glucagon. These hormones are manufactured and secreted from cell clusters called the islets of Langerhans. Glucagon and insulin regulate the amount of sugar that is present in the bloodstream. Glucagon is a potent counter-regulatory hormone that raises the blood sugar by fostering the release of glucose from stores in the liver. Insulin stimulates glucose uptake by peripheral tissues, inhibits lipolysis, and inhibits hepatic glucose production.

Type 1 Diabetes Mellitus

 EVIDENCE BASE Hamilton, H., Knudsen, G., Vaina, C., et al. (2017). Children and young people with diabetes: Recognition and management. *British Journal of Nursing, 26*(6), 340–347.

Nierengarten, M. (2016). Pitfalls in pediatric type 1 diabetes management. *Contemporary Pediatrics, 33*(4), 16–20.

Diabetes mellitus (DM) is a disorder of glucose intolerance caused by deficiency in insulin production and action, resulting in hyperglycemia and abnormal carbohydrate, protein, and fat metabolism. In younger and school-age children, most cases are type 1, formerly called juvenile-onset or insulin-dependent DM. Type 1 DM affects as many as 1 in 500 children. As of 2014, there has been a 21% increase in type 1 diabetes when compared to 2007 rates. Females and males are equally impacted. The prevalence of type 1 diabetes varies with race and ethnicity. The incidence is highest in non-Hispanic white children.

Type 2 DM (formerly called adult-onset or noninsulin-dependent DM) traditionally was found in only about 2% of cases of diabetes in children and adolescents. This is rapidly changing, and type 2 diabetes now accounts for up to 40% of cases of diabetes diagnosed in adolescents. Etiology suggests morbid obesity, sedentary lifestyle, high caloric intake, and family history of diabetes. There is also an increased risk in black, Hispanic, and Native American populations. The onset of pubertal development and the insulin resistance that is characteristic of puberty may be a factor in the onset of type 2 diabetes in susceptible adolescents. Type 2 DM is discussed in Chapter 25.

Pathophysiology and Etiology

1. Etiology for type 1 DM suggests genetic and environmental or acquired factors, association with certain human leukocyte antigen types, and abnormal immune responses, including autoimmune reactions.
2. Autoimmune destruction of the islets of Langerhans in the pancreas that secrete insulin, resulting in insulin deficiency.
3. Because insulin facilitates glucose transport into cells, glucose builds up in the bloodstream, causing hyperglycemia.
4. As the kidneys attempt to lower blood glucose levels, glycosuria and polyuria result, with electrolyte excretion.
5. Because the body cells are unable to use glucose for energy, protein and fat are broken down.
6. Fat metabolism results in a buildup of ketones and acidosis.

7. Diabetic ketoacidosis (DKA) occurs in 20% to 40% of patients at the time of diagnosis. Also, DKA at diagnosis is more common in children under 5 years of age and in children who have limited or no access to medical care. It is a potentially fatal condition characterized by hyperglycemia, ketonemia, ketonuria, and metabolic acidosis (pH less than 7.3, bicarbonate less than 15 mEq/L) and caused by insulin deficiency. In children with established T1DM, there is an increased incidence of DKA in those individuals with poor metabolic control, children who omit insulin doses or when caregivers omit doses of their child's insulin, children with psychiatric or eating disorders, peripubertal or adolescent girls, and interruption or failure of insulin pump therapy.

Clinical Manifestations

Onset is rapid (usually over a period of a few weeks).

Major Symptoms
1. Increased thirst.
2. Increased urination, enuresis.
3. Increased food ingestion.
4. Weight loss.
5. Fatigue.

Minor Symptoms
1. Skin infections.
2. Dry skin, poor wound healing.
3. Monilial vaginitis in adolescent females.

Diabetic Ketoacidosis
1. Hyperglycemia, polyuria, and polydipsia.
2. Dehydration, decreased skin turgor.
3. Nausea, vomiting, generalized malaise, weakness.
4. Kussmaul respirations (rapid, deep, sighing), fruity or acetone breath odor, altered level of consciousness (LOC), confusion.

Diagnostic Evaluation

1. Criteria for diagnosis of type 1 and type 2 DM are the same: fasting blood glucose of more than 126 mg/dL on two occasions (different day); random blood glucose of more than 200 in the presence of symptoms (polydipsia, polyphagia, polyuria); glucose greater than 200 following 2 hour oral glucose tolerance test; random hemoglobin A1C ≥ 6.5% (less sensitive and has not been validated in children).
2. Glycosuria or ketonuria on routine examination may arouse suspicion of diabetes.
3. Evaluation for metabolic acidosis with acute presentation (pH less than 7.3 and bicarbonate less than 14 mEq/L).
4. Hemoglobin A1c testing every 3 months to determine long-term plasma glucose control is dependent on age. Children, especially young children, are at high risk for hypoglycemia and are at low risk for complications prior to puberty. Goals are age dependent.
   a. Toddlers, children less than 6 years: less than 8.5% (less than 8% if hypoglycemia is avoided).
   b. Children ages 6 to 12 years: less than 8%.
   c. Adolescents ages 13 to 19 years: less than 7.5%. (A lower goal may be reasonable if excessive hypoglycemia does not result.)
5. Screening for celiac disease should be done at the time of diagnosis and if disease is detected, child should be referred to a pediatric gastroenterologist. A gluten-free diet is recommended for children with celiac disease.
6. Thyroid function is also recommended at the time of diagnosis.

EVIDENCE BASE Chan, C., McFann, K., Newnes, L., et al. (2014). Hemoglobin A1c assay variations and implications for diabetes screening in obese youth. *Pediatric Diabetes, 15*(8), 557–563.

Management

1. Insulin therapy (see Table 50-2).
   a. New insulin analogs provide more options for insulin duration and frequency of administration. Basal insulins, such as glargine and detemir, provide a duration of up to 24 hours without a pronounced peak of action. Rapid-acting insulins, such as lispro, glulisine, and aspart, offer rapid onset with shorter duration.
   b. Dosage needs are based on the child's weight, diet, and level of activity. Dosages are adjusted through daily monitoring of blood glucose levels.
   c. Insulin pump therapy, consisting of a continuous subcutaneous infusion of insulin that can be programmed to give bolus and basal rates, may be used by some children.
2. Treatment of DKA (see Box 50-2).
   a. IV fluid therapy to increase perfusion and glucose uptake in the periphery, which will reduce hyperglycemia; also increases glomerular filtration and reverses acidosis.
   b. Regular IV insulin administration at a rate of 0.1 U/kg/hour after initial fluid replacement. Provide IV dextrose solution as plasma glucose decreases, titrate rate of insulin infusion to achieve a rate of glucose decline of 50 to 150 mg/dL per hour.
   c. Bicarbonate is not indicated; acidosis will correct with adequate insulin infusion.
   d. Close monitoring of vital signs, electrocardiogram, mental status, and neurologic system.
   e. Replacement of electrolytes—sodium, potassium, ionized calcium.
3. Balanced diet with controlled carbohydrates and adequate protein and fat to meet energy and growth requirements.

EVIDENCE BASE Brink, S. (2014). Paediatric and adolescent diabetic ketoacidosis. *Practical Diabetes, 31*(8), 342–347.

Table 50-2	Types of Insulin and Their Effects		
TYPE OF INSULIN	**ONSET (MINUTES)**	**MAXIMAL ACTIVITY (HOURS)**	**DURATION (HOURS)**
Aspart	10–20	1–3	3–5
Glulisine	2–5	1	2
Lispro	<15	0.5–1.5	6–8
Regular	30–60	2–4	6–8
Semilente	30–60	2–4	10–12
NPH	120	4–12	24
Lente	120	8–10	24
Ultralente	4–8 hours	14–20	36
Detemir	Slow	3–6	6–11
Glargine	≥60	N/A	≥24

N/A, not applicable.

Complications

Acute

1. Usually reversible.
2. DKA accounting for 70% of diabetes-related deaths in children younger than age 10 years.
3. Cerebral edema—related to treatment of DKA; thought to be due to a rapid decline in blood glucose causing a fluid shift in the brain.
4. Hyperglycemia (untreated or undertreated).
5. Hypoglycemia (insulin reaction).

Subacute

Develops over a short period.

1. Lipohypertrophy (localized tissue buildup from giving injections in the same site)—repeated injections in the same area; can cause abnormal absorption.
2. Skeletal and joint abnormalities—limited joint mobility.
3. Growth failure and delayed sexual maturation due to underinsulinization.

Chronic

Very rarely seen in children, but develop after years to decades with inadequate treatment.

1. Retinopathy/cataracts—may cause blindness.
2. Neuropathy—peripheral and autonomic.
3. Nephropathy—proteinuria/renal failure.
4. Cardiopathy—heart failure.

Nursing Assessment

1. When the child first presents with suspected DM:
   a. Obtain history of onset of signs and symptoms of clinical manifestations.
   b. Assess for levels of dehydration and weight loss with level of appetite.
   c. Check for sores that are slow to heal.
   d. Identify any fruity smell to breath—acetone breath due to ketosis.
   e. Assess abdominal pain—may mimic appendicitis.
2. For child with DKA:
   a. Assess for potential cerebral edema (diminished LOC) on presentation and when fluid replacement is initiated. Fluid replacements precede and are then concurrent with insulin therapy.
   b. Assess cardiac function—tachycardia with dehydration, arrhythmias related to potassium imbalances.
   c. Assess renal function—urine output with intake and output, ketonuria, glycosuria.
   d. Watch for hypoglycemia—overtreatment of insulin; glucose level correction should be slow. IV replacements frequently contain glucose to prevent large osmotic fluid shifts leading to cerebral edema.
3. During treatment/routine follow-up:
   a. Assess growth parameters—excessive weight gain may indicate overtreatment of insulin (child eats because of constant hunger). Loss or lack of weight gain may indicate underinsulinization (losing calories that are not metabolized).
   b. Review blood glucose diaries and glucose monitor for level of control and need for insulin adjustments. (Check for appropriate adjustments of insulin made by parents.) Glucose should be checked before meals (preprandial) and at bedtime. Optimal levels are age related.

BOX 50-2 Treatment of Diabetic Ketoacidosis

INITIATE INTRAVENOUS FLUIDS

- Start with 0.9% normal saline (NS) solution.
- Estimate fluid deficit by amount of weight loss (2.2 lb [1 kg] equals 1 L of fluid). Infuse fluids to replace one half of estimated loss plus maintenance needs (10 to 20 mL/kg) over first 8 to 12 hours; second half plus maintenance needs over next 16 to 36 hours.
- When blood glucose falls below 250 mg/dL, change to 5% glucose in 0.45% NS solution.
- Closely monitor vital signs, electrocardiogram (ECG), and intake and output, and obtain laboratory values, including urine and blood glucose, electrolytes, blood urea nitrogen and creatinine, serum osmolarity, arterial or venous pH, serum and urine ketones, calcium, and phosphorus every 1 to 4 hours as condition warrants.

NURSING ALERT Avoid infusion of hypertonic solutions because ketoacidosis is accompanied by a profound free water deficit. Replace fluids slowly to prevent rapid decline in serum osmolarity, which may precipitate cerebral edema.

ADMINISTER INSULIN

- Give IV bolus of 0.1 unit/kg of regular insulin if no intermediate-acting insulin has been given in the past 6 to 8 hours.
- Provide continuous IV drip of regular insulin at rate of 0.1 unit/kg/hour.
- Continue IV insulin until metabolic acidosis is corrected (pH greater than 7.3 and bicarbonate greater than 13 to 15) and bowel sounds have returned and oral fluids can be taken.
- When meals are tolerated, begin subcutaneous short-acting or rapid-acting insulin at least 30 minutes before discontinuing IV insulin.
- When stabilized, return to previous insulin regimen or begin therapy using conventional dosing (intermediate-acting insulin with short-acting insulin) or basal-bolus therapy (basal insulin with rapid-acting insulin)

NURSING ALERT Flush IV tubing with insulin solution before infusion and change tubing with each bag because insulin will bind to the plastic tubing, changing concentration.

POTASSIUM AND BICARBONATE REPLACEMENT

- Initial serum K levels will be normal or high even though intracellular levels are low. Serum levels will fall as insulin therapy drives K into the cells.
- Begin replacement of K when urine output and renal function have been established.
- Add KCl 20 to 40 mEq to each liter of fluid.
- Monitor T waves on ECG for peaking (hyperkalemia) or flattening (hypokalemia).
- Bicarbonate administration is controversial in correcting acidosis but may be indicated for respiratory depression, decreased myocardial contractility, or refractory, severe acidosis.

---

    i. Toddlers and children under age 6: 100 to 180 mg/dL preprandial; 110 to 200 mg/dL at bedtime.
    ii. Children ages 6 to 12: 90 to 180 mg/dL preprandial; 100 to 180 mg/dL at bedtime.
    iii. Adolescents ages 13 to 19: 90 to 130 mg/dL preprandial; 90 to 150 mg/dL at bedtime.
  c. Obtain history of any hypoglycemic reactions—be specific to time of day, dietary record, and exercise and activity.
  d. Assess injection sites—look for signs of lipohypertrophy.
  e. Assess for signs of hyperglycemia—polyuria, polydipsia. Does the child need to get up during the night to go to the bathroom?

Nursing Diagnoses

- Deficient Fluid Volume related to osmotic diuresis and vomiting.
- Imbalanced Nutrition: Less Than Body Requirements due to metabolic catabolism due to lack of insulin.
- Deficient Knowledge related to insulin management.
- Deficient Knowledge related to blood glucose monitoring.
- Risk for Unstable Blood Glucose.
- Fear/Anxiety of child and family related to diagnosis, treatment, and management procedures.

Nursing Interventions

Restoring Fluid Balance

1. Administer IV fluids, as ordered.
2. Monitor intake and output, BP, serum electrolyte results, and daily weight.
3. Report abnormal sodium and potassium results promptly.
4. Assess for signs of dehydration—dry skin and mucous membranes, constipation.
5. Encourage oral fluids when able.

Meeting Nutritional Requirements

1. Provide an adequate diet for the child and teach the family about the diet.
  a. The most common meal plan is one based on carbohydrate counting. This type of meal plan offers flexibility and a wide variety of choices. Total carbohydrate requirements will be calculated, then labels can be read and charts consulted to determine grams of carbohydrate per serving of food eaten. Insulin dosage is based on the total amount of carbohydrates eaten; for example, 1 unit of short-or rapid-acting insulin for every 15 g of carbohydrate.
  b. Occasionally, a more rigid, strictly controlled diet is necessary.
  c. The diet should be composed of approximately 55% carbohydrate, 30% fat, and 15% protein.

i. Some diets are restricted in carbohydrates, saturated fats, and cholesterol and may be based on the exchange method as recommended by the American Diabetes Association.

ii. Approximately 70% of the carbohydrate content should be derived from complex carbohydrates such as starch.

iii. Foods with high fiber content should be encouraged.

iv. All diets must supply sufficient caloric intake for activity and growth, sufficient protein for growth, and the required vitamins and minerals.

d. Foods are distributed throughout the day to accommodate varying peak action of insulin. Distribution may be adjusted for increased or decreased amounts of exercise.

e. Include fluids containing sugar (sodas, juices, milk) in carbohydrate count.

f. Determine the child's usual dietary habits so that adherence to the controlled diet will be easier.

g. Include the child and parents in meal planning as soon as possible.

h. Allow the child normal activity while hospitalized so that the observed result of the dietary control will be valid. Because the child's activity level usually decreases during the hospital stay, the child and family must understand that the insulin and dietary needs will alter on discharge.

i. Allow the child to eat with other children.

j. Make certain that the child adheres to the prescribed diet and understands the rationale for it.

k. Refer family to a dietitian for additional planning and education.

Increasing Knowledge About Insulin Administration

1. Insulin should be given, as directed. Rapid-acting insulin analogues lispro and aspart begin to work immediately and should be given right before the meal. If taking regular insulin, the child should not eat until 20 to 30 minutes after injection is given.

2. Be aware of the major types of insulin and their effects.

3. Develop a systematic plan for injections that emphasizes rotation of sites (Figure 50-3).

a. The upper arms and thighs are the most acceptable sites for injection in children, but the outer areas of the abdomen or hips may also be used.

b. Subsequent injections are given about 1 inch (2.5 cm) apart.

c. Guidelines for site location:

i. Arms—begin below the deltoid muscle and end one handbreadth above the elbow. Begin at the midline and progress outward laterally, using the external surface only.

ii. Thighs (see Figure 50-4, page 1350)—begin one handbreadth below the hip and end one handbreadth above the knee. Begin at the midline and progress outward laterally, using only the outer, anterior surface.

iii. Abdomen—avoid the beltline and 1 inch (2.5 cm) around the umbilicus.

iv. Buttocks—use the upper outer quadrant of the buttocks.

4. Be certain that the measuring scale of the syringe matches the unit strength on the bottle of insulin. U-100 insulin is preferred because it allows the smallest possible amount to be given. Other concentrations of insulin are rarely used.

5. Opened bottles of insulin may be stored at room temperature or in the refrigerator. Open bottles should be discarded after 28 days. Use insulin that is at room temperature.

a. The bottle in use may be kept at room temperature for approximately 1 month without losing appreciable strength.

b. Extra bottles should be stored in the refrigerator.

6. Insulin pens (either prefilled or using insulin cartridges) are increasing in popularity. Pens are generally kept at room temperature once opened and discarded after 28 days; check the manufacturer's directions. All insulin pens require an "air shot" (clearing air from pen) prior to giving *each* dose.

7. Mix insulin solutions, such as NPH and Ultralente, thoroughly by shaking the bottle (rolling may not be effective).

8. Administer insulin subcutaneously. Do not aspirate.

9. Observe the skin closely for signs of irritation. Avoid the injection site for several weeks if signs of local irritation are observed.

10. Observe the skin for a rash indicating an allergic reaction to the insulin (rare with newer preparations). Notify the health care provider immediately if there is an allergic reaction.

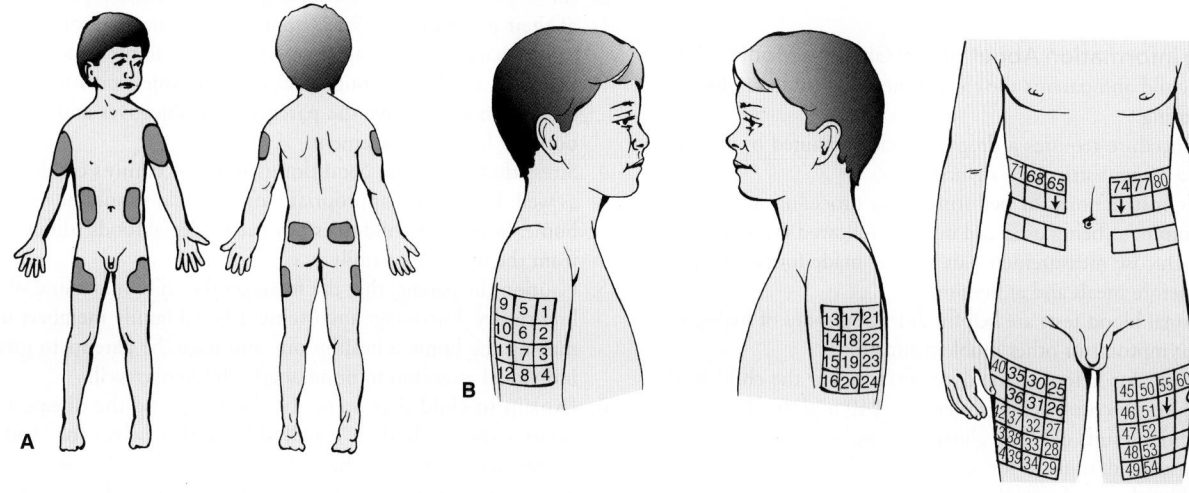

Figure 50-3. (A) Insulin injection sites are the upper outer portions of the arms, the thighs, and the abdominal area. **(B)** Injection sites are rotated, with subsequent injections given about 1 inch (2.5 cm) apart.

Figure 50-4. Insulin injection by a child.

11. Be aware of factors that vary the need for and utilization of insulin, particularly exercise and infection.
    a. Exercise tends to lower the blood sugar level. Encourage normal activity, regulated in amount and time.
    b. Infection or illness increases the child's insulin requirement (insulin is still administered during illness). Be alert for signs of infection and dehydration.
12. Encourage the child to express feelings about the injections. The child may be helped to master fear of injections by gaining control of the situation through play and active participation in the procedure.

 DRUG ALERT None of the basal insulins (detemir, glargine, or glusiline) have been approved by the Food and Drug Administration for mixing with any other insulin.

Providing Information About Blood Glucose Monitoring

1. Teach child and parents the chosen method for blood glucose monitoring.
2. The procedure requires a drop of blood (obtained by fingerstick), a reagent strip, and a glucometer.
3. Specific instructions for performing the procedure vary with the equipment being used and must be followed explicitly.
4. Blood glucose measurements are usually made four times per day—before meals and at bedtime.
5. Additional blood tests are helpful during episodes of hypoglycemic symptoms or other problem situations.
6. Urine tests for ketones should be performed if the child is ill or if blood glucose level is greater than 240 mg/100 dL.
7. Record the results of blood glucose testing accurately.
    a. Use a standard form for recording so that the information will be clear and readily available.
    b. Help the child to understand how the disease is controlled by teaching the child to test his or her own blood, record

results, and report information to health care personnel or parents.

Identifying and Controlling Hypoglycemia

1. Have glucagon available for injection if a hypoglycemic reaction occurs and the child is unconscious, has a seizure or is unable to swallow liquids safely, or is combative. Administer 0.5 to 1 mg IM or subcutaneously and assess response.
2. Teach family the causes, signs and symptoms, and treatment for hypoglycemia.
    a. Common causes:
        i. Overdose of insulin.
        ii. Reduction in diet or increased exercise without sufficient caloric coverage.
    b. Symptoms:
        i. Trembling, shaking, dizziness.
        ii. Sweating, apprehension.
        iii. Tachycardia.
        iv. Hunger, weakness.
        v. Drowsiness, unusual behavior.
        vi. Mental confusion.
        vii. Seizures, coma.
    c. Be prepared to give glucose tablets, orange juice, sugar cubes, or another food containing readily available simple sugars.
3. Watch for a pattern of activity or time of day that precedes hypoglycemic reactions and work with family to alter behavior to prevent reactions.
4. If prescribed, teach the child and family how to use an emergency glucagon injection kit.
5. If glucagon is not available and the child is unresponsive, activate the emergency response system (911).

Reducing Fear and Anxiety

1. Explain the need and purpose of every test to child and parents. Allow child to vent feelings and cry if fearful. When appropriate, demonstrate procedures on yourself first (eg, fingersticks for glucose testing, allowing parent to give saline injection for practice of insulin injection).
2. Teach family the pathophysiology of diabetes. Understanding the disease process aids in understanding the treatment and signs and symptoms. Assess knowledge level of teaching by having family verbalize knowledge of disease management.
3. Allow parents to verbalize feelings related to the expectations of their performance. Stress that the learning is through the actual "hands-on" management. Assist the parents in performing the needed tasks (fingersticks, insulin injections) to build their confidence. Give the parents clear objectives and directions for home management.
4. Stress that the child's condition is now the family's condition as well. Only foods appropriate for the child should be in the home. Stress that child does not need "special foods" different from the rest of the family.
5. Caution the parents that the focus on the child may cause sibling rivalry. Encourage involvement by all family members in making the home a healthy one and urge the parents to give individual attention to nondiabetic children as well.
6. Explain to child that he or she did not cause the disease to occur—young children usually blame themselves for "bad" things that happen to them. Help the child understand that good management is the key to participating in all usual activities. The perspective should be that he or she is a "child with diabetes," not a "diabetic child."

Community and Home Care Considerations

1. Perform home assessment for adequate nutritional resources.
2. Reteach and assess family's adherence to insulin administration and blood glucose monitoring.
3. Reteach and assess family's ability to respond to hypoglycemia.
4. Make sure that school is able to follow through with management plan for insulin administration, planned exercise and mealtimes, and responding to hypoglycemia.
5. When child is ill, evaluate for dehydration, hyperglycemia, and ketonuria. Teach family how to monitor condition, maintain insulin coverage, and notify the health care provider. (See "Diabetes sick-day guidelines," page 748.)

Family Education and Health Maintenance

Patient or parental education is one of the most important aspects in the nursing care of the child with diabetes. Thorough instruction is essential in the following areas:

1. Influence of exercise, emotional stress, and other illnesses on insulin and diet needs.
2. Recognition of the symptoms of insulin shock and diabetic acidosis and knowledge of related emergency management.
3. Prevention of infection:
   a. Attend to regular body hygiene, with special attention to foot care.
   b. Report any breaks in the skin. Treat them promptly.
   c. Use only properly fitted shoes; do not wear vinyl or plastic, which do not permit ventilation. Avoid calluses and blisters. Teach child not to walk barefoot.
   d. Dress the child appropriately for the weather.
   e. See that the child receives regular dental checkups and maintenance every 6 months.
   f. Follow routine immunizations according to the recommended schedule; receive yearly flu vaccination.
4. Precautionary measures:
   a. Have the child carry an identifying card that states that he or she has diabetes and includes name, address, telephone number, and health care provider's name and telephone number.
   b. Suggest a simple, convenient source of sugar that can be carried easily by the child or parents in a pocket, purse, or backpack to have available for hypoglycemic symptoms. A good example is glucose tablets, glucose gel, five sugar cubes, or cake decorating gel that comes in a tube.
   c. Help the family discuss the child's disease with the school nurse and other responsible adults who are in close contact with the child (eg, teachers, scout leaders).
   d. Advise parents that vials of insulin should be kept on one's person when traveling because baggage may be subjected to extreme temperatures and pressures incompatible with the stability of insulin. If necessary, a thermos can be used to keep the insulin at the appropriate temperature.
5. Follow up with the primary care provider or pediatrician for immunizations, all regular health checkups, and growth and development evaluations.
6. For additional information and support, refer to agencies, such as American Diabetes Association, ATTN: National Call Center, 2451 Crystal Drive, Suite 900 Arlington, VA 22202, 1-800-DIABETES (800-342-2383), www.diabetes.org; and Juvenile Diabetes Research Foundation International, 26 Broadway, 14th floor, New York, NY 10004; 800-JDF-CURE (212-785-9595), www.jdrf.org.

Evaluation: Expected Outcomes

- No signs of dehydration.
- Parents and child describe consistent meal plan.
- Child and parents demonstrate correct insulin administration technique.
- Child and parents demonstrate correct glucose monitoring technique.
- Child and parents verbalize causes, signs and symptoms, and treatment for hypoglycemia.
- Child and parents speak openly about diabetes, ask appropriate questions, display no crying.

 TRANSITIONAL CARE ALERT After the stress of having a hospitalized child, families will need support in the transition to home or another aftercare location. It is crucial that they have complete and understandable care instructions on home care, and medications and follow up appointments. If arrangements have been made for nursing care in the home, families should be aware of the agency providing services and when they can expect communication regarding care arrangements. Families should have thorough written (and if necessary to assist understanding, pictorial) instructions on signs and symptoms to monitor for worsening of status. Children with metabolic and endocrine disorders require careful monitoring with frequent laboratory assessments. Family caregivers may need additional instructions and monitoring equipment to continue optimal care in the home setting.

Management of metabolic and endocrine disorders may likely require modifications to daily routine in school and the work place (for older teens and young adults). Nurses should be aware of state and federal guidelines for IEP and 504 documentation for accommodation of the needs to maintain the best outcomes of these conditions.

SELECTED REFERENCES

Acerini, C., Albanese, F., Casey, A., et al. (2012). Initiating growth hormone therapy for children and adolescents. *British Journal of Nursing*, 21(18), 1091–1097.

Adis Medical Writers. (2018). Diagnose and treat paediatric hypothyroidism promptly to achieve optimal growth and developmental outcomes. *Drugs & Therapy Perspectives, 34*(3), 116–120.

Alois, C., & Rizzolo, D. (2017). Diabetic ketoacidosis: Heralding type 1 diabetes in children. *Journal of the American Academy of Physician Assistants*, 30(7), 20–23.

Alvar, C., Coddington, J., Foli, K., et al. (2017). Depression in the School-Aged Child with Type 1 Diabetes: Implications for Pediatric Primary Care Providers. *Journal of Pediatric Health Care*, 32(1), 43–52.

Amedro, P., Tahhan, N., Bertet, H., et al. (2017). Health-related quality of life among children with Turner syndrome: Controlled cross-sectional study. *Journal of Pediatric Endocrinology and Metabolism*, 30(8), 863–868.

American Association of Diabetes Educators. (2016). *Management of children with diabetes in the school setting.* AADE Position Statement. Available: *https://www.diabeteseducator.org/docs/default-source/practice/practice-resources/position-statements/diabetes-in-the-school-setting-position-statement_final.pdf*

Barry, S., Teplitsky, L., Wagner, D., et al. (2017). Partnering with Insurers in Caring for the Most Vulnerable Youth with Diabetes: NICH as an Integrator. *Current Diabetes Report*, 17(4), 26.

Brink, S. (2014). Paediatric and adolescent diabetic ketoacidosis. *Practical Diabetes*, 31(8), 342–347.

Chan, C., McFann, K., Newnes, L., et al. (2014). Hemoglobin A1c assay variations and implications for diabetes screening in obese youth. *Pediatric Diabetes*, 15(8), 557–563.

Collin, J., Whitehead, A., & Walker, J. (2016). Educating children and families about growth hormone deficiency and its management: Part 1. *Nursing Children and Young People*, 28(1), 32–37.

Collin, J., Whitehead, A., & Walker, J. (2016). Educating children and families about growth hormone deficiency and its management: Part 2. *Nursing Children and Young People*, 28(2), 30–36.

Copeland, K., Silverstein, J., Moore, K., et al. (2013). Clinical practice guideline: Management of newly diagnosed type 2 diabetes mellitus (T2DM) in children and adolescents. *Pediatrics*, 131(2), 364–382. Available: *http://pediatrics.aappublications.org/content/early/2013/01/23/peds.2012-3493*

Cremonesini, L. (2017). Type 2 diabetes in children and its association with obesity. *Independent Nurse*, 7, 17–20.

D'Adamo, E., & Caprio, S. (2011). Type 2 diabetes in youth: Epidemiology and pathophysiology. *Diabetes Care*, 34(Suppl. 2), S161–S165.

Davies, K. (2015). Understanding clinical investigations in children's endocrinology. *Nursing Children and Young People*, 27(8), 26–36.

Di Iorgi, N., Allegri, A., Napoli, F., et al. (2014). Central diabetes insipidus in children and young adults: Etiological diagnosis and long-term outcome of idiopathic cases. *Journal of Clinical Endocrinology and Metabolism*, 99(4), 1264–1272.

Erlichman, I., Mimouni, F., Erlichman, M., et al. (2016). Thyroxine-Based Screening for congenital Hypothyroidism in Neonates with Down Syndrome. *Journal of Pediatrics*, 173, 165–168.

Fuhrman, B., & Zimmerman, J. (2016). *Pediatric critical care* (5th ed.). Philadelphia, PA: Elsevier.

Garvey, K., Wolpert, H., Rhodes, E., et al. (2012). Health care transition with patients with type 1 diabetes: Young adult experiences and relationship to glycemic control. *Diabetes Care*, 35(8), 1716–1722.

Gravholt, C., Andersen, N., Conway, G., et al. (2017). Clinical practice guidelines for the care of girls and women with Turner syndrome: Proceedings from the 2016 Cincinnati International Turner Syndrome Meeting. *European Journal of Endocrinology*, 177(3), G1–G70.

Hamilton, H., Knudsen, G., Vaina, C., et al. (2017). Children and young people with diabetes: Recognition and management. *British Journal of Nursing*, 26(6), 340–347.

Hilton, L. (2017). HbA1C predictive of pediatric diabetes. *Contemporary Pediatrics*, 34(2), 30–32.

Hunter, F., & Calikoglu, A. (2016). Etiological and clinical characteristics of central diabetes insipidus in children: a single center experience. *International Journal of Pediatric Endocrinology*, 2/11/2016, 1–5.

Ilkowitz, J., Choi, S., Rinke, M., et al. (2016). Pediatric Type 1 Diabetes: Reducing Admission Rates for Diabetes Ketoacidosis. *Quality Management in Health Care*, 25(4), 231–237.

Jacob, H., & Peters, C. (2015). Screening, diagnosis and management of congenital hypothyroidism: European Society for Paediatric Endocrinology Consensus Guideline. *Archives of Disease in Childhood*, 100(5), 260–263.

Kearsey, I., Hutson, J., & Hutson, J. M.. (2017). Disorders of sex development (DSD): Not only babies with ambiguous genitalia: A practical guide for surgeons. *Pediatric Surgery International*, 33(3), 355–361.

Kirk, J. (2012). Indications for growth hormone therapy in children. *Archives of Disease in Childhood*, 97(1), 63–68.

Le Gresley, H., Palmer, S., & Paul, S. (2016). Diagnostic dilemma. *Emergency Nurse*, 24(8), 14.

Marathe, P., Gao, H., & Close, K. (2017). American Diabetes Association of Medical Care in Diabetes 2017. *Journal of Diabetes*, 9(4), 320–324.

Moloney, S., Murphy, N., & Collin, J. (2015). An overview of the nursing issues involved in caring for a child with adrenal insufficiency. *Nursing Children and Young People*, 27(7), 28–36.

Morris, A. (2017). Genetics: New insights into Turner syndrome. *Nature Review Endocrinology*, 13(8), 439.

Nierengarten, M. (2016). Hypothyroidism in children. *Contemporary Pediatrics*, 33(5), 29–33.

Nierengarten, M. (2016). Pitfalls in pediatric type 1 diabetes management. *Contemporary Pediatrics*, 33(4), 16–20.

Palmert, M., & Dunkel, L. (2012). Delayed puberty. *New England Journal of Medicine*, 355(5), 443–453

Pierce, J., Kozikowski, C., Lee, J., et al. (2017). Type 1 diabetes in very young children: A model of parent and child influences on management and outcomes. *Pediatric Diabetes*, 18(1), 17-25.

Rechenberg, K., Whittemore, R., Grey, M., et al. (2016). Contribution of income to self-management and health outcomes in pediatric type 1 diabetes. *Pediatric Diabetes*, 17(2), 120–126.

Rechenberg, K., Whittenmore, R., & Grey, M. (2017). Anxiety in youth with type 1 diabetes. *Journal of Pediatric Nursing*, 32, 64–71.

Rose, S., Cook, D., & Fine, M. (2014). Growth hormone therapy guidelines: Clinical and managed care perspectives. *American Journal of Pharmacological Benefits*, 6(5), e134–e146.

Rothkopf, A., & John, R. (2014). Understanding disorders of sexual development. *Journal of Pediatric Nursing*, 29(5), 23–24.

Silva, N., Bullinger, M., Sommer, R., et al. (2018). Children's psychosocial functioning and parents' quality of life in paediatric short stature: The mediating role of caregiving stress. *Clinical Psychology & Psychotherapy*, 25(1), e017–e118.

Skinner, T., Lange, K., Hoey, H., et al. (2018). Targets and teamwork: Understanding difference in pediatric diabetes centers treatment outcomes. *Pediatric Diabetes*, 19(3), 559–565.

Sy, V. (2016). Empowering staff nurses as primary educators to children with type 1 diabetes. *Pediatric Nursing*, 42(5), 247–251.

Tishelman, A., Shumer, D., & Nahata, L. (2017). Disorders of Sex Development: Pediatric Psychology and the Genital Exam. *Journal of Pediatric Psychology*, 42(5), 530–543.

U.S. Preventive Services Task Force. (2008). *Screening for congenital hypothyroidism in newborns: Clinical summary of U.S. Preventive Services Task Force recommendation* (AHRQ Publication No. 08-05109-EF-3). Rockville, MD: Agency for Healthcare Research and Quality. Available: *www.ahrq.gov/clinic/uspstf08/conhyposum.htm*

Villamor, E., & Jansen, E. (2016). Nutritional Determinants of the Timing of Puberty. *Annual Review of Public Health*, 37, 33–46.

Waddell, J. (2017). An update on type 2 diabetes management in primary care. *Nurse Practitioner*, 42(8), 20–29.

Williams, J., Paul, D., & Bisset, G. (2013). Thyroid disease in children: Part 1: State-of-the-art imaging in pediatric hypothyroidism. *Pediatric Radiology*, 43(10) 1244–1253

51

Pediatric Oncology

PEDIATRIC ONCOLOGIC DISORDERS

EVIDENCE BASE American Cancer Society. (2018). Cancer facts and figures. Atlanta, GA. Available: https://www.cancer.org/content/dam/cancer-org/research/cancer-facts-and-statistics/annual-cancer-facts-and-figures/2018/cancer-facts-and-figures-2018.pdf.

Cancer is the leading cause of death from disease in children ages 1 to 14. Cancer incidence in the United States has slowly increased by 0.6% per year since 1975 among children ages 1 to 14 with an estimated 10,270 new cases predicted in 2017. In contrast, childhood cancer deaths have continued to decline by more than two thirds from 1969 (6.5 per 100,000) to 2014 (2.0 per 100,000) annually in the United States. Approximately 1,190 will die from the disease in 2017. There are few known risk factors for childhood cancer; however, the incidence of specific cancers is related to age, gender, ethnic background, and geographical region.

Common types of cancer in children (in order of frequency) include leukemia (29%), brain and central nervous system (CNS) cancers (26%), neuroblastoma (6%), Wilms tumor (5%), lymphoma (8%), rhabdomyosarcoma (3%), osteosarcoma (2%), retinoblastoma (2%), and bone cancer (1%). Childhood cancers are treated with surgery, radiation and chemotherapy, blood and marrow transplant, immunotherapy, and gene therapy.

Cancers in adolescents (15 to 19 years) differ somewhat from those in children in terms of type and distribution. For example, brain and other nervous system tumors (21%) and lymphoma (20%) are equally common. Leukemia is third (13%), followed by germ cell and gonadal tumors (11%) and thyroid carcinoma (11%). Melanoma of the skin accounts for 4% of the cancers diagnosed in adolescents.

Acute Lymphocytic Leukemia

EVIDENCE BASE Hunger, S. P., & Mullighan, C. G. (2015). Acute lymphoblastic leukemia in children. *New England Journal of Medicine, 373*(16), 1541–1552.
National Cancer Institute. (2017). Childhood acute lymphoblastic leukemia treatment (PDQ)—Health professional version. Available: www.cancer.gov/types/leukemia/hp/child-all-treatment-pdq.

Acute lymphocytic leukemia (ALL) is a primary disorder of the bone marrow in which the normal marrow elements are replaced by immature or undifferentiated blast cells. When the quantity of normal marrow is depleted below the level necessary to maintain peripheral blood elements within normal ranges, anemia, neutropenia, and thrombocytopenia occur. ALL is the most common malignancy in children, representing more than a quarter of all pediatric cancers (29%). The peak incidence in children is ages 2 to 5 years, and incidence subsequently decreases with age. The annual incidence of ALL within the United States is 3.7 to 4.9 cases per 100,000 children ages 0 to 14. Advances in cancer treatment have led to marked improvements in survival rates among children greater than 80%. It is more common among white and Hispanic children and is more common in boys than in girls.

Pathophysiology and Etiology

1. The exact cause of ALL is unknown.
2. Environmental factors, as well as genetic factors and chromosomal abnormalities are suspected in some cases.
3. ALL results from the growth of an abnormal type of nongranular, fragile leukocyte in the blood-forming tissues, particularly in the bone marrow, spleen, and lymph nodes.
4. The abnormal lymphoblast has little cytoplasm and a round, homogeneous nucleus (see Figure 51-1).
5. ALL is classified according to the cell type involved: T-lymphoblastic leukemia or B-lymphoblastic leukemia.
6. Normal bone marrow elements may be displaced or replaced in this type of leukemia.
7. The changes in the blood and bone marrow result from the accumulation of leukemic cells and from the deficiency of normal cells.
   a. Red blood cell (RBC) precursors and megakaryocytes from which platelets are formed are decreased, causing anemia, prolonged and unusual bleeding, tendency to bruise easily, and petechiae.
   b. Normal white blood cells (WBCs) are significantly decreased, predisposing the child to infection.
   c. The bone marrow is hyperplastic, with a uniform appearance caused by leukemic cells.
8. Leukemic cells may infiltrate into lymph nodes, spleen, and liver, causing diffuse adenopathy and hepatosplenomegaly.
9. Expansion of marrow or infiltration of leukemic cells into bone causes bone and joint pain.
10. Invasion of the CNS by leukemic cells may cause headache, vomiting, cranial nerve palsies, convulsions, coma, papilledema, and blurred or double vision.

Figure 51-1. Abnormal lymphoblast in acute lymphocytic leukemia.

11. Weight loss, muscle wasting, and fatigue may occur when the body cells are deprived of nutrients because of the immense metabolic needs of the proliferating leukemic cells.

Clinical Manifestations

1. Manifestations depend on the degree to which the bone marrow has been compromised and the location and extent of extramedullary infiltration.
2. Presenting symptoms:
   a. Fatigability.
   b. General malaise, listlessness.
   c. Persistent fever of unknown cause.
   d. Recurrent infection.
   e. Petechiae, purpura, and ecchymosis after minor trauma.
   f. Pallor.
   g. Generalized lymphadenopathy.
   h. Abdominal pain caused by organomegaly.
   i. Bone and joint pain.
   j. Headache and vomiting (with CNS involvement).
3. Presenting symptoms may be isolated or in any combination or sequence.

Diagnostic Evaluation

1. May have altered peripheral blood counts. Blood studies may show the following:
   a. Low hemoglobin level, RBC count, hematocrit, and platelet count.
   b. Decreased, elevated, or normal WBC count.
2. Bone marrow examination and stained peripheral smear examination show large numbers of lymphoblasts and lymphocytes.
3. Lumbar puncture to assess for lymphoblasts in CNS to determine CNS involvement.
4. Renal and liver function studies determine contraindications or precautions for chemotherapy.
5. Chest x-ray determines whether a mediastinal mass or pneumonia is present.
6. Varicella and cytomegalovirus titer determine risk of infection.
7. The CNS and testes are sites of "sanctuary"; CNS treatment and surveillance is standard and testes are evaluated with physical examinations.

Management

1. Supportive therapy is indicated to control such disease complications as hyperuricemia, electrolyte imbalance, infection, anemia, bleeding, pain, nausea/vomiting, and fatigue.
2. Specific therapy is warranted to eradicate malignant cells and to restore normal marrow function.
3. Chemotherapy is used to achieve complete remission, with restoration of normal peripheral blood and physical findings; it is administered through an indwelling central catheter or implantable port. (See Table 51-1.)
4. Although no universally accepted standard therapy for the treatment of children with ALL exists, most facilities have similar protocols that use a combination of drugs.
5. Components of therapy:
   a. Induction, the initial course of therapy designed to achieve complete remission, usually lasts 4 to 6 weeks. For those who do not achieve complete remission by the end of induction therapy, an allogeneic bone marrow transplant is usually pursued. Induction usually includes a combination of vincristine, L-asparaginase, and corticosteroids. A fourth drug, such as daunorubicin, doxorubicin, or cytosine arabinoside, may be added.
   b. Consolidation treatment, a period of intensified treatment immediately after remission induction, attempts

Table 51-1	Commonly Used Chemotherapeutic Agents to Treat Acute Lymphocytic Leukemia
CHEMOTHERAPEUTIC AGENT	**COMMON SIDE EFFECTS**
Asparaginase	Pain at injection site Allergic reaction Increased plasma ammonia level Clotting factor abnormalities Fatigue, weakness Diarrhea
Cytarabine	Nausea, vomiting Fever Headache
Methotrexate	Nausea, vomiting Headache Elevated liver enzymes Mucositis Nephrotoxicity
Vincristine	Hair loss Neuropathy Constipation
Daunorubicin	Nausea, vomiting Hair loss Red urine Bone marrow suppression Cardiac dysfunction
Cytoxan	Nausea, vomiting Hair loss Loss of appetite Gonadal dysfunction Bone marrow suppression Nephrotoxicity
Mercaptopurine	Bone marrow suppression
Thioguanine	Bone marrow suppression

total eradication of residual leukemic cells. Consolidation treatment usually lasts approximately 6 to 9 months, but can vary in length based on different protocols. It usually includes a combination of methotrexate, 6-mercaptopurine, etoposide, thioguanine, cytosine arabinoside, cyclophosphamide, prednisone, vincristine, L-asparaginase, and doxorubicin or daunorubicin.

c. Maintenance or continuation therapy is the final and often longest stage of treatment in childhood ALL. The goal of maintenance therapy is to lower the risk of relapse once remission has been achieved, and typically lasts 2 to 3 years. Boys require longer maintenance therapy to prevent testicular relapse in some protocols. It usually includes daily oral administration of 6-mercaptopurine and weekly oral or IM administration of methotrexate with intermittent administration of other drugs, such as monthly vincristine, corticosteroids, cyclophosphamide, cytosine arabinoside, or daunorubicin.

d. Reinduction therapy induces remission if relapse occurs and usually includes the same initial drugs. Sometimes, however, additional agents may be added.

e. If testicular relapse occurs, radiation therapy to the testicles is administered.

f. CNS disease prophylaxis generally consists of intrathecal administration of methotrexate alone or in combination with intrathecal or systemic therapy that can cross the blood–brain barrier including cytarabine and hydrocortisone. Craniospinal irradiation may also be used to treat CNS disease.

g. The role of allogeneic hematopoietic stem cell transplant (HSCT) is considered for those patients with very high risk of relapse and/or treatment failure. Components of this therapy usually include total body irradiation (TBI) and chemotherapy agents in the preparative regiment and undergo transplant from either a matched sibling or alternate donor sources.

6. Current standards of treatment are designed on risk-based criteria; patients with worse prognostic indicators receive more intensive therapy.

7. Blood and marrow transplantation has been used successfully to treat children who fail to respond to conventional treatment.

 DRUG ALERT Assess the patient and monitor vital signs after administration of L-asparaginase–type drugs for signs of anaphylaxis. Have emergency drugs and equipment at the bedside (oxygen, epinephrine, antihistamines, and steroids). If administering in the outpatient setting, observe patients for at least 1 hour.

Prognosis

1. At least 98% of children with ALL can be expected to achieve an initial remission if treated in a specialized facility.
2. Overall 5-year survival is 90%.
3. The prognosis becomes poorer with each relapse the child experiences.
4. Relapse is rare after 7 years from diagnosis.
5. Factors associated with prognosis:
   a. Initial WBC count (WBC count greater than 50,000 has worse prognosis).
   b. Age (younger than age 2 years and older than 10 years have poorer prognosis, and infants younger than 1 year of age have even worse prognosis).

c. Extramedullary involvement (poorer prognosis).
d. Type of leukemia cytogenetic factors and immunophenotype (DNA index, karyotype).

Complications

1. Infection—most frequently occurs in the blood, lungs, GI tract, or skin. Patients with central lines are at increased risk.
2. Hemorrhage—usually caused by thrombocytopenia.
3. CNS involvement.
4. Bony involvement.
5. Testicular involvement.
6. Urate nephropathy (rarely seen except in induction).
7. Acute complications of treatment (eg, cardiomyopathy).
8. Late effects of treatment (treatment specific). Most frequent long-term complication is neurocognitive dysfunction causing school difficulty.

Nursing Assessment

1. Obtain a history.
   a. When taking the history, focus on symptoms that led to the diagnosis and previous symptoms for the past 2 weeks. For example, inquire about fatigue, headache, nausea, vomiting, pallor, bleeding, pain, or fever.
   b. Ask about past history of varicella zoster infection (chickenpox), which could lead to disseminated infection if acquired during immunosuppression. Also ask about recent exposures, including sibling exposures.
2. Perform a physical examination, including:
   a. Examination of skin for petechiae, purpura, and ecchymosis.
   b. Palpation of lymph nodes for enlargement, tenderness, and mobility.
   c. Palpation of spleen and liver for enlargement.
   d. Examination of fundi to detect papilledema with CNS disease.
   e. Inspection of skin for areas of infection, including indwelling catheter sites.
   f. Auscultation of lungs for crackles or rhonchi, indicative of pneumonia.
   g. Temperature for fever.
3. Assess family coping mechanisms and use of resources such as support systems.

 NURSING ALERT Report changes in behavior or personality, persistent nausea, vomiting, headache, lethargy, irritability, dizziness, ataxia, convulsions, or alterations in state of consciousness. These may be signs of CNS disease or relapse. CNS relapse is usually caught on routine screening.

Nursing Diagnoses

- Anxiety of parents related to learning of diagnosis.
- Risk for Infection and hemorrhage related to bone marrow suppression caused by chemotherapy and disease.
- Disturbed Body Image related to alopecia associated with chemotherapy.
- Imbalanced Nutrition: Less than Body Requirements related to anemia, anorexia, nausea, vomiting, pain, stress, inflammation, psychological problems, taste aversion, and mucosal ulceration secondary to chemotherapy or radiation.

- Acute Pain related to diagnostic procedures, progression of the disease, and adverse effects of treatment.
- Activity Intolerance related to fatigue that results from the disease and treatment.
- Anxiety of child related to hospitalization and diagnostic and treatment procedures.

Nursing Interventions

Decreasing Parental Anxiety

1. Be available to the parents when they want to discuss their feelings.
2. Offer kindness, concern, consideration, and sincerity toward the child and parents; be a source of consolation.
3. Contact the family's clergyman or the hospital chaplain.
4. Obtain the services of a social worker, as appropriate, to help the family use appropriate community resources.
5. Offer hope that therapy will be effective and will prolong life.
6. Have parents speak with parents of a child currently on therapy.
7. Encourage parents to participate in activities of daily living to help them feel a part of their child's care.
8. Assess family dynamics and coping mechanisms and plan interventions accordingly.
9. Help the parents to deal with anticipatory grief.
10. Help the parents to deal with other family members and friends.
11. Encourage the parents to discuss concerns about limiting their child's activities, protecting child from infection, disciplining child, and having anxieties about the illness.
12. Facilitate communication with the clinic nurse or clinical specialist who may interact with the child during the entire course of illness.
13. Encourage parents to continue established family patterns, including school attendance, social life, and family activities, as medically indicated.

Preventing Infection and Hemorrhage

EVIDENCE BASE Linder, L., Gerdy, C., Abouzelof, R., et al. (2017). Using practice-based evidence to improve supportive care practices to reduce central line-associated bloodstream infections in a pediatric oncology unit. *Journal of Pediatric Oncology Nursing, 34*(3), 185–195.

1. Monitor complete blood count (CBC), as ordered.
2. Provide adequate hydration.
   a. Maintain parenteral fluid administration.
   b. Offer small amounts of oral fluids, if tolerated.
3. Observe renal function carefully.
   a. Measure and record urine output.
   b. Check specific gravity.
   c. Observe the urine for evidence of gross bleeding.
   d. Use lab sticks to determine if occult urinary bleeding is present.
4. Protect the child from infection sources.
   a. Never use a rectal thermometer, suppositories, or enemas when caring for a neutropenic patient.
   b. Family, friends, personnel, and other patients who have infections should not visit or care for the child. Discuss care of siblings while the child is on therapy.
   c. Private rooms are preferred, but if it is necessary to share, do not place a child with an infection in the same room with a child with leukemia.

d. Good hand washing is the most important way to control infection.
5. Observe the child closely and be alert for signs of impending infection.
   a. Observe broken skin or mucous membrane for signs of infection.
   b. Report fever of more than 101°F (38.3°C).
   c. Assess central line site for redness or tenderness.
6. Administer growth factors, such as granulocyte colony–stimulating factor, to stimulate the production of neutrophils and to decrease the incidence of severe infections in the child after high-dose chemotherapy.
7. Administer IV antibiotics, as ordered.
8. Administer PCP prophylaxis, such as cotrimoxazole, if ordered, twice daily three times per week to prevent infection with *Pneumocystis carinii*. (Dapsone and pentamidine are also given for patients unable to take cotrimoxazole.)
9. Record vital signs and report changes that may indicate hemorrhage, including:
   a. Tachycardia.
   b. Lowered blood pressure.
   c. Pallor.
   d. Diaphoresis.
   e. Increasing anxiety and restlessness.
10. Observe for GI bleeding and Hematest all emesis and stool.
11. Move and turn the child gently because hemarthrosis may occur and may cause pain.
    a. Handle the child in a gentle manner.
    b. Turn the child frequently to prevent pressure ulcers.
    c. Place the child in proper body alignment in a comfortable position.
    d. Allow the child to be out of bed in a chair if this position is more comfortable.
    e. Encourage the child to ambulate, if possible.
12. Avoid IM injections, if possible; if not possible, ensure platelet count has been obtained prior to injection and hold pressure to the area for at least 5 minutes.
13. Handle catheters and drainage and suction tubes carefully to prevent mucosal bleeding.
14. Protect the child from injury by monitoring activities and exposure to environmental hazards, such as slippery floors or uneven surfaces.
15. Be aware of emergency procedures for control of bleeding:
    a. Apply local pressure carefully so as not to interfere with clot formation.
    b. Administer leukocyte-poor, irradiated, packed RBCs and platelets, as ordered.

NURSING ALERT Patients with low WBC count may not respond to infection with usual signs and symptoms (ie, fever and purulent drainage from infected wound).

Promoting Acceptance of Body Changes

1. Prepare the patient for potential changes in body image (alopecia, weight loss, muscle wasting) and help the child cope with related feelings.
2. Engage child life therapist for medical play and support.
3. Contact the school nurse and teacher to help them prepare for the child's return to school. Discuss the bodily changes that have occurred and that may happen in the future.

Promoting Optimal Nutrition

EVIDENCE BASE Arpaci, T., Toruner, E., & Altay, N. (2018). Assessment of nutritional problems in pediatric patients with cancer and the informational needs of their parents: A parental perspective. *Asia-Pacific Journal of Oncology Nursing, 5*(2), 231–236.

1. Provide a highly nutritious diet as tolerated by the child.
   a. Determine the child's food likes and dislikes.
   b. Offer frequent, small meals.
   c. Offer high-calorie, high-protein supplemental feedings.
   d. Encourage the parents to assist at mealtime.
   e. Allow the child to eat with a group at a table if his or her condition allows.
   f. Avoid foods high in salt while the child is taking steroids.
   g. Administer enteral and parenteral feeds, as ordered.
2. Give careful oral hygiene; the gums and mucous membranes of the mouth may bleed easily.
   a. Use a soft toothbrush.
   b. If the child's mouth is bleeding or painful, clean the teeth and mouth with a moistened cotton swab or sponge-tipped swab.
   c. Use a nonirritating rinse for the mouth (no alcohol-containing mouthwash or sodium bicarbonate).
   d. Apply petroleum to dry, cracked lips.
   e. Assess for mucositis and provide appropriate mouth rinse.
3. Be alert for nausea and vomiting.
   a. Administer antiemetic drugs on a round-the-clock, regular schedule (eg, serotonin antagonist, dexamethasone).
   b. Become knowledgeable about chemotherapeutic agents and adjust antiemetic therapy for those drugs with delayed nausea and vomiting.
   c. Monitor strict intake and output.
   d. Maintain parenteral fluid administration and assess for signs of dehydration or overhydration.
   e. Administer antiemetic drugs for patients who receive radiation to the chest, abdomen, pelvis, or craniospinal axis.
   f. Suggest relaxation techniques or guided imagery for patients who experience anticipatory nausea and vomiting.

Relieving Pain

EVIDENCE BASE Mercadante, S., & Giarratano, A. (2014). Pharmacological management of cancer pain in children. *Critical Reviews in Oncology/Hematology, 91*(1), 93–97.
Wiffen, P. J., Cooper, T. E., Anderson, A. K., Gray, A. L., Grégoire, M. C., Ljungman, G., & Zernikow, B. (2017). Opioids for cancer-related pain in children and adolescents. *The Cochrane Library,* (7), CD012564.

1. Position the child for comfort.
2. Assess the child's pain using a developmentally appropriate pain scale at regular intervals.
3. Administer drugs on a preventive schedule before pain becomes intense. Continuous infusion pumps for opioid administration are commonly used.
4. Manipulate the environment, as necessary, to increase the child's comfort and to minimize unnecessary exertion.
5. Prepare the child for treatment and diagnostic procedures.
   a. Use knowledge of growth and development to prepare the child for such procedures as bone marrow aspirations, spinal taps, blood transfusions, and chemotherapy.
   b. Provide a means for talking about the experience. Play, storytelling, or role-playing may be helpful.
   c. Convey to the child an acceptance of fears and anger.
   d. Use anesthetic cream at spinal tap, injection, and bone marrow sites to decrease pain.
   e. Administer conscious sedation before procedures and monitor pulse, BP, respirations, and pulse oximetry during and after procedures.
6. Consider implementing complementary and alternative medicine (CAM) interventions for pain control as well as for management of nausea, vomiting, and anxiety. CAM strategies to consider include the following:
   a. Hypnosis/self-hypnosis.
   b. Imagery.
   c. Distraction/relaxation techniques.
   d. Cognitive-behavioral therapy.
   e. Music therapy.
   f. Massage.

Conserving Energy

1. Assess the child's energy level and space needed activities accordingly. Allow the child to rest, if necessary.
2. Encourage the child to limit strenuous activity after such diagnostic procedures as bone marrow aspirations and spinal taps.

Reducing the Child's Anxiety

1. Provide for continuity of care.
2. Encourage family-centered care.
3. Facilitate play activities for the child and use opportunities to communicate through play.
4. Maintain some discipline, placing calm limitations on unacceptable behavior.
5. Provide appropriate diversional activities.
6. Encourage independence and provide opportunities that allow the child to control his or her environment.
7. Explain the diagnosis and treatment in age-appropriate terms.

Community and Home Care Considerations

EVIDENCE BASE Brandowicki, P., Vessey, J., Temple, K., et al. (2016). Building bridges from hospital to home. *Journal of Pediatric Oncology Nursing, 33*(5), 370–377.

1. Begin to develop a home care plan before the child leaves the hospital.
2. Communicate with health care provider, hospital nurses, family, and others familiar with the case to gather information about the child's illness, treatment plan, and specific needs in the home.
3. Arrange schedule for blood draws and how results will be managed.
4. Contact the child's school and arrange a meeting with the school nurse, principal, appropriate teachers, and other relevant school personnel to explain child's diagnosis, treatment, and potential time away from school.
5. Discuss with patient the possibility of making a visit to the classroom; explain about cancer and the adverse effects of chemotherapy to facilitate school reentry in a manner that would be understood by classmates.
6. Collaborate with primary care provider regarding immunization schedule and the contraindication for children on immunosuppressive therapy.
7. Make sure that parents or caregivers can demonstrate the proper technique for care of venous access, such as dressing changes, flushing, and assessing for infection.

8. Ensure parents or caregivers receive education for home medications, including medication schedule, side effects, and indications for scheduled and PRN medications.

Family Education and Health Maintenance

1. Teach parents about normal CBC values and expected variations caused by therapy.
2. Instruct parents about leukemia and adverse effects of chemotherapy.
3. Tell parents to call the health care provider if the child has a fever of more than 101°F (38.3°C), which may indicate overwhelming infection and impending septic shock, bleeding, and signs of infection. Parents should also immediately report if the child has been exposed to chickenpox. Immunosuppressed children are in danger of developing disseminated varicella and may be treated prophylactically with varicella immune globulin.
4. Teach preventive measures, such as hand washing and isolation from children with communicable diseases.
5. Reinforce that parents are *never* to use a rectal thermometer.
6. Refer parents to such agencies as Candlelighters (*www.candlelighters.org*) or the Leukemia and Lymphoma Society (*www.leukemia-lymphoma.org*).

Evaluation: Expected Outcomes

- Parents discuss their feelings about the child's diagnosis and treatment.
- Remains afebrile, no signs of localized infection or bleeding.
- Maintains a positive body image.
- Eats enough calories to maintain weight.
- Experiences relief from pain (no crying or expression of pain).
- Rests at intervals.
- Acts out feelings in play; participates in age-appropriate activities.

Brain Tumors in Children

EVIDENCE BASE National Cancer Institute. (2017). Childhood astrocytomas treatment (PDQ)—Health professional version. Available: *www.cancer.gov/types/brain/hp/child-astrocytoma-treament-pdq*.

Paul, S. P., Perrow, R., & Webster, M. A. (2014). Brain tumours in children: Reducing time to diagnosis: Siba Prosad Paul and colleagues discuss the role of emergency nurses in the acute management of brain tumours in children and young people. *Emergency Nurse, 22*(1), 32–36.

Brain tumors are abnormal and uncontrollable growth of cells in the brain. Approximately 25% of the malignant tumors that occur in children are brain tumors, with an incidence rate of 4.84 per 100,000 children age 0 to 19 years. Tumors occurring in the CNS are the most common cause of death from childhood cancers. Of the children that do survive a brain tumor, approximately 60% will be left with a life-altering disability. Four main types of brain tumors appear in children. Glial cell tumors, including *astrocytoma* and *diffuse pontine glioma*, can grow at any location in the brain and account for approximately 30% to 40% of all pediatric brain tumors. *Medulloblastoma* is a type of embryonal tumor, which is highly malignant and rapidly growing, usually found in the cerebellum. Embryonal tumors are the most common tumors of the CNS in children. *Ependymoma* is a tumor derived from the ependyma, or lining of the central canal of the spinal cord and cerebral ventricles. It frequently arises on the floor of the fourth ventricle, causing obstruction of the flow of cerebrospinal fluid (CSF). Ependymomas represent approximately 5%

to 10% of all primary childhood CNS tumors. *Germ cell tumors* are midline tumors typically diagnosed in children age 6 to 14 years with a higher incidence in parts of Asia, specifically Japan.

Pathophysiology and Etiology

1. The etiology of brain tumors is unknown. Triggers that are found to be associated with increased risk of brain tumors include certain genetic syndromes and environmental factors.
2. Symptoms are associated with the location of the tumor, size of the tumor, rate of growth, and chronologic and developmental age of the child.
3. Astrocytomas typically present in the infratentorial region, producing increased intracranial pressure (ICP). It is classified according to its malignancy, from grade I (least malignant) to grade IV (most malignant). More than 80% of astrocytomas located in the cerebellum are low grade I. Surgery and radiation are the primary therapies.
4. Medulloblastoma grows rapidly and produces evidence of increased ICP progressing during several weeks. It is classified as standard risk or high risk depending on tumor histology. Combination therapy of surgery, radiation, and chemotherapy is usually required.
5. Germ cell tumors grow in the midline of the brain and the majority present in the suprasellar or pineal regions. The growth rate varies, but frequently symptoms precede diagnosis by several months.
6. Ependymomas grow with varying speed. Because of location, tumors can invade the cardiorespiratory center, cerebellum, and spinal cord. They are graded according to degree of differentiation.

Clinical Manifestations

Glial Cell Tumors
Onset and growth is related to stage of tumor.
1. Evidence of increased ICP—especially ataxia, vomiting, or headache.
2. Cerebellar signs—ataxia, dysmetria (inability to control the range of muscular movement), and nystagmus.
3. Behavioral changes.
4. Seizures.
5. Precocious puberty.
6. Vision and hearing problems.

Medulloblastoma
Fast growing, malignant, and invasive.
1. The child may present with unsteady gait, anorexia, vomiting, and early morning headache.
2. May later develop ataxia, nystagmus, papilledema, drowsiness, increased head circumference, head tilt, and cranial nerve palsies. May develop obstructive hydrocephalus.

Germ Cell Tumor
Signs of midline shifts.
1. Visual disturbances.
2. Personality and sleep pattern alterations.
3. Dramatic weight loss.
4. Hydrocephalus.
5. Endocrinopathies.
6. Seizures.

Ependymoma of the Fourth Ventricle
1. Signs of increased ICP.
   a. Nausea or vomiting.
   b. Headache.
2. Unsteady gait or ataxia; dysmetria.
3. Focal motor weakness, vision disturbances, seizures.

Diagnostic Evaluation

Determined by the type of tumor that is suspected; usually includes many or all of the following procedures to localize and determine extent of the tumor:

1. Computed tomography (CT).
2. Magnetic resonance imaging (MRI).
3. Fluid-attenuated inversion recovery imaging.
4. Positron emission tomography (PET).
5. Lumbar puncture with CSF cytologic evaluation (not commonly performed).
6. Angiography (occasional).

Management

1. Surgery is performed to determine the type of tumor, to assess the extent of invasiveness, and to excise as much of the lesion as possible.
2. Radiation therapy is usually initiated as soon as the diagnosis is established and the surgical wound is healed.
3. Chemotherapy is used to treat chemoresponsive tumors and is particularly important in children who are too young to receive radiation therapy.
4. A ventriculoperitoneal shunt is usually necessary for children who develop hydrocephalus.
5. The use of immunotherapy is being investigated for potential for future treatment.
6. Prognosis is improved in cases that involve early diagnosis and adequate therapy. Five-year survivors are increasing, especially in children with low-grade astrocytomas or ependymomas. However, there are still tumors such as diffuse intrinsic pontine glioma that have no known cure.

Complications

1. Brain stem herniation.
2. Hydrocephalus.
3. Permanent neurological disabilities.
4. Increased risk for bone fractures.
5. Increased risk of developing other tumors later in life.

Nursing Assessment

Assess the child's neurologic status to help locate the site of the tumor and the extent of involvement as well as to identify signs of disease progression.

1. Obtain a comprehensive nursing history from the child and parents, particularly data related to normal behavioral patterns and presenting symptoms.
2. Perform portions of the neurologic examination, as appropriate. Assess muscle strength, coordination, gait, posture, and how well the senses and reflexes work.
3. Observe for the appearance or disappearance of the clinical manifestations previously described. Report these to the health care provider and record each of the following in detail:
   a. Headache—onset, beneficial and provoking factors, duration, location, severity, and impact.
   b. Vomiting—onset, amount, presence of blood, color, frequency, and foods eaten in the past 24 hours.
   c. Seizures—activity before seizure, type of seizure, areas of body involved, behavior and level of consciousness (LOC) during and after seizure, duration, changes to skin, heart rate, and respiratory status.
4. Monitor vital signs frequently, including BP and pupillary reaction.

5. Monitor ocular signs. Check pupils for size, equality, reaction to light, and accommodation.
6. Observe for signs of brain stem herniation—should be considered a neurosurgical emergency. This complication occurs when brain tissue, CSF, and blood vessels are pressed or shifted from their usual position inside of the skull.
   a. Abnormal posturing (opisthotonis) caused by muscle spasms. (see figure 51-2.).
   b. Tilting of the head; neck stiffness.
   c. Poorly reactive and dilated pupils.
   d. Increased BP; widened pulse pressure.
   e. Change in respiratory rate and nature of respirations.
   f. Irregular pulse or decreased pulse rate.
   g. Alterations of body temperature.

> **! NURSING ALERT** Signs of brain stem herniation, especially opisthotonos, are ominous and considered a medical emergency. The health care provider should be called immediately, and the child should be prepared for ventricular tap to relieve pressure. Resuscitation equipment needs to be readily available.

Nursing Diagnoses

- Anxiety of parents related to the nature of the diagnosis and the need for surgery.
- Fear of child related to hospitalization and to diagnostic and treatment procedures.
- Acute Pain related to increased ICP and surgery.
- Imbalanced Nutrition: Less than Body Requirements related to nausea and vomiting associated with increased ICP, chemotherapy, and radiation.
- Risk for Infection postoperatively.
- Disturbed Body Image related to appearance of the incision, shaved head, or changes caused by radiation, chemotherapy, and steroids.

Nursing Interventions

Reducing Parents' Anxiety

1. Continue to keep the parents updated about their child's progress and be honest about differential diagnoses.
2. Encourage the parents to ask questions and to understand fully the risks and benefits of surgery and other interventions.
3. Prepare the parents for the postoperative appearance of their child and for the fact that the child might be comatose immediately following surgery.
4. Provide emotional support for the parents during the postoperative period. They may be frightened, shocked, anxiety, and upset by the appearance of their child and by necessary emergency procedures.

Figure 51-2. Opisthotonos, a sign of brain stem herniation.

5. Facilitate the return of normal parent–child relationships.
   a. The parents may be overprotective.
   b. Help the parents to see the child's increasing capabilities and clinical progression.
   c. Encourage parents to foster independence with their child.
   d. Help the parent prepare to adjust to the transition from an inpatient setting to outpatient, follow-up care.
   e. Direct the parent to services and resources that may support them with the financial costs associated with care and treatment.

EVIDENCE BASE American Cancer Society. (2017). Children diagnosed with cancer: Returning to school. Atlanta, GA. Available: *www.cancer.org/treatment/children-and-cancer/when-your-child-has-cancer/returning-to-school.html*.

TRANSITIONAL CARE ALERT It is important for children with cancer to return to school as soon as they can as it provides them with a clear message that they have a future and potential for full recovery. Their lives become more normal, and it allows opportunity for social interaction with peers.

Reducing the Child's Fear

1. Prepare the child for surgery in realistic terms, but at the appropriate developmental level. Involve the child life therapist and social worker in the preparation process.
2. Encourage the child to ask questions and express concerns.
3. Determine the plan regarding shaving of the child's head, bandages, and other procedures. Prepare the child accordingly.
4. Prepare the child for postoperative expectations (eg, may feel sleepy, have a headache, will need to remain flat, and will see IV tubes, drainage tubes, and machines attached to him or her). Arrange visit to pediatric intensive care unit before surgery to prepare for environment.
5. Bring a comfort item (eg, special blanket or favorite toy) for the child to have in possession postoperatively.

Reducing Pain Postoperatively

1. Administer opioids, as ordered, in the immediate postoperative period, assessing the child's LOC prior to administration as well as the child's response to opioid administration.
2. Keep the child as comfortable as possible by repositioning.
3. Apply nonpharmacological techniques for pain management in combination with opioid administration.

Maintaining Nutritional Status

1. Feed the child after vomiting. (Vomiting is not usually associated with nausea.)
2. Allow the child to participate in the selection of foods.
3. Maintain IV hydration or hyperalimentation and intralipids, if indicated.
4. Encourage the child to eat progressively larger meals as he or she recovers.
5. If the child cannot eat, provide tube feedings. A gastrostomy tube may be inserted.
6. Be aware that children taking steroids to decrease swelling may have increased appetite.
7. Monitor weight and laboratory values daily to ensure efficacy of nutritional support.

Preventing Infection and Other Complications Postoperatively

1. Position the child according to surgeon's request—usually on unaffected side with head level with body.
   a. Raising the foot of the bed may increase ICP and bleeding.
   b. Post a sign above the bed, noting the exact position of the head.
2. Check the dressing for bleeding and for drainage of CSF.
3. Monitor the child's temperature closely.
   a. A significant rise in temperature may be caused by trauma, disturbance of the heat-regulating center, or intracranial edema.
   b. If hyperthermia occurs, administer antipyretics and use cooling techniques, as ordered. Temperature should not be reduced too rapidly.
4. Observe the child closely for signs of shock, increased ICP, seizure activity, and alterations in LOC.
5. Assess the child for edema of the head, face, and neck.
6. Carefully regulate fluid administration and blood pressure to prevent increased cerebral edema.
7. Change the child's position frequently and provide meticulous skin care to prevent hypostatic pneumonia and pressure ulcers.
   a. Move the child carefully and slowly, being certain to move the head in line with the body.
   b. Support paralyzed or spastic extremities with pillows, rolls, or other devices.
8. Have equipment readily available for cardiopulmonary resuscitation, respiratory assistance, oxygen inhalation, blood transfusion, ventricular tap, and other potential emergency situations.
9. Report fever or sign of infection.
10. If the child is receiving chemotherapy or radiation, assess for fever greater than 101°F (38.3°C) or nausea and vomiting unrelated to chemotherapy.

Promoting Acceptance of Body Changes

1. Encourage the child to express feelings regarding the threat to body image.
2. Reassure the child that a wig or a hat can be worn after recovery. Refer parents to *www.locksoflove.org* or *www.wigsforkids.org*.
3. If the child's hair has not been totally shaved, comb it so that the area of baldness is not evident.
4. Reassure the child that hair will grow back after surgery and chemotherapy (hair does not grow back at site of radiation therapy).
5. Prepare the child and family for cushingoid changes (moon face, edema) if long-term steroids are required.

Family Education and Health Maintenance

1. Provide parents with written information regarding the child's needs—medications, activity, care of the incision, and follow-up appointments.
2. Teach the parents about radiation and chemotherapy and their adverse effects.
3. If a child has a ventriculoperitoneal shunt, teach parents to report fever, nausea, vomiting, irritability, or a bulging anterior fontanelle.
4. Initiate a referral to a home health nurse to provide care and teaching at home and to maintain therapeutic support for the family.
5. Encourage parents to contact the child's teacher and the school nurse before the child returns to school so that they can prepare classmates for child's return and help them to deal with their feelings.

6. Provide the parents with the phone number of the clinic or nursing unit so that they may call if questions occur after discharge. For additional resources, refer family to such agencies as the American Brain Tumor Association (*www.abta.org*), Mikey's Way (*www.mikeysway.org*), Children's Tumor Foundation (*www.ctf.org*), The Lily Fund (*www.thelilyfund.org*), or Candlelighters (*www.candlelighters.org*).

Evaluation: Expected Outcomes

- Parents discuss feelings about the child's diagnosis and surgery.
- Child demonstrates decreased fear and anxiety through verbalization, play, or other age-appropriate activities.
- Child verbalizes relief from pain.
- Child maintains weight through adequate intake.
- Vital signs are stable, afebrile, and lungs are clear.
- Child verbalizes acceptance of physical appearance and desire to visit with friends.

Neuroblastoma

 EVIDENCE BASE National Cancer Institute. (2017). Neuroblastoma treatment (PDQ)—Health professional version. Available: *www.cancer.gov/types/neuroblastoma/hp/neuroblastoma-treatment-pdq*.

Pinto, N. R., Applebaum, M. A., Volchenboum, S. L., Matthay, K., et al. (2015). Advances in risk classification and treatment strategies for neuroblastoma. *Journal of Clinical Oncology, 33*(27), 3008–3017.

Salazar, B. M., Balczewski, E. A., Ung, C. Y., & Zhu, S. (2016). Neuroblastoma, a Paradigm for Big Data Science in Pediatric Oncology. *International Journal of Molecular Sciences, 18*(1), 37.

Neuroblastoma refers to a malignant tumor that arises from the sympathetic nervous system. It is the third most common childhood cancer, with a prevalence of 1 in 7,000 children in the United States. It primarily affects infants and young children under the age of 5 years, with the highest rate of diagnosis in the first month of life. Neuroblastoma occurs slightly more frequently in boys than in girls, and is more fatal in blacks.

Pathophysiology and Etiology

1. Etiology is unknown; no strong risk factors have been identified.
2. Tumors arise from embryonic neural crest cells anywhere along the craniospinal axis. A type of small, round, blue cell tumor.
3. Histologic picture varies greatly from tumor to tumor and even within the same tumor; racial differences in tumor biology.
4. Tumors are staged primarily by extent of disease; International Neuroblastoma Staging System:
   a. Stage 1 (tumor confined to the organ or structure of origin with complete surgical resection) to stage 4 (remote disease involving the skin, skeleton, parenchymal organs, soft tissue, distant lymph nodes, or bone marrow).
   b. Stage 4S refers to cases that would otherwise be stage 1 or 2 but that have dissemination limited to the liver, skin, or bone marrow in a patient less than 1 year of age.
5. Neuroblastoma is one of the few tumors that may demonstrate spontaneous remission.

Clinical Manifestations

1. Symptoms depend on the location of the tumor and the stage of the disease.

2. Most tumors are located within the abdomen and present as firm, nontender, irregular masses that may or may not cross the midline.
3. Other common signs:
   a. Bowel or bladder dysfunction that results from compression by a paraspinal or pelvic tumor.
   b. Neurologic symptoms, such as paralysis and Horner syndrome, because of compression by the tumor on nerve roots or because of tumor extension.
   c. Supraorbital ecchymosis, periorbital edema, and exophthalmos that results from metastases to the skull bones and retrobulbar soft tissue.
   d. Lymphadenopathy, especially in the cervical area.
   e. Bone pain with skeletal involvement.
   f. Swelling of the neck or face, wheezing, dyspnea, and cough with thoracic masses.
   g. Symptoms of bone marrow failure, such as anemia, bleeding, or infection.
   h. General symptoms of pallor, bluish skin discoloration, anorexia, fever, weight loss, and weakness with widespread metastasis.

Diagnostic Evaluation

Workup done to document the extent of the disease throughout the body include:

1. Chest and skeletal x-rays.
2. Bone scan.
3. Bone marrow aspiration and biopsy.
4. CBC, platelet count, ferritin.
5. Twenty-four-hour urine collection—elevated excretion of homovanillic acid (HVA) and vanillylmandelic acid (VMA).
6. Liver and kidney function tests.
7. Histologic confirmation.
8. Additional studies:
   a. CT of primary site and chest.
   b. MRI—areas above diaphragm.
   c. Ultrasound examination.
   d. Liver and spleen scan.
   e. Metaiodobenzylguanidine (MIBG) scan
9. Genetic indicators of poor prognosis include n-myc oncogene amplification, hyperdiploid karyotype, and chromosome deletion.

Management

1. Surgery—role is diagnostic and therapeutic. Either primary (before chemotherapy or radiation) or delayed/secondary (after therapy).
2. When complete surgical resection of a stage I tumor is possible, this may be the only treatment required.
3. Children with other than stage I disease generally receive a combination of surgery, radiation therapy, and chemotherapy. Drugs of choice include vincristine, topotecan, irinotecan, cyclophosphamide, doxorubicin, cisplatin, carboplatin, ifosfamide, and etoposide. See Table 51-2.
4. Survival rate for early stages is as high as 95%; advanced stages, 40%.
5. Influencing factors for prognosis:
   a. Stage of disease—the earlier the stage, the better the prognosis.
   b. Age—infants younger than age 1 demonstrate the best survival.
   c. Site of primary tumor—children with tumors above the diaphragm appear to do better than children with abdominal tumors.

CHEMOTHERAPEUTIC AGENT	COMMON SIDE EFFECTS
Carboplatin	Nausea, vomiting Bone marrow suppression Electrolyte imbalance
Cytoxan	Nausea, vomiting Hair loss Loss of appetite Gonadal dysfunction Bone marrow suppression Nephrotoxicity
Doxorubicin	Nausea, vomiting Hair loss Red urine Bone marrow suppression Cardiac dysfunction
Etoposide	Nausea, vomiting Hair loss Weakness Bone marrow suppression Nephrotoxicity Hepatotoxicity
Irinotecan	Diarrhea, abdominal cramping, runny nose, tearing, salivation, sweating, photophobia Nausea, vomiting Loss of appetite Bone marrow suppression Fever Weakness Elevated liver enzymes Elevated eosinophils
Temozolomide	Bone marrow suppression Nausea, vomiting Constipation Loss of appetite

Table 51-2 Commonly Used Chemotherapeutic Agents to Treat Neuroblastoma

d. Pattern of metastasis—children with metastasis to the bone marrow, liver, and skin have better prognosis than those with radiographic bone involvement.
e. Genetic and histologic factors.
6. Autologous stem cell transplantation, newer chemotherapy drugs, retinoid therapy, and immunotherapy such as Interleukin-2 may also be a part of the treatment regimen.

Complications

1. Metastasis to the liver, soft tissue, bones, lymph nodes, bone marrow, and skin.
2. Neurologic deficits due to nerve compression.

Nursing Assessment

 EVIDENCE BASE Kline, N. (Ed.). (2014). *Essentials of pediatric oncology nursing: A core curriculum* (4th ed.). Glenview, IL: Association of Pediatric Hematology/Oncology Nurses.

1. Obtain a history.
   a. Inquire about when symptoms began. Focus on decrease in appetite, weakness, pain, abdominal distention, or change in bowel and bladder function.
   b. Symptoms exhibited depend on the location of the primary tumor.
2. Perform a physical examination, including:
   a. Examination of skin for signs of increased bruising or petechiae.
   b. Palpation of liver and spleen for enlargement.
   c. Palpation of abdominal mass or other primary site of tumor.
   d. Auscultation of lungs.
   e. Palpation of lymph nodes.
   f. Blood pressure monitoring for detection of hypertension.
   g. Temperature for fever caused by infection or disease.
   h. Assessment of bones and joints for pain or swelling.
   i. Neurologic examination for signs of compression by tumor. Nerves involved depend on location of tumor.
3. Assess coping mechanisms of family.

Nursing Diagnoses

- Anxiety of parents related to learning of diagnosis.
- Fear of child related to diagnostic procedures and surgery or biopsy.
- Activity Intolerance related to fatigue from tumor growth and bone marrow suppression.
- Constipation or Bowel and Bladder Incontinence related to pressure of tumor.
- Risk for Infection related to bone marrow suppression from chemotherapy and radiation.
- Acute Pain related to tumor, surgery, or progression of disease.
- Disturbed Body Image related to hair loss.

Nursing Interventions

Reducing Parents' Anxiety
See previous sections, pages 1356 and 1359.

Reducing Child's Anxiety and Fear
See previous sections, pages 1357 and 1360.

Increasing Activity Tolerance
See previous section, page 1357.

Regaining Normal Bowel and Bladder Function
1. Assess normal elimination patterns the child had before the illness began.
2. Keep careful intake and output records.
3. Assess for urinary overflow incontinence and loss of bowel function, depending on the child's age.
4. Notify health care provider if these should occur.

Preventing Infection
See previous sections, pages 1356 and 1360.

Observe the surgical incision for erythema, drainage, or separation of the incision. Report these changes.

Relieving Pain
See previous sections, pages 1357 and 1360.

Monitor for increasing or new location of pain, indicating progression of disease (eg, fracture due to bone involvement).

Promoting Acceptance of Body Changes
See previous section, pages 1356 and 1360.

Family Education and Health Maintenance

1. Teach parents about the laboratory tests and imaging studies needed at diagnosis and periodically throughout therapy.
2. Instruct parents about chemotherapy drugs used and their potential adverse effects.
3. Inform parents about potential treatment methods, such as radiation therapy and bone marrow transplantation.
4. Advise parents to use good hand washing technique and to prevent exposure to children with communicable diseases.
5. Refer families to resources such as Candlelighters (*www. candlelighters.org*).

Evaluation: Expected Outcomes

- Parents and child discuss their feelings about diagnosis and treatment.
- Participates in play and expresses feelings through play.
- Maintains normal activity level.
- Resumes normal voiding and bowel patterns.
- Remains afebrile, lungs clear, no signs of localized infections.
- Rests without crying or guarding of surgical incision; good pain control according to developmentally appropriate scale.
- Interacts with others, seems comfortable with self.

Rhabdomyosarcoma

 EVIDENCE BASE Bekiesinska-Figatowska, M., Duczkowska, A., Duczkowski, M., et al. (2017). CNS metastases from bone and soft tissue sarcomas in children, adolescents, and young adults: Are they really so rare? *BioMed Research International, 2017.* doi: 10.1155/2017/ 1456473.

National Cancer Institute. (2017). Childhood rhabdomyosarcoma treatment (PDQ)—Health professional version. Available: *www.cancer.gov/types/soft-tissue-sarcoma/hp/ rhabdomyosarcoma-treatment-pdq.*

Parida, L. (2014). Nonurological malignancies in children. *Journal of Indian Association of Pediatric Surgeons, 19*(1), 31.

Rhabdomyosarcoma is a highly malignant soft tissue tumor that arises from the immature mesenchymal cells that form striated muscle. The incidence is approximately 4.5 per 1 million children in the United States and rhabdomyosarcoma accounts for 3.5% of all malignant disease in children younger than age 14 years and 2% of the cases among adolescents and young adults aged 15 to 19 years. It has bimodal distribution with a peak between 2 and 6 years old and again between 10 and 18 years old. Children aged 1 to 9 years have the best prognosis, whereas those younger and older fare less well. Rhabdomyosarcoma can occur anywhere in the body, the most common sites are the head and neck, genitourinary (GU) tract, and extremities.

Pathophysiology and Etiology

1. Etiology is unknown in most cases.
2. Certain genetic and environmental factors have been associated with its development.
3. Two major variants are embryonal and alveolar, with embryonal more common in infants and young children and alveolar more common in adolescents. Alveolar rhabdomyosarcoma tends to grow faster than embryonal and usually requires more intensive treatment.
4. Tumor spreads either by local extension or by metastasis via the venous and lymphatic system.

5. The lung is the most common site of metastasis.
6. Tumor staging is based on the extent of the disease:
   a. Stage/group I: localized tumor, completely resected; often in the orbit, head and neck, GU tract, and bile ducts.
   b. Stage/group II: local tumor resected, microscopic residual disease; often in the bladder or prostate, arm or leg, and a parameningeal site.
   c. Stage/group III: localized disease, with gross residual disease after resection; tumor is 5 cm across and may or may not have spread to nearby lymph nodes.
   d. Stage/group IV: metastatic disease at diagnosis.

Clinical Manifestations

1. Commonly presents as an asymptomatic painless lump noted by the patient or parent.
2. Signs and symptoms are variable and reflect the location of the tumor and metastasis.
   a. Orbit—ptosis, ocular paralysis, exophthalmos, impaired vision.
   b. Nasopharynx—epistaxis, pain, dysphagia, nasal voice, airway obstruction.
   c. Sinuses—swelling, pain, discharge, sinusitis.
   d. Middle ear—pain, chronic otitis, facial nerve palsy.
   e. Neck—hoarseness, dysphagia.
   f. Trunk, extremities, testicular areas—enlarging soft tissue masses.
   g. Prostate, bladder—urinary tract symptoms.
   h. Retroperitoneal tumors—GI and urinary tract obstruction, weakness, paresthesia, pain.
   i. Vaginal—abnormal vaginal bleeding or mass.

Diagnostic Evaluation

To document the extent of the disease and to provide objective criteria for measuring response to therapy:

1. Open biopsy of the primary tumor—definitive diagnostic procedure.
2. CT of the chest and primary lesion.
3. MRI.
4. Bone marrow aspiration and biopsy.
5. Bone scan or skeletal survey.
6. Ultrasonography.
7. Chest x-ray.
8. PET.
9. CBC, liver and renal function tests, electrolytes, serum calcium and phosphorus, uric acid.
10. Monoclonal antibody assays.
11. Urinalysis.
12. Lumbar puncture—for children with cranial lesions.

Management

1. Surgery—to biopsy the lesion, determine the stage of the disease, and completely remove or reduce the primary tumor. Increasingly, chemotherapy and radiation therapy are used before surgery to avoid the disability associated with radical surgery for selected anatomic sites (head, neck, and pelvis).
2. Radiation—high-dose radiation is generally recommended for the primary tumor and metastasis.
3. Chemotherapy:
   a. Used for all patients, usually in combination with irradiation (see Table 51-3).

Table 51-3 Commonly Used Chemotherapeutic Agents to Treat Rhabdomyosarcoma

CHEMOTHERAPEUTIC AGENT	COMMON SIDE EFFECTS
Cytoxan	Nausea, vomiting Hair loss Loss of appetite Gonadal dysfunction Bone marrow suppression Nephrotoxicity
Dactinomycin	Nausea, vomiting Bone marrow suppression
Vincristine	Hair loss Neuropathy Constipation

b. Commonly used drugs include dactinomycin, vincristine, cyclophosphamide, doxorubicin, cisplatin, etoposide, ifosfamide, irinotecan, melphalan topotecan, paclitaxel, and docetaxel.

4. Survival rates have improved considerably in recent years. Survival for stage I, with favorable histology, is greater than 90%; and survival for stage IV tends to be between 20% and 40%.

5. Prognosis is related to the stage of the disease at diagnosis, the location of the primary tumor, and the age at diagnosis.

Complications

1. Direct tumor extension to CNS with cranial nerve palsy, brain stem compromise with bradypnea and bradycardia.

2. Metastasis to the bone, bone marrow, lung.

Nursing Assessment

1. Obtain a history.
   a. Ask about recent illness history and when the child became symptomatic.
   b. Obtain review of systems to help identify the primary tumor and metastasis present.

2. Perform physical examination, including:
   a. Palpation of lymph nodes for enlargement, tenderness, and mobility.
   b. Palpation of the liver and spleen to detect hepatosplenomegaly.
   c. Palpation of primary site of tumor and suspected areas of metastasis.
   d. Auscultation of lungs to assess breath sounds or abnormality caused by the spread of the tumor.

3. Assess family coping, resources, and emotional state of the child and parents.

Nursing Diagnoses

- Risk for anxiety among parents related to learning of diagnosis.
- Fear of child related to diagnostic procedures and surgery or biopsy.
- Imbalanced Nutrition: Less than Body Requirements related to anemia, anorexia, nausea, vomiting, and mucosal ulceration secondary to chemotherapy or radiation.
- Acute Pain related to surgery or possible progression of disease.
- Disturbed Body Image related to alopecia associated with chemotherapy.
- Risk for Infection related to bone marrow suppression from chemotherapy or radiation.

Nursing Interventions

Reducing Parents' Anxiety
See previous sections, pages 1356 and 1359.

Reducing the Child's Fear and Anxiety
See previous sections, pages 1357 and 1360.

Promoting Optimal Nutrition
See previous sections, pages 1357 and 1360.

Relieving Pain
See previous sections, pages 1357 and 1360.

Promoting Acceptance of Body Changes
See previous sections, pages 1356 and 1360.

Preventing Infection
See previous sections, pages 1356 and 1360.

Family Education and Health Maintenance

1. Teach the parents about laboratory diagnostic tests that will be done periodically to follow the child's condition.

2. Instruct the parents about treatment methods, including chemotherapy and radiation protocols postoperatively, and their adverse effects.

3. Stress the importance of follow-up care so that recurrence can be detected early and appropriate treatment can be instituted.

4. Refer families to such resources as Candlelighters (*www.candlelighters.org*). Assist patients in coordinating care with an orthopedic surgeon, a medical or pediatric oncologist, a radiation oncologist, a pathologist, and a physiatrist.

Evaluation: Expected Outcomes

- Parents verbalize understanding of diagnosis.
- Child plays, interacts with others, and asks questions.
- Eats sufficient calories to maintain weight.
- Verbalizes reduced pain.
- Verbalizes acceptance of self; looks in mirror.
- Remains afebrile, no signs of localized infection.

Wilms Tumor

 EVIDENCE BASE American Cancer Society (2018). Atlanta, GA. What are the key statistics about Wilms tumor? Available: *https://www.cancer.org/cancer/wilms-tumor/about/key-statistics.html.*

National Cancer Institute. (2016). Wilms' tumor and other childhood kidney tumors treatment (PDQ)—Health professional version. Available: *www.cancer.gov/types/kidney/hp/wilms-treatment-pdq.*

Wilms tumor, also known as nephroblastoma, is a malignant renal tumor and is the most common renal neoplasm in children. It constitutes approximately 7% of all childhood tumors, but in the 15- to 19-year age group, most tumors are renal cell carcinoma. Incidence is approximately 8 cases per 100,000 children younger than age 15 years. About 500 cases are diagnosed each year in the United States; 75% of cases occur before the child is age 5 years. The average age a diagnosis is about 3 to 4 years. Most commonly a unilateral disease, but in 5%, both kidneys are involved. It may appear as swelling in the abdomen below the costal margin. In the United States, girls have a slightly higher risk of Wilms tumor than do boys, and the risk is slightly higher in African American children and lowest among Asian American children.

Pathophysiology and Etiology

1. The etiology is not known.
2. Genetic inheritance has been documented in 1% to 2% of cases.
3. Children with Wilms tumor may have associated anomalies.
4. Wilms tumor has a capacity for rapid growth and usually grows to a large size before it is diagnosed.
5. The effect of the tumor on the kidney depends on the site of the tumor.
6. In most cases, the tumor expands the renal parenchyma and the capsule of the kidney becomes stretched over the surface of the tumor, which is encapsulated at the time of surgery.
7. Wilms tumors present various histologic patterns and are grouped into two general categories: favorable histology and unfavorable histology.
8. The neoplasms metastasize either by direct extension or by way of the bloodstream. They may invade perirenal tissues, lymph nodes, the liver, the diaphragm, abdominal muscles, and the lungs. Invasions of bone and brain are less common.
9. Staging of Wilms tumor is done based on clinical and anatomic findings. It ranges from stage I (tumor is limited to the kidney and is completely excised) to stage IV (metastasis is present in the liver, lung, bone, or brain). Stage V includes those cases that include bilateral involvement, either initially or subsequently.

Clinical Manifestations

1. A firm, nontender upper quadrant abdominal mass is usually the presenting sign; it may be on either side. (It is usually first observed by the parents.)
2. Abdominal pain, which is related to rapid growth of the tumor, may occur. As the tumor enlarges, pressure may cause constipation, vomiting, abdominal distress, anorexia, weight loss, and dyspnea.
3. Less common are hypertension, fever, hematuria, and anemia.
4. Associated anomalies:
   a. Hemihypertrophy.
   b. Aniridia (without the iris of the eyes).
   c. Genitourinary tract abnormalities.
   d. Overgrowth syndromes (Beckwith-Wiedemann syndrome).
   e. Mental retardation.

Diagnostic Evaluation

1. Abdominal ultrasound to show the tumor and assess the status of the opposite kidney.
2. Radiography of chest to identify metastases.
3. CBC and peripheral smear to determine baseline data.
4. Urinalysis to detect for hematuria.
5. Blood chemistries, especially serum electrolytes, uric acid, renal function tests (blood urea nitrogen and creatinine), and liver function tests (bilirubin, alanine aminotransferase, aspartate aminotransferase, lactate dehydrogenase [LD], total protein, albumin, and alkaline phosphatase) may show abnormalities.
6. Urinary VMA and HVA to distinguish from neuroblastoma.
7. MRI or CT of the abdomen to evaluate local spread to lymph nodes or adjacent organs.
8. Renal biopsy to confirm diagnosis.
9. Real-time ultrasonography.

Management

1. Accurate staging and assessment of tumor spread is first conducted.

2. The standard treatment for stages I and II tumors is surgery (eg, partial nephrectomy, simply nephrectomy, or radical nephrectomy) followed by chemotherapy.
3. The standard treatment for stages III and IV is the same as for stages I and II but includes radiation.
4. If both kidneys are removed, which is the treatment for stage V, the patient will require dialysis until a transplant is possible.
5. Radiation or chemotherapy may be administered preoperatively to patients with advanced tumors or risky intravascular extension to reduce tumor burden.
6. Radiation therapy may be given to the tumor bed postoperatively to render nonviable all cells that have escaped locally from the excised tumor. Children who have stage III and IV Wilms tumor, or who have an unfavorable histology, usually receive this treatment.
7. Whole-lung radiation is used to treat stage IV tumors with lung metastasis.
8. Late effects of radiation therapy to the abdomen include scoliosis and underdevelopment of soft tissues and possible organ dysfunction in radiation field.
9. Chemotherapy is initiated postoperatively to achieve complete eradication of tumor cells (see Table 51-4).
10. Overall survival rates for Wilms tumor are among the highest for all childhood cancers—greater than 90% survival at 4 years.
11. Prognosis is based on histologic tumor features, lymph node involvement, age, tumor size, and possible chromosomal factors.

Complications

1. Metastasis to the lungs, lymph nodes, liver, bone, and brain.
2. Complications from radiation therapy include bowel obstruction, hepatic damage, nephritis, sterility in girls, interstitial pneumonia, and scoliosis.
3. Cumulative incidence of second malignancy is 1.6% after 15 years, with radiation being the greatest risk factor.

Nursing Assessment

1. Obtain a history.
   a. Ask how tumor was first discovered.
   b. Ask whether the child has history of other GU anomalies or whether there is a family history of cancer.
   c. Determine whether the child has had hematuria, dysuria, constipation, abdominal pain, decreased appetite, or fever before hospitalization and ask how these were treated.

Table 51-4	Commonly Used Chemotherapeutic Agents to Treat Wilms Tumor
CHEMOTHERAPEUTIC AGENT	**COMMON SIDE EFFECTS**
Vincristine	Hair loss Neuropathy Constipation
Dactinomycin	Nausea, vomiting Bone marrow suppression
Doxorubicin	Nausea, vomiting Hair loss Red urine Bone marrow suppression Cardiac dysfunction

2. Perform a physical examination that includes the following:
   a. Assessment for associated anomalies: aniridia, hemihypertrophy of the spine, or cryptorchidism.
   b. Palpation of lymph nodes for enlargement, tenderness, and mobility.
   c. Palpation of the liver and spleen for enlargement.
   d. Palpation of the abdomen to determine the size and location of the tumor.
   e. Auscultation of the lungs to assess breath sounds or abnormality because of spread of tumor.
3. Assess coping, resources, and emotional state of the family.

NURSING ALERT Avoid indiscriminate manipulation of the abdomen preoperatively and postoperatively to decrease the danger of metastasis. Because the tumor is soft and highly vascular, seeding may occur with excessive palpation or handling of the child's abdomen.

Nursing Diagnoses

- Anxiety of parents related to learning of diagnosis.
- Fear of child related to surgery and diagnostic tests.
- Risk for Deficient Fluid Volume postoperatively.
- Acute Pain related to surgery and possible progression of the disease.
- Imbalanced Nutrition: Less than Body Requirements related to anemia, anorexia, nausea, vomiting, and mucosal ulceration secondary to chemotherapy or radiation.
- Disturbed Body Image related to alopecia associated with chemotherapy.
- Activity Intolerance related to fatigue that results from the size of the tumor and treatment.
- Risk for Infection and hemorrhage related to bone marrow suppression caused by chemotherapy.

Nursing Interventions

Reducing Parents' Anxiety
See previous sections, pages 1356 and 1359.

Reducing the Child's Fear and Anxiety
See previous sections, pages 1357 and 1360.

Preventing Fluid Volume Deficit and Other Complications
1. Insert a nasogastric tube, as ordered. Many children require gastric suction postoperatively to prevent distention or vomiting.
2. Monitor gastric output accurately and replace it with the appropriate IV fluids, as ordered.
3. When bowel sounds have returned, begin with small amounts of clear fluids.
4. Keep accurate intake and output record.
5. Monitor vital signs as the child's condition warrants and check the surgical dressing frequently for drainage.

Relieving Pain
See previous sections, pages 1357 and 1360.

Promoting Optimal Nutrition
See previous sections, pages 1357 and 1360.

Promoting Acceptance of Body Changes
See previous sections, pages 1356 and 1360.

Increasing Activity Tolerance
See previous section, page 1357.

Preventing Infection
See previous sections, pages 1356 and 1360.

Family Education and Health Maintenance

1. Teach parents of children with one kidney the signs and symptoms of kidney disease.
2. Advise parents to call the health care provider if the child has a fever of more than 101°F (38.3°C), bleeding, signs of infections, or has been exposed to chickenpox.
3. Teach measures to prevent infection, such as hand washing and isolation from children with communicable disease.
4. Refer families to resources such as Candlelighters (*www.candlelighters.org*).

Evaluation: Expected Outcomes

- Parents discuss their feelings about diagnosis and treatment.
- Expresses feelings during play and participates in playroom activities.
- Has no abdominal distention or vomiting, vital signs stable.
- Verbalizes relief from pain.
- Eats adequate calories to maintain weight, nausea relieved by antiemetics.
- Plays with others without notice to alopecia.
- Participates in all normal daily activities without fatigue.
- Remains afebrile, no signs of local infection.

Osteosarcoma

 EVIDENCE BASE American Cancer Society. (2018). Atlanta, GA. Osteosarcoma: Early detection, diagnosis, and staging. Available: *https://www.cancer.org/cancer/osteosarcoma/detection-diagnosis-staging.html*.
Rothermundt, C., Seddon, B. M., Dileo, P., Strauss, S. J., et al. (2016). Follow-up practices for high-grade extremity osteosarcoma. *BMC Cancer, 16*(1), 301.

Osteosarcoma is a malignant tumor of the bone. It is the most commonly diagnosed primary malignant bone cancer in pediatrics, affecting about 400 children and adolescents ages 0 to 19 years annually. The incidence of osteosarcoma increases with age throughout childhood and adolescents, but then decreases. It commonly affects adolescents during the growth spurt when bones and soft tissue are already vulnerable because of the developmental process, with the majority of cases occurring between the ages of 8 and 25 years. Osteosarcoma is very rare among children younger than 5 years of age. The 5-year relative survival rate of osteosarcoma is 70%. It is the most common secondary malignancy among retinoblastoma survivors. The incidence of osteosarcoma is slightly higher in males than in females, and also higher in African American and Latino children compared with white and Asian/Pacific Islander children. It is somewhat more likely to affect males than females.

Pathophysiology and Etiology

1. Etiology is unknown. Risk factors may include prior radiation treatment for another tumor, taller children, and genetic syndromes.
2. Presumably arises from bone-forming mesenchymal tissue.
3. Produces malignant spindle cell stroma, which gives rise to malignant osteoid tissue.
4. Common sites of occurrence are in the metaphysis of long bones, such as distal femur, proximal tibia, and proximal humerus. Less common sites include the skull, pelvis, phalanges, and jaw.
5. Most commonly metastasizes to lungs and other bones.

Clinical Manifestations

1. Sporadic pain in the affected site, frequently causing limp, stiffness, or limited range of motion.
2. Pain may worsen at night or with activity.
3. A painless swelling or noticeable and palpable, tender, fixed bony mass often in the arm or leg.
4. A broken bone that occurs without injury.
5. Additional symptoms related to site of metastasis, if present.

Diagnostic Evaluation

1. Radiographic examination of lesion is conducted to visualize the tumor.
2. A biopsy of the lesion is conducted to confirm the diagnosis and to provide histologic data for the selection of a treatment plan.
3. CT and MRI are helpful to assess internal tumor composition and to evaluate local extent of disease prior to surgery.
4. Chest x-ray may be done to detect pulmonary metastases.
5. Bone scan is helpful in detecting the initial extent of malignancy, planning therapy, and evaluating effects of treatment.
6. Renal and liver function tests should be monitored to observe for elevated serum lactate dehydrogenase (LD).
7. Arteriography may be a possibility if limb salvage procedure is a consideration.

Management

1. Surgery—procedures fall into two categories:
   a. Limb salvage procedure is priority—greater than 80% of tumors can be treated with limb salvage surgery.
   b. Radical amputation of the affected extremity and, commonly, the joint proximal to the involved area.
2. The type of surgery performed depends on tumor location, size, extramedullary extent, distant metastasis, age of child, skeletal development, as well as preferences regarding lifestyle and quality of life.
3. Chemotherapy is necessary following surgery because the majority of patients treated with local therapy alone develop distant metastases within several years. Chemotherapy agents, such as methotrexate with leucovorin, cyclophosphamide, cisplatin, doxorubicin, and ifosfamide, are also used preoperatively for patients who undergo resection surgery and for the treatment of metastatic disease (see Table 51-5).
4. Survival has greatly improved with the aggressive use of multimodal therapy.
5. With current treatment, the 5-year survival rate for people with localized osteosarcoma is approximately 70% for those who undergo surgery followed by chemotherapy.
6. Important prognostic factors are extent of disease at diagnosis, age, gender, serum LD, and amount of tumor necrosis at the time of surgery. Osteosarcomas arising in previously irradiated areas have a worse prognosis.
7. Limb salvage surgery has improved the quality of life for many survivors.
8. Patients with relapse to lung may still be curable with surgical excision.

Complications

1. Metastasis to the lung and bones.
2. Later metastasis to the CNS and lymph nodes.
3. Treatment-induced hearing loss.
4. Physical limitations resulting from surgical resection.

Table 51-5	Commonly Used Chemotherapeutic Agents to Treat Osteosarcoma
CHEMOTHERAPY	**COMMON SIDE EFFECTS**
Doxorubicin	Nausea, vomiting Hair loss Red urine Bone marrow suppression Cardiac dysfunction
Cisplatin	Nausea, vomiting Bone marrow suppression Hypomagnesemia Loss of appetite Hearing loss Renal dysfunction
Methotrexate	Elevated liver enzymes Mucositis Nephrotoxicity
Etoposide	Nausea, vomiting Hair loss Weakness Bone marrow suppression
Ifosfamide	Nausea, vomiting Hair loss Bone marrow suppression Gonadal dysfunction Renal dysfunction

Nursing Assessment

1. Obtain a history.
   a. Inquire about how and when symptoms first presented as well as the duration of symptoms.
   b. Determine whether the child has pain or limitation of motion in the affected area.
2. Perform a physical examination, including:
   a. Palpation of the mass to determine the size and location. (Determine whether the mass is tender or is fixed to the bone.)
   b. Palpation of other bones to check for metastasis.
   c. Auscultation of the lungs to assess breath sounds or other abnormalities caused by spread of tumor.
3. Assess family coping, resources such as support systems, and emotional state of the patient and parents.
4. Assess degree of mobility, especially for lower extremity tumors.

Nursing Diagnoses

- Anxiety of parents related to learning of diagnosis.
- Fear of child or adolescent related to surgery, diagnostic tests, and treatment.
- Disturbed Body Image related to surgery and possible amputation and alopecia associated with chemotherapy.
- Acute Pain related to surgery and possible progression of the disease.
- Imbalanced Nutrition: Less than Body Requirements related to anemia, anorexia, nausea, vomiting, and mucosal ulceration caused by chemotherapy.
- Risk for Infection related to surgery or bone marrow suppression secondary to chemotherapy.
- Impaired Mobility due to surgery or disease.
- Risk for Injury due to pathologic fractures related to the diagnosis.

Nursing Interventions

Reducing Parents' Anxiety

1. Involve the parents in the teaching plan and make sure they know what to expect before going to surgery.
2. Explain to the parent about the disease process and available treatment options.
3. Provide parents with strategies related to effective coping with the diagnosis and postoperative care.
4. Provide parents with positive reinforcement, honesty, and transparency in the care process.
5. Encourage the parent to participate in the care process to prepare for discharge.

Reducing the Adolescent's Fear and Anxiety

1. Incorporate the adolescent's developmental level when explaining diagnostic tests and postoperative care.
2. Support and prepare the child for routine surgical care or care of the amputated limb.
3. If an amputation will be done, teach the child about the need for physical therapy for exercises and to learn crutch walking and the need for a prosthesis.
4. If limb salvage surgery will be done, reinforce the importance of physical therapy exercises following surgery to restore as much function as possible to the affected bone and/or joint.
5. Nursing care of the adolescent with osteosarcoma is the same as care of the adult.

Promoting Acceptance of New Self-Image

1. Understand that adolescents need time and support to accept the diagnosis and the surgery and to grieve for their lost body part if an amputation is done.
2. Try to introduce the adolescent to another adolescent with the same diagnosis who has undergone similar treatment.
3. Suggest the selection of clothing that will camouflage the prosthesis and be fashionable and appealing.
4. Suggest wigs, scarves, or hats for adolescents who experience hair loss because of chemotherapy.
5. Encourage visits by peers and help the child to deal with questions and reactions from peers.

Relieving Pain

See previous sections, pages 1357 and 1360.

Promoting Optimal Nutrition

See previous sections, pages 1357 and 1360.

Preventing Infection and Hemorrhage

See previous sections, pages 1356 to 1357 and 1360.

Community and Home Care Considerations

1. Assess the home for accessibility of adolescent who has had an amputation.
2. Educate parents about changes they may need to make in the home.
3. Encourage the parents to contact the school system to arrange for a tutor for a student who needs to remain out of school for a lengthy period.
4. Assist the parents in contacting the school nurse to facilitate reentry into the classroom.
5. Identify any financial concerns that may be associated with care and treatment and refer patients to a social worker or case manager to access community services and resources.

Family Education and Health Maintenance

1. Teach adolescents and parents about infection control measures, such as good hand washing and preventing exposure to children with communicable diseases, because chemotherapy is usually long term.
2. Parents and adolescents should be instructed about chemotherapy medications used and their potential adverse effects.
3. Teach parents and adolescents about the radiation procedure and effects.
4. Advise the adolescent to protect a leg that has received radiation treatment by avoiding excessive pressure on the leg through sports. Consult orthopedic specialist for appropriate activity limitations.
5. Teach parents measures to ensure safety of patient throughout treatment and convalescence.
6. Refer families to resources such as Candlelighters (*www.candlelighters.org*).

Evaluation: Expected Outcomes

- Parents and child (if age appropriate) discuss feelings about surgery and chemotherapy treatments.
- Parents and child (if age appropriate) verbalizes feelings about surgery and asks questions.
- Looks in mirror, touches amputation site.
- Parents and child (if age appropriate) verbalizes relief from pain.
- Maintains an adequate eating pattern, nausea relieved by antiemetics.
- Remains afebrile, vital signs stable, no signs of bleeding.
- Maintains skin integrity.

Retinoblastoma

 EVIDENCE BASE Chantada, G., & Schaiquevich, P. (2015). Management of retinoblastoma in children: Current status. *Pediatric Drugs, 17*(3), 185–198.
Mendoza, P. R., & Grossniklaus, H. E. (2016). Therapeutic options for retinoblastoma. *Cancer Control, 23*(2), 99–109.
National Cancer Institute. (2018). Retinoblastoma treatment (PDQ)—Health professional version. Available: *https://www.cancer.gov/types/retinoblastoma/hp/retinoblastoma-treatment-pdq*.

Retinoblastoma is a malignant, congenital tumor, arising in the retina of one or both eyes. It accounts for about 3% of the cancers occurring in children younger than 15 years, and approximately 1 in 14,000 to 18,000 live births; this rate of diagnosis is consistent worldwide. Median age of diagnosis is age 2 years and it is rarely diagnosed after age 6 years.

Pathophysiology and Etiology

1. Most cases appear sporadically and have been associated with advanced paternal age; there is also an inherited form of the disease.
   a. Nonhereditary somatic mutations account for approximately 70% to 75% of all retinoblastomas; always demonstrate unilateral involvement.
   b. All bilateral cases are heritable.
      i. Mode of inheritance is autosomal dominant.
      ii. Offspring of affected individuals have a 50% chance of inheriting the disease.
2. Can be associated with chromosomal aberrations.
3. Usually arise in multiple foci rather than a single tumor from any of the nucleated retinal layers.
4. Some tumors (endophytic type) arise in the internal nuclear layers of the retina and grow forward into the vitreous cavity.

5. Some tumors (exophytic type) arise in the external nuclear layer and grow into the subretinal space, with detachment of the retina.
6. Most tumors have a combination of endophytic and exophytic growth.
7. Extension of the tumor may occur into the choroid, sclera, and optic nerve.
8. "Trilateral retinoblastoma" is the presence of bilateral retinoblastoma in addition to an intracranial midline neuroblastic tumor.
9. Hematogenous spread of the tumor may occur to the bone marrow, skeleton, lymph nodes, and liver.
10. Tumor staging reflects the extent of the disease and the probability of preserving useful vision in the affected eye, from group I (very favorable) to group V (very unfavorable).

Clinical Manifestations

1. Signs and symptoms of an intraocular tumor depend on its size and position.
2. "Cat's-eye reflex"—whitish appearance of the pupil (leukocoria) represents visualization of the tumor through the lens as light falls on the tumor mass—most common sign. Also characterized by the absence of red reflex on photographs.
3. Strabismus—second most common presenting sign.
4. Other occasional presenting signs:
   a. Orbital inflammation, eye pain.
   b. Hyphema, bulging of the eye.
   c. Fixed pupil.
   d. Heterochromia iridis—different colors of each iris or in the same iris.
5. Vision loss is not a symptom because young children do not complain of unilaterally decreased vision.
6. Symptoms of distant metastasis—anorexia, weight loss, vomiting, headache, bone pain.

Diagnostic Evaluation

1. Bilateral indirect ophthalmoscopy under general anesthesia.
2. Ultrasonography and CT or MRI of head and eyes to visualize tumor.
3. Bone marrow aspiration and lumbar puncture under anesthesia to determine metastasis.

Management

1. Depends on the stage of the disease at the time of diagnosis.
2. Unilateral tumors in stages I, II, or III are usually treated with intraocular and systemic chemotherapy.
   a. Goal of treatment is to eradicate the tumors, prevent systemic metastasis, promote resolution of retinal detachment, preserve useful vision, if possible, and control the malignancy to prevent enucleation or eye removal.
   b. Most common chemotherapies are carboplatin, cyclophosphamide, doxorubicin, platinum, etoposide, and vincristine (see Table 51-6). Melphalan is often the medication of choice for intra-arterial chemotherapy for children with advanced disease.
   c. Periocular injections of topotecan can also reduce retinoblastoma tumor burden when given systemically, via intra-arterial, or via intravitreal injections because it avoids the retinal toxicity of other chemotherapy agents.
3. Surgery (enucleation) is the treatment of choice for advanced tumor growth, especially with optic nerve involvement when no hope exists for useful vision.

Table 51-6	Commonly Used Chemotherapeutic Agents to Treat Retinoblastoma
CHEMOTHERAPEUTIC AGENT	**COMMON SIDE EFFECTS**
Carboplatin	Nausea, vomiting Bone marrow suppression Electrolyte imbalance
Vincristine	Hair loss Neuropathy Constipation

4. Bilateral disease usually requires enucleation of the severely diseased eye and treatment of the least affected eye.
   a. Every attempt is made to salvage whatever vision there may be.
   b. Bilateral enucleation is indicated with extensive bilateral retinoblastoma when no hope of vision exists.
5. Focal laser treatments such as photocoagulation, plaque brachytherapy, thermotherapy, and cryotherapy are sometimes used to treat small, localized tumors.
6. External beam radiotherapy can be used to treat eyes unresponsive to other treatments.
7. Novel treatment options are being explored, including gene therapy and autologous stem cell rescue. Gene therapy is a type of therapy that introduces a viral or bacterial gene into tumor cells, thus allowing the conversion of a nontoxic compound into a lethal drug to kill the tumor cells. However, it is unlikely that this type of gene therapy could be used as first-line treatment for retinoblastoma.
8. Overall survival rate is high (90%).
9. Heritable retinoblastoma and bilateral retinoblastoma are associated with a high incidence of spontaneous and radiation-related new tumors, particularly sarcomas.

Complications

1. Spread to brain and other eye.
2. Metastasis to bone, bone marrow, liver, and lymph nodes.
3. Risk for secondary tumors, including osteosarcomas, soft tissue sarcomas, and melanomas.

Nursing Assessment

1. Obtain a history.
   a. Ask about a family history that is positive for retinoblastoma or other types of cancer.
   b. Inquire about when symptoms began and strabismus, cat's-eye reflex, orbital inflammation, vomiting, or headache.
2. Perform a physical examination.
   a. Assess pupils for reactivity of light, size, and leukocoria.
   b. Evaluate strabismus when checking muscle balance.
   c. Assess eyes for associated signs, such as erythema, inflammation of the orbit, hyphema, and heterochromia iridis.
3. Assess family's ability to cope, to use support systems, and to communicate feelings.

Nursing Diagnoses

- Anxiety of parents related to the diagnosis, treatment, and genetic implications of the diagnosis.
- Impaired Tissue Integrity related to skin changes, loss of lashes, fat atrophy, impaired bone growth, and dryness caused by radiation.
- Fear of child related to hospitalization and to diagnostic and treatment procedures.

- Disturbed Body Image and Ineffective Coping related to enucleation and need for an eye prosthesis.
- Impaired Sensory Perception (Visual) related to disease process or enucleation.

Nursing Interventions

Decreasing Parental Anxiety and Guilt

1. Listen to the parental feelings of guilt about transmitting the disease to the child or because they did not notice symptoms earlier.
2. Discuss the benefit of consultation about the probability of having another affected child.
   a. Risk ranges from approximately 1% to 10%, depending on family history and whether the affected child had unilateral or bilateral disease.
   b. The reportedly high lifelong cancer burden among retinoblastoma patients may also be important to parents in making informed decisions.
   c. Refer for genetic counseling and support parental decisions regarding future pregnancies.
3. Encourage the parents to seek genetic counseling for the affected child when he or she reaches puberty.
   a. The risk to offspring is from 1% to 50%, depending on family history and whether disease was unilateral or bilateral.
   b. Among affected offspring, there is a high probability (greater than 50%) of bilateral disease.

Preserving Tissue Integrity

1. Administer sedatives or assist with anesthesia for intraocular chemotherapy, if necessary.
   a. Administer the medication in a timely manner so that sedation is adequate for positioning of the child.
2. Observe for possible adverse effects of chemotherapy and prepare the parents for their occurrence.
   a. Swelling and edema surrounding the intraocular chemotherapy site.
   b. Nausea and vomiting with systemic chemotherapy.

Reducing the Child's Anxiety and Fear

See also previous sections about reducing child's anxiety and fear.
1. Encourage the parents to room in and participate in the child's care to minimize separation anxiety.
2. Prepare the child and parents for all diagnostic procedures.
3. Describe the surgery and anticipated postoperative appearance of the child. Draw pictures or use a doll, if one is available.
   a. A surgically implanted sphere maintains the shape of the eyeball.
   b. The child's face may be edematous and ecchymotic.
4. Offer the family the opportunity to talk with another parent who has gone through the experience or to see pictures of another child with an artificial eye.
5. See "Nursing management of eye enucleation," pages 439 to 440.

Promoting Acceptance of Prosthesis

1. Explain to the child the changes related to losing the diseased eye, having a bandaged orbit until it heals after surgery, and receiving a prosthetic eye.
2. Explain that the prosthesis will be made for him or her and will look like the removed eye.
3. Tell parents to expect the child to grieve the loss and to help him or her by talking about it, but to treat the child as the same person.

Minimizing Effects of Vision Loss

1. Maintain a safe, uncluttered environment for the child.
2. Orient the child to the surrounding environment.
3. Hold the child frequently and stand close, within child's field of vision, while speaking or providing care.
4. Encourage the use of touch and other senses for exploring.
5. Set environmental limits so that the child feels safe and can obtain help easily.

Family Education and Health Maintenance

1. Teach care of the orbit.
2. Teach care of the prosthesis—initial instructions are provided by the ocularist and should be reinforced by the nurse.
3. Advise protection of the remaining eye from accidental injury, such as wearing safety glass for sports, not putting sharp objects near eye, treating eye infections promptly.
4. Encourage maintenance of routine checkups for eye and medical care.
5. Stress need to have subsequent children carefully evaluated for retinoblastoma.
   a. An ophthalmologic examination under anesthesia is usually recommended at approximately age 2 months.
   b. The child should receive frequent examinations thereafter until judged safe from developing retinoblastoma, usually approximately age 3 years.
6. Refer families to resources such as Candlelighters (*www.candlelighters.org*).

Evaluation: Expected Outcomes

- Parents discuss feelings openly, show affection to the child.
- Parents describe possible adverse effects of radiation and how to care for skin around eyes.
- Demonstrates lessened anxiety by participating in age-appropriate activities.
- Shows acceptance of the prosthesis and not inhibited in behavior.
- Moves about environment with ease.

SELECTED REFERENCES

American Cancer Society. (2014). Cancer facts and figures: Special section: Cancer in children and adolescents. Available: *https://www.cancer.org/content/dam/cancer-org/research/cancer-facts-and-statistics/annual-cancer-facts-and-figures/2014/special-section-cancer-in-children-and-adolescents-cancer-facts-and-figures-2014.pdf*

American Cancer Society. (2018). Cancer facts and figures. Atlanta, GA. Available: *https://www.cancer.org/content/dam/cancer-org/research/cancer-facts-and-statistics/annual-cancer-facts-and-figures/2018/cancer-facts-and-figures-2018.pdf*

American Cancer Society. (2018). Retinoblastoma: Early detection, diagnosis, and staging. Atlanta, GA. Available: *https://www.cancer.org/cancer/retinoblastoma/detection-diagnosis-staging.html*

American Cancer Society. (2018). What are the key statistics about Wilms tumor? Atlanta, GA. Available: *https://www.cancer.org/cancer/wilms-tumor/about/key-statistics.html*

Arpaci, T., Toruner, E., & Altay, N. (2018). Assessment of Nutritional Problems in Pediatric Patients with Cancer and the Informational Needs of Their Parents: A Parental Perspective. *Asia-Pacific Journal of Oncology Nursing, 5*(2), 231–236.

Barbel, P., & Peterson, K. (2015). Recognizing subtle signs and symptoms of pediatric cancer. *Nursing, 45*(40), 30–37.

Bekiesinska-Figatowska, M., Duczkowska, A., Duczkowski, M., et al. (2017). CNS metastases from bone and soft tissue sarcomas in children, adolescents, and young adults: Are they really so rare? *BioMed Research International, 2017.* doi: 10.1155/2017/1456473.

Bozlu, G., & Çıtak, E. Ç. (2018). Evaluation of renal tumors in children. *Turkish journal of urology, 44*(3), 268–273.

Brandowicki, P., Vessey, J., Temple, K., et al. (2016). Building bridges from hospital to home. *Journal of Pediatric Oncology Nursing, 33*(5), 370–377.

Caselli, D., Tamburini, A., LaTorre, A., et al. (2014). High dose chemotherapy with autologous stem cell rescue for treatment of retinoblastoma: Report of five cases. *Pediatric Transplantation, 18*(6), 631–636.

Chantada, G., & Schaiquevich, P. (2015). Management of retinoblastoma in children: Current status. *Pediatric Drugs, 17*(3), 185–198.

Fabian, I. D., Onadim, Z., Karaa, E. E., et al. (2018). The management of retinoblastoma. *Oncogene, 37*(12), 1551–1560.

Haddox, C. L., Han, G., Anijar, L., et al. (2014). Osteosarcoma in pediatric patients and young adults: a single institution retrospective review of presentation, therapy, and outcome. *Sarcoma,* 2014. doi: 10.1155/2014/402509.

Hunger, S. P., & Mullighan, C. G. (2015). Acute lymphoblastic leukemia in children. *New England Journal of Medicine, 373*(16), 1541–1552.

Jaradat, I., Mubiden, R., Salem, A., et al. (2012). High-dose chemotherapy followed by stem cell transplantation in the management of retinoblastoma: a systematic review. *Hematology/oncology and stem cell therapy, 5*(2), 107–117.

Kline, N. (Ed.). (2014). *Essentials of pediatric oncology nursing: A core curriculum* (4th ed.). Glenview, IL: Association of Pediatric Hematology/Oncology Nurses.

Linder, L., Gerdy, C., Abouzelof, R., et al. (2017). Using practice-based evidence to improve supportive care practices to /reduce central line-associated bloodstream infections in a pediatric oncology unit. *Journal of Pediatric Oncology Nursing, 34*(3), 185–195.

Margonari, H., & Hannah, M. (2017). Quality improvement initiative on pain knowledge, assessment, and documentation skills of pediatric nurses. *Pediatric Nursing, 43*(2), 65–70.

Meel, R., Radhakrishnan, V., & Bakhshi, S. (2012). Current therapy and recent advances in the management of retinoblastoma. *Indian Journal of Medical and Paediatric Oncology, 33*(2), 80.

Mendoza, P. R., & Grossniklaus, H. E. (2016). Therapeutic options for retinoblastoma. *Cancer Control, 23*(2), 99–109.

Mercadante, S., & Giarratano, A. (2014). Pharmacological management of cancer pain in children. Critical Reviews in Oncology/Hematology, *91*(1), 93–97.

National Cancer Institute. (2017). Childhood acute lymphoblastic leukemia treatment (PDQ)—Health professional version. Available: *www.cancer.gov/types/leukemia/hp/child-all-treatment-pdq*.

National Cancer Institute. (2017). Childhood astrocytomas treatment (PDQ)—Health professional version. Available: *www.cancer.gov/types/brain/hp/child-astrocytoma-treatment-pdq/*.

National Cancer Institute. (2017). Neuroblastoma treatment (PDQ)—Health professional version. Available: *www.cancer.gov/types/neuroblastoma/hp/neuroblastoma-treatment-pdq*.

National Cancer Institute. (2018). Retinoblastoma treatment (PDQ)--Health professional version. Available: *https://www.cancer.gov/types/retinoblastoma/hp/retinoblastoma-treatment-pdq*.

National Cancer Institute. (2017). Childhood rhabdomyosarcoma treatment (PDQ)—Health professional version. Available: *www.cancer.gov/types/soft-tissue-sarcoma/hp/rhabdomyosarcoma-treatment-pdq*.

National Cancer Institute. (2016). Wilms' tumor and other childhood kidney tumors treatment (PDQ)—Health professional version. Available: *www.cancer.gov/types/kidney/hp/wilms-treatment-pdq*.

Palma, J., Sasso, D. F., Dufort, G., et al. (2012). Successful treatment of metastatic retinoblastoma with high-dose chemotherapy and autologous stem cell rescue in South America. *Bone Marrow Transplantation, 47*(4), 522–527.

Parida, L. (2014). Nonurological malignancies in children. *Journal of Indian Association of Pediatric Surgeons, 19*(1), 31.

Paul, S. P., Perrow, R., & Webster, M. A. (2014). Brain tumours in children: Reducing time to diagnosis: Siba Prosad Paul and colleagues discuss the role of emergency nurses in the acute management of brain tumours in children and young people. *Emergency Nurse, 22*(1), 32–36.

Pinto, N. R., Applebaum, M. A., Volchenboum, S, et al. (2015). Advances in risk classification and treatment strategies for neuroblastoma. *Journal of Clinical Oncology, 33*(27), 3008–3017.

Romao, R. L., & Cox, A. (2018). Urological issues arising after treatment of pediatric malignancies. *Canadian Urological Association Journal, 12*(4 Suppl 1), S37–S41.

Rothermundt, C., Seddon, B. M., Dileo, P., et al. (2016). Follow-up practices for high-grade extremity osteosarcoma. *BMC Cancer, 16*(1), 301.

Salazar, B. M., Balczewski, E. A., Ung, C. Y., et al. (2016). Neuroblastoma, a Paradigm for Big Data Science in Pediatric Oncology. *International Journal of Molecular Sciences, 18*(1), 37.

Selwood, K., Hemsworth, S., & Rigg, J. (2013). Children with cancer: Quality of information for returning to school: Karen Selwood and colleagues discuss the importance of reintegration and why families need consistent guidance from healthcare professionals. *Nursing Children and Young People, 25*(5), 14–18.

Skalet, A. H., Gombos, D. S., Gallie, B. L., et al. (2018). Screening children at risk for retinoblastoma: Consensus report from the American association of ophthalmic oncologists and pathologists. *Ophthalmology, 125*(3), 453–458.

Ward, E., DeSantis, C., Robbins, A., et al. (2014). Childhood and adolescent cancer statistics, 2014. *CA: A Cancer Journal for Clinicians, 64*(2), 83–103.

Wiffen, P. J., Cooper, T. E., Anderson, A. K., et al. (2017). Opioids for cancer-related pain in children and adolescents. *The Cochrane Library,* (7), CD012564.

52

Pediatric Hematologic Disorders

PEDIATRIC HEMATOLOGIC DISORDERS

Anemia

 EVIDENCE BASE Cadet, M. (2018). Iron deficiency anemia: A clinical case study. *MEDSURG Nursing*, 27(2), 108–120.

Anemia refers to lower than normal number of red blood cells (RBCs) or hemoglobin (Hb) in the blood. Hb is a main part of the red blood cell and binds oxygen. Anemia results in decreased oxygen-carrying capacity of the red blood cell. It is the most frequent hematologic disorder encountered in children. Approximately 2% of the normal population is anemic.

Pathophysiology and Etiology

1. RBCs and Hb are normally formed at the same rate at which they are destroyed. The function of the RBC is to deliver oxygen from the lungs to the tissues and carbon dioxide from the tissues to the lung. This is accomplished by the use of hemoglobin. In anemia, there is a decrease in the number of RBCs transporting oxygen and carbon dioxide.
2. May be caused by blood loss related to:
   a. Trauma and ulceration.
   b. Decreased production of platelets.
   c. Increased destruction of platelets.
   d. Decreased number of clotting factors.
3. May be caused by impairment of RBC production caused by nutritional deficiency. This impairment includes poverty, malnutrition (including strict vegan and vegetarian diets), and certain intestinal/medical conditions.
   a. Iron deficiency—the most common type of anemia in ages 6 months to 3 years.
   b. Folate deficiency—causes formation of large RBCs with abnormal nuclear maturation (megaloblastic anemia).
   c. Vitamin B_{12} deficiency—causes megaloblastic anemia (deficiency in vitamin B_{12}, folate, or both); called *pernicious anemia* if because of lack of intrinsic factor for

absorption of vitamin B_{12}; intestinal diseases such as celiac disease.
   d. Vitamin B_6 deficiency.
   e. Excessive milk intake.
   f. Certain prescription medications (ie, antiseizure drugs, antacids).
   g. Lead poisoning—lead absorbed by the bone marrow attaches to newly formed RBCs and inhibits synthesis of heme. This results in the decrease in circulating Hb.
   h. Vitamin C deficiency.
4. May be caused by decreased erythrocyte production. This occurs in the bone marrow and stem cells.
   a. Pure RBC anemia.
   b. Secondary hemolytic anemias associated with chronic infection, renal disease, and drugs. In anemia of chronic infection and inflammation, the life span of the RBC is moderately decreased, and the ability of the bone marrow to produce RBCs is significantly decreased.
   c. Bone marrow depression—leukemia, aplastic anemias, and transient erythrocytopenia of childhood.
5. May be caused by increased erythrocyte destruction.
   a. Extrinsic factors:
      i. Drugs and chemicals (ie, acetaminophen, ibuprofen, antibiotic such as penicillin's).
      ii. Infections—transient erythroblastopenia of childhood caused by parvovirus (fifth disease), usually between ages 6 months and 4 years.
      iii. Antibody reactions—passively acquired antibodies against Rh, A, or B isoimmunization (transfusion of ABO incompatible blood), autoimmune disorders, burns, and poisons (including lead poisoning).
   b. Intrinsic factors:
      i. Abnormalities of the RBC membrane.
      ii. Enzymatic defects—glucose-6-phosphate dehydrogenase deficiency.
      iii. Abnormal Hb synthesis—sickle cell disease and thalassemia syndromes. These result in defective RBC production.

c. In hemolytic anemias, the RBCs are destroyed at abnormally high rates, primarily by the spleen. The normal life span of an RBC is 120 days. RBCs are sequestered and destroyed in the spleen.

   i. The activity of the bone marrow increases to compensate for the shortened survival time of the RBCs.

   ii. The bone marrow hypertrophies and occupies a larger than normal share of the inner structure of the bones.

   iii. Products of RBC breakdown increase with hemolysis. If chronic, this may lead to increased excretion of bilirubin into the biliary tract causing gallstones.

   iv. Jaundice results when the conversion of Hb to bilirubin exceeds the liver's capacity.

   v. Iron builds up (hemosiderosis) and may deposit on body tissues.

6. May result from chronic illness such as rheumatoid arthritis, Crohn disease, lupus, and other inflammatory disorders (anemia of chronic disease).

7. "Physiologic anemia" occurs in term infants at ages 8 to 12 weeks; Hb should be between 9 and 11 g/dL. In mild anemia of prematurity, recovery may occur 3 to 6 months after birth.

Clinical Manifestations

1. Condition may be acute or chronic. The more slowly the onset of anemia, the less likely the patient will be symptomatic.
2. Early symptoms:
   a. Fatigue and loss of energy.
   b. Dizziness or lightheadedness.
   c. Low appetite.
3. Late symptoms:
   a. Pallor.
   b. Weakness.
   c. Tachycardia.
   d. Palpitations.
   e. Tachypnea and shortness of breath on exertion.
   f. PICA.
   g. Insomnia.
   h. Cold hands and feet.
   i. Leg cramps.
   j. Tingling or numbness in hands and/or feet.
   k. Jaundice (with hemolytic anemias).

Diagnostic Evaluation

1. Complete blood count (CBC) with mean corpuscular volume (MCV), mean corpuscular hemoglobin concentration (MCHC), and iron indices—vary with types of anemia (see Table 52-1).

2. Serum iron and total iron-binding capacity—ratio of less than 0.2.
3. Serum ferritin—less than 12 g/dL.
4. Lead—greater than 10 g/dL.
5. Free erythrocyte protoporphyrin—greater than 35 g/dL.
6. B_{12}, B_6, and folate levels—may be decreased.
7. Hb electrophoresis—may show Hb S or other abnormalities.
8. Parvovirus B19 titer—may be elevated in transient erythroblastopenia.
9. Coombs test—shows whether your body is making antibodies to destroy RBCs.
10. Haptoglobin, bilirubin, and liver function tests.
11. Testing for G6PD deficiency.
12. Hemoglobin electrophoresis.

Management

Iron Deficiency Anemia

1. Oral iron at a dose of 3- to 6-mg elemental iron/kg per day divided one to three times daily. Reticulocyte count should increase in 7 to 10 days; Hct increases in approximately 4 weeks. Should not be given on an empty stomach; should be given 1 to 2 hours before or after meals; do not give with milk. Vitamin C–containing juice may improve absorption but is not essential.
2. Dietary: decrease milk intake to 16 to 24 ounces per day; include iron-fortified cereals and bread products; increase consumption of red meat; include foods rich in vitamin C; increase green, leafy vegetables.
3. Good sources of iron: red meat, beans, egg yolks, whole grain products, nuts, seafood, spinach, and dark green leafy vegetables.
4. Typically requires a minimum of 3 months of therapy. Treatment on average is 3 to 6 months.
5. Blood transfusion through an IV is not recommended in the setting of chronic anemia other than in hemoglobinopathy patients (genetic mutation of Hb molecule).

Anemia of Chronic Lead Poisoning

See page 1136.

1. Early detection of high lead levels through patient questionaires and blood tests. The CDC defines elevated blood level as greater than or equal to 5 mg/dL.
2. Maintenance of a well-balanced diet, high in calcium and vitamin D.
3. Administration of chelating agents such as edetate disodium calcium, dimercaprol, or succimer according to recommendations of the Centers for Disease Control and Prevention. Only used when blood levels are greater than 45 secondary to depletion of essential nutrients such as calcium, iron, and zinc.

Table 52-1	Blood Tests in Anemia by Cause				
	MCV	**MCHC**	**RETICULOCYTE**	**FERRITIN**	**FEP**
Iron deficiency	Low	Low	Low	Low	High
Lead poisoning	Low	Low	Low	Normal	High
β-Thalassemia	Low	Low	Low	Normal	Normal
Folate deficiency	High	Normal	Low	Normal	Normal
B_{12} deficiency	High	Normal	Low	Normal	Normal
Sickle cell disease	Normal	Normal	High	Normal	Normal

FEP, free erythrocyte protoporphyrin; MCHC, mean corpuscular hemoglobin concentration; MCV, mean corpuscular volume.

4. Use of lead-free paints and gasoline. (Lead paint was predominantly used in homes built between 1940 and 1959.)
5. Testing of house and soil.
6. Removal of individuals from unsafe environment.
7. Universal screening of children in vulnerable populations (ie, children who are Medicaid eligible).

Megaloblastic Anemia
1. Folate deficiency—administration of folic acid orally.
2. B_{12} deficiency—administration of B_{12} (cyanocobalamin) IM.

Hemoglobinopathies
1. Sickle cell anemia (see page 1376).
2. Thalassemia (see page 1381).

Transient Erythroblastopenia of Childhood:
1. Median age of presentation is 18 to 26 Months.
2. Spontaneous recovery in 4 to 8 weeks.
3. Packed RBC (PRBC) transfusion recommended in patients with severe signs of clinical decompensation including hemodynamic instability, exercise intolerance, or altered mental status.
4. Usually, unless cardiac failure occurs, supportive care, not therapy, is provided.

Anemia from Blood Loss or Bone Marrow Suppression
PRBC transfusions may be necessary (see page 775).

Complications
1. Mental sluggishness, as a result of decreased oxygen and energy for normal neural activity, usually associated with a decreased attention span, decreased intelligence, and lethargy.
2. Decrease in IQ and neurological development.
3. Long-term behavioral changes.
4. Growth retardation related to anorexia and decreased cellular metabolism.
5. Delayed puberty related to growth retardation.
6. Iron overload.
7. Aplastic crises (in patients with chronic hemolytic anemia).
8. Hypersplenism.
9. Cerebral infarction.
10. Ischemic stroke—most prevalent in children with sickle cell disease.
11. Cardiac enlargement related to muscle hypertrophy because of increased strain on the heart, attempting to compensate for increased oxygen demand by the tissues, and eventually results in heart failure.
12. Studies suggest prolonged lead poisoning can lead to violent and criminal behavior later in life.
13. Death from cardiac failure related to circulatory collapse and shock.

Nursing Assessment
1. Obtain history of potential causes.
   a. Dietary history: including the amount of milk and meat consumed, include vegetarianism, lack of red meat, animal products, or green leafy vegetables.
   b. Family history for genetic causes including blood disorders or diseases.
   c. Medication history: some can increase risk of GI blood loss; others can cause vitamin deficiencies.
   d. Past medical history including chronic diseases that can cause anemia.
   e. Persistent infection, fever, or chronic disease.
   f. Symptoms of shortness of breath, palpitations, fatigue, and headache.
   g. Exercise and athletic endeavors/intolerance.
   h. Cold intolerance.
   i. Pica—craving and consuming nonfood items (eg, paint chips, paper).
   j. Changes in bowel movement habits—constipation, diarrhea, and changes in color and consistency of stool.
   k. Prolonged or heavy menstrual bleeding.
   l. In older children and adolescents—history of alcohol intake.
   m. Socioeconomic status—most common in individuals with low socioeconomic status.
2. Obtain a baseline assessment.
   a. Observe skin and mucous membranes for pallor and jaundice.
   b. Obtain height and weight and plot on growth curve. Observe for tachycardia and tachypnea.
   c. Measure vital signs, including blood pressure (BP).
   d. Assess child's functional level—level of exercise tolerance/intolerance and mental functioning.
   e. Assess attainment of developmental milestones.
   f. Review medication history.
   g. Review history of recent illnesses and surgeries.
3. Observe for fatigue, listlessness, and irritability.
4. Observe for blood loss: bruising, bleeding, hematuria, or hematochezia (blood in stool). Assess for excessive menstrual bleeding in adolescent females.

 NURSING ALERT Be alert for children at risk for iron deficiency anemia—children in rapid growth stages (toddlers and adolescents) and pregnant or lactating adolescents.

Nursing Diagnoses
- Activity Intolerance related to tissue hypoxia.
- Imbalanced Nutrition: less than body requirements of recommended daily dietary allowances and decreased knowledge of nutritional needs.
- Risk for Infection related to decreased hemoglobin.
- Impaired Gas Exchange related to ventilation–perfusion.
- Ineffective Breathing Pattern related to fatigue.
- Anxiety related to hospitalization and painful diagnostic procedures (venipunctures, finger sticks).
- Delayed Growth and Development related to decreased energy.

Nursing Interventions
Minimizing Fatigue
1. Plan nursing care to allow for lengthy periods when the child is not disturbed by hospital routines, procedures, and treatments; set priorities.
2. Observe for early signs of fatigue, such as irritability, hyperactivity, and listlessness.
3. Establish balance between activities and rest.
4. Maintain a well-balanced diet.
5. Maintain hydration by drinking water throughout the day. May drink sports drinks during exercise. Water and sports drinks during exercise prevent dehydration, electrolyte loss, and muscle fatigue.
6. Gradually increased endurance and intensity of exercise.
7. Allow for rest and recovery after exercising.
8. Administer oxygen and position upright if dyspnea is present.
9. Transfuse packed RBCs, as directed.

NURSING ALERT Monitor transfusion for signs and symptoms of reaction: headache, anxiety, chills, dyspnea, chest pain, hypotension, flank pain, rash, hives, bronchospasm, pruritus, hypertension, and more than 1 degree increase in baseline temperature.

Providing Adequate Nutritional Intake

1. Be aware of the child's food preferences and plan diet accordingly.
2. Provide nutritional guidance as to foods that are rich in iron.
3. Offer small amounts of food at frequent intervals.
4. Reward the child for positive attempts to eat.
5. Allow the child to participate in selection of foods.
6. Avoid tiring activities and unpleasant procedures at mealtime.
7. Make mealtime as pleasurable as possible.
8. If iron is ordered, give between meals (2 hours before or after meals) and with orange juice (iron is absorbed best in an acidic environment).
9. Limit milk and milk products to 16 to 24 ounces per day. Milk products inhibit the absorption of oral iron.
10. Administer liquid iron with a dropper or straw or dilute with water or fruit juice to prevent staining the teeth.
    a. If administered by dropper, make sure that liquid iron is deposited in the back of the mouth.
    b. Dental stains can be removed by brushing the teeth with baking soda paste. If the child is resistant, you can put baking soda on a washcloth and rub on the teeth.
11. Be alert for adverse effects of iron supplements—gastric distress, colicky pain, diarrhea, or constipation; may call for decreased dose.
12. Advise family that child's stool may turn dark green or black.
13. Stress the importance of continuing iron therapy according to health care provider's directions, even though the child may not appear to be ill.
14. Inform parents that iron overdoses can be harmful or fatal.

Preventing Infection

1. Teach and assist with good hygiene practices, such as handwashing and mouth care.
2. Avoid exposure to others with colds and infections.
3. Wash vegetable and fruits well before eating.
4. Cook meat until it is well done.
5. Make sure that staff, family, and visitors always wash hands thoroughly.
6. Keep children away from turtles, snakes, and lizards which can carry *Salmonella*.
7. Keep immunizations up to date.
8. Report temperature elevation or other signs of infection.

Impaired Gas Exchange

1. Monitor respiratory rate, depth, and effort.
2. Monitor behavior and mental status for restlessness, agitation, or confusion.
3. Monitor oxygen saturation.
4. Position child with head of bed elevated to improve perfusion.
5. Encourage use of oxygen when necessary. Allow for play therapy to encourage compliance.

Ineffective Breathing Pattern

1. Assess for signs and symptoms of ineffective breathing pattern, that is, shallow respirations and tachypnea.
2. Provide calm and restful environment to reduce fear and anxiety.
3. Provide analgesics if child is in pain.
4. Teach deep breathing techniques through use of incentive spirometer or bubbles.
5. Increase activity as tolerated.
6. Consult a respiratory therapist if necessary.

Reduce Anxiety

1. Provide a calm and supportive environment.
2. Allow the child to handle equipment used for tests and procedures (tourniquets, syringes).
3. Explain all tests, procedures, and the treatment plan in age-appropriate manner.
4. Encourage verbalization of fear and anxiety.
5. Include parents in teaching sessions to encourage their support of the child.

Promoting Normal Growth and Development

1. Make sure that nutrition is adequate for age and activity level.
2. Encourage participation in age-related activities.
3. Encourage bedtime ritual and appropriate hours of sleep.
4. Encourage doing homework and tutored activities.
5. Encourage peer socialization.
6. Promote age-appropriate play and therapeutic play.
7. Provide a support system for child and parents.
8. Perform periodic growth chart evaluation and developmental testing.
    a. Share results with parents and explain the association between diet/anemia and growth and development.
    b. Notify health care provider and make referrals, as indicated.

Family Education and Health Maintenance

1. Stress to the parents the importance of continuing the iron therapy according to the provider's directions even though the child may not appear ill.
2. Stress the need for regular medical and laboratory follow-up to evaluate disease progression and response to therapy.
3. Initiate and reinforce good dietary habits.
    a. Foods rich in iron include dark green leafy vegetables, fortified cereals, dried fruits, nuts, and red meats.
    b. Limit milk intake to 16 to 24 ounces per day. Promote iron-containing foods.
    c. Provide vitamin supplements, if necessary. Vitamin C appears to enhance the absorption of iron.
    d. Explain the reasons for diet change to parents and child in a language they can understand. Visual aids and pictures may be helpful.
    e. Assist the parents to select iron-rich foods that are acceptable to the child, within the family's food budget, and culturally acceptable.
    f. Recognize cultural aspects related to food preference and preparation.
4. Initiate a nutritional consultation, as indicated.
5. Discuss with parents any of the social, economic, and environmental problems that may contribute to the child's disease.
6. Emphasize to the parents the benefits of a referral to a community health nurse if it appears that the family will need support in dealing with the child's chronic disease.
7. Discuss general health measures, including adequate rest, diet, sunshine, and fresh air activity.
8. Encourage regular medical and dental evaluations. Encourage the need for immunizations according to recommended schedule. Emphasize the need for appropriate follow-up visits.
9. Educate regarding infection prevention.

10. Teach the parents how to administer medication.
11. Alert the parents to signs of disease progression—increased fatigue, pallor, weakness, developmental delays, and poor performance in school and activities.
12. Prepare for possible adverse GI effects, including constipation and change in stool color.

 DRUG ALERT Much variation exists in elemental iron content of commercially available liquid preparations that contain iron. For clarity, dosages should be expressed in terms of elemental iron to ensure proper amounts.

Evaluation: Expected Outcomes

- Increasing activity without fatigue noted.
- Nutritional intake will provide a more balanced, iron-containing diet.
- Remains free from infection; normal temperature.
- Maintains growth curve; manages age-appropriate developmental activities.
- Cognitive performance at school and job (for older adolescents) will improve.
- Attendance at school, job (for older adolescents) and other social obligations will improve.
- Maintain compliance with medication regimen and lab monitoring.

Sickle Cell Disease (Sickle Cell Anemia)

 EVIDENCE BASE Shook, L., Farrell, C., Kalinyak, S., et al. (2016). Translating sickle cell guidelines into practice for primary care providers with Project ECHO. *Medical Education Online, 24*(21), 33616.

Sickle cell disease is a group of inherited red blood cell disorders. It is a severe hereditary form of anemia in which a mutational form of Hb distorts the RBCs into a crescent shape at low oxygen levels. The crescent-shaped "sickled" cell blocks the flow of cells through the blood vessels and interrupts the delivery of oxygen to the tissues. The most common form of sickle cell disease in North America is homozygous HbSS disease, an autosomal recessive disorder. In the United States, approximately 100,000 people have sickle cell disease. It occurs in about 16,300 Hispanic American births. Approximately 1 in 3 black or African Americans has sickle cell trait, accounting for about 3 million people.

Pathophysiology and Etiology

1. Genetically determined and inherited as an autosomal recessive condition (see Figure 52-1).
2. Each person inherits one gene from each parent, which governs the synthesis of Hb (see Table 52-2).
3. The sickle cell mutation reflects a single change in the amino acid building blocks of Hb.
4. Hb is a complex protein molecule made up of four subunits of globin.
5. Hb has two proteins that allow it to carry and release oxygen, alpha globin and beta globin.
6. The alpha globin is normal in sickle cell disease. The beta globin has the amino acid valine at position 6 instead of glutamic acid.

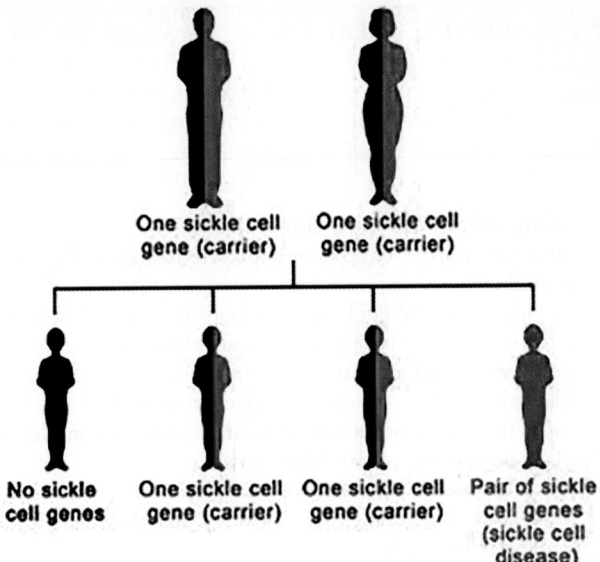

Figure 52-1. Transmission of sickle cell disease.

7. If only one of the beta genes is the sickled gene and the other is normal, the person is a carrier and has sickle cell trait.
8. If both beta gene codes are sickled, the person has sickle cell disease.
9. Sickle cell Hb aggregates into elongated crystals under conditions of low oxygen concentration, acidosis, and dehydration.
10. This distorts the membrane of the RBC, causing it to assume a crescent or sickle shape. The cells easily become entangled and enmeshed, leading to increased blood viscosity, vessel occlusion, and tissue necrosis.
11. Sickled RBCs are fragile and are rapidly destroyed in the circulation; they can live as little as 4 days versus 120 days for normal RBCs.
12. Anemia results when the rate of destruction of RBCs is greater than the rate of production.
13. Increased sequestration of RBCs occurs in the spleen.

Clinical Manifestations

Usually present since the first year of life. Affected infants do not develop symptoms in the first few months of life because the Hb produced by the developing fetus, fetal Hb, protects RBCs from sickling. The fetal Hb is absent in RBCs produced after birth so that by 5 months of age, sickling of RBCs is prominent and symptoms can begin.

Table 52-2	Transmission of Sickle Cell Disease		
GENOTYPE OF PARENTS	PROBABILITY OF ABNORMAL HEMOGLOBIN IN OFFSPRING		
	NORMAL	TRAIT	DISEASE
One parent with trait	50%	50%	0
Both parents with trait	25%	50%	25%
One parent with trait; one parent with disease	0	50%	50%
Both parents with disease	0	0	100%

Prenatal diagnosis is possible using amniocentesis or chorionic villus sampling. All 50 states, the District of Columbia, and all US territories require every baby be tested for sickle cell anemia on the newborn screening.

Signs of Anemia
Vary from person to person and may change over time.
1. Hb level—6 to 9 g/dL, average of 8 g/dL.
2. Loss of appetite.
3. Pallor.
4. Tiredness.
5. Easily fatigued.
6. Irritability.
7. Shortness of breath.
8. Have a feeling of heart racing.
9. Jaundice; increased hemolysis results in hemosiderosis (increased iron storage in the liver).

Precipitating Factors of Crisis
1. Dehydration.
2. Infection.
3. Stress.
4. Strenuous physical exertion.
5. Extreme fatigue.
6. Cold exposure.
7. Temperature extremes.
8. Humidity.
9. Air quality.
10. Nutritional deficiencies.
11. High altitude.
12. Exposure to low doses of carbon monoxide.
13. Socioeconomic factors.
14. Surgery.
15. Pregnancy.

Sickle Cell (Vaso-occlusive) Crisis
1. Most common form of crisis. Typically lasts 3 to 14 days. Most common sites are the lower back, leg, hip, abdomen, or chest. Usually occurs in one or more locations.
   a. Small blood vessels are occluded by the sickle-shaped cells, causing distal ischemia and infarction. This can cause severe pain and permanent damage to the brain, heart, lungs, kidney, liver, bones, and spleen (see Figure 52-2).
2. Extremities:
   a. Bony destruction—related to erythroid hyperplasia of the marrow, leading to osteoporosis or ischemic necrosis.
   b. Aseptic necrosis—results from poor blood supply to an area of the bone, causing localized bone death.
   c. Bone infarction—bone tissue dies due to lack of sufficient blood supply.
   d. Dactylitis ("hand–foot" syndrome)—swelling and inflammation of hands and feet caused by injury to the bones of affected digits by repeated episodes of inadequate blood circulation; commonly first vaso-occlusive event seen in infants and toddlers and children up to age 8.
   e. Arthritis—can accompany dactylitis—presents with pain, swelling, tenderness, and limited range of motion (ROM).
3. Spleen:
   a. Abdominal pain.
   b. Splenomegaly—initially enlarges because of increased activity at the site of RBC hemolysis; increased size results in discomfort. The spleen usually does not work after 4 to 6 months of age. Enlargement usually seen up to 5 years of age.
   c. After multiple episodes of splenic vaso-occlusion, the spleen becomes fibrotic and atrophied.

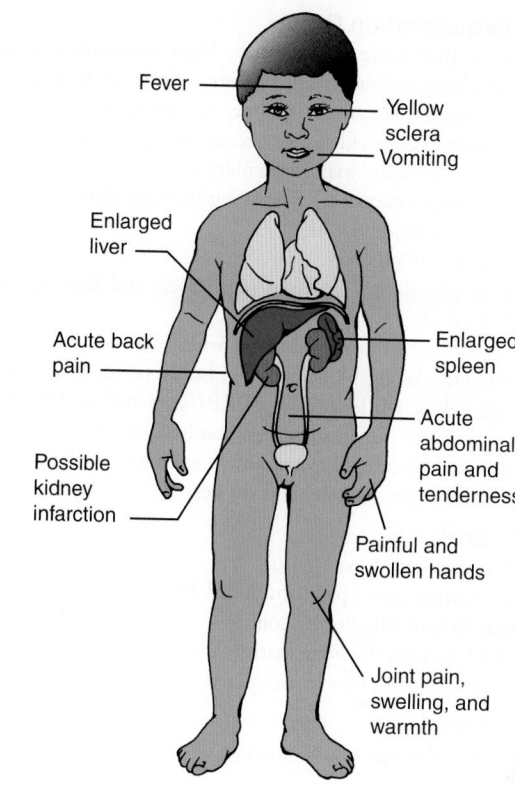

Figure 52-2. Sickle cell crisis signs and symptoms.

Labels: Fever; Yellow sclera; Vomiting; Enlarged liver; Enlarged spleen; Acute back pain; Acute abdominal pain and tenderness; Possible kidney infarction; Painful and swollen hands; Joint pain, swelling, and warmth

   d. Decreased splenic function increases the risk of infection.
   e. Important for protection against germs; serious, life-threatening infections occur secondary to damage to the spleen.
4. Cerebral occlusion:
   a. Stroke—most common killer of patients over age 3 years; between 8% and 10% of patients suffer from a stroke, typically at around age 7 years.
   b. Hemiplegia.
   c. Retinal damage, leading to blindness.
   d. Seizures.
   e. Aneurysms—common and often located where they cannot be surgically treated.
5. Pulmonary:
   a. Acute chest syndrome—more likely to occur after infection, sickle cell crisis, general anesthesia, blood clot, and heavy doses of opiates for pain; lowers levels of oxygen in the blood; and can cause lung damage and be life-threatening.
   b. Pulmonary hypertension—occurs when pressure in the arteries of the lungs increases; seen mostly in adult population.
   c. Infarction—triggered by dehydration; results in cycle of deoxygenation which exacerbates sickling leading to small vessel occlusions and ultimately infarction of areas of the pulmonary parenchyma.
6. Altered renal function—enuresis, hematuria, difficulty concentrating urine, protein loss in the urine, and increased risk of kidney disease.
7. Impaired liver function—may develop iron overload secondary to frequent need for blood transfusion.
8. Priapism—abnormal, recurrent, prolonged, painful penile erection; blood flow out of the erect penis is blocked by sickled cells; can lead to permanent damage and lead to impotence.
9. Infections—most common include *Chlamydia pneumoniae*, *Mycoplasma pneumoniae*, and Gram-negative bacteria; may develop leg ulcers as a result of infectious process.

Splenic Sequestration Crisis

Can be a life-threatening emergency. Most commonly seen in children between 5 months and 4 years of age. If first episode occurs under age 2 years, there is higher risk for recurrence.

1. Large amounts of sickled cells become trapped in the spleen.
2. The spleen becomes massively enlarged.
3. Hemoglobin decreases by at least 2 g/dL secondary to sudden, large drop in blood count.
4. Increase in reticulocytes.
5. Signs of circulatory collapse (eg, shock and hypotension) develop rapidly.
6. Frequent cause of death in infants with sickle cell disease.
7. Restore circulating blood volume; bolus 10 to 20 mL/kg of normal saline while awaiting PRBCs; transfuse 10 mL/kg PRBCs; do not transfuse higher than baseline Hb.
8. Sequestered blood will eventually re-enter circulation increasing risk for hyperviscosity and strokes.

Aplastic Crisis

1. Increased risk with parvovirus.
2. Bone marrow ceases production of RBCs only.
3. Results in low reticulocyte counts.
4. After a few days, the bone marrow usually recovers on its own.
5. Blood transfusion may be necessary.

Chronic Symptoms

Chronic organ damage results in organ dysfunction.

1. Jaundice.
2. Gallstones.
3. Progressive impairment of kidney function.
4. High risk of infection.
5. Growth retardation of the long bones and spine deformities.
6. Delayed growth and puberty.
7. Cardiac decompensation related to chronic anemia (may develop heart failure).
8. Chronic, painful leg ulcers related to decreased peripheral circulation and unrelated to injury; may take months to heal or may not heal without intense therapy, including blood transfusions and grafting.
9. Deep vein thromboses.
10. Pulmonary emboli.
11. Stroke.
12. Malnutrition.
13. Increased risk of renal medullary carcinoma later in life.
14. Altered bony structures—aseptic necrosis of the bones, especially the femoral and humoral heads.
15. Decreased life span.

Diagnostic Evaluation

1. Ante-/perinatal testing via amniocentesis or chorionic villus sampling.
2. Newborn screening—done in all 50 states, the District of Columbia, and all US territories.
3. Those needing further testing:
   a. Immigrants who were not tested in their home country.
   b. Children moving state to state who have not been tested.
   c. Anyone displaying symptoms.
4. Hemoglobin S solubility test and sodium metabisulfite test.
   a. Done by finger or heel stick.
5. Hemoglobinopathy evaluation
   a. Hemoglobin electrophoresis.
   b. Hemoglobin fractionation by HPLC.
   c. Isoelectric focusing—highly sensitive, used at large laboratories

6. DNA analysis—used to investigate alterations and mutations in the genes that produce hemoglobin components.
   a. Requires venipuncture.

Management

Preventing Sickling

1. Promote adequate oxygenation and hemodilution.
   a. Encourage increased intake of fluids—at least eight 8-ounce glasses of water daily.
   b. Avoid high altitudes and other low-oxygen environments.
   c. Exercise regularly but not so much that you become really tired.
   d. Reduce or avoid stress.
   e. Avoid extreme heat or cold. Wear warm clothes in cold weather, stay in air conditioning in hot weather, and do not swim in cold water.
   f. Treat infection as soon as it occurs.
   g. Only travel in commercial pressurized airplanes.
   h. Avoid alcohol, soda, and caffeine—their ingredients make the kidneys excrete more water into the urine increasing the risk of dehydration.
   i. Do not smoke.
   j. Routine blood transfusions (increase number of normal RBCs) (see page 775). Lowers the hemoglobin S circulating in the blood.

Acute Management

Supportive and symptomatic care depends on the type of crisis.

1. Aplastic episode—supportive care and blood transfusions to maintain adequate hematocrit until marrow activity is restored.
2. Splenic sequestration—intravenous fluids and transfusion required to maintain intravascular volume. One or more episodes may require splenectomy, though this is still debated.
3. Hemolytic episode—usually requires only hydration. May occur with splenic sequestration, aplastic, and painful episodes, which are then treated accordingly. Transfusions are required if a significant drop in Hb occurs.
4. Vaso-occlusive or painful episode—must determine if the painful event is a manifestation of an underlying illness (infection) or of an inflammatory condition. Most commonly caused by increased sickling, resulting from hypoxemia and acidosis. Often requires an inpatient stay.
   a. Hydration—this is accomplished by increased oral and parenteral fluid intake of up to two times of fluid maintenance needs.
   b. Analgesics—administered on fixed schedule, not to extend beyond the duration of the pharmacologic effect. IV opioids, such as morphine, are preferred for severe pain, either as a continuous infusion or on a patient-controlled analgesia pump to reach desired effects. Other agents, such as nonsteroidal anti-inflammatory drugs (NSAIDs) and acetaminophen, are used for milder pain or to increase the analgesic effects of opioids.
   c. Alternative pain management techniques—behavior modification programs, relaxation therapy, hypnosis, music therapy, and massage.
   d. Those with chronic or severe vaso-occlusive crises may benefit from monthly blood transfusions, which will improve anemia and decrease total amount of sickle hemoglobin; however, iron overload is a possible complication.
   e. Use of hydroxyurea on a daily basis—hydroxyurea increased the amount of fetal Hb in RBCs allowing the cells to travel more easily through the blood vessels; best used on patients who have had recurrent episodes of pain crises.

f. If there is an HLA matched sibling without sickle cell disease, an allogeneic transplant is standard of care prior to the presentation of symptoms and disease complications.

g. New research on gene therapy as a cure is currently being investigated.

5. Infection—most common cause of morbidity and mortality.

a. Most serious include *S. pneumoniae*, *H. influenzae*, *Salmonella* species, *Mycoplasma pneumoniae*, *Chlamydia pneumoniae*, *Escherichia coli*, and *Klebsiella pneumoniae*.

b. Infection of any type is more difficult to eradicate in patients with sickle cell and commonly exacerbates crises such as aplastic episodes caused by parvovirus (fifth disease), increases the rate of hemolysis, and precipitates vaso-occlusive episodes.

c. Prevention is most important—give usual primary immunizations as well as pneumococcal, *Haemophilus* b conjugate, hepatitis, meningococcal, and trivalent influenza vaccines.

d. Antibiotic prophylaxis—penicillin prophylaxis is recommended in children less than 5 years of age and older children with a previous history of severe pneumococcal infection or have functional/surgical asplenia.

e. Patients with unexplained fever should be cultured thoroughly. If clinical condition suggests septicemia, broad-spectrum antibiotics should be initiated after complete culturing. Patients with septicemia can expire in only a few hours.

6. Stroke prevention:

a. Transcranial Doppler (TCD) screening for all children with sickle cell anemia from age 2 to 16. TCD should be repeated annually if normal and every 6 months if questionable.

b. Children with abnormal TCD should be kept on a chronic maintenance transfusion program to keep their Hb S less than 30%.

c. Stroke risk has decreased from 11% to 1% with use of TCD.

Complications

1. Chronic hemolytic anemia. Characterized by anemia, jaundice, periodic crises, splenomegaly, and gallstones. Symptoms worsen during crises.

2. Main causes of death in children from sickle cell anemia were infection and acute splenic sequestration.

3. Common causes of death for older individuals with sickle cell anemia are intercurrent infections, acute chest syndrome, pulmonary emboli, infarction of a vital organ, and renal failure.

4. Life expectancy is variable; however, it is improving with new forms of treatment. Survival has steadily increased to greater than 50 years of age.

Nursing Assessment

1. Observe for pallor and jaundice, changes in vital signs (elevated temperature, tachycardia, hypotension, tachypnea), change in mental status, swelling of extremities, ulcers or skin lesions, or signs of dehydration (decreased elasticity of the skin, dry mucous membranes, decreased urine output, increased urine concentration, and specific gravity).

2. Examine for enlarged liver and spleen and tenderness of hands or feet.

3. Discuss symptoms and duration of pain, dyspnea, fever, pallor, and lethargy.

4. Discuss precipitating factors for crises, that is, fever, travel, and procedures.

5. Discuss history of chest crises and management.

6. Discuss any comorbidities that may exist, for example, asthma.

7. Discuss usual treatment protocol including chronic transfusions and use of hydroxyurea.

8. Evaluate growth and development.

Nursing Diagnoses

- Acute Pain related to tissue anoxia from chronic disease process.
- Altered Tissue Perfusion related to increased blood viscosity and sickling of hemoglobin.
- Risk for Dehydration related to inadequate fluid intake.
- Risk for Infection related to chronic disease and fibrotic changes in the spleen.
- Activity Intolerance related to anemia.
- Interrupted Family Processes related to frequent medical care, hospitalization, and chronic illness.
- Knowledge Deficit related to lack of understanding about cause and treatment of sickle cell disease.

 EVIDENCE BASE Smith, K., Reinman, L., Schatz, J., et al. (2018). Parent perspectives on pain management in preschool-age children with sickle cell disease. *Journal of Pediatric Oncology Nursing*, 35(1), 16–24.

Relieving Pain

1. Identify and use effective measures to alleviate pain, such as:

a. Carefully position and support painful areas. Joints and extremities can be extremely painful.

b. Hold or rock the infant; handle gently.

c. Provide distractions by singing, reading stories, providing appropriate play activities, or television or videos.

d. Provide familiar objects.

e. Bathe the child in warm water, applying local heat or providing massage.

f. Administer opioid analgesics as ordered. Continuous IV infusion is used for the duration of a painful crisis.

2. Communicate effective methods of reducing pain with other staff members and family.

3. Patients with chronic pain may not display typical pain behavior; remember, "pain is what the patient says it is."

4. Assess physical and psychological effectiveness of intervention.

Increasing Tissue Perfusion

1. Avoid physical exertion, emotional stress, and low-oxygen environments to reduce the body's need for oxygen.

2. Administer blood transfusions as ordered.

3. Perform caregiving activities in groups to provide for optimum rest.

4. Administer oxygen to increase diffusion of gas across membranes.

5. Educate family regarding the need for prophylactic transfusions to lower risk of cardiovascular accident.

Risk of Dehydration

1. Calculate and educate family with regard to child's daily fluid requirements.

2. Assess mucous membranes for signs of dehydration.
3. Record daily intake and output to assure adequate fluid intake.

Reducing Infection

1. Ensure adequate nutrition through high-calorie, high-protein diet.
2. Ensure immunizations are up to date.
3. Isolate child from sources of infection if possible.
4. Administer antibiotics, as prescribed.
5. Provide meticulous care to leg ulcers and other open wounds.
6. Use and demonstrate good handwashing and meticulous technique with all procedures.

Activity Intolerance

1. Assess child's level of mobility and activity tolerance.
2. Encourage adequate rest periods throughout the day.
3. Prioritize tasks when episodes of activity intolerance occur.
4. Encourage good eating habits, sleep, and relaxation.
5. Encourage verbalization of feelings regarding limitations.

Normalizing Family Processes

1. Encourage parents to talk about their child, the illness, and how they feel about it.
2. Expect such feelings as guilt, shock, frustration, depression, and resentment.
3. Accept negative feelings, but try to build on positive coping mechanisms.
4. Provide factual information to child and parents about their concerns.
5. Encourage role-playing and play activities to identify fears.
6. Assure adolescents that although sexual development is delayed, they will eventually catch up with their peers.
7. Stress the normalcy of the child despite having sickle cell disease.
   a. Sickle cell disease does not affect intelligence; the child should go to school and keep up with classwork while stable.
   b. Between periods of crisis, the child can usually participate in peer group activities, with the exception of some strenuous sports.
   c. The child needs the same discipline as other children in the family.

Knowledge Deficit

1. Review basics of sickle cell disease with family and child.
2. Teach the family about signs and symptoms of crises.
3. Educate the family as to when immediate medical care is essential.
4. Teach the importance of balanced, healthy nutrition, hydration, sleep, and periods of rest.
5. Arrange for genetic counseling and testing for sickle cell trait in family members.

Community and Home Care Considerations

Home care nurses and school nurses can be instrumental in the care of patients with sickle cell anemia by ensuring that their primary health care needs are met. A reliable medical home is essential for patients with sickle cell anemia.

1. The following examinations should be done as indicated:
   a. Regularly scheduled medical checkups: every 2 to 4 months from birth to 24 months, every 6 months from 2 to 12 years of age, and every 6 to 12 months from age 12 and above.
   b. CBC—yearly.
   c. Quantitative electrophoresis—at birth, repeat between age 1 and 2.
   d. RBC antigen testing—between age 1 and 2 or prior to first transfusion.
   e. LFTs/bilirubin/renal bloodwork—annually.
   f. Urinalysis—annually in older children and adolescents.
   g. Ophthalmology examinations—annually after age 10.
   h. Hearing tests—only if clinical concern, secondary to prolonged and frequent use of antibiotics.
   i. PFTs—oxygen saturation testing at each visit and baseline PFT in adolescence.
   j. A tuberculin skin test every 2 to 3 years (every year in at-risk populations). Any positive findings should be followed up promptly.
   k. All routine childhood immunizations, as well as the hepatitis B series, pneumococcal conjugate vaccine, pneumococcal polysaccharide vaccine, meningococcal, *H. influenzae* type B, and yearly trivalent influenza.
   l. Dental checkups and teeth cleaning every 6 months.
2. Educate parents, teachers, and daycare providers involved in the care of children with sickle cell disease about their common problems and special needs:
   a. Frequent absences because of pain and illness.
   b. Fatigue and inattention, caused by anemia or ischemia of central nervous system tissue.
   c. Need for adequate hydration throughout the course of the day.
   d. Inability to concentrate urine, requiring frequent restroom breaks.
   e. Permanent learning disabilities or delays, requiring individualized teaching plans.
   f. Need for a controlled environment to prevent sickling, avoiding temperature extremes, dehydration, and excessive stress.
   g. Need for moderate physical exercise, with avoidance of rough contact sports and activities.
   h. Desire to feel "normal" and have opportunities and environmental stimulation similar to other children their age.
3. Assess the child's home environment for protection from infection and injury, adequate nutritional resources, transportation to medical appointments, and emotional support. Initiate social service and other referrals, as needed.
4. Consider/explore possible complementary and alternative therapies.

Family Education and Health Maintenance

1. Discuss the genetic implications of sickle cell disease and offer genetic counseling to the family.
2. Instruct the parents in ways that they can help their child to avoid sickling episodes.
   a. Do not allow the child to become chilled or to wear tight clothing that might impede circulation.
   b. Provide adequate fluids and notify health care provider if excessive fluids are lost through vomiting, diarrhea, fever, and excessive sweating.
   c. Limit excessive exercise and offer frequent breaks with activity.
   d. Avoid extreme temperature settings.
3. Instruct parents how to recognize signs of dehydration (dry skin and mucous membranes, decreased urine output; irritability or listlessness in the infant).
4. Encourage parents to seek prompt treatment of cuts, sores, and mosquito bites and to notify the health care provider if the child is exposed to a communicable disease.

5. Encourage good dental hygiene and twice yearly dental check-ups to avoid dental infections.
6. Instruct on preventive care, including all the recommended childhood immunizations and screening tests.
7. Encourage a calm, emotionally stable environment.
8. Warn against trips to the mountains or against trips in unpressurized airplanes that will decrease oxygen concentration.
9. Provide sexually active adolescents with information on contraception and sexually transmitted disease.
10. Teach signs of a mild crisis:
    a. Fatigue.
    b. Yellowish color of the skin and whites of eyes.
    c. Decreased appetite.
    d. Irritability.
    e. Low-grade fever.
    f. Painful swelling of hands and/or feet.
    g. Teach parents to palpate the spleen.
11. Instruct on home management of mild crisis.
    a. Encourage fluids.
    b. Administer antipyretic medications, as directed by health care provider familiar with the condition.
    c. Encourage rest.
    d. Keep the child warm.
    e. Apply warm compresses to the painful area.
    f. Hospitalization may be required for the child if pain becomes severe or if IV hydration is required.
12. Teach the signs of severe crisis and whom to notify:
    a. Pallor.
    b. Lethargy and listlessness.
    c. Severe pain in the abdomen, chest, bones, and/or joints.
    d. Swelling in hands and feet.
    e. Abdominal swelling.
    f. Weakness is the face, arms, or legs.
    g. Trouble walking or talking.
    h. Visual disturbance.
    i. Numbness.
    j. Fever of 102°F (38.9°C)—report immediately.
    k. Decreased appetite and dehydration.
13. Instruct the parents to have emergency information available to those involved in the child's care (school nurse, teacher, babysitter, family members).
    a. Name and phone number of health care provider or clinic.
    b. Closest emergency facility and ambulance phone number.
    c. Child's blood type, allergies, medications, and medical records number.
    d. Name of informed neighbor or relative to be notified in an emergency.
14. Stress the benefit of wearing a MedicAlert bracelet.
15. For additional information and support, refer to Sickle Cell Foundation (*www.scdfc.org*).

Evaluation: Expected Outcomes

- Able to drink enough fluids and eat a well-balanced diet.
- Pain well controlled or absent.
- Less pallor without the need for oxygen.
- Afebrile without signs of infection.
- Respirations within normal limits for age; uses incentive spirometer hourly.
- Ambulates throughout the day for short intervals with minimal or no pain.
- Parents verbalize concerns about chronic illness.

Thalassemia Major (Cooley's Anemia)

 EVIDENCE BASE de Dreuzy, E., Bhukhai, K., Leboulch, P., et al. (2016). Current and future alternative therapies for beta-thalassemia major. *Biomedical Journal, 339*(1), 24–38.

Thalassemia major is the most severe of the beta-thalassemia syndromes and represents the homozygous form of the disease. Beta-thalassemia (β-thalassemia) refers to a group of inherited genetic disorders characterized by a reduction or absence of the β-globulin chain in Hb synthesis. Classification and severity grading are based on spontaneous Hb level and clinical tolerance. Patients with thalassemia major have Hb concentrations between 3 and 7 g/dL and exhibit severe anemia. It was first discovered in the Mediterranean basin and is highly prevalent in countries also affected by malaria. It manly affects people of Mediterranean, Southern Asia, Southeast Asia, and Middle Eastern origin. In the United States, it affects approximately 1,000 people.

Pathophysiology and Etiology

1. Genetically determined, inherited autosomal recessive disorder (see Figure 52-3).
2. Defect can be a complete absence of the β-globin protein or severely reduced synthesis of the β-globin protein.
3. The resulting RBCs are abnormally small, are not produced in normal amounts, and do not contain enough functional Hb, leading to severe hemolytic anemia and resultant chronic hypoxia.
4. The abnormalities result in quantitative changes in globin's as opposed to the qualitative or functional changes seen in hemoglobinopathies.
5. Erythroid activity is significantly increased in an attempt to overcome the increased rate of destruction. This results in:
    a. An enormous expansion of the bone marrow and thinning of the bony cortex.
    b. Skeletal deformities: frontal and maxillary bossing.
    c. Growth retardation.
    d. Deformities of the long bones of the leg.
    e. Massive hepatosplenomegaly.
6. Decreased erythropoietic drive and increased iron load result in higher hepcidin levels. These higher levels moderate dietary absorption and causes macrophages to retain iron. This causes body iron stores to increase because of the inability to excrete the iron and leads to tissue damage.

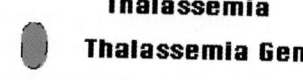

Figure 52-3. Transmission of thalassemia.

7. Hemoglobin F (Hb F) amount to less that 1% of Hb by 6 to 12 months of age: in genetic disorders such as thalassemia major, there is a persistent presence of Hb F because of alteration of the β-globin cluster; Hb F does not hold oxygen well.

Clinical Manifestations

1. Infants exhibit symptoms within the first 2 years of life, often between 3 and 6 months after birth.
2. Symptoms are primarily related to the progressive anemia, expansion of the marrow cavities of the bone, hepatosplenomegaly, and extramedullary hematopoiesis in the chest and abdomen.
3. Early symptoms commonly include failure to thrive, feeding difficulties, pallor, diarrhea, irritability or fussiness, recurrent fevers, and mild jaundice.
4. Further signs of progressive anemia include headache, bone pain, exercise intolerance, jaundice, and protuberant abdomen caused by hepatosplenomegaly.
5. If untreated, it can cause abnormal expansion of the bone marrow causing bones to become thinner, wider, and brittle; this can cause frontal bossing, prominent malar eminence, and depressed bridge of the nose and hypertrophy of maxilla; also see increased risk of fracture of the long bones.

Diagnostic Evaluation

1. CBC with differential—determines number of RBCs and how much Hb is in them; evaluates red cell indices including MCV.
2. Peripheral blood smear—looks at a layer of the blood with a microscope and can assess number and type of white blood cells, platelets, and RBCs.
3. Iron studies—iron, ferritin, unsaturated iron-binding capacity (UIBC), total iron-binding capacity (TIBC), and percent saturation of transferrin.
4. DNA analysis—confirms mutation in the alpha and beta globin–producing gene.
5. Amniocentesis—can be done perinatally if increased risk is a concern.

Management

1. Frequent and regular blood transfusions of packed RBCs to maintain Hb levels between 9 and 10 g/dL.
   a. All children starting regular transfusions should be vaccinated against hepatitis B as early as possible.
   b. Children on chronic transfusion regimens should have an extended red cell phenotype/genotype prior to or as soon as possible after commencing therapy.
   c. RBC component of transfusions: in children less than 4 months of age, PRBCs should be compatible with maternal and neonatal ABO and D group and clinically significant maternal antibodies; in children over 4 months of age, PRBCs should be compatible with recipients ABO and D group and any red cell alloantibodies.
   d. Washed, packed RBCs are usually used to minimize the possibility of transfusion reactions. If unavailable, leukofiltered cells can be substituted.
   e. Goal of transfusion is to shut off erythropoiesis as much as possible; should be given at 3- to 4-week interval.
   f. Target Hb should be between 9 and 10 g/dL; in patients with cardiac insufficiency, higher levels of 10 to 12 g/dL should be maintained.

2. Iron chelation therapy reduces the toxic adverse effects of excess iron and increases iron excretion through urine and feces. Iron chelation is usually started at 2 to 4 years of age after 20 to 25 units of PRBCs is transfused and a serum ferritin level of greater than 1,000 μg/dL and a liver iron concentration (LIC) of greater than 3 mg/iron/g dry weight measured by liver biopsy or hepatic T2 MRI are achieved.
   a. Deferoxamine: IV, IM, or SQ formulation of iron-chelating agent; in IV formulations, it is administered over at least 8 to 12 hours 5 to 7 days per week—should not exceed 60 mg/kg/day; if given SQ, administered at 30 to 60 mg/kg/day over 8 to 12 hours 5 to 7 days per week; vitamin C increases the excretion of iron in the presence of deferoxamine—after 1 month of chelation therapy, should take 2 to 4 mg/kg/day of vitamin C soon after infusion is complete.
   b. Deferasirox: oral iron chelation agent; initial dosing at 10 mg/kg/day—can be adjusted up to 40 mg/kg/day; must be mixed in apple juice, orange juice, or water—for dosing less than 1,000 mg, mix in ½ cup fluid, and in dosing greater than 1,000 mg, must be mixed in 1 cup of fluid; no antacids containing aluminum should be given while on deferasirox.
   c. The new tablet formulation of deferasirox (Jadenu) has demonstrated improved compliance with therapy.
3. Splenectomy. Optimal clinical management from the time of diagnosis may delay or prevent hypersplenism. Increased efficiency of transfusion therapy may reduce the need for splenectomy. Splenectomy should be considered if:
   a. Annual blood requirement is greater than 1.5 times that of splenectomized patients.
   b. Increased iron stores despite good chelation therapy.
   c. Splenic enlargement is accompanied by left upper quadrant pain, early satiety, or concern for splenic rupture.
   d. Leucopenia or thrombocytopenia because of hypersplenism causes recurrent bacterial infections or bleeding.
   e. Prior to splenectomy, the child should be immunized against *Streptococcus pneumoniae*, *Haemophilus influenza B*, and *Neisseria meningitidis*.
   f. Oral penicillin prophylaxis is necessary (250 mg bid) post splenectomy.
   g. Family should be educated that urgent medical attention is required for fever greater than 101°F.
   h. Should be avoided under age 5 secondary to increased risk for fulminant postsplenectomy sepsis.
4. Supportive management of complications.
5. Hematopoietic stem cell transplants are the only known cure. Young patients with few complications are the best candidates.
6. Prognosis is poor; life expectancy is 17 years of age, but most children die before their 13th birthday.

Complications

1. Splenomegaly—usually requires splenectomy; major long-term risk after splenectomy is overwhelming sepsis.
2. Growth retardation in the second decade. Growth is usually normal until 9 to 10 years of age. Multifactorial including hemosiderosis-induced damage of the endocrine glands, chronic anemia, hypoxia, chronic liver disease, vitamin and nutritional deficiencies, use of chelating agents, endocrinopathies, low IGF-1 levels, and emotional factors.
3. Endocrine abnormalities:
   a. Hypogonadism—most obvious clinical consequence of iron overload.

b. Delayed puberty.

c. Hypothyroidism.

d. Disturbed calcium homeostasis—results in osteopenia and/or osteoporosis.

e. Hypoparathyroidism.

f. Growth hormone deficiency.

g. Diabetes mellitus—presents after the age of 10 years.

h. Adrenal insufficiency.

4. Skeletal complications—become less common because of early transfusion therapy and maintenance of Hb levels above 10 g/dL:

a. Frontal and parietal bossing (enlarging).

b. Maxillary hypertrophy, leading to malocclusion.

c. Increased risk of osteopenia and osteoporosis.

d. Pathologic fractures of the long bones and vertebral collapse, especially in the lumbar region.

5. Cardiac complications:

a. Arrhythmias—EKG changes specifically increased QTc and QTd intervals.

b. Cardiomyopathy secondary to cardiac iron overload.

c. Increase in left ventricular septal and posterior wall thickness.

d. Premature vascular aging including abnormal vascular stiffening noted as patients live longer.

e. Heart failure—usual cause of death.

6. Liver disease:

a. Chronic infection develops in 70% to 80% of patients leading to chronic liver disease.

b. Liver fibrosis and cirrhosis.

c. Hepatocellular carcinoma—develops in 1% to 5% of individuals over the age of 20.

7. Gallbladder disease—gallstones develop secondary to chronic anemia. Up to two thirds of patients with thalassemia major develop gallstones; most patients remain asymptomatic; cholecystectomy is rarely required.

8. Megaloblastic anemia—caused by sporadic folic acid and vitamin B_{12} deficiency from increased use by hyperplastic marrow. Folic acid supplementation is recommended for all patients.

9. Skin—pruritus and xerosis seen frequently and jaundice secondary to iron overload.

10. Leg ulcers.

Nursing Assessment

1. Review family medical history especially those associated with anemia.

2. Perform whole-body examination to assess for anemia and systemic complications of thalassemia.

3. Observe for signs and symptoms of anemia.

4. Measure growth and development parameters.

Nursing Diagnoses

- Ineffective Tissue Perfusion related to abnormal Hb and oxygen delivery to cells.
- Chronic Pain related to progression of disease in the bone.
- Imbalanced Nutrition related to lack of appetite and nutritional deficiencies.
- Activity Intolerance related to bone pain, cardiac dysfunction, and anemia.
- Risk for Infection related to progressive anemia and splenectomy.
- Deficient Knowledge related to iron chelation therapy.

- Disturbed Body Image related to endocrine and skeletal abnormalities.
- Ineffective Family Coping related to poor prognosis.

Nursing Interventions

Inadequate Tissue Perfusion

1. Blood transfusion

a. Mainstay of treatment.

b. Prevents most of the serious complications associated with thalassemia.

c. Signs and symptoms indicative of the need for transfusion include increased cardiac effort or tachycardia, sweating, poor appetite, poor growth, and inability to maintain daily activities.

d. Must rule out infectious/septic etiology.

e. Observe for signs of transfusion reaction (increased chance caused by frequency):

i. Fever.

ii. Chills.

iii. Hives.

iv. Edema.

v. Pain or burning in the abdomen, chest, or back.

vi. Sense of doom.

vii. Breathing problems.

viii. Swelling/bruising at transfusion site.

ix. Nausea, vomiting, and/or diarrhea.

f. Reaction may occur within 15 to 20 minutes of start of transfusion, although delayed reactions may occur up to several months later.

2. Monitor cardiovascular status for complications.

a. Monitor vital signs: apical pulse, BP, and respirations.

b. Assess for edema.

c. Auscultate heart sounds for gallop and lungs for rales.

d. Assess extremities for ulcer formation.

e. Increased risk of pulmonary hypertension.

f. Major complication of transfusions is iron overload in the heart. Starting chelation early is essential in preventing life-threatening complications.

Chronic Bone Pain

1. Bone pain is a characteristic feature of thalassemia major.

2. Monitor CBC for hemoglobin values less than 10 g/dL.

3. Use warm packs—can reduce muscle spasms and reduce inflammation.

4. Eat a healthy diet that includes calcium and vitamin D to help keep bones as strong as possible.

5. Administer and teach proper administration of NSAIDs, such as ibuprofen or naproxen. Use carefully and monitor liver enzymes in patients with liver complications.

Activity Intolerance

1. Encourage participation in activities that do not require significant strenuous activity. Full participation in some activities, especially with peers, will increase self-esteem. Allow for periods of rest during such activities.

2. Facilitate physical and occupational therapy to develop an acceptable exercise plan.

3. Involve the parents' and child's school in developing a plan of gym activities, classes, and rest periods that allow the greatest level of participation and slowly develop endurance.

4. Advise parents that during the week of the scheduled transfusion, the fatigue will be greatest, so gym and other exertional activities should be modified.

5. Discourage participation in contact or other sports that increase the child's risk of a fracture (skateboarding, football, soccer).

Infection Risk

1. Maintain and teach good handwashing techniques.
2. Minimize exposure to infectious illnesses.
3. After splenectomy, the child has increased susceptibility to infection and should be maintained on oral penicillin prophylaxis.
4. Vaccinate child against *H. influenzae*, pneumococcal, and meningococcal infections before splenectomy and encourage yearly trivalent influenza vaccination.
5. Encourage prompt medical attention for fever or signs of infection. Fever of 102°F (38.9°C) should be reported immediately and IV broad-spectrum antibiotics initiated.

Knowledge Deficit

1. Explain the importance of chelating (binding) agents to decrease iron deposits in tissues and to increase iron excretion through urine and feces.
2. Administer IV deferoxamine as prescribed:
   a. Infuse slowly, during 8 to 24 hours, through peripheral line or implanted infusion device or via volumetric pump.
   b. Have emergency resuscitation equipment nearby in case a severe allergic reaction occurs.
3. Review administration of oral deferasirox and encourage adherence to the medication schedule.
4. Ocular and auditory disturbances are seen in long-term use. Periodic visual and audiometric testing is recommended.

NURSING ALERT Because of the excess iron deposition in children with thalassemia, dietary iron should be decreased as much as possible.

Improving Body Image

1. Explore the child's feelings of being different from other children.
2. Encourage the child to express feelings through the use of play: art and role playing.
3. Give positive reinforcement regarding appearance.
4. Encourage socialization and peer interaction.
5. Encourage endocrine consultation for delayed growth and puberty.
6. Encourage craniofacial specialist evaluation for bony abnormalities.
7. Suggest support group or individual counseling, as needed.

Improving Family Coping Strategies

1. Alleviate the child's anxieties about illness by providing explanation based on developmental level.
2. Use role-playing and play activities to identify concerns.
3. Assist in strengthening coping mechanisms, such as support network and problem solving.
4. Help identify resources for financial support, medical supplies, respite care, etc.
5. Encourage involvement in school and after-school activities.
6. Encourage parents to set limits and to provide discipline for the child that is consistent with that for other children in the family.
7. Provide supportive care to the dying child.
8. Encourage bereavement support for parents, siblings, and family.

Family Education and Health Maintenance

1. Discuss the genetic implications of thalassemia and refer for genetic counseling.
2. Provide a detailed instruction about:
   a. Prevention and prompt treatment of infections.
   b. Medications.
   c. Home chelation therapy.
   d. Dietary modifications to limit iron intake.
   e. Activity restrictions, including avoidance of activities that increase the risk of fractures.
   f. Signs of complications.
3. Encourage parents to provide information about the child's condition to significant adults who are involved with the child (teacher, school nurse, babysitter, scout leader).
4. For additional information and support, refer to Cooley's Anemia Foundation (*www.thalassemia.org*).

Evaluation: Expected Outcomes

- Vital signs stable.
- Skin integrity intact without evident edema.
- No edema evident.
- Rates pain as less than 4 out of 10 on developmentally appropriate scale.
- Attends school on a regular basis.
- Reports increased participation in activity and less fatigue.
- No febrile illnesses reported. Immunizations up to date.
- Parent has good understanding of and is proficient in administration of chelation agents.
- Child verbalizes interest in appearance and positive statements about self.
- Family participates in support groups.
- Parents discuss illness with child and siblings.

Hemophilia

EVIDENCE BASE Moort, I., Joosten, M., Maat, M., et al. (2017). Pitfalls in the diagnosis of hemophilia severity: What to do? *Pediatric Blood & Cancer, 64*(4), 3.

Hemophilia is one of a group of inherited X-linked recessive bleeding disorders that cause abnormal or exaggerated bleeding and poor blood clotting. It is most commonly used to refer to two specific conditions, hemophilia A and hemophilia B. Hemophilia A is caused by a deficiency of clotting factor VIII. Hemophilia B is caused by a deficiency of clotting factor IX. Males are commonly affected and females are usually carriers of the disease. Hemophilia A occurs in 1 in 5,000 live births and is four times as common as hemophilia B. There are an estimated 20,000 individuals in the United States with hemophilia. Worldwide incidence is estimated at more than 400,000.

- 80% to 85% have factor VIII deficiency or hemophilia A (classic hemophilia).
- 15% to 20% have factor IX deficiency or hemophilia B (Christmas disease).
- Few have factor XI deficiency or hemophilia C.

EVIDENCE BASE Lillicrap, D. (2013). von Willebrand disease: advances in pathogenetic understanding, diagnosis, and therapy. *Blood, 122,* 3735–3740.

Table 52-3	Transmission of Hemophilia					
GENOTYPE OF PARENTS	**PROBABILITY OF ABNORMALITY IN OFFSPRING**					
	FEMALE			**MALE**		
	NORMAL	CARRIER	HEMOPHILIAC	NORMAL	HEMOPHILIAC	
Female carrier/normal male	50%	50%	0	50%	50%	
Noncarrier female/hemophiliac male	0	100%	0	100%	0	
Female carrier/hemophiliac male	0	50%	50%	50%	50%	

von Willebrand disease (pseudohemophilia) is the most common inherited bleeding disorder (in the hemophilia category) caused by deficiency or abnormality in von Willebrand factor (VWF), a key protein that helps clotting. von Willebrand disease shows no geographical or ethnic predilection. Both sexes inherit the genetic mutation with equal frequency, although females outnumber males (2:1). The prevalence of von Willebrand disease is 0.6% to 1.3% of the population.

Pathophysiology and Etiology

1. Hereditary (approximately 80% of patients) (Table 52-3).
   a. Autosomal dominant pattern—in rare cases, inherited can see autosomal recessive pattern.
   b. Three types exist—1, 2, and 3:
      i. Type 1—mild to moderate reduction in functional normal VWF—accounts for 65% to 80% of affected individuals.
      ii. Type 2—involves expression of functionally abnormal VWF—occurs in 20% to 35% of affected individuals.
      iii. Type 3—absence of VWF—affects 1 in 1 million people.
   c. Those who inherit one copy of the mutated gene will develop type 1 or 2.
   d. Those who inherit a mutated gene from both parents will develop type 3.
   e. May appear in females if a female carrier bears offspring with a male hemophiliac, although this is rare (see Figure 52-4).
2. Spontaneous mutations may occur when the family history is negative for the disease. Although not initially inherited, it can be passed on to the affected person's children.
3. The basic defect is in the intrinsic phase of the coagulation cascade. The blood clotting factors are necessary for the formation of prothrombin activator, which acts as a catalyst in the conversion of prothrombin to thrombin.
   a. When damage to the vessel wall occurs, bleeding starts and platelets are activated to the site of the injury resulting in platelet aggregation.
   b. Clotting proteins, such as factors VIII and IX, are activated on the surface of the platelets to form a meshlike fibrin clot.
   c. These proteins work in a domino-like reaction known as the coagulation cascade. If the protein is absent, the chain reaction is broken, either preventing clot formation or resulting in slower clot formation.
4. The result is an unstable fibrin clot.
5. Coagulation factors are involved in hemostasis and the formation of clots. PTT is used to measure coagulation factors, including factors VIII and IX.

6. Platelet number and function are normal; therefore, small lacerations and minor hemorrhages are usually not a problem.
7. Patients do not bleed more rapidly; rather, there is delayed or abnormal clot formation.

Clinical Manifestations

1. In majority of patients, hemophilia is diagnosed at birth because of family history, although in approximately 1/3 of patients, the occurrence of hemophilia represents a new mutation.
2. Approximately 30% of male infants with hemophilia have bleeding with circumcision.
3. In those patients who do not have a family history, diagnosis is often made when the child begins to walk or crawl.
4. Varies in severity, depending on the plasma level of the coagulation factor involved.
   a. Level of less than 1% of normal—severe hemophilia; commonly severe clinical bleeding with minimal or unknown trauma and often experience unprovoked muscle and joint bleeding one to six times monthly (factor level less than 0.01 µ/mL).

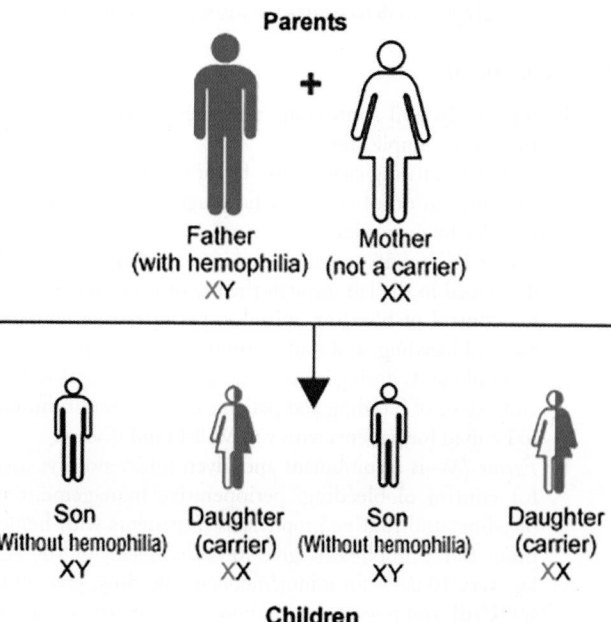

Inheritance of Hemophilia
Father With Hemophilia and Mother Who Is Not a Carrier

Figure 52-4. Transmission of hemophilia.

b. Level of 1% to 5% of normal—moderately afflicted; may be free from spontaneous bleeding and may not manifest severe bleeding until trauma occurs (factor level less than 0.02 to 0.05 μ/mL).

c. Level of 6% to 40% of normal—mildly afflicted; patients usually lead normal lives and bleed only with severe injury or surgery (factor level greater than 0.05 μ/mL).

d. Degree of severity tends to be constant within a given family. Within an individual, severity does not vary over time unless inhibitor (autoantibody to infused factor) develops.

5. Signs and symptoms of abnormal bleeding include:

a. History of prolonged bleeding episodes such as after circumcision.

b. Easily bruised.

c. Oral bleeding.

d. Spontaneous soft tissue hematomas.

e. Hemorrhages into the joints (hemarthrosis)—especially the elbows, knees, and ankles, causing pain, swelling, and limitation of movement.

f. Hematuria.

g. Black, tarry stools.

h. Heavy or long menstrual bleeding, often with blood clots greater than 1 inch.

i. Excessive bleeding from an injury.

j. Head trauma, resulting in intracranial hemorrhage.

Diagnostic Evaluation

1. Prothrombin time and bleeding time—measures clotting ability of factors I, II, VII, and X—normal.

2. Partial thromboplastin time—measures clotting ability of factors VIII, IX, XI, and XII—prolonged.

3. Fibrinogen—assesses patients' ability to form a blood clot.

4. Assays for specific clotting factors—measures levels of factor VIII and IX—abnormal.

5. VWF—helps to diagnose von Willebrand disease and distinguish between types of disease—persons with O type blood have VWF levels 25% less than other blood types.

6. Gene analysis—to detect carrier state, for prenatal diagnosis.

Management

1. Prompt, early, and appropriate treatment is the key to preventing most complications.

2. Must replace missing coagulation factor (VIII or IX) through the administration of type-specific coagulation concentrates during bleeding episodes.

a. *Factor VIII*—75% of the factor is recombinant, which is developed in the lab through the use of DNA technology; for control of bleeding episodes, perioperative management of bleeding, and routine prophylaxis in patients with hemophilia A; dosing is intravenous and based on location and extent of bleeding and patients clinical condition; not to be used for patients with von Willebrand disease.

b. *Factor IX*—is recombinant and given intravenously; used for control of bleeding, perioperative management of bleeding, and routine prophylaxis in patients with hemophilia B; for prophylaxis, give 50 IU/kg weekly or 100 IU/kg every 10 days; for minor/moderate bleeding, give 30 to 60 IU/dL and repeat every 48 hours as necessary; for major bleeding, give 80 to 100 IU/dL, repeat in 6 to 10 hours, and then give every 24 hours for 3 days and then every 48 hours until healing is achieved.

3. No viral inactivated concentrate exists for hemophilia C; fresh frozen plasma is given to supply factor XI.

4. Mild and moderate factor VIII–deficient hemophiliacs and some patients with von Willebrand disease may respond to desmopressin, which causes the release of factor VIII from the endothelial stores. Treatment is started in case of bleeding or before an intervention, that is, dental work. Dosing can be intravenously to intranasally. IV dosing is 0.3 μg/kg and intranasally 150 μg per nostril. It can be repeated every 12 to 24 hours depending on response. Patients receiving desmopressin should restrict fluids during use to prevent hyponatremia and seizures.

5. Plasma-derived VWF—use dependent on predicted amount of bleeding and intervention to be performed for patients with von Willebrand disease; dosing is concentrate dependent; recombinant von Willebrand concentrate has been developed and shown increased activity compared to plasma derived factor but was approved by the FDA in 2015 only for adults.

6. Antifibrinolytics, such as aminocaproic acid and tranexamic acid, are given as adjunctive therapy for dental procedures and for nose and mouth bleeding; it is administered orally.

7. Activated prothrombin complex concentrates that have activated factors VII, IX, and X are used when inhibitors (autoantibodies) have developed to bypass factor VIII or IX.

8. Supportive therapies:

a. NSAIDs are used to decrease inflammation and arthritic-like pain associated with chronic hemarthroses. They must be used with caution because some types and higher doses interfere with platelet adhesion. Should only be used when prescribed by licensed practitioner who is familiar with bleeding disorders.

b. Physical therapy to prevent contractures and muscle atrophy. This includes exercise, whirlpool, and icing.

c. Orthotics to prevent injury to affected joint and to help resolve hemorrhages.

9. Synovectomy—orthopedic surgical intervention to remove damaged synovium in chronically involved joints.

a. Open procedure provides direct visualization of joint and removal of damaged tissue.

b. Arthroscopic—visualization and removal of the joint synovium through the use of an arthroscope.

c. Radionucleotide—instillation of radioisotope P32 into the joint, which removes stops excessive growth of the synovium, decreases amount of bleeding, and decreases potential for arthritis; done through a needle with x-ray guidance.

10. Gene therapy research—genetic copies of sequenced factor VIII and IX molecules are inserted into the body via some type of vector cell to find their way into the human host genetic machinery and begin to produce either factor VIII or factor IX in deficient patients.

11. Patients with bleeding disorders should avoid aspirin and aspirin-containing products, nonsteroidal anti-inflammatories, and blood thinners such as warfarin and heparin.

Complications

1. Airway obstruction caused by hemorrhage into the neck and pharynx.

2. Joint disease—secondary to repetitive bleeding into the joints, often results in arthritis, and may require joint replacement therapy.

3. Intestinal obstruction caused by bleeding into intestinal walls or peritoneum.

4. Compression of nerves with paralysis caused by hemorrhaging into deep tissues, known as *compartment syndrome*.

5. Intracranial bleeding, resulting in serious neurologic impairments.

6. Inhibitor development—30% of patients with hemophilia A and 2% to 3% of patients with hemophilia B develop inhibitors to factor replacements.

7. Viral infections—risk from plasma-derived factor concentrates—less often now that recombinant forms of factor are available.

8. Death may result from exsanguination after any serious hemorrhage, such as intracranial, airway, or other highly vascular areas.

9. Life span—varies based on whether they receive proper treatment; without proper treatment, many die before reaching adulthood; with proper treatment, life expectancy is about 10 years less than those without hemophilia: children can expect to have a normal life expectancy.

Nursing Assessment

1. Obtain history of and observe for unusual bleeding—ecchymosis, prolonged bleeding from mucous membranes and lacerations, hematomas, hemarthroses, hematuria, and rectal and GI bleeding. Determine time frame of most recent bleeding episode.

2. Obtain history of whether patient has inhibitors and, if so, what their titer is.

3. Assess for acute or chronic bleeding.

4. Priority assessment of joints for swelling, warmth, tenderness, ROM, contractures, and surrounding muscle atrophy.

5. Check for hematuria and bleeding from the mouth, lips, gum, and rectum.

6. Check vision, hearing, and neurological development.

7. Obtain information on prior treatment with blood products.

8. Assess family resources and coping skills.

Nursing Diagnoses

- Risk for Deficient Fluid Volume related to hemorrhage.
- Risk for Bleeding related to inability of blood to clot.
- Impaired Physical Mobility related to repeated hemarthroses.
- Acute Pain related to bleeding into joints and muscles.
- Ineffective Family Coping related to disabling and life-threatening disease.

Nursing Interventions

Preventing Hypovolemia Through Control of Bleeding

1. Provide emergency care for bleeding.
   a. Apply pressure and cold to the injury site to assist in clot formation. Immobilize and elevate injured area. This should be done especially after venipuncture or injection.
   b. Do not aspirate hematomas or joints.
   c. Suturing and cauterization should be avoided.

2. Immobilize the affected part and elevate above the level of the heart.

3. Recognize early and late signs of a joint bleed. Early signs include tingling and bubbling sensation but no real pain or tightness and pain without visible signs of a bleed. Late signs include swelling at the joint, warmth of the skin to touch, pain when bending or extending the joint, and increased difficulty with mobilization.

4. Administer recombinant factor VIII or factor IX coagulation concentrate.
   a. Administration should be slow IV push; usually 2 to 3 mL/minute; consult package inserts.
   b. In the case of head trauma, administer factor replacement immediately and prior to obtaining imaging—waiting to administer factor can have serious neurologic effects.
   c. Cryoprecipitate and fresh frozen plasma are not recommended because of their lack of viral inactivation treatment. They may be only treatment of choice in some countries.
   d. Stop the transfusion if hives, headaches, tingling, chills, flushing, or fever occurs.

5. Apply fibrinolytic agents to wound for oral bleeding. Popsicles also work for minor mouth bleeding. Do not use fibrinolytic agents for hematuria.

6. Attempt to keep child relaxed and quiet during treatment to decrease pulse and rate of bleeding.

7. Monitor vital signs and treat for shock if child becomes hypotensive.

Providing Protection Against Bleeding

1. For patients with severe hemophilia, administer prophylactic factor IX or XIII two to three times weekly to prevent spontaneous bleeds.

2. Avoid obtaining rectal temperatures; insert thermometer probe gently and use axillary, oral (if age-appropriate), or external ear route.

3. Use soft toothbrush and encourage regular dental checkups.

4. Avoid injections, if possible.
   a. Administer medications orally whenever possible.
   b. Subcutaneous route is preferred over IM.
   c. Apply pressure to injection site for 10 to 15 minutes. Then apply a pressure dressing with self-adhesive gauze.

5. Maintain a safe environment and teach parents safety measures.
   a. Protect child with kneepads, elbow pads, and helmets when riding bicycles or tricycles.
   b. Use safety belts and straps in high chairs, car seats, and strollers.
   c. Infants should have appropriate padding in cribs or playpen to prevent injury.
   d. Supervise toddlers as they learn to walk.
   e. Remove or pad furniture with sharp corners.
   f. Keep small and sharp objects out of reach.
   g. Check play equipment and outdoor play areas for possible hazards.
   h. Child should wear a MedicAlert bracelet.
   i. Be aware of safe activities that your child can enjoy including swimming, biking, and walking.

 DRUG ALERT Children with hemophilia should not receive aspirin, compounds containing aspirin, or nonsteroidal anti-inflammatory agents because these medications affect platelet function and prolong bleeding time.

Preserving Mobility

1. Treat hemarthrosis or muscle bleed as soon as possible.

2. Provide supportive care for hemarthrosis.
   a. Immobilize the joint in a position of slight flexion.
   b. Elevate the affected part above the level of the heart.
   c. Factor, if readily available, should be administered before ice is applied to the joint.

3. For severe hemarthroses, continue factor administration at home until joint pain and immobility have resolved.
4. For less severe hemarthroses, begin gentle, passive exercise 48 hours after the acute phase to prevent joint stiffness and fibrosis. Progress to active exercises.
5. Short course of corticosteroids has shown clinical effectiveness in the treatment of hemarthrosis.
6. Physiotherapy is an essential adjunct for joint bleeding.
7. Hydrotherapy can reduce pain and instability in target joints and improve ROM and muscle tone.

Relieving Pain

1. Be aware that increased pain usually means that bleeding continues and further replacement therapy may be needed.
2. Assess for further swelling of joints and limitation of movement.
3. Administer or teach administration of acetaminophen during acute phase. NSAIDs may be used for chronic pain, but cautiously, to prevent interference with platelet function.
4. Administer opioids sparingly, as ordered, for severe, acute pain.
5. If pain persists for a prolonged duration, referral to a Pain Management Center is recommended.

Enhancing Family Coping

1. Acknowledge parents' feeling of guilt or anger with regard to diagnosis.
2. Use play therapy to help the young child and siblings adjust to illness.
3. Encourage the parents to allow the child to participate in as many normal activities as possible within the realm of safety.
4. Have child wear a MedicalAlert bracelet that also includes clotting factor that is best used in an emergency.
5. Make sure anyone involved in caring for your child is aware of your child's condition.
6. Encourage the child's education. Involve teacher, principal, and assistants in understanding disease process and limitations that need to be enforced for child's safety.
7. Refer to social worker for counseling and identification of resources for financial concerns and emotional support.
8. Encourage avoidance of overprotection. This can place too many restrictions on the child's normal development. This can result in the child becoming overly dependent or becoming defiant and engaging in risky behaviors or activities.
9. Encourage involvement in support group.

Community and Home Care Considerations

1. Perform a home safety survey (inside and outside) to identify potential hazards to the hemophiliac child.
2. Provide teaching and referrals to initiate an infusion therapy program at home when hemorrhage begins.
3. Have child participate in regular exercise program to help strengthen joints which helps prevent damage or pain from internal bleeding.
4. Make sure that primary health care needs are being met by facilitating the following:
   a. Regular visits to primary care provider for preventive health maintenance to address growth and development, behavior, and psychosocial issues.
   b. Dental examinations and teeth cleaning every 6 months.
   c. All the recommended childhood immunizations, plus hepatitis A, to prevent infection from blood-borne pathogens.

5. Provide education to family and all caregivers about recognizing and treating bleeds appropriately.
6. Provide emotional support through the provision of educational materials, information about support groups, and a list of resources within the community.
7. Educate teachers and other school faculties about the child's special needs.
   a. These children can have permanent mental or physical disabilities from old hemorrhages, necessitating individualized plans.
   b. Avoidance of rough or contact sports and activities.
   c. All injuries must be taken seriously. The school nurse should be notified so that proper first aid and treatment can be initiated.
   d. Although they have a chronic illness, these children have a strong desire to be "normal," with the same opportunities and environmental stimulation as other children.

Family Education and Health Maintenance

1. Review safety measures to prevent or minimize trauma.
2. Encourage education by parents to teachers, babysitters, and others involved in child's care so that they can be responsive in an emergency.
3. Advise wearing a MedicAlert bracelet.
4. Teach emergency treatment for hemorrhage.
   a. Immobilize the part with splints or an elastic compression bandage. (These materials should be immediately available in the home.)
   b. Apply ice packs. Parents should keep two or three plastic bags of ice immediately available in the freezer. Popsicles can be used for minor mouth bleeding.
   c. Consult the child's health care provider and initiate additional recommended therapy.
5. Encourage regular medical and dental supervision.
   a. Preventive dental care is important. Soft-bristled or sponge-tipped toothbrushes should be used to prevent bleeding. Factor replacement therapy is necessary for extensive dental work and extractions.
   b. Hepatitis B vaccine is necessary to protect against the rare occurrence of hepatitis B from blood transfusions.
6. Teach healthy diet to avoid obesity, which places additional strain on the child's weight-bearing joints and predisposes to hemarthroses.
7. Assist the parents in helping the child to understand the exact nature of the illness as early as possible. Special attention should be given to the signs of hemorrhage, and the child should be told of the need to report even the slightest bleeding to an adult immediately.
8. Advise families that genetic counseling and family planning are available for parents and adolescent patients.
9. For additional information and support, refer to National Hemophilia Foundation (*www.hemophilia.org*).

TRANSITIONAL CARE ALERT Provide written discharge summaries understandable to parents regarding course of treatment during hospitalization. Ensure that discharge instructions include written medication plans, with medication name, reason for use, dosage, and times of administration. If PRN medications are prescribed, ensure understanding of when and how often these medications can be administered. Allow parents time to process information and address any questions or concerns. Provide contact numbers for parents for emergencies that require immediate attention. Schedule follow up appointments within 1 week of discharge at outpatient clinic or with primary care provider.

SELECTED REFERENCES

Abu shosha, G., & Al Kalaldeh, M. (2018). Challenges of having a child with thalassaemia major: a phenomenological study. *Journal of Research in Nursing, 23*(1), 9–20.

Acharya, S. (2013). Rare bleeding disorders in children: Identification and primary care management. *Pediatrics, 132*(5), 882–892.

Amid, A., & Odame, I. (2014). Improving outcomes in children with sickle cell disease: Treatment considerations and strategies. *Pediatric Drugs, 15*(3), 255–266.

Bertamino, M., Riccardi, F., et al. (2017). Hemophilia care in the pediatric age. *Journal of Clinical Medicine, 6*(5), 54.

Bhatnagar, Neha and Hall, Georgia W. (2018). Major bleeding disorders diagnosis, classification, management and recent developments in haemophilia. *Archives of Disease in Childhood, 103*, 509–513.

Cadet, M. (2018). Iron deficiency anemia: A clinical case study. *MEDSURG Nursing, 27*(2), 108–120.

Chakravorty, S., & Williams, T. (2015). Sickle cell disease: A neglected chronic disease of increasing global health importance. *Archives of Disease in Childhood, 100*(1), 48–53.

Darbari, D., Ballas, S., & Clauw, D. (2014). Thinking beyond sickling to better understand pain in sickle cell disease. *European Journal of Haematology, 93*(2), 89–95.

de Dreuzy, E., et al. (2016). Current and future alternative therapies for beta-thalassemia major. *Biomedical Journal, 339*(1), 24–38.

DeLoughery, T. (2014). Microcytic anemia. *New England Journal of Medicine, 371*(14), 1324–1331.

Fijnvandraat, K., et al. (2012). Diagnosis and management of hemophilia. *British Medical Journal, 334*, e2707.

Jauregui-Lobera, I. (2014). Iron deficiency and cognitive functions. *Neuropsychiatric Disease, 10*, 2087–2095.

Kassim, A., et al. (2015). How I treat and manage strokes in sickle cell disease. *Blood, 125*(22), 3401–3410.

Keane, B. (2016). Supported or stigmatized? The impact of sickle cell disease on families. *Community Practitioner, 89*(6), 44–47.

Leebeek, F., & Eikenboom, J. (2016). Von Willebrand's disease. *The New England Journal of Medicine, 375*, 2067–2080.

Lillicrap, D. (2013). von Willebrand disease: Advances in pathogenetic understanding, diagnosis, and therapy. *Blood, 122*, 3735–3740.

Manwani, D., & Frenette, P. (2013). Vaso-occlusion in sickle cell disease: Pathophysiology and novel targeted therapies. *Blood, 122*, 3892–3898.

Neutze, D., & Roque, J. (2016). Clinical evaluation of bleeding and bruising in primary care. *American Family Physician, 93*(4), 279–286.

Orkin, S., et al. (2014). *Nathan and Oski's hematology and oncology of infancy and childhood* (8th ed.). Elsevier Health Sciences.

Parise, L., & Berlinger, N. (2016). Sickle cell disease: Challenges and progress. *Blood, 127*, 789.

Parkin, P., et al. (2016). Severe iron-deficiency anaemia and feeding practices in young children. *Public Health Nutrition, 19*(4), 1260–1269.

Piel, F. B., Steinberg, M. H. & Rees, D. C. (2017). Sickle cell disease. *New England Journal of Medicine, 376*, 1561–1573.

Powers, J., & Buchanan, G. (2017). Potential for improved screening, diagnosis, and treatment for iron deficiency and iron deficiency anemia in young children. *Journal of Pediatrics, 588*, 8–10.

Powers, J., McCavit, T., & Buchanan, G. (2015). Management of iron deficiency anemia: A survey of pediatric hematology/oncology specialists. *Pediatric Blood Cancer, 62*(5), 842–846.

Saunders, N., et al. (2016). Iron status of young children from immigrant families. *Archives of Disability in Childhood, 101*(12), 1130–1136.

Sayed, S., et al. (2013). The early cardiac involvement in patients with B thalassemia major. *The Egyptian Heart Journal, 65*(3), 243–249.

Shinde, S., Bakshi, A., & Shikhande, A. (2015). Infections in sickle cell disease. *International Archives of Integrated Medicine, 2*(11), 26–34.

Shook, L., et al. (2016). Translating sickle cell guidelines into practice for primary care providers with Project ECHO. *Medical Education Online, 24*(21), 33616.

Singh, P., & Seth, A. (2017). Growth and endocrine issues in children with thalassemia. *Pediatric Hematology Oncology Journal, 2*(4), 98–106.

Smith, K., Reinman, L., Schatz, J., et al. (2018). Parent perspectives on pain management in preschool-age children with sickle cell disease. *Journal of Pediatric Oncology Nursing, 35*(1), 16–24.

Tantiworawit, A., et al. (2016). Iron overload in non-transfusion-dependent thalassemia: Association with genotype and clinical risk factors. *Journal of Hematology, 103*(6), 643–648.

Tewari, S., et al. (2015). Environmental determinants of severity in sickle cell disease. *Hematologica, 100*(9), 1108–1116.

Wacharasin, C., Phaktoop, M., & Sananreangsak, S. (2015). Examining the usefulness of a family empowerment program guided by the illness beliefs model for families caring for a child with thalassemia. *Journal of Family Nursing, 21*(2), 295–321.

Wang, M. (2016). Iron deficiency and other types of anemia in infants and children. *American Family Physician, 93*(4), 270–278.

Zuffo, C. R. K., Osorio, M. M., et al. (2016). Prevalence and risk factors of anemia in children. *Jornal de Pediatria, 92*(4), 353–360.

53

Pediatric Immunologic Disorders

IMMUNOLOGIC DISORDERS

Pediatric Human Immunodeficiency Virus/Acquired Immunodeficiency Syndrome

Human immunodeficiency virus (HIV) infection for infants, children, and adolescents is represented by a continuum of immunologic and clinical classifications ranging from no to severe immunologic suppression and asymptomatic to severely symptomatic. *Acquired immunodeficiency syndrome (AIDS)* is the end stage of the continuum. Also see Chapter 29, HIV Infection and AIDS, page 808.

Epidemiology

EVIDENCE BASE UNAIDS Fact Sheet World AIDS Day 2017. Available: *www.unaids.org/sites/default/files/media_asset/UNAIDS_FactSheet_en.pdf.* Accessed May 2018.

Centers for Disease Control and Prevention. HIV Surveillance Report, 2016; vol. 28. Available: *http://www.cdc.gov/hiv/library/reports/hiv-surveillance.html.* Published November 2017. Accessed [May 20, 2018]

1. HIV is a pandemic, affecting people all over the world; the World Health Organization estimated 30.8–42.9 million people living with HIV (in 2016).
2. Children under age 15 account for 1.8 million infected with HIV worldwide (end 2015). In North America, UNAIDS reported there were more than 1.2 million people living with the virus in 2013, of which 13% are unaware they are infected.
3. HIV is transmitted through sexual contact with an infected person; through exposure to infected blood and blood components (sharing needles via IV drug use, tattooing, piercing, and unsterilized medical equipment); or from an HIV-infected mother to her baby before or during birth or through breastfeeding.
4. In the United States, sexually acquired HIV remains the main mode of transmission. It is estimated that youth aged 13 to 24 represent the second highest rate of newly acquired HIV.
5. Globally, 76% (60–88%) of all pregnant HIV-infected women are treated to prevent vertical transmission, which has contributed to the greater than 47% decline in new infections among children, since 2010.
6. In the US, prenatally acquired HIV infection has dramatically decreased from about 25% to less than 1% of pediatric cases.
7. This decrease reflects concerted efforts to provide improved preconception counseling; HIV testing for all pregnant women; initiation the use of combination antiretroviral therapy (cART) as early as possible; with the goal of full viral suppression to the limits of detection; providing prophylaxis medication to the infant; and exclusive formula feeding.
   a. If viral load is suppressed, HIV-infected women can deliver vaginally while continuing to take their oral antiretrovirals during delivery. The HIV-exposed infant will be given 4 weeks of zidovudine as prophylaxis.
   b. If viral load is not suppressed during delivery (greater than 1,000 copies/mL), additional steps can be taken to reduce the risk of transmission: scheduled caesarean delivery, use of intrapartum IV zidovudine, and use of combination antiretroviral prophylaxis for the infant.
      i. Consultation with a pediatric HIV specialist is highly recommended in cases where cART may be required for the infant.
8. An HIV-infected mother can have a child who is infected and subsequent children who are uninfected. Likewise, one infant in a multiple birth can be infected, whereas the other infant(s) are not.
9. Children born to mothers with a high HIV viral load and low CD4+ lymphocyte counts and with severely symptomatic HIV disease are at greater risk for infection.
   a. Infants born to such mothers and who become infected appear to be at increased risk for more rapid disease progression.
   b. Infants born to mothers who seroconvert during pregnancy are at an increased risk for becoming infected.
10. With the advent of HAART, the morbidity and mortality in HIV-infected children has decreased significantly. Thus, in those who have access to medication and who are adherent to therapy, HIV has become a chronic, manageable illness.

EVIDENCE BASE Panel on Treatment of HIV-Infected Pregnant Women and Prevention of Perinatal Transmission. (2018). Recommendations for use of antiretroviral drugs in pregnant HIV-1-infected women for maternal health and interventions to reduce perinatal HIV transmission in the United States. Available: *http://aidsinfo.nih.gov/contentfiles/lvguidelines/PerinatalGL.pdf*.

Pathophysiology and Etiology

EVIDENCE BASE American Academy of Pediatrics. (2015). Section 3: Summaries of infectious diseases. In D. Kimberlin, M. Brady, M. A. Jackson, S. S. Long, (Eds.), *Red Book: 2015 Report of the Committee on Infectious Diseases* (30th ed., pp. 453–475). Elk Grove Village, IL: American Academy of Pediatrics.

1. The causative agent is a retrovirus that damages the immune system by infecting and depleting the CD4+ lymphocytes (T4 helper cells). These CD4+ lymphocytes play a central role in the regulation of the immune system.
2. There are also abnormalities in the function of cellular and humoral immunity (B cells, CD8+ cells, natural killer cells, monocytes, macrophages, and specific antibodies).
3. Progressive destruction of the immune system leads to:
   a. Increased incidence of serious bacterial infections, such as bacteremia, bacterial pneumonias, and osteomyelitis.
   b. Opportunistic infections, which commonly include *Pneumocystis jirovecii* pneumonia (PCP), esophageal candidiasis, and *Mycobacterium avium* infection.
   c. More aggressive forms of viral infections, such as severe varicella, disseminated zoster, and cytomegalovirus pneumonitis.
   d. Cancers, especially lymphomas.
   e. Wasting syndromes and encephalopathy.
4. Multisystem organ involvement results in cardiomyopathies; nephropathies; neurologic impairment; GI dysfunction; endocrine disorders; dermatologic manifestations; musculoskeletal abnormalities; ocular impairments; ear, nose, and throat problems; and hematologic disorders.
5. An AIDS diagnosis occurs when a child presents as severely symptomatic (Category C) or with lymphoid interstitial pneumonitis (LIP from Category B) along with severe immunosuppression (see Tables 53-1 and 53-2).
6. Once an AIDS diagnosis is made, it is not reversed even with reconstitution of the immune system and recovery from the opportunistic infection.

Clinical Manifestations of Disease Progression

1. Generalized lymphadenopathy, especially in less common sites, such as epitrochlear and axillary areas.
2. Persistent, recurrent oral candidiasis.
3. Failure to thrive.
4. Developmental delays or loss of previously acquired milestones.
5. Hepatomegaly.
6. Splenomegaly.
7. Persistent diarrhea.
8. Hypergammaglobulinemia or hypogammaglobulinemia (elevated or diminished levels of immunoglobulin [Ig] G, IgM, IgA).
9. Parotitis.
10. Unexplained anemias, thrombocytopenia.
11. Unexplained cardiac or kidney disease.
12. Recurrent mild or serious bacterial infections.

EVIDENCE BASE Panel on Antiretroviral Therapy and Medical Management of HIV-Infected Children. Guidelines for the use of antiretroviral agents in pediatric HIV infection. Available: *http://aidsinfo.nih.gov/contentfiles/lvguidelines/pediatricguidelines.pdf*. Accessed May 20,2018 [pages B1, C1, 6, 7, D1–2, E1–3, F1–7, H1–3, J1–2.

Diagnostic Evaluation

1. All pregnant women in the United States should have HIV antibody testing (ELISA enzyme–linked immunoassay) as standard of care.
2. Antibody testing in children less than 18 months is not reliable for diagnosis. A positive ELISA test may only be an indication of the presence of circulating maternal antibodies.
3. HIV-DNA PCR (polymerase chain reaction) assay is the most sensitive, specific, and preferred method for detecting HIV infection in a child less than 18 months. The 2016 Centers for Disease Prevention and Control (CDC) guidelines recommend testing for infants using PCR at ages 14 to 21 days, 1 to 2 months, and 4 to 6 months.

Table 53-1 Pediatric HIV Classification*

	CLINICAL CATEGORIES			
IMMUNOLOGIC CATEGORIES	**N: NO SIGNS/ SYMPTOMS**	**A: MILD SIGNS/ SYMPTOMS**	**B:† MODERATE SIGNS/ SYMPTOMS**	**C:† SEVERE SIGNS/ SYMPTOMS**
1: No evidence of suppression	N1	A1	B1	C1
2: Evidence of moderate suppression	N2	A2	B2	C2
3: Severe suppression	N3	A3	B3	C3

*Children whose HIV infection status is not confirmed are classified by using the above grid with a letter E (for perinatally exposed) placed before the appropriate classification code (eg, EN2).
†Category C and lymphoid interstitial pneumonitis in Category B are reportable to state and local health departments as acquired immunodeficiency syndrome.
Centers for Disease Control and Prevention. (1994). 1994 revised classification system for human immunodeficiency virus infection in children less than 13 years of age. Morbidity and Mortality Weekly Report, 43(RR-12), 1–10. Available: www.cdc.gov/mmwr/preview/mmwrhtml/00032890.htm.

Table 53-2	Immunologic Categories Based on Age-Specific CD4+ T-lymphocyte Counts and Percentage of Total Lymphocytes					
	AGE OF CHILD					
	YOUNGER THAN AGE 12 MONTHS		**AGES 1–5**		**AGES 6–12**	
IMMUNOLOGIC CATEGORY	MM³	(%)	MM³	(%)	MM³	(%)
	≥1,500	(≥25)	≥1,000	(≥25)	≥500	(≥25)
1: No evidence of suppression						
2: Evidence of moderate suppression	750–1,499	(15–24)	500–999	(15–24)	200–499	(15–24)
3: Severe suppression	<750	(<15)	<500	(<15)	<200	(<15)

Centers for Disease Control and Prevention. (1994). 1994 revised classification system for human immunodeficiency virus infection in children less than 13 years of age. Morbidity and Mortality Weekly Report, 43(RR-12), 1–10. Available: www.cdc.gov/mmwr/preview/mmwrhtml/00032890.htm.

4. Residual maternal HIV antibodies may still be present in children 18 to 24 months; thus, diagnosis use of HIV-DNA PCR should be used.

5. After age 24 months, HIV antibody assays can be used for testing because maternal antibodies should not be present by this age. As with adults, a reactive ELISA must be followed by a confirmatory Western blot test.

6. In known infected children or at-risk infants (those born to an HIV-infected mother but whose own status is still indeterminate), computed tomography scanning or magnetic resonance imaging of the head may be indicated if there is evidence of neurologic impairment, falling rate of head growth, or developmental delays or regression.

Management

HIV-Exposed Infant

1. Additional laboratory studies requiring monitoring on the HIV-exposed infant include complete blood count (CBC) with differential (diff) to monitor for anemia and neutropenia and lymphocyte subsets (CD4+ counts), lactate and cognitive

HIV Infected

2. At the time of diagnosis, baseline CD4, HIV RNA (viral load), drug resistance (genotypic and phenotypic resistance should be used) should be performed. Child should have a complete age-appropriate medical history (including immunization history) and physical exam and additional laboratory evaluations for HIV-associated conditions: CBC with

differential, chemistry of glucose, liver and renal function, and urinalysis and serologic evaluation for coinfections and immunities. HLA-B*5701 is used to assess potential for abacavir hypersensitivity. In addition, a baseline echocardiogram and chest x-ray should be done and repeated yearly.

3. Child needs ongoing laboratory assessment; CBC with differential, platelet counts, serum chemistries, serial CD4+ counts, and HIV RNA (viral load) should be done every 3 to 6 months (depending on previous results and the stage of disease).

4. Initiation of PCP prophylaxis is indicated when low CD4+ counts occur, with the exception that all infants born to HIV-infected women should be started on PCP prophylaxis at age 4 to 6 weeks, regardless of their CD4+ count (see Table 53-3).

   a. The first drug of choice is co-trimoxazole.

   b. Pentamidine, atovaquone, and dapsone are alternative choices.

   c. PCP prophylaxis should be discontinued in infants whose infection has been reasonably excluded on the basis of two or more negative viral diagnostic tests performed at greater than 4 weeks and greater than 8 weeks of age. Some experts may choose not to give prophylaxis to infants in whom antenatal and peripartum management has been appropriate and in whom the risk of infection is very low.

   d. Infants confirmed infected should remain on PCP prophylaxis until at 1 year of age and then reassessed based on their CD4 count.

5. Antiretroviral therapy is recommended for all HIV-infected children less than 1 year of age and in older children who have clinical symptoms of HIV or evidence of immunosuppression

Table 53-3	Recommendations for PCP Prophylaxis and CD4+ Monitoring for HIV-Exposed Infants and HIV-Infected Children, by Age and HIV Infection Status	
AGE/HIV INFECTION STATUS	**PCP PROPHYLAXIS**	**CD4+ MONITORING**
Birth to ages 4–6 weeks, HIV exposed	No prophylaxis	1 month
Ages 4–6 weeks to 4 months, HIV exposed	Prophylaxis	3 months
Ages 4–12 months, HIV infected or indeterminate	Prophylaxis	6, 9, and 12 months
Under ages 4–12 months, HIV infection reasonably excluded	No prophylaxis	None
Ages 1–5, HIV infected	Prophylaxis if: CD4+ count is <500 cells/L or CD4+ percentage is <15%	Every 3–4 months
Ages 6–12, HIV infected	Prophylaxis if: CD4+ count is <200 cells/L or CD4+ percentage is <15%	Every 3–4 months

Adapted from Centers for Disease Control and Prevention. (1995). 1995 revised guidelines for prophylaxis against Pneumocystis carinii pneumonia for children infected with or perinatally exposed to human immunodeficiency virus. Morbidity and Mortality Weekly Report, 44(RR-4), 1–11. Available: www.cdc.gov/mmwr/preview/mmwrhtml/00037275.htm.

regardless of the age of the child or HIV PCR level (viral load). Although new guidelines recommend early initiation of treatment for all HIV-infected individuals, many factors need to be considered for children greater than 1 year of age before starting. Factors such as the severity of disease progression, appropriate medication (availability, cost, dose, formulation, taste, side effects, and complexity of regimen), resistance pattern, and coinfection are but a few.

Clinical trial data from both adults and children have demonstrated that antiretroviral therapy in symptomatic patients slows clinical and immunologic disease progression and reduces mortality.

Six classes of antiretrovirals (ARVs) have been approved for use in children: nucleoside reverse transcriptase inhibitors (NRTIs), non–nucleoside reverse transcriptase inhibitors (NNRTIs), protease inhibitors (PIs), integrase inhibitor, CCR5 antagonist, and fusion inhibitor.

Combination therapy is now standard care, using at least three ARVs from at least two drug classes.

6. Adherence is the basis for successful viral suppression; strategies should be developed to encourage adherence. Adherence is essential to prevent viral resistance; particularly, NNRTI resistance develops rapidly with even slight fluctuations in drug levels.
7. Use of IV immunoglobulin is still recommended for HIV-infected children who have had two or more serious bacterial infections within 1 year and for the treatment of HIV-related thrombocytopenia or immunoglobulin deficiency.
8. Use of antifungal drugs, such as nystatin, ketoconazole, fluconazole, itraconazole, and clotrimazole, for persistent or recurrent oral candidiasis.
9. Use of antivirals, such as acyclovir, valacyclovir, ganciclovir, and cidofovir, for suppression or treatment of recurrent viral infections.
10. Aggressive, prompt assessment and treatment of febrile illnesses.
11. Nutritional support.
12. Evaluation and treatment of developmental delays and regression.
13. Adequate pain management in advanced or end-stage disease.
14. Support and interventions for the child and family (including all caregivers) with issues of disclosure, parental guilt, long-term care, and bereavement.

 DRUG ALERT Test for the presence of ARV drug-resistant virus in both experienced and naive patients before initiating ARV combination therapy, thus ensuring the most effective regimen.

 DRUG ALERT Lack of adherence to prescribed antiretroviral regimens and subtherapeutic drug levels increase the possibility that a resistant virus will develop. Strict adherence (more than 95%) to combination regimens is critical in ensuring sustained response to treatment.

 NURSING ALERT Families can find out about clinical treatment trials available for their child by calling (800) TRIALS-A or visiting *www.clinicaltrials.gov.*

Complications

1. Untreated or inadequately treated HIV:
   a. Repeated, overwhelming infections and certain cancers, particularly lymphomas.
   b. Hearing loss, tooth and gum disease, acute and chronic ear, nose, and throat infections.
   c. Opportunistic infections.
   d. Reactive airway disease.
   e. Cardiomyopathy.
   f. Failure to thrive, malabsorption, wasting.
   g. Chronic atopic dermatitis and other skin reactions.
   h. Nephropathy.
   i. Neuropathy, myopathy.
   j. Anemia, thrombocytopenia, neutropenia.
   k. Loss of treatment options related to the development of drug resistance.
   l. Developmental delay.
   m. Learning disabilities.
   n. Psychological challenges for children and caregivers, including multiple losses, issues of disclosure, fear, discrimination, stigmatization, and isolation.
   o. Death.
2. Complications of HIV treatment:
   a. NRTIs—anemia, neutropenia, lactic acidosis, pancreatitis, abacavir hypersensitivity reaction, peripheral neuropathy, lipodystrophy/lipoatrophy, renal dysfunction, osteopenia, headache, nausea, potential for vascular dysfunction.
   b. NNRTIs—psychological changes, sleep disturbances/nightmares, neural tube defects (fetal exposure), hepatitis, rash.
   c. PIs—dyslipidemia, GI upset, diarrhea.
   d. Fusion inhibitors—injection site reactions.

 DRUG ALERT Because some liquid preparations are unpalatable, nonadherence to the drug regimen is common. Suggestions to overcome this would include using Popsicle just before administration to numb the taste buds, followed by a teaspoon of chocolate/strawberry syrup, jam, or peanut butter immediately after. Speak to pharmacist about other ways to mask the taste.

Nursing Assessment

1. Review maternal records to identify infants who may be at risk for HIV disease. Infected infants are not easily identifiable by outward appearance.
2. Review records of at-risk or known infected children to determine nutritional status, growth and development, frequency of serious bacterial infections, presence or risk of opportunistic infections, laboratory values, and immunization status.
3. Assess growth, development, lymph nodes, hepatomegaly, splenomegaly, and oropharynx for presence of oral candidiasis and dental caries.
4. Assess the family's understanding of the child's condition, care needs, prognosis, and medical care plan.
5. Assess the family's coping mechanisms, comfort with disclosure issues, and long-term plans for care including transition plans for the child to an adult care program.
6. Assess the health of primary caregiver and discuss long-term care plans for respite and permanent alternative caregivers (including guardianship issues), as appropriate.

7. Assess the child's understanding of health condition and medications.
8. In children with advanced or end-stage disease, assess the level of pain and discomfort.
9. Assess the child's coping and response to the frequent painful and invasive procedures experienced as part of the ongoing diagnosis and management of the disease.
10. Assess for animal contact.
11. Take a thorough travel history to evaluate risk of coinfections, such as tuberculosis (TB), malaria, or other parasitic infections. Also evaluate potential travel plans, particularly to developing countries.
12. In the adolescent, assess increased at-risk behaviors, such as substance use, piercing, or sexual activity. Also determine methods of birth control, as appropriate.

 NURSING ALERT Always discuss with the primary caregiver how much the child knows about his/her own HIV status or about other family members' status. Never assume anyone knows the child's HIV status; other family, friends, daycare, or school not even the child may know.

 DRUG ALERT Some antiretrovirals interact with the effect of birth control pills and may reduce efficacy or increase hormonal-related side effects. *For more information, see CDC's U.S. Medical Eligibility Criteria for Contraceptive Use, 2016, www.cdc.gov/mmwr/volumes/65/ rr/pdfs/rr6503.pdf. Current perinatal guidelines do not restrict the use of efavirenz during pregnancy.*

Nursing Diagnoses

- Risk for Infection related to immunodeficiency, neutropenia.
- Ineffective Therapeutic Regimen Management related to insufficient knowledge of HIV, noncompliance, and limited resources.
- Imbalanced Nutrition: Less than Body Requirements related to malabsorption, anorexia, or pain.
- Impaired Oral Mucous Membranes related to candidiasis and herpes stomatitis.
- Diarrhea related to enteric pathogens, disease process, and medications.
- Hyperthermia related to HIV infection and secondary infection.
- Delayed Growth and Development related to HIV central nervous system (CNS) infection.
- Pain related to advanced or end-stage HIV disease.
- Anxiety/Fear related to frequent invasive procedures, diagnosis, stigmatization, transmission to others, and separation from others.
- Denial related to learned response patterns—cultural factors, personal/family value system; fear of rejection/stigma.
- Ineffective Coping by child related to unresolved issues around disclosure, hospitalization, and losses; negative role modeling or inadequate support.
- Ineffective Family Coping related to parental guilt; excessive demands on individual and family; stigma.
- Social isolation related real or feared rejection and discrimination.
- Powerlessness related to loss of control, stigmatization.
- Alteration in body image related to effects of medication and disease.

Nursing Interventions

Preventing Infection

 EVIDENCE BASE Centers for Disease Control and Prevention. Recommended immunization schedules for children and adolescents aged 18 or younger, United States 2017. Available: *www.cdc.gov/ vaccines/schedules/hcp/child-adolescent.html.*

1. Monitor viral load, CD4 count, and CBC with differential.
2. Monitor other lab values to assess for side effects, that is, significant drop in absolute neutrophil count.
3. Use aseptic techniques when performing invasive procedures.
4. Administer or teach caregiver the importance of giving pharmacologic agents that may help prevent opportunistic infections. *See Management.*
5. Assess and maintain skin integrity
6. Monitor immunization status and advocate for completion of all recommended childhood immunizations (see Table 53-4). Also see page 1119 for routine pediatric

Table 53-4	Vaccination of Individuals with HIV Based on the Canadian Immunization Guide	
VACCINE	**HIV/AIDS**
Inactivated Vaccines	
Dtap, Tdap, Td	Routine use*
IPV	Routine use
Hib	Routine use
Influenza	Recommended
Pneumococcal	Recommended
Meningococcal	Routine use
Hep A	Recommended (MSM, IDU)
Hep B	Recommended/routine use†
Human papillomavirus	Recommended
Live Vaccines	
MMR	Routine use‡ (if no significant compromise)
Varicella	Consider in asymptomatic and mild symptomatic disease
OPV	Contraindicated (alternate available)
Oral typhoid	Contraindicated (alternate available)
BCG	Contraindicated
Yellow fever	Contraindicated**
Oral cholera	Contraindicated

*Routine vaccination schedules should be followed with age-appropriate booster doses.
†Hep B vaccine (HB) is now recommended for all infants.
‡Most HIV-positive children can receive the first MMR vaccine without significant risk. Administration of the second MMR dose (particularly in adults) must be evaluated on a case-by-case basis.
**Consultation with an expert is recommended.
© All rights reserved. Canadian Immunization Guide. Public Health Agency of Canada, modified in 2017. Adapted and reproduced with permission from the Minister of Health, 2018. Available: www.phacaspc.gc.ca/publicat/ cig-gci/p03-07-eng.php.

immunization information based on the CDC. In general, live vaccines should be used with caution in children with HIV infections.

- a. The measles, mumps, rubella (MMR), and varicella vaccines are recommended for HIV-infected children who are not severely immunocompromised.
- b. Oral polio vaccine should be avoided because there is an alternative injectable inactivated polio vaccine available.
- c. Yellow fever vaccine should be avoided unless the risk of exposure is extremely high; consultation with an expert is recommended.
- d. In the United States, the bacille Calmette-Guérin vaccine is also not recommended.
- e. Yearly influenza vaccine and a 3- to 5-year pneumococcal vaccine are also recommended in addition to the standard childhood immunization schedule.
- f. An annual TB skin test should also be administered.
7. Have a high index of suspicion for secondary infection even when clinical manifestations are subtle or absent.
8. Provide appropriate chemoprophylaxis following exposure to communicable diseases.
9. Educate family/patient on the importance of prevention of secondary infections.
    - a. Maintain cleanliness of the environment and teach family members the essentials of environmental sanitation.
    - b. Routine handwashing with soap and water.
    - c. Oral hygiene and assessment for dental carries.
    - d. Skin care to prevent break down.
    - e. Safe food preparation and clean water use.
    - f. Risk associated with handling animals; cats may transmit *toxoplasmosis or bartonella*, birds may transmit *Cryptococcus neoformans* or *M. avium*, and reptiles may transmit *Salmonellosis*. Good hand washing with soap and water after handling animals; contact with animal feces should be avoided.
    - g. Attend Travel Medicine Clinic before traveling, particularly to developing or tropical countries, to prevent infections such as malaria or typhoid.
    - h. How to use condoms to prevent sexually transmitted diseases such as syphilis or chlamydia.

DRUG ALERT Uninfected children living with HIV-infected parents or siblings should not receive the oral polio vaccine, but rather the injectable inactivated polio vaccine. This is due to the prolonged shedding of the virus from the live oral vaccine, which may prove to be hazardous for immunocompromised individuals.

Maximizing Adherence to HAART

EVIDENCE BASE Panel on Antiretroviral Therapy and Medical Management of HIV-Infected Children. Guidelines for the use of antiretroviral agents in pediatric HIV infection. Available: *http://aidsinfo.nih.gov/contentfiles/lvguidelines/pediatricguidelines.pdf.* Accessed April 17, 2017.
NOTE: Use of antiretrovirals in pediatric patients is evolving rapidly. These guidelines are updated regularly to provide current information. The most recent information is available at *http://aidsinfo.nih.gov.*
Centers for Disease Control and Prevention, Health Resources and Services Administration, National Institutes of Health, American Academy of HIV Medicine, Association of

Nurses in AIDS Care, International Association of Providers of AIDS Care, the National Minority AIDS Council, and Urban Coalition for HIV/AIDS Prevention Services.
Center for Disease Control and Prevention. (2014). Recommendations for HIV prevention with adults and adolescents with HIV in the United States, 2014. Available: *https://www.cdc.gov/hiv/guidelines/recommendations/personswithhiv.html.* pp. 83–96.

1. Develop a trusting relationship with the patient by maintaining a nonjudgmental attitude to maintain open communication and assist in assessing barriers to adherence.
2. Assess drug readiness and strategies to maximize adherence before initiating therapy.
3. Provide the simplest regimen possible; for example, least number of pills (combination therapies), least often (once daily), based on viral resistance.
4. Stress the need for adherence at every visit.
5. Use several strategies for evaluating adherence (eg, viral load, pill count, self-reporting, and pharmacy refill checks).
6. Collaborate with patient to determine what reminder tools may work the best (pill box, calendar, stickers, alarm, associating pill-taking with daily routine).

Maintaining Adequate Nutrition
1. Carefully monitor growth parameters (height, weight, head circumference).
2. Consult with a dietitian to develop strategies for nutritional care, including additional calories, nutritional supplements while reducing cholesterol.
3. Teach the family to prepare high-calorie, nutritious meals that are pleasing and acceptable to children.
4. As age appropriate, involve the child in meal planning.
5. Encourage small, frequent meals if the child is experiencing absorption problems.

Maintaining Oral Mucosa and Dental Integrity
1. Include regular examinations of the oral mucosa and teeth in the physical assessment of the child.
2. Administer prescribed antifungal and antiviral therapy.
3. Offer fluids and pureed foods to minimize chewing and facilitate swallowing; avoid highly seasoned or acidic foods.
4. Encourage regular dental hygiene and dental visits.

Minimizing Effects of Diarrhea
1. Monitor for the presence or development of diarrhea.
2. Monitor daily weight when diarrhea is present.
3. Monitor intake and output and assess skin and mucous membranes for turgor and dryness.
4. Use enteric precautions.
5. Avoid foods that increase intestinal motility.
6. Administer IV hydration, as indicated.
7. Plan a regimen of skin care, including cleansing/blot drying of the anal area and application of ointment or skin barrier cream.
8. Teach the family safe food preparation techniques to minimize contamination of food.
9. Administer medications, as directed, for relief of severe diarrhea and enteric infections.

Detecting and Controlling Fever
1. Monitor for fever and report any core temperature over 101°F (38.3°C).
2. Institute comfort measures, such as sponge baths, dry clothing and linens, and antipyretics, as ordered.

3. Teach the family how to accurately monitor the child's rectal temperature.
4. Teach the family to promptly report any febrile episode over 101°F rectally.
5. Administer antipyretics.

Promoting Developmental Goals

1. Assess the child's developmental status on a regular basis.
2. Report regression or delay in achieving developmental milestones.
3. Make appropriate referrals for more in-depth developmental evaluation when delays and regression are noted.
4. Teach the family appropriate developmental stimulation activities for their child.
5. Implement recommendations for developmental stimulation (including school-based programs) and assist the family in doing likewise.
6. Facilitate successful transition to adult care (see Box 53-1).

 EVIDENCE BASE Children's HIV Association (CHIVA). (2017). *CHIVA guidance on transition for adolescents living with HIV*. London: Author. Available: www.chiva.org.uk/guidelines/tr.

Promoting Effective Family Coping

1. Practice within a framework of family-centered care.
2. Assess the family's coping mechanisms, strengths, and weaknesses.
3. Provide emotional support to the family.
4. Refer the family to appropriate community resources for grief counseling and legal assistance (eg, wills, custody issues).
5. Help the family set realistic goals and expectations for the child.
6. Maintain a nonjudgmental attitude and nonprejudicial approach.
7. Allow the family to use denial as a protective mechanism because this gives them some sense of control.
8. Explain all care and treatment plans to the family.
9. Involve the family in planning for the care and management of their child.
10. Give strategies and guidance to families regarding *partial truth telling* so they can answer child's questions as honestly as possible.
11. Provide support to new mothers who grieve the loss of not being able to breastfeed. Provide strategies on how to deflect questions about the choice not to breastfeed.
12. Encourage parent to allow adolescent to start taking increased responsibility for own health care, including individual time alone with health care provider and self-advocacy.
13. Provide family and disclosed patient with hopeful information about the future, such as continuing education or, possibly, getting married and having a family.
14. Refer the family to community resources for home care, daycare of other siblings, transportation services, school-based services, respite care, and hospice.

BOX 53-1	**Transition to Adult Care**

Transition is the purposeful, planned movement of adolescents and young adults with chronic illness/disabilities from child-centered to adult-oriented systems. With the advent of highly active antiretroviral therapy, children with human immunodeficiency virus (HIV) are surviving and living well into adulthood. As they become adults, they are graduating from pediatric health care programs—with parents the child's advocate—to adult programs where individual care becomes the focus, with the young adult becoming his or her own advocate.

It is imperative for the pediatric health care team to prepare children and families for the changes and challenges of adolescence, with a focus on increased autonomy and self-reliance and independence.

The transition into adolescence is a normal part of growth and development; however, special considerations need to be addressed when caring for a teenager with a chronic illness.

KEY ELEMENTS OF TRANSITION
- Focus the orientation on the future and keep it proactive and flexible.
- Start as early as possible.
- Build on knowledge about HIV and issues of confidentiality and disclosure.
- Make sure your approach fosters personal and medical interdependence and creative problem solving.
- Provide opportunities for own consultations during clinic visit.
- Have open, honest, age-appropriate sexual health discussions.
- Develop a written transition policy—agreed upon by all members of the multidisciplinary team and target adult services—posted for families and young adults to see.

- Discuss different care models and possible settings in which the young adult can access care as an adult.
- Provide liaison personnel in both pediatric and adult health care centers.
- Coordinate an initial meeting for teen to meet adult care provider and staff.
- Ensure a flexible policy on the timing of events, with anticipation of change.
- Provide an education program for young people and their families that addresses medical, psychosocial, and educational/vocational aspects of care.
- Develop an individualized health care transition plan by age 14, in collaboration with the young adult and his or her family, and continuously update, as needed.
- Identify a network of relevant community agencies and adult primary and subspecialty care providers.
- Implement a training program for pediatric and adult providers on transition and adolescent issues.
- Provide for appropriate primary preventive care.
- Ensure affordable continuous health and medication insurance coverage.

 EVIDENCE BASE Boudreau, M., & Fisher, C. (2012). Providing effective medical and case management services to HIV-infected youth preparing to transition to adult care. *Journal of the Association of Nurses in AIDS Care, 23*(4), 318–328.

Strengthening Coping Skills of the Child

 EVIDENCE BASE Evangeli, M., Kagee, A. (2016). A model of caregiver paediatric HIV disclosure decision-making. *Psychology, Health & Medicine, 21*(3), 338–353.

Penn, C. (2015). "Too much for one day": a case study of disclosure in the paediatric HIV/AIDS clinic. *Health Expectations, 18* (4), 578–589.

1. Introduce the subject of disclosure of diagnosis to the child with the family. Offer the family guidelines as to age-appropriate approaches.
2. Accept that some families may not be able to disclose the nature of the disease to their child, even after much support and guidance.
   a. Explore with families how they want you to address questions the child may present to you.
   b. The illness and its impact can be effectively handled without actually telling the child about the HIV disease or AIDS status, if the family refuses to disclose it.
3. Answer the child's questions as honestly as possible within parental constraints that may be present.
4. Actively involve the child in as much of the care as possible, such as by having the child decide where to place the IV line, cleaning off skin for needle insertion, and so forth.
5. Use therapeutic play techniques (age appropriate), such as drawing, playing with dolls, playing with medical equipment, and storytelling, to allow the child to express himself or herself in less verbal ways.
6. Refer the child and family for counseling if the child's coping skills do not progress or there appears to be regression in handling the issue of illness and chronic health care needs. Signs indicating possible need for additional in-depth interventions include more acting out by the child, withdrawn behavior, and difficulty in school (either behaviorally or academically).
7. Recommend and facilitate peer support groups.

Minimizing Discomfort

1. Assess for signs of pain in the child. In the infant or nonverbal child, such signs include restlessness, crying, withdrawn behavior, and changes in vital signs.
2. Discuss concerns over pain issues with the primary health care provider and team providing care for the child. Initiate or request referral to a pain management team if the child does not experience relief.
3. Stress to the parent or guardian the need for adequate pain management in children; many people do not acknowledge that infants or children suffer from pain and that this needs to be alleviated.
4. Use appropriate techniques to assess the level of pain or discomfort a child is experiencing.

Minimizing Fear

1. Make sure that all painful and invasive procedures are done in a location other than the child's bed in the hospital.
2. Monitor central line if used for venous access. Central line access may be less traumatic over time than repeated peripheral access attempts. Some children with HIV will need long-term, probably lifelong, IV therapies and blood monitoring, and a central line greatly eliminates the pain and anxiety associated with these procedures.
3. Make sure that the parent/caregiver realizes that most clinic visits will involve blood tests so that they do not falsely reassure the child that "no needle sticks" will occur.
4. Use diversionary techniques, such as bubble-blowing, for distraction during painful procedures. Practice first with the child and tell him or her this is an activity that you will help with during the procedure. Children can also be taught other relaxation techniques.
5. Offer small rewards (such as stickers, small toy items) after painful procedures to reduce anxiety. Such rewards should be given regardless of how the child reacted. The reward is not for "not crying" but acknowledges difficulty in going through painful and invasive procedures on a regular basis.
6. Involve the child in the procedure as much as possible (age appropriate). Such involvement can include selecting a possible site for accessing or receiving IV medications, cleaning the site, or selecting a special bandage for after the procedure. Use topical anesthetic.

Community and Home Care Considerations

1. Assess home environment for resources, such as nutritious foods and safe food preparation; adequate water, heat, electricity, and space; developmentally appropriate toys; and supplies needed for care and hygiene.
2. Assess caregiver's correct administration of medications.
3. Draw blood samples using universal precautions and careful transport of blood and used equipment.
4. Perform developmental assessment periodically.
5. Act as liaison among family, specialists, school officials, and other team members.

Family Education and Health Maintenance

1. Teach families and other caregivers of the child universal precautions. In caring for HIV-infected infants and children, gloves are recommended when handling potentially contaminated body fluids (such as blood) but are not considered necessary for routine diaper-changing unless bloody diarrhea or hematuria exists.
2. Facilitate supply of adequate numbers of latex (or nonlatex, if necessary) gloves to families to use, as indicated.
3. Facilitate education as well as a supply of latex condoms and other forms of birth control for teens who are sexually active or about to become sexually active.
4. Offer guidance as to how to initiate discussion of their child's HIV status with schools and daycare settings. The "need-to-know" principle serves as a guideline when deciding to whom disclosure should be made (generally the principal, school nurse, and classroom teacher). It is not currently required that schools and daycare centers be advised, but is generally encouraged because this alerts the school to notify the parent promptly in the event of an outbreak of infectious disease that could pose a threat to the HIV-infected child (such as varicella).
5. Offer guidance to teens about how to initiate disclosure of HIV status to sexual partners or peers. Provide support during the process and offer to help facilitate the disclosure in the clinical setting.
6. Give families concrete guidelines as to when to notify health care provider about their child's condition. Signs and symptoms of illness require prompt notification, all fevers over 101°F (38.3°C) should be reported, and any adverse

experiences or suspected adverse experiences with medications need prompt reporting.

7. Assess whether the parents are receiving care for themselves. Typically, parents will neglect their own care to provide for their child. As a result, the parents' immune status may become more quickly compromised.

8. Refer families to a social worker or social services agency. Children with HIV may qualify for certain entitlement programs that help with their health care and the family's financial situation. Many states have initiated case management programs for people with HIV.

9. Provide guidance using a childhood chronic illness model that addresses such psychosocial issues as disclosure and parental guilt as well as such medical issues as multiorgan involvement and likelihood of exacerbations of a variety of related conditions (eg, infections and nutritional deficiencies).

10. Assist parents in obtaining the latest information regarding treatment protocols of pediatric HIV. Such information can be obtained through (800) TRIALS-A or *www.aidsinfor.nih.gov*.

Evaluation: Expected Outcomes

- Absolute neutrophil count within normal limits; aseptic technique maintained.
- Maintains medication regimen; keeps follow-up appointments; achieves an undetectable viral load.
- Nutritional intake adequate to meet body requirements; growth curve maintained.
- Oral mucous membranes without ulceration, good dentition.
- Two to three loose stools per day; perianal skin without irritation.
- Afebrile; parent or caregiver demonstrates accurate monitoring of temperature.
- Achieves normal growth patterns as evidenced by height, weight, and developmental tasks.
- Parents discuss their feelings about the diagnosis of HIV; family seeks help through community resources.
- Child participates in care, asks questions; adolescent successfully transitions to an adult care program without disruption in care.
- Reports increase in comfort level.
- Practices distraction techniques during procedures; reports reduced fear.

Primary Immunodeficiencies

Primary immunodeficiencies (PID) encompass more than 300 types of disorders that affect distinct components of the innate and adaptive immune systems. The overall incidence of PID is estimated to be 1:2,000. The most common presentation of an immunodeficiency is increased frequency of infections or infections that are unusual or difficult to treat. PID diseases are often undiagnosed or have a significant delay in diagnosis, which can lead to significant end-organ damage from recurrent infections. Increasingly, it is recognized that PID may present in other ways, such as multiple autoimmune manifestations and some types of malignancies.

 EVIDENCE BASE Picard, C., Gaspar, B., Bousfiha, A., et al. (2018). International Union of Immunological Societies: 2017 Immunodeficiency Diseases Committee Report on Inborn Errors of Immunity. *Journal of Clinical Immunology, 38*(1), 96–128.

Pathophysiology and Etiology

 EVIDENCE BASE Younger, E., Epland, K., Zampelli, A., & Hintermeyer, M. (2015). Primary immunodeficiency diseases: a primer for PCP's. *The Nurse Practitioner, 40*(2), 1–7.

1. PID diseases are due to genetic alterations in the immune system. Inheritance may be X-linked, autosomal recessive, or autosomal dominant depending on the type. The genetic mutation may be de novo with no prior family history.

2. About three quarters of PID diseases are caused by humoral or combined humoral and cellular abnormalities, with the remainder being defects in phagocytic or complement components of the immune system.

3. Risk factors for PID diseases include a family history of immunodeficiency, early infant deaths, parental consanguinity, autoimmunity, and increased incidence of lymphoid malignancy in family members.

Clinical Manifestations

1. Hallmark of PID diseases is susceptibility to infection, including recurrent pneumonia, sinusitis, otitis, sepsis, meningitis, recurrent or resistant candidiasis, or infection with an opportunistic organism. Course of infection may be unusual with a need for intravenous antibiotics and/or hospitalization to clear infections. See Table 53-5.
2. Chronic diarrhea.
3. Nonhealing wounds.
4. Extensive skin lesions.
5. Failure to gain weight or grow normally (failure to thrive).
6. Complications from a live viral vaccine.
7. Unexplained autoimmunity or fevers.
8. Absence or enlargement of lymphoid tissue, including tonsils, spleen, and liver.

Diagnostic Evaluation

Specific Evaluation for Immunodeficiency

1. Complete blood count with differential to look for decreased numbers of lymphocytes and evidence of abnormalities in other cell lines, such as decreased platelets, neutrophils, or hemoglobin.
2. Immunoglobulin levels (IgG, IgA, IgM, and IgE) include total protein and albumin to rule out protein loss.
3. Antibody titers to previously administered vaccines to evaluate the ability to produce functional specific antibodies to infectious agents. Measurement of isoagglutinins (isoantibodies to blood groups) in children older than 2 years.
4. Measurement of the classical (CH50) and alternate pathway (AH50) of the complement system to rule out a complement deficiency.
5. Lymphocyte subset analysis by flow cytometry including CD3 (total T cells), CD4 (T helper), CD8 (T cytotoxic), CD19 or CD20 (B cells), and CD16/56 (natural killer cells) for suspected T cell, B cell, or combined immunodeficiency.
6. Lymphoproliferative assays to assess the cellular function.
7. Measurement of phagocytic oxidative responses (neutrophil oxidative burst index [NOBI] by flow cytometry) if a phagocytic disorder is suggested, such as chronic granulomatous disease.
8. Genetic testing for suspected cause of immunodeficiency.

Table 53-5 Infections Associated with Subtypes of PID Diseases

TYPE	TYPES OF INFECTIONS	ORGANISMS	OTHER FEATURES
Humoral (B cell)	Sinopulmonary, otitis media, gastrointestinal, cellulitis, meningitis, osteomyelitis	Encapsulated bacteria: *Haemophilus*, pneumococci, streptococci Parasites: *Giardia lamblia*, *Cryptosporidium* Virus: *Enterovirus*	Autoimmunity GI problems including malabsorption
Cellular (T cell or combined T and B cells)	Pulmonary, gastrointestinal, skin	Fungal: *Candida* species, *Pneumocystis jiroveci* Viral: CMV, EBV, RSV, parainfluenza, adenovirus, viral GI disease mycobacterium species	Failure to thrive Oral thrush Skin: rashes, dermatitis Postvaccination disease from live viral vaccines
Phagocytic disorders	Severe skin and visceral infections by common pathogens	Bacteria: *Staphylococcus aureus*, *Pseudomonas* species, *Serratia* species, *Klebsiella* species Fungi: *Candida*, *Nocardia*, *Aspergillus*	Granuloma formation, including granulomatous enteritis Poor wound healing Abscesses Oral cavity infections Anorectal infections
Complement disorders	Meningitis Septicemia	*Neisseria* infections: meningococcal, pneumococcal	Rheumatoid disorders: lupus-like syndrome Angioedema

CMV, cytomegalovirus; EBV, Epstein-Barr virus.

Other Tests

1. Evaluation for infection, including inflammatory markers (C-reactive protein, sedimentation rate), appropriate cultures, radiological image of the site of suspected infections.
2. Electrolytes, glucose, urea, creatinine, arterial blood gases, if indicated.
3. Advanced immunologic evaluations, T-cell repertoire by v-betas, T-cell receptor incision circles (TREC, a measure of mature cells from the thymus).
4. PCR testing for suspected infectious agents if there is concern that the patient may not produce functional antibodies from PI disease. CD45 RA/RO to evaluate naïve versus memory T cells.
5. Newborn screen for severe combined immunodeficiency (SCID) by TREC if available.

Management

1. Prompt recognition and treatment of infections. Empiric antibiotic therapy pending culture results should be instituted.
2. May consider preventive antibiotic treatment for some PID diseases.
3. Avoidance of live viral vaccines, as they may be disease-causing in PID patients.
4. Postexposure infectious prophylaxis may be necessary following exposure to varicella.
5. For suspected T-cell immunodeficiency, blood products must be irradiated to eliminate leukocytes and screened for cytomegalovirus.
6. *Pneumocystis jirovecii* prophylaxis for T-cell immunodeficiencies.
7. Antibody replacement therapy with intravenous or subcutaneous gammaglobulin for combined and antibody deficiencies (X-linked agammaglobulinemia, common variable immunodeficiency, CD40 ligand or CD40 deficiency, selective antibody deficiency, SCID and peritransplant).
8. Bone marrow transplant (BMT) to replace the defective immune system in severe PID diseases (severe combined immunodeficiency, combined immunodeficiencies, Wiskott-Aldrich syndrome, chronic granulomatous disease, and others). Indications for BMT in PID diseases are constantly expanding, as new genes are identified.
9. Gene therapy is an experimental option for some PID diseases: adenosine deaminase deficiency (a type of severe combined immunodeficiency), Wiskott-Aldrich syndrome, and chronic granulomatous disease.

Complications

1. Organ damage from infection, particularly the lungs, gastrointestinal tract, and joints.
2. Chronic lung disease (bronchiectasis).
3. Granulomatous lesions in the skin, liver, spleen, and lungs (common variable immunodeficiency and chronic granulomatous disease).
4. Gastrointestinal malabsorption because of infection or from bacterial overgrowth.
5. Autoimmunity.
6. Early death (less than 1 year of age for severe combined immunodeficiency).
7. Malignancy (especially lymphoma and leukemia).
8. Psychological and social reactions to chronic disease.

Nursing Assessment

1. Focus history on infections including age of onset, sites, number, frequency, types, duration, and response to treatment.
2. Detailed family history including focus on unexplained infant deaths, recurrent miscarriages, consanguinity, malignancies, and autoimmunity in other members.
3. Review of immunization record and history to determine complications from vaccines and to ensure that immunizations are given at proper intervals.
4. Focus physical examination on the site of infections, such as lung air entry, as well as vital signs, growth and development,

presence or absence of lymphoid tissue, examination of the skin for evidence of candidiasis or other skin abnormalities.

5. Assess the family and child's understanding of the condition, care needs, prognosis, and plan of care.
6. Assess the family's coping mechanisms and resources, particularly for patients that may require bone marrow transplant or lifelong treatment with immunoglobulins.

Nursing Diagnoses

- Risk for Infection related to immunodeficiency.
- Imbalanced Nutrition: Less than Body Requirements related to infections, malabsorption, or autoimmune gastrointestinal diseases.
- Impaired Oral Mucous Membranes related to candidiasis or other infections.
- Ineffective Therapeutic Regimen Management related to insufficient knowledge, nonadherence, and limited resources.
- Delayed Growth and Development related to infection or specific PID disease.
- Ineffective Family Coping related to diagnosis of immunodeficiency.
- Impaired Family Processes due to chronic diseases.

Nursing Interventions

Preventing Infection

1. Educate families about signs and symptoms of infection that specific PID disease is susceptible to and when to seek health care advice.
2. Administer or teach caregiver to administer prescribed pharmacologic agents including treatment protocols for gammaglobulin therapy, if indicated.
3. Adhere to infection control policies for protection of severe T-cell immunodeficiencies when hospitalized.
4. Avoid administration of live viral vaccines for suspected PID (oral polio, measles, mumps, rubella, varicella, yellow fever, rotavirus, inhaled influenza, and bacilli Calmette-Guérin [BCG] vaccine).
5. Encourage yearly influenza vaccine for patients and family members.
6. Administer and teach family good infectious control techniques including handwashing and skin care to avoid infection.

Maintaining Adequate Nutrition

1. Carefully monitor growth parameters including height, weight, and head circumference.
2. Consult with a dietician to develop nutritional plan of care, including adequate caloric intake and parental teaching.
3. Administer and teach families to administer supplemental feeds via NG or G-tube if indicated.

Maintaining Oral Mucosa

1. Include assessment of oral mucosa in routine physical assessments.
2. Administer and teach families to administer prescribed antifungal or antiviral medications.
3. Promote good dental hygiene and dental care.

Promoting Therapeutic Regime Management

1. Teach patients and families about prescribed medications and treatments. Review teaching periodically.
2. For patients on gammaglobulin treatment, doses should be adjusted to reflect increased weight, so as to ensure adequate

replacement of antibodies. For patients on subcutaneous gammaglobulin, periodically assess patient adherence to infusion protocol and re-educate, as necessary.

Promoting Growth and Development

1. Assess for normal growth and development.
2. Make appropriate referrals for more in-depth developmental assessments and adhere to treatment programs instituted (important for prolonged admissions, such as bone marrow transplant).
3. Teach the family appropriate developmental activities for their child.
4. Facilitate successful transition to adult care.

Promote Effective Family Coping

 EVIDENCE BASE Hernandez-Trujillo, V., Scalchunes, C., Hernandez-Trujillo, H., et al. (2015). Primary Immunodeficiency diseases: an opportunity in pediatrics for improving patient outcomes. *Pediatrics*, 54(13), 1265–1275.

1. Assess family coping skills including strengths and weaknesses.
2. Provide emotional support and counseling, as necessary.
3. Refer the family for genetic counseling, as diagnosis may impact other family members or future pregnancies.
4. Encourage families to allow children to take increased responsibility for their care as they mature.
5. Provide continuous teaching about disease process and treatment. It is particularly important for children diagnosed at very young ages to learn as they grow—lifelong diseases.

Normalizing Family Processes

1. Refer to community resources and support groups.
2. Encourage family and child to verbalize feelings about diagnosis and treatment.
3. Encourage attendance at school, participation in activities, and socialization with peers as much as possible.
4. Encourage parents to spend time with siblings and each other, as well as affected child.

Community and Home Care Considerations

1. Assess home environment for resources, such as nutritious foods, developmentally appropriate toys, and supplies needed for care and hygiene.
2. Assess caregivers' correct administration of medications.
3. Ensure that patient has a community care practitioner.
4. For PID patient requiring gammaglobulin treatment, assess ability of parents to adhere to infusion regime for IVIG treatment. For SCIG treatment, assess home for adequate storage of gammaglobulin products and supplies.
5. Provide education to school nurses so that individual educational plans are implemented and maintained.

Family Education and Health Maintenance

1. Give families guidelines as to when to notify health care provider about their child's condition. Signs and symptoms of illness require prompt notification, all fevers over 101°F (38.3°C) should be reported, and any adverse experiences or suspected adverse events to medications require prompt reporting.
2. Assess family coping and refer to social worker or social services, as required.

3. Refer families to immunodeficiency patient support agencies so as to provide ongoing PID disease-specific education to patients and families.

Evaluation and Expected Outcomes

- Reduced incidence of infections.
- Adequate intake for child's age and developmental stage.
- No oral lesions, denies oral discomfort.
- Adherence to treatment regimes.
- Achieves normal growth, as evidenced by height, weight, and developmental tasks.
- Child and family seek appropriate support and resources, as required.
- Child and parents verbalize feelings about the illness; include siblings in activities.

CONNECTIVE TISSUE DISORDERS
Juvenile Idiopathic Arthritis

 EVIDENCE BASE McKeever, A., & Kelly, M. (2015). Growing up with Juvenile Idiopathic Arthritis. *The American Journal of Maternal Child Nursing*, 40(1), 8–15.

Juvenile idiopathic arthritis (JIA) has replaced the terms "juvenile chronic arthritis" and "juvenile rheumatoid arthritis" as the commonly agreed-upon terminology to describe arthritis in children. JIA is defined as persistent arthritis for longer than 6 weeks in children ≤16 years of age. The disease is a heterogeneous disease that has been further classified into seven subtypes with similar presentation, clinical features, disease course, and outcomes.

JIA is a chronic disease affecting approximately 1 in 1,000 children (1.7 to 8.4 million children worldwide, most of these children undiagnosed) and often persisting into the adult years. There are epidemiological differences between sexes and age of onset that are specific to subtype.

Pathophysiology and Etiology

 EVIDENCE BASE Petty, R. E., Laxer, R. M, Lindsley, C. B., et al. (Eds.). (2016). *Textbook of pediatric rheumatology* (7th ed.). Philadelphia, PA: Elsevier.

1. The cause of JIA is unknown. It is likely multifactorial and variable between subtypes. Hypotheses suggest that environmental stimuli trigger disease in genetically predisposed children during a time of susceptibility.
   a. Genetic risk factors—associations with specific human leukocyte antigen (HLA) class I (B27) and class II genes, protein tyrosine phosphatase N22 gene, and interleukin-2 receptor alpha gene have been well established.
   b. Immune dysregulation of the adaptive and innate immune system. Autoantibodies including antinuclear antibody (ANA); rheumatoid factor (RF); T-lymphocytes and cytokines, tissue necrosis factor (TNF) of adaptive immunity as well as neutrophils and interleukin (IL)-1, IL-6 of innate immunity are present in sera and synovial fluids.
   c. Infection as a trigger to immune dysregulation is suspected but has not been clearly established.
   d. Hormonal factors.

2. Arthritis is inflammation of one or more synovial joints. Immune complexes trigger the inflammatory response, causing:
   a. The synovium to become thickened from congestion and edema.
   b. Increased production of intra-articular fluid exhibited as a joint effusion. It is not uncommon for synovial cysts to develop (Baker cyst).
   c. Development of periarticular soft tissue edema.
   d. Extension of the inflammatory process to the tendons, tendon sheaths, and entheses results in inflammatory changes similar to the synovial tissues.
   e. Weakness and atrophy of muscle surrounding affected joints leading to flexion contractures.
   f. Growth centers in long bones may undergo either premature epiphyseal closure or accelerated epiphyseal growth. The result is overgrowth or shortening of the affected limb.

3. Long-term disease activity can result in joint destruction and eventual joint failure, necessitating joint replacement.
   a. Degrading enzymes released during synovial inflammation result in chondrolysis and osteolysis; erosion of the articular cartilage and bone.
   b. Following destruction, the overgrowth of granulation tissue may result in the formulation of new cartilage and bone, leading to ankylosis.
   c. Joint destruction is characterized by joint space narrowing, erosions, deformities, subluxation, and ankylosis.
   d. Generalized osteopenia is common, increasing the risk for fracture.

Clinical Manifestations

Clinical manifestations include joint and extra-articular features that vary among subtypes (see Table 53-6, page 1402).
1. The inflamed joint is characterized by four of the five cardinal signs of inflammation: swelling, pain, heat, loss of function. Erythema occurs in some cases.
   a. Joint stiffness in the morning or after prolonged inactivity (gelling) is common.
   b. Pain may not be expressed verbally; the child may alter activities to protect the painful joint.
2. Extra-articular features include fever, rash, fatigue, weight loss, altered growth, subcutaneous nodules, and uveitis.
   a. Fevers occur in systemic JIA and occasionally at the onset of polyarticular JIA. In systemic JIA, fevers are daily, usually above 102.2°F (39°C), following a quotidian pattern of one or two spikes with a rapid return to baseline and accompanied by a classic salmon-pink rash.
   b. Altered growth includes localized growth abnormalities and poor linear growth.
      i. Overgrowth or undergrowth of bones in sites affected by arthritis result in leg length discrepancy, shortened limbs, and micrognathia and or/retrognathia (receding chin) with arthritis of the temporomandibular joint (TMJ).
      ii. Poor linear growth is attributed to the inhibitory affects chronic inflammation and circulating cytokines have on growth.
   c. Uveitis associated with arthritis is found in 20% to 40% of cases. It is commonly asymptomatic at onset requiring frequent examinations by an eye specialist. An exception is the patient with subtype enthesitis-related arthritis (ERA), who presents with redness, pain, photophobia, headache, and decreased visual acuity.

Table 53-6 Characteristics of Juvenile Idiopathic Arthritis

ILAR SUBTYPE	OLIGOARTICULAR • PERSISTENT • EXTENDED	POLYARTICULAR (RF NEGATIVE)	POLYARTICULAR (RF POSITIVE)
% Total JIA patients	40%–50%	20%–25%	5%
Age of Onset	Early childhood; 1–3 years	2 peaks: 2–4 years and 6–12 years	Early adolescence
Sex	F > M	F > M	F > M
Typical Joint Involvement	≤4 joints in first 6 months Large joints: knees, ankles, wrist Extended disease: involves >4 joints after first 6 months	≥5 joints Symmetric distribution Knees, wrists, ankles TMJ can be affected	≥5 joints Small and large joints Symmetric C-spine and TMJ affected Erosive joint disease
Laboratory Tests	ANA 60%–80% positive	ANA 50% positive	ANA 75% positive RF positive
Occurrence of Uveitis	Common (30%) Usually asymptomatic	Common (15%)	Rare (<1%)
Other Features	Leg length discrepancies Contractures	Fatigue	Rheumatoid nodules Fever and constitutional signs at onset of disease

ILAR, International League for Associations of Rheumatology; F, female; M, male; ANA, antinuclear antibody; HLA, human leukocyte antigen; RF, rheumatoid factor.
Adapted with permission from Pediatric Clinics of North America, 59(2), Gowdie P. and Tse S, Juvenile idiopathic arthritis, 301–327, Copyright 2012, with permission from Elsevier.

Diagnostic Evaluation

1. Laboratory studies cannot exclusively confirm diagnosis. They are used to support diagnosis, measure disease activity, predict prognoses, and monitor toxicity of therapy.
   a. Elevated erythrocyte sedimentation rate (ESR).
   b. Leukocytosis, thrombocytosis, anemia.
   c. Elevated serum immunoglobulins.
   d. Elevated C-reactive protein.
   e. Presence of ANA, RF, and anticyclic citrullinated peptide (anti-CCP) antibodies. ANA is associated with high incidence of uveitis. Anti-CCP is an early predictor of erosive disease in polyarticular JIA.
2. Radiographic studies.
   a. Early x-ray changes include soft tissue swelling, osteopenia, and effusions.
   b. Late x-ray changes include erosions, joint space narrowing, boutonniere or swan neck deformity of the fingers, early maturation of cartilage, and subluxations.
   c. Ultrasound for detection of tenosynovitis.
   d. Magnetic resonance imaging (MRI) is most sensitive to detect specific joint disease, including TMJ and sacroiliac.
3. Ophthalmologic examination.
   a. Slit-lamp examination to monitor for uveitis is required within 1 month of diagnosis and every 3 to 12 months, depending on age, presence of ANA, and duration of illness.

Management

1. There is no cure for JIA.
2. Management of JIA should be provided by a multidisciplinary team in a family-centered approach.
3. The primary goal of treatment is to facilitate disease remission.
   a. In the process of working toward remission, other goals of therapy include control pain and maintain range of motion, muscle strength, and function.
   b. To promote normal growth.
   c. To support normal psychological and social development.
4. Goal attainment requires nonpharmacologic and pharmacologic approaches.
5. Nonpharmacologic approaches to treatment include:
   a. Occupational and physical therapies that employ strength and stretching exercises, splinting, serial casting, orthotics, and thermal modalities to reduce stiffness or pain and to protect function.
   b. Strengthening and aerobic-based exercise are safe in children with JIA. Studies have demonstrated improved physical function and quality of life.
   c. Nutritional and vitamin supplementation are required to promote growth, maintain bone mineralization, and prevent toxicity from medication. Vitamin D, calcium, iron, and folic acid may be prescribed.
   d. Orthopedic surgery may be performed to manage joint complications; tendon lengthening for severe contractures;

SYSTEMIC	ENTHESITIS-RELATED ARTHRITIS	PSORIATIC ARTHRITIS	UNDIFFERENTIATED
5%–10%	5%–10%	5%–10%	10%
Throughout childhood	Late childhood and adolescence	2 peaks: 2–4 years and 9–11 years	
F = M	M ≥ F	F ≥ M	
Oligoarticular or Polyarticular distribution Progressive and destructive arthritis	Weight-bearing joints: hip, feet Axial and sacroiliac joint involvement Enthesitis	Asymmetric or symmetric small or large joints Dactylitis Enthesitis	
ANA 5%–10% positive	HLA–B27 positive		
Rare (<1%)	Symptomatic; acute onset, painful red eye Unilateral	Common (10%)	
Daily quotidian fever ≥2 week Evanescent rash Lymphadenopathy Hepatosplenomegaly Serositis Macrophage activation syndrome is life-threatening complication	Association with inflammatory bowel disease	Nail pits, onycholysis Psoriasis	Does not fulfill criteria for any of the other categories or fulfills criteria for >1 category

tenosynovectomy to treat trigger finger; total joint replacements, particularly hips and knees.

6. Pharmacologic therapies are introduced in a systematic step-wise approach targeted to the specific subtypes of JIA. Refer to Table 53-7, page 1404. Recently, a more aggressive progression through the steps is advocated, as evidence suggests rapid control of inflammation may positively influence prognosis.

   a. Nonsteroidal anti-inflammatory drugs are the first line of therapy aimed at symptom relief.

   b. Disease-modifying antirheumatic drugs (DMARDs) are second-line immunosuppressive agents that can achieve disease control and influence the course of disease.

   c. Newer biologic agents are selected when DMARDs fail. They target very specific immune responses responsible for inflammation. Biologics offer treatment options for children with refractory arthritis.

   d. Corticosteroids are potent anti-inflammatories used mainly as a bridging therapy until other treatments begin to take effect. Steroids have not been shown to be disease modifying. They can be administered by oral, intramuscular, intravenous, intra-articular, or intraocular route and should be administered at the lowest effective dose. With the exception of intra-articular steroid injections, which are well tolerated, steroids can lead to serious toxic side effects including weight gain, edema, acne, fatigue, growth suppression, decreased bone density, hypertension, hyperglycemia, glaucoma, and cataracts.

7. Children receiving the immunosuppressive therapies used to treat arthritis require special considerations.

   a. Close monitoring for signs of infection.

   b. Screening for tuberculosis prior to initiation of corticosteroid or biologic therapy. Testing should be repeated annually for those taking biologics and/or those travelling to endemic areas or close contact with visitors from these areas. Steroids can alter the result of tuberculin skin testing. Biologic therapy can reactivate latent tuberculosis.

   c. Children receiving DMARDs, corticosteroids, or biologics should not receive live vaccines (varicella, measles, mumps, and rubella). When considering treatment with methotrexate, varicella immunization may be recommended prior to starting therapy in susceptible children. In such circumstances, methotrexate cannot be started for 28 days post immunization.

   d. Regular blood monitoring for toxicity.

   e. Regular clinical examinations to assess for adverse effects. In 2008, the FDA reported several cases of malignancies in children receiving biologic therapy. Recent studies have both supported and refuted possible links between cancer and biologic therapy.

8. The course and outcome of JIA has changed dramatically with early intervention and more successful therapies. However, active disease continues into adulthood in 50% to 70% of children with polyarticular and systemic JIA, 40% to 50% of oligoarticular JIA. Current research in biomarkers, genetics and immunology to help predict response or nonresponse to therapy choices (treat to target) will guide and advance care within the next decade

Table 53-7 Pharmacologic Treatment for Juvenile Idiopathic Arthritis

	MEDICATION	INDICATION	DOSING
NSAIDs	COX-1, COX-2 inhibitors, naproxen, ibuprofen, indomethacin, celecoxib	First-line therapy for all subtypes of JIA; symptom management	PO variable dose frequency
DMRADs	Methotrexate	Second-line therapy for all sub-types except systemic JIA	PO or sc once weekly 15 mg/m^2/dose (maximum 25 mg) Therapeutic effect in 6–12 weeks
	Sulfasalazine	Oligoarticular JIA; polyarticular JIA; ERA	PO 50 mg/kg/day divided bid. Therapeutic effect in 6–12 weeks
	Leflunomide	Oligoarticular; polyarticular	PO once daily 10–20 mg/day Therapeutic effect in 6–12 weeks
Glucocorticoids	Methylprednisolone, prednisone, prednisolone, triamcinolone, hexacetonide	Used for quick anti-inflammatory effect or bridging agent for all subtypes of JIA	IV, IM, PO, intra-articular, topical, intraocular for uveitis Dose/frequency depends on route and severity of inflammation
Biologics	TNF inhibitors: Etanercept Infliximab Adalimumab Golimumab	Used when fail second-line agents Effective to treat uveitis	SC (Etanercept, adalimumab) IV (infliximab) Dose/frequency variable Therapeutic effect reported after three doses
	IL inhibitors: Anakinra (IL-1) Canakinumab (IL-1β) Tocilizumab (IL-6)	Systemic JIA Tocilizumab under study for other forms of JIA	Anakinra sc once/day Canakinumab sc q4 weeks Tocilizumab IV q2 weeks
	T-cell costimulatory modulators: Abatacept	JIA except systemic subtype	IV 10 mg/kg/dose Give at 0, 2 weeks then q4 weeks Therapeutic effect reported as early as second infusion

IM, intramuscular; IV, intravenous; JIA, juvenile idiopathic arthritis; PO, oral; SC, subcutaneous.

 EVIDENCE BASE Klotsche, J., Niewerth, M., Haas, J., et al. (2016). Long-term safety of etanercept and adalimumab compared to methotrexate in patients with juvenile idiopathic arthritis (JIA). *Annals of the Rheumatic Diseases, 75*, 855–861.

Hinze, C., Gohar, F., & Foell, D. (2015). Management of juvenile idiopathic arthritis: hitting the target. *Nature Reviews Rheumatology, 11*, 290–300.

Complications

1. Bone and growth changes:
   a. Growth disturbance, short stature.
   b. Osteopenia, osteoporosis.
   c. Cervical spine and TMJ problems (micrognathia/retrognathia).
   d. Leg length discrepancies.
   e. Joint contractures.
2. Psychological and social reactions to illness.
3. Cataracts, glaucoma, or blindness secondary to uncontrolled, chronic uveitis.
4. Pericarditis.
5. Macrophage activation syndrome—a life-threatening complication of systemic JIA characterized by massive activation of T cells and macrophages; features include sustained fever, hepatosplenomegaly, anemia, liver function abnormalities, coagulopathy, encephalopathy, sudden drop in ESR, extreme elevation of ferritin, and marked elevation of D-dimers.

ADVERSE EFFECTS	MONITORING	CONSIDERATIONS
Gastritis; pseudoporphyria; hepato-toxicity; renal toxicity	CBC, liver enzymes, creatinine at baseline then q6 months	Pseudoporphyria most commonly seen in fairskinned children
GI upset; mouth ulcers; hepatotoxic-ity; teratogenicity	CBC, liver enzymes at baseline, 1 month then q3–4 months on stable dose	Provide folate supplement Avoid live vaccines Give VZIG within 96 hours for chicken pox exposure Avoid alcohol Avoid pregnancy Interaction with the antibiotics sulfa-methoxazole and trimethoprim (bone marrow suppression)
GI upset; rash; bone marrow sup-pression; hepatotoxicity; allergy	CBC, liver enzymes at baseline, then q4–12 weeks	Inquire about sulfa allergies Avoid live vaccines Beware of additive hepatotoxicity in combination with methotrexate
GI upset; rash; hepatotoxicity; teratogenicity	CBC, liver enzymes at baseline, then q4–12 weeks	Use when methotrexate not tolerated Cholestyramine used to enhance elimination Avoid pregnancy Avoid alcohol Avoid live vaccines
Increased appetite; GI upset; mood changes; hypertension; acne; straie; Cushing syndrome; growth suppres-sion; osteoporosis; hyperglycemia; cataracts; glaucoma	Dependent on route of adminis-tration and length of treatment	Monitor BP; urine for glycosuria Annual bone mineral density Delay immunization schedule Give VZIG within 96 hours for chicken pox exposure
Allergic reaction; infection; demy-elinating disease; possible risk for malignancy	CBC, liver enzymes, creatinine at baseline then q3–6 months Tuberculosis screen prior to start then yearly	Assess for family history of multiple sclerosis; if positive then MRI prior to start
Injection site or infusion reactions; infection	Tuberculosis screen prior to start then yearly	Monitor for infection Avoid live vaccines
Infection	Tuberculosis screen prior to start then yearly	Monitor for infection Avoid live vaccines Monitor for infection Avoid live vaccines Avoid pregnancy

Nursing Assessment

1. History should include a thorough musculoskeletal inquiry including location, onset, duration of joint pain and stiffness; alleviating and exacerbating factors; activity limitations; medication and other nonpharmacologic treatments used; review of systems to look for associated symptoms and complications of JIA and side effects of medication; most recent ophthalmology examination; immunizations; and tuberculosis screening.
2. Physical examination focused on the clinical manifestations of the different subtypes of JIA including joint and gait assessment, vital signs, growth parameters, and a pain assessment using a developmentally appropriate tool.
3. Gather data for psychosocial assessment including inquiry into the impact of this chronic, painful disease on the child's self-esteem and coping and the family's coping.

Nursing Diagnoses

- Acute and Chronic Pain related to joint inflammation.
- Impaired Physical Mobility related to joint inflammation and pain.
- Delayed Growth and Development related to chronic inflammation and side effects of medication.
- Impaired Family Processes related to caring for a child with a chronic, painful illness.

Other Nursing Diagnoses may include:

- Disturbed Sleep Pattern related to pain.
- Fatigue related to inflammation.
- Disturbed Body Image related to short stature; leg length discrepancy; side effects of prednisone (stretch marks, weight gain, acne), micrognathia.
- Risk for Chronic Low Self-Esteem related to changes in body image and physical capabilities.
- Impaired Nutrition: Less Than Body Requirements related to increased metabolic activity associated with inflammation.
- Risk for Imbalanced Nutrition: More Than Body Requirements related to side effect of medication.
- Deficient Knowledge related to potential adverse effects of medications.

Nursing Interventions

Minimizing Discomfort

1. Administer or teach parents to administer medications to reduce inflammation and control pain. When inflammation and pain are controlled, a child is more willing and able to do exercises to improve joint strength and prevent loss of movement.
2. Encourage a warm bath or shower to relieve morning stiffness. Use other thermal modalities such as soaking or warm, moist pads or ice packs to soothe inflamed joints. Some children respond to heat and some to cold.
3. Use assistive devices to make mobility and activities of daily living (ADL) easier. Examples include splints; orthotics; special adaptors for pencils, doorknobs, or utensils; or Velcro or zipper pulls.

Preserving Joint Mobility

1. Encourage compliance with physical therapy regimen to strengthen muscles and mobilize joints. Assist with range of motion (ROM) exercises, as indicated.
2. Splint joints to maintain proper position (joint extension) and decrease pain and deformity.
3. Encourage prone position with a thin pillow or no pillow and firm mattress.
4. Encourage therapeutic play (swimming, throwing, and bike riding).
5. Encourage child to do own ADL to maintain joint mobility. Refer to occupational therapy for provision of adaptation devices to facilitate completion of daily activities (velcro closures, utensils, and self-care implements with enlarged handles).
6. Schedule rest periods to maximize energy; discourage complete immobilization or lengthy inactivity because they increase stiffness.

Promote Normal Growth and Development

1. Identify developmental tasks appropriate to age of child. Educate parents and work with child and family to set goals with necessary adaptations to promote successful achievement.
2. Encourage attendance in school, participation in activities, and socialization with peers as much as possible.
3. Encourage compliance with treatment plan to prevent complications related to prolonged inflammation.
4. Promote healthy diet; obtain diet history; make referral to dietician, as necessary.

Normalizing Family Processes

1. Refer to community resources and support groups.
2. Encourage child and family to verbalize feelings.
3. Remind parents to devote time to other children themselves and each other because the disease affects the whole family.

Family Education and Health Maintenance

1. Educate (consider cultural/language barriers and literacy) and motivate parents child to continue program of treatment at home. This is a chronic disease with an unpredictable course; however, compliance with prescribed treatment is important to improve functional outcome and to allow the child to grow and develop to his or her full potential.
2. Encourage medication compliance by helping to create a medication calendar or suggesting weekly pill boxes or strategies to reduce side effects such as taking NSAIDs with food or taking methotrexate on the weekends before bed.
3. Encourage open communication with school authorities. Child should receive accommodations such as use of school elevator, two sets of textbooks so child does not need to carry heavy backpack to and from school, use of a computer for difficulties with writing, and allowance to move around during prolonged periods of sitting.
4. Educate the family about the importance of a daily exercise routine to maintain ROM, muscle strength, and function. Periodically re-evaluate need for physical and occupational therapy.
5. Provide nutritional counseling to promote a balanced diet with special attention given to the intake of calcium, vitamin D, folic acid, and iron. Portion control and healthy snacks should be encouraged to prevent obesity.
6. Stress the need for routine follow-up care and ophthalmologic evaluation.
7. Educate families about the special considerations required when their child is receiving immunosuppressive medications: seek prompt medical attention for fever and other signs of infection; child and family members should receive annual influenza vaccine; live vaccinations need to be postponed until child is no longer receiving immunosuppression.
8. Refer family to community agencies such as the Arthritis Foundation (*www.arthritis.org*).

Evaluation: Expected Outcomes

- Reports decreased pain.
- ROM, muscle strength, and joint function is preserved.
- Growth and development parameters, including psychological and social are appropriate for age.
- Parents seek additional resources.

Systemic Lupus Erythematosus

Systemic lupus erythematosus (SLE) is a systemic multisystem, chronic autoimmune disease that has the potential to affect any organ or organ system. Disease onset in childhood occurs in 10% to 20% of all SLE cases. Although the disease manifestations and disease course of flares and remissions is similar across the lifespan, pediatric systemic lupus erythematosus (pSLE) patients have a more severe disease requiring more aggressive treatment with immunosuppression. The incidence is higher in females than in males (4.5 to 5:1) with higher rates in Hispanic, Afro-Caribbean, Aboriginal, and Asian populations.

Pathophysiology and Etiology

1. Cause is unknown. Involves a complex interaction between genetic predisposition and the environment. Etiologic factors include:
   a. Immune system dysregulation of both innate and adaptive immunity.
   b. Genetic susceptibility—associations with certain HLA types, complement deficiencies, and TNF polymorphisms.
   c. Environmental factors.
   d. Hormonal factors—presence of estrogen; low levels of androgens
2. Possible factors that trigger or unmask initial symptoms:
   a. Ultraviolet radiation (ultraviolet B-light)—photosensitivity
   b. Viral infection—herpes family viruses; cytomegalovirus
   c. Stress, extreme fatigue.
   d. Vaccination
   e. Chemical exposure—cigarette smoke, pesticides, heavy metals.
   f. Medications—drug-induced lupus is a lupus-like syndrome that presents after several months of specific medication use. Complete resolution of symptoms happens weeks to months after discontinuation
3. SLE is characterized by the production of autoantibodies and the deposition of immune complexes in tissues and organs throughout the body.
   a. Spontaneous hyperactivity of B lymphocytes leads to increased antibody production. Additionally, the life of the B lymphocytes is abnormally prolonged, enhancing antibody production.
   b. These antibodies combine with antigen to form immune complexes, which deposit in tissue.
   c. The immune complexes activate the complement cascade, leading to inflammation (recruitment of inflammatory cells and production of oxidants, proteases, prostaglandins, and cytokines).
   d. Long-term inflammation can lead to irreversible cell destruction and tissue and organ damage.
4. Antiphospholipid syndrome (APS) produces a variety of antibodies against phospholipids and may occur in pSLE. The primary event resulting from APS is thrombolytic in nature.
5. Neonatal lupus erythematosus (NLE) is a separate entity from SLE. It is a disease of the developing fetus and neonate as the result of transplacental passage of maternal autoantibodies (anti-SSA/Ro or anti-SSB/L).
   a. Infant may or may not develop clinical symptoms.
   b. The most common clinical manifestations of NLE are cardiac, dermatologic, hematologic, and hepatic.
   c. The most serious manifestation is congenital heart block (CHB), requiring pacemaker insertion as an infant or child.
   d. The skin, liver, and hematologic symptoms resolve by 1 year of age as the maternal antibodies clear, with few long-term effects.

Clinical Manifestations

The presentation of the manifestations of SLE in children is diverse involving any organ system and may be gradual or acute.

1. Constitutional symptoms: fever, weight loss, fatigue, loss of appetite.
2. Mucocutaneous disease:
   a. Malar rash (butterfly rash), which is present over the bridge of nose and cheeks sparing the nasolabial folds; rash may vary from a faint blush to scaly erythematous papules; most often a photosensitive. Rash may spread from face and scalp to neck, chest, and extremities. Scarring is rare.
   b. Raynaud phenomenon; triphasic color change of fingers and toes in response to cold; may also be induced by emotions. Tip of nose, ears, and penis may also be affected.
   c. Mucosal ulceration or erythema of hard palate, tongue, or nose. Lesions are usually painless.
   d. Hair loss.
3. Musculoskeletal disease:
   a. Arthritis, most commonly of small joints of hands; rarely associated with erosive disease.
   b. Reduced bone density secondary to both active disease and treatment with steroids.
4. Cardiovascular disease:
   a. Early atherosclerosis—children with lupus have been shown to have unfavorable lipid profiles.
   b. Pericarditis, endocarditis, myocarditis.
5. Renal disease (lupus nephritis):
   a. Nephritis is leading cause of morbidity and mortality; prevalence of 20% to 80% of children with 18% to 50% progressing to end-stage kidney disease.
   b. 80% to 90% develop nephritis within the first year of diagnosis.
   c. Hematuria, proteinuria, and hypertension may be evident.
6. Neuropsychiatric disease:
   a. CNS involvement manifested by psychosis (visual and/or auditory hallucinations), depression, headache (severe, unremitting), cerebrovascular disease (stroke), cognitive impairment (worsening school performance), and seizures.
   b. More frequent in children.
7. Hematologic involvement:
   a. Coombs positive autoimmune hemolytic anemia caused by destruction of red cells in the spleen.
   b. Leukopenia involving lymphocytes and neutrophils.
   c. Thrombocytopenia—low platelets can commonly be the initial presentation; immune thrombocytopenic purpura (ITP) can precede lupus by 10 years.
   d. Low complement levels C3 and C4 are an important laboratory measurement of disease activity.
8. Pulmonary involvement with pleural effusion and lupus pneumonitis.

Diagnostic Evaluation

1. Diagnosis is made by both clinical manifestations and specific laboratory findings (see Box 53-2).
2. Laboratory studies:
   a. Autoantibodies, antinuclear antibody (ANA)—nonspecific but positive in 90% of people with SLE.
   b. Other antibodies such as anti-ds DNA, anti-Sm, anti-Ro/SSA, anti-La/SSB, anti-ribonucleoprotein (anti-RNP) are all common in SLE. Anti-dsDNA and anti-Sm are highly specific for lupus.
   c. ESR—elevated.
   d. Serum complements studies—decreased.
   e. CBC—leukopenia, hemolytic anemia, thrombocytopenia.

BOX 53-2 | **Criteria for Diagnosis of Systemic Lupus Erythematosus**

According to the American College of Rheumatology, the presence of four or more criteria must be documented to diagnose SLE.

- Malar (butterfly) rash.
- Discoid lupus rash.
- Photosensitivity.
- Oral or nasal mucocutaneous ulcerations.
- Nonerosive arthritis.
- Nephritis*:
  - Proteinuria greater than 0.5 g/day.
  - Cellular casts.
- Encephalopathy*:
  - Seizures.
  - Psychosis.
- Pleuritis or pericarditis.
- Hemolytic anemia, leukopenia, thrombocytopenia.
- Positive immunoserology*:
  - Antibodies to double-stranded DNA.
  - Antibodies to Sm nuclear antigen.
  - Positive finding of antiphospholipid antibodies based on immunoglobulin (Ig)G or IgM anticardiolipin antibodies, lupus anticoagulant, or confirmed false-positive serologic test for syphilis for at least 6 months.
- Positive antinuclear antibody.

Any one item satisfies this criterion.

---

   f. Evaluation for APS—elevated prothrombin time, partial thromboplastin time; false-positive syphilis tests such as VDRL; elevated anticardiolipin antibodies; and elevated dilute Russell viper venom time. The presence of one or more suggests APS and an increased risk for thrombosis.

   g. Serum chemistry and urine studies to detect kidney and other body system involvement.

3. Renal biopsy—verifies lupus nephritis and classification.
4. Electrocardiogram and other cardiac testing.
5. Bone mineral density.

Management

1. There is no cure for SLE. Course is unpredictable, is usually progressive, and may terminate in death, if untreated. Therapy is based on the extent and severity of disease. SLE may be classified as:
   a. Mild (fever, arthritis, rash).
   b. Moderate (clinically significant but non–life-threatening involvement of the kidneys or other major organs).
   c. Severe (substantial renal, pulmonary, hematologic, or neurologic disease).
2. Goal of treatment is to control disease activity and to prevent organ damage using the least toxic therapies.
3. Management of SLE should be provided by a multidisciplinary team in a family-centered approach.
4. Nonpharmacologic approaches include:
   a. Nutritional counseling and vitamin supplementation to control disease, promote growth, maintain bone mineralization, and prevent toxicity from medication. Reduced sodium and potassium diets, fluid restrictions for kidney

disease. Vitamin D, calcium, iron, and folic acid may be supplemented.
   b. Mental health and social support for the child and family to manage the issues of chronic disease.
   c. Education about sun protection including avoidance of midday sun, use of protective clothing, application of daily sunscreen 30 minutes prior to going outside.
   d. Vaccination against pneumococcal infection; annual influenza vaccine as well as routine inactivated vaccines.
   e. Regular adequate sleep and exercise.
5. Pharmacologic therapies:
   a. NSAIDs are used to relieve musculoskeletal symptoms, fever, fatigue, and pain. Avoid NSAID use in children with renal insufficiency.
   b. Methotrexate may be used for joint/skin symptoms or as a steroid-sparing agent.
   c. Antimalarials, such as hydroxychloroquine and chloroquine, are used to:
      Relieve joint symptoms and skin rash.
      Manage thrombocytopenia.
      Improve dyslipidemia.
      Maintain remission.
   d. Corticosteroids are required for almost all children with SLE and are administered either orally as prednisone or via IV line as methylprednisolone.
      Low-dose oral steroids are usually used to control arthritis, fever, dermatitis, or serositis.
      High-dose oral or IV steroids are used to treat moderate or severe SLE, especially in the presence of CNS involvement, pulmonary disease, hemolytic anemia, and nephritis.
   e. Immunosuppressive agents, such as azathioprine, cyclophosphamide, cyclosporine, mycophenolate mofetil, tacrolimus, and rituximab—used in severe disease including nephritis and neuropsychiatric disease.
   f. Treatment of complications with antibiotics, antihypertensives, anticonvulsants, antipsychotics, anticoagulation.
6. Dialysis and renal transplantation as adjunctive therapy for severe lupus nephritis.

 DRUG ALERT IV glucocorticoid "pulse" therapy has been known to cause hypertension or hypotension, tachycardia, blurring of vision, flushing, sweating, and metallic taste in the mouth. Close monitoring of temperature, pulse rate, respiratory rate, and blood pressure (BP) is indicated.

Complications

1. Infection—primarily resulting from steroid and immunosuppressive therapy.
2. Renal—hypertension, renal failure.
3. Cardiac—atherosclerosis, myocardial infarction, and valvular disease.
4. Growth disturbance; obesity and short stature secondary to inflammation and steroid therapy.
5. Musculoskeletal—osteopenia/osteoporosis, avascular necrosis, and compression fractures (resulting from steroid therapy).
6. Ocular—cataracts, glaucoma secondary to steroid therapy; retinal toxicity secondary to hydroxychloroquine therapy.
7. Macrophage activation syndrome—a life-threatening complication of SLE.

Nursing Assessment

1. History should include a thorough review of systems aimed at symptoms, complications, and medication side effects; current medications; immunizations; recent ophthalmology examination; auditory/visual hallucinations; and medication adherence.
2. Perform a complete physical examination, focusing on signs that might indicate major organ involvement including vital signs, growth parameters, and neuromental health assessment.
3. Assess psychosocial status to evaluate child's and family's coping with chronic illness, school performance, and socialization.

Nursing Diagnoses

Systemic lupus erythematosus has the potential to affect any organ system. The list of potential nursing diagnosis will vary extensively with each individual depending on the type and severity of disease as well as the individual's experience with treatment side effects.

- Fatigue related to chronic inflammation.
- Impaired Sleep Pattern related to side effects of glucocorticoid therapy.
- Acute and chronic Pain related to arthritis.
- Risk for Electrolyte Imbalance related to impaired kidney function.
- Excess Fluid Volume related to kidney disease.
- Risk for Unstable Blood Glucose related side effects of glucocorticoid therapy.
- Hyperthermia related to disease process.
- Risk for Injury related to CNS involvement (seizures).
- Risk for Acute Confusion related to Neuropsychiatric manifestations of lupus.
- Risk for Infection related to treatment.
- Impaired Urinary Elimination related to kidney involvement.
- Imbalanced Nutrition: Less than Body Requirements related to increased metabolic activity associated with inflammation and oral ulcers.
- Risk for Overweight related to side effects of glucocorticoid therapy.
- Disturbed Body Image related to manifestations of disease or medication side effects.
- Risk for Caregiver Role Strain related to having a child with a chronic disease.
- Interrupted Family Processes related to hospitalization, frequent clinic visits.

Nursing Interventions

Minimizing Fatigue

1. Intersperse periods of rest between activities.
2. Caution to resume school activities slowly. Parents should negotiate with the school to implement accommodations to minimize fatigue (ie, second set of textbooks, rest area, and extra time to complete assignments). Consider half days at school until fatigue is diminished. The child may also be a candidate for homeschooling.
3. Maintain good sleep hygiene.

Promoting Comfort

1. Administer or teach parents to administer analgesics, NSAIDs, steroids, and other medications, as prescribed. Review medication side effects with family. Provide written medication aids.
2. For child on steroids, monitor for glycosuria and check blood test results for hyperglycemia, hypokalemia, and hyperlipidemia.
3. Encourage a warm bath or shower to relieve morning stiffness associated with arthritis.
4. Provide diversional activities appropriate for age.

Controlling Fever

1. Monitor temperature every 4 hours and document pattern.
2. Administer or teach parents to administer antipyretics, as prescribed; note results.
3. Encourage increased fluids by mouth when feverish. Dress in lightweight clothing.

Protecting from Injury because of Neuropsychiatric Disease

1. Institute seizure precautions, if indicated.
2. Monitor during seizure and postictal state.
3. Minimize noxious stimuli for patients experiencing hallucinations.
4. Implement safety measures during altered mental state.

Protecting from Adverse Reactions

1. While administering IV glucocorticoid therapy, monitor pulse and BP every 15 minutes for 1 hour and then every 30 minutes for 1 hour.
2. Slow the rate or discontinue infusion if there are significant changes in BP or pulse.
3. Notify the health care provider and continue to monitor vital signs frequently until they return to normal.

Maintaining Urinary Elimination

1. Monitor laboratory tests for signs of renal abnormalities: blood for creatinine, urine for specific gravity, blood and protein.
2. Monitor intake and output.
3. Monitor BP; watch for development of edema.

Promoting Appropriate Nutritional Intake

1. Allow child to help in selecting and preparing foods. Family members should set an example for healthy diet and consider complying with the same diet plan as has been recommended for the child.
2. Apply topical medication to oral ulcers or give analgesics before meals.
3. Monitor food intake and weight. Consider consultation with a dietician to assist with healthy food choices.
4. Low-sodium and low-potassium diet for those with nephritis and those on high-dose steroid therapy.
5. Encourage food high in calcium and vitamin D to decrease risk of low bone density.

Improving Self-Image

1. Encourage contact with peers and family.
2. Allow child to vent feelings about bodily changes and chronic illness.
3. Allow child to be involved in planning care and making decisions.
4. Consider a referral for counseling for adolescents to help with the development of coping strategies, if required.

Family Education and Health Maintenance

1. Teach ways to prevent exacerbations and complications of the disease. Teaching points include:
    a. Get enough rest; try not to overexert.
    b. Minimize stress and anxiety.
    c. Encourage adherence to medication schedule through use of medication calendar, pill boxes; understand adverse medication effects and strategies to reduce them; check with health care provider prior to using over-the-counter drugs or therapies found on the Internet.
    d. Avoid contact with people with infectious diseases; get pneumococcal and flu vaccine and keep routine immunizations up to date.
    e. Provide nutritional counseling to promote a balanced diet with special attention given to portion control and the intake of calcium, vitamin D, and when indicated iron, potassium, folic acid, and sodium content.
    f. Seek medical attention at times of illness or stress.
    g. Minimize sun exposure through protection with sunscreen, hats, and long clothing.
    h. Recognize warning signs of exacerbation such as fatigue, weight loss, joint pain, hair loss, new rashes, mouth sores, headaches, trouble with concentration, seizures, shortness of breath, chest pain, abdominal pain, fever, and urinary changes.
2. Educate parents about normal growth and development, emphasizing issues such as adolescent body image, peer relationships, and the impact of chronic illness on the child and the family.
3. Teach the importance of continual medical follow-up.
    a. Disease management requires frequent re-evaluation; medications and laboratory parameters require frequent monitoring to prevent complications and identify disease flares.
    b. Transition to adult care should begin in early adolescence. Teenagers should know their medications; understand their disease; learn to advocate for themselves with their doctor.
4. Advise family that all children with SLE need annual ophthalmologic exams. Those taking hydroxychloroquine require more frequent ophthalmologic evaluation to identify retinal changes early.
5. Refer to agencies such as the Lupus Foundation of America (*www.lupus.org*).

Evaluation: Expected Outcomes

- Participates in activities with peers without fatigue; attends school full time.
- Reports reduced level of pain.
- Remains afebrile, knows what to do if febrile.
- Seizure precautions maintained.
- No changes in vital signs during glucocorticoid infusion.
- Urine output adequate.
- Appropriate dietary intake, weight stable.
- Compliant with medication regime.
- Prepared for transition to adult care.

Henoch-Schönlein Purpura

Henoch-Schönlein purpura (HSP) is an immune-mediated vasculitis with IgA deposition and subsequent inflammatory reaction around capillaries and arterioles. It is considered a small-vessel vasculitis. HSP can affect the skin, intestines, joints, kidneys, and nervous system. Incidence is higher in males than in females (2:1). Onset generally is between ages 3 and 15; it is seen most commonly in winter and can occur in clusters. Higher rate has been noted in those children diagnosed with familial Mediterranean fever.

Pathophysiology and Etiology

1. Cause is unknown; however, theories include an immunologic reaction to a variety of antigenic stimuli, in a genetically prone individual such as infection (viral, bacterial or fungal), dietary allergens, insect bites, and drugs.
2. Acute vasculitis develops.
    a. Swelling and edema of capillaries, small venules, and arterioles.
    b. Fibrin is deposited in the glomeruli of the kidney.
3. Vasculitis results in skin manifestations (nonthrombocytopenic palpable purpura), arthritis, GI (abdominal pain, GI bleeding), and renal symptoms.

Clinical Manifestations

1. Rash—sudden onset may precede or follow other manifestations.
    a. Typical rash begins with palpable maculopapular erythematous or urticarial rash.
    b. These lesions become less raised and purpuric in character and do not fade with pressure. They blanch initially and then progress to ecchymotic areas until they fade.
    c. Several stages of the rash may be present at one time.
    d. Rash appears primarily on the buttocks, lower back, and extensor aspects of the arms, legs, and face and then disappears.
    e. Localized subcutaneous edema in dependent and periorbital area is common.
2. Arthritis occurs in 50% to 80% of patients, primarily affecting the knee and ankle joints; the wrists, elbows, and finger joints may also be affected, although this is rare.
    a. The arthritis is moderately severe, with painful swelling because of periarticular edema and limitation of motion.
    b. The arthritis is self-limited and does not cause permanent sequelae.
3. Orchitis in 2% to 35% of male children.
4. Colicky abdominal pain—from submucosal and subserosal hemorrhage and edema in two thirds of children. May be accompanied by intussusception and GI bleeding.
5. Nausea, vomiting, malaise, low-grade fever.
6. Renal disease—proteinuria and hematuria.
7. Rarely, CNS involvement, such as headache, seizure, or cerebral hemorrhage.
8. Symptoms may appear acutely or gradually and vary in intensity and duration.

Diagnostic Evaluation

1. Blood studies (not diagnostic, but support clinical evidence):
    a. IgA may be elevated (more than 50% of cases).
    b. Coagulation studies and platelet count are typically normal in presence of purpura.
    c. ESR and WBC count may be elevated.
    d. Anemia is possible.
    e. Elevated BUN and creatinine with severe kidney involvement.
2. Urine studies show proteinuria, microscopic hematuria, and casts.
3. Stools may show occult or gross blood.

4. Abdominal ultrasound or x-rays may help confirm bowel involvement.

Management

Treatment is primarily symptomatic and supportive. Hydration, rest, and adequate pain relief are the goals of treatment.

1. Bed rest until the child is able to ambulate and can do so without increasing edema of the lower extremities, genital area, and buttocks.
2. Antibiotic therapy if acute episode was preceded by infection, especially streptococcal.
3. Management of complicating abdominal or renal involvement and arthritis.
   a. Steroid use is controversial. Suggested for use if symptoms prevent adequate oral intake or if the child has challenges with ambulation or performing ADL.
   b. Immunosuppressive therapy, such as azathioprine or cyclophosphamide, may be given to stabilize persistent renal involvement (rare).
   c. High-dose immunoglobulin has been recommended for severe cases.
4. Provide comfort measures and analgesics, such as acetaminophen or NSAIDs.

Complications

1. Acute nephritis or nephrosis that may lead to chronic nephritis. Ninety percent of children who develop serious renal involvement will do so within 2 months of diagnosis.
2. Intussusception (approximately 5% incidence).
3. Significant GI bleeding may require a transfusion (rare).
4. Neurologic vasculitis with headaches, seizures, and neuropathies.

 NURSING ALERT Be alert for signs of intussusception—sudden onset of paroxysmal, colicky abdominal pain, blood in stools, vomiting, and increasing abdominal distention and tenderness—report immediately.

Nursing Assessment

1. Obtain a complete history. There is some suggestion of allergy to insect bites or medications as a basis for development of the disease. Also controversial is association with streptococci, viruses, and vaccination.
2. Perform physical assessment of renal, integumentary, musculoskeletal, and GI systems.
3. Determine impact of illness on the psychosocial well-being of the child and family.

Nursing Diagnoses

- Acute Pain related to arthritis and abdominal pain.
- Activity Intolerance related to fatigue and pain.
- Risk for Impaired Skin Integrity related to rash and itching.
- Impaired Urinary Elimination related to renal involvement.
- Fear related to discomfort, hospitalization, and lack of knowledge.

Nursing Interventions

Reducing Discomfort

1. Monitor pain level and location. Use appropriate developmental pain scales to determine level of pain.

2. Administer or teach parents to administer pain medications, as prescribed, and monitor child's response.
3. Apply warm or cool compresses to joints or abdomen for 30-minute periods to help soothe painful areas.
4. Provide diversional activities in accordance with the child's age.

Increasing Participation in Activities

1. Monitor completion of daily and diversional activities; offer choice.
2. Alternate activities with rest periods.

Maintaining Skin Integrity

1. Assess skin condition and turgor.
2. Maintain adequate fluids.
3. Provide loose, comfortable clothing.
4. Administer or teach parents to administer antipruritics, if necessary.
5. Avoid soap, scratching, or dry skin that may exacerbate rash.

Maintaining Urinary Output

1. Record intake and output, vital signs, weight, urine-specific gravity, and level of edema.
2. Check urine for protein, hematuria, and color; monitor creatinine
3. Report or teach parents to report changes promptly.

Alleviating Fear

1. Allow child and family to verbalize feelings about hospitalization and illness.
2. Monitor anxiety level of child and family. Ensure information is given at the child's level of understanding.
3. Offer realistic encouragement. The long-term outlook is good when renal involvement is minimal.
4. Encourage the family and peers to visit the hospitalized child and bring in familiar items from home.
5. Allow child to make age-appropriate decisions and become involved in planning care.

Family Education and Health Maintenance

1. Reassure the parents that symptoms are usually self-limiting.
2. Make sure that parents and child understand the disease and the need to report changes in urine or signs of intussusception.
3. Educate the parents about the importance of continued care. Long-term follow-up of urinalysis will be necessary to evaluate renal function.

Evaluation: Expected Outcomes

- Reports relief from pain.
- Participates in activity for longer period each day.
- Rash resolved, skin intact.
- Urine output adequate, negative protein.
- Child verbalizes feelings about illness.

Kawasaki Disease

Kawasaki disease (KD) is a common vasculitis of childhood affecting medium and small blood vessels. Coronary arteries are the most common site of damage, giving KD the potential to cause severe morbidity and even death without early diagnosis and treatment. It is characterized by multisystem inflammation including fever, conjunctivitis, lymphadenopathy, and changes in blood vessels. It is the leading cause of acquired heart disease in children in the United States.

Pathophysiology and Etiology

EVIDENCE BASE Yeung, R. S. M. (2012). Vasculitis: Kawasaki disease. In A. Y. Elzouki, H. A. Harfi, H. Nazer, et al. (Eds.), *Textbook of clinical pediatrics* (2nd ed., pp. 1675–1684). New York: Springer.

1. KD is a disease of early childhood with 85% of affected children under 5 years of age. It occurs in children of all origins, although those of Asian descent have the highest incidence.
2. Etiology is unknown, although most investigators believe the disease is related to an infectious or environmental trigger in a genetically susceptible host. The result is a prolonged immune response targeted at vessel walls of medium and small arteries.
3. Infection as a trigger is supported by the fact that KD is endemic with seasonal fluctuations (winter and early spring). It is further hypothesized that super antigens, proteins present in certain organisms (*Staphylococci, Streptococci, Mycobacterium, Mycoplasma*, Epstein-Barr virus), are responsible for the prolonged inflammation through stimulation of large numbers of T cells.
4. Genetic predisposition to KD is evident in the observations that siblings have 10-fold higher risk of developing the disease and the children of parents who had KD have a twofold increase in risk than the general population.
5. Researchers have not found associations between exposure to drugs, environmental toxins, pesticides, chemicals, or heavy metals and KD.
6. KD is a generalized systemic vasculitis involving blood vessels throughout the body. The full extent of the inflammatory process leading to aneurysm formation is not understood. Marked elevation in the cytokine TNF is thought to activate matrix metalloproteinase enzymes capable of breaking down elastin in arterial vessel walls. This breakdown leads to loss of integrity and ballooning and aneurysm formation.
7. Aneurysms, the result of prolonged inflammation, usually develop in the 2nd to 8th week of the illness. The most common site for development is the coronary artery although other sites such as celiac, mesenteric, femoral, iliac, renal, and axillary may be affected. Early treatment following the recommended protocol of Intravenous gamma globulin (IVIG) and aspirin has reduced aneurysm development by 85%.

EVIDENCE BASE Son, M., & Sundel, R. (2016). Kawasaki disease. In R. E. Petty, R. M. Laxer, et al. (Eds.), *Textbook of pediatric rheumatology* (7th ed., pp. 285–317). Philadelphia, PA: Elsevier.

Clinical Manifestations

Kawasaki disease is divided into three phases, each with distinct clinical features. See Figure 53-1.

Acute Phase (First 10 to 14 Days of Illness)
1. During the acute phase, the children exhibit classic signs of inflammation (redness, swelling, and heat) presented as multisystem changes. They appear ill and irritable.
2. The diagnostic criteria of Kawasaki disease occur during the acute phase. See Box 53-3. Fever, in addition to four out of

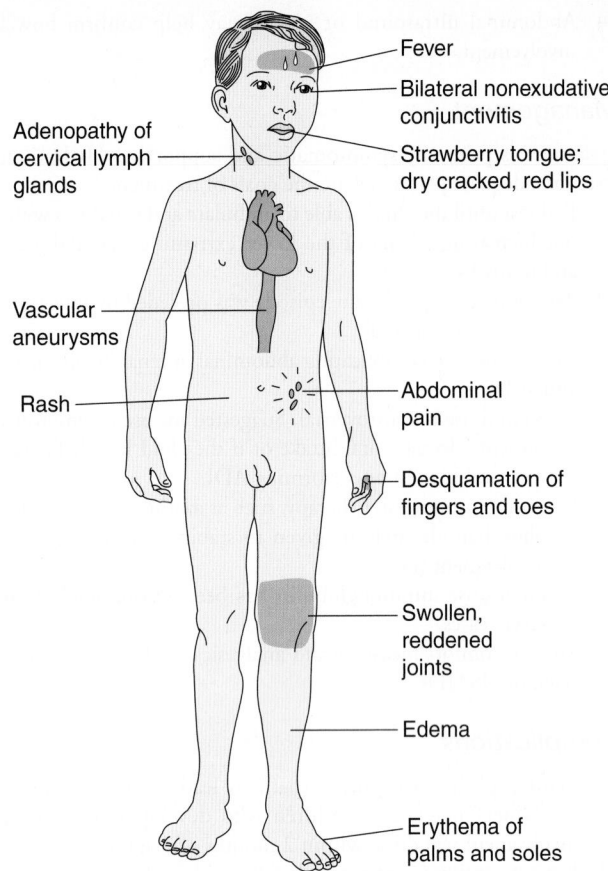

Figure 53-1. Clinical manifestations of acute Kawasaki disease.

five of the other features, is required for diagnosis; not all features occur at a single point in time.
3. Other associated findings:
   a. Cardiovascular—early tachycardia, myocarditis, pericarditis, S3 gallop; reduced contractibility may progress to signs of heart failure.
   b. Aseptic meningitis; anterior uveitis—children extremely irritable; photophobic.
   c. Arthritis—painful; usually large joints; short duration with rapid response to standard treatment for KD.
   d. Gastrointestinal—diarrhea, vomiting, abdominal pain, hepatomegaly, hydrops of the gallbladder.

BOX 53-3	American Heart Association Diagnostic Features for Kawasaki Disease

Persistent fever for at least 5 days. Fever is high (generally greater than 102.2°F [39°C]). Four out of the following five features:

- Bilateral conjunctival injection.
- Changes of the lips and oral cavity.
- Cervical lymphadenopathy.
- Polymorphous exanthema.
- Changes in the peripheral extremities (swelling of the hands or feet) or perineal area.

Cervical lymphadenopathy; at least one node greater than 1.5 cm; usually unilateral.

EVIDENCE BASE Paul, S., Paul, P., & McAllister, T. (2016). Clinical update: common cardiovascular conditions in children. *Community Practitioner, 89*(7), 33–37.
Singh, S., Vignesh, P., & Burgner, D. (2015). The epidemiology of Kawasaki disease: a global update. *Archives of Disease in Childhood, 100*(11), 1084–1088.

Subacute Phase (11 to 25 Days after Onset of Illness)

1. The classic inflammatory features of the acute phase resolve and the temperature returns to normal. If treated, many children are asymptomatic. If untreated or unresponsive to treatment, then fever, oral changes, and conjunctivitis may be present until 3rd or 4th week. Arthritis may be present.
2. Desquamation of toes and fingers in classic distribution starting in periungual region.
3. Coronary artery aneurysm is detected.
4. Thrombocytosis peaks at about 14 days.

Convalescent Phase

1. The acute-phase reactants (ESR and platelets) return to normal.
2. The child appears well.
3. Transverse grooves present on fingernails and toenails (Beau lines).
4. Vessels undergo healing, remodeling, fibrosis, and scarring. Pre-existing small aneurysms may resolve, and large aneurysms may develop thrombosis, leading to complications including myocardial infarction, dysrhythmias, or death.

Diagnostic Evaluation

1. There are no specific diagnostic tests for Kawasaki disease. The diagnosis is based on the clinical manifestations occurring in phases. There is a subset of children, usually the very young or old, who do not meet the diagnostic criteria for KD, yet present with prolonged fever and two or three of the features. They are a challenge to diagnose and are the group who has the highest risk for developing coronary aneurysms.
2. Although there are no specific laboratory tests, the following may help support diagnosis or rule out other diseases:
   a. CBC—leukocytosis; mild normochromic, normocytic anemia.
   b. Platelet count (from 500,000 to 1 million/mm^3)—increased during 2nd to 4th week of illness.
   c. ESR (usually greater than 40 mm/hour).
   d. C-reactive protein (usually greater than 3.0 mg/dL).
   e. Albumin—low levels associated with more severe and prolonged disease.
   f. Liver enzymes (AST, ALT)—moderately elevated.
   g. Serum lipids—reduced high-density lipoprotein levels; elevated triglyceride and low-density lipoprotein levels during the subacute phase.
3. Lumbar puncture often performed because of the degree of child's irritability demonstrates aseptic meningitis; cerebral spinal fluid analysis shows elevated white blood cell count; normal protein; normal glucose.
4. Echocardiogram—should be performed as soon as the diagnosis is suspected and at 2 weeks and at 6 to 8 weeks after diagnosis. More frequent assessment may be required for complicated cases.
5. Cardiac catheterization and angiocardiography may be required for more complex cardiac abnormalities.

Management

EVIDENCE BASE Singh, S., Vignesh, P., & Burgner, D. (2015). The epidemiology of Kawasaki disease: a global update. *Archives of Disease in Childhood, 100*(11), 1084–1088.
Williams, K. (2017). Preventing long-term cardiac damage in pediatric patients with Kawasaki disease. *Journal of Pediatric Healthcare, 31*(2), 196–202.

1. The goal of treatment is to prevent the long-term sequelae associated with KD by controlling inflammation.
2. The American Heart Association recommends that children with KD should be treated with IVIG and aspirin within 10 days of illness to reduce aneurysm formation. Treatment before day 5 has not shown any effect on coronary outcome and may increase the requirement for a second treatment.
   a. IVIG should be given as a single infusion at a dose of 2 g/kg. Most infusion protocols run very slow with stepwise increases in rate for a total infusion time of 8 to 12 hours.
   b. Ten to 20% of children will have persistent fever or recurrence of fever within the first 36 hours after treatment with IVIG. Experts agree that these children should be retreated with a single infusion of 2 g/kg.
   c. Aspirin therapy—the anti-inflammatory dose of 80 to 100 mg/kg/day divided into four doses is recommended during the acute phase. The length of treatment varies from 24 to 72 hours after fever resolves to 2 weeks. The aspirin is then reduced to antiplatelet dosing of 3 to 5 mg/kg/day, which is continued until laboratory measures of inflammation have returned to normal and the echocardiogram at 6 to 8 weeks shows no sign of coronary aneurysm. Children with aneurysms will continue aspirin for life.
3. In more complicated aneurysms, other anticoagulant and thrombolytic medications may be required.
4. Rarely, coronary artery bypass surgery or cardiac catheterization techniques are indicated.
5. Supportive measures:
   a. Maintain fluid and electrolyte balance.
   b. Give nutritional support.
   c. Provide comfort.
6. Follow-up by pediatric cardiologist with serial echocardiograms is necessary to monitor aneurysms.

DRUG ALERT Inflammation of the child's heart may compromise the heart's ability to handle the fluid challenge associated with IVIG. The infusion may need to be of longer duration.

DRUG ALERT Risk of Reye syndrome exists for children on aspirin therapy if they develop varicella or influenza. For children who are not immune to chickenpox, aspirin may need to be withheld after an exposure. Families should be instructed to receive annual influenza vaccines to minimize the risk for influenza.

Complications

1. Coronary aneurysm.
2. Aspirin toxicity.
3. Mortality is less than 0.3%.

Nursing Assessment

1. A thorough history to document data that support the diagnosis of Kawasaki disease; features of KD do not always present simultaneously.
2. Perform physical examination focusing on clinical features, hydration, and cardiovascular status. Document vital signs including accurate temperature, BP, heart rate, rhythm, heart sounds, respiratory rate.
3. Perform pain assessment using age-appropriate pain scale.

Nursing Diagnoses

- Acute Pain related to conjunctival inflammation; swollen, cracked lips; and joint inflammation.
- Risk for Decreased Cardiac Tissue Perfusion related to inflammation of coronary blood vessels.
- Impaired Oral Mucous Membrane related to oral vessel inflammation.
- Risk for Impaired Skin Integrity related to edema, dehydration, and desquamation of digits.
- Deficient Fluid Volume related to hyperthermia, anorexia, and oral changes.
- Fear of Parents and Child related to severity of illness and hospitalization.

Other Nursing Diagnoses may include:

- Hyperthermia related to inflammatory pathology of disease.
- Risk for Ineffective Peripheral Tissue Perfusion related to inflammation of blood vessels.
- Imbalanced Nutrition: Less Than Body Requirements related to anorexia, oral changes, increased metabolic requirements of inflammatory state.

Nursing Interventions

Reducing Discomfort

1. Offer pain medication on a scheduled basis rather than as needed during acute phase. Monitor pain level and child's response to analgesics.
2. Conjunctivitis and associated uveitis can cause photosensitivity; darken the room; offer sunglasses; apply cool compresses.
3. Use age-appropriate diversional techniques such as relaxation breathing, guided imagery, and distraction.

Maintaining Cardiac Output

1. Implement continual cardiac monitoring during acute-phase hospitalization.
2. Assess the child for signs of myocarditis and heart failure (tachycardia, gallop rhythm, chest pain, dyspnea, nasal flaring, grunting, retractions, cyanosis, orthopnea, crackles, moist respirations, distended neck veins, edema).
3. Closely monitor intake and output. Calculate fluid balance. Administer oral and IV fluids, as ordered.
4. If administering IVIG, give premedication, as directed, and monitor closely for adverse effects.

 DRUG ALERT Infusion of IVIG has been known to cause a precipitous drop in BP mimicking anaphylaxis. Monitor BP and heart rate at the start of infusion, after 15 and 30 minutes, and then hourly until infusion is complete. Slow the infusion and have patient evaluated for any drop in BP. Give premedication as prescribed to help prevent adverse effects. Make sure medications to treat anaphylaxis are readily available.

Preserving Oral Mucous Membranes

1. Offer and encourage frequent cool liquids (ice chips and ice pops). Avoid acidic, sugary, or carbonated beverages; progress to soft, bland foods.
2. Give mouth care every 1 to 4 hours; use soft toothbrush.
3. Apply petroleum to dry, cracked lips.
4. Observe the mouth frequently for signs of infection.
5. Monitor food and fluid intake for nutrition appropriate for age.

Improving Skin Integrity

1. Avoid the use of soap to prevent drying; apply emollients to skin, as ordered.
2. Elevate edematous extremities.
3. Use sheepskin, convoluted foam mattress, and smooth sheets.
4. Encourage soft flannel or terry cloth loose-fitting clothing; change damp garments and linens frequently when febrile.
5. Protect peeling skin; observe for signs of infection.

Maintaining Fluid Balance

1. Offer fluids at least every hour when child is awake; monitor and document fluid intake and output.
2. Monitor hydration status by checking skin turgor, daily weight, urine output, presence of tears and moist mucous membranes, and urine-specific gravity.
3. Pay attention to insensible loss during febrile stage. Monitor temperature every 4 to 8 hours and administer antipyretics, as directed. Maintain temperature graph chart.

Reducing Fear

1. Use play therapy (passive and active) to help the child express feelings. Consult a Child Life therapist, as needed.
2. Explain all procedures and treatment plans to the child and family. Encourage the parents and child to verbalize their concerns, fears, and questions.
3. Provide respite for parents during irritable stage of illness when child may be inconsolable. Provide emotional support, as necessary.
4. Keep family informed of progress and reinforce information about stages and prognosis.

Family Education and Health Maintenance

1. Advise parents to take child's temperature daily for 2 weeks post discharge. Call health practitioner for temperatures over 101°F (38.3°C).
2. Ensure family is aware of plan for follow-up. Emphasize the need for long-term care. Complications can occur during the convalescent period months after the acute illness.
3. Advise parents that IVIG is pooled immunoglobulin. Immunizations, although not harmful, may not mount a protective response after IVIG administration. Live vaccinations are not recommended for 6 months post treatment. Catch-up vaccinations may be needed.
4. Advocate for compliance with the prescribed level of physical activity. Activity will be restricted if child is receiving anticoagulant therapy or if child has cardiac complications identified on stress testing.
5. Encourage family members to learn cardiopulmonary resuscitation.
6. Teach parents to report the possible development of salicylate toxicity—tinnitus, nausea and vomiting, GI distress, blood in stool, and increased respirations.
7. For children without physical activity limitations, educate parents that children may be fatigued for several weeks. They may require naps, shorter school days, and special accommodations by school.

8. Provide anticipatory guidance about child's behavior.
   a. Do not overprotect the child. Discuss with parents the grief process of denial, anger, bargaining, depression, and acceptance they may be going through because of the illness.
   b. Discuss regression that often occurs during stresses such as hospitalization and illness.
9. Refer to community organizations such as the American Heart Association (*www.heart.org*).

Evaluation: Expected Outcomes

- Reports improved comfort level.
- Vital signs stable, no signs of reduced cardiac output.
- Eating and drinking without difficulty, reports no oral discomfort.
- No pain or signs of infection with desquamation.
- Child expresses feelings about illness; parents report confidence in ability to manage care.

 TRANSITIONAL CARE ALERT Adherence to treatment for patients with primary immunologic diseases is challenging due to the large number of complex medication regimens and costs that may not be covered by insurance. Nurses should explore patient and parental understanding with recommendations for calendars and computer applications that may prove helpful. If specialized skills are required for administration, initial training and verification on subsequent visits should be required if necessary. Parents and patients should have an understanding of when they should contact their primary care provider or their medical specialist for questions.

SELECTED REFERENCES

American Academy of Pediatrics. (2015). Section 3: Summaries of infectious diseases. In D. Kimberlin, M. Brady, M. A. Jackson, S. S. Long (Eds.), *Red book: 2015 report of the Committee on Infectious Diseases* (30th ed., pp. 453–475) Elk Grove Village, IL: American Academy of Pediatrics.

Burke, L., Kirkham, J., Arnott, J., et al. (2018). The transition of adolescents with juvenile idiopathic arthritis or epilepsy from paediatric health care services to adult health care services: A scoping review of the literature and a synthesis of the evidence. *Journal of Child Health Care,* January 21, 2018.

Centers for Disease Control and Prevention. Recommended immunization schedules for children and adolescents aged 18 or younger, United States 2017. Available: *www.cdc.gov/vaccines/schedules/hcp/child-adolescent.html*

Centers for Disease Control and Prevention. HIV Surveillance Report, 2016; vol. 28. *http://www.cdc.gov/hiv/library/reports/hiv-surveillance.html.* Published November 2017. Accessed May 20, 2018.

Children's HIV Association (CHIVA). (2017). *CHIVA guidance on transition for adolescents living with HIV.* London: Author. Available: *www.chiva.org.uk/guidelines/tr/*

Couture, J., & Silverman, E. D., (2016). Update on the pathogenesis and treatment of childhood-onset systemic lupus erythematosus. *Current Opinion in Rheumatology, 28*(5), 488–496.

Daniels, L., Gordon, J., Burns, J. (2012). Kawasaki disease: Late cardiovascular sequelae. *Current Opinion in Cardiology, 27*(6), 572–577.

EULAR Standing Committee. (2008). EULAR recommendations for the management of systemic lupus erythematosus. Report of a Task Force of the EULAR Standing Committee for International Clinical Studies Including Therapeutics. *Annals of Rheumatic Disease, 67*(2), 195–205.

Evangeli, M., & Kagee, A. (2016). A model of caregiver paediatric HIV disclosure decision-making. *Psychology, Health & Medicine, 21*(3), 338–353.

Foster, H., Minden, K., Clemente, D., et al. (2017) EULAR/PReS standards and recommendations for the transitional care of young people with juvenile-onset rheumatic diseases. *Annals of the Rheumatic Diseases. 76,* 639–646.

Hahn, B., McMahon, M., Wilkinson, A., et al. (2012). American College of Rheumatology guidelines for screening, treatment and management of lupus nephritis. *Arthritis Care and Research, 64,* 797–808.

Hernandez-Trujillo, V., Scalchunes, C., Hernandez-Trujillo, H., et al. (2015). Primary immunodeficiency diseases: An opportunity in pediatrics for improving patient outcomes. *Pediatrics, 54*(13), 1265–1275.

Hinze, C., Gohar, F., Foell, D. (2015). Management of juvenile idiopathic arthritis: Hitting the target. *Nature Reviews Rheumatology, 11,* 290–300.

Klein-Gitelman, M., & Lane, J. (2016). Systemic lupus erythematosus. In R. E. Petty, R. M. Laxer, et al. (Eds.), *Textbook of Pediatric Archaeology* (7th ed., pp. 285–317). Philadelphia: Elsevier.

Klotsche, J., Niewerth, M., Haas, J., et al. (2016). Long-term safety of etanercept and adalimumab compared to methotrexate in patients with juvenile idiopathic arthritis (JIA). *Annals of the Rheumatic Diseases, 75,* 855–861.

Knight, A., Vickery, M. E., Muscal, E., et al. (2016). Identifying targets for improving mental healthcare of adolescents with systemic lupus erythematosus: Perspectives from pediatric rheumatology clinicians in the United States and Canada. *The Journal of Rheumatology, 43*(6), 1136–1145.

Kuo, H., Yang, K., Chang, W., et al. (2012). Kawasaki disease: An update on diagnosis and treatment. *Pediatrics and Neonatology, 53*(1), 4–11.

Lima, G. L., Paupitz, J., Aikawa, N. E., et al. (2016). Vitamin D supplementation in adolescents and young adults with juvenile systemic lupus erythematosus for improvement in disease activity and fatigue scores: A randomized, double-blind, placebo-controlled trial. *Arthritis Care & Research, 68*(1), 91–98.

McCrindle, B., Rowley, A., Newburger, J. et al. (2017). Diagnosis, treatment and long-term management of Kawasaki disease: A scientific statement for health professionals from the American Heart Association. *Circulation, 135,* E1–E73.

McKeever, A., & Kelly, M. (2015). Growing up with juvenile idiopathic arthritis. *The American Journal of Maternal Child Nursing, 40*(1), 8–15.

McLellan, M. C., & Baker, A. L. (2011). At the heart of the fever: Kawasaki disease. *American Journal of Nursing, 111*(6), 57–63.

Panel on Antiretroviral Therapy and Medical Management of HIV-Infected Children. Guidelines for the use of antiretroviral agents in pediatric HIV infection. Available: *http://aidsinfo.nih.gov/contentfiles/lvguidelines/pediatricguidelines.pdf.* Accessed May 20, 2018.

Panel on Treatment of HIV-Infected Pregnant Women and Prevention of Perinatal Transmission. (2018). Recommendations for use of antiretroviral drugs in pregnant HIV-1-infected women for maternal health and interventions to reduce perinatal HIV transmission in the United States. Available: *http://aidsinfo.nih.gov/contentfiles/lvguidelines/PerinatalGL.pdf.* Accessed May 20, 2018 (pages C-1, D-1).

Paul, S., Paul, P., & McAllister, T. (2016). Clinical update: common cardiovascular conditions in children. *Community Practitioner, 89*(7), 33–37.

Penn, C. (2015). "Too much for one day": A case study of disclosure in the paediatric HIV/AIDS clinic. *Health Expectations, 18* (4), 578–589.

Petty, R. E., Laxer, R. M., Lindsley, C. B., et al. (Eds.). (2016). *Textbook of pediatric rheumatology* (7th ed.). Philadelphia, PA: Elsevier.

Pibernat, A., Pibernat, E., Rodriguez, F., et al. (2015). The important role of nursing in primary care exploring knowledge about human immunodeficiency virus and other sexually transmitted diseases in adolescents. *Journal of Adolescent Health, 56*(6), 681–682.

Picard, C., Gaspar, B., Bousfiha, A., et al. (2018). International Union of Immunological Societies: 2017 Immunodeficiency Diseases Committee Report on Inborn Errors of Immunity. *Journal of Clinical Immunology, 38*(1), 96–128.

Singh, S., Vignesh, P., Burgner, D. (2015). The epidemiology of Kawasaki disease: A global update. *Archives of Disease in Childhood, 100*(11), 1084–1088.

Siok Hoon, L., Pullenayegum, E., Feldman, B., et al. (2018). From childhood to adulthood: Disease activity trajectories in childhood-onset systemic lupus erythematosus. *Arthritis Care & Research, 70*(5), 750–757.

Son, M., & Sundel, R. (2016). Kawasaki disease. In R. E. Petty, R. M. Laxer, et al. (Eds.), *Textbook of pediatric rheumatology* (7th ed., pp. 285–317). Philadelphia, PA: Elsevier.

Son, M. B., Sergeyenko, Y., Guan, H., et al. (2016). Disease activity and transition outcomes in a childhood-onset systemic lupus erythematosus cohort. *Lupus, 25,* 1431–1439.

Tektonidou, M., Lewandowski, L., Hu, J., et al. (2017) Survival in adults and children with systemic lupus erythematosus: A systematic review and Bayesian meta-analysis of studies from 1950 to 2016. *Annals of Rheumatic Diseases, 76*(12), 2009–2016.

UNAIDS *Fact Sheet World AIDS Day* 2017. Available: *www.unaids.org/sites/default/files/media_asset/UNAIDS_FactSheet_en.pdf.* Accessed May 2018.

Wheeler, T. (2010). Systemic lupus erythematosis: The basics of nursing care. *British Journal of Nursing, 19*(4), 249–253.

Williams, K. (2017). Preventing long-term cardiac damage in pediatric patients with Kawasaki disease. *Journal of Pediatric Healthcare, 31*(2), 196–202.

Yeung, R. S. M. (2012). Vasculitis: Kawasaki disease. In A. Y. Elzouki, H. A. Harfi, H. Nazer, et al. (Eds.), *Textbook of clinical pediatrics* (2nd ed., pp. 1675–1684). New York: Springer.

Younger, E., Epland, K., Zampelli, A., & Hintermeyer, M. (2015). Primary immunodeficiency diseases: A primer for PCP's. *The Nurse Practitioner, 40*(2), 1–7.

54
Pediatric Orthopedic Problems

ORTHOPEDIC PROCEDURES

 See additional online content: Procedure Guidelines 54-1 and 54-2.

Immobilization: Casts, Braces, Splints, and External and Internal Fixators

 EVIDENCE BASE Tho Hang, B., Gross, C., Otero, H, et al. (2017). An Update on Common Orthopedic Injuries and Fractures in Children: Is Cast Immobilization Always Necessary? *Clinical Pediatric Emergency Medicine, 18*(1), 62–73.
Hill, C. E., Masters, J. P., & Perry, D. C. (2016). A systematic review of splinting versus complete plaster casts for the management of childhood buckle fractures of the wrist. *Journal of Pediatric Orthopedics, 25*(2), 183–190.

Casting, bracing, and splinting are all means of immobilizing an injured or diseased body part, primarily bones and musculature. Internal and external fixators have been utilized to provide stability and immobilization of bones, which are fractured or in the process of reconstruction. The length of time for use of these various devices can vary from a few days to several months. Also see pages 860–866, but realize that the management of children who are immobilized requires age-appropriate adaptation and support.

Types of Fixators

1. Fractures that require open reduction, such as those that do not align, include more than one broken area of the bone or involve attaching long bones in reconstructive surgery that can be managed with open reduction internal fixation (ORIF).
2. External fixators involve pins and screws placed through the skin and into the bone to stabilize a fracture. External fixation can include types of traction. They are also used when osteotomies are required or for limb-lengthening procedures.

Complications of Immobilization

1. Peripheral neurovascular compromise.
2. Alteration in skin integrity because of pressure or friction.
3. Loss of efficient use of affected extremity because of noncompliance.

Traction

Traction is the application of a pulling force to an injured or diseased part of the body or an extremity, whereas a countertraction pulls in the opposite direction. Traction may be used to reduce fractures or dislocations, maintain alignment and correct deformities, decrease muscle spasms and relieve pain, promote rest of a diseased or injured body part, and promote exercise. Advances in nailing and rodding, along with use of internal and external fixators for fractures and spinal curvatures, have reduced the use of traction overall. Interest in ambulation for children is another consideration when surgeons decide between traction and other methods of immobilization. Currently, traction is still a very viable option especially for femur and femoral shaft fractures and hip and cervical fractures but remains an effective process for other immobilization requirements. Types of traction include reference to the mechanism and also specific named types such as Russell or Bryant traction for femoral fractures or halo traction with the use of Crutchfield tongs for stabilization of spinal fractures or injuries. Complications of traction include injury to the cranial nerves and other neurologic injuries.

Types of Traction

1. Manual—direct pulling on the extremity or body part. Usually, it is used to reduce fractures before treatment or immobilization.
2. Skin—force is applied directly to the skin by means of traction strips or tapes secured by elastic bandages or by means of traction boots, usually of short-term duration and commonly used in children in whom small amounts of force are required.
3. Skeletal—force is applied to the body part through fixation directly into or through the bone by means of a traction pin or screw. This allows for greater force over longer periods or used when skin traction is not feasible, as in soft tissue injury or damage.

4. Continuous or intermittent—traction forces should be disrupted only in accordance with the health care provider's orders.

Complications of Traction

1. Neurovascular compromise to extremity.
2. Skin and soft tissue injury.
3. Pin or screw tract infection and osteomyelitis (with skeletal traction).

COMMON ORTHOPEDIC DISORDERS IN CHILDREN

 See additional online content: Patient Education Guidelines 54-1.

Fractures

A *fracture* is a break or disruption in the continuity of the bone. Fractures in children differ from those in adults because of the differences in anatomy, biomechanics, and physiology of the child's skeleton compared to that of an adult. Involvement of the epiphysis or metaphysis can disrupt the epiphyseal plate, interfering with growth (see Figure 54-1). Fractures are extremely common in children, with an estimated 42% of boys and 27% of girls sustaining fractures during childhood.

 EVIDENCE BASE Baker, R., Orton, E., Tata, L. J., et al. (2015). Risk factors for long bone fractures in children up to five years of age: A nested case-controlled study. *Archives of Disease in Children, 100*(5), 432–437.

Sameer, N., Erali, R., Warner, W., et al. (2016). Epidemiology of pediatric fractures presenting to the emergency department in the United States. *Journal of Pediatric Orthopaedics. 36*(4), E45–E46.

Servaes, S., Brown, S. D., Choudhary, et al. (2016). The etiology and significance of fractures in infants and young children: A critical multidisciplinary review. *Pediatric Radiology, 46*(5), 591–600.

Epiphysis — Articular cartilage
Metaphysis — Cancellous bone
— Epiphyseal plate
— Blood vessel
— Compact bone
Diaphysis
— Medullary (marrow) cavity
Metaphysis
Epiphysis

Figure 54-1. Structure of a bone.

Pathophysiology and Etiology

1. Most fractures in children are a result of low-velocity trauma such as a fall.
   a. Up to the age of 2 years, most fractures are sustained as a result of the child being injured by another person.
   b. Fractures in neonates and infants are commonly the result of child maltreatment, which should be suspected when evaluating and treating fractures in this age group.
2. A bone fractures when the force applied to it exceeds the amount the bone can absorb.
   a. Children's long bones are more resilient than those of adults. They are able to withstand greater deflection without fracturing.
   b. The majority of children who are at risk for long bone fractures are over the age of 1 year.
   c. The bones of children have thick periosteum, as compared to adults, providing a protective membrane to help prevent incidence of fractures.
3. The involvement of growth plates (epiphyseal plate) is unique to fractures in children. Cartilaginous growth plates are present at each end of the long bones and at one end of metacarpals and metatarsals. The plate is weaker than surrounding ligaments, tendons, and joint capsules and is disrupted before these tissues are injured.
   a. Damage to the growth plate may result in cessation of or a disturbance in bone growth (depending on the extent of damage sustained at the growth plate).
   b. On the other hand, acceleration in bone growth commonly occurs after a fracture in the long bones of children.
4. Children's fractures heal more rapidly than adult fractures. The younger the child, the more rapidly the bone heals.
5. Children's fractures remodel more completely and actively than adult fractures and usually result in less disability and deformity.

Sites of Fractures in Children

 EVIDENCE BASE Franklin, C. C., Wren, T., Ferkel, E., et al. (2014). Predictors of conversion from conservative to operative treatment of pediatric forearm fractures. *Journal of Pediatric Orthopedics, 23*(2), 150–154.

Goodell, P. B., & Bauer, A. (2016). Problematic pediatric hand and wrist fractures. *Journal of Bone and Joint Surgery, 4*(5), 1–9.

Shuh, A. M., Whitlock, K. B., & Klein, E. J. (2016). Managing toddler fractures in the pediatric emergency room. *Pediatric Emergency Care, 32*(7), 452–454.

As children grow, the fracture rate increases, with the peak incidence occurring in early adolescence. Forearm fractures are the most common injury.

Forearm and Wrist Fractures

1. The most common site of fracture in children, occurring more frequently in children older than the age of 5 years.
2. Major categories of classification include fracture dislocations, midshaft fractures, and distal fractures.
3. Most common cause is from a fall on an outstretched arm.

Epiphyseal or Growth Plate Injuries

1. Constitute approximately 15% to 25% of all skeletal injuries in children.
2. The most frequent site of physeal injuries (excluding phalangeal fractures) is the distal radius and ulna.

3. The 11- to 15-year-old age group tends to sustain the majority of physeal injuries to the distal radius and ulna.
4. The mechanism of injury is usually a fall on an outstretched arm.

Clavicle Fractures
1. Frequent site of fracture in children.
2. The shaft of the clavicle is the most common site of injury.
3. A fall on the shoulder or excessive lateral compression of the shoulder as in a difficult vaginal delivery in a newborn is usually the mechanism of injury.
4. Treatment involves support in the form of immobilization with a sling.
5. Reduction of clavicle fractures in children occurs only in instances of extreme displacement.

Humerus Fractures
1. The mechanism of injury for the majority of humeral fractures is a fall onto an outstretched arm or hand.
2. Supracondylar fractures are the most common fractures of the humerus and may be associated with acute vascular injury.
3. Approximately 10% of all humeral fractures occur at the shaft of the humerus; they are usually a result of twisting injuries in infants and toddlers. Direct trauma to the humeral shaft is the most common mechanism of injury in older children.
4. Distal humeral fractures occur more often in the lateral epicondyle than the medial epicondyle.
5. Less than 1% of fractures occur at the proximal humerus.

Spinal Fractures
1. Rare in children.
2. Mechanism of injury is due to significant trauma, such as a fall from a significant height, athletic activities, assault, or pedestrian–motor vehicle accident.
3. Most spinal fractures involve the cervical spine.

Pelvic Fractures
1. Pelvic fractures are uncommon in children and adolescents; they are commonly the result of high-energy trauma or a crush-type injury.
2. Associated injuries are present in approximately 75% of children with pelvic fractures and include hemorrhage and damage to the abdominal wall and pelvic organs.

Hip Fractures
1. Hip fractures in children are uncommon but may occur from motor vehicle accidents, bicycle accidents, falls from significant heights, or child maltreatment (in children under age 3).
2. Hip fractures can result in avascular necrosis of the femoral head and damage to the physis resulting in growth arrest, malunion, and nonunion.
3. Pelvic avulsion fractures are more common, especially in boys ageing 12 to 14 years.

Femur Fractures
1. Common in children. Peak incidence occurs in two age groups—children aging 2 to 3 years and adolescents.
2. Fractures of the femoral shaft (diaphysis) are uncommon in children but are the most common location in this area.
3. Usually the result of high-energy trauma, such as a motor vehicle accident or fall from a significant height; most common cause in children younger than age 1 is child maltreatment.

Tibial Fractures
1. The most common lower extremity fracture in children occurs in the tibial and fibular shaft—constitutes 10% to 15% of all pediatric fractures.

2. Most diaphyseal tibia fractures in children ages 5 to 6 are nondisplaced or minimally displaced spiral or oblique fractures. A rotational mechanism of injury to the lower leg is the most common cause of tibial fractures in children under age 3 (toddler's fracture or CAST [childhood accidental spiral tibial]).
3. Greater force is required to injure the tibia in older children; motor vehicle accidents and sports injuries are the most common causes of tibial fractures in children and adolescents.

Ankle Fractures
1. Represent approximately 5% of all pediatric fractures.
2. Involve the growth plate in approximately one of six injuries.
3. Greatest incidence is in males ages 10 to 15 years.
4. Usually the result of direct trauma.
5. Mortise view as well as anteroposterior (AP) and lateral x-rays should be obtained.

Foot Fractures
1. Foot fractures account for approximately 6% of all fractures in children and 50% of foot fractures occur at the metatarsals.
2. Most metatarsal and phalangeal fractures are nondisplaced.
3. Mechanism of injury is usually a direct or indirect trauma, such as from falls, jumping from heights, object falling on foot, and twisting injuries.

Classification of Fractures

1. Open fractures: underlying fracture in the bone communicates with an external wound; usually the result of high-energy trauma or penetrating wounds.
2. Closed fractures: underlying fracture with no open wound.
3. Plastic deformation: a bending of the bone in such a manner as to cause a microscopic fracture line that does not cross the bone. When the force is removed, the bone remains bent. Unique to children and most common in the ulna (see Figure 54-2A).
4. Buckle (torus) fractures: fracture on the tension side of the bone near the softer metaphyseal bone; crosses the bone and buckles the harder diaphyseal bone on the opposite side, causing a bulge (see Figure 54-2B).

Figure 54-2. Common fractures in children. **(A)** Plastic deformation (bend). **(B)** Buckle (torus). **(C)** Greenstick. **(D)** Complete.

5. Greenstick fracture: the bone is bent and the fracture begins but does not entirely cross through the bone (see Figure 54-2C).
6. Complete fractures (see Figure 54-2D):
   a. Spiral—from a rotational force.
   b. Oblique—diagonally across the diaphysis.
   c. Transverse—usually diaphyseal.
   d. Epiphyseal—through the physis.

Clinical Manifestations

1. Inability to stand, walk, or use injured part.
2. Limb deformity (visible or palpable).
3. Ecchymosis.
4. Pain, described as point tenderness.
5. History of injury or trauma (may not be the case with pathologic fractures).
6. Spontaneous onset of pain (usually seen with pathologic fractures).
7. Local swelling and marked tenderness.
8. Movement between bone fragments.
9. Crepitus or grating.
10. Muscle spasm.

Diagnostic Evaluation

1. X-rays of suspected limb fractures should include the joint above and below the injury.
   a. Should always include a minimum of two views at 90-degree angles to each other (AP and lateral).
   b. Comparison views of the opposite extremity are frequently needed. They help to distinguish the fracture line from the growth plate.
   c. In some situations, oblique x-rays are warranted to help identify a fracture that is difficult to detect.
2. Further radiologic studies may be indicated in certain instances to evaluate a fracture: ultrasound, tomography, magnetic resonance imaging (MRI), computed tomography (CT) scan, bone scan, and fluoroscopy.
3. Vascular assessment may include the use of:
   a. Doppler studies.
   b. Compartment pressure monitoring.
   c. Angiography.

Management

Treatment is dependent upon the type of fracture, its location, and the age of the child.
1. Treatment may consist of:
   a. Immobilization by cast, splint, external fixator, or brace.
   b. Closed reduction followed by a period of immobilization in a cast or splint.
   c. Open reduction with or without internal fixation and usually followed by a period of immobilization in a cast or splint.
   d. Closed reduction and percutaneous pinning followed by a period of immobilization.
   e. Closed or open reduction and application of an external fixator.
   f. Traction (skin, skeletal) followed by a period of immobilization.
2. Most pediatric fractures heal in 12 weeks or less. Simple fractures that are closed and nondisplaced can heal enough to be free from immobilization within 3 weeks.

Complications

1. Infection and avascular necrosis.
2. Delayed union, nonunion, and malunion.
3. Shortening—epiphyseal arrest (deformities in angulation or limb length).
4. Vascular injuries.
5. Nerve injuries—palsies.
6. Visceral injuries.
7. Tendon and joint injuries.
8. Fat embolism.
9. Compartment syndrome (orthopedic emergency).
10. Osteoarthritis (occurs later).
11. Reflex sympathetic dystrophy.

Nursing Assessment

1. Follow the basic assessment for the trauma victim (see page 945).
2. Obtain history from child, parents, and others to include accident or trauma details, noting the position of the extremity at impact.
3. Perform physical examination for location of deformity, swelling, ecchymosis, and pain, vital signs, and neurovascular assessment.
4. Assess child's support mechanisms/social situation with consideration of discharge needs.

Nursing Diagnoses

- Acute Pain related to tissue trauma and reflex muscle spasms secondary to fracture.
- Ineffective Peripheral Tissue Perfusion related to swelling and immobilization.
- Impaired Skin Integrity related to mechanical trauma (eg, fixation device, traction, casts, other orthopedic devices).
- Ineffective Coping related to separation from family and home.
- Impaired Physical Mobility related to fracture and external immobilization device (eg, cast, splint, external fixator).
- Bathing/Dressing/Feeding/Toileting/Self-Care Deficit related to external devices (eg, cast, splint).
- Risk for Infection related to trauma (fracture) and surgery.
- Risk for Peripheral Neurovascular Dysfunction related to restrictive envelope secondary to cast or splint.

Nursing Interventions

Also see page 868 for orthopedic surgery.

Promoting Comfort

1. Monitor and assess pain level using an age-appropriate pain scale (eg, Oucher or FACES scale).
2. Properly position, align, and support affected body part.
3. Administer analgesics, as indicated, and monitor effectiveness of analgesia.
4. Use nontraditional methods of pain relief—music therapy, diversionary activities, relaxation techniques, therapeutic touch, and play therapy.

Maintaining Tissue Perfusion

1. Frequently assess perfusion of limb by checking temperature, color, sensation, and pulses.
2. Elevate extremity above heart level to prevent edema.
3. Encourage movement of digits on affected limb.

4. Remove compressive bandages (eg, elastic bandages, splints) that restrict flow of circulation.

Maintaining Skin Integrity

1. Assess for and relieve pressure caused by tight bandages, casts, and splints.
2. Provide periodic cleaning, thorough drying, and lubrication to pressure points if in traction.
3. Encourage frequent position changes as allowed.
4. Assess skin condition on a regular basis.
5. Massage healthy skin around affected area to stimulate circulation.
6. Protect the skin at risk with special dressings or products (eg, barrier cream, moisture-permeable dressing).
7. Discourage the use of sticks, pens or pencils, or small toys or other objects to scratch itchy skin.
8. Promote a diet high in protein, carbohydrates, and calcium.

Promoting Effective Coping

1. Assess the child's and parents' response to events; provide reassurance and emotional support.
2. Explain condition, treatment, and rehabilitation goals, as indicated.
3. Refer to community-based support agencies (eg, social services, home care nursing), if indicated.
4. Structure the child's day with routine, activities, and therapy to keep him or her busy.
5. Encourage child to express feelings and emotions through writing (eg, journal), drawing, or play therapy.

Promoting Mobility

1. Encourage exercise of uninvolved limbs regularly throughout the day.
2. Collaborate with physical and occupational therapist to teach appropriate ambulation techniques using aids such as crutches, walkers, or wheelchairs, as indicated.
3. Teach safety precautions when using an ambulatory aid.

Attaining Independence

1. Assess family situation for ability to care for child at home.
2. Allow child to care for self, and participate in care when able.
3. Encourage parents and siblings to assist only as needed.
4. Evaluate child's ability to participate in self-care activities.

Preventing Infection

 EVIDENCE BASE Schroeder, N. O., Seeley, M. A., Hariharan, A., et al. (2017). Utility of postoperative antibiotics after percutaneous pinning of pediatric supracondylar humerus fracture. *Journal of Pediatric Orthopedics, 37*(6), 363–367.

Trionfo, A., Cavanaugh, P. K., & Herman, M. J. (2016). Pediatric open fractures. *Orthopedic Clinics of North America, 47*(3), 565–578.

1. Assess wounds, including pin sites, frequently for warmth, erythema, swelling, tenderness, or purulent drainage.
2. Pin site care and the use of dressings are indicated by the orthopedist or institution. A cleansing ritual with chlorhexidine or other antiseptic is beneficial, which includes gentle massage to remove superficial drainage.
3. Report signs of infection.
4. Provide appropriate wound care for open injuries and surgical wounds.
5. Administer antibiotics, as ordered.

6. Encourage child to eat and maintain good caloric and protein intake to promote healing.
7. Teach good handwashing technique to child and parents.

Preventing Peripheral Neurovascular Dysfunction

1. Assess the neurovascular status of affected limb every hour for the first 24 hours (or as indicated by hospital protocol)—compare with unaffected limb.
2. Assess for nerve injury (eg, abduct all fingers, touch thumb to small finger, plantar flexion, dorsiflexion).
3. Assess for the presence of numbness, tingling, "pins and needles," and excessive pain (disproportionate to injury and analgesia administered).
4. Encourage range of motion (ROM) exercises in fingers, toes, and unaffected limbs.
5. Teach child and parents signs and symptoms of neurovascular compromise and advise them to contact the health care provider immediately if signs of compromise occur.

 TRANSITIONAL CARE ALERT Inpatient rehabilitation or home care nursing visits may be necessary in the initial postoperative stage. Rehabilitation facilities provide occupational and physical therapy and education for the child to return to function. Home nursing care provides assessment of family coping with the care of their immobilized child. In either situation, reinforcement is needed to help reassure the parents that they are able to care for their child. Make sure the parents and caregivers know who to contact if they have any questions about a possible complication.

Community and Home Care Considerations

1. Assess the skin for signs of breakdown and condition of cast.
2. Assess neurovascular status of affected limb.
3. Assess traction device to make sure it is intact and maintained.
4. Assess child's nutritional status and bowel and bladder routine.
5. Assess coping ability of child and family members and answer questions parents may have about the care of their immobilized child.
6. Teach patient and family about care of their child's pin site care and adjustment of screws. Have them do a return demonstration for evaluation of teaching.
7. Teach the child and family about signs and symptoms of infection and whom to contact should an infection occur.

Family Education and Health Maintenance

1. Teach proper care of casts, splints, and immobilization devices.
2. Teach safety measures and prevention of further injuries.
   a. Advise use of bicycle helmets and knee, elbow, and wrist pads.
   b. Emphasize importance of supervising young children while playing.
   c. Teach safety measures, such as placing gates at stairs and installing top-opening windows on second floors.
3. Teach family and child the natural history of fracture healing (eg, presence of fracture bump, gradual recovery of ROM, predicted time frame for healing).

Evaluation: Expected Outcomes

- Reports acceptable level of comfort.
- Extremity warm with good color sensation, pulses, and capillary refill.

- No skin breakdown noted.
- Parents comfort child; child responds appropriately.
- Uses ambulatory aids and ambulates independently.
- Bathes and feeds self with minimal assistance.
- No fever or signs of infection surrounding wound.
- Denies numbness and tingling.

Osteomyelitis

 EVIDENCE BASE Godley, D. R. (2015). Managing musculoskeletal infections in children in the era of increasing antibiotic resistance. *Journal of the American Academy of Physician Assistants, 28*(4), 24–29.
Pyles, V. (2015). Pediatric Acute Hematogenous Osteomyelitis. *Continuing Education Topics & Issues, 17*(1), 14–18.

Osteomyelitis is a pyogenic infection of the bone and surrounding soft tissues. It occurs mostly in children between ages 3 and 12 years and is primarily a disease of growing bones. Long bones are frequently involved, and the characteristic site of involvement is the metaphyseal region. Males are afflicted two times as frequently as females.

Pathophysiology and Etiology

Etiologic Agents and Risk Factors
1. Microorganisms that cause osteomyelitis vary and are related to the age of the child.
   a. The most commonly identified pathogenic organism in acute osteoarticular infections is *Staphylococcus aureus*, with this organism responsible for about 70% of cases; methicillin-resistant *S. aureus* infections have risen in the last several years.
   b. Group A beta-hemolytic streptococcus, *Enterobacter, Escherichia coli*, and *Streptococcus pneumoniae* are other etiologic agents.
   c. Vertebral infections are increasingly a result of Gram-negative microorganisms.
2. Classification based on pathogen's mode of entry:
   a. Hematogenous osteomyelitis (through the bloodstream)—occurs primarily in children.
   b. Contiguous osteomyelitis—caused by pathogenic spread from outside the body or by progressive spread of infection from tissue adjacent to the bone.
3. Risk factors include:
   a. Impetigo.
   b. Furunculosis.
   c. Direct trauma to area adjacent to site of osteomyelitis.
   d. Infected burns.
   e. Prolonged use of an intravenous (IV) line or intraosseous needle.
   f. Immunizations, especially with bacille Calmette-Guérin (BCG).
   g. Intravenous drug addiction.
   h. Sickle cell disease.

Pathophysiologic Changes
1. When the site is inoculated, the invading pathogen provokes the following responses:
   a. Inflammatory response.
   b. Pus formation.
   c. Edema.
   d. Vascular congestion.
   e. Leukocyte activity.
   f. Abscess formation.
2. Small terminal vessels thrombose and exudate the bone's canaliculi.
   a. Inflammatory exudate extends into the metaphyseal and marrow cavity and through small metaphyseal openings into the cortex.
3. Exudate reaches outer surface of the cortex, forming abscesses that lift periosteum off the underlying bone, disrupting blood vessels and entering the bone through periosteum, thereby causing deprivation of blood supply to the bone. This leads to necrosis and death of the infected bone.
4. Sequestrum or devitalized bone is produced.
5. Intense osteoblastic response is stimulated upon lifting of the periosteum.
6. New bone is lain down by osteoblasts that partially or completely surround infected bone.
7. New bone, also known as *involucrum*, is formed.
8. Exudate escapes into surrounding soft tissue through openings in the involucrum, from which it escapes though the skin via sinus tracts.
9. Acute osteomyelitis is an abrupt onset of inflammation. Failure to halt acute osteomyelitis can lead to chronic osteomyelitis.
10. Chronic osteomyelitis:
    a. Signs and symptoms are usually vague.
    b. Infection is silent between exacerbations.
    c. Small abscesses or fragments containing microorganisms produce occasional flare-ups of acute osteomyelitis.
    d. Inadequate or inappropriate therapy and drug-resistant microorganisms can result in progression of acute osteomyelitis to chronic osteomyelitis.

Clinical Manifestations
1. Infants—involvement of multiple sites within the same bone or in multiple bones.
   a. Acute illness characterized by fever and failure to move affected limb.
2. Children—usually affects long bones but can affect the pelvis and spine.
   a. Abrupt onset of fever and systemic signs of toxicity.
   b. Swelling, redness, and discrete tenderness over the affected area.
   c. Decreased ability to bear weight as well as decreased ROM of affected limb.
3. Adolescents (less affected)—affects long bones but may involve vertebrae.
   a. Back pain.
   b. Signs and symptoms described above for children.

Diagnostic Evaluation
1. Blood cultures (positive in about 50% of cases) should be obtained before initiation of antibiotic therapy to help identify the causative pathogen.
2. Needle aspiration of soft tissue should be done to identify the causative agent.
   a. Gram stain, culture, and sensitivity of specimen once obtained.
   b. Negative aspirate does not always rule out infection.
3. Complete blood count—marked leukocytosis and low hemoglobin.

4. Erythrocyte sedimentation rate (ESR) and C-reactive protein (CRP)—elevated.
5. X-ray:
   a. Detects deep soft tissue swelling and loss of normal fat planes.
   b. Detects presence of bone resorption and periosteal new bone formation.
   c. Comparison films of one limb with another can be done.
6. Ultrasound—has become useful for both diagnosis and in guiding aspiration as the ultrasound detects soft tissue changes in periosteum and surrounding soft tissue.
7. Bone scan in children younger than age 1 is required to determine multisite involvement.
   a. Localizes area of skeleton with altered physiology but does not identify the cause.
8. MRI—superior to CT and most useful in showing anatomic detail in many planes as well as detecting pathologic changes within marrow and soft tissues.
9. CT scan—can be used to detect focal areas of bone destruction and to delineate soft tissue abscesses associated with the bone infection.
   a. Unable to detect early stages of osteomyelitis and radiation poses high risk to young children.

Management

1. Aspiration is necessary to confirm the diagnosis of osteomyelitis and to identify the responsible microorganism to treat with the appropriate antibiotic. Aspiration is also needed to determine if surgical debridement is required.
   a. Aspirated fluid is sent for culture and Gram stain.
2. IV antibiotics:
   a. Broad-spectrum antibiotics such as vancomycin or clindamycin, targeting Gram + organisms until sensitivity is obtained.
   b. Treatment is recommended based on the IV antibiotics for 3 to 6 weeks and based on symptoms and CRP level (there are no established guidelines for duration of therapy).
   c. May require placement of a central intermittent infusion catheter (eg, midline or peripherally inserted central catheter [PICC] line).
   d. After course of IV antibiotics, a switch to oral antibiotic is made.
3. Surgical debridement—helps to stop further tissue destruction, thereby allowing a shorter course of antibiotic therapy.
4. Bed rest and immobilization to help with pain management.

Complications

 EVIDENCE BASE Funk, S. S., & Copley, L. A. (2017). Acute Hematogenous Osteomyelitis in Children: Pathogenesis, Diagnosis, and Treatment. *Orthopedic Clinics of North America, 48*(2), 199–208.

Complications of osteomyelitis are reported in about 6% of children and include:
1. Chronic osteomyelitis.
2. Pathologic fracture.
3. Growth arrest.
4. Osteonecrosis and avascular necrosis.
5. Recurrence of infection.
6. Septic arthritis.
7. Systemic infection—life-threatening if unrecognized and untreated.
8. Bone or muscle abscess.

Nursing Assessment

1. Obtain a detailed history, including recent infections (ear, tonsils, chest, urinary tract), trauma, and onset of symptoms.
2. Obtain history of current or recent antibiotic therapy and its effect.
3. Perform physical assessment for signs of primary infection as well as osteomyelitis.
4. Assess coping mechanisms and resources of family.

Nursing Diagnoses

- Acute Pain related to swelling, hyperthermia, and infectious process of the bone.
- Hyperthermia related to inflammatory response secondary to osteomyelitis.
- Impaired Physical Mobility related to pain in affected limb secondary to inflammatory response or surgical treatment.
- Readiness for Enhanced Self-Health Management related to IV drug therapy.

Nursing Interventions

Maintaining Comfort and Reducing Temperature
1. Assess pain characteristics and use age-appropriate pain measurement tools.
2. Assess temperature every 4 hours and increase fluid intake to prevent dehydration.
3. Maintain rest and immobilization of affected part.
4. Administer analgesics/antipyretics, as indicated, and monitor their effectiveness.

Preventing Complications of Immobility
1. Instruct on allowable activities—generally no weightbearing on affected limb and remain on bed rest during acute phase.
2. Encourage use and exercise of unaffected limbs and joints through play.
3. Provide ambulatory aids if indicated (eg, crutches, walker) and instruct on safe and proper use.

Promoting Compliance with Therapeutic Regimen
1. Instruct patient and family on the need for maintaining serum levels of antibiotics after discharge, even after signs and symptoms of infection improve.
2. Initiate appropriate home care referrals for administration and monitoring of IV therapy and wound care.
3. Evaluate response to treatment through periodic laboratory tests (ESR, CRP, serum drug levels if indicated) and follow-up.
4. Teach family about proper maintenance and care of vascular access device (eg, midline, PICC line).
5. Teach family and patient about oral antibiotic and importance of compliance with therapy.

Community and Home Care Considerations

1. Teach parents and child (if appropriate) about signs and symptoms of an infection.
2. Teach parents how to prepare the antibiotic for IV administration.
3. Teach parents how to administer the IV antibiotic.
4. Teach parents about the antibiotic being administered.
5. Teach parents and child about maintenance of the vascular access device.

6. Teach parents and child how to care for the child's wound.
7. Teach parents and child about potential complications after discharge.
8. Assess parents' and patient's coping abilities.
9. Reinforce teaching to parents on a frequent basis. Employ the use of return demonstrations to assess parental ability to administer IV antibiotics and care for their child's wound.
10. Provide the family with the phone number of a nurse whom they may contact for advice or if they have concerns.

 TRANSITIONAL CARE ALERT Ongoing home visits may be necessary to make sure parents are comfortable with the child's vascular access device. Coaching about medication administration, maintenance of the device, and wound care can prevent readmission.

Family Education and Health Maintenance

1. Instruct the family on the signs and symptoms of recurrent or chronic infection.
2. Stress the importance of compliance with treatment.
3. Encourage parents to seek early medical intervention for subsequent infections.

Evaluation: Expected Outcomes

- Reports reduced pain or no pain.
- Remains afebrile.
- Exercises unaffected limbs.
- Surgical wounds without signs of infection; child and parents demonstrate proper techniques for care of IV access device and infusion.

Developmental Dysplasia of the Hip

Developmental dysplasia of the hip (DDH) is the term used to describe abnormalities of the developing hip, including subluxation, dislocation, and dysplasia of the hip joint. DDH may be associated with other congenital anomalies; its incidence is 1 out of every 1,000 live births in the United States. White infants are affected more frequently than blacks. Bilateral involvement occurs in more than 50% of cases, and the left hip is more frequently involved than the right hip. Females are afflicted four to eight times more frequently than males.

Pathophysiology and Etiology

1. Risk factors include breech birth, first born, large infants, oligohydramnios, female gender, positive family history of DDH, ethnic background, lower limb deformity, torticollis, metatarsus adductus, hip asymmetry, and other congenital musculoskeletal abnormalities.
2. Subluxed hip—maintains contact with the acetabulum but not fully located within the hip joint.
3. Dislocated hip—no contact between the femoral head and acetabulum; sometimes located but may be dislocated easily.
4. Dysplasia—acetabulum is shallow or sloping instead of cup shaped (see Figure 54-3).

Clinical Manifestations

Physical findings change as the child ages; the presence of one or more of the following should be noted (see Figure 54-4).
1. Thigh asymmetry or thigh gluteal folds (present in 10% of normal infants).

Figure 54-3. Developmental dysplasia of the hip. (Anatomical Chart Company.)

2. Limited hip abduction.
3. Positive Barlow test (dislocation).
4. Positive Ortolani test (reduction).
5. Shortening of affected femur (Galeazzi sign).
6. Abnormal gait patterns—Trendelenburg gait (downward tilt of the pelvis on affected side).
7. Pain in older children.

Diagnostic Evaluation

 EVIDENCE BASE Shaw, B. A., Segal, L. S.; Section on Orthopaedics, American Academy of Pediatrics (AAP). (2016). Evaluation and Referral for Developmental Dysplasia of the Hip in Infants. *Pediatrics, 138*(6).

1. Ultrasound examination (with a skilled technician)—yields a high degree of accuracy in diagnosing DDH in children younger than the age of 6 months.
   a. Enables visualization of the femoral head and outer lip of the acetabulum.
   b. The AAP published guidelines for both ultrasonography indications and referral to orthopedist based on physical exam, clinical findings, and history.
2. X-rays—cartilaginous femoral head is difficult to visualize in the newborn. As the child ages, the ossification center can be better viewed and the efficiency of x-ray improves, usually after the age of 6 months. It can be useful in ruling out other pelvic, spinal, and femoral anomalies.

Management

 EVIDENCE BASE Larson, J. E., Patel, A. R., Weatherford, B., et al. (2017). Timing of Pavlik harness initiation: Can we wait? *Journal of Pediatric Orthopedics.* Epub ahead of print.
Murphy, R. F., & Kim, Y-J. (2016). Surgical management of pediatric developmental dysplasia of the hip. *Journal of the American Academy of Orthopedic Surgeons, 24*(9), 615–623.

The aim is to restore as closely as possible the anatomic alignment of the hip. Methodology depends on the age of the child at presentation. More than 80% of clinically unstable hips at birth have been shown to resolve spontaneously.

Figure 54-4. Signs of developmental dysplasia of the hip. **(A)** Unequal thigh folds; **(B)** apparent short femur (Galeazzi sign); **(C)** limited abduction of affected hip; **(D)** downward tilt of the pelvis on affected side (Trendelenburg sign); and **(E)** adduction and depression of the femur dislocate hip (Barlow test), and a "click" is felt when dislocated hip is abducted and relocated (Ortolani sign). (Jackson, D. B., & Saunders, R. B. [1993]. Child health nursing. Philadelphia: Lippincott Williams & Wilkins.)

Birth to Age 6 Months
1. Subluxable hips:
   a. Observe for 3 weeks.
   b. If persistent, treat with Pavlik harness (see Figure 54-5).
2. Dislocated or dislocatable hips:
   a. Pavlik harness—frequent follow-up is needed to check position, make strap adjustments, and determine hip stability.
   b. Ultrasound to determine if the hip was reduced.
   c. Infant will wear harness on a full-time basis until clinical and ultrasound examinations are normal.

Ages 6 to 18 Months
1. Hip subluxation and dislocation in children between ages 6 and 9 months:
   a. Treatment with the Pavlik harness requires frequent evaluation and may continue for 4 months or until the child is able to stand in the harness.
   b. When the child is standing, the harness is exchanged for an abduction brace until the hip is normal.
   c. Closed reduction and hip spica application if harness treatment is unsuccessful.

Figure 54-5. Pavlik harness.

2. Hip subluxation and dislocation in children ages 9 to 18 months—follow-up continues until age of skeletal maturity.

Ages 18 to 36 Months

1. Dislocated hip:
   a. Closed reduction.
   b. Application of hip spica cast for 3 months to maintain the reduction.
2. Failure of closed reduction and casting:
   a. Open reduction and innominate osteotomy.
   b. Hip spica cast application.
   c. Abduction bracing.
3. Follow-up continues until age of skeletal maturity.

Ages 3 and Older

1. Subluxation or dislocation of the hip—treated surgically by open reduction.
2. Follow-up continues until age of skeletal maturity.

Adolescents

1. Acetabular dysplasia:
   a. Use of nonsteroidal anti-inflammatory drugs and an ambulation device (eg, crutches, cane) to limit weightbearing on the affected limb.
   b. Usually need surgical correction.

Complications

1. Avascular necrosis.
2. Redislocation or subluxation.
3. Loss of ROM.
4. Leg length discrepancy.
5. Early osteoarthritis.
6. Recurrent dislocation or unstable hip.
7. Femoral nerve palsy.
8. Iatrogenic hip dislocation.

Nursing Assessment

1. Obtain a family history, including hip pathology.
2. Obtain an obstetric history for the presence of risk factors, such as breech presentation and firstborn status.
3. Perform a physical assessment for ROM, appearance of Trendelenburg sign, Barlow test, Ortolani test, and examination for asymmetric thigh folds.
4. Assess family's response to the diagnosis.

Nursing Diagnoses

- Risk for Impaired Parenting related to ineffective adaptation to stressors associated with a diagnosis of DDH and the prescribed therapeutic regimen.
- Risk for Impaired Skin Integrity related to perineal soiling secondary to confinement in an orthopedic device (eg, Pavlik harness, hip spica cast).
- Impaired Physical Mobility related to external device (eg, hip spica cast).

Nursing Interventions

Also see page 868 for orthopedic surgery.

Promoting Effective Parenting

1. Explain the condition and treatment in terms the family can understand.
2. Encourage holding the child with abduction of the hips while handling.

3. Advise parents to avoid swaddling the infant.
4. Reassure parents that effective outcome depends on early intervention and compliance.
5. Demonstrate application of Pavlik harness and make sure that parents know and feel comfortable in applying it.
6. Stress the importance of keeping follow-up appointments and strict compliance with prescribed treatment.
7. Provide parents with the name and number of a contact person if they have concerns about their child's care.

Maintaining Skin Integrity

See page 1420.

Preventing Complications of Immobility

1. Stimulate the child with games and activities to exercise upper body and feet as able.
2. Turn the child frequently and encourage ambulation as able. Support the head and legs to reposition.
3. Encourage deep breathing exercises at intervals to prevent atelectasis and hypostatic pneumonia. Children can blow bubbles, party favors, and cotton balls across the table as appropriate.
4. Encourage fluids and a high-fiber diet to prevent constipation.

Community and Home Care Considerations

1. An initial home care visit may be required to assess the child in a Pavlik harness.
2. For children in a hip spica cast, see the "Community and Home Care Considerations" section under "Fractures."
3. Carefully assess parental role development and educate them on normal care of infant as well as special care needed by their child, such as safety measures and positioning.

Family Education and Health Maintenance

1. If the child is to be treated with an abduction splint, explain its purpose and demonstrate its application and removal to the parents.
   a. Instruct the parents as to if and when the device can be removed.
   b. Instruct the parents to check fit of abduction splint at every diaper change.
   c. Allow the parents to demonstrate their ability to properly place the device on the child.
   d. Provide the parents with written instructions whenever possible.
2. Instruct the parents on skin care and to report any skin breakdown or disruption of the cast, brace, or splint.
3. Encourage regular follow-up evaluations and regular health maintenance visits.

Evaluation: Expected Outcomes

- Parents hold child and participate in care (eg, applying Pavlik harness).
- No perineal skin breakdown.
- Lungs clear with good aeration bilaterally.

Congenital Clubfoot (Talipes Equinovarus)

Clubfoot is a congenital anomaly characterized by a three-part deformity of the foot, consisting of inversion of the heel (hindfoot varus), adduction and supination of the forefoot, and ankle equinus. Clubfoot typically points down and twists inward.

The bone, muscle, ligaments, nerves, and blood vessels below the knee may all be displaced. Other congenital disorders of the foot and ankle occur but are less common. Incidence of clubfoot is 1 to 3 in 1,000 live births. It is bilateral in 30% to 50% of afflicted children, and the ratio of occurrence in males to females is 2.5:1.

Pathophysiology and Etiology

1. Equinovarus type (forefoot adduction, about 95% of cases)—foot is plantar flexed (talipes equinus) and inverted (talipes varus). See Figure 54-6.
2. Calcaneovalgus type (reverse clubfoot, about 5% of cases)—foot is dorsiflexed and everted (talipes valgus).
3. Exact etiology is unknown. Suggested theories point to vascular, viral, genetic, anatomic, and environmental factors; may also result from position in utero.

Clinical Manifestations

1. Deformity usually is obvious at birth with varying degrees of rigidity and ability to correct position. May range from a mild postural clubfoot to severe neuromuscular clubfoot that coexists with various diagnoses such as arthrogryposis and spina bifida.
2. Deformity becomes fixed if untreated, which can lead to:
   a. Child bearing weight on lateral border of the foot.
   b. Awkward gait.
   c. Development of callosities and bursae over the lateral side of the foot.

Diagnostic Evaluation

1. Clinical presentation and physical examination.
2. X-rays determine bony anatomy and assess treatment efficiency.

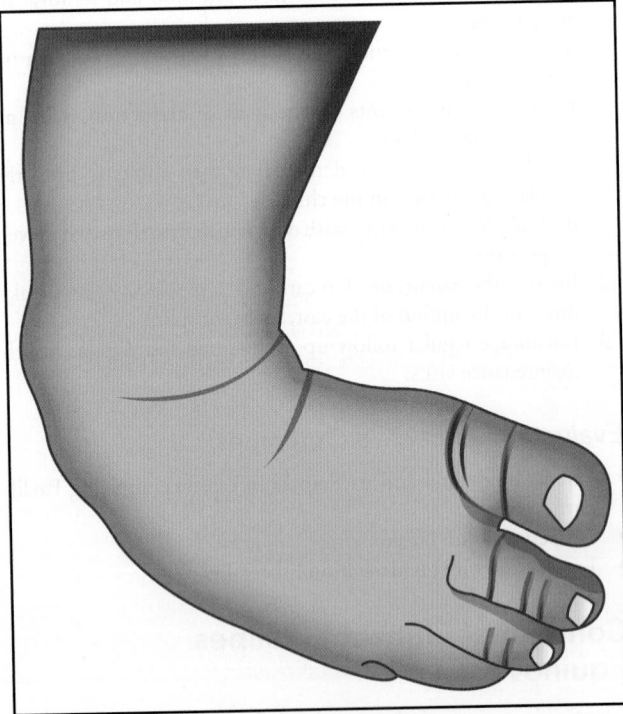

Figure 54-6. Equinovarus-type clubfoot. (Pansky, B. & Gest, T. R. [2011] Lippincott Concise Illustrated Anatomy. Philadelphia: Lippincott Williams & Wilkins.)

Management

EVIDENCE BASE Batti, S. E., Solla, F., Clement, J., et al. (2016). Initial treatment of congenital, idiopathic clubfoot: Prognostic factors. *Orthopaedics and Traumatology, Surgery and Research, 102*(8), 1081–1085.

Management should begin as soon after birth as possible, with the goal to establish a functional, pain-free foot that can be fit with standard footwear. Despite management, however, the child will always have a small calf and foot on the affected side. Nonoperative management, including manipulation, stretching, and serial casting, is currently the treatment of choice.

1. The Ponseti method is the initial method for treatment and incorporates gentle stretching and manipulation, followed by cast immobilization to promote relaxation and softening of tissues and remodeling of abnormal joint surfaces.
   a. Consists of weekly casting for approximately 6 weeks, followed by an Achilles tenotomy performed under local anesthetic and subsequent wearing of orthotic boots for 23 to 24 hours per day for 3 to 4 months.
   b. Treatment is completed with daytime ankle–foot orthoses (AFOs) and nighttime boots situated on a bar for 2 years.
2. Other nonoperative treatment includes cast changes and foot manipulation, which is usually done on a weekly basis for 6 weeks.
   a. After 6 weeks of weekly manipulation and casting, the foot is then manipulated and casted every 2 weeks.
   b. After the initial period (approximately 3 months of casting), an evaluation is performed to determine whether to continue with manipulation and casting, perform a percutaneous tenotomy, or proceed to use corrective shoes—with or without a Denis-Browne bar or the more recent Wheaton brace or Bebax shoe.
3. Surgical treatment may be required for some children to achieve correction of the deformity; usually performed within the second 6 months of life so that the child is free from postoperative immobilization before beginning walking.
4. Surgical treatment may also be required following nonoperative treatment, consisting of medial plantar release, posterior release, lateral release, or reduction and fixation—depending on the extent of the deformity.
5. The child who presents late or has a recurrent or residual deformity may require an aggressive surgical procedure to stabilize the bony structures and balance the muscle and tendons by a combination of fusions, releases, lengthening, and transfers.
6. Postoperative routines usually include a period of cast immobilization of up to 12 weeks, followed by a brace (AFO) or corrective shoe for a period of 2 to 4 years.

Complications

1. "Rocker bottom" deformity from excessive dorsiflexion and "breaking through" the midtarsal bones.
2. Disturbances in epiphyseal plates from overaggressive manipulation.
3. Recurrent or residual deformity.

Nursing Assessment

1. Obtain a family history of foot deformities.
2. Obtain an obstetric history for risk factors.

3. Perform a physical assessment for the presence of other anomalies and classic foot position and ROM. If late presentation, perform a thorough neurologic examination to rule out causative factors.
4. Assess family coping and resources available for lengthy treatment.

Nursing Diagnoses

- Risk for Impaired Parenting related to ineffective adaptation to stressors associated with a diagnosis of clubfoot and the intense therapeutic regimen.
- Risk for Impaired Skin Integrity related to serial casting.
- Ineffective Peripheral Tissue Perfusion related to postoperative edema or casting.
- Acute Pain related to tissue and muscle trauma secondary to surgery.

Nursing Interventions

Also see page 868 for orthopedic surgery.

Promoting Effective Parenting
1. Provide an accurate description of deformity and the importance of treatment in terms the parents can understand.
2. Provide opportunity for parents to verbalize questions and concerns.
3. Reinforce causative factors and the fact that it was not anyone's fault that the child has clubfoot.
4. Encourage parents to hold and play with child and participate in care.
5. Provide parents with a contact family that has been through the treatment process for support.

Protecting Skin Integrity
1. Assess fit of cast, splint, orthotic device, or special shoes. Advise parents that because of rapid growth rate of the infant, the cast or splint may need to be replaced to prevent skin breakdown.
2. Assess and teach assessment of excessive pressure on the skin—redness, excoriation, foul odor from underneath cast, or pain.

Preserving Tissue Perfusion
1. Perform frequent neurovascular assessments after tenotomy and surgery, including color, warmth, sensation, capillary refill, pulses, and presence of pain.
2. Elevate the extremity to prevent edema in the postoperative period.
3. Protect and assess foot for injury.

Relieving Pain
1. Assess for signs of discomfort, such as irritability, crying, poor feeding and sleeping, tachycardia, and increased blood pressure.
2. Administer analgesics regularly for 24 to 48 hours after surgery.
3. Provide comfort measures, such as soft music, pacifier, teething ring, and rocking and cuddling with parent.
4. Encourage parents to administer analgesics after discharge from hospital (when needed). Discuss dosage and administration and dispel misconceptions about addiction.

Family Education and Health Maintenance
1. Teach parents to remove cast at home before weekly manipulation and recasting by soaking in water and vinegar mixture.

2. Teach the parents when orthotic devices may be removed—usually for bathing. Stress that devices must be worn as prescribed.
3. Advise parents that infant's sleep may be disturbed initially due to wearing of brace at night and that he or she may be irritable while awake because of fatigue.
4. Instruct parents on providing a safe environment for the ambulatory child.
5. Discuss the importance of long-term and frequent follow-up and assist parents with special needs such as transportation, flexible appointment times, and financing orthotic equipment.
6. Teach parents to check color, warmth, capillary refill, movement of toes, and position of cast (make sure cast does not slip to hide the toes).
7. Encourage parents to comply with treatment regimen to achieve the best possible outcome.

Evaluation: Expected Outcomes
- Parents hold infant, participating in care.
- No signs of skin breakdown.
- Neurovascular status of affected foot intact.
- Rests and feeds well.

Legg-Calvé-Perthes Disease

Legg-Calvé-Perthes (LCP) disease is a self-limiting condition of the proximal femur characterized by a temporary loss of blood supply, which leads to avascular necrosis of the femoral head. The incidence of LCP is .2 to 20 per 100,000 in the general population. It occurs most commonly in children between ages 4 and 8. Ratio of occurrence in males to females is 5:1, and it is frequently found in Whites and Asians. It is bilateral in 10% to 20% of cases. There is a 30% to 40% familial occurrence

 EVIDENCE BASE Cook, P. C. (2014). Transient synovitis, septic hip, and Legg-Calve-Perthes disease: An approach to the correct diagnosis. *Pediatric Clinics of North America, 61*(1), 1109–1118.
Fornari, E. D., Karkenny, A., & Schulz, J. (2015). Legg-Calve-Perthes disease. *Pediatric Orthopaedics, 26*(5), 487–493.

Pathophysiology and Etiology
General Information
1. Etiology is unknown and may be due to factors such as secondhand smoke, poverty, hyperactivity, delayed bone age, short stature, mechanical dysfunction, and metabolic disorders.
2. Interruption of the vascular supply to the femoral head leads to the death of the bone. Deformity can occur with loss of the spherical nature of the femoral head during the disease process. The disease progresses through four identifiable stages.

Stage I (Avascularity)
1. Spontaneous interruption of the blood supply to the upper femoral epiphysis.
2. Bone-forming cells in the epiphysis die and the bone ceases to grow.
3. Slight widening of the joint space.
4. Swelling of the soft tissues around the hip.
5. The first stage lasts only a few weeks.

Stage II (Revascularization or Fragmentation)

1. The femoral head is flattened and fragmented. Growth of new vessels supplies the area of necrosis; bone resorption and deposition take place.
2. The new bone lacks strength and pathologic fractures may occur.
3. Abnormal forces on the weakened epiphysis may produce progressive deformity.
4. This stage lasts several months to 1 year.

Stage III (Reossification)

1. The head of the femur gradually reforms.
2. Nucleus of the epiphysis breaks up into a number of fragments with cystlike spaces between them.
3. New bone starts to develop at the medial and lateral edges of the epiphysis, which becomes widened.
4. Dead bone is removed and is replaced with a new bone, which gradually spreads to heal the lesion.
5. This stage lasts 2 to 4 years.

Stage IV (Healing)

1. Without treatment:
   a. Head of the femur flattens and becomes mushroom shaped.
   b. Incongruity between the head of the femur and the acetabulum persists and worsens.
2. With treatment:
   a. Head of the femur remains near spherical.
   b. Acetabulum appears normal.
   c. Width of the neck of the femur is normal.

Clinical Manifestations

1. Child presents with limp or pain in the hip, may be intermittent initially or may last for several months.
2. Referred pain to knee, inner thigh, and groin—usually with activity and often resolved with rest.
3. Limited abduction and internal rotation of the hip.
4. Mild to moderate muscle spasm on rotation of the hip in extension, limited internal rotation flexion, and abduction.
5. Trendelenburg gait—dip on the opposite side of the pelvis when weightbearing on the affected limb.
6. History of related trauma.

Diagnostic Evaluation

1. X-rays (AP and frog leg lateral) allow assessment of the extent of epiphyseal involvement and stage of disease—early findings may be normal.
2. MRI has been useful in detecting infarction but is not accurate in showing the stages of healing.
3. Bone scan is used to help diagnose LCP in the early stage of the disease, where the diagnosis is questionable.
4. Ultrasound may show early joint effusion.
5. Arthrograms may be useful in evaluating sphericity of the femoral head.

Management

 EVIDENCE BASE Smith, C. (2014). Increasing awareness of Legg-Calve-Perthes disease. *British Journal of School Nursing, 9*(1), 21–23.
    Hailer, Y., Haag, A., & Nilsson, O. (2014). Legg-Calve-Perthes disease: Quality of life, physical activity, and behavior pattern. *Journal of Pediatric Orthopedics, 34*(5), 514–521.

The goal of management is to preserve and restore the femoral head and to relieve pain.

1. Restore motion—initial relief of synovitis, muscle spasm, and pain in the joint:
   a. Salicylates (with caution) and anti-inflammatory medications.
   b. Limitation of activities and bed rest with or without activity modification.
2. Monitor progress of the disease and make sure the hip remains congruent through serial x-rays.
3. Surgical intervention, now rarely done, may vary but generally involves varus osteotomy, innominate osteotomy, osteotomy of the proximal femur or pelvis, or a combination of these, if the femoral head becomes subluxed or incongruent with the acetabulum before the reparative process.
4. Treatment outcome depends on age of the child, extent of necrosis, stage of disease at time of treatment, and congruence of joint with skeletal maturity.

Complications

1. Early degenerative joint disease.
2. Residual deformity.
3. Loss of motion or function of involved hip.
4. Persistent pain and gait disturbance.

Nursing Assessment

1. Obtain a detailed history, including onset of symptoms and characteristics of pain.
2. Perform a physical assessment to include evaluation of gait, ROM, and presence of any contractures.

Nursing Diagnoses

- Acute Pain secondary to disease process.
- Impaired Physical Mobility related to pain on ambulation.

Nursing Interventions

Also see page 868 for orthopedic surgery.

Promoting Comfort

1. Monitor and assess pain level using age-appropriate pain measurement tool.
2. Instruct child and parents as to which activities can be continued and which to avoid (eg, contact sports or high-impact sports).
3. Administer analgesics, as indicated, and monitor effectiveness.

Promoting Mobility

1. Encourage activities to maintain ROM (eg, swimming, bicycle riding).
2. Encourage parents to allow activities that involve unaffected body parts within restriction guidelines.
3. Provide equipment to assist with mobility (eg, wheelchair, walker).

Family Education and Health Maintenance

1. Teach proper care of assistive ambulatory aids and the need to remain compliant with usage.
2. Stress the need to remain active within restrictions and to promote positive body image.
3. Reinforce to child that he or she is only temporarily restricted. Stress remaining positive aspects of activity.

4. Explain the disease process to parents and child, emphasizing the importance of compliance with treatment.
5. Allow child to voice concerns and ask questions about his or her treatment.
6. Encourage attendance at regular follow-up appointments.

Evaluation: Expected Outcomes

- Pain is adequately managed.
- ROM and function maintained.

Structural Scoliosis

Scoliosis is lateral curvature of the spine of greater than 10 degrees. The different types of scoliosis vary by age of onset and structure of the spine.

Pathophysiology and Etiology

1. Idiopathic scoliosis—80% of scoliosis in children; possible causes include genetic factors, vertebral growth abnormality, or central nervous system abnormality. Three classifications (based on age at time of diagnosis) include:
    a. Infantile—birth to age 3, less than 1% of all idiopathic scoliosis.
    b. Juvenile—presentation between ages 3 and 10 or before onset of adolescence.
    c. Adolescent—presentation at adolescence (greater than 10 years):
        i. Partially familial, affects 2% of the population.
        ii. Prevalence for curves greater than 30 degrees is less common—1½ to 3 per 1,000; severe curvatures are rare.
        iii. Progressive curves are more prevalent in females than in males (7:1 females to males for curves greater than 25 degrees). Progression is greatest during adolescent growth spurt, just prior to onset of menses.
2. Congenital scoliosis—congenital malformation of one or more vertebral bodies that results in asymmetric growth.
    a. Type I—failure of vertebral body formation (eg, isolated hemivertebra, wedged vertebra, multiple wedged vertebrae, multiple hemivertebrae).
    b. Type II—failure of segmentation (eg, unilateral unsegmented bar, bilateral block vertebra).
    c. Type III—failure of segmentation along with failure of formation.
        i. More than 50% of patients with congenital scoliosis have another associated anomaly commonly associated with other congenital anomalies in other systems (eg, Klippel-Feil syndrome, genitourinary tract abnormalities, VACTERL syndrome, and others).
3. Neuromuscular scoliosis: can be neuropathic or myopathic, most severe in nonambulatory patients. Occurs in children with cerebral palsy, muscular dystrophy, spinal muscular dystrophy, and others.
4. Miscellaneous factors that can cause scoliosis include osteopathic conditions, fractures, arthritic conditions, spinal irradiation, endocrine disorders, postthoracotomy, and nerve root irritation.
5. In all types of scoliosis, the vertebral column develops lateral curvature.
    a. The vertebrae rotate to the convex side of the curve, which rotates the spinous processes toward the concavity.
    b. Vertebrae become wedge-shaped.
    c. Disk shape is altered, as are the neural canal and posterior arch of the vertebral body.
6. As the deformity progresses, changes in the thoracic cage increase. Respiratory and cardiovascular compromise can occur in cases of severe progression.
    a. Changes in the thoracic cage, ribs, and sternum lead to further characteristic deformities such as the "rib hump."
    b. Neurologic compromise in idiopathic scoliosis is rare.

Clinical Manifestations

1. Physical characteristics (see Figure 54-7):
    a. Poor posture.
    b. Increased or decreased thoracic kyphosis or lumbar lordosis.
    c. Leg length discrepancy.
    d. Shoulder asymmetry.
    e. Scapular prominence.
    f. Truncal imbalance (relationship of trunk over pelvis).
    g. Lump (rib hump) on back.
    h. Uneven waistline.
    i. Uneven breast size.
2. Back pain may be present but is not a routine finding in idiopathic scoliosis.

Diagnostic Evaluation

 EVIDENCE BASE Defelice, F., Fabio, Z., Danzelli, S. and Negrini, S. (2018) The natural history of idiopathic scoliosis during growth: A Meta-analysis. *American Journal of Physical Medicine and Rehabilitation.* 97(5), 346–356.
Yi-Fang, L., & Yu-Chu, H. (2017). Bracing in adolescent idiopathic scoliosis. *Journal of Nursing,* 64(2), 117–123.

1. Thorough history should include onset of menses, recent growth spurt, and family history of scoliosis.
2. Physical examination—the American Academy of Pediatrics recommends screening for girls at ages 10 and 12 years and boys at ages 13 and 14 years. Adams forward bending test is

Figure 54-7. Characteristic truncal imbalance and scapular prominence with scoliosis.

used to screen for scoliosis. A scoliometer can be used to measure rotational deformity. Risser classification is used to grade skeletal maturity based on the level of bone ossification and fusion of the iliac crest apophyses.

3. Thorough neurologic evaluation:
   a. Evaluate balance, motor strength, sensation, and reflexes (including abdominal).
   b. Skin exam for café au lait spots, axillary freckles, etc. to indicate neurologic problem.
   c. Exam for the presence of a hairy patch or other lesions in the lumbosacral area.
   d. Examination for limb length difference that could cause the appearance of scoliosis.
4. Radiologic assessment of the spine in the upright position, preferably posterior–anterior and lateral views on one long (36-inch [91-cm]) plate—shows characteristic curvature.
5. CT scan may be used to further define anatomy. MRI is indicated for all patients with early-onset scoliosis and is often used prior to surgery to rule out other deformities.
6. Pulmonary function tests for those with compromised respiratory status.
7. Clinical photographs to assist with documenting the appearance of the spine over time.
8. Workup for associated renal abnormalities with a congenital scoliosis because of a high correlation between the two.

 EVIDENCE BASE Brooks, J. T., & Sponseller, P. D. (2016). What's new in the management of neuromuscular scoliosis? *Journal of Pediatric Orthopedics,* *36*(6), 627–633.

Management

Goal of management is to stop progression of the existing curve by nonoperative means. When this fails, the goal of operative management should be to correct the scoliosis as much as possible and balance and stabilize the spine by fusion to prevent further progression.

Medical Management

1. Observation—periodic (usually every 6 months) physical and radiographic examinations to detect curve progression.
   a. Child is not skeletally mature.
   b. Curves less than 25 degrees.
2. Brace management—the goal is to prevent progression of the curve.
   a. Requires faithful compliance on the part of the child for success; recommended 23 hours per day.
   b. Some curves progress despite brace wear.
   c. Bracing is for skeletally immature children with curves that are about 25 to 40 degrees.
3. Types of braces include:
   a. Boston orthosis for low thoracic and thoracolumbar curves. This is an underarm molded orthosis.
   b. Milwaukee brace for thoracic or double major curves. Standard brace has neck ring with chin rest.
   c. Charleston bending brace has been tried for nighttime usage in selected patients. Results have been positive in some centers, but widespread acceptance has not occurred.
4. Exercise therapy has been promoted to help maintain flexibility in the spine and prevent muscle atrophy during prolonged bracing by strengthening back muscles.

Surgical Correction

 EVIDENCE BASE Fletcher, N., Glotzbecker, M., Marks, M., et al. (2017). Development of consensus-based best practice guidelines (BPG) for postoperative care following posterior spinal fusion for adolescent idiopathic scoliosis. *Spine,* *42*(9), E547–E554.

Martus, J., Otsuka, N., & Kelly, D. (2016). What's new in pediatric orthopaedics. *Journal of Bone and Joint Surgery American Volume,* *98*(7), 317–324.

1. Stabilization of the spinal column is the goal. This is usually accomplished with a spinal fusion and one of several methods of instrumentation.
2. Indications for surgical correction vary, but generally accepted principles include:
   a. Progression of the curve over a short period in a curve greater than 45 degrees despite bracing.
   b. Management with a brace is not possible.
   c. Cosmetic.
3. Surgical approach and techniques may be anterior or posterior with various instrumentation methods.
4. Strategies have evolved from body cast fixation to nonsegmental rods, such as the Harrington; to segmental wire fixation, such as the Luque, Drummond instrumentation, or segmental hook fixation, and Cotrel-Dubousset instrumentation; to current techniques, such as segmental screw fixation.
5. Segmental fixation systems provide a three-dimensional correction of coronal, sagittal, and rotational deformities.
   a. Posterior fusion is the standard approach, which allows correction and instrumentation of the majority of curves and levels.
   b. Stainless or titanium rods with segmental hooks (see Figure 54-8) and pedicle screw fixation are currently the instrumentation systems of choice.
   c. A reduction in the number of vertebrae requiring fusion may be achieved with anterior fusion.
   d. Combined anterior and posterior fusion may be used to correct severe curves.

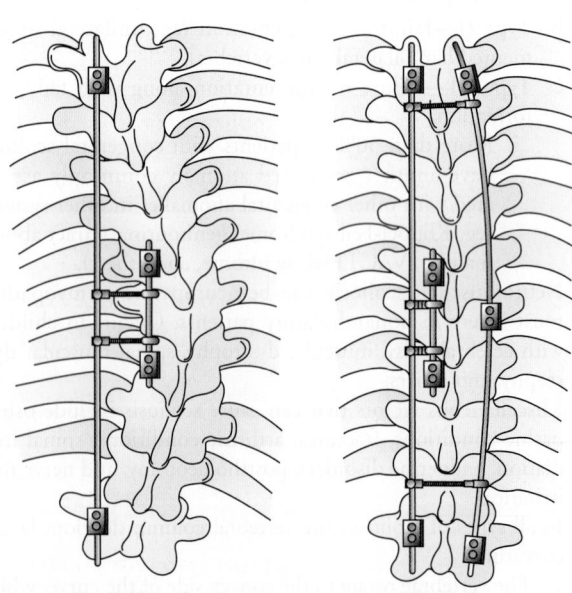

Figure 54-8. Cotrel-Dubousset rods to correct scoliosis. A short distraction rod is linked to a longer one to correct the major curve.

e. Perioperative halo-gravity traction may be used in rare cases when risk of neurologic compromise from rapid correction exists.

f. Vertical, expandable prosthetic titanium ribs may be used to lengthen and expand a constricted hemithorax and allow for growth of thoracic spine and rib cage in thoracic insufficiency. Once the child's lungs have fully developed, a spinal instrumentation and fusion can be performed.

Nursing Assessment

1. Assess respiratory, cardiovascular, and neurologic systems.
2. Perform a physical examination in the upright and forward bending positions and observe physical characteristics, such as leg lengths, gait, hips, shoulders, and overall development.

Nursing Diagnoses

- Disturbed Body Image related to negative feelings about spinal deformity and appearance in brace.
- Risk for Impaired Skin Integrity related to mechanical irritation of brace.
- Risk for Injury related to postoperative complications.
- Ineffective Therapeutic Regimen (Family) related to chronicity and complexity of treatment regimen.

Nursing Interventions

Also see page 868 for orthopedic surgery.

Promoting Positive Body Image

1. Encourage child to express feelings and concerns about body image.
2. Encourage child to express concerns about wearing a brace and offer comfortable options for wearing it and disclosing condition with classmates.
3. Encourage child to discuss scoliosis with peers, or provide a peer support person to discuss positive outcomes and expected future care.

Preserving Skin Integrity

1. Assess skin integrity and proper fit of brace at every follow-up appointment.
2. Teach proper skin care to patient and family.
3. Instruct patient to wear cotton shirt under brace to avoid rubbing.

Preventing Postoperative Complications

1. Prepare patient for surgery by teaching deep breathing and coughing exercises and explaining positioning, patient-controlled analgesia, or another method of pain control.
2. Following surgery, encourage frequent logrolling side to side to prevent skin breakdown and respiratory complications. Medicate for pain prior to repositioning and ambulation.
3. Perform frequent neurovascular assessments and monitor vital signs frequently. Encourage early ambulation (1–2 days if stable).
4. Monitor drainage or bleeding from incision site.
5. Maintain indwelling urinary catheter as indicated. Monitor intake and output, but remove as soon as possible to prevent urinary infection.
6. Engage physical therapy assistance for patient mobility to be out of bed, sit in chair, and begin ambulation.
7. Active bowel sounds should be present before diet is advanced. Patients should have bowel regimen ordered and adjusted based on stool frequency and consistency. Lack of mobility and opioid use may contribute to constipation.

Promoting Compliance with Treatment

1. Explain scoliosis and the treatment options to the child in a language she or he can understand.
2. Explain the importance of complying with treatment and possible outcomes with noncompliance.
3. Encourage the child and family to discuss concerns and questions they may have about scoliosis and the prescribed treatment.
4. Assist with social service referral for financial, transportation, and other needs.

Family Education and Health Maintenance

1. Provide adequate information on condition and treatment.
2. Instruct parents to examine brace daily for fit or breakage. Also instruct them to contact orthotist when repairs or adjustments are needed.
3. Teach family to inspect skin for irritation under brace.
4. Ensure that child can be transported safely in vehicles with potential modification in safety restraints.
5. Suggest to family to discuss child's treatment with teachers and school officials, so child can receive tutoring or homeschooling to keep up with grade requirements if out for surgery.

Evaluation: Expected Outcomes

- Child makes positive comments about self.
- Skin without signs of breakdown.
- Neurovascular status intact; no bleeding noted; bowel sounds present; pain is adequately managed.
- Wears brace as prescribed, following up as directed.

Slipped Capital Femoral Epiphysis

EVIDENCE BASE Thawrani, D. P., Feldman, D. S., & Sala, D. A. (2016). Current Practice in the Management of Slipped Capital Femoral Epiphyis. *Journal of Pediatric Orthopedics, 36*(3), e27–e37.

Hosseinzadeh, P., Iwinski, H. J., Salava, J., et al. (2017). Delay in the diagnosis of stable slipped capital femoral epiphysis. *Pediatric Orthopaedics, 37*(1), e19–e22.

Slipped capital femoral epiphysis (SCFE) is the most common hip disorder in adolescents, which occurs in puberty just before the physis (growth plate) closes. It is characterized by a slipping of the epiphysis and metaphysis because of weakening of the perichondral ring of the physis. The epiphysis slips downward and backward. Incidence is 10 per 100,000 and it is three times more common in males than in females. Approximately 20% of patients present with bilateral slips at time of presentation, and 20% to 30% will develop a contralateral slip within 12 to 18 months of initial slip.

Pathophysiology and Etiology

1. Skeletally immature and obese adolescents are at greatest risk.
2. Left hip is most frequently affected.
3. Exact etiology is unknown; possible risk factors include:
   a. Sedentary lifestyle.
   b. Rapid growth spurt.
   c. Overweight and obesity.
   d. African American ethnicity.

4. Femoral neck slips off the proximal femoral epiphysis and is contained within the acetabulum.
5. Classified by duration of symptoms:
   a. Acute—sudden onset, symptoms for less than 3 weeks.
   b. Chronic—symptoms lasting more than 3 weeks.
6. Approximately 85% of children have stable slips.
7. Because of vague symptoms, diagnosis is often delayed, which can result in complications.

Clinical Manifestations

1. Pain in the groin, medial thigh, or knee (referred pain).
2. Decreased ROM in affected hip.
3. Sudden onset of pain (acute SCFE).
4. Inability to bear weight (acute SCFE).
5. Limp when walking (usually found in chronic cases).
6. Intermittent pain.
7. Trendelenburg gait.
8. External rotation of the lower limb; involved limb may be shortened.

Diagnostic Evaluation

1. X-rays confirm diagnosis—AP and frog leg lateral views.
2. Bone scan—rules out the presence of avascular necrosis.
3. MRI or CT scan—helps to define extent of slip, used primarily in severe slips.

Management

1. Goal is to prevent progressive slippage and minimize deformity while avoiding necrosis of cartilage (chondrolysis) and avascular necrosis.
2. Treatment is surgical—in situ pinning with one or two screws is usually done within 24 to 48 hours.

Complications

1. Chondrolysis over the femoral head resulting in permanent loss of ROM.
2. Avascular necrosis of the femoral head.
3. Osteoarthritis.

Nursing Assessment

1. Obtain a detailed history, including onset of symptoms and characteristics of pain.
2. Perform a physical assessment and include evaluation of gait and ROM in the hips.

Nursing Diagnoses

• Acute and Chronic Pain related to disease process.
• Impaired Physical Mobility related to disease process.
• Deficient Diversional Activity related to activity restriction.

Nursing Interventions

Also see page 868 for orthopedic surgery.

Promoting Comfort
1. Monitor and assess pain level using age-appropriate pain measurement tools.
2. Instruct child and parents as to which activities can be continued and which to avoid (eg, contact sports, high-impact activities).
3. Administer analgesics, as indicated, and monitor effectiveness.

Promoting Mobility
1. Facilitate bed rest or other activity restrictions, as directed.
2. Provide equipment to assist with mobility (eg, wheelchair, crutches).

Promoting Diversional Activities
1. Be alert to the needs of adolescents to socialize with peers. Encourage visitation and communication with friends and family.
2. Encourage family to provide books, magazines, games, and electronics for the adolescent to use.
3. Provide support for the family and reinforce the importance of following activity restrictions to prevent permanent damage to the femur.

Family Education and Health Maintenance

1. Teach proper use of mobility devices (eg, crutches).
2. Stress the need to maintain activity within restrictions and to promote positive body image.
3. Encourage follow-up during active treatment and following surgery. About 25% of children later develop the same condition in the opposite hip, so careful attention must be paid to both legs at follow-up.

Evaluation: Expected Outcomes

• Child reports feeling little or no pain.
• Child follows activity restriction.
• Child maintains socialization with friends and partakes of hobbies in the room.

 TRANSITIONAL CARE ALERT Many children discharged from the hospital diagnosed with orthopedic conditions will have extensive discharge needs. Families will need support in the transition to home or another aftercare location. It is crucial that they have complete and understandable care instructions on home care, equipment, medications, and follow-up appointments. If arrangements have been made for nursing care in the home, families should be aware of the agency providing services and when they can expect communication regarding care arrangements. Families should have thorough written (and if necessary to assist understanding, pictorial) instructions on signs and symptoms to monitor for that could suggest worsening of status. Families may also need extensive instructions on necessary equipment to ensure safe mobility including ambulation for the child. Health providers should ensure that the child has safe and appropriate means for transport from the hospital to the home. The bulk of casts and other orthopedic equipment may necessitate changes for car safety as the child may no longer fit in the prior car restraint system. Instructions should include clear understanding of acceptable discharge expectations as many children may be in different phases if a continued surgical repair is necessary. Parents should be aware of when and where they should seek further emergency care if the child's condition deteriorates.

SELECTED REFERENCES

Baker, R., Orton, E., Tata, L. J., et al. (2015). Risk factors for long bone fractures in children up to five years of age: A nested case-controlled study. *Archives of Disease in Childhood, 100*(5), 432–437.

Batti, S. E., Solla, F., Clement, J., et al. (2016). Initial treatment of congenital, idiopathic clubfoot: Prognostic factors. *Orthopaedics and Traumatology, Surgery and Research, 102*(8), 1081–1085.

Brooks, J. T., & Sponseller, P. D. (2016). What's new in the management of neuro-muscular scoliosis? *Journal of Pediatric Orthopedics, 36*(6), 627–633.

Cook, P. C. (2014). Transient synovitis, septic hip, and Legg-Calve-Perthes disease: An approach to the correct diagnosis. *Pediatric Clinics of North America, 61*(1), 1109–1118.

Defelice, F., Fabio, Z., Danzelli, S., & Negrini, S. (2018). The natural history of idiopathic scoliosis during growth: A Meta-analysis. *American Journal of Physical Medicine and Rehabilitation, 97*(5), 346–356.

Divi, S., & Bielski, R. (2016). Legg-Calve-Perthes. *Pediatric Annals, 45*(4), e144–9.

Fletcher, N., Glotzbecker, M., Marks, M., et al. (2017). Development of Consensus-Based Best Practice Guidelines (BPG) for Postoperative care following posterior spinal fusion for Adolescent Idiopathic Scoliosis. *Spine, 42*(9), E547–E554.

Fornari, E. D., Karkenny, A., & Schulz, J. (2015). Legg-Calve-Perthes disease. *Pediatric Orthopaedics, 26*(5), 487–493.

Franklin, C. C., Wren, T., Ferkel, E., et al. (2014). Predictors of conversion from conservative to operative treatment of pediatric forearm fractures. *Journal of Pediatric Orthopedics, 23*(2), 150–154.

Funk, S. S., & Copley, L. A. (2017). Acute Hematogenous Osteomyelitis in Children: Pathogenesis, Diagnosis, and Treatment. *Orthopedic Clinics of North America, 48*(2), 199–208.

Godley, D. R. (2015). Managing musculoskeletal infections in children in the era of increasing antibiotic resistance. *Journal of the American Academy of Physician Assistants, 28*(4), 24–29.

Goodell, P. B., & Bauer, A. (2016). Problematic pediatric hand and wrist fractures. *Journal of Bone and Joint Surgery, 4*(5), 1–9.

Hailer, Y., Haag, A., & Nilsson, O. (2014). Legg-Calve-Perthes disease: Quality of life, physical activity, and behavior pattern. *Journal of Pediatric Orthopedics, 34*(5), 514–521.

Hill, C. E., Masters, J. P., & Perry, D. C. (2016). A systematic review of splinting versus complete plaster casts for the management of childhood buckle fractures of the wrist. *Journal of Pediatric Orthopedics, 25*(2), 183–190.

Hosseinzadeh, P., Iwinski, H. J., Salava, J., et al. (2017). Delay in the diagnosis of stable slipped capital femoral epiphysis. *Pediatric Orthopaedics, 37*(1), e19–e22.

Larson, J. E., Patel, A. R., Weatherford, B., et al. (2017). Timing of Pavlik harness initiation: Can we wait? *Journal of Pediatric Orthopedics,* Jan 16, 1–4.

Madhuri, V., Dutt, V., Gahukamble, A. D., et al. (2014). Interventions for treating femoral shaft fractures in children and adolescents. *Evidence Based Child Health, 9*(4), 753–856.

Martus, J., Otsuka, N., & Kelly, D. (2016). What's new in pediatric orthopaedics. *Journal of Bone and Joint Surgery (American Volume), 98*(7), 317–324.

Murphy, R. F., & Kim, Y-J. (2016). Surgical management of pediatric developmental dysplasia of the hip. *Journal of the American Academy of Orthopedic Surgeons, 24*(9), 615–623.

Pyles, V., Osafo, D., ed. (2015). Pediatric acute hematogenous osteomyelitis. *Continuing Education Topics and Issues,* January 14–18.

Pyles, V. (2015). Pediatric acute hematogenous osteomyelitis. *Continuing Education Topics & Issues, 17*(1), 14–18.

Sameer, N., Erali, R., Warner, W., et al. (2016). Epidemiology of pediatric fractures presenting to the emergency department in the United States. *Journal of Pediatric Orthopaedics. 36*(4), E45–E46.

Schroeder, N. O., Seeley, M. A., Hariharan, A., et al. (2017). Utility of postoperative antibiotics after percutaneous pinning of pediatric supracondylar humerus fracture. *Journal of Pediatric Orthopedics, 37*(6), 363–367.

Servaes, S., Brown, S. D., Choudhary, A. K., et al. (2016). The etiology and significance of fractures in infants and young children: A critical multidisciplinary review. *Pediatric Radiology, 46*(5), 591–600.

Shaw, B. A., Segal, L. S.; Section on Orthopaedics, American Academy of Pediatrics (AAP). (2016). Evaluation and Referral for Developmental Dysplasia of the Hip in Infants. *Pediatrics, 138*(6).

Shuh, A. M., Whitlock, K. B., & Klein, E. J. (2016). Managing toddler fractures in the pediatric emergency room. *Pediatric Emergency Care, 32*(7), 452–454.

Smith, C. (2014). Increasing awareness of Legg-Calve-Perthes disease. *British Journal of School Nursing, 9*(1), 21–23.

Thawrani, D. P., Feldman, D. S., & Sala, D. A. (2016). Current Practice in the Management of Slipped Capital Femoral Epiphyis. *Journal of Pediatric Orthopedics, 36*(3), e27–e37.

Tho Hang, B., Gross, C., Otero, H., et al. (2017). An update on common orthopedic injuries and fractures in children: Is cast immobilization always necessary? *Clinical Pediatric Emergency Medicine, 18*(1), 62–73.

Trionfo, A., Cavanaugh, P. K., & Herman, M. J. (2016). Pediatric Open Fractures. *Orthopedic Clinics of North America, 47*(3), 565–578.

Yi-Fang, L., & Yu-Chu, H. (2017). Bracing in Adolescent Idiopathic Scoliosis. *Journal of Nursing, 64*(2), 117–123.

55

Pediatric Integumentary Disorders

BURNS

Management of Burns in Children

Burns are common childhood injuries. They may be caused by heat, electrical energy, or chemicals. Long-term surgical and psychological sequela often follows a serious burn injury and may include reconstruction and issues related to posttraumatic stress disorder. Serious burns may include:

1. Partial-thickness (second-degree) burns of 12% to 15% or more of body surface area.
2. Full-thickness burns.
3. Burns of the face, hands, feet, perineum, or joint surfaces.
4. Electrical burns.
5. Burns in the presence of other injuries.
6. Any burn that cannot be cared for adequately at home.

Epidemiology

1. Burns are the fourth leading cause of accidental death in children 17 years old and younger, with the highest incidence of burns occurring in children younger than age 5.
2. Children at high risk are of lower socioeconomic status and of single parents. However, any child, supervised or unsupervised, is at risk for a burn injury.
3. Scalds are the leading cause of injury in children, followed by flame burns.
4. Burns from a hot liquid are most common in children younger than age 5.
   a. Tap water temperature above 120°F (48.9°C) (at 130°F [54.4°C]) takes only 30 seconds to produce a full-thickness injury in adult skin—less time in the very young; at 155°F (68.3°C), tap water will cause a full-thickness injury in a child in 1 second.
   b. Child left unsupervised in tub turns on hot water tap.
   c. Child placed in tub of hot water that has not been tested.
   d. Spilling of hot liquid, such as coffee or tea, on child. Spilling occurs especially when pot handles stick out on top of stove, when hot liquids and foods are removed from microwave oven, and when child grabs or pulls items from surfaces.
   e. Ingestion and aspiration of hot foods and liquids from microwave oven as well as scald burns to skin and palate from hot formula.

5. Burns from open flames:
   a. House fires.
   b. Child climbing on stove, resulting in ignited clothing.
   c. Children playing with lighters, especially 3- to 10-year-olds.
   d. Playing or working with gasoline.
   e. Automobile accidents with subsequent fire.
   f. Juvenile fire-setters.
6. Electrical burns in children are not as common but most often caused by:
   a. Child playing with electrical outlets or appliances.
   b. Child playing with extension cords; children commonly bite through the cord.
   c. Child playing on railroad tracks; climbing trees and touching high-tension wires; struck by lightening.
7. Other causes:
   a. Caustic acid or alkali burns, often of the mouth and esophagus.
   b. Chemical burns of the skin—child playing with gasoline or chemical cleaning agents.
   c. Burns inflicted on the child as a result of neglect or abuse (immersion and contact burns are most common).
   d. Smoke inhalation and inhalation from products of combustion of synthetics, such as plastics and rayon, may yield cyanide and formaldehyde.
   e. Radiation burns—sunburn most common, may be secondary to cancer radiation therapy.
   f. Contact burns from touching hot surfaces, such as radiators, woodburning stoves, fireplaces, or open ovens.
   g. Fireworks burns, typically as a result of misuse and lack of adult supervision; may be combined with explosive hand injuries.
   h. Friction burns such as those seen with exercise treadmills in the home.

 NURSING ALERT With combined injury, management of trauma takes precedence over the burn.

Pathophysiology and Etiology

See "Burns in Adults," page 919.

Clinical Manifestations

Characteristics of Burn Wounds

1. See page 924 for characteristics of superficial, partial-thickness, and full-thickness burns.
2. Electrical burns:
   a. Especially of the mouth in a child younger than age 2 years; may chew or suck on live wire.
   b. Are progressive and may take up to 3 weeks to fully manifest the extent of injury.

Symptoms of Shock

Symptoms of hypovolemic shock are dependent upon the size and thickness of the burn. Hypovolemic shock may develop in large surface size burns within the first 1 to 2 hours of the injury.

1. Rapid pulse and low blood pressure.
2. Subnormal temperature.
3. Pallor, cyanosis, and prostration.
4. Failure to recognize parents or other familiar people.
5. Poor muscle tone and flaccid extremities.

Upper Respiratory Tract Injury

Causes inflammation or edema of the glottis, vocal cords, and upper trachea and is characterized by symptoms of upper airway obstruction and immediate attention to securing and maintaining the airway takes precedence over the burn injury. Signs of inhalation are:

1. Dyspnea, tachypnea, and hoarseness.
2. Stridor, substernal and intercostal retractions, and nasal flaring.
3. Restlessness, drooling, cough, and increasing hoarseness.
4. Carbonaceous sputum.
5. Facial burns and/or edematous lips.
6. Black nasal or oral secretions.
7. Hypoxemia.
8. History of burn within a closed space.

 NURSING ALERT Increasing hoarseness, drooling, and stridor are leading indicators for immediate intubation.

Smoke Inhalation

Smoke inhalation may cause no initial symptoms other than mild bronchial obstruction during the initial phase after the burn. Within 6 to 48 hours, the child may develop sudden onset of the following conditions:

1. Bronchiolitis.
2. Pulmonary edema (acute respiratory distress syndrome)—of noncardiac origin.
3. Severe airway obstruction. Larger surface area burns and extensive facial burns increase the risk of airway edema.
4. Delayed damage: up to 7 days after the burn injury.

Suspicious Burns in Children

Mechanism of injury is an important assessment when a burn injury involves a child. If the mechanism of injury seems out of proportion to the injuries of the child, notification to law enforcement is mandated by all nursing practice acts. Be alert for the following characteristics that may require further investigation by law enforcement:

1. Burns that are bilateral and symmetrical and have clearly demarcated lines without splash patterns.
2. History and physical findings inconsistent with the burn injury.

3. Burn injuries incompatible with child's developmental level.
4. Burn to the buttocks, perineum, or genitals.
5. Burns involving immersion into hot water. Typical findings reveal the back of the knees will be spared of burn injury, with entire feet and lower legs burned.
6. Multiple and new and old burns in different stages of healing.
7. Burns that are circular in nature, likely because of cigarette burns.
8. Presence of other nonburn injuries such as bruises, scrapes, or previous fractures.

Diagnostic Evaluation

Calculation of the Burn Area

1. Rule of nines (used in assessment of the extent of burns in adults) has not been proven to be exact when applied to young children; it may be acceptable to use in child older than age 10 years. It is not recommended for hospital use; the Lund and Browder chart is recommended. Total body surface area (TBSA) is based on age, thus compensating for changes in body surface area that change during growth (see Figure 55-1).
   a. During infancy and early childhood, the relative surface area of different parts of the body varies with age.
   b. The younger the child, the greater is the proportion of the surface area constituted by the head and the lesser is the proportion of the surface area constituted by the legs.
2. A rough estimate can be obtained by using the child's hand (palm, with fingers extended), which is equal to 1%.

Categorization of Severity of Burn

1. Total area injured, depth of injury, and location of injury.
2. Age of child.
3. Condition of patient (ie, level of consciousness). Confusion is the hallmark of an anoxic brain.
4. Medical history (ie, comorbidities, chronic disease).
5. Additional injuries.

Schematic Classification of Burn Severity

1. Minor burn—10% TBSA or less; first- and second-degree burn.
2. Moderate burn:
   a. 10% to 20% TBSA; second-degree burn.
   b. 2% to 5% TBSA; third-degree burn not involving the eyes, ears, face, genitals, hands, or feet or circumferential burns.
3. Major burn:
   a. 20% TBSA or greater; second-degree burn.
   b. All third-degree burns greater than 10%; depending on the age of child, 5% is sometimes used.
   c. All burns involving the hands, face, eyes, ears, feet, or genitals.
   d. All electrical burns.
   e. Complicated burn injuries involving fracture or other major trauma.
   f. All poor-risk patients (ie, head injury, cancer, lung disease, diabetes).

Management

Fluid Resuscitation: Intravenous (IV) Fluid Replacement

Note: Controversy exists regarding fluid resuscitation solution and amount. Not all pediatric patients require fluid resuscitation. Children with burns 15% TBSA or less may be treated with oral rehydration therapies and supplemental maintenance IV fluids.

AREA OF BODY	RELATIVE PERCENTAGE OF BODY SURFACE (VARIES BY AGE)					ESTIMATED PERCENTAGE OF BODY AREA WITH:	
	0–1 Years	1–4 Years	5–9 Years	10–15 Years	Adult	2nd-degree burns	3rd- and 4th-degree burns
Head	19	17	13	10	7		
Neck	2	2	2	2	2		
Anterior trunk	13	13	13	13	13		
Posterior trunk	13	13	13	13	13		
Right buttock	2	2	2	2	2		
Left buttock	2	2	2	2	2		
Genitalia	1	1	1	1	1		
Right upper arm	4	4	4	4	4		
Left upper arm	4	4	4	4	4		
Right lower arm	3	3	3	3	3		
Left lower arm	3	3	3	3	3		
Right hand	2	2	2	2	2		
Left hand	2	2	2	2	2		
Right thigh	5	6	8	8	9		
Left thigh	5	6	8	8	9		
Right lower leg	5	5	5	6	7		
Left lower leg	5	5	5	6	7		
Right foot	3	3	3	3	3		
Left foot	3	3	3	3	3		
					TOTAL:	+	=

Figure 55-1. The Lund and Browder chart is used to determine the extent of burns in children because it is based on age, thus compensating for changes based on growth.

1. Fluid loss from transcapillary leakage is greatest during the first 12 hours after injury. Fluid loss after 48 hours is due to vaporization of water from the wound.
2. Replacement usually consists of lactated Ringer solution, an isotonic electrolyte solution. Lactated Ringer solution has a much lower sodium content than 0.9% saline (130 mEq/L vs. 154 mEq/L), has a much higher pH (6.5 vs. 6.0), and has 28 mmol/L of lactate, which is used as a buffering agent.
3. The consensus formula is commonly used to determine the fluid needed for resuscitation for burns greater than 15% TBSA (see page 925). Children up to 30 kg should receive a maintenance containing formula with dextrose to prevent hypoglycemia (5% dextrose or D5LR).
    a. One half of the requirements are given during the first 8 hours.
    b. The remainder is given over the next 16 hours.

Burn Treatment

1. Burns are most commonly treated by the closed method. Using the closed method is preferred as it allows children to be more mobile when a burn injury is covered and because they experience less pain.
2. Hydrotherapy is the treatment of choice for cleaning wounds. The use of a handheld shower to facilitate the loosening and removal of sloughing tissue, eschar, exudate, and topical medications is gaining popularity. The shower—water about 90°F (32.2°C)—flows over the child; debridement is then performed.
3. Children should be encouraged to participate with washing off cream whenever possible. A gentle soap or shampoo can be used to wash the burned and nonburned parts of the body and hair. Tub or shower treatments are usually done daily unless a longer-acting dressing is in place between hydrotherapy sessions.
4. Use pharmaceutical and psychological interventions, unique to each child and appropriate for their developmental stage and comfort needs, to ensure appropriate pain and anxiety management.
5. See page 925 for wound cleaning and debridement, hydrotherapy, topical antimicrobials, surgical management, and burn wound grafting. It is important to use bacitracin ophthalmic ointment on a child's face because touching or rubbing the face may get ointment into the eyes. Topical bacitracin will cause conjunctivitis if it gets into the eyes.

Complications

Vary according to severity of burn injury; commonly occur, especially with severe burn injury.

Acute

1. Infection, burn wound sepsis, pneumonia, urinary tract infection (UTI), and phlebitis, and toxic shock syndrome.
2. Curling (stress) ulcer and GI hemorrhage; rarely seen now that histamine-2 (H_2) blockers are commonly used prophylactically, especially in burns greater than 20% TBSA.
3. Acute gastric dilation, paralytic ileus; occurs especially in child younger than age 2 with greater than 20% injury and develops early in postburn period, lasting 2 to 3 days.
4. Renal failure.
5. Respiratory failure; severe inhalation injury is the insult most likely to cause death.
6. Hypertension.
7. Central nervous system dysfunction.
8. Vascular ischemia.
9. Anxiety and complex pain (acute to chronic presentations).
10. Anemia and malnutrition; may resolve when the burn area is covered.
11. Constipation and fecal impaction.
12. Labile moods secondary to hospitalization, repeated procedures, and changing body image.

Long Term

1. Growth and development delays secondary to malnutrition, hospitalization, and complexities of injury and recovery.
2. Developmental regression.
3. Scarring, disfigurement, and contractures.
4. Impact of psychological trauma.

Nursing Assessment

1. Initially, perform emergency assessment of the burn patient to determine priorities of care.
    a. Airway, breathing, and circulation: airway may be compromised with inhalation injury.
    b. Extent of burn injury.
    c. Additional injuries. (Although establishing a patent airway always comes first, trauma takes precedence over the burn.)
2. Obtain a history of the injury—for example, when the injury occurred; what first aid was given; location of the child; if smoke was present, was child in a closed space; who was supervising the child; what the specific mechanism of injury was; what other factors need to be considered in terms of the context of the injury; and consider if additional injuries may exist.
3. Obtain a complete medical history, including childhood diseases, immunizations (especially tetanus status), current medications, allergies, recent infections, and general health and developmental status.
4. Assess level of pain and emotional status; provide pain relief and reassurance while performing assessment and determining priorities.
5. Subsequently, focus assessment on fluid volume balance, condition of the burn wounds, and signs of infection (burn wound, pulmonary, urinary).
6. Remain vigilant for signs of sepsis. Although not completely supported by all expert clinicians, the American Burn Association 2007 consensus guidelines are the most recent available and provide definitions for sepsis and common infections in burn patients. Additional markers such as procalcitonin, C-reactive protein, and erythrocyte sedimentation rate can be used. Sepsis occurs in children when at least three of the following occur:
    a. Temperature above 102.2°F (39°C) or below 97.7°F (36.5°C).
    b. Progressive tachycardia more than 2 standard deviations (SD) above age-specific norms.
    c. Progressive tachypnea more than 2 SD above age-specific norms.
    d. Thrombocytopenia (not applicable until 3 days after initial resuscitation) less than 2 SD below age-specific norms.
    e. Hyperglycemia (in the absence of pre-existing diabetes mellitus).
        i. Untreated plasma glucose greater than 200 mg/dL.
        ii. Insulin resistance.

f. Inability to continue enteral feedings for more than 24 hours.
  i. Abdominal distention.
  ii. Enteral feeding intolerance.
  iii. Uncontrollable diarrhea.
7. In addition, it is required that infection be documented by positive culture, pathologic tissue source identified, or clinical response to antimicrobials observed.

 EVIDENCE BASE Vyles, D., Sinha, M., Rosenberg, D. I., et al. (2014). Predictors of serious bacterial infections in pediatric burn patients with fever. *Journal of Burn Care and Research, 35*(4), 291–295.

Nursing Diagnoses

- Decreased Cardiac Output related to fluid shifts and hypovolemic shock.
- Risk for Infection related to altered skin integrity, decreased circulation, and immobility.
- Impaired Gas Exchange related to inhalation injury, pain, and immobility.
- Imbalanced Nutrition: Less Than Body Requirements related to hypermetabolic response to burn injury.
- Dysfunctional Gastrointestinal Motility related to paralytic ileus and stress.
- Ineffective Peripheral Tissue Perfusion related to edema and circumferential burns.
- Risk for Imbalanced Fluid Volume related to fluid resuscitation and subsequent mobilization 3 to 5 days postburn.
- Impaired Skin Integrity related to burn injury and surgical interventions (donor sites).
- Impaired Urinary Elimination related to indwelling catheter.
- Ineffective Thermoregulation related to loss of skin microcirculatory regulation and hypothalamic response.
- Impaired Physical Mobility related to edema, pain, dressings, and splints.
- Acute Pain related to burn wound and associated treatments.
- Disturbed Body Image related to cosmetic and functional sequelae of burn wound.
- Fear and Anxiety related to pain, treatments, procedures, and hospitalization.
- Impaired Parenting related to crisis situation, prolonged hospitalization, and disfigurement.
- Disturbed Sleep Pattern related to unfamiliar surroundings and pain.

Nursing Interventions

Supporting Cardiac Output

1. Be alert to the symptoms of shock that occur shortly after a severe burn—tachycardia, hypothermia, hypotension, pallor, prostration, shallow respirations, and anuria.
2. Monitor the administration of IV fluids because major burns are followed by a reduction in blood volume because of outflow of plasma into the tissues.
3. Maintain and record intake and output to provide an accurate measure of volume.
   a. Record time and amount of all fluids given.
   b. Measure urine output every hour and report diminished output, as ordered (0.5 mL/kg/hour is considered minimally acceptable urine output; however, 1 mL/kg/hour is preferable).
   c. Check urine specific gravity to determine concentration or dilution.
4. With severe burn injuries, insert an indwelling catheter.
5. Weigh patient daily to help evaluate fluid balance.
6. Monitor sensorium, pulse, pulse pressure, capillary refill, and blood gas values.
7. Provide a rich oxygen environment to combat hypoxia, as necessary.
8. Monitor electrolyte and hematocrit results as a guide to fluid replacement.
9. Maintain a warm, humidified ambient environment (especially with burns of 20% TBSA) to maintain body temperature and decrease fluid needs.

Preventing Infection

1. Wash hands with antibacterial cleansing agent before and after all patient contact and use appropriate precautions.
   a. Use barrier garments—isolation gown or plastic apron—for all care requiring contact with the patient or the patient's bed.
   b. Cover hair and wear mask when wounds are exposed or when performing a sterile procedure.
   c. Use sterile examination gloves for all dressing changes and all care involving patient contact.
2. Be alert for reservoirs of infection and sources of cross-contamination in equipment and assignment of personnel.
3. Observe burn wounds with each dressing change: assess drainage for color, odor, and amount; necrosis; increase in pain; and surrounding erythema, warmth, swelling, and tenderness, which may indicate infection.
4. Administer topical antimicrobials and systemic antibiotics, as ordered.
5. Provide meticulous skin care to prevent infection and promote healing.
6. Be alert for early signs of septicemia, including changes in mentation, tachypnea, and decreased peristalsis as well as later signs, such as increased pulse, decreased blood pressure (BP), increased or decreased urine output, facial flushing, increased and later decreased temperatures, increasing hyperglycemia, and malaise. Report to health care provider promptly.
7. Obtain urine, sputum, and blood cultures for two or more consecutive temperatures of 103°F (39.4°C) or a single temperature of 104°F (40°C).
8. Promote optimal personal hygiene for the patient, including daily cleansing of unburned areas, meticulous care of teeth and mouth, shampooing of hair every other day, and meticulous care of IV and urinary catheter sites.
9. Prevent the child from scratching by administering antipruritics and applying protective devices to his or her hands.
10. Be alert for the development of pneumonia or UTI related to immobility and invasive procedures. Encourage coughing, turning, deep breathing, ambulation, and early discontinuation of indwelling catheter to minimize complications.
11. Ensure that appropriate nutrition and enteral feeding are in place within 6 to 8 hours of injury to prevent translocation of bacteria in the gut.
12. Administer tetanus prophylaxis based on immunization history.
   a. If primary series is complete (or at least three doses of tetanus toxoid are obtained) and last injection was within past 5 years, it is not necessary.
   b. If at least three doses are obtained and last injection was more than 5 years, give tetanus toxoid.
   c. If two or fewer doses are obtained, give tetanus immunoglobulin and tetanus toxoid.

NURSING ALERT Even with meticulous skin care, the burn wound is fully colonized in 3 to 5 days. A warm, moist environment becomes an excellent medium for bacterial growth, especially of *Pseudomonas*.

Optimizing Gas Exchange

1. Be alert for and report symptoms of respiratory distress—dyspnea, stridor, tachypnea, restlessness, cyanosis, coughing, increasing hoarseness, and drooling.
2. Younger children, those with larger burn injuries, and those with extensive facial burns are at higher risk of airway compromise from edema.
3. Administer supplemental humidified oxygen.
4. Monitor arterial blood gas (ABG) levels as necessary.
5. Evaluate the carboxyhemoglobin on ABG results (because of inhalation of carbon monoxide, a product of combustion) and be prepared to support ventilation if signs of hypoxemia and respiratory failure develop.
6. Assist with pulmonary function and bronchoscopy, as indicated.
7. Have intubation supplies readily available. If unable to intubate the child, then tracheostomy may be necessary. If unable to extubate in 14 to 21 days, then may be converted to tracheostomy for continuous pulmonary management. The current trend is to use the earlier time frame.
8. Prevent atelectasis and pneumonia through chest physical therapy, postural drainage, meticulous pulmonary technique, and, if indicated, tracheostomy care.

Ensuring Adequate Nutrition for Healing and Growth Needs

1. Be aware that hypernutrition is important because of the extreme hypermetabolism related to large burn injuries.
   a. Twice the predicted basal metabolic rate in calories, based on ideal weight, may be necessary. Caloric recommendation is 1,800 kcal/m² total body surface for maintenance, plus 2,000 kcal/m² of burned surface area.
   b. Hypermetabolic state generally subsides when the majority of the wounds are grafted or healed.
   c. High caloric intake to support hypermetabolic state; protein synthesis; calories should come from carbohydrates.
   d. High-protein intake to replace protein lost by exudation; support synthesis of immunoglobulins and structural protein; prevent negative nitrogen balance.
   e. Vitamin and mineral supplement needed, particularly vitamins B and C, iron, and zinc.
2. Maintain ambient temperature at 82.4°F to 90°F (28°C to 32.2°C) to minimize metabolic expenditure by maintaining core temperature.
3. Minimize anorexia to increase caloric intake.
   a. Offer small amounts of food, perhaps four to five feedings rather than three per day.
   b. Give choice of foods; determine favorites.
   c. Provide high-calorie, high-protein oral or nasogastric (NG) supplementation, as necessary.
   d. Consider long-term use of G-tube or NJ tube for supplemental nutrition.
   e. Make meals a pleasant time, unassociated with treatments or unpleasant interruptions. Maintain oral intake as much as possible.
4. Monitor dietary compliance with dietary goals and adjust, as needed.

5. Administer total parenteral nutrition, if necessary.
6. Administer serum albumin or fresh frozen plasma to combat hypoalbuminemia when burn area exceeds 20% TBSA.
7. Monitor nutritional status through weight gain, wound healing, serum transferrin, and serum albumin.

Relieving Gastric Dilation and Preventing Stress Ulcer

1. Be alert for the development of gastric distention, especially with burns greater than 20% TBSA, associated injury, or tachypnea.
2. Maintain nothing-by-mouth status if distention or decreased bowel sounds develop.
   • Insert NG tube, as indicated, to prevent vomiting, aspiration, and paralytic ileus.
3. Monitor the return of bowel sounds after NG extubation and before reinstituting oral feeding.
4. Administer H₂ blockers such as cimetidine to prevent Curling ulcer development.

Promoting Peripheral Perfusion

1. Remove all jewelry and clothing.
2. Elevate extremities.
3. Monitor peripheral pulses hourly. Use Doppler, as necessary.
4. Prepare the patient for escharotomy if circulation is impaired.
5. Avoid tight constrictive dressings.
6. Observe for and report signs of thrombophlebitis or catheter-induced infections.

Facilitating Fluid Balance

1. Titrate fluid intake as tolerated. The initial resuscitation formula is only a guide.
2. Maintain accurate intake and output records.
3. Weigh the patient daily.
4. Monitor results of serum potassium and other electrolytes.
5. Be alert to signs of fluid overload, especially during initial fluid resuscitation and immediately afterward, when fluid mobilization is occurring.
6. Administer diuretics, as ordered.

Protecting and Reestablishing Skin Integrity

1. Cleanse wounds and change dressings once or twice daily. The size of the burn and the stage of wound healing can be considered when determining the frequency of dressing changes. Use an antimicrobial solution or mild soap and water. Dry gently. This may be done in the hydrotherapy tank, in the bathtub, in the shower, or at the bedside.
2. Perform debridement of dead tissue at this time. May use gauze, scissors, or forceps, as appropriate. Try to limit time to 20 to 30 minutes depending on the patient's tolerance. Additional analgesia may be necessary. Consider having an appropriate time interval to premedicate before debridement for best pain management.
3. Apply topical bacteriostatic agents, as directed. Cream or ointment is applied ⅛-inch (3-mm) thick.
4. Dress wounds, as appropriate, using conventional burn pads, gauze rolls, or any combination. Dressings may be held in place, as necessary, with gauze rolls or netting.
5. For grafted areas, use extreme caution in removing dressings; observe for and report serous or sanguineous blebs or purulent drainage. Redress grafted areas according to facility protocol.
6. Observe all wounds daily and document wound status on the patient's record.
7. Promote healing of donor sites by:
   a. Preventing contamination of donor sites that are clean wounds.

b. Opening to air for drying postoperatively if gauze or impregnated gauze dressing is used. If exudate occurs after the first 24 hours, swab the area for culture and apply an antimicrobial topical cream. If the culture is positive, treatment will be in accord with sensitivities.

c. Following health care provider's or manufacturer's instructions for care of sites dressed with synthetic materials.

d. Allowing dressing to peel off spontaneously.

e. Cleansing healing donor site with mild soap and water when dressings are removed; lubricating site twice daily and as needed.

8. Inspect unburned skin carefully for signs of pressure and breakdown.

Preventing Urinary Infection

1. Maintain closed urinary drainage system and ensure patency. Use a catheter impregnated with an antimicrobial agent whenever possible.
2. Frequently observe color, clarity, and amount of urine.
3. Empty drainage bag per facility protocol.
4. Provide catheter care per facility protocol.
5. Encourage removal of catheter and use of urinal, bedpan, or commode as soon as frequent urine output determinations are not required.

Promoting Stable Body Temperature

1. Be efficient in care; do not expose wounds unnecessarily.
2. Maintain warm ambient temperatures.
3. Use radiant warmers, warming blankets, or adjustment of the bed temperature to keep the patient warm.
4. Obtain urine, sputum, and blood cultures for temperatures above 102°F (38.9°C) rectal or core temperature or if chills are present.
5. Provide a dry top layer for wet dressings to reduce evaporative heat loss.
6. Warm wound cleansing and dressing solutions to body temperature.
7. Use blankets in transporting patient to other areas of the hospital.
8. Administer antipyretics, as prescribed.

Preserving Mobility

1. Make sure that physical and occupational therapy are begun early to facilitate rehabilitation.
2. Child Life Professionals can also assist in making therapy and routines child-friendly, thereby increasing the child's participation and ultimately preserving and improving mobility.
3. Encourage range-of-motion exercises, ambulation, and position changes to minimize joint and skin complications.
4. Position joint in opposite direction of expected contracture. Reassess positioning regularly; reconfigure patient room or positioning of bed or television to encourage different positions if patient is bedridden.
5. Apply splints to aid joint positioning and decrease skin contractures and hypertrophy.
6. Apply pressure garments to aid circulation, protect newly healed skin, and prevent and treat hypertrophic scar formation by promoting dermal collagen fiber growth in parallel direction. Encourage the use of pressure garments for as long as 12 to 18 months after injury, until the healed skin has matured.
7. Medicate for pain before therapy or exercise to minimize discomfort.
8. Use play opportunities to help the child accept the therapy program (eg, tricycle riding may be used as a form of exercise).

Controlling Pain

 EVIDENCE BASE Baartmans, M., de Jong, A., van Baar, M., et al. (2016). Early Management in children with burns: Cooling, wound care and pain management. *Burns, 42*(4), 777–782.

1. Assess for signs of pain, such as irritability, crying, increased BP, tachycardia, decreased mobility, and inability to sleep using reliable and valid assessment measures.
2. Use principles of the WHO analgesic ladder using combinations of analgesic where one type is ineffective alone until pain relief is achieved.
   a. Step 1: Nonopioids.
   b. Step 2: Mild opioids.
   c. Step 3: Strong opioids.
3. Acetaminophen has been shown to safely manage background pain in pediatric burns and is considered the first step in managing such pain.
4. Regular nonsteroidal anti-inflammatory drugs should also be prescribed unless contraindicated.
5. Opioid analgesia is the gold standard for burn pain and should be dosed for each individual with concurrent laxative treatment provided. Strong (morphine) versus mild (codeine) opioids should be considered for severe pain.
6. In severe burns, analgesia should be given via IV line because of lack of absorption of IM injections during the emergency phase. Emphasis is on maintaining an alert, reasonably comfortable child. Monitor child closely when using IV opioids and sedatives.
7. Other adjunctive medications, such as antiemetics and sedatives, should be considered to increase comfort and decrease distress.
8. The use of benzodiazepines for continuous infusions in the severely burned child should be approached with caution. Although more research is needed in the pediatric population, there is significant evidence that the development of delirium in mechanically ventilated adult patients is associated with benzodiazepine administration. Use a therapeutic surface to relieve pressure and provide comfort.
9. Maintain warmth and prevent chilling.
10. Provide diversional activities appropriate for age to distract from focus on pain.
11. Teach simple relaxation techniques, such as relaxation breathing and guided imagery.
12. Recognize that fear may exacerbate discomfort; assess anxiety and child temperament. Provide reassurance and empathy. Develop a plan to minimize anxiety and fear. Collaborate with other health care professionals, such as a Child Life therapist.
13. Ensure an adequate sleep routine and establish good sleep hygiene as possible to minimize sleep disturbances.

Addressing Body Image Disturbance

1. Encourage the child to talk about the way he or she feels and looks; let the child set the pace for discussions.
   a. The child may feel guilty and think that the burn is a punishment for some wrong deed.
   b. Small children may be fearful of the appearance of bandages, scars, or pressure garments; offer reassurance.
   c. Encourage the use of play with dolls or puppets, role-playing, or picture drawing to help the child express feelings and fears.
2. Treat the child with warmth and affection and encourage parents to continually express their love and provide physical and emotional comfort.
3. Support child in viewing self in a mirror when ready and encourage the presence of family members.

4. Encourage early contact with other children. Maintain connections with siblings, friends, and community where possible.
5. Suggest psychiatric consultation and work with psychosocial resources for anticipatory guidance and ongoing adjustment and adaptation to burn injury. Specific requests may be related to heightened anxiety, alterations in mood, or problems manifesting as:
   a. Refusal to eat.
   b. Developmental regression.
   c. Resistance to procedures.
   d. Aggressive behaviors, excessive sadness, or withdrawal.
   e. Increasing isolation or resisting socialization.
6. Advise parents that returning to home and community routines and separation from the hospital environment, caregivers, and other patients can produce excessive anxiety or disruption in the child's coping. Consider a plan to develop a graduated discharge process with time-limited home passes (overnight, weekend), as well as plan for aftercare to support the transition home.
7. If the child is school age, help prepare for school re-entry; contact teacher or discuss with parents the need to prepare peers for what to expect.
8. Discuss and plan for issues of social re-entry, such as responding to questions and stares from strangers and perceived rejection by friends.
   a. Ensure enrollment in an aftercare (follow-up) program, ideally one that is targeted at both child and family adjustment.
   b. Refer to a support group or peer mentor where possible.
   c. Refer to a burn camp—usually this may be the first opportunity for the child to wear a swimsuit after the injury.
9. Initiate family consultation with a plastic surgeon about future scar revision.
10. Encourage the older child to engage in long-term follow-up to address issues of concern as they arise at various developmental stages. Some children and teens may wish to experiment with clothing and consult with a burn cosmetic specialist to enhance appearance and body image.

Reducing Fear and Anxiety

1. Explain procedures, surgeries, and treatments to the child according to age and level of understanding.
2. Allow the child to express fears through puppets, dolls, water play, clay, and drawings.
3. Expect regression because of the physical pain and psychological trauma the child is experiencing.
4. Encourage parents to stay with a young child as much as possible.
5. Teach parents how to engage their child to foster development of coping skills.
6. Encourage involvement with treatment plan and self-care activities.

Promoting Effective Parenting

1. Be alert to signs of depression or stress syndromes in parents and encourage counseling for them to promote a healthier family.
2. Encourage parents to assess the effects on siblings at home; they may have needs that are unrecognized or neglected as a result of this crisis.
3. Attempt to have parents become actively involved in the child's care when they are ready to do so.

   a. Provide training for parents to effectively participate in treatments and respect their wishes not to participate if the situation is too distressful—the focus for parents is on their ability to comfort their child.
   b. Advise parents that their visits and involvement can have a positive effect on the child's survival and recovery.
   c. If the parents are unable to visit, telephone calls and family photographs are helpful. New technologies like videoconferencing can also be helpful to maintain connections with family and community supports.
4. Give the parents the opportunity to discuss their feelings.
   a. Parents commonly express guilt regarding their lack of supervision when the accident occurred.
   b. Typically, burn injury is associated with actual or perceived parental neglect. Remember that this type of injury is sudden and acute, placing the family in a state of crisis.
5. Keep the parents informed of the child's progress.
   a. Begin initial teaching at admission with supportive words and limited technical information.
   b. Education and orientation to the facility and the burn injury will decrease some anxiety and begin to build rapport on which future support can be based.
   c. Encourage meetings with other parents who have coped with trauma.
   d. Refer families for aftercare programs intended to support adjustment over time.

Sleep Pattern Disturbance

1. Allow a parent to stay with the patient.
2. Provide a structured environment. Perform dressing changes, therapy, and meals at the same time daily.
3. Combine interventions so that child can get longest possible intervals of uninterrupted sleep.
4. Minimize noise and lights within the room.
5. Ensure adequate pain relief and comfort measures at bedtime or naptime.

Community and Home Care Considerations

1. Make routine home visits to perform, teach, and supervise burn wound care and rehabilitation program.
2. Inspect the wounds for signs of infection at every visit.
3. Assess coping ability of child and family to care for child and provide psychological support and counseling referrals, as needed.
4. Make sure that parents can:
   a. Discuss and demonstrate treatments, procedures, and dressing changes.
   b. Obtain equipment necessary to perform treatment at home.
   c. Understand reason for and adverse effects of medications as well as dietary requirements.
   d. Follow up at appropriate intervals with the designated health care provider.
5. Encourage the use of smoke alarms on every floor in the home, a fire extinguisher, and an emergency fire escape plan. Assist parents to review strategies for childhood safety.

Family Education and Health Maintenance

1. Teach the family that special skin care is necessary after burn injury.
   a. Avoid exposure to sunlight; use sunscreen with sun protection factor (SPF) 30 or higher and apply frequently.

b. Use pressure garments to prevent hypertrophic scar formation—worn 23 of 24 hours each day for effectiveness for 1 to 2 years depending on the maturation of the scar.

c. Use lotions and creams to prevent skin from drying, cracking, and itching; topical or oral antihistamines or antipruritics may be necessary to reduce itching.

d. Burn area has decreased sensation to touch, heat, and pressure; take precautions to prevent injury to the area.

2. Advise the family that adjustment after burn is usually prolonged and painful. Adjustment can ebb and flow with developmental stages. Encourage ongoing family and individual psychological and social support.

3. Encourage continued physical therapy to prevent and minimize contractures and preserve function.

4. Monitor outcomes over time in keeping with the Health Outcomes Burn Questionnaire for infants and children 5 years of age and younger; burn size and visible scarring are not predictive of psychological adaptation.

5. Initiate home health, psychiatric referral, physical and occupational therapy, financial assistance, and other referrals, as necessary.

6. Teach parents and children the prevention of burn injury as well as other safety measures (see page 1127).

7. Teach first aid emergency care for burn injury (ie, cool burned area with cool water, remove clothing, seek medical assistance).

8. Teach children how to stop, drop, and roll if their clothes catch fire and how to crawl to safety if a fire occurs in the house.

Evaluation: Expected Outcomes

- Absence of shock: stabilization of vital signs and normal serum and electrolyte values.
- Absence of infection: normal laboratory values, clean wound, and normal temperature.
- No respiratory distress: stable vital signs, respiratory status, and ABG levels.
- Adequate nutritional status: weight gain and wound healing.
- No GI complications: normal bowel sounds and ability to tolerate oral feeding.
- Tissue perfusion.
- No signs of fluid overload and weight stable.
- Donor site and burn wounds healing without signs of infection.
- Urine output adequate via catheter.
- Temperature remains below 102°F (38.9°C).
- Improved mobility: involved in play and other activities.
- Minimal discomfort: stable vital signs, verbalization, and involved in play.
- Positive body image: verbalization, socialization, and ability to look in the mirror.
- Relief of fear: able to play and participates in care.
- Effective parenting: involved in child's care, accurate discussion of child's progress, and treatment plan.
- Sleeping between treatments through the night and napping for 1-hour intervals during the day.

DERMATOLOGIC DISORDERS

Atopic Dermatitis (Infantile and Childhood Eczema)

Atopic dermatitis, the most common cause of eczema in childhood, is a highly pruritic chronic inflammatory skin disorder affecting 15% to 25% of the pediatric population. Peak prevalence is age 6 months to 8 to 10 years. Ninety-five percent of children with atopic dermatitis have asthma or allergic rhinitis. It is an abnormal immune response to environmental allergens in a genetically susceptible individual. These individuals tend to have dry skin and a lower threshold for itching. Itching leads to scratching, which causes lichenification or skin thickening, creating increased sensitivity to renewed itching. Many children with atopic dermatitis have a personal or family history of disorders in the atopic triad (allergic rhinitis, asthma, and atopic dermatitis). During the past three decades, the incidence of atopic dermatitis has increased, especially in industrialized nations. Possible causes include urban migration, increased antibiotic use, and decreased incidence of early childhood infections.

Atopic dermatitis has a typical age-related morphology and distribution and a chronic or chronically relapsing nature. By age 5, 90% of patients who will develop atopic dermatitis have already manifested the disease. The appearance and location of the lesions change with age in a characteristic manner. Atopic dermatitis usually improves or resolves by adolescence but can persist in some form throughout adulthood.

Pathophysiology and Etiology

1. Although it has both immunologic and genetic components, the etiology of atopic dermatitis is unknown. Approximately 80% of children with atopic dermatitis have elevated immunoglobulin (Ig) E levels and increased rates of sensitization to common allergens. Histamine release from basophils is increased, and hyperreactive cutaneous T cells, which secrete proinflammatory cytokines, cause increased Th2 and decreased Th1 cytokine responses. There is also a hereditary component. When both parents have a history of atopic dermatitis, there is an 80% chance a child will be affected. When only one parent is affected, the prevalence drops to 50%. A number of genes have been tentatively linked to atopic dermatitis.

2. Atopic dermatitis causes breakdown of the stratum corneum, which allows allergens and bacteria to penetrate deeper layers, causing inflammation and possible infection.

3. Atopic dermatitis is known as the "itch that rashes." The skin is dry and becomes pruritic when exposed to common environmental allergens, such as wool; occlusive synthetic fabrics, soaps, and detergents; perspiration; extremes of temperature and humidity; and emotional stress.

4. Food allergies contribute to atopic dermatitis in up to 30% of infants and very young children with moderate to severe disease. Eggs, milk, peanut, soy, wheat, tree nuts, fish, and shellfish account for more than 90% of the reactions. The most common offender is eggs.

5. One third to one half of children with atopic dermatitis are allergic to house dust mites, animal dander, weeds, and molds.

6. Children with atopic dermatitis are at increased risk for developing allergic rhinitis or asthma, known as the "atopic march" or "atopic triad."

Clinical Manifestations

Age and Distribution of Lesions

Atopic dermatitis is divided into three phases based on the age of the patient and the distribution of the lesions. These are referred to as the infant, childhood, and adult phases.

1. Infant (ages 2 months to 3 years):
   a. The onset is between ages 2 and 6 months. One half of affected infants have spontaneous resolution by age 2 or 3.

Figure 55-2. Characteristic rash of infant atopic dermatitis of the head (**A**) and of the limbs (**B**).

b. Characterized by intense itching, erythema, papules, vesicles, oozing, and crusting (see Figure 55-2).

c. The rash usually begins on the cheeks, forehead, or scalp and then extends to the trunk or extremities in scattered, commonly symmetric patches. The perioral, paranasal, and diaper areas are usually spared (see Figure 55-3).

2. Childhood (ages 4 to 10 years):

a. Affected people in this age group are less likely to have exudative and crusted lesions. Eruptions are characteristically more dry and papular and commonly occur as circumscribed scaly patches. There is a greater tendency toward chronicity and lichenification.

b. The typical areas of involvement are the face, including the perioral and paranasal areas, neck, antecubital and popliteal fossae, wrists, and ankles. May have severe pruritus.

3. Adult (puberty to old age):

a. Predominant areas of involvement include the flexor folds, face, neck, upper arms, back, dorsa of the hands and feet, fingers, and toes.

Figure 55-3. Distribution of infant atopic dermatitis occurs primarily on the face but may develop on symmetrical areas of the body. Diaper areas are usually clear.

b. The eruption appears as thick, dry lesions, confluent papules, and large lichenified plaques. Weeping, crusting, and exudation can occur, but they are usually the result of superimposed external irritation or infection.

Clinical Appearance

Atopic dermatitis is also divided into three stages based on the clinical appearance of the lesions. The acute, subacute, and chronic stages can occur in infants, children, and adults.

1. Acute (see Figure 55-4A)—moderate to intense erythema, vesicles, a wet surface, and severe itching.

2. Subacute:

a. Erythema and scaling are present in various patterns with indistinct borders. The redness may be faint or intense. The surface is dry. There are varying degrees of pruritus.

b. The subacute stage may be an initial stage or may follow an acute inflammation or exacerbation of a chronic stage. Irritation, allergy, or infection can convert a subacute process into an acute one.

3. Chronic (see Figure 55-4B)—the inflamed area thickens and the surface skin markings become more prominent. Thick plaques with deep parallel skin markings are called *lichenified*. Lichenification is the hallmark of chronic eczema. The surface of the skin is dry and the border of the lesion well defined. There is moderate to intense itching. There may be postinflammatory hypopigmentation.

Diagnostic Evaluation

1. There is no single clinical, laboratory, or histologic marker that will definitively diagnose atopic dermatitis. It is a clinical diagnosis based on the evaluation of the aggregate of signs, symptoms, stigmata, course, and associated familial findings. The presence of pruritus, recurring symptoms, and age-specific morphology and distribution is the most important diagnostic feature. Several sets of clinical diagnostic criteria have been established. See Box 55-1.

2. Although not diagnostic for atopic dermatitis, prick skin testing, patch testing, and radioallergosorbent test may be helpful in the identification of food and aeroallergen triggers in infants and young children with moderate to severe disease. Negative skin prick sensitivity tests eliminate the possibility of IgE-mediated food allergy. Positive tests, which predict 30% to 50% of food allergies, may be useful. To avoid

Figure 55-4. **(A)** Acute atopic dermatitis. **(B)** Chronic atopic dermatitis.

unnecessary dietary restrictions, positive tests should be confirmed by controlled food challenges, elimination diets, or atopy patches.

Treatment

EVIDENCE BASE Conceicao, V. (2016). The nursing management of infantile eczema. *Journal of Community Nursing, 30*(5), 12–14.

Daily skin care is the cornerstone of prevention and treatment, including proper cleansing, moisturizing, and avoidance of triggers.

Acute
1. Open, wet dressings, such as Burow solution, for 1 to 3 days.
2. Avoidance of known allergen or trigger. Atopic dermatitis patients have decreased threshold to irritants.

BOX 55-1 | Clinical Criteria for Atopic Dermatitis

MAJOR FEATURES: THREE OR MORE
- Pruritus.
- Eczematous changes.
- Typical and age-specific morphology and location.
- Face, neck, and extensor surfaces in infants/children.
- Flexural lesions in older children/adults.
- Chronicity or chronically relapsing.
- Personal or family history of atopy (allergic rhinitis, asthma, atopic dermatitis).

MINOR FEATURES: THREE OR MORE
- Early age of onset.
- Elevated serum immunoglobulin E.
- Itching with sweating.
- Intolerance to wool and lipid solvents.
- Immediate (type 1) skin test reactivity.
- Tendency toward skin infections.
- Facial pallor or erythema.
- Food intolerance.
- Xerosis (very dry skin).
- Ichthyosis/palmar hyperlinearity/keratosis pilaris.
- Hand or foot dermatitis.
- Pityriasis alba (white patches on the face).
- Conjunctivitis.
- Severity of symptoms influenced by environmental or emotional factors.

---

3. Management of secondary infection.
4. Topical corticosteroids:
   a. Topical corticosteroids are the mainstay of drug therapy. These agents are ranked into seven groups according to potency. Group 1 contains the most potent topical steroids and group 7 the least potent agents. The concentration listed on the medication does not correlate with its potency or safety but is merely a statement of its specific chemical formulation. Adverse effects are related to the potency rating of the compound, the duration of use, and the thickness of the skin to which it is applied.
   b. Group 1 topical corticosteroids are avoided in children younger than age 12 because of greater skin absorption.
5. Oral medications to relieve itching—hydroxyzine, diphenhydramine, or promethazine—often are sedating. Mild sedation may be desirable to allow sleep.

DRUG ALERT Topical corticosteroids of adequate strength should be used two times per day for a specific length of time, such as 7 to 21 days, to achieve control and avoid adverse effects. Long-term use of topical corticosteroids can cause striae, cutaneous atrophy, telangiectasia, acne, growth retardation, adrenal suppression, Cushing syndrome, and cataracts.

Subacute and Chronic
1. Prevention of dry skin:
   a. Reduce the frequency and duration of bathing.
   b. Use mild soap or hydrophilic cleanser.
   c. Lubricate the skin with emollients. Apply within 3 minutes after exiting bath. Apply over, not under, topical corticosteroids. Newer barrier repair moisturizers contain the skin lipid ceramides and help rebuild/repair skin. (Some over-the-counter products are CeraVe, Cetaphil Restoderm, and Eucerin Professional Repair.)
   d. Maintain environmental humidity above 40% during winter months.
   e. Tar preparations may be added to bath water; however, they are rarely used because of odor and staining.
2. Avoidance of known allergens or triggers.
3. Management of secondary infection.
4. Topical corticosteroids as described above. Apply the least potent topical corticosteroid that provides adequate control.

Topical corticosteroids may be applied under occlusion, which is under plastic wrap to increase absorption, for short-term therapy.

5. Topical immunomodulators, also called *calcineurin inhibitors*, are approved for the short-term and intermittent long-term treatment of subacute and chronic atopic dermatitis for patients age 2 and older when conventional therapies are inadvisable, ineffective, or not tolerated.
    a. Tacrolimus 0.03% ointment and pimecrolimus 1% cream.
    b. These agents do not cause skin atrophy (which corticosteroids may cause) and can be used on the face and neck. However, their long-term safety is unknown.
    c. Active viral, bacterial, or fungal skin infections must be cleared before use.
    d. Topical immunomodulators should be discontinued if lymphadenopathy of unknown etiology develops.
6. Phosphodiesterase-4 (PDE4) inhibitor is the newest class of topical medications approved for treatment of mild to moderate atopic dermatitis in patients aging 2 years and older.
    a. Crisaborole 2% ointment.
    b. Considered relatively safe as the only known adverse effect is application site burning or stinging that resolves after the first 1 to 2 days of use.
    c. No contraindications (except hypersensitivity reaction) to long-term use.

 DRUG ALERT The U.S. Food and Drug Administration issued a black box warning for *calcineurin inhibitors* stating long-term safety has not been established. Although causal relationship has not been proven, rare cases of malignancy (skin and lymphoma) have been reported. Drugs should be used for short-term, second-line therapy for patients over 2 years of age.

Complications

1. Increased risk of secondary infection by bacterial, viral, or fungal agents. Bacterial infections are typically caused by *Staphylococcus aureus*. Rate of infection with methicillin-resistant *S. aureus* is increasing. Infections secondary to papillomaviruses (warts), *Molluscum contagiosum*, herpes simplex, tinea, and candida are more common.
2. Adverse effects from topical corticosteroids (folliculitis, skin atrophy) or topical immunomodulators (local reactions, acne).

Nursing Assessment

1. Take a nursing history focusing on clinical manifestations:
    a. Onset and duration of rash.
    b. Location, course, and distribution of lesions.
    c. Change in morphology of lesions.
    d. Previous episodes of rashes.
    e. Local and systemic symptoms, especially itching.
    f. Exposure to possible allergens or triggers, especially wool, occlusive synthetic fabrics, soaps, detergents, perspiration, extremes of temperature and humidity, emotional stress, and certain foods in infants and toddlers.
    g. Personal history of allergies, asthma, or allergic rhinitis.
    h. Family history of eczema, asthma, or allergic rhinitis.
    i. Medications, treatments tried, and their effect.
    j. Diet for possible triggers.

2. Perform a physical assessment.
    a. Examine the entire skin in an orderly fashion with specific attention to the type of lesion (ie, macule, papule, or vesicle), its appearance (shape, border, color, texture, and surface), and its distribution (areas of the body involved).
    b. Note associated symptoms, such as scratching, fever, or drainage.
    c. Assess patient for signs of other atopic disorders, including nasal congestion, mouth breathing, cough, or wheezing.
    d. Palpate for lymphadenopathy.
3. Document findings:
    a. Describe skin findings using dermatologic terminology.
    b. Draw pictures to facilitate communication.
    c. Document the presence or absence of associated signs or symptoms.

Nursing Diagnoses

- Impaired Skin Integrity or Risk for Impaired Skin Integrity related to skin pathology and scratching.
- Deficient Knowledge related to trigger avoidance.
- Impaired Comfort related to itching.
- Risk for Infection related to increased bacterial colonization of the skin and possible break in defensive barrier.

Nursing Interventions

The nurse may perform the following interventions or teach patient and/or family to do them.

Improving Skin Integrity

1. Reduce inflammation during the acute stage with the topical application of open wet dressings.
    a. Use a soft, lightweight cloth, such as a handkerchief, a thin cloth diaper, or strips of bed sheeting. Do not use gauze (adheres to skin), washcloths, or towels (too heavy). Warm moist pajamas layered under dry pajamas are effective and soothing.
    b. Open wet dressings should be clean. In certain situations, they should be sterile to prevent contamination.
    c. Solutions should be lukewarm or at body temperature to soothe the skin and prevent chilling.
    d. Compresses should be moderately wet, not dripping, and removed after 20 minutes, unless otherwise directed. They should be reapplied three to four times per day.
    e. After the compress, a topical corticosteroid may be applied to further reduce itching and inflammation.
    f. Observe the skin for changes in response to therapy.
2. Prevent dry skin during the subacute and chronic stages.
    a. Decrease the frequency and duration of bathing. Long, hot tub baths should be avoided.
    b. Avoid hot water and harsh soaps. Patients should bathe in lukewarm water using mild soap with a neutral pH (eg, Dove, Neutrogena); avoid bubble baths; rinse well and pat skin dry with towel.
    c. If bath water stings, add 1 cup of table salt.
    d. Apply unscented emollients (eg, Eucerin, Keri, Aquaphor, and Lubriderm) within 3 minutes of bathing, when the skin is still slightly moist. Apply over topical medications. This traps water in the skin. Creams and ointments are more effective than lotions because they are better at preventing evaporation of water from the skin.

e. Some patients may benefit from soaking in a tar bath for 15 to 20 minutes daily, preferably in the evening. Add to bath water as directed. Instructions must include the ability to stain the skin and clothing and cause sunlight sensitivity.

f. For patients with extremely dry skin, clean with a hydrophilic cleanser (eg, Cetaphil). Apply without water until light foam occurs. Remove by wiping with soft cotton cloth or cleansing tissue.

g. Keep environmental humidity above 40% during winter months. Use a humidifier.

h. Observe the skin for changes in response to therapy.

> **NURSING ALERT** Apply unscented emollients to the skin within 3 minutes of bathing when the skin has been patted dry but is still moist to maintain a high level of hydration to the epidermis.

Patient and Caregiver Education to Improve Avoidance of Triggering Factors

1. Follow recommended guidelines related to preventing food allergies.
   a. Encourage breastfeeding during the first 6 months. For infants not breastfed, extensively or partially hydrolyzed formulas (Nutramigen, Alimentum) are preferable to cow's milk formula.
   b. Follow the current American Academy of Pediatrics guidelines related to timing of the introduction of new foods, especially dairy, eggs, peanuts, tree nuts, seafood, and other highly allergenic foods.
2. Eliminate trigger foods for infants and toddlers with known or suspected food allergies.
   a. Observe skin for flare-ups after exposure to potential allergens.
   b. Suggest referral to allergy specialist for infants and young children with moderate to severe atopic dermatitis.
   c. Be aware of the results of skin prick sensitivity, patch testing, or blood testing.
   d. Record known allergens on chart and care plan.
   e. Notify dietary department, caregivers, and school personnel of food allergies.
   f. Consult with dietitian to ensure a balanced diet that excludes identified allergens.
   g. Check food for known allergens before feedings.
   h. Prevent accidental ingestion by informing visitors of food allergies and keeping offending foods from patient.
   i. Teach parents and caregivers to read food labels for the elimination of offending food proteins.
   j. Assess compliance with prescribed diet and relief of symptoms.
3. Be aware of environmental triggers.
   a. Maintain a warm climate with moderate humidity and avoid exposure to excessive heat and cold or humidity extremes.
   b. Dress child in soft, lightweight cotton clothing and avoid wool and occlusive synthetic fabrics. A new type of non-irritating, antimicrobial fabric impregnated with silver is useful as a sleep garment. Infants should not be allowed to crawl on wool carpeting.
   c. Participation in strenuous athletic activities that promote sweating. Activities should be modified according to the needs of the child. Swimming is recommended in chlorinated pools (although bromine in pool water may be irritating).
   d. Irritating/harsh soaps, perfumes, detergents, chemicals, and fabric softeners.
   e. Bathing in hot water.
   f. Smoking around child.
   g. Avoid harsh soap and hot water. Avoid fabric softeners. Use fragrance-free and dye-free detergents.
   h. Discourage smoking in child's presence.
4. Try to alleviate stress.
   a. Encourage parents to stay with young child as much as possible.
   b. Involve child in age-appropriate diversional activities.

Table 55-1 Common Pediatric Skin Problems

DISORDER/ORGANISM	CLINICAL MANIFESTATIONS

Impetigo
Bacterial infectious disease affecting the superficial layers of the skin and characterized by the formation of vesicles, honey-colored crusts, or bullae.
Etiology and incidence:
• Caused by *Staphylococcus aureus* and *Streptococcus pyogenes*. Occurs most commonly when personal hygiene is poor.
• Common in children younger than age 10.
• Spread by close contact—easily conveyed from person to person via hands, nasal discharge, shared towels and toys, plastic wading pools in summer—when water is not replaced and no disinfectant is used; highly contagious.
• An abrasion of the skin may serve as a portal of entry.
Diagnosis:
• Usually clinical.
• Rarely, a culture of the lesion's exudate is indicated to confirm the diagnosis.
	• Incubation period is 1–10 days.
	• Lesion first appears as pink–red macules that quickly change to vesicles, which, in turn, rupture, develop crusts, and leave a temporary superficial erythematous area.
	  • Bullous (neonate and older child)—large, thin-roofed blisters break to form thin, light-brown crusts. Lesions may occur anywhere on the body but are more common on the face, axillae, and groin.
	  • Crusted (preschool age—seen more commonly in summer on exposed body parts)—lesions appear with thick, yellow crusts; skin around crusts is red and weeping with satellite lesions.
	• Regional lymphadenopathy is common with secondary infection of insect bites, eczema, poison ivy, and scabies.
	• Autoinoculation is the major cause of spreading.
	• Pruritus may occur.

Controlling Pruritus

1. Apply topical medications as ordered by the health care provider.
   a. Assess for possible contraindications to medication before use. Check skin for active viral, bacterial, or fungal infection and for lymphadenopathy.
   b. Apply a thin layer of topical medication to the affected skin two to four times per day, as directed by the health care provider. Use only for the duration prescribed.
   c. Do not apply to wet or occluded skin.
   d. Apply emollients over top of medication.
   e. Observe for possible adverse effects including burning, itching, and erythema at application site and from long-term use of topical medications such as striae, cutaneous atrophy, telangiectasia, and acne because of topical corticosteroid use.
2. Note scratching and apply age-appropriate interventions to address avoidance of scratching.
3. Consider interventions such as cool compresses and bleach baths as described above.
4. Administer prescribed oral antipruritic medications, monitor for side effects, and provide related medication teaching as needed.

Preventing Secondary Infection

1. Discourage and prevent scratching per interventions described above.
2. Assess and treat secondary infection.
   a. Observe the skin for signs of bacterial, viral, or fungal infection (discharge, oozing, crusts, increased redness, fever). Report any positive findings.
   b. Administer medications, as prescribed.
   c. Loosen exudate and crusts with water or wet dressings, unless otherwise specified.
   d. Note changes in the skin in response to therapy.

Family Education and Health Maintenance

1. Teach patient and family to avoid potential triggering factors.
2. Use fragrance-free and dye-free detergents and soaps.
3. Bathe/shower in tepid water and apply emollients immediately after bathing. The child should bathe/shower after swimming and exposure to other irritants or triggering factors.
4. Avoid stressful situations, when possible.
5. Follow the American Academy of Pediatrics guidelines related to the introduction of new and solid foods.
6. Make sure that the child and/or family know to avoid common triggers, prevent dry skin, recognize signs of flares or secondary infection, apply topical medications, and follow up for routine appointments.
7. Recommend consultation with dermatology specialist for children with severe or persistent atopic dermatitis.
8. Provide resources for additional information from the following websites:
   a. American Academy of Dermatology (*www.aad.org*).
   b. American Academy of Pediatrics (*www.aap.org*).
   c. National Eczema Society (*www.eczema.org*).
9. Stress the importance of regular health maintenance examinations, immunizations, and preventive practices.

 NURSING ALERT Advise family that fresh water (pond, lake, river) should be avoided if child has breaks in skin integrity, because of risk of infection.

Evaluation: Expected Outcomes

- Skin intact with minimal erythema and lichenification.
- Names common triggers and avoidance measures.
- Verbalizes less itching and less scratching observed.
- No signs of secondary infection.

Other Dermatologic Disorders

See Table 55-1.

TREATMENT/PREVENTION	NURSING CONSIDERATIONS

Based on etiology and type of infection.
• Gently wash affected area with soap and water three times per day.
• Crusts and debris can be removed from the affected area by gentle soaking or wet compresses. Use tap water, normal saline, or 1:20 Burow solution.
* If indicated, obtain drainage or debris for culture before antibiotics are provided.
• Apply topical antibacterial medication, such as bacitracin or mupirocin ointment or retapamulin.
• Systemic antibiotics (cephalosporins, erythromycin, or dicloxacillin) if widespread or recurrent.
• Methicillin-resistant *S. aureus* infection is common.
• Prevention—close contact with other children should be avoided until 24 hours after treatment is initiated.
	• Assess the child's skin condition and document the location and appearance of lesions. Note new lesions.
	• Initiate and teach measures to prevent the spread of infection.
	  • Engage in frequent handwashing. Use separate towels.
	  • Daily bathing with soap and water. Regular laundering for contaminated bed linens, towels, and clothing.
	  • Observe drainage and secretion precautions for 24 hours after the start of therapy.
	  • Isolate the child from direct contact with other children (school or day care) until 24 hours after treatment has started.
	  • Trim fingernails and toenails. Apply small amount of bacitracin or mupirocin ointment under the fingernails to prevent the spread of infection.
	  • Engage the child in diversional activities to discourage scratching.
	• Be aware that the patient with streptococcal impetigo has an increased risk of acute glomerulonephritis.

(continued)

Table 55-1   Common Pediatric Skin Problems (*Continued*)

DISORDER/ORGANISM	CLINICAL MANIFESTATIONS
Ringworm of the Scalp (Tinea Capitis) (See page 910 for ringworm of the body [Tinea corporis]) A fungal infection of the scalp and hair follicles *Etiology and incidence:* • Most ringworm of the scalp is caused by *Trichophyton tonsurans*. *Microsporum canis* and *Microsporum audouinii* are also causative agents. • Is seen primarily in children before puberty (usually ages 3–10). • May be spread through child-to-child contact as well as through the common use of towels, pillows, combs, brushes, and hats. Cats and dogs may also be the source of the infection. *Diagnosis:* • Hair or skin scrapings for microscopic evaluation or fungal culture, obtained by rubbing a swab or toothbrush over the affected area. *Differential diagnosis:* • Tinea amiantacea, lichen planopilaris, and perifolliculitis capitis abscedens et suffodiens must be ruled out clinically or histologically. Woods lamp inspection has limited benefit.	• The lesions appear on the scalp in a variety of ways: • One or more patchy areas of dandruff-like scaling with little or extensive alopecia (hair loss). • One or more discrete areas of alopecia with tiny broken hairs. • Numerous discrete pustules or excoriations with little alopecia. • A kerion or boggy, tender, inflammatory mass that produces edema and pustules. • Pruritus usually occurs in the involved area.
Pediculosis Infestation of humans by lice. *Etiology:* • Three types of lice affect human beings: • *Pediculosis capitis* (head lice)—commonly infests school-age children. • *Pediculosis corporis* (body lice)—rare in the United States. • *Pediculosis pubis* (pubic or crab lice)—common in sexually active adolescents or adults—can be found on pubic hair, chest hair, axillary hair, eyebrows, eyelashes, and beards. • Each type of louse generally remains in the area designated by its name. • Lice are transmitted by personal contact with people harboring them or through contact with articles that temporarily harbor them (clothing or bed linens). • Head and pubic lice are not health hazards or signs of uncleanliness. Only body lice can transmit disease. *Diagnosis:* • Identification of lice or their eggs with the naked eye confirmed by using a hand lens or microscope. • In active infection of head or pubic lice, nits and eggs are found on the hair shaft within 1 cm of the skin and are difficult to remove. • Body lice and their eggs are found in the seams of undergarments.	• Itching in the area affected is the primary symptom of pediculosis. Scratch marks may be evident in these areas. However, not all affected people itch. • Other signs of infestation are pillows or clothing that looks unusually dirty. • Infested scalp areas may become secondarily infected from scratching. • Crusts, lice, nits, eggs, and dirt may combine to cause a foul odor and matted hair. • Body lice may produce minute red lesions.

TREATMENT/PREVENTION	NURSING CONSIDERATIONS

• Micronized griseofulvin—an antifungal antibiotic that is administered orally, 15–20 mg/kg/day (maximum 1 g) in a single dose with a high-fat food for 4–12 weeks. Some children may require higher doses or micronized griseofulvin 20–25 mg/kg/day or ultramicronized griseofulvin 5–10 mg/kg/day (maximum 750 mg).
 	
• Topical antifungal medicines are not effective. Selenium sulfide lotion 2.5% used twice per week decreases fungal shedding and may curb the spread of infection.
 	
• Treatment should be continued for 2 weeks after clinical resolution.
 	
• Treatment with oral itraconazole, oral terbinafine, or oral fluconazole is effective, but only terbinafine has been approved by the Food and Drug Administration for this disorder.
	• Assess the scalp for characteristic lesions.
	• Administer or teach the patient and family to administer medications as prescribed.
	• Be aware of adverse effects, such as headache, heartburn, nausea, epigastric discomfort, diarrhea, urticaria, photosensitivity, and possible granulocytopenia caused by griseofulvin.
	• Griseofulvin is absorbed more efficiently with a fatty meal. Children can be given the medicine once per day with ice cream or peanut butter.
	• Liver function monitoring may be required for prolonged treatment (greater than 6 months) or for children with baseline abnormal liver function.
	• Teach the child and family methods to prevent further episodes.
	  • Teach general hygiene measures—regular shampooing and bathing.
	  • Advise them to avoid sharing hats, combs, brushes, pillows.
	  • Routine cleaning of heavily contaminated articles, such as pillowcases, sheets, towels, hats, bike helmets, combs, brushes.
	  • All family members and close contacts should be screened for tinea infections. The child's school should be notified to facilitate the screening of classmates.
	• Hair loss is usually temporary, except in some cases with a kerion, when the hair follicles may have been destroyed.
	• Child may attend school after treatment has been initiated. Hats are not necessary.

• Pediculosis capitis and pediculosis pubis may be treated with over-the-counter agents, such as permethrin or natural pyrethrin-based products. Lindane 1% (Rx) is indicated for second-line therapy only. Natural pyrethrin-based products and lindane may be reapplied 7–10 days later. Lindane should be avoided in children younger than age 2, people with known seizures, and pregnant or lactating women.
 	
• For infestation of eyelashes by crab lice, petroleum jelly applied twice daily to the eyelashes for 8 to 10 days is effective.
 	
• Pediculicides are not necessary for the treatment of pediculosis corporis. Washing infested clothing and linens, where the lice harbor, in hot water and machine drying (on hot cycle) is adequate.
 	
• Because pediculicides kill lice shortly after application, the detection of living lice on scalp inspection 24 hours or more after treatment suggests incorrect use, reinfection, or resistance. Immediate retreatment with a different pediculicide followed by a second application 7 days later is recommended.
 	
• A suffocation-based pediculicide (DSP) lotion applied and then blown dry with a hair dryer weekly for up to 3 weeks effectively treats 95% of head lice. The hair can be shampooed 8 hours after application. The lotion is not visible and the hair can be styled.
 	
• Studies of the efficacy of suffocation of lice by the application of occlusive agents, such as petroleum jelly, olive oil, or mayonnaise, have not been performed. Cotrimoxazole and ivermectin have been shown to be effective, but neither is approved by the FDA as a pediculicide.
 	
• "No nit" policies requiring children to be free from nits for the return to school do not reduce transmission and are not recommended.
 	
• Shaving head is not necessary.
	• Administer or teach administration of antiparasitic as directed. Natural pyrethrin-based products work best on dry hair. Avoid shampoo, cream rinses, and conditioners before application.
	• Although both pyrethrins and permethrin are quite safe, limit exposure to the skin by rinsing the hair in a sink rather than the shower and use cool water to minimize absorption from vasodilation.
	• Removal of nits with a fine-tooth comb may be attempted for aesthetic reasons or to decrease diagnostic confusion. However, mechanical removal of nits after treatment does not prevent spread.
	• Inspect the scalp (or have the family inspect the scalp) 24–48 hours after treatment to see what lice remain. The presence of large lice may mean that the treatment was ineffective or that the lice are resistant.
	• Provide appropriate teaching for the family to prevent recurrences.
	  • Wash clothing, bed linens, and towels in hot water and machine dry (on hot cycle). Temperature above 128.3°F (53.5°C) for 5 minutes will kill lice and eggs. Dry cleaning or simply storing contaminated articles in a well-sealed plastic bag for 10 days is also effective.
	  • Teach children not to share combs, brushes, headgear or hats. Combs and brushes can be disinfected by soaking in hot water for 10 minutes or washing with a pediculicide shampoo.
	  • Environmental insecticide sprays are not helpful. Vacuuming carpets and car seats is a safe alternative.
	  • Household, other close contacts, and classmates of the child with head lice should be screened for parasites and treated if affected. Prophylactic treatment of head lice is unnecessary and may increase resistance. Notify the child's school or day care so classmates can be screened.
	  • Children should be allowed back to school or day care the morning after their first treatment. "No nit" policies for the return to school are unnecessary.
	  • Prophylactic treatment of all sexual contacts of adolescents and adults with pubic lice is warranted because of the high coinfection rate.

(continued)

Table 55-1   Common Pediatric Skin Problems (*Continued*)

DISORDER/ORGANISM	CLINICAL MANIFESTATIONS
Scabies A disease of the skin produced by the burrowing action of a parasitic mite in the epidermis, resulting in irritation and the formation of burrows, vesicles, or pustules. *Etiology*: • The mite, *Sarcoptes scabiei*, is the cause of this disorder. • Occurs in people of all socioeconomic levels, regardless of personal hygiene standards. • Is transmitted by direct skin contact with infected people or by indirect contact through soiled bed linens, clothing. *Diagnosis*: • Identification of a mite, ova, or feces from skin scrapings. • Often based on clinical presentation.	• Itching, particularly at night, is the primary symptom. The onset of itching is usually insidious. • Secondary skin infection is common and may confuse the diagnosis. • Systemic manifestations are absent, unless they result from the secondary infection. • The burrow, a gray or white, tortuous, threadlike line, is seen most commonly in older children and adults between the fingers, in the wrists, in the axillary and buttock folds, along the belt line, on the male genitalia, on the female breasts, and on the knees, elbows, and ankles. • In infants and small children, the lesions may occur on any part of the body and are usually widespread. Vesicles on the palms and soles are characteristic. • Incubation period in children without previous exposure is 4–6 weeks.
Oral Candidiasis (Thrush) Oral candidiasis is a mycotic stomatitis characterized by the appearance of white plaques on the oral mucous membranes, gums, and tongue. (Chronic mucocutaneous candidiasis may be associated with endocrine diseases or immunodeficiency disorders or use of systemic antibiotic or inhaled corticosteroids.) *Etiology*: • Caused by *Candida albicans*. • Maternal vulvovaginitis is the primary source of neonatal thrush. Evaluate for endocrine diseases or immunodeficiency disorders if thrush occurs after 6 months of life or is chronic. • Nipples, pacifiers may be reservoirs.	• The infant develops small plaques on the oral mucous membranes, tongue, or gums. These plaques look like curds of milk but cannot be wiped out of the mouth. • Most infants with thrush appear to have little pain or discomfort, unless the case is severe and there are erosion and ulceration of the mucosa. • The mouth may be dry. • Occasionally, the infant may appear to have some difficulty swallowing or may eat less vigorously. • Enteric infection is usually associated with oral thrush.
Diaper Dermatitis Candidal diaper dermatitis—a rash characterized by bright red, sharply circumscribed but moist patches with pustular satellite lesions. *Etiology*: • 80% of diaper rashes present for 3 or more days are caused by *Candida albicans*. • Most commonly seen in infants and toddlers who wear diapers. • May be associated with oral candidiasis.	• Buttock rash consisting of erythematous maculopapular eruption with perianal distribution. • Generally causes discomfort, especially with wetting and cleanings. Lesions last approximately 2 weeks, desquamate, and resolve without scarring.

TREATMENT/PREVENTION	NURSING CONSIDERATIONS
• Application of a scabicide to the skin: • The drug of choice is 5% permethrin. Alternative drugs are lindane 1% and crotamiton. Permethrin should be removed after 8–14 hours by bathing, lindane after 8–12 hours, and crotamiton after 48 hours. • Lindane can cause neurotoxicity from absorption through the skin. It should be avoided in children younger than age 2, people with known seizures, pregnant and lactating women, and people with extensive dermatitis. • Infected children and adults should apply the scabicidal lotion or cream on the entire body from the neck down. The entire head, neck, and body of infants and young children should be treated. Bathing immediately before treatment should be avoided. • Oral ivermectin at 200 mcg/kg/dose is not FDA-approved but has been shown to be effective.	• People caring for affected children should wear gloves. • Contagion is unlikely 24 hours after treatment. Children may return to school or day care. • Teach the patient and family to launder all clothing, bed linens, and towels used by the patient during the 4 days prior to therapy with hot water and hot drying cycle to kill mites. Clothing that cannot be laundered can be stored in a plastic bag for 1 week. Further environmental disinfection is rarely necessary. • Itching may continue 2–3 weeks after successful therapy because of a hypersensitivity reaction to the mites. The use of oral antihistamines and topical corticosteroids can help relieve symptoms. • All household and close contacts should be treated prophylactically and at the same time to prevent reinfection. Caretakers with prolonged skin-to-skin contact with infected patients may also benefit from prophylactic treatment. Manifestations of scabies can occur as late as 2 months after exposure.
• Topical administration of nystatin in suspension three to four times daily is the treatment of choice. Apply ½ doses to each side of the mouth after feeding. • Retain in the mouth as long as possible before swallowing. Allow the child to swallow any medication to treat any lesions along the GI tract. • Clotrimazole troches can be used in children older than age 3. • Amphotericin B, clotrimazole, ketoconazole, fluconazole, and newer antifungal agents are used for candidiasis resistant to nystatin. Not all of these drugs are approved for use in infants and children.	• Recognize the appearance of thrush. • Be aware of the infant or child who is particularly susceptible to the development of this condition, especially normal infants younger than age 6 months, low-birth-weight infants, immunocompromised or debilitated hosts, and people on prolonged, broad-spectrum antibiotics. • Teach parents to inspect the child's mouth before every feeding for the presence of thrush and report the appearance of thrush.

• Keep the affected area clean and dry by frequent diaper changes.
• Clean the skin with water-based, alcohol-free baby wipes with a pH of 5.5 or with water.
• Use disposable diapers with sodium polyacrylate polymers in the diaper core that form a gel when hydrated to keep liquid away from the skin or a breathable diaper.
• Topical application of nystatin, clotrimazole, or miconazole cream or ointment after gentle cleaning of the affected area. If no improvement in 2 days, consider nonadherence, failure to relieve aggravating factors, or need for a different drug.
• Nystatin may be given orally if rash is persistent.
• Burow solution compresses for severe inflammation or vesiculation.
• Low-potency topical corticosteroids for short-term use may be added.
	• Teach parents the general principles of prevention.
	  • Change diaper as soon as possible after wetting or soiling. Prolonged contact of feces with the skin promotes the development of candidal diaper dermatitis. Check diaper frequently (every 3–4 hours). Encourage use of disposable diapers.
	  • Wash the entire diaper area with warm water or use water-based, alcohol-free baby wipes.
	  • If using cloth diapers, use a second hot rinse when washing diapers to neutralize ammonia produced when infant urinates; use vinegar, Borax, or Diaparene in wash.
	  • Avoid powder and oil, which tend to clog pores and cake on skin, retaining bacteria.
	  • Avoid occlusive plastic coverings and tightly pinned or double diapers, all of which tend to increase production and retention of body heat and moisture.
	  • Allow the infant to go without a diaper for short periods to leave area open to air.
	• Diaper rashes present for 3 or more days should be evaluated by a health care provider.

SELECTED REFERENCES

American Burn Association. (2016). *Advanced burn life support provider manual.* Chicago, IL: American Burn Association.

Baartmans, M., de Jong, A., van Baar, M., et al. (2016). Early Management in children with burns: Cooling, wound care and pain management. *Burns, 42*(4), 777–782.

Comeau, O., Heffernan, J., Sheaffer, J., et al. (2014). Rising to the challenge. *Critical Care Nursing Quarterly, 37*(3), 336–343.

Conceicao, V. (2016). The nursing management of infantile eczema. *Journal of Community Nursing, 30*(5), 12–14.

Eichenfield, L. F., Tom, W. L., Berger, T. G., et al. (2014). Guidelines of care for the management of atopic dermatitis: Section 2. Management and treatment of atopic dermatitis with topical therapies. *Journal of the American Academy of Dermatology, 71*(1), 116–32.

Fenster, D. (2015). Scratching the surface: A review of skin and soft tissue infections in children. *Current Opinion in Pediatrics, 27*(3), 303–307.

Fore, S., Munchel, E., Goldstein, S., et al. (2016). Comparison of pediatric burn wound colonization and the surrounding environment. *Comprehensive Child & Adolescent Nursing, 39*(2), 154–160.

Greenhalgh D. G. (Ed.). (2016). *Burn care for general surgeons and general practitioners.* Switzerland: Springer International Publishing.

Hall, B. J., & Hall, J. C. (2017). *Sauer's manual of skin diseases* (11th ed.). Philadelphia, PA: Lippincott Williams & Wilkins.

Herndon, D. (2017). *Total Burn Care* (5th ed.). Philadelphia: Elsevier.

James, W. D., Berger, T., & Elston, D. M. (2016). *Andrews' diseases of the skin clinical dermatology* (12th ed.). Philadelphia, PA: W.B. Saunders.

Jennings, P., Cullen, M., Mark, R., et al. (2015). Developing a Pediatric Burn Treatment Program in a Community Hospital. *Pediatric Nursing, 41*(5), 219–225.

Kraft, R., Herndon, D. N., Finnerty, C. C., et al. (2014). Occurrence of multi-organ dysfunction in pediatric burn patients—Incidence and clinical outcome. *Annals of Surgery, 259*(2), 381–387.

Lawton, S. (2015). Identifying common skin infections and infestations. *Journal of Community Nursing, 29*(1), 41–46.

Lyons, J., Milner, J., & Stone, K. (2015). Atopic dermatitis in children. *Immunology and Allergy Clinics of North America, 35*(1), 161–183.

Moore, E. R., Bennett, K., Dietrich, M. S., et al. (2015). The Effect of Directed Medical Play on Young Children's Pain and Distress during Burn Wound Care. *Journal of Pediatric Health Care, 29*(3), 265–273.

National Center for Injury Prevention and Control. Center for Disease Control. Available: *https://webappa.cdc.gov/sasweb/ncipc/leadcause.html*

Oszukowska, M., Michalak, I., Gutfreund, K., et al. (2015). Role of primary and secondary prevention in atopic dermatitis. *Advances in Dermatology and Allergology, 32*(6), 409–420.

Paller, A. S., & Mancini, A. J. (2016). *Hurwitz clinical pediatric dermatology* (5th ed.). Philadelphia, PA: Elsevier.

Parker, J., & Jacob, S. (2017). Crisaborole topical ointment, 2%. *Journal of the Dermatology Nurses Association, 9*(4), 205–207.

Penzer, R. (2015). Prescribing for children with atopic eczema in primary care. *Nurse Prescribing, 13*(7), 326–334.

Rimmer, R. B., Bay, R. C., Alam, N. B., et al. (2015). Measuring the burden of pediatric burn injury for parents and caregivers: Informed burn center staff can help to lighten the load. *Journal of Burn Care and Research, 36*(3), 421–427.

Rosenberg, M., Ramirez, M., Epperson, K., et al. (2015). Comparison of long-term quality of life of pediatric burn survivors with and without inhalation injury. *Burns, 41*(4), 721–726.

Rowan, M. P., Cancio, L. C., Elster, E. A., et al. (2015). Burn wound healing and treatment: Review and advancements. *Critical Care, 19*(1), 243.

Singleton, A., Preston, R. J., & Cochran, A. (2015). Sedation and analgesia for critically ill pediatric burn patients: The current state of practice. *Journal of Burn Care and Research, 36*(3), 440–445.

Starnes, C., Bailey, E., Calvert, C., et al. (2016). Development of a Pediatric Educational Tool: Helping Burns Heal…An Adventure for Kids with Burns. *Journal of Pediatric Surgical Nursing, 5*(2), 50–59.

Szabo, M. M., Ferris, K. A., Urso, L., et al. (2017). Social competence in pediatric burn survivors: A systematic review. *Rehabilitation Psychology, 62*(1), 69–80.

Van Onselen, J. (2017). Dermatology prescribing update: Eczema. *Nurse Prescribing, 15*(7), 324–329.

Van Onelson, J. (2018). Treating eczema in children in general practice. *Practice Nursing, 29*(5), 223–229.

Vyles, D., Sinha, M., Rosenberg, D. I., et al. (2014). Predictors of serious bacterial infections in pediatric burn patients with fever. *Journal of Burn Care and Research, 35*(4), 291–295.

Watkins, J. (2015). Common causes of itching in children. *Practice Nursing, 26*(7), 345–359.

World Health Organization. (2012). *WHO's pain ladder.* Geneva: Author. Available: *www.who.int/cancer/palliative/painladder/en.*

Yamamoto, L. (2017). Treatment of skin and soft tissue infections. *Pediatric Emergency Care, 33*(1), 49–55.

56
Developmental Disabilities

OVERVIEW AND ASSESSMENT

The spectrum of developmental disabilities is a group of interrelated chronic neurodevelopmental disorders. It includes cerebral palsy, mental retardation, autism, learning disabilities, communication disorders, anxiety disorders, and attention deficit disorders. These conditions are suspected or noticed at varying stages during childhood. Some conditions, such as Down syndrome, can be recognized prenatally or at birth; other conditions, such as cerebral palsy or autism, may not present themselves until the child fails to meet typical developmental milestones. This phenomenon makes the nurse's role in developmental assessment crucial. The pediatric nurse who understands that the development of the child occurs in an orderly, predictable manner and who knows what the milestones should be may be the first person to recognize the deviation and raise the suspicion to the parent or pediatrician. Because there are many confusing and overlapping characteristics for many of these conditions, it is important for the health care provider and family to refer to clinicians who are experienced and knowledgeable in typical and atypical child development to arrive at an accurate diagnosis and coordinate an appropriate care plan. Nurses can play a significant role in supporting the family in navigating the complex needs of many of these disorders.

When a known condition exists, the nurse should be aware of the predisposing health issues associated with the condition and the resources available to promote optimal growth and development of the child within the family.

 NURSING ALERT Normal child development is predictable and sequential. The nurse who is knowledgeable about normal development may be the first person to raise the question that a developmental disability exists.

Signs of Developmental Delay

Criteria for Referral

Communication and Feeding
1. Feeding difficulties—weak sucking or poor coordination of suck–swallowing to sustain normal weight gain.
2. No social smile by age 4 months.
3. No babbling (*ga-ga*, *da-da*) by age 9 months.
4. No *mama* and *dada* (specific) by age 14 months.
5. No name of object (one word) by age 14 months.
6. At least 10 words by age 18 months (not just repeating).
7. Combines words (eg, *me outside*, *more milk*) and uses pronouns by age 24 months.
8. Regression in language or social responses at any age.
9. Unresponsive to name.

 NURSING ALERT Do not simply reassure the family that normal development "should" or "probably will" develop. Make sure that the child is referred for an appropriate evaluation to properly assess the suspected delay and establish a diagnosis, if possible. In the presence of a developmental delay, a comprehensive vision and hearing evaluation should also be included.

Motor Delay
1. Asymmetrical movements and poor tone are noted.
2. Not rolling over by age 6 months.
3. Not sitting by age 9 months.
4. Not walking by age 15 months.
5. Not stair climbing by age 2 years.

See Chapter 40 for normal pediatric growth and development.

Care of the Child with a Developmental Disability

Nursing Assessment
1. Review the child's record including the prenatal and birth history to determine existing health problems that may cause or affect the developmental disability. Always rule out a vision or hearing impairment.
2. Review the family history, if available, to determine if there are any family members with a history of developmental disabilities. If possible, assess when parents and siblings of the patient reached specified developmental milestones.
3. Assess the family's understanding of the diagnosis and its ramifications. The parents' experiences, cultural beliefs, attitudes toward disabilities, cognitive ability, stage of grief, and

their own health affect their ability to assimilate information provided. It will be necessary to repeat the information. (For example, a woman who has just given birth to a child with Down syndrome may have difficulty processing much information shortly after birth.) If possible, provide the family with written information that reinforces verbal information given at the visit. Provide resources with careful consideration of information overload. Additional information and resources may be better introduced at subsequent visits.

4. Determine the developmental age of the child. The pediatric nurse should be familiar with normal developmental milestones (see Chapter 40, page 1080), noting the child's strengths and areas presenting challenges, for example, the communication skills are at a 12-month level and the gross motor skills are at a 36-month level. Children who are found to be functioning at one half or less of their chronological age have a moderate to severe developmental delay.

5. Administer a developmental tool such as the Clinical Adaptive Test–Clinical Linguistic Auditory Milestone Scales (CAT–CLAMS). It is a reliable tool that nurses can be trained to use to assess cognitive and communicative development in children at the 1- to 36-month developmental level. It has been found to be more sensitive than the Denver Developmental Screening Scale because language development is the best early predictor of cognitive abilities.

6. Assess the functional level of the child. The WeeFIM is a tool used to track functional independence in children. It has had multiple revisions and is reliable and valid. It uses the following categories to describe function: completely dependent, needs some physical assistance, can physically perform the task but needs verbal cues and coaching, and completely independent. Functional areas to assess include:
   a. Feeding.
   b. Grooming and bathing.
   c. Dressing.
   d. Mobility.
   e. Problem solving.
   f. Communication.

7. Assess parents' perception of the child's development level and the appropriateness of parental expectations. Use such questions as, "Do you have any concerns regarding things your child is doing or should be doing?" "Is your child progressing like your other children have?"

8. Assess parent–child interaction. Observe and explore bonding and attachment, ability to set appropriate limits, management of behavioral problems, and methods of discipline.

9. Assess the need for additional resources, such as financial aid, transportation, and counseling, for long-term support of child and family.

 NURSING ALERT Be aware of the diversity of cultural norms that may affect developmental milestones.

 EVIDENCE BASE Lynch, B., Weaver, A., Starr, S., et al. (2015). Developmental screening and follow-up by nurses. *MCN: The American Journal of Maternal Child Nursing, 40*(6), 388–393.
Williams, A., Cormack, C., Chike-Harris, K., et al. (2015). Pediatric developmental screenings: A primary care approach. *Nurse Practitioner, 40*(4), 34–39.

Nursing Diagnoses

- Impaired Parenting related to birth and diagnosis of developmentally disabled child.
- Interrupted Family Processes related to multiple needs of child and difficult bonding.
- Ineffective Infant Feeding Pattern related to protruding tongue, poor muscle tone, and weak sucking.
- Delayed Growth and Development related to impaired cognitive and motor functioning.
- Social Isolation related to developmental differences from other children.
- Risk for Injury related to neurologic impairment and developmental delay.

Nursing Interventions

Promoting Adjustment

1. Allow the parents access to the infant at all possible times to promote bonding when parents appear ready.
2. Focus on the positive aspects of the infant and serve as a role model for handling and stimulating.
3. Be cognizant of the grieving process (loss of the anticipated and planned-for "normal child") that families experience when a diagnosis is made, and be aware that spouses can be at different stages.
4. Accept all questions and reactions nonjudgmentally, offering verbal and written explanations.
5. Provide the family a quiet place to discuss their questions with each other and someone knowledgeable about the condition (primary care provider, clinical nurse specialist) to support their concerns.
6. Offer the family the option to take advantage of counseling. A social worker or psychologist can help families deal with immediate reactions. Many parents benefit from continuous or periodic support of counseling professionals.

 NURSING ALERT Children with developmental disabilities and chronic illness are at greater risk for experiencing divorce, child abuse, and neglect than the general population.

Strengthening the Role of the Family

1. Help the family to realize what strengths they have in caring for their child. The role of the parents is critical; a nurturing, loving environment gives the child the best chance at maximizing potential. An individual who grows up at home has markedly higher adaptive abilities and an increased life span compared with those raised in residential care facilities.
2. Enlist the help of family and siblings, who can offer valuable support to the parents and child and assist with stimulation activities. Including siblings in the care can help them feel needed and involved, thus strengthening the family.
3. If sibling issues arise, suggest family counseling to address the needs of all family members.
4. Identify resources available to the family, such as parent support groups, early intervention programs, specialty clinics, pediatrician or primary health care provider, respite care, financial support programs, and advocacy groups for individuals with developmental disabilities.
5. For those parents concerned with their ability to care for the child, explore with them their options of foster care, adoption, and residential placement in a nonjudgmental manner.
6. Ensure that the family has adequate respite services to prevent exhaustion and mental fatigue.

Establishing Effective Feeding Techniques

 EVIDENCE BASE Hurley, K., Yousafzai, A., & Lopez-Boo, F. (2016). Early child development and nutrition: A review of the benefits and challenges of implementing integrated interventions. *Advances in Nutrition,* 7(2), 357–363.

Zuckerman,K., Chavez, A., & Reeder, J., (2017). Decreasing Disparities in Child Development Assessment: Identifying and Discussing Possible Delays in the Special Supplemental Program for Women, Infants, and Children (WIC). *Journal of Developmental & Behavioral Pediatrics,* 38(5), 301–309.

1. Be aware that the presence of hypotonia, as in children with many genetic syndromes and metabolic disorders, or hypertonia, as in children with cerebral palsy, can interfere with feeding by compromising sucking and swallowing.
2. Demonstrate proper feeding positioning, with the infant's head elevated, and encourage the parents to always hold the infant during feedings with his or her head elevated and supported in arms.
3. Try different nipples, bottles, and positions to find the easiest for the infant to use without leakage or danger of aspiration.
4. Allow adequate time for feeding and increase frequency of feedings if infant tires easily.
5. Offer support and guidance for breastfeeding. Refer to lactation consultant, if needed.
6. Consider referral for a feeding evaluation to a speech therapist or to an occupational therapist who has experience working with children and families.
7. Be aware of and anticipate the need for initiation of tube feeding (nasogastric or gastrostomy) so that early referral and education of the parents about feeding options can be discussed.
8. Assess for signs of feeding intolerance and gastroesophageal reflux disease, which is common in children with hypotonia; implement management strategies to optimize feeding and minimize risk of aspiration, such as upright position after feedings.
9. Frequently assess growth (length or height, weight, and head circumference) to ensure adequate dietary intake, and be aware that growth in children with neurologic impairment and genetic syndromes may be slower or limited in relation to the general pediatric population and standard growth charts.
10. Monitor bowel and elimination patterns of children with neurologic impairment, especially those with generalized hypotonia, as they are at risk for poor gastric motility and constipation. Dietary measures, such as increased fiber and fluid intake, or pharmacologic agents to promote adequate elimination may be needed.

Promoting Optimum Growth and Development

1. Refer parents to the early intervention program administered by their county so that they can take advantage of the educational and support services available for children from birth to age 3 years.
2. If the condition is identified after age 3 years, refer parents to the school district in which they reside.
3. Help the parents to understand the concept of developmental age and identify the functional level of the child.
4. Determine whether there is consistency between the developmental age of the child and degree of independence. Cognitive and physical limitations may interfere with emerging independence; however, parents may "baby" or overindulge a child who has a disability.

5. Work with parents to set reasonable expectations and to break down tasks into simple, achievable steps. Care should be taken not to address too many areas at one time so as not to overwhelm the family.
6. Use appropriate discipline and behavior modification techniques, such as extinction, time-out, and reward, to achieve cooperation and success.
7. Demonstrate and encourage play with the child at the appropriate level to provide stimulation and work toward achieving developmental milestones.
8. Provide parents with information and links to community, regional, or national associations for children with special needs, and refer to parent support groups. These resources are frequently found online and can be easily accessed to provide an ongoing source of information and support to families.
9. Ensure that the child's physical well-being is optimized to promote optimal development and self-esteem. Any congenital defects should be considered for repair (ie, orthopedic, cardiac, craniofacial, etc), and attention should be paid to dental health and restorative orthodontic procedures that can improve facial appearance.
10. Consider any pertinent cultural and ethnic impact on health care.

Providing Opportunities to Develop Social and Self-Care Skills

1. Be aware that feeding, toileting, dressing, and grooming are important aspects of socialization and development of self-esteem. These tasks should be taught in a developmentally appropriate manner to children with a focus on maximizing independence. Many adaptive devices are available, and an occupational therapist can guide families in effective techniques to help children with developmental disabilities master these important self-care skills.
2. Make parents aware that recreational and leisure-time experiences are valuable in building social skills and self-esteem. Rehearse and role-play desirable social behaviors—such as waving goodbye, saying "hello," taking turns, saying "please" and "thank you," and responding to their name—will help build social confidence and acceptance within the child's peer group.
3. Offer suggestions that will be enjoyable and developmentally appropriate for the child. Interaction with developmentally delayed and nondevelopmentally delayed peers is desirable. The Special Olympics is one example of an adaptive program. Local programs are also available in many areas.
4. Praise the child for participation in activities, regardless of whether the child succeeds.

Maintaining Safety

1. When handling the infant, provide adequate support with a firm grasp because the infant may be floppy because of poor muscle tone.
2. If hypotonia is accompanied by poor head control and neck strength, position the infant to prevent aspiration should vomiting occur.
   a. Support the infant with a diaper roll, if needed, to maintain position.
   b. Change the infant's position frequently.
   c. Continuously check the environment for the safety needs of the child.
3. Be aware that hypotonia can also lead to increased heat loss as more surface area is exposed; therefore, infants may need

close attention paid to swaddling and environmental control to maintain thermoregulation.

4. Advise the parents to:
   a. Maintain appropriate surveillance of the child when cooking or exposing him or her to other potential hazards that he or she may be able to get into but not understand.
   b. Help the child to read words, such as *danger* and *stop*.
   c. Teach the child how to call and ask for help.
   d. Teach the child to say no to strangers.
   e. Teach the child appropriate and socially acceptable sexual behaviors to prevent exploitation.
   f. Teach sex education, with practical information about anatomy, physical development, and contraception, in a way the child and adolescent can understand.
5. Ensure that parents and caregivers have the knowledge and resources to transport their child safely.

 NURSING ALERT Teach caregivers to base safety needs on the developmental, not the chronological, age of the child.

Family Education and Health Maintenance

1. Remind the parents to recognize the child's routine health care needs and maintain regular follow-up with a primary care provider.
   a. Immunizations.
   b. Regular dental checkups.
   c. Vision and hearing examinations.
   d. Anticipatory guidance related to developmental stages, safety, behavior, and transition planning.
2. Provide guidance and support to parents with their child's multidimensional treatment plan. Make sure parents know whom to contact when problems arise. Encourage parents to develop and maintain a notebook with a calendar to keep track of agencies, subspecialists, and professionals who will be involved with their child. It should include such information as business cards, names, addresses, phone numbers, appointment dates, health providers' orders, and insurance information.
3. Teach parents the benefits of a therapeutic home environment.
   a. Develop optimum sleeping, eating, working, and playing routines.
   b. Ensure adequate nutrition.
   c. Divide tasks and expectations into small, manageable parts. Give only one or two instructions at a time.
   d. Set firm but reasonable limits on behavior and carry through with consistent discipline.
   e. Avoid situations that cause excessive excitement, stimulation, or fatigue.
   f. Provide an energy outlet through physical activity and outdoor play, as well as vocal outlet.
   g. Channel the need for movement into safe, appropriate activities.
4. Discuss preparation for independent living, when appropriate.
   a. Help the parents identify areas of home responsibilities that may be delegated to the cognitively impaired child.
   b. Guide development of social skills that will be an asset to later vocational life.
   c. Help the child to develop a set of attitudes and behaviors that will increase motivation.
   d. Refer for vocational assistance to ARC (formerly Association of Retarded Citizens) or other rehabilitative agencies.

   e. Begin planning for transition from pediatric care providers to adult providers well in advance of when eligibility for services will run out to ensure appropriate provider(s) can be established in a timely way and to avoid gaps in health care.
5. Refer for genetic consultation for information about genetics of the disorder, risk in subsequent pregnancies (parents) or risk to offspring (patient), or risk to other relatives as it is warranted by the diagnosis.

 EVIDENCE BASE Milen, M., & Nicholas, D. (2017). Examining transitions from youth to adult services for young persons with autism. *Social Work in Health Care, 56*(7), 636–648.
Castillo, M., Clark, D., Schaller, E., et al. (2018). Descriptive assessment of problem behavior during transitions of children with intellectual and developmental disabilities. *Journal of Applied Behavior Analysis, 51*(1), 99–117.

Evaluation: Expected Outcomes

- Parents hold infant frequently and seek information from health care provider.
- Family members feed, assist with care, and bond with child.
- Parents and health care providers monitor nutrition, growth, and development closely, with ongoing assessment of most effective feeding techniques and management of any feeding-related problems.
- Parents describe developmental level of child and have realistic goals for attainment of next milestones in collaboration with their health care team and occupational, speech, and physical therapists.
- Parents seek out support and resources that enable them to share their experience in raising a child with special needs and gain information needed to optimize the child's developmental and health outcomes throughout childhood.
- Child remains safe through careful handling and appropriate supervision.

DEVELOPMENTAL DISABILITIES
Cognitive Developmental Delay

Cognitive developmental delay, also known as *intellectual disabilities*, refers to the most severe, general lack of cognitive and problem-solving skills. The American Association on Intellectual and Developmental Disabilities defines intellectual disabilities as a disability characterized by significant limitations both in intellectual functioning and in adaptive behavior, which covers many everyday social and practical skills. This disability originates before the age of 18 years. There are many causes and a wide range of impairments. Up to 7.7 million people in the United States have at least a mild developmental disability that impacts their daily functioning. One in six children (or about 15%) aged 3 through 17 years have one or more developmental disabilities.

Pathophysiology and Etiology

1. No identifiable organic or biologic cause can be found for 50% of children with cognitive delays.
2. Identifiable causes include:
   a. Genetic causes, such as Down syndrome, fragile X syndrome, Angelman syndrome, and inborn errors of metabolism such as phenylketonuria (PKU).

b. Congenital anomalies, including brain malformations, hydrocephalus, and microcephaly.

c. Intrauterine influences, such as alcohol and drug exposure, congenital infections, and teratogens.

d. Perinatal trauma—birth hypoxia and intracranial hemorrhage.

e. Postnatal trauma—acquired brain injury from falls, automobile accidents, near drownings, and child abuse (shaken baby syndrome).

f. Postnatal infections and diseases (meningitis, encephalitis, sepsis, hypoxia, brain tumors).

g. Environmental exposure to toxins such as lead, environmental deprivation, and neglect.

3. The malfunctioning brain is poorly understood in most cases, but physiologic alterations identified in some cases include:

a. Congenital brain malformations, brain tissue damage, or underdevelopment of the brain as shown by normal results of computed tomography (CT) scan or magnetic resonance imaging (MRI).

b. Biochemical errors or errors of metabolism, in which an absence of an enzyme or hormone produces abnormal brain function or formation, as in PKU or hypothyroidism.

4. IQ is 75 or below; classification has been recently changed to mild and severe and includes both cognitive and functional abilities.

a. The more severe types of intellectual developmental disability tend to be diagnosed in early infancy, especially when they coexist with an identifiable syndrome or congenital anomaly.

b. Milder forms of intellectual developmental disability tend to be diagnosed in the preschool years, when language and behavioral concerns call attention to slower development.

5. Limitations in adaptive ability occur in communication, self-care, home living, social skills, community use, self-direction, health and safety, functional academics, leisure, and work.

Clinical Manifestations

Developmental delays (failure to achieve age-appropriate skills) are evident to some degree in almost all areas.

Infancy

1. "Poor feeder"—a weak or uncoordinated suck results in poor breast- or bottle-feeding, leading to poor weight gain.

2. Delayed or decreased visual alertness and curiosity with poor visual tracking of the face or objects.

3. Decreased or lack of auditory response.

4. Decreased spontaneous activity or asymmetric activity.

5. Delayed head and trunk control.

6. Floppy (hypotonic) or spastic (hypertonic) muscle tone.

 NURSING ALERT Although 75% of individuals with intellectual developmental disabilities have no physical signs, they typically achieve motor milestones at a slower rate.

Toddler

1. Delayed independent sitting, crawling, pulling to stand, and independent ambulation.

2. Delayed communication—failure to develop receptive and expressive language milestones. Almost 50% of children with intellectual developmental disability are identified after age 3 years, when speech delays manifest themselves.

3. Failure of the child to make progress or show interest in the area of independence in self-feeding, dressing, and toilet training may reflect cognitive impairment.

4. Short attention span and distractibility.

5. Behavioral disturbances.

6. Decreased muscle coordination.

Diagnostic Evaluation

Federal law (PL 94-142, Education for All Handicapped Children, and PL 101-476, Individuals with Disabilities Education Act [IDEA]) ensures that each child with a delay or suspected of having a delay has a comprehensive evaluation by a multidisciplinary team. Part C of PL 105-17 calls for the creation of statewide, coordinated, multidisciplinary interagency programs for the provision of early intervention services. Each state has its own definitions and organizational framework to provide these services. No single test can diagnose intellectual developmental disabilities. The multidisciplinary evaluation should be individually tailored to the child.

1. Rule out sensory deficits by assessment of vision and hearing, even if neonate hearing screen was normal.

2. Medical evaluation should include prenatal history, developmental history, sequential developmental assessments, family history including genetic assessment, and physical examination. The positive findings determine the direction of the individual evaluation and any diagnostic testing.

a. Unusual appearance (dysmorphic features) warrants evaluation by a genetic specialist.

b. History consistent with loss of developmental milestones and positive family history warrant workup for presence of an inborn error of metabolism (diagnosed by blood, urine, or DNA analysis) or lead poisoning.

c. Children with macrocephaly, microcephaly, or neurologic abnormalities may require imaging studies, such as CT scan or MRI.

d. EEG is indicated for children with seizures.

3. Psychological testing (appropriate tests selected by a child psychologist):

a. The Bayley Scales are used to assess children ages. This test is weighted on nonlanguage items and is used to assess fine motor, gross motor, language skills, and visual problem solving.

b. The McCarthy Scale offers a "general cognitive index" that is roughly equivalent to an IQ score.

c. The Stanford-Binet Intelligence Scale is used to test the mental abilities of children aged 2 and older.

d. The Wechsler Preschool and Primary Scale of Intelligence-Fourth Edition (WPPSI-IV) measures mental age of 2 years and 6 months to 7 years and 7 months.

e. The Wechsler Intelligence Scale for Children-Fifth Edition (WISC-V) tests children whose functional age is above a 6-year level.

f. The Vineland Scale tests social-adaptive abilities—self-help skills, self-control, interaction with others, and cooperation; the Adaptive Behavior Scale is similar to Vineland but also measures adjustment.

Complications and Associated Findings

1. Seizures.

2. Cerebral palsy.

3. Sensory deficits.

4. Communication disorders (speech and language).

5. Neurodevelopmental disorders.
6. Psychiatric illness.
7. Specific learning disabilities.
8. Emotional and behavioral problems (self-injury, hyperactivity, aggression).

Management

1. An interdisciplinary team evaluation by a developmental pediatrician, clinical psychologist, and counselor is usually the initial step in the management of mental delays. This type of evaluation can be obtained through a state or private diagnostic and evaluation center, public school, or university-affiliated program.
2. Associated medical problems, such as seizures, feeding difficulties and poor nutrition, sensory deficits, or dental problems, must be treated to allow the child to maximize his or her potential.
3. If a treatable cause is identified, such as an inborn error of metabolism, a therapeutic diet can be instituted. Hypothyroidism can be treated with thyroid hormone.
4. A family assessment is essential to address:
   a. Financial stressors—financial aid may be available through social security, Medicaid, or state and local programs to help families with children with developmental delays.
   b. Family functioning and coping abilities.
   c. Support for parents, siblings, and extended family.
   d. Respite services.
   e. Support groups.
   f. Recreational programs, such as the Special Olympics and summer camps.
   g. Identification of other affected or at-risk people and the need for genetic counseling for recurrence risk.
5. The initial evaluation usually leads to recommendations for more targeted evaluations, such as physical therapy, occupational therapy, and social work assessment.

See "Care of the Child with a Developmental Disability," page 1453.

Down Syndrome

EVIDENCE BASE Crawford, D. (2016) Down's syndrome. *Nursing Children & Young People, 28*(9), 17. Khatri, S., & Carlisle, J. (2016). Down syndrome. *Contemporary Pediatrics, 33*(8), 30–46.

Down syndrome was first described in 1866. It is the most common genetic cause of intellectual disability and is also referred to as trisomy 21. According to the National Down Syndrome Society, the incidence of this error in cell division is about 1 in 700 live births, about 6,000 infants each year. Down syndrome occurs when an individual has a full or partial extra copy of chromosome 21. Each child with Down syndrome has a unique set of genes, besides the effects of the extra genes on chromosome 21, and the child will need individualized evaluation. The most common life experience of a child with Down syndrome is to live with the family, participate in infant stimulation and preschool programs, and attend school while receiving support from special education services. Adults with Down syndrome can function in supported employment or supervised programs. These adults may live in small residential group homes, with their families or in environments with supervision. Life expectancy depends on the presence of medical complications; when there are no complications, life expectancy is slightly shorter than average, approximately 60 years.

Pathophysiology and Etiology

See Chapter 4, page 29.

Clinical Manifestations and Associated Problems

1. Characteristic facies—brachycephaly; oblique palpebral fissures; epicanthal folds; flat nasal bridge; protruding tongue; small, low-set ears; and simian crease of palms (see Figure 56-1).
2. Congenital heart defects (seen in up to 50% of infants with Down syndrome, compared to 0.8% in the general population), most commonly ventricular septal defects and patent ductus arteriosus.
3. Mental delays.
4. Hypotonia.
5. Growth retardation.
6. Dry, scaly skin.
7. Table 56-1, pages 1459 to 1460, provides a comprehensive list of potential problems that occur with Down syndrome. Some are identified at birth; others arise and cause difficulties later in the life cycle. Percentages are listed that represent occurrence within the Down syndrome population.

Diagnosis and Management

1. See "Care of the Child with a Developmental Disability," page 1453, for a general approach to assessment.
2. See Table 56-1, pages 1459 to 1460, for specific conditions requiring medical management related to Down syndrome, such as otolaryngologic, endocrine, orthopedic, gastrointestinal, and cardiac problems.
3. Alternative therapies—nutritional and supplemental vitamin therapy for Down syndrome remains controversial and effects have not been medically proven.

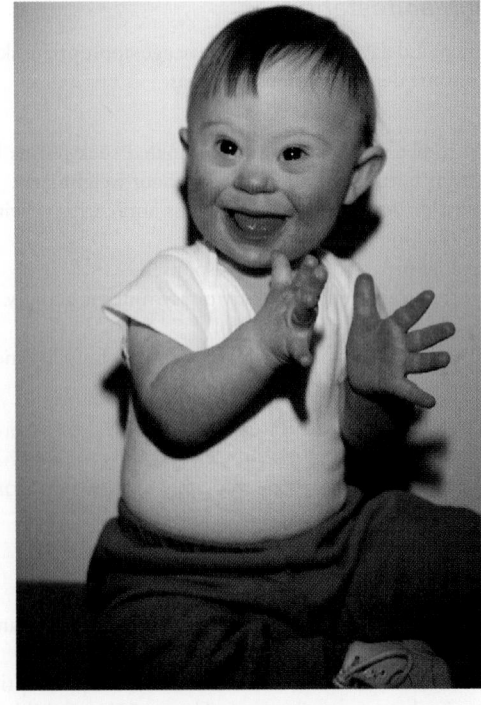

Figure 56-1. A 1-year-old child with Down syndrome, recently diagnosed with hypothyroidism.

Table 56-1   Down Syndrome (DS)

POTENTIAL PROBLEMS	EVALUATION	MANAGEMENT
Congenital heart malformations (ie, AV canal, VSD, PDA, and tetralogy of Fallot) (40%)	• Observe for color changes, pulse, and respiratory rate at rest and with stress. Assess tolerance of feeding for early tiring or frequent interruptions in feeding. Echocardiogram is usually done during neonatal period on all infants with DS.	• Early identification and treatment can prevent heart failure and decompensation or poor growth. Medical or surgical intervention correction has minimized mortality from simple cardiac defects.
Congenital GI malformations (12%) • Pyloric stenosis • Duodenal atresia, tracheoesophageal fistula	• Observe for coughing or vomiting, especially with feeding: bile-stained vomitus suggests lower tract abnormalities; partially digested contents suggest upper tract problem. Observe bowel movements and for abdominal distention. • Radiographic studies are done.	• GI reflux (spillage of material from the esophagus into the trachea) can cause arching during feedings, poor weight gain, chronic respiratory problems, allergy and asthma symptomatology, pneumonia, and aspiration. Medication management and, if needed, surgical intervention can occur in the early neonatal period.
Hypothyroidism (10%–20%)	• Monitor for weight gain, hair loss, lethargy, short stature, voice changes, and depression (can develop at any time over life cycle). Neonatal screening includes T_3, TSH, and T_4 biannually.	• Thyroid hormone replacement.
Visual defects • Refractive errors (70%) • Strabismus (50%) • Nystagmus (35%) • Cataracts (3%)	• Observe for indication of vision problems, such as head tilt or poor visual tracking. Use Teller activity as a visual screen tool for those who cannot cooperate with Snellen chart. • Positive findings in the first year of life warrant immediate referral to ophthalmologist. All individuals should be seen by a pediatric ophthalmologist (or one who is skilled in evaluating children) at age 1, and vision evaluations should continue throughout life.	• Undetected visual deficits can cause failure to achieve developmental milestones and cause permanent loss of vision.
Hearing defects (60%–90%): • Mild to moderate conductive hearing loss • Enlarged adenoids • Sleep apnea	• Assess for curiosity and response to sounds of varying quality. Auditory brain stem response assesses hearing in infants. Sound field testing for children older than age 1. • Tympanometry to assess middle ear function.	• Narrow ear canals and subtle immunodeficiencies can cause chronic middle ear infections. Enlarged adenoids can cause upper airway obstruction, especially during sleep. • Treatment can range from antibiotics for simple otitis media to myringotomy tubes, adenoidectomy, or hearing loss.
Hypotonia of infants (100%)	• Observe for floppiness, poor head control, and poor oral motor function. Infant should be placed on abdomen periodically while being observed and monitored for potential for suffocation.	• Physical, occupational, and speech therapy. Adaptive equipment gives extra support to the head and neck when handling neonate. Always keep head elevated for at least 1 hr after meals. Change position regularly.
Atlanto-occipital and atlantoaxial subluxation (dislocation of the upper spine because of joint laxity) (15%)	• Assess for head tilt; increasing clumsiness, limping, or refusal to walk; and weakness of the arms. X-ray of cervical spine to evaluate for atlantoaxial dislocation at age 2 and then every 5 yr during childhood. Precise measurements are taken to document alignment of the skull and vertebrae. Shifting of the two can cause compression and neurologic damage. Participation in Special Olympics and other activities that may require neck flexion should warrant a baseline evaluation.	• If present, participation in contact sports and gymnastics is contraindicated. In severe cases, surgery to fuse the vertebrae and occiput and stabilize the spinal column.
Gait abnormalities (15%)	• Monitor for onset of limp, leg length discrepancy. Hip x-rays can document dislocation or subluxation.	• Physical therapy and, sometimes, orthopedic surgery are necessary.
Failure to thrive	• Monitor growth on DS growth chart. Monitor feedings for length of feeding, feeding schedule, loss of feeding by vomiting, or poor seal on nipple. Monitor type of formula and caloric content.	• Nutritionist can advise on formula adjustments. Therapists can help with positioning and types of nipples used to counteract effects of weak sucking reflex and large, protruding tongue.

(continued)

Table 56-1 Down Syndrome (DS) *(Continued)*

POTENTIAL PROBLEMS	EVALUATION	MANAGEMENT
Short stature (100%)	• Plot growth on DS growth chart. Monitor stages of puberty. Delayed puberty may warrant further investigation.	• Use of human growth hormone may be considered; this is still controversial.
Obesity (50%)	• Monitor thyroid hormone levels. Serial monitoring of weight. Monitor for amount of exercise and caloric intake.	• Overindulgence by adults or use of food in behavior management increases risk of overeating. Lack of social involvement leads to decreased activity. Behavior modification is necessary.
Malocclusions (60%–100%)	• Assess for malocclusions, periodontal disease, and delayed eruption of teeth. Regular dental checkups begin at age 1 yr or when teeth erupt.	• Encourage good oral hygiene with proper toothbrushing.
Mental retardation with varying degrees from mild to moderate (100%)	• Routine developmental assessment using standardized tools of measurement.	• Special education and training.
Alzheimer disease after age 40 (15%–30%)	• Assess for decreased cognitive function and loss of memory. MRI or CT scan shows areas of plaque.	• Increased supervision is needed.
Seizures (6%)	• Onset of seizures is seen primarily during adolescence and middle age.	• Neurologic evaluation and appropriate antiseizure medications.
Other problems • Communication disorders • Alopecia (10%) • Leukemia (1%)		

AV, atrioventricular; CT, computed tomography; GI, gastrointestinal; MRI, magnetic resonance imaging; PDA, patent ductus arteriosus; TSH, thyroid-stimulating hormone; T3, triiodothyronine; T4, levothyroxine; VSD, ventricular septal defect.

Considerations for Adult Patients with Down Syndrome

 EVIDENCE BASE Esbensen, A. (2016). Sleep problems and associated comorbidities among adults with Down syndrome. *Journal of Intellectual Disability Research, 60*(1), 68–79.

Silva, V., Campos, C., Sa, A., et al. (2017). Wii-based exercise program to improve physical fitness, motor proficiency and functional mobility in adults with Down syndrome. *Journal of Intellectual Disability, 61*(8), 755–765.

Infants born with Down syndrome today are expected to live well into their 50s. Adults with Down syndrome experience accelerated aging and have a higher incidence of dementia. Other medical problems more prevalent in this population include spinal and neck problems, pulmonary hypertension, hypothyroidism, testicular cancer, sleep apnea, and dermatologic problems. Mental health disorders can include depression and obsessive–compulsive disorder. Annual health exams are crucial, and every attempt should be made to find a health care provider that is comfortable with these patients and knowledgeable of the specific health maintenance concerns.

Fragile X Syndrome

Fragile X syndrome is the second most common identifiable cause of intellectual developmental disability as well as the most common inherited cause. About 80% of boys with fragile syndrome demonstrate intellectual disabilities compared to about one third of females. The fragile X phenotype is nonspecific and commonly becomes more apparent with age; therefore, diagnosis usually is not made until midchildhood or later. This syndrome can cause a wide range of cognitive and behavioral characteristics, ranging from mild to severe. Chromosome analysis reveals that the long arm of the X chromosome is constricted and appears fragile, but this cannot be detected in all cases; thus, deoxyribonucleic acid (DNA) analysis is preferred for diagnosis. Fragile X is more common in males, occurring in 1 in 2,500 to 4,000 boys and 1 in 7,000 to 8,000 girls. Genetic counseling and testing of family members are necessary to evaluate recurrence risks.

Pathophysiology and Etiology

See Chapter 4, page 30.

Clinical Manifestations and Associated Problems

1. Mild to moderate developmental delays (IQ range 41 to 88).
2. Elongated face, prominent ears, macrocephaly, high-arched palate, dental crowding, epicanthal folds (fold of the skin on either side of the nose), hypertelorism (increased distance between the eyes), and flattened nasal bridge.
3. Macroorchidism (enlarged testicles) after puberty.
4. Delay in both expressive and receptive language and perseverative or repetitive speech.
5. Delay in adaptive behavior skills.
6. Autistic-like communication disorders.
7. Attention deficit and hyperactivity.
8. Self-stimulating and self-injurious behaviors such as hand biting.
9. Associated problems, including mitral valve prolapse, seizures, joint laxity or hyperextensibility, and feeding problems.
10. Adult patients may develop tremors and ataxia.
11. Women are at risk for premature ovarian failure and early menopause.

Diagnosis and Management

1. See "Care of the Child with a Developmental Disability," page 1453, for a general approach to management.
2. See Table 56-2, for specific medical issues related to fragile X syndrome.

Turner Syndrome

Turner syndrome is a genetic disorder found in females. The incidence of this syndrome is approximately 1 in 2,000 female live births. The most severe phenotype occurs in approximately 50% of females with the absence of an X chromosome. There are typically mosaic variations seen with Turner syndrome and the clinical effects can vary between individuals. It is important to note that most girls will present with short stature and/or ovarian failure, but the other syndrome characteristics may not be present or may be present in mild form, causing a delay in diagnosis. The cognitive impairments and phenotype can be nonspecific in early childhood, and a diagnosis is commonly not made until failure of pubertal development is noted.

Pathophysiology and Etiology

See Chapter 4, page 30.

Clinical Manifestations and Associated Problems

1. The most prevalent characteristics of Turner syndrome include:
   a. Short stature, webbed neck, low posterior hairline, and edema of the hands and feet (see Figure 56-2).
   b. Congenital cardiac defects.

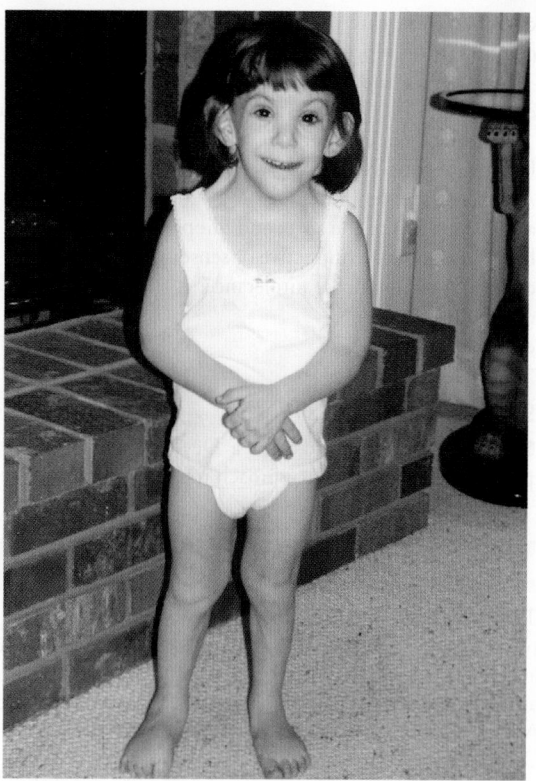

Figure 56-2. A 3-year-old child with Turner syndrome. Note the webbed neck.

Table 56-2	Fragile X Syndrome	
POTENTIAL PROBLEMS	**EVALUATION**	**MANAGEMENT**
Hypotonia of infancy	• Assess ability to control the head and assume upright posture. • Assess feeding for efficient suck and coordination of suck/swallow.	Physical therapy, stimulation program, feeding adaptations.
Seizures (20% of cases)	• Assess for muscle tremors, deviation of the eyes to one side, rhythmic jerking of the body, and loss of consciousness.	Referral to a neurologist for diagnosis and anticonvulsants to treat seizures.
Mitral valve prolapse (80% of males)	• Assess dyspnea, cyanosis, and murmur. Echocardiogram to evaluate valve function.	Antibiotics for prophylaxis before invasive procedures to prevent endocarditis. Treatment of heart failure; surgical repair may be necessary.
Self-stimulating behavior	• Rule out source of pain (ie, otitis media, tooth pain) that may be causing behavior. Rule out sensory deficits.	Behavior management techniques: Focus on replacing undesirable behaviors with purposeful, meaningful ones, with emphasis on positive reinforcement and extinguishing negative reinforcement.
Hyperactivity, attention deficits	• Assess activity of attention span within the context of the developmental age of the child.	Behavior management and special educational techniques.
Discipline problems	• Assess social skills.	Males tend to do best in self-contained classrooms for children with similar degrees of mental retardation.
Communication disorders	• Assess language development (usually weakest area of development).	Speech–language therapy can be beneficial.
Poor auditory memory; auditory reception	• Assess how child lets needs be known: cries, gestures, single words, or sentences.	Speech therapy, behavior modification.
Cognitive dysfunction • Short-term memory deficits • Poor problem-solving skills • Functional limitations in self-care	• Assess for appropriateness of educational placement and child's reaction to situation.	Specialized training and education, assisted living.

c. Broad chest with inverted or underdeveloped nipples.

d. Immature reproductive organs, delayed puberty, and primary amenorrhea.

e. Hypothyroidism, obesity, type II diabetes, osteoporosis, and fractures in adulthood.

f. Learning disabilities.

2. Associated problems include:

a. Coarctation of the aorta and idiopathic hypertension.

b. Hearing loss—conductive or sensorineural.

c. Obesity and glucose intolerance.

d. Feeding problems.

e. Renal anomalies.

Diagnosis and Management

1. See "Care of the Child with a Developmental Disability," page 1453, for a general approach to assessment.

2. See Table 56-3, for specific medical issues related to Turner syndrome.

3. Diagnosis may occur prenatally through an amniocentesis, with genetic testing, or any time after birth. A preliminary diagnosis may be made based on physical characteristics. This should then be confirmed by genetic testing. A diagnosis is often not made until there is a failure to begin menstruation.

Fetal Alcohol Spectrum Disorder

Fetal alcohol spectrum disorder (FASD) is a significant problem. Children with FASD have a wide range of physical, mental, behavioral, and/or learning disabilities that put them at risk. FASD is the leading known preventable cause of intellectual developmental disabilities in developed countries.

Table 56-3	Turner Syndrome	
POTENTIAL PROBLEMS	**EVALUATION**	**MANAGEMENT**
Congenital heart malformations: • Increased incidence of left-sided heart anomalies • Aortic valve anomalies • Coarctation of the aorta	Observe for color changes, pulse, and respiratory rate at rest and with stress. Monitor blood pressure. Assess tolerance of feeding for early tiring or frequent interruptions in feeding. An electrocardiogram should be done in the neonatal period. A yearly echocardiogram or magnetic resonance imaging should also be done.	Early identification and treatment can prevent secondary problems. If needed, prophylactic antibiotic for subacute bacterial endocarditis. Referral to a cardiologist.
Renal and renovascular anomalies: • Horseshoe kidney • Duplicated renal pelvis • Vascular anomalies	Renal sonogram should be done to rule out anomalies. Routine urinalysis and culture to screen for urinary tract infection and glycosuria.	Referral to a nephrologist if a renal anomaly is present. Monitor for the development of diabetes mellitus.
Edema in the hands and feet	Edema may persist for months or may recur; if recurrence, monitor for renal or cardiac causes.	—
Dysmorphic features: webbed neck, face, ears	Parents may elect plastic surgery to minimize the visible defects.	Enhances the socialization of females with Turner syndrome in school. May need additional support or therapy.
Nutrition: failure to thrive in the infant period and obesity in childhood	Infants may have inefficient sucking and swallowing reflexes. Monitor growth utilizing a Turner syndrome growth chart.	Nutrition counseling and encouragement of exercise to maintain appropriate weight.
Hearing loss	Hearing loss may be conductive or sensorineural. Routine screening should be performed.	Otitis media should be treated aggressively to minimize potential hearing loss.
Short stature and failure to develop secondary sex characteristics	—	Endocrine therapy may be indicated for growth and development. Hormonal therapy may enhance the development of secondary sex characteristics.
Infertility	Ovaries are not developed. Usually no need for testing.	Infertility is generally expected in Turner syndrome. Infertility techniques may be able to assist with childbearing.
Hypothyroidism	Periodic laboratory testing.	Thyroid hormone replacement therapy.
Behavioral problems, learning disabilities	—	Behavioral management. Special education.
Strabismus	If detected, referral to an ophthalmologist is recommended.	Patching or surgical repair.
Cognitive function	Average to slightly below-average intelligence. Problem areas include spatial perception and math functions.	Special education.

Pathophysiology and Etiology

1. According to the National Institute on Alcohol Abuse and Alcoholism of the NIH, the prevalence of FASD in the general population ranges from 0.2 to 7 cases per 1,000 children and 2% to 5% for the entire continuum of FASD. It is caused by use or abuse of alcohol during pregnancy. The alcohol ingested by the mother passes easily across the placenta to the fetus.
   a. There is no "safe" level of alcohol use during pregnancy and a pregnant woman who drinks any amount of alcohol is at risk.
   b. Larger amounts of alcohol and binge drinking appear to cause more significant risk to the fetus.
   c. Alcohol use in the first trimester is more problematic.

Clinical Manifestations and Associated Problems

 EVIDENCE BASE Pei, J., Baugh, L., & Andrew, G. (2017). Intervention recommendations and subsequent access to services following clinical assessment for fetal alcohol spectrum disorders. *Research in Developmental Disabilities, 60,* 176–186.

1. Intrauterine growth delay.
2. Decreased muscle tone and poor coordination.
3. Delayed development and problems in three or more major areas: cognitive, speech, motor, or social skills.
4. Hyperactivity and attention deficits.
5. Vision or hearing problems.
6. Heart defects such as ventricular septal defect or atrial septal defect.
7. Craniofacial abnormalities including narrow, small eyes with large epicanthal folds, small head, small upper jaw, smooth groove in the upper lip, and smooth and thin upper lip.
8. The average IQ is 65 with a range from 20 to 120, with many of these children qualifying for special education services.
9. Many will go on to have disrupted school progress, criminal offenses, and alcohol- and drug-related problems.

Diagnosis and Management

1. Diagnosis is usually made with history and clinical presentation. Ultrasounds during pregnancy may demonstrate physical features. Brain imaging studies (CT and MRI) may be performed later to document neuroabnormalities.
2. Management includes evaluation and regular monitoring of growth and nutrition. Ongoing management of symptoms related to other medical issues is a priority.
3. Nurses should be knowledgeable of educational and community resources that may be necessary for the child to reach his or her maximum potential. See "Care of the Child with a Developmental Disability," page 1453.

PERVASIVE DEVELOPMENTAL DISORDER OR AUTISM SPECTRUM DISORDER

Autism spectrum disorders refer to a group of pervasive developmental disorders including autism, Asperger disorder (AD), and disorders noted as pervasive developmental disorder not otherwise specified. This disorder has been identified in 1 in 42 males and 1 in 189 females averaging 1 in 68 children.

Autism

 EVIDENCE BASE Celia, T., Freysteinson, W., & Frye, R. (2016). Concurrent medical conditions in autism spectrum disorders. *Pediatric Nursing, 42*(5), 230–234.

Autism is a complex neurobiological developmental disorder that most typically appears during the first 2 years of life. The diagnosis of autism is based on a persistent deficit in social communication and social interaction across multiple contexts as manifested in the time of exam or by history. Autism is a lifelong disorder defined by the individual's interactive difficulties, which can range from mild to severely impaired. It is four to five times more common in males than in females, but affected females tend to be more severely impaired.

Approximately 50% of people with autism are cognitively impaired, with a wide range of potential IQs. Autism is seen in approximately 60 to 70 per 10,000 live births.

Pathophysiology and Etiology

1. A clear cause has not been identified; however, evidence suggests a genetic predisposition, but no specific mutation has been identified.
2. Studies have shown that measles, mumps, and rubella vaccine do *not* cause autism. Likewise, thimerosal, a preservative found in many vaccines, does *not* cause autism.
3. Before diagnosis, parents may be initially concerned about their infant's social interactions, delayed or unusual speech development, and reactions to various stimuli (ie, tactile defensiveness).
4. Individuals with ASD have neuroanatomical differences, including small neuron cell size, increased cell packing, relative macrocephaly, and large third ventricles.

Clinical Manifestations

1. In general, the features present with the diagnosis include problems with social interactions, communication, and language skills.
2. Patients with autism have abnormalities in relating to people, objects, and events. They have abnormal responses to sensory stimuli, usually sound.
3. The stereotypical behaviors of autism are restricted and repetitive, like the commonly known symptom of echolalic speech.

Diagnosis and Management

 EVIDENCE BASE Bacon, E., Courchesne, E., Barnes, C., et al. (2017). Rethinking the idea of late autism spectrum disorder onset. *Developmental Psychopathology, 14,* 1–17.
Kaufmann, W., Kidd, S., Andrews, H., et al. (2017). Autism spectrum disorder in fragile X syndrome concurring conditions and current treatment. *Pediatrics, 139*(Suppl 3), 194–206.

1. Early diagnosis leads to earlier interventions, resulting in improved outcomes for these children.
2. The two major diagnostic challenges in the evaluation of ASD include making the differential diagnosis and searching for the

etiologic disorder associated with ASD (fragile X syndrome is the most common known single gene cause of ASD).

3. Comprehensive standardized assessment tools specific for ASD usually require specialized training; these tools include Childhood Autism Rating Scale (CARS), Diagnostic Interview of Social and Communication Disorders (DISCO), Autism Diagnostic Interview (ADI), Autism Diagnostic Interview Schedule (ADIS), and Checklist for Autism in Toddlers (CHAT).

4. Alternative treatments such as nutrition and vitamin therapy are being investigated, but no definitive research has been conclusive to date.

5. Many children with ASD also have psychiatric comorbidities with such conditions as obsessive–compulsive disorder, attention deficit/hyperactivity disorder (ADHD), depression, mood disorders, and Tourette syndrome. These conditions can be challenging to diagnose as it may be difficult to assess the child with communication and behavioral problems. Indeed, health care providers need to be vigilant in screening and monitoring for these comorbidities to ensure optimal functioning of the child with ASD.

6. Treatment is focused on management of symptoms. Medications may be helpful in treating some of the more disruptive behavioral symptoms. The most commonly used medications include select serotonin reuptake inhibitors, atypical antipsychotic/neuroleptics, stimulants, and alpha agonists.

7. Medical comorbidities are also common in children with ASD, including seizure disorders, sleep disturbances, GI disorders, and dental problems. As with psychiatric comorbidities, health care providers need to be vigilant in their assessment, as it can improve behavior and functioning of the child with ASD.

8. A multidisciplinary team—including primary care provider; medical subspecialists; occupational, speech, and physical therapists; and educational specialist—is essential for optimal care. See "Care of the Child with a Developmental Disability," page 1453.

Childhood Disintegrative Disorder

Childhood disintegrative disorder follows a period of normal development. This normal developmental period may last from ages 2 to 10 years, with the most common age of onset being 3 and 4 years of age. The child begins to experience a significant loss of previously acquired skills. Areas that may be affected include expressive and receptive language, social skills or adaptive behavior, bowel and bladder control, and motor skills. The loss of these skills generally reaches a point at which they do not disintegrate further. At such point, some limited improvements may be seen. This condition differs from autism in the pattern of onset, course, and outcome.

Pathophysiology and Etiology

Etiology is unknown. Childhood disintegrative disorder appears to be more common in males. The incidence of this disorder is rare.

Diagnosis and Management

See "Care of the Child with a Developmental Disability," page 1453, for a general approach to assessment.

Asperger Disorder

Asperger disorder is considered a milder form of autism and is characterized by poor peer relationships, lack of empathy, and the tendency to be overfocused on certain topics.

Asperger disorder is one of several developmental disabilities associated with normal intelligence. Academic and functional underachievement in the preschool and school-age child with normal intelligence is the common picture. Proper diagnosis, utilizing a cooperative team effort from several individuals, is imperative to develop an individualized treatment plan.

Pathophysiology and Etiology

The etiology is unknown. Asperger disorder is commonly not diagnosed until the child reaches school age. The prevalence estimates vary widely with many individuals never being formally diagnosed.

Clinical Manifestations

1. Child does not seek spontaneous interpersonal interactions.
2. Average to above-average intelligence and development of normal language skills with regard to vocabulary and grammar.
3. No significant delays in the areas of cognitive development, development of age-appropriate self-help skills, adaptive behavior, and curiosity about the environment.
4. Limited range of interests, strict adherence to routines and rituals, and repetitious motor movements or sequences.
5. May have obsessional interests and appear "eccentric" to others.

Diagnosis and Management

1. Complete medical review, family history, and physical examination, including vision and hearing assessment and neurologic evaluation, to rule out other disorders.
2. Genetic evaluation and counseling to identify the presence of recurrence risks.
3. Psychological testing to determine the exact nature of cognitive and perceptual dysfunctions.
4. Behavioral and social assessment.
5. Assessment of academic performance.
6. MRI and other testing to determine underlying neurologic abnormality, if appropriate.
7. Occupational and physical therapy and speech and language evaluations, as necessary.
8. School evaluation—involves IQ testing and achievement testing (teacher's input is also essential).
   a. The focus of a school evaluation is to determine eligibility for services. Most school systems will provide services only when moderate to severe problems exist.
   b. It may be necessary for the family to provide remediation for problems considered mild or outside of the educational setting.
9. Because the disorder may include health manifestations as well as behavioral and educational implications, the school nurse should be prepared to provide guidance on complex management.

 EVIDENCE BASE Ward, B. (2016). Sibling Experiences: Living with Young Persons with Autism Spectrum Disorders. *Pediatric Nursing, 42*(2), 69–76.

Pervasive Developmental Disorder, Not Otherwise Specified

Pervasive developmental disorder, not otherwise specified (PDD-NOS) was used when the child meets some but not all criteria for the diagnosis of autism. A diagnosis may be made at a later date because of the appearance of additional manifestation. The DSM-5 notes that individuals with a well-established diagnosis of autistic disorder, Asperger disorder, or pervasive developmental disorder not otherwise specified should be given the diagnosis of autism spectrum disorder. This suggests that there is a spectrum of developmental disorders with common features, which may range widely in severity and represent a range of genetically influenced impairments.

ATTENTION DISORDERS AND LEARNING DISABILITIES

Attention disorders and learning disabilities are separate but overlapping problems and may need specific approaches based on the nature of the disability. An estimated 5% to 10% of children (ranging up to 30%) have attention deficit disorder (ADD); learning disabilities are reportedly present in 12.6% of children by the end of the second grade. Learning disabilities and ADD commonly occur together.

Pathophysiology and Etiology

1. Multiple hypotheses exist because the exact causes are unknown and may be genetic.
   a. A family trait—other members of the family have similar difficulties.
   b. Characteristic of inborn errors of metabolism.
   c. Sex chromosome abnormalities commonly exhibit these traits.
2. Not shown to be associated with a history of birth trauma or brain damage.
3. Exposure to prenatal and postnatal factors that might adversely affect brain development and function—lead, alcohol, cocaine, central nervous system (CNS) infections, low birth weight, and prematurity.
4. May coexist with other disabling conditions, such as spina bifida, cerebral palsy, or seizure disorders.
5. May have biomedical, emotional, social, and environmental components.
6. ADD is an alteration in the response-inhibition mechanisms of the brain controlled by the frontal cortex and reticular activating system and alteration in neurotransmitter.
7. Learning disabilities—authorities are investigating abnormalities in the parietal lobe of the brain and in the central visual pathways located in the occipital lobe.
8. Although emotional and environmental factors play a role, serotonin deficiency may serve as a physiologic basis for these disorders.

Attention Disorders

 EVIDENCE BASE Ahmann, E. (2017). Interventions in children and teens: A focus on ADHD coaching. *Pediatric Nursing, 43*(3), 343–349.

Attention disorders are characterized by a cluster of symptoms, including developmentally inappropriate short attention span, impulsivity, and distractibility. The classification system identifies three subtypes of attention disorders: predominantly inattentive, predominantly hyperactive–impulsive, and combined. Attention disorders are more common in boys than in girls by a ratio of 3 to 1. Females are much more likely to have inattentive type, showing more symptoms of attention deficit rather than hyperactivity.

There is no specific laboratory test or radiographical test that can diagnose attention disorders. The best way to diagnose attention disorders is through careful history from parents, child, and teachers; use of standardized questionnaires or rating scales; and observation. There are a number of behavior rating scales that

are used to establish the diagnosis of ADD and ADHD. Examples of rating scales include the Conners Rating Scale, the Brown Attention Deficit Disorder Scale for Children and Adolescents, and the Vanderbilt ADHD Rating Scale.

Clinical Manifestations and Diagnostic Evaluation

General Behavior

 EVIDENCE BASE Burns, C. (2017). Cognitive-perceptual disorders. In C. Burns, A. Dunn, M. Brady, et al. (Eds.), *Pediatric primary care* (pp. 393–409). Philadelphia, PA: Elsevier.

Behavior varies slightly based on the child's age. Some impairments across the life span can include:

1. Childhood: Needs for special education, grade retention, classroom behavior management issues, and behavioral difficulties at home and other settings.
2. Adolescence: School failure and dropout, social difficulties with peer relationships, substance abuse (in untreated), high comorbidity with other psychiatric disorders, and involvement in juvenile criminal activities.
3. Adult: Fewer employment possibilities and frequent job hopping; high risk of tobacco, drug, and alcohol use; high risk of motor vehicle accidents; marital problems and higher divorce rates; and increased incidence of criminal activity.

Diagnostic Criteria for ADHD

Diagnostic criteria are outlined in the *Diagnostic and Statistical Manual of Mental Disorders, Fifth Edition*, Text Revision (DSM-5) criteria for attention deficit/hyperactivity disorder. In this edition, the core symptoms reflect how the disorder presents in school-age children, as well as older adolescents and adults. Examples of questions include:

1. Does the child often fidget with hands or feet or squirm in seat?
2. Does the child have difficulty remaining seated when required to do so?
3. Is the child easily distracted by extraneous stimuli?
4. Does the child have difficulty awaiting his or her turn in games or group situations?
5. Does the child often blurt out answers to questions before they have been completed?
6. Does the child often have difficulty following instructions from others?
7. Does the child have difficulty sustaining attention in tasks or play activities?
8. Does the child often shift from one uncompleted activity to another?
9. Does the child have difficulty playing quietly?
10. Does the child often talk excessively?
11. Does the child often interrupt or intrude on others?
12. Does the child often not seem to listen to what is being said to him or her?
13. Does the child often lose things necessary for tasks or activities at school or at home?
14. Does the child often engage in physically dangerous activities without considering possible consequences?

Management

Multidisciplinary Approach

A multidisciplinary approach, including environmental and behavioral approaches, is the treatment of choice.

Pharmacologic Treatment

1. CNS stimulants are effective for 70% to 80% of children with attention disorders.
   a. Effective in decreasing motor activities and increasing attention span and concentration, thereby allowing the child to be more available to learn.
   b. Medications generally include stimulant medications, but nonstimulant medications may also be effective, especially in adults. Examples include methylphenidate, dextroamphetamine, amphetamine, lisdexamfetamine, and atomoxetine.
2. Adverse effects:
   a. Insomnia may result from increased dosage or if administered too late in the day.
   b. Anorexia, weight loss, hair loss, and temporary growth retardation.
   c. Increased pulse and respiratory rates, nervousness, nausea, and stomachache.
   d. Altered effects of many antiseizure drugs and tricyclic antidepressants.
   e. Do not cause euphoric effect or addiction in children.

Nursing Responsibilities and Family Education

1. Administer the drug before breakfast and lunch (sustained-release forms may not require a second dose).
2. Work with school system to make sure that the lunch dose is given.
3. Consider "drug holidays" during vacations and on weekends to monitor effectiveness and the need for a dosage change; this is especially recommended at the start of each academic school year.
4. "Drug holidays" may be difficult in the older adolescent population as the medication may be necessary for optimal functioning in employment and while driving motor vehicles.
5. Based on the newest evidence, it appears that children without cardiac disease who receive stimulant therapy are not at increased cardiovascular events compared with the general population, so cardiac evaluations are not routinely ordered.
6. Stimulant drugs are not usually given to children younger than age 6.
7. The child is usually started on a small dose, which is gradually increased until the desired response is achieved.
8. Evaluate the child's response to the drug by direct observation and consultation with others, such as parents and teachers.

 DRUG ALERT Stimulant drugs for attention disorders should be used in conjunction with a comprehensive therapeutic regimen and not as the sole method of treatment. Stimulant drugs require monitoring and feedback from the parents and teachers who directly observe the effects.

Learning Disability

Difficulties with academic achievement fall under a broad category of learning problems. The cause or influencing factors can be biomedical, developmental, behavioral, emotional, social, environmental, and family issues. The problem may be in the area of reading, math, written expression, motor skills, and communication disorders. Attention deficit, anxiety, and behavioral disorders must be ruled out.

Clinical Manifestations

1. Signs of learning disabilities include:
   a. School achievement significantly lower than potential.
   b. Perceptual–motor impairments.
   c. Emotional lability.
   d. Speech and language disorders.
   e. Coordination deficits.
2. There can be a wide range of cognitive ability from mild retardation to above-average intelligence.

Areas of Learning Disabilities

Auditory Perception

Auditory perception is characterized by difficulty distinguishing between similar sounds or words. This includes the inability to process the sounds into words that have a meaning at a rapid enough rate to be able to follow conversations.

Visual Perception

Visual perception difficulties involve problems interpreting what is seen. This may include problems recognizing shapes and positions of letters or words. Depth perception may pose a problem to some children with visual perception disorders.

Integrative Processing

Integrative processing disabilities encompass, to varying degrees, the inability to sequence events or facts, comprehend abstract ideas or implied meanings, and organize learned information and apply it to what has been previously acquired.

Memory

Disabilities generally affect short-term memory, which stores information that has just been perceived for a brief period before it is either discarded or stored in long-term memory.

Expressive Language

An *expressive language* disorder affects the child's verbal communication. Characteristics depend on the child's age and the severity of the disorder. Language skills in terms of vocabulary, grammatical content, fluency, and language formulation can be affected.

Motor

Motor disabilities can affect either gross motor or fine motor muscle groups. A disability affecting the gross motor development can cause children to be "clumsy." These children have a tendency to fall or bump into things and have difficulty running and playing sports. Fine motor disabilities affect muscles for detailed tasks, such as writing, using scissors, and painting.

Management and Special Teaching Strategies

1. For visual perceptual deficit—present material verbally; use hands-on experience; tape-record teaching sessions.
2. For auditory perceptual deficit—provide materials in written form; use pictures; provide tactile learning.
3. For integrative deficit—use multisensory approaches; print directions while you verbalize them; use calendars and lists to organize tasks and activities.
4. For motor and expressive deficits—break down skills and projects into their multiple component parts; verbally describe the component parts; provide extra time to perform; allow the child to type work rather than use cursive writing.
5. For highly distractible child—provide a structured environment; have child sit in the front of the class; place child away from doors or windows; decrease clutter on his or her desk.

NURSING ALERT Historically, preschool and kindergarten screening tools have not been accurate in predicting learning disabilities; newer tests of language and memory are better predictors.

RESOURCES AND SUPPORT GROUPS

Agencies that may provide information, support, and additional resources include:

The ARC of the United States (formerly Association for Retarded Citizens of the United States)
1825 K Street NW, Suite 1200
Washington, DC 20006
(800) 433-5255
www.thearc.org

Autism Society
4340 East-West Hwy, Suite 350
Bethesda, MD 20814
www.autism-society.org

Children and Adults with Attention Deficit/Hyperactivity Disorder (CHADD)
4601 Presidents Drive, Suite 300
Landover, MD 20706
(301) 306-7070
www.chadd.org

Council for Learning Disabilities
11184 Antioch Road
P.O. Box 405
Overland Park, KS 66210
(913) 491-1011
www.cldinternational.org

The Joseph P. Kennedy Jr. Foundation
1325 G St. NW
Washington, DC 20005
(202) 393-1250
www.jpkf.org

Learning Disabilities Association of America
4156 Library Road, #1
Pittsburgh, PA 15234-1349
(412) 341-1515
www.ldanatl.org

National Down Syndrome Congress
30 Mansell Court, Suite 108
Roswell, GA 30076
(800) 232-NDSC
www.ndsccenter.org

National Down Syndrome Society
8 E 41st Street, 8th floor
New York, New York 10017
(800) 221-4602
www.ndss.org

National Fragile X Foundation
2100 M St NW #170
Washington, DC 20037
https://fragilex.org

 TRANSITIONAL CARE ALERT After the stress of having a hospitalized child, families will need support in the transition to home or another aftercare location. It is crucial that they have complete and understandable care instructions on home care, medications, and follow-up appointments. If arrangements have been made for nursing care in the home, families should be aware of the agency providing services and when they can expect communication regarding care arrangements. Families should have thorough written (and if necessary to assist understanding, pictorial) instructions on signs and symptoms to monitor for that could suggest worsening of status, especially if the child is nonverbal and cannot relay symptoms to the caregivers. Children with developmental disorders may be discharged to home requiring oxygen or other procedures (like suctioning) or both. Nurses responsible for discharging children should ensure that families understand (and can demonstrate care if possible) proper use of necessary treatments. If the child is cared for in a residence other than that of the family caregiver, health care providers should ensure that the individuals caring for the child after the hospitalization are knowledgeable and comfortable providing necessary care.

SELECTED REFERENCES

Ahmann, E. (2017). Interventions in children and teens: A focus on ADHD coaching. *Pediatric Nursing, 43*(3), 343–349.

American Psychiatric Association. (2013). *Diagnostic and statistical manual of mental disorders* (5th ed.). Washington, DC: Author.

Bacon, E., et al. (2017). Rethinking the idea of late autism spectrum disorder onset. *Development and Psychopathology, 14,* 1–17.

Bennett, E., et al. (2017). Treatment of obesity among youth with intellectual and developmental disabilities: An emerging role for telenursing. *Western Journal of Nursing Research, 39*(8), 1008–1027.

Bergstrom, S., et al. (2016). Trends in congenital heart defects in infants with Down syndrome. *Pediatrics, 138*(1), e20160123, Epub.

Blows, E., Teoh, L., & Paul, S. (2016). Recognition and management of learning disabilities in early childhood by community practitioners. *Community Practitioner, 89*(5), 32–37.

Bricker, D., Macy, M., Squires, J., & Marks, K. (2013). *Developmental screening in your community: An integrated approach for connecting children with services.* Baltimore, MD: Brookes.

Brown, N., Finch, J., Obradovic, J., et al. (2017). Maternal care mediates the effects of nutrition and responsive stimulation interventions on young children's growth. *Child: Care, Health & Development, 43*(4), 577–587.

Bunt, C., & Bunt, S. (2014). Role of the family physician in the care of children with Down syndrome. *American Family Physician, 90*(12), 851–858.

Burns, C. (2017). Genetic disorders. In C. Burns, A. Dunn, M. Brady, et al. (Eds.), *Pediatric primary care* (pp. 1032–1054). Philadelphia, PA: Elsevier.

Castillo, M., Clark, D., Schaller, E., et al. (2018). Descriptive assessment of problem behavior during transitions of children with intellectual and developmental disabilities. *Journal of Applied Behavior Analysis, 51*(1), 99–117.

Celia, T., Freysteinson, W., & Frye, R. (2016). Concurrent medical conditions in autism spectrum disorders. *Pediatric Nursing, 42*(5), 230–234.

Challinor, G., Baggley, J., & Finney, A. (2017). Making a difference for patient with learning disabilities. *Practice Nurse, 47*(3), 26–30.

Crawford, D. (2016) Down's syndrome. *Nursing Children & Young People, 28*(9), 17.

DeVeney, S., Hoffman, L., & Cress, C. (2012). Communication-based assessment of developmental age for young children with developmental disabilities. *Journal of Speech, Language, and Hearing Research, 55*(3), 695–709.

Esbensen, A. (2016). Sleep problems and associated comorbidities among adults with Down syndrome. *Journal of Intellectual Disability Research, 60*(1), 68–79.

Esbenson, A., Boshkoff, E., Amaral, J., et al. (2016). Differentiating aging among adults with Down syndrome and comorbid dementia or psychopathology. *American Journal on Intellectual & Developmental Disabilities, 121*(1), 13–24.

Frolli, A., Piscopo, S., & Conson, M. (2015). Developmental changes in cognitive and behavioral functioning of adolescents with fragile-X syndrome. *Journal of Intellectual Disability Research, 59*(7), 613–621.

Heslam, S. (2011). Health issues for adults with Down's syndrome. *Learning Disability Practice, 14*(6), 26–27.

Hurley, K., Yousafzai, A., & Lopez-Boo, F. (2016). Early child development and nutrition: A review of the benefits and challenges of implementing integrated interventions. *Advances in Nutrition, 7*(2), 357–363.

Ibrahim, K., & Donyai, P. (2015). Drug holidays from ADHD medication: International experience over the past four decades. *Journal of Attention Disorders, 19*(7), 551–568.

Ibrahim, K., Vogt, C., & Donyai, P. (2016). Caught in the eye of the storm: A qualitative study of views and experiences of planned drug holidays form methylphenidate in child and adolescent ADHD treatment. *Child and Adolescent Mental Health, 21*(4), 192–2000.

Inoune, M., et al. (2017). Fetal alcohol spectrum disorder information dissemination by health care professions. *Journal of Social Work Practice in the Addictions, 17*(3), 275–290.

Ivan, D., & Cromwell, P. (2014). Clinical practice guidelines for management of children with down syndrome: Part 1. *Journal of Pediatric Health Care, 28*(1), 105–110.

Jones, P. (2016). Thoughtfulness and grace: End-of-life decision making for children with severe developmental disabilities. *American Journal of Bioethics, 16*(2), 72–73.

Kaufmann, W., et al. (2017). Autism spectrum disorder in fragile X syndrome concurring conditions and current treatment. *Pediatrics, 139*(Suppl 3), 194–206.

Khatri, S., & Carlisle, J. (2016). Down syndrome. *Contemporary Pediatrics, 33*(8), 30–46.

King, E., Esposito, C., & Sollazzo, L. (2017). Providing end-of-life care for developmentally disabled individuals. *Journal of the New York State Nurses Association, 45*(1), 1–10.

Kleinman, R., & Greer, F. (2014). Nutritional support for children with developmental disabilities. In *Pediatric nutrition* (7th ed., pp. 883–906). Elk Grove Village, IL: American Academy of Pediatrics.

Kryszak, E., Mulick, J., & Butler, E. (2017). Autism. In T. McInerny, H. Adam, D. Campbell, et al. (Eds.), *American Academy of Pediatrics textbook of pediatric care.* Elk Grove Village, IL: American Academy of Pediatrics.

Kwiatek, E., Powell, H., & Mathieson, A. (2016). Supporting students to care for people with learning disabilities. *Learning Disability Practice, 19*(3), 24–27.

Lauderdale-Littin, S., & Blacher, J. (2017). Young adults with severe intellectual disability: Culture, parent, and sibling impact. *Journal of Intellectual & Developmental Disability, 42*(3), 230–239.

Lee, C., Walter, G., & Cleary, M. (2012). Communicating with children with autism spectrum disorder and their families: A practical introduction. *Journal of Psychosocial Nursing and Mental Health Services, 50*(8), 40–44.

Lehmann, K., Hales, L., & Glackin, M. (2015). Regular medication reviews for children and young people with ADHD. *Nurse Prescribing, 13*(11), 562–568.

Leigers, K., Kleinert, H., & Carter, E. (2017). "I never truly thought about them having friends": Equipping schools to foster peer relationships. *Rural Special Education Quarterly, 36*(2), 73–83.

Lovette, B. (2008). Safe transportation for children with special needs. *Journal of Pediatric Health Care, 22*, 323–328.

Lynch, B., et al. (2015). Developmental screening and follow-up by nurses. *MCN: The American Journal of Maternal Child Nursing, 40*(6), 388–393.

McIntosh, C., Thomas, C., & Brattain, C. (2016). Nurses identify education and communicating among professionals as essential in service ASD children. *NASN School Nurse, 31*(3), 164–169.

McKenzie, K., et al. (2017). Out of school and into distress: Families of young adults with intellectual and developmental disabilities in transition. *Journal of Applied Research in Intellectual Disabilities, 30*(4), 774–781.

Milbrandt, T., & Thomas, E. (2013). Turner syndrome. *Pediatrics in Review, 34*(9), 420–421.

Milen, M., & Nicholas, D. (2017). Examining transitions from youth to adult services for young persons with autism. *Social Work in Health Care, 56*(7), 636–648.

Miller, H., et al. (2017). An exploratory study of the knowledge of personal safety skills among children with developmental disabilities and their parents. *Journal of Applied Research in Intellectual Disabilities, 30*(2), 290–300.

Mills, S., & Black, L. (2014). Ensuring children with Down's syndrome reach their full potential. *British Journal of School Nursing, 9*(2), 97–99.

Murphy, C., et al. (2016). Sex education and intellectual disability: Practices and insight from pediatric genetic counselors. *Journal of Genetic Counseling, 25*(3), 552–560.

Natale, R., Camejo, S., Asfour, L., et al. (2017). Promoting healthy weight among children with developmental delays. *Journal of Early Intervention, 39*(1), 51–65.

Nguyen, T., Henderson, D., & Steward, D. (2016). You never transition alone! Exploring the experiences of youth with chronic health conditions, parents and healthcare providers on self-management. *Child Care, Health and Development, 42*(4), 464–472.

Patel, A., et al. (2017). Care provision and prescribing practices of physicians treating children and adolescents with ADHD. *Psychiatric Services, 68*(7), 681–688.

Pei, J., Baugh, L., & Andrew, G. (2017). Intervention recommendations and subsequent access to services following clinical assessment for fetal alcohol spectrum disorders. *Research in Developmental Disabilities, 60*, 176–186.

Ptomey, L., & Wittenbrook, W. (2015). Position of the academy of nutrition and dietetics: Nutrition services for individuals with intellectual and developmental disabilities and special health care needs. *Journal of the Academy of Nutrition and Dietetics, 115*(4), 593–608.

Ryan, C., Kramer, J., & Cohn, E. (2016). Exploring the self-disclosure process in peer mentoring relationships for transition-age youth with developmental disabilities. *Intellectual and Developmental Disabilities, 54*(4), 245–259.

Sarkar, T. (2015). Intellectual and developmental disability: Transition to adulthood and decision making process. *Child Health and Human Development, 8*(4), 517–527.

Silva, V., et al. (2017). Wii-based exercise program to improve physical fitness, motor proficiency and functional mobility in adults with Down syndrome. *Journal of Intellectual Disability, 61*(8), 755–765.

Sooben, R. (2015). Breastfeeding of newborns with Down's syndrome. *Learning Disability Practice, 18*(6), 26–28.

Srour, M., & Shevell, M. (2014). Genetics and the investigation of developmental delay/intellectual disability. *Archives of Disease in Childhood, 99*(4), 386–389.

Ward, B. (2016). Sibling experiences: Living with young persons with autism spectrum disorders. *Pediatric Nursing, 42*(2), 69–76.

Williams, A., et al. (2015). Pediatric developmental screenings: A primary care approach. *Nurse Practitioner, 40*(4), 34–39.

Wolf-Fordham, S., et al. (2015). Emergency preparedness of families of children with developmental disabilities: What public health and safety emergency planners need to know. *Journal of Emergency Management, 13*(1), 7–18.

Zaal-Schuller, I., et al. (2016). How parents and physicians experience end-of-life decision-making for children with profound intellectual and multiple disabilities. *Research in Developmental Disabilities, 59*, 283–293.

Zuckerman, K., Chavez, A., & Reeder, J., (2017). Decreasing disparities in child development assessment: Identifying and discussing possible delays in the special supplemental program for women, infants, and children (WIC). *Journal of Developmental & Behavioral Pediatrics, 38*(5), 301–309.

Problems of Mental Health

PART FIVE

PSYCHIATRIC NURSING

57
Problems of Mental Health

ANXIETY-RELATED DISORDERS
Anxiety

 EVIDENCE BASE American Psychiatric Association. (2013). *Diagnostic and statistical manual of mental disorders* (5th ed.). Washington, DC: Author.

Anxiety disorders are the most common of all psychiatric disorders. An individual with one of these disorders experiences physiologic, cognitive, and behavioral symptoms of anxiety. The physiologic manifestations are related to the "fight-or-flight" response and result in cardiovascular, respiratory, neuromuscular, and gastrointestinal (GI) stimulation. The cognitive symptoms include subjective feelings of apprehension, uneasiness, uncertainty, or dread. Behavioral manifestations include irritability, restlessness, pacing, crying and sighing, and complaints of tension and nervousness. The common theme among anxiety disorders is that the individual experiences a level of anxiety that interferes with functioning in personal, occupational, and social areas. *Note: obsessive–compulsive disorder is no longer classified as an anxiety disorder. It is considered part of the class of body dysmorphic and hoarding disorders, which are not covered in this book because of space constraints; however, anxiety is a key feature.*

Classification

1. Panic disorder.
2. Agoraphobia.
3. Specific phobia.
4. Social anxiety disorders.
5. Generalized anxiety disorder.
6. Anxiety disorder because of a general medical condition.
7. Substance-induced anxiety disorder.
8. Anxiety disorder not otherwise specified.

Pathophysiology and Etiology

The underlying etiology of anxiety disorders as well as any of the psychiatric disorders is complex, having multiple factors that interact. Therefore, it is essential to examine the biochemical, genetic, psychosocial, and sociocultural factors.

Biochemical Factors

1. The limbic system, which is called the *emotional brain*, regulates emotional responses. Anxiety disorders are associated with abnormalities within this system (including the frontal cortex, hypothalamus, amygdala, hippocampus, brainstem, and the autonomic nervous system).
2. Neurotransmitters and their specific receptor sites function to transmit inhibiting or stimulating messages across the synapses between nerve cells in the brain. Abnormalities in the neurotransmitters or the receptor sites have been associated with multiple psychiatric disorders, including anxiety disorders.
3. Norepinephrine is a stimulating neurotransmitter, which is released as part of the fight-or-flight response and is associated with the cardiovascular and respiratory effects of anxiety. Serotonin is a neurotransmitter that regulates multiple responses, including sleep and alertness and sensations of hunger and satiation. Genetic variation resulting in a decrease in the number of select serotonin receptors (particularly 1A) may be associated with the development of panic disorder.
4. Panic disorders may be related to the reception of a false signal from the brain that there is a shortage of oxygen or an increase in carbon dioxide (suffocation alarm theory). Those who have panic attacks have also been reported to have higher levels of norepinephrine.
5. Positron emission tomography (PET) and computed tomography (CT) scanning have shown abnormalities in glucose metabolism in the frontal and prefrontal cortex and the basal ganglia of the brains of individuals with panic disorder.

Genetic Factors

1. First-degree relatives of individuals with panic disorder have a four to seven times greater chance of developing this disorder. Twin studies demonstrate a higher concordance rate for monozygotic than dizygotic twins.
2. Approximately 20% of first-degree relatives of people with agoraphobia also have agoraphobia.
3. Approximately 25% of first-degree relatives with generalized anxiety disorder are also affected by generalized anxiety disorder.

Psychosocial Factors

1. Psychodynamic theory describes unconscious conflicts having early childhood origin and resulting from repressed wishes

and drives. These conflicts cause guilt and shame, which lead to anxiety and associated symptoms.

2. Interpersonal theory implicates early relationships, which directly affect development of self-concept and self-esteem. Individuals with poor self-concept and decreased self-esteem have increased susceptibility to anxiety-related disorders.

3. Behavioral theory describes anxiety and associated symptoms as a conditioned response to internal and external stressors.

4. Cognitive theory describes faulty thinking patterns that lead to an individual's misperceiving events affecting self, the future, and the world. These faulty thinking patterns contribute to the subjective experience of anxiety.

Sociocultural Factors

1. Anxiety disorders and ritualistic behaviors are commonly seen in high-technology societies.

2. There is a higher incidence of anxiety disorders in urban communities than in rural communities.

Clinical Manifestations

Generalized Anxiety Disorder

1. A pattern of worrying or anxiety that results in increased autonomic activity persisting for a period of at least 6 months.

2. An examination and history would reveal symptoms from three of four categories:
   a. Motor (eg, trembling, restlessness, inability to relax, and fatigue).
   b. Autonomic hyperactivity (eg, sweating, palpitations, cold clammy hands, urinary frequency, lump in the throat, pallor or flushing, increased pulse, and rapid respirations).
   c. Apprehensiveness (eg, worry, dread, fear, rumination, insomnia, and inability to concentrate).
   d. Hypervigilance (eg, feeling edgy, scanning the environment, and distractibility).

Panic Disorder

1. The presence of recurrent unexpected anxiety attacks for at least 1 month with a sudden onset of feelings of intense apprehension and dread.

2. These feelings result in sympathetic activation that manifests through the appearance of at least four of the following symptoms: chest discomfort or pain, dyspnea, palpitations, syncope, diaphoresis, trembling, hot or cold flashes, and dizziness.

Phobias

1. A phobia is a persistent irrational fear of an object or situation that the person may recognize as being unreasonable.

2. Exposure to the feared object or situation may result in a panic attack.

3. An example is agoraphobia, which is a fear of being alone in open or public places where escape might be difficult.

Diagnostic Evaluation

1. Measurement tools for anxiety:
   a. Hamilton Rating Scale for Anxiety.
   b. State–Trait Anxiety Inventory.

2. Measurement tools for panic disorders:
   a. Acute panic inventory.
   b. Sheehan Client-Rated Anxiety Scale.

3. Sodium lactate infusion or carbon dioxide inhalation will likely produce a panic attack in a person with panic disorder.

4. Increased arousal may be measured through studies of autonomic functioning (ie, heart rate, electromyography, sweat gland activity) in a person with posttraumatic stress disorder (PTSD).

5. Dexamethasone suppression test (DST) may be used to demonstrate heightened glucocorticoid feedback in individuals with PTSD.

6. Measurement tools for dissociation:
   a. Dissociation Impulsivity Scale (DIS).
   b. Dissociative Experiences Scale (DES).
   c. Dissociative Disorders Interview Schedule (DDIS).

Management

 EVIDENCE BASE Baldwin, D. S., Anderson, I. M., Nutt, D. J., et al. (2014). Evidence-based pharmacological treatment of anxiety disorders, post-traumatic stress disorder and obsessive-compulsive disorder: A revision of the 2005 guidelines from the British Association for Psychopharmacology. *Journal of Psychopharmacology, 28*(5), 403–439.
Jones, A. M., West, K. B., & Suveg, C. (2017). Anxiety in the school setting: A framework for evidence-based practice. *School Mental Health.* 2017, 1–11. Available: *doi. org/10.1007/s12310-017-9235-2.*

1. Various levels and sites of care can be provided: psychiatric inpatient, outpatient, or home care. Most care is provided on an outpatient basis. Site of care is based on many factors, including degree of disability of affected individual, community services available, and insurance and managed care considerations. Generally, the recommended treatment is a combination of drugs and psychotherapy, along with education of the individual and family.

2. Psychoeducational strategies:
   a. Relaxation techniques.
   b. Progressive muscle relaxation.
   c. Guided imagery or visualization exercises.
   d. Stress management.
   e. Assertiveness training.

3. Psychotherapy:
   a. Psychodynamic—assists people in understanding their experiences by identifying unconscious conflicts and developing effective coping behaviors.
   b. Behavioral—focuses on the individual problematic behavior and works to modify or extinguish the behavior. One form of behavioral therapy effective in management of phobic disorders is systematic desensitization.
   c. Cognitive—assists patient to question faulty thought patterns (reframing) and examine alternatives. In treatment of PTSD and dissociative disorders, reframing is used to help the patient view self as a survivor rather than a victim.
   d. Hypnotherapy—can be used as part of therapy for those suffering dissociative disorders.
   e. Support group therapy—useful in providing a supportive and psychoeducational approach for patients with anxiety or dissociative disorders.

4. Somatic therapies:
   a. Biofeedback—relaxation through biofeedback is achieved when a person learns to control physiologic mechanisms that are not ordinarily within one's awareness. Awareness and control are accomplished by monitoring body processes, including muscle tone, heart rate, and brain waves.

Table 57-1   Dosage and Adverse Reactions of Antianxiety Drugs

DRUG: CLASS/GENERIC/TRADE NAME	ADULT THERAPEUTIC DOSAGE RANGE (MG/DAY)	ADVERSE REACTIONS
Benzodiazepines		For all benzodiazepines:
Alprazolam	0.75–1 mg	• Drowsiness, sedation, and dizziness
Chlordiazepoxide	15–75 mg	• Possibility of dependence
Clonazepam	0.5–2 mg	
Clorazepate	15–60 mg	
Diazepam	4–40 mg	
Lorazepam	2–6 mg	
Oxazepam	30–120 mg	
Tetracyclic Agent		
Mirtazapine	15–45 mg	• Somnolence, increased appetite, weight gain, dry mouth, constipation
Selective Serotonin Reuptake Inhibitors (SSRIs)		
Citalopram	20–60 mg	• Nausea, dry mouth, diarrhea, fatigue, drowsiness, ejaculatory delay, impotence
Duloxetine	40–60 mg	• Nausea, dry mouth, dizziness, constipation, diarrhea, fatigue, increased sweating
Escitalopram	10–20 mg	• Nausea, ejaculatory delay, impotence
Fluoxetine	20–80 mg	• Delayed orgasm, headache, nervousness, insomnia, anxiety, tremor, dizziness, nausea, diarrhea, anorexia, dry mouth
Fluvoxamine	50–300 mg	• Nausea, vomiting, drowsiness, anorexia, constipation, tremor, insomnia
Paroxetine	10–50 mg	• Nausea, dry mouth, headache, somnolence, insomnia, diarrhea, constipation, tremor

b. Psychopharmacologic—traditionally, drugs used to treat anxiety-related disorders were those that would increase GABA (benzodiazepines), regulate serotonin levels (antidepressants), or reduce physiologic effects of anxiety by causing peripheral beta-adrenergic blockade (beta-adrenergic blockers). Currently, selective serotonin reuptake inhibitors are prescribed as first-line treatment for managing several anxiety-related disorders because of their safety and tolerability. See Table 57-1.

Complications

1. Undiagnosed medical reasons for anxiety could lead to physical deterioration and a delay in obtaining appropriate medical care. It is important to screen for coexisting medical illness.
2. If panic and phobic disorders are left untreated, they can lead to increasing social withdrawal and isolation, which may severely impair the person's social and work life.
3. Undiagnosed or untreated PTSD or acute stress disorder can lead to substance abuse or dependence, aggressive or violent behavior and, possibly, suicide.
4. If a person with a dissociative disorder goes untreated, aggressive behavior may develop toward self or others. Such behaviors may include assaults, depression, PTSD, psychoactive substance abuse disorder, rape, self-mutilation, and suicide attempts.

Nursing Assessment

1. Assess psychological, cognitive, and behavioral symptoms.
   a. Defense mechanisms or coping measures used.
   b. Mood.
   c. Suicide potential.
   d. Thought content and process.
   e. Severity of subjective experience of anxiety.
   f. Understanding of specific disorder.
2. Explore social functioning.
   a. Ability to function in social and work situations.
   b. Impact of symptoms on patient's relationships, especially work and family relationships.
   c. Diversional and recreational behavior.
   d. Identification of stressors related to self-concept, role performance, life values, social status, and support systems.
   e. Benefits (primary and secondary gains) and risks of the presenting symptoms.

Nursing Diagnoses

- Anxiety related to unexpected panic attacks or related to reexperiencing traumatic events.
- Acute Confusion related to severe anxiety.
- Impaired Social Interaction related to avoidance behavior or related to embarrassment and shame associated with symptoms.
- Ineffective Role Performance related to inability to function in usual social and occupational situations secondary to anxiety-related symptoms.
- Disturbed Personal Identity related to a traumatic event.
- Risk for Injury related to anxiety-related behavior.

Nursing Interventions

Reducing Symptoms of Anxiety

1. Help patient identify anxiety-producing situations and plan for such events.
2. Assist patient to develop assertiveness and communication skills.

3. Practice stress reduction techniques with patient.
4. Teach patient to monitor for objective and subjective manifestations of anxiety.
   a. Tachycardia, tachypnea.
   b. Signs and symptoms associated with autonomic stimulation—perspiration, difficulty concentrating, insomnia.
5. Promote use of stress reduction techniques in managing symptoms of anxiety.
6. Encourage patient to verbalize feelings of anxiety.
7. Administer prescribed anxiolytics to decrease anxiety level.

 DRUG ALERT Benzodiazepines are associated with tolerance and dependence and are appropriate for short-term use. Withdrawal symptoms may occur when drug is abruptly discontinued. Gradual dosage reduction is necessary. Overdose or taking benzodiazepines with alcohol or other central nervous system (CNS) depressants can cause respiratory depression requiring emergency intervention.

Improving Concentration

1. Use short, simple sentences when communicating with patient.
2. Maintain a calm, serene manner.
3. Use adjuncts to verbal communication, such as visual aids and role-playing, to stimulate memory and retention of information.
4. Teach relaxation techniques to diminish distress that interferes with concentration ability.

Increasing Social Interaction

1. Encourage discussion of reasons for and feelings about social isolation.
2. Help patient identify specific causes and situations that produce anxiety that inhibits social interaction.
3. Recommend participation in programs directed at specific conflict areas or skill deficiencies. Such programs may focus on assertiveness skills, body awareness, managing multiple role responsibilities, and stress management.

Encouraging Independence

1. Identify secondary benefits, such as decreased responsibility and increased dependency, that inhibit patient's move to independence.
2. Provide experiences in which patient can be successful.
3. Explore alternative methods of meeting dependency needs.
4. Explore beliefs that support a helpless or dependent mode of behavior.
5. Teach and role-play assertive behaviors in specific situations.
6. Provide instruction in decision-making skills, allowing opportunities for practice and rehearsal of techniques in role-play situations.
7. Assist patient to improve skills based on performance.
8. Encourage family members to avoid fostering dependency.

Strengthening Identity

1. Develop an honest, nonjudgmental relationship with patient.
2. Try to establish open communication.
3. Do not overwhelm patient.
4. Teach patient containment techniques to assist in coping with the painful memories becoming conscious (eg, visualizing a safe environment, recall of past successes in dealing with anxiety, focusing on slowing of physiologic responses).

Reducing Harm from Behavior

1. Encourage patient to set limits on ritualistic behavior as part of established treatment plan.

2. Assist patient in listing all objects and places that trigger anxiety as part of exposure–response prevention program.
3. Use cognitive strategies, such as reframing, to assist patient in placing thoughts and feelings in a different perspective.
4. Participate as member of treatment team in establishing program for systematic desensitization.
5. Intervene as needed and obtain emergency assistance when patient is in immediate danger.

Community and Home Care Considerations

1. Patients with anxiety-related disorders are generally treated in an outpatient setting. Many of these patients may not see a mental health professional but will be treated by their family health care provider, utilizing pharmacologic therapy. Nurses who encounter patients taking prescribed drugs for anxiety should assess effectiveness and patient knowledge base regarding safe use of these drugs. Patients should be encouraged to utilize anxiety reduction techniques.
2. Because anxiety disorders will affect family functioning, the nurse should provide support for the family, including teaching family members about the disorder and treatment measures.
3. Patients may elect to utilize alternative and complementary therapies to obtain relief from symptoms. Advise patients not to use nutritional supplement or "natural" remedy, such as St. John wort or kava kava, without discussing it with a health care provider; many drug interactions exist.
4. Several community support groups are available to provide patient with continued support. Patient may also be able to learn further techniques for the management of anxiety through participation in these programs. Such programs may also provide patient with an opportunity to practice previously learned skills in a supportive environment.

 TRANSITIONAL CARE ALERT Medication monitoring for effectiveness and adverse reactions is of utmost importance to keep the patient safe, reduce inpatient admission and readmission, and improve outcomes. Be aware that cost may affect adherence, and some medications require a period of 2 to 3 weeks until a desired effect is seen.

Family Education and Health Maintenance

1. Teach patient and family members about anxiety.
   a. Define anxiety and differentiate it from fear.
   b. Explain causes of anxiety.
   c. Identify events that can trigger anxiety.
   d. Identify relevant signs and symptoms of anxiety.
2. Describe the drug regimen, including significant action, adverse effects, dosage considerations, and any food or drug interactions.
3. Identify, describe, and practice deep muscle relaxation techniques, relaxation breathing, imagery, and other relaxation therapies (see page 25).
4. Teach family to give positive reinforcement for use of healthy behaviors.
5. Teach family not to assume responsibilities or roles normally assigned to patient.
6. Teach family to give attention to patient, not patient's symptoms.

7. Teach alternative ways to perform activities of daily living (ADLs) if physical or emotional disability inhibits function and performance.

8. For additional information and support, refer to such agencies as the Anxiety and Depression Association of America (*https://adaa.org*).

9. Many Web sites provide support for individuals and family members. Some examples include Agoraphobics Building Independent Lives, *www.anxietysupport.org* (for sufferers from anxiety disorders), and the National Alliance on Mental Illness, *www.nami.org*.

Evaluation: Expected Outcomes

• Identifies stressors and demonstrates normal heart rate, respirations, sleep pattern, and subjective feelings of anxiety.

• Demonstrates improved concentration and thought processes through improved ability to focus, think, and solve problems.

• Reports increased participation and enjoyment in family- and community-related events.

• Reports going to work, keeps appointments.

• Uses coping strategies in situations that are anxiety provoking.

• Does not injure self or others.

Stress- and Trauma-Related Disorders

EVIDENCE BASE American Psychiatric Association. (2013). *Diagnostic and statistical manual of mental disorders* (5th ed.). Washington, DC: Author.

Burges-Watson, I. P., Brune, M., & Bradley, A. J. (2016). The evolution of the molecular response to stress and its relevance to trauma and stressor-related disorders. *Neuroscience & Biobehavioral Reviews, 68*, 134–147.

Stress- and Traumatic-Related Disorders are characterized by exposure to an event perceived as traumatic or stressful. These disorders were previously classified underneath the umbrella of anxiety orders, primarily because of the association of fear and anxiety with responses to the exposure event. Over time, it has become apparent that the responses to stressful events can result in variable symptomology and distress. As a result, a category of stress-related disorders was created. These disorders still share a significant number of features with anxiety and related disorders, primarily the expression of fear.

Classification

1. Acute stress disorder
2. Posttraumatic stress disorder
3. Reactive attachment disorder
4. Disinhibited social engagement disorder
5. Adjustment disorders

Pathophysiology and Etiology

Fear responses lead to activation of the amygdala and other parts of the brain involved with the interpretation of environmental stimuli. This leads to a condition response to events that may share features with the original event. This results in hypervigilance as the individual remains alert for events that pose a danger. Sympathetic hyperarousal results from exposure to events triggering the fear response.

Biochemical Factors

1. Gamma-aminobutyric acid (GABA) is an inhibitory neurotransmitter that normally acts to decrease anxiety responses. An individual who genetically produces lower amounts of GABA may have an increased likelihood of developing anxiety- or stress-related disorders (eg, PTSD).

2. Suppression of cortisol through administration of dexamethasone has been associated with PTSD, suggesting heightened glucocorticoid feedback sensitivity.

Genetic Factors

1. Reduced hippocampal volumes are believed to contribute vulnerability to PTSD.

2. Deficits in the expression of a protein (FKBP5) associated with immune responses are found tied to stress disorders.

3. Variants in a gene that regulates the breakdown of catecholamines may lead to prolonged catecholamine activity increasing the risk for development of stress-related disorders.

Clinical Manifestations

1. Conscious or unconscious efforts to avoid stimuli related to the triggering event lead to hypervigilance and avoidant behaviors.

2. Signs and symptoms may include elements of dissociation manifesting as flashbacks.

3. Affect and emotions often appear negative, and the individual could display a sense of numbness, a lack of emotional responses, feelings of depersonalization or derealization, a feeling of confusion, and a loss of memory for aspects of the original event.

Acute Stress and Posttraumatic Stress Disorders

1. Acute stress and posttraumatic stress disorder (PTSD) share several symptoms, with the major difference between the two conditions being the time frame in which symptoms develop.

2. For acute stress, symptoms develop within 1 month of the traumatic event and last for 2 days to 3 weeks, whereas for PTSD, the symptoms are more enduring and have lasted for at least 1 month at the time of diagnosis.

3. During the initial traumatic event, the individual needs to have displayed an initial response of horror, accompanied by intense feelings of helplessness to meet criteria for each of these disorders.

4. Both disorders share a cluster of dissociative symptoms with attempts to avoid stimuli associated with the original trauma while also reexperiencing intrusive memories and recollections of the traumatic event.

5. An examination and history would elicit findings that would include three or more of the following: a sense of numbness, a lack of emotional responses, feelings of depersonalization or derealization, a feeling of confusion, and a loss of memory for aspects of the original event.

6. There will also be increased sympathetic activation, hypervigilance, and a pattern of reexperiencing the event through intrusive dreams, flashbacks, or increased anxiety when presented with stimuli associated with the traumatic event. Increased sympathetic activation associated with anxiety is demonstrated through insomnia, difficulty concentrating, feelings of restlessness, and hypervigilance.

Reactive Attachment Disorder

A stress-related disorder occurring in children younger the 5 years of age. Believed to results from environments characterized by emotional or social neglect. Situations in which the primary caregiver has frequently changed are also related to development of the condition through a lack of opportunities for the child to learn appropriate social relations. The child exhibits a lack of emotional engagement with others, manifesting as decreased interaction with adults and reduced responsiveness to attempts from adults to engage or comfort the child.

See pages 1471 to 1474 for diagnostic evaluation, management, and the nursing process.

Dissociative Disorders

Dissociative disorders are conditions in which the anxiety associated with a stressful or traumatic event induces a subjective feeling of being not connected to one's body or to reality. These conditions are viewed as unconscious defense mechanisms that result in a disorder when the ability to function in social or work environments is significantly impaired because of feelings of dissociation. These conditions were previously grouped under the umbrella of anxiety disorders but are now considered a separate but interrelated diagnostic category.

 EVIDENCE BASE American Psychiatric Association. (2013). *Diagnostic and statistical manual of mental disorders* (5th ed.). Washington, DC: Author.
Lemche, E. Surguladze, S. A., Brammer, M. J., & Phillips, M. L. (2016). Dissociable brain correlates for depression, anxiety, dissociation, and somatization in depersonalization-derealization disorder. *CNS Spectrums, 21*(1), 35–42.

Classification/Clinical Manifestations

1. Depersonalization/derealization disorder—a persistent or recurrent experience of feeling detached from oneself. A common sensation is of being an outside observer of one's body. This experience can cause significant impairment in daily function.
2. Dissociative amnesia—one or more episodes of inability to recall important information, usually of a traumatic or stressful nature.
3. Dissociative identity disorder—previously known as multiple personality disorder, this disorder is evidenced by the presence of two or more distinct identities, each with its own patterns of relating, perceiving, and thinking. At least two of these identities take control of the person's behavior.

Pathophysiology

1. Associated with traumatic events, often in childhood.
2. Individual responds by "splitting off" or dissociating the self from the memory of the trauma.
3. Dissociative identity disorder may result from severe physical, sexual, or psychological abuse in early childhood.

See pages 1471 to 1474 for diagnostic evaluation, management, and the nursing process.

Somatic Symptoms and Related Disorders

 EVIDENCE BASE American Psychiatric Association. (2013). *Diagnostic and statistical manual of mental disorders* (5th ed.). Washington, DC: Author.
Katz, J., Rosenbloom, B. N., Fashier, S. (2015). Chronic pain, psychopathology, and DSM-5 somatic symptom disorder. *Canadian Journal of Psychiatry, 60*(4), 160–167.

Somatic symptom and related disorders are characterized by physical symptoms that cannot be explained by known physical mechanisms. These disorders have in common the belief that physical symptoms are real despite evidence to the contrary. The affected individual experiences changes or loss in physical function. The physical symptoms are not under the individual's voluntary control. Significant impairment occurs in social or occupational functioning.

Classification

1. Somatic symptom disorder.
2. Factitious disorder.
3. Conversion disorder.
4. Illness anxiety disorder.
5. Somatic symptom and related disorder not otherwise specified.

Pathophysiology and Etiology

The underlying etiology of somatoform disorders is difficult to define. The following factors may interact in the individual with these disorders.

Biochemical Factors

1. An individual with a somatoform disorder may experience high levels of physiologic arousal (increased awareness of somatic sensations).
2. The phenomenon of alexithymia, or deficient communication between brain hemispheres, may result in difficulty expressing emotions directly, and therefore, distress may be expressed as physical symptoms.
3. The concept of somatosensory amplification, in which there is the tendency to experience somatic sensation as intense, noxious, and disturbing, may be related to the development of somatoform disorders.

Genetic Factors

1. Somatization disorder has been found to have a 10% to 20% frequency in first-degree female biological relatives of women with this disorder.
2. Twin studies have validated some increased risk in conversion disorder in monozygotic twins.
3. The genetic basis for other somatoform disorders is not well established.

Psychosocial Factors

1. Psychodynamic theory—the psychological source of ego conflict is denied and finds expression through displacement of anxiety onto physical symptoms. Both primary gain (anxiety relief) and secondary gains (increased dependence and relief from normal responsibilities) are common to these disorders.
2. Behavioral theory—the child learns from parent to express anxiety through somatization; secondary gains reinforce symptoms.
3. Cognitive theory—the individual has cognitive distortions in which benign symptoms are magnified and interpreted as serious disease.
4. Family theory—a family system that is overly enmeshed may utilize dysfunction in one person as a means to handle anxiety. In such families, the individual may not see self as a separate and distinct person; instead, the person may view him- or herself as an extension of the family.

Sociocultural Factors

1. Incidence of somatoform disorders is highest in rural populations and in low socioeconomic groups.
2. Somatic symptoms are more common in cultures that view direct expression of emotions as unacceptable.
3. Women may experience certain chronic pain conditions more commonly than men (this may have more of a cultural than a genetic basis).

Clinical Manifestations

Somatic disorders are psychiatric conditions that manifest in the appearance of, or preoccupation with, symptoms that reflect medical illnesses or injuries. For the diagnosis of these conditions to be made, other physical health issues must be ruled out. As with other mental health conditions, these problems lead to problems with the ability to perform necessary ADLs.

Somatic Symptom Disorder
1. This disorder is characterized by presentation of at least one somatic symptom (pain, fatigue, etc.) that is distressing in nature or leads to a significantly impairment in daily function.
2. The individual displays recurrent and intrusive thoughts or behaviors related to the symptom.
3. A significant level of anxiety may occur.
4. The symptoms must manifest over a period of 6 months, although they may not be constant during that period.
5. Based on the number of symptoms, the disorder may be classified as mild, moderate, or severe.

Factitious Disorder
1. The individual fakes or otherwise falsifies the signs of symptoms of a disease or injury.
2. The falsified disease may be physical or psychological.
3. The individual claims to be ill or impaired to others.

Conversion Disorder
1. With this condition, the individual develops symptoms compatible with a neurological disorder.
2. Examples include loss of vision, deafness, peripheral neuropathy, or bladder and bowel dysfunction. Some patients may exhibit paralysis or seizure activity.
3. These symptoms cannot be associated with a physical illness for the diagnosis of this disorder.

Illness Anxiety Disorder
1. A fixed preoccupation the individual has a serious medical condition.
2. This belief often persists in spite of medical tests or procedures that do not find any physical condition.
3. The condition must exist for at least 6 months; however, the nature of the preoccupation may change during that time.
4. This preoccupation often leads to significant problems with daily function.

Diagnostic Evaluation
1. Individuals with somatic disorders will present in the medical rather than the psychiatric setting because of their belief that the problems are medical.
2. The individual should receive a thorough medical evaluation (if possible, avoiding repeating tests that have already had negative results).
3. The diagnosis of somatoform disorder will be made after a thorough medical evaluation in which no organic basis for the symptoms is found.

Management
1. Level and setting of care to be provided is determined. In general, the individual will be treated on an outpatient basis, unless underlying mood disorder is present leading to risk for self-harm.
2. Referral to psychiatric treatment is generally rejected by the individual with a somatoform disorder; therefore, the goal of management is to maintain a long-term relationship with a specific health care provider to prevent patient from seeking multiple providers with multiple recommendations for testing, treatments, and drugs.
3. Psychotherapy:
   a. Psychodynamic—assist the individual to express conflicts and emotions verbally rather than displacing them onto physical symptoms.
   b. Behavioral—establish a program whereby adaptive behavior is reinforced and illness behaviors do not receive secondary gains.
   c. Cognitive—restructure belief system that perpetuates illness-related behaviors.
   d. Family therapy—assist family members to define appropriate boundaries and support patient in increasing self-responsibility.
4. Somatic therapies: somatic disorders are usually not treated with psychopharmacologic drugs because these patients are susceptible to dependency on drugs used.
5. Mood disorders, especially depression, are a common comorbid problem in individuals with somatic disorders. Antidepressant drugs may be used to treat the mood disorder.

Complications
1. A patient with a known history of a somatic disorder may have a coexisting medical condition that could go undiagnosed. Careful screening is essential to rule out medical problems.
2. Increased risk of suicide and substance use disorder is possible in patient with an untreated somatic disorder.

Nursing Assessment
1. Assess physical complaints.
   a. Current and past history as well as duration of problems.
   b. Diagnostic testing completed.
   c. Number of health care providers consulted.
   d. Types and amounts of drugs as well as whether self-medicating (over the counter) or prescribed.
2. Assess psychological processes.
   a. Perception of illness and current stressors.
   b. Self-concept and body image.
   c. Secondary gains from physical symptoms.
   d. Mood.
   e. Suicide potential.
3. Explore social functioning (see page 1472).

Nursing Diagnoses
- Anxiety related to multiple physical symptoms and belief that serious disease exists.
- Ineffective Coping related to preoccupation with physical symptoms.

Other nursing diagnoses and nursing interventions under anxiety disorders may apply.

Nursing Interventions

Encouraging Recognition of Anxiety
1. Discuss current life stressors in the areas of social, occupational, and family functioning.
2. Assist patient to identify anxiety-producing situations and plan coping strategies.

3. Avoid focus on physical symptoms (after appropriate screening to rule out physical etiology).
4. Maintain focus on feelings and emotional responses rather than on somatic symptoms.

Improving Coping

1. Teach and reinforce problem-solving approach to stressors.
2. Practice use of stress reduction techniques with patient.
3. Encourage use of support groups.
4. Set limits on manipulative behaviors in a matter-of-fact manner.
5. Decrease reinforcement of secondary gains for physical symptoms.
6. Help patient identify and use positive means to meet emotional needs.

Community and Home Care Considerations

1. Encourage patient to cooperate with referrals for psychiatric or psychotherapy treatments.
2. Promote patient attendance and participation at community support groups.
3. Teach patient and family the importance of remaining with one health care provider to ensure continuity of care.
4. Nurses who encounter patients with somatoform disorders in the community should maintain a matter-of-fact attitude to decrease emphasis on dramatic symptoms. Any approach to patient should include a focus on patient's strengths and capabilities rather than on disability.

Family Education and Health Maintenance

1. Teach patient and family about the relationship between stressors, anxiety, and physical symptoms.
2. Family should expect person to function despite physical symptoms; doing things and making decisions for patient will increase dependent behaviors.
3. Encourage family therapy, which may be helpful to clarify roles, communication, and expectations.

Evaluation: Expected Outcomes

- Verbalizes anxiety about specific problems rather than expressing anxiety with physical symptoms.
- Makes decisions on own; demonstrates less dependence on family and friends.

MOOD DISTURBANCES
Depressive Disorders

Depressive disorders are considered mood disorders. A mood is a sustained emotion that, when extreme, affects the person's view of the world. Mood disorders are characterized by disturbances in feelings, thinking, and behavior. These disorders may occur on a continuum ranging from severe depression to severe mania (hyperactivity). A depressive illness is painful and can be psychophysiologically debilitating. Depression is much more than just sadness; it affects the way one feels about the future and can alter basic attitudes about the self. A depressed person can become so despairing as to express hopelessness. When moods become severe or prolonged or interfere with a person's interpersonal or occupational functioning, this may signal a mood disorder.

Pathophysiology and Etiology

The exact causes for depressive disorders have not been established. These disorders are thought to result from complex interactions among various factors.

Biochemical Factors

1. Biogenic amine theory proposes that there is a norepinephrine and serotonin deficiency in individuals with a depressive disorder. Changes in quantity and sensitivity of receptor sites for these neurotransmitters may also be important.
2. Kindling theory describes a process whereby external environmental stressors activate internal physiologic stress responses, which trigger the first depressive episode. Subsequent episodes can occur with less stress in response to the electrophysiologic sensitivity that was established in the brain from the initial episode.
3. Neuroendocrine dysfunction:
   a. Hypothalamic–pituitary–adrenal axis dysfunction may be present in some individuals. Abnormalities include increased cortisol levels, resistance of cortisol to suppression by dexamethasone, and blunted adrenocorticotropin hormone response to corticotropin-releasing factor.
   b. Subclinical hypothyroidism has been associated with depression, especially in women.
   c. Dysfunction of circadian rhythms has been theorized related to depression. Abnormal sleep EEGs have been demonstrated in many individuals. Increased early morning awakening is common, as are multiple nighttime awakenings.

Genetic Factors

1. Risk of developing a mood disorder is 1½ to 3 times greater in individuals with a first-degree relative with a mood disorder.
2. Twin studies reveal a higher rate of concordance in monozygotic twins than in dizygotic twins.
3. Mood states are associated with activation of several neuroendocrine pathways within the central and peripheral nervous systems. These pathways involve a number of neurochemical processes that involve activation of a particular binding protein identified as cyclic AMP response-binding protein 1 (CREB-1). Genetic profiles of individuals with depression have found evidence that genes involved in the cellular signaling pathways utilizing CREB-1 are associated with major depression. There then may be alleles (coding genes) that are related to the development of mood disorder.
4. Genetic variation in a certain region of the serotonin transporter gene (5-HTT) has been found to interact with the perception of stressful events (possibly through neuroendocrine pathways) to produce higher levels of depression and suicidality than in individuals without this variation.
5. Although genetic evidence has supported conceptualizations of neurochemical and biologic alteration in the development of mood and other psychiatric disorders, no one single gene or factor has appeared to emerge as the main culprit. Most likely, a number of different genes and disposing factors are involved. Possible genes include 5-HTT, brain-derived neurotrophic growth factor, and the monoamine oxidase A gene.

Medical Factors

1. Many drugs have the adverse effect of depression, including hormones, cardiovascular drugs, psychotropic drugs, and anti-inflammatory and antiulcer drugs.
2. Clinically significant depressive symptoms are detected in approximately 12% to 36% of individuals with a nonpsychiatric general medical condition.

Psychosocial Factors

1. Psychodynamic theory describes the occurrence of a significant loss (object loss) that is associated with anger and aggression, which is turned inward and leads to negative feelings

about self. The negative feelings about the self, including shame and guilt, then lead to depression.

2. Life events and environmental stress, such as loss of a family member through death, divorce, or separation; lack of social support; and significant health problems have all been associated with the onset of depression.

3. Cognitive theory describes how faulty thought patterns, including negative distortions of life experiences, produce negative self-evaluation, pessimistic thinking, and hopelessness.

4. Learned helplessness theory posits that a person who internalizes the belief that an unwanted event is his or her own fault and that nothing can be done to avoid or change it is prone to developing depression.

Clinical Manifestations

EVIDENCE BASE American Psychiatric Association. (2013). *Diagnostic and statistical manual of mental disorders* (5th ed.). Washington, DC: APA.

Depression

1. A major depressive disorder reflects a level of depression that persists over a 2-week period.

2. The severity of depression may be classified as mild, moderate, or severe depending on the number of symptoms.

3. Certain qualifying terms can be used that indicate whether the depression is associated with a change in the seasons (with seasonal pattern) or follows the birth of an infant (with peripartum onset).

4. Should delusions or hallucinations exist, the depression would be said to have psychotic features.

5. Major depression results in a significant change in ability to work or participate in social activities.

6. Physical examination and history findings should reveal at least five or more symptoms that include the following:
   a. Depressed mood, fatigue.
   b. Insomnia or an increased need for sleep.
   c. Lack of interest in pleasurable activities (anhedonia).
   d. Recent gain or loss of weight that represents at least 5% of body weight.
   e. Feelings of worthlessness.
   f. Inability to concentrate or make a decision.
   g. Suicidal ideation.

Persistent Depressive Disorder

1. A chronic, less intense level of depressed mood characterized by the same symptoms as seen in major depression and that lasts for at least 2 years in adults, at least 1 year in children and adolescents. Previously known as dysthymia.

2. A major distinguishing feature is that depression does not alter the ability to participate in social or work-related functions to the extent of major depressive disorder.

Diagnostic Evaluation

1. Rating scales of depression—to determine presence and severity of the problem:
   a. Zung Depression Scale.
   b. Raskin Depression Rating Scale.
   c. Hamilton Rating Scale for Depression.
   d. Beck Depression Inventory.

2. Laboratory studies:
   a. Thyroid function tests and thyrotropin-releasing hormone stimulation test—to detect underlying hypothyroidism, which may cause depression.
   b. DST—to evaluate depression that may be responsive to antidepressant or electroconvulsive therapy (ECT).
   c. Twenty-four–hour urinary 3-methoxy-4-hydroxyphenylglycol (MHPG)—may show slightly lower level in unipolar depression than in bipolar depression.

3. Polysomnography—an increase in the overall amount of rapid eye movement (REM) sleep and shortened REM latency period in patients with major depression.

4. Additional diagnostic tests to evaluate physical conditions, such as CT scan or magnetic resonance imaging (MRI), complete blood count (CBC), chemistry panel, rapid plasma reagin (RPR), human immunodeficiency virus (HIV) test, EEG, vitamin B_{12} and folate levels, and toxicology studies.

Management

1. Patients may receive treatment in acute inpatient psychiatric hospitals or in the community in an outpatient program. Decision about treatment setting is made according to the severity of patient's illness, with primary concern being the risk of self-harm (suicide) as well as the presence of symptoms that are severely disabling.

2. Inpatient treatment is directed toward drug management and supportive psychotherapy using milieu management.

3. Somatic therapies:
   a. Psychopharmacologic: drugs used to treat depression are those that will increase serotonin and norepinephrine (see Table 57-2, page 1479). Another agent, a selective norepinephrine reuptake inhibitor (reboxetine) has seen used in Europe but is not yet approved for use in the United States.
   b. ECT may be used to treat severe depression that is unresponsive to antidepressant drugs.
   c. Ultraviolet light therapy may be recommended for depression that occurs during fall and winter months (seasonal affective disorder).

4. Patient may select complementary and alternative treatments. The use of herbal supplements, especially St. John wort, is a popular alternative for antidepressant drugs. However, use of nutritional or herbal supplements should be discussed with the health care provider because of the potential for drug interactions.

5. Psychotherapy:
   a. *Psychodynamic therapy* helps patient to become aware of unconscious anger directed toward object loss and "work through" these feelings to alleviate depression.
   b. *Cognitive therapy* is the recommended psychotherapeutic approach for depression. This approach includes identifying and challenging the accuracy of patient's negative thought patterns and encouraging behaviors designed to counteract depressive symptoms.
   c. *Family therapy* assists patient and family members in developing a sense of self that is separate from that of the family as a whole. Patient is then encouraged to take responsibility for his or her own actions.

DRUG ALERT Antidepressant drugs have many interactions, which may lead to serotonin syndrome, a state of excessive serotonin in the synaptic cleft. Symptoms include insomnia, confusion, agitation, hyperreflexia, involuntary movements, and hypotension. Hypertensive crisis can occur if patients take a monoamine oxidase inhibitor antidepressant in combination with a sympathomimetic drug or eat foods high in tyramine.

Table 57-2 Dosage and Adverse Reactions of Antidepressant Drugs

DRUG: CLASS/GENERIC/ TRADE NAME	ADULT THERAPEUTIC DOSAGE RANGE (MG/DAY)	ADVERSE REACTIONS
Tricyclic Agents		
Amitriptyline (Elavil, Endep)	50–300 mg	*For all tricyclic and tetracyclic agents:*
Clomipramine (Anafranil)	25–250 mg	• Possibility of triggering a manic episode in bipolar patients
Desipramine	75–300 mg	• Anticholinergic effects. Dry mouth, constipation, blurred vision, urine retention
Doxepin	75–300 mg	• Sedative effects
Imipramine	75–300 mg	• Autonomic effects: orthostatic hypotension, sweating, palpitations, and increased blood pressure
Nortriptyline	25–150 mg	• Cardiac effects: tachycardia, T-wave flattening, prolonged QT interval
Protriptyline	15–60 mg	• Twitch, extrapyramidal movement effects
Trimipramine	75–200 mg	
Tetracyclic Agent		
Mirtazapine	15–45 mg	*See tricyclic agents:*
		• Somnolence, increased appetite, weight gain, dry mouth, constipation
Bicyclic Agent		
Venlafaxine	75–375 mg	• Nervousness, weight loss, dizziness, hypertension
Desvenlafaxine	50–100 mg	• Nausea, headache, dry mouth, insomnia, fatigue, dizziness
Selective Serotonin Reuptake Inhibitors (SSRIs)		
Citalopram	20–60 mg	• Nausea, dry mouth, diarrhea, fatigue, drowsiness, ejaculatory delay, impotence
Duloxetine	40–60 mg	• Nausea, dry mouth, dizziness, constipation, diarrhea, fatigue, increased sweating
Escitalopram	10–20 mg	• Nausea, ejaculatory delay, impotence
Fluoxetine	20–80 mg	• Delayed orgasm, headache, nervousness, insomnia, anxiety, tremor, dizziness, nausea, diarrhea, anorexia, dry mouth
Fluvoxamine	50–300 mg	• Nausea, vomiting, drowsiness, anorexia, constipation, tremor, insomnia
Paroxetine	10–50 mg	• Nausea, dry mouth, headache, somnolence, insomnia, diarrhea, constipation, tremor
Sertraline	50–150 mg	• Insomnia, diarrhea, nausea, weight loss
Vilazodone	40 mg	• Nausea, vomiting, insomnia, diarrhea
Monoamine Oxidase Inhibitors (MAOIs)		
Isocarboxazid	30–50 mg	For all MAOIs:
Phenelzine	45–90 mg	• Orthostatic hypotension, weight gain, edema, insomnia, sexual dysfunction, myoclonus, muscle pains, paresthesia, anticholinergic effects
Tranylcypromine	20–60 mg	• Food and beverages containing tyramine in combination with MAOIs as well as combining sympathetic drugs with an MAOI can cause hypertensive crisis
Selegiline	10 mg	
Dibenzoxazepine Agent		
Amoxapine	100–600 mg	• Dizziness, orthostatic hypotension, reflex tachycardia, extrapyramidal movement disorders
Unicyclic Agent		
Bupropion	225–450 mg	• Dry mouth, constipation, headache, insomnia, restlessness, agitation, menstrual irregularities, increased seizure risk
Triazolopyridine Agent		
Trazodone	150–600 mg	• Sedation, orthostatic hypotension, dizziness, headache, nausea, priapism
Phenylpiperazine Agent		
Nefazodone	200–600 mg	• Orthostatic hypotension, anxiety, nervous tremor, agitation
Combination Therapies		
Amitriptyline and chlordiazepoxide	2.5–5 mg/10–25 mg	• Blurred vision, dizziness, drowsiness, fatigue, tremor
Fluoxetine and olanzapine	3–12 mg/25–50 mg	• Dry mouth, fatigue, somnolence, increased appetite, and increased weight
Perphenazine and amitriptyline	2–4 mg/10–25 mg	• Extrapyramidal reactions are possible because of the presence of perphenazine

Complications

1. An undiagnosed medical condition causing depressive symptoms could lead to physical deterioration and delay in obtaining appropriate treatments.
2. Untreated depressive illness can lead to suicide.
3. Use of alcohol or drugs to "feel better" or numb dysphoric feelings.

 NURSING ALERT During the first 60 days of antidepressant therapy, young adults and children (those under age 24) are considered to be at increased risk for suicidal thinking and behavior. The Food and Drug Administration has issued black box warnings of this risk for most antidepressants. Those taking these medications require additional monitoring and supervision during this period. The evidence does not support the need for this type of monitoring in those over age 24.

 EVIDENCE BASE Gibbons, R. D., Perraillion, M. C., Hur, K., Conti, R. M., Valuck, R. J., & Brent, D. A. (2014). Antidepressant treatment and suicide attempts and self-inflicted injury in children and adolescents. *Pharmacoepidemiology and Drug Safety, 24*(2), 208–214.

Nursing Assessment

1. Assess posture and affect for:
   a. Poor or slumped posture.
   b. Appearance of being older than stated age.
   c. Facial expression of sadness, dejection.
   d. Episodes of weeping.
   e. Anhedonia—inability to experience pleasure.
2. Assess thought processes:
   a. Identify the presence of suicidal thoughts.
   b. Poor judgment, indecisiveness.
   c. Impaired problem solving, poor concentration.
   d. Negative thoughts.
3. Explore feelings for:
   a. Anger and irritability.
   b. Anxiety, guilt.
   c. Worthlessness.
   d. Helplessness, hopelessness.
4. Assess physical behavior for:
   a. Psychomotor agitation or retardation.
   b. Vegetative signs of depression.
      i. Change in eating patterns.
      ii. Change in sleeping patterns.
      iii. Change in elimination patterns.
      iv. Change in level of interest in sex.
      v. Change in personal hygiene.
5. Assess for evidence of "masked depression":
   a. Hypochondriasis.
   b. Psychosomatic disorders.
   c. Compulsive gambling.
   d. Compulsive overwork.
   e. Accident proneness.
   f. Eating disorders.
   g. Addictive illnesses.
6. Assess for risk of suicide.

 NURSING ALERT All mentally ill individuals, especially those who are depressed, should be assessed for suicide risk and referred for crisis intervention if they are deemed at risk.

Nursing Diagnoses

- Hopelessness related to depressive thoughts.
- Risk for Injury related to hopelessness and impaired problem solving.
- Bathing and Dressing Self-Care Deficit related to lack of motivation and poor concentration.
- Disturbed Sleep Pattern related to insomnia.

Nursing Interventions

Strengthening Coping and Sense of Hope

1. Initiate interaction with patient at a regularly scheduled time.
2. Be clear and honest about your own feelings related to patient's behavior.
3. Encourage verbal expression of feelings.
4. Validate feelings that are appropriate to the situation.
5. Explore with patient what is producing and maintaining the feeling of depression.
6. Encourage patient to identify events that cause unpleasant emotional responses.
7. Assess significant losses patient has experienced.
8. Identify cultural and social factors that may contribute to how patient copes with loss and feelings.
9. Assess patient's support network.

Maintaining Safety

1. Assess current suicide risk.
2. Implement appropriate level of observation based on a focused suicide assessment (eg, constant observation or 15-minute checks).
3. Explain observation precautions to patient.
4. Remove harmful objects from patient's possession and assess environmental safety of patient's room and unit.
5. Encourage patient to negotiate a "no-self-harm and no-suicide" agreement with the staff.
6. Monitor need to revise level of observation.
7. Provide additional structure by keeping patient involved in therapeutic and psychorehabilitative activities.

Encouraging Participation in ADLs

1. Collaborate with occupational and physical therapists to determine patient's functional capacity to accomplish ADLs.
2. If patient cannot accomplish ADLs independently, provide hygiene activities in collaboration with patient.
3. Acknowledge and reinforce patient's efforts to maintain appearance; do not rush patient when self-care is slow.
4. Reinforce what patient can do rather than what patient cannot do without assistance.
5. Remain with patient during mealtimes to determine the level of need for assistance or cueing in the ability to eat.

Facilitating Sleep

1. Determine patient's past and current sleep patterns and sleep hygiene.
2. Ask what strategies patient has already used to improve sleep and elicit which ones have been successful.
3. Consider decreasing the amount of daytime sleep by encouraging participation in an activity.

4. Discuss alternative methods for facilitating sleep:
   a. Avoid caffeine and nicotine.
   b. Avoid emotionally charged or upsetting discussions before bedtime.
   c. Avoid exercise 30 minutes to 1 hour before bed.
   d. Increase physical activity within functional limits.
   e. Use relaxation techniques.
   f. Try a warm bath or warm milk.
5. Administer prescribed drugs that cause sleepiness at bedtime; avoid giving drugs that cause insomnia at night.

Community and Home Care Considerations

1. Mood disorders tend to be chronic, with acute episodes that may require inpatient treatment. In the home or community setting, patient will require ongoing monitoring regarding the use of drugs as well as support and education in terms of the disorder.
2. Community health care providers, including nurses, must be aware of the need for primary and secondary prevention programs directed at education as well as early case finding and prompt treatment.

Family Education and Health Maintenance

1. Instruct patient and family members about symptoms of depression.
2. Instruct patient and family members about purpose of antidepressant drugs, effects, adverse effects, and their management, and how to recognize early signs and symptoms of relapse.
3. Instruct patient and family members about the effect of a depressive disorder on the family system.
4. Provide patient and family members with written material on coping with depression.
5. Provide patient and family members with information about appropriate community-based programs and support groups. Contact the National Foundation for Depressive Illness (*www.depression.org*).

Evaluation: Expected Outcomes

- Reports improvement in mood and increased interest in daily living.
- Remains free from self-harm.
- Accomplishes ADLs in an independent manner.
- Obtains a minimum of 5 hours of uninterrupted sleep.

Bipolar and Related Disorders

Bipolar disorders, also considered *mood disorders*, include the occurrence of depressive episodes and one or more elated mood episodes. An elated mood can include a range of affect, from normal mood to hypomania to mania. In the most intense presentation, the person with bipolar disorder experiences altered thought processes, which can produce bizarre delusions.

Pathophysiology and Etiology

Genetic Factors

1. Twin studies reveal a concordance rate of 65% in monozygotic twins for bipolar disorder.
2. Risk of developing bipolar disorder is increased 4% to 24% in first-degree relatives of people with bipolar disorder.
3. Current research indicates that defective genes located within chromosomes 18 and 21 may be related to bipolar disorder.

Biochemical Factors

1. Patients with bipolar disorders may have lower plasma norepinephrine, urinary MHPG, and platelet serotonin uptake and higher red blood cell/plasma lithium rates than do unipolar populations.
2. Pathology of the limbic system, basal ganglia, and hypothalamus is proposed to contribute to the development of mood disorders.

Psychosocial Factors

1. Psychosocial stressors appear to have an important role early in the illness, in concert with the electrical kindling and behavioral sensitization models.
2. Mania and hypomania have been viewed by psychoanalytic theorists as a defense against depression.

Clinical Manifestations

 EVIDENCE BASE American Psychiatric Association. (2013). *Diagnostic and statistical manual of mental disorders* (5th ed.). Washington, DC: Author.

Mood disorders are often characterized by varying degrees of mania that can alternate with periods of depression. The distinguishing characteristic between forms of bipolar disorder is the degree of mania, with or without the signs of depression. Mania is an elevation of mood that persists for at least 1 week.

Bipolar I Disorder

1. Physical examination and history findings for bipolar I disorder are the presence of a single manic episode generally without the individual also meeting the criteria for a major depressive episode.
2. Severity of the disorder can be classified mild, moderate, or severe depending on the number of symptoms present.
3. A mixed episode refers to the symptoms of mania and depression coexisting across the course of 1 week.
4. Mania is characterized by a cluster of at least three symptoms across the course of at least 1 week that result in a disruption in daily function. These behaviors can include the following:
   a. Excessive or pressured speech.
   b. Difficulty in maintaining concentration or focus.
   c. A reduced need for sleep and an increase in either goal-directed or pleasure-seeking behaviors.

Bipolar II Disorder

1. In bipolar II disorder, there has been an episode of hypomania along with an episode of major depression.
2. Hypomania is a less intense form of mania (increased energy does not result in significant changes in functional ability) with duration of at least 4 days, but less than a week.

Cyclothymic Disorder

1. A chronic alteration in mood that persists over a 2-year period of time during which there are several episodes of hypomania and depressed mood but no episodes of major depression.
2. In children and adolescents, a 1-year time frame is used.
3. During the course of the 2 years, symptoms cannot have abated for more than 2 months.

Diagnostic Evaluation

1. Rating scale assessment tools:
   a. Young Mania Rating Scale.
   b. Manic State Rating Scale.

2. There appear to be no laboratory features that distinguish major depressive episodes found in major depressive disorder from those in bipolar I or bipolar II disorder.
3. Complete psychophysiologic examination.
4. Complete assessment to rule out medical conditions.

Management

 EVIDENCE BASE Fountoulakis, K. N., Lakshmi, Y., Grunze, H., Vieta, E., et al. (2017). The International College of Neuro-Psychopharmacology (CINP) Treatment Guidelines for Bipolar Disorder in Adults (CINP-BD-2017), Part 2: Review, Grading of the Evidence, and a Precise Algorithm. *International Journal of Neuropsychopharmacology, 20*(2), 121–179.

1. Patients may receive treatment in acute inpatient psychiatric hospitals or in the community in an outpatient program. The decision about treatment setting is made according to severity of patient's illness, including degree of mania or depression as well as risk of self-harm or harm to others.
2. Inpatient treatment is directed toward drug management as well as supportive psychotherapy to alleviate the acute manic symptoms.
3. Pharmacologic treatment for acute mania and bipolar disorder consists of:
   a. Lithium carbonate.
   b. Anticonvulsants, such as carbamazepine and valproate, for mood-stabilizing properties.
   c. Neuroleptic agents, such as risperidone, for acute psychotic thinking.
   d. Benzodiazepines, such as clonazepam or lorazepam, for acute agitation.
   e. Combination therapies, often incorporating an antipsychotic (perphenazine or olanzapine) along with an antidepressant (amitriptyline or fluoxetine). Another approach involves combining a benzodiazepine (chlordiazepoxide) with an antidepressant (amitriptyline) to combat comorbid depression and anxiety.
4. Psychotherapy is used as described above in the section related to depression.
5. Psychiatric home care nursing to facilitate compliance with drugs and therapeutic interventions.
6. Community-based support group participation.

 DRUG ALERT Patients taking lithium can develop toxicity related to elevated levels in the blood; therefore, lithium blood levels must be monitored periodically. Initial therapy requires daily monitoring until a safe, therapeutic level is attained; weekly and then monthly monitoring is then recommended. Lithium toxicity is related to decreased serum sodium levels and inadequate hydration. Therefore, patients taking lithium must have normal sodium intake and drink 2 L of water daily.

Complications

1. Untreated bipolar disorder can lead to physical exhaustion.
2. Poor judgment and risk-taking behavior can lead to financial problems.
3. Alcohol and drug abuse problems can develop and cause disruption in the family.
4. Concurrent medical conditions may be exacerbated.

Nursing Assessment

1. Assess mood for stability; range of affect, from elation to irritability to severe agitation; laughing, joking, and talking continuously; uninhibited familiarity with interviewer.
2. Assess behavior for constant activity, starting many projects but finishing few, mild to severe hyperactivity, spending large sums of money, increased appetite, indiscriminate sexual behavior, minimal to no sleeping, outlandish or bizarre dress, poor concentration.
3. Assess thought processes for flight of ideas; pressured speech, usually with content that is sexually explicit; clang associations (sound of word, rather than its meaning, directs subsequent associations); delusions; hallucinations.

Nursing Diagnoses

- Ineffective Impulse Control related to biological changes as demonstrated by agitation, hyperactivity, and inability to concentrate.
- Disturbed Sleep Pattern related to hyperactivity and perceived lack of need for sleep.
- Compromised Family Processes related to role changes, economic strain, and lack of knowledge about patient's illness.
- Imbalanced Nutrition: Less than Body Requirements related to hyperactivity.

Nursing Interventions

Improving Impulse Control and Decreasing Disturbed Thoughts

1. Assess patient's degree of distorted thinking.
2. Redirect patient when you are unable to follow thought processes.
3. Use brief explanations.
4. Remain consistent in approach and expectations.
5. Frequently orient patient to reality; speak in a clear, simple manner.
6. Provide patient with a relaxing area with decreased environmental stimulation.
7. Assist patient with a gradual and progressive integration into the social environment while observing for behavioral changes that indicate readiness for participation in further activities.

Improving Sleep Pattern

1. Establish a distraction-free environment at bedtime.
2. Help patient avoid the intake of caffeine and nicotine.
3. Administer prescribed drugs, as ordered, and monitor patient's response.

Improving the Effect of Bipolar Illness on Family

1. Assess family's external support network and encourage participation in family therapy and support groups.
2. Assess communication and boundaries within family.
3. Observe and assess interaction patterns within family and discuss their influence on patient and family functioning.
4. Provide patient and family with information about bipolar disorder and the treatment plan, prognosis, and aftercare plan.

Ensuring Adequate Nutrition

1. Maintain accurate documentation of food and fluid intake.
2. Offer small, frequent meals of high-calorie foods. Include foods that patient likes and that can be eaten "on the move."
3. Serve patient meals in a low-stimulus environment.
4. Monitor patient's serum electrolyte and albumin levels and weigh patient every other day.
5. Monitor patient's vital signs.

Family Education and Health Maintenance

1. Instruct patient and family about bipolar illness, including symptoms of relapse.
2. Instruct patient and family members about psychopharmacologic treatment, including its purpose, effects, adverse effects, and management.
3. Advise patient and family members about community-based support groups or health care agencies that are relevant to his or her care.
4. For additional information, refer them to such organizations as the National Association on Mental Illness (*www.nami.org*).

Evaluation: Expected Outcomes

- Improved thought processes demonstrated by clear sentences with no evidence of flight of ideas and completion of simple tasks.
- Sleeps for at least 5 hours at night.
- Family members verbalize realistic, goal-directed thinking related to patient's abilities, recovery, and control of condition.
- No weight loss noted.

THOUGHT DISTURBANCES (PSYCHOTIC DISORDERS)
Schizophrenia, Schizophreniform, and Delusional Disorders

Schizophrenia, schizophreniform, and delusional disorders are conditions in which there is a disruption of thought process and/or perception. These conditions are often defined by the presence of psychotic symptoms. Psychotic symptoms are produced by a loss of ego boundaries or a gross impairment in reality testing, which includes prominent hallucinations and delusions, disorganized speech, and grossly disorganized or catatonic behavior. Schizophrenia can be classified as having positive or negative symptoms, although most patients have a mixture. The positive symptoms include hallucinations, delusions, loose associations, and bizarre or disorganized behavior. The negative symptoms include restricted emotion (flat affect), anhedonia (lack of interest in pleasurable activities), avolition (lack of motivation or initiative), alogia (lack of speech or content), and social withdrawal.

Pathophysiology and Etiology

The exact cause of these disorders remains unclear. The current consensus is that they result from complex interactions among various factors.

Schizophrenia, Schizophreniform Disorder
1. Genetic factors:
   a. Studies of monozygotic twins reveal a 50% concordance rate with a 15% rate with dizygotic twins.
   b. If one parent is affected with schizophrenia, a 12% rate is demonstrated in the children, while having two parents with the disorder increases the risk to 35% to 39%.
   c. Research is focused on a number of different genes that may be related to the development of schizophrenia. An increased risk of schizophrenia is seen in individuals with genetic variation in the catechol-*O*-methyltransferase gene, which is involved in the manufacture of an enzyme that metabolizes neurotransmitters. Other current candidate genes include GRM3, DISC1, dysbindin, and neuregulin.

2. Biochemical and structural brain factors:
   a. Dopamine hypothesis—hyperactivity in the dopaminergic system, possibly because of receptor neurons that are functionally hyperactive.
   b. Norepinephrine, serotonin, glutamate, and GABA may also play a role in modulating the symptoms of schizophrenia.
   c. Endogenous dysfunction of *N*-methyl-D-aspartate receptor–mediated neurotransmission could lead to the development of schizophrenia.
   d. Neuroanatomic studies—cerebral ventricular enlargement; sulcal enlargement; cerebellar atrophy; decreased cranial, cerebral, and frontal size; abnormalities in basal ganglia; structural abnormalities at the cellular level, particularly in the limbic and periventricular regions.
   e. Functional and metabolic studies—regional cerebral blood flow studies demonstrated hypofrontality: schizophrenic patients were unable to increase blood flow to their frontal lobes during a task thought to increase frontal lobe functions; PET studies also consistently found evidence for a relative hypofrontality.
   f. Electrophysiologic studies—EEG findings in schizophrenic patients demonstrated decreased alpha and increased delta activity; changes in evoked potential studies and amplitude reduction may occur in responses reflecting selective attention and stimulus evaluation. P300 response (reduced amplitude to unexpected stimuli using auditory and visual parameters) is the most pronounced and is prolonged. This defect leads to information or sensory overload and an inability to "screen out" irrelevant stimuli.
   g. Research evidence supports speculation that schizophrenia is a neurodevelopmental disorder that may result from brain injury occurring early in life and interfering with normal developmental events.

3. Psychosocial factors:
   a. Psychodynamic theory proposes that the essential feature of schizophrenia is a defect in interpersonal relationships because of a withdrawal of the libido into the self.
   b. Interpersonal theory proposes that the lack of a warm, nurturing relationship in the early years of life contributes to the lack of self-identity, reality misperception, and relationship withdrawal that is apparent in the disorder.
   c. Family theory related to the role of the family in the development of schizophrenia has not been validated by research. An area of family functioning that has been implicated is increased relapse risks in families characterized by high expressed emotion. This characteristic is described as emotional overinvolvement along with hostile and critical feedback.

Delusional Disorder
1. Little has been established about the etiology of delusional disorder.
2. There is no demonstrated genetic linkage.
3. It is possible that psychosocial stressors have a role in the etiology of delusional disorder in some people. This is illustrated in some of the rarer conditions such as shared psychotic disorder.

Clinical Manifestations

 EVIDENCE BASE American Psychiatric Association. (2013). *Diagnostic and statistical manual of mental disorders* (5th ed.). Washington, DC: Author.

Thought disorders are characterized by the appearance of positive and negative symptomatology. Positive symptomatology refers to the presence of delusions or hallucinations, whereas negative is the lack of personality traits that should normally be present. A lack of affect, interest in daily activities, and an inability to attend to daily hygiene or self-care reflect negative symptomatology. Distinguishing between the various thought disorders requires careful attention to the presence and duration of positive and negative symptomatology. As with other psychiatric disorders, the symptoms must be severe enough to alter daily function.

Schizophrenia

Previously schizophrenia was classified into five different forms. Currently, for diagnosis, the individual must display at least one positive symptom.

1. Positive symptoms include delusional thinking, disorganized speech, and hallucinations.
2. Symptoms must be present for at least 1 month with a total duration of illness for a period of at least 6 months. The 6-month period may include periods of active symptoms and remission.
3. Symptoms must lead to a significant disruption of the individual's ability to function in social or social settings, or impact ability to attend ADLs.
4. The diagnosis may indicate whether this is an acute episode or if the individual is in remission.
5. Severity can be rated on a five-point scale from zero to four. A rating of four would indicate the presence of severe and active symptoms, while a zero indicates that symptoms are not currently present.

Schizophreniform Disorder

1. The primary difference between schizophreniform disorder and schizophrenia is a period of symptom duration of less than 6 months but more than 1 month.
2. Those with this disorder can appear schizophrenic with the presence of positive and/or negative symptomatology.
3. Diagnostic criteria include delusions, hallucinations, and patterns of disorganized behavior or speech along with negative symptoms.

Schizoaffective Disorder

1. A psychiatric condition in which there is a comorbid thought and mood disorder.
2. Those with this disorder may display signs and symptoms of depression or mania along with the positive and negative symptoms of schizophrenia.

Other Psychotic Disorders

1. Delusional disorders encompass nonbizarre delusions of at least 1 month's duration but no positive or negative symptoms of schizophrenia present.
2. Psychotic disorder because of a general medical disorder contains prominent hallucinations that may last longer than the course of the underlying disorder.
3. Brief psychotic disorders contain one or more of the following: delusions, disorganized speech, grossly disorganized or catatonic behavior, hallucinations. Duration is at least 1 day and less than 1 month, then return to previous level of functioning.
4. Shared psychotic disorder occurs in an individual with an already established delusion who develops another delusion similar to another's in the context of a close relationship with that person.
5. Substance-induced psychotic disorder contains prominent hallucinations and delusions associated with substance intoxication or withdrawal but not exclusively during the course of underlying drug use.

Diagnostic Evaluation

1. Clinical diagnosis is developed on historical information and thorough mental status examination.
2. No laboratory findings have been identified that are diagnostic of schizophrenia.
3. Routine battery of laboratory tests may be useful in ruling out possible organic etiologies, including CBC, urinalysis, liver function tests, thyroid function tests, RPR, HIV test, serum ceruloplasmin (rules out an inherited disease, Wilson disease, in which the body retains excessive amounts of copper), PET scan, CT scan, and MRI.
4. Rating scale assessment:
   a. Scale for the Assessment of Negative Symptoms.
   b. Scale for the Assessment of Positive Symptoms.
   c. Brief Psychiatric Rating Scale.

Management

 EVIDENCE BASE Samara, M. T., Dold, M., Gianatsi, M., et al. (2016). Efficacy, acceptability, and tolerability of antipsychotics in treatment-resistant schizophrenia: A network meta-analysis. *JAMA Psychiatry, 73*(3), 199–210.

Schizophrenia and Schizophreniform Disorder

1. Patients may receive treatment in inpatient settings or in community-based outpatient programs or psychiatric home care. The level of care depends on the severity of symptoms and the risk of harm to self and others.
2. These disorders generally require long-term treatment; therefore, a case management approach is important to coordinate multiple services.
3. Pharmacologic therapy with either the typical or atypical neuroleptics (antipsychotics) is the mainstay of treatment (see Table 57-3, page 1485).
   a. The typical neuroleptics have multiple adverse effects that require careful management (see Table 57-4, page 1486).
   b. The atypical neuroleptics have fewer adverse effects and may also be more effective in decreasing the negative symptoms of schizophrenia.
   c. Pharmacologic therapy with both the typical and atypical neuroleptics can include the use of long-lasting, or depot, injections. The use of such injections is increasing. Five drugs are currently available in depot formulations, haloperidol, fluphenazine, olanzapine, paliperidone, and risperidone.
4. Psychosocial treatments (social skills training, ADL instruction).
5. Supportive therapy that is reality oriented and pragmatic.
6. Family therapy.
7. Psychoeducational individual, group, and family support.
8. Support groups in the community.
9. Community-based partial hospitalization programs.
10. Psychiatric home care nursing.
11. Vocational and social skills education.

Delusional Disorder

1. Neuroleptic drugs have demonstrated some success in reducing the intensity of the delusion.
2. Individual psychotherapy.
3. Hospitalization for comprehensive assessment for diagnostic purposes or if suicidal or homicidal.

Table 57-3	Dosage and Adverse Reactions of Antipsychotic Drugs	
DRUG: CLASS/GENERIC/ TRADE NAME	**ADULT THERAPEUTIC DOSAGE RANGE (MG/DAY)**	**ADVERSE REACTIONS**
Butyrophenone		
Haloperidol	2–40 mg	Extrapyramidal adverse effects are common. Decreased incidence of orthostatic hypotension as compared with phenothiazines
Aliphatic Phenothiazine		
Chlorpromazine	30–800 mg	Orthostatic hypotension, sedation, dry mouth, extrapyramidal adverse effects, agranulocytosis, ocular changes
Piperidine Phenothiazine		
Thioridazine	200–800 mg	Sedation, orthostatic hypotension, fewer extrapyramidal symptoms than other phenothiazines
Piperazine Phenothiazine		
Fluphenazine	2.5–40 mg	Extrapyramidal symptoms and lower incidence of orthostatic
Perphenazine	8–64 mg	hypotension than with other phenothiazines
Trifluoperazine	15–40 mg	
Dibenzoxazepine		
Loxapine	60–250 mg	Extrapyramidal adverse effects, hypotension, dizziness
Thioxanthene		
Thiothixene	20–60 mg	Extrapyramidal adverse effects, hypotension, tachycardia, insomnia
Atypical Antipsychotics		Extrapyramidal adverse effects can occur with the use of any of the atypical antipsychotics, although the incidence of occurrence usually is less than that seen with other classes of antipsychotic medications
Aripiprazole	10–30 mg	Headache, anxiety, insomnia, nausea, vomiting, dizziness, and drowsiness
Asenapine	10–20 mg	Extrapyramidal adverse effects, drowsiness, oral hypoesthesia, weight gain
Clozapine	150–600 mg (requires careful titration)	Seizure, agranulocytosis (obtain weekly white blood cell count), hypotension, tachycardia, cardiac dysrhythmia, drowsiness, sedation, increased salivation
Iloperidone	12–24 mg	Extrapyramidal adverse effects, orthostatic hypotension, weight gain
Lurasidone	40–160 mg	Extrapyramidal adverse effects primarily akathisia and pseudoparkinsonism, nausea, somnolence
Olanzapine	5–20 mg	Orthostatic hypotension, tachycardia, drowsiness, agitation, akathisia, constipation
Paliperidone	3–6 mg	Extrapyramidal adverse effects, tremor, muscle stiffness
Pimozide	1–10 mg	Orthostatic hypotension, tachycardia, drowsiness, sedation, akathisia, akinesia
Quetiapine	200–800 mg	Orthostatic hypotension, tachycardia, drowsiness, dizziness, dry mouth
Risperidone	4–16 mg	Orthostatic hypotension, tachycardia, drowsiness, dizziness, dry mouth
Ziprasidone	20–80 mg	Dysrhythmia, drowsiness, dizziness, nausea, restlessness, constipation

Complications

1. If left undiagnosed, untreated, or ineffectively treated, schizophrenia can lead to profound inability to function and contributes to the problem of homelessness in our society.
2. Neglect of other medical conditions; therefore, complications because of untreated medical illness are common.
3. Depression and suicide.
4. Substance use, abuse, or dependency.

Nursing Assessment

Assess for positive symptoms of schizophrenia. These symptoms reflect aberrant mental activity and are usually present early in the first phase of the schizophrenic illness.

Alterations in Thinking

1. Delusion—false, fixed belief that is not amenable to change by reasoning. The most frequent elicited delusions include the following:
   a. Ideas of reference.
   b. Delusions of grandeur.
   c. Delusions of jealousy.
   d. Delusions of persecution.
   e. Somatic delusions.
2. Loose associations—the thought process becomes illogical and confused.
3. Neologisms—made-up words that have a special meaning to the delusional person.
4. Concrete thinking—an overemphasis on small or specific details and an impaired ability to abstract.

Table 57-4	Management of Adverse Effects of Neuroleptic Drugs
SYMPTOM	**MANAGEMENT**
Orthostatic Hypotension	Assess for orthostatic blood pressure changes and dizziness and teach the patient: • When rising from bed or chair, get up slowly. • Sit at side of bed for a few minutes, dangling legs. • Do ankle pumps before standing. • Once standing, move slowly. • Do not twist or turn quickly. • Use assistive devices, hand rails, canes, walkers when necessary for functional deficits. • Do not drive or operate machinery when dizzy.
Peripheral Anticholinergic Effects Dry mouth and nose, blurred vision, constipation, urine retention	*Dry mouth:* • Brush teeth after each meal with a fluoridated toothpaste. • Rinse mouth frequently. • Limit caffeinated or alcoholic drinks because they can be dehydrating. • Stop smoking because of the irritation of oral mucosa. • Suck on sugarless candy or gum; avoid sugared candy to decrease the risk of fungal infections and dental caries. • Avoid dry or spicy foods. • Drink fluids between meals unless on a specific fluid restriction. • Avoid acidic beverages because of potential irritation. • Use dressing, juices, or sauces (if allowed) to moisten food. *Constipation:* • Drink fluids (within prescribed limits set by health care provider). • Eat roughage: fruits, vegetables (raw leafy types) to increase bulk and help soften stool. • Eat dried fruits, such as prunes or dates, for laxative effect. • Maintain activity level within functional limits. • Consult with health care provider to determine appropriate use of over-the-counter laxatives or stool softeners. *Urine retention:* • Void at regular intervals. • Ensure privacy.
Extrapyramidal Adverse Effects **Short term** Akathisia: restless legs, jitters, nervous energy, motor agitation	• Reassure patient. • Differentiate between agitation and akathisia. • Consider reducing dosage. • Consider switching patient to another class of antipsychotic.
Akinesia: weakness (hypotonia), fatigue, painful muscles, anergy (lack of energy), absence of movement	• Assess functional ability. • Dose reduction or cessation should improve movement if problems are due to akinesia vs. psychotic symptoms.
Dystonias, dyskinesias: grimacing, torticollis, intermittent spasms, opisthotonos, oculogyric crises, head-neck stiffness, myoclonic twitches, laryngeal–pharyngeal dystonia	• Consider prophylaxis with anticholinergic medications. • Treat with IM or IV anticholinergics, as prescribed.
Parkinsonian effects: muscle stiffness, cog wheel rigidity, shuffling gait, stooped posture, drooling	• Treat with anticholinergics, as prescribed. • Stop the antipsychotic, as directed.
Long term *Tardive dyskinesia:* a delayed effect of neuroleptic drugs usually occurring after 6 months of treatment involving abnormal, involuntary, irregular, and choreoathetoid movements of the muscles of the head, limbs, and trunk	• Complete regular objective rating/assessment of the movement disorder. • Reduce or stop neuroleptic, as directed. • Consider clozapine or risperidone. • Comprehensive medical psychiatric assessment necessary with close monitoring of movement disorder.

5. Echolalia—pathologic repeating of another's words.
6. Clang associations—the meaningless rhyming of a word in a forceful way.
7. Word salad—a mixture of words that is meaningless to the listener.

Alterations in Perceiving

1. Hallucinations—sensory perceptions that have no external stimulus. The most common are auditory, visual, gustatory, olfactory, and tactile.

2. Loss of ego boundaries—lack a sense of their body and how they relate to the environment.
   a. Depersonalization is a nonspecific feeling or sense that a person has lost his or her identity or is unreal.
   b. Derealization is the perception by a person that the environment has changed.

Alterations in Behavioral Responses
1. Bizarre behavioral patterns.
   a. Motor agitation and restlessness.
   b. Automatic obedience or robot-like movement.
   c. Negativism.
   d. Stereotyped behaviors.
   e. Stupor.
   f. Waxy flexibility (allowing another person to reposition extremities).
2. Agitated or impulsive behavior.
3. Negative symptoms of schizophrenia that reflect a deficiency of mental functioning.
   a. Alogia—lack of speech.
   b. Anergia—inability to react.
   c. Anhedonia—inability to experience pleasure.
   d. Avolition—lack of motivation or initiation.
   e. Poor social functioning.
   f. Poverty of speech.
   g. Social withdrawal.
   h. Thought blocking.
4. Associated symptoms of schizophrenia.
   a. Substance use, abuse, or dependence.
   b. Depression.
   c. Fantasy.
   d. Violent or aggressive behavior.
   e. Water intoxication.
   f. Withdrawal.

Nursing Diagnoses
- Acute Confusion related to perceptual and cognitive distortions, as demonstrated by suspiciousness, defensive behavior, and disruptions in thought.
- Social Isolation related to an inability to trust.
- Activity Intolerance related to adverse reactions to psychopharmacologic drugs.
- Ineffective Coping related to misinterpretation of environment and impaired communication ability.
- Risk for Self-Directed or Other-Directed Violence related to delusional thinking and hallucinatory experiences.

Nursing Interventions
Strengthening Differentiation Between Delusions and Reality
1. Provide patient with honest and consistent feedback in a nonthreatening manner.
2. Avoid challenging the content of patient's behaviors.
3. Focus interactions on patient's behaviors.
4. Administer drugs, as prescribed, while monitoring and documenting patient's response to the drug regimen.
5. Use simple and clear language when speaking with patient.
6. Explain all procedures, tests, and activities to patient before starting them, and provide written or video material for learning purposes.

Promoting Socialization
1. Encourage patient to talk about feelings in the context of a trusting, supportive relationship.

2. Allow patient time to reveal delusions to you without engaging in a power struggle over the content or the reality of the delusions.
3. Use a supportive, empathic approach to focus on patient's feelings about troubling events or conflicts.
4. Provide opportunities for socialization and encourage participation in group activities.
5. Be aware of patient's personal space and use touch judiciously.
6. Help patient to identify behaviors that alienate significant others and family members.

Improving Activity Tolerance
1. Assess patient's response to prescribed antipsychotic drug.
2. Collaborate with patient and occupational and physical therapy specialists to assess patient's ability to perform ADLs.
3. Collaborate with patient to establish a daily, achievable routine within physical limitations.
4. Teach strategies to manage adverse effects of antipsychotic drug that affect patient's functional status, including:
   a. Change positions slowly.
   b. Gradually increase physical activities.
   c. Limit overdoing it in hot, sunny weather.
   d. Use sun precautions.
   e. Use caution in activities if extrapyramidal symptoms develop.

Improving Coping with Thoughts and Feelings
1. Encourage patient to express feelings.
2. Focus on patient's feelings and behavior.
3. Provide honest perceptions of reality and feedback about symptoms and behaviors.
4. Encourage patient to explore adaptive behaviors that increase abilities and success in socializing and accomplishing ADLs.
5. Decrease environmental stimuli.

Ensuring Safety
1. Monitor patient for behaviors that indicate increased anxiety and agitation.
2. Collaborate with patient to identify anxious behaviors as well as the causes.
3. Tell patient that you will help with maintaining behavioral control.
4. Establish consistent limits on patient's behaviors and clearly communicate these limits to patient, family members, and health care providers.
5. Secure all potential weapons and articles from patient's room and the unit environment that could be used to inflict an injury.
6. To prepare for possible continued escalation, form a psychiatric emergency assist team and designate a leader to facilitate an effective and safe aggression management process.
7. Determine the need for external control, including seclusion or restraints. Communicate the decision to patient and put plan into action.
8. Frequently monitor patient within the guidelines of facility's policy on restrictive devices and assess patient's level of agitation.
9. When patient's level of agitation begins to decrease and self-control is regained, establish a behavioral agreement that identifies specific behaviors that indicate self-control against a reescalation of agitation.

Community and Home Care Considerations
1. Patients with these disorders may be in supportive housing, such as transitional living halfway houses, foster homes, and board and care homes. Supervision and drug management

are important areas of concern for the nurse working in the community.

2. Psychosocial rehabilitation approach may be used in the community setting, where skills necessary for independent living are taught. Patient who has been symptomatic since early adulthood may not have learned these skills. The nurse working in the community setting may work as a member of the treatment team using this approach.

Family Education and Health Maintenance

1. Instruct patient and family members in disease process and how to recognize and cope with relapse symptoms.
2. Instruct patient and family members about the uses, actions, and adverse effects of prescribed drugs.
3. Provide instruction on when to notify primary care provider regarding adverse drug effects or increased disease symptomatology.
4. Instruct patient and family about community resources, support groups, and possible use of psychiatric home care nursing.
5. For additional information and support, refer patient and family to such agencies as the Brain and Behavior Research Foundation (*www.bbrfoundation.org*) or *Schizophrenia*. The National Alliance on Mental Illness *www.nami.org* has a 24 hour helpline 800-950-6264.

Evaluation: Expected Outcomes

- Exhibits improved reality orientation, concentration, and attention span, as demonstrated through speech and behavior.
- Communicates with family and staff in a clear manner without evidence of loose, dissociated thinking.
- Independently maintains personal hygiene without fatigue.
- Attends group activities.
- Remains free from harm or violent acts.

NEUROCOGNITIVE DISORDERS
Delirium, Dementia, and Amnestic Disorders

Neurocognitive disorders reflect states where cognitive impairment is the primary issue. This category encompass specific disorders that produce either temporary or permanent neuronal damage, resulting in psychological or behavioral dysfunction, such as delirium, dementia, and amnestic disorder, as described in DSM-5. Although dementia is recognized as a term reflecting chronic disruption, the preferred diagnosis is neurocognitive disorder.

Delirium is an acute disturbance of consciousness and a change in cognition that develops over a brief period and is often reversible. *Dementia or neurocognitive disorder* is a chronic, progressive disturbance involving multiple cognitive deficits, including memory impairment. Impairment can be classified as mild or major based on degree of cognitive decline and whether symptoms interfere with daily function. For major neurocognitive disorder, symptoms must interfere with the ability of the individual to be independent in ADLs. *Amnestic disorder* is characterized by memory impairment in the absence of other significant cognitive impairments.

Pathophysiology and Etiology

Delirium

Can be caused by numerous pathophysiologic conditions. Some of the major possibilities include the following:

1. CNS pathology: head trauma, hypertensive cerebral changes, seizures, tumors.
2. Endocrinopathies: hyper- or hypothyroidism, hyper- or hypoparathyroidism.
3. Hypoxemia.
4. Hypothermia or hyperthermia.
5. Substance intoxication or abstinence and withdrawal states.
6. Exposure to certain metals, toxins, or drugs.
7. Metabolic: diabetic acidosis, hypoglycemia, acid–base imbalances.
8. Hepatic encephalopathy.
9. Thiamine deficiency.
10. Postoperative states.
11. Psychosocial stressors: relocation stress, sensory deprivation or overload, sleep deprivation, immobilization.

Mild or Major Neurocognitive Disorder (Dementia)

1. Neurodegenerative Disease—psychotic features may occur.
   a. Alzheimer disease.
   b. Lewy body disease.
   c. Vascular disease.
2. Infection-related dementias.
   a. Acquired immunodeficiency syndrome.
   b. Chronic meningitis.
   c. Creutzfeldt-Jakob disease.
   d. Progressive multifocal leukoencephalopathy.
   e. Postencephalitic dementia syndrome.
   f. Syphilis.
   g. Subacute sclerosing panencephalitis.
   h. Tuberculosis.
3. Subcortical degenerative disorders.
   a. Huntington disease.
   b. Parkinson disease.
   c. Wilson disease.
   d. Thalamic dementia.
4. Hydrocephalic dementias.
5. Vascular dementias.
6. Traumatic conditions, such as posttraumatic encephalopathy and subdural hematoma.
7. Neoplastic dementias.
   a. Glioma.
   b. Meningioma.
   c. Meningeal carcinomatosis.
   d. Metastatic deposits.
8. Inflammatory conditions, such as sarcoidosis, systemic lupus erythematosus, and temporal arteritis.
9. Toxic conditions, such as alcohol-related syndrome and iatrogenic dementias (anticonvulsant, anticholinergic, antihypertensive, psychotropic drugs).
10. Metabolic disorders.
    a. Anemias.
    b. Deficiency states (minerals and vitamins).
    c. Cardiac or pulmonary failure.
    d. Hepatic encephalopathy.
    e. Porphyria (deficiency in enzymes involved in heme synthesis).
    f. Uremia.
11. Genetic factors:
    a. Familial Alzheimer disease is associated with abnormal genes on chromosomes 1, 14, and 21, particularly with genes located on these chromosomes (1 and 14) that encode for amyloid precursor protein, which leads to accumulation of the amyloid beta-peptide in plaques.
    b. A specific cholesterol-bearing protein, apolipoprotein E4 (Apo E4), is found on chromosome 19 twice as often in people with Alzheimer's disease as in the general population.

12. Biochemical and brain structural factors:
    a. The neurotransmitter acetylcholine has been implicated in terms of relative deficit or receptor abnormalities as related to Alzheimer disease.
    b. Autopsy findings reveal presence of brain changes, that is, the presence of amyloid plaques and neurofibrillary tangles associated with nerve cell destruction.
    c. Additional areas of investigation include the following:
        i. Slow viral infection.
        ii. Autoimmune processes.
        iii. Head trauma.

Amnestic Disorder

1. Posttraumatic amnesia: head trauma is the most common cause of amnesia.
2. Poststroke amnesia: damage to the fornix or hippocampus.
3. Neoplasms.
4. Anoxic states.
5. Herpes simplex encephalitis.
6. Hypoglycemic states.
7. Epileptic seizures.
8. Electroconvulsive therapy.
9. Substance induced.

Clinical Manifestations

See Table 57-5.

Table 57-5	Clinical Manifestations of Neurocognitive Disorders
DISORDER	**CLINICAL MANIFESTATIONS**
Delirium	
(severe impairment in functioning)	• Fluctuating levels of awareness • Clouding of consciousness (confused and disoriented) • Perceptual disturbances (illusions and hallucinations) • Memory, especially recent memory, is disturbed • Alteration in sleep–wake cycle • EEG changes • Abrupt onset may last about 1 week • Reversible when underlying cause has been treated
Dementia (Neurocognitive Disorder)	
(severe impairment in functioning)	• Slow, insidious onset • Impaired long- and short-term memory • Deterioration of cognitive abilities—judgment, abstract thinking • Often irreversible, based on cause • Personality changes • No or slow EEG changes
Amnestic Syndrome	
(moderate to severe impairment in functioning)	• Impairment in short- and long-term memory • Inability to learn new material • Remote memory better than that of recent events • Confabulation • Apathy, lack of initiative • Emotionally bland

Diagnostic Evaluation

Various diagnostic tests may be done to determine the cause. A comprehensive neuropsychiatric evaluation must be completed to make an accurate diagnosis.

1. Basic laboratory examination, including CBC with differential, chemistry panel (including blood urea nitrogen, creatine, and ammonia), arterial blood gas values, chest x-ray, toxicology screen (comprehensive), thyroid function tests, and serologic tests for syphilis.
2. Additional tests may include CT scan, MRI, additional blood chemistries (heavy metals, thiamine, folate, antinuclear antibody, and urinary porphobilinogen), lumbar puncture, PET/single photon emission CT scans.
3. Complete mental status examination.
4. Comprehensive physical examination.

Management

 EVIDENCE BASE Theleritis, C., Siarkos, K., Katirtzoglou, E., & Politis, A. (2016). Pharmacological and nonpharmacological treatment for apathy in Alzheimer disease. *Journal of Geriatric Psychiatry and Neurology, 30*(1), 26–49.

Delirium

1. Treatment generally occurs in acute hospital-based setting where the goal is diagnosis to identify specific reversible causes of the delirium so that treatment is focused on ameliorating the causative factors.
2. Pharmacologic therapy is dependent on underlying causes. Additional drugs may be used that are directed toward the reduction of the acute symptoms of delirium. These include the following:
    a. Benzodiazepines, such as lorazepam, for substance withdrawal states.
    b. Neuroleptics, such as risperidone and haloperidol, for agitation.
    c. Combined administration of haloperidol and lorazepam for agitated and psychotic symptomatology.
3. Environmental management:
    a. Safe, structured environment.
    b. Orientation facilitated by clocks, calendars, and other visual cues.
4. Family teaching about the nature of the disorder.
5. Family participation in the treatment plan to assist in the management of behavior.

Dementia

1. Treatment is generally community focused; the goal of treatment is to maintain the quality of life as long as possible despite the progressive nature of the disease. Effective treatment is based on:
    a. Diagnosis of primary illness and concurrent psychiatric disorders.
    b. Assessment of auditory and visual impairment.
    c. Measurement of the degree, nature, and progression of cognitive deficits.
    d. Assessment of functional capacity and ability for self-care.
    e. Family and social system assessment.
2. Environmental strategies to assist in maintaining the safety and functional abilities of patient as long as possible.

Table 57-6 Dosage and Adverse Reactions of Drugs used in the Treatment of Dementia

DRUG: CLASS/GENERIC/TRADE NAME	ADULT THERAPEUTIC DOSAGE RANGE (MG/DAY)	ADVERSE REACTIONS
Cholinesterase Inhibitors		
Donepezil	10–23 mg	Nausea, diarrhea, anorexia, fatigue
Galantamine	8–24 mg	Nausea, diarrhea, dizziness, fatigue
Rivastigmine	6–12 mg	Nausea, vomiting, anorexia, dizziness
NMDA Receptor Antagonist		
Memantine	10–20 mg	Fatigue, dizziness, headache

3. Pharmacologic therapy used for the person with Alzheimer disease is directed toward the use of anticholinesterase drugs to slow the progression of the disorder by increasing the relative amount of acetylcholine. Available drugs include donepezil, galantamine, and rivastigmine. An NMDA receptor antagonist memantine may be provided in an attempt to improve cognition (see Table 57-6). Other drugs may be used for behavioral control and symptom reduction.
   a. Agitation management: neuroleptic drugs.
   b. Psychosis: neuroleptic drugs.
   c. Depression: select antidepressants such as citalopram, duloxetine, escitalopram, fluoxetine, fluvoxamine, paroxetine, and mirtazapine; ECT.
4. Hypertension management in vascular dementia is important in reducing the severity of symptoms.
5. Family education is a treatment strategy because statistics indicate that family caregivers provide care for patients with Alzheimer disease in 7 out of 10 cases. The family and the treatment team collaborate in the delivery of care.

Complications

1. Without accurate diagnosis and treatment, dementia resulting from another disease states may result in permanent cognitive deficits.
2. Falls with serious orthopedic or cerebral injuries.
3. Self-inflicted injuries.
4. Aggression or violence toward self, others, or property.
5. Wandering events, in which the person can get lost and potentially suffer exposure, hypothermia, injury, and even death.
6. Serious depression is demonstrated in caregivers who receive inadequate support.
7. Caregiver stress and burden may result in patient neglect or abuse.

Nursing Assessment

See Table 57-7.
1. Assess the onset and characteristics of symptoms (determine type and stage of disorder).
2. Establish cognitive status using standard measurement tools.
3. Determine self-care abilities.
4. Assess threats to physical safety (eg, wandering, poor reality testing).
5. Assess affect and emotional responsiveness.
6. Assess ability and level of support available to caregivers.

Nursing Diagnoses

- Impaired Verbal Communication related to cerebral impairment as demonstrated by altered memory, judgment, and word finding.
- Bathing and Dressing Self-Care Deficit related to cognitive impairment as demonstrated by inattention and inability to complete ADLs.
- Risk for Injury related to cognitive impairment and wandering behavior.
- Impaired Social Interaction related to cognitive impairment.
- Risk for Violence: Self-Directed or Other-Directed related to suspicion and inability to recognize people or places.

Nursing Interventions

Improving Communication
1. Speak slowly and use short, simple words and phrases.
2. Consistently identify yourself and address the person by name at each meeting.
3. Focus on one piece of information at a time. Review what has been discussed with patient.

Table 57-7 Nursing Assessment for Delirium, Dementia, and Amnestic Disorder

	DELIRIUM	DEMENTIA	AMNESTIC DISORDER
Onset	Acute	Slow, insidious	Sudden
Course	Usually brief	Progresses over years	Transient or chronic
Mood	Fearfulness, anxiety, irritability	Mood labile, personality traits accentuated	Apathy, agitation, emotional blandness, shallow range of affective expression
Perception	Auditory, visual, tactile hallucinations; illusions	Hallucinations not a prominent feature	No hallucinatory experiences
Memory	Short-term memory impaired	Short-term memory deficit followed by long-term memory deficit	Impaired ability to learn new information; unable to recall previously learned information or past events
Communication	Slurred speech; confabulation	Normal—early stage: progressive aphasia and confabulation	Confabulation

4. If patient has vision or hearing disturbances, have him or her wear prescription eyeglasses or a hearing device.
5. Keep environment well lit.
6. Use clocks, calendars, seasonal decorations, and familiar personal effects in patient's view.
7. If patient becomes verbally aggressive, identify and acknowledge feelings.
8. If patient becomes aggressive, shift the topic to a safer, more familiar one.
9. If patient becomes delusional, acknowledge feelings and reinforce reality. Do not attempt to challenge the content of the delusion.

Promoting Independence in Self-Care
1. Assess and monitor patient's ability to perform ADLs.
2. Encourage decision-making regarding ADLs as much as possible.
3. Label clothes with patient's name, address, and telephone number.
4. Use clothing with elastic and Velcro for fastenings rather than buttons or zippers, which may be too difficult for patient to manipulate.
5. Monitor food and fluid intake.
6. Weigh patient weekly.
7. Provide food that patient can eat while moving.
8. Sit with patient during meals and assist by cueing.
9. Initiate a bowel and bladder program early in the disease process to maintain continence and prevent constipation or urine retention.

Ensuring Safety
1. Discuss restriction of driving when recommended.
2. Assess patient's home for safety: remove throw rugs, label rooms, and keep the house well lit.
3. Assess community for safety.
4. Alert neighbors about patient's wandering behavior.
5. Alert police and have current pictures taken.
6. Provide patient with a MedicAlert bracelet.
7. Install complex safety locks on doors to outside or basement.
8. Install safety bars in bathroom.
9. Closely observe patient while he or she is smoking.
10. Encourage physical activity during the daytime.
11. Give patient a card with simple instructions (address and phone number) in case he or she gets lost.
12. Use nightlights.
13. Install alarm and sensor devices on doors.

Improving Socialization
1. Provide magazines with pictures as reading and language abilities diminish.
2. Encourage participation in simple, familiar group activities, such as singing, reminiscing, doing puzzles, and painting.
3. Encourage participation in simple activities that promote the exercise of large muscle groups.

Preventing Violence and Aggression
1. Respond calmly and do not raise your voice.
2. Remove objects that might be used to harm self or others.
3. Identify stressors that increase agitation.
4. Distract patient when an upsetting situation develops.

Community and Home Care Considerations
1. Multidisciplinary team approach is important, along with collaboration among professionals in nursing, medicine, psychiatry, nutrition, social work, pharmacy, and rehabilitative specialties.
2. Nurses involved in community care need to utilize case-finding approach as well as provide long-term support for family members involved in caregiving.
3. Adult day care and respite care may be utilized to provide the level of care needed by patient as well as allow the family to continue to maintain normal functioning.

Family Education and Health Maintenance
1. Instruct family about the process of the disorder, whether delirium, dementia, or amnestic disorder.
2. Instruct family about safety measures, environmental supports, and effective interventions for common symptoms to provide care in the home.
3. Instruct about and refer family members to community-based groups (adult day care centers, senior assessment centers, home care, respite care, and family support groups).
4. For additional information and support, refer to Alzheimer's Association (*www.alz.org*) or National Institutes of Health, National Institute on Aging, Alzheimer's Disease Education and Referral Center (800-438-4380; *https://www.nia.nih.gov/health/alzheimers*). For information on caregiving tips and advice with referral to local community groups, consult Today's Caregiver (*https://caregiver.com*) or AlzOnline Caregiver Support Online (800-677-1116; *http://alzonline.phhp.ufl.edu*).

Evaluation: Expected Outcomes
- Demonstrates decreased anxiety and increased feelings of security in supportive environment.
- Maintains maximum degree of orientation and self-care within level of ability.
- Safety precautions and close surveillance maintained; no injury.
- Attends group activities; sings, exercises with group.
- Decreased occurrence of acting-out behaviors.

ADDICTION AND SUBSTANCE-RELATED DISORDERS
Substance Use

The use of alcohol and other psychoactive substances has become an endemic problem throughout all levels of society. In terms of substance use, a substance can be defined as a prescribed drug, an illegal drug, or a substance used in an unintended manner to produce mood or mind-altering effect (eg, inhalants, glues, or steroids). Continued substance use may arise unintentionally from the initial use of a substance for its approved purpose. The individual commonly faces not only the psychological ramifications of a substance-related disorder but also physiologic consequences resulting from substance use.

Current criteria for diagnosing substance use disorder recognize elements of abuse and dependence. The criteria reflect dynamics of inability to control use of a substance, use in situations that may put the individual at risk, and a centering of daily activities around the use or obtaining of a substance. These criteria reflect a pattern of use that has led to the development of one or more life problems.

Classification

 EVIDENCE BASE American Psychiatric Association. (2013). *Diagnostic and statistical manual of mental disorders* (5th ed.). Washington, DC: Author.

A substance use disorder includes elements of abuse and possible dependence within the criterion. The defining characteristic of a disorder is when there is impairment of ability to perform social roles in the home, school, or work setting. Substance use can occur in relation to use of any of 10 categories of substance: caffeine, tobacco, opioids, alcohol, hallucinogens, sedatives, stimulants, anxiolytics, inhalants, and hypnotics. Additionally, the severity of substance use can be specified as mild, moderate, or severe based on the number of symptoms present.

- Substance (specify) use.
- Substance (specify)-induced disorders.
- Substance (specify) intoxication.

A number of disorders can be induced through the use of a particular substance; in such cases, the symptoms cannot be explained by another condition or disorder and are related to substance use. Such substance-induced disorders include the following:

- Substance-induced intoxication.
- Substance-induced withdrawal.
- Substance or medication-indicated mental disorders.

Dual diagnosis is defined as the presence of a substance-related diagnosis along with another psychiatric disorder.

Pathophysiology and Etiology

As with the development of other psychiatric conditions and disorders, the development of substance-related disorders reflects a complex interaction of biological, genetic, sociologic, and psychological factors. Several theoretical approaches have been developed to describe the process of abuse and dependence.

Biochemical Factors

1. Dopamine is one of the primary neurotransmitters within the CNS and is known to be involved in the integration of environmental stimuli with physiologic responses. Cannabis, cocaine, and alcohol increase the dopamine level, thereby producing a strong association between physiologic effects and behavior.
2. Dopamine is also involved in CNS pathways that mediate feelings of pleasure. Opioids indirectly increase dopamine activity by modulation of the mesolimbic system, leading to reinforcement of substance use.
3. Neurons in the mesolimbic system can become sensitized to the presence of amphetamine and cocaine. Such sensitization is the reverse of tolerance, with the development of an enhanced neuronal response upon repeated exposure. These responses appear to be associated with the development of substance dependence.

Genetic Factors

1. Alcoholism is strongly associated with a familial history of alcoholism. In these individuals, a genetic disposition (attention deficit/hyperactivity disorder [ADHD] allele) to alcoholism combines with a learning environment in which patient develops certain beliefs about the use of a substance and its effects. The presence of genetic disposition, in the absence of parental alcoholism, does not result in a significantly higher risk of alcoholism than in those individuals without such disposition. These findings provide support for models focusing on genetic and environmental interaction in the etiology of substance abuse.
2. Genetic variation in gene regulation resulting in lower levels of serotonin in the CNS may be associated with the development of alcoholism.

Psychosocial Factors

1. An individual learns to use substances in certain situations with certain expectations as to the effects of the substance (eg, relaxation, disinhibition). As the individual experiences the desired effects, this may reinforce the desire to use the substance.
2. Use may begin with an attempt to fit in with a larger peer group as a means of boosting self-esteem.
3. Substances may be used to relieve anxiety or as a means of coping with other traumatic events (self-medication).

Sociocultural Factors

1. Societies around the world use psychoactive substances for a number of reasons. The individual learns the approved use of the substance within the societal or familial structure and may consider such use to be appropriate.
2. The society in which an individual resides may consider dependence on certain substances to be a minor issue, thereby providing a justification for continued use.

Clinical Manifestations

 EVIDENCE BASE American Psychiatric Association. (2013). *Diagnostic and statistical manual of mental disorders* (5th ed.). Washington, DC: Author.

Overview

1. Substance use disorder is characterized by a loss of control.
2. A pattern of substance use must be sustained over a period of 12 months and impair ADLs.
3. Whether the pattern is one of steady or binge use, activities related to substance use must interfere with daily functioning, in terms of time off work or curtailing of social activities to provide more time to participate in, or recover from, substance use.
4. A differentiating factor between abuse and dependence is that dependence is characterized by the development of tolerance with the appearance of substance-specific withdrawal symptomatology in the absence of use.

 TRANSITIONAL CARE ALERT The complications of substance abuse such as injuries and liver disease may be treated in the hospital, but the underlying substance abuse may not be known or addressed by the medical staff. Nurses should monitor for the presence of substance use and withdrawal symptoms during and following hospitalization so that the medical condition does not worsen and appropriate referrals can be made.

Substance Abuse

Physical examination and history findings compatible with substance abuse includes at least one of the following:

1. Continued use even in the face of an inability to meet major life obligations.
2. Use in situations that pose a danger of harm to self or others (ie, driving while intoxicated).
3. Continued use regardless of legal issues associated with use (ie, continued driving while intoxicated after suspension of a license) or continued use after the development of problems in social relationships (ie, an impending divorce brought about by substance use).

Substance Dependence

Physical examination and history findings include meeting at least three diagnostic criteria, which include the following:

1. Tolerance to substance-related effects.
2. Withdrawal in the absence of the substance.
3. Unsuccessful attempts to reduce or halt use.
4. Cutting down or avoiding social obligations or work responsibilities to spend time in substance-related activity (eg, obtaining, using, recovering from).
5. Continued use despite the development of significant life problems (ie, loss of job).

Diagnostic Evaluation

A number of tools have been designed to assess for the presence of substance-related disorders in specific populations (eg, adolescents, pregnancy). The tool used should be specific to patient being assessed.

1. Measurement tools for alcohol abuse or dependence:
   a. CAGE.
   b. Michigan Alcohol Screening Test (MAST).
   c. Alcohol Use Disorders Identification Test (AUDIT).
2. Measurement tools for other substance abuse and dependence:
   a. CAGE-AID.
   b. Drug Abuse Screening Tool (DAST).
3. Laboratory testing of blood, saliva, sweat, and hair for the presence of a substance or metabolite. The period of effective measurement varies based on the procedure and the substance.
4. States of drug intoxication or withdrawal can be identified through the presence of physiologic and behavioral symptoms associated with the use of a particular substance.
5. Additional screening and testing is recommended for the presence of other disease conditions or illnesses (HIV, hepatitis) that may have resulted from risk-taking behavior while under the influence of substances or may have resulted from the physiologic effects of the substance (as in cardiac dysrhythmia in the case of cocaine use).

Management

For the treatment of substance overdose and alcohol-related delirium, see Chapter 35, pages 957 to 960.

1. The management of substance use includes outpatient and inpatient treatment modalities. Inpatient modalities include programs of detoxification and therapy sessions designed to aid in the recognition of a substance-related disorder. Outpatient therapies include support groups, continued therapy sessions, and the use of pharmacologic drugs to aid in the maintenance of sobriety.
2. Initial detoxification is typically provided through inpatient hospitalization. Detoxification protocols are unique to each substance. Benzodiazepine taper is utilized during detoxification from alcohol. The treatment of cocaine withdrawal may include administration of prescribed drugs that can reduce craving, such as amantadine or bromocriptine. The treatment of heroin withdrawal generally involves transdermal clonidine along with oral administration, as necessary.
3. Drugs may also be used in the treatment of alcohol abuse.
   a. Disulfiram is used as aversion therapy. It leads to accumulation of acetaldehyde in the blood system, causing flushing, tachycardia, vomiting, nausea, and chest pain if alcohol is consumed.
   b. A nonaversion therapy, acamprosate sodium, may be used in attempts to ensure abstinence from alcohol. It interacts with the GABA neurotransmitter system to restore balance between neuronal excitation and inhibition.
   c. Topiramate, an anticonvulsant, may reduce craving for alcohol. Clinical trials have demonstrated that ondansetron may aid in reducing drinking.
4. Drug therapy in the treatment of opiate withdrawal includes several classes.
   a. Administration of an opioid antagonist, such as naloxone and naltrexone, reverses the effects of opioids. Injectable sustained-release formulations of naltrexone may also be used.
   b. Outpatient detoxification is typically focused on the administration of the opioid agonist, methadone, or levo-alpha-acetylmethadol, a longer-lasting formulation, to substitute for the illicit drug.
   c. Another opioid agonist, buprenorphine, is available in the outpatient treatment of opioid addiction. An injectable form is used in the treatment of chronic pain. It is also available in sublingual and transdermal formulations and often blended with naloxone to prevent euphoria from intravenous injection of oral formulations.
5. Psychosocial support through the use of 12-step or other treatment programs such as Rational Recovery.
6. Psychoeducational therapy to understand triggers of substance use and prevention of relapse.
7. Family support and educational groups.

Complications

1. The physiologic complications of substance-induced disorders are specific to the substance involved. Physiologic complications can also result from exposure to other substances (eg, talcum powder, strychnine) that are mixed with cocaine or heroin.
2. Psychological complications include increased potential for risk-taking and suicidal behavior.
3. Individuals under the influence of substances are more likely to experience automobile or other accidents.
4. Suicide rates increase in the presence of substance use. This includes accidental overdose related to the substance.
5. The physiologic complications or consequences associated with alcohol abuse involve each organ system and include the development of GI ulcers, liver disease, malnutrition, anemia, and dehydration.
6. Complications associated with the use of cocaine or amphetamines include cardiac dysrhythmia, seizures, dehydration, and acute renal failure. Mood lability and psychosis are commonly associated with the use of amphetamines and cocaine.
7. Heroin use can result in respiratory complications and the development of infectious disease through the sharing of needles. Endocarditis, skin abscesses, and other infectious sequelae may result.
8. The use of 3,4-methylenedioxymethamphetamine (Ecstasy) can have complications similar to those associated with amphetamine use. Research has also demonstrated effects on short- and long-term memory through neurotoxic effects on serotonergic pathways, with possible additional effects on dopamine pathways in the CNS.

Nursing Assessment

1. Assess physiologic stability.
   a. Elevated or decreased blood pressure.
   b. Cardiac abnormalities.

c. Confusion, memory deficits, ataxia, nystagmus (Wernicke encephalopathy, a thiamine deficiency).

d. Lasting memory deficits (Korsakoff amnestic disorder).

e. Lung congestion or diminished breath sounds.

f. Fever.

g. Mood lability.

2. Assess for evidence of medical complications.

a. Hepatic disease.

b. Renal disease.

c. Anemia.

d. Sexually transmitted disease.

e. Anxiety and depression.

3. Identify risk-taking behaviors.

a. Participation in criminal activities.

b. Sexual activity and behaviors, including use of protective devices.

c. Motor vehicle violations.

d. Participation in hazardous sports or activities.

4. Gather information regarding substance use.

a. Substances used and amounts.

b. Method of use (eg, injection, inhalation).

c. Previous attempts to reduce or stop use.

d. Prior history of withdrawal symptoms.

e. Longest previous period of sobriety.

f. Prior treatment programs attended.

g. Familial history of substance abuse.

h. Precipitating events to substance use.

5. Examine coping mechanisms and behaviors.

a. Denies presence of a substance-related problem.

b. Does not recognize the presence of physical or emotional health problems.

c. Blames others for the presence of problems.

d. Uses substance in stress-provoking situations.

e. Justifies use of substance.

f. Prior psychiatric history.

6. Monitor for withdrawal symptoms.

a. Agitation, mood lability, paranoia, or mania (cocaine, amphetamines).

b. Dehydration, nutritional deficiencies, hallucinations, seizures, GI disturbances (alcohol and other substances).

c. Nausea, vomiting, flulike symptoms, diarrhea, and muscle pain (opioids).

Nursing Diagnoses

The following is a partial list of nursing diagnoses that may be appropriate in working with an individual with a substance-related disorder.

- Ineffective Denial related to substance use.
- Compromised Family Coping related to roles and relationships.
- Risk for Injury related to effects of the substance.
- Readiness for Enhanced Coping related to life stressors.

Other nursing diagnoses may apply depending on the particular substance involved and may include the following:

- Risk for Self-Directed or Other-Directed Violence.
- Powerlessness.
- Self-Care Deficit.
- Imbalanced Nutrition: Less than Body Requirements.

Nursing Interventions

Facilitate Recognition of Substance-Related Disorder

1. Approach patient in a direct, nonjudgmental manner.

2. Assess patient's level of knowledge about substance.

3. Have patient identify situations preceding substance use.

4. Discuss consequences of substance use.

5. Reinforce desire for change.

Encourage Participation of Family and Significant Others

1. Provide support to family and significant others while acknowledging substance-related disorder of patient.

2. Encourage family to attend supportive and educational group meetings.

3. Have family members identify effects of substance use on family functioning.

4. Discuss role relationships with family that may be related to substance-seeking behavior.

Ensuring Safety

1. Monitor patient for symptoms of substance withdrawal.

2. Provide prescribed medications, as indicated, for the treatment of withdrawal symptomatology.

3. Educate patient on relationship between symptoms and substance use.

4. Monitor hydration and nutritional status.

5. Reduce level of stimulation, as appropriate.

6. Assess for presence of agitation or mood lability.

Enhancing Coping Strategies

1. Aid in identifying triggers to use.

2. Have patient develop a list of personal strengths.

3. Help patient develop an understanding of dependence as an illness.

4. Assist patient in developing alternative coping strategies through participation in role-playing activities and groups.

5. Identify alternative methods of participating in social situations without resorting to use of substance.

6. Reinforce need for ongoing attendance of support group meetings.

Community and Home Care Considerations

1. Assist in resource finding for inpatient or outpatient program. Provide referral and information about community-based programs and activities that can aid in the maintenance of sobriety. The individual may benefit from placement in a residential treatment program or halfway house that provides supportive services and continued programs of treatment in a community setting.

2. Assist in educating and encouraging adherence to drug therapy regimen. Provide information about medication therapy, as appropriate, including known adverse effects and means of obtaining prescribed drugs, as necessary (eg, methadone).

Family Education and Health Maintenance

1. Instruct patient and family about adverse physiologic and psychological effects of substance use.

2. Discuss health maintenance practices to minimize potential effects of substance use (eg, vitamin use, proper diet).

3. Explain the potential for injury from risk-taking behaviors.

4. Reinforce the need for aftercare groups and activities.

5. For general information and support, consult such agencies as the National Institute on Drug Abuse, National Institutes of Health (*www.drugabuse.gov*), or National Institute on Alcohol Abuse and Alcoholism, National Institutes of Health (*www.niaaa.nih.gov*). General information can also be obtained from Substance Abuse & Mental Health Services Administration (*https://www.samhsa.gov*) or Alcoholics Anonymous (*www.aa.org*).

Evaluation: Expected Outcomes

- Acknowledges the presence of a substance-related disorder.
- Identifies negative effects of substance use or abuse on family, work, and other relationships.
- Describes negative effects of substance use or abuse on physical and emotional health.
- Continues to attend treatment programs; refrains from substance use.

CHILD AND ADOLESCENT PROBLEMS

Children and adolescents are capable of developing the same psychiatric disorders seen in adult populations, such as major depression, bipolar disorder, and substance-related disorders. In addition, children and adolescents face a number of developmental and age-specific mental health issues. A child faced with a traumatic situation may engage in a pattern of destructive or deviant behavior. Working with such a child can be frustrating to both health care personnel and parents. The intent of this section is to provide a brief overview of a select group of mental health issues specific to pediatric populations. For further information, the reader is strongly encouraged to seek out texts and materials dedicated to pediatric mental health and child development.

 EVIDENCE BASE American Psychiatric Association. (2013). *Diagnostic and statistical manual of mental disorders* (5th ed.). Washington, DC: Author.

Psychiatric disorders specific to child populations, as defined by the *DSM-5*, include the following:
1. Attentional deficit and autism spectrum disorders (see Chapter 56, page 1465).
2. Behavioral disorders.
   a. Conduct disorder.
   b. Oppositional defiant disorder.
3. Elimination disorders.
   a. Encopresis—incontinence of feces not caused by organic process.
   b. Enuresis—involuntary voiding during sleep; may be physiologic during early childhood.

Other psychiatric disorders already discussed in this chapter may appear in childhood and adolescence and persist into adulthood. Eating disorders commonly begin during the adolescent years and continue well into adulthood (see Chapter 20, page 576).

Behavioral Disorders

Conduct disorder and oppositional defiant disorder may arise in children of all ages. The most significant difference between the two is that in conduct disorder, the child or adolescent is violating societal norms and rules. With oppositional defiant disorder, the child or adolescent is displaying disruptive and negative behavior primarily toward authority figures, without violation of societal norms.

Pathophysiology and Etiology

The development of a psychiatric disorder commonly reflects a complex interaction of several etiologic factors.
1. Twin studies have provided some evidence that conduct disorder may have a genetic predisposition.
2. Other genetic studies have indicated that regions located on chromosomes 2 and 19 may be associated with the development of conduct disorder.
3. These predisposing genetic factors most likely interact with environmental influences, such as household violence, neglect, and other situational variables, in contributing to the development of behavioral or attentional disorders.

Clinical Manifestations

1. Conduct disorder is a pattern of persistent behavior during which the individual violates either the rights of another person or accepted societal norms. Behavioral criteria incorporates four possible domains, across which three or more behaviors must be observed within a 12-month period:
   a. Aggression toward people or animals (threatening behaviors, physical cruelty, initiating of physical confrontations, or weapon use).
   b. Aggression toward property (intentional fire-setting or destruction of property).
   c. Theft or deceitfulness (breaking into property of others, stealing of items).
   d. Violation of rules (before age 13, staying out late at night, regardless of parental instruction; running away from home, absence from school).
2. If the individual does not violate societal norms but engages in a pattern of hostile, defiant, and negative behavior toward authority figures or adults in general, oppositional defiant disorder may be considered. This pattern of behavior must endure for at least 6 months, during which time at least four of the following behaviors are exhibited:
   a. Frequently loses temper.
   b. Often argues with adults.
   c. Often refuses to comply with, or actually defies, rules.
   d. Often blames others for behavior or mistakes.
   e. Intentionally provokes others on a frequent basis.
   f. Often appears easily annoyed or irritated by others.
   g. Often appears angry or resentful toward others.
   h. Frequently engages in spiteful and vindictive behavior.
3. The behavioral disorders have been found to have a significant degree of comorbidity. These disorders may also coexist with attention deficits such as ADHD.

Diagnostic Evaluation

1. The evaluation of a child and adolescent ideally incorporates information from patient, parents, other family members, and teachers.
2. Evaluation should also include a detailed physical and nutritional assessment.
3. Depending on patient's age, play activities may be incorporated into the interview to facilitate trust and patient expression. Younger children may be more capable of depicting family dynamics and their own feelings through play or art.

Management

1. Care of the individual with a behavioral disorder may initially involve treatment in a structured inpatient program that incorporates many behavioral modification techniques, including a level system, a token economy, and close monitoring.
2. Residential or partial hospitalization treatment programs may also be employed.
3. Treatment of a behavioral disorder includes family therapy, parental and patient education, and, ideally, teacher

interaction. Family counseling and education are essential aspects of any treatment modality.

4. Drugs may be employed in the treatment program, based on the presence of comorbidities and behavioral severity.

Nursing Diagnoses

Any of the following may be individualized to the child or adolescent:

- Chronic Low Self-Esteem.
- Compromised Family Coping.
- Impaired Parenting.
- Risk for Injury.
- Risk for Suicide.
- Readiness for Enhanced Coping.
- Readiness for Enhanced Parenting.
- Readiness for Enhanced Self-Concept.

Nursing Interventions

Interventions should be selected that encourage the verbal expression of feelings and provide alternatives to destructive behavior. Interventions should also be included that address parental education. Interventions to be considered include the following:

1. Aid patient in identifying events that trigger inappropriate behavioral responses.
2. Assist patient in developing communication skills.
3. Teach alternative behaviors and methods of expression.
4. Provide consistent limits and consequences for inappropriate behaviors.
5. Provide positive feedback for appropriate behaviors.
6. Monitor behavior for violence directed toward self or others.
7. Utilize role-play to practice alternative behavioral responses.
8. Teach parenting skills to parents or primary caregivers.
9. Teach parents appropriate limit setting and emphasize need to clearly state expectations.

Evaluation: Expected Outcomes

- Reduction in frequency and intensity of outbursts while interacting with others.
- Uses alternative coping strategies in situations in which he or she would previously have been angered or engaged in destructive behavior.
- Attends school on consistent basis.
- Does not injure self or others

SELECTED REFERENCES

American Psychiatric Association. (2013). *Desk reference to the diagnostic criteria from DSM-5.* Washington, DC: American Psychiatric Publishing.

American Psychiatric Association & DSM-5 Task Force. (2013). *Diagnostic and statistical manual of mental disorders: DSM-5* (5th ed.). Washington, DC: American Psychiatric Association.

Baldwin, D. S. Anderson, I. M., Nutt, D. J., et al., (2014). Evidence-based pharmacological treatment of anxiety disorders, post-traumatic stress disorder and obsessive-compulsive disorder: A revision of the 2005 guidelines from the British Association for Psychopharmacology. *Journal of Psychopharmacology, 28*(5), 403–439.

Bass, C., & Halligan, P. (2016). Factitious disorders and malingering in relation to functional neurologic disorders. *Handbook of Clinical Neurology, 139,* 509–520.

Birur, B., Math, S. B., & Fargason, R. E. (2017). A review of psychopharmacological interventions post-disaster to prevent psychiatric sequelae. *Psychopharmacology Bulletin, 47*(1), 8–26.

Blumberger, D. M., Hsu, J. H., & Daskalakis, Z. J. (2015). A review of brain stimulation treatments for late-life depression. *Current Treatment Options in Psychiatry, 2*(4), 413–421.

Borisovskaya, A., Bryson, W. C., Buchholz, J., et al. (2016). Electroconvulsive therapy for depression in Parkinson's disease: systematic review of evidence and recommendations. *Neurodegenerative Disease Management, 6*(2), 161–176.

Brown, R. J. (2016). Dissociation and functional neurologic disorders. *Handbook of Clinical Neurology, 139,* 85–94.

Cessak, G., Rokita, K., Dabrowska, M., et al. (2016). Therapeutic equivalence of antipsychotics and antidepressants—A systematic review. *Pharmacological Reports, 68*(2), 217–223.

Deeley, Q. (2016). Hypnosis as therapy for functional neurologic disorders. *Handbook of Clinical Neurology, 139,* 585–595.

Edgcomb, J. B., Tseng, C. H., & Kerner, B. (2016). Medically unexplained somatic symptoms and bipolar spectrum disorders: A systematic review and meta-analysis. *Journal of Affective Disorders, 204,* 205–213.

Fiest, K. M., Walker, J. R., Bernstein, C. N., et al. (2016). Systematic review and meta-analysis of interventions for depression and anxiety in persons with multiple sclerosis. *Multiple Sclerosis and Related Disorders, 5,* 12–26.

Goldstein, L. H., & Mellers, J. D. (2016). Psychologic treatment of functional neurologic disorders. *Handbook of Clinical Neurology, 139,* 571–583.

Hilt, R. J., Nussbaum, A. M., & American Psychiatric Association. (2016). *DSM-5 pocket guide for child and adolescent mental health.* Arlington, VA: American Psychiatric Association Publishing.

Huguet, A., Rao, S., McGrath, P. J., et al. (2016). A systematic review of cognitive behavioral therapy and behavioral activation apps for depression. *PLOS One, 11*(5), e0154248.

Jones, A. M., West, K. B., & Suveg, C. (2017). Anxiety in the school setting: A framework for evidence-based practice. *School Mental Health.* 2017, 1–11. Available: *doi.org/10.1007/s12310-017-9235-2.*

Keil, M. F., Briassoulis, G., Stratakis, C. A., & Wu, T. J. (2016). Protein kinase A and anxiety-related behaviors: A mini-review. *Frontiers in Endocrinology (Lausanne), 7,* 83.

Kerr, I. B., Finlayson-Short, L., McCutcheon, L. K., et al. (2015). The 'self' and borderline personality disorder: Conceptual and clinical considerations. *Psychopathology, 48*(5), 339–348.

Krause-Utz, A., Frost, R., Winter, D., & Elzinga, B. M. (2017). Dissociation and alterations in brain function and structure: Implications for borderline personality disorder. *Current Psychiatry Reports, 19*(1), 6.

Lam, R. W., Kennedy, S. H., Parikh, S. V., et al. (2016). Canadian Network for Mood and Anxiety Treatments (CANMAT) 2016 clinical guidelines for the management of adults with major depressive disorder: Introduction and methods. *Canadian Journal of Psychiatry, 61*(9), 510–523.

Lehn, A., Gelauff, J., Hoeritzauer, I., et al. (2016). Functional neurological disorders: mechanisms and treatment. *Journal of Neurology, 263*(3), 611–620.

Malas, N., Ortiz-Aguayo, R., Giles, L., & Ibeziako, P. (2017). Pediatric somatic symptom disorders. *Current Psychiatry Reports, 19*(2), 11.

Matte, D. L., Pizzichini, M. M., Hoepers, A. T., et al. (2016). Prevalence of depression in COPD: A systematic review and meta-analysis of controlled studies. *Respiratory Medicine, 117,* 154–161.

Morrell, C. J., Sutcliffe, P., Booth, A., et al. (2016). A systematic review, evidence synthesis and meta-analysis of quantitative and qualitative studies evaluating the clinical effectiveness, the cost-effectiveness, safety and acceptability of interventions to prevent postnatal depression. *Health Technology Assessment, 20*(37), 1–414.

Petry, N. M. (2016). *Behavioral addictions : DSM-5® and beyond.* Oxford; New York: Oxford University Press.

Remes, O., Brayne, C., van der Linde, R., & Lafortune, L. (2016). A systematic review of reviews on the prevalence of anxiety disorders in adult populations. *Brain and Behavior, 6*(7), e00497.

Schmeltzer, S. N., Herman, J. P., & Sah, R. (2016). Neuropeptide Y (NPY) and posttraumatic stress disorder (PTSD): A translational update. *Experimental Neurology, 284,* 196–210.

Smith, E. K., Gopalan, P., Glance, J. B., & Azzam, P. N. (2016). Postpartum depression screening: A review for psychiatrists. *Harvard Review of Psychiatry, 24*(3), 173–187.

Staniloiu, A., & Markowitsch, H. J. (2014). Dissociative amnesia. *Lancet Psychiatry, 1*(3), 226–241.

Tsui, P., Deptula, A., & Yuan, D. Y. (2017). Conversion disorder, functional neurological symptom disorder, and chronic pain: Comorbidity, assessment, and treatment. *Current Pain and Health Reports, 21*(6), 29.

van der Linde, R. M., Dening, T., Stephan, B. C., et al. (2016). Longitudinal course of behavioural and psychological symptoms of dementia: systematic review. *British Journal of Psychiatry, 209*(5), 366–377.

Vilagut, G., Forero, C. G., Barbaglia, G., & Alonso, J. (2016). Screening for depression in the general population with the center for epidemiologic studies depression (CES-D): A systematic review with meta-analysis. *PLoS One, 11*(5), e0155431.

APPENDICES AND INDEX

Appendix A
Diagnostic Studies and Interpretation

BOX A-1 Selected Abbreviations Used in Appendices

CONVENTIONAL UNITS

kg = kilogram
g = gram
mg = milligram
μg = microgram
μμg = micromicrogram
ng = nanogram
pg = picogram
dL = 100 milliliters
mL = milliliter
mm³ = cubic millimeter
fL = femtoliter
mM = millimole

nM = nanomole
mOsm = milliosmole
mm = millimeter
μm = micron or micrometer
mm Hg = millimeters of mercury
U = unit
mU = milliunit
μU = microunit
mEq = milliequivalent
IU = International Unit
mIU = milliInternational Unit

SI UNITS

g = gram
L = liter
mol = mole
mmol = millimole
μmol = micromole
nmol = nanomole
pmol = picomole

Table A-1 Reference Ranges—Hematology and Coagulation

| LABORATORY TEST | NORMAL ADULT REFERENCE RANGE | | CLINICAL SIGNIFICANCE |
	CONVENTIONAL UNITS	SI UNITS	
Bleeding Time	3–10 minutes	3–10 minutes	• Prolonged in thrombocytopenia, defective platelet function, and aspirin therapy
D-Dimer	<250 mg/mL	<0.25 mg/L	• Increased in disseminated intravascular coagulation, malignancy, and arterial and venous thrombosis
Erythrocyte Count Males	4,600,000–6,200,000/mm³	4.6–6.2 × 10¹²/L	• Increased in severe diarrhea and dehydration, polycythemia, acute poisoning, and pulmonary fibrosis
Females	4,200,000–5,400,000/mm³	4.2–5.4 × 10¹²/L	• Decreased in all anemias in leukemia and after hemorrhage, when blood volume has been restored
Erythrocyte Indices Mean corpuscular volume (MCV)	84–96 μm³	84–96 fL	• Increased in macrocytic anemia; decreased in microcytic anemia
Mean corpuscular hemoglobin (MCH)	28–34 μμg/cell	28–34 pg	• Increased in macrocytic anemia; decreased in microcytic anemia
Mean corpuscular hemoglobin concentration (MCHC)	32%–36%	Concentration fraction: 0.32–0.36	• Decreased in severe hypochromic anemia

Table A-1 Reference Ranges—Hematology and Coagulation (Continued)

LABORATORY TEST	NORMAL ADULT REFERENCE RANGE		CLINICAL SIGNIFICANCE
	CONVENTIONAL UNITS	SI UNITS	
Erythrocyte Sedimentation Rate (ESR)—Westergren Method			
Males younger than age 50	<15 mm/hour	<15 mm/hour	• Increased in tissue destruction, whether inflammatory or degenerative; during menstruation and pregnancy; and in acute febrile diseases
Males older than age 50	<20 mm/hour	<20 mm/hour	
Females younger than 50	<20 mm/hour	<20 mm/hour	
Females older than age 50	<30 mm/hour	<30 mm/hour	
Hematocrit			
Males	42%–52%	Volume fraction: 0.42–0.52	• Decreased in severe anemia, anemia of pregnancy, and acute massive blood loss
Females	37%–47%	Volume fraction: 0.37–0.47	• Increased in erythrocytosis of any cause and in dehydration or hemoconcentration associated with shock
Hemoglobin			
Males	13–18 g/dL	2.02–2.79 mmol/L	• Decreased in various anemias, in pregnancy, in severe or prolonged hemorrhage, and with excessive fluid intake
Females	12–16 g/dL	1.86–2.48 mmol/L	• Increased in polycythemia, chronic obstructive pulmonary disease, failure of oxygenation due to heart failure, and normally in people living at high altitudes
Leukocyte Count			
Total	5,000–10,000/mm^3	5–10 × 10^9/L	• Total is elevated in acute infectious diseases, predominantly in the neutrophilic fraction with bacterial diseases, and in the lymphocytic and monocytic fractions in viral diseases
Basophils	0%–0.5%	Number fraction: 0.6–0.7	• Elevated in acute leukemia, following menstruation, and following surgery or trauma
Eosinophils	1%–4%	Number fraction: 0.01–0.04	• Eosinophils elevated in collagen disease, allergy, and intestinal parasitosis
Lymphocytes	20%–30%	Number fraction: 0.00–0.05	• Depressed in aplastic anemia, in agranulocytosis, and by toxic chemotherapeutic agents used in treating malignancy
Monocytes	2%–6%	Number fraction: 0.2–0.3	
Neutrophils	60%–70%	Number fraction: 0.02–0.06	
Platelet Count	140,000–400,000/mm^3	0.14–0.4 × 10^{12}/L	• Increased in malignancy, myeloproliferative disease, rheumatoid arthritis, and postoperatively; about 50% of patients with unexpected increase of platelet count will be found to have a malignancy
			• Decreased in thrombocytopenic purpura, acute leukemia, and aplastic anemia and during cancer chemotherapy
Reticulocytes	0.5%–1.5% of red blood cells	Number fraction: 0.005–0.015	• Increased with any condition stimulating increase in bone marrow activity (infection, blood loss [acute and chronically following iron therapy in iron deficiency anemia], and polycythemia vera)
			• Decreased with any condition depressing bone marrow activity, acute leukemia, and late stage of severe anemias

Laboratory values may vary according to the techniques used in different laboratories.

Table A-2 Reference Ranges—Serum, Plasma, and Whole Blood Chemistries

LABORATORY TEST	NORMAL ADULT REFERENCE RANGE		CLINICAL SIGNIFICANCE	
	CONVENTIONAL UNITS	SI UNITS	INCREASED	DECREASED
Alkaline Phosphatase Adults	40–150 IU/L	40–150 IU/L	• Conditions reflecting increased osteoblastic activity of bone • Rickets • Hyperparathyroidism • Hepatic disease	• Malnutrition • Cretinism • Severe anemia • Celiac disease
Alanine Aminotransferase (ALT)	5–40 IU/L	5–40 IU/L	• Liver disease • Muscle trauma • MI	• Azotemia • Chronic dialysis
Aspartate Aminotransferase (AST)	5–40 IU/L	5–40 IU/L	• Same as ALT	—
Bilirubin Total Direct (conjugated) Indirect (unconjugated)	0.1–1.2 mg/dL 0.1–0.2 mg/dL 0.1–1 mg/dL	2–20 µmol/L 0–4 µmol/L 1.7–17.1 µmol/L	• Hemolytic anemia (indirect) • Biliary obstruction and disease • Hepatocellular damage (hepatitis) • Pernicious anemia • Hemolytic disease of the newborn	—
Calcium	8.6–10.3 mg/dL	2.15–2.57 mmol/L	• Tumor or hyperplasia of parathyroid • Hypervitaminosis D • Multiple myeloma • Nephritis with uremia • Malignant tumors • Sarcoidosis • Hyperthyroidism • Skeletal immobilization • Excess calcium intake: milk-alkali syndrome	• Hypoparathyroidism • Diarrhea • Celiac disease • Vitamin D deficiency • Acute pancreatitis • Nephrosis • After parathyroidectomy
Carbon Dioxide, Venous Adults Infants	22–30 mEq/L 18–24 mEq/L	22–30 mmol/L 18–24 mmol/L	• Respiratory acidosis (CO_2 retention) • Metabolic alkalosis (vomiting)	• Respiratory alkalosis (hyperventilation) • Metabolic acidosis (diabetic ketoacidosis)
Chloride	98–106 mEq/L	98–106 mmol/L	• Nephrosis • Nephritis • Urinary obstruction • Cardiac decompensation • Anemia	• Diabetes • Diarrhea • Vomiting • Pneumonia • Heavy metal poisoning • Cushing syndrome • Intestinal obstruction • Febrile conditions
Creatinine	0.7–1.4 mg/dL	62–124 µmol/L	• Renal insufficiency, muscle disease • Chronic renal disease	• Advanced liver disease
Glucose Fasting Postprandial (2 hours)	60–99 mg/dL 65–140 mg/dL	3.3–6.05 mmol/L 3.58–7.7 mmol/L	• Diabetes • Cushing disease • *Note:* 100–126 is impaired fasting glucose; >126 fasting is diagnostic for diabetes	• Hyperinsulinism/insulinemia • Addison disease • Insulin therapy
Potassium (K)	3.5–5 mEq/L	3.5–5 mmol/L	• Renal failure • Acidosis • Cell lysis • Tissue breakdown or hemolysis	• GI losses • Diuretic administration

Table A-2 Reference Ranges—Serum, Plasma, and Whole Blood Chemistries (*Continued*)

| LABORATORY TEST | NORMAL ADULT REFERENCE RANGE | | CLINICAL SIGNIFICANCE | |
	CONVENTIONAL UNITS	SI UNITS	INCREASED	DECREASED
Protein, Total	6–8 g/dL	60–80 g/L	• Hemoconcentration • Shock • Multiple myeloma (globulin fraction) • Chronic infections (globulin function) • Liver disease (globulin)	• Malnutrition • Hemorrhage • Loss of plasma from burns • Proteinuria
Albumin	3.5–5 g/dL	35–50 g/L		
Globulin	1.5–3 g/dL	15–30 g/L		
Sodium	135–145 mEq/L	135–145 mmol/L	• Hemoconcentration • Diabetes insipidus	• Diuretic therapy • Water intoxication
Urea Nitrogen, Blood (BUN)	10–20 mg/dL	3.6–7.2 mmol/L	• Acute glomerulonephritis • Obstructive uropathy • Mercury poisoning • Nephrotic syndrome	• Severe hepatic failure • Pregnancy

Appendix B
Conversion Tables

Metric Units and Symbols, 1502
Celsius (Centigrade) and Fahrenheit
   Temperature Formulas, 1502

Nomogram for Estimating Surface Area of
Infants and Young Children, 1503

Nomogram for Estimating Surface Area of
Older Children and Adults, 1504

Table B-1   Metric Units and Symbols

QUANTITY	UNIT	SYMBOL	EQUIVALENT
Length	Millimeter	mm	1,000 mm = 1 m
	Centimeter	cm	100 cm = 1 m
	Decimeter	dm	10 dm = 1 m
	Meter	m	1,000 m = 1 km
Volume	Cubic centimeter	cc or cm^3	1,000 cc = 1 cm^3 or liter
	Milliliter	ml or mL	1,000 mL = 1 liter
	Cubic decimeter	dm^3	1,000 dm^3 = 1 m^3
	Liter	L	1,000 L = 1 m^3
Mass	Microgram	µg	1,000 µg = 1 mg
	Milligram	mg	1,000 mg = 1 g
	Gram	g	1,000 g = 1 kg
	Kilogram	kg	1,000 kg = 1 metric ton (t)

To convert from pounds to kilograms, divide by 2.2.
To convert from kilograms to pounds, multiply by 2.2.

Table B-2   Celsius (Centigrade) and Fahrenheit Temperature Formulas

To convert °F to °C: Subtract 32, then divide by 1.8. Example: 97°F − 32 = 65, 65 divided by 1.8 = 36°C.
To convert °C to °F: Multiply by 1.8, then add 32. Example: 37°C × 1.8 = 66.6, 66.6 + 32 = 98.6°F.

HEIGHT		SURFACE AREA	WEIGHT	
feet	centimeters	in square meters	pounds	kilograms

Figure B-1. Nomogram for estimating surface area of infants and young children. To determine the surface area of the patient, draw a straight line between the point representing the patient's height on the left vertical scale and the point representing the patient's weight on the right vertical scale. The point at which this line intersects the middle vertical scale represents the surface area in square meters. (Courtesy of Abbott Laboratories.)

HEIGHT		SURFACE AREA	WEIGHT	
feet	centimeters	in square meters	pounds	kilograms

Figure B-2. Nomogram for estimating surface area of older children and adults. To determine the surface area of the patient, draw a straight line between the point representing the patient's height on the left vertical scale and the point representing the patient's weight on the right vertical scale. The point at which this line intersects the middle vertical scale represents the surface area in square meters. (Courtesy of Abbott Laboratories.)

Appendix C
Pediatric Laboratory Values

Table C-1 Blood Chemistries			
LABORATORY TEST	**QUALIFICATION**	**CONVENTIONAL UNITS**	**SI UNITS**
Carbon Dioxide (CO_2) Content	Cord blood	14–22 mmol/L	14–22 mmol/L
	Child	20–24 mmol/L	20–24 mmol/L
	Adult	24–30 mmol/L	24–30 mmol/L
Chloride	—	99–111 mEq/L	99–111 mmol/L
Creatinine (Serum)	**Age (years)**	**Upper Limits, mg/dL (µmol/L)**	
		Males	**Females**
	1	0.6 (53)	0.5 (44)
	2–3	0.7 (62)	0.6 (53)
	4–7	0.8 (71)	0.7 (62)
	8–10	0.9 (80)	0.8 (71)
	11–12	1.0 (88)	0.9 (80)
	13–17	1.2 (106)	1.1 (97)
	18–20	1.3 (115)	1.1 (97)
	Adult	1.2 (106)	1.4 (124)
Potassium	<age 10 days	4–6 mEq/L	4–6 mmol/L
	>age 10 days	3.5–5 mEq/L	3.5–5 mmol/L
Sodium	Premature	130–140 mEq/L	130–140 mmol/L
	Older	135–148 mEq/L	135–148 mmol/L
Urea Nitrogen	—	7–22 mg/dL	2.5–7.9 mmol/L

Table C-2   Normal Values—Hematology

AGE	HEMOGLOBIN (G/DL)	HEMATOCRIT (%)	MEAN CORPUSCULAR VOLUME (FL)	MEAN CELL HEMOGLOBIN CONCENTRATION (G/DL RBC)
	MEAN (−22 SD)	MEAN (−22 SD)	MEAN (−22 SD)	MEAN (−22 SD)
26–30 Weeks' Gestation*	13.4 (11)	41.5 (34.9)	118.2 (106.7)	37.9 (30.6)
28 Weeks' Gestation	14.5	45	120	31
32 Weeks' Gestation	15	47	118	32
Term† (Cord)	16.5 (13.5)	51 (42)	108 (96)	33 (30)
1–3 Days	18.5 (14.5)	56 (45)	108 (95)	33 (29)
2 Weeks	16.6 (13.4)	53 (41)	105 (88)	31.4 (28.1)
1 Month	13.9 (10.7)	44 (33)	101 (91)	31.8 (28.1)
2 Months	11.2 (9.4)	35 (28)	95 (84)	31.8 (28.3)
6 Months	12.6 (11.1)	36 (31)	76 (68)	35 (32.7)
6 Months–2 Years	12 (10.5)	36 (33)	78 (70)	33 (30)
2–6 Years	12.5 (11.5)	37 (34)	81 (75)	34 (31)
6–12 Years	13.5 (11.5)	40 (35)	86 (77)	34 (31)
12–18 Years				
Male	14.5 (13)	43 (36)	88 (78)	34 (31)
Female	14 (12)	41 (37)	90 (78)	34 (31)

*Values are from fetal samplings.
†Younger than age 1 month, capillary Hb exceeds venous: age 1 hour, 3.6 g difference; age 5 days, 2.2 g difference; age 3 weeks, 1.1 g difference.
‡Mean (95% confidence limits).
Used from Kahl, L., & Hughes, H. (Eds.). (2018). The Harriet Lane handbook (21st ed.). Philadelphia, PA: Elsevier/Mosby, with permission.

Table C-3   Sample Conversions of Pounds and Ounces to Grams*

POUNDS	OUNCES								
	0	1	2	3	4	5	6	7	8
0	—	28	57	85	113	142	170	198	227
1	454	482	510	539	567	595	624	652	680
2	907	936	964	992	1,021	1,049	1,077	1,106	1,134
3	1,361	1,389	1,417	1,446	1,474	1,503	1,531	1,559	1,588
4	1,814	1,843	1,871	1,899	1,928	1,956	1,984	2,013	2,041
5	2,268	2,296	2,325	2,353	2,381	2,410	2,438	2,466	2,495
6	2,722	2,750	2,778	2,807	2,835	2,863	2,892	2,920	2,948

*1 ounce = approximately 30 g.

RETICULOCYTE COUNT (%)	WHITE BLOOD CELL/MM³ × 100 MEAN (−2 SD)	PITS (10³/MM³) MEAN (±2 SD)
—	4.4 (2.7)	254
(5–10)	—	(180–327)
(3–10)	—	275
(3–7)	18.1 (9–30)‡	290
(1.8–4.6)	18.9 (9.4–34)	290
—	11.5 (5–20)	192
(0.1–1.7)	10.8 (5–19.5)	252
—	—	—
(0.7–2.3)	11.9 (6–17.5)	—
—	10.6 (6–17)	(150–350)
(0.5–1.0)	8.5 (5–15.5)	(150–350)
(0.5–1.0)	8.1 (4.5–13.5)	(150–350)
(0.5–1.0)	7.8 (4.5–13.5)	(150–350)
(0.5–1.0)	7.8 (4.5–13.5)	(150–350)

9	10	11	12	13	14	15
255	283	312	340	369	397	425
709	737	765	794	822	850	879
1,162	1,191	1,219	1,247	1,276	1,304	1,332
1,616	1,644	1,673	1,701	1,729	1,758	1,786
2,070	2,098	2,126	2,155	2,183	2,211	2,240
2,532	2,551	2,580	2,608	2,637	2,665	2,693
2,977	3,005	3,033	3,062	3,090	3,118	3,147

Appendix D
Pain

GUIDE TO GENERAL PAIN MANAGEMENT

Overview and Assessment

Types of Pain

1. Somatic pain—caused by direct tumor involvement of sensory receptors in cutaneous and deep tissues.
   a. Usually described as dull, sharp, aching, and throbbing; usually constant and localized.
   b. Most common somatic pain is bone pain caused by metastasis.
   c. Can usually be controlled with NSAIDs or oral opioids.
2. Neuropathic pain.
   a. Results from nerve injury or compression.
   b. Includes phantom pain and postherpetic neuralgia.
   c. Described as burning, shooting, electric, and lancinating. (It can be constant or sporadic.)
   d. Usually associated with paresthesia.
   e. Treatment usually includes combinations of antidepressants, anticonvulsants, and opioids.
3. Visceral pain.
   a. Usually described as deep, dull, aching, squeezing, or pressure sensation. It can be vague or ill defined and can be referred to cutaneous sites, making it difficult to differentiate from somatic pain.
   b. Usually caused by abnormal stretching of smooth muscle walls, ischemia of visceral muscle, and serosal irritation.
   c. Can be treated with oral opioids or surgery to remove the cause.

Other Clinical Manifestations

1. Fatigue from sleep disturbances—most patients have not slept for extended periods.
2. Loss of appetite, weight loss.
3. Anxiety and depression.
4. Change in self-concept and quality of life.

Pain Assessment

1. Screen for pain at each visit. Evaluate objectively the nature of the patient's pain, including location, duration, quality, and impact on daily activities. Pain self-assessment is the most reliable guide to both cause of the pain and the effectiveness of pain treatment.
   a. Explore pain interventions that have been used and their effectiveness.
   b. Determine whether the intensity of the pain correlates with the prescribed analgesic.
2. Assess patient history and physical examination findings and laboratory values to differentiate expected pain from pain due to a new problem, a complication, or worsening of the underlying process.
3. Use a pain intensity scale of 0 (no pain) to 10 (worst possible pain) or other pain scale as appropriate. Take careful history of prior and present medications, response, and adverse effects.
   a. Ask the patient, "On a scale of 0 to 10, what would be your pain rating if 0 means no pain and 10 means the worst pain you can imagine?"
4. Assess relief from medications and duration of relief. (Use the same measuring scale every time.) Reevaluate the pain frequently. The requirement for analgesia should decrease as a condition improves due to healing or if other treatment is given, such as physical therapy or radiation therapy.

Management of Pain

 EVIDENCE BASE Chou, R., Gordon, D. B., de Leon-Casasola, O. A., et al. (2016). Management of Postoperative Pain: A Clinical Practice Guideline from the American Pain Society, the American Society of Regional Anesthesia and Pain Medicine, and the American Society of Anesthesiologists' Committee on Regional Anesthesia, Executive Committee, and Administrative Council. *Journal of Pain*, 17(2), 131–157.

Paice, J. A., Portenoy, R., & Lacchetti, C. (2016). *Management of chronic pain in survivors of adult cancers*. Alexandria, VA: American Society of Clinical Oncology. Available: *https://www.asco.org/practice-guidelines/quality-guidelines/guidelines/patient-and-survivor-care#/13021*.

Principles of Pain Management

1. The goal of pain management is complete relief of pain.
2. Placebos are never indicated for the treatment of pain.
3. Physical dependence and tolerance commonly occur; patients may require escalating doses of medications to control pain.
4. It is essential that physicians and nurses do not confuse addiction with tolerance. Addiction is an unrelated medical disorder with behavioral components. These facts must also be stressed with patients who are reluctant to take medications.
5. Multimodal therapies are often most effective, utilizing several classes of medication, and adding nonpharmacologic

therapies. Cognitive behavioral therapies and transcutaneous elective nerve stimulation can be effective adjuncts to pharmacological therapies.

Pharmacologic Management

Nonopioid Analgesics

1. Acetaminophen—a centrally acting analgesic; does not have anti-inflammatory or antiplatelet activities. May be effective for children and adults as a component of a multimodal therapy.
2. NSAIDs.
   a. Produce analgesia by decreasing levels of inflammatory mediators such as prostaglandins at the site of tissue injury.
   b. Suppress platelet function, decrease creatinine clearance, and interfere with the protective effect of prostaglandins on the gastric mucosa.
   c. Used to treat mild to moderate pain; examples include ibuprofen, 400 to 800 mg PO tid; nabumetone, 500 to 1,000 mg PO bid; indomethacin, 25 to 50 mg PO tid.
   d. COX-2 inhibitors are NSAIDs that are somewhat selective for cyclooxygenase 2 (COX-2) compounds, present in most tissues but less present than COX-1 in gastric mucosa. COX-2 is induced in response to inflammation and converts arachidonic acid to prostaglandin. COX-2 inhibitors inhibit prostaglandins at the site of inflammation but cause less GI irritation and bleeding. Examples include celecoxib 100 to 200 mg PO bid or meloxicam 7.5 to 15 mg PO bid.
3. Corticosteroids—may decrease inflammation and edema associated with acute musculoskeletal injuries, rheumatologic conditions, and tumor invasion in cancer.
   a. Examples include dexamethasone, 4 to 10 mg PO qd (dosage varies); prednisone, 5 to 60 mg PO qd (dosage varies).
4. Bisphosphonates—used for lytic bone lesions to prevent fractures and may help control bone pain. Examples include zoledronic acid, 4 mg IV every 3 to 4 weeks; pamidronate, 90 mg IV every 4 weeks.
5. Anticonvulsants and antidepressants for neuropathic pain—used to enhance the effect of opioids. Examples include amitriptyline, 25 to 100 mg PO every h.s. (may cause drowsiness); gabapentin, 300 to 600 mg qid to tid; pregabalin, 100 to 300 mg/day.

Opioid Analgesics

1. Oral route is preferred unless the patient cannot swallow or absorb medications through the GI tract. Doses should be adjusted to achieve pain relief with an acceptable level of adverse effects.
2. Most important to administer on a schedule rather than on an as-needed basis.
3. Optimal treatment approach is to treat with long-acting drugs to control baseline pain, paired with short-acting drugs, as needed, for breakthrough pain.
4. Oral opioids—primary course of treatment for moderate to severe pain; produce analgesia by binding to specific opiate receptors in the brain and spinal cord.
   a. Short-acting opioids—may be used for breakthrough pain, with relief lasting 3 to 4 hours. Examples include morphine, oxycodone, or hydromorphone.
   b. Long-acting opioids—should be equivalent to daily dose of short-acting opiates. Examples include morphine and oxycodone. Should be prescribed every 8 to 12 hours.

   c. Fentanyl—transdermal patch applied to the skin that is changed every 3 days. The peak effect is delayed for up to 3 days after applying. Should be used for patients with stable opioid requirements.
5. Parenteral administration of opioids is used for patients who cannot tolerate oral opioids or who are in an acute pain crisis.
   a. Patient-controlled analgesia (PCA)—administered by either SC or IV route using a computer-assisted drug delivery system.
   b. SC infusion of morphine should not exceed 5 mL/hour.
6. Intraspinal administration of opiates for management of acute or chronic pain:
   a. A catheter is placed into spinal epidural or subarachnoid (intrathecal) space.
   b. Catheter may be placed percutaneously and sutured in site or tunneled subcutaneously to the abdominal wall and exteriorized, or the pump system may be implanted.
   c. Catheter is positioned as near as possible to the spinal segment where the pain is projected.
   d. Preservative-free sterile morphine or other analgesic or local anesthetic drug is injected into the system at specified intervals.
   e. May be delivered by PCA pump or by continuous or intermittent infusion.
   f. Spinally administered local anesthetics produce their effects predominantly by action on axons of spinal nerve roots; produce long-lasting pain relief with relatively low doses with little or no blunting of patient's level of responsiveness.
   g. Complications of intraspinal administration include respiratory depression, urine retention, pruritus, infection, leakage, technical problems, and development of tolerance.

Nursing Interventions

1. Base the initial analgesic choice on the patient's report of pain.
2. Administer drugs orally whenever possible; avoid IM injection.
3. Administer analgesia "around the clock" rather than as needed.
4. Convey the impression that the patient's pain is understood and that the pain can be controlled.
5. Use alternative measures to relieve pain such as guided imagery, relaxation, and biofeedback.
6. Provide ongoing support and open communication. It is estimated that 40% of cancer survivors experience persistent pain.
7. Assess for side effects of medication.
   a. Respiratory depression is a potentially life-threatening adverse effect of opioids; be alert for shallow respirations and hypoxemia in patients who are opioid naïve.
   b. Constipation is expected with opioids and is treated prophylactically.
   c. Nausea is usually transitory and controllable with prophylactic antiemetics.
   d. Sedation is common initially and is transitory.
8. Suggest referral to a pain specialist for intractable pain.
9. Ensure that the least effective dose is used for the shortest amount of time, and that refills are not given without repeated assessment.
10. Assess the risk of adverse effects of opioids used in pain management and incorporate universal precautions to minimize abuse, addiction, and adverse consequences.
11. Follow specific state regulations that allow access to medical cannabis or cannabinoids for patients with chronic pain, if such treatment is prescribed.

INDEX

Note: Page numbers with b indicate boxes; those with f indicate figures; and those with t indicate tables.